Current Practice of Clinical Electroencephalography

THIRD EDITION

Current Practice of Clinical Electroencephalography

THIRD EDITION

Editors

John S. Ebersole, M.D.

Professor of Neurology and Director
Adult Epilepsy Center
Department of Neurology
The University of Chicago
Chicago, Illinois

Timothy A. Pedley, M.D.

Henry and Lucy Moses Professor of Neurology
Chairman, Department of Neurology
Columbia University
and
Neurologist-in Chief
Neurological Institute of New York
Columbia University Medical Center
New York, New York

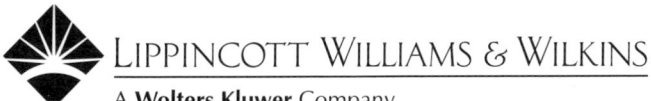

LIPPINCOTT WILLIAMS & WILKINS
A **Wolters Kluwer** Company
Philadelphia · Baltimore · New York · London
Buenos Aires · Hong Kong · Sydney · Tokyo

Acquisitions Editor: Charles W. Mitchell
Developmental Editor: Keith Donnellan
Supervising Editor: Steven P. Martin
Production Service: Bermedica Production, Ltd.
Manufacturing Manager: Colin J. Warnock
Cover Designer: Christine Jenny
Compositor: Lippincott Williams & Wilkins Desktop Division
Printer: Edwards Brothers

© 2003 by LIPPINCOTT WILLIAMS & WILKINS
530 Walnut Street
Philadelphia, PA 19106 USA
LWW.com

Library of Congress Cataloging-in-Publication Data

Current practice of clinical electroencephalography / editors, John S. Ebersole, Timothy A. Pedley.—3rd ed.
p. ; cm.
Includes bibliographical references and index.
ISBN 0-7817-1694-2
1. Electroencephalography. 2. Brain—Diseases—Diagnosis. I. Ebersole, John S. II. Pedley, Timothy A.
[DNLM: 1. Electroencephalography. WL 150 C976 2002]
RC386.6.E43 C87 2002
616.8′047547—dc21   2002030191

Care has been taken to confirm the accuracy of the information presented and to describe generally accepted practices. However, the authors, editors, and publisher are not responsible for errors or omissions or for any consequences from application of the information in this book and make no warranty, expressed or implied, with respect to the currency, completeness, or accuracy of the contents of the publication. Application of this information in a particular situation remains the professional responsibility of the practitioner.

The authors, editors, and publisher have exerted every effort to ensure that drug selection and dosage set forth in this text are in accordance with current recommendations and practice at the time of publication. However, in view of ongoing research, changes in government regulations, and the constant flow of information relating to drug therapy and drug reactions, the reader is urged to check the package insert for each drug for any change in indications and dosage and for added warnings and precautions. This is particularly important when the recommended agent is a new or infrequently employed drug.

Some drugs and medical devices presented in this publication have Food and Drug Administration (FDA) clearance for limited use in restricted research settings. It is the responsibility of the health care provider to ascertain the FDA status of each drug or device planned for use in their clinical practice.

10 9 8 7 6 5 4 3 2 1

Dedication

*To Gilbert H. Glaser, founding Chairman of the Department of Neurology
at Yale University, who introduced us to the role and possibilities of EEG
in neurological research and practice
and
To our wives, Susan and Barbara,
for their seemingly inexhaustible patience, support, and encouragement.*

PREFACE

This is the third edition of a textbook that first appeared in 1978 with Donald W. Klass and David D. Daly as editors. Daly remained an editor of the second edition, published in 1990, but Timothy A. Pedley succeeded Klass. Now, in the third edition of *Current Practice of Clinical Electroencephalography*, John S. Ebersole follows Daly, who died unexpectedly shortly after publication of the previous edition.

But there have been other, more important changes that reflect the continued evolution of electroencephalography (EEG) and clinical neurophysiology, and their relevance to clinical practice. This new edition is therefore not simply a revised version of the previous one. The second edition had 23 chapters; the third has 31, and 23 of these are entirely new. We are now firmly in the digital era, and the book strongly reflects this new reality. Advanced display and analytical techniques have extended the utility of EEG beyond the traditional EEG laboratory or epilepsy monitoring unit to the operating room and intensive care unit. New methods of source modeling and detection software are aiding seizure recognition and localization of epileptogenic brain regions. EEG in its broadest sense continues to play a vital role in the study of normal cerebral function and in conditions traditionally categorized as neurological, psychiatric, or psychological but now properly viewed more broadly as brain disorders.

Like its predecessors, this edition of *Current Practice* is not meant to be read from cover to cover following the chapter order listed in the Table of Contents. Residents in neurology and postdoctoral fellows in clinical neurophysiology will have different interests and needs than attending physicians or experienced investigators. We hope, therefore, that the topics and their coverage serve the needs of both novice and expert alike, and as an initial general reference source in the majority of matters related to EEG. Bibliographic citations include both historical and "classical" papers as well as recent publications describing new methods, revised interpretations of EEG data, and new or extended applications. We believe that in-depth knowledge of basic EEG recording methods, normal EEG patterns and phenomena (including changes resulting from development and aging), and the data base of clinical EEG abnormalities are essential to advanced and new applications. To this end, we have aimed to provide a systematic and critical approach to EEG interpretation so that clinical–electrographic correlations are not some mysterious assemblage of meaningless words but rather have practical clinical utility because they are soundly based on physiological principles and evidence from clinical studies.

Because multiauthored textbooks present an array of challenges that sometimes seem insurmountable, we are deeply grateful to our many contributors who generously shared their time, knowledge, and experience. We thank them too for their patience, as this volume has had a much longer gestation than anyone anticipated. We remarked in the second edition that, for those who wonder how editors in the trenches feel, it is useful to recall one of Abraham Lincoln's stories. Lincoln once told of a man who had been tarred and feathered and, while being ridden out of town on a rail, was heard to remark: "If it weren't for the honor, it wouldn't be worth it." We think it was worth it, and we are pleased with the final results; we hope our fellow authors are also.

In closing, we acknowledge with gratitude the many past contributions of David Daly and John Knott, both now sadly deceased, whose earlier work shaped the form of this edition. We also value the tireless efforts and understanding support of Charles Mitchell and Keith Donnellan at Lippincott Williams & Wilkins. Their role has been largely behind the scenes but no less important.

John S. Ebersole, M.D.
Timothy A. Pedley, M.D.

CONTENTS

CONTRIBUTING AUTHORS

David C. Adams, M.D.
Associate Professor of Anesthesiology
University of Vermont College of Medicine;
Attending Anesthesiologist
Fletcher Allen Health Center
Burlington, Vermont

Carl W. Bazil, M.D., Ph.D.
Assistant Professor
Department of Neurology
Columbia University;
Assistant Attending Neurologist
The Neurological Institute
New York-Presbyterian Hospital
New York, New York

A.G. Christina Bergqvist, M.D.
Assistant Professor of Neurology and Pediatrics
University of Pennsylvania School of Medicine;
Attending Physician
Division of Neurology
The Children's Hospital of Philadelphia
Philadelphia, Pennsylvania

Thomas P. Bleck, M.D., F.C.C.M.
The Louise Nerancy Professor of Neurology and
Professor of Neurological Surgery and Internal
*   Medicine;*
Director, Neuroscience Intensive Care Unit
Department of Neurology
University of Virginia
Charlottesville, Virginia

Richard P. Brenner, M.D.
Professor, Departments of Neurology and
*   Psychiatry*
University of Pittsburgh;
Director, EEG Lab
University of Pittsburgh Medical Center
*   Western Psychiatric Institute and Clinic*
Pittsburgh, Pennsylvania

György Buzsáki, M.D., Ph.D.
Professor, Center for Neuroscience
Rutgers University
Newark, New Jersey

Gian-Emilio Chatrian, M.D.
Professor Emeritus
Laboratory Medicine (Electroencephalography
*   and Clinical Neurophysiology) and*
*   Neurological Surgery*
University of Washington School of Medicine
*   and*
University of Washington Medical Center
Seattle, Washington

Robert R. Clancy, M.D.
Professor of Neurology and Pediatrics
University of Pennsylvania School of
*   Medicine;*
Director, Pediatric Regional Epilepsy Program
Division of Neurology
The Children's Hospital of Philadelphia
Philadelphia, Pennsylvania

Mary B. Connolly, M.B., F.R.C.P.(C)
Clinical Associate Professor
Division of Neurology
Department of Pediatrics
University of British Columbia;
Children's & Women's Hospital
Vancouver, British Columbia, Canada

Roger Q. Cracco, M.D.
Chairman, Department of Neurology
State University of New York Health Science
*   Center at Brooklyn*
State University of New York Downstate Medical
*   Center*
Brooklyn, New York

Stephen D. Cranstoun, M.S.E.E.
Department of Bioengineering
University of Pennsylvania
Philadelphia, Pennsylvania

Darryl C. De Vivo, M.D.
Sidney Carter Professor of Neurology and
*   Professor of Pediatrics*
Columbia University College of Physicians and
*   Surgeons;*
Director, Pediatric Neuroscience, Emeritus
Columbia-Presbyterian Medical Center
New York, New York

Dennis J. Dlugos, M.D.
Assistant Professor of Neurology and Pediatrics
University of Pennsylvania School of Medicine;
Section Head, Clinical Neurophysiology
Division of Neurology
The Children's Hospital of Philadelphia
Philadelphia, Pennsylvania

John S. Ebersole, M.D.
Professor of Neurology and Director
Adult Epilepsy Center
Department of Neurology
The University of Chicago
Chicago, Illinois

Ronald G. Emerson, M.D.
Professor, Department of Neurology
Columbia University College of Physicians and
*   Surgeons;*
Attending, Neurology Service,
The Neurological Institute of New York
Columbia-Presbyterian Medical Center
New York, New York

Charles M. Epstein, M.D.
Professor, Department of Neurology and
Director, Operating Room and Intensive Care
*   Unit Monitoring*
Emory University
Atlanta, Georgia

C. William Erwin, M.D.
Professor of Psychiatry Emeritus
Departments of Psychiatry and Medicine
*   (Neurology)*
EEG and Evoked Potential Laboratories
Duke University Medical Center
Durham, North Carolina

Bruce J. Fisch, M.D.
Professor, Department of Neurology
Louisiana State University;
Director, Epilepsy Center
Memorial Medical Center
New Orleans, Louisiana

Douglas S. Goodin, M.D.
Professor, Department of Neurology
University of California, San Francisco and
Medical Director
University of California, San Francisco
*   Multiple Sclerosis Center*
San Francisco, California

Jean Gotman, Ph.D.
Professor, Montrèal Neurological
*   Institute;*
Department of Neurology and
*   Neurosurgery*
McGill University
Montrèal, Quèbec, Canada

Susan T. Herman, M.D.
Assistant Professor of Neurology
University of Pennsylvania
Philadelphia Pennsylvania

Aatif M. Husain, M.D.
Assistant Professor
Department of Medicine (Neurology)
Duke University
Director, Evoked Potentials Laboratory
Duke University Medical Center
Durham, North Carolina

Akio Ikeda, M.D., D.M.S.
Lecturer, Department of Neurology
Kyoto University School of Medicine;
Staff Neurologist
Department of Neurology
Kyoto University Hospital
Kyoto, Japan

John R. Ives, B.Sc.
Associate Professor of Neurology
Harvard Medical School;
Technical Director
Clinical Neurophysiology
*   Laboratory*
Department of Neurology
Beth Israel Deaconess Medical Center
Boston, Massachusetts

Kenneth G. Jordan, M.D., F.A.C.P.
Associate Clinical Professor of
*   Neurology*
Biomedical Services (Neurology)
University of California, Riverside,
*   California;*
Director, Clinical Neurology and Neurodiagnostic
*   Services*
Arrowhead Regional Medical Center
Colton, California

Peter Kellaway, Ph.D.
Professor of Neurology
Section of Neurophysiology
Department of Neurology
Baylor College of Medicine
Houston, Texas

George H. Klem, R.EEG T.
Supervisor, Epilepsy and Sleep Disorders
Department of Neurology
The Cleveland Clinic Foundation
Cleveland, Ohio

Linda D. Leary, M.D.
Assistant Professor
Department of Neurology and Pediatrics
Columbia University College of Physicians and
  Surgeons:
Attending Physician
Division of Pediatric Epilepsy
Children's Hospital of New York Presbyterian
  Hospital
New York, New York

Ronald P. Lesser, M.D.
Professor, Department of Neurology
The Johns Hopkins University School of Medicine
Baltimore, Maryland

Brian Litt, M.D.
Assistant Professor
Departments of Neurology and Bioengineering
University of Pennsylvania;
Director, EEG Laboratory
Department of Neurology
Hospital of the University of Pennsylvania
Philadelphia, Pennsylvania

Hans O. Lüders, M.D., Ph.D.
Professor and Chairman
Department of Neurology
The Cleveland Clinic Foundation
Cleveland, Ohio

Omkar N. Markand, M.D.
Professor Emeritus
Department of Neurology
Indiana University School of Medicine;
Director, Clinical Neurophysiology
Department of Neurology
University Hospital
Indianapolis, Indiana

Anil Mendiratta, M.D.
Assistant Clinical Professor of Neurology
Department of Neurology
Columbia University;
The Comprehensive Epilepsy Center
The Neurological Institute of New York
Columbia-Presbyterian Medical Center
New York, New York

Eli M. Mizrahi, M.D.
Professor of Neurology and Pediatrics
Section of Neurophysiology
Department of Neurology and
Section of Pediatric Neurology
Department of Pediatrics
Baylor-Methodist Comprehensive Epilepsy Center
Baylor College of Medicine,
The Methodist Hospital and
Texas Children's Hospital
Houston, Texas

Douglas R. Nordli, Jr., M.D.
Associate Professor of Pediatrics
Northwestern University Medical School;
Lorna S. and James P. Langdon
Chair of Pediatric Epilepsy
Children's Memorial Hospital
Chicago, Illinois

Marc R. Nuwer, M.D., Ph.D.
Professor, Department of Neurology
University of California, Los Angeles;
Department Head
Department of Clinical Neurophysiology
University of California, Los Angeles, Medical
  Center
Los Angeles, California

Timothy A. Pedley, M.D.
Henry & Lucy Moses Professor of Neurology
Chairman, Department of Neurology
Columbia University;
Neurologist-in-Chief
Neurological Institute of New York
Columbia University Medical Center
New York, New York

Rodney A. Radtke, M.D.
Professor of Medicine (Neurology)
Duke University Medical School;
Director, Sleep Disorders Center
Duke University Medical Hospital
Durham, North Carolina

Donald L. Schomer, M.D.
Professor of Neurology
Harvard Medical School;
Director, Comprehensive Epilepsy Center and
Chief, Clinical Neurophysiology Laboratory
Beth Israel Deaconess Medical Center
Boston, Massachusetts

Frank W. Sharbrough, M.D.
Professor of Neurology Emeritus
Department of Neurology
Mayo Clinic
Rochester, Minnesota

Elson L. So, M.D.
Professor of Neurology
Department of Neurology
Mayo Clinic and Mayo Medical School;
Director, Section of Electroencephalography
Mayo Medical Center
Rochester, Minnesota

Michael R. Sperling, M.D.
Professor, Department of Neurology
Thomas Jefferson University;
Director, Clinical Neurophysiology Laboratory
Thomas Jefferson University Hospital
Philadelphia, Pennsylvania

Roger D. Traub, M.D.
Professor of Physiology, Pharmacology, and
*   Neurology*
State University of New York Health Science
*   Center at Brooklyn*
Brooklyn, New York

Giorgio S. Turella, M.D., Col.M.C.
Chief, Neurophysiology Laboratory
Department of Neurology
Madigan Army Medical Center
Tacoma, Washington

Anne C. Van Cott, M.D.
Assistant Professor
Department of Neurology
University of Pittsburgh;
Assistant Professor
Department of Neurology
Veterans Affairs Pittsburgh Health Care System
Pittsburgh, Pennsylvania

Thaddeus S. Walczak, M.D.
Associate Clinical Professor of Neurology
University of Minnesota;
Director of Clinical Neurophysiology
MINCEP Epilepsy Care
Minneapolis, Minnesota

Barbara F. Westmoreland, M.D.
Professor of Neurology
Department of Neurology
Mayo Clinic
Rochester, Minnesota

Peter K.H. Wong, B.Eng., M.D., F.R.C.P.(C)
Professor, Department of Pediatrics
University of British Columbia;
Director, Department of Diagnostic
*   Neurophysiology*
Children's & Women's Health Center
Vancouver, British Columbia, Canada

Benjamin G. Zifkin, M.D., C.M., F.R.C.P.(C).
Professeur Adjoint de Clinique
Faculté de Mèdecine
Université de Montrèal;
Neurologist, Epilepsy Clinic
Montrèal Neurological Hospital
Montrèal, Quèbec, Canada

Chapter 1

The Cellular Basis of EEG Activity[1]

György Buzsáki, Roger D. Traub, and Timothy A. Pedley

Sources of Extracellular Current Flow
  Fast (Na^+) Action Potentials
  Synaptic Activity
  Calcium Spikes
  Voltage-Dependent Intrinsic Oscillations
**Intrinsic Spike Afterhyperpolarizations: Their
  Contribution to Cortical Delta Waves**

Other Nonsynaptic Neuronal Effects
  Neuron–Glia Communication
  Ultrafast Cortical Rhythms
Summary
References

At this time, three methods can provide high temporal resolution of neuronal interactions at the network level: electric field recording (electroencephalogram [EEG]), magnetoencephalogram (MEG) (51,70), and optical images (32,86). Each of these has its advantages and shortcomings. MEG is not practical for experimental work on freely moving subjects, because of the large size of magnetic sensors. A major obstacle of the optical imaging method is that its "view" is confined to surface events. Because most of the network interactions occur at the level of the synapses, much of this in the depths of the brain, a search for alternative methods is warranted. In addition, research in both MEG and optical imaging fields faces the same fundamental questions as those that arose decades ago in connection with scalp-recorded EEG: the "reverse engineering" problem of signal interpretation (14,31,63) (see Chapter 4).

Membrane currents generated by neurons pass through the extracellular space. These currents can be measured by electrodes placed outside the neu-rons. The field potential (i.e., local mean field), recorded at any given site, reflects the linear sum of numerous overlapping fields generated by current sources (current from the intracellular space to the extracellular space) and sinks (current from the extracellular space to the intracellular space) distributed along multiple cells. This macroscopic state variable can be recorded with electrodes as a field potential or EEG or with magnetosensors (superconducting interference devices [SQUIDs]) as a MEG. These local field patterns therefore provide experimental access to the spatiotemporal activity of afferent, associational, and local operations in a given neural structure. To date, field potential measurements provide the best experimental and clinical tool for assessing cooperative neuronal activity at high temporal resolution. However, without a mechanistic description of the underlying neuronal processes, scalp or depth EEG is simply a gross correlate of brain activity rather than a predictive descriptor of the specific functional and anatomical events. The essential experimental tools for the exploration of EEG generation have yet to be developed. This chapter provides a

[1]Supported by the National Institutes of Health (NS34994, MH54671) and the Wellcome Trust.

basic description of field potential generation in the mammalian archicortex and neocortex and summarizes progress and future directions.

A straightforward approach to decompose the surface (scalp) recorded event is to study electrical activity simultaneously on the surface and at the sites of the extracellular current generation. Electrical recording from deep brain structures by means of wire electrodes is one of the oldest recording methods in neuroscience. Local field potential measurements, or "micro-EEG" (66), combined with recording of neuronal discharges is the best experimental tool available for studying the influence of cytoarchitectural properties, such as cortical lamination, distribution, size, and network connectivity of neural elements on electrogenesis. However, a large number of observation points combined with decreased distance between the recording sites are required for high spatial resolution and for enabling interpretation of the underlying cellular events. Progress in this field should be accelerated by the availability of micromachine silicon-based probes with numerous recording sites (60). Information obtained from the depths of the brain will then help clinicians interpret the surface-recorded events. Such a task clearly requires collaborative work among the fields of neuroscience, silicon nanotechnology, micromachinery, electric engineering, mathematics, and computer science. The stakes are high, because interpretation of macrosignals such as those obtained with EEG, MEG, fast magnetic resonance imaging (MRI), positron emission tomography (PET), or optical imaging methods will still require interpretation of the cellular-synaptic interactions at the network (submillimeter) level.

In principle, every event associated with membrane potential changes of individual cells (neurons and glia) should contribute to the perpetual voltage variability of the extracellular space. Until recently, synaptic activity was viewed as the exclusive source of extracellular current flow or EEG potential. As discussed later, however, synaptic activity is only one of the several membrane voltage changes that contribute to the measured field potential. Progress during the 1990s revealed numerous sources of relatively slow membrane potential fluctuations, not directly associated with synaptic activity. Such nonsynaptic events may also contribute significantly to the generation of local field potentials. These events include calcium spikes, voltage-dependent oscillations, and spike afterpotentials observed in various neurons.

SOURCES OF EXTRACELLULAR CURRENT FLOW

Fast (Na$^+$) Action Potentials

The largest amplitude intracellular event is the sodium-potassium spike, referred to as the fast (Na$^+$) action potential when it occurs at the intracellu-

lar level, and as unit activity when it occurs at the extracellular level. Individual fast action potentials are usually not considered to contribute significantly to scalp-recorded EEG potentials, mainly because of their short duration (<2 milliseconds). An additional factor is the high-pass frequency filtering (capacitive) property of the extracellular medium, which attenuates spatial summation of high-frequency events. As a result, the voltage of extracellular unit activity decreases much more rapidly with distance between the cell membrane and the recording site than is the case for slower membrane events. However, when a microelectrode is placed close to the cell body layer of cortical structures, the recorded field potentials contain both extracellular units and summed synaptic potentials. Furthermore, when action potentials from a large number of neighboring neurons occur within a short time window, such as in response to electrical stimulation of afferents, during epileptic activity, or even during synchronous physiological patterns, these "population spikes" can be recorded with relatively large electrodes and in a larger volume (Color Fig. 1.1) (4,9,25).

Synaptic Activity

In most physiological situations, synaptic activity is clearly the most significant source of the extracellular current flow that produces EEG potentials. The notion that synaptic potentials contribute to the generation of EEG potentials stems from the recognition that for the summation of extracellular currents from numerous individual compartments, the events must be relatively slow (39). The dendrites and soma of a neuron form a tree consisting of an electrically conducting interior surrounded by a relatively insulating membrane with tens of thousands of synapses on it. Each synapse acts as a small battery to drive current, always in a closed loop. Depending on the chemical nature of the neurotransmitter released in the synaptic cleft, the postsynaptic membrane is depolarized (excitatory postsynaptic potential [EPSP]) or hyperpolarized (inhibitory postsynaptic potential [IPSP]). Excitatory currents, involving Na$^+$ or Ca^{2+} ions, flow inwardly toward an excitatory synapse (i.e., from the activated postsynaptic site to the other parts of the cell) and outwardly away from it. The outward current is referred to as a *passive return current* from the intracellular milieu to the extracellular space. Inhibitory loop currents, involving Cl$^-$ or K$^+$ ions, flow in the opposite direction. The current flowing across the external resistance of the cortex sums with the loop currents of neighboring neurons to constitute a local mean field (see Fig. 1.1). Viewed from the perspective of the extracellular space, membrane areas where current flows into or out of the cells are termed *sinks* or *sources,* respectively. The active or passive nature of the sinks and sources is ambiguous, unless the location and types of synapses, involved in the current generation, are identified. Supplementary information may come from simultaneous intracellular recording from neurons dominantly involved in the current generation. Alternatively, extracellular recording of the action potentials and their cross-correlation with the laminar distribution of the field event can provide the necessary clues for the identification of a sink, as opposed to a passive return (inward) current of an active inhibitory source (outward). Cross-correlation of the interneuronal discharges with the field potential in question may further decrease the ambiguity regarding the passive versus active nature of the sink-source dipole (16).

Identification of Synaptic Currents in the Archicortex

Figure 1.1 illustrates the necessary steps in identifying network mechanisms of evoked and spontaneous field events. The example is taken from the hippocampus because it is a simple, three-layered structure consisting of orderly arranged principal cells (pyramidal and granule cells) and interneurons. Therefore, the synaptic interpretation of the extracellular current is much simpler than in multilayered structures. The termination zones of the excitatory paths and the inhibitory connections in the hippocampus are also well studied (14,85). Activation of the excitatory associational input by indirect, trisynaptic electrical stimulation depolarizes the midapical and basal dendrites of pyramidal cells (shown in blue in Fig. 1.1). The passive return current flows out of the cells at the level of the neuronal bodies and distal apical dendrites (shown in red in Fig. 1.1). This change in voltage is reflected by the characteristic distribution of field potentials in different depths. The extracellular voltage is negative close to the excitatory synapse and positive in the cell body layer. The reason for this is the large depolarization of the dendrite and the gradual decrease of intracellular depolarization toward the soma. This synaptic activity–induced intracellular voltage difference between the dendrites and soma (a dipole)–results in a current flow across the membrane (arrows in Fig. 1.1*F*). Simultaneous events in many neighboring pyramidal cells will linearly summate and produce an extracellular voltage fluctuation, which can be measured with closely spaced electrodes. After the impedance characteristics of the extracellular space are determined, the voltage change can be converted into current change (28).

Increased afferent discharge also activates interneurons, some of which terminate on the cell bodies of the pyramidal cells. The discharging basket cells release γ-aminobutyric acid (GABA) and activate Cl^- channels with resulting hyperpolarization of the pyramidal cell somata. Somatic hyperpolarization, in turn, creates a voltage gradient between the soma and dendrites (inhibitory dipole). The created intracellular voltage difference is the driving force of charges across the cell membrane and the consequent spatially distributed current flow in the surrounding extracellular fluid (see Fig. 1.1). Note that the direction of current flow is the same as that when the driving force is apical dendritic depolarization (active sink). Because the directions of current flow are identical for dendritic excitation and somatic inhibition, the excitatory and inhibitory currents sum in the extracellular space, resulting in large-amplitude field potentials.

The contribution of $GABA_A$ receptor-mediated inhibitory currents, however, is believed to be small, because the Cl^- equilibrium potential is close to the resting membrane potential. Thus, the change of the transmembrane voltage is limited. However, in actively spiking neurons, when the cell body is depolarized, the transmembrane potential, mediated by $GABA_a$ synapses, can be large. Another cautionary note is that inhibition may operate also on the dendrites, causing current flow opposite to the direction of excitatory currents. For the identification of excitatory and inhibitory components, represented by the extracellular current flow, a precise knowledge about the anatomical network is essential. Physiological experiments, including recordings from interneurons and pyramidal cells and differential pharmacological blockage of the excitatory and inhibitory synapses, can then provide the necessary knowledge as to which cell types are involved when the associational pathways are electrically activated. These extracellular and intracellular events therefore provide circumstantial evidence that the same neuronal machinery is activated during spontaneously occurring sharp waves (SPWs) as during electrical stimulation of the associational afferent fibers.

Identification of Synaptic Currents in the Neocortex

The strategy just described is, in principle, applicable to any other *a priori* identified rhythmic or sparse EEG event. Complications arise when several dipoles are involved in the generation of the same EEG patterns, especially when these dipoles are phase shifted, as is the case in the generation of the numerous neocortical patterns (10,80,81).

Of the neocortical EEG patterns, two conspicuous low-frequency (<15 Hz) rhythms, the physiological sleep spindles and the spike-and-wave discharges associated with petit mal epilepsy, have been studied most extensively (10,13,44,55,77,81). It is widely accepted that the source of rhythm generation for both patterns is the interplay between the GABAergic reticular nucleus and corticopetal nuclei of the thalamus (10,13,79,81). It is less clear, however, whether synaptic currents of the thalamocortical afferents can fully account for these rhythms or whether intracortical circuitries are significantly involved in their generation (40). Initially, the "recruiting" response, evoked by repetitive stimulation of intralaminar thalamic nuclei, was thought to be the evoked equivalent of spontaneous spindle waves and spike-and-wave patterns (19,24,41,59,67). Subsequent studies, however, have suggested that spindle waves are more similar to the "augmenting" response, a pattern evoked by repetitive simulation of sensorimotor thalamic nuclei (58,75,76). From the point of EEG generation, this distinction is important because recruiting and augmenting responses have different voltage-versus-depth profiles in the cortex. Thus, a critical issue is the identity of synapses and neurons involved in the generation of these rhythmic patterns. If the thalamocortical synapses are the major source of the extracellular synaptic current, then the major sinks are expected to correspond to the anatomical targets of the corticopetal thalamic fibers.

Use of the approach just described for the hippocampus helped clarify these issues (Color Fig. 1.2) (44). The most striking aspects of the experiment shown in Fig. 1.2 is the general similarity of the spontaneous and evoked field events, which is independent of the initiating conditions. The spatial position of the major current sinks or sources are similar, independently which thalamic nucleus or hemisphere is being stimulated. The differences are expressed mainly in the latencies of the large sink-source pairs. Therefore, the similar spatiotemporal distribution of the main sinks and sources suggest that the major current flow derives from the activity of the intracortical circuitry. The neocortex, in essence, functions as a powerful amplifier during these oscillatory events. Because the thalamocortical network is in a metastable state during reduced activities of the brainstem and basal forebrain (55,77), a weak thalamic or callosal input is capable of recruiting a large population of intracortical neurons. The triggering input may even remain undetectable in the field, and the spread of activity reflects primarily the connectivity and excitability of the cortical circuitry rather than the nature of the initiating input (16,17).

The current source density (CSD) map and the associated multiple-site unit analysis also revealed that at least three dipoles were involved in the generation of the rhythmic field events (Color Fig. 1.3) (44). The most consistent dipole was characterized by a major sink in layer IV (dipole 2). When a surface-positive field component was present, it was associated with a major sink in layer VI and a source in layers II to III (dipole 1). The third, delayed dipole was represented by a surface-negative spike component and a corresponding sink in layers II to III (dipole 3). The relative strength of these respective sinks varied within single episodes of high-wave spike-and-

voltage discharge (HVS) (see Fig. 1.3). Although the numerous cell types and the complexity of the intracortical circuitry makes identification of the cellular-synaptic origin of neocortical EEG potentials less accessible, these findings indicate that the use of simultaneous recording of field and unit activity is a proper method for the revelation of the synaptic-cellular mechanisms of extracellular current flow in the neocortex.

Calcium Spikes

In addition to the fast Na^+ spike, an important nonsynaptic event in neurons is a wide Ca^{2+}-mediated action potential. These Ca^{2+} spikes are generated in dendrites and do not propagate to the soma (89). It is believed that their major roles are to boost synaptic inputs and assist plastic modification of synapses (42,53,54,91). Ca^{2+} spikes represent an inward dendritic current and are large in amplitude (20 to 50 mV). They can occur synchronously with dendritic EPSPs, and for this reason they cannot be simply revealed or separated from EPSPs with extracellular recordings. Because Ca^{2+} spikes are activated by a voltage-dependent mechanism, intradendritic depolarization can trigger them.

Figure 1.4 illustrates *in vivo* recording from a distal dendrite of a hippocampal CA1 pyramidal neuron during theta oscillation (43). As the dendrite is progressively depolarized by intracellular current injection, the rhythmic synaptic potentials are superseded by large-amplitude Ca^{2+} events. Are such Ca^{2+} spikes triggered by physiological stimuli? There is evidence that this may well be the case. Patterned stimulation of the visual system evoked putative Ca^{2+} events in layer V pyramidal neurons of area 17 (37). Furthermore, intradendritic recordings during spontaneous SPW bursts revealed that the amount of depolarization, brought about by the converging active presynaptic afferent fibers to CA1 pyramidal cells, is sufficient to trigger voltage-dependent Ca^{2+} spikes (42). This new information, of course, indicates the need for the reinterpretation of the extracellular events illustrated in Fig. 1.1. Provided that Ca^{2+} spikes occur simultaneously in several neurons near the recording electrodes, these large inward currents can significantly contribute to the field sinks observed in the dendritic layers.

To date, the quantitative contribution of dendritic Ca^{2+} spikes to the field EEG has not been determined. They may be quite important in highly synchronous events, such as epilepsy, because synchronous Ca^{2+} spikes in neighboring neurons may be reflected in the field as large sinks. A complicating factor is that, in contrast to EPSPs, Ca^{2+} spikes can actively propa-

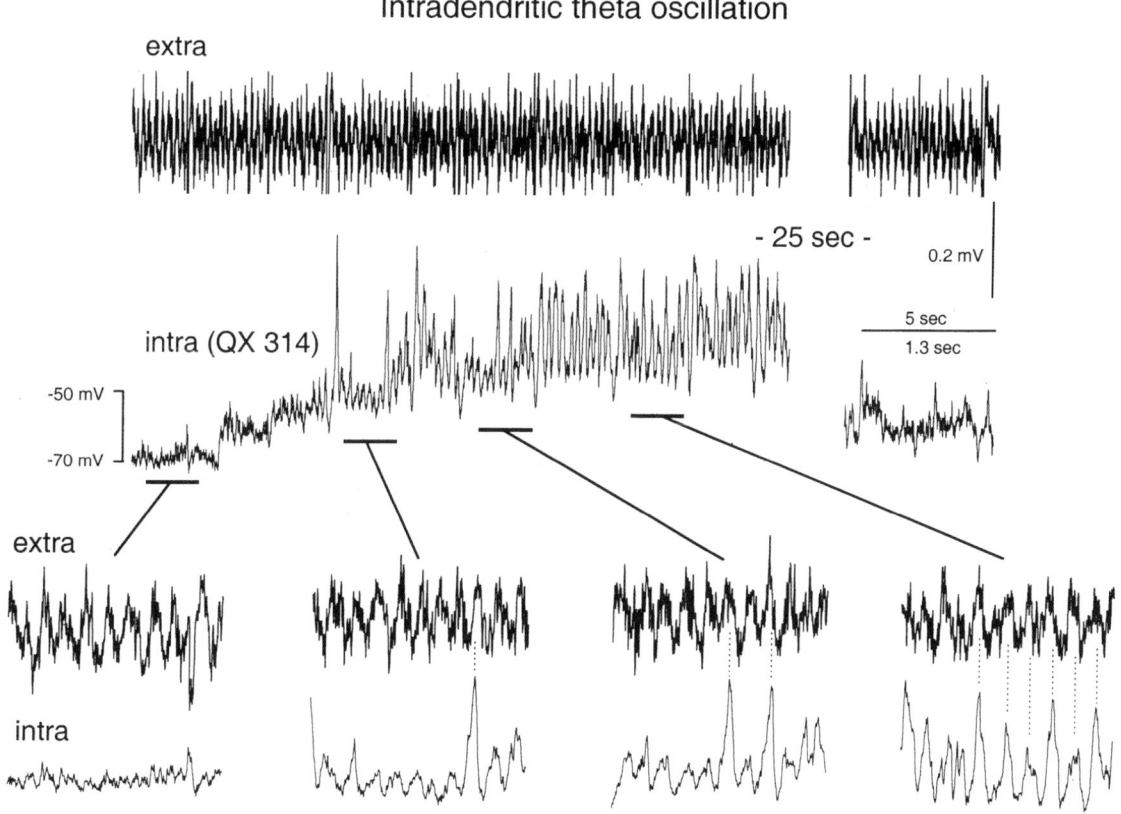

FIG. 1.4. Voltage-dependence of theta frequency oscillation in a hippocampal pyramidal cell dendrite. Continuous recording of extracellular (extra) and intradendritic (intra) activity in a CA1 pyramidal cell. Holding potential was manually shifted to progressively more depolarized levels by intradendritic current injection (0 to 0.8 nA). The marked epochs (*horizontal bars*) are shown at faster speed in the bottom records. The recording electrode also contained QX-314 to block Na+ spikes (20 mM). Note large increase of intradendritic theta oscillation amplitude upon depolarization. The relationship of the putative high-threshold calcium spikes to the phase of extracellular theta waves in the CA1 pyramidal layer is indicated by *dotted lines.* (From Kamondi A, Acsády L, Wang X-J, et al. Theta oscillations in somata and dendrites of hippocampal pyramidal cells *in vivo:* activity dependent phase-precession of action potentials. *Hippocampus* 1998;8:244–261.)

gate, and large dendritic segments and dendritic locations distant from the initiating site may therefore also be involved.

Voltage-Dependent Intrinsic Oscillations

Experiments similar to that shown in Fig. 1.4 revealed that when intradendritic depolarization is sufficiently strong, the resonant property of the membrane may give way to a self-sustained oscillation of the voltage in the theta frequency range, even in the absence of network-driven theta activity. Intrinsic, voltage-dependent slow oscillations and theta frequency resonance have also been observed in somatic recordings of hippocampal pyramidal

cells (49), thalamocortical neurons (63), stellate cells of the entorhinal cortex (2), and layer V pyramidal cells of the neocortex (73). In stellate cells, the main driving force of the oscillation is a persistent Na+ current (2), whereas another depolarizing current (I_h), in conjunction with the low threshold Ca^{2+} current (I_T), is responsible for the maintenance of the cellular rhythm in thalamic neurons (6).

Voltage-dependent oscillatory activation of ionic channels has been shown also in the gamma frequency range. The membrane potential of sparsely spiny inhibitory interneurons in cortical layer IV can sustain a 40-Hz oscillation by sequential activation of a persistent Na+ current, followed by a slowly inactivating K+ conductance (50,51). Similar intrinsic oscillatory properties have been shown in the intralaminar thalamocortical nuclei and GABAergic neurons of the nucleus reticularis *in vivo* (81) and in the dendrites of hippocampal pyramidal cells (65).

In most neurons, the voltage-dependent oscillation is below the threshold to trigger action potentials. However, when action potentials do occur, they are phase locked to the depolarizing portion of the oscillatory cycle. Because these intrinsic, oscillatory membrane fluctuations can occur simultaneously in a number of nearby neurons, their contribution to the extracellular EEG may be substantial. This is perhaps best illustrated in the "low-Ca^{2+}, high Mg^{2+}" model of epilepsy, in which all synaptic activity is completely blocked and the large rhythmic extracellular field potentials are caused exclusively by the voltage-dependent fluctuation of pyramidal cells, coordinated by ephaptic (nonsynaptic) transmembrane effects (33).

INTRINSIC SPIKE AFTERHYPERPOLARIZATIONS: THEIR CONTRIBUTION TO CORTICAL DELTA WAVES

In addition to voltage changes, perturbation of the intracellular concentration of one ion species may trigger influx of other ions by activation of ligand-gated channels. The large Ca^{2+} influx, in association with a dendritic Ca^{2+} spike, is followed by the suppression of fast spikes and hyperpolarization of the membrane caused by activation of Ca^{2+}-mediated increase of K^+ conductance (38,72). These burst-induced afterhyperpolarizations (AHPs) are frequently larger in amplitude and of longer duration than synaptic events. A logical progression of thought is to conclude that they should also be considered important source of the extracellularly recorded EEG potential.

Slow, large-amplitude delta waves (1 to 4 Hz) have been among the most frequently studied neocortical EEG patterns. These irregular, semirhythmic or rhythmic patterns are most frequently observed during stage 4 sleep in the normal brain. The rhythmicity of the cortical delta waves is explained by the triggering effect of the periodic quasisynchronous thalamocortical inputs (22,78). The thalamus can maintain a rhythmic oscillation in the delta range because of the intrinsic properties of thalamocortical neurons and their network connectivity with the GABAergic reticular nucleus (22,78). In short, the "rhythm generator" of delta waves is the thalamus, whereas the "voltage generator" is the neocortex; this situation is analogous to that for sleep spindles and spike-and-wave patterns, discussed earlier.

Delta waves occur with largest amplitude in deep (layer V) cortical layers, and they are recorded as negative waves on the neocortical surface or the scalp. Depth profile measurements in the neocortexes of the cat (15,40,71), rabbit (68), and rat (10,87) revealed that surface negative–deep positive delta waves during slow-wave sleep correlate with the suppression or cessation of discharges of layer V pyramidal neurons. At the intracellular level, the deep positive waves are correlated with hyperpolarization of pyramidal cells (21).

The depth profile of the slow delta waves and the associated unit activity are compatible with the hypothesis that the extracellularly recorded delta waves reflect inhibition of pyramidal cells mediated by GABAergic interneurons (3,69,74). GABA released at the somata of layer V pyramidal cells would open the Cl^- channels and produce an active outward current whose extracellular spatial summation corresponds to deep positivity. A simultaneously occurring passive inward current at the distal dendrites would set up extracellular (surface) negativity. Indeed, with their widespread action, GABAergic interneurons may play an important role in affecting large numbers of pyramidal cells, as discussed earlier. Because subcortical inputs also terminate on GABAergic interneurons (29,30), the subcortical afferents may globally affect the whole neocortical mantle.

A major problem with this "classic" model of delta wave generation is the lack of direct supportive evidence. An explicit prediction of the GABA-interneuron-pyramidal cell model of slow wave generation is that GABAergic cells should fire during the deep positive delta waves. However, experiments directly addressing this issue have failed to find such a correlation in the rat neocortex (10). All putative, physiologically identified neocortical interneurons decreased their firing rates during the deep positive slow waves. Although the duration of the GABA effect may outlast the action potentials by tens of milliseconds (23), the effect may be too short for the postulated delta wave–associated GABA-mediated somatic hyperpolarization. $GABA_B$-receptor–mediated IPSPs may be a possible candidate for producing this hyperpolarization.

An alternative nonsynaptic explanation of the origin of delta wave generation is based on the summation of long-lasting AHPs of layer V pyramidal neurons (10,77). During sleep, pyramidal cells of the neocortex often fire bursts in response to rhythmic thalamic volleys (22,78), and these bursts, in turn, can trigger Ca^{2+}-mediated K^+-conductance changes. The long-lasting nature of AHPs favors the summation of outward somatic currents of individual pyramidal cells, which results in a local positive field in deep layers. Such extracellularly summated currents were hypothesized to form the basis of slow delta EEG waves recorded during sleep (14). Delta waves occur only during slow-wave sleep because subcortical neurotransmitters, such as basal forebrain and brainstem cholinergic neurons, locus ceruleus cells, neurons of the raphe nuclei, and hypothalamic histaminergic neurons (1,5,10,34,77), are released mostly in the awake brain, and the common property of these neurons is to reduce the calcium-mediated potassium conductance (20,33,52). These actions of subcortical neurotransmitters at the cellular level therefore result in the blockade of delta waves. Using whole-cell recordings *in vivo,* Metherate and Ashe (57) could differentiate between IPSPs and AHPs in cortical neurons of the intact brain. First, they showed, by intracellular injection of cesium, that a large part of the delta EEG wave results from a K^+ current. Second, stimulation of the cholinergic nucleus basalis caused an effect that mimicked the cesium effect. Third, cesium injection blocked the nucleus basalis stimulation effect. These findings directly support the suggestion that delta wave–concurrent hyperpolarizations result from the calcium-activated K^+ current, rather than from GABA-mediated IPSPs. Overall, these examples illustrate that knowledge of the intrinsic properties of the neurons is as important for the identification of sources of the extracellular ion flow as knowledge of synaptic potentials and anatomical circuitry.

OTHER NONSYNAPTIC NEURONAL EFFECTS

Synchronous discharge of large neuronal populations is often associated with large-amplitude extracellular potentials (millivolts to tens of millivolts) and steep voltage-versus-depth gradients. These large field currents, in turn, can influence the activity of nearby neurons by changing their transmembrane voltage (ephaptic effects). Measurement of transmembrane potential changes (as opposed to potentials relative to a distant ground) indicated that such extracellular current loops can depolarize neurons to spike threshold under certain conditions (33,83). Computer simulations of multiple neurons, embedded in a conductive medium, show that such a mechanism is plausible with observed estimates of extracellular resistivity (84). Of importance is that the voltage gradient across pyramidal cell bodies during physiological SPWs and especially during epileptic or interictal spikes is larger than experimentally induced voltage gradients that are known to affect cellular excitability. It is possible, although direct experimental evidence is not available yet, that ephaptic effects could recruit neurons to fire that are otherwise not sufficiently activated by synaptic inputs alone (9,33).

Neuron–Glia Communication

The glial syncytium (astrocytes) is connected through gap junctions, which allow the direct spread of current and the diffusion or transport of small molecules. Although the role of concerted changes in membrane potentials of glial cells in the generation of extracellular currents under physiological conditions has not been studied extensively, work on neuron–glia interactions indicate that the glial syncytium may contribute to the slow field patterns in an important way. Intercellular coupling through gap junctions is required for both propagating Ca^{2+} waves and spreading depression (62). The traveling Ca^{2+}, waves, in turn, can trigger calcium influx into neurons (61,62). The neuron–glia dialogue *in vivo* may be responsible for postictal depression (8,26,35,36,48,82). The increased $[K^+]_O$, resulting from intensive neuronal activity during epileptic afterdischarge, may trigger propagating waves in the astrocytic network, which are reflected by the slowly spreading sustained potentials. In turn, astrocytes at the front of the propagating depolarization wave release more K^+ (47,56), resulting in a large depolarization of neurons. The ensuing depolarization block of spike generation contributes to the termination of the afterdischarge and is regarded as the cause of the consequent "postictal depression" of the EEG (8,82).

Direct currents (DC) or ultraslow change of the extracellular voltage cannot be recorded with conventional EEG devices with high pass-filtered inputs. Nevertheless, the relatively quick changes in the DC level, such as epilepsy-associated spreading depression (8), could be identified mistakenly as slow delta or faster "waves," because of the differential effect of the high-pass filters.

Neuron–glia communication may also contribute to physiological EEG patterns. Sensory evoked responses in scalp recordings with DC amplifiers and nonpolarizing electrodes often contain reliable and relatively long-lasting DC changes, usually referred to as *Bereitschaftpotential* (46) or *contingent negative variation* (88). It remains to be revealed whether and to what extent glial depolarization contributes to these evoked patterns.

Ultrafast Cortical Rhythms

SPW-associated depolarization of hippocampal CA1 neurons sets into motion a short-lived, dynamic interaction between interneurons and pyramidal cells. The product of this interaction is an oscillatory field potential (ripple) within the stratum pyramidale hippocampi and a phase-locked discharge of the CA1 network at 200 Hz in the rat (11). SPW-related ripples are also present in higher mammals, including humans (7). The specific synaptic currents, mediating the high-frequency oscillation, are largely mediated by rhythmic, synchronized IPSPs near the soma of CA1 neurons. The mechanism by which highly coherent discharge of pyramidal cells is

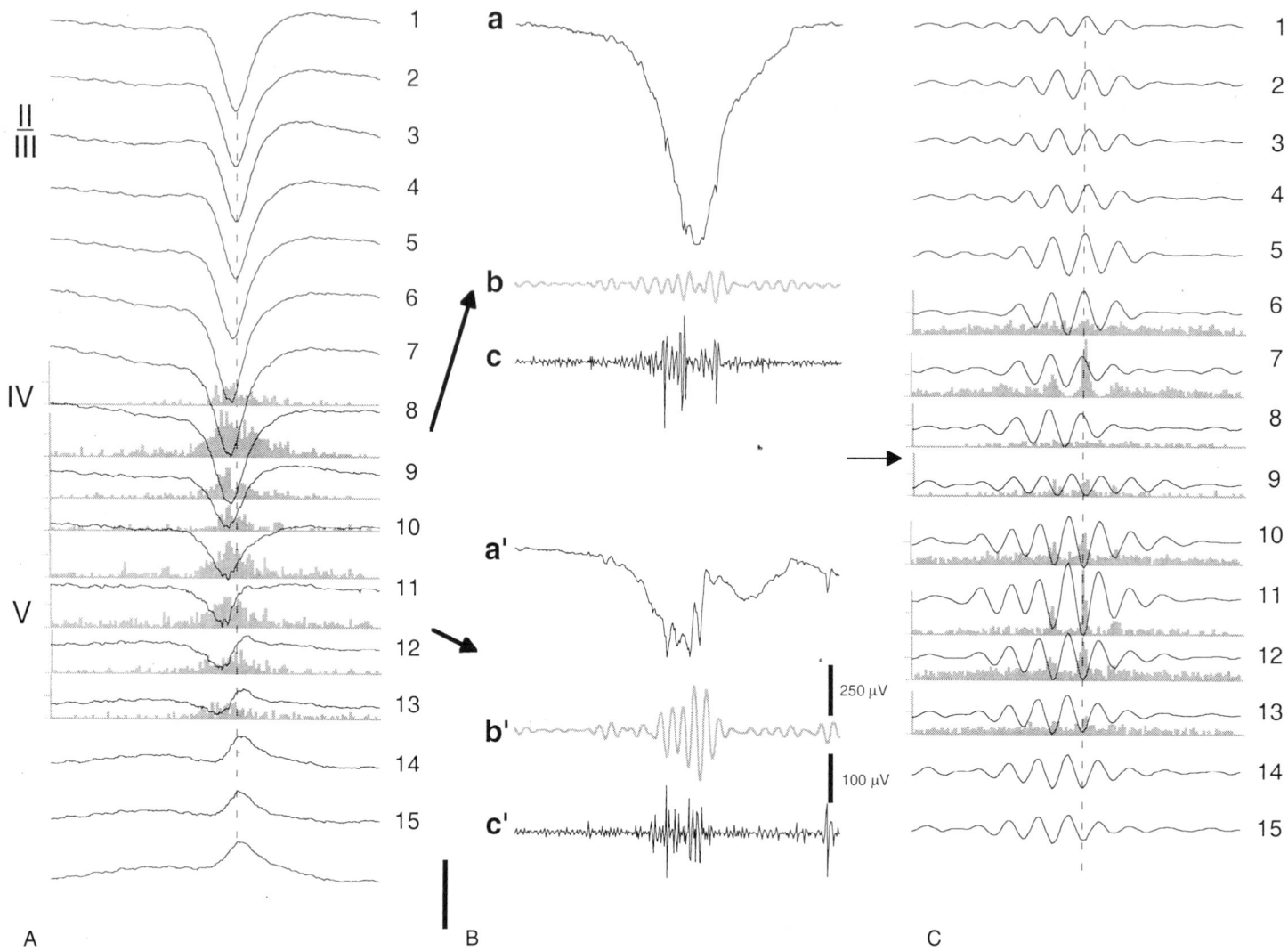

FIG. 1.5. High-wave spike-and-voltage (HVS) pattern—induced fast field oscillation (400- to 500-Hz ripple). **A:** Averaged HVS and associated unit firing histograms from layers IV to VI. **B:** Wide-band (a and a'; 1 to 5 kHz), filtered field (b and b'; 200 to 800 Hz), and filtered unit (c and c'; 0.5 to 5 kHz) traces from layer IV and layer V. **C:** Averaged fast waves and corresponding unit histograms. The field ripples are filtered (200- to 800-Hz) derivatives of the wide-band signals recorded from 16 sites. Note sudden phase-reversal of the oscillatory waves (*arrow*) and phase-locked discharges of units in all cortical layers (*dashed line*). (From Kandel A, Buzsáki G. Cellular-synaptic generation of sleep spindles, spike-and-wave discharges and evoked thalamocortical responses in the neocortex of the rat. *J Neurosci* 1997;17:6783–6797.)

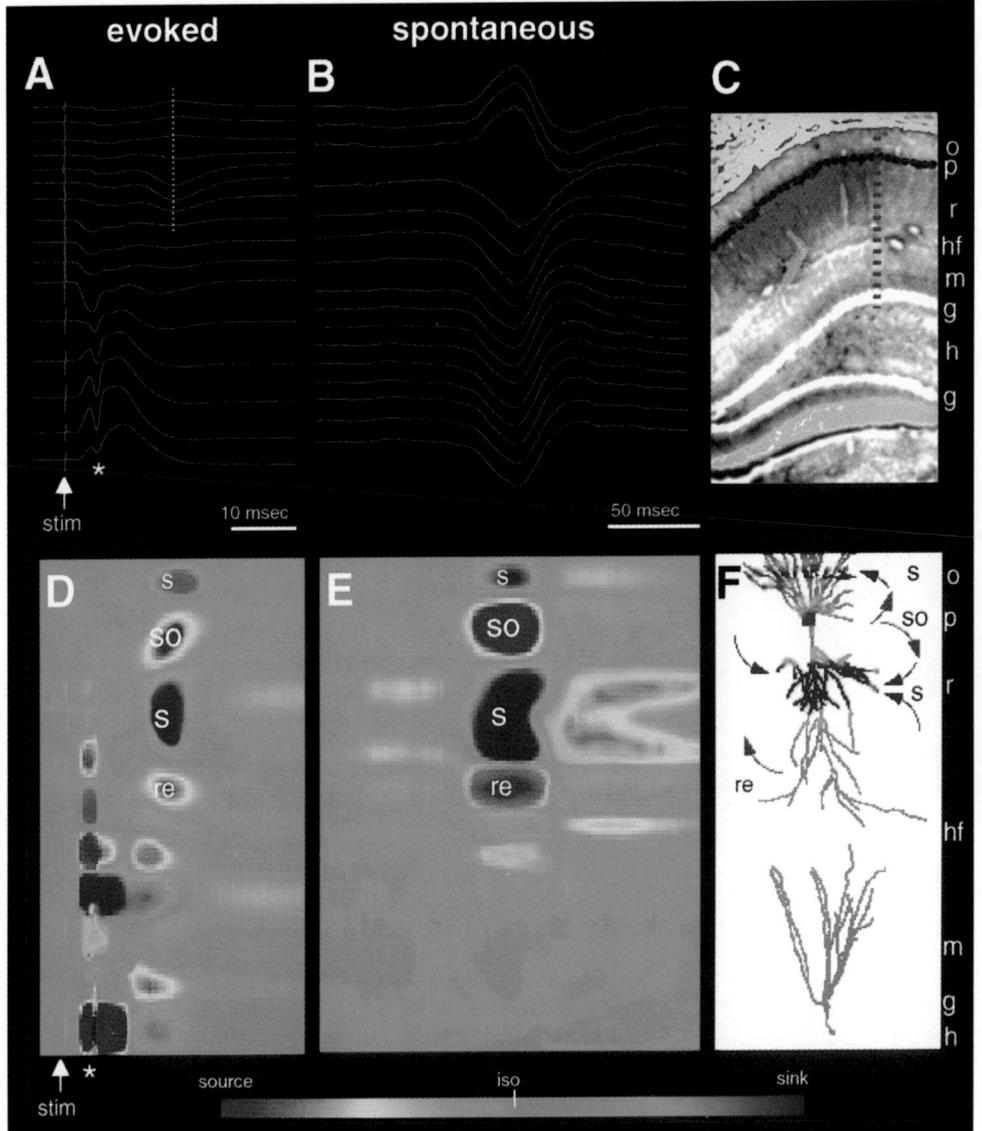

FIG. 1.1. Generation of extracellular field potentials. The time scale in A and D, B and E are the same. **A:** Simultaneously recorded evoked field responses in the CA1-dentate gyrus axis of the rat hippocampus in response to stimulation of the entorhinal input (stim). The *asterisk* indicates population discharge of the monosynaptically activated granule cells. Their discharge, in turn, activates CA3 pyramidal cells (not shown) whose associational collaterals will depolarize CAI pyramidal cells and interneurons. This trisynaptic activation of CAI pyramidal cells is reflected as a late field event (*vertical dashed line*). **B:** Spontaneously occurring sharp wave recorded during immobility. The traces are averages of 40 individual events. **C:** A frontal section of the hippocampus, indicating the contact sites of the recording silicon probe (*small squares*). o, stratum oriens; p, pyramidal layer; r, stratum radiatum; hf, hippocampal fissure; g, granule cell layer; h, hilar region. **D and E:** Current source density (CSD) maps of evoked field responses to perforant path stimulation (D) and of the spontaneous sharp wave (SPW) pattern. Sinks (s, inward currents) and sources (so, outward currents) are indicated by cold and warm colors, respectively. iso, zero current flow. **F:** Interpretation of the current sinks and sources on the basis of anatomical connectivity. Recorded layers are shown on the right of the pyramidal cell (above) and granule cell (below). Putative active currents are indicated on the right and passive return (re) currents on the left of the pyramidal neuron. Note identical current sink-source distribution of the evoked and spontaneous events in the CAI region (compare parts *D* and *E*). Sinks in the stratum radiatum hippocampi and the stratum oriens hippocampi reflect excitation of the apical and basal dendrites of CA1 pyramidal cells, respectively, by the associational (Schaffer) collateral fibers of the CA3 region. The large source in the pyramidal layer is a combination of active outward current caused by hyperpolarization of the soma by the simultaneously activated basket cells (not shown) and passive return currents from the sinks generated in the basal and apical dendrites. The source in the distal apical dendrites (re) is assumed to represent a passive return current caused by the active sink in the middle of the stratum radiatum hippocampi. In addition to excitatory postsynaptic potentials (EPSPs), dendritic Ca^{2+} spikes may also contribute to the sinks in the stratum oriens hippocampi and the stratum radiatum hippocampi (see Fig. 1.4). (From Buzsáki G, Traub RD. Generation of EEG. In: Engel J Jr, Pedley TA, eds. *Epilepsy: a comprehensive textbook.* Philadelphia: Lippincott-Raven, 1996.)

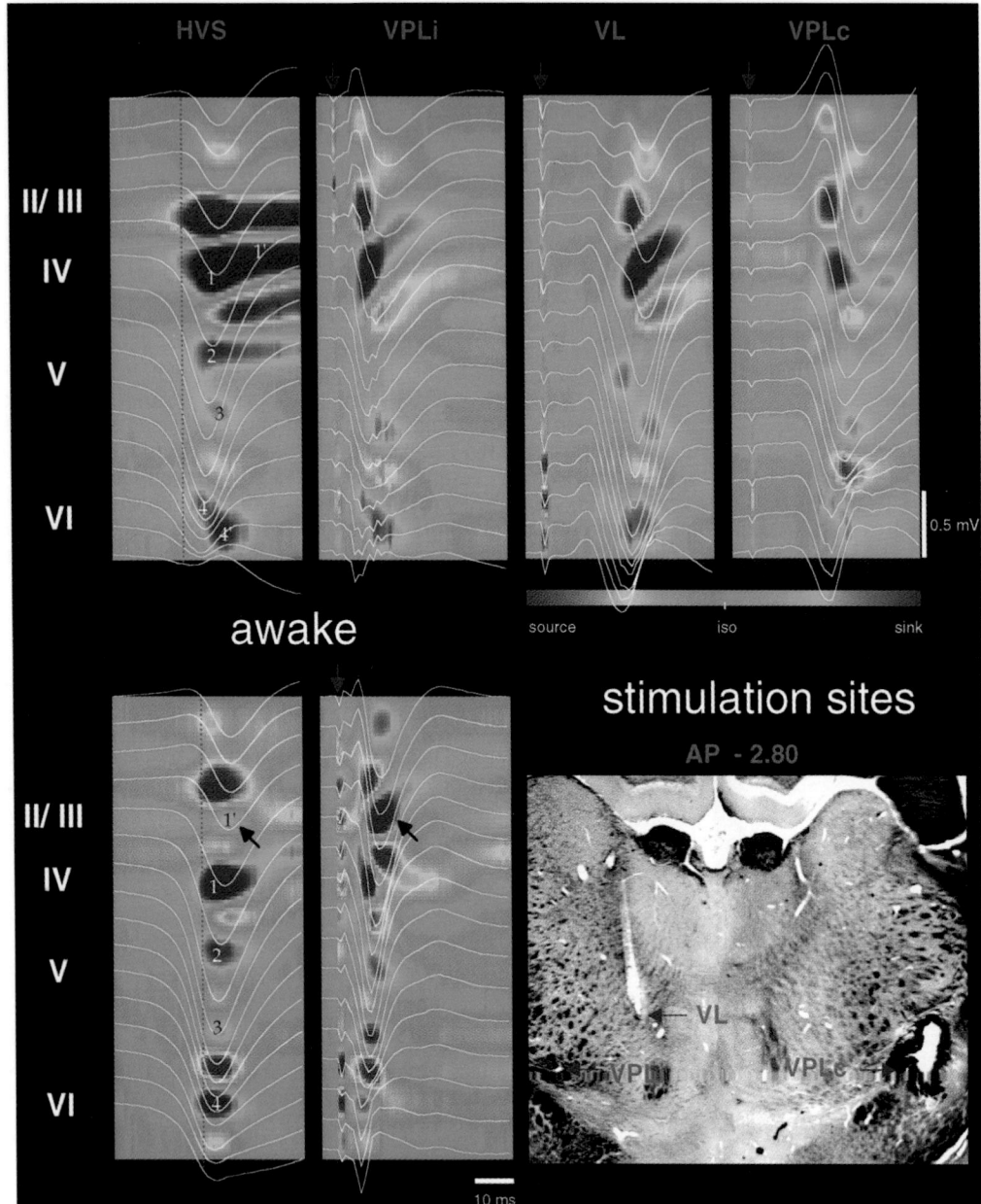

FIG. 1.2. Voltage versus depth profiles superimposed onto current source density (CSD) maps of high-voltage spike-and-wave (HVS) patterns and thalamic evoked responses in the rat under ketamine-induced anesthesia and in the awake rat. The 16-site recording probe was located in the somatosensory area. The approximate position of the different layers are indicated left of the CSD maps. Note the overall similarity of the major sinks and sources of the averaged HVS patterns, and evoked responses. Major sinks are numbered (1 to 4 in HVS patterns). *Vertical dashed lines* help identify the earliest sinks and sources. VPLi, primary response; VL and VPLc, augmenting responses 200 milliseconds after the primary response (not shown). In VL, weak early sinks can be identified in layer VI and layer V, followed by major sinks at similar locations, as in the other CSD maps. Stimulating sites are shown in the histological section. The tip of the ipsilateral VPL (VPLi) was two sections (120 μm) posterior to the VL site. An electrolytic lesion was produced at the contralateral VPL (VPLc) stimulating site. Voltage and current calibrations are identical in all panels. iso, baseline isopotential. (From Kandel A, Buzsáki G. Cellular-synaptic generation of sleep spindles, spike-and-wave discharges and evoked thalamocortical responses in the neocortex of the rat. *J Neurosci* 1997;17:6783–6797.)

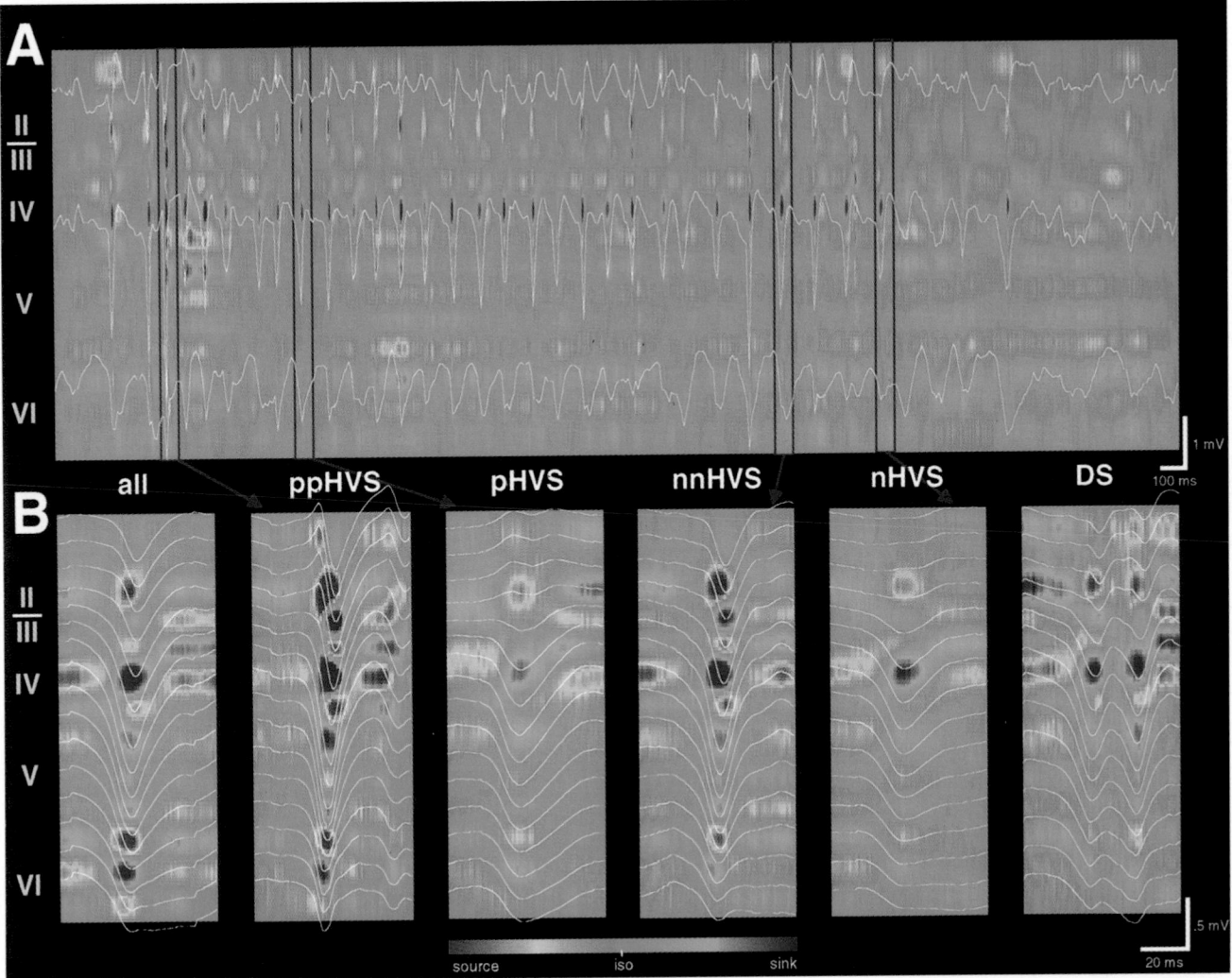

FIG. 1.3. Variations in the voltage-versus-depth profiles and current source density (CSD) maps of high-voltage spike-and-wave (HVS) patterns in the awake rat. **A:** CSD map of a single HVS episode (3-second sweep). The superimposed field traces were recorded from layers II, IV, and VI. Note the consistent presence of the layer IV sink but large variability of sinks and sources at other depth locations. **B:** Selected averages of HVS traces and corresponding CSD maps. All represent averages of 200 successive events. Note a prominent delayed sink in layers II to III in ppHVS and nnHVS. Averages from 40 to 50 traces selected from a 5-minute recording session. Representative single events of the averages are indicated by *vertical lines* in part *A*. DS, average HVS with double-spike components at short interspike intervals; iso, baseline isopotential; nHVS, average HVS with negative spike component in layer IV; nnHVS, average HVS with dominant surface-negative spike component and large sink in layers II to III; pHVS, average HVS with less pronounced surface-positive component; ppHVS, average HVS with prominent surface-positive spike component. (From Kandel A, Buzsáki G. Cellular-synaptic generation of sleep spindles, spike-and-wave discharges and evoked thalamocortical responses in the neocortex of the rat. *J Neurosci* 1997; 17:6783–6797.)

brought about over the entire dorsal hippocampus during the ripple is not understood (18). Three hypotheses have been advanced to explain the spatial coherence of fast ripples. According to the first, the CA3 output produces a voltage-dependent fast discharge in the interneurons, and synchronization of the interneurons is mediated by gap junctions (45). The second explanation, which is based on the reciprocal connections between the interneuronal and pyramidal cell populations, is that fast oscillatory discharges in interneurons would, again, be brought about by the ramp-like depolarizing CA3 output. Chance discharge of just a few CA1 pyramidal cells within approximately 1 millisecond, is hypothesized to reset ongoing oscillatory spiking in the target interneurons and generate a short-lived coherent discharge (90). According to the third hypothesis, zero time lag synchronization of pyramidal neurons is brought about by assumed gap junctions between their axons (25).

Fast field oscillations (300 to 500 Hz) are also present in the neocortex, particularly in association with sleep spindles and spike-and-wave patterns (Fig. 1.5) (44). The maximum amplitude of the field oscillation occurs in layer V, and the ripple waves reverse in phase in the upper part of layer V. The discharge of pyramidal cells are phase locked to the ripples. The physiological significance of the fast ripples has yet to be clarified. It may be that the fast oscillation of interneurons during a strong network drive provides a dissipative mechanism to decelerate and limit population synchrony of pyramidal cells and to prevent the all-or-none discharge of the activated pyramidal cells by protracting the recruitment process and limiting the number of participating neurons.

Because conventional EEG devices are limited in their frequency response, these fast events are often impossible to discern reliably from human scalp recordings (21a). In addition, volume conduction of these fast events is quite limited because of the low-pass filtering properties of lipid membranes, as discussed earlier. Nevertheless, their detection may be of clinical importance because fast oscillatory events may herald the spread or termination, or both, of epileptic activity (8,27).

SUMMARY

Field potential measurements provide an excellent tool for the exploration of network activity in the intact brain. The various rhythms and intermittent EEG potentials can be regarded as time reference points to relate neuronal discharges of single cells. These field potentials (local or global EEG potentials) emerge as a result of synchronous (i.e., simultaneous) changes of the membrane potential of neighboring neurons. Synchronous membrane potential changes can be brought about by synaptic activity (EPSPs and IPSPs) or Ca^{2+} spikes, or they can emerge as a result of intrinsic neuronal patterns (oscillations, burst-induced afterpotentials). The isolated cortical tissue maintains burst discharges of pyramidal cells, followed by long-lasting afterhyperpolarization. The synchronous hyperpolarizations in neighboring pyramidal cells can be measured as slow waves in the extracellular space (synchronization). In addition, these subcortical neurotransmitters induce a gamma frequency oscillation (desynchronized pattern) by activating networks of inhibitory interneurons.

REFERENCES

1. Abercrombie ED, Jacobs BL. Single-unit response of noradrenergic neurons in the locus coeruleus, of freely moving cats. I. Acutely presented stressful and nonstressful stimuli. *J Neurosci* 1987;7:2837–2843.
2. Alonso A, Llinás RR. Subthreshold Na+-dependent theta-like rhythmicity in stellate cells of entorhinal cortex layer 11. *Nature* 1989;342:175–177.
3. Amzica F, Steriade M. Electrophysiological correlates of sleep delta waves. *Electroencephalogr Clin Neurophysiol* 1998;107:69–83.
4. Andersen P, Bliss TV, Skrede KK. Unit analysis of hippocampal polulation spikes. *Exp Brain Res* 1971;13:208–221.
5. Aston-Jones G, Bloom FE. Norepinephrine-containing locus coeruleus neurons in behaving rats exhibit pronounced responses to non-noxious environmental stimuli. *J Neuroscience* 1981;1:887–900.
6. Bal T, Von Krosigk M, McCormick DA. Synaptic and membrane mechanisms underlying synchronized oscillations in the ferret lateral geniculate nucleus *in vitro*. *J Physiol (Lond)* 1995;483:641–663.
7. Bragin A, Engel J Jr, Wilson CL, et al. Hippocampal and entorhinal cortex high-frequency oscillations (100–500 Hz) in human epileptic brain and in kainic acid–treated rats with chronic seizures. *Epilepsia* 1999;40:127–137.
8. Bragin A, Penttonen M, Buzsáki G. Termination of epileptic afterdischarge. *Neuroscience* 1997;17:2567–2579.
9. Buzsáki G. Hippocampal sharp waves: their origin and significance. *Brain Res* 1986;398:242–252.
10. Buzsáki G, Bickford TG, Ponomareff G, et al. Nucleus basalis and thalamic control of neocortical activity in the freely moving rat. *Neuroscience* 1988;8:4007–4026.
11. Buzsáki G, Horvath Z, Urioste R, et al. High-frequency network oscillation in the hippocampus. *Science* 1992;256:1025–1027.
12. Buzsáki G, Leung L, Vanderwolf CH. Cellular bases of hippocampal EEG in the behaving rat. *Brain Res Rev* 1983;6:139–171.
13. Buzsáki G, Smith A, Berger S, et al. Petit mal epilepsy and parkinsonian tremor: hypothesis of a common pacemaker. *Neuroscience* 1990;36:114.
14. Buzsáki G, Traub RD. Generation of EEG. In: Engel J Jr, Pedley TA, eds. *Epilepsy: a comprehensive textbook*. Philadelphia: Lippincott-Raven, 1996:819–830.
15. Calvet J, Valvet MC, Scherrer J. Etude stratigraphique corticale de l'activité EEG spontanee. *Electroencephalogr Clin Neurophysiol* 1964;17:109–125.
16. Castro-Alamancos MA, Connors BW. Spatiotemporal properties of short-term plasticity in sensorimotor thalamocortical pathway in the rat. *J Neurosci* 1996;16:2767–2779.

17. Castro-Alamancos MA, Connors BW. Short-term plasticity of a thalamocortical pathway dynamically modulated by behavioral state. *Science* 1996b;272:274–277.

18. Chrobak JJ, Buzsáki G. High-frequency oscillations in the output networks of the hippocampal-entorhinal axis of the freely moving rat. *J Neurosci* 1996;16:3056–3066.

19. Clare HM, Bishop GH. Potential wave mechanism in cat cortex. *Electroencephalogr Clin Neurophysiol* 1956;8:583–602.

20. Cole AE, Nicoll RA. Characterization of a slow cholinergic postsynaptic potential recorded *in vitro* from rat hippocampal pyramidal cells. *J Physiol (Lond)* 1984;352:173–188.

21. Creutzfeldt O, Watanabe S, Lux HD. Relations between EEG phenomena and potentials of single cortical cells. 1. Evoked responses after thalamic and epicortical stimulation. *Electroencephalogr Clin Neurophysiol* 1966;20:1–18.

21a.Curio G. Linking 600Hz "spikelike" EEG/MEG wavelets ("σ bursts") to cellular-substrates. *J Clin Neurophysiol* 2000;17:377–396.

22. Curro Dossi R, Nunez A, Steriade M. Electrophysiology of a slow (0.5–4 Hz) intrinsic oscillation of CAT thalamocortical neurones *in vivo. J Physiol (Lond)* 1992;447:215–234.

23. De Koninck Y, Mody I. Noise analysis of miniature IPSCs in adult rat brain slices: properties and modulation of synaptic GABAA receptor channels. *J Neurophysiol* 1994;71:1318–1335.

24. Demsey EW, Morison RS. The mechanism of thalamo-cortical augmentation and repetition. *Am J Physiol* 1942;138:297–308.

25. Draguhn A, Traub RD, Schmitz D, et al. Electrical coupling underlies high-frequency oscillations in the hippocampus *in vitro. Nature* 1998;394:189–192.

26. Fertziger AP, Ranck JB Jr. Potassium accumulation in interstitial space during epileptiform seizures. *Exp Neurol* 1970;26:209–218.

27. Fisher RS, Webber WRS, Lesser RP, et al. High frequency EEG activity at the start of seizures. *J Clin Neurophysiol* 1992;9:441–448.

28. Freeman JA, Nicholson C. Experimental optimization of current source-density technique for anuran cerebellum. *J Neurophysiol* 1975;38:369–382.

29. Freund TF, Antal M. GABA-containing neurons in the septum control inhibitory interneurons in the hippocampus. *Nature* 1988;336:170–173.

30. Freund TF, Gulyas A, Acsady L, et al. Serotonergic control of the hippocampus via local inhibitory interneurons. *Proc Natl Acad Sci U S A* 1990;87:8501–8505.

31. Gevins AS, Schaffer RE, Doyle JC, et al. Shadows of thought: rapidly changing, asymmetric, brain potential patterns of a brief visuomotor task. *Science* 1983;220:97–99.

32. Grinvald A, Frostig R, Lieke E, et al. Optical imaging of neuronal activity. *Physiol Rev* 1988;68:1285–1366.

33. Haas HL, Jefferys JGR. Low-calcium field burst discharges of CA1 pyramidal neurones in rat hippocampal slices. *J Physiol* 1984;354:185–201.

34. Haas HL, Konnerth A. Histamine and noradrenaline decrease calcium-activated potassium conductance in hippocampal pyramidal cells. *Nature* 1983;302:432–434.

35. Haglund MM, Schwartzkroin PA. Role of Na-K pump potassium regulation and IPSPs in seizures and spreading depression in immature rabbit hippocampal slices. *J Neurophysiol* 1990;63:225–239.

36. Heinemann U, Lux HD, Gutnick MJ. Extracellular free calcium and potassium during paroxysmal activity in cerebral cortex of the cat. *Exp Brain Res* 1977;27:237–243.

37. Hirsch JA, Alonso JM, Reid RC. Visually evoked calcium action potentials in cat striate cortex. *Nature* 1995;378:612–616.

38. Hotson JR, Prince DA. A calcium-activated hyperpolarization follows repetitive firing in hippocampal neurons. *J Neurophysiol* 1980;43:409–419.

39. Humphrey DR. Re-analysis of the antidromic cortical response. I. Potentials evoked by stimulation of the isolated pyramidal tract. *Electroencephalogr Clin Neurophysiol* 1968;24:116–129.

40. Jasper H, Stefanis C. Intracellular oscillatory rhythms in pyramidal tract neurones in the cat. *Electroencephalogr Clin Neurophysiol* 1965;18:541–553.

41. Jasper HH, Drooglever-Fortuyn J. Experimental studies on the functional anatomy of petit mal epilepsy. *Res Publ Ass Res Nerv Ment Dis* 1947;26:272–298.

42. Kamondi A, Acsády L, Buzsáki G. Dendritic spikes are enhanced by cooperative network activity in the intact hippocampus. *J Neurosci* 1998;18:3919–3928.

43. Kamondi A, Acsády L, Wang X-J, et al. Theta oscillations in somata and dendrites of hippocampal pyramidal cells in vivo: activity dependent phase-precession of action potentials. *Hippocampus* 1998;8:244–261.

44. Kandel A, Buzsáki G. Cellular-synaptic generation of sleep spindles, spike-and-wave discharges and evoked thalamocortical responses in the neocortex of the rat. *J Neurosci* 1997;17:6783–6797.

45. Katsumaru H, Kosaka T, Heizmann CW, et al. Gap junctions on GABAergic neurons containing the calcium-binding protein parvalbumin in the rat hippocampus (CA1 region). *Exp Brain Res* 1988;72:363–370.

46. Kornhuber HH, Becker W, Taumer R, et al. Cerebral potentials accompanying voluntary movements in man: readiness potential and reafferent potentials. *Electroencephalogr Clin Neurophysiol* 1969;26:439.

47. Kuffler SW. Neuroglial cells: physiological properties and a potassium mediated effect of neuronal activity on the glial membrane potential. *Proc R Soc Lond B Biol Sci* 1966;168:1–21.

48. Leao AAP. Spreading depression of activity in the cerebral cortex. *J Neurophysiol* 1944;7:359–390.

49. Leung LS, Yim CY. Intrinsic membrane potential oscillations in hippocampal neurons *in vitro. Brain Res* 1991;553:261–274.

50. Llinás RR. The intrinsic electrophysiological properties of mammalian neurons: insight into central nervous system. *Science* 1988;242:1654–1664.

51. Llinás RR, Ribary U, Joliot M, et al. Content and context in temporal thalamocortical binding. In: Buzsáki G, Llinás RR, Singer W, et al., eds. *Temporal coding in the brain.* Berlin: Springer-Verlag, 1994.

52. Madison DV, Nicoll RA. Actions of noradrenaline recorded intracellularly in rat hippocampal CA1 pyramidal neurons, *in vitro. J Physiol (Lond)* 1986;321:175–177.

53. Magee JC, Johnston D. A synaptically controlled, associative signal for Hebbian plasticity in hippocampal neurons. *Science* 1997;275:209–213.

54. Markram H, Lübke J, Frotscher M, et al. Regulation of synaptic efficacy by coincidence of postsynaptic APs and EPSPs. *Science* 1997;275:213–215.

55. McCormick DA. Neurotransmitter actions in the thalamus and cerebral cortex and their role in neuromodulation of thalamocortical activity. *Prog Neurobiol* 1992;39:337–388.

56. MacVicar BA. Voltage-dependent calcium channels in glial cells. *Science* 1984;226:1345–1347.

57. Metherate R, Ashe JH. Ionic flux contributions to neocortical slow waves and nucleus basalis-mediated activation: whole-cell recordings *in vivo. J Neurosci* 1993;13:5312–5323.

58. Morin D, Steriade M. Development from primary to augmenting responses in the somatosensory system. *Brain Res* 1981;205:49–66.

59. Morison RS, Dempsey EW. A study of thalamo-cortical relations. *Am J Physiol* 1942;135:281–292.

60. Nadasdy Z, Csicsvari J, Penttonen M, et al. Extracellular recording and analysis of electrical activity: from single cells to ensembles. In: Eichenbaum H, Davis JL, eds. *Neuronal ensembles: Strategies for recording and decoding.* New York: Wiley-Liss, 1998:17–55.

61. Nedergaard M. Direct signaling from astrocytes to neurons in cultures of mammalian brain cells. *Science* 1994;263:1768–1771.

62. Nedergaard M, Cooper AJ, Goldman SA. Gap junctions are required for the propagation of spreading depression. *J Neurobiol* 1995;28:433–444.

63. Nunez PL. *Electrical fields of the brain: the neurophysics of EEG.* New York: Oxford University Press, 1981.

64. Pedroarena C, Llinás R. Dendritic calcium conductances generate high-frequency oscillation in thalamocortical neurons. *Proc Natl Acad Sci U S A* 1997;94:724–728.

65. Penttonen M, Kamondi A, Sik A, et al. Gamma frequency oscillation in the hippocampus: intracellular analysis *in vivo*. *Eur J Neurosci* 1998;10:718–728.

66. Petsche H, Pockberger H, Rappelsberger P. On the search for the sources of the electroencephalogram. *Neuroscience* 1984;11:1–27.

67. Ralston B, Ajmone-Marsan C. Thalamic control of certain normal and abnormal cortical rhythms. *Electroencephalogr Clin Neurophysiol* 1956;8:559–583.

68. Rappelsberger P, Pockberger H, Petsche H. The contribution of the cortical layers to the generation of the EEG: field potential and current source density analyses in the rabbit's visual cortex. *Electroencephalogr Clin Neurophysiol* 1982;53:254–269.

69. Ribak CE. Aspinous and sparsely spinous stellate neurons in the visual cortex of rats contain glutamic acid decarboxylase. *J Neurocytol* 1978;7:461–478.

70. Ribary U, Ioannides AA, Singh KD, et al. Magnetic field tomography (MTF) of coherent thalamo-cortical 40-Hz oscillations in humans. *Proc Natl Acad Sci U S A* 1991;88:11037–11041.

71. Schaul N, Gloor P, Ball G, et al. The electrophysiology of delta waves induced by systemic atropine. *Brain Res* 1978;143:475–486.

72. Schwartzkroin PA, Stafstrom CE. Effect of EGTA on the calcium activated afterhyperpolarization in CA3 pyramidal cells. *Science* 1980;210:1125–1126.

73. Silva LR, Amital Y, Connors BW. Intrinsic oscillations of neocortex generated by layer five pyramidal neurons. *Science* 1991;251:432–435.

74. Somogyi P, Kisvarday ZL, Martin KAC, et al. Synaptic connections of morphologically identified and physiologically characterized large basket cells in the striate cortex of the cat. *Neuroscience* 1983;10:261–294.

75. Spencer WA, Brookhart JM. Electrical patterns of augmenting and recruiting waves in depth of sensorimotor cortex of cat. *J Neurophysiol* 1961;24:26–49.

76. Spencer WA, Brookhart JM. A study of spontaneous spindle waves in sensorimotor cortex of cat. *J Neurophysiol* 1961;24:50–65.

77. Steriade M, Buzsáki G. Parallel activation of the thalamus and neocortex. In: Steriade M, Biesold D, eds. *Brain cholinergic system.* Oxford, UK: Oxford University Press, 1991.

78. Steriade M, Curro Dossi R, Nunez A. Network modulation of a slow intrinsic oscillation of cat thalamocortical neurons implicated in sleep delta waves: cortically induced synchronization and brainstem cholinergic suppression. *J Neurosci* 1991;11:3200–3217.

79. Steriade M, Deschénes M, Domich L, et al. Abolition of spindle oscillation in thalamic neurons disconnected from nucleus reticularis thalami. *J Neurophysiol* 1985;54:1473–1497.

80. Steriade M, Gloor P, Llinás RR, et al. Basic mechanisms of cerebral rhythmic activities. *Electroencephalogr Clin Neurophysiol* 1990;76:481–508.

81. Steriade M, McCormick DA, Sejnowski TJ. Thalamocortical oscillations in the sleeping and aroused brain. *Science* 1993;262:679–685.

82. Sypert GW, Ward AA. Unidentified neuroglia potentials during propagated seizures in the neocortex. *Exp Neurol* 1971;33:239–255.

83. Taylor CP, Dudek FE. Excitation of hippocampal pyramidal cells by an electrical field effect. *J Neurophysiol* 1984;52:126–142.

84. Traub RD, Dudek FE, Snow RW, et al. Computer simulations indicate that electrical field effects contribute to the shape of the epileptiform field potential. *Neuroscience* 1985;15:947–958.

85. Traub RD, Jefferys JGR, Whittington MA. *Fast oscillations in cortical circuits.* Cambridge, MA: MIT Press, 1999.

86. Ts'o D, Frostig R, Lieke E, et al. Functional organization of primate visual cortex revealed by high resolution optical imaging. *Science* 1990;249:417–420.

87. Vanderwolf CH. Cerebral activity and behavior: control by central cholinergic and serotonergic systems. *Int Rev Neurobiol* 1988;30:225–340.

88. Walter WG. The contingent negative variation: an electro-cortical sign of sensorimotor reflex association in man. *Proc Brain Res* 1968;22:364–377.

89. Wong RK, Prince DA, Basbaum AI. Intradendritic recordings from hippocampal neurons. *Proc Natl Acad Sci U S A* 1979;76:986–990.

90. Ylinen A, Bragin A, Nádasdy Z, et al. Sharp wave associated high frequency oscillation (200 Hz) in the intact hippocampus: network and intracellular mechanisms. *J Neurosci* 1995;14: 30–46.

91. Yuste R, Denk W. Dendritic spines as a basic unit of synaptic integration. *Nature* 1995;375: 682–684.

Chapter 2

Cortical Generators and EEG Voltage Fields

John S. Ebersole

THE SOURCE OF ELECTROENCEPHALOGRAPHIC POTENTIALS

Cerebral sources of electroencephalographic (EEG) potentials are three-dimensional volumes of cortex. These sources produce three-dimensional potential fields within the brain. From the surface of the scalp, these can be recorded as two-dimensional fields of time-varying voltage. In order to localize and characterize cortical generators of the EEG, the physical and functional factors that determine the voltage fields that these sources produce must be appreciated. In Chapter 1, the cellular mechanisms underlying brain electrical activity were reviewed. This chapter changes the scale from the microscopic to the macroscopic, for the EEG can reveal cortical activity only at a macroscopic level. When considering the combined electrical activity of approximately 10^8 neurons in a cortical area of several square centimeters, rather than a single cell or cortical column, it is neces-

sary to understand several important concepts in order to interpret an EEG properly.

The principle generators of EEG fields that are measured on the surface of the brain or at the scalp are graded synaptic potentials: namely, excitatory postsynaptic potentials (EPSPs) and inhibitory postsynaptic potentials (IPSPs), of pyramidal neurons (4,6,10,11,13). At the synaptic site of an EPSP, there is an active current sink. Positive ions rush into the cell to depolarize the local membrane. At the same time, at a more distal portion of the cell, a passive current source, consisting of current flow out of the cell, completes a closed circuit. The current flows in the opposite direction with an IPSP. A local active current source is coupled with a distant passive current sink. These currents, generated by synaptic activity, pass through the extracellular and intracellular spaces and set up a potential field around the cell. Near a current sink, the extracellular space is relatively negative, whereas near a current source, it is positive (Fig. 2.1). The current flow and associ-

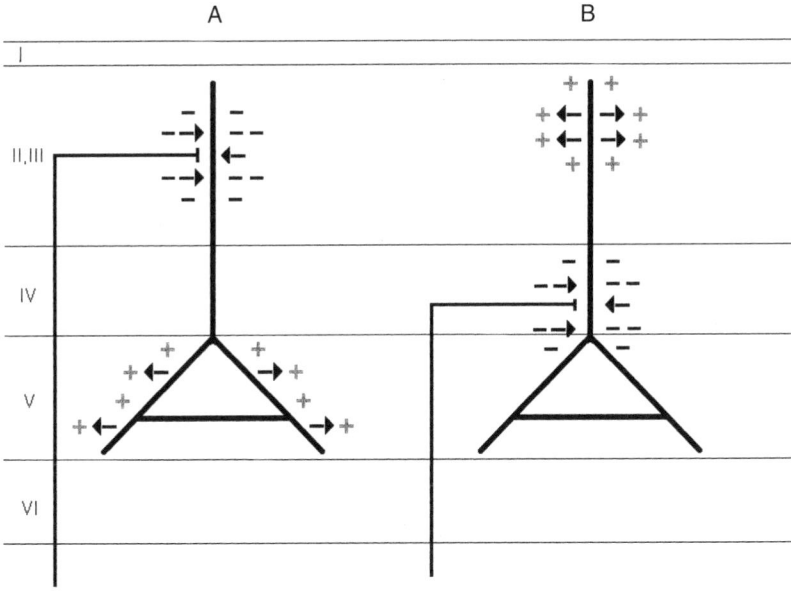

FIG. 2.1. Generation of extracellular voltage fields from graded synaptic activity. **A:** Excitatory postsynaptic potential (EPSP) at the apical dendrite is associated with a flow of positive ions into the cell (an active current sink) and an extracellular negative field. A passive current source at the level of the cell body and basal dendrites is associated with an extracellular positive field. **B:** EPSP on the proximal apical dendrite at the level of cortical layer IV is associated with an active current sink and an extracellular negative field. A passive current source at the distal apical dendrite in layers II and III is associated with an extracellular positive field.

ated field potential around individual cells are very small, and they would not be recordable at the scalp except for the fact that the pyramidal cells are all aligned perpendicular to the surface of the cortex. Because of this geometric arrangement, the voltage fields produced by individual cells can summate to produce a potential large enough to be recorded some distance from the generators, if the activity is synchronous. Summation of potential fields as a result of synaptic currents can more readily occur than can that resulting from fast sodium action potentials because the former events are relatively long in duration (10).

To a first approximation, EEG fields are generated by the large, vertically oriented pyramidal neurons located in cortical layers III, V, and VI. For example, an EPSP at an apical dendrite of a large pyramidal cell that extends through several cortical laminae would produce an active current sink and a negative local field potential superficially in the cortex, whereas the passive current source at the cell body or basal dendrites would result in a positive field potential in the deeper cortical laminae (see Fig. 2.1A). The same synaptic event is thus viewed as potentials with opposite polarity, depending on the location of the recording electrode. This juxtaposition of negative and positive charge and resultant current flow is similar to that of a dipole. Pyramidal cells can be thought of as a population of vertically oriented dipoles. Therefore, voltage fields recorded on the surface of the head usually have a dipolar configuration–that is, two maxima: one negative and one positive. The amplitude and the polarity of the potential recorded from the same event likewise depend on the location of the electrode in relation to the dipole source.

The cortex is a multilaminar structure. Current sinks and sources can arise in different locations, depending on the type of input into the cortex. Excitatory input into layer IV, a primary sensory receiving lamina, would produce a local negativity that is reflected in a cortical surface positivity (see Fig. 2.1B). Thus, the early components of normal sensory evoked potentials, for example, are commonly surface positive. Epileptic spikes, on the other hand, are commonly surface negative because of depolarization of the superficial laminae (see Fig. 2.1A). Electrodes in deeper cortical layers, in the underlying white matter, or even on the scalp at the opposite side of the head record a positive potential. Subsequent repolarization and depolarization cycles, often caused by recurrent excitation and inhibition among laminae, result in the typical sequence of a negative spike followed by a positive afterpotential, which is in turn followed by a negative wave. Spikes that originate in deeper cortical layers may show an initial surface positivity. Propagation of activity from one layer to another also changes the laminar arrangement of extracellular voltage. Mechanistically, a large population of active neurons can be thought of as a collection of oscillating dipoles.

PHYSICAL FACTORS DETERMINING SCALP ELECTROENCEPHALOGRAPHIC PATTERNS

A number of factors determine whether the extracellular voltage field produced by a region of cortex can be recorded from scalp EEG electrodes. These factors are both physical and functional. Physical factors include source location, orientation, and area. Functional factors include potential amplitude, frequency, and synchrony. A transient potential, such as an epileptic spike, serves as a good example for appreciating these relationships between source character and EEG fields.

It is both logical and correct that the scalp EEG voltage field should be related to the location of its cortical source. However, this relationship is not straightforward. An unfortunately simplistic assumption in traditional EEG interpretation is that the source of an EEG potential must necessarily underlie the electrode recording it; hence the practice of referring to epileptic discharges by the name of the electrode recording the maximal potential. This assumption is true only in limited cases. That a negative field maximum is recorded from a particular electrode does not necessarily mean that the spike source is beneath it, as discussed in detail later.

The importance of source area in determining whether cortical activity will be recordable on the scalp EEG has been appreciated for some time. Using a simulated cortical source beneath a piece of fresh skull, Cooper et al. (3) determined that 6 cm^2 of synchronously active area are probably necessary to produce a scalp-recordable field. Gloor (7,8) also discussed the importance of source area in appreciating EEG fields at the scalp in his dissertation of the "solid angle" theory. In essence, only when a cortical region subtends a large enough solid angle, from the perspective of a given electrode, will that electrode record the potential generated by it. Ebersole and Pacia (5,12), in a series of simultaneous intracranial and scalp recordings, showed that for individual epileptic spikes, the 6 cm^2 estimate was accurate (Figs. 2.2 and 2.3). What was demonstrated in addition, however, was that the area of sources for typical scalp interictal spikes is often substantially larger, often encompassing 20 cm^2 or more of gyral cortex (see Figs. 2.13 and 2.14).

Because of the attenuating properties of the intervening skull, spatial summation of cortical activity is critical for producing a voltage field recordable from the scalp. As commonly observed in candidates implanted for epilepsy surgery, most of the cortical activity recorded from subdural or depth electrodes is not evident in the scalp EEG (1,9). This is not necessarily because the amplitude of the individual cortical potentials is too small; more often, it is because the area of the cortical generator is not large enough. Although they are not well appreciated, this factor, source area, and a closely related factor, source orientation, are the two most important variables in determining whether cerebral potentials are recordable from the scalp. The EEG can detect small and remote sources, but this usually requires the averaging of hundreds to thousands of repetitive signals, such as potentials evoked by sensory stimuli.

Spatial summation of the voltage field generated by multiple cortical sources is three-dimensional. If adjacent active cortical areas have the same orientation, their voltage fields combine, and the resultant voltage field measured at the scalp is the linear sum of the fields of both sources. If, however, adjacent active regions of cortex have a different orientation, the voltage fields summate in relation to the geometry of their respective field vectors. For example, if two cortical areas have an opposite orientation, such as the two sides of a sulcus, cancellation occurs, and no voltage field from them is evident at the scalp (Fig. 2.4, source 3).

Source area is maximal for a given electrode (and the solid angle is maximal) when the orientation of the active cortical region is face-on. This is usually the case when the resultant voltage field is radial and the electrode is directly above the source (see Fig. 2.4, source 2). In this instance, the electrode records the field maximum. As the orientation of a cortical source becomes progressively less radial and more tangential to a recording electrode, that electrode is able to record a voltage field of progressively less amplitude. If the source is directly below an electrode but it is oriented perfectly tangential to the recording electrode, the electrode records no potential, because this location is on the zero isopotential line of the source's scalp field (see Fig. 2.4, source 1 and 4). To summarize the concepts illustrated in Fig. 2.4, cortical sources 4-2 and 4-3 produce voltage fields with a net radial orientation, and, correspondingly, they have a negative field maximum on the scalp directly above them. Sources 4-1 and 4-4 result in a tangential field. The zero isopotential line is located on the scalp immediately above these sources, whereas negative and positive maxima are displaced on either side. In general, midline interhemispheric and basal cortical sources tend to be tangential; lateral convexity cortical sources tend to be radial. Sources on one bank of a sulcus in the lateral cortex may be tangential; however, epileptiform sources are commonly so large that both banks of the sulcus are activated. These opposing fields cancel, as depicted in source 4-3, which leaves only the radial field from the sulcus bottom to predominate.

Taken from the broader perspective of electrodes over the entire head, a radial source produces one field maximum directly above it and another field maximum of opposite polarity on the diametrically opposite side of the head. For a superficial cortical source, the scalp maximum nearest the source is significantly greater in amplitude than that on the opposite side of the head. The negative field voltage gradient is steeper, and the negative

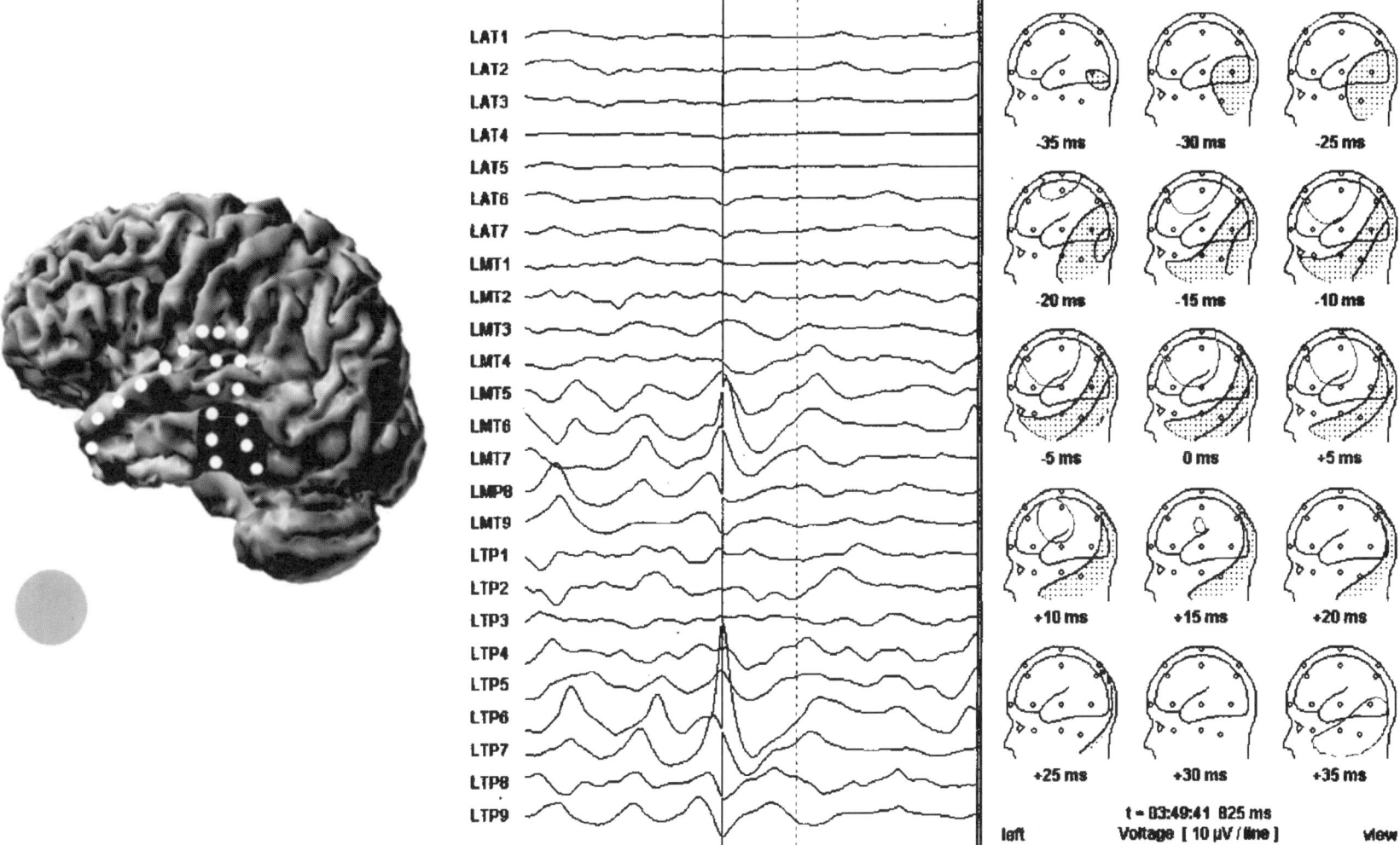

FIG. 2.2. Left: Three-dimensional magnetic resonance imaging (MRI) reconstruction of the brain, illustrating the subdural electrode placements in a patient with left temporal lobe epilepsy. The shaded cortical area represents an estimate of the spike source at the time of the cursor. The shaded circle defines 6 cm². **Right:** Intracranial electroencephalogram showing a negative (up) spike involving subdural electrode contacts LMT 5 to 7 and LTP 5 to 7. the map sequence depicts simultaneous scalp voltage topography at 5-millisecond intervals, centered on the cursor, spanning 70 milliseconds. Note that there is no appropriate scalp field associated with the cortical spike.

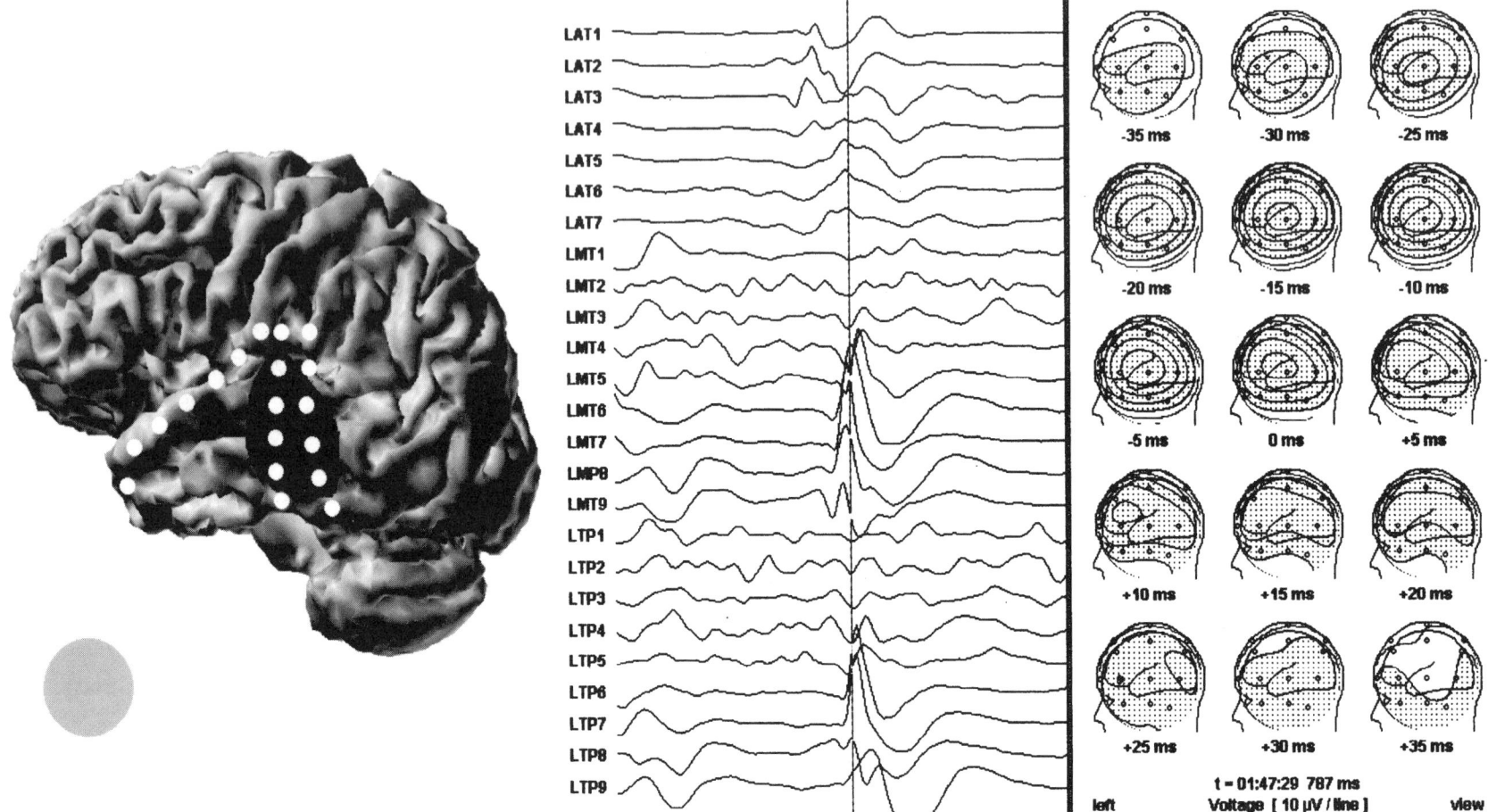

FIG. 2.3. **Left:** Illustration of subdural electrode placements as in Fig. 2.2. The shaded cortical area is an estimate of the spike source at the time of the cursor. **Right:** Intracranial electroencephalogram showing a negative spike (up) involving subdural electrode contacts LMT 6 to 9 and LTP 6 to 8. Map sequence depicts simultaneous scalp voltage topography at 5-millisecond intervals, centered on the cursor, spanning 70 milliseconds. Note that the cortical spike source area is larger than in Fig. 2.2 and that a voltage field with a midtemporal negative maximum is recorded from the scalp.

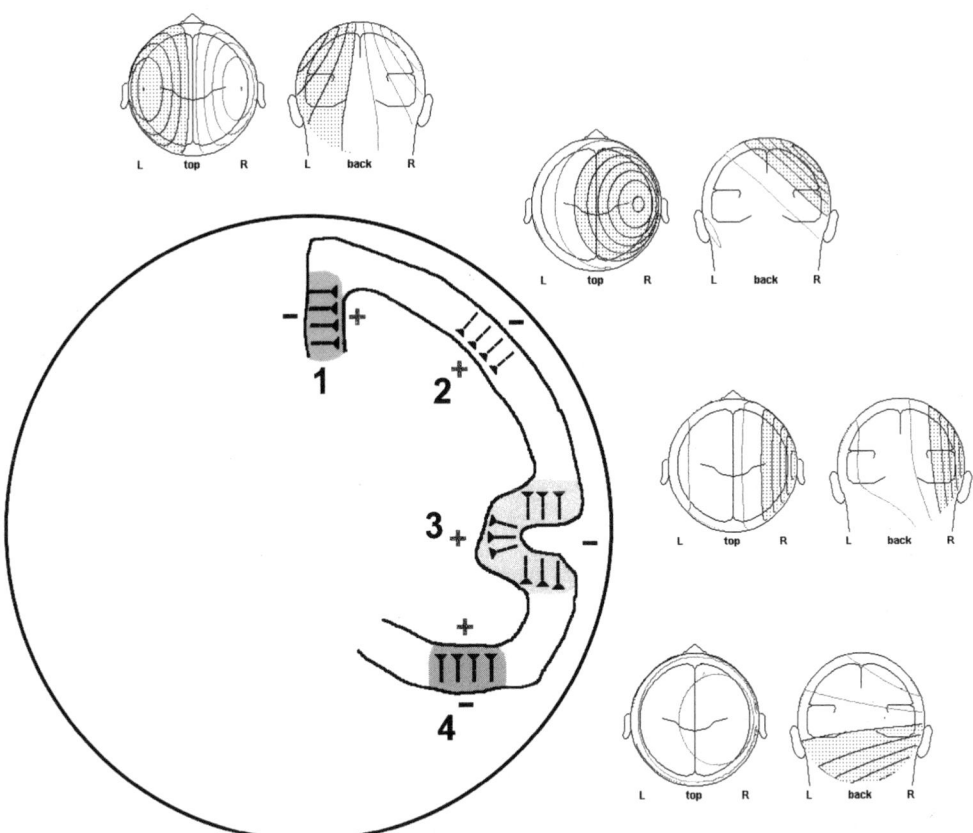

FIG. 2.4. Schematic of a brain cross-section, illustrating four representative cortical electroencephalographic (EEG) sources. Note that the alignment of the pyramidal cells (and thus the EEG voltage field) is orthogonal to the orientation of the cortical surface. Minus (–) and plus (+) signs depict the polarity of the epileptiform potentials generated by these sources. Top and back views of the head show the scalp voltage field generated by each source. The shaded area denotes field polarity (speckled represents negative). Sources 2 and 3 produce radial fields, and the negative voltage maximum is directly above them. Fields from opposing sulcal walls cancel each other in source 3, leaving the radial component from the sulcus bottom to dominate. Sources 1 and 4 produce tangential fields. No voltage is recorded directly above them; instead, negative and positive voltage maxima are displaced to either side.

field size is smaller than for a deeper radial source (Fig. 2.5). In the case of a spike, for example, the negative field maximum above the source is of greater amplitude than is the positive maximum on the other side of the head. For cortical sources whose net orientation is progressively more tangential, the nearest field maximum is progressively displaced away from the region directly above the source. Conversely, the field maximum of opposite polarity moves progressively closer (Fig. 2.6). For a source that is tangential to the skull, both maxima are displaced equally in opposite directions on either side of the source, and the fields are of equal amplitude. The distance between the two maxima is dependent on the depth of the source: The deeper the source, the farther apart are the maxima, and vice versa (Fig. 2.7). The simplistic assumption that the cortical generator underlies the voltage field maximum is not true for tangentially oriented sources. This is a very important concept. Localization and even lateralization are commonly false when cortical sources have an orientation that is even partially tangential.

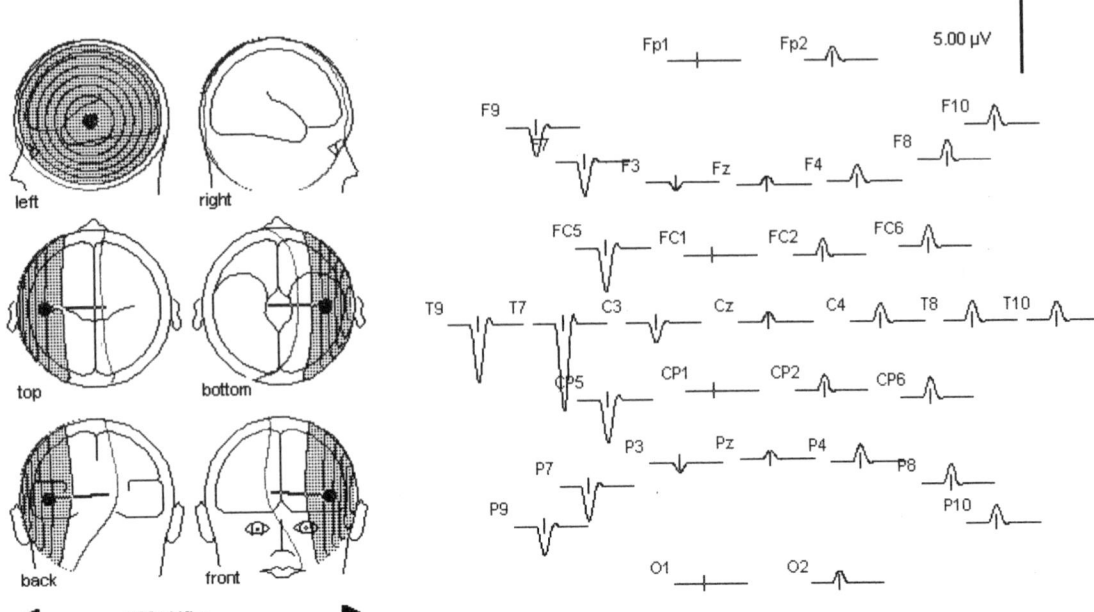

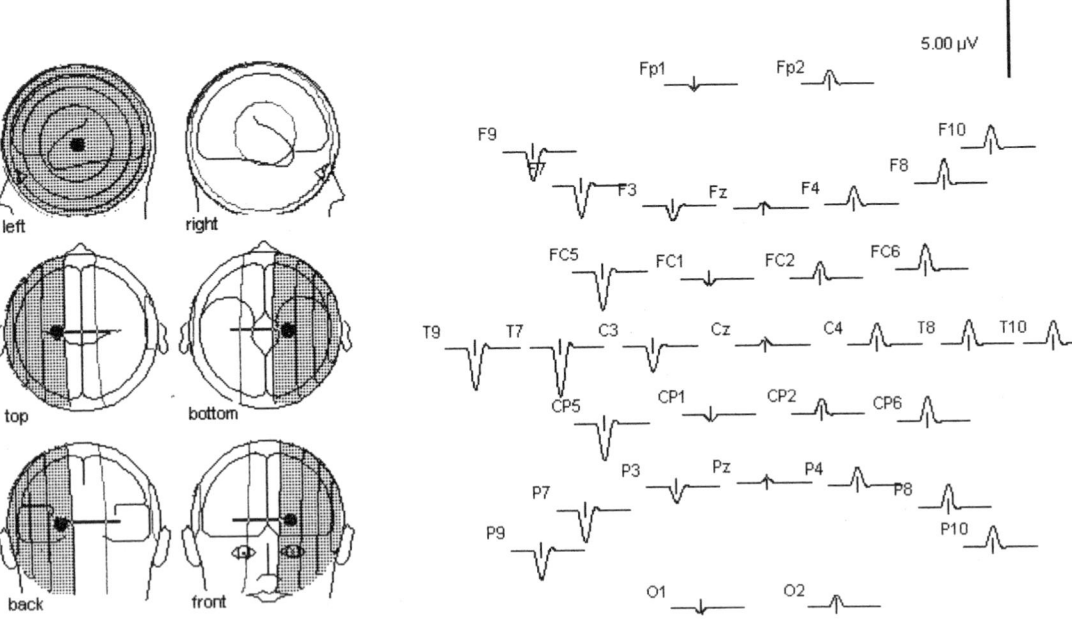

FIG. 2.5. A: Computer simulation of the scalp spike voltage field produced by a superficial, radially oriented dipole source (*dot* represents dipole source; *vector* from dot represents source orientation) in the left temporal lobe. Note that the negative field (hatched area) has a steep voltage gradient and a maximum directly above the source. A weak positive field with a shallow voltage gradient exists on the opposite side of the head. Electroencephalographic (EEG) traces of the simulated spike are shown at right. Note the high-amplitude left temporal negative spike (downward deflection in this and following simulations) and low-amplitude right temporal positive potential (upward deflection). (Simulation of EEG traces and voltage field by a forward dipole solution through a three-shell head model was accomplished with "Dipole Simulator" by P. Berg and M. Scherg, see Chapter 23.) **B:** Similar computer simulation of the scalp voltage field produced by a deeper, radially oriented dipole source. Note that the negative field is larger and has a less steep voltage gradient, but the maximum remains directly above the source. The positive field on the opposite side of the head is now of higher amplitude. EEG traces show a lower amplitude left temporal spike and a higher amplitude positive potential.

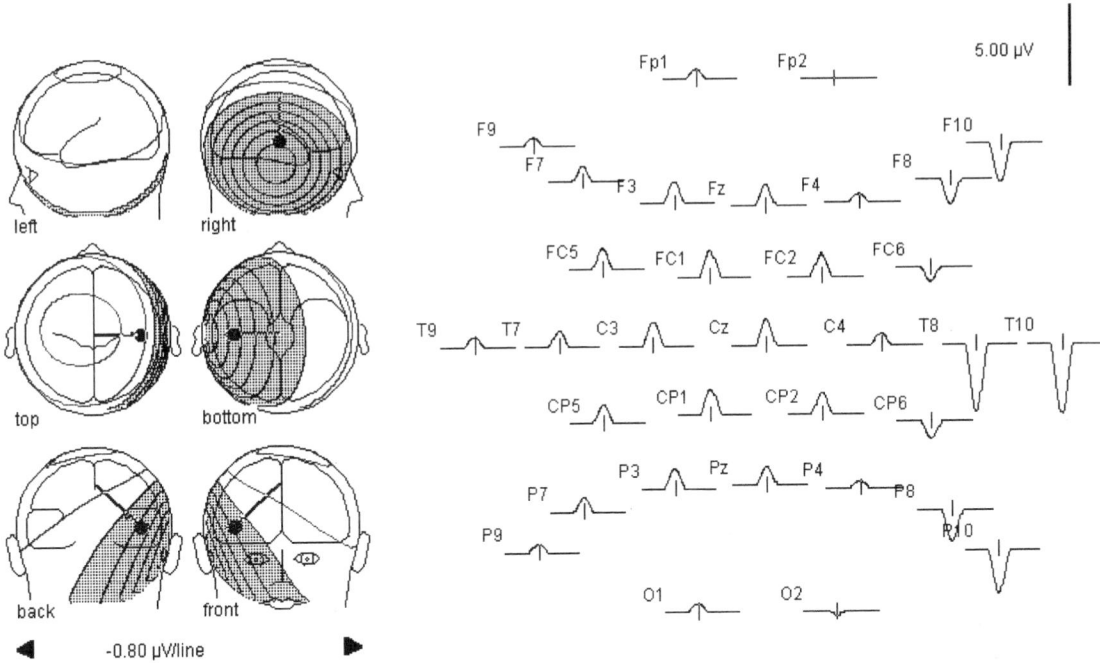

FIG. 2.6. Computer simulation of the scalp spike voltage field produced by a superficial oblique-oriented dipole source (*dot* represents dipole source; *vector* from dot represents source orientation) in the right temporal lobe. Note that the negative field (hatched area) has a steep voltage gradient and a maximum that is displaced downward onto the subtemporal scalp region. A weaker positive field with a shallow voltage gradient has a vertex-located maximum. Electroencephalogram (EEG) traces of the simulated spike are shown at right. Note high-amplitude right subtemporal and temporal negative spike (downward deflection) and the lower amplitude, more widespread vertex positive potential (upward deflection). (Simulation of EEG traces and voltage field by a forward dipole solution through a three-shell head model was accomplished with the "Dipole Simulator" by P. Berg and M. Scherg, see Chapter 23.)

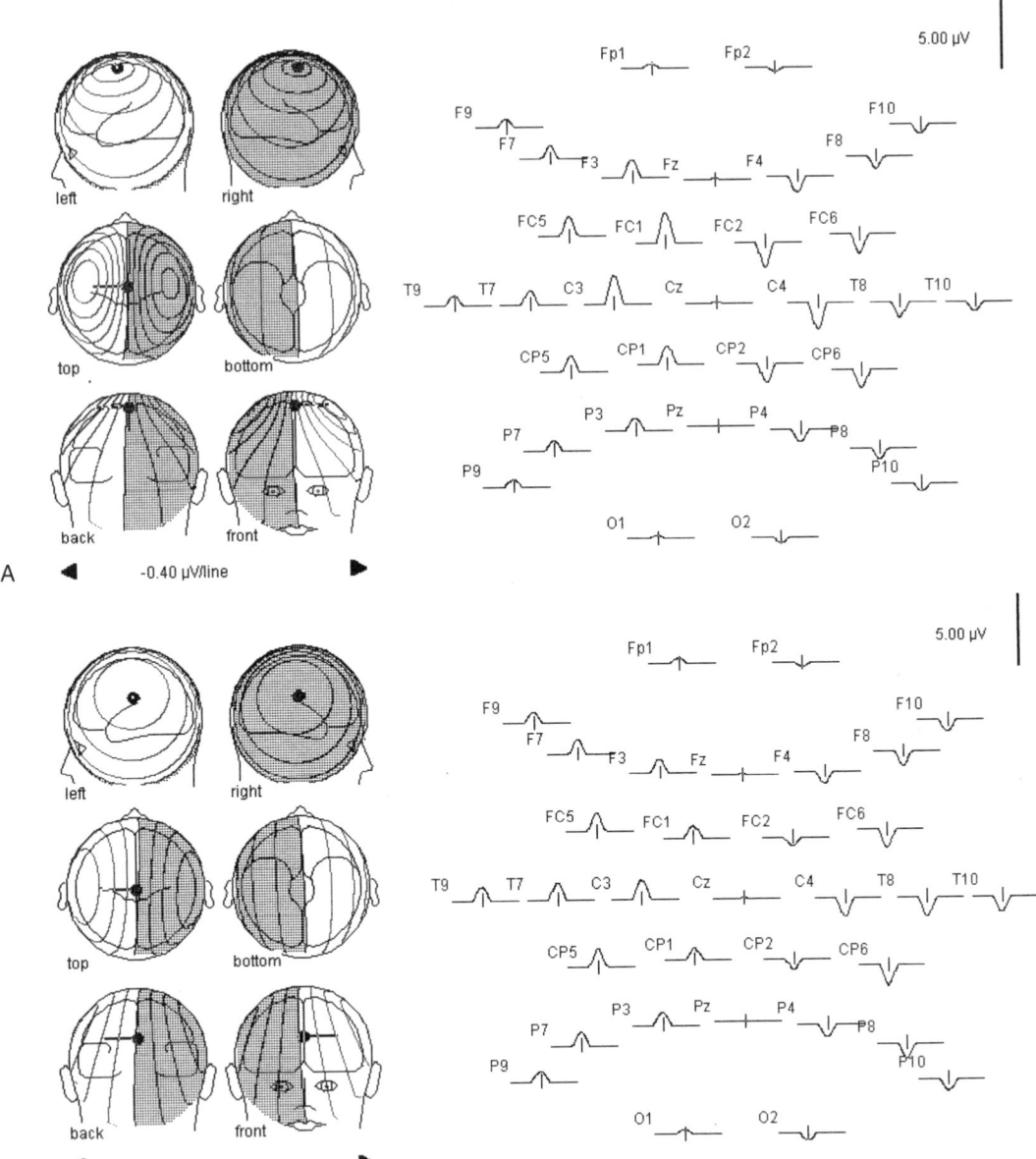

FIG. 2.7. A: Computer simulation of the scalp spike voltage field produced by a superficial tangentially oriented dipole source (*dot* represents dipole source; *vector* from dot represents source orientation) in the interhemispheric region. Note that both negative (hatched area) and positive fields have a steep voltage gradient and that their maxima are relatively close together and symmetrically displaced on either side of the fissure. Electroencephalogram (EEG) traces of the simulated spike are shown at right. Note high-amplitude right central negative spike (downward deflection) and left central positive spike (upward deflection). Midline Cz electrode directly above the source records no significant activity. (Simulation of EEG traces and voltage field by a forward dipole solution through a three-shell head model was accomplished with "Dipole Simulator" by P. Berg and M. Scherg, see Chapter 23.) **B:** Similar computer simulation of the scalp voltage field produced by a deeper, tangentially oriented dipole source. Note that both the negative and positive fields have a less steep voltage gradient and that their maxima are farther apart and symmetrically displaced on either side of the fissure. EEG traces show a lower amplitude negative and positive spikes and no significant midline voltage.

ELECTROENCEPHALOGRAPHIC SOURCE LOCALIZATION PRINCIPLES

In view of the previous discussion, it becomes obvious that a single voltage field maximum cannot be used to define the location or orientation of a cortical EEG generator. In all instances, except for a purely radial source, the EEG field maxima are displaced from a position directly above it. To characterize a cortical source, the location of both field maxima, negative and positive, and their relative strengths must be taken into consideration. Noting the relative location of these two voltage field maxima provides the easiest and most accurate assessment of source orientation. A three-dimensional line drawn between the two maxima identifies the orientation of the field. Accordingly, the net orientation of the cortex generating the field is orthogonal to this line (see Figs. 2.5, 2.6, and 2.7). As a first approximation, the center of the cortical source should lie somewhere along this three-dimensional line. The amplitude and gradient of the field maxima determines this location–that is, the depth of the source. The source should be proportionately closer to the field maximum of greater amplitude. In the case of sources with tangentially oriented fields, the separation of the negative and positive maxima is dependent on the depth of the source. A three-dimensional line connecting the maxima will travel deeper through the head when the maxima are farther apart (see Fig. 2.7). The center of the source should, again, lie along this line proportionately closer to the field maximum of greater amplitude. Thus, by simply inspecting the scalp voltage topography of any EEG potential, much can be learned about the cortical source generating it.

DEEP SOURCES AND SCALP ELECTROENCEPHALOGRAPHY

Whether an EEG from sources deeper than the most superficial cortex can be recorded continues to be debated (2,7). Recording scalp potentials from deep structures depends on the same factors, and the more important are, again, source area and orientation. Because physiological signals from the cortex are limited in amplitude, effective source area becomes increasingly more important as source depth increases. This argument is particularly relevant in the discussion of the origin of temporal lobe spikes in mesial temporal epilepsy. Because the hippocampus is a rather small and deep structure that is curved in shape, properties that would tend to minimize a voltage field, it is unlikely that potentials isolated to this region could be recordable from the scalp. Simultaneous scalp and intracranial EEG recordings (4,11) have confirmed this assertion (Fig. 2.8). However, propagation of spike activity from the hippocampus into adjacent basal temporal cortex is common. This cortex has a larger area and a net orientation that would allow for summation of voltage fields. Because the basal temporal cortex is tangential to the lateral surface of the skull, voltage fields from this source are not well recorded from standard temporal electrodes. Instead, the negative field maximum is recorded from subtemporal electrodes.

Another factor that favors recording deep sources is the shielding effect of the skull. Ironic as it may seem, signal attenuation produced by the skull improves the chances of identifying deeper activity by affecting superficial sources to a greater extent. If there was no skull and the head was a homogeneous volume conductor, the amplitude of an EEG potential would diminish as the square of the distance from the source. However, the intervening skull has the same effect on EEG signals as would moving cerebral sources farther from the recording electrodes by shrinking the brain to only 60% of the radius of the head (13) (Fig. 2.9). All EEG potentials are reduced in amplitude (Fig. 2.10), but a relatively greater attenuation of surface events makes deep activity more discernible.

FUNCTIONAL FACTORS DETERMINING SCALP ELECTROENCEPHALOGRAPHIC PATTERNS

Several functional factors also affect what can be recorded on a scalp EEG. Amplitude of cortical activity is important, but it has a physiological upper limit. Normal background rhythms and evoked potentials may generate potentials at the brain's surface of several hundred microvolts, and pathological potentials, such as epileptic spikes, may be greater than a millivolt in amplitude. Other functional factors may become equally or more important in determining the eventual scalp voltage field. The synchrony of cortical activity is crucial. The EEG is the measure of spatially and temporally averaged activity of a large population of neurons. The EEG emphasizes the contribution of synchronously oscillating dipolar sources, whereas asynchronous activity may cancel itself despite of its amplitude (Fig. 2.11). Synchronization of cortical neurons may, however, be limited to relatively small regions of cortex. In this case, summation of their voltage fields may not be great enough to produce a field recordable from the scalp. Regions of cortical synchronization commonly become larger with certain pathological

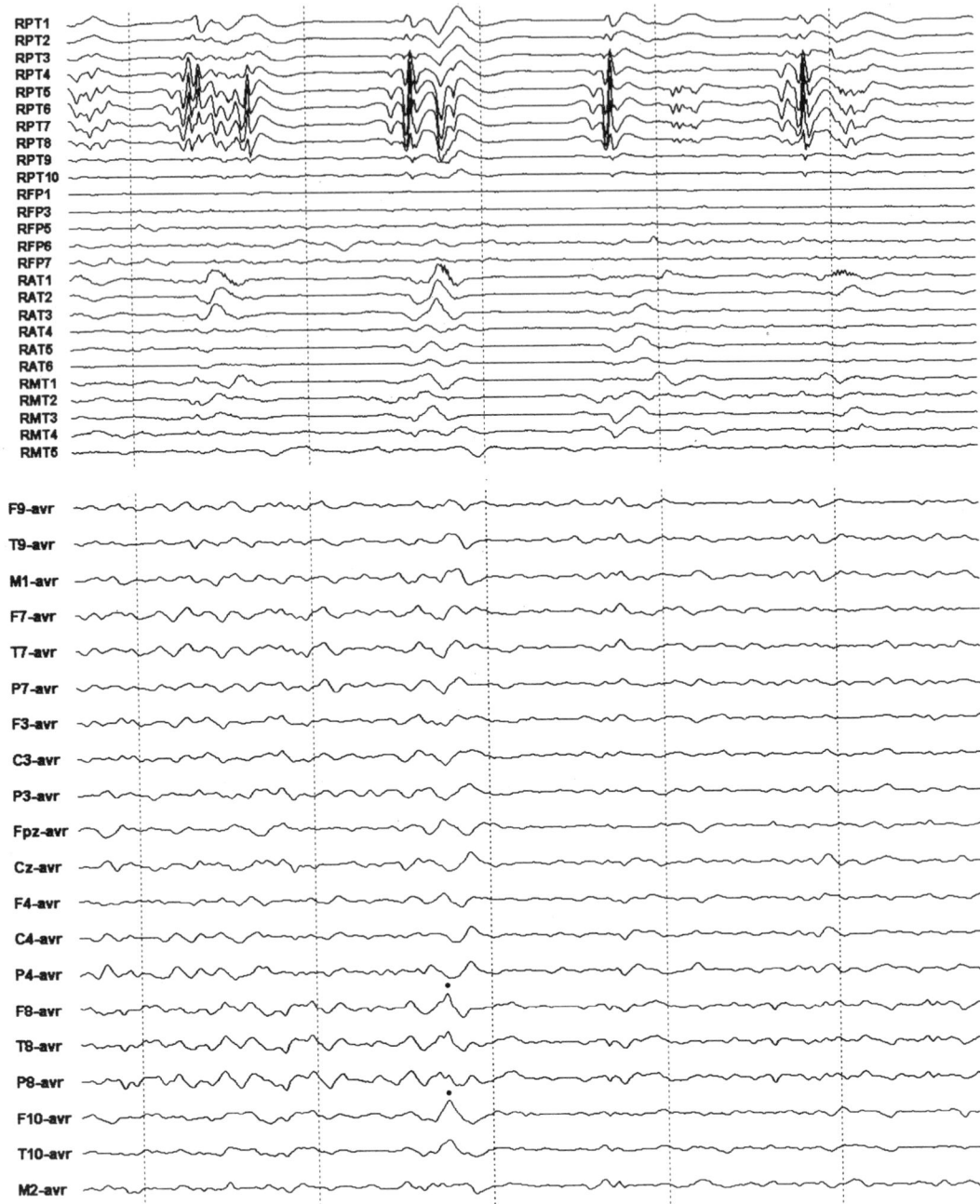

FIG. 2.8. Simultaneous intracranial and scalp electroencephalographic (EEG) recording. Prominent hippocampal spikes are recorded from depth electrode contact RPT4 to 8. No scalp EEG spikes or sharp waves are associated with these spikes unless there are related sharp waves from inferior temporal cortex sources of sufficient size (contacts RAT 1 to 5, RMT 1 to 3). Note that the maximal scalp sharp wave amplitude (*dot marker*) is recorded from the subtemporal electrode, F10.

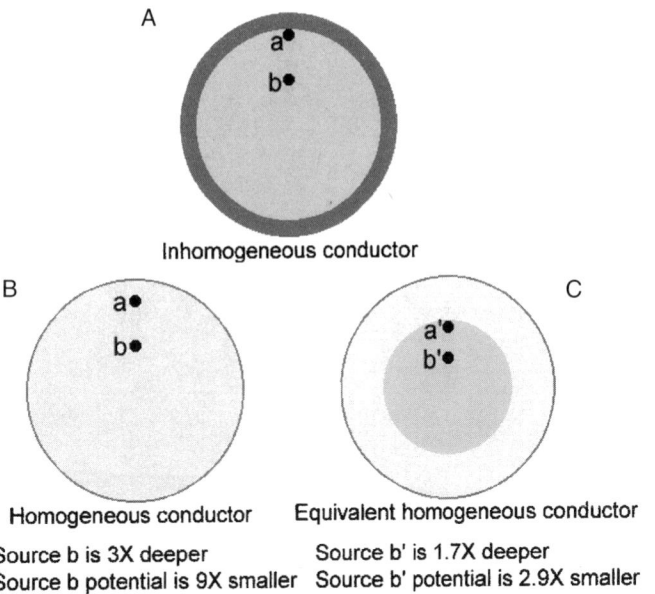

FIG. 2.9. Shielding effect of the skull. **A:** The skull, in particular, makes the head, which is modeled here as a sphere, an inhomogeneous volume conductor. The brain normally occupies approximately 85% of the radius of the head. Brain electroencephalographic (EEG) sources *a* and *b* are superficial and deep, respectively. **B:** If the head were a homogeneous conductor, the amplitude of surface EEG potentials would diminish as the square of the distance (i.e., depth) of the sources. Source *b* is three times deeper than source *a*. Its surface potential for the same activity would be one-ninth the size of source *a*. **C:** The shielding effect of the skull is equivalent to shrinking the brain to 60% of the head's radius. Source *b'* is now 1.7 times deeper than source *a'*. Its surface potential for the same activity would be 1/2.9 the size of source *a'*.

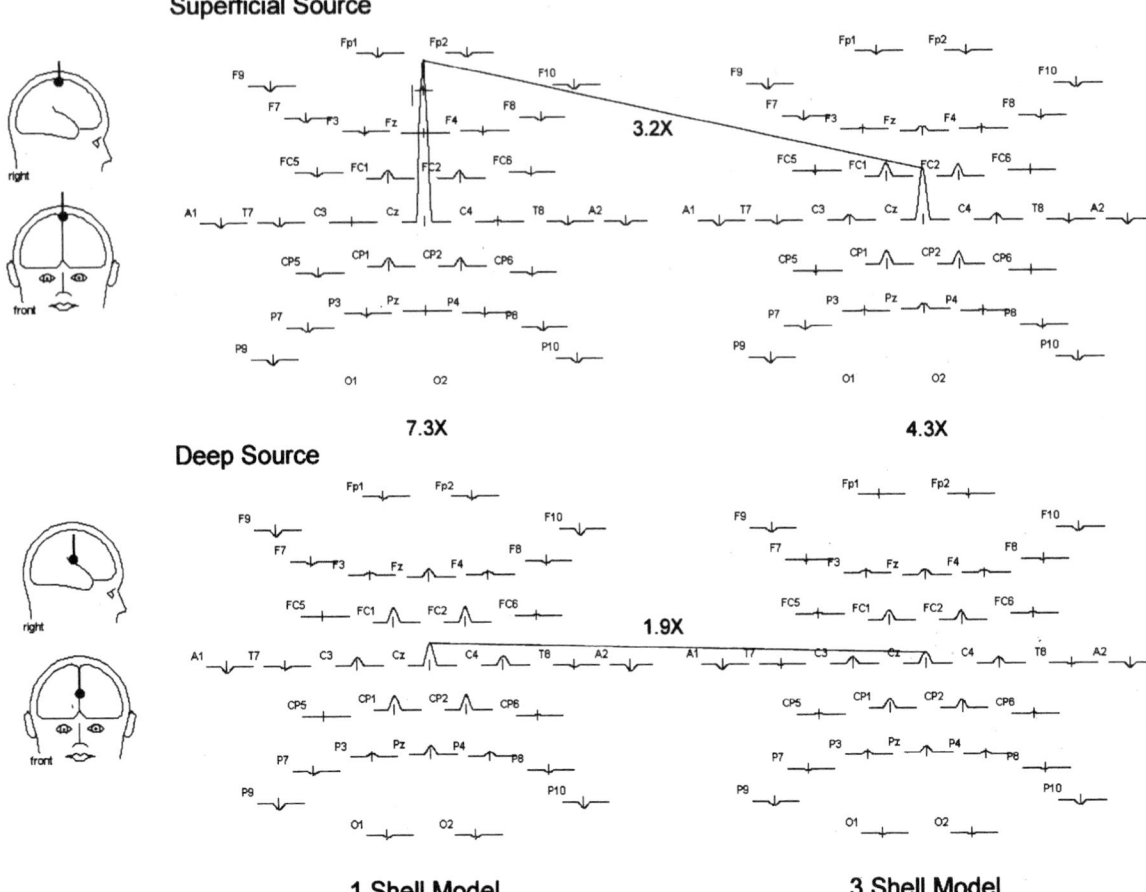

FIG. 2.10. The shielding effect of the skull on the electroencephalogram (EEG) from superficial and deep sources is demonstrated in this computer simulation ("Dipole Simulator" by P. Berg and M. Scherg, see Chapter 23), with the use of a forward solution of a dipole source potential onto the scalp through a one-shell (no skull) and three-shell (with skull) head model. Because the same superficial radial source is below electrode Cz, the presence of a skull reduces the amplitude of the recorded scalp potential by a factor of 3.2. For the same source that is 4 cm deeper, the skull reduces the amplitude of the recorded potential only by a factor of 1.9. Viewed alternatively, without a skull (one-shell model), the scalp EEG potential from the deep source is 1/7.3 the size of the superficial source. However, with a skull (three-shell model), the scalp electroencephalographic potential from the deep source is 1/ 4.3 the size of that from the superficial source. Although the skull reduces the amplitude of the EEG, potentials from deep sources are relatively less attenuated.

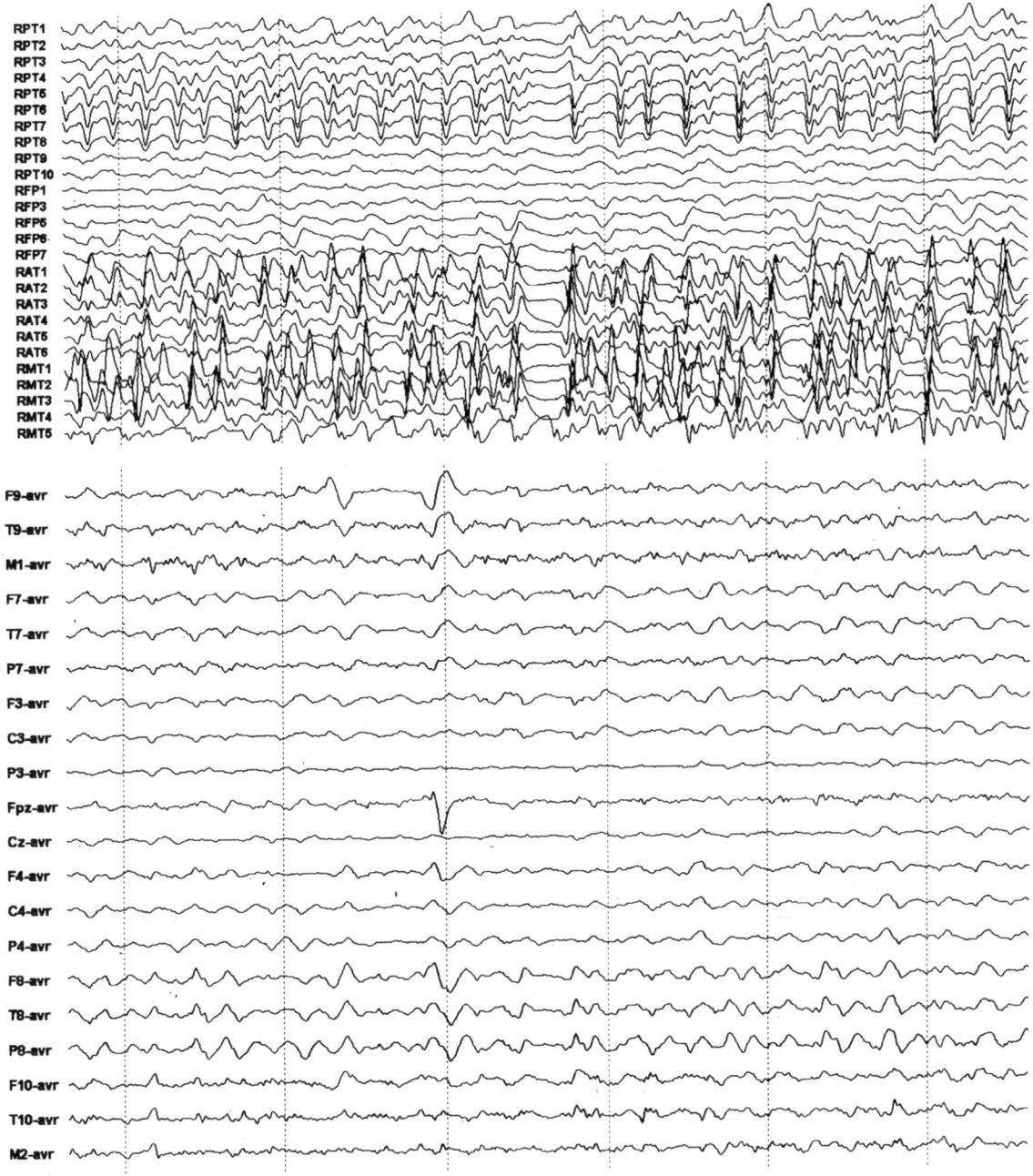

FIG. 2.11. Simultaneous intracranial and scalp electroencephalogram (EEG) recording of a temporal lobe seizure. Although the seizure rhythm from the hippocampus is synchronous (depth electrode contact RPT 4 to 8), seizure rhythms from the temporal neocortex are relatively asynchronous (subdural strip electrode contacts RAT1 to 6 and RMT1 to 5). The scalp EEG shows a poorly developed seizure rhythm despite the high-amplitude cerebral activity.

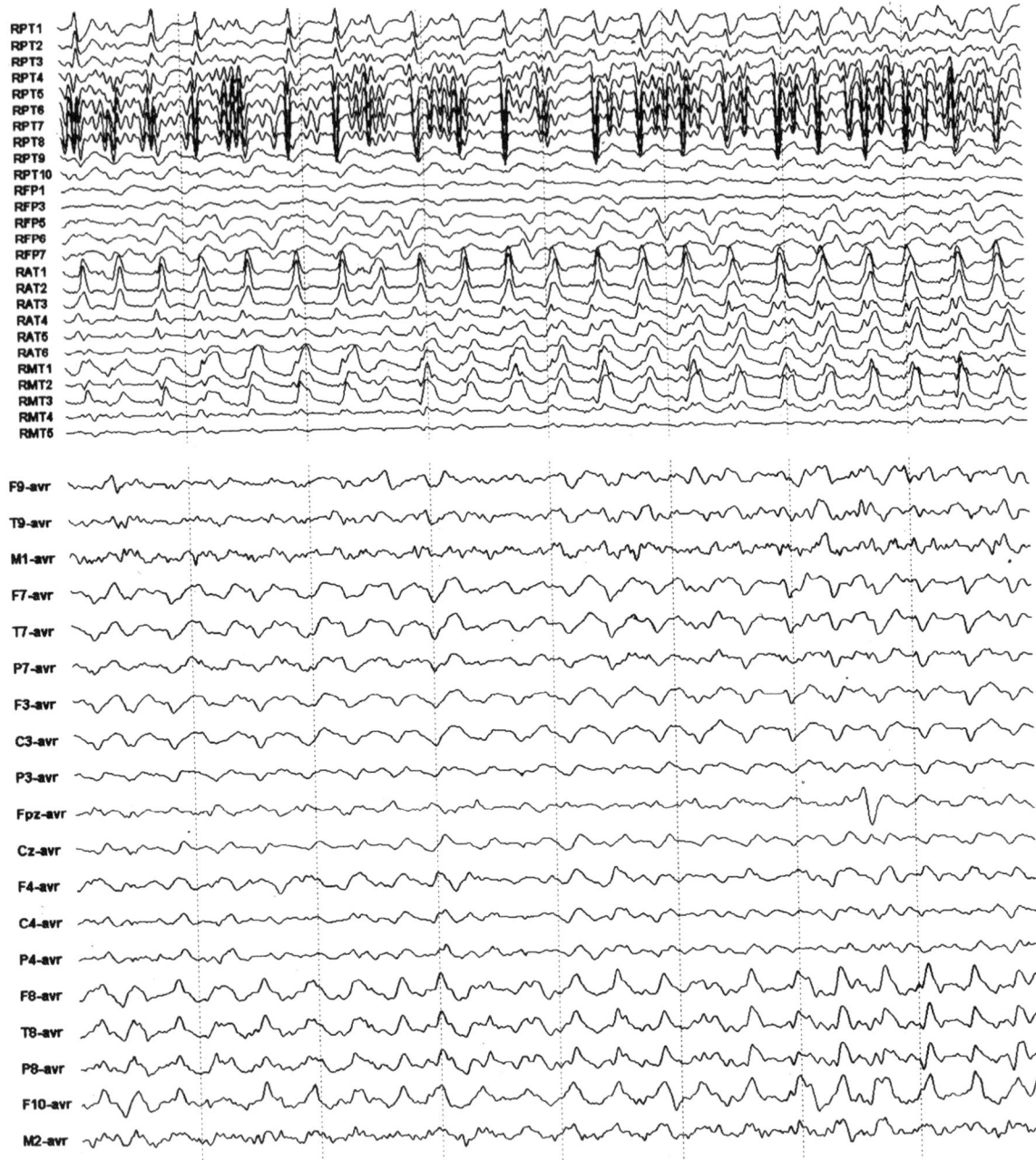

FIG. 2.12. Simultaneous intracranial and scalp electroencephalographic (EEG) recording of a temporal lobe seizure. The seizure rhythm from the temporal neocortex is relatively synchronous (subdural electrode contacts RAT1 to 6 and RMT1 to 4) but of less amplitude than that depicted in Fig. 2.11. The scalp EEG, however, shows a well-developed seizure rhythm.

potentials, such as epileptic spikes or seizures, which makes them easily appreciated on the scalp EEG (Fig. 2.12). Transient patterns of longer duration and thus lower frequency have a greater chance of having at least a partial overlap in activity and thus some summation of their fields.

PROPAGATION

If cortical activation remains localized to one area, which undergoes the usual depolarization and repolarization sequence, the resultant voltage fields on the scalp rises and falls in amplitude and reverses in polarity, but the location of the maxima does not change; nor does the overall shape of the fields. If, however, activity propagates into adjacent cortical regions, the overall geometry of the source changes. A new location to the overall center of activity and a new net orientation of the source cortex exist. These changes result in a different voltage field. Movement of scalp field maxima or change in the shape of the fields over tens of milliseconds suggests propagation of source activity. This is particularly common with epileptiform spikes or seizures (5). Such changes in voltage fields can provide important information concerning propagation direction and extent.

An example illustrating all these relationships is shown in Figs. 2.13 and 2.14. Figure 2.13 illustrates simultaneous EEG recordings from intracranial and scalp electrodes, as well as the scalp EEG voltage topography at the time of the cursor. Note in the intracranial EEG traces the progressive delay of the spike potential, which originates in the mesial temporal tip (LAT1) and propagates posteriorly over basal and lateral temporal surfaces to contacts LAT7 and LMT9. The first recordable scalp field, shown in the topographical maps, has a frontopolar negative maximum that is appropriate for a temporal tip source orientation. The locations of the subdural electrodes are depicted in Fig. 2.14 on a three-dimensional magnetic resonance imaging (MRI) reconstruction of the patient's brain. Also illustrated is the approximate area of cortex undergoing depolarization at five instances during the spike. Shown as well are the five scalp voltage fields produced by this propagating cortical source. As this area of activated cortex propagates posteriorly and laterally, the corresponding scalp EEG field maxima move appropriately for the net source location and orientation. Note also the eventual large size of the cortical source, which approximates 20 cm². This example confirms that the voltage field recorded from scalp electrodes is directly related to geometrical features of the cortical spike source. Because of this systematic relationship, source models of scalp EEGs can be used to estimate the location, orientation, and propagation of cortical generators. (See Chapter 23.)

EFFECT OF REFERENCE ON ELECTROENCEPHALOGRAPHIC FIELDS

The measurement of EEG potentials is relative to a reference. Polarity and amplitude are dependent on this comparison. There has been considerable debate about the effect of choice of reference on the appearance of EEG traces and on voltage field maps (see Chapter 4). Most authorities now agree that varying the reference does not alter the contours or gradients of the voltage fields (i.e., the relative differences) or the information concerning source character. What is altered is simply the display of the same data. In fact, EEG source models, such as dipoles, in which topographic voltage distributions are used as raw data for calculation, are reference independent.

The easiest way to appreciate the effect of the recording reference is to think of EEG voltage topography as geographical topography: namely, mountains of one polarity and valleys of another. The reference in this model would be the level of a coexisting ocean that covers part of this landscape. Everything above sea level has an altitude of one polarity, and everything below sea level has a depth of the opposite polarity. With a different sea level, the altitudes and depths of particular points on the landscape change, but the shape of the mountains or the undersea valleys does not change. If the highest mountaintop or deepest ocean valley is chosen to be the reference and all points on the landscape are of one polarity or the other, but the underlying structure has not changed. The same is true for changes in EEG recording reference (Fig. 2.15).

Any reference can be used and data interpreted properly, if the effect of reference on the EEG display is appreciated. There is no such thing as an "inactive" reference, because any point on the head or body carries some electrical potential. Traditionally, reference electrodes were thought to be "active" only when they were within the negative field of a spike. This notion resulted in part from the misconception that outside of this negative field there was no other activity related to the spike. Spikes were commonly thought to have only a negative field maximum, except for the "horizontal dipoles" of benign Rolandic epilepsy. In fact, all spikes have, by electromagnetic necessity, both negative and positive field maxima. Depending on source location and orientation, both maxima may not be recorded in standard 10 to 20 montages, as discussed earlier. Because positive field maxima

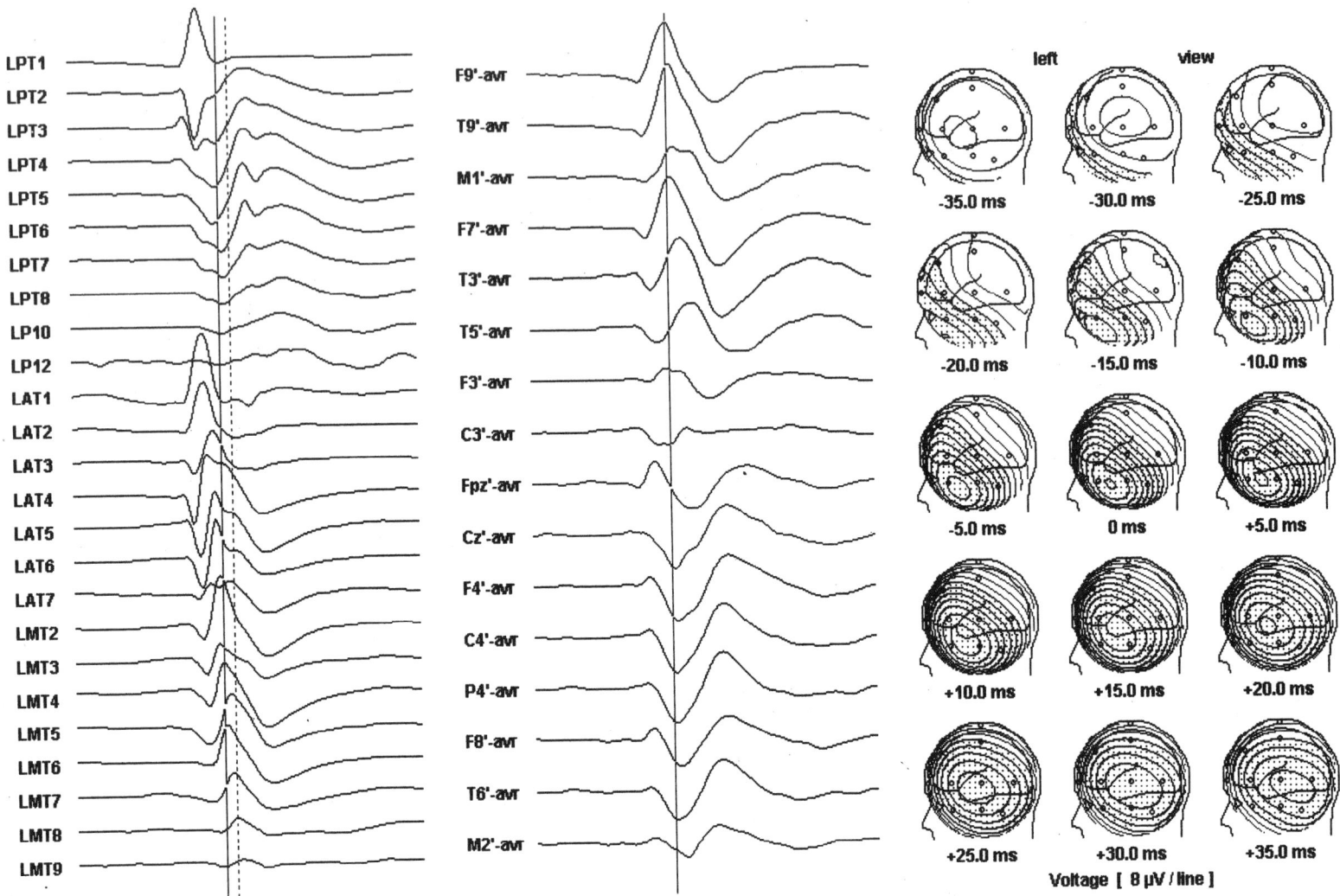

FIG. 2.13. Left: Simultaneous intracranial and scalp electroencephalographic (EEG) recording of a left temporal spike. Subdural electrode placements are illustrated in Fig. 2.14. The intracranial EEG was referenced to the contralateral mastoid; negative polarity is upward deflection of traces. The scalp EEG is displayed in common average reference. **Right:** Map sequence depicts simultaneous scalp voltage topography at 5-millisecond intervals, centered on the cursor, spanning 70 milliseconds. Voltage map shading denotes field polarity (speckled area is negative). Isopotential lines indicate field strength. Note spike onset in temporal tip cortex (LAT 1, LAT 2, and LPT 1), followed by mesial to lateral propagation across temporal tip subdural contacts (LAT 1 to LAT 7) and then midtemporal subdural contacts (LMT 2 to LMT 8). LPT is a longitudinal mesial temporal depth probe. Contact 1 is most anterior; contacts 4 to 7 are located in the hippocampus. Note that the initial scalp voltage field is inferior frontopolar, which is appropriate for an inferior temporal tip source. Over 70 milliseconds, as the spike propagates, the negative field maximum progressively moves into an anterior inferior temporal and eventually into a midtemporal location.

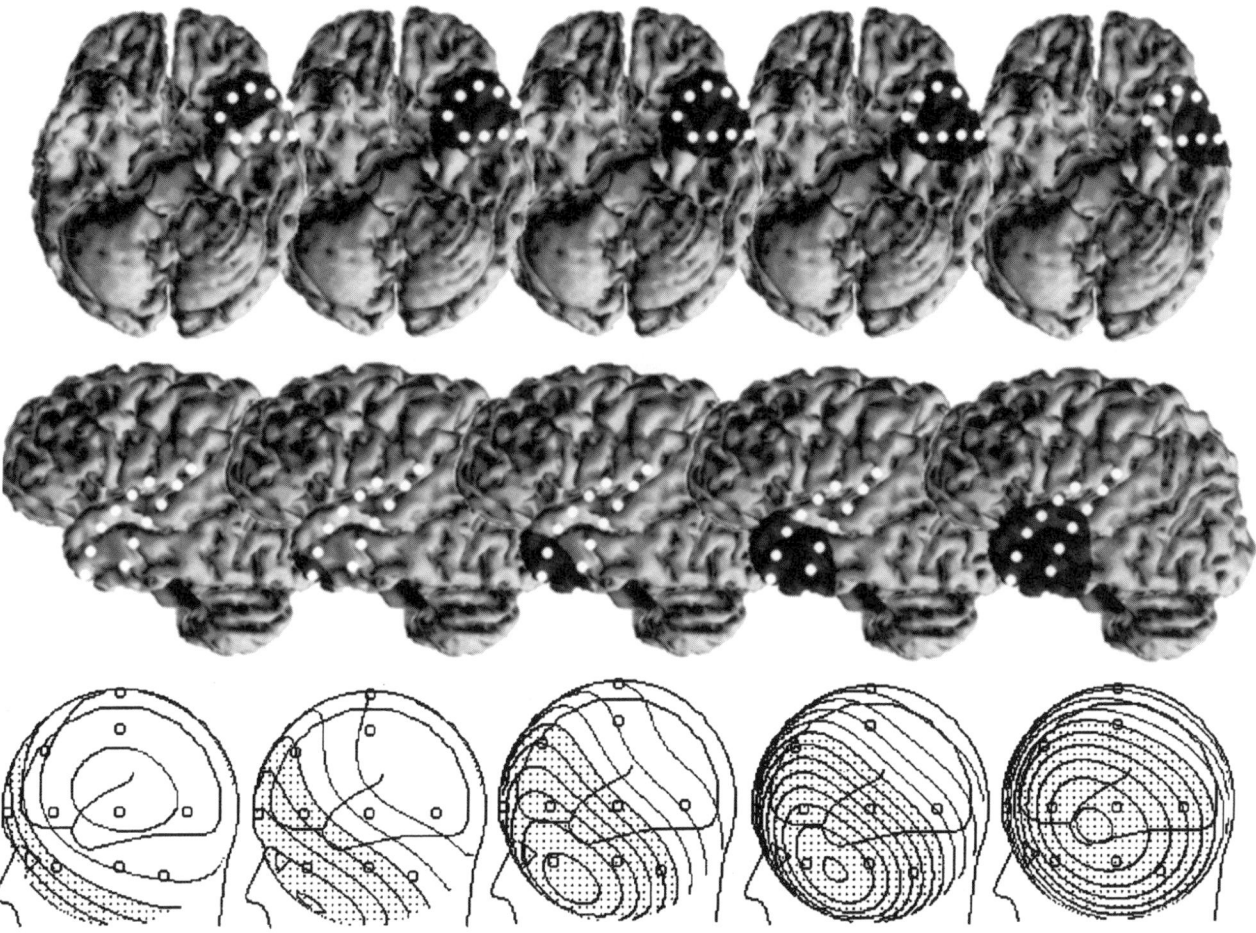

FIG. 2.14. Three-dimensional magnetic resonance imaging (MRI) reconstruction of brain and subdural electrode contacts from patient whose data were depicted in Fig. 2.13. The most anterior strip is LAT. Contact 1 is most mesial; contact 7 is most lateral and superior. The more posterior strip is LMT. Contact 2 is most mesial; contact 9 is most lateral and superior. The darkened cortical area denotes estimated region of concurrent cortical depolarization (negative potential) during propagation of the spike. Source estimate derived from intracranial electroencephalogram of Fig. 2.13. Five time points at 15-millisecond intervals are illustrated, corresponding to latencies −30 to 30 milliseconds in Fig. 2.13. Scalp voltage topography at these times is shown at the bottom. Note the relatively large area of the spike source, its propagation over time, and the close relationship between source geometry and the scalp voltage field. The negative scalp maximum moves from frontopolar to subtemporal to temporal location over 60 milliseconds.

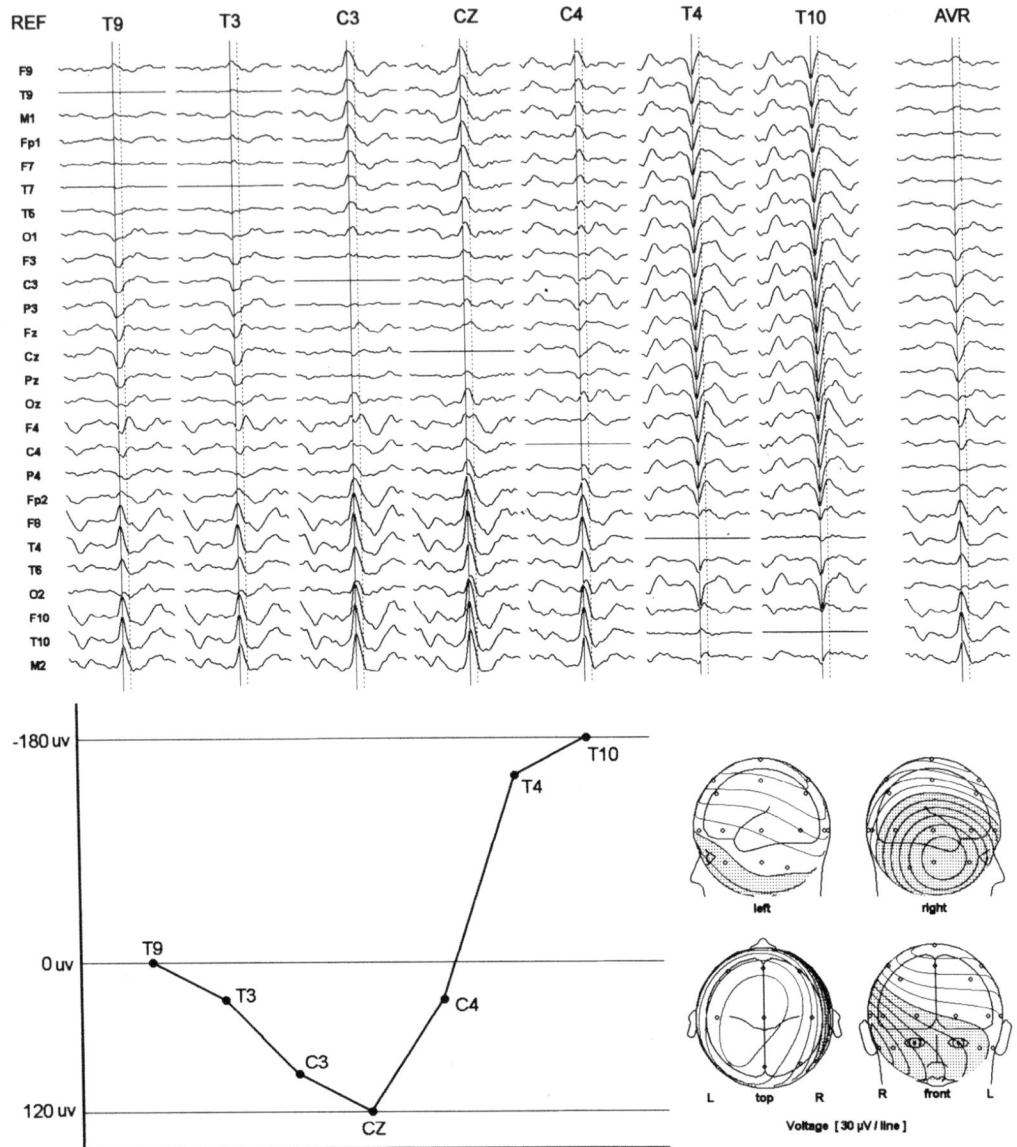

FIG. 2.15. Bottom: The magnitude and polarity of a right temporal spike recorded in common average reference from a midcoronal chain of electrodes is graphed into a two-dimensional landscape. The voltage topography of this spike is illustrated at the right. Isopotential lines are drawn at every 30 μV; the hatched area is negative. **Top:** Electroencephalographic (EEG) traces of this spike are displayed, with each electrode in the midcoronal chain in succession used as the common reference. Note that changing reference alters only where the zero voltage line is placed. The relative voltage differences among electrodes remains unchanged. When T10, the negative field maximum, is the reference, all EEG deflections are positive (downward). When Cz, the positive field maximum, is the reference, all EEG deflections are negative (upward). When T9 is the reference, the EEG deflections are similar to that of the common average reference because this electrode lays on the common average reference zero isopotential line.

were not thought to be present in most spikes, reference manipulations were often performed to eliminate the appearance of positive potentials whenever they did occur.

For example, common average reference derivations were often calculated only after removal of the electrodes recording the largest negative potentials. If the electrodes were not removed, it was said, positive potentials might appear on the opposite side of the head. These were thought to be reference artifacts, rather than the true opposite-polarity field maximum that is produced by any dipolar source. Deleting electrodes with the most negative potential from the average simply shifted the reference "sea level" in a positive direction so that the true positive field would appear to have less amplitude (see Fig. 2.15).

As discussed earlier, however, maximal information about source character can be obtained only by identifying both field maxima. A simple and yet very effective way to do this is to use a common average reference made up from all recording electrodes. If the mean potential recorded from all electrodes is used as a zero reference level, then by necessity both relatively more negative and more positive fields are accentuated and thus more easily identified. This type of reference also makes physical sense. By the laws of physics, the net charge or net potential over the surface of the head from any source should be zero (i.e., positivity balancing negativity). The mean of all recording electrodes is an approximation of this. Obviously, the more electrodes used, particularly from undersampled regions of the head, the more such a reference approximates the true zero potential. To the untrained eye, such a reference may initially cause confusion because fields of both polarities are emphasized. Focal negative spikes from one hemisphere or lobe are accompanied by positive potentials, commonly from the opposite hemisphere. This distribution does not represent bilateral spike sources; rather, it represents the normal dipolar field of any cerebral generator. The greater amplitude and steeper voltage gradient of the negative maximum identifies the source as being nearer to it, whereas its geometrical relationship to the positive maximum conveys the overall field orientation and thus the net orientation of the generating cortex, which is orthogonal to that of the field (see Figs. 2.4, 2.5, 2.6, and 2.7).

CONCLUSIONS

Too often the EEG is thought of as simply time-varying potentials, or wiggles, that supposedly reflect the activity of brain under the recording electrodes. Recognition of the pattern of these wiggles has been the foundation of EEG education. Fortunately, this is not all there is to EEG recording. It is a multidimensional signal and a carrier of abundant information, much of which is not routinely used. Limitations of traditional EEG recording are often artificial and imposed, in part, by simplistic interpretation methods. Practitioners of modern EEG recording must go beyond one dimensional to multidimensional thinking, if more information is to be extracted from the EEG. In order to take EEG interpretation beyond simple description toward an analysis of source location and character, it is essential that the interpreter appreciate the relationships between cortical sources and the EEG voltage fields that they produce.

REFERENCES

1. Abraham K, Ajmone-Marsan C. Patterns of cortical discharges and their relationship to routine scalp electroencephalography. *Electroencephalogr Clin Neurophysiol* 1958;10:447–461.
2. Alarcon G, Guy CN, Binnie CD, et al. Intracerebral propagation of interictal activity in partial epilepsy: implications for source localization. *J Neurol Neurosurg Psychiat* 1994;57:435–449.
3. Cooper R, Winter AL, Crow HJ, et al. Comparison of subcortical, cortical and scalp activity using chronically indwelling electrodes in man. *Electroencephalogr Clin Neurophysiol* 1965;18:217–228.
4. Creutzfeldt O, Houchin J. Neuronal basis of EEG waves. In: Creutzfeldt O, ed. *Handbook of Electroencephalography and Clinical Neurophysiology, vol 2C.* Amsterdam: Elsevier, 1974: 5–55.
5. Ebersole JS. Defining epileptogenic foci: past, present, and future. *J Clin Neurophysiol* 1997; 14:470–483.
6. Eccles JC. Interpretation of action potentials evoked in the cerebral cortex. *Electroencephalogr Clin Neurophysiol* 1951;3:449–464.
7. Gloor P. Neuronal generators and the problem of localization in electroencephalography: application of volume conductor theory to electroencephalography. *J Clin Neurophysiol* 1985;2: 327–354.
8. Gloor P. Contributions of electroencephalography and electrocorticography to the neurosurgical treatment of the epilepsies. In: Purpura DP, Penry JK, Walter RD, eds. *Advances in neurology, vol. 8: neurosurgical management of the epilepsies.* New York: Raven Press, 1975:59–105.
9. Goldensohn ES. Neurophysiologic substrates of EEG activity. In: Klass DW, Daly DD, eds. *Current practice of clinical electroencephalography.* New York: Raven Press, 1979:421–439.
10. Humphrey DR. Re-analysis of the antidromic cortical response: II. On the contribution of cell discharge and PSPs to the evoked potential. *Electroencephalogr Clin Neurophysiol* 1968;25: 421–442.
11. Li CH, Jasper H. Microelectrode studies of the electrical activity of the cerebral cortex in the cat. *J Physiol* 1953;121:117–140.
12. Pacia SV, Ebersole JS. Intracranial EEG substrates of scalp ictal patterns from temporal lobe foci. *Epilepsia* 1997;38:642–653.
13. Purpura DP, Grundfest H. Nature of dendritic potentials and synaptic mechanisms in cerebral cortex of cat. *J Neurophysiol* 1956;19:573–595.
14. Scherg M. Fundamentals of dipole source potential analysis. In: Grandori F., Hoke M, Romani GL, eds. *Auditory evoked magnetic fields and potentials. Advances in audiology.* Basel: Karger, 1990:40–69.

Chapter 3

Engineering Principles

Brian Litt and Stephen D. Cranstoun

Electroencephalography (EEG) involves recording and analyzing electrical signals generated by the brain. These signals are small and surrounded by a variety of large electrical potentials originating in the environment. Resolving true electrical brain activity requires three elements: good equipment, meticulous recording technique, and informed interpretation of the data. Improper technique may, in the worst case, lead to injury of a patient from improper grounding or stray electrical currents. This chapter reviews principles of electricity and electronics relevant to EEG technology.

New to this chapter is a review of the basic technical principles underlying digital EEG. Because of the increasing availability of low-cost microcomputers and digital electronic technology, cumbersome banks of amplifiers and chart writers on wheels are rapidly yielding way to portable, paperless personal computer–driven machines, some requiring no more than a notebook computer, a headbox, and some cabling. Reams of remotely warehoused EEG paper and days filled with ink stains and paper cuts are being replaced by high-density, accessible digital storage media, such as recordable compact disks (CDs) and digital video disks (DVD), and by networked computer reading stations. More than just a new fad, digital EEG technology offers great improvements over analog technology, including lower cost; increased diagnostic yield; less environmental pollution and less consumption of natural resources; access to quantitative and automated analysis tools for EEG; and remote transfer, monitoring, and interpretation of EEG records. Clearly, digital EEG is a permanent tool. Every electroencephalographer, medical student, and medical technologist should be familiar with the science and engineering underlying clinical EEG, now supplemented with a practical knowledge of digital computers, principles of digital signal processing, computer networking, and data bases.

ELECTRICAL BASICS

The standard clinical (surface) EEG records potential differences (voltage) between two points, one or both of which are on the scalp. The signals of the EEG are based on the movement of electrical charges in biological tissue. Charge, represented by the symbol Q, is quantized. It exists in units that correspond to the charge of elementary particles, such as protons and electrons. The charge of a single electron is very small; in practice, much larger units of charge are used. In the metric meter-kilogram-second (MKS) system, charge is measured in coulombs (C). One coulomb is approximately equal to the charge of 6×10^{18} electrons (14). Movement of charge is called *current,* usually denoted by I, and is measured in units of amperes (A). One ampere of current represents a flow of 1 C of charge per second (for review, see Purcell [26]). Current flows when electrons move or in association with movement of negative ions (e.g., Cl^-, anionic proteins) or positive ions (e.g., cations Na^+, K^+, or Ca^+). Electron flow is more important in electronic devices, and ionic flow is more important in biological systems. Current flow is conventionally defined from positive to negative. For example, Na^+ ions moving from left to right (or Cl^- ions moving from right to left) would generate a positive current to the right.

According to a fundamental principle of electricity, like charges repel and opposite charges attract. Thus, a collection of freely moving charges will arrange itself in a uniform distribution so that (a) positive and negative charges are as near to each other as possible and (b) positive-positive and negative-negative charge pairs are as far apart as possible. Other physical forces such as gravity, friction, magnetism, moving mass, and nuclear forces can oppose these electrical attractions and repulsions. This results in a separation of charges into more positive and negative areas. Such a system stores electrical potential energy. This energy is released when charges move to restore regional electrical neutrality. The unit of energy in the MKS system is the joule (J). One joule, defined in terms of kinetic energy, is the energy required to accelerate a 1-kg mass by 1 m per square second over a distance of 1 m. This is approximately equivalent to the energy a person would feel after dropping a lemon on his or her foot from waist high. Voltage (V; or E, for electromotive force) is defined as energy per unit charge. One joule of energy is expended when 1 C of charge is moved across a potential difference of 1 V. Voltages are always measured between two points in space. It makes no more sense to say that a single point in an electrical circuit is 5 V than it does to say that a ball is "5 m." In some circumstances, the reference point for height or for voltage differences is implicit. This implicit location of a reference potential is called *ground* ("physical ground" in a discussion of the height of a ball, or "electrical ground" in the case of a voltage difference). The precise meaning of electrical ground is elusive, because two places in the earth are rarely at identical potential with regard to any third point. Nevertheless, potential differences between a circuit element and either ground rod typically are large in comparison with potential differences between two ground points. Exceptions and cautions regarding possible voltages between two different grounds are reviewed near the end of this chapter, in the section on electrical safety.

Table 3.1 lists typical voltages and currents for a few commonly encountered systems.

TABLE 3.1. *Examples of voltage and current for circuits of interest*

System	Volts	Amps
Lightening	100,000,000	10,000
Hoover Dam	50,000	2,000
Static from carpet	2,000	0.000001
Household light bulb	110	1
Car battery	12	200
Flashlight battery	1.5	0.6
Electrocardiogram	0.0015	0.00001
Scalp EEG	0.00005	0.000001

Note: Numbers are rough approximations, for illustrative purposes only. EEG, electroencephalography.

CIRCUIT ELEMENTS

Combinations of a few simple elements can serve as models for many important electrical circuits, simple and complex: resistors, capacitors, inductors, and power sources. These elements are described in detail in numerous electronics texts; only a brief overview is given here (14).

Resistors

In the real world, energy transfer is never completely efficient: Energy carried by currents dissipates into heat by resistance of the conducting medium. Resistance is measured in joule-seconds per coulombs squared, or ohms (Ω). One ohm is the resistance that will cause 1 J of energy to dissipate when a current of 1 A flows through it for a period of 1 second.

Figure 3.1 shows a hydraulic analogy to an electrical circuit. In this system, electrical potential difference is represented by the difference in gravitational potential energy (proportional to the difference in height) between points A and B; current is represented by the flow of water (I), and the resistor is the paddle wheel (R). As resistance increases (done by increasing the paddle wheel radius or by making it more difficult to rotate), flow decreases in an inverse proportional relationship for the same potential difference. This is a statement of Ohm's law:

$$V = I \cdot R$$

where V (or E, for electromotive force) represents the voltage, I represents the current, and R represents the resistance. According to this law, the potential difference across a resistance is equal to the current flowing through it, multiplied by its resistance.

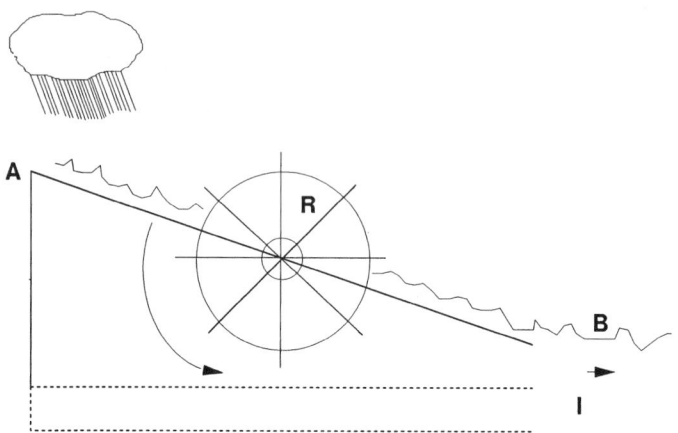

FIG. 3.1. Fluid analog of Ohm's law. A-B is the change in height (which determines difference in gravitational potential energy) driving water flow. I, paddle wheel; R, resists water flow.

Figure 3.2 shows a simple circuit consisting of a voltage source (e.g., a battery) of 10 V and a 100-ω resistor. According to Ohm's law,

$$V = I \cdot R$$
$$10\ V = I \cdot 100\Omega$$
$$I = 10V/100\Omega = 0.1A$$

In this circuit diagram, the symbol represents a voltage source, with the positive terminal (or anode) drawn as the long line and the negative terminal (cathode), or ground, drawn as the shorter line. The symbol is used to represent a resistor.

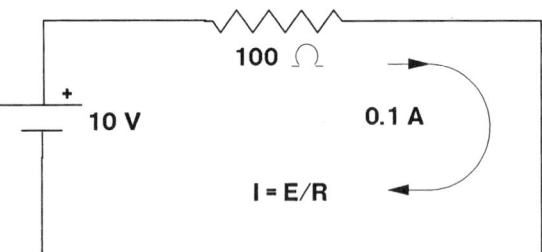

FIG. 3.2. Simple circuit illustrating Ohm's law. $I = V/R = 10\ V/100\ \Omega I = 1/10$ A, where V is a 10-V battery and R is a 100-ω resistor.

Electrical circuit resistors are usually made from materials whose atoms do not easily release electrons, such as carbon. Materials of very high resistance (e.g., rubber, glass, or air) are referred to as *insulators.* Resistive elements in the circuit created during EEG recording include the subject's body, scalp-electrode interface, electrode, wiring, and internal circuitry of the EEG machine.

Resistors may be adjustable to different resistance values. A straightforward example is a potentiometer, in which a dial adjusts the length of a resistive substance through which current must pass. Modern electronic circuits and several important biological circuits (e.g., electrically excitable neuronal membranes) involve the use of resistors whose resistances change as a function of voltage.

Capacitors

A capacitor is a device that stores separated charges. It can be thought of as two conducting plates that are very close together but separated by a thin insulator, so that no charge can flow between the plates. When a potential difference is placed across a capacitor, positive charges accumulate on the plate at the positive end of the circuit. This attracts negative charges toward the other plate. Movement of charges on the plates toward the boundary between them causes a current to flow on both sides of the capacitor, without charges actually flowing across the plates. When repulsion by like charges on each plate of the capacitor balances the force from the applied potential, no more current flows. It is intuitive that a large plate allows more charge accumulation before crowding and mutual repulsion halt currents. Similarly, closer proximity of the plates increases attractive force across plates and thereby increases the currents. The third determinant of capacitance is the type of insulator material between the plates, known as the *dielectric.* In mathematical terms,

$$C = Q/V$$

where capacitance (C) is defined as the amount of charge that a particular device can store for a given potential difference; Q represents the charge (in coulombs); and V represents the potential difference (in volts). The unit of capacitance is the farad (F): 1 F is the capacitance that stores 1 C of charge when a potential difference of 1 V is applied across the two plates of the capacitor. A 1-F capacitor is enormously large and is found only in very specialized applications. Most circuits use capacitors of 10^{-6} F (microfarads, or μF) or of 10^{-12} F (picofarads, or pF).

If the voltage across a capacitor remains constant, charge accumulation on the plates eventually stops current flow. This property can be recognized

quantitatively by differentiating the equation $C = Q/V$ with regard to time and by assuming C is a constant:

$$\frac{dC}{dt} = 0 = -\frac{Q}{V^2}\frac{dV}{dt} + \frac{1}{V}\frac{dQ}{dt}$$

$$\frac{dQ}{dt} = \frac{Q}{V}\frac{dV}{dt}$$

$$I = C\frac{dV}{dt}$$

Current is equal to capacitance multiplied by the change in voltage with regard to time. Again, in circumstances in which potential difference does not change in time, there is no current flow because of capacitors. Changing voltages induces current flow in circuits containing capacitors. As an example, Fig. 3.3 displays the capacitor voltage versus time when the switch

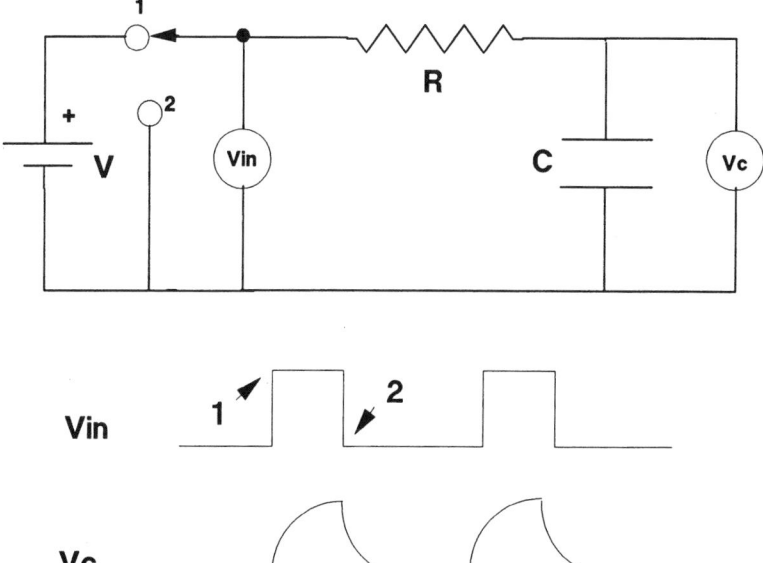

FIG. 3.3. Resistor-capacitor circuit (used as a high-frequency filter) containing voltage source (V), resistance (R), capacitance (C), and voltmeters measuring voltage at input (V_{in}) and across the capacitor (V_c). The switch allows generation of square-wave input shown at bottom of figure (V_{in}). Capacitor charges and discharges exponentially with time constant: $\tau = R \cdot C$.

moves between positions 1 and 2 in the circuit shown. The capacitor serves to "smooth out" and delay the voltage pulse introduced into the circuit. It is evident then that capacitors can serve as resistive elements (resisting current flow), depending on how rapidly current is changing. Capacitors will "pass" alternating current (AC) and block direct (unidirectional) current (DC), after an initial current flow when the DC is first applied. This "resistance" to current flow is called *capacitive reactance* and is usually designated by X_c. Capacitive reactance is inversely proportional to the frequency of an AC and is inversely proportional to the capacitance of the capacitor. The formal formula is

$$X_c = 1/(2\pi fC)$$

where X_c represents the reactance (in ohms); π is approximately 3.14; f is frequency of AC (in hertz [Hz], or cycles per second); and C is capacitance in farads. Energy "lost" in capacitive reactance is not really lost as it is in heat dissipated by a resistor; rather, it is mostly converted to potential energy in the form of charge separation.

Several biological elements have capacitance that alters the EEG signal. These include cerebrospinal fluid, the skull, and the scalp. The electrodes used to connect the patient to the EEG machine also alter the EEG signal. If a train of 1-Hz delta waves in the EEG were led to a capacitor of 1 μF, reactance would be $1/(6.28 \times 1 \times 10^{-6})$, or 159,236 Ω. If a train of 20-Hz beta waves were led to the same capacitor, then the reactance would be approximately 7,962 Ω. In this way, the capacitance of the scalp-electrode interface offers more resistance to current flow at low frequencies than at high frequencies.

Inductors

Inductance is a magnetic phenomenon. Charge in motion generates a magnetic field; therefore, electric current flow produces a magnetic field. A voltage is induced in any conductor that encircles a time-varying magnetic field. This finding is the basis for power generation in hydroelectric plants, in which falling water from a dam or natural waterfall spins a magnet surrounded by a coil of wires, inducing substantial voltages in the connecting circuits.

An inductor is made of coils of wire that encircle the magnetic field that is generated by current flowing in the wire itself. Coils of wire, consisting of many turns, are employed in inductors in order to encircle the magnetic field many times, increasing the induced voltage. In addition, increasing the number of turns of wire increases the magnetic field strength for a given current. Inductance is proportional to the square of the number of turns in the coil.

Magnetic induction is the basis for transformers, which convert one voltage level to another (Fig. 3.4).

The voltage across an inductor is proportional to the derivative, with regard to time, of the current passing through it. The constant of proportionality is called the *inductance*. Inductance is measured in henrys (H) and is conventionally designed by the letter L. Inductance has the same relationship to current that capacitance does to voltage. It is governed by the equation

$$V = L\frac{dI}{dt}$$

A potential difference of 1 V placed across a 1-H inductance causes the current through it to increase at a rate of 1 A per second. Induction may thus be conceived as a form of electrical inertia. "Resistance" of an inductor to current flow is referred to as *inductive reactance,* usually designated by X_L Inductive reactance is proportional to inductance and to the frequency of the current through it. The formula is

$$X_L = 2\pi fL$$

where X_L represents the inductive reactance (in ohms); f represents the frequency (in hertz); and L represents the inductance (in henrys). Energy "lost" to inductance is actually stored in the magnetic field.

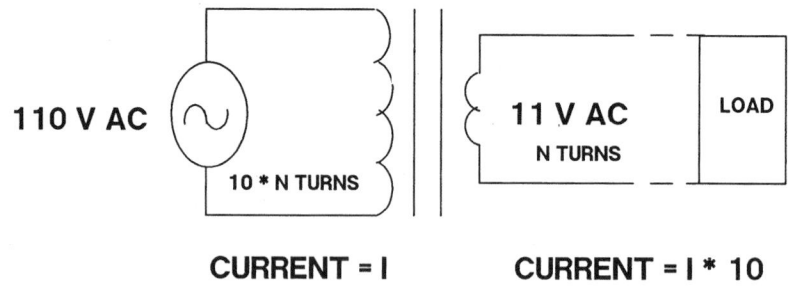

FIG. 3.4. Transformer uses two inductors to change 110 V of alternating current (AC) with current *I* (through 10 · *N* turns) to 11 V of AC with current 10 · *I* (through *N* turns). Note that power (*I* · *V*) is conserved.

Inductance is an important concept in electrical circuits; however, the magnitude of inductive reactance is usually small in circuits relevant to clinical electroencephalography.

Power Sources

Power (P) is energy per unit time, expressed in joules per second, or watts (W). In an electrical circuit, power is calculated as voltage multiplied by current: *VI*. For a resistor, from Ohm's law, this translates to I^2R, or V^2/R. Power corresponds approximately to the colloquial impression of "strength." A high-voltage, low-current shock does not have much power, just as a high-pressure spray from a garden hose with a very low water flow rate does not have much strength. To continue the hydraulic analogy, a high flow rate in a garden hose with little water pressure produces a soothing wash. Fire hoses combine high water pressure with high flow rates to produce a powerful stream. It is fortunate that high voltages alone cannot kill, or the human race would long ago have been destroyed by static electricity. As discussed later, currents are more dangerous to patients than are voltages.

The two most commonly available sources of electrical power in modern society are batteries and wall sockets. Batteries produce power by chemical interactions between two metals immersed in an acid and produce DC. An everyday wall socket is an AC power source that delivers a sinusoidal voltage at the conventional frequency (in the United States) of 60 Hz. Line voltage may be expressed as

$$V(t) = V_p \sin(\omega t + \theta)$$

where $V(t)$ represents the voltage as a function of time; V_p represents the peak amplitude of the voltage; ω represents the angular frequency (in radians/second), equal to $2\pi f$ (frequency in hertz); t represents the time (in seconds); and θ represents the phase angle (in radians), which corresponds to the amount of offset from the beginning of the sine wave cycle that exists at time = 0. Figure 3.5 reviews some basic characteristics of sine waves.

Most AC voltages are described by the root mean square (RMS) voltage and not by the peak value. The RMS voltage is effective and produces the same average power as would a DC voltage of the same value. For a sinusoid, the RMS value is equal to the peak value divided by the square root of 2. Thus, a wall socket that provides 110 V of AC (VAC) RMS actually delivers peak voltages of 156 V. Most AC voltmeters measure RMS volts.

Electronic circuits usually operate from DC power; however, they usually employ a power supply circuit that converts commonly available AC

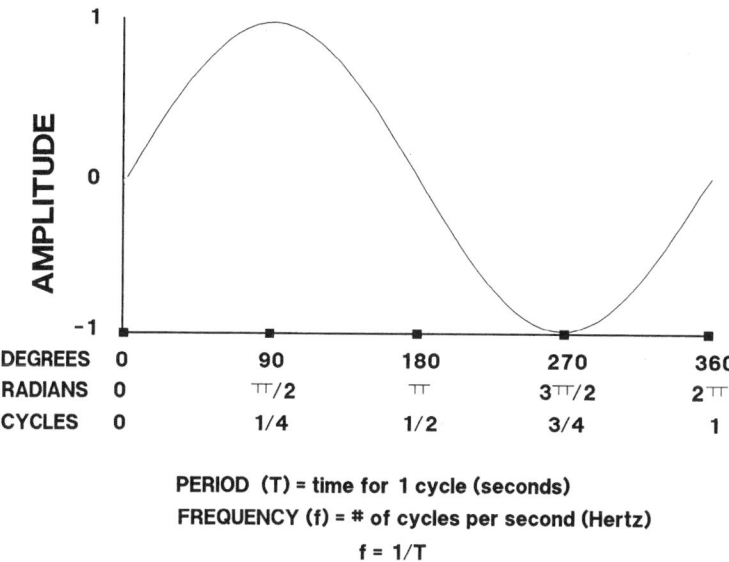

PERIOD (T) = time for 1 cycle (seconds)
FREQUENCY (f) = # of cycles per second (Hertz)
f = 1/T
PHASE = amount wave is shifted horizontally
(in degrees, radians or cycles)

FIG. 3.5. Sine wave demonstrates relationship among degrees, radians, cycles and among period, frequency, and phase.

power into DC. AC power sources are commonly provided because of their advantages in production, storage, and delivery to consumers, in comparison with DC.

Table 3.2 summarizes definitions, symbols, and useful formulas pertaining to common electrical terminology.

TABLE 3.2. *Electrical terms and symbols*

Term	Units	Symbol	Comments
Charge	Coulombs (C)	Q	6×10^{18} electrons
Current	Amperes (A)	I	$I = dQ/dt$
Voltage	Volts (V)	V, EMF, E	Joules/coulomb
Energy (work)	Joules (J)	E (or W)	$kg \times m^2/s^2$
Resistance	Ohms (R)	Ω	$V = I \times R$
Capacitance	Farads (F)	C	$I = C \times dV/dt$
Inductance	Henrys (H)	L	$V = L \times dI/dt$
Reactance (capacitance)	Ohms	X_C	$X_C = 1/(2\pi fC)$
Reactance (inductance)	Ohms	X_L	$X_L = 2\pi fL$
Power	Watts (W)	P	$P = I \times V$

Active Circuit Elements

Active circuit elements, which include vacuum tubes, transistors, and integrated circuits, serve as fundamental building blocks for most modern electronic devices, particularly amplifiers and oscillators. Active components add power to a system and provide voltage amplification. Space does not permit discussion of active circuit elements. Information may be found in any standard electronics text (e.g., see Budak [2] and Horowitz and Hill [14]).

CIRCUITS

Sustained current flow requires a closed circuit; otherwise, the circuit functions as a very inefficient capacitor, with charges accumulating at the open circuit ends and inhibiting further charge flow. Circuits comprise the various elements detailed earlier. Even the simplest real-life circuit—for example, a battery with its positive and negative poles connected by a strand of wire—exhibits a certain (small) amount of resistance, capacitance, and inductance. Most circuits contain elements with more explicit resistive, capacitive, or inductive components. Several circuit properties are important for the understanding of EEG technology.

Circuit Elements in Series and in Parallel

Resistors and capacitors can be placed end to end (i.e., in series) or side by side (i.e., in parallel) or in other configurations less pertinent to EEG technology. Any number of resistors in series can be represented by a single resistor of value equal to the sum of all of the series resistors:

$$R = R_1 + R_2 + \ldots + R_n$$

Resistors in parallel can be represented by a single resistor of value equal to the reciprocal of the sum of the reciprocals:

$$R = \cfrac{1}{\cfrac{1}{R_1} + \cfrac{1}{R_2} + \ldots + \cfrac{1}{R_n}}$$

Figure 3.6 gives some examples of series and parallel resistors and their equivalents.

A similar relation holds for multiple capacitors in a circuit, except that capacitors are additive when positioned in parallel:

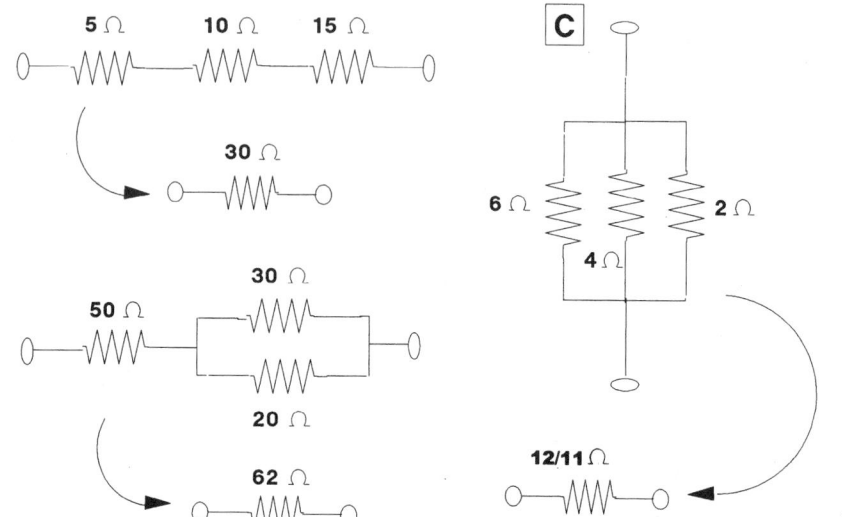

FIG. 3.6. Demonstration of equivalent resistance. **A:** Three resistances in series reduce to one resistance equal to their sum. **B:** Two parallel resistances equal the reciprocal of the sum of the reciprocals of resistances (12 Ω), which adds to 50 Ω resistance in series. **C:** Three parallel resistances reduce to the reciprocal of the sum or the reciprocal (12/11 Ω).

$$C = C_1 + C_2 + \ldots + C_n$$

Capacitors in series decrease total capacitance by the formula

$$C = \cfrac{1}{\cfrac{1}{C_1} + \cfrac{1}{C_2} + \ldots + \cfrac{1}{C_n}}$$

It is possible to construct an endless number of complex circuits from a voltage source, resistors, and capacitors, if they can be arranged in serial and parallel combinations. Three basic rules of electrical circuits are useful in analysis of current flow and potential difference across any circuit element:

1. *Thévenin's theorem* states that any system made up of resistors and voltage sources enclosed in a box with two terminals protruding can be exactly modeled by a system composed of one voltage source and one resistor in series. The value of the equivalent voltage source is found

from the voltage appearing at the terminals when no current is drawn from the terminals. The value of the equivalent resistance can be found by dividing the equivalent voltage by the current that flows when the terminals are short-circuited.

2. *Kirchhoff's voltage law* states that the sum of the voltages across circuit elements in a complete loop (starting and finishing in the same place) must be zero. Because of this, all elements in parallel have the same voltage across them.

3. *Kirchhoff's current law* asserts that the net current flow into a node (junction point) anywhere in a circuit must be zero; that is, total current exiting a node equals total current entering a node. This means that all elements in series have the same current passing through them.

In Fig. 3.7 these laws are applied to analyze simple circuits used in EEG machinery. Figure 3.7 shows a circuit made up of an ideal voltage source and two resistors in series. To analyze the circuit, Ohm's law is first applied:

$$V = I \cdot R$$
$$V_{in} = (R_1 + R_2) \cdot I$$
$$I = \frac{V_{in}}{(R_1 + R_2)}$$
$$V_1 = I \cdot R_1 = V_{in} \cdot \frac{R_1}{(R_1 + R_2)}$$

$$V_2 = I \cdot R_2 = V_{in} \cdot \frac{R_2}{(R_1 + R_2)}$$

Assume that

$$V_{in} = 11V, R_1 = 1\Omega, \text{ and } R_2 = 10\Omega$$

Therefore,

$$V_1 = 11V \cdot \frac{1\Omega}{(1\Omega + 10\Omega)} = \frac{11V \cdot \Omega}{11\Omega}$$
$$V_1 = 1V$$

and

$$V_2 = 11V \cdot \frac{10\Omega}{(1\Omega + 10\Omega)} = \frac{110V \cdot \Omega}{11\Omega}$$
$$V_2 = 10V$$

This circuit is called a voltage divider. It can be used to produce smaller voltages in any ratio desired, depending on the ratio of the resistances.

Figure 3.8 illustrates a more complex voltage divider with two switches. This circuit, which is actually the sensitivity setting circuit from an EEG amplifier, allows selection between two resistors with switch 1 and allows selection among 12 resistors with switch 2 (32).

Analysis of circuits containing multiple capacitors is analogous to the exercises above.

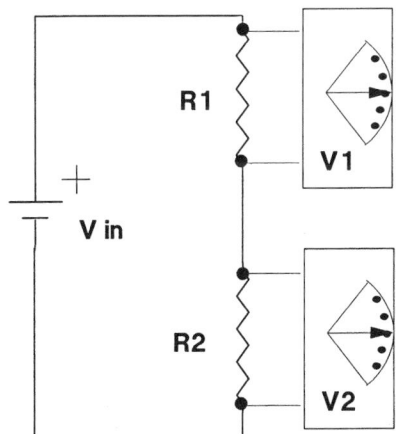

FIG. 3.7. Simple voltage divider. If *R*1 and *R*2 are selected appropriately, V_{in} can be divided up into V_1 and V_2 in any ratio desired. $V_1 = V_{in} \cdot R1/(R1 + R2)$; $V_2 = V_{in} \cdot R2/(R1 + R2)$.

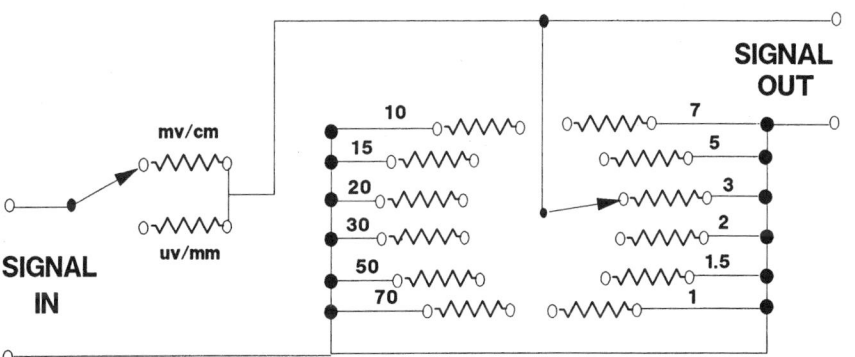

FIG. 3.8. Electroencephalographic sensitivity switch circuit. A voltage divider with selectable values for *R*1 and *R*2 via two switches. This circuit governs output voltage amplitude to the electroencephalogram pen system.

Time Constants

Figure 3.9 shows a capacitor and a resistor in series with a power source connected via a switch. The input voltage (V_{in}) and the output voltage across the resistor (V_c) are measured, as shown, by two imaginary voltmeters. This circuit does not pass DC because of capacitive reactance. As discussed earlier, it resists current flow in inverse proportion to the frequency. A point less evident is that the resistor-capacitor (RC) circuit will also alter the timing of applied electrical signals. The bottom of Figure 3.9 shows what happens when a square-wave voltage is applied to the circuit at V_{in}. By Kirchhoff's voltage law, voltage across the capacitor and the resistor must sum to the voltage generated by the power supply. When the switch is in position 1, electrons travel to the right plate (P_R) of the capacitor and begin to charge that plate negatively. In the first small slice of time, few negative charges on the left plate (P_L) of the capacitor are repelled from this charge buildup, and thus there is little voltage across the capacitor. The entire voltage therefore appears across the resistor. Later in time, P_R becomes more negatively charged, and more negative charges are repelled from P_L. A voltage appears across the capacitor, and less is measured across the resistor. Later still, electrons slow their migration to P_R, because they are repelled in proportion to the number of electrons already there. The equation to describe a process whose rate is dependent on its amount is called an *exponential* equation, and the inverse (reversed axes) is a *logarithmic* equation. Many processes in nature are exponential or logarithmic: for example, unrestricted population growth, cooling of a brick, radioactive decay, and the wearing away of a stone's surface in a stream. The process of charging the capacitor in the RC circuit is exponential, so that the rate of charging is inversely proportional to how much it is already charged.

The formula for the voltage across the resistor (V_c) is

$$V(t) = Ae^{-t/\tau}$$

where $V(t)$ represents the voltage across the resistor at time t; A is a constant representing maximum voltage; and τ is called the *time constant*. The term e represents the base of natural logarithms (approximately 2.718) and is also the one constant for which the proportionality between the rate of change of an exponential process and the process itself is unity.

The inverse equation may be obtained by taking the logarithm of each side:

$$\ln(V(t)) = \ln(A) - t/\tau$$

Theoretically, the capacitor in an RC circuit never becomes fully charged; instead, it only approaches the full battery voltage in ever-decreasing increments (the more it is already charged, the less it charges in the next time slice). Consequently, a convenient convention is needed to describe how long it takes an RC circuit to charge. One possibility would be to use the $t_{1/2}$, the time required to charge a capacitor to halve its final value. Engineers prefer to use the natural logarithm as a yardstick and to utilize $1/e$, which is approximately $1/(2.718)$, which equals 0.368, or approximately 37%, as a standard measure rather than the 50% point. Conventionally, the time constant of a series RC circuit, τ, is the time required for the voltage across the resistor to fall to 37% of the initial value. This is arithmetically equivalent to the time required to charge the capacitor to 63% of its final value. The time constant of an RC circuit can be calculated as the product of the resistance and capacitance:

$$\tau = R \cdot C$$

The bigger the resistor, the smaller the amount of current that is delivered to the capacitor (by Ohm's law) and the longer it takes to fully charge. The

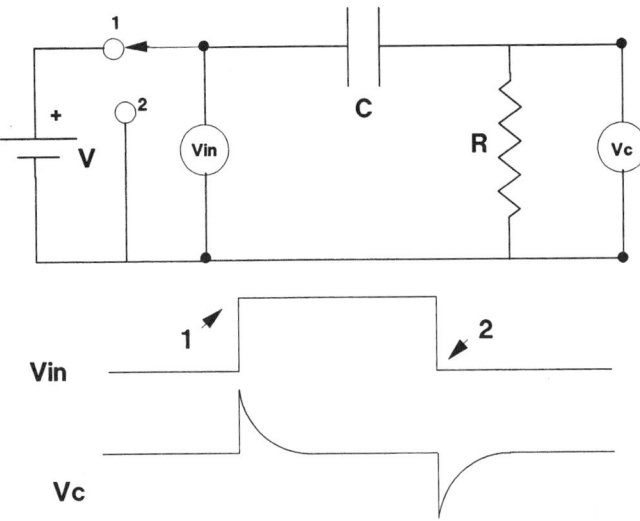

FIG. 3.9. Resistor-capacitor circuit employed as a low-frequency filter, demonstrating exponential decay of output to square-wave input signal. Circuit contains voltage source (*V*), capacitance (*C*), resistance (*R*) and voltmeters measuring voltage across the input (*V$_{in}$*) and across the resistor (*V$_c$*). Output at *V$_c$* illustrates low frequency filtering (and differentiation) of input (*V$_{in}$*).

larger the capacitor, the longer the first plate takes to "fill" with electrons and develop a repulsive force on the second plate.

Once the capacitor in an RC circuit is nearly fully charged (this being an exponential process), a switch may be opened to prevent the charge from leaking off. If the charged capacitor is then removed from the circuit and placed in series with a resistor, then as soon as a complete circuit is formed, the capacitor will discharge through the resistor. The rate of discharge is also exponential (or logarithmic, depending on which axis in the voltage-time relation is chosen as the independent variable). Initially, charges rush off each plate, repelled by like charges on the same plate and attracted by opposite charges on the other plate. As charges redistribute more equally, there is progressively less force driving the movement of charge. The time constant, τ, also defines the time required for the charge to decline to 37% of the initial value. To avoid confusion over 63% versus 37% and charging versus discharging, it is useful to remember that time constants represent a "majority" of the appropriate change: (a) an increase to 63% of maximum voltage on charging or (b) a decrease to 37% of initial voltage on discharging. The direction of current flow is, of course, opposite to that of the initial charging period, and voltage measured across the resistor therefore jumps to a negative value (see Fig. 3.9).

A circuit with a 1×10^6 Ω (1 MΩ) resistor in series with a 1-μF capacitor would have a time constant of 1 second. Any constant stepped voltage drop applied across the resistor would decrease voltage to 37% of its final value in 1 second. Similarly, a circuit with a 100-Ω resistor in series with a 1-μF capacitor would exhibit a time constant of 0.0001 second. Applied voltage steps downward would decline to tiny fractions of their initial values within a few hundred microseconds.

If there are several circuits like the one in Fig. 3.9 (employed as a low-frequency filter) in series, then the overall time constant is less than any individual time constant and may be estimated by the reciprocal of the sum of reciprocals of the time constants of each circuit (6,14):

$$\tau = \frac{1}{\dfrac{1}{\tau_1} + \dfrac{1}{\tau_2} \ldots + \dfrac{1}{\tau_n}}$$

Simple Filters

The analysis of an RC circuit demonstrates that low frequencies are filtered by recording across the resistor of the circuit. How much filtering is done depends on (a) the frequency content of the input voltage and (b) the time constant of the circuit. Low-frequency filtering is used in every clinical EEG recording in order to prevent DC potentials (e.g., tissue-electrode polarization) from overwhelming the biological signals. Figure 3.10 shows examples of calibration voltage pulses passed through EEG circuitry with time constants corresponding to filters with cutoff frequencies of 0.1, 0.3, 1.0, and 5.0 Hz. Note that on many EEG machines, the time constants are given in seconds. The time constant in seconds is calculated from the following equation, which governs its relation to the cutoff frequency. The shorter the time constant is, the more attenuated the low-frequency components of the signal become. A low-frequency filter is sometimes referred to as a *high-pass filter,* because it allows high-frequency signals to pass. Another way to characterize a low-frequency filter is by specifying the frequency (assuming a pure sine wave input) at which output is reduced to a fixed fraction of the input. This frequency, called the *cutoff frequency,* is inversely related to the time constant and multiplied by a factor of $1/(\pi)$ (to convert from frequency in radians to cycles per second):

$$f_{cutoff} = \frac{1}{2\pi RC} = \frac{1}{2\pi\tau} = \frac{0.16}{\tau}$$

With a time constant of 1 second, the cutoff frequency is 0.16 Hz. A time constant of 5 seconds yields a cutoff frequency of 0.03 Hz. A τ of 0.1 second corresponds to a cutoff of 1.6 Hz. High-pass (low-frequency) filters pass at least 70% (more precisely, $1/\sqrt{2}$) of the signal amplitude for inputs of frequencies higher than the cutoff frequencies.

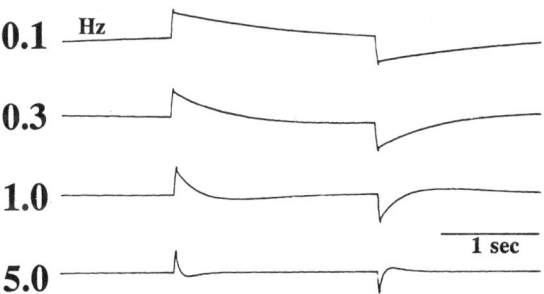

FIG. 3.10. Response of low-frequency filters to 50-μV square-wave calibration input, with respective cutoff frequencies of 0.1-, 0.3-, 1.0-, and 5.0-Hz.

Low-frequency filtering causes an advance in the timing of voltage peaks for a sinusoidal input signal. One way to envision the mechanism of this phase shift is to recognize that the later portions of a slow wave occur at a time when the filter capacitor is resisting accumulation of additional charge on the plates. The later portions of the slower waves are therefore attenuated, and the peak of the wave is shifted to the left (i.e., the filter *differentiates* the input voltage with regard to time). At the cutoff frequency, the peak is shifted earlier by $\pi/4$ radians (45°, or one-eighth of a cycle) (32). This can be very significant in practice if filtering is applied to one channel and not another. For example, assume a 5-Hz theta wave is recorded in two different EEG channels having low-frequency filters set to different cutoff frequencies. If channel 1 has a cutoff of 0.1 Hz and channel 2 has a cutoff frequency of 5 Hz, then the wave in channel 2 will appear to have occurred 25 milliseconds before the wave in channel 1, even though they both came from the same source. If the EEG reader is not aware of these filter settings, he or she may misinterpret this type of record.

High-frequency filtering may be obtained from an RC circuit by taking the output across the capacitor. Rapidly changing input voltages (high frequencies) generate little potential difference across the capacitor and thus generate little output. Slowly changing currents, in contrast, build up substantial voltages across the capacitor plates (the capacitor has time to charge). A high-frequency filter is a low-pass filter. The cutoff frequency is defined as the reciprocal of $2\pi\tau$ ($1/[2\pi\tau]$), just as with high-pass filters. Figure 3.11 shows the

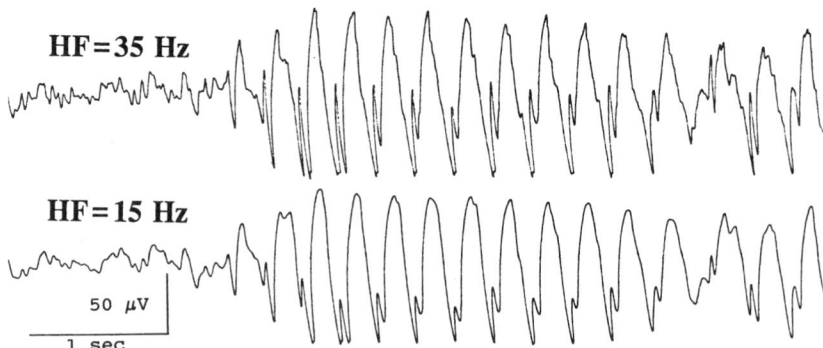

FIG. 3.11. High-frequency filtering of spike waves to show attenuation of spike component with 15-Hz high-frequency cutoff. Data are reproduced from an ambulatory cassette electroencephalographic (EEG) monitor played back to a standard EEG machine for paper output.

effect of two high-frequency filters having cutoff frequencies of 35 Hz and 15 Hz on a spike-and-wave discharge. Spike amplitudes become noticeably attenuated at a lower high-frequency cutoff; slow waves are barely altered, except that they are made smoother.

High-frequency filtering also produces phase shifts in the timing of sinusoidal (or approximately sinusoidal) signals, because it takes time for a capacitor to charge and develop a voltage across the two plates. In this case, the phase shift causes a delay in the peak of the waveform. This delay becomes significant only for high-frequency signals. At the cutoff frequency, a sine wave is delayed by one-eighth (45°, or $\pi/4$ radians) of a cycle (32).

Impedance

Impedance is a term used for the combined effects of resistance, capacitive reactance, and inductive reactance. The formula for calculating the impedance of a series circuit is

$$Z = \sqrt{R^2 + (X_C + X_L)^2}$$

where Z is in ohms and the remaining terms are as defined earlier. Inductive reactance is subtracted from the capacitive reactance, because their values have opposite phase. In the practice of EEG, inductive reactance can usually be ignored. Impedance, represented by Z, replaces resistance in the analysis of AC circuits. In AC circuits, Ohm's law takes the form

$$V = I \cdot Z$$

This equation describes only the amplitudes of the waveforms considered. V, I, and Z are each a function of frequency, and they may be shifted in phase in comparison with one another. These phase shifts can have significant effects on the behavior of AC circuits; however, a proper treatment of this subject requires complex mathematics that are beyond the scope of this discussion.

Impedance can be significant in several aspects of EEG. The most important of these is probably safety considerations (see later section on electrical safety): dangerously low circuit impedances can allow high currents to pass through tissue with potentially disastrous consequences. Impedance is also important in comparing amplitudes in different EEG channels. High impedance (typically in a poorly affixed electrode) causes the EEG machine amplifiers to work improperly and distorts the resulting signal in that channel. Impedance is also an important factor in coupling the output of one amplification stage to another. The EEG machine is designed so that electrodes should have impedances in the range of a few thousand ohms, whereas the input impedance of the machine is in millions of ohms. If the impedance of the input is too low, the second stage may draw significant current from the primary stage and distort the measurement. Suppose, for example, that a 100-μV EEG signal is inputted into a circuit with a 1,000-Ω resistor. Assume that the input impedance of the EEG machine is $10^6\ \Omega$ and therefore in a position to draw negligible current from the circuit. Current through the circuit will be 0.1 nA (10^{-9} A). In contrast, now suppose that the EEG machine has an input impedance of 1,000 Ω. Total circuit impedance is now 2,000 Ω, and current through the circuit is 50 nA. Because of the low-input impedance, the output signal is attenuated and measured as 50 μV rather than 100 μV, as in the first case. This illustrates that the high-input impedance of a good amplifier produces its output voltage largely independently of electrode impedance. It is essentially the voltage divider seen earlier in this chapter, with one resistance being *much* larger than the other. As a result of this design, the electrode impedance during normal EEG recording can vary by a factor of almost 10, with only minor alterations in the quality of the EEG. Very high electrode impedances, which approach those of the EEG machine input, cause the phenomenon called *impedance mismatch,* which results in signal attenuation, as demonstrated in the example earlier.

THE DIGITAL WORLD

Introduction to Digital Computers

The rapid and continuing spread of computers into all aspects of people's personal and professional lives requires that much information gathering, storage, and communication be converted to their language, the language of numbers. Properly referred to as *digital* computers, these devices primarily manipulate, store, and display numbers, or their equivalents, in various forms. Their strength lies in the fact that they perform these tasks extremely fast, executing simple commands at speeds measured in millions of instructions per second (*mips*) and performing calculations measured in millions of floating point operations per second (*megaflops*). Conceptually, a digital computer can be envisioned as a group of individual devices, such as a calculator (central processing unit [CPU]), information archive area (hard disk), computer monitor, floppy disk drive, keyboard, printer, and temporary memory storage area in which data are temporarily kept for manipulation (random access memory [RAM]).

These devices are all connected both to each other, by a communication cable called a *bus,* and to a clock. Each device is assigned a priority, according to its importance, and an interrupt flag, which is turned on when the device needs to do something and turned off when it is waiting for instructions. Figure 3.12 depicts a schematic of this arrangement. The clock keeps track of time, so that events can occur in a synchronized manner. In a typical instruction cycle in a computer's life, the clock ticks, and the CPU goes looking around the bus to determine which devices need to be serviced. It checks the devices in order of priority around the bus to determine which get served first. The CPU services the devices as necessary before moving on to the next request. If an instruction is given to copy data from the floppy drive to the hard disk, the floppy drive sets its interrupt flag to "on" and asks for service. The CPU, cycling around devices on the bus, notices this and moves a piece or pieces of data from the floppy drive to the hard disk, as requested, all the while taking brief periods to look around the bus for other tasks to complete, which it prioritizes. If no other devices need service, it may continue this operation until the file is copied and then turn the flag on the floppy drive to "off." If other devices with higher priority request attention, then the floppy drive will wait until

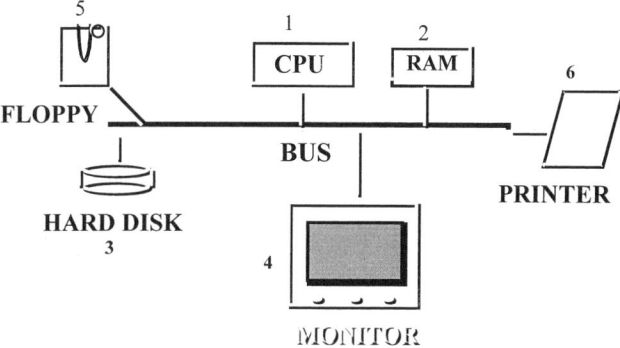

FIG. 3.12. Schematic diagram of personal computer architecture. A fast clock is built into the central processing unit (CPU), which is connected to random access memory (RAM), peripheral structures (such as the floppy and hard drives, printer, and fax machine), and computer monitor. State-of-the-art machines have a variety of other design features and peripheral devices, such as "burst cache" memory, network access, and digital video disk (DVD) drives. Despite these tremendous advances, the basic machine design reduces to the operations described in the text.

the more important tasks are completed. Devices with lower priority may wait until the current job is finished before they are serviced. If many devices request attention at one time, as frequently happens, then the CPU may take turns servicing them, but it distributes service time according to device priority. The faster the clock ticks (as of this writing, personal computers have clock speeds of over a billion cycles per second [gigahertz]), and the larger the capacity of the bus, the faster and more efficiently the computer operates. As computers become even faster, this rule breaks down somewhat as the rate-limiting steps in some processes change; for instance, they may change to time it takes for the reading heads to access the hard disk drive or transfer information to and from memory. More ingenious ways of speeding up these processes continue to be dreamed up by engineers, such as "burst cache", an ultra-fast hard-wired section of memory that holds critical information for brief periods, and putting more and more microscopic devices on the machine's CPU chip, so that transfer distances and times are minimized. Because theoretical limits to the density of integration of these chips are approached, completely new types of computing strategies, even using living cells to store information, are under development.

Computer programs that directly access machine hardware and allow users to give commands to this system via the keyboard or to run programs are called *operating systems* or software *platforms* (e.g., Windows, Macintosh Operating System (MOS), Disk Operating System (DOS), UNIX, and LINUX). The actual machines and their individual components together form *hardware platforms*. Other computer programs that run on these computers and can be started or stopped by commands through the operating system are called *applications*. The computer programs that provide interfaces, displays, and commands through which users interact with digital EEG machines are examples of such applications. In most cases, however, the hardware platforms that constitute these machines are the same standard personal computers that are used to balance checkbooks or surf the Internet, with the exception of some specialized hardware, which is discussed later. The easy-to-use graphical windows through which these programs are run are called GUIs (pronounced "gooeys"), for graphical user interfaces.

Analog and Digital Signals

The basic currency of EEG is electrical activity generated by the brain and recorded by scalp electrodes after it is conducted through the inter-vening tissues. On a standard EEG machine, filters and amplifiers process brain signals so that they can be conducted to pens, which transfer these signals in a continuous flow of ink to the EEG paper that scrolls beneath them. Throughout this process, brain activity, although transformed, remains continuous and uninterrupted. In this scheme, brain activity remains an *analog* signal, as it is analogous to the source signal, and every point in time can be mapped back to every point in the source signal if one knows the "recipe" for transformation is known. A *digital* signal is different in that it is discontinuous, consisting of a sampling of the source signal in time with spaces left between the data points. Rather than begin a smooth, continuous line drawn on paper, a digitized signal can be written as a table of numerical values. When these values are plotted on a graph, they form a representation of the original signal, with spaces between the data points. Engineering theory provides mathematical rules, which determine how many points, or *samples,* are necessary to uniquely resolve a particular kind of signal or waveform. These rules, to some degree, are governed by what clinicians wish to do with the data and are discussed later. Table 3.3 reviews a number of common items that can be represented in analog or digital form.

TABLE 3.3. *Analog and digital comparisons*

Reference	Analog machine	Digital machine	Comments
Time	Pendulum clock	Digital clock	The pendulum clock has smoothly moving hands; the digital clock has discrete numbers.
Music	Long-playing vinyl record	Compact disk	The stylus traces groves in vinyl records, generating an electrical signal that is carried to the speakers. Numbers burned onto a compact disk are read by a laser, generating discrete voltages sent to speakers.
Art	Oil painting	Newspaper photograph	The painting has smooth, continuous brush strokes. Dots or pixels compose the newspaper photograph; they can be seen through a magnifying glass.

Analog-to-Digital Converters

The heart of a digital EEG machine is the *analog-to-digital converter* (ADC). This device usually consists of a circuit board installed in a computer and is composed of several conceptual parts: (a) a clock, (b) a voltmeter or series of voltmeters, and (c) very rapidly accessible memory storage. The signal from a single EEG channel is inputted into a corresponding channel in the ADC board, the voltage across the input in the board is measured, and its numerical value is written down in memory. The clock ticks off a certain measure of time, and the process is repeated at regular intervals, yielding a table of evenly spaced numbers. The number of times per second that the voltage is measured is called the *sample rate* and is measured in samples per second (hertz). The higher the sample rate, in general, the better the reproduction of the input signal. ADC boards are measured (and priced) according to their number of input channels; their *throughput,* or the total number of samples per second that can be acquired by the entire device; and their resolution (described later). The throughput can usually be directed to and divided among any number of channels in the device. This number may be only one channel, if very fast sampling is required, or the total number of channels available, depending on the application. For example, if an ADC board has 32 input channels and a total throughput of 6,400 samples per second (6.4 kilohertz [kHz]), it can sample each of 32 channels at a maximum of 200 Hz each. The device could also sample two channels at 3.2 kHz each.

ADCs are also distinguished by their design for data sampling, including boards that sample each channel in turn and stagger them in time (it takes at least a few milliseconds to sample each channel), sample-and-hold devices that sample sequentially and then align data points in time, and devices that sample all channels simultaneously. Another important characteristic of ADCs is their *resolution* or *precision.* This is a measure of how finely the voltage can be subdivided when measured (e.g., to 1, 0.1, or 0.01 V). This precision is measured in *bits,* each bit being a place in a binary number. The total number of voltage values that can be resolved is 2^n, where n is the number of bits. If V_r is the maximum range of the board, then the input is resolved in steps, whereby ΔV is $V_r/2^n$. For example, if the board can resolve only two bits and is measuring on a scale of -100 to 100 μV, then there are 2^2, or four, possible values for the EEG signal, each data point being rounded to the nearest 50 μV. At this resolution, such a signal would look very rough, as measurements are rounded to the nearest 50 μV, without any possible values in between. This type of resolution is far different from the smooth lines drawn by pens on paper that are used with analog machines. Bits are used to measure resolution because the language of computers is *binary* numbers, in which each bit is a little electrical switch that is turned either on (a value of 1) or off (a value of 0). When these switches grouped together (usually in multiples of 8, 16, 32, or 64 at a time), they become binary numbers. For example, in the number 101 in binary, the first place on the right has the decimal value of $1 \cdot 1 = 1$, the 0 in the middle (twos) place has the decimal value $0 \cdot 2 = 0$, and the 1 in the most leftward (fours) place has a decimal value of $1 \cdot 4 = 4$. Therefore, the binary number 101 is equal to $(1 \cdot 4) + (0 \cdot 2) + (1 \cdot 1)$, or 5, in the decimal system. The number of bits, *n,* in a binary number can then resolve into a maximum of 2^n divisions. ADC used in early digital EEG machines were eight-bit devices, able to resolve EEG signals into $2^8 = 256$ divisions. Therefore, in a range -150 to $+150$ μV, steps of $300/256$ μV, or 1.17 μV, can be resolved. This initial resolution partially contributed to slow acceptance of these new devices because the tracings did not look as good as on paper. Most current EEG machines have 16-bit resolution and, for an input range of ±150 μV, can resolve $300/65,536$ μV, or 0.00457 μV. Table 3.4 depicts the resolution of a voltage range of -1.0 to 1.0 V as a function of the number of bits of the ADC.

Of importance is that the input voltage (2,000 μV in this case) is not the actual input voltage that is divided up by the ADC. Rather, all brain activity, once brought into the machine, is amplified by a certain multiplier (called *gain;* the inverse of this is *sensitivity,* the term commonly used to refer to controls to adjust amplitude on the EEG) that brings it into the standard input range of the ADC device (a typical range is ±5 V). In the earlier case, recording $\pm1,000$ μV would require a gain of 5,000 to bring it to ±5 V.

Although it may not seem at first that a typical electroencephalographer can tell the difference between 8-, 12-, and 16-bit resolution, these differences, particularly at the lower end of resolution, are easily apparent on rou-

TABLE 3.4. *Voltage steps for digitizers of various resolutions*

No. bits	No. levels	ΔV for V_r = 2000 μV
1	$2^1 = 2$	1,000 μV
2	$2^2 = 4$	500 μV
3	$2^3 = 8$	250 μV
4	$2^4 = 16$	125 μV
8	$2^8 = 256$	7.8 μV
12	$2^{12} = 4,096$	0.49 μV
16	$2^{16} = 65,536$	0.031 μV

tine reading of clinical records. For this reason, digital EEG technology was not widely used until 12- and 16-bit machines became available.

Visual Resolution: How The Electroencephalogram Looks to the Reader

As noted earlier, a frequent criticism of digital EEG, particularly when this technology first became available, was that it just did not look as good as on paper. At first glance, this is true. Paper EEGs are larger than most early computer monitors, the tracings are continuous waveforms in dark black ink, and large areas of the paper are devoted to each channel with, in general, plenty of space between channels. Digital EEG systems initially used 15-inch monitors; channels were often crammed together with little space between them, depending on the number of channels; and waveforms just did not appear as crisp as paper EEGs. Newer digital systems have improved a great deal on these early systems, making use of larger monitors with higher resolution and with better and more flexible graphical displays. A number of important characteristics should be kept in mind in assessing how a digital EEG tracing looks to a reader. Many of these parameters can be adjusted to improve the appearance of the EEG, although some may be hard-wired into the EEG machine.

Data Sample Rate

Low data sample rates may leave considerable spaces between data points, when tracings are magnified to rapid paper speeds on digital displays. Higher sample rates give an EEG recording the appearance of a smoother, connected line in the horizontal (time) dimension.

Data Resolution

Data resolution, mentioned earlier in the context of ADC, is a function of the ADC and consists of the number of bits in which the EEG signal is recorded. The more bits of data resolution there are, the better the signal looks, because smaller incremental changes in voltage are displayed, giving the appearance of a smooth, connected line rather than a jumpy, step-like tracing in the vertical dimension. On older eight-bit EEG machines, this stepwise quality to EEG tracings was sometimes quite evident. On newer systems, this is much rarer, inasmuch as tracings are viewed on standard gain settings with multiple channels displayed on the screen at one time; however, it is possible to adjust display parameters so as to allow the reader

to view the limitations of a given data resolution—in many cases, primarily by spreading smaller epochs of time over the screen (e.g., 1 to 2 seconds) at high gains (see later discussion).

Monitor Resolution

This feature, sometimes neglected in discussions of digital EEG display, is, along with monitor size and dot pitch, an important determinant of how a digital signal looks when the EEG pattern appears on a monitor. Monitor resolution is the number of pixels in each direction that can be used to fill in points on the EEG tracing. For example, a common resolution of computer monitors is $1,024 \times 768$ pixels. If 10 seconds of the EEG are displayed (for the time being, without regard to pixels dedicated to channel labels, screen borders, and so forth), then each second of the EEG on the horizontal axis has 102 pixels devoted to its display. If the EEG is sampled at 250 Hz, then less than every other data point can be displayed. In the vertical direction, there is a more severe restriction, because typical EEG tracings may have 32 channels or more. In this case, again without regard to pixels devoted to borders or labels, each channel may have only 24 pixels devoted to it in the vertical direction. If the EEG has a dynamic range of $300\mu V$, then very sharp waveforms, such as spikes, which may change by 150 μV over a fraction of a second, may look quite choppy. Larger monitors may help to better visualize tracings and allow space for each channel, in comparison with paper. This increased size of the viewing area should also be coupled with higher resolution, when possible (and affordable), so that the increased size does not serve to emphasize the distance between data points and does not further accentuate the noncontinuous nature of digital waveforms. Smaller monitors have the advantage of crowding each channel in such a way as to make it appear more continuous to the eye, but this is overridden by the disadvantage of making the reader strain to make out what can turn into a jumble of waveforms crammed into a small space.

Other Items: Dot Pitch and Color

Other items that can affect the appearance of the EEG are the dot pitch of the monitor and how color is applied to tracings. Their effect is, in general, smaller than that of the items just described. Dot pitch is the diagonal distance between display pixels. The smaller the pitch is, the higher the screen resolution is and the greater the number of pixels that the screen can contain. Changes in color for different groups of channels are sometimes used for ease of reading, although less commonly by more seasoned electroencephalographers. The authors' preference is to make the tracings black against a white or easy-to-read light background, but choice of colors and tracing displays are usually a matter of personal preference.

Recording "The Right Stuff": Nyquist's Theorem and Aliasing

A few important engineering rules govern how digital EEG signals must be acquired in order to guarantee that the EEG records the appropriate signals. The most important of these is called *Nyquist's Theorem*, which states that, in order to reliably digitize a signal of a given frequency, F, the signal must be sampled at a rate of more than two times F. For example, if the signal to be recorded has components of interest at 100 Hz, then a sample rate of greater than 200 samples per second (also properly stated as 200 Hz) is required. The reason for this sampling requirement is something called *aliasing*. Aliasing occurs when a signal of a certain frequency is sampled too slowly to resolve its frequency content, so that the resulting samples, when put together, compose a signal whose frequency is lower than that of the source signal. The true frequency of the signal "folds back" on one-half the sampling frequency, giving the aliased frequency. Once this aliasing has taken place, it is impossible to recover the original signal from the samples. This is best demonstrated by an example. Suppose an electroencephalographer wants to record a brain rhythm that occurs at 75 Hz, which requires a minimum sampling rate of 150 Hz, but the bargain-basement device that the purchasing department acquired for the electroencephalographer has a maximum sampling rate of 100 Hz per channel. Not believing in Nyquist's theorem, the electroencephalographer records the activity. An aliased signal of 25 Hz will therefore be recorded, introducing error into the data. Figure 3.13 depicts this phenomenon for a 5-Hz sine wave sampled at 8 Hz, which is less than the Nyquist frequency of 10 Hz. The sine wave reconstructed from the samples is only 3 Hz. Just as the term "alias" in common speech means a false name, so is an aliased signal a false representation of the source signal.

One method to significantly reduce aliasing is through the use of *antialiasing* filters. These simply are low-pass filters whose cutoff frequencies are equal to or less than one-half the sampling rate, the highest frequency component of the signal that can be resolved without aliasing. This ensures that higher frequency components are eliminated before digitization. Another way to be sure that a signal is not aliased is to *oversample*, which is sampling at a rate higher than that required by Nyquist's theorem. For example, most commercial EEG machines have sampling rates of at least 250 Hz to sample a bandwidth of 0.1 to 100 Hz. There are many practical reasons for doing this.

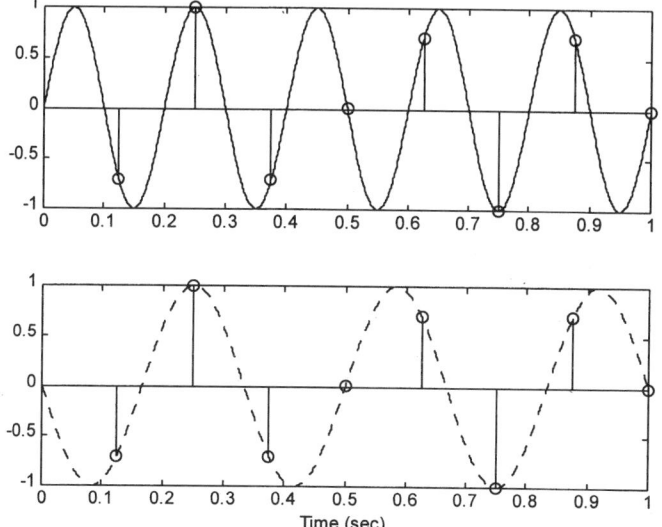

FIG. 3.13. Example of aliasing in an under sampled signal. ***Top:*** The original analog signal, a 5-Hz sine wave, and the discrete points sampled at eight times per second (*open circles*). ***Bottom:*** The analog sine wave reconstructed from the samples. Note that the frequency of the reconstructed signal is only 3 Hz.

Most important is that most commercial filters, such as those used in antialiasing, remove only approximately 37% (30% on Grass machines) of signal power at the cutoff frequency. This means that there is still significant power higher than the cutoff allowed into the EEG. Oversampling prevents this portion of the source signal from being aliased. When oversampling is combined with antialiasing filters, the aliasing can be eliminated.

Referential Recording

One important difference between analog and digital EEG machines is that digital machines use the principle of "referential recording." In this scheme, a separate electrode, called the *reference*, or a combination of electrodes such as the ear or mastoid electrodes (A1 and A2, or linked ears), are used as the second input ("grid 2" in older EEG language) into the differential amplifier for each channel. In this recording convention, the potential difference at the reference is subtracted from each electrode location (e.g., Fp1 − ref, Fp2 − ref), so that each data point stored in memory consists of

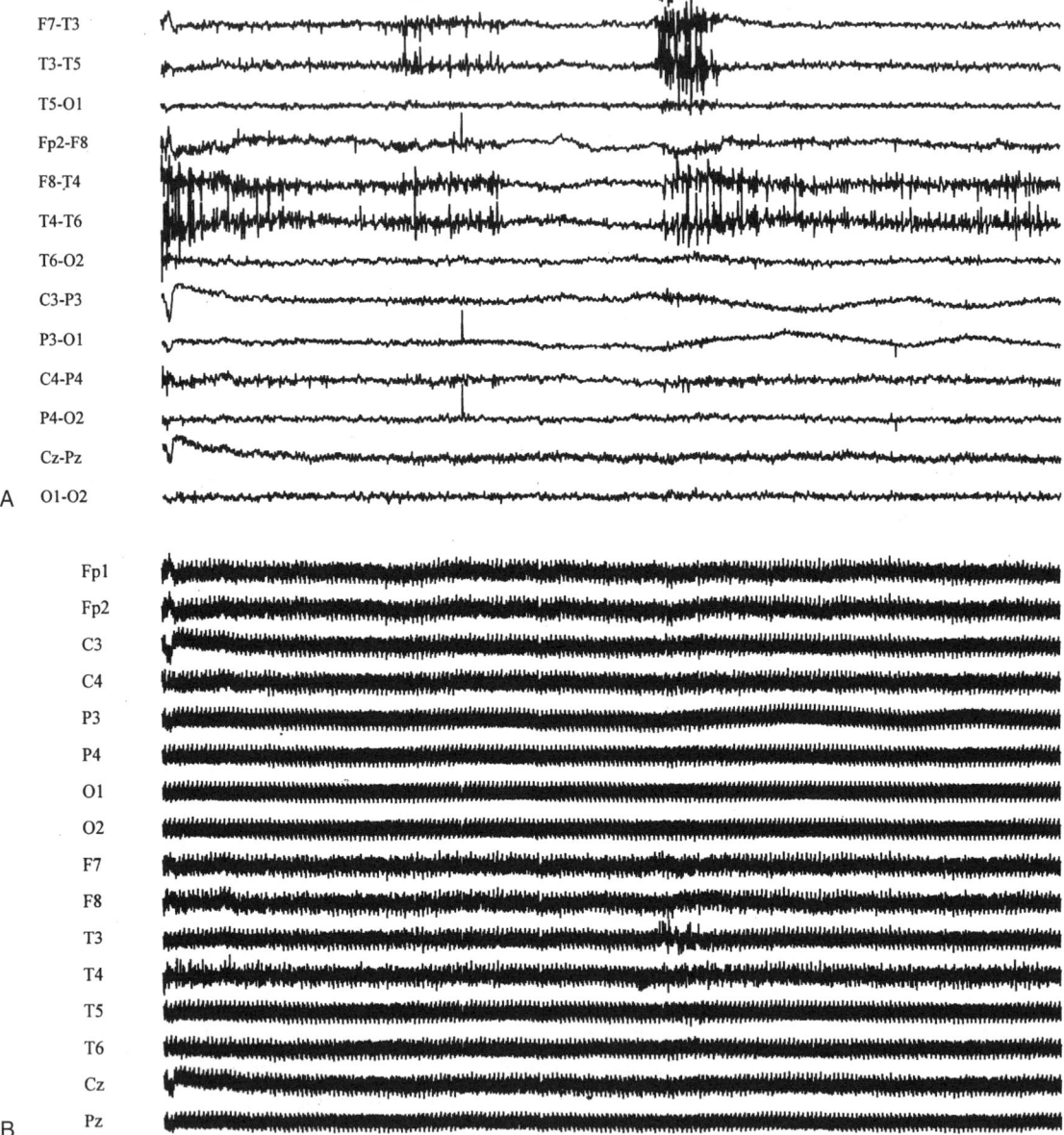

FIG. 3.14. Example of a referential digital recording, viewed in both a bipolar montage **(A)** and then the "machine reference" montage **(B),** with the potential at each electrode location minus the reference displayed. In this case, with the references (lined ears) off the patient, the bipolar record appears to demonstrate low voltage and muscle artifact (a). On the machine reference, notice the 60-Hz artifact in all channels, which indicates that the reference is either of high impedance or off the patient. The data viewed in *A* are not physiological.

the voltage derived by subtracting the potential at each electrode location minus the reference. This convention allows the reader to convert this simply by subtracting or adding channels appropriately. For example, to get the channel Fp1 – Fp2, the technician needs only to take the data in memory for the channel Fp1 – ref and subtract Fp2 – ref:

$$(Fp1 - ref) - (Fp2 - ref) = Fp1 - ref - Fp2 + ref = Fp1 - Fp2$$

The reference channel activity thus cancels, and the result is Fp1 – Fp2. In this way, simply adding and subtracting the appropriate channels can yield any conceivable montage. This is to be distinguished from bipolar recording, in which the montages remain fixed and can be changed only by physically changing the wiring in the machine, which may be accomplished through the channel selector or montage selector on analog machines (see later discussion). Referential recording has numerous advantages over bipolar recording in that it allows the reader to revise the montage at will when examining a particular section of the EEG to get numerous views of a particular discharge. In addition, referential recording allows use of a variety of computed references, such as an "average reference," Laplacian reference, or individualized custom references for each patient by combining signals from multiple channels mathematically. One potential disadvantage of referential recording is that the data in all channels may be compromised if the reference electrode or electrodes are disrupted or are of high impedance, particularly in the presence of significant external noise. In these cases, the noise may overwhelm the signal in all channels, leaving the reader a tracing of very low amplitude with little to no signal content. A quick review of EEG data on the machine reference montage demonstrates high-amplitude 60 Hz artifact in all channels, indicating the reference problem. For this reason, the authors recommend that each digital tracing be viewed briefly both during recording by the technologist and later on review by the reader first on a "machine reference" montage (each channel minus the reference) to check for high impedance in the reference electrode (see Figure 3.14). The authors have personally seen records misinterpreted as low voltage with little normal background because of such technical difficulties.

THE ELECTROENCEPHALOGRAPHIC MACHINE: AN OVERVIEW

The EEG machine has been the subject of study, development, and use since the 1920s. Although the basic elements are similar to those employed in the days of Hans Berger, many of the components and circuits have been vastly improved. One-channel machines have expanded to machines with 8, 16, 20, 24, 32, 64, 128, and even more channels. Vacuum tube–based amplifiers have given way to transistorized amplifiers and then to integrated circuits of increasing complexity and smaller size. The electronics that once constituted machines of several hundred pounds that were pushed around the hospital by burly EEG technologists now can be worn on a patient's belt. Paper output has persisted for a surprisingly long time, arguably because electroencephalographers tend to be very conservative and concrete. Nevertheless, oscilloscopic output devices and methods for computerized signal analysis have been around for decades and steadily attract devotees. The paperless EEG is in a race with the paperless office. In the next section, the major components of a typical modern EEG machine are considered in view of the engineering principles described earlier, with new emphasis on integration of digital signal technology. Figure 3.15 shows a block diagram of the circuit containing the patient and EEG machine, which consists of both

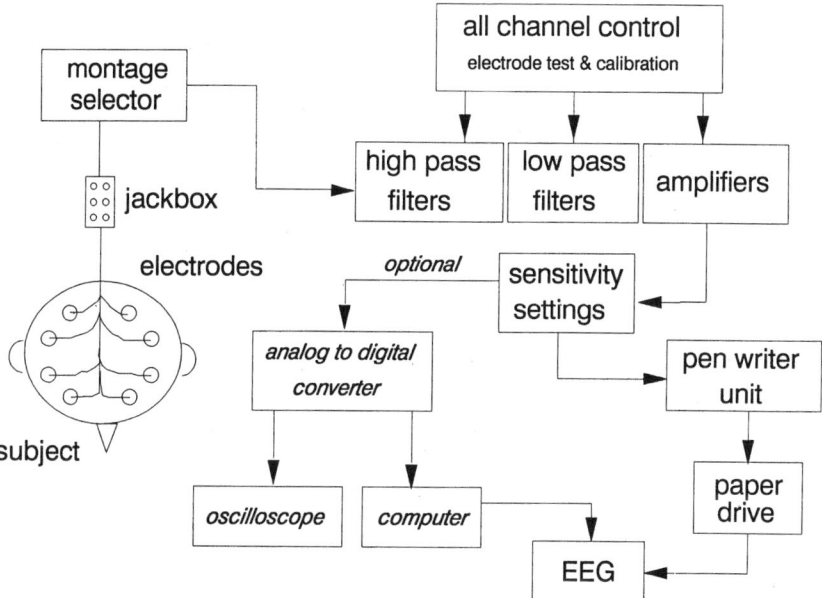

FIG. 3.15. Block diagram of major functional units of the electroencephalographic (EEG) machine. Filters and amplifiers are contained in EEG amplifier units. Paper, ink, and drive train are replaced in digital EEG machines by an analog-to-digital converter, a computer monitor (oscilloscope), and a computer.

digital and analog components. The machine's main functional units are defined in individual blocks.

Just as the function of an automobile is to serve its driver, the function of an EEG machine is to serve the patient. The entirety of EEG technology is devoted to faithful representation of the electrical signals generated by a patient's brain. These signals arise primarily from spontaneous synaptic activity in cerebral cortex. Regional voltage differences in brain are communicated via the conductive components of the head to the scalp. At that site, biology meets technology.

Electrodes

Electrodes conduct electrical potentials from patient to the EEG machine, usually with help from a conductive paste connecting skin to electrode. The electrically conducting paste that is used to couple the electrode and the skin serves two functions: It transmits potentials from the brain to the EEG machine, and it decreases movement artifacts. Electrodes are made of metal, but not all metals make equally good EEG electrodes. Proper electrodes must be good electrical conductors (an indicator of available mobile charge) and must make good contact with the electrolyte paste that covers the skin. Electrodes establish this contact through double layers of charge.

When metals are placed into a conducting solution, such as a solution that contains free ions to carry current flow, there is the opportunity for charge to move between the metal and the solution. Diffusion of ions leads to a separation of metal ions from the metal electrode. How far the charge strays and how great a potential difference is developed depend on the balance between an ion's mobility in solution and the retarding force from charge separation. In the steady state, a layer of charge is established on the metal surface, and a layer with opposite polarity is established in the solution near the metal. This system resembles the charged plates of a capacitor. If a voltmeter is connected across the solution by connecting one lead to the metal and another to the solution, a small potential is measured. This indicates that a small steady-state current of ions is flowing between the metal and solution. The potential measured in this manner is called the *electrode potential.* Electrode potentials may be measured in the range of up to 1 V: that is, four to five orders of magnitude larger than the voltage of the EEG (6).

When a voltage (such as that from the EEG machine) is applied to an electrode and an electrolyte solution, the double layer between the two is disturbed, and current flows between the electrolyte solution and the electrode. This current is added to the steady-state electrode-electrolyte current. If the electrode potential is large in comparison to the signal of interest, the electrode is said to be *polarized* or *nonreversible.* Such electrodes have large resistances and capacitances, which distort the EEG pattern. In order to detect the EEG signal with polarized electrodes, low-frequency filtering to remove the DC electrode potential is required. Furthermore, the electrode itself serves as a low-frequency filter because of capacitance at the double layer.

Reversible electrodes are electrodes that do not easily become polarized. One way to produce such electrodes is to deposit a metallic salt containing an ion in common with the conducting solution on the electrode. An example of this is the silver chloride (AgCl) electrode. Such an electrode may be fabricated by immersing silver wire in a solution of electrolyte-containing chloride and placing a positive voltage across the electrode. Chloride ions migrate to the surface of the silver and impart a distinctive gray color. When a chloride-treated silver electrode comes into contact with NaCl solution on the skin, currents of Cl^- ions flow freely between the electrode and the solution and prevent the electrode from becoming polarized. Polarization is avoided because the electrode and the solution can communicate with ions (namely, Cl^- ions from electrode and electrolyte, respectively) that exhibit identical mobilities in solution. Silver chloride electrodes are useful for recording DC and potentials of very low frequency.

Reversible electrodes can also be constructed from noble metals, such as platinum and iridium. For a more in-depth consideration of these electrodes, see Cooper (5), Cooper et al. (6), or Weyer (33).

The ability of different kinds of electrodes to reproduce a square-wave test voltage is illustrated in Figure 3.16, taken from Cooper et al. (6). In this illustration, the distortion of the waveforms results from the electrode impedance, which is a function of the electrode capacitance and resistance. Notice that the silver chloride electrode best reproduces the waveform. Figure 3.17, adapted from Niedermeyer (24), shows a simple circuit that models the interface between electrode and skin. In this diagram, R_{eq} is the resistance resulting from the electrode-skin junction. R_D and C_D are the resistance and capacitance of the electrode double layer, and R_d and C_d are the frequency-dependent resistance and capacitance of the system related to diffusion, which compose the Warburg impedance (10,25).

Large electrode resistances, greater than 5,000 Ω for skin electrodes or 15,000 Ω for needle electrodes, can result in noise artifacts in the EEG recording (6,30). This happens because strong electric fields present around the EEG machine induce small currents in the electrodes where they meet large impedances (e.g., at the scalp-electrode junction). By Ohm's law ($V = I \cdot Z$), high electrode impedance leads to high voltages, even in the presence of small

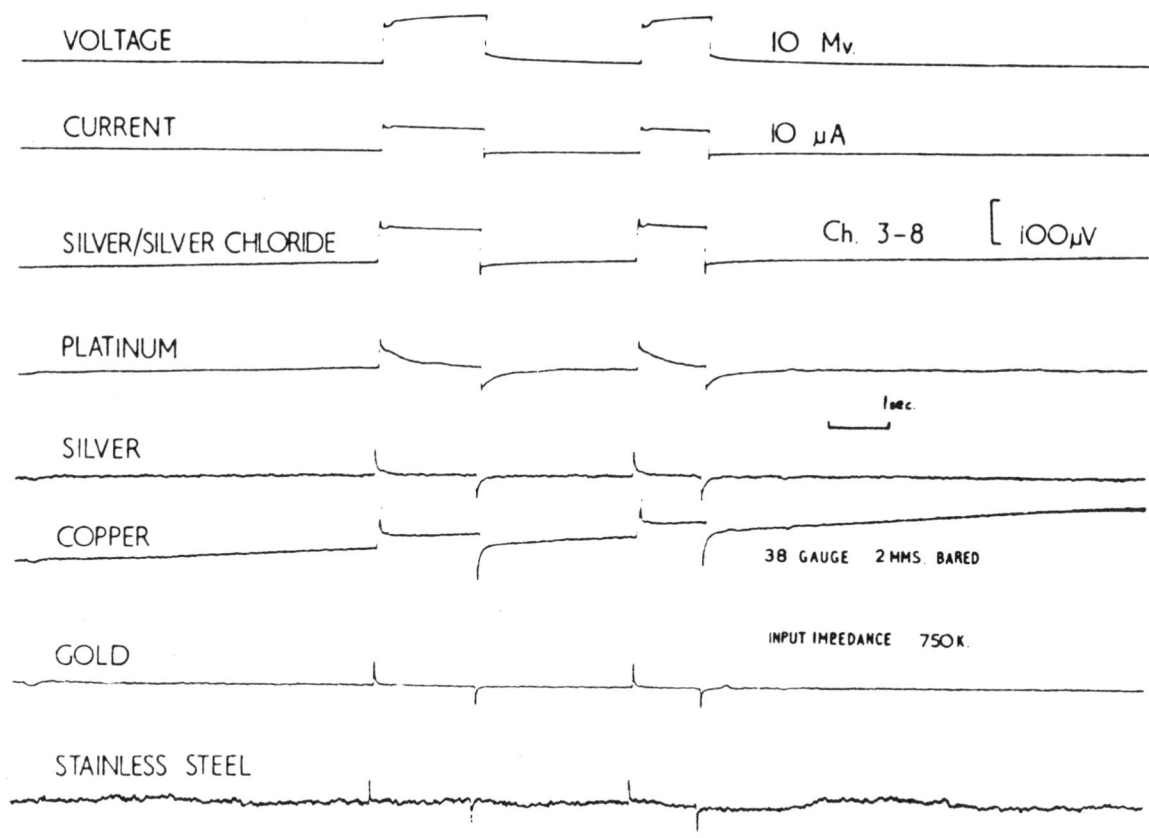

VOLTAGE   10 Mv.

CURRENT   10 μA

SILVER/SILVER CHLORIDE   Ch. 3-8 [100μV

PLATINUM

SILVER

COPPER   38 GAUGE 2 MMS. BARED

GOLD   INPUT IMPEDANCE 750 K.

STAINLESS STEEL

FIG. 3.16. Ability of various types of commonly used electroencephalographic electrodes to reproduce a 10-mV, 10-mA square-wave input. (Adapted from Cooper R, Osselton JW, Shaw J. *EEG technology.* London: Butterworths, 1980.)

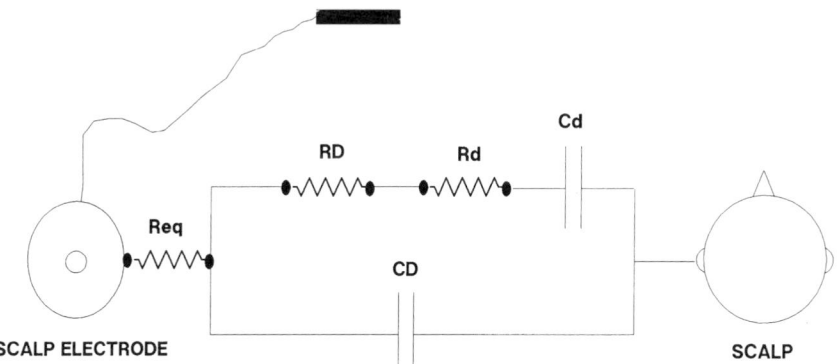

SCALP ELECTRODE

Req   RD   Rd   Cd   CD   SCALP

FIG. 3.17. A simplified model of the electrode-tissue interface. R_{eq} is the resistance of electrolyte material (e.g., gel) between tissue and metal; R_D and C_D are the resistance and capacitance of the electrode double layer; R_d and C_d are the time and frequency dependent diffusion impedances (these are very large if electrode becomes polarized). (Adapted from Niedermeyer E, Lopes da Silva FH, eds. *Electroencephalography: basic principles, clinical applications, and related fields,* 4th ed. Baltimore: Williams & Wilkins, 1999.)

currents. Because of a small area of contact with the subject, a needle electrode has high impedance and is more susceptible to line (60-Hz) artifacts. In certain circumstances (e.g., the use of needle sphenoidal electrodes to record activity from the anterior-inferior temporal lobe), the benefits of a needle electrode may outweigh the drawback of high impedance. Electrode impedances are tested after application by ohmmeters. These devices pass a small constant current through the electrode circuit and a remote reference (e.g., *on* the forehead or ear) attached to the patient. Voltage change is measured, and Ohm's law is used to calculate impedance. Impedance is frequency dependent, and the ohmmeter should therefore use frequencies in a range relevant to the EEG, such as 10 to 30 Hz. DC ohmmeters induce polarizations in electrodes and invalidate the measurement. High DC currents can also cause discomfort for the patient.

Before placement of an electrode, the scalp must be prepared by being rubbed vigorously with alcohol or with a skin preparation agent. This action removes dirt and oil from the electrode site and lowers the impedance of the scalp-electrode junction. Obviously, excessive cleaning can be irritating to the patient. Similarly, some patients are sensitive to paste containing salt solutions or bentonite. Several varieties of electrode attachment media, including sodium chloride pastes or gels, conducting sponges, and other specialized electrolytes, are available. Scalp electrodes are usually cupped, with a hole at the peak, to facilitate contact with electrode paste. Electrodes may be held in place by viscous gels, by mechanical restrictions (bands or rubber caps), or by collodion. Collodion is a glue formulated from pyroxylin (an element of gunpowder) in ether, alcohol, or camphor; it is liquid when applied, but it is able to dry to a strong adhesive within minutes. It is suitable for patients who cannot keep still or who need electrodes in place for more than a few hours. Ether is highly flammable. Flames, excessive heat, or pure oxygen should not be near collodion applications, and collodion should be used only in well-ventilated areas. It must be remembered that collodion is not an adequate conductive medium: Conductive gel must be injected into the cup electrodes and refreshed periodically. A blunt needle is usually employed for this task. Collodion is removed with acetone scrubs (6).

Common Types of Electrodes

Each of the commonly used electrodes has a simple design: a metal contact surface, flexible and insulated wire, and a connecting pin to mate with the headbox or jackbox of the EEG machine. Wires are usually color-coded for easy tracing in troubleshooting (4).

Scalp electrodes (Fig. 3.18*A*) are suitable for most routine recordings and are usually of the reversible type. They are most often made of chloride treated silver disks 4 to 10 mm in diameter. Electrodes fabricated from platinum, gold, or tin are sometimes used. Properly applied electrodes demonstrate resistances of a few hundred ohms. Resistances smaller than this usually indicate a short circuit in the electrode. According to the international standards for the EEG, electrode resistances should be less than 5,000 Ω and greater than 100 Ω (1). Positioning of scalp electrodes and methods for constructing montages of electrode pairs are considered elsewhere in this book.

Subdermal electrodes (see Fig. 3.18*B*) are fine metal electrodes made from stainless steel or platinum and are approximately 10 mm long and 0.5 mm in diameter. Skin is cleaned with a presurgical scrub such as iodophor or benzalkonium chloride (Zephiran), and the electrodes are inserted through the horny layer of the skin into the subdermis. Insertion is made to the needle hub, in a direction nearly parallel to the scalp. Subdermal electrodes are attached quickly and simple to use, but their disadvantages are many. First, they are painful and consequently are best used on comatose patients. They have a high resistance (generally 10,000 to 15,000 Ω), which makes them more susceptible to noise. Subdermal electrodes can cause infection and must be sterilized before each use; therefore, in the era of serious, transmissible viral illnesses, such as hepatitis, Jakob-Creutzfeldt disease, and acquired immunodeficiency syndrome (AIDS), the use of subdermal electrodes should generally be avoided. In the rare occasions when they are employed, most institutions require that they be discarded after a single use.

Clip electrodes (see Fig. 3.18*C*) are cup electrodes filled with conducting paste and clipped to the earlobes, usually for referential recordings. Their properties are similar to those of scalp electrodes. Because of their location, these electrodes are prone to movement artifacts. Some electroencephalographers prefer to place the A1 and A2 electrodes (left and right ears, respectively) over the mastoid processes (sometimes they are then labeled M1 and M2), obviating the need for clip electrodes.

Nasopharyngeal electrodes (see Fig. 3.18*D*) have historically been used in conjunction with standard scalp electrodes in order to improve detection of inferior temporal or frontal discharges. They are made from a 10- to 15-cm-long segment of flexible insulated wire with an uninsulated 2-mm gold tip. Nasopharyngeal electrodes can be purchased or fabricated from insulated silver wire by stripping 5 mm of insulation from the tip and heating the wire with a match. The silver melts, forming a little ball at the tip. A pin connector is soldered at the proximal end. The wire may then undergo chloride treatment by immersion in 1N HCl or NaCl and passage of 1.5 to 9 V of pos-

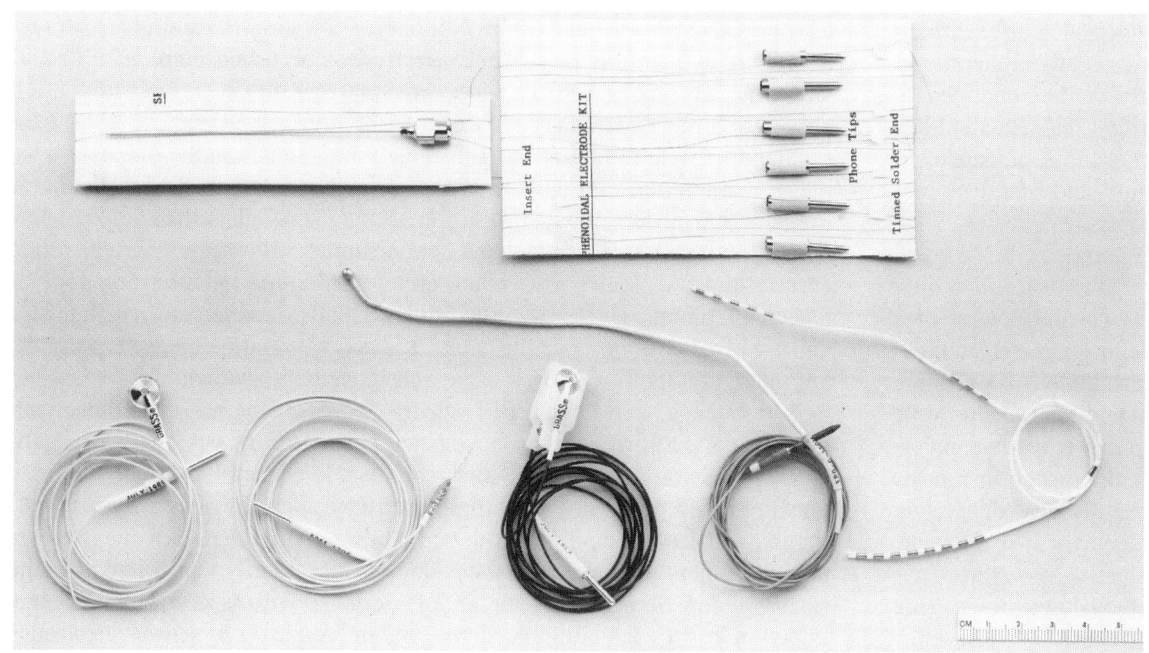

FIG. 3.18. Photograph of commonly used electro-encephalographic electrodes. **A:** Scalp cup electrode. **B:** Subdermal or "needle" electrode. **C:** Clip electrode for recording from the earlobe. **D:** Nasopharyngeal electrode. **E:** Sphenoidal electrode with needle introducer. **F:** Depth electrode, with eight recording contacts.

itive battery current through the wire until it is evenly gray. A 1,000- to 10,000-Ω resistor should be placed in series with the silver wire to limit current flow (if current flow is too high, chloride deposition may be uneven). Any thick-gauge wire can serve as a reference in the solution. Electrodes should then be thoroughly washed and sterilized. A physician or an experienced technologist inserts one electrode in each of the patient's nostrils. Wires are bent into an "S" shape, threaded along the nasopharynx, and rotated outward to their position within 2 cm of the anterior mesial surface of the temporal lobes. Insertion technique was reviewed in detail by MacLean (23). Nasopharyngeal electrodes may increase the yield of interictal spike detection, but only by about 5% (28). Unfortunately, they are uncomfortable for the patient and highly prone to respiratory motion artifact. Nasopharyngeal electrodes are now rarely used clinically, having been replaced by a ring of subtemporal electrodes (e.g., T1, T2, and cheek) or sphenoidal electrodes, which substantially increase the ability to record anterior and deeper temporal discharges without being subject to the same respiratory and motion artifact seen in nasopharyngeal electrodes.

Sphenoidal electrodes (see Fig. 3.18*E*), as initially described by Silverman in 1960 (29), are used to record discharges from the anterior tip of the temporal lobe. Electrodes are usually made from thin, straight insulated stainless steel wire about 50 mm long and 0.5 mm in diameter, with a small uninsulated ball at the tip. Sphenoidal electrodes are introduced through a needle cannula into the temporal and masseter muscles; the insertion point is between the zygoma and sigmoid notch of the mandible. Penetration is directed slightly anteriorly so that the tip rests lateral to the foramen ovale at the greater wing of the sphenoid bone. In theory, there is risk of injury to branches of the trigeminal and facial nerves, and rare complications have been reported; in practice, however, these electrodes are well tolerated. Infection is a potential risk but is very rare. Sphenoidal electrodes were traditionally sterilized after each use and destroyed after use on a patient with a known or suspected transmissible viral infection. At present, these electrodes are disposable, and it is rare that they are reused, even after sterilization. Some authors have held that sphenoidal electrodes are more sensitive than scalp or nasopharyngeal electrodes (31), but others have disputed this

(13,28). More recent studies claim that sphenoidal electrodes offer limited advantages over cheek electrodes in detecting and localizing temporal epileptiform discharges (19), although many epilepsy centers continue to use them as part of initial (phase I) epilepsy monitoring (18). Other studies report that introducing these electrodes under fluoroscopic guidance, to ensure exact placement, can maximize the diagnostic yield of sphenoidal electrode recording (9,16,17).

Tympanic electrodes (not shown in Fig. 3.18) are another type of basal electrode used for recording from the mesial temporal lobe or for recording brainstem auditory evoked potentials. The electrodes usually consist of a thin insulated conducting wire with an uninsulated 7-mm-diameter stainless steel, gold, or platinum ball wrapped in felt. The electrode tip is soaked in a conducting solution and threaded through the external auditory meatus to lie next to the tympanic membrane. A conservative approach is recommended, stopping the procedure as soon as the patient senses any discomfort in the internal auditory canal. These electrodes must be carefully placed, to avoid trauma to the eardrum, and must be sterilized between uses. In practice, these electrodes are rarely used.

Wieser and Moser (34,35) have described foramen ovale electrodes (not shown) for recording mesial temporal or frontal discharges. These electrodes are fine silver wires insulated with polytef (Teflon) and mounted on a stainless steel wire 0.1 mm in diameter. The external diameter of the array is 0.33 mm. Up to four contact points, separated by 15 mm, are recommended. Electrode impedances range from 200 to 700 Ω. Electrodes can inserted with the use of local or general anesthesia, in meticulous sterile procedure. A guide needle punctures the cheek 3 cm lateral to the corner of the mouth and is aimed as directed (34). The foramen ovale and the subarachnoid space are penetrated by the introducer, after which the electrode is inserted into the caudal end of the ambient cistern. In this study (34,35), two of 37 patients experienced transient sensory deficits, and about half of the patients experienced minor discomfort.

Depth electrodes (see Fig. 3.18F) are arrays of electrodes designed for introduction directly into the substance of the brain by a neurosurgeon. They are used to detect and localize voltages not visible with scalp EEG recording. Typically, depth electrodes are composed of a fine array of thin stainless steel, platinum, or gold insulated wires of different lengths, ending in uninsulated tips. The electrodes most commonly used at present consist of plastic-encased wires with 1- to 3-mm uninsulated bands exposed at regular intervals, so as to allow spatial sampling along the mesial and neocortical temporal structures. Chloride-treated silver can irritate brain tissue after direct contact for several days. In contrast, stainless steel, gold, and platinum are relatively inert and safe. Depth electrodes are usually implanted stereotactically (according to a three-dimensional coordinate reference frame), although some experienced neurosurgeons prefer to place the electrodes freehand or with radiographic guidance, under sterile protocol. Electrodes may remain in place for days or weeks. Orientation, targets, and methods for implantation differ among institutions. Other chapters in this text review various approaches. The amygdala, hippocampus, entorhinal or orbitofrontal cortex, and supplementary motor areas of the frontal lobe are popular placement targets. Depth EEG recordings usually demonstrate excellent signal-to-noise ratio, because these electrodes have relatively low impedance, are relatively unaffected by muscle and movement artifact, and bypass the high-resistance skull. Depth EEG clearly increases the ability to detect and localize epileptiform activity in selected patients (30), but it has disadvantages. First, not all deep brain sites can be studied with this technique, and thus there is a possibility of sampling error. Epileptiform activity originating in a particular depth electrode only indicates that the electrode is closer than the others to the seizure focus and not necessarily that it is within the seizure focus. Second, the technique is invasive, with risks for hemorrhage, infection, reactive meningitis edema, and headache. Use of these electrodes should be restricted to experienced centers.

The current explosion in research on implantable devices to treat neurological conditions, such as movement disorders (Parkinson's disease, tremor) and now epilepsy requires that the use of depth and cortical electrodes be used not only to record the EEG but also for stimulation in deep brain structures (e.g., the thalamus) and on the cortical surface itself. Although these applications have not resulted in drastically new designs for intracranial electrodes, they are now available in a wide variety of configurations, with different electrode spacing and geometries, depending on the intended site of implantation. The development of new designs, materials, and implementations of chronic indwelling electrodes for brain recording and stimulation is expected to evolve considerably over the coming years.

Cortical electrodes (Fig. 3.19) are used to record directly from the surface of the brain during neurosurgical procedures (12). The technique is usually referred to as *electrocorticography* (ECoG). Epileptiform events can be localized in relation to brain anatomy, enabling a "tailoring" of the resection during epilepsy surgery. Unfortunately, the relatively brief time available for recording, the need to restrict recording to the craniotomy site, and EEG suppressant effects of most anesthetics limit the practical value of ECoG. Some investigators believe that location of corticographically recorded discharges at

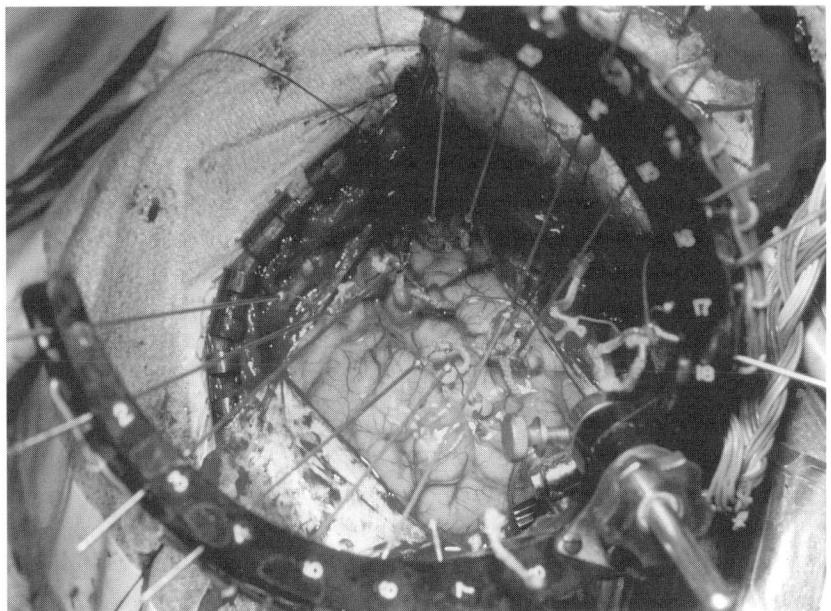

FIG. 3.19. Intra-operative photograph of electrocorticography (EcoG) apparatus with cotton wick electrodes soaked in sterile saline. Electrodes are held in place by a metal halo attached to the surgical table. This apparatus is mainly of historical interest, inasmuch as most corticography is now performed with subdural grids moved from place to place during surgical procedures. (Photograph courtesy of Dr. Sumio Uematsu.)

the time of surgery, and persistence of these discharges after resection, may have prognostic value for surgical outcome (15), although this is debated.

An old cotton wick ECoG apparatus, now mostly of only historical interest, is shown in Fig. 3.19. In this apparatus, cortical electrodes are usually made from stainless steel, silver, or platinum. Although metal ball electrodes may be placed directly on the cortex, brain pulsations can make this hazardous. In the past, it was common to make electrodes in this manner, connected to the brain by cotton wicks soaked in a sterile isotonic saline solution. Electrodes were held in an adjustable halo frame anchored to the skull or surgical table. Such equipment has been replaced by moving subdural strips and grids of electrodes over the cerebral cortex (see following discussion). Recording in the operating room with these electrodes is now standard practice in most institutions.

Subdural electrodes (Fig. 3.20) are designed to be in contact with cortical tissue of conscious, cooperative patients for periods of a few days to a few weeks. The goal of subdural recording is localization of seizure foci in relation to important functional areas of brain (11,21). In the epilepsy surgery of the past several decades, this facilitated the critically important distinction between "bad brain" (epileptogenic areas) and "good brain" (normal areas). Seizure discharges are identified and localized by recording. Areas of cortex involved in sensorimotor, speech, reading, or cognition are identified by stimulation through pairs of adjacent electrodes, which causes transient suspension of function in these regions. Benefits and risks of this technique are discussed elsewhere in this book. In order to study a large region of cortex, subdural grids may be assembled in an approximately hand-sized array, with up to eight rows and eight columns of electrodes. These electrodes are usually flat 3-mm disks fabricated from stainless steel or platinum. Electrodes are embedded in a sheet of flexible plastic, usually with center-to-center electrode separation of 1 cm (see Fig. 3.20). Grids may be cut to size during implanta-

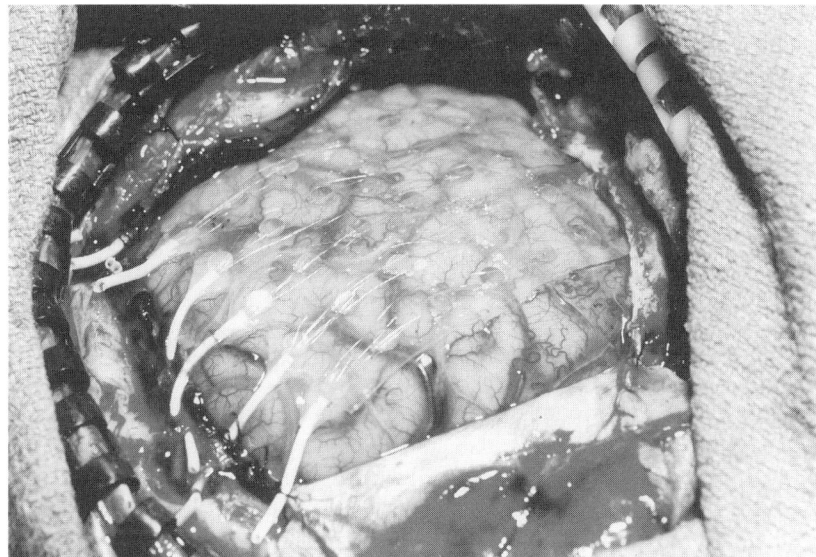

FIG. 3.20. Subdural stimulating-recording grid of electrodes photographed just before anterior temporal lobectomy. An 8 × 5 array of electrodes is illustrated. Cut wires, visible in the upper left, connect to a 2 × 8 array of electrodes placed inferiorly to the temporal lobe. (Photograph courtesy of Dr. Sumio Uematsu.)

tion. Placement requires a full craniotomy. Aggressive surgical resection of regions demonstrating early onset of seizures outside of the temporal lobe has declined somewhat, as a result of only fair clinical outcomes and newer ideas related to the role of neuronal networks in the generation of focal seizure onsets. Despite this change in thinking, implantation of intracranial electrodes, grids, strips, and depth electrodes continues to be common, although surgical resection is somewhat more limited to cases with focal lesions or functional abnormalities in which the chances of a good outcome are high.

Epidural electrodes in single or double-row strips are less invasive than subdural grids (they can be placed through a burr hole) and often provide important information about seizure foci (36). Because a smaller area is covered, the true focus of seizure onset is less likely to be in the field of recording. In addition, epidural electrical stimulation is painful, unless dural nerves are cut (12).

THE ELECTROENCEPHALOGRAPH MACHINE: PRACTICAL ISSUES

Over the years, EEG recording devices have evolved into many different forms, each uniquely addressing the challenge of presenting the electrical activity of the brain to the electroencephalographer in a faithful and useful manner. Special credit is due the Grass Corporation for their historical efforts to further EEG technology. The following section traces a signal through an EEG machine, from patient to paper (and digital computer screen; see Fig. 3.12). The purpose of this review is to develop in the student an appreciation for the function of the different components of a generic EEG machine. Discussion of specific machines can be found in the manuals distributed with them. Such manuals are not only a technical necessity for proper operation and maintenance of an EEG machine but are also a useful source of general information about EEG technology.

Jackbox and Montage Selector

The EEG signal is conducted from the subject through conducting electrodes to the electrode board, also called the *electrode box* or *jackbox*. Electrodes are identified on the jackbox in accordance with the International 10-20 system electrode nomenclature. All electrodes except midline electrodes are identified by a number and a letter; all midline electrodes carry the subscript "Z" instead of a number. Odd-numbered electrodes are on the left side of the head, and even-numbered electrodes are on the right. Electrodes are labeled according to the brain region proximate to their location: frontopolar electrodes are labeled "Fp"; frontal, "F"; central, "C"; temporal, "T"; parietal,

"P"; and occipital, "O." Ear or aural electrodes are labeled "A," and mastoid electrodes are labeled "M." It is important to note that only the F7 and F8 electrodes may appear to be misnamed, inasmuch as they record more from the anterior temporal than frontal regions. The jackbox contains an additional input for a ground electrode; a scalp electrode affixed to the midline forehead or other relatively neutral site connects to this input. Numbered inputs are available on most jackboxes to accommodate special electrodes or transducers. Safety issues pertaining to proper grounding are considered later in the chapter. A jackbox may be electrically or optically isolated to limit the possibility of passing current to the patient (4,32).

The jackbox for digital EEG machines has additional components that are not seen in analog machines. For example, there is one or more additional inputs for the reference electrode. This electrode is often placed somewhere between Fpz and Fz in single reference devices, although it can be located in any place that is relatively noise free and where a good contact with the scalp can be maintained. In some machines, two electrodes, usually A1 and A2 (linked ears) are used together to form the reference. As explained earlier, in digital EEG machines, each channel is stored as G1-Ref, where G1 (grid one) is a particular electrode of interest and Ref is the potential at the reference electrode. It is important to note here a vulnerability specific to digital EEG machines that can render recordings devoid of information. If the reference electrode becomes detached in the presence of an electromagnetically noisy environment, this noise may actually saturate the recording amplifier in the reference channel. In this instance, the EEG signal in each channel (each channel being G1-Ref) is overwhelmed by noise. When individual channels are subtracted in a typical display montage (e.g., longitudinal bipolar), the record appears to be very low voltage and with little activity. This pattern can be hard to recognize as a technical artifact for technicians who are not familiar with this problem. For this reason, it is the authors' opinion that EEG technologists should always look at the machine reference montage for a short time at the beginning of the record (each channel minus the reference) to see whether the reference is detached or of very high impedance. This is usually demonstrated by the presence of high-voltage line artifact (60-Hz noise) in every channel. It is remarkable that in most cases in which the reference is of high impedance, the EEG record can appear completely normal on other montages, unless the reference amplifier is saturated, although the machine reference montage demonstrates widespread 60-Hz artifact (see Fig. 3.14).

Another important feature of digital EEG machines is that ADCs and amplifiers are frequently reduced in size and installed as part of the jackbox itself. This requires a little more careful handling of the jackbox than seasoned EEG technicians are used to with their analog predecessors. Again, it is important to consult individual machine manuals to determine the design and care of particular pieces of equipment.

From the jackbox, the EEG electrode inputs are carried to the montage selector board of the EEG machine, a two-dimensional array of pushbuttons. Each row across the board contains one button per jackbox input. Vertically, the array is organized into channels, with two rows of buttons per channel. Each channel's output is equal to the potential of the electrode selected in row 1 minus the potential of the electrode selected in row 2. The top input of the pair is sometimes referred to as "grid 1" (G1) and the bottom as "grid 2" (G2), from the days of vacuum tube technology; more recently, they have been referred to as "input 1" and "input 2." For example, in channel 1, if the O1 button is depressed in the first row and the O2 button is depressed in the second row, then the output of channel 1 will be O1 minus O2. One electrode's potential can be an input into more than one channel. With 21 electrodes and 16 channels, there are 21^{16}, or 1.43×10^{21}, possible montages. This impractical number calls for a certain choice of a limited number of montages in a recording session. Reasons for choosing particular montages are discussed in other chapters. Once a montage is determined, it may be programmed into the EEG hardware (usually by boards inserted into slots) so that it can be implemented with a single-switch selection. This master electrode selector switch spares the technologist from having to specify each channel of each montage with each recording.

Montage selection and recording are quite different in digital EEG machines. Because all recording is performed referentially, simple addition and subtraction are performed to derive any montage without requiring selections of particular recording configurations in advance. Remontaging is performed at the click of a mouse or touch of a button, which changes only the way that the computer displays prerecorded information or information being recorded. This scheme also makes available other computer-calculated montages, which may enhance information embedded but not readily visible in the EEG. Such examples include average reference and Laplacian montages, in which global or local averages of the potential at specified electrode locations are used to provide a more balanced reference or to enhance local features of the EEG in particular regions.

Amplifiers

From the montage selector board, EEG signals move on to amplifiers. Amplifiers in EEG machines are compound devices and should be distin-

guished from an amplifier whose sole function is to increase voltage. EEG amplifiers also contain filters, voltage dividers, input and output jacks, and calibration devices. Amplifiers designed to receive small inputs (e.g., microvolts or millivolts) are often called *preamplifiers,* and those designed to receive large inputs (volts) are called *amplifiers;* however, this distinction is arbitrary. An amplifier multiplies an input voltage by a constant. Because EEG signals are very small, the assumption is that this constant will be a number greater than 1, usually in the range of 2 to 1,000; however, step-down amplifiers are also available. The amplification factor is referred to as *gain* and may be expressed as V_{out}/V_{in}. More commonly, gain is expressed as a logarithmic ratio in order to compress representation of the wide range of possible input voltages. The unit of gain is the *decibel* (dB):

$$decibels \ (dB) = 20 \cdot log \left(\frac{V_{out}}{V_{in}} \right)$$

An amplifier that increases input voltage by a factor of 10 has a gain of 20 dB.

Amplifiers are designed to receive input voltages within a certain range, called the *dynamic range.* Inputs smaller than this range may be lost in background noise. Voltages exceeding the maximum recommended input may be distorted or may cause damage to the equipment. Flexible control of the dynamic range is achieved with a sensitivity setting on an EEG machine. Sensitivity has units of either millivolts per centimeter or microvolts per millimeter and is defined as the amount of voltage required to deflect the recording pens a given distance. A typical sensitivity setting for the EEG is 7 µV per millimeter, leading to pen deflections of 3 to 20 mm for typical EEG input voltages. An electrocardiographic monitoring channel, in contrast, may require a sensitivity of 1 or 10 mV per centimeter. The sensitivity control switch is a voltage divider, which attenuates the input to a level consistent with faithful reproduction by the EEG amplifiers and output system. In practice, an EEG technologist adjusts the sensitivity of the EEG machine so that EEG signals of interest produce a pen deflection large enough to read, but not so large that it runs into the pen output of adjacent channels.

Figure 3.21 shows an EEG signal at several sensitivities. To increase the amplitude of the pen deflection, the voltage to the writer-unit must be increased by increasing the gain. Inexperienced technicians are sometimes confused by the concept that to increase the gain, they must use a sensitivity setting with a smaller numerical value. A moment's thought clarifies this. At a sensitivity of 5 µV per millimeter, a 100-µV signal deflects the pen 20 mm (100 ÷ 5). At a sensitivity of 10 µV/mm, the pen deflects only 10 mm

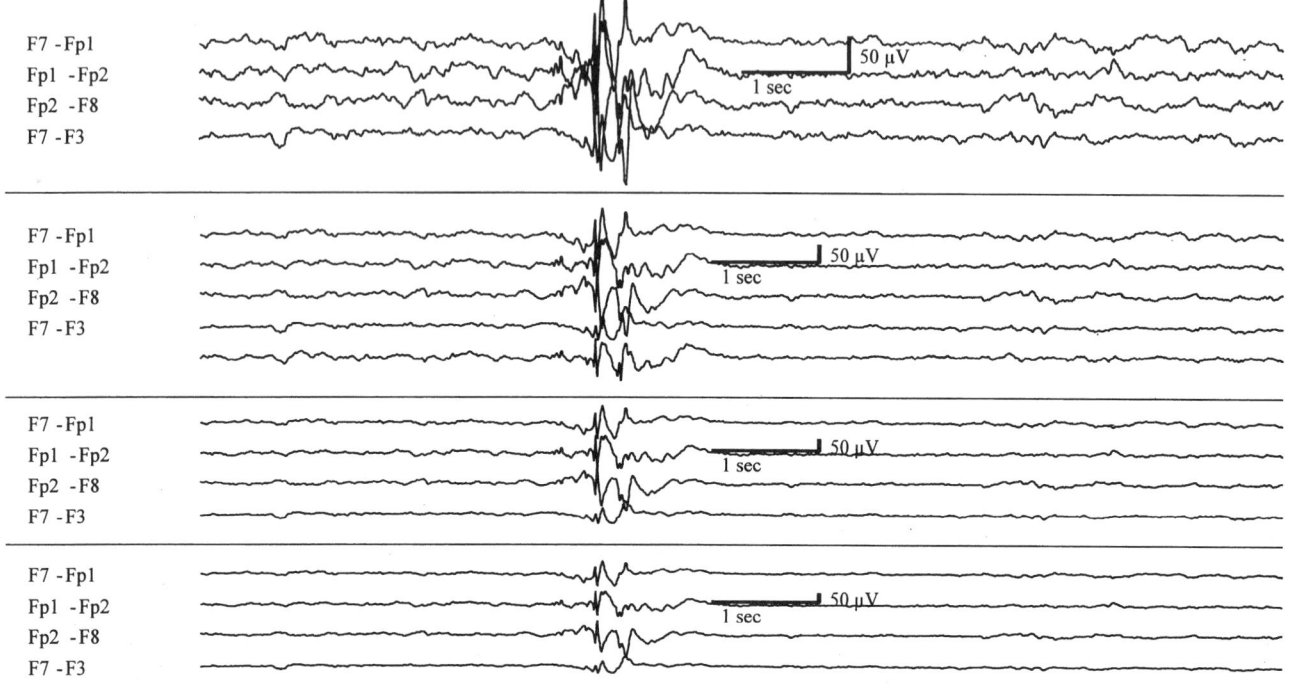

FIG. 3.21. Illustration of effect of sensitivity setting on electroencephalographic (EEG) tracing. The same EEG input is displayed at sensitivities of 5, 10, 15, and 20 μV per millimeter. As sensitivity is increased, the waveform, which initially appeared to be some sort of artifact, is revealed to be a generalized, high-voltage spike and slow-wave discharge. Before the era of digital EEG, such discharges passed without a chance of definitive interpretation, unless the technologist was very fast or the discharge was repeated.

(100 ÷ 10). At the beginning of every recording, to verify the accuracy of amplification, the technologist calibrates each channel with a known standard voltage, typically 50 μV for a sensitivity of 7 μV per millimeter. At the end of the recording, the technologist documents an appropriate voltage calibration for every sensitivity setting used (e.g., 50 μV for a sensitivity of 7 μV per millimeter, 100 μV for a sensitivity of 10 μV per millimeter, or 200 μV for a sensitivity of 20 μV per millimeter).

Of importance is that this type of calibration loses much of its meaning for digital EEG machines. In this case, amplifiers may be testable by the machines that would put a known current pulse into the inputs of the amplifiers and verify that they, the ADC, and the analog and digital filters are functioning properly. In machines that synthesize only a pretended calibration signal and display it, this process serves little or no purpose.

The EEG amplifier itself has a frequency response that is linear over a wide range of input voltages. In practice, the settings that the technologist chooses for the filters determine the range of linear frequency response. Figure 3.22 displays the relationship between frequency and amplification for a typical EEG amplifier (4). It is important to choose an amplifier whose frequency response is linear over the expected range of input voltages so that high- or low-frequency components will not cause distortion. Thus, amplifiers for EEGs and amplifiers for evoked responses differ substantially in amplification and settings for filters (see later discussion).

Signals from each electrode are led to a differential amplifier, which subtracts one signal's voltage, in relation to some reference electrode (the isolated ground electrode [isoground] on the scalp in most machines), from another signal, in relation to the same reference, and amplifies the difference signal. This process removes voltages (e.g., noise) common to both electrodes. Although one of the input pairs could be connected to the machine's ground circuit, this would expose the signal to massive amounts of noise generated by line current and electrical appliances. The two inputs for each channel are therefore kept isolated (floating) from the system ground. When a distant electrode is chosen as the common reference for

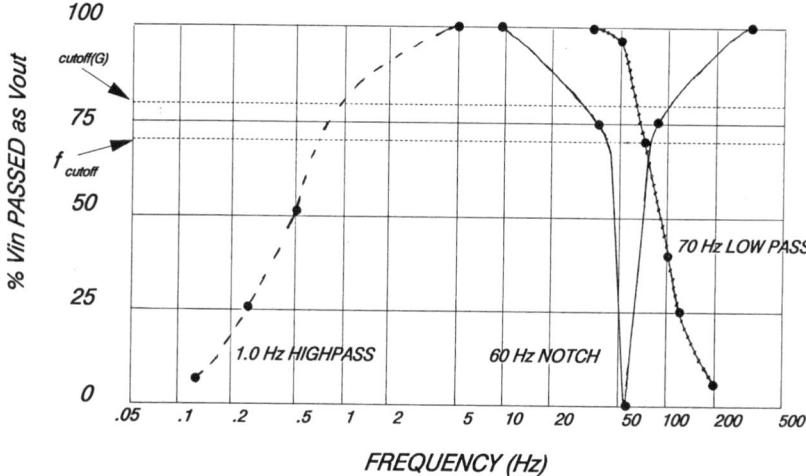

FIG. 3.22. Frequency response of 1.0-Hz high-pass, 60-Hz notch, and 70-Hz low-pass filters. The conventional cutoff frequency, at which input is attenuated by approximately 30%, is marked "cutoff." The cutoff frequency of this particular machine, defined by the manufacturer to be the point at which the input is attenuated by 20%, is marked "cutoff (G)." (Adapted with permission from Grass Instruments® EEG machine instruction manual.)

several channels, the montage is said to be *referential*. The older term *monopolar* is inaccurate, because a voltage must always be recorded between two points. Montages linking nearby electrodes are called *bipolar*. Referential montages are more sensitive to regional changes in EEG potential. Bipolar montages, which are configured to record more localized potentials, are less disturbed by noise. Both types of montage should be used in a clinical EEG recording.

Signals common to both inputs of a differential amplifier are canceled. Such signals are said to be *in phase*, or *common mode*, which implies that they vary together over time. Noise from a 60-Hz line current is an example of a signal likely to be in phase at all inputs. Unfortunately, differential amplifiers are not perfect and do not completely cancel common-mode signals. The ability of an amplifier to reject in-phase and amplify out-of-phase potentials is measured by the common-mode rejection ratio (CMRR) of the amplifier. The CMRR can be measured by connecting a voltage source to two amplifier inputs so that each input "sees" the same signal. The output voltage, which should be close to zero, forms the denominator of the

CMRR. This is compared to the output voltage when the voltage source is connected to one input and the machine ground is connected to the other (the numerator of the CMRR). The ratio of these output voltages is the CMRR. Good EEG amplifiers have CMRRs of at least 1,000, and many have CMRRs of 10,000. Under ideal circumstances, CMRRs of 100,000 may be achieved. It is important to note that common-mode rejection is effective only over a limited range of common-mode voltages. It is possible that in extreme circumstances (e.g., if an electrode falls off the head), the voltage of common-mode signals may exceed the amplifier's input range. In this case, the output is unpredictable. It is also important that the reference electrode used be reasonably close to the recording electrodes. This maximizes chances that major noise signals will be common mode and canceled. If the reference electrode is placed at a distant location (on the leg, for example), the widely spaced electrodes may act as an antenna and pick up signals that may exceed the common-mode range of the amplifiers.

When recording is done with differential amplifiers, the polarity convention for display of EEG signals is that negative waveforms cause an upward deflection and positive waveforms cause a downward deflection. For example:

1. If input 1 is negative with regard to input 2 (i.e., input 1 minus input 2 is negative), the pen (or waveform displayed on the computer monitor) deflects up. If input 1 is positive with regard to input 2 (i.e., input 1 minus input 2 is positive), the pen or monitor waveform deflects down.
2. If input 2 is negative with regard to input 1 (i.e., input 1 minus input 2 is positive), the pen or monitor waveform deflects down. If input 2 is positive with regard to input 1 (i.e., input 1 minus input 2 is negative), the pen or monitor waveform deflects up.

This convention leads to the principle of *phase reversal* of the EEG signal, by which negative potentials can be localized to an electrode demonstrating phase reversal between two channels sharing a common electrode. Figure 3.23 illustrates this principle. The montage in this instance is a simplified, linked bipolar montage. Channel 1 represents the differential voltage between Fp1 (electrode 1) and F7 (electrode 2). Channel 2 shows a differential input from F7 (electrode 1) and T3 (electrode 2). Because the pen deflects down in channel 1, F7 is negative with regard to Fp1. Because the pen deflects up in channel 2, F7 is also negative with regard to T3. At F7 there is therefore a local maximum of extracellular negativity. Such extracellular negativity occurs during interictal spikes near an epileptic focus, as a result of sudden influx of positive ions (sodium and calcium) into the depolarizing neurons. Of course, many other EEG events, including those

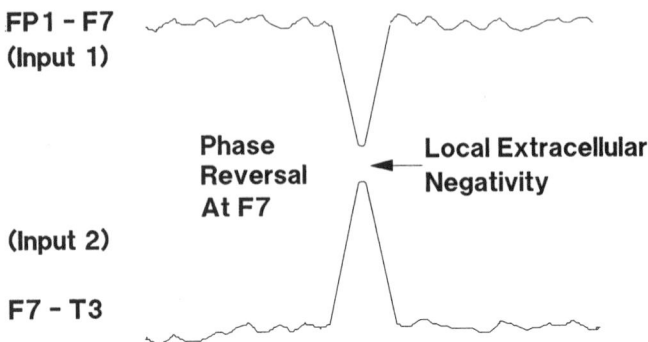

FIG. 3.23. Schematic drawing of a phase reversal, representing site of local extracellular negativity, which in this illustration is at the F7 electrode.

pass filter attenuates components of the signal that have frequencies less than a specified value; the low-pass filter removes components with frequencies higher than a certain value. A special filter, a 60-Hz notch filter, is available to remove electrical noise generated by line current. The ideal in EEG recording is to minimize the use of filters—for example, by using a low cutoff frequency of 0.1 Hz and a high cutoff frequency of 70 Hz. Filters distort both the amplitude and the interchannel phase of signals. In some circumstances, high-frequency artifacts from muscle and low-frequency artifacts from movement or sweat potentials mandate use of more stringent filtering. Figure 3.24 illustrates how filtering can rescue a nearly uninterpretable tracing. The use of filters should always be documented on the EEG recording, so that the electroencephalographer can interpret their possible influence.

derived from normal spontaneous brain activity, may result in instances of local extracellular negativity. In practice, electroencephalographers first identify potentials with the morphology of interictal spikes or sharp waves and then attempt to determine a physiological field, perhaps including a phase reversal, for the potential. The electrode common to the two channels showing phase reversal may be assumed to be near the origin of the discharge. Extracellularly positive potentials (generally of less practical importance to electroencephalographers) cause phase reversals with pen deflections away from each other in adjacent channels. These are seen on occasion on scalp EEGs, usually in the case of transversely oriented dipoles in the generating tissue. This method of localizing discharges is applicable only to recordings with linked bipolar montages.

Outputs of one amplifier may be used as input to another. This allows a series of amplifiers, each with a limited dynamic range, to boost the EEG signal substantially. As the signal becomes amplified, it becomes large in relation to ambient noise, and differential amplification may no longer be required. Internal amplifiers may thus be single ended (one active input measured with regard to ground). The principles of differential amplifiers and common mode rejection explained earlier are central to most systems for recording clinical EEGs and unchanged in digital EEG machines.

Electroencephalogram Filters

After EEG signals are subtracted and amplified, the output is filtered to remove specified frequency components, as described earlier. The high-

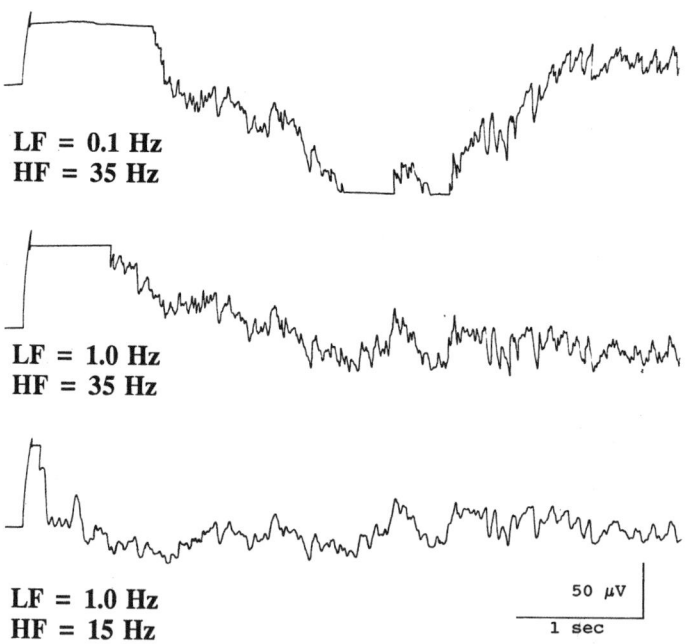

FIG. 3.24. Effects of different low- and high-filter cutoff frequencies on a noisy electroencephalographic (EEG) tracing. Note enhanced readability at the expense of lost detail in the most severely filtered tracing at the bottom. Data reproduced from an ambulatory cassette EEG monitor played back to paper output.

Of importance is that the principles of filtering remain the same in digital EEG machines, except that most filtering is performed post hoc—that is, after the signal has been acquired and stored. Most digital EEG machines record and store EEG broad band—that is, with the filters open as wide as possible, without introducing aliasing, artifacts, or severe distortion into the data. Because the data are to be displayed, computer programs are used to filter the data as they are projected to the computer monitor. In reality, the source data, recorded with less stringent filtering (e.g., 0.01 to 100 Hz), remains untouched by digital filtering. Of importance is that digital filters induce the same changes into the EEG, such as phase shifts, as do analog filters, although the digital environment allows for correction of these changes, if desired, because this requires only numerical manipulation of the digital data.

Ancillary Electroencephalographic Controls

Typical EEG machines offer several controls to validate proper functioning of electrodes and amplifiers and to provide flexibility in presentation of data. A few of the more important controls are considered as follows:

Individual channel controls: It is a convenience to use the *all-channel control* to set gain and filters for all channels; however, this is not practiced if input signals vary widely, as is the case when cardiac, electromyographic, or movement monitors (or transducers) are used to measure respiration or intracranial pressure, or during recording from invasive electrodes. Such circumstances require individualizing of gain and filters for each channel. In the digital environment, channels can be individually displayed, filtered, and manipulated numerically post hoc, after acquisition.

Calibration signal: A calibration signal is an internally or externally generated input of known voltage. The operator chooses a calibration voltage (square-wave pulse) ranging from 1 to 10 mV or more. This signal is passed through all stages of EEG signal processing, from the first stage of amplification to pen output. In addition to serving as a voltage reference, the calibration procedure can (a) show differences in channel amplitude or pen alignment that might introduce artifact and (b) show the effect of filter settings on a square-wave input. No EEG tracing is complete without a voltage calibration signal for each filter and sensitivity setting used during the recording session. As mentioned earlier, the actual implementation of calibration signals varies from one digital EEG machine to another. It is important to consult the manual for individual EEG

machines to understand the details of how this procedure is performed for any given piece of hardware.

Electrode test switch: The electrode test switch conducts an artificial (e.g., 30-Hz sine wave) signal through each electrode to the pens. Electrodes with impedances less than approximately 1,000 Ω produce no pen response. Electrodes of higher resistance generate pen deflections of about 0.5 mm for each 1,000 Ω of resistance (Fig. 3.25). Testing electrodes entails passing current through electrodes to the patient. This is of theoretical concern with cortical or depth electrodes. The test current is, however, very small and is probably below a level able to produce biological effects. For the Grass Model 8 EEG machine, test current is 0.035 μA (9). In digital EEG machines, this procedure is performed the same way as in analog devices, but impedances are usually displayed as numbers, in ohms or kilohms on the EEG machine screen. Some digital machines do not record these numbers as part of the EEG record, which

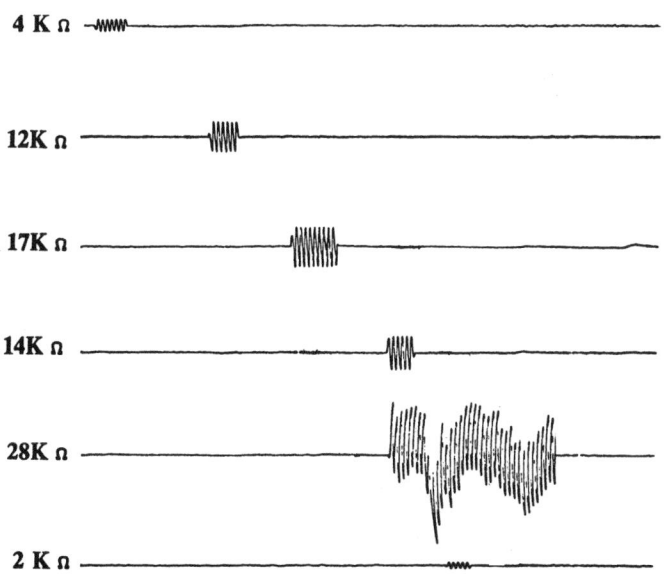

FIG. 3.25. Illustration of electrode test output from six electroencephalographic electrodes. The resistance of each electrode is marked to the left of its tracing (assuming a resistance of 2,000 Ω per millimeter). Electrodes 2 to 5 would need to be reaffixed before resumption of recording, because their resistances are more than 5,000 Ω.

is a disadvantage with regard to later interpretation. Electrode tests should be performed at the beginning and end of each recording session, according to accepted EEG standards (1).

Baseline adjustment: The baseline adjustment for each channel is used to set the pen tracing baseline to coincide with the 0-V line on the EEG paper. This permits maximum travel of the pen. There is no equivalent control in digital EEG machines.

Sensitivity adjustment: As an EEG machine ages, the amplification factors for individual channels may drift out of the specified range. The sensitivity adjustment is a turn-screw used to set the sensitivity in conjunction with the all-channel calibration signal. The sensitivity of each channel can be adjusted to produce equal output for the same input signal. Amplifiers in digital EEG machines must also be checked and calibrated in a similar manner over time. The Biomedical Engineering section of hospital facilities that service this type of equipment usually undertakes this responsibility. Procedures for testing and adjusting this equipment vary between manufacturers.

Event markers: Event marker buttons provide a quick and convenient way for the technologist to annotate time of occurrence for an event of interest. On digital EEG machines, this feature is usually more sophisticated, allowing technologists to type specific comments into the record, with the computer keyboard or with a light pen that allows them to write longhand on the computer screen, or to display a variety of preset comments from a series of "hot keys" programmed on the computer keyboard.

Trace restore: High-amplitude, low-frequency signals cause the pens to deflect and slowly return to baseline. If the return to baseline requires several seconds, EEG information may be lost. The trace restore button quickly neutralizes amplifier blocking so that recording can continue. This feature is usually omitted in digital EEG machines; however, many digitally controlled amplifiers have preprogrammed features to suppress these types of artifacts.

Output and input jacks: When output other than paper tracing is desired, it is necessary to have a means of transmitting the EEG signal to another output device. Examples of such outputs are analog tape recordings, oscilloscopes, and analog-to-digital devices for computer input. Some EEG machines provide several outputs in order to facilitate impedance matching of the output and input equipment. Similarly, EEG machines may have input jacks to allow playback of external signals in the machine circuitry. This input may be before or after the initial stage of amplification and filtering. One com-

monly employed input is a marker for photic stimulation. Attention must be given to the proper range of input voltages for each input jack. The high-quality amplifiers used in analog EEG machines still offer the advantage that their output signals can be digitized at very high rates, with the appropriate filters in place; thus, they are very important in the basic science community, in which they remain extremely popular in research on biological signals. Many digital EEG machines provide an analog output to allow playing the recording back into a standard paper EEG machine to generate old-fashioned paper tracings. With the growing acceptance of digital EEGs and the widespread availability of affordable universal reader software for the majority of EEG programs and manufacturers, it is expected that this feature will be used less over time.

Penmanship

The final link between the patient and a legible EEG tracing is the writer. Most EEG machines involve the use of a pen-ink-paper system in which pen tips move back and forth in proportion to voltage while EEG paper is transported by rollers at a constant velocity under the pens. Several varieties of ink-writing systems are available. The most common system uses a coil of wire to generate a magnetic field in proportion to the applied voltage. This field is opposed by the field of a nearby stationary magnet, which results in deflection of the pen. This type of apparatus is called a *galvanometer.* Mechanical force from a spring on the pen mounting restores the pen position to baseline.

Because the pen moves in an arc rather than in a straight line, there is a small error in representing the amplitude and time to reach the peak of particular waveforms in the EEG signal. In addition, the pens are mechanical devices with mass and friction, which exert effects on the paper as it scrolls by. They are thus filters, unable to respond with perfect fidelity to EEG signals. Pens are high-frequency filters because of mass, and they usually cannot respond to frequencies higher than approximately 90 Hz. Pens may be low-frequency filters because of friction. Friction is usually considered more of a problem at low frequencies than at higher ones, because it takes more energy to initiate movement in an object than to keep an object moving. The effect of pen friction is to decrease and delay response to low frequencies. Finally, the resonance of the system is a function of both the electrical and mechanical characteristics of the pen writing system. A sensitive system might respond quickly to an input, but it may oscillate when the input pulse is very sharp, as with a square wave or a spike. At the other extreme, a pen system can be overdamped, with little or no oscillation in response to very sharp input signals but with substantial attenuation and delay of the input signal (see Cooper et al. [6] for a detailed discussion).

In routine practice of EEG, pen-writing systems are entirely satisfactory, despite the qualifications just listed. In special applications involving high-frequency recordings, alternative methods are needed. Such methods include rectilinear ink jet recorders, oscilloscopic data presentation, analog tape, and digital recording of the EEG. Again, with the increasing popularity of digital EEGs, these factors will likely become less important over time. Of historical interest is that experienced EEG technologists often rely on the sound that the pens make on paper to detect certain conditions: for example, the 3-Hz waveforms of absence epilepsy. This sound was thought to be so important in the past that early digital EEG machines actually synthesized the sound of pens writing on paper while the EEG scrolled by on the computer screen, so as to preserve these auditory cues.

Paper Transport

The writer unit is the final part of the EEG machine to influence the EEG record. This is the system by which the paper is pulled below the pens in order to provide a written tracing of the EEG. The writer unit consists of a small rotating wheel (pressure roller) connected to a motor. The switch controlling the writer is usually a lever with three settings: "off" (no paper or pen movement), "chart" (allows the paper to move, but the pens do not conduct the EEG signal to the paper), and "chart and pens" (the paper moves and the pens conduct the EEG signal to the paper). On most machines, at least three speeds are offered: 15, 30, and 60 mm per second. The slowest time setting is used to conserve paper or to highlight slow activity. The setting of 30 mm per second is standard in the United States, although 15 mm per second is common in other parts of the world. The 60-mm per second chart speed is used to examine fast activity or interchannel latency relationships that are not easily discerned at slower paper speeds. This setting serves to draw out the tracing, thereby allowing the reader to see more detail. Figure 3.26 shows some examples of an EEG tracing containing ictal activity seen on three different paper speeds. One area in which digital EEGs demonstrate superiority over analog EEG is in the ability to replay segments of the EEG at different gains and paper speeds. Single events that may occur

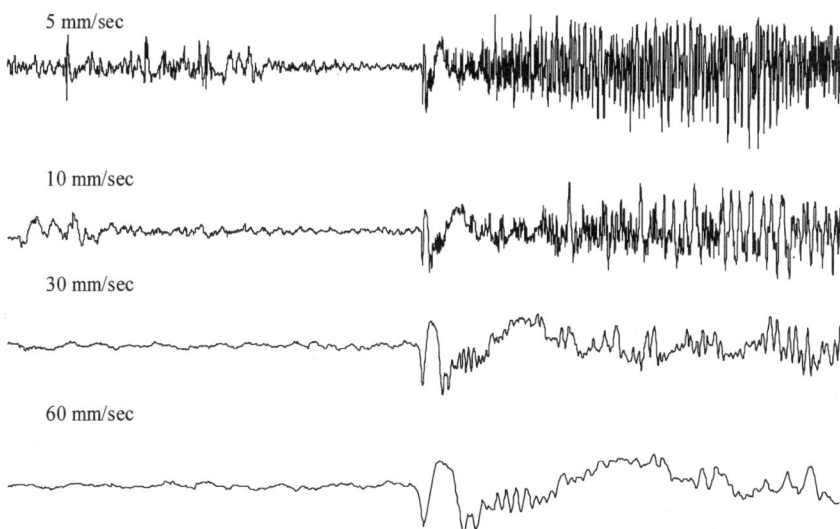

FIG. 3.26. Electroencephalogram from a single channel at the start of a complex partial seizure recorded at several paper speeds. This recording was obtained digitally. At slower paper speeds, more of the event, including its evolution, can be discerned. At faster speeds, more detail over shorter periods of time becomes apparent.

suddenly and be uninterpretable when written on paper may be diagnostic of a variety of conditions when they can be reviewed post hoc after being stored digitally.

Processing During and After Data Acquisition

Because digitally acquired EEGs are stored as numerical data, a wide variety of computer programs and algorithms can be used to analyze, extract features from, and display data in many different forms. These methods have utility in both clinical and research applications. Examples of clinical uses include compressed spectral array displays of long-term EEG data, such as for intraoperative, intensive care unit or anesthesia monitoring; seizure detection algorithms used for inpatient epilepsy monitoring (27); and automated sleep staging systems. Research applications include such investigations as functional brain mapping with the use of focal cortical desynchronization in electrocorticographic recordings during cognitive tasks (7,8) and investigation into seizure precursors and prediction (20,22). Details related to this topic are covered in other sections of this book.

Networking, Data Storage, and Report Generation

As mentioned earlier, one of the most useful aspects of digital EEG technology is the ability to connect acquisition machines, which collect data from the patient, to computer networks. This allows for transmission, interpretation, and archival of recordings to remote sites and availability for review at many locations at one time. With the development of broader band networks (e.g., those capable of carrying more data per unit time), typical 16-bit records 20 to 40 Mb in length can be transferred in minutes to locations that are sometimes miles away from the patient. Urgent studies can be read rapidly in these systems and, with appropriate bandwidth access at home (e.g., cable modem or DSL line), after a transfer time of just a few minutes. Transmission of such large files over more standard modems on telephone lines (e.g., 56 K baud) remains impractical for this purpose for now, requiring up to 3 hours to transfer a typical digital EEG record.

Figure 3.27 depicts a typical "high end" network system for a comprehensive center performing routine EEG, epilepsy monitoring, and EEG during Wada testing, positron emission tomographic scanning, intraoperative monitoring, and record review in multiple locations. In this scheme, the EEG machines, also called "collectors," are placed in a variety of inpatient and outpatient locations. At each site, the machine is plugged into a network jack, and studies are transmitted to the hospital server. Epilepsy monitoring unit (EMU) data are kept locally for review and clipping before transfer to the hospital server, because of the large volume of EEG and digital video data that are continuously collected. Data on the server can then be reviewed, and reports can be generated and sent to remote archives on CD, DVD, or other media. In the authors' laboratory, it is protocol never to delete a study from the collector unless a report has been generated and the data are verified to be intact in the archive. Remote sites can be monitored in real time, such as in the operating room, intensive care unit, or elsewhere, although at present, this usually requires the use of third-party software (e.g., PC Anywhere, NetMeeting) for network communication. Home access provides its own challenges, particularly with regard to patient confidentiality and adherence to Health Care Finance Administration and other federal and local standards, which are being considered and put into place at this

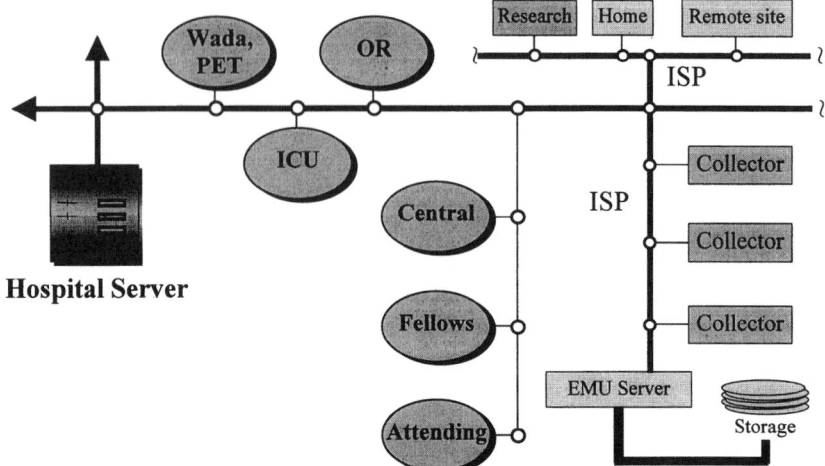

FIG. 3.27. Schematic of computerized electroencephalographic (EEG) network in a tertiary hospital. "Collectors" are digital EEG recording units, with or without digital video; "Central, Fellows and Attending" are reading station areas; "OR" stands for operating room, "ICU" for intensive care unit, and "EMU" for epilepsy monitoring unit. "Research, Home and Remote site" are areas away from the central hospital where data may be reviewed or copied. "ISP" stands for Internet service provider, which provides the link for Internet access to remote locations outside the hospital network.

time. Most comprehensive EEG systems contain both local area networks (LANs), such as in the EMU and outpatient EEG laboratories, and wide area networks (WANs), which cover entire medical centers. The network architecture that makes the most sense for a particular laboratory is a complex issue, often best left to professional designers. It is a function of institutional resources, hardware, usage, and policy and regulations.

Data Storage, Media, Universal Readers, and Report Generation

EEG data, whether paper or digital, have an associated cost of acquisition and storage, in view of regulations that require, in most states, keeping documentation of medical studies for at least 7 years. Table 3.5 lists media and storage costs per year for paper and several types of digital media. Because there are no microfilm, clipping, or remote storage costs for digital media, in addition to environmental considerations, the cost savings of digital stud-

TABLE 3.5. *Cost of storage media per electroencephalographic study*

Paper and microfilm*	$10.54
Optical (1GB)	$4.50
CD-ROM (700MB)	$0.03
DAT (7GB)	$0.12
DLT (15GB)	$0.12
Video tape	$0.31
Jaz Drive (1GB)	$6.00
DVD (4.7GB)†	$0.13

*Does not include off-site storage costs.
†May increase to 20 GB.
CD-ROM, compact disk, read-only memory; DAT, digital audio tape; DLT, digital linear tape; DVD, digital video disk.

ies are easy to see. Of importance is that the costs of digital media continue to drop; for example, a CD at the time of writing this chapter cost about $1.00 and as low as $0.75 when purchased in bulk.

One issue of importance to digital electroencephalographers is having the ability to read data from EEG machines manufactured by different companies on a single platform (e.g., a universal reading station). This is important in cases in which patients are referred for evaluation and bring digital records from other laboratories. The American Society for Testing and Materials is composed of representatives from the EEG community and industry dedicated to working out a universal storage format to enable this type of record exchange. Several software manufacturers also provide universal reading platforms that accept data from *most* manufacturers. Both of these efforts are works in progress but show promise of success in accomplishing this task in the long run.

An added benefit of using digital EEG machines is the ability to read records on a personal computer, which can also be loaded with data base and word-processing software to enable rapid generation of reports and searchable archives for clinical, research, and continuous quality assessment purposes. In such systems, as the authors and others have implemented them, technologists input data that they would normally write on a cover sheet, such as the patient's identifying information, conditions of the record, and medical history, into fields in a data base record residing on the laboratory server. The recording is performed and sent to the server for remote review, and the reading physician inputs features of the record and impressions into the same data base record. In addition to quality information, the need to review the record at conference and technical issues are flagged in the

appropriate fields. Finally, when completed, the reader generates a report through a mail-merge program, which takes fields from the data base and inserts them into the body of a report form that has been previously constructed. The process is quite streamlined, except for very difficult records, and is usually time and cost efficient. Reports are then uploaded to the laboratory server, where they can be accessed throughout the hospital through the EEG laboratory's web site. Some manufacturers are currently including data base and report generation software as part of their digital EEG software. Other third-party programs to accomplish this task are becoming available for use, as the popularity of digital systems continues to rise.

EVOKED POTENTIALS

Routine EEG investigates spontaneous electrical activity of the brain. A relatively new and growing area involves study of EEG potentials evoked by sensory signals (visual, auditory, or somatosensory evoked potentials) or by motor tasks (motor evoked potentials). Electrical principles and technological requirements underlying recording of evoked potentials are similar to those underlying recording of the spontaneous EEG, with a few exceptions. Evoked potentials recorded are usually very brief and occur at short latencies, after the evoking stimuli. Rapid data acquisition and storage are thus needed. Evoked EEG signals are sampled at very fast acquisition rates and digitized to facilitate mathematical manipulation. Evoked potentials are small and are subject to poor signal-to-noise ratios. This is overcome by averaging several responses. With such averaging, random noise and other signals that are uncorrelated with the stimulus cancel, leaving only an evoked response (or correlated artifact) related to the stimulus. If N is the number of trials averaged, then the signal-to-noise ratio of an evoked potential is improved by a factor of $\sqrt{N}$. Figure 3.28 shows a typical brainstem auditory evoked potential with 1, 100, 500, and 2,000 averaged trials. The pen-ink-paper method is not conducive to signal averaging; therefore, virtually every modern evoked potential machine entails the use of oscilloscope or computer screen outputs, with the capacity to print studies to a laser or similar printer.

Evoked potential amplifier and filter settings differ substantially from parameters used for routine EEG. In the recording of brainstem auditory evoked potentials gain is set to 200,000 to 500,000. Low-frequency filter cutoffs are usually set at 50 to 150 Hz, high-frequency cutoffs are usually set at 3,000 Hz, and the minimum sampling rate is 10,000 samples per second. Detailed discussions of technique and interpretation of evoked potentials can be found in later chapters in this book, as well as in other standard texts (3).

NUMBER OF AVERAGES

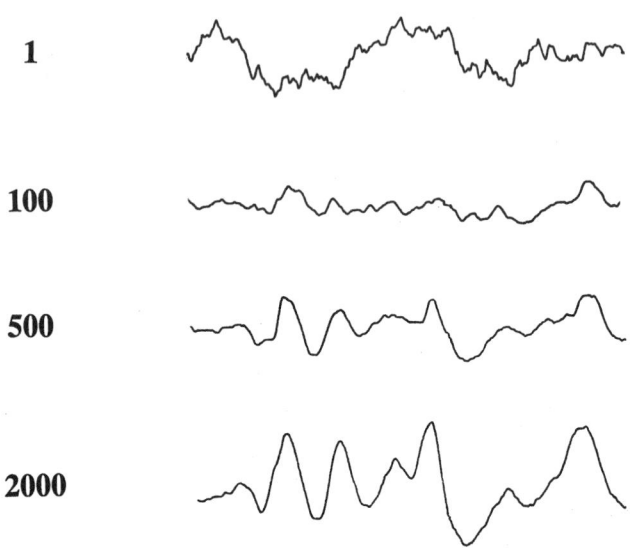

1

100

500

2000

FIG. 3.28. Record of brainstem auditory evoked potential with 1, 100, 500, and 2,000 signal averages. As number of averages is increased, the resolution of the normal waveform increases. Time displayed is 10 milliseconds. The gain of the first tracing is half that of the lower three tracings, to prevent saturation of amplifier by noise.

ELECTRICAL SAFETY

EEG is an extremely safe procedure, but a small possibility of injury does exist. It is imperative that the technologist and electroencephalographer understand how to minimize this risk. Current is the most important predictor of electrical injury. It can cause pain and burns if applied to the skin. Seizures can result from certain types of current applied directly to the brain or to the scalp. Current can electroplate irritating metals from intracranial electrodes into brain tissue. Current can even kill, by inducing ventricular fibrillation. Injury risk can be discussed in terms of three groups with different types of relationships to EEG equipment. The safest group comprises persons who are simply near and possibly touching an electrical device but not intentionally connected to it. The second group comprises people with electrodes attached to skin, in the absence of other medical instrumentation.

TABLE 3.6. *Effects of various currents at 60 Hz*

Current for 1 second	Effect
0.1 mA	Ventricular fibrillation if applied to the heart
0.3 mA	Sensory threshold
1.0 mA	Pain threshold
5 mA	Maximal harmless level
15 mA	Muscle tetany
50 mA	Tissue injury
100 mA	Fibrillation or death

Adapted from Tyner F, Knott J, Mayer WJ. *Fundamentals of EEG technology.* New York: Raven Press, 1983.

The third group contains patients at higher risk, such as neonates and patients with intravascular catheters or other medical instrumentation.

Table 3.6, adapted from Tyner et al. (32), summarizes effects of various currents at 60 Hz on normal persons (group I described earlier).

There are several potential sources of dangerous currents that may flow through patients connected to EEG machines and cause them harm. These sources are described as follows.

Improper grounding

Improper grounding can result from a disruption of the ground circuit inside the EEG machine or from use of a two-prong socket. The cylindrical contact (green wire) on the three-prong plug is the ground contact. Should a short circuit occur in the machine and a current-bearing element make contact with the chassis of the machine, this current should immediately be shunted to the ground contact, because this is the path of lowest resistance. This would quickly blow a fuse or circuit breaker in the EEG machine, which would sense the abnormally high current flow through the now very low resistance of the short circuit. This would not happen immediately, and some current might flow through the patient even if the proper safety mechanisms were intact during a short circuit. If the machine ground contact is not intact, substantial current (possibly life-threatening) may pass through the patient.

EEG machines should never be powered by an inadequately grounded circuit: Three-prong to two-prong adapters should not be used. Machines must always be protected with regulation fuses. Fuses should not be defeated: There is always a reason when a fuse stops working, and it is important to discover that reason rather than subject the patient to an electrical hazard. Hospital-grade power outlets should be used whenever possible for EEG machines (or for any other machines that are to be connected to patients).

These outlets are labeled with a green dot and indicate a higher standard of safety and quality of construction than do other outlets (32). A schedule of preventive maintenance on the EEG machine and outlets should be enacted.

Leakage currents

Leakage currents arise from two main sources: stray capacitance and stray inductance. Stray capacitance usually arises from wires connected to a wall socket or to the EEG machine power supply. Capacitance is a function of the construction of the power cords and of their length. Nearby wires in a power cord are insulated from each other and therefore can function as a capacitor. AC current flows through the "hot" (black) wire in the cord and induces small capacitive currents in the neutral (white) and ground (green) wires as they alternately charge and discharge with the AC current. This leakage current is usually shunted directly to the ground contact; however, if the ground connection is not properly made, this current may flow through the patient. Extension cords should not be used with EEG machines, because they increase the capacitive current to a potentially dangerous amount. Because wires are inefficient capacitors, capacitive currents from an EEG machine are generally far less than 0.1 mA and may be only a few microamperes. Nevertheless, if applied directly to the heart, 0.1 mA could cause ventricular fibrillation.

Each wire carrying current to and through the EEG machine induces a magnetic field that, in turn, creates currents in other wires, including neutral and ground wires. These currents are usually shunted directly to the ground contact, but, again, they may be conducted through the patient should some ground malfunction (ground fault) occur. Stray inductances generally are of less magnitude than stray capacitances.

According to Hill and Dolan (cited in Cooper et al. [6]), maximum leakage currents allowed for the three groups defined earlier are 500 µA for those having casual contact with a medical device; 100 µA for those connected to electrical devices; and 10 µA for the group at high risk.

Double-grounding

If a patient is connected to an EEG machine and to another electrical instrument, there is probably be more than one ground connection. This creates a situation referred to as double-grounding or a ground loop. Because no two ground connections are at identical potential, current may flow from one ground connection to the other through the patient. There are several potential sources of ground-loop currents. Short circuits in the machine or other circuit faults can deliver massive current to a ground loop. Less dangerous but more common are currents in the ground circuit as a result of stray capacitance and stray inductance. Additional currents may be induced in the ground wires by nearby magnetic fields. In this case, the induced potentials in question are small, but the resistances of the ground paths are also small. By Ohm's law, large currents could flow from one ground circuit to another through the patient.

Double-grounding is of particular concern in areas where patients are connected to multiple devices, such as intensive care units and operating rooms. It is not unusual to observe patients connected to EEG machines, electrocardiographic monitors, temperature monitors, electric blood pressure cuffs, ventilators, pulse oximeters, warming or cooling blankets, electric beds, arterial and venous catheters, intracranial pressure monitors, and a variety of other hardware. In such circumstances, the presence of a ground loop is virtually guaranteed. The solution is to connect all devices attached to the patient to a common ground connection plugged into the same wall outlet. If necessary, a grounding bar can be used to gang together the various ground connections. This provides only one low-resistance ground path (not through the patient) for stray currents.

The EEG technologist must remember the principle of single-grounding when an accessory ground connection is necessary to eliminate 60-Hz interference. All ground connections should travel to one point. If the patient is already grounded by another device, it is not necessary (and is potentially dangerous) to attach another ground connection to the patient. Avoidance of multiple ground connections, in addition to being a requirement for patient safety, improves recording quality.

In high-risk circumstances, such as when patients have intravenous catheters, special isolation jackboxes should be employed. These boxes use optical isolation or solid-state variable resistors to separate the patient from any currents generated in the EEG machine (12,32).

Switch sparking

Whenever the power switch on the EEG machine or on the pens is enabled, a small spark occurs inside the machine. This was an explosive and shock hazard in the past (when volatile anesthetics such as ether were in common use) but is not a major concern in most modem recording environments.

Exacerbating Factors

Predicting the consequences of an electric shock is difficult, because several factors influence the biological response. In the clinical setting, the

TABLE 3.7. *Safety rules for performing electroencephalography (EEG)*

Maintain machinery to avoid faulty circuits
Always use a grounded (three-prong) plug to power
Properly fuse the EEG machine
Use one ground connection to patient or ground to a common point
Use an isolation jackbox in high-risk situations

most important factor is instrumentation. A transvenous pacemaker or a central venous pressure catheter provides a low-resistance route for stray currents to travel directly to the heart. Ventricular fibrillation can result from currents that would not even be perceived through intact skin. Skin wounds or excessive abrasion with cleaning paste may increase the risk for injury by a given current at those sites. Good general health may be a factor in resisting effects of electric shock, but many hospitalized patients are ill (6,32). Table 3.7 summarizes important safety rules in EEG recording.

CONCLUSIONS

It is easy to see how the engineering and electronics technology behind EEG continue to evolve as fast digital computers free electroencephalographers and technologists from paper and ink and provide opportunities for quantitative analysis of neurally generated signals. Nonetheless, the basic core technology remains the same as it was when discovered during the 1930s. Postsynaptic potentials generated by large functional masses of neuronal tissue, filtered by and conducted through the cerebrospinal fluid, dura, skull, scalp, and skin are transduced by surface electrodes, amplified, and filtered for review. Unfortunately, as the understanding of brain function and dysfunction increases, the limitations of this empirically discovered technology become more apparent. Functional activity generated by deep structures central to clinical epilepsy, such as the mesial temporal lobe and deep frontal lobe, remain inaccessible for EEG recording. Patterns generated by metabolic encephalopathies are often indistinguishable from those of subtle or nonconvulsive status epilepticus. Seizures that are not directly on the brain surface are often obscured, poorly localized, or even invisible on surface EEGs, sometimes even after placement of intracranial electrodes. These common problems highlight the need for a new type of EEG technology, designed specifically for modern clinical epileptology and neuroscience research, to replace what has been the gold standard for assessing electrophysiologic function in the central nervous system since the early twentieth

century. Just as potent "designer" compounds have replaced the less effective naturally occurring substances, which spawned their development in the pharmaceutical armamentarium, so may a new technology devoted to real-time assessment of brain function supplant the current form of EEG. This may well be a long time in coming, because it will be hard to improve upon the immediate accessibility, portability, relatively low cost, and excellent reliability of current EEG technology.

ACKNOWLEDGMENTS

The authors are greatly indebted to Robert Fisher, M.D., Ph.D., for his wonderful and witty input to this chapter in the previous edition. We are also grateful to the late Dr. Sumio Uematsu for the intraoperative photographs reproduced in this chapter. He continues to be missed by the many of us who worked with him. The thoughts expressed in this chapter reflect past experiences and continued learning with many wonderful electroencephalographers throughout training and practice, such as Bob Fisher, Alan Krumholz, Tom Henry, Chip Epstein, Jacqueline French, John Ebersole, Bob Webber, and others too many to be named. Finally, a large measure of gratitude is due Ernst Niedermeyer for providing teaching and mentoring over the years about the importance of a meticulously recorded and judiciously interpreted EEG.

ELECTROENCEPHALOGRAPHIC TECHNOLOGY KEY POINTS

1. EEG current is approximately 1 μA, voltage is approximately 2 to 300 μV.
2. $V = IR$ (volts, amperes, ohms)
3. Voltage law:
   Total of all voltages around a closed circuit is zero
   OR
   V input = total of voltage drops in circuit
   OR
   V input − total of voltage drops in circuit = 0.
4. Current law:
   Total current into a node equals total current out of a node
   OR
   Total current at any junction is zero.
5. For capacitors:

$$Q = CV \qquad \text{(coulombs, farads, volts)}$$

$$I = C \, dV/dt$$

Current = capacitance (a constant) · change in voltage over time.

6. Capacitive reactance (like resistance, but frequency dependent):

$$X_c = 1/(2\pi f C)$$

where f is frequency in cycles per second, or hertz, and C is capacitance, in farads.

NOTE: Capacitors resist current flow more at lower frequencies.

7. Inductance (L, measured in henrys) (not very important to EEG).

$$\text{Inductive reactance} = X_L = 2\pi f L.$$

8. Power $= I^2 R = \dfrac{V^2}{R}$ (measured in watts).

9. Alternating current (AC) comes out of wall socket:

$$V(t) = V_p \cdot \sin(\omega t + \tau)$$

where ω is angular frequency (in radians per second) and τ is phase angle (in radians).

radians per second $= 2\pi f$ (frequency in Hz).

10. Direct current (DC) comes out of a battery and has no frequency content.

11. Root mean square (RMS) is equivalent DC voltage of an AC voltage:

$$\text{RMS (sine wave)} = \frac{\text{peak voltage}}{\sqrt{2}}$$

Wall socket delivers 110 V RMS = $110 \cdot \sqrt{2}$ = 156 V amplitude.

12. Resistances in series: $ADD = R1 + R2 + R3 \ldots$
Resistances in parallel: reciprocal of sum of reciprocals $= 1/(1/R1 + 1/R2 + 1/R3 \ldots)$.

13. Capacitances in series: reciprocal of sum of reciprocals $= 1/(1/C1 + 1/C2 + 1/C3 \ldots)$

$$\text{Capacitances in parallel: } ADD = C1 + C2 + C3. \ldots$$

14. Time constant $= \tau = R \cdot C$

τ = time it takes for voltage across resistor to fall to approximately 37% ($1/e$) of initial value, or for a capacitor to charge to 63% ($1 - 1/e$) of maximum value in an RC circuit.

NOTE: e is approximately 2.718.

NOTE: Avoid confusion: percentage is major change in direction of charge or discharge (up to 63% charging, or down to 37% discharging).

15. Cutoff frequency of a filter (frequency at which $1/\sqrt{2}$ or approximately 70% of signal is passed) is related to the time constant τ by the formula

$$f_{\text{cutoff}} = 1/(2\pi\tau) = 1/(2\pi RC) = 0.16/\tau$$

16. In low-frequency filters, the voltage across the resistor is

$$V(t) = Ae^{-t/\tau}$$

17. Time constants are related to cutoff frequency:

$$\tau = 1/(2\pi f_{\text{cutoff}})$$

Time constant is in seconds, cutoff frequency is in Hz. The cutoff frequency is the frequency at which $1/\sqrt{2}$ of signal is passed (approximately 70%).

18. Low-frequency filtering advances the timing of voltage peaks for the sinusoidal signal. High-frequency filtering delays the timing of voltage peaks. At the cutoff frequency timing, the change is a phase shift of 45° $= \pi/4$ radians = one-eight of the cycle.

19. Ohm's law for *AC*:

$$V = I \cdot Z \qquad \text{where } Z \text{ is impedance}$$

$$Z = \sqrt{(R^2 + (X_C - X_L)^2}$$

20. Reversible electrodes do not easily become polarized, which means they have low electrode potentials, which in turn means they produce signals better.

21. Decibels (dB):

$$\text{dB} = 20 \cdot \log(V_{out}/V_{in})$$

22. Frequency response of a filter: how the signal is altered as a function of frequency. Rolloff is how steep slope of curve is when amplitude plotted against log (frequency). Measured in decibels/(factor of 10 in frequency) = decibels/octave.

23. Common-mode rejection ratio (CMRR): a measure of how well a differential amplifier filters out signals common to both inputs:

$$CMRR = \frac{\text{voltage when input 1} = \text{V and input 2} = \text{ground}}{\text{input 1} = \text{V and input 2} = \text{V}}$$

24. Electrode impedance: 30-Hz sine wave is sent by machine through elec-

trodes. Impedance = 1 or 2 kΩ (machine dependent) per 1 mm of pen deflection.

25. Pen frequency response is limited to about 90 Hz before there is significant arcing.

26. Paper speed is commonly 30 mm per second in the United States; elsewhere, 15 mm per second is used. Slower paper speeds for operative monitoring (and usually for sleep) are sometimes used. Faster speeds help analyze fast events.

27. Analog signal: no spaces between data points, a continuous waveform (e.g., electrical current).

28. Digital signal: An analog signal is sampled at intervals measured in samples per second (= sample rate).

29. Nyquist's law: in order to resolve a waveform of frequency X cycles per second (= X Hz), the signal must be sampled at more than $2 \cdot X$/second (= Nyquist frequency).

30. Aliasing: If a signal of frequency X is sampled at the Nyquist frequency or lower, it can look like a signal of a lower frequency, corrupting the data. This process is called *aliasing*. The signal is said to be aliased.

31. To prevent aliasing, all frequencies that are higher than the band of interest should be filtered out, and sampling at slightly higher than the Nyquist frequency (called oversampling) should be performed just to be sure of accuracy. It should be remembered that filters have a frequency response curve, not just a vertical cutoff (infinite slope).

32. Digital storage: Resolution of a digital signal is a function of the voltage range being sampled (typically ±10 V), the sample rate, number of bits in ADC, the number of bits used for storage, and the resolution of the computer screen used for display.

33. The number of bits (n) used to store digital data divides the voltage range into 2^n increments. The more bits used, the better the resolution of the data. For example:
    1 bit allows data to be 0 or 1
    2 bits allows $2^2 = 4$ increments
    3 bits allows $2^3 = 8$ increments
    4 bits allows $2^4 = 16$ increments
    8 bits allows $2^8 = 256$ increments
    12 bits allows $2^{12} = 4,096$ increments

34. Safety:
    I. Three risk groups
       A. Bystanders
       B. Subjects connected to machine
       C. High risk: patients connected to intravenous catheters and other devices; neonates
    II. Potential sources of danger
       A. Improper grounding: more than one ground, three prongs converted to two, defeated fuses
       B. Leakage currents: capacitance of long wires (no extension cords) or nearby cords
       C. Switch sparking (not a "turn on")
       D. Working in puddles (e.g., in the operating room)
    III. Rules to follow:
       A. Use green dot outlets (hospital standard)
       B. Regular maintenance
       C. Proper fusing
       D. No extension cords
       E. One common ground
       F. Isolation jackbox for high-risk circumstances
    IV. Injury table: effects of various currents at 60 Hz

Current for 1 second	Effect
0.1 mA	Ventricular fibrillation if applied to the heart
0.3 mA	Sensory threshold
1.0 mA	Pain threshold
5 mA	Maximal harmless level
15 mA	Causes muscle tetany
50 mA	Causes tissue injury
100 mA	Causes fibrillation or death

    V. Leakage current limits
       Devices standing alone   500 μA
       If patients are connected   100 μA
       Patients at high risk (e.g., with   intravenous catheters)   10 μA

REFERENCES

1. Barlow JS, Kamp A, Morton HB, et al. EEG instrumentation standards: Report of the committee on EEG instrumentation standards of the International Societies for Electroencephalography and Clinical Neurophysiology. *Electroencephalogr Clin Neurophysiol* 1974;37:539–553.
2. Budak A. *Circuit theory fundamentals and applications.* Englewood Cliffs, NJ: Prentice-Hall, 1978.
3. Chiappa KH. *Evoked potentials in clinical medicine,* 3rd ed. Philadelphia: Lippincott-Raven, 1997:ix, 709.
4. Company GI. *Grass model 8 instruction manual.* Quincy, MA: Grass Instrument Company. 1974.

5. Cooper R. Electrodes. *Am J EEG Technol* 1963;3:91–101.

6. Cooper R, Osselton JW, Shaw J. *EEG technology.* London: Butterworths, 1980.

7. Crone NE, Miglioretti DL, Gordon B, et al. Functional mapping of human sensorimotor cortex with electrocorticographic spectral analysis. I. Alpha and beta event–related desynchronization. *Brain* 1998;121:2271–2799.

8. Crone NE, Miglioretti DL, Gordon B, et al. Functional mapping of human sensorimotor cortex with electrocorticographic spectral analysis. II. Event-related synchronization in the gamma band. *Brain* 1998;121:2301–2315.

9. Fenton DS, Geremia GK, Dowd AM, et al. Precise placement of sphenoidal electrodes via fluoroscopic guidance. *AJNR Am J Neuroradiol* 1997;18:776–778.

10. Geddes L, Baker L. *Principles of applied biomedical instrumentation.* New York: John Wiley & Sons, 1968.

11. Goldring S, Gregorie EM. Surgical management of epilepsy using epidural recordings to localize the seizure focus. Review of 100 cases. *J Neurosurg* 1984;60:457–466.

12. Graf M, Niedermeyer E, Schiemann J, et al. Electrocorticography: information derived from intraoperative recordings during seizure surgery. *Clin Electroencephalogr* 1984;15:83–91.

13. Homan RW, Jones MC, Rawat S. Anterior temporal electrodes in complex partial seizures. *Electroencephalogr Clin Neurophysiol* 1988;70:105–109.

14. Horowitz P, Hill W. *The art of electronics.* New York: Cambridge University Press, 1981.

15. Jasper H, Arfel-Capdevielle G, Rasmussen T. Evaluation of EEG and cortical electrographic studies for prognosis of seizures following surgical excision of epileptogenic lesions. *Epilepsia* 1961;2:130–137.

16. Kanner AM, Jones JC. When do sphenoidal electrodes yield additional data to that obtained with antero-temporal electrodes? *Electroencephalogr Clin Neurophysiol* 1997;102:12–19.

17. Kanner AM, Ramirez L, Jones JC. The utility of placing sphenoidal electrodes under the foramen ovale with fluoroscopic guidance. *J Clin Neurophysiol* 1995;12:72–81.

18. King DW, So EL, Marcus R, et al. Techniques and applications of sphenoidal recording. *J Clin Neurophysiol* 1986;3:51–65.

19. Krauss GL, Lesser RP, Fisher RS, et al. Anterior "cheek" electrodes are comparable to sphenoidal electrodes for the identification of ictal activity. *Electroencephalogr Clin Neurophysiol* 1992;83:333–338.

20. Lehnertz K. Non-linear time series analysis of intracranial EEG recordings in patients with epilepsy—an overview. *Int J Psychophysiol* 1999;34:45–52.

21. Lesser RP, Luders H, Klem G, et al. Extraoperative cortical functional localization in patients with epilepsy. *J Clin Neurophysiol* 1987;4:27–53.

22. Litt B, Esteller R, Echauz J, et al. Epileptic seizures may begin hours in advance of clinical seizures: a report of five patients. *Neuron* 2001;30:51–64.

23. MacLean P. A nasopharyngeal lead. EEG. *Clin Neurophysiol* 1949;1.

24. Niedermeyer E. Depth electroencephalography. In: Niedermeyer E, Lopes da Silva FH, eds. *Electroencephalography: basic principles, clinical applications, and related fields,* 3rd ed. Baltimore: Williams & Wilkins, 1993:593–617.

25. Niedermeyer E, Lopes da Silva FH, eds. *Electroencephalography: basic principles, clinical applications, and related fields,* 4th ed. Baltimore: Williams & Wilkins; 1999:xi, 1258.

26. Purcell E. *Electricity and magnetism.* New York: McGraw-Hill, 1965.

27. Qu H, Gotman J. A patient-specific algorithm for the detection of seizure onset in long-term EEG monitoring: possible use as a warning device. *IEEE Trans Biomed Eng* 1997;44:115–122.

28. Sadler RM, Goodwin J. Multiple electrodes for detecting spikes in partial complex seizures. *Can J Neurol Sci* 1989;16:326–329.

29. Silverman D. The anterior temporal electrode and the ten-twenty system. *Electroencephalogr Clin Neurophysiol* 1960;12:735–737.

30. Spencer SS, Spencer DD, Williamson PD, et al. The localizing value of depth electroencephalography in 32 patients with refractory epilepsy. *Ann Neurol* 1982;12:248–253.

31. Sperling MR, Mendius JR, Engel J. Mesial temporal spikes: a simultaneous comparison of sphenoidal, nasopharyngeal, and ear electrodes. *Epilepsia* 1986;27:81–86.

32. Tyner F, Knott J, Mayer WJ. *Fundamentals of EEG technology.* New York: Raven Press, 1983.

33. Weyer E. Bioelectrodes. *Ann N Y Acad Sci* 1968;148:221.

34. Wieser HG, Elger CE, Stodieck SR. The "foramen ovale electrode": a new recording method for the preoperative evaluation of patients suffering from mesio-basal temporal lobe epilepsy. *Electroencephalogr Clin Neurophysiol* 1985;61:314–322.

35. Wieser HG, Hajek M. Foramen ovale and peg electrodes. *Acta Neurol Scand Suppl* 1994;152:33–35.

36. Wyler AR, Ojemann GA, Lettich E, et al. Subdural strip electrodes for localizing epileptogenic foci. *J Neurosurg* 1984;60:1195–1200.

Chapter 4

Electrical Fields and Recording Techniques

Mary B. Connolly, Frank W. Sharbrough, and Peter K. H. Wong

Electroencephalography (EEG) enables clinicians to study and analyze electrical fields of brain activity by recording amplified voltage differences between electrodes placed on the scalp, directly on the cortex (e.g., with subdural electrodes), or within the brain (with depth electrodes). For each electrical field, the clinician attempts to determine the nature, location, and configuration of the generator of EEG patterns and whether they are normal or abnormal and epileptiform or nonepileptiform. The clinical interpretation of the EEG findings must correspond to the patient's symptoms, findings on physical examination, and results of other investigations, such as brain imaging.

The traditional and universally accepted method of scalp electrode placement is the international 10-20 system (17,18). The spatial distribution of a changing electrical field requires orderly arrangement of multiple channels, termed a *montage*. Within a montage, different derivations record activity from different spatial intervals.

CEREBRAL GENERATORS OF ELECTROENCEPHALOGRAPHIC POTENTIALS

EEG signals represent the summated electrical activity generated by large populations of neurons (10^5 or more) (12) (see Chapter 1 for a more detailed

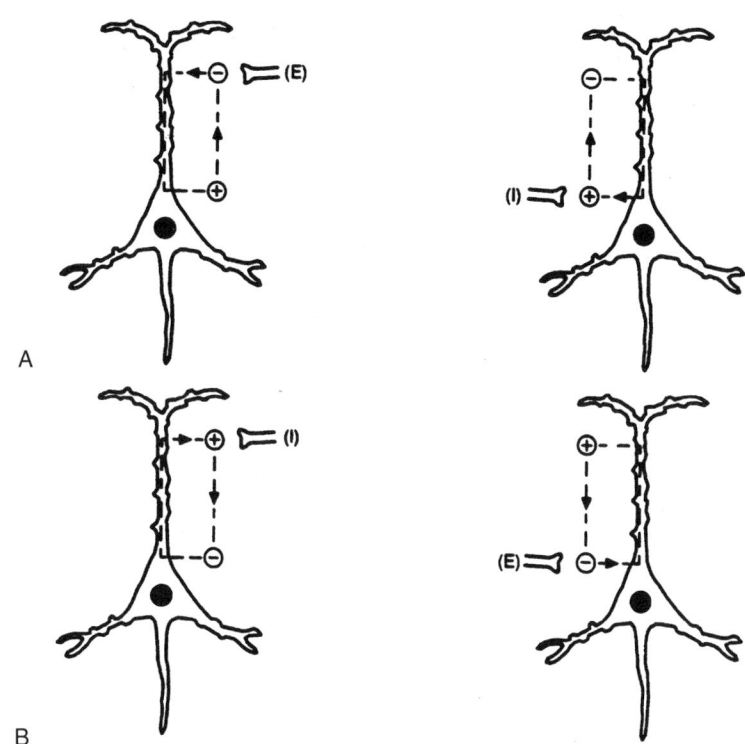

FIG. 4.1. A: A pyramidal cell dipole that is surface negative and depth positive can be produced either by excitatory synaptic input at the surface or by inhibitory synaptic input in the depths. **B:** Conversely, a pyramidal cell dipole that is surface positive and depth negative can be produced by inhibitory activity at the surface-positive end of the pyramidal cell or excitatory activity at the negative end. See also Fig. 4.4.

discussion). The main sources of EEG potentials are cortical neurons, which are arranged in layers beneath the cortical surface. Within each layer, neurons are aligned in bundles oriented perpendicular to the cortical surface and activated by synapses on soma-dendritic membranes. EEG signals are continuous variations of summated cellular electrical potentials as a function of time and location. All generators of scalp-recorded electrical activity, whether cerebral or extracerebral in origin, behave like a "dipole": that is, a generator with positive and negative poles. Pyramidal cells are the major source of synaptic potentials and are radially oriented. Synaptic activity at one end of the pyramidal cell produces an active ionic current as a result of changes in membrane permeability. The current loop is completed passively through neuronal mem-

branes at distant, relatively inactive sites. This means that synaptic input at one end of a pyramidal neuron causes current flow through the neural membrane whose direction at the surface is opposite its direction in the depth. This produces polarization shifts in opposite directions at the surface and in the depth; therefore, electrically, the neuron behaves as an extracellular, transcortical, surface-to-depth, radially oriented dipole (see Chapter 2 for detailed discussion).

Although a measurement of polarization extracellularly at the cortical surface predicts opposite extracellular polarization in the depth, it does not permit determination of whether the polarization changes result from excitatory or inhibitory synaptic activity (Fig. 4.1). Thus, it is difficult to determine the three-dimensional intracranial location and configuration of cerebral generators from scalp EEG activity alone (the so-called inverse problem). However, by using intracellular recordings from experimental animals or tissue slices, it is theoretically possible to predict the two-dimensional location and configuration of the scalp potential field for any type of activity. This is the *forward EEG projection* or problem (24,26,27). It is more common in clinical practice to try to determine the (unknown) EEG generators on the basis of the pattern of activity recorded at the surface; thus, the inverse problem is of clinical interest.

ELECTRODE PLACEMENT

Since EEG was first recorded from humans by Hans Berger, who used two electrodes applied on the front and back of the head, various systems have been used over the years (2,21). The Committee of the International Federation of Societies for Electroencephalography and Clinical Neurophysiology (IFSECN) recommended a specific system of electrode placement under standard conditions for use in all laboratories (Fig. 4.2A) (17). This is the system now known as the international 10-20 system. Specific measurements from bony landmarks are used to determine the placement of electrodes. From these anatomical landmarks, specific measurements are made, and then 10% to 20% of a specified distance is used as the electrode interval. This enables replication consistently over time and between laboratories. The American Clinical Neurophysiology Society (formerly the American Electroencephalographic Society) has recommended using a minimum of 21 electrodes in the international 10-20 system. Odd-numbered electrodes are placed on the left side of the head, and even-numbered electrodes, on the right side of the head. Specific letters designate the anatomical area; for example, "F" means frontal.

In 1991, the American Electroencephalographic Society added nomenclature guidelines that designate specific identifications and locations of 75 electrode positions along five anterior-posterior planes, lateral to the mid-

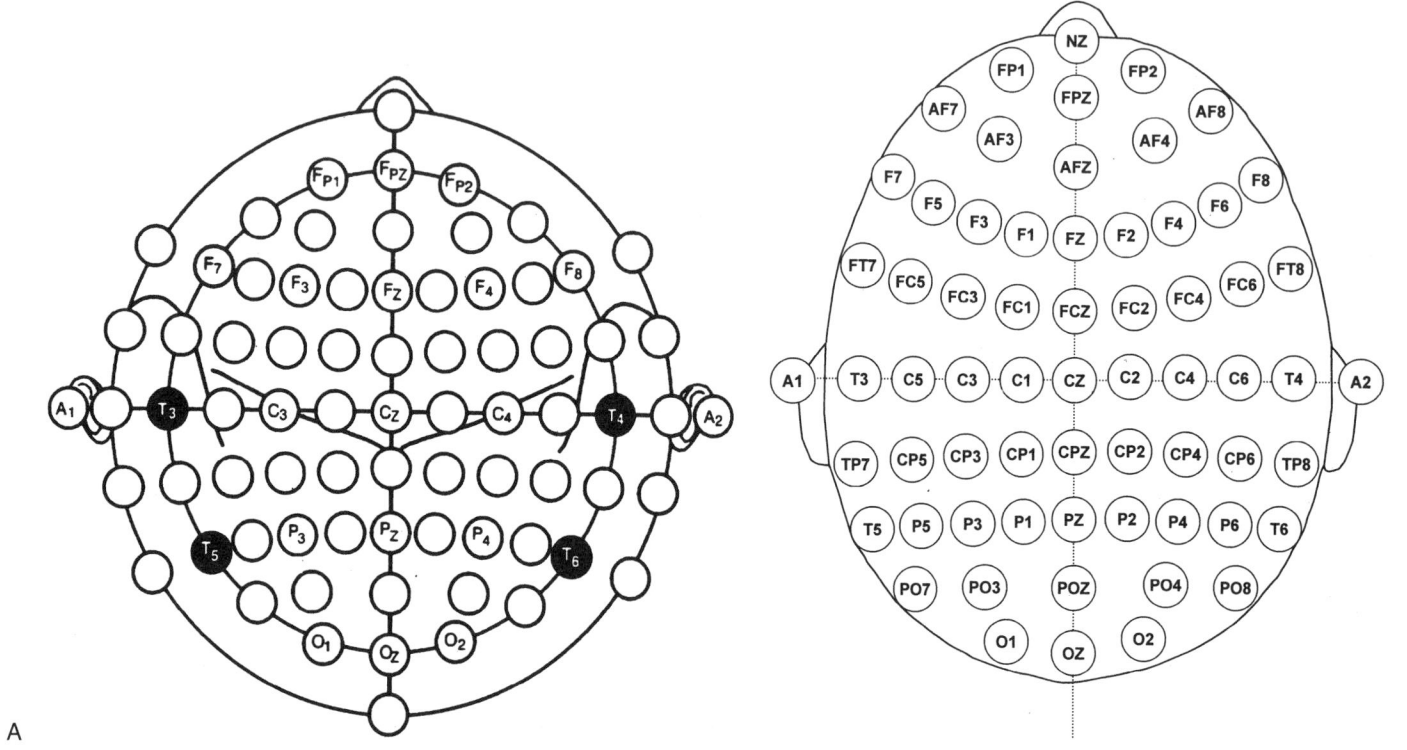

FIG. 4.2. A: Electrode nomenclature of the 19 most commonly used electrodes, according to the International Federation of Clinical Neurophysiology 10-20 system. **B:** Electrode nomenclature in the International Federation of Clinical Neurophysiology 10-20 system with additional electrodes (this is the 10% system).

line chain of 11 specific sites (see Fig. 4.2*B*). In addition, four coronal chains lie anterior, and four posterior, to the chain of 13 electrode sites between the earlobe electrodes along the midline at the Cz electrodes. Several electrodes have different names in the 10-20 system and the extended nomenclature. The electrodes T3 and T4 in the 10-20 system are referred to as T7 and T8 in the expanded system, and T5 and T6 are referred to as P7 and P8 under the new nomenclature. Currently, there is inconsistency among laboratories in identifying these electrodes (6,7,25,26).

For infants, fewer electrodes are used, and the number varies from laboratory to laboratory. For neonates, a 12.5% to 25% system is used in the Children's Hospital of British Columbia (Fig. 4.3). Specific issues related to recording EEG activity in newborns are discussed in Chapter 6.

In certain situations, additional electrodes can be applied to increase the yield from EEG recordings. These include, for example, sphenoidal, T1, and T2 electrodes in patients with known or suspected temporal lobe epilepsy. Sadler and Goodwin (28) recorded simultaneously from nasopharyngeal, sphenoidal, minisphenoidal, mandibular notch, surface, T1, and T2 electrodes. Like Binnie et al. (3), they found that T1 and T2 electrodes were as effective as sphenoidal and minisphenoidal electrodes and were significantly superior to nasopharyngeal electrodes. T1 and T2 are placed according to Silverman's (29) recommendations: 1 cm above one-third of the distance from the external auditory meatus to the external canthus (nearer to the former). If there is a question of a medial frontal focus, additional electrodes can be usefully applied near the midline (F1, F2, FC1, FC2, FCz).

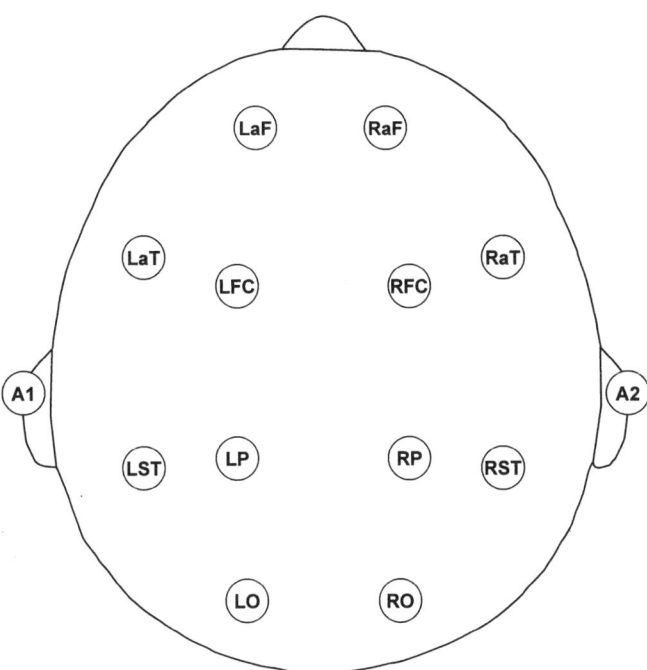

FIG. 4.3. Diagram illustrating the neonatal electrode placements used routinely (12.5% to 25%) at British Columbia Children's Hospital. 1: Measure from nasion to inion and from ear to ear, and mark position one-eighth up from ears, nasion, and inion. 2: Measure head circumference; calculate one-sixteenth, and mark to the left and right of the Fpz position; calculate one-eighth and mark the remainder of the circumference positions. 3: Measure the distance between the anterior temporal electrodes and divide into three parts; repeat for the posterior temporal area. 4: Measure from the frontal-polar to the occipital region, and divide by three.

ELECTROENCEPHALOGRAPHIC DERIVATIONS, POLARITY CONVENTIONS, CALIBRATION, SENSITIVITY, AND FILTER SETTINGS

Derivations

The amplified and filtered output from one recording channel documents the EEG voltage over time across one spatial interval in a relatively undistorted, continuous, and direct display. This appears on paper or video display as a graph of voltage over time. With traditional EEG machines, this potential difference appears in an analog manner as a pen deflection. The direction of the pen, up or down, depends on a polarity convention that is based on whether one input of the amplifier is more positive or negative than the other input.

Polarity Conventions

The two inputs of a differential amplifier are designated *input 1* and *input 2*. In the past, the terms "G1" and "G2" were used, in reference to actual grids in vacuum tubes that were used in the past. The IFSECN has recommended using the terms "input terminal 1" and "input terminal 2" (5). By convention, upward pen deflection occurs either when input 1 is more negative than input 2 or when input 2 is more positive than input 1 (Fig. 4.4). Downward pen deflection occurs if input 1 is more positive than input 2 or if input 2 is more negative than input 1. The polarity convention also specifies that the 10-20 electrode symbols, separated by a dash, designate electrodes connected to the two inputs of an amplifier (e.g., F3-C3 or F4-A2) and that the electrode whose symbol lies to the left of the dash (F3 or F4 in the example) connects to input 1; the amplifier input is indicated by the sign at the top of the calibration signal. Similarly, the electrodes whose symbol lies to the right of the dash (C3

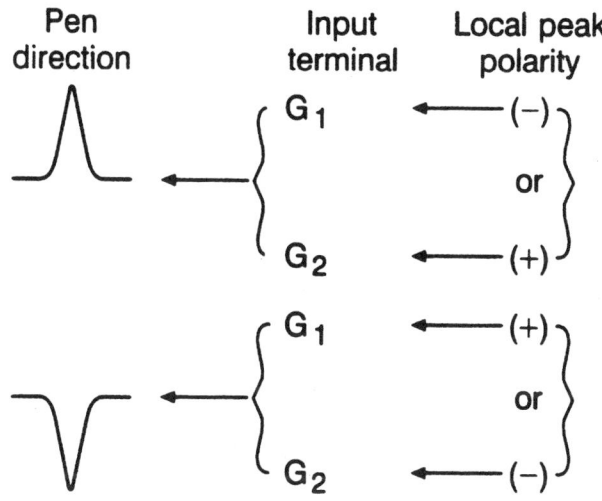

FIG. 4.4. According to the standard polarity convention, an upward signal deflection results if input 1 is more negative than input 2 or if input 2 is more positive than input 1. Conversely, a downward signal deflection results if input 1 is more positive than input 2 or if input 2 is more negative than input 1.

and A2 in the example) are connected to input 2. A single differential amplifier cannot determine absolute polarity. Recording with multiple electrode pairs and displaying EEG activity in several montages enables delineation of the field and determination of the polarity of a given potential.

Calibration and Sensitivity

Individual EEG channels have adjustable controls that allow variation of sensitivity and frequency response. An amplifier's sensitivity (or gain) control changes output voltage; that is, it attenuates the output voltage equally for all input frequencies. Sensitivity is expressed in microvolts per millimeter, which is the input voltage necessary to produce a given amount of vertical deflection and is indicated by a voltage specification placed beside a vertical calibration mark. The EEG instrument's dynamic range specifies the range of input voltages that can be measured accurately from the least to the maximum. The dynamic range is affected not only by the sensitivity setting used but also by the mechanical properties of the display system. During recordings, the technologist should adjust the sensitivity setting as necessary to maintain EEG activity within the system's dynamic range (Fig. 4.5). For ink-writing analog EEG machines, the most important part of calibration is that deflections are measured and carefully observed in all channels, before the start of the EEG recording. For traditional analog paper EEG recordings, the calibration signal also checks pen alignment and time axis. When pen alignment has been adequately adjusted, a sharp signal change applied to every channel should produce a tracing on paper that is exactly synchronized in all channels and of identical deflection amplitude. Obviously, video displays do not use pens and have no alignment problems. In this sense, as in many others, digital EEG systems are considerably more convenient, flexible, and accurate.

A small calibrating voltage, such as a 5-μV input, displayed with a sensitivity of 7 or 7.5 μV per millimeter, produces a very small deflection, less than 1 mm. This should be assessed to determine whether the onset of the wave is rounded or whether the deflection is absent in any channel. An additional biological calibration is essential to ensure that all the amplifiers respond equally and correctly to a variety of frequencies and not just to a direct current signal. This form of calibration is more sensitive to amplifier malfunction. It is also recommended that a second calibration be performed at the end of the EEG recording, with all of the sensitivities and filter settings that were employed during the recording (American Electroencephalographic Society recommendation, 1986). In the particular setting of electrocerebral inactivity, there is a requirement to calibrate with a 1- or 2-μV calibration signal.

With digital technology, calibration need be performed only once, and amplifier gain and direct current offset can be corrected automatically by the system's software to yield the same gain across channels. Calibration at different frequencies can be a built-in automatic function, and this eliminates the need for manual biocalibration (32).

Filters

The range of neurophysiological activity within the brain ranges from between 0.25 and 0.3 Hz to as high as 2,000 Hz (in the cerebellum). Under certain circumstances, as in studies of the contingent negative variation or negative direct current shift and pre-ictal activity, frequencies even slower than 0.25 Hz may be recorded. In studies of evoked potentials, a very broad frequency band is required. The broader the frequency band of the recording is, the greater the fidelity with which the actual neurophysiological activity is reproduced. However, a wide frequency band increases the amount of outside interference and unwanted noise. For this reason, filters are used to preserve, to the greatest extent possible, brain wave activity of interest while minimizing extraneous signals. For routine clinical use, it is usually not necessary to record activity greater than 50 Hz; this is in sharp contrast to evoked potentials, whose signal components reach as high as 5,000 Hz. Filters are components in the amplifier that eliminate unwanted frequencies. A filter is described by the frequency range in which signals are amplified without significant distortion. For EEG activity, more than 70% attenuation of a particular frequency component by a filter results in significant distortion. In addition, conventional pen writing mechanisms are incapable of recording activity above 100 Hz accurately.

The instrument's frequency response capabilities are adjustable (19,30). The high-frequency filter, also referred to as the low-pass filter, affects high-frequency activity. A commonly used high-frequency filter setting is 70 Hz; on occasion, 35 Hz is used. The number refers to the particular frequency that has been reduced or attenuated in amplitude. The percentage attenuation varies with the filter characteristic called "rolloff." Thus, a 70-Hz filter affects the designated 70-Hz frequency by 20% to 60% (depending on roll-off) but has much less effect on lower frequencies. In contrast, frequencies above 70 Hz are attenuated to a much greater degree. In the context of epileptiform activity, it is critical that the filters be set so that fast components represented in spikes are not attenuated or distorted. For example, too low a high-frequency filter setting results in spikes that have the appearance of beta activity (Fig. 4.6).

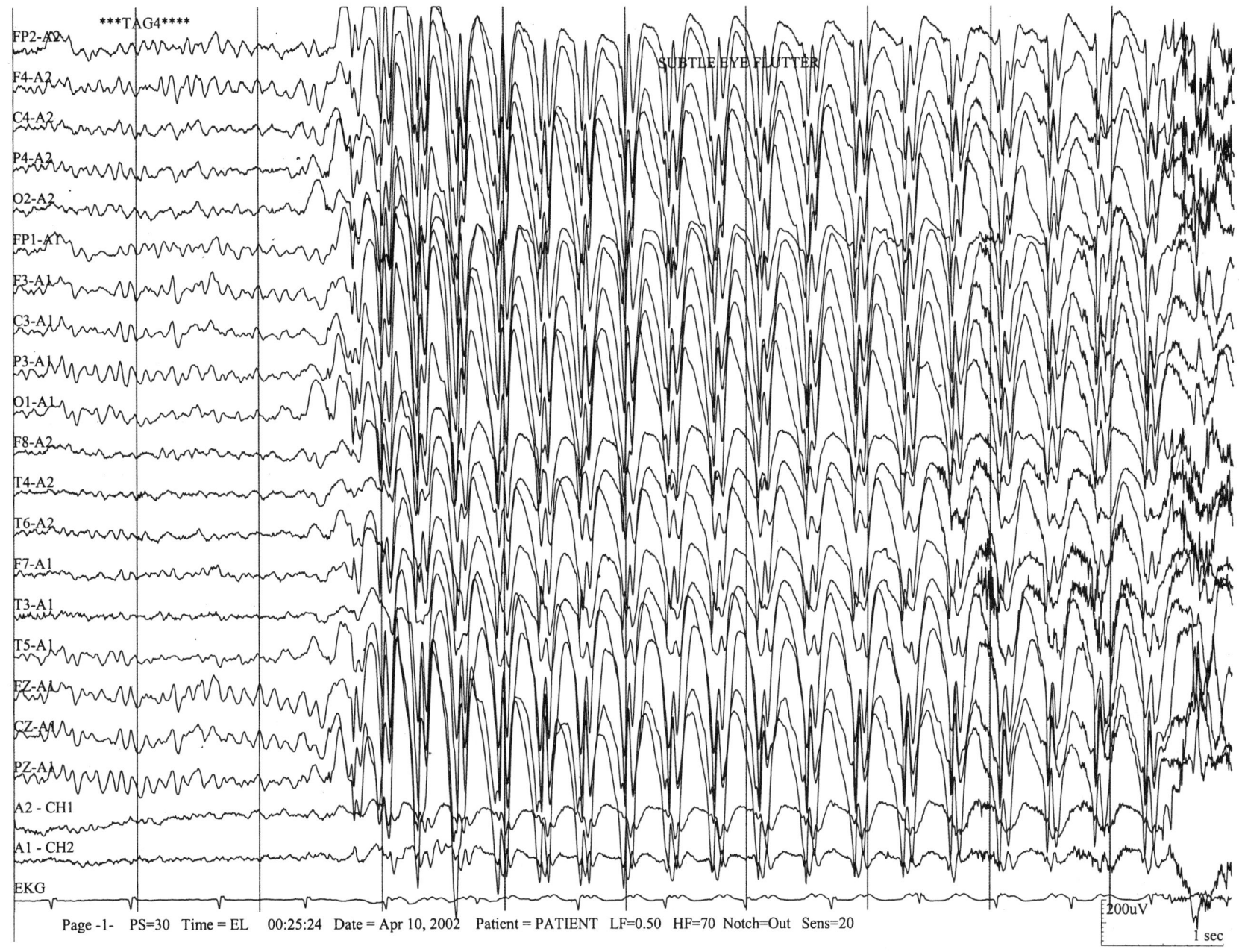

FIG. 4.5. **A:** Generalized 3-Hz spike-wave recorded at a sensitivity of 20 μV/mm; this setting results in clipping of the wave component. **B:** Similar burst of a 3-Hz spike-wave activity as in part *A* but displayed with a sensitivity of 50 μV/mm. (*Figure continues.*)

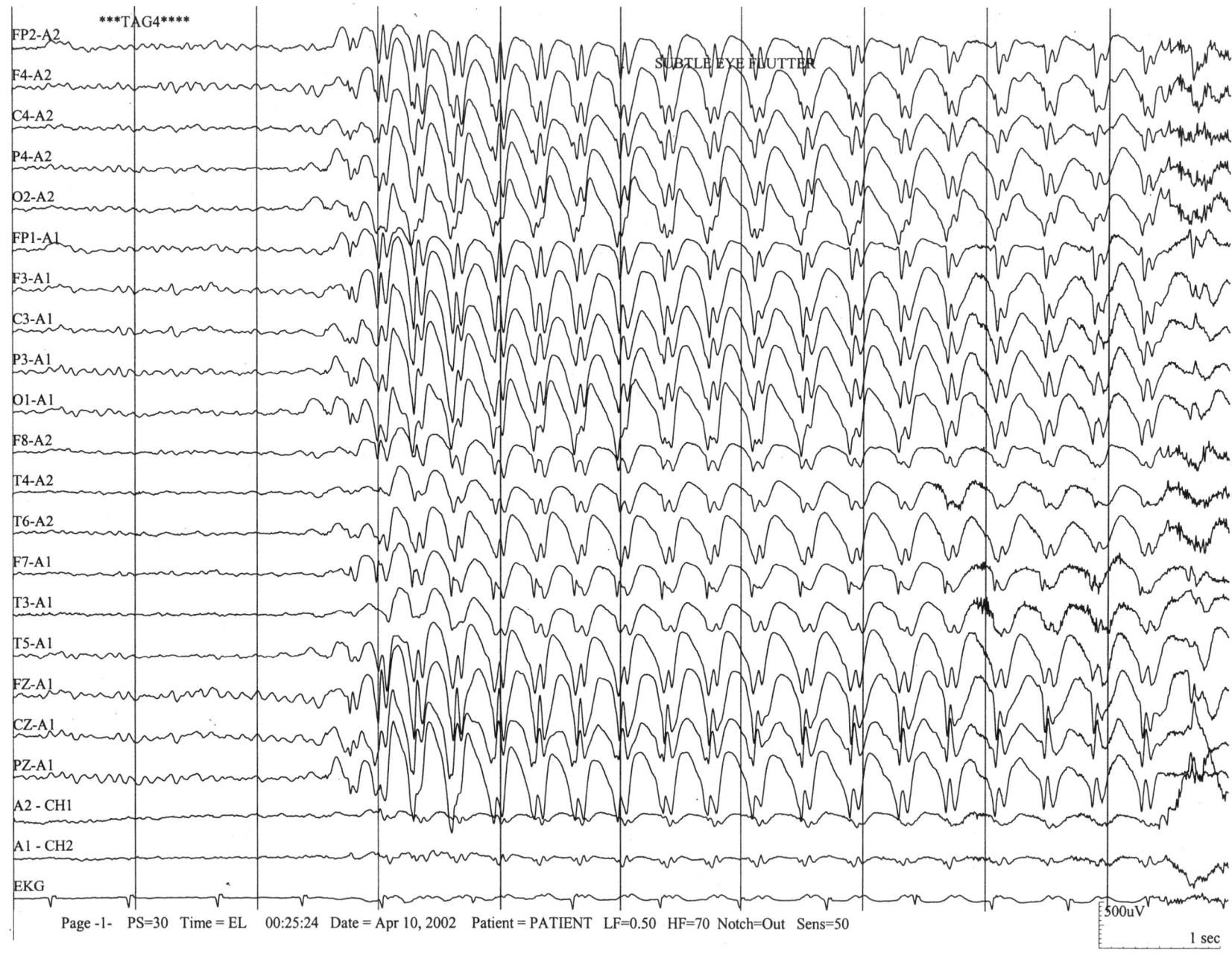

FIG. 4.5. *Continued.*

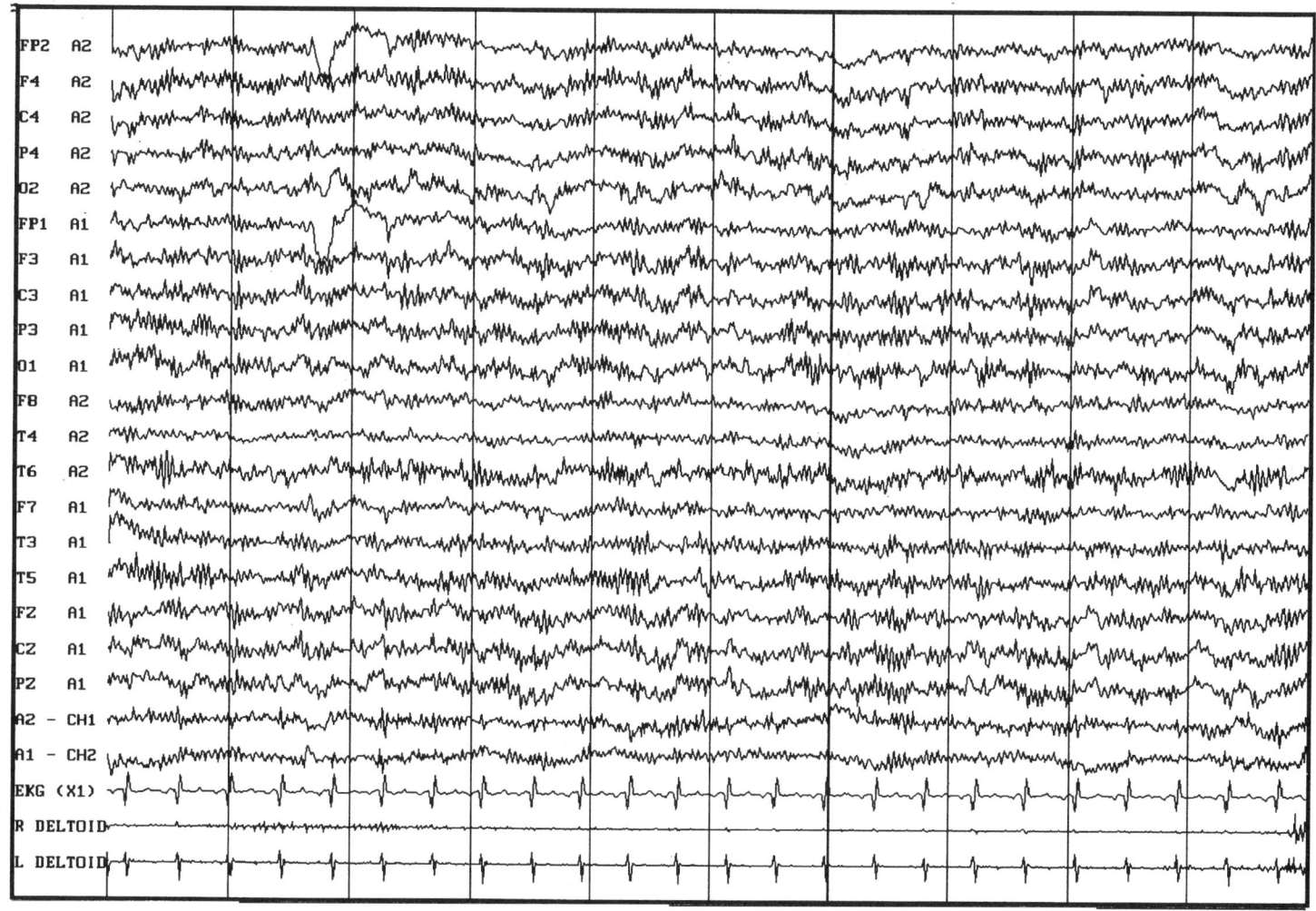

FIG. 4.6. A: Generalized beta activity recorded with sensitivity of 15 µV/mm, a high-frequency filter setting of 70 Hz, and a low-frequency filter setting of 0.5 Hz. **B:** Generalized beta activity displayed with sensitivity and low-frequency filter settings the same as in part A but with a high-frequency filter setting of 35 Hz. This results in attenuation of some beta activity. **C:** Generalized beta activity displayed with sensitivity and low-frequency filter settings as in part A but with a high-frequency filter setting of 15 Hz. There is even more marked attenuation of beta activity and distortion, resulting in spike-like transients. (*Figure continues.*)

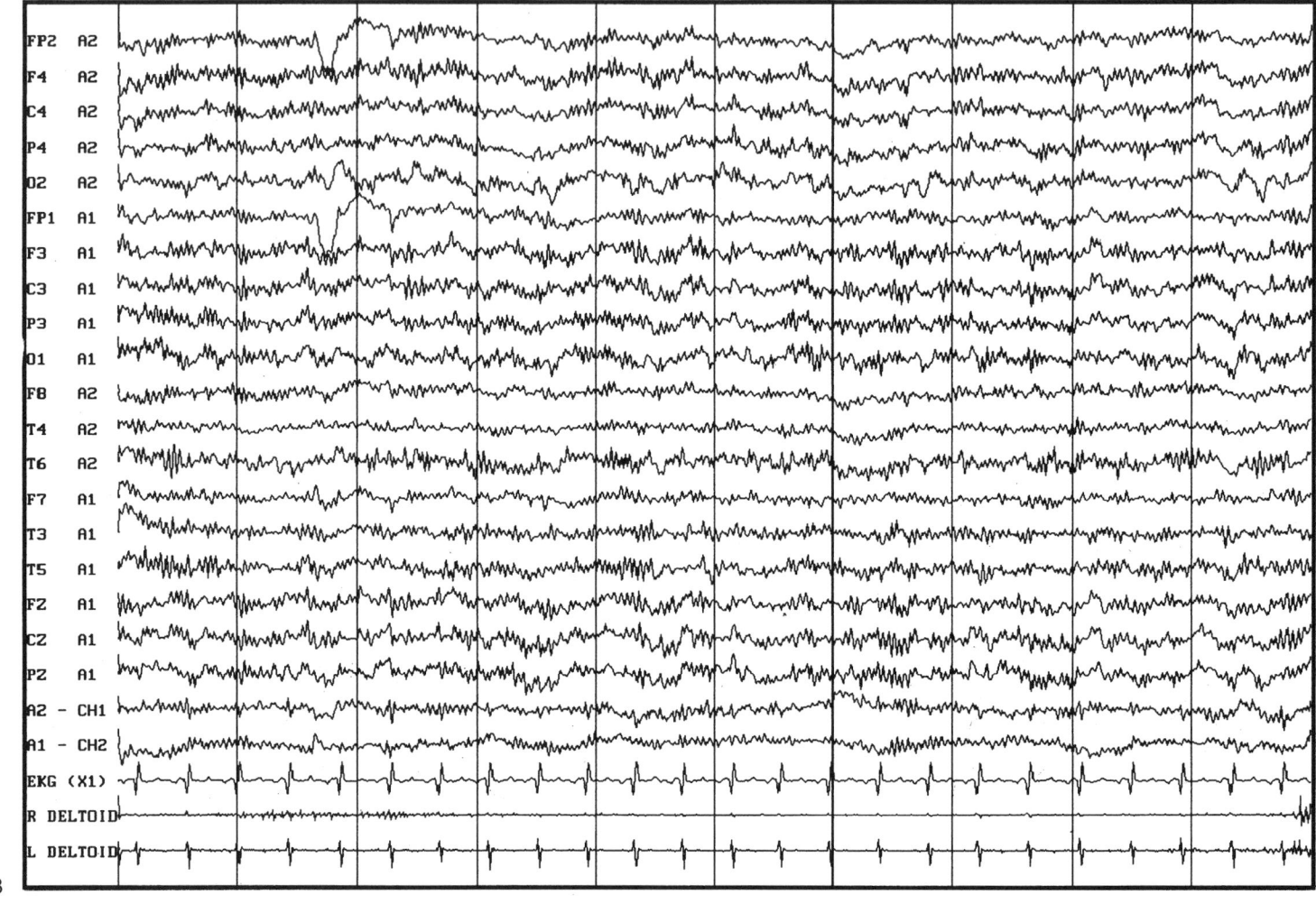

FIG. 4.6. *Continued.*

Low-frequency filter settings identify the lower frequency limits below which the amplifier progressively attenuates and distorts physiological signals. Above this limit, the amplifier does not distort signals to a significant degree. Low-frequency filters are also referred to as high-pass filters because they allow higher frequencies above the specified frequencies to pass largely unchanged. The effect of a low-frequency filter is determined by its time constant. In the simple traditional amplifier, one time constant (TC) is calculated by multiplying resistance by capacitance. Time constant can also be defined as the time it takes for a square-wave deflection to decline 63% from its peak or as the time it takes for a square-wave signal deflection to drop within 37% of the baseline. The terms *time constant* and *low frequency* are used interchangeably in practice to describe a low filter's

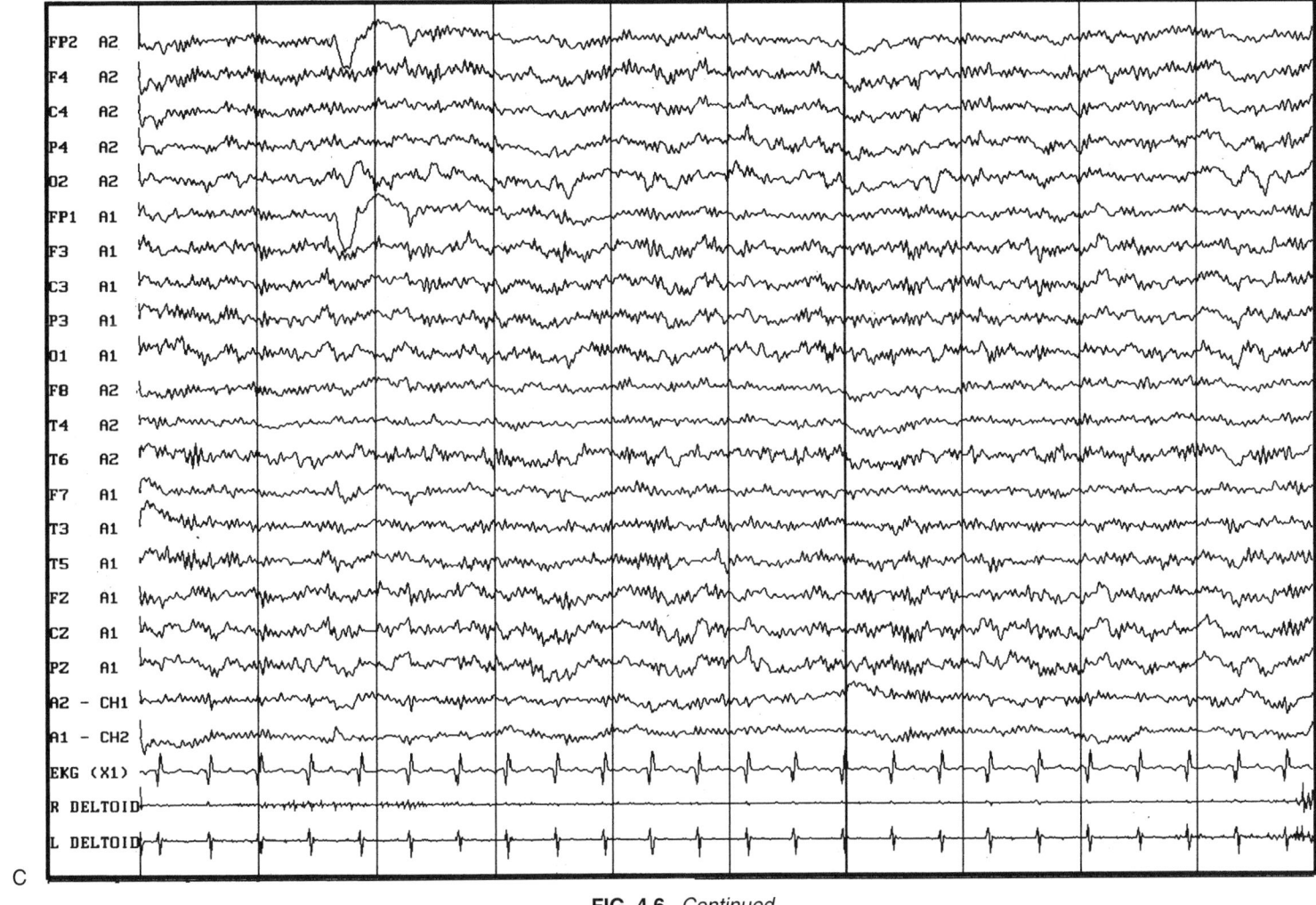

FIG. 4.6. *Continued.*

effect on slower activity, but they are distinct terms and are specified differently. For example, a time constant of 1 second represents a low-frequency filter of 0.1 or 0.16 Hz, depending on the filter roll-off involved; a time constant of 0.3 seconds represents a low-frequency filter of 0.5 Hz. Knowledgeable use of the low-frequency filter increases the yield of important clinical information. For example, in a record dominated by slow activity, short time constants or narrow low-frequency filters attenuate most delta activity (Fig. 4.7) but allow faster frequencies to be displayed more clearly. This may facilitate recognition of asymmetries of faster frequency patterns, such as sleep spindles or beta activity.

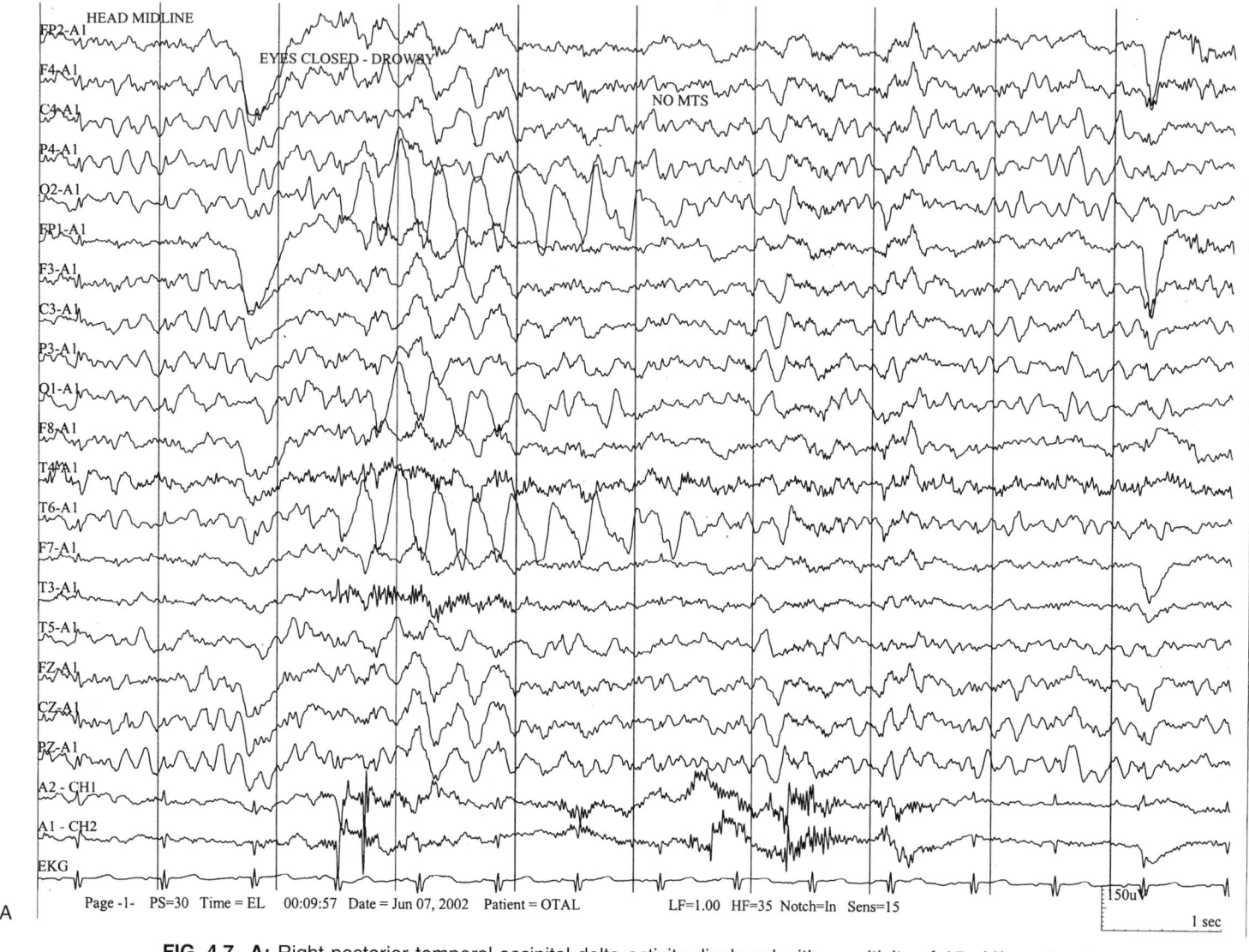

FIG. 4.7. A: Right posterior temporal-occipital delta activity displayed with sensitivity of 15 μV/mm, low-frequency filter setting of 1 Hz, and high-frequency filter setting of 35 Hz. **B:** Same delta activity displayed with low-frequency filter setting of 3 Hz and with sensitivity and high-frequency filter settings as in part *A*. Note mild attenuation of right posterior delta activity. **C:** Same EEG sample but with low-frequency filter setting of 10 Hz and high-frequency filter and sensitivity settings as in part *A*. There is now marked attenuation of right posterior delta activity. **D:** The right posterior delta activity is enhanced with a display speed of 15mm/sec (sensitivity of 20 μV/mm in this example). (*Figure continues.*)

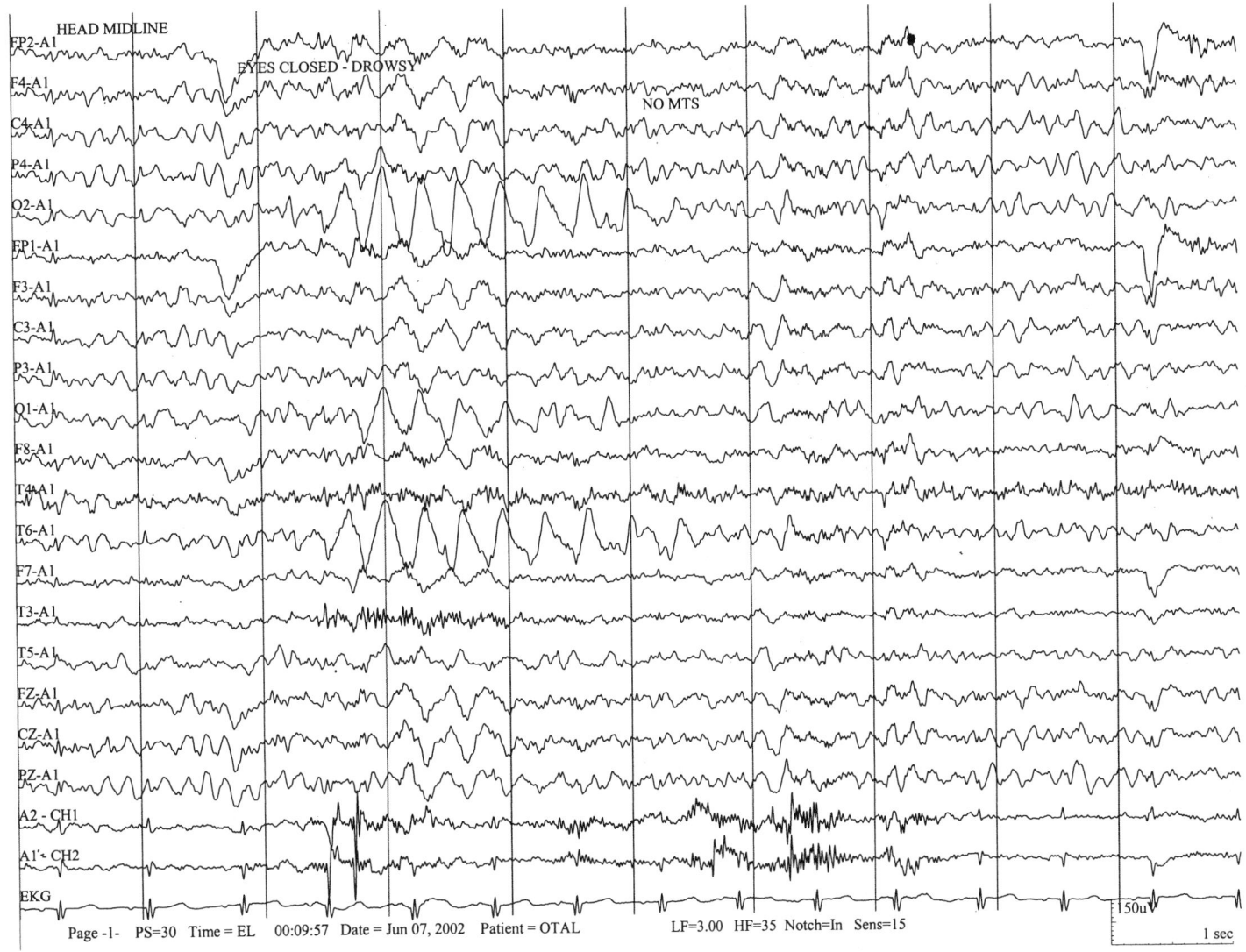

FIG. 4.7. *Continued.*

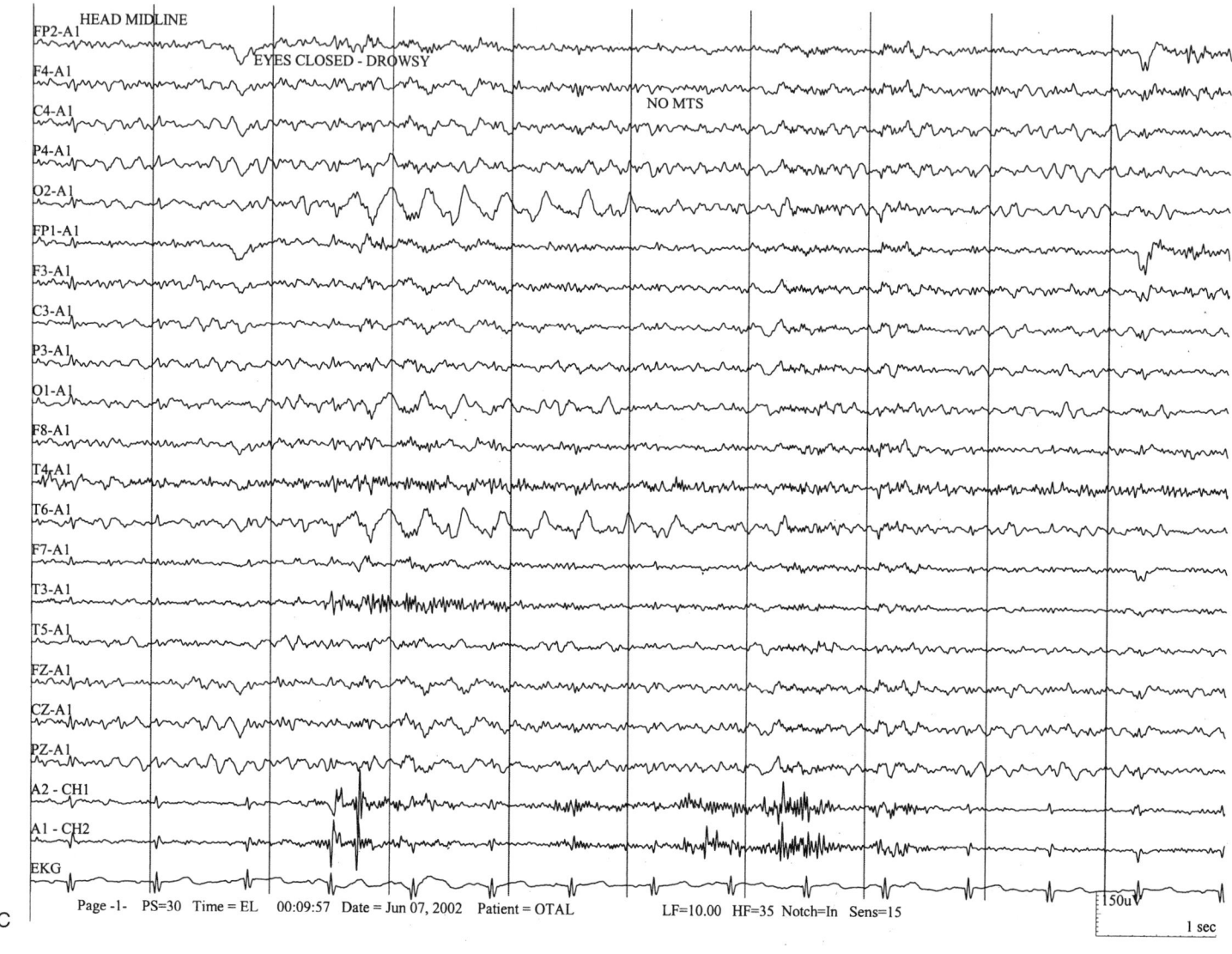

FIG. 4.7. *Continued.*

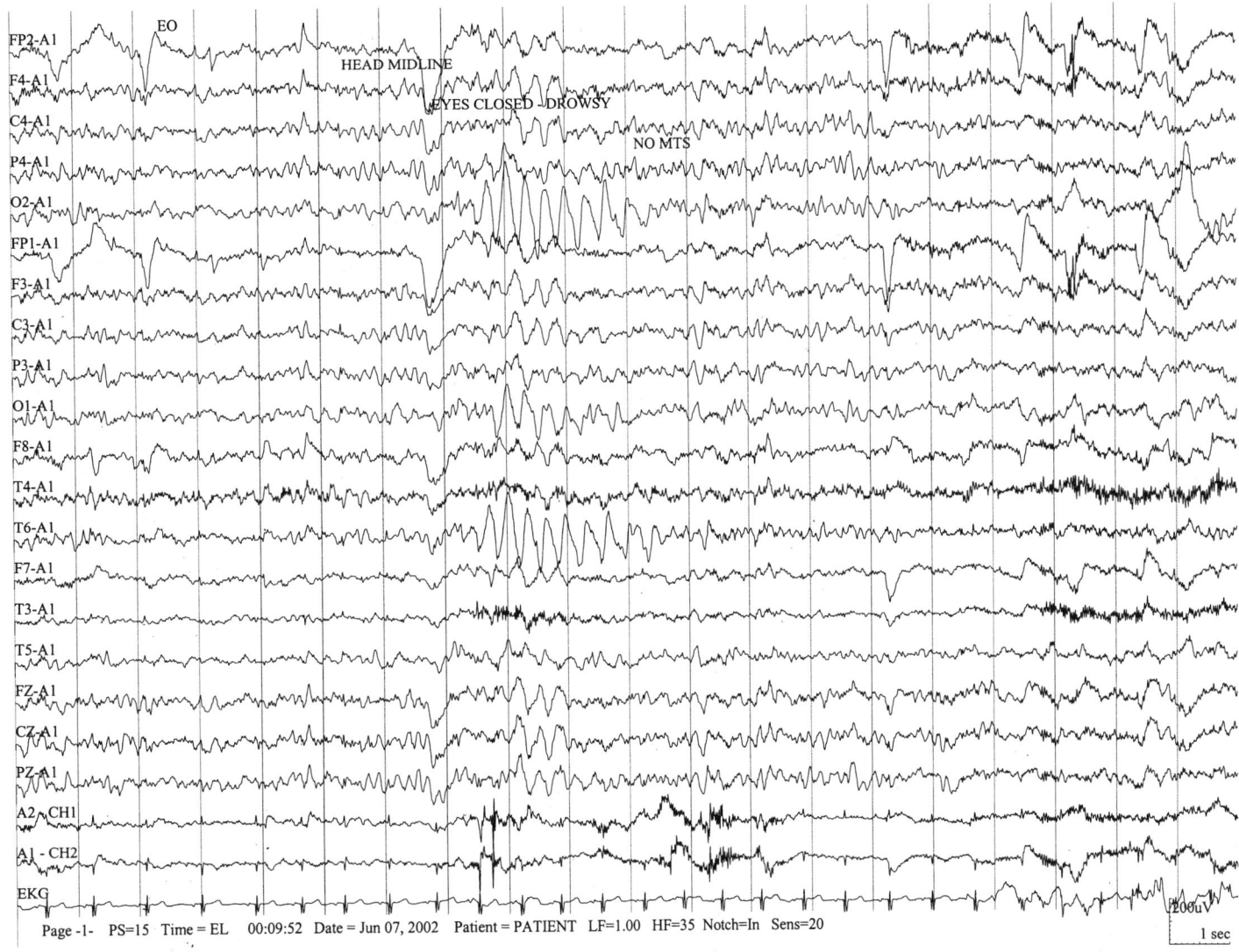

FIG. 4.7. *Continued.*

MONTAGES

Common conventional montages, even with logically organized series of channels, distort spatial information by converting complex patterns of EEG activity originating in three dimensions to a series of channels whose output displays are horizontal, spatially discontinuous, and variable. Spatial delineation of fields has improved steadily as advances in technology have led to a steady increase in the number of recording channels available, but spatial sampling, although vastly improved, is still fraught with problems even today. In addition, the electroencephalographer infers the spatial distribution of EEG activity only indirectly, by cross-comparing activity from different channels. Even this presentation is distorted, however, because a grid of electrodes, each with up to four neighbors (anterior and posterior sagittally and left and right coronally), appears as a series of channels with only two vertical (upper and lower) neighbors on a typical EEG display. Thus, EEG montages unavoidably distort spatial relations among electrodes, because the visual presentation has fewer dimensions that the reality that it depicts (consider the analogous distortions that occur in maps based on Mercator projections of the earth).

Like other inherent mapping distortions, a given EEG montage tends to preserve spatial relationships of electrodes in one direction better than in others. Therefore, a montage is classified as longitudinal if it preserves spatial relations best between electrodes in the sagittal direction and as transverse if it better preserves spatial relations in the coronal direction.

Montages may be classified as unpaired, electroanatomical paired-group, or paired-channel and as referential, bipolar, or laplacian (source derivation). In longitudinal montages, channels are arranged along sagittal lines. Adjacent channels within a sagittal line may either link in bipolar chains or connect to a reference. In transverse montages, channels are arranged in coronal lines.

Unpaired, Paired-Group, and Paired-Channel Montages

In unpaired longitudinal or transverse montages, channels are arranged in anatomical neighboring sequences: for example, sequentially from front to back or from left to right. These are often referred to as *electroanatomical* groupings (19). In paired-group montages, electrodes are arranged from homologous areas of the scalp by placing together left and right temporal, or left and right parasagittal, linkages. Paired-group arrangements apply only to longitudinal montages because the brain does not have functional or anatomical symmetry in the coronal direction. In paired-channel montages, channels from homologous brain areas are paired. Left and right pairs are then subgrouped together in longitudinal lines (e.g, a line of temporal pairs and a line of parasagittal pairs). Midline electrodes cannot be paired.

The characteristics of these montage arrangements are different in terms of the accuracy of voltage representation (distortion) and display of any asymmetry:

Unpaired	Least distortion, worst display of symmetry
Paired-group	Fair distortion, fair display of symmetry
Paired-channel	Most distortion, best display of symmetry

Display Conventions

In montages, electrodes are arranged in anterior-posterior sequences. For longitudinal montages, this means that frontal electrodes precede central, parietal, and occipital electrodes; anterior temporal electrodes precede midtemporal and posterior temporal electrodes. For transverse montages, electrodes are also displayed in a front-to-back sequence. The left-right convention dictates that for unpaired longitudinal montages, left-sided channels are placed above right-sided channels. In transverse montages, each line of channels proceeds from left to right. For paired longitudinal montages, left-sided channels appear above the homologous grouping of right-sided channels. These left-right displays are used widely throughout North America and conform to the guidelines of the American Electroencephalographic Society (1). However, the reverse convention of "right over left" is used routinely in Europe and is recommended by the IFSECN (18).

Referential, Bipolar, and Laplacian Montages

Localizing voltage peaks within a potential field requires a line of electrodes crossing the field's maximal potential. For longitudinal or transverse linkages, the clinician attempts to identify one or more electrodes that register the peak potential more than other electrodes within the field. More precise localization requires identifying the maximally involved electrode or electrodes in both sagittal and coronal directions. Such multiple direction readings give information about the topography of the peak. This means that for any voltage peak, the potential recorded by that electrode is greater than the potentials seen simultaneously by its four immediate neighbors. For example, a right frontal potential field can be localized to F4 if the voltage peak at F4 is larger than the voltage change seen simultaneously at FP2, C4, FZ, and F8. Problems in localization arise if peaks lie at the perimeter of an electrode grid (end of the chain) (Fig. 4.8). Localization is commonly achieved with appropriate combinations of referential and bipolar montages (Fig. 4.9). The laplacian source derivation method may also be helpful (9,14,15,23,24,27,28).

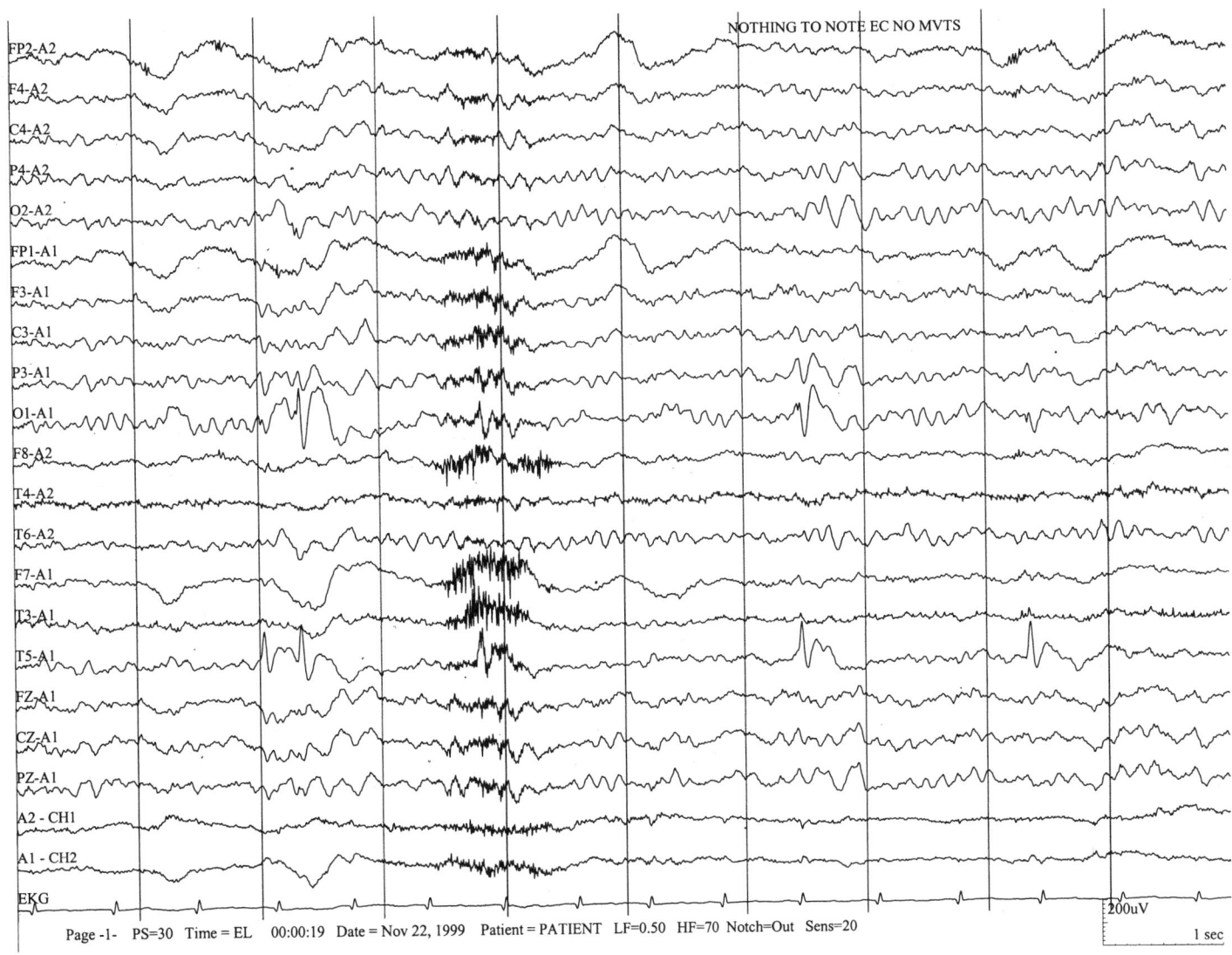

FIG. 4.8. A: Left occipito-temporal spikes displayed with sensitivity of 15 µV/mm, low-frequency filter setting of 1 Hz, and high-frequency filter setting of 70 Hz. **B:** Same spikes as in part *A*, displayed in a bipolar longitudinal montage, which enables accurate localization to the T5 and O1 electrodes. (*Figure continues.*)

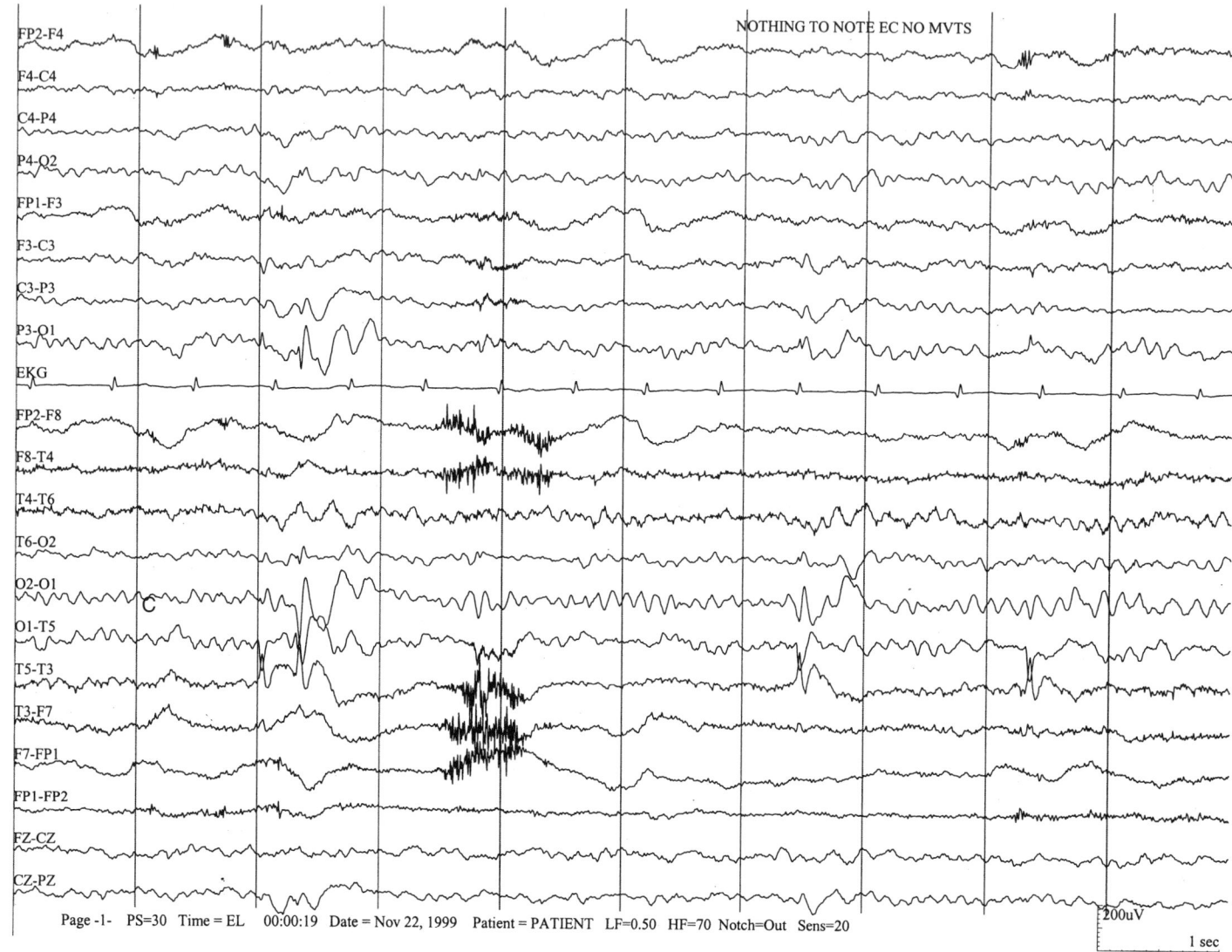

FIG. 4.8. *Continued.*

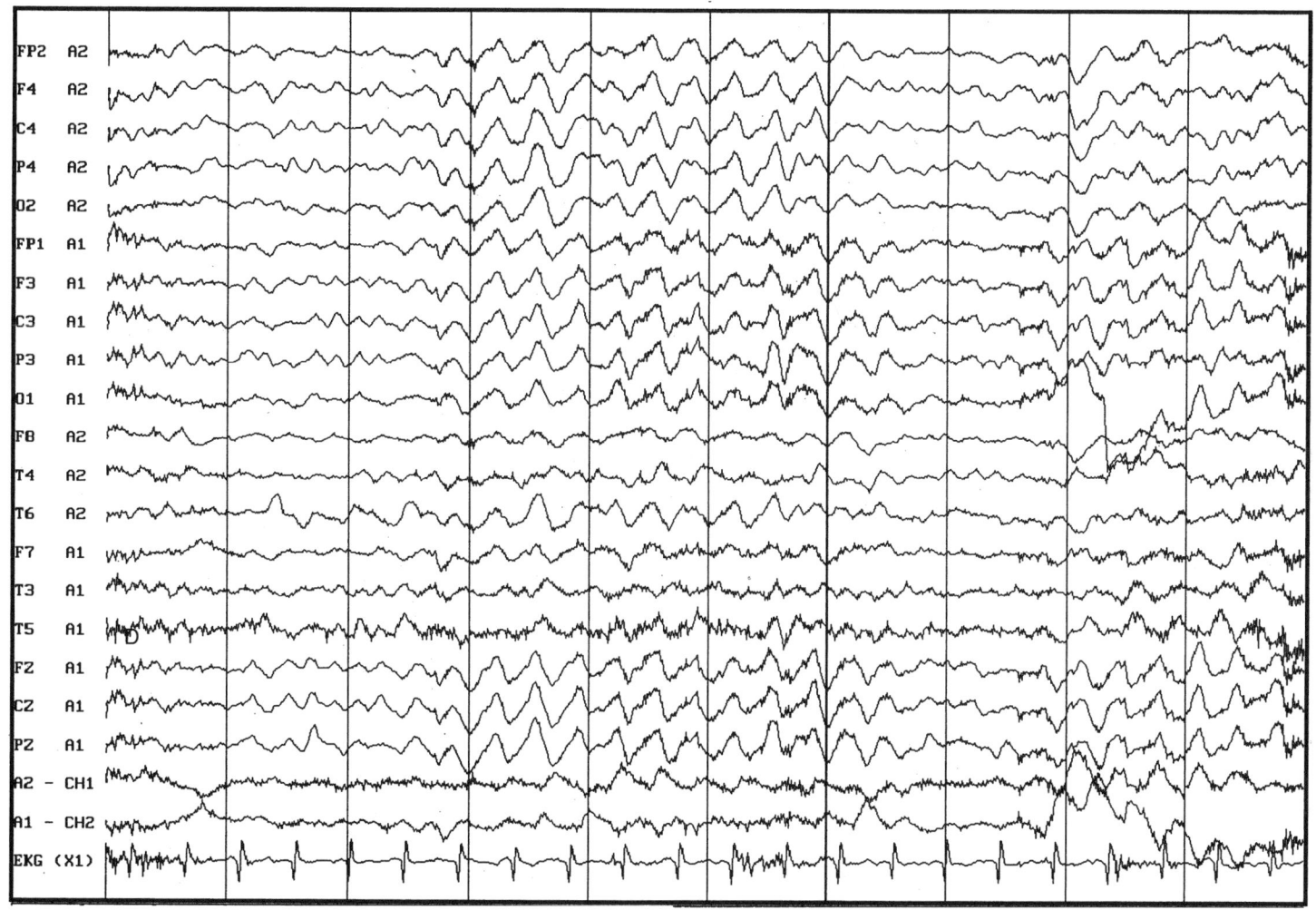

A

FIG. 4.9. A: Temporal delta activity recorded with an ipsilateral ear reference montage, a sensitivity of 50 μV/mm, a low-frequency filter setting of 0.5 Hz, and a high-frequency filter setting of 70 Hz. Delta activity in both temporal regions makes A1 and A2 active and thus poor references. **B:** Temporal delta activity in part *A* displayed on a bipolar montage, which permits accurate localization. (*Figure continues.*)

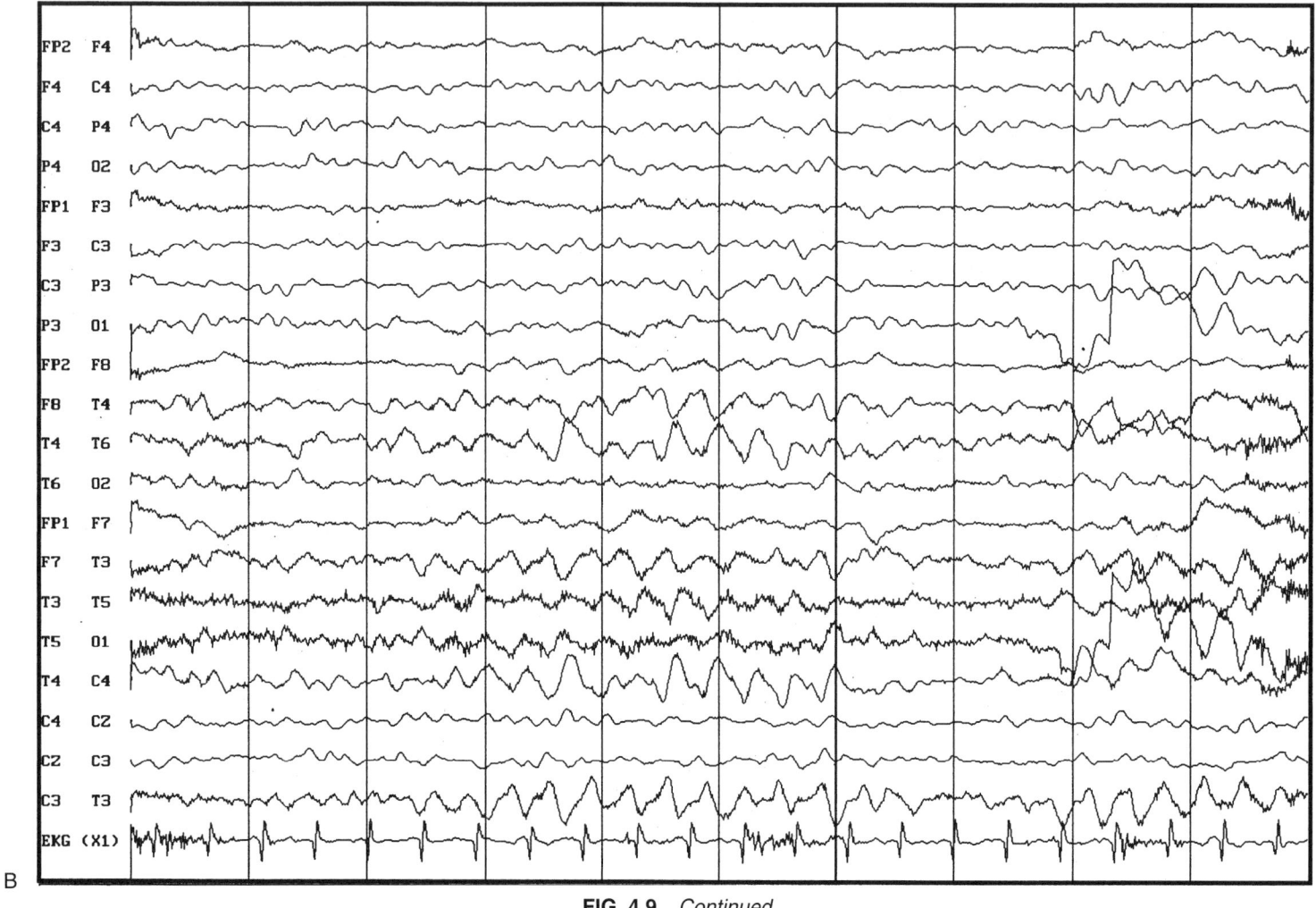

FIG. 4.9. *Continued.*

Referential Montages

In referential montages, a common reference electrode is connected to input 2 of each amplifier. Ideally, for each pair of electrodes in a channel, only one (input 1) is active. This situation is never achieved in real life, because the common reference site is always active to some degree and therefore invari-

ably contributes to the output signal (19). In the past, referential recording was also referred to as *monopolar* recording. The types of reference electrodes used include A1 and A2 ("ipsilateral ears"); A1 plus A2 ("linked ears") (28); Cz, a balanced noncephalic reference such as the neck-chest region; and the average reference ("Goldman-Offner"). The average reference is traditionally derived electronically by interconnecting all active scalp electrodes (all those of input 1) (13). The clinician can delete selectively from the average one or more electrodes that may contribute disproportionately high voltage activity to the reference, such as frontal leads showing prominent eye movements or electrodes over an area of focal slowing or epileptiform activity.

With digital recordings, a true average reference can be created with any combination of two or more electrodes. As long as electrodes connected to input 1 are more active than the input 2 common reference, a referential montage clearly displays a potential's polarity and voltage field. Selection of a reference site is important. If the selected reference site lies within the field of interest, it is "active"; this makes it difficult or impossible to determine polarity and spatial distribution of the field. A major advantage of digital recording techniques is that they allow reformatting of the EEG with different montages, including those uniquely created for individual patients. The following are examples:

1. A left temporal discharge contaminating the left ear reference and reformatted with the contralateral ear as a reference. The field and amplitude of the discharge can be more readily determined (Figs. 4.10*A* and *B*).
2. A left temporal spike contaminating an ear reference. This can be eliminated by changing the reference to bipolar (see Fig. 4.10*C*) and enhanced by increasing the paper speed (see Fig. 4.10*D*).

Bipolar Montages

In bipolar recordings, both input 1 and input 2 are connected to active recording electrodes. No single electrode is common to input 1 or input 2. Bipolar montages link sequential pairs of electrodes in longitudinal or coronal lines. In linked chains, a single electrode becomes common to two adjacent channels, but it is connected to input 2 in the first channel and to input 1 in the second channel. The site of maximal voltage within a field appears as a phase reversal; that is, simultaneous deflections in two channels sharing a common electrode occur in opposite directions. The direction of the phase reversal (deflections coming together for local negative peaks or diverging for local positive peaks) assists in determining polarity. If the voltage peaks involve two adjacent electrodes equally—for example, F4 and C4—they are equipotential. If equipotential electrodes connect to input 1 and input 2, there is *in-phase* cancellation, and no output appears in that channel. Localizing by phase reversal is possible only if bipolar montages fully encompass the site of maximal voltage in both longitudinal and transverse directions. A phase reversal does not occur unless the electrode chain fully encompasses a local voltage peak. For example, a negative voltage gradient increasing from C3 to P3 to O1 (as with an occipital spike) does not show a phase reversal, and only a downward deflection is seen. Addition of a suboccipital electrode may reveal a phase reversal if the discharge is maximal at O1.

Bipolar montages are most useful in defining localized potential gradients. Of importance, however, is that the deflection in a particular channel is greatest when the voltage gradient between the two electrodes is steepest, *not* necessarily when the absolute voltage is largest. This is an important distinction between bipolar and referential recordings. Other advantages of bipolar montages include (a) eliminating the effect of contaminated references (see Fig. 4.10); (b) easy localization of relatively discrete focal abnormalities by phase reversal; and (c) avoiding problems that can arise from unbalanced amplifier inputs with a common reference. On the other hand, it is possible only to infer (and not compare directly) activity from individual electrodes, and voltage and polarity determinations are always positive. Referential recordings allow clear characterization of widespread or complex potential fields, unambiguous determinations of voltage polarity, and less distortion of EEG patterns exhibiting time lags across the scalp. The major disadvantage of referential recording is that no single reference electrode or method is optimal for all situations, inasmuch as no reference is truly inactive; thus, it is crucial to select an appropriate reference for a particular situation (34). Using the same reference routinely and without thought largely invalidates the advantages offered by a referential recording. With regard to the relation between bipolar and referential montages, it is helpful to remember that they are simply mathematical transformations of one another. For example, converting absolute voltage-to-voltage difference is only a matter of computing the voltage gradient of spatially continuous voltage fields (the first spatial derivative) inferred from longitudinal and transverse electrode arrays displaying discrete fields. Bipolar-to-referential transformation is analogous to integrating an electrical field's voltage gradient in relation to a fixed site to obtain the voltages at individual electrodes. This conceptual parallel between manipulations of spatially discontinuous EEG data and spatially continuous electrical field data assists in understanding laplacian source derivations.

Laplacian Montages

In the laplacian source derivation, voltages at each electrode site are compared with a local average of voltages at immediately surrounding electrodes. Operationally, this means that each channel measures the voltage difference between the electrode of interest (input 1) and a reference (input 2) derived from the average voltage of its nearest neighbor. For example, for F4, the simplest value of the local average would consist of

$$(FP2 + C4 + FZ + F8)/4$$

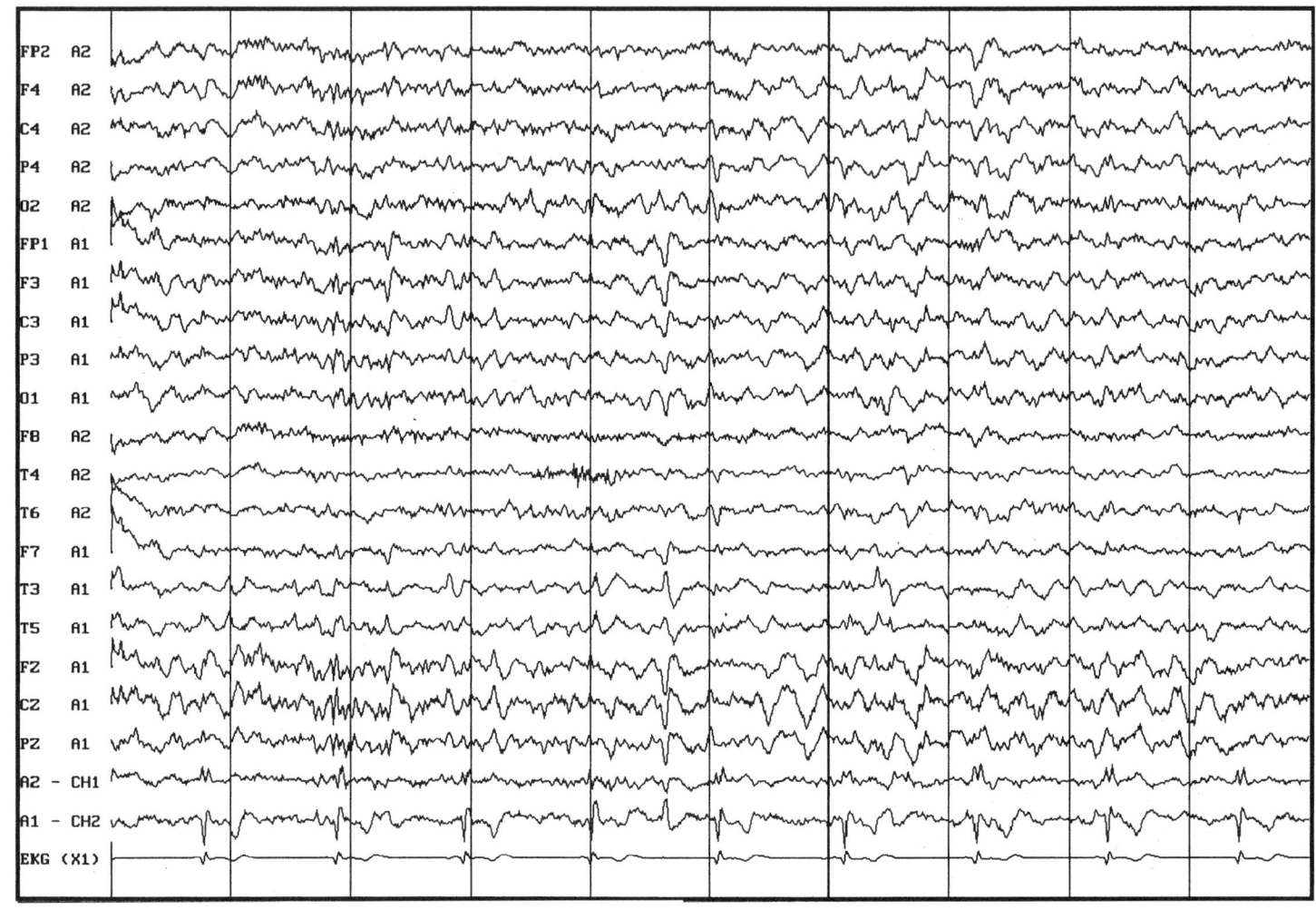

A

FIG. 4.10. A: Left mid-temporal spike makes A1 active when used as a reference. **B:** Left mid-temporal spike displayed with A2 as the reference. **C:** Same left mid-temporal spike displayed on a bipolar montage allows localization by phase reversal. **D:** Same left mid-temporal spike as in B displayed with paper speed of 60mm/sec. (*Figure continues.*)

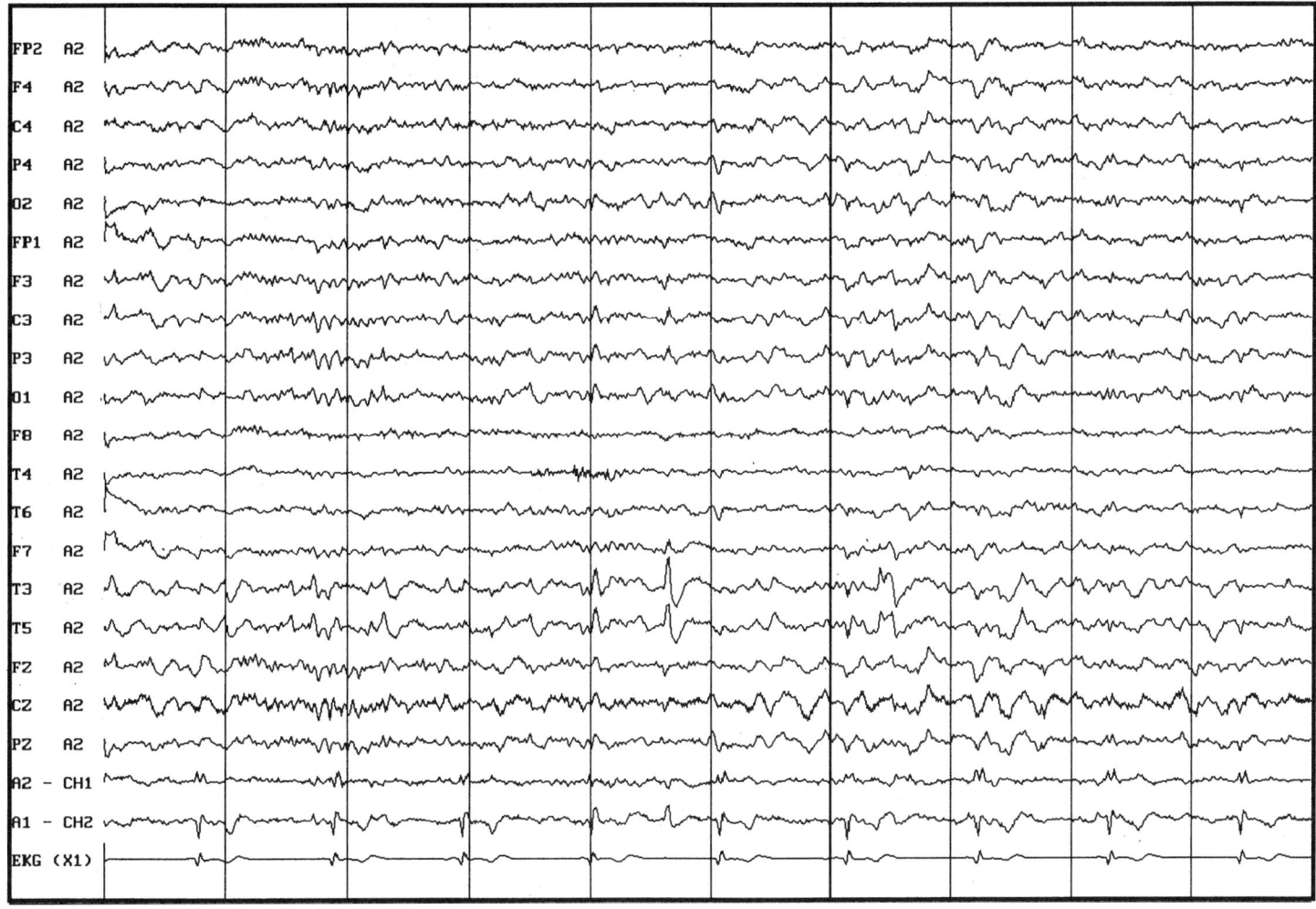

FIG. 4.10. *Continued.*

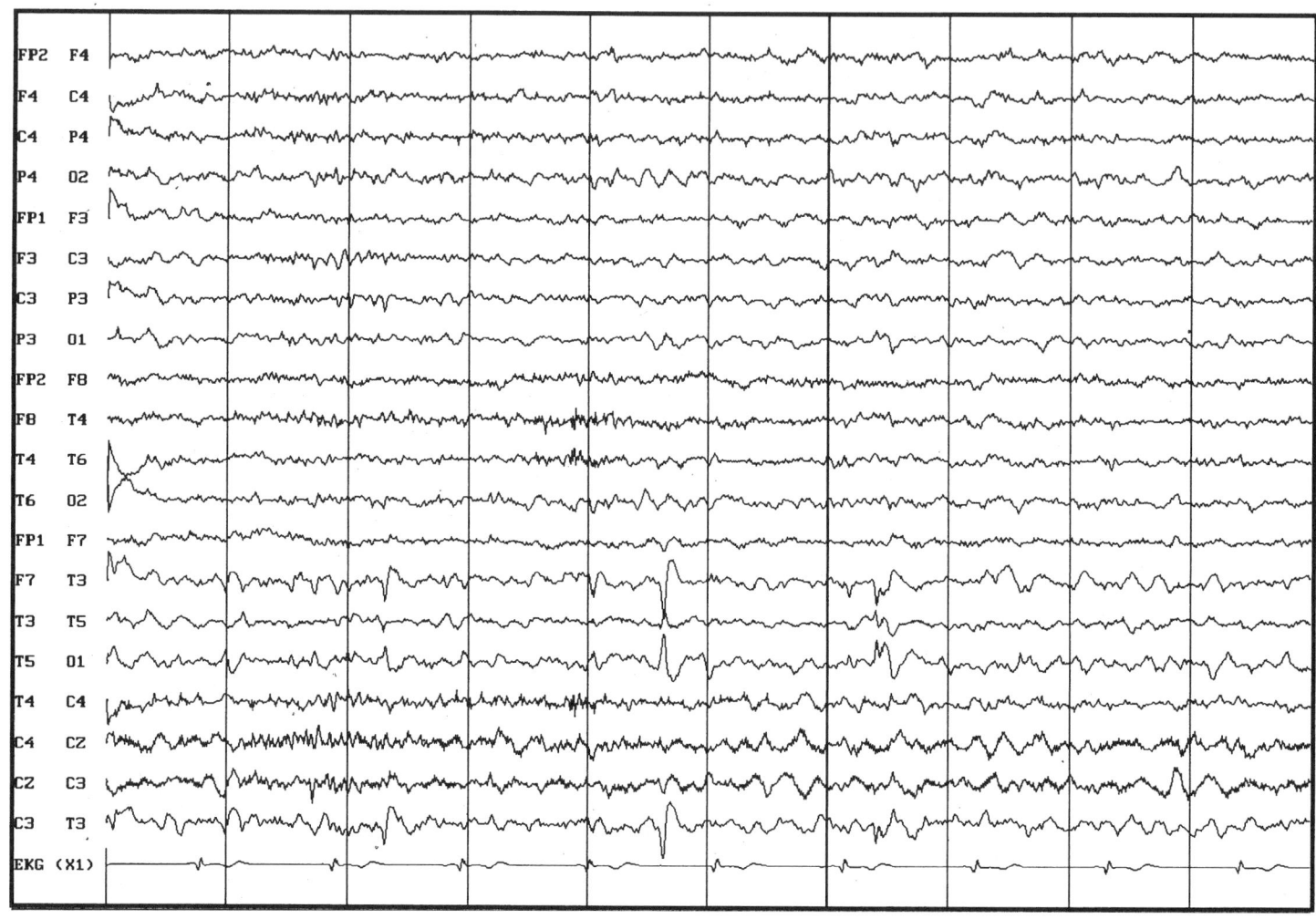

C

FIG. 4.10. *Continued.*

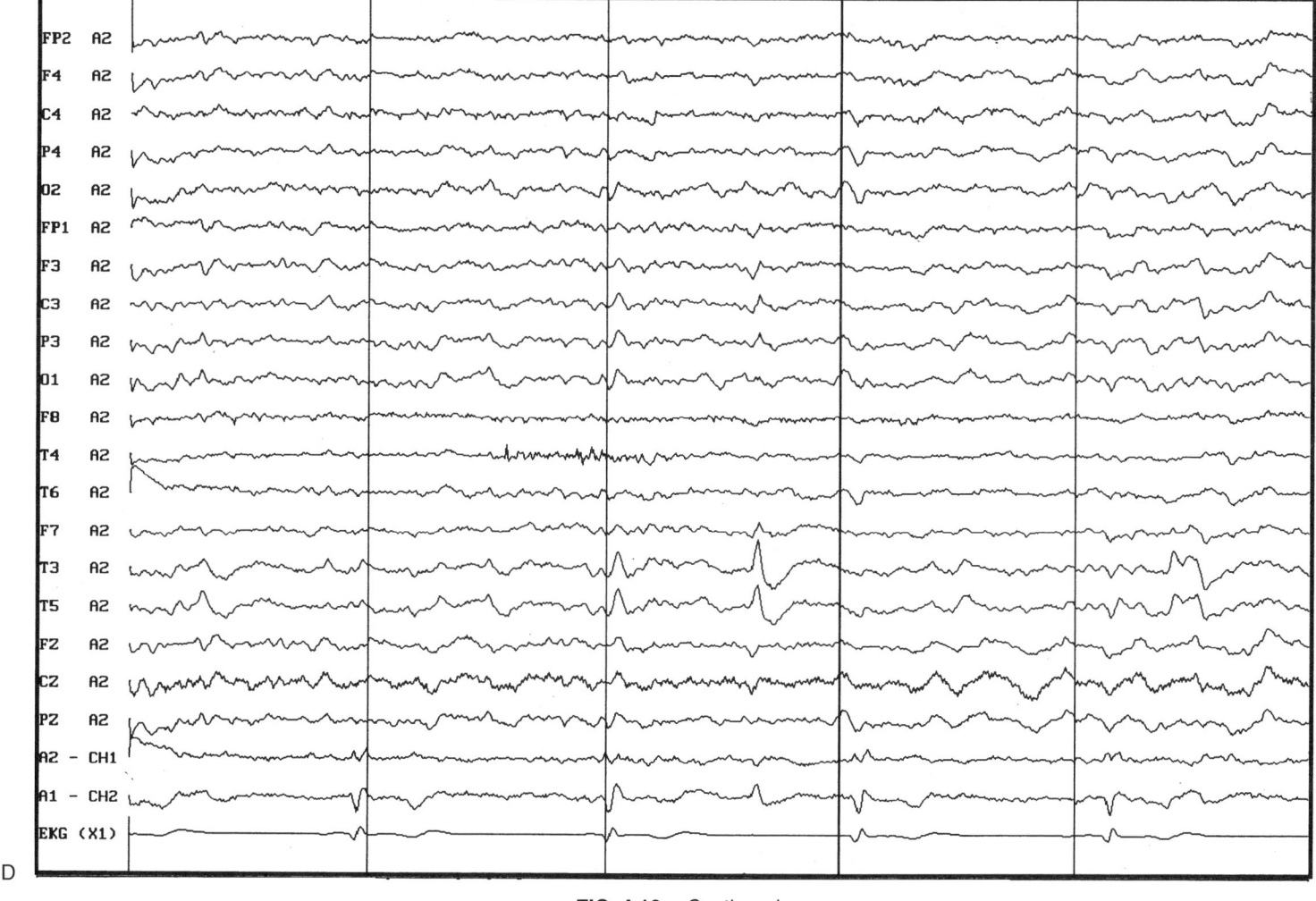

D

FIG. 4.10. *Continued.*

Because it involves discontinuous measurements from closely spaced electrodes, the source derivation only *approximates* the true mathematical laplacian display of the electrical field, which is a continuous mathematical function representing the second spatial derivative of the field. The output of any channel is proportional to the intensity of local current sources or sinks. Consequently, source derivation combines attributes of both bipolar and referential recording methods. Source derivation montages emphasize regions of local voltage peaks and deemphasize widely distributed activity, much as do bipolar derivations. Voltage peaks are localized to the channel of maximal deflection, and polarity is accurately indicated by direction of signal movement, as with common reference recording. True laplacian source derivations eliminate concern for an active reference. In practice, however, neighborhood average approximations with large interelectrode distances (approximately 5 cm, as seen with 21 scalp channels) and without symmetry among nearest neighbors (as with edge electrodes such as Fp1/2, F7/8, and O1/2) cause spatial aliasing, the equivalent of an active reference (9,14,15,24,26). This may result in falsely localized voltage peaks, spurious phase reversals, and inaccurate inferences about field distribution. These limitations are lessened, although not eliminated, by the use of more electrodes to provide a denser array (e.g., 128 scalp electrodes).

Hjorth (14,15) addressed the interelectrode distance problem by including in the local average some additional electrodes lying on lines diagonal to the electrode of interest and weighting their contribution as a function of distance. For electrodes of a grid (e.g., Fp1/2, F7/8) with only three neighbors, adding inferior electrodes minimizes spatial aliasing in the laplacian estimate. The mathematical basis of the laplacian transform, as well as the derivation of the laplacian operator, is quite complex and beyond the scope of this discussion. Nunez (23) discussed this quantitatively. The practical use of laplacian derivations has been limited because of difficulty in applying them to conventional EEG hardware. However, with the computer-based EEG machines now widely available, coupled with denser electrode arrays, laplacian derivations are easier to apply.

Selection of Montages

The three types of montages just described can be viewed as three types of input to input 2: (a) Input 2 is the nearest neighboring electrode and changes from channel to channel (bipolar derivation); (b) input 2 is a distant electrode common to all channels (common reference); or (c) input 2 is computed (A1 plus A2 average, common average, and laplacian reference). The "averaged ears" reference and common average reference remain the same in all channels; the laplacian reference differs from channel to channel. Each type of montage has advantages and disadvantages. Optimal EEG recording combines referential and bipolar methods. Comprehensive and accurate assessment of potential fields requires combining all methods intelligently (16,19,22).

Table 4.1 lists eight logical arrangements for referential and bipolar montages. The American Electroencephalographic Society recommended that each laboratory routinely use one of several alternatives from each major group: longitudinal referential, longitudinal bipolar, and transverse bipolar montages. This recommendation does not, of course, preclude using other montages required by individual laboratories, for special purposes, or in particular recording circumstances, but it does establish standards (1). For the

TABLE 4.1. *Montage arrangements*

Montage arrangement	Longitudinal	Transverse
Unpaired	Referential and bipolar	Bipolar and referential
Paired-group	Referential and bipolar	
Paired-channel	Referential and bipolar	

standard longitudinal referential montage, the American Encephalographic Society Guidelines proposed choosing among unpaired, paired-group, and paired-channel options. For the longitudinal bipolar montage, the Guidelines recommended using either unpaired or paired-group arrangements as the interlaboratory standard. A paired-channel longitudinal bipolar montage was not recommended, because phase reversals localizing a voltage maximum occur in alternate, not adjacent, channels. The Guidelines recommended only bipolar options for the transverse montage. This reflects difficulty in choosing a suitable, unbiased reference for transverse arrays. Source derivations, with their inherent advantage of less biased reference, may well increase in popularity with the availability of digital EEG and an increased number of scalp channels.

INVERSE OR "BACKWARD" ELECTROENCEPHALOGRAPHIC PROJECTION

Two questions frequently arise:

1. What are the shape and location of the potential field on the surface (which is curved and two-dimensional) of the cerebral cortex?
2. What are the shape and location of the cerebral generator within the three-dimensional volume of the cerebral cortex?

These questions form the so-called inverse, or "backward," EEG projection problem.

The first question has a unique answer if information about electrical properties of tissues intervening between scalp and cortex is sufficient. Spatial deconvolution (24) is the general method of predicting cortical electrical fields (which can later be validated by corticography) from scalp-recorded EEG. However, these predicted cortical fields are simpler than those actually recorded from the brain's surface, because many low-voltage and fast-frequency components of the corticogram attenuate so markedly that they do not appear at the scalp and therefore cannot be reconstructed.

Also, skull thickness varies over the head, which makes it difficult to estimate resistance accurately. New algorithms based on realistic head models created from high-resolution magnetic resonance imaging (MRI) scans take these variables into account (10,11,20). In this new approach, scalp EEG signals are used to estimate the electrocorticogram (ECoG), as if it had been recorded from surgically implanted subdural grid electrodes (4,8,35) (see also Chapter 2 for a more detailed discussion).

The second question lacks a unique solution (9,23,24,27) because information in the two-dimensional scalp EEG is insufficient to specify the shape and location of the specific generators within the brain. By analogy, a common problem in algebra may clarify the matter. Predicting the two-dimensional cortical surface field from scalp EEG data is like using two independent equations to solve two unknowns. In contrast, predicting the form and location of specific cerebral generators is like trying to solve for three or more unknowns with only two equations. In the latter case, only a family of possible solutions can be specified. An example of this can be found in the so-called dipole localization method (DLM), which tries to fit a mathematically acceptable generator (or source) configuration to the scalp EEG information, on the basis of an assumed number of localized discrete sources (or dipoles) (see Chapter 2 for a more detailed discussion). In practice, the segment of EEG containing the discharge of interest is fitted to a head model (commonly a sphere, but preferably, and increasingly, a realistic head shape), and the location of this dipole that provides the best mathematical fit is computed. An arrow depicting the dipole and placed at this location represents the physical neuronal generator.

Usually the location and direction of a single dipole are accurate enough to be clinically meaningful, if the actual cortical generator is discrete and not diffuse or multifocal. It must be remembered that this solution represents only one possibility of many. If two or more dipoles are used in the model, even better mathematical solutions will be obtained. Although it is tempting to view these as superior to the single-dipole model, multiple-dipole models must be used with great understanding and caution, because they can lead to mathematically perfect but clinically meaningless results. Examples of DLM can be found elsewhere in this volume (33).

ELECTROCAP SYSTEMS

When applied according to the international 10-20 system, the usual complement of 21 scalp electrodes has interelectrode distances of approximately 5 cm, with an electrode position error of approximately 0.5 cm or less, depending on how fastidiously the head is measured. For large numbers of electrodes, such as 64, it becomes increasingly difficult to position each individual electrode accurately. The authors have found that when 64 or more electrodes are needed, the use of a commercial elastic cap with embedded electrodes both is easier and yields more accurate results. One reason for this is that the elastic mesh ensures a uniform interelectrode distance throughout. It is thus necessary to measure the exact location of only a few key electrodes, because the rest are predictable by a simple mathematical formula. One such system is available from the MANSCAN Equipment (SAM Technology Inc., San Francisco). With practice, it is possible to apply a cap containing 128 electrodes with good impedance in 2 to 2.5 hours. Having the scalp and hair freshly washed is helpful.

Because of differences in head size and shape, there are various sizes and elastic stretch characteristics suitable for fitting children as well as adults. By measuring electrode locations with reference to fiduciary skull positions (nasion, pre-auricular points), all electrodes can be positioned precisely. This system allows coregistration of physiological data with anatomical images provided by high-resolution MRI (see later discussion). Visualization of electrodes in relation to the underlying cortex provides a much higher degree of anatomical correlation.

Increasing electrode density results in smaller interelectrode distances. It has been estimated that synchronous activation of approximately 6 cm^2 of cortex, or a circle 2.8 cm in diameter, is required to produce an EEG potential that is recordable on the scalp. Cerebral sources of smaller area would not be recorded, and separate sources closer than this distance may not produce two distinct EEG fields. Theoretically, a greater number of electrodes should be able to record more detailed cortical activity, until the interelectrode distance is reduced to 2.8 cm. For average head sizes, this requires between 128 and 256 evenly spaced scalp electrodes (36).

THREE-DIMENSIONAL DEVICES

Traditional EEG recordings provide information about the location, topography, and waveform morphology of abnormal signals arising from unknown intracranial generators. For specific clinical applications, such as lesion localization and determining boundaries of an epileptogenic region, it would be very helpful to obtain accurate three-dimensional localization of the generators of the EEG abnormalities. The outcome would be the ability to specify the actual anatomical structure or area that is responsible for the abnormal EEG pattern, rather than indicating the location by electrode position. This difference is important because the international 10-20 system provides only approximate correlation to underlying brain structures, and these correlations may vary from individual to individual. The coregistration of electrode positions and MRI data sets would be a first step toward this goal, because brain anatomy in would be displayed relation to gyral markings and other abnormalities.

In practice, the simplest coregistration procedure would involve the following steps:

1. Application of scalp electrodes.
2. Measurement of each electrode's position and three fiduciary skull landmarks (nasion, right and left pre-auricular points) with reference to a fixed coordinate system.
3. Making a three-dimensional plot that includes each electrode position in relation to the coordinate system.
4. Performing MRI, using thin cuts with physical markers placed at the same fiduciary points.

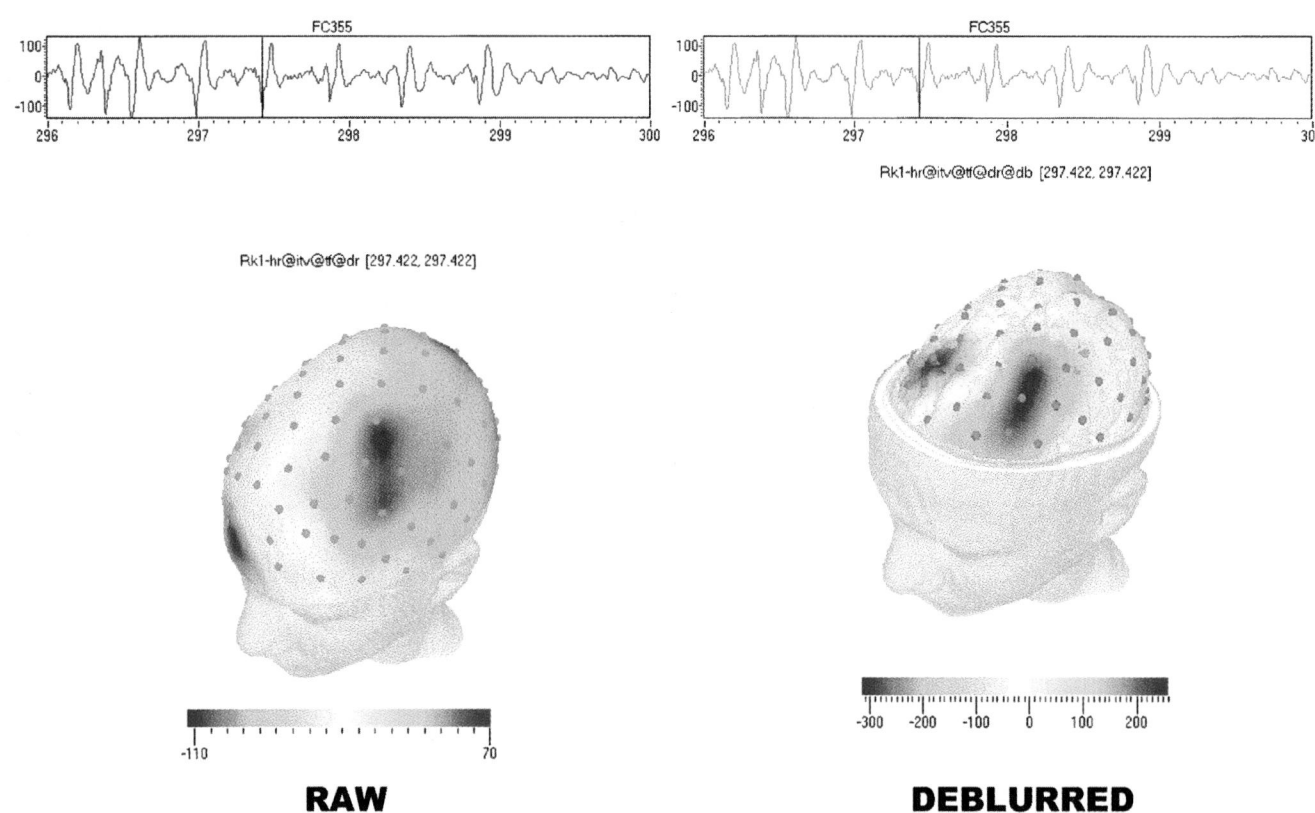

RAW   **DEBLURRED**

FIG. 4.11. Seizure 1 (Ref: Ears, filter: 1-35 Hz)A single channel of raw **(left)** and deblurred **(right)** electroencephalographic samples of the negative peak of the same spike. The topographic maps are color-coded for voltage, with the maximum negativity localized to the left frontal region in both examples. Unfortunately, the color-coding does not translate correctly to black and white, although the only areas of positivity are on the right hemisphere and should be ignored.

5. Merging the MRI data set with the plot of the electrode positions by using the three common fiduciary points as locking markers (this can be done with a suitable graphical software program).

This results in a coregistered plot of the patient's head and applied electrode positions, which can be rotated and sized at will in order to clarify the relationship of each scalp electrode to underlying brain anatomy. By further graphical manipulation (a process called *segmentation*), software can remove unwanted layers of tissue, revealing the structures beneath (virtual reality craniotomy). For example, selective removal of scalp, skull, and meningeal tissues can create a window to reveal the underlying cortical anatomy and gyral markings (10).

Figure 4.11 shows an epileptogenic focus, displayed as an EEG tracing, a scalp topographic map of the negative spike peak, and superimposed brain anatomy. Although the raw and deblurred maps represent the same negative spike peak, their topographies are different: the cortical peak location is displaced more laterally than might be suggested in the scalp map.

Measurements of individual electrode positions can be made simply by using three-dimensional electromagnetic devices that are based on magnetic coils and sensors, if the instrument is kept away from large ferrous metal structures, which tend to distort magnetic measurements. An alternative with electrode caps is to use caliper measurements to estimate the locations of each of the electrodes in relation to the fiduciary points.

REFERENCES

1. American Electroencephalographic Society Guidelines in EEG and Evoked Potentials. Guideline seven: A proposal for standard montages to be used in clinical EEG. *J Clin Neurophysiol* 1986;3(Suppl 1):26–33.
2. Berger H. On the electroencephalogram of man. *Arch Psychiatr Nervenkrenkh* 1929;87:527–570.
3. Binnie CD, Marston D, Polkey CE, et al. Distribution of temporal spikes in relation to the sphenoidal electrode. *Electroencephalogr Clin Neurophysiol* 1989;73:403–409.
4. Bjornson B, Giaschi D, Cochrane D, et al. Non-invasive mapping of sensorimotor cortex in a child with a cavernous angioma: fMRI and high resolution EEG compared with surgical mapping. *Neuroimage* 1999;9(6II):S696.
5. Chatrian GE, Bergamini L, Dondey M, et al. A glossary of terms most commonly used by clinical electroencephalographers. *Electroencephalogr Clin Neurophysiol* 1974;37:538–548.
6. Chatrian GE, Lettich E, Nelson PL. Ten percent electrode system for topographic studies of spontaneous and evoked EEG activities. *Am J EEG Technol* 1985;25:83–92.
7. Chatrian GE, Lettich E, Nelson PL. Modified nomenclature for the "10%" electrode system. *J Clin Neurophysiol* 1988;5:183–186.
8. Dougherty R, Au Young S, Giaschi D, et al. Comparison of visual activation measured by fMRI and high resolution EEG. *Neuroimage* 1998;7(4II):S309.
9. Fender DH. Source localization of brain activity. In: Gevins AS, Rémond A, eds. *Handbook of electroencephalography and clinical neurophysiology: revised series, vol. 1: Methods of analysis of brain electrical and magnetic signals.* Amsterdam: Elsevier, 1987:355–403.
10. Gevins A, Le J, Martin N, et al. High resolution EEG: 124-channel recording, spatial Deblurring and MRI integration methods. *EEG Clin Neurophysiol* 1994;90:337–358.
11. Gevins A, Le J, Smith S. Deblurring. *J Clin Neurophysiol* 1999;16:204–213.
12. Gloor P. Neuronal generators and the problems of localization in electroencephalography: application of volume conductor theory to electroencephalography. *J Clin Neurophysiol* 1985;2:327–354.
13. Goldman D. The clinical use of the "average" electrode in monopolar recording. *Electroencephalogr Clin Neurophysiol* 1950;2:211–214.
14. Hjorth B. An on-line transformation of EEG scalp potentials into orthogonal source derivations. *Electroencephalogr Clin Neurophysiol* 1975;39:526–530.
15. Hjorth B. Multichannel EEG preprocessing: analog matrix operations in the study of local effects. *Pharmakopsychiatr Neuropsychopharmakol* 1979;12:111–118.
16. Jasper HH. Electroencephalography. In: Penfield W, Erickson T, eds. *Epilepsy and cerebral localization.* Springfield, IL: Charles C Thomas, 1941:391.
17. Jasper HH. The ten-twenty electrode system of the International Federation. *Electroencephalogr Clin Neurophysiol* 1958;10:371–373.
18. Jasper HH. The ten-twenty electrode system of the International Federation. In: *International Federation of Societies for Electroencephalography and Clinical Neurophysiology: recommendations for the practice of clinical neurophysiology.* Amsterdam: Elsevier, 1983:3–10.
19. Knott JR. Further thoughts on polarity, montages and localization. *J Clin Neurophysiol* 1985;2:63–75.
20. Le J, Gevins A. Method to reduce blur distortion from EEG's using a realistic head model. *IEEE Trans on Biomed Eng* 1993;40(6):517–528.
21. Lehmann D. Principles of spatial analysis, In: Gevins AS, Rémond A, eds. *Handbook of electroencephalography and clinical neurophysiology: revised series, vol. 1: Methods of analysis of brain electrical and magnetic signals.* Amsterdam: Elsevier,1987:309–354.
22. Lesser RP, Luders H, Dinner DS, et al. An introduction to the basic concepts of polarity and localization. *J Clin Neurophysiol* 1985;2:45–61.
23. Nunez PL. *Electrical fields of the brain: the neurophysics of EEG.* New York: Oxford University Press, 1981.
24. Nunez PL. Methods to estimate spatial properties of the dynamic cortical source activity. In: Pfurt-Scheller G, Lopes da Silva F, eds. *Functional brain imaging.* Berlin: Springer-Verlag, 1988:3–10.
25. Nuwer MR. Recording electrodes site nomenclature. *J Clin Neurophysiol* 1987;4:121–133.
26. Pernier J, Perrin F, Bertrand O. Scalp current density fields: concepts and properties. *Electroencephalogr Clin Neurophysiol* 1988;69:385–389.
27. Perrin F, Bertrand O, Pernier J. Scalp current density mapping: value and estimation from potential data. *IIIE Trans Biomed Eng* 1988;BME-34:283–288.
28. Sadler RM, Goodwin J. Multiple electrodes for detecting spikes in partial complex seizures. *Can J Neurol Sci* 1989;16:326–329.
29. Silverman D. The anterior temporal electrode and the ten-twenty system. *Electroencephalogr Clin Neurophysiol* 1960;12:735–737.
30. Tyner FS, Knott JR, Mayer WB Jr. *Fundamentals of EEG technology, vol. 1: Basic concepts and methods.* New York: Raven Press, 1983.
31. Walter WG, Shipton HW. A new toposcopic display system. *Electroencephalogr Clin Neurophysiol* 1951;3:281–292.
32. Wong PKH. *Digital EEG in clinical practice.* Philadelphia: Lippincott-Raven, 1996.
33. Wong PKH. Potential fields, EEG maps, and cortical spike generators. *Electroencephalogr Clin Neurophysiol* 1998;106:138–141.
34. Wong PKH. Routine clinical protocol. *J Clin Neurophysiol* 1998;15(6):481–484.
35. Wong PKH, Bjornson B, Connolly M, et al. High resolution electroencephalography (HR-EEG) and seizure localization. *Neuroimage* 1999;9(6II):S601.
36. Wong PKH, Brenner RP, Chiappa K, et al. New developments. *J Clin Neurophysiol* 1998;15(6):489–492.

Chapter 5

Orderly Approach to Visual Analysis: Elements of the Normal EEG and Their Characteristics in Children and Adults

Peter Kellaway

INTRODUCTION TO THE VISUAL ANALYSIS OF THE ELECTROENCEPHALOGRAM

Analysis of the electroencephalogram (EEG) is a rational and systematic process requiring a series of orderly steps characterizing the recorded electrical activity in terms of specific descriptors and measurements. The elements of this analysis are listed in Table 5.1. For example, in the hypothetical case of an 8-year-old child, some 2-Hz waves are identified in the awake EEG. This activity must then be characterized according to their location, voltage, waveform, manner of occurrence (random or rhythmic, intermittent or continuous), frequency, amplitude modulation (smooth, variable, unchanging, paroxysmal), synchrony and symmetry in homologous derivations on the two sides, and reactivity (e.g., to eye opening). A sustained occipital alpha rhythm of 8.5 Hz is present. The maximum voltage of the 2-Hz waves varies from 40 to 70 μV, approximating the voltage of the occipital alpha rhythm. The slow waves occur randomly and block with the alpha waves when the eyes are open; they tend to occur synchronously and fairly symmetrically on the two sides.

Taken as a whole, these descriptors fit those of a normal EEG slow pattern that occurs commonly in this age group: namely, "posterior slow waves of youth" (2,165). A variance in any of these descriptors might entirely change the significance of the 2-Hz waves; a different locus, a much higher voltage, a more complex waveform, a failure to block with eye opening, or any combination of these may render the findings abnormal. For instance,

TABLE 5.1. *Essential characteristics of electroencephalographic analysis*

1. Frequency or wavelength
2. Voltage
3. Waveform
4. Regulation
   a. Frequency
   b. Voltage
5. Manner of occurrence (random, serial, continuous)
6. Locus
7. Reactivity (eye opening, mental calculation, acapnia, sensory stimulation, movement, affective state)
8. Interhemispheric coherence (homologous areas)
   a. Symmetry
      i. Voltage
      ii. Frequency
   b. Synchrony
      i. Wave
      ii. Burst

2-Hz, 40- to 76-μV random waves in the frontal, rather than occipital, derivations in an awake 8-year-old child is an abnormal finding, the significance of which may be entirely different if the slow waves are rhythmic rather than random, if the waveform are complex, and if the voltage regulation are paroxysmal rather than variable within a narrow range.

The only clinical information required before the EEG analysis is begun is the patient's *age and state.* The age is listed on the patient's data sheet, which should be part of the EEG record.[1] The younger the patient, the more critical it is that age information be precise. In the newborn, age should be specified in days since delivery (chronological age); in infants aged 1 to 3 months, it should be specified in weeks; and in those aged 3 to 36 months, it should be specified in months. This progressively decreasing degree of precision reflects the fact that the landmarks of ontogenetic development of the EEG in the newborn are clearly differentiated in weekly or biweekly epochs but become progressively less sharply delineated with increasing age; for example, there are clearly defined differences between the EEG of a premature infant with a conceptional age of 35 weeks and that of an infant with a conceptional age of 36 weeks, but there are no important or sharply delineated differences between the EEG of a 3-year-old child and that of a 4-year-old child.

The "state" of the patient refers to the clinical assessment of the patient's general state of consciousness; this should be specified in such terms as "alert," "lethargic," "stuporous," and "semicomatose" on the clinical data sheet that accompanies the record. The patient's state also refers to the physiological variations of alertness and levels of sleep that occur during the recording, which are noted by the technologist.

Although these two items of information (the patient's age and state of consciousness) are essential for an accurate interpretation of the EEG, it is a good teaching exercise and a test of analytic acumen to read a record occasionally when only one or neither of these two items is known. Attempting to determine the patient's age or, more easily, physiological state according to the characteristics of the EEG activity sharpens analytic technique and subjective criteria.

That *age* is an important determinant of the characteristics of the EEG has been known since Hans Berger's early studies in 1932. The electrical activity of the brain—awake, asleep, and in response to stimuli—varies considerably with age; a particular activity or pattern that is normal at one age may be quite abnormal at another.

In the premature infant, the age factor is critical. In reading the records of such infants, the initial step is to determine whether the conceptional age

---

[1]Both age and birth date should be recorded.

(gestational age plus time since delivery) can be determined from the characteristics of the EEG. Absence or distortion of features that normally make this possible is evidence of abnormality, as are differences between the maturational characteristics of the various stages of the awake/sleep cycle in the same infant (dyschronism). At the other end of the age spectrum, EEG features such as focal, episodic, temporal theta activity may be within the normal range for an elderly person but are outside the normal range for a young adult.

The *state of alertness* or of altered levels of consciousness (physiological and pathological) is also a critical factor in EEG interpretation. The obvious situations are the well-known alpha-type record and the spindle sleep-like patterns that may be seen in comatose patients, which, in spite of their "normal" appearance, have precise pathological significance in the altered states of consciousness in which they may be found. Less well recognized are the dramatic EEG changes sometimes seen in young children in association with changes in affective state and with subtle physiological alterations of cerebral state that are antecedent to the onset of clinically evident sleep.

FEATURES OF THE NORMAL ELECTROENCEPHALOGRAM

Reactivity

Before the various features of the normal EEG of adults and children are described and discussed, it is important to recognize that the identification of a particular activity or phenomenon may depend on its "reactivity" (see Table 5.1). An important element of the recording and its analysis is the testing of the reactions, or responses, of the various components of the EEG to certain physiological changes or provocations. These include eye opening and closing, repetitive movements of the extremities, visual scanning, sensory stimulation, and hypocapnia produced by hyperventilation.

Specification of the reactivity of a given activity, rhythm, or pattern is essential for the identification and subsequent analysis of the activity and may clearly differentiate it from another activity with similar characteristics. For example, occipital slow waves intermixed with the alpha rhythm, which block with the alpha rhythm when the eyes are opened, may be a normal finding in a child, but similar slow waves that do not block may be pathological. Similarly, a series of rhythmic, high-voltage, monomorphic 3- to 4-Hz waves in the frontal leads occurring in association with arousal in a young child may be normal, but a similar burst occurring spontaneously and not associated with arousal may be abnormal.

Alpha Rhythm

The occipital alpha rhythm should be the starting point for visual analysis. The initial questions should be the following: Is an occipital alpha rhythm present, and are its characteristics appropriate for age? If there is little or no occipital alpha rhythm, is it because the patient's eyes are open (reactivity) or because the patient is drowsy or asleep (state)? Is it an idiosyncrasy of a normal adult (genetic)? Or is it an abnormal finding?

Some persons (adults; rarely children) who are apparently normal show no alpha activity, at least under the conditions of a routine clinical recording. Other persons, also apparently normal, may show brief episodes of occipital alpha activity only during hyperventilation or, transiently, on arousal from sleep.

In addition to providing clues concerning the patient's affective state (e.g., anxiety) or level of arousal, the presence and character of the occipital alpha rhythm are critical determinants in evaluating the significance of other activities present. Thus, the presence of some low-voltage, 5- to 6-Hz rhythmic frontocentral activity in an adult may, in the transient absence of an occipital alpha rhythm, merely signify the patient's drowsiness; in the total absence of an occipital alpha rhythm, however, such activity may have pathological significance. Similarly, the presence of the frontocentral theta activity would be more ominous if the occipital alpha rhythm itself were slow (e.g., 7 Hz). It is important to remember that the occipital alpha rhythm may be preserved in conditions that produce marked slowing of the activity in anterior derivations. Thus, a slow occipital alpha rhythm usually denotes a more serious change than if its frequency were maintained.[2] Conversely, preservation of the occipital alpha rhythm despite marked slowing elsewhere is a favorable finding.

Normal Characteristics

The normal range for the frequency of the occipital alpha rhythm in adults is usually given as 8 to 13 Hz. The distribution curve for the mean alpha rhythm frequency in a series of 200 selected men (141) is shown in Fig. 5.1. Note that the incidence of an occipital alpha rhythm as slow as 8 Hz is less than 1%. Although population studies indicate that an 8-Hz alpha rhythm may be found in normal asymptomatic young adults, in clinical practice this should always raise the suspicion that the alpha rhythm has slowed, which, statisti-

---

[2]There are exceptions: A notable example is the slowing of the occipital alpha rhythm that may be an early sign of intoxication with phenytoin.

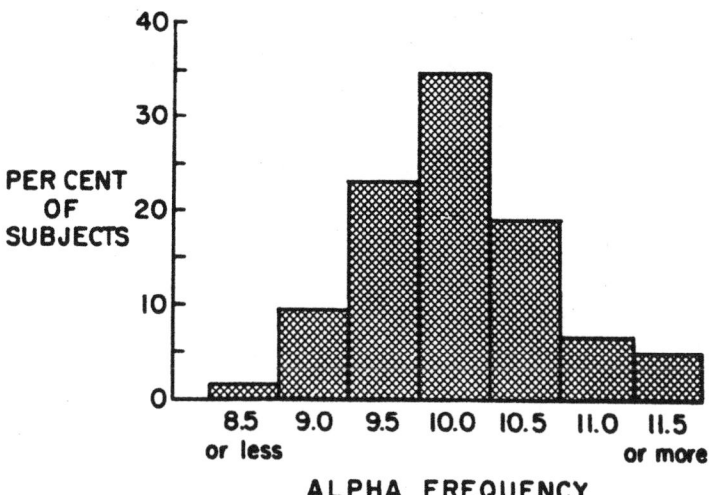

FIG. 5.1. Distribution of the mean alpha frequency in a series of 200 volunteer flight personnel, aged 24 to 35 years, on active duty in the United States Air Force (144 pilots and 56 navigators).

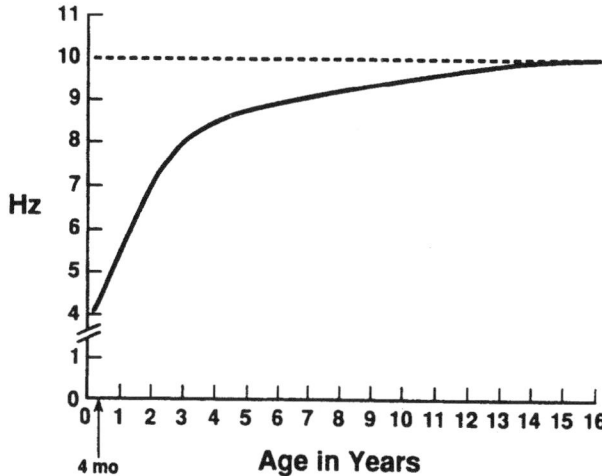

FIG. 5.2. Curve showing the development of the occipital alpha rhythm between the ages of 4 months and 16 years. Some rhythmic 3- to 4-Hz activity is present in the electroencephalograms of awake infants aged 2 to 4 months, but it is not reactive to eye opening. From the time rhythmic activity that is reactive to eye opening first appears, the frequency increases rapidly, reaching 5 to 6 Hz by 12 months and 8 Hz by 36 months. At that age, there is a sharp inflection in the rate curve, and the frequency increases only 2 Hz over the next 6 years. (From Kellaway P, Noebels JL, eds. *Problems and concepts in developmental neurophysiology.* Baltimore: The Johns Hopkins University Press, 1989.)

cally, is more likely. The maturational curve for occipital alpha rhythm frequency (Fig. 5.2) shows that the lower limit of the adult range is usually reached by the age of 3 years. The curve has an overall parabolic course, with the rate of change diminishing after late adolescence. In late life, the frequency of the occipital alpha rhythm tends to decrease, and this change appears to be related to changes in cerebral metabolic rate (57,84,154–157,182).

It has been shown that the frequency of the occipital alpha rhythm is closely related to cerebral blood flow; it has also been shown that if cerebral perfusion falls below a certain critical level, the occipital alpha rhythm slows. This relationship of alpha rhythm frequency to the adequacy of cerebral perfusion has been demonstrated repeatedly in patients with cardiac failure: Pacemaker or cardiac implants may result in an increase of as much as 2 Hz in alpha rhythm frequency (188).

When certain drugs (particularly phenytoin) approach toxic levels, the alpha rhythm slows without other changes in the EEG (175a). Consequently, if alpha rhythm frequencies are at the low end of the normal spectrum for age in patients who are taking such drugs, the possibility of toxic effects should be considered. Carbamazepine, at therapeutic levels, may slow the alpha rhythm in children (59).

Frequency in Children

The relationship of the occipital alpha rhythm frequency to age in normal control subjects is shown in Fig. 5.2. Occipital rhythmic activity that is responsive to eye opening appears in approximately 75% of normal infants between the third and fourth months after (full-term) birth. Initially, this activity is not well sustained and has a frequency of approximately 3.5 to 4.5 Hz. The frequency increases rapidly, reaching 5 to 6 Hz in approximately 70% of children by 12 months of age. At age 36 months, 82% of normal children born at full term show a mean occipital alpha rhythm frequency of 8 Hz (range, 7.5 to 9.5 Hz). By the age of 9 years, the mean alpha rhythm frequency is 9 Hz in 65% of controls; in the same percentage of persons, the mean is 10 Hz by the age of 15 (48,165).

In infants and young children, the occipital alpha rhythm may totally block with the eyes open, and slower activity may be mistaken for the occipital alpha rhythm. For this reason, a portion of the awake EEG should be recorded during passive eye closure. Infants and very young children usually do not close their eyes until they become drowsy and are ready to fall asleep; at that time, the occipital rhythm may slow before disappearing.

Frequency in the Elderly

For many years, it was commonly thought that the frequency of the dominant posterior rhythm decreased, with normal aging, to the lower end of the alpha activity range or even below it. Extrapolation from the parabolic curve describing the age–alpha frequency relation indicates that a decline in frequency might be expected at about age 58 years (48,165). The weight of the evidence derived from studies of healthy elderly persons indicates that although there may be a decrease in alpha frequency in some normal persons in later life, the mean frequency is maintained at or above 9 Hz (57,84,100,154–157,168,182,191). In another study of selected healthy subjects with a mean age of 68 years, the mean alpha frequency was 9.7 Hz, and only two subjects had an alpha rhythm as slow as 8 Hz (3).

Voltage

Absence of an alpha rhythm (or even a very-low-voltage alpha rhythm) is not encountered when recordings are made directly from appropriate regions of the brain in unanesthetized persons. Indeed, a number of alpha rhythm generators exist in the cortex and the depths of the brain, and they produce remarkably high voltage rhythms (181). On the other hand, the voltage of the alpha rhythm as recorded at the scalp in apparently healthy persons (73) may barely exceed the noise level of the amplifiers.

Normative studies have shown that 6% to 7% of healthy adults have alpha rhythm voltages of less than 15 μV at the scalp (141). It must be kept in mind, however, in considering the voltage characteristics of a given activity, that interelectrode distance is a factor that influences the actual voltage measured, depending on the size of the potential field and the position of the electrodes in relation to that field (Fig. 5.3). In discussing voltage, the electrode placements used in measuring the voltage should be specified. In one series in which the P4-O2 derivation was used, 75% of normal adults were found to have alpha rhythm voltages of 15 to 45 μV (141). The relationship between interelectrode distance and the amplitude of activity recorded in the

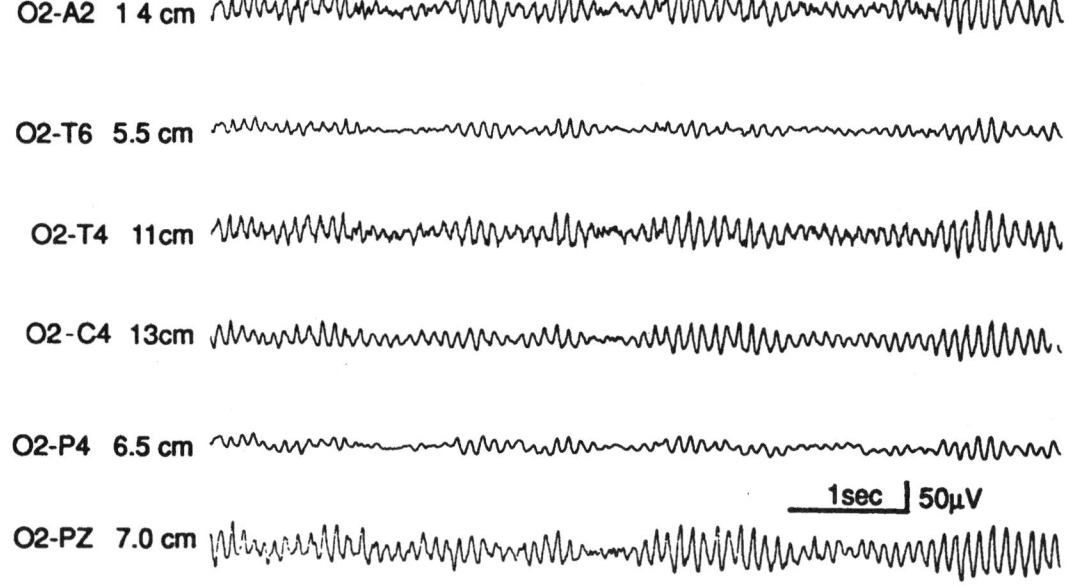

O2-A2 14 cm

O2-T6 5.5 cm

O2-T4 11cm

O2-C4 13cm

O2-P4 6.5 cm

1sec 50μV

O2-PZ 7.0 cm

FIG. 5.3. Effect of interelectrode distance on recorded amplitude of alpha rhythm. Note that this is not the only factor determining amplitude; the geometry of the potential field is also a factor. For example, although the interelectrode distance between O2 and PZ is half that between O2 and A2, the recorded amplitude is actually somewhat greater.

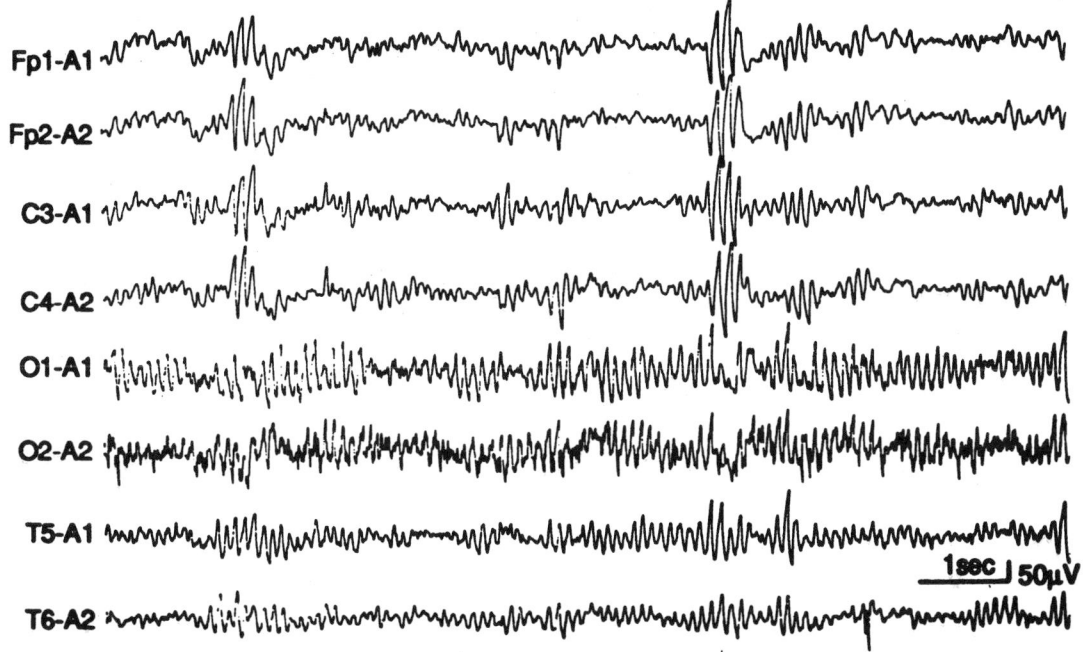

FIG. 5.4. Paroxysmal generalized 8-Hz rhythmic activity in a 21-year-old man with an initial buildup of rhythmic, frontal-dominant but generalized high-voltage 8- to 10-Hz activity.

scalp EEG can be accurately characterized by an exponential function (52); the increase in potential difference is proportional to the square of the distance up to about 10 cm.

Children rarely show low-voltage (less than 30 µV) alpha rhythms. In their control group, Petersén and Eeg-Olofsson (165), using the T5-O1 derivation, found no children with voltages less than 20 µV; only 1.3% of the children had voltages of 20 to 30 µV, and all of those were older than 12 years.

In this same series, the average alpha rhythm voltage in children aged 3 to 15 years was 50 to 60 µV. Approximately 9% of the children of this age group (predominantly those aged 6 to 9 years) showed alpha rhythm voltages of 100 µV or more. High voltage should never, in itself, be considered an abnormal finding; however, paroxysmal bursts of 9- to 12-Hz activity having a wider area distribution than the occipital alpha rhythm (Fig. 5.4) are abnormal (63). This pattern, associated with epilepsy, can be clearly differentiated from a normal alpha rhythm on the basis of its distribution, paroxysmal features, and lack of reactivity to eye opening.

The voltage of the occipital alpha rhythm diminishes with increasing age; this probably, in large part, reflects (a) changes in the density of the bone and (b) increased electrical impedance of the intervening tissue, rather than a decrease in the voltage of the electrical activity of the brain. This impression is based on the observation that during electrocorticography, the voltage is not appreciably reduced in older patients who showed low-voltage alpha rhythms at the scalp. The relation between EEG voltage and the impedance of the intervening tissues is discussed in more detail in the later section on bilateral voltage symmetry.

Regulation

Good regulation of frequency[3] and voltage[4] of the occipital alpha rhythm is characteristic of the EEGs of approximately 80% of young adults (48,165). With increasing age, there is a tendency for alpha activity to become less well regulated.

---

[3]"Good regulation" of frequency is defined as follows: a sustained rhythm in which the mean frequency does not vary more than ±0.5 Hz (as measured during any 2-second epoch in which the activity is sustained).

[4]Regulation in terms of voltage refers to the smoothness of the envelope of the waxing and waning of voltage that the alpha rhythm typically shows.

As mentioned earlier, the peak frequency of the occipital alpha rhythm is remarkably constant and, in healthy persons, shows virtually no variation throughout the day or over long periods (37,51,177,193). Precise computer analytic techniques have demonstrated that the peak alpha rhythm frequency may increase in women during the initial phase of the menstrual cycle, but the change is so small (0.3 Hz) that it escapes notice in routine visual analysis (37,51,177,193). The *stability* of frequency regulation of the alpha rhythm does fluctuate somewhat throughout the day and in relation to certain physiological changes (e.g., the menstrual cycle). Regulation is also affected in some persons by mental activity and anxiety. Thus the general comments concerning "regulation" of the alpha rhythm refer to conditions of recording that approach the optimal conditions for "good" regulation: a quiet, nonstressful environment; eyes closed; the subject at rest but still alert.

Both voltage regulation and frequency regulation of the occipital alpha rhythm are "good" from the ages of approximately 6 months through 3 years. During this period, the occipital activity may be almost monorhythmic, and the voltage variation on the EEG is usually smoothly contoured (Fig. 5.5). From the ages of 3 to 14 years, poor regulation (particularly of

voltage) is common in normal subjects, and the regulation in approximately 33% of children in this age group is poorer on the low-voltage side (48,165).

Distribution

The occipital region is the site of maximal alpha rhythm voltage in 65% of adults and 95% of children. However, in some normal persons, the amplitude of the alpha activity in the central and temporal regions is equal to or greater than that in the occipital derivations. In about 32% of normal young adults, the alpha activity is widely distributed; it may be predominantly central or temporal, or it may be essentially equal in both areas (141). Studies with implanted electrodes have shown that multiple alpha generators exist in the human brain, not only in the occipital region but also in central and temporal regions (163). These generators overlap and influence each other; therefore, what is recorded at the scalp at any locus reflects an "averaged" field pattern.

Bilateral Symmetry

Asymmetry of the occipital alpha rhythm voltage on the two sides occurs in 60% of adults; in 50%, the right side shows the higher voltage (without

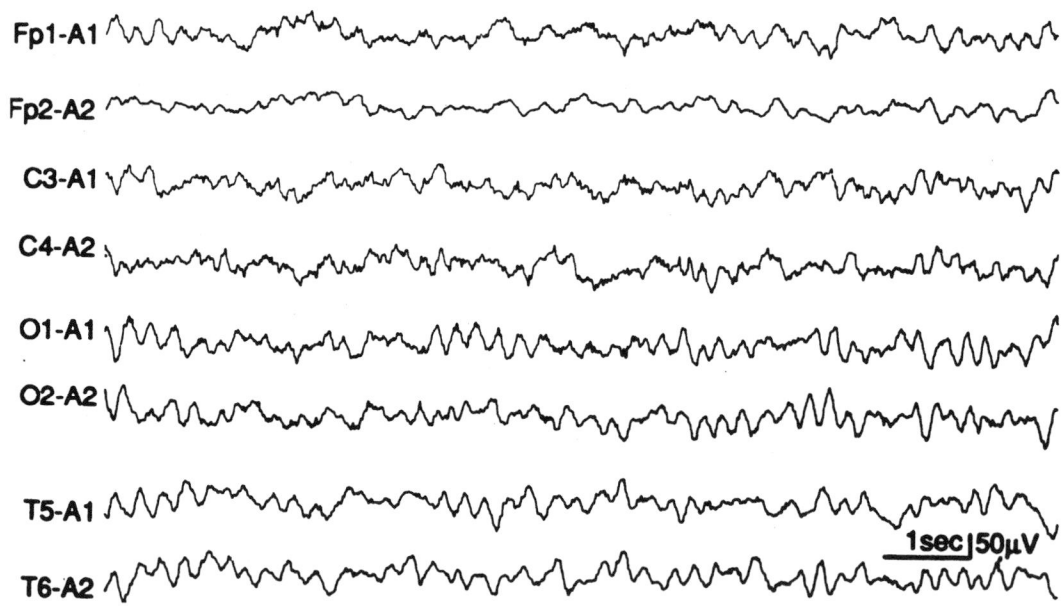

FIG. 5.5. Normal electroencephalogram of an awake, asymptomatic 9-month-old infant, eyes closed. The almost monorhythmic occipital activity with little or smoothly contoured amplitude modulation is typical of the 4- to 24-month age group.

consistent correlation with handedness). The asymmetry between sides is generally less than 20%[5]; only 17% of normal adults show differences greater than this. In only 1.5% is the asymmetry more than 50% (141).

In practice, an asymmetry of 50% or more should be regarded as clinically significant until proved otherwise. An additional consideration is the side of the low voltage. Because there is a statistical probability that the alpha rhythm has a higher voltage on the right side in a given individual, asymmetries of 35% to 50% should be considered suspect if the right side has the low voltage.

In 95% of normal children, the alpha rhythm voltage has an asymmetry between sides of up to 20%. In 98% of these children, the lower voltage is on the left side, and there is no relationship to handedness. In the 5% of children with asymmetries of more than 20%, none showed a difference of more than 50%. The same rule mentioned above for adults should be used in the assessment of asymmetries in children when the low voltage appears on the right side, because the likelihood that the right side should be the high-voltage side is 98:2 (48,165).

A difference in skull thickness on the two sides may be a major factor in determining the presence of voltage asymmetry. Through the use of an ultrasonic-pulse technique, it was shown that a difference in skull thickness of more than 33% in homologous regions of the two sides may be present in normal persons; the left is more commonly the thicker side (approximately 72% of cases). Differences in skull thickness of this degree can account for voltage asymmetries of 20% to 70% (129). Thus, a difference in bone thickness on the two sides not only may account for asymmetries seen in normal subjects but also may mask or simulate abnormality. In the absence of actual measurements of bone thickness, asymmetries of less than 50% probably are diagnostically insignificant. The clinician should be especially attentive to the presence of subgaleal swelling caused by hematoma and for leakage during an infusion into a scalp vein, because these also greatly reduce the apparent voltage of the EEG activity recorded by overlying electrodes.

Asymmetry of the mu rhythm (a central rhythm of alpha activity frequency, discussed in detail later in this chapter) and of temporal alpha activity is the rule rather than the exception, and predominance of the activity on one side is not uncommon in asymptomatic persons. For these reasons, asymmetry of the mu and temporal alpha activity should be interpreted with caution, especially in children. In prolonged (36-hour) and serial studies in children, the mu rhythm sometimes showed higher voltage on one side (even

to the point that it appears unilateral) for prolonged periods and then showed predominance on the opposite side (34,67). Such findings may well be significant in terms of subtle brain functions, but the clinical electroencephalographer should not conjecture about the presence of focal cortical lesions. Admittedly, there appear to be cases, such as those that Gastaut et al. (67) originally described, in which the mu rhythm appears to be enhanced at or near the site of a craniocerebral injury, but the greatest percentage of unilaterally predominant mu rhythms are not associated with evident cortical lesions. It must also be remembered that high voltage of the mu rhythm on one side may result from an underlying or subjacent skull defect (e.g., bur hole) that provides a low-resistance pathway for activity in the cortex underlying the region of absence of bone. Mu rhythms are often enhanced during and after hyperventilation, and this may further mislead the inexperienced electroencephalographer to an assumption of abnormality.

Temporal alpha activity in young adults is usually fairly symmetrical on the two sides. However, elderly persons, in whom the voltage of this temporal activity may be greater than that of the occipital alpha rhythm, may show alternating voltage lateralization; in 80%, the left side shows higher voltage. (This is discussed further later in this chapter in relation to temporal slow activity in the elderly.)

Reactivity

The reactivity (i.e., blocking) of the alpha rhythm to conditions other than eye opening is variable. Hans Berger found early on that an individual's alpha rhythm diminished in amplitude or "blocked" during periods of concentrated mental effort, such as making calculations. However, in 24% of the normal young adults studied by Maulsby et al. (141), no alpha blocking was detected in a controlled test situation. Failure of the alpha activity on one side to attenuate during concentrated mental effort is evidence of cerebral dysfunction or lesion of the nonreactive side (212). In some apparently healthy persons, the alpha rhythm seems to be blocked almost continuously, appearing only very briefly (1 second or less) in certain situations (e.g., upon arousal or starting hyperventilation). It has been suggested, although not proved, that in some subjects the alpha rhythm may be "blocked" or diminished in amplitude by "anxiety."

Alpha Variants

A characteristic of the occipital alpha rhythm is that it may show what seem to be abrupt phase reversals, so that the resultant wave or waves have

---

[5]The asymmetry is the difference between the two sides, expressed as the percentage of the high-voltage side.

a frequency of half that of the ongoing alpha activity and in some instances have a greater amplitude. This phenomenon was first described by Goodwin in 1947 (76). He also described a "bifurcation" in the individual alpha waves, so that a superimposed harmonic rhythm of twice the basic frequency was produced. He noted that both the subharmonic and harmonic patterns blocked with eye opening, along with the alpha rhythm. He referred to the two patterns, respectively, as "slow" and "fast" alpha variants. In different people, these two patterns vary in their degree of expression, from a random, sporadic occurrence to a predominant feature of the occipital activity. All degrees occur in apparently normal persons. The current concept of alpha variants is that they are a "physiological variation of the basic cortical rhythm" and that they "have no correlation with any clinical entity or with increased convulsive susceptibility" (2).

An early report indicated that the slow alpha variant pattern is much more common in persons with "symptoms usually associated with emotional instability" (2) or with "psychoneurosis" (76) than in normal persons. However, more rigorous investigation is needed before this can be established as fact, and even if such a correlation were established, its meaning would have to be determined before the findings had any clinical utility.

Several other rare occipital slow patterns of unknown significance have been seen in adults referred for EEG studies. One of these patterns may be related to the slow alpha variant, because it seems to evolve from it. The typical slow alpha variant configuration progressively changes to a simple monomorphic wave with a frequency of half that of the alpha rhythm. The new rhythm may persist for several seconds and then be replaced by a return of the alpha rhythm. This sequence of events may occur several times over a period of several minutes. Aird and Gastaut (2) found only one case that approached this type of pattern in their study of 500 "normal" young adults aged 19 to 22 years, and Maulsby et al. (141) found three cases in their study of 200 highly selected male subjects aged 24 to 36 years.

Mu Rhythm

The mu rhythm,[6] a central rhythm of alpha activity frequency (usually 8 to 10 Hz) (Fig. 5.6) in which the individual waves have an arch-like shape,

---

[6]Synonymous with wicket, comb, and arcade rhythms and *rythme en arceaux,* these names were derived from the distinctive waveform of this activity. The Greek letter mu (μ) now designates this rhythm because the symbol resembles the waveform and conforms with the practice of using Greek letters to name specific EEG activities.

is present as a visually detectable rhythm in 17% to 19% of young adults (65,141,167). It is less common in the elderly and in children. A clearly defined mu rhythm occurs in only 5% of normal children younger than 4 years, and the incidence increases little up to the age of 8 years. Between 8 and 16 years, the incidence increases from about 7% to the adult figure of 18%. It is more common in girls than in boys throughout childhood and adolescence; the incidence is approximately twice as high in girls at age 14 (48,165).

The voltage characteristics of the mu rhythm resemble those of the occipital alpha rhythm. The mu rhythm does not block with eye opening but blocks unilaterally with movement of the opposite extremity. Its presence relates to the level of attention and is enhanced by immobility (28).

The mu rhythm is particularly labile (26–28): It is suppressed by fatigue, by somatosensory and sensorimotor stimulation (26,27,118), and, to some degree, by mental arithmetic (25,27) and problem solving (36). However, because it commonly occurs when an alpha rhythm is present in the central region, it may be difficult to differentiate by visual inspection (119).

The mu rhythm may be present one day and undetectable the next (personal observations from prolonged monitoring studies; see also Schoppenhorst et al. [179]). Its degree of expression may also vary from time to time during the same day (20). The true incidence of the mu rhythm in normal persons is obscured by all these factors, which would tend to produce significant sampling errors in any study group.

According to established facts and personal experience in recording electrocorticograms from the sensorimotor cortex of unanesthetized patients during surgery, the mu pattern is a *ubiquitous rhythm of the sensorimotor cortex at rest,* a concept first enunciated by Shoppenhorst et al. (179). However, it is the central beta rhythm recorded directly from the prerolandic region that shows a strong blocking response to movement of the extremities on the opposite side (95).

Routine clinical studies have shown that the mu rhythm may be quite asymmetrical and asynchronous on the two sides, even though the subject is motionless and at rest (119). It may be present on only one side in persons with no clinical or other laboratory evidence of organic brain disease. Very-high-voltage mu activity may be recorded in the central region over a bone defect (e.g., bur hole), and its sharp configuration, mixed with slower frequency activities that may be present, may mislead the clinician to a presumption of a potentially epileptogenic focal process (32,119).

In infants whose occipital alpha rhythm is still less than 6 Hz, a well-organized and fairly well-sustained 8- to 10-Hz activity may be present in the

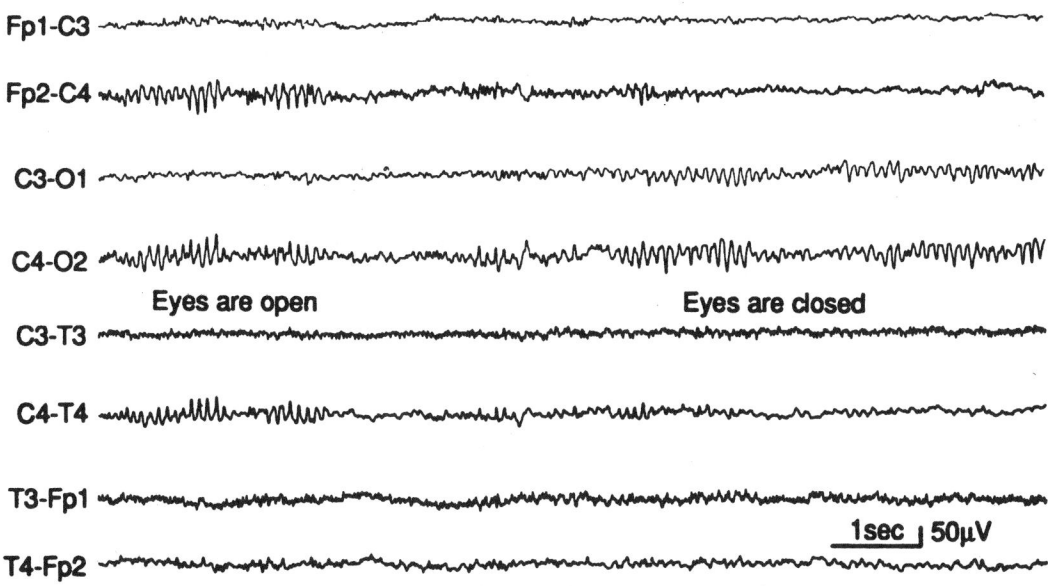

Fp1-C3

Fp2-C4

C3-O1

C4-O2

Eyes are open   **Eyes are closed**

C3-T3

C4-T4

T3-Fp1

T4-Fp2

1sec 50μV

FIG. 5.6. Episode of mu rhythm occurring during a period when the eyes are open and the occipital alpha rhythm is blocked. Electroencephalogram of asymptomatic 25-year-old woman. Mu-rhythm asymmetries of this degree are not uncommon in normal subjects.

central regions bilaterally. It lacks the characteristic waveform of the mu rhythm but may be ontogenetically related to it. This activity was originally described by Pampiglione in 1977 (158):

> "In the rolandic area of each hemisphere and at the vertex some rhythmic activity kept on appearing in most infants, at somewhat irregular intervals, in the form of 8–10 per sec waves of the order of 20–40 microvolts, with variable lateralization, often occurring independently over the right or the left side. . . . This activity would often diminish or disappear altogether when the baby used his hands or played with toys, but it would increase when the baby was at rest with his arms and hands relaxed. . . . Distribution, frequency and behavior were similar to those of the mu rhythm in older children and adults."

Beta Activity

Activities with frequencies higher than 13 Hz are commonly present in the EEGs of normal adults and children. Three distinct frequency bands in the beta activity range may be distinguished: a common 18- to 25-Hz band, a less common 14- to 16-Hz band, and a rare 35- to 40-Hz band. High-voltage activity in the first two frequency bands is present at the cortex in unanesthetized humans, particularly in the prerolandic and postrolandic cortex. This fast activity is greatly attenuated in the scalp EEG. In 97% to 98% of normal awake adults and children, the voltage in the EEG is less than 20 μV; in 70%, it is 10 μV or less (recorded between closely spaced scalp electrodes) (48,141,165).

Beta activity with a voltage of 25 μV or more in the clinical EEG has been considered abnormal. Although such findings are statistically outside the range of normal variation, little is known about the significance of beta activity. The early literature documents a significantly higher percentage of "fast" EEGs in epileptic patients than in normal controls and implies that a fast EEG (a record with much beta activity with a voltage of 25 μV or more) may be considered supportive evidence for a diagnosis of epilepsy. However, "fast" EEGs also occur with a greater incidence than in normal controls in a number of other, nonepileptic conditions (89,201,204), and fast EEGs have no correlation with epilepsy in children (46,61,62,88,185).

The presence of beta activity at amplitudes of 25 μV or more is currently of little or no diagnostic utility (except when drug ingestion is suspected). Thus, if a patient with a differential diagnosis of syncope versus epilepsy is referred for EEG studies, the finding of excessive voltage and a prevalence of beta activity in no way clarifies the diagnosis. Similarly, the impression that high-voltage beta activity may have some specific significance for the diagnosis of minimal brain dysfunction, dyslexia, behavior disorder, or hyperactivity (attention deficit hyperactivity disorder) has no established basis; the finding neither proves nor illuminates the diagnosis.

There is evidence that beta activity is a multifactorial genetic trait and that an age factor is responsible for its penetrance (203); however, the relationship to age is complicated. For example, whereas beta activity is a predominant feature of the EEG of premature and full-term infants, it is barely evident in the EEGs of young children. It may be increased in voltage and persistent in the precentral region in middle-aged and elderly women, but it tends to have a low voltage during old age, especially in men (57,84,154–157,182).

In evaluating beta activity, it should be kept in mind that many commonly used drugs (e.g., barbiturates, benzodiazepines, chloral hydrate) increase the amplitude, and thus apparently the amount, of beta activity (58). Because the incidence of beta rhythms with amplitudes much above 20 μV is statistically low in normal persons, the presence of such activity suggests the possibility of drug ingestion. Although the 18- to 25-Hz band is the one most generally affected, some drugs also increase the 14- to 16-Hz activity.

In the presence of skull defects, beta activity in the area of the defect or adjacent to it may be enhanced as a consequence of the low-impedance pathway. Defects of dura, bone, and scalp enhance beta activity more than other, lower frequency activity (99), which has led to erroneous identification of so-called foci of fast activity in patients with surgical or traumatic skull defects.

Beta activity of 18 to 25 Hz usually increases in amplitude during drowsiness, light sleep, and rapid-eye-movement (REM) sleep, and it usually decreases during deep sleep. When a barbiturate or other beta-enhancing drug is administered to promote sleep during the EEG examination, the resultant fast activity increases with the onset of light sleep, decreases markedly during deep sleep, and then remains prominent after the patient is aroused. This effect of sedation is particularly pronounced in children.

Beta activity should have the same frequency on both sides. However, even in normal persons, there may be a voltage asymmetry, with the activity being as much as 35% lower on one side. Such asymmetries may result from differences in skull thickness, as described earlier for the alpha rhythm. On the other hand, a consistently low voltage on one side (greater than 35%), whether focal, regional, or hemispheric, is often a useful diagnostic feature; it indicates cortical injury (e.g., acute contusion, acute ischemia, or the presence of a subdural or epidural fluid collection). Focal, regional, or

hemispheric depression of beta activity may also occur transiently after a focal epileptic seizure. Beta activity is generally the first to show diminished voltage in the presence of a cortical injury or subdural or epidural fluid collection; therefore, its presence on the low-voltage side can be helpful in assessing the significance of a voltage asymmetry of other background activity in the same region (if the asymmetry is borderline in degree). In this regard, it must be remembered that beta activity amplitude is particularly susceptible to the presence of subgaleal fluid, and special care should be taken by the technologist to note the presence of scalp swelling: its location, extent, and degree.

Beta activity, especially when frontocentral in origin, is predominantly out of phase in the two hemispheres; consequently, its amplitude is greater in the paired interhemispheric frontal derivation than in either frontal electrode paired with an "indifferent" electrode or with another adjacent scalp electrode (Fig. 5.7).

Beta activity in the 14- to 16-Hz band is usually most marked in the frontocentral region but may show maximum voltage elsewhere, even in the occipital region. The location of the maximum potential field does not appear to have particular physiological or pathophysiological significance. Beta activity in this band, when present, is usually enhanced by hyperventilation and indeed may become clearly evident only during this activity. It may be present during sleep but should be distinguished from sigma activity, which, by definition, occurs only in bursts.

Activity in the 35- to 40-Hz band is rarely seen in clinical EEGs. Only one report has described activity of this frequency; it was seen only in adults and was reported to be associated with "organic psychosis" or "dull psychopathy" (70). Such activity has not been reported in any series of normal adults or children, and the frequency response of some EEG amplifiers precludes the possibility of recording activity of this frequency even if present.

Although frequencies above 25 Hz are rarely seen in scalp recordings, depth electrode studies in humans have revealed cortical activities with frequencies up to 50 Hz and voltages of 15 to 70 μV (163).

The 18- to 25-Hz activity in the EEG during wakefulness is usually enhanced during stages 1 and 2 sleep, and tends to decrease during the deeper sleep stages.[7] In infants older than 6 months, the onset of sleep is

---

[7]REM sleep is rarely documented in routine clinical EEG recordings of adults and children because time and other factors often do not allow this stage to be reached. However, when REM sleep is recorded, beta activity equal to or greater than that seen in the record during wakefulness is usually present.

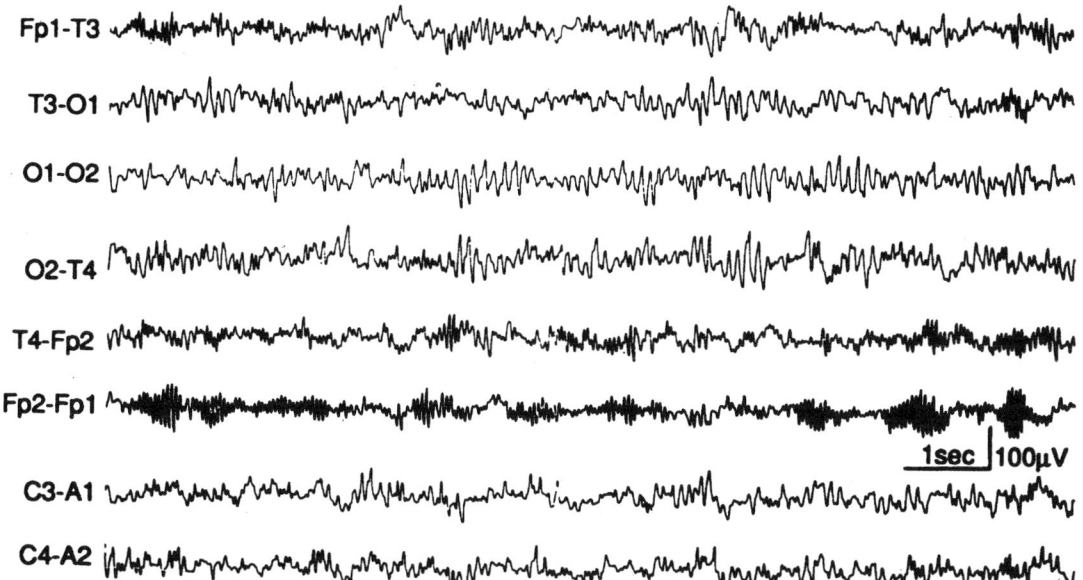

FIG. 5.7. Frontal beta activity in a 12-year-old boy, referred for abdominal pain and receiving diphenoxylate and atropine (Lomotil). Note the high amplitude of the beta activity in paired frontal derivation in comparison with ipsilateral derivations.

marked by increased beta activity in the central and postcentral regions (110). The frequency of this activity is usually 20 to 25 Hz; in infants aged 12 to 18 months (the age at which beta activity is usually maximally expressed), it may have a maximum amplitude of 60 μV (Fig. 5.8). This activity diminishes in both incidence and voltage with increasing age, and beta activity amplitudes exceeding 5 to 10 μV are rare after the age of 6 years. Again, the diagnostic utility of beta activity during sleep is limited.

Focal, regional, or hemispheric depression (defined as being at least 50% lower on one side) of beta activity is a reliable indicator of abnormality, and it is usually accompanied by depression of other background activity on the same side. It is a sign of either cortical depression (contusion, ischemia, atrophy, or cystic defect) or the presence of an intervening fluid collection somewhere between the cortex and the electrode sites. Conversely, high-voltage, generalized but anterior-dominant, fast activity may be a sign of brain damage. In children, a mixture of 18- to 25-Hz and 14- to 16-Hz beta activity with sigma activity of 10 to 14 Hz may occur during sleep in a pattern that has been called "continuous spindling and fast activity" (101). This abnormal finding is seen in certain cases of cere-

bral palsy and mental retardation. The continuous sigma activity may be the predominant feature of the pattern and has led to the name *extreme spindles,* which has been applied to essentially the same phenomenon (69). The interpretation of pronounced fast rhythms (but not so pronounced as to qualify as "continuous fast activity and spindling") in children during sleep is an unresolved problem. Whatever the voltage and duration of the beta activity, consideration must be given to the effects of any drugs the patient may have been taking; consideration must also be given to the effects of any drugs used to promote sleep for the purpose of the EEG study. The electrographic effects of a given drug dose are different in different persons, even if dose-weight schedules are used. There have been no definitive studies to determine whether these differences are related to the drug level in the blood or to differences in the response of the brain to equivalent levels. In children given sedation for sleep in the EEG laboratory, beta activity may become very pronounced if sleep does not ensue after a reasonable period (approximately 35 minutes). Similarly, beta activity may become greatly enhanced in the postsleep record when the child is awakened.

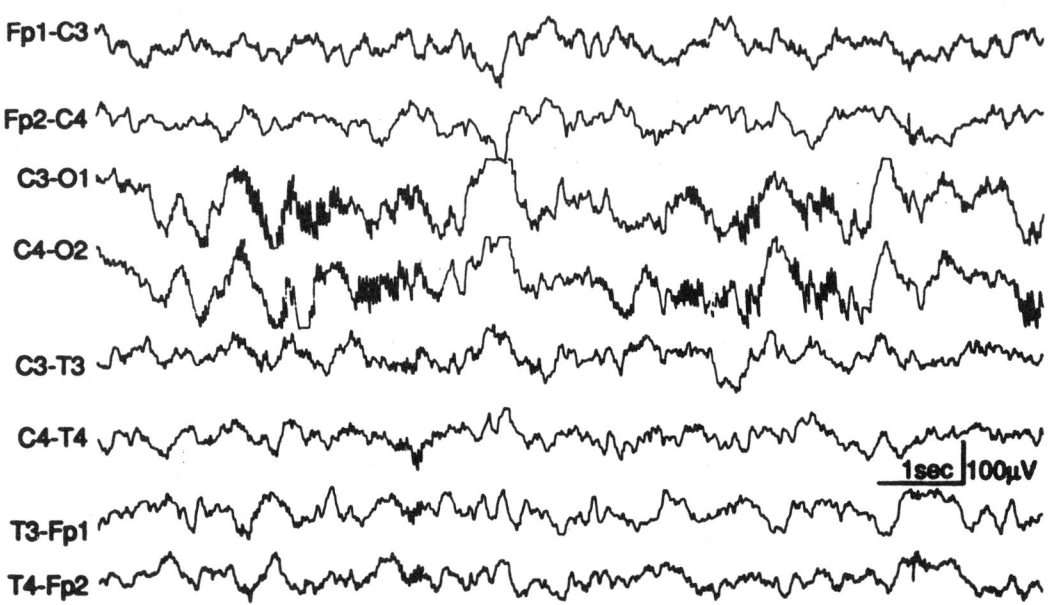

FIG. 5.8. Posterior 20- to 22-Hz activity present almost continuously but tending to show bursts of high voltage, in an asymptomatic 18-month-old girl.

Theta Activity

Frontal and Frontocentral Theta Activity

Most normal young adults show traces of 6- to 7-Hz random activity but show no activity slower than this. In approximately 35%, some low-voltage (less than 15 µV) 6- to 7-Hz waves may be present in the frontal or frontocentral region with the eyes closed and in the presence of a well-sustained occipital alpha rhythm (141,216). The 6- to 7-Hz activity in the frontocentral region tends to become sustained and higher in voltage with the onset of drowsiness, but this effect can usually be recognized because the occipital alpha rhythm concomitantly becomes intermittent or disappears. In patients whose alpha rhythm is low in voltage or poorly sustained, the onset of drowsiness can be determined objectively by using eye electrodes to detect the slow, pendular eye movements that accompany the onset of the drowsy state (141).

In young adults, and particularly in children, heightened emotional states enhance frontal rhythmic theta activity in the 6- to 7-Hz range (24,33,54,60, 93,122,123,150,210). Moreover, some normal persons show marked frontocentral rhythmic theta activity (with the eyes open) while performing certain tasks (218). It has not been established whether this latter effect results from a change in affective state related to the task or is a concomitant of some other aspect of brain function.

Because the routine clinical EEG examination generally does not encompass evaluation of "affective state" or even of "vigilance" during the recording, the presence of some 6- to 7-Hz random or rhythmic activity in the routine EEG cannot be regarded as having pathological significance. As mentioned earlier, approximately 35% of young, nondrowsy, asymptomatic adults show some very-low-voltage (less than 15-µV) 6- to 7-Hz activity in the frontal or frontocentral region in the environment of a quiet, smoothly operating, clinical EEG laboratory. In 10%, the voltage is 15 to 25 µV, and the activity tends to occur in rhythmic serials. The extent to which more sustained, higher voltage (greater than 15-µV), 6- to 7-Hz rhythms reflect the patient's emotional state (24,33,54,60,93,122,123,150,210) or some other physiological condition cannot be assessed properly unless specific procedures are carried out. Hence, there is no clear-cut end point at which frontal theta activity can be specified as abnormal. This problem is particularly important in children, who are especially prone to increased theta activity in highly emotional states and in whom frontal theta activity was once identified as an abnormality having a specific association with behavior disorders. Indeed, the presence of this "abnormality" in the EEG was originally thought to be "evidence of the organic nature of the behavior disorder present" (96). Clearly, enhanced theta activity in such children might result from emotional upsets engendered by the behavior problem and its consequences rather than from pathologically altered brain function. The clinical interpretation of anterior theta rhythms in the EEGs of children was overly influenced by a series of early reports, beginning with that of Jasper et al. in 1938 (96), who stated that such activity was more pronounced and more prevalent in children with behavior problems than in normal, age-matched controls. It is clear that Jasper et al. and subsequent investigators regarded this theta activity as evidence of fundamental brain pathology. Lindsley and Cutts (133), for example, reported that although occasional brief runs of 5- to 8-Hz waves in the frontal and central regions are not unusual in normal subjects, they should be considered abnormal "if they are present as much as 10% of the time in well-organized `runs' or `bursts.'" This concept has been reiterated ever since (usually without critical reappraisal) as a criterion of abnormality in children. However, the runs of 6-Hz activity shown in Fig. 5.9 are comparable to those that Lindsley and Cutts described as abnormal. The tracing in this figure is from the EEG of an asymptomatic 19-year-old man. Such rhythmic activity appears in approximately 15% to 20% of asymptomatic children and adolescents between the ages of 8 and 16 years; serial studies indicate that the occurrence of such rhythms is age-related, appearing in a given child at a certain age, increasing to a peak voltage at approximately the age of 8 years, and tending to diminish and finally disappear thereafter (48,165). Thus, age and ontogenetic processes are factors in the appearance of this type of anterior theta rhythm. Evidence also indicates that genetic factors may play a role (43). The problem is: At what point do frontal 6- to 7-Hz rhythms—because of high voltage, unusual persistence, or paroxysmal regulation—qualify as evidence of abnormal function?

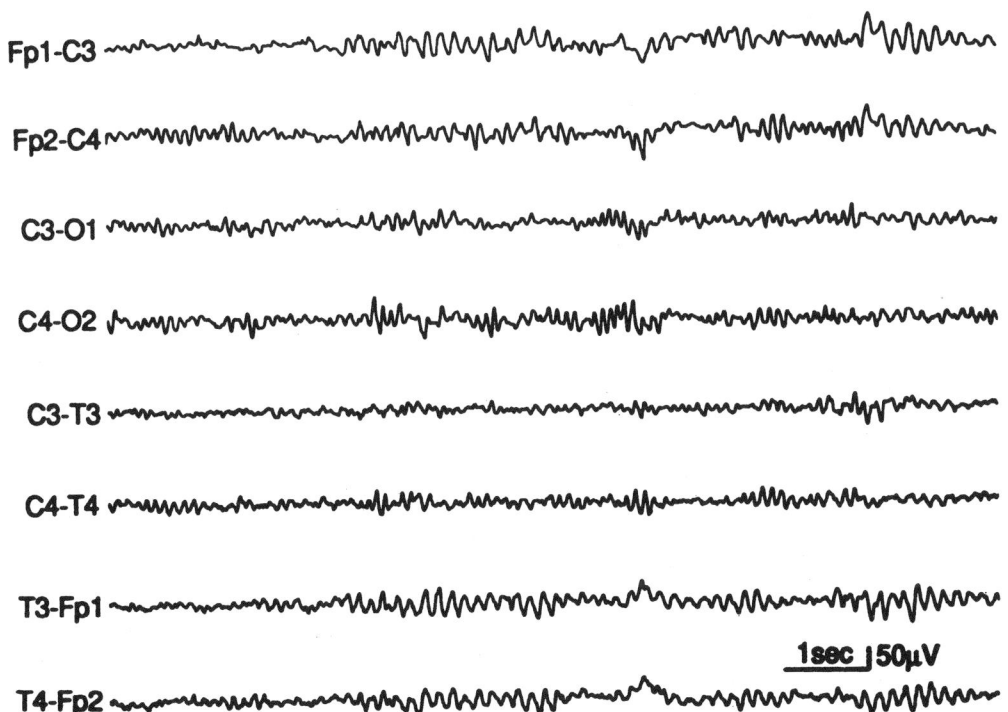

FIG. 5.9. Monomorphic, rhythmic 6- to 7-Hz moderate-voltage activity, occurring in fairly prolonged runs in the frontal leads in an asymptomatic 19-year-old pilot. Theta activity of this degree occurs in asymptomatic young adults but usually not so continuous or so pronounced at this age as in this subject.

Monomorphic, rhythmic 6- to 7-Hz activity occurring in high-voltage (greater than 100-µV) paroxysmal bursts in the frontal or frontocentral region (Fig. 5.10) is not typically seen in normal children (zero incidence in controls). The two extremes of rhythmic theta activity occurrence are shown in Figs. 5.9 and 5.10; however, all degrees of theta activity may be encountered in pediatric practice. At what rate of amplitude change, maximum voltage attained, or degree of persistence, or in what combination of these, does such activity have diagnostic significance? The problem is compounded by the fact that such rhythms are potentiated during drowsiness and by hyperventilation, and what may be a "baseline" rhythm awake and at rest may become paroxysmal during stage I sleep or during overbreathing. Clearly, the true meaning of such rhythms must await development of a more sophisticated knowledge of neuropsychiatry. In clinical practice, the electroencephalographer should not be misled by poorly controlled studies that purport to show that monomorphic frontocentral activity of 4 to 6 Hz (which interrupts and exceeds in peak amplitude the background activity) is correlated with clinical epilepsy. Activity of this description is seen as often in children referred for problems other than epilepsy. Nor should the electroencephalographer be led into false syllogistic thinking—that is, that because a significant incidence of such theta rhythms has been reported in epileptic patients, other disorders that display such rhythms must be epileptic in character.

The problem of interpretation of pronounced theta rhythms in children has been compounded by the reports of Doose et al. (42,43,45,80,81), who equated such rhythms with susceptibility to convulsions and particularly with "clinically manifest epilepsy" (44). They described the pattern as consisting of runs of bilaterally synchronous, monomorphic 4- to 7-Hz rhythmic activity shown most clearly by referential recording from the central regions. The runs

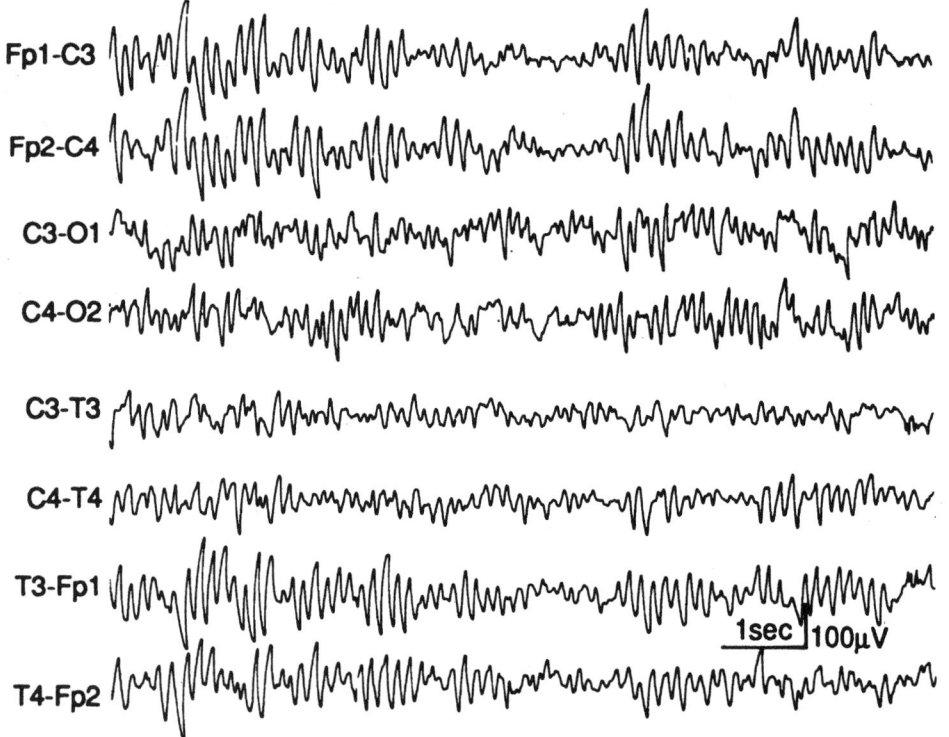

FIG. 5.10. Monomorphic, rhythmic, high-voltage 6- to 7-Hz activity in a 9-year-old boy. Rhythmic 6- to 7-Hz activity, similar to that seen in Fig. 5.9, occurs commonly in this age group but usually not so continuously as in this subject. This high-voltage, frontal theta activity is outside the range of normal variation for any age.

of rhythmic 4- to 7-Hz monomorphic waves often have a spindle shape, tend to spread to the frontal and posterior regions, and tend to dominate the EEG. The rhythm occurs predominantly in children aged 2 to 6 years.

The examples these authors used to illustrate this activity (e.g., Fig. 1 of Doose and Gundel [44]) are typical of what normal children of this age may show in the hypnagogic state. They dismissed this point, however, with the inaccurate assumption that hypnagogic activity occurs "predominantly as a paroxysmal generalized phenomenon," whereas the theta rhythms that they described "are less paroxysmal and tend to be localized in the parietal regions" (see Fig. 1of Doose and Gundel [44]). They also dismissed the hypnagogic state as a possible explanation, because children who show the rhythm "may show no evidence of being sleepy." Yet the term *hypnagogic* was originally used, instead of the term *drowsy waves,* to describe the hypersynchrony prodromal to sleep so as to convey the important fact that the infant or young child showing the pattern *may have the appearance of being fully awake.*

Doose et al. (42,43,45,80,81) presented evidence that the 4- to 7-Hz rhythm that they described "is not only characteristic of primary epilepsies of early childhood but may be found in secondary epilepsies with focal symptomatology" and "in a relatively high percentage of controls" (44). The author's experience with EEGs of many thousands of young children (both normal and with wide-ranging complaints) has led him to believe that the theta pattern as described by Doose et al. is a ubiquitous pattern related to age, not to dysfunction.

Midline Central Theta Activity

A midline central (Cz) theta rhythm has been described in children and adults (31,148,211). As described by Westmoreland and Klass (211), it consists of trains of rhythmic waves of sinusoidal or mu-like form having a consistent frequency within the 4- to 7-Hz range. The rhythm, which is predominantly 6 or 7 Hz, occurs episodically in trains that have a duration of 4 to 20 seconds. It is present only in the awake state, is not related to drowsiness, and is a different rhythm from the bilateral rhythmic central theta activity that is a common finding in sleep. The rhythm has a high correlation with epilepsy but is not related to any particular type (148,211). It is, however, not specifically related to epilepsy, inasmuch as about 25% of the persons who show this pattern have other disorders.

It is not seen in normal subjects at any age, but it is mentioned here so that it may be clearly differentiated from the midline *frontal* theta rhythm that may occur in adults during mental tasks (218), such as reading.

Posterior Slow Waves

Perhaps no EEG finding has been more misunderstood and misevaluated to the detriment of the patient than slow activity in the parieto-occipital and occipitotemporal regions. The interpretation of such activity in children, adolescents, and young adults continues to be fraught with difficulties. Perhaps the problem can be clarified by reviewing how some of the difficulties arose.

In 1938, Jasper et al. (96), beginning with the premise that "the important electrical signs of brain dysfunction given by the electroencephalogram might contribute to our understanding" of certain primary behavior disorders, studied 71 children between the ages of 2 and 16 years who had been admitted to the Bradley Home with a primary diagnosis of behavior problem. For controls, a comparison was made with the EEGs of "40 normal children of comparable age, 70 normal adults, and 219 patients with other nervous or mental disorders." As a pioneer effort, this study was important chiefly in terms of its heuristic value. The authors' conclusion that "abnormal brain function as revealed by the electroencephalogram is an important component in the majority of a group of problem children whose disorder had been considered as primarily psychogenic previous to using this method of diagnosis" was to have a far-reaching influence on future studies, and for a long time no systematic attempt was made to examine this concept or its implications. A long series of papers reported similar findings and reached similar conclusions, each tending to repeat the errors in the research design of the original study without, however, the extenuating circumstance of being the first to deal with the subject.

The errors of experimental design in the original study of Jasper et al. (96) were largely a reflection of the lack of knowledge at this very early point in the history of clinical electroencephalography. Thus, although the authors were concerned about the intelligence of the subjects, they did not control for state (e.g., drowsiness, alertness) and did not appear to make significant adjustments of EEG criteria in terms of age. Consequently, although the study included children as young as 2 years, the authors considered, for the purpose of their study, that the EEG was abnormal if the waves below 7 Hz occurred in more than 10% of at least 100 seconds of record.

The fundamental limitations of this original study (and of many subsequent studies) were the small size of the control group and the basis of the criteria of abnormality. Furthermore, in all the studies, there was the pervading concept that the "abnormalities" are signs of damage. The evidence for this concept was not conclusive (only circumstantial) and included some statistical conceptualizations of questionable validity.

The occipital slow activity seen by Jasper et al. (96), by Lindsley and Cutts (133), and by other early workers who studied children with behavior problems was not well characterized and, in fact, consisted of several types, ranging from continuous delta activity with no alpha rhythm to episodic delta activity with a continuous superimposed alpha rhythm of normal frequency. Clearly, several varieties of occipital or posterior slow activity may be present in children; furthermore, there are numerous permutations of amplitude, waveform, incidence, and posterior areal distribution that cannot be combined into a single category of abnormality without regard for age and state.

The weight of the statistical evidence (33,87,95,133,161) seems to confirm a greater incidence of posterior slow activity in children with behavior disorders than in selected controls of the same age. The character of the deviation and its degree vary considerably, however, and probably do not reflect a unitary pathophysiological mechanism, even in terms of brain damage or lack of it. The evidence of Aird and Gastaut (2), Wiener et al. (216),

and Sutter and Harrelson (190) suggests that asymptomatic children with no antecedent history of brain insult may show posterior slow activity, and this slow activity appears to be age-related. It is likely that some of the types of posterior slow activity described in problem children reflect simply that the subjects are children of a certain age.

The interpretation of posterior slow activity can be made coherent only if its characteristics are clearly defined in terms of the analysis schema outlined in the first two sections of this chapter. First, some posterior slow activity, intermixed with the alpha rhythm, is present in the EEGs of 7% to 10% of highly selected normal young adults (18 to 30 years of age). The type of activity present in 90% of these persons consists of moderate-voltage (defined as no more than 120% of the alpha rhythm voltage) fused waves intermixed with the alpha rhythm (which is often superimposed on them). These waves have been called *polyphasic waves* (48,165) or *posterior slow waves of youth* (2). An example of this type of activity in a normal young adult is shown in Fig. 5.11. This type of posterior slow activity is rare

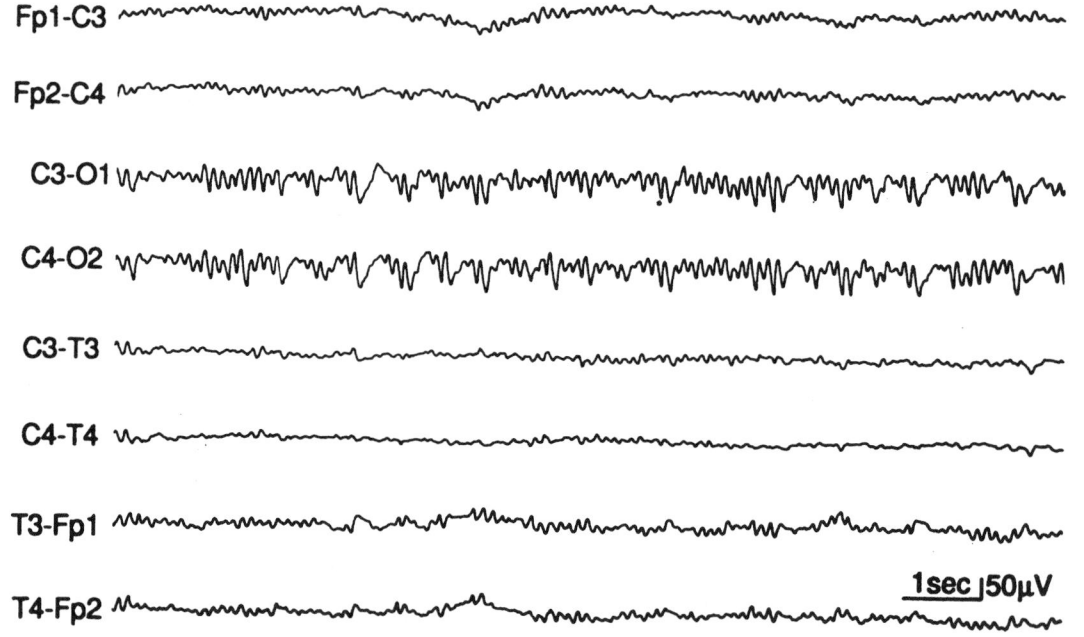

FIG. 5.11. "Posterior slow waves of youth" in an 18-year-old asymptomatic woman. Long interelectrode distances and the central-occipital derivations emphasize this type of slow activity.

in normal adults after age 21 years but has a 15% incidence in persons aged 16 to 20 years (48,165).

Such waves are uncommon in children younger than 2 years, but they are maximally expressed (in amplitude and incidence) in children aged 8 to 14 years (see Fig. 5.16*B*); they occur more often in girls than in boys. It is common for the amplitude and incidence of posterior polyphasic waves in a child to diminish as the recording proceeds. The basis for this change is not clear; it may reflect a change in the anxiety or stress level of the child (24,33,54,60,93,122,123,150,151,210).

A practical point to remember is that the potential field of posterior polyphasic waves is such that they appear to be much more pronounced when recorded from C3–O1 or C4–O2 than from scalp-to-ear derivations (e.g., O2–A2). These waves block with eye opening and disappear with the alpha rhythm during drowsiness and light sleep. They are not always symmetrical or synchronous on the two sides, but the asymmetry should not consistently be more than 50%. They are accentuated by overventilation and, possibly, by stress (24,33,54,60,93,122,123,150,151,210).

If polyphasic or fused waves were the only type of occipital slow activity encountered in children, the difficulty of interpreting children's EEGs would be considerably lessened. However, occipital slow activity may be present in numerous permutations of amplitude, waveform, occurrence, and topography, which renders it difficult to distinguish between normal and abnormal findings.

In terms of manner of occurrence, there is an occipital slow activity that is semirhythmic in character and is a normal finding between the ages of 1 and 15 years (48,165); this is discussed in detail later. Except for this age-related finding, in the awake state there should be no *rhythmic* component in the occipital regions that has a frequency slower than that of the normal range (for age) of the occipital alpha rhythm.

Random, occipital slow activity may be present in normal children in a wide range of waveforms, voltages, and wavelengths, and interpreting the meaning of such activity is complicated by the fact that, in children, the occipital region appears to be a common site for the EEG expression of disordered function. Thus, after closed-head injury or hypoxia or in the various encephalitides, occipital slow activity may be the initial and the last persisting EEG sign of dysfunction resulting from the brain insult. However, because of the wide range of normal variation in the amount and character of occipital slow activity in normal children of various ages and under various conditions, it is often difficult to assess the significance of random occipital slow waves. Nevertheless, it is possible to provide some guidelines for interpretation on the basis of (a) studies of normal children and (b) the experience gained from prospective serial studies of children with various types of brain insult.

Serial observations dating from the time a brain insult is incurred allow definition of certain features of occipital slow activity that are more characteristic of abnormal than of normal function. Thus, when the slow activity deviates from that commonly seen in normal children, the deviation or deviations can be characterized in terms of (a) complexity and variability of waveform, (b) incidence (how often slow waves occur within a given time epoch, such as 10 seconds),[8] (c) voltage ratio (e.g., whether the voltage of the slow activity is greater than 1.5 times the voltage of the occipital alpha rhythm), (d) persistence (whether the occipital slow activity persists with the eyes open), (e) synchrony (whether the occipital slow activity is synchronous on the two sides), and (f) symmetry (whether the occipital slow activity is predominant on one side) (Figs. 5.12 and 5.13).

Any or all of these factors and their degree of expression may be used to formulate an index of abnormality. When this index is high, there should be no difficulty with evaluation. A definitive statement of normal or abnormal cannot be made, however, about many EEGs encountered in clinical practice. The term *borderline* is sometimes applied in this situation, but the clinical utility of this designation is doubtful.

When serial EEGs are obtained after brain injury (147) or in patients with various disease states (e.g., encephalitis), this index of abnormality can be employed effectively. It is much less useful if the EEG is an isolated diagnostic study. In the latter circumstance, even if the electroencephalographer can conclude with confidence that occipital slow activity present on an EEG is outside the range of normal variation, the diagnostic significance (or clinical meaning) of such a finding is not clearly evident *ipso facto.* If, for example, the patient is referred to the EEG laboratory because of "possible seizures," does the presence of an occipital dysrhythmia—or, for that matter, any nonspecific dysrhythmia—help establish a diagnosis of epilepsy? Occipital slow dysrhythmia, as an isolated finding, occurs as often in children who are referred for behavior disorder or learning disability and who

---

[8]In children aged 6 to 24 months, awake, occipital activity is monorhythmic, and with the eyes closed, there should be no random slow waves with a duration exceeding 0.25 second aftnd an amplitude more than 1.5 times that of the alpha rhythm. This is not true of light sleep, in which random delta waves characterize the occipital derivations (110).

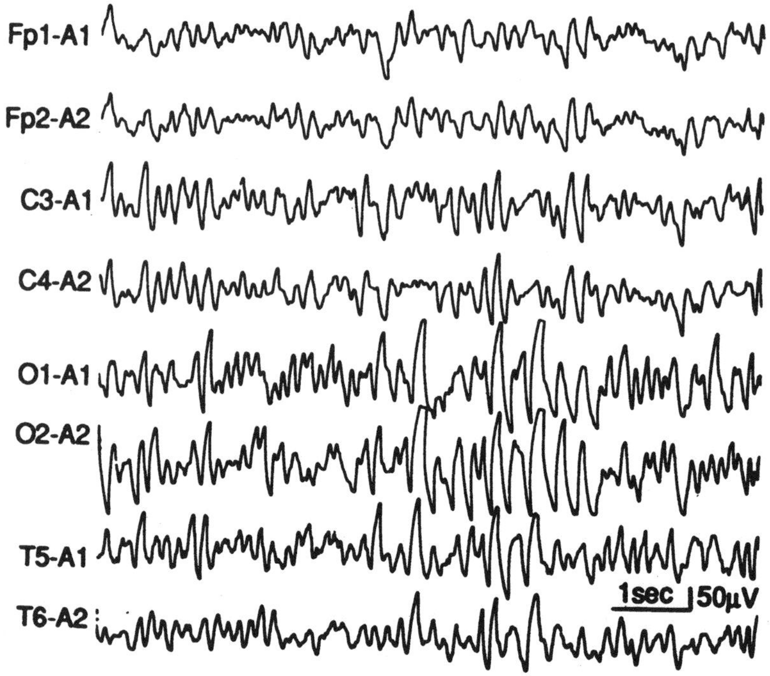

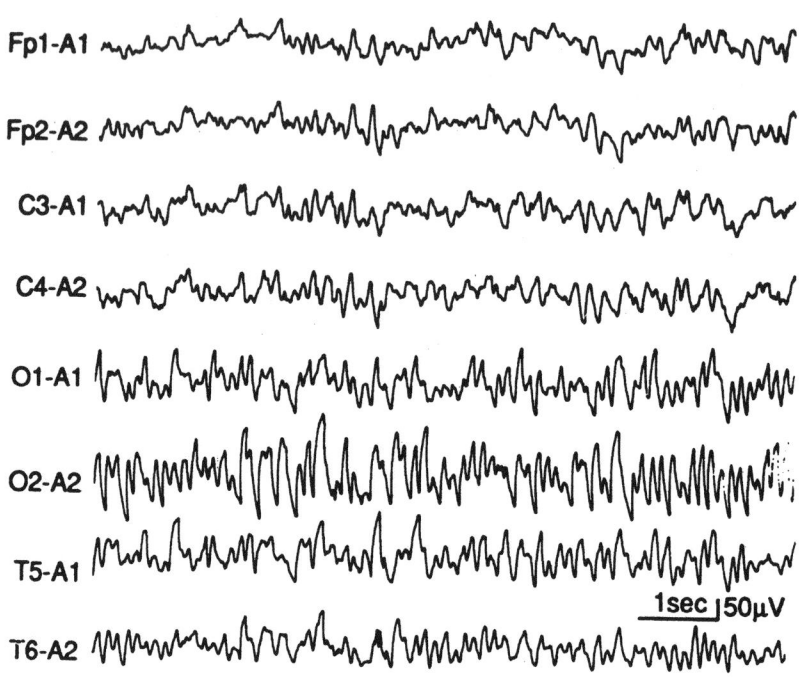

Fp1-A1

Fp2-A2

C3-A1

C4-A2

O1-A1

O2-A2

T5-A1

T6-A2

1sec 50µV

A

Fp1-A1

Fp2-A2

C3-A1

C4-A2

O1-A1

O2-A2

T5-A1

T6-A2

1sec 50µV

B

Fp1-A1

Fp2-A2

C3-A1

C4-A2

O1-A1

O2-A2

T5-A1

T6-A2

1sec 50µV

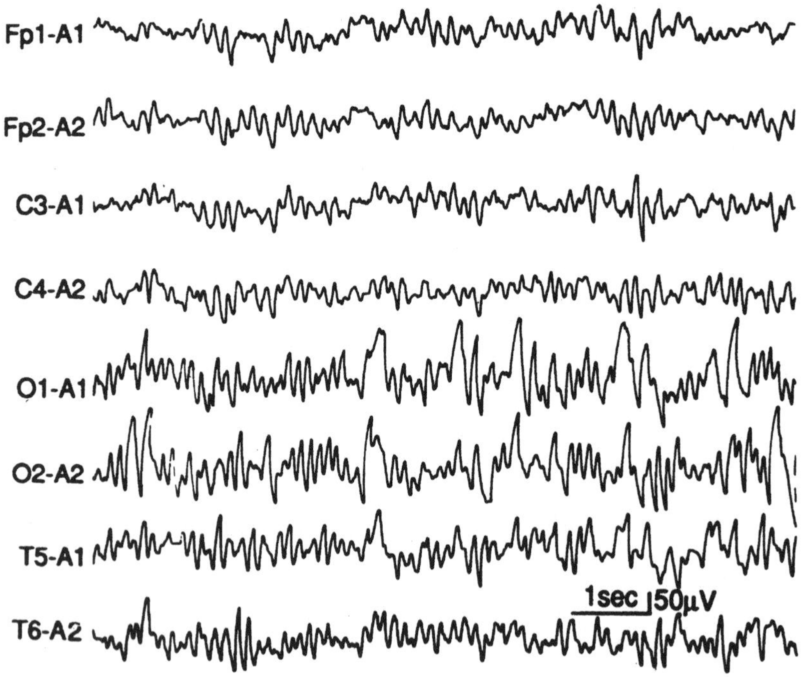

C

FIG. 5.12. A: This EEG is outside the range of normal variation for age (8 years, 1 month) because of high-voltage (three times that of the alpha rhythm), rhythmic 4-Hz waves, which are not seen in normal children. **B:** This occipital slow activity is chiefly 5 to 6 Hz; although it sometimes exceeds the voltage of the occipital alpha rhythm, it is within the range of normal variation for age (8.5 years). Occipital slow activity is usually of higher voltage on the right side; this degree of asymmetry causes no concern. In view of the amount, frequency, and voltage of the occipital activity, this EEG is slightly slow. **C:** The occipital slow activity (3 to 4 Hz) is polymorphic, asynchronous, and over 300 µV. These features are outside the range of normal variation for age (8 years); however, the slow activity in anterior derivations is well within the range of normal. (*Figure continues.*)

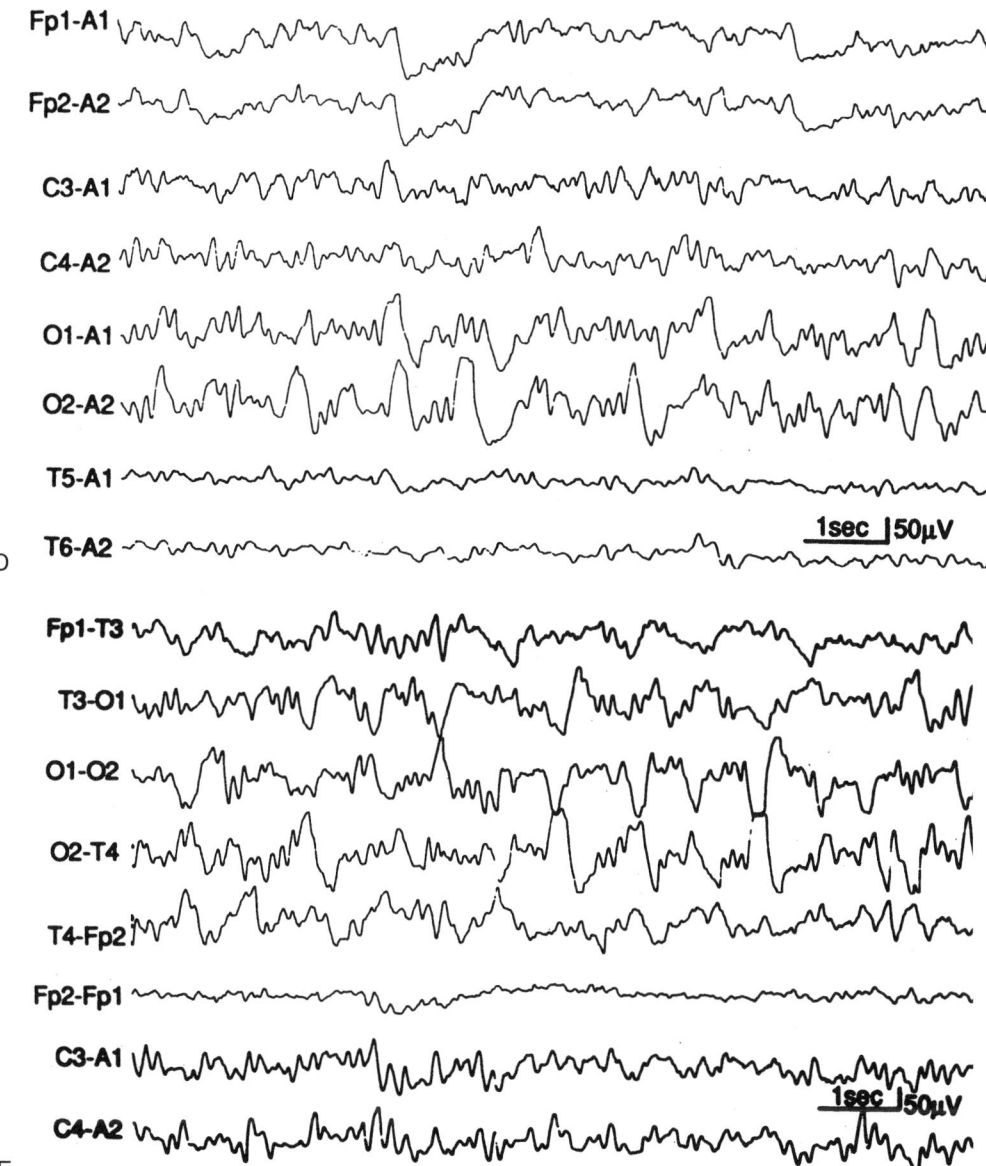

FIG. 5.12. *Continued.* **D:** In an 8-year-old child with meningitis, these high-voltage, random, 2.5- to 3.0-Hz asynchronous waves in the occipital derivations are abnormal, even though the slow activity in anterior derivations is within the range of normal variation. **E:** From the same patient as in part *D.* In scalp-to-scalp derivations, the amount and degree of occipital slow activity are obvious. Note that the duration of some waves exceeds 0.75 seconds. (*Figure continues.*)

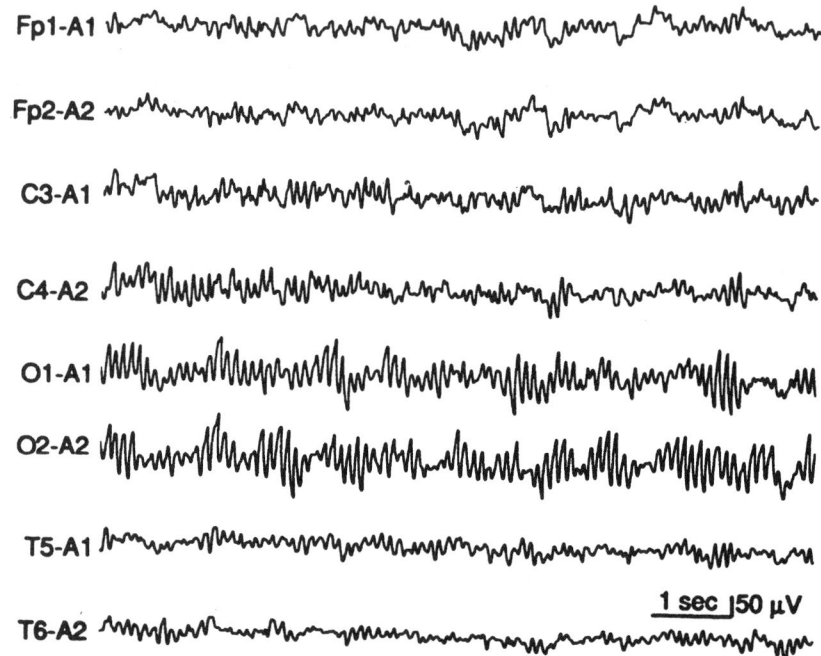

F

FIG. 5.12. *Continued.* **F:** For comparison, a "supernormal" electroencephalogram in a boy aged 7 years, 9 months. Occipital slow activity is minimal and masked by a continuous alpha rhythm. The amount of slow activity seen in anterior derivations is within the range of normal variation up to age 16 years.

do not have seizures as it does in epileptic children (Table 5.2). Even in instances of known epilepsy, the finding of an occipital slow dysrhythmia does little to illuminate the diagnosis. The occipital dysrhythmia may be bilateral, but even this does not establish that the patient has a "generalized" epilepsy. The patient may also have an occult focus not revealed in the EEG. In such a case, it is possible that the occipital dysrhythmia does not relate directly to the patient's epilepsy, but instead occurs as a result of some other intercurrent factor (e.g., phenytoin intoxication).

The foregoing is prelude to a plea: The criteria for what is considered abnormal in children and indicative of disease or disorder must be improved. Also, more caution must be exercised in assigning significance to such findings. Examples of various degrees and types of slow activity encountered in children of a given age are shown in Fig. 5.12. The samples illustrate the range from supernormal to clearly abnormal. It would be more useful if the various types of occipital slow activity could be illustrated for each age. In addition to *random* slow waves, occipital or "posterior" *rhythmic* slow waves are seen in normal children (48,165). Episodic rhythmic, 2.5- to 4.5-Hz, monomorphic

and polymorphic low- to moderate-voltage waves (<100 μV) occur in the parieto-occipitotemporal region (usually maximal at O1 and O2) in approximately 25% of normal awake children aged 1 to 15 years. Such activity is most prominent in those 5 to 7 years of age. Runs of this activity rarely last more than 3 seconds and are present only 2% of the time (48,165). Hyperventilation generally causes this activity to become more continuous and higher in voltage.

Rhythmic occipital slow activity of various types and frequencies that does not seem to reflect an insult or to have an established genetic origin has been reported in the EEGs of adults (2,6,120,166). These rhythms are perhaps of some interest as EEG anomalies, but they are important in the discussion of the characteristics of the normal EEG only in that they can be recognized as being outside the range of normal variation but having no known pathophysiological significance.

Posterior Slow-Wave Transients Associated with Eye Movements. In some young children (aged 6 months to about 10 years), some eye blinks or eye movements are associated with a single monophasic or diphasic slow transient that has a duration of 200 to 400 milliseconds and an amplitude of

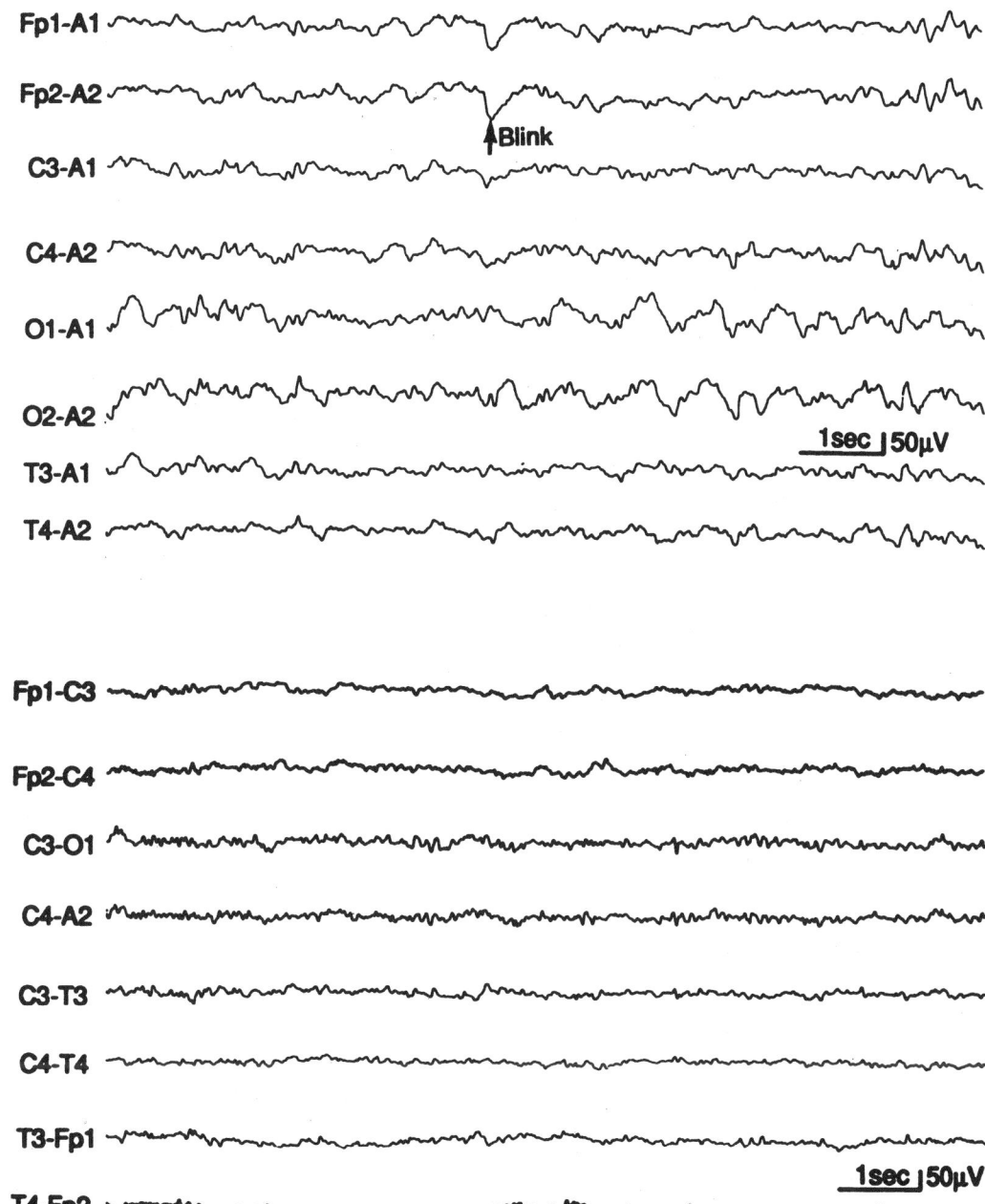

Fp1-A1

Fp2-A2

↑Blink

C3-A1

C4-A2

O1-A1

O2-A2

1sec ⌐50μV

T3-A1

T4-A2

A

Fp1-C3

Fp2-C4

C3-O1

C4-A2

C3-T3

C4-T4

T3-Fp1

1sec ⌐50μV

B T4-Fp2

FIG. 5.13. A: Polymorphic slow activity in the occipital leads is often difficult to evaluate if low in voltage and random in occurrence, as in a 14-year-old boy. The slow activity is different from that shown in Fig. 5.11 (normal for the age of 18 years) and from that in Fig. 5.16*B* (normal for the age of 10 years). The occipital slow activity in this tracing, made 6 hours after injury, typifies that seen soon after closed-head injury (concussion) occurring in late childhood or adolescence. This slow activity usually resolves within 10 days. **B:** From the same patient as in part *A,* 7 days after injury. Note that the occipital slow waves have disappeared. The alpha rhythm is somewhat slow, poorly sustained, and poorly organized, but it is "normal" for age.

TABLE 5.2. *Electroencephalographic (EEG) findings in children with known seizures compared with other children commonly referred for EEG studies (age group: 3–16 years)**

EEG findings	Epilepsy (%) (N = 3,046)	Primary behavior disorders (%) (N = 2,626)	Learning and communication disorders (%) (N = 3,148)	Questionable seizures (%) (N = 1,163)
Normal	39.6	66.9	65.8	64.0
Nonspecific dysrhythmias	19.0	19.9	21.0	24.0
Foci	29.8	7.5	8.0	8.7
Spike-and-wave	4.8	1.8	1.9	3.0
Other	7.8	0	0	0.3

*Note that the incidence of nonspecific dysrhythmias is approximately the same for all groups and is similar to the incidence (16%) given by Wiener et al. (216) for normal children.

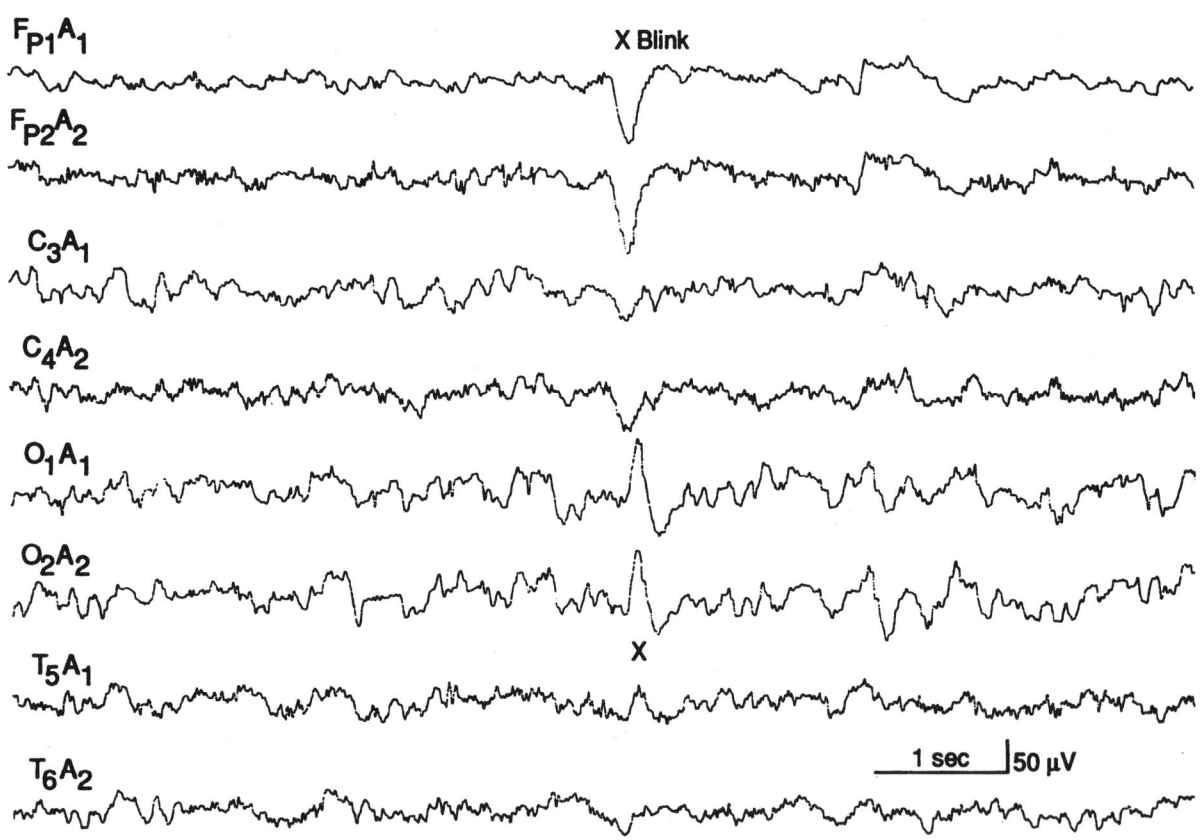

FIG. 5.14. Occipital sharp transient associated with eye blink in a 13-month-old boy, awake.

up to 200 μV. These transients are usually confined to the occipital region and occur with a latency of 100 to 500 milliseconds after the blink or eye movement (Fig. 5.14).

The initial component of these transients is surface positive, and it and the ascending phase of the next surface-negative component have a steep wave front. The descending phase of the second component is much less steep. These transients are often asymmetrical on two sides and do not occur with every eye movement or blink. They are seen most frequently in children aged 2 to 3 years (213).

These posterior slow-wave transients that follow an eye movement or blink are normal phenomena but may be mistaken for abnormal activity, par-

ticularly if they seem to occur in the absence of eye movements or blinks. To establish an association between these events, it may be necessary to record horizontal and oblique as well as vertical eye movements, because the former may not be detected easily in frontal EEG derivations.

Anterior Slow Activity in Children

It has long been known that the amount of slow activity in the EEGs of children decreases with increasing age and that the persistence and frequency of the slow activity vary in different areas. Both of these facts are clearly illustrated in Fig. 5.15, a graphic representation of the findings of an

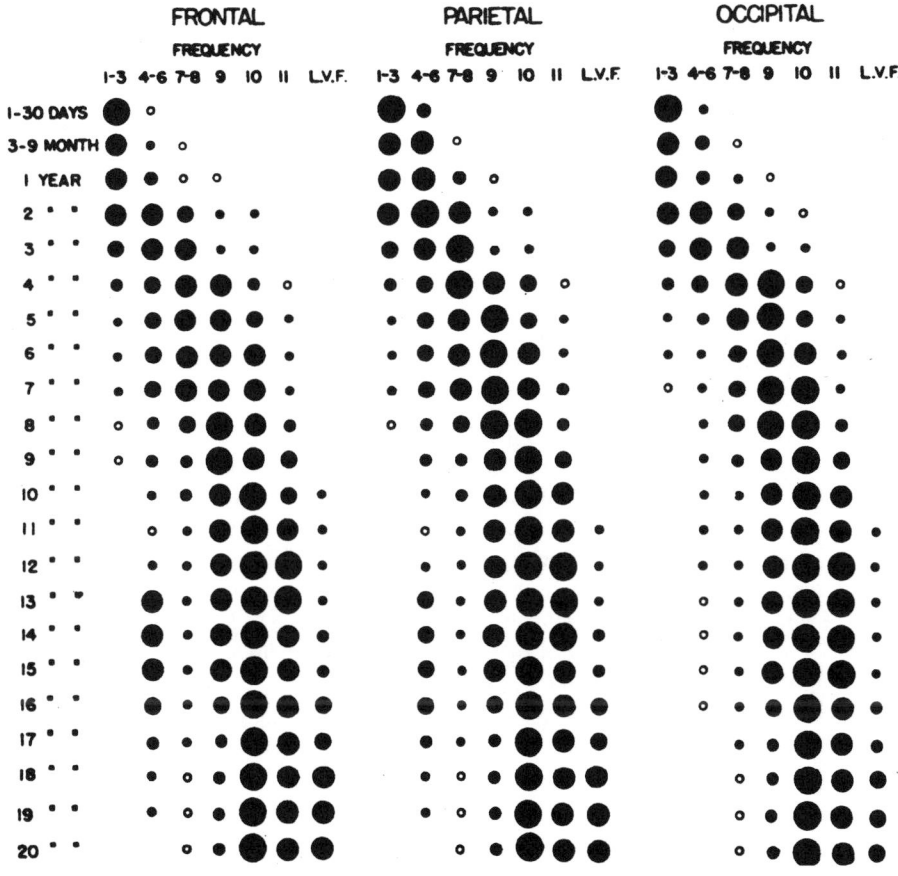

FIG. 5.15. Graphic summary of early frequency-analysis study of Gibbs and Knot (75). The designation of "Parietal" refers to the parietal bone of the skull. Actual electrode locations are approximately those of the C3 and C4 positions. At the time this study was made, temporal derivations were not used routinely by this group. L.V.F., low-voltage fast activity.

early frequency-analysis study by Gibbs and Knott (75). This figure may be regarded as a fairly good approximation of the frequencies present and their degree of expression in various regions at different ages. It does not, however, provide information concerning the waveform of the activity, its voltage, or the manner of its occurrence (e.g., random, continuous runs), all of which are critical elements of visual analysis and are essential to clinical evaluation of the EEG.

Another important aspect of assessing the amount of slow activity in the EEG is the frequency:voltage ratio. It has become the practice for clinical electroencephalographers to rate an activity as having high or low voltage in relation to its frequency. Thus, at the two ends of the EEG frequency spectrum, a 25-Hz activity is regarded as being high in voltage if its amplitude is 30 μV, but a 1- to 2-Hz wave of similar amplitude is considered low in voltage. This convention grew out of the everyday experience of recording the EEGs of human subjects: Beta activity is generally much lower than 25 μV in amplitude; hence, anything higher is "high voltage." On the other hand, 1- to 2-Hz waves of over 800 μV are common during physiological (sleep) and in abnormal conditions in humans. The convention has significance in terms of the power-spectral characteristics of the EEG. The clinical electroencephalographer assesses the significance of slow activity in relation to its voltage; this frequency:voltage ratio is an important component of the set of mental templates (one for each age range) that must be developed in order to have a consistent basis for evaluation. The age range to which each such template can be applied varies with age, because the *range* of normal variation is different at different age levels.

In evaluating the amount and duration of slow activity present in relation to the age of the patient, it is helpful to use the concept of the "ideal" EEG for each age as a standard of comparison. "Ideal" is not used to convey perfection (particularly in a clinical sense) but is, instead, employed in the platonic sense of "prototype." The "ideal" is based on what 75% of asymptomatic children of a given age show in terms of the slow activity present in the various derivations. Approximately 5% of normal children (same age) show less slow activity than the ideal, and their EEGs more closely approximate the adult pattern (these are sometimes called "supernormal" EEGs) (48,165). Another 15% of normal children show slightly greater amounts of slow activity than the ideal, and 5% show moderately increased amounts of slow activity. These general concepts have been adopted, modified, and expanded by the author's colleagues and collaborators in Sweden and underlie their categorizations of "slightly increased slow" and "moderately increased slow" (48,165). These benchmark papers of Eeg-Olofsson and

Petersén provide the essential data on which the kind of mental template required for the evaluation of children's EEGs can be developed.

Eeg-Olofsson and Petersén (48,165) rated the amount of nonrhythmic (random) slow activity in the EEGs of children in their normal series as "minute," "normal," "slightly increased (SIL)," and "moderately increased (MIL)" for age. Of their highly selected healthy children, approximately 87% had random slow activity in an amount rated as normal for age. Approximately 8% had lesser amounts of slow activity than this, and 4.3% had slightly greater amounts of nonrhythmic slow activity; in 0.5% of the series, the random slow activity was MIL. This compares with the concept of the "ideal" EEG and the range of normal variation that was developed from studies of asymptomatic but not highly selected children. Eeg-Olofsson and Petersén found that the incidences of SIL and MIL were greatest in children between 6 and 11 years of age and were significantly higher in girls than in boys.[9]

Comparison of Eeg-Olofsson and Petersén's prototypic EEG samples of "normal," "slightly increased," and "moderately increased" slow activity with the author's own prototypes indicates that the highly selected healthy children in the Gothenburg series (48,165) showed lesser amounts of random slow activity than did the author's unselected asymptomatic children. If the criteria offered by the Gothenburg study of highly selected children are used as a basis of interpretation in routine clinical practice, considerable caution must be exercised in categorizing an EEG of a given child as "outside" the range of normal variation; care should be taken here because the "pathological" significance of an abnormal EEG, which is too readily equated with brain "damage" (or, at best, "dysfunction"), is often based on simplistic reasoning. The talent of the clinical electroencephalographer is measured not so much by an ability to make a visual analysis of the tracing but by an ability to determine what the findings mean in a particular patient under particular circumstances in relation to a particular clinical history. The characteristics of the EEG are determined by numerous influences, not the least of which may be the uniqueness of the laboratory environment. Factors that determine the characteristics of an individual's EEG at any time are discussed in the final section of this chapter. It is beyond the scope of this chapter to attempt to convey the "ideal" and the "range of normal variation" for each age. Figure 5.16 illustrates the concept for a single age level.

---

[9]This finding is in accord with the concept that the *range* of normal variation itself varies with age.

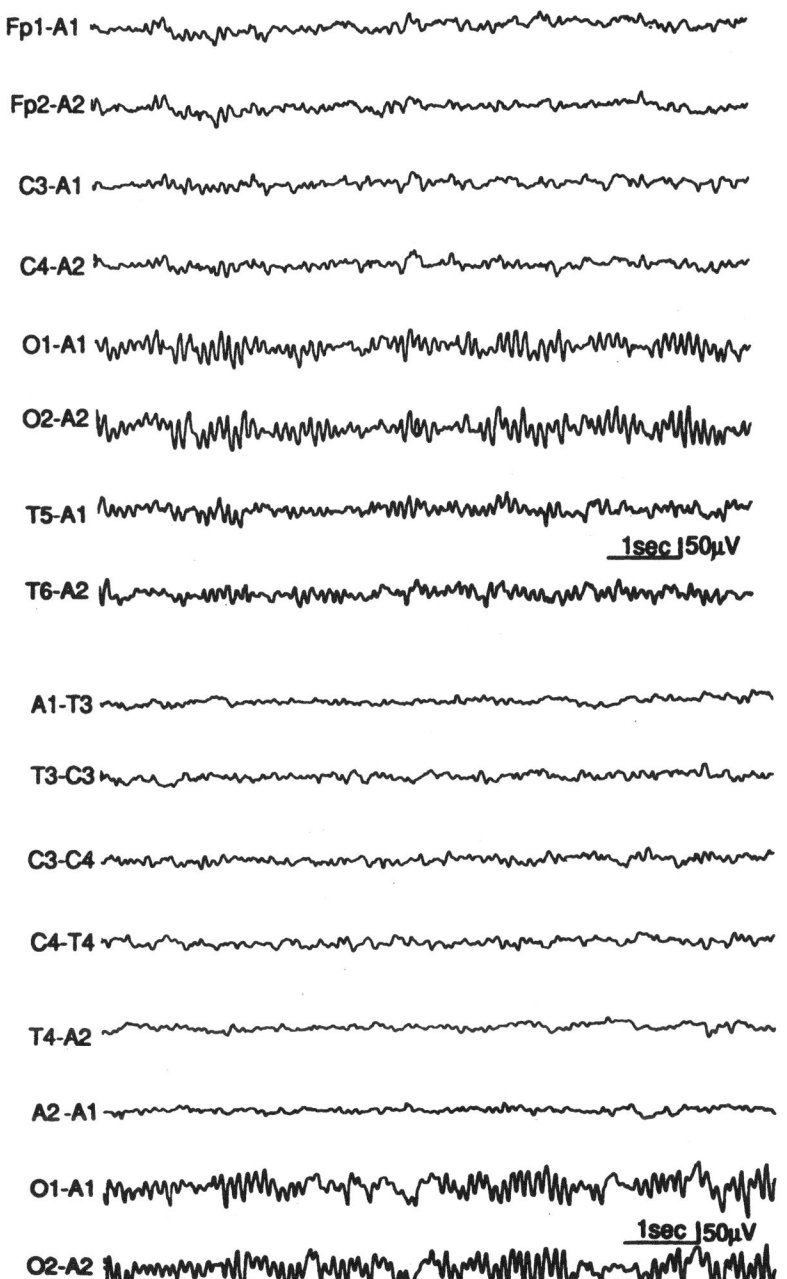

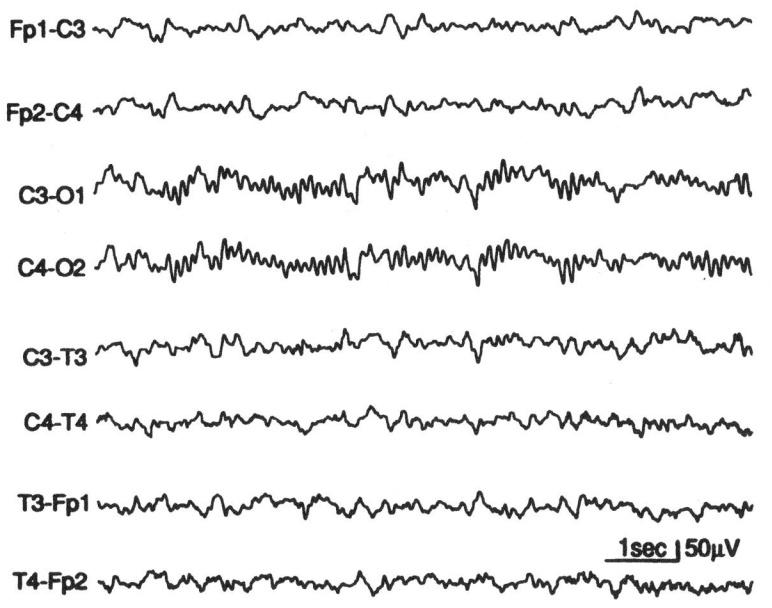

FIG. 5.16. A: "Supernormal" electroencephalogram (EEG) for age (10-year-old girl). Greater amounts of slow "fused" (polyphasic) activity could appear in the occipital leads, as in part *B,* or greater amounts on random 4- to 6- Hz moderate-voltage activity could appear in the anterior leads and yet remain within the range of normal for age. **B:** This EEG, from an asymptomatic boy aged 10 years, 2 months, shows greater amounts of "posterior slow waves of youth" than in part *A* but has slightly smaller amounts of anterior slow activity. **C:** Moderately increased slow activity; random moderate-voltage, 4- to 6-Hz activity; and some slower low-voltage fused forms in anterior derivations. Occipital derivations show moderate amounts of polyphasic slow activity. The subject was 9 years, 8 months old.

Lambda Waves

When an individual's eyes are open, especially if the room is well illuminated, sharp waves with a duration of 160 to 250 milliseconds may be recorded in the occipital regions bilaterally. These sharp transients, designated *lambda waves,* are particularly likely to be present if the patient is visually scanning a complex picture. The necessary condition for generation of these waves is saccadic movements of the eyes (4,56). Gastaut (68) initially described them as "biphasic or triphasic potential variations with a small initial positive phase and a prominent subsequent negative phase." More recent studies, involving the use of computer techniques, have shown that the most prominent phase in the occipital region is surface negative (132,174). However, most of the studies concerning lambda waves recorded from the scalp in human subjects (4,53,79,173,176,180,194) describe them as predominantly surface positive at the occipital electrodes (Fig. 5.17). Routine experience indicates that the duration and waveform of lambda waves vary considerably among individuals and that, particularly in children, the highest amplitude and sharpest component are generally surface negative in the occipital derivations. Lambda waves are much more commonly seen in children aged 2 to 15 years than in adults; they are rarely seen in the routine EEGs of elderly people. With long interelectrode distances (e.g., C3 to O1), lambda waves with amplitudes as high as 65 µV may be seen in children (Fig. 5.18).

In a routine clinical EEG, lambda waves may be quite asymmetrical on the two sides and, in fact, may be present on only one side. This asymmetry may lead to the misinterpretation of lambda waves as a focus of abnormal activity. This is especially likely to occur if the technologist or electroencephalographer fails to note that the waves occur only during the eyes-open condition. If there is any doubt concerning the nature of the activity, then eye closure, diminution of illumination, or having the patient stare at a blank white card should eliminate lambda waves but should have no effect on the incidence or amplitude of abnormal occipital sharp waves.

The amplitude of lambda waves, and hence the likelihood that they will be seen in routine EEGs, is greatly influenced by the complexity of the sensory field, by the intensity of illumination of the sensory field, and by its proximity. There are also marked individual differences in the ease with which such waves may be detected (28,56,180).

In children, and less commonly in young adults, scanning of a complex geometric pattern may produce lambda waves, which are predominantly surface negative and have a spike-like configuration (see Figs. 18*A* and *B*).

These are a normal finding even when asymmetric on the two sides. When present unilaterally, they may be mistaken for an abnormal focus of spike discharge, but the distinction can easily be made by simply replacing the geometric image with a blank surface. These observations (105) were confirmed by Sunku et al. (189).

Temporal Slow Activity: A Normal Finding in the Elderly?

With increasing age, a significant number of persons show episodic, irregular slow activity in the temporal regions, usually with maximum voltage in the midsylvian region. A 50-year-old subject may typically show a series of EEG changes in the temporal regions during the next 15 years of life. The sequence of changes may be as follows: the first new activity to appear might be episodic, temporal 8- to 10-Hz waves of higher voltage than the occipital alpha rhythm. With time, some episodic activity that is usually a subharmonic frequency (4 to 5 Hz) of the alpha rhythm may then appear. This mixed alpha/theta activity is usually more marked on the left side, is enhanced by overventilation, and may persist when the occipital alpha rhythm blocks with eye opening or with drowsiness. The episodes are usually quite brief, ranging from two to three waves to rarely more than six or seven. Overventilation increases their voltage and persistence. Enhanced temporal alpha activity is not a constant feature. Episodic temporal theta activity of this type, designated *sylvian theta activity* by Gastaut et al. (64), may remain unchanged for many years (up to 20 years in the author's experience), or it may become higher in voltage, more polymorphic, and more persistent.

Because independent temporal focal slow activity may be seen in aged but asymptomatic persons, Obrist et al. (154–156) and Kooi et al. (117) suggested that it is a normal accompaniment of the aging process. Others (21,64,66,112,196), beginning with Gastaut et al. (64), suggested that temporal EEG changes are associated with cerebrovascular insufficiency. A group of persons with evidence of cerebrovascular insufficiency was compared with an age-matched group of controls who had no evidence of such disease; the age incidence of temporal slow activity was shifted to the left in the insufficiency group, and there was a greater overall incidence of this type of activity (Crawley and P. Kellaway, unpublished observations). Furthermore, in a series of subjects aged 50 to 70 years, a comparison of the persons who show temporal slow activity with those who do notrevealed a 35% higher incidence of hypertension, coronary insufficiency, peripheral artery occlusion, and other evidence of systemic vascular disease in those

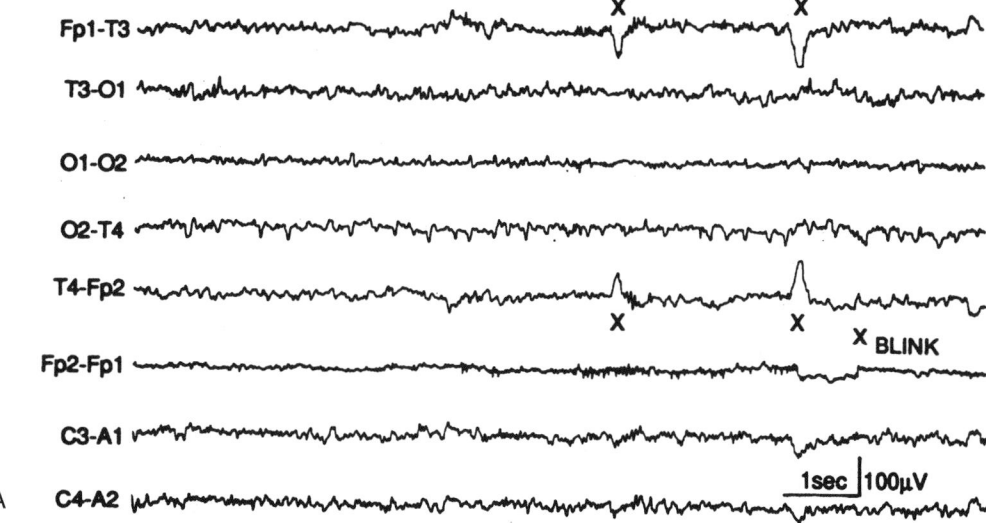

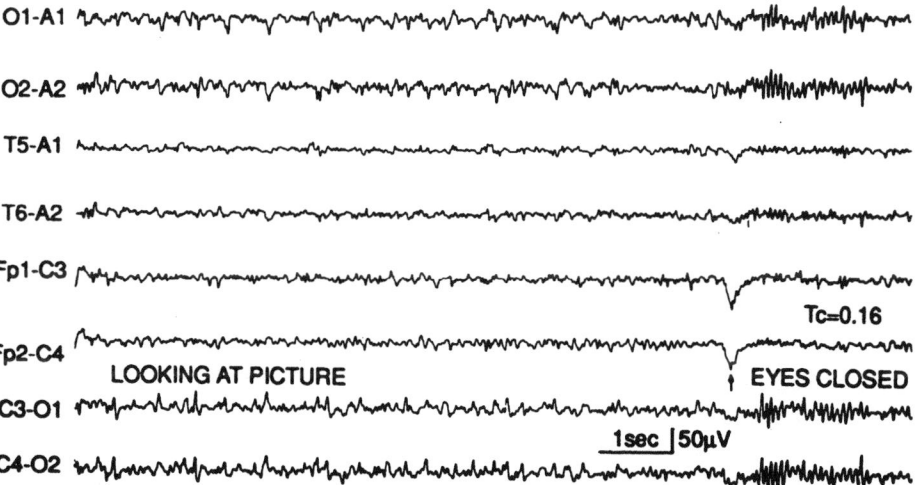

FIG. 5.17. A: Lambda waves in an asymptomatic 25-year-old woman looking at a pattern (e.g., ceiling tile). **B:** Recording designed to provide greater definition of lambda waves In an asymptomatic girl, aged 12 years. Note that lambda waves are often polyphasic, and in this child the predominant phase is positive at the occipital electrode.

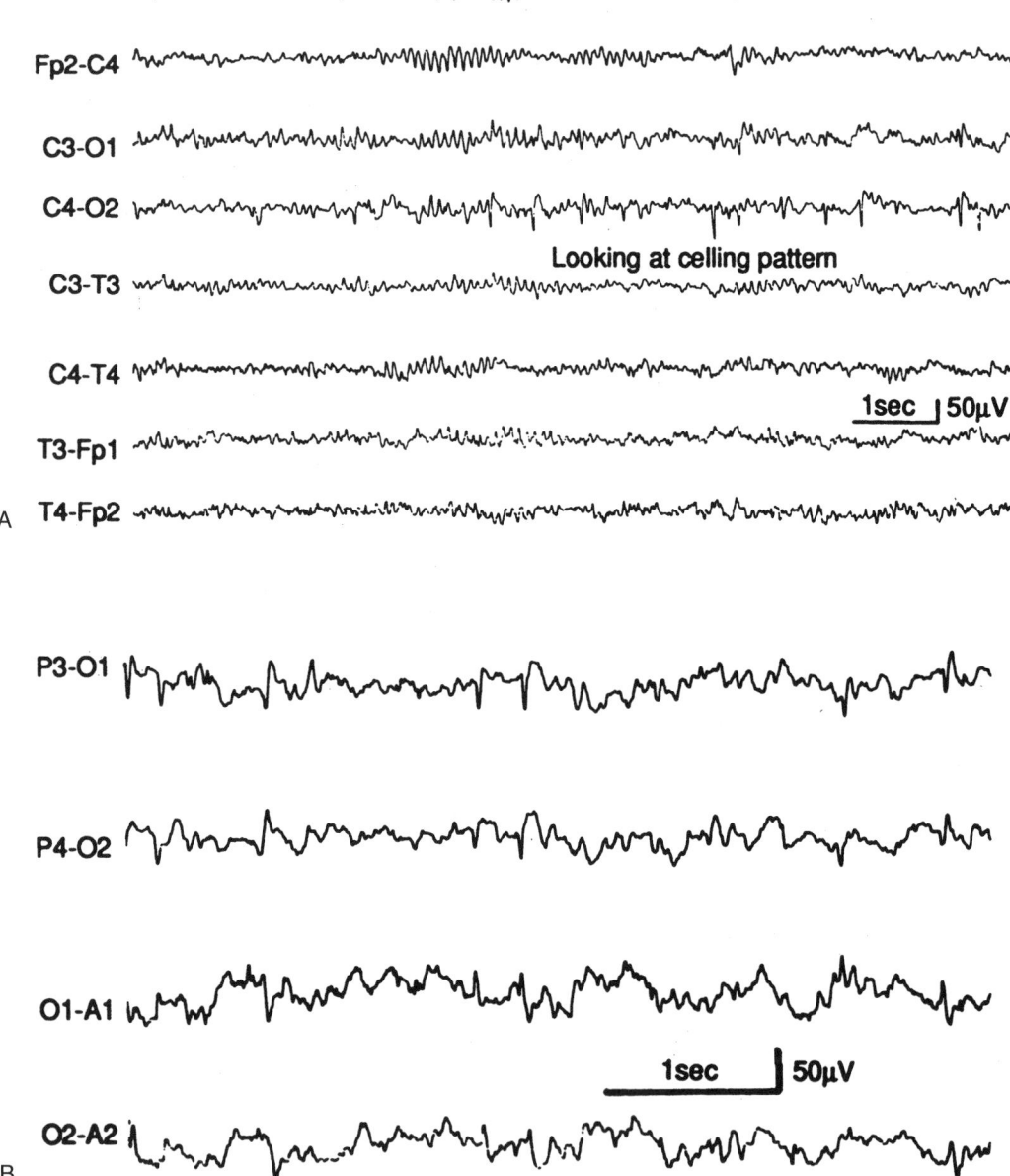

Fp1-C3

Fp2-C4

C3-O1

C4-O2

Looking at ceiling pattern

C3-T3

C4-T4

1sec ⌐ 50μV

T3-Fp1

A   T4-Fp2

P3-O1

P4-O2

O1-A1

1sec ⌐ 50μV

O2-A2

B

FIG. 5.18. A: High-voltage lambda waves in an asymptomatic 15-year-old, with the maximum amplitude phase negative at the occipital electrode. Note that lambda waves are quite "sharp," are of short duration, and occur almost entirely on the right side. **B:** Lambda waves occurred bilaterally while the subject, a normal child aged 10 years, 7 months, was looking at a pattern in the ceiling tile. Note that the waves have a sharp negative phase.

with the temporal slow activity (Crawley and P. Kellaway, unpublished observations). However, the predominantly left lateralization of the temporal slow activity appeared to have no relationship to the side on which the first or any subsequent transient ischemic attack or completed stroke might occur. These observations, made over a period of 20 years, are based on presurgical and postsurgical EEGs of more than 1,800 patients with insufficiency and on serial EEGs of a group of 200 executives aged 45 to 75 years. However, a well-designed prospective and longitudinal study with quantitative methods has not been performed, and so the descriptive data just mentioned have not been published. To be useful, such a study would have to include measurements of regional blood flow, quantitative EEGs, and neuropsychological evaluations. In the absence of such data, the clinical electroencephalographer faces the problem of interpreting the significance, if any, of various degrees of temporal slow activity seen in a high percentage of middle-aged and elderly patients. It is common practice to report some temporal theta waves and possibly a few temporal delta waves as normal findings in elderly patients. The problems of how much slow activity is allowed and how old the patient must be for the findings to be considered normal are currently being neglected; as a consequence, there is enormous variability in the way individual electroencephalographers evaluate this type of finding.

When episodic 4- to 5-Hz, low- to moderate-voltage waves are present in the temporal leads bilaterally or with a marked predominance on one side (usually the left) in persons aged 50 years or older, it is reasonable to report their presence and to note that such activity may occur in asymptomatic persons in this age group. When the activity is present in younger adults, or if there is episodic temporal delta activity, the suspicion of clinically significant abnormality is increased. It is important also to recognize that, because temporal slow activity occurs in asymptomatic elderly persons, such findings in patients of this age group who are referred because of head injury or possible cerebral metastases are *unlikely* to be related to these etiologies and therefore carry the same meaning here as would a normal EEG.

A case in point concerns a 65-year-old man who was in the hospital for gallbladder surgery. He fell out of bed one morning and bruised his forehead; he was not unconscious but seemed confused for several minutes after getting back into bed. The EEG (made on the afternoon of the same day) showed a well-regulated 9-Hz occipital alpha rhythm, with some episodic, low-voltage 3- to 5-Hz waves in the left temporal region and some rare activity of similar frequency that occurred independently in the right temporal region. Statistically, there is a high likelihood that such EEG findings in a man of this age predated the injury; also, focal episodic left-lateralized temporal theta activity is an unlikely consequence of an acute closed-head injury. Follow-up EEGs 5 and 10 days later showed no change.

Another case concerns a 72-year-old woman with a history of breast cancer and bilateral mastectomy, referred for EEG studies because of attacks of dizziness and headaches. The tentative diagnosis was cerebral metastasis. The EEG showed an 8-Hz alpha rhythm, with some moderate-voltage (85 μV maximum) 4- to 5-Hz waves that appeared episodically in the left and right temporal regions independently but were much more marked on the left side, where there were also occasional low-voltage 3- to 4-Hz waves. The EEG report indicated that these findings were probably not related to the presence of cerebral metastasis but that a follow-up study at 4 weeks might be helpful in this regard. Over a period of 18 months, the patient continued to complain of headache and dizziness, but several EEGs failed to show any change. Over the next 3 years, the patient's symptoms showed some fluctuation but no progression and no evidence of cerebral metastasis. The EEG remained essentially unchanged.

Torres et al. (191) found a significantly higher percentage of focal slow activity in volunteer elderly subjects "who showed no signs or symptoms of central nervous system disease" than in patients with known cardiovascular disease. However, in another series of elderly patients "rigorously selected for neuropsychiatric normality," Katz and Horowitz (100) found a very low incidence of focal temporal slow activity, and one study (200) reported that temporal slowing is correlated with subtle speech problems and computed topographic scan changes.

The more that temporal slow activity differs from the simple prototype shown in Fig. 5.19, the more it should be regarded with suspicion. The slower the activity, the greater the voltage, and the more complex and (particularly) the more continuous the waveform is, the less reasonable it becomes to regard the finding as being within the range of normal variation for age.

The definition of temporal slow activity is critically important. The slow activity must be characterized in terms of frequency, amplitude, mode of occurrence, precise location, and percentage of time during which the subject is awake. All studies of elderly patients have found low-voltage intermittent temporal theta activity in a percentage of asymptomatic elderly persons; an incidence of about 35% has been reported by several different groups (3,23,91,191). Paroxysmal bursts or long trains of rhythmic theta

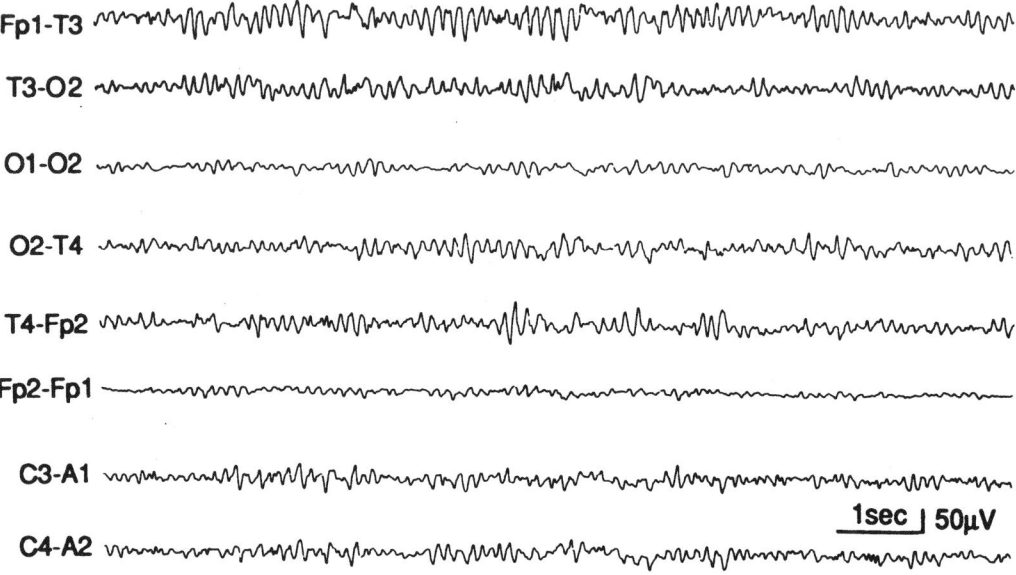

FIG. 5.19. Temporal alpha and fused slow activity on the left side and occasionally independently on the right in a 60-year-old man with occlusive carotid disease, more marked on the right.

activity in the temporal region are not seen in normal elderly persons. Episodic focal temporal delta activity occurs in only 12% to 18% of such persons (3,100,191). The slower the activity, the higher its voltage, the greater its persistence, and the more strongly lateralized it is, the less likely that it will be found in normal elderly subjects.

Episodic delta activity occurring focally in the temporal regions, synchronously or asynchronously on the two sides, is an abnormal finding in elderly persons (162,196); moreover, the correlation with vascular insufficiency, particularly with small-vessel disease, is much greater than it is with temporal theta activity (P. Kellaway and Crawley, unpublished observations).

Hyperventilation Response

Throughout the literature of pediatric electroencephalography, the response to hyperventilation is cited repeatedly as partial or complete supporting evidence of brain abnormality in children. Historically, this concept originated in the early report of Lindsley and Cutts (133):

> Overbreathing in some cases produced what we have called a "hyperventilation effect." This is defined as a distinct change (usually abrupt) in the electroen-

cephalogram, consisting of a sequence of slow waves, ranging in frequency from 2 to 8 per second and usually of a magnitude considerably above anything of similar frequency occurring in the records before hyperventilation. The "hyperventilation effect" may persist as a continuous series of rhythmic slow waves or may consist of repeated bursts of slow waves at irregular intervals. Two measurements were made, one of the duration from the beginning of hyperventilation to the onset of the "effect," the other of the duration from the cessation of hyperventilation to the disappearance of the "effect."

Lindsley and Cutts's subjects spent 1.5 minutes hyperventilating unless a marked effect appeared before that time, in which case subjects were told to stop overbreathing and to remain quiet until the record returned to the original state. Lindsley and Cutts found that children with behavior problems showed a more abrupt and greater buildup of slow activity and more prolonged effects after cessation of hyperventilation than did normal controls. The subjects were instructed "how to hyperventilate or overbreathe at a relatively uniform depth and constant rate," but no measurements were made to determine the blood carbon dioxide tension (PCO_2) or pH changes, nor were the blood-glucose levels measured at the time of the test. It is now known that all of the measures of the "hyperventilation effect" used by Lindsley and Cutts (i.e., abruptness of the change, amplitude and slowness of the waves produced, and degree of persistence of the effect after overbreathing stopped) are determined by the effectiveness of the overbreathing in producing a change in blood PCO_2 as well as by the level of blood glucose at the time of the test. It is difficult to judge the degree of hypocapnia (blood PCO_2 reduction) produced by a given hyperventilation effort (9), particularly in children; the rate, depth, and consistency of the respiratory effort are extremely difficult to gauge and compare without measuring the respiratory exchange or blood PCO_2 changes. Even if attempts are made to standardize the performance of overbreathing, the effect on blood chemistry is unpredictable (149); furthermore, an uncertain relation exists between the levels of peripheral and cerebral blood gases because of cerebral vasoconstriction and resulting in hypoxia, which, until recently, has been considered the main basis for the effect on the EEG (77,160). A critical review of the world literature on the subject (156) has not yielded unequivocal evidence for the idea that cerebral hypoxia is the critical factor in producing this response. It has been shown that hypocapnia produces decreased activity of the of the mesencephalic reticular formation (10) and that lesions that disconnect the cortex from the anterior part of the reticular ascending activating system abolish the hypersynchronous slowing effect of hyperventilation (10,183).

The blood-glucose level is important in determining the degree of response to hyperventilation (17,18,41). Most routine EEG studies of children do not control for this factor; however, even in adults, a low blood glucose level (<80 mg per 100 mL) favors the appearance of slow waves, and a high level (>120 mg per 100 mL) tends to inhibit or prevent such an effect (41).

If effective overventilation is obtained in children, slow waves appear much more abruptly and are more pronounced than in adults, and the slowing outlasts the overbreathing for a longer time in children (74). The degree and abruptness of the response seem to relate directly to age (19,74,78,206). Indeed, when the blood PCO_2 change produced by overbreathing is measured, there is a linear relationship between age and the effect produced (38,39). Practically speaking, under routine laboratory conditions, in which respiratory effort and effect are not measured, the most pronounced responses to overventilation usually occur in children 8 to 12 years of age (19,55,165) (Fig. 5.20).

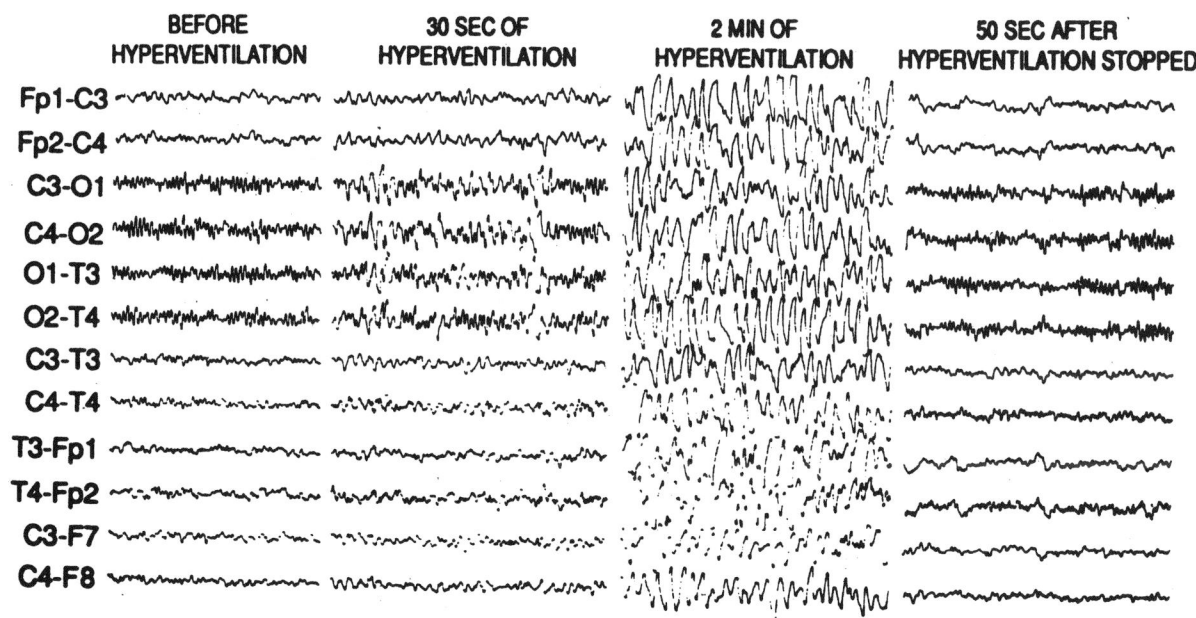

FIG. 5.20. Example of pronounced overventilation response that may occur in children 8 to 12 years of age. The subject was a girl aged 9 years, 6 months, at time of the electroencephalographic study, with serum glucose level of 110 mg/dL. She had no history of seizures or evidence of central nervous system disease. Note that initial posterior slowing, typically seen in children, is quite marked after only 30 seconds of overventilation. Some frontal delta activity continues 50 seconds after overventilation stopped.

Practical experience has shown that in routine diagnostic electroencephalography, interpretation must allow wide latitude for the degree of slowing and for the abruptness and duration of the hyperventilation effect. Only the elicitation of *abnormal wave complexes (spike-and-slow-wave, sharp-and-slow-wave) or clear focal or lateralizing changes* can be considered unequivocal evidence of abnormality. Even paroxysmal slow bursts are not acceptable evidence of abnormality, because these may be elicited in normal children under certain circumstances (48,165). Nonetheless, "susceptibility to hyperventilation" (7) and other characterizations of pronounced overventilation responses have been used as diagnostic measures in the evaluation of children (92).

Although prominent slow activity occurs less commonly in adults than in children, it too should be regarded with the same degree of caution. An abrupt, pronounced, or prolonged buildup of slow waves should never, in itself, be considered a basis for classifying an EEG in an adult as abnormal and certainly should *never* be considered a criterion for the diagnosis of epilepsy. If the blood glucose is near normal and the pronounced or prolonged slowing persists, there may be some reason to suspect abnormal brain function. However, in the absence of direct measurement of the blood PCO_2 level, only elicitation of a focal abnormality or production of an abnormal wave pattern can reliably indicate disordered brain function.

Activity of Drowsiness, Arousal, and Sleep

Activity of Drowsiness (Stage I Sleep)

Monorhythmic Slow Activity. The state termed drowsiness in adults and children—a condition characterized by slow, pendular eye movements—is classically associated with the disappearance of the occipital alpha rhythm and the appearance of some rhythmic and semirhythmic theta activity in the central or frontocentral regions. A comprehensive study of drowsiness has shown that there may be several variations of this pattern, including some persistence of the occipital alpha activity into the drowsy state (178). The various EEG patterns are not detailed here but are well documented in Santamaria and Chiappa's book (178), which is devoted entirely to this subject. Many of the patterns described have been recognized as state-related and not abnormal findings by experienced electroencephalographers, without benefit of the rigorously derived data that this book provides. The findings reported in this book are critical to the interpretation of the EEG and, as the authors stated in their preface, will be of great utility to electroencephalographers, polysomnographers, and investigators involved in psychophysical studies that use EEG and evoked potentials.

Drowsiness is usually defined as a presleep state, or a prodromal or twilight condition between being fully awake and asleep. In infants and young children, overt signs of drowsiness may not be evident even though the EEG shows changes indicating that the child is falling asleep. "Drowsiness" commonly conjures up a certain vision of a "heavy-lidded" appearance and, on the contrary, infants may have their eyes wide open and may be irritable and restless during a variable period before onset of clinical and electrographic sleep. For that reason, the author and colleagues have used the less common term *hypnagogic* to refer to this state (110). A smooth transition from the hypnagogic state to sleep may not occur, especially in the strange environment of the EEG laboratory; instead, the child's condition may fluctuate between sleep, arousal, and transitional states. A steady state of slow-wave sleep (stages II, III, and IV) may not appear under ordinary conditions in the EEG laboratory for intervals ranging from a few minutes to an hour or more.

In order not to be misled by the sometimes dramatic changes in the EEG that occur during the transition between wakefulness and sleep, the clinical electroencephalographer must know the EEG patterns and their variations that may occur during this state in children of various ages. The electroencephalographer can better understand and interpret what transpires if the entire process of falling asleep is recorded. The irrational, if economical, practice of turning off the instrument while waiting for the child to fall asleep may also result in loss of critical data: An important electrographic event may occur only once or only during one stage of the sleep cycle. Furthermore, the child sometimes drops precipitously into deep sleep, with a consequent omission of the productive stages II and III of sleep.

The changes that take place in the transient stage between wakefulness and sleep are best understood in view of the changes with increasing age from birth onward: once a sustained, rhythmic, occipital activity appears at approximately 3 months of age, the onset of the hypnagogic state is marked by sustained, monorhythmic, slow generalized activity. When this activity first appears, the frequency is 3 to 4 Hz, and it increases in older children to 4 or 5 Hz. Approximately 30% of 3-month-old infants show this hypnagogic hypersynchrony; the degree of its expression and duration vary in a single infant at different times and on different days. It may be seen in normal children up to the age of 12 or 13 years but is increasingly rare after the age of 11 years, when it appears in only 10% of healthy children. Figure 5.21 shows the incidence of this drowsy pattern in the author's own series of 1,000 healthy children. The relation to age resembles that reported by Gibbs and Gibbs in asymptomatic children (71) and by Eeg-Olofsson et al. in highly selected normal subjects (49).

In some children, the occipital alpha rhythm may slow as drowsiness ensues (Fig. 5.22), and at a time when anterior derivations show the more usual 4- to 5-Hz hypnagogic hypersynchrony, the occipital derivations may show some high-voltage, less regulated, slower (3- to 4-Hz) activity. The latter effect occurs in not more than 3% of healthy children before the onset of sleep, but it occurs in approximately 6% after arousal. It commonly occurs during a transient episode of arousal. In the author's series of healthy controls, all children with this pattern were younger than 4 years.

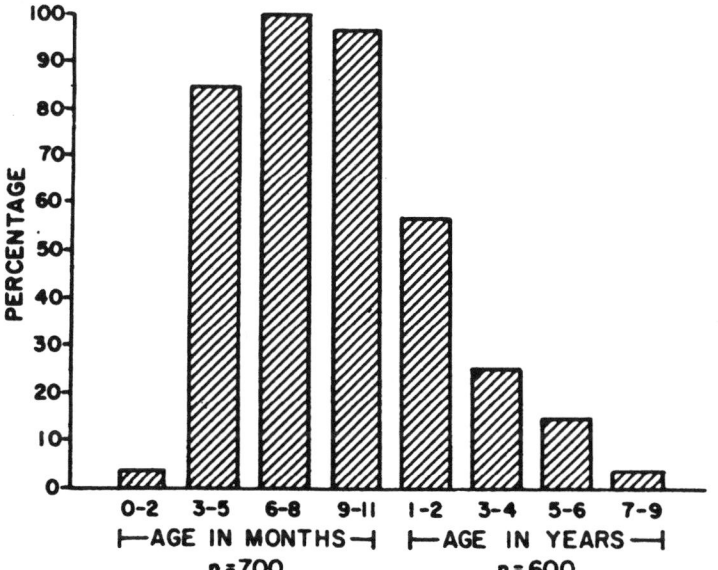

FIG. 5.21. Age distribution and incidence of sustained monorhythmic slow-activity drowsiness in asymptomatic children.

More commonly, as a shift toward sleep takes place, the occipital alpha rhythm becomes less persistent, and a central or frontocentral rhythm of 4-6 Hz develops; this rhythm may have a high voltage (200 µV). Examples of monorhythmic drowsy patterns in children of various ages are shown in Figs. 5.22 and 5.23.

Paroxysmal Slow Activity. Gibbs and Gibbs (71) and Kellaway and Fox (110) were the first to describe paroxysmal slow bursts during drowsiness in normal children. The latter authors described it as follows:

"The onset of the hypnagogic phase is signaled by a general reduction in the amplitude and rhythmicity of the activity of all areas. This relative 'quiet' may then be broken by paroxysmal bursts of high voltage sinusoidal waves which involve all leads but which are greater in amplitude in the precentral or central regions and generally more strongly expressed in the frontal than in the occipital regions."

"These paroxysmal bursts may reach extremely high voltages when maximally expressed (in excess of 350 microvolts) and therefore constitute a possible source of error both for the interpretation of sleep where this is sought and for the interpretation of waking records where the oscitant state may intervene without true sleep ensuing....The appearance of such bursts in the period just preceding true sleep, or at its onset, or at a time when the electrogram shows other evidence of the hypnagogic state, is never considered an epileptiform manifestation unless accompanied by spike discharges in some form. Long experience has shown that if a patient with established petit mal epilepsy shows abnormal paroxysmal activity during sleep the spike component is always strongly in evidence and the epileptiform serials persist into fairly deep levels of sleep. A distinguishing characteristic then of the pre-oscitant paroxysmal episodes is that they make a brief appearance at the onset of sleep and do not persist into deeper stages."

The example of paroxysmal drowsy waves illustrated in the report of Kellaway and Fox (110) is shown in Fig. 5.24. The paroxysmal activity in this sample, which they considered representative for age (35 months), has a frequency of 4.0 to 4.5 Hz, shows maximum voltage in the central regions, and shows a spindle-like waxing and waning of amplitude typical of the drowsy patterns seen in their series of asymptomatic children.

More complex waveforms, slower wave bursts, and a more frontal dominant distribution of the activity may also be seen in normal children. The example of paroxysmal slow activity illustrated by Gibbs and Gibbs (71)

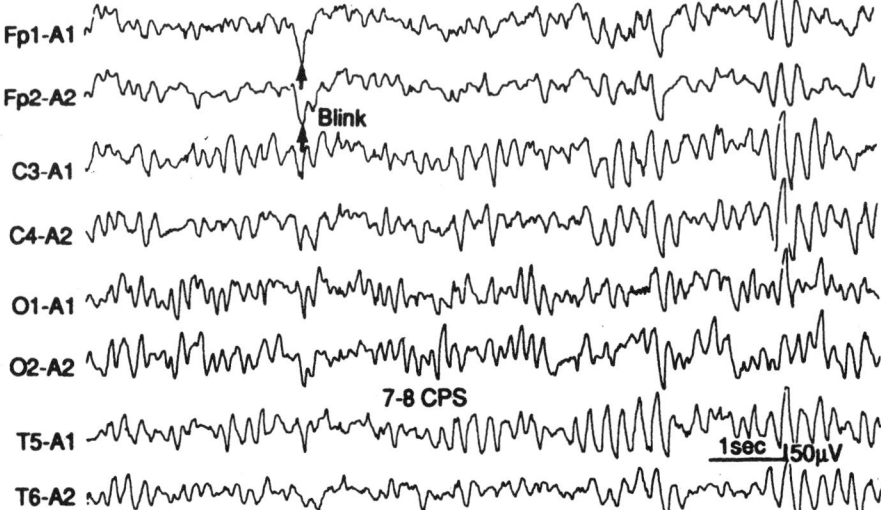

A

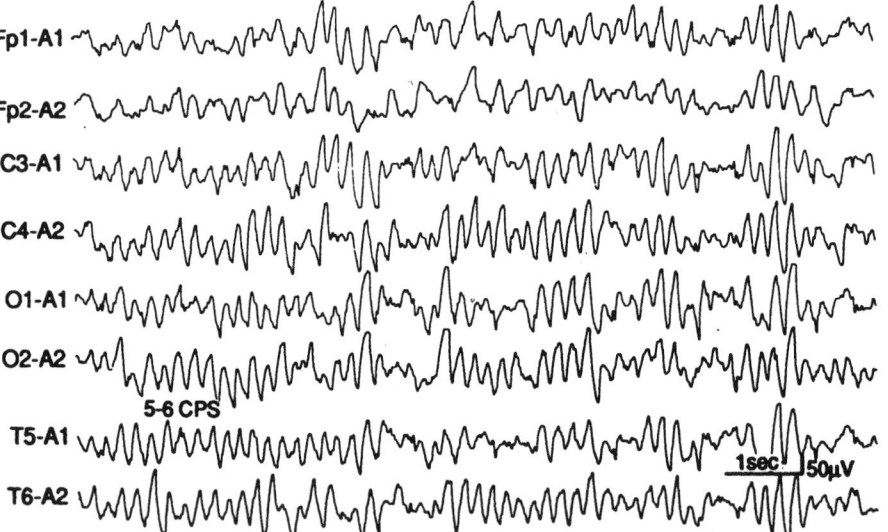

B

FIG. 5.22. A and **B:** Slowing of the occipital alpha rhythm as the record shifts from the awake state (first two-thirds of part *A*) to the drowsy state (last third of part *A* and all of part *B*) in an asymptomatic girl aged 28 months.

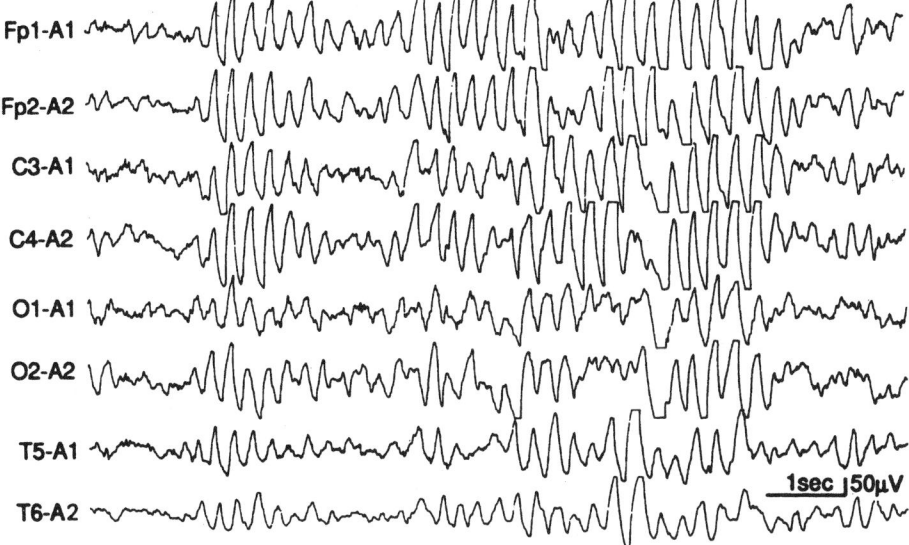

A

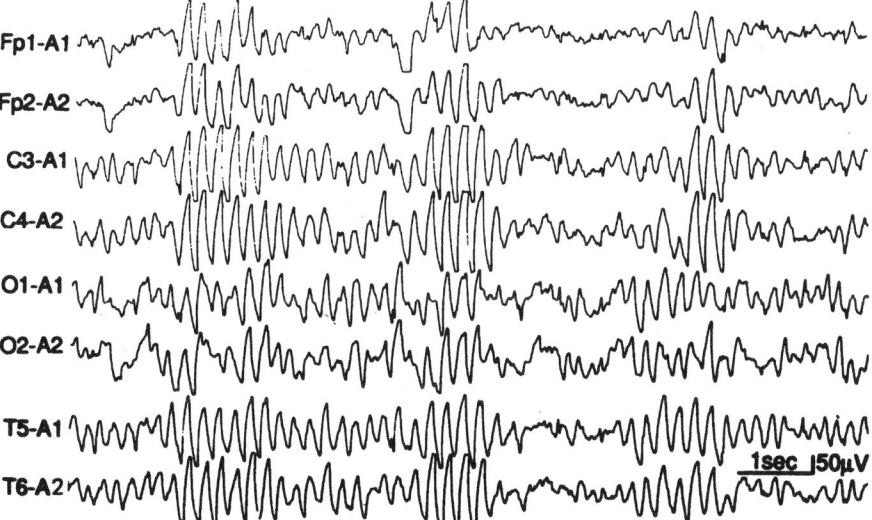

B

FIG. 5.23. A: Almost continuous "hypnagogic hypersynchrony" in an asymptomatic 6-month-old infant. **B:** Continuous "drowsy" pattern in an asymptomatic 12-month-old infant.

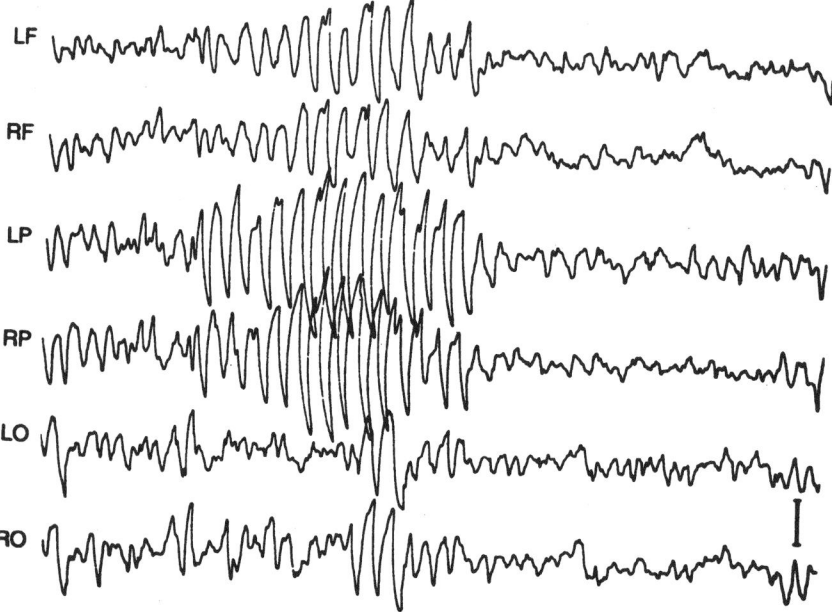

FIG. 5.24. Paroxysmal "hypnagogic hypersynchrony" in an asymptomatic girl aged 35 months. (From Kellaway P, Fox BJ. Electroencephalographic diagnosis of cerebral pathology in infants during sleep. I. Rationale, technique, and the characteristics of normal sleep in infants. *J Pediatr* 1952;41:262–287.)

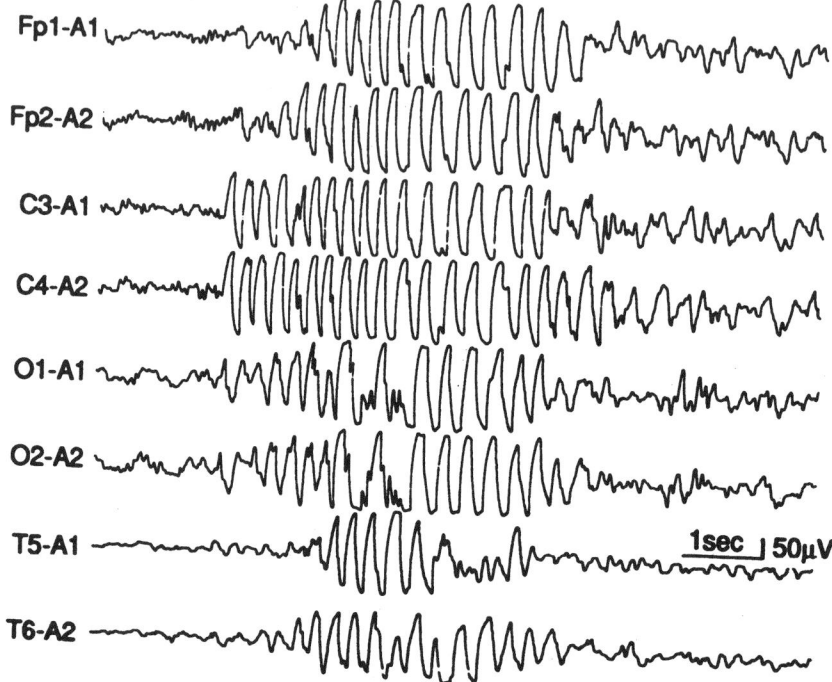

FIG. 5.25. Paroxysmal "hypnagogic hypersynchrony" in a 14-year-old girl, asymptomatic at the time of the electroencephalographic study and during the 20 years after the tracing was made. There was no family history of seizures. Complex, paroxysmal slow bursts of this type, occurring only in drowsiness, are rare at this age (see Fig. 5.27).

shows (a) some waves at the end of the bursts as slow as 2.5-3.0 Hz, and (b) some complex waveforms with faster components superimposed on, or intermixed with, the slow waves. Figures 5.25 and 5.26 show examples of activity of this type in drowsy asymptomatic children. It is difficult to distinguish between such bursts and a pattern described by Gibbs and Gibbs (72) which they designated "pseudo petit mal." They characterized the pattern as "paroxysmal diffuse 3–4 per second slow waves, with a poorly developed spike in the positive trough between the slow waves, occurring in drowsiness only...and most prominent in the parietal [central: C3–C4] areas." Gibbs and Gibbs saw this pattern only in children between the ages of 3 months and 9 years and only in 0.1% of normal children aged 0 to 14 years. Eeg-Olofsson et al. (49), however, found similar activity during drowsiness in 7.9% of 599 highly selected normal children aged 1 to 16

years. The highest incidence (12%) was in children aged 4 to 5 years. Gibbs and Gibbs described this "drowsy" pattern as consisting of bursts of 2- to 4-Hz waves of 100 to 300 μV, with a spike or spike-like component appearing briefly, early or late, in the burst. The pattern disappeared as soon as drowsiness was replaced by deeper sleep. A wide diversity of patterns of paroxysmal drowsy bursts, , ranging from a common type with occasional notching of the slow waves to bursts with polyspike-like components, may occur in normal children (see Fig. 5.26).

Figure 5.27 illustrates the incidence of "paroxysmal hypnagogic hypersynchrony" in asymptomatic children of different ages. The hatched bars

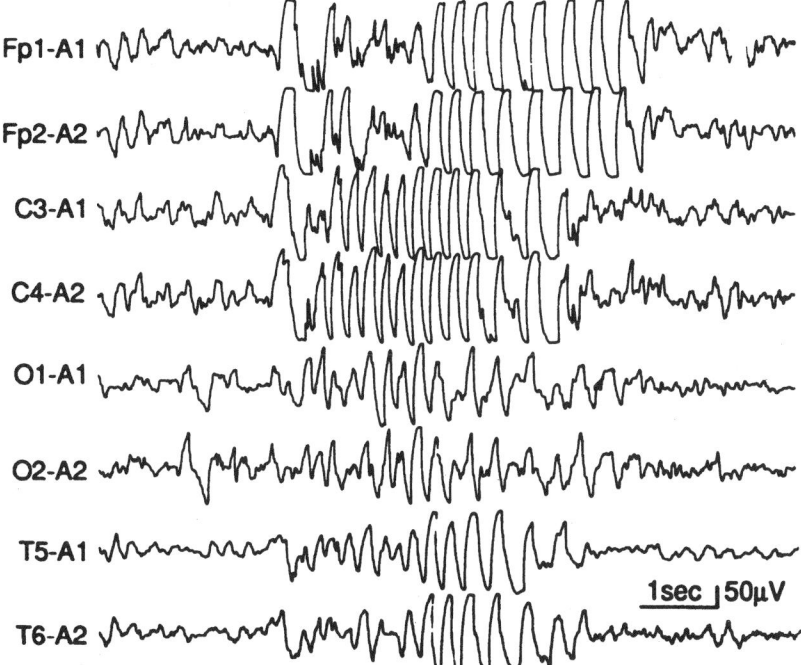

FIG. 5.26. Complex wave configurations such as in O1 and O2, as well as low-voltage, spike-like components seen in other derivations, are most common in drowsy, asymptomatic children between the ages of 4 and 9 years. The subject was an asymptomatic 7-year-old boy.

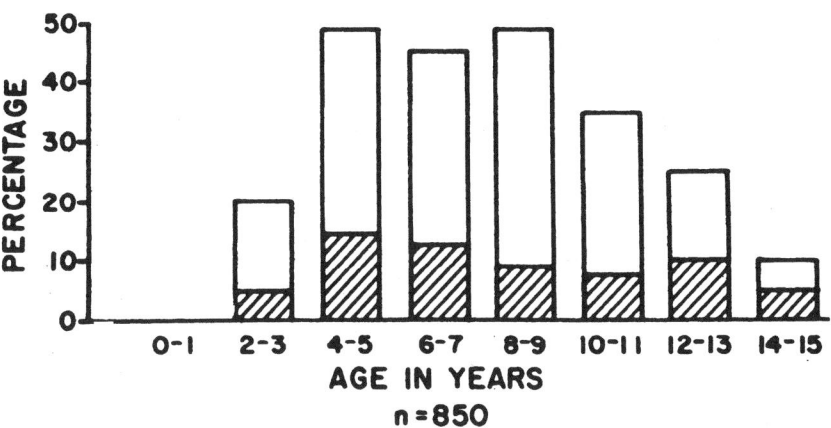

FIG. 5.27. Percentages of asymptomatic children of various ages who show paroxysmal slow bursts in drowsiness. Hatched areas show percentages having sharp or spike-like components intermixed with slow waves, as in Figs. 5.25 and 5.26.

show the incidence of what Brandt and Brandt (12) called the "severe" type (i.e., slow bursts with sharp or "spike-like" components). The percentage approximates that found by Eeg-Olofsson et al. (49) in their highly selected normal children.

In routine clinical practice, if such bursts occur only during drowsiness or at the onset of sleep, they cannot be considered evidence of abnormal function and certainly cannot support a clinical diagnosis of epilepsy. Even bursts with a clearly defined spike component fitting Gibbs and Gibbs's (72) definition of "pseudo petit mal" have only a tenuous association (10%) with febrile convulsions. According to Gibbs and Gibbs, the incidence of epilep-

tic (other than febrile) convulsions is only 7% greater in children with "pseudo petit mal" bursts than in children with normal EEGs, a difference that is not statistically significant.

From the ages of 3 months to 6 years, patterns of drowsiness may vary from time to time in the same child. If sleep begins abruptly, little hypersynchrony of any type may be seen. If there is a delay in the onset of true sleep, continuous, rhythmic, high-voltage slow or paroxysmal slow activity may persist for prolonged periods. Transient arousals (Fig. 5.28) frequently elicit a paroxysmal type of slow pattern; thus, it is important for the technologist to make note of such arousals and for the electroencephalographer to watch for artifacts associated with such a change of state.

Arousal from any level of sleep in infants and children is generally associated with a paroxysmal change. This may be a single, high-voltage, sharp-wave transient similar to that in adults, or it may be a complex three-phase change, which, if unexpected or unrecognized as an arousal event, may be misinterpreted as abnormal.

In general, the ages with pronounced arousal patterns coincide with those for hypersynchronous slow drowsy patterns.

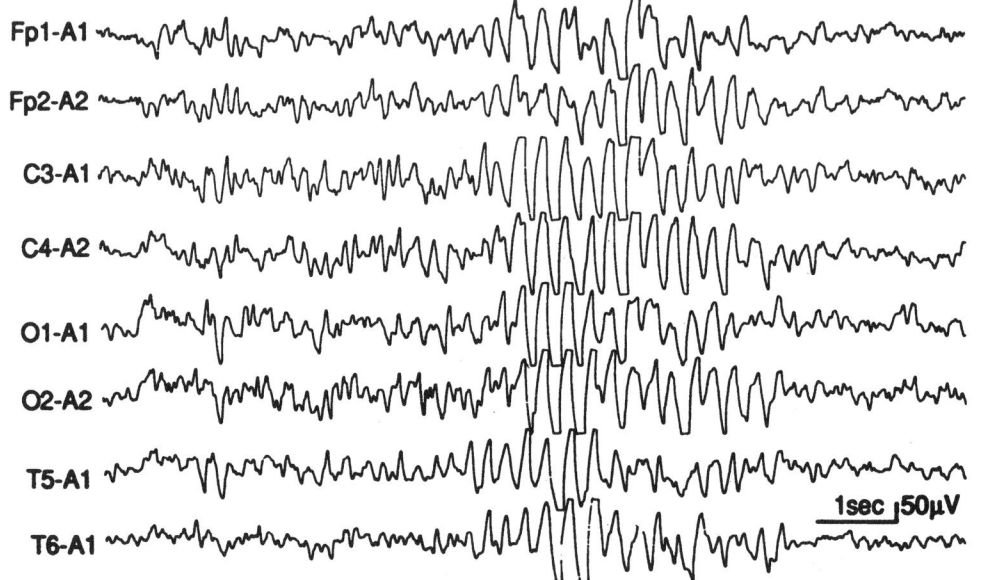

Fp1-A1

Fp2-A2

C3-A1

C4-A2

O1-A1

O2-A2

T5-A1

T6-A1

1sec | 50μV

FIG. 5.28. Transient arousal in an asymptomatic boy, aged 7 years. Just before the beginning of the sample, the child had been asleep (stage II). A brief period of desynchronization is followed by some central and occipital alpha activity lasting 2.0 to 2.5 seconds and, in turn, by a high-voltage, central-dominant, "drowsy" burst lasting about 3 seconds; then sleep resumes.

Activity of Arousal

Loomis et al. (135) were the first to show that reactive arousal involved a more or less complex electrographic pattern, rather than a simple and immediate transition from sleep to waking activity. In adults, they observed an initial diphasic slow wave followed by a series of rapid oscillations of about 8 to 14 per second, the total pattern occurring maximally in the central regions "but appearing at lower amplitude in the frontal, occipital, and temporal areas also."

This phenomenon appears prominently in children but varies somewhat in character and degree with age. The initial slow component, sometimes erroneously referred to as the *K complex,* is discussed later in relation to the spontaneous, bilateral central sharp-wave transients seen in light sleep. The fast component represents, as the original workers hinted, a process associated with a greater degree of arousal. Thus, the slow-transient component may represent the only response to a stimulus (e.g., a loud sound), with no clinical signs of arousal and, in fact, no transition to a lighter stage of electrographic sleep (Fig. 5.29*A*). The fast component

FIG. 5.29. Response to stimulus, and phases of arousal response, in a normal child, aged 6 years. **A:** Hand-clap elicits only a vertex transient, with no clinical or electroencephalographic evidence of arousal. Calling the child's name results in a full sequence of arousal, as follows: **B:** The first phase is the central dominant fast component. **C:** In the next phase, the central fast component is replaced by generalized slow activity, with rhythmic monomorphic delta activity in the frontal regions and slower, less rhythmic, activity in posterior derivations. **D:** The last phase of the arousal pattern before the normal alpha rhythm reappears consists of posterior rhythmic and semirhythmic delta activity. The child appears to be awake as soon as phase C (frontal delta activity) occurs. The calibration is the same for all four tracings. Arousal in a child may be aborted at any of these phases, with a reversion to sleep. The degree of arousal may alternate between phases two or more times before an awake state is sustained.

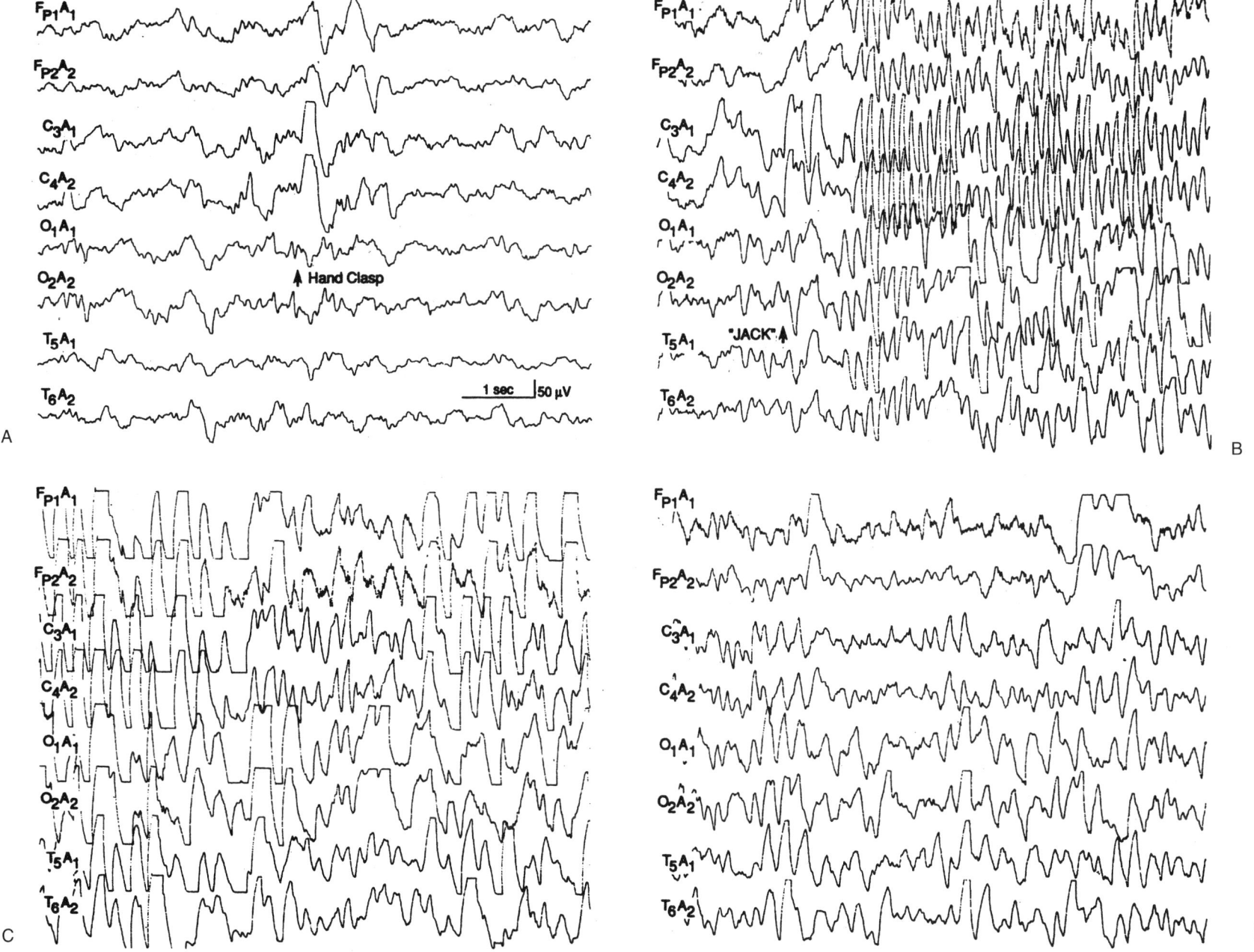

(see Fig. 5.29*B*) may also occur without further EEG or clinical evidence of arousal but is often *followed* by such evidence.

Neither component of the electrographic arousal reaction is clearly defined before the age of 2 months. During the first 8 weeks after birth, and especially during the first 6 weeks, the transition from sleep to waking is characterized only by a degree of desynchronization. Sometime between the eight and twelfth week, rudimentary diphasic slow-wave responses to applied stimuli may occur; also, at about this time, the first signs of a definite rhythmic hypersynchrony, similar to that of the drowsy state, appear in the immediate postarousal state. However, the slow component of the arousal reaction is rarely well defined before the age of 3 months.

The faster component of the arousal reaction usually does not appear before the age of 7 months. Initially rudimentary, it consists of a few moderately high voltage sinusoidal waves of 4.0 to 4.5 Hz in the frontocentral region, superimposed on a slower, irregular background activity.

With increasing age, this fast component of arousal increases in frequency until it reaches the adult rate of 8 to 10 Hz. In children, it is maximal in the central region (C3 to C4), and its field is such that its voltage is higher at F3 and F4 than at P3 and P4. Its appearance is transitory, and its duration is usually no more than 4 to 5 seconds. Occasionally, runs of this activity may last as long as 30 seconds (110).[10]

Postarousal Hypersynchrony

In children, the fast component of the arousal pattern is quickly followed by what in adults would be called a "paradoxical arousal response." Thus, as the child awakens, a high-voltage, monomorphic, quite slow rhythm (2.5 to 3.5 Hz) appears in the frontal regions (see Fig. 5.29*C*); and as further arousal ensues, the rhythmic slow activity becomes less slow and moves posteriorly, with the voltage and persistence of the rhythm progressively diminishing in anterior derivations (see Fig. 5.29*D*). In infants and children in whom continuous "monorhythmic slow" or "paroxysmal slow" activity occurs during drowsiness, there may be similar episodes of postarousal hypersynchronous slow activity of similar frequency (110).[11]

The various components of arousal and awakening patterns in children shown in Fig. 5.29 may be aborted at any point in the process. If an external

---

[10]This is probably the same arousal rhythm that White and Tharp (214) reported in a series of children with "minimal brain dysfunction"; they did not study its incidence in a matched control group.

[11]In infants, when this phase of postarousal slow activity is over, passive eye closure should be done in order to determine the frequency of the occipital alpha rhythm.

stimulus triggers the arousal (if there is a sudden sound, if the child's name is called, or if the child is touched), a diphasic sharp-wave transient appears in the region of the vertex; if no arousal effect is produced, the background EEG activity reverts immediately to its prestimulation character (as in Fig. 5.29*A*). Presumably, a further degree of arousal is signaled by the appearance of the fast central component (as in Fig. 5.29*B*), and overt signs of arousal (e.g., movement or eye opening) do not occur until the hypersynchronous slow activity appears (see Fig. 29*C*). *Spontaneous* arousal may occur without the appearance of the diphasic central (vertex) sharp-wave transient.

In adults, the arousal pattern depends on the level of sleep that preceded the arousal. Arousal from stage I (drowsiness) is not associated with any change other than a reversion to the awake alpha rhythm pattern (Fig. 5.30). Once the spindle stage has been reached, an attenuated form of the arousal patterns seen in children may occur: There may be an initial diphasic central sharp-wave transient, followed by a brief train of waves of alpha activity frequency that occur *in the frontocentral region,* and there may be one or two high-voltage, frontal slow waves (1.5 to 3.0 Hz). Examples of adult arousal patterns are illustrated in Figs. 5.30 and 5.31.

A postarousal, frontocentral burst of 4- to 5-Hz waves of brief duration may occur in young adults and is fairly common in adolescents. The only data on the incidence of this type of postarousal burst in asymptomatic subjects are those of Gibbs and Gibbs (71), who found the bursts in at least 40% of subjects 10 to 14 years of age.

Perspective on Patterns of Drowsiness and Arousal

Episodes of drowsiness and arousal are common in routine EEG studies and are expected aspects of prolonged EEG monitoring. For the clinical neurophysiologist, they constitute a paradox: Their occurrence is to be sought because they may reveal abnormal rhythms or discharges not otherwise manifest; however, transient episodes of drowsiness, particularly if recurrent throughout the record, are a common hazard for misinterpretation. Similarly, transient episodes of arousal or semiarousal may be mistaken for paroxysmal abnormalities. Santamaria and Chiappa, in their monograph on the subject (178), made an excellent case for using eye-movement monitoring for the detection of drowsiness and arousal. They showed that, in addition to the better known slow, pendular movements that signal the oscitant state, there occur more rapid phasic movements of the eyes and eyelids that may facilitate recognition of the drowsy state.

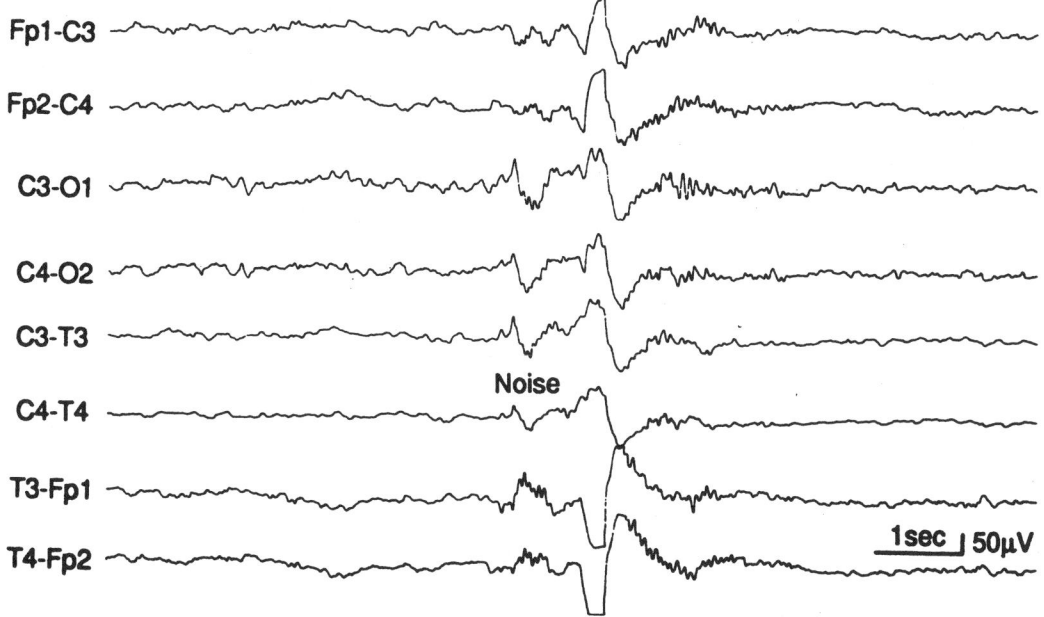

Fp1-C3

Fp2-C4

C3-O1

C4-O2

C3-T3

C4-T4

Noise

T3-Fp1

T4-Fp2

1sec 50μV

FIG. 5.30. In stage I sleep, arousal is associated with an immediate return of the waking pattern without an initial high-voltage, slow-wave transient.

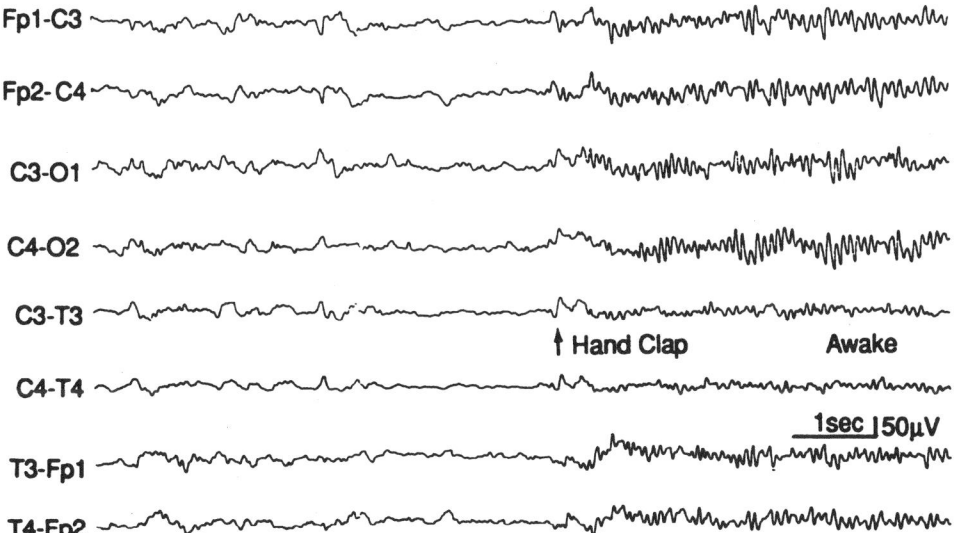

Fp1-C3

Fp2-C4

C3-O1

C4-O2

C3-T3

↑ Hand Clap   Awake

C4-T4

1sec 50μV

T3-Fp1

T4-Fp2

FIG. 5.31. Abortive-arousal response consisting of a slow-wave transient, maximum in voltage in the frontal leads, followed by a train of 9- to 14-Hz waves; the subject was a normal adult. Vertex transient and low-voltage spindle (sigma) activity occur before the abortive-arousal response. Such arousal patterns may occur spontaneously.

A wide range of patterns associated with drowsiness and arousal were seen in a small sample of normal subjects (55 adults, aged 22 to 79 years). These patterns differed from those generally recognized by electroencephalographers as being characteristic of normal drowsiness or arousal (178). In routine practice, whether frontocentral or central 3- to 5-Hz activity seen in an adult's EEG is related to drowsiness can be determined with the aid of hyperventilation. The constant urging to greater or sustained effort has the effect of keeping the subject alert and thus decreasing slow activity that is associated with drowsiness; at the same time, abnormal slow activity is accentuated as a result of hypocapnia produced by the hyperventilation.

The complex and varied EEG patterns of sleep and arousal are not well understood. Transitions through the various stages of sleep and from sleep to arousal involve changes in the activity and interaction of brainstem systems and in the noradrenergic and cholinergic modulation of cortical activity (187,198). The diverse EEG patterns that reflect these complex functional changes may therefore contain important information concerning physiological and pathophysiological processes. They have already yielded useful insights concerning pathophysiological mechanisms in epilepsy (108). As Santamaria and Chiappa (178) suggested, the less common patterns of drowsiness (and, perhaps, of arousal) and their relationship to eye movements and other behavioral phenomena may have significance in dysfunctional terms for disorders of sleep and cognition and for aberrations of the aging process.

It is regrettable that in this new era of diagnostic imaging, interest in electroencephalographic phenomena should be waning long before the significance of the many varied electrical patterns associated with sleep has been explored, much less determined.

Activity of Sleep

Vertex Sharp-Wave Transients. The onset of stage II sleep is signaled by the appearance of bilaterally synchronous sharp-wave transients in the central region (Fig. 5.32). Although maximal in voltage in the C3 and C4 electrode positions, when they are of high voltage, as they sometimes are in young children, they may be evident over a wide area of the frontocentral region. These sharp waves are usually diphasic, with an initial surface-negative deflection followed by a low-voltage, surface-positive phase. The sharp wave may be followed by a slow, surface-negative wave and/or a sleep spindle.

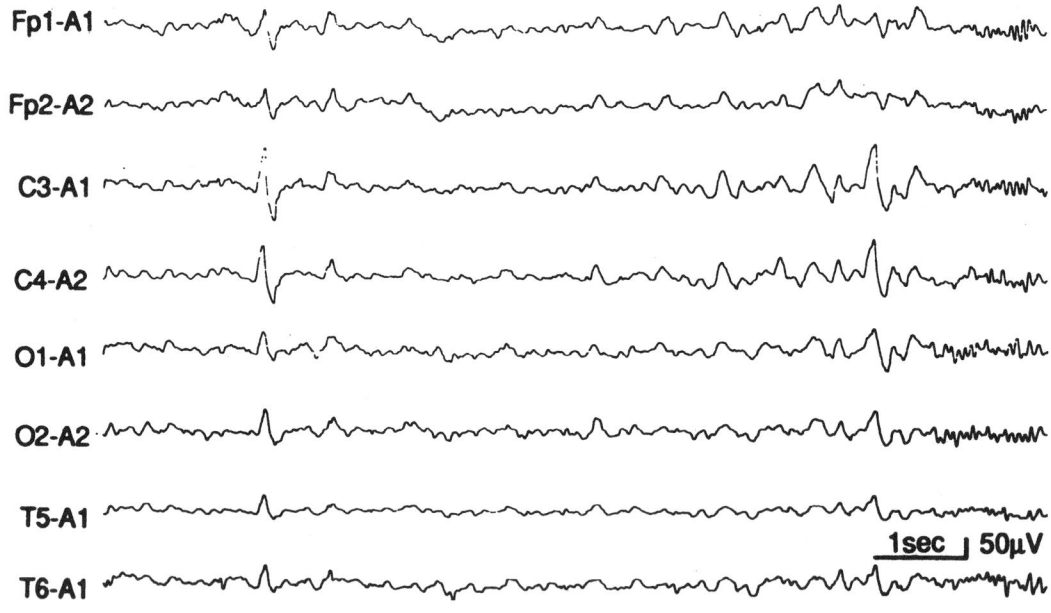

FIG. 5.32. Example of bilateral vertex transients in an asymptomatic 12-year-old girl. Note the diphasic waveform in central derivations.

From the time these waves first appear (at approximately 8 weeks post term), they are bilaterally synchronous and essentially symmetrical on the two sides. With persistent asymmetry of more than 20%, a lesion on the low side should be suspected. Some variable voltage difference between the two sides is not uncommon in young children, but if the low voltage always appears on the same side, it should be regarded as significant. Unlike other sleep activity (e.g., spindles), vertex transients are always bilaterally synchronous in normal persons. A breakdown of this synchrony is usually a sign of increased intraventricular pressure (obstructive hydrocephalus). Asynchrony should be distinguished from the situation not uncommonly seen in children in which the vertex transients do not occur on both sides each time. In this situation, one or the other side may show more vertex transients (and spindles), but whenever they occur bilaterally, they are symmetrical on the two sides. Although this phenomenon—in which an occasional vertex transient (and spindle) may be missing on one side—occurs in apparently healthy children, it is comparatively rare (<3%) and may indeed be pathophysiologically significant.

The very high voltage that vertex transients may attain in children aged 2 to 4 years may come as a surprise to the electroencephalographer not accustomed to children's records. The high voltage and sharply peaked waveform must not lead to an incorrect interpretation of abnormality. Similarly, these vertex transients in children, in contrast to the situation in adults, may occur in quick succession (every 1 to 2 seconds), and an "interference pattern" may result, giving these waves a complex configuration that seems abnormal (Fig. 5.33).

The voltage and, to some degree, the configuration of successive vertex transients in any series may fluctuate considerably, and in a given montage, it may be difficult to distinguish the vertex transients (Fig. 5.34) from abnormal sharp-wave discharges arising unilaterally or bilaterally from foci in this region (rolandic spikes). The problem often can be solved by mapping the fields of the various sharp waves present.

K Complexes and Vertex Transients. The term K complex was originally used by Loomis et al. (134,135) to denote a series of waves that could be detected in the EEG during sleep in response to an auditory stimulus (see Fig. 5.31). As the word "complex" implies, the term was not meant to describe a single transient or sharp wave, although the term K complex has often been applied to the spontaneous vertex transients of sleep. The electrical field of the slow component of the K complex at the scalp is essentially similar to that of the vertex transient, and the initial component may have a similar waveform. It has, in fact, been suggested that vertex transients constitute EEG responses to afferent stimuli arising from interoceptors.

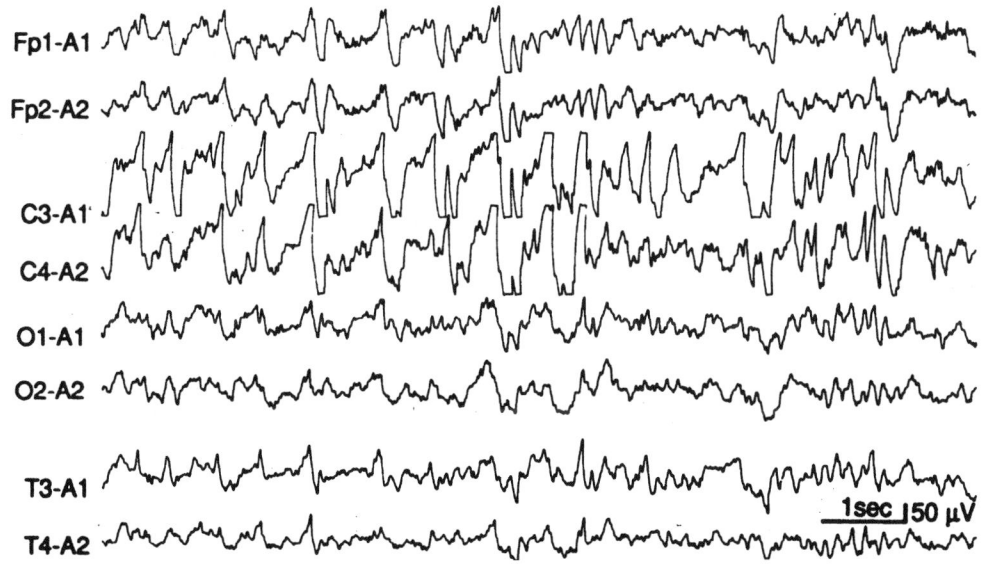

FIG. 5.33. Vertex transients occurring in repetitive sequence in an asymptomatic 11-year-old boy. Note the variable and often sharp waveform. The higher-voltage transients cause blocking at normal gain.

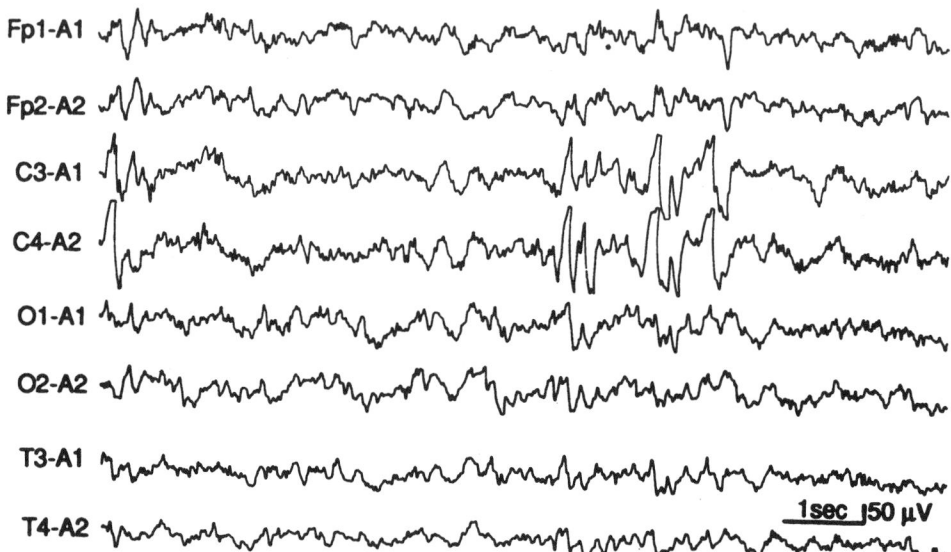

FIG. 5.34. Characteristically "sharp" appearance of some vertex transients in children is increased in this montage by the admixture of electrocardiographic artifact and fast activity. The sample is from an asymptomatic girl aged 9 years 6 months with no evidence of central nervous system disease.

Once stage II sleep has been reached, a single "click" stimulus will elicit a sharp, diphasic wave in the central region bilaterally that is indistinguishable in waveform, amplitude, and field from the spontaneously occurring vertex transient in the same individual. The spontaneous vertex transients may occur in relatively quick succession, as shown in Fig. 5.33, and appear in quick succession (every 1 to 2 seconds) throughout stages 2 to 4 of non—rapid-eye-movement (NREM) sleep; however, the central sharp-wave transients elicited by a stimulus show a relatively long refractory period and may disappear if the stimulus is repeated at short intervals over a period of 30 seconds or more. This accommodation effect can be overcome simply by changing to a novel stimulus: for example, by substituting the calling of the child's name for one of the clicks (personal observations). The duration of the refractory period in which a second stimulus (e.g., a click) is not effective has not been measured precisely, but it is estimated to be at least 5 seconds.

Spindles. Sleep spindles are bilaterally asynchronous at the time of their first appearance at 6 to 8 weeks post term (110) (Fig. 5.35), and they become increasingly more synchronous during the first year of life; thus by the eighteenth month, most spindles are bilaterally synchronous. Before the age of 2 years, asynchrony of sleep spindles cannot be considered evidence of abnormality. The waveform and duration of sleep spindles in infants differ from those in adults: The spindles may be 2 to 4 seconds in duration and lack the typical fusiform amplitude modulation that gives the adult type of sleep spindle its name. The individual waves of the spindle may be sharply peaked (reminiscent of the mu rhythm) in the surface-negative phase (110) (see Fig. 5.35).

Three types of spindles may be distinguished by their frequency characteristics and potential field. The most common, and usually the only type seen in adults, has a frequency of approximately 14 Hz, and the center of the field coincides closely with the C3 and C4 electrode placements. The spindles are characteristic of stages II and III sleep, but they are also the distinguishing characteristic of "spindle coma" or "coma sleep" (29). Unilateral slowing of spindle frequency may occur in the presence of lesions of the ipsilateral hemisphere (172).

Spindles that have a fundamental frequency of approximately 10 to 12 Hz and a more anterior locus of origin occur in 5% of normal children aged 3 to 12 years (Fig. 5.36). These "frontal" spindles, which are seldom more than 3 seconds in duration, should be clearly differentiated from "continuous spindling" or "exaggerated" spindles, which are an abnormal finding seen in children with certain types of cerebral palsy and mental retardation. Frontal 10-Hz spindling that is almost continuous can result from drug

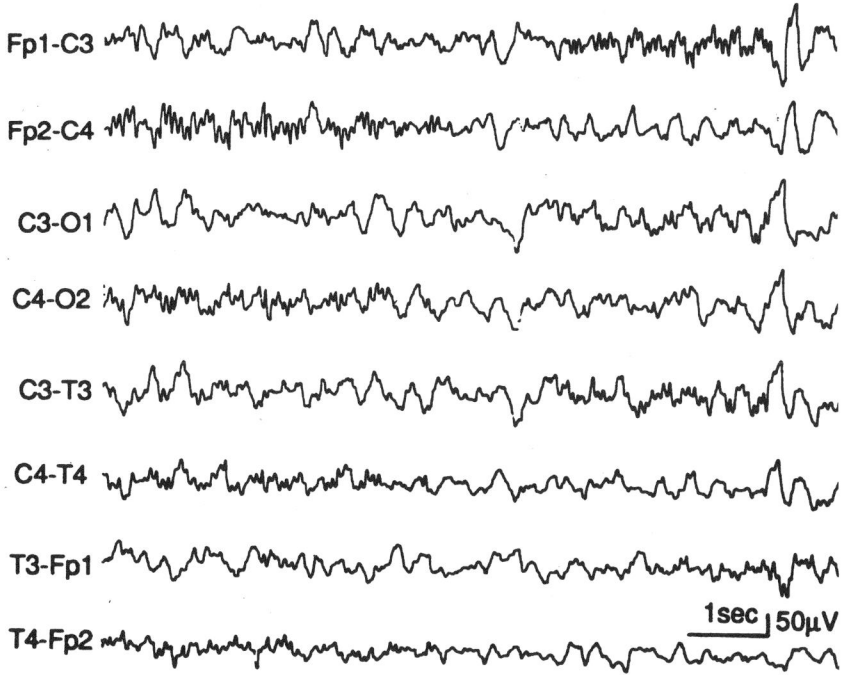

FIG. 5.35. Typical infant sleep spindles. Note the asynchrony (attenuation) between the two sides, prolonged duration (>4 seconds), lack of fusiform amplitude modulation, and mu-like waveform.

action (e.g., morphine and halothane anesthesia), but the unremitting character of the activity and the lack of reactivity to intense stimuli clearly distinguish it from the frontal dominant 10-Hz spindles of sleep (Fig. 5.37).

Fusiform bursts of 18- to 22-Hz activity in sleep should not be confused with sleep spindles (sigma activity). Most commonly, these bursts are effects of medication, particularly the phenothiazines and barbiturates (Fig. 5.38), but they are also associated with certain pathological conditions in the absence of drugs.

Fast Activity. Sometime between the fifth and sixth month, many infants begin to show low-voltage fast activity during the early stages of sleep. This activity occurs in all derivations but is most pronounced in the central or postcentral region (see Fig. 5.8). The frequency averages approximately 28 Hz, but it varies as much as ±6 Hz in different subjects. When the fast activity first occurs, its amplitude is very low (5 μV or less), but relatively high amplitudes (30 μV maximum) may be seen by the twelfth to eighteenth month, when it seems to reach its maximum expression. After the age of 30

to 36 months, pronounced fast activity during early sleep is less common, and in general, the amplitudes seen are not as great as in children aged 12 to 18 months. Older children are much less likely to show fast activity during early sleep, and after the age of 7, it is relatively uncommon (110).

When sedation with a barbiturate or other fast activity–inducing drug is used to promote sleep, fast activity is increased in the awake and asleep EEG. This fast activity has a frequency chiefly in the range of 18 to 22 Hz and a predominantly anterior distribution. When sedatives are administered at some point just before or during the recording, the fast activity induced displays maximum voltage during light sleep (stages 1 and 2) and is greatly diminished during deeper sleep. Upon arousal, the fast activity increases again and becomes much more pronounced than in the presleep record— unless there was an inordinate delay in the onset of sleep. Fast activity induced by chronic medication, or by a drug administered a long time before the recording, shows the same diminution during the deep sleep stages but is *equal* during the pre-sleep and post-sleep *awake* tracings.

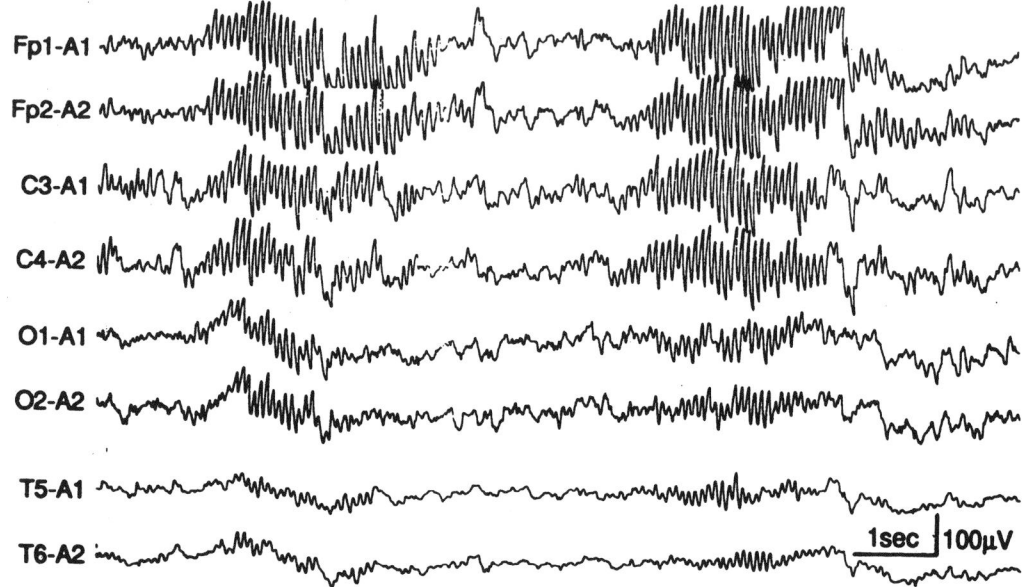

A

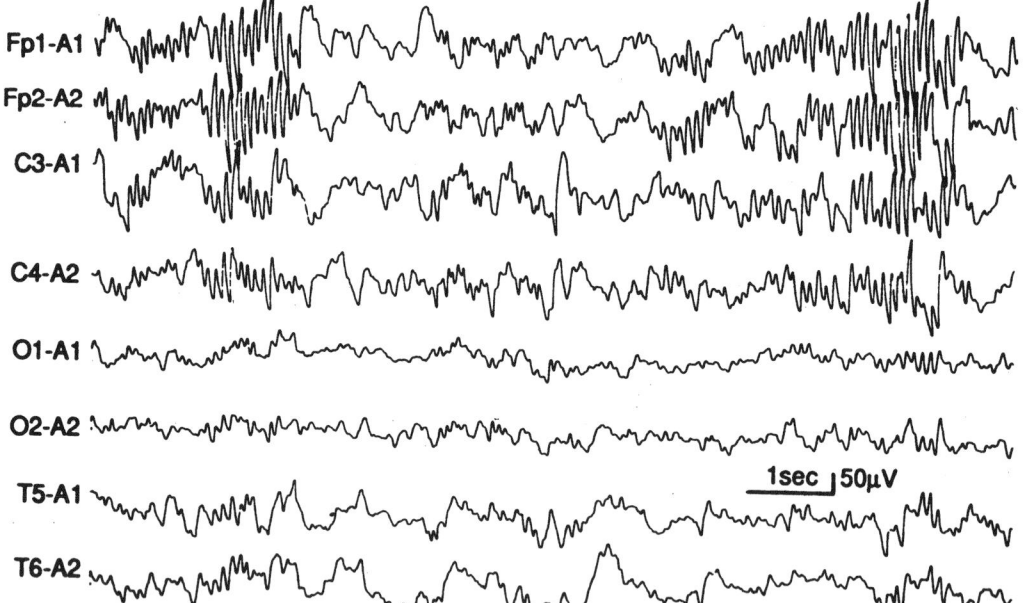

B

FIG. 5.36. A: Example of 12-Hz frontal-dominant spindles in stage II sleep in an asymptomatic male, aged 10 years, 10 months. These spindles are often high in voltage in comparison with 14-Hz central spindles and have a larger potential field. **B:** Example of 10-Hz frontal-dominant spindles in an asymptomatic 6-year-old boy.

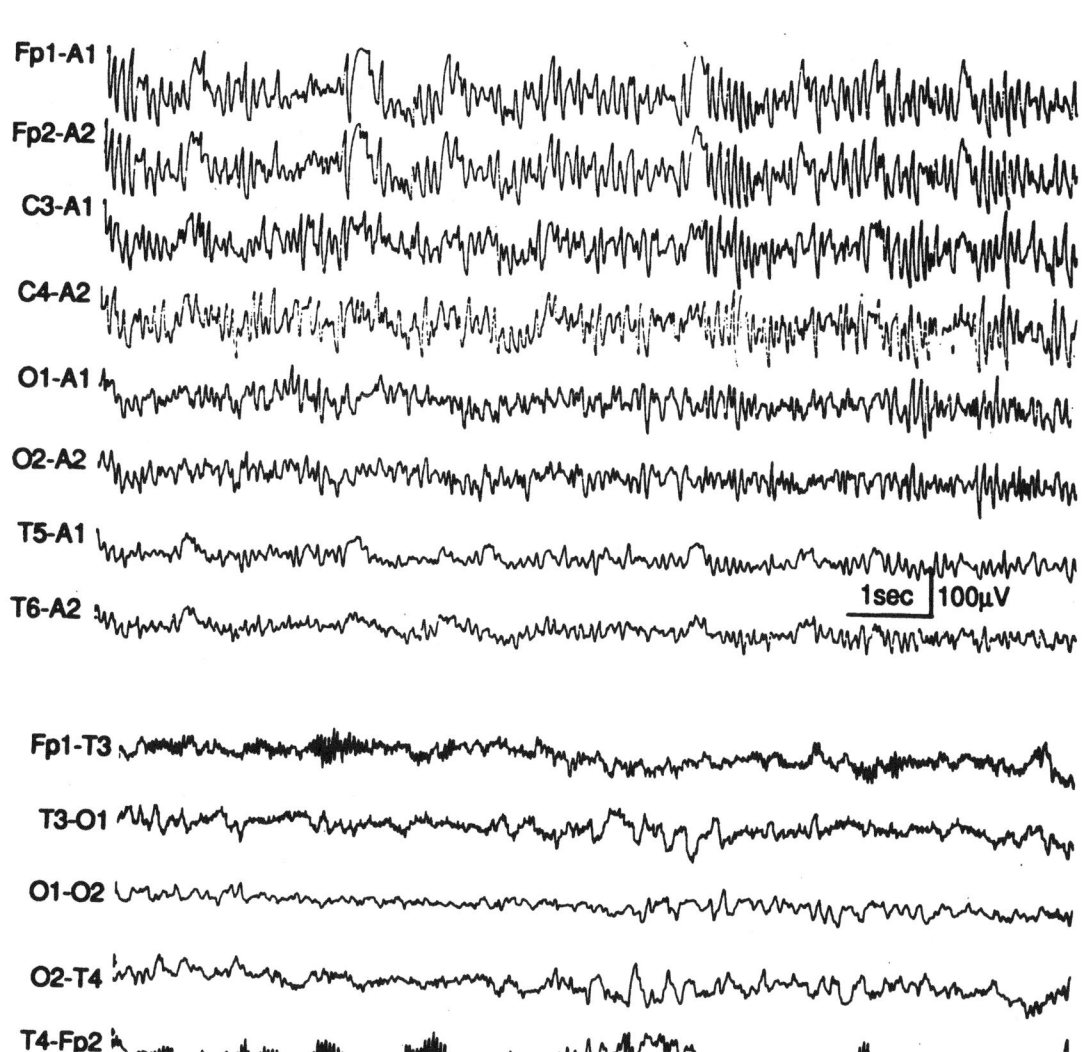

FIG. 5.37. Almost continuous 10- to 12-Hz, moderately high voltage, frontal-dominant activity showing a spindle-like amplitude modulation in a woman aged 52 years who was stuporous from a diazepam overdose.

FIG. 5.38. Barbiturate "spindles" such as those in this figure are sometimes confused with physiological sleep spindles. Note the greater amplitude of paired frontal derivation in comparison to homolateral frontal derivations; this is a common finding with barbiturate spindles but is not characteristic of sleep spindles. The subject was a boy aged 13 years, 4 months, with generalized seizures and taking phenobarbital (150 mg per day). Fast activity was not present before treatment. The sample is from stage I sleep.

The voltage of both natural and induced fast activity should be essentially the same bilaterally. With a consistent difference of more than 30%, an abnormality on the low-voltage side should be suspected, except when the fast activity is confined to a circumscribed focal area, in which case it may be associated with a focal lesion in that region (94). (Beware, however, of the pitfall mentioned elsewhere: the low-resistance pathway provided by a bone defect in the skull.)

Fast activity of cortical origin is particularly susceptible to the effects of ischemia, hypoxia, contusion, and the presence of subdural fluid. Thus, its depression or absence focally or unilaterally may be a useful sign on the EEG, particularly in relation to other findings (e.g., the presence of a slow-wave focus).

Positive Occipital Sharp Transients. Surface-positive sharp transients, occurring singly or, more commonly, in runs of 4 to 5 Hz, are often seen in routine EEG sleep recordings (Fig. 5.39). These interesting waves are commonly seen in the EEG laboratory because they are prone to occur during daytime naps and particularly if the patient has been partially aroused and quickly returns to sleep. The pattern occurs in persons aged 4 to 50 years and is most common and best expressed in those aged 15 to 35 years. The individual waves show a sharp, surface-positive peak, followed in some instances by a low-voltage, surface-negative peak. The initial deflection of each wave has a somewhat slower time course than the ascending phase, and so the resultant waveform may have a checkmark-like shape; some authors refer to them as occipital V waves of sleep.

Positive occipital sharp transients of sleep (POSTs) (199) are always bilaterally synchronous but are commonly asymmetrical on the two sides (Fig. 5.40); voltage differences as great as 60% are seen in normal persons. This may lead to misinterpretation of POSTs as abnormal sharp-wave activity in one or the other occipital region. In this regard, it is important to remember that POSTs may occur at a time when the background activity has an amorphous character that might be thought to represent drowsiness or a slightly slow awake pattern (Fig. 5.41).

The helpful distinguishing characteristics of POSTs are (a) their surface positivity (abnormal surface-positive cerebral spikes are rare), (b) the fact that they tend to occur in trains with a repetition rate of 4 to 5 Hz, and (c) their predominantly monophasic checkmark-like waveform.

Occipital Slow Transients. In children, the transition from light to deep sleep may be associated with the bilateral appearance of high-voltage slow transients in the occipital regions (110). These waves vary from a cone-shaped configuration (Fig. 5.42) to a diphasic slow transient (Fig. 5.43) rem-

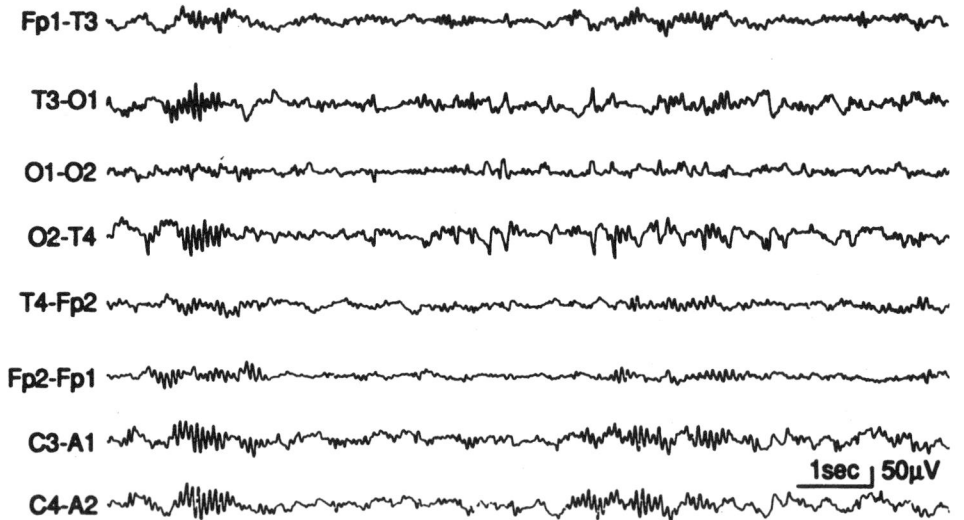

FIG. 5.39. Positive occipital sharp transients of sleep (POSTs) during stage II sleep (note presence of 14-Hz spindles) in an asymptomatic 14-year-old boy.

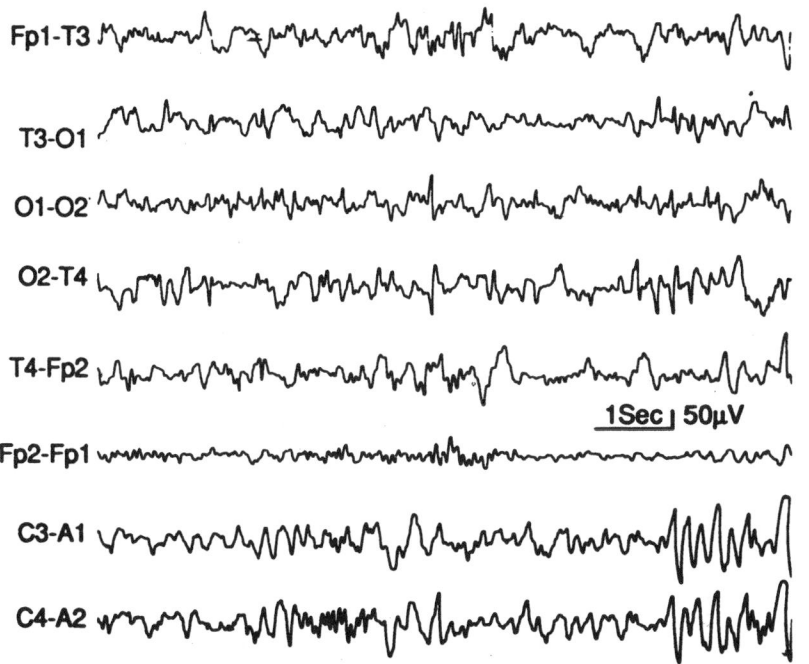

Fp1-T3

T3-O1

O1-O2

O2-T4

T4-Fp2

1Sec | 50µV

Fp2-Fp1

C3-A1

C4-A2

FIG. 5.40. Asymmetrical positive occipital sharp transients of sleep (POSTs) in a healthy girl aged 11 years. Note considerable voltage difference between sides, especially of the isolated sharp wave (POST) near the center of the sample. The facts that the series shows a repetition rate of about 5 Hz at the right side of sample and that the sharp waves are positive at O2 provide clues to their identity. However, although positive sharp waves or spikes rarely signify abnormal activity, electrodes near the midline (e.g., O1 or O2) may reveal only the positive end of a dipole, presumably because the negative end lies on the mesial surface of the hemisphere.

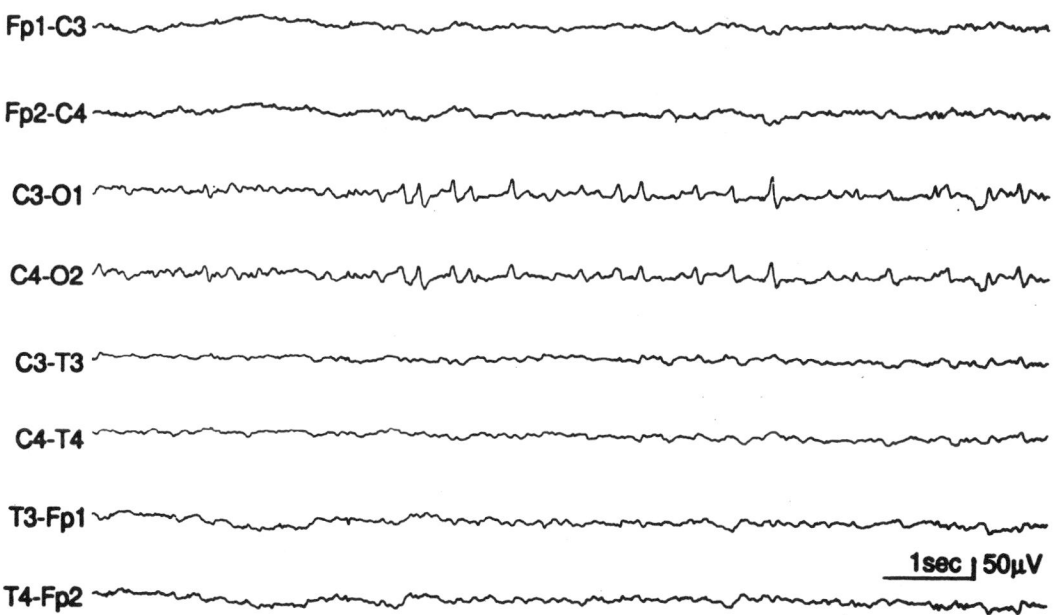

Fp1-C3

Fp2-C4

C3-O1

C4-O2

C3-T3

C4-T4

T3-Fp1

1sec | 50µV

T4-Fp2

FIG. 5.41. Positive occipital sharp transients of sleep (POSTs), occurring after drowsiness but before spindle sleep had been reached, in an asymptomatic 17-year-old girl. Note the low-voltage, slightly slow or "drowsy" appearance of the record. POSTs are often seen during daytime naps that may occur during routine studies in the typical electroencephalograph laboratory.

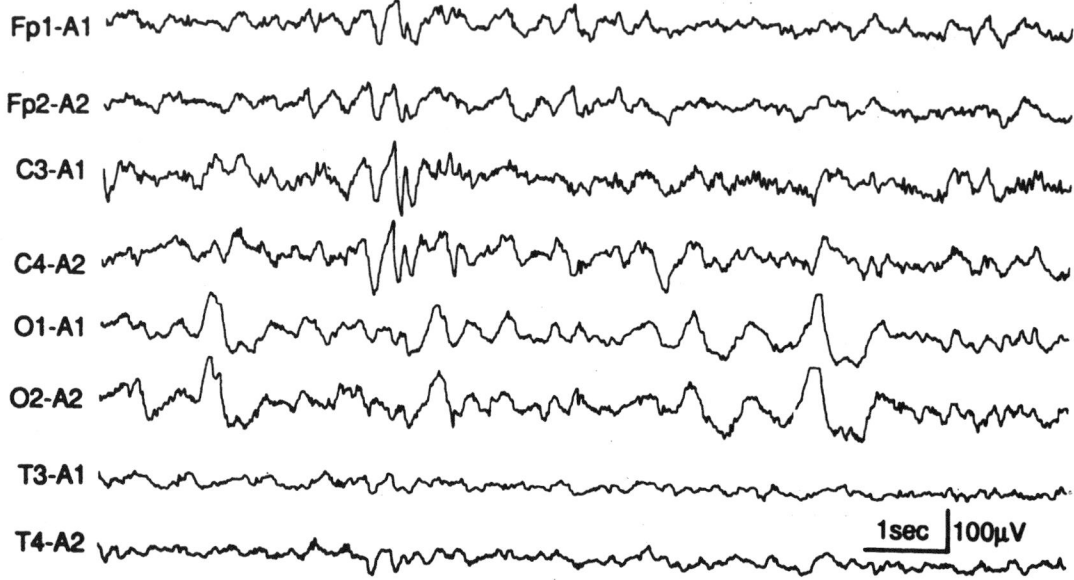

FIG. 5.42. Cone-shaped, posterior slow transients during light sleep in an asymptomatic 35-month-old boy.

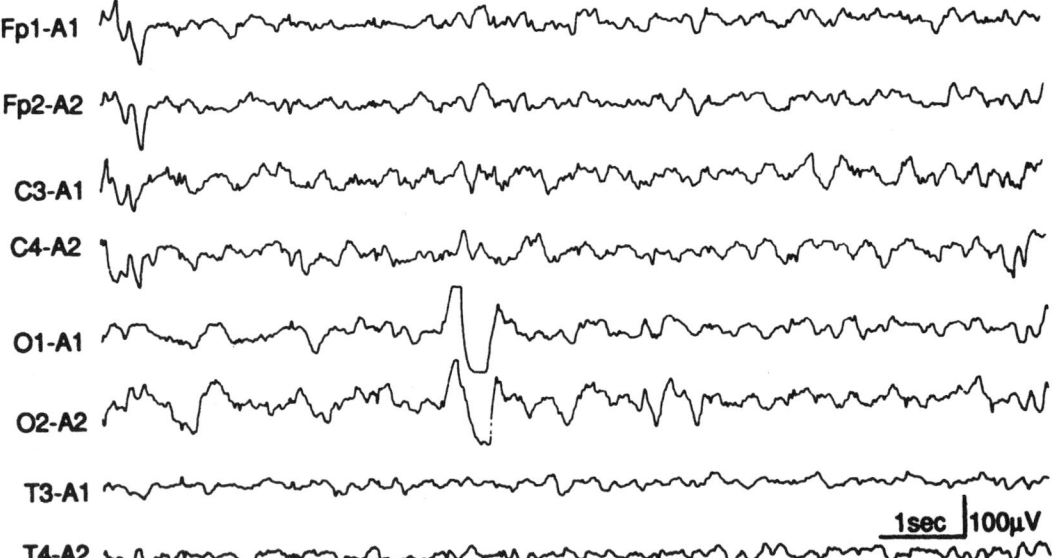

FIG. 5.43. Diphasic slow-wave transients in the occipital derivations in light sleep in the same subject as in Fig. 5.42.

iniscent of a prolonged vertex transient. At first, during light sleep, these transients occur every 3 to 6 seconds; with deepening sleep, they appear more frequently and seem to meld into the continuous, occipital-dominant, random, very slow delta waves of stage IV sleep.

THE CLINICAL REPORT

Visual analysis in terms of the specific descriptors as set forth in Table 5.1 provides the basis for the initial part of the formal EEG report, namely the *technical description.* The next aspect of the report, the *technical impression,* comprises a summary statement of the overall analysis (e.g., paroxysmal generalized 3-Hz spike and wave dysrhythmia with normal background activity for age). Finally, an assessment is made of the significance of the EEG findings in relation to the clinical history and the patient's clinical state: the *clinical impression.*

THE MEANING OF "NORMAL" AND THE SIGNIFICANCE OF DEVIATIONS FROM THE NORM

The purposes of this chapter are to delineate the processes involved in an orderly approach to visual analysis and to provide information concerning the elements of the "normal" EEG in adults and children. The latter endeavor, if it is to be anything more than a pedagogical exercise, requires some discussion of the meaning of "normal." Perhaps more important is that some thought should be directed toward the meaning of deviations from normative data. Do such deviations always imply *abnormality?* Do they imply that the brain has suffered some sort of insult? Does their presence necessarily mean that they have a causative relationship with the symptoms or signs for which the patient was referred? The history of clinical electroencephalography has certainly not been distinguished by thoughtful analysis of these problems or even by a critical sense of their significance. Perhaps this has been the natural outcome of the quest for laboratory techniques that can provide "penny in the slot" diagnoses: the kind of explicit certainty that computed tomography and magnetic resonance imaging are apparently now providing, at a somewhat higher price, for diseases with a morphological signature.

From its inception, there has been a tendency in electroencephalography to view minor deviations from the norm as objective evidence of disordered brain function,[12] the result of some past or ongoing pathological process. To

---

[12]Minor dysrhythmias have been used to "prove" the already tenuous clinical diagnosis of minimal brain damage.

some electroencephalographers, many EEG findings automatically mean epilepsy; to others, certain findings (e.g., a spike focus) always imply the presence of a palpable brain lesion. Such concepts are now undergoing reappraisal (106,107). It is gradually becoming recognized that the EEG characteristics of a given individual are the product of diverse internal and external influences, acting on a genetically determined substrate. These influences may be conceptualized diagrammatically in terms of their interactions. Figure 5.44 represents an attempt to specify the factors that determine the characteristics of the EEG and to illustrate their interplay (109).

Many years ago, Kennard (113,114) suggested that the total EEG pattern may ultimately result from all the stabilizing and disruptive influences brought to bear on cerebral function. The validity of this concept is being clarified only now.

The Individuality and Stability of the Human EEG

Fortunately for clinical electroencephalography, the EEG of an adult shows remarkable stability over time. This was originally noted by Travis (192,193)

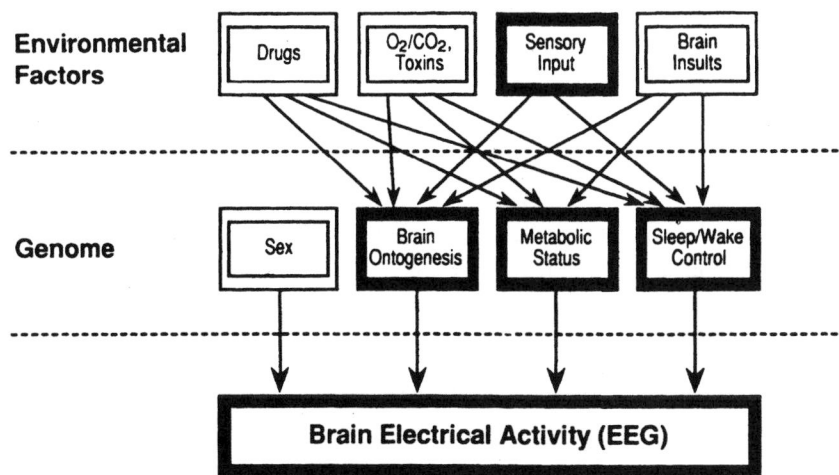

FIG. 5.44. Schematic representation of the factors and their interactions that determine the characteristics of brain electrical activity. (From Kellaway P. Introduction to plasticity and sensitive periods. In: Kellaway P, Noebels JL, eds. *Problems and concepts in developmental neurophysiology.* Baltimore: The Johns Hopkins University Press, 1989:3–28.)

in the very early days of electroencephalography and has been confirmed by several more recent studies (8,116,139,197). With the application of modified techniques of communication theory with multivariate statistical analysis, it has been shown that an individual can be recognized by his EEG spectral pattern with a confidence probability of about 90%. The stability of the individual's spectral pattern holds for different conditions such as eyes open, eyes closed, auditory stimulation, and task performance. This specific individuality of the human EEG provides strong presumptive evidence that the characteristics of the EEG are determined primarily by genetic factors.

The Genetic Substrate

After the individuality and stability of the EEG had been established, there was an effort to determine EEG similarity within pairs of monozygotic and dizygotic twins (40,85,130,131,171,201,203). Analysis of the EEGs of 110 pairs of monozygotic twins of various ages revealed only one pair with dissimilar awake EEGs and four pairs with dissimilar sleep EEGs. Of 98 dizygotic pairs, in contrast, only 17 were found to be similar. The rate of maturation of the EEG was similar for the monozygotic twins but different for the dizygotic ones (201,203). Striking similarities in the spectral features of the resting EEGs of monozygotic twins have been found by several different groups (47,136,137,219). The similarity of the EEGs of monozygotic twins has been shown in such twins who were reared apart in different environments (97,98,184).

A finding with dual significance in this regard is that alcohol has similar effects on the EEGs of monozygotic twins, but the EEGs of fraternal twins become more dissimilar after alcohol ingestion (169,170). This indicates that the effect of alcohol on the EEG is under genetic control and reflects genetic differences in the sensitivity of the target organ. A common observation in routine clinical electroencephalography is the very great difference in the amount and amplitude of beta activity that may be seen in persons of similar ages and with similar blood levels of barbiturates, benzodiazepines, and other drugs that increase fast activity. Thus, the findings of the alcohol study may, as the authors suggest, be generalized to all centrally acting substances.

The possibility that each of the spontaneous rhythms of the human brain might constitute heritable traits now seems fully confirmed. However, although there is strong evidence for apparent polygenic transmission of some spectral frequency patterns, no specific gene locus for a specific EEG rhythm has yet been identified in humans. Researchers have obtained unambiguous evidence in mice that a spontaneous and predominant EEG rhythm can be expressed as a hereditary trait under the control of a single recessive locus (124,152).

Kennard (113,114) was the first to suggest the possibility that familial or inherited tendencies may be important in the genesis of some of the deviations from normal (e.g., nonspecific dysrhythmias) seen in children. A significant familial factor has been established for certain abnormal or specific patterns of the child's EEG: 3-Hz spike-and-wave activity (83,143–146), rolandic spikes (13–16,151a), and 14- and 6-Hz positive spikes (164,175, 202). The most provocative and surprising finding is the genetic or familial factor associated with focal EEG abnormality (5,14). Clearly, it appears that deviations from "normal" may be the "neurophysiological consequence of a genetically controlled biosynthetic pathway" (145).

Ontogenetic Plasticity

Although the emergence and differentiation of the electrical activity of the brain are initially dependent on the genetic substrate, the character of the activity is also vitally influenced by environmental factors. For example, the maturational evolution of the brain, which continues for some time after birth, is currently conceived as an orderly sequence of interactions between the genome and the milieu. The fine-tuning of cortical properties is governed to a certain extent by the external environment so as to adapt the organism to the characteristics of that environment. If these requirements exceed the limits set by genetic rules, the respective functional characteristics are eliminated (for review, see Kellaway and Noebels [111]).

This plasticity is possible only when processes of organization are taking place. In general, the period of life in which the organism is maximally susceptible to lasting structural and functional changes coincides with the period of fastest neuronal growth (35). However, there is evidence that some modification of structure and function by subtle environmental factors may be possible, at least in the visual system, up to the age of 2 to 3 years (86,205).

Afferent input (in terms of the entire sensory environment) is a critical factor in the ontogenesis of the electrical activity of the brain; aberrations of sensory input early in life may profoundly alter the character of the EEG. Thus, persons deprived of visual input from birth have no occipital alpha activity, and deprivation or incongruity of input from the two eyes occurring within a very early epoch after birth may result in the development of occipital spikes (109).

As stated previously, age is a primary factor in determining the characteristics of the EEG: The younger the individual, the more critical the age factor.

In premature infants, an age difference of a week may be associated with markedly different EEG characteristics, but there is little difference between the EEG characteristics of an infant at term and those of one aged 4 to 5 weeks. The EEG of an 8-year-old child may be indistinguishable from that of an 11-year-old. The ontogenetic evolution of the EEG throughout infancy, childhood, and adolescence has been well documented (48,103,165).

Less clearly understood is the role played by age—degree of cerebral development—in determining the characteristics of the EEG in response to a brain insult or injury, particularly during very early life. For example, it has been shown repeatedly that when a significant injury is sustained during the perinatal period, the EEG initially may manifest abnormality, become normal and remain so throughout early childhood, and then become abnormal again during middle or late childhood. Thus, brain damage may not be revealed in the EEG recorded at a given age even though it is in fact present (104,109).

The effect of a given insult or injury on the immature brain may be determined in part by the stage of development at the time of the injury. For example, hypsarrhythmia, and the characteristic infantile spasms that accompany it, may be a manifestation of a wide variety of diffuse cerebral insults operant during the perinatal period and early infancy (90,102,121). If the same degrees and types of insult are sustained later in the course of cerebral maturation, they do not produce the same types of EEG changes or the same types of clinical seizures. Hypsarrhythmia and infantile spasms constitute the response of the brain to a nonspecific insult at a certain critical stage of development.

The rate of maturation set by genetic instruction may be retarded or arrested by the effects of various brain insults, and the timing of such an insult determines the characteristics of the EEG both acutely and in the long term. Walter (208,209) suggested that many of the lesser dysrhythmias of childhood may simply reflect delayed cerebral maturation. He hypothesized that such a delay might occur, even in the absence of a causative brain insult, as a result of "less than optimal trophic influences or systemic growth promoting endocrine and chemical influences" (209).

The suggestion has been made, and evidence adduced to support it, that differences in the EEGs of control children and, for example, children of a similar age with behavior problems may reflect maturational differences rather than damage or dysfunction (11,115,140). Common experience also suggests that maturational factors are significantly related to minor dysrhythmias, but the nature of this relationship remains obscure. Thus, the slow rhythms (e.g., frontal theta activity and posterior slow waves) tend to disappear with increasing age. This was documented in serial studies (P. Kellaway, unpublished observations) and can be inferred from samplings of different age groups (48,165). In practical terms, if minor dysrhythmias are important for the diagnosis and evaluation of behavior disorders, learning disabilities, and so forth (as has been suggested), they must then be progressively less so with increasing age.

Epidemiological studies (125–128) of behavior disorders in children yielded some interesting findings that have a bearing on this point. In a study of 482 children selected randomly from households systematically sampled in Buffalo, New York, Lapouse (126) found "a strikingly high prevalence of so-called symptomatic behavior" and pointed out that its "excessive presence in younger as contrasted with older children, and the weak association between those behaviors and adjustment, give rise to the question *whether behavior deviations are truly indicative of psychiatric or organic brain disorder or whether they occur as transient developmental phenomena* in essentially normal children" (emphasis added). It seems likely that parallel deviations may occur in the behavior and EEG patterns at a certain time in the life of a young child as coincident manifestations of a transient, ontogenetically determined influence.

Gender

The normative studies of Eeg-Olofsson and Petersén (48,165) showed statistically significant sex differences in the incidence of certain EEG patterns or in their characteristics (e.g., a much higher incidence of mu rhythms and a significantly higher frequency of the occipital alpha rhythms in girls and women). Some of these are mentioned elsewhere in this chapter.

Metabolic and Homeostatic Factors

The influences of homeostatic and metabolic factors have been well documented and have been discussed in several reviews (e.g., Harding and Thompson [82]). These factors become more important when deranged, and it is essential that the electroencephalographer recognize that disease states may affect the EEG secondarily through these factors rather than directly. For example, the frequency of the occipital alpha rhythm may be decreased by any condition that impairs cerebral metabolism. Thus, slowing of the alpha rhythm may result from chronic pulmonary insufficiency, chronically diminished cardiac output, or profound hypothyroidism. It was enlightening, in the early days of heart transplantation and implantation of cardiac pacemakers, to observe increases in alpha frequency of up to 2 Hz after normal cardiac output was restored, with the brain no longer subjected to chronic hypoperfusion.

Sleep and Wakefulness

The characteristics of the EEG, in subjects awake and asleep, are considered briefly in terms of their interpretation in clinical EEG practice. More extensive treatment of the transformations of the EEG that occur during normal sleep is available in several monographs (159,217).

Psychoaffective State

Kennard (113,114) suggested that anxiety or tension states might influence the EEG characteristics of a child in important ways. This possibility has been espoused most persistently by Lairy (122,123) and Igert and Lairy (93). They drew attention to the fact that occipital slow activity (or "posterior slow activity of youth") appears responsive to psychological factors, and Cohn and Nardini (33) speculated that posterior slow waves constitute "a conditioned response of a disordered brain to the exigencies of interpersonal experiences." Werre (210) reported evidence that, even in adults, posterior slow waves are sensitive to frustration; and Garcia-Badaracco (60) adduced circumstantial evidence to support his view that posterior slow waves are the consequence of frustration as well as evidence of what he called a "quasi-constitutional sensitivity to frustrations." Speculations aside, it is a common observation that the amount and amplitude of this slow activity may vary throughout a recording, generally being more pronounced at the beginning of the recording period and diminishing with time. Many factors could account for this phenomenon; there have been no controlled studies in this area, but the obvious suggestion is that the slow activity diminishes as the child becomes more accustomed to the unique and unfamiliar circumstances of the laboratory procedure. Carels (24) reported an increase in posterior slow waves in a young adult neurotic patient with each "social encounter," the EEG becoming more normal in a hospital (protective) environment.

Lairy (123) maintained that posterior slow activity in children with behavior disorders and learning disturbances may reflect adaptation to stress and that certain EEG abnormalities may be interpreted as a sign of impaired adaptation. The prognostic significance of the findings "depends upon the degree of impaired control and the possibilities of recovering equilibrium." In her view, the presence of posterior slow activity implies a more favorable prognosis for therapy than does a "normal" EEG, inasmuch as she believed that the latter is a sign of "hyperadaptation, which leaves little hope for functional secondary readaptation." Lairy's hypothesis appears to be based largely on intuitional or circumstantial evidence and on inferences drawn from her own and others' clinical observations. In spite of the fact that these concepts have yet to be proved by systematic research, they are of heuristic importance and should not be dismissed lightly.

Of all areas of the brain sampled during scalp electroencephalography, the occipitotemporal regions in the child are the most sensitive to hyperventilation (38,39; P. Kellaway, unpublished data); after hypoxia, head injury, or encephalitis in children, the slowing effect persists longest in the occipital region (147). Similarly, in children with leukemia, posterior or occipital slowing of undetermined origin occurs during the acute phase and with exacerbation (138). Each of these findings indicates a sensitivity or high reactivity of this part of the brain in children. A similar high reactivity to emotional factors may also be present, as suggested by the findings of Werre (210) in a single subject.

Several investigators have reported an association between emotional state and theta activity. Walter (208), for example, reported that he induced bursts of this activity by depriving young children of pleasurable stimuli. Similarly, frustration, annoyance, and embarrassment have been reported to cause enhancement of theta activity (54), even in adult subjects (150). Adey et al. (1) and Burch et al. (22) reported increased theta activity in the EEG of an astronaut during launch and the initial hours of space flight, and similar findings have been reported during space flights conducted by the Russians (186). The Russian scientists (207) interpreted the findings as a reflection of a "high level" of psychoemotional reactions during the early phases of the flight. Adey et al. (1) believed that more fundamental physiological substrates—concerned primarily with alerting and orientation—were involved. Whether the anterior theta rhythms in humans are responsive simply as part of an alerting or orienting mechanism or are elements of a psychoaffective response has not been clearly established by experimental studies such as those of Walter (208,209) or Melin (142), who exposed young adults to shocking and horrifying movies and found increases in the theta and occasionally the delta components of the subjects' EEGs.

That EEG patterns are indeed plastic and responsive to functional factors appears to be established; it has yet to be proved, however, that persistent aberrations of the EEG of the child may be a consequence of prolonged emotional stress (e.g., chronic anxiety or frustration). Nordland (153) attempted to answer the question by comparing the EEGs of maladjusted children who had histories of chronic psychological stress (e.g., conflict, insecurity, or anxiety) with a group in whom these factors were not significant. Her results indicated that "an abnormal EEG may be a symptom of protracted states of psychological tension"; but, as Nordland herself pointed out, the study does not provide conclusive answers to the question. Nevertheless, the evidence is sufficient (50) to give pause to those who maintain the view that the dysrhythmic EEG is always evidence of organic dysfunction acquired through infection, injury, or other organic insult (30,215).

Extrinsic Factors

Extrinsic factors (e.g., drugs, trauma, infection) are considered in various other chapters of this book.

ACKNOWLEDGMENT

This work was supported in part by grant NS11535 from the National Institute of Neurological Disorders and Stroke, National Institutes of Health, United States Public Health Service.

REFERENCES

1. Adey WR, Kado RT, Walter DO. Computer analysis of EEG data from Gemini flight GT-7. *Aerospace Med* 1967;38:345–359.
2. Aird RB, Gastaut Y. Occipital and posterior electroencephalographic rhythms. *Electroencephalogr Clin Neurophysiol* 1959;11:637–656.
3. Arenas AM, Brenner RP, Reynolds CF III. Temporal slowing in the elderly revisited. *Am J EEG Technol* 1986;26:105–114.
4. Barlow JS, Cigánek L. Lambda responses in relation to visual evoked responses in man. *Electroencephalogr Clin Neurophysiol* 1969;26:183–192.
5. Barslund I, Danielsen J. Temporal epilepsy in monozygotic twins. *Epilepsia* 1963;4:138–150.
6. Belsh JM, Chokroverty S, Barabas G. Posterior rhythmic slow activity in EEG after eye closure. *Electroencephalogr Clin Neurophysiol* 1983;56:562–568.
7. Berges J, Netchine S, Lairy GC. Quelques aspects particuliers du trace E.E.G. chez l'enfant présentant des troubles de la psychomotricité. *Rev Neurol (Paris)* 1963;109:238–246.
8. Berkhout J, Walter DO. Temporal stability and individual differences in the human EEG: an analysis of variance of spectral values. *IEEE Trans Biomed Eng* 1968;15:165–168.
9. Blinn KA, Noell WK. Continuous measurement of alveolar CO_2 tension during the hyperventilation test in routine electroencephalography. *Electroencephalogr Clin Neurophysiol* 1949;1:333–342.
10. Sherwin I. Differential effects of hyperventilation on the excitability of intact and isolated cortex. *Electroencephalogr Clin Neurophysiol* 1965;18:599–607.
11. Bosaeus E, Matousek M, Petersén I. Correlation between paedopsychiatric findings and EEG-variables in well-functioning children of ages 5–16 years. *Scand J Psychol* 1977;18:140–147.
12. Brandt S, Brandt H. The electroencephalographic patterns in young healthy children from 0 to five years of age. *Acta Psychiatr Scand* 1955;30:77–89.
13. Bray PF, Wiser WC. A modified concept of idiopathic epilepsy. *Trans Am Neurol Assoc* 1964;89:140–142.
14. Bray PF, Wiser WC. Evidence for a genetic etiology of temporal-central abnormalities in focal epilepsy. *N Engl J Med* 1964;271:926–933.
15. Bray PF, Wiser WC. The relation of focal to diffuse epileptiform EEG discharges in genetic epilepsy. *Arch Neurol* 1965;13:223–237.
16. Bray PF, Wiser WC, Wood MC, et al. Hereditary characteristics of familial temporal-central focal epilepsy. *Pediatrics* 1965;36:207–212.
17. Brazier MAB, Finesinger JE, Schwab RS. Characteristics of the normal electroencephalogram. II. The effect of varying blood sugar levels on the occipital cortical potentials in adults during quiet breathing. *J Clin Invest* 1944;23:313–317.
18. Brazier MAB, Finesinger JE, Schwab RS. Characteristics of the normal electroencephalogram. III. The effect of varying blood sugar levels on the occipital cortical potentials in adults during hyperventilation. *J Clin Invest* 1944;23:319–323.
19. Brill NQ, Seidemann H. The electroencephalogram of normal children: effect of hyperventilation. *Am J Psychiat* 1941;98:250–256.
20. Brockmeier D, Prüll G. Langzeituntersuchungen der rhythmischen variation spektralanalytisch gewonnener EEG-Merkmale. *EEG -EMG Z Elektroenzephalogr Elektromyogr Verwandt Geb* 1975;6:42.
21. Bruens JH, Gastaut H, Giove G. Electroencephalographic study of the signs of chronic vascular insufficiency of the sylvian region in aged people. *Electroencephalogr Clin Neurophysiol* 1960;12:283–295.
22. Burch NR, Dossett RG, Vorderman AL, et al. *Period analysis of the electroencephalogram from the orbital flight of Gemini VII.* Final report. Washington, DC: National Aeronautics and Space Administration, 1967.
23. Busse EW, Obrist WD. Pre-senescent electroencephalographic changes in normal subjects. *J Gerontol* 1965;20:315–320.
24. Carels G. Les ondes lentes postérieures de l'électroencéphalogramme d'un jeune adulte et leur variation quantitative dans le temps. *Acta Neurol Belg* 1959;59:409–413.
25. Chatrian GE. Characteristics of unusual EEG patterns: incidence; significance. *Electroencephalogr Clin Neurophysiol* 1964;17:471–472.
26. Chatrian GE. The mu-rhythm. In: Rémond A, ed. *Handbook of Electroencephalography and clinical neurophysiology, vol. 6, part A: The EEG of the waking adult.* Amsterdam: Elsevier, 1976:46–49.
27. Chatrian GE, Petersén MC, Lazarte JA. The blocking of the rolandic wicket rhythm and some central changes related to movement. *Electroencephalogr Clin Neurophysiol* 1958;10:771–772.
28. Chatrian GE, Petersén MC, Lazarte JA. The blocking of the rolandic wicket rhythm and some central changes related to movement. *Electroencephalogr Clin Neurophysiol* 1960;11:497–510.
29. Chatrian GE, White LE Jr, Daly D. Electroencephalographic patterns resembling those of sleep in certain comatose states after injuries to the head. *Electroencephalogr Clin Neurophysiol* 1963;15:272–280.
30. Chess S. *An introduction to child psychiatry.* New York: Grune & Stratton, 1969.
31. Cigánek L. Theta-discharges in the middle-line: EEG symptom of temporal lobe epilepsy. *Electroencephalogr Clin Neurophysiol* 1961;13:669–673.
32. Cobb WR, Guiloff R, Cast J. Breach rhythm: the EEG related to skull defects. *Electroencephalogr Clin Neurophysiol* 1979;47:251–271.
33. Cohn R, Nardini JE. The correlation of bilateral occipital slow activity in the human EEG with certain disorders of behavior. *Am J Psychiat* 1958;115:44–54.
34. Covello A, De Barros-Ferreira M, Lairy GC. Etude telemetrique des rythmes centraux chez l'enfant. *Electroencephalogr Clin Neurophysiol* 1975;38:307–319.
35. Cragg BS. The development of synapse in the visual system of the cat. *J Comp Neurol* 1975;160:147–166.
36. Creutzfeldt O, Grünewald G, Simonova O, et al. Changes of the basic rhythms of the EEG dur-

ing the performance of mental and visuomotor task. In: Evans C, Mulholland T, eds. *Attention in neurophysiology.* London: Butterworths, 1969:148–168.

37. Creutzfeldt OD, Arnold P-M, Becker D, et al. EEG changes during spontaneous and controlled menstrual cycles and their correlation with psychological performance. *Electroencephalogr Clin Neurophysiol* 1976;40:113–131.

38. Daute K-H, Frenzel J, Klust E. Über den unspezifischen hyperventilationseffekt im EEG des gesunden kindes. I. Stärkegrad. *Z Kinderheilkd* 1968;104:197–207.

39. Daute K-H, Klust E, Frenzel J. Über den unspezifischen hyperventilationseffekt im EEG des gesunden kindes. II. Strukturbesonderheiten, schlussfolgerungen. *Z Kinderheilkd* 1968;104:208–217.

40. Davis H, Davis PA. Action potentials of the brain in normal persons and in normal states of cerebral activity. *Arch Neurol Psychiat* 1936;36:1214–1224.

41. Davis H, Wallace WMcL. Factors affecting changes produced in electroencephalogram by standardized hyperventilation. *Arch Neurol Psychiat* 1942;47:606–625.

42. Doose H, Gerken H, Völzke E. Genetics of centrencephalic epilepsy in childhood. *Epilepsia* 1968;9:107–115.

43. Doose H, Gerken H, Völzke E. On the genetics of EEG-anomalies in childhood. I. Abnormal theta rhythms. *Neuropaediatrie* 1972;3:386–401.

44. Doose H, Gundel A. 4 to 7 CPS rhythms in the childhood EEG. In: Anderson VE, Hauser WA, Penry JK, et al., eds. *Genetic basis of the epilepsies.* New York: Raven Press, 1982:83–93.

45. Doose H, Petersén CE, Völzke E, et al. [Fever cramps and epilepsy. I. Etiology, clinical picture and course of the so-called infection or fever cramps.] *Arch Psychiatr Nervenkr* 1966;208:400–432.

46. Dumermuth G. *Elektroencephalographie im kindesalter.* Stuttgart: Thieme, 1965.

47. Dumermuth G. Variance spectra of electroencephalograms in twins. In: Kellaway P, Petersén I, eds. *Clinical electroencephalography of children.* Stockholm: Almqvist & Wiksell, 1968:119–154.

48. Eeg-Olofsson O. The development of the electroencephalogram in normal adolescents from the age of 16 through 21 years. *Neuropaediatrie* 1971;3:11–45.

49. Eeg-Olofsson O, Petersén I, Selldén U. The development of the EEG in normal children from the age of 1 to 15 years: paroxysmal activity. *Neuropaediatrie* 1971;4:375–404.

50. Ellingson RJ. The incidence of EEG abnormality among patients with mental disorders of apparently nonorganic origin: a critical review. *Am J Psychiat* 1954;111:263–274.

51. Engel GL, Romano J, Ferris EB. Variations in the normal electroencephalogram during a five-year period. *Science* 1947;108:600–601.

52. Epstein CM, Brickley GP. Interelectrode distance and amplitude of the scalp EEG. *Electroencephalogr Clin Neurophysiol* 1985;60:287–292.

53. Evans CC. Spontaneous excitation of the visual cortex and assocation areas—lambda waves. *Electroencephalogr Clin Neurophysiol* 1953;5:69–74.

54. Faure J, Guérin A. Au sujet de l'électroencéphalogramme des enfants caractériels. *Rev Neurol (Paris)* 1958;99:209–219.

55. Fiedlerová D. Der einfluss der hyperventilation yon 3 minuten auf das EEG-bild bei gesunden kindern im alter yon 7 bis 11 jahren. *Sborn Lek* 1967;4:417–422.

56. Fourment A, Calvert J, Bancaud J. Electrocorticography of waves associated with eye movements in man during wakefulness. *Electroencephalogr Clin Neurophysiol* 1976;40:457–469.

57. Frey TS, Sjögren H. The electroencephalogram in elderly persons suffering from neuropsychiatric disorders. *Acta Psychiatr Scand* 1959;34:438–450.

58. Frost JD Jr, Carrie JRG, Borda RP, et al. The effects of Dalmane (flurazepam hydrochloride) on human EEG characteristics. *Electroencephalogr Clin Neurophysiol* 1973;34:171–175.

59. Frost JD Jr, Glaze DG, Hrachovy RA, et al. EEG and neuropsychological changes associated with carbamazepine therapy in children with partial seizures. *J Clin Neurophysiol* 1988;5:336–337.

60. Garcia-Badaracco J. *EEG et psychisme: Les entretiens psychiatriques 1953.* Paris: Collection Psyché, Arche, 1953:140–165.

61. Garsche R. Die beta-aktivität im EEG des kindes. I. Mitteilung erscheinungsformen bei gesunden kindern. *Z Kinderheilkd* 1956;78:441–457.

62. Garsche R. Die beta-aktivität im EEG des kindes. II. Mitteilung erscheinungsformen bei cerebralen erkrankungen. *Z Kinderheilkd* 1956;78:458–479.

63. Gastaut H, Broughton R. *Epileptic seizures: clinical and electrographic features, diagnosis and treatment.* Springfield, IL: Charles C Thomas, 1972.

64. Gastaut H, Bruens JH, Roger J, et al. Étude électroencéphalographique des signes d'insuffisance circulatoire sylvienne chronique. *Rev Neurol (Paris)* 1959;100:59–65.

65. Gastaut H, Lee MC, Laboureur P. Comparative EEG and psychometric data for 825 French naval pilots and 511 control subjects of the same age. *Aerospace Med* 1960;31:547–552.

66. Gastaut H, Poirier F. The electroencephalogram in cerebrovascular diseases. *Neurology* 1960;11:110–111.

67. Gastaut H, Terzian H, Gastaut Y. Etude d'une activité électroencéphalographique méconnue: le "rythme rolandique en arceau." *Marseille Med* 1952;89:296–310.

68. Gastaut Y. Un signe électroencéphalographique peu connu: les pointes occipitales survenant pendant l'ouverture des yeux. *Rev Neurol (Paris)* 1951;84:640–643.

69. Gibbs EL, Gibbs FA. Extreme spindles: correlation of electroencephalographic sleep pattern with mental retardation. *Science* 1962;138:1106–1107.

70. Gibbs EL, Lorimer FM, Gibbs FA. Clinical correlates of exceedingly fast activity in the electroencephalogram. *Dis Nerv Syst* 1950;11:323–326.

71. Gibbs, FA, Gibbs EL. *Atlas of electroencephalography, vol. 1: Normal controls.* Cambridge, MA: Addison-Wesley, 1950.

72. Gibbs FA, Gibbs EL. *Atlas of electroencephalography, vol. 2: Epilepsy.* Cambridge, Addison-Wesley, 1952.

73. Gibbs FA, Gibbs EL, Lennox WG. Electroencephalographic classification of epileptic patients and control subjects. *Arch Neurol Psychiat* 1943;50:111–128.

74. Gibbs FA, Gibbs EL, Lennox WG. Electroencephalographic response to overventilation and its relation to age. *J Pediatr* 1943;23:497–505.

75. Gibbs FA, Knott JR. Growth of the electrical activity of the cortex. *Electroencephalogr Clin Neurophysiol* 1949;1:223–229.

76. Goodwin JE. The significance of alpha variants in the EEG, and their relationship to an epileptiform syndrome. *Am J Psychiat* 1947;104:369–379.

77. Gotoh F, Meyer JS, Takagi Y. Cerebral effects of hyperventilation in man. *Arch Neurol* 1965;12:410–423.

78. Götze W. Änderung des himstrombildes bei hyperventilation yon hirngesunden kindern. *Zbl Neurochir* 1942;7:202–207.

79. Green J. Some observations on lambda waves and peripheral stimulation. *Electroencephalogr Clin Neurophysiol* 1957;9:691–704.

80. Gundel A, Baier W, Doose H. Spectral analysis of EEG in the late course of primary generalized myoclonic-astatic epilepsy. II. Cluster analysis of the power spectra. *Neuropediatrics* 1980;12:110–118.

81. Gundel A, Baier W, Doose H, et al. Spectral analysis of EEG in the late course of primary generalized myoclonic-astatic epilepsy. I. EEG and clinical data. *Neuropediatrics* 1980;12:62–74.

82. Harding GFA, Thompson CRS. EEG rhythms and the internal milieu. In: Lairy GC, ed. *Handbook of electroencephaloqraphy and clinical neurophysiology, vol. 6: The normal EEG throughout life, part A: The EEG of the waking adult.* Amsterdam: Elsevier Scientific, 1975:176–194.

83. Harvald B. *Heredity in epilepsy.* Copenhagen: Munksgaard, 1954.

84. Harvald B. EEG in old age. *Acta Psychiatr Scand* 1958;33:193–196.

85. Heuschert D. EEG-untersuchungen an eineiigen zwillingen im höheren lebensalter. *Z Menschl Vererb Konstitutionsl* 1963;37:128–172.

86. Hickey TL. Postnatal development of the human lateral geniculate nucleus: relationship to a critical period for the visual system. *Science* 1977;198:836–838.

87. Hill D. Cerebral dysrhythmia: its significance in aggressive behavior. *Proc R Soc Med* 1944; 37:317–330.

88. Hirsch W, Belitz H, Geipel G, et al. Genetische-klinische studien an abnormalen und cerebral geschädigten kindern. *Monatsschr Kinderheilkd* 1958;106:209–221.

89. Hirt HR. Zur diagnostischen bedentung der pathologischen beta-aktivität im EEG des kindes und jugendlichen. *Fortschr Neurol Psychiat* 1968;36:412–433.

90. Hrachovy RA, Frost JD Jr. Infantile spasms: a disorder of the developing nervous system. In: Kellaway P, Noebels JL, eds. *Problems and concepts in developmental neurophysiology.* Baltimore: The Johns Hopkins University Press, 1989:131–147.

91. Hughes JR, Cayaffa JJ. The EEG in patients at different ages without organic cerebral disease. *Electroencephalogr Clin Neurophysiol* 1977;42:776–784.

92. Hughes JR, Park GE. The EEG in dyslexia. In: Kellaway P, Petersén I, eds. *Clinical electroencephalography of children.* Stockholm: Almqvist & Wiksell, 1968:307–327.

93. Igert CI, Lairy GC. Intérêt pronostique de l'EEG au cours de l'évolution des schizophrènes. *Electroencephalogr Clin Neurophysiol* 1962;14:183–190.

94. Jaffe R, Jacobs L. The beta focus: its nature and significance. *Acta Neurol Scand* 1972;48: 191–203.

95. Jasper HH, Penfield W. Electrocorticograms in man: effect of voluntary movement upon electrical activity of precentral gyrus. *Arch Psychiat* 1949;183:163–174.

96. Jasper HH, Solomon P, Bradley C. Electroencephalographic analyses of behavior problem children. *Am J Psychiat* 1938;95:641–658.

97. Juel-Nielsen N. Individual and environment: a psychiatric-psychological investigation of MZ twins reared apart. *Acta Psychiatr Scand* (Suppl) 1965:183.

98. Juel-Nielsen N, Harvald B. The electroencephalogram in uniovular twins brought up apart. *Acta Genet (Basel)* 1958;8:57–64.

99. Jung R, Riechert R, Meyer-Mickeleit RW. Über intracerebrale himpotentialableitungen bei hirnchirurgischen eingriffen. *Dtsch Z Nervenheilk* 1950;162:52–60.

100. Katz RI, Horowitz GR. Electroencephalogram in the septuagenarian: studies in a normal geriatric population. *J Am Geriatr Soc* 1982;30:273–275.

101. Kellaway P. The development of sleep spindles and of arousal patterns in infants and their characteristics in normal and certain abnormal states. *Electroencephalogr Clin Neurophysiol* 1952;4:369.

102. Kellaway P. Neurologic status of patients with hypsarhythmia. In: Gibbs FA, ed. *Molecules and mental health.* Philadelphia: Lippincott, 1959:134–149.

103. Kellaway P. *Ontogenic evolution of the electrical activity of the brain in man and animals.* Rapport du Premier Congrés International des Sciences Neurologigues, Bruxelles, 1967:141–154.

104. Kellaway P. Afferent input: a critical factor in the ontogenesis of brain electrical activity. In: Burch N, Altshuler HL, eds. *Behavior and brain electrical activity.* New York: Plenum Press, 1975:391–420.

105. Kellaway P. An orderly approach to visual analysis: parameters of the normal EEG in adults and children. In: Klass DW, Daly DD, eds. *Current practice of clinical electroencephalography.* New York: Raven Press, 1979:69–147.

106. Kellaway P. The incidence, significance and natural history of spike foci in children. In: Henry CE, ed. *Current clinical neurophysiology: update on EEG and evoked potentials.* New York: Elsevier/North-Holland, 1981:151–175.

107. Kellaway P. Genetic, ontogenetic, and biorhythmic factors in epilepsy. In: Appel SH, ed. *Current neurology, vol. 5.* New York: John Wiley & Sons, 1984:259–284.

108. Kellaway P. Sleep and epilepsy. *Epilepsia* 1985;26(Suppl. 1):15–30.

109. Kellaway P. Introduction to plasticity and sensitive periods. In: Kellaway P, Noebels JL, eds. *Problems and concepts in developmental neurophysiology.* Baltimore: The Johns Hopkins University Press, 1989:3–28.

110. Kellaway P, Fox BJ. Electroencephalographic diagnosis of cerebral pathology in infants during sleep. I. Rationale, technique, and the characteristics of normal sleep in infants. *J Pediatr* 1952;41:262–287.

111. Kellaway P, Noebels JL, eds. *Problems and concepts in developmental neurophysiology.* Baltimore: The Johns Hopkins University Press, 1989.

112. Kendel K, Koufen H. EEG veränderungen bei cerebralen gefabinsulten des hirnstamms. *Dtsch Z Nervenheilk* 1970;197:42–55.

113. Kennard MA. Inheritance of electroencephalogram patterns in children with behavior disorders. *Psychosom Med* 1949;11:151–157.

114. Kennard MA. Significance of abnormal EEGs in disorders of behavior. *Electroencephalogr Clin Neurophysiol* 1949;1:118–119.

115. Kennard MA. EEG abnormality in first grade children with "soft" neurological signs. *Electroencephalogr Clin Neurophysiol* 1969;27:544.

116. Kennard M, Schwartzman AE. A longitudinal study of electroencephalographic frequency patterns in mental hospital patients and normal controls. *Electroencephalogr Clin Neurophysiol* 1957;9:263–275.

117. Kooi KA, Guvener AM, Tupper CJ, et al. Electroencephalographic patterns of the temporal region in normal adults. *Neurology* 1964;14:1029–1035.

118. Koshino Y, Niedermeyer E. Enhancement of rolandic mu-rhythm by pattern vision. *Electroencephalogr Clin Neurophysiol* 1975;38:535–538.

119. Kozelka JW, Pedley TA. Beta and mu rhythms. *J Clin Neurophysiol* 1990;7:191–207.

120. Kuhlo W, Heintel H, Vogel F. The 4-5 c-sec rhythm. *Electroencephalogr Clin Neurophysiol* 1969;7:613–618.

121. Lacy JR, Penry JK. *Infantile spasms.* New York: Raven Press, 1976.

122. Lairy GC. E.E.G. et neuropsychiatrie infantile. *Psychiatr Enfant* 1961;3:525–608.

123. Lairy GC. L'EEG comme moyen d'investigation des modalité individuelles d'adaptation aux situations de stress. *Electroencephalogr Clin Neurophysiol* Suppl 1967;25:282–298.

124. Lane PW, Deol MS. Mocha, a new coat color and behavior mutation on chromosome 10 of the mouse. *J Hered* 1974;65:362–364.

125. Lapouse R. The relationship of behavior to adjustment in a representative sample of children. *Am J Public Health* 1965;55:1130–1141.

126. Lapouse R. The epidemiology of behavior disorders in children. *Am J Dis Child* 1966;111: 594–599.

127. Lapouse R, Monk MA. An epidemiologic study of behavior characteristics in children. *Am J Public Health* 1958;48:1134–1144.

128. Lapouse R, Monk MA, Street E. A method for use in epidemiologic studies of behavior disorders in children. *Am J Public Health* 1964;54:207–222.

129. Leissner P, Lindholm L-E, Petersén I. Alpha amplitude dependence on skull thickness as measured by ultrasound technique. *Electroencephalogr Clin Neurophysiol* 1970;29:392–399.

130. Lennox WG, Gibbs EL, Gibbs FA. The brain-wave pattern, an hereditary trait: evidence from 74 "normal" pairs of twins. *J Hered* 1945;36:233–243.

131. Lennox WG, Gibbs FA, Gibbs EL. Twins, brain waves, and epilepsy. *Arch Neurol Psychiat* 1942;47:702–704.

132. Lesêvre, N. Étude de réponses moyennes recueillies sur la région postérieure du scalp chez l'homme au cours de l'exploration visuelle ("complexe lambda"). *Psychol Franc* 1967;12:26–36.

133. Lindsley DB, Cutts KK. Electroencephalograms of "constitutionally inferior" and behavior problem children: comparison with those of normal children and adults. *Arch Neurol Psychiat* 1940;44:1199–1212.

134. Loomis AL, Harvey EN, Hobart G. Brain potentials during hypnosis. *Science* 1936;83: 239–241.

135. Loomis AL, Harvey EN, Hobart G. Distribution of disturbance patterns in the human electroencephalogram with special reference to sleep. *J Neurophysiol* 1938;1:413–430.

136. Lykken DT, Tellegen A, Iacono WG. EEG spectra in twins: evidence for a neglected mechanism of genetic determination. *Physiol Psychol* 1982;1:245–259.

137. Lykken DT, Tellegen A, Thorkelson K. Genetic determination of EEG frequency spectra. *Biol Psychol* 1974;1:245–259.

138. Mahoney DH Jr, Britt CW, Kellaway P, et al. Childhood leukemia: implications of EEG findings at time of diagnosis. *J Pediatr* 1981;98:437–440.

139. Matousek M, Arvidsson A, Friberg S. Serial quantitative electroencephalography. *Electroencephalogr Clin Neurophysiol* 1979;49:614–622.

140. Matousek M, Petersén I. *Objective measurement of maturation defects and other EEG abnormalities by means of frequency analysis.* Fifth World Congress of Psychiatry proceedings, Mexico City, Excerpta Medica Series no. 274 VII. Amsterdam: Excerpta Medica, 1971: 759–765.

141. Maulsby RL, Kellaway P, Graham M, et al. *The normative electroencephalographic data reference library.* Final report, contract NAS 9-1200. Washington, DC: National Aeronautics and Space Administration, 1968.

142. Melin K-A. The EEG in infancy and childhood. *Electroencephalogr Clin Neurophysiol Suppl* 1953;4:205–211.

143. Metrakos JD, Metrakos K. Genetics of convulsive disorders. I. Introduction, problems, methods, and base lines. *Neurology* 1960;10:228–240.

144. Metrakos JD, Metrakos K. Childhood epilepsy of subcortical ("centrencephalic") origin. *Clin Pediatr (Phila)* 1966;5:536–542.

145. Metrakos JD, Metrakos K. Discussion: genetic studies in clinical epilepsy. In: Jasper HH, Ward AA Jr, Pope A, eds. *Basic mechanisms of the epilepsies.* Boston: Little, Brown, 1969:700–708.

146. Metrakos K, Metrakos JD. Genetics of convulsive disorders. II. Genetic and electroencephalographic studies in centrencephalic epilepsy. *Neurology* 1961;11:474–483.

147. Mizrahi EM, Kellaway P. Cerebral concussion in children: assessment of injury by electroencephalography. *Pediatrics* 1984;73:419–425.

148. Mokrán V, Cigánek L, Kabátnik Z. Electroencephalographic theta discharges in the midline. *Eur Neurol* 1971;5:288–293.

149. Morrice JKW. Slow wave production in the EEG, with reference to hyperpnoea, carbon dioxide and autonomic balance. *Electroencephalogr Clin Neurophysiol* 1956;8:49–72.

150. Mundy-Castle AC. Theta and beta rhythm in the electroencephalograms of normal adults. *Electroencephalogr Clin Neurophysiol* 1951;3:477–486.

151. Netchine S, Lairy GC. The EEG and psychology of the child. In: Lairy GC, ed. *Handbook of electroencephalography and clinical neurophysiology, vol. 6: The normal EEG throughout life. Part B: The evolution of the EEG from birth to adulthood.* Amsterdam: Elsevier Scientific, 1975:69–104.

151a. Neubauer BA, Fiedler B, Himmelein B, et al. Centrotemporal spikes in families with rolandic epilepsy: linkage to chromosome 15q14. *Neurology* 1998;51:1608–1612.

152. Noebels JL, Sidman RL. Persistent hypersynchronization of neocortical neurons in the mocha mutant of mouse. *J Neurogenet* 1989;6:53–56.

153. Nordland E. Conflict state and abnormal EEG: a study of boys with behavior disturbances and abnormal EEG. *Scand J Educ Res* 1969;13:199–221.

154. Obrist WD. The electroencephalogram of normal aged adults. *Electroencephalogr Clin Neurophysiol* 1954;6:235–244.

155. Obrist WD, Busse EW, Eisdorfer C, et al. Relation of the electroencephalogram to intellectual function in senescence. *J Gerontol* 1962;17:197.

156. Obrist WD, Sokoloff L, Lassen NA, et al. Relation of EEG to cerebral blood flow and metabolism in old age. *Electroencephalogr Clin Neurophysiol* 1963;15:610–619.

157. Otomo E. Electroencephalography in old age: dominant alpha pattern. *Electroencephalogr Clin Neurophysiol* 1966;21:489–491.

158. Pampiglione G. Development of rhythmic EEG activities in infancy (waking state). *Rev Electroencephalogr Neurophysiol Clin* 1977;7:327–334.

159. Passouant P, ed. *Handbook of electroencephalography and clinical neurophysiology, vol. 7: Physiological correlates of EEG. part A: EEG and sleep.* Amsterdam: Elsevier Scientific, 1975.

160. Patel VM, Maulsby RL. How hyperventilation alters the EEG: a review of controversial viewpoints emphasizing neurophysiological mechanisms. *J Clin Neurophysiol* 1987;4:101–120.

161. Pavy R, Metcalfe J. The abnormal EEG in childhood communication and behavior abnormalities. *Electroencephalogr Clin Neurophysiol* 1965;19:414.

162. Pedley TA, Miller JA. Clinical neurophysiology of aging and dementia. In: Mayeux MD, Rosen W, eds. *Advances in neurology. Vol. 38: The dementias.* New York: Raven Press, 1983:31–49.

163. Perez-Borja C, Chatrian GE, Tyce FA, et al. Electrographic patterns of the occipital lobe in man: a topographic study based on use of implanted electrodes. *Electroencephalogr Clin Neurophysiol* 1962;14:171–182.

164. Petersén I, Akesson HO. EEG studies of siblings of children showing 14 and 6 per second positive spikes. *Acta Genet (Basel)* 1968;18:163–169.

165. Petersén I, Eeg-Olofsson O. The development of the electroencephalogram in normal children from the age of 1 through 15 years—non-paroxysmal activity. *Neuropaediatrie* 1971;2:247–304.

166. Petersén I, Sörbye R. Slow posterior rhythm in adults. *Electroencephalogr Clin Neurophysiol* 1962;14:161–170.

167. Picard P, Navarranne P, Laboureur P, et al. Confrontations des données de l'électroencéphalogramme et de l'examen psychologique chez 309 candidats pilotes a l'aéronautique. *Electroencephalogr Clin Neurophysiol Suppl* 1957;6:304–314.

168. Prinz PN, Peskind ER, Vitaliano PP, et al. Changes in the sleep and waking EEGs of nondemented and demented elderly subjects. *J Am Geriatr Soc* 1982;30:86–93.

169. Propping P. Genetic control of ethanol action in the central nervous system. An EEG study in twins. *Hum Genet* 1977;35:309–334.

170. Propping P, Krueger J, Abdellatif J. Effect of alcohol on genetically determined variants of the normal electroencephalogram. *Psychiat Res* 1980;2:85–98.

171. Raney ET. Brain potentials and lateral dominance in identical twins. *J Exp Psychol* 1939;24:21–39.

172. Reeves AL, Klass DW. Frequency asymmetry of sleep spindles associated with focal pathology. *Electroencephalogr Clin Neurophysiol* 1998;106:84–86.

173. Rémond A, Lesêvre N. Remarques sur les conditions d'apparition et l'importance statistique des ondes lambda chez les individus normaux. *Rev Neurol (Paris)* 1994;94:160–161.

174. Rémond A, Lesêvre N, Torres F. Étude chrono-topographique de l'activité occipitale moyenne recueilli sur le scalp chez l'homme en relation avec le déplacement du regard (complexe lambda). *Rev Neurol (Paris)* 1965;113:193–226.

175. Rodin EA. Familial occurrence of the 14 and 6/sec positive spike phenomenon. *Electroencephalogr Clin Neurophysiol* 1964;17:556–570.

176. Roth M, Green J. The lambda wave as a normal physiological phenomenon in the human electroencephalogram. *Nature* 1953;172:864–866.

177. Rubin MA. The distribution of the alpha rhythm over the cerebral cortex of normal man. *J Neurophysiol* 1938;1:313–323.

178. Santamaria J, Chiappa KE. *The EEG of drowsiness.* New York: Demos Publications, 1987.

179. Schoppenhorst M, Brauer F, Freund G, et al. The significance of coherence estimates in determining central alpha and mu activities. *Electroencephalogr Clin Neurophysiol* 1980;48:25–33.

180. Scott DF, Groetheysen UC, Bickford RG. Lambda responses in the human electroencephalogram. *Neurology* 1967;17:770–778.

181. Sem-Jacobsen CW, Petersén MC, Dodge HW, et al. Electroencephalographic rhythms from the depths of the parietal, occipital and temporal lobes in man. *Electroencephalogr Clin Neurophysiol* 1956;8:263–278.

182. Sheridan FP, Yeager CL, Oliver WA, et al. Electroencephalography as a diagnostic and prognostic aid in studying the senescent individual: a preliminary report. *J Gerontol* 1955;10:53–59.

184. Shields J. *Monozygotic twins brought up apart and brought up together.* London: Oxford University Press, 1962.

185. Simonova O, Roth B, Stein J. Veränderungen der physiologischen und pathologischen EEG-aktivität bei geistiger tätigkeit und aufmerksamkeit. *Arch Psychiatr Nervenkr* 1968;211:460–469.

186. Sisakyan NM, Yazdovskiy VI. *First group flight into outer space.* U.S. Department of Commerce, Joint Publications Research Service, Translation TT: 64-31567. 1964:91.

187. Steriade M, Llinás RR. The functional states of the thalamus and the associated neuronal interplay. *Physiol Rev* 1988;68:649–742.

188. Sulg IA, Cronqvist S, Schuller H, et al. The effect of intracardial pacemaker therapy on cerebral blood flow and electroencephalogram in patients with complete atrioventricular block. *Circulation* 1969;39:487–494.

189. Sunku AJ, Donat JF, Johnston JA, et al. Occipital responses to normal pattern stimulation. *Electroencephalogr Clin Neurophysiol* 1997;103;28p.

190. Sutter C, Harrelson AB. Occipital slowing in the EEG of 5–15 year olds (teenage slow): a report on this finding in 237 child psychiatric patients. *Electroencephalogr Clin Neurophysiol* 1966;20:624–625.

191. Torres F, Faoro A, Loewenson R, et al. The electroencephalogram of elderly subjects revisited. *Electroencephalogr Clin Neurophysiol* 1983;56:391–398.

192. Travis LE. Do brain waves have individuality? *Science* 1936;84:532–533.

193. Travis LE, Gottlober AB. How consistent are an individual's brain potentials from day to day? *Science* 1937;85:223–234.

194. Tsai H-J, Liu S-Y. [Lambda waves of human subjects of different age levels.] *Acta Psychol Sin* 1965;4:343–352. (Translated from Chinese by Barlow JS. Contemporary brain research in China. New York: Consultants Bureau, 1971:50–61.

195. Tyner FS, Knott JR, Mayer WB Jr. *Fundamentals of EEG technology, vol. 2. Clinical correlates.* New York: Raven Press, 1989:49–58.

196. Van der Drift JHA. Ischemic cerebral lesions. *Angiology* 1961;12:401–418.

197. van Dis H, Corner M, Dapper R, et al. Individual differences in the human electroencephalogram during quiet wakefulness. *Electroencephalogr Clin Neurophysiol* 1979;47:87–94.

198. Vertes RP. Brainstem control of the events of REM sleep. *Prog Neurobiol* 1984;22:241–288.

199. Vignaendra V, Matthews RL, Chatrian GE. Positive occipital sharp transients of sleep: relationships to nocturnal sleep cycle in man. *Electroencephalogr Clin Neurophysiol* 1974;37:239–246.

200. Visser SL, Hooijer C, Jonker C, et al. Anterior temporal focal abnormalities in EEG in normal aged subjects: correlations with psychological and CT brain scan findings. *Electroencephalogr Clin Neurophysiol* 1987;66:1–7.

201. Vogel F. *Über die erblichkeit des normalen elektroencephalogramms.* Stuttgart: Thieme, 1958.

202. Vogel F. "14 and 6/sec positive spikes" in schlaf-EEG yon jugendlichen ein- and zweierigen zwillingen. *Humanagenetik* 1965;1:390–391.

203. Vogel F. The genetic basis of the normal human electroencephalogram (EEG). *Humangenetik* 1970;10:91–114.

204. Vogel F, Götze W. Statistische betrachtungen über die β-wellen im EEG des menschen. *Dtsch Z Nervenheilk* 1962;184:112–136.

205. von Senden M. *Space and sight. The perception of space and shape in the congenitally blind before and after operation.* Glencoe, IL: Free Press, 1960.

206. Von Simkova D. Das EEG bei gesunden kindern im alter yon 7 bis 10 jahren. *Psychiatr Neurol Med Psychol (Leipzig)* 1965;17:66–71.

207. Voskrenzenskiy AD, Gazenko OG, Izosimov GV, et al. Working ability of cosmonauts during orbital flight. In: *Problems of space biology (U.S.S.R.).* Washington, DC: U.S. Library of Congress, Aerospace Technology Division, 1965;4(91):79.

208. Walter WG. The function of the electrical rhythms in the brain. *J Ment Sci* 1950;96:1–31.

209. Walter WG. Intrinsic rhythms of the brain. In: Field J, Magoun HW, Hall VE, eds. *Handbook of physiology. Section 1: Neurophysiology, vol. 1.* Washington, DC: American Physiological Society, 1959:279–298.

210. Werre PF. *The relationships between electroencephalographic and psychological data in normal adults.* Leiden: Universitaire Presse Leiden, 1957.

211. Westmoreland BF, Klass DW. Midline theta rhythm. *Arch Neurol* 1986;43:139–141.

212. Westmoreland BF, Klass DW. Defective alpha reactivity with mental concentration. *J Clin Neurophysiol* 1998;15:424–428.

213. Westmoreland BF, Sharbrough FW. Posterior slow wave transients associated with eye blinks in children. *Am J EEG Technol* 1975;15:14–19.

214. White JC, Tharp B. An arousal pattern in children with organic cerebral brain dysfunction. *Electroencephalogr Clin Neurophysiol* 1974;37:265–268.

215. White RW. *The abnormal personality.* New York: Ronald Press, 1964.

216. Wiener JM, Delano JC, Klass DW. An EEG study of delinquent and nondelinquent adolescents. *Arch Gen Psychiatry* 1966;15:144–150.

217. Williams RL, Karacan I, Hursch CJ. *Electroencephalography (EEG) of human sleep: clinical applications.* New York: John Wiley and Sons, 1974.

218. Yamaguchi, Y., Ishihara, T., and Mizuki, Y. (1985): Frontal midline theta rhythm (FmO). *Electroencephalogr. Clin Neurophysiol* 1985;60:38.

219. Young JP, Lader MH, Fenton GW. A twin study on the genetic influences on the electroencephalogram. *J Med Genet* 1972;9:13–16.

Chapter 6

Neonatal Electroencephalography

Robert R. Clancy, A.G. Christina Bergqvist, and Dennis J. Dlugos

Unaided clinical neurological examination of the healthy or sick newborn has severe, inherent limitations. The natural functional repertoire of the immature central nervous system (CNS) is modest. The bedside neurological examination is performed to assess the state of consciousness or arousal, to judge the amount and quality of motor activity, to evaluate active and passive tone, and to observe primitive and postural reflexes. The clinical examination, per se, does not directly measure higher cortical function, preservation of which is key to a healthy neurological future.

Although the actual generators of the neonatal electroencephalogram (EEG) are not specifically known, they are presumed to arise directly from neurons in the cerebral cortex, under the modulation of critical "deep gray" structures such as the thalami. The neonatal EEG is one of the few objective methods of measuring the functional integrity of the immature cortex and its connections. Empirically, it is most commonly used to measure the impact of a known medical or neurological insult on the brain and to detect or confirm the presence of seizures (17). Neonatal EEG is best employed as a supplement to a comprehensive evaluation of the patient that assimilates the clinical, neuroimaging, and electrophysiological viewpoints. EEG is rarely used to determine precisely the cause of an encephalopathy. Rather, it is performed to determine the severity of the brain injury and the likelihood that a permanent neurological condition will persist. As such, neonatal EEG is a premier prognostic tool when performed by an experienced electroencephalographer.

Although the basic electrophysiological principles that underlie neonatal EEG interpretation are similar to those used to read EEGs of older children, there is a different approach to interpreting and understanding tracings recorded in the very young infants. During infancy, brain maturation occurs at a rapid pace, accompanied by parallel changes in the appearance of the neonatal EEG. This is a challenge to the interpreter, who must be knowledgeable about the normal appearances of the EEG for a variety of ages, behavioral states, and medical conditions of the patients.

Routine bedside EEG examinations are sometimes supplemented or supplanted by the use of cerebral functional monitors, intended for long-term detection of electrographic seizure activity or to record global, simple measures of EEG trends over time (such as "amplitude integrated EEG") (1,5,9,26,39,40,66,94). The intention of this chapter is to provide a useful, broad perspective on conventional neonatal EEG examinations so that meaningful interpretations may be made even by those who are not highly experienced in reading newborns' records. Although there are abundant publications of highly detailed descriptions of the subtle nuances of neonatal EEG interpretation (19,56), the focus of this chapter is to provide a pragmatic, orderly approach to visual EEG analysis.

TECHNICAL ASPECTS OF NEONATAL ELECTROENCEPHALOGRAPHIC RECORDING AND INTERPRETATION

The international 10-20 system of electrode placement has been modified for neonatal EEG recording because of infants' small head size and the relative lack of EEG activity in the extreme frontopolar regions (Fig. 6.1). The standard neonatal montage includes electrodes Fp3 (halfway between Fp1 and F3), Fp4 (halfway between Fp2 and F4), C3, C4, T3, T4, 01, 02, Fz, Cz, Pz, A1, and A2 (19). If the earlobes are too small, mastoid leads (M1 and M2) may be substituted. Fp3 and Fp4 electrodes are used because electrographic background activity and frontal physiological sharp waves are better visualized there than at the usual frontopolar locations (Fp1 and Fp2) (88).

A single montage, which includes both anterior-posterior and transverse arrays with coverage across the central vertex (Cz), is acceptable for most neonatal recordings (Fig. 6.2). Recording montages that include vertex

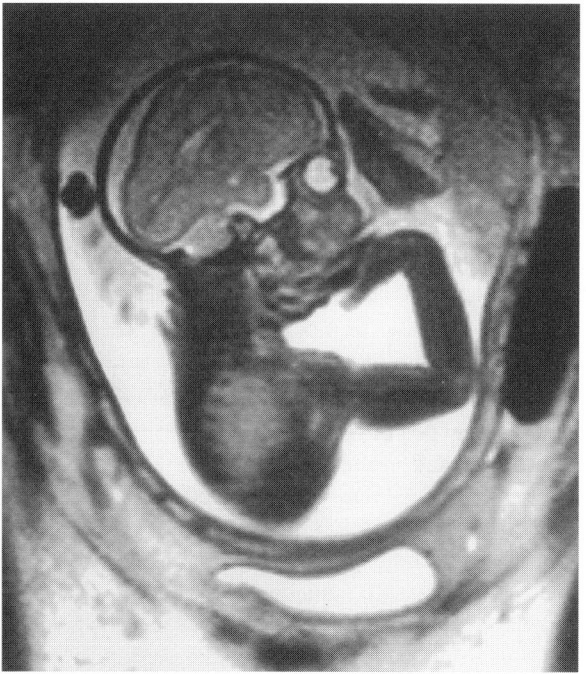

FIG. 6.1. Intrauterine magnetic resonance imaging examination of fetus 30 weeks of estimated gestational age. Notice the relatively simple convolutional markings of the frontal lobes in comparison with the occipital cortices.

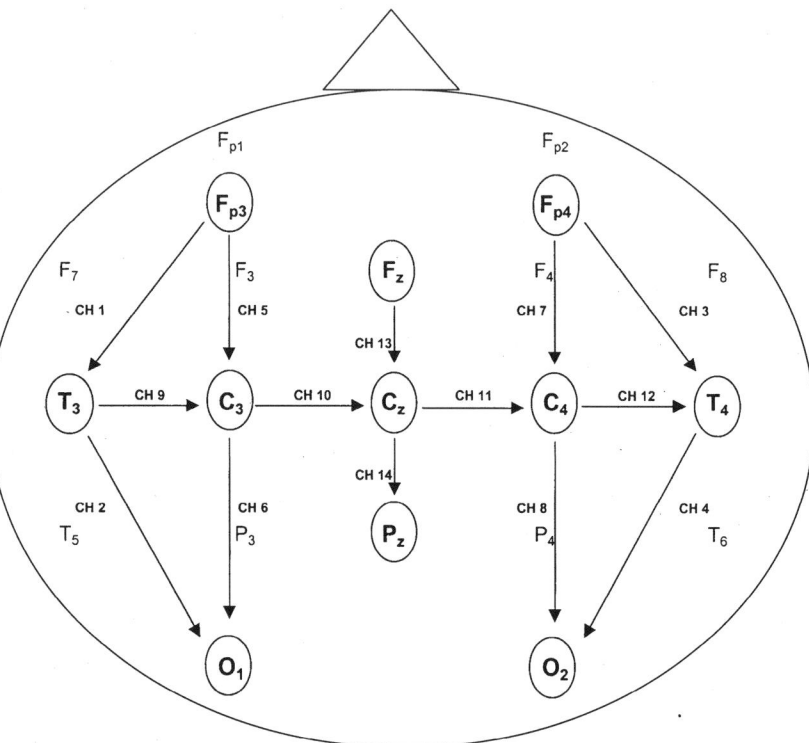

FIG. 6.2. Modification of the international 10-20 system commonly used in neonates. A single montage includes anteroposterior, transverse, and midline arrays. Fp3 and Fp4 replace the usual Fp1 and Fp2 electrode locations.

regions are highly recommended. Some important EEG transients such as positive vertex sharp waves, negative vertex sharp waves, and electrographic patterns of seizures may be confined to those regions and missed if midline electrodes are not included in the recording montage (79). Extra recording electrodes or other montages may be employed to clarify localized abnormalities if necessary. Eighteen EEG channels are typically needed to allow for the standard neonatal montage and noncerebral electrodes. Thus, eight-channel recording machines are inadequate for a comprehensive evaluation of simultaneous EEG and physiological variables such as heart rate and respiration. The presence of scalp intravenous catheters in neonates may disrupt the usual placement of EEG electrodes. The electrode should be placed adjacent to the catheter site, as close as possible to the usual scalp location. The corresponding contralateral electrode should be placed in a symmetrical scalp location.

Noncerebral electrodes provide crucial information about the behavioral state of the infant and assist in the recognition of artifacts. In neonates, at least two channels must be devoted to noncerebral electrodes (2). The following noncerebral electrodes are commonly employed:

1. A respiratory monitor is usually placed on the abdomen or chest to detect respiratory motion. The sensitivity should be adjusted to yield a clearly visible vertical deflection when a low-frequency filter setting of 0.3 to 0.6 Hz is used. These monitors help identify the deep, slow, and regular respiratory pattern of quiet sleep, the more rapid and irregular pattern of wakefulness and active sleep, periodic breathing and apneas.
2. Eye monitors are used so that both vertical and horizontal eye movements (including eye blinks, nystagmus, and rapid eye movements [REMs]) can be identified and distinguished from cerebral electrical activity in the frontal regions. Two electrodes are placed obliquely across either eye: one on the nasion and the other inferior to the outer canthus. The sensitivity setting in the eye channels should be the same as the cerebral electrodes.
3. The electrocardiogram (ECG) monitor detects electrocardiographic activity and assists in identification of movement artifacts. Pulse artifact may be seen over the anterior fontanel in electrodes Fz, Cz, or Pz and can be temporally correlated with the QRS complexes.
4. An optional electromyogram (EMG) electrode may be placed under the chin to monitor submental muscle tone. If recorded, the ECG channel may be omitted because the R wave is usually visible in the submental channel. A sensitivity of 3 mV per millimeter, a low-frequency filter setting of 5 Hz, and a high-frequency filter setting of 70 Hz are often optimal for this channel. Although submental EMG activity per se is unreliable in identifying sleep states in neonates, the channel can be helpful in confirming the extracerebral nature of movement artifacts. In patients being supported with extracorporeal membrane oxygenation (ECMO), the EMG channel can be attached to the ECMO pump to time pump cycles and monitor pump flow artifact. Surface electrodes may also be placed on involved limbs if tremors or clinical seizure manifestations are present.

Paper speed may be set at the standard speed of 30 mm per second or at the "slow paper speed" of 15 mm per second. Recording at 15 mm per second may be advantageous because it *compresses* the recording and facilitates visual recognition of delta activity, the dominant frequency in neonatal EEG. This principle is also used to optimize the recognition of slow activity in tracings of older persons. Slow paper speed also helps to visually assess the degree of discontinuity and interhemispheric synchrony in discontinuous recordings. All EEG samples illustrated in this chapter were recorded at a paper speed of 15 mm per second.

Electrode impedance less than 5 kΩ can be obtained regularly, although higher impedances may be allowed to avoid excessive abrasion of delicate infant skin. Marked differences in impedance between electrodes should be avoided. Sensitivity for cerebral electrodes is initially set at 7 μV per millimeter and adjusted as needed to visualize low-voltage fast activity. Higher sensitivity may also be helpful in patients with apparent low-voltage records from scalp edema. The low-frequency filter is usually set at 0.3 to 1.0 Hz to capture the full complement of delta activity in the neonatal EEG. The high-frequency filter is set at 50 to 70 Hz.

Accurate, abundant clinical data and behavioral notations by the EEG technologist are critical for adequately interpreting the neonatal EEG. Estimated gestational age (EGA), legal age, conceptional age, medical status, medications, mechanical ventilation or ECMO, and other relevant observations should be recorded. During the recording, frequent notations of eye opening and closing are necessary to recognize state changes. Notations regarding head position, scalp edema, small and large body movements, breathing patterns, apnea, hiccups, sucking, and "patting" by caregivers also provide information about the context of the recording session and help to identify artifacts. Clinical descriptions of the presence of unusual behavior such as tonic posturing, sustained eye deviation, nystagmus, clonic jerking, myoclonic activity, apnea, color changes, and vital sign fluctuations allow for clinical correlation with electrographic seizure activity.

At the end of the recording, the technologist should stimulate the infant vigorously and long enough to demonstrate the presence or absence of EEG reactivity. Stimulation is especially important in patients with a depressed mental status; in patients with an invariant, excessively discontinuous EEG; and in those who are therapeutically paralyzed. Auditory and somatosensory stimuli should be applied and notations made regarding behavioral or electrographic changes. Photic stimulation is rarely clinically useful in neonates and is not strongly recommended (2).

The length of a neonatal EEG varies with the clinical situation. Ideally, the full gamut of wakefulness, active sleep, transitional sleep, quiet sleep, and arousal are all recorded (31). Thirty minutes is the minimum duration for a record, but records often extend for 60 minutes or more if there is a strong clinical suspicion for seizures that have not been recorded.

Recording Artifacts

Various extracerebral artifacts complicate the interpretation of neonatal EEGs. Many artifacts can be identified in accordance with the same principles applied to adult EEG interpretation. For example, the simultaneous presence of unusual-appearing activity in extracerebral electrodes (e.g., the ECG or respiratory channel) or an activity of peculiar morphology (e.g., electrode pops) suggest artifact. Genuine electrographic seizures typically evolve in morphology, frequency, and amplitude. Some sustained rhythmic artifacts superficially mimic electrographic seizures (e.g., ECG, pulse, and respiratory artifacts) but do not show the physiological progression of ictal waveforms. In older patients, identifying a plausible "potential field" of an event may help distinguish genuine cerebral activity from some extracerebral activity, but this principle is less helpful in some neonates. Some normal and abnormal EEG transients in neonates have restricted electrical fields. For example, abnormal positive vertex sharp waves may be exquisitely confined to a single electrode without "physiological spread" to neighboring regions.

Muscle artifact may be prominent in the temporal bipolar derivations, but it is typically too fast to be confused with cerebral activity. EMG artifact reduces when the infant calms down or falls asleep. Sucking artifact, a unique form of neonatal muscle activity (Fig. 6.3), typically results in high-amplitude, very sharp potentials in both temporal regions, without spread to adjacent scalp regions. Notations by the technologist should clarify the situation. Hiccups produce movement artifact occasionally with striking regularity in both cerebral and extracerebral electrodes (Fig. 6.4).

Eye movement artifact may be confused with frontal EEG activity, and eye monitor electrodes aid in their recognition. Eye movements generate deflections that are "out of phase" between the eye channels (Fig. 6.5), whereas frontal cerebral activity is "in phase" between the eye channels.

ECG, pulse, ballistocardiographic, and respiratory artifacts are also identified with the aid of extracerebral electrodes. ECG artifact (Fig. 6.6) can dominate the tracing in a low-voltage recording and is especially prominent as a cardiac "dipole" across the temporal regions. The ECG potentials reflected over the scalp surface are coincident with the QRS complexes in the ECG channel. Pulse artifact may occur at any location, but it is often prominent over the anterior fontanel, especially in the Cz electrode. Intermittent pulsations of the fontanel are transmitted to cerebral EEG electrodes, causing rhythmic deflections that may mimic focal rhythmic delta activity or an electrographic seizure. There is a slight but consistent delay between a QRS complex and its coupled pulse artifact. In some infants, cardiac motion causes recoil of the infant's entire body, leading to ballistocardiographic artifact (Fig. 6.7), which may be present in all electrodes or limited to the dependent (e.g., occipital) leads. Respiratory artifact (Fig. 6.8) may also occur at any location. Mechanical ventilation with high-frequency jet ventilators (which generate respiratory rates up to 400 breaths per

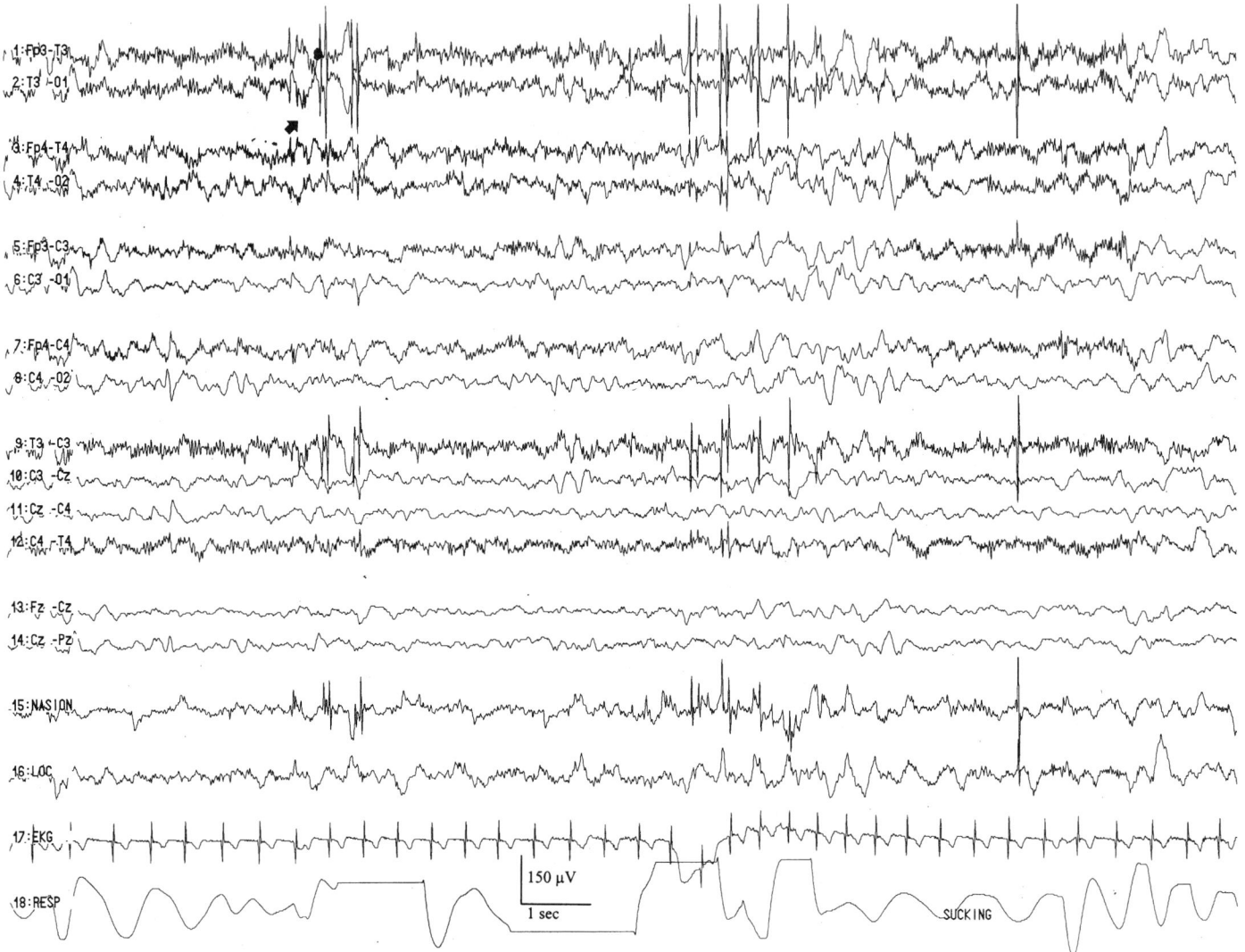

FIG. 6.3. Sucking artifact in an infant 46 weeks of conceptional age with a history of hypoxic ischemic encephalopathy (HIE) and seizures. Sucking artifact (*arrow*) is clearly evident over both temporal regions, the left more than the right.

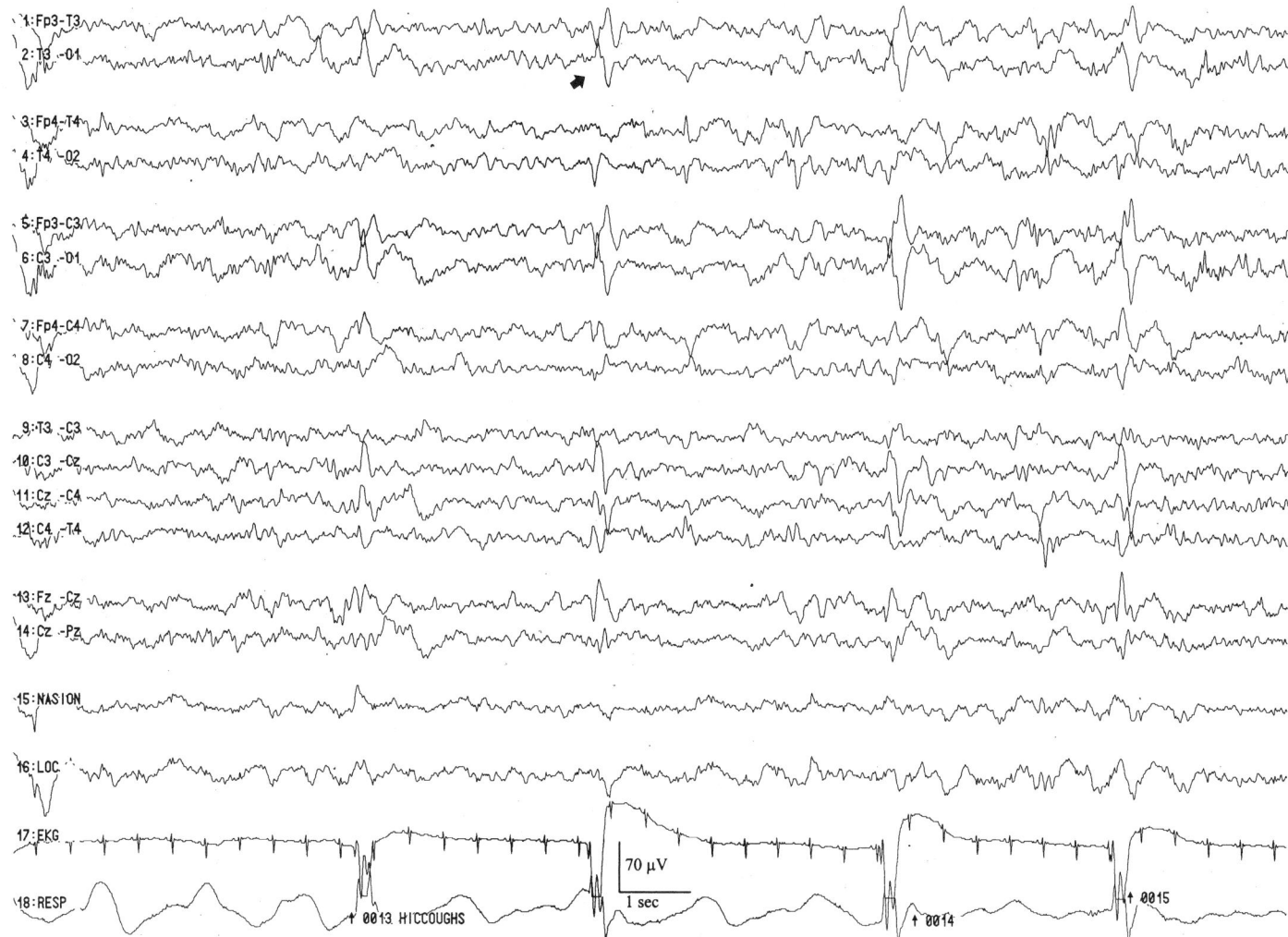

FIG. 6.4. Hiccup artifact in an infant 41 weeks of conceptional age with meningitis. Typical hiccup artifacts (*arrow*) are present, which impart a "periodic" appearance to the record. Note the prominent movement artifact contaminating the electrocardiogram and respiratory channels, which confirms its extracerebral origin.

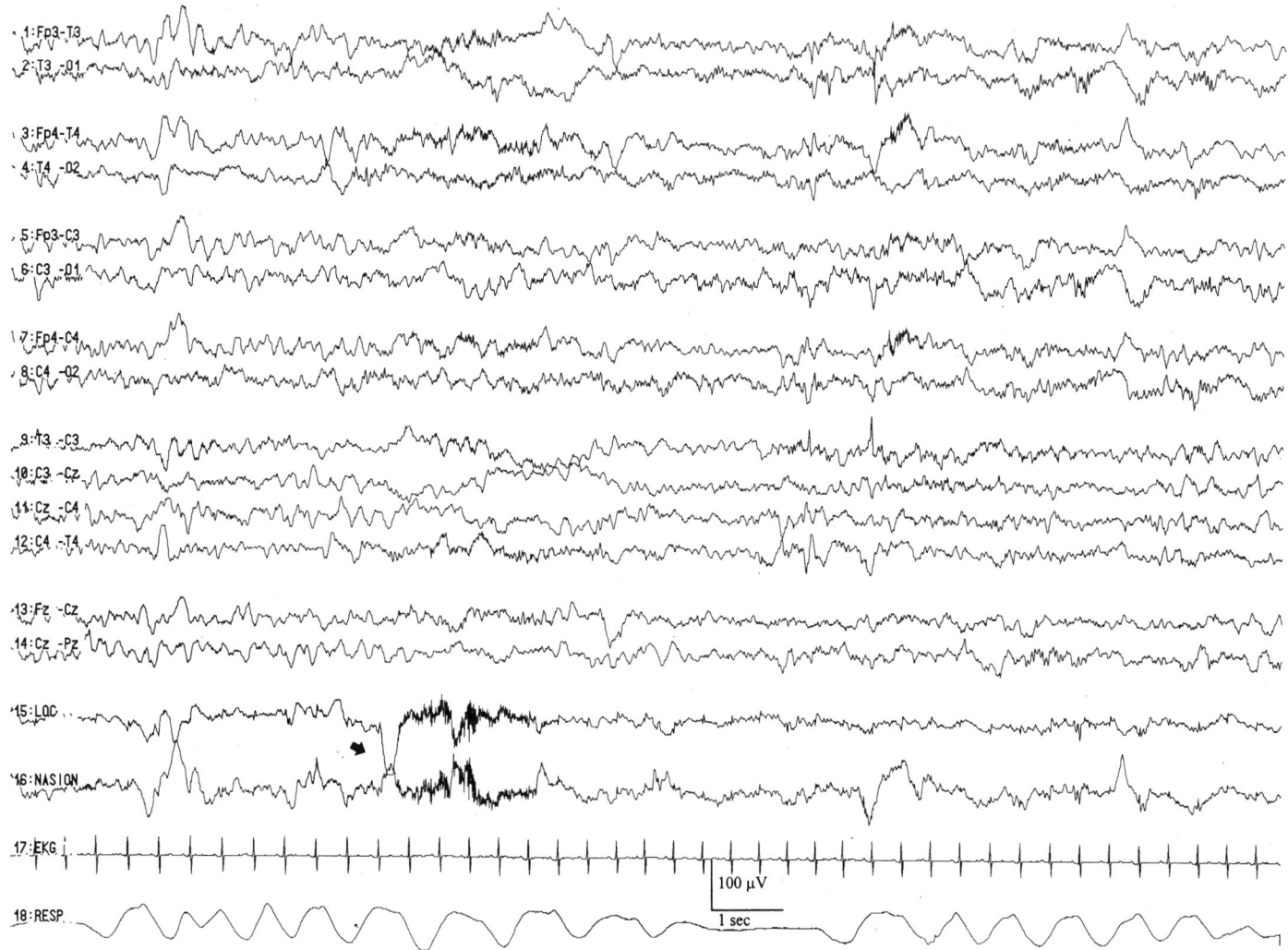

FIG. 6.5. Eye movements in an infant 40 weeks of conceptional age with gastroesophageal reflux. Out-of-phase activity is present in the two eye channels (*arrow*), which confirms extraocular movement activity.

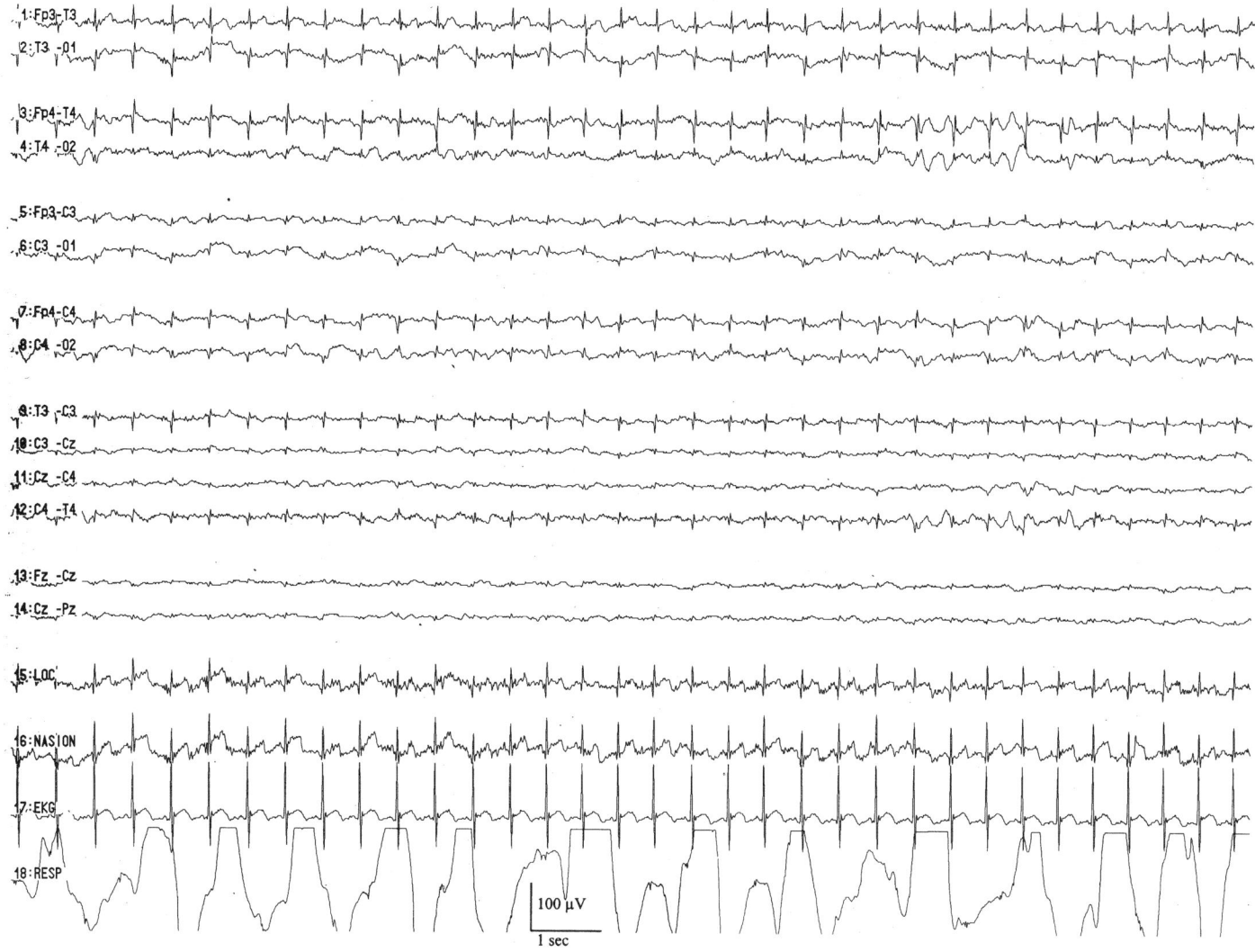

FIG. 6.6. Electrocardiogram (ECG) artifact in an infant 46 weeks of conceptional age with Klippel-Trenaunay-Weber syndrome and seizures. ECG artifact is present throughout the electroencephalographic background. Note the positive T3 and negative T4 dipole of the QRS complex.

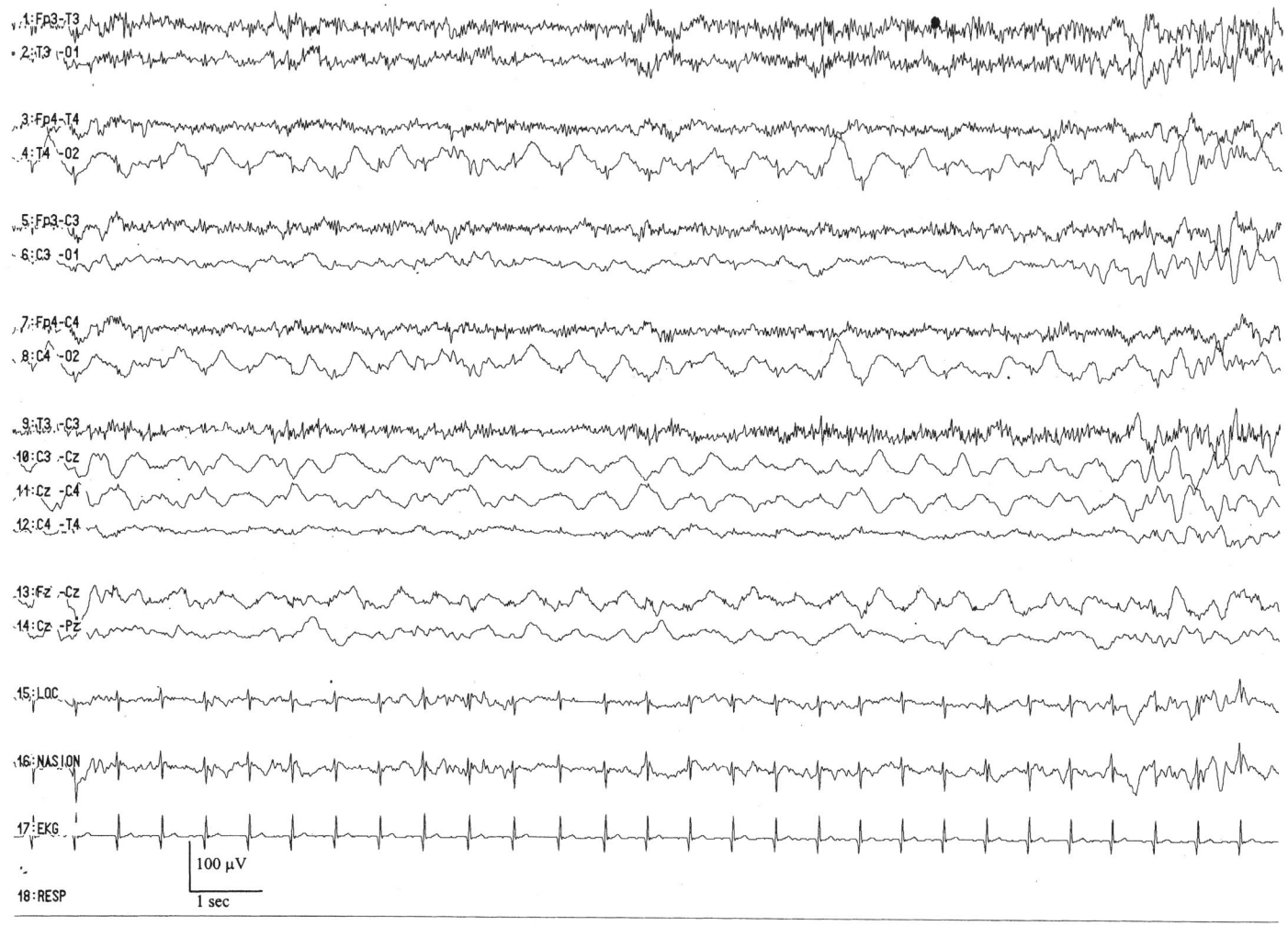

FIG. 6.7. Ballistocardiographic artifact in an infant 44 weeks of conceptional age with left ventricular hypertrophy. The head was turned to the right. Cardiac recoil motion resulted in rhythmic movement artifact at O2 and Cz.

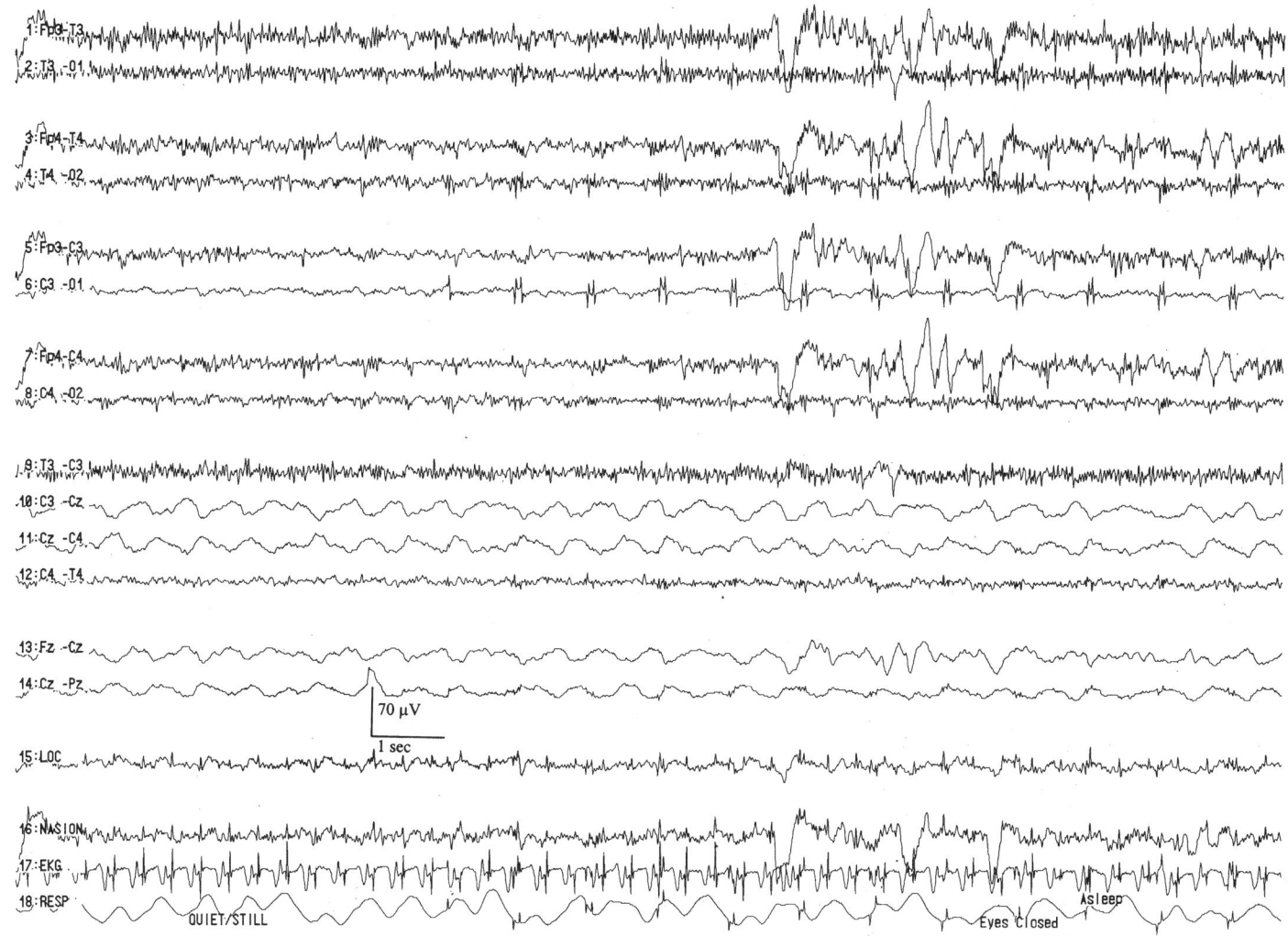

FIG. 6.8. Respiratory artifact in an infant 41 weeks of conceptional age with head trauma. Rhythmic activity at Cz correlated with respirations.

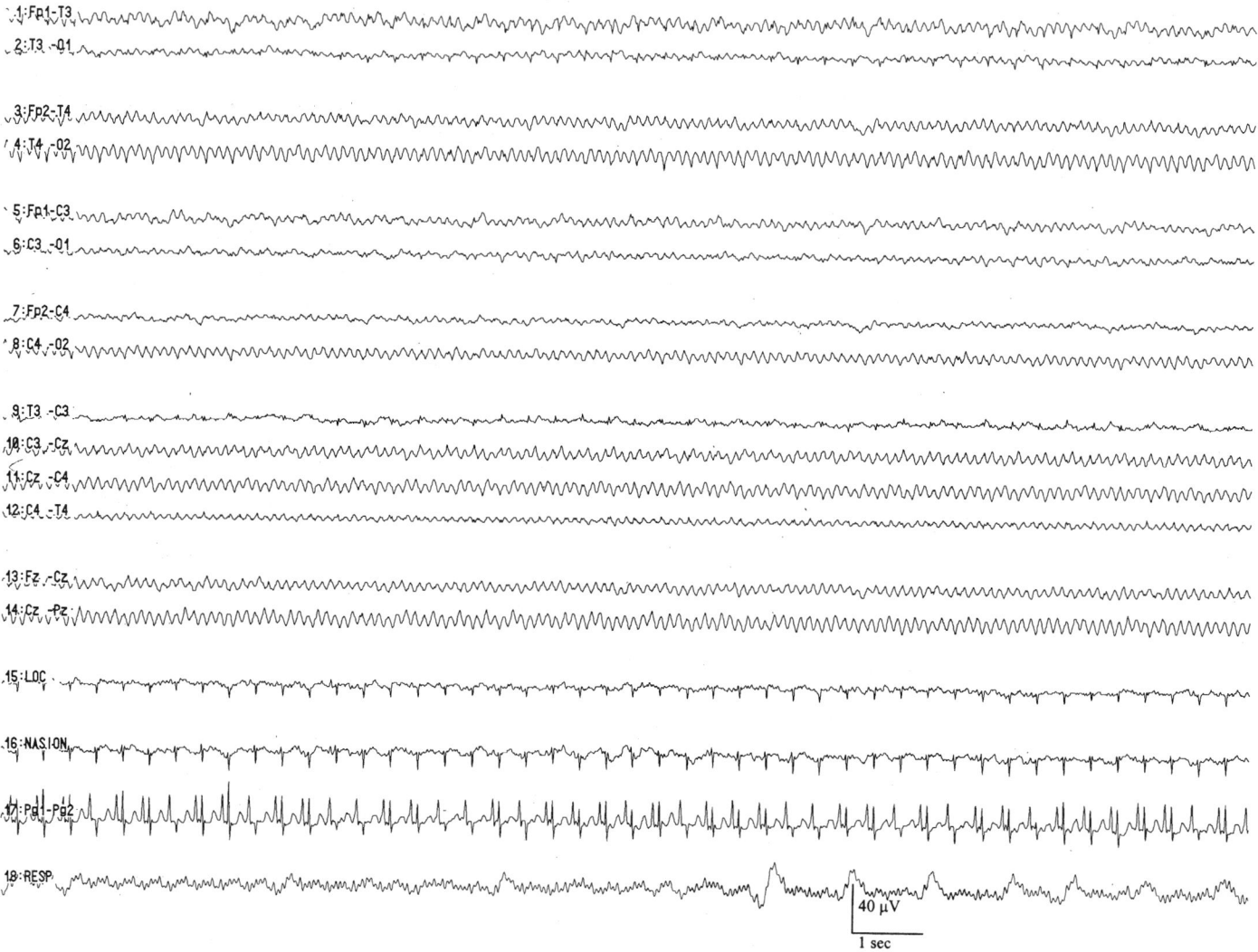

FIG. 6.9. High-frequency ventilator artifact in an infant 40 weeks of conceptional age with persistent pulmonary hypertension. Invariant, rhythmic, sinusoidal artifact from the ventilator is widely reflected throughout the tracing.

minute) and oscillating ventilators cause the infant's entire body to vibrate, which results in focal or diffuse rhythmic artifact (Fig. 6.9). Correlation of the rhythmic EEG activity with the respiratory monitor allows for identification. ECMO pump artifact is usually conspicuously constant and invariant throughout the record.

"Patting the baby" artifact may mimic electrographic seizure activity (Fig. 6.10), and the technologist's notations are critical for correct interpretation. Crescendo clonic limb movements in a jittery baby (Fig. 6.11) may generate rhythmic movement artifact that is transmitted to cerebral electrodes, causing deflections that sometimes mimic focal electrographic

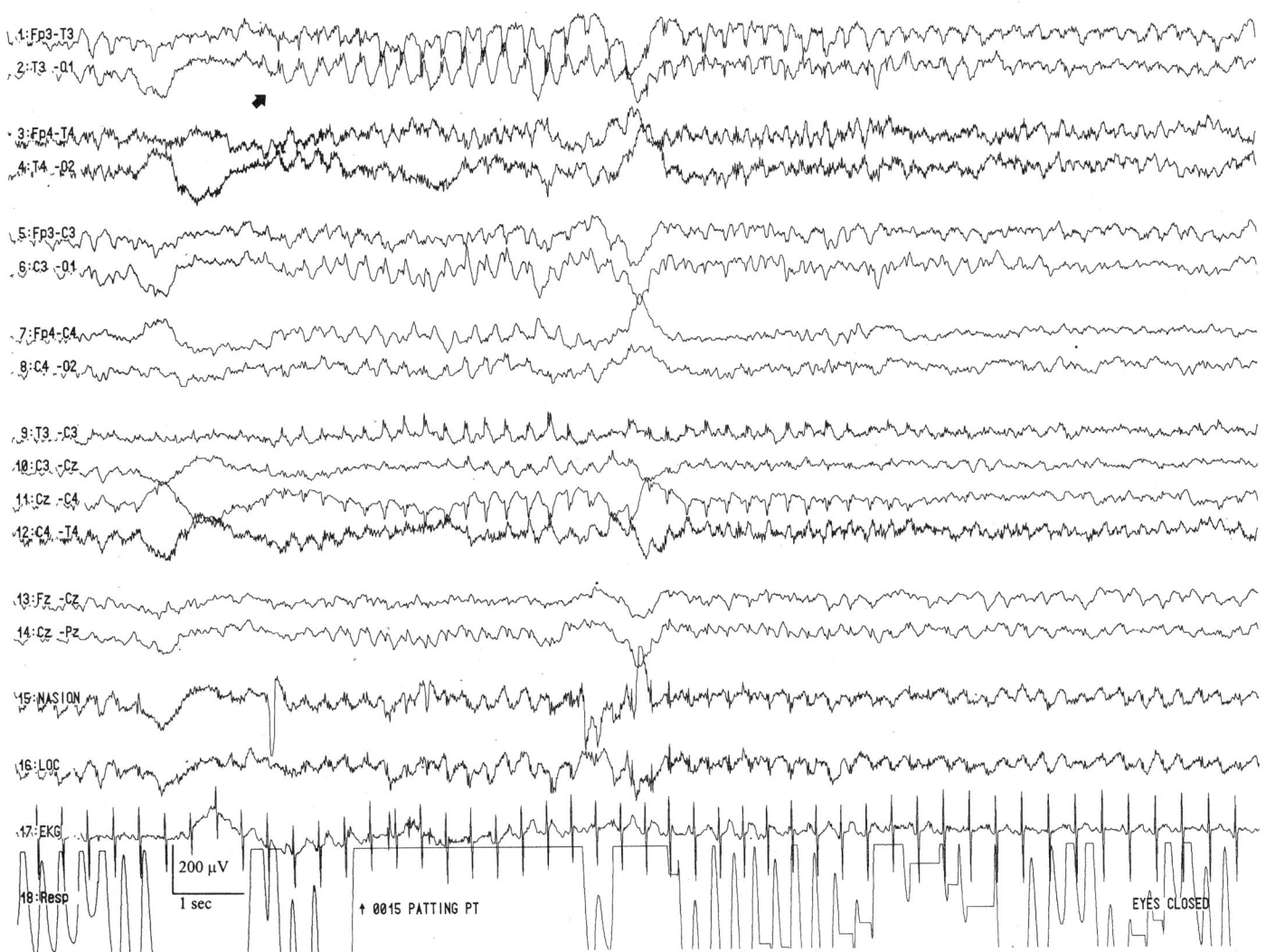

FIG. 6.10. Patting artifact in an infant 44 weeks of conceptional age with sepsis, apnea, and seizures. Patting artifact (*arrow*) can mimic an electrographic seizure.

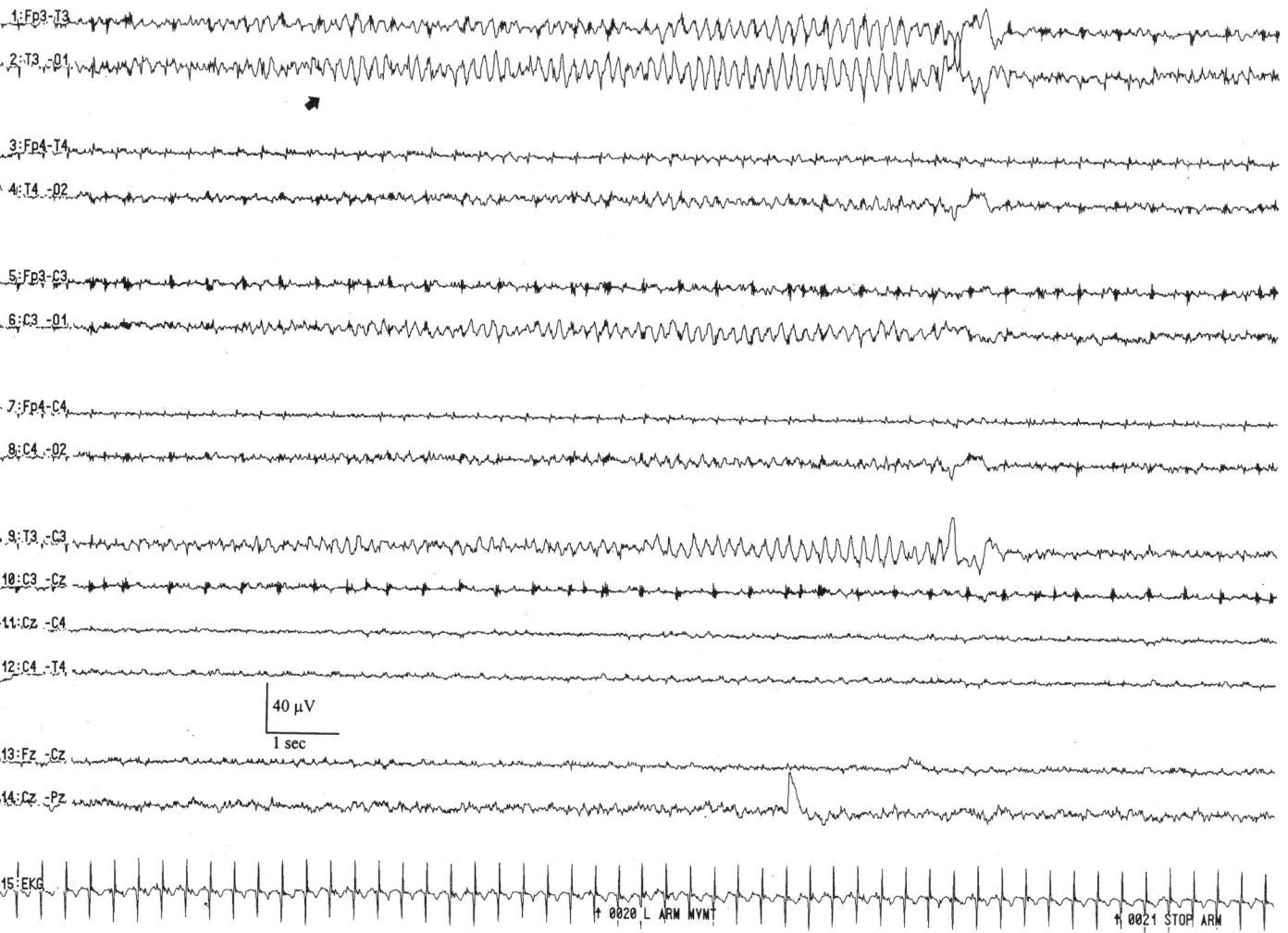

FIG. 6.11. Clonic limb movement artifact in an infant 47 weeks of conceptional age who had recently suffered cardiac arrest. Clonic movement of the left arm mimicked an electrographic seizure (*arrow*). When the technologist restrained the left arm, the artifactual "seizure" ceased.

seizure activity. In most cases, the frequency of the movement is relatively invariant, and the EEG does not show the typical frequency evolution of seizure activity. If the technologist briefly restrains the shaking extremity, the movement artifact "seizure" subsides, allowing for interpretation of background cerebral activity.

Single electrode "pops" (Fig. 6.12) may be confused with pathological positive sharp waves, but the initial deflection is nearly vertical—similar to the discharge of a charged capacitor and too rapid to be of cerebral origin.

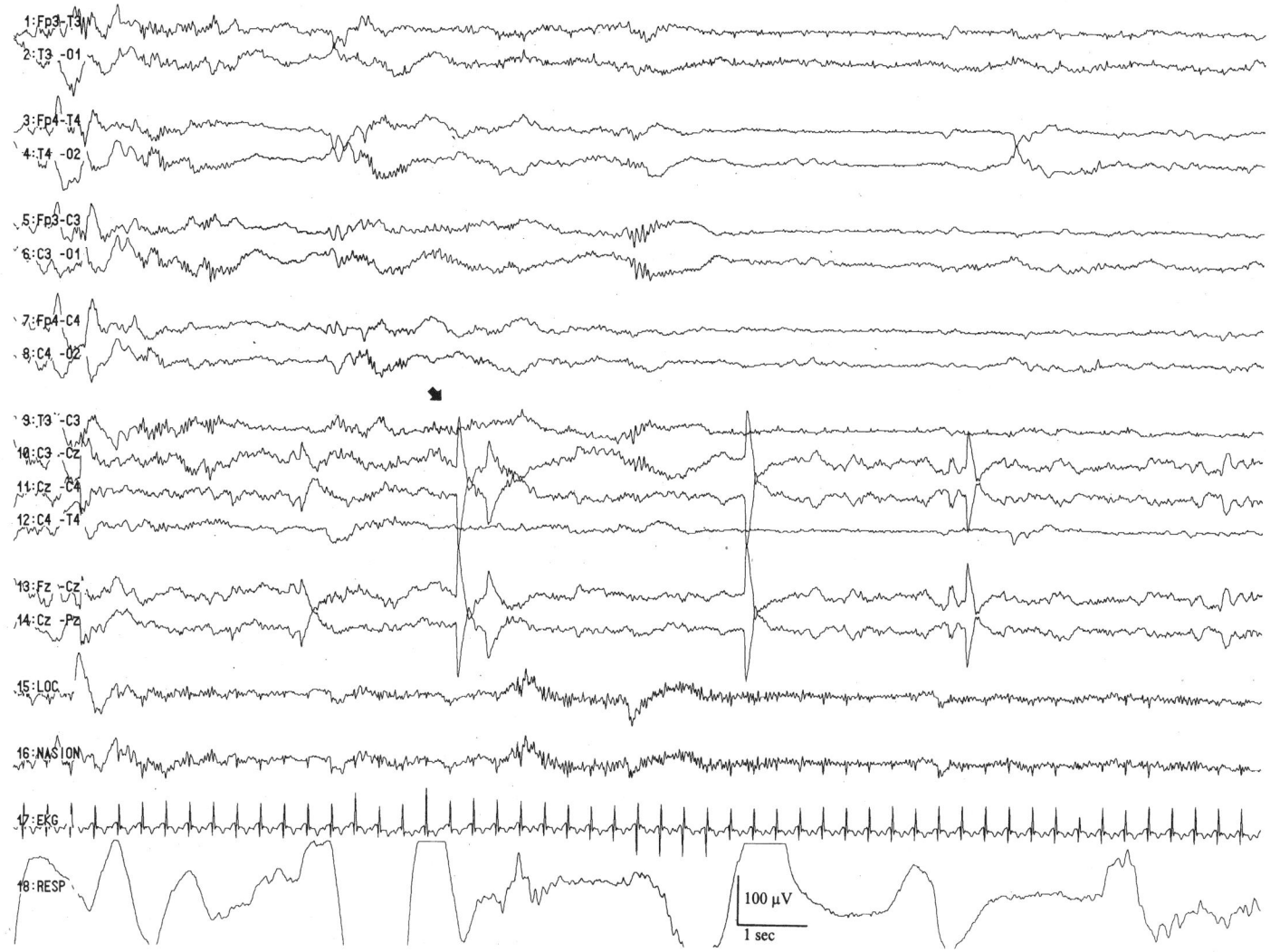

FIG. 6.12. Electrode artifacts-in an infant 34 weeks of conceptional age with complex congenital heart disease. Electrode pops (*arrow*) can be confused with genuine positive sharp waves. Note that the initial deflection is nearly vertical—too rapid to be of cerebral origin.

VISUAL ANALYSIS OF THE NORMAL NEONATAL ELECTROENCEPHALOGRAPHIC BACKGROUND

Conceptional Age, State, and Medical Status

Conceptional Age

It is necessary to know several relevant definitions of *age* in order to properly understand and interpret the neonatal EEG. The estimated gestational age (EGA) is the age of the fetus since conception. This is typically determined by calculation of the length of the gestation from the time of the mother's last menstrual period (LMP) to the day of the infant's birth. If the LMP is unknown or the mother's menses are irregular, gestational age can be estimated by fetal ultrasound examinations early in the pregnancy or by the Ballard examination of physical maturity (6,13), performed shortly after birth. Newborns are considered premature if born before the 37th week of the gestation. Full-term infants are born between the 37th and 42nd weeks of gestation, and post-term infants are born after 42 weeks of gestation.

An infant's legal age is simply the age since birth. For example, if an infant was born 2 weeks ago, the legal age is 2 weeks. Age since conception (conceptional age) is determined by adding the legal age and EGA. Thus, both a 1-week-old (legal age) infant born at 39 weeks of EGA and a 13-week-old (legal age) infant born prematurely at 27 weeks of EGA have a conceptional age of 40 weeks. Conceptional age is the key observation when interpreting the neonatal EEG. EEG maturity is principally determined by the conceptional age, because neurological development is thought to proceed at the same rate during intrauterine and extrauterine life. On occasion, careful assessment of the EEG background can be used to estimate the conceptional age within ±2 weeks if there is no information from other sources about EGA or legal age (43).

State

In the newborn infant, biobehavioral state is simply determined by the operational definitions of *wakefulness* and *sleep*. In sleep, the eyes are closed, and in wakefulness, the eyes are open. This operational definition of state is not applicable to the extremely premature infant born before the eyelids are unfused (which typically occurs at approximately 23 to 24 weeks of EGA). In children and adults, state can be further characterized by a constellation of behavioral and physiological variables that determine the presence of full alertness, drowsiness, active or rapid-eye-movement (REM) sleep, and light to deep quiet (non-REM) sleep. In healthy older infants, there is a predictable and well-defined agreement (*concordance*) in various sleep states between behavioral and physiological observations (e.g., phasic movements of the limbs during REM sleep) accompanied by a specific appearance of the EEG. However, this concordance between the clinical and electrographic expressions of state is not well developed in very premature infants; it evolves in a predictable manner as term approaches.

In a well-developed infant in active sleep, the infant's eyes are closed. There are a variety of small and large body movements, sucking, and even crying behaviors that are punctuated by bursts of predominantly horizontal rapid eye movements—the REM phase of active sleep. Brief apneas are relatively common, especially before term. During active sleep, the EEG background resembles the low-voltage, continuous EEG of quiet wakefulness. Newborn infants often enter into active sleep from wakefulness, thus mimicking the sleep patterns of "narcoleptic" older persons. This pattern of sleep onset continues until about 4 months post-term, at which time quiet sleep precedes active sleep.

In a well-developed infant in quiet sleep, the eyes are closed and there are few head, trunk, or limb movements. Respirations are exquisitely regular, deeper, and slower. Apnea is uncommon. Occasional startles or arousals may briefly interrupt quiet sleep, but usually the infant settles back down quickly unless the arousal was sufficient to provoke a change longer than a minute and a transition to wakefulness or active sleep. Quiet sleep is the state in which the infant's EEG is most vulnerable to adverse medical or neurological conditions. In sick newborns, the amount of time spent in well-defined quiet sleep diminishes at the cost of increasing the percentage of time in indeterminate sleep. In EEG recording, it is essential to try to capture quiet sleep because it may be the only sleep state in which some EEG abnormalities may be detected. In infants with some mild encephalopathies, the awake and active sleep recording may appear normal, but quiet sleep recordings reveal previously unrecognized abnormalities.

Even in healthy newborns, much of sleep is *indeterminate* or *transitional:* That is, even with a good-quality EEG and careful behavioral observation, it is not possible to determine precisely whether the child is in active or quiet sleep. This is clearly the case when the infant transits from one behavioral state to another (transitional sleep), but it also applies when an exact designation of active or quiet sleep cannot be assigned. A large proportion of total sleep time is indeterminate at term and increases in the setting of medical or neurological illness (Fig. 6.13) (98).

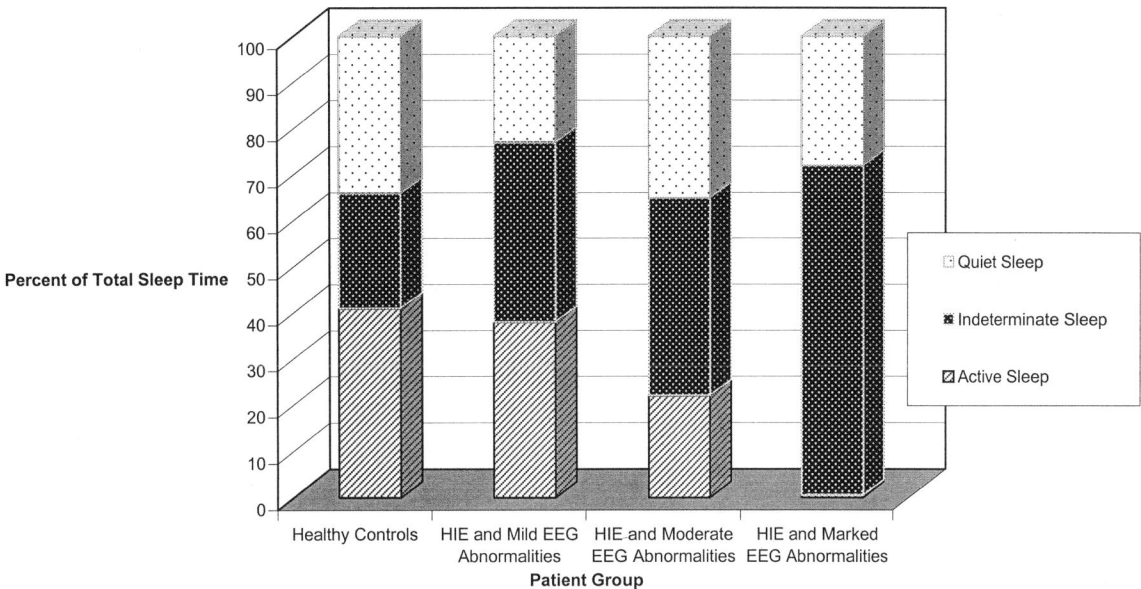

FIG. 6.13. The percentage of total sleep time occupied by indeterminate sleep is significantly increased in sick newborns with abnormal electroencephalographic backgrounds. (Adapted from Watanabe K, Miyazaki S, Hara K, et al. Behavioral state cycles, background EEGs and prognosis of newborns with perinatal hypoxia. *Electroencephalogr Clin Neurophysiol* 1980;49:618–625.)

Medical Status

Knowledge of the overall medical/neurological status of the newborn is also vital for properly interpreting the results of the EEG examination. Medically sick infants are exposed to a wide variety of conditions such as shock, respiratory failure, sepsis, and metabolic disturbances. Just as nonspecific EEG background abnormalities may be recorded in medically ill older persons, mild to moderate degrees of abnormalities may be observed in sick neonates. Often, these are reflections of the presence of medical disease and do not necessarily imply the existence of fixed, permanent brain dysfunction or damage. Likewise, the administration of medications intended to reduce pain (e.g., fentanyl, morphine), agitation (e.g., diazepam, lorazepam), or seizures (e.g., phenobarbital) may introduce unknown, hard-to-quantify effects into the EEG. Some newborns with critical cardiorespiratory conditions are given neuromuscular blocking agents (e.g., pancuronium, vecuronium) to achieve therapeutic paralysis. This obscures the clinical assessment of biobehavioral state and creates an additional challenge to the EEG interpretation. Critically ill neonates may undergo ECMO to prevent cardiocir-culatory collapse. These infants are often given both neuromuscular paralyzing drugs and long-term inhalation anesthetics (e.g., isoflurane). "Third-spacing" of fluid accumulates within a few days, and significant scalp edema develops. Because the right carotid artery is preferred for ECMO cannulation, the infant's head position is maintained to face to the left; therefore, the scalp edema is asymmetrical, greater on the dependent left side. It can be a considerable challenge to interpret the EEGs of such patients.

Timing of Electroencephalographic Examinations

The timing of EEG examinations may have a substantial impact on their meaningful interpretation. It is generally inadequate to simply record a single study near the end of the patient's hospital course. Substantial "nonspecific" normalization may occur after the peak of an illness (the time when the EEG is likely to reveal its maximal degree of abnormality, which is important in formulating a prognosis), and the EEG may show substantial improvement in parallel with early clinical signs of neurological recovery

(92,93) (Fig. 6.14). Because EEGs are most commonly obtained in an acute medical or neurological crises, it is critical that one or more studies be obtained when the infant is likely to display the most revealing prognostic information. If, when the infant is sickest, the worst EEG is still relatively well preserved and normal, it is reasonable to conclude that the illness has not severely affected CNS function. On the other hand, if, at the height of the illness, the EEG background demonstrates severe disturbances, it is reasonable to conclude that brain function has been adversely affected, and the prognosis is substantially worse. A note of caution, however, is in order: EEGs obtained in the *immediate* wake of a brief acute event (cardiac arrest, seizure, drug administration) may be misleading. The record may initially appear very abnormal but quickly show substantial improvement in just a few hours. It is desirable to repeat the examination the next day to determine whether the severe abnormalities are lasting or have resolved.

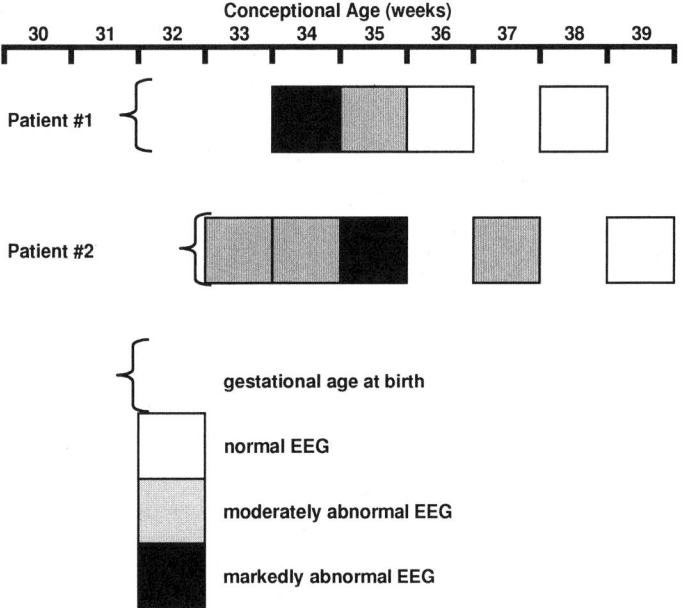

FIG. 6.14. Substantial, nonspecific normalization of the electroencephalographic (EEG) background may occur over time. Neurological prognosis is based on the most abnormal of serial EEG examinations. (Adapted from Tharp B, Scher M, Clancy R. Serial EEGs in normal and abnormal infants with birth weights less than 1200 grams—a prospective study with long term follow-up. *Neuropediatrics* 1989;20:64–72.)

The other consideration about EEG timing pertains to serial EEG examinations in premature infants. The sequential changes in EEG background during brain maturation should progress at the same rate whether the child is inside or outside the uterus. Thus, in the infants of very low birth weight, it would be reassuring to demonstrate that the tracings sequentially mature at the proper tempo from preterm birth until the conceptional age approaches full term. This is especially true in preterm infants with chronic lung disease (bronchopulmonary dysplasia), in whom clinical and electrographic maturity may be delayed (36,37,42,55,57,70,80,90–92).

General Properties of the Electroencephalographic Background

Continuity

The earliest vestiges of EEG activity are believed to arise after the eighth week of gestation. The EEG tracing appears as a completely discontinuous recording in which brief periods of electric activity ("bursts") are interrupted by periods of quiescence ("interburst" intervals). As such, the overall signal is a series of EEG bursts separated by flat or low-voltage interburst intervals (IBIs). With the development of CNS maturity and the increased influence of the deep grey structures that modulate cortical function, the duration of the burst (burst interval [BI]) increases, whereas the length of the IBI decreases.

EEG signals that regularly vary between the high-amplitude "on" periods of the bursts and low-amplitude "off" periods of the IBI are called *discontinuous* EEGs. Those that display a relatively steady amplitude are considered *continuous*.

The duration of the IBIs is a semiquantitative measurement of one aspect of the neonatal EEG. A typical, representative portion of the discontinuous portion of the EEG is selected for review, and the duration of the IBIs is measured and counted over a specific period of time: for example, a 10-minute sample. In that representative portion of time, numerous measurements of the IBI are made and the mean, median, and longest IBI values can be measured. The prime determinant of measures of the IBI is the infant's conceptional age. A typical median IBI at the conceptional age of 24 weeks is 10 seconds; this gradually decreases at older conceptional ages to values around 2 to 4 seconds (Fig. 6.15) (10,22,29,31,33,35,42,44,57,88,93).

In a study of mortality in premature infants, those whose IBIs decreased with advancing conceptional age had a much higher chance of survival than those whose IBIs remained constant or increased with conceptional

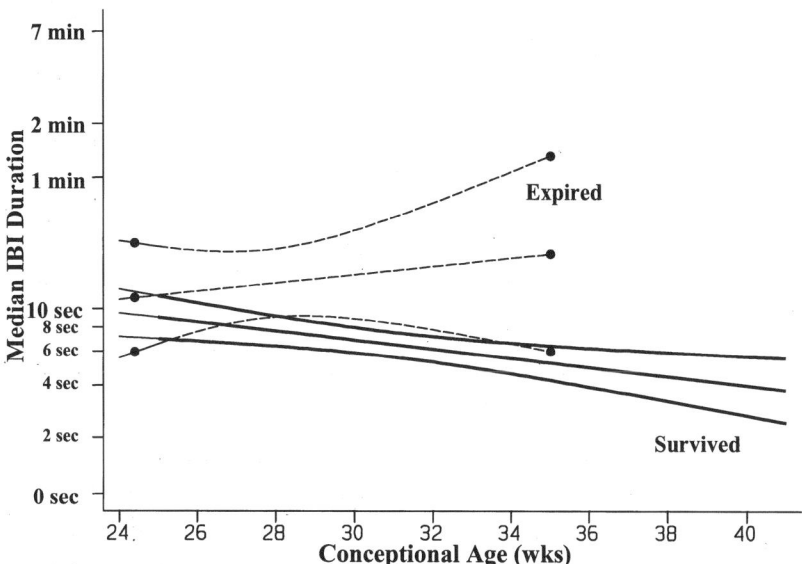

FIG. 6.15. Median interburst interval (IBI) duration decreases with advancing conceptional age in survivors of prematurity. The premature infants who died are characterized by IBIs that are significantly longer in duration than the IBIs of survivors. (Adapted from Clancy R, Rosenberg H, Bernbaum J, et al. Survival outcome prediction in premature infants with IVH by cranial ultrasonography and EEG. *Ann Neurol* 1994;36:489.)

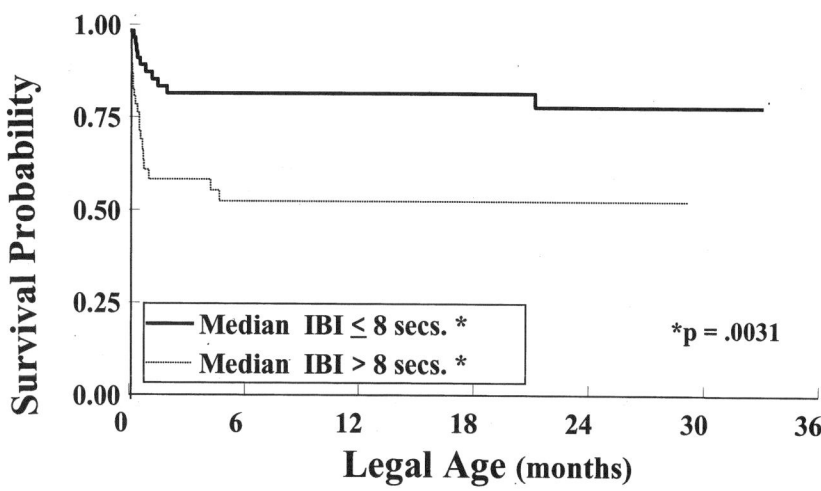

FIG. 6.16. Kaplan-Meier survival curve shows that premature infants with median interburst intervals (IBIs) of 8 seconds or less had a significantly higher incidence of survival than did those with longer duration IBIs. (Adapted from Clancy R, Rosenberg H, Bernbaum J, et al. Survival outcome prediction in premature infants with IVH by cranial ultrasonography and EEG. *Ann Neurol* 1994;36:489.)

age. In general, infants at a conceptional age of 30 weeks and older with median IBIs of 8 seconds or less had a significantly higher incidence of survival than those with longer median IBIs (22) (Fig. 6.16). In an individual infant, IBI can be affected by transient influences such as noxious stimulation, arousals, hypoxia, drug administration (e.g., lorazepam), and seizure. The duration of the IBIs may correlate with measures of medical illness. Prolonged IBIs have been associated with elevated serum ammonia levels in citrullinemia (18) (Fig. 6.17) and with transient hypoxia in respiratory distress syndrome (30,89) (Fig. 6.18). Measurement of the IBIs in a brief sample of EEG is thus a simple approach for quantifying one aspect of neonatal EEG.

Earlier investigators reported a wide range of possible IBI values for premature infants. However, because IBI are dependent not just on conceptional age but also on medical status (e.g., degree of hypoxia and hypercarbia in respiratory distress syndrome), interpretation of IBI data from older

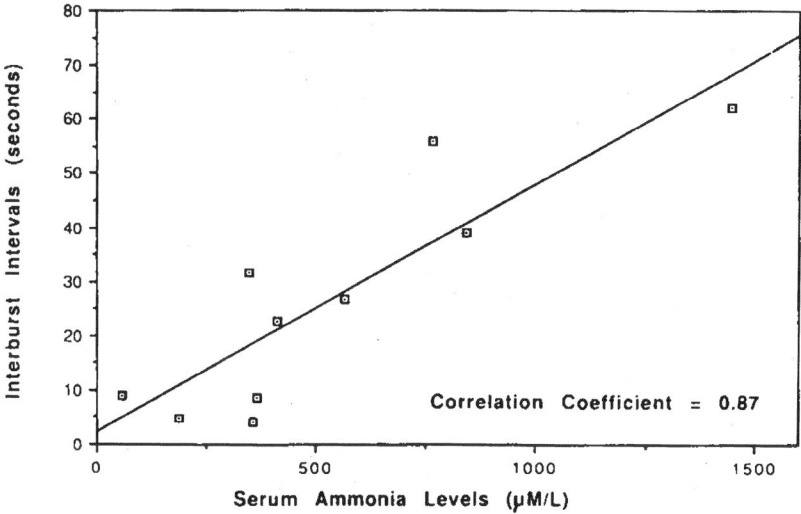

FIG. 6.17. There is a significant linear relationship between the serum ammonia levels and the interburst interval in this group of three neonates with citrullinemia. (Adapted from Clancy R, Chung H. EEG changes during recovery from acute severe neonatal citrullinemia. *Electroencephalogr Clin Neurophysiol* 1991;78:222–227.)

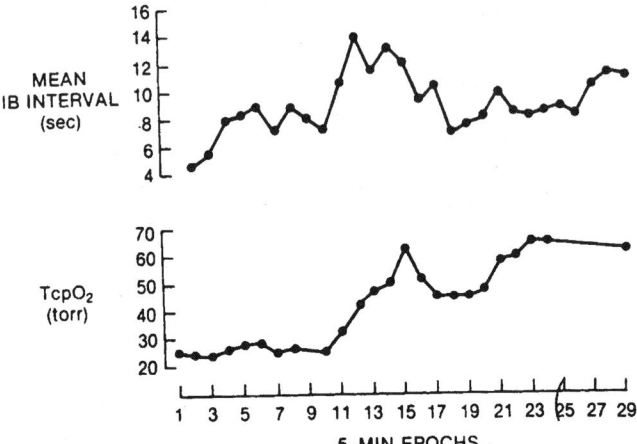

FIG. 6.18. The relationship between oxygenation and the mean interburst interval in a premature infant with hypoxic-ischemic encephalopathy and pulmonary hypertension. (Adapted from Tharp B. Intensive video/EEG monitoring of neonates. In: Gumnit R, ed. *Advances in neurology, vol. 46: Intensive neurodiagnostic monitoring.* New York: Raven Press, 1986:114.)

studies should be tempered by the knowledge that their measurements also reflected the medical conditions of their patients at that time. For example, Lombroso (55) reported that IBIs of up to 2 minutes can be "normal". Perhaps this should now be interpreted to mean that some infants with IBIs of this duration may be fortunate to survive with a good outcome, but an IBI of 2 minutes is no longer considered normal in current practice. Advances in high-risk neonatal care progress rapidly, and normative values will require renormalization as innovations such as artificial surfactant, high-frequency jet ventilation, ECMO, and nitric oxide administration are made more widely available.

Symmetry

Normal EEG activity arising between the two hemispheres or homologous brain regions should be essentially symmetrical. There are two facets of background symmetry to be judged: *amplitude* and *waveform composition* (Figs. 6.19 and 6.20). Amplitude symmetry implies that, in a suitably large sample of cerebral electrical activity, the background voltages between the hemispheres or specific regions are approximately equal. There is no

universal agreement as to what amount of amplitude asymmetry constitutes an electrographic abnormality. A useful interpretation guideline is that an abnormality may be suspected if the amplitude difference between two regions exceeds a 2:1 ratio (3,55–57).

Interhemispheric Synchrony

Synchrony and asynchrony also reflect CNS maturation in the developing neonate. Interhemispheric synchrony and asynchrony are *temporal* electrographic features that can be measured during the discontinuous portions of the EEG. *Asynchrony* is defined as bursts of morphological similar of EEG activity in homologous head regions separated by more than 1.5 to 2.0 seconds in time (Fig. 6.21). Somewhat paradoxically, infants at a conceptional age of less than 30 weeks exhibit hypersynchrony, whereby the majority of bursts arising within the two hemispheres appear at the same time (Fig. 6.22). The physiological basis for interhemispheric hypersynchrony is unknown. After the conceptional age of 30 weeks, hypersynchrony gives way to the appearance of asynchronous bursts of cerebral electrical activity between the two hemispheres. About 70% of bursts during quiet sleep are synchronized at the conceptional age of 31 to 32 weeks, increasing to 80% at 33 to 34 weeks, 85% between 35 and 36 weeks, and 100% after 37 weeks (55,57,88,90).

Overview of Electroencephalographic Ontogeny

The development of the fetal brain undergoes explosive changes with regard to its overall anatomic appearance, synaptic connectivity, time-dependent genetic expression of neurotransmitter receptor subunits, and their consequent functional abilities. In parallel with these anatomical and functional changes is an orderly, predictable pattern of neonatal EEG characteristics that emerge simultaneously with advancing maturity of the fetal brain (Fig. 6.23). For practical reasons, the discussion of EEG ontogeny begins with the infant at 24 weeks EGA, near the current boundary of fetal viability (33).

24 to 29 Weeks of Conceptional Age

EEGs obtained from the very premature infant are, for the most part, discontinuous recordings. The normal record consists of brief periods of moderate-amplitude cerebral electrical activity (composed of recognizable,

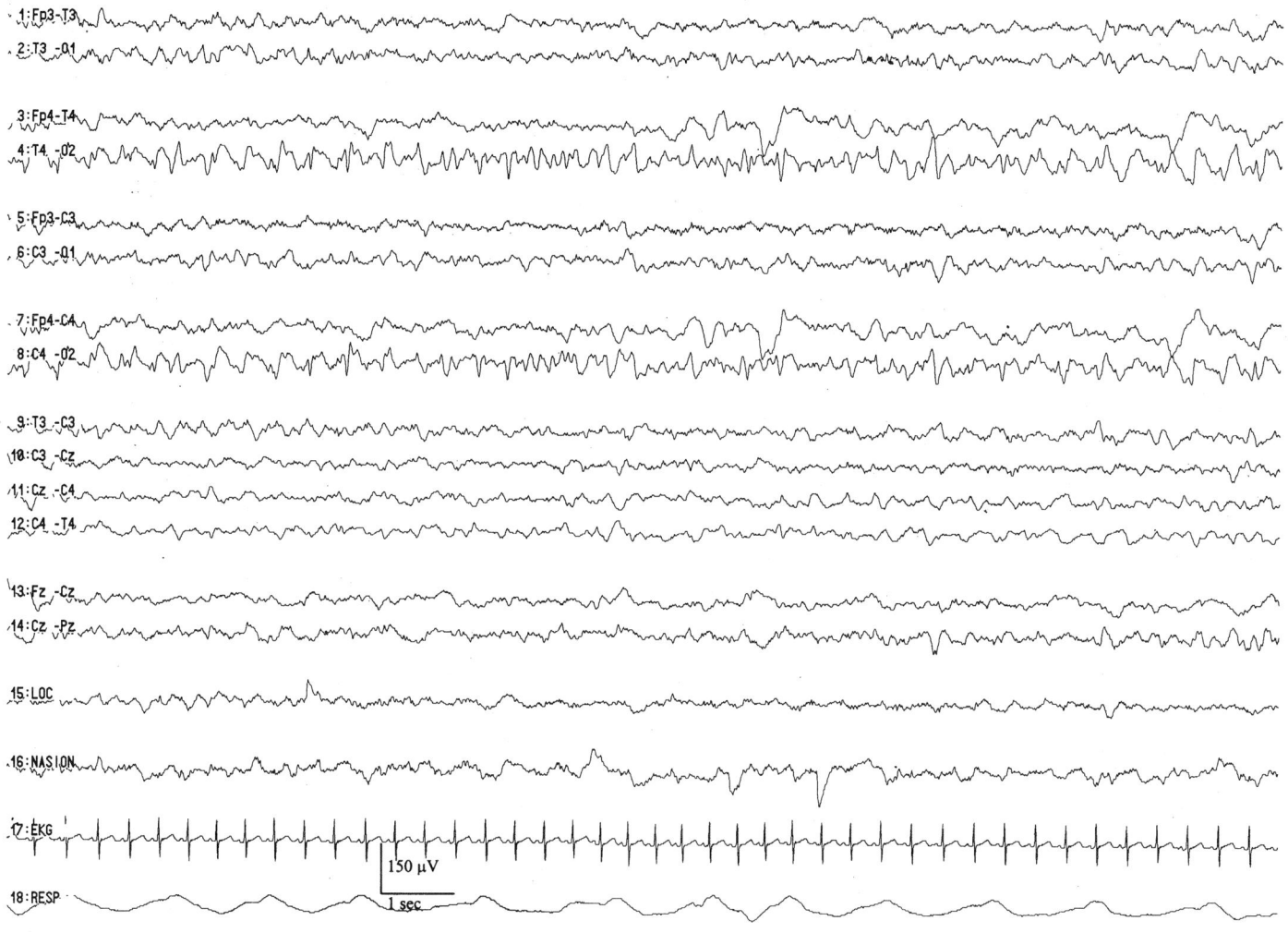

FIG. 6.19. Asymmetry secondary to cerebral pathology in an infant 41 weeks of conceptional age with Sturge-Weber syndrome affecting the right hemisphere. The right occipital region is slow and contains sharp waves, in comparison with the normal-appearing left hemisphere.

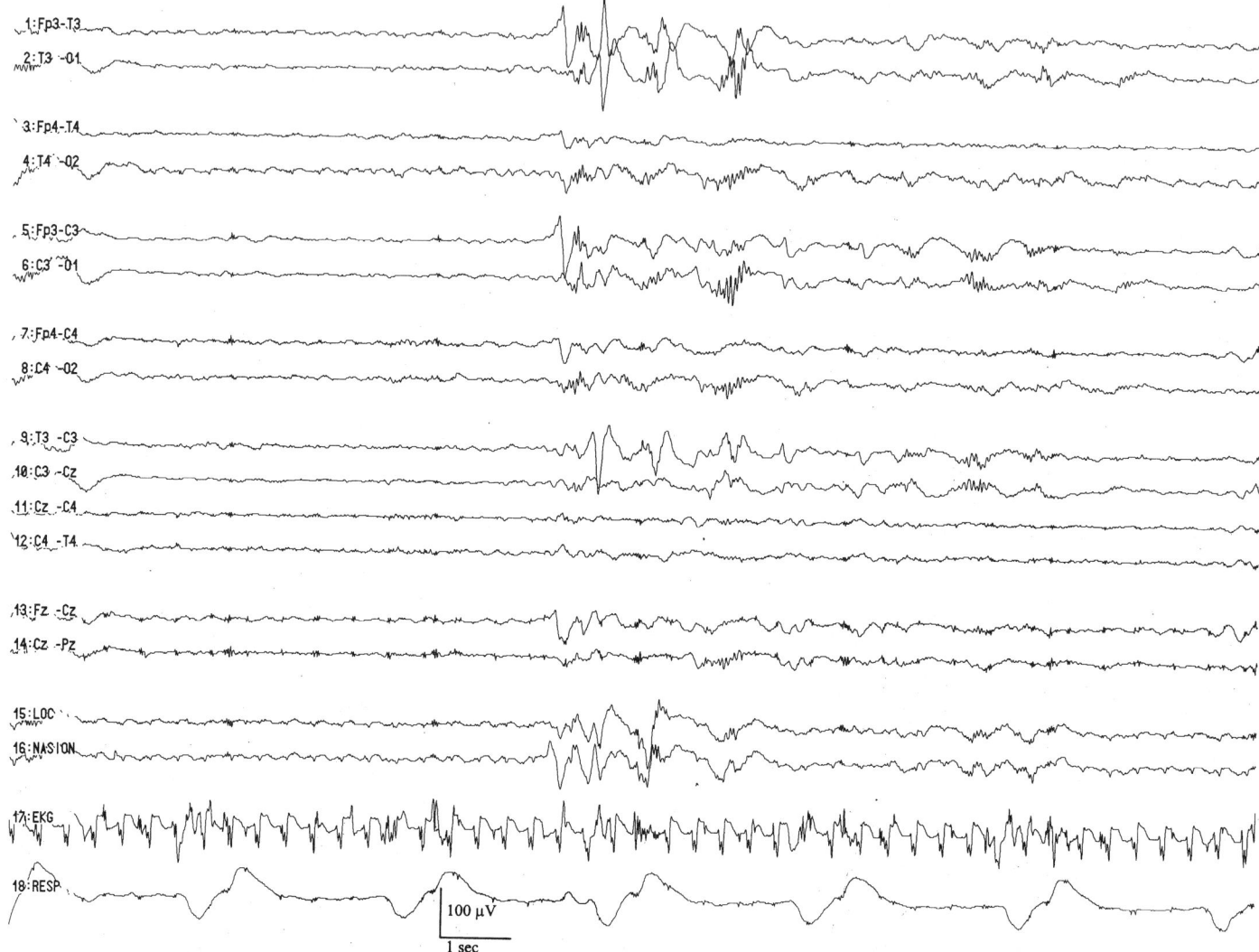

FIG. 6.20. Asymmetry secondary to scalp edema in an infant 41 weeks of conceptional age with tetralogy of Fallot and seizures. The infant's head was turned to the right, and marked right scalp edema was present. The amplitude is decreased on the right side, but the background composition is similar to the that of the left. The asymmetry disappeared after the scalp edema resolved.

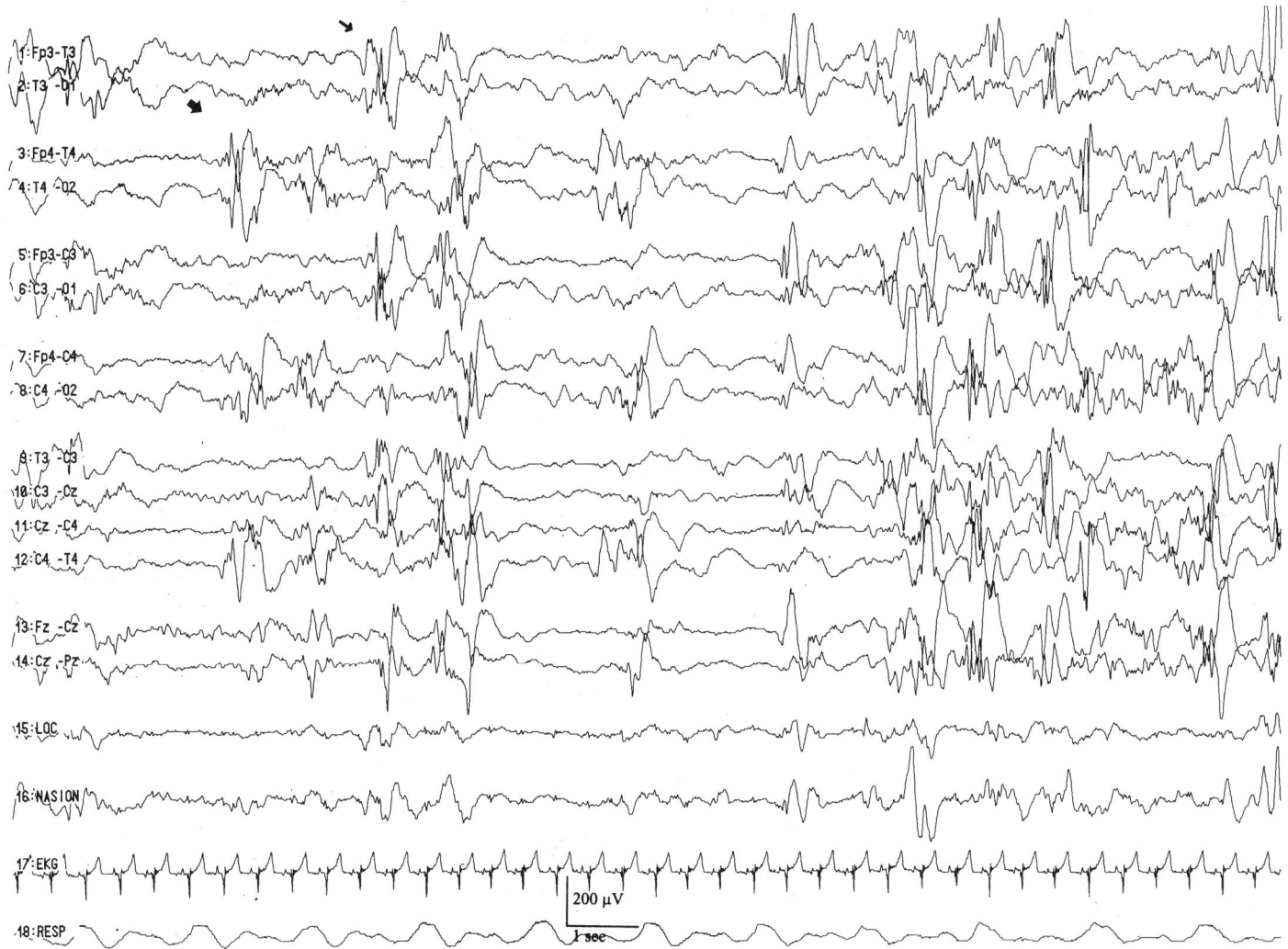

FIG. 6.21. Excessive asynchrony in an infant 46 weeks of conceptional age infant with nonketotic hyper-glycinemia. Bursts of right (*large arrow*) and left (*small arrow*) hemispheric activity are not synchronized.

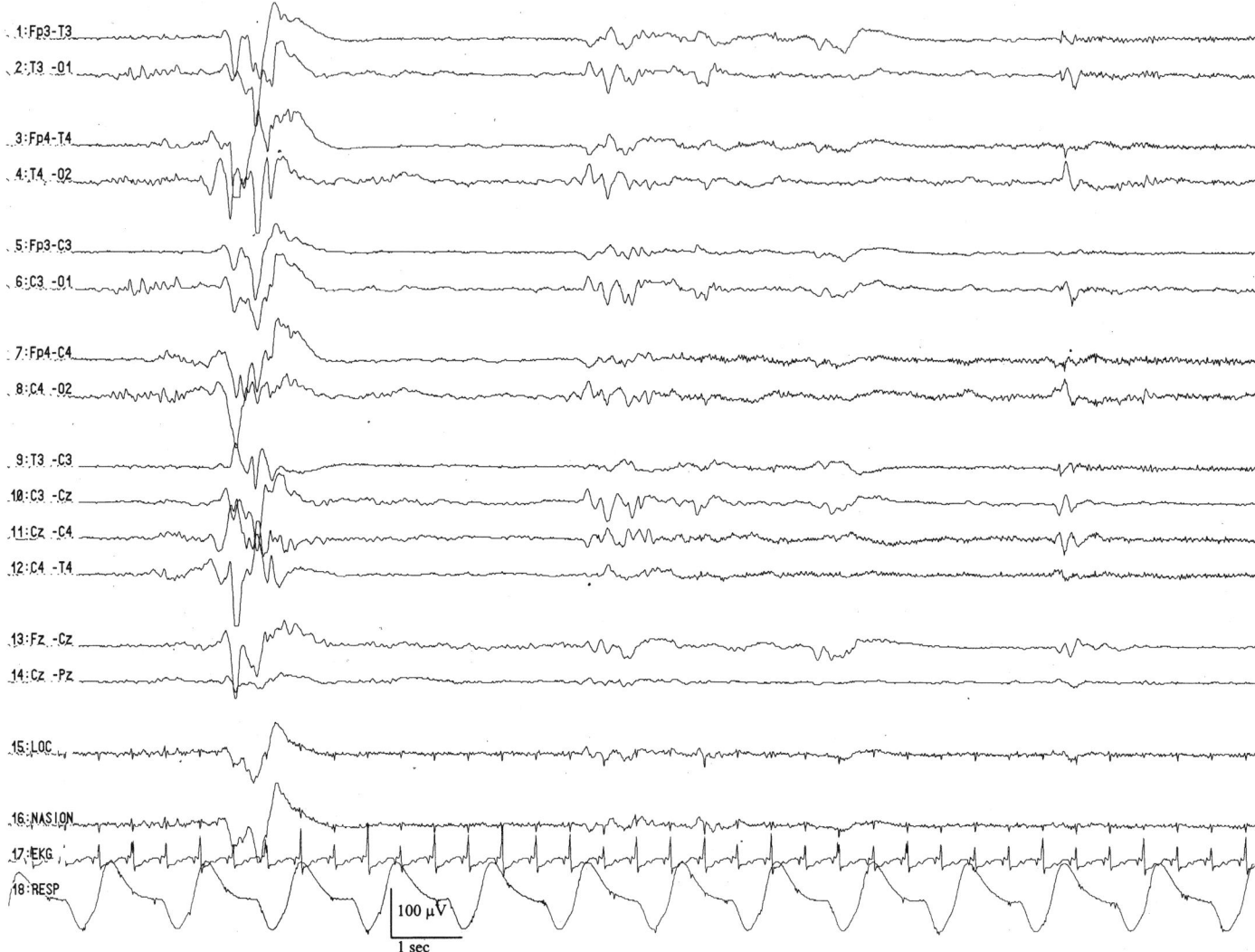

FIG. 6.22. Synchrony in a premature infant 27 weeks of conceptional age with dysmorphic facial features. Cerebral activity is well synchronized between the hemispheres.

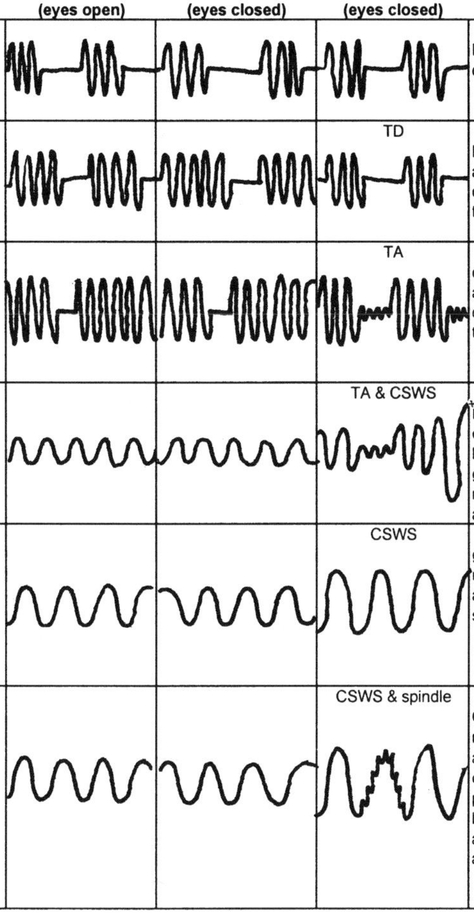

Conceptional Age (CA)	EEG Schematic for the Biobehavioral States			Clinical and EEG Concordance	Reactivity	Continuity	Burst Composition	Burst Synchrony	Interburst Interval Duration	Interburst Interval Amplitude
	Awake (eyes open)	Active Sleep (eyes closed)	Quiet Sleep (eyes closed)							
24-29 weeks				EEG appears the same while awake, or asleep	No change in EEG with stimulation	no sustained continuity	monorhythmic occipital delta; rhythmic theta activity in occipital and temporal areas; delta brushes	nearly 100% synchronized "hypersynchrony"	6-12 secs	<2 mV
30-34 weeks			TD	EEG appears the same awake and AS with longer periods of continuity; completely discontinuous in QS (trace discontinu-TD).	some change in EEG with stimulation while awake or AS	few periods of longer continuous EEG	monorhythmic occipital delta; bursts of rhythmic theta in occipital and temporal; more delta brushes in AS than QS.	about 70-80%	5-8 secs	<25 mV
35-36 weeks			TA	definitely distinguishable awake and AS record (activite moyenne) compared to discontinuous trace alternans (TD) pattern of QS	stimulation during discontinuous QS tracing provokes voltage flattening and more continuity	low to moderate amplitude, mixed frequency, continuous in awake/AS	symmetric, mixture of all EEG frequencies; rthymic temporal theta; more delta brushes in QS than AS	about 85%	4-6 secs	>25 mV
37-40 weeks			TA & CSWS	EEG is mostly indeterminate during transitions between biobehavioral states; otherwise good agreement between activite moyenne (awake/AS) and trace alternans (quiet sleep)	consistent reaction of EEG background to internal or external stimulation	completely continuous during wakefullness and AS	activite moyenne, comprised of continuous, low to moderate amplitude mixed frequency activity. More delta activity in bursts that comprise trace alternans. Some CSWS in QS.	about 100%	2-4 secs	50-75 mV
40-44 weeks			CSWS	good agreement between activite moyenne (awake/AS) and trace alternans or continuous slow wave sleep (quiet sleep)	EEG can be stimulated to alter within quiet sleep and between QS and awake/AS	continuous while awake/AS and during the CSWS portion of QS	activite moyenne and TA as above. In CSWS, continuous delta activity, best developed posteriorly. Delta brushes predominate in QS.	100% in TA portion of record	2-4 secs	75-100 mV
44-46 weeks			CSWS & spindle	CSWS gradually replaces less mature TA. Low-moderate amplitude awake EEG clearly different from higher amplitude, predominantly delta frequency CSWS background. Distinct sllep spindles at 12-14 Hz from midline-central areas in CSWS.	stimulation during CSWS produces prompt EEG change with voltage attenuation and reduction of delta activity.	continuous in all bio-behavioral states	activite moyenne in wake/AS record. Delta brushes dissappear from QS and tracing matures from TA to CSWS. Sleep spindles first appear from midline and spread into central regions.	not applicable	not applicable	not applicable

FIG. 6.23. Overview of development of electroencephalographic background between 24 and 46 weeks of conceptional age.

named patterns such as the delta brush, monorhythmic occipital delta activity, and bursts of rhythmic occipital and temporal theta activity) that are regularly punctuated by low-voltage (<25-μV) quiet periods. The duration of the low-voltage IBIs varies with age, being longer in the youngest patient and decreasing in duration as the brain matures. The typical IBI averages about 6 to 12 seconds in physically healthy infants at this age. Most of the EEG bursts are well synchronized, appearing simultaneously (within 1.5 to 2.0 seconds) between the left and right cerebral hemispheres. Although infants clinically cycle through awake/asleep periods with eye opening (i.e., wakefulness) and eye closure (i.e., sleep), there is qualitatively little difference in the appearance of the EEG background. The EEG appears essentially monotonous with no definite state organization regardless of the infant's clinical status. There is little concordance (agreement) between the clinical and electrographic expressions of the biobehavioral state at this conceptional age.

30 to 32 Weeks of Conceptional Age

By this conceptional age, there first appears some differentiation of the EEG pattern that distinguishes wakefulness (or REM/active sleep) from non-REM, or quiet, sleep. There is some concordance between the appearance of the background EEG and behavioral state. During wakefulness or active sleep , the EEG begins to "fill in" some of the low-voltage IBIs that had previously remained monotonously invariant. The awake/active sleep EEG is relatively more continuous, with longer duration BIs. The actual composition of the bursts still largely resembles that at earlier gestational ages, dominated by the synchronized, monorhythmic occipital delta activity, some of which are incorporated into posterior delta brushes. The brief bursts of rhythmic theta activity have migrated more from the occipital to the temporal areas. There are still many portions of the record that are discontinuous, even during wakefulness and active sleep, but the IBIs are a little briefer, about 5 to 8 seconds on average. During well-developed quiet sleep, the record is persistently discontinuous and is distinguishable from the awake/active sleep tracing. The term *trace discontinu* (discontinuous tracing) is first applied to this early form of a healthy quiet sleep recording in which bursts of normal cerebral electric activity are regularly interspersed with low-voltage (<25 μV) periods of quiescence. The record may be marginally reactive to external stimulation: if the patient is provoked during quiet sleep, there is a visible change of the actual EEG background (not just EMG or movement artifact from patient motion) with the appearance of a more continuous background resulting from the arousal.

33 to 34 Weeks of Conceptional Age

By this conceptional age, there is further consolidation of the biobehavioral states: active and quiet sleep are more clearly distinguishable both clinically and electrographically, and the concordance between the appearance of the EEG and behavioral state is easier to recognize. Less of the EEG is indeterminate—that is, lacking in the distinguishing characteristics that allow definitive classification into specific biobehavioral states. In the awake and active sleep record, the background is more continuous with further filling in of the gaps between the EEG bursts. The IBIs are fewer and briefer than before. The monorhythmic occipital delta activity is fading, and most of the bursts of rhythmic theta activity appear in the temporal regions. Up to this conceptional age, there are more delta brushes per minute in the awake and active sleep portions of the recording than during quiet sleep. Trace discontinu continues to be the quiet sleep pattern, and the IBIs range from 5 to 8 seconds, but the synchrony of the bursts is, paradoxically, less than at earlier conceptional ages. Only about 70% to 80% of the bursts in the discontinuous portions of the study are synchronized, occurring within 1.5 to 2.0 seconds between the two hemispheres.

35 to 36 Weeks of Conceptional Age

By this conceptional age, biobehavioral states are easily distinguished, and the EEG shows definite and reproducible reactivity to external stimulation. In wakefulness and active sleep, the EEG is essentially continuous and is composed of low- to moderate-amplitude, mixed-frequency activity. This normal pattern that typifies the awake and active sleep record is commonly called *activité moyenne* ("average activity"). There is little left of the high-amplitude monorhythmic occipital delta and only few remnants of the rhythmic theta bursts. The signal is composed of admixed, coexisting frequencies ranging from delta to beta frequencies and a few delta brushes in the occipital, central, and temporal areas. The quiet sleep record remains discontinuous, but the amplitude of the IBI gradually increases as the duration further declines. At this point, the typical IBI duration is about 4 to 6 seconds, and its amplitude clearly exceeds 25 μV. The name of this normal immature, discontinuous quiet sleep pattern is *trace alternant,* indicating a pattern that alternates between high-amplitude burst intervals and low-amplitude IBIs.

These bursts are typically more synchronized than at the prior conceptional age; about 85% appear simultaneously between the two hemispheres. Delta brushes are more abundant in quiet sleep than in active sleep, and much of the record can be assigned to definite sleep categories.

37 to 40 Weeks of Conceptional Age

In healthy full-term infants, there are clearly and easily recognizable periods of wakefulness/active sleep and quiet sleep. About 25% of total sleep time is occupied by indeterminate sleep (98). Once quiet sleep is established, trace alternant first appears with typical IBIs of 2 to 4 seconds, and essentially all of the bursts arise synchronously. If the infant remains asleep for awhile, trace alternant gives way to a moderate- to high-amplitude, uninterrupted delta activity, the earliest expression of continuous slow-wave sleep (CSWS). This sets the stage for the EEG background that typifies quiet sleep for the rest of the life span. Trace alternant and CSWS comingle at this age. Delta brushes remain more abundant in quiet sleep than in active sleep, and the amplitude of background delta activity is highest posteriorly, an early expression of a frequency-amplitude gradient (86).

41 to 44 Weeks of Conceptional Age

In healthy infants of this conceptional age, *activité moyenne* continues to constitute the background during wakefulness/active sleep, whereas delta brushes gradually disappear by 44 weeks. On occasion, the awake EEG displays broad biphasic lambda waves in the occipital regions bilaterally, coincident with visual fixation. In quiet sleep, CSWS gradually replaces trace alternant, except at the onset of quiet sleep. The bursts of activity in trace alternant are well synchronized, but the IBI durations are quite brief, typically less than 2 to 4 seconds, and their amplitudes exceed 50 μV. By the end of this epoch, all of the discontinuous portions of quiet sleep have been "filled in" and trace alternant is completely replaced by CSWS.

45 to 46 Weeks of Conceptional Age

The distinguishing characteristic of this period is the first appearance of *sleep spindles* in CSWS (31,50). Once they arise, they appear with their usual frequency (about 12 to 14 Hz) and are typically centered over the midline (Fz-Cz region), spreading to the neighboring left or right central regions (C3 or C4). In the course of the entire quiet sleep record, there are about the same numbers of sleep spindles spreading into the left and right central regions (i.e., they are symmetric), but they are not well synchronized. Indeed, they do not achieve full synchronization until about the age of 2 years.

Composition of Electroencephalographic Background Activity (Named Patterns)

EEG background refers to the presence of all the aggregated patterns, waveforms, and frequencies that collectively constitute the ongoing cerebral electric activity. As such, it represents an infrastructure or stage that may be punctuated by fleeting EEG transients (physiological or pathological sharp waves) or electrographic seizures. The appearance and composition of the background varies with state and conceptional age, but the predominant frequencies that constitute the neonatal EEG are represented by theta and delta activity. There are, however, several specific components appearing in premature and full-term infants that warrant individual description and illustration.

Monorhythmic Occipital Delta Activity

This activity represents a conspicuous, stereotyped run of monomorphic, high-amplitude, surface polarity–positive, 0.5- to 1-Hz delta waves, often appearing synchronously in the occipital scalp regions (Fig. 6.24). A run of monorhythmic occipital delta activity can last from 2 to 60 seconds and appears relatively symmetrically and synchronized bilaterally. It is present at the conceptional age of 23 to 24 weeks, peaks in abundance between 31 and 33 weeks, and then significantly fades by 35 weeks. Persistence of well-developed monorhythmic delta activity after 35 weeks conceptional age is often considered evidence of electrographic "immaturity." This pattern represents the dominant rhythmic activity in the posterior brain regions and serves as the delta constituent of occipital delta brushes (see later discussion). This is also a sturdy rhythm in that it may persist in the presence of severe, acute encephalopathies, long after other specific patterns have disappeared.

Rhythmic Occipital Theta Activity

This specific pattern appears as brief (2- to 10-second) bursts of stereotyped, rhythmic, sinusoidal 4-Hz theta activity in the occipital regions (Fig. 6.25), sometimes spreading into the temporal regions. These bursts

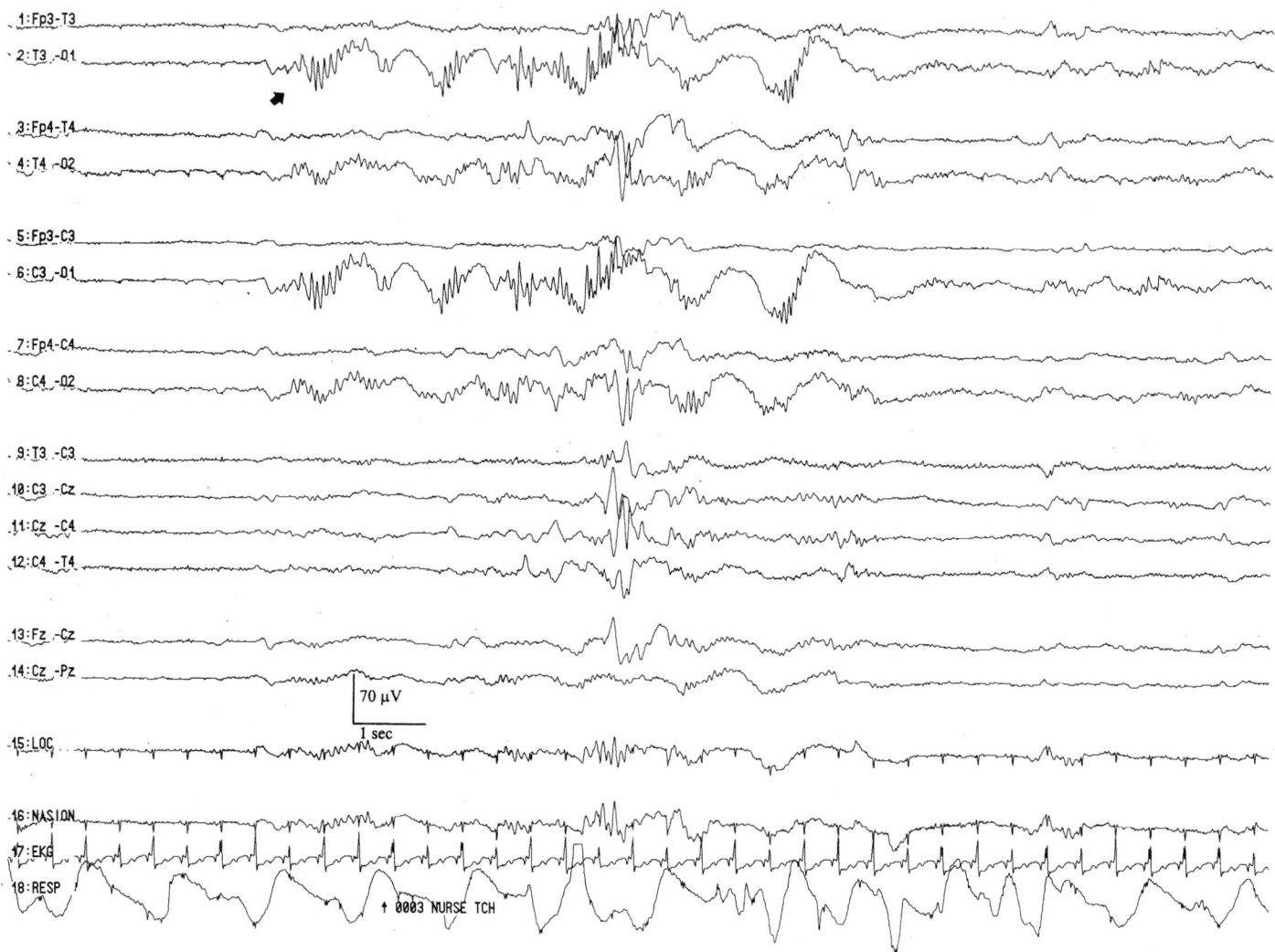

FIG. 6.24. Monorhythmic occipital delta activity in an infant 31 weeks of conceptional age with apnea. Occipital delta activity with delta brushes (*arrow*) is present. Note that the occipital delta transients are synchronized between the two hemispheres.

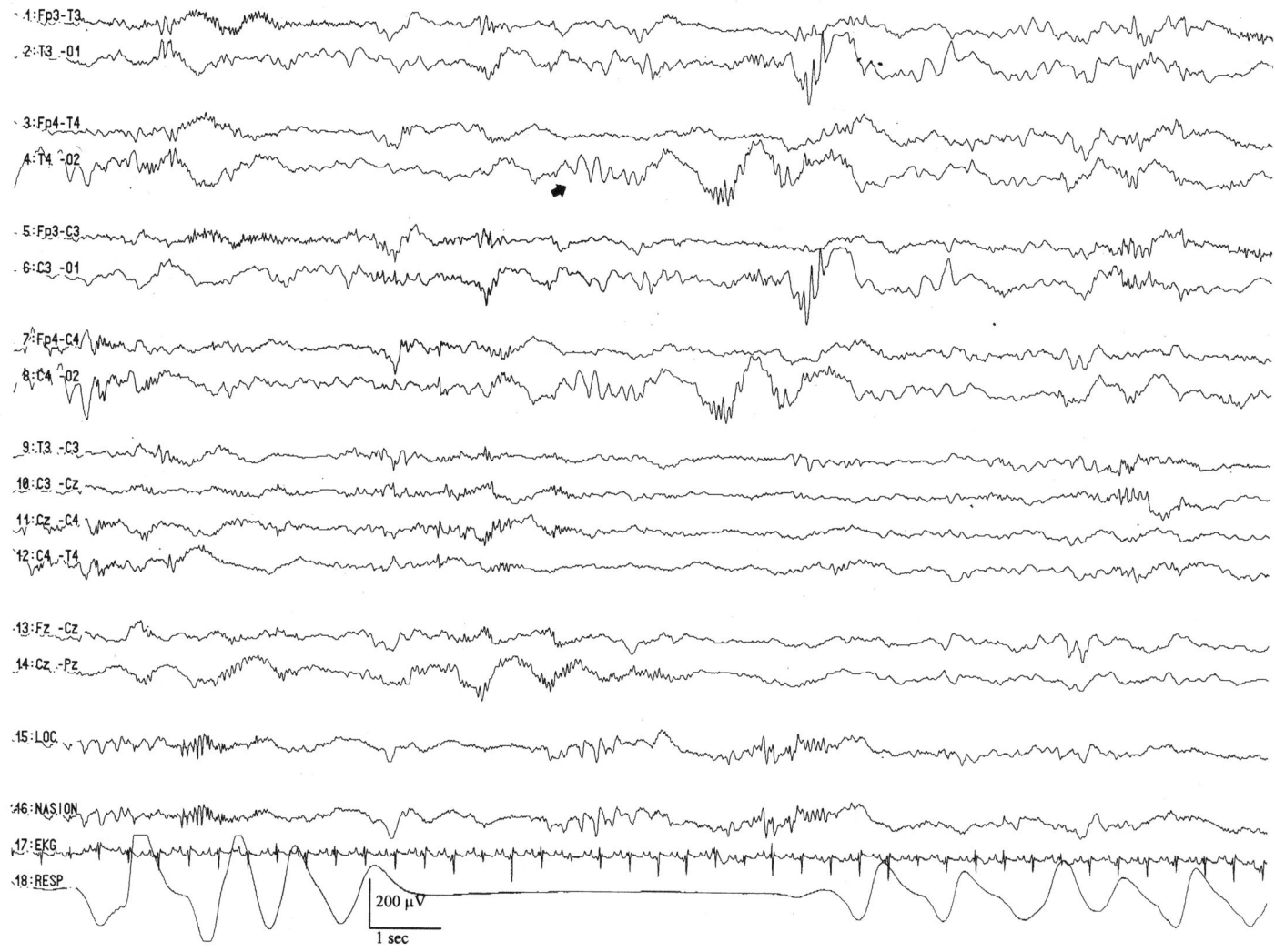

FIG. 6.25. Rhythmic occipital theta activity in an infant 30 weeks of conceptional age who underwent fetal surgery for repair of myelomeningocele. Bilateral rhythmic occipital theta activity (*arrow*) is present, although more on the right side than on the left.

commonly mingle or superimpose on coincident monorhythmic occipital delta activity. They are present in the awake or sleeping infant and are apparent at the conceptional age of 23 to 24 weeks. They peak in abundance by 30 weeks and then fade from the occipital areas by 33 weeks; the rhythmic theta pattern migrates anteriorly to the temporal areas at older ages.

Rhythmic Temporal Theta Activity

This pattern is morphologically similar to that arising in the occipital regions. It peaks between the conceptional ages of 31 and 33 weeks. It appears as brief paroxysms simultaneously or independently in the temporal areas (Fig. 6.26). However, over a long time period, these bursts are equally represented bilaterally. They are occasionally "sharply" contoured, which raises the concern that they are a brief ictal discharge, but they do not evolve in morphology or frequency. On occasion, an abortive or larval burst of this pattern gives rise to a "sharp wave," but close examination shows that it is merely a morphological fragment of an abbreviated run of rhythmic temporal theta activity.

Centrotemporal Delta Activity

This pattern is represented by the intermittent appearance of sustained trains of conspicuous, 0.5- to 2-Hz delta activity, often with a prominent surface-positive polarity in the C3-C4 to T3-T4 areas (Fig. 6.27). They may appear semirhythmically, but they are not usually as regular and well modulated as monorhythmic occipital delta activity. This pattern serves as the delta wave foundation for rolandic and temporal brushes. It peaks by the conceptional age of 30 weeks and fades after 33 weeks.

Delta Brushes

These patterns (also called "brushes," "ripples of prematurity," and "spindle-like fast rhythms") are often considered the premier electrographic signature of the premature infant. The pattern is composed of a combination of a specific delta frequency transient with a superimposed "buzz" of 8- to 20-Hz activity (see Figs. 6.24 and 6.27). Brushes are symmetrically represented between the two hemispheres and homologous brain regions. They are not commonly displayed synchronously except when they arise in concert with runs of monorhythmic occipital delta activity. They appear in awake and sleeping infants, and so they should not be considered a type of precursor of the "spindle" of mature quiet sleep, which first appears around the conceptional age of 46 weeks. Up to the conceptional age of 33 weeks, there are more brushes per minute in active sleep than in quiet sleep. After the conceptional age of 34 weeks, brushes are more numerous in quiet sleep. Brushes may appear in any scalp region but are scarce in the frontal areas. In the youngest premature infants, brushes are mostly expressed in the rolandic regions. At their peak expression (during the conceptional ages of 32 to 34 weeks), they arise mostly in the occipital, central, and temporal areas. By term, brushes may still persist in immature trace alternant but have largely vanished from the awake and active sleep portions of the recording. By 1 month post term, they are no longer in evidence.

Anterior Dysrhythmia

This pattern appears as paroxysmal, brief bursts of frontally dominant, 50- to 100-μV, semirhythmic delta activity (Fig. 6.28). Their morphological features may subtly evolve over a few seconds and acquire a sharp contour, commonly admixing and blending with a related rhythm, *encoche frontale*. Runs of anterior dysrhythmia tend to arise symmetrically and synchronously between the frontal regions and may be present in all behavior states. They are most conspicuous in the transition from active to quiet sleep but scarce in the period of active sleep immediately after quiet sleep. Despite the usual connotation of the "dys-" prefix, anterior dysrhythmia is a normal developmental electroencephalographic pattern. However, in the wake of definite encephalopathies such as hypoxia-ischemia or meningitis, its excessive presence may be considered a nonspecific electrographic abnormality (14,30,42). Marked and persistent asymmetries of their number, morphology or amplitude may also represent an electrographic abnormality. Its counterpart pattern, frontal sharp waves (*encoches frontales*) are described later.

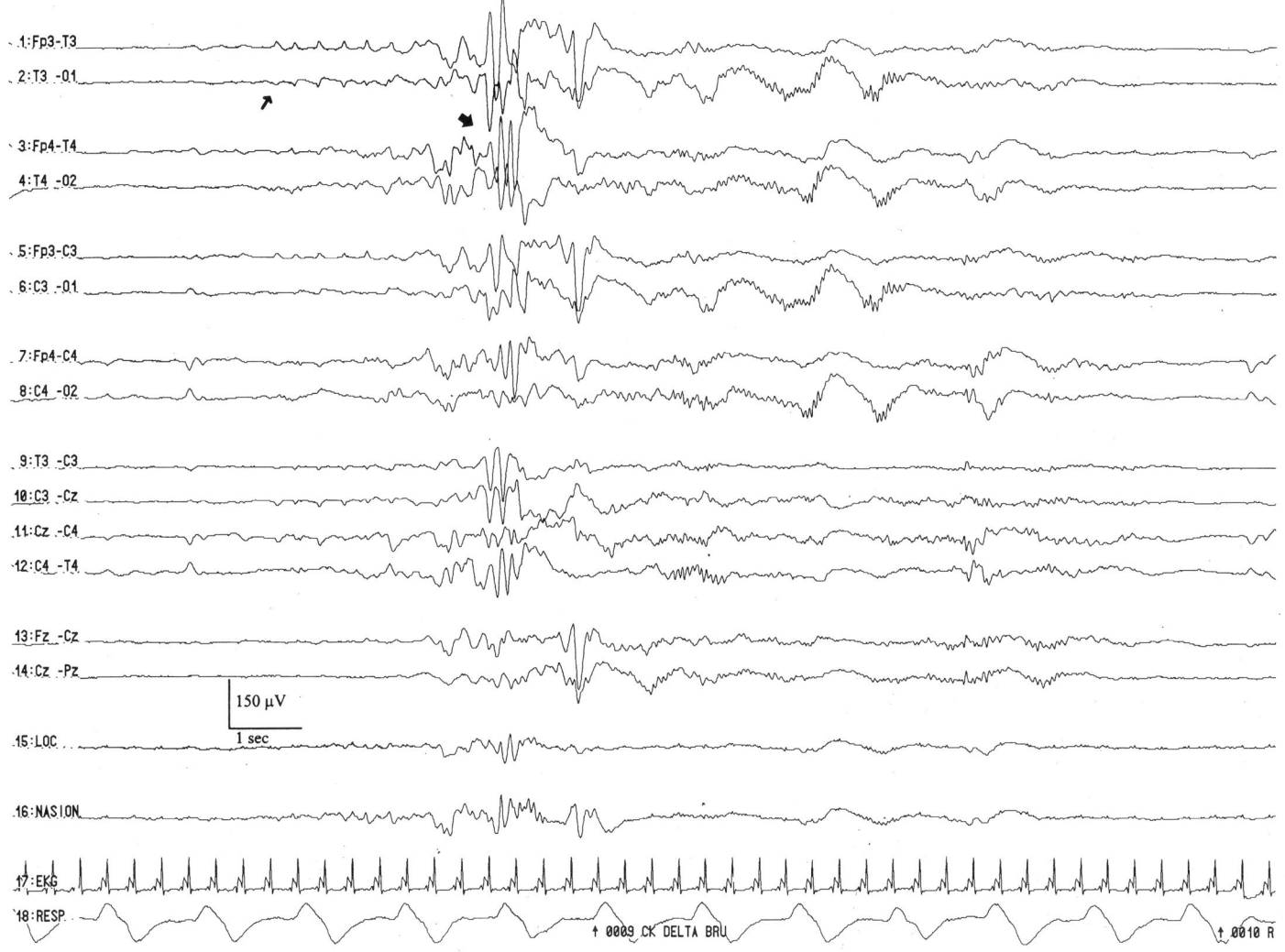

FIG. 6.26. Rhythmic temporal theta activity in an infant 31 weeks of conceptional age with pneumonia. Sharply contoured rhythmic temporal theta activity (*large arrow*) is present. Also, note a run of low-amplitude, positive left temporal sharp waves (*small arrow*), which are considered normal transients for age.

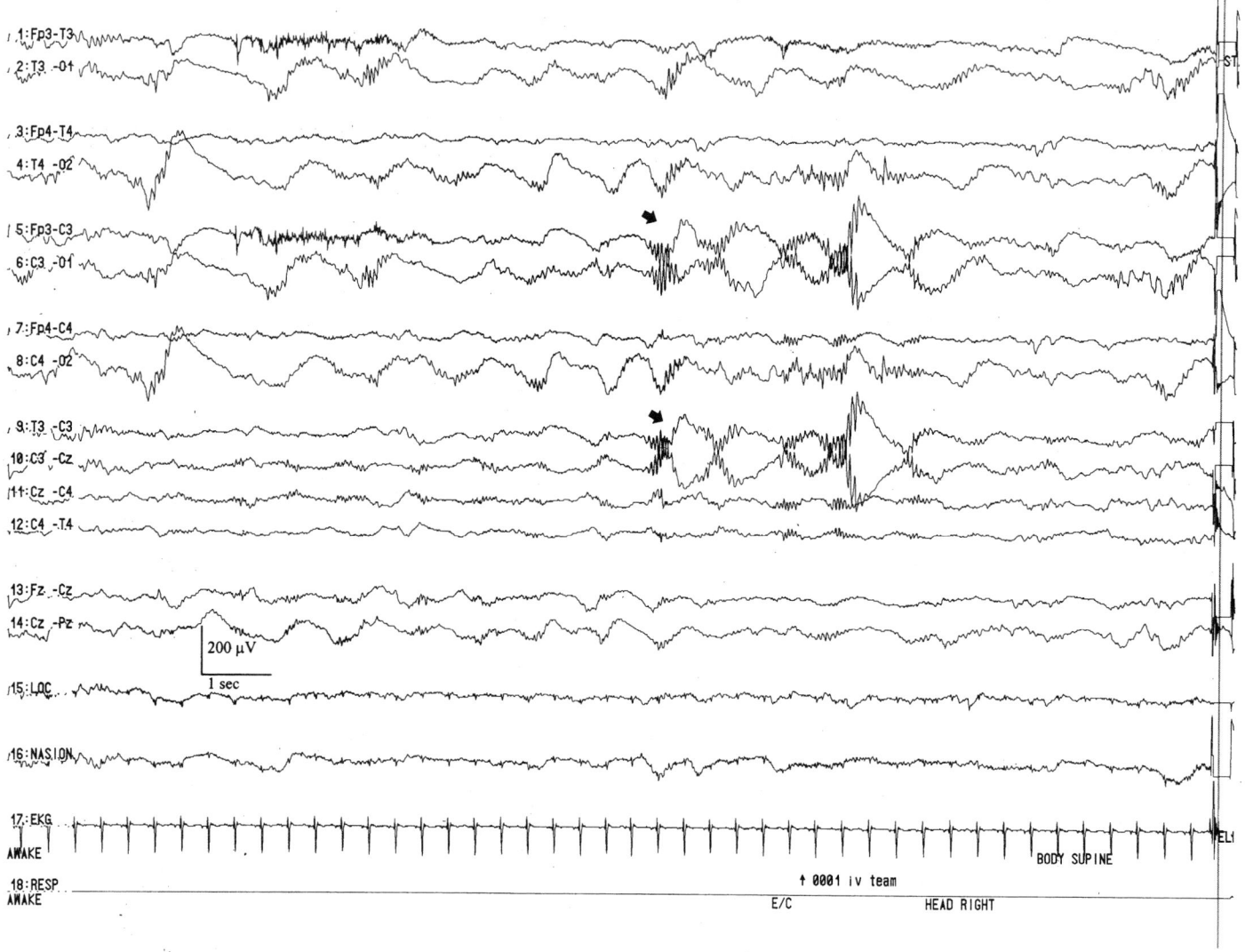

FIG. 6.27. Rhythmic centrotemporal delta activity in an infant 31 weeks of conceptional age with dysmorphic facial features. *Arrows* indicates left centrotemporal delta activity admixed with delta brushes.

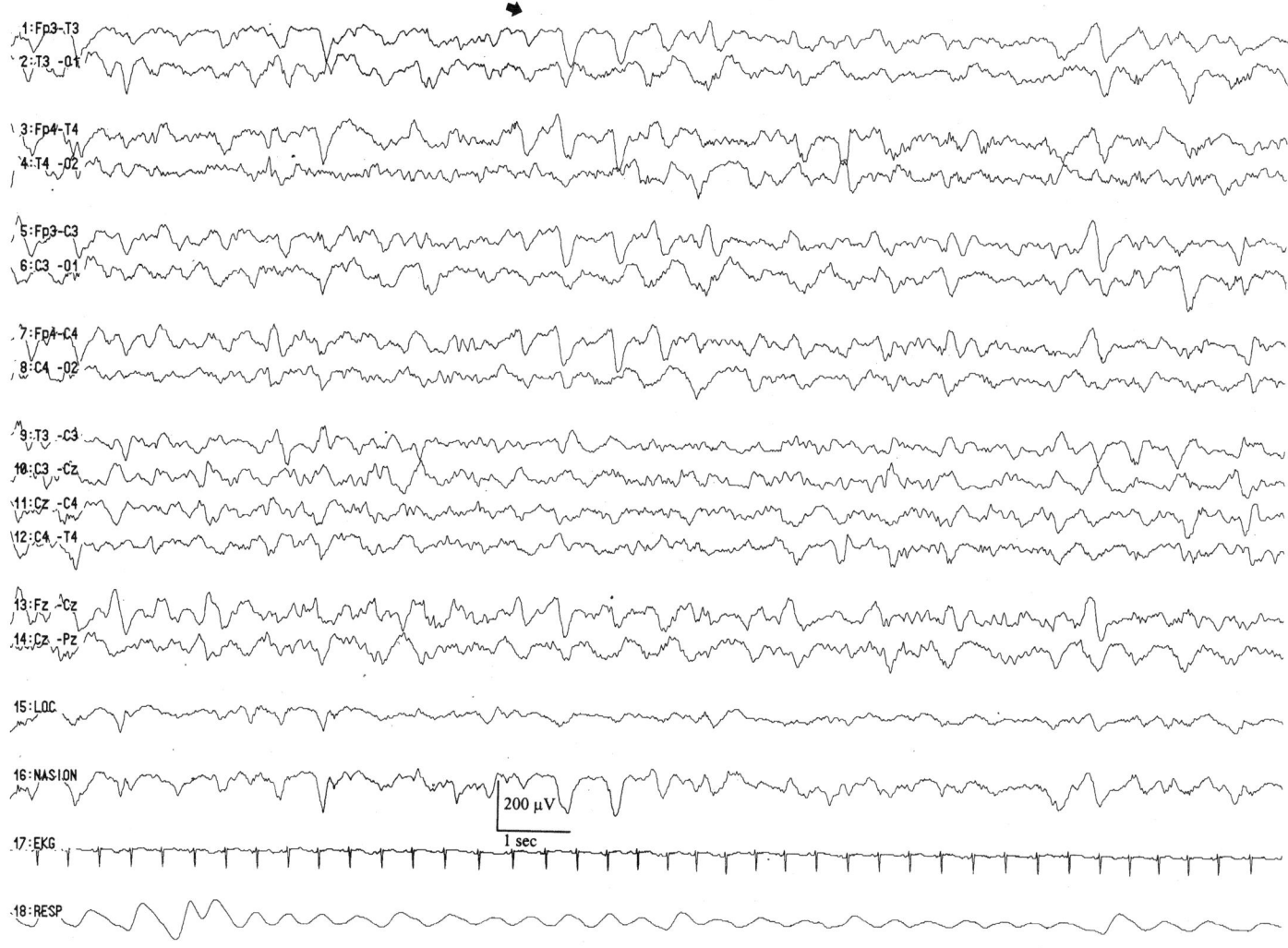

FIG. 6.28. Anterior dysrhythmia in an infant 40 weeks of conceptional age with pneumonia. Bilateral frontal anterior dysrhythmia (*arrow*) is admixed with poorly formed *encoches frontales*.

Specific Neonatal Electroencephalographic Background Patterns and State

Wakefulness and Active Sleep

The waking EEG resembles the background of the onset of active sleep, composed of low-amplitude (<25-μV), predominantly 4- to 7-Hz theta and low-amplitude delta activity (Fig. 6.29). There are two basic active sleep patterns in neonates older than 36 weeks of conceptional age.

Neonates usually enter their sleep cycle in active sleep, and the duration of active sleep cycles vary between 10 and 45 minutes. As the infant enters active sleep the first time, the background is composed of moderate-amplitude (25- to 50-μV) irregular theta and delta activity with relatively few frontal transients (encoches frontales) (Fig. 6.30) (29). Subsequent cycles of active sleep have lower amplitude, more theta activity, and less delta activity and resemble the EEG of the awake state (activité moyenne).

Trace Discontinu

Trace discontinu is an important EEG maturational milestone, inasmuch as it is the first EEG pattern to emerge that differentiates wakefulness from sleep in the premature infant. With the development of trace discontinu, there is, for the first time, some concordance between the infant's clinical state and the EEG background. During quiet sleep, the trace discontinu pattern develops; it consists of bursts of high-amplitude (≤200-μV) activity separated by periods of relative quiescence with amplitudes of less than 25 μV (Fig. 6.31). The bursts are composed of normal theta and delta activity, and the acceptable range of the IBIs durations is determined by the conceptional age.

By 32 to 34 weeks of conceptional age, the trace discontinu pattern is well developed. Wakefulness and active, quiet, and indeterminate (transitional) sleep EEG stages emerge with improved clinical concordance. Trace discontinu remains the EEG pattern of quite sleep until 36 weeks of conceptional age, when the IBI amplitude exceeds 25 μV, which defines the more mature pattern of quite sleep, trace alternant.

Trace Alternant

Between 34 and 36 weeks of conceptional age, the trace discontinu pattern of normal quiet sleep begins to evolve into the more mature pattern of trace alternant (Fig. 6.32) (29). In both trace discontinu and trace alternant, the tracing is discontinuous. The fundamental distinction between trace discontinu and trace alternant lies in the amplitude of the IBI. In trace discontinu, it is less than 25 μV, whereas in trace alternant, it is greater than 25 μV. The bursts of cerebral activity in trace alternant consist of symmetrical delta activity, admixed with faster frequencies, with amplitudes of 50 to 300 μV. The duration of the bursts varies considerably but typically is more than 2 seconds. The composition of the IBI of trace alternant resembles the EEG during wakefulness and active sleep and consists of mixed frequencies with amplitudes of 25 to 50 μV. The duration of the IBI shortens as term approaches and normally does not exceed 2 to 4 seconds by 38 to 40 weeks of conceptional age (89). Trace alternant itself begins to wane by 38 to 40 weeks of conceptional age, although fragments may persist until 44 to 46 weeks of conceptional age. Trace alternant is gradually replaced by the more mature pattern of CSWS (31,97).

Continuous Slow-Wave Sleep

CSWS is the final major stage developed in the ontogeny of the EEG in quiet sleep. CSWS consists of nonstop delta and theta activity with amplitudes of 50 to 300 μV; it resembles stage 3 and 4 sleep seen in older patients. Discontinuity with BIs and IBIs are no longer present. The first fragments of CSWS emerge around 35 weeks of conceptional age. In one study, CSWS accounted for about 10% of total quiet sleep time at 36 weeks of conceptional age, 40% at 40 weeks, and 100% by 44 to 45 weeks (97). (Fig. 6.33)

Sleep spindles (Fig. 6.34) first appear between 44 and 49 weeks of conceptional age and consist of 12- to 14-Hz activity at the Cz, C3, or C4 electrode. Spindles are only rare at first but are well developed by 3 months post term, occurring at a mean rate of 4.2 spindles per minute (31). Spindles in infancy are typically asynchronous between the two hemispheres and remain so until the age of 2 years.

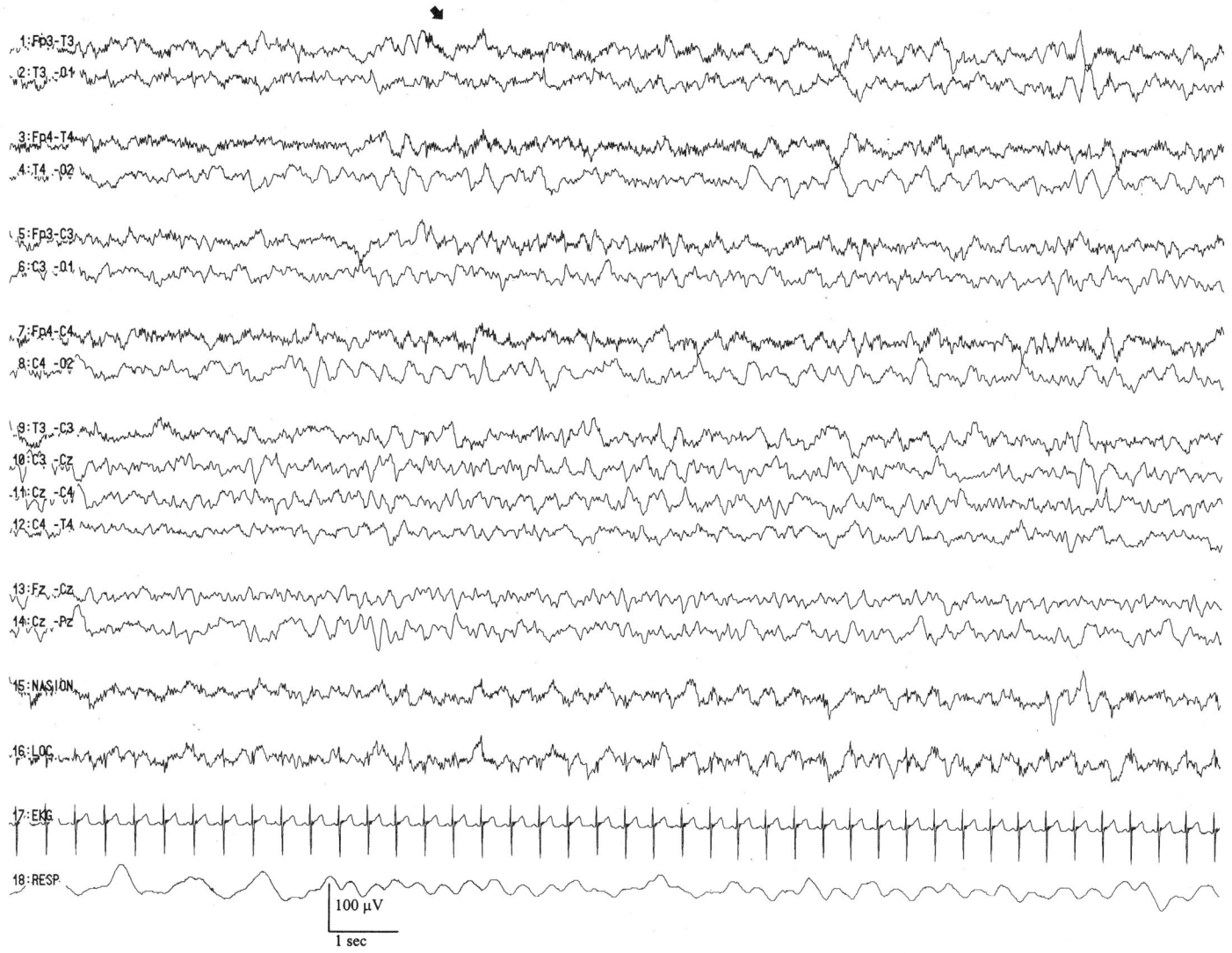

FIG. 6.29. Wakefulness in an infant 41 weeks of conceptional age evaluated for staring episodes. The tracing consists of continuous, mixed-frequency activity of low to medium amplitude (*activité moyenne*). Muscle activity (*arrow*) suggests wakefulness and helps to distinguish this pattern from that of active sleep.

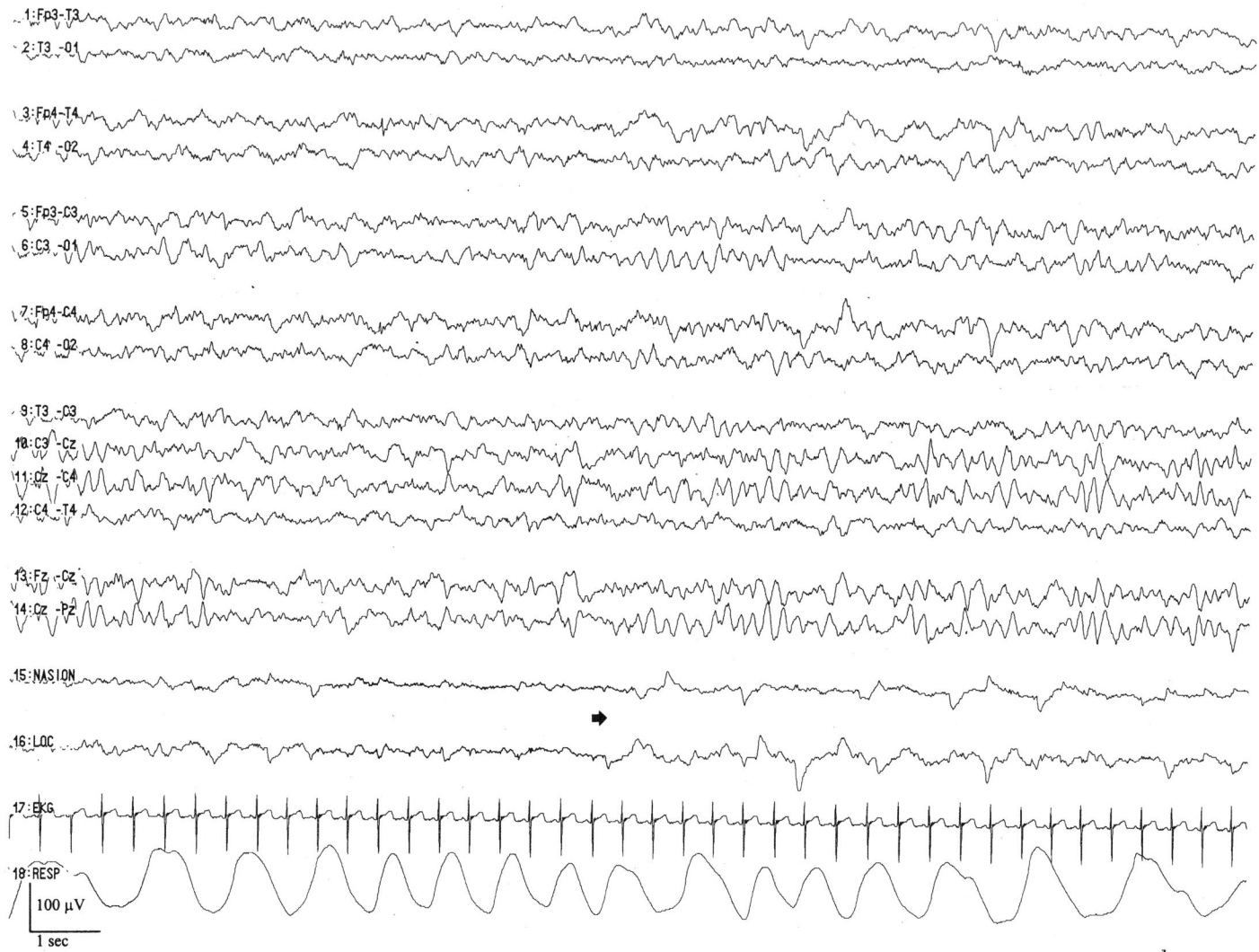

FIG. 6.30. Active sleep-in the same infant as in Fig. 6.29. The tracing also consists of continuous activity of low to moderate amplitude (*activité moyenne*). Rapid eye movements (*arrow*) and the lack of tonic muscle activity indicate active sleep.

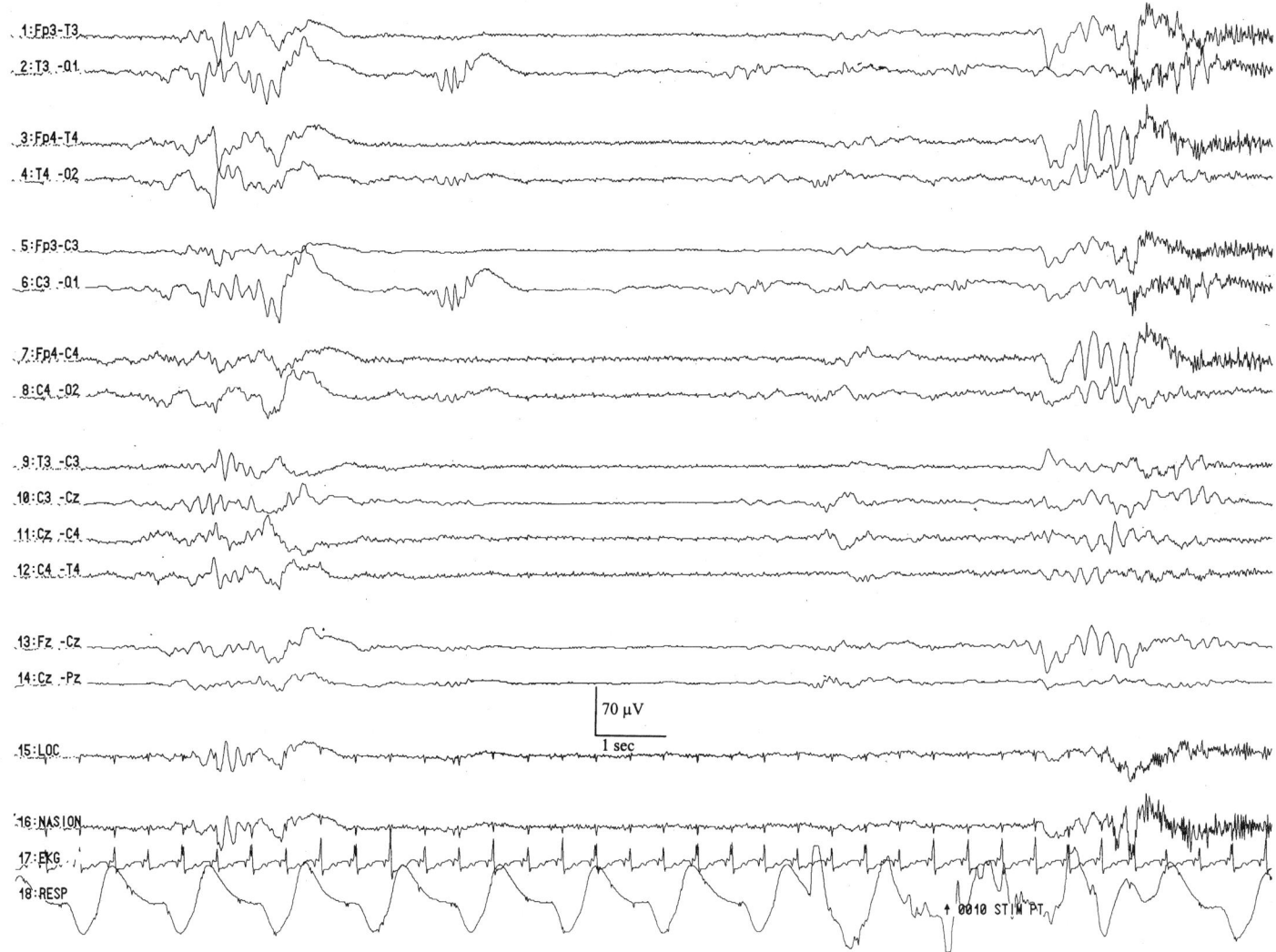

FIG. 6.31. Trace discontinu in an infant 31 weeks of conceptional age with apnea. The tracing is discontinuous. Bursts of activity are composed of normal patterns for age, and the amplitude of the interburst interval is less than 25 μV.

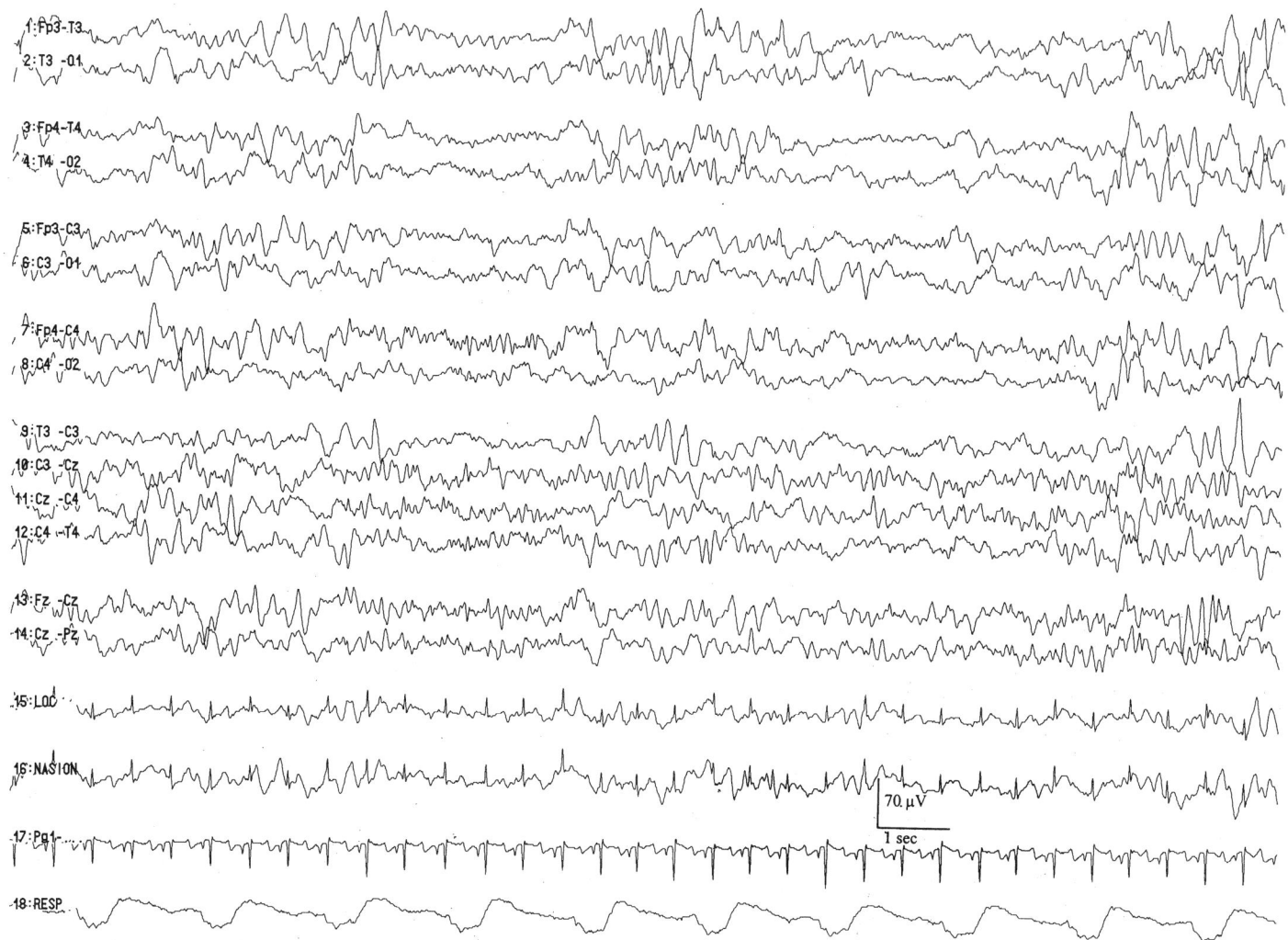

FIG. 6.32. Trace alternant in an infant 37 weeks of conceptional age with hypotonia. The tracing is discontinuous. Bursts of higher amplitude patterns, which are normal for age, *alternate* with lower amplitude activity. The amplitude of the interburst intervals exceeds 25 μV.

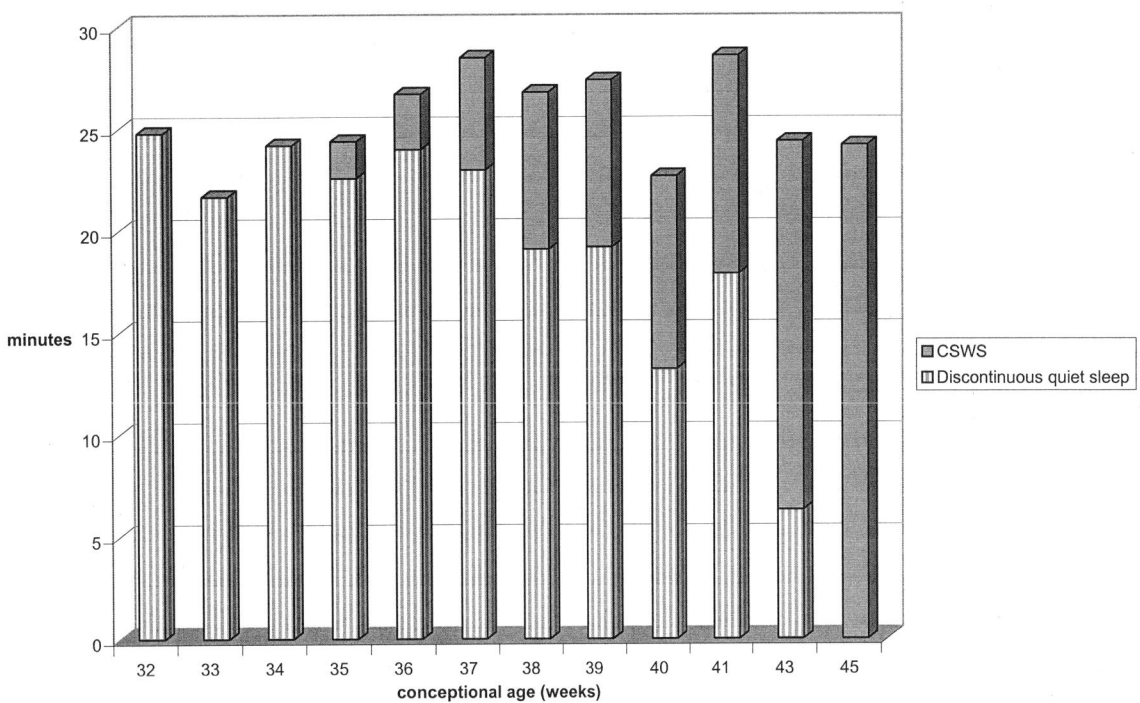

FIG. 6.33. Evolution of quiet sleep from immature trace alternant to continuous slow-wave sleep (CSWS) in normal infants. At 32 weeks of conceptional age, all quiet sleep is discontinuous. By 46 weeks, all quiet sleep in CSWS. (Adapted from Watanabe K, Iwase K, Hara, K. Development of slow-wave sleep in low-birthweight infants. *Dev Med Child Neurol* 1974;16:23–31.).

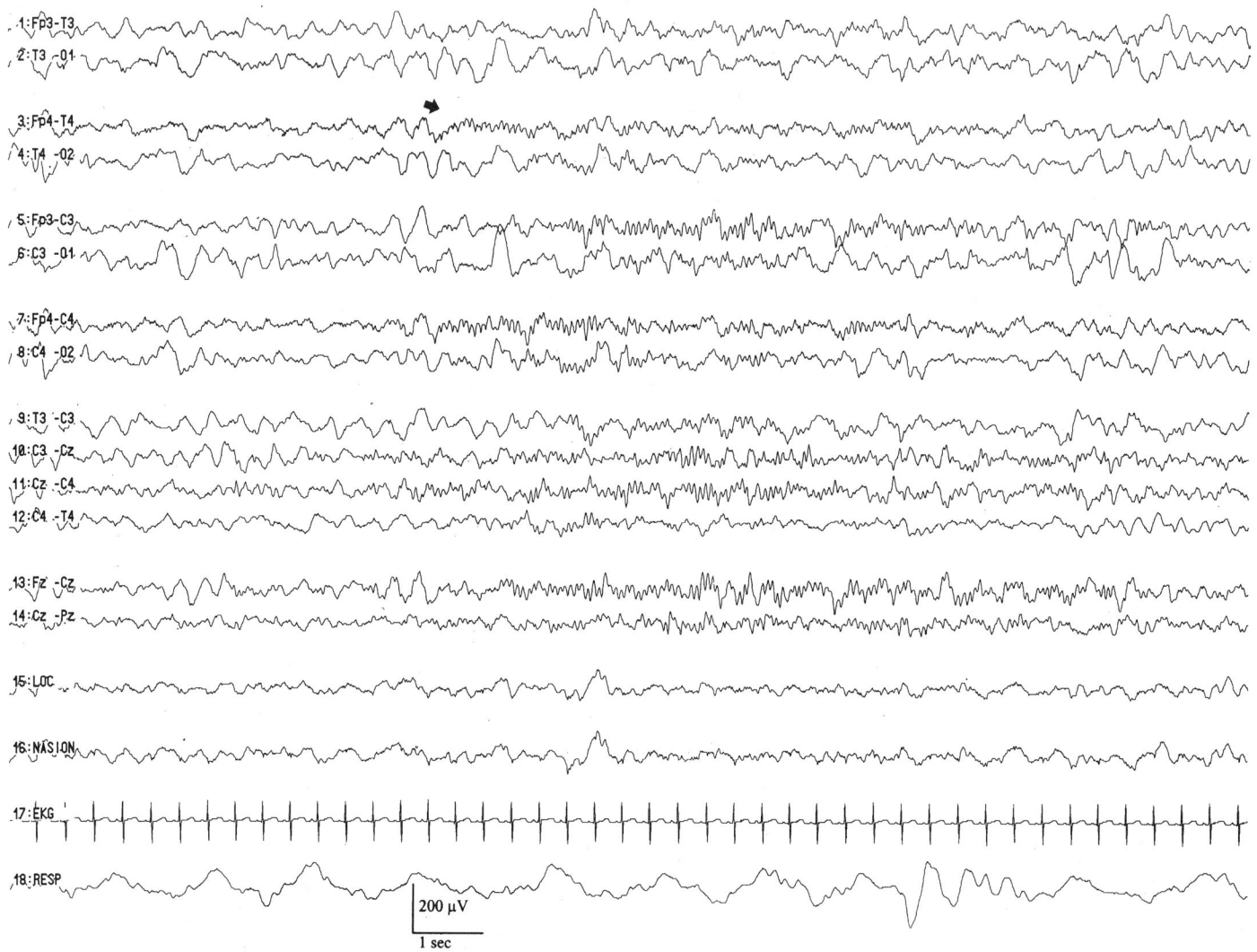

FIG. 6.34. Continuous slow-wave sleep with sleep spindles in an infant 48 weeks of conceptional age with episodes of staring and stiffening. *Arrow* indicates sleep spindles, arising asynchronously between the two hemispheres.

TYPES AND SIGNIFICANCE OF ABNORMAL ELECTROENCEPHALOGRAPHIC BACKGROUNDS

Just as the characteristics of the normal neonatal EEG background may be described in terms of continuity, synchrony, composition, and voltage, abnormal EEGs may also be judged from similar perspectives. Abnormal EEGs commonly display multiple, overlapping pathological features such as low voltage, excessive discontinuity, and poorly developed patterns and rhythms. The major characteristics of each type of abnormality are considered separately.

Excessive Discontinuity

A discontinuous EEG is an appropriate finding in the premature infant. With increasing conceptional age, the discontinuous EEG is confined to behavioral quiet sleep, and by 44 to 46 weeks of conceptional age, even quiet sleep is composed entirely of CSWS as the remnants of trace alternant disappear. EEGs that have inappropriately long IBIs or an overrepresentation of discontinuous activity are *excessively discontinuous* for conceptional age (Fig. 6.35). Because trace discontinu and trace alternant are normal, age-specific EEG patterns in healthy infants, the terms are inappropriate to apply to tracings that are abnormal and excessively discontinuous for conceptional age recorded from encephalopathic or medically ill neonates.

When the EEG appears excessively discontinuous, it is important to scrutinize the composition of the bursts. If the burst activity is well preserved and demonstrates a rich variety of the patterns and rhythms appropriate for the conceptional age, the excessive discontinuity may have relatively little significance. However, if the tracing is excessively discontinuous and if the bursts are poorly developed and lack normal background patterns, greater pathological significance can be presumed.

Burst-Suppression Pattern

The most extreme degree of discontinuity is burst-suppression (Fig. 6.36), characterized by an invariant, excessively discontinuous background with prolonged IBIs of very low voltage (<5 μV) that are interrupted by brief (1- to 10-second) bursts of paroxysmal higher voltage theta, delta, and other frequencies. These synchronous or asynchronous bursts may be admixed with sharp waves. Differentiation among biobehavioral states is lost. Burst suppression should not be confused with the immature quiet sleep patterns of tracé discontinu and tracé alternant. Burst-suppression tracings are *excessively* discontinuous and invariant. The IBI duration may be exceedingly long—30 minutes or more. The discontinuity is completely unreactive to noxious stimulation, and no spontaneous cycling of state is apparent. Furthermore, in burst-supresion, the burst periods themselves are devoid of the anticipated conceptional age–specific patterns (34).

It is important to be able to confidently recognize burst-suppression because it is commonly seen in severe encephalopathies and has clear unfavorable prognostic implications for both premature and full-term infants. Only exceptional infants enjoy a normal outcome in the wake of burst suppression. However, confirmation of a persistent burst-suppression pattern with serial EEGs is recommended before a definitive unfavorable prognosis is rendered. Tharp's (93) prospective study of 81 at-risk newborns of low birth weight (<1,200 g) included 41 EEGs with burst-suppression patterns. The 5-year follow-up revealed that 85% (35 of 41) had a very poor outcome, including eight deaths. In the full-term infant, burst suppression is also a nonspecific pattern of a severe degree of encephalopathy that may be caused by numerous conditions, including asphyxia, stroke, encephalitis or meningitis, metabolic disorders, inborn errors of metabolism such as non-ketotic hyperglycinemia, and cerebral dysgenesis. The rate of poor outcome for full-term infants with burst suppression is also high, ranging from 85% to 100% in recent studies (64,72,87,91,92).

Excessive Discontinuity for Conceptional Age

Some critically ill, very young premature infants may not display all of the usual criteria for burst suppression. The presence of discontinuity per se may be appropriate, even though the duration of the IBIs is usually quite excessive. The bursts themselves may still preserve a few of the named background premature patterns, especially delta brushes or monorhythmic occipital delta activity. Although such tracings fall short of the criteria for burst suppression, they also carry an ominous prognosis.

Less disturbed EEG backgrounds that also do not fulfill the criteria for burst suppression may nonetheless be judged abnormal by excessive discontinuity for conceptional age, determined by measuring the mean or median duration of IBIs or the duration of the record's longest IBI measurement. After 30 weeks of conceptional age, those with a *median* IBI duration of less than 8 seconds fared better than those with longer IBIs (22). Hahn et al. (35) provided useful data concerning the values of the single *longest* acceptable IBI duration for different conceptional ages (Table 6.1). There

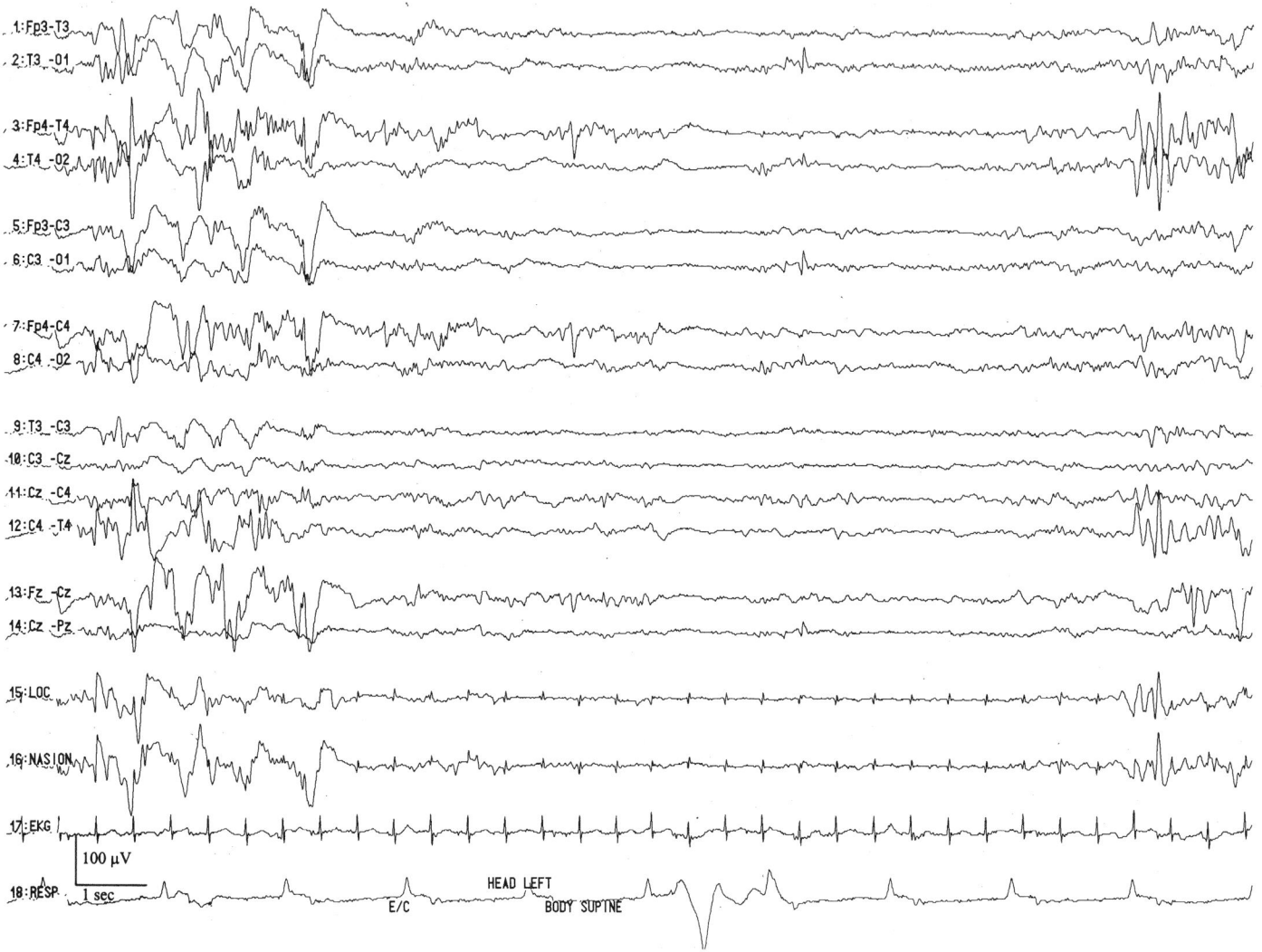

FIG. 6.35. Excessive discontinuity for age in an infant 37 weeks of conceptional age with cervical teratoma. The interburst interval is 11 seconds, which is excessive for an infant of this age.

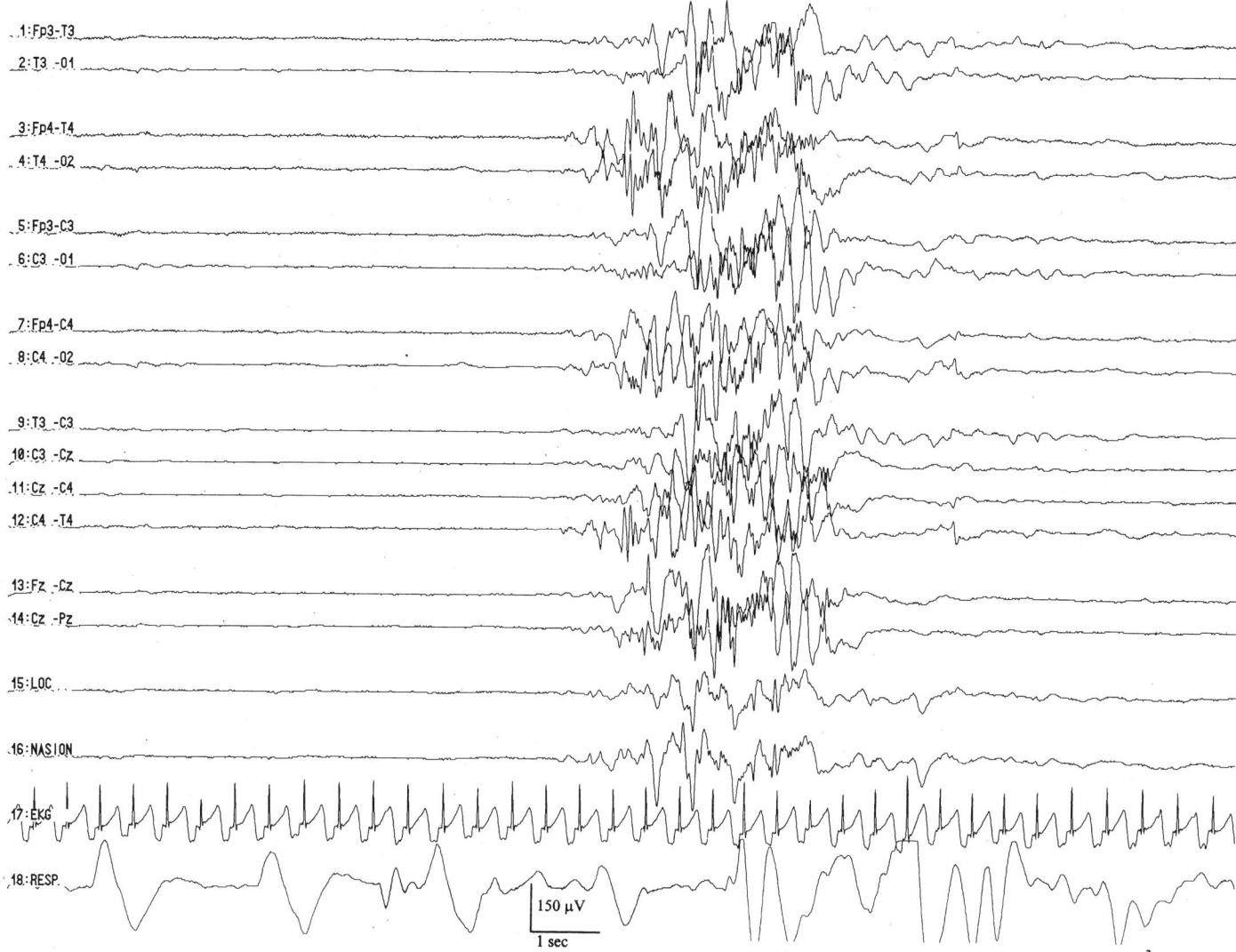

FIG. 6.36. Burst suppression in an infant 38 weeks of conceptional age with multiple contractures and dysmorphic features. The burst of activity is clearly abnormal and contains obvious sharp waves and spikes. The interburst interval is very low amplitude. This pattern persisted for the duration of the recording and did not react to noxious stimulation.

TABLE 6.1. *Longest acceptable single interburst interval (IBI) duration values for conceptional age*

Conceptional age	<30 weeks	31–33 weeks	34–36 weeks	37–40 weeks
Maximal IBI	30–35 s	20 s	10 s	6 s

Adapted from Hahn J, Monyer H, Tharp B. Interburst interval measurements in the EEGs of premature infants with normal neurological function. *Electroencephalogr Clin Neurophysiol* 1989;73:410–4.

are no universally agreed-upon IBI duration criteria that define the exact boundaries of "mildly," "moderately," or "markedly" excessive discontinuity for conceptional age. Previous studies (90–93) suggested that 30-second IBIs were moderately prolonged for a conceptional age of less than 30 weeks or 45 seconds for a conceptional age of 30 weeks or more. Typical IBIs exceeding 60 seconds were markedly abnormal for any conceptional age. However, these earlier criteria have not been revalidated for contemporary practice and are possibly outdated. Certainly, 30-second IBIs would be considered prolonged by today's standards. Like burst suppression, excessive discontinuity is an etiologically nonspecific EEG background abnormality.

Abnormal Voltage

The voltage or amplitude of a normal neonatal EEG regularly and predictably varies with conceptional age and biobehavioral state. For example, the voltages of the EEG bursts during quiet sleep in a premature infant are quite robust, whereas those during active sleep after quiet sleep are much lower in full-term infants. Several descriptions of background abnormalities caused by low voltage have been proposed. Other than the isoelectric recording, no single proposal has been universally accepted.

Persistent Low Voltage

The background in a persistently low-voltage record is attenuated and usually composed of 5- to 15-μV activity during wakefulness and 10- to 25-μV activity during quiet sleep (64). Faster frequencies may be especially "depressed" or of low voltage, but the EEG should otherwise have the normal states, patterns, and frequencies expected for conceptional age. This pattern has been described in some full-term newborns and is prognostically significant only if it persists into the third week after term.

Depressed and Undifferentiated

In this abnormal pattern, the term *depressed and undifferentiated* describes the reduction of rich, complex, faster "polyfrequency" background EEG patterns and does not directly imply a depression of voltage, even though many records of this variety are, in fact, of very low amplitude (<10 μV) (Figs. 6.37 and 6.38). These records may also be excessively discontinuous and do not change with state or stimulation. Low-amplitude, poorly organized electrographic seizures of the "depressed brain type" may be recorded. This is a nonspecific pattern that may be present in many severe conditions, including asphyxia, cerebral hemorrhage, overt dysgenesis, CNS infections, and inborn errors of metabolism. However, postictal states, hypothermia, high drug levels, and very abnormal acid-base status may briefly cause similar EEG patterns and should therefore be ruled out before a prognosis is made.

Isoelectric

When the neonatal EEG is performed in accordance with the established technological criteria to determine electrocerebral silence (ECS) in cases of suspected brain death, the absence of any definite cerebral electrical activity greater than 2 μV constitutes an *isoelectric* tracing (Fig. 6.39). The challenge is to distinguish the ubiquitous recording artifacts in the electronically hostile environment of the neonatal intensive care unit from genuine cerebral electrical activity. Unfortunately, different recording sensitivity criteria have historically been used to define this pattern in neonates. Reported amplitudes in isoelectric recordings have ranged from less than 2 to 10 μV, depending on the investigator. However, the absence of discernible background activity with the sensitivity set at 2 μV in a continuously nonreactive record remains the formal criteria of the American Electroencephalographic Society (2).

Abnormal Asymmetry

A persistent interhemispheric amplitude asymmetry of more than 50% is considered an electrographic abnormality (4,52,55). Persistent amplitude asymmetries may be broadly attributable to excessively high amplitudes in one area or excessively low amplitudes in another. In individual patients, it may be difficult to decide which hemisphere is "abnormal" on the basis of amplitude criteria alone. Neonatal EEG activity is commonly classified in

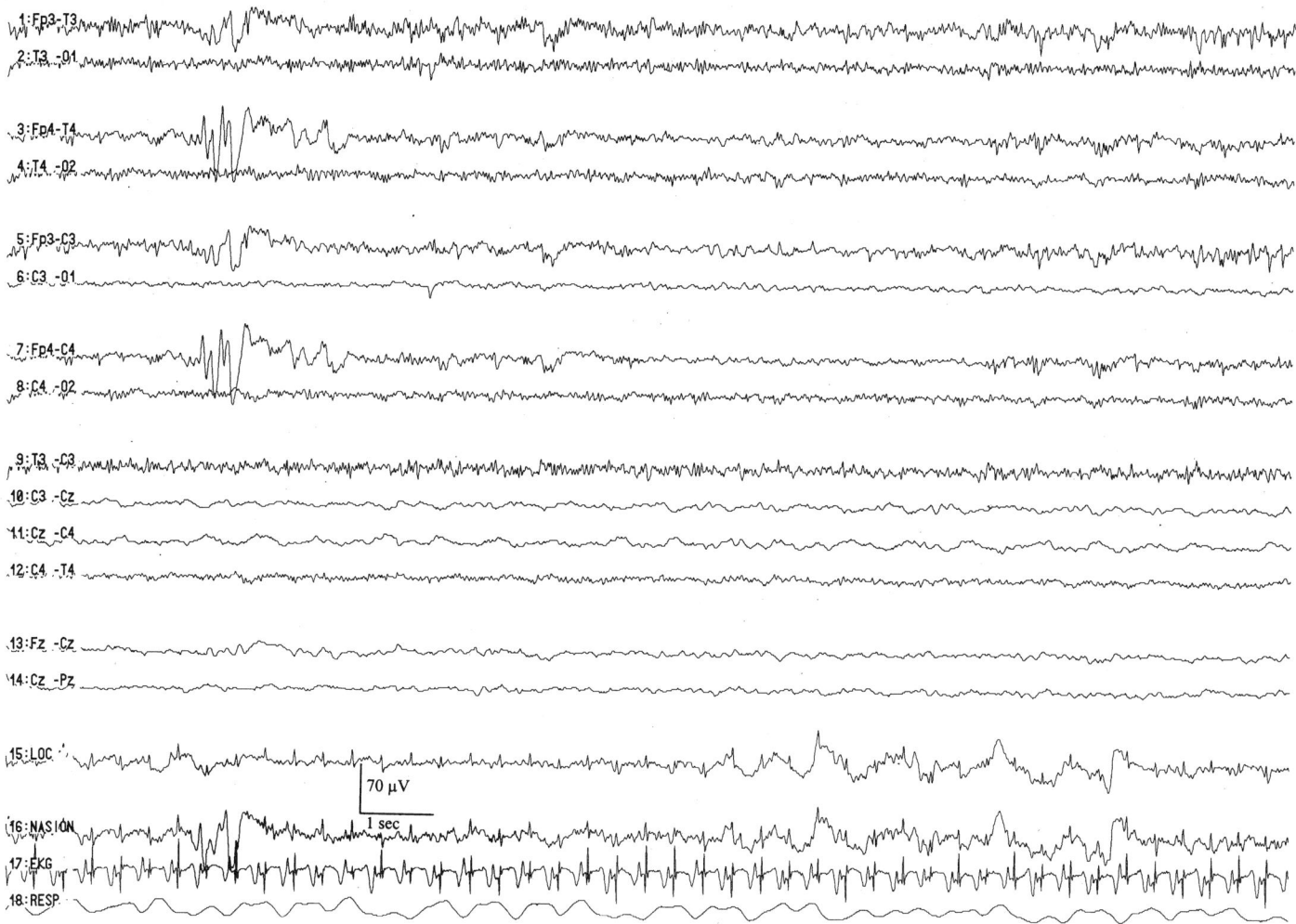

FIG. 6.37. Depressed and undifferentiated background in an infant 41 weeks of conceptional age with birth trauma. The background shows little of the rich, polyfrequency activity expected in a healthy infant of this age.

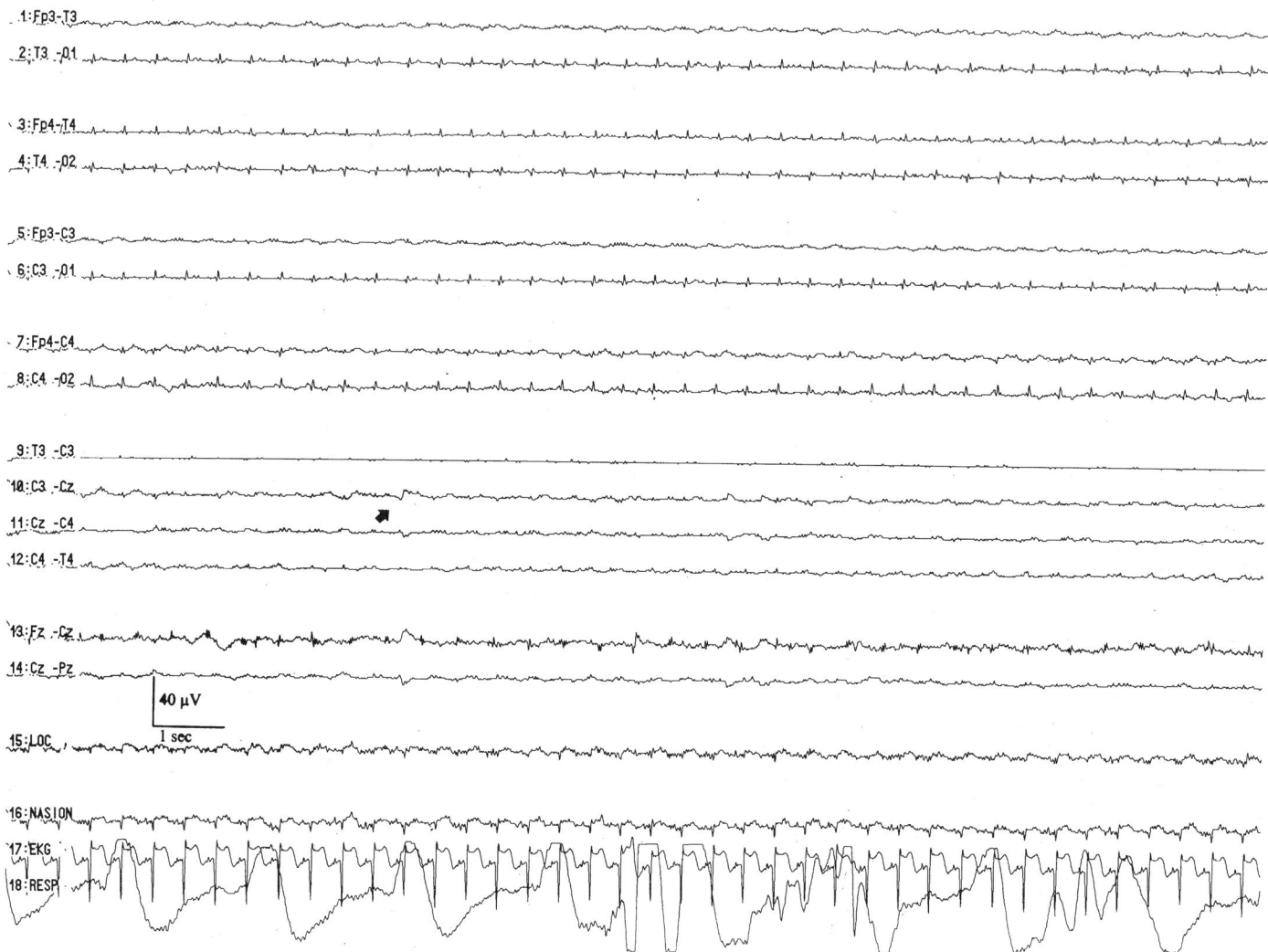

FIG. 6.38. Extreme low voltage background in an infant 39 weeks of conceptional age with severe hypoxic-ischemic encephalopathy. Cerebral activity is nearly absent, except for some minimal slow activity at Cz (*arrow*).

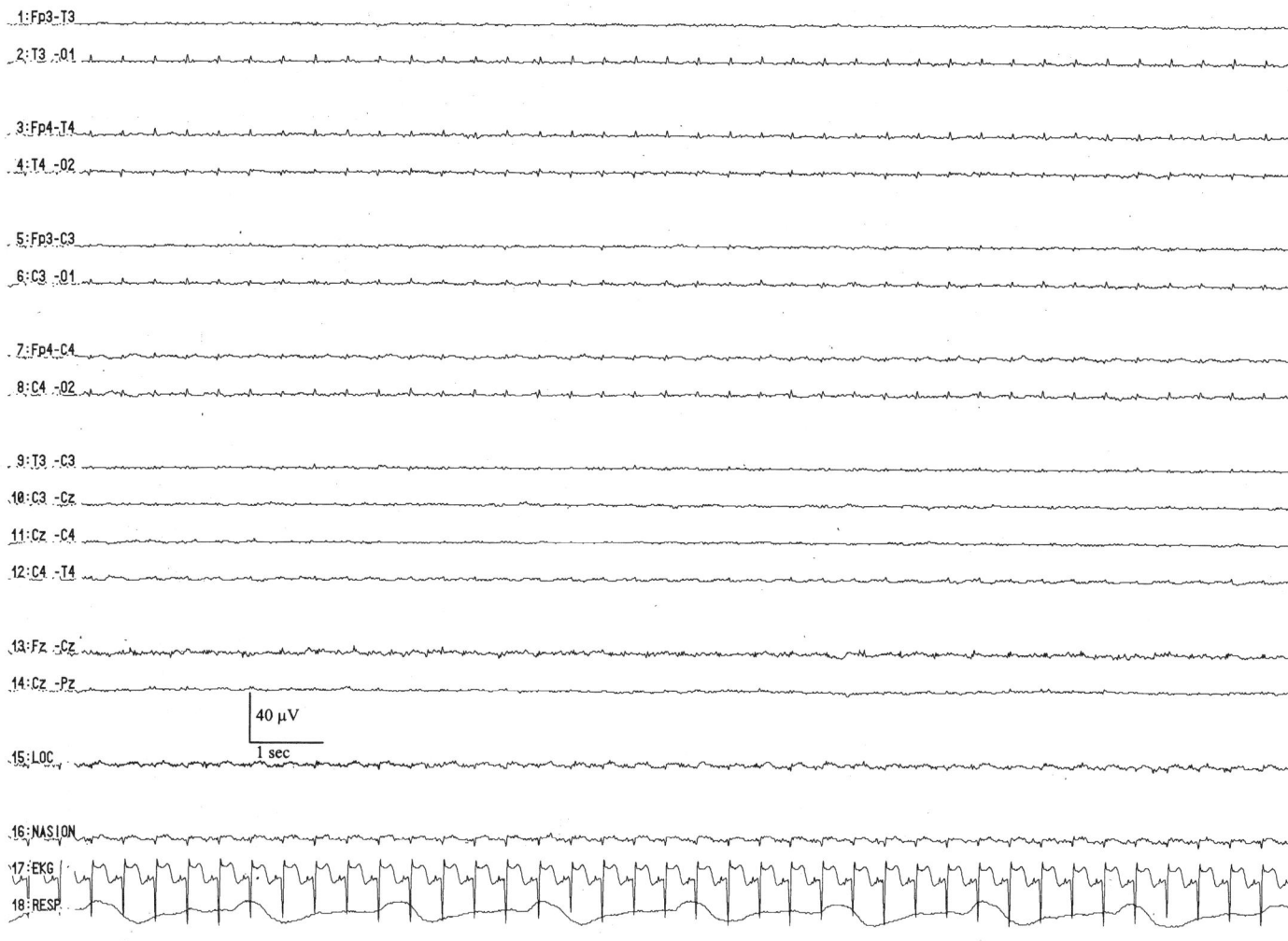

FIG. 6.39. Isoelectric or electrocerebral silence (ECS) in an infant 39 weeks of conceptional age with clinical brain death from severe hypoxic-ischemic encephalopathy. No definite cerebral activity is seen at maximal recording sensitivity. Electrocardiographic artifact is present.

bipolar montages as low (<25 μV), medium (25 to 50 μV), and high (50 to 200 μV) in amplitude. Although extremely high or low amplitudes may themselves technically constitute an abnormality, the interpreter should carefully inspect the EEG background composition before making the definitive determination of abnormal asymmetry.

Most causes of acute encephalopathy in the neonate arise from diffuse pathological conditions such as global hypoxia-ischemia, metabolic abnormalities, or sepsis with meningitis, and EEGs recorded in these circumstances display symmetric abnormalities. Focal brain injury may be caused by localized cerebral infarction (stroke), venous or dural sinus thrombosis, abscess, restricted hemorrhage, contusion, or similar pathological processes. The EEG asymmetries in these circumstances often appear as a voltage reduction (from loss of signal generators), seizures arising from a limited number of brain regions, depression of normal background patterns, focal slowing, or sharp waves (see Fig. 6.19). On the other hand, when the electrographic asymmetry is purely a loss of voltage (see Fig. 6.20), with preservation of the composition of the background, a technical problem (e.g., electrode spacing or asymmetrical scalp edema) or possible subdural fluid collection could be responsible.

The unfavorable prognostic significance of this abnormality has been reported by several authors (3,4,52,55,95). In the setting of meningitis, Chequer et al. (14) reported that persistent EEG asymmetries correlated well with specific localized injuries such as abscess or large vessel infarction. Tharp et al. (91) noted that in nine patients with more than 50% amplitude asymmetry persisting in all states, the prognosis was poor, including death or definite neurological handicaps. In contrast, neonates with less than 50% interhemispheric asymmetry with an otherwise normal EEG for conceptional age enjoyed a favorable prognosis, even if the abnormality persisted throughout the record.

Abnormal Interhemispheric Asynchrony

Synchrony is typically determined by analyzing 5 minutes of the discontinuous portion of the EEG (64,93). Interhemispheric bursts separated by more than 1.5 to 2 seconds of each other are considered asynchronous. The percentage of EEG bursts that are synchronized approach 100% in the healthy full-term infant. Gross asynchrony of the EEG is rarely encountered in isolation; instead, it is usually accompanied by other obvious background abnormalities such as excessive discontinuity or burst suppression. Excessive asynchrony can be seen in a variety of *acute* causes of encephalopathy, such as hypoxic-ischemic encephalopathy (HIE) or meningitis, and in *chronic* conditions, such as cerebral dysgenesis. Neuropathological findings in infants with an abnormally asynchronous EEG include periventricular leukomalacia, intraventricular hemorrhage, and any developmental abnormality of the corpus callosum (4). Aicardi's syndrome is confined to girls and characterized by distinctive retinal colobomas, agenesis of the corpus callosum, occasional interhemispheric cysts, striking degree of interhemispheric EEG asynchrony, and refractory, early-onset seizures that include infantile spasms (88).

Abnormal Maturation

In the setting of acute encephalopathies such as HIE or trauma, the common EEG background abnormalities of excessive discontinuity, depressed background composition, and impaired reactivity are useful yardsticks for measuring the impact of the disease on functional CNS integrity. However, infants exposed to subacute, prolonged illness may never experience a sudden, sentinel clinical event; rather, they are neurologically stressed over extended time frames. Examples of such infants are premature infants who require long-term mechanical ventilation because of bronchopulmonary dysplasia and full-term infants affected with congestive heart failure from a congenital heart defect. In these infants, the CNS may not mature at the appropriate rate. Such chronically ill infants experience an actual delay or arrest of physical brain development that can be reflected as "immaturity" in serial EEG examinations (37,93).

A neonatal EEG record is considered immature or dysmature (Fig. 6.40) if it contains patterns that indicate that its current maturity is 2 or more weeks younger than the stated conceptional age (52). Interpretative criteria used to determine dysmaturity include the degree of discontinuity during quiet sleep, the degree of interhemispheric asynchrony, the frequency and location of delta brushes during active sleep and quiet sleep, the presence of *encoches frontales,* and the number of temporal theta bursts. Rating an EEG as dysmature is relatively subjective, although normative scales have been suggested to aid with the diagnosis (11,35,54,69). The pathological correlate of a persistently immature EEG is actual CNS dysmaturity, visible as inappropriately delayed neuronal migration and maturation. Transient dysmaturity is not correlated with a poor prognosis, although persistent dysmaturity on serial EEGs can be associated with an unfavorable outcome.

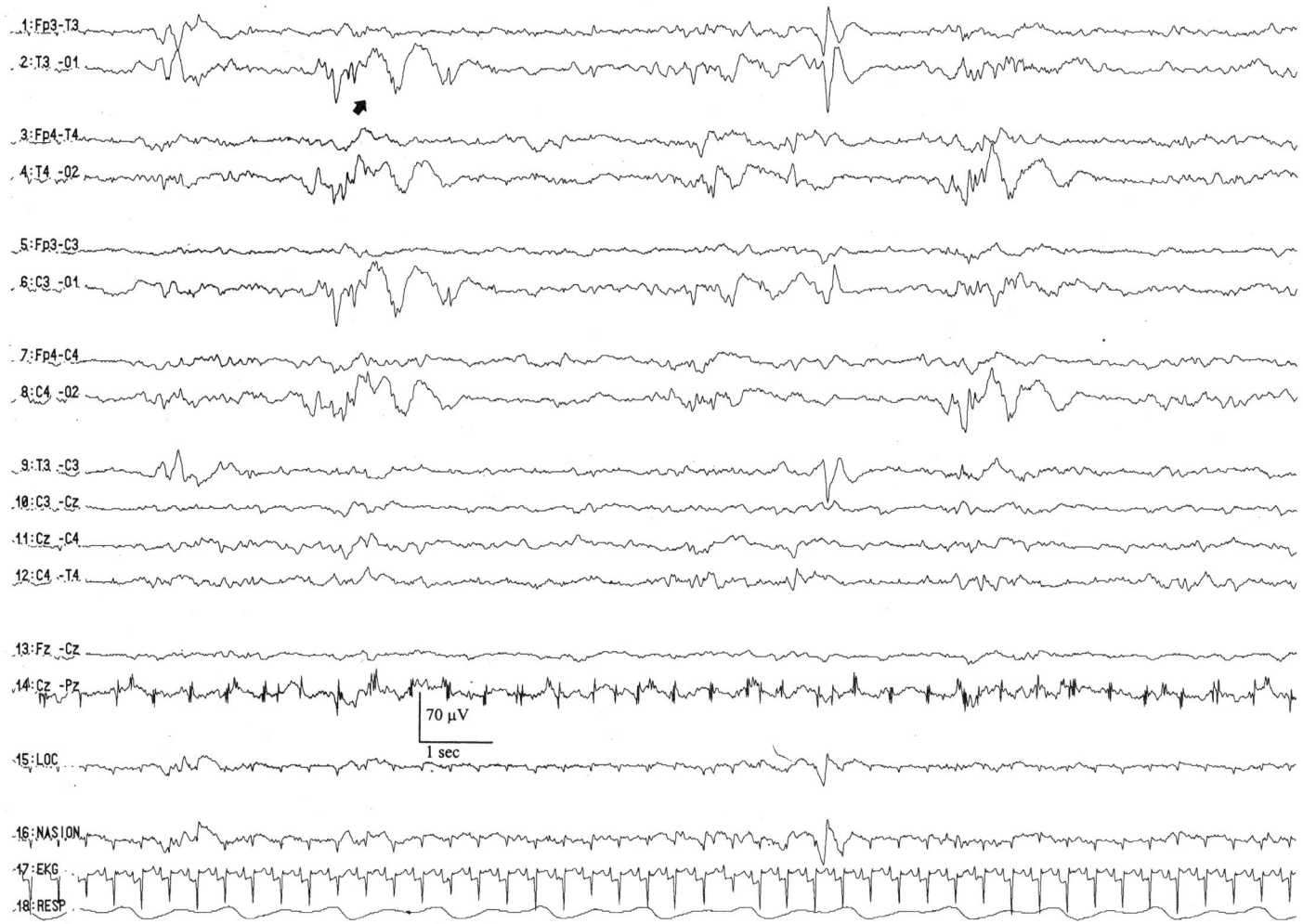

FIG. 6.40. Immature background for age in an infant 42 weeks of conceptional age with complex congenital heart disease. Rhythmic occipital delta activity (*arrow*) is not normally present in infants of this conceptional age.

Classification of the Electroencephalographic Background and Its Implications

The EEG background correlates strongly with a neonate's clinical neurological status, prognosis, and eventual neurological outcome. Several grading systems of the neonatal EEG background have been suggested (24,25,41, 53,64,91,92,98). Although there are minor differences among the grading scales, the main features are similar and broadly classify tracings as normal or mildly, moderately, or markedly abnormal according to criteria describing continuity, voltage, reactivity, and background composition (Table 6.2).

TABLE 6.2. *Classification of electroencephalographic background activity*

1. Normal
2. Transient or persistent immaturity (dysmaturity)
3. Mildly abnormal
   a. Mildly excessive discontinuity during the discontinuous portions of the tracing
   b. Mildly excessive interhemispheric asynchrony for conceptional age
   c. Poor concordance between clinical and electrographic sleep states
   d. Mild poverty of anticipated background rhythms for conceptional age (e.g., mild decrease in monorhythmic occipital delta activity, rhythmic occipital or temporal theta activity, brushes)
   e. Mild focal abnormalities (e.g., excessive sharp waves in temporal or central regions, focal voltage attenuation)
4. Moderately abnormal
   a. Moderately excessive discontinuity during the discontinuous portions of the tracing
   b. Moderately excessive interhemispheric asynchrony for conceptional age
   c. Poverty of anticipated background rhythms for conceptional age
   d. Definite focal abnormalities (e.g., persistent focal delta activity or focal depression of expected background patterns such as brushes)
   e. Persistent low voltage (generalized reduction of voltage <25 µV for all states)
5. Markedly abnormal
   a. Markedly excessive discontinuity for age, despite the preservation of some age-appropriate background patterns
   b. Burst suppression pattern
   c. Gross interhemispheric asynchrony
   d. Extremely low voltage (<5 µV)
   e. Depressed and undifferentiated
   f. Isoelectric

Adapted from Clancy R, Tharp B. Positive rolandic sharp waves in the electroencephalograms of premature neonates with intraventricular hemorrhage. *Electroencephalogr Clin Neurophysiol* 1984;57:395–404.

Most infants with markedly abnormal EEG backgrounds have an abnormal mental status (lethargy or coma) caused by the severe, diffuse acute encephalopathy and face a very high risk of an unfavorable outcome such as death or permanent neurological disability (84). Infants with an *unexplained,* grossly abnormal EEG background may harbor an unexpected cerebral dysgenesis such as holoprosencephaly. Infants with normal serial EEGs usually have normal mental status, as assessed by examination, and were exposed to mild or minimal diffuse pathological processes or to definite but restricted injuries. For example, an infant with an acute embolic stroke usually has a normal mental status and a well-preserved overall EEG, although focal abnormalities may be evident (21). Most infants with normal or mildly abnormal tracings have a favorable outcome. However, those with genetic disorders such as Down's syndrome who have not experienced any type of acute encephalopathy also display nearly normal records, despite the realistic expectation for an abnormal neurological outcome. Moderately abnormal EEGs fall between these two extremes with regard to the coincident mental status, the cause or causes of the encephalopathy, and the chances of an adverse outcome.

The prognostic value of serial EEGs in premature infants has been shown in many studies, including the study by Tharp et al. (92) of 81 infants younger than 36 weeks of EGA. Markedly abnormal EEGs were associated with a 96% incidence of death or adverse outcome. Worsening on serial EEGs was seen in 41% of the children with major neurological sequelae but only in 3% of patients with normal outcome and 15% of those with minor sequelae. Tharp et al. (93) investigated infants weighing less than 1,200 g who were admitted to their neonatal intensive care unit and found that EEG was better than the clinical neurological examination at predicting poor outcome (72% versus 39%). Normal outcome was predicted with equal accuracy by the clinical examination and the EEG. In the study by Clancy et al. (22) of 101 premature infants with EEG and head ultrasound (HUS) examinations, survival rates were significantly better among those with normal or mildly abnormal recordings (Fig. 6.41). The prognostic value of serial EEG has also been investigated in full-term infants. Watanabe et al. (98) assessed 173 full-term infants after HIE and found that infants with mild background abnormalities that lessened over the first few days of life had a good outcome. Poorer outcome was noted if markedly abnormal abnormalities persisted more than 4 days or if milder abnormalities lasted many days.

What are the neuropathological correlates of the abnormal EEG? Few investigators have attempted to address this important question by directly

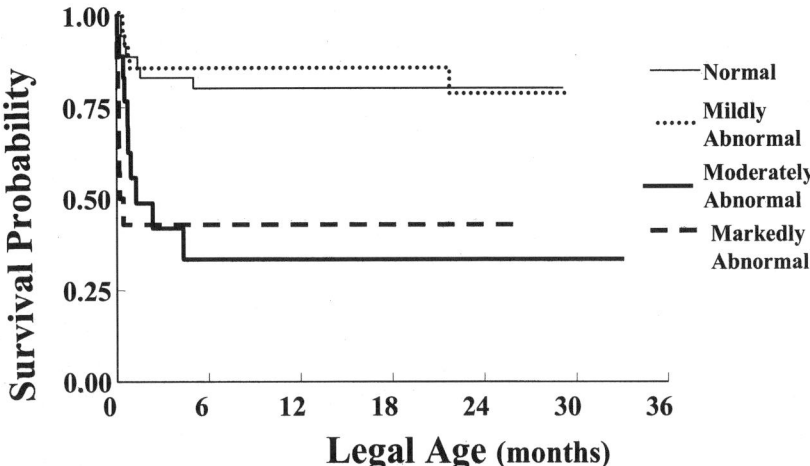

 # p < .00005: normal/mildly vs moderately/markedly abnormal

FIG. 6.41. Kaplan-Meier survival curve shows significantly greater survival in premature infants with normal or mildly abnormal electroencephalographic backgrounds than in those with moderately or markedly abnormal tracings. (Adapted from Clancy R, Rosenberg H, Bernbaum J, et al. Survival outcome prediction in premature infants with IVH by cranial ultrasonography and EEG. *Ann Neurol* 1994;36:489.)

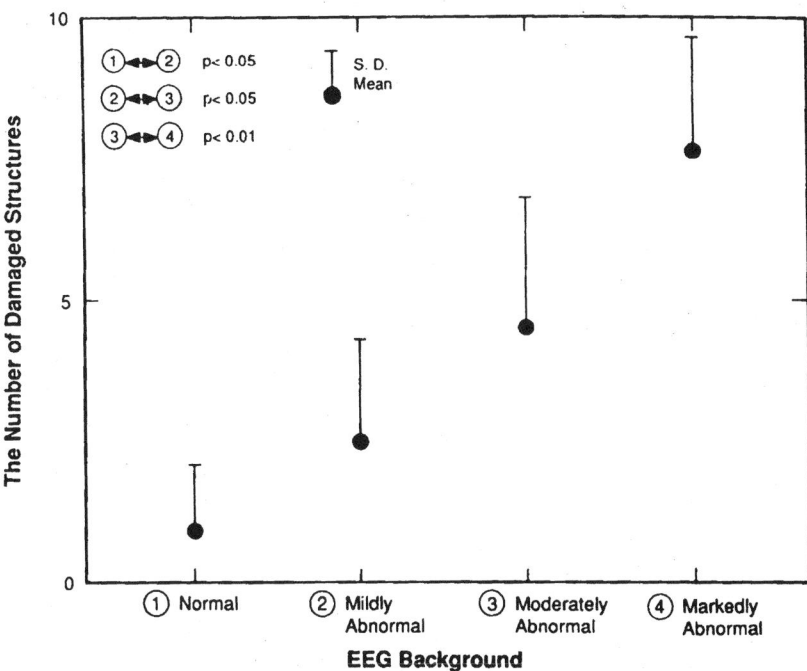

FIG. 6.42. The correlation between the electroencephalographic background and the number of neuropathological lesions. (Adapted from Aso K, Scher M, Barmada M. Neonatal electroencephalography and neuropathology. *J Clin Neurophysiol* 1989;6:103–123.)

associating the varieties and severities of EEG background patterns with the results of postmortem brain examinations (3,4,73,92). Because markedly abnormal EEGs empirically confer an adverse neurological outcome, it is reasonable to attempt to understand its neuropathological basis. In the largest study of its type, Aso et al. (3) analyzed 107 EEGs in 47 infants who later died during the neonatal period and on whom autopsy was performed. Macroscopic and microscopic examinations were performed in selected anatomical structures: the cerebral cortex, subcortical white matter, corpus callosum, thalamus, hypothalamus, corpus striatum, midbrain, pons, and medulla. Normal EEGs correlated with histologically normal brains, whereas progressively abnormal EEGs were associated with more extensive and severe neuropathological processes. The degree of EEG abnormality significantly correlated with the number of damaged brain regions counted at autopsy (Fig. 6.42). Some interesting electrographic-neuropathological associations were also revealed. Isoelectric EEGs were correlated consistently with widespread encephalomalacia and, commonly, with ischemic

necrosis of the cortex, thalamus, corpus striatum, midbrain, and pons. Burst suppression patterns were also associated with multifocal lesions, including widespread neuronal necrosis but variably present intraventricular hemorrhage (IVH), periventricular leukomalacia, cerebral infarctions, and pontosubicular necrosis. There was no single lesion present in all infants with burst suppression. Interhemispheric amplitude asymmetries of more than 50% were correlated with localized cerebral lesions, including infarctions and IVH. The hemisphere with more EEG attenuation was the worst affected pathologically. Excessive asynchrony was identified in 9 of 18 patients older than 31 weeks of conceptional age. Their anatomical abnormalities were mild to moderate in severity but specifically involved the corpus callosum in only two. Conversely, no child with normal synchrony had a callosal lesion. Positive rolandic sharp waves (PRSs) were always associated with white matter lesions but did not consistently correlate with any other type of neuropathology. PRSs were a highly specific but insensitive marker, inasmuch as the incidence of PRS was only 32% in those with proven white matter lesions.

SHARP ELECTROENCEPHALOGRAPHIC TRANSIENTS

Sharp EEG transients (SETs) are defined as sharply contoured waves of brief duration that are clearly distinguishable from the ongoing background activity. In the neonatal EEG, the definitions of a sharp wave and a spike are slightly different from those used in pediatric and adult EEG. SETs with a duration between 100 and 500 milliseconds are called *sharp waves,* whereas those with a duration of 100 milliseconds or less are *spikes.* The polarity of sharp waves or spikes may be monophasic, biphasic, or polyphasic. SETs may appear in any scalp location. Just as SETs in older persons may be innocent (e.g., lambda waves or small sharp spikes) or pathological, a similar situation exists in the interpretation of neonatal EEGs. Interpretative criteria to assist in the discrimination between physiological and pathological SETs have been proposed.

Frontal Sharp Electroencephalographic Transients

Morphologically, physiological frontal sharp waves (*encoches frontales*) are high-amplitude (>150-µV), broad, biphasic (negative-positive) transients seen maximally in the frontal regions (Fp3 and Fp4). They generally appear symmetrically, bilaterally, and synchronously; however, when they first appear at around 34 weeks of conceptional age, they may arise somewhat asynchronously. *Encoches frontales* may appear alone or may intermingle with runs of slow 2- to 4-Hz waves (anterior dysrhythmia) (Fig. 6.43). Frontal sharp waves are most abundant during the transition from active sleep to early quiet sleep and are scarce in the period of active sleep that immediately follows arousal from quiet sleep. They persist until about 4 weeks after birth, at which point they begin to disappear (29). *Encoche frontales* are normal, physiological, age-dependent SETs that do not suggest a "lowered seizure threshold."

Several characteristics of pathological frontal sharp waves distinguish them from the innocent *encoches frontales.* A clearly excessive amount of frontal slowing and *encoches frontales* in active sleep/wakefulness may be seen in the context of resolving or mild HIE, meningitis, or metabolic encephalopathies. Frontal SETs that are atypical in morphology (e.g., true spikes) or are markedly asymmetrical may also be considered electrographic abnormalities (Fig. 6.44).

Temporal and Central Negative Sharp Electroencephalographic Transients

The initial and predominant deflection of negative SETs is surface polarity negative in standard bipolar derivations. They may be found in any scalp region but are most frequent in the temporal and central regions. Negative centrotemporal SETs are best evaluated during the low-voltage, continuous portions of the tracing, which correspond to wakefulness and active sleep. It is difficult to quantitatively evaluate sharp waves that may occur during the bursts of activity in immature quiet sleep, because many infants generate "spikey" or sharp-quality quiet sleep bursts. Few data describing SETs before the conceptional age of 33 to 34 weeks are available.

The significance of abnormal negative sharp waves is controversial. Some authors consider them a nonspecific electrographic finding that may occur in a variety of pathological conditions without a clear relationship to clinical or electrographic seizures (55,56). This situation has a counterpart in adult EEGs in that sharp waves may be seen in uremia, hypoxia with ischemia, and drug withdrawal without the presence of clinical or electrographic seizures and may be interpreted as nonspecific electrographic abnormalities (23). However, there is also evidence in neonates that some characteristics of negative, centrotemporal SETs are epileptiform and are encountered more commonly in infants with seizures. Clancy (16) examined the EEG backgrounds and characteristics of SETs in 78 EEGs from 30 neonates with confirmed electrographic seizures and compared them with the EEG characteristics of SETs recorded from 69 healthy neonates without seizures. Both the EEG background and specific features of negative SETs were contrasted in the seizure and comparison groups. In the seizure group, 41 (52.6%) of 78 tracings had EEG backgrounds classified as moderately or severely abnormal, in comparison with 0 of 69 abnormal backgrounds in the comparison group. Centrotemporal SETs were characterized in terms of *abundance* (number of SETs counted during a 10-minute continuous EEG epoch), *morphology* (spike versus sharp wave), *repetitive behavior,* and *spatial distribution* (among locations C3, C4, T3, and T4).

In infants without seizures, centrotemporal SETs (Fig. 6.45*A* and *B*) occurred at a rate of less than one per minute (Fig. 6.46) and were evenly distributed between both hemispheres (T3 and C3 versus T4 and C4), both

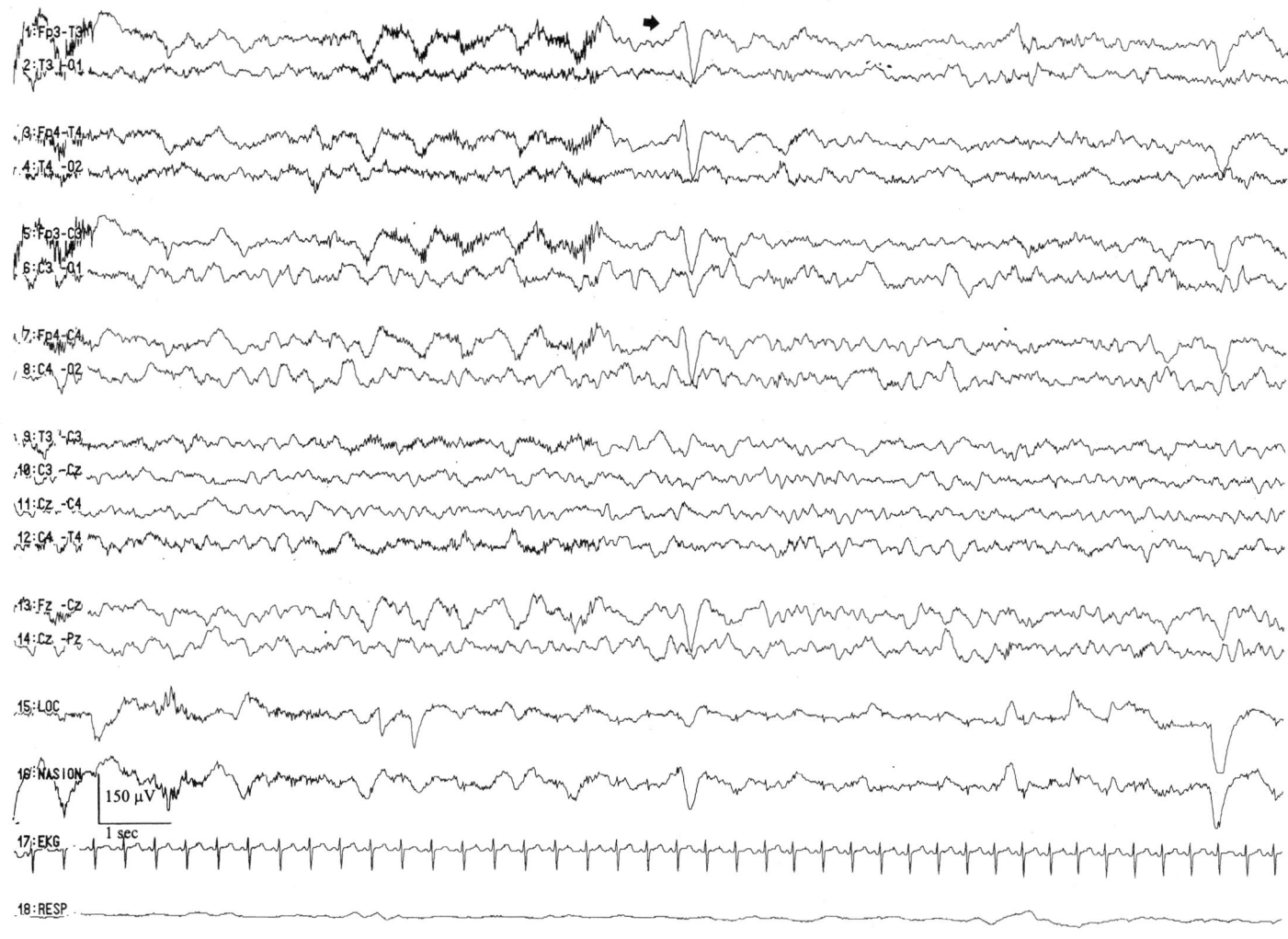

FIG. 6.43. *Encoches frontales* in an infant 40 weeks of conceptional age with clinically suspected seizures. Normal frontal sharp waves—*encoches frontales*—(*arrow*) are admixed with anterior dysrhythmia.

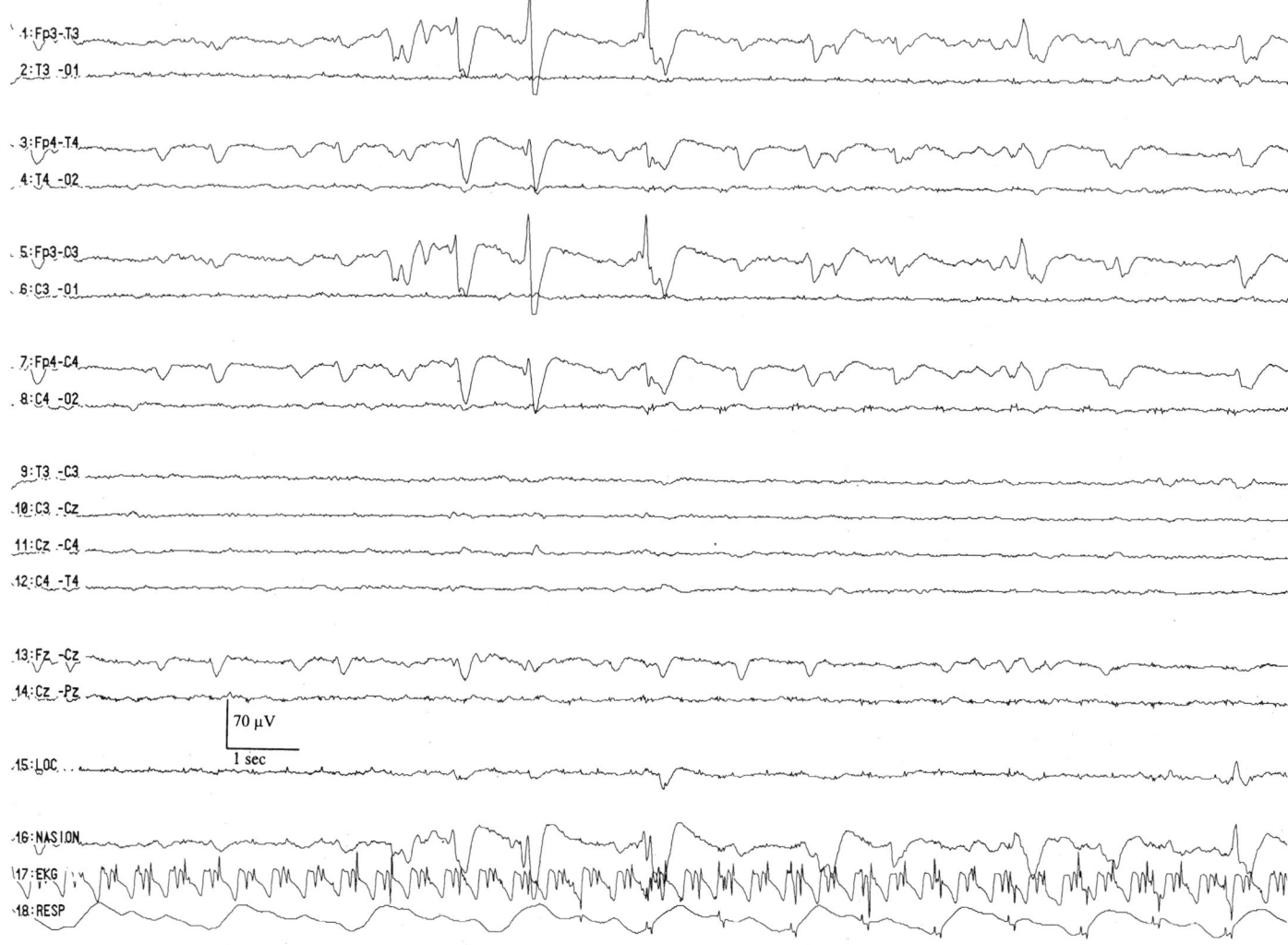

FIG. 6.44. Abnormal frontal sharp waves in an infant 41 weeks of conceptional age with head trauma. Frontal sharp waves are excessively sharp and superimposed on a featureless background.

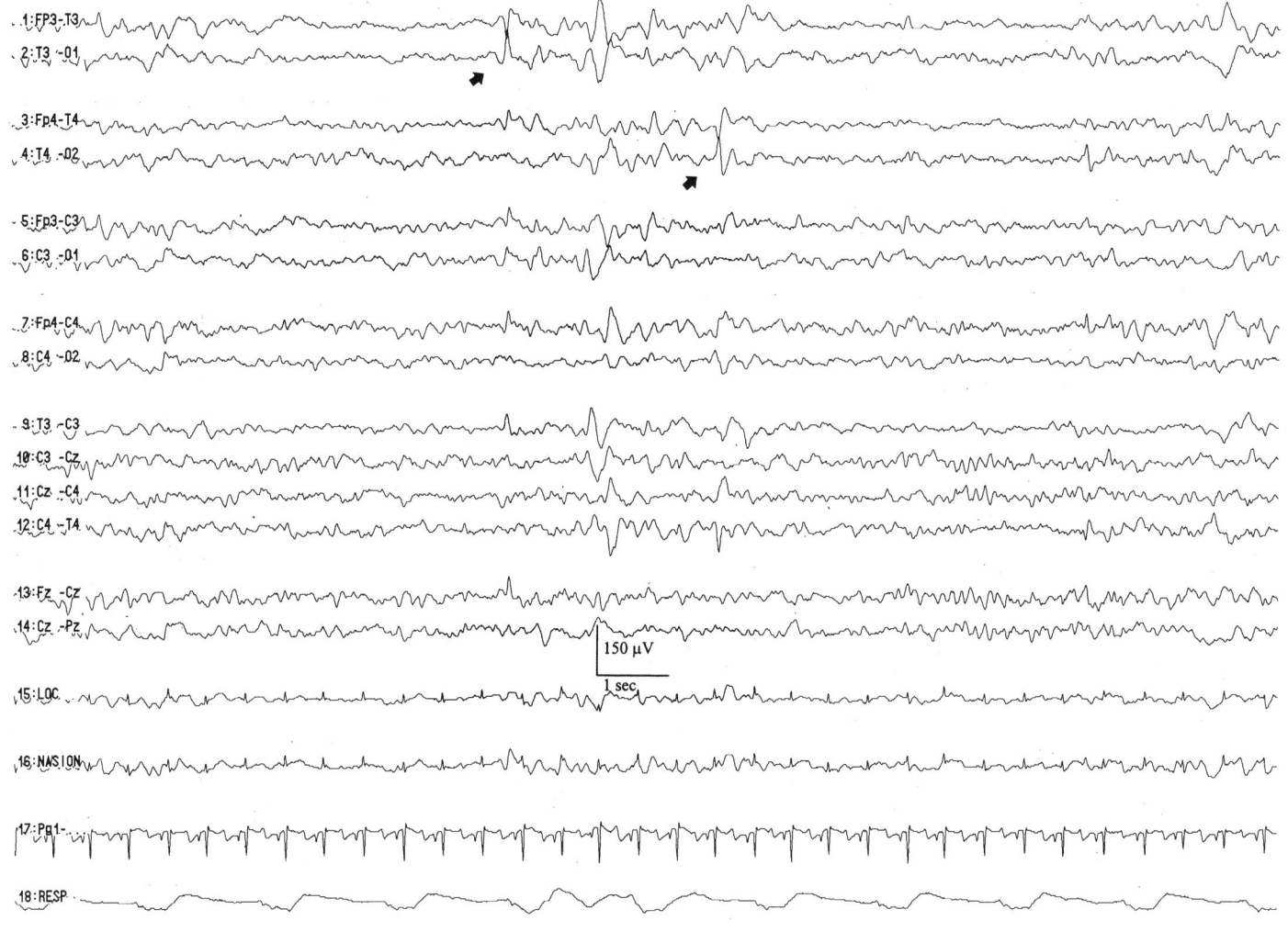

A

FIG. 6.45. A: Normal temporal sharp electrographic transients (SETs) in an infant 43 weeks of conceptional age with pneumonia. Right and left temporal SETs (*arrows*) are present. In this tracing, SETs were infrequent and were equally distributed between both temporal regions. (*Figure continues.*)

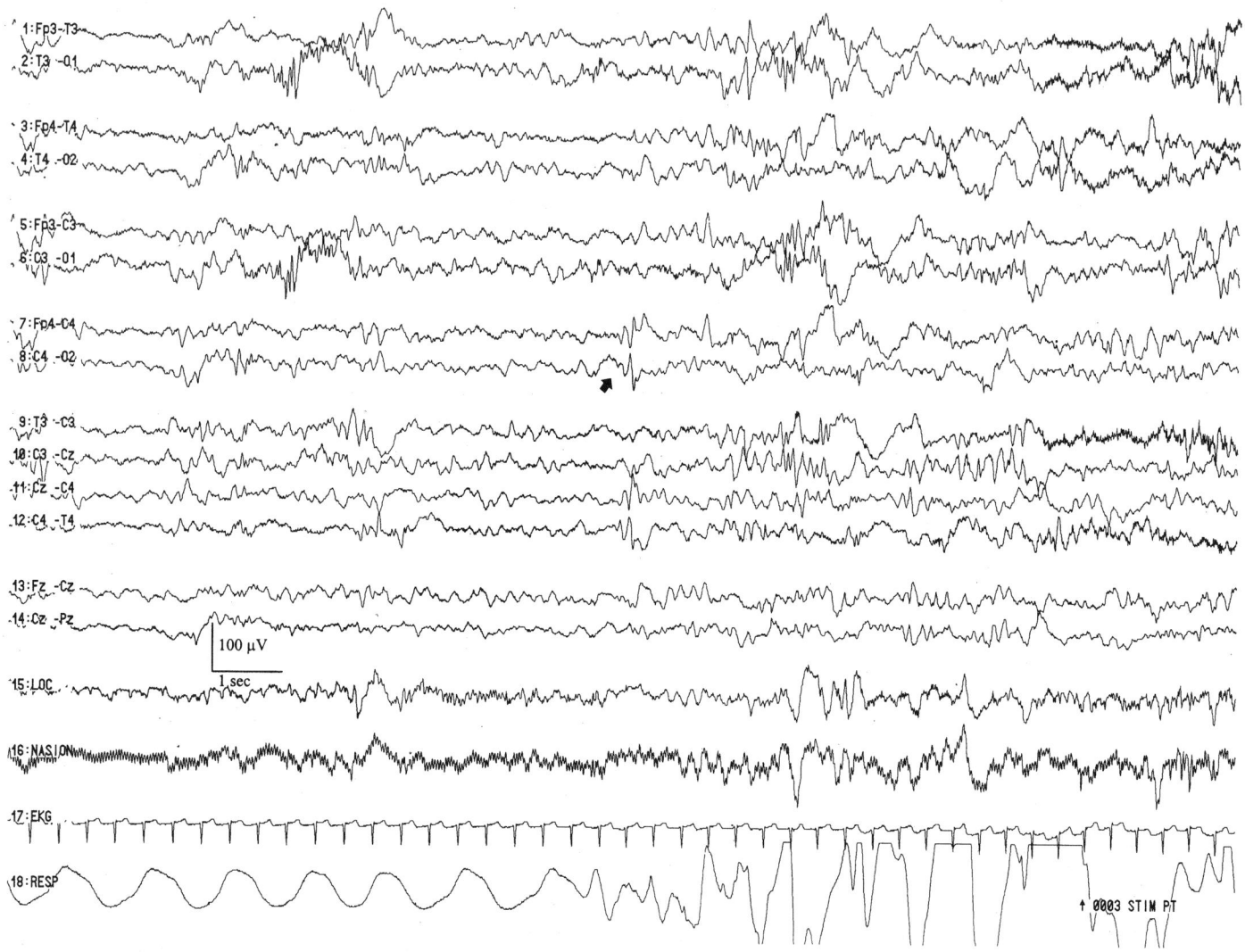

B

FIG. 6.45. *Continued.* **B:** Normal central SETs in an infant 39 weeks of conceptional age with Pierre Robin syndrome. *Arrow* indicates a normal-appearing right central negative sharp wave. Rare right and left temporal and central negative sharp waves were present in this record.

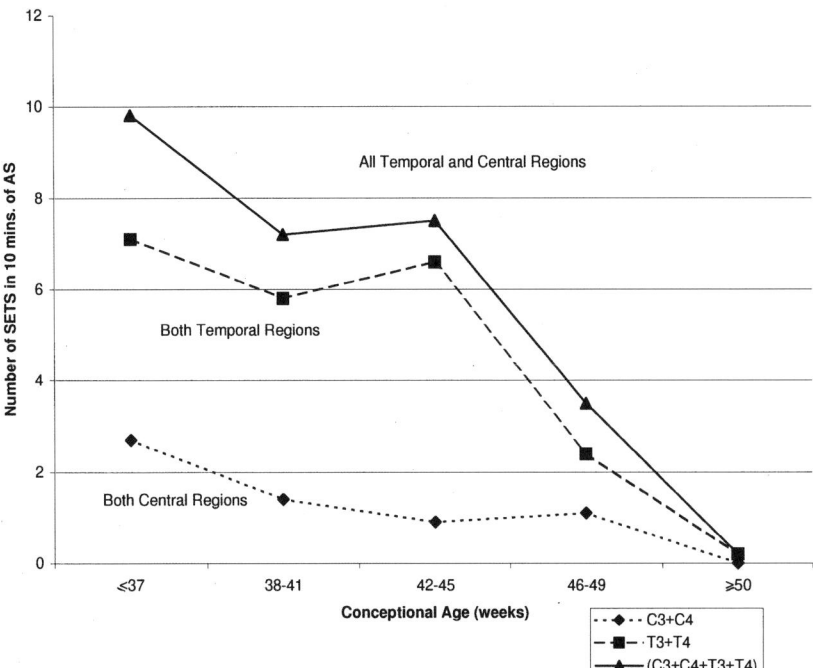

FIG. 6.46. Normal abundance of sharp electroencephalographic transients by location and conceptual age. (Adapted from Clancy R. Interictal sharp EEG transients in neonatal seizures. *J Child Neurol* 1989;4:30–38.)

characterized by abnormal backgrounds and excessive spikes or sharp waves that sometimes recurred in brief runs and were distributed nonrandomly in the temporal and central regions.

This study has implications for interpreting EEG abnormalities in infants with seizures that are suspected but not specifically confirmed by recording electrographic seizures. Neonates with abnormal backgrounds and abnormal negative SETs are considered to display patterns of abnormalities similar to those in infants with electrographically confirmed seizures. They may be considered to have EEG characteristics of a "lowered seizure threshold" at that time. However, this constellation of interictal EEG findings is not diagnostic of neonatal seizures. In contrast, neonates with abnormal backgrounds and normal negative SETs have nonspecific cerebral dysfunction. But this does not exclude the possibility of neonatal seizures.

Neonates with normal backgrounds and abnormal SETs are relatively uncommon. However, in the context of the "well neonate" with seizures who has a normal EEG background with abnormal SETs, the diagnostic possibilities should include conditions such as simple hypocalcemia, in which excessive sharp waves tend to arise in the central or central vertex regions (96), and mild subarachnoid hemorrhage, which may "irritate" the cortex.

Negative Sharp EEG Transients in Other Locations

Just as electrographic neonatal *seizures* can arise from any scalp regions, abnormal negative spikes or sharp waves may arise from any or many areas. Multifocal SETs may be recorded from some infants with diffuse encephalopathies, including those involving the midline (Fz, Cz, or Pz) and occipital regions (Figs. 6.48 and 6.49). However, the significance of finding excessive SETs that are limited to the occipital and midline areas is unclear, inasmuch as few studies have systematically examined them (32,61,82).

Positive Sharp Waves (Rolandic, Vertex, and Temporal)

Positive sharp waves may appear in the sick neonate as sharp EEG transients (duration, less than 400 to 500 milliseconds) (7,8,12,15,19, 24,25,27,28,45,59,60,67,68) with an initial and predominant surface-positive polarity. They may arise from the rolandic regions (PRSs) (Fig. 6.50), the central vertex (positive vertex sharp wave [PVS]) (Fig. 6.51), and the

temporal regions (T3 versus T4), and both central regions (C3 versus C4). SETs were more abundant in the temporal areas than in the central areas (Fig. 6.46). In this group, SETs consisted of sharp waves and only rare spikes; runs or bursts of SETs were not seen. In the seizure group, centrotemporal SETs usually occurred more frequently than two per minute, were often spikes (rather than sharp waves), and often recurred in repetitive runs. In the seizure group, SETs were more often nonrandomly distributed: significantly distributed to favor one location or hemisphere more than others (Fig. 6.47). These distinctions between the groups, however, were not absolute. Of 78 EEGs from the seizure group, 16 (21%) had relatively normal backgrounds and SETs that behaved similar to those of the comparison group. Most neonates with EEG-confirmed seizures had interictal tracings

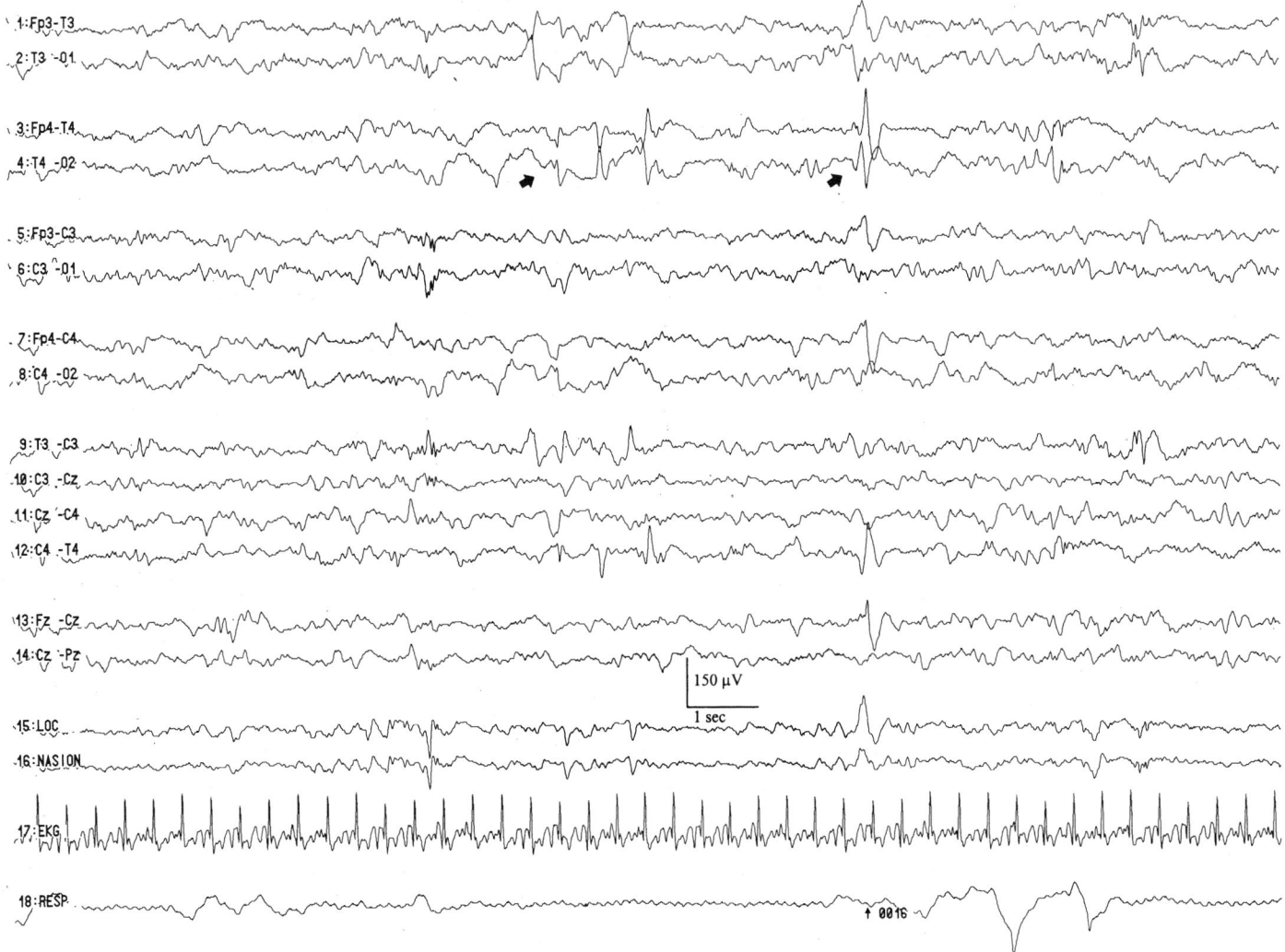

FIG. 6.47. Abnormal temporal sharp electrographic transients (SETs) in an infant 38 weeks of conceptional age with persistent pulmonary hypertension and seizures. Multiple right temporal sharp waves are present (*arrow*). In this record, left temporal sharp waves are rare.

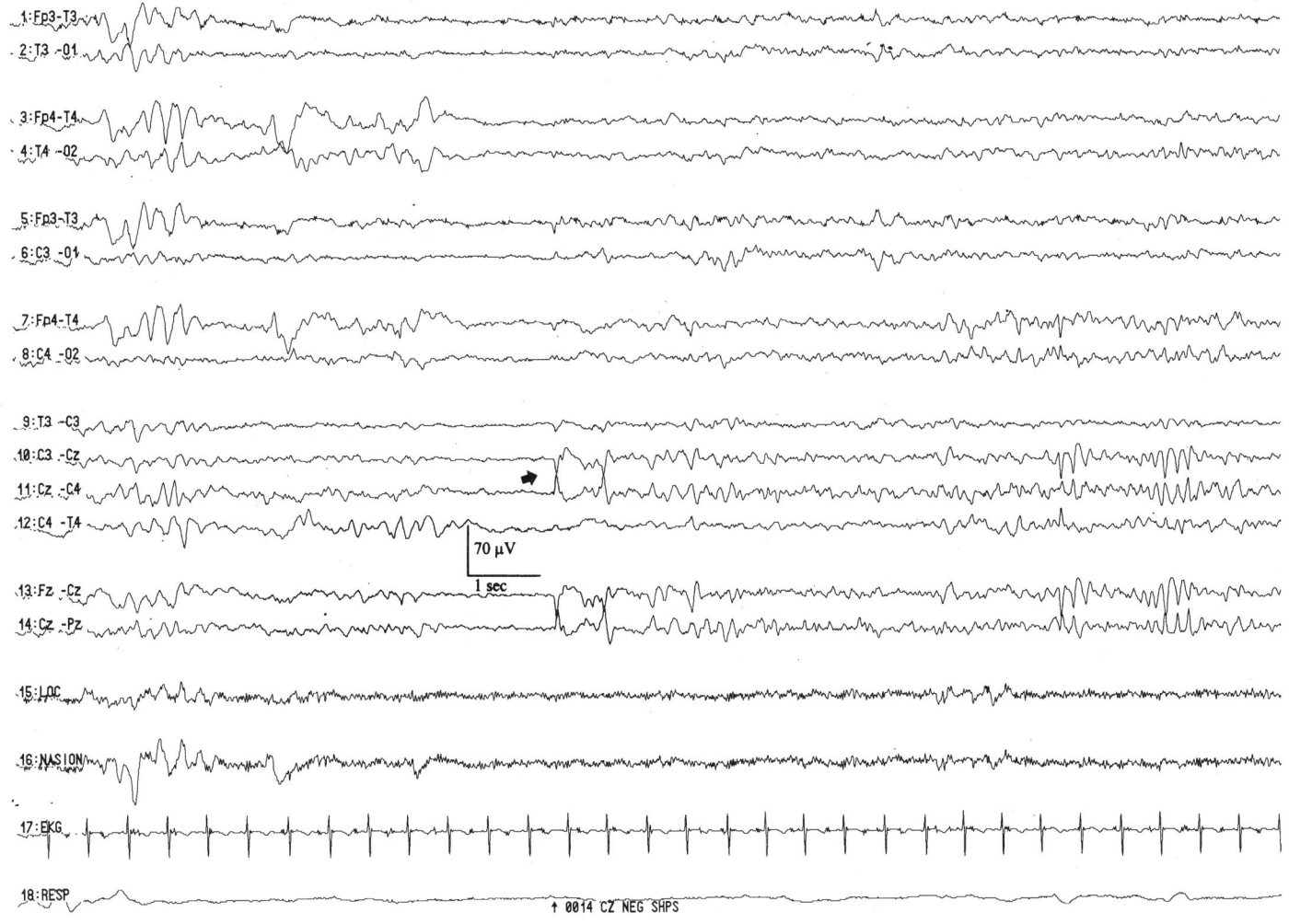

FIG. 6.48. Abnormal vertex sharp electrographic transients (SETs) in an infant 43 weeks of conceptional age with seizures. Sharp waves isolated to the central vertex are seen (*arrow*). If electrode Cz had been omitted from the montage, these SETs would have been missed.

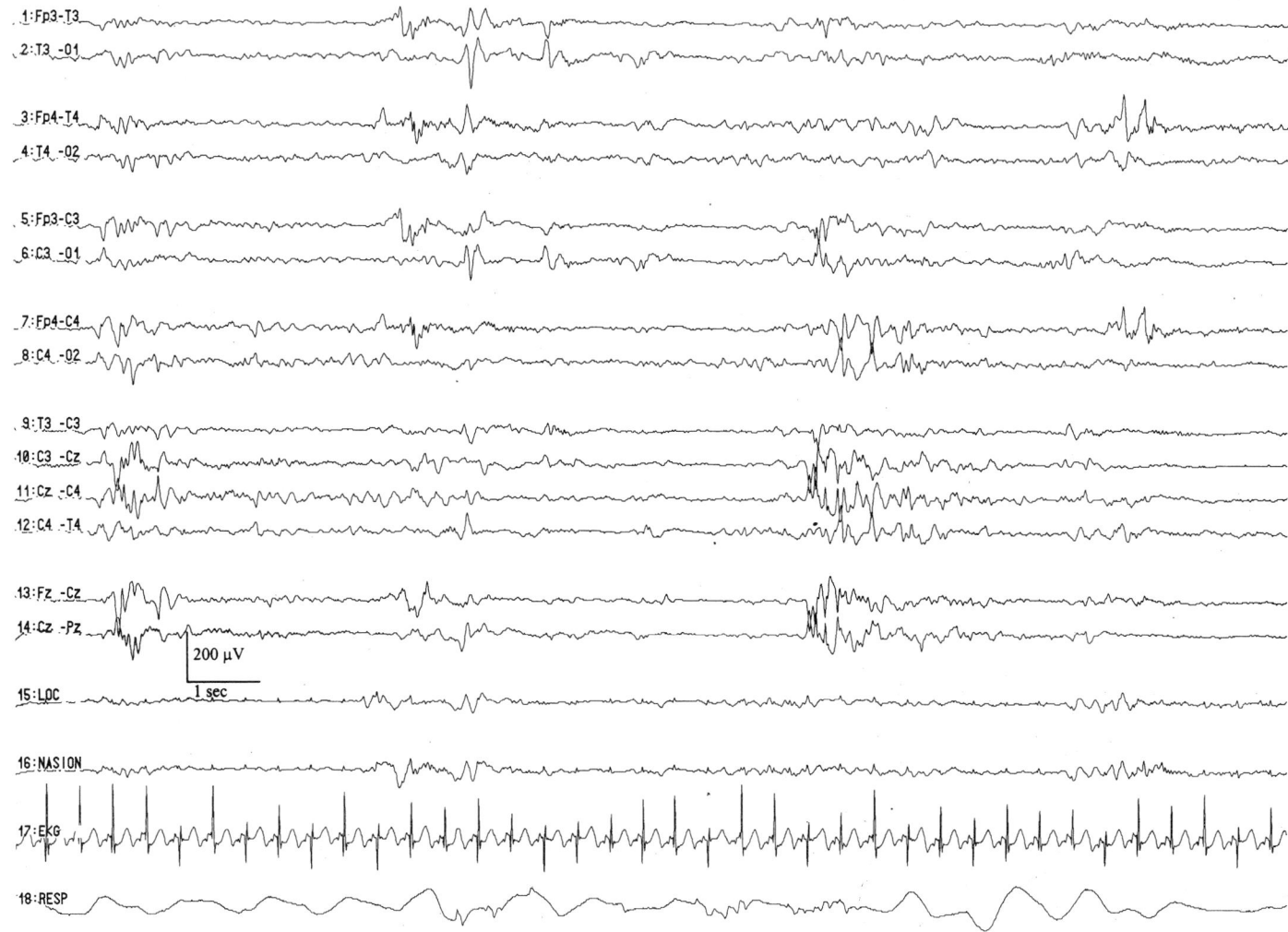

FIG. 6.49. Multifocal negative sharp waves in an infant 37 weeks of conceptional age with hypoxic-ischemic encephalopathy and seizures. Abnormal sharp EEG transients are present at T3, C3, C4, and Cz.

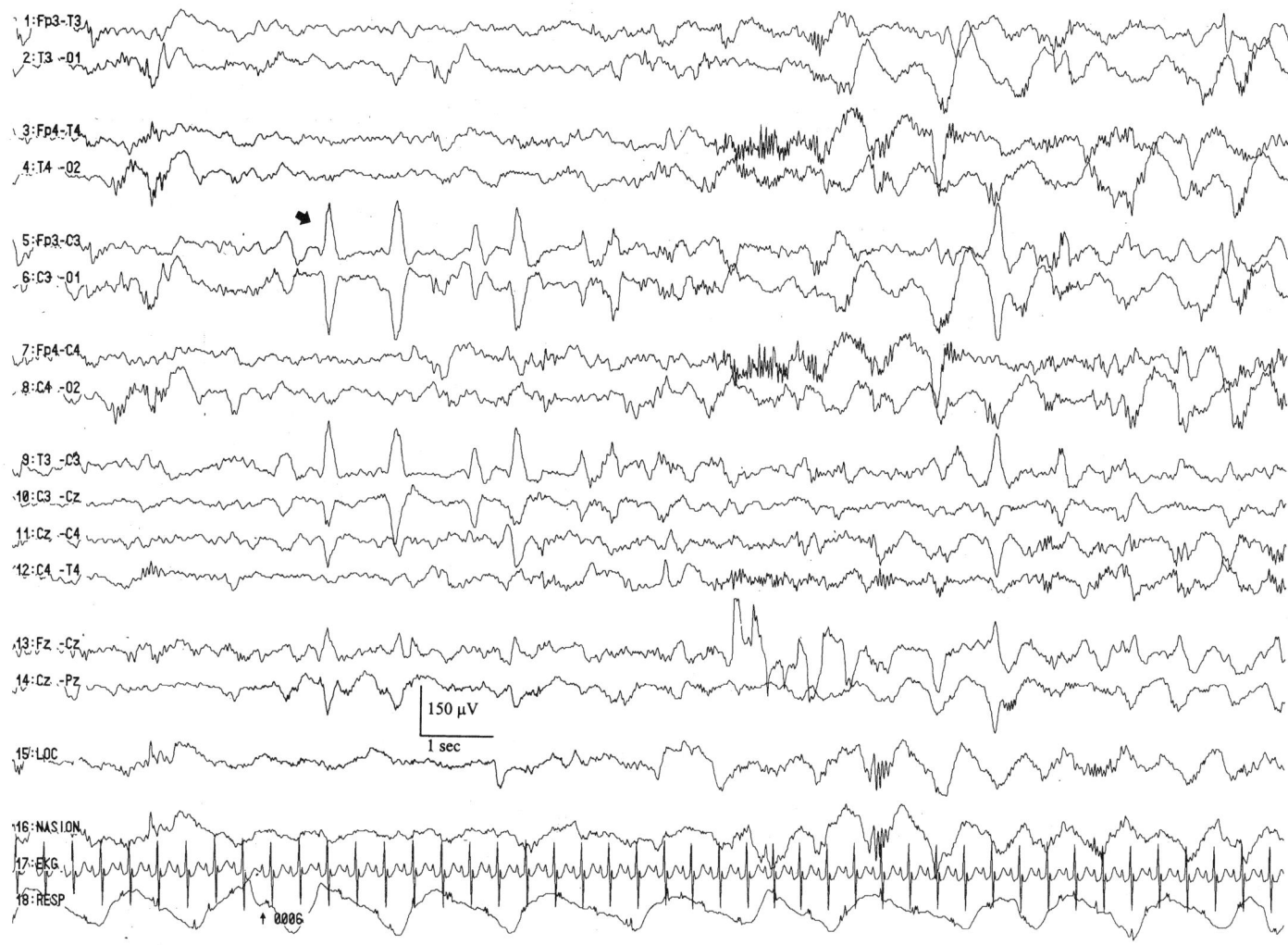

FIG. 6.50. Positive rolandic sharp waves in an infant 34 weeks of conceptional age with left-sided grade IV intraventricular hemorrhage. Repetitive positive rolandic sharp waves are seen at C3 (*arrow*).

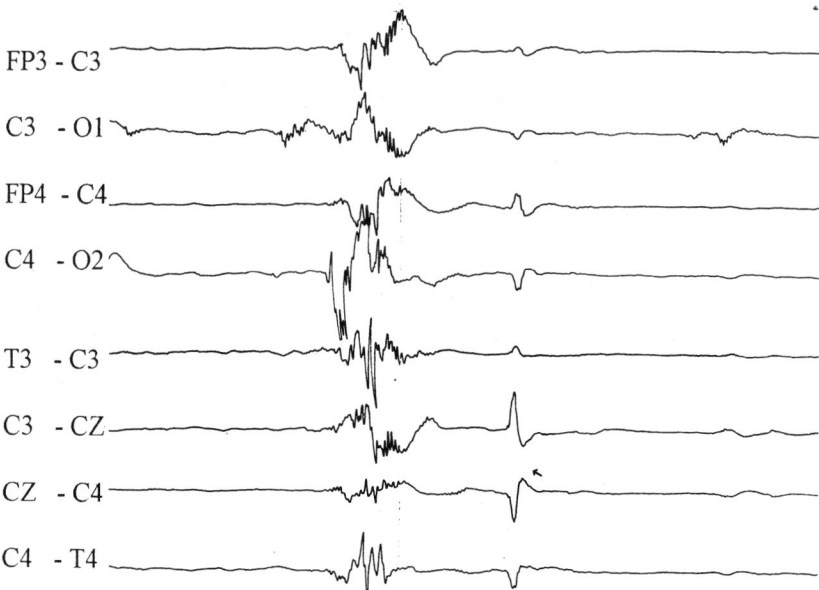

FIG. 6.51. Positive vertex sharp waves in an infant 29 weeks of conceptional age with right-sided grade III intraventricular hemorrhage. Positive vertex sharp waves are seen at Cz (*arrows*). In this case, a recording montage that included Cz was necessary to record these abnormal transients.

temporal regions (positive temporal sharp waves [PTS]) (Fig. 6.52). These pathological waveforms are not indicative of a "lowered seizure threshold" but rather are electrographic markers of parenchymal brain injuries, especially in the deep cerebral white matter, and can be seen in a variety of conditions, including periventricular leukomalacia, IVH, hydrocephalus, meningitis, inborn errors of metabolism, and HIE. The usual locations of pathological positive sharp waves in the premature infant are the midline vertex (Cz) and rolandic (C3 and C4) regions. PVSs and PRSs occur singly or in brief runs with moderate to high voltages (50 to 250 µV) and sometimes are comingled with beta activity.

The clinical significance of identifying PRSs and PVSs in premature infants has been investigated by several authors. Clancy et al. (24) investigated 44 infants with IVH verified by computed tomography or autopsy. PRSs were present in 13 infants with IVH and in 22 of the 30 EEGs. How-

ever, PRSs were present in only one premature infant without IVH. Clancy et al. concluded that PRSs have low sensitivity but high specificity for destructive IVH. Among infants with larger hemorrhages (grades 3 and 4), there was a higher incidence (69.2%) of PRSs than among infants with lower grade hemorrhages (31.8%). PRSs and PVSs were most commonly observed between the fifth and eighth postnatal day of life and gradually disappeared by 3 or 4 weeks of age. It is difficult to ascertain the prognostic significance of these patterns per se, because they are often observed in the context of substantially abnormal EEG backgrounds, which themselves forecast adverse outcomes. However, they may be best considered electrographic signs of underlying structural brain abnormalities.

PTSs (see Fig. 6.52) in full-term infants are maximally expressed in the midtemporal regions (T3 and T4) (15,28). They have received less attention than PRSs and PVSs but share similar morphological features and also appear to be linked to structural brain lesions, including periventricular leukomalacia, intracerebral hemorrhages, and infarctions. In the study of Chung and Clancy (15), more than 1,000 neonatal EEGs were reviewed for the presence of PTSs. Forty-six EEGs from 31 full-term infants were found to have "excessive" PTSs, "excessive" being defined as greater than one PTS per minute during the low-voltage, continuous portions of the tracing. EEG backgrounds were normal in nine records and abnormal in the others. In 25 of the 31 infants, a neuroimaging study or an autopsy was performed; 16 (64%) of the 25 patients were found to have focal or diffuse structural lesions, the most common of which were infarction and hemorrhage. In patients with focal lesions, the side of the lesion correlated with the laterality of the PTS. PTSs appeared within 2 to 3 days of the acute illness and disappeared within 4 to 5 weeks. Other studies (7,45,68) have also found PTSs to be correlated with hypoxia-ischemia or structural brain pathological processes. Some authors, however, have questioned the significance of isolated PTS in the absence of other EEG background abnormalities (56). There is agreement, however, that PTS are not specifically epileptiform and are not directly associated with neonatal seizures.

Little is known about the significance of PTSs in the premature infant. PTSs of low to moderate amplitude have been noted in the EEGs of healthy premature infants, with a frequency of 15% at 33 to 34 weeks of conceptional age, decreasing to 0.75% by 39 to 40 weeks of conceptional age (80). The morphological features and amplitudes of these benign PTSs differed from those of the pathological PTSs noted in full-term infants (see Fig. 6.52).

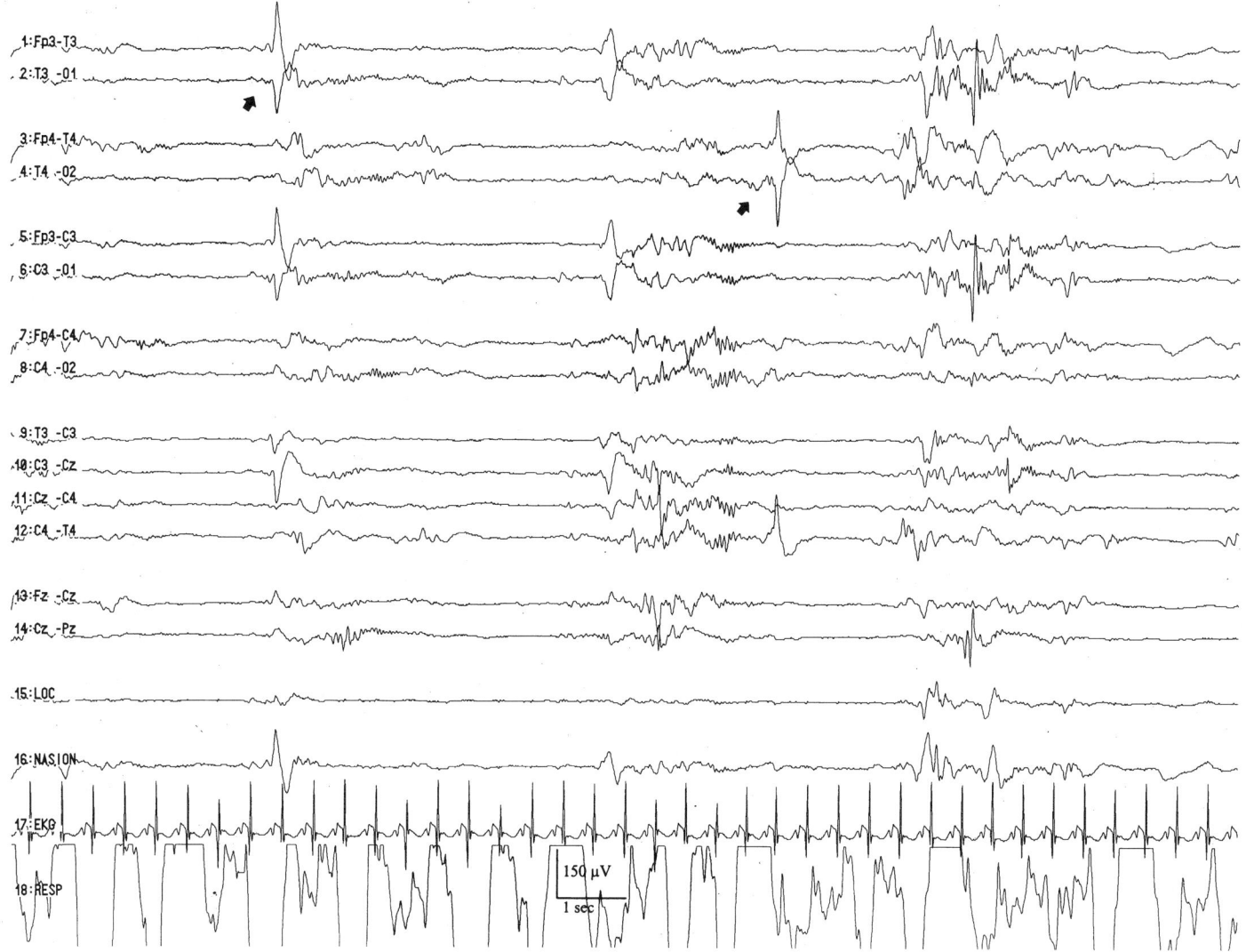

FIG. 6.52. Positive temporal sharp waves in an infant 40 weeks of conceptional age with hypoxic-ischemic encephalopathy and seizures. Left- and right-sided positive temporal sharp waves (*arrows*) are present.

ELECTROGRAPHIC NEONATAL SEIZURES AND CLINICAL CORRELATIONS

It is a challenge for all involved in the care of neonates to distinguish epilepsy-based neonatal seizures from the wide array of nonepileptic paroxysmal behaviors that may occur in healthy or sick infants. The essential role of video-EEG monitoring for accurate diagnosis of suspected neonatal seizures was established by Mizrahi and Kellaway (62), who analyzed video-EEGs from 349 neonates between the conceptional ages of 28 and 44 weeks in whom there was a clinical suspicion of seizures. A total of 415 paroxysmal clinical events were found in 71 patients, but only 119 (29%) of these events in 23 patients had a close temporal association with an ictal EEG discharge; another 11 patients had occult seizures, which are electrographic seizures without conspicuous clinical signs. Other studies have found significantly higher numbers of neonates with occult seizures (71,99). For example, Scher et al. (81) found that 92 (2.3%) of 4,020 neonates admitted to an intensive care nursery over a 4-year period had an electrographic neonatal seizure (ENS), but clinical signs accompanied these seizures in only 28 (45%) of 62 preterm infants and 16 (53%) of 30 full-term infants.

The hallmark of an ENS is the sudden appearance of a repetitive discharge event consisting of a definite beginning, middle, and end. ENS evolve in frequency, morphological appearance, and amplitude (Fig. 6.53) (19,20,48,99,100). An interpretative pitfall for the electroencephalographer is to distinguish ENS from rhythmic extracerebral artifacts, which are typically monomorphic and do not evolve in frequency, morphological appearance, or amplitude. The characteristics of ENS can be described in terms similar to those used for pediatric and adult electrographic seizures: location, duration, morphological appearance, and amplitude.

Location. The overwhelming majority of ENSs are focal in onset. Generalized, bilateral, synchronous spike and slow-wave discharges have only rarely been described. An ENS may be recorded from any scalp region, but the central and temporal regions are the most common sites of origin. Repetitive ENSs originating from a single scalp region are termed unifocal, whereas recurrent ENSs arising from multiple scalp regions are termed multifocal. Recurrent ENSs arising from a single scalp region should raise the suspicion of a focal or lateralized structural lesion such as an infarction from an embolism (21), but not all unifocal ENSs are accompanied by localized abnormalities on neuroimaging studies. Both unifocal and multifocal ENSs may propagate to adjacent or distant scalp locations (see Fig. 6.53). Simultaneous and independent ENSs may arise from multiple scalp regions (Fig. 6.54).

Duration. A minimum ictal duration of 10 seconds is conventionally (and perhaps arbitrarily) required for the designation of ENS in most studies. The average duration of an ENS is brief. In one study of 487 ENSs (20), 230 (47%) lasted less than 1 minute, and 90 (18%) lasted between 1 and 2 minutes; the finding of a mean duration of 2.25 minutes in this study was influenced by rare prolonged seizures that lasted up to 46 minutes. Discharges lasting less than 10 seconds and showing typical evolution in frequency, morphological appearance, or amplitude have been termed brief ictal rhythmic discharges (BIRDs) (85) and are of unclear significance. BIRDs (Fig. 6.55) clearly suggest a lower seizure threshold and may have the same significance as the longer duration ENS. It is uncommon to encounter a single electrographic seizure in most routine ictal recordings. Instead, multiple ENSs are usually encountered (Fig. 6.56). The precise difference between multiple ENSs and status epilepticus in the neonate is unknown. It is difficult to apply the traditional definitions of status epilepticus (continuous seizure activity for 30 minutes or recurrent seizures without full recovery of consciousness) to neonates. An alternative definition of neonatal status epilepticus used in some studies is (a) total seizure duration exceeding 30 minutes or (b) the sum of the duration of individual seizures exceeding 50% of the tracing (72). According to these criteria, status epilepticus was present in 22 (27%) of 81 neonates with EEG-proven seizures (72).

Morphological Appearance. ENSs are characterized by a rich variety of ictal morphological appearances, both between patients and in a given individual. All frequencies (delta, theta, alpha, and beta) are represented (Figs. 6.57 and 6.58). Ictal waveforms range from simple sinusoidal patterns to complex, bizarre ictal patterns. Evolution of morphological appearance within an ENS is helpful in distinguishing ENS from artifact.

Amplitude. Just as ENSs display evolution of waveform morphological appearance, they also typically evolve in amplitude. ENSs commonly first appear at relatively low amplitudes, which gradually increase as the seizure evolves (Fig. 6.59).

It is challenging to design a clinically useful approach for the use of EEG in the high-risk neonate. One strategy is to limit the use of serial tracings to tracings with clinically suspected seizures. This approach risks the underdiagnosis of ENS, in view of the high frequency of occult seizures in this age group. Another strategy, outlined by Laroia et al. (47), is to use the initial EEG background to decide which high-risk infants would benefit from subsequent prolonged monitoring. In the study validating that approach, 51 infants with risk factors for seizures (such as HIE or meningitis) underwent a 30- to 60-minute screening EEG, followed by continu-

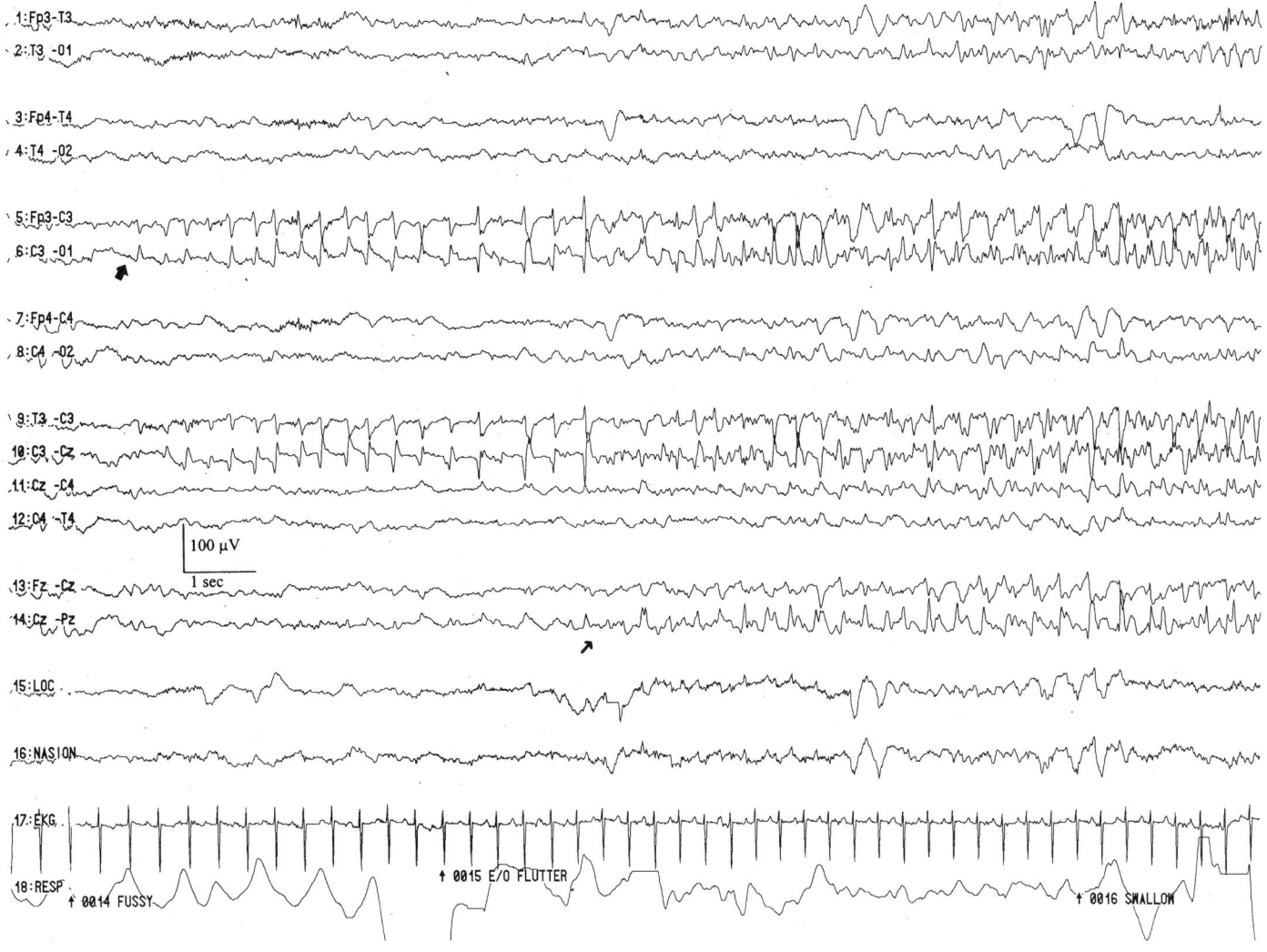

FIG. 6.53. Ictal onset and propagation in an infant 40 weeks of conceptional age with hypoxic-ischemic encephalopathy and seizures. Ictal onset is seen over the left central region (*large arrow*), with subsequent propagation to the central vertex region (*small arrow*). Eventually, ictal activity is also seen in the left temporal region.

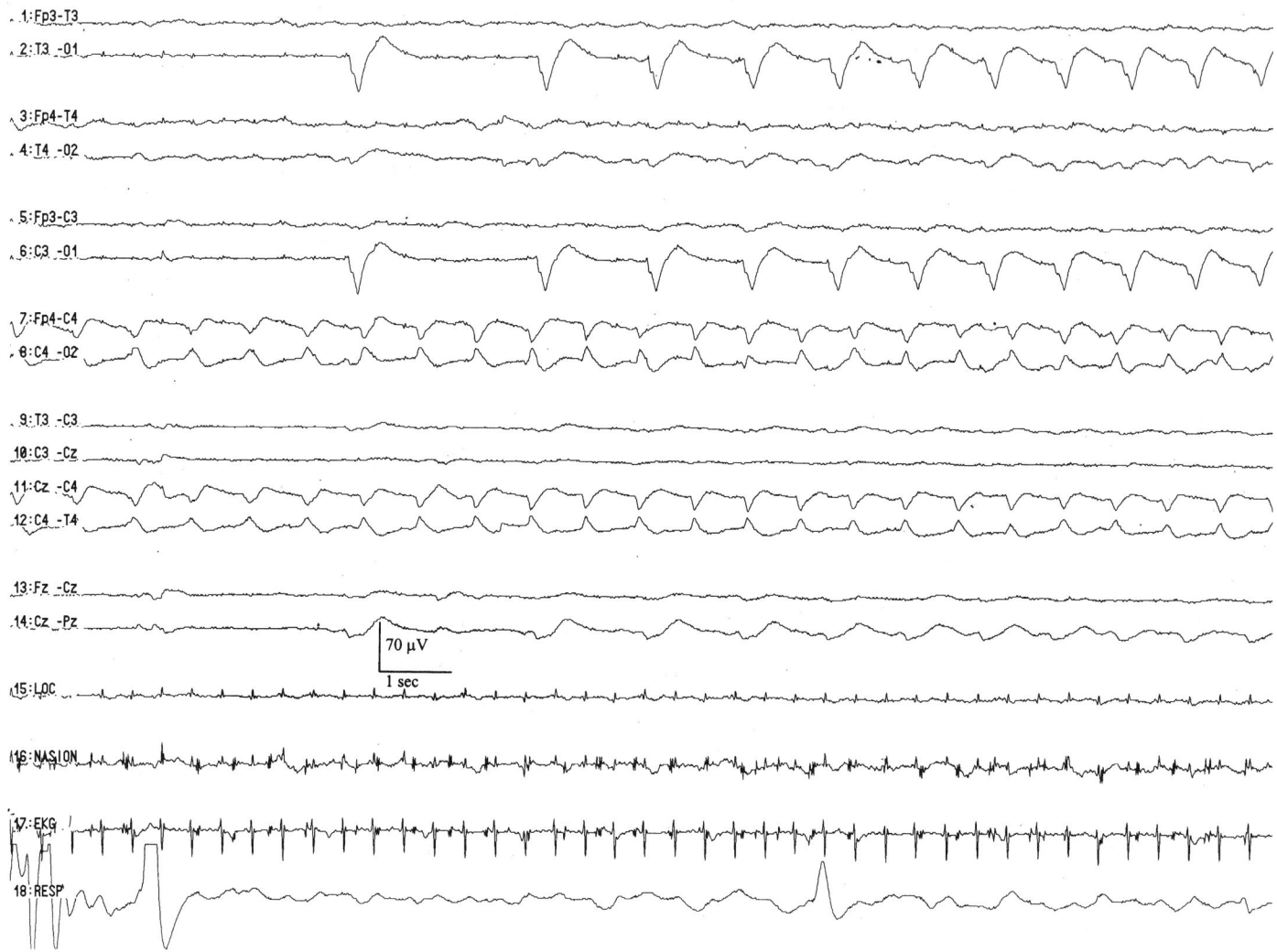

FIG. 6.54. Simultaneous, independent seizures in an infant 37 weeks of conceptional age with hypoxic-ischemic encephalopathy and seizures. Independent seizures are present simultaneously at C4 and O1.

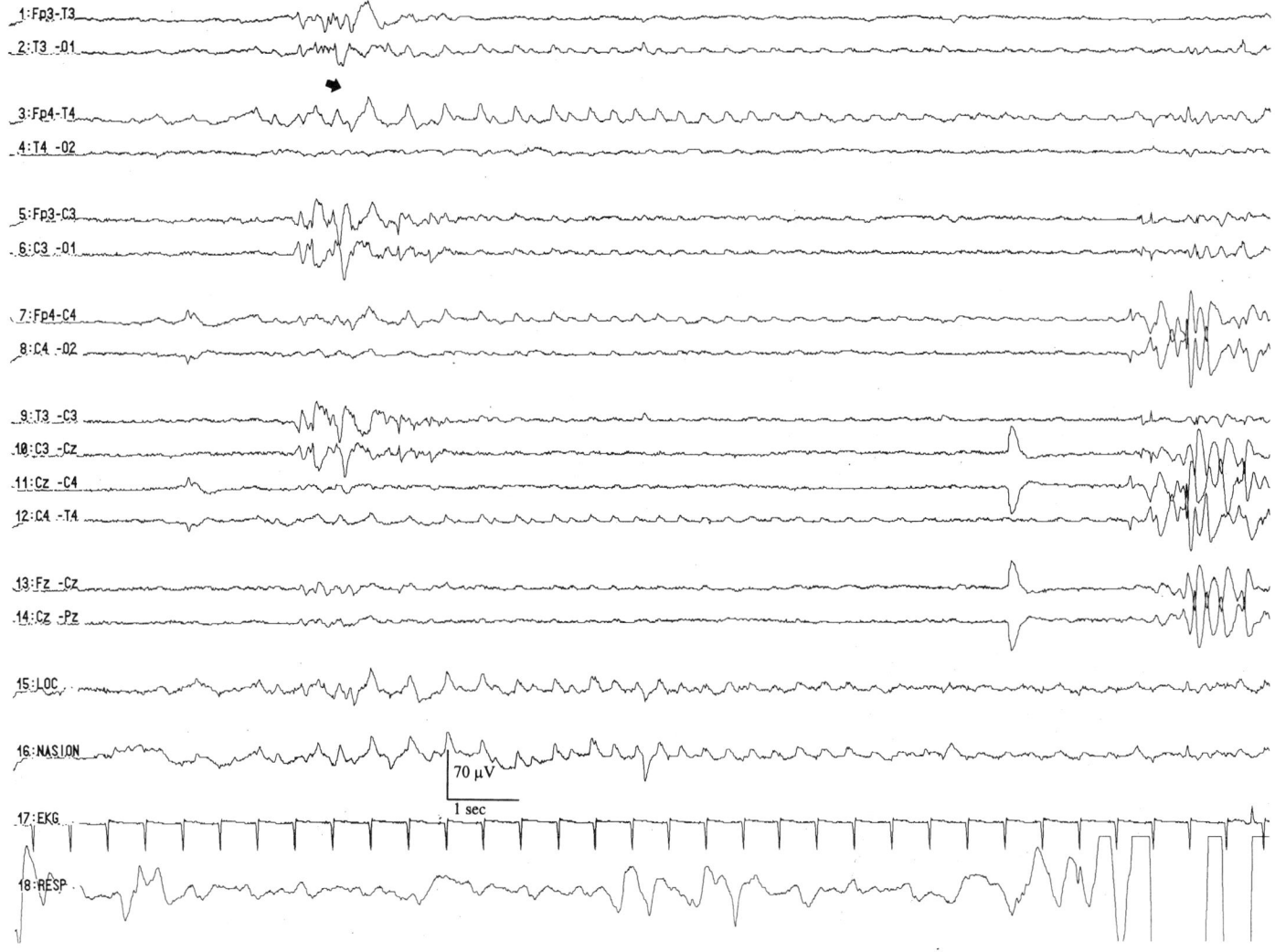

FIG. 6.55. Brief ictal rhythmic discharge (BIRD) in an infant 42 weeks of conceptional age with double-outlet right ventricle and a history of cardiac arrest. A BIRD is present at Fp4 (*arrow*) and T4. The evolution in morphological appearance and amplitude and the presence of a physiological field distinguishes this BIRD from artifact.

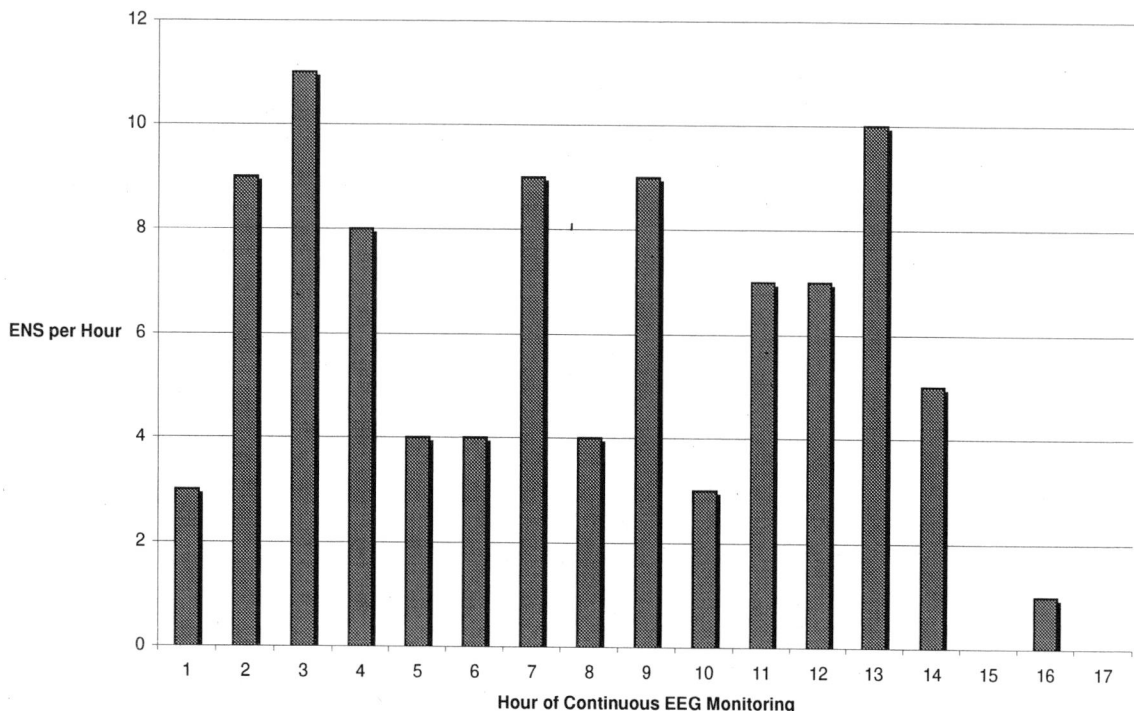

FIG. 6.56. Continuous video-electroencephalographic monitoring of an infant 40 weeks of conceptional age with birth trauma revealed numerous electrographic seizures each hour until the infant was treated vigorously with thiopental. Many acutely ill neonates experience multiple seizures.

ous EEG monitoring for 18 to 24 hours. The EEG background of the initial tracing was classified as normal, immature for age, mildly abnormal, moderately abnormal, or severely abnormal. Only 1 (4.2%) of 24 infants with normal or immature EEG backgrounds had subsequent ENSs. However, 22 (81%) of 27 infants with abnormal EEG backgrounds had ENSs. Thus, a normal or immature initial EEG background predicted the absence of seizures in the subsequent 18 to 24 hours with a sensitivity of 96% and a specificity of 81% (Table 6.3).

A developing strategy is the use of automated, computer-based ENS detection algorithms. Such systems are highly sensitive when used to detect seizures in older children and adults (46) but are more challenging to design for use in neonates because of the different ictal waveform frequencies and characteristics. Brief, low-amplitude ENS are especially difficult to detect. Nonetheless, computer-aided detection systems with sensitivities of 71% to 84% have been reported (51,76).

The impact of ENS per se on subsequent neurological outcome is difficult to determine. Outcome is heavily dependent on the underlying cause of the seizures and the degree of background abnormality. Those with benign neonatal seizures fare well (58,78), whereas infants whose seizures are provoked by acute illness face a much higher risk of permanent neurological handicap. In general, neonates with seizures superimposed on a normal EEG background have lower risks of adverse outcomes, whereas those with ENS and a moderately or severely abnormal background have worse outcomes (83). In their classic study of 137 full-term neonates with *clinically diagnosed seizures,* Rose and Lombroso (75) found that 67 (78%) of 85 infants with normal backgrounds or a unifocal abnormality on initial EEG had normal outcomes, whereas only 4 (8%) of 52 patients with multifocal abnormalities and low-amplitude or periodic backgrounds had normal outcomes. In a later study, Rowe et al. (77) examined outcome after clinically diagnosed seizures in 74 preterm and full-term infants. Normal or mildly

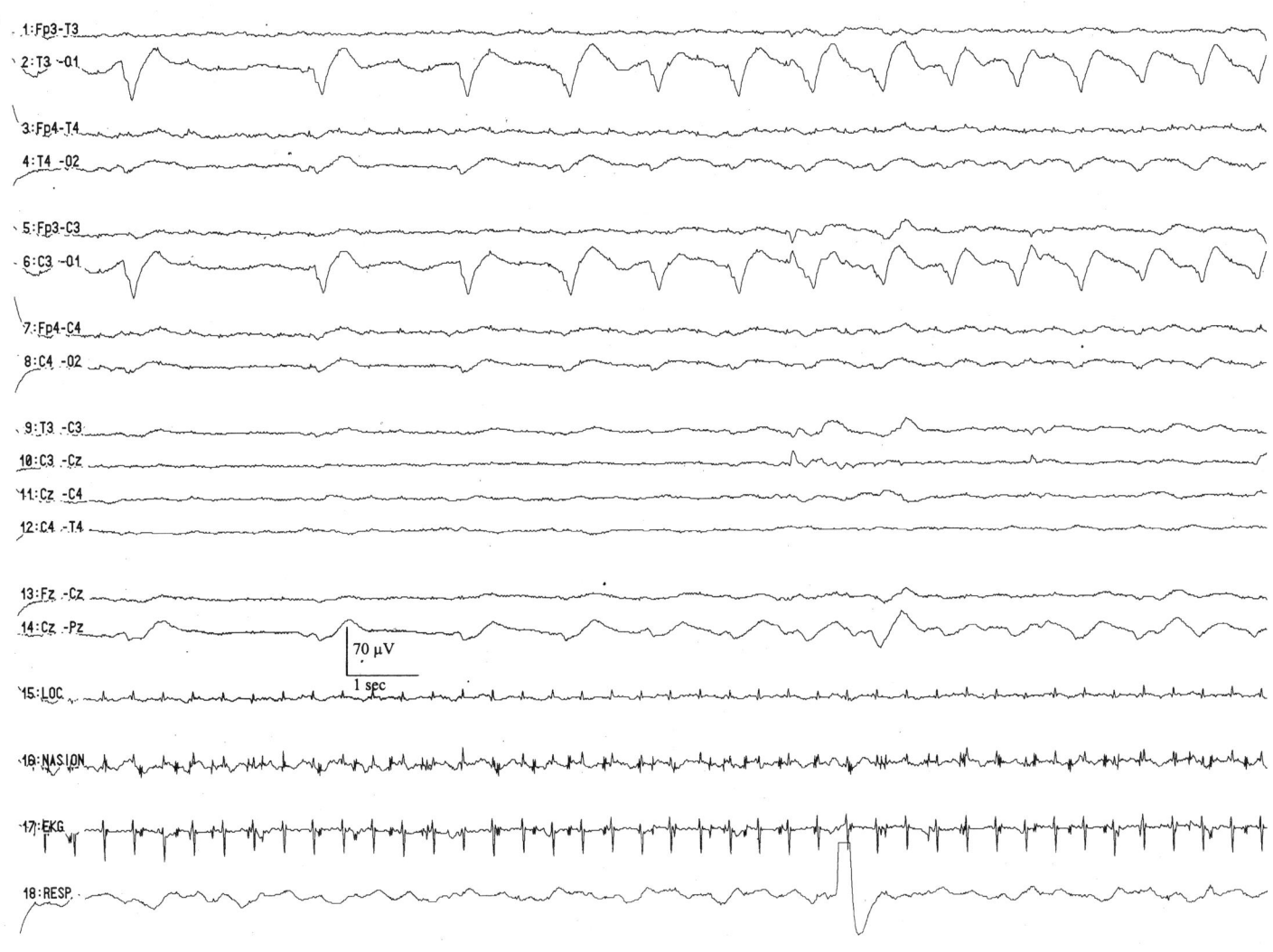

FIG. 6.57. Delta frequency seizure in an infant 37 weeks of conceptional age with hypoxic-ischemic encephalopathy and seizures. A delta frequency seizure is seen to evolve from O1.

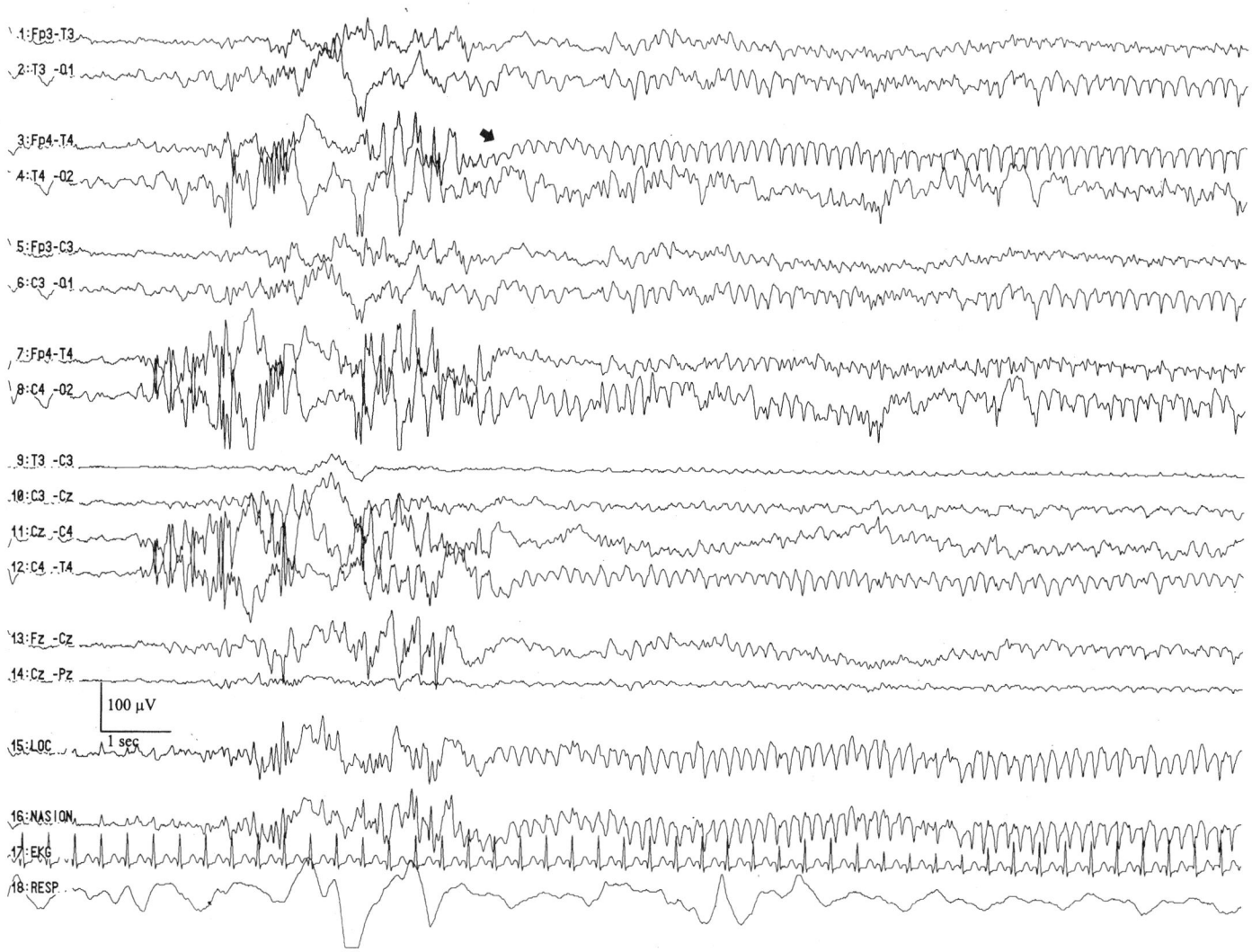

FIG. 6.58. Theta frequency seizure in an infant 36 weeks of conceptional age who had recently suffered cardiac arrest. After a burst of cerebral activity, an ictal discharge with a frequency of 5 Hz begins over the right frontal region (*arrow*).

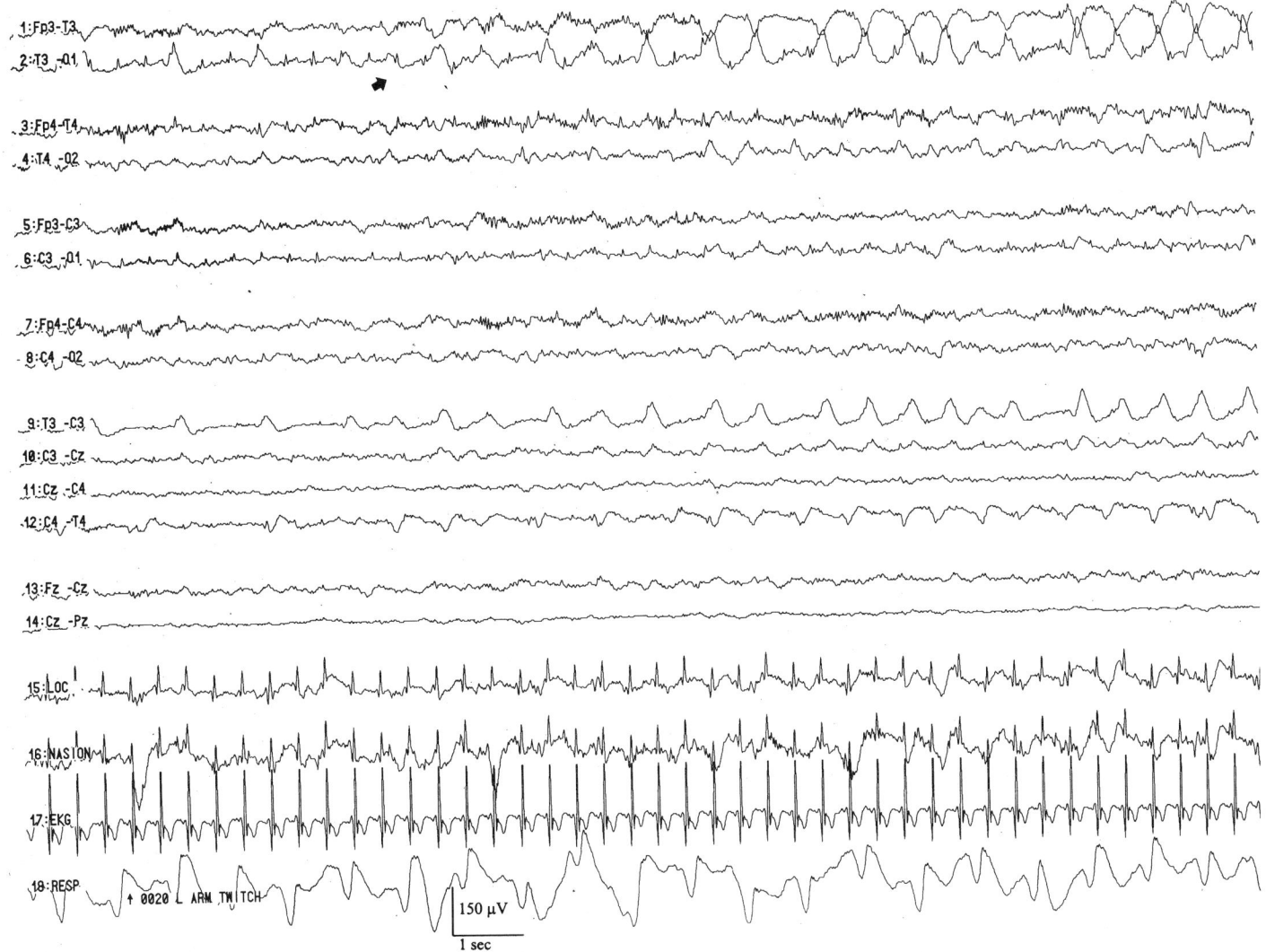

FIG. 6.59. Amplitude evolution of an electrographic seizure in an infant 40 weeks of conceptional age with respiratory syncytial virus pneumonia. A seizure is evolving in amplitude at T3 (*arrow*).

TABLE 6.3. *Association of electroencephalographic (EEG) background and electrographic neonatal seizures*

	Normal or immature EEG background	Abnormal EEG background
No electrographic seizures	23	5
Electrographic seizures	1	22

Adapted from Laroia N, Guillet R, Burchfiel J, et al. EEG background as predictor of electrographic seizures in high-risk neonates. *Epilepsia* 1998;39: 545–551.

abnormal outcomes were found in 22 (85%) of 26 infants with normal EEG backgrounds, in 5 (45%) of 11 infants with moderately abnormal backgrounds, and in 1 (2.7%) of 37 infants with severely abnormal backgrounds. In two other studies, researchers examined outcome after *EEG-confirmed* neonatal seizures. Scher et al. (81) reported that 56 (61%) of 92 neonates with EEG-confirmed seizures survived. Normal outcome was documented in 9 (25%) of 36 preterm infants and in 12 (60%) of 20 full-term infants. Legido et al. (49) monitored outcomes in 40 neonates with EEG-confirmed seizures. Twenty-seven (68%) survived, but outcome was unfavorable in 70% of those survivors. Factors associated with unfavorable outcome included etiology (such as asphyxia, meningitis, or cerebral dysgenesis), moderately or severely abnormal EEG background, and higher seizure frequency.

AN ORGANIZED APPROACH TO VISUAL ANALYSIS OF THE NEONATAL ELECTROENCEPHALOGRAM AND COMMON INTERPRETATION PITFALLS

This final section intends to serve as a template to review a typical neonatal EEG examination, emphasizing the common high points for interpretation and identifying areas that commonly introduce interpretative difficulties. Before beginning the inspection of the neonatal EEG, several pieces of historical data are needed to prepare a mental picture of the expected range of anticipated findings by which to judge the actual EEG while it is produced. The two main facts are the *conceptional age* at the time the EEG was recorded and the patient's *biobehavioral state* (awake, transitional, indeterminate sleep, active sleep, and quiet sleep). The accurate clinical assessment of *state* requires ample notes from the recording technologists describing whether the eyes are open or closed, the presence of REMs and large or small body movements. It is also necessary to distinguish artifacts introduced by the handling of the patient by health care providers. Information about medical and neurological status can also help create the proper context in which to interpret the patient's EEG. Infants who are known to have systemic illnesses can be reasonably expected to show at least mild disturbances of the EEG background, which do not necessarily imply fixed and lasting CNS insults. Commonly, the EEG improves or normalizes after the correction of the underlying medical illness. Specifically, conditions such as mild hypoxia or hypercarbia from respiratory disease, congenital heart defects, sepsis, simple metabolic disorders such as hyponatremia, and the administration of CNS-active drugs (for pain, agitation, or sedation) can all introduce mild, transient background abnormalities that have no special prognostic significance. Finally, the condition of the infant's scalp should be known. Increased thickness of the scalp usually attenuates the apparent amplitude, and the EEG may appear underdeveloped or "washed out" in a generalized or localized region. Scalp thickness may be increased from local or generalized swelling caused by a caput succedaneum, cephalohematoma, or the tremendous third spacing of fluid during sepsis, ECMO, or hydrops fetalis. Collectively, these considerations broadly provide the context in which to anticipate the expected background composition and continuity or discontinuity of the record.

In a typical patient, the beginning of the EEG may show a brief period of wakefulness, because the patient has just been stimulated by the technologist with measuring, marking, and rubbing the scalp surface. The patient may then be calmly awake for a brief period before the eyes close and the infant transitions from the awake to a sleeping state. At the onset of sleep in neonates, active sleep usually emerges first, and there is little qualitative change in the background between the awake and the active sleep states. *Continuity* is determined first. In very young premature infants, the background is discontinuous, even when the infant is awake, and it is necessary to count several representative IBIs in seconds to decide whether the discontinuity is excessive. There is a range of counted values with some unusually brief or long IBIs, but the typical IBIs should not exceed the values found in Table 6.1. The tracing is considered excessively discontinuous if the patient's typical IBIs clearly exceed the norms for age. After the continuity of the record is judged, the composition of the tracing is evaluated. What are the patterns, rhythms, and frequencies that constitute the background? Are there specific, named, identifiable normal patterns present, such as monorhythmic occipital delta activity, bursts of rhythmic theta activity in the occipital or temporal regions, delta brushes in the occipital or centrotemporal regions, and runs of anterior dysrhythmia and *encoches frontales? Symmetry* is judged as an overall impression of the amount, amplitude, and composition of background activity contrasted between homologous areas and both hemispheres. Even major interhemispheric asymmetries that arise just transiently have little significance. A *persistent* difference of at least 50% is usually necessary to declare a background abnormality on the basis of asymmetry alone. More often, significant asymmetries are detected in the company of other background abnormalities such as excessive discontinuity or an abnormal profile of sharp EEG transients.

After a brief portion of active sleep, perhaps 15 to 20 minutes, the undisturbed infant may make another transition to quiet sleep. It is important to continue the study long enough to capture some quiet sleep because in some infants, electrographic abnormalities may be observed only during this specific state. During transitional sleep, the EEG background is indeterminate and does not conform entirely to the characteristics of wakefulness, active sleep, or quiet sleep. Once definite quiet sleep has emerged, it is possible to compare the appearance of the earlier awake/active sleep EEG to that of quiet sleep. In older neonates, there should be easily distinguishable differences between the awake/active sleep and quiet sleep segments of the study. The degree of discontinuity is again judged by counting or estimating the duration of typical IBIs and comparing these with norms. At the end of the study, it is important to vigorously stimulate the patient in quiet sleep to demonstrate that the observed discontinuity is reactive.

Sharp EEG transients are very common in the neonatal EEG. Virtually all healthy infants display the ubiquitous *encoches frontales* admixed with anterior dysrhythmia. In the central and temporal regions, SETs are relatively common, up to 1 per minute in wakefulness or active sleep, appearing as solitary transients that are about equally distributed between the left and right temporal areas and are much rarer in the central areas. In discontinuous quiet sleep, many infants have a sharp or "spikey" quality to the bursts, but this has no known significance. Electrographic seizures should be recognized as a sustained event that evolves in amplitude, frequency, and morphological appearance.

The report of the EEG examination should comment on the appearance of the overall background, whether it is appropriately mature for the stated conceptional age, and the degree of background abnormality and possible prognostic significance, if any. If clinically warranted, a follow-up examination may be suggested to monitor the progress of the infant's encephalopathy and electrocerebral maturation. If the study is technically limited, the examination should be repeated. Abnormalities of the EEG background provide limited insight into the cause of the encephalopathy. This fact can be recognized in the report by statements such as "Such EEG abnormalities are not specific from the viewpoint of etiology." If electrographic seizures are present, it is helpful to the clinician to note whether any or all of the ENSs are accompanied by distinctive clinical signs so that the bedside observer might have an indication of how accurate visual quantification may be for a specific patient. In some infants, virtually none of the ENSs are accompanied by clinical seizures, and the clinician should be alerted to that information. In patients with abnormal backgrounds who display a clear excess of SETs, it can be stated that such patterns raise the concern for a lowered seizure threshold, even if no actual clinical or electrographic seizure has been detected. Positive sharp transients in the temporal, central, or midline vertex regions are not associated with seizures but rather with underlying structural abnormalities such as periventricular leukomalacia, stroke, or hemorrhage. Naturally, the presence of structural CNS abnormalities is best determined by specific neuroimaging techniques such as ultrasonography, computed tomography, or magnetic resonance imaging.

There are several common pitfalls of the neonatal EEG examination: (a). Neonatal EEG examinations are not commonly performed and interpreted in some laboratories. Consequently, each time a patient is examined, the process seems uncertain and unfamiliar. One solution is to maintain a small "reference library" of normal EEGs at several conceptional ages that can be reviewed as needed to compare with those of the patient undergoing an examination. These serve as quick reminders of the normal EEG appearance at a variety of developmental ages. (b) Inadequate use of the polygraphic aspects of neonatal EEG makes interpretation very difficult. The neonatal EEG is a specialized kind of sleep study that can be understood only when the patient's state and behaviors are clearly known. It is critical that the patient be stimulated adequately during the examination to produce a state change and electrographic reactivity (not just EMG artifact from nonspecific muscle activity). (c) Serial EEG examinations, including those conducted during the peak of the infant's medical or neurological illness, are necessary to capture the electrographic findings of greatest prognostic significance. (d) It is very tempting to "overcall" physiological sharp EEG transients as *pathological* unless the interpreter is comfortable with the relatively broad range of normal sharp EEG transients that can be encountered in the healthy neonate. On the other hand, electrode "pops" can remarkably resemble some pathological positive waves. Genuine PTSs, PRSs, and PVSs may be exquisitely confined to the T3 and T4, C3 and C4, or Cz electrodes without field spread to adjacent electrodes. (e) Rhythmic EEG artifacts from limb tremors, hiccups, ECMO pump artifact, and pulse can, in the occasional patient, create a very convincing recording pattern that at least superficially resembles an electrographic seizure. The diagnosis of neonatal seizures mandates an immediate and thorough diagnostic evaluation by the clinician, often including lumbar puncture, transportation outside the safer confines of the nursery to a brain scanner, and the administration of medications. These steps may be unnecessary if the seizure was actually an innocent electrographic artifact!

REFERENCES

1. Al Naqeeb N, Edwards AD, Dowan FM, et al. Assessment of neonatal encephalopathy by amplitude-integrated electroencephalography. *Pediatrics* 1999;103:1263–1271.
2. American Electroencephalographic Society Guidelines in Electroencephalography, Evoked Potentials, and Polysomnography. *J Clin Neurophysiol* 1994;11:1–147.
3. Aso K, Abdab-Barmada M, Scher M. EEG and the neuropathology in premature neonates with intraventricular hemorrhage. *J Clin Neurophysiol* 1993;10:304–313.
4. Aso K, Scher M, Barmada M. Neonatal electroencephalography and neuropathology. *J Clin Neurophysiol* 1989;6:103–123.
5. Azzopardi D, Guarino I, Brayshaw C, et al. Prediction of neurological outcome after birth asphyxia from early continuous two-channel electroencephalography. *Early Hum Dev* 1999;55:113–123.
6. Ballard J. A simplified assessment of gestational age. *Pediatr Res* 1977;11:374.
7. Barlow J, Holmes G. Positive sharp waves: an electroencephalographic marker for recent hypoxia-ischemia in the neonate. *Ann Neurol* 1990;28:454–455.
8. Baud O, d'Allest A, Lacaze-Masmonteil T. The early diagnosis of periventricular leukomalacia in premature infants with positive rolandic sharp waves on serial electroencephalography. *J Pediatr* 1998;132:813–817.
9. Bell A, McClure B, Hicks E. Power spectral analysis of the EEG of term infants following birth asphyxia. *Dev Med Child Neurol* 1990;32:990–998.
10. Benda G, Engel R, Zhang Y. Prolonged inactive phases during the discontinuous pattern of prematurity in the electroencephalogram of very-low-birthweight infants. *Electroencephalogr Clin Neurophysiol* 1989;72:189–197.
11. Biagioni E, Bartalena L, Boldrini A, et al. Background EEG activity in preterm infants: correlation of outcome with selected maturational features. *Electroencephalogr Clin Neurophysiol* 1994;91:154–161.
12. Blume W, Dreyfus-Brisac C. Positive rolandic sharp waves in neonatal EEG: types and significance. *Electroencephalogr Clin Neurophysiol* 1982;53:277–282.
13. Brazelton T. Neonatal behavioral assessment scale. In: *Clinics in Developmental Medicine, No. 50*. London: Heinemann, Spastics International Medical Publications, 1973.
14. Chequer R, Tharp B, Dreimane D, et al. Prognostic value of EEG in neonatal meningitis: retrospective study of 29 infants. *Pediatr Neurol* 1992;8:417–422.
15. Chung H, Clancy R. Significance of positive temporal sharp waves in the neonatal electroencephalogram. *Electroencephalogr Clin Neurophysiol* 1991;79:256–263.
16. Clancy R. Interictal sharp EEG transients in neonatal seizures. *J Child Neurol* 1989;4:30–38.
17. Clancy R. The contribution of EEG to the understanding of neonatal seizures. *Epilepsia* 1996;37:S52–S59.
18. Clancy R, Chung H. EEG changes during recovery from acute severe neonatal citrullinemia. *Electroencephalogr Clin Neurophysiol* 1991;78:222–227.
19. Clancy R, Chung H, Temple J. *Neonatal electroencephalography*. Amsterdam: Elsevier, 1993:1–7.
20. Clancy R, Legido A. The exact ictal and interictal duration of electroencephalographic neonatal seizures. *Epilepsia* 1987;28:537–541.
21. Clancy R, Malin S, Laraque D, et al. Focal motor seizures heralding stroke in full-term neonates. *Am J Dis Child* 1985;139:601–606.
22. Clancy R, Rosenberg H, Bernbaum J, et al. Survival outcome prediction in premature infants with IVH by cranial ultrasonography and EEG. *Ann Neurol* 1994;36:489.
23. Clancy R, Spitzer A. Cerebral cortical function in infants at risk for sudden infant death syndrome. *Ann Neurol* 1985;18:41–47.
24. Clancy R, Tharp B. Positive rolandic sharp waves in the electroencephalograms of premature neonates with intraventricular hemorrhage. *Electroencephalogr Clin Neurophysiol* 1984;57:395–404.
25. Clancy R, Tharp B, Enzman D. EEG in premature infants with intraventricular hemorrhage. *Neurology* 1984;34:583–590.
26. Connell J, de Vries L, Oozeer R, et al. Predictive value of early continuous electroencephalogram monitoring in ventilated preterm infants with intraventricular hemorrhage. *Pediatrics* 1988;82:337–343.
27. Cukier F, Andre M, Monod N, et al. Apport de l'EEG au diagnostic des hemorragies intra-ventriculaires du premature. *Rev Electroencephalogr Neurophysiol Clin* 1972;2:318–322.
28. Da Costa J, Lombroso CT. Neurophysiological correlates of neonatal intracerebral hemorrhage. *Electroencephalogr Clin Neurophysiol* 1980;50:183–184.
29. Dreyfus-Brisac C. Ontogenesis of sleep in human prematures after 32 weeks of conceptual age. *Dev Psychobiol* 1970;3:91–121.
30. Eaton D, Wertheim D, Oozeer R, et al. Reversible changes in cerebral activity associated with acidosis in preterm neonates. *Acta Paediatr* 1994;83:486–492.
31. Ellingson RJ, Peters JF. Development of EEG and daytime sleep patterns in normal full-term infant during the first 3 months of life: longitudinal observations. *Electroencephalogr Clin Neurophysiol* 1980;49:112–124.
32. Fischer R, Clancy R. Midline foci of epileptiform activity in children and neonates. *J Child Neurol* 1987;2:224–228.
33. Goto K, Wakayama K, Sonoda H, et al. Sequential changes in electroencephalogram continuity in very premature infants. *Electroencephalogr Clin Neurophysiol* 1992;82:197–202.
34. Grigg-Damberger M, Coker S, Halsey C, et al. Neonatal burst suppression: its developmental significance. *Pediatr Neurol* 1989;5:84–92.
35. Hahn J, Monyer H, Tharp B. Interburst interval measurements in the EEGs of premature infants with normal neurological outcome. *Electroencephalogr Clin Neurophysiol* 1989;73:410–418.
36. Hahn J, Tharp B. They dysmature EEG pattern in infants with bronchopulmonary dysplasia and its prognostic implications. *Electroencephalogr Clin Neurophysiol* 1990;76:106–113.
37. Hayakawa F, Okumura A, Kato T, et al. Dysmature EEG pattern in EEGs of preterm infants with cognitive impairment: maturation arrest caused by prolonged mild CNS depression. *Brain Dev* 1997;19:122–125.
38. Hellstrom-Westas L, Rosen I, Svenningsen N. Silent seizures in sick infants in early life. *Acta Paediatr Scand* 1985;74:741–748.
39. Hellstrom-Westas L, Rosen I, Svenningsen N. Cerebral function monitoring during the first week of life in extremely small low birthweight (ESLBW) infants. *Neuropediatrics* 1991;22:27–32.
40. Hellstrom-Westas L, Rosen I, Svenningsen N. Predictive value of early continuous amplitude integrated EEG recordings on outcome after severe birth asphyxia in full term infants. *Arch Dis Child Fetal Neonatal Ed* 1995;72:F34–F38.

41. Holmes G, Rowe J, Hafford J, et al. Prognostic value of the electroencephalogram in neonatal asphyxia. *Electroencephalogr Clin Neurophysiol* 1982;53:60–72.

42. Holmes H, Lombroso C. Prognostic value of background patterns in the neonatal EEG. *J Clin Neurophysiol* 1993;10:323–352.

43. Howard J, Parmelee J, Arthur H, et al. A neurologic comparison of pre-term and full-term infants at term conceptional age. *J Pediatr* 1976;88:995–1002.

44. Hughes J, Fino J, Gagnon L. Periods of activity and quiescence in the premature EEG. *Neuropediatrics* 1983;14:66–72.

45. Hughes J, Kuhlman D, Hughes C. Electro-clinical correlations of positive and negative sharp waves on the temporal and central areas in premature infants. *Clin Electroencephalogr* 1991; 22:30–39.

46. Kim H, Clancy R. Sensitivity of a seizure activity detection computer in childhood video/EEG monitoring. *Epilepsia* 1997;38:1192–1197.

47. Laroia N, Guillet R, Burchfiel J, et al. EEG background as predictor of electrographic seizures in high-risk neonates. *Epilepsia* 1998;39:545–551.

48. Legido A, Clancy R, Berman P. Recent advances in the diagnosis, treatment, and prognosis of neonatal seizures. *Pediatr Neurol* 1988;4:79–86.

49. Legido A, Clancy R, Berman P. Neurologic outcome after electroencephalographically proven neonatal seizures. *Pediatrics* 1991;88:583–596.

50. Legido A, Clancy R, Spitzer A, et al. Electroencephalographic and behavioral-state studies in infants of cocaine-addicted mothers. *Am J Dis Child* 1992;146:748–752.

51. Liu A, Hahn JS, Heldt GP, et al. Detection of neonatal seizures through computerized EEG analysis. *Electroencephalogr Clin Neurophysiol* 1992;82:30–37.

52. Lombroso C. Neurophysiological observations in diseased newborns. *Biol Psychiat* 1975;10: 527.

53. Lombroso C. Convulsive disorders in newborns. In: Thompson R, Green J, eds. *Pediatric neurology and neurosurgery.* New York: Spectrum Publications, 1978:202–239.

54. Lombroso C. Quantified electrographic scales on 10 pre-term healthy newborns followed up to 40–43 weeks of conceptional age by serial polygraphic recordings. *Electroencephalogr Clin Neurophysiol* 1979;46:460–474.

55. Lombroso C. Neonatal polygraphy in full-term and preterm infants: a review of normal and abnormal findings. *J Clin Neurophysiol* 1985;2:105–155.

56. Lombroso C. Neonatal electroencephalography. In: Niedermeyer E, Lopes da Silva F, eds. *Electroencephalography: basic principles, clinical applications and related fields,* 3rd ed. Baltimore: Williams & Wilkins, 1993:599–637.

57. Lombroso C. Neonatal EEG polygraphy in normal and abnormal newborns. In: Niedermeyer E, Lopes da Silva F (eds). *Electroencephalography: basic principles, clinical applications and related fields,* 3rd ed. Baltimore: Williams & Wilkins, 1993:803–875.

58. Malafosse A, Beck C, Bellet H, et al. Benign infantile familial convulsions are not an allelic form of the benign familial neonatal convulsions gene. *Ann Neurol* 1994;35:479–482.

59. Marret S, Parain D, Jeannot E, et al. Positive rolandic sharp waves in the EEG of the premature newborn: a five year prospective study. *Arch Dis Child* 1992;67:948–951.

60. Marret S, Parain D, Samson-Dollfus D. Positive rolandic sharp waves and periventricular leukomalacia in the newborn. *Neuropediatrics* 1986;17:199–202.

61. McCutchen C, Coen R, Iragui V. Periodic lateralized epileptiform discharges in asphyxiated neonates. *Electroencephalogr Clin Neurophysiol* 1984;61:210–217.

62. Mizrahi E, Kellaway P. Characterization and classification of neonatal seizures. *Neurology* 1987;37:1837–1844.

63. Mizrahi E, Kellaway P. The response of electroclinical neonatal seizures to antiepileptic drug therapy. *Epilepsia* 1992;33:114.

64. Monod N, Pajot N, Guidasci S. The neonatal EEG: statistical studies and prognostic value in full-term and pre-term babies. *Electroencephalogr Clin Neurophysiol* 1972;32:529–544.

65. Murat I. *Interet discriminatif des pointes positives rolandiques. Contribution au diagnostic des hemorragies intraventriculaires.* Thesis for the Doctor of Medicine, Academy of Paris, University René Descartes, Faculty of Medicine Cochin Port Royal, Paris, 1978.

66. Murdoch Eaton D, Toet M, Livingston J, et al. Evaluation of the Cerebro Trac 2500 for monitoring of cerebral function in the neonatal intensive care. *Neuropediatrics* 1994;25:122–128.

67. Novotny E, Tharp B, Coen R, et al. Positive rolandic sharp waves in the EEG of the premature infant. *Neurology* 1987;37:1481–1486.

68. Nowack W, Janati A, Angtuaco T. Positive temporal sharp waves in neonatal EEG. *Clin Electroencephalogr* 1989;20:196–201.

69. Nunes M, Da Costa J, Moura-Ribeiro M. Polysomnographic quantification of bioelectrical maturation in preterm and full term newborn at matched conceptual ages. *Electroencephalogr Clin Neurophysiol* 1997;102:186.

70. Obrecht R, Pollock M, Evans S, et al. Prediction of outcome in neonates using EEG. *Clin Electroencephalogr* 1982;13:46–49.

71. Olmos-Garcia de Alba G, Mora E, Valdez J, et al. Neonatal status epilepticus II: electroencephalographic aspects. *Clin Electroencephalogr* 1984;15:197–201.

72. Ortibus E, Sum J, Hahn J. Predictive value of EEG for outcome and epilepsy following neonatal seizures. *Electroencephalogr Clin Neurophysiol* 1996;98:175–185.

73. Pezzani C, Radvanyi-Bovet M, Relier J, et al. Neonatal electroencephalography during the first twenty-four hours of life in full-term newborn infants. *Neuropediatrics* 1986;17:11–18.

74. Roessgen M, Zoubir A, Boashash B. Seizure detection of newborn EEG using a model-based approach. *IEEE Trans Biomed Eng* 1998;45:673–685.

75. Rose A, Lombroso C. What is a neonatal seizure? Problems in definition and quantification for investigative and clinical purposes. *J Clin Neurophysiol* 1970;7:315–368.

76. Rosenblatt B, Gorman J. Computerized EEG monitoring. *Semin Pediatr Neurol* 1999;6: 120–127.

77. Rowe J, Holmes G, Hafford J, et al. Prognostic value of the electroencephalogram in term and preterm infants following neonatal seizures. *Electroencephalogr Clin Neurophysiol* 1985;60: 183–196.

78. Ryan S, Wiznitzer M, Holman C, et al. Benign familial neonatal convulsions: evidence for clinical and genetic heterogeneity. *Ann Neurol* 1991;29:469–473.

79. Scher M. Midline electrographic abnormalities and cerebral lesions in the newborn brain. *J Child Neurol* 1988;3:135–146.

80. Scher M. Positive temporal sharp waves on EEG recordings of healthy neonates: a benign pattern on dysmaturity in pre-term infants at post-conceptional term ages. *Electroencephalogr Clin Neurophysiol* 1994;90:173–178.

81. Scher M, Aso K, Beggarly M, et al. Electrographic seizures in preterm and full-term neonates: clinical correlates, associated brain lesions, and risk for neurologic sequelae. *Pediatrics* 1993; 91:128–134.

82. Scher M, Beggarly M. Clinical significance of focal periodic discharges in neonates. *J Child Neurol* 1989;4:175–185.

83. Scher M, Painter M, Bergman I, et al. EEG diagnoses of neonatal seizures: clinical correlations and outcome. *Pediatr Neurol* 1988;5:17–24.

84. Selton D, Andre M. Prognosis of hypoxic-ischaemic encephalopathy in full-term newborns—value of neonatal electroencephalography. *Neuropediatrics* 1997;28:276–280.

85. Shewmon D. What is a neonatal seizure? Problems in definition and quantification for investigative and clinical purposes. *J Clin Neurophysiol* 1990;7:315–368.

86. Slater G, Torres F. Frequency-amplitude gradient, a new parameter for interpreting pediatric sleep EEGs. *Arch Neurol* 1979;36:465–470.

87. Takeuchi T, Watanabe K. The EEG evolution and neurological prognosis of neonates with perinatal hypoxia neonates. *Brain Dev* 1989;11:115–120.

88. Tharp B. Neonatal and pediatric electroencephalography. In: Aminoff M, ed. *Electrodiagnosis in clinical neurology,* 2nd ed., vol. 2. New York: Churchill Livingstone, 1986:77–124.

89. Tharp B. Intensive video/EEG monitoring of neonates. In: Gumnit R, ed. *Advances in*

neurology, vol. 46: Intensive neurodiagnostic monitoring. New York: Raven Press, 1986: 114.

90. Tharp B. Electrophysiological brain maturation in premature infants: an historical perspective. *J Clin Neurophysiol* 1990;7:302–314.

91. Tharp B, Cukier F, Monod N. Valeur prognostique de l'EEG du premature. *Rev Electroencephalogr Neurophysiol* 1979;7:386–391.

92. Tharp B, Cukier F, Monod N. The prognostic value of the electroencephalogram in premature infants. *Electroencephalogr Clin Neurophysiol* 1981;51:219–236.

93. Tharp B, Scher M, Clancy R. Serial EEGs in normal and abnormal infants with birth weights less than 1200 grams—a prospective study with long term follow-up. *Neuropediatrics* 1989; 20:64–72.

94. Thornberg E, Ekström-Jodal B. Cerebral function monitoring: a method of predicting outcome in term neonates after severe perinatal asphyxia. *Acta Paediatr* 1994;83:596–601.

95. Van Lieshout H, Jacobs J, Rotteveel J, et al. The prognostic value of the EEG in asphyxiated newborns. *Acta Neurol Scand* 1995;91:203–207.

96. Watanabe K, Hara K, Miyazaki S, et al. Neurophysiological study of newborns with hypocalcemia. *Neuropediatrics* 1982;13:34–38.

97. Watanabe K, Iwase K, Hara, K. Development of slow-wave sleep in low-birthweight infants. *Dev Med Child Neurol* 1974;16:23–31.

98. Watanabe K, Miyazaki S, Hara K, et al. Behavioral state cycles, background EEGs and prognosis of newborns with perinatal hypoxia. *Electroencephalog Clin Neurophysiol* 1980;49: 618–625.

99. Watanabe K, Negoro T, Inokuma K, et al. Subclinical delta status in the newborn—an unfavorable prognostic sign. *Clin Electroencephalogr* 1984;15:125–131.

100. Weiner S, Painter M, Geva D, et al. Neonatal seizures: electroclinical dissociation. *Pediatr Neurol* 1991;7:363–368.

Chapter 7

Benign Electroencephalographic Variants and Patterns of Uncertain Clinical Significance[1]

Barbara F. Westmoreland

Rhythmic Patterns
    Rhythmic Temporal Theta Bursts of Drowsiness
        (Psychomotor Variant Pattern)
    Alpha Variant
    Subclinical Rhythmic Electrographic (Theta)
        Discharge in Adults
    Midline Theta Rhythm
    Frontal Arousal Rhythm

Benign Patterns with an Epileptiform Morphology
    Fourteen- and Six-Hertz Positive Bursts
    Small Sharp Spikes (SSS)
    Six-Hertz Spike-and-Wave Bursts ("Phantom
        Spike and Wave")
    Wicket Spikes
    Breach Rhythm
Conclusion
References

There are several benign variants of electroencephalographic (EEG) activity, including variations of normal rhythms, rhythmic patterns, and patterns with an "epileptiform" morphology, which the electroencephalographer should recognize to avoid overinterpreting them with regard to their significance.

Some patterns represent a superimposition of background frequencies producing activity that may simulate "epileptiform-like" discharges, and one must consider the context of the background activity from which the waveform is arising (20). Other EEG patterns have an epileptiform appearance but are non-epileptogenic in that they have no established association with clinical seizures. Although there is controversy and difference of opinion regarding some of these patterns, most of the nonepileptogenic epileptiform patterns described in this chapter are now considered to be normal variants or patterns of uncertain clinical significance (20,25,32,33). These can be subdivided into rhythmic patterns and patterns with an epileptiform morphology.

RHYTHMIC PATTERNS

Rhythmic patterns consist of rhythmic activity that may be in the theta, alpha, or beta frequency ranges. They may also consist of a mixture of two or more frequencies or be a reflection of harmonic frequencies. The rhythmic patterns consist of rhythmic temporal theta bursts of drowsiness (RTTD), the alpha variant patterns, the midline theta rhythm, the frontal arousal rhythm (FAR), and subclinical rhythmic electrographic discharge of adults (SREDA).

Rhythmic Temporal Theta Bursts of Drowsiness (Psychomotor Variant Pattern)

The term *psychomotor variant pattern* was originally used (9,10) because of the occurrence of this pattern over the temporal regions and because of its rhythmic nature, which seemed to resemble a "psychomotor" or temporal lobe seizure discharge. It has also been called "rhythmic midtemporal discharges" (RMTDs) (17). The preferred term is now *rhythmic temporal theta bursts of drowsiness* (1). The temporal theta pat-tern of drowsiness (4,6,9,10,17,22,32,39) is characterized by bursts or serial trains of rhythmic theta waves ranging from 5 to 7 Hz with a flat-topped, sharp-contoured, or notched appearance. The notching occurs as a result of either (a) a superimposition of faster frequencies or (b) harmonics of the resting background frequency (Fig. 7.1). The bursts occur predominantly over the temporal regions and are usually maximal in the midtemporal electrodes. There can be some spread to the parasagittal regions. The temporal theta bursts occur bilaterally or independently over the two hemispheres, or they show a shifting emphasis from side to side. The trains usually begin and end with a gradual increase and decrease in amplitude. The pattern differs from a true seizure discharge in that it is usually a monomorphic or monorhythmic pattern that does not evolve into other frequencies or waveforms. It occurs predominantly during relaxed wakefulness and drowsiness and is seen mainly in adolescents and adults. Gibbs et al. (10) reported an incidence of approximately 0.5%, whereas Maulsby (25) found the pattern in 2% of selected normal adults. Although some authors have related this pattern to various symptoms, it is now considered a non-specific finding in the EEG that has no significance with regard to seizures or other neurological symptoms (20).

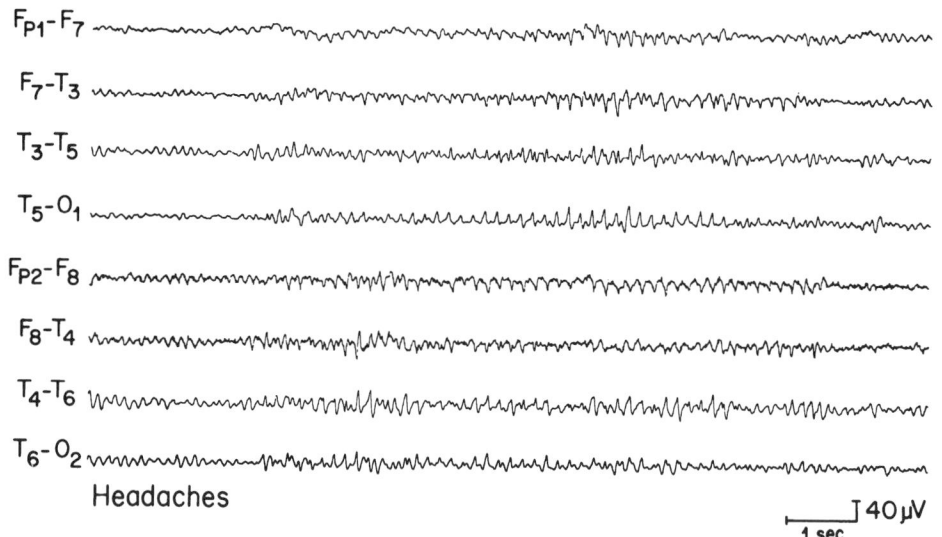

FIG. 7.1. Rhythmic temporal theta bursts of drowsiness in a 40-year-old woman. (From Westmoreland BF. EEG in the evaluation of headaches. In: Klass DW, Daly DD, eds. *Current practice of clinical electroencephalography.* New York: Raven Press, 1979:381–394, with permission of Lippincott Williams & Wilkins.)

Alpha Variant

Alpha variant patterns consist of activity over the posterior head regions that have a harmonic relationship to the alpha rhythm and show similar reactivity and distribution (11).

Slow Alpha Variant Pattern

The slow alpha variant pattern is a subharmonic of the alpha rhythm that has a frequency about half that of the alpha rhythm, usually in the range of 4 to 5 Hz. The waveforms usually have a sinusoidal or notched appearance and can alternate or be admixed with the regular alpha activity (1,11) (Fig. 7.2). The alpha variant pattern is seen mainly in adults during relaxed wakefulness and is considered a physiological variant of the alpha rhythm. The slow alpha variant sometimes has a notched appearance and may resemble the RTTD, except that it occurs over the posterior head regions.

Fast Alpha Variant

The fast alpha variant pattern has a frequency that is usually twice that of the resting alpha rhythm and ranges from 16 to 20 Hz, with a voltage of 20–40 μV; it alternates or is admixed with the alpha rhythm (1). It arises from the posterior head regions, and its reactivity resembles that of the alpha rhythm.

Subclinical Rhythmic Electrographic (Theta) Discharge in Adults

This uncommon pattern is seen mainly in people older than 50 years (26,28,29,46,48). SREDA may occur at rest or during drowsiness, and occasionally occurs mainly during hyperventilation. The pattern is a distinctive one and consists of mixed-frequency components in the delta and theta frequency ranges that evolve into a rhythmic pattern consisting of sharp-contoured components 5–7 Hz (Figs. 7.3 and 7.4) (30,46,48). SREDA usually occurs in a widespread distribution with maximal amplitude over the parietal–posterior temporal head regions. Usually it is bilateral, but it may occur in a more focal or asymmetric fashion. The duration of the SREDA pattern may range from 20 seconds to a few minutes; however, the average duration is 40–80 seconds. In half the patients, SREDA may have an abrupt onset in which the background activity is suddenly replaced by repetitive monophasic sharp waveforms (Fig. 7.3). In other patients, the discharge begins with a single, high-voltage, monophasic

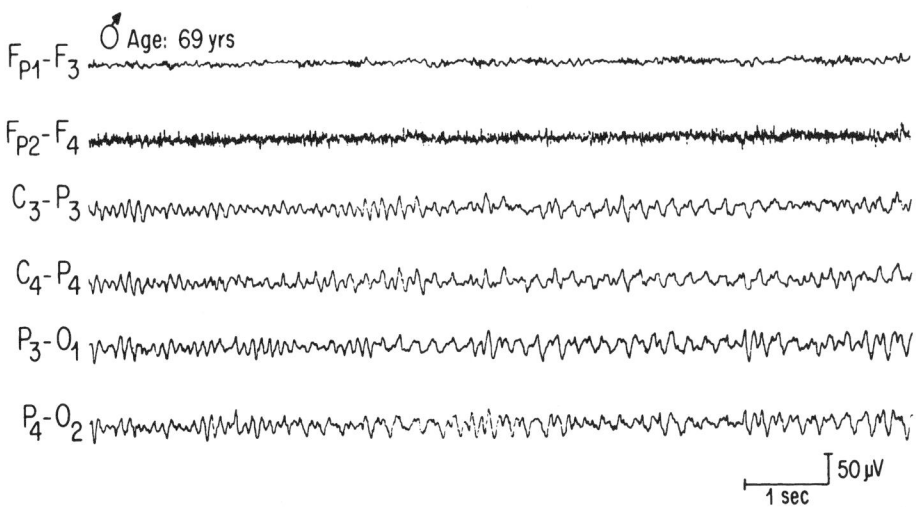

FIG. 7.2. Example of slow alpha variant pattern in a 69-year-old man.

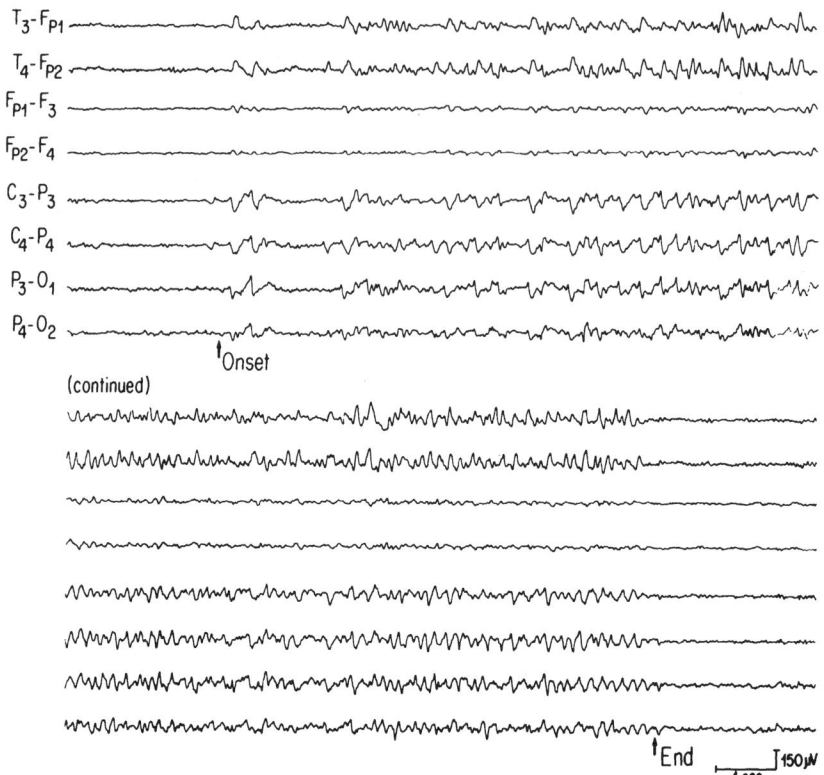

FIG. 7.3. Subclinical rhythmic electrographic discharge (SREDA) in a 52-year-old woman. (From Westmoreland BF. Benign EEG variants and patterns of uncertain clinical significance. In: Daly DD, Pedley TA, eds. *Current practice of clinical electroencephalography*, 2nd ed. New York: Raven Press, 1990:243–252, with permission of Lippincott Williams & Wilkins.)

change in bloodflow. The authors concluded that this provided evidence that SREDA was not an "epileptic pattern" (43). SREDA has been seen in patients with diverse clinical complaints. No clinical alteration is associated with the pattern, and the patient does not complain of any subjective symptoms while the pattern is present. Although its mechanism of origin remains uncertain, SREDA seems to represent a benign EEG phenomenon that has little or no diagnostic significance (26,30,46,48).

Midline Theta Rhythm

The midline theta rhythm occurs as a focal rhythm over the midline region and usually is most prominent in the central vertex (Cz) lead (47) (Fig. 7.5). Occasionally, there is some spread to adjacent electrodes. It consists of a rhythmic train of 5–7 Hz activity and usually has a smooth, sinusoidal, arciform, spiky, or mu-like appearance. The midline rhythm is of variable duration and tends to wax and wane. It is present during wakefulness and drowsiness and shows variable reactivity to eye opening, alerting, and limb movement.

The pattern was originally described by Cigánek (2) as "theta discharges in the middle line." Cigánek initially saw this in patients with temporal lobe epilepsy and believed that it occurred predominantly in such patients. Later, Mokrán et al. (27) reviewed a less selected group of patients and found that this rhythm was also present in patients without epilepsy. A more recent review has shown that a midline theta rhythm can occur in a heterogeneous group of patients, and, although its mechanism is uncertain, the midline rhythm appears to represent a nonspecific variant of theta activity (47).

sharp- or slow-wave component that is followed 1 second or several seconds later by other sharp waves, progressively recurring at shorter intervals and then increasing in frequency to merge into a sustained, rhythmic, sinusoidal pattern of 5–7 Hz (26,46,48) (Figs. 7.4 and 7.5). Although the pattern may resemble a subclinical EEG seizure discharge, it does not have any correlation with clinical seizures. A single-photon emission computed tomographic (SPECT) study was performed on a patient with a focal SREDA pattern involving the right occipitotemporal region and showed no

Frontal Arousal Rhythm

FAR, a rhythm that was initially described by White and Tharp (51), occurs in children following arousal from sleep. The pattern consists of trains of 7- to 20-Hz waveforms that occur predominantly over the frontal regions in runs lasting up to 20 seconds (Fig. 7.6). There may be varying harmonics, which give the pattern a notched appearance and a superficial resemblance to a rhythmic discharge pattern. FAR, however, usually disappears once the child is fully awake. Although FAR was initially described in children with minimal cerebral dysfunction (51), it is considered to be more a nonspecific pattern of no clinical significance.

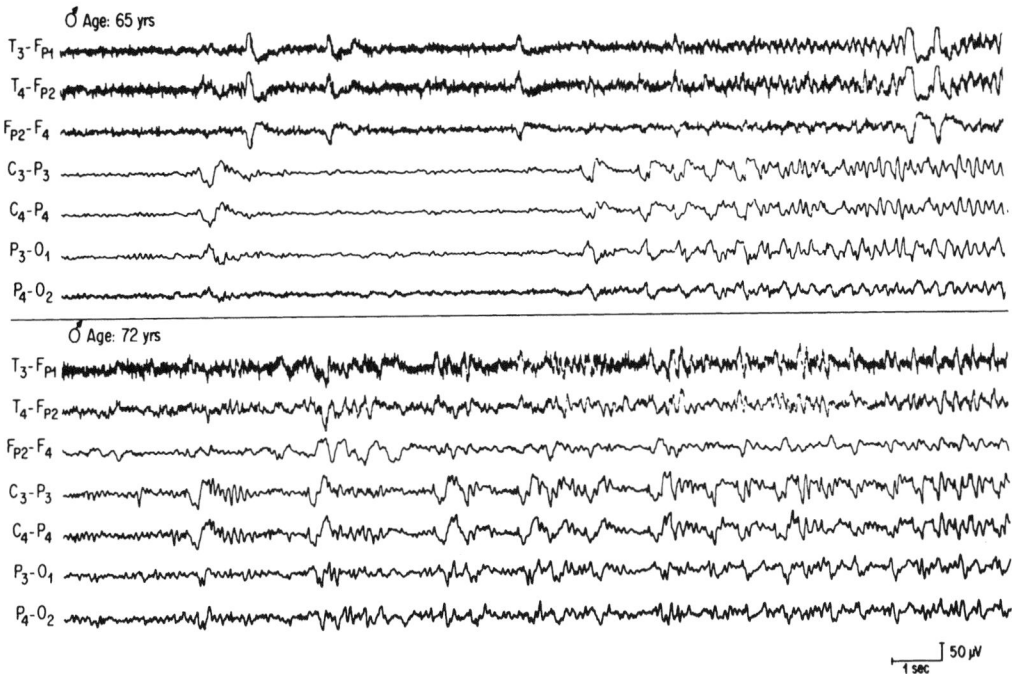

FIG. 7.4. Onset of SREDA in two patients. **Top:** An initial sharp wave complex, followed several seconds later by repetitive sharp waves that merge into a sustained theta rhythm. **Bottom:** Repetitive sharp waves gradually increasing in frequency to a repetitive theta rhythm. (From Westmoreland BF. Benign EEG variants and patterns of uncertain clinical significance. In: Daly DD, Pedley TA, eds. *Current practice of clinical electroencephalography*, 2nd ed. New York: Raven Press, 1990:243–252, with permission of Lippincott Williams & Wilkins.)

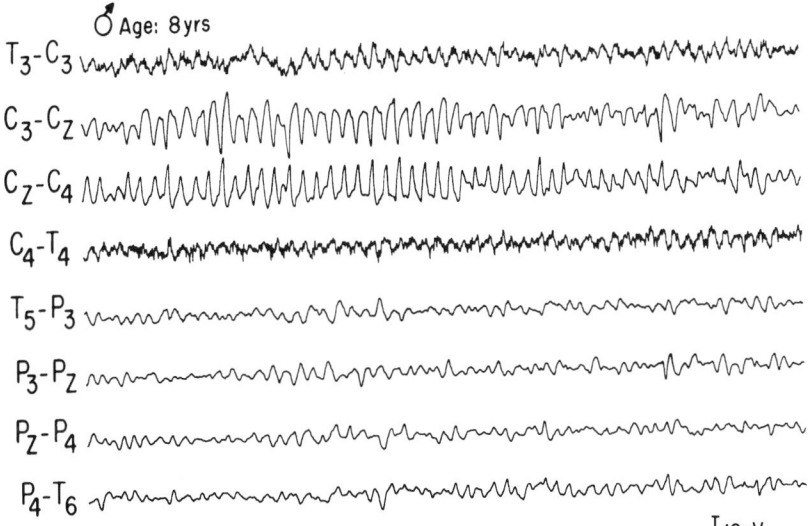

FIG. 7.5. Midline theta rhythm (seen predominantly in the CZ electrode) in an 8-year-old boy. (From Westmoreland BF. Benign EEG variants and patterns of uncertain clinical significance. In: Daly DD, Pedley TA, eds. *Current practice of clinical electroencephalography*, 2nd ed. New York: Raven Press, 1990:243–252, with permission of Lippincott Williams & Wilkins.)

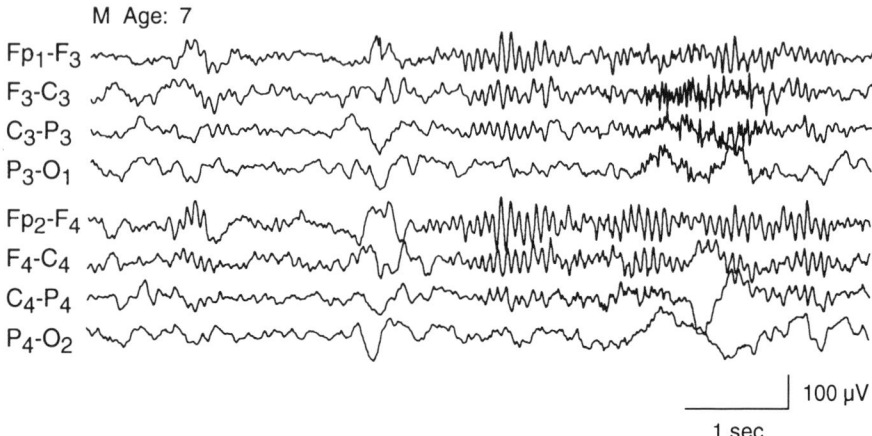

FIG. 7.6. Frontal arousal rhythm in a 7-year-old boy.

BENIGN PATTERNS WITH AN EPILEPTIFORM MORPHOLOGY

These patterns have an epileptiform appearance but are not epileptogenic; that is, they are not associated with seizures. They include 14- and 6-Hz positive bursts, small sharp spikes (SSS), 6-Hz spike-and-wave bursts, wicket waves, and the breach rhythm.

Fourteen- and Six-Hertz Positive Bursts

These bursts were originally called "14- and 6-Hz positive spikes"; the term *ctenoids* (23) had also been used for this phenomenon (1,4,5,7–9, 12,14,18,20,23,25,32–34,37–39,52). The preferred term now is *14- and 6-Hz positive bursts* .

These bursts occur predominantly during drowsiness and light sleep and consist of short trains of arch-shaped waveforms with alternating positive spiky components and a negative, smooth, rounded waveform that resembles a sleep spindle with a sharp positive phase (Fig. 7.7). The bursts occur at a rate of 14 Hz or 6–7 Hz and last from 0.5 to 1 second. Usually, the faster frequency is the more prevalent, but the slower rate can occur either independently or in association with a train of 14-Hz positive bursts. The waveform is best displayed on a long-distance or referential montage to the ear. It usually has maximal amplitude over the posterior temporal region. The bursts can occur asynchronously or independently over the two

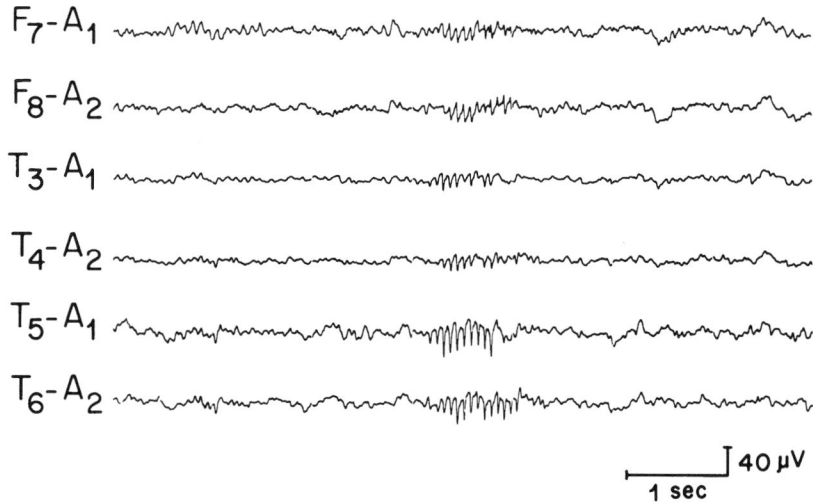

FIG. 7.7. A 14- and 6-Hz positive burst, on a referential montage, in a 29-year-old woman. (From Westmoreland BF. EEG in the evaluation of headaches. In: Klass DW, Daly DD, eds. *Current practice of clinical electroencephalography*. New York: Raven Press, 1979:381–394, with permission of Lippincott Williams & Wilkins.)

sides but may preferentially involve one side; they may also shift from side to side in predominance.

In a normal population, 14- and 6-Hz positive bursts begin to appear in children between 3 and 4 years old, are maximally expressed in the adolescent age group (with a peak at age 13–14 years), and then progressively decrease in incidence with increasing age (20).

In the past, this pattern has been associated with various clinical symptoms, including headaches, dizziness, vertigo, abdominal complaints, emotional instability, rage, violence, and "thalamic" or "hypothalamic" epilepsy. However, 14- and 6-Hz positive bursts occur in normal control populations and in asymptomatic persons. Moreover, depending on the study, these bursts were present in 10%–58% of subjects. Differences in the incidence may be due to the age group studied, the amount of EEG recorded during drowsiness and light sleep, and the montage used (20,32). Most authorities now regard this as a benign variant of no clinical significance.

Small Sharp Spikes (SSS)

"Small sharp spikes" (7,9,16,19–21,25,32–34,36,38,40,45,49,50) is the original name used by Gibbs and Gibbs (7,9). The pattern has also been referred to as "benign epileptiform transients of sleep" (BETS) (50) and "benign sporadic sleep spikes" (BSSS) (20). SSS are seen mainly in adults during drowsiness and light sleep. They are generally of low voltage, usually less than 50 μV; however, they occasionally may have a higher amplitude (Fig. 7.8). SSS are of short duration, usually less than 50 milliseconds. The waveform usually consist of single monophasic or diphasic spike with an abrupt ascending limb and a steep descending limb (Fig. 7.8). SSS have a single aftercoming slow-wave component or may be associated with an aftercoming dip in the background; however, they do not have the prominent aftercoming slow wave that temporal spikes have, and they do not occur in repetitive trains. The morphology varies from patient to patient and with different types of montages, so not all SSS have a stereotyped appearance (20,49). Because SSS have a broad, sloping potential field, they are seen best in derivations with long interelectrode distances and are displayed most clearly in the temporal and ear leads (20).

SSS occur predominantly as a unilateral waveform. However, provided that the EEG recording is of sufficient length, SSS are almost always are bilaterally represented, either occurring independently or having some reflection to the opposite hemisphere (Fig. 7.8). In addition, the field sometimes corresponds to an oblique transverse dipole across the two hemispheres, with oppo-

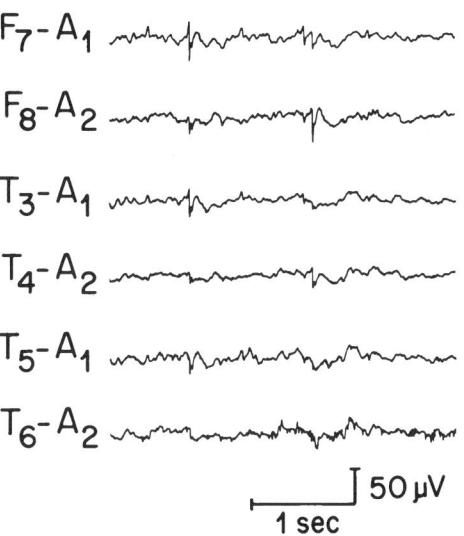

FIG. 7.8. Examples of small sharp spikes (benign sporadic sleep spikes) occurring over the left and right temporal regions, as seen on a referential montage. (From Westmoreland BF. Benign EEG variants and patterns of uncertain clinical significance. In: Daly DD, Pedley TA, eds. *Current practice of clinical electroencephalography,* 2nd ed. New York: Raven Press, 1990:243–252, with permission of Lippincott Williams & Wilkins.)

site polarity on the two sides of the head, a topography that is unusual for spikes of cerebral origin (19–21,36). The two phases of the same discharge also may vary in distribution in an anteroposterior direction (20). Unlike the more significant epileptogenic discharges that can arise from the temporal areas, SSS usually do not distort the background, are not associated with rhythmic slow-wave activity, do not occur in trains, and tend to diminish or disappear with deeper levels of slow-wave sleep.

The incidence of SSS in a normal control population or in asymptomatic subjects is approximately 20%–25% (20,50). In a study on the significance of this phenomenon, White and associates (50) found BETS (or SSS) in 24% of normal subjects and in 20% of unselected patients. The current consensus is that SSS have no significance in the diagnosis of epileptic seizures (20,32–34,36). In addition, the bilateral occurrence of the BSSS should not be misinterpreted as representing bilateral epileptogenic foci (20).

Six-Hertz Spike-and-Wave Bursts ("Phantom Spike and Wave")

The 6-Hz spike-and-wave discharges (1,7,9,13,15,24,31,39,41,42) have a repetition rate of 6 Hz, with a range of 5–7 Hz (Fig. 7.9). The bursts are usually brief, lasting 1 or 2 seconds, although rarely they persist for 3 or 4 seconds. The pattern has also been called the "phantom spike and wave" (1,44) because of the evanescent nature of the spike, which is usually very brief and small in amplitude, in contrast to the more prominent slow-wave component, which has a higher amplitude and a more widespread distribution. At times, the spike may be difficult to see.

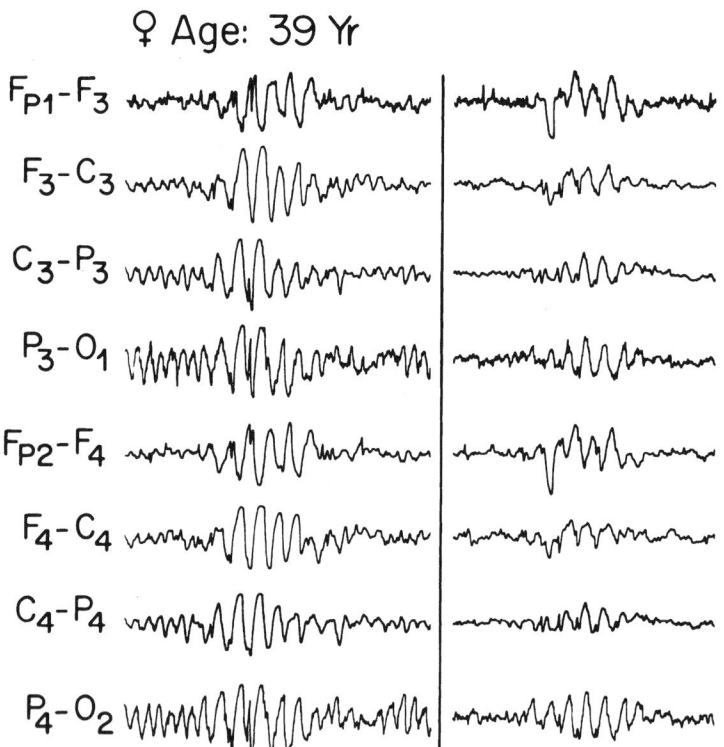

FIG. 7.9. Six-Hertz spike-and-wave bursts in a 39-year-old woman. (From Westmoreland BF. EEG in the evaluation of headaches. In: Klass DW, Daly DD, eds. *Current practice of clinical electroencephalography.* New York: Raven Press, 1979:381–394, with permission of Lippincott Williams & Wilkins.)

The 6-Hz spike-and-wave pattern is seen in both adolescents and adults, with an overall incidence of 2.5%. It occurs mainly during relaxed wakefulness and drowsiness and disappears during deeper levels of sleep.

The 6-Hz spike-and-wave bursts usually occur in a bilaterally synchronous and diffuse manner, although the bursts can occur in an asymmetrical fashion or predominate over the anterior and posterior head regions. There may be some resemblance to the 6-Hz positive bursts described above, and there may be a transition between the two types of waveforms, which can occur in the same person (37).

Although there is still some difference of opinion about the exact significance of the 6-Hz spike-and-wave burst, it has not proved to be a reliable indicator of seizures (20,42). One of the problems may be the difficulty in distinguishing the atypical forms of 6-Hz spike-and-wave discharge from fragments of more significant spike-and-wave complexes. Two types of 6-Hz spike-and-wave discharges have been described by Hughes (13), who used the acronyms of FOLD and WHAM to describe the two variants. FOLD (female occipital-predominant low amplitude and drowsiness) describes the characteristics seen with the more benign variant of the 6-Hz spike-and-wave pattern, and WHAM (wake high-amplitude anterior predominance in male) refers to the variant that is more likely to be associated with seizures. Seizures are more likely if the spike discharges are high in amplitude and the rate is less than 5 or 6 Hz. Another helpful way of making the distinction is that the benign 6-Hz spike-and-wave burst tends to disappear during sleep, whereas more significant types of spike-and-wave discharges tend to persist or even become more prominent with deeper levels of sleep (20).

Wicket Spikes

These waveforms, described in detail by Reiher and Lebel (35), consist of intermittent trains or clusters of monophasic arciform waveforms or single spike-like waveforms that look like a Greek mu or wicket (Fig. 7.10). When they occur as a single waveform, wicket spikes can be mistaken for a temporal spike discharge; however, if the single waveform is analyzed and compared with a train of wicket spikes, the wicket spikes have a morphology similar to that of a train of wicket-like activity. Another feature that distinguishes a wicket spike from the more pathological spike is that it is not associated with either (a) an aftercoming slow-wave component or (b) a distortion or slowing of the background that occurs with a true temporal spike.

Wicket spikes are seen mainly during drowsiness and light sleep. They may be present during the awake recording but are often masked by other

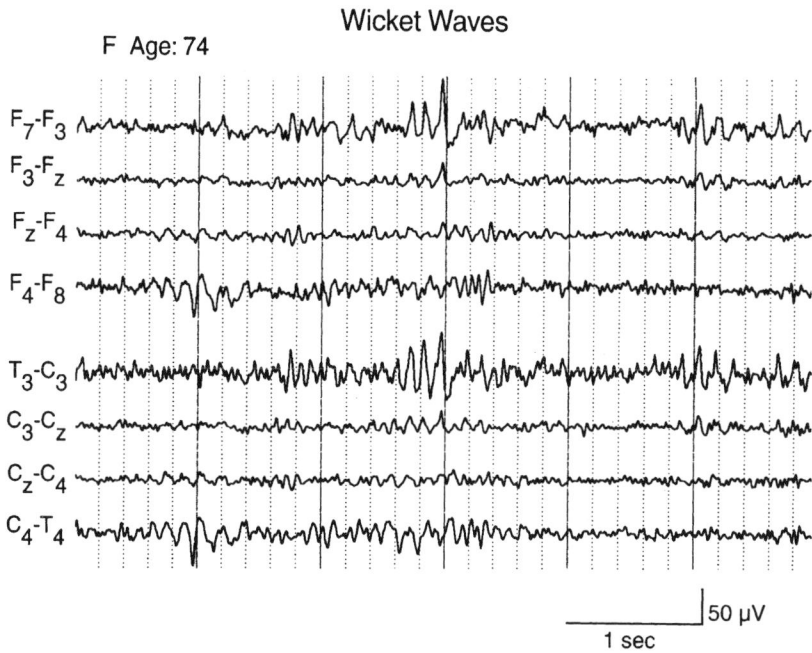

FIG. 7.10. Wicket spikes in a 74-year-old woman.

background rhythms and usually emerge or become apparent during drowsiness, when the alpha and other awake patterns disappear. Wicket spikes are seen predominantly over the temporal regions and occur bilaterally or independently over the two temporal regions. They may have a shifting predominance or may be more consistently evident on one side. Wicket spikes usually occur with a frequency of 6–11 Hz and have an amplitude ranging from 60 to 200 μV. They are seen predominantly in adults older than 30 years and have an incidence of 0.9% (35). They likely represent fragments of so-called "temporal alpha activity."

Breach Rhythm

The breach rhythm was described by Cobb and associates (3) in 1979 and refers to high-voltage activity that occurs in the region of a skull defect. The breach rhythm frequently has a spiky appearance and consists of sharply contoured arciform waveforms that usually have a frequency of 6–11 Hz but may sometimes be associated with faster or slower wave activity. The breach rhythm is most prominent when recorded over the central and temporal regions, and, at times, it may have a threefold increase in amplitude compared with activity in other regions (Fig. 7.11). The activity over the central regions often reflects mu activity and, like mu activity, responds to touch or movement. The other prominent location for the breach rhythm is over the temporal areas, where wicket spikes and other spike-like activity can be quite prominent. The breach rhythm usually is easily recognizable when it occurs in serial trains. A problem may arise when one sees single spike-like or sharp-contoured waveforms that may be mistaken for potentially epileptogenic activity. It is helpful to compare this with the waveforms of the rhythmic activity constituting the breach rhythm to determine whether these are distinct waveforms or whether they are similar to the activity that constitutes the breach rhythm. Other factors that help make the distinction between a breach rhythm and more significant epileptogenic abnormalities are the absence of aftercoming slow-wave components and lack of spread to other areas. The presence of the breach rhythm should not be considered an indicator of epilepsy or recurrence of a tumor or underlying lesion.

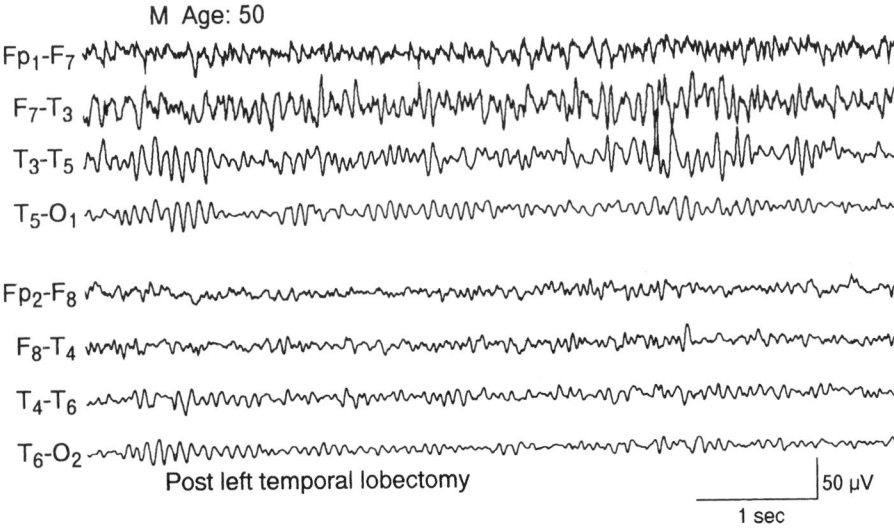

FIG. 7.11. Breach rhythm over the left midtemporal region following a left temporal lobectomy in a 50-year-old man.

Although bone reabsorption or absence of bone in the area of the skull defect has a major role in the prominence of the breach rhythm, other factors may also be involved (see Chapter 11 for additional discussion).

CONCLUSION

This chapter has discussed some of the EEG patterns that represent benign variants of EEG activity or activity of uncertain significance. None should be considered abnormal. These patterns can occur in normal or asymptomatic persons, or in patients with various complaints, and they should be differentiated from true epileptogenic or abnormal activity. In making the distinction, the electroencephalographer needs to consider various parameters of EEG activity, including the morphology, topography, distribution, phase relations, amplitude, duration, frequency, coexisting background from which the activity is arising, reactivity, and state of the patient (20,32,33). Critical evaluation of the various types of EEG activity is important in making the distinction between patterns that are benign and those that are associated with epilepsy.

REFERENCES

1. Chatrian GE, Bergamini L, Dondey M, et al. A glossary of terms most commonly used by clinical electroencephalographers. *Electroencephalogr Clin Neurophysiol* 1974;37:538–548.
2. Cigánek L. Theta-discharges in the middle-line—EEG symptom of temporal lobe epilepsy. *Electroencephalogr Clin Neurophysiol* 1961;13:669–673.
3. Cobb WA, Guiloff RJ, Cast J. Breach rhythm: the EEG related to skull defects. *Electroencephalogr Clin Neurophysiol* 1979;47:251–271.
4. Dondey M, Gaches J. Seminology in clinical EEG. In: Rémond A, ed. *Handbook of electroencephalography and clinical neurophysiology*, Vol 11, Part A. Amsterdam: Elsevier Science, 1977:25–79.
5. Eeg-Olofsson O. The development of the electroencephalogram in normal children from the age of 1 through 15 years: 14 and 6 Hz positive spike phenomenon. *Neuropadiatrie* 1971;2: 405–427.
6. Garvin JS. Psychomotor variant pattern. *Dis Nerv Syst* 1968;29:307–309.
7. Gibbs FA, Gibbs EL. *Atlas of electroencephalography*, Vol 2. Cambridge, MA: Addison Wesley, 1952.
8. Gibbs FA, Gibbs EL. Fourteen and six per second positive spikes. *Electroencephalogr Clin Neurophysiol* 1963;15:553–558.
9. Gibbs FA, Gibbs EL. *Atlas of electroencephalography*, Vol 3. Reading, MA: Addison Wesley, 1964.
10. Gibbs FA, Rich CL, Gibbs EL. Psychomotor variant type of seizure discharge. *Neurology (Minneap)* 1963;13:991–998.
11. Goodwin JE. Significance of alpha variants in EEG, and their relationship to epileptiform syndrome. *Am J Psychiatry* 1947;104:369–379.
12. Henry CE. Positive spike discharges in the EEG and behavior abnormality. In: Glaser GH, ed. *EEG and behavior*. New York: Basic Books, 1963:315–344.
13. Hughes JR. Two forms of the 6/sec spike and wave complex. *Electroencephalogr Clin Neurophysiol* 1980;48:535–550.
14. Hughes JR. A review of the positive spike phenomenon: recent studies. In: Hughes JR, Wilson WP, eds. *EEG and evoked potentials in psychiatry and behavioral neurology*. Boston: Butterworth-Heinemann, 1983:295–324.

15. Hughes JR. A review of the 6/sec spike and wave complex. In: Hughes JR, Wilson WP, eds. *EEG and evoked potentials in psychiatry and behavioral neurology*. Boston: Butterworth-Heinemann, 1983:325–346.

16. Hughes JR. A review of small sharp spikes. In: Hughes JR, Wilson WP, eds. *EEG and evoked potentials in psychiatry and behavioral neurology*. Boston: Butterworth-Heinemann, 1983: 347–359.

17. Hughes JR, Cayaffa JJ. Is the "psychomotor variant"–"rhythmic mid-temporal discharge" an ictal pattern? *Clin Electroencephalogr* 1973;4:42–49.

18. Hughes JR, Cayaffa JJ. Positive spikes revisited—in the adult. *Clin Electroencephalogr* 1978; 9:52–59.

19. Klass DW. Electroencephalographic manifestations of complex partial seizures. *Adv Neurol* 1975;11:113–140.

20. Klass DW, Westmoreland BF. Nonepileptogenic epileptiform electroencephalographic activity. *Ann Neurol* 1985;18:627–635.

21. Lebel M, Reiher J, Klass D. Small sharp spikes (SSS): electroencephalographic characteristics and clinical significance. *Electroencephalogr Clin Neurophysiol* 1977;43:463(abst).

22. Lipman IJ, Hughes JR. Rhythmic mid-temporal discharges: an electro-clinical study. *Electroencephalogr Clin Neurophysiol* 1969;27:43–47.

23. Lombroso CT, Schwartz IH, Clark DM, et al. Ctenoids in healthy youths: controlled study of 14- and 6-per-second positive spiking. *Neurology* 1966;16:1152–1158.

24. Marshall C. Some clinical correlates of the wave and spike phantom. *Electroencephalogr Clin Neurophysiol* 1955;7:633–636.

25. Maulsby RL. EEG patterns of uncertain diagnostic significance. In: Klass DW, Daly DD, eds. *Current practice of clinical electroencephalography*. New York: Raven Press, 1979: 411–419.

26. Miller CR, Westmoreland BF, Klass DW. Subclinical rhythmic EEG discharge of adults (SREDA): further observations. *Am J EEG Technol* 1985;25:217–224.

27. Mokrán V, Cigánek L, Kabatnik Z. Electroencephalographic theta discharges in the midline. *Eur Neurol* 1971;5:288–293.

28. Naquet R, Franck G, Vigouroux R. Données nouvelles sur certaines décharges paroxystiques du carrefour pariéto-temporo-occipital, rencontrées chez l'homme. *Zentralbl Neurochir* 1965; 25:153–180.

29. Naquet R, Louard C, Rhodes J, et al. Apropos of certain paroxysmal discharges from the temporo-parieto-occipital junction: their activation by hypoxia [in French]. *Rev Neurol (Paris)* 1961;105:203–207.

30. O'Brien TJ, Sharbrough FW, Westmoreland BF, et al. Subclinical rhythmic electrographic discharges of adults (SREDA) revisited: a study using digital EEG analysis. *J Clin Neurophysiol* 1998;15:493–501.

31. Olson SF, Hughes JR. The clinical symptomatology associated with the 6 c-sec spike and wave complex. *Epilepsia* 1970;11:383–393.

32. Pedley TA. EEG patterns that mimic epileptiform discharges but have no association with seizures. In: Henry CE, ed. *Current clinical neurophysiology: update on EEG and evoked potentials*. New York: Elsevier Science, 1980:307–336.

33. Pedley TA. Interictal epileptiform discharges: discriminating characteristics and clinical correlations. *Am J EEG Technol* 1980;20:101–119.

34. Reiher J, Klass DW. Two common EEG patterns of doubtful clinical significance. *Med Clin North Am* 1968;52:933–940.

35. Reiher J, Lebel M. Wicket spikes: clinical correlates of a previously undescribed EEG pattern. *Can J Neurol Sci* 1977;4:39–47.

36. Reiher J, Lebel M, Klass DW. Small sharp spikes (SSS): reassessment of electroencephalographic characteristics and clinical significance. *Electroencephalogr Clin Neurophysiol* 1977;43:775(abst).

37. Silverman D. Phantom spike-waves and the fourteen and six per second positive spike pattern: a consideration of their relationship. *Electroencephalogr Clin Neurophysiol* 1967;23:207–213.

38. Small JG. Small sharp spikes in a psychiatric population. *Arch Gen Psychiatry* 1970;22:277–284.

39. Small JG, Sharpley P, Small IF. Positive spikes, spike-wave phantoms, and psychomotor variants: a survey of these EEG patterns in psychiatric patients. *Arch General Psychiatry* 1968;18:232–238.

40. Small JG, Small IF. EEG spikes in non-epileptic psychiatric patients. *Dis Nerv Syst* 1967; 28:523–525.

41. Tharp BR. The 6-per-second spike and wave complex: the wave and spike phantom. *Arch Neurol* 1966;15:533–537.

42. Thomas JE, Klass DW. Six-per-second spike-and-wave pattern in the electroencephalogram: a reappraisal of its clinical significance. *Neurology* 1968;18:587–593.

43. Thomas P, Migneco O, Darcourt J, et al. Single photon emission computed tomography study of subclinical rhythmic electrographic discharge in adults. *Electroencephalogr Clin Neurophysiol* 1992;83:223–227.

44. Walter WG. Epilepsy. In: Hill D, Parr G, eds. *Electroencephalography: a symposium on its various aspects*. London: Macdonald, 1950:228–272.

45. Westmoreland BF. EEG in the evaluation of headaches. In: Klass DW, Daly DD, eds. *Current practice of clinical electroencephalography*. New York: Raven Press, 1979:381–394.

46. Westmoreland BF, Klass DW. A distinctive rhythmic EEG discharge of adults. *Electroencephalogr Clin Neurophysiol* 1981;51:186–191.

47. Westmoreland BF, Klass DW. Midline theta rhythm. *Arch Neurol* 1986;43:139–141.

48. Westmoreland BF, Klass DW. Unusual variants of subclinical rhythmic electrographic discharge of adults (SREDA). *Electroencephalogr Clin Neurophysiol* 1997;102:1–4.

49. Westmoreland BF, Reiher J, Klass DW. Recording small sharp spikes with depth electroencephalography. *Epilepsia* 1979;20:599–606.

50. White JC, Langston JW, Pedley TA. Benign epileptiform transients of sleep. Clarification of the small sharp spike controversy. *Neurology* 1977;27:1061–1068.

51. White JC, Tharp BR. An arousal pattern in children with organic cerebral dysfunction. *Electroencephalogr Clin Neurophysiol* 1974;37:265–268.

52. Wiener JM, Delano JG, Klass DW. An EEG study of delinquent and nondelinquent adolescents. *Arch General Psychiatry* 1966;15:144–150.

Chapter 8

Activation Methods

Bruce J. Fisch and Elson L. So

Electroencephalographic (EEG) activation as defined by the International Federation of Clinical Neurophysiology Societies (75) includes any procedure designed to enhance or elicit normal or abnormal EEG activity, especially epileptiform abnormalities. Activation stimuli include various sensory modalities, electrical and pharmacological stimulation, and changes in behavioral state and consciousness. Activation procedures used routinely in the EEG laboratory are hyperventilation, photic stimulation, and sleep. Hyperventilation and photic stimulation are most useful for activating epileptiform abnormalities, whereas drowsiness and sleep are useful for activating all forms of EEG abnormalities as well as normal epileptiform patterns (so-called pseudoepileptiform patterns). In addition to these routine activating procedures, other procedures are used in patients with abnormal paroxysmal behaviors that can be triggered by a specific stimulus. Examples of the latter include reading (reading-induced myoclonus or seizures), music (musicogenic epilepsy), mental calculation (calculation-induced seizures), and even immersion in water (so-called hot tub seizures). Direct electrical activation of the brain is performed using either needle, subdural, or depth electrodes to evoke afterdischarges or electrographic seizures. Pharmacological activating procedures include the withdrawal of antiepileptic drugs (AEDs) and the administration of convulsant medications such as pentylenetetrazol. Behavioral activation procedures, in contrast to EEG activation procedures, are performed during EEG recording to activate behavioral events that do not typically elicit epileptiform abnormalities. Examples include postural changes in patients with movement disorders or generalized or localized orthostatic ischemia (e.g., limb-shaking transient ischemic attacks [TIAs]), emotional changes in infants with possible breath-holding spells, or a variety of suggestion techniques in individuals with suspected psychogenic pseudoseizures. Procedures used for the activation of epileptiform abnormalities are summarized in Table 8.1.

EEG reactivity procedures are distinguished from activating procedures as being intended to verify the presence or absence of normal EEG responses to exogenous sensory or endogenous cognitive stimulation. Examples of routine reactivity procedures include eye opening and closure in alert patients to demonstrate the alpha rhythm, or vigorous stimulation in patients in coma to demonstrate evidence of cortical responsiveness. Pharmacological reactivity procedures include the quantitative EEG analysis of drug-induced beta activity (e.g., diazepam) or EEG monitoring during intracarotid amobarbital (Wada) testing. This chapter focuses on activation methods used to provoke EEG abnormalities.

TABLE 8.1. *Activation methods known to induce epileptiform activity*

Visual Stimulation
Visual exploration
Stroboscopic flash stimulation
Pattern stimulation
Television
Eye closure
Somatosensory Stimulation
Tactile
Electrical
Water immersion
Auditory Stimulation
Nonspecific sounds
Music
Sleep
Pharmacologically induced
Spontaneous
Sleep deprivation
Hyperventilation
Pharmacological Agents
Anticonvulsant medication withdrawal
Pentylenetetrazol
Pentylenetetrazol and photic stimulation
Bemegride
Methohexital
Metabolic Toxicity
Hypoglycemia
Hypoxia
Special Stimuli
Startle
Reading
Writing
Mental calculation
Mental imagery
Eating

HYPERVENTILATION

Hyperventilation is the oldest EEG activating procedure. In 1934, Hans Berger was the first to describe the effect of hyperventilation on the human EEG (13). Using a polygraphic four-channel recorder with EEG, respiration, and electrocardiogram (ECG) (Fig. 8.1), he demonstrated that "The alpha waves increase in amplitude and merge into separate groups of 0.3–0.5 second duration."(58) Berger's findings on the effects of hyperventilation were published in the same year that Adrian and Matthews confirmed his claim that the human EEG could be recorded from the scalp (5). The initial use of hyperventilation as an EEG activating procedure arose from the discovery in 1924 that epileptic seizures could be triggered by hyperventilation (49,129). The year after Berger's report on hyperventilation, Frederick Gibbs, Hallowell Davis, and their colleagues (56,57) provided a more detailed description of the effects of hyperventilation. The effectiveness of hyperventilation in inducing generalized epileptiform activity was quickly established (108), and remains clinically important in this context.

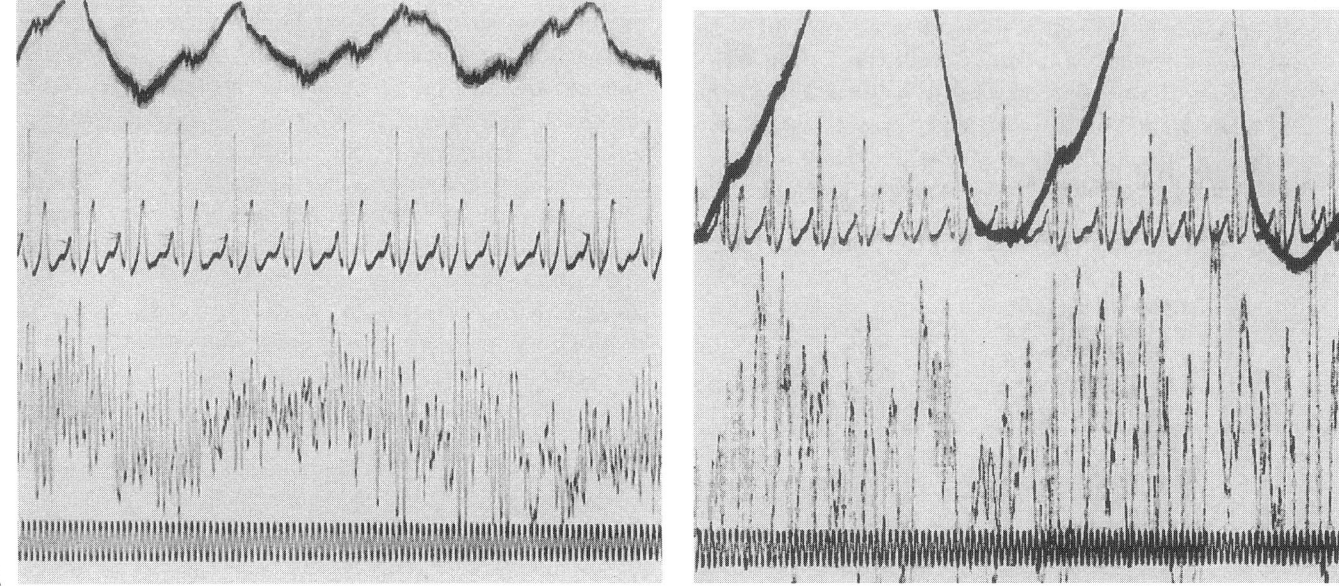

A   B

FIG. 8.1. First EEG recorded in a human during hyperventilation. **A:** Normal respiration in a 33-year-old woman with idiopathic epilepsy. Top channel is respiration, followed by ECG, EEG, and time marker with 1- to 10-second cycles. Recorded from the forehead and occiput with chlorided needle electrodes. **B:** Hyperventilation in the same subject several minutes after onset. Note higher amplitude and slower respiratory effort and slowing and increased amplitude of the EEG activity. (From Gloor P. Hans Berger on the electroencephalogram of man: fourteen original reports on the human electroencephalogram. *Electroencephalogr Clin Neurophysiol Suppl* 1969;28, with permission.)

Normal Response to Hyperventilation

The typical hyperventilation response consists of a buildup of medium- to high-amplitude, bisynchronous delta and theta waves and an increase in amplitude of theta and alpha waveforms. The distribution of delta and theta activity is typically anterior dominant in adolescents and adults but can be either anterior or posterior dominant in children. The hyperventilation response often includes frontal intermittent rhythmic delta activity (FIRDA; Fig. 8.2) or, particularly in children, occipital intermittent rhythmic delta activity (OIRDA; Fig. 8.3). Although spontaneously occurring FIRDA or OIRDA indicates the presence of a diffuse cerebral dysfunction, their isolated appearance in hyperventilation is considered normal. Simi-

larly, occasional sharply contoured components may be intermixed with FIRDA or OIRDA patterns (particularly if the EEG contains prominent alpha and beta waveforms) that can be misinterpreted as generalized epileptiform activity. As noted above, alpha frequency activity often increases in amplitude (33). Moreover, the alpha rhythm may first appear clearly in the recording only after hyperventilation, perhaps because of its relaxing effects. Technologists should therefore be instructed to perform hyperventilation early in the recording if a well-defined alpha rhythm is not apparent. In normal individuals, the record usually returns to baseline less than 1 minute after hyperventilation ends. The magnitude of the hyperventilation response depends on several factors, including effort, age, posture, and blood sugar. Younger individuals tend to produce the

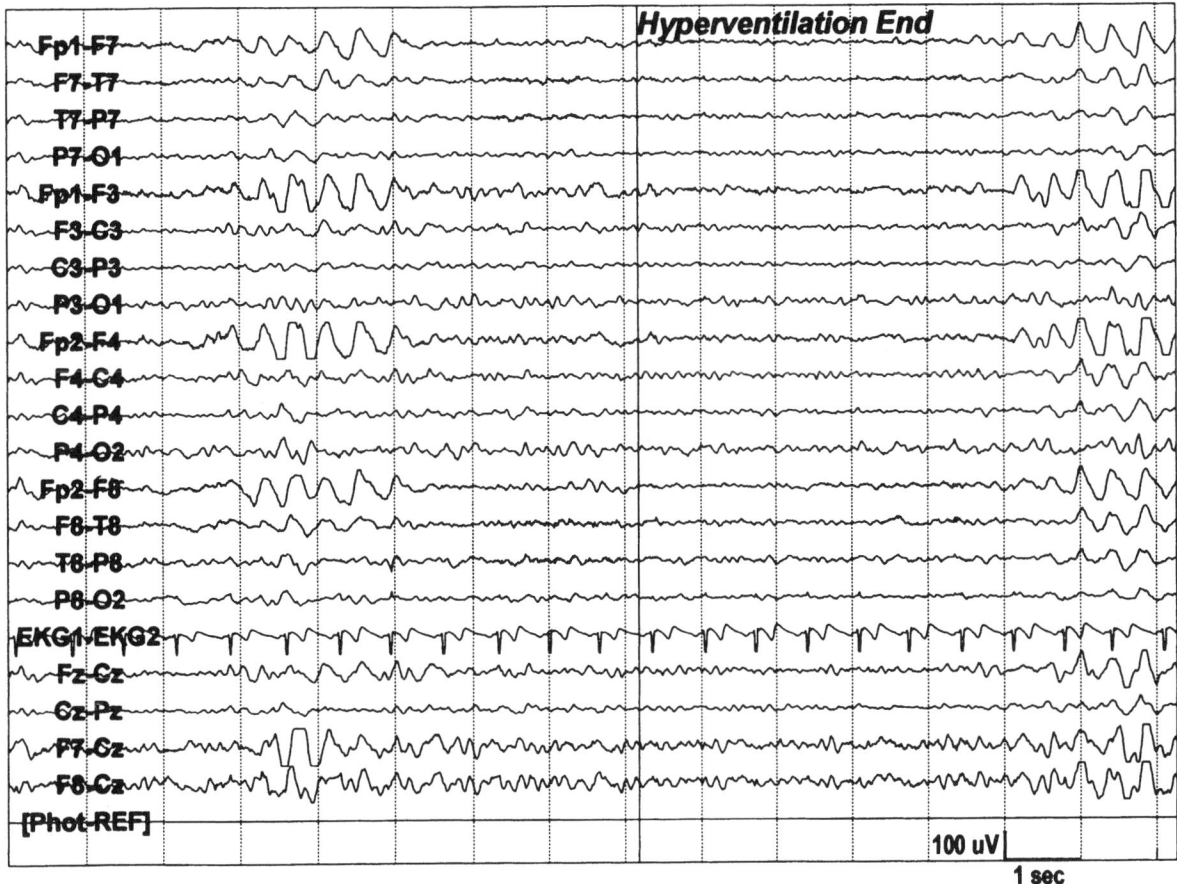

FIG. 8.2. Frontal intermittent delta activity produced by hyperventilation in an adolescent referred for the evaluation of possible migraine headache. Note the persistence of FIRDA immediately following the instruction to end hyperventilation.

largest responses, whereas elderly individuals often fail to show any EEG change (170).

The first quantitative EEG study of hyperventilation was performed by Gibbs and colleagues (55). Their observations mirrored those of routine visual inspection. They found that, as CO_2 measured from the internal jugular vein fell with increasing hyperventilation, the overall amount of EEG measured as total spectral power (i.e., the total area between the EEG waveforms and the zero baseline) increased and the mean frequency of the EEG decreased. A comparison of more recent quantitative studies suggests that the older the subject is, the more likely hyperventilation will produce an overall increase in EEG amplitude without decreasing the mean frequency (1,84). This may be partly due to the overall greater magnitude of response that occurs in children compared to adults. By routine visual EEG inspection, over 70% of children show a clear response to hyperventilation, whereas, in adults, a response may

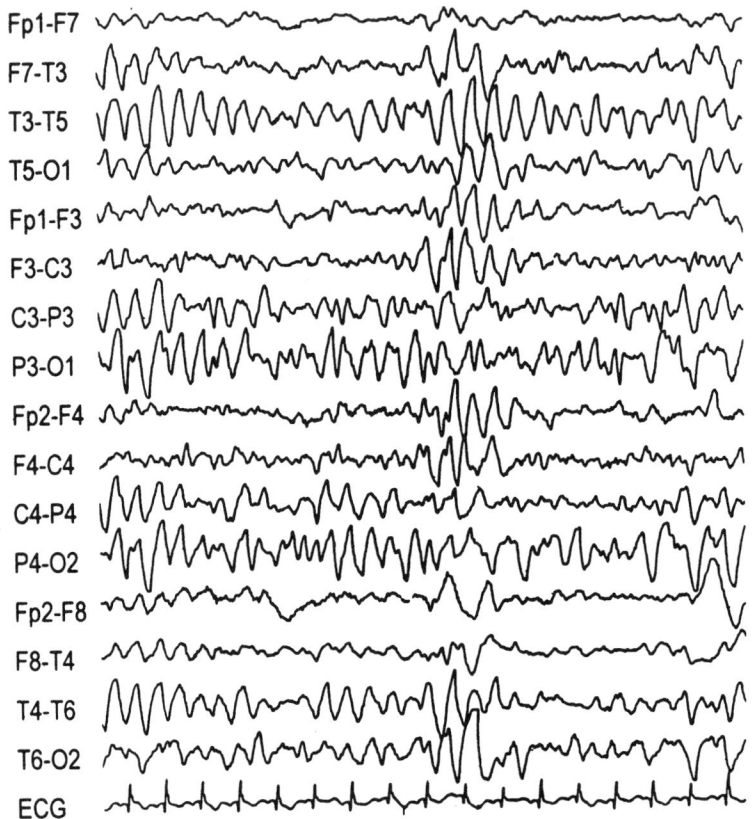

FIG. 8.3. Posterior delta activity produced by hyperventilation in a 6-year-old boy. Older adolescents and adults typically show anterior-dominant slowing in response to hyperventilation.

be seen in less than 10% of individuals during routine EEG laboratory testing (54). The maximum frequency of response occurs between the ages of 8 and 12 years, when up to 85% of subjects have some type of hyperventilation response; interestingly, this is about the same age range in which most individuals with idiopathic epilepsy and photosensitivity develop photosensitivity (see below) (23,115). In a study of 37 normal children ages 6–17 years in which ventilation, partial pressure of oxygen (PO_2), and partial pressure of carbon dioxide (PCO_2) were measured, Konishi (84) found a nearly inverse relationship between EEG slowing and age using a standardized hyperventi-

lation protocol. The effect of hyperventilation on the EEG begins earlier in children than adults and is apparent in 50% of cases within the first minute and 90% within the first 2 minutes (34).

Hyperventilation Procedure

Hyperventilation is routinely performed by asking the patient to overbreathe for at least 3 minutes. The recording technologist should encourage deep breathing over rapid shallow breathing to enhance air exchange and decrease in PCO_2. It is often helpful if the EEG technologist intermittently places a hand in front of the patient's mouth to monitor the level of effort and provide encouragement. Young children can be encouraged to hyperventilate by asking them to blow on a colorful pinwheel. In general, more vigorous and prolonged hyperventilation is desirable for activating seizures. A minimum 1-minute baseline recording is made before starting hyperventilation.

Blood gas monitoring is not routinely performed during hyperventilation, but the standardization of hyperventilation using blood gas monitoring appears to significantly enhance the likelihood of detecting EEG changes. Zwiener and colleagues (171) found that, when volunteers underwent standardized hyperventilation (in which PCO_2 was maintained at 15 mm Hg), a nearly sixfold increase in delta frequency band power was produced compared to nonstandardized hyperventilation. Remarkably, there have been no recent attempts to correlate blood gas changes with the activation of epileptiform patterns or with the effects of anticonvulsant medications on activated patterns. Unless blood gas monitoring is used, it is impossible to know if hyperventilation has been adequately performed, particularly in patients with absent or minimal responses.

The importance of continuing the EEG recording for at least 6 minutes following hyperventilation has been emphasized by Achenbach-Ng and colleagues (1). In a study of nine normal adult subjects, they found that PCO_2 fell continuously during hyperventilation and then immediately began to increase. In contrast, PO_2 increased during hyperventilation but then decreased to an average of 25 mm Hg below baseline at 5.2 minutes following the cessation of hyperventilation. The posthyperventilation decline in PO_2 that is presumably related to hypocapnia-induced hypopnea also occurs in children (170). Although Zwiener and colleagues (171) failed to find a significant decline in posthyperventilation PO_2, the time course of declining PO_2 found in these other studies more closely parallels EEG slowing in patients with moyamoya disease. Indeed, in individuals with borderline cerebral perfusion disorders, hyperventilation can be deleterious because of hypocapnia-induced ischemic vasoconstriction and shunting effects, posthyperventilation hypoxia, or both. As recommended by the American Clinical Neurophysiology Society (formerly the American Electroencephalographic Society), hyperventilation should not be performed in certain clinical settings, including acute stroke, recent intracranial hemorrhage, large-vessel severe stenosis and associated TIA (e.g., limb-shaking attacks), documented moyamoya disease, severe cardiopulmonary disease, and sickle cell disease or trait.

Response testing is used to document lapses in consciousness at the time of hyperventilation-induced epileptiform activity. The simplest form of response testing consists of asking the patient to repeat or recall words presented during the abnormal activity. A more precise method consists of having the patient press a button to mark the EEG record in response to the presentation of an auditory signal given by the technologist. The electroencephalographer must take care not to misinterpret the clinical significance of response testing during hyperventilation, particularly in children. The significance of impaired responsiveness is most likely to occur during generalized high-amplitude 2- to 3-Hz activity—a phenomenon referred to as *pseudo-absence seizures*. Epstein and colleagues (42) found that 12 of 12 normal children tested demonstrated an impairment of verbal memory, and 8 of those 12 failed to respond to repeated auditory clicks during periods of hyperventilation-induced slowing that was greater than 100-μV voltage and consisted of 3- to 5-Hz waveforms lasting 3 seconds or longer, using an average reference montage. None of the children manifested automatisms or abnormal motor activity. It is also well known that episodic changes of consciousness or awareness, numbness, dizziness, tingling, transient blurring of vision, and ringing in the ears are common manifestations of hyperventilation attacks that can occur in the absence of EEG slowing—possibly as a result of increased autonomic activation (51,106). Therefore, response testing alone should not be used to classify an EEG change as an epileptiform abnormality during hyperventilation. Impaired responsiveness during hyperventilation can be confidently interpreted as a manifestation of a seizure only if: (a) an abnormal EEG pattern is combined with motor phenomena (e.g., automatisms or convulsive movements) or (b) the EEG contains well-defined electrographic seizure activity.

Physiological Basis of the EEG Response to Hyperventilation

Alteration of PCO_2, rather than pH or PO_2, is the most important factor in producing the EEG response to hyperventilation, whereas the most obvious and dramatic physiological effect of hyperventilation is decreased cerebral blood flow. EEG hyperventilation changes are more likely to occur with blood sugar levels below 80 mg per 100 mL and less likely to occur with levels over 120 mg per 100 mL. All of these observations led Davis and Wallace (36) to propose that the EEG changes that accompany hyperventilation are caused by ischemic cerebral hypoxia. Their view is supported by the observation that the hyperventilation response is reduced by hyperbaric oxygen (117,125). An alternative explanation was proposed by Gibbs and colleagues (54), who believed that cerebral hypoxia sufficient to cause EEG slowing cannot occur because the vasodilatory effects of anoxia should override the constrictive effects of hypocapnia. Instead, they concluded that cerebral hypocapnia is directly responsible for the typical EEG changes. As noted by Patel and Maulsby (114), several observations support the idea that EEG slowing results from the direct effects of hypocapnia on the brainstem: (a) hyperventilation does not modify the EEG in animals in the *cerveau isole* preparation (22), (b) the effects of hyperventilation on chemically induced spike foci, electrical afterdischarges, and cortical responsiveness are interrupted or dampened by surgically isolating the cortex (137), and (c) the hyperventilation effect can be blocked by lesions of the anterior thalamus (138). In the brainstem model of hyperventilation, it remains to be determined if hypoxia of the brainstem or of other subcortical structures is most critical.

Abnormal EEG Responses to Hyperventilation

Hyperventilation produces three main kinds of EEG abnormalities: (i) lateralized or localized slowing, (ii) delayed symmetrical or lateralized slowing, and (iii) epileptiform patterns.

Hyperventilation may increase or provoke localized slowing in the presence of an underlying lesion or localized area of cortical dysfunction, but it does not produce abnormal slowing or significant-amplitude background asymmetries in normal individuals. Abnormal slowing usually begins within the first 2 minutes of hyperventilation and may either persist or sometimes become more obvious after hyperventilation ceases. A buildup of slowing several minutes after hyperventilation ends is highly suggestive of moyamoya disease (Fig. 8.4) (83). As noted above, the time course of the onset of slowing roughly parallels the decline of PO_2 caused by posthyperventilation reduced ventilatory drive (1,78,148). The delayed buildup of slowing in moyamoya disease is often maximal approximately 5 minutes after hyperventilation ends. It may be unilateral or bilateral. Because of the remote risk of stroke, hyperventilation is avoided in patients with known moyamoya disease.

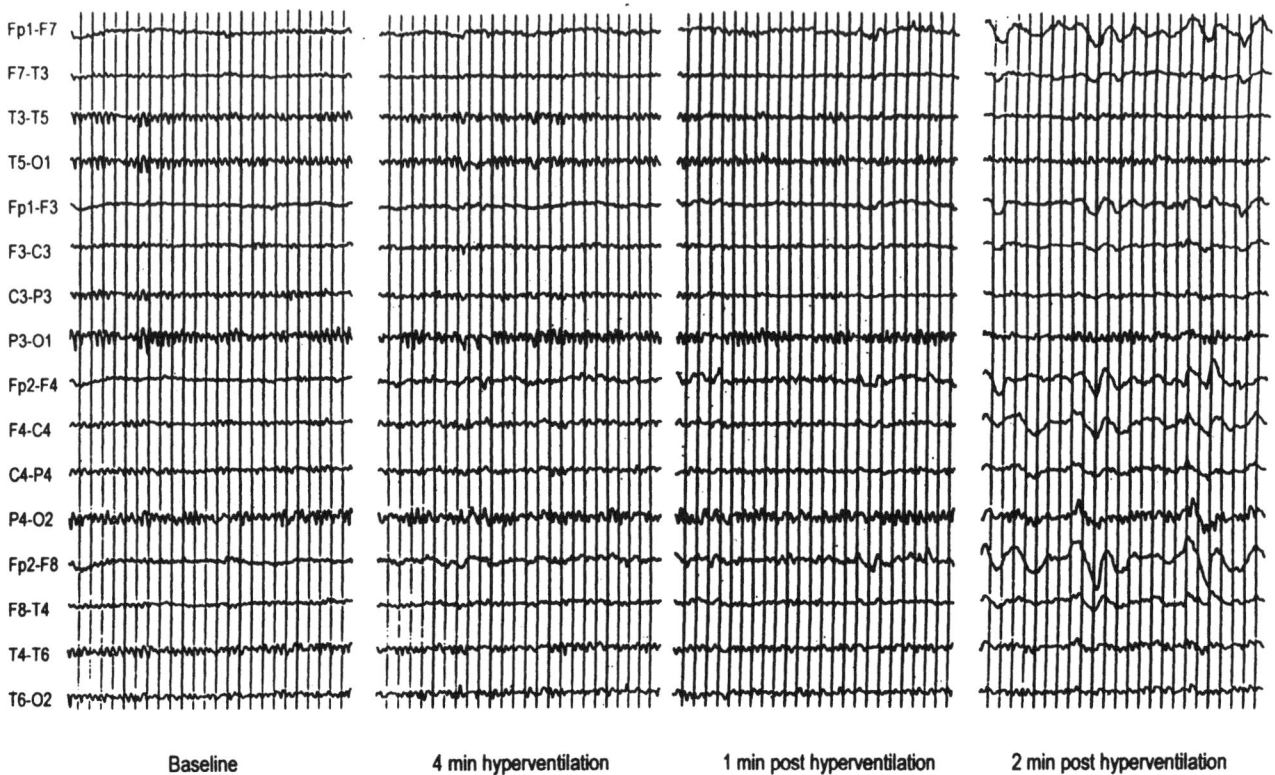

FIG. 8.4. Typical pattern of delayed hemispheric slowing after hyperventilation in a 15-year-old with moyamoya disease.

Hyperventilation is the most effective method for activating ictal and interictal epileptiform activity associated with typical absence seizures. According to Dalby (32), hyperventilation will activate seizures in over 80% of untreated children with absence seizures. As demonstrated by Adams and Lueders (4), hyperventilation is more effective than a 6-hour passive recording in detecting the typical 3-Hz spike-and-wave pattern in children with absence seizures. Indeed, in an untreated child, if hyperventilation evokes prominent slowing, or PCO_2 monitoring shows a substantial decline to a level of less than 20 mm Hg, and epileptiform activity does not appear, then the diagnosis of absence seizures becomes doubtful. Approximately 35% of children with absence seizures demonstrate prolonged, spontaneous runs of localized rhythmic 2.5- to 3.5-Hz occipital-dominant delta activity. During hyperventilation, this activity may evolve directly into the typical anterior-dominant 3-Hz spike-and-wave epileptiform pattern. Although this occipital pattern in the absence of 3-Hz spike and wave may be quite striking, only 30%–40% of children who have it actually have epilepsy. Yet virtually all children who have the occipital pattern and also have absence seizures will demonstrate typical 3-Hz spike-and-wave discharges with prolonged hyperventilation. Cobb and colleagues (29) found that children with epilepsy with this pattern usually stopped having seizures between the ages of 10 and 12 years.

Hyperventilation is most likely to produce epileptiform activity in patients with typical absence seizures, but it may activate almost any type of seizure or interictal epileptiform activity (46). The overall effectiveness of hyperventilation in epilepsy is currently difficult to assess because, as previously noted, uniform methods employing a similar duration of effort with monitoring to control for variations in blood gases have not been used. With routine hyperventilation (i.e., without blood gas monitoring) approximately 50% of those patients with generalized slow spike-and-wave patterns who are able to perform hyperventilation demonstrate activation of epileptiform patterns (21,97). Miley and Foerster reported that hyperventilation activated focal interictal epileptiform activity in greater than 6% of 255 patients with complex partial seizures and clinical seizures in over 4% (101). Even higher rates of activation in patients with partial seizures have been reported more recently (71,135). In our experience, hyperventilation rarely if ever activates partial seizures, but various investigators have emphasized the need for long duration and intensive hyperventilation, particularly in patients with partial seizures (135). Until CO_2 monitoring is used to verify the efficacy of effort, the potential usefulness of hyperventilation in epilepsy will remain unclear.

Hyperventilation rarely provokes paroxysmal attacks in patients with multiple sclerosis (109,156). The EEG is usually unchanged or shows a mild, normal activation pattern. The attacks typically last 1–2 minutes and may include tonic spasms. When the manifestations include ataxia, diplopia, or dysarthria, then a seizure disorder is highly unlikely. Individuals with paroxysmal attacks of any kind that are triggered by emotional upset are often suspected of having psychogenic pseudoseizures. However, it should be remembered that, during episodes of crying or panic attacks, hyperventilation occurs and may trigger an epileptic seizure in susceptible individuals. Thus a strong association between emotional attacks and seizures alone should not lead to the conclusion that the attacks represent psychogenic pseudoseizures.

Pathophysiological Basis of Ictal and Interictal Epileptiform Activation

The mechanism underlying the activation of ictal and interictal epileptiform activity during hyperventilation is probably central nervous system excitation combined with altered thalamocortical function. The scalp-recorded negative direct current (DC) shift that commonly accompanies excitatory phenomena, such as an electrographic seizure, is also produced during hyperventilation in humans, and its amplitude may be reduced by pretreatment with anticonvulsant medications (127). Evidence for corticospinal excitation has been reported by Kukumberg and colleagues (86) and Seyal

and colleagues (136). Both groups found that hyperventilation increased the amplitude of transcranial magnetic motor evoked potentials, whereas Seyal and colleagues (136) found that hyperventilation to an end-tidal PCO_2 of 15 mm Hg also shortened the latency of transcranial magnetic motor evoked potentials and increased the amplitude of F waves. In some individuals, the role played by hypocapnia has been questioned because activation can occur so quickly after the onset of hyperventilation. Interestingly, this observation is consistent with the rapid onset of a substantial (10%) decrease in the cortical (but not white matter) functional magnetic resonance imaging (MRI) signal in the first 20 seconds of hyperventilation reported by Posse and colleagues (118). However, in their study, MRI signal changes were delayed in comparison to PCO_2 changes. Positron emission tomography scan activation of corticospinal motor pathways also occurs with hyperventilation, with a significant increase in activity of the frontal premotor and primary motor cortices compared to that of the temporal, occipital, or parietal lobes (73). As noted previously, hyperventilation can induce changes in consciousness (42,51,106), and it can also reduce the amplitude of long-latency auditory and somatosensory evoked potentials (72). It is reasonable, therefore, to consider that, as in the corticoreticular model of primary generalized epilepsy, cortical excitation and altered thalamocortical function combine to facilitate epileptiform activity and seizures during hyperventilation.

PHOTIC STIMULATION

Richard Caton (1842–1926) is credited with the discovery of spontaneous electrical brain activity in mammals (26). In his original experiments, he also tested the electrical reactivity of the brain to various stimuli. Among the various sensory stimuli he tested, the strongest EEG reaction was consistently produced by retinal light stimulation (26). Adrian and Matthews (5) performed the first investigation of the effects of light stimulation on the human EEG. Following the discovery that light stimulation could trigger seizures, the modern technique of stroboscopic photic stimulation was developed by Walter and colleagues (161). Since that time, stroboscopic stimulation has become part of routine screening for photosensitive epilepsy in laboratories throughout the world. Seizures activated by photic stimulation are the most common form of reflex epilepsy, accounting for nearly one-third of such cases. Photic stimulation is most effective for provoking generalized epileptiform activity or generalized seizures; rarely, focal epileptiform activity or partial seizures with occipital onset can be activated (77).

Photic Stimulation Procedure

Photic stimulation is routinely performed with a stroboscopic diffuse light flash at frequencies ranging between 1 and 30 Hz. A generally accepted protocol is described in Table 8.2 (14,80). If an abnormal epileptiform response occurs during stimulation, then the stimulus train is repeated to verify that the abnormal activity is temporally related to the flash stimulus. Repetition using the same frequency of stimulus train should not be repeated immediately because there is evidence that habituation with blocking of the response will occur (155). Therefore, either more than 30 seconds of nonstimulation should separate trials of the same frequency of stimulation or the interposition of a different frequency stimulus train is recommended before repeating the activating flash frequency.

The effectiveness of diffuse light stimulation is determined by flash frequency, stimulus intensity (luminance), level of consciousness, and direction of gaze. Photic stimulation is less effective when performed during sleep. The intensity of ambient lighting may also play a role in the effectiveness of the stimulus in some individuals. Unilateral monocular stimulation or stimulation during conjugate ocular deviation away from the stimulus is less effective than binocular gaze–directed stimulation.

The stimulator should be placed directly in front of the patient's eyes at a distance of no more than 30 cm. The patient is usually instructed to begin with the eyes open, but stimulation may also be performed with the eyes closed, particularly if the light source is too irritating. In addition to stimulating at fixed frequencies, some investigators believe that using flash stimuli that gradually increase or decrease in frequency during the stimulus train is activating in some patients. Technologists performing this procedure must be skilled in identifying epileptiform patterns so that stimulation can be immediately terminated at the onset of an epileptiform pattern. Otherwise a generalized tonic–clonic seizure (GTCS) may be provoked. Surprisingly, many commercially available photostimulators lack the features essential to effective photostimulation, including a high-intensity flash, a large circular surface area, and a fairly consistent luminance at different flash frequencies from 1 to 60 Hz (see Table 8.2).

Following the seminal studies of Grey Walter and colleagues (161), it was found that diffuse light stimulation produces three main categories of electrographic response: (i) photic driving, (ii) the photomyogenic (formerly referred to as photomyoclonic) response, and (iii) the photoepileptiform response (PER) (also referred to as the photoparoxysmal response [PPR]).

TABLE 8.2. *Standardization of screening methods for photosensitivity*

Photostimulator Characteristics (equivalent to setting 4 on a Grass model PS22)
A maximal intensity > 100 Nit-s per flash
Circular field diameter of 13 cm
Granular diffuser producing light diffusion similar to that of the Grass stimulator
Central fixation point on diffuser
Attachment of patterns available
Single flashes or trains that can be delivered with constant intensity from 1 to 60 Hz
Procedure
IPS should not be performed during or within 3 min of hyperventilation
Nasion-to-lamp distance of 30 cm
Longitudinal bipolar or common reference montage
Flash trains of 10 s with at least 7-s intervals
Eyes open for first 5 s of IPS and then closed
Eyes fixated on center of stimulator
IPS frequencies: 1, 2, 3, 4, 6, 8, 10, 12, 14, 16, 18, 20, 60, 50, 40, 30, 25
IPS is stopped abruptly if a PPR appears

IPS, intermittent photic stimulation; PPR, photoparoxysmal response.
Adapted from Kasteleijn-Nolst Trenite DG, Binnie CD, Harding GF, et al. Photic stimulation: standardization of screening methods. *Epilepsia* 1999;40[Suppl 4]: 75–79.

Photic Driving Response

The photic driving response consists of rhythmic, occipital-dominant waveforms that either show a one-to-one relationship with each flash or appear as a harmonic (an integer multiple) or subharmonic (an integer dividend) of the flash frequency. The term *photic driving* describes an induced rhythm, not the isolated visual flash evoked potentials that occur with very slow rates (< 5 Hz) of stimulation. Driving is typically seen at stimulation rates between 5 and 30 Hz. Large positive occipital sharp transients of sleep (POSTS) and lambda waves in response to scanning a complex pattern are predictive of a prominent driving response. The onset of the occipital response usually occurs with a 70- to 150-millisecond delay from the onset of the flash stimulus. Higher amplitude driving responses usually appear at frequencies that are close to the frequency of the ongoing posterior background rhythm. This apparent entrainment of the background activity may briefly outlast the flash stimulus. At slower flash rates (< 5 Hz), the photic response consists of a diffuse light evoked potential (Fig. 8.5).

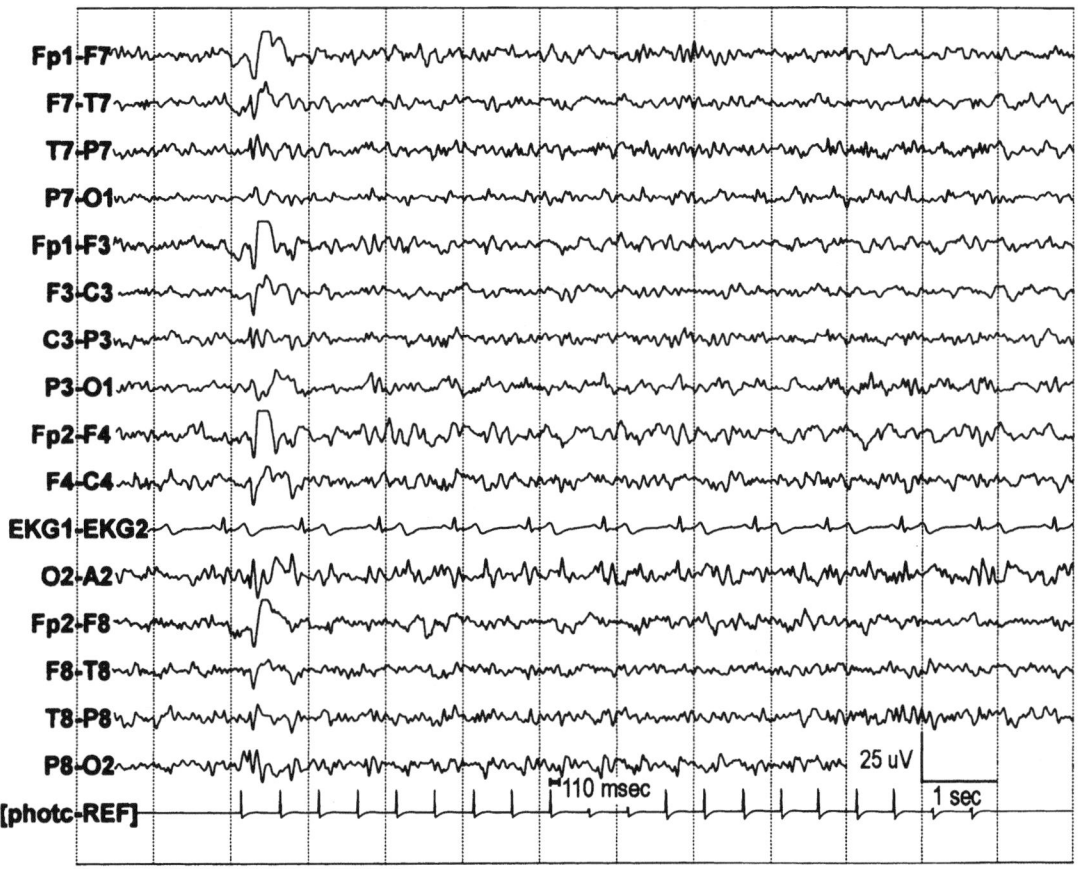

FIG. 8.5. "On effect" at the beginning of 4-Hz photic stimulation. At slow rates of stimulation, the photic response, when present, consists of flash evoked potentials. As indicated in the figure, the initial positivity occurs with a delay of approximately 110 milliseconds.

Abnormal Responses in Specific Cerebral Disorders

Just as POSTS or lambda waves may be strikingly asymmetrical in normal individuals, an asymmetrical driving response is considered normal unless accompanied by other EEG abnormalities (30). In normal individuals, asymmetrical POSTS or lambda waves are usually associated with a similar asymmetry of the driving response (46). Cortical epileptogenic lesions or skull defects can enhance the amplitude of the photic driving response ipsilaterally, whereas destructive lesions can attenuate it ipsilaterally (14). In some abnormal individuals with unilateral photic driving, the only other EEG abnormality may be a failure of the contralateral alpha rhythm to attenuate with eye opening (i.e., Bancaud's phenomenon)(46).

Adults who have abnormal background slowing and who demonstrate high-amplitude photic driving at very slow flash rates usually suffer from progressive degenerative cerebral disorders. Similarly, individuals at any age who demonstrate high-amplitude epileptiform spikes time locked to very slow photic flash rates often suffer from either progressive degenerative or acute structural brain disorders (Fig. 8.6). High-voltage occipital spikes that occur in a time-locked fashion in response to slow rates of stimulation in individuals in late infancy or childhood with intellectual decline, myoclonus, and optic

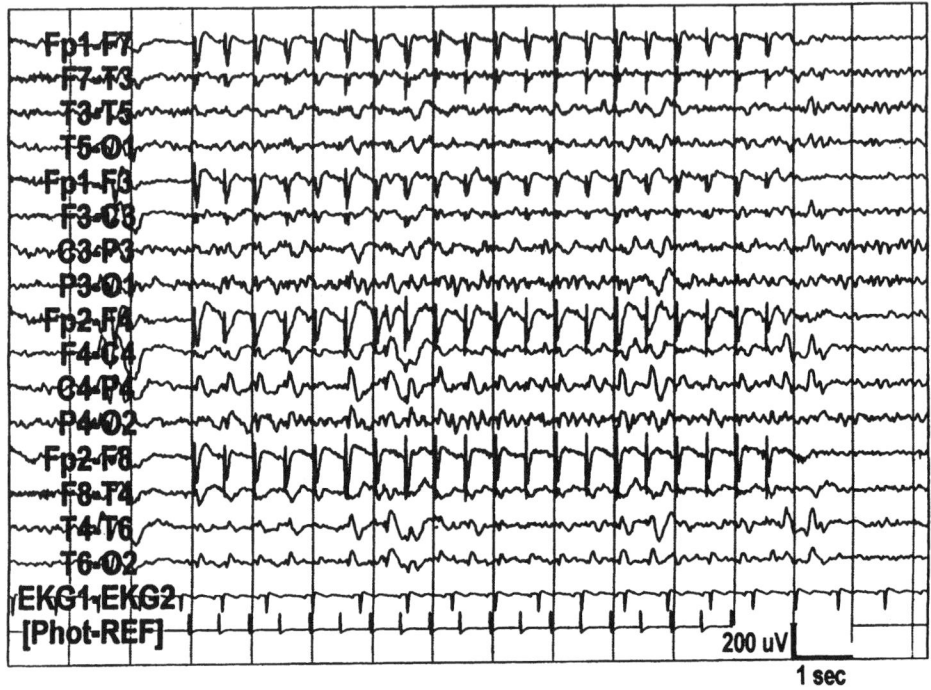

FIG. 8.6. Prominent right parieto-occipital sharp waves evoked by 2-Hz photic stimulation in an adult woman during an exacerbation of MELAS (mitochondrial myopathy, encephalopathy, lactic acidosis, and stroke-like episodes).

atrophy are virtually pathognomonic for the late infantile form of ceroid lipofuscinosis (Bielschowsky-Jansky form of Batten's disease) (110,116).

Victor and Brausch (160) originally described the photoparoxysmal response (see below) occurring in the majority of patients in alcohol withdrawal. Fisch and colleagues (47) subsequently studied photic responses to diffuse light and patterned stroboscopic stimulation in patients undergoing untreated alcohol withdrawal. None of their patients had a PPR, or any form of PER. Therefore, it is now generally accepted that patients in alcohol withdrawal without delirium tremens have little or no increased risk of developing a PPR. Whether or not there is an increased incidence of PPR in delirium tremens remains unknown.

Photomyogenic Response

The photomyogenic (photomyoclonic) response (Fig. 8.7) consists of electromyographic potentials time locked to the flash frequency. It was first described by Gastaut and Remond (53). Bickford and colleagues (16) provided a more detailed description and coined the term *photomyoclonic response* to describe its frequent association with photically induced myoclonus. Typically, muscle artifact time locked to the flash stimulus builds in intensity as the stimulation continues and ceases immediately with the termination of stimulation. Indeed, it is the immediate cessation of the response at the end of stimulation and prominent electromyographic activity that help to distinguish the photomyogenic response from an abnormal photoepileptiform response. It usually appears prominently over the anterior head regions as a result of involvement of the frontalis and orbicularis oculi muscles. Observable movements include stimulus time-locked contraction of the periocular muscles, myoclonic movements of the face, and less often myoclonic movements of the upper body. Rarely, a photomyogenic response may progress to a GTCS. It may be enhanced or provoked by heightened emotional tone or tension or metabolic/toxic states associated with reflex hyperactivity. A prominent, clinically observable response probably occurs

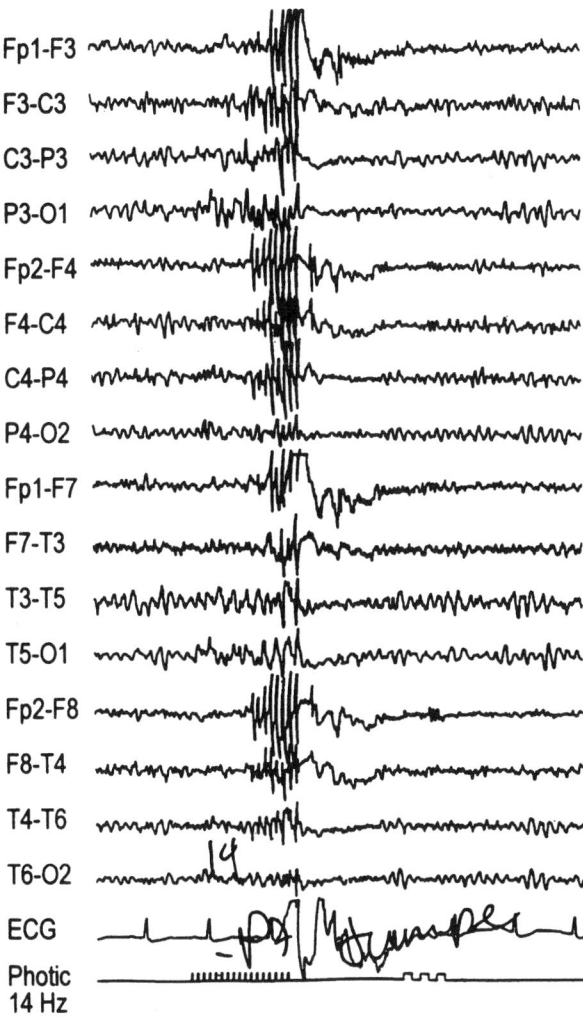

FIG. 8.7. Photomyogenic (photomyoclonic) response to 14-Hz photic stimulation. Prominent frontalis and temporalis myogenic potentials time locked to the flash stimulus end with a whole-body jerk.

in less than 0.1% of normal individuals and less than 1% of individuals with epilepsy (85,100,124,141). Although its appearance is sometimes dramatic and always statistically unusual, the photomyogenic response has no known clinical significance and is therefore considered a normal variant (105).

Photoepileptiform and Photoparoxysmal Responses

Photoepileptiform responses (PERs) are epileptiform patterns that are activated consistently by photic stimulation. Their association with epilepsy varies according to their topography, which can be divided into three main distributions:

1. Anterior dominant or generalized; bisynchronous and approximately symmetrical
2. Occipital dominant; bisynchronous and approximately symmetrical
3. Occipital dominant and localized; unilateral or strongly lateralized

Very rarely, unilateral anterior-dominant spikes are activated. Approximately 40% of bilateral PERs (categories 1 and 2) demonstrate asymmetries, particularly at the onset (17). One form of PER, the photoparoxysmal response (PPR) (formerly referred to as the photoconvulsive response) (Fig. 8.8), is defined as a generalized or anterior-dominant epileptiform pattern (category 1) (27). Although some authors refer to any bilaterally symmetrical and bisynchronous PER (i.e., categories 1 and 2) as highly epileptiform, posterior-dominant responses are far less likely to be associated with epilepsy than generalized or anterior-dominant responses (93,105). This topographical distinction is also found with pattern viewing and television or video game stimulation (64,125). In the closest animal model of human photosensitivity—the photosensitive baboon—photically induced epileptiform activity appears first in the frontorolandic cortex, not the occipital cortex (48). Thus, although the occipital cortex is believed to be involved in the generation of the PPR (18), generalized or anterior-dominant patterns are most closely associated with epilepsy.

The weak correlation between posterior PER and seizures often leads to difficulties in distinguishing between a posterior-dominant PER and an atypical photic driving response. There are no uniformly agreed on criteria for making this distinction, but three features that help to identify a normal variant are (i) a posterior-dominant response that is time locked or appears as a subharmonic or harmonic of the flash frequency, regardless of the amplitude or apiculate appearance; (ii) a prominent posterior response that occurs while photic stimulation is being terminated but ceases abruptly

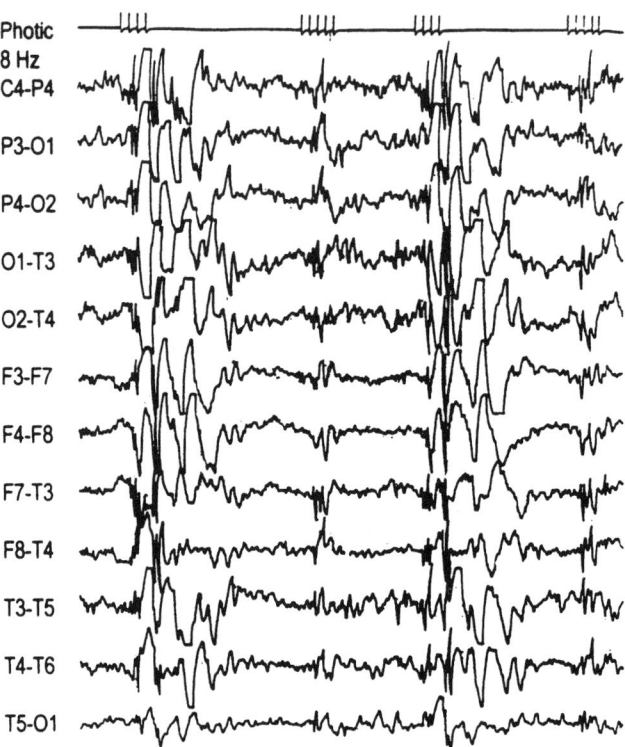

FIG. 8.8. Photoparoxysmal response to 8-Hz photic stimulation in a 6-year-old girl. Note the irregular spike-and-wave complexes and greater amplitudes in more anterior derivations.

within 150 milliseconds of the last flash stimulus; and (iii) a widespread sharp- or spike-and–slow wave complex restricted to the onset or cessation of the stimulus train (the "on response" and "off response," respectively; see Fig. 5) (77). The most suggestive features of a posterior-dominant PER are (i) a response that contains medium- to high-amplitude spikes or sharp waves and persists well beyond (> 200 milliseconds) the termination of the flash stimulus, and (ii) posterior response–associated clinical convulsive or nonconvulsive seizure activity.

Photoparoxysmal patterns are associated with three types of generalized seizure activity: (i) tonic–clonic, (ii) myoclonic, and (iii) absence. Most photoparoxysmal patterns consist of repetitive generalized irregular spike and multiple spike-and–slow wave complexes (see Fig. 8.8). During a self-lim-

ited discharge, there may be a slight impairment of consciousness that can be easily documented by a well-trained technologist. As the discharge persists, it becomes more organized and rhythmic at nearly 3 Hz in patients who have photosensitive absence seizures (Fig. 8.9), whereas those who have convulsive attacks often show persistent irregular spike-and–slow wave complexes. If the epileptiform pattern continues, the patient may develop an absence attack or symmetrical myoclonus, or progress directly into the tonic phase of a GTCS. PPRs are most often elicited at flash frequencies of 10–20 Hz (77), with the majority of investigators finding stimulation frequencies between 15 and 20 Hz to be the most effective (77,82,155). In some individuals, the PPR may be enhanced by stimulation with eyes open or with eyes closed or with eye opening and closure during stimulation (111). As previously noted, photosensitivity is reduced by sleep.

Although it is widely held that PPRs that outlast the stimulus are more likely to be associated with epilepsy compared to self-limited PPRs (124), other investigators have not found this to be a discriminating feature (76,142). As noted by Binnie (18), it is highly likely that any well-defined PPR obtained in an EEG laboratory in a patient with suspected epilepsy will be associated with seizures. Electrographic features that may increase the clinical significance of the PPR include an anterior-dominant or generalized response that is easily and consistently elicited, that lasts more than several seconds, and that clearly persists more than 200 milliseconds beyond the termination of the flash stimulation.

Approximately 4% of all individuals with epilepsy have a PPR (167), and between 70% and 77% of individuals with PPRs have epilepsy (76,162). The likelihood of encountering a typical PPR in the normal population is remote. In a study of 13,658 men in the Air Force, Gregory et al. (61) found a PPR that persisted beyond the termination of the flash stimulus in only 5 individuals, and only 1 developed epilepsy. Binnie (18) has estimated the likelihood of a PPR in a normal individual to be approximately 1 in 4,000. Most PPRs occur in adolescents and teenagers, coincident with the peak onset of idiopathic epilepsy syndromes associated with photosensitivity. In Great Britain, approximately 2% of all cases of epilepsy were found to manifest a PPR on the initial EEG (121). However, among those patients between the ages of 7 and 19, the incidence reaches 10%. Similarly, in a prospective study, Jeavons and Harding (77) found that photosensitive epilepsy most often begins at puberty. PPRs have a maximal incidence between 6 and 15 years of age and occur frequently in siblings of identified probands— whether or not the proband has epilepsy. Thus, in most cases, the PPR occurs as phenotypic expression of a genetic process that is variably associ-

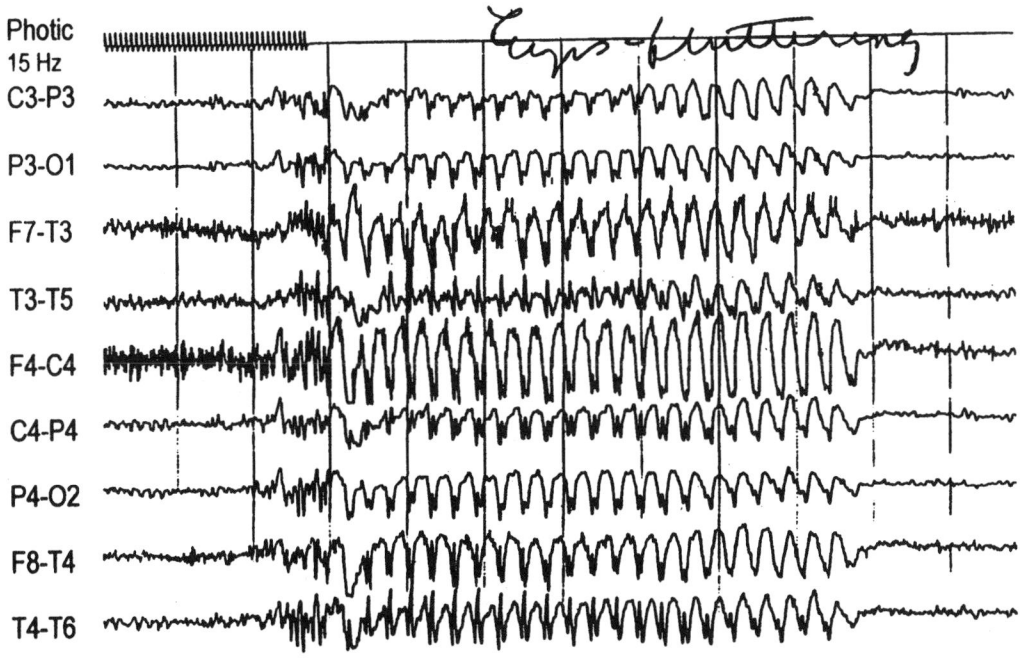

FIG. 8.9. Photoparoxysmal response to 15-Hz photic stimulation with initial fast activity evolving into a typical generalized 3-Hz spike-and-wave pattern. Eye fluttering typical of a myoclonic absence seizure was observed.

ated with the genetic determinant of seizures. In patients with known or suspected seizures, a generalized PPR strongly suggests that the patient has a genetically determined form of primary generalized epilepsy.

At least 30% of individuals with PPRs lose their photosensitivity by age 24, although there is no way of predicting which individuals will do so (63). As the PPR disappears, it is sometimes replaced by a more simplified pattern, lower in amplitude and without prominent spike components. Harding and Jeavons (66) have also shown that AED treatment, particularly with sodium valproate, can produce a similar effect: photosensitivity is diminished to the point where stimulation activates brief bursts of generalized slow-wave activity with absent or rare epileptiform components. It is therefore likely that this pattern of degraded photic activation represents latent photosensitivity. Unfortunately, a degraded PPR can only be identified with confidence in individuals who have previously demonstrated typical PPRs. Its value for predicting the risk of continuing seizures in patients undergoing AED treatment warrants further study.

Pure photosensitive epilepsy occurs in individuals who only have seizures in response to a visual stimulus. It accounts for nearly 40% of all photo-

sensitive individuals with seizures. Seizure types include tonic–clonic (> 80%), absence (6%), partial (2.5%), and myoclonic (1.5%) seizures (18). Juvenile myoclonic epilepsy (JME) is also closely associated with photosensitivity. In a study of 181 patients with JME, PPRs occurred in 38%. Ninety-four percent of all the patients with JME had grand mal seizures, and 24% of all patients had absence seizures (75). In contrast, the syndrome of childhood absence epilepsy (pyknolepsy) with typical absence seizures and infrequent GTCSs is not associated with photosensitivity. Similarly, the syndrome of childhood epilepsy with occipital spikes is not associated with PPR to stroboscopic photic stimulation. Instead, darkness or eye closure activates the PER, whereas visual fixation or photic stimulation may inhibit it (92,112).

Pattern-Activated Photoparoxysmal Responses

In some patients the PPR is more likely to be evoked by stroboscopic pattern stimulation than by diffuse stroboscopic stimulation (64,87). In such patients abnormalities occurring in response to patterned stimulation may signify the persistence of photosensitive epilepsy, whereas abnormalities occurring in response to diffuse stimulation indicate that the patient is at immediate risk for seizures. Once photosensitivity is identified, it can be diminished by avoiding rapidly varying light sources or by reducing light stimulation by various means (e.g., wearing sunglasses).

The likelihood of patients with a diffuse-light PPR having responses to stationary pattern viewing is probably between 5% and 22% (15,150). Pattern-evoked PERs should not be confused with the normal response to pattern viewing that occurs in some patients with prominent lambda waves (Fig. 8.10). The most effective activating patterns for either stroboscopic pattern stimulation or stationary pattern viewing consist of vertical parallel lines with high contrast (Fig. 8.11) (82). Moving patterns that oscillate between 15 and 20 Hz appear to be more effective than stationary ones and may elicit PPRs in the majority of photosensitive individuals with epilepsy. According to Harding and Fylan (64), responsive-

ness to stationary stimuli is found in individuals with PPRs, but not in those who have occipital spikes. As noted by Binnie (18), stationary pattern–induced photosensitivity has never been described in a normal individual. Moreover, it is extremely unusual for an individual to have pattern sensitivity without having stroboscopic pattern or diffuse light sensitivity, particularly with repeated testing. Because of the greater overall sensitivity of stroboscopic pattern stimulation, some investigators have recommended its routine use in laboratory testing. Clearly, all large institutional- and university-based laboratories should be equipped to perform pattern stimulation.

Typical absence is the most commonly activated seizure type among individuals with self-induced photosensitive epilepsy or pattern-sensitive epilepsy (113). The goal of identifying pattern sensitivity is the removal of certain patterns (in clothing, flooring, wallpaper, etc.) from the patient's environment. This can be particularly effective in preventing seizures in children.

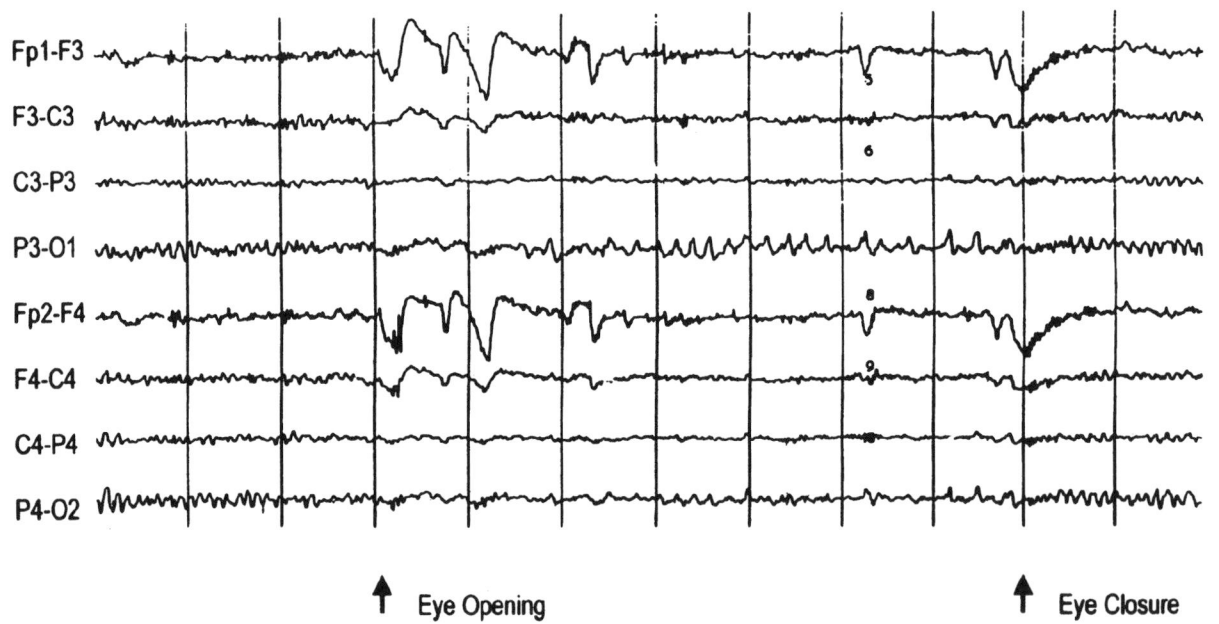

FIG. 8.10. Prominent lambda waves evoked by visual scanning of a complex object. Positive sharp waves arising from the occipital electrodes have the same morphology and topography as positive occipital sharp transients of sleep.

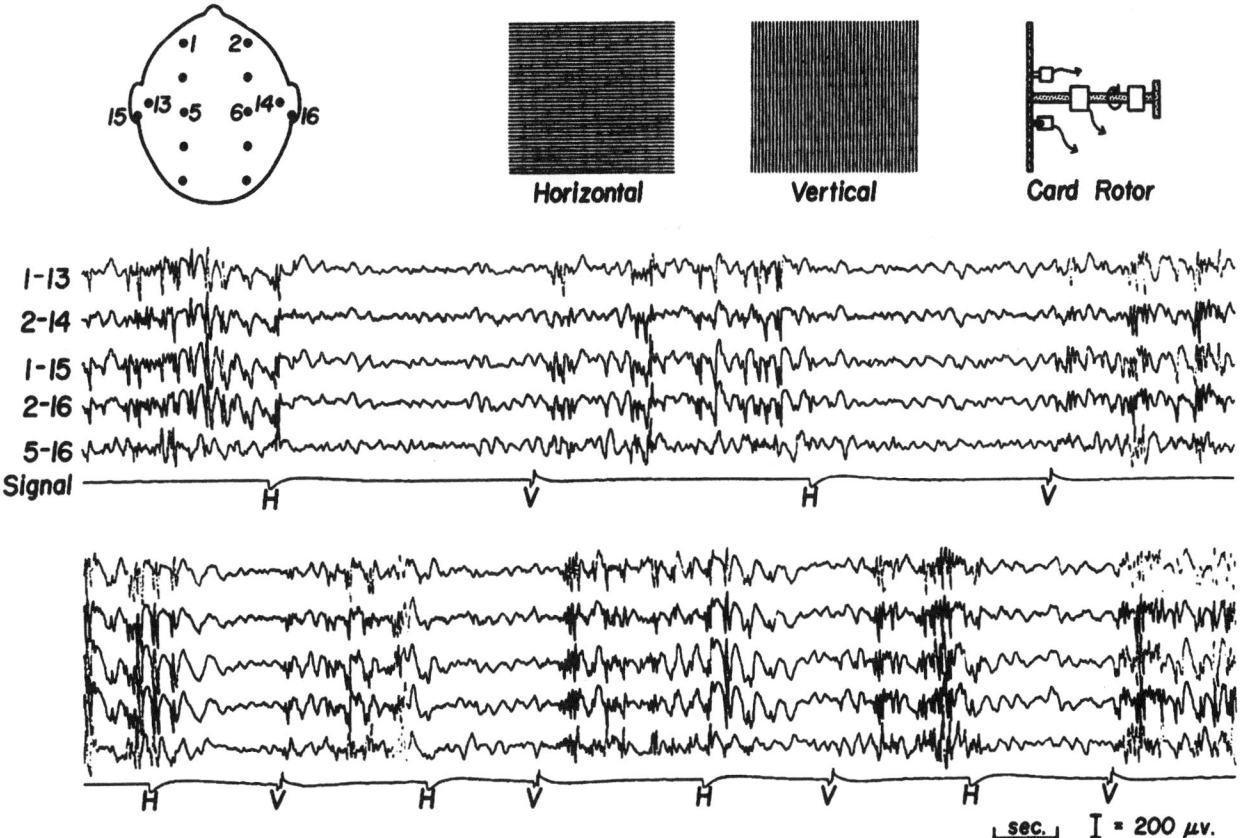

FIG. 8.11. Photoparoxysmal response to stationary pattern viewing of parallel lines. Specificity of vertical line sensitivity over horizontal line sensitivity is demonstrated. (From Bickford RG, Klass DW. Sensory precipitation and reflex mechanisms. In Jasper HH, Ward AA Jr, Pope A, eds. *Basic mechanisms of the epilepsies.* Boston: Little, Brown and Company, 1969:543–564, with permission.)

Photoepileptiform Responses and Partial Seizures

Photic stimulation rarely activates focal or unilateral occipital spikes. In such instances, there is almost always a lesion involving the occipital, parietal, or posterior temporal lobe (see Fig. 8.6). Focal occipital spikes are occasionally activated by other visual stimuli, including simple eye closure (Fig. 8.12).

It has been suggested that a PPR that is equally elicited by left or right hemifield stimulation is most likely due to a genetic disorder, whereas unequal responses are more typical of acquired lesions (149). The activation of a focal seizure by photic stimulation is also an unusual occurrence. The first occipital seizure induced by photic stimulation was not reported until 1951 (103). Ludwig and Marsan (90) found that only 3 of 54 patients with occipital lobe

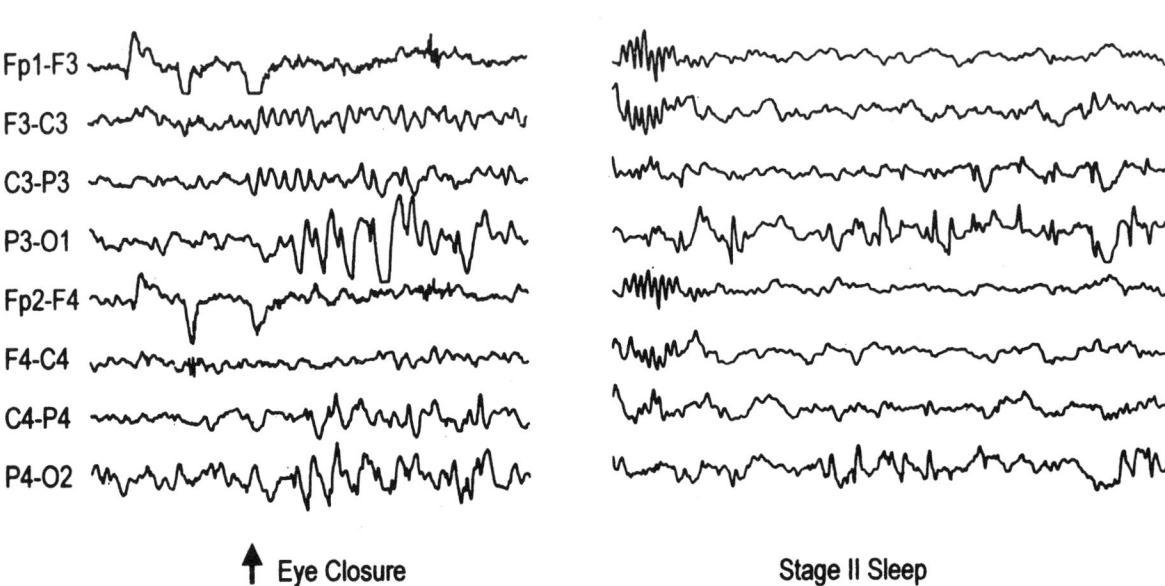

4 y.o. male   Occipital Epileptiform Spikes Activated by Eye Closure and Sleep

↑ **Eye Closure**   **Stage II Sleep**

FIG. 8.12. Left occipital epileptiform spikes activated by sleep and eye closure in a 4-year-old boy with partial seizures.

epilepsy developed seizures during photic stimulation. Wolf and Goosses (169) were unable to activate seizures in any of 12 patients with a history of photosensitivity and partial seizures. Photically activated occipital lobe seizures have been demonstrated in patients with absence seizures who have no evidence of occipital lobe lesions, in patients without spontaneous seizures who have migraine, and in patients with benign partial epilepsy with extreme somatosensory evoked potentials (126). Patients with occipital seizures may also have a history of seizures provoked by a variety of light stimuli, including eye opening or closure, sunlight, sudden exposure to or withdrawal from a bright room, car lights, and television (9,11,68,139,152). In a tertiary referral center for epilepsy, Binnie and colleagues (19) found photosensitivity in only 2.8% of individuals with partial epilepsy compared to 21% of those with idiopathic generalized epilepsy. Less than 10% of patients with epilepsy with a PPR have partial seizure disorders. Therefore, a photoparoxysmal pattern in a patient with generalized seizures argues strongly for primary generalized epilepsy.

During epilepsy monitoring, particularly presurgical evaluations, it is important to note that partial seizures activated by photic stimulation may be a manifestation of genetically determined epilepsy (77). Several authors have described a syndrome of idiopathic, localized, age-related, photosensitive occipital lobe epilepsy with occipital unilateral or bilateral electrographic ictal onset (62). Triggering stimuli include photic stimulation, television, and computer monitors. The interictal epileptiform activity is limited to the occipital lobes.

SLEEP ACTIVATION

Activation during Sleep

Sleep is a highly effective method for eliciting both generalized and focal interictal epileptiform discharges (IEDs) (7,107,133). In as many as one-third of patients with complex partial epilepsy, IEDs may not be present during wakefulness but appear only during sleep (107). Epileptiform discharges are also often more easily detected during sleep. Recordings during wakefulness are often obscured by muscle and movement artifacts, especially in children and adults who are unable to cooperate or relax during the recording. Nearly all patients with IEDs during daytime nap recording have their first discharge within 15–30 minutes of sleep onset (123,143). Thus outpatient EEGs in patients with suspected seizures should always include sleep, but the actual sleep recording generally does not have to exceed 30 minutes in duration. Epilepsy syndromes that commonly show activation with sleep are listed in Table 8.3.

When a sleep EEG recording is clinically indicated and the patient is unable to fall asleep, a short-acting sedative can be used to help induce sleep. Short-acting barbiturates and chloral hydrate are two agents that have been used for this purpose. Chloral hydrate is generally preferred because, unlike barbiturates, it does not induce beta-frequency activity in the background EEG. Every patient considered for sedation should be medically assessed for the risk of sedation. Patients should also be counseled about restricting their activities until the effect of sedation has worn off (see discussion under "Activation by Sleep Deprivation").

The detection and localization of IEDs are both important in routine diagnosis, as well as in presurgical epilepsy evaluations, particularly in the most common type of epilepsy surgery, anterior temporal lobectomy for intractable epilepsy (122). Temporal lobe IEDs during non–rapid-eye-movement (REM) sleep have been observed to become multifocal or more diffuse in distribution than IEDs recorded when the patient is awake. In contrast, IEDs during REM sleep apparently resemble awake IEDs more closely in location and distribution (132,163). Compared with IEDs during non-REM sleep, the location of

TABLE 8.3. *Epileptic syndromes with seizures or interictal epileptiform activity activated by sleep*

Continuous spike-and-wave pattern during slow-wave sleep (electrographic status epilepticus in sleep) (151)
Benign occipital epilepsy in infancy (10)
Generalized tonic seizures in chronic childhood epileptic encephalopathies (e.g., Lennox-Gastaut syndrome) (52)
Nocturnal epileptic myoclonus (99)
Benign epilepsy with centrotemporal spikes (benign rolandic epilepsy) (20)
Benign juvenile myoclonic epilepsy (i.e., on awakening) (8)
Epilepsy with generalized tonic–clonic seizures on awakening (74)
Frontal lobe epilepsy (168)
Autosomal dominant nocturnal frontal lobe epilepsy (134)

IEDs recorded during either wakefulness or REM sleep generally corresponds better with the location of the surgical epileptogenic zone. However, because outpatient sleep EEG recordings are usually no longer than 30 minutes, they consist of mostly non-REM sleep and rarely of REM sleep. Nonetheless, a recent study showed that a non-REM sleep EEG of about 25 minutes' duration correctly disclosed lateralizing IEDs in 75% of temporal lobectomy candidates whose EEG during wakefulness had either bilateral or no IEDs (2). However, in patients undergoing presurgical monitoring, special attention should be paid to epileptiform activity during REM sleep.

In many patients, seizures, IEDs, or both occur either exclusively or predominantly during sleep. Table 8.3 lists the epilepsy syndromes in which seizures or IEDs are more likely to occur during sleep. Routine EEG with recording of sleep activity is valuable when any of these syndromes is clinically suspected. Nighttime sleep recording maybe indicated when the daytime nap recording is inconclusive.

Activation by Sleep Deprivation

Sleep deprivation is an effective method for activating interictal discharges in many individuals with epilepsy (39). When the initial baseline EEG does not contain IEDs, a repeat EEG recording with sleep deprivation has between a 30% and a 70% probability of showing IEDs. Following sleep deprivation, IEDs may appear even when the patient is awake (50,119, 143,159). Thus the appearance of IEDs on the EEG following sleep deprivation is somewhat independent of the occurrence of sleep during the recording. In addition to sleep deprivation, the placement of additional electrodes may further enhance IED detection (143). In patients whose epilepsy diagnosis is clinically established or whose prior EEG has already revealed IEDs, sleep deprivation is unlikely to alter clinical management (39,159).

Although the effectiveness of sleep deprivation in activating seizures has not been objectively demonstrated by EEG recordings, a study of the effect of stressful life events on seizure frequency clearly showed sleep deprivation to be a significant factor (104). When seizures have not occurred in the first day or two of prolonged video-EEG monitoring, we sleep deprive our patients at least every other night, permitting only about 4 hours of sleep until seizures begin to appear.

Opinions regarding the need to routinely record sleep activity have not been uniform among clinicians. Some prefer to initially attempt recording spontaneous sleep activity (40). If this fails in a patient whose treatment may be altered by the detection of epileptiform abnormalities, sleep deprivation or pharmacological sedation is then employed for a separate EEG procedure. However, when a second EEG procedure is not practical (e.g., patients who reside far from the laboratory), partial sleep deprivation and pharmacological sedation can both be used for the initial outpatient recording. Patients who have been sleep deprived or pharmacologically sedated for their EEG should be asked to restrict activities such as driving until they have recovered from the effects of sleep deprivation or sedation. Neither sleep deprivation nor pharmacological sedation should ever be used in those patients who cannot observe this precaution.

PHARMACOLOGICAL ACTIVATION

Discontinuing AEDs

There are three main clinical situations in which AEDs are withdrawn: (i) entering a medication-free state after a 1- to 2-year seizure remission (12); (ii) switching from one AED to another AED (38); and (iii) discontinuing the AED for the purpose of increasing the probability of interictal and ictal abnormalities occurring during long-term video-EEG recording. The rate of AED withdrawal varies in these situations. When a medication-free state of seizure remission is being attempted, gradual withdrawal over 2–3 months is recommended. In contrast, AED use is usually terminated abruptly or over a few days in inpatients undergoing video-EEG monitoring. When switching from one AED to another, the rate of AED withdrawal is determined by the urgency of the clinical situation and the pharmacokinetic properties of the AED involved. Our discussion is confined to the rapid withdrawal of an AED for the purpose of recording interictal and ictal events during long-term monitoring.

Activation of Interictal Epileptiform Discharges

Although 1%–2% of individuals without epilepsy have IEDs on their EEG (131), the detection of IEDs is still important in supporting a clinical suspicion of epileptic seizure disorder. As many as 40% of newly diagnosed epilepsy patients do not have IEDs on their initial EEG recordings (6). IEDs can also be absent in a considerable proportion of chronic epilepsy patients. According to Chung et al., approximately 10% of candidates for epilepsy surgery do not have IEDs despite long-term monitoring (28), although this percentage is far lower in our experience. The location of IEDs in epilepsy surgery patients is valuable in predicting the focus of ictal EEG onset (70) and the degree of postsurgical seizure control (122). Indeed, the value of IEDs in predicting the outcome of anterior temporal lobectomy is independent of the MRI findings (122).

The use of AEDs has long been suspected to suppress IEDs. Ludwig and Marsan (91) reported that 10 of 13 patients who had no EEG discharges while on AEDs developed spikes after abrupt drug withdrawal. Fifty-seven percent of all their patients reportedly developed a discrete epileptiform focus after drug withdrawal. Rodin and colleagues (128) also observed that IEDs become less frequent when phenytoin is taken. Intravenous phenytoin can suppress generalized IEDs, but the effect is only transient, lasting 10–20 minutes (102). Paroxysmal EEG activities have been observed in association with barbiturate withdrawal in addicted nonepileptic persons (165), but many of the reported EEG findings are nonepileptiform.

Most studies, including those referred to above, have not considered the role of nonpharmacological factors and have failed to evaluate study variables quantitatively using statistical analysis (158). In addition, serum AED concentrations were unavailable or were not used. More recently, using serum AED concentrations, Gotman and Marciani (60) found no correlation between AED withdrawal and the spiking rate of IEDs. Their findings are consistent with an earlier study of carbamazepine withdrawal in primates with partial epilepsy that failed to show an intensification of spike discharges (35). As yet, the most convincing effect of AEDs on IEDs is that of valproate on generalized spike-and-wave discharges (65). Both animal and clinical studies have demonstrated that valproate suppresses generalized IEDs, and that these discharges reappear after the drug is withdrawn. It is likely that the same findings pertain to other AEDs in patients with absence epilepsy that is successfully controlled.

The occurrence of seizures is a major factor in determining the likelihood and rate of IEDs in patients undergoing long-term video-EEG monitoring during AED withdrawal. Gotman and Marciani (60) found that spiking activity was enhanced after seizure occurrence, and that the effect could last several days. They used a continuous and automated method of spike detection and quantitation during long-term EEG recording. Using the same method of EEG analysis, their observations were duplicated in a kindling model of focal epileptic activity. Their findings raise concerns about the validity of previous studies of AED withdrawal that failed to consider the activating effects of seizures.

Activation of Epileptic Seizures

The abrupt discontinuation of AEDs is well known to exacerbate seizures in persons with active epilepsy. Seizure exacerbation in these patients has been attributed to a transient "rebound" phenomenon, or to a loss of therapeutic effect of the AED that was withdrawn. A rebound phenomenon similar to that seen in abstinence syndromes of drug addiction (44,69) was suspected by Marciani and colleagues (96), who observed that seizure frequency increased early as the AED dose or the concentration declined, but not when the dose became minimal. The exacerbation of seizure frequency was also self-limited—it did not always persist toward the end of the AED tapering process. Theodore and colleagues (154) also observed that seizure attack rates were highest when serum concentrations passed below 15 μg per milliliter, but not when concentrations were much lower.

There is also evidence to support a loss of therapeutic effect, rather than a rebound phenomenon, as the basis for increased seizures during AED withdrawal. Studies (24,98) have shown that that seizure frequency increases when serum drug concentrations become subtherapeutic, but not as levels are falling from their baseline values. A comparative assessment of studies in the literature is difficult because the AEDs tapered were not the same between studies, and the order and rate of AED withdrawal were not uniform. The definition of the withdrawal and the baseline periods were mostly dissimilar or unstated. Furthermore, the schedule of serum AED measurement also differed between studies. Thus it is currently not possible to determine with certainty whether a rebound phenomenon or the loss of therapeutic effect is responsible for increased seizure frequency after abrupt AED withdrawal.

Despite difficulty in attributing withdrawal seizure exacerbation to a rebound phenomenon, abrupt discontinuation of barbiturates (44) or benzodiazepines (69) is unequivocally known to produce an abstinence syndrome with withdrawal seizures in individuals without epilepsy. The seizures are almost always generalized convulsive episodes without focal onset, and they mainly occur during the period of the abstinence syndrome. Animal studies suggest that these seizures are subcortical in origin (43). This raises the theoretical possibility of nonlocalizing rebound seizures confounding the identification of the onset of seizures recorded during long-term monitoring in patients undergoing barbiturate or benzodiazepine withdrawal. However, rebound seizures occur in patients abruptly withdrawing from prolonged exposure to very high doses of barbiturates and benzodiazepines. Most cases also involve short-acting barbiturates (e.g., secobarbital and pentobarbital) that are not used for chronic treatment of epilepsy. In epilepsy patients taking clinically appropriate doses, the long half-life of phenobarbital probably prevents acute abstinence syndrome and rebound seizures from developing. In fact, seizures may not increase until several weeks after phenobarbital is discontinued (154), whereas rebound seizures in persons addicted to barbiturates occur within days or hours following medication withdrawal (44).

Localizing Value of EEG Abnormalities Activated by AED Withdrawal

Epileptiform discharges that occur as a result of postictal enhancement have been observed to be more widespread or contralateral to the focus of seizure onset (59). Caution should be exercised when using these IEDs to help localize the focus for epilepsy surgery. Localization of the surgical focus should not be based solely on the location of IEDs, particularly those seen in the hours immediately following seizures.

Drug withdrawal may occasionally unmask a seizure focus that is different from the location where habitual seizures originate (95,147). Spencer and colleagues (147) evaluated the video and depth electrode recordings of 71 baseline and 89 withdrawal seizures in 18 patients. During AED withdrawal, four patients had seizures with EEG or clinical features that were not typical of habitual seizures. One of the four had a poor surgical outcome despite habitual seizures having originated from a single area. It is doubtful that drug withdrawal could activate a de novo seizure focus that was not preexistent. Notably different seizures can also occur when an AED is not yet withdrawn (98). Also, bilaterally independent foci of EEG discharges are often present even before the AED is withdrawn (95). GTCSs occur in nearly half of all partial epilepsy patients undergoing AED withdrawal during long-term monitoring, including many who previously have never had generalized seizures (96). As a rule, these seizures also begin clinically and electrographically as partial seizures that are no different from the patients' habitual seizures (95). The duration of either partial or secondarily generalized seizures is usually unaffected by AED dose reduction (144,153). There is no evidence that AED withdrawal alters the pattern of ictal discharges at the onset of these seizures.

Regardless of the status of AED medication and the number of foci detected, seizures recorded in an epilepsy monitoring unit should always be reviewed and verified with the patient and family, friends, or caretakers to ensure that they are the same as habitual seizures. Multiple seizures should be recorded when localizing the seizure focus for epilepsy surgery, especially in patients whose clinical history or MRI is not consistent with the electrophysiological data. Video-EEG monitoring should be extended to ensure that another epileptogenic focus is not overlooked. One study (67) shows that, in patients with bilateral foci, seizures that occur close to each other in time are more likely to arise from the same hemisphere than seizures that occur farther apart from each other (more than 8 hours in between). The discovery of multiple ictal foci does not preclude surgery, if it can be established that habitual seizures originate from one surgically resectable area (41,145).

Potential Complications of AED Withdrawal and Their Prevention

The most important risk of AED withdrawal is the development of status epilepticus (45,140). More commonly, injuries such as fractures, joint dislocations, and external or internal soft tissue injuries result from isolated seizure episodes. The elderly are especially susceptible to vertebral compression fractures (94).

Most complications of AED withdrawal can be prevented if patients are under the care of experienced staff. Table 8.4 lists measures that can be employed to reduce the risk of AED withdrawal in the video-EEG monitoring environment. Theodore and colleagues (153) observed that GTCSs that stop spontaneously usually do so within 2 minutes. Unless medically contraindicated, intravenous lorazepam should be given for GTCSs that persist more than 2 minutes. If necessary, this can be followed by nonloading doses of fosphenytoin. Rectal diazepam is also appropriate for treating seizure

---

TABLE 8.4. *Recommended measures of reducing risk of AED withdrawal in the setting of video-EEG monitoring*

General Measures
1. Incorporate safety features when designing patient areas, such as padding furniture and bathroom fixtures and providing ample space for ambulation.
2. Ensure availability of qualified staff, equipment, and medication for cardiopulmonary resuscitation.
3. Accompany patients when they are ambulating. Use head-protection gear for those at high risk of falling.
4. Evaluate the patient when a seizure occurs, to ensure that ictal and postictal events do not compromise the patient's safety or vital functions.
5. Note the time of occurrence and the severity of each seizure.

Pharmacological Measures
1. Establish and maintain intravenous access throughout the drug withdrawal period.
2. When two or more generalized epileptic convulsions occur within 12 h, consider resuming oral AED or using rectal diazepam.
3. When two or more generalized epileptic convulsions occur within 2 h, consider giving intramuscular or intravenous fosphenytoin. If fosphenytoin is contraindicated, consider phenobarbital, lorazepam, or valproic acid.
4. When epileptic convulsion lasts 2 min or longer, administer intravenous lorazepam if seizure is persisting at the time of administration.
5. In patients with epilepsy, resume oral therapy with the AED withdrawn or with a new AED before discharge from the hospital.
6. When appropriate, check the serum concentration of the AED that the patient will be taking, to ensure that the concentration is in the "therapeutic" range before discharge from the hospital.

---

clusters (89), and sublingual lorazepam has also been reported to be effective in controlling seizure clusters in adults (94). In instances when the threat of status epilepticus is not high and there is no immediate need to prevent seizure recurrence, resumption of the oral AED that was withdrawn may be sufficient. Van der Meyden and colleagues (157) have demonstrated that, in 80% of the patients who were not taking phenytoin or carbamazepine, "therapeutic" serum concentrations could be achieved in 4 hours after oral loading with phenytoin and in 8 hours after carbamazepine loading.

Benzodiazepines and short-acting barbiturates should be cautiously withdrawn. Seizures and other withdrawal symptoms may be particularly severe in persons who have been taking either medication at a high dose (44,146). A state of agitation and dysphoria can follow carbamazepine withdrawal (37). Temporary resumption of carbamazepine or the use of an oral benzodiazepine can alleviate the symptoms.

A postictal psychiatric disturbance has been reported to occur in nearly 8% of patients in the video-EEG monitoring unit. Half of these patients never had previous psychiatric disorders (79). Complications of prolonged inactivity can occur during video-EEG monitoring. The complications include venous thromboembolic disorders and postural hypotension. They can be minimized by having the patient exercise on a treadmill or a stationary bike under close supervision. The patient can also exercise in a recumbent position by using a pedaling device attached to the bed frame. In most centers, the risk of major complications can be kept below 1% (94,96).

AED Withdrawal Procedure for Long-Term Monitoring

The schedule of drug withdrawal should be individualized to optimize the probability of recording seizures without undue risk of injury. Because of the concern of injury from unattended seizures, drug tapering is often deferred until after admission or at least one concurrent AED is maintained until admission. After admission, all AEDs can be simultaneously reduced by a third of the maintenance dose every day. Simultaneous withdrawal of AED is advisable because peak activation of seizures can be delayed for weeks if some AEDs are maintained (24).

Abrupt discontinuation of valproate may be appropriate in the setting of video-EEG monitoring because studies have shown that the pharmacological effect of valproate persists beyond its complete elimination from the serum (65,130). Because of the possibility of platelet dysfunction associated with valproate usage (88), we prefer that valproate be withdrawn before epilepsy surgery is performed.

A slower taper of AEDs is warranted when the patient's history suggests that activation of status epilepticus is highly probable, or when the risk of convulsion-related complications is unacceptable. AEDs do not need to be withdrawn if the patient is experiencing daily seizures at the time of admission.

Activation with Parenteral Drugs

Before long-term video-EEG monitoring became technically feasible and clinically practical, there was a much greater need for parenteral drugs to induce interictal and ictal discharges. Intravenous drugs previously used to induce EEG discharges include pentylenetetrazole (31), methohexital (166), and bemegride (Megimide) (164). A study of 133 patients with depth EEG recordings revealed that only 60% of the pharmacologically induced seizures were localized to the same foci as those localized by spontaneous seizures. Moreover, the risk of failure in seizure control with resection of a focus that was localized by drug-induced seizures is two times higher than that with resection of a spontaneous seizure focus (164). The failure rate of resection of drug-induced seizure foci was 39%, compared with 18% with resection of spontaneous seizure foci. For these reasons, drugs are no longer used to induce seizures for localization in epilepsy surgery.

Intravenous alfentanil hydrochloride has been demonstrated to be effective in inducing temporal lobe spikes for intraoperative electrocorticographic and depth electrode recording (25). Alfentanil hydrochloride is a short-duration opioid analgesic used to augment intraoperative anesthesia. It is not used with extraoperative EEG recording because of the need for respiratory support when it is administered.

REFERENCES

1. Achenbach-Ng J, Diao TCP, Mavroudakis N, et al. Effects of routine hyperventilation on PCO2 in normal subjects: implications for EEG interpretation. *J Clin Neurophysiol* 1994;11:220–225.
2. Adachi N, Alarcon G, Binnie C, et al. Predictive value of interictal epileptiform discharges during non-REM sleep on scalp EEG recordings for the lateralization of epileptogenesis. *Epilepsia* 1998;39:628–632.
3. Adams DJ, Luders H, Pippenger C. Sodium valproate in the treatment of intractable seizure disorders: a clinical and electroencephalographic study. *Neurology* 1978;28:152–157.
4. Adams DJ, Lueders H. Hyperventilation and 6-hour EEG recording in evaluation of absence seizures. *Neurology* 1981;31:1175–1177.
5. Adrian ED, Matthews BHC. The Berger rhythm: potential changes from the occipital lobes in man. *Brain* 1934;57:355–385.
6. Ajmone Marsan C, Zivin L. Factors related to the occurrence of typical paroxysmal abnormalities in the EEG records of epileptic patients. *Epilepsia* 1970;11:361–381.
7. Angeleri F. Partial epilepsies and nocturnal sleep. In: Levin P, Koella W, eds. *Sleep 1974*. Basel: Karger, 1975:196–203.
8. Asconape J, Penry J. Some clinical aspects of benign juvenile myoclonic epilepsy. *Epilepsia* 1984;25:108–114.
9. Aso K, Watanabe K, Negoro T, et al. Visual seizures in children. *Epilepsy Res* 1987;1:246–253.
10. Beaumanoir A. Infantile epilepsy with occipital spikes and good prognosis. *Eur Neurol* 1983;22:43–52.
11. Beaumanoir A, Capizzi G, Nahory A, et al. Scotogenic seizures. In: Beaumanoir A, Gastaut H, Naquet R, eds. *Colloquium on reflex epilepsy*. Geneva: Edition Medicine et Hygiene, 1989: 219–223.
12. Berg A, Shinnar S. Relapse following discontinuation of antiepileptic drugs: a meta-analysis. *Neurology* 1994;44:601–608.
13. Berger H. Uber das elektrenkephalogramm des menschen. *Arch Psychiatr Nervenkr* 1934;102: 538–557.
14. Bickford R. Activation procedures and special electrodes. In: Klass DW, Daly DD, eds. *Current practice of electroencephalography*. New York: Raven Press, 1979:269–305.
15. Bickford R, Klass DW. Sensory precipitation and reflex mechanisms. In: Jasper HH, Ward AA, Pope A, eds. *Basic mechanisms of the epilepsies*. Boston: Little, Brown and Company, 1969: 543–564.
16. Bickford RG, Sem-Jacobsen GW, White PT, et al. Some observations on the mechanism of photic and photometrazol activation. *Electroencephalogr Clin Neurophysiol* 1952;4:275–282.
17. Binnie CD. Human and simian photosensitivity. In: Wolf P, ed. *Epileptic seizures and syndromes*. London: John Libbey, 1994:49–54.
18. Binnie CD. Simple reflex epilepsies. In: Engel J Jr, Pedley TA, eds. *Epilepsy: a comprehensive textbook*. Philadelphia: Lippincott–Raven Publishers, 1997:2489–2505.
19. Binnie CD, Darly CE, Kasteleijn-Nolst Trenite DGA, et al. Photosensitive epilepsy: clinical features. In: Beaumanoir A, Gastaut H, Naquet R, eds. *Colloquium on reflex epilepsy*. Geneva: Edition Medicine et Hygiene, 1989:241–243.
20. Blom S, Heijbel J. Benign epilepsy of children with centro-temporal EEG foci: discharge rate during sleep. *Epilepsia* 1975;16:133–140.
21. Blume WT, David RB, Gomez MR. Generalized sharp and slow wave complexes: associated clinical features and long-term follow-up. *Brain* 1973;96:289–306.
22. Bonvallet M, Dell P. Reflections on the mechanisms of the action of hyperventilation upon the EEG. *Electroencephalogr Clin Neurophysiol* 1956;8:170.
23. Brill NQ, Seidemann H. The electroencephalogram of normal children: effect of hyperventilation. *Am J Psychiatry* 1941;98:250–256.
24. Bromfield E, Dambrosia J, Devinsky O, et al. Phenytoin withdrawal and seizure frequency. *Neurology* 1989;39:905–909.
25. Cascino G, So E, Sharbrough F, et al. Alfentanil-induced epileptiform activity in patients with partial epilepsy. *J Clin Neurophysiol* 1993;10:520–525.
26. Caton R. The electric currents of the brain. *Br Med J* 1875;2:278.
27. Chatrian GE, Bergamini L, Dondey M, et al. A glossary of terms most commonly used by clinical electroencephalographers. *Electroencephalogr Clin Neurophysiol* 1974;37:538–548.
28. Chung M, Walczak T, Lewis D, et al. Temporal lobectomy and independent bitemporal activity: What degree of lateralization is sufficient? *Epilepsia* 1991;32:195–201.
29. Cobb WA, Gordon N, Matthews C, et al. The occipital delta rhythm in petit mal. *Electroencephalogr Clin Neurophysiol* 1961;13:142–143.
30. Coull BM, Pedley TA. Intermittent photic stimulation: clinical uses of non-convulsive responses. *Electroencephalogr Clin Neurophysiol* 1978;44:353–363.
31. Cure C, Rasmussen T, Jasper H. Activation of seizures and electroencephalographic abnormalities in epileptic and in control subjects with "Metrazol". *Arch Neurol Psychiatry* 1948;59:691–717.
32. Dalby MA. Epilepsy and 3 per second spike and wave rhythms: a clinical, electroencephalographic and prognostic analysis of 346 patients. *Acta Neurol Scand Suppl* 1969;40:1–80.
33. Darrow CW, Pathman JH. The role of blood pressure in electroencephalographic changes during hyperventilation. *Fed Proc Am Soc Exp Biol* 1943;2:9.

34. Daute KH, Klust E, Frenzel JL. Ueber den unspezifischen hyperventilationseffekt im EEG des gesunden kindes. II. Strukturbensonderheiten. Schlussfolgerungen. *Z Kinderheilkd* 1968;104: 208–217.

35. David J, Grewal R. Effect of carbamazepine (Tegretol) on seizure and EEG patterns in monkeys with alumina-induced focal motor and hippocampi foci. *Epilepsia* 1976;17:415–422.

36. Davis H, Wallace WM. Factors affecting changes produced in the electroencephalograms by standardized hyperventilation. *Arch Neurol Psychiatry* 1942;47:606–625.

37. Duncan J, Shorvon S, Trimble M. Withdrawal symptoms from phenytoin, carbamazepine and sodium valproate. *J Neurol Neurosurg Psychiatry* 1988;51:924–928.

38. Duncan J, Shorvon S, Trimble MR. Discontinuation of phenytoin, carbamazepine, and valproate in patients with active epilepsy. *Epilepsia* 1990;31:324–333.

39. Ellingson R, Wilken K, Bennet D. Efficacy of sleep deprivation as an activation procedure in epilepsy patients. *J Clin Neurophysiol* 1984;1:83–101.

40. Engel J Jr. A practical guide for routine EEG studies in epilepsy. *J Clin Neurophysiol* 1984;1: 109-142.

41. Engel J Jr, Crandall PH. Falsely localizing ictal onsets with depth EEG telemetry during anticonvulsant withdrawal. *Epilepsia* 1983;24:344–355.

42. Epstein MA, Duchowny M, Jayakar T, et al. Altered responsiveness during hyperventilation-induced EEG slowing: a non-epileptic phenomenon in normal children. *Epilepsia* 1994;35: 1204–1207.

43. Essig C. Convulsive and sham rage behaviors in decorticate dogs during barbiturate withdrawal. *Arch Neurol Psychiatry* 1962;7:471–475.

44. Essig C. Clinical and experimental aspects of barbiturate withdrawal convulsions. *Epilepsia* 1967;8:21–30.

45. Fagan K, Lee S. Prolonged confusion following convulsion due to generalized nonconvulsive status epilepticus. *Neurology* 1990;40:1689–1694.

46. Fisch BJ. *Fisch and Spehlmann's primer of analog and digital EEG*. Amsterdam: Elsevier Science, 1999.

47. Fisch BJ, Hauser WA, Brust JCM, et al. The EEG response to diffuse and patterned photic stimulation during acute untreated alcohol withdrawal. *Neurology* 1989;39:434–436.

48. Fischer-Williams M, Poncet M, Riche D, et al. Light-induced epilepsy in the baboon Papio papio: cortical and depth recordings. *Electroencephalogr Clin Neurophysiol* 1968;25:557–569.

49. Foerster O. Hyperventilationsepilepsie. *Dtsch Z Nerv* 1924;1:347–356.

50. Fountain N, Kim J, Lee S. Sleep deprivation activates epileptiform discharges independent of the activating effects of sleep. *J Clin Neurophysiol* 1998;15:69–75.

51. Fried R. *The hyperventilation syndrome*. Baltimore: Johns Hopkins University Press, 1987.

52. Gastaut H, Broughton R. Tonic seizures. In: Gastaut H, Broughton R, eds. *Epileptic seizure: clinical and electroencephalographic features; diagnosis and treatment*. Springfield, IL: Charles C Thomas Publisher, 1972:37–47.

53. Gastaut H, Remond A. L'activation de l'electroencephalogramme dans les affections cerebrales non epileptogenes (vers une neurophysiologie clinique). *Rev Neurol (Paris)* 1949;81:594–598.

54. Gibbs FA, Gibbs EL, Lennox WG. Electroencephalographic response to overventilation and its relation to age. *J Pediatr* 1943;23:497–505.

55. Gibbs FA, Williams D, Gibbs EL. Modification of the cortical frequency spectrum by changes in CO_2, blood sugar and O_2. *J Neurophysiol* 1940;3:49.

56. Gibbs GA, Davis H. Changes in the human electroencephalogram associated with loss of consciousness. *Am J Physiol* 1935;113:49.

57. Gibbs GA, Davis H, Lennox WG. The electroencephalogram in epilepsy and in conditions of impaired consciousness. *Arch Neurol Psychiatry* 1935;34:1133.

58. Gloor P. Hans Berger on the electroencephalogram of man: fourteen original reports on the human electroencephalogram. *Electroencephalogr Clin Neurophysiol Suppl* 1969;28.

59. Gotman J, Koffler D. Interictal spiking increases after seizures but does not after decrease in medication. *Electroencephalogr Clin Neurophysiol* 1989;72:7–15.

60. Gotman J, Marciani M. Electroencephalographic spiking activity, drug levels, and seizure occurrence in epileptic patients. *Ann Neurol* 1985;17:597–603.

61. Gregory RP, Oates T, Merry RTG. Electroencephalogram epileptiform abnormalities in candidates for aircrew training. *Electroencephalogr Clin Neurophysiol* 1993;86:75–77.

62. Guerrini G, Dravet A, Genton P, et al. Idiopathic photosensitive occipital lobe epilepsy. *Epilepsia* 1995;36:883–891.

63. Harding GF, Edson A, Jeavons PM. Persistence of photosensitivity. *Epilepsia* 1997;38:663–669.

64. Harding GF, Fylan F. Two visual mechanisms of photosensitivity. *Epilepsia* 1999;40:1446–1451.

65. Harding G, Herrick C, Jeavons PM. A controlled study of the effect of sodium valproate on photosensitivity and its prognosis. *Epilepsia* 1978;19:555–556.

66. Harding GFA, Jeavons PM. *Photosensitive epilepsy, new edition*. London: MacKeith Press, 1994.

67. Haut S, Legatt A, O'Dell C, et al. Seizure lateralization during EEG monitoring in patients with bilateral foci: the cluster effect. *Epilepsia* 1997;38:937–940.

68. Hishikawa Y, Yamamoto J, Furuya E, et al. Photosensitive epilepsy: relationships between the visual evoked responses and the epileptiform discharges induced by intermittent photic stimulation. *Electroencephalogr Clin Neurophysiol* 1967;23:320–334.

69. Hollister L, Motzenbecker F, Degan R. Withdrawal reactions from chlordiazepoxide ("Librium"). *Psychopharmacologia* 1961;2:63–68.

70. Holmes M, Dodrill C, Wilensky A, et al. Unilateral focal preponderance of interictal epileptiform discharges as a predictor of seizure origin. *Arch Neurol* 1996;53:228–232.

71. Hufnagel A, Elger CE, Durwen HF, et al. Activation of the epileptic focus by transcranial magnetic stimulation of the human brain. *Ann Neurol* 1990;27:49–60.

72. Huttunen J, Tolvanen H, Heinonen E, et al. Effects of voluntary hyperventilation on cortical sensory responses: electroencephalographic and magnetoencephalographic studies. *Exp Brain Res* 1999;125:248–254.

73. Ishii K, Sasaki M, Yamaji S, et al. Cerebral blood flow changes in the primary motor and premotor cortices during hyperventilation. *Ann Nucl Med* 1998;12:29–33.

74. Janz D. The grand mal epilepsies and the sleep-waking cycle. *Epilepsia* 1962;3:69–109.

75. Janz D, Durner M. Juvenile myoclonic epilepsy. In: Engel J Jr, Pedley TA, eds. *Epilepsy: a comprehensive textbook*. Philadelphia: Lippincott–Raven Publishers, 1997:2389–2400.

76. Jayakar P, Chiappa KH. Clinical correlations of photoparoxysmal responses. *Electroencephalogr Clin Neurophysiol* 1990;75:251–254.

77. Jeavons PM, Harding GFA. *Photosensitive epilepsy*. London: Heinemann, 1975.

78. Kameyama M, Shirane R, Tsurumi Y, et al. Evaluation of cerebral blood flow and metabolism in childhood moyamoya disease: an investigation into "re-build-up" on EEG by positron CT. *Childs Nerv Syst* 1986;2:130–133.

79. Kanner A, Stagno S, Kotagal P, et al. Postictal psychiatric events during prolonged video-electroencephalographic monitoring studies. *Arch Neurol* 1996;53:258–262.

80. Kasteleijn-Nolst Trenite DG, Binnie CD, Harding GF, et al. Photic stimulation: standardization of screening methods. *Epilepsia* 1999;40[Suppl 4]:75–79.

81. Kasteleijn-Nolst Trenite DGA, van Emde Boas W, Binnie CD. Photosensitivity as an age related disorder. In: Wolf P, ed. *Epileptic seizures and syndromes*. London: John Libbey, 1994:41–48.

82. Klass DW, Fischer-Williams M. Sensory stimulation, sleep and sleep deprivation. In: Remond A, ed. *Handbook of electroencephalography and clinical neurophysiology*, Vol 3D. Amsterdam: Elsevier Science, 1976:5–73.

83. Kodama N, Aoki Y, Hiraga H, et al. Electroencephalographic findings in children with moyamoya disease. *Arch Neurol* 1979;36:16–19.

84. Konishi T. The standardization of hyperventilation on EEG recording in childhood. II. The quantitative analysis of build-up. *Brain Dev* 1987;9:21–25.

85. Kooi K, Thomas MH, Mortenson FN. Photoconvulsive and photomyoclonic responses in adults: an appraisal of their clinical significance. *Neurology* 1960;10:1051–1058.

86. Kukumberg P, Benetin J, Kuchar M. Changes of motor evoked potential amplitudes following magnetic stimulation after hyperventilation. *Electromyogr Clin Neurophysiol* 1996;36:271–273.

87. Leijten FS, Dekker E, Spekreijse H, et al. Light diffusion in photosensitive epilepsy. *Electroencephalogr Clin Neurophysiol* 1998;106:387–391.

88. Loiseau P. Sodium valproate, platelet dysfunction and bleeding. *Epilepsia* 1981;22:141–146.

89. Lombroso C. Intermittent treatment of status and clusters of seizures. *Epilepsia* 1989;30[Suppl 2]: S11–S14.

90. Ludwig BI, Marsan CA. Clinical ictal patterns in epileptic patients with occipital electroencephalographic foci. *Neurology* 1975;25:463–471.

91. Ludwig BI, Marsan CA. EEG changes after withdrawal of medication in epileptic patients. *Electroencephalogr Clin Neurophysiol* 1975;39:173–181.

92. Lugaresi E, Crignotta F, Montagna P. Occipital lobe epilepsy with scotosensitive seizures: the role of central vision. *Epilepsia* 1984;25:115–120.

93. Maheshwari MC, Jeavons PM. The clinical significance of occipital spikes as a sole response to intermittent photic stimulation. *Electroencephalogr Clin Neurophysiol* 1975;39:93–95.

94. Malow B, Blaxton T, Stertz B, et al. Carbamazepine withdrawal: effects of taper rate on seizure frequency. *Neurology* 1993;43:2280–2284.

95. Marciani M, Gotman J. Effects of drug withdrawal on location of seizure onset. *Epilepsia* 1986;27:423–431.

96. Marciani M, Gotman J, Andermann F, et al. Patterns of seizure activation after withdrawal of antiepileptic medication. *Neurology* 1985;35:1537–1543.

97. Markand ON. Slow spike-wave activity in EEG and associated clinical features: often called 'Lennox' or 'Lennox-Gastaut' syndrome. *Neurology* 1977;27:746–757.

98. Marks D, Katz A, Scheyer R, et al. Clinical and electrographic effects of acute anticonvulsant withdrawal in epileptic patients. *Neurology* 1991;41:508—512.

99. Meier-Ewert K, Broughton R. Photomyoclonic response of epileptic subjects during wakefulness, sleep and arousal. *Electroencephalogr Clin Neurophysiol* 1967;23:142–151.

100. Melsen S. The value of photic stimulation in the diagnosis of epilepsy. *J Nerv Ment Dis* 1959;128:508–519.

101. Miley CE, Foerster FM. Activation of partial complex seizures by hyperventilation. *Arch Neurol* 1977;34:371–373.

102. Milligan N, Oxley J, Richens A. Acute effects of intravenous phenytoin on the frequency of inter-ictal spikes in man. *Br J Clin Pharmacol* 1983;16:285–289.

103. Mundy-Castle AC. A case in which hallucinations related to past experience were evoked by photic stimulation. *Electroencephalogr Clin Neurophysiol* 1951;3:353–356.

104. Neugebauer R, Paik M, Hauser W, et al. Stressful life events and seizure frequency in patients with epilepsy. *Epilepsia* 1994;35:336–343.

105. Newmark ME, Penry JK. *Photosensitivity and epilepsy: a review*. New York: Raven Press, 1979.

106. Niedermeyer E. Nonepileptic attacks. In: *Electroencephalography: basic principles, clinical applications, and related fields*, 3rd ed. Baltimore: Williams & Wilkins, 1993:Ch 29.

107. Niedermeyer E, Rocca U. The diagnostic significance of sleep electroencephalograms in temporal lobe epilepsy: a comparison of scalp and depth tracings. *Eur Neurol* 1972;7:119–129.

108. Nims LF, Gibbs EL, Lennox WG, et al. Adjustment of acid-base balance of patients with petit mal epilepsy to overventilation. *Arch Neurol Psychiatry* 1940;43:262–269.

109. Ostermann PO, Westerberg CE. Paroxysmal attacks in multiple sclerosis. *Brain* 1975;98:189–202.

110. Pampiglione G, Harden A. So-called neuronal ceroid lipofuscinosis: neurophysiological studies in 60 children. *J Neurol Neurosurg Psychiatry* 1977;323:330.

111. Panayiotopoulos CP. Effectiveness of photic stimulation on various eye-states in photosensitive epilepsy. *J Neurol Sci* 1974;23:165–173.

112. Panayiotopoulos CP. Inhibitory effect of central vision on occipital lobe seizures. *Neurology* 1981;31:1331–1333.

113. Panayiotopoulos CP. Epilepsies characterized by seizures with specific modes of precipitation (reflex epilepsies). In: Wallace S, ed. *Childhood epilepsy*. London: Chapman and Hall, 1996: 355–375.

114. Patel VM, Maulsby RL. How hyperventilation alters the electroencephalogram: a review of controversial viewpoints emphasizing neurophysiological mechanisms. *J Clin Neurophysiol* 1987;4:101–120.

115. Petersen I, Eeg-Olofsson O. The development of the electroencephalogram in normal children from age 1 through 15 years—nonparoxysmal activity. *Neuropaediatrie* 1971;2: 247–304.

116. Pinsard N, Livet MO, Saint-Jean M. A case of cerebral lipidosis with an atypical presentation. *Rev Electroencephalogr Neurophysiol Clin* 1978;8:175–179.

117. Plum F, Posner JB, Smith WW. Effect of hyperbaric-hyperoxic hyperventilation on blood, brain and CSF lactate. *Am J Physiol* 1968;215:1240–1244.

118. Posse S, Olthoff U, Weckesser M, et al. Regional dynamic signal changes during controlled hyperventilation assessed with blood oxygen level-dependent functional MR imaging. *Am J Neuroradiol* 1997;18:1763–1770.

119. Pratt K, Mattson R, Weikers N, et al. EEG activation of epileptics following sleep deprivation: a prospective study of 114 cases. *Electroencephalogr Clin Neurophysiol* 1968;24: 11–15.

120. Quirk JA, Fish DR, Smith SJM, et al. First seizures associated with playing electronic screen games: a community-based study in Great Britain. *Ann Neurol* 1995;37:733–737.

121. Quirk JA, Fish DR, Smith SJM, et al. Incidence of photosensitive epilepsy: a prospective national study. *Electroencephalogr Clin Neurophysiol* 1995;95:260–267.

122. Radahkrishnan K, So E, Silbert P, et al. Predictors of outcome of anterior temporal lobectomy for intractable epilepsy: a multivariate study. *Neurology* 1998;51:465–471.

123. Raroque H, Karnaze D, Thompson S. What is the optimum duration of sleep recording? *Epilepsia* 1989;30:717(abstr).

124. Reilly EW, Peters JF. Relationship of some varieties of electroencephalographic photosensitivity to clinical convulsive disorders. *Neurology* 1973;23:1040–1057.

125. Reivich M, Dickson J, Clark J, et al. Role of cerebral hypoxia in cerebral circulatory and metabolic changes during hypocarbia in man: studies in hyperbaric milieu. *Scand J Clin Lab Invest Suppl* 1968;102:IV:B.

126. Ricci S, Vigevano F. Occipital seizures provoked by intermittent light stimulation: ictal and interictal findings. *J Clin Neurophysiol* 1993;10:197–209.

127. Rockstroh B. Hyperventilation-induced EEG changes in humans and their modulation by an anticonvulsant drug. *Epilepsy Res* 1990;7:146–154.

128. Rodin E, Rim C, Rennick P. The effects of carbamazepine on patients with psychomotor epilepsy: results of a double-blind study. *Epilepsia* 1974;15:546–561.

129. Rosett J. The experimental production of rigidity, of abnormal involuntary movements and of abnormal states of consciousness. *Brain* 1924;47:293.

130. Rowan A, Binnie C, Warfield C, et al. The delayed effect of sodium valproate on the photoconvulsive response in man. *Epilepsia* 1979;20:61–68.

131. Sam M, So E. A community-based study of the significance of epileptiform discharges in nonepileptic persons. *Neurology* 1998;50[Suppl 4]:A224.

132. Samaritano M, Gigli G, Gotman J. Interictal spiking during wakefulness and sleep and the localization of foci in temporal lobe epilepsy. *Neurology* 1991;41:290–297.

133. Sato S, Dreifuss F, Penry J. The effect of sleep on spike wave discharges in absence seizures. *Neurology* 1973;23:1335–1345.

134. Scheffer I, Bhatia K, Lopes-Cendes I, et al. Autosomal dominant nocturnal frontal lobe epilepsy: a distinctive clinical disorder. *Brain* 1995;118[Pt 1]:61–73.

135. Schuler P, Claus D, Stefan H. Hyperventilation and transcranial magnetic stimulation: two methods of activation of epileptiform EEG activity in comparison. *J Clin Neurophysiol* 1993; 10:111–115.

136. Seyal M, Mull B, Gage B. Increased excitability of the human corticospinal system with hyperventilation. *Electroencephalogr Clin Neurophysiol* 1998;109:263–267.

137. Sherwin I. Differential effects of hyperventilation on the excitability of intact and isolated cortex. *Electroencephalogr Clin Neurophysiol* 1965;18:599–607.

138. Sherwin I. Alterations in the non-specific cortical afference during hyperventilation. *Electroencephalogr Clin Neurophysiol* 1967;23:532–538.

139. Shuper A, Vining EPG. Photosensitive complex partial seizures aggravated by phenytoin. *Pediatr Neurol* 1991;7:471–472.

140. Simon R. Physiologic consequences of status epilepticus. *Epilepsia* 1985;26[Suppl 1]:S58–S66.

141. Small JG. Photoconvulsive and photomyoclonic responses in psychiatric patients. *Electroencephalogr Clin Neurophysiol* 1971;2:78–88.

142. So EL, Ruggles KH, Ahmann PA, et al. Prognosis of photoparoxysmal responses in nonepileptic patients. *Neurology* 1993;43:1719–1722.

143. So EL, Ruggles KH, Ahmann PA, et al. Yield of sphenoidal recordings in sleep-deprived outpatients. *J Clin Neurophysiol* 1994;11:226–230.

144. So N, Gotman J. Changes in seizure activity following anticonvulsant drug withdrawal. *Neurology* 1990;40:407–413.

145. So N, Olivier A, Andremann F, et al. Results of surgical treatment in patients with bitemporal epileptiform abnormalities. *Ann Neurol* 1989;25:432–439.

146. Specht U, Boenigk H, Wolf P. Discontinuation of clonazepam after long-term treatment. *Epilepsia* 1989;30:458–463.

147. Spencer S, Spencer D, Williamson P, et al. Ictal effects of anticonvulsant medication withdrawal in epileptic patients. *Epilepsia* 1981;22:297–307.

148. Sunder TR, Erwin CW, Dubois PJ. Hyperventilation induced abnormalities in the electroencephalogram of children with moyamoya disease. *Electroencephalogr Clin Neurophysiol* 1980;49:414–420.

149. Takahashi T. Activation methods. In: *Electroencephalography: basic principles, clinical applications, and related fields*, 3rd ed. Baltimore: Williams & Wilkins, 1993:Ch 15.

150. Takahashi T, Tsukahara Y. Photoconvulsive response induced by use of "visual stimulator." *Tohoku J Exp Med* 1980;130:273–281.

151. Tassinari C, Bureau M, Della-Bernardina B, et al. Epilepsy with continuous spike and waves during slow wave sleep. In: Roger J, Dravet C, Bureau M, et al, eds. *Epileptic syndromes in infancy, childhood and adolescence*. London: John Libbey, 1985:194–204.

152. Tassinari CA, Rubboli G, Plasmati R, et al. In: Beaumanoir A, Gastaut H, Naquet R, eds. *Colloquium on reflex epilepsy*. Geneva: Edition Medicine et Hygiene, 1989:241–243.

153. Theodore W, Porter R, Albert P, et al. The secondarily generalized tonic-clonic seizure: a videotape analysis. *Neurology* 1994;44:1403–1407.

154. Theodore W, Porter R, Raubertas R. Seizures during barbiturate withdrawal: relation to blood level. *Ann Neurol* 1987;22:644–647.

155. Topalkara K, Alarcon G, Binnie CD. Effects of flash frequency and repetition of intermittent photic stimulation on photoparoxysmal responses. *Seizure* 1998;7:249–255.

156. Twomey JA, Espir ML. Paroxysmal symptoms as the first manifestations of multiple sclerosis. *J Neurol Neurosurg Psychiatry* 1980;43:296–304.

157. Van der Meyden C, Kruger A, Muller F, et al. Acute oral loading of carbamazepine-CR and phenytoin in a double-blind randomized study of patients at risk of seizures. *Epilepsia* 1994;35:189–194.

158. Van Weiringen A. Effects of antiepileptic drugs on the electroencephalogram background and epileptiform activity. In: Wada J, Ellingson R, eds. *Handbook of electroencephalography and clinical neurophysiology*, Vol 4. Amsterdam: Elsevier Science, 1990:433–456.

159. Veldhuizen R, Binnie C, Beintema D. The effect of sleep deprivation on the EEG in epilepsy. *Electroencephalogr Clin Neurophysiol* 1983;55:505–512.

160. Victor M, Brausch C. The role of abstinence in the genesis of alcoholic epilepsy. *Epilepsia* 1967;8:1–20.

161. Walter WG, Dovey VJ, Shipton H. Analysis of the electrical response of the human cortex to photic stimulation. *Nature* 1949;158:540–541.

162. Waltz S, Christen HJ, Doose H. The different patterns of the photoparoxysmal response—a genetic study. *Electroencephalogr Clin Neurophysiol* 1992;83:138–145.

163. Weiser H. Temporal lobe epilepsy, sleep and arousal: stereo-EEG findings. In: Degen R, Niedermeyer E, eds. *Epilepsy, sleep and sleep deprivation*. Amsterdam: Elsevier Science, 1984:137–167.

164. Weiser H, Bancaud J, Talairach J, et al. Comparative value of spontaneous and chemically and electrically induced seizures in establishing the lateralization of temporal lobe seizures. *Epilepsia* 1979;20:47–59.

165. Wikler A, Fraser H, Isbell H, et al. Electroencephalograms during cycles of addiction to barbiturates in man. *Electroencephalogr Clin Neurophysiol* 1955;7:1–13.

166. Wilder B. Electroencephalogram activation in medically intractable epileptic patients. *Arch Neurol* 1971;25:415–426.

167. Wilkins AJ, Binnie CD, Darby CE, et al. Inferences regarding the visual precipitation of seizures, eye strain, and headaches. In: Avoli M, Gloor P, Kostopoulos G, et al, eds. *Generalized epilepsy: neurobiological approaches*. Boston: Birkhauser, 1990:314–328.

168. Williamson P. Frontal lobe epilepsy: some clinical characteristics. In: Jasper H, Riggio S, Goldman-Rakic P, eds. *Epilepsy and the functional anatomy of the frontal lobe*. New York: Raven Press, 1995:127–152.

169. Wolf P, Gooses R. Relation of photosensitivity to epileptic seizures. *J Neurol Neurosurg Psychiatry* 1986;49:1386–1391.

170. Yamatani M, Konishi T, Murakami M, et al. Hyperventilation activation on EEG recording in childhood. *Epilepsia* 1994;335:1199–1203.

171. Zwiener U, Lobel S, Rother M, et al. Quantitative topographical analysis of EEG during nonstandardized and standardized hyperventilation. *J Clin Neurophysiol* 1998;15:521–528.

Chapter 9

Artifacts

George H. Klem

Physiological Artifacts
    Eye Movements
    Electrocardiographic Artifacts
    Electromyographic Artifacts
    Glossokinetic Artifact
    Galvanic Skin Response
    Physiological Movements

Nonphysiological Artifacts
    Instrumental Artifacts
    Electrode Artifacts
    Environmental
    Digital
References

The recording of any physiological activity is always plagued with having to differentiate between genuine activity and that which is introduced through a variety of extraneous influences. These artifacts may affect the outcome of the recording procedure. Artifacts originate from a variety of sources, and their recognition, identification, and possible elimination are a primary responsibility of the electroencephalographic (EEG) technologist. Even the most expert technologist cannot always eliminate all artifacts. However, it is always a major goal to identify the artifactual activity and to offer proof to the electroencephalographer that it is not of cerebral origin and should not be misinterpreted as such. This can be accomplished in many ways. First one must understand that most recorded physiological activity will have a logical topographic field of distribution with an expected falloff of voltage potentials. Therefore, one must have a firm understanding of the principals of localization and use this knowl-

edge in a logical way, not relying just on pattern recognition (11,13). Whenever something unusual or unexpected occurs during any EEG recording, the source of the activity must be determined. The unusual or unexpected may be something localized to a single electrode, multiple electrodes or channels, and will usually have an illogical distribution that defies the principles of localization mentioned earlier. The source of this activity is usually noncerebral (Table 9.1). Frequently these artifacts will appear genuine and, if unrecognized, can lead to misinterpretation of the recordings.

Artifacts are generally divided into two groups: physiological and nonphysiological (3,16). Physiological artifacts usually arise from generator sources within the body but not necessarily the brain (see Table 9.1). Bioelectrical generators present in the body may produce artifacts when an EEG recording is made directly from the surface of the brain (electrocorticogra-

TABLE 9.1. *Artifact sources*

Physiological	Nonphysiological
Eye Movements	**Instrumental Artifacts**
Horizontal eye movements	Amplifier & electronic components
Vertical eye movements	Sixty cycle (line frequency) (fifty cycle)
Oblique eye movements	Capacitive
"Glass eye" asymmetries	Inductance
Eyelid flutter	Magnetic
Nystagmus	Electrostatic
Electroretinogram	
Electrocardiographic Artifacts	**Electrode Artifacts**
Normal high-voltage QRS complex	"Electrode pop"
Extra systoles	Intermittent contact
Pulse artifacts	Impedance-related artifacts
Ballistocardiographic artifacts	Electrolytes
Pacemaker	Electrode movement
Arrhythmia	Electrode placement
Defibrillators	
Electromyographic Artifacts	**Environmental Artifacts**
Lateral rectus	Radiofrequency artifacts
Single motor units	Line isolation scanners
Frontalis EMG	Bipolar coagulators
Temporalis EMG	Impedance mismatches
Occipital EMG	Multiple ground artifacts
Swallowing, chewing	IV drip, IV pumps
Glossokinetic Artifact	Sequential pressurized stockings
Tongue movements	Static
Galvanic Skin Response	**Digital Artifacts**
Perspiration	DC offset
Salt bridge	Aliasing
Physiological Movements	**Multiplexing Artifacts**
Tremors	
Hypnic jerks	
Nocturnal leg movements	

phy). Nonphysiological artifacts come from a variety of sources, and some of these are also listed in Table 9.1. A good rule to remember is that if the activity in question is limited to a single channel or electrode, it must be assumed to be artifactual in origin until proved otherwise. As technology expands and additional equipment is developed and put into clinical use, novel artifacts will appear. It will remain essential that technologists and electroencephalographers develop the skills necessary to recognize them and thereby avoid misinterpretation (2).

PHYSIOLOGICAL ARTIFACTS

Eye Movements

The eye movements recorded by standard 10-20 electrode placements are generated by the corneoretinal potential. This generator produces a direct current (DC) potential of approximately 50–100 mV. The electrodes involved are the ones closest to the eyeball: Fp1, Fp2, F7, and F8. This potential is best regarded as a dipole with the positive pole localized to the cornea and the negative pole to the retina (18). The electrical potential detected by the electrodes surrounding the eyeball is a positive potential, and the voltage is usually greater than the cerebral potential generated by the brain. The artifact created by this generator is detected whenever there is movement of the eyes. When the eyes are closed, the movement of eyeballs is in a natural upward position (Bell's phenomenon), and this upward movement is detected by a positive potential recorded at the supraorbital electrodes placed at Fp1 and Fp2. As with most physiological potentials, the activity will have a falloff recorded at the next electrode (15). The activity recorded at F3 and F4 will be smaller in amplitude (Fig. 9.1). When the eyeball moves in a downward direction, the inverse occurs.

When the eye moves to the left, the activity recorded at Fp1 and Fp2 remains steady, with no change in potential, because the positive pole of the eyeball position remains constant relative to these electrodes. However, the positive potential is detected by the electrode F7, and it becomes more positive than other electrodes connected to it in the montage. Because the eyes usually move conjugately, the cornea is moving away from the F8 electrode and it becomes less positive, or more negative, because the retina is now closer to this electrode. This horizontal movement to the left produces a positive phase reversal with maximal positive potential at F7, and a negative phase reversal with maximal negative potential recorded at F8. This is shown in the bipolar montage seen in Figure 9.1.

Monitoring vertical and horizontal eye movement is best accomplished by placing electrodes near both the left and right outer canthi and above and below the eyes. The electrodes should be placed close to the eye and will record potentials greater in amplitude than the standard electrodes placed according to the "10-20" international placement system.

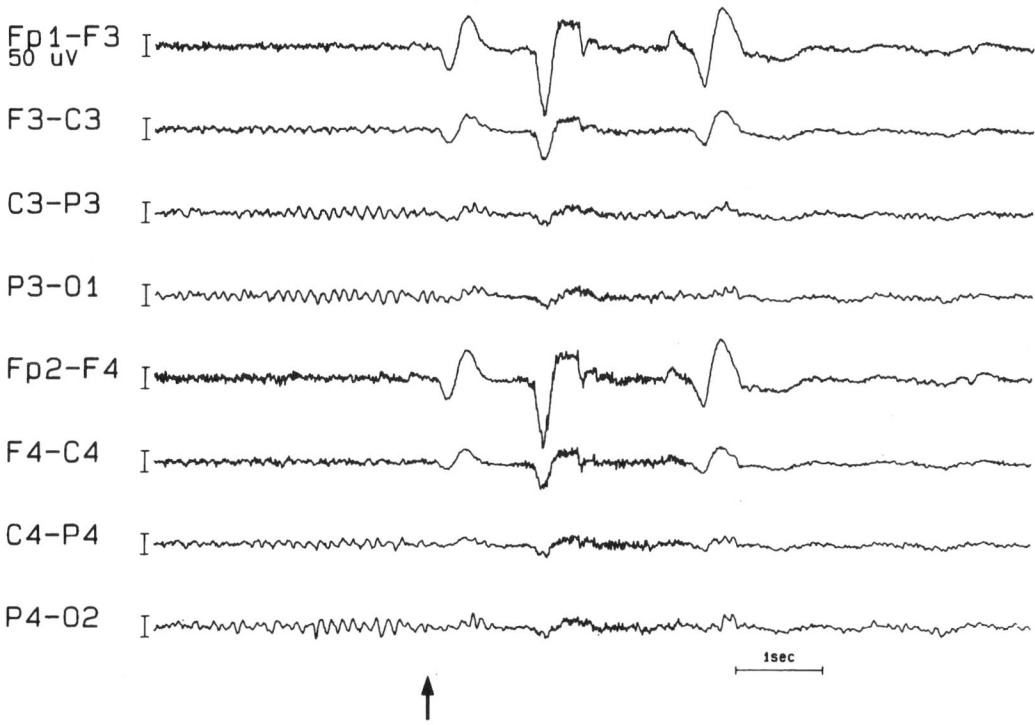

FIG. 9.1. The most common physiological artifact seen in EEG recordings is eye movement. This sample demonstrates the natural falloff of voltages seen with opening of the eyes, and also demonstrates the blocking of the alpha rhythm when this occurs.

Oblique eye movements may be more difficult to detect and are not infrequently misinterpreted as focal abnormalities. An eye movement upward and to the left would generate an equal positive potential recorded in a bipolar montage recording from electrodes Fp1-F7, and a large upward deflection on the channel recording Fp2-F8. This occurs because the positive potential (cornea) involves both Fp1 and F7 relatively equally, and the potential difference recorded with a differential amplifier approximates zero.

The potential difference recorded from the derivation of Fp2-F8 is negative at Fp2 and positive at F8, creating an upward deflection on that channel. This is due to the rules of localization (if input 1 is more negative than input 2, an upward deflection will be recorded). This example is only correct if there is a true 45-degree oblique eye movement. Of course this rarely occurs, and one must be cautious in interpreting this without the use of eye-monitoring electrodes as described above.

Asymmetric eye movements can occur for several reasons (18). The first problem to be looked for is asymmetrical placement of the electrodes. A small deviation from the standard placement can lead to slight asymmetries in the recording. The next most obvious cause for this type of artifact is unilateral enucleation and a prosthetic eye replacement. Patients with a third cranial nerve palsy or external ophthalmoplegia will be unable to produce conjugate upward gaze and will have an asymmetrical eye blink with decreased amplitude, (a smaller deflection) on the side of the paralysis. Asymmetry of eye movement may also be due to a skull defect, usually a craniotomy. Here the eye blink (vertical) artifact will have greater amplitude on the side contralateral to the cranial defect when recorded in a bipolar anterior–posterior derivation. This is, in effect, a "breach" artifact (see Chapter 7). The frontal pole (Fp1) electrode will record the greatest voltage potential because it is closest to the generator source. The frontal electrode (F3) will record a very similar response as a result of the defect in the skull, and, when the frontal pole and frontal electrodes are connected, they will show a cancellation effect because the two electrodes are recording similar-amplitude eye movements. The homologous electrodes contralateral to the defect record the difference in voltages, with a higher amplitude recorded from the frontal pole electrode and the usual voltage gradient recorded from the frontal electrode.

Eyelid flutter is less easy to evaluate. The patient will frequently produce rhythmic activity, typically at a frequency of 5–8 Hz, that will be intermittent but occurs for many seconds at a time. This activity may mimic intermittent rhythmic slow (IRS) activity in the theta or even delta range. However, it usually consists of low-voltage slowing and is often detected at only the Fp1 and Fp2 electrodes. There may not be a falloff of the voltage detected at F3 or F4 or even at FZ because of the low-voltage of the flutter. This activity can be felt by lightly placing one's fingers over the eyelids and then noting on the recording the presence or absence of the eye movements. The typical monitoring for this type of activity is to record it from electrodes placed on the left or right side above (L/RAE) and under (L/RUE) one eyeball using a bipolar montage.

Horizontal nystagmus normally occurs bilaterally, but it is often only detected unilaterally. The electrode recording this movement is either F7 or F8, and the movement may be recorded only by the electrode on the side of the fast direction of the nystagmus because of the larger positive voltage produced by the proximity of the cornea to that electrode. This artifact will often mimic a calibration square wave with a low-frequency cutoff of 0.12 seconds' duration (Fig. 9.2). Vertical nystagmus is rarely detected from the Fp1 and Fp2 electrodes because of the low voltage generated by this movement and the distance of these electrodes from the eyeball. When seen, it typically follows an eye closure and will produce a positive signal when recorded from Fp1-F3 and Fp2-F4. It is usually semirhythmic and

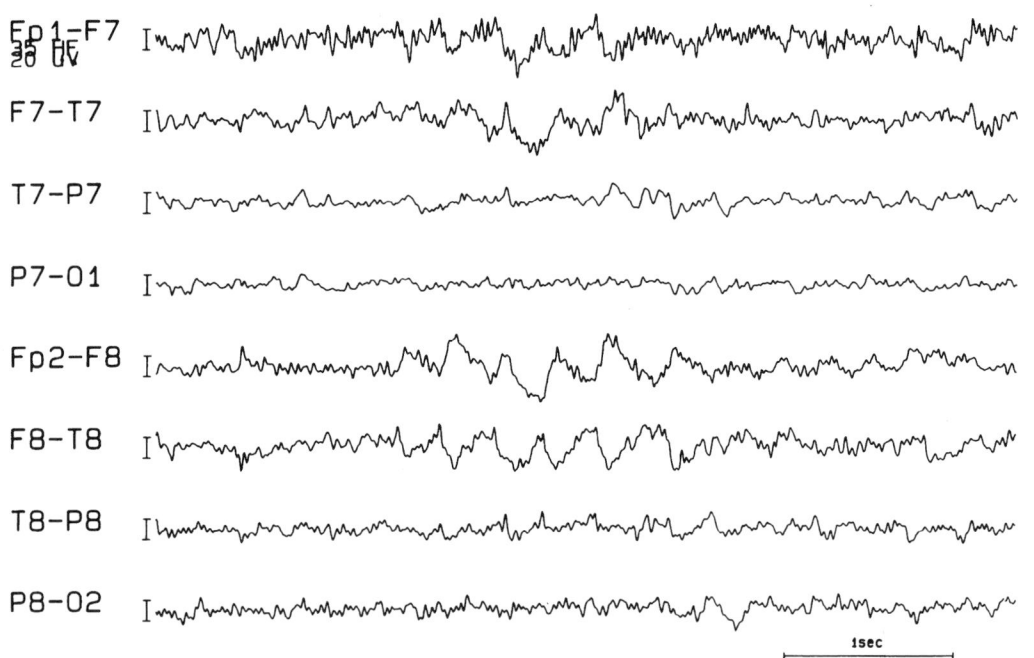

FIG. 9.2. Horizontal nystagmus to the right. There is a positive phase reversal at the F8 electrode as the cornea comes closer to that electrode. There is a lesser negative phase reversal at the same time as the F7 electrode becomes less positive as a result of the cornea moving away from the left temporal area.

may appear to be IRS activity, highly localized to the frontal poles. Rotary nystagmus is rarely detected in the outpatient EEG laboratory. It is more often seen in hospitalized patients requiring bedside recordings. In all cases, monitoring of the nystagmus with extraocular eye electrodes is essential to identify the movements accurately.

The electroretinogram (ERG) is a low-voltage response to light stimulus of the retina. In normal subjects, the voltage typically recorded during an evoked potential ERG is usually less than 50 μV using a contact lens electrode placed directly on the eyeball. The activity consists of two peaks, an A peak and a B peak, that occur approximately 12 and 35 milliseconds following a bright light stimulus (i.e., photic stimulation) (Fig. 9.3). This response is usually obscured by normal EEG activity recorded from the frontal poles, especially when recorded as an analog signal at paper speeds

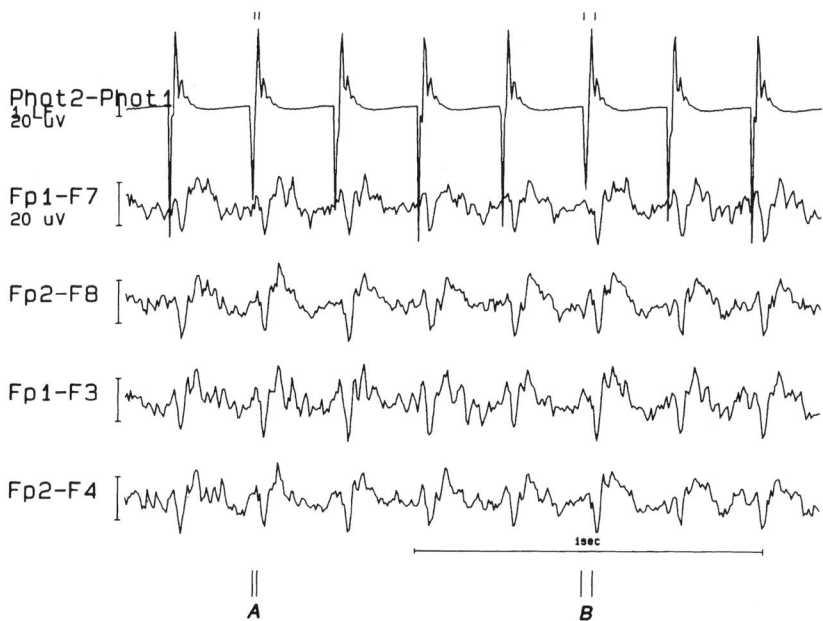

FIG. 9.3. ERG recorded in a bipolar montage. Note that the time scale is increased to measure the latency of the response from the stimulus artifact seen in the first channel. Time at "A" shows a 13-millisecond latency, while the latency at "B" is 33 milliseconds. These correspond to the "a and b" wave of the ERG.

of 30 mm per second. During recordings to determine electrocerebral inactivity (ECI), the background activity is by definition of extremely low voltage, and the retinal response can be seen during photic stimulation. This normal physiological response can be confused with an electrode artifact generated by a silver electrode reacting to the light source (19). To determine which source is causing the artifact, the technologist can simply drive the photic stimulator to produce a signal of approximately 30 flashes per second. If the response recorded maintains a constant amplitude, the source is a faulty electrode. If the amplitude of the response diminishes, it is due to the retinal response being physiologically unable to respond to the faster flash rates. If the response is constant, with no delay to the stimuli, and no decrease in amplitude, then the artifact is most likely due to the silver metal of the electrode being exposed. This can be caused by a chip in the plating of the electrode. This artifact can be identified by shielding the frontal electrodes with an opaque covering that prohibits the light source from being recorded by a faulty electrode.

Electrocardiographic Artifacts

The normal cardiac QRS complex is an easily monitored artifact. It is best recorded by applying electrodes to the chest. Usually two electrodes are attached, one to the left chest and another to the right chest. These electrodes are then connected in a bipolar fashion. The resultant signal is a high-voltage response generated by the electrical field of the heart. This signal is then recorded as an additional channel to the usual montage. In evoked potential terms, ECG recorded at the scalp represents a "far-field" potential. The artifact is most often detected by referential montages, especially those using the ear electrodes as a reference. The field of the heart is oriented to produce a negative polarity signal from one side of the head, detected by the electrode A1 or A2, and a positive polarity artifact from the remaining reference electrode, A2 or A1. ECG is particularly prevalent in obese patients, patients with short necks, and babies, in whom the head is close to the thorax. It can sometimes be detected at the occipital electrodes when a "neck roll" issued to extend the head off the bed. The artifact is especially prominent in ECI recordings (4). It may be possible to reduce the amount of this artifact by changing the head position relative to the position of the thorax.

Extra systoles and cardiac arrhythmias are frequently detected in the temporal chain of bipolar montages but not in the parasagittal derivations, because the temporal electrodes are closer to the electrical field of the heart. These cardiac beats often mimic cerebral sharp waves, spikes, or even temporal theta activity and may be misinterpreted because the field of electrical activity can have a logical distribution, or electrical field (Fig. 9.4).

Pulse artifact is usually confined to a single electrode and appears as a slow-wave potential (2,10). It occurs when an electrode is placed over surface arteries and is most prominent when the electrode is loosely applied. It is easily monitored by using an electrocardiogram (ECG) lead and recorded close to the artifact. The ECG signal will be time locked to the slow wave and always occurs at the same location in respect to the slow wave (Fig. 9.5).

Another artifact typically seen in ECI recordings is the ballistocardiographic potential. This artifact is more prevalent during repeat studies for

ECI than on the first study. It is troublesome to the technologist because, even with good electrode technique, it is difficult to correct, and the artifact frequently obscures the entire recording. Cardiac monitoring demonstrates the relationship of the cardiac signal to these pulsations, although they are not always time locked to any particular phase of the signal. These vibratory pulsations often mimic low-voltage theta, alpha, and beta frequencies, and mixtures of these low-voltage frequencies often resemble cerebral activity.

Pacemaker-generated artifact introduces high-voltage, short-duration spike activity that precedes the usual cardiac signal and is easily monitored with electrodes placed on the chest. This artifact may be continuous or intermittent, depending on the type of pacemaker (continuous or demand).

Cardiac arrhythmias are frequently recorded from the same electrode derivations described above and can be misinterpreted as ictal events,

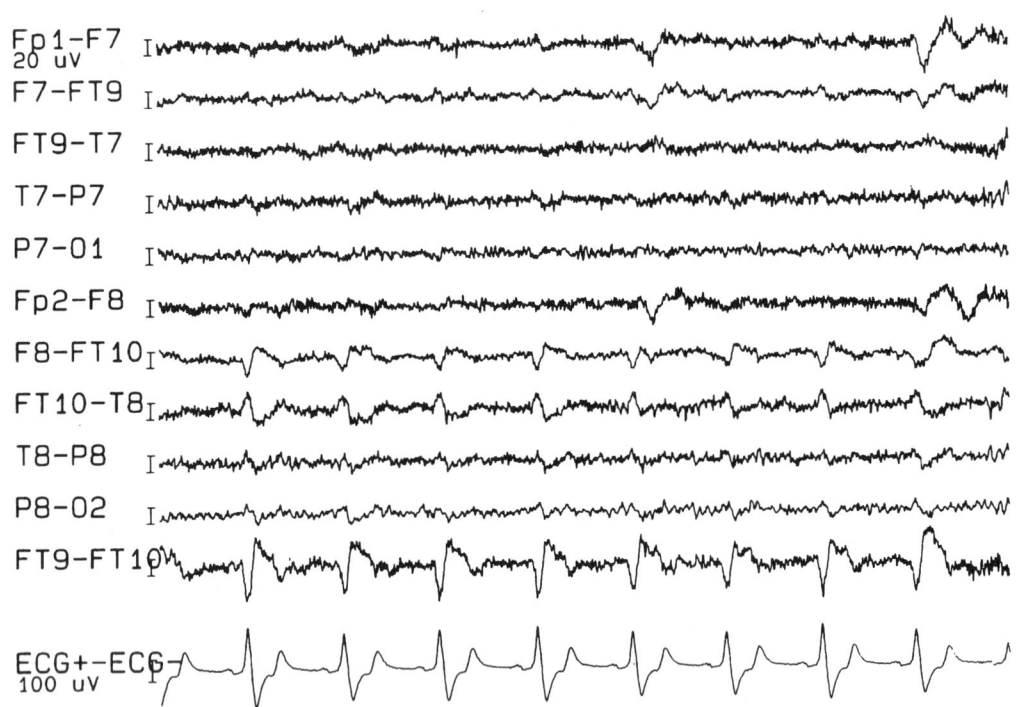

FIG. 9.4. ECG artifact that is recorded from electrodes on the right temporal bipolar montage and mimics a periodic pattern. Without an ECG monitoring channel, one might find it difficult to call this an artifact.

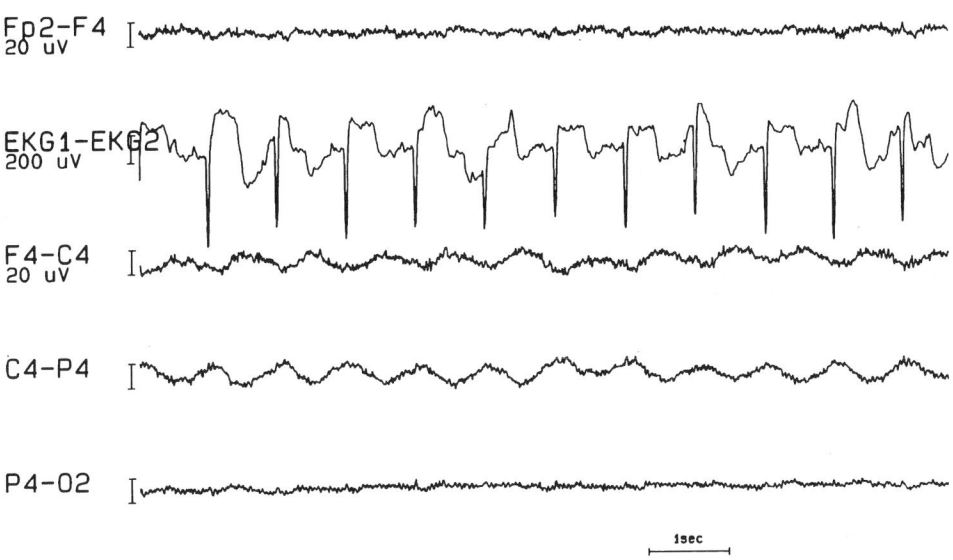

FIG. 9.5. Pulse artifact recorded from the C4 electrode. With digital EEG, it is easy to reformat any montage; in this case the ECG monitoring channel was changed to record the ECG close to the artifact.

because they may present as an evolving pattern. These patterns are easily monitored by recording from electrodes attached to the chest (19).

Electromyographic Artifacts

Lateral rectus artifacts are generated by low-voltage motor unit potentials localized to the lateral rectus muscles (3,19). They are typically recorded from the F7 and F8 surface electrodes, and the positive component is most commonly seen. When recorded in a bipolar montage, the activity is best seen at the electrode closest to the lateral rectus muscle being contracted. The lateral rectus potential appears with a sharp positive deflection of very short duration with a slow falloff as the muscle relaxes. It mimics the appearance of a calibration signal. The activity is usually not seen from the corresponding contralateral electrode.

Single motor units may be recorded from any electrode placed over one of the scalp muscles (19). They appear as repetitive negative or positive deflections that have a comb-like appearance and are typically recorded from a single electrode. Although usually repetitive, they may occur in iso-lated single deflections that seem random. This artifact is generally not reproduced at adjoining electrodes, and even recording from an electrode placed next to the electrode in question may not produce the same activity.

The frontalis electromyogram (EMG) is recorded from the frontal electrodes and is typically seen in patients who are contracting these muscles, as when tightly closing their eyes. The frontalis muscles are often activated by photic stimulation, and a photomyoclonic response is recorded. This activity occurs approximately 50 milliseconds following each flash. The amplitude of the response can be very large and may thus be recorded from several electrodes because of the natural electrical gradient. At times it may obscure EEG activity and even be confused with a photoconvulsive response (13).

The temporalis EMG is recorded from the electrodes placed over the temporal lobe: F7/8, T7/8, and P7/8. The artifact is seen when patients tightly close their jaws or make chewing movements (Fig. 9.6) and are frequent in patients with oral automatisms prior to or during an ictal event or who have orofacial dyskinesias (Fig. 9.7). EMG actiivity recorded over the frontal and occipital areas are common in tense individuals.

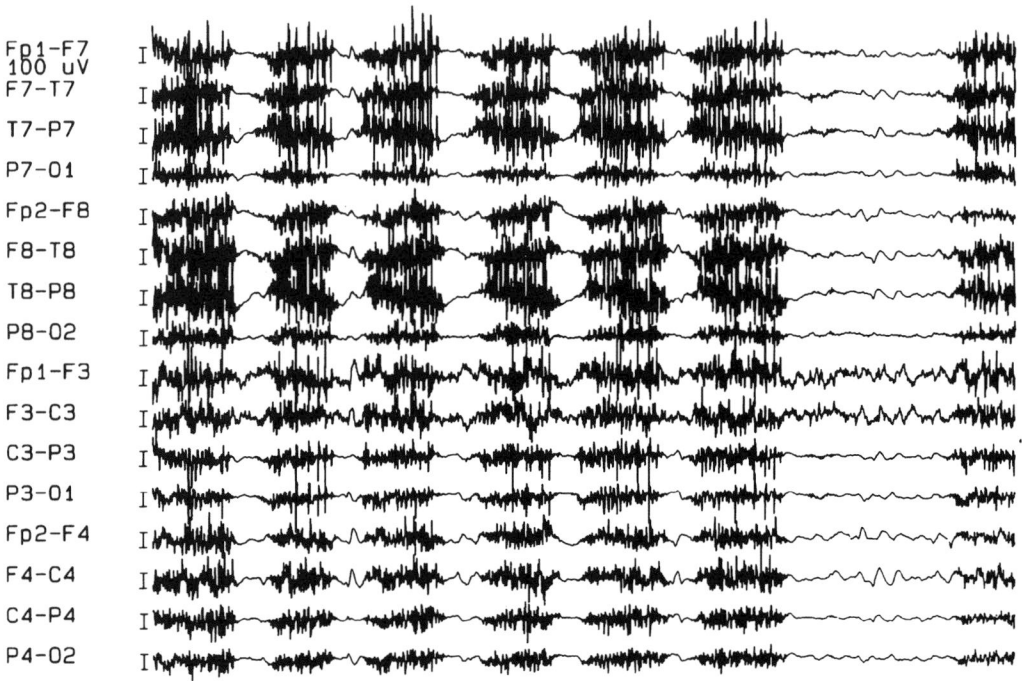

FIG. 9.6. EMG artifact recorded while the patient is eating lunch in a monitoring unit. This artifact is reminiscent of the EMG artifact seen during a temporal lobe seizure with oral automatisms (see Fig. 9.7).

Most EMG artifacts can be reduced or eliminated with the use of relaxation techniques, such as reassuring the patient, comforting the patient, or simply massaging the muscle groups (9). The use of high-frequency filters to eliminate the artifact should be avoided, because these filters rarely eliminate the high frequency; rather, they alter its appearance from a sharp or spike wave to a more sinusoidal frequency that may look more like cerebral beta activity.

Glossokinetic Artifact

Movement of the tongue produces a DC potential similar to the one associated with movement of the eye. The tip of the tongue is negative in polarity with respect to its base, and the potentials generated are frequently recorded as slow movements from the temporal electrodes (19,20). The electrical field generated by these tongue movements is extensive and can be recorded broadly over the entire face or from frontal and temporal scalp areas. The activity may be unilateral or bilateral depending on the direction of the tongue movements. Monitoring the activity is done by placing an electrode on the cheek and another on the submental muscle of the lower jaw (Fig. 9.8). The activity recorded from these electrodes will have greater amplitude than the activity recorded from the standard scalp electrodes, and the frequency will be time locked. The artifact may be reproduced by having the patient repeat words or phrases that produce active tongue movements, such as la-la-la or ta-ta-ta.

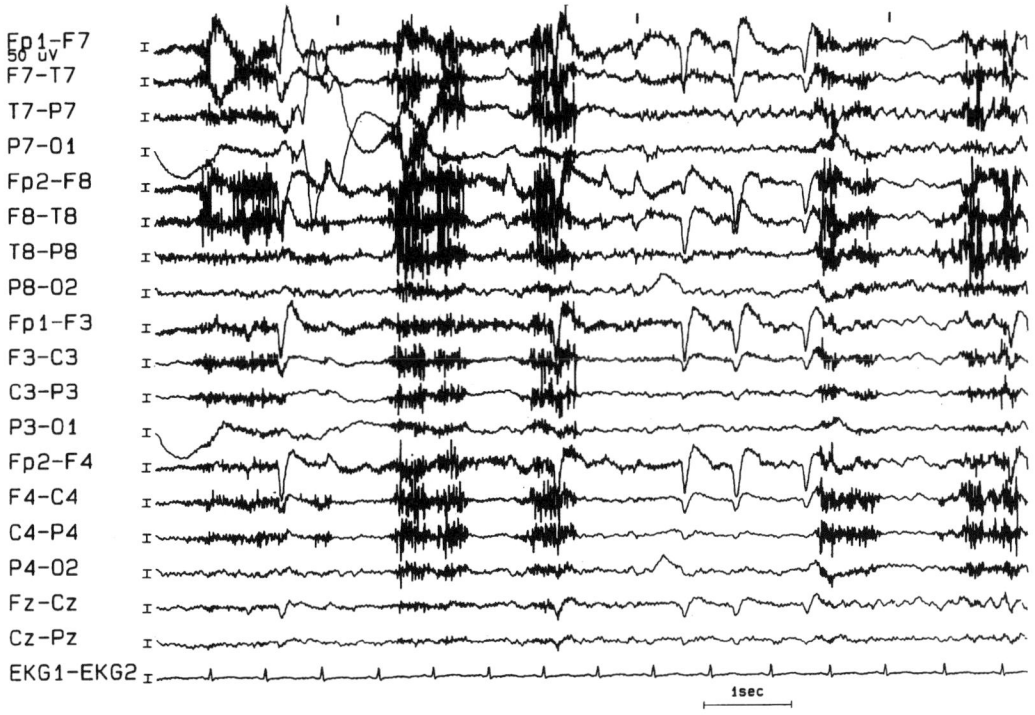

FIG. 9.7. Oral automatisms seen during a clinical seizure, prior to any EEG detectable seizure pattern.

Galvanic Skin Response

Perspiration artifacts are recorded as high-amplitude, very slow potentials. The use of standard low-frequency filters generally reduces the amount of this artifact. They can be recorded from infants as they change states from waking to drowsy or sleep; from babies and children who have been crying during the electrode application; from any febrile patient; and when the room temperature is too high. The amount of this activity may be reduced by cooling the patient or reducing the room temperature, or by use of a cooling fan or air conditioning. Patients resting on perspiration-soaked pillows may display a voltage asymmetry created by a salt bridge that shorts two electrodes contacting the perspiration. This can be eliminated by cooling the patient and taking his or her head off the pillow by using a neck roll (Fig. 9.9).

Physiological Movements

A variety of physiological movements may produce potentials recorded by standard scalp electrodes. The localization of these artifacts is usually related to the movement of the body part involved, the strength of the movement, and the relative location of the electrode wires. Familial essential tremor and the tremor of Parkinson's disease can involve the head, the arms and hands, or both (19). Tremor movement is most often between 4 and 6

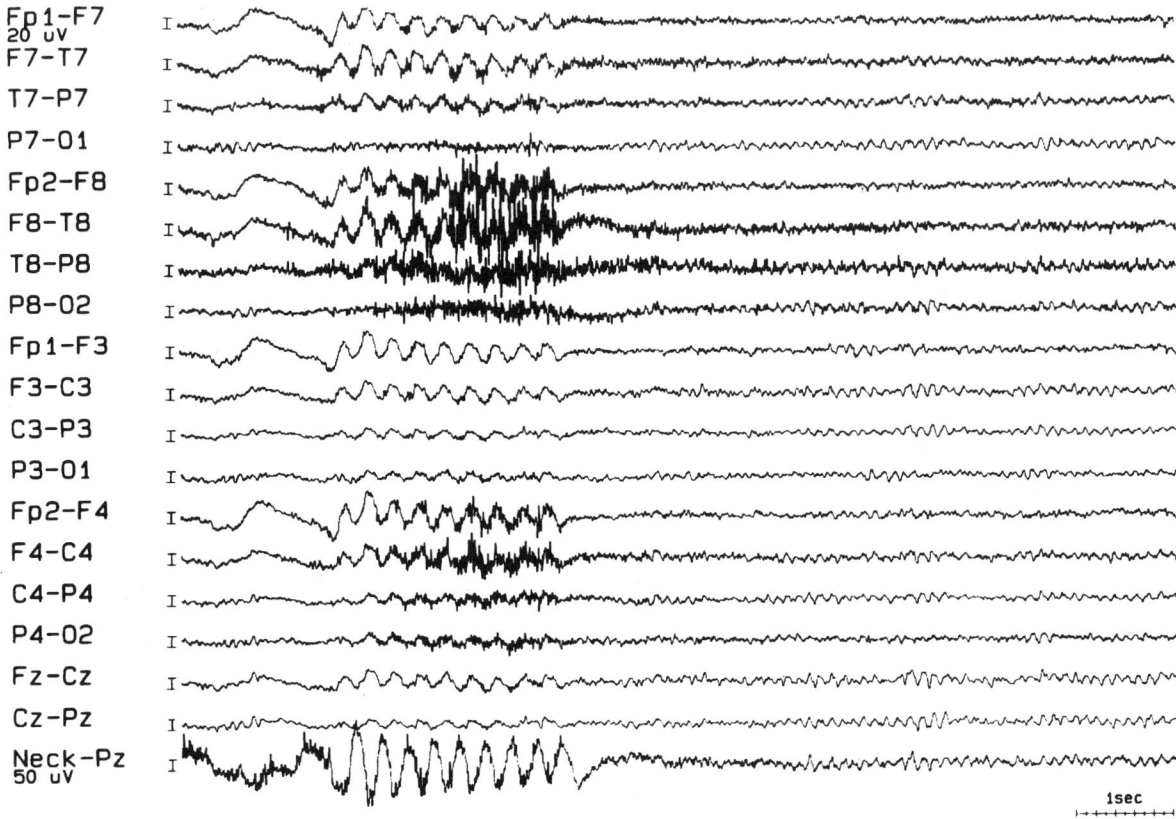

FIG. 9.8. Glossokinetic artifact generated by tongue movement as the patient is instructed to say "la, la, la, la." This is monitored by an electrode placed on the submental muscle and in this case referred to a PZ reference.

Hz. The artifact is caused by movement of the head electrodes in contact with the bed or pillow. If the tremor occurs in the upper limbs, it may be intense enough to cause movement of the head and body especially if there is nuchal rigidity. Tremor artifact may be monitored by placing two electrodes in close proximity on the moving limb or the neck muscles and recording the movements using a bipolar derivation.

Myoclonic limb movements, nocturnal leg movements, hypnic jerks, and even the Mayo reflex of infants can produce enough body movement to move the electrodes or the head, producing a potential in the recording. These movements can be monitored by placing a pair of electrodes on the muscle producing the movement and recording the activity.

NON-PHYSIOLOGICAL ARTIFACTS

Non-physiological artifacts are generated externally or in the environment and come from a vast variety of sources. Many of these originate within the

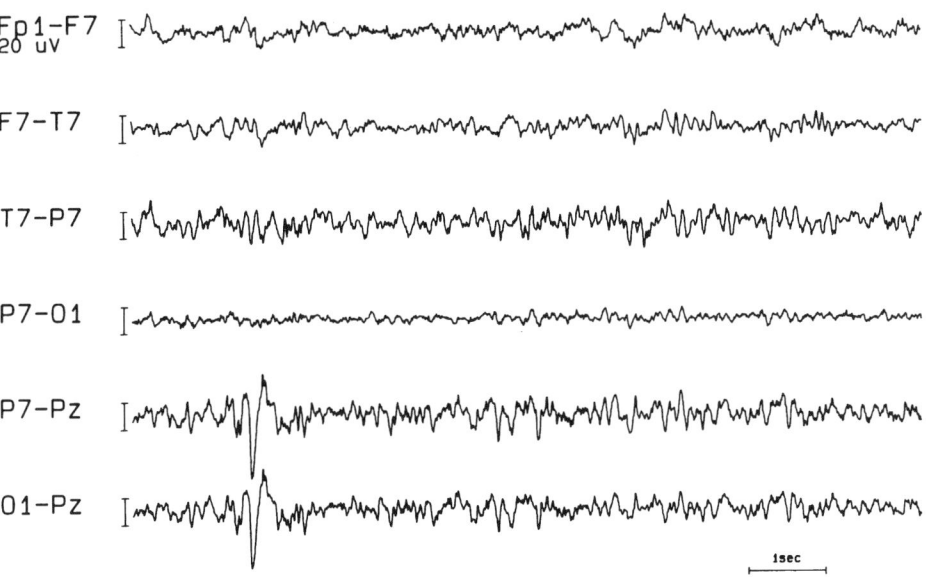

FIG. 9.9. Salt bridge artifact seen in the fourth channel; this is confirmed by recording the electrodes independently to a common reference. Minor differences in amplitude and frequencies seen in channels 5 and 6 are reflected in the fourth channel of the bipolar recording.

equipment used to record the EEG. Others are generated by the actual recording electrodes and environmental sources.

Instrumental Artifacts

Electronic noise generated by moving electrons within the recording amplifiers can be evident at high-gain settings. This high-frequency noise is inherent in all electronic components but generally is a problem only when recording for ECI or in evoked potential records requiring high-frequency responses in the range of several thousand hertz (5).

Sixty-cycle interference recorded in an EEG generally results from poor electrode application. The artifact is often due to high-impedance electrodes that, when connected to the recording device, affect the input circuitry of the amplifier, and also common mode rejection when impedances are not equal. Ensuring impedance measurements of less than 5 kilohms will usually eliminate such line-frequency artifact (1,6,17). Modern EEG amplifiers have greatly reduced the amount of 60-cycle interference seen as a result of the much higher input impedances of the ampli-

fiers compared to earlier models. However, one should be aware that the presence of 60-cycle artifact in all channels of a recording may represent a problem with electrical safety and should be investigated, with particular attention being given to the safety of the patient. In all EEG recordings, care must be taken to avoid ground loops, or double grounding, of any patient (5). This is especially true in recordings made outside of the usual laboratory setting.

Capacitive, inductive, magnetic, and electrostatic artifacts are similar in origin and are usually related to movement of the electrode wires, the electrode input cable, or the alternating current power cable. Of course, all of these affect the recording through the electrodes, but the electrode–disk interface will not be a problem in this case. The most common cause of capacitive artifacts is someone stepping on the input cable. This cable acts as a capacitor because of the multiple insulated wires enclosed in the insulated cable. Moving or stepping on this cable causes the capacitor to discharge, resulting in a relatively high-voltage, transient recorded on the EEG. It should always be obvious that this transient is artifactual, because it will never have a logical distribution of its electrical field.

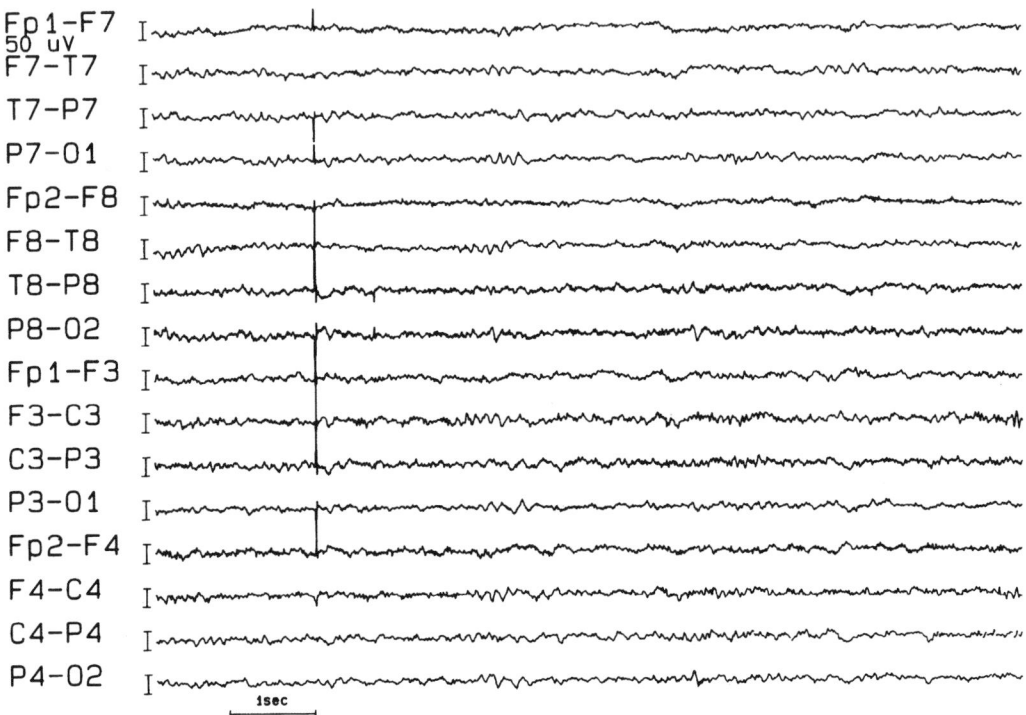

FIG. 9.10. Electrostatic artifact created by IV fluid drip falling near the electrode wires. Notice that there is no logical distribution to this artifact.

Few artifacts are related to inductance. However, the drip artifact frequently seen when recording from patients with intravenous (IV) infusions is produced by an individual drop of IV fluid falling near the electrode wires, producing a change in potentials associated with the arrangement of the electrode wires on the patient's bed (12) (Figs. 9.10 and 9.11). This artifact is relatively rare because IVs are now mostly regulated as micro-drips rather than macro-drips.

Electrostatically induced artifacts, caused by static electricity stored on a variety of clothing and bedding manufactured of synthetic fibers, remain a problem. This voltage may be discharged by touching a metal bed rail, or even passed from person to person. The artifact is again a high-voltage spike transient that will again have an illogical distribution of its electrical field because it is likely to affect the recording electrodes closest to the source.

There will be no need to monitor the artifact: Often the technologist is the recipient of the discharge and will automatically know its origin.

Electrode Artifacts

A variety of electrode artifacts can be seen in any EEG recording, and are easily identified by an experienced EEG technologist. Any unusual event that is confined to a single or common electrode must be considered artifactual and monitored to verify its source, with replacement or adjustment made to correct the problem. The proper application of electrodes is one of the most important tasks for any technologist, and particular care and time must be devoted to ensure proper and accurate recordings. Most electrode artifacts will be related to one of several causes: poorly attached electrodes,

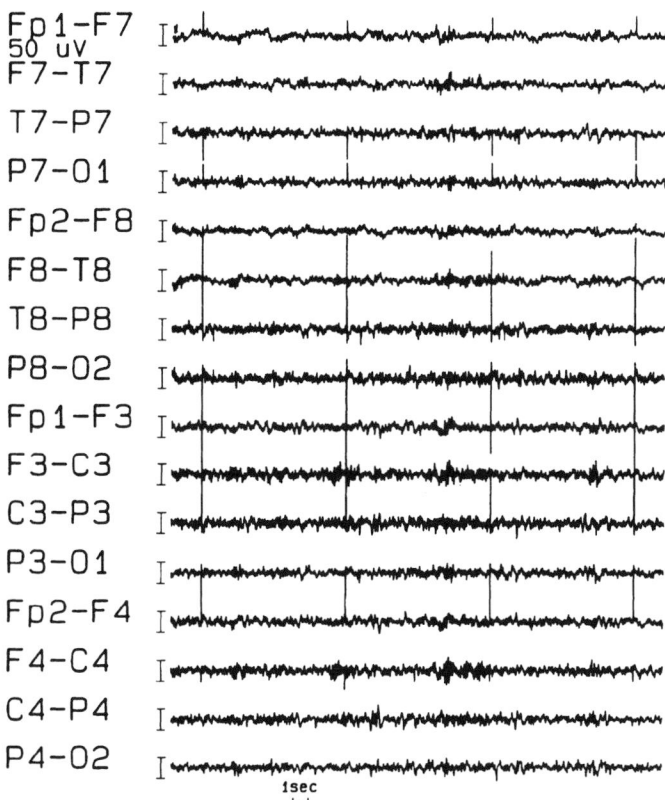

FIG. 9.11. Using the same electrostatic artifact shown in Figure 9.10, the recording has been compressed to show regularity and distribution of the artifact, which allows for easier recognition and identification by the technologist.

high resistance, a broken wire, or changes in the lead–scalp interface, usually caused by a change in the electrolytic gel used to complete this interface (7,8). In the latter case, an artifact may result from the electrolyte drying, or a change in potential related to an air bubble under the electrode causing a discharge. A good general rule when dealing with an electrode artifact is to note it the first time it occurs, determine the source of the artifact the second time it occurs, and replace the electrode or at least reapply it on the third occurrence (Figs. 9.12 and 9.13).

Environmental

Of all the artifacts typically seen in any EEG recording, the most troublesome by far are those classified as environmental. They are troublesome for a variety of reasons, but perhaps primarily because they are not easily controlled by the EEG technologist. Thus, although many of them can be identified, and some of them can be monitored, they may be difficult to eliminate. This adds an additional degree of complexity to the interpretation of recordings in which they are present. Some of these are generated by radiofrequency waves, a high-frequency signal that may be continuous or intermittent and can affect only a few or all channels of the recording. The source may be a microwave oven in a kitchen or lounge located anywhere within the vicinity of the EEG recording location. Clues to the origin of this artifact include the specific time of the day during which it occurs (i.e., lunchtime for microwaves). Another possible source is activity occurring in adjacent rooms. For example, while the technologist is recording an EEG in one operating room, high-frequency cautery may be in use in any of the adjacent rooms producing interference in the EEG recording (14). Occasionally radiofrequency artifact can be reduced or even eliminated by changing the position or orientation of the recording equipment relative to the patient.

Other environmental artifacts include line isolation scanners. These devices, which are common to intensive care units and operating rooms, often generate a particular frequency while scanning electrical outlets for leakage currents. These signals commonly produce a very low-voltage output that can be detected using the increased EEG sensitivity settings often required in these areas. Multiple ground artifacts (60-cycle artifacts) have been discussed above, but one must be aware that the interference recorded may not be from the EEG instrument, but derive instead from another electrical device connected to the patient. There are many other sources of environmental artifacts, too numerous to mention here. A good technologist will be aware of the environment and other equipment in use within the area, and must be cognizant of the fact that they all may be potential sources of extraneous signals contaminating the EEG recording.

Digital

Digital artifacts are unique to the system in use. The term *digital artifacts* is, in fact, misleading, because these artifacts are commonly related not to digital technology, but to failure of various components used in the acquisi-

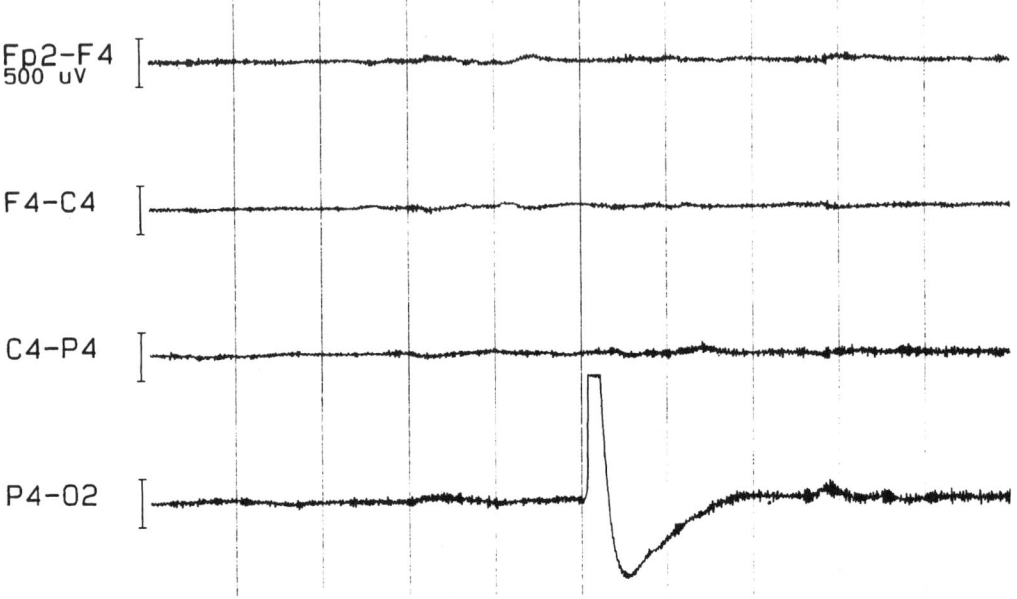

FIG. 9.12. Electrode "pop" artifact. In addition to demonstrating one of the most common artifacts seen in EEGs, this recording demonstrates that the high-voltage deflection actually exceeds the limits of the individual channel sensitivity recording capabilities and blocks or "squares off" at the top.

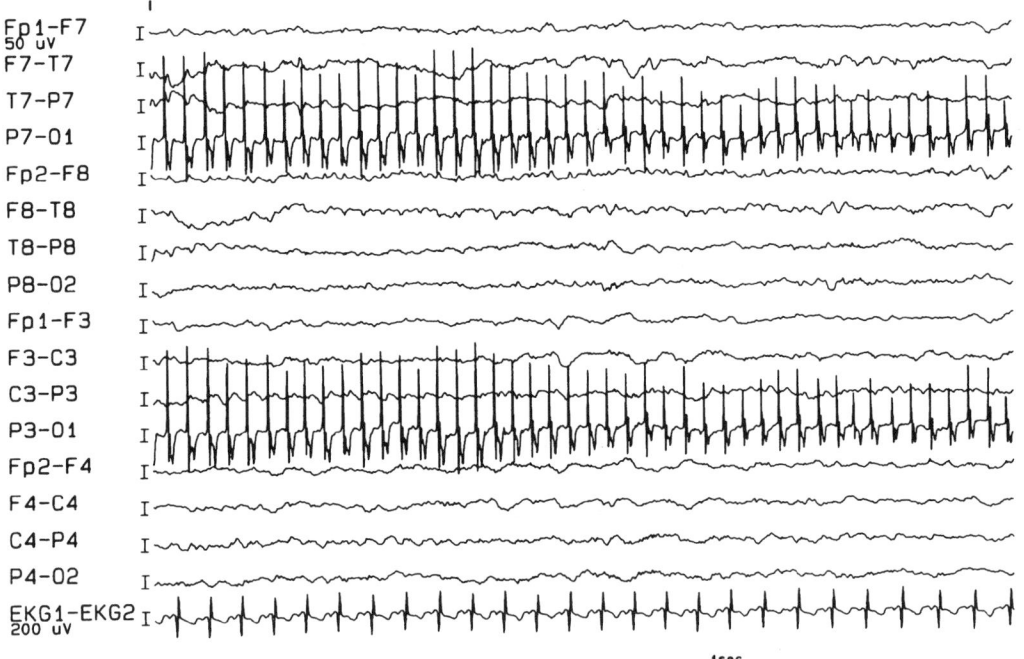

1sec

FIG. 9.13. Electrode artifact at the O1 electrode. The frequency of the discharge mimics the ECG signal on the last channel. The artifact and the ECG signal are not time locked, as they should be if the artifact were related to the heart. The technologist noted that the mother of the patient was patting the baby's back during the recording.

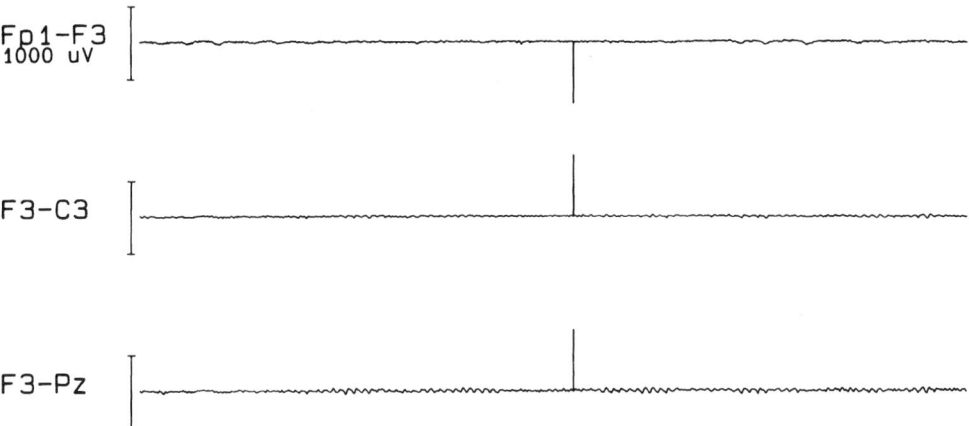

FIG. 9.14. Digital artifact produced at electrode F3 is a result of missed sampling of one data point in the channel recording F3-P3.

tion of EEG data (5,14). For example, failure of the analog-to-digital converter to accurately sample data points on a regular basis may produce something called a "sticky bit," which will result in a display like that seen in Figure 9.14. This represents a true digital artifact.

Similarly, artifacts related to aliasing (sampling at a rate that is less than twice the frequency of the high-frequency filter) will result in an error in the actual display of the acquired data. Because most commercial digital EEG instruments sample at a rate of at least 200 samples per channel per second, and most sample at a higher rate, it is uncommon to see aliasing artifacts in routine EEGs. However, the recorded photic stimulus signal often is composed of a much higher frequency, and aliasing may be present on the channel displaying the input stimulus, as seen in Figure 9.15.

Multiplexing artifacts may be seen in any type of amplifier used in digital EEG, but they are more common in amplifiers with 64 or even 128 chan-

nels. An example is seen in Figure 9.16, where the amplifier recorded 32 channels and the sampling was done in groups of 16 channels. Notice that the first 16 channels were switched with the second group of 16 channels, which was clearly seen by observing the position of the ECG monitoring channel. Digital artifacts, like other nonphysiological artifacts, often produce recordings that do not make sense. They will always lack a logical distribution of recorded activity.

In most instances, digital EEG has made it easier for the technologist to record EEG. With the ability to make changes in sensitivity, filtering, and remontaging off line, improper montages are eliminated, because the electroencephalographer can always modify the montage. Pen blocking is never a problem during high-voltage 3-Hz spike-and-wave discharges, as the display can always be changed to reduce high-voltage discharges after the recording is complete. Filtering also can always be changed after the

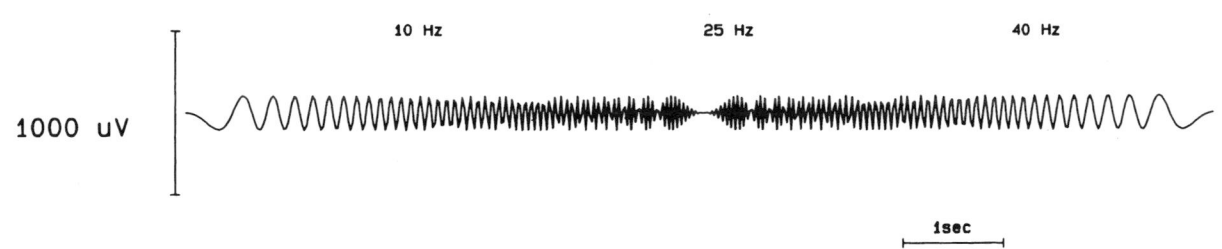

FIG. 9.15. Effect of aliasing caused by inadequate sampling rate. This sine wave recording sweeps through a frequency range of 0–50 Hz at a constant voltage and a sampling rate of 50 Hz. Notice the effect on the 25-Hz frequency.

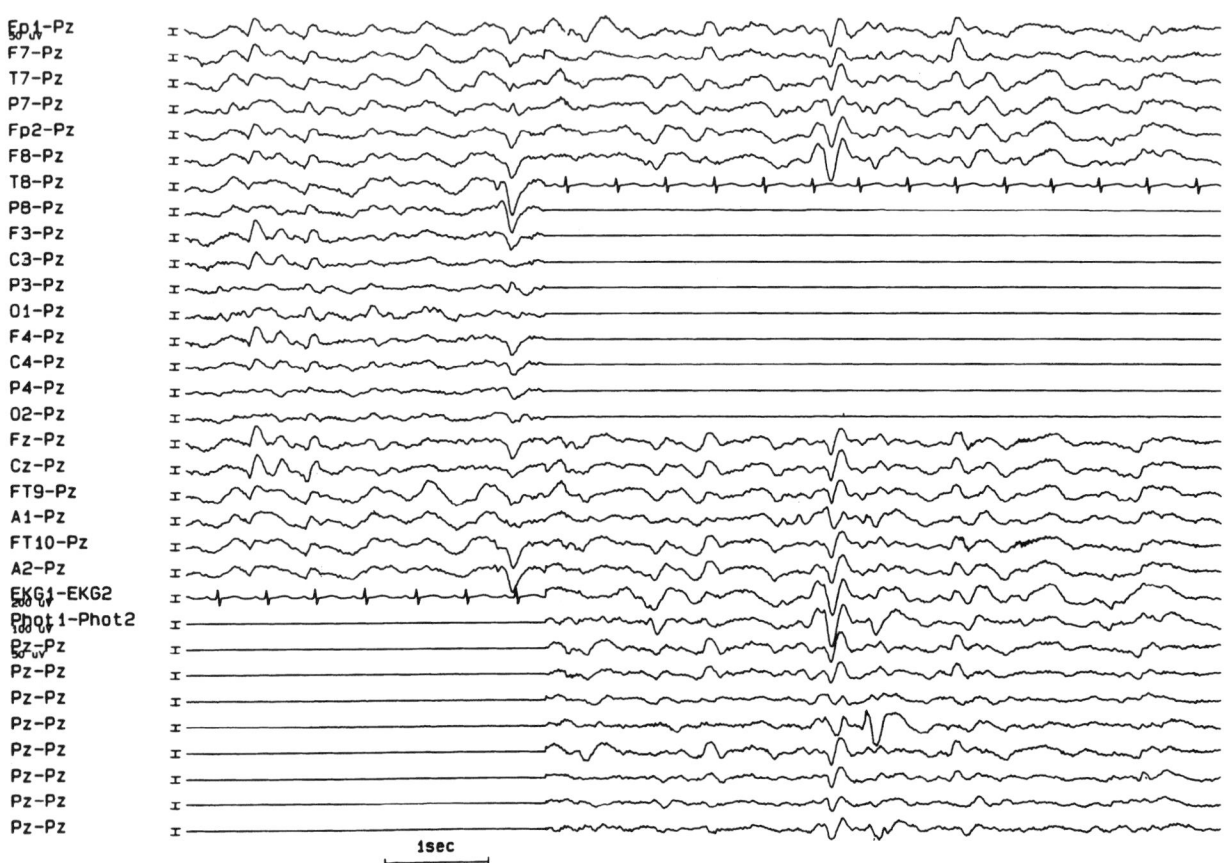

FIG. 9.16. This multiplexing artifact results when sampling is done on 16 channels at a time instead of sampling the entire 32-channel amplifier simultaneously. A timing error occurs and the groups of 16 channels invert. This is clearly seen by observing the position of the ECG monitoring channel.

recording is complete. Digital EEG does not eliminate artifacts, however, and the technologist, as well as the electroencephalographer, must still be aware of the variety of known physiological and nonphysiological artifacts that may be present in any recording. It has always been the technologist's responsibility to recognize artifacts, identify them with monitoring, and eliminate them whenever possible. Digital EEG has not altered this in any way; it has created an entirely new collection of artifacts that must be recognized.

REFERENCES

1. American Electroencephalographic Society. Guidelines in electroencephalography, evoked potentials, and polysomnography. *J Clin Neurophysiol* 1994;11:10–13.
2. Brittenham D. Recognition and reduction of physiological artifact. *Am J EEG Technol* 1973; 13:158–165.
3. Brittenham D. Artifacts. In Daly DD, Pedley TA, eds. *Current practice of clinical electroencephalography*, 2nd ed. New York: Raven Press, 1990:85–105.
4. Chatrian GE. Electrophysiological evaluation of brain death: a critical appraisal. In: Aminoff MJ, ed. *Electrodiagnosis in clinical neurology*. New York: Raven Press, 1986:669–736.

5. Cooper R, Osselton JW, Shaw JC. *EEG technology*, 3rd ed. London: Butterworth-Heinemann, 1990:111–114.
6. Ford RG. A practical guide to EEG recording technique. *Am J EEG Technol* 1981;21:79–101.
7. Geddes LA. Bioelectrodes, part I. *Am J EEG Technol* 1973;13:195–203.
8. Geddes LA. Bioelectrodes, part III. *Am J EEG Technol* 1975;15:99–106.
9. Johnson TL, Feldman RG, Sax DS. Reduction of muscle artifact in electroencephalographic recording. *Am J EEG Technol* 1973;13:13–25.
10. Jurko MF, Foshee DP. Tremor: considerations in recording techniques. *Am J EEG Technol* 1962;2:82–89.
11. Lesser RP, Lüders H, Dinner DS, et al. An introduction to the basic concepts of polarity and localization. *J Clin Neurophysiol* 1985;2:45–61.
12. Lininger AW, Volow MR, Gianturco DT. Intravenous infusion artifact. *Am J EEG Technol* 1981;21:167–173.
13. Lüders HO, Noachtar S. *Atlas and classification of electroencephalography*. Philadelphia: WB Saunders, 2000;119–193.
14. Nuwer MR. Basic electrophysiology: evoked potentials and signal processing. In: Nuwer MR, ed. *Evoked potential monitoring in the operating room*. New York: Raven Press, 1986:5–49.
15. Peters JF. Surface electrical fields generated by eye movements. *Am J EEG Technol* 1967;7:27–40.
16. Saunders MG. Artifacts: activity of noncerebral origin in the EEG. In: Klass DW, Daly DD, eds. *Current practice of clinical electroencephalography*. New York: Raven Press, 1979:37–67.
17. Seaba PC. Differential amplifiers and their limitations. *Am J EEG Technol* 1984;24:11–23.
18. Shafer MA. Problem record of the month: asymmetrical eye-blink artifact. *Am J EEG Technol* 1970;10:153–156.
19. Tyner FS, Knott JR, Mayer WJ Jr. *Fundamentals of EEG technology*, Vol 1. New York: Raven Press, 1983:83–119.
20. Westmoreland FF, Espinosa RE, Klass WW. Significant prosopoglossopharyngeal movements affecting the EEG. *Am J EEG Technol* 1973;13:59–70.

Chapter 10

An Orderly Approach to the Abnormal Electroencephalogram

Benjamin G. Zifkin and Roger Q. Cracco

It is an obvious but important truism that the electroencephalogram (EEG) evaluates brain function, not structure. Although many different pathological processes disturb brain function, the repertoire of resulting EEG abnormalities is limited. As with other physiological tests, EEG abnormalities, although reliable indicators of brain dysfunction, cannot, except in rare instances, distinguish etiology or pathology. Advances in neuroimaging have fortunately reduced dependence on the EEG for information that it cannot reliably provide, while new methods of data processing have led to further development of its usefulness in examining brain physiology (see Chapters 4, 22, 23, and 24).

In this chapter we present a systematic approach to visual analysis of the abnormal EEG, complementing that of Chapter 5. As when analyzing a normal EEG, the electroencephalographer must (a) see abnormalities in the recording; (b) systematically characterize them in terms of morphology, topography, temporal characteristics, reactivity, and state sensitivity; and (c) retain these characteristics in mind while composing the description and interpretation. The electroencephalographer must describe abnormalities accurately, fully, and succinctly. The glossary of the Committee on Terminology of the International Federation of Societies for Electroencephalography and Clinical Neurophysiology (7) provides a common vocabulary and helps us to avoid errors of logic (e.g., referring to interictal spikes as "spike seizure discharges") and jargon (e.g., referring to triphasic waves as "liver waves"). Consistently used, this approach will sharpen the electroencephalographer's powers of observation and ensure that no abnormality goes unmentioned in the report.

This approach additionally benefits the electroencephalographer by providing a framework for evaluating articles and reports on EEG. Anyone who regularly reads journal articles inevitably encounters some that lack illustrations and whose texts contain undefined terms ("a slight to moderate degree of diffuse slow-wave activity") or empty sentences ("slow tracings contained activity below 8 cps in sufficient quantities to warrant positive interpretation"). Such style should immediately alert the reader's critical faculties and lead to judicious appraisal before acceptance of any conclusions made by the author(s). Even more troubling are articles in which illustrations and text are discrepant, not a rare occurrence. An electroencephalographer whose "eye" has been sharpened by systematic analysis will quickly recognize such discrepancies and draw his or her own conclusions.

We divide our discussion into the following topics:

1. Abnormal changes in normal rhythms
2. Abnormal slow activity
3. Distinctive abnormal patterns (e.g., pseudoperiodic patterns)
4. Interictal and ictal abnormalities

Although the notion of abnormality is, strictly speaking, a statistical concept, in clinical practice an abnormal EEG is one that contains some feature known to be associated with cerebral dysfunction. An EEG may be abnormal if normal patterns are altered or if certain abnormal patterns occur. Very often, both types of abnormality are seen in the same recording, as shown in Figures 10.1 and 10.4 later in this chapter. Certain waveforms are unusual, and their appearance may be striking; however, they are seen as often in the EEGs of asymptomatic subjects as in those of patients. Accurate visual assessment of the EEG requires a systematic approach that incorporates (a) knowledge of the age and state of the subject and (b) critical assessment of voltage, frequency, rhythmicity, distribution, reactivity, and persistence of waveforms. In abnormal EEGs, each of these may be altered alone or in combination, and these changes may be localized, lateralized, or diffuse.

ABNORMAL CHANGES IN NORMAL RHYTHMS

Abnormal Alpha Rhythms

Absent or scanty posterior alpha rhythm may be due to eye opening, attention, anxiety, or drowsiness. Some asymptomatic individuals normally have little or no alpha rhythm, perhaps on a genetic basis. These factors must be considered before concluding that an apparent bilateral absence of alpha activity is abnormal. Absence of alpha rhythm, therefore, cannot be regarded necessarily as abnormal. In patients with brain pathology, bilateral absence of alpha rhythm is usually accompanied by other bilateral abnormalities, such as widespread voltage attenuation or diffuse slow activity. Clinically, such cases usually represent diffuse encephalopathies. In stupor or coma, the alpha rhythm is absent, and other rhythmic activities can be reduced or lost. This loss can be reversible (e.g., with severe barbiturate intoxication) or irreversible (e.g., with hypoxia). The prognostic value of a single EEG is therefore small, but serial recordings are helpful in evaluating improvement or deterioration.

Some asymmetry of alpha and beta rhythms, not caused by technical factors, is common and may be due to differences in skull thickness (36). Alpha activity is statistically more likely to be of higher voltage over the right side. Asymmetry of the alpha rhythm of more than 20% (expressed as a percentage of the higher side) is unusual in normal adults (40), and a consistent asymmetry of 50% or more should be regarded as clinically significant. In view of the common and normal slight right-sided predominance, asymmetries of 35%–50% may be significant and considered abnormal when the lower voltage is on the right side (33).

Localized or lateralized relative flattening or obliteration of alpha activity (Fig. 10.1) can occur ipsilateral to cortical lesions, a finding confirmed by electrocorticography (43). When this is observed in the scalp EEG, local abnormal slow activity or other localized abnormalities should be sought. This combination over the same hemisphere is a reliable sign of a focal cerebral lesion (1). Ipsilateral reduction in the amount of alpha rhythm has also been reported with unilateral thalamic tumors (32) and in a case of unilateral thalamic infarction involving predominantly the anterior and lateral thalamus (24). The presence of particular associated abnormalities such as focal paroxysmal or slow activity may help to determine (a) the severity and extent of a unilateral disturbance of alpha activity and (b) the structures most likely to be involved (see below).

Drowsiness must be excluded before attributing pathological significance to a slow background rhythm, especially in children, whose dominant occipital rhythm may slow before drowsiness is clinically evident. Alerting tasks given by the technologist (counting, repeating phrases) will be helpful. The

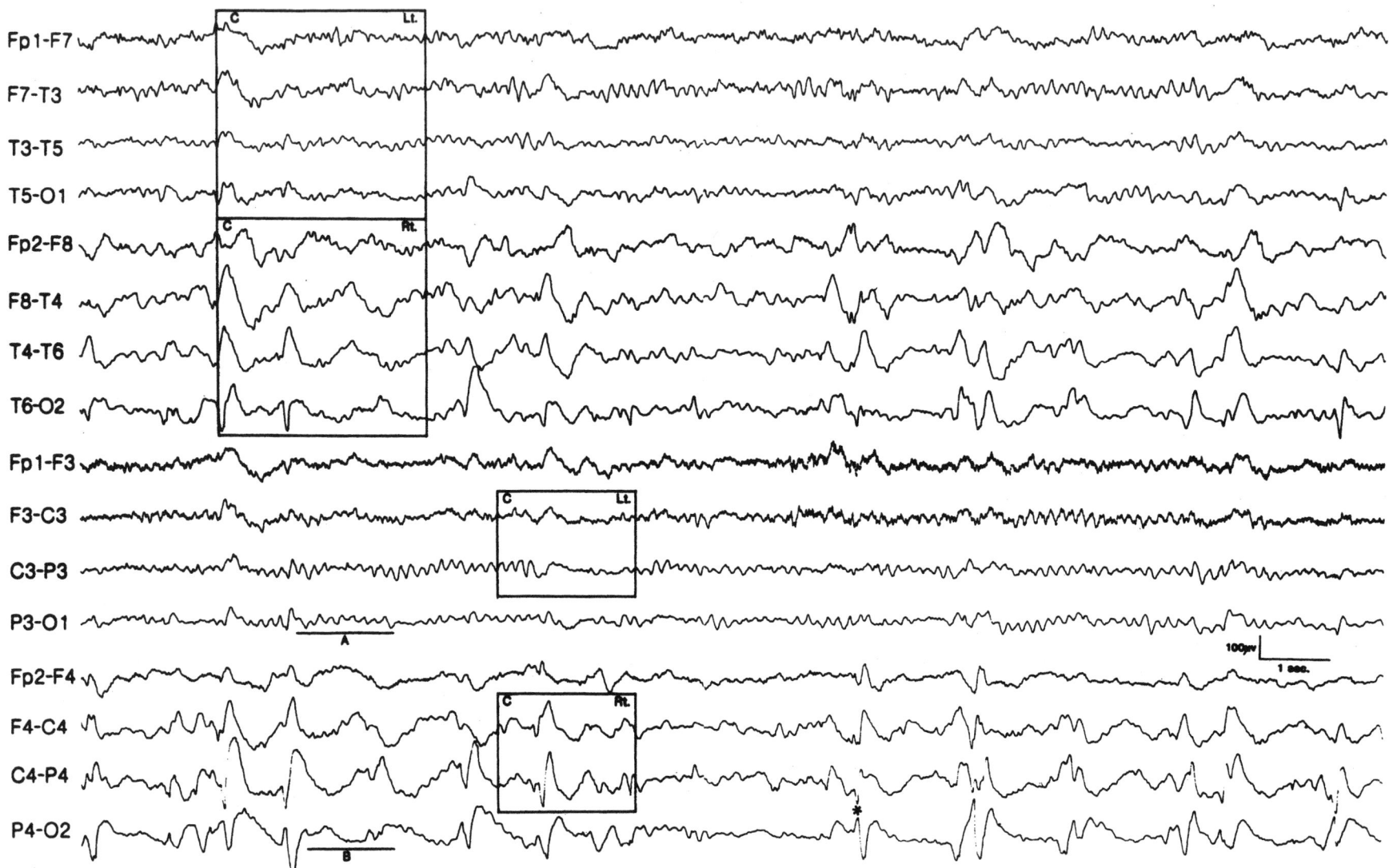

FIG. 10.1. Waking EEG of a 19-year-old man with chronic left hemiparesis, seizures, and developmental delay. Careful examination of this apparently complex recording can resolve it into its component abnormalities. **A** and **B**: Background rhythm is abnormally slow over the right occipital region; moreover, there is a significant asymmetry, with the background rhythm over the right occipital region being scanty or absent. **C**: Rhythmic activity is significantly reduced over the right hemisphere compared to the left, and right-sided arrhythmic delta activity is almost continuous. The *asterisk* indicates localized epileptiform activity over the right parietal region. (This localization must be confirmed by recording with other montages.)

frequency of the alpha rhythm does not fall below normal limits in normal aging. Slowing below 8–8.5 Hz (see Chapter 5) is a sensitive but nonspecific indication of disturbed cerebral activity. Indeed, normative studies in adults suggest that an alpha frequency of 8 Hz is more likely to be slowed from some faster frequency than to be a normal constitutional finding (33). Reduced cerebral blood flow reduces alpha frequency (49); moreover, slowed dominant occipital rhythm, often in the theta band, is seen early in many toxic and metabolic encephalopathies, including anticonvulsant drug toxicity. This finding is etiologically nonspecific but is functionally and clinically significant.

Focal slowing of alpha activity is a rare finding in cases of localized disturbances such as tumor or head trauma. A persistent difference of at least 1.5 Hz should be interpreted as being significant. Serial studies may be useful, because this abnormality may be transient and can be followed by a local amplitude asymmetry.

Whereas the normal alpha rhythm is predominant posteriorly and reacts with attenuation in response to eye opening or alerting, nonreactive monorhythmic diffuse activity in the alpha frequency band occurs in some cases of severe encephalopathy with coma, a pattern called "alpha coma" (55). When caused by hypoxia, the alpha coma pattern has been associated with a poor neurological prognosis, although this has been disputed (2). Alpha coma has been reported with good outcomes in a few cases of drug overdose (6), but this cause can usually be distinguished by the greater admixture of faster frequencies and less underlying delta activity in such cases.

The rare Bancaud's phenomenon (3) is a unilateral failure of alpha rhythm to attenuate with bilateral eye opening. The abnormal hemisphere is the one over which the alpha rhythm does not attenuate. A pattern of higher amplitude alpha rhythm and reduced reactivity over an affected hemisphere is also rare and of similar significance (25). Unilateral eye opening does not normally affect alpha rhythm, but may produce contralateral attenuation in patients with albinism, possibly as a result of misrouting of visual pathways (48).

Abnormal Delta Rhythms

Children normally develop sleep spindles in the first 6–8 weeks of post-term life, and well-formed spindles are bilaterally synchronous before the age of 2 years (Fig. 10.2*B*). Although bilateral absence of sleep spindles indicates a cerebral disturbance (31), the interpreter must be certain that the patient is in the appropriate stage of sleep for spindle occurrence (29). This is especially true for children and the elderly, in whom state changes may be rapid, frequent, and clinically hard to detect.

Stage 2 sleep in children from 6 months to 6 years of age is normally marked by high-voltage occipital delta activity. Voltage predominance often shifts from side to side, but an anterior–posterior voltage gradient should be evident (47). Delay or failure of this pattern to develop, or bilateral loss of this normal sleep-related occipital delta activity, is a sensitive but nonspecific indicator of cerebral dysfunction in early childhood.

A lateralized but shifting asymmetry of sleep spindles can occur in normal subjects. Persisting asymmetries of more than 50%, especially if the amplitude of other rhythms is also reduced on the same side, should suggest an abnormality affecting thalamocortical pathways ipsilateral to the side of the lower voltage. Coexisting localized arrhythmic delta activity (see below) indicates, moreover, that thalamocortical white matter is also involved. The normal posterior slow waves of sleep in children can be deceiving and should not be mistaken for abnormal delta activity. If significantly asymmetrical, the abnormal side is that of the lower voltage if craniotomy flaps or other bone defects are excluded. Transient asymmetries of vertex sharp waves are common and normal, especially in children and near the beginning of sleep, when these waves may be grouped and very prominent (Fig. 10.3*A*). An asymmetry that persists throughout sleep is abnormal and suggests a cerebral disturbance lateralized to the side of the lower voltage.

Bilateral spindles characteristic of slow-wave sleep may occur in the diurnal EEGs of some comatose patients. In these cases, spindles persist without reactivity and without being part of a periodic sleep cycle (9). This pattern has been called "spindle coma." Its prognostic value is unclear, but some EEG change after arousal stimuli (such as pain or loud sound) is believed to be a favorable prognostic sign in such patients.

High-voltage, exaggerated sleep spindles ("extreme spindles") were described by Gibbs and Gibbs (20) as a common abnormality in mentally retarded persons (see Fig. 10.2*A*). Our own experience agrees with this. The pattern consists of 100- to 400-μV spindles of 8- to 15-Hz activity over anterior head regions that are more continuous than normal spindles. In more severely retarded subjects, this pattern is often present in both wakefulness and sleep. It is not associated with epilepsy. Extreme spindles must be distinguished from fast activity of early sleep (see Fig. 10.3*A*), which is part of the normal sleep EEG in children, and from the expected increase in beta activity seen with certain psychoactive drugs, especially barbiturates and benzodiazepines. Extreme spindles indicate a marked diffuse cerebral disturbance but are not specific, and other abnormalities suggesting a diffuse encephalopathy would be expected in an EEG showing this pattern.

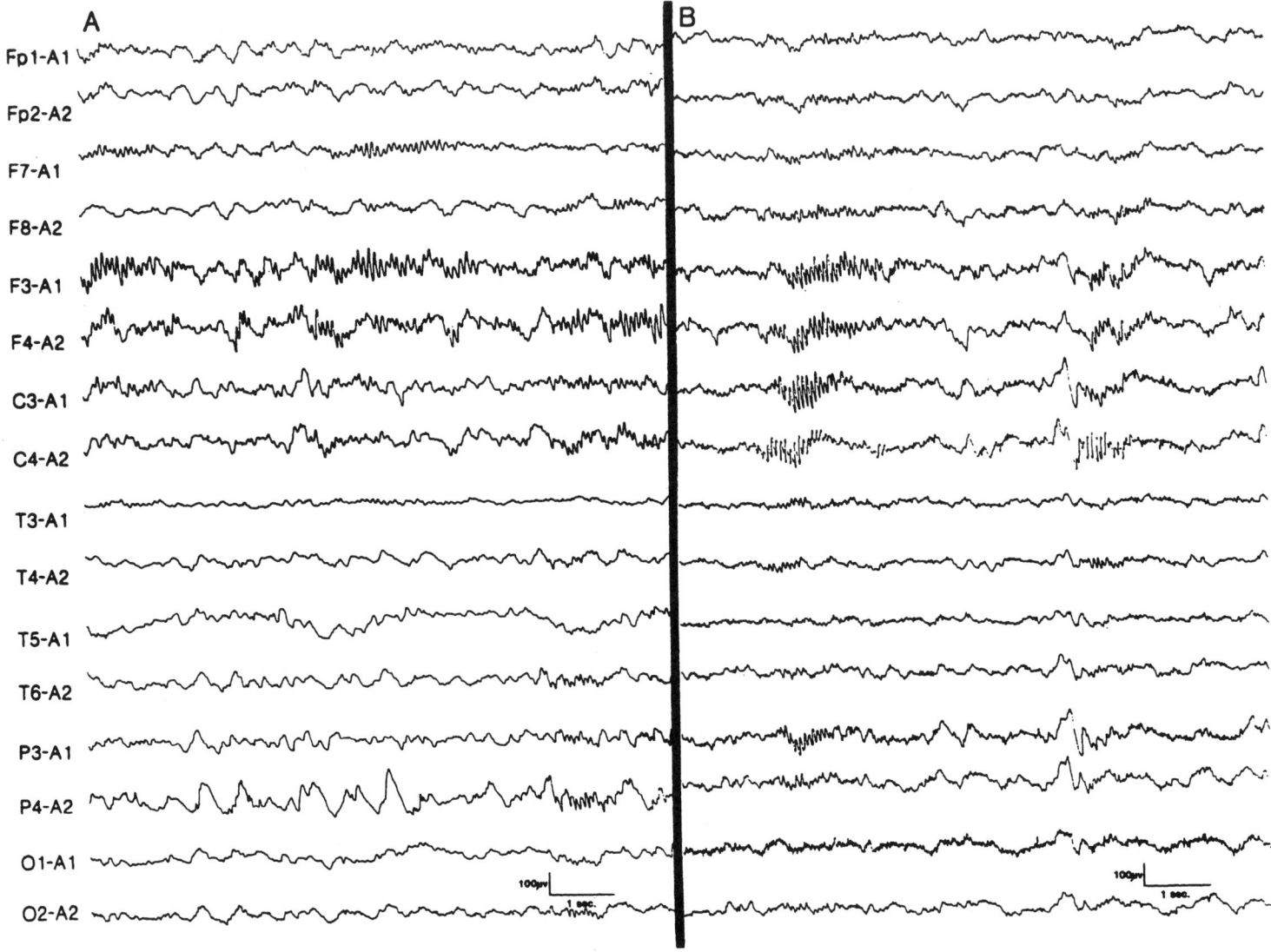

FIG. 10.2. A: Sleep recording in an 8.5-year-old mentally retarded boy. High-amplitude anterior spindles are virtually continuous throughout the EEG and do not form part of a normal sleep cycle (extreme spindles). **B:** Normal sleep recording in a 2-year-old girl. High-amplitude spindles may be seen at this age, but they are not continuous and are usually frontocentral. They form part of a pattern of cycling sleep stages as seen later in this recording.

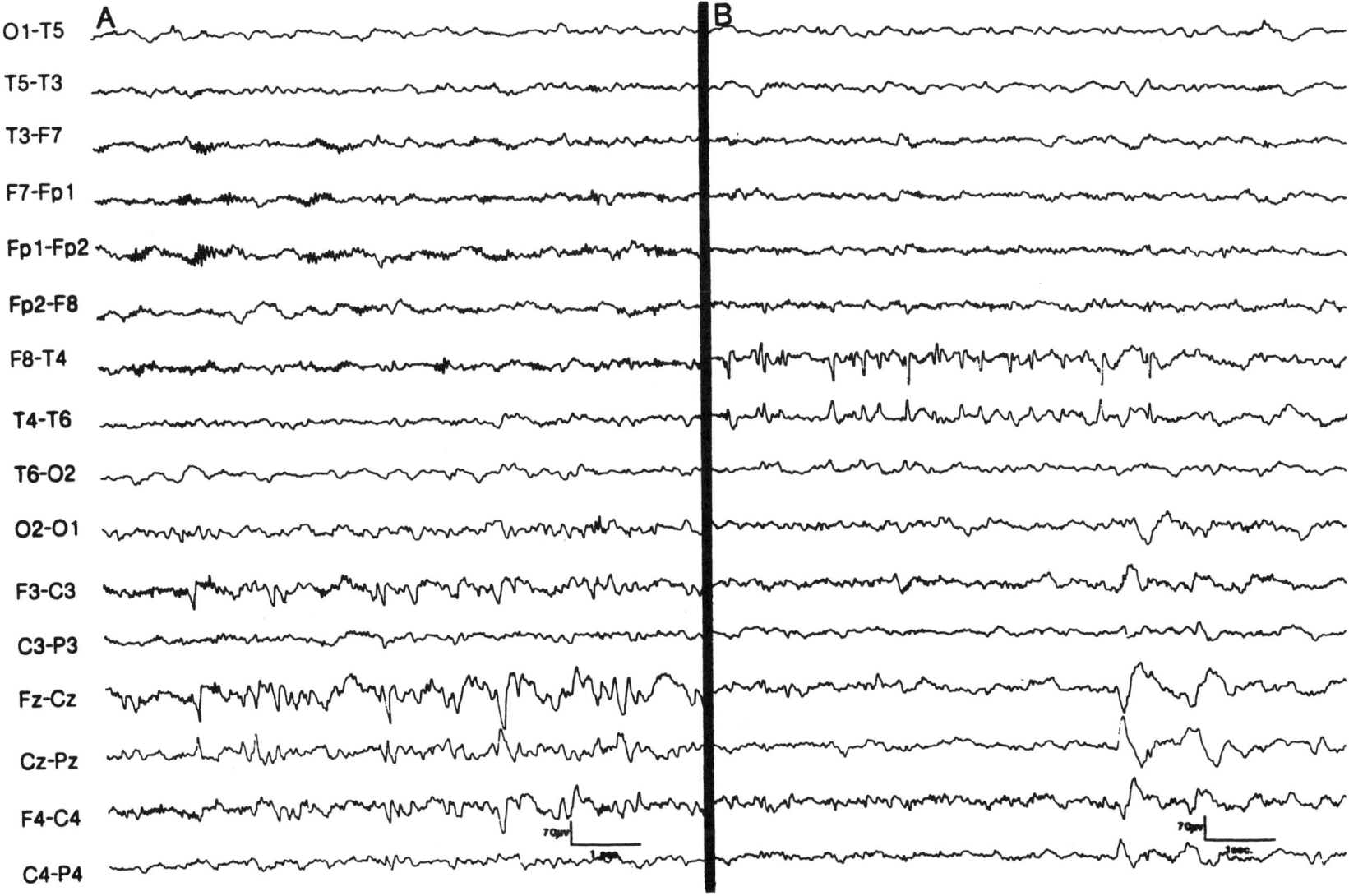

FIG. 10.3. A: Early sleep in a 9-year-old boy. Fast activity of early sleep is seen over both anterior head regions. Vertex sharp waves (channels 13 and 14) are prominent and repetitive and must be distinguished from epileptiform potentials. **B:** Later in the same recording, localized spikes are seen (channels 7 and 8) over the right temporal region, with a vertex sharp wave recorded in the sixth second of this segment.

Abnormal Beta Rhythms

The occurrence of unusually abundant symmetrical beta activity in an otherwise normal EEG is of little clinical value except to raise the question of possible sedative, hypnotic or anxiolytic drug use. It should not be interpreted as an abnormality. Rhythmic activity that is unusually fast for the subject's age, and often of unusually high amplitude in routine bipolar montages, has been reported with a variety of dysplastic cortical lesions. Localized or regional abnormal fast rhythmic activity has been reported with regional dysplastic lesions. Diffuse abnormal fast rhythmic activity is seen with diffuse lesions such as agyria (lissencephaly) or pachygyria. This may not be beta activity at first: Sustained rhythmic theta or alpha activity is abnormal in the neonate. Unusual high-amplitude, unreactive anterior or diffuse alpha and later beta activity typically develops in these children over several months (12,16).

Beta activity in normal controls may be up to 35% lower on one side, but a greater asymmetry, especially if combined with other abnormalities, is a sensitive indicator of cortical injury underlying the region of lower amplitude (see Fig. 10.1). Such an asymmetry may localize a lesion even if the associated abnormalities are more widespread. A transient localized or lateralized reduction in beta activity may also be seen following a partial seizure with or without secondary generalization.

Other Abnormal Rhythms

Rarely, patients with hemisphere lesions may have increased voltage of alpha rhythm or local beta activity on the side of the lesion (1). Green and Wilson (22) found locally diminished beta activity in patients with stroke but noted increased beta activity over some tumors.

Localized or lateralized voltage asymmetries of normal cerebral activity must be carefully evaluated before concluding that they are abnormal. Technical factors, including calibration errors, must be excluded. The technician should examine the scalp for local swelling and should check interelectrode distances, noting these procedures on the EEG. Voltage asymmetries in bipolar montages should be confirmed by referential recording using special care to select a reference electrode that is not near the region in question.

Asymmetries of lambda waves, positive occipital sharp transients of sleep (POSTS), positive slow waves of youth, and mu rhythm are common and should not be interpreted as being abnormal in the absence of associated abnormalities.

Probably the most common reason for an asymmetrical regional increase in EEG voltage is the presence of a skull defect. This is seen in scalp EEGs performed before replacement of a bone flap, but it often persists after replacement of the flap and healing of the scalp. Voltage increases may also be observed at or near isolated bur holes. The patient's history and the technician's observation of the scalp during preparation for recording should reveal such a defect, and a sketch of the location of bur holes and craniotomy scars should form part of the technician's report. "Breach rhythm" is typically a sharply contoured central or midtemporal pattern often resembling a high-voltage mu rhythm, mixed with prominent beta activity and attenuated by actual or intended movement of the contralateral hand. Breach rhythm indicates that the subject has a bone defect, but its occurrence seems to be purely the result of physical effects of the skull changes on the recording of cortical potentials rather than the result of changes in the underlying brain, though other theories have been proposed (11,15,18,30) (see also Chapter 7). The asymmetry is usually persistent, but it may be reduced after cranioplasty with bone or acrylic. After craniotomy, high-voltage regional activity that is otherwise normal should not be reported as abnormal. Because the waveforms near skull defects or bur holes are usually very sharp or "spiky," interpretation of possible spikes should be exceptionally conservative. If there is underlying brain pathology, abnormal local patterns may coexist (26). Progression of a lesion beneath the flap or bur hole should be suspected if serial EEGs show (a) attenuation of preexisting high-amplitude rhythm and/or (b) the presence of local slow waves.

ABNORMAL SLOW ACTIVITY

Delta activity was first recognized and named by Walter (56) because of its association with *d*isease, *d*egeneration, and *d*eath. Arrhythmic or polymorphic delta activity consists of delta waves that are irregular in shape and have a variable duration and frequency without a stable predominant frequency. Rhythmic delta activity consists of delta waves that are regular in shape and have a fairly constant duration and stable predominant frequency. The description and subsequent interpretation of abnormal slow activity requires study of its frequency, distribution over the scalp, temporal features, abundance, and reactivity. A single recording may contain two or more different abnormal delta activities, each with its own characteristics.

Thus delta activity may be localized, unilateral with or without focal predominance, or generalized, sometimes with a varying degree of localized or lateralized predominance. It may be continuous or intermittent. Intermittent delta activity may be random or may occur in bursts (paroxysmally); moreover, it may be bilaterally synchronous or independent over each hemisphere or homologous scalp regions. The amplitude and amount of delta activity must also be considered, as well as whether or not it reacts to external stimuli.

Delta activity can be seen with localized, lateralized, or diffuse encephalopathies and is a very significant, but nonspecific, sign of disturbed cerebral activity. It has been found empirically that qualitative differences in delta activity are clinically significant, especially in serial recordings from a single patient. Lower frequency, higher amplitude, and greater abundance are all signs of a more acute or severe abnormality, and they are consistent in serial recordings with a progressing disturbance. A reversal of these trends indicates improvement.

Localized Arrhythmic Delta Activity

The original definition of delta activity included activity slower than 8 Hz; indeed, focal arrhythmic theta activity has the same significance as delta activity but suggests a less severe or less acute disturbance. Localized arrhythmic delta activity (ADA) is characteristic of supratentorial hemispheric lesions involving white matter (21,41). It commonly occurs with other EEG indications of localized cortical disturbance, such as reductions in amplitude and amount of faster rhythmic activity (see Fig. 10.1). As a sign of locally disordered cerebral function, localized ADA is not confined to gross structural lesions. It can be seen transiently as a postictal phenomenon and in disorders such as complicated migraine (27) and head trauma. The potential field of localized ADA may be quite extensive and is typically larger than the underlying lesion as judged by computed tomography. This can be due to other functional changes assessed by the EEG, such as local reduced blood flow, or to the shallow, broad potential gradient characteristic of a deep-seated lesion. Arfel and Fischgold (1) found that the most reliable EEG localization of cerebral tumors was indicated by lower voltage delta activity without intermixed faster frequencies.

Diffuse and/Bilateral Arrhythmic Delta Activity

Diffuse ADA, or generalized slow activity, reflects a diffuse but etiologically nonspecific disturbance of cerebral activity. It is seen most commonly with various metabolic and toxic encephalopathies and varies with the severity of the underlying disorder. Assessing bilateral arrhythmic slow activity requires (a) analyzing frequency, amplitude, distribution, persistence, and reactivity; and (b) searching for associated findings that may indicate an underlying lateralized or localized disturbance. Because these characteristics are related to the severity of the encephalopathy, which may itself evolve, serial studies usually prove to be more valuable than a single recording. Initially, or in mild disturbances, slowing of the dominant occipital

rhythm occurs, perhaps mixed with some bilateral irregular theta activity. It may be difficult to distinguish this pattern from that of drowsiness, especially in children. The technologist may help by noting the EEG response to state changes or arousal stimuli. With more severe encephalopathies, the amount of diffuse slow activity increases, the frequency slows, and the amplitude increases. Reactivity, demonstrated by attenuation of the slow activity following arousal stimuli, disappears with progressive obtundation and the onset of coma. Bilateral diffuse ADA may also be seen with thalamic or midbrain dysfunction caused by bilateral lesions or compression from herniation.

The most common metabolic disorders producing diffuse ADA are hypoglycemia, hypoxia or global cerebral ischemia, uremia or hepatic disease, and disordered osmolarity. A common toxic etiology is drug toxicity or overdose, in which diffuse beta activity mixed with the slow waves may suggest sedative drugs as the cause. Diffuse white matter encephalopathies such as leukodystrophies (21) can produce this pattern, as can encephalitis, meningitis, and subarachnoid hemorrhage.

Bilateral ADA may be so prominent as to mask focal EEG abnormalities that would indicate a lateralized hemisphere lesion as the underlying cause of the diffuse encephalopathy. Such ADA therefore should not be interpreted as excluding a lateralized lesion. One example of this is an expanding supratentorial mass compressing the thalamus and midbrain.

Intermittent Rhythmic Delta Activity

Cobb (10) was the first to describe bilaterally synchronous delta or theta activity, usually with anterior predominance, as an abnormal pattern in the waking adult EEG. It consists of regular delta waves with a relatively constant frequency in any one EEG. Van der Drift and Magnus (52) named it "frontal intermittent rhythmic delta activity" (FIRDA). Intermittent rhythmic delta activity (IRDA) need not be confined to the frontal regions, and indeed it is often more diffuse. Sometimes the bursts may include theta activity (Fig. 10.4). IRDA may be asymmetrical, lateralized, or even unilateral. Its onset is abrupt, and it is clearly distinguished from the surrounding EEG activity. Although bifrontal predominance is typical in adults, occipital predominance is usual in children; this seems to be related to maturation rather than to any morphological abnormality (14).

Vertical eye blinks may be distinguished from FIRDA by recording simultaneously from infraorbital and frontal scalp electrodes connected to a common reference (see Chapter 9). The electrooculogram will be 180 degrees out of phase, whereas FIRDA will be in phase, in recordings taken from

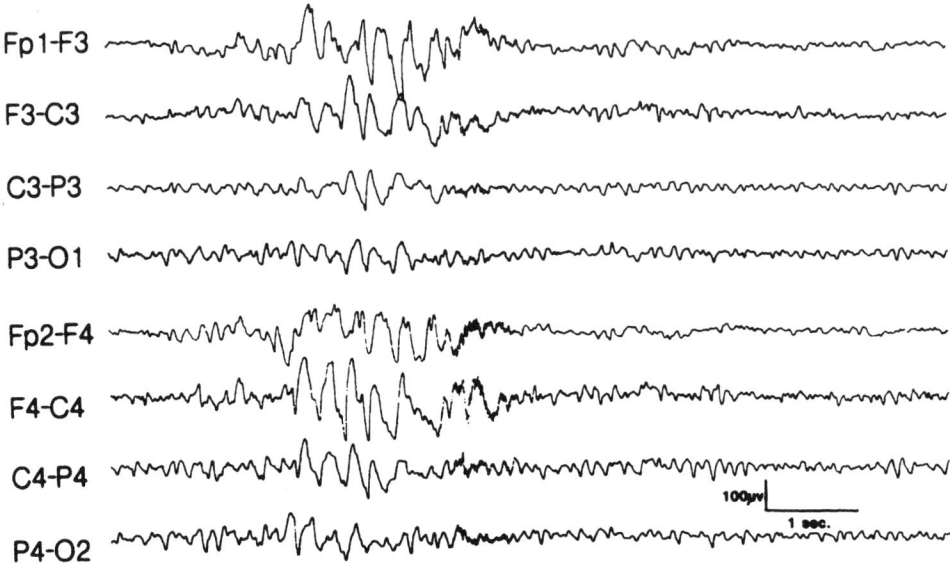

FIG. 10.4. EEG of a 26-year-old man. Bilateral intermittent rhythmic delta activity can be mixed with other frequencies and associated with other abnormalities. Background rhythm is also somewhat slow in this subject with Down's syndrome, without any evidence of a midline lesion or increased intracranial pressure.

above and below the eye. The normal response to hyperventilation, as well as the paroxysmal pattern of drowsiness in childhood (hypnagogic hypersynchrony), can be very striking and must be differentiated from abnormal bursts of rhythmic waves. Sleep-deprived normal adults may show occasional bilateral paroxysmal slow activity (42) of no clinical importance except as evidence of sleep deprivation. The pattern may also occur occasionally in the EEG of an asymptomatic elderly subject (50).

IRDA is clearly abnormal in adults and is observed with many types of cerebral dysfunction. Although paroxysmal, it is not epileptiform or predictive of epilepsy. Although IRDA may be seen with structural brain lesions (13,53), it is more often associated with diffuse encephalopathies as a nonspecific finding. IRDA is commonly a temporary pattern in the course of a cerebral disturbance. When it occurs alone in an otherwise normal EEG, it suggests a mild to moderate, diffuse, nonspecific disturbance of brain function (44,45). In metabolic encephalopathies, a common setting in which these bursts occur, background rhythm is usually abnormal as well, and consciousness is often altered (28). FIRDA is more commonly seen with anterior hemispheric lesions than with posterior ones (53). Focal EEG abnormalities such as localized ADA must be carefully sought as more reliable clues to a possible localized lesion responsible for the FIRDA.

Interpretation of this pattern should be based on its lack of specificity. It does not necessarily indicate the presence of a subcortical lesion, increased intracranial pressure, or a deep midline lesion, although these correlations have been made. Although a diffuse encephalopathy is most likely, the electroencephalographer must identify and comment on any lateralized or localized EEG signs as clues to an underlying localized lesion.

OTHER DISTINCTIVE ABNORMAL PATTERNS

Pseudoperiodic Patterns

EEG patterns consisting of spikes, sharp waves, and slow waves, or combinations of these that repeat regularly (or nearly so), are called "periodic" or, more strictly, "pseudoperiodic." They are paroxysmal, standing out from the surrounding EEG activity. Barring general anesthesia or barbiturate coma, they occur with a variety of severe encephalopathies. Other abnormalities are also found in such EEGs. Routine visual analysis of such patterns requires knowledge of the age and state of the patient. The electroencephalographer must then evaluate the pattern in terms of (a) its form; (b) its distribution over the scalp; (c) its relation to wakefulness, sleep, or pathologically altered consciousness; and (d) its reactivity to external stimuli. EEG activity between the pseudoperiodic events must also be assessed. Any association between the paroxysmal activity and possible clinical manifestations, at times helpful in differential diagnosis, should be noted by the technologist and scrutinized by the interpreter. Additional electrodes or other devices, such as an accelerometer to document myoclonic jerks, may be helpful.

Such a systematic approach to visual analysis of these transients will usually lead to clear differentiation among them. This is important because several of these patterns have strong and diagnostically important clinical correlations. Their salient characteristics are summarized in Table 10.1.

TABLE 10.1. *Periodic and pseudoperiodic abnormal EEG patterns, along with EEG characteristics and clinical correlation*

Pattern	Form	Scalp distribution	Interparoxysm interval	Relation to state	Interburst EEG	Clinical correlation	Chapter to see
Pseudoperiodic generalized sharp waves	Diphasic or triphasic sharp waves or spikes	Generalized: may be lateralized in early stages	<2.5 s; shortens with progression sof disease; usually <1 s	In wakefulness and/or sleep	Relatively featureless	Creutzfeldt-Jakob disease; eventually seen in almost all patients	12, 13
Pseudoperiodic bilaterally synchronous and–slow sharp-wave discharges	Irregular high-voltage slow waves or sharp-and–slow wave complexes	Diffuse, bilaterally synchronous	5–10 s; very regular in a single recording	May be evoked with hyperventilation or sleep in early stages	Diffuse, lower voltage delta activity	Subacute sclerosing panencephalitis; almost always seen except early or late in the disease	12
Pseudoperiodic lateralized epileptiform discharges (PLEDS)	Biphasic or triphasic sharp waves, spikes, or polyspikes	Hemispheric; lateralization may shift	1–2 s	Consciousness often impaired, except in children; PLEDS persist in sleep	Diffuse, abnormal slow activity; may be locally predominant	Early, acute, severe lateralized encephalopathy; may correlate with focal seizurest; transient in adults, may persist in children	11
Pseudoperiodic slow complexes with temporal predominance	Sharp or triphasic waves mixed with paroxysmal slow activity; may resemble PLEDS	Unilateral temporal predominance	1–4 s	Consciousness impaired	Localized or diffuse slow activity	Herpes simplex encephalitis; may occur before abnormality on computed tomography scan	11
Burst-suppression	Brief bursts of mixed spikes, slow waves, and sharp waves, interrupted by longer periods of relative EEG flattening	Bilateral; may be synchronous and/or asymmetrical	Variable	Coma; pattern not reactive to applied stimuli; does not form part of sleep cycle	Diffuse relative flattening	Severe diffuse encephalopathy, often anoxic; may be reversible (e.g.,with drug intoxication); distinct from neonatal quiet sleep	14, 15
Triphasic waves	High-amplitude deflections, typically negative–positive–negative	Bilaterally synchronous; anterior predominance with anterior–posterior lag of 25–140 ms in bipolar EEG	Groups or runs of 1.5- to 2.5-Hz waves	Impairment of consciousness	Slowed background rhythms	Toxic or metabolic encephalopathy, especially hepatic	12, 15

Unusual Asymmetrical Abnormal Activity and Dysplastic Brain Lesions

Patients with extensive unilateral dysplastic brain lesions may have characteristic interictal EEG findings. In particular, hemimegalencephaly is associated with typical interictal abnormalities lateralized to the abnormal side (54). Their morphology depends on the age of the subject: A newborn may have unilateral burst suppression, but unilateral hypsarrhythmia may be recorded several months later. The EEG over the affected hemisphere is also asymmetrical later, with higher amplitude and frequency in wakefulness and sleep, an asymmetry that may also be found with less evident lateralized malformations. EEG electrodes must be carefully placed to avoid false lateralizations resulting from the abnormal hemisphere that extends across the midline. Hemimegalencephaly often occurs with abundant interictal epileptiform activity and very frequent lateralized ictal patterns and clinical seizures from the neonatal period. Although the diagnosis must be made by neuroimaging, magnetic resonance imaging may be impractical in the critically ill newborn and is not rapidly available in many areas outside the United States. These EEG patterns are thus useful in diagnosis.

INTERICTAL AND ICTAL ABNORMALITIES

Interictal Epileptiform Activities

Epileptiform pattern, an interpretative term, refers to "distinctive waves or complexes, distinguished from background activity, and resembling those recorded in a proportion of human subjects suffering from epileptic disorders."(7). The "distinctive waves" are spikes or sharp waves, and distinguishing these specific epileptiform transients from sharply contoured waves of normal or abnormal background activity is critical but sometimes difficult. Several criteria are used in making this distinction (for a review, see ref. 39), including the form of the transient and the surrounding activity from which it arises, but the sharpness of the wave at its peak seems to provide the best differentiation. Expressing this concept in mathematical terms of a second-order differential equation underlies attempts at computerized analysis of epileptiform activity (see Chapter 22). In everyday visual analysis, in order to extract maximal information, the electroencephalographer must systematically analyze and describe epileptiform activity in terms of temporal features, morphology, and topography.

Distinguishing spikes from sharp waves is ultimately arbitrary and of limited physiological utility. By convention, spikes last more than 20 milliseconds and less than 70 milliseconds, and sharp waves last more than 70 milliseconds and less than 200 milliseconds. The transient may occur alone, but more often a slow wave follows, forming a spike-and–slow wave complex (subsequently in this discussion, "spike" and "sharp wave" are used interchangeably). The slow wave comprises the major temporal component of spike-and–slow wave complexes, lasting from 150 to 350 milliseconds (Fig. 10.5A). Spikes or complexes may occur once or repetitively. With repetitive complexes, the repetition rate carries important information. The electroencephalographer must determine if one complex immediately succeeds another (rhythmic burst), or if complexes recur at intervals that are constant (periodic discharges) or slightly varying (pseudoperiodic discharges).

If epileptiform discharges occur widely over the head, particularly over the left and right sides, the electroencephalographer must determine if the discharges are simultaneous and bisynchronous, or so temporally separated as to be considered independent and asynchronous (see Fig. 10.5). Because the potential field of a single large generator may extend across the midline, only transverse montages can distinguish such a generator from two discrete, but bisynchronous, generators. Two generators sometimes occur within one hemisphere and also produce asynchronous discharges.

"Morphology" describes the very brief temporal characteristics of a spike. The discharge (Fig. 10.5B) may abruptly leave the baseline and return (monophasic); cross the baseline and return (biphasic); or cross, recross, and return (triphasic), after which counting ceases (polyphasic). The polarity of a spike has equal importance. In most instances the predominant component is surface negative (see Fig. 10.3B). The voltage topography of spikes on the scalp reflects a dipole-like source (see Chapters 2 and 23). For cortical generators with a radial orientation, the negative EEG field maximum is directly above the source, and it is of much higher amplitude than the positive field maximum on the opposite side of the head. For spike generators with a tangential orientation, field maxima on the scalp are displaced on either side of the source, and they may be of nearly the same amplitude. Spikes with voltage fields suggesting a tangential dipole generator have most commonly been associated with benign rolandic epilepsy of childhood (23) (see Chapters 16 and 17), but now these are known to occur commonly in other focal seizure disorders (see Chapter 23). Correctly assessing the location and orientation of spike sources requires an appreciation for how different montages display scalp voltage fields, in particular how the choice of reference can alter this display (see Chapters 2 and 4). Surface-positive spikes rarely occur in patients with epilepsy but can occur in healthy persons as a "benign" normal variant, 14- and 6-Hz positive bursts (see Chapter 7).

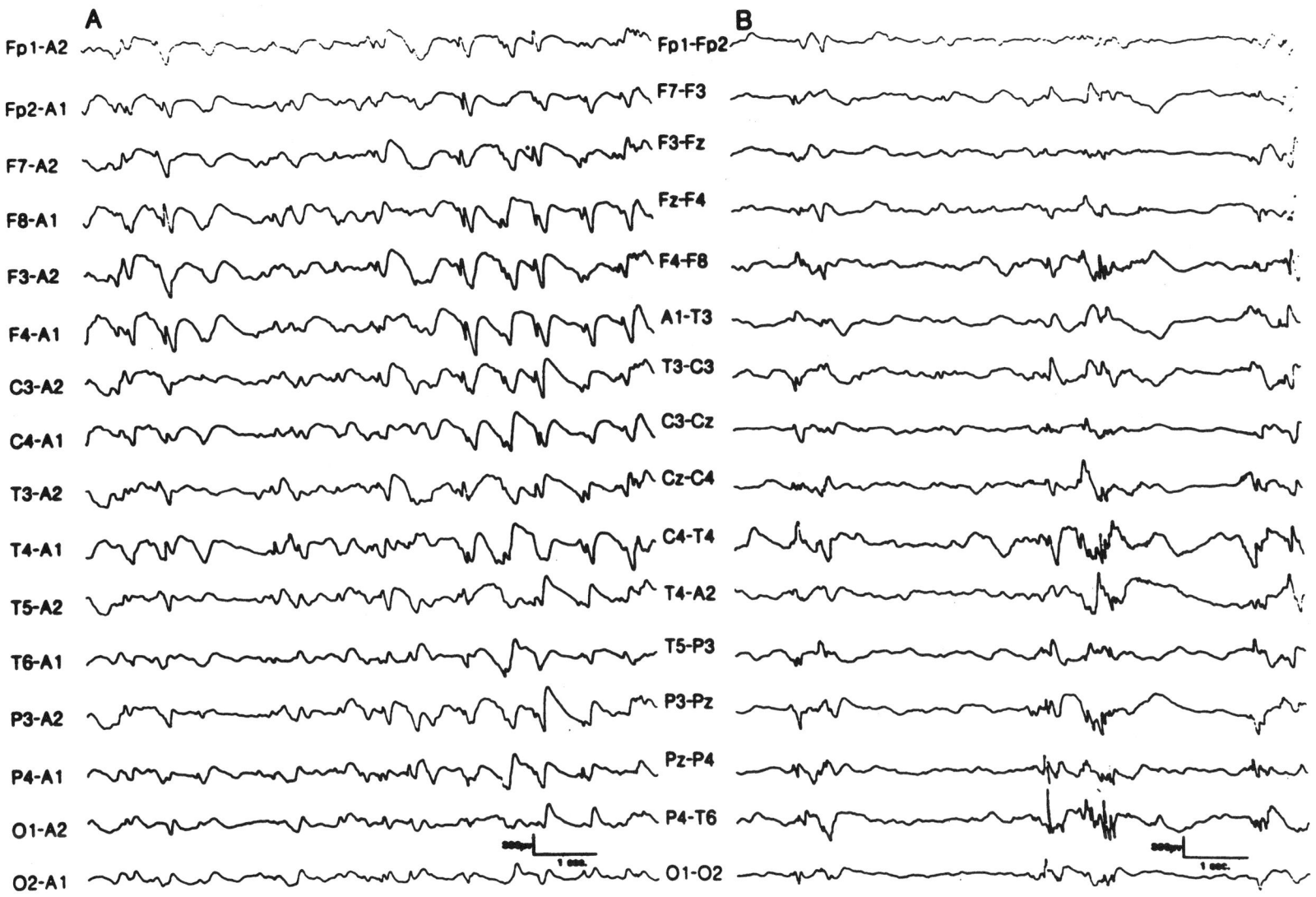

FIG. 10.5. Sedated sleep tracing of a 1-year-old girl with a diffuse encephalopathy. Many different epileptiform patterns can be recorded in a single EEG when recordings are of adequate length. **A:** Sharp waves and repetitive spike-and–slow wave complexes. The right-sided predominance of the epileptiform activity is difficult to appreciate easily in this montage. **B:** Later, spikes of varying morphology are seen, including triphasic and polyphasic spikes. The right-sided predominance is more evident.

Aftercoming slow waves are surface negative and may represent prolonged hyperpolarization caused by secondary inhibition in a large neuronal population (see Chapter 1).

As with other abnormalities, epileptiform discharges may be (a) localized (at times exquisitely so); (b) unilateral with or without focal preponderance (e.g., periodic lateralized epileptiform discharges); (c) multifocal and, usually, asynchronous; (d) generalized with shifting lateralization (e.g., 2.5-Hz sharp-and–slow wave discharges), or (e) generalized and symmetrical (e.g., 3-Hz spike-and–slow wave discharges). Particularly in children, the topography of focal spikes varies over time, appearing in serial EEGS in three or more locations (51). The bisynchronous spike components of 3-Hz spike-and–slow wave complexes typically show maximal negativity at F3 and F4; however, during non–rapid-eye-movement (NREM) sleep, isolated complexes may occur with maximal negativity over one or the other frontal region. Thus one should not assume that spikes unvaryingly arise immediately subjacent to a scalp electrode or, even less, that they signify local pathological changes. Indeed, it is common for fragments of a generalized spike-and-wave discharge to appear transiently "focal" or "asymmetrical".

Distinguishing Nonepileptiform from Epileptiform Discharges

Because a strong, but not absolute, correlation exists between epileptiform discharges in the EEG and epilepsy, certain normal bioelectrical potentials must not be confused with epileptiform discharges. Mu rhythms have asymmetrical waveforms, perhaps as a result of intermixing with quasi-harmonic beta rhythms; the negative half of the wave changes voltage more rapidly, giving it a sharp or "spiky" appearance in contrast with the sinusoidal positive half. Mu rhythms are readily distinguished from spikes by (a) a consistent frequency of 8–10 Hz, (b) voltage modulation in spindles, and (c) reactivity to contralateral actual or imagined motor acts (see Chapter 5).

In younger children (see Fig. 10.3), vertex sharp transients appearing in stage 2 NREM sleep have surprisingly high amplitudes, exhibit sharp peaks, and occur repetitively; however, their ascending and descending limbs are more symmetrical than those of spikes, their duration is somewhat longer, and they lack an aftercoming slow wave. POSTS occur at the occipital pole, appear in stage 1 NREM sleep, and disappear on arousal; these features readily distinguish them from the usual surface-negative epileptogenic occipital spikes.

"Lateral rectus spikes" are single motor unit potentials, best detected in F7 and F8 electrodes during lateral deviation of the eyes. They ride on the slower potential caused by movement of the globe (see Chapter 9). These normal rhythms are best recognized by "the company they keep": location, physiological state, reactivity, and age of the patient.

Finally, one must remember that electrode artifact can simulate most types of electrocerebral activity, both normal and abnormal. If undetected and uncorrected, it usually ultimately reveals itself by (a) abrupt discontinuities, (b) "pops," and (c) other bizarre, clearly noncerebral features.

Epileptiform Discharges and Seizures

In carefully screened populations of healthy persons, a very small percentage will have EEGs with epileptiform discharges. There is thus a strong, but not absolute, correlation between epileptiform discharges and seizures, and EEG reports should recognize this. Nonetheless, having carefully analyzed and described the discharges in terms of morphological, temporal, and topographic features, the electroencephalographer can integrate these with the clinical data and interpret them in terms of known "electroclinical" associations.

A few examples suffice (Chapter 17 provides extended discussions). In children, the topography of focal spikes correlates with their epileptogenicity: 91% of children with anterior temporal spikes have seizures, whereas only 38% of children with rolandic spikes have seizures (34). Children whose EEGs show 3-Hz spike-and–slow wave bursts and independent bursts of occipital intermittent rhythmic delta activity (OIRDA) have a better than 50% chance of spontaneous remission within 10 years and are unlikely to develop tonic–clonic seizures. In contrast, if the EEG lacks OIRDA but shows photoparoxysmal responses, such children are more likely to develop tonic–clonic seizures, and only 6% will have spontaneous remission (38).

Ictal Patterns

In the ordinary course of events, EEG laboratories infrequently record seizures, except for those laboratories associated with epilepsy centers. Those seizures that do occur are likely to overrepresent a narrow band (e.g., absence seizures) in the broader spectrum of seizures. Consequently, many electroencephalographers are relatively unfamiliar with the widely varying types of transition from interictal to ictal patterns. The simplest transition is persistent, repetitive interictal epileptiform discharges. A burst may contain a single complex or repeating complexes; if the burst persists long enough, behavioral changes appear (see Chapter 17 for further discussion). In a meticulous study of focal seizures, Blume et al. (4) found that slightly less than one-half began with repetitive spikes or sharp waves; the remainder began with rhythmic, sinusoidal waves. Thus, in focal seizures, "prolongation" of the interictal epileptiform discharge is not the most common transition.

Furthermore, in the study of Blume et al. (4), when clinically apparent seizures occurred, two-thirds began with rhythmic waves. Geiger and Harner (19) have reported similar findings in a more heterogeneous population of patients with seizures, of whom only 40% had long-standing epilepsy. Rhythmic discharges are the hallmark of ictal transition in certain generalized epilepsies. Chatrian et al. (8) reported the EEGs of 35 patients with tonic–autonomic seizures; 28 had Lennox-Gastaut syndrome: "The most characteristic feature of our patients' electrical seizures was ... bilaterally synchronous generalized rhythmic discharge." The discharges were usually of high frequency, faster than 15 Hz in 85% of patients. With focal seizures, Geiger and Harner (19) have noted similar findings, with seizures being initiated by rhythmic discharges that were faster than 13 Hz in 50% of patients. Seizures beginning with frequencies in the alpha range, sometimes referred to as the "epileptic recruiting rhythm" (17), occurred less often, ranging from 8% (4) to 16% (8). In patients with tonic seizures, rhythms slower than 8 Hz did not occur; however, in patients with focal seizures, rhythms of 4–7 Hz appeared in 46%, whereas those of less than 4 Hz appeared in 20%.

Seizures may begin with "attenuation," a sudden diminution of voltage. Sporadic interictal epileptiform discharges may abruptly cease several seconds before attenuation occurs. Blume et al. (4) noted attenuation in 10% of focal seizures; Chatrian et al. (8) found a similar incidence in patients with tonic–autonomic seizures. Attenuation occurs so commonly as a part of infantile spasms that some have called them "electrodecremental" seizures. In a study of ictal EEG patterns in 5,042 infantile spasms, Kellaway et al. (35) found attenuation as part of the seizure in 71% and as the sole manifestation in 12%.

Finally, seizures may begin in cortical regions not readily accessible to scalp electrodes. Studies using simultaneous recordings from scalp and depth electrodes have clearly documented this for seizures arising in the medial temporal lobe (37). However, if the seizure evolves to altered awareness and automatism, the scalp EEG usually alters (see Chapters 17 and 18 for further discussion).

Although suddenly appearing seizure patterns may alert the EEG technologist, determining whether the seizure is purely an electrical event ("subclinical seizure") or a behavioral event ("clinical seizure") poses significant problems in the laboratory (see also Chapters 17 and 18). In research laboratories, studies of children with absence seizures have shown that reaction time reliably alters within 0.5 seconds after onset of a 3-Hz spike-and–slow wave burst (5). Comparable evidence suggests that, with focal spikes, altered responses may occur during the aftercoming slow wave with intervals as short as 200 milliseconds (46). Obviously, in the usual laboratory setting, epileptic patterns of brief duration may elude adequate behavioral testing. Conversely, certain paroxysmal patterns that seemingly qualify as ictal patterns may show no evidence whatsoever for behavioral change (e.g., subclinical rhythmic EEG discharge of adults) (see Chapter 7).

CONCLUSION

Visual assessment of the abnormal EEG requires a knowledge of normal patterns, their range of variation, and the abnormalities that altered normal patterns may represent. Other abnormal patterns may coexist with these or may appear alone. A systematic approach to the abnormal EEG requires examination of (a) the type or types of abnormality, (b) their distribution in time and space, (c) reactivity, and (d) associated findings. Assessment of the course of an abnormality in serial recordings can be particularly valuable. This approach permits interpretation that is useful and clinically relevant. Although EEG abnormalities are usually etiologically nonspecific, competent and prudent EEG interpretation can provide information of differential diagnostic value.

REFERENCES

1. Arfel G, Fischgold H. EEG-signs in tumours of the brain. *Electroencephalogr Clin Neurophysiol Suppl* 1961;19:36–50.
2. Austin EJ, Wilkus RJ, Longstreth W Jr. Etiology and prognosis of alpha coma. *Neurology* 1988;38:773–777.
3. Bancaud J, Hécaen H, Lairy GC. Modifications de la réactivité EEG, troubles de fonctions symboliques et troubles confusionnels dans les lésions hémispheriques localisées. *Electroencephalogr Clin Neurophysiol* 1955;7:179–192.
4. Blume WT, Young GB, Lemieux JF. EEG morphology of partial epileptic seizures. *Electroencephalogr Clin Neurophysiol* 1984;57:295–302.
5. Browne TR, Penry JK, Porter RJ, et al. Responsiveness before, during, and after spike-wave paroxysms. *Neurology* 1974;24:659–665.
6. Carroll WM, Mastaglia FL. Alpha and beta coma in drug intoxication uncomplicated by cerebral hypoxia. *Electroencephalogr Clin Neurophysiol* 1979;46:95–105.
7. Chatrian GE, Bergamini L, Dondey M, et al. A glossary of terms most commonly used by clinical electroencephalographers. *Electroencephalogr Clin Neurophysiol* 1974;37:538–548.
8. Chatrian GE, Lettich E, Wilkus RJ, et al. Polygraphic and clinical observations on tonic-autonomic seizures. *Electroencephalogr Clin Neurophysiol Suppl* 1982;35:101–124.

9. Chatrian GE, White LE Jr, Daly D. Electroencephalographic patterns resembling those of sleep in certain comatose states after injuries to the head. *Electroencephalogr Clin Neurophysiol* 1963;15:272–280.

10. Cobb WA. Rhythmic slow discharges in the electroencephalogram. *J Neurol Neurosurg Psychiatry* 1945;8:65–78.

11. Cobb WA, Guiloff RJ, Cast J. Breach rhythm: the EEG related to skull defects. *Electroencephalogr Clin Neurophysiol* 1979;47:251–271.

12. Dalla Bernardina B, Perez-Jimenez A, Fontana E, et al. Electroencephalographic findings associated with cortical dysplasias. In: Guerrini R, Andermann F, Canapicchi R, et al, eds. *Dysplasias of cerebral cortex and epilepsy*. Philadelphia: Lippincott–Raven Publishers, 1996:235–245.

13. Daly D, Whelan JL, Bickford RG, et al. The electroencephalogram in cases of tumors of the posterior fossa and third ventricle. *Electroencephalogr Clin Neurophysiol* 1953;5:203–216.

14. Daly DD. Genesis of abnormal activity. In: Rémond A, ed. *Handbook of electroencephalography and clinical neurophysiology*, Vol 14. Amsterdam: Elsevier Science, 1975:5–10.

15. Fischgold H, Pertuiset B, Arfel-Capdeville G. Quelques particularités électroencéphalographiques au niveau des brèches et des volets neurochirurgicaux. *Rev Neurol (Paris)* 1952;86:126–132.

16. Gastaut H, Pinsard N, Raybaud C, et al. Lissencephaly (agyria-pachygyria): clinical features and serial EEG studies. *Dev Med Child Neurol* 1987;29:167–180.

17. Gastaut H, Tassinari CA. The significance of the EEG and ictal and interictal discharges with respect to epilepsy. In: Rémond A, ed. *Handbook of electroencephalography and clinical neurophysiology*, Vol 13, Part A. Amsterdam: Elsevier Science, 1975:3–6.

18. Gastaut H, Terzian H, Gastaut Y. Étude d'une activité électroencéphalographique méconnue: 'le rhythme rolandique en arceau'. *Marseille Méd* 1952;89:296–310.

19. Geiger LR, Harner RN. EEG patterns at the time of focal seizure onset. *Arch Neurol* 1978;35:276–286.

20. Gibbs EL, Gibbs FA. Extreme spindles: correlation of electroencephalographic sleep pattern with mental retardation. *Science* 1962;138:1106–1107.

21. Gloor P, Kalabay O, Giard N. The electroencephalogram in diffuse encephalopathies: electroencephalographic correlates of grey and white matter lesions. *Brain* 1968;91:779–802.

22. Green RL, Wilson WP. Asymmetries of beta activity in epilepsy, brain tumor, and cerebrovascular disease. *Electroencephalogr Clin Neurophysiol* 1961;13:75–78.

23. Gregory DL, Wong PK. Topographical analysis of the centrotemporal discharges in benign rolandic epilepsy of childhood. *Epilepsia* 1984;25:705–711.

24. Hammond EJ, Wilder BJ, Ballinger WE Jr. Electrophysiologic recording in a patient with a discrete unilateral thalamic infarction. *J Neurol Neurosurg Psychiatry* 1982;45:640–643.

25. Hess R. Localization of cerebral tumors. In: Rémond A, ed. *Handbook of electroencephalography and clinical neurophysiology*, Vol 14, Part C. Amsterdam: Elsevier Science, 1975:17–28.

26. Hess R. Postoperative controls. In: Rémond A, ed. *Handbook of electroencephalography and clinical neurophysiology*, Vol 14, Part C. Amsterdam: Elsevier Science, 1975:56–65.

27. Hockaday JM, Whitty CW. Factors determining the electroencephalogram in migraine: a study of 560 patients, according to clinical type of migraine. *Brain* 1969;92:769–788.

28. Hooshmand H. The clinical significance of frontal intermittent rhythmic delta activity (FIRDA). *Clin Electroencephalogr* 1983;14:135–137.

29. Hughes JR. Sleep spindles revisited. *J Clin Neurophysiol* 1985;2:37–44.

30. Jaffe R, Jacobs L. The beta focus: its nature and significance. *Acta Neurol Scand* 1972;48:191–203.

31. Jankel WJ, Niedermeyer E. Sleep spindles. *J Clin Neurophysiol* 1985;2:1–35.

32. Jasper HH, Van Buren J. Interrelationship between cortex and subcortical structures: clinical electroencephalographic studies. *Electroencephalogr Clin Neurophysiol* 1953;5:33–40.

33. Kellaway P. An orderly approach to visual analysis: the parameters of the normal EEG in adults and children. In: Klass DW, Daly DD, eds. *Current practice of clinical electroencephalography*, New York: Raven Press, 1979:69–148.

34. Kellaway P. The incidence, significance and natural history of spike foci in children. In: Henry CE, ed. *Current clinical neurophysiology: update on EEG and evoked potentials*. Amsterdam: Elsevier Science, 1980:151–175.

35. Kellaway P, Hrachovy RA, Frost JD Jr, et al. Precise characterization and quantification of infantile spasms. *Ann Neurol* 1979;6:214–218.

36. Leissner P, Lundholm L-E, Petersen I. Alpha amplitude dependence on skull thickness as measured by ultrasound technique. *Electroencephalogr Clin Neurophysiol* 1970;29:392–399.

37. Lieb JP, Walsh GO, Babb TL, et al. A comparison of EEG seizure patterns recorded with surface and depth electrodes in patients with temporal lobe epilepsy. *Epilepsia* 1976;17:137–160.

38. Loiseau P, Pestre M, Dartigues JF, et al. Long-term prognosis in two forms of childhood epilepsy: typical absence seizures and epilepsy with rolandic (centrotemporal) EEG foci. *Ann Neurol* 1983;13:642–648.

39. Maulsby RL. Some guidelines for assessment of spikes and sharp waves in EEG tracings. *Am J EEG Technol* 1971;11:3–16.

40. Maulsby RL, Kellaway P, Graham M, et al. *The normative electroencephalographic data reference library*. Final report, Contract NAS9-1200, National Aeronautics and Space Administration, 1968.

41. Rhee RS, Goldensohn ES, Kim RC. EEG characteristics of solitary intracranial lesions in relationship to anatomic location. *Electroencephalogr Clin Neurophysiol* 1975;38:553P(abst).

42. Rodin EA, Luby ED, Gottlieb JS. The electroencephalogram during prolonged experimental sleep deprivation. *Electroencephalogr Clin Neurophysiol* 1962;14:544–551.

43. Scarff JE, Rahm WE Jr. Human electrocorticogram: report of spontaneous cerebral potentials obtained from exposed human brain. *J Neurophysiol* 1941;4:418–426.

44. Schaul N, Gloor P, Gotman J. The EEG in deep midline lesions. *Neurology* 1981;31:157–167.

45. Schaul N, Lueders H, Sachdev K. Generalized, bilaterally synchronous bursts of slow waves in the EEG. *Arch Neurol* 1981;38:690–692.

46. Shewmon DA, Erwin RJ. The effect of focal interictal spikes on perception of reaction time. I. General considerations. *Electroencephalogr Clin Neurophysiol* 1988;69:319–337.

47. Slater GE, Torres F. Frequency-amplitude gradient: a new parameter for interpreting pediatric sleep EEGs. *Arch Neurol* 1979;36:465–470.

48. Smith SA, Wong PK, Jan JE. Unilateral alpha reactivity: an electroencephalographic finding in albinism. *J Clin Neurophysiol* 1998;15:146–149.

49. Sulg IA, Cronqvist S, Schuller H, et al. The effect of intracardial pacemaker therapy on cerebral blood flow and electroencephalogram in patients with complete atrioventricular block. *Circulation* 1969;39:487–494.

50. Torres F, Faoro A, Loewenson R, et al. The electroencephalogram of elderly patients revisited. *Electroencephalogr Clin Neurophysiol* 1983;56:391–398.

51. Trojaborg W. Changes in spike foci in children. In: Kellaway P, Petersen I, eds. *Electroencephalography in children*. New York: Grune & Stratton, 1968:213–226.

52. Van der Drift JH, Magnus O. The value of the EEG in the differential diagnosis of cases with cerebral lesions. *Electroencephalogr Clin Neurophysiol Suppl* 1961;19:183–196.

53. Van der Drift JHA. *The significance of electroencephalography for the diagnosis and localization of cerebral tumours*. Leiden: H. E. Stenfert-Kroese, 1957.

54. Vigevano F, Fusco L, Granata T, et al. Hemimegalencephaly: clinical and EEG characteristics. In: Guerrini R, Andermann F, Canapicchi R, et al, eds. *Dysplasias of cerebral cortex and epilepsy*. Philadelphia: Lippincott–Raven Publishers, 1996:285–294.

55. Vignandra V, Wilkus RJ, Copass MK, et al. Electroencephalographic rhythms of alpha frequency in comatose patients after cardiopulmonary arrest. *Neurology* 1974;24:582–588.

56. Walter WG. The location of cerebral tumours by electroencephalography. *Lancet* 1936;2:305–308.

Chapter 11

Focal Electroencephalographic Abnormalities

Carl W. Bazil, Susan T. Herman, and Timothy A. Pedley

HISTORICAL BACKGROUND

Before the introduction of modern brain imaging methods, electroencephalography (EEG) was routinely used to identify and localize intracranial pathology. In 1936, Walter (178) first described localized delta activity with tumors of the cerebral hemispheres, and EEG quickly became a standard test for localization of focal cerebral lesions. Theta rhythm was subsequently associated with subcortical abnormalities (179); focal attenuation of background activity as a feature of tumors was reported in 1944 (94). Over the ensuing decades, electroencephalographers refined these findings and became adept at using them to localize superficial cerebral lesions. EEG remained of limited utility for deeply located lesions, especially those located in the posterior fossa, because findings in such cases were typically nonspecific and diffuse.

In recent years, of course, computed tomography (CT) and magnetic resonance imaging (MRI) have replaced EEG as diagnostic tests of choice for detecting and localizing cerebral lesions. Both are superior to EEG for these indications, and also provide useful information about etiology. EEG, however, is still useful and can be complementary to imaging studies. Unlike CT and MRI, EEG provides information about the physiological function of the brain. Such information can be important in estimating the extent of *functional* (not anatomical) impairment, recognizing a coexisting metabolic or toxic encephalopathy, and indicating the lesion's epileptogenic potential. Occasionally, as in acute ischemia, EEG changes may precede or outlast imaging abnormalities. Combining imaging studies and EEG, therefore, will often give a more complete pathophysiological picture than will either study alone.

In this chapter, we discuss specific focal EEG abnormalities. The emphasis is on nonepileptiform abnormalities; epileptiform patterns are discussed in detail in Chapter 17. The description of each type of focal finding is illustrated by a discussion of specific neurological conditions that may be associated with the EEG abnormality. Keep in mind, however, that many neurological conditions are accompanied by several EEG findings. For example, focal slowing may be seen with attenuation of fast-frequency activity and absence of the alpha rhythm. In this chapter, conditions are discussed under the most prevalent EEG abnormality noted in each. The final section of the chapter briefly discusses the use of EEG in the intensive care unit (ICU) and operating room to identify focal abnormalities of brain function.

NON-EPILEPTIFORM ABNORMALITIES

Changes in the EEG produced by focal brain lesions may be categorized as either epileptiform or nonepileptiform. Epileptiform abnormalities include spikes, sharp waves, spike-and-wave or sharp-and–slow wave discharges, and periodic discharges (see Chapter 17 for further discussion of epileptiform patterns). Nonepileptiform abnormalities are of several types. First, localized slow activity is the most prevalent abnormality associated with focal brain lesions; the slowing is further classified as arrhythmic (polymorphic) or rhythmic (e.g., frontal intermittent rhythmic delta activity [FIRDA]). Second, there can be alteration in normally present cerebral rhythms such as frontal beta activity or the alpha rhythm. Third, background activity can be attenuated locally. Finally, widespread or diffuse abnormalities also occur with focal lesions, especially those located in the subfrontal regions or thalamus or that produce hydrocephalus.

Changes in Normal Rhythms

A complex mixture of different background rhythms and frequencies are present in the EEGs of normal individuals. These include beta frequencies (typically most prominent over the frontal regions), alpha rhythm and other posterior-dominant rhythms, mu rhythm, and normal features of sleep such as spindles and vertex waves. These different activities are evaluated routinely in terms of voltage, frequency, persistence, symmetry, and reactivity. Because the characteristics and normal variability of these patterns in healthy individuals are well established, changes in any of the foregoing measures are useful in identifying focal or regional abnormalities. Voltage asymmetries alone, however, are common in normal persons and should be interpreted conservatively—or even ignored—in the absence of other, more specific findings indicating an abnormality. (See Chapter 5 for detailed descriptions of normal EEG patterns and their variations.)

Focal Enhancement of Beta Activity

Anterior beta activity is normal in healthy adults (121), and it can be enhanced in voltage, rhythmicity, and quantity by many sedative, tranquilizing, or hypnotic medications, including benzodiazepines, barbiturates, and chloral hydrate (9,10,58). These drugs are frequently used by patients referred to EEG laboratories for treatment of epilepsy or other nervous disorders, or as sedation for the test itself. In such cases, fast activity is enhanced symmetrically. This bilateral and usually diffuse increase in normal beta activity should not be interpreted as abnormal; rather, it should be considered as being consistent with a clinically insignificant medication effect. Occasionally, prominent rhythmic beta activity recorded in the absence of known therapeutic drug use raises the possibility of illicit drug use.

Persistent asymmetry of beta activity indicates focal cortical dysfunction, which is often due to a cerebral lesion. The most common cause of focally enhanced beta activity is the "breach rhythm" (Fig. 11.1). This is usually the consequence of intracranial surgery requiring a craniotomy or burr hole. Less often, the breach rhythm results from a skull fracture. Skull defects enhance the voltage of frontal fast rhythms as much as threefold (28,80). This is most evident at C3/4 or T3/4 electrode sites because of their proximity to underlying mu rhythms or temporal rhythmic activity in the alpha frequency range. Although the enhanced beta activity is maximal nearest a burr hole or craniotomy margin, there is typically a broad voltage distribution.

Focally enhanced beta activity is rare in other circumstances. It has been described with brain abscess (139,175), stroke, arteriovenous malformations, tumors (13,68,80), and focal cortical dysplasia (142,145). Localized *attenuation* of beta activity is much more common in these conditions than enhancement.

Normal beta activity that has a predominant rhythmic frequency has a waxing and waning quality but remains more or less constant in a given state and over the course of the recording. Paroxysmal beta activity (also referred

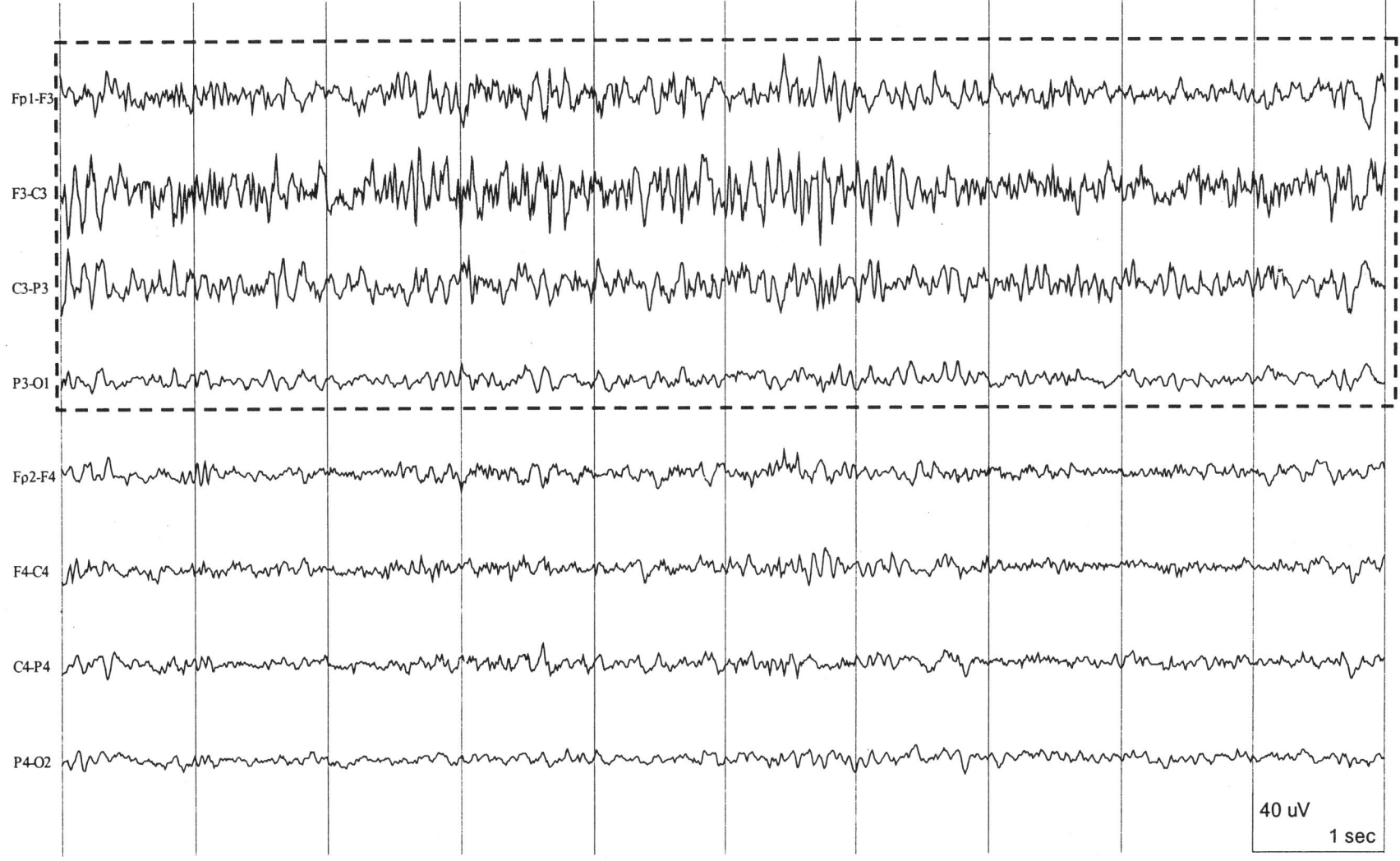

FIG. 11.1. EEGs of a 79-year-old man who had had a left subdural hematoma evacuated. **A:** Waking EEG demonstrates a breach rhythm in the left parasagittal region and focal polymorphic mixed theta and delta activity. (*Figure continues.*)

A

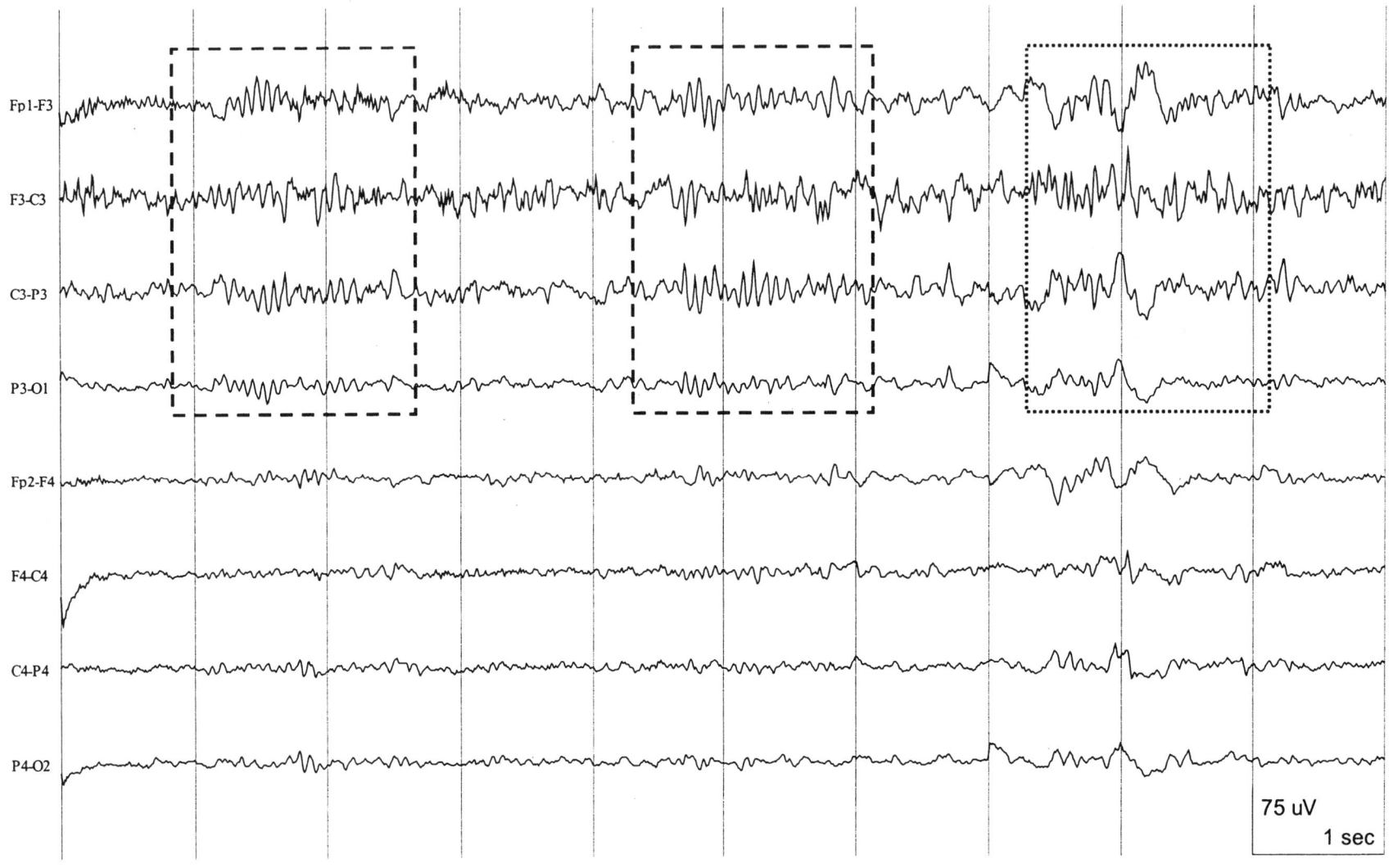

FIG. 11.1. *Continued.* **B:** Sample from stage 2 sleep illustrating higher voltage K complexes and sleep spindles (*boxed areas*) in the region of the skull defect.

to as paroxysmal fast activity), in contrast, is typically seen in epileptic encephalopathies, such as Lennox-Gastaut syndrome, where it is often an ictal pattern that accompanies tonic seizures (see also Chapter 17). Nealis and Duffy (125) reported nine patients with focal paroxysmal beta activity, all of whom had epilepsy. Most also had other focal EEG findings, such as sharp waves or slow-frequency activity, in the same area as the paroxysmal fast activity (Fig. 11.2).

Focal Attenuation of Beta Activity

Asymmetrical beta activity should be considered abnormal if there is a persistent voltage difference of 35% or more between homologous areas of the two sides. Frontal beta activity tends to occur out of phase on the left and right sides, and a voltage asymmetry can therefore be enhanced using bipolar montages that connect homologous areas. Focal attenuation of beta activity is a reliable sign of a cortical abnormality.

Focal attenuation of beta activity is seen in a number of conditions, including brain abscess (139,175), stroke (68), arteriovenous malformations (78), and brain tumors (13,68). Green and Wilson concluded that beta activity seems to be diminished with vascular lesions and enhanced by tumors (68). Barbiturates have been used to bring out a beta asymmetry, because focal structural lesions often diminish the usual enhancing effect of such drugs (134,135).

Beta activity is also attenuated by subdural, epidural, or subgaleal fluid collections (96). These selectively suppress higher frequency activity, much like a fast-frequency filter. Focal slowing usually accompanies parenchymal lesions but not fluid collections, a point that is sometimes helpful for interpretation. However, when extraaxial blood or cerebrospinal fluid results from a head injury, the underlying cortex is often injured as well, invalidating this distinction.

Abnormalities of the Alpha Rhythm and Photic Driving Response

Focal cerebral lesions can alter the alpha rhythm, even when they do not directly involve the occipital lobes and adjacent posterior brain regions (Fig. 11.3). Changes that can result from focal lesions include unilateral (a) slowing of frequency (1 Hz or more difference between the sides); (b) loss of reactivity; (c) loss of modulation; and (d) voltage attenuation. Unilateral attenuation or absence of alpha rhythm usually occurs with lesions of the occipital cortex and anteroventral thalamus (83). Unilateral failure of the alpha rhythm to attenuate with eye opening (Bancaud's phenomenon) occurs with posterior subcortical lesions (3). Voltage asymmetry, by itself, is only rarely an indication of focal abnormality. In contrast, asymmetries of frequency and reactivity are abnormal and reliably indicate the side of the lesion.

Skull defects result in higher voltage alpha rhythm, a difference that can be two to three times that of the normal side (28). Rarely, the alpha rhythm is higher on the side of a brain tumor (38,89), but in such cases the alpha rhythm is also usually less reactive and poorly modulated.

Asymmetries in the response to intermittent photic stimulation may result from lesions on the side of lower voltage, but responses can also be consistently lateralized in some normal individuals (31). Therefore, voltage asymmetries in photic driving should not be interpreted as abnormal in the absence of corroborative findings such as focal slowing or localized attenuation of background rhythms on the same side. Rarely, epileptogenic lesions result in responses to photic stimulation that are of higher voltage on the side of the lesion (Fig. 11.4).

Changes in Other Normal Rhythms

A unique precentral alpha-frequency rhythm was first recognized by Jasper and Andrews (82) and later characterized by Gastaut and coworkers (55) as "*le rythme rolandique en arceau.*" They described a 7- to 11-Hz arch-shaped rhythm over one or both rolandic areas that was unaltered by eye opening but attenuated with contralateral sensory stimuli or movement, either passive or active. The "parietal focal theta rhythm" described by Cobb (27) was probably similar activity. Fishgold et al. (47) first reported on the effects of bone defects on EEG activity. These investigators concluded that bone defects resulted in higher voltage alpha rhythm, but they were probably describing the effect on mu rhythm (28). Cobb and colleagues (28) recorded EEGs from 33 patients before and after replacement of a bone flap. Electrode location was controlled by radiography. Most recordings with the bone absent showed asymmetrical 6- to 11-Hz waves that were maximal over the rolandic region (usually C3/4) and blocked by fist clenching. They termed this a "breach rhythm." Although it usually had a limited field, the breach rhythm could be identified several centimeters from the bone edge. In most patients, replacing the bone flap either attenuated the breach rhythm significantly or eliminated it completely. The breach rhythm is mu activity made especially prominent (long duration, high voltage, and sharp contour) by a skull defect (see Fig. 11.1). Like all mu activity, it attenuates with real

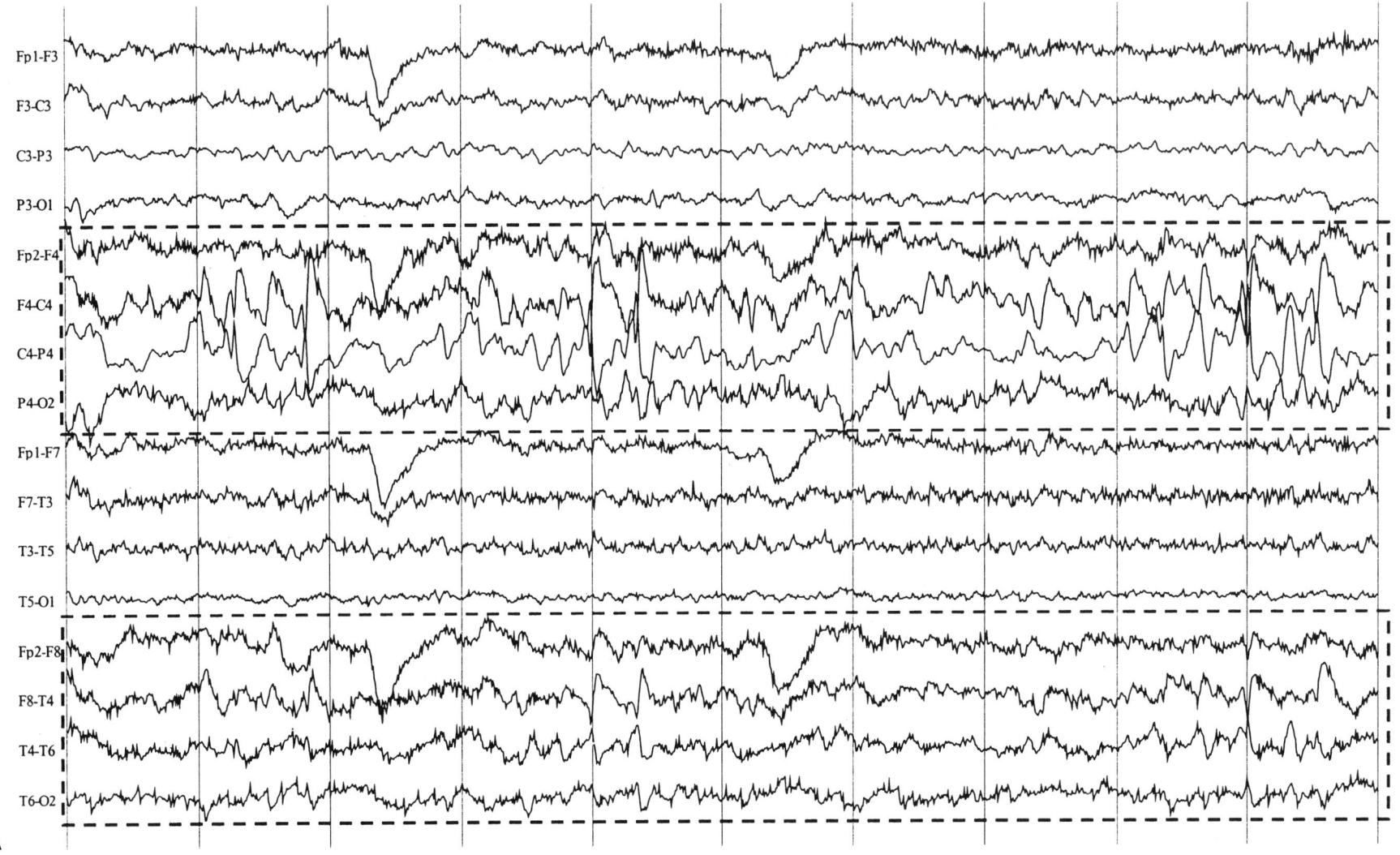

A

FIG. 11.2. EEGs of a 47-year-old man who had a right parietal intracerebral hemorrhage evacuated recently. Afterward, he developed confusional episodes secondary to frequent nonconvulsive seizures. **A:** There is focal polymorphic delta activity, attenuation of faster organized frequencies, and epileptiform discharges over the right central-parietal region. Rhythmic theta activity is higher voltage on the right because of the craniotomy. *(Figure continues.)*

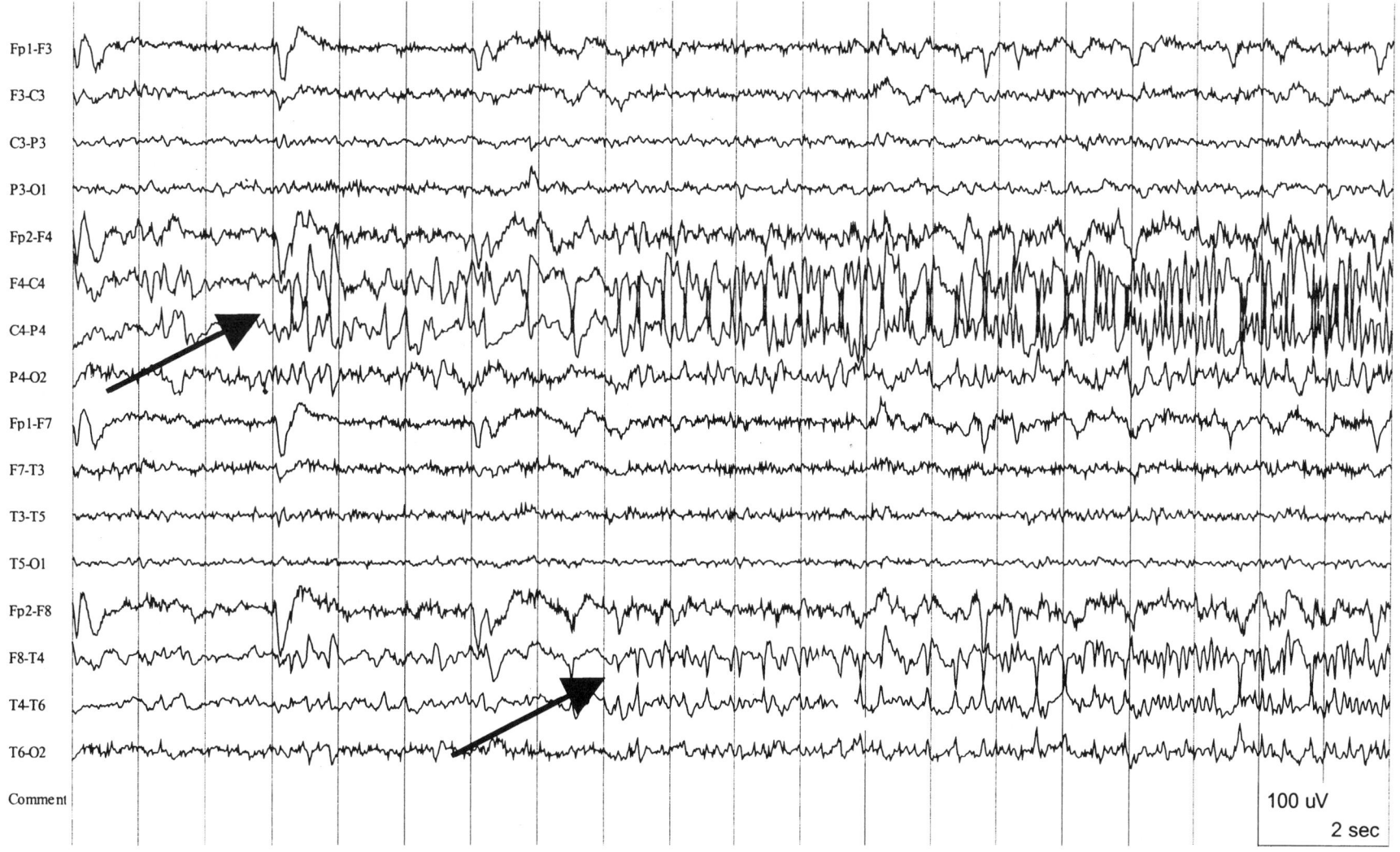

FIG. 11.2. *Continued.* **B:** Interictal–ictal transition in the right central epileptogenic brain region. Note that individual epileptiform discharges first increase in frequency (*higher arrow* on left) and then evolve into an ictal pattern consisting of rhythmic 12- to 14-Hz waves that spread to involve the adjacent right temporal area (*lower arrow* on right).

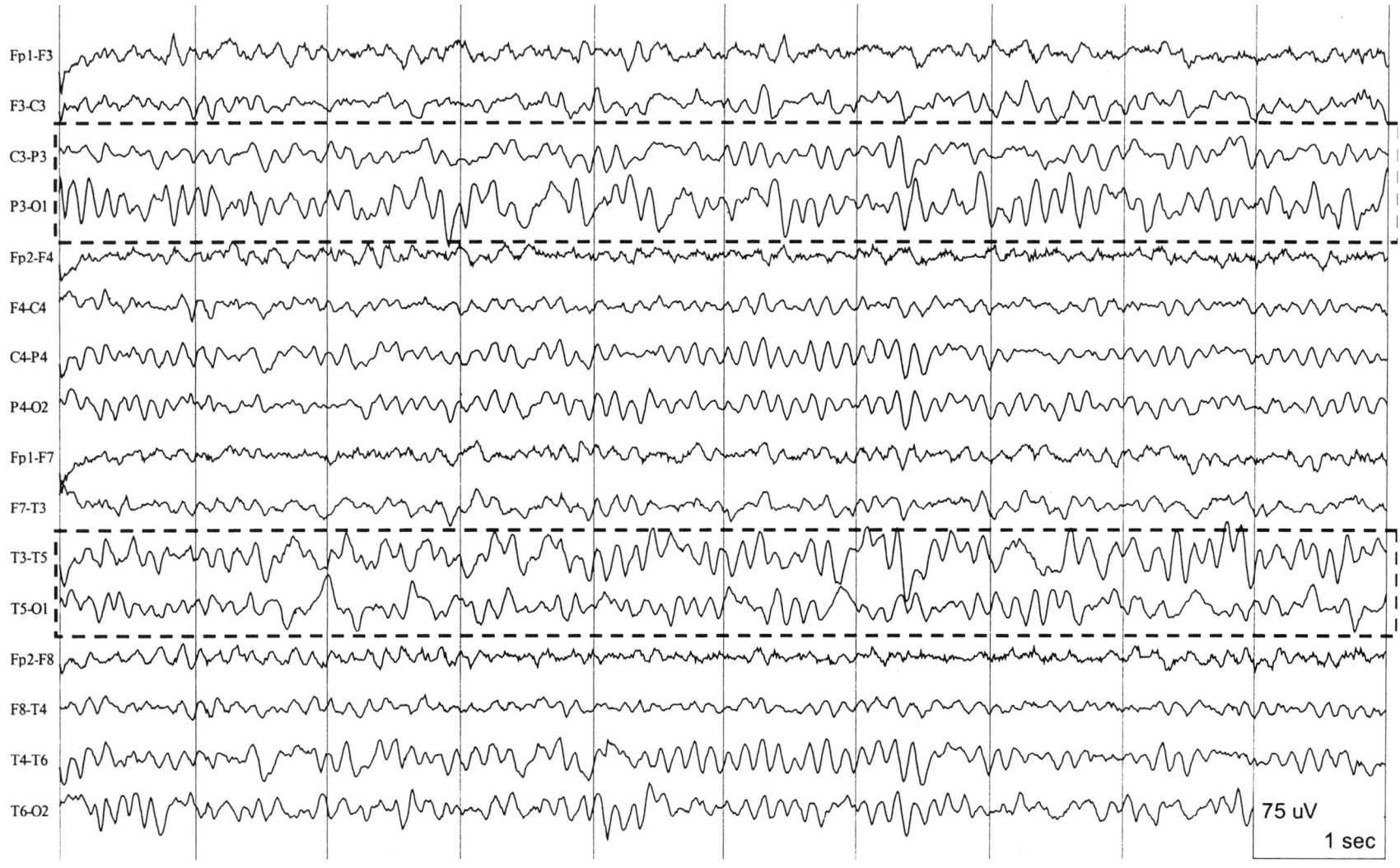

FIG. 11.3. EEG of a 31-year-old man with a left occipital arteriovenous malformation. There is continuous focal polymorphic delta activity over the left parieto-occipital–posterior temporal areas. The alpha rhythm on the left is 1–1.5 Hz slower and paradoxically of higher voltage on the left.

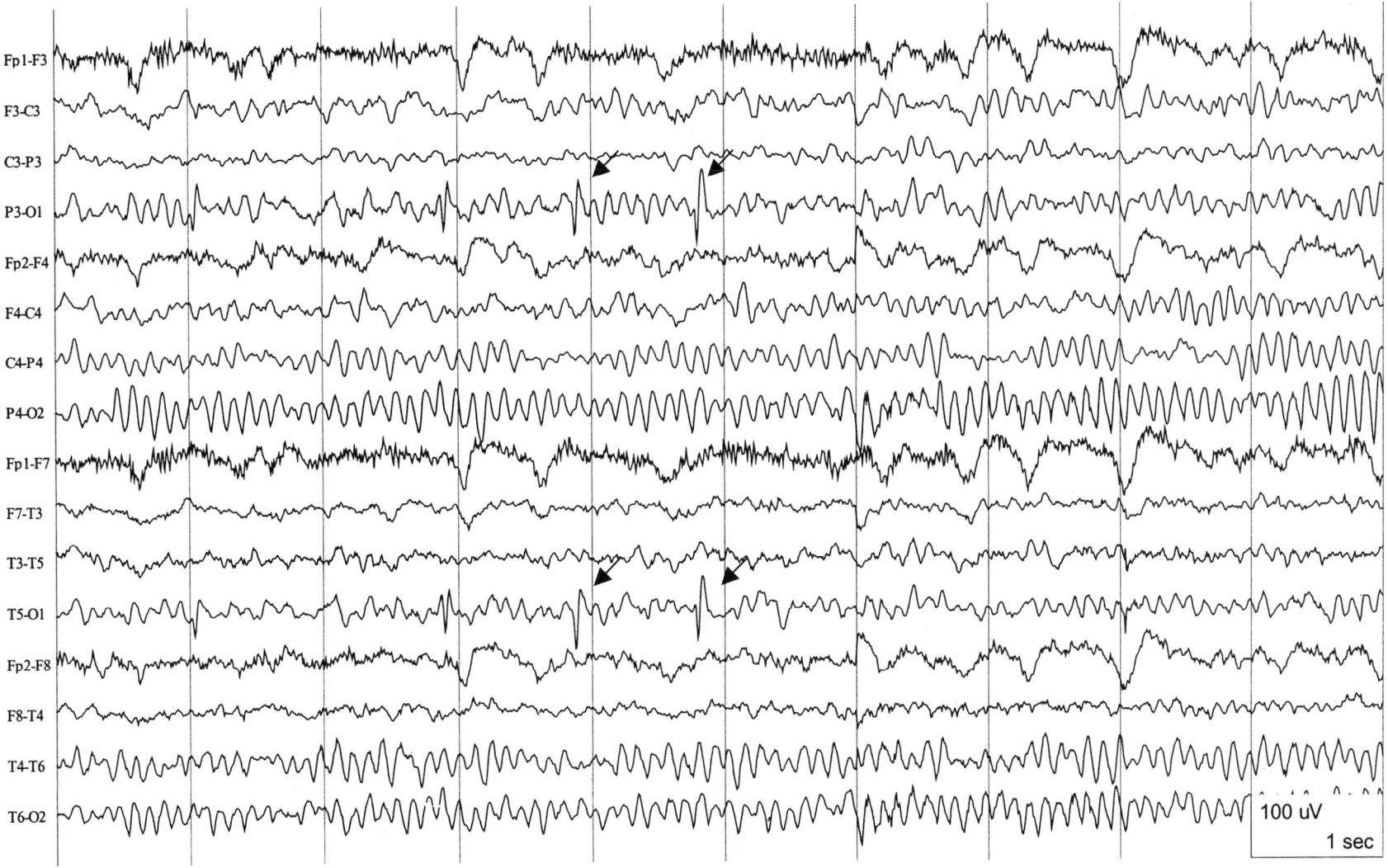

A

FIG. 11.4. EEGs of a 6-year-old boy with intractable epilepsy and left occipital cortical dysplasia on MRI scan. **A:** Asymmetry of the alpha rhythm, which is normal on the right but greatly attenuated and poorly regulated on the left. There are frequent left occipital (O1) epileptiform discharges (*arrows*). (*Figure continues.*)

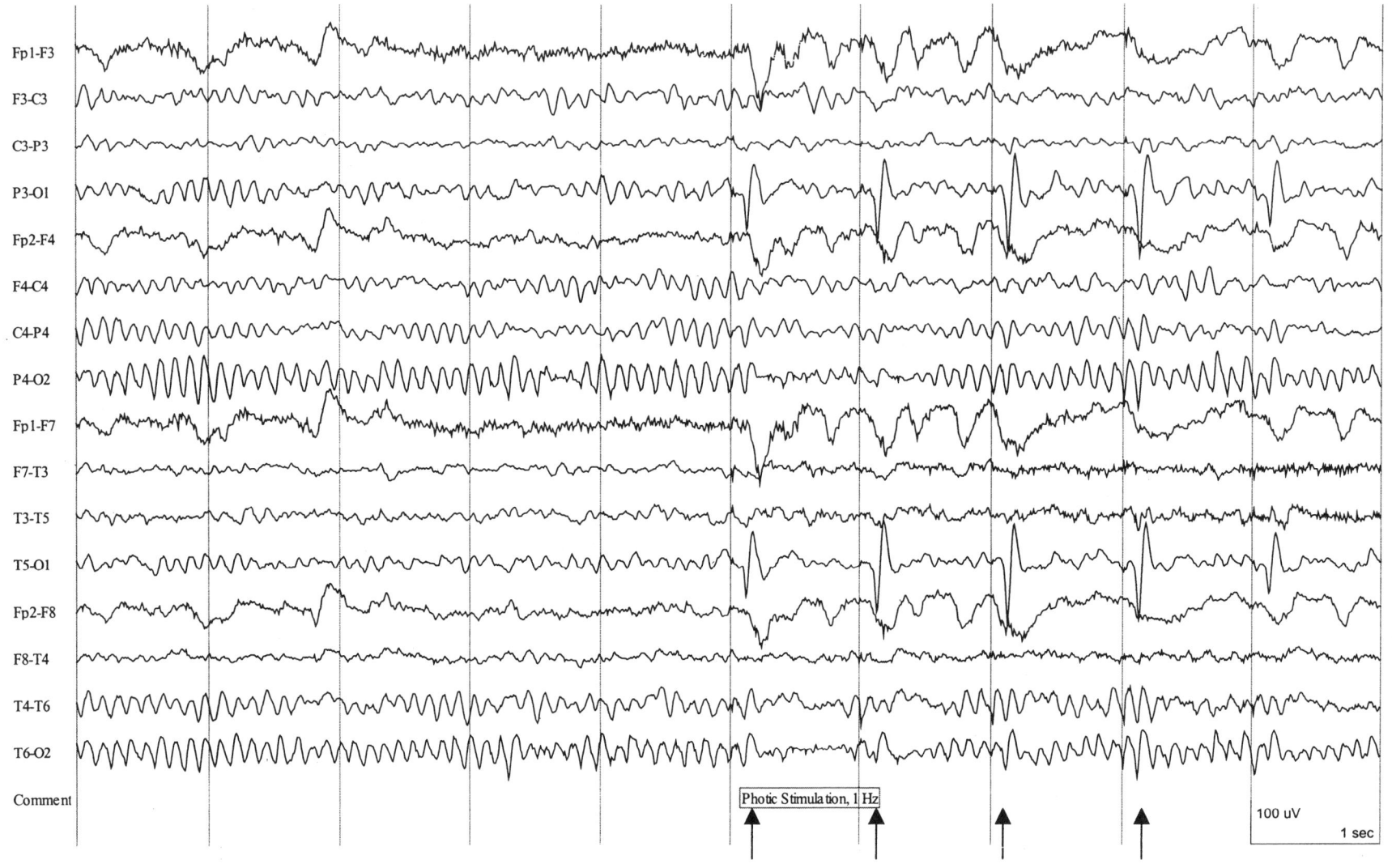

FIG. 11.4. *Continued.* **B:** Paradoxical enhancement of photic responses to 1-Hz light flashes on the left (*arrows* indicate typical examples in channels 4[P3-01] and 12[T5-01]).

or imagined movement of the contralateral hand. It probably results primarily from physical factors related to removing a portion of high-impedance calvarium. Development of adhesions that act as low-impedance bridges between cortex and dura or skull may also play a role (47). A postoperative mu or breach rhythm has no clinical implications, and one must exercise caution in not overinterpreting sharply contoured fragments of such activity as epileptiform.

Although both the unilateral appearance and absence of mu activity were at one time thought to indicate focal cerebral pathology (15,155), this has not been substantiated. It is now recognized that asymmetries of mu rhythm are common (mu is unilateral in about 30% of normal people) and of no clinical significance.

Normal sleep patterns, especially sleep spindles and vertex waves, can be affected by cerebral lesions. Once stage 2 sleep is well established, persistent asymmetry of spindles indicates an abnormality on the side of lower voltage. Lesions of the parietal lobe or thalamus can attenuate sleep spindles (17,34). Thalamic lesions can also result in interhemispheric asynchrony of spindles, affect regulation of spindle frequency, or, rarely, lead to the appearance of spindle-like rhythms during the waking state (75). Skull defects enhance the scalp-recorded voltage of sleep spindles and vertex waves (see Fig. 11.1).

Focal Slow-Wave Activity

Slow-wave activity is classified as rhythmic or arrhythmic, intermittent or continuous, and focal or generalized. Focal polymorphic (arrhythmic) delta activity is slow-frequency activity (< 4 Hz) that lacks sustained rhythmicity; it is characterized by a constantly changing morphology, frequency, and voltage. Continuous focal polymorphic delta activity is highly correlated with a localized structural lesion (149,178), such as a tumor, stroke, abscess, intraparenchymal hematoma, or contusion (Fig. 11.5). Such delta activity usually persists during changes in physiological state. The clinical correlations of intermittent polymorphic slow-wave activity are less well defined, as are those of delta waves that attenuate with eye opening (or other alerting maneuvers) or disappear with sleep. Voltage of focal polymorphic delta activity is usually higher than ongoing background activity, but it can vary, depending in large part on the proximity of the lesion to the cortical surface and recording electrodes. Typical voltage of focal polymorphic delta activity is 100–150 µV in adults and up to 500 µV in children.

Focal polymorphic delta activity is often, but by no means always, maximal over the lesion. If sufficient destruction of the cortex and adjacent white matter has occurred, however, the voltage of the delta activity is actually reduced over the area of maximal cerebral involvement by the lesion (3). It is particularly important to pay attention to areas of relative inactivity ("flat" or "smooth" polymorphic delta activity), in which the voltage of both slow waves and faster background rhythms is depressed. In these cases, the voltage will be higher in the areas bordering the lesion (64). The localizing value of focal polymorphic delta activity is greatest when it is topographically discrete and associated with depression of superimposed faster background frequencies (3,64). Superficial lesions tend to produce more restricted EEG changes, whereas deep cerebral lesions can result in hemispheric, or even bilateral, delta activity. Focal delta activity associated with lesions of the frontal lobe typically spreads to homologous contralateral areas, where it typically is of lower voltage and has a smaller field than slowing ipsilateral to the lesion. Lesions involving the posterior frontal and parietal lobes often produce delta activity that is falsely localized to the temporal areas.

Clinical (63,127) and experimental (62) data indicate that polymorphic delta activity results primarily from lesions affecting cerebral white matter. Involvement of superficial cortex is not essential; indeed, lesions restricted to the cortical mantle do not generally produce significant focal delta activity. Cerebral edema, by itself, does not make a substantial contribution to production of delta waves (56,62,127). Brain tumors, abscesses, and areas of infarction are electrically silent (48,153). The EEG changes produced by these lesions, therefore, probably reflect alterations in cortical electrogenesis caused (a) directly by anatomic disruption of neurons and their local networks or by locally impaired blood flow, cellular metabolism, and the microenvironment; and (b) indirectly by modifying input onto cortical neurons. EEG is generally not useful in distinguishing among different types of brain lesions. This is largely because there are only a limited number of ways the brain can react to injury; therefore, a few electrographic changes are seen with a wide variety of conditions affecting the central nervous system.

Although experimental, clinical, and brain imaging studies have demonstrated the strong correlation between localized anatomical pathology and focal polymorphic delta activity, they also illustrate that delta activity can occur in the absence of a demonstrable lesion (60). This is most likely to occur when the polymorphic slowing is intermittent and contains substantial amounts of intermixed theta activity (Fig. 11.6). In these cases, the underlying cerebral dysfunction is often reversible. Examples include migraine, trauma, encephalitis, and postictal dysfunction. Focal arrhythmic theta activity can be seen early in the course of benign or well-differentiated brain tumors and during resolution of acute lesions caused by stroke or head trauma.

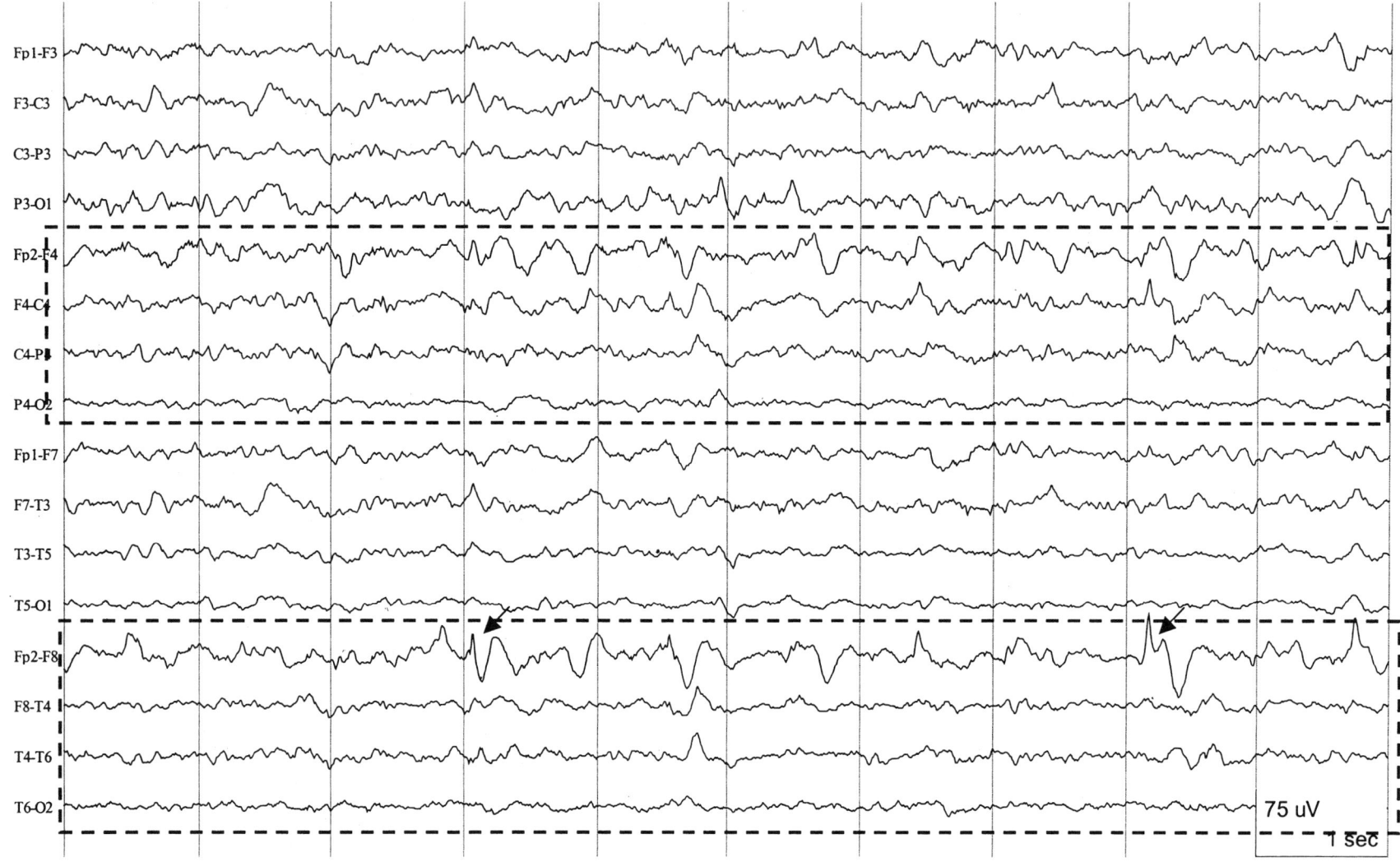

FIG. 11.5. EEG of a 79-year-old man with focal seizures secondary to multiple right hemisphere infarcts (frontal gyrus rectus, thalamus, and occipital lobe). There is continuous right frontal polymorphic delta activity, which spreads to the left frontal areas intermittently. There are also right frontal polar epileptiform discharges (*arrows*). Background activity is diffusely slowed and poorly differentiated.

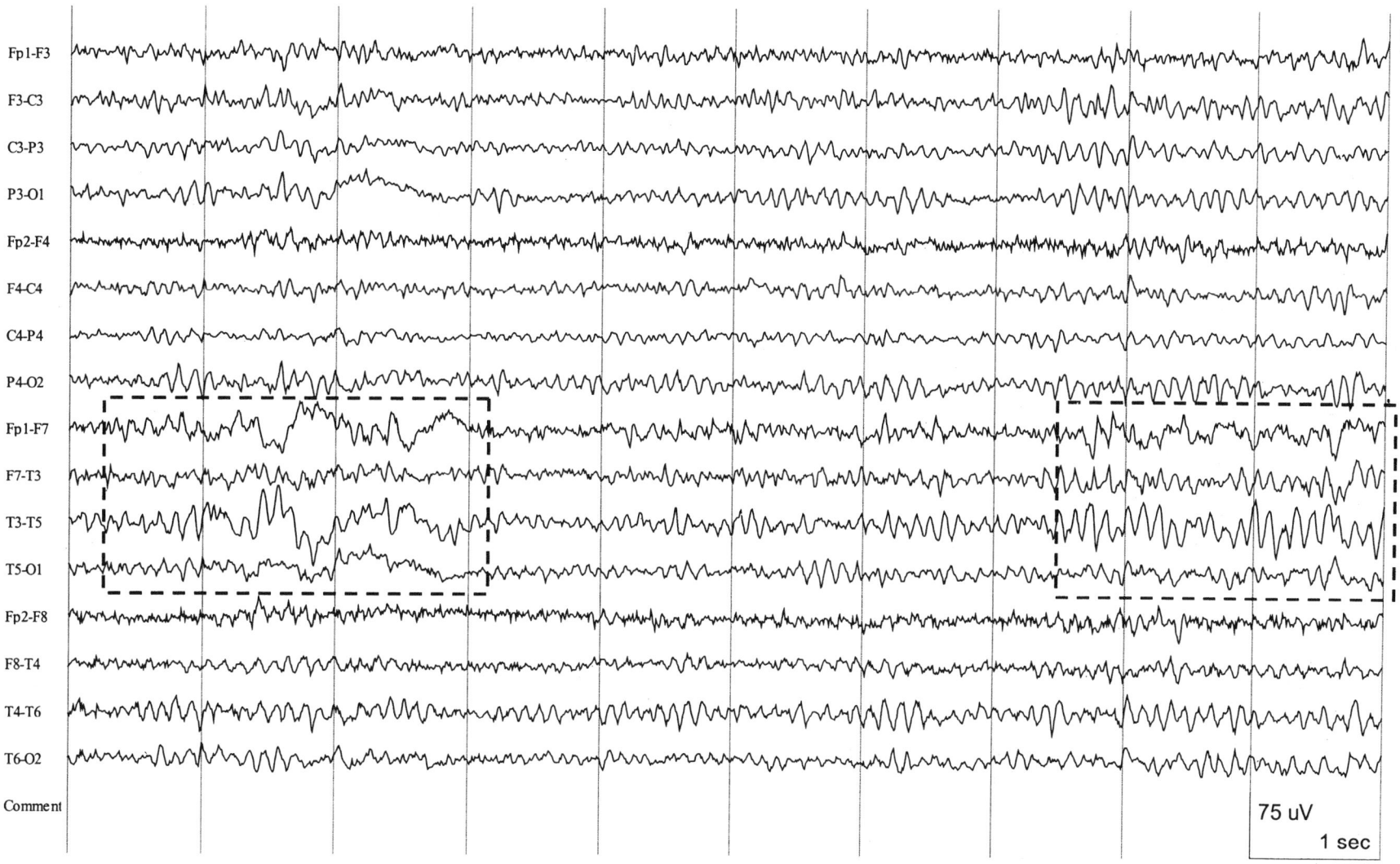

FIG. 11.6. EEG of a 57-year-old woman with a left temporal subcortical lesion and aphasia secondary to neu-rosarcoidosis. There is intermittent focal polymorphic delta activity in the left temporal area (*boxed channels*) that is relatively isopotential in the F7-T3 channel. Note that faster frequencies are preserved, riding on the delta waves.

Focal Voltage Attenuation

The value of voltage attenuation was referred to in the foregoing section. Berger (9) first described localized areas of low voltage in the EEG. These indicate either loss of normal cortical electrical activity (as with cerebral atrophy, invasion by tumor, or ischemia) or signal attenuation by fluid collections such as subdural hematoma (2).

Hemispheric voltage attenuation occurs with congenital lesions (e.g., infantile hemiplegia syndrome resulting from cerebral infarction), porencephaly, or Sturge-Weber disease (Fig. 11.7). Focal voltage attenuation occurs most often in combination with focal polymorphic delta activity, as described in the foregoing section of this chapter. Attenuation results from injury to, or destruction of, cortex as well as the subjacent white matter, as occurs with large cerebral infarctions and malignant brain tumors. Subdural hematoma, subgaleal fluid accumulation, and parasagittal meningioma also attenuate faster frequency activity, because they act as high-frequency filters. EEG alone cannot reliably distinguish among these possibilities.

Intermittent Rhythmic Delta Activity

Intermittent rhythmic delta activity (IRDA) was first described by Cobb (27) and later by Jasper and Van Buren (83) and Daly et al. (33). Although intermittent rhythmic theta activity also occurs, most studies and textbooks have emphasized IRDA that is maximal over the frontal regions (FIRDA). For many years, electroencephalographers tried to correlate IRDA with lesions involving deep midline or posterior fossa structures. It is now clear that most bilateral rhythmic slow-wave patterns are not reliably associated with localized structural pathology or specific anatomical locations.

IRDA is characterized by bursts and runs of high-voltage, bisynchronous, well-formed slow waves of relatively fixed frequency (about 2.5 Hz) and waveform. It usually increases with hyperventilation and during drowsiness, attenuates with eye opening, and disappears during stage 2 and deeper sleep (34). Interestingly, IRDA can reappear during rapid-eye-movement sleep (158). In children under the age of 15 years, IRDA appears most prominently over the occipital areas (OIRDA) (34). This age-related variability in voltage field is most likely the result of maturational factors, not differences in etiology of the IRDA.

The pathophysiology of IRDA is not well understood. The final common pathway may be abnormal thalamocortical interactions (62,64,83). However, it is likely that generation of IRDA requires pathological dysfunction, not complete disruption, of thalamocortical connections. This is supported by the observation of spindle-like rhythms seen both experimentally after isolated thalamic lesions (62) and clinically (but only rarely) in children with thalamic brain tumors (75). The dorsal medial nucleus of the thalamus has been implicated as being particularly important in generating IRDA, because rhythmic slow waves are seen when this nucleus is partially, but not completely, destroyed (30,83). IRDA occurs in a wide variety of neurological disorders with both structural and physiological etiologies (43,150). Historically, subfrontal, diencephalic, or infratentorial lesions have all been associated with IRDA. Schaul and coworkers (154) reviewed EEGs from 154 patients with diencephalic or posterior fossa lesions. Only 12% of those with diencephalic lesions had normal EEGs, whereas 60% of patients with lower brainstem and 73% of patients with cerebellar pathology had normal EEGs. Lateralized IRDA has a high correlation with ipsilateral deep lesions (Fig. 11.8). When IRDA occurs in patients with posterior fossa lesions, it is most often due to obstructive hydrocephalus. In fact, FIRDA and OIRDA are relatively nonspecific in regard to etiology. In a general EEG laboratory's referral population, FIRDA is seen much more often in the setting of metabolic disorders or other diffuse encephalopathies and idiopathic epilepsy than with focal lesions, regardless of location. OIRDA is especially common in children ages 6–10 years who have absence seizures (32).

Temporal intermittent rhythmic delta activity (TIRDA) (Fig. 11.9) is associated with complex partial seizures and temporal lobe epilepsy (147) (see Chapter 17). Like FIRDA, zeta waves are more prominent during drowsiness and light sleep.

Finally, Magnus and Van der Holst (106) described an unusual form of rhythmic delta slowing in which the waveform is characterized by an initial negativity followed by a steep positivity crossing the baseline, then a slow return to baseline. They designated these waveforms as *zeta waves* because of their appearance. Zeta waves have been associated with particularly severe brain lesions, especially those due to trauma, but not stroke.

Activating Techniques

This topic is covered extensively in Chapter 8. We discuss it here only as it relates to focal abnormalities. Hyperventilation is useful in accentuating focal slowing that is low voltage and intermittent at baseline. Intermittent photic stimulation has no effect on focal slowing. The effect of sleep on focal polymorphic delta activity relates to the severity of the abnormality. Sleep has little effect on continuous polymorphic delta activity. Its effect on intermittent polymorphic delta activity is more variable. When slowing is caused by a structural

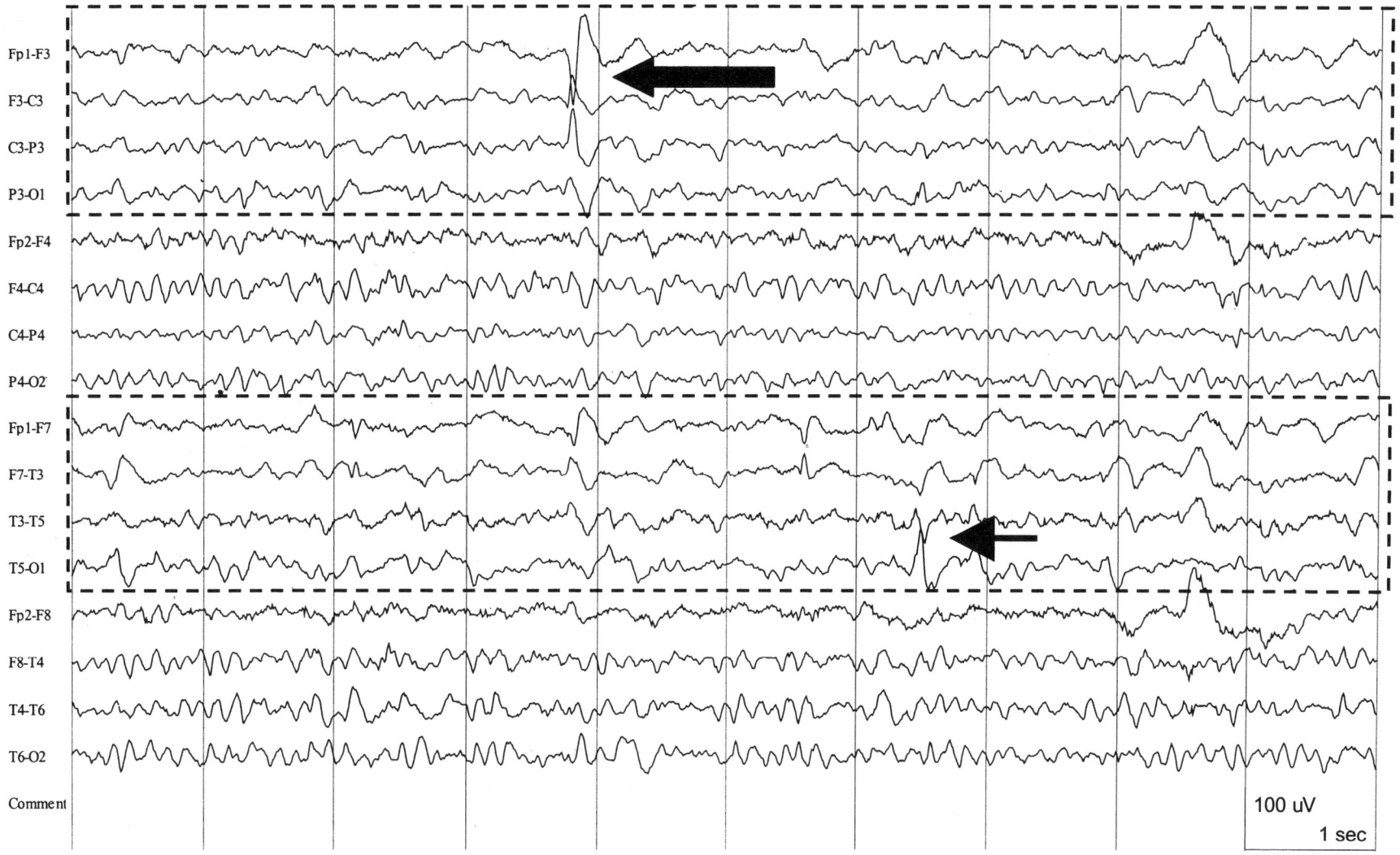

FIG. 11.7. EEG of a 40-year-old woman with right hemiparesis and intractable epilepsy secondary to a congenital left hemisphere stroke. There is continuous polymorphic delta activity over the entire left hemisphere, with attenuation of faster frequencies and nearly complete loss of the alpha rhythm. There are multifocal epileptiform sharp waves (left frontal and left posterior temporal discharges are indicated by *arrows*).

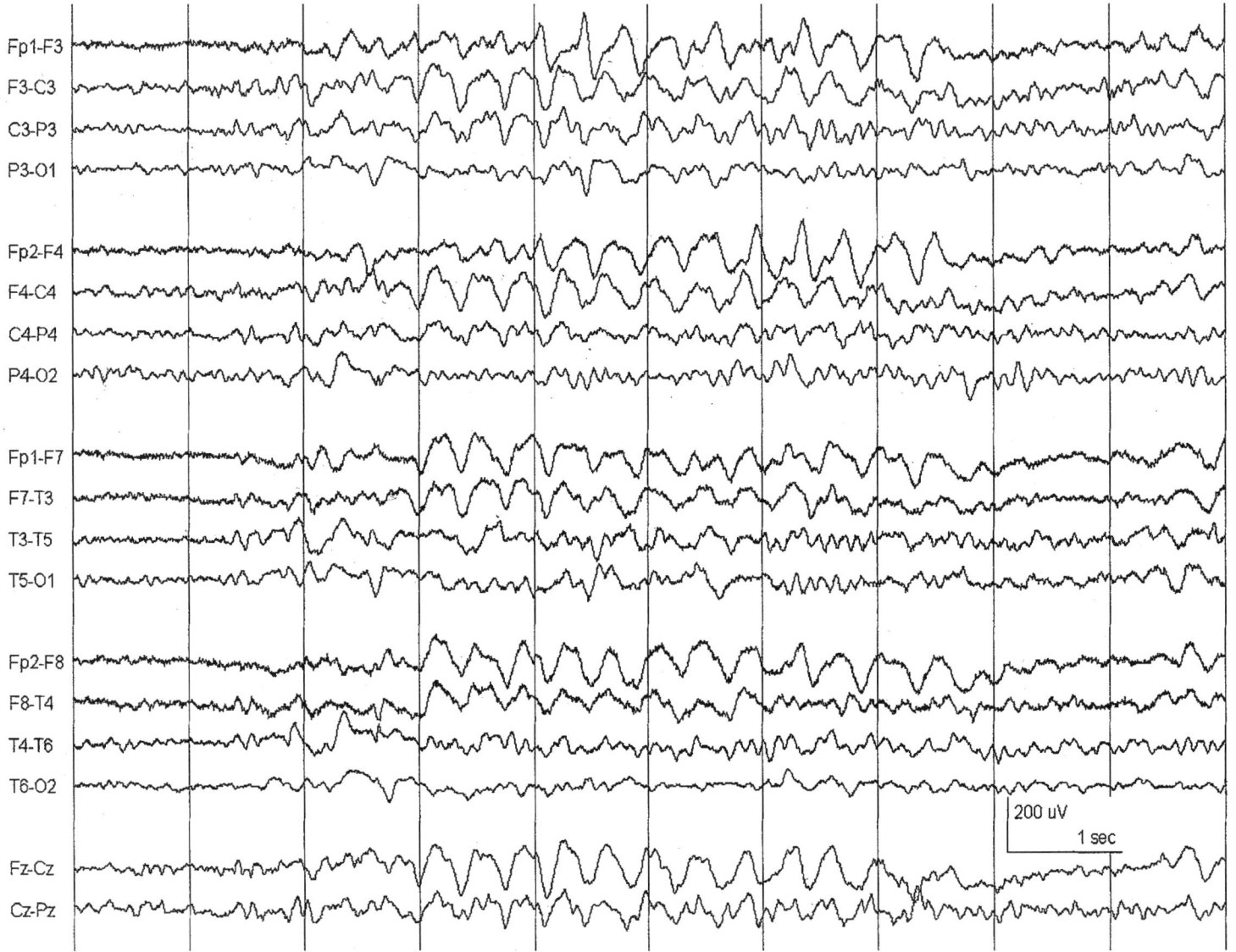

FIG. 11.8. EEG of a 67-year-old woman with bilateral thalamic and basal ganglia infarcts. Note runs of rhythmic 2.5 Hz activity, seen maximally in the frontal region bilaterally (FIRDA). The intervening background shows only mild diffuse theta frequency slowing.

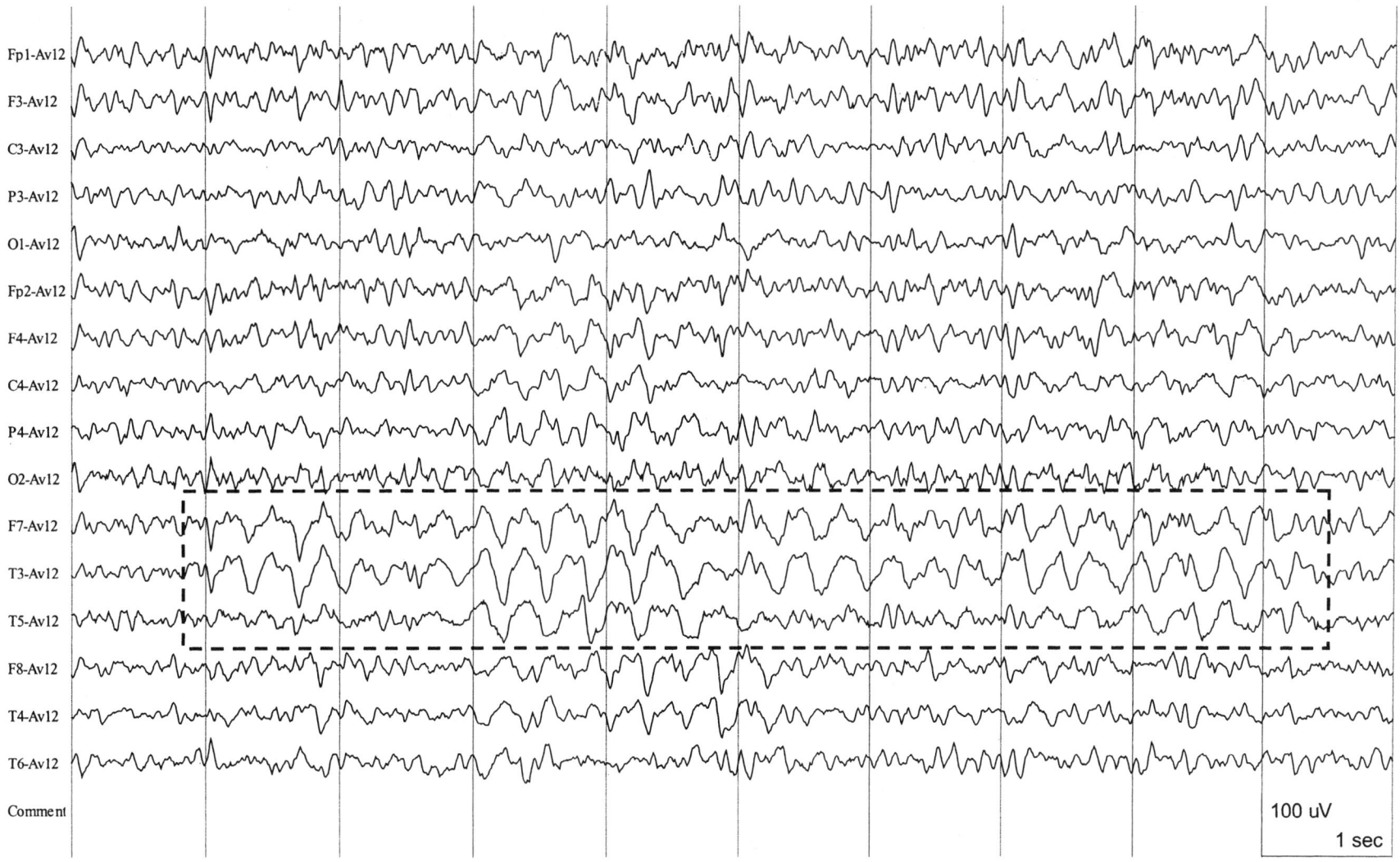

FIG. 11.9. EEG of a 44-year-old man with paroxysmal atrial fibrillation and new-onset seizures. There are frequent runs of intermittent rhythmic temporal delta activity (TIRDA) (*boxed channels*) that are not associated with epileptiform discharges.

brain lesion, sleep has little effect. However, with reversible, nonstructural etiologies, sleep may attenuate focal intermittent slowing. Hypoglycemia activates slowing associated with structural lesions (6,113) and epilepsy (67,155). In areas where the blood–brain barrier has been compromised, high doses of intravenous penicillin can activate focal epileptiform activity (148).

EPILEPTIFORM ABNORMALITIES

Seizures are a common symptom of chronic or slowly progressive focal lesions, so it should not be surprising that interictal epileptiform discharges are frequently present in the EEGs of such patients (see Fig. 11.7) (91). Epileptiform activity (spikes or sharp waves) is common in EEGs of patients with well-differentiated glioma, traumatic cicatrix, brain abscess, medial temporal sclerosis, and cortical dysplasia. In patients with benign or very slowly progressive tumors, focal epileptiform discharges sometimes antedate the appearance of focal slow-wave activity by months or years (72). In general, however, patients with brain tumors usually have other EEG abnormalities (focal slowing, voltage attenuation) in addition to spikes or sharp waves (14). Epileptiform discharges are less common with acute cerebral infarction or hemorrhage. Although these typically occur ipsilateral to the infarct, they can be seen rarely contralateral to an acute stroke (173). A complete discussion of epileptiform abnormalities is provided in Chapter 17.

Acute destructive lesions such as stroke, tumor, abscess, and viral (especially herpes simplex) encephalitis can result in periodic lateralized epileptiform discharges (PLEDs) (23,35,36,98,108,143,157,164,177) (Fig. 11.10). Although the most common cause of PLEDs is stroke, their occurrence in this condition is infrequent (90). PLEDs have also been reported early in the course of Creutzfeldt-Jakob disease (50) and in patients with subdural hematoma (26), MELAS (mitochondrial myopathy, encephalopathy, lactic acidosis, and stroke-like episodes) (49), nonketotic hyperglycemia (160), and, occasionally, chronic lesions, especially in the presence of a superimposed metabolic abnormality. Electrolyte abnormalities and nonketotic hyperglycemia have also been postulated as factors that contribute to PLEDs appearing after acute stroke (126). Specific etiologies associated with epileptiform activity are described in the following sections.

SPECIFIC ETIOLOGIES

Trauma

Routine EEG has little role to play in management of acute head injury. Following closed head trauma with concussion, the EEG most often shows diffuse, nonspecific slow-wave activity. The degree of slowing and the extent to which normal background rhythms are lost (e.g., loss or slowing of the posterior dominant rhythm) are proportional to the severity of trauma and the patient's level of consciousness at the time the EEG is recorded. Focal abnormalities indicate cerebral contusion or hemorrhage. Sometimes focal changes are present and persist even in the absence of abnormalities on brain imaging, indicating that functional injury can occur without identifiable anatomical changes. Transient focal changes are often multifocal.

Brain Tumors

Tumors are a common cause of focal slow-wave activity in the EEG (Figs. 11.11 and 11.12). Among EEGs showing focal polymorphic delta activity, tumors account for 13% (60) to 40% (180) depending on the laboratory's referral population. The character and distribution of EEG changes produced by a tumor, as with any focal lesion, depend on its size, its distance from the cortical surface, and the anatomical structures involved. With brain tumors, the degree of malignancy, reflected in rapidity of growth and acute or subacute mass effect, is an additional factor. Tumors having substantial mass effect that results in shift of midline structures, compression of the lateral ventricle, and downward pressure on the thalamus and upper brainstem produce IRDA and bilateral arrhythmic slowing as well as focal slowing. When severe, these secondary bilateral and diffuse features may partially obscure focal indicators of the underlying lesion.

The EEG is normal in up to 40% of brain tumors (11), but this statement must be qualified. Normal EEGs actually occur in only about 5% of hemispheric tumors, which account for the majority of brain tumors in adults. In contrast, EEGs are normal in at least 25% of deep midline, basal, and infratentorial tumors (33,72,111), and this figure is undoubtedly higher in the absence of obstructive hydrocephalus and increased intracranial pressure. Unlike supratentorial intraparenchymal tumors, parasagittal meningiomas may be relatively silent electrically (92,170). Early on, they tend to produce localized attenuation of beta activity and focal spikes or sharp waves, but focal polymorphic delta activity is not usually prominent until there is sufficient tumor bulk to compress the underlying cortex and adjacent white matter. Rarely, hemispheric brain tumors produce focal enhancement of alpha (38) or beta (74) activity. Thus brain tumors can be associated with any or all of the EEG abnormalities seen with focal lesions.

Isolated spikes and sharp waves are rare as the sole electrographic manifestation of a neoplasm (11). Sharp waves are said to be more common than

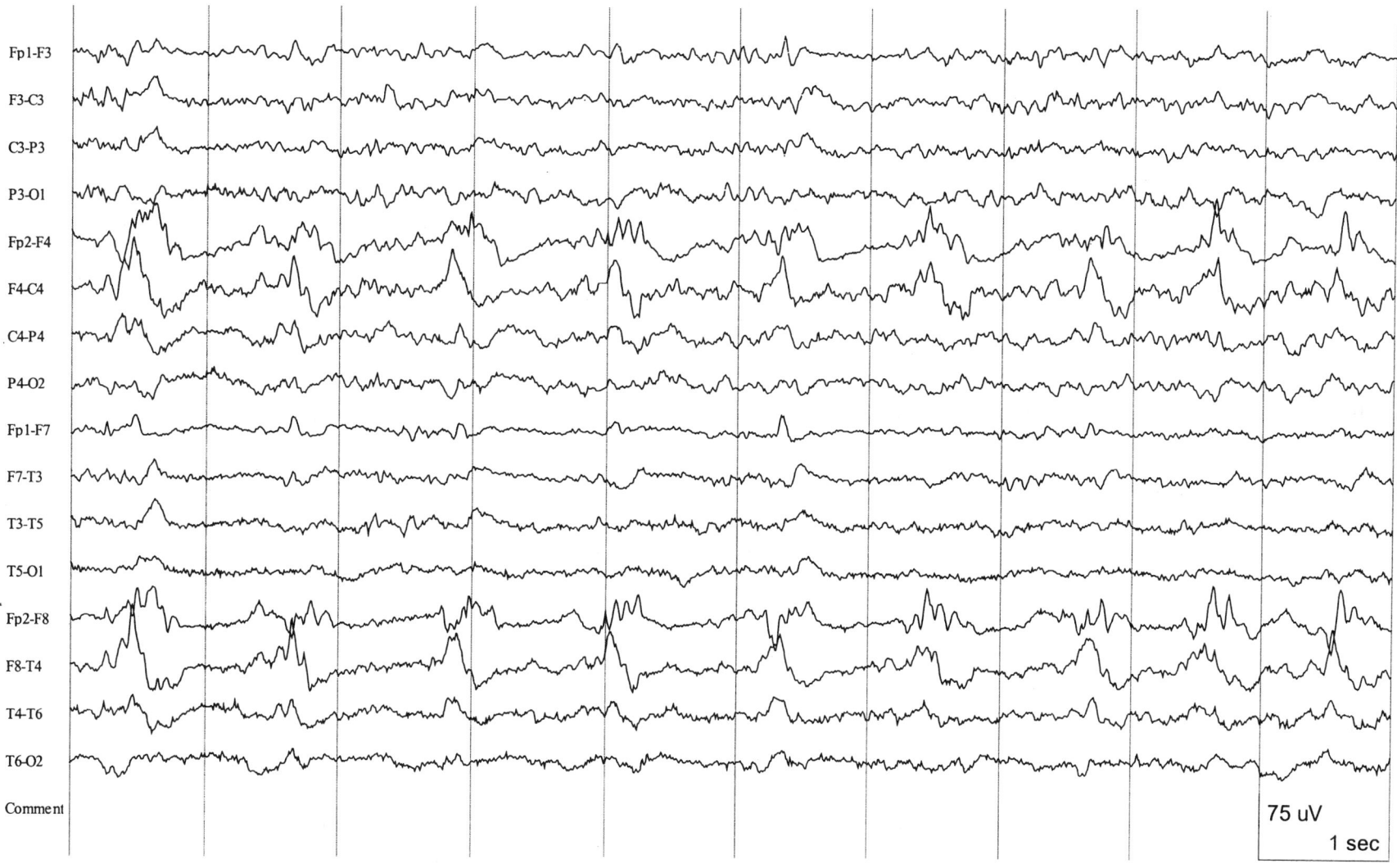

FIG. 11.10. EEG of a 90-year-old man with acute infarcts involving right anterior and middle cerebral artery territories. There are right frontal–temporal PLEDS occurring with a repetition rate of about 1.5 Hz. Note associated diffuse slowing of background rhythms, which is continuous and generally more pronounced on the right.

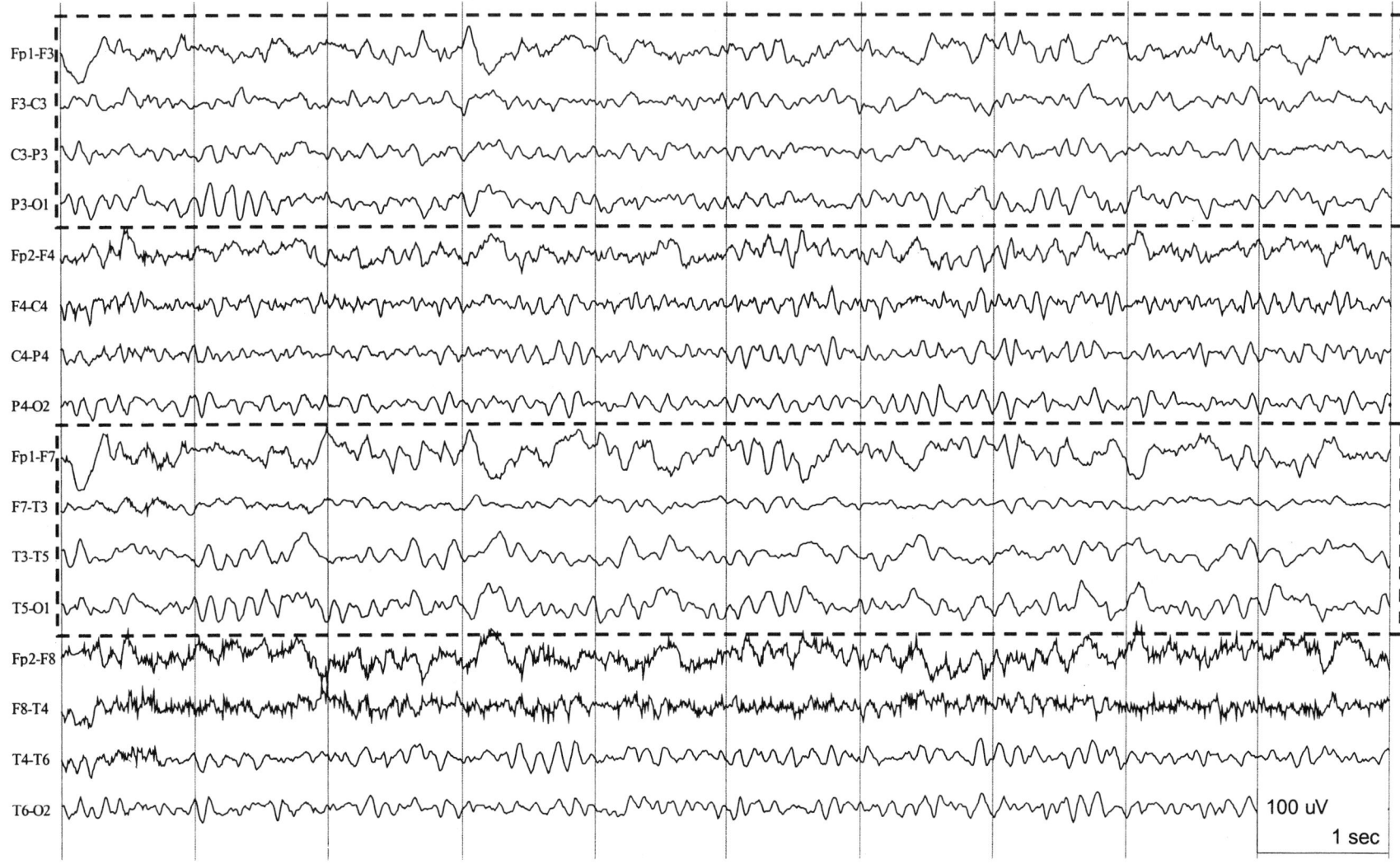

FIG. 11.11. EEG of a 44-year-old man with a large suprasellar meningioma extending mainly to the left, compressing subfrontal and temporal regions. There is widespread polymorphic delta activity over the left hemisphere with attenuation of faster background frequencies. In this bipolar montage, the slowing is isopotential in the F7-T3 channel.

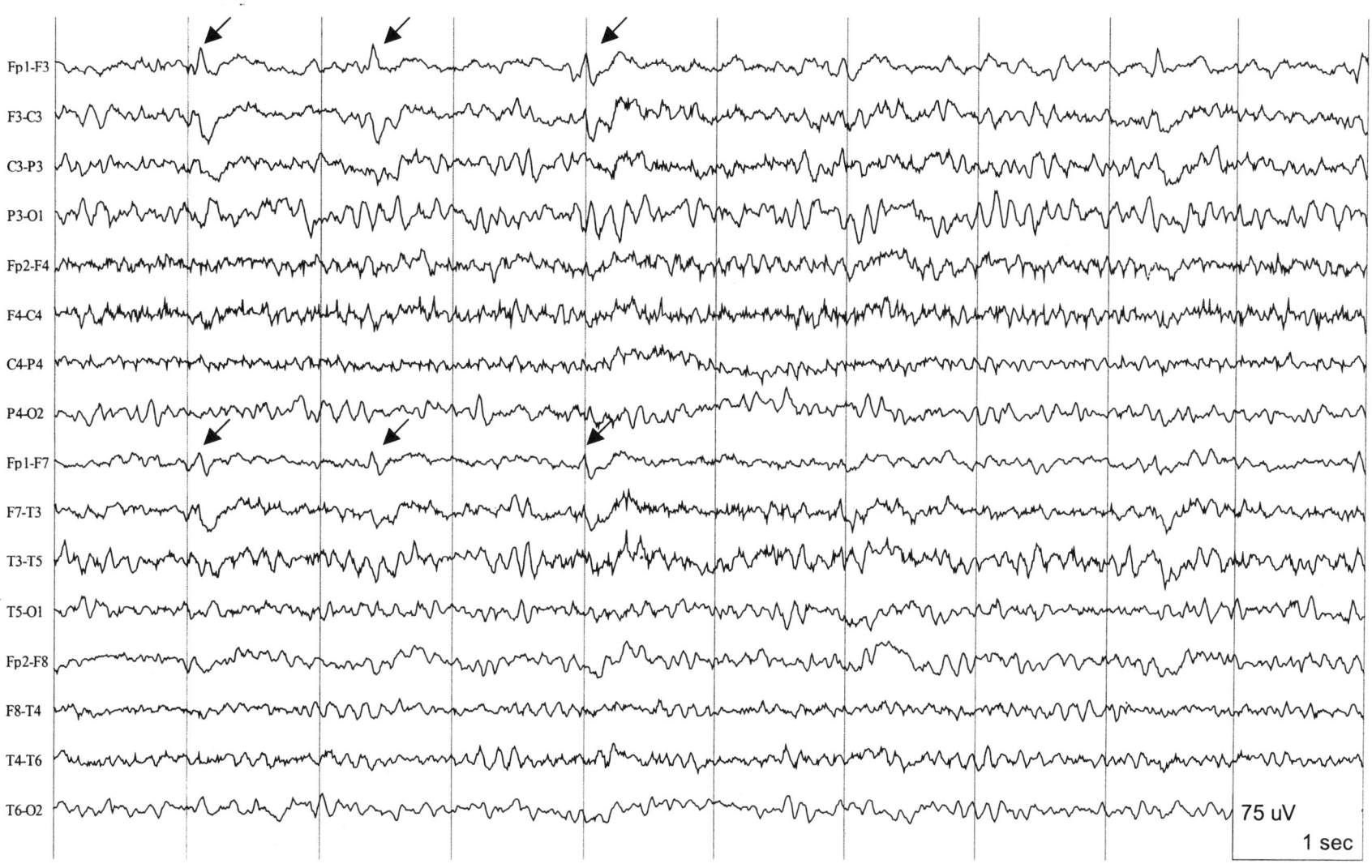

FIG. 11.12. This 80-year-old woman has esophageal carcinoma and new-onset twitching of right facial muscles, dysarthria, and confusion secondary to metastasis involving the left frontal calvarium with infiltration of the underlying meninges and cortex. The EEG shows left frontal polymorphic delta activity, which spreads intermittently to the right frontal area, attenuation of fast-frequency activity over the left frontal region, and left frontal epileptiform discharges (*arrows*).

spikes with oligodendroglioma and astrocytoma, but they do not correlate with clinical seizures (89,91). FIRDA is historically associated with subcortical tumors (27,169), but this statement must be qualified, as discussed above in the section on "Intermittent Rhythmic Delta Activity."

Although EEG can usually lateralize tumors accurately, more precise localization is often not possible (see Fig. 11.12). In addition to factors that produce more widespread changes in the EEG, such as mass effect and hydrocephalus, it has long been recognized empirically that EEG abnormalities are often "displaced" in relation to the tumor's anatomical location. Thus maximal delta activity may be more anterior, and the effect on alpha rhythm more posterior, than the lesion itself (46,85). In addition, abnormalities may have a temporal emphasis regardless of tumor location (166).

It is obviously not possible to determine the type of tumor by EEG, but several generic observations provide useful guidelines. Slow-growing extraaxial lesions, such as meningiomas, usually produce the least changes in the EEG. Rapidly growing intraparenchymal lesions, such as glioblastomas and malignant gliomas, result in the most pronounced abnormalities in terms of focal continuous polymorphic delta activity and localized attenuation of background rhythms (81). Bilateral but lateralized slow-wave activity is characteristic of frontal lobe tumors. Subfrontal and diencephalic tumors are most likely to produce bilateral but asymmetrical IRDA. Bilateral arrhythmic slowing with bursts of IRDA reflects hydrocephalus or mass effect with shift. Parasellar and hypothalamic tumors do not cause EEG changes unless they obstruct the third ventricle or extend into the temporal lobe on one side (124).

Gastaut and colleagues (56) studied 127 cases of brain tumor using both CT and EEG. They included both malignant and benign tumors. Intermittent or continuous focal delta activity occurred in 62% of the EEGs. The presence of surrounding edema, even when extensive, did not affect EEG findings. Other investigators have also found that cerebral edema does not contribute significantly to EEG findings (62,127). More recent studies using quantitative EEG analysis provide further evidence that vasogenic edema does not contribute to delta activity (44,45).

Intracranial Hemorrhage

Subdural hematomas that are not associated with significant compression or shift of the underlying brain produce little effect on the EEG. As with meningiomas, large subdural collections produce ipsilateral voltage attenuation, especially for faster frequency activity and variable amounts of arrhythmic slow-frequency activity (103) (Fig. 11.13). Very large lesions produce bilateral, sometimes generalized findings that are most pronounced on the side of the subdural hematoma (171).

EEG changes with acute subarachnoid hemorrhage (SAH) generally parallel the Hunter and Hess grading scale: grade I SAH may not be associated with any EEG abnormalities, whereas grade IV or V SAH produces severe, bilateral delta activity consistent with the patient's stupor or coma. Focal slow-wave activity indicates parenchymal extension of the hemorrhage or onset of vasospasm with ischemia corresponding to the affected vascular territory (117,172).

Acute intracerebral hemorrhage into the basal ganglia or centrum semiovale results in ipsilateral hemispheric polymorphic delta activity with more localized voltage attenuation and loss of faster frequencies over the hematoma (Fig. 11.14) (172). With large hemorrhages that produce midline shift and compression of diencephalic structures, there is bilateral slowing and bursts of ipsilateral IRDA (76). EEG effects of thalamic hemorrhages depend very much on lesion size. Small hemorrhages produce restricted or more widespread ipsilateral slowing depending on their location within the thalamus. Involvement of the ventrobasal thalamus attenuates sleep spindles and sometimes affects their frequency regulation. Lesions affecting the anteromedial thalamus attenuate the ipsilateral alpha activity (83) and usually produce frontotemporal delta activity as well. EEG findings with brainstem hemorrhage also depend on size and location, but tend to be similar to the range of effects described below for ischemic stroke.

Stroke

Because of its incidence and prevalence, stroke is the most common cause of continuous focal polymorphic delta activity (60,84).

Transient Ischemic Attacks

The EEG is usually normal in patients with transient ischemic attacks (41). However, if the EEG is performed at, or in close proximity to, the time a patient is symptomatic, there will often be focal slowing in the appropriate vascular territory, even though CT or routine MRI scans are likely to be normal (105,110). Chronic ischemia within the middle cerebral artery (MCA) territory is associated with intermittent, low-voltage delta or theta activity, mainly over the temporal areas (19,54). When focal

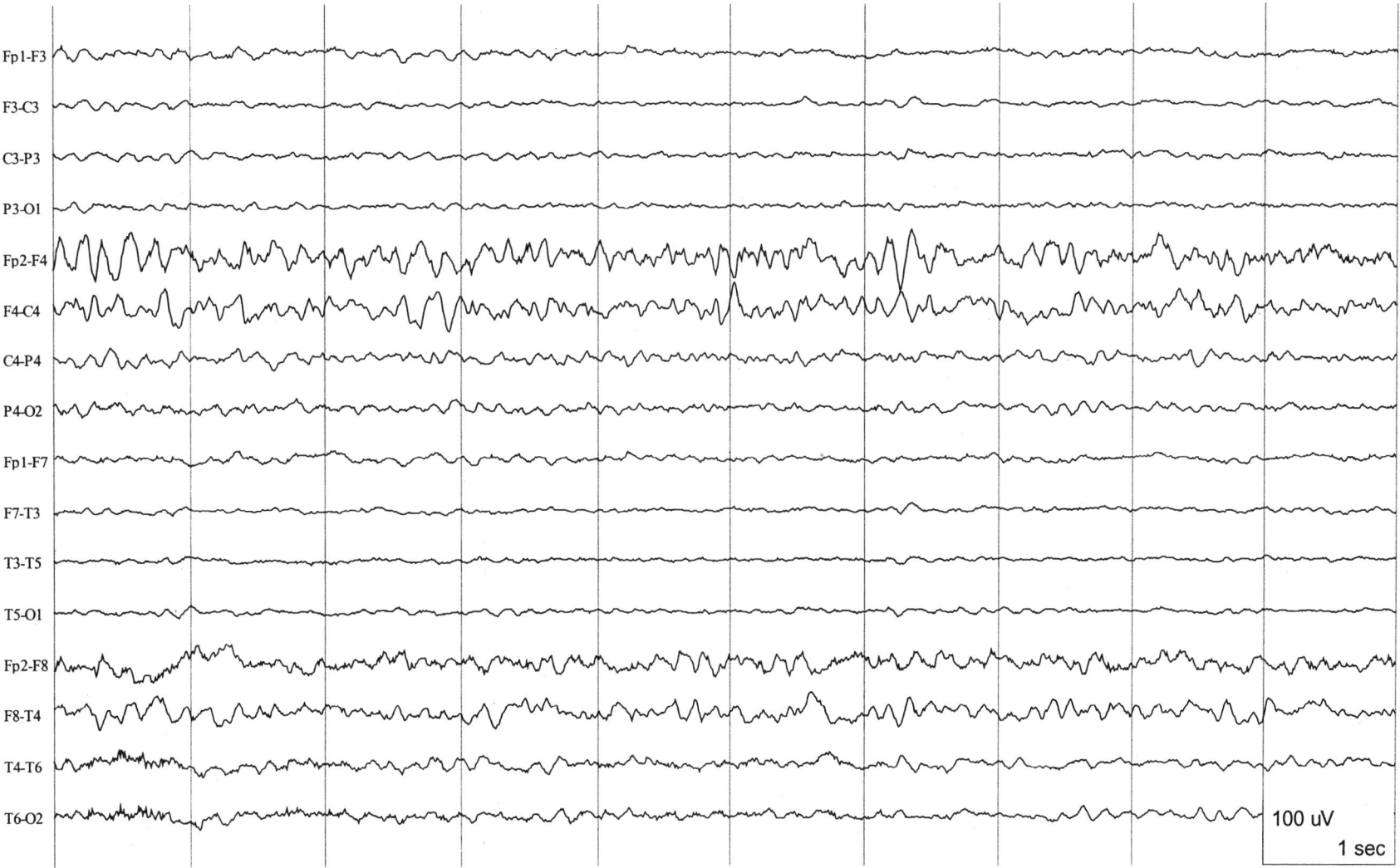

FIG. 11.13. EEG of an 81-year-old man following evacuation of a right subdural hematoma, who then developed an acute left-sided subdural hematoma. There is marked voltage attenuation and loss of faster frequency activity over the entire left hemisphere. There is continuous rhythmic and arrhythmic slowing over the right frontal region accompanied by enhanced voltage of both 6-Hz rhythmic activity and mixed-frequency beta activity in the same area. The increased voltage on the right is a postcraniotomy effect (breach rhythm).

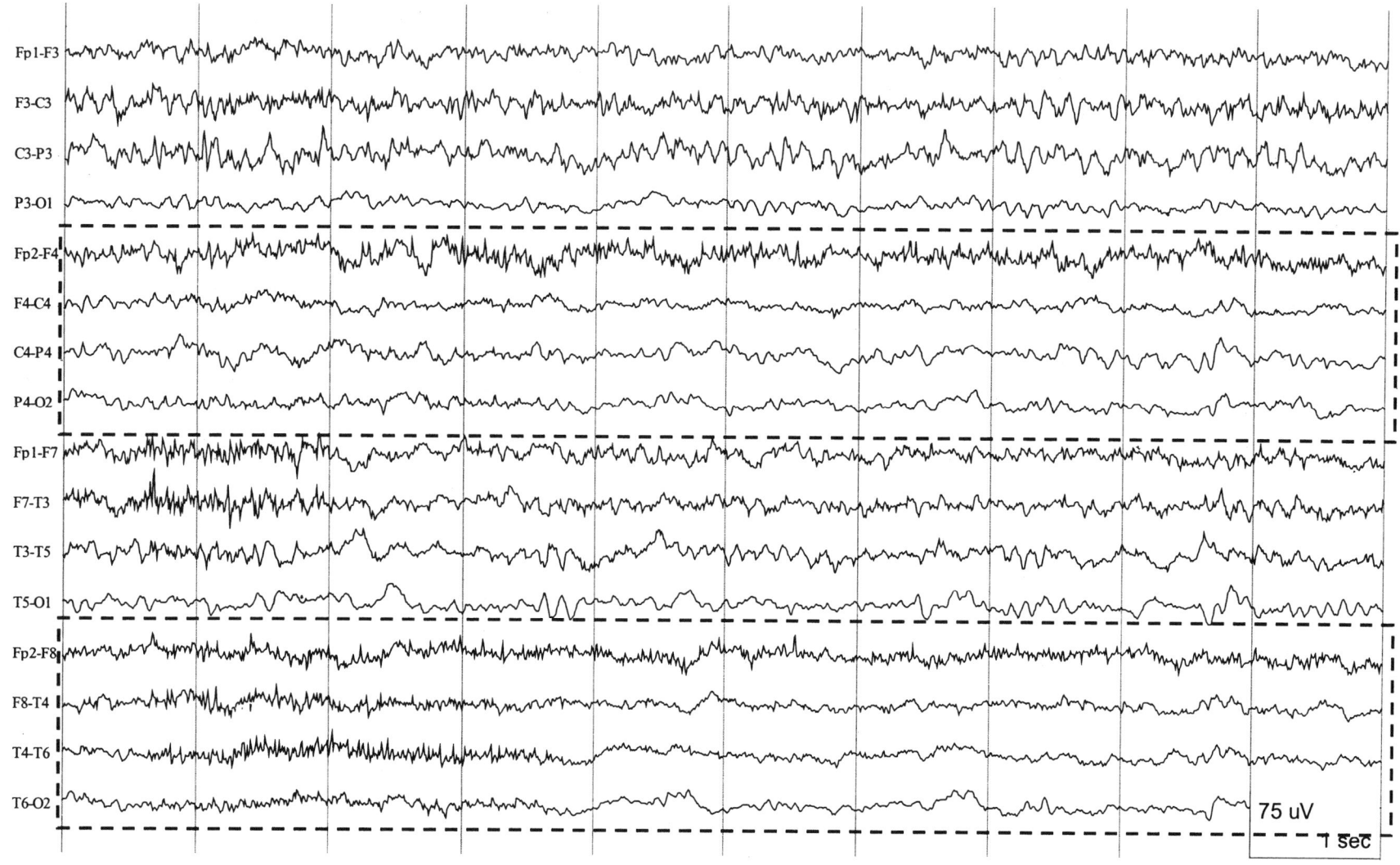

FIG. 11.14. EEG of a 67-year-old man with an acute hemorrhage into the right frontal lobe. Head CT showed the hemorrhage with a small right-to-left midline shift. There is nearly continuous arrhythmic delta activity over the right frontal and temporal regions with marked voltage attenuation of faster frequencies, especially in the right temporal area (*boxed channels*). There is also procedure slowing over the right hemisphere, but overall background activity is better preserved. The more rhythmic delta waves on the right spread to homologous regions on the left side.

or lateralized slow-wave activity is pronounced and of new onset, but the patient has no symptoms or signs, there is risk of vascular occlusion and impending infarction (182).

Ischemic Stroke: Large Infarcts

The major cause of ischemic stroke is occlusion of the internal carotid artery (ICA), the MCA, or one of its branches. Following acute occlusion of the ICA or MCA, there is widespread attenuation of all EEG activity for the first few hours (171). Polymorphic delta activity appears that is maximal over the anterior and midtemporal regions and, to a somewhat lesser extent, over the frontal area (Fig. 11.15). The alpha rhythm may be attenuated or show decreased reactivity on the side of the stroke. FIRDA is common, and this may paradoxically be of higher voltage contralaterally because of voltage attenuation on the ischemic side (171). Large infarcts are accompanied by cerebral edema and mass effect, which increase over the first 72 hours. PLEDs (see Fig. 11.10) and other epileptiform discharges occur in a minority of patients. These acute changes diminish and evolve over the next few weeks (171) (Fig. 11.16). Polymorphic slow activity becomes intermittent, and more theta frequencies appear as the amount of delta activity decreases. Faster frequencies and the overall complexity of background activity reappear to the extent that viable cortex remains. PLEDs are always a transient phenomenon and, if present, disappear over 2–3 weeks.

Strokes involving the anterior cerebral artery are less common than those involving the MCA. The EEG in such cases demonstrates delta activity over the ipsilateral frontal area, usually with attenuation of faster background frequencies. Infarctions within the territory supplied by the posterior cerebral artery produce focal slowing that is maximal over the ipsilateral posterior temporal, parietal, and occipital regions. There is usually complete loss or marked disruption of the alpha rhythm on the same side.

Uncomplicated strokes or other lesions of the lower pons and medulla (e.g., Wallenberg's syndrome) are not accompanied by EEG abnormalities. Lesions of the rostral pons and midbrain have variable effects on the EEG, largely dependent on the extent to which the reticular activating system is damaged. For example, patients with infarcts that affect the ventral pons but spare the pontine tegmentum produce the "locked-in syndrome," in which the patient is mute and quadriplegic because of disruption of descending motor pathways but fully conscious with a normal EEG because the reticular activating system is spared (71,107). When the reticular activating system in the rostral pons, midbrain, or thalamus is involved, patients are comatose, and their EEGs show various types of diffuse background abnormalities, including both rhythmic and arrhythmic frequencies, widespread paroxysmal theta and delta waves, and abnormal or absent reactivity to various stimuli (Fig. 11.17) (154). Rarely, lesions of the rostral brainstem show diffuse, monorhythmic alpha frequency activity that is a variation of the "alpha coma" pattern (181).

Frequency analysis and topographic EEG mapping may be superior to routine EEG in detecting and localizing focal abnormalities following stroke (129). These methods also seem to correlate more closely with regional cerebral blood flow (122,123,167).

Ischemic Strokes: Lacunar Infarction

Single lacunae or other discrete, small subcortical lesions usually produce little or no change in the EEG acutely: only 9% (104) to 13% (138) of lacunar infarctions are accompanied by ipsilateral slow-wave activity. Although 53% of patients with lacunar infarcts will have mild EEG abnormalities, most of these reflect previous strokes or are unexplained (86,138).

Role of the EEG in Stroke

Today, EEG plays only a limited role in management of patients with stroke. In the first 48–72 hours, the degree of focal slowing generally correlates with the clinical deficit. Clinical worsening as a result of stroke progression or the consequences of developing edema and mass effect is accompanied, and sometimes preceded, by deterioration in EEG activity. Marked hemispheric slowing following a transient ischemic attack, especially when routine head CT or brain MRI is normal, likely indicates marginal perfusion and chronic ischemia. This finding adds urgency to the evaluation and to the consideration of surgical or endovascular intervention. EEG monitoring during carotid endarterectomy can be helpful, because EEG changes (attenuation of cortical faster frequencies, with or without focal polymorphic delta activity) appear before irreversible ischemic injury occurs. If prolonged or severe, such changes are strongly associated with postoperative clinical deficits (29). EEG monitoring can help distinguish epileptic from ischemic causes of episodic neurological dysfunction. Epileptiform discharges, including PLEDs, are highly correlated with clinical seizures occurring during the first few weeks following a stroke (77). Finally, EEG is essential to identify patients who, although completely paralyzed and unable to speak, are conscious and aware (the locked-in syndrome).

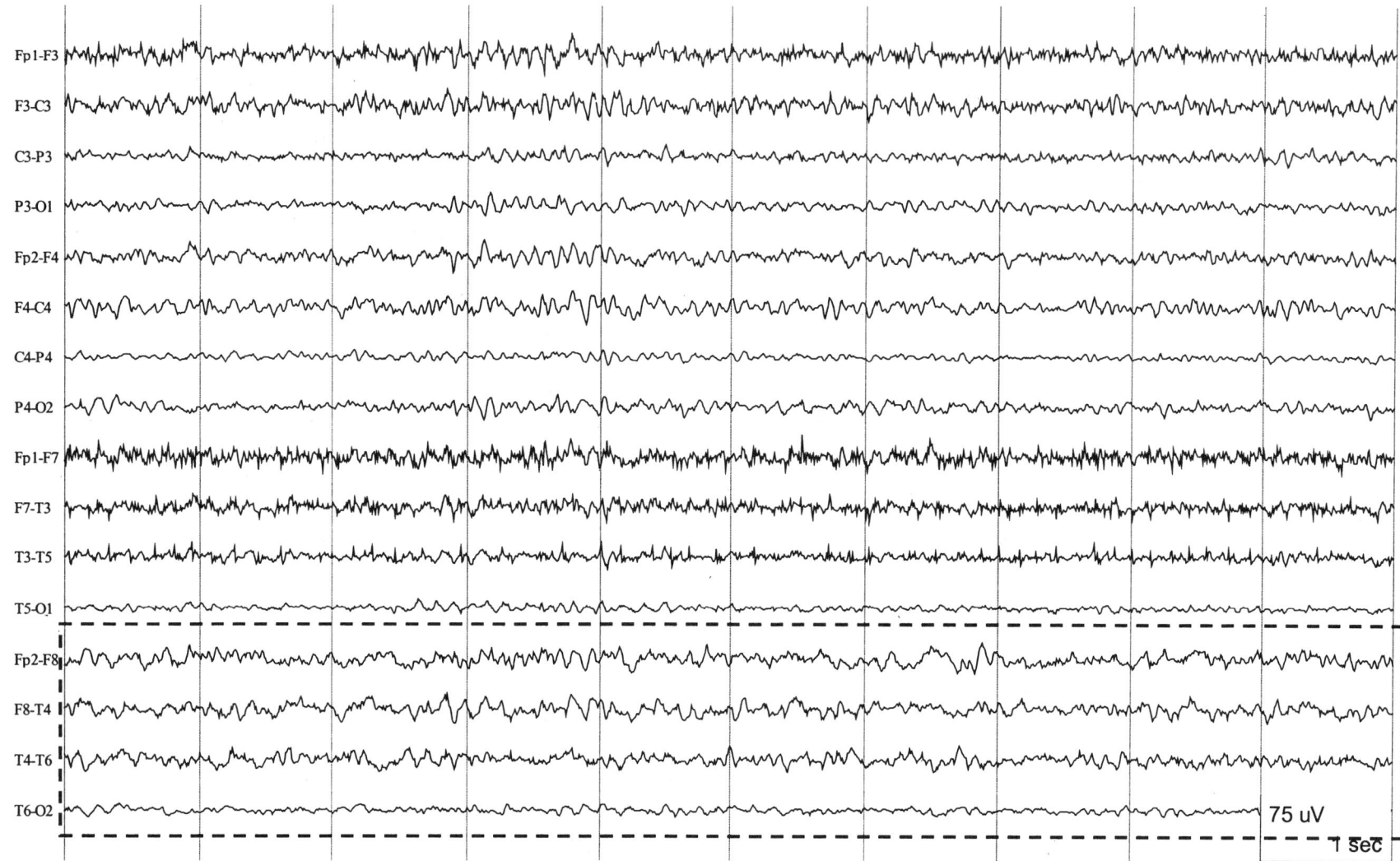

A

FIG. 11.15. EEGs of an 82-year-old woman with subacute infarction involving the right middle cerebral artery territory. **A:** With the patient awake, there is continuous polymorphic delta activity with voltage attenuation of all frequencies over the right hemisphere. **B:** With the patient asleep, note absence of sleep spindles over the right hemisphere. (*Figure continues.*)

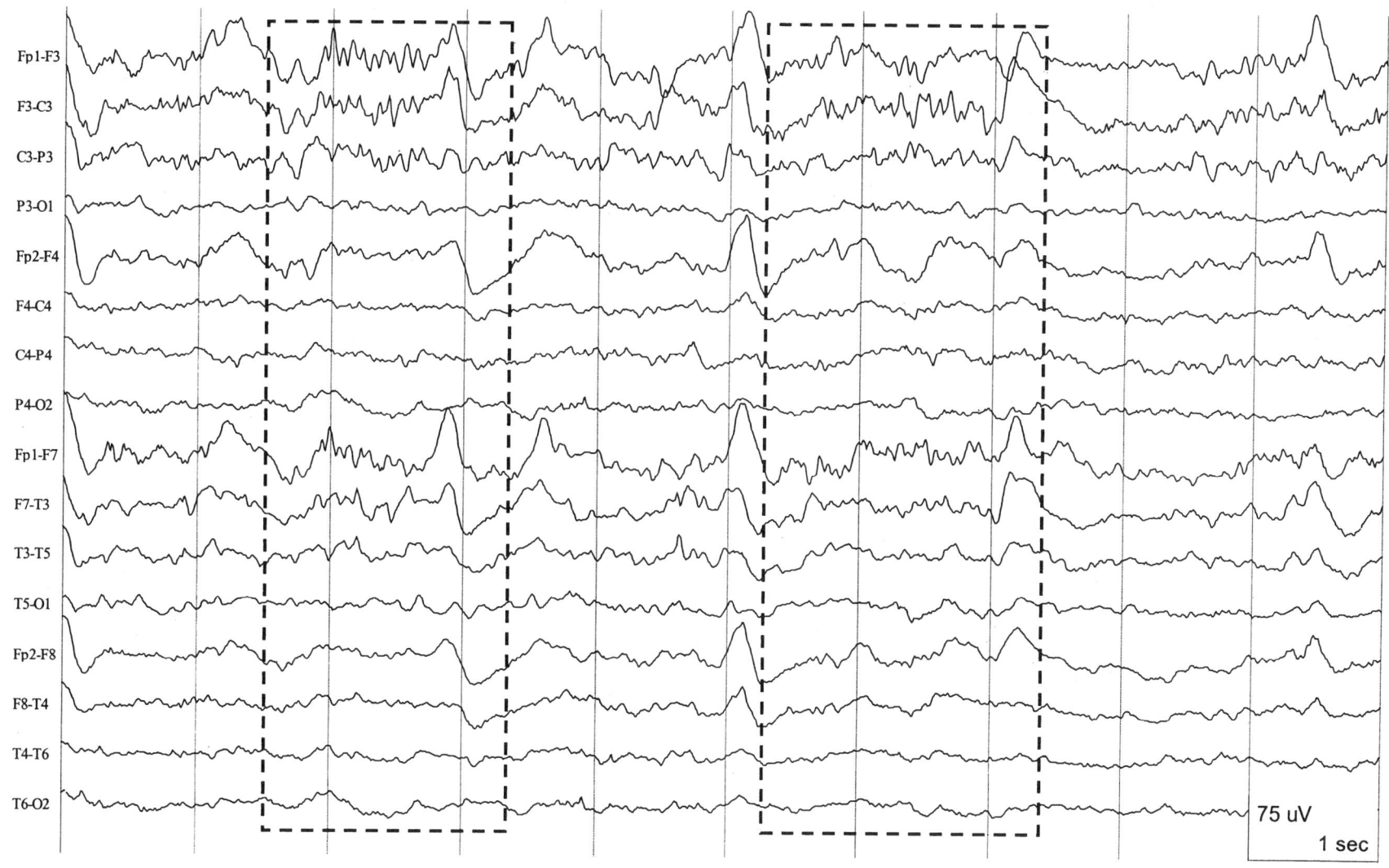

B

FIG. 11.15. *Continued.*

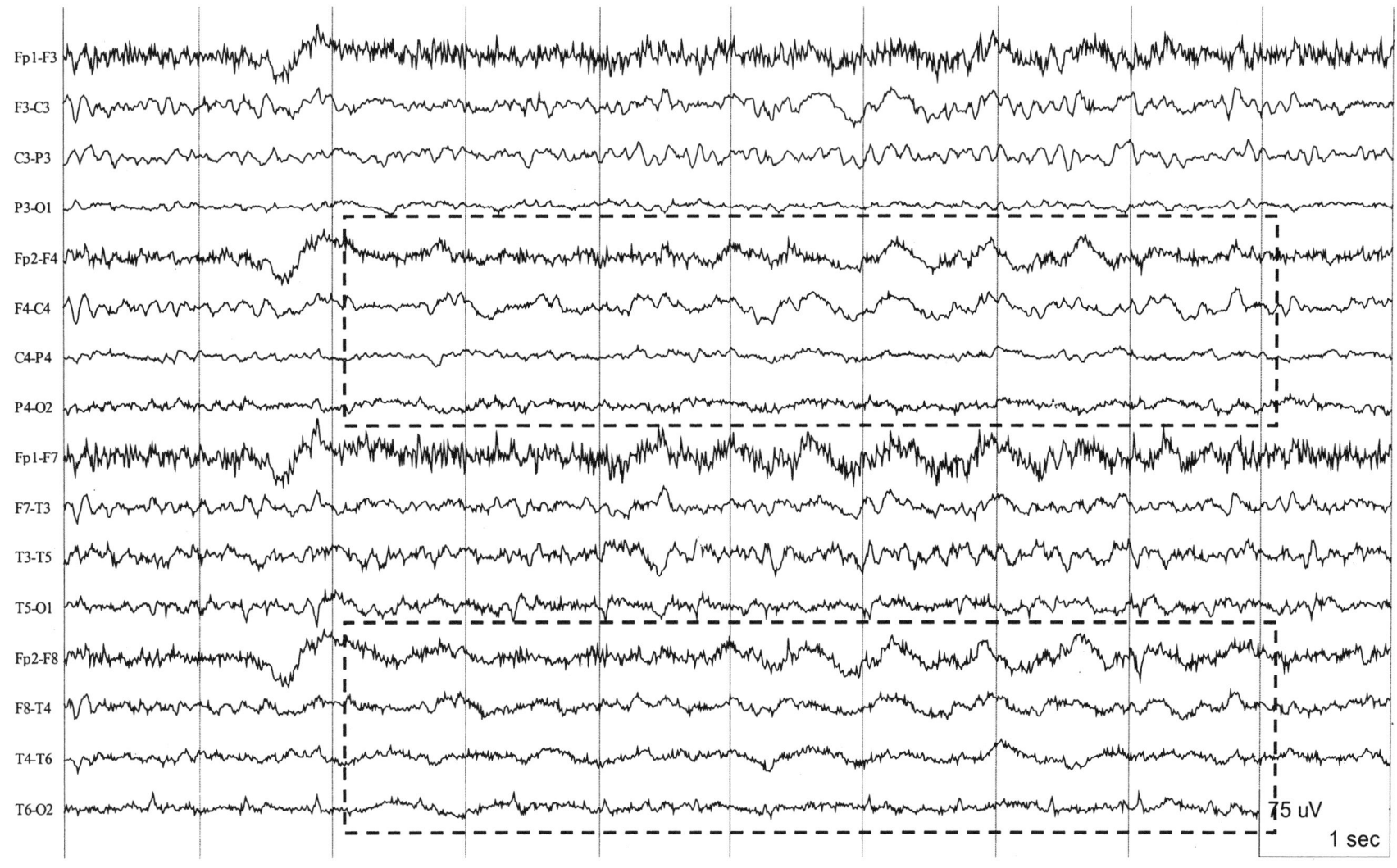

FIG. 11.16. EEG of an 82-year-old woman with an old right middle cerebral artery stroke. There is continuous focal polymorphic delta activity over the right temporal region.

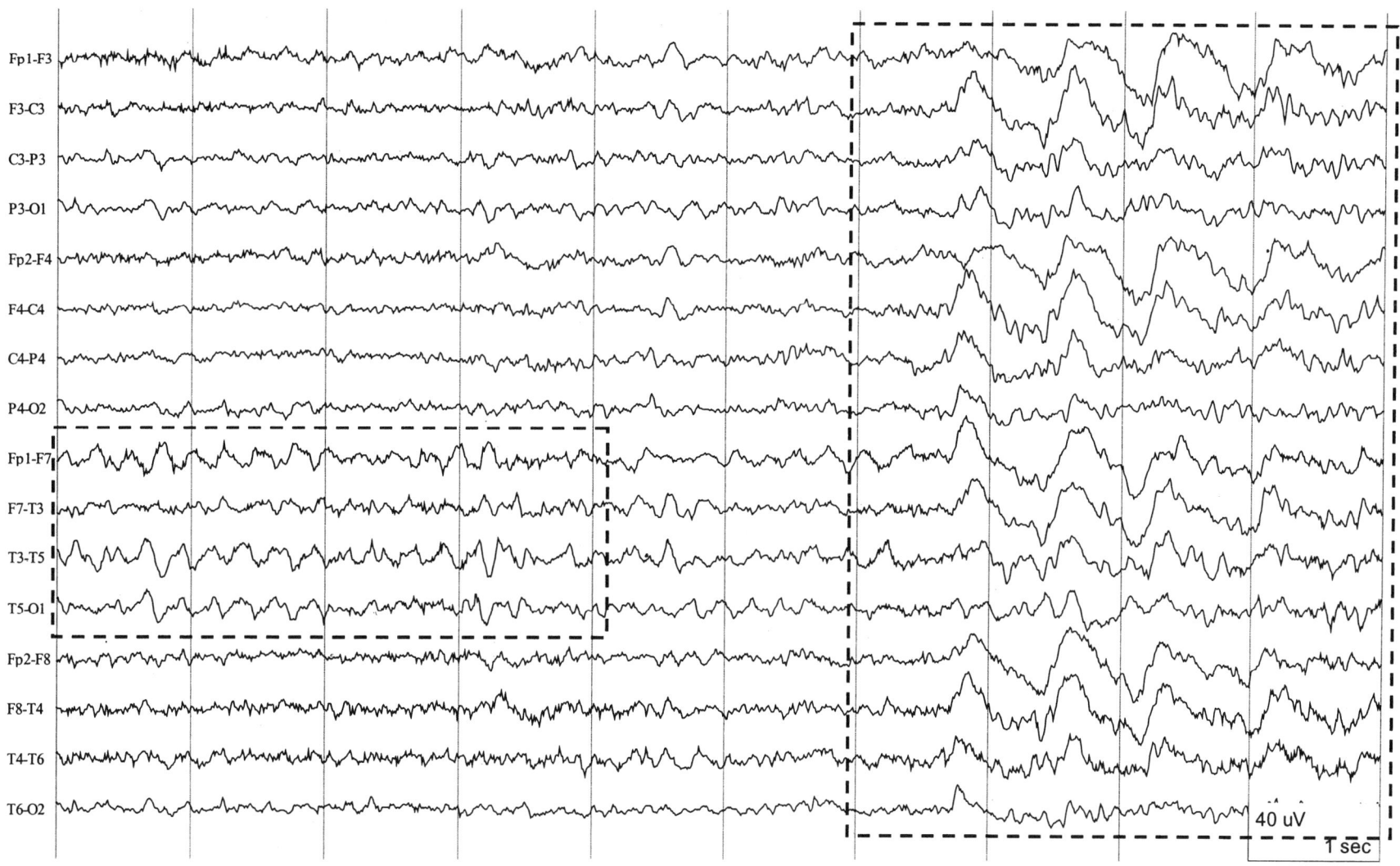

FIG. 11.17. This 70-year-old man has acute infarcts of the left basal ganglia and right thalamus. An EEG with the patient drowsy shows runs of intermittent rhythmic 4- to 5-Hz activity over the left temporal region (*left boxed area*) and bursts of 1.5- to 2-Hz FIRDA (*right boxed area*).

Brain Abscess

EEG findings caused by cerebral abscess are similar to those seen with brain tumors (Fig. 11.18). Focal polymorphic delta activity is the most common finding (5,37,114,139,184), and this tends to be both very slow (0.5–2 Hz) and of high voltage (140). As with tumors, EEG changes are related not just to the lesion itself, but also to mass effects that may be present. Edema, per se, does not play a significant role (114). Epileptiform discharges occur frequently and are often abundant around bacterial abscesses, and seizures occur in nearly three-fourths of patients. PLEDs occur but are rare (114). Epileptiform activity at the time of diagnosis and treatment does not predict later epilepsy (101). Most EEG changes disappear following surgery, although residual focal slow-wave activity will persist, declining over several years following treatment (101).

Focal Cortical Dysplasia

Focal cortical dysplasia is a common cause of epilepsy, especially in children. Raymond et al. (146) studied 22 patients with localized cortical dysgenesis and seizures beginning in childhood (age 3 weeks to 10 years). The main EEG findings were (a) generally preserved, age-appropriate background rhythms; (b) localized slow-wave activity in half of the patients; and (c) epileptiform discharges in 20 of 22 patients. A distinctive feature of the epileptiform activity was that it was either continuous or nearly so. Other reports have also emphasized the presence of focal polymorphic delta activity (15) and rhythmic epileptiform discharges (51,145) in these patients. A minority of patients have had abnormal focal fast-frequency activity (142,145) (Fig. 11.19).

Epilepsy

Focal slowing is frequently present in patients with localization-related epilepsy; it occurs both with and without associated sharp waves (Fig. 11.20). Epilepsy is the most common cause of continuous focal polymorphic delta activity in patients with nonlesional brain imaging studies (60,110). In the great majority of cases, focal delta activity is ipsilateral to the epileptogenic brain area, although rarely the delta activity is maximal on the contralateral side (128,137). Intermittent focal polymorphic delta activity localized to the temporal region is a common finding in patents with medial temporal lobe epilepsy and hippocampal sclerosis (95,137). Such slowing most likely reflects multiple factors, including microscopic changes in the epileptogenic tissue (neuron loss, abnormal neuron morphology, gliosis) and nonepileptic

physiological dysfunction within the epileptogenic cortex. When the scalp-recorded delta activity is rhythmic, chronically implanted depth electrodes occasionally reveal ictal discharges restricted to deep structures.

Migraine

A variety of abnormalities have been reported in migraine, including generalized or focal slowing, exaggerated responses to hyperventilation and photic stimulation, excessive fast activity, changes in the alpha rhythm, and epileptiform discharges. These have been reviewed by Gronseth and Greenberg (69). However, much of this literature is difficult to interpret because control groups were usually not included, definitions of "normal" and "abnormal" have changed, and recording techniques were inconsistent (69,156). During classical visual auras, the EEG can be normal, show posterior delta activity, or demonstrate loss of the normal alpha rhythm (8,152). Enhanced photic driving is frequently cited as being typical of migraine (161,163), but there is, in fact, little convincing evidence to support significant differences in photic responses between migraineurs and healthy individuals without migraine (65). Beaumanoir and Jekiel (8) described repetitive spike discharges that disappeared with onset of headache. There does appear to be a slightly increased incidence of nonspecific abnormalities such as intermittent focal (usually temporal) or generalized slow-frequency activity during and after common or classical migraine attacks, but these are the exception, not the rule (66).

During hemiplegic migraine, there is contralateral delta activity, which is sometimes accompanied by attenuation of beta activity (57,73,183). EEGs obtained during attacks of basilar migraine, which can present as a confusional state in children, sometimes show generalized slow-frequency activity and extended runs of high-voltage rhythmic delta waves over the posterior head regions (52,100). Occipital spikes have been reported in some patients with basilar migraine (121,136), and Gastaut (53) found that about one-third of children with benign focal epilepsy of childhood with occipital spikes had migraine-like headaches (see Chapter 17 for further discussion). Migraine is common, however, and its coexistence with other disorders (e.g., epilepsy) or epileptiform EEG findings (12,61) should not be unexpected (7,109).

Because there are no EEG findings that are diagnostic of migraine or that distinguish different types of headache, there is little justification for obtaining EEGs routinely as part of the evaluation of patients with headache. The exception to this is the small subgroup of patients with atypical headache, and in whom the differential diagnosis includes both migraine and epilepsy (69,141). In such cases, EEG may aid in making a diagnosis of epilepsy.

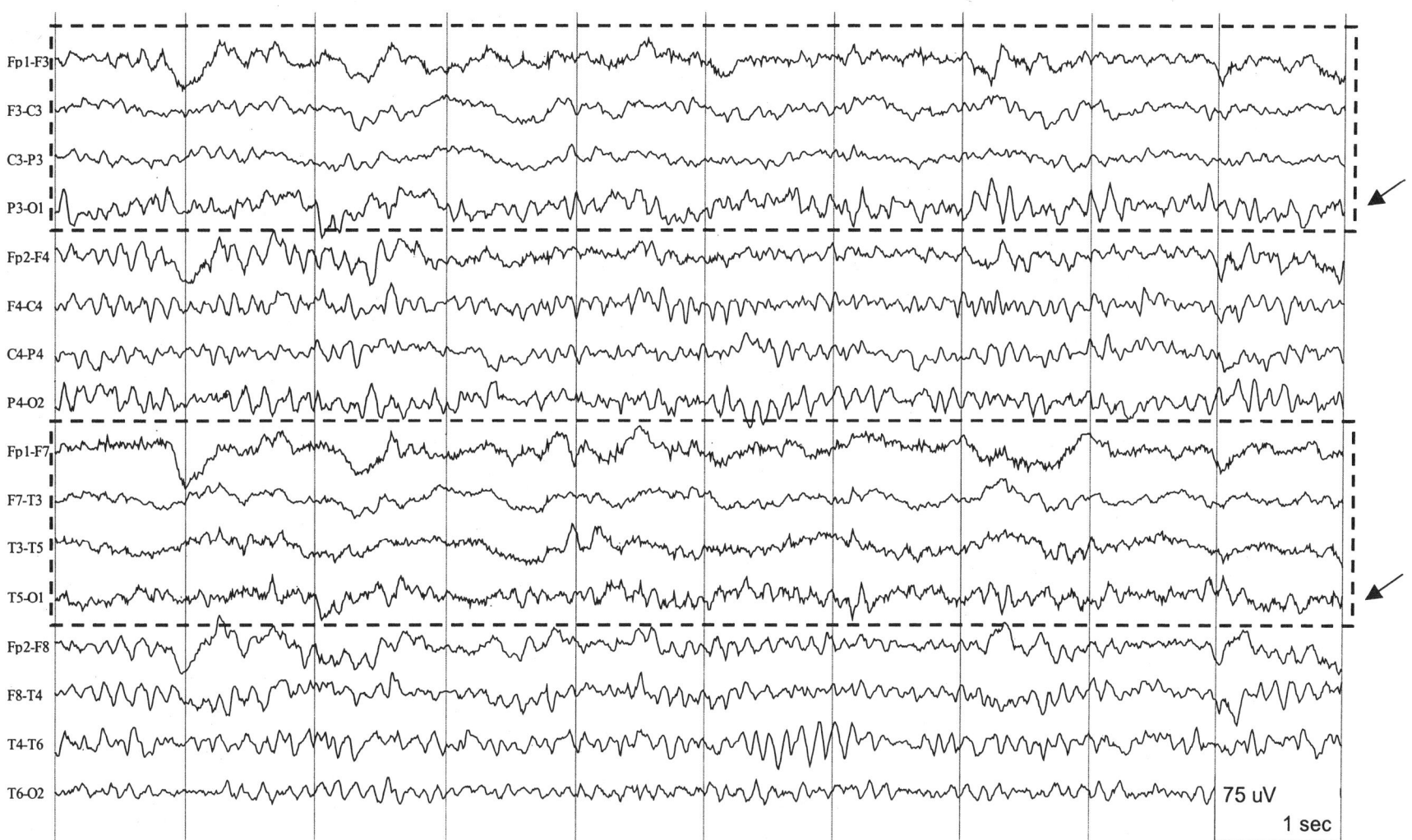

FIG. 11.18. EEG of a 36-year-old woman with a history of ulcerative colitis and abscesses involving the left frontal lobe. She has a right hemiparesis and aphasia. Note continuous arrhythmic delta activity over the left temporal and frontal areas. Faster frequencies are attenuated in the same region. The parieto-occipital regions are relatively uninvolved, although the alpha rhythm is disorganized and poorly modulated on the left.

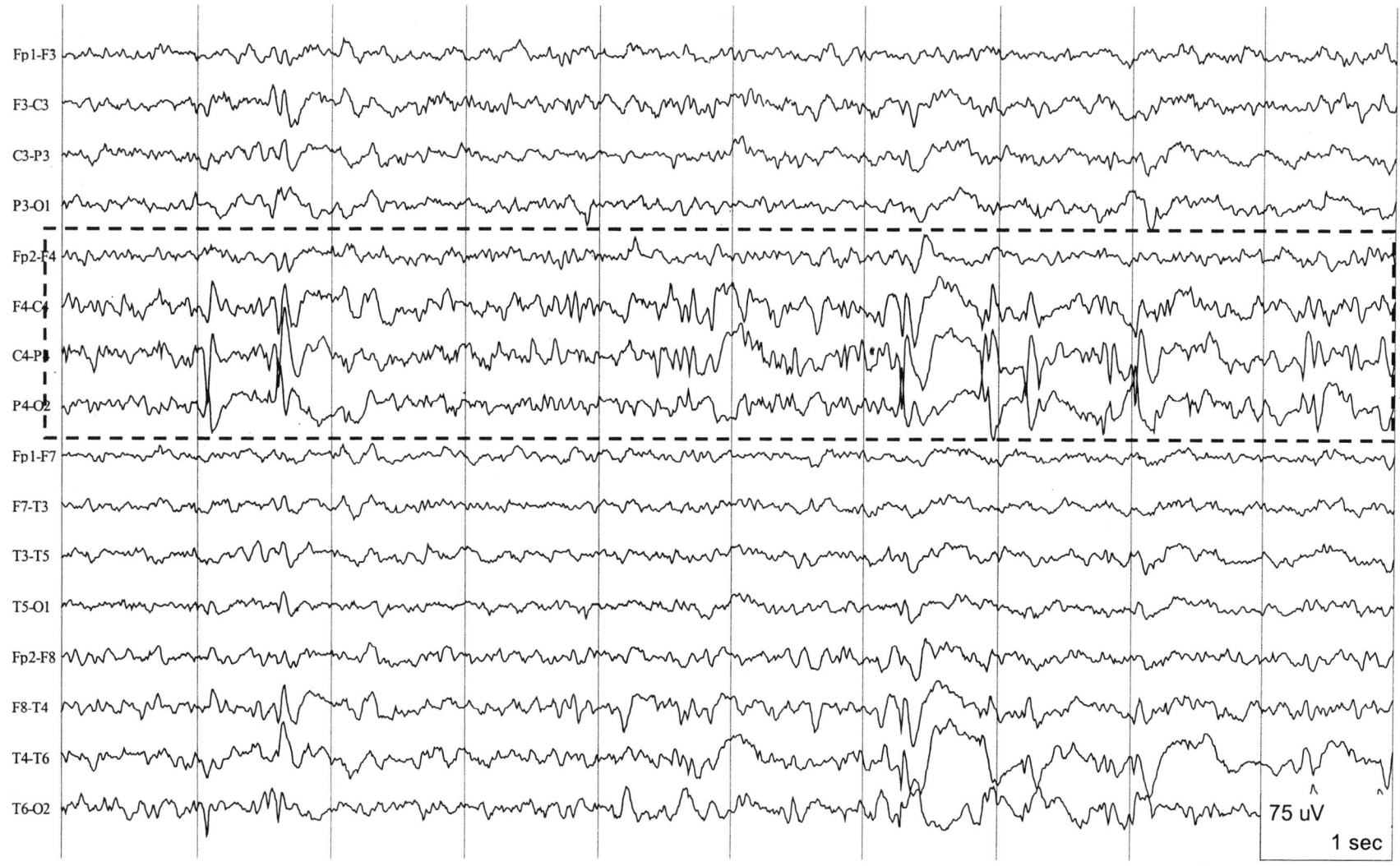

A

FIG. 11.19. EEGs of a 12-year-old girl with intractable nocturnal secondarily generalized seizures and cortical dysplasia involving the right parietal lobe. **A:** There are frequent spikes in the right parietal region that also involve the posterior temporal and occipital areas on that side. (*Figure continues.*)

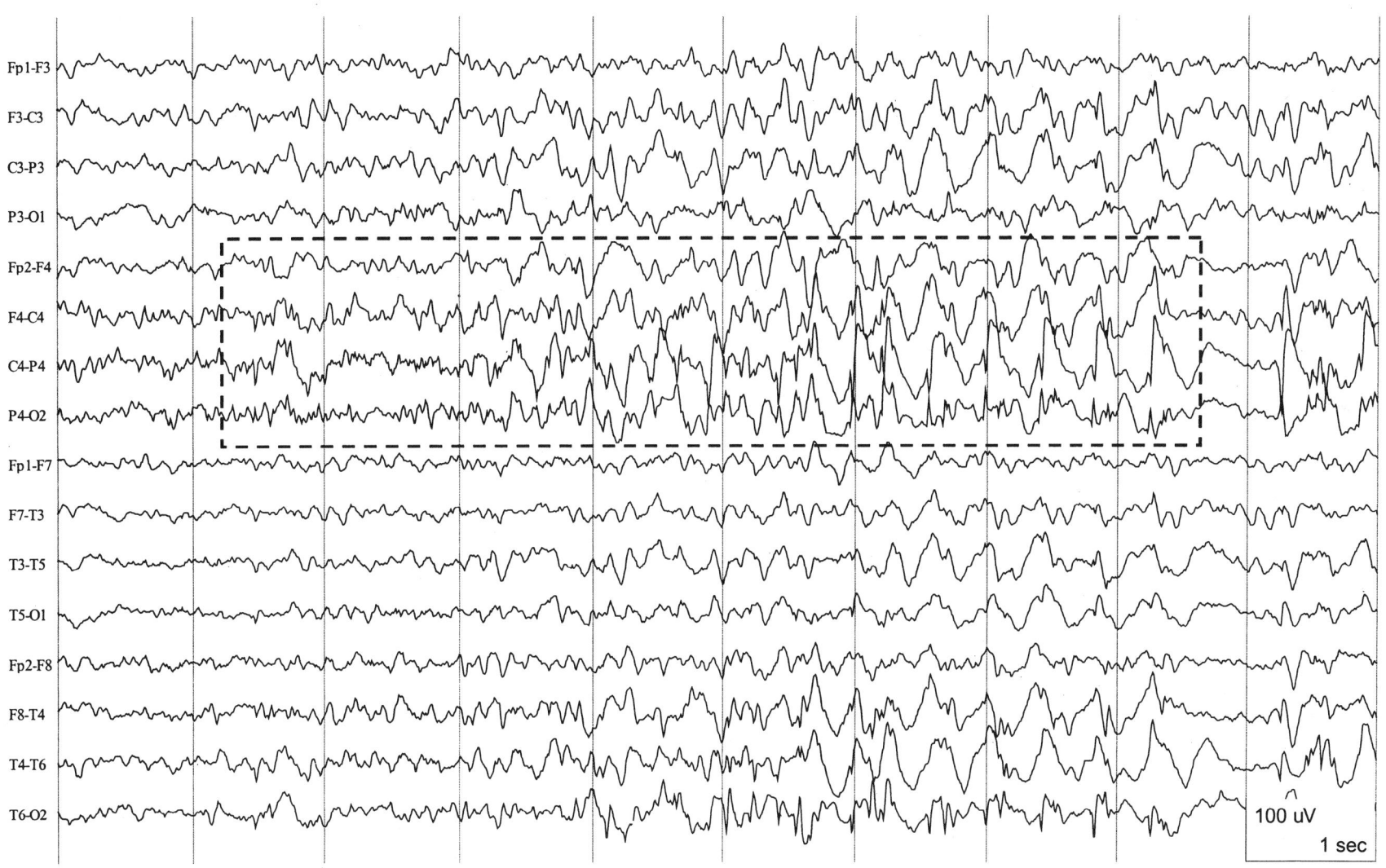

FIG. 11.19. *Continued.* **B:** A brief ictal episode arising from the right parietal region with buildup of spikes and rhythmic 5-Hz activity that slows to 2.5-Hz activity. There is contralateral spread. There were no clinical manifestations. (*Figure continues.*)

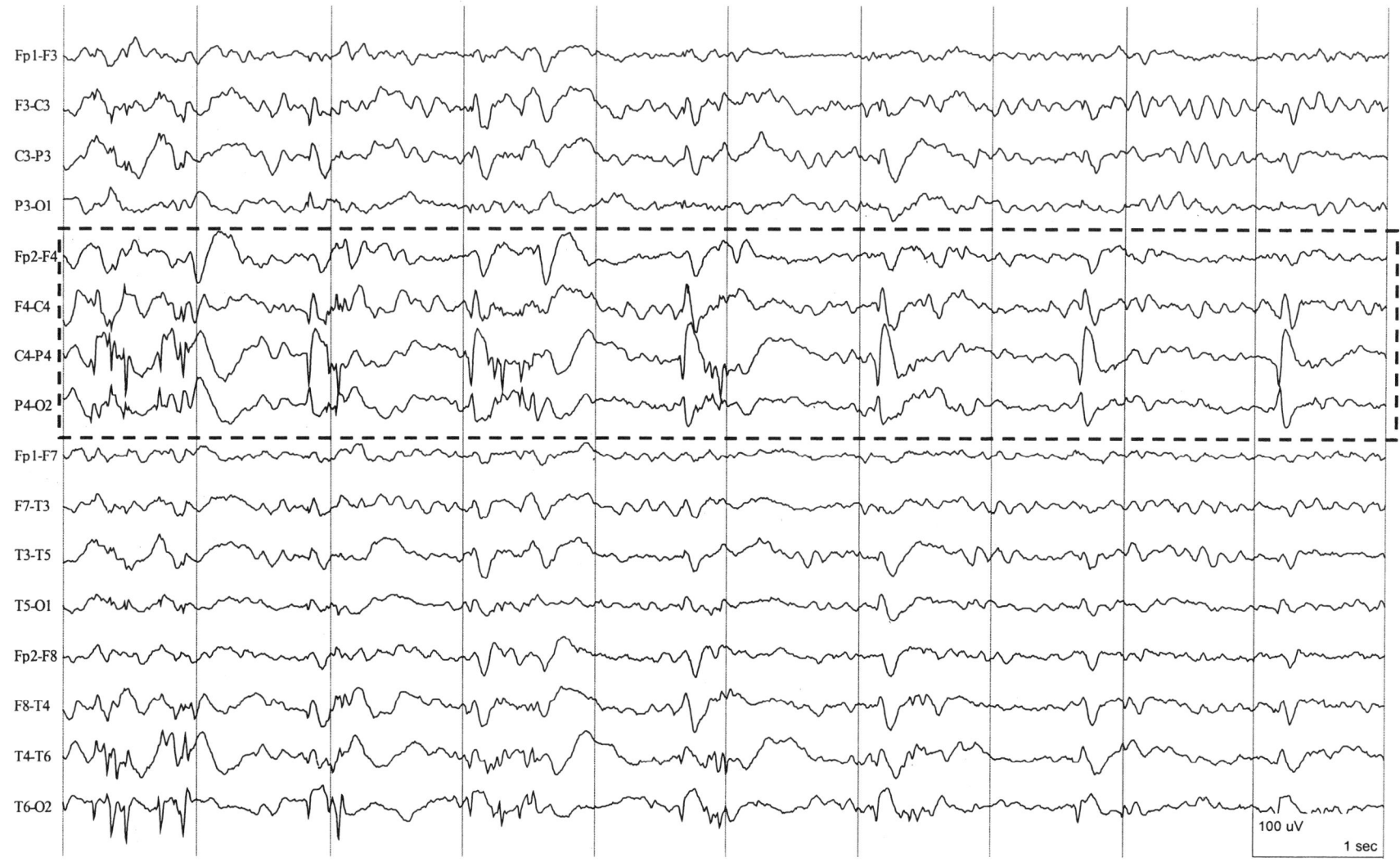

FIG. 11.19. *Continued.* **C:** This subclinical seizure ends with bursts of semirhythmic spikes and multiple spikes associated with voltage attenuation of background activity. (*Figure continues.*)

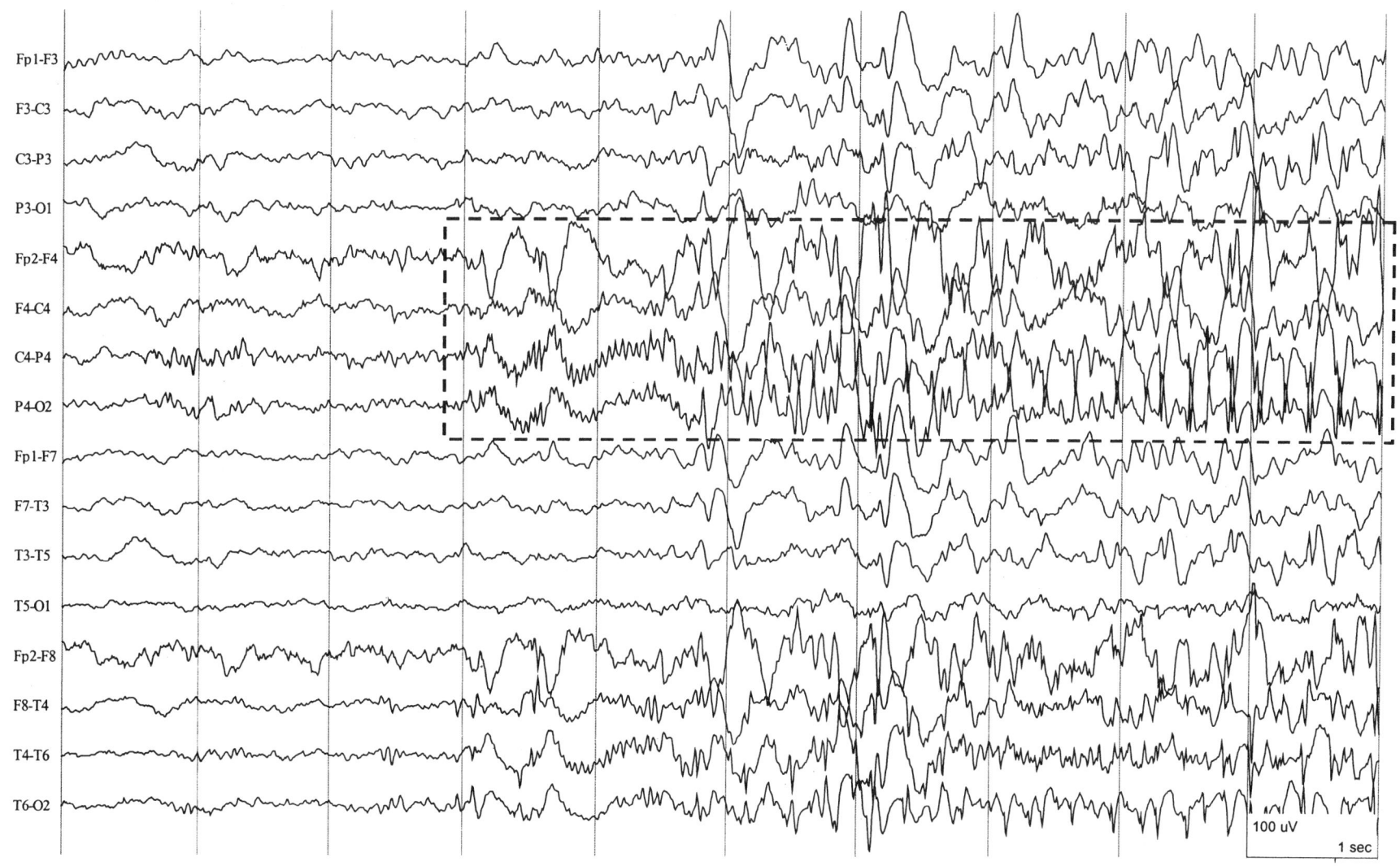

FIG. 11.19. *Continued.* **D:** A clinical seizure begins with paroxysmal beta activity in the right parietal region followed by rhythmic 6- to 8-Hz spikes at P4 that gradually slow to about 5 Hz in the last 3 seconds of the page. There is spread of rhythmic slow waves to the left side, and intermittent spikes occur at P3 and T5.

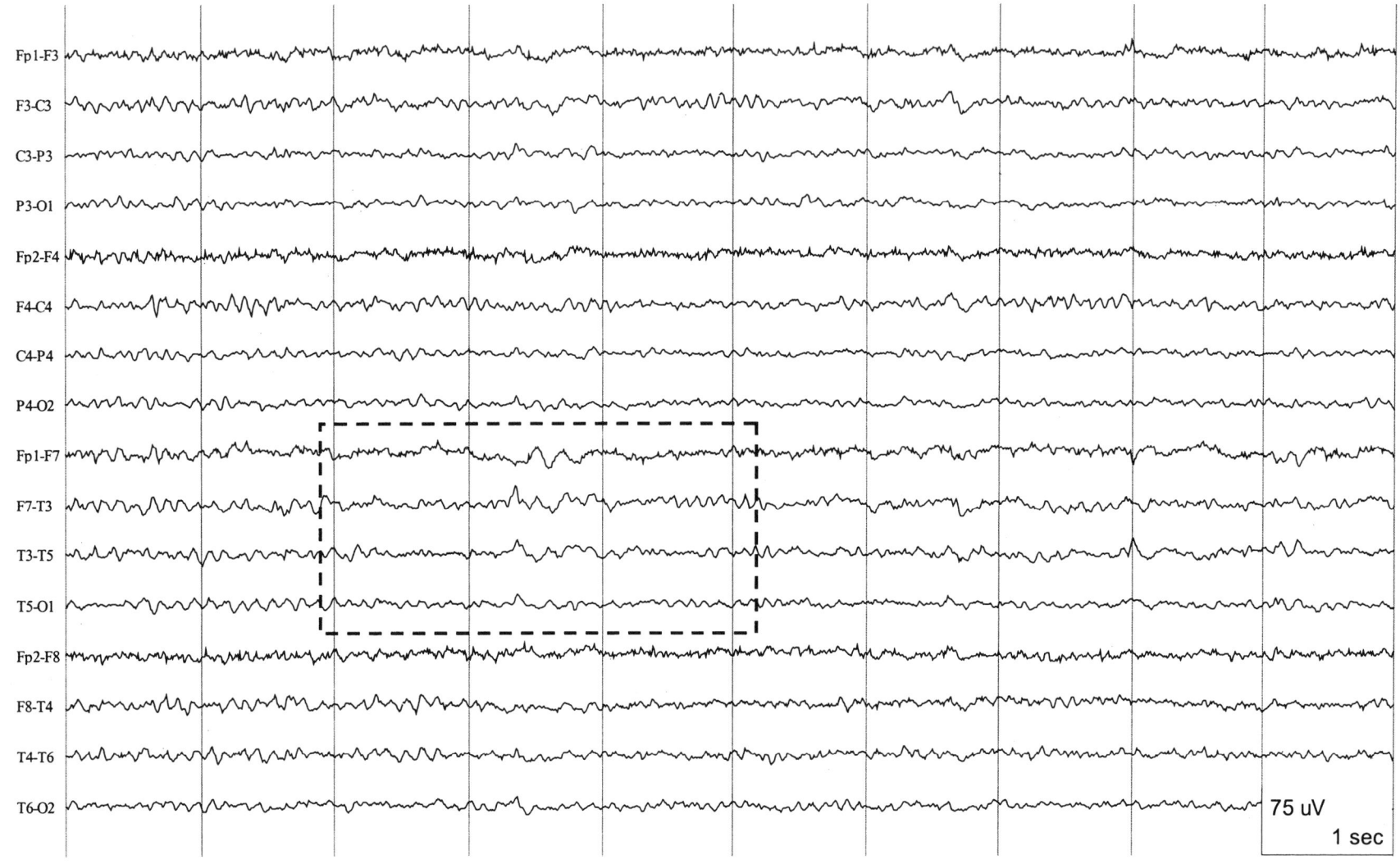

A

FIG. 11.20. EEGs of a 66-year-old man with a 10-year history of episodes he characterized as "loss of time."
A: There is intermittent arrhythmic slowing over the left temporal region during drowsiness (*boxed channels*).
(*Figure continues.*)

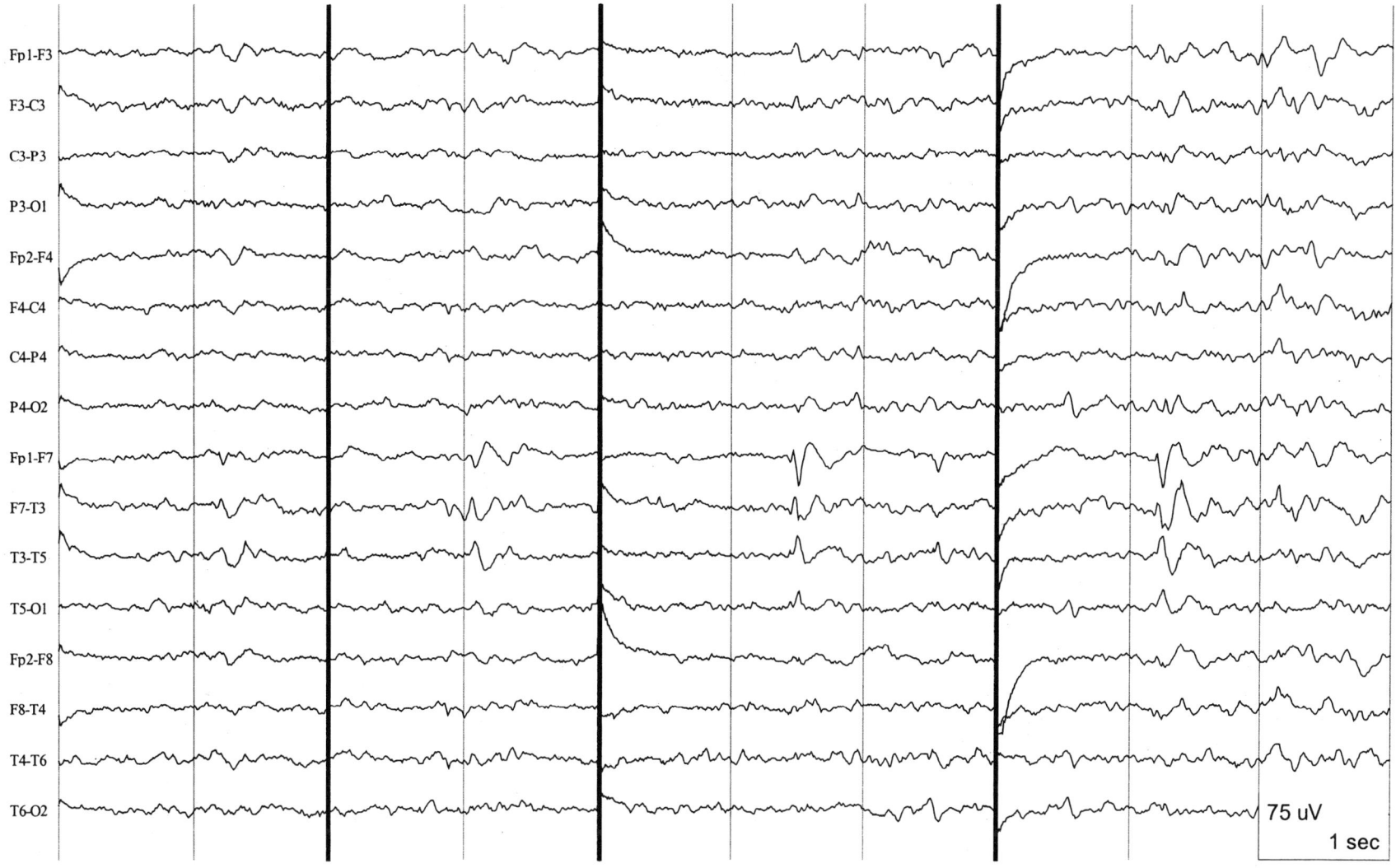

75 uV

1 sec

B

FIG. 11.20. *Continued.* **B:** During stage 2 sleep, there are frequent spikes and sharp waves in the same area.

Temporal Slowing in the Elderly

The amount of both diffuse and focal slow-frequency activity increases with age, and the degree of these changes correlates with impaired cognition and decreased longevity (120,159). This correlation is best for moderate or severe changes, because mild slowing of EEG activity does not preclude normal intellectual function (130,131). Focal theta and delta activity is common over the temporal regions, especially the left, in persons over the age of 60 (93,132,159). In a study of 424 volunteers of all ages, Busse and Obrist (20) found that 20% of people between the ages of 40 and 59 years had focal theta activity over the temporal areas; this was maximal on the left in 80% of cases. In persons between 60 and 79 years of age, focal theta and delta activity was seen in 40%. Kooi and colleagues (93) studied 218 "neurologically intact" adults; 37 of these were over 60 years of age. Two-thirds of this group had temporal theta activity, and one-third had temporal delta activity. The slowing was enhanced by drowsiness. There was no medical or other historical explanation for the slow-frequency activity.

Some earlier investigators had argued that these changes indicate subclinical pathology and should not be attributed to "normal aging" (130). Subsequent studies of carefully selected neurologically and psychologically normal elderly persons supported this view. Katz and Horowitz (87) studied healthy septuagenarians and found that focal slow-wave activity in the theta range occurred in only 17% of EEG records and, when present, occupied no more than 1% of waking background activity. Delta activity was rare and consisted only of random, single transients. In studying normal subjects 65 years of age and older, Visser and coworkers (176) reported that temporal delta activity correlated with decreased performance on a verbal fluency test consistent with temporal lobe dysfunction.

What conclusions can be drawn from these observations, and how should they affect interpretation of focal slow-wave activity in elderly individuals? First, there are people over 60–65 years of age who have few of the EEG findings traditionally attributed to normal aging. Second, focal slow-wave activity over one or both temporal regions is nonetheless common in older persons who are functioning normally at home and in their communities, and whose routine neurological examinations are normal. Third, the more prominent the focal slowing in terms of frequency (delta), voltage, and persistence, the more likely it is to be associated with focal dysfunction and symptoms. Finally, it is useful to define, for practical clinical purposes, focal slow-wave activity that is "benign" and of little use in drawing infer-

ences that are helpful in diagnosis or management. Such benign focal slow-wave activity of the elderly is temporal in location, predominantly in the theta frequency range, intermittent, and either rhythmic or arrhythmic. It occurs mainly in drowsiness, but sometimes appears when patients are alert. Focal slowing that meets these criteria should be interpreted conservatively and not considered strongly indicative of structural pathology.

Viral Encephalitis

EEG findings are particularly important in the diagnosis of encephalitis caused by herpes simplex virus, type 1 (HSV-1), and some reports have suggested that a normal EEG excludes the diagnosis (1,39,99). Many types of abnormalities have been described, including focal or diffuse slow-wave activity, focal epileptiform discharges, electrical seizure patterns, localized attenuation of background activity, and PLEDs (1,24,70, 79,116,168). Because HSV-1 causes severe hemorrhagic necrosis mainly of the inferior and medial parts of the temporal lobes and the orbital frontal regions, focal or lateralized findings that are maximal in these areas are highly suggestive of herpes encephalitis and can also be helpful in determining the best site for brain biopsy (24,99) (Fig. 11.21). The acute destructive nature of the lesions probably accounts for the frequency with which PLEDs are seen. PLEDs appear in the acute phase of the illness, usually between the fifth and twelfth day after onset of neurological symptoms (99). They consist of 100- to 500-μV sharply contoured slow waves or polyphasic spikes that typically recur at 1.5- to 2.5-second intervals, although both slower and faster rates can be seen (1,22,99,116,144, 170). The periodic complexes are usually unilateral, but they can be bilateral and occur either independently or time locked on the two sides (162). PLEDs usually appear before changes on head CT (18,42,88) but not before abnormalities on brain MRI.

Although the periodic pattern is usually seen in adults with herpes simplex encephalitis, it has been reported in infants and children (22,162). Some authors have reported that periodic complexes are associated with increased mortality (24,40), whereas others have disputed this (79,99).

Herpes simplex virus, type 2, causes encephalitis in neonates, and this is also associated with a distinctive periodic EEG pattern (115,118,151). The periodic discharges are not restricted to the temporal areas and are often multifocal. Each site of discharge has its own morphology and periodic interval. Focal spikes and seizures are also common. Other forms of focal encephalitis cause focal slowing and spikes, but PLEDs are rare.

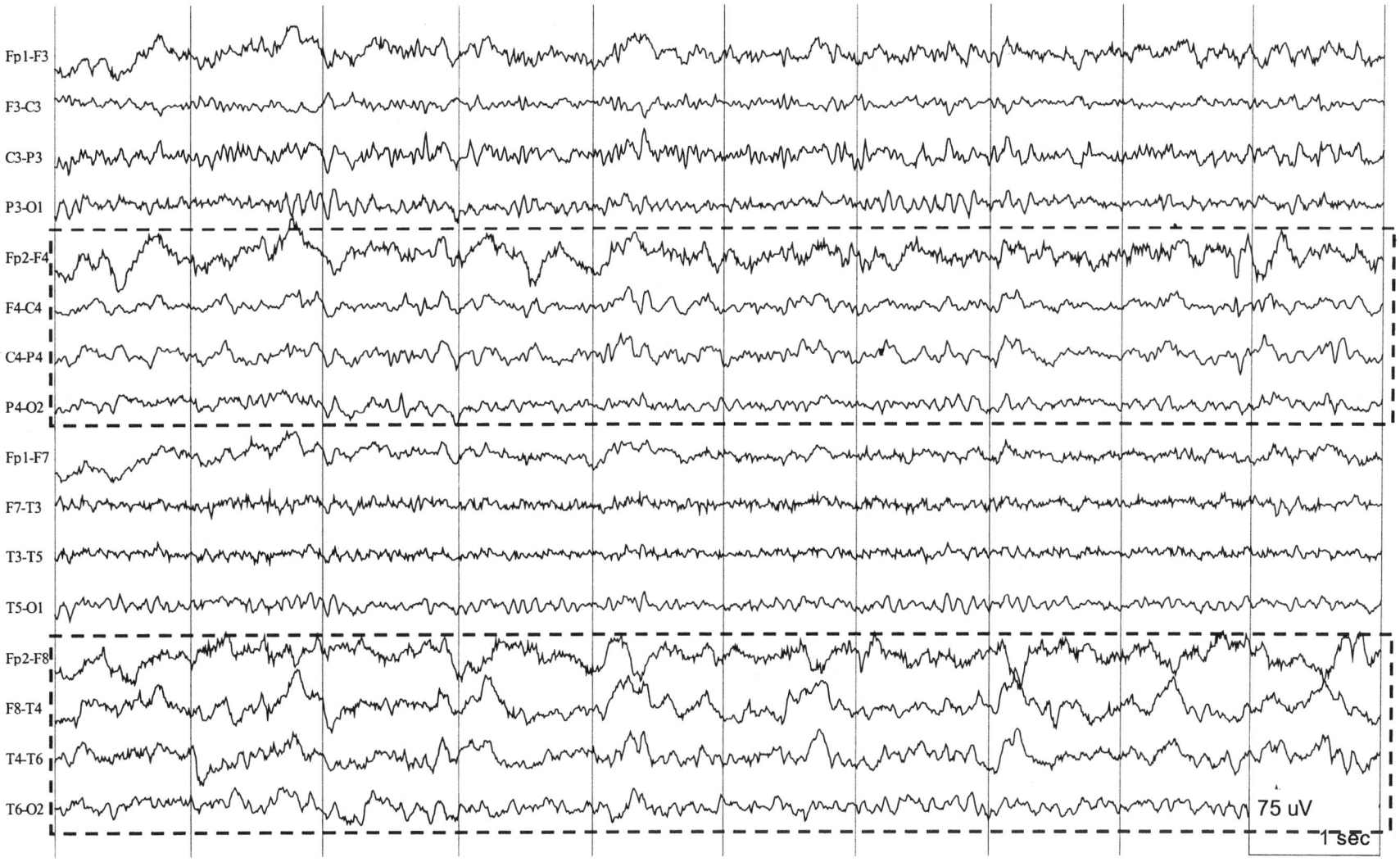

FIG. 11.21. EEG of a 64-year-old woman with herpes simplex encephalitis affecting mainly the right temporal lobe and orbital region of the right frontal lobe. There is continuous arrhythmic and semirhythmic delta activity of medium to high amplitude over the right temporal, frontal, and frontal-polar regions. Lower voltage polymorphic delta and theta activity are seen over the entire right hemisphere, and the alpha rhythm is largely absent on that side. Although the right frontal slow activity spreads to contralateral homologous regions, left hemisphere activity is otherwise relatively well preserved.

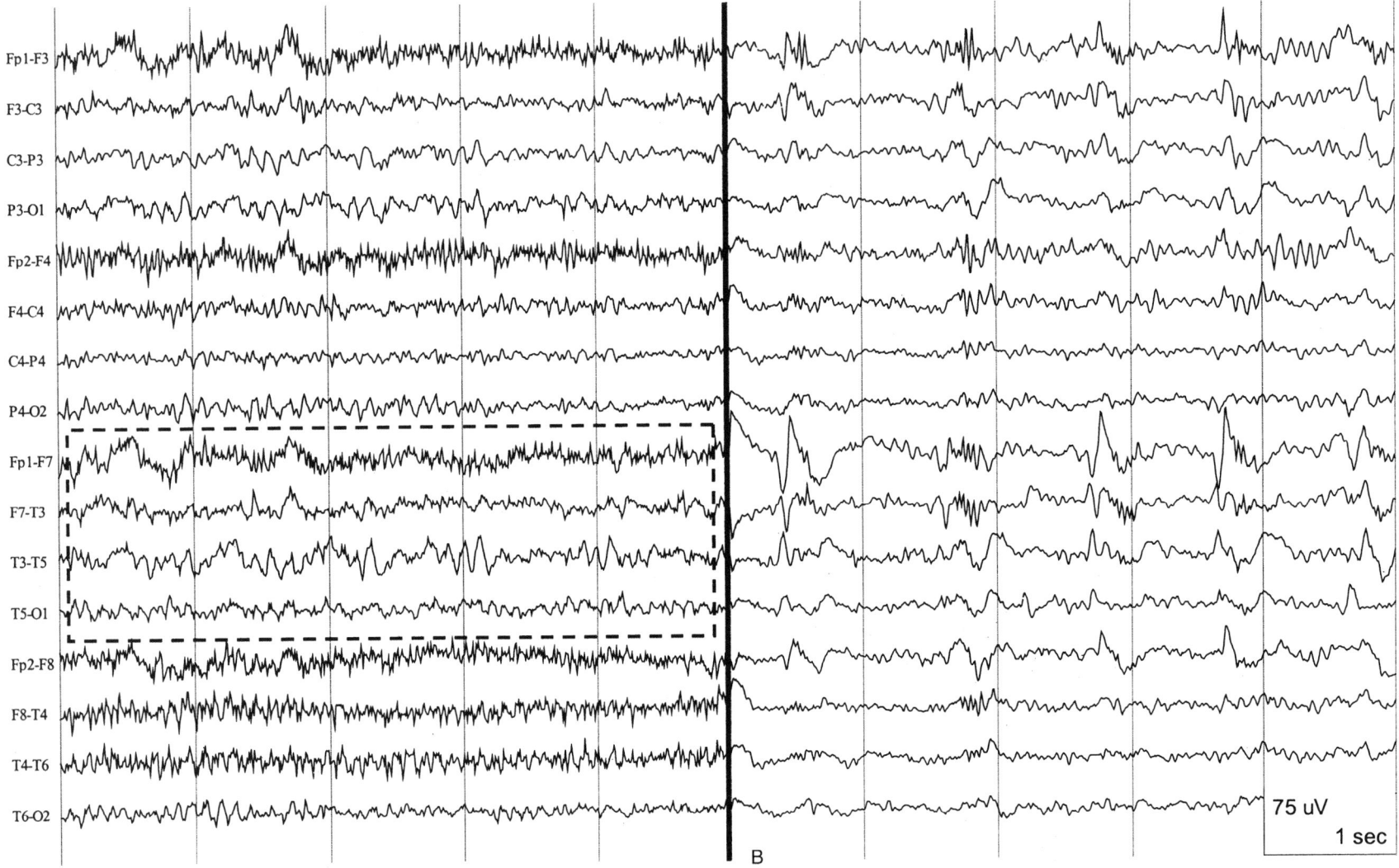

FIG. 11.22. EEGs of a 47-year-old man with neurocysticercosis and new-onset seizures. MRI demonstrated multiple ring-enhancing lesions, with the largest involving the left posterior hippocampus and adjacent cortex. **A:** Awake EEG. There is intermittent polymorphic delta activity over the left temporal region (*boxed area*) with spread to the suprasylvian and parasagittal areas. **B:** Sleep EEG. There are periodic complexes over the left midtemporal region consisting of a sharp wave followed by paroxysmal fast activity lasting 200–400 milliseconds. The paroxysmal fast activity spreads to the frontopolar region.

Other Conditions

EEG abnormalities are common in multiple sclerosis, especially as the disease progresses (59). All are nonspecific and include focal and diffuse slow-wave activity, and voltage attenuation (102). Sturge-Weber syndrome, which includes "tramline" calcification within layers of the parieto-occipital cortex, is associated with focal voltage attenuation and epileptiform discharges (17). In cysticercosis, there are focal or multifocal spikes accompanied by focal or multifocal delta activity (112) (Fig. 11.22). Generalized slow-wave activity also occurs. Cerebral arteriovenous malformations may have no effect on the EEG, but, if large or associated with ischemia or hemorrhage, they produce focal polymorphic delta activity, often accompanied by localized voltage attenuation (133) (see Fig. 11.3).

USE OF EEG IN THE ICU AND OPERATING ROOM

The sensitivity of EEG to acute focal brain dysfunction makes it a useful tool to monitor cerebral physiological function. Scalp EEG has been used for this purpose during carotid endarterectomy to make decisions about the need for shunting (25,97,119). Arnold and others (4) used EEG and transcranial Doppler ultrasound to monitor 82 patients undergoing carotid endarterectomy. EEG had a high correlation with decreased velocity of blood flow, but there were many false positives. Consequently, these authors concluded that EEG did not add additional useful information in these cases. Others, however, disagree with this conclusion (see Chapter 31 for a full discussion). EEG has also been used during endovascular embolization of arteriovenous malformations. The procedure generally used is to inject low doses of sodium amobarbital through an intra-arterial catheter into the feeding artery(ies). Neurological and EEG assessment during this reversible period of anesthesia is used to predict the functional effects of permanently occluding the feeding artery(ies). When embolization has been performed despite EEG changes during a preceding amobarbital test, clinically important deficits have resulted (133).

Continuous EEG monitoring is increasingly used in the neonatal ICU to detect ischemic changes caused by vasospasm following subarachnoid hemorrhage (174) and to identify subclinical seizures. Because of the large volume of acquired data, the use of compressed spectral array (CSA) can aid in detecting clinically significant changes. CSA uses power spectra to summarize data over time and indicate trends related to improvement or deterioration in focal, hemispheric, or bilateral cerebral function. CSA can never fully replace raw EEG. Conventional displays of EEG activity must be available for each patient to determine the meaning of CSA patterns. A complete discussion of ICU monitoring is contained in Chapter 25.

REFERENCES

1. Adams JH, Jennett WB. Acute necrotizing encephalitis: a problem in diagnosis. *J Neurol Neurosurg Psychiatry* 1967;30:248–260.
2. Aird RB, Shimuzu M. Neuropathological correlates of low-voltage EEG foci. *Arch Neurol* 1970;22:75–80.
3. Arfel G, Fischgold H. EEG-signs in tumors of the brain. *Electroencephalogr Clin Neurophysiol Suppl* 1961;19:36–50.
4. Arnold M, Sturznegger M, Schaffler L, et al. Continuous intraoperative monitoring of middle cerebral artery blood flow velocities and electroencephalography during carotid endarterectomy. *Stroke* 1997;28:1345–1350.
5. Arseni C, Howat HL, Maretsis M, et al. EEG alterations in cerebral abscesses. *Electroencephalogr Clin Neurophysiol* 1964;17:589.
6. August JT, Hiatt HH. Severe hypoglycemia secondary to a non-pancreatic fibrosarcoma with insulin activity. *N Engl J Med* 1958;258:17–22.
7. Bazil CW. Migraine and epilepsy. *Neurol Clin* 1995;12:115–128.
8. Beaumanoir A, Jekiel M. Electrographic observations during attacks of classical migraine. In: Andermann F, Lugaresi E, eds. *Migraine and epilepsy*. Boston: Butterworth-Heinemann, 1987:163–180.
9. Berger H. Über das elektrenkephalogramm des menschen. *J Psychol Neurol* 1930;40:160–179.
10. Berger H. Über das elektrenkephalogramm des menschen. 8. *Arch Psychiatr Nervenkr* 1934;101:452–469. (English translation: Gloor P. Hans Berger on the electroencephalogram of man. *Electroencephalogr Clin Neurophysiol Suppl* 1969;28:210–216.
11. Bickford RG. Electroencephalographic diagnosis of brain tumors. *Am J Surg* 1957;93:946–951.
12. Bladin PF. The association of benign rolandic epilepsy with migraine. In: Anderman F, Lugaresi E, eds. *Migraine and epilepsy*. Boston: Butterworth-Heinemann, 1987:145–152.
13. Blume WT, David RB, Gomez MR. Generalized sharp and slow wave complexes, associated clinical features, and long term follow up. *Brain* 1973;96:289–306.
14. Blume WT, Girvin JP, Kaufmann JCE. Childhood brain tumors presenting as uncontrolled focal seizure disorders. *Ann Neurol* 1982;12:538–541.
15. Bogart K, Smith D. Clinical correlates of unilateral mu. *Clin Electroencephalogr* 1978;9:181–185.
16. Brazier M, Finesinger J. Action of barbiturates on the cerebral cortex: electroencephalographic studies. *Arch Neurol Psychiatry* 1945;53:51–58.
17. Brenner RP, Sharbrough FW. Electroencephalographic evaluation in Sturge-Weber syndrome. *Neurology* 1976;26:629–632.
18. Brodtkorb E, Lindqvist M, Jonsson M, et al. Diagnosis of herpes simplex encephalitis: a comparison between electroencephalography and computed tomography findings. *Acta Neurol Scand* 1982;66:462–471.
19. Bruens JH, Gastaut H, Gioive G. Electroencephalographic study of the signs of chronic vascular insufficiency of the Sylvian region in aged people. *Electroencephalogr Clin Neurophysiol* 1960;12:283–295.
20. Busse EW, Obrist WD. Pre-senescent electroencephalographic changes in normal subjects. *J Gerontol* 1965;20:315–320.
21. Camfield PR, Metrakos K, Andermann F. Basilar migraine, seizures and severe epileptiform EEG abnormalities. *Neurology* 1978;28;584–588.

22. Carmon A, Behar A, Beller A. Acute necrotizing encephalitis presenting clinically as a space-occupying lesion: a clinicopathological study of six cases. *J Neurol Sci* 1965;2:328–343.

23. Chatrian GE, Shae GM, Leffman H. The significance of periodic lateralized epileptiform discharges: an electroencephalographic, clinical, and pathological study. *Electroencephalogr Clin Neurophysiol* 1964;17:177–193.

24. Ch'ien LT, Boehm RM, Robinson H, et al. Characteristic early electroencephalographic changes in herpes simplex encephalitis. *Arch Neurol* 1977;34:361–364.

25. Cho I, Smullens SN, Streletz LJ, et al. The value of intraoperative EEG monitoring during carotid endarterectomy. *Ann Neurol* 1986;20:508–512.

26. Chu NS. Acute subdural hematoma and the periodic lateralized epileptiform discharges. *Clin Electroencephalogr* 1979;10:145–150.

27. Cobb WA. Rhythmic slow discharges in the electroencephalogram. *J Neurol Neurosurg Psychiatry* 1945;8:65–78.

28. Cobb WA, Guiloff RJ, Cast J. Breach rhythm: the EEG related to skull defects. *Electroencephalogr Clin Neurophysiol* 1979;47:251–271.

29. Collice M, Arena O, Fontana RA, et al. Role of EEG monitoring and cross-clamping duration in carotid endarterectomy. *J Neurosurg* 1986;65:815–819.

30. Cordeau JP. Monorhythmic frontal delta activity in human electroencephalogram: a study of 100 cases. *Electroencephalogr Clin Neurophysiol* 1959;11:733–746.

31. Coull BM, Pedley TA. Intermittent photic stimulation: clinical usefulness of non-convulsive responses. *Electroencephalogr Clin Neurophysiol* 1978;44:353–363.

32. Dalby MA. Epilepsy and 3 per second and wave rhythms. *Acta Neurol Scand Suppl* 1969;40:1–183.

33. Daly D, Whelan JL, Bickford RG, et al. The electroencephalogram in cases of tumors of the posterior fossa and third ventricle. *Electroencephalogr Clin Neurophysiol* 1953;5:203–216.

34. Daly DD. The effect of sleep upon the electroencephalogram in patients with brain tumors. *Electroencephalogr Clin Neurophysiol* 1968;25:521–529.

35. Dauben RD, Adams AH. Periodic lateralized epileptiform discharges in EEG: a review with special attention to etiology and recurrence. *Clin Electroencephalogr* 1977;8:116–124.

36. de la Paz D, Brenner RP. Bilateral independent periodic lateralized epileptiform discharges: clinical significance. *Arch Neurol* 1981;38:713–715.

37. Dimitrov V. The diagnostic value of EEG in brain abscesses. *Electroencephalogr Clin Neurophysiol* 1964;17:708.

38. Duensing F. Die alphawellenaktivierung als herdsymptom im electroenzephalogramm. *Nervenarzt* 1948;19:544–552.

39. Dutt MK, Johnston IDA. Computed tomography and EEG in herpes simplex encephalitis: their value in diagnosis and prognosis. *Arch Neurol* 1982;39:99–102.

40. Elian M. Herpes simplex encephalitis: prognosis and long-term follow-up. *Arch Neurol* 1975;32:39–43.

41. Engel S, Lechner H, Logar C, et al. Clinical value of EEG in transient ischemic attacks. In: Lechner H, Aranibar A, eds. *EEG and clinical neurophysiology*. Amsterdam: Excerpta Medica, 1980:173–180.

42. Enzmann DR, Ransom B, Norman D, et al. Computed tomography of herpes simplex encephalitis. *Radiology* 1978;129:419–425.

43. Fariello RG, Orrison W, Blanco G, et al. Neuroradiological correlates of frontally predominant intermittent rhythmic delta activity (FIRDA). *Electroencephalogr Clin Neurophysiol* 1982;54:194–202.

44. Fernandez-Bouzas A, Harmony T, Galan L, et al. Comparison of Z and multivariate statistical brain electromagnetic maps for the localization of brain lesions. *Electroencephalogr Clin Neurophysiol* 1995;95:372–380.

45. Fernandez-Bouzas A, Harmony T, Marosi E, et al. Evolution of cerebral edema and its relationship with power in the theta band. *Electroencephalogr Clin Neurophysiol* 1997;102:279–285.

46. Fischgold H. Quelques causes l'erreurs dans la localisation des tumeurs des hemispheres. *Sem Hop Paris* 1950;26:2631–2633.

47. Fischgold H, Pertuiset B, Arfel-Capdeveille G. Quelques particularites electroencephalographiques au niveau des breches et des volets neurochirurgicaux. *Rev Neurol (Paris)* 1952;86:126–132.

48. Foerster O, Altenburger H. Electrobiologische vorgange an der menschlichen hirnrinde. *Dtsch Z Nervenheilkd* 1935;135:277–288.

49. Funakawa I, Yasuda T, Terao A. Periodic lateralized epileptiform discharges in mitochondrial encephalomyopathy. *Electroencephalogr Clin Neurophysiol* 1997;103:370–375.

50. Furlan AJ, Henry CE, Sweeney PHJ, et al. Focal EEG abnormalities in Heidenhain's variant of Jakob-Creutzfeldt disease. *Arch Neurol* 1981;38:213–214.

51. Gambardella A, Palmini A, Andermann F, et al. Usefulness of focal rhythmic discharges on scalp EEG of patients with focal cortical dysplasia and intractable epilepsy. *Electroencephalogr Clin Neurophysiol* 1996;98:243–249.

52. Gascon G, Barlow C. Juvenile migraine presenting as an acute confusional state. *Pediatrics* 1970;45:628–635.

53. Gastaut H. A new type of epilepsy: benign partial epilepsy of childhood with occipital spike-waves. *Clin Electroencephalogr* 1982;13:13–22.

54. Gastaut H, Bruens JH, Roger J, et al. Etude electroencephalographique des signes d'insuffisiance circulatoire syvienne chronique. *Rev Neurol (Paris)* 1959;100:59–65.

55. Gastaut H, Terzian H, Gastaut Y. Etude d'une activite electroencephalographique meconnue: "le rythme rolandique in arceau". *Marseille Med* 1952;89:296–310.

56. Gastaut JL, Michel B, Hassan S, et al. Electroencephalography in brain edema (127 cases of tumor investigated by cranial computerized tomography). *Electroencephalogr Clin Neurophysiol* 1979;46:239–255.

57. Gastaut JL, Yermenos E, Bonnefoy M, et al. Familial hemiplegic migraine: EEG and CT scan study of two cases. *Ann Neurol* 1981;10:392–395.

58. Gibbs F, Gibbs E, Lennox W. Effect on the electroencephalogram of certain drugs which influence nervous activity. *Arch Intern Med* 1937;60:154–166.

59. Gibbs FA, Becka D. Reappraisal of the electroencephalogram in multiple sclerosis. *Dis Nerv Sys* 1968;29:589–592.

60. Gilmore PC, Brenner RP. Correlation of EEG, computerized tomography, and clinical findings: study of 100 patients with focal delta activity. *Arch Neurol* 1981;38:371–372.

61. Giovanardi Rossi P, Santucci M, Gobbi G, et al. Epidemiological study of migraine in epileptic patients. In: Andermann F, Lugaresi E, eds. *Migraine and epilepsy*. Boston: Butterworth-Heinemann, 1987:312–322.

62. Gloor P, Ball G, Schaul N. Brain lesions that produce delta waves on EEG. *Neurology* 1977;27:326–333.

63. Gloor P, Kalabay O, Giard N. The electroencephalogram in diffuse encephalopathies: EEG correlates of gray and white matter lesions. *Brain* 1968;91:779–802.

64. Goldensohn ES. Use of the EEG for evaluation of focal intracranial lesions. In: Klass D, Daly D, eds. *Current practice of clinical electroencephalography*. New York: Raven Press, 1979.

65. Golla FL, Winter AL. Analysis of cerebral response to flicker in patients complaining of episodic headache. *Electroencephalogr Clin Neurophysiol* 1959;11:539–549.

66. Gorman MJ, Welch KMA. Cerebral blood flow and migraine. In: Phillips JW, ed. *The regulation of cerebral blood flow*. Boca Raton, FL: CRC Press, 1993:399–410.

67. Green JB. The activation of EEG abnormalities by tolbutamide-induced hypoglycemia. *Neurology* 1963;13:192–200.

68. Green RL, Wilson WP. Asymmetries of beta activity in epilepsy, brain tumor and cerebrovascular disease. *Electroencephalogr Clin Neurophysiol* 1961;13:75–78.

69. Gronseth GS, Greenberg MK. The utility of the electroencephalogram in the evaluation of patients presenting with headache: a review of the literature. *Neurology* 1995;45:1263–1267.

70. Gupta PC, Seth P. Periodic complexes in herpes simplex encephalitis: a clinical and experimental study. *Electroencephalogr Clin Neurophysiol* 1973;35:67–74.

71. Hawkes CH, Bryan-Smyth L. The electroencephalogram in the "locked-in" syndrome. *Neurology* 1974;24:1015–1018.

72. Hess R. Brain tumors and other space-occupying processes. In: Remond A, ed. *Handbook of electroencephalography and clinical neurology*, Vol 14, Part C. Amsterdam: Elsevier Science, 1975:11–28.

73. Heyck H. Varieties of hemiplegic migraine. *Headache* 1973;12:135–142.

74. Hill D. Psychiatry. In: Hill D, Parr G, eds. *Electroencephalography: a symposium on its various aspects*. London: Macdonald, 1950:319–363.

75. Hirose G, Lombroso CT, Eisenberg H. Thalamic tumors in childhood. *Arch Neurol* 1975;32:740–744.

76. Hirose G, Saeki M, Kosoegawa H, et al. Delta waves in the EEGs of patients with intracerebral hemorrhage. *Arch Neurol* 1981;38:170–175.

77. Holmes GL. The electroencephalogram as a predictor of seizures following cerebral infarction. *Clin Electroencephalogr* 1980;11:83–86.

78. Hooshmand H, Morganroth R, Corredor C. Significance of focal and lateralized beta activity in the EEG. *Clin Electroencephalogr* 1980;11:140–144.

79. Illis LS, Taylor FM. The electroencephalogram in herpes simplex encephalitis. *Lancet* 1972;1:718–721.

80. Jaffe R, Jacobs L. The beta focus: its nature and significance. *Acta Neurol Scand* 1972;48:191–203.

81. Jallon P, Constant P, Caille JM, et al. Encephalotomographie axiale transverse et EEG dans les tumeurs cerebrales. *Rev EEG Neurophysiol* 1976;6:421.

82. Jasper H, Andrews H. Electroencephalography. III. Normal differentiation of occipital and precentral regions in man. *Arch Neurol Psychiatry* 1938;39:96–115.

83. Jasper H, Van Buren J. Interrelationships between cortex and subcortical structures: clinical electroencephalographic studies. *Electroencephalogr Clin Neurophysiol Suppl* 1953;4:168–188.

84. Joynt RJ, Cape CA, Knott JR. Significance of focal delta activity in adult electroencephalogram. *Arch Neurol* 1965;12:631–638.

85. Jung R. Neurophysiologische untersuchungsmethoden. In: Bergmann G, Frey W, Schwiegk H, eds. *Handbuch der inneren medizin*, Vol 1, 1. Berlin: Springer-Verlag, 1953:1216–1325.

86. Kappelle LJ, van Huffelen AC, van Gijn J. Is the EEG really normal in lacunar stroke? *J Neurol Neurosurg Psychiatry* 1990;53:63–66.

87. Katz RI, Horowitz GR. The septuagenarian EEG: studies in a selected normal geriatric population. *J Am Geriatr Soc* 1982;3:273–275.

88. Kaufman DM, Zimmerman RD, Leeds NE. Computed tomography in herpes simplex encephalitis. *Neurology* 1979;29:1392–1396.

89. Kershman J, Conde A, Gibson WC. Electroencephalography in differential diagnosis of supratentorial tumors. *Arch Neurol Psychiatry* 1949;62:255–268.

90. Kilpatrick CJ, Davis SM, Tres BM, et al. Epileptic seizures in acute stroke. *Arch Neurol* 1990;47:157–160.

91. Kirstein L. The occurrence of sharp waves, spikes and fast activity in supratentorial tumors. *Electroencephalogr Clin Neurophysiol* 1953;5:33–40.

92. Klass DW, Daly DD. Electroencephalography in patients with brain tumor. *Med Clin North Am* 1960;44:1041–1051.

93. Kooi KA, Guvener AM, Tupper CJ, et al. Electroencephalographic patterns of the temporal regions in normal adults. *Neurology* 1964;14:1029–1035.

94. Kornmuller AE. *Klinische elektroenzephalographie*. Munich: JF Lehmann, 1944.

95. Koutroumanidis M, Binnie CD, Elwes RDC, et al. Interictal regional slow activity in temporal lobe epilepsy correlates with lateral temporal hypometabolism as imaged with 18FDG PET: neurophysiological and metabolic implications. *J Neurol Neurosurg Psychiatry* 1998;65:170–176.

96. Kozelka JW, Pedley TA. Beta and mu rhythms. *J Clin Neurophysiol* 1990;7:191–207.

97. Kresowik TF, Worsey MJ, Khoury MD, et al. Limitations of electroencephalographic monitoring in the detection of cerebral ischemia accompanying carotid endarterectomy. *J Vasc Surg* 1991;13:439–443.

98. Kuroiwa Y, Celesia G. Clinical significance of periodic EEG patterns. *Arch Neurol* 1980;37:15–20.

99. Lai C, Gragasin ME. Electroencephalography in herpes simplex encephalitis. *J Clin Neurophysiol* 1988;5:87–103.

100. Lapkin MS, French JH, Golden GS, et al. The electroencephalogram in childhood basilar artery migraine. *Neurology* 1977;27:580–583.

101. Legg NJ, Gupta PC, Scott DF. Epilepsy following cerebral abscess: a clinical and EEG study of 70 patients. *Brain* 1973;96:259–268.

102. Levic ZM. Electroencephalographic studies in multiple sclerosis: specific changes in benign multiple sclerosis. *Electroencephalogr Clin Neurophysiol* 1978;44:471–478.

103. Lusins J, Jaffe R, Bender MB. Unoperated subdural hematomas: long term follow-up study by brain scan and electroencephalography. *J Neurosurg* 1976;44:601–607.

104. Macdonell RAL, Donnan GA, Bladin PF, et al. The electroencephalogram and acute ischemic stroke. *Arch Neurol* 1988;45:520–524.

105. Madkour O, Elwan O, Hamdy H, et al. Transient ischemic attacks: electrophysiological (conventional and topographic EEG) and radiological (CCT) evaluation. *J Neurol Sci* 1993;119:8–17.

106. Magnus O, Van der Holst M. Zeta waves: a special type of slow delta waves. *Electroencephalogr Clin Neurophysiol* 1987;67:140–146.

107. Markand ON. EEG in the 'locked-in' syndrome. *Electroencephalogr Clin Neurophysiol* 1976;40:529–534.

108. Markand ON, Daly DB. Pseudoperiodic lateralized paroxysmal discharges in the electroencephalogram. *Neurology* 1971;21:975–981.

109. Marks DA, Ehrenberg BL. Migraine-related seizures in adults with epilepsy, with EEG correlation. *Neurology* 1993;43:2476–2483.

110. Marshall DW, Brey RL, Morse MW. Focal and/or lateralized polymorphic delta activity: association with either 'normal' or 'nonfocal' computed tomographic scans. *Arch Neurol* 1988;45:33–35.

111. Martinius J, Matthes A, Lombroso CT. Electroencephalographic features in posterior fossa tumors in children. *Electroencephalogr Clin Neurophysiol* 1968;25:128–139.

112. McCormick GF, Zee C-S, Heiden J. Cysticercosis cerebri: review of 127 cases. *Arch Neurol* 1982;39:534–539.

113. Meyer JS, Portnoy HA. Localized cerebral hypoglycemia simulating stroke. *Neurology* 1958;8:601–604.

114. Michel B, Gastaut JL, Bianchi L. Electroencephalographic cranial computerized tomographic correlations in brain abscess. *Electroencephalogr Clin Neurophysiol* 1979;46:256–273.

115. Mikati MA, Feraru E, Krishnamoorthy K, et al. Neonatal herpes simplex encephalitis: EEG investigations and clinical correlates. *Neurology* 1990;40:1433–1437.

116. Millar JHD, Coey A. The EEG in necrotizing encephalitis. *Electroencephalogr Clin Neurophysiol* 1959;2:582–585.

117. Miller JHP. The electroencephalogram in cases of subarachnoid hemorrhage. *Electroencephalogr Clin Neurophysiol* 1953;5:165–168.

118. Mizrahi E, Tharp B. A characteristic EEG pattern in neonatal herpes simplex encephalitis. *Neurology* 1982;32:1215–1220.

119. Mola M, Collice M, Levati A. Continuous intraoperative electroencephalographic monitoring in carotid endarterectomy. *Eur Neurol* 1986;25:53–60.

120. Muller HF, Schwartz G. Electroencephalograms and autopsy findings in geropsychiatry. *J Gerontol* 1978;33:504–513.

121. Mundy-Castle AC. Theta and beta rhythm in the electroencephalograms of normal adults. *Electroencephalogr Clin Neurophysiol* 1951;3:477–486.

122. Nagata K, Mizukami M, Araki G, et al. Topographic electroencephalographic study of cerebral infarction using computed mapping of the EEG. *J Cereb Blood Flow Metab* 1982;2:79–88.

123. Nagata K, Yunoki K, Araki G, et al. Topographic electroencephalographic study of transient ischemic attacks. *Electroencephalogr Clin Neurophysiol* 1984;58:291–301.

124. Nau HE, Bock WJ, Clar HE. Electroencephalographic investigations in sellar tumors. *Acta Neurochir (Wien)* 1978;44:207–214.

125. Nealis JGT, Duffy FH. Paroxysmal beta activity in the pediatric electroencephalogram. *Ann Neurol* 1978;4:112–116.

126. Neufeld MY, Vishnevskaya S, Treves TA, et al. Periodic lateralized epileptiform discharges (PLEDs) following stroke are associated with metabolic abnormalities. *Electroencephalogr Clin Neurophysiol* 1997;102:295–298.

127. Newmark ME, Theodore WH, Sato S, et al. EEG, transmission computed tomography, and positron emission tomography with fluorodeoxyglucose [18]F. *Arch Neurol* 1983;40:607–610.

128. Nuwer MR. Frequency analysis and topographic mapping of EEG and evoked potentials in epilepsy. *Electroencephalogr Clin Neurophysiol* 1988;69:118–126.

129. Nuwer MR, Jordan SE, Ahn SS. Evaluation of stroke using EEG frequency analysis and topographic mapping. *Neurology* 1987;37:1153–1159.

130. Obrist WD. The electroencephalogram of normal aged adults. *Electroencephalogr Clin Neurophysiol* 1954;6:235–244.

131. Obrist WD. Problems of aging. In: Remond A, ed. *Handbook of electroencephalography and clinical neurophysiology*, Vol 6, Part A. Amsterdam: Elsevier Science, 1976:275–292.

132. Otomo E, Tsubaki T. Electroencephalography in subjects sixty years and over. *Electroencephalogr Clin Neurophysiol* 1966;20:77–82.

133. Paiva T, Campos J, Baeta E, et al. EEG monitoring during endovascular embolization of cerebral arteriovenous malformations. *Electroencephalogr Clin Neurophysiol* 1995;95:3–13.

134. Pampiglione G. Induced fast activity in the EEG as an aid in the location of cerebral lesion. *Electroencephalogr Clin Neurophysiol* 1952;4:79–82.

135. Pampiglione G. Very short acting barbiturate (methohexital) in the detection of cortical lesions. *Electroencephalogr Clin Neurophysiol* 1965;19:314.

136. Panayiotopoulos CP. Basilar migraine? Seizures and severe epileptic EEG abnormalities. *Neurology* 1980;30:1122–1125.

137. Panet-Raymond D, Gotman J. Asymmetry in delta activity in patients with focal epilepsy. *Electroencephalogr Clin Neurophysiol* 1990;75:474–481.

138. Petty GW, Labar DR, Fisch BJ, et al. Electroencephalography in lacunar infarction. *J Neurol Sci* 1995;134:47–50.

139. Pine I, Atoynatan TH, Margolis G. The EEG findings in eighteen patients with brain abscess: case reports and a review of the literature. *Electroencephalogr Clin Neurophysiol* 1952;4:165–179.

140. Puech P, Lerique-Koechlin A. L'EEG dans les abces du cerveau. *Rev Neurol (Paris)* 1944;76:303–305.

141. Quality Standards Subcommittee of the American Academy of Neurology: Practice Parameter: The electroencephalogram in the evaluation of headache. *Neurology* 1995;45:1411–1413.

142. Quirk JA, Kendall B, Kingsley DPE, et al. EEG features of cortical dysplasia in children. *Neuropediatrics* 1993;24:193–199.

143. Raroque HG, Gonzales PC, Jhaveri HS, et al. Defining the role of structural lesions and metabolic abnormalities in periodic lateralized epileptiform discharges. *Epilepsia* 1993;34:279–283.

144. Rawls WE, Dyck PK, Klass DW, et al. Encephalitis associated with herpes simplex virus. *Ann Intern Med* 1966;64:104–115.

145. Raymond AA, Fish DR. EEG features of focal malformations of cortical development. *J Clin Neurophysiol* 1996;13:495–506.

146. Raymond AA, Fish DR, Boyd SG, et al. Cortical dysgenesis: serial EEG findings in children and adults. *Electroencephalogr Clin Neurophysiol* 1995;94:389–397.

147. Reiher J, Beaudry M, Leduc CP. Temporal intermittent rhythmic delta activity (TIRDA) in the diagnosis of complex partial epilepsy: sensitivity, specificity and predictive value. *Can J Neurol Sci* 1989;16:398–401.

148. Remler MP, Marcussen WH. EEG monitoring of focal lesions of the blood-brain barrier. *Acta Neurol Scand* 1982;65:51–58.

149. Rohmer F, Gastaut Y, Dell MB. L'EEG dans la pathologie vasculaire du cerveau. *Rev Neurol (Paris)* 1952;87:93–144.

150. Rowan AJ, Rudolf N de M, Scott DF. EEG prediction of brain metastases. *J Neurol Neurosurg Psychiatry* 1974;37:888–893.

151. Sainio K, Stenberg D, Keskimaki I, et al. Visual and spectral EEG analysis in the evaluation of the outcome in patients with ischemic brain infarction. *Electroencephalogr Clin Neurophysiol* 1983;56:117–124.

152. Sand T. EEG in migraine: a review of the literature. *Funct Neurol* 1991;6:7–22.

153. Scarf JE, Rahm WE. The human electrocorticogram: a report of spontaneous electrical potentials obtained from the exposed brain. *J Neurophysiol* 1941;4:418–426.

154. Schaul N, Gloor P, Gotman J. The EEG in deep midline lesions. *Neurology* 1981;31:157–167.

155. Schnell R, Klass D. Further observations on the rolandic arceau rhythm. *Electroencephalogr Clin Neurophysiol* 1966;20:95.

156. Schoenen J. Clinical neurophysiology of headache. *Neurol Clin* 1997;15:85–105.

157. Schwartz MS, Prior PF, Scott DF. The occurrence and evolution in the EEG of lateralized periodic phenomenon. *Brain* 1973;96:613–622.

158. Scollo-Lavizzari A. The effect of sleep on EEG abnormalities at a distance from the lesion: all night study of 30 cases. *Eur Neurol* 1970;3:65–87.

159. Silverman AJ, Busse EW, Barnes RH. Studies in the processes of aging: electroencephalographic findings in 400 elderly subjects. *Electroencephalogr Clin Neurophysiol* 1955;7:67–74.

160. Singh BM, Gupta DR, Strobos RJ. Nonketotic hyperglycemia and epilepsia partialis continua. *Arch Neurol* 1973;29:187–190.

161. Slater KH. Some clinical and EEG findings in migraine. *Brain* 1968;91:85–98.

162. Smith JB, Westmoreland BF, Reagan TJ, et al. A distinctive clinical EEG profile in herpes simplex encephalitis. *Mayo Clin Proc* 1975;50:469–474.

163. Smyth VOG, Winter AL. The EEG in migraine. *Electroencephalogr Clin Neurophysiol* 1964;16:194–202.

164. Snodgrass SM, Tsuburaya K, Ajmone-Marsane C. Clinical significance of periodic lateralized epileptiform discharges: relationship with status epilepticus. *J Clin Neurophysiol* 1989;6:159–172.

165. Sperling MR. Hypoglycemic activation of focal abnormalities in the EEG of patients considered for temporal lobectomy. *Electroencephalogr Clin Neurophysiol* 1984;58:506–512.

166. Strauss H, Ostrow M, Greenstein L, et al. Temporal slowing as a source of error in electroencephalographic localization. *Electroencephalogr Clin Neurophysiol Suppl* 1953;3:67.

167. Tolonen U, Sulg IA. Comparison of quantitative EEG parameters from four different analysis techniques in evaluation of relationships between EEG and CBF in brain infarction. *Electroencephalogr Clin Neurophysiol* 1981;51:177–185.

168. Upton A, Gumpert J. EEG in diagnosis of herpes simplex encephalitis. *Lancet* 1970;1:650–652.

169. Van der Drift JHA. *The significance of electroencephalography for the diagnosis and localisation of cerebral tumors.* Leiden: Stenfert Kroese NV, 1957.

170. Van der Drift JHA. The EEG in cerebrovascular disease. In: Vinken PJ, Bruyn GW, eds. *Handbook of clinical neurology*, Vol 11. Amsterdam: North-Holland, 1972:267–291.

171. Van der Drift JHA, Magnus O. The EEG in cerebral ischemic lesions: correlations with clinical and pathological findings. In: Meyer JS, Gastaut H, eds. *Cerebral anoxia and the electroencephalogram.* Springfield, IL: Charles C Thomas Publisher, 1961:180–196.

172. Van der Drift JHA, Magnus O. Intracranial hemorrhage. In: Magnus O, Storm van Leeuwen W, Cobb WA, eds: *Electroencephalography and cerebral tumors.* Amsterdam: Elsevier Science, 1961:141–159.

173. Verma NP, Kooi KA. Contralateral epileptiform transients in stroke (CETS). *Epilepsia* 1986;27:437–440.

174. Vespa PM, Nuwer MR, Juhasz C, et al. Early detection of vasospasm after acute subarachnoid hemorrhage using continuous EEG ICU monitoring. *Electroencephalogr Clin Neurophysiol* 1997;103:607–615.

175. Vignaendra V, Ghee LT, Chawla J. EEG in brain abscess: its value in localization compared to other diagnostic tests. *Electroencephalogr Clin Neurophysiol* 1975;38:611–622.

176. Visser SL, Hooijer C, Jonker C, et al. Anterior temporal focal abnormalities in EEG in normal aged subjects: correlations with psychopathological and CT brain scan findings. *Electroencephalogr Clin Neurophysiol* 1987;66:1–7.

177. Walsh JMW, Brenner RP. Periodic lateralized epileptiform discharges—long term outcome in adults. *Epilepsia* 1987;28:533–536.

178. Walter WG. The localization of cerebral tumors by electroencephalography. *Lancet* 1936;2:305–308.

179. Walter WG, Dovey VJ. Delineation of subcortical tumors by direct electroencephalography. *Lancet* 1946;1:5–9.

180. Weisberg LA, Nice C, Katz M. Seizure disorders and correlation with specific EEG patterns. In: *Cerebral computed tomography*. Philadelphia: WB Saunders, 1978:291–292.

181. Westmoreland BF, Klass DW, Sharbrough FW, et al. "Alpha coma": electroencephalographic, clinical, pathological and etiological correlation. *Arch Neurol* 1975;32:713–718.

182. Yanagihara T, Houser DW, Klass DW. Computed tomography and EEG in cerebrovascular disease. *Arch Neurol* 1981;38:597–600.

183. Young GF, Leon-Barth CA, Green J. Familial hemiplegic migraine, retinal degeneration, deafness, and nystagmus. *Arch Neurol* 1970;23:201–209.

184. Ziegler DK, Hoeffer PF. EEG and clinical findings in 28 verified cases of brain abscess. *Electroencephalogr Clin Neurophysiol* 1952;2:41–44.

Chapter 12

Metabolic, Infectious, and Hereditary Encephalopathies

Akio Ikeda, George H. Klem, and Hans O. Lüders

TABLE 12.1. *Types of diffuse encephalopathies*

Metabolic encephalopathies
Anoxic encephalopathies
Endocrine encephalopathies
Nutritional deficiencies
Infectious and inflammatory encephalopathies
Hypertensive encephalopathies
Neurodegenerative and hereditary diseases (adult onset only)
   Progressive myoclonic epilepsy syndromes
   Leukodystrophies of adult onset
   Mucopolysaccharidoses
   Niemann-Pick disease
   MELAS

TABLE 12.2. *EEG abnormalities frequently seen in diffuse encephalopathies*

Background slow activity
Diffuse intermittent slow activity
Diffuse intermittent rhythmic slow activity
Diffuse continuous slow activity
Periodic patterns and PLEDs/ BiPLEDs
Triphasic waves
Burst suppression
Diffuse background suppression
Special EEG patterns seen in patients in coma
   Alpha coma
   Spindle coma
   Beta coma
   Delta/theta coma
   Electrocerebral inactivity

Electroencephalography (EEG) is a sensitive and reliable test to assess cerebral dysfunctions, and occasionally it can detect abnormalities even before clinical symptoms appear. The degree of EEG abnormality usually parallels the severity of the brain damage, and can therefore provide an objective measurement of the severity of a diffuse encephalopathy. Most encephalopathies produce nonspecific EEG abnormalities, but there are selected exceptions, such as Creutzfeldt-Jakob disease (CJD), that are associated with highly specific EEG patterns. The EEG usually cannot differentiate between acute and chronic states of diffuse encephalopathies even if acute insults in general tend to produce relatively more severe EEG abnormalities for any given insult. In this chapter, we describe EEG findings of diffuse encephalopathies caused by various etiologies as listed in Table 12.1. Drug effects and toxic encephalopathy, specific progressive pediatric syndromes, and EEG changes with organic brain syndrome are described elsewhere in this book.

ABNORMAL EEG PATTERNS FREQUENTLY SEEN IN DIFFUSE ENCEPHALOPATHIES

This section provides a description of the EEG abnormalities most commonly seen in diffuse encephalopathies (81) (Table 12.2). Most of these EEG patterns are nonspecific but, as mentioned above, tend to reflect the severity of cerebral dysfunction. The abnormalities described below are listed according to degree of EEG abnormality, starting with the least abnormal patterns.

Background Slow Activity

Background slow activity is defined as slowing of the main rhythmical posterior background activity (Fig. 12.1). It is a very sensitive index of a nonspecific diffuse encephalopathy, and occurs in almost all diffuse encephalopathies of mild or moderate degree. The degree of background slowing is also a function of the degree of cerebral dysfunction. Background slow activity frequently also occurs in association with some of the other abnormal EEG findings listed below.

Diffuse Intermittent Slow Activity

Diffuse intermittent slow (IS) activity is defined as excessive slow activity (exceeding the physiological slowing) that appears in an intermittent fashion (Fig. 12.2). The posterior dominant background rhythms are usually well preserved but may be abnormally slow (background slow activity). When occurring in isolation, diffuse IS activity usually reflects a mild, diffuse, and nonspecific cortical or subcortical dysfunction.

Diffuse Intermittent Rhythmic Slow Activity

Diffuse intermittent rhythmic slow (IRS) activity is a subclass of diffuse IS activity in which the slow waves appear grouped in bursts and consist of

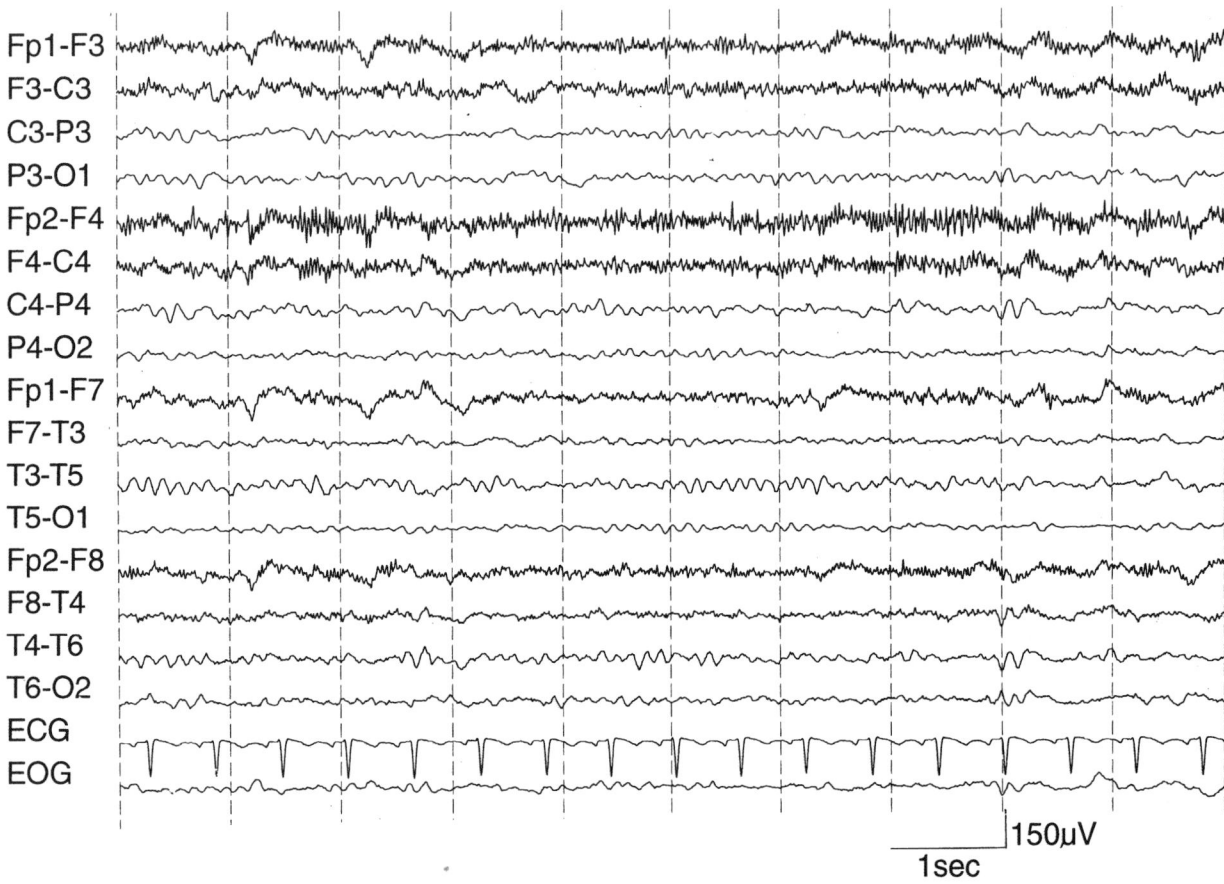

FIG. 12.1. Background slow activity in an 84-year-old man with dementia and confabulation 1 month after subarachnoid hemorrhage. The alpha rhythm is about 7 Hz, and there is also a diffuse, low-amplitude delta activity.

relatively rhythmic waves. Diffuse IRS activity is usually maximal over the anterior head regions in adults (frontal intermittent rhythmic delta activity [FIRDA]) (Fig. 12.3) and over the posterior head regions in children below 10 years (occipital intermittent rhythmic delta activity, or OIRDA).

It often shows shifting asymmetries, and not infrequently is associated with background slow and/or diffuse continuous slow (CS) activity as described below. It is usually an expression of a nonspecific, diffuse encephalopathy of any cause. Less frequently it occurs in patients with mesial frontoparietal cortical lesions or focal subcortical gray matter lesions (destructive processes involving subcortical gray matter structures, such as third ventricle tumors or increased intraventricular pressure).

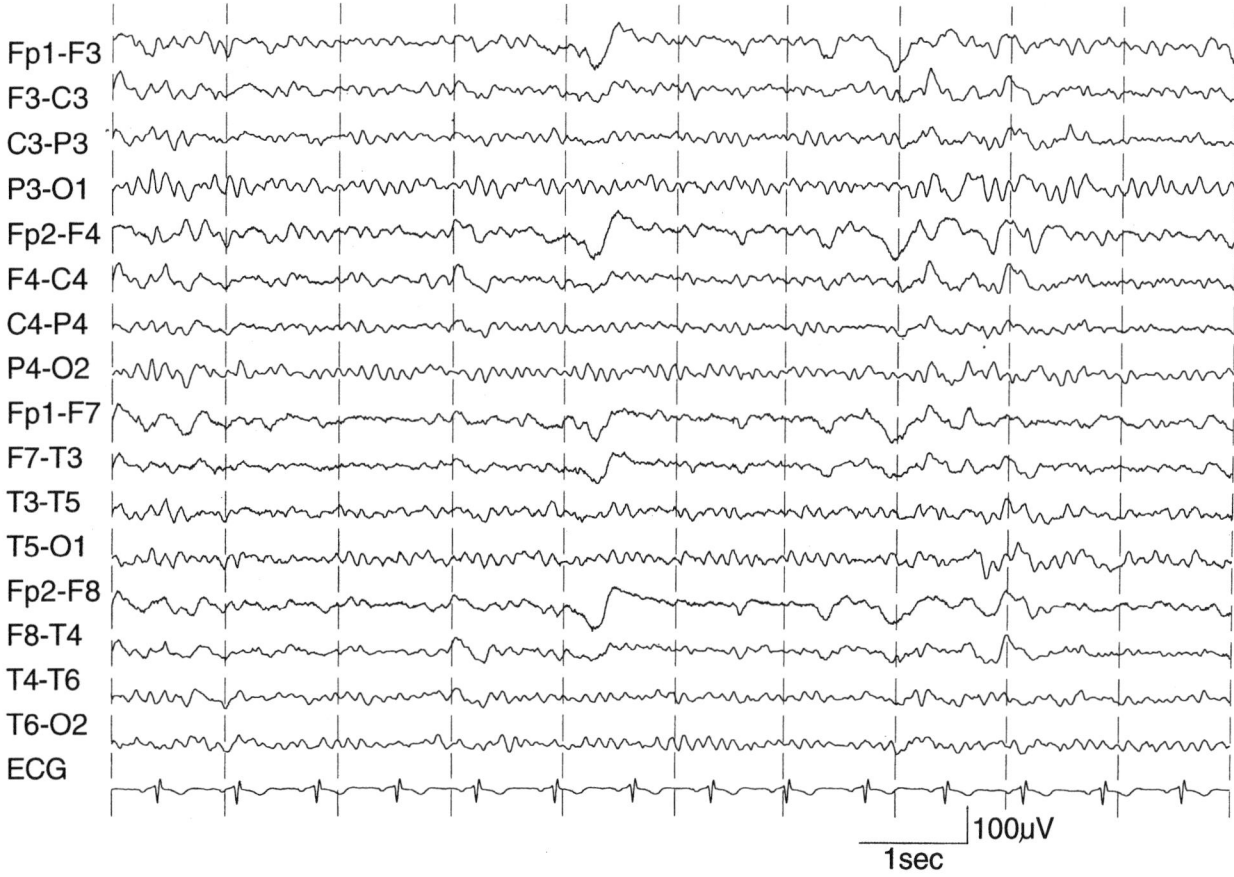

FIG. 12.2. Diffuse intermittent slow activity in a 26-year-old man with acute viral encephalitis.

Diffuse Continuous Slow Activity

Diffuse continuous slow (CS) activity consists of continuous, nonrhythmic, irregular (polymorphic) slow activity that is nonreactive to external stimuli, and exceeds the amount of CS activity that is physiologically appropriate for the age of the patient (Fig. 12.4). Variable degrees of disturbance of interneuronal connections or the biochemical environment of cortical neurons lead to diffuse CS. Gloor et al. (44) observed that polymorphic delta activity (PDA) was less common in pure cortical and subcortical gray matter disease in which white matter was relatively preserved. Their studies suggest that cortical deafferentation is an important cause of diffuse CS activity. The degree of slowing and its amount tend to be a function of the

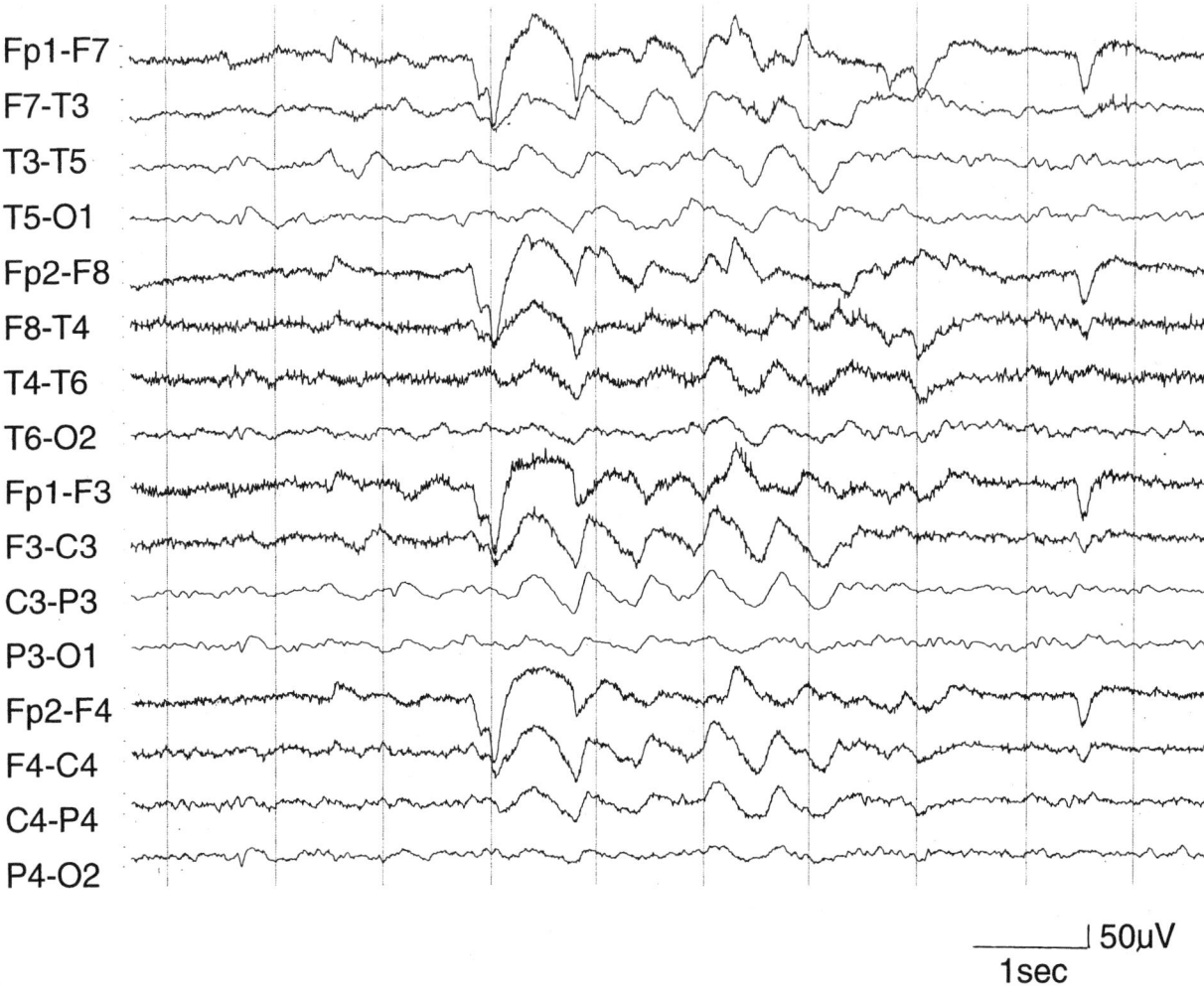

FIG. 12.3. Diffuse intermittent rhythmic slow activity maximal in the frontal areas. This is also termed frontal intermittent rhythmic delta activity (FIRDA).

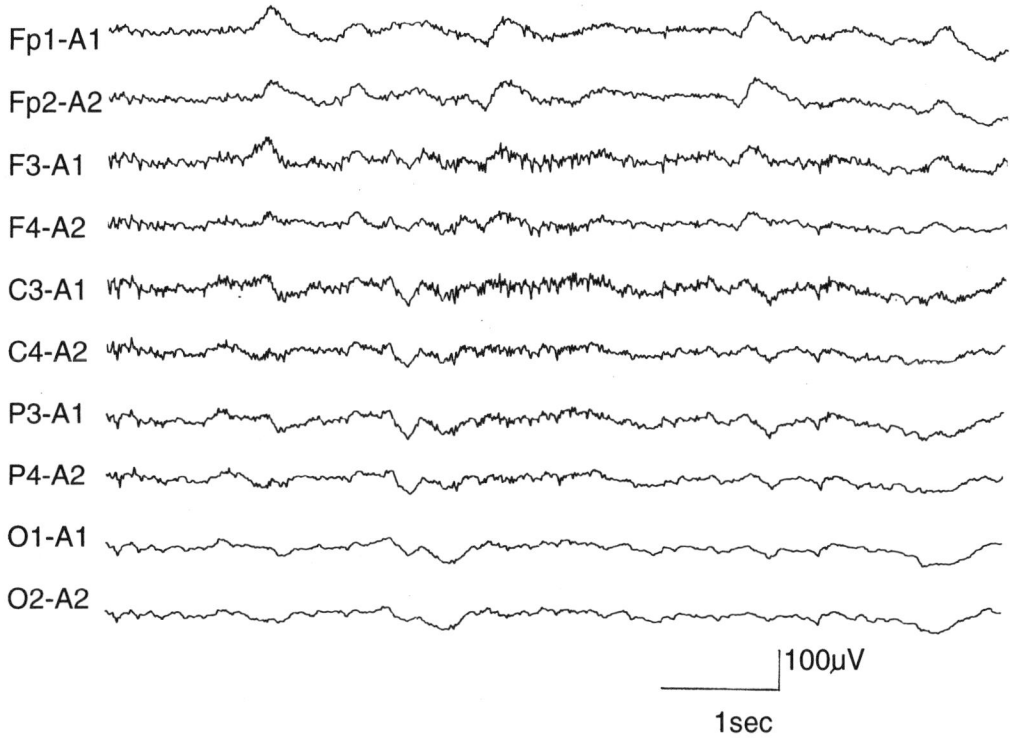

FIG. 12.4. Diffuse continuous slow activity in a 54-year-old man in stupor from acute meningoencephalitis and acute renal failure.

severity of diffuse encephalopathy. However, diffuse CS activity occurring with no remaining rhythmic background activity is usually an expression of a severe diffuse encephalopathy, such as that in patients with stupor or coma. Moderate or even mild degrees of CS activity may occur when rhythmic background activity is still preserved.

Periodic Patterns

Periodic patterns consist of relatively stereotyped waveforms (frequently sharp waves) that appear in a periodic or quasiperiodic fashion. They are usually indicative of an acute or subacute, severe, diffuse encephalopathy. The repetition rate and waveform of the periodic complexes are relatively characteristic for encephalopathies of different etiologies. A repetition rate of more than once every 2 seconds is most frequently seen in CJD in adults and in lipidosis in infants and children. Periodic patterns with a much slower repetition rate, from 4 to 10 seconds, characteristic of subacute sclerosing panencephalitis (SSPE) (18) (Fig. 12.5).

As one of the nondiffuse periodic patterns, periodic lateralized epileptiform discharges (PLEDs) are defined as sharp transients, including sharp waves or spikes, that have a lateralized distribution and appear in a periodic or quasiperiodic fashion (Fig. 12.6). They may be unilateral (PLEDs) or may have a bilateral distribution (bilateral periodic lateralized epileptiform discharges [BiPLEDs]) (26) (Fig. 12.7). These patterns are seen in (a) acute or subacute,

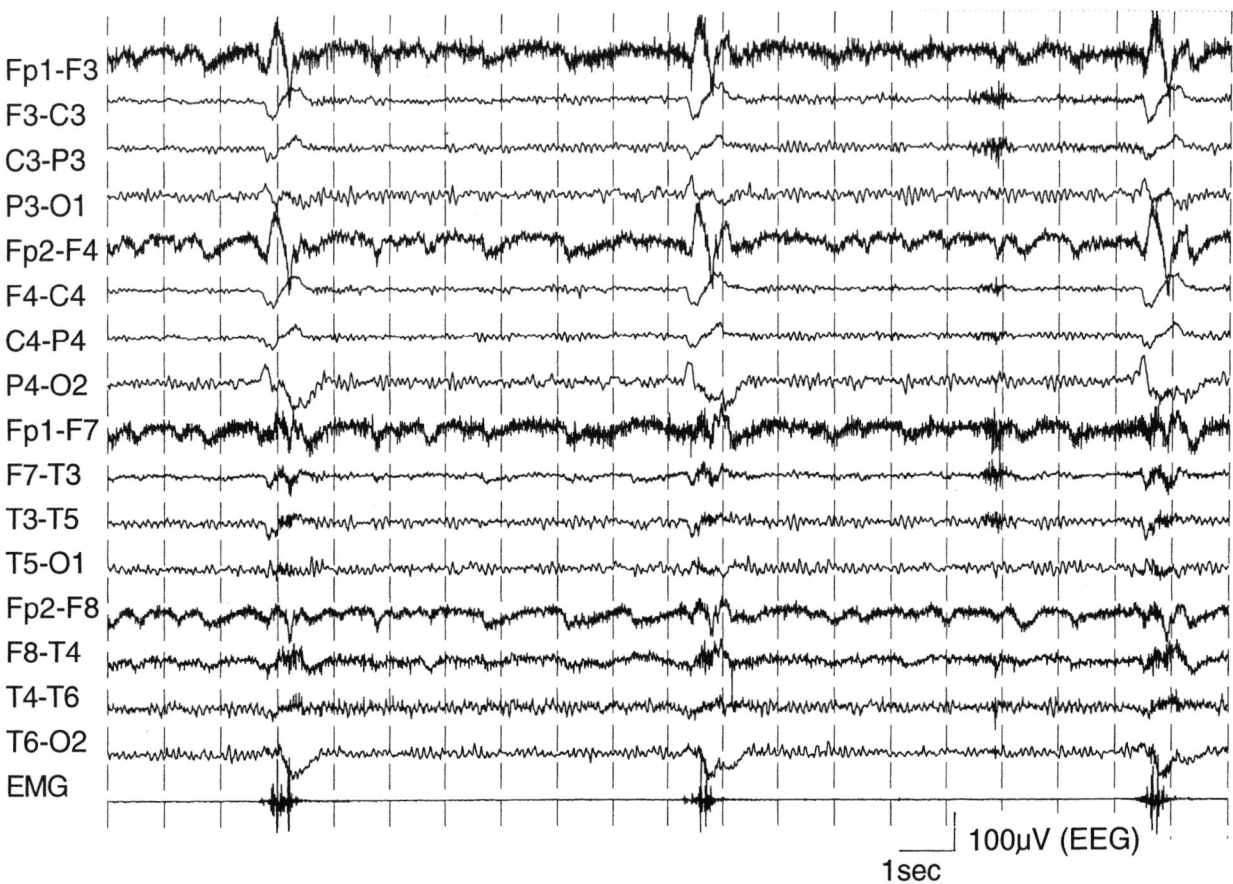

FIG. 12.5. Diffuse periodic discharges every 7–8 seconds in a 19-year-old woman with the early stage of SSPE. Posterior dominant rhythms of 9 Hz are well preserved. Electromyogram of the right extensor carpi radialis is shown in the last channel.

severe, focal destructive lesions (most often acute hemorrhagic infarcts, fast-growing tumors, or herpes simplex encephalitis); or (b) focal epileptogenic lesions not necessarily associated with an acute underlying structural pathology. In both conditions, focal pathology is frequently associated with a diffuse encephalopathy. PLEDs may occur in patients with diffuse encephalopathies with focal manifestation, such as herpes simplex encephalitis.

Triphasic Waves

Triphasic waves consist of high-voltage (> 70 μV), positive sharp transients that are preceded and followed by negative waves of relatively lower amplitude (Fig. 12.8). They have a diffuse, usually anterior-dominant, distribution and a periodic repetition rate of approximately 1–2 Hz (16).

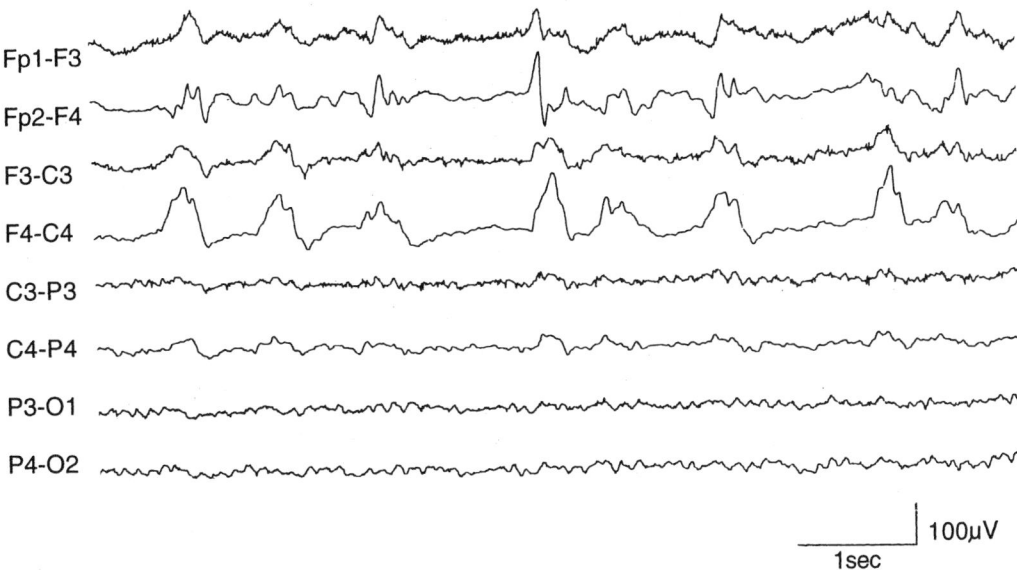

Fp1-F3

Fp2-F4

F3-C3

F4-C4

C3-P3

C4-P4

P3-O1

P4-O2

| 100µV

1sec

FIG. 12.6. PLEDs in a 52-year-old woman with acute onset of delirium who had a liver transplant 6 months ago.

Triphasic waves are usually due to a metabolic encephalopathy, and although they are particularly frequent in hepatic encephalopathy, they may be seen in other toxic/metabolic conditions, such as uremia, severe hyponatremia, and lithium toxicity. Triphasic waves usually occur in patients with a mild alteration of consciousness but not in conditions as severe as stupor or coma. Occasionally, triphasic waves and generalized slow spike-and-wave epileptiform discharges are difficult to distinguish (35).

Burst-Suppression

Burst-suppression constitutes a subgroup of periodic patterns in which the activity between the complexes (spikes and sharp waves mixed with nonspecific waves of variable amplitude, frequency, and waveform) is almost completely attenuated (less than 10 µV) (Fig. 12.9). Generalized burst-suppression EEGs occur in patients with a severe degree of toxic or anoxic encephalopathy and constitute the EEG pattern that immediately precedes electrocerebral inactivity (ECI) in patients who are deteriorating progressively. Patients who show diffuse burst-suppression in their EEGs are always in coma.

Diffuse Background Attenuation

This pattern is defined as absence of electrical brain activity greater than 10 µV. It is seen in patients in coma or deep stupor, and it is always indicative of a severe diffuse encephalopathy. However, some normal individuals have EEG activity that may not exceed 10 µV. Therefore, this pattern should only be considered abnormal if the patient is in stupor or coma (1).

Special EEG Patterns Seen in Patients in Coma

For a more detailed discussion of EEG changes in coma and brain death, see Chapter 14.

Alpha Coma

Alpha coma refers to by an EEG in which the predominant rhythmic activity is in the alpha range and occurs in patients who are in coma. The alpha activity most frequently has a diffuse distribution with frontal pre-

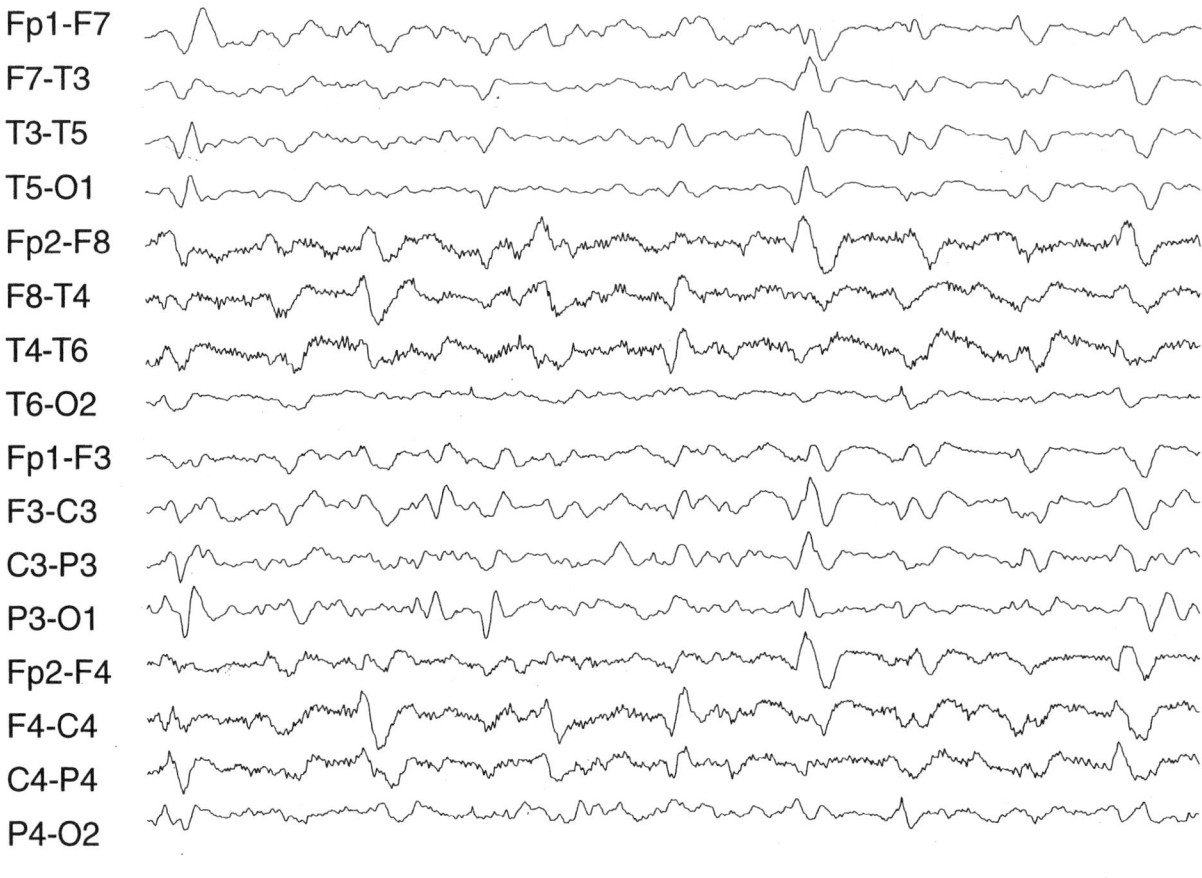

Fp1-F7
F7-T3
T3-T5
T5-O1
Fp2-F8
F8-T4
T4-T6
T6-O2
Fp1-F3
F3-C3
C3-P3
P3-O1
Fp2-F4
F4-C4
C4-P4
P4-O2

50µV

1sec

FIG. 12.7. BiPLEDs in a 74-year-old woman with encephalitis.

dominance and is nonreactive to external stimuli. This EEG pattern is most frequently seen in severe anoxic encephalopathy and is associated with an extremely poor prognosis. Less frequently, this pattern is seen in patients with more limited lesions at the pontomesencephalic level. It has been reported that patients with alpha coma resulting from anoxia due to respiratory arrest and high-voltage electrical injury tend to have a better outcome than those with alpha coma occurring after cardiac arrest (45,46).

Spindle Coma

Spindle coma is a term used when diurnal EEG activity in comatose patients contain features of stage 2 sleep, including prominent spindle-like activity (73). It can occur in patients with nonprogressive conditions such as a posttraumatic or postencephalitic encephalopathy, but most frequently it is an expression of a high mesencephalic lesion. This EEG pattern usually carries a good prognosis.

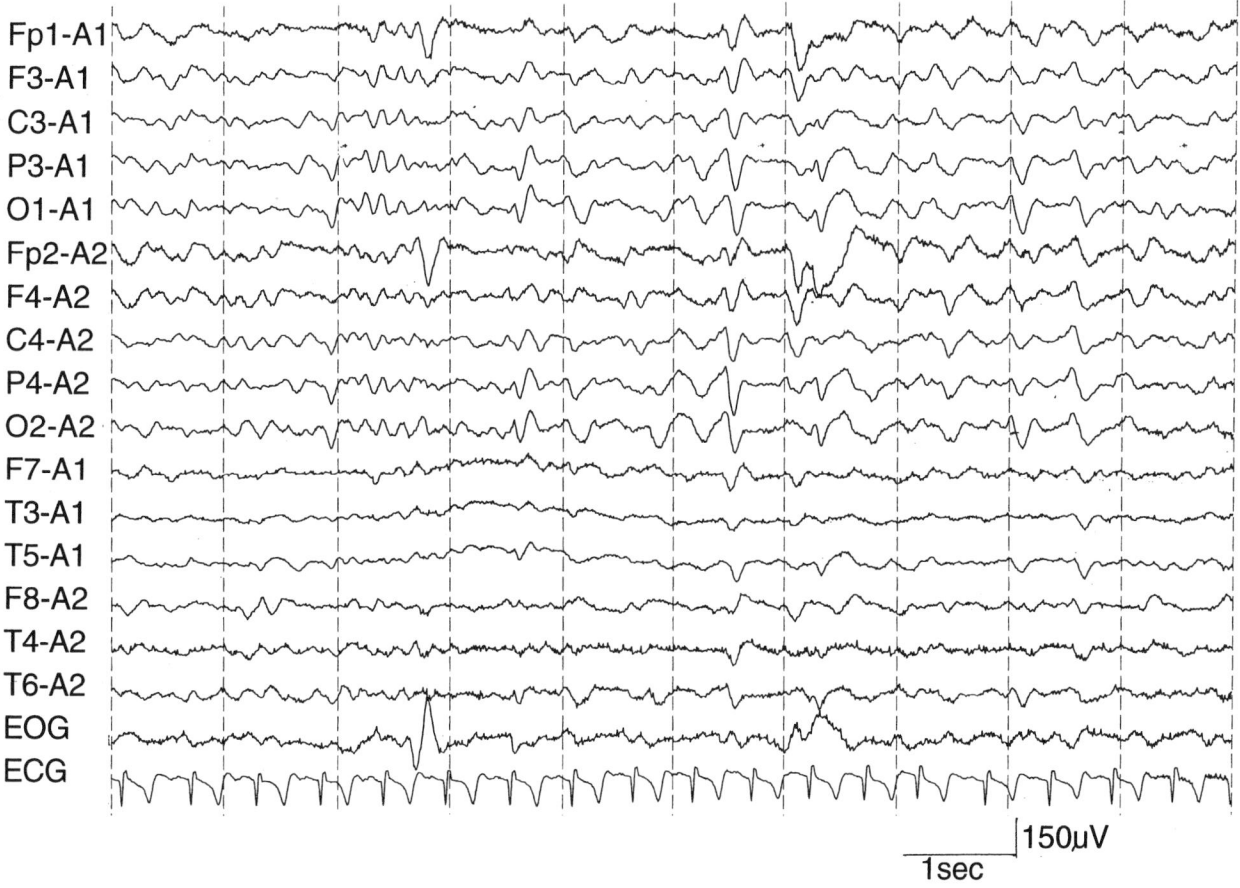

FIG. 12.8. Triphasic waves in a 61-year-old woman with hepatic encephalopathy.

Beta Coma

Beta coma EEGs consist of high-amplitude beta activity (usually > 30 μV) in patients who are in coma. It is usually seen in diffuse encephalopathies caused by drug intoxication, and therefore represents a potentially reversible EEG abnormality. It may also occur in acute brainstem lesions (98).

Delta/Theta Coma

Delta/theta coma EEGs show delta or theta activity as the predominant background activity in patients who are in coma. It is seen in patients with diffuse encephalopathies of diverse etiologies, and is a potentially reversible EEG pattern. The prognosis depends mainly on the reversibility of the underlying cause(s) of the encephalopathy (19).

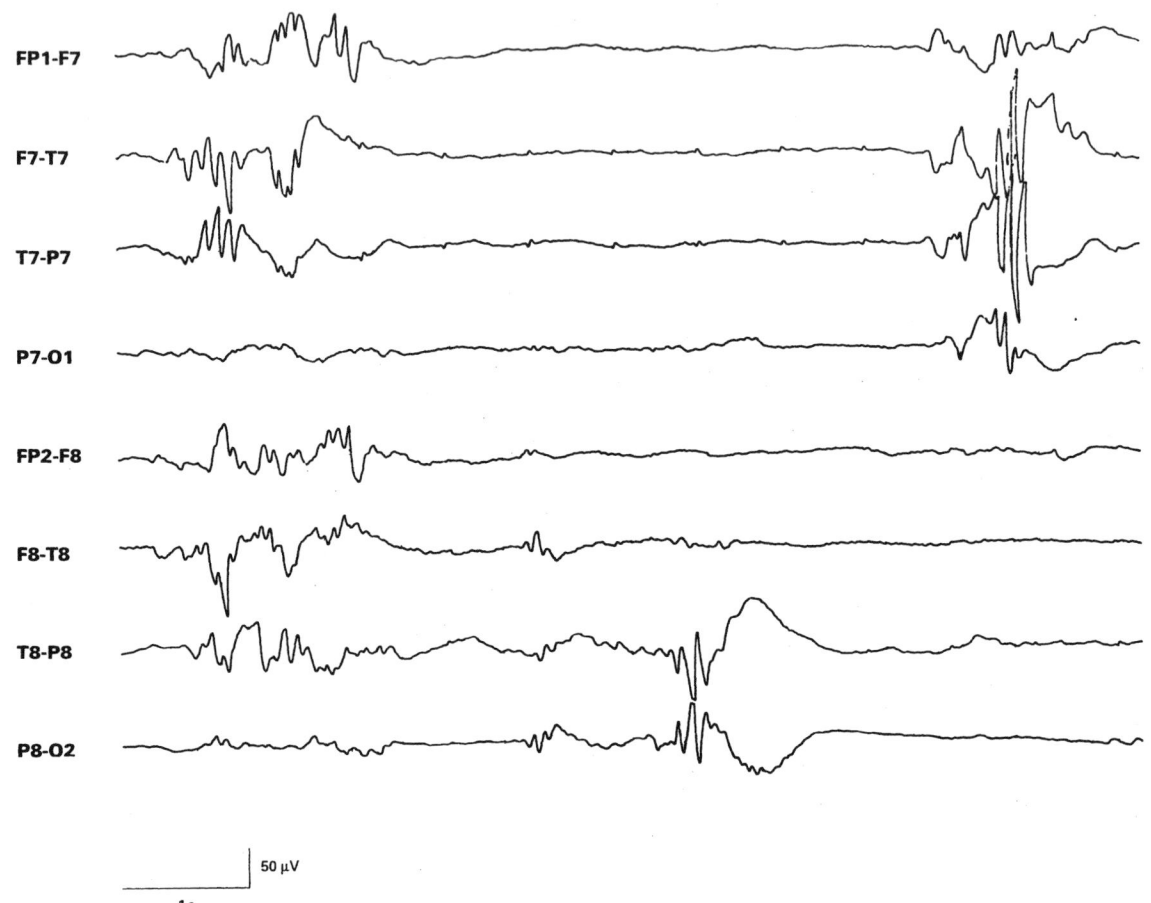

FIG. 12.9. Burst-suppression in a 3-year-old boy with severe anoxic encephalopathy. (From Lüders HO, Noachtar S. *Atlas and classification of electroencephalography*. Philadelphia: WB Saunders, 1999, with permission.)

Electrocerebral Inactivity

ECI is defined as no electrical brain activity exceeding 2 μV in EEGs recorded from scalp electrodes following the minimal technical standards proposed by the American Electroencephalographic Society (2) (Fig. 12.10). With very few exception it is an expression of brain death.

Encephalopathies involving mainly cortical regions are associated with seizures with generalized epileptiform discharges, changes in background rhythms, and amplitude attenuation of background activity, whereas those mainly involving white matter are correlated with arrhythmic, polymorphic slow activity in the theta and delta frequencies. Most diffuse encephalopathies, however, affect both the gray and white matter, and lead to all the EEG abnormalities listed above. Fluctuations of the EEG pattern over time, such as normal sleep-wave changes and reactivity to external stimuli, indicate less severe brain dysfunction than when no variability or reactivity is present. In contrast, the presence of a constant EEG pattern that does not change over time and does not react to external stimuli indicates a more severe disturbance. Serial EEG recordings are useful because the evolution

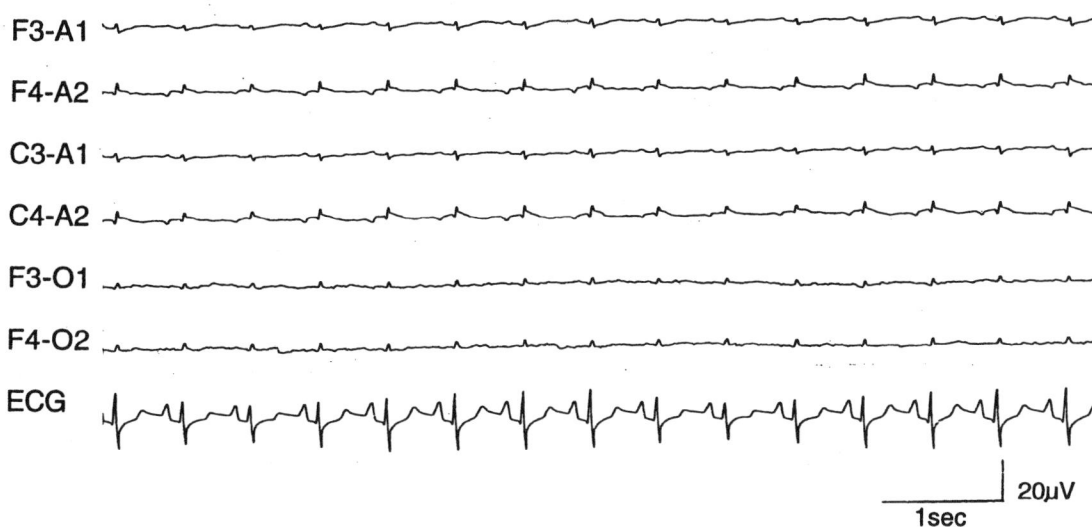

FIG. 12.10. Electrocerebral inactivity in a 19-year-old woman who 6 days ago had suffered a severe head injury in a traffic accident.

of the EEG pattern not infrequently allows more precise evaluation of the prognosis of a diffuse encephalopathy.

METABOLIC ENCEPHALOPATHIES

Hepatic Encephalopathy

EEG changes in hepatic encephalopathy vary from mild abnormalities such as background slow and diffuse IRS activity to severe, diffuse CS activity, seen usually in patients who are in coma. Triphasic waves are seen in moderate stages of encephalopathy usually associated with somnolence and mild stupor (see Fig. 12.8). Triphasic waves resemble spike-and-wave complexes in morphology, as earlier suggested by Foley et al. (35), who identified them as "blunt spike-wave" discharges. Triphasic waves are no longer regarded as a specific EEG abnormality for hepatic encephalopathy, as they can be seen in a variety of other metabolic encephalopathies such as renal failure, anoxia, hyperosmolar state, hypoglycemia, hyponatremia, hypercalcemia, and hyperthyroidism. However, there are reports suggesting that triphasic waves occur relatively more commonly in hepatic encephalopathy than in metabolic encephalopathies of other causes (34).

Triphasic waves can be classified into "typical" (bilaterally symmetrical and synchronous, anterior predominance, fronto-occipital time lag, occurrence in groups or runs) and "atypical" (lack of at least one of the four features specified for typical triphasic waves). According to Reiher (106), typical triphasic waves occur almost exclusively in patients with hepatic encephalopathy, although this has been disputed by Fisch and Klass (34).

In patients who undergo liver transplantation, the frequency of the posterior background activity tends to increase significantly (31). This improvement is apparently correlated with changes in cerebral blood flow in the frontal areas (25). It has also been reported that survival at 18 months after liver transplantation is strongly associated with higher frequencies of the background activity at baseline (31). Epileptiform abnormalities in EEGs from patients after orthotopic liver transplantation have been associated with serious, often irreversible brain damage, and most probably are the result of metabolic, electrolyte, and toxic alterations superimposed on structural brain changes (138).

In patients under age 20, triphasic waves do not accompany hepatic encephalopathy (29). In children with Reye's syndrome (acute childhood toxic encephalopathy), which is always associated with hepatic dysfunction of varying severity, EEG findings range from minimal background slow activity to burst-suppression or background attenuation. Triphasic waves, however, are extremely rare. Interestingly, 14- and 6-Hz positive spikes are seen not infrequently. Focal or multifocal epileptiform discharges and EEG seizure activity can be seen in the later stages of the disease (4).

Uremic Encephalopathies

Acute renal failure is more frequently associated with clinical encephalopathy than is chronic renal failure, and epileptic seizures are seen in more than 30% of patients with acute renal failure. This is a significantly higher incidence than in other metabolic encephalopathies (80). In milder degrees of uremic encephalopathy, only background slow or diffuse IRS activity occurs, whereas triphasic waves and diffuse CS activity occur in more severe stages. Myoclonus (labeled as polymyoclonus because of its multifocal character), asterixis (negative myoclonus), and generalized seizures are frequent. Focal seizures may also occur, most often in patients with previous focal brain lesions. Epileptiform discharges are rare, but photic stimulation often elicits photoparoxysmal and photomyoclonic responses (63). These observations are consistent with animal experiments in which urea infusion can produce myoclonus that rapidly progresses into uncontrollable generalized tonic–clonic convulsions (92,142). The myoclonus observed in these animal experiments most probably arises from the brainstem reticular formation, and it has been suggested that it is mediated by glycine (23).

In chronic renal failure, the EEG tends to be less abnormal than in acute renal failure. However, generalized epileptiform discharges have been reported in 8%–9% of patients (58). In "dialysis dysequilibrium syndrome," patients may deteriorate and even have seizures during or immediately after hemodialysis. The symptoms of dialysis dysequilibrium syndrome are due to a sudden normalization of some major biochemical blood abnormalities. The EEG in this syndrome shows diffuse IRS activity (69). The syndrome is rare with modern dialysis methods.

"Dialysis dementia" (also called progressive dialysis encephalopathy) is seen in patients who have been on hemodialysis for 3–4 years and is characterized by dysarthria, myoclonus, dementia, and eventually seizures and death. Sudden onset of hesitant, nonfluent speech is the most common characteristic and usually the earliest sign. The EEGs are more abnormal than would be expected from the clinical findings, showing high-voltage spike-and-wave patterns intermixed with abundant slow activity. This combination of clinical and EEG features is virtually pathognomonic (79). Aluminum intoxication is probably a major contributor to this syndrome. It was preva-

lent during the 1970s, but it is now extremely infrequent, most probably as a result of the use of an aluminum-free dialysate (20).

Encephalopathies Related to Alterations of Glucose Metabolism

Hypoglycemia

Level of consciousness and blood sugar levels do not necessarily parallel each other. However, the degree of EEG changes (background slow, diffuse IS, diffuse CS activity) in hypoglycemia tends to correlate closely with the severity of cerebral dysfunction. Epileptiform activity can be associated with diffuse slowing (94), and patients may clinically show confusion, stupor, coma, and even generalized convulsions.

Hyperglycemia

In diabetic coma, which is usually associated with acidosis and electrolyte imbalance, the EEG usually shows diffuse CS activity. In nonketotic hyperglycemia, localized epileptic phenomena such as PLEDs occur in association with partial seizures or epilepsia partialis continua (51,84). Ketotic hyperglycemia, in contrast, is much less frequently associated with seizures, most probably because of the antiepileptic effects of ketosis (67).

Encephalopathies Related to Electrolyte and Fluid Balance Alterations

Drowsiness, confusion, stupor, and coma, as well as generalized seizures and other neurological abnormalities, may occur with derangements of electrolyte or fluid balance (i.e., hypo- and hypernatremia, hypo- and hypercalcemia, hypophosphatemia, and hypomagnesemia). In these conditions, the EEG shows nonspecific, generalized slowing consistent with the degree of diffuse encephalopathy. Usually the *rate* of changes of electrolyte concentration is more important than the absolute degree of electrolyte abnormality as a factor responsible for developing clinical and EEG abnormalities, especially epileptic seizures.

Hyponatremia (usually of less than 125 mEq per liter) tends to be associated with hypo-osmolarity, which leads to cellular dehydration and brain edema. The syndrome of inappropriate antidiuretic hormone secretion is a frequent cause of hyponatremia that complicates many neurological disorders such as head trauma, meningitis, encephalitis, subarachnoid hemorrhage, and neoplasm. In this syndrome, alpha activity is replaced by high-voltage slow waves. These EEG abnormalities tend to persist even after correcting the hyponatremia, most probably because of a delay in equilibration of extracellular and intracellular water and electrolytes or because of acute cellular damage (97). Hypernatremia is associated with brain volume reduction, and the EEG usually only shows mild, nonspecific slowing.

Hypomagnesemia (less than 1.4 mEq per liter) can be caused by reduced intestinal absorption of magnesium (malabsorption syndrome, bowel resection, etc.) and excessive use of diuretics. No detailed studies of the EEG changes in hypomagnesemia have been reported. Magnesium deficiency has an inhibitory effect on the parathyroid gland, leading to secondary hypocalcemia. Hypomagnesemia produces generalized or partial seizures together with neuromuscular irritability (action or intention tremor, myoclonic jerks, startle response). A direct correlation between low plasma magnesium concentrations and seizure frequency has been demonstrated (10). Hypo- and hypercalcemia are described in the section on "Endocrine Encephalopathies" further on.

Encephalopathies Related to Alterations in Body Temperature

With hypothermia, depending on its severity, EEG changes can vary from diffuse slowing to burst-suppression and ECI. Burst-suppression occurs at 20–22°C, and ECI appears with body temperatures below 18°C (103). During cooling for open-heart surgery, sporadic spikes and periodic patterns may occur. In assessing ECI, especially at body temperatures below 32.2°C (90°F), potentially reversible EEG abnormalities produced by hypothermia should be considered (131). A mean increase in background frequency from 9 to 13 Hz has been described when the body temperature rises by 3.5°C (55), whereas relatively low-voltage and slow EEGs occur with temperature elevation to 42°C (107).

Acute Intermittent Porphyria

This autosomal dominant disease is characterized by attacks of abdominal pain, acute polyneuropathy, and cerebral dysfunction (confusion, delirium, visual defects, and seizures). The EEG in severe states of acute intermittent porphyria shows nonspecific diffuse slowing and epileptiform discharges (28).

Eclampsia

Eclampsia is a multisystem disorder associated with hypertension, proteinuria, edema, hemoconcentration, hypoalbuminemia, and diffuse encephalopathy with generalized, and occasionally also partial, seizures. These symptoms are most likely due to an extensive vasculopathy or vasospasm secondary to an exaggerated vascular responsiveness to circulating angiotensin II and catecholamines. Brain computed tomography and magnetic resonance imaging (MRI) show cerebral edema in the white matter mainly in posterior brain areas. EEG findings include diffuse slow activity and epileptiform discharges (126). These abnormalities disappear relatively quickly after clinical recovery. The EEG, clinical, and imaging findings in eclampsia are similar to those seen in hypertensive encephalopathy (118,127).

ANOXIC ENCEPHALOPATHY

During complete interruption of cerebral blood flow, predictable sequential EEG changes occur (39,88). No clinical or EEG changes occur in the first 6 seconds. Between 7 and 13 seconds, diffuse CS activity or FIRDA is recorded as consciousness is lost. When the arrest of circulation is prolonged, background attenuation occurs. Total cerebral anoxia of more than 5 minutes in a normothermic subject causes irreversible cerebral damage.

The EEG patterns that Prior (103) and Hockaday et al. (56) observed after a cardiopulmonary arrest can be subdivided into the following five grades:

Grade 1: dominant alpha activity (with or without scattered theta activity)
Grade 2: dominant theta activity (with rare alpha activity and diffuse IS activity of delta frequency)
Grade 3: diffuse CS activity, with little activity of faster frequency; spontaneous variability and reactivity of the EEG to stimuli are present
Grade 4: low-amplitude unreactive diffuse CS activity of delta frequency
Grade 5: background attenuation, burst-suppression, or ECI

Grade 1 indicates an excellent prognosis for recovery, whereas grades 4 and 5 are usually associated with a permanent neurovegetative state or death. Patients with EEGs of grades 2 and 3 show more variable outcomes. However, patients with ECI in the first hour after cardiopulmonary arrest may recover. Therefore, for prognostic purposes, it is recommended to obtain an EEG 5–6 hours after the time of cardiopulmonary arrest (99,103). Serial EEGs showing progressive deterioration or progression toward normalization are of great value for correct prognosis.

In addition to the above nonspecific EEG findings, several special EEG patterns can be seen in patients who have suffered from cardiopulmonary arrest. The following EEG patterns occur in patients who are comatose and carry a bad prognosis:

1. Generalized periodic spikes or sharp waves, at intervals of 0.5–2 seconds (75). Clinically these patients have bilateral, multifocal or generalized status myoclonicus (21), and at times electrographic status epilepticus in the absence of conspicuous somatic motor manifestations (119,120). The EEGs in these patients resemble triphasic waves and occasionally resemble those seen in patients with CJD.
2. Bilateral PLEDs consisting of periodically repetitive sharp-wave discharges occurring asynchronously over the two hemispheres.
3. Alpha coma pattern.

Patients with apallic syndrome show marked EEG attenuation during the day when they are "active" (Fig. 12.11), and at night two EEG patterns, suggesting rapid-eye-movement (REM) and non-REM sleep, can be distinguished (86). Normal slow-wave sleep is absent.

Postanoxic myoclonus is an action or intention myoclonus frequently associated with other neurological symptoms, including cerebellar ataxia, gait disturbance, postural lapse, and generalized seizures (Lance-Adams syndrome) (78). This myoclonus is of cortical origin and is associated with epileptiform discharges that, when not observed by direct visual analysis,

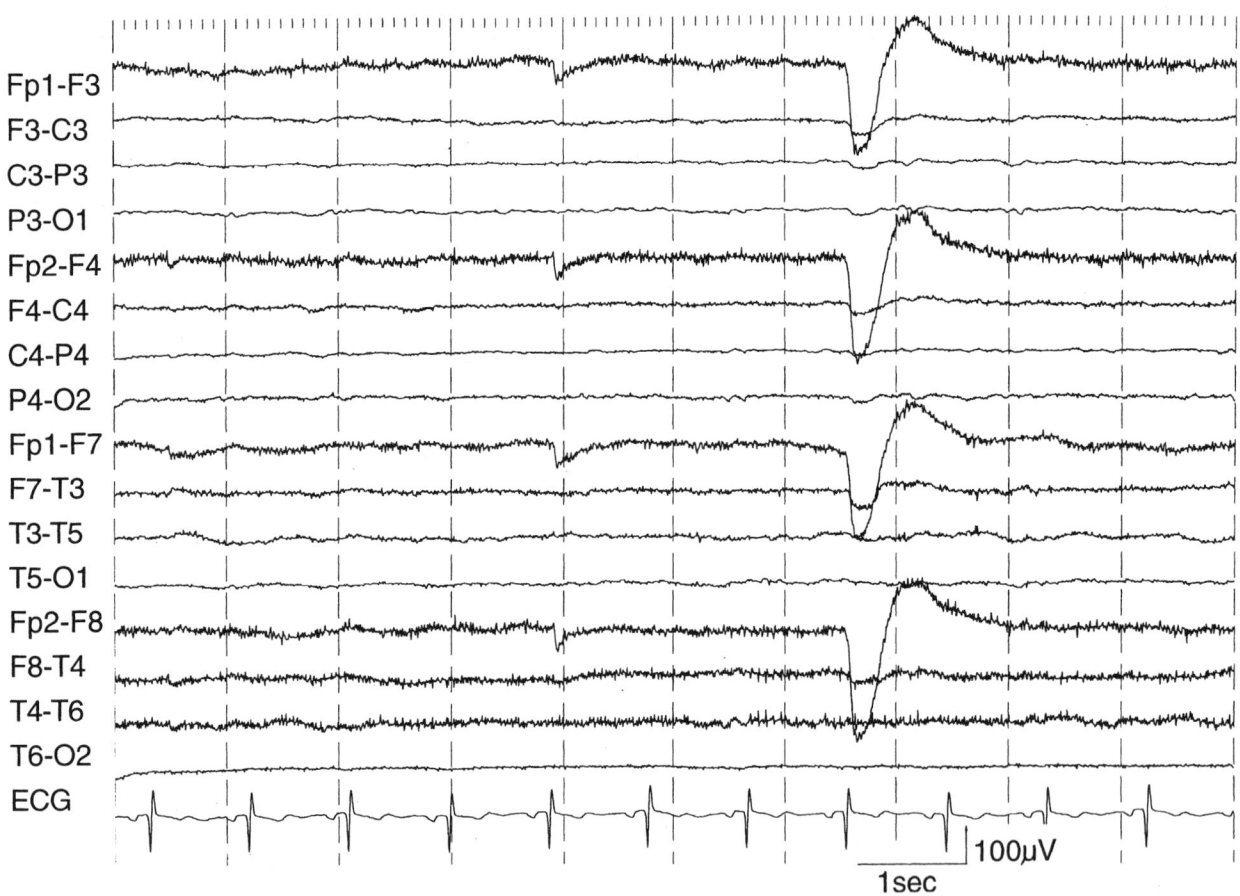

FIG. 12.11. Low-voltage EEG in a 54-year-old man who had a severe anoxic encephalopathy 6 months ago and now has severe cognitive deficits.

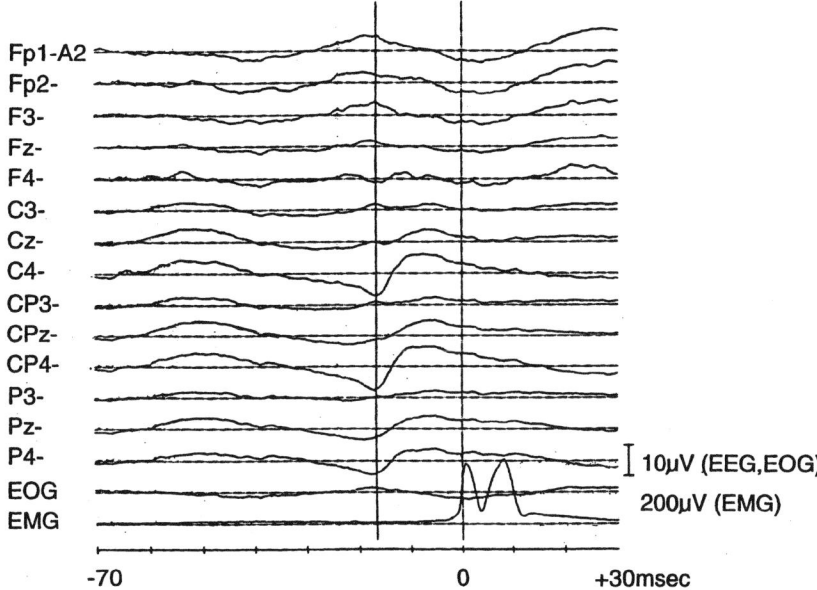

FIG. 12.12. Jerk-locked back-averaging in an 18-year-old man with severe action myoclonus (Lance-Adams syndrome). A positive potential maximum at C4 and CP4 preceding the action myoclonus at the left extensor carpi radialis by 16.7 milliseconds (shown by the left vertical line) can be distinguished by the back-averaging. Average of 250 trials. EEG recording referential to A2.

can be uncovered by jerk-locked back-averaging technique (112) (Fig. 12.12).

ENDOCRINE ENCEPHALOPATHIES

Thyroid Disorders

Hyperthyroidism is associated with a slight acceleration of alpha rhythm, enhancement of fast activity, and augmentation of rolandic mu rhythms (137). Bursts of epileptiform discharges and clinical seizures can occur, and epilepsy patients with hyperthyroidism respond poorly to anticonvulsants. In thyrotoxicosis and Hashimoto's encephalopathy, which is most likely caused by an immune-mediated cerebral vasculitis, diffuse slowing, FIRDA, sharp waves, and occasional triphasic waves have been reported (50,102).

Hypothyroidism in adults is associated with low-amplitude and diffusely slowed EEGs, and an absent or poor alpha blocking response. As expected, the EEG slowing becomes much more prominent in myxedematous coma. Seizures in hypothyroidism are associated with prolonged postictal recovery (32). In myxedematous infants, a EEG development, especially of sleep spindles, may be delayed (111).

Calcium Abnormalities

Hypocalcemia increases Na^+ conductance, which leads to membrane depolarization and repetitive neuron firing. This produces tetanic manifestations of peripheral origin. Hypocalcemia with calcium levels of 5–6 mg/dL also produces epileptic seizures of both generalized and partial origin, and epileptiform activity in the EEG. In addition, the EEG also shows irregular high-voltage delta activity that is enhanced by hyperventilation (43).

In hypercalcemia, epileptic activities usually do not occur. However, EEG changes consisting of diffuse slowing, diffuse IS activity, and sometimes triphasic waves appear when the calcium level reaches 13 mg/dL (57).

Adrenal Gland Abnormalities

Adrenocortical insufficiency (Addison's disease) can be associated with background slow, diffuse IS, and CS activity, depending on the severity of the disease. In severe cases, loss of reactivity to eye opening, increased sensitivity to hyperventilation, and decreased beta activity also appear (131). Usually no epileptic activity is seen.

EEG changes in adrenal cortical hyperfunction (Cushing's syndrome) tend to be less prominent than in Addison's disease. There are isolated reports that therapeutic dosages of adrenocorticotropic hormone (ACTH) may produce enhanced seizure susceptibility (101). This is in contrast to the well-recognized antiepileptic effect of ACTH in children with infantile spasms and hypsarrhythmia (108).

Pheochromocytomas produce extremely high blood pressure values, but the EEG shows no or little change except for those cases in which hypertensive encephalopathy occurs.

Pituitary Gland Abnormalities

Hypopituitarism, as seen in patients with postpartum necrosis of the anterior lobe of the pituitary gland (Sheehan's syndrome) is associated with diffuse IS or CS activity accompanied by alteration of consciousness. These clinical and EEG changes are most probably due to secondary hypofunction of the adrenal cortex (70). Pituitary adenomas may also cause similar EEG dysfunction secondary to hypopituitarism. In these patients, seizures may also occur related to an extension of the tumor to the uncinate gyrus and the mesial temporal region (5).

NUTRITIONAL DEFICIENCY ENCEPHALOPATHIES

Thiamine (vitamin B_1) deficiency gives rise to Wernicke's syndrome (disturbance of consciousness, gaze palsy, cerebellar ataxia, nystagmus) with or without Korsakoff's psychosis (amnestic–confabulatory encephalopathy). EEG findings parallel the severity of the neurological symptoms, and epileptiform discharges occur in severe cases (37).

Pellagra (nicotinic acid deficiency) manifests with dermatitis, diarrhea, depression, and dementia, and the EEG shows only nonspecific diffuse slowing (122).

Pyridoxine (vitamin B_6) deficiency can cause polyneuropathy and seizures. Seizures are particularly severe in neonates and infants with vitamin B_6 deficiency. Pyridoxine dependency is a rare, autosomal recessive, vitamin-responsive aminoacidopathy. It is characterized by early onset of convulsions (even in utero), failure to thrive, hypertonia–hyperkinesia, irritability, tremulous movements, and exaggerated auditory startle response, and leads to irreversible psychomotor retardation if not treated. There are decreased levels of pyridoxal 5-phosphate and γ-aminobutyric acid in the brain, and daily oral supplement of pyridoxine controls the symptomatology and permits normal development. The EEG in infants shows paroxysmal and epileptiform patterns consisting of generalized bursts of bilateral, asynchronous, high-amplitude, 1- to 4-Hz waves intermixed with spikes similar to the hypsarrhythmia pattern (89).

In vitamin B_{12} deficiency (pernicious anemia), besides subacute combined degeneration of the spinal cord and polyneuropathy, mental signs (irritability, apathy, somnolence, confusion, depressive psychosis, intellectual deterioration) and visual impairment (centrocecal scotoma and optic atrophy) occur in a minority of patients. Diffuse EEG slowing and focal epileptiform discharges occur frequently (71,132). These neurological and EEG findings are not secondary effects of anemia but are rather directly related to the effects of vitamin B_{12} deficiency on the central and peripheral nervous systems.

INFECTIOUS AND INFLAMMATORY ENCEPHALOPATHIES

Meningitis

In patients with meningitis, the EEG shows various degrees of slow activity depending on the type of meningitis and the associated degree of involvement of the brain parenchyma. In aseptic meningitis, the EEG shows no or little slowing, and any EEG changes return to normal in days to a few weeks. In meningitis associated with infectious mononucleosis, the EEG shows mild to moderate slowing. In acute purulent meningitis, moderate to severe diffuse slowing occurs, but with effective treatment resolves in several weeks (134). Haemophilus influenzae type B used to be the most frequent cause of acute purulent meningitis in children, but after introduction of conjugate vaccine for this bacterium in the United States, five other pathogens (Streptococcus pneumoniae, Neisseria meningitidis, group B streptococcus, Listeria monocytogenes, and H. influenzae) have become the major causes of meningitis in the United States (110). In tuberculous meningitis, severe inflammation with proliferative changes and vasculitis can lead to clinical symptoms such as level of consciousness disturbance ranging from stupor to coma, cranial nerve involvement, hydrocephalus, hemiplegia, and epileptic seizures. The EEG shows at least moderate diffuse slowing with or without focal findings and epileptiform discharges, depending on the severity of the clinical symptoms. The mortality rate is more than 50% in patients with tuberculosis meningitis who present with stupor or coma (76).

Acute Encephalitis

In acute encephalitis, the EEG is always abnormal because the inflammatory process predominantly affects the brain parenchyma. The degree of EEG abnormality is more pronounced than in meningitis (see Fig. 12.2).

In acute viral encephalitis, both diffuse abnormalities (generalized convulsions, delirium, stupor, coma, etc.) and focal findings (aphasia, mutism, hemiparesis, focal seizures, ataxia) occur. The EEG is always abnormal, showing at least diffuse slowing. Leukoencephalitides caused by non-neurotropic viruses (e.g., measles, rubella) and the postvaccinal state are associated with more severe EEG changes than those encephalitides caused by neurotropic viruses (e.g., mumps, equine encephalomyelitis, St. Louis encephalitis), which affect predominantly the gray matter (71). This is consistent with the experimental observation (44) that polymorphic delta activity is primarily produced by dysfunction of the white matter. During the acute stage of uncomplicated childhood viral infections such as measles, mumps, rubella, chickenpox, and scarlet fever, diffuse EEG slowing can be observed even when there was no clinically overt evidence of nervous system involvement (42). Acute bacterial encephalitides (e.g., those caused by Mycoplasma pneumonia, L. monocytogenes, and Legionella pneumophila) also show similar non-specific diffuse slowing, as well as focal abnormalities if focal lesions develop.

Herpes simplex encephalitis (HSE) is frequently associated with characteristic EEG findings consisting of unilateral or bilateral periodic complexes

(PLEDs or BiPLEDs) (130). HSE usually gives rise to intense hemorrhagic necrosis of the inferior and mesial parts of the temporal lobes and the orbital parts of the frontal lobes. The earliest changes in HSE consist of background slow and irregular slow activity appearing in a focal or lateralized fashion with predominance over the involved temporal areas (Fig. 12.13). Focal or lateralized sharp- and/or slow-wave complexes then appear over the temporal regions, and rapidly evolve to periodic patterns occurring every 1–3 seconds (PLEDs or BiPLEDs). Background activity between periodic discharges is usually attenuated (see Fig. 12.7). The periodic patterns tend to develop within several days after the clinical onset, frequently as BiPLEDs

occurring synchronously, either in a bilateral time-locked relationship with one another or independently (77). The periodic patterns are generally transient, lasting only 3–4 days, and almost always disappearing in a week regardless of whether there is clinical deterioration or improvement. EEGs in neonates with HSE also show periodic or quasiperiodic complexes, electrical seizures, slowing, and attenuation of background rhythms (91). As already mentioned, PLEDs reflect acute destructive cortical lesions and, therefore, are not pathognomonic for the diagnosis of HSE. However, the presence of this EEG pattern in combination with clinical findings suggesting HSE strongly supports the diagnosis.

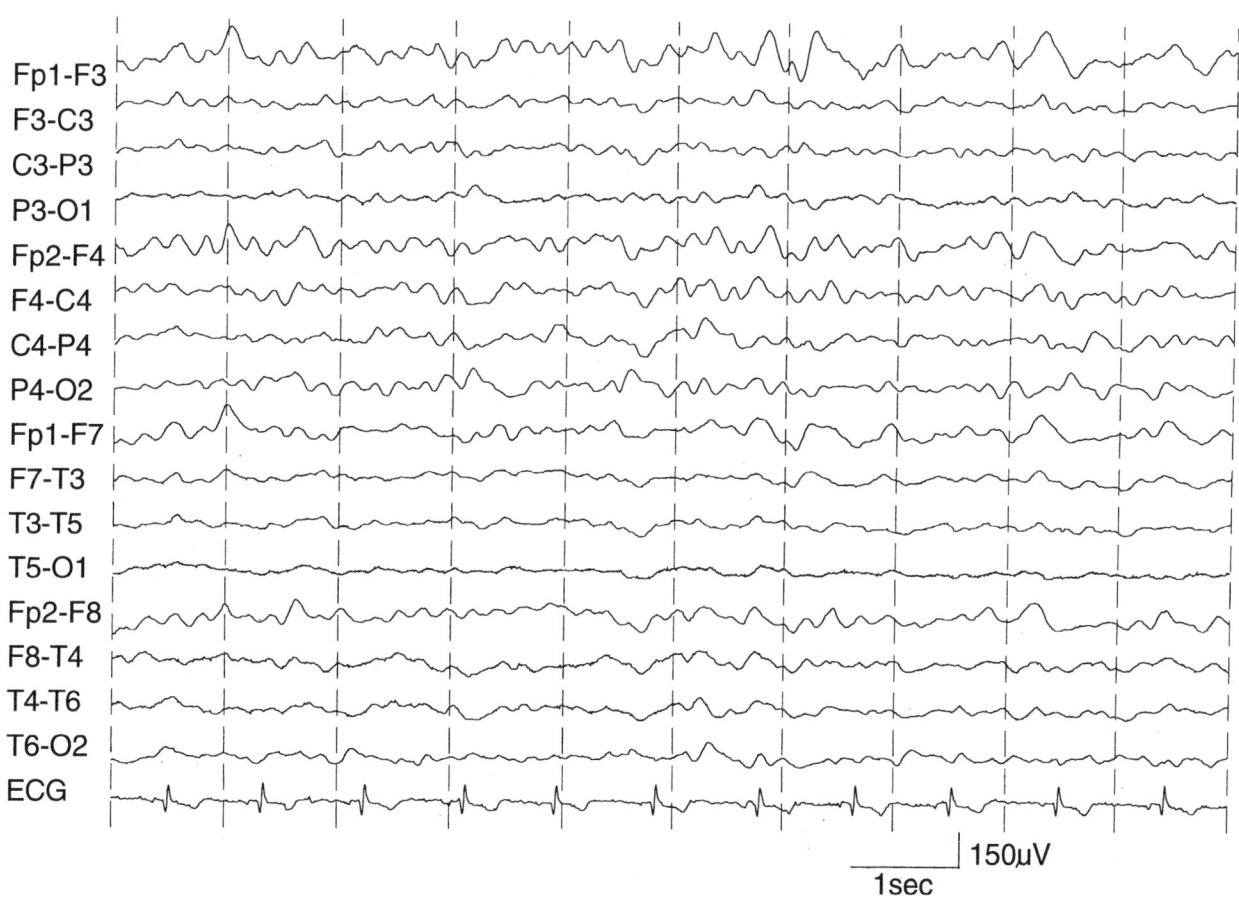

FIG. 12.13. Diffuse continuous slow activity, more on the right, in a 16-year-old boy with dementia and frequent generalized seizures who had herpes simplex encephalitis 1 year ago.

Subacute and Chronic Encephalitis

SSPE is a chronic measles infection that has almost disappeared in countries where routine measles vaccination has been introduced. The EEG pattern in SSPE is one of the most characteristic and specific in EEG (24). The pathology of SSPE involves the cerebral cortex and white matter of both hemispheres and also the brainstem. Clinically, several stages can be identified (62):

Stage I: personality changes and intellectual disturbance
Stage II: progressive intellectual deterioration with convulsions, myoclonus, and ataxia
Stage III: rigidity, hyperactive reflexes
Stage IV: decorticate state

High-voltage (300–1,500 µV) repetitive polyspike- and sharp-and–slow wave complexes of 0.5–2 seconds in duration, recurring every 4–15 seconds, occur in stage I or II. Initially this periodic pattern can be seen with normal background activity, and the complexes recur at irregular intervals (see Fig. 12.5). At this stage, EEG complexes can often be evoked by external stimuli. Later, however, the complexes occur at regular intervals and are no longer influenced by external stimuli (24). These periodic EEG complexes are usually associated with slow myoclonic jerks or dystonic myoclonus. During sleep, the periodic EEG discharges remain, although clinical myoclonus disappears. In the later stages, background activity between the periodic discharges becomes slow, and there is shortening of the intervals between the complexes. In the final stage, background activity is greatly attenuated and periodic discharges disappear (85).

Subacute measles encephalitis usually occurs in patients with defective cellular immunity, such as those with acquired immunodeficiency syndrome (AIDS). Symptoms (seizures, myoclonus, stupor, and coma) occur 1–10 months after measles, and epileptic discharges have been observed. Periodic EEG patterns, like as those with SSPE, have not been reported (40).

Progressive rubella encephalitis is very rare, and may appear as long as 10 years after exposure to rubella or in congenital rubella. Dementia, ataxia, and myoclonic seizures occur. The clinical picture is similar to that of SSPE, but EEG abnormalities and myoclonus are not as prominent as in SSPE (133).

Progressive multifocal leukoencephalopathy, caused by JC virus, is almost always a complication of chronic immunosuppression. It is characterized by widespread demyelinating lesions of the cerebral hemispheres, as well as the brainstem and cerebellum. Diffuse delta activity, most prominent in the posterior head regions, is common; epileptiform discharges with seizures and myoclonus are rare (33).

Transmissible Spongiform Encephalopathies (Prion Diseases)

CJD (sporadic and familial types), Gerstmann-Sträussler-Scheinker syndrome (GSS), fatal familial insomnia, and the new variant of CJD are classified as prion diseases transmissible between humans (49,65). Because these diseases do not cause an immune response, they simulate degenerative diseases.

CJD usually occurs in persons after the age of 50 years, and clinically is characterized by progressive dementia, myoclonic jerks, and various focal neurological deficits (e.g., ataxia, aphasia, visual loss, amyotrophy). The disease progresses to akinetic mutism, and at the later stages even the myoclonic jerking subsides. Early in the disease the EEG can be normal or show only mild non-specific slowing. As the disease progresses, typical periodic complexes appear (Fig. 12.14). For the diagnosis of CJD, these periodic complexes have a specificity and sensitivity of 67% and 86%, respectively (123). However, if repeated EEGs are obtained, more than 90% of patients show the characteristic periodic pattern (22). Myoclonic jerks are frequently, but not always, time-locked to the periodic EEG discharges, suggesting that there are both cortical and subcortical generator mechanisms for the myoclonic jerks (116). The periodic EEG pattern may disappear in the terminal phase, when the myoclonus also subsides (see Chapter 13 for further details).

GSS is usually a familial, slowly progressive disorder characterized by cerebellar ataxia, dysarthria, diminished tendon reflexes, and dementia, a phenotype similar to hereditary ataxia. Usually myoclonic jerks are absent and no periodic EEG pattern occurs (36), although a patient with sporadic GSS, confirmed by prion protein gene analysis (Pro102Leu mutation), was reported to show a periodic EEG pattern (60).

Fatal familial insomnia is characterized by progressive insomnia, hypovigilance, attention deficits, dysautonomia (tachycardia, sweating, hypertension), focal motor signs, and cognitive decline. The main pathological changes occur in the thalamus. Patients with fatal familial insomnia cannot generate a normal sleep pattern, and the awake EEG shows diffuse slowing (82,83).

A "new variant" of CJD in humans was reported in 1996 in the United Kingdom. This has been attributed to transmission from diseased cattle with bovine spongiform encephalopathy (mad cow disease). The new variant of CJD differs from sporadic CJD in several ways: (a) patients are young, with a mean age of 29 years; (b) the initial symptoms are often behavioral changes, ataxia, and peripheral sensory disturbances; and (c) the EEG abnormality is not periodic. In this prion disease, the EEG only shows non-specific diffuse slowing (136,141).

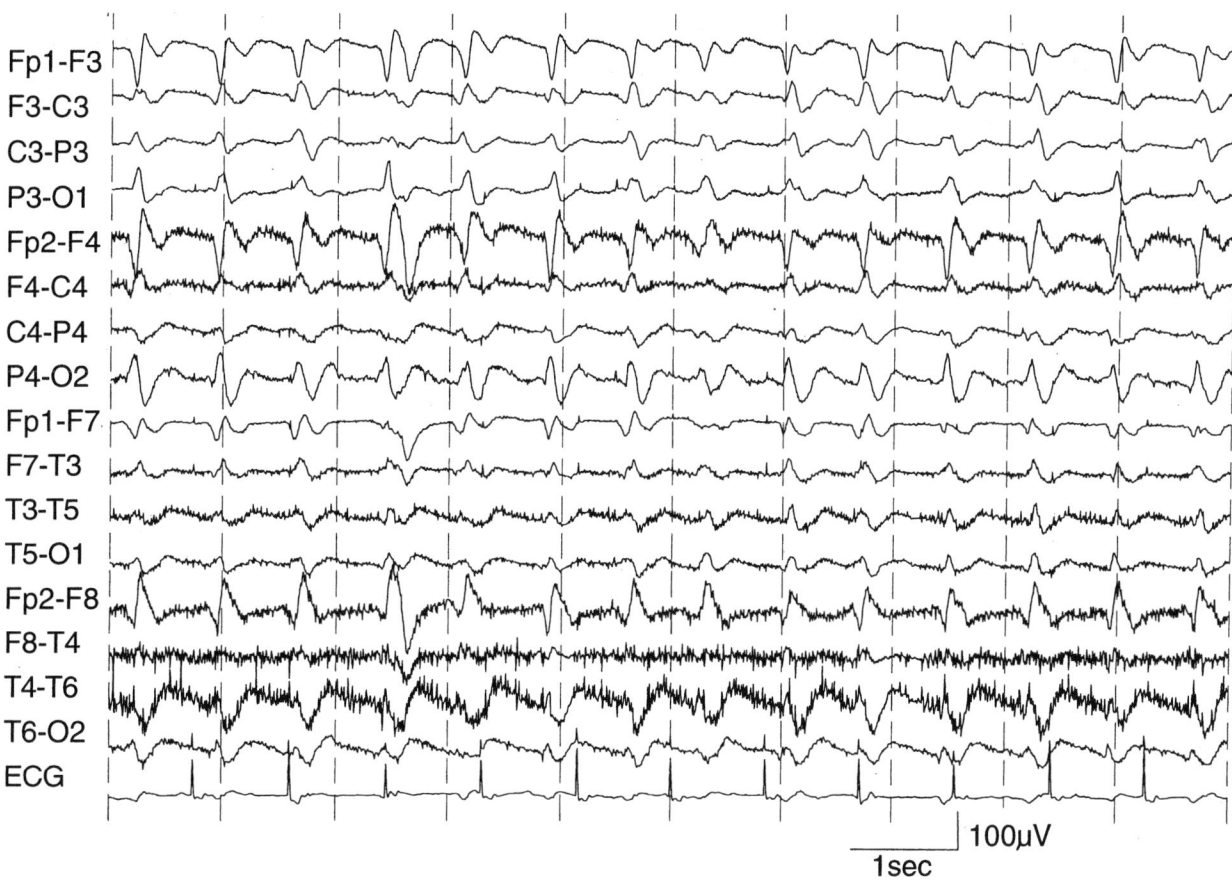

FIG. 12.14. Diffuse periodic pattern clearly dominant in the right hemisphere in a 72-year-old woman with CJD. The periodic discharges have a repetition rate of slightly more than 1 Hz.

AIDS and Human Immunodeficiency Virus Infection

Acute neurological manifestations of human immunodeficiency virus (HIV) infection may take the form of a meningoencephalitis, myelopathy, or neuropathy. Most patients recover from the acute illness, which usually precedes seroconversion. After seroconversion, as immunodeficiency appears and worsens, patients become vulnerable to opportunistic infections causing focal (brain abscess, toxoplasmosis, neurosyphilis, tuberculoma) as well as non-focal (cytomegalovirus, varicella-zoster virus, herpes simplex virus)

brain disease, primary central nervous system (CNS) lymphoma, and AIDS dementia complex (subacute chronic HIV encephalitis). Neurological abnormalities occur in one-third of patients with AIDS, although at autopsy, the nervous system is affected in nearly all patients.

EEGs in HIV symptomatic infection and AIDS usually show nonspecific abnormalities; epileptiform discharges are rare (38,48). Epileptic seizures occur in less than 5% of the HIV-infected population at any stage of the disease (76) but may affect 10% of more of those with advanced disease (131a). Quantitative EEG analysis studies also show no significant EEG abnormalities in patients with asymptomatic HIV infection (93,96). There is an isolated report of action myoclonus of cortical origin demonstrated by JLA technique in HIV-positive patients (68). In AIDS dementia complex, low-avoltage slow activity (47) and myoclonic jerks associated with triphasic waves (125) have been reported. Over time, there is further voltage attenuation and de-differentiation of EEG activity (47).

Multiple Sclerosis and Other Autoimmune Diseases

The incidence of EEG abnormalities in multiple sclerosis (MS) varies from 20% to 50%, depending on the location, size, and number of lesions, the duration and stage of the disease, and the rate of progression (71). EEG abnormalities consist most often of diffuse irregular slow activity; some patients also show diffuse rhythmic slowing. Focal EEG abnormalities may correlate with the area of maximal cerebral involvement, but more often, there is little correlation between EEG findings and clinical signs or symptoms (61,71). Epileptiform discharges are rarely observed, consistent with the low incidence of seizures (less than 2%) in MS (41).

In acute disseminated encephalomyelitis (ADEM), convulsions, confusion, stupor, and myoclonus occurs. The EEG in ADEM shows non-specific, diffuse, high-voltage slowing with epileptiform discharges; and focal slow activity can also occur. Spindle coma and alternating patterns may occur in patients who recover (17).

Miller-Fisher syndrome, characterized by acute ophthalmoplegia, ataxia, and areflexia, usually has a good outcome. It is associated with anti-GQ1b Iqg antibodies (94,136a). Non-specific EEG abnormalities (diffuse slow activity) may occur transiently in the acute stage of the disease (9,114). Coma has been reported in one patient (85a).

Systemic autoimmune diseases such as systemic lupus erythematosus (SLE) and polyarteritis nodosa can produce EEG abnormalities resulting from cerebral vasculitis or immune-complex neuronal dysfunction. The EEG is abnormal in 50% of patients with SLE, including those without symptomatic cerebral involvement, and both diffuse and focal slow activity, as well as epileptiform discharges, may occur (52). Seizures are most commonly seen in patients with SLE and with primary granulomatous angiitis of the brain (74).

Celiac Disease

Celiac disease is primarily a gastrointestinal disease with gluten-sensitive enteropathy and malabsorption. In about 10% of cases, neurological symptoms appear several years after the onset of enteropathy in the absence of vitamin E deficiency. Neurological manifestations include peripheral neuropathy, myelopathy, encephalopathy, cerebellar ataxia, progressive multifocal leukoencephalopathy, cerebral atrophy, and dementia. Seizures and polymyoclonus of cortical origin may occur (15), and, in these patients, the EEG usually shows multifocal epileptiform discharges (72). From a clinical standpoint, these cases may be regarded as a form of progressive myoclonic epilepsy or progressive myoclonic ataxia.

HYPERTENSIVE ENCEPHALOPATHY

Encephalopathy can complicate hypertension of any cause, such as chronic renal disease, acute glomerulonephritis, pheochromocytoma, and Cushing's disease but it is most often caused by rapid worsening of essential hypertension. Eclampsia is thought by some to share pathophysiological mechanisms similar to those of hypertensive encephalopathy. The symptoms, caused by rapid development of malignant hypertension, consist of headache, nausea, vomiting, visual disturbances, convulsions, and, in advanced stages, stupor and coma. MRI shows increased T2-weighted signal abnormalities in the white matter, usually in the posterior hemispheres. This is not due to infarction but is the result of fluid accumulation with little or no mass effect. Scattered, punctate lesions occur in a watershed distribution. This clinical picture has been labeled as reversible posterior leukoencephalopathy syndrome (53), because the MRI changes disappear with clinical recovery. Focal occipital seizures may be the main symptomatology in mild cases (6). The EEG shows diffuse slow activity with or without focal abnormalities in the occipital areas. Patients with profound slow activity in the EEG tend to have more grand mal seizures and more prolonged disturbance in consciousness than those with less amount of slow activity (139).

NEURODEGENERATIVE AND HEREDITARY DISEASES

Many progressive neurological diseases once thought to be neurodegenerative in nature are now known to be genetically determined. The specific diagnosis in a given condition is made by testing for an enzyme defect, a gene mutation or abnormal protein product, a biochemical marker, or a pathognomonic pathological abnormality. In diseases affecting primarily white matter, such as leukodystrophies, the most prominent clinical and EEG features are due to the dysfunction and interruption of white matter tracts (corticospinal, corticobulbar, cerebellar peduncle, sensory, medial longitudinal fasciculi, and visual pathways). Seizures, myoclonus, and epileptiform discharges are less frequently initial manifestations, whereas diffuse polymorphic and rhythmic slow activity tends to be prominent (44). In diseases affecting mainly cerebral gray matter (poliodystrophies), as in the progressive myoclonic epilepsy (PME) syndromes, seizures, myoclonus, chorea, dystonia, ataxia, and tremor occur frequently. In these cases, the EEG is characterized by epileptiform discharges (hypsarrhythmia in infants or children) in addition to diffuse irregular slow activity. However, in advanced stages, white and gray matter diseases are difficult to differentiate, and both evolve to an undifferentiated, attenuated pattern.

PME Syndromes

PME syndromes are familial disorders characterized by cortical myoclonus (mainly action and intention types), epileptic seizures (generalized tonic–clonic, myoclonic, or absence seizures), and progressive neurological deterioration (usually dementia and ataxia) (11,12,14,112,113). Specific disorders manifesting as PME syndrome are listed in Table 12.3. Common EEG findings consist of (a) background slowing with diffuse IS activity; (b) gener-

TABLE 12.3. *Age of onset, mode of inheritance, and causes of progressive myoclonic epilepsy syndromes*

	Age at onset (yr)	Mode of inheritance[c]	Diagnosis or causes
Common			
Unverricht-Lundborg disease	10–20	AR	Gene for cystatin B
Lafora body disease	10–20	AR	Mutation of *EPM2A*
Neuronal ceroid lipofuscinoses		AR	
Late infantile classical (Jansky-Bielschowsky disease)	1.5–4		*CLN2* gene (lysosomal pepstatin-sensitive protease)
Late infantile variant	2–7		*CLN5, -6, -7* genes
Juvenile (Spielmeyer-Vogt-Sjögren disease)	5–10		*CLN3* gene
Progressive epilepsy with mental retardation	5–10		*CLN8* gene
Adult (Kufs' disease)	10–40	(AD also)	*CLN4* gene
Sialidosis	7–20	AR	
Type I (cherry-red spot myoclonus syndrome)			α-*N*-Acetylneuraminidase deficiency
Type II (galactosialidosis)[a]			Neuraminidase & β-galactosidase deficiency
Myoclonic epilepsy with ragged red fibers (MERRF)	10–40	Sporadic or familial	Point mutation of mitochondrial DNA
Rare			
G$_{M2}$ gangliosidosis		AR	β-*N*-Acetylhexosaminidase subunits
Tay-Sachs disease	6 mo		
Juvenile	1–4		
Adult variant	15–20		
Gaucher's disease (noninfantile form)	10–40	AR	β-Glucocerebrosidase
Juvenile neuroaxonal dystrophy	9–10	AR	Axon spheroid in peripheral and central nerves
Action myoclonus-renal failure syndrome[b]	19	AR	
Dentatorubral-pallidoluysian atrophy[a]	5–60	AD	DNA triplet (CAG) repeat expansion
Familial cortical myoclonic tremor[a]	30–50	AD	
Celiac disease		nh	Gluten-sensitive enteropathy

[a]Mainly reported in Japan.
[b]Mainly reported in Canada.
[c]AD, autosomal dominant; AR, autosomal recessive; nh, nonhereditary.
Modified from Berkovic et al. (12), Shibasaki (112), and Bate and Cardiner (7).

alized polyspikes and spike-wave complexes and focal (particularly occipital), at times multifocal, independent epileptiform discharges; (c) photoparoxysmal responses (Fig. 12.15); and (d) enhanced cortical components of short latency evoked potentials such as "giant" somatosensory evoked potentials (SEPs) (Fig. 12.16). Action or intention myoclonus is often associated with clear epileptiform discharges in the EEG, and jerk-locked back-averaging techniques consistently reveal spikes over the sensorimotor area in the con-

tralateral hemisphere. These precede the jerk by 15–20 milliseconds, even in patients who do not show spikes in a single EEG record. This finding supports a cortical origin for the myoclonus (115). Patients with PME frequently have enhanced long-loop reflexes with giant SEPs, also suggesting a cortical "reflex" myoclonus (117) (Fig. 12.16).

Unverricht-Lundborg disease (ULD), common in Finland, is also found sporadically worldwide. In ULD, myoclonus is very severe and generalized

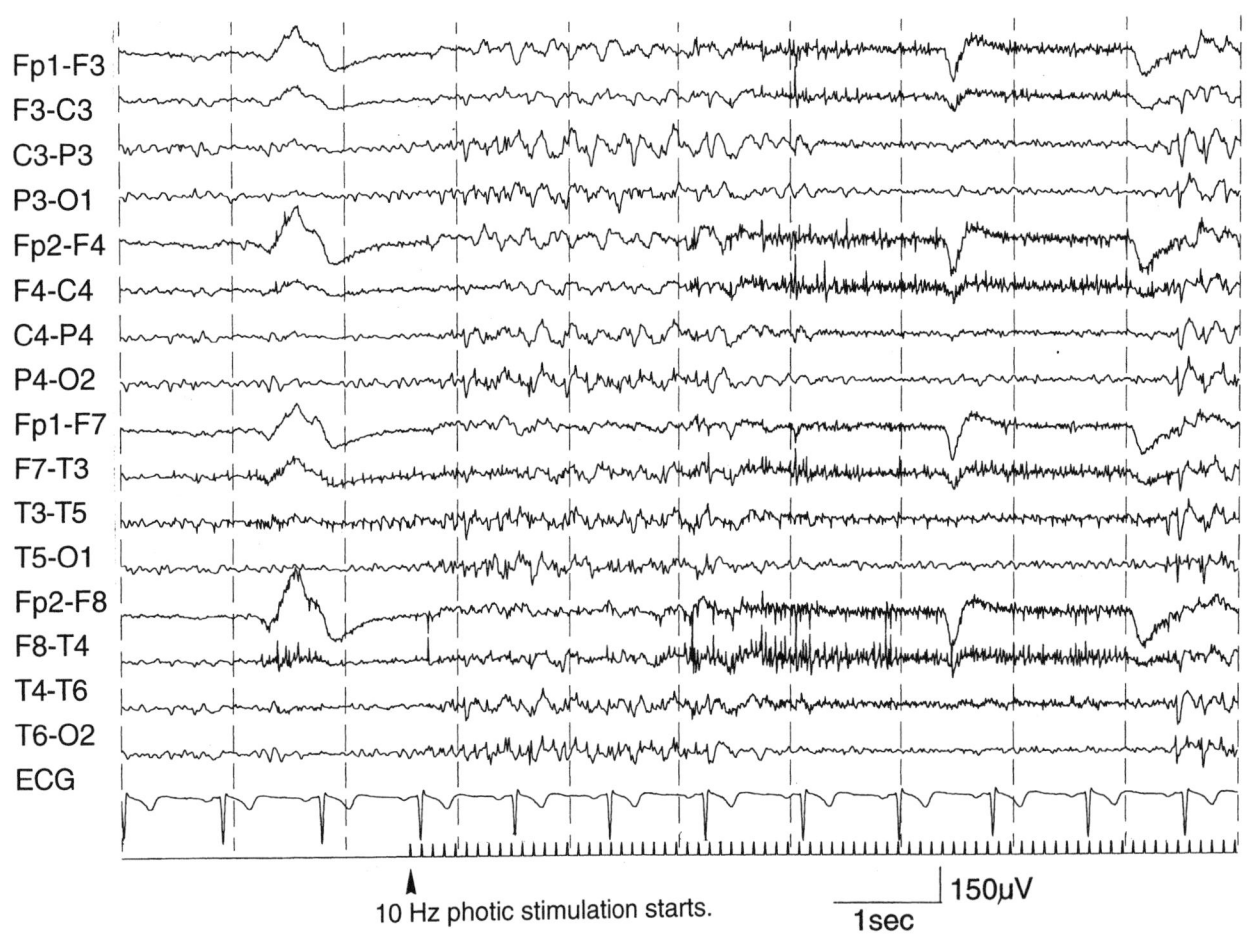

10 Hz photic stimulation starts.

150μV

1sec

FIG. 12.15. High-amplitude, widespread photoparoxysmal responses in a 38-year-old man with familial cortical myoclonic tremor.

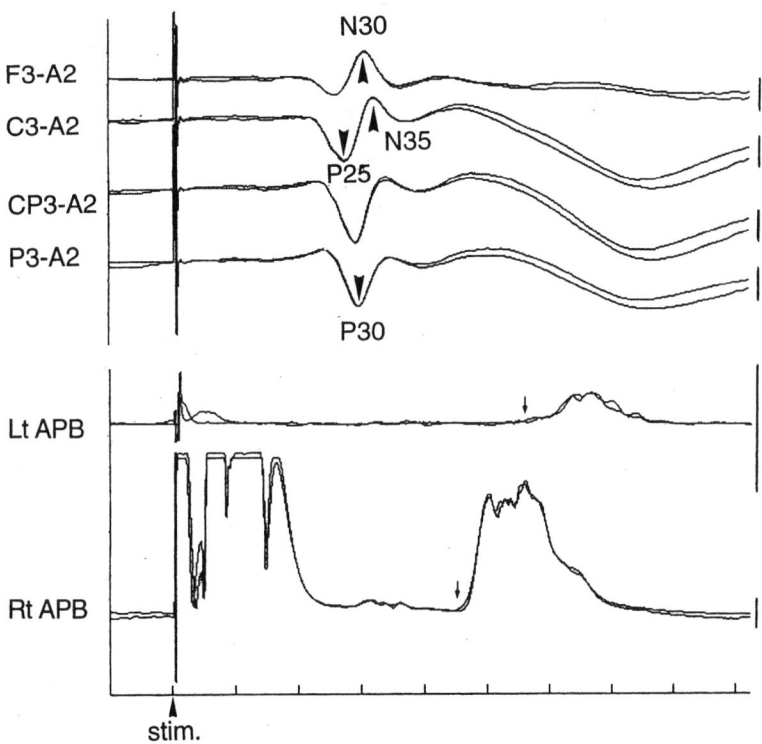

FIG. 12.16. Giant SEPs (P25, N30, P30, N35) (the peaks shown by *large arrows*) and enhanced C reflexes (the onsets shown by *small arrows*) in response to electric stimulation of the right median nerve at the wrist in a 74-year-old woman with familial cortical myoclonic tremor. *APB*, abductor pollicis brevis muscle. Vertical bars correspond to 20 μV, and one horizontal division corresponds to 10 milliseconds. (Modified from Terada K, Ikeda A, Mima T, et al. Familial cortical myoclonic tremor as a unique form of cortical reflex myoclonus. *Mov Disord* 1997;12:370–377.)

clinical features. The EEG findings are similar to the ones described in ULD. Focal spikes in Lafora disease are also particularly frequent in the occipital areas (128) (Fig. 12.17). Spike-wave complexes are not enhanced during sleep in Lafora disease (14).

Neuronal ceroid lipofuscinoses occur worldwide and are divided into at least five forms; all are characterized by the accumulation of abnormal lipopigment in the lysosomes. The late infantile type of lipofuscinosis (Jansky-Bielschowsky disease; *CLN2* gene) is characterized by seizures, ataxia, psychomotor regression, visual failure, and progressive spasticity. EEG photosensitivity is characteristic, and visual evoked potentials (VEPs) are of high voltage (135). A late infantile variant of lipofuscinosis is similar to the classical infantile form, except that the onset is later and progression occurs earlier. Abnormally large VEPs are also similar, but tend to decrease in amplitude as the disease progresses (109). In juvenile lipofuscinosis (Spielmeyer-Vogt-Sjögren disease; *CLN3* gene), visual failure occurs early, followed by dementia and extrapyramidal signs. Seizures are a relatively minor symptom. Photosensitivity is not present, and VEPs are of low voltage (100,135). Adult lipofuscinosis (Kufs' disease; *CLN4* gene) is very rare, and characterized clinically by dementia and extrapyramidal and cerebellar signs. Blindness does not occur. EEG shows poly-spike-wave complexes with marked photosensitivity (13).

Sialidosis is divided into type I (occurring mainly in Italy) and type II (occurring mainly in Japan). Type I sialidosis (cherry-red spot myoclonus syndrome) is characterized by severe myoclonus, gradual visual loss, ataxia, and typical retinal cherry-red spots. There is no dementia (105). Type II sialidosis (galactosialidosis) includes, in addition to the clinical features characteristic of type I sialidosis, gargoyle-like facial features, hearing loss, vertebral dysplasia, corneal opacity, and limited intellect (129). In both type I and type II sialidosis, EEG background activity shows low-amplitude fast activity and trains of vertex-positive, 10- to 20-Hz, small spikes associated with myoclonic EMG discharges. Generalized spike-wave complexes are not observed (30).

Myoclonic epilepsy with ragged red fibers (MERRF) is probably the most common form of PME today. It is characterized by myoclonus and myopathy with ragged red fibers on skeletal muscle biopsy. Generalized tonic–clonic seizures, dementia, and ataxia are also common. Less often, there is neuropathy, deafness, and optic atrophy. The EEG shows progressive background slowing, generalized spike-wave or polyspike-wave complexes, and sporadic focal spikes. VEPs are usually normal (121).

In non-infantile Gaucher's disease, apraxia of horizontal eye movements and splenomegaly are present in addition to other clinical features of PME.

seizures may be difficult to control, but progression of ataxia and dementia is relatively mild. The EEG shows progressive background slow activity, generalized spike-wave complexes, generalized polyspike-wave complexes, and focal occipital spikes.

Lafora disease, which used to be reported mainly in Southern Europe, is now found worldwide. Partial seizures, particularly of occipital origin, rather mild myoclonus, and relatively severe dementia are characteristic

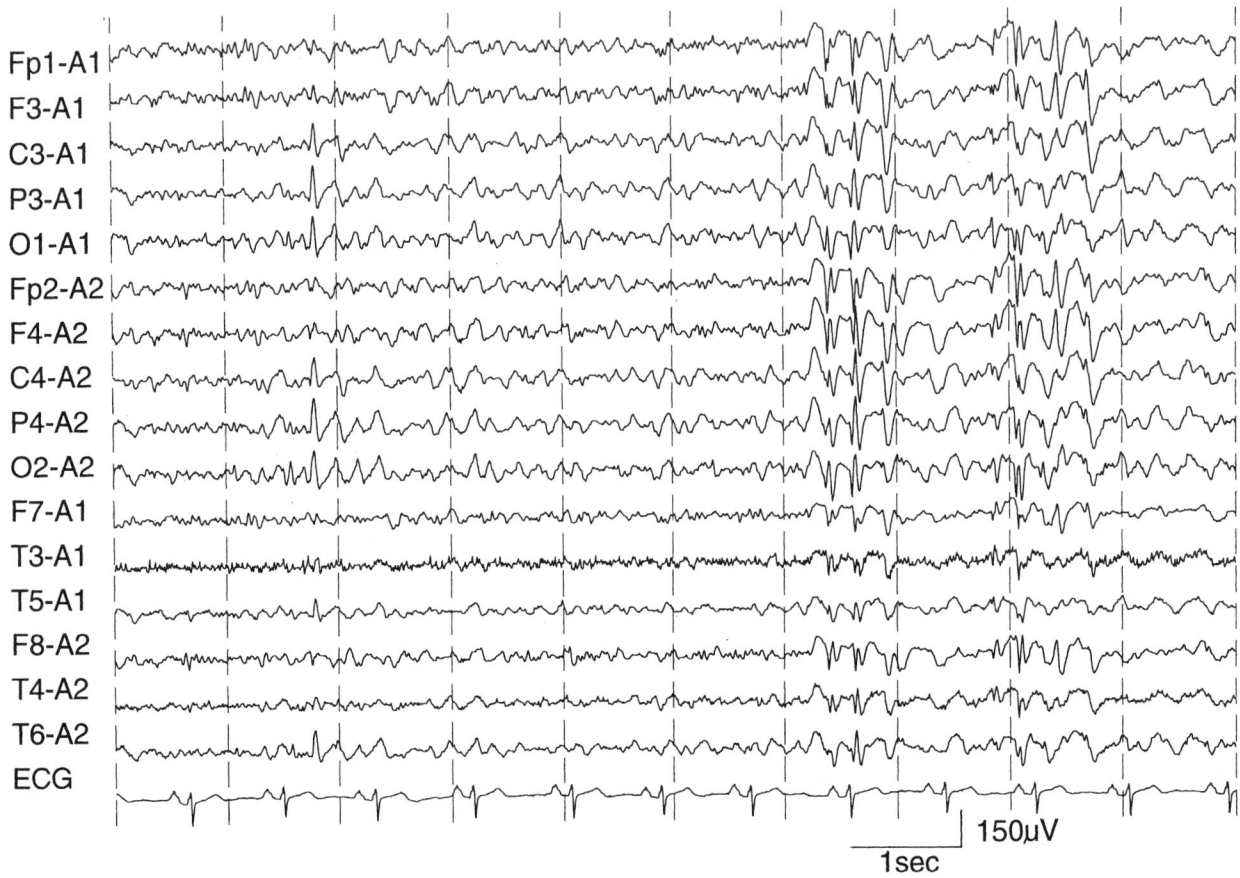

FIG. 12.17. Generalized spike-and-wave complexes with regional spike-and-wave complexes maximal either anteriorly or posteriorly in a 19-year-old man with Lafora disease.

The EEG shows generalized spike-wave complexes and bursts of 6- to 9-Hz spikes or sharp waves over the central and posterior head regions (95).

Juvenile neuroaxonal dystrophy manifests as chorea and peripheral neuropathy in addition to the clinical features of PME. The EEG shows generalized polyspikes and polyspike-wave discharges. Sporadic and induced occipital spikes are often seen (27).

Action myoclonus–renal failure syndrome is characterized by tremor, action myoclonus, generalized seizures, and proteinuria associated with progressive renal failure; dementia does not occur (3). The EEG shows the typical features of PME with marked photosensitivity (87). In this syndrome, CNS dysfunction progresses even if renal failure is controlled by dialysis or transplantation.

Dentatorubral-pallidoluysian atrophy (DRPLA), mainly reported in Japan, has a variety of clinical phenotypes (PME, ataxic choreoathetosis, choreo-dementia). The EEG in PME-type DRPLA shows slowing of background activity, frequent generalized polyspike-wave complexes, and multifocal spikes. Photosensitivity is prominent. However, the SEP amplitude is always relatively small in spite of the giant VEPs, frequent myoclonus, and generalized seizures. The photosensitivity is most likely due to a severe disturbance in the afferent pathways above the lemniscus medialis (90).

Familial cortical myoclonic tremor (124), called also cortical tremor (59) or benign adult familial myoclonic epilepsy (140), is a frequent cause of PME in adults in Japan, where it has been reported exclusively. It is characterized by rhythmic postural and action myoclonus involving distal limbs (thus resembling essential tremor), absence of ataxia and dementia, rare generalized tonic–clonic seizures, and no or only minimal progression. The EEG usually shows normal background activity with only occasional epileptiform discharges. Photosensitivity is seen in some patients (see Fig. 12.15). In addition, giant SEPs and, by back-averaging, spikes preceding the tremor-like EMG discharges can be observed (see Fig. 12.16). Familial cortical myoclonic tremor should be differentiated from familial essential myoclonus, which has similar clinical characteristics except for the absence of epileptic seizures and no evidence of cortical hyperexcitability either on EEG or SEPs (104).

Leukodystrophies of Adult Onset

Leukodystrophies of adult onset include metachromatic leukodystrophy (MLD) (an autosomal recessive, sphingolipid storage disease caused by arylsulfatase deficiency, resulting in sulfatide accumulation mainly in the white matter); globoid body leukodystrophy (Krabbe's disease) (an autosomal recessive disease caused by galactocerebrosidase deficiency, resulting in the accumulation of galactocerebroside, particularly in the white matter); and adrenoleukodystrophy (ALD) (X-linked autosomal recessive disease caused by impaired peroxisomal oxidation of very-long-chain fatty acids, leading to their accumulation in the brain and adrenal glands). Krabbe's disease usually occurs in infancy, and MLD and ALD are seen most frequently in childhood. However, all three leukodystrophies can also occur in adults. Because these diseases affect white matter primarily, the most prominent clinical signs and symptoms are due to the interruption of white matter tracts (corticospinal, corticobulbar, cerebellar peduncle, sensory, medial longitudinal fasciculi, and visual pathways). Epileptic seizures and myoclonus are infrequent. The EEG usually shows high-amplitude, continuous, polymorphic slow waves (44), which in ALD are most prominent posteriorly (8), in good agreement with the predominant involvement of the white matter in the posterior hemispheres shown by MRI and the frequent occurrence of cortical blindness. Epileptiform discharges are infrequent (Fig. 12.18).

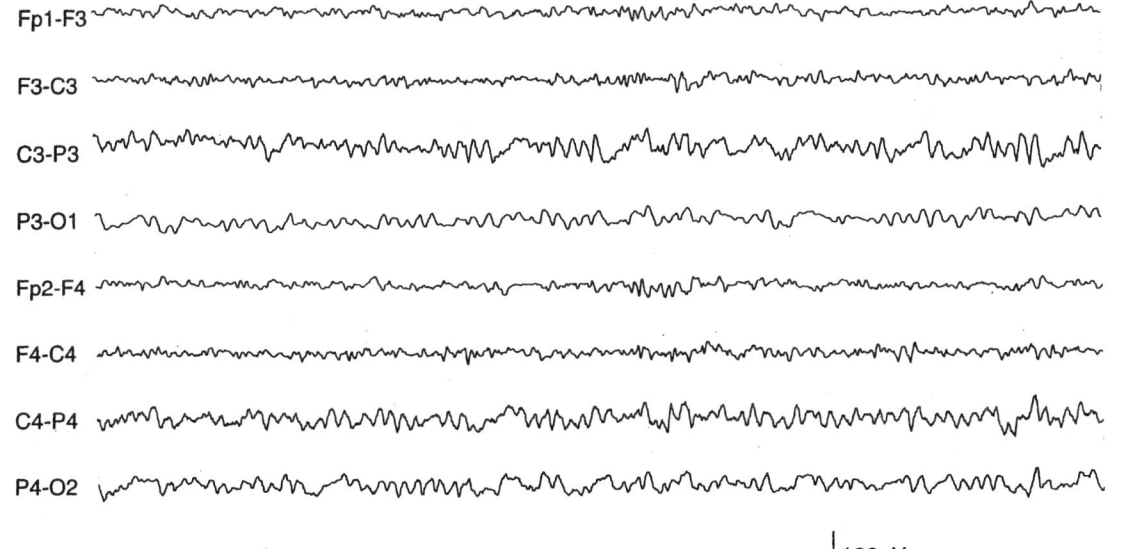

FIG. 12.18. Diffuse continuous slow activity most prominent in the posterior hemispheres in a 28-year-old man with diffuse leukodystrophy of unknown etiology.

Other Inherited Metabolic Diseases of Adult Onset

Mucopolysaccharidoses are mainly autosomal recessive diseases in which acid mucopolysaccharides (glycosaminoglycans) are degraded and accumulate within lysosomes in neurons (brain, spinal cord), connective tissues, heart, viscera, and bone because of enzyme defects. Obstructive hydrocephalus secondary to skeletal deformity and thickening of the base of the skull is a frequent complication. The EEG shows non-specific slowing consistent with the degree of impaired cerebral function.

Niemann-Pick disease (autosomal recessive disease with increased sphingomyelin due to sphingomyelinase deficiency) can occur in adolescents, and cataplexy has been described in a variant of this disease(66).

MELAS (mitochondrial myopathy, encephalopathy, lactic acidosis, and stroke-like episodes) is a mitochondrial disease characterized by metabolic strokes, encephalopathy (seizures, dementia), mitochondrial dysfunction with lactic acidosis, and ragged red fibers. Myopathic weakness, exercise intolerance, myoclonus, ataxia, short stature, and hearing loss are also common. The disease can be due to several types of mitochondrial DNA point mutations. Because of the metabolic strokes, the EEG most often shows focal rather than diffuse abnormalities. Focal and generalized epileptiform discharges may occur in association with, respectively, focal and generalized seizures (54). Kojewnikoff's syndrome (epilepsia partialis continua) may also be seen in patients with MELAS.

ACKNOWLEDGMENTS

This study was partly supported by Grants-in-Aid for Scientific Research (C) 10670583 and (C2) 13670640 from the Japan Ministry of Education, Science, Sports and Culture, and JSPS-RFTF97L00201 from the Research for the Future Program from the Japan Society for the Promotion of Science. The authors thank Mrs. M. Yoshikawa (REEG T) for providing Figure 12.8.

REFERENCES

1. Adams A. Studies on flat electroencephalograph in man. *Electroencephalogr Clin Neurophysiol* 1959;11:34–41.
2. American Electroencephalographic Society. Guideline three: technical standards for EEG recording in suspected cerebral death. *J Clin Neurophysiol* 1994;11:10–13.
3. Andermann E, Andermann F, Carpenter S, et al. Action myoclonus-renal failure syndrome: a previously unrecognized neurological disorder unmasked by advances in nephrology. *Adv Neurol* 1986;43:87–103.
4. Aoki Y, Lombroso CT. Prognostic value of electroencephalography in Reye's syndrome. *Neurology* 1973;23:333–343.
5. Bairamian D, Di Chiro G, Blume H, et al. Pituitary adenoma with seizures: PET demonstration of reduced glucose utilization in the medial temporal lobe. *J Comput Assist Tomogr* 1986;10:529–532.
6. Bakshi R, Bates VE, Mechtler LL, et al. Occipital lobe seizures as the major clinical manifestation of reversible posterior leukoencephalopathy syndrome: magnetic resonance imaging findings. *Epilepsia* 1998;39:295–299.
7. Bate L, Cardiner M. Genetics of inherited epilepsies. *Epileptic Disord* 1999;1:7–19.
8. Battaglia A, Harden A, Pampiglione G, et al. Neurophysiological studies in 13 patients with adrenoleukodystrophy. *Electroencephalogr Clin Neurophysiol* 1981;51:53P(abst).
9. Becker WJ, Watters GV, Humphreys P. Fisher syndrome in childhood. *Neurology* 1981;31:555–560.
10. Benga I, Baltescu V, Tilinca R, et al. Plasma and cerebrospinal fluid concentrations of magnesium in epileptic patients. *J Neurol Sci* 1985;67:29–34.
11. Berkovic SF. Progressive myoclonic epilepsies. In: Engel J Jr, Pedley TA, eds. *Epilepsy: a comprehensive textbook*. Philadelphia: Lippincott–Raven Publishers, 1997:2455–2468.
12. Berkovic SF, Andermann F, Carpenter S, et al. Progressive myoclonic epilepsies: specific causes and diagnosis. *N Engl J Med* 1986;315:296–305.
13. Berkovic SF, Carpenter S, Andermann F, et al. Kufs' disease: a critical appraisal. *Brain* 1988;111:27–62.
14. Berkovic SF, So NK, Andermann F. Progressive myoclonic epilepsies: clinical and neurophysiological diagnosis. *J Clin Neurophysiol* 1991;8:261–274.
15. Bhatia KP, Brown P, Gregory R, et al. Progressive myoclonic ataxia associated with coeliac disease: the myoclonus is of cortical origin, but the pathology is in the cerebellum. *Brain* 1995;118:1087–1093.
16. Bickford RG, Butt HR. Hepatic coma: the electroencephalograph pattern. *J Clin Invest* 1955;34:790–799.
17. Bortone E, Bettoni L, Buzio S, et al. Spindle coma and alternating pattern in the course of measles encephalitis. *Clin Electroencephalogr* 1996;27:210–214.
18. Brenner RP, Schaul N. Periodic EEG patterns: classification, clinical correlation, and pathophysiology. *J Clin Neurophysiol* 1990;7:249–267.
19. Britt CW Jr, Saulus D, Armstrong S. "Theta coma"—clinical, electroencephalographic, and physiologic features. *Neurology* 1981;31[Pt 2]:89.
20. Burn DJ, Bates D. Neurology and the kidney. *J Neurol Neurosurg Psychiatry* 1998;65:810–821.
21. Celesia GG, Grigg MM, Ross E. Generalized status myoclonicus in acute anoxic and toxic-metabolic encephalopathies. *Arch Neurol* 1988;45:781–784.
22. Chiofalo N, Fuentes A, Galvez S. Serial EEG findings in 27 cases of Creutzfeldt-Jakob disease. *Arch Neurol* 1980;37:143–145.
23. Chung EY, Van Woert MH. Urea myoclonus: possible involvement of glycine. *Adv Neurol* 1986;43:565–568.
24. Cobb W. The periodic events of subacute sclerosing leukoencephalitis. *Electroencephalogr Clin Neurophysiol* 1966;21:278–294.
25. Dam M, Burra P, Tedeschi U, et al. Regional cerebral blood flow changes in patients with cirrhosis assessed with 99mTc-HM-PAO single-photon emission computed tomography: effect of liver transplantation. *J Hepatol* 1998;29:78–84.
26. de la Paz D, Brenner RP. Bilateral independent periodic lateralized epileptiform discharges: clinical significance. *Arch Neurol* 1981;38:713–715.
27. Dorfman LJ, Pedley TA, Tharp BR, et al. Juvenile neuroaxonal dystrophy: clinical, electrophysiological, and neurophysiological features. *Ann Neurol* 1978;3:419–428.
28. Dow RS. The electroencephalographic findings in acute intermittent porphyria. *Electroencephalogr Clin Neurophysiol* 1961;13:425–437.
29. Drury I. 14-and-6 positive bursts in childhood encephalopathies. *Electroencephalogr Clin Neurophysiol* 1989;72:479–485.

30. Engel J Jr, Rapin I, Giblin DR. Electrophysiological studies in two patients with cherry red spot–myoclonus syndrome. *Epilepsia* 1977;18:73–87.
31. Epstein CM, Riecher AM, Henderson RM, et al. EEG in liver transplantation: visual and computerized analysis. *Electroencephalogr Clin Neurophysiol* 1992;83:367–371.
32. Evans EC. Neurological complications of myxedema: convulsions. *Ann Intern Med* 1960;52:434–444.
33. Farrell DF. The EEG in progressive multifocal leukoencephalopathy. *Electroencephalogr Clin Neurophysiol* 1969;26:200–205.
34. Fisch BJ, Klass DW. The diagnostic specificity of triphasic wave pattern. *Electroencephalogr Clin Neurophysiol* 1988;70:1–8.
35. Foley JM, Watson CW, Adams RD. Significance of the electroencephalographic changes in hepatic coma. *Trans Am Neurol Assoc* 1950;75:161–165.
36. Foncin JF, Cardot JL, Martinet Y, et al. Gerstmann-Sträussler Scheinker disease: anatomoclinical genealogical study. *Rev Neurol (Paris)* 1982;138:123–135.
37. Fournet A, Lanternier M. Constatations électroencéphalographiques dans 17 cas d'encephalopathie de Gayet-Wernicke. *Rev Neurol (Paris)* 1956;94:644–645.
38. Gabuzda D, Levy S, Chiappa K. EEG in AIDS and AIDS-related complex. *Clin Electroencephalogr* 1988;19:1–6.
39. Gastaut H, Fischer-Williams M. Electroencephalographic study of syncope: its differentiation from epilepsy. *Lancet* 1957;2:1018–1025.
40. Gazzola P, Cocito L, Cappello E, et al. Subacute measles encephalitis in a young man immunosuppressed for ankylosing spondylitis. *Neurology* 1999;52:1074–1077.
41. Ghezzi A, Montanini R, Basso PF, et al. Epilepsy in multiple sclerosis. *Eur Neurol* 1990;30:218–223.
42. Gibbs FA, Gibbs EL, Carpenter PR, et al. Electroencephalographic abnormality in "uncomplicated" childhood diseases. *JAMA* 1959;171:1050–1055.
43. Glaser GH, Levy LL. Seizures and idiopathic hypoparathyroidism: a clinical-electroencephalographic study. *Epilepsia* 1960;1:454–465.
44. Gloor P, Kalabay O, Giard N. The electroencephalogram in diffuse encephalopathies: electroencephalographic correlates of grey and white matter lesions. *Brain* 1968;91:779–802.
45. Grindal AB, Suter C. "Alpha pattern" coma in high voltage electrical injury. *Electroencephalogr Clin Neurophysiol* 1975;38:521–526.
46. Grindal AB, Suter C, Martinez AJ. Alpha-pattern coma: 24 cases with 9 survivors. *Ann Neurol* 1977;1:371–377.
47. Harden CL, Daras M, Tuchman AJ, et al. Low amplitude EEGs in demented AIDS patients. *Electroencephalogr Clin Neurophysiol* 1993;87:54–56.
48. Harrison MJ, Newman SP, Hall-Craggs MA, et al. Evidence of CNS impairment in HIV infection: clinical, neuropsychological, EEG, and MRI/MRS study. *J Neurol Neurosurg Psychiatry* 1998;65:301–307.
49. Haywood AM. Transmissible spongiform encephalopathies. *N Engl J Med* 1997;337:1821–1828.
50. Henchey R, Cibula J, Helveston W, et al. Electroencephalographic findings in Hashimoto's encephalopathy. *Neurology* 1995;45:977–981.
51. Hennis A, Corbin D, Fraser H. Focal seizures and non-ketotic hyperglycemia. *J Neurol Neurosurg Psychiatry* 1992;55:195–197.
52. Hietaharju A, Jäntti V, Korpela M, et al. Nervous system involvement in systemic lupus erythematosus, Sjögren syndrome and scleroderma. *Acta Neurol Scand* 1993;88:299–308.
53. Hinchey J, Chaves C, Appignami B, et al. A reversible posterior leukoencephalopathy syndrome. *N Engl J Med* 1996;334:494–500.
54. Hirano M, Pavlakis SG. Mitochondrial myopathy, encephalopathy, lactic acidosis, with stroke-like episodes (MELAS): current concepts. *J Child Neurol* 1994;9:4–13.
55. Hoagland H. Temperature characteristics of the "Berger rhythm" in man. *Science* 1936;83:84–85.
56. Hockaday JM, Potts F, Epstein E, et al. Electroencephalographic changes in acute cerebral anoxia from cardiac or respiratory arrests. *Electroencephalogr Clin Neurophysiol* 1965;18:575–586.
57. Honigsberger L. Blood calcium and the EEG. *Electroencephalogr Clin Neurophysiol* 1969;26:539–540.
58. Hughes JR. EEG in uremia. *Am J EEG Technol* 1984;24:1–10.
59. Ikeda A, Kakigi R, Funai N, et al. Cortical tremor: a variant of cortical reflex myoclonus. *Neurology* 1990;40:1561–1565.
60. Imaiso Y, Mitsuo K. Gerstmann-Sträussler Scheinker syndrome with a Pro102Leu mutation in the prion protein gene and atypical MRI findings, hyperthermia, tachycardia, and hyperhidrosis [abstract in English]. *Clin Neurol (Tokyo)* 1998;38:920–925.
61. Iragui-Madoz VJ. Electrophysiology in multiple sclerosis. In: Day DD, Pedley TA, eds. *Current practice of clinical electroencephalography*, 2nd ed. New York: Raven Press, 1990:707–738.
62. Jabbour JT, Garcia JH, Lemmi H, et al. Subacute sclerosing panencephalitis: a multidisciplinary study of eight cases. *JAMA* 1969;207:2248–2254.
63. Jacob JC, Gloor P, Elwan OH, et al. Electroencephalographic changes in chronic renal failure. *Neurology* 1965;15:419–429.
64. Jamal GA, Ballantyne JP. The localization of the lesion in patients with acute ophthalmoplegia, ataxia and areflexia (Miller Fisher syndrome): a serial multimodal neurophysiological study. *Brain* 1988;111:95–114.
65. Johnson RT, Gibbs CG Jr. Creutzfeldt-Jakob disease and related transmissible spongiform encephalopathies. *N Engl J Med* 1998;339:1994–2004.
66. Kandt RS, Emerson RG, Singer HS, et al. Cataplexy in variant forms of Niemann-Pick disease. *Ann Neurol* 1982;12:284–288.
67. Kaplan PW. Metabolic and endocrine disorders resembling seizures. In: Engel J Jr, Pedley TA, eds. *Epilepsy: a comprehensive textbook*. Philadelphia: Lippincott–Raven Publishers, 1997:2661–2670.
68. Kapoor R, Griffin G, Barrett G, et al. Myoclonic epilepsy in an HIV positive patient: neurophysiological findings. *Electroencephalogr Clin Neurophysiol* 1991;78:80–84.
69. Kennedy AC, Linton AL, Luke RG, et al. Electroencephalographic changes during haemodialysis. *Lancet* 1963;1:408–411.
70. Kennedy JM, Thomson AP, Whitfield IC. Coma and electroencephalographic changes in hypopituitarism. *Lancet* 1955;2:907–908.
71. Kiloh LG, McComas AJ, Osselton JW. *Clinical electroencephalography*, 3rd ed. London: Butterworth-Heinemann, 1972.
72. Kinney HC, Burger PC, Hurwitz BJ, et al. Degeneration of the central nervous system associated with celiac disease. *J Neurol Sci* 1982;53:9–22.
73. Klass D, Daly D, eds. *Current practice of clinical electroencephalography and clinical neurophysiology*. New York: Raven Press, 1979.
74. Koppel B. Connective tissue diseases. In: Engel J Jr, Pedley TA, eds. *Epilepsy: a comprehensive textbook*. Philadelphia: Lippincott–Raven Publishers, 1997:2597–2604.
75. Kuroiwa Y, Celesia GG. Clinical significance of periodic EEG pattern. *Arch Neurol* 1980;37:15–20.
76. Labar DR, Harden C. Infection and inflammatory diseases. In: Engel J Jr, Pedley TA, eds. *Epilepsy: a comprehensive textbook*. Philadelphia: Lippincott–Raven Publishers, 1997:2587–2596.
77. Lai CW, Gragasin ME. Electroencephalography in herpes simplex encephalitis. *J Clin Neurophysiol* 1988;5:87–103.
78. Lance JW, Adams RD. The syndrome of intention or action myoclonus as a sequel to hypoxic encephalopathy. *Brain* 1963;86:111–136.
79. Lederman RJ, Henry CE. Progressive dialysis encephalopathy. *Ann Neurol* 1978;4:199–204.
80. Locke J, Merrill JP, Tyler HR. Neurologic complications of uremia. *Arch Intern Med* 1961;108:519–530.

81. Lüders HO, Noachtar S. *Atlas and classification of electroencephalography.* Philadelphia: WB Saunders, 1999.

82. Lugaresi E, Medori R, Montagna P, et al. Fatal familial insomnia and dysautonomia with selective degeneration of thalamic nuclei. *N Engl J Med* 1986;315:997–1003.

83. Lugaresi E, Tobler I, Gambetti P, et al. The pathophysiology of fatal familial insomnia. *Brain Pathol* 1998;8:521–526.

84. Maccario MJ, Messis CP, Vastola EF. Focal seizures as a manifestation of hyperglycemia without ketoacidosis. *Neurology* 1965;15:195–206.

85. Markand ON, Panszi JG. The electroencephalogram in subacute sclerosing panencephalitis. *Arch Neurol* 1975;32:719–726.

85a. Matsumoto H, Kobayashi O, Tamura K, et al. Miller Fisher syndrome with transient coma: comparison with Bickerstaff's encephalitis. *Brain Dev* 2002;24:98–101.

86. Matsuo F. EEG features of the apallic syndrome resulting from cerebral anoxia. *Electroencephalogr Clin Neurophysiol* 1985;61:113–122.

87. Mervaala E, Andermann F, Quesney LF, et al. Common dopaminergic mechanism for epileptic photosensitivity in progressive myoclonus epilepsies. *Neurology* 1990;40:53–56.

88. Meyer JS, Sakamoto K, Akiyama M, et al. Monitoring cerebral blood flow, metabolism and EEG. *Electroencephalogr Clin Neurophysiol* 1967;23:497–508.

89. Mikati MA, Trevathan E, Krishnamoorthy KS, et al. Pyridoxine-dependent epilepsy: EEG investigations and long-term follow-up. *Electroencephalogr Clin Neurophysiol* 1991;78:215–221.

90. Miyazaki M, Hashimoto T, Nakagawa R, et al. Characteristic evoked potentials in childhood-onset dentatorubral-pallidoluysian atrophy. *Brain Dev (Tokyo)* 1996;18:389–393.

91. Mizrahi EM, Tharp BR. A characteristic EEG pattern in neonatal herpes simplex encephalitis. *Neurology* 1982;32:1215–1220.

92. Muscatt R, Rothwell J, Obeso J, et al. Urea-induced stimulus-sensitive myoclonus in the rat. *Adv Neurol* 1986;43:553–563.

93. Newton TF, Leuchter AF, Miller EN, et al. Quantitative EEG in patients with AIDS and asymptomatic HIV infection. *Clin Electroencephalogr* 1994;25:18–25.

94. Niedermeyer E. *Epilepsy guide: diagnosis and treatment of epileptic seizure disorders.* Baltimore: Urban & Schwarzenberg, 1983.

95. Nishimura R, Omos-Lau N, Ajmone-Marson C, et al. Electroencephalographic findings in Gaucher disease. *Neurology* 1980;30:152–159.

96. Nuwer MR, Miller EN, Visscher BR, et al. Asymptomatic HIV infection does not cause EEG abnormalities: results from the Multicenter AIDS Cohort Study (MACS). *Neurology* 1992;42:1214–1219.

97. Okura M, Okada H, Nagoumi I, et al. Electroencephalographic changes in acute water intoxication. *Jpn J Psychiatry Neurol* 1990;44:729–734.

98. Otomo E. Beta wave activity in the electroencephalogram in cases of coma due to acute brainstem lesion. *J Neurol Neurosurg Psychiatry* 1966;29:383–390.

99. Pampiglione G, Harden A. Resuscitation after cardiopulmonary arrest: prognostic evaluation of early electroencephalographic findings. *Lancet* 1968;1:1261–1263.

100. Pampiglione G, Harden A. So-called neuronal ceroid lipofuscinosis: neurophysiological studies in 60 children. *J Neurol Neurosurg Psychiatry* 1977;40:323–330.

101. Pine I, Engel FL, Schwartz TB. The electroencephalogram in ACTH and cortisone treated patients. *Electroencephalogr Clin Neurophysiol* 1951;3:301–310.

102. Primavera A, Brusa G, Novello P. Thyrotoxic encephalopathy and recurrent seizures. *Eur Neurol* 1990;30:186–188.

103. Prior PF. *The EEG in acute cerebral anoxia.* Amsterdam: Excerpta Medica, 1973.

104. Przuntek H, Muhr H. Essential familial myoclonus. *J Neurol* 1983;230:153–162.

105. Rapin I, Goldfischer S, Katzman R, et al. The cherry-red-spot myoclonus syndrome. *Ann Neurol* 1978;3:234–242.

106. Reiher J. The electroencephalogram in the investigation of metabolic comas. *Electroencephalogr Clin Neurophysiol* 1970;28:104.

107. Reilly EL. Electrocerebral inactivity as a temperature effect: unlikely as an isolated etiology. *Clin Electroencephalogr* 1981;12:69–71.

108. Riikonen R. Infantile spasm: modern practical aspect. *Acta Paediatr Scand* 1984;73:1–12.

109. Santavuori P, Rapola J, Sainio K, et al. A variant of Jansky-Bielschowsky disease. *Neuropediatrics* 1982;13:135–141.

110. Schuchat A, Robinson K, Wenger JD, et al. Bacterial meningitis in the United States in 1995. *N Engl J Med* 1997;337:970–976.

111. Schultz M, Schulte FJ, Akiyama Y, et al. Development of electroencephalographic sleep phenomena in hypothyroid infants. *Electroencephalogr Clin Neurophysiol* 1968;25:351–358.

112. Shibasaki H. Progressive myoclonic epilepsy. In: Lüders H, Lesser RP, eds. *Epilepsy: electroclinical syndromes.* London: Springer-Verlag, 1987:187–206.

113. Shibasaki H. Overview and classification of myoclonus. *Clin Neurosci* 1996;3:189–192.

114. Shibasaki H, Igisu H, Kuroiwa Y. EEG abnormality in Fisher's syndrome. *Folia Psychiatr Neurol Jpn* 1972;36:201–207.

115. Shibasaki H, Kuroiwa Y. Electroencephalographic correlates of myoclonus. *Electroencephalogr Clin Neurophysiol* 1975;39:455–463.

116. Shibasaki H, Motomura S, Yamashita Y, et al. Periodic synchronous discharge and myoclonus in Creutzfeldt-Jakob disease: diagnostic application of jerk-locked averaging method. *Ann Neurol* 1981;9:150–156, 1981.

117. Shibasaki H, Yamashita T, Neshige R, et al. Pathogenesis of giant somatosensory evoked potentials in progressive myoclonic epilepsy. *Brain* 1985;108:225–240.

118. Sibai BM, Spinnato JA, Watson DL, et al. Eclampsia. IV. Neurological findings and future outcome. *Am J Obstet Gynecol* 1985;152:184–192.

119. Simon RP, Aminoff MJ. Electrographic status epilepticus in fatal anoxic coma. *Ann Neurol* 1986;20:351–355.

120. Snyder BD, Hauser A, Loewenson RB, et al. Neurologic prognosis after cardiopulmonary arrest: III. Seizure activity. *Neurology* 1980;30:1292–1297.

121. So N, Berkovic SF, Andermann F, et al. Myoclonus epilepsy and ragged-red fibers (MERRF) 2. Electrophysiological studies and comparison with the other progressive myoclonic epilepsies. *Brain* 1989;112:1261–1276.

122. Srikantia SG, Veeraraghava-Reddy M, Krishnaswamy K. Electroencephalographic patterns in pellagra. *Electroencephalogr Clin Neurophysiol* 1968;25:386–388.

123. Steinhoff BJ, Räcker S, Herrendorf G, et al. Accuracy and reliability of periodic sharp wave complexes in Creutzfeldt-Jakob disease. *Arch Neurol* 1996;53:162–166.

124. Terada K, Ikeda A, Mima T, et al. Familial cortical myoclonic tremor as a unique form of cortical reflex myoclonus. *Mov Disord* 1997;12:370–377.

125. Thomas P, Borg M. Reversible myoclonic encephalopathy revealing the AIDS-dementia complex. *Electroencephalogr Clin Neurophysiol* 1994;90:166–169.

126. Thomas SV. Neurological aspects of eclampsia. *J Neurol Sci* 1998;155:37–43.

127. Thomas SV, Somanathan N, Radhakumari R. Interictal EEG changes in eclampsia. *Electroencephalogr Clin Neurophysiol* 1995;94:271–275.

128. Tinuper P, Aguglia U, Pellissier JF, et al. Visual ictal phenomena in a case of Lafora disease by skin biopsy. *Epilepsia* 1983;24:214–218.

129. Tsuji S, Yamada T, Tsutsumi A, et al. Neuraminidase deficiency and accumulation of sialic acid in lymphocytes in adult type sialidosis with partial b-galactosidase deficiency. *Ann Neurol* 1982;11:541–543.

130. Upton A, Gumpert J. EEG in diagnosis of herpes simplex encephalitis. *Lancet* 1970;1:650–652.

131. Vas GA, Cracco JB. Diffuse encephalopathies. In: Day DD, Pedley TA, eds. *Current practice of clinical electroencephalography*, 2nd ed. New York: Raven Press, 1990:371–399.

131a. Van Paesschen W, Irazo A, Marti-Fabregas J, et al. Prospective study of new-onset seizures in patients with human immunodeficiency virus seropostive patients. *Epilepsia* 1995;36:146–150.

132. Walson JN, Kiloh LG, Osselton JW, et al. The electroencephalogram in pernicious anaemia and

subacute combined degeneration of the spinal cord. *Electroencephalogr Clin Neurophysiol* 1954;6:45–64.

133. Weil MI, Itabashi HH, Cremer NE, et al. Chronic progressive panencephalitis due to rubella virus simulating subacute sclerosing panencephalitis. *N Engl J Med* 1975;292:994–998.

134. Westmoreland BF. The EEG in cerebral inflammatory processes. In: Niedermeyer E, Lopes da Silva, eds. *Electroencephalography: basic principles, clinical applications, and related fields*, 4th ed. Philadelphia: Lippincott Williams & Wilkins, 1999:302–316.

135. Westmoreland BF, Groover RV, Shabrough FW. Electrographic findings in three types of cerebromacular degeneration. *Mayo Clin Proc* 1979;54:12–21.

136. Will RG, Ironside JW, Zeidler M, et al. A new variant of Creutzfeldt-Jakob disease in the UK. *Lancet* 1996;347:921–925.

136a. Willison HJ, O'Hanlon GM. Immunopathogenesis of Miller Fisher syndrome. *J Neuroimmunol* 1999;100:3–12.

137. Willson WP, Johnson JE. Thyroid hormone and brain function. I. The EEG in hyperthyroidism with observations on the effect of age, sex and reserpine in the productions of abnormalities. *Electroencephalogr Clin Neurophysiol* 1964;16:321–328.

138. Wszolek JK, Aksamit AJ, Ellington RJ, et al. Epileptiform electroencephalographic abnormalities in liver transplant recipient. *Ann Neurol* 1991;30:37–41.

139. Yap HK, Low PS, Lee BW, et al. Factors influencing the development of hypertensive encephalopathy in acute glomerulonephritis. *Child Nephrol Urol* 1988;9:147–152.

140. Yasuda T. Benign adult familial myoclonic epilepsy (BAFME). *Kawasaki Med J* 1991; 17:1–13.

141. Zeidler M, Stewart GE, Barraclough CR, et al. New variant Creutzfeldt-Jakob disease: neurological features and diagnostic test. *Lancet* 1997;350:903–907.

142. Zuckermann EC, Glaser GH. Experimental urea-induced myoclonic seizures: mechanism and sites of action. *Trans Am Neurol Assoc* 1971;96:101–105.

Chapter 13

Organic Brain Syndromes and Dementias

Omkar N. Markand and Richard P. Brenner

There has been a change in the classification of organic disorders characterized by cognitive or memory deficits as employed in the *Diagnostic and Statistical Manual of Mental Disorders, Fourth Edition* (DSM-IV) of the American Psychiatric Association (4). The previous edition (DSM-III) distinguished two major disorders: organic brain syndrome and organic mental disorders. The former term referred to the disorder without reference to etiology (e.g., delirium, dementia, etc.), whereas the latter designated disorder with known or presumed etiology (Alzheimer's disease [AD], multi-infarct dementia [MID], etc.). In the DSM-IV, the term *organic mental disorder* has been eliminated because it incorrectly implies that "nonorganic" mental disorders do not have a biological basis. The disorders with significant deficits in cognition or memory compared to the previous level of functioning are now placed into three subgroups: delirium, dementia, and amnesic or other cognitive disorders.

Organic brain syndrome is a term commonly used by the medical community to refer collectively to these three subgroups. Delirium or acute confusional state refers to an acute but reversible disturbance of fluctuating consciousness. Dementia is characterized by global impairment of cognitive functions that is more or less persistent. Amnesic disorders comprise conditions with selective memory impairment in the absence of other cognitive deficits.

Because electroencephalography (EEG) measures cortical activity, it can help in diagnosis and prognosis of organic brain syndromes. Although EEG changes are usually nonspecific (e.g., generalized slowing of background activity), EEG can play an important discriminative role in several circumstances:

1. EEG can alert physicians to unexpected toxic-metabolic causes for changes in mental state displaying distinctive EEG patterns (e.g., tripha-

sic waves in hepatic or renal encephalopathy, or fast rhythms superimposed on slow activity in sedative-hypnotic drug ingestion).

2. EEG is indispensable in diagnosing nonconvulsive status epilepticus producing acute confusional states.

3. By demonstrating periodic discharges, EEG is often the first test to suggest certain encephalitides, such as Creutzfeldt-Jakob disease (CJD).

Selected reviews that discuss EEG in diffuse encephalopathies include those by Markand (113), Brenner (15), and Rosen (169).

EEG CHANGES WITH NORMAL AGING

Because organic brain syndromes, particularly dementias, are common in older age groups, it is essential to discuss EEG in normal elderly subjects. An important feature of the EEG is the frequency of the alpha rhythm, which in adults ranges from 8 to 13 Hz. During the seventh decade and particularly during the eighth, normal subjects show a shift to slower frequencies posteriorly compared to younger adults (84). In subsequent studies (7,93,205), the mean alpha frequency approached 10 Hz in carefully selected normal elderly subjects. A number of earlier studies, which reported slower alpha frequencies, included a variety of different subject groups, ranging from normal volunteers living in the community to institutionalized subjects, some with significant neurological and/or medical disease (212). This variation in selection criteria yielded discrepant findings of dominant alpha frequencies in elderly subjects (93). Arenas et al. (7) found that, in 42 healthy, elderly subjects who had a well-developed alpha rhythm, only 6 had frequencies less than 9.0 Hz and in no subject was the frequency less than 8.0 Hz. Pedley and Miller (148) considered an alpha frequency, while alert, of less than 8.5 Hz as abnormal. Katz and Horowitz (93) considered a dominant frequency of less than 8.0 Hz as abnormal in elderly subjects (up to 80 years of age), and this is probably true in the "old old" (> 80 years) as well (83,143).

Oken and Kaye (141) found that the posterior peak frequency (PF), determined by computerized EEG frequency analysis (which in almost all cases was within 0.5 Hz of the PF determined visually), was maintained above 8 Hz in all subjects under age 84. However, it was between 7 and 8 Hz in 5 of 22 subjects over 84. All subjects were extremely healthy and cognitively intact. Soininen and Riekkinen (185) studied 52 subjects ages 20–91 years and found that aging was not associated with slowing. Relative power of delta, theta, alpha, and beta activity did not differ across age. In addition,

Brenner et al. (19) in a study of older individuals found that, although the parasagittal mean frequency decreased with age, changes were not significant when subjects were grouped by decade (ages 60–87 years).

Another finding in the elderly, long recognized (26), is that EEGs of normal elderly subjects often contain focal slowing consisting of delta and theta activity. This focal slowing in normal subjects is limited to the temporal regions and is present considerably more often over the left side (Fig. 13.1). There is enormous variation in the way electroencephalographers evaluate such activity in this age group. In addition, Torres et al. (205) reported that 52% of EEGs of asymptomatic healthy elderly individuals would be called abnormal if judged on the basis of standards usually applied to young adults. Thus there is a need to modify these standards when interpreting EEGs of the aged.

In a study of 50 carefully selected healthy elderly (60 years or greater) subjects, without evidence of neurological or psychiatric disorders, Arenas et al. (7) found that intermittent focal slowing in the temporal area during wakefulness occurred in 36% of subjects. This finding was similar to that of other studies (26–28,84). Like other investigators, Arenas et al. (7) found the slowing to be predominantly left sided (72%). The explanation for this left-sided dominance remains unclear. As regards the amount of slow (delta-theta) activity, Arenas et al. (7), found that the percentage of recording time of such activity ranged from 0.2 to 10.2; however, excluding one subject, slow activity did not exceed 1.8%. Similar results have been reported in a study of healthy septuagenarians by Katz and Horowitz (93), who found that slowing, predominantly in the delta (< 4 Hz) frequency, did not occupy more than 0.6% of the total recording time in any subject. The following is a summary of the characteristics of "benign temporal transients of the elderly" (95):

They occur chiefly at ages greater than 60 years.

They are confined to the temporal regions and, within these regions, are maximal anteriorly.

They occur more frequently on the left side.

They do not disrupt background activity and are not associated with an abnormal asymmetry of the alpha rhythm.

Their morphology is usually rounded but occasionally irregular.

Their voltage is usually greater than 60–70 μV.

They are attenuated by mental alerting and eye opening, and their prevalence is increased by drowsiness and hyperventilation.

They occur sporadically as single waves or in pairs, not in longer rhythmic trains.

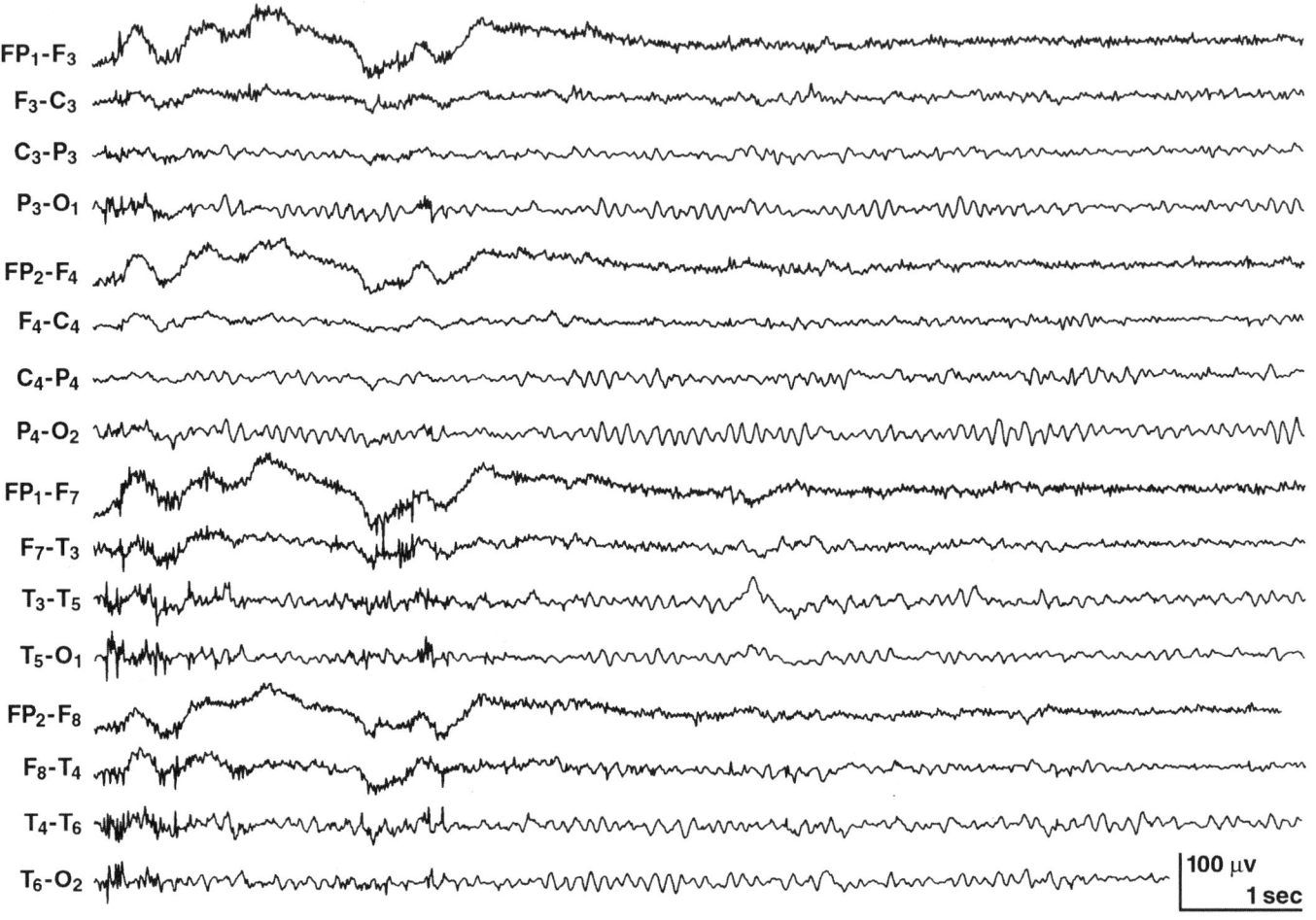

FIG. 13.1. EEG of a 78-year-old person showing intermittent slow transients in the left temporal region.

They are present for only a very small proportion (up to > 1%) of the recording time.

Temporal theta activity is also increased in the elderly and usually occupies a higher percentage of recording time than does delta activity (7,148). Pedley and Miller (148) allowed 10%–15% before considering it abnormal.

Arenas et al. (7) found approximately 2%, except for one subject with approximately 10%.

The clinical significance of mild temporal slowing is uncertain, and most studies have not shown a correlation between these focal abnormalities and neurological deficits (139–141). However, one study reported that a subgroup of normal elderly subjects whose EEGs showed left temporal slowing performed poorly on a fluency test compared to those normal elderly subjects without temporal slowing (208). The etiology of the slowing is uncertain, although vascular factors have often been invoked. Oken and Kaye (141) found intermittent temporal slowing in 17 (52%) of 33 subjects over age 65 years. Its presence was related to the presence of white matter hyperintensities on magnetic resonance imaging (MRI) but not to blood pressure or cognitive function.

State-related changes are important in the interpretation of EEGs in any age group. However, there are some findings in the elderly that are noteworthy. Aside from the slowing of the dominant rhythm (seen in all ages during drowsiness), as well as the increase of temporal slowing that accompanies drowsiness and is seen particularly in the aged, the elderly also have bursts of generalized rhythmic delta activity, maximal anteriorly, during drowsiness (Fig. 13.2). Katz and Horowitz (94) termed this pattern *sleep*

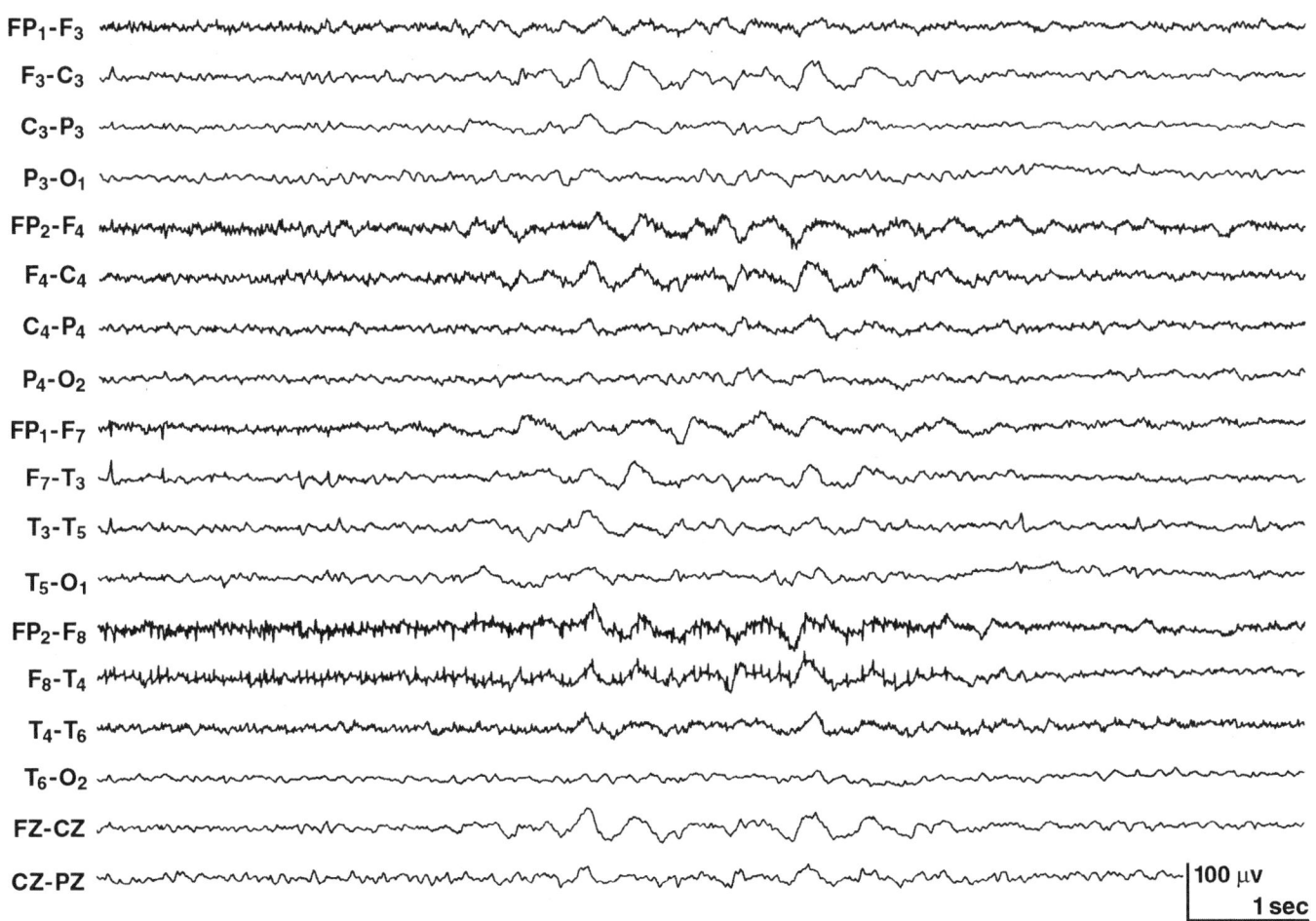

FIG. 13.2. EEG of a 66-year-old man showing frontal intermittent rhythmic delta activity at sleep onset, a normal finding in elderly subjects.

onset–FIRDA (frontal intermittent rhythmic delta activity) to help distinguish it from FIRDA that is abnormal and not limited only to drowsiness. FIRDA during wakefulness is present in a wide variety of diffuse disturbances, most often toxic-metabolic encephalopathies (172). Thus, in the interpretation of frontal delta activity on the EEG in the elderly, one has to consider whether this pattern occurs only during drowsiness and is normal, or is clearly present during wakefulness and is abnormal. Other clues to detect drowsiness include a decrease in frequency of the alpha rhythm, appearance of slow lateral eye movements, decrease in myogenic artifact, and clinical appearance of the subject. In addition, the bursts need to be distinguished from noncerebral activity such as artifacts related to vertical eye movement or tongue movement (glossokinetic potential).

DELIRIUM (ACUTE CONFUSIONAL STATE)

"Delirium" in the DSM-IV refers to an acute but transient development of altered consciousness that tends to fluctuate during the course of the day, accompanied by difficulty in sustaining/shifting attention, and one or more evidences of abnormal behavior, such as perceptual disturbance, impaired memory, incoherent speech, altered psychomotor activity (agitation or lethargy), and disturbed sleep–wake cycle. Neurologists often distinguish acute confusional state from delirium, using the former term in a generic manner and restricting the term delirium to a more florid confusional state with psychomotor hyperactivity (agitation, restlessness, combativeness). This difference is probably unwarranted because psychomotor activity can shift from one extreme to the other over the course of a day.

Early studies by Engel and Romano (45,168) have demonstrated that changes in EEGs paralleled degree of behavioral impairment. In early stages, slowing of alpha rhythms appeared, succeeded by medium- to high-voltage generalized slow activity in the theta-delta range. Resolution of delirium was reflected by reversal of these changes, although (particularly in the elderly) resolution lagged behind behavioral recovery.

Obrecht et al. (137) reported on the value of EEG in 95 patients with acute confusional state; 83 had abnormal EEGs, 52 with marked and 31 with mild disturbance of the background activity. Patients who had intracranial pathology often showed asymmetries of delta activity and paroxysmal discharges. Quantitative EEG (qEEG) was performed in 51 elderly delirious patients and compared to that of 19 controls in a study by Koponen et al. (96). Delirious patients showed significant reduction of alpha percentage, increased theta-delta activity, and slowing of the PF and mean frequency.

The reduction in the alpha percentage and various ratio parameters correlated significantly with score on the Mini-Mental State Examination, whereas delta percentage and mean frequency correlated with the lengths of delirium and hospitalization. Similar spectral abnormalities have been reported in elderly delirious patients by Jacobson et al. (85). The paper by Brenner (15) provides a review of the utility of the EEG in delirium in the elderly.

Although excessive slowing in the theta-delta frequency and decreased to absent alpha rhythm constitute major EEG findings in the acute confusional state, low-voltage fast (beta frequency) activity may dominate the EEG in some delirious patients (159). These patients have usually been hyperactive and agitated, with apparently heightened levels of arousal (delirium tremens) often marked by fear and anxiety. Such EEGs have been most often described in patients withdrawing from sedative drugs such as alcohol. In such cases, the EEG probably cannot be labeled abnormal during delirium without establishing a significant change through serial EEG studies, because approximately 10% of normal adults may show low-amplitude tracings.

Spehr and Stemmler (186) used spectral power density analysis and Hjorth's time-domain descriptors to study 48 patients with chronic alcoholism within 2 days after cessation of delirium tremens (54%) or impending delirium (34%) and 18 days later after clinical recovery. In the acute phase after florid delirium, EEGs showed prominent beta activity and sparse amounts of relatively normal-frequency alpha rhythm. A second group showed persistent, rather slow delta activity and little beta or alpha activity. This group drank twice the amount of alcohol and had significant electrolyte disturbances, and perhaps were medically more sick.

DEMENTIA

The hallmark of dementia is global impairment of cognitive function without alteration of consciousness. Major clinical features are memory impairment, poor judgment, personality change, decreased capacity for abstraction, aphasia, agnosia, and apraxia, which lead to social and occupational disability. In the past two decades, some neurologists have attempted to distinguish between cortical and subcortical dementia. Patients with progressive supranuclear palsy (PSP), Huntington's disease, and parkinsonism were said to have "subcortical" dementia with impaired memory and learning associated with slow intellectual function, depression, and apathy but without impaired language, perception, or praxis, the latter three symptoms putatively characterizing "cortical" dementia. The concept of subcortical dementia was further expanded to include Wilson's disease, normal-pressure hydrocephalus (NPH), and acquired immunodeficiency syndrome (AIDS) dementia. A clamorous debate has ensued regarding the validity of this subdivision. Whitehouse (215) has critically reviewed the problem and has found "little support for this classification system, although adequate systematic studies have not been performed."

The separation of dementias into subcortical and cortical types has no firm basis on either clinical or pathological grounds. The neuropathology of AD—a prototype of cortical dementia—shows subcortical involvement, and the so-called subcortical dementias have significant neuronal degeneration in the cerebral cortex. Paulsen et al. (147) demonstrated distinctive cognitive profiles in neuropsychological tests in cortical (AD) and subcortical (Huntington's disease) dementias at all levels of dementia severity. However, the clinical and pathological overlap makes the distinction between cortical and subcortical dementias less relevant.

There are numerous inadequacies in earlier studies attempting to correlate EEG changes and behavioral changes in dementia. While making obeisance to the maxim that only neuropathological examination can confirm the diagnosis of AD, most early studies (61,62,101,106,138) did not address accuracy of diagnosis. Earlier epidemiological studies of clinically diagnosed AD documented an agreement between clinical and pathological diagnosis in only 55%–70% of patients (166,195), although the accuracy of clinical diagnosis of AD has improved to 75%–100%, according to most recent reports (119,211). Also, lack of uniform psychometric testing procedures makes comparison across different studies impossible. Lack of behavioral measures of severity and rate of progression have rendered most studies a grab bag of patients having various degrees of dementia progressing at varying rates. Some well-conceived prospective studies have addressed these problems (34,35,149).

Another problem encountered in EEG investigation of dementia has been lack of an appropriate control group or the use of an ill-defined one. Criteria for what constitutes an appropriate control group for dementia have varied among studies, with relevant subject variables such as age, sex, race, and socioeconomic status all being important in defining the comparative group.

In addition to this morass of methodological problems, EEG studies have been plagued by a lack of uniformity in describing and categorizing EEG changes. Some studies lack clear descriptions of EEG criteria (183); other studies have relied on qualitative visual evaluation and used broad categories such as (a) normal, (b) excessive beta activity, (c) predominant theta activity, or (d) predominant delta activity (164). One study reporting on patients with AD, Pick's disease, and MID did not distinguish between focal and generalized slowing (89).

Finally, in analyzing the EEGs of patients with dementia, one must consider age-specific changes that occur in healthy elderly persons (*vide supra*). Quantitative EEG studies (35,57,149) have shown that changes with age in a healthy population are distinct from those seen in patients with dementia associated with AD. With these extensive caveats in mind, we now review EEGs in various types of dementia.

Alzheimer's Disease

Epidemiological studies around the world suggest that AD occurs in about 2%–6% of people age 65 years or older (166). Autopsy studies of dementia at all ages have found that 50%–60% of cases result from AD (198,204). Most patients with AD lack an obvious family history and are classified as sporadic. A small proportion of cases, particularly with early onset, have a positive family history and an autosomal dominant inheritance. Some of them have a specific genetic mutation of the amyloid precursor protein (*APP*) gene on chromosome 2 (60). Other mutations have been mapped to chromosome 14 (173) or chromosome 19 (150). In late-onset familial and sporadic AD patients, the e4 allele of the *APOE* gene has been found to manifest at a higher frequency than in controls; the frequency is 50% in late-onset familial and 36% in sporadic cases compared to 16% in controls (171,193).

The EEG changes in AD are generalized, as reported in several studies (61,62,101,106,138,183). Alpha rhythm is slow or may be absent, and diffuse low- to medium-amplitude irregular theta activity appears. Theta activity later becomes the dominant background activity, and irregular diffuse delta waves may occur randomly (Figs. 13.3 through 13.7). Runs of large-amplitude generalized, irregular or semirhythmic delta activity may also appear, often more prominently over the frontotemporal regions (88,138). Spontaneous or barbiturate-induced beta activity, normally seen over the frontocentral regions, is reduced or absent. Sleep potentials may be disorganized, with poorly developed spindles; K complexes may be difficult to evoke (101). Rarely, patients with AD may develop myoclonus, but their EEGs lack the periodic complexes characteristic of CJD. Many studies (89,106,121,164,183) have found a positive correlation between (a) the severity of intellectual impairment in demented patients and (b) abnormalities on visual inspection of the EEG.

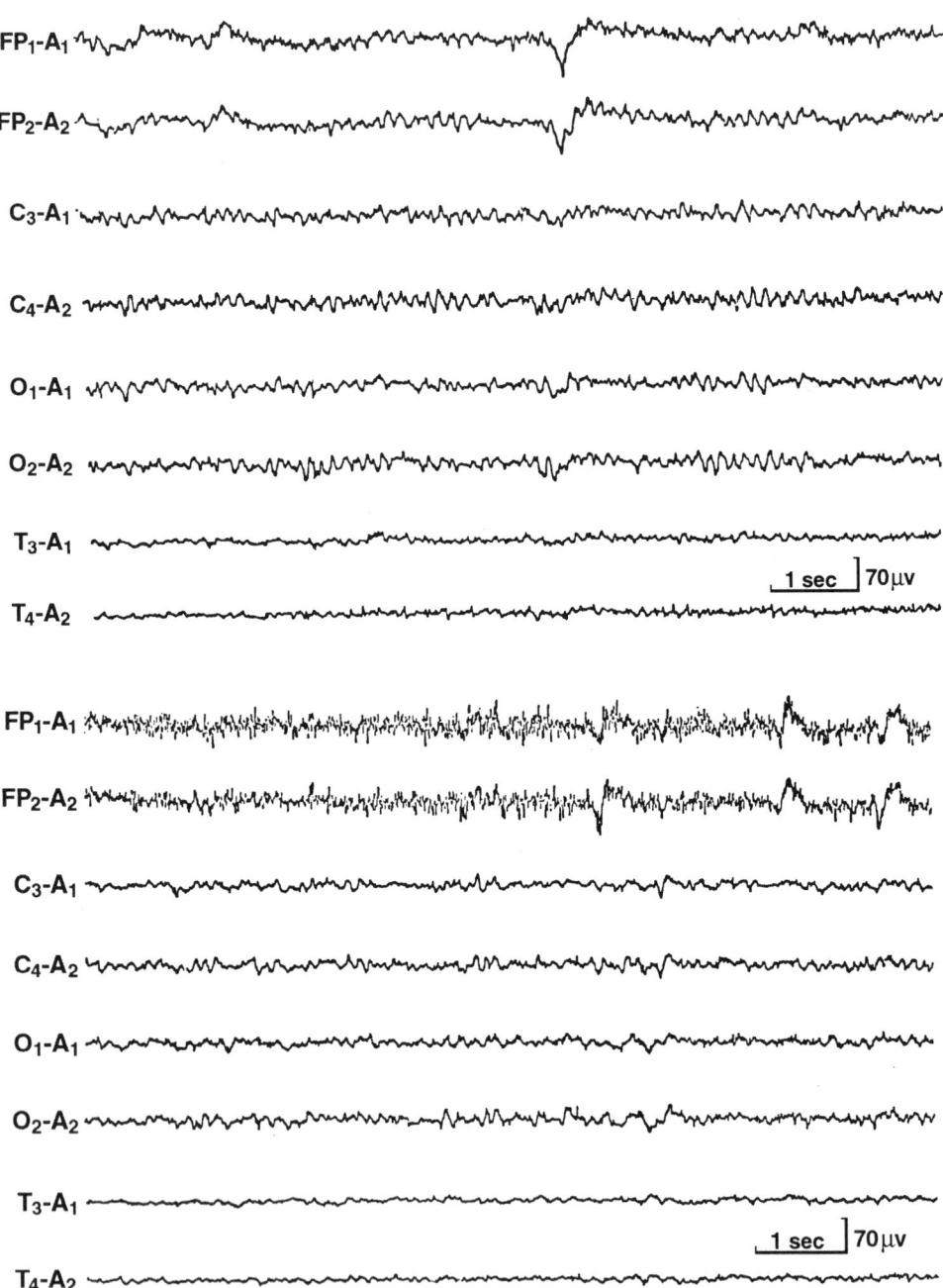

FIG. 13.3. Initial EEG of a 59-year-old woman with Alzheimer's dementia 1 year after onset of mild difficulty with memory and calculations. Alpha rhythm is at lower limit of normal frequency, 8 Hz. Note frontocentral 7-Hz theta rhythms. (From Markand ON. Electroencephalography in diffuse encephalopathies. *J Clin Neurophysiol* 1984;1:357–407, with permission).

FIG. 13.4. EEG 2 years later in the same patient as in Figure 13.3 shows alpha rhythm replaced with background of low-amplitude theta and delta activity. At that time, she had moderate dementia: She was unable to prepare meals, shop, or balance her checkbook. (From Markand ON. Electroencephalography in diffuse encephalopathies. *J Clin Neurophysiol* 1984;1:357–407, with permission).

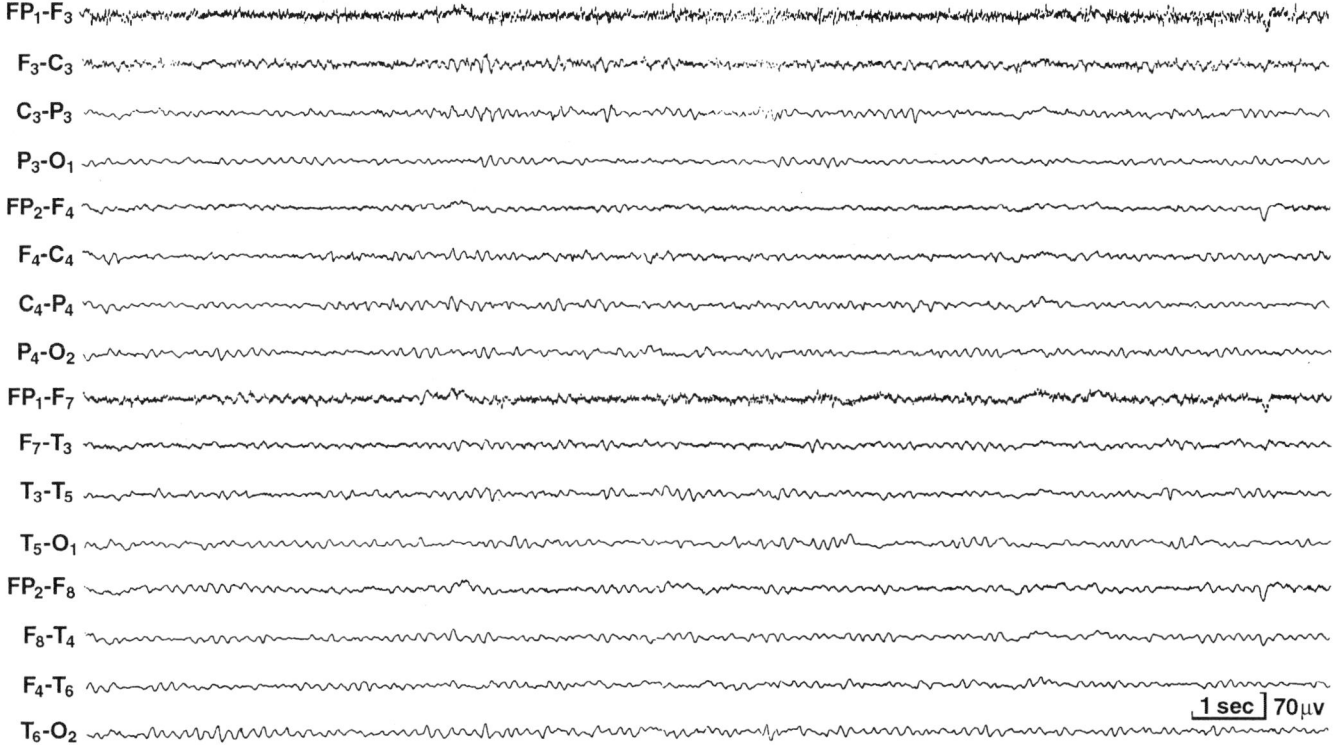

FIG. 13.5. EEG of an 80-year-old man with a history of depression, progressive intellectual impairment, and episodes of confusion for 2 years resulting from dementia. Note absence of alpha rhythm and diffuse rhythmic 6-Hz theta activity.

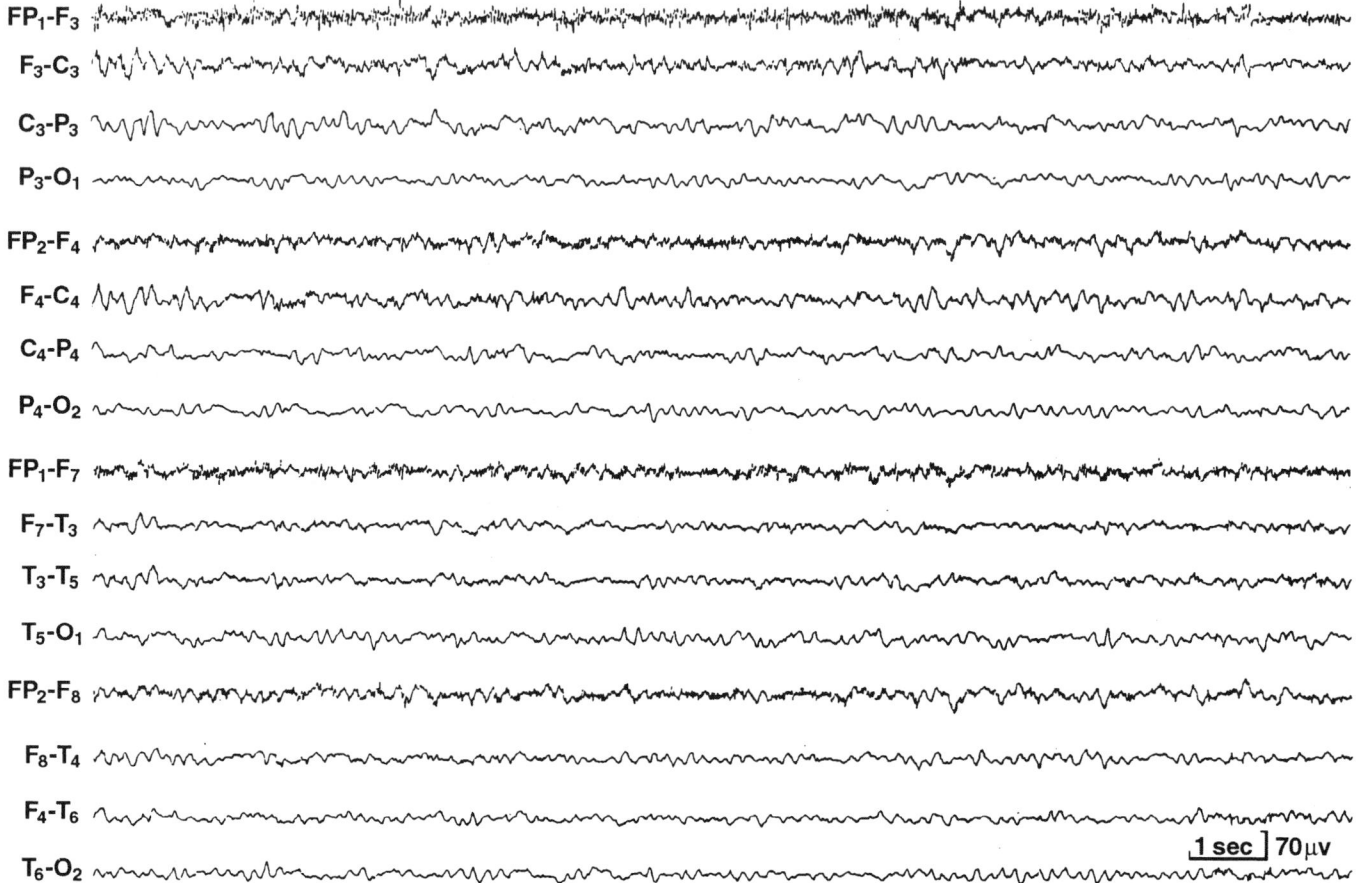

FIG. 13.6. EEG of same patient as in Figure 13.5 recorded 13 months later shows further deterioration with absence of alpha rhythm, slower (5-Hz) and higher amplitude theta rhythms, and arrhythmic centroparietal delta activity.

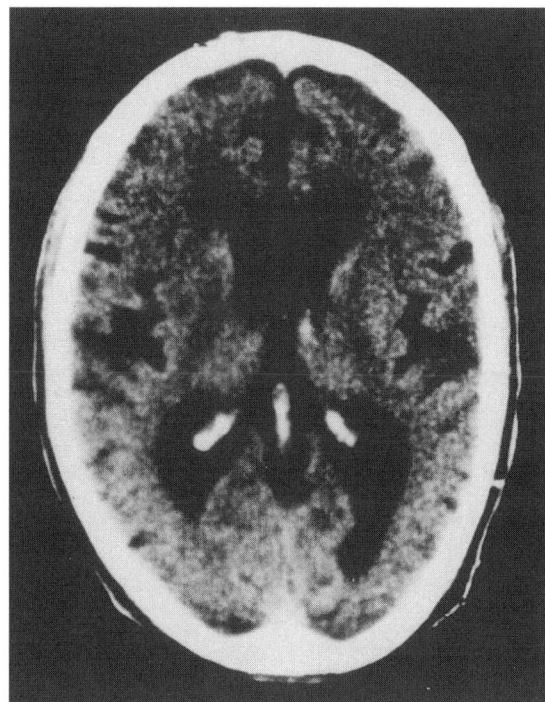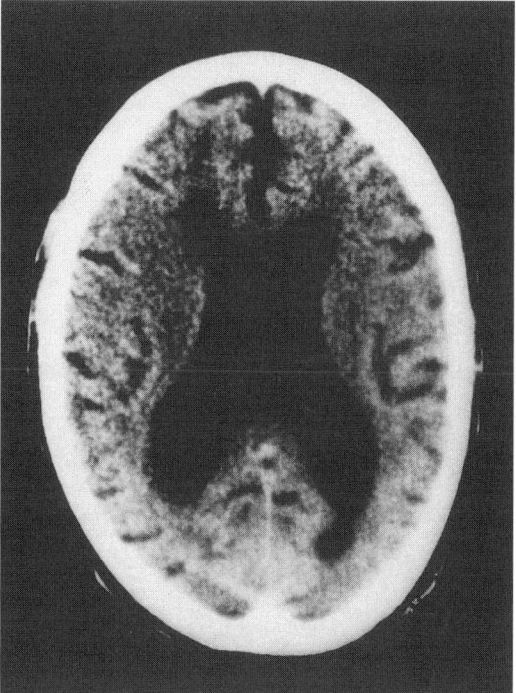

FIG. 13.7. CT scan of same patient as in Figures 13.5 and 13.6 made at time of second EEG shows dilated ventricles and prominent sulci, indicating cerebral atrophy.

Epileptiform discharges are rare even if epileptic seizures are part of the clinical picture. Muller and Kral, in 1967 (125), described sharp or triphasic waves usually occurring over posterior head regions in severely demented patients (Fig. 13.8). More recently, others (13,155,161) have reported similar waveforms in dementia. Rae-Grant et al. (161) found 15 of 268 EEGs in patients with AD, and Primavera and Traverso (155) found 15 of 114 patients with probable AD, showing triphasic waves. Triphasic waves are usually associated with a severe degree of dementia and are posterior dominant in most such patients (13,125,155), compared to their usual frontal dominance in acute metabolic encephalopathies. They may occasionally be quasiperiodic in their occurrence (13,42,155) but usually lack the persistence and regular periodicity seen in CJD (*vide infra*). Myoclonus can occur in late stages of the disease. Hallett and Wilkins (72) have described small multifocal jerks of muscles in distal parts of the extremities: "EEG was slow often with some epileptic activity that could not be readily correlated with the jerks." However, back-averaging EEG activity from myoclonic jerks revealed focal negativity in the contralateral rolandic area 20–40 milliseconds before the jerk, suggesting cortical myoclonus.

Although many authors have reported abnormal EEGs with slowing of background rhythms in almost all cases of AD (62,88,101,138), this statement is true only for those patients with moderate to severe dementia. Systematized blind interpretation of EEGs in 86 patients with AD showed abnormal findings in 87.2% at the initial examination and 92% at the follow-up (165); a normal EEG had a predictive value of 0.825 for the diagnosis of AD. In early stages, however, when cognitive difficulties first develop, EEGs may be normal, with alpha rhythms well over 8 Hz (see Fig. 13.3). Using strict criteria for EEG abnormalities (e.g., moderate diffuse slowing) such that most normal subjects are correctly classified, a high false-negative rate occurs in patients with AD, especially in the early stages (16,20).

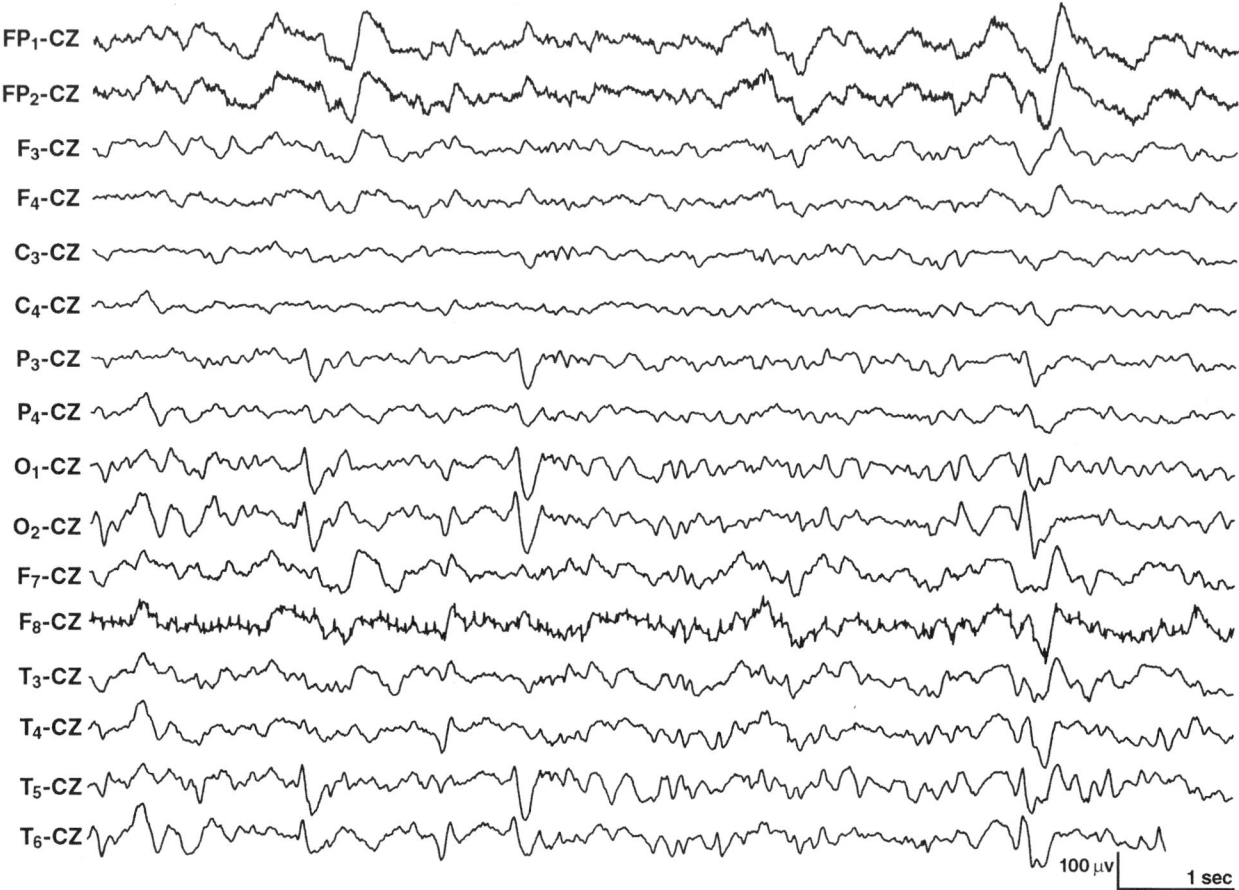

FIG. 13.8. EEG of an 82-year-old woman with advanced dementia shows diffuse slow activity and posterior hemispheric sharp (triphasic) waves.

In the hope of increasing the diagnostic value of EEG, interest has developed in computerized EEG spectral analysis, which provides more quantitative data than does conventional visual EEG analysis. Findings with spectral analysis are similar to those reported with conventional EEG analysis. Several studies (20,34,35,57,123,174,209) have shown a shift of the spectrum to slower frequencies, with an increase in theta activity and a decrease in beta activity, in patients with AD compared to normal elderly subjects. There is

a correlation between spectral EEG measures, such as mean frequency and severity of dementia (20,29,39,149,179,191). In mild dementia, there is an increase in theta and a decrease in beta activity (34,35), whereas with greater severity of dementia there are also decreases in alpha and increases in delta activity (35,43,78,123,149,182,190).

In a study comparing the diagnostic efficacy of computerized spectral versus visual EEG analysis in elderly normal and AD subjects, Brenner et al. (16) found that spectral analysis afforded only modest advantages over visual EEG analysis in differentiating AD patients from elderly controls. Because the degree of spectral and visual EEG abnormalities correlated with the severity of dementia, both tests more often correctly classified those AD patients with lower Mini-Mental State Examination (49) scores. Also, both tests identified primarily the same patients. The authors did not find the computer to be more sensitive than the eye in the identification of AD patients with mild impairment, and such patients, who are more difficult to diagnose clinically, may not be identified by EEG criteria. However, computerized spectral data were derived from only 4 channels, while 16 channels and a longer recording time were used for visual analysis. Strijers et al. (192), utilizing 19 channels for visual analysis and 12 channels for computerized data, which included both frequency analysis and coherence, also found that accuracy in identifying demented patients was comparable between visual analysis and qEEG. However, only nine AD patients were studied.

Soininen et al. (184) also thought that the value of spectral analysis of the EEG in the diagnosis of AD in its early stages had limitations. Using a T6-O2 derivation, they found that in 50% of early AD cases there were no EEG alterations or worsening at 1-year follow-up. Similarly, Coben et al. (33), using an occipital-vertex derivation, reported only modest sensitivity (about 20%) of the EEG to detect individuals with mild AD when compared to normal subjects. However, the specificity was 100%. Although Hooijer et al. (82) found a slight advantage in visual analysis over quantitative analysis, Schreiter-Gasser et al. (175) found quantitative data, particularly absolute power of delta activity, to be the best predictor of degree of dementia. Both qEEG and visual EEG analysis were highly correlated with degree of dementia, but computed tomography (CT) scans were not.

In addition to spectral analysis, qEEG studies have also evaluated coherence, which is a measure of the synchronizational neuronal activity between two cortical sites. Several studies (10,40) reported decreased coherence in AD patients, suggesting fewer neuronal connections. Whether coherence provides any useful information beyond the known frequency analysis changes per se is uncertain, because relatively few studies have been performed. Furthermore, there is not a prospective validation of the clinical utility for coherence testing in patients with dementia (135).

Currently, although both visual analysis of EEG and qEEG compare favorably to other laboratory tests, such as CT, MRI, single-photon emission CT (SPECT), and positron emission tomography, in the evaluation of dementia (76,90,165), for mild degrees of dementia the specificity and sensitivity are limited. This may be improved with further development of quantitative techniques and mathematical manipulations, such as discriminant analysis and artificial neural networks (5,11,158). At present, the clinical usefulness of qEEG in dementia is limited, because most changes can be seen in routine EEG testing (135). Unlike Jonkman (90), we do not believe that qEEG is the preferred study, and concur with Nuwer (134) that qEEG should not be employed separately from routine EEG. Furthermore, even with improvements in qEEG techniques, it is possible that in early dementia the sensitivity and specificity of these tests may be mediocre compared to other routine kinds of medical testing, such as neuropsychometric testing (134).

There have been several longitudinal EEG studies of AD patients. Coben et al. (35) found overall changes in power spectra (increases in delta and theta and decreases in beta, alpha, and mean frequencies) over a 2.5-year period. Sloan and Fenton (179) did not find significant power spectra changes in an 18-month follow-up of AD patients. Hooijer et al. (82) found visual analysis to be better for showing a progression of slowing of the EEG in AD patients than power spectral analysis. However, with progression of disease, the conventional EEG does not invariably worsen in all AD patients (161).

What is the role of the EEG as a predictor of progression in dementia? Berg et al. (9), using spectral measures, did not find this test to be predictive of progression of dementia in AD patients at a 1-year follow-up. Helkala et al. (77), using both conventional visual EEG analysis and spectral measures, found that AD patients with an abnormal EEG at an early stage of the disease had a different pattern of cognitive decline than AD patients (matched for severity of dementia) with a normal EEG. Those with deteriorating EEGs during the initial 1-year follow-up subsequently showed a greater decline in praxic functions, as well as a tendency toward a higher frequency of extrapyramidal symptoms and a greater risk of institutionalization, than AD patients with stable EEGs during the first year. Lopez et al. (107) found more marked EEG abnormalities (conventional visual and spectral analysis) in AD patients with delusions and hallucinations compared to AD patients matched for severity of dementia, but without delusions and hallucinations. Patients with these psychotic symptoms had a more rapid rate of decline as measured by the Mini-Mental State Examination (49). In a subsequent study, Lopez et al. (108) found both abnormal EEG and psychosis to be independent predictors of disease progression. Rodriguez et al. (167), in a pilot study of 31 AD patients, thought that qEEG may have prognostic relevance and be useful for clinical purposes such as predicting loss of activities of daily living, incontinence, and death, whereas Forstl et al. (51) did not find qEEG a predictor for cognitive performance.

The magnitude of disease-related changes in ventricular size and dilation of sulci correlates roughly with cognitive deficits, particularly in advanced stages of dementia (38,121). However, most authors have found no correlation between (a) diffuse EEG abnormalities in dementia and (b) magnitude of cerebral atrophy (164,188). Because EEG reflects disordered function rather than loss of neural tissue, this lack of relationship is less surprising. The degree of background slowing correlates better with severity of cognitive impairment (89,92,154) and severity of pathological changes at autopsy (126) in demented patients. Kaszniak et al. (92) have shown further that EEG slowing better predicted mortality and related more closely to widely disrupted cognitive functions than did degree of cerebral atrophy. Therefore, the effects on both cognition and survival appear to be more severe when the brain is electrophysiologically abnormal than when there is only simple tissue loss.

A number of investigators have evaluated sleep in patients with primary degenerative dementias (156,157,162,163). Demented patients nap frequently in the daytime and awaken frequently during the night, resulting in decreased sleep efficiency as compared with normal elderly persons. Sleep architecture shows several changes: (a) decreased rapid-eye-movement (REM) sleep time and REM activity, (b) decreased amount of delta sleep, (c) normal or slightly increased latency to REM sleep, and (d) increased percentage of time awake in bed. Comparing demented patients and normal elderly subjects yields statistically significant differences only for certain variables (162). Sleep maintenance and sleep efficiency are reduced in demented patients. EEGs show poorly developed sleep spindles and K complexes; thus scoring of stage 2 non-REM sleep in dementia becomes difficult.

Although some changes of sleep overlap in demented and depressed patients, certain major differences exist. Both demented and depressed patients demonstrate diminished sleep efficiency; however, inability to maintain sleep particularly marks depressed patients, who awaken frequently and consequently have lower sleep maintenance percentage. Delta sleep diminishes in both demented and depressed patients, but REM sleep increases in elderly depressed (as compared to demented) patients. Depressed patients have also shorter REM latency, often less than 30 minutes. An interesting shift of REM sleep time and REM intensity occurs in depressed patients during the first part of the night's sleep. Duration of first REM period, as well as REM activity during this period, increases compared

to that of normal elderly or demented patients. In patients with depression, the first REM period may increase to more than 18 minutes. Despite these differences in REM sleep parameters, usefulness of polysomnography in early diagnosis of dementia or in separating organic dementias from pseudododementia remains limited because of significant overlaps in abnormalities.

Pick's Disease

Pick's disease occurs less commonly and is characterized by circumscribed atrophy of the frontal and temporal lobes. It constitutes one of the subtypes under the broad category of "frontal" or "frontotemporal" dementias (128). Terry (197) has reported a ratio of 1:50 for Pick's disease compared to AD. Munoz-Garcia and Ludwin (127) have identified two subgroups among sporadic Pick's disease; the first group (classical) had predominantly cortical atrophy, whereas the second group (generalized) showed subcortical as well as cortical atrophy. Familial cases occur, although usually the disease appears sporadically. In a study of a kinship with 25 cases, EEGs in 13 patients were within normal limits in 11 while 2 patients had excessive frontoparietal theta activity, although alpha rhythm was of normal frequency (67). Similarly, only one of three patients reported by Gordon and Sim (62), two of ten patients reported by Tissot et al. (203), and three of seven patients reported by Johannesson et al. (89) had abnormalities in the EEG. More recently, Yener et al. (218) compared conventional and quantitative EEG in 26 patients with AD and 13 patients with frontotemporal dementia (all had confirming findings on SPECT studies). In the majority of patients with frontotemporal dementia, there was a well-preserved alpha rhythm, which was not the case in AD patients. Thus a majority of patients with Pick's disease or frontotemporal dementia show mild EEG abnormalities, consisting of low- to medium-amplitude slow activity over anterior hemispheric areas, while alpha rhythm may remain normal even with severe dementia (Fig. 13.9).

There have been relatively few qEEG studies in frontotemporal dementia. Like visual analysis, qEEG studies have found EEG changes to be less severe in this group of patients than in those with AD (50,218).

Huntington's Disease

This autosomal dominant disease manifests at age 20–40 years with chorea, mental disorders, and progressive dementia. The rare juvenile form

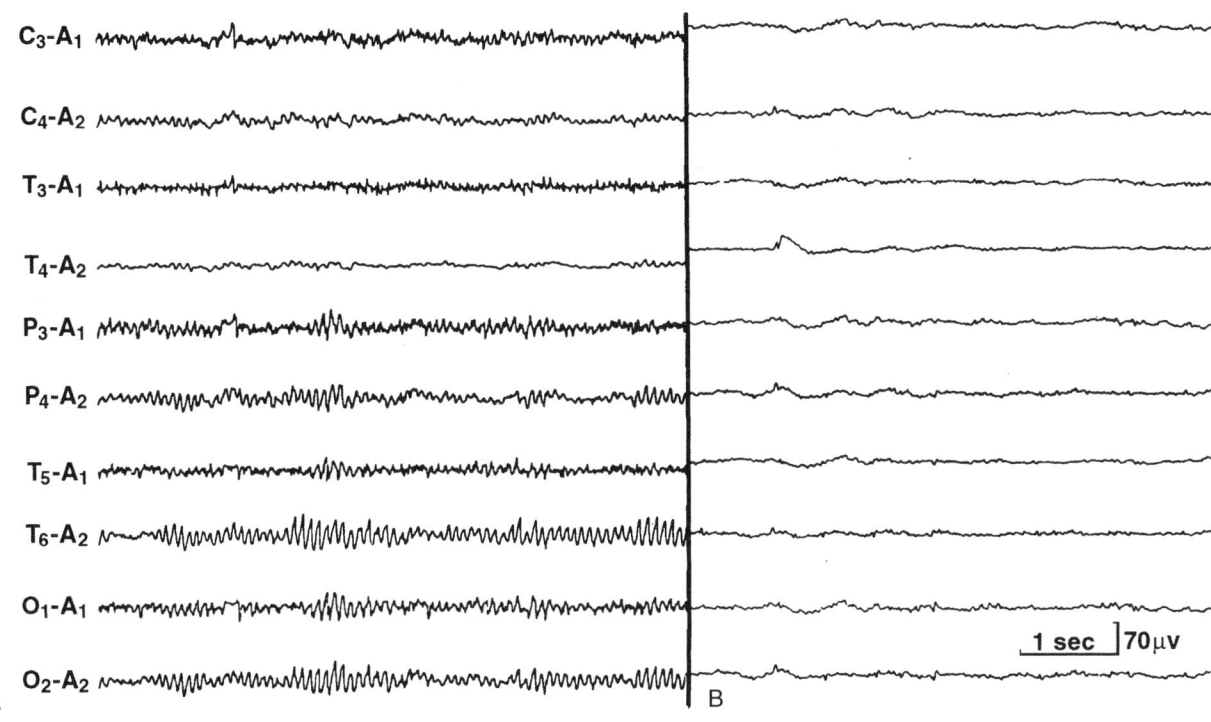

C₃-A₁

C₄-A₂

T₃-A₁

T₄-A₂

P₃-A₁

P₄-A₂

T₅-A₁

T₆-A₂

O₁-A₁

O₂-A₂

A   B

1 sec 70µV

FIG. 13.9. EEGs in a 27-year-old patient with rapidly progressive Pick's disease, proven by brain biopsy. Patient had a 2-month history of aphasia, difficulty in simple calculations, memory deficits, and personality change. **A:** Initial EEG is normal, with 80–90 µV, 11-Hz alpha rhythm. **B:** Nine months later, EEG shows loss of alpha rhythm along with very low-amplitude (15 µV), irregular slow activity. By now, patient had no evident cognitive functions and led a virtually vegetative existence.

shows parkinsonian rigidity, rather than chorea, and epileptic seizures. The disorder has been demonstrated to be due to expanded trinucleotide (cytosine, adenine, and guanine) repeats involving the Huntington gene on chromosome 4. Controls have 12–36 such repeats compared to over 40 (as high as 80) in patients with Huntington's disease (69). EEGs characteristically have very low-voltage ("flat") background activity (52,79) (Fig. 13.10), a finding reported by Margerison and Scott (112) in 60% of patients; others (142) have reported a much lower incidence, particularly in early stages when diagnosis often is difficult. Adams (2) has investigated clinical correlates of "flat" EEGs, defined as alpha rhythm voltage less than 20 µV, and has found flat tracings in 10% of adults without neurological or psychiatric disorders and in 13% of various neurological and psychiatric conditions afflicting patients ages 40–70 years. He has concluded that flat EEGs lack diagnostic significance. In a detailed study of 95 patients with Huntington's disease, Scott et al. (176) have used more stringent criteria for flat EEGs,

designating an EEG "positive" only if it lacked any activity exceeding 10 µV. Such tracings, not found in normal subjects, occurred in one-third of Huntington's disease patients. Hyperventilation tends to increase amplitude and persistence of rhythmic activity in normal subjects with flat EEGs, but caused no change in patients with Huntington's disease. In a more recent study of 16 patients, Sishta et al. (178) found 10 with "positive" EEGs by the criteria of Scott et al. (176); another 4 had mean amplitudes below 10 µV, although they occasionally showed activity exceeding 10 µV. Of additional interest was universally abnormal sleep patterns with diminished or absent vertex sharp waves, sleep spindles, and K complexes. Although EEGs of less than 10 µV are not peculiar to Huntington's disease, they occur infrequently with other neurological or psychiatric disorders and never occur in normal subjects.

Myoclonus is rare but has been reported as a major feature in a few families with Huntington's disease. EEG in some of them may show bisynchro-

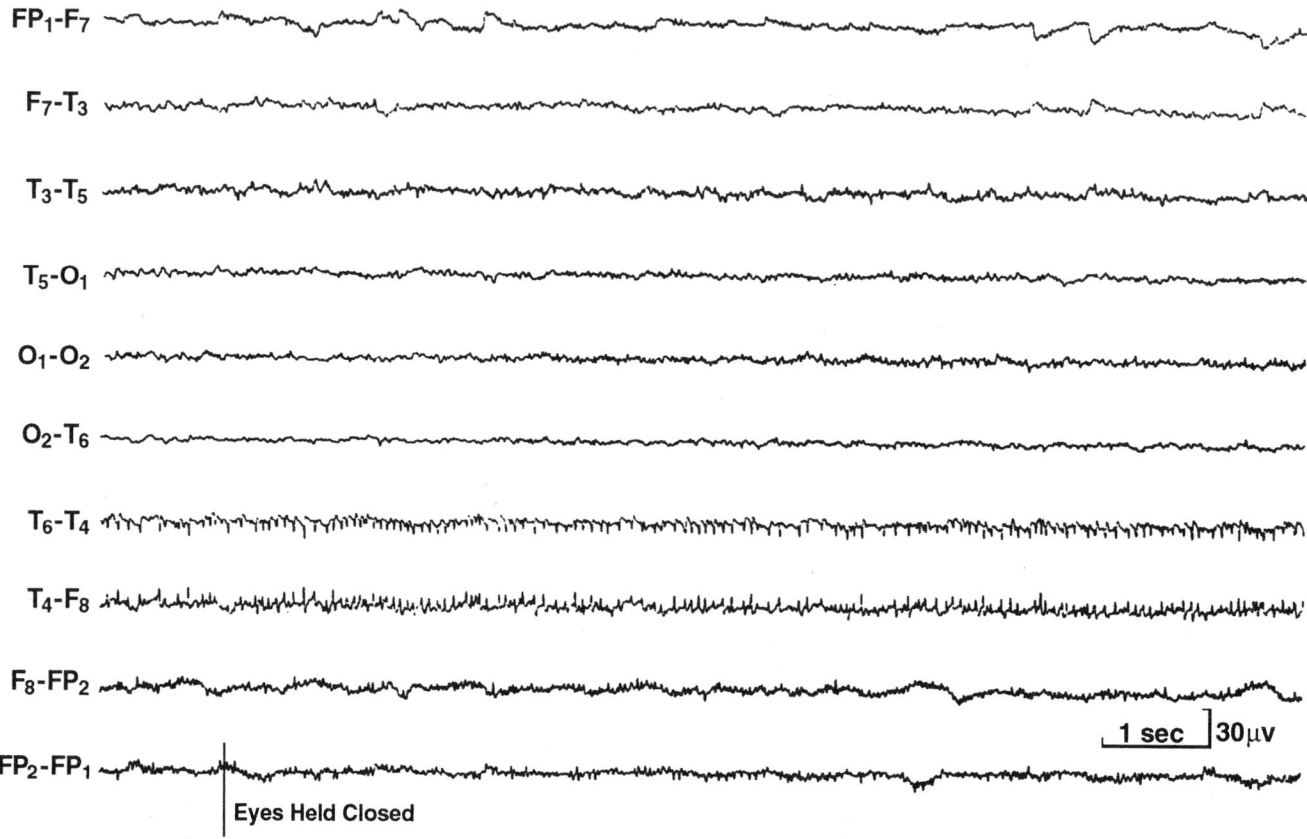

FIG. 13.10. EEG of a 53-year-old patient with Huntington's disease shows low-amplitude (10 μV) scattered theta-delta activity.

nous generalized spike-waves or polyspike-waves that may be enhanced by photic stimulation (210). Epileptiform discharges are more likely to occur in juvenile patients with seizures (12,64).

Low-amplitude tracings in Huntington's disease remain unexplained, although Scott et al. (176) have claimed a significant correlation between low-amplitude EEGs and generalized cortical atrophy.

Attempts to detect presymptomatic carriers of the gene for Huntington's disease have failed. In 26 at-risk persons from nine families with Huntington's chorea, Patterson et al. (146) had predicted, on the basis of slow-wave activity, development of the disease in 19. In 1966, Chandler (31) reported

follow-up studies on 23 of the 26 individuals. Prediction based on EEG findings was correct in 11 and incorrect in 12 at-risk cohort members! Streletz et al. (191), using computerized analysis, found increased theta and decreased alpha activity in patients with Huntington's disease; quantitatively similar changes were found in patients with AD.

Parkinson's Disease

In 1959, England et al. (46) reported abnormal EEGs in 39 of 75 patients from a clinic for Parkinson's disease, abnormalities characterized as bilateral theta or mixed theta-delta activity predominantly over posterior head regions. Patients were withdrawn from drugs for only 36–48 hours before EEG, an interval not sufficient to eliminate drug effects. Ganglberger (56) reported abnormality in 34.6% of patients with parkinsonism; in most patients (32.2%), abnormality consisted of alpha rhythm of less than 8 Hz. Sirakov and Mezan (177) reported on 100 patients selected from a population of "several hundred" on the basis of "technically good records." In 64 patients, EEGs were regarded as normal; the majority of the remaining patients showed slight to moderate degrees of "diffuse slow-wave activity" (Fig. 13.11). Yeager et al. (217) have reported on EEGs of 223 patients with parkinsonism who were candidates for stereotactic surgery; subsequently, 118 underwent operation. EEGs of 142 patients were interpreted as normal; 41 showed diffuse slowing; 22, focal slowing; and 18, focal and diffuse slowing. The authors recognized sampling bias in that all patients were candidates for surgical treatment, presumably reflecting more intractable and disabling parkinsonism. From these earlier studies, one can conclude that the majority of patients with parkinsonism probably have normal EEGs. In a minority (approximately one-third) of patients, probably representing more advanced stages of parkinsonism, slowing of alpha rhythm to below 8

Hz and generalized slow activity in the theta or theta-delta range occur; some of these changes could represent drowsiness induced by drugs or could reflect direct effects of drug toxicity.

There has been increasing awareness of dementia in idiopathic Parkinson's disease, with the incidence varying in different studies from 20% to 81% (116,153). A few more recent studies have therefore compared the EEG findings (visual analysis or qEEG) in patients with and without dementia. In a study of 128 patients, Neufeld et al. (131) reported abnormal EEGs characterized by slowing of the background in 7 of 43 (16%) nondemented and 35 of 80 (44%) demented patients with Parkinson's disease, a statistically significant difference ($p < 0.005$). In this study, the EEG slowing was also related to motor disability. There was a strong suggestion that the two factors—cognitive and motor status—affected the EEG independently because, in the nondemented patients, increased motor disability correlated significantly with increased slowing of the EEG. In studies using frequency analysis on one channel (181) and on multiple channels (130) in controls, nondemented parkinsonian patients, and demented parkinsonian patients, findings have been largely similar to those of unaided visual analysis of the EEG. Parkinsonian patients without dementia showed more ampli-

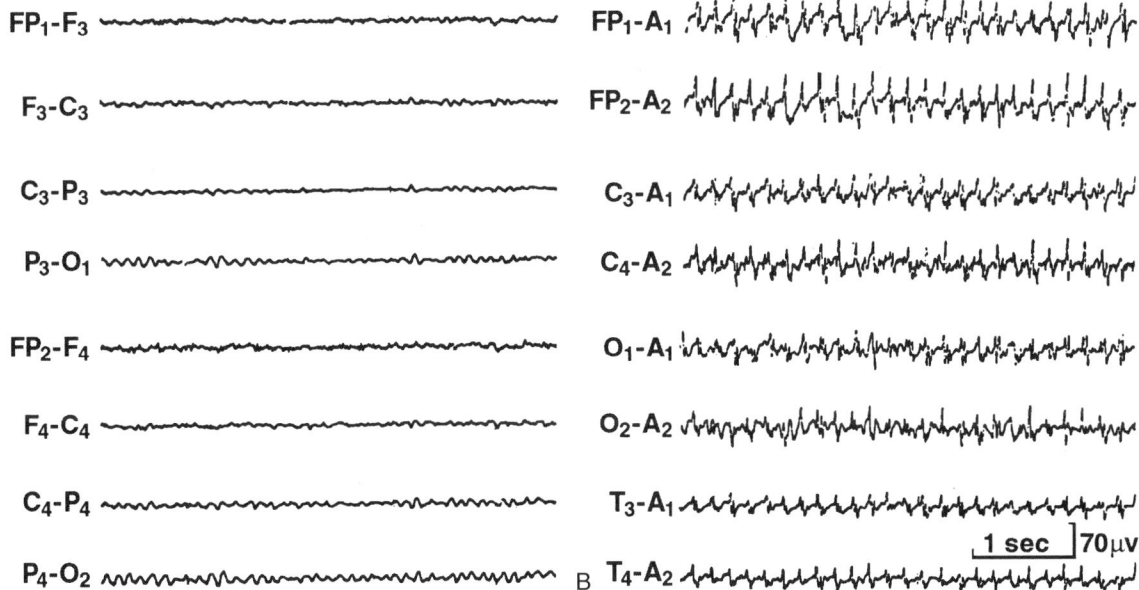

FIG. 13.11. EEG of a 57-year-old patient with Parkinson's disease shows slight slowing of the background activity **(A)** and characteristic 4- to 6-Hz, rhythmic tremor artifact **(B)**. (From Markand ON. Electroencephalography in diffuse encephalopathies. *J Clin Neurophysiol* 1984;1:357–407, with permission).

tude in the theta frequency band and diminution in the amplitude of alpha band activity. The demented patients showed a further increase in the theta and delta amplitudes compared to the nondemented patients.

Stereotactic surgery has significant, often permanent, effects on the EEG as shown by Ganglberger (56) and Yeager et al. (217). After stereotactic surgery, EEG abnormalities developed in 50% of patients even if none existed preoperatively. Postsurgical changes include diffuse or focal theta-delta slowing, or both. Focal or lateralized slowing usually occurs ipsilateral to the side of surgery. Slowing may be diffuse immediately postoperatively but later usually remains confined to the side of surgery. No relationship exists between target site (globus pallidus or lateral-ventral thalamus) or side (right or left) and severity of EEG abnormalities. Dopa therapy may improve preexisting abnormalities (63) but can also induce seizures and paroxysmal EEG abnormalities (110). Neufeld (129) described four parkinsonian patients who developed levodopa-induced encephalopathy, with their EEGs showing quasiperiodic generalized triphasic waves. The clinical condition and EEG cleared following levodopa reduction or discontinuation.

Parkinsonism–dementia syndrome occurs in endemic form among Chamorro Indians on Guam. EEGs have been abnormal in 12 patients studied (80). Alpha rhythms may be 8–9 Hz or slower. Scattered diffuse theta activity and, at times, focal arrhythmic delta activity appear in the frontotemporal regions. Severity of EEG abnormalities appears to correlate with degree of mental deterioration. Although this syndrome clinically resembles CJD, EEG findings differ in that they lack periodic complexes.

Progressive Supranuclear Palsy

Steele et al. (187) have described PSP, a heterogeneous system degeneration, and distinguished it from Parkinson's disease. Lesions are largely confined to diencephalic and brainstem nuclei. Su and Goldensohn (194) reported EEG findings in 12 patients. In the initial stages, alpha rhythms have normal frequencies. In five of eight patients, initially normal EEGs became abnormal over 3 months to 7 years. Abnormalities were varied: Focal arrhythmic delta activity occurred in three patients, whereas intermittent rhythmic delta activity occurred in five. As the illness progressed, EEGs deteriorated, showing increased slowing—and eventually disappearance—of alpha rhythm. In two series (53,111), EEGs were normal in over one-half of patients. The remainder had excessive diffuse or bitemporal theta activity, minor asymmetries of slow activity, low-voltage tracings, or frontal intermittent rhythmic delta activity.

Montplaisir et al. (124) evaluated quantitative EEG and sleep architecture in six patients with PSP and compared those findings with results in age-matched controls. qEEG demonstrated more severe slowing in the frontal region rather than temporal areas, a finding in accordance with the imaging and neuropsychological studies showing impairment of frontal lobes in PSP. These authors also confirmed the earlier reported abnormalities in the sleep architecture (68) in patients with PSP. Patients with PSP show a shorter total sleep time, lower sleep efficiency, a drastic reduction in sleep spindles, an atonic slow-wave sleep, and a marked reduction in REM sleep with reduction both in the number of REM periods and the mean duration of a REM period. REM sleep abnormalities are consistent with the known PSP-associated degeneration of the pedunculopontine tegmentum—a critical structure in REM sleep generation.

Creutzfeldt-Jakob Disease

CJD was once regarded as a neurodegenerative disorder, but it has been firmly established that it is due to a transmissible agent attributed to prior infection (160). Prion diseases can be sporadic, familial, or iatrogenic. They are characterized by abnormal metabolism of the prion protein PrP, leading to accumulation of an abnormal infectious prion protein, scrapie (PrP^{sc}), which is an isoform of normal cellular PrP. Human prion diseases include CJD, Gerstmann-Sträussler-Scheinker (GSS) syndrome, kuru, and fatal familial insomnia; CJD is the most common. Although most cases of CJD are sporadic, 5%–15% are clustered in families (23,117). The clinical picture is similar in sporadic and familial patients. Three clinical stages are recognized. The first is characterized principally by progressive dementia or a wide variety of focal symptoms indicating lesions in various parts of the brain. In the second stage, the focal features tend to disappear as a picture of progressive dementia, bilateral rigidity, pyramidal signs, and widespread myoclonus evolves. In the third stage, the patient becomes bedbound with deepening stupor, increasing rigidity, and weakness of the limbs that proceeds relentlessly to death. Markand (114) has reviewed the EEG findings in CJD.

In the first phase, EEG changes are limited to a progressive disorganization of background rhythms and increased amounts of generalized slow (theta-delta) activity (24). These changes may be more marked anteriorly or posteriorly, or over one hemisphere or part of a hemisphere (Fig. 13.12A, B). Such focal or lateralized features may suggest a tumor or even a stroke, but sooner or later EEG activity becomes bilaterally slow.

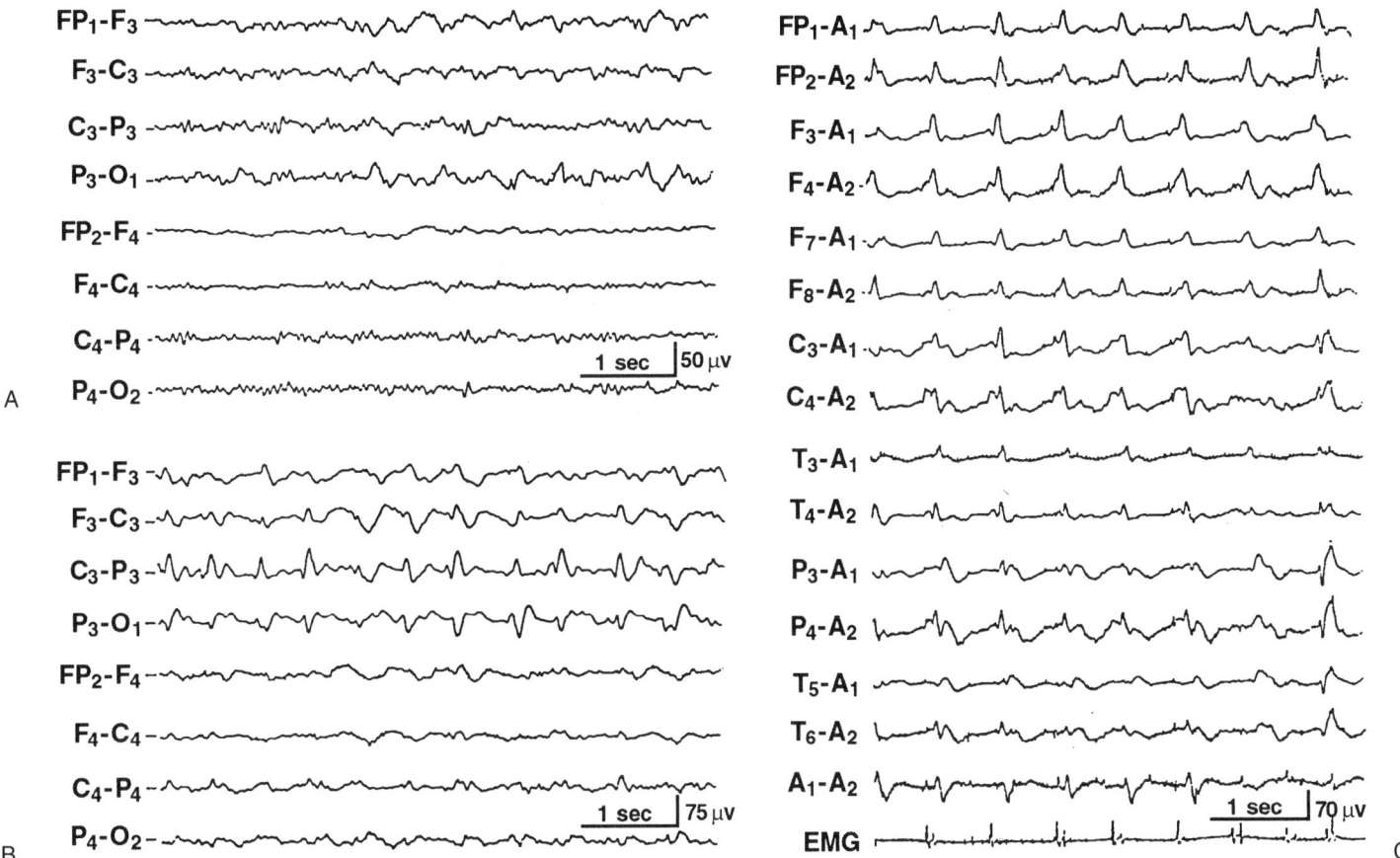

FIG. 13.12. EEGs of a 62-year-old patient with Creutzfeldt-Jakob disease. **A:** The earliest EEG, taken 2 months after the onset of dementia and right hemiparesis, shows lateralized abnormality consisting of widespread delta activity over the left hemisphere. **B:** Two weeks later, the EEG shows periodic lateral epileptiform discharges on the left side. There is more deterioration of background activity over both sides. **C:** EEG obtained 5 months after the onset of Creutzfeldt-Jakob disease shows generalized periodic sharp waves recurring every second. Patient had rhythmic jerks of the left arm, which are monitored on the last channel. The channel next to last (A1-A2) records the electrocardiogram. The periodic complexes have a close temporal relationship to the myoclonic jerks but are independent of the cardiac activity. (From Markand ON. Electroencephalography in diffuse encephalopathies. *J Clin Neurophysiol* 1984;1:357–407, with permission).

During the second phase of CJD, the EEG is characterized by periodic, bilaterally synchronous potentials (1,24). The periodic potentials take the form of diphasic or triphasic sharp waves, 200–500 milliseconds in duration and up to 300 μV in amplitude. As the disease progresses, some patients exhibit more complex discharges with multiphasic or polyspike configuration (3). The frequency of the periodic complexes is close to 1 per second; the interval between successive discharges varies from 0.5 to 1.6 seconds. There is a fairly close, but not precise, relationship between the periodic complexes and the myoclonic jerks: The jerks may occur a few milliseconds before or after the electrical event (Fig. 13.12C). The periodic sharp-wave complexes (PSWCs) in the EEG may occur without associated myoclonic jerks. This is particularly true during sleep or late in the course of the disease, when the myoclonic jerks decrease or disappear while the PSWCs persist (1).

This periodic pattern continues into the third (i.e., final) phase of CJD. Many authors (1,3,14) describe a progressive lengthening of the interval between periodic complexes with advancing disease, but others (24) have reported a remarkable consistency of the frequency even into the terminal stages. Finally, the amplitude of the background activity decreases, which results in an undifferentiated low-voltage tracing from which rhythmic discharges emerge.

The characteristic periodic pattern has been reported in 75%–94% of patients with CJD (24,32). From original data and review of the literature, Levy et al. (105) affirmed that lack of periodic abnormalities in EEGs after an illness of 12 weeks weighs strongly against CJD. However, at least a few patients with CJD, particularly those with forms considered atypical (e.g., ataxic or amyotrophic variety or with long duration), may not show periodic EEG activity at any point in the entire illness (3,22,219).

No comprehensive evaluation of EEGs has been carried out in familial cases of CJD. It appears, however, that PSWCs are less common in familial than in sporadic CJD, although the clinical characteristics are not dramatically different. Tietjen and Drury (201) reported an absence of myoclonus and PSWCs in serial EEGs of four members of a kindred with pathologically verified CJD.

In the early stages of CJD, periodic discharges may be present only for 5–10 seconds at a time or may appear only a few times in a single EEG. Also, before the periodic pattern is fully established, the EEG may show state-dependent variability.

During periods of drowsiness or sleep, the PSWCs may virtually disappear and be replaced by medium-amplitude generalized theta-delta activity.

Also during this state, the myoclonic jerks often disappear, heart and respiratory rates are reduced, and periods of apnea may occur (14,91). Periodic complexes reappear during the periods when the patient is aroused and more alert. The EEG may thus show a cyclic alternating pattern, that is, alternation of the two stereotyped EEG patterns (PSWC pattern alternating with diffusely slow EEG).

Another characteristic feature of the PSWCs, particularly in the early stages, is their reactivity to alerting stimuli or to the administration of drugs. Before the PSWCs are well established, or when they occur only intermittently, acoustic or other alerting stimuli may trigger the periodic pattern when delivered during a diffusely slow EEG phase (14). In some patients, intermittent photic stimulation (IPS) may elicit tight coupling of periodic complexes to flashes, particularly when the rate of stimulation is close to that of the periodic complexes (3,14). In the terminal stages of CJD, when the PSWCs are nearly absent, IPS may be able to initiate the onset of time-locked triphasic waves coincidental to each stimulus (14). Administration of 10 mg of diazepam intravenously, in contrast, may be followed by a transient disappearance of PSWCs and myoclonus that restarts after several minutes in response to acoustic stimuli (14).

The periodic discharges of CJD are classically bilaterally symmetrical and generalized in distribution. However, focal or lateralized periodic sharp waves (i.e., a PLEDs pattern) may occur in the early stages of the disease (8,41,54), as illustrated in Figure 13.12B. With progression of the disease, the periodic events become bilaterally symmetrical.

The *Heidenhain variant of CJD* is characterized by predominant involvement of the occipital cortex, often resulting in cortical blindness early in the disease. The EEG may show slowing of the background activity and PSWCs over the posterior head region. The complexes may be focal or unilateral initially but become bilateral over the posterior regions as the disease progresses (54).

GSS disease is a rare familial variant of CJD, characterized by spinocerebellar ataxia, diminished reflexes, myoclonus, and a longer course (2–15 years) than CJD (100). The EEG is characterized by variable slowing of the background activity, but, unlike CJD, periodic complexes are absent.

The localization of the PSWCs corresponding to the site of maximum involvement (occipital cortex) in the Heidenhain variant of CJD and the absence of PSWCs in the ataxic variant of CJD with maximum cerebellar involvement suggest that cortical pathology is a critical substrate for the production of PSWCs in CJD. The pathogenesis of PSWCs, however, remains unknown. They may derive from mechanisms intrinsic to affected neurons that become electronically coupled because of virus-induced membrane fusion (206).

Similar EEG patterns consisting of sharp waves occurring regularly every 1.0–1.5 seconds may rarely occur in other encephalopathies (cerebral anoxia, subtle status epilepticus, hepatic/renal encephalopathies, lithium and baclofen intoxication, etc.) (18,133). A few authors (42,213) have also described a similar EEG picture in rapidly progressive AD, but the resemblance was only superficial. These cases showed frequently occurring sharp waves that had random, not periodic, intervals—even when frequently repetitive. This confusion stresses the need for a more strict definition of periodicity in EEG. Not every frequently recurring paroxysmal discharge in the EEG should be called "periodic." This category should be reserved only for those discharges for which a modal value of intervals can be established at a minimal range of variation around that value (59).

ACQUIRED IMMUNODEFICIENCY SYNDROME

Markand (114) discussed EEG findings in AIDS. Infection by the human immunodeficiency virus, type 1 (HIV-1), results in a spectrum of central nervous system (CNS) complications. The best known are the opportunistic infections and neoplasia of the brain secondary to immunodeficiency. A devastating but poorly understood consequence of HIV-1 infection is a progressive encephalopathy that results in the AIDS dementia complex, HIV-1–associated cognitive–motor complex, or HIV-1 dementia. Approximately 15%–20% of all patients with AIDS will develop dementia. Although some cases of dementia are probably due to subacute encephalitis caused by HIV-1, in others the pathological changes are relatively minor. It has been suggested that neurotoxic viral proteins or the biological activities of cytokines released from HIV-activated macrophages cause CNS dysfunction (152). The pathological changes and the MRI-demonstrated atrophy involve both cortex and basal ganglia; the most severe changes occur in the basal ganglia, especially the caudate nucleus (37).

The EEG is invariably abnormal in well-established cases of HIV-1 dementia. The abnormalities include a slow or absent posterior rhythm and intermittent or continuous theta-delta slowing, which is either generalized or predominantly anterior (55,97,145,202). There is a good correlation between the severity of the EEG abnormalities and the severity of HIV-1 dementia. Some patients with advanced dementia have low-voltage (< 20 μV), slow EEGs (73), not unlike that reported in Huntington's disease (176). Periodic sharp or triphasic waves, 1.5–2.0 cycles per second, over both frontocentral regions have also been described in a patient with HIV-1 dementia similar to the characteristic EEG pattern of CJD (200). This patient had myoclonic jerks; the periodic EEG pattern and the myoclonus both responded dramatically to zidovudine therapy.

An interesting aspect of the EEG in HIV infection has been the reports of EEG abnormalities even in asymptomatic HIV-1–infected individuals (44,55,97,145). It is proposed that these EEG abnormalities (usually background slowing) provide the earliest indicator of subclinical CNS dysfunction (97) and may predict subsequent development of HIV-1–related neurological disease (144). Parisi et al. (144) reported computer-analyzed EEG abnormalities in 50 of 185 (27%) asymptomatic or lymphadenopathy-only individuals infected with HIV-1. Inclusion of intravenous drug users in the HIV-seropositive group and absence of matched seronegative controls make it difficult to ascribe EEG abnormalities specifically to the HIV infection. A well-controlled study by Nuwer et al. (136) reported no significant difference in either clinical or computer-analyzed EEG between HIV-seronegative (*n* = 86) and HIV-seropositive (*n* = 114) asymptomatic men. They found that 22% of the seropositive and 26% of the seronegative men showed abnormal or borderline EEGs; rates were higher in both groups (45% in seronegative and 36% in seropositive men) when neuropsychological abnormalities coexisted. The incidence of EEG abnormalities thus failed to correlate with the serostatus but correlated with an impaired neuropsychological status in HIV-infected patients as well as controls. If risk factors such as intravenous drug abuse (which increases the incidence of EEG abnormalities) are excluded, the incidence of EEG abnormalities among the asymptomatic HIV-infected group is probably less than 7%, a rate comparable to that of uninfected controls (132).

CEREBROVASCULAR DISEASE

Hachinski et al. (71) introduced the term *multi-infarct dementia* to characterize relatively global cognitive impairments resulting from multiple infarcts (none of which alone would cause dementia) and to emphasize that the dementia reflects cumulative effects of multiple infarcts. Roberts et al. (164) have compared EEG findings in 48 patients with "nonvascular" dementia and 33 patients with "vascular" dementia. They used four EEG categories: normal (type I), excess beta activity (type II), theta activity predominant (type III), and delta activity predominant (type IV). In vascular dementia, types I and II occurred in 33% of patients, type III in 61%, and type IV in only 6%. In nonvascular dementia, however, type III represented only 46% while type IV represented 19%. Most striking was a prevalence of focal EEG abnormalities in 74% of patients with vascular dementia as opposed to 19% with nonvascular dementia. Subsequent studies reported by Harrison et al. (74), Soininen et al. (183), and Erkinjuntti et al. (47) have also stressed the occurrence of focal and paroxysmal findings in vascular dementia. Thus, in general, focal slow waves in EEG and focal neurological signs help to distinguish vascular from degenerative dementias.

There is no consensus on the utility of quantitative EEG in differentiating AD patients from those with MID (90). Spectral studies have compared AD and MID. Erkinjuntti et al. (47) found a decline in the percentage of alpha power and a concomitant increase in theta and delta power relative to the degree of dementia for both groups. Furthermore, there were no significant group differences. However, Leuchter et al. (103) reported that 22 of 24 (92%) subjects with either AD or MID were accurately classified using discriminant analysis of both EEG frequency and coherence. Leuchter and Walter (104) subsequently reported topographic mapping findings in 40 subjects: 15 with AD, 13 with MID, and 12 age-matched controls. Functional images using spectral ratios showed that subjects with AD had a characteristic left temporoparietal deficit that distinguished them from subjects with MID and from control subjects. More recently, Leuchter et al. (102), using a ratio of coherence from corticocortical–corticosubcortical networks divided by coherence from long corticocortical tracts, correctly classified 76% of subjects into AD or MID categories. Sloan and Fenton (179) also found some spectral differences, with AD patients having more delta and theta power and less alpha power than MID patients matched for severity of dementia.

A rare form of dementia, *Binswanger's disease*, reflects subcortical arteriosclerotic encephalopathy. Despite preserved cortical architecture, dementia is prominent, presumably as a result of lesions in white matter disrupting corticipetal and corticocortical fibers. Caplan and Schoene (30) have reported on 11 cases, 5 confirmed by autopsy. EEGs of six patients showed "diffuse slowing" (not otherwise described), two showed "focal slowing," and three were normal. Single case reports have described triphasic or sharp waves with a tendency toward periodicity (25,214). The findings differ from the periodic discharges in CJD in that the sharp waves were lateralized and occurred only for brief periods.

Dementia Resulting from Other Causes

Normal-Pressure Hydrocephalus

NPH classically presents with gait difficulty, urinary incontinence, and progressive dementia; it results from known or presumed obliteration of subarachnoid spaces, impairing absorption of spinal fluid. Brown and Goldensohn (21) have reported on 11 patients with NPH. Six had normal EEGs. Four had focal or diffuse theta-delta slowing against a well-preserved alpha rhythm, whereas the remaining patients demonstrated both slowing of the alpha rhythm and focal delta slowing. Subsequent authors have reported a higher incidence of abnormal EEGs among patients with NPH: Wood et al. (216) reported 27 of 32 patients; Hashi et al. (75), 12 of 13 patients; and Greenberg et al. (65), 61 of 67 patients. The reported EEG abnormalities have been focal or diffuse theta-delta slowing superimposed on a normal or slightly slow background. Of particular interest are the "projected" rhythms, which signify, among other processes, raised intraventricular pressure. Paroxysmal monorhythmic theta or delta activity has been reported in a few patients with NPH (75,151). Follow-up EEG studies after a shunting procedure are likely to show significant improvement in the EEG (75).

Neurosyphilis

Once the leading cause of dementia, general paresis resulting from neurosyphilis is now uncommon. Over two-thirds of patients have abnormal EEGs with slowing of the alpha rhythm and generalized slow activity of theta-delta frequency (6). EEGs are more abnormal when neurosyphilis is active, but they may improve with successful therapy (48). In "burnt out" disease, on the other hand, EEGs may be normal or minimally affected even in the face of severe residual neurological deficits.

Alcoholism

Alcoholism is common, and dementia occurs in 3% of chronic alcoholic patients, which accounts for 7% of patients admitted for evaluation of progressive intellectual impairment (36,115). Krauss and Niedermeyer (98) reported on the EEG findings in 213 patients with chronic alcoholism, 152 of whom were referred to the EEG laboratory for epileptic seizure and remaining 61 for delirium or other causes. The majority (almost two-thirds) had normal tracings if one included low-voltage tracing as a normal variant in adults. Approximately 30% had nonlocalized slowing, 2% focal slowing, and 4% focal epileptiform abnormalities. The most common EEG finding was a low-voltage (< 25 µV) tracing recorded in one-half of the patients (106 of the 213) compared to a 13.9% incidence of such tracings in the nonalcoholic "control" group. Unlike the low-amplitude EEG encountered at times in anxious patients, the low amplitude in chronic alcoholics persisted during hyperventilation and even during sleep. Presence of cortical atrophy on CT scan was one of the factors that correlated with low-amplitude tracings. Even though the incidence of low-amplitude tracings is significantly higher in chronic alcoholics, this does not constitute an EEG abnormality except in infancy and childhood. Focal or diffuse slowing and epileptiform abnormalities seen in a minority are related to alcohol-related complications such as metabolic encephalopathy, brain injury, and the like.

PSEUDODEMENTIA

Pseudodementia refers to cognitive impairments associated with severe depression. Characteristically, these patients have prominent subjective, as opposed to objective, changes in memory, which distinguishes them from patients with organic dementia. Pseudodementia accounts for 10% of patients presenting with a clinical picture of dementia (180). Because changes in EEG are subtle in early dementia (*vide supra*), the EEG may contribute little to differential diagnosis. By the time abnormalities in EEG become evident, dementia is equally evident. Mildly demented patients may also have reactive depressive episodes, further confounding the problems of diagnosis.

Brenner et al. (17) reported EEG findings in 33 elderly patients with mixed symptoms of depression and dementia who were followed longitudinally to confirm the diagnosis. Two groups of patients, those with dementia with depressive features and those with depressive pseudodementia, were defined. There were significant group differences on waking EEGs between those "mixed" patients who did well after treatment for depression (depressive pseudodementia) and those with dementia with secondary depression. Most patients with dementia with secondary depression had abnormal EEGs, with approximately one-third having moderate or severe abnormalities. In contrast, patients with depressive pseudodementia had EEGs that usually were normal or showed only mild abnormalities.

AMNESIC SYNDROMES

Transient Global Amnesia

Since its first description, transient global amnesia (TGA) has aroused the interest of electroencephalographers, but conflicting reports of normal EEGs, epileptiform activity, and focal slow-wave activity have clouded the picture. In an early study, Jaffe and Bender (87) reported normal EEGs in 26 of 27 patients; the only exception was a patient who showed nonspecific temporal slowing during and after TGA. Subsequently, there have been reports of a small group of patients with TGA in whom interictal EEGs demonstrated spike-and–sharp wave abnormalities (58,66,109,170,189,199). These studies led to the suggestion that TGA may represent an epileptic seizure involving mesial temporal structures involved with recent memory. The evidence for epileptic etiology has been largely based on the presence of interictal EEG abnormality over the temporal region or a good response to antiepileptic medication. Not only is this evidence weak, but also in many studies the illustrations showed a variety of nonspecific benign variants, such as benign epileptiform transients of sleep, that have no correlation with epileptic seizures.

An EEG has rarely been recorded during an actual episode of TGA. In a large series of 117 patients with TGA, Miller et al. (122) had 13 EEG recordings made during episodes of TGA; 8 showed no abnormality, 1 had subclinical rhythmic electrographic discharge of adults, and the remaining 4 had nonspecific theta-delta slowing, either generalized or focal. None contained epileptiform abnormalities during TGA. Only a few patients have been reported who, during a supposed TGA, had an ictal pattern recorded over the temporal region (86,120,196).

Large case–control studies on TGA in recent years have concluded that TGA is commonly related either to cerebral ischemia (thromboembolic or hemodynamic) (70,99) or to migraine (81,118). In only one large series on TGA (81), comprising 114 patients, did a significant minority (7%) develop epilepsy, usually within 1 year of presentation. One can make a valid conclusion that, in most patients with TGA, the EEG both interictally and during the episodes is normal or shows nonspecific slow-wave abnormalities; only on occasion do epileptic seizures masquerade as TGA.

Korsakoff's Syndrome

Korsakoff's syndrome, a chronic amnesic state, usually follows an acute episode of Wernicke's encephalopathy. In the acute phase, EEGs are abnormal in about 50% of patients, with the abnormality consisting of background slowing in the theta-delta range (207). When Korsakoff's syndrome emerges, the EEG usually has become normal.

CONCLUSIONS

In evaluating changes in mental state, EEG has definite advantages counterbalanced by significant limitations. Bearing these in mind, electroencephalographers can offer help to clinicians in certain circumstances. In patients with abrupt onset of confusional or catatonic-like states, EEG can confirm or refute the occurrence of nonconvulsive status epilepticus, which can develop at any time from childhood to old age. In patients in whom mental changes emerge more gradually, EEG may suggest (a) a metabolic basis such as chronic uremia or hepatic encephalopathy or (b) a focal cerebral lesion such as subdural hematoma. With relatively rapidly developing dementia, EEG may provide the first laboratory evidence for CJD, with its characteristic periodic discharges. In the early stage of AD, overlap with healthy elderly persons and depressed patients reduces the specificity of EEG. EEG has value in the differential diagnosis of clinically established dementia. Preserved alpha rhythms characterize Pick's or frontotemporal dementia, as opposed to AD or PSP dementia. "Flat" EEGs with background activity voltages less than 10 μV occur in a majority of demented patients with Huntington's disease. Thus, although most of the EEG abnormalities in dementia are "nonspecific," the available clinical information can enable electroencephalographers to give balanced, useful appraisals.

REFERENCES

1. Abbott J. The EEG in Jakob-Creutzfeldt's disease. *Electroencephalogr Clin Neurophysiol* 1959;11:184–185(abst).
2. Adams A. Studies on the flat electroencephalogram in man. *Electroencephalogr Clin Neurophysiol* 1959;11:35–41.
3. Aguglia U, Farnarier G, Tinuper P, et al. Subacute spongiform encephalopathy with periodic paroxysmal activities: clinical evolution and serial EEG findings in 20 cases. *Clin Electroencephalogr* 1987;18:147–158.
4. American Psychiatric Association. *Diagnostic and statistical manual of mental disorders*, 4th ed. Washington, DC: American Psychiatric Association, 1994.
5. Anderer P, Saletu B, Kloppel B, et al. Discrimination between demented patients and normals based on topographic EEG slow wave activity: comparison between Z statistics, discriminant analysis and artificial neural network classifiers. *Electroencephalogr Clin Neurophysiol* 1994; 91:108–117.
6. Arantsen K, Voldby H. Electroencephalographic changes in neurosyphilis. *Electroencephalogr Clin Neurophysiol* 1952;4:331–337.
7. Arenas AM, Brenner RP, Reynolds CF. Temporal slowing in the elderly revisited. *Am J EEG Technol* 1986;26:105–114.
8. Au WJ, Gabor AJ, Viyan N, et al. Periodic lateralized epileptiform complexes (PLEDs) in Creutzfeldt-Jakob disease. *Neurology* 1980;30:611–617.
9. Berg L, Danziger WL, Storandt M, et al. Predictive features in mild senile dementia of the Alzheimer type. *Neurology* 1984;34:563–569.
10. Besthorn C, Forstl H, Geiger-Kabisch C, et al. EEG coherence in Alzheimer disease. *Electroencephalogr Clin Neurophysiol* 1994;90:242–245.
11. Besthorn C, Zerfass R, Geiger-Kabisch C, et al. Discrimination of Alzheimer's disease and normal aging by EEG data. *Electroencephalogr Clin Neurophysiol* 1997;103:241–248.
12. Bittenbender JB, Quadfasel FA. Rigid and akinetic forms of Huntington's chorea. *Arch Neurol* 1962;7:275–288.
13. Blatt I, Brenner RP. Triphasic waves in a psychiatric population: a retrospective study. *J Clin Neurophysiol* 1996;13:324–329.
14. Bortone E, Bettoni L, Giorgi C, et al. Reliability of EEG in the diagnosis of Creutzfeldt-Jakob disease. *Electroencephalogr Clin Neurophysiol* 1994;90:323–330.
15. Brenner RP. Utility of electroencephalography in delirium: past views and current practice. *Int Psychogeriatr* 1991;3:211–229.
16. Brenner RP, Reynolds CF III, Ulrich RF. Diagnostic efficacy of computerized spectral versus visual EEG analysis in elderly normal, demented and depressed subjects. *Electroencephalogr Clin Neurophysiol* 1988;69:110–117.
17. Brenner RP, Reynolds CF III, Ulrich RF. EEG findings in depressive pseudodementia and dementia with secondary depression. *Electroencephalogr Clin Neurophysiol* 1989;72: 298–304.
18. Brenner RP, Schaul N. Periodic EEG patterns: classification, clinical correlation and pathophysiology. *J Clin Neurophysiol* 1990;7:249–267.
19. Brenner RP, Ulrich RF, Reynolds CF. EEG spectral findings in healthy, elderly men and women—sex differences. *Electroencephalogr Clin Neurophysiol* 1995;94:1–5.
20. Brenner RP, Ulrich RF, Spiker DG, et al. Computerized EEG spectral analysis in elderly normal, demented and depressed subjects. *Electroencephalogr Clin Neurophysiol* 1986;64: 483–492.
21. Brown DG, Goldensohn ES. The electroencephalogram in normal pressure hydrocephalus. *Arch Neurol* 1973;29:70–71.
22. Brown P, Cathala F, Castaigne P, et al. Creutzfeldt-Jakob disease: clinical analysis of a consecutive series of 230 neuropathologically verified cases. *Ann Neurol* 1986;20:597–602.
23. Brown P, Cathala F, Raubertas RF, et al. The epidemiology of Creutzfeldt-Jakob disease: conclusion of a 15 year investigation in France and review of the world literature. *Neurology* 1987; 37:895–904.
24. Burger LJ, Rowan J, Goldenshon E. Creutzfeldt-Jakob disease. *Arch Neurol* 1972;26:428–433.
25. Burger PC, Burch JG, Kunze U. Subcortical arteriosclerotic encephalopathy (Binswanger's disease): a vascular etiology of dementia. *Stroke* 1976;7:626–631.
26. Busse EW, Barnes RH, Silverman AJ, et al. Studies of the process of aging: factors that influence the psyche of elderly persons. *Am J Psychiatry* 1954;100:897–903.
27. Busse EW, Obrist WD. Significance of focal electroencephalographic changes in the elderly. *Postgrad Med* 1963;34:179–182.
28. Busse EW, Obrist WD. Pre-senescent electroencephalographic changes in normal subjects. *J Gerontol* 1965;20:315–320.
29. Canter NL, Hallett M, Growdon JH. Lecithin does not affect EEG spectral analysis or P300 in Alzheimer disease. *Neurology* 1982;32:1260–1266.
30. Caplan LR, Schoene WC. Clinical features of subcortical arteriosclerotic encephalopathy (Binswanger disease). *Neurology* 1978;28:1206–1215.
31. Chandler JH. EEG prediction of Huntington's chorea: an 18 year followup. *Electroencephalogr Clin Neurophysiol* 1966;21:79–80.
32. Chiofalo N, Fuentes A, Galvez S. Serial EEG findings in 27 cases of Creutzfeldt-Jakob disease. *Arch Neurol* 1980;37:143–145.
33. Coben LA, Chi D, Snyder AZ, et al. Replication of a study of frequency analysis of the resting awake EEG in mild probable Alzheimer's disease. *Electroencephalogr Clin Neurophysiol* 1990;75:148–154.

34. Coben LA, Danziger WL, Berg L. Frequency analysis of the resting awake EEG in mild senile dementia of Alzheimer type. *Electroencephalogr Clin Neurophysiol* 1983;55:372–380.

35. Coben LA, Danziger W, Storandt M. A longitudinal EEG study of mild senile dementia of Alzheimer type at 1 and at 2.5 years. *Electroencephalogr Clin Neurophysiol* 1985;61:101–112.

36. Cutting J. Alcoholic dementia. In: Benson DF, Blumer D, eds. *Psychiatric aspects of neurologic disease*, Vol 2. New York: Grune & Stratton, 1982:149–164.

37. Dal Pan GJ, McArthur JH, Aylward E, et al. Pattern of cerebral atrophy in HIV-1-infected individuals: results of a quantitative MRI analysis. *Neurology* 1992;42:2125–2130.

38. De Leon MJ, George AE. Computed tomography in aging and senile dementia of the Alzheimer's type. In: Mayeux R, Rosen WG, eds. *The dementias*. New York: Raven Press, 1983:103–122.

39. Duffy FH, Albert MS, McAnulty G. Brain electrical activity in patients with presenile and senile dementia of the Alzheimer type. *Ann Neurol* 1984;16:439–448.

40. Dunkin JJ, Osato S, Leuchter AF. Relationships between EEG coherence and neuropsychological tests in dementia. *Clin Electroencephalogr* 1995;26:47–59.

41. Eggertson DE, Pillay N. Creutzfeldt-Jakob disease: correlation of focal electroencephalographic abnormalities and clinical signs. *Can J Neurol Sci* 1986;13:120–124.

42. Ehle AL, Johnson PC. Rapidly evolving EEG changes in a case of Alzheimer's disease. *Ann Neurol* 1977;1:593–595.

43. Elmstahl S, Rosen I, Gullberg B. Quantitative EEG in elderly patients with Alzheimer's disease and healthy controls. *Dementia* 1994;5:119–124.

44. Elovaara I, Saar P, Valle SL, et al. EEG in the early HIV-1 infection is characterized by anterior dysrhythmicity of low maximal amplitude. *Clin Electroencephalogr* 1991;22:131–140.

45. Engel GL, Romano J. Delirium, a syndrome of cerebral insufficiency. *J Chronic Dis* 1959;9:260–277.

46. England AC, Schwab RS, Peterson E. The electroencephalogram in Parkinson's syndrome. *Electroencephalogr Clin Neurophysiol* 1959;11:723–731.

47. Erkinjuntti T, Larsen T, Sulkava R, et al. EEG in the differential diagnosis between Alzheimer's disease and vascular dementia. *Acta Neurol Scand* 1988;77:36–43.

48. Finley KH, Rose AS, Solomon HC. Electroencephalographic studies on neurosyphilis. *Arch Neurol Psychiatry* 1942;47:718–736.

49. Folstein MF, Folstein SE, McHugh PR. "Mini-mental state": a practical method for grading the cognitive state of patients for the clinician. *J Psychiatr Res* 1975;12:189–198.

50. Forstl H, Besthorn C, Hentschel F, et al. Frontal lobe degeneration and Alzheimer's disease: a controlled study on clinical findings, volumetric brain changes and quantitative electroencephalography data. *Dementia* 1996;7:27–34.

51. Forstl H, Sattel H, Besthorn C, et al. Longitudinal cognitive, electroencephalographic and morphological brain changes in aging and Alzheimer's disease. *Br J Psychiatry* 1996;168:280–286.

52. Foster DB, Bagchi BK. Electroencephalographic observations in Huntington's chorea. *Electroencephalogr Clin Neurophysiol* 1949;1:247–248.

53. Fowler CJ, Harrison MJG. EEG changes in subcortical dementia: a study of 22 patients with Steele-Richardson-Olszewski (SRO) syndrome. *Electroencephalogr Clin Neurophysiol* 1986;64:301–303.

54. Furlan A, Henry CE, Sweeny PJ, et al. Focal EEG abnormalities in Heidenhain's variant of Jakob-Creutzfeldt disease. *Arch Neurol* 1981;38:312–314.

55. Gabuzda DH, Levy SR, Chiappa KH. Electroencephalography in AIDS and AIDS-related complex. *Clin Electroencephalogr* 1988;19:1–6.

56. Ganglberger JA. The EEG in parkinsonism and its alteration by stereotaxically produced lesions in pallidum or thalamus. *Electroencephalogr Clin Neurophysiol* 1961;13:828(abst).

57. Giaquinto S, Nolfe G. The EEG in the normal elderly: a contribution to the interpretation of aging and dementia. *Electroencephalogr Clin Neurophysiol* 1986;63:540–546.

58. Gilbert GJ. Transient global amnesia: manifestation of medial temporal lobe epilepsy. *Clin Electroencephalogr* 1978;9:147–152.

59. Gloor P. EEG characteristics in Creutzfeldt-Jakob disease [Letter]. *Ann Neurol* 1980;8:341.

60. Goate A, Chartier-Harlan MC, Mullan M, et al. Segregation of a missense mutation in the amyloid precursor protein gene with familial Alzheimer's disease. *Nature* 1991;349:704–706.

61. Gordon EB. Serial EEG studies in presenile dementia. *Br J Psychiatry* 1968;114:779–780.

62. Gordon EB, Sim M. The EEG in presenile dementia. *J Neurol Neurosurg Psychiatry* 1967;30:285–291.

63. Green J, Haycool WM. Electroencephalographic changes in parkinsonian patients treated with levodopa and levodopa-amantadine in combination. *Clin Electroencephalogr* 1971;2:28–34.

64. Green JB, Dickinson ES, Gunderman JR. Epilepsy in Huntington's chorea: clinical and neurophysiological studies. In: Barbeau A, Chase TN, Paulson GW, eds. *Huntington's chorea*. New York: Raven Press, 1973:105–114.

65. Greenberg JO, Shenkin HA, Adam R. Idiopathic normal pressure hydrocephalus—a report of 73 patients. *J Neurol Neurosurg Psychiatry* 1977;40:336–341.

66. Greene HH, Bennett DR. Transient global amnesia with a previously unreported EEG abnormality. *Electroencephalogr Clin Neurophysiol* 1974;36:409–413.

67. Groen JJ, Endtz LJ. Hereditary Pick's disease: second re-examination of a large family and discussion of other hereditary cases with particular reference to electroencephalography and computerized tomography. *Brain* 1982;105:443–459.

68. Gross RA, Spehlmann R, Daniels JC. Sleep disturbances in progressive supranuclear palsy. *Electroencephalogr Clin Neurophysiol* 1978;45:16–25.

69. Group HDCR. A novel gene containing a trinucleotide repeat that is expanded and unstable on Huntington's disease chromosomes. *Cell* 1993;72:971–983.

70. Guidotti M, Anzalone N, Morabito A, et al. A case control study of transient global amnesia. *J Neurol Neurosurg Psychiatry* 1989;52:320–323.

71. Hachinski VC, Lassen NA, Marshall J. Multi-infarct dementia, a cause of mental deterioration in the elderly. *Lancet* 1974;2:207–210.

72. Hallett M, Wilkins DE. Myoclonus in Alzheimer's disease and minipolymyoclonus. In: Fahn S, Marsden CD, Van Woert M, eds. *Myoclonus.* New York, Raven Press, 1986:399–405.

73. Harden CL, Daras M, Tuchman AJ, et al. Low amplitude EEGs in demented AIDS patients. *Electroencephalogr Clin Neurophysiol* 1993;87:54–56.

74. Harrison MJ, Thomas DJ, Du-Boulay GM, et al. Multi-infarct dementia. *J Neurol Sci* 1979;40:97–103.

75. Hashi K, Nishimura S, Kondo A, et al. The EEG in normal pressure hydrocephalus. *Acta Neurochir* 1976;33:23–35.

76. Hegerl U, Moller H-J. Electroencephalography as a diagnostic instrument in Alzheimer's disease: reviews and perspectives. *Int Psychogeriatr* 1997;9:237–246.

77. Helkala E-L, Laulumaa V, Soininen H, et al. Different pattern of cognitive decline related to normal or deteriorating EEG in three year follow-up study with patients of Alzheimer's disease. *Neurology* 1991;41:528–532.

78. Hier DB, Mangone CA, Ganellen R, et al. Quantitative measurement of delta activity in Alzheimer's disease. *Clin Electroencephalogr* 1991;22:178–182.

79. Hill D. Discussion of the electroencephalogram in organic cerebral disease. *Proc R Soc Med* 1948;41:242–248.

80. Hirano A, Kurland LT, Krooth RS, et al. Parkinsonism-dementia complex, an endemic disease on the island of Guam. I. Clinical features. *Brain* 1961;84:642–661.

81. Hodges JR, Warlow CP. The etiology of transient global amnesia: a case-control study of 114 cases with prospective follow-up. *Brain* 1990;113:639–657.

82. Hooijer C, Jonker C, Posthuma J, et al. Reliability, validity and follow-up of the EEG in senile dementia: sequelae of sequential measurement. *Electroencephalogr Clin Neurophysiol* 1990;76:400–412.

83. Hubbard O, Sunde D, Goldensohn ES. The EEG in centenarians. *Electroencephalogr Clin Neurophysiol* 1976;40:407–417.

84. Hughes JR, Cayaffa JJ. The EEG in patients at different ages without organic cerebral disease. *Electroencephalogr Clin Neurophysiol* 1977;42:776–784.

85. Jacobson S, Leuchter AF, Walter DO. Conventional and quantitative EEG in the diagnosis of delirium among the elderly. *J Neurol Neurosurg Psychiatry* 1993;56:153–158.

86. Jacome DE. EEG features in transient global amnesia. *Clin Electroencephalogr* 1989;20:183–192.

87. Jaffe R, Bender MB. EEG studies in the syndrome of isolated episodes of confusion with amnesia. *J Neurol Neurosurg Psychiatry* 1966;29:472–474.

88. Johannesson G, Brun A, Gustafson I, et al. EEG in presenile dementia related to cerebral blood flow and autopsy findings. *Acta Neurol Scand* 1977;56:89–103.

89. Johannesson G, Hagberg B, Gustafson L, et al. EEG and cognitive impairment in presenile dementia. *Acta Neurol Scand* 1979;59:225–240.

90. Jonkman EJ. The role of the electroencephalogram in the diagnosis of dementia of the Alzheimer type: an attempt at technology assessment. *Neurophysiol Clin* 1997;27:211–219.

91. Jonkman EJ, Ponsen L. A review of Creutzfeldt-Jakob disease. *J Electrophysiol Technol* 1981;7:68–79.

92. Kaszniak AW, Fox J, Gandell DL, et al. Predictors of mortality in presenile and senile dementia. *Ann Neurol* 1978;3:246–252.

93. Katz RI, Horowitz GR. Electroencephalogram in the septuagenarian: studies in a normal geriatric population. *J Am Geriatr Soc* 1982;3:273–275.

94. Katz RI, Horowitz GR. Sleep-onset frontal rhythmic slowing in a normal geriatric population. *Electroencephalogr Clin Neurophysiol* 1983;56:27P(abst).

95. Klass DW, Brenner RP. EEG of the elderly. *J Clin Neurophysiol* 1995;12:116–131.

96. Koponen H, Partanen J, Paakkonen A, et al. EEG spectral analysis in delirium. *J Neurol Neurosurg Psychiatry* 1989;52:980–985.

97. Koralnik IJ, Beaumanoir A, Hausler R, et al. A controlled study of early neurologic abnormalities in men with asymptomatic human immunodeficiency virus infection. *N Engl J Med* 1990;323:864–870.

98. Krauss GL, Niedermeyer E. Electroencephalogram and seizures in chronic alcoholism. *Electroencephalogr Clin Neurophysiol* 1991;78:97–104.

99. Kushner MJ, Hauser WA. Transient global amnesia: a case-controlled study. *Ann Neurol* 1985;18:684–691.

100. Kuzuhara S, Kanazawa I, Sasaki H, et al. Gerstmann-Straussler-Scheinker's disease. *Ann Neurol* 1983;14:216–225.

101. Letemendia F, Pampiglione G. Clinical and EEG observation in Alzheimer's disease. *J Neurol Neurosurg Psychiatry* 1958;21:167–172.

102. Leuchter AF, Newton TF, Cook IA, et al. Changes in brain functional connectivity in Alzheimer-type and multi-infarct dementia. *Brain* 1992;115:1543–1561.

103. Leuchter AF, Spar JE, Walter DO, et al. Electroencephalographic spectra and coherence in the diagnosis of Alzheimer's-type and multi-infarct dementia. *Arch Gen Psychiatry* 1987;44:993–998.

104. Leuchter AF, Walter DO. Diagnosis and assessment of dementia using functional brain imaging. *Int Psychogeriatr* 1989;1:63–71.

105. Levy SR, Chiappa KH, Burke CJ, et al. Early evolution and incidence of electroencephalographic abnormalities in Creutzfeldt-Jakob disease. *J Clin Neurophysiol* 1986;3:1–21.

106. Liddell DW. Investigation of EEG findings in presenile dementia. *J Neurol Neurosurg Psychiatry* 1958;21:173–176.

107. Lopez OL, Becker JT, Brenner RP, et al. Alzheimer's disease with delusions and hallucinations: neuropsychological and electroencephalographic correlates. *Neurology* 1991;41:906–912.

108. Lopez OL, Brenner RP, Becker JT, et al. EEG spectral abnormalities and psychosis as predic-

tors of cognitive and functional decline in probable Alzheimer's disease. *Neurology* 1997;48:1521–1525.

109. Lou HOC. Repeated episodes of transient global amnesia. *Acta Neurol Scand* 1968;44:612–618.

110. MacPherson A. Convulsive seizures and electroencephalographic changes in the patients during levo-dopa therapy. *Neurology* 1970;12[Suppl 2]:41–45.

111. Maher ER, Lees AJ. The clinical features and natural history of Steele-Richardson-Olszowski syndrome (progressive supranuclear palsy). *Neurology* 1986;36:1005–1008.

112. Margerison JH, Scott DF. Huntington's chorea: clinical EEG and neuropathological findings. *Electroencephalogr Clin Neurophysiol* 1965;19:314(abst).

113. Markand ON. Electroencephalography in diffuse encephalopathies. *J Clin Neurophysiol* 1984;1:357–407.

114. Markand ON. EEG in the diagnosis of CNS infections. In: Roos KL, ed. *Central nervous system infectious diseases and therapy*. New York: Marcel Dekker, 1997:667–689.

115. Marsden CD, Harrison MJG. Outcome of investigation of patients with presenile dementia. *Br Med J* 1972;2:249–252.

116. Martin WE, Loewenson RB, Resch JA, et al. Parkinson's disease: clinical analysis of 100 patients. *Neurology* 1973;23:783–790.

117. Masters CL, Harris JO, Gajdusek DC, et al. Creutzfeldt-Jakob disease: patterns of worldwide occurrence and the significance of familial and sporadic clustering. *Ann Neurol* 1979;5:177–188.

118. Melo TP, Ferro JM, Ferro H. Transient global amnesia: a case control study. *Brain* 1992;115:261–270.

119. Mendez MF, Mastri AR, Sung JH, et al. Clinically diagnosed Alzheimer's disease: neuropathological findings in 650 cases. *Alzheimer Dis Assoc Disord* 1992;6:35–43.

120. Meo R, Bilo L, Striano S, et al. Transient global amnesia of epileptic origin accompanied by fever. *Seizure* 1995;4:311–317.

121. Merskey H, Ball MJ, Blume WT, et al. Relationships between psychological measurements and cerebral organic changes in Alzheimer's disease. *Can J Neurol Sci* 1980;7:45–49.

122. Miller JW, Yanagihara T, Petersen RC, et al. Transient global amnesia and epilepsy. *Arch Neurol* 1987;44:629–633.

123. Miyauchi T, Hagimoto H, Ishii M, et al. Quantitative EEG in patients with presenile and senile dementia of the Alzheimer type. *Acta Neurol Scand* 1994;89:56–64.

124. Montplaisir J, Petit D, Decary A, et al. Sleep and quantitative EEG in patients with progressive supranuclear palsy. *Neurology* 1997;49:999–1003.

125. Muller HF, Kral VA. The electroencephalogram in advanced senile dementia. *J Am Geriatr Soc* 1967;15:415–426.

126. Muller HF, Schwartz G. Electroencephalograms and autopsy findings in geropsychiatry. *J Gerontol* 1978;33:504–513.

127. Munoz-Garcia D, Ludwin SK. Classic and generalized variants of Pick's disease: a clinicopathological, ultrastructural and immunocytochemical comparative study. *Ann Neurol* 1984;16:467–480.

128. Neary D, Snowden JS, Mann DMA, et al. Clinical and neuropathological criteria for frontotemporal dementia. *J Neurol Neurosurg Psychiatry* 1994;57:416–418.

129. Neufeld MY. Periodic triphasic waves in levodopa-induced encephalopathy. *Neurology* 1992;42:444–446.

130. Neufeld MY, Blumen S, Aitkin I, et al. EEG frequency analysis in demented and nondemented parkinsonian patients. *Dementia* 1994;5:23–28.

131. Neufeld MY, Inzelberg R, Korczyn AD. EEG in demented and nondemented parkinsonian patients. *Acta Neurol Scand* 1988;78:1–5.

132. Newton TF, Leuchter AF, Miller EN, et al. Quantitative EEG in patients with AIDS and asymptomatic HIV infection. *Clin Electroencephalogr* 1994;25:18–25.

133. Nilsson BY, Olsson Y, Sourander P. Electroencephalographic and histopathological changes

resembling Jakob-Creutzfeldt disease after transient cerebral ischemia due to cardiac arrest. *Acta Neurol Scand* 1972;48:416–426.

134. Nuwer MR. Quantitative EEG analysis in clinical settings. *Brain Topogr* 1996;8:201–208.
135. Nuwer MR. Assessment of digital EEG, quantitative EEG, and EEG brain mapping: report of the American Academy of Neurology and the American Clinical Neurophysiology Society. *Neurology* 1997;49:277–292.
136. Nuwer MR, Miller EN, Visscher BR, et al. Asymptomatic HIV infection does not cause EEG abnormalities: results from the Multicenter AIDS Cohort Study (MACS). *Neurology* 1992;42: 1214–1219.
137. Obrecht R, Okhomina FOA, Scott DF. Value of EEG in the acute confusional states. *J Neurol Neurosurg Psychiatry* 1979;42:75–77.
138. Obrist WD. The electroencephalogram of normal aged adults. *Electroencephalogr Clin Neurophysiol* 1954;6:235–244.
139. Obrist WD. EEG and intellectual function in the aged. *Electroencephalogr Clin Neurophysiol* 1972;33:253(abst).
140. Obrist WD, Busse EW, Eisdorfer C, et al. Relation of the electroencephalogram to intellectual function in senescence. *J Gerontol* 1962;17:197–206.
141. Oken BS, Kaye JA. Electrophysiologic function in the healthy, extremely old. *Neurology* 1992; 42:519–526.
142. Oltman JE, Friedman S. Comments on Huntington's chorea. *J Med Genet* 1961;3:298–314.
143. Otomo E. Electroencephalography in old age: dominant alpha pattern. *Electroencephalogr Clin Neurophysiol* 1966;21:489–491.
144. Parisi A, Di Perri G, Strosselli M, et al. Usefulness of computerized electroencephalography in diagnosing, staging and monitoring AIDS-dementia complex. *AIDS* 1989;3:209–213.
145. Parisi A, Strosselli M, Di Perri G, et al. Electroencephalography in the early diagnosis of HIV-related subacute encephalitis: analysis of 185 patients. *Clin Electroencephalogr* 1989; 20:1–5.
146. Patterson RM, Bagchi BK, Test A. The prediction of Huntington's chorea. *Am J Psychiatry* 1948;104:786–797.
147. Paulsen JS, Butters N, Sadek JR, et al. Distinctive cognitive profiles of cortical and subcortical dementia in advanced illness. *Neurology* 1995;45:951–956.
148. Pedley TA, Miller JA. Clinical neurophysiology of aging and dementia. *Adv Neurol* 1983;38: 31–49.
149. Penttila M, Partanen JV, Soininen H, et al. Quantitative analysis of EEG in different stages of Alzheimer's disease. *Electroencephalogr Clin Neurophysiol* 1985;60:1–6.
150. Pericak-Vance MA, Bebout JL, Gaskell PC, et al. Linkage studies in familial Alzheimer's disease: evidence for chromosome 19 linkage. *Am J Hum Genet* 1991;48:1034–1050.
151. Peterson RC, Mokri B, Laws ER Jr. Surgical treatment of idiopathic hydrocephalus in elderly patients. *Neurology* 1985;35:307–311.
152. Petito CK. What causes brain atrophy in human immunodeficiency virus infection? *Ann Neurol* 1993;34:128–129.
153. Pollock M, Hornabrook RW. The prevalence, natural history and dementia in Parkinson's disease. *Brain* 1966;89:429–448.
154. Primavera A, Norello P, Finocchi C, et al. Correlation between mini-mental state examination and quantitative electroencephalography in senile dementia of the Alzheimer's type. *Neuropsychobiology* 1990;23:74–78.
155. Primavera A, Traverso F. Triphasic waves in Alzheimer's disease. *Acta Neurol Belg* 1990;90: 274–281.
156. Prinz PN, Peskind E, Vitaliano PP, et al. Changes in the sleep and waking EEGs of nondemented and demented elderly subjects. *J Am Geriatr Soc* 1982;30:86–93.
157. Prinz PN, Vitaliano PP, Vitiello MV, et al. Sleep, EEG and mental function changes in senile of the Alzheimer's type. *Neurobiol Aging* 1983;3:361–370.
158. Pritchard WS, Duke DW, Coburn KL, et al. EEG-based, neural-net predictive classification of Alzheimer's disease versus control subjects is augmented by non-linear EEG measures. *Electroencephalogr Clin Neurophysiol* 1994;91:118–130.
159. Pro JD, Wells CE. The use of electroencephalogram in the diagnosis of delirium. *Dis Nerv Syst* 1977;38:804–808.
160. Prusiner SB, Hsiao KK. Human prion diseases. *Ann Neurol* 1994;35:385–395.
161. Rae-Grant A, Blume W, Lau C, et al. The electroencephalogram in Alzheimer-type dementia: a sequential study correlating the electroencephalogram with psychometric and quantitative pathologic data. *Arch Neurol* 1987;44:50–54.
162. Reynolds CF, Kupfer DJ, Taska LS, et al. EEG sleep in elderly depressed, demented and healthy subjects. *Biol Psychiatry* 1985;20:431–442.
163. Reynolds CF, Spiker DG, Hanin I, et al. EEG, sleep, aging, and psychopathology: new data and state of the art. *Biol Psychiatry* 1983;18:139–155.
164. Roberts MA, McGeorge AP, Caird FI. Electroencephalography and computerized tomography in vascular and nonvascular dementia in old age. *J Neurol Neurosurg Psychiatry* 1978;41: 903–906.
165. Robinson D, Merskey H, Blume W, et al. Electroencephalography as an aid in the exclusion of Alzheimer's disease. *Arch Neurol* 1994;51:280–284.
166. Rocca WA, Amaducci LA, Schoenberg BS. Epidemiology of clinically diagnosed Alzheimer's disease. *Ann Neurol* 1986;19:415–424.
167. Rodriguez G, Nobil F, Arrigo A, et al. Prognostic significance of quantitative electroencephalography in Alzheimer patients: preliminary observations. *Electroencephalogr Clin Neurophysiol* 1996;99:123–128.
168. Romano J, Engel GL. Delirium. I. Electroencephalographic data. *Arch Neurol Psychiatry* 1944;51:356–377.
169. Rosen I. Electroencephalography as a diagnostic tool in dementia. *Dement Geriatr Cogn Disorder* 1997;8:110–116.
170. Rowan AJ, Protass LM. Transient global amnesia: clinical and electroencephalographic findings in 10 cases. *Neurology* 1979;29:869–872.
171. Saunders AM, Strittmatter WJ, Schmechel D, et al. Association of apolipoprotein E allele epsilon 4 with late onset familial and sporadic Alzheimer's disease. *Neurology* 1993;43:1467–1472.
172. Schaul N, Lueders H, Sachdev K. Generalized, bilaterally synchronous bursts of slow waves in the EEG. *Arch Neurol* 1981;38:690–692.
173. Schellenberg GD, Bird TD, Wijsman EM, et al. Genetic linkage evidence for a familial Alzheimer's disease locus on chromosome 14. *Science* 1992;258:668–671.
174. Schreiter-Gasser U, Gasser T, Ziegler P. Quantitative EEG analysis in early onset Alzheimer's disease: a controlled study. *Electroencephalogr Clin Neurophysiol* 1993;86:15–22.
175. Schreiter-Gasser U, Gasser T, Ziegler P. Quantitative EEG analysis in early onset Alzheimer's disease: correlations with severity, clinical characteristics, visual EEG and CCT. *Electroencephalogr Clin Neurophysiol* 1994;90:267–272.
176. Scott DF, Heathfield KWG, Toone B, et al. The EEG in Huntington's chorea: a clinical and neuropathological study. *J Neurol Neurosurg Psychiatry* 1972;35:97–102.
177. Sirakov AA, Mezan IS. EEG findings in parkinsonism. *Electroencephalogr Clin Neurophysiol* 1963;15:321–322.
178. Sishta SK, Troupe A, Marszalek KS, et al. Huntington's chorea: an electroencephalographic and psychometric study. *Electroencephalogr Clin Neurophysiol* 1974;36:387–393.
179. Sloan EP, Fenton GW. EEG power spectra and cognitive change in geriatric psychiatry: a longitudinal study. *Electroencephalogr Clin Neurophysiol* 1993;86:361–367.
180. Smith JS, Kilow LG. The investigation of dementia: results of 200 consecutive admissions. *Lancet* 1981;1:824–827.
181. Soikkeli R, Partanen J, Soininen H, et al. Slowing of EEG in Parkinson's disease. *Electroencephalogr Clin Neurophysiol* 1991;79:159–165.
182. Soininen H, Partanen JV. Quantitative EEG in the diagnosis and follow-up of Alzheimer's disease. In: Giannitrapani D, Murri L, eds. *The EEG of mental activities*. Basel: Karger, 1988:42–49.

183. Soininen H, Partanen JV, Helkola EL, et al. EEG findings in senile dementia and normal aging. *Acta Neurol Scand* 1982;65:59–70.

184. Soininen H, Partanen J, Laulumaa V, et al. Longitudinal EEG spectral analysis in early stages of Alzheimer's disease. *Electroencephalogr Clin Neurophysiol* 1989;72:290–297.

185. Soininen H, Riekkinen PJ. EEG in diagnostics and follow-up of Alzheimer's disease. *Acta Neurol Scand* 1992;139[Suppl]:36–39.

186. Spehr W, Stemmler G. Post-alcoholic diseases: diagnostic relevance of computerized EEG. *Electroencephalogr Clin Neurophysiol* 1985;60:106–114.

187. Steele JC, Richardson JC, Olszewski J. Progressive supranuclear palsy. *Arch Neurol* 1964;10:333–359.

188. Stefoski D, Bergen D, Fox J, et al. Correlation between diffuse EEG abnormalities and cerebral atrophy in senile dementia. *J Neurol Neurosurg Psychiatry* 1976;39:751–755.

189. Steinmetz EF, Vroom FQ. Transient global amnesia. *Neurology* 1972;22:1193–1200.

190. Stigsby B, Johannesson G, Ingvar DH. Regional EEG analysis and regional cerebral blood flow in Alzheimer's and Pick's diseases. *Electroencephalogr Clin Neurophysiol* 1981;51:537–547.

191. Streletz LJ, Reyes PF, Zalewska M, et al. Computer analysis of EEG activity in dementia of the Alzheimer's type and Huntington's disease. *Neurobiol Aging* 1990;11:15–20.

192. Strijers RLM, Scheltens PH, Jonkman EJ, et al. Diagnosing Alzheimer's disease in community-dwelling elderly: a comparison of EEG and MRI. *Dement Geriatr Cogn Disord* 1997;8:198–202.

193. Strittmatter WJ, Saunders AM, Schmechel D, et al. Apolipoprotein E: high affinity binding to βA amyloid and increased frequency of type A allele in familial Alzheimer's. *Proc Natl Acad Sci U S A* 1993;90:1977–1981.

194. Su P, Goldensohn ES. Progressive supranuclear palsy: electroencephalographic studies. *Arch Neurol* 1973;29:183–186.

195. Sulkova R, Haltia M, Paetau A, et al. Accuracy of clinical diagnosis in primary degenerative dementia: correlation with neuropathological findings. *J Neurol Neurosurg Psychiatry* 1983;46:9–13.

196. Tassinari CA, Ciarmatori C, Alesi C, et al. Transient global amnesia as a postictal state from recurrent partial seizures. *Epilepsia* 1991;32:882–885.

197. Terry RD. Dementia, a brief and selective review. *Arch Neurol* 1976;33:1–4.

198. Terry RD, Katzman R. Senile dementia of the Alzheimer type. *Ann Neurol* 1983;14:497–506.

199. Tharp BR. The electroencephalogram in transient global amnesia. *Electroencephalogr Clin Neurophysiol* 1969;26:96–99.

200. Thomas P, Borg M. Reversible myoclonic encephalopathy revealing the AIDS-dementia complex. *Electroencephalogr Clin Neurophysiol* 1994;90:166–169.

201. Tietjen GE, Drury I. Familial Creutzfeldt-Jakob disease without periodic EEG activity. *Ann Neurol* 1990;28:585–588.

202. Tinuper P, DeCarolis P, Galeotti M, et al. Electroencephalogram and HIV infection: a prospective study in 100 patients. *Clin Electroencephalogr* 1990;21:145–150.

203. Tissot R, Constantinidis J, Richard J. *La maladie de Pick*. Paris: Masson, 1975:80–81,84–85.

204. Tomlinson BE, Blessed G, Ruth M. Observations on the brains of demented old people. *J Neurol Sci* 1970;11:205–242.

205. Torres F, Faoro A, Loewenson R, et al. The electroencephalogram of elderly subjects revisited. *Electroencephalogr Clin Neurophysiol* 1983;56:391–398.

206. Traub RD, Pedley TA. Virus induced electronic coupling hypothesis of the mechanism of periodic EEG discharges in Creutzfeldt-Jakob disease. *Ann Neurol* 1981;10:405–410.

207. Victor M, Adams RD, Collins GH. The Wernicke-Korsakoff syndrome. In: *Contemporary neurology series*, Vol 7. Philadelphia: FA Davis, 1971:72.

208. Visser SL, Hooijer C, Jonker C, et al. Anterior temporal focal abnormalities in EEG in normal aged subjects: correlations with psychological and CT brain scan findings. *Electroencephalogr Clin Neurophysiol* 1987;66:1–7.

209. Visser SL, Van-Tilburg W, Hooijer C, et al. Visual evoked potentials in senile dementia (Alzheimer type) and in non-organic behavioral disorder in the elderly: comparison with EEG parameters. *Electroencephalogr Clin Neurophysiol* 1985;60:115–121.

210. Vogel CM, Drury I, Terry LC, et al. Myoclonus in adult Huntington's disease. *Ann Neurol* 1991;29:213–215.

211. Wade JPH, Mirsen TR, Hachinski VC, et al. The clinical diagnosis of Alzheimer's disease. *Arch Neurol* 1987;44:24–29.

212. Wang HS, Busse EW. EEG of healthy old persons—a longitudinal study. I. Dominant background activity and occipital rhythm. *J Gerontol* 1969;24:419–426.

213. Watson CP. Clinical similarity of Alzheimer's and Creutzfeldt-Jakob disease. *Ann Neurol* 1979;6:368–369.

214. White JC. Periodic EEG activity in subcortical arteriosclerotic encephalopathy (Binswanger's type). *Arch Neurol* 1979;36:485–489.

215. Whitehouse PJ. The concept of subcortical and cortical dementia: another look. *Ann Neurol* 1986;19:1–6.

216. Wood JH, Barlet D, James AE, et al. Normal pressure hydrocephalus: diagnosis and patient selection for shunt surgery. *Neurology (Minneap)* 1974;24:517–526.

217. Yeager CL, Alberts WW, Delattree LD. Effects of stereotaxic surgery upon electroencephalographic status of Parkinson's patients. *Neurology* 1966;16:904–910.

218. Yener GG, Leuchter AF, Jenden D, et al. Quantitative EEG in frontotemporal dementia. *Clin Electroencephalogr* 1966;27:61–68.

219. Zochodne DW, Young GB, McLachlan RS, et al. Creutzfeldt-Jakob disease without periodic sharp wave complexes: a clinical, electroencephalographic and pathologic study. *Neurology* 1988;38:1056–1060.

Chapter 14

Electrophysiological Evaluation of Coma, Other States of Diminished Responsiveness, and Brain Death

Gian-Emilio Chatrian and Giorgio S. Turella

ELECTROPHYSIOLOGICAL EVALUATION OF COMA: ASSOCIATED ELECTROENCEPHALOGRAPHIC PATTERNS

Early work considered bilateral high-voltage slow waves to be the electroencephalographic (EEG) manifestations of coma, which, in turn, was regarded as equivalent to deep sleep (114,178). However, it was soon realized that, as coma deepened, the EEG commonly underwent changes that were different from those of sleep and were associated with increasingly altered and ultimately abolished effects of external stimuli ("EEG reactivity") (159). Distinct EEG patterns were also identified in comatose patients that included "triphasic waves" (TWs) (45), alpha rhythms commonly associated with wakefulness (297), other patterns of alpha frequency (474), and spindles and other waveforms characteristically seen in various stages of normal sleep (86). Special efforts were made and are still in progress to determine the relations between EEG patterns and reactivity and other variables, including etiology and duration of coma and other unresponsive states, underlying pathological lesions, and clinical outcome.

EEG patterns displayed by comatose patients are not unchanging and mutually exclusive features, but instead often transiently express mutable pathological influences. They may also evolve into one another during successive examinations or may occur in the same recording (159). Thus the description of distinct EEG patterns that follows is at least partly artificial and primarily serves descriptive purposes.

Among the EEG patterns variably associated with comatose states, the following deserve special consideration: intermittent rhythmic delta activity (IRDA); alternating pattern; continuous high-voltage delta activity; pseudo-periodic patterns; interictal and ictal epileptic discharges; low-voltage, slow, unreactive EEG; unilateral, lateralized, or focal abnormalities; TWs; sleep patterns; and rhythms of alpha frequency.

Intermittent Rhythmic Delta Activity

IRDA may appear in early stages of coma simultaneously with or after disorganization or loss of alpha rhythm and development of scattered theta and delta waves. IRDA (Fig. 14.1) consists of bursts of high-voltage, regular,

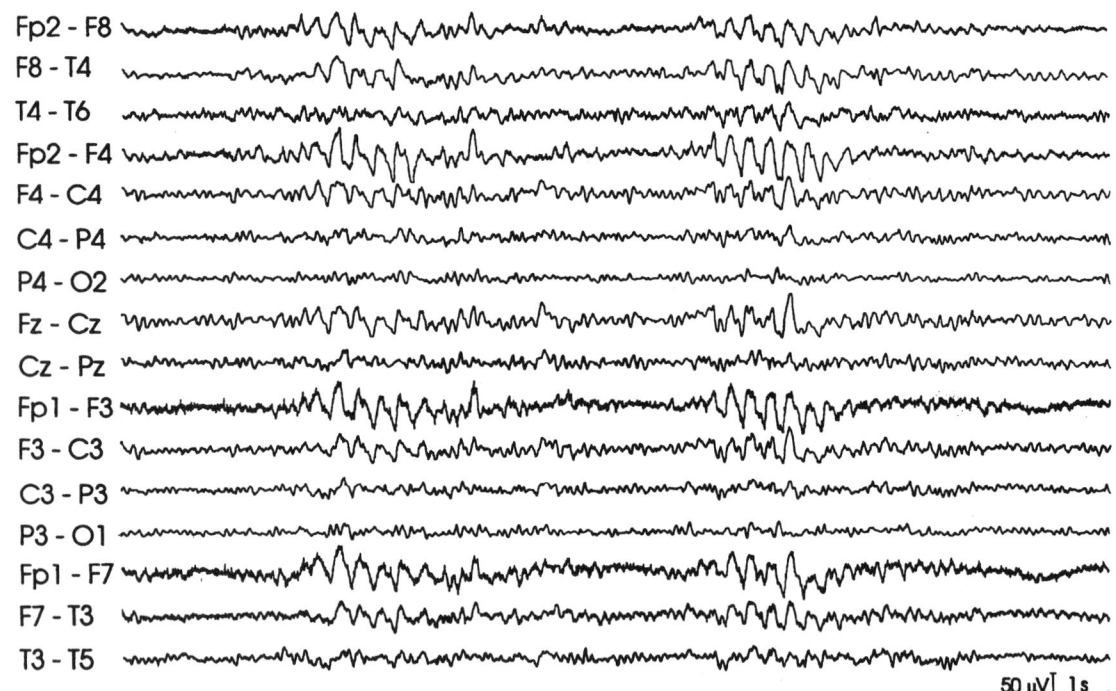

50 µV ⌐ 1s ⌐

FIG. 14.1. Bursts of high-voltage bilaterally synchronous frontal intermittent rhythmic delta activity in a 41-year-old lethargic patient with uremic encephalopathy. (From Chatrian G-E. Electrophysiological evaluation of brain death: a critical appraisal. In: Aminoff MJ, ed. *Electrodiagnosis in clinical neurology.* New York: Churchill Livingstone, 1980:525–588, with permission.)

quasi-sinusoidal waves, mostly at 2–3 Hz. Bursts may be bilateral or unilateral. When bilateral, they are typically synchronous but may be either symmetrical or asymmetrical (148). IRDA is characteristically most prominent over the frontal regions in adults but over occipital areas in children. Bursts may be blocked by eye opening. Some alteration of consciousness is especially common with bilateral, fairly persistent IRDA. This pattern occurs in a wide variety of conditions, including (a) supratentorial hemispheric or midline lesions (113,148,221), with increased pressure within the third ventricle (113,221); (b) toxic or metabolic encephalopathies (213); and (c) widespread structural brain disease predominantly involving both subcortical and cortical gray matter (183). It is commonly believed that IRDA is an expression of abnormal interactions between cortical and subcortical (thalamic) neuronal systems (181,403). Why IRDA generally prevails over the frontal areas in adults and over the occipital regions in children is unclear.

Alternating Pattern

The alternating pattern consists of alternating periods of high-voltage, widespread delta activity and lower voltage irregular potentials. These two EEG features are accompanied by characteristic autonomic and muscular changes (20,141,159). Noxious and other stimuli delivered during periods of low-voltage activity tend to be followed by high-voltage delta waves, whereas the opposite often occurs with excitations delivered in the presence of high-voltage delta activity (20,159). According to some (141), reactivity of this pattern to noxious and other excitations tends to be associated with favorable clinical outcome.

Continuous High-Voltage Delta Activity

In many comatose states there is continuous or nearly continuous high-voltage, mostly arrhythmic, 1- to 2-Hz activity over all head regions (114,178) (Fig. 14.2). In early stages of coma, this activity may be attenuated by external stimuli, but more commonly it is unaffected. Reactivity to noxious and other stimuli generally is lost in deeper stages of coma (293,414). This pattern tends to be associated with an unfavorable clinical outcome (141). Widespread continuous delta activity is common in patients with encephalopathies caused by structural lesions primarily involving subcortical white matter (183), and localized delta activity appears in the cor-

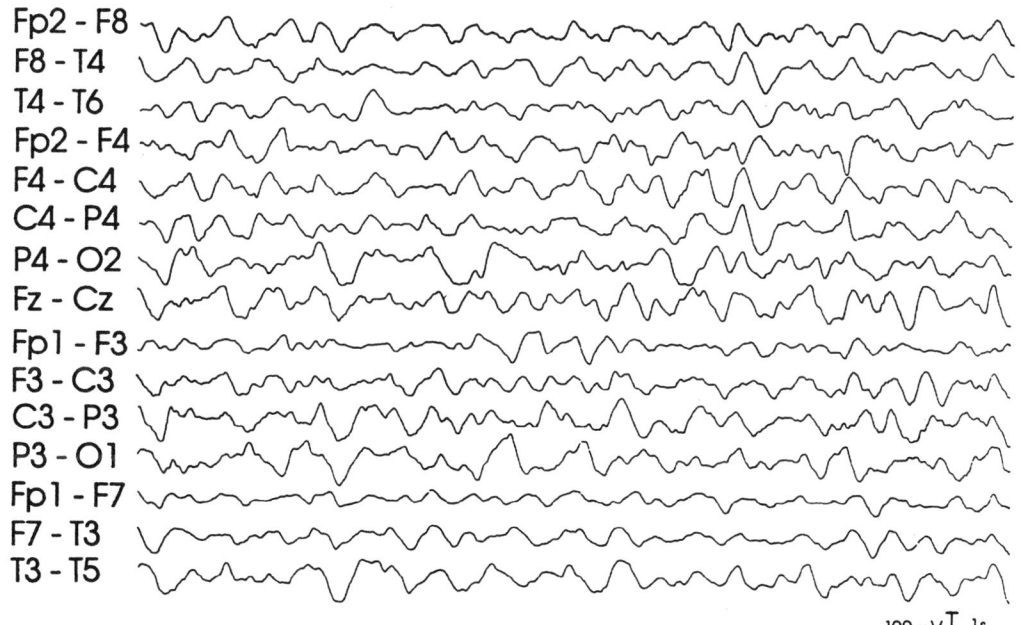

100 µV | 1s

FIG. 14.2. Widespread high-voltage arrhythmic delta activity in a 36-year-old man 13 hours after head injury sustained in a motor vehicle accident. The patient was deeply comatose and artificially ventilated, with midposition fixed pupils, poor oculocephalic and caloric responses, and bilateral extensor posturing with noxious stimulation. He died 5 days later. (From Chatrian G-E. Electrophysiological evaluation of brain death: a critical appraisal. In: Aminoff MJ, ed. *Electrodiagnosis in clinical neurology.* New York: Churchill Livingstone, 1980:525–588, with permission.).

tex overlying a circumscribed white matter lesion in animals (182). Thus it has been suggested that cortical deafferentation may play a major role in generating continuous widespread delta activity in comatose individuals (182,403).

Pseudoperiodic Patterns

Some comatose patients display bilateral widespread pseudoperiodic patterns in their EEGs. These include burst-suppression and periodic generalized epileptiform discharges.

Burst-suppression (Fig. 14.3) consists of somewhat stereotyped bursts of bilaterally synchronous, widespread high-voltage delta and theta waves with or without intermixed spikes and sharp waves. These bursts are separated by intervals during which the EEG shows no activity discernible at usual instrumental sensitivities or low-voltage potentials of delta and theta frequency. Interburst intervals commonly last from 2 to 10 seconds, although durations of several minutes or longer are occasionally observed. Myoclonic jerks

may occur during bursts (257,299,384) or without consistent relationships to them. Clinical conditions most commonly producing coma with EEG burst-suppression include (a) acute intoxication with drugs depressing central nervous system (CNS) function (48,206,252,311,441,489); (b) severe anoxic encephalopathies (223,281,283,365,377,384,415) (Fig. 14.3); (c) severe hypothermia (361); and (d) anesthesia produced by various agents (237,248,317,381,508).

Pseudoperiodic generalized epileptiform discharges (PGEDs) (Fig. 14.4) consist of spikes, multiple spikes, or sharp waves occurring bilaterally synchronously over all head regions, generally at 0.5–1 Hz, with intervening periods of apparent inactivity or low-voltage slow activity. Bilateral myoclonic jerks are often present and show close, variable, or no apparent gross temporal relations to the EEG discharges. PGEDs occur most commonly in comatose patients following acute, severe cerebral anoxia (235,308,365,449) and in Creutzfeldt-Jakob disease (1,53,99,291,324), although they may be absent in the terminal stages of the latter condition when consciousness is most impaired. They have also been reported in metabolic and toxic encepha-

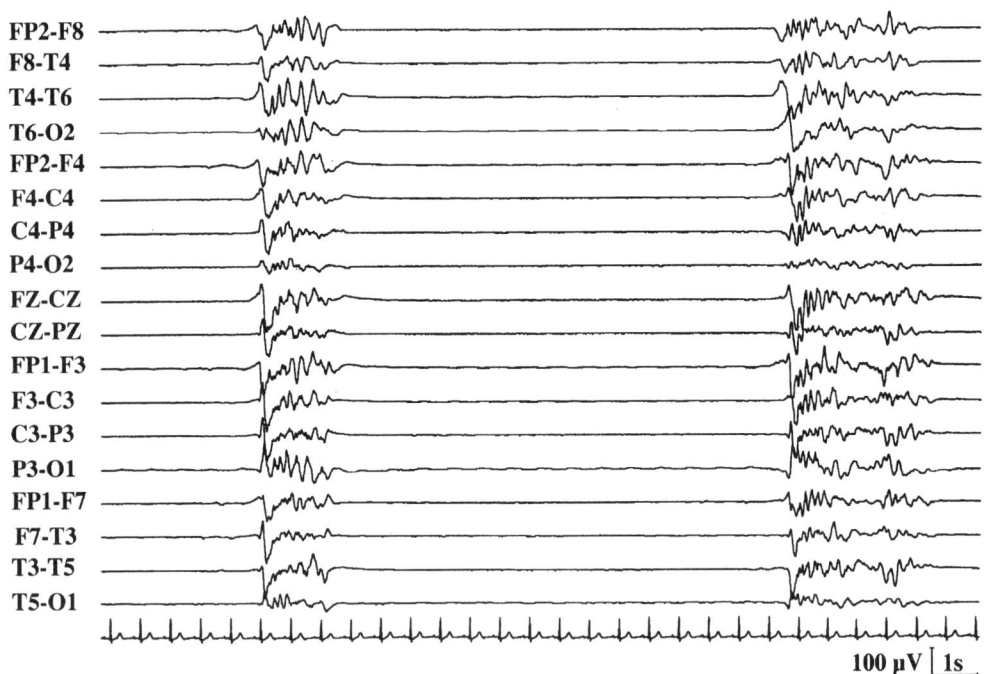

FIG. 14.3. Burst-suppression pattern in a 73-year-old woman 24 hours after a 20-minute cardiac arrest. The patient was comatose, artificially ventilated, and given pancuronium bromide to suppress bilateral myoclonic jerks associated with the bursts. Death occurred 72 hours later. Same patient as in Figure 14.6.

100 µV   1s

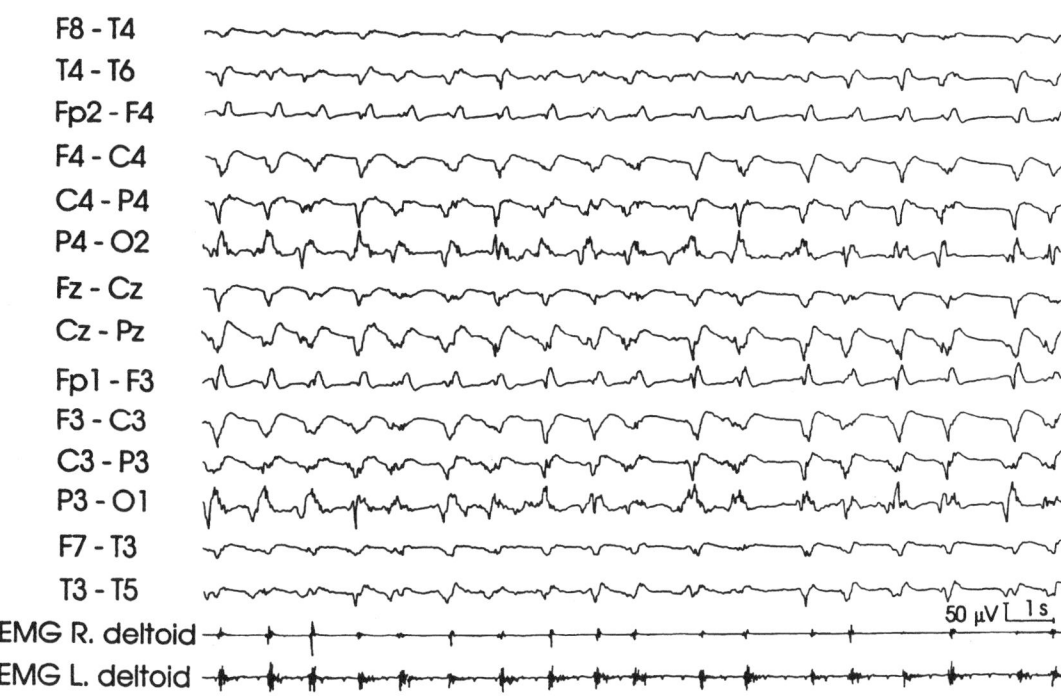

F8 - T4
T4 - T6
Fp2 - F4
F4 - C4
C4 - P4
P4 - O2
Fz - Cz
Cz - Pz
Fp1 - F3
F3 - C3
C3 - P3
P3 - O1
F7 - T3
T3 - T5
EMG R. deltoid
EMG L. deltoid

50 µV ⌐ 1 s.

FIG. 14.4. Pseudoperiodic generalized sharp waves and spikes repeating at 1–1.5 Hz. EEG discharges show gross temporal relationships to muscular jerks involving the chin and both shoulders. This 66-year-old man was comatose as a result of alcoholic liver disease with cirrhosis complicated by bowel infarction, recent bowel resection, and respiratory alkalosis. He died 12 days later. (From Chatrian G-E. Electrophysiological evaluation of brain death: a critical appraisal. In: Aminoff MJ, ed. *Electrodiagnosis in clinical neurology.* New York: Churchill Livingstone, 1980:525–588, with permission.)

lopathies such as those induced by lithium (419) and baclofen (147,226). Some authors (235) categorize atypical TWs associated with toxic-metabolic encephalopathies as PGEDs, although this pattern has no clearly established relation to epilepsy. Occasionally, patients comatose from acute anoxia display unremitting bilaterally synchronous spike-and–slow wave complexes occurring rhythmically at 2–3.5 Hz (37,69,299,417) (Fig. 14.5).

Most comatose patients with postanoxic burst-suppression pattern or PGEDs die, but a few survive, generally with major neurological disabilities (223,257,365,377,495,512). In contrast, a substantial number of individuals with burst-suppression caused by drug intoxication recover, often without neurological sequelae (48,311,439). Characteristically, as a patient's condition worsens, bursts become shorter, simpler in form, and lower in voltage, and periods of suppression become longer until electrocerebral inactivity (ECI) supervenes. In contrast, shortened suppression intervals, prolonged bursts, and gradual reappearance of physiological rhythms characterize clinical recovery.

Intracellular recordings during burst-suppression produced by anesthetic agents in cats have demonstrated the occurrence of a characteristic sequence of phasic depolarization of cortical neurons associated with the EEG burst and sustained hyperpolarization of the same elements associated with the interburst interval. Simultaneous recordings from thalamic neurons suggested that thalamic networks might trigger the recurrent EEG bursts (432). However, cortical slabs isolated from all subcortical (as well as cortical) connections characteristically display burst-suppression in both animals and humans (138,217). Evidence has been produced that the mechanisms underlying postanoxic burst-suppression might differ in some respect from those operating in drug-induced burst-suppression (44). Subcortically triggered cortical excitatory events alternating with prolonged inhibitory events have also been postulated by some to account for the PGEDs occurring following cerebral anoxia and in Creutzfeldt-Jakob disease (54,72,183,432). Other investigators have hypothesized that, in Creutzfeldt-Jakob disease, fusion of neuronal processes, particularly dendrites, may lead to abnormal electro-

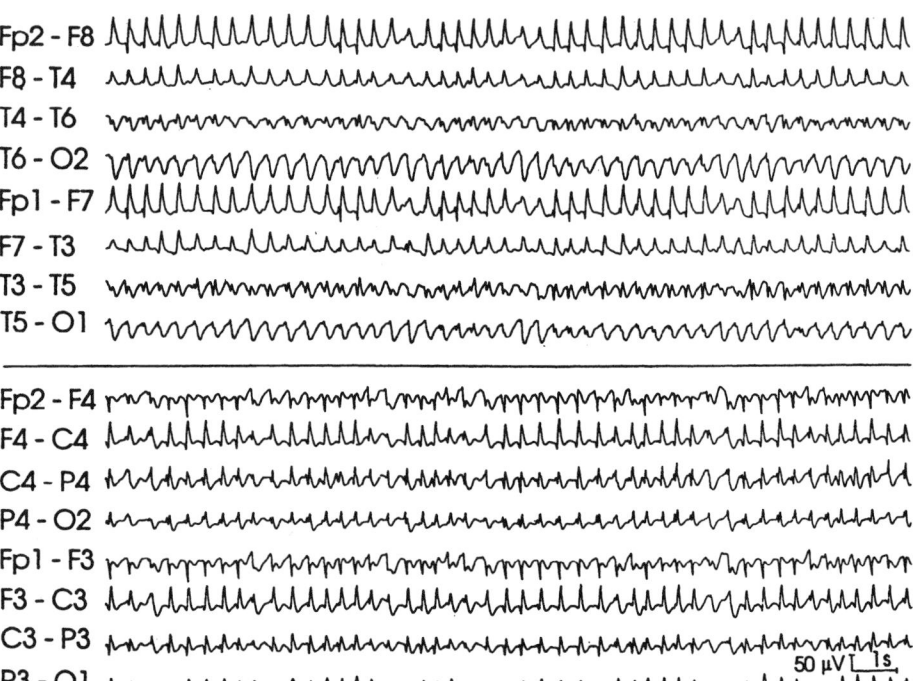

Fp2 - F8
F8 - T4
T4 - T6
T6 - O2
Fp1 - F7
F7 - T3
T3 - T5
T5 - O1

Fp2 - F4
F4 - C4
C4 - P4
P4 - O2
Fp1 - F3
F3 - C3
C3 - P3
P3 - O1

50 µV | 1s

FIG. 14.5. Unremitting generalized 2.5- to 3-Hz spike-and–slow wave complexes in a 78-year-old man. Following a cardiac arrest resulting from myocardial infarction, he was comatose with midposition pupils sluggishly reactive to light, had faint corneal and absent oculocephalic reflexes, and demonstrated intermittent fluttering of the eyelids. Noxious stimuli elicited extensor posturing. He died 4 weeks later. (From Chatrian G-E. Electrophysiological evaluation of brain death: a critical appraisal. In: Aminoff MJ, ed. *Electrodiagnosis in clinical neurology.* New York: Churchill Livingstone, 1980:525–588, with permission.)

tonic coupling between cells, providing the basis for powerful excitatory interactions that cause large neuronal aggregates to burst in near-synchrony (464).

Periodic lateralized epileptiform discharges (PLEDs) (85) sometimes occur over variable extents of one hemisphere (with frequent reflection over the homologous areas of the opposite side) and occasionally appear over both hemispheres independently (117). PLEDs are found in patients with a variety of hemispheric lesions, including acute infarction, hemorrhage, tumors, and infections (85,313), especially when associated with metabolic abnormalities (85,347), infections such as herpes simplex encephalitis (97), long-standing lesions such as old infarcts (85), and chronic seizure disorders (85,371).

Periodic generalized slow-wave complexes that repeat at intervals of 4–14 seconds and are associated with myoclonic jerking characterize patients with subacute sclerosing panencephalitis (102,103), and periodic lateralized slow-wave complexes, also accompanied by focal jerking, occur with vari-

ous hemispheric lesions (85). These patients' consciousness may be variously impaired.

Interictal Epileptiform Discharges and Seizure Discharges

Interictal epileptiform and seizure discharges, whether focal or generalized, can occur in comatose patients, especially with cortical contusions, intracerebral hematomas (107,436,449), systemic metabolic derangements such as uremic (213) and hepatic (151) encephalopathies, and acute brain anoxia (308,417,449).

Low-Voltage, Slow, Unreactive EEG

A low-voltage, slow, unreactive EEG (Fig. 14.6), consists of arrhythmic potentials in the delta and theta ranges generally not exceeding 20 µV that are unmodified by sensory stimuli. Such a pattern is common among

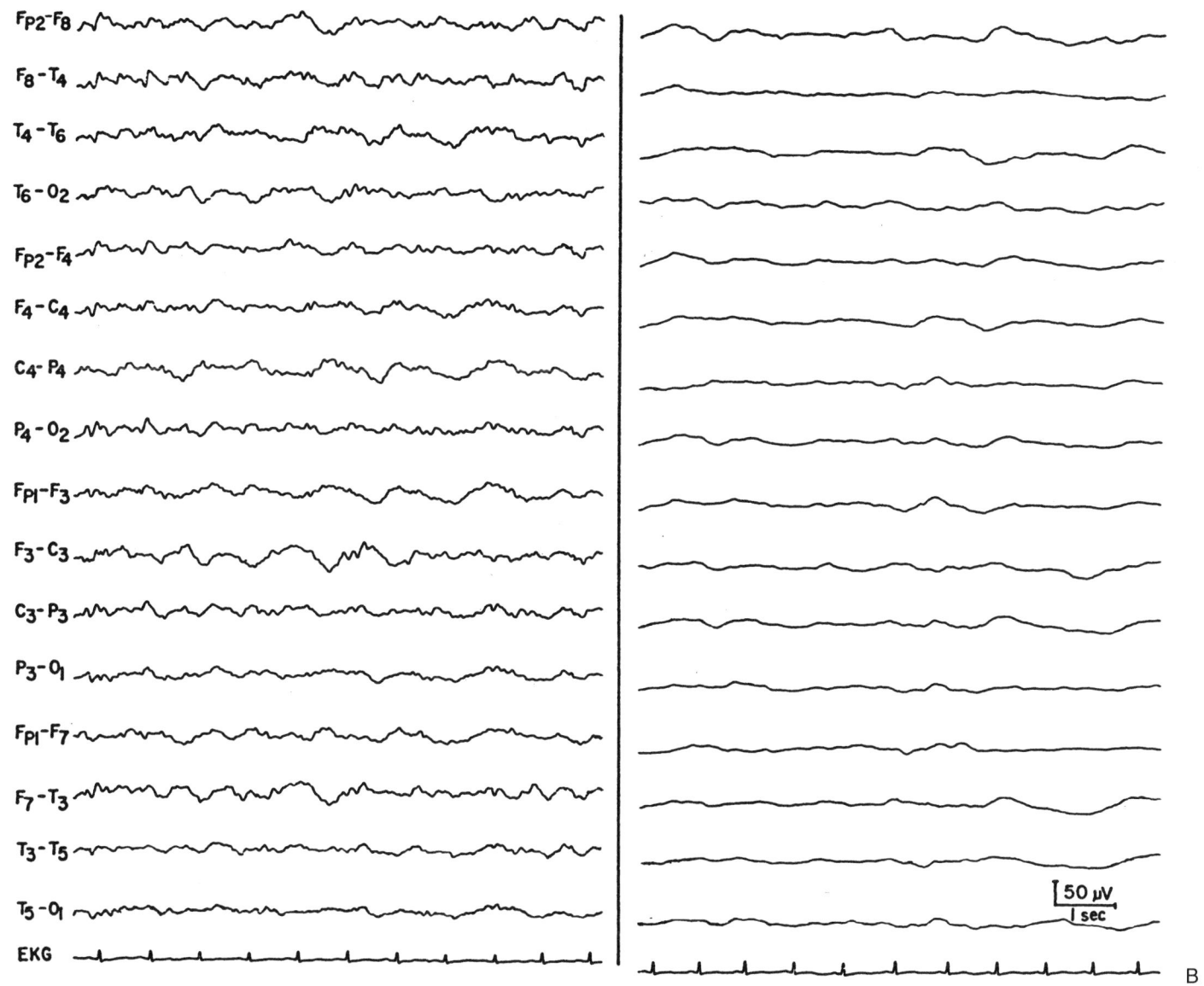

FIG 14.6. Widespread arrhythmic 1- to 2-Hz activity intermixed with 5- to 7-Hz potentials **(A)** evolving into a low-voltage, slow, unreactive pattern **(B)**. This 24-year-old patient was comatose following an episode of ventricular fibrillation that occurred after strenuous exercise. **A:** On admission, he had spontaneous respiration and preserved corneal and oculocephalic reflexes. **B:** Ten days later, he required artificial ventilation and his corneal reflexes could no longer be elicited. He survived 15 days. (From Chatrian G-E. Electrophysiological evaluation of brain death: a critical appraisal. In: Aminoff MJ, ed. *Electrodiagnosis in clinical neurology*. New York: Churchill Livingstone, 1980:525–588, with permission.)

comatose patients with severe, widespread cortical damage, who either die or survive in a vegetative state. One must distinguish this low-voltage, slow, unreactive pattern from the low-voltage EEG found in some healthy subjects. The latter type consists of diffuse activity not exceeding 20 μV, composed of mixed beta, theta, and, to a lesser degree, delta activity, with or without alpha rhythm. Unlike the low-voltage, slow, unreactive EEG of comatose patients, this normal record changes with certain physiological stimuli, hyperventilation, sleep, and pharmacological agents (76).

Unilateral, Lateralized, or Focal Alterations

In some circumstances, large unilateral lesions of the cerebral hemispheres producing coma may cause unilateral, lateralized, or, less frequently, focal EEG changes. These occur ipsilaterally to the lesion and consist of one or more of the following:

Arrhythmic delta activity distinguishable from more widespread slow waves because of slower frequency, higher voltage, or both
Diminished voltage of continuous or intermittent delta activities
Decreased amplitude of intermixed fast activity
Decreased voltage of EEG responses to external stimuli (20)
Diminished amplitude of characteristic EEG patterns such as TWs (154) or sleep patterns (61)
Interictal or ictal epileptic discharges, including PLEDs as noted above (85,107,371,435,449)

Generally, unilateral alterations are especially obvious in lighter stages of altered responsiveness and become less apparent or disappear with deepening coma. They sometimes occur in toxic-metabolic encephalopathies, including nonketotic hyperosmolar diabetic coma, in the absence of hemispheric lesions (213,305). In patients who have undergone surgery, spurious asymmetries may result from apparently augmented voltages over skull defects.

Triphasic Waves

Early studies reported the occurrence of bursts of characteristic complexes in the EEGs of patients with hepatic coma. These waveforms, first described as 2 per second "blunt spike and wave" because of their appearance in referential montages (162), were later renamed "triphasic waves" (45) based on their form in bipolar derivations. TWs consist of a high-volt-

age "positive" potential preceded and followed by "negative" deflections of lower voltage (45) (Figs. 14.7 and 14.8). They were originally described as bilaterally synchronous, generalized, and maximal over the frontal or, less frequently, the occipital or temporal areas. TWs were said to appear first over anterior regions and later over posterior areas. The fronto-occipital "phase lag" of the major "positive" component varies from 25 to 140 milliseconds (45). In subsequent studies, TWs predominated on anterior regions in 60% of records and posteriorly or diffusely in 40%. They were lateralized in 9% of patients, mostly with structural hemispheric lesions. Phase lags were less apparent in referential (27%) than in bipolar longitudinal (73%) montages (154). The triphasic morphology varies considerably. Some complexes have an especially sharp, spike-like first component, whereas other waves are monophasic, diphasic, or quadriphasic (307,413). Morphological congruence over homologous areas is also mutable. Repetition rate of TWs is mostly about 2 Hz but is occasionally slower (29).

Relation to Diminished Consciousness

Some investigators have reported that, as consciousness declined in patients with hepatic encephalopathy, EEGs successively displayed widespread theta activity, TWs, arrhythmic delta activity, and, finally, generalized "suppression." Patients in the triphasic and delta stages were "semicomatose or completely unresponsive" (45) or were in grades II–III of hepatic coma, characterized by somnolence and stupor (306). However, other researchers observed a wider range of altered consciousness, and some even reported normal responsiveness in patients with TWs from various causes (29,62,154,214,307,374,413,418). EEG reactivity was also variable (154).

Etiological Specificity and Prognostic Significance

The diagnostic specificity of TWs has been the subject of controversy (3,45). Reiher (385) distinguished "typical" TWs having the features described by Bickford and Butt (45) from "atypical" TWs not meeting all criteria. He regarded the former as "pathognomonic" for hepatic coma, whereas the latter could appear in both hepatic and other metabolic encephalopathies, CNS degenerative disorders, cerebrovascular lesions, and supratentorial and infratentorial tumors. This distinction did not win general acceptance. At present, most electroencephalographers agree that TWs, whether typical or atypical, can occur in various toxic-metabolic encepha-

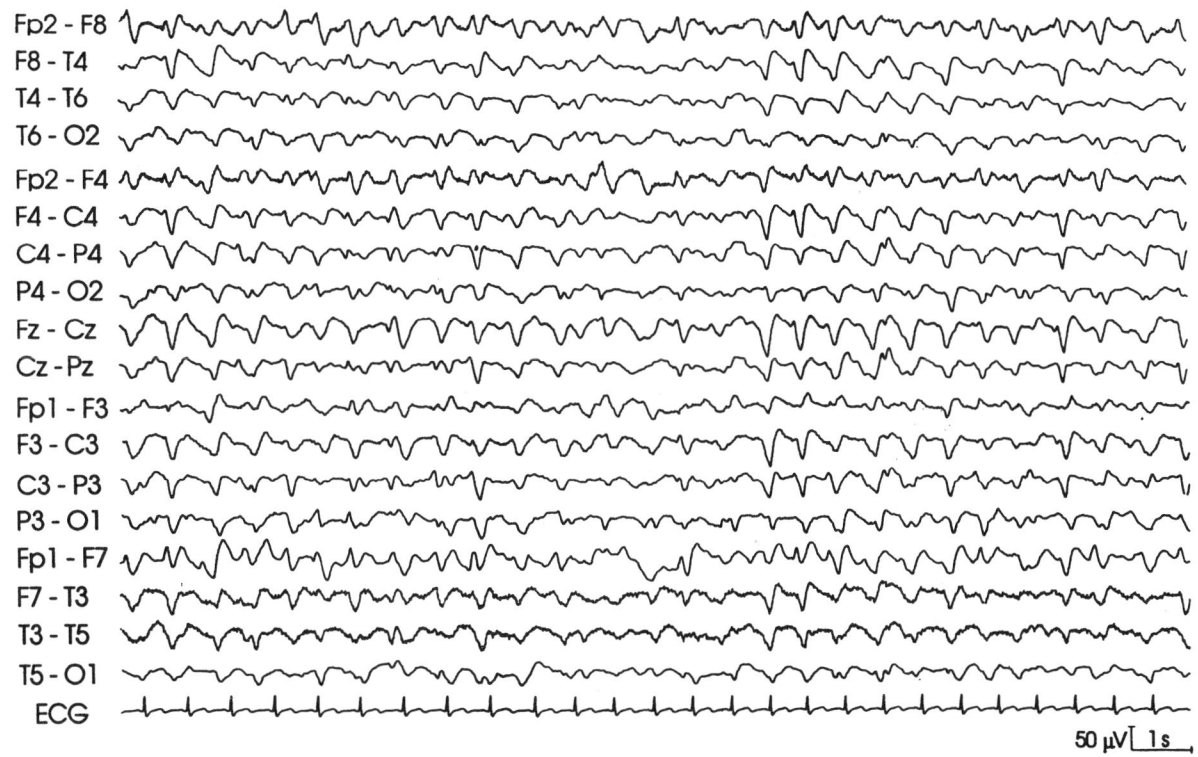

Fp2 - F8
F8 - T4
T4 - T6
T6 - O2
Fp2 - F4
F4 - C4
C4 - P4
P4 - O2
Fz - Cz
Cz - Pz
Fp1 - F3
F3 - C3
C3 - P3
P3 - O1
Fp1 - F7
F7 - T3
T3 - T5
T5 - O1
ECG

50 µV ⌐ 1s ⌐

FIG. 14.7. Triphasic waves in a 53-year-old lethargic woman with hepatic encephalopathy. (From Chatrian G-E. Electrophysiological evaluation of brain death: a critical appraisal. In: Aminoff MJ, ed. *Electrodiagnosis in clinical neurology*. New York: Churchill Livingstone, 1980:525–588, with permission.)

lopathies whether the latter are due to hepatic failure (Fig. 14.7) or other causes. These include uremia (29,154,213,214,306,498); valproic acid–induced hyperammonemic encephalopathy (269); severe water and electrolyte imbalance (29,214,266); hypercalcemia (452); anoxia (29,154, 214,452,498) (Fig. 14.8); hypoglycemia (29,214,266); hyperthyroidism (374,376,472); myxedema (391); Hashimoto's encephalopathy (216); accidental hypothermia (390); intoxication with CNS depressant and other drugs (280), including baclofen (226), levodopa (346), and pentobarbital (284); and serotonin syndrome (127). Currently, there is widespread agreement that no single feature or combination of features of TWs distinguishes hepatic from other metabolic encephalopathies or nonmetabolic conditions (29,154,307,418).

Investigators have described TWs in awake, confused patients with Alzheimer's disease and other dementias (50,376,447) and in individuals with vascular, degenerative, neoplastic, infectious, or traumatic brain pathologies (5,154,159,330,385,413,414,446,509) and even in subdural hematomas (307,488). In some publications, it is difficult to determine whether concurrent systemic metabolic derangements existed and whether the EEG patterns were TWs, waveforms superficially resembling TWs, or even triphasically shaped epileptiform discharges. Differentiating TWs from epileptiform patterns is complicated by the finding of TWs in uremic and other encephalopathies frequently associated with seizures (79), and the detection of variously triphasic sharp-and–slow wave complexes in some ictal (353) or postictal (357) stuporous states. To our knowledge, TWs have not been reported in children (306).

Mortality is high among patients with TWs who suffer from metabolic disorders and severe anoxia (29,266,306), whereas it varies in other conditions depending on etiology.

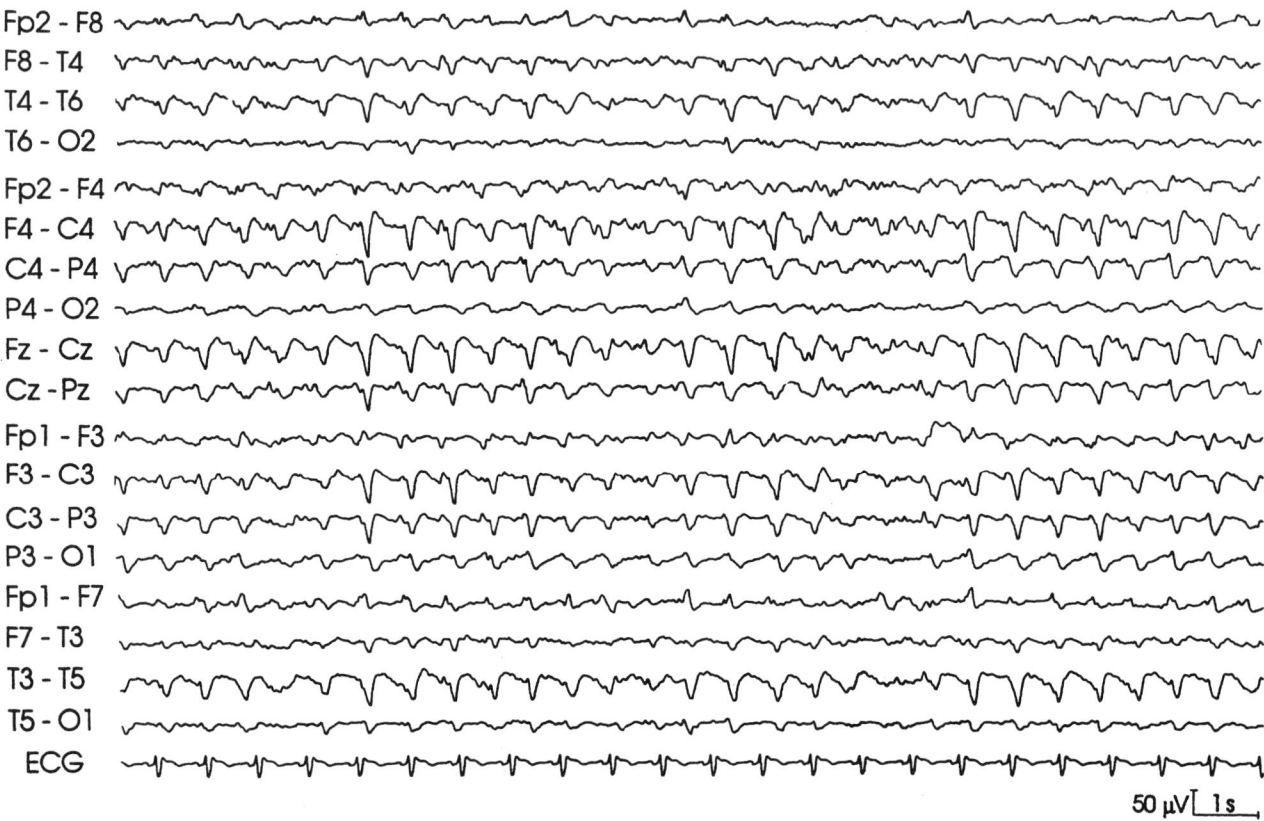

FIG. 14.8. Triphasic waves in a 66-year-old comatose man 2 days after cardiac arrest resulting from myocardial infarction. Following resuscitation, the patient remained comatose and developed episodes of twitching of the face with hiccup and upward deviation of the eyes that subsided with phenytoin and phenobarbital treatment. (From Chatrian G-E. Electrophysiological evaluation of brain death: a critical appraisal. In: Aminoff MJ, ed. *Electrodiagnosis in clinical neurology.* New York: Churchill Livingstone, 1980:525–588, with permission.)

Pathophysiological Interpretations

Factors responsible for TWs are poorly understood. It seems plausible that, in patients with systemic metabolic derangements, this pattern reflects primary biochemical disturbances. The finding that elevated blood ammonia levels cause TWs in patients with hepatic insufficiency (374) remains unconfirmed (413). It seems more likely that TWs in hepatic coma are due to multiple metabolic alterations (306) recently summarized by Young and DeRubeis (511).

In bipolar montages, a fronto-occipital lag of the main "positive" component of TWs suggested a traveling wave sweeping the scalp front to back at about 1.5 m per second (45). However, in referential montages, this phase shift is frequently lacking (45,154,418). To account for this discrepancy, Harner and Simsarian (214) proposed a longitudinal dipole model of TWs, interpreting the apparent anteroposterior delays in bipolar derivations as being due to "differential recording of activity which was synchronous, but 180 degrees out of phase in anterior and posterior locations." However, Fisch and Klass (154) observed more complex phase relationships.

Some authors (45,162,266) hypothesized that TWs reflected disturbed thalamocortical relays recruiting metabolically impaired cortical neurons. Similar interpretations were offered by other investigators (306). In the absence of animal models of TWs (306), these interpretations remain speculative.

Sleep Patterns

In Diurnal EEGs

Diurnal EEGs of some comatose individuals display patterns of sleep including spindles and vertex sharp waves intermixed with widespread delta and theta activity (Figs. 14.9 and 14.10A). In most patients, loud auditory or noxious stimuli elicit K complexes or bilateral bursts of delta activity, often mixed with rhythmic waves of theta and alpha frequency over posterior areas (Fig. 14.9) (37,40,46,57,61,65,75,86,87,112,141,210,220,229–231,236,245, 298,344,377,398,399,414,434,435,449,454,475). Occasionally, changes occur during an individual EEG that mimic transitions from stages 1 to 4 of non–rapid-eye-movement (NREM) sleep, although consciousness does not appear to vary (87).

In Nocturnal Polygraphic Records

Some individuals who are comatose or vegetative following head injury demonstrate some or all of the nocturnal polygraphic patterns and behav-

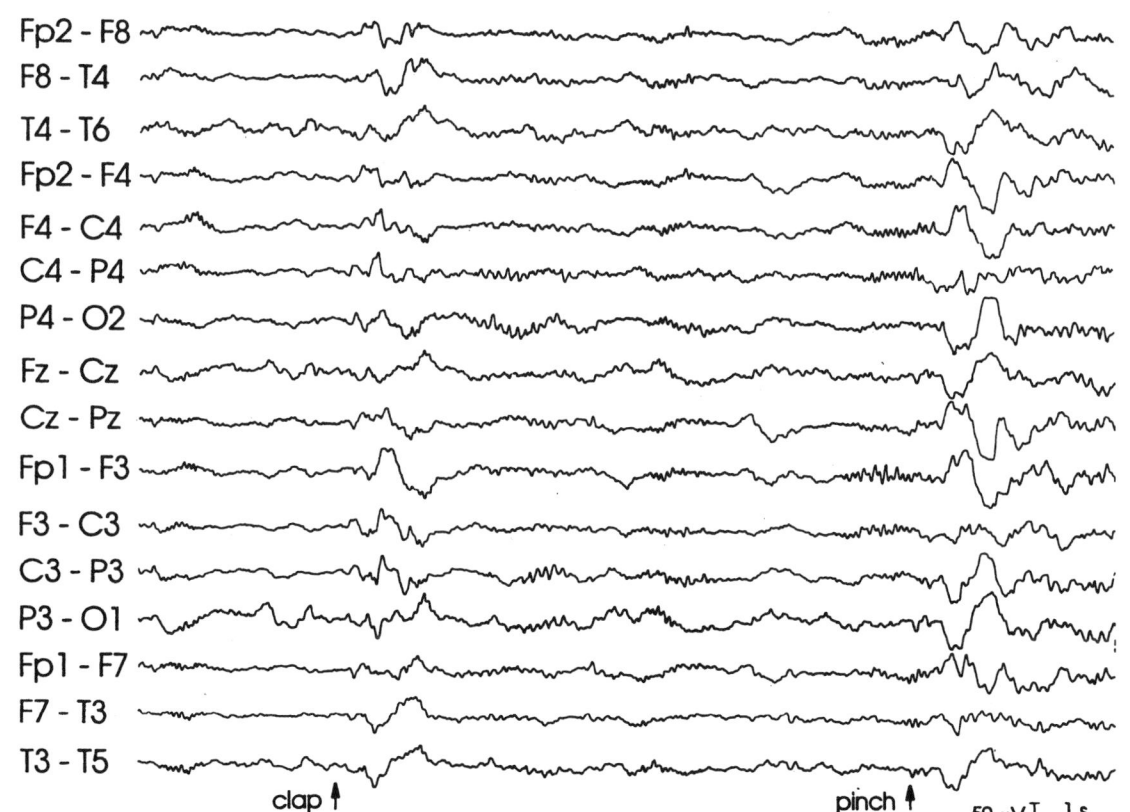

FIG. 14.9. EEG patterns of sleep, including spindles, and K complexes in response to auditory and noxious stimuli. Twelve hours after head injury, this 17-year-old girl was stuporous and demonstrated anisocoria, left pupil larger than right, and left Babinski's sign. Noxious stimulation elicited inconstant withdrawal movements and agitation. The patient recovered with slight left upper extremity paresis. (From Chatrian G-E. Electrophysiological evaluation of brain death: a critical appraisal. In: Aminoff MJ, ed. *Electrodiagnosis in clinical neurology*. New York: Churchill Livingstone, 1980:525–588, with permission.)

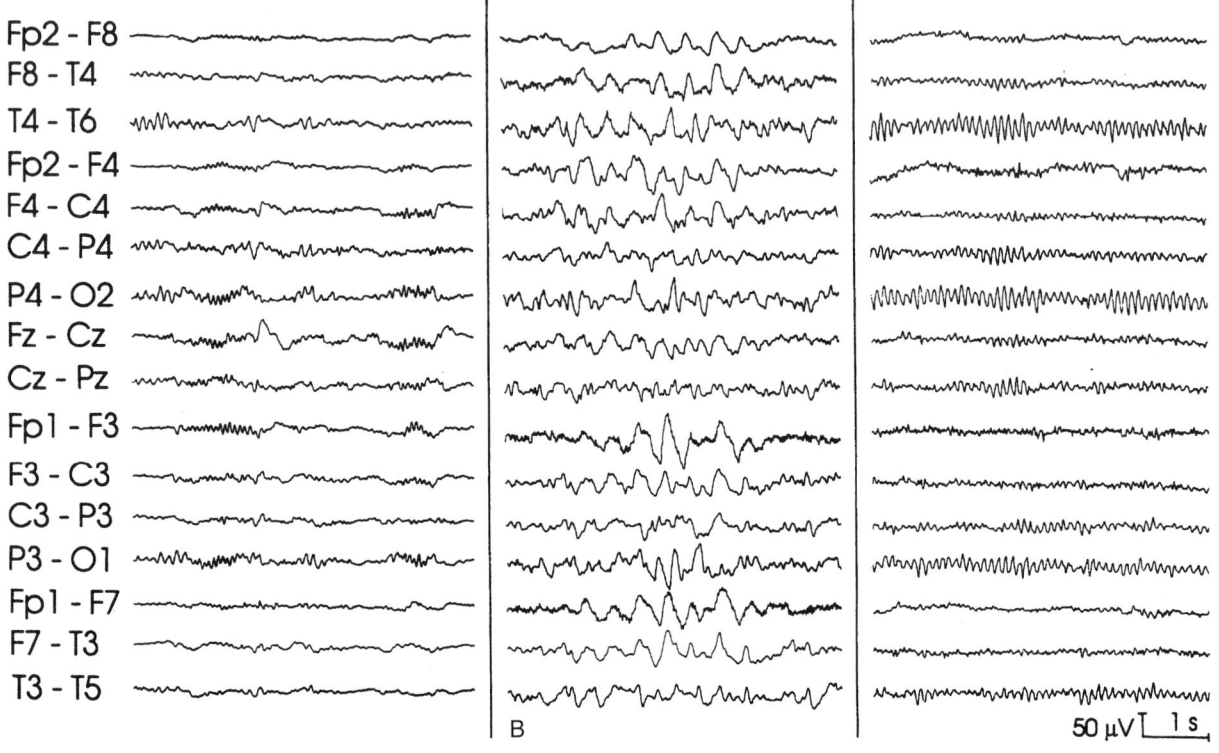

Fp2 - F8
F8 - T4
T4 - T6
Fp2 - F4
F4 - C4
C4 - P4
P4 - O2
Fz - Cz
Cz - Pz
Fp1 - F3
F3 - C3
C3 - P3
P3 - O1
Fp1 - F7
F7 - T3
T3 - T5

A   B   50 μV ⌐ 1 s ⌐   C

FIG. 14.10. Serial EEGs recorded in the same patient as in Figure 14.9. **A:** Patient stuporous with sleep spindles 12 hours after injury. **B:** Patient alert but agitated 4 days after the accident. **C:** Patient alert and quiet 18 days after trauma. (From Chatrian G-E. Electrophysiological evaluation of brain death: a critical appraisal. In: Aminoff MJ, ed. *Electrodiagnosis in clinical neurology.* New York: Churchill Livingstone, 1980:525–588, with permission.)

ioral signs of sleep (39,40,56,57). In certain subjects, no EEG sleep patterns are detected. Some of these latter patients display "biphasic" nocturnal patterns consisting of alternating periods of high-voltage slow and low-voltage faster activities, whereas a "monophasic" pattern consisting exclusively of slow activity appears in other individuals (39,40,57).

Prevalence and Etiology

Many studies of comatose states associated with spindles and other patterns of sleep in diurnal EEGs were conducted on patients who had suffered head injury (37,39,46,57,59,63,75,86,87,106,136,141,210,220,229,230, 236,298,344,377,398,399,414,434,435,449,454,475). However, other etiologies were associated with coma and EEG patterns of sleep. These included tumors principally involving the floor of the third ventricle or mid-

brain but sparing the thalamus (245); acute cerebral anoxia (61,210,231, 377); viral encephalitis (52,112); cerebral, thalamic, brainstem, or cerebellar hemorrhage or infarction (61,210); subarachnoid hemorrhage (61); drug intoxication (61,264); metabolic encephalopathies; postictal state; and other or multiple etiologies.

Pathophysiological Interpretations and Pathological Findings

An early study hypothesized that a transient, reversible functional derangement of the midbrain reticular formation was responsible for the impaired responsiveness and the sleep EEG patterns observed in some patients following head injury (87). Other works suggested that sleep spindles in daytime recordings expressed a functional disturbance or anatomical lesion(s) involving (a) the hypothalamus and midbrain (245); (b) the midbrain (398); (c) deep-seated structures below the diencephalon (414); (d) rostral parts of the brainstem (220); and (e) the pontomesencephalic reticular formation (301). Regrettably, pathological observations confirming these interpretations are few and scanty. Luecking (301) reported "minimal lesions in the reticular formation of the midbrain" in an unspecified number of patients who had suffered head injury and died from extracerebral causes. Prior (377) described generalized edema, as well as a "rather soft and almost necrotic" brainstem, in an individual following cerebral anoxia. In the patients studied by Hansotia et al. (210), lesions of unspecified nature and extent were found scattered in the cerebral hemispheres, diencephalon, midbrain, and pontomedullary and cerebellar regions. Also, a hemorrhage was demonstrated by computed tomography in the rostral midbrain of a patient in posttraumatic coma with spindles (63). Whatever their nature and location, the structural alterations responsible for the manifestation of sleep patterns in comatose patients appear to be compatible with a considerable degree of functional preservation of the cerebral hemispheres. It is conceivable that preeminent functional alterations of critical brainstem structures may also account for the manifestation of sleep EEG patterns in patients rendered comatose by more widespread disorders such as metabolic, infectious, and anoxic encephalopathies.

Bricolo et al. (57) attempted to explain results of overnight polygraphic records of "prolonged post-traumatic" (presumably vegetative) patients by postulating lesions or combinations of lesions at various brainstem, diencephalic, and cortical levels, but these conjectures were not supported by pathological observations.

Relations to Duration, Depth, and Functional Levels of Coma

Short diurnal (399,475), polygraphic nocturnal (39,57), and spectrally analyzed (58) recordings determined that spindles and other EEG patterns of sleep and organized nocturnal sleep cycles were more common in short-lasting than in long-lasting comatose states resulting from head injury. Spindles progressively decreased as depth of coma increased, becoming distorted and asymmetrical and finally disappearing (398,399,414,475). Also, typical spindles, vertex sharp waves, and K complexes diminished as patients in posttraumatic coma underwent clinically assessed rostrocaudal deterioration (398).

EEG Evolution, Clinical Outcome, and Prognostic Value

Several authors have reported that posttraumatic comas with EEG patterns of sleep in diurnal EEGs had relatively benign outcomes (39,40,56,

57,87,344,475). EEG reactivity, including elicitation of K complexes, was similarly associated with favorable outcome (141,236,399). In many instances, recovery of alertness was first associated with confusion, disorientation, intermittent restlessness, hallucinations, and appearance of widespread high-voltage rhythmic delta waves (see Fig. 14.10B). Subsequently, mental status and EEG gradually cleared, although some neurological deficits often persisted (87) (Fig. 14.10C). Other investigators broadened their observations to include comas with spindles of various etiologies. In the National Institute of Neurological and Communicative Disorders (NINCDS) Collaborative Study, only a few individuals who were comatose and apneic from various causes and demonstrated spindles in their EEGs at one time or another survived (229), an outcome not surprising in such a selection-biased group. Another investigation of patients with comas from traumatic or nontraumatic causes failed to find any relationships among (a) presence and features of spindles and other EEG patterns of sleep, (b) improved sleep organization in successive records, (c) EEG reactivity, (d) duration and depth of coma, and (e) final outcome. Death rates did not significantly differ in comatose individuals with and without spindles (210). In contrast, an individual study reported that deeply comatose patients with impaired brainstem motor functions and spindles in their EEGs had unfavorable evolutions (61). More recently, metaanalysis of the available literature showed an overall mortality of 23% in patients in coma with spindles compared to mortalities exceeding 65% in comas associated with other EEG patterns, including burst-suppression, periodic patterns, and alpha-frequency comas (265). Death or a vegetative state occurred in 73% of patients with structural lesions of the brainstem and cerebrum, 33% of individuals with hypoxia and cardiorespiratory arrest, 15% of subjects with head trauma, and none of the patients with toxic-metabolic encephalopathies or postictal states. (265). We interpret these findings as suggesting that etiology is the prime determinant of outcome in these particular comatose states.

Evoked Potentials

Limited information is available on evoked potentials (EPs) in comatose patients with EEG patterns of sleep. Short-latency somatosensory evoked potentials (SL-SEPs) (321), brainstem auditory evoked potentials (BAEPs), and visual evoked potentials (VEPs) (445) were normal in a few infants and children with comas of various etiologies. In contrast, a child with imipramine overdose had prolonged II–V BAEP interpeak intervals (IPIs), which subsequently returned to normal (378). These patients recovered without neurological sequelae.

Rhythms of Alpha Frequency

The EEGs of some unresponsive patients consist primarily of rhythmic activity of alpha frequency. The term *alpha coma*, coined by Westmoreland et al. (491), has popularized this notion but has done little to clarify the fundamental concept that distinctive alpha patterns characterize clinically and pathologically different entities, including some that superficially resemble, but that must be distinguished from, coma.

Unresponsive states showing EEG rhythms of alpha frequency include (a) coma secondary to acute diffuse brain anoxia or other structural pathology, (b) coma from toxic or metabolic causes, and (c) deefferented states resulting from brainstem lesions.

Widespread Alpha Activity in Coma Resulting from Acute Diffuse Brain Anoxia

The occurrence of a rhythm of alpha frequency in patients with diffuse cerebral anoxia resulting from cardiac or respiratory arrest was briefly alluded to in early reports (47,60,223,286,377). Subsequent detailed accounts described this pattern as typically consisting of a rhythm of 8–13 Hz and 10–50 µV that is detected in patients rendered comatose by acute cerebral anoxia (11,28,33,53,100,161,193,264,423,468,474,491,510). Sometimes this rhythm has a lower frequency (4–7 Hz) or consists of potentials in both the alpha and the theta ranges (264,448,453,455,510) ("theta" or "alpha-theta" coma). Most commonly the alpha activity detected in anoxic coma is sinusoidal, varies little in amplitude, and is distributed widely over the head but dominates frontally (Fig. 14.11). In our experience, this widespread rhythm is rarely modified by manual eye opening or by photic, auditory, tactile, and noxious stimuli. However, in one series, reactivity of the alpha-frequency pattern to noxious excitations was observed more frequently than in earlier studies (264).

The EEG often shows variable amounts of intermixed theta or delta waves, generally widespread but occasionally focal. The prevalence of patients with alpha activity while comatose after cardiorespiratory arrest varies from 13.3% (474) to 25.8% (28). This pattern occurs not only in adults of all ages but also in infants and children (105,225,244,336,515).

EEG Evolution and Clinical Course

The alpha-frequency pattern generally was detected within a few hours to 4 days, but occasionally as long as 6–9 days, after onset of coma (100). In

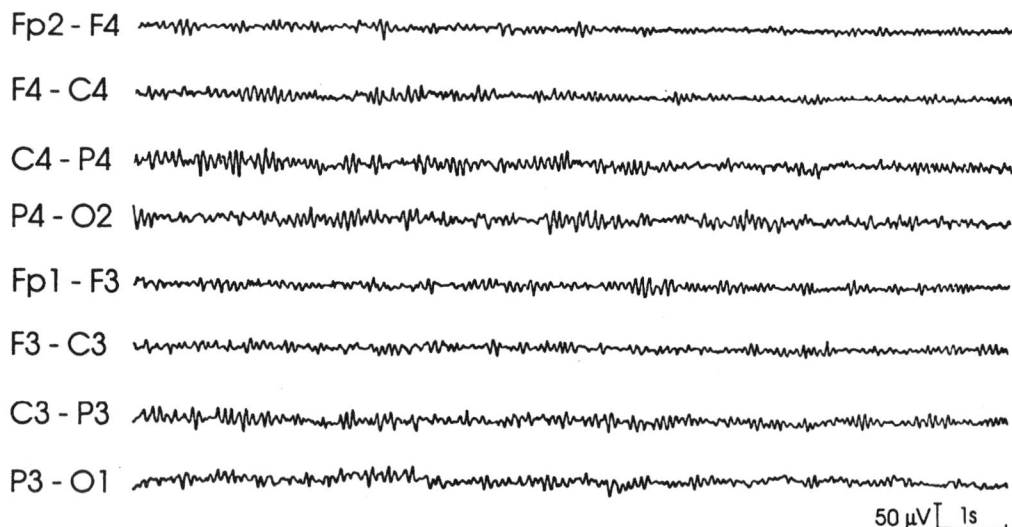

Fp2 - F4

F4 - C4

C4 - P4

P4 - O2

Fp1 - F3

F3 - C3

C3 - P3

P3 - O1

50 µV ⌐ 1s ⌐

FIG. 14.11. Widespread alpha activity unaltered by sensory stimuli in a 29-year-old man 3 days after cardiopulmonary arrest resulting from accidental strangulation. The patient was comatose and exhibited extensor rigidity, small reactive pupils, and spontaneous hyperventilation. He survived 5 days. (Modified from Vignaendra V, Wilkus RJ, Copass MK, et al. Electroencephalographic rhythms of alpha frequency in comatose patients after cardiopulmonary arrest. *Neurology* 1974;24:582–588.)

serial recordings, sometimes this activity preceded, accompanied, or followed other patterns, including EEGs described as displaying no electrocortical activity (60,100) but probably not fulfilling contemporary criteria for ECI, burst-suppression (193,286,491), low-voltage unreactive activity (166) with discernible potentials in the delta and theta (423) or beta (218) ranges, widespread theta and delta activity of higher voltage (100,218,455), and generalized sharp waves and spike-and–slow wave complexes (193). Sleep (100,244,423,474) and burst-suppression (515) patterns coexisted, although exceptionally, with alpha activity.

Deteriorating clinical state often was associated with the following: diminishing voltage of theta and delta activities (193,218); manifestation of multifocal electrical seizures (225), pseudoperiodic sharp waves (490), and burst-suppression (11,218,510); and ultimately ECI (60,100,355,515). Klem and Henry (273) observed such an evolution in a single recording. In contrast, lightning of coma and gradual neurological recovery generally were first accompanied by widespread theta waves mixed with residual alpha activity unreactive to stimuli (192,335) and were later associated with gradually appearing physiological rhythms. These included alpha rhythms that were frequently low in voltage, posterior in distribution (105,192,193,423, 455), and reactive to eye opening (192,193). Photic driving response and patterns of sleep generally appeared at this time (192). However, widespread or focal abnormalities persisted to varying degrees in some patients (242).

Prognostic Significance

Opinions have varied on the prognostic significance of postanoxic alpha activity. Some authors believe that it has a grave prognostic significance (11,47,335,355,461,474,491). Other investigators challenged this notion (193), and some even found longer survivals and better recoveries in individuals with anoxic coma who displayed widespread alpha-frequency activity, compared to other EEG patterns (423). A review of some published reports disclosed that 73% of patients who demonstrated widespread alpha-frequency activity while in coma following cardiopulmonary arrest died without recovering consciousness, 5% regained consciousness but subsequently died during the hospitalization, 19% survived with neurological sequelae of varying severity, and only 3% had nearly total or total recovery (79). Similar results were obtained in a more recent analysis of the literature (264). Thus the risks of never regaining consciousness and dying in the hospital or surviving with severe neurological deficits are high among patients with this EEG pattern while in postanoxic coma (79). However, it has been shown that there is no significant difference in outcome between patients in postanoxic coma with and without alpha-frequency pattern in their EEGs (28). Thus it seems likely that these patients' outcome is related to the severity of the anoxic insult rather than to the finding of widespread alpha-frequency activity. There is evidence that the outcome tends to be better when this alpha pattern appears and resolves within 24 hours of onset of anoxic coma than when it is detected on or after the second day (242). It has also been suggested that reactivity of the EEG patterns occurring after subsidence of alpha activity may be more prognostically significant than the alpha pattern itself (510).

Pathological Findings

Pathological studies revealed changes typical of brain anoxia (430). Alterations in neocortex ranged from mild and patchy to severe and extensive, especially in deeper cortical layers. The hippocampus and cerebellum were markedly involved, whereas alterations of the thalamus, basal ganglia, midbrain, and pons were inconsistent (100,193,218,474,491). A completely necrotic "respirator brain" occurred in only one patient (100). There is no indication that these anoxic alterations differ in patients with and without an alpha-frequency EEG pattern.

Pathophysiological Mechanisms

A fundamental issue is whether the alpha activity seen in comatose patients with diffuse brain anoxia represents a paradoxically retained "normal" alpha rhythm or a newly generated, abnormal activity of alpha frequency (491). To answer this question, one should consider three lines of evidence:

1. Alpha activity in postanoxic comatose states differs sharply from the alpha rhythm of normal, awake, resting subjects. With some notable exceptions, the former is (a) widely distributed, frequently anteriorly predominant; (b) poorly modulated; (c) unreactive to sensory, including noxious, stimuli; and (d) not associated with a photic driving response. In contrast, as a rule, alpha rhythms of normal, awake, resting subjects are (a) best developed posteriorly, (b) better modulated and slightly faster in frequency, (c) frequently attenuated by eye opening, and (d) often associated with photic driving. These differences appear clearly when comparing EEGs in comatose patients with widespread unreactive alpha activity to EEGs in the same patients before onset (166,242) or after resolution (192,242,455) of coma.

2. The alpha-activity pattern observed in postanoxic infants and children often has a frequency inappropriately fast for age (105,225,244,336, 515). On recovery, an alpha rhythm of slower frequency consistent with the patient's age becomes apparent (105).

3. Computer analyses of the EEG have demonstrated differences between alpha activities detected in comatose patients compared to normal subjects. These include reduced coherence of alpha activity between homologous regions of the two hemispheres (325) and more variable "dimensionality" of alpha activity over different temporal EEG segments in comatose patients compared to normal subjects (270). The evidence strongly suggests that the alpha-frequency pattern of patients in anoxic coma is not a paradoxically retained normal alpha rhythm but newly generated abnormal activity (105,161,242) sharing with the alpha rhythm of normal subjects only the frequency range.

One must assume that preserved neuronal systems within the cerebral hemispheres, diencephalon, or brainstem generate this widely synchronized alpha activity. However, the identity of the generators and the mechanisms producing this rhythm are still unclear. Gurvitch et al. (200) suggested that alpha activity of human postanoxic states may be analogous or identical to spindle bursts recorded in dogs following resuscitation from induced circulatory arrest. Although the amygdaloid nuclei would give raise to these spindles, other subcortical structures, especially the thalamus and caudate nucleus, would play a role in their generalization (200,201). In humans, the relative continuous occurrence and unvarying voltage of alpha activity in postanoxic coma distinguishes it from these intermittent and highly modulated canine amygdaloid spindles. Moreover, the amygdaloid nucleus is relatively smaller in humans than in dogs. Thus the amygdaloid origin of alpha activity in comatose humans remains unproved (79). Multiple mechanisms may be responsible for generating this pattern. It seems likely that subcortical structures, including the thalamus, play a role in producing this rhythmic activity in individuals with acute, widespread cortical anoxic alterations.

Widespread Alpha Activity in Coma Resulting from Toxic-Metabolic Causes

Some patients in coma resulting from acute drug intoxication or high-dose therapeutic sedation show rhythmic activity of 8–12 (and occasionally 12–16) Hz and 20–50 µV mixed with theta and delta waves (Fig. 14.12).

Generally, these alpha and slow beta potentials are distributed widely, maximally over the anterior head regions, and are unreactive to manually opening the eyes and to auditory and noxious stimuli (28,43,71,119,120,140,161, 187,193,202,219,244,264,279,280,282,288,327,378,468).

Substances causing these comatose states include sedative-hypnotic drugs such as barbiturates (279,280,327) and the benzodiazepines (71,119,202, 219); imipramine (378); meprobamate (328); and various anesthetic agents such as fentanyl, isoflurane, and nitrous oxide (28), among others. Similar alpha-frequency activity has also been reported in patients with severely disturbed glucose metabolism (27,503).

The prevalence of alpha or low beta frequencies in patients with acute drug intoxication varies from 7% (264) to 29% (279). A few reports have described this pattern in children (288,378).

Clinical Outcome, EEG Evolution, and Prognostic Value

There is general agreement that most patients with drug-induced coma and alpha-frequency pattern in their EEGs recover promptly except when cardiac arrest has occurred, causing severe cerebral anoxia. A published mortality of 8% among these patients included cases complicated by anoxia (264). Clinical recovery is paralleled by evolution of mixed alpha and beta waves into widely distributed theta activity with intermixed beta potentials, in turn succeeded by an alpha rhythm of normal (posterior) distribution and reactivity (71,119,140,282,288). Because both frequently reversible drug intoxication and often-lethal severe cerebral anoxia can be associated with a widespread alpha-frequency pattern, the EEG cannot differentiate between drug intoxication with and without superimposed cerebral anoxia and cannot predict outcome.

Pathophysiological Mechanisms

Most authors emphasize that a widespread, maximally frontal distribution and lack of reactivity to stimuli distinguish alpha activity in coma caused by acute drug intoxication from the alpha rhythm characteristic of normal, awake subjects. These differences strongly suggest that alpha activity of drug-induced coma, like the alpha-frequency pattern of postanoxic patients, is not a persistent normal rhythm but newly generated abnormal activity. Some investigators have postulated pharmacological depression of reticulothalamic pathways with increased, widespread cortical synchronization (71), but no direct evidence supports this conjecture.

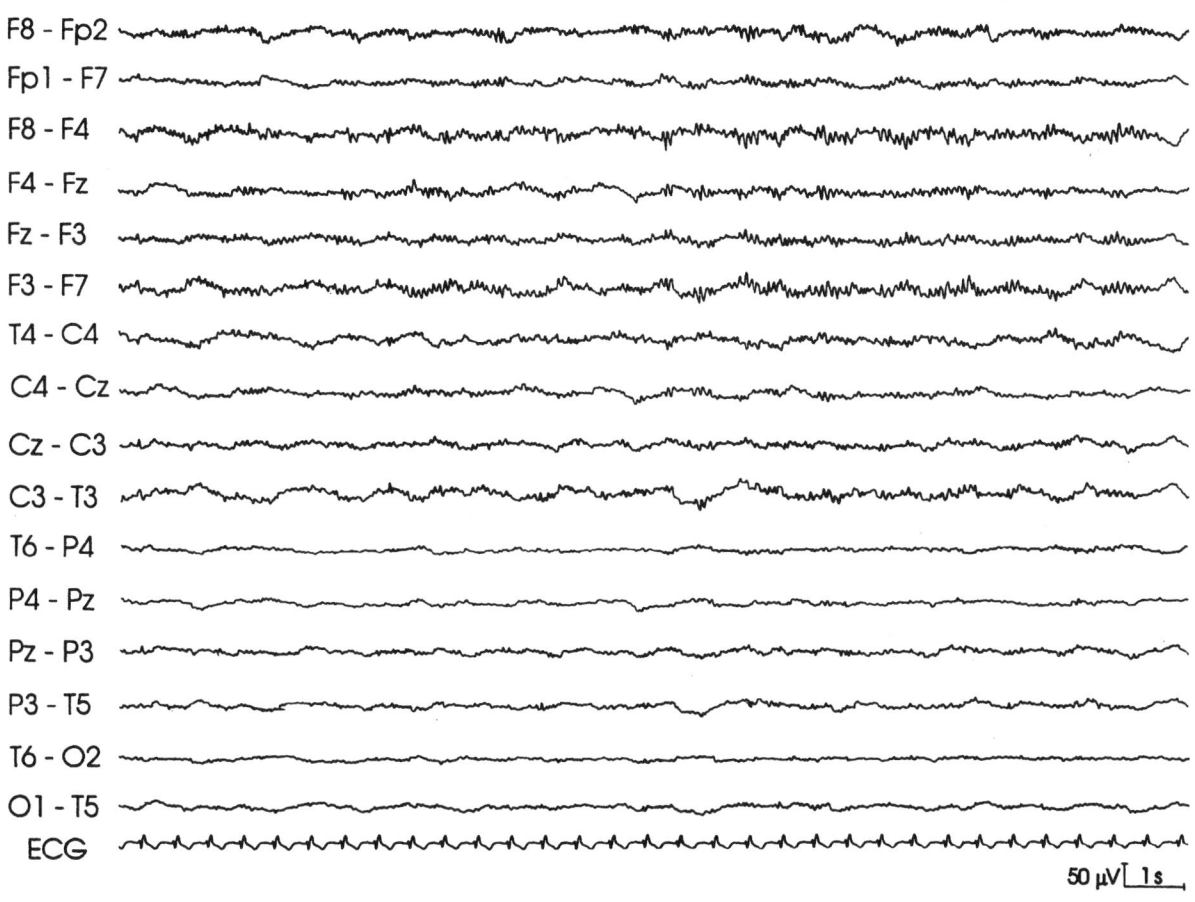

FIG. 14.12. Widespread unreactive 10-Hz rhythm recorded on a 40-year-old man who was comatose 1 day after head trauma. At the time of recording, the patient was receiving high-dose pentobarbital because of elevated intracranial pressure. He survived 9 days. (From Chatrian G-E. Electrophysiological evaluation of brain death: a critical appraisal. In: Aminoff MJ, ed. *Electrodiagnosis in clinical neurology.* New York: Churchill Livingstone, 1980:525–588, with permission.)

Alpha Rhythm in Deefferented ("Locked-In") States

The term *deefferented states* describes individuals who are quadriplegic and mute but demonstrate substantially normal mental functions when properly tested. Usually, these patients have paralysis of lower cranial nerves but have variably preserved vertical eye and eyelid movements that allow them to communicate to some extent. This condition (487) is commonly referred to as the *"locked-in" syndrome* (370). Some "incompletely locked-in" (34) patients have remnants of voluntary movement besides vertical eye and eyelid movements. Still other patients have lost all avenues of communication.

In the latter individuals, one cannot determine clinically whether they are comatose or "totally locked in" (34,496), that is, aware of internal and external stimuli but unable to make responses.

Pathological Findings

Patients in deefferented states have various lesions, usually infarcts or hemorrhages (367), destroying the ventral pons bilaterally. There is either substantial sparing of pontine and mesencephalic tegmentum ("ventral pontine syndrome") (409) or variable extension of the lesion to pontine tegmentum without or with only unilateral involvement of the midbrain tegmentum and thalamus (34,74,88,161,205,215,230,297,303,312,316,352,356,491, 497). Limited bilateral midbrain (268,322,373) or internal capsule (93) infarcts have also been described in a few patients. Nonvascular etiologies include tumors (92), trauma (64,160), abscesses (342), multiple sclerosis (163), *Borrelia burgdorferi* meningitis (329), brainstem encephalitis (367), central pontine myelinolysis (367), and heroin abuse (367). Mute paralyzed patients suffering from severe acute polyneuropathy or polyradiculoneuropathy may also appear locked in (71,135).

EEG Findings and Clinical Outcome

The EEGs of deefferented ("locked-in") patients show alpha activity with most or all features of the alpha rhythm of normal individuals (Fig. 14.13). Typically, this rhythm is most prominent over the posterior head regions and is attenuated by eye opening, whether voluntary or passive (Fig. 14.14), and a photic driving response is variably present. However, lower frequencies (6–7 Hz), higher voltage (up to 100 μV), lack of clear posterior preponderance of this rhythm, absence of reactivity to sensory stimuli (205,243), or low-voltage recordings with only intermittent alpha activity can also occur.

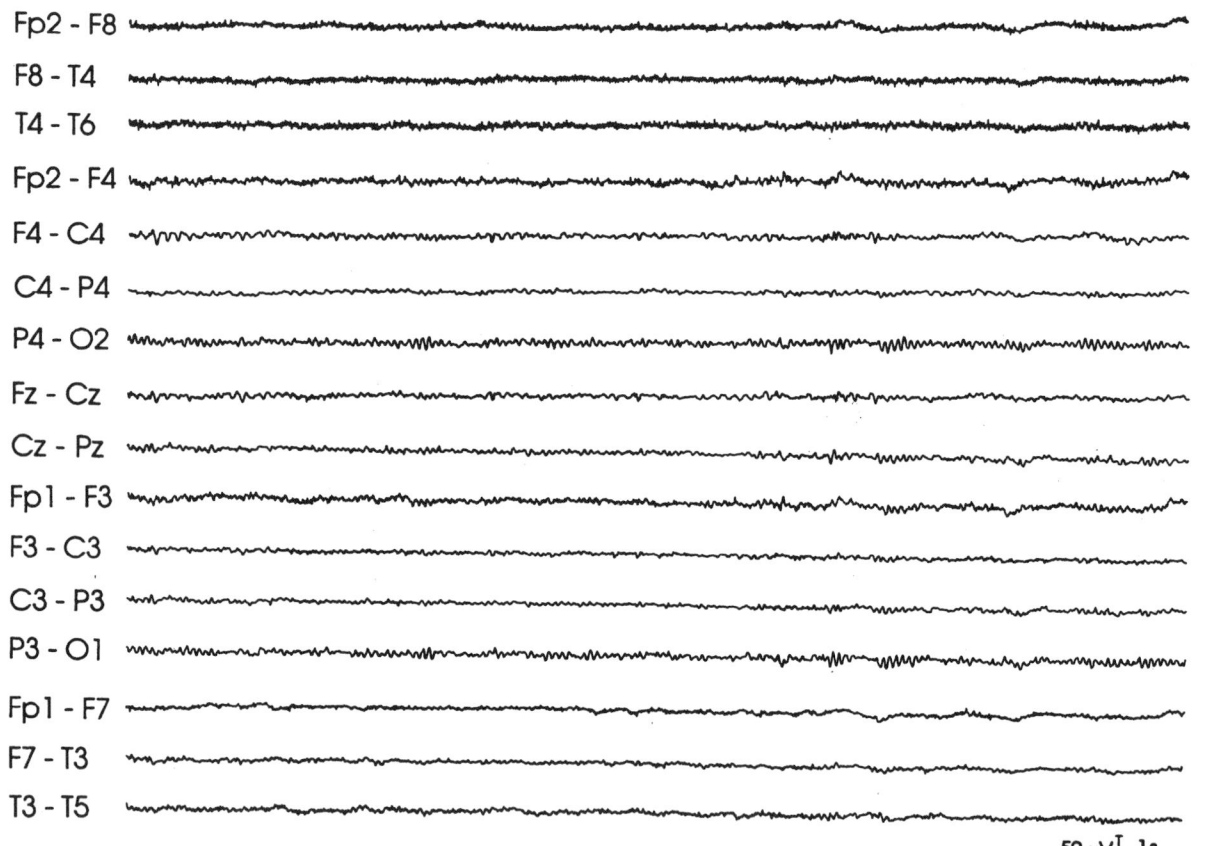

FIG. 14.13. Ten-Hz alpha rhythm in a 65-year-old man who collapsed and became unresponsive after 1 week of dizziness, right hemiparesis, and dysarthria. When the EEG was recorded 2 days later, he was mute and quadriplegic, with bilateral weakness of lower face, tongue, and palate; left gaze paralysis; and right-sided flexor posturing in response to noxious stimulation. He could open his eyes and make slow vertical movements. This patient's "locked-in" state was a result of extensive pontine infarction transecting the pons up to its junction with the midbrain. He survived 2 months. (From Chatrian G-E. Electrophysiological evaluation of brain death: a critical appraisal. In: Aminoff MJ, ed. *Electrodiagnosis in clinical neurology*. New York: Churchill Livingstone, 1980:525–588, with permission.)

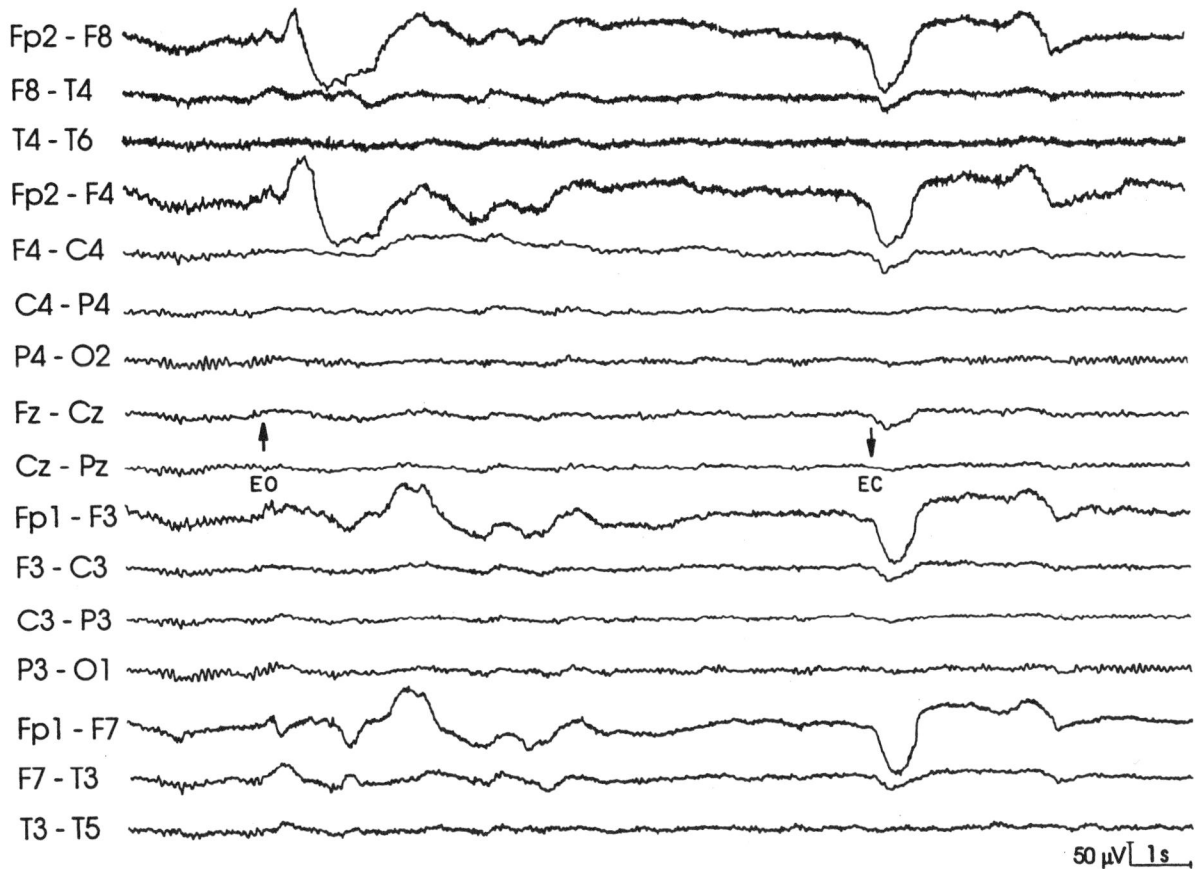

Fp2 - F8
F8 - T4
T4 - T6
Fp2 - F4
F4 - C4
C4 - P4
P4 - O2
Fz - Cz
Cz - Pz
EO   EC
Fp1 - F3
F3 - C3
C3 - P3
P3 - O1
Fp1 - F7
F7 - T3
T3 - T5

50 μV ⌐ 1 s ⌐

FIG. 14.14. Attenuation of the alpha rhythm by eye opening on command in the same patient and recording as in Figure 14.13. (From Chatrian G-E. Electrophysiological evaluation of brain death: a critical appraisal. In: Aminoff MJ, ed. *Electrodiagnosis in clinical neurology.* New York: Churchill Livingstone, 1980:525–588, with permission.)

Some deefferented patients also demonstrate variable amounts of theta and delta waves, which may be diffuse, lateralized, or focal and are often most prominent over the frontal or temporal areas (34,65,73,74,88,149,150,161, 205,209,212,215,230,243,258,260,276,296,297,303,312,351,352,355,356, 367,407,438,491,497). Prolonged polygraphic studies of some deefferented patients give variable results, including (a) complete loss or marked diminution of rapid-eye-movement (REM) sleep (314,497); (b) moderate to marked decrease in total sleep time, with loss of REM sleep (110,497) and diminished or normal percentage of REM sleep (149,165); and (c) preserved REM and NREM sleep with sleep architecture described as normal or nearly normal (110,276,314,358). The hypothesis that in most deefferented individuals altered sleep may be related to lesions interfering with the functions of the raphe nuclei in the pons and midbrain (165,314) has been called into question (358).

A review of the literature revealed that 60% of deefferented patients died. Among survivors, recovery was faster and more complete in individuals with nonvascular lesions (367).

Pathophysiological Mechanisms

The topography and reactivity of the alpha rhythm of most deefferented patients indicates that this is a preserved normal awake alpha rhythm rather than newly generated abnormal alpha activity such as characterizes anoxic and drug-intoxicated patients. In addition, the location of the pathology in deefferented individuals confirms the notion that, in humans, not only lesions transecting the brainstem up to the pontomesencephalic junction (337) but also extensive unilateral lesions of the midbrain and thalamus and discrete bilateral lesions of the midbrain (74,322,491) are compatible with a preserved alpha rhythm.

We conclude that the concept that the alpha rhythm that characterizes awake humans can occur in coma is wrong. A true alpha rhythm—usually predominant posteriorly, often reactive to eye opening, and frequently associated with photic driving—can occur in individuals with structural brain lesions that have rendered them mute and quadriplegic. These patients are unable to communicate except by eye movement, if at all, but can demonstrate normal mental function in appropriate circumstances. Thus they are deefferented rather than comatose. In contrast, rhythmic activity of alpha frequency, usually widely distributed but maximal over anterior areas and unreactive to alerting stimuli, appears in some truly comatose patients suffering from acute anoxic or toxic-metabolic encephalopathies. The general term *alpha coma* does not differentiate between these two fundamentally different groups of conditions.

In apparently unresponsive patients, demonstrating a posterior alpha rhythm such as characterizes awake normal subjects is of major importance. Provided psychogenic unresponsiveness is ruled out, such a finding suggests that these individuals may be aware of themselves and of the external environment, that is, that they may be deefferented rather than comatose (215). However, in some instances the alpha rhythm of deefferented patients lacks clear posterior predominance, reactivity to external alerting stimuli, or both. Similarly, in some individuals with anoxic or toxic-metabolic comas, alpha-frequency activity exhibits posterior preponderance, reactivity, or both (205,243,264). In these cases, the EEG gives no indication as to whether the patient's failure to respond is due to deefferentation or coma.

Evoked Potentials

Median nerve SL-SEP findings, known in a limited number of deefferented patients with or without pathologically controlled pontine infarcts, include the following: (a) normal responses to stimulation of either median nerve (144,463); (b) altered responses to the same stimulus (32); (c) abolished N$\overline{20}$ cortical component in response to stimulation of either

median nerve (351,463); and (d) N$\overline{20}$ potential preserved in response to stimulation of the median nerve or the fingers of one side but diminished in voltage and prolonged in latency in response to excitation of the same structures contralaterally, and similar findings with posterior tibial nerve stimulation. A report (355) described fully developed responses to stimulation of either median nerve shortly after onset of the locked-in syndrome in a patient also displaying an EEG alpha rhythm. As death neared and high-voltage delta activity developed, all response components disappeared except for a single positive wave. Autopsy demonstrated infarction of the rostral two-thirds of the basis pontis bilaterally with scattered ischemic lesions in the tegmentum.

In deefferented patients, BAEPs have been variously described as (a) normal (32,66,157,209,437,463); (b) abnormal (32,66,73,179,212,260,407, 433); (c) initially normal in response to stimulation of either ear but subsequently abnormal (65,260,433); and (d) initially abnormal with later return to normal (438). When present, BAEP abnormalities consisted of prolonged I–V IPIs (73,179,260,438) resulting from lengthened I–III (260) or III–V (65,179,407) intervals; prolonged latencies of all waves (260); and loss of all components, excluding (212,260) or including (65,260,441) wave I. Prolonged latencies and IPIs were frequently associated with diminished amplitudes and altered waveforms (441).

VEPs were elicited in a locked-in individual (79) and in an unresponsive, presumably completely deefferented patient with a pontine infarct and intact cerebrum (497). In one study, motor evoked potentials (MEPs) normally elicited in upper limb muscles by magnetic transcranial stimulation of the motor cortex were either absent or present in deefferented individuals, and these findings were related to motor recovery (32). In another work, MEPs were initially absent and subsequently normal on one side and present although altered in latency and amplitude contralaterally (144).

Highly heterogeneous results of auditory and somatosensory stimulations reflect the variability of the direct and indirect effects of the pathology causing the locked-in syndrome. Normal BAEPs and SL-SEPs suggest a lesion largely confined to the basis pontis and selectively interrupting the corticospinal pathways. In contrast, delayed or abolished BAEPs and SL-SEPs indicate extension into, or indirect effects on, auditory tracts and nuclei of the medial lemniscus. Preserved MEPs in paralyzed limbs may suggest reversible functional changes. Hence, EPs may help in understanding and evaluating deefferented patients, in whom it is difficult to assess the extent of sensory impairment and to forecast the likelihood of motor recovery. In addition, a P$\overline{300}$ (P$\overline{3}$) cognitive evoked potential (CEP) has been recorded in some locked-in patients (359). Unlike conventional sensory EPs, which primarily depend on the physical characteristics of the stimulus, long-latency CEPs elicited with particular "oddball" stimulus paradigms mostly reflect cerebral processing of incoming signals related to certain cognitive functions (i.e., higher cerebral activity; see Chapter 30). Demonstrating a P$\overline{300}$ was interpreted as evidence of "ongoing cognitive activity" (359). This information is valuable in individuals whose abilities to communicate are dramatically reduced, if not absent, although the P$\overline{300}$, like other CEPs, does not indicate to what extent full cognitive capacities are preserved or have been recovered (see "Cognitive Evoked Potentials" later in this chapter).

GOALS OF ELECTROPHYSIOLOGICAL TESTING IN COMATOSE STATES

The goals of EEG and EP studies of comatose patients generally include one or more of the following:

1. Providing objective measures of brain dysfunction
2. Determining the etiology of coma, specifically differentiating between toxic-metabolic causes and structural lesions
3. Localizing structural lesions, specifically differentiating between hemispheric and brainstem lesions and establishing the rostrocaudal level of brain dysfunction
4. Determining depth of coma and predicting clinical outcome
5. Following the course of comatose states
6. Distinguishing coma from diminished responsiveness resulting from seizure activity or psychogenic factors
7. Continuously monitoring brain function in the intensive care unit (ICU)

The availability of multiple potentially useful techniques requires that decisions should be made on the choice of the method, or combination of methods, best suited to each clinical situation. This decision demands a clear understanding of the strengths and weaknesses of each approach. The following generalizations are intended to help in this choice.

Providing Objective Measures of Brain Dysfunction

Because the EEG reflects cerebral cortical activity modulated by diencephalic and brainstem influences, it is potentially useful in providing measures of brain dysfunction in coma and other states of diminished responsiveness. However, these conditions are associated with a wide variety of EEG patterns that are not readily amenable to quantification. In contrast, EP measures can contribute exquisitely quantitative information on neural function at multiple levels within the brain that is well suited for statistical analysis and easily related to other physiological and clinical indices.

Establishing the Etiology of Coma: Differentiating between Toxic-Metabolic Causes and Structural Lesions

In rare instances, a single EEG can suggest the nature of the underlying disorder. For example, finding TWs may raise the suspicion of a metabolic encephalopathy, and the finding of fast intermixed with slow potentials suggests the possibility of drug intoxication. However, most EEG patterns provide no dependable information on the cause of coma. This lack of etiological specificity is perhaps best illustrated by noting that many EEG patterns, including burst-suppression, PGEDs, widespread unreactive activity of alpha or theta frequencies, low-voltage unreactive recordings, and ECI, may occur in patients rendered comatose by brain anoxia as well as in comatose individuals intoxicated by or treated with high doses of CNS depressants. Lack of specificity of individual EEGs is only partly overcome by serial recordings.

Even more than the EEG, EPs lack etiological specificity. However, when used with due caution, SL-SEPs and BAEPs can contribute to broadly differentiating between toxic-metabolic encephalopathies, in which they were traditionally believed to remain unchanged (348,439), and lesions involving the central somatosensory and auditory pathways, which abolish or markedly alter them. However, one should be aware that barbiturate concentrations substantially exceeding those commonly employed in ICUs (134), the intravenous administration of high doses of phenytoin (222,323), and the combined administration of two or more medications (170,320) may variously alter the latencies, amplitudes, and waveforms of both SL-SEPs and BAEPs. In addition, it has long been known that alcohol intoxication (426) and, especially, hypothermia (315,440) can cause prolongations of SL-SEP and BAEP latencies and IPIs that closely resemble those associated with certain structural lesions. Although most marked at esophageal temperatures below 32.5°C, alterations produced by hypothermia may already appear at temperatures as high as 35.5°C. In addition, quantifiable EP alterations occur in certain systemic metabolic derangements. Patients with chronic renal failure as a group demonstrate delayed pattern reversal and flash VEPs (104,375,394, 484), prolonged latencies of BAEPs with minimal but significant increases of I–V IPIs (375,483,484), and increased latencies of peripheral and central components of SL-SEPs with no central conduction time (CCT) changes (484). These alterations suggested both peripheral and central effects of chronic renal failure. In contrast, progressive prolongation and eventual loss of cortical components of median nerve SEPs of latency with increased IPIs, but normal CCTs, and unaltered BAEPs, characterized hepatic encephalopathy, suggesting dysfunction largely confined to the cerebral cortex (101,198,505).

The notion itself that SL-SEPs and BAEPs are abolished or markedly altered by structural lesions of the brainstem deserves critical consideration. These EP changes generally only occur with brainstem lesions sufficiently extensive to cause coma with loss of cephalic reflexes and spontaneous respiration that are most likely to involve somatosensory and auditory pathways. In contrast, SL-SEPs and BAEPs may persist and may be even normal in individuals with more discrete brainstem lesions causing clinical signs of less global brainstem dysfunction and sparing the somatosensory and auditory pathways (439).

Localizing Structural Lesions: Differentiating between Hemispheric and Brainstem Lesions and Determining Rostrocaudal Levels of Brain Dysfunction

Localization of lesions causing coma is most commonly achieved by neuroimaging techniques that are capable of depicting in detail most structural pathological processes. However, the EEG can provide some information on the location of cerebral hemispheric lesions, and EPs can help differentiate between cerebral hemispheric and brainstem lesions and determine level of dysfunction within the brainstem.

Unilateral loss or marked abnormality of the cortical N20 component of SL-SEPs is most commonly associated with hemispheric pathology, specifically focal lesions of the parietal cortex or thalamocortical radiations (320). Similarly, unequal ("asymmetrical") CCT prolongation favors primary hemispheric over brainstem pathology, whereas the opposite is true of bilaterally equal ("symmetrical") CCT prolongation (320). Loss of wave V of BAEPs, prolonged I–V and especially III–V IPIs, and diminished V:I amplitude ratio provide evidence of a brainstem lesion. In contrast, a recording showing loss of wave I and of all subsequent waves cannot differentiate

between lesion or dysfunction of peripheral auditory structures with substantially intact brainstem, loss of function of both peripheral and brainstem auditory pathways as can be seen with basilar artery occlusion, or global loss of function of peripheral, brainstem, and cerebral auditory structures as in brain death.

Broad relationships have been described between EEG patterns and clinically assessed levels of brain dysfunction in coma. Specifically, it has been reported that, as head-injured patients with central herniation syndrome undergo craniocaudal deterioration (370), the amount of widespread delta activity increases and the range of EEG patterns, the presence of alternating and sleep patterns, and the EEG reactivity to alerting stimuli diminish until slow EEG activity and finally ECI ensue (397,398).

Early studies suggested that, in individuals rendered comatose by severe head injury or acute anoxia, BAEP alterations were closely related to clinically assessed levels of dysfunction within the brainstem (427,469,470). However, less precise relationships were subsequently reported (274,321,466). In particular, Mauguière et al. (321) found that BAEPs persisted in patients with intact brainstem reflexes, whereas they disappeared in individuals in whom these reflexes were abolished. Closer relations between BAEP changes and levels of brainstem dysfunction could not be demonstrated. However, sequential, orderly loss of BAEP components generated at progressively lower levels of the brainstem were repeatedly observed in serial recordings of patients with clinical evidence of rostrocaudal deterioration culminating in brain death (197,406,427, 436,471) (Fig. 14.15).

FIG. 14.15. BAEPs in response to monaural clicks at 65 dB sound level in a patient who had suffered an anoxic episode. *D4* and *D10* refer to day of hospitalization. Two records were taken on days 7 and 8. On day 4, the patient was comatose but withdrew in response to noxious stimuli and had spontaneous respiration and preserved cephalic reflexes. One day earlier his EEG had shown widespread delta activity. On the seventh day, cephalic reflexes were no longer present, there was extensor posturing in response to noxious stimuli, and low-voltage delta activity was present in the EEG. Lack of spontaneous breathing and EEG demonstrating ECI were noted on day 8. On day 10, all responses to noxious stimuli were absent. The patient expired 14 days after admission. Sequential loss of BAEPs of progressively shorter latency paralleled the craniocaudal deterioration of the patient's clinical status. (Modified from Starr A. Auditory brain stem responses in brain death. *Brain* 1976;99:543–554.)

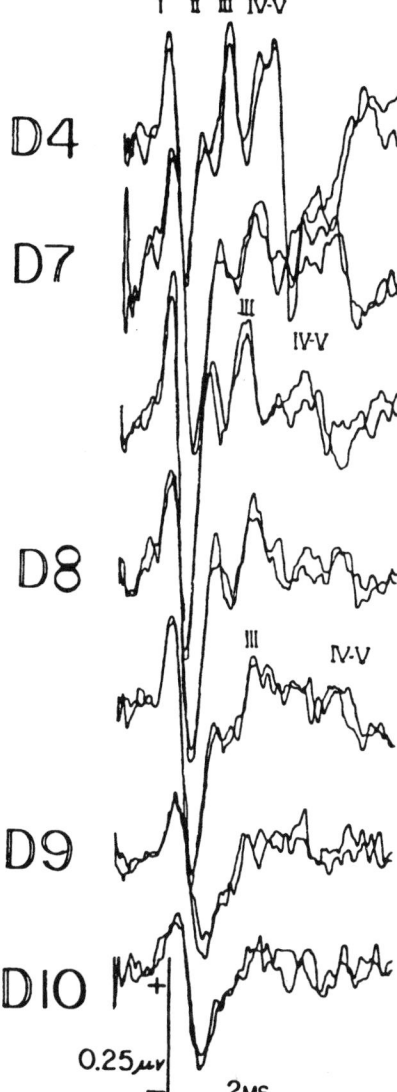

Determining Depth and Predicting Clinical Outcome of Coma

The EEG as a Measure of Depth of Coma and a Predictor of Outcome

Early work established that broad relationships exist between EEG patterns and reactivity to alerting stimuli and clinically assessed depth of coma, but recognized that discrepancies between these features were often observed (20,159). More controversial is the notion, discussed earlier in this chapter, that some particular EEG patterns displayed by unresponsive patients, such as sleep patterns and activities of alpha frequency, can predict clinical outcome.

Some studies reported signifcant statistical associations between graded EEG abnormality and final clinical status of comatose adults (31,59,91,223, 265a,377,380,396,405,453,454,468,504,513,513a,513b) as well as neonates and children (410a). Of special interest is Prior's (377) early study of patients with comas of various, but mostly anoxic, etiologies. She found 85% concordance between the first EEG rating and clinical outcome, and computer-aided discriminant function analysis of large numbers of variables further increased prognostic accuracy. Subsequent work suggested that, in individuals rendered comatose by acute brain anoxia, mild, graded EEG abnormalities were predictive of survival (91,405,454,468,504). There is widespread agreement at present that in anoxic comas the most severe grades of abnormality, such as ECI, burst suppression, and delta activity of very low voltage show strong statistical association with death or a vegetative state. Mortalities of 81–98% have been reported among patients demonstrating these extreme EEG alterations (26,31,91,396,453,468,513a,513b,514). In contrast, the belief that in anoxic comas, mild, graded EEG abnormalities were predictive of favorable outcome (91,405,454,468,504) has met with skepticism (31,396,410a).

Some investigators focused on posttraumatic coma and found strong statistical associations between graded EEG alterations and ultimate clinical state (59,263,379,380,398,454), but a report contended that this relation only applied to recordings of ECI and other severely abnormal EEGs (236). Other studies emphasized the preeminent importance of EEG reactivity to alerting stimuli in forecasting outcome of coma resulting from head injury (9,203,236) or anoxia (264). In a small series, all postanoxic comatose patients with nonreactive alpha-frequency rhythms in their EEGs died (264). We believe that EEG reactivity may deserve more attention in the study of coma than it has received so far. However, determining the presence or absence of reactivity in retrospectively reviewed EEGs carries some imprecision. This phenomenon is influenced to a considerable degree by the tenacity of the technologist seeking to demonstrate it and the type and intensity of stimuli delivered, which are difficult to standardize in routine examinations. The frequent occurrence of noises in busy ICUs and the possible existence of major sensory deficits in the patients may also variously interfere with the assessment of EEG reactivity (198).

The prognostic relevance of computer analyses of the EEGs of comatose patients (9,263,458) warrants further study.

Evoked Potentials as Predictors of Outcome

Somatosensory Evoked Potentials

Abnormalities of median nerve SEPs the prognostic value of which has been investigated in comatose patients, include (a) bilateral loss of the N$\overline{20}$ early cortical potential (b) bilateral preservation of the N$\overline{20}$ potential (c) unilateral loss of the N$\overline{20}$ potential and (d) prolonged somatosensory central conduction time, and (e) alterations of the middle- and long-latency SEPs.

Bilateral loss of the early cortical potential N$\overline{20}$ (or N$\overline{20}$-P$\overline{27}$ complex) with preservation of peripheral N$\overline{9}$, spinal N$\overline{13}$, brainstem P$\overline{14}$ and subcortical N$\overline{18}$ (Fig. 14.16) indicates severe cortical dysfunction. Abolition of the N$\overline{20}$ potential bilaterally has been reported in patients rendered comatose by severe brain anoxia (6,26,31,67,68,91,184,310,354,395,396,396a,508, 513,514,514a), head trauma (26,35,137,204,227,256,396a) (Fig. 18.3), nontraumatic (116,169), and miscellaneous (95,168,185,505) etiologies. Its prognostic value of this finding varies depending on the etiology of coma.

Meta-analyses of the literature have determined that 100% of adults who demonstrate bilaterally absent N$\overline{20}$ potential within 48 hours (31) or 1 week (514a) of onset of coma caused by brain anoxia die or remain vegetative. Their brains disclose widespread ischemic changes of of cerebral (396a) and cerebellar cortices and thalamus (68). In the available literature, only three patients who were comatose following cardiac arrest occurring during anesthesia (197) or heroin overdose (265a) (Kaplan, personal commnuication) and demonstrated bilateral extinction of the N$\overline{20}$ potential regained con-

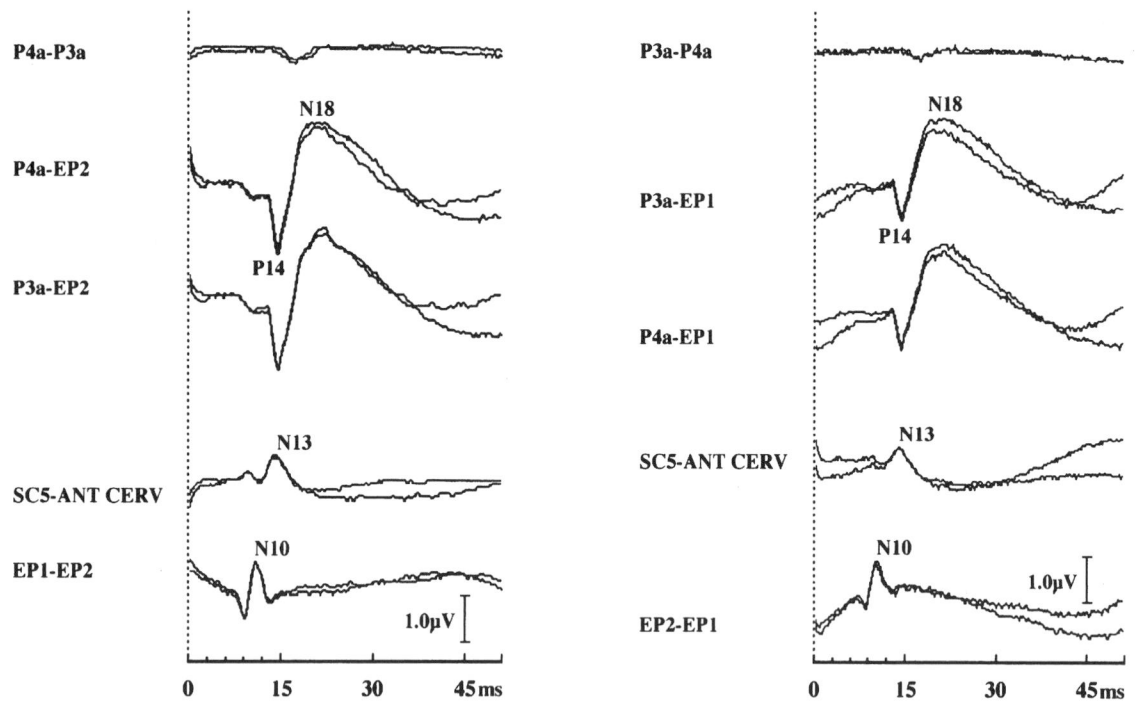

FIG. 14.16. SL-SEPs in response to electrical stimulation of the left **(A)** and right **(B)** median nerves. Electrode P4a (right postcentral) was halfway between standard positions P4 and C4 while electrode P3a (left postcentral) was midway between standard positions P3 and C3. In A and B, recordings demonstrate Erb's point N$\overline{10}$, spinal N$\overline{13}$, brainstem P$\overline{14}$ and bilateral subcortical N$\overline{18}$ potentials but no N$\overline{20}$ contralateral cortical response. Same patient as in Figure 14.3.

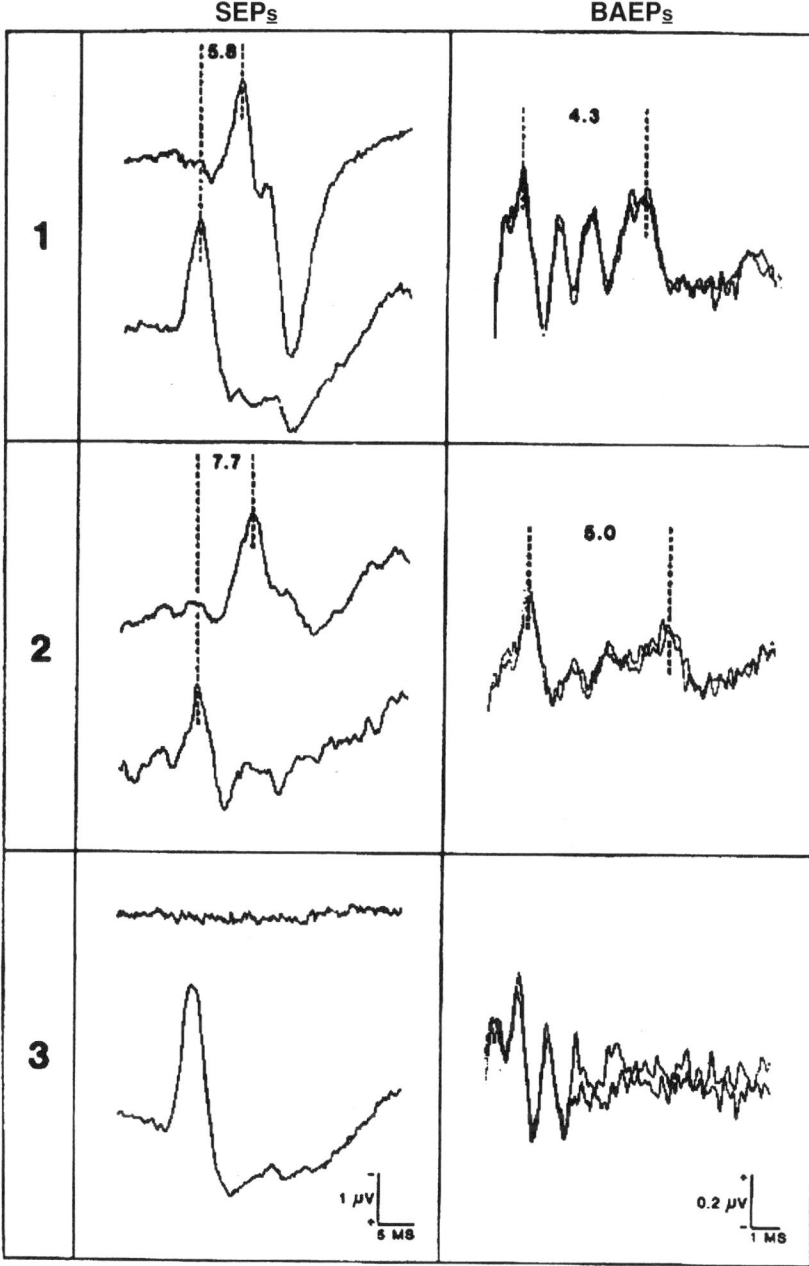

SEPs

BAEPs

1

2

3

FIG. 14.17. Median nerve SEPs and BAEPs recorded in three patients within 4 days of onset of posttraumatic coma. SEPs 1–3 were recorded over the contralateral central scalp (**top**) and the second cervical vertebra (**bottom**) using a mid-forehead reference. BAEPs 1–3 were detected between the vertex and the ipsilateral earlobe. Grade 1 SEPs demonstrated normal $N\overline{13}$-$N\overline{20}$ CCT and grade 1 BAEPs showed normal I–V CCT. Grade 2 SEPs and BAEPs were characterized by abnormally prolonged CCTs. Grade 3 responses displayed lack of $N\overline{20}$ potentials of SEPs and wave V of BAEPs. In this study, graded SEPs but not graded BAEPs reliably predicted both bad and good outcomes. (Modified from Cant BR, Hume AL, Judson JA, et al. The assessment of severe head injury by short-latency somatosensory and brain-stem auditory evoked potentials. *Electroencephalogr Clin Neurophysiol* 1986;65:188–195.)

sciousness, two with abnormal neurological function (197). Hence, in adults with coma caused by severe brain anoxia, bilateral obliteration of the $N\overline{20}$ potential is virtually 100% specific for death or vegetative survival. However substantial numbers of patients rendered comatose by severe brain anoxia who die or remain vegetative demonstrate variously preserved, rather than bilaterally abolished, $N\overline{20}$ potential. Specifically, the sensitivity of bilateral obliteration of the $N\overline{20}$ response to these unfavorable outcomes varied from 28% to 73% in different series of individuals in post-anoxic coma (514a). Additional studies are needed to confirm that bilateral loss of the $N\overline{20}$ potential also predicts death or vegetative survival in children and infants who suffered severe anoxic insults (163a,410a).

Bilaterally absent $N\overline{20}$ potential has lower predictive value in comas related to causes other than brain anoxia. About 90% of patients with coma of traumatic origin (396a) or of predominantly traumatic or cerebrovascular origin (320) who had bilaterally extinguished $N\overline{20}$ potential died or became vegetative. Most of the remaining individuals had severe neurologic disabilities, but few recovered fully and showed gradual restoration of the $N\overline{20}$ response (197).

According to recent guidelines for the practice of EEG and EPs (198), in patients with alpha coma unrelated to sedative drugs, bilateral loss of the $N\overline{20}$ potential would be associated with lack of recovery, whereas preservation of this response would presage a favorable outcome. Evidence substantiating this belief is desirable.

One should be aware that bilateral loss of $N\overline{20}$ potential may be caused by a reversible brainstem lesion or a preexisting neurological condition involving the somatosensory pathways (320) and occasionally it may be mimicked by bilateral subdural hematomas (35).

Comatose individuals with *bilaterally preserved N20 (and P27) potentials* (whether normal or delayed) have variable outcomes that are strongly influenced by the etiology of their condition (15,31,68,91,189,233,234, 295,309,319,396,396a,401,484). Pooling data from various series (396a) indicates that 64% of patients who were comatose after suffering severe anoxia but retained the N20 potential bilaterally died or remained vegetative as opposed to 22% of individuals who demonstrated the same pattern while comatose following head trauma. The remaining patients regained consciousness, most of them with various degrees of neurologic disability. In another review, 35% of individuals with comas of predominantly traumatic or cerebrovascular origin (320) and bilaterally demonstrable N20 potential died, remained vegetative, or had severe neurological neurologic defects.

It appears that the prognosis of coma is more hopeful in patients with bilaterally preserved N20 potential than in individuals in whom this response is bilaterally absent, but carries considerable uncertainty and is strongly influenced by the etiology of coma. Abnormally prolonged latency of bilaterally preserved N20 has been said to decrease substantially the probability of favorable outcome (396a).

Unilateral loss of the N20 (and P27) potential most commonly results from damage to the parietal cortex, the thalamo-parietal radiations, or both (320) whereas it is rare in comas caused by brain anoxia. Pooling published results revealed that 74% of patients with comas of mostly traumatic or cerebrovascular origin who had unilateral obliteration of the N20 potential remained vegetative or severely neurologically disabled whereas 26% had moderate disability or good recovery (320). Similar unfavorable outcomes characterized a substantial portion of patients with comas of various etiologies who demonstrated unilaterally abolished N20 response (94,485).

Determining loss or preservation of cortical SEPs in comatose patients requires sound technique. This should be designed to detect responses generated at several levels from sensory periphery to cerebral cortex, and to differentiate between subcortically generated N18 and early cortical N20 potentials (14a) (Fig. 14.16). In addition, interpretation of test results demands intimate knowledge of temporal and spatial features, and putative sources of each response component.

Initial studies (233) reported that, within 3½ days after head injury, the spinal N13–cortical N20 IPI or *somatosensory "central conduction time"* (232) correctly predicted outcome measured by the Glasgow Outcome Scale (GOS) (250) in 78% of patients. In successive examinations performed up to 500 days after onset of coma, CCT predicted final state in 84% of individuals. This measure recovered exponentially over many months, although differences persisted between patients with good recovery and disabled individuals. The association between CCT and outcome was confirmed by subsequent investigations of comas resulting from various causes, including brain anoxia (15,142,146,203,256,262,294,304,310,400,401,485). However, the strength of this relationship varied in different reports. Lumping the results of several studies of coma of predominantly traumatic or cerebrovascular origin determined that a prolonged CCT was associated with death, vegetative state, or severe neurological disability in 58.5% of patients, whereas the remaining 41.5% demonstrated moderate disability or good recovery (320). Some authors concluded that CCT measurement improved only minimally the predictive power of SL-SEPs (294) and was of little clinical value (294,310). In contrast, other investigators pointed out that serial CCT measurements predicted final status more reliably than did single measurements during the acute stage of coma (233,234,349,401).

A few reports (111,197) suggested that additional information of prognostic value could be obtained in coma by including in the SEP analysis one or more cortical components topographically distinct from the parietal N20-P27 complex, specifically the centrofrontal P22, the central P45, and the frontocentral N60 potentials (124,125,204,205). These components are best demonstrated by sequential mapping techniques (see Chapter 24).

Extending the analysis to include *middle-latency and long-latency SEPs (ML-SEPs and LL-SEPs)* in the 30- to 200-millisecond latency range was said to substantially increase the predictive power of median nerve SEPs (118,189,295,309,369,401). Normal potentials with these latencies were associated with good recovery or moderate disability in 86% of patients with coma of predominantly traumatic or cerebrovascular origins. Only 14% of these individuals died, remained vegetative, or demonstrated severe disability (320). In contrast, because ML-SEPs and LL-SEPs were highly variable and were altered by sedative drugs, their absence had little prognostic significance (320).

Auditory Evoked Potentials

BAEP findings most commonly considered in prognosticating the outcome of comatose states include (a) absence of all BAEPs following wave I or waves I and II, (b) absence of wave V or waves III and V, and (c) normal BAEPs.

Bilateral absence of all BAEPs following wave I or waves I and II strongly predicts an unfavorable outcome irrespective of etiology

(15,55,172,185,259,267,304,360,406,466,471). In a review of several studies, 98.2% of patients with coma of traumatic or cerebrovascular origin who displayed this abnormality died or remained vegetative, and the remaining 1.8% survived with severe disability (320). Nevertheless, the possibility of a preexisting neurological condition causing dysfunction of the brainstem auditory pathways should always be considered and investigated.

Bilateral or even unilateral absence (or extreme amplitude reduction) of wave V (or waves III and V) with preserved wave I in a comatose patient presages almost invariably death or a vegetative state, much as does the absence of all BAEP components (15,26,70,267,294,366).

According to some authors, *abnormally prolonged I–V IPIs* (see Fig. 14.17) are associated with variable outcome of coma (185,263,304,360, 471,502), whereas closer associations of this measure to the patient's final state were reported by others (111,458). Other investigators reported empirically determining cutoff values of I–V (145,401,424) and III–V (401) IPIs, which allowed discrimination between individuals who succumbed or remained severely disabled and those with more favorable outcomes. The III–V IPI ("auditory brainstem conduction time") was found to be an especially valuable measure, unaffected by peripheral auditory disorders (401).

Normal BAEPs recorded during the acute phase of coma of traumatic or cerebrovascular origin were associated with good recovery or mild neurological sequelae in about 70% of patients, but death, a vegetative state, or severe disability occurred in the remaining 30% of individuals studied by various authors (320). These unfavorable outcomes also characterize a substantial proportion of patients who display normal BAEPs in the acute period of anoxic coma (90,122,393). In contrast, persistently normal BAEPs following this period would indicate increased likelihood of survival (126,188,406), at least in the absence of hemispheric lesions such as intracerebral hemorrhage or hemorrhagic infarction (171).

Several authors extended their search for prognostically useful indicators to middle-latency and long-latency auditory evoked potential (AEP) components *(ML-AEPs and LL-AEPs)* (156,158,190,208,259,295). These studies indicated that demonstration of a normal Pa component of ML-AEPs strongly predicted return of consciousness (158). However, this potential was detected in only few patients (158) and was very vulnerable to CNS depressants. Similarly, presence of $\overline{N100}$ (158,198) and $\overline{P200}$ (198) LL-AEP components was significantly associated with recovery of consciousness. In contrast, absence of ML-AEPs or LL-AEPs had no prognostic value.

VEPs and MEPs

Except for some early studies (41,486), most investigations of the prognostic value of EPs in coma have used VEPs primarily in conjunction with other EPs. Normal compound MEPs in response to transcranial magnetic stimulation of the motor cortex did not reliably predict good outcome (517), and absent MEPs were even significantly associated with false pessimistic predictions (142).

Multimodality Evoked Potentials

EP testing of two or more sensory modalities (multimodality evoked potentials [MMEPs]) yields greater prognostic power than does the examination of a single modality. In early prospective investigations of severely head-injured patients, Greenberg et al. (188) graded SEPs, AEPs, and VEPs on a 4-point scale according to the number of wave peaks detected, with grades I–IV indicating increasing loss of peaks. One to 7 days after injury, only SEPs were significantly associated ($p < 0.001$) with clinical outcome graded according to the GOS (250). Specifically, patients with grade I–II SEP abnormalities had 90% probability of good recovery or only moderate disability. Eight to 30 days after trauma, BAEPs also showed significant but weaker association with outcome ($p < 0.005$). VEPs correlated least with the patient's final state. Graded MMEPs predicted outcome even 1 year after injury with about 80% accuracy (188). Combining these three-modality EPs yielded 91% correct predictions with no falsely pessimistic errors. These findings indicated that the prognostic power of MMEPs exceeded that of the clinical data, the computed tomography scan, and the intracranial pressure (345). However, other investigations concluded that MMEPs improved only slightly the predictions based on clinical indices (295). Several studies confirmed that SEPs provided earlier and more accurate prognostic information in traumatic coma than did AEPs (15,146,295,382), whereas the value of VEPs remained controversial (90,152,445).

Joint SEP-AEPs with or without VEPs were said to be good predictors of outcome not only in traumatic comas but also in comas caused by brain anoxia (30,196,197,422) and intracerebral hemorrhage (143,146). In an individual study, BAEPs and brainstem trigeminal potentials jointly allowed 84% correct predictions, which increased to 93% when clinical data were included (424). Combined SL-SEPs–MEPs were found by some to improve outcome prediction and to facilitate the assessment of sensorimotor dysfunction (142).

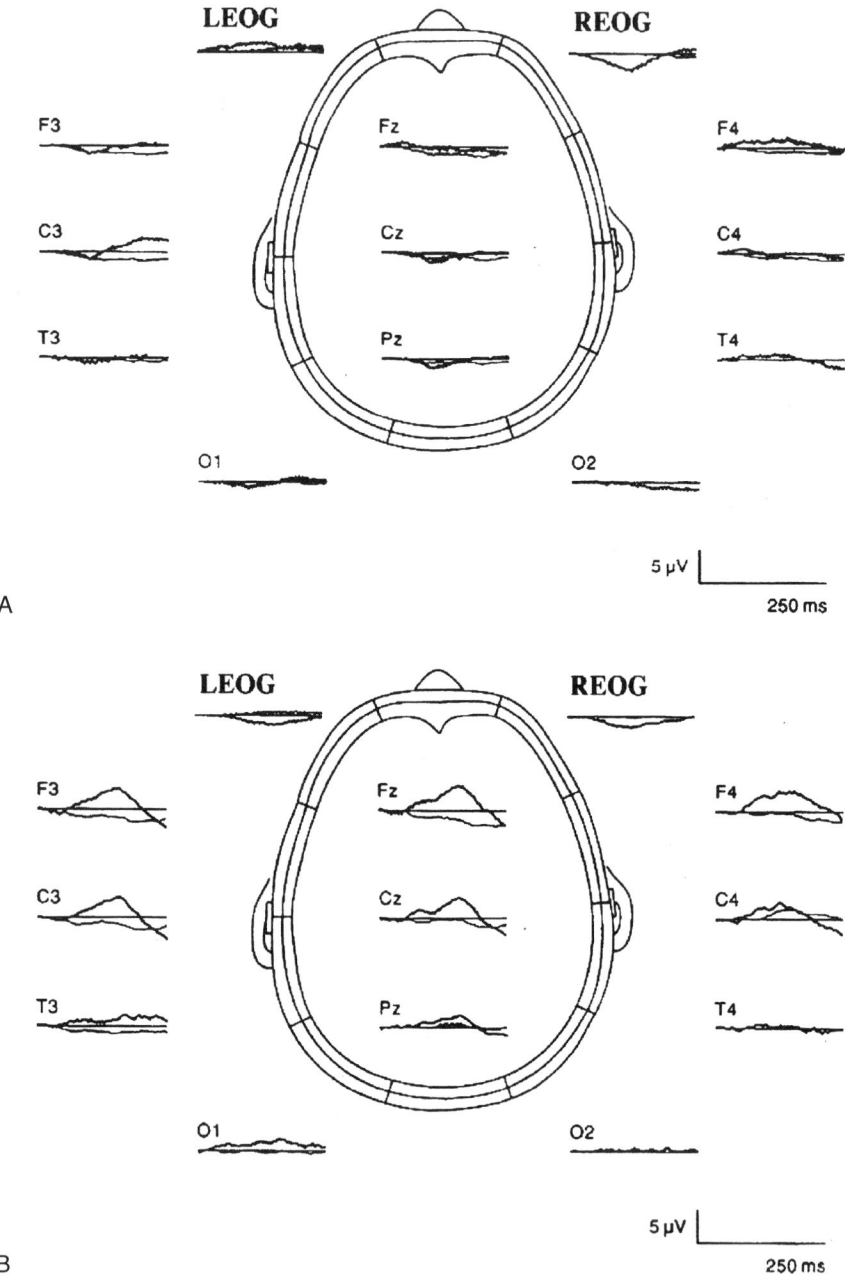

However, others contended that joint SL-SEPs–MEPs as well as SL-SEPs–BAEPs added only minimally to the prognostic value of the neurological examination (294) or were even inferior to it (380,506).

Guérit et al. (197) have developed two graded indices of brain function: an index of global cortical function (IGCF) based on presence or absence and latency of VEP and SEP components, and an index of brainstem conduction based on IPIs of BAEP and SEP. Unfavorable outcome was predicted by both indices in traumatic coma and by the IGCF in anoxic coma, whereas neither measure proved adequate to prognosticate favorable outcome.

Cognitive Evoked Potentials

Several authors have succeeded in eliciting long-latency CEPs in comatose patients. A P$\overline{300}$-like wave was recorded in individuals with comas of various etiologies (158,186,262,343,412,507), but the proportion of patients with this response who recovered consciousness varied in these studies from 50% to 100%.

Of special interest is the demonstration of another CEP, the "mismatch negativity" (MMN) (Fig. 14.18B), in the initial examination of a proportion (22%–42%) of comatose individuals (158,261,262) most of whom (91%–100%) regained consciousness within 1 or more days (158,261,262), averaging 6.3 days in one study (158). A highly significant association was found between the latency of the MMN and the 90-day outcome (262). In contrast, the absence of MMN in the initial examination of comatose patients was followed by death or lack of recovery of consciousness in a variable proportion of individuals (32%–76%) (158,261,262). When serially studied, most of the remaining patients with no initially demonstrable MMN who subsequently developed this response regained consciousness (261) (Fig. 14.18A and B). Similar results were reported in the study of a highly variable positive–negative CEP complex detected acutely in a small proportion of comatose patients (199).

It appears that the detection of a MMN predicts awakening from coma with a degree of specificity that substantially exceeds that of other CEPs. However,

FIG. 14.18. A: Absent MMN response in an unconscious patient (Glasgow Coma Scale [GCS] score = 4) following severe head injury. **B:** Subsequent manifestation of this response in the same comatose individual (GCS score = 5) prior to the recovery of consciousness. (Modified from Kane NM, Curry SH, Rowlands CA, et al. Event-related potentials—neurophysiological tools for predicting emergence and early outcome from traumatic coma. *Intensive Care Med* 1996;22:39–46.)

a relatively limited number of comatose patients display this response in their initial examination when prognostication of outcome is most needed, and somewhat elaborate techniques are required to demonstrate it beyond doubt (158). In addition, the detection of a MMN provides no information on the quality of functional recovery as well as the restoration of full cognitive capacities (158,261). Thus, in ordinary clinical circumstances, eliciting a MMN (as other CEPs) may provide intriguing insights into disordered brain functions in comatose states but is of questionable practicality.

Summary and Conclusions

Of all electrophysiological measures investigated, bilateral obliteration of the earliest cortical response to median nerve stimulation, the $N\overline{20}$ (or $N\overline{20}$-$P\overline{27}$ complex) during the first week of coma has emerged as the most reliable predictor of unfavorable outcome in patients rendered comatose by acute, severe brain anoxia: virtually 100% of these individuals who demonstrate bilateral loss of the $N\overline{20}$ potential die or remain vegetative (514). However, a meta-analysis of the available literature (514) indicates that, following severe brain anoxia, absence of the pupillary light reflex or motor responses to noxious stimuli predicts death or vegetative survival with the same specificity as the bilateral absence of the $N\overline{20}$ potential, although with a slightly lower sensitivity (531). It follows that, when either or both of these clinical signs are demonstrated 72 hours after onset of anoxic coma (514a), bilateral loss of the $N\overline{20}$ potential strongly confirms the clinical prediction of unfavorable outcome but is largely redundant (278). In contrast, demonstrating bilateral abolition of the $N\overline{20}$ potential provides valuable information on the likelihood of death or vegetative survival when conditions exist that limit or preclude the clinical examination, such as facial or other injuries or the effects of sedative or paralyzing drugs. However, caution should be exercised in using individual neurophysiological prognostic indices in isolation to justify the withdrawal of supportive measures (31,514a). Combinations of clinical, neurophysiologic, and other indices may increase the accuracy of prediction of outcome from anoxic coma in the future (514a).

As opposed to the utility of bilaterally extinguished $N\overline{20}$ potential in prognosticating death or vegetative survival in post-anoxic coma, no electrophysiological measure allows at present confident prognostication of unfavorable outcome from comas due to causes other than anoxia, or of favorable outcome from coma of any etiology. Overcoming these limitations is a major challenge for future investigations.

Following the Evolution of Comatose States

Although EEGs, EPs, and CEPs potentials can be useful in following the evolution of comatose states, prompt assessment and management of rapidly evolving comas requires continuously monitoring the EEG, EPs, and systemic functions, often combined with each other. Continuous electrophysiological monitoring in the ICU is reviewed in Chapter 25.

Distinguishing Coma from Other Conditions of Diminished Responsiveness

This chapter has already described EEG features that help distinguish comatose from locked-in states. Other potentially confounding conditions include frequent seizure activity and psychogenic unresponsiveness. In some instances, frequent seizure activity is responsible for or contributes to the patient's diminished responsiveness, and may cause additional brain damage, especially in patients with borderline cerebral perfusion. This ictal activity may be associated with minimal or no detectable clinical manifestations, especially when paralyzing agents are used. Thus its demonstration by EEG, especially continuous monitoring, is crucially important in devising the appropriate treatment and preventing complications. In contrast, EPs are not helpful in detecting epileptic activity (79,198).

Psychogenic unresponsiveness is said to account for 1% of comas "of unknown etiology" (370). A normal EEG with a well-developed alpha rhythm attenuated by sensory stimuli more likely suggests psychogenic, rather than structural or metabolic, causes (370). However, faced with such an EEG, one must take care to exclude a deefferented state mimicking coma. Moreover, the EEGs of psychogenically unresponsive patients may show changes caused by psychotropic and other drugs. EPs may also contribute to differentiation between psychogenic and structural causes of diminished responsiveness.

ELECTROPHYSIOLOGICAL EVALUATION OF OTHER STATES OF DIMINISHED RESPONSIVENESS

Selective Failure of Forebrain or Brainstem Function

The "irreversible loss of function of the brain, including the brain stem" characterizes brain death (389). However, failure may involve the forebrain,

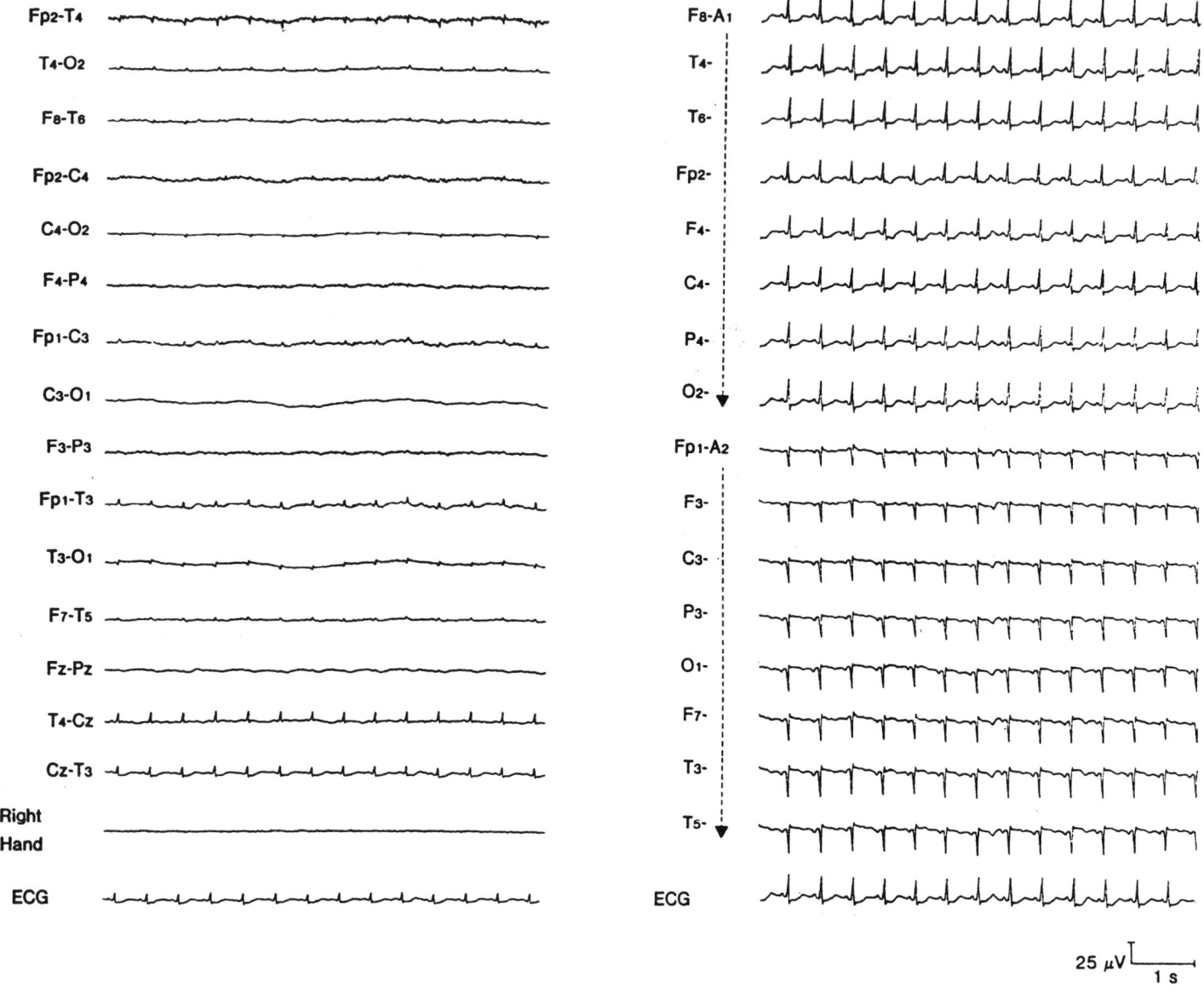

FIG. 14.19. ECI in a 45-year-old woman 3 days after an episode of ventricular fibrillation following coronary artery bypass graft. The patient was comatose with no withdrawal responses to noxious stimuli and was artificially ventilated but exhibited intermittent spontaneous respiration and intact brainstem reflexes. She died 6 days later. Her brain demonstrated pseudolaminar necrosis of the whole cerebral cortex and necrosis of other forebrain structures, with relative preservation of brainstem and spinal cord. (Modified from Wytrzes LM, Chatrian G-E, Shaw C-M, et al. Acute failure of forebrain with sparing of brain stem function: electroencephalographic, multimodality evoked potentials, and pathologic findings. *Arch Neurol* 1989;46:93–97.)

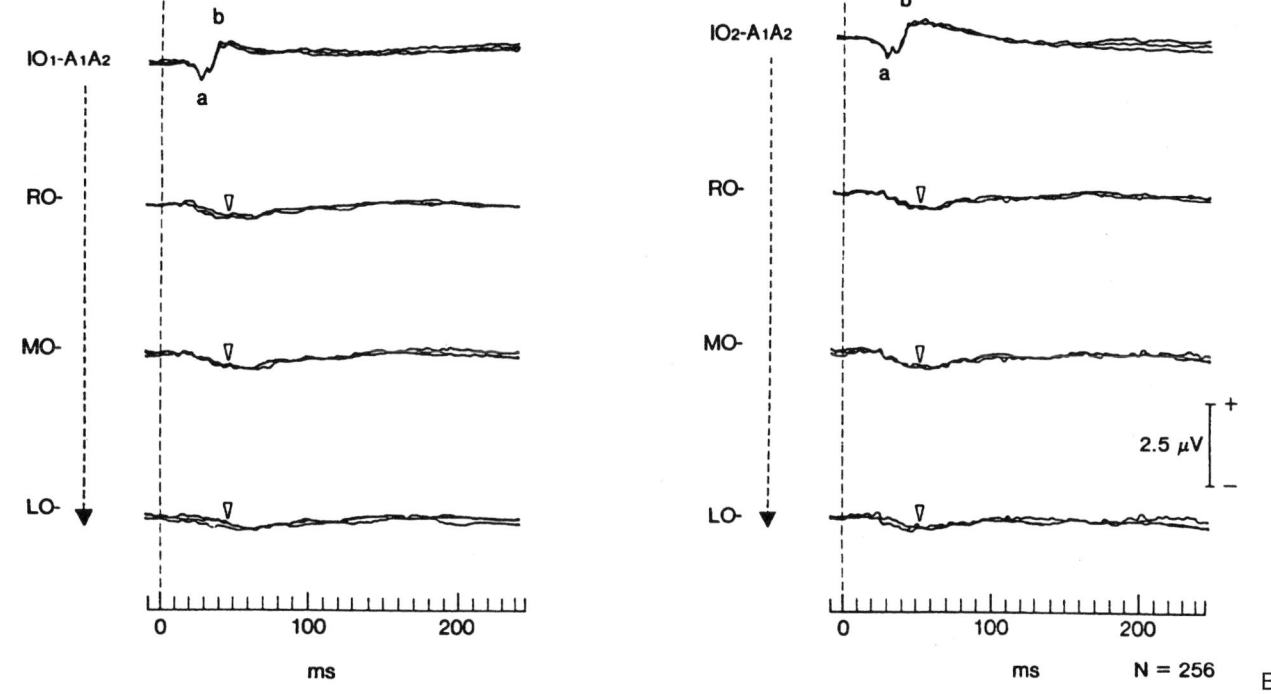

FIG. 14.20. Retinal, but no cerebral, responses to flash stimulation of the left **(A)** and right **(B)** eyes in the same patient as in Figure 14.19. ERGs (waves *a* and *b*) were detected between left (*Io1*) and right (*IO2*) infraorbital electrodes and linked earlobe reference (*A1A2*). Slow downgoing potential (*clear arrows*) in recordings from right (*RO*), midline (*MO*), and left (*LO*) occipital electrodes was interpreted as an ERG detected by the A1-A2 reference. SL-SEPs showed similar abolition of cortical N20 potential with preserved brainstem P14 and spinal N13 components. Same patient as in Figure 14.19. (Modified from Wytrzes LM, Chatrian G-E, Shaw C-M, et al. Acute failure of forebrain with sparing of brain stem function: electroencephalographic, multimodality evoked potentials, and pathologic findings. *Arch Neurol* 1989;46:93–97.)

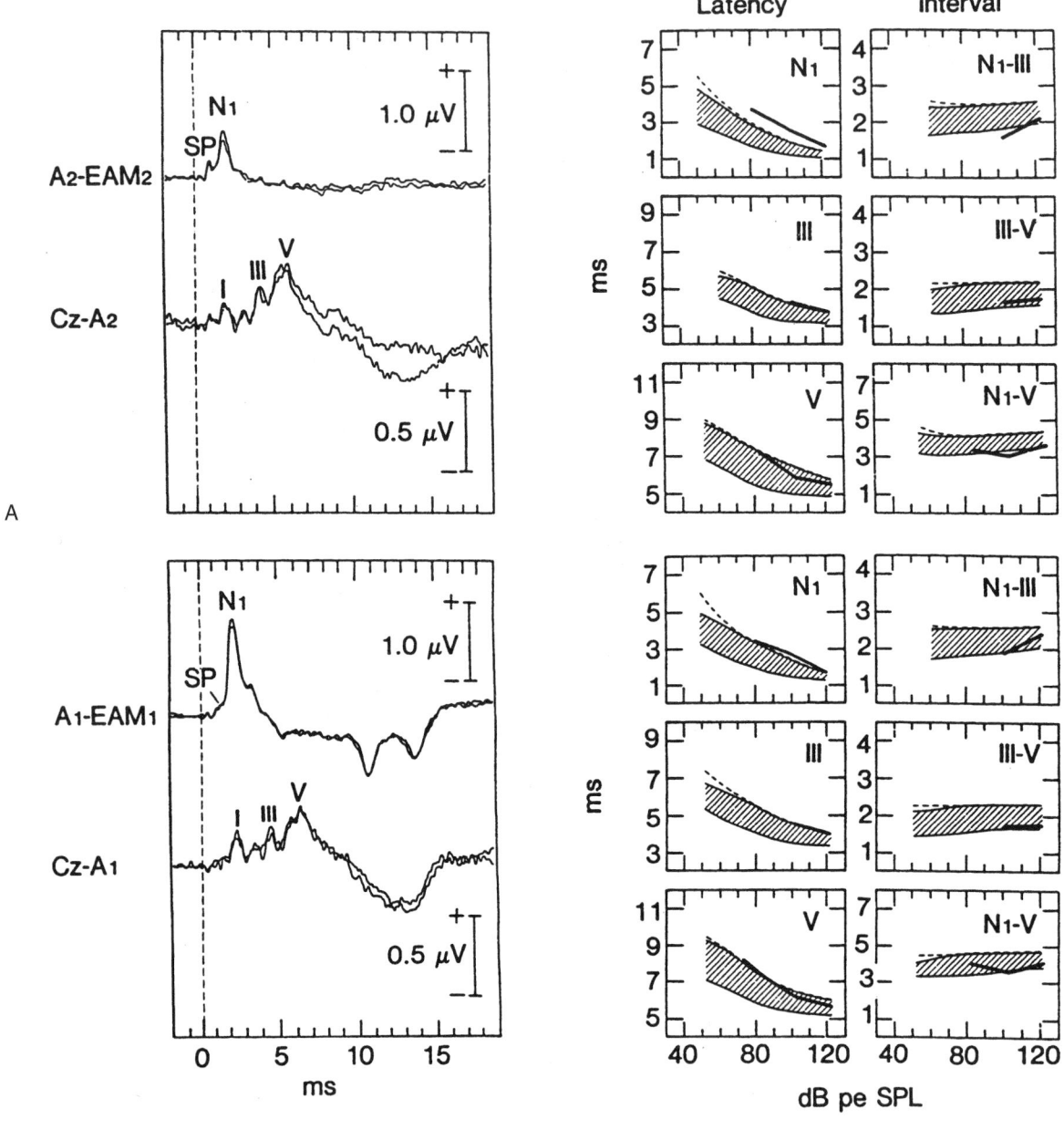

FIG. 14.21. Electrocochleograms (ECochGs) (*top trace*) and BAEPs (*bottom trace*) in response to stimulation of right **(A)** and left **(C)** ears with clicks of alternating polarity at 120 dB sound pressure level and dB peak-equivalent sound pressure level (pe SPL) of 8.3 per second. *EAM2* and *EAM1*, right and left auditory meatuses. **B** and **D:** Plots of latency– and interval–intensity functions for major response components shown in **A** and **C**, respectively. *Shaded areas*, 2 standard deviations; *dashed lines*, 95% tolerance limits for 95% of normal population of the same age; *heavy solid lines*, functions computed in this patient. All IPIs were within normal limits. Same patient as in Figures 14.19 and 14.20. (Modified from Wytrzes LM, Chatrian G-E, Shaw C-M, et al. Acute failure of forebrain with sparing of brain stem function: electroencephalographic, multimodality evoked potentials, and pathologic findings. *Arch Neurol* 1989;46: 93–97.)

with substantially preserved brainstem function, or, conversely, it may involve the brainstem with relative sparing of the forebrain. Clinical states resulting from these failures differ from brain death.

Acute Forebrain Failure (Cortical Death)

Patients studied shortly after resuscitation sometimes have acute failure of the forebrain with variable sparing of brainstem function (501) or "cortical death," described in earlier publications as "neocortical death" (60,333,395), "partial brain death" (372), and "apallic syndrome" (238). This condition, characterized by deep coma with variably preserved brainstem reflexes, differs from vegetative states (251,340) that result from chronic forebrain failure and are manifested by alternating wakefulness and sleep without cognitive awareness. However, acute forebrain failure may evolve into a vegetative state (240).

The EEGs of patients with acute forebrain failure most commonly demonstrate an EEG pattern of ECI (Fig. 14.19) or slow activating of very low voltage. Occasionally they display widespread, frontally dominant alpha activity or burst-suppression later evolving into ECI (60,239,395,501).

EP findings are variable. Median nerve–elicited cortical $\overline{N20}$-$\overline{P27}$ ($\overline{P25}$) potentials are abolished bilaterally in some subjects (68,69,184,395,485, 501). In other individuals, $\overline{N20}$ is present and normal bilaterally but the subsequent $\overline{P27}$ ($\overline{P25}$) component may be normal, altered, or absent (67, 68,137,184,485,501). In the majority of cases, the $\overline{P14}$ brainstem potential is preserved (68). Pathological changes in these patients are variable. In individuals with normal cortical SL-SEPs, histological lesions are commonly restricted to Sommer's sector of the hippocampus (CA1) and Purkinje cells of the cerebellum, which are known to be highly vulnerable to anoxia (67,68). In contrast, the brains of individuals with no recordable cortical SL-SEPs demonstrate anoxic-ischemic alterations involving diffusely cerebral cortex, thalamus, and cerebellum with no or with minor brainstem and spinal cord changes (184,395,501). An exception is the finding of a structurally normal brain in one patient who died few hours after cardiac arrest (184). It thus appears that the variability of cortical SL-SEPs in patients with acute forebrain failure closely reflects the extent and severity of anoxic damage, which, in turn, partly depends on the duration of survival after onset of coma. The predilection of the pathology for the hippocampus is somewhat difficult to reconcile with the appellation "neocortical death" (60). The term *cortical death* describes more accurately this condition.

Generally, no cerebral VEPs can be elicited in patients with acute forebrain failure (Fig. 14.20), whereas BAEPs are most commonly normal (395,501) (Fig. 14.21). The occasional finding in these individuals of absent BAEPs, including wave I, and preserved cortical SL-SEPs suggests hypoxic cochlear damage, precluding the activation and assessment of central auditory pathways (67).

Brainstem Failure (Brainstem Death)

Cases described in the literature as "brainstem " (121,392) or "rhombencephalic" (440) death mostly consisted of individuals who had lesions transecting the brainstem at the pontine level but sparing the midbrain, preserved EEG, and loss of BAEPs. Because these individuals were completely deefferented, it is impossible to determine clinically whether they were comatose or totally locked-in (i.e., aware of stimuli but unable to respond) (34,497).

On occasion, whole-brain death may be mimicked by a lesion destroying the reticular core of the midbrain and causing unresponsiveness and brainstem deficits. Ingvar and co-workers (240,241) described a patient whose acute unresponsiveness evolved into persistent coma culminating in death. In this individual, initial "general depression" of the EEG with unilaterally preserved alpha activity was followed by the development of widespread low-voltage delta waves associated with markedly reduced hemispheric blood flow and cerebral oxygen consumption. Cortical biopsy 18 months after onset of unresponsiveness showed no neuronal loss. Pathological findings 17 months later included a cystic hemorrhagic lesion in the dorsal midbrain destroying most of the periaqueductal gray matter, an infarct in the right posterior thalamus and the adjacent areas of the internal capsule and globus pallidus, and marked cortical atrophy with laminar loss of nerve cells. The authors hypothesized that nearly complete destruction of the midbrain reticular core severely depressed cerebral metabolism and blood flow, causing diffuse low-voltage, slow activity in the EEG.

Vegetative States

Clinical Criteria

As time elapses after onset of coma, some patients neither die nor regain consciousness but rather evolve into a "vegetative state" (251). The Multi-Society Task Force on PVS (340) defined as vegetative states a group of conditions having in common "complete unawareness of the self and the

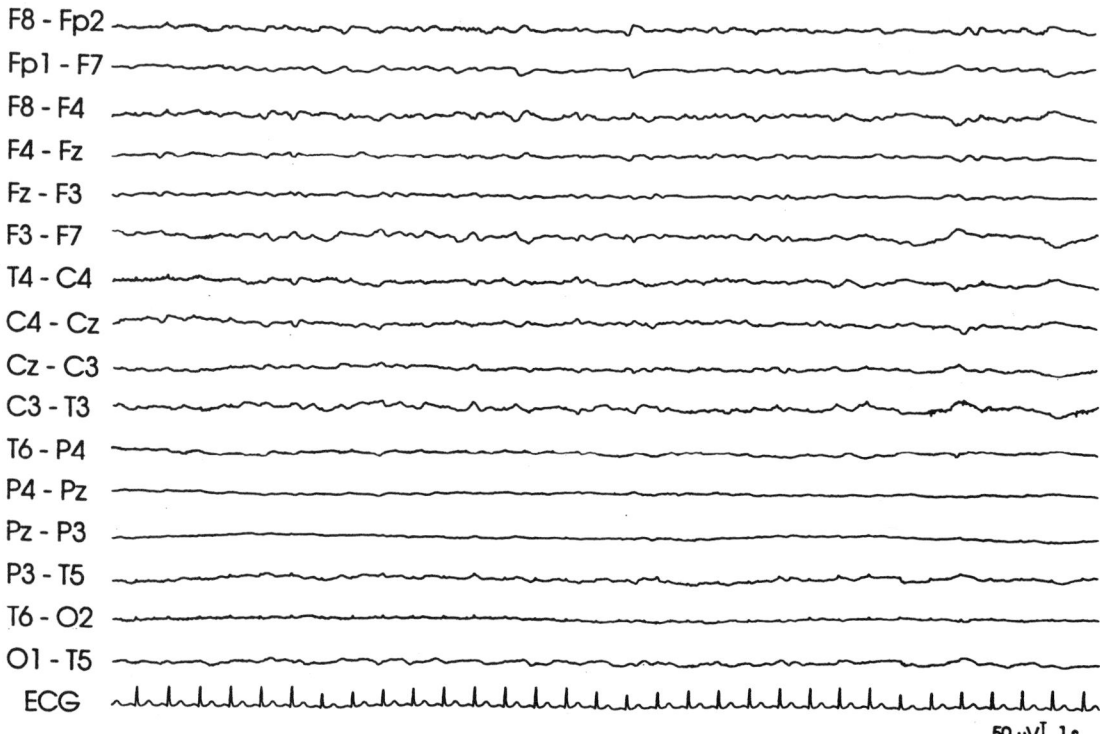

FIG. 14.22. Widespread 1- to 5-Hz activity best developed over the anterior and middle head regions in a 47-year-old woman. The patient had suffered retroperitoneal hemorrhage with circulatory collapse and loss of consciousness following earlier total pelvic exenteration for recurrent adenocarcinoma of the cervix. One month after the onset of coma, she was in a vegetative state. (From Chatrian G-E. Electrophysiological evaluation of brain death: a critical appraisal. In: Aminoff MJ, ed. *Electrodiagnosis in clinical neurology.* New York: Churchill Livingstone, 1980:525–588, with permission.)

environment accompanied by sleep-wake cycles with either complete or partial preservation of hypothalamic and brain stem autonomic functions." Observation of these individuals indicates that they are incapable of "sustained, reproducible, purposeful, or voluntary behavioral responses to visual, auditory, tactile, or noxious stimuli" and give "no evidence of language comprehension or expression" (340). Terms employed in the past to describe this condition or states resembling it have included "apallic syndrome" (277), "coma vigil" (7), "noncognitive states" (275), and "akinetic mutism," among others.

A vegetative state was observed in 12% of individuals 1 month after onset of nontraumatic coma of various etiologies (290) and in 1%–14% of comatose patients following severe head injury (340). In some patients the vegetative state is transient and reversible (175,176,340), whereas in other individuals it persists for months or years (292,340) ("persistent" and "permanent" vegetative states) (340).

Mortality is high among vegetative patients and is greater in adults than in children and following nontraumatic than traumatic brain injuries (340). A review of earlier reports concluded that average life expectancy for vegetative adults was 2–5 years and that the possibility of survival beyond 15 years after injury was exceedingly small (< 1 in 15,000–75,000) (340), but improved standards of care may modify this outlook (289).

Changing concepts and definitions of vegetative states (12,16,177,340) and studies suggesting a high rate of misdiagnosis of these conditions (98) make it difficult to analyze reported clinical, pathological, and electrophysiological findings.

EEG Findings

In the past, EEGs of some vegetative patients were described as electrocerebrally inactive (37,60,109,175,239). In retrospect, it appears likely that

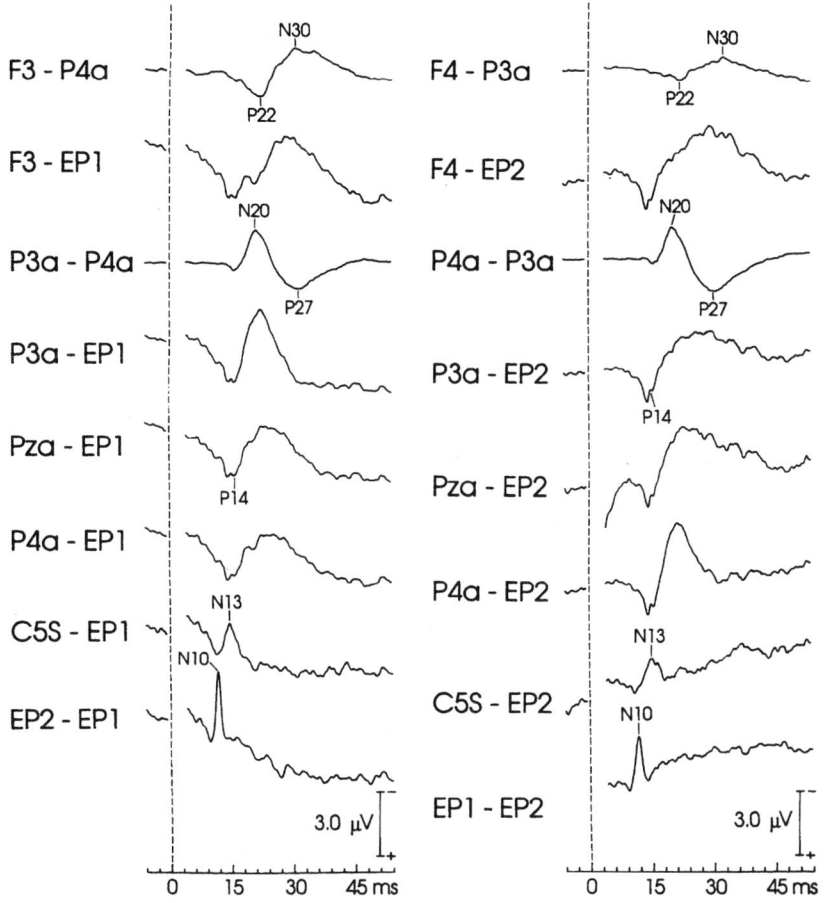

FIG. 14.23. SL-SEPs in response to electrical stimulation of the right **(A)** and left **(B)** median nerves at the wrist. *F3 and F4*, left and right frontal electrodes; *P3a, Pza, and P4a*, electrodes halfway between P3 and C3, Pz and Cz, and P4 and C4 of the 10-20 system; *EP1 and EP2*, left and right Erb's points electrodes; *C5S*, C5 spine electrode. Responses, including early cortical postcentral (N20-P27) and frontal (P22-N30) potentials, had normal latencies and IPIs. Same patient as in Figure 14.22. Nine days after onset of coma, neurological status remained unchanged. (Modified from Wytrzes LM, Chatrian G-E, Shaw C-M, et al. Acute failure of forebrain with sparing of brain stem function: electroencephalographic, multimodality evoked potentials, and pathologic findings. *Arch Neurol* 1989;46:93–97.)

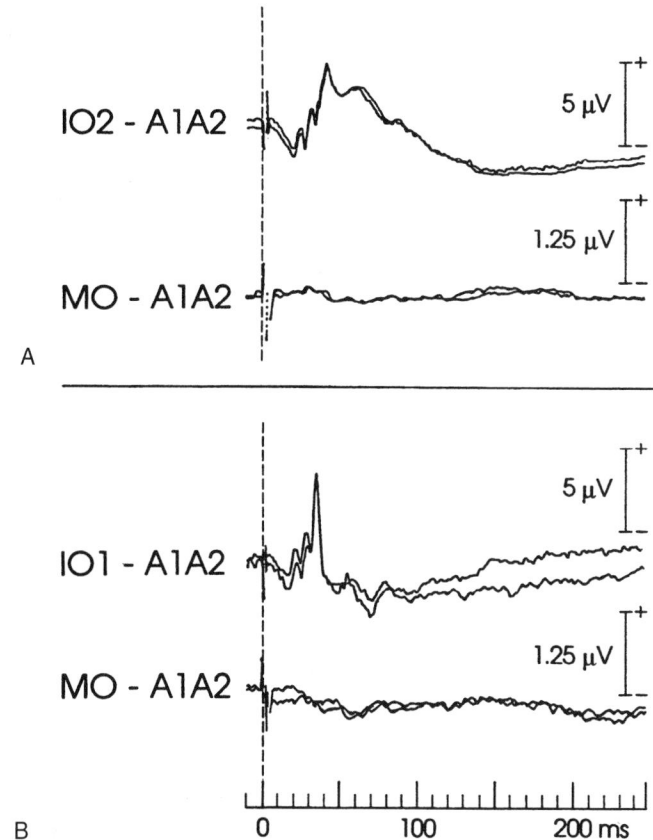

FIG. 14.24. Asymmetrical ERGs (waves *a* and *b*), but no cerebral responses, following flash stimulation of the right **(A)** and left **(B)** eyes. Recording technique and abbreviations are the same as in Figures 14.22 and 14.23. Same patient as in Figure 14.22, 15 days after onset of unresponsiveness. Neurological status remained unchanged.

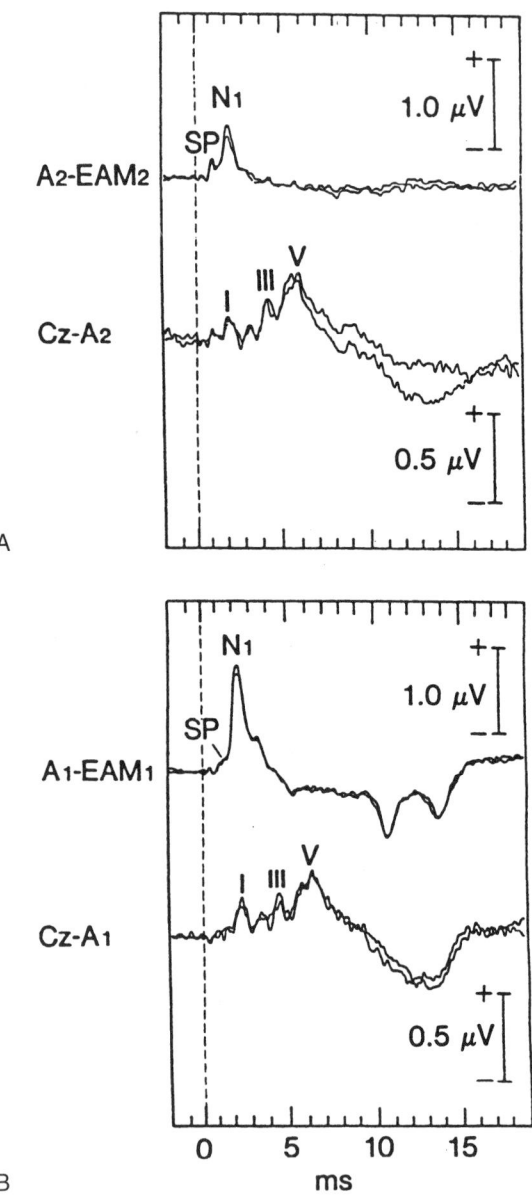

A

B

N = 2048

most of these records demonstrated low-voltage, slow, unreactive activity rather than ECI as currently defined (14). More recent reports have established that vegetative individuals demonstrate a wide variety of EEG patterns, including widespread, slow, unreactive activity often of low voltage (Fig. 14.22); burst-suppression; bilateral pseudoperiodic complexes; epileptiform discharges; diffuse unreactive alpha or theta activity; and even highly organized waking and sleep patterns regarded as only mildly abnormal (4,37, 38,56,57,108,174,175,211,239,255,287,300,302,318,372,411,475). Thus individual diurnal EEGs are of little value in diagnosing vegetative states.

Some studies indicated that recovery from the vegetative state was paralleled by diminution of delta and theta activity when present in earlier EEGs, reappearance of a reactive alpha rhythm (247,300), progressive restoration of organized sleep EEG patterns and nocturnal sleep cycles, and recovery of REM sleep (8,174). Extreme variability of findings precludes the use of the EEG to predict the clinical outcome of vegetative states. However, spectral analysis of the EEG was said to indicate that "slow monotonous spectrograms" were mostly associated with death, whereas "changeable spectrograms" had a more favorable prognosis (467).

Evoked Potential Findings

Just as with EEGs, EP findings are extremely variable in vegetative patients. The $N\overline{20}$ cortical component of median nerve SL-SEPs may be normal (Fig. 14.23), although CCTs may be increased or may be variously altered or absent with variably preserved brainstem $P\overline{14}$ potential (196,211, 372,383). Similarly, cortical VEPs may be variously abnormal (196,383) or absent (196,372) (Fig. 14.24). BAEPs are reportedly normal in many vegetative patients (Fig. 14.25), although brainstem conduction time may be prolonged, but demonstrate various alterations in other individuals (196,211,372,383,470). Heterogeneity of results hinders the use of EPs as predictors of outcome of vegetative states.

Because CEPs are related to certain aspects of cognitive behavior, it seems natural that they should be called on to assess the preservation and to predict the restoration of cognitive capacities in vegetative patients. Thus,

FIG. 14.25. Electrocochleograms and BAEPs in response to click stimulation of the right **(A)** and left **(B)** ears. Recording technique and abbreviations are the same as in Figures 14.23 and 14.24. Latencies and IPIs were normal. Same subject as in Figures 14.22, 14.23, and 14.24.

Guérit et al. (196) suggested that preservation of these faculties could be tested in vegetative individuals by attempting to elicit somatosensory CEPs. Unfortunately, the patient substantiating this belief was capable of following simple orders and producing behavioral responses to various stimuli, at variance with the definition of vegetative state. Another study has claimed that the majority of vegetative patients displaying $\overline{N200}$ and $\overline{P300}$ cognitive potentials eventually regained consciousness, whereas all individuals in whom these responses could not be elicited did not (180). Confirmation of these suggestive findings is desirable.

Neuropathological Findings and Conclusions

Neuropathological changes in vegetative patients are variable. Extensive multifocal or diffuse, laminar cortical necrosis follows acute global hypoxia and ischemia, causing virtual decortication. Scattered small areas of infarction or neuronal loss may be additionally present in the basal ganglia, hypothalamus, or brainstem (129,239). Extensive subcortical axonal injury is caused by shearing of nerve fibers by acute trauma (2,443,444). These last changes cause virtual cortical isolation (249). In patients with head injury complicated by acute circulatory or respiratory failure, axonal injury may be associated with diffuse laminar necrosis (340). Severe brainstem abnormalities are infrequent and primarily follow transtentorial herniation during the early stage of illness (340). Vegetative patients with degenerative disorders and developmental abnormalities display the pathological changes characteristic of their underlying conditions (341). In a highly publicized individual case of "persistent" vegetative state, extensive, bilateral thalamic scarring by far exceeded damage in the cortex, basal ganglia, and cerebellum (272). The fact that in individual patients pathological lesions may primarily involve cerebral cortex, cerebral hemispheric white matter, and thalamic or brainstem structures to a variable degree and in various combinations likely accounts for the remarkable variability of EEG, EP, and CEP findings reported in vegetative states.

ELECTROPHYSIOLOGICAL EVALUATION OF BRAIN DEATH

Brain Death in Adults

Concept, Clinical Criteria, and Confirmatory Tests

The concept of brain death has evolved since it was first formulated and has been the subject of controversy (78). Recent U.S. guidelines define brain death as "the irreversible loss of function of the brain, including the brainstem" (389). The same guidelines specify that the diagnosis of brain death in the adult is established by demonstrating the clinical signs of unresponsiveness, absent brainstem reflexes, and apnea established by a strictly standardized apnea test. Repetition of clinical testing after an interval such as 6 hours is advisable but not required. The application of these clinical criteria is contingent on (a) the demonstration by clinical and neuroimaging studies of an acute CNS catastrophe compatible with brain death and (b) the exclusion of confounding medical conditions that may reversibly cause clinical manifestations mimicking brain death. These complicating conditions include hypothermia with core temperature below 32°C (89.6°F), drug intoxication or poisoning, and severe metabolic derangements and endocrine crises (389,492,493). Brain death as defined excludes other states of diminished responsiveness such as deefferented (locked-in) states (370) and vegetative states (340).

Current U.S. standards emphasize that the diagnosis of brain death in adults can be made in ordinary circumstances by good history and competent clinical examination supplemented by routine laboratory tests and neuroimaging studies. They recommend, but do not mandate, that a confirmatory test should be performed when, after a period of observation exceeding 24 hours, not all prerequisites for clinical testing are satisfied or specific components of clinical testing cannot be reliably performed or evaluated (389,492,494). Such standards vary in other countries; in France (331,332), confirmatory tests are required by law, whereas in the United Kingdom they are regarded as unnecessary (364,429,499). Substantial numbers of small hospitals in developed countries and most hospitals in the developing world lack the instrumentation and skills required to perform and interpret ancillary studies designed to corroborate the clinical diagnosis of irreversible loss of brain viability. In these circumstances, unless the patient can be safely transported to a properly equipped medical center, there are no alternatives but to establish the diagnosis of brain death by clinical observation alone. However, we believe that, whenever the diagnosis of brain death is in doubt and the appropriate resources are available, no effort should be spared to decrease the chances of error, expedite the diagnosis, provide objective proof of irreversible extinction of brain function, and increase the opportunities for removal of viable organs for life-saving transplantation. The following is a critical review of the role currently played by electrophysiological testing in the diagnosis of brain death in the adult.

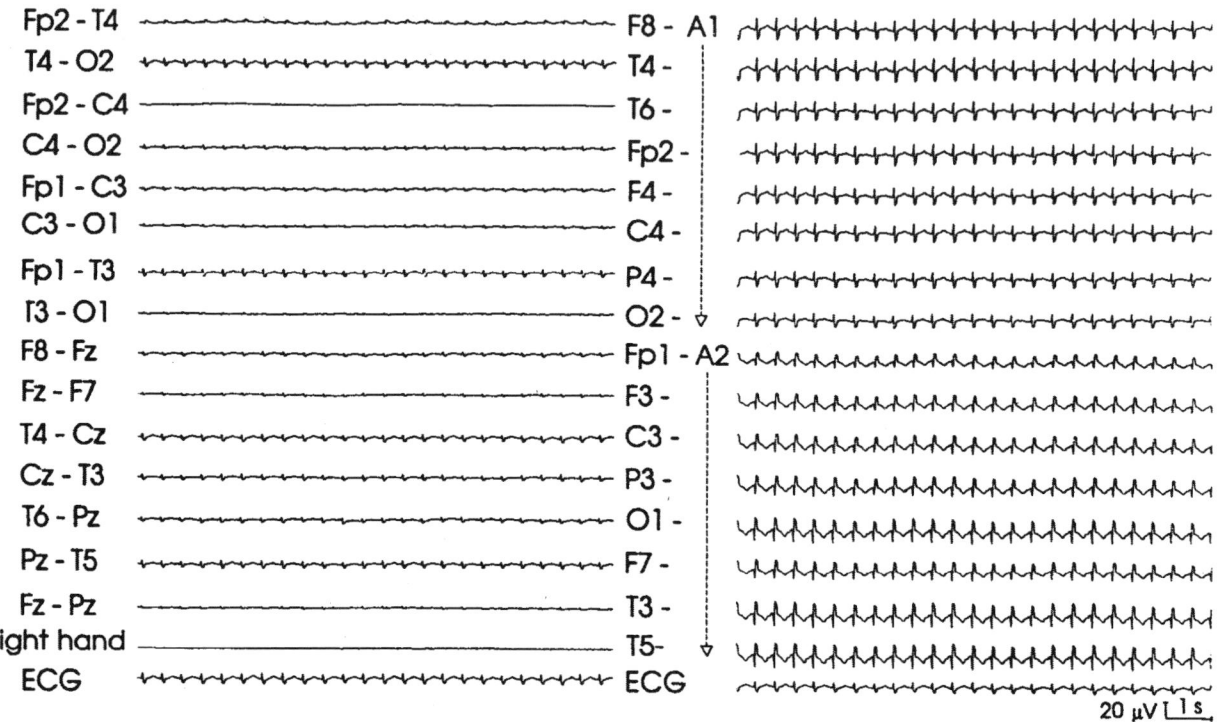

FIG. 14.26. ECI in a 23-year-old hypertensive woman 2 days after intracerebral hemorrhage. The patient was unresponsive to stimuli and had no spontaneous respiration, no cephalic reflexes, and dilated pupils. ECG artifact was especially prominent at high sensitivities and in referential derivations.

The EEG as a Confirmatory Test

ECI: Definition

In a substantial proportion of patients who are clinically brain dead (about 80%) (191), scalp recordings show absence of demonstrable EEG potentials. Such a state of "electrocerebral inactivity" is defined as "absence over all regions of the head of identifiable electrical activity of cerebral origin, whether spontaneous or induced by physiological stimuli and pharmacological agents" (350) (Fig. 14.26). Electrical activity of cerebral origin is identified when it exceeds an assumed instrumental noise of 2 μV. Other terms used in the literature to describe ECI include "electrocerebral silence" and "isoelectric," "flat," and "null" EEG, among others. Our definition of ECI *excludes*

Recordings displaying burst-suppression, which are commonly found in conditions including acute intoxications with CNS depressants, severe anoxic encephalopathies, and deep hypothermia and anesthesia

Low-voltage, slow, generally unreactive EEGs consisting primarily of delta and theta potentials, which usually occur in comatose patients with severe widespread cortical damage

Recordings showing no detectable electrocerebral activity over limited areas of the scalp

TABLE 14.1. *Requirements for demonstrating electrocerebral inactivity in the adult*

1. Sixteen or more EEG channels should be recorded simultaneously (83,389).
2. In addition to all electrodes of the 10-20 system (246) and a ground electrode, two electrodes should be routinely placed on the arms, shoulders, or chest for ECG monitoring, and two should be applied 6–7 cm apart on the dorsum of the right hand to monitor artifacts from the surroundings (14,83).
3. The use of other electrodes may be required, including special transducers for monitoring respiration and related artifacts (14,83).
4. Interelectrode impedance should be below 10,000 but above 1,000 ohms (14,83).
5. The integrity of the entire recording system should be checked (14).
6. Instrumental sensitivities should be no less than 2 µV/mm for at least 30 min of recording time, and calibrations should use appropriate voltages (14,83).
7. Low frequency cutoffs (–3 dB) should be at approximately 0.5 Hz (corresponding to a time constant of 0.3 s). However, in the presence of excessive slow artifacts, the use of low-frequency filters at about 1.5 Hz (corresponding to a time constant of 0.1 s) during part of the recording is justified. High-frequency filter cutoffs should be at approximately 70 Hz. Cutoffs at 50 or even 35 Hz during part of the recording are justified in the presence of irreducible electromyographic activity when pharmacological neuromuscular blockade is contraindicated (83).
8. The recording should include bipolar (anteroposterior and transverse) and referential montages. Bipolar montages should primarily consist of large- (double-) distance electrode linkages (14,83).
9. Requirements 6 through 8 above apply to recordings obtained with analog recorders. When using digital recorders, the same requirements should be fulfilled for on-line data display and off-line data review. Digital instruments offer the advantage that the recording, typically obtained referentially and stored electronically, can be reviewed with different sensitivities, filters, montages, and paper speeds without altering the parameters of the signal stored. This attractive capability does not justify decreasing the overall recording time because of the danger of missing EEG activity that occurs intermittently at long intervals (83).
10. To test EEG reactivity, stimuli, especially noxious excitations, should be delivered with prudence because they can produce marked fluctuations in intracranial pressure or cardiovascular changes that are potentially harmful to individuals with borderline brain perfusion and may cause prolonged electromyographic contamination of the EEG (82,83).
11. The examination should be conducted or closely supervised by a qualified technologist experienced in ICU recordings and working under the direction of an experienced clinical neurophysiologist (14,82,83). The latter should be present during at least part of the recording and should provide prompt interpretation of the test.
12. When doubt exists about whether or not the test demonstrates ECI, the entire procedure should be repeated after an interval such as 6 h (14).
13. Special precautions should be taken against electrical hazard, transmission of infection, and harmful effects of manipulations, especially head lifting and stimulation (83).
14. The minimal duration of actual, interpretable recording should be 30 min or longer (389,492,494).
15. Following resuscitation from circulatory arrest, at least 8 h should elapse between the onset of coma and the EEG examination (253).

Modified from Chatrian G-E. Electrophysiologic evaluation of brain death: a critical appraisal. In: Aminoff MJ, ed. *Electrodiagnosis in clinical neurology.* New York: Churchill Livingstone, 1999:681–705.

Low-voltage reactive EEGs displaying "activity of amplitude not greater than 20 μV over all head regions" (84), which are found among normal persons

Problems and Pitfalls in Demonstrating ECI

Whenever EEG confirmation of the clinical diagnosis of brain death is requested, the procedure should begin with a brief preliminary recording using all electrodes of the 10-20 system (246) and those instrumental settings and montages that are commonly used in the individual laboratory for the study of comatose patients. If this preliminary sampling suggests absent or questionable electrocerebral activity, the recording technique should be promptly modified to demonstrate ECI. Basic requirements for these recordings are summarized in Table 14.1.

Artifacts often contaminate EEG records designed to demonstrate ECI. These spurious electrical events include potentials generated by instruments near or connected to the patient, such as electrocardiographic (ECG) monitors, pacemakers, warming blankets, and dialysis units, as well as biopotentials of cardiovascular, muscular, and respiratory origin (37).

The most frequent and disturbing of all biological artifacts is the ECG, especially prominent in ear reference montages. ECG potentials occasionally resemble sharp-and–slow wave complexes or TWs. Premature ventricular contractions or ventricular tachycardia may produce potentials appearing as sharp transients or theta or delta rhythms, respectively. In addition, rhythms of mostly alpha frequency occasionally result from head vibrations caused by the systolic pulse wave (ballistocardiogram) (37). Disconnecting ECG monitors, repositioning the patient's head, and selecting montages less prone to EEG pickup may reduce, but frequently do not eliminate, ECG arti-

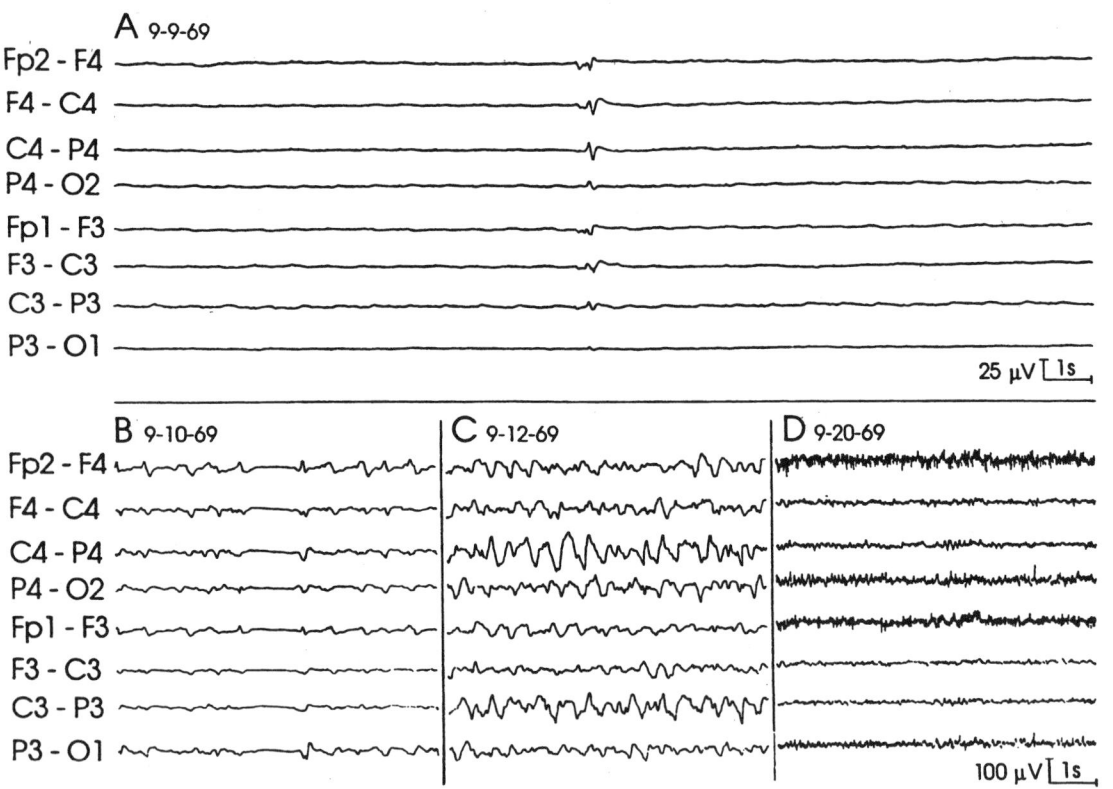

FIG. 14.27. Serial EEGs of a 30-year-old woman with secobarbital overdose. **A:** Second day of hospitalization. The patient was comatose and artificially ventilated, with a blood barbiturate level of 35 mg per 100 milliliters. The EEG showed isolated sharp-and–slow wave complexes separated by periods of suppression lasting up to 22 seconds. **B:** One day later, her clinical condition was unchanged. The EEG showed bilateral asymmetrical pseudoperiodic sharp waves at 1–2 Hz. **C:** Four days after admission, the patient was withdrawing in response to noxious stimuli, with pupils reacting to light. The EEG showed high-voltage bilateral 2- to 3-Hz activity. **D:** Eight days later, the patient was alert and responsive to verbal commands. The EEG showed 9- to 10-Hz posterior reactive rhythm. (From Chatrian G-E. Electrophysiological evaluation of brain death: a critical appraisal. In: Aminoff MJ, ed. *Electrodiagnosis in clinical neurology.* New York: Churchill Livingstone, 1980:525–588, with permission.)

fact. Thus, having attempted these and other maneuvers, the technologist generally can do little but accept this artifact and try to prove its origin by monitoring the ECG simultaneously with the EEG. Methods proposed to remove the ECG artifact from the EEGs of patients suspected of being brain dead (42) are of questionable practicality (78).

Electromyographic potentials may obscure possible electrocerebral activity unless neuromuscular blocking agents, such as pancuronium bromide (425) or succinylcholine (449,450), are given. However, caution is suggested by a report of cardiac arrest and death following administration of succinylcholine to reduce myogenic artifact (473).

It is sometimes more difficult to identify the origin of respiration-related artifacts. Respirators delivering a bolus of air to the patient through flexible tubes may cause the tubes to vibrate and to produce rhythmic activity of alpha or other frequencies, and head movements associated with respiration may generate large transients resembling periodic paroxysmal discharges (37). Monitoring with appropriate transducers can distinguish these artifacts from EEG potentials. On occasion, it may even be necessary to briefly stop the respirator to assess questionable activity (37). However, whenever this test is carried out over minutes, adequate oxygenation must be provided to avoid additional anoxic damage (83).

Technical Requirements for Demonstrating ECI

Obtaining in the ICU recordings that satisfy stringent technical requirements for demonstrating brain death often seriously challenges the competence, experience, ingenuity, and determination of the EEG technologist. In the NINCDS Collaborative Study, 22.3% of recordings required special efforts to identify and eliminate artifacts, although only 5.2% were considered technically unsatisfactory (37). Additional delays are caused by the prudent preparation of patients hovering between life and death and by interruptions of the EEG examination to allow performance of essential therapeutic maneuvers (83). Thus the production of at least 30 minutes of interpretable recording that fulfills present technical requirements may take as long as 2 hours and sometimes longer (368).

Recordings made by means of electrodes directly applied on the cerebral cortex or implanted within the brain have been advocated (479) but are of questionable utility and carry substantial risks (78).

Prerequisites for the EEG Confirmation of Brain Death: Significance of ECI. The demonstration of ECI in adult patients with clinical diagnosis of brain death indicates absence of cerebral cortical function, but does not imply that this functional loss is permanent unless confounding pathological conditions that may cause reversible extinction of electrocerebral activity have been ruled out. These conditions include drug intoxication, hypothermia, profound hypotension, and severe metabolic and endocrine derangements—that is, those same disorders that may reversibly cause the clinical manifestations of brain death.

Patients rendered comatose by overdoses of CNS depressants most frequently display a burst-suppression pattern in their EEGs. In some instances, electrocerebral activity is reduced to brief bursts or isolated waves of low voltage separated by intervals lasting several minutes (Fig. 14.27A). Most early reports of ECI persisting 24 hours or longer in patients who were drug intoxicated described EEGs that probably were not electrocerebrally inactive by present standards. However, other evidence of the occurrence of ECI in short-term EEGs of patients with overdoses of CNS depressants is more credible (37,479). Only sparse information is available on the blood levels of CNS depressants causing ECI in adults, who often are under the influence of multiple drugs and suffer from local or systemic conditions that alter the blood–brain barrier. Thus, caution should be exercised in interpreting the significance of ECI in adults with evidence of even small amounts of CNS depressants in their blood. Hypothermia with core temperature below 32.3°C (90°F) can cause reversible extinction of electrocerebral activity (388). The EEG may also be abolished by cardiovascular shock with low cerebral perfusion pressure and may be restored when blood pressure is raised above 80 mm Hg (479). Severe metabolic and endocrine disorders that can cause or contribute to the generation of ECI (388) include profound abnormalities of blood serum electrolytes, acid–base balance, blood gases, and the alterations resulting from severe dysfunction of the liver, kidneys, and pancreas.

Meticulous serial studies by Jørgensen and Malchow-Møller determined that ECI developed immediately in patients who suffered circulatory arrest of primary cardiovascular etiology. EEG activity, first intermittent and then continuous, recovered from 10 minutes to 8 hours after resuscitation in those individuals who subsequently regained consciousness (253) and from 11 to 128 hours after resuscitation in those patients who remained unconscious 1 year later (254). It follows that, at variance with current guidelines (14), no less than 8 hours should elapse after circulatory arrest before an EEG seeking confirmation of brain death is recorded.

Whenever the confounding conditions just alluded to are ruled out in an adult patient at least 8 hours (253,254) after an acute, catastrophic insult to the brain, the combination of the EEG pattern of ECI with the clinical signs of coma, absent brainstem reflexes, and apnea attests to a global failure of brain function that is highly likely to be permanent (14,37,79–82,388,416,479).

Persistence of EEG Activity in Adults Who Satisfy All Preconditions and Clinical Criteria of Brain Death

As many as 20% of patients who satisfy all preconditions and clinical criteria for brain death do not demonstrate ECI but display some electrocerebral activity in their EEGs several hours to several days after death of their brains has been diagnosed clinically (191). This activity often consists of multifocal bursts of potentials of variable amplitude and duration. It has been conjectured that islands of relatively preserved brain tissue may still be capable of generating this aberrant electrical activity in brain-dead adults (78,191). This contention is partly supported by pathological findings indicating that remnants of EEG activity most commonly characterize patients whose brains show only patchy swelling, edema, infarction, and necrosis (285,338,481), whereas patients with ECI have a significantly higher incidence of swollen brains, cerebral herniations, and "respirator brains" (271,481). Individuals with EEGs classified as equivocal display pathological changes intermediate between these two groups.

Preservation of minimal EEG activity in clinically brain-dead patients is most likely incompatible with both lasting survival and any form of residual sentience, and does not justify the continuation of life-supporting measures (78,81,82). However, how much EEG activity is compatible with brain death and justifies cessation of life-supporting measures has not been established. In these circumstances, justifiably hesitant EEG interpretations are often greeted with understandable impatience by transplant teams.

Neuropathological Alterations and EEG Changes

The neuropathological changes in brain death are remarkably diverse (49,271,285,338,481). No statistically significant association was demonstrated between ECI and any specific pathology, although there was a tendency for this pattern to be more common in cases with hemorrhage, edema, and necrosis than with other types of lesions (481,482). Some patients with ECI who died less than 24 hours after onset of coma had minimal or no pathological alterations. Changes of "respirator brain" developed 12–36 (usually about 24) hours after onset of coma and apnea (229,285,478,480). Contrariwise, patients with some preserved EEG activity in their last recording sometimes revealed a respirator brain. However, in general, severity of EEG changes as measured by preserved electrocerebral activity in all, some, or none of the EEGs was said to be related to the degree of pathological changes in the brain. Additionally, progression to ECI, loss of brainstem reflexes, and evidence of herniation showed significant association with the presence of a "respirator brain" (285). In contrast, no significant association was demonstrated between ECI and site of primary pathology: 63% of patients with brainstem lesions exhibited ECI, as did 60% of individuals with diffuse cerebral lesions and 60% of patients with focal cortical lesions (479,481).

Suitability of EEG as a Confirmatory Test

In some countries, including the United States, the EEG has long enjoyed the status of test of choice for confirming the clinical diagnosis of brain death in adults. In other countries such as France, the performance of an EEG for the determination of brain death is even mandated by law (332). Yet growing recognition of limitations and pitfalls of the EEG indicates that primary reliance on this test is no longer justified (81,82,155,198). EEGs recorded according to current rigorous standards on adults suspected of being brain dead are difficult, cumbersome, time-consuming procedures that require a high degree of specialized technical and professional expertise, are subject to failures and misinterpretations, and have low specificity and sensitivity (78,81,82,362,363). In particular, ECI can be reversibly caused by those same conditions that may also transiently cause clinical manifestations of global loss of brain function (i.e., drug intoxication, hypothermia, profound hypotension, and severe metabolic or endocrine disorders). This is a major limitation because laboratory confirmation of irreversible failure of brain function is especially needed when the existence of these conditions hinders the clinical diagnosis (80–82). In addition, the consideration that, in the absence of these confounding conditions, ECI shows a high degree of statistical association with brain death (14) should not obscure the finding that a substantial number (about 20%) of clinically brain-dead patients do not demonstrate ECI but rather various amounts of residual EEG activity the relations of which to brain death are less clearly established (191). The tendency to identify the specificity of the particular EEG pattern of ECI in the absence of complicating conditions with the specificity of the EEG method in general in the context of brain death is a major source of confusion in official recommendations (389) and individual publications (494). We believe that medically sound and cost-effective management requires that, when available, tests other than the EEG should be

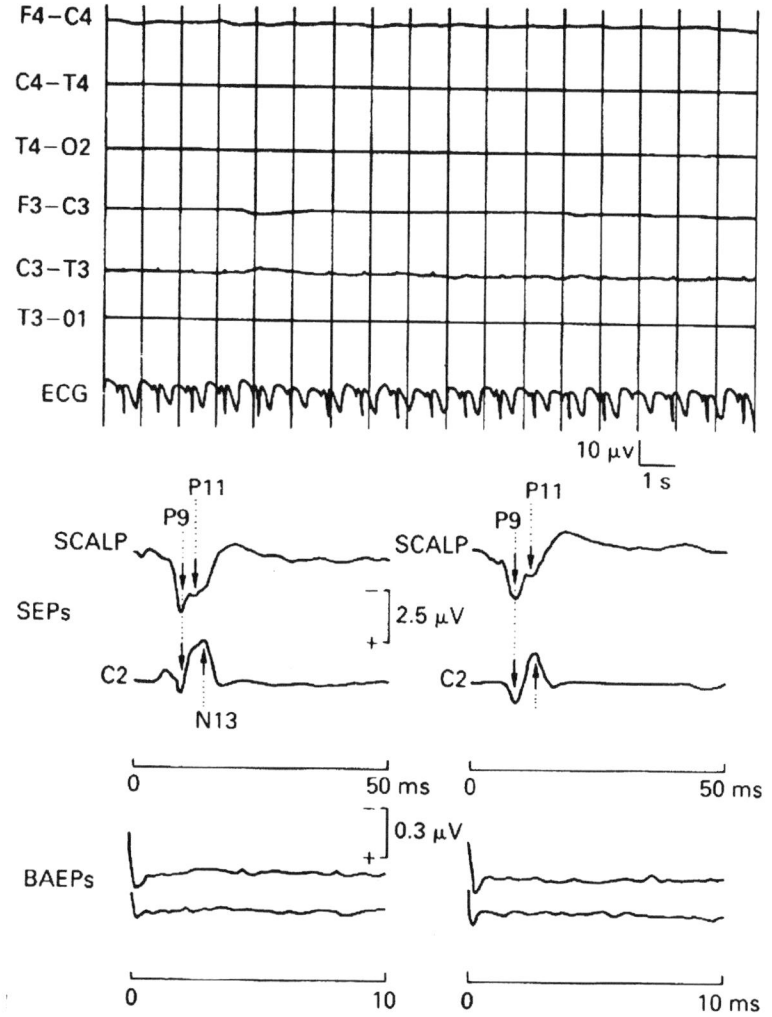

FIG. 14.28. Electrophysiological studies in a 20-year-old clinically brain-dead woman with absent cephalic reflexes. **Top:** The EEG demonstrated ECI. **Middle:** SL-SEPs showed peripheral P9 and spinal P11 and N13 components, while brainstem P14 and cortical N20-P27 potentials are bilaterally absent. **Bottom:** BAEPs showed absence of all response components, including wave I. (Modified from Mauguière F, García-Larrea L, Murray NMF, et al. Evoked potential diagnostic strategies: EPs in coma. In: Osselton JW, ed. *Clinical neurophysiology. Vol. 1. EMG, nerve conduction, and evoked potentials.* Oxford, England: Butterworth-Heinemann, 1995:482–522.)

used as first choices to corroborate the clinical diagnosis of brain death. These procedures continue to evolve rapidly as new technologies become available. At present, methods designed to demonstrate absence or critical deficit of brain perfusion, although not entirely free of shortcomings, deserve special consideration (81,82,198).

Evoked Potentials as Confirmatory Tests

Short-Latency SEPs

In clinically brain-dead individuals, SL-SEPs in response to electrical stimulation of the median nerve show (a) bilateral obliteration of cortical N20 and subsequent components of SL-SEPs (17,36,184,194,321,400,401, 465); (b) loss of medullary P14 potential; (c) inconstant preservation of spinal N13 potential; and (d) frequent persistence of N9 brachial plexus potential (17,184,194) (Fig. 14.28, middle section). Reports of variable preservation of the P14 potential in some brain-dead individuals (36,321) are of uncertain significance. It has been suggested that, in patients who gradually evolve from deep coma to brain death, the medial lemniscus that presumably generates the P14 potential undergoes gradual rostrocaudal destruction. Occasional transient functional preservation of caudal portions of this structure at a time when brain death is already clinically apparent would result in a P14 potential of reduced amplitude in scalp-noncephalic reference derivations (477). In these circumstances, a simultaneous mid-frontal scalp-nasopharyngeal recording would demonstrate loss of the P14 potential from rostral portions of the medial lemniscus. This last finding has been said to differentiate brain-dead from deeply comatose patients in whom the rostral component of the P14 potential would be preserved (477).

SL-SEPs (as well as BAEPs) are extremely resistant to barbiturates and other CNS depressants causing coma or used in the treatment of coma (134,173,233,420,428,441,451). However, they are profoundly altered by hypothermia (207,315,441). Cortical SL-SEPs may also be abolished or altered by peripheral nerve, brachial plexus, cervical root, and spinal cord injury; dysfunction of somatosensory pathways as a result of preexisting conditions such as multiple sclerosis, degenerative diseases, and Arnold-Chiari malformation (320); and extensive brainstem lesions. On occasion, myogenic contamination may complicate them (194). In addition, recordings of median nerve SL-SEPs taken between the Fz (scalp) and C2 (spine) electrodes (184) pose special interpretive problems. These are overcome by derivations utilizing a noncephalic or ipsilateral ear reference (123,139,198,462).

Brainstem Auditory Evoked Potentials

Brain death is associated with obliteration of all BAEP components with or without preservation of waves I or I and II (184,259,274,321,334,406, 431,439,456,469–471,491) (see Fig. 14.28, lower section). A review of the available literature (79) found that loss of all BAEPs including wave I occurred in 57% of brain-dead patients, loss of all waves except I in 37%, and absence of all waves except I and II in 6%.

A major limitation of BAEPs in the study of patients with suspected brain death is that obliteration of wave I (the auditory nerve compound action potential) and all subsequent BAEP components attests to loss or severe impairment of peripheral (cochlear and auditory nerve) function. This deficit precludes the activation of central auditory pathways. Thus loss of wave I and of all subsequent BAEPs is compatible with, but cannot be taken as evidence of, loss of function of the auditory pathways in the brainstem such as occurs in brain death. In patients with suspected irreversible extinction of brain function, obliteration of wave I and all subsequent BAEPs can result from a variety of causes, including cochlear ischemia secondary to arrest of the intracranial circulation (67,184,319) and deafness or profound hearing loss, whether preexisting or caused by trauma or meningitis. In head-injured patients, in particular, cochlear or auditory nerve damage secondary to fracture of the temporal bone, injury to the middle ear or the tympanic membrane, and blood in the external auditory canal may result in complete absence of BAEPs. The detection of BAEPs may be further hindered by protracted nasotracheal intubation and positive-pressure ventilation, which can cause obstruction of the eustachian tubes and middle ear effusions resulting in conductive deficits. Because absence of wave I limits the utility of BAEPs in corroborating the clinical diagnosis of brain death, this finding should be scrutinized with special care. To this end, the possibility that failure of the stimulus or the recording circuit may be responsible for failure to demonstrate this wave (and all subsequent BAEPs) must be tested and excluded. The use of sufficiently high stimulus intensities and of recording electrodes in the external auditory meatus is also suggested to maximize the chances of detecting wave I (89,96).

Visual Evoked Potentials

Cerebral VEPs (in response to flash stimulation) are abolished in individuals fulfilling clinical criteria of brain death (19,194,427,465,486). In contrast, VEPs (and the EEG) are preserved in patients with large brainstem lesions who are deefferented and have lost both SL-SEPs and BAEPs. These findings help to differentiate between brain death and deefferented states.

A major limitation of VEPs in the corroboration of brain death is that they are highly vulnerable to the effects of CNS depressants and hypothermia (386,402). Moreover, because the retina is more resistant than the brain to anoxia, flash stimulation may elicit electroretinograms (ERGs) over the anterior head regions in the absence of cerebral responses. Preservation of the ERG is irrelevant to the outcome of clinically brain dead patients (77). Thus, when attempting to average cerebral VEPs in patients suspected of being brain dead, the possibility that the ERG may simulate them should be carefully assessed (18,77,79,82,465).

Motor Evoked Potentials

In patients with irreversibly extinguished brain function, MEPs are absent in response to magnetic (or electrical) transcranial stimulation of the motor cortex but are preserved in response to cervical excitation (153). However,

TABLE 14.2. *Types of studies and observation periods for determining brain death in children*[a,b]

Patient's age	Types of studies and observation periods
2 mo to 1 yr	Two physical examinations and two EEGs demonstrating ECI at least 24 hr apart ; or a physical examination, an EEG demonstrating ECI, and a cerebral radionuclide angiogram demonstrating nonvisualization of cerebral arteries.
Over 1 yr	Assuming demonstration of irreversible cause of coma, two physical examinations 24 hr apart should fulfill the criteria of brain death when laboratory testing is not to be performed. The period of observation should be prolonged by at least 24 hr if the extent and irreversibility of brain damage are uncertain (especially in hypoxic-ischemic encephalopathy), or it may be reduced if the EEG demonstrates ECI or if cerebral radionuclide angiography does not visualize cerebral arteries.

EEG, electroencephalogram; ECI, electrocerebral inactivity.
[a]Summary of the Report of Special Task Force on Brain Death in Children (387). (From Chatrian G-E. Electrophysiologic evaluation of brain death: a critical appraisal. In: Aminoff MJ, ed. *Electrodiagnosis in clinical neurology*. New York: Churchill Livingstone, 1999:681–705, with permission.)
[b]*Note:* The above guidelines have been seriously questioned, as indicated in the text.

TABLE 14.3. *Physical examination and laboratory criteria for determining brain death in children[a,b]*

Physical examination	EEG	Cerebral angiography
1. Coma and apnea. 2. Absence of brainstem function. 3. Lack of significant hypothermia or hypotension for age. 4. "Flaccid tone and absence of spontaneous or reflex movements excluding spinal myoclonus." The above findings should remain constant throughout the observation period.	Electrocerebral inactivity over a 30-minute period according to American Electroencephalographic Society guidelines. In small children, "inter-electrode distances should be decreased proportional to the patient's head size." "Drug concentrations should be insufficient to suppress EEG activity.	Lack of visualization of intracranial arterial circulation in cerebral radionuclide angiography or lack of blood flow to brain in contrast angiography. Value of cerebral radionuclide angiography in infants under 2 months is under investigation.

[a]Summary of the Report of Special Task Force on Brain Death in Children (387). (From Chatrian G-E. Electrophysiologic evaluation of brain death: a critical appraisal. In: Aminoff MJ, ed. *Electrodiagnosis in clinical neurology*. New York: Churchill Livingstone, 1999:681–705, with permission.)
[b]*Note:* The above guidelines have been seriously questioned, as indicated in the text.

experience with the routine clinical use of this method to confirm brain death is limited so far.

Summary and Conclusions

When all confounding conditions have been excluded, abolished EPs—including median nerve SL-SEPs after $N\overline{12}$, BAEPs with or without preserved waves I or I and II, VEPs with or without preserved ERGs, and transcranially elicited MEPs—indicates widespread failure of brain function, and adds substance to the clinical diagnosis of brain death. Because of limitations and pitfalls inherent in the study of a single neural pathway, exploring multiple sensory modalities is highly desirable in patients suspected of being brain dead (195). However, special emphasis should be placed on the study of SL-SEPs. BAEPs are of more uncertain assistance in confirming brain death, and VEPs are indicated primarily to differentiate between brain death and deefferented states caused by brainstem lesions that obliterate SL-SEPs and BAEPs. Although multimodality EPs can confirm that brain functions are irreversibly extinguished, their performance in the ICU is a time-consuming task that requires technical expertise and interpretive skills not available in all medical centers.

Methods chosen to confirm irreversible extinction of brain functions in the adult may vary according to the instrumentation and the technical and professional skills available in each medical center, and are dictated in some countries by governmental regulations. The nature of these tests is in constant evolution as new technologies become available. At present, techniques designed to demonstrate absence or critical deficit of brain perfusion, including radioisotope scintigraphy and Doppler ultrasonography, although not entirely free of shortcomings, are most commonly used in the United States to routinely confirm brain death in adults.

Brain Death in Neonates, Infants, and Small Children

Doubts have long been expressed that standards established for adults may be applicable to young patients. Guidelines issued in the United States by a Special Task Force for the Determination of Brain Death in Children (387) warned that establishing cessation of cerebral and brainstem functions and determining its irreversibility following severe brain insults was not possible in newborns earlier than 7 days after term. Clinical criteria of brain death applicable after this age did not differ from those recommended for adults. However, between the ages of 7 days and 1 year, the validity of these clinical standards depended on their persistence over specified periods of time and on their confirmation by EEG, cerebral radionuclide or contrast angiography, or both. No such constraints were advocated after the age of 1 year (Tables 14.2 and 14.3). These recommendations drew sharp criticism from Freeman and Ferry (164) and from Shewmon (410), who thought that the proposed standards were premature and based on combined clinical criteria and laboratory tests none of which had been validated. Perhaps in keeping with these objections, a survey of diverse pediatric ICUs in the United

TABLE 14.4. *Suggested requirements for demonstrating electrocerebral inactivity in children*

Patient age	Requirements
7 d–2 mo	Multiple physiological measures (typically eye movements, mental, electromyographic, respiration, and ECG) should be monitored in addition to the EEG (13).
	Numbers and locations of electrodes, and montages should meet guidelines for recordings in neonates and young infants (13).
	Effective recording time should be no less than 1 hr (13).
	The technologist obtaining the recording and the physician interpreting it should have special expertise in the EEG of neonates and young infants.
	Recordings demonstrating ECI should be repeated after a suitable interval to ensure persistent lack of electrocerebral activity (387).
> 2 mo–1 yr	Recording technique does not differ substantially from that recommended for adults. However, EEGs demonstrating ECI should be repeated after a suitable interval to ensure persistent lack of electrocerebral activity (387).
> 1 yr	Recording technique does not differ substantially from that recommended for adults.

Modified from Chatrian G-E. Electrophysiologic evaluation of brain death: a critical appraisal. In: Aminoff MJ, ed. *Electrodiagnosis in clinical neurology.* New York: Churchill Livingstone, 1999:681–705.

States (326) revealed only scant adherence to the guidelines of the Special Task Force. In the United Kingdom, a Working Party of the British Paediatric Association (500) thought that the concept of brain ("brainstem") death was itself "inappropriate" before 37 weeks' gestation and that confident diagnosis of this condition was "rarely possible" between the ages of 37 weeks' gestation and 2 months of age. For children older than 2 months, the assessment of brain death should be "approached in an unhurried manner" to ensure that all preconditions and clinical criteria are satisfied. The Working Party also denied the need to perform EEG, EP, angiographic, radioisotope, and Doppler studies to confirm the diagnosis of brain death in the developing child.

Clinical Criteria

There is general agreement that unique problems are met in attempting to determine by clinical observation and ancillary methods that brain functions have ceased in newborns and young infants and in establishing that this functional failure is irreversible. The clinical criteria of deep coma, absent brainstem reflexes, and apnea have limitations as indicators of loss of brain function in neonates and young infants, and periods of observation longer than in older patients are essential to establish their irreversibility (22,476).

The EEG as a Confirmatory Test

Technical and Interpretive Requirements

The EEGs of children have peculiar features (see Chapters 5 and 6) that evolve particularly rapidly from prematurity to 2 months after term. Neonatal EEGs are characteristically discontinuous; that is, they display bursts of activity separated by periods of apparent inactivity or generalized voltage attenuation that decrease in duration with increasing age. Widespread voltage depression, burst-suppression, and ultimately ECI readily develop in these recordings under the influence of a variety of factors, including hypoxia, hypotension, hypothermia, drug intoxication, and metabolic disorders (131–133,228,442). These particular features and the small head size of these young patients require substantial modifications of the recording technique used to demonstrate ECI in the adult (Table 14.4) as well as special interpretive skills that are uncommon even among pediatric neurologists. These requirements received little consideration in the report of the Special Task Force (387).

Reliability

Newborns up to 7 days after term with clinically diagnosed brain death may display in their EEGs either a pattern of ECI or variously preserved electrocerebral activity irrespective of whether cerebral blood flow is abolished, critically diminished, or preserved (21,23,25). Early reports of restoration of EEG activity following ECI in young patients were not documented beyond doubt in the absence of hypothermia, hypotension, CNS-depressant drugs (339,421), cerebral malformations, and the postictal state. It is now apparent that, however infrequently, recovery of EEG activity did occur in neonates with ECI who had none of these complicating conditions (23,228). In most instances, ECI was followed by other abnormal EEG patterns and the patients demonstrated neurological sequelae. However, a few neonates were said to survive over 2 years while continuing to display ECI (228).

ECI was reported in newborns in the presence of cerebral blood flow (23,25,460), and at least some electrocerebral activity was observed in the absence of demonstrable flow (21,23–25,130,224,459), although repeated EEG recordings ultimately demonstrated ECI in some of these patients (21,23–25,130). Conflicting results of these ancillary methods, and discrepancies between either of them and the clinical diagnosis, suggest that the EEG (and probably also cerebral perfusion tests) are of questionable assistance in confirming brain death in the immediate postnatal period (81,82). However, a review by Ashwal and Schneider (23) affirmed the notion that ECI persisting over 24 hours in the absence of complicating conditions in a neonate who remains clinically brain dead confirms that brain function has been irreversibly lost.

Evidence has been adduced by Alvarez et al. (10) that EEG recordings demonstrating ECI are more helpful in confirming the clinical diagnosis of brain death in patients older than 2–3 months. Their retrospective study showed that even a single EEG demonstrating ECI in the absence of hypothermia, hypotension, and toxic or metabolic disorders was sufficient to confirm permanent loss of brain viability above the age of 3 months. However, an appreciable proportion of patients of the same age suspected of being brain dead display some electrocerebral activity in their recordings. Incongruent results of EEG and brain perfusion tests also occur, although less commonly than in neonates, in small infants between the ages of 7 days and 2 months (21,23–25,130,459,460), and even in older infants and children up to the age of 5 years (21,23–25,51,167,224,459). Hence, special caution should be exercised in assessing the results of EEGs even after the age of 2–3 months. In particular, the detection of some electrocerebral activity in the face of persistent clinical manifestations of extinguished brain function, especially if associated with absent cerebral blood flow, should not be viewed as inconsistent with brain death and as encouraging the continu-ation of life-supporting measures in neonates, infants, and young children (21,22,130,224,404,476), as in adults (80,191,285,338,478). However, the amount of EEG activity that is compatible with brain death in these young patients is even less clear than in adults.

Evoked Potentials as Confirmatory Tests

Limited and primarily anecdotal data have been reported on EPs in neonates, infants, and children with suspected loss of brain function. Obliteration of cortical SL-SEPs and BAEPs was described in a limited number of patients of these ages in whom brain death had been diagnosed (115,130,408,431,457). However, loss of BAEPs occurred transiently following hypoxic episodes in a few newborns, infants, and small children who did not fulfill criteria of brain death and survived, although mostly with neurological sequelae (115,130,431,457).

CONCLUSIONS

Assessing the literature on the EEG in the developmental period poses major problems. These include extreme paucity of published data and their mostly anecdotal and retrospective nature; the use of EEG techniques often not or incompletely described or inadequate by present standards to demonstrate ECI, especially in neonates and small infants; and the heterogeneity of constantly evolving cerebral perfusion tests performed in conjunction with the EEG (81). In our opinion, these limitations justify some of the reservations expressed by concerned physicians regarding the guidelines issued by the Special Task Force for the Determination of Brain Death in Children (387) as well as the caution inspiring the report of the Working Party of the British Paediatric Association (500). We also believe that, until much additional information becomes available, EPs should not be routinely relied on to confirm irreversible loss of brain viability in young patients (79–82).

REFERENCES

1. Abbott J. The EEG in Jakob-Creutzfeldt's disease. *Electroencephalogr Clin Neurophysiol* 1959;11:184–185(abst).
2. Adams JH, Graham DI, Murray LS, et al. Diffuse axonal injury due to nonmissile head injury in humans: an analysis of 45 cases. *Ann Neurol* 1982;12:557–563.
3. Adams RD, Foley JM. The neurologic disorder associated with liver disease. *Res Publ Assoc Res Nerv Ment Dis* 1953;32:198–237.
4. Agardh CD, Rosen I, Ryding E. Persistent vegetative state with high cerebral blood flow following profound hypoglycemia. *Ann Neurol* 1983;14:482–486.

5. Aguglia U, Gambardella A, Oliveri RL, et al. Triphasic waves and cerebral tumors. *Eur Neurol* 1990;30:1–5.
6. Ahmed I. Can somatosensory evoked potentials predict outcome from coma? *Clin Electroencephalogr* 1992;23:126–131.
7. Alajouanine T. Les altérations des états de conscience causées par les désordres neurologiques. *Acta Med Belg* 1957;2:19–41.
8. Alexandre A, Rubini L, Nortempi P, et al. Sleep alterations during post traumatic coma as a possible predictor of cognitive defects. *Acta Neurochir Suppl (Wien)* 1979;28:188–192.
9. Alster J, Pratt H, Feinsod M. Density spectral array, evoked potentials, and temperature rhythms in the evaluation and prognosis of the comatose patient. *Brain Inj* 1993;7:191–208.
10. Alvarez LA, Moshé SL, Belman AL, et al. EEG and brain death determination in children. *Neurology* 1988;38:227–230.
11. Alving J, Møller M, Sindrup E, et al. 'Alpha pattern coma' following cerebral anoxia. *Electroencephalogr Clin Neurophysiol* 1979;47:95–101.
12. American Congress of Rehabilitation Medicine. Recommendations for the use of uniform nomenclature to patients with severe alterations in consciousness. *Arch Phys Med Rehabil* 1995;76:205–209.
13. American Electroencephalographic Society Guidelines in Electroencephalography, Evoked Potentials, and Polysomnography, Guideline Two: Minimum technical standards for pediatric electroencephalography. *J Clin Neurophysiol* 1994;11:6–9.
14. American Electroencephalographic Society Guidelines in Electroencephalography, Evoked Potentials, and Polysomnography, Guideline Three: Minimum technical standards for EEG recording in suspected cerebral death. *J Clin Neurophysiol* 1994;11:10–13.
14a. American Electroencephalographic Society Guidelines in Electroencephalography, Evoked Potentials, and Polysomnography. Guidline Nine: Guidelines of Evoked Potentials. *J Clin Neurophysiol* 1994;11:40–73
15. Anderson DC, Bundlie S, Rockswold GL. Multimodality evoked potentials in closed head trauma. *Arch Neurol* 1984;37:222–225.
16. Andrews K, Murphy L, Munday R, et al. Misdiagnosis of the vegetative state: retrospective study in a rehabilitation unit. *BMJ* 1996;313:13–16.
17. Anziska BJ, Cracco RQ. Short-latency somatosensory evoked potentials in brain dead patients. *Arch Neurol* 1980;37:222–225.
18. Arfel G. Stimulations visuelles et silence cérébral. *Electroencephalogr Clin Neurophysiol* 1967;23:172.
19. Arfel G. *Problèmes électroencéphalographiques de la mort.* Paris: Masson, 1970.
20. Arfel G. Introduction to clinical and EEG studies in coma. In: Rémond AE, ed. *Handbook of electroencephalography and clinical neurophysiology*, Vol 12. Amsterdam: Elsevier Science, 1975:5–23.
21. Ashwal S, Schneider S. Failure of electroencephalography to diagnose brain death in comatose children. *Ann Neurol* 1979;6:512–517.
22. Ashwal S, Schneider S. Brain death in children: Part I. *Pediatr Neurol* 1987;3:5–11.
23. Ashwal S, Schneider S. Brain death in the newborn. *Pediatrics* 1989;84:429–437.
24. Ashwal S, Schneider S, Thompson J. Xenon computed tomography measuring cerebral blood flow in the determination of brain death in children. *Ann Neurol* 1989;25:539–546.
25. Ashwal S, Smith AJK, Torres F, et al. Radionuclide bolus angiography: a technique for verification of brain death in infants and children. *J Pediatr* 1977;91:722–728.
26. Attia J, Cook DJ. Prognosis in anoxic and traumatic coma. *Crit Care Clin* 1998;14:497–511.
27. Austin EJ, Bhagat A, Dodrill CB, et al. EEG rhythms of alpha frequency in a patient with hyperosmolar diabetic coma followed by partial recovery. *Electroencephalogr Clin Neurophysiol* 1984;57:61P(abst).
28. Austin EJ, Wilkus RJ, Longstreth WT Jr. Etiology and prognosis of alpha coma. *Neurology* 1988;38:773–777.
29. Bahamon-Dussan JE, Celesia GG, Grigg-Damberger MM. Prognostic significance of EEG triphasic waves in patients with altered state of consciousness. *J Clin Neurophysiol* 1989;6:313–319.
30. Barelli A, Valente MR, Clemente A, et al. Serial multimodality-evoked potentials in severely head-injured patients: diagnostic and prognostic implications. *Crit Care Med* 1991;19:1374–1381.
31. Bassetti C, Bomio F, Mathis J, et al. Early prognosis in coma after cardiac arrest: a prospective clinical, electrophysiological, and biochemical study of 60 patients. *J Neurol Neurosurg Psychiatry* 1996;61:610–615.
32. Bassetti C, Mathis J, Hess CW. Multimodal electrophysiological studies including motor evoked potentials in patients with locked-in syndrome: report of six patients. *J Neurol Neurosurg Psychiatry* 1994;57:1403–1406.
33. Bauer G, Aichner F, Klinger K. Aktivitäten im Alpha-Frequenzbereich und Koma. *EEG EMG* 1982;13:28–33.
34. Bauer G, Gerstenbrand F, Rumpl E. Varieties of the locked-in syndrome. *J Neurol* 1979;221:77–91.
35. Beca J, Cox PN, Taylor MJ, et al. Somatosensory evoked potentials for prediction of outcome in acute severe brain injury. *J Pediatr* 1995;126:44–49.
36. Belsh JM, Chokroverty S. Short-latency somatosensory-evoked potentials in brain-death patients. *Electroencephalogr Clin Neurophysiol* 1987;68:75–78.
37. Bennett DR, Hughes JR, Korein J, et al, eds. *Atlas of electroencephalography in coma and cerebral death: EEG at the bedside or in the intensive care unit.* New York: Raven Press, 1976.
38. Beresford HR. The Quinlan decision: problems and legislative alternatives. *Ann Neurol* 1977;2:74–81.
39. Bergamasco B, Bergamini L, Doriguzzi T. Clinical value of the sleep electroencephalographic patterns in post-traumatic coma. *Acta Neurol Scand* 1968;44:495–511.
40. Bergamasco B, Bergamini L, Doriguzzi T, et al. EEG sleep patterns as a prognostic criterion in post-traumatic coma. *Electroencephalogr Clin Neurophysiol* 1968;24:374–377.
41. Bergamasco B, Bergamini L, Mombelli AM, et al. Longitudinal study of visual evoked potentials in subjects in post-traumatic coma. *Schweiz Arch Neurol Neurochir Psychiatr* 1966;97:1–10.
42. Berger EL, Stockard JJ, Aung MH, et al. Removal of EKG artifact from EEG in brain death and other recordings. *Electroencephalogr Clin Neurophysiol* 1974;37:202.
43. Bermejo Pareja F, Martinez Martin P, Alvarez Tejerina J. "Coma alfa": analisis de una serie de 19 casos. *Arch Neurobiol* 1979;42:243–262.
44. Beydoun A, Yen CE, Drury I. Variance of interburst intervals in burst suppression. *Electroencephalogr Clin Neurophysiol* 1991;79:435–439.
45. Bickford RG, Butt HR. Hepatic coma: the electroencephalographic pattern. *J Clin Invest* 1955;34:790–799.
46. Bickford RG, Klass DW. Acute and chronic EEG findings after head injury. In: Caveness WF, Walker AE, eds. *Head injury.* Philadelphia: JB Lippincott, 1966:63–88.
47. Binnie CD, Prior PF, Lloyd DSL, et al. Electroencephalographic prediction of fatal anoxic brain damage after resuscitation from cardiac arrest. *Br Med J* 1970;4:265–268.
48. Bird TD, Plum F. Recovery from barbiturate overdose coma with a prolonged isoelectric electroencephalogram. *Neurology* 1968;18:456–460.
49. Black PM. Brain death (second of two parts). *N Engl J Med* 1978;299:393–401.
50. Blatt I, Brenner RP. Triphasic waves in a psychiatric population: a retrospective study. *J Clin Neurophysiol* 1996;13:324–329.
51. Bode H, Sauer M, Pringsheim W. Diagnosis of brain death by transcranial Doppler sonography. *Arch Dis Child* 1988;63:1474–1478.
52. Bortone E, Bettoni L, Buzio S, et al. Spindle coma and alternating pattern in the course of measles encephalitis. *Clin Electroencephalogr* 1996;27:210–214.
53. Bortone E, Bettoni L, Giorgi C, et al. Reliability of EEG in the diagnosis of Creutzfeldt-Jakob disease. *Electroencephalogr Clin Neurophysiol* 1994;90:323–330.

54. Brenner RP, Schaul N. Periodic EEG patterns: classification, clinical correlation, and pathophysiology. *J Clin Neurophysiol* 1990;7:249–267.

55. Brewer CC, Resnick DM. The value of BAEP in assessment of the comatose patients. In: Nodar RH, Barber D, eds. *Evoked potentials II*. London: Butterworth-Heinemann, 1984: 578–581.

56. Bricolo A, Gentilomo A, Rosadini G, et al. Akinetic mutism following cranio-cerebral trauma: physiopathological considerations based on sleep studies. *Acta Neurochir (Wien)* 1968;18: 68–77.

57. Bricolo A, Gentilomo A, Rosadini G, et al. Long lasting post-traumatic unconsciousness: a study based on nocturnal EEG and polygraphic recording. *Acta Neurol Scand* 1968;44: 512–532.

58. Bricolo A, Turazzi S, Faccioli F, et al. Clinical applications of compressed spectral array in prolonged coma. *Electroencephalogr Clin Neurophysiol* 1978;45:211–225.

59. Bricolo A, Turella G. Electroencephalographic patterns of acute traumatic coma: diagnostic and prognostic value. *J Neurosurg Sci* 1973;17:278–285.

60. Brierley JB, Adams JH, Graham DI, et al. Neocortical death after cardiac arrest: a clinical, neurophysiological, and neuropathological report of two cases. *Lancet* 1971;2:560–565.

61. Britt CW Jr. Nontraumatic "spindle coma": clinical, EEG, and prognostic features. *Neurology* 1981;31:393–397.

62. Britt CW Jr, Morris HHI. Triphasic waves in a fully alert patient with liver disease. *Clin Electroencephalogr* 1979;10:72–74.

63. Britt CW Jr, Raso E, Gerson LP. Spindle coma, secondary to primary traumatic midbrain hemorrhage. *Electroencephalogr Clin Neurophysiol* 1980;49:406–408.

64. Britt RH, Herrick MK, Hamilton RD. Traumatic locked-in syndrome. *Ann Neurol* 1977;1: 590–592.

65. Britt RH, Herrick MK, Mason RT, et al. Traumatic lesions of the pontomedullary junction. *Neurosurgery* 1980;6:623–631.

66. Brown RH, Chiappa KH, Brooks E. Brainstem auditory evoked responses in 22 patients with intrinsic brain stem lesions: implications for clinical interpretations. *Electroencephalogr Clin Neurophysiol* 1981;51:38P(abst).

67. Brunko E, Delecluse F, Herbaut AG, et al. Unusual pattern of somatosensory and brain stem auditory evoked potentials after cardio-respiratory arrest. *Electroencephalogr Clin Neurophysiol* 1985;62:338–342.

68. Brunko E, Zegers de Beyl D. Prognostic value of early cortical somatosensory evoked potentials after resuscitation from cardiac arrest. *Electroencephalogr Clin Neurophysiol* 1987;55: 15–24.

69. Calhoun CL, Ettinger MG. Unusual EEG in coma after cardiac arrest. *Electroencephalogr Clin Neurophysiol* 1966;21:385–388.

70. Cant BR, Hume AL, Judson JA, et al. The assessment of severe head injury by short-latency somatosensory and brain-stem auditory evoked potentials. *Electroencephalogr Clin Neurophysiol* 1986;65:188–195.

71. Carroll WM, Mastaglia GL. Alpha and beta coma in drug intoxication uncomplicated by cerebral hypoxia. *Electroencephalogr Clin Neurophysiol* 1979;46:95–105.

72. Celesia GG. Pathophysiology of periodic EEG complexes in subacute sclerosing panencephalitis (SSPE). *Electroencephalogr Clin Neurophysiol* 1973;35:293–300.

73. Chang B, Morariu MA. Transient traumatic 'locked-in' syndrome. *Eur Neurol* 1979;18: 391–394.

74. Chase TN, Moretti L, Prensky AL. Clinical and electroencephalographic manifestations of vascular lesions of the pons. *Neurology* 1968;18:357–368.

75. Chatrian GE. Electrographic and behavioral signs of sleep in comatose states. In: Rémond A, ed. *Handbook of electroencephalography and clinical neurophysiology*, Vol 12. Amsterdam: Elsevier Science, 1975:63–77.

76. Chatrian GE. The low voltage EEG. In: Rémond A, ed. *Handbook of electroencephalography and clinical neurophysiology, Vol 6, Part A. The EEG of the waking adult*. Amsterdam: Elsevier Science, 1976:77–89.

77. Chatrian G-E. Electrophysiological evaluation of brain death: a critical appraisal. In: Aminoff MJ, ed. *Electrodiagnosis in clinical neurology*. New York: Churchill Livingstone, 1980: 525–588.

78. Chatrian G-E. Electrophysiologic evaluation of brain death: a critical appraisal. In: Aminoff MJ, ed. *Electrodiagnosis in clinical neurology*, 2nd ed. New York: Churchill Livingstone, 1986:669–736.

79. Chatrian G-E. Coma, other states of altered responsiveness, and brain death. In: Daly DD, Pedley TA, eds. *Current practice of clinical electroencephalography*, 2nd ed. New York: Raven Press, 1990:425–487.

80. Chatrian G-E. Electrophysiologic evaluation of brain death: a critical appraisal. In: Aminoff MJ, ed. *Electrodiagnosis in clinical neurology*, 3rd ed. New York: Churchill Livingstone, 1992: 737–793.

81. Chatrian G-E. Diagnosis of brain death. In: Collins GM, Dubernard JM, Land W, et al, eds. *Procurement, preservation and allocation of vascularized organs*. Dordrecht: Kluwer Academic Publishers, 1997:23–46.

82. Chatrian G-E. Electrophysiologic evaluation of brain death: a critical appraisal. In: Aminoff MJ, ed. *Electrodiagnosis in clinical neurology,* 4th ed. New York: Churchill Livingstone, 1999: 681–705.

83. Chatrian G-E, Bergamasco B, Bricolo A, et al. IFCN recommended standards for electrophysiologic monitoring in comatose and other unresponsive states: report of an IFCN committee. *Electroencephalogr Clin Neurophysiol* 1996;99:103–122.

84. Chatrian GE, Bergamini L, Dondey M, et al. A glossary of terms most commonly used by clinical electroencephalographers. *Electroencephalogr Clin Neurophysiol* 1974;37:538–548.

85. Chatrian GE, Shaw C-M, Leffman H. The significance of periodic lateralized epileptiform discharges in EEG: an electrographic, clinical and pathological study. *Electroencephalogr Clin Neurophysiol* 1964;17:177–193.

86. Chatrian GE, White LE Jr. Sleep EEG patterns in certain comatose states following brain concussion. *Electroencephalogr Clin Neurophysiol* 1961;13:661(abst).

87. Chatrian GE, White LE Jr, Daly D. Electroencephalographic patterns resembling those of sleep in certain comatose states after injuries to the head. *Electroencephalogr Clin Neurophysiol* 1963;15:272–280.

88. Chatrian GE, White LE Jr, Shaw CM. EEG pattern resembling wakefulness in unresponsive decerebrate state following traumatic brainstem infarct. *Electroencephalogr Clin Neurophysiol* 1964;16:285–289.

89. Chatrian GE, Wirch AL, Lettich E, et al. Click-evoked human electrocochleogram: noninvasive recording method, origin, and physiological significance. *Am J EEG Technol* 1982;22: 151–174.

90. Cheliout-Héraut F, Durand MC, Clair B, et al. Importance of evoked potentials in the evolutive prognosis of coma during cerebral anoxia in adults. *Neurophysiol Clin* 1992;22:269–280.

91. Chen R, Bolton CF, Young GB. Prediction of outcome in patients with anoxic coma: a clinical and electrophysiologic study. *Crit Care Med* 1996;24:672–678.

92. Cherington M, Stears J, Hodges J. Locked-in syndrome caused by a tumor. *Neurology* 1976; 26:180–182.

93. Chia L-G. Locked-in state with bilateral internal capsule infarcts. *Neurology* 1984;34: 1365–1367.

94. Chiappa KH, Hill RA. Evaluation and prognostication in coma. *Electroencephalogr Clin Neurophysiol* 1998;106:149–155.

95. Chiappa KH, Hoch DB. Electrophysiologic monitoring. In: Ropper AH, ed. *Neurological and neurosurgical intensive care*, 3rd ed. New York: Raven Press, 1993:147–183.

96. Chiappa KH, Parker SW. A simple needle electrode technique for improved registration of wave I in brainstem auditory potentials. In: Starr A, Rosemberg C, Don M, et al, eds. *Sensory*

evoked potentials, 1. An international conference on standards in auditory brainstem response testing. Milan: Edizioni Tecniche, 1984:137–139.

97. Chien LT, Boehm RM, Robinson H, et al. Characteristic early electroencephalographic changes in herpes simplex encephalitis. *Arch Neurol* 1977;34:361–364.

98. Childs NL, Mercer WN, Childs HW. Accuracy of diagnosis of persistent vegetative state. *Neurology* 1993;43:1465–1467.

99. Chiofalo N, Fuentes A, Galves C. Serial findings in 27 cases of Creutzfeldt-Jakob disease. *Arch Neurol* 1980;37:143–145.

100. Chokroverty S. "Alpha-like" rhythms in electroencephalograms in coma after cardiac arrest. *Neurology* 1975;25:655–663.

101. Chu N-S, Yang S-S, Liaw Y-F. Evoked potentials in liver diseases. *J Gastroenterol Hepatol* 1997;12:S288–S293.

102. Cobb W. The periodic events of subacute sclerosing leucoencephalitis. *Electroencephalogr Clin Neurophysiol* 1966;21:278–294.

103. Cobb W, Hill D. Electroencephalogram in subacute progressive encephalitis. *Brain* 1950;73:392–404.

104. Cohen SN, Syndulko K, Rever B, et al. Visual evoked potentials and long latency event-related potentials in chronic renal failure. *Neurology* 1983;33:1219–1222.

105. Collins AT, Chatrian GE. EEG rhythms of alpha frequency in a 22-month-old child after strangulation. *Neurology* 1980;30:1316–1319.

106. Courjon J, Naquet R, Baurand D, et al. Valeur diagnostique et prognostique de l'EEG dans les suites immédiates des traumatismes crâniens. *Rev Electroencephalogr Neurophysiol Clin* 1971;1:133–150.

107. Courjon J, Scherzer E. Traumatic disorders. In: Rémond A, ed. *Handbook of electroencephalography and clinical neurophysiology*, Vol 14, Part B. Amsterdam: Elsevier Science, 1972:8–39.

108. Cravioto H, Silverman J, Feigin I. A clinical and pathologic study of akinetic mutism. *Neurology* 1960;10:10–21.

109. Crow HJ, Winter A. Serial electrophysiological studies (EEG, EMG, ERG, evoked responses) in case of 3 months' survival with flat EEG following cardiac arrest. *Electroencephalogr Clin Neurophysiol* 1969;27:332–333.

110. Cummings JL, Greenberg R. Sleep patterns in the "locked-in" syndrome. *Electroencephalogr Clin Neurophysiol* 1977;43:270.

111. Cusumano S, Paolin A, Di Paola F, et al. Assessing brain function in post-traumatic coma by means of bit-mapped SEPs, BAEPs, CT, SPET and clinical scores: prognostic implications. *Electroencephalogr Clin Neurophysiol* 1992;84:499–514.

112. Dadmehr N, Pakalnis A, Drake ME. Spindle coma in viral encephalitis. *Clin Electroencephalogr* 1987;18:34–37.

113. Daly D, Whelan JL, Bickford RG, et al. The electroencephalogram in cases of tumors of the posterior fossa and third ventricle. *Electroencephalogr Clin Neurophysiol* 1953;5:203–216.

114. Davis PH, Davis PA. The electrical activity of the brain: its relation to physiological states and to states of impaired consciousness. *Res Publ Assoc Res Nerv Ment Dis* 1939;19:50–80.

115. Dear PRF, Godfrey DJ. Neonatal auditory brainstem response cannot reliably diagnose brainstem death. *Arch Dis Child* 1985;60:17–19.

116. De Giorgio CM, Rabinowicz A, Gott PS. Predictive value of P300 event-related potentials compared with EEG and somatosensory evoked potentials in non-traumatic coma. *Acta Neurol Scand* 1993;87:423–427.

117. de la Paz D, Brenner RF. Bilateral independent periodic lateralized epileptiform discharges: clinical significance. *Arch Neurol* 1981;38:713–715.

118. de la Torre JC, Trimble JL, Beard RT, et al. Somatosensory evoked potentials for the prognosis of coma in humans. *Exp Neurol* 1978;60:304–317.

119. Deleu D, De Keyser J. Flunitrazepam intoxication simulating a structural brainstem lesion. *J Neurol Neurosurg Psychiatry* 1987;50:236–237.

120. Deleu D, Ebinger G. Alpha coma with sedative overdose. *Neurology* 1989;39:156–157.

121. Deliyannakis E, Ioannou F, Davaroukas A. Brain stem death with persistence of bioelectric activity of the cerebral hemispheres. *Clin Electroencephalogr* 1975;6:75–79.

122. De Meirleir LJ, Taylor MJ. Evoked potentials in comatose children: auditory brainstem responses. *Pediatr Neurol* 1986;2:31–34.

123. Desmedt JE, Cheron G. Central somatosensory conduction in man: neural generators and interpeak latencies of the far-field components recorded from neck and right or left scalp and earlobes. *Electroencephalogr Clin Neurophysiol* 1980;50:382–403.

124. Desmedt JE, Nguyen TH, Bourguet M. The cognitive P40, N60, P100 components of somatosensory evoked potentials and the earliest signs of sensory processing in man. *Electroencephalogr Clin Neurophysiol* 1983;56:272–282.

125. Desmedt JE, Nguyen TH, Bourguet M. Bit-mapped color imaging of human evoked potentials with reference to the N20, P22, P27 and N30 somatosensory responses. *Electroencephalogr Clin Neurophysiol* 1987;68:1–19.

126. De Weerd AW, Groeneveld C. The use of evoked potentials in the management of patients with severe cerebral trauma. *Acta Neurol Scand* 1985;72:489.

127. Dike GL. Triphasic waves in serotonin syndrome [Letter]. *J Neurol Neurosurg Psychiatry* 1997;62:200.

128. Dolce GE, Kaemmerer E. Contributo anatomico ed elettroencefalografico alla conoscenza della sindrome apallica: studio dell'evoluzione dell'EEG da sonno in 5 casi. *Sist Nerv* 1967;29:12–23.

129. Dougherty JH, Rawlinson DG, Levy DE, et al. Hypoxic-ischemic brain injury and the vegetative state: clinical and neuropathologic correlation. *Neurology* 1981;31:991–997.

130. Drake B, Ashwal S, Schneider S. Determination of cerebral death in the pediatric intensive care unit. *Pediatrics* 1986;78:107–112.

131. Dreyfus-Brisac C. L' électroencéphalogramme: critère d'âge conceptionnel du nouveau-né à terme et du prématuré. *Biol Neonat* 1962;4:154–173.

132. Dreyfus-Brisac C, Flescher J, Plassart E. The electroencephalogram of the premature infant and full-term newborn: normal and abnormal development of waking and sleeping patterns. In: Kellaway P, Petersén I, eds. *Neurological and electroencephalographic correlative studies in infancy*. New York: Grune & Stratton, 1964:186–206.

133. Dreyfus-Brisac C, Larroche J-C. Discontinuous EEGs in prematures and full-term neonates. *Electroencephalogr Clin Neurophysiol* 1972;32:575.

134. Drummond JC, Todd MM, U HS. The effect of high dose sodium thiopental on brain stem auditory and median nerve somatosensory evoked responses in man. *Anesthesiology* 1985;63:249–254.

135. Drury I, Westmoreland BF, Sharbrough FW. Electroencephalographic studies in a locked in and locked out state due to severe acute inflammatory polyradiculoneuropathy. *Electroencephalogr Clin Neurophysiol* 1986;64:27P(abst).

136. Dusser A, Navelet D, Devictor D, et al. Short and long term value of the electroencephalogram in children with severe head injury. *Electroencephalogr Clin Neurophysiol* 1989;73:85–93.

137. Ebner A, Zentner J. Prognostic value of somatosensory and motor evoked potentials in comatose patients with severe head injury. In: Rossini PM, Marsden CD, eds. *Non-invasive stimulation of brain and spinal cord: fundamentals and clinical applications*. New York: Alan R. Liss, 1988:313–319.

138. Echlin FA, Arnett V, Zoll J. Paroxysmal high voltage discharges from isolated and partially isolated human and animal cerebral cortex. *Electroencephalogr Clin Neurophysiol* 1952;4:147–164.

139. Emerson RG, Pedley TA. Somatosensory evoked potentials. In: Daly DD, Pedley TA, eds. *Current practice of clinical electroencephalography*, 2nd ed. 1990:679–705.

140. Endo M, Hirano M, Nakamura I, et al. Two cases of alpha-pattern coma caused by large amounts of hypnotica and neuroleptica. *Folia Psychiatr Neurol Jpn* 1980;34:451–458.

141. Evans BM, Bartlett JR. Prediction of outcome in severe head injury based on recognition of

sleep related activity in the polygraphic electroencephalogram. *J Neurol Neurosurg Psychiatry* 1995;59:17–25(abst).

142. Facco E, Baratto F, Munari M, et al. Sensorimotor central conduction time in comatose patients. *Electroencephalogr Clin Neurophysiol* 1991;80:469–476.

143. Facco E, Behr AU, Munari M, et al. Auditory and somatosensory evoked potentials in coma following spontaneous cerebral hemorrhage: early prognosis and outcome. *Electroencephalogr Clin Neurophysiol* 1998;107:332–338.

144. Facco E, Caputo P, Fiore D, et al. Sensorimotor and auditory central conduction time in locked-in syndrome. *Electroencephalogr Clin Neurophysiol* 1989;73:552–556.

145. Facco E, Martini A, Zuccarello M, et al. Is the auditory brain stem response (ABR) effective in the assessment of post-traumatic coma? *Electroencephalogr Clin Neurophysiol* 1985;62: 332–337.

146. Facco E, Munari M, Baratto F, et al. Multimodality evoked potentials (auditory, somatosensory and motor) in coma. *Neurophysiol Clin* 1993;23:237–258.

147. Fakhoury T, Abou-Khalil B, Blumenkopf B. EEG changes in intrathecal baclofen overdose: a case report and review of the literature. *Electroencephalogr Clin Neurophysiol* 1998;107: 339–342.

148. Faure J, Droogleever-Fortuyn J, Gastaut H, et al. De la génèse et de la signification des rythmes recueillis à distance dans les cas de tumeurs cérébrales. *Electroencephalogr Clin Neurophysiol* 1951;3:429–434.

149. Feldman MH. Physiological observations in a chronic case of "locked-in" syndrome. *Neurology* 1971;21:459–477.

150. Ferguson JM, Bennett DR. Sleep in a patient with a pontine infarction. *Electroencephalogr Clin Neurophysiol* 1974;36:210–211(abst).

151. Ficker DM, Westmoreland BF, Sharbrough FW. Epileptiform abnormalities in hepatic encephalopathy. *J Clin Neurophysiol* 1997;14:230–234.

152. Firsching R, Frowein RA. Evoked potentials and early prognosis in comatose patients. *Neurosurg Rev* 1990;13:141–146.

153. Firsching R, Wilhelms S, Cséscei G. Pyramidal tract function during onset of brain death. *Electroencephalogr Clin Neurophysiol* 1992;84:321–324.

154. Fisch BJ, Klass DW. The diagnostic specificity of triphasic wave patterns. *Electroencephalogr Clin Neurophysiol* 1988;70:1–8.

155. Fischer C. EEG recording in the diagnosis of brain death. *Neurophysiol Clin* 1997;27: 373–382.

156. Fischer C, Ibañez V, Jourdan C, et al. Potentiels évoqués auditifs précoces (PEAP), auditifs de latence moyenne (PALM) et somesthésiques (PES) dans le prognostic vital et fonctionnel des traumatismes crâniens graves en réanimation. *Agressologie* 1988;29:359–363.

157. Fischer C, Mauguière F, Echallier JF, et al. Contribution of brainstem auditory evoked potentials to diagnosis of tumors and vascular diseases. In: Courjon J, Mauguière F, Revol M, eds. *Clinical applications of evoked potentials in neurology.* New York: Raven Press, 1982: 177–185.

158. Fischer C, Morlet D, Bouchet P, et al. Mismatch negativity and late auditory evoked potentials in comatose patients. *Clin Neurophysiol* 1999;110:1601–1610.

159. Fischgold H, Mathis P. *Obnubilations, comas et stupeurs: etudes électroencéphalographiques.* Electroencephalogr Clin Neurophysiol. Paris: Masson, 1959.

160. Fitzgerald LG, Simpson RK. Locked-in syndrome resulting from cervical spine gunshot wound. *J Trauma* 1997;42:147–149.

161. Flügel KA. Alphakoma, Pseudoalphakoma and Alpha-Pseudokoma: zur Differentialdiagnose des sogennanten Alpha-Komas. *Fortschr Neurol Psychiatr* 1982;50:371–386.

162. Foley JM, Watson CW, Adams RD. Significance of the electroencephalographic changes in hepatic coma. *Trans Am Neurol Assoc* 1950;75:161–165.

163. Forti A, Ambrosetto G, Amore M, et al. Locked-in syndrome in multiple sclerosis with sparing of the ventral portion of the pons. *Ann Neurol* 1982;12:393–394.

163a. Frank LM, Furgiuele TL, Etheridge JE. Prediction of chronic vegetative state in children using evoked potentials. *Neurology* 1985;35:931–934.

164. Freeman JM, Ferry PC. New brain death guidelines in children: further confusion. *Pediatrics* 1988;81:301–303.

165. Freemon FR, Salinas-Garcia RF, Ward JW. Sleep patterns in a patient with a brainstem infarction involving the raphe nucleus. *Electroencephalogr Clin Neurophysiol* 1974;36:657–660.

166. Fung PC, Tucker RP. Alpha rhythm and alpha-like activity in coma. *Clin Electroencephalogr* 1984;15:167–172.

167. Furgiuele TL, Frank LM, Riegle C, et al. Prediction of cerebral death by cranial sector scan. *Crit Care Med* 1984;12:1–3.

168. Ganes T, Lundar T. EEG and evoked potentials in comatose patients with severe brain damage. *Electroencephalogr Clin Neurophysiol* 1988;69:6–13.

169. Ganji S, Peters G, Frazier E. Somatosensory and brainstem auditory evoked potentials studies in nontraumatic coma. *Clin Electroencephalogr* 1988;19:55–67.

170. García-Larrea L, Artru F, Bertrand O, et al. Transient drug-induced abolition of BAEPs in coma. *Neurology* 1988;38:1487–1489.

171. García-Larrea L, Artru P, Bertrand O, et al. The combined monitoring of brain-stem auditory evoked potentials and intracranial pressure in coma: a study of 57 patients. *J Neurol Neurosurg Psychiatry* 1992;55:792–798.

172. García-Larrea L, Bastuji H, Mauguière F. Mapping study of somatosensory evoked potentials during selective spatial attention. *Electroencephalogr Clin Neurophysiol* 1991;80:201–214.

173. García-Larrea L, Bertrand O, Artru F, et al. Brain-stem monitoring. II. Preterminal BAEP changes observed until brain death in deeply comatose patients. *Electroencephalogr Clin Neurophysiol* 1987;68:445–457.

174. Gentilomo A, Rivano C, Rosadini GE. Studio elettroclinico longitudinale del coma cerebrale evolvente verso la sindrome apallica. *Rass Arch Chir* 1966;4:816–832.

175. Gerstenbrand F. *Das traumatische apallische Syndrom: Klinik, Morphologie, Pathophysiologie und Behandlung.* New York: Springer-Verlag, 1967.

176. Gerstenbrand F. The symptomatology of the apallic syndrome. In: Dalle Ore G, Gerstenbrand F, Lücking CH, et al, eds. *The apallic syndrome.* Berlin: Springer-Verlag, 1977.

177. Giacino JT, Zasler ND, Katz DI, et al. Development of practice guidelines for assessment and management of the vegetative and minimally conscious states. *J Head Trauma Rehabil* 1997; 12:79–89.

178. Gibbs FA, Gibbs EL. *Atlas of electroencephalography.* Cambridge, MA: Cummins, 1941.

179. Gilroy J, Lynn GE, Ristow GE, et al. Auditory evoked brain stem potentials in a case of "locked-in" syndrome. *Arch Neurol* 1977;34:492–495.

180. Glass I, Sazbon L, Groswasser Z. Mapping "cognitive" event-related potentials in prolonged postcoma unawareness state. *Clin Electroencephalogr* 1998;29:19–30.

181. Gloor P. Generalized and widespread paroxysmal abnormalities. In: Rémond A, ed. *Handbook of electroencephalography and clinical neurophysiology*, Vol 11, Part B. Amsterdam: Elsevier Science, 1976:52–87.

182. Gloor P, Ball G, Schaul N. Brain lesions that produce delta waves in the EEG. *Neurology* 1977; 27:326–333.

183. Gloor P, Kalabay O, Giard N. The electroencephalogram in diffuse encephalopathies: electroencephalographic correlates of grey and white matter lesions. *Brain* 1968;91:779–802.

184. Goldie WD, Chiappa KH, Young RR, et al. Brainstem auditory and short-latency somatosensory evoked responses in brain death. *Neurology* 1981;31:248–256.

185. Goodwin SR, Friedman WA, Bellefleur M. Is it time to use evoked potentials to predict outcome in comatose children and adults? *Crit Care Med* 1991;19:518–524.

186. Gott PS, Rabinowicz AL, De Giorgio CM. P300 auditory event-related potentials in nontraumatic coma. *Arch Neurol* 1991;48:1267–1270.

187. Gottschalk PG, Hansotia P, Berendes J. Alpha coma: report of eleven cases. *Electroencephalogr Clin Neurophysiol* 1978;44:122(abst).

188. Greenberg RP, Becker DP, Miller JD, et al. Evaluation of brain function in severe human head trauma with multimodality evoked potentials. Part 2: Localization of brain dysfunction and correlation with posttraumatic neurological conditions. *J Neurosurg* 1977;47:163–177.

189. Greenberg RP, Ducker TB. Evoked potentials in the clinical neurosciences. *J Neurosurg* 1982; 56:1–18.

190. Greenberg RP, Newlon PG, Hyatt MS, et al. Prognostic implication of early multimodality evoked potentials in severely head-injured patients: a prospective study. *J Neurosurg* 1981;55: 227–236.

191. Grigg MM, Kelly MA, Celesia GG, et al. Electroencephalographic activity after brain death. *Arch Neurol* 1987;44:948–954.

192. Grindal AB, Suter C. "Alpha-pattern coma" in high voltage electrical injury. *Electroencephalogr Clin Neurophysiol* 1975;38:521–526.

193. Grindal AB, Suter C, Martinez AJ. Alpha-pattern coma—24 cases with 9 survivors. *Ann Neurol* 1977;1:371–377.

194. Guérit JM. Unexpected myogenic contaminants observed in the somatosensory evoked potentials recorded in one brain-dead patient. *Electroencephalogr Clin Neurophysiol* 1986;64:21–26.

195. Guérit JM. Evoked potentials: a safe brain-death confirmatory tool? *Eur J Med* 1992;1: 233–243.

196. Guérit JM. The interest of multimodality evoked potentials in the evaluation of chronic coma. *Acta Neurol Belg* 1994;94:174–182.

197. Guérit JM, de Tourtchaninoff M, Soveges L, et al. The prognostic value of three-modality evoked potentials (TMEPS) in anoxic and traumatic comas. *Neurophysiol Clin* 1993;23: 209–226.

198. Guérit J-M, Fischer C, Facco E, et al. Standards of clinical practice of EEG and EPs in comatose and other unresponsive states. *Electroencephalogr Clin Neurophysiol Suppl* 1999; 52:117–131.

199. Guérit JM, Verougstraete D, de Tourtchaninoff M, et al. ERPs obtained with the auditory oddball paradigm in coma and altered states of consciousness: clinical relationships, prognostic value, and origin of components. *Clin Neurophysiol* 1999;110:1260–1269.

200. Gurvitch AM, Zarzhetsky YV, Mutuskina YA. Neuro-physiological mechanisms of post-resuscitation brain pathology. *Resuscitation* 1979;7:237–248.

201. Gurvitch AM, Zarzhetsky YV, Trush VD, et al. Experimental data on the nature of postresuscitation alpha frequency activity. *Electroencephalogr Clin Neurophysiol* 1984;58:426–437.

202. Guterman B, Sebastian P, Sodha N. Recovery from alpha coma after lorazepam overdose. *Clin Electroencephalogr* 1981;12:205–208.

203. Gütling E, Gonser A, Imhof H-G, et al. EEG reactivity in the prognosis of severe head injury. *Neurology* 1995;45:915–918.

204. Gütling E, Gonser A, Regard M, et al. Dissociation of frontal and parietal components of somatosensory evoked potentials in severe head injury. *Electroencephalogr Clin Neurophysiol* 1993;88:369–376.

205. Gütling E, Isenmann S, Wichmann W. Electrophysiology in the locked-in-syndrome. *Neurology* 1996;46:1092–1101.

206. Haider I, Matthew H, Oswald I. Electroencephalographic changes in acute drug poisoning. *Electroencephalogr Clin Neurophysiol* 1971;30:23–31.

207. Hall JW, Mackey-Hargadine JR, Allen SJ. Monitoring neurologic status of comatose patients in the intensive care unit. In: Jacobson JT, ed. *The auditory brainstem response*. San Diego: College-Hill Press, 1985:253–283.

208. Hall JW, Mackey-Hargadine JR, Kim EE. Auditory brain-stem response in determination of brain death. *Arch Otolaryngol* 1985;111:613–620.

209. Hammond EJ, Wilder BJ. Short latency auditory and somatosensory evoked potentials in a patient with "locked-in" syndrome. *Clin Electroencephalogr* 1982;13:54–56.

210. Hansotia P, Gottschalk P, Green P, et al. Spindle coma: incidence, clinico-pathologic correlates, and prognostic value. *Neurology* 1981;31:83–87.

211. Hansotia PL. Persistent vegetative state: review and report of electrodiagnostic studies in eight cases. *Arch Neurol* 1985;42:1048–1052.

212. Hari R, Sulkava R, Haltia M. Brainstem auditory evoked responses and alpha-pattern coma. *Ann Neurol* 1982;11:187–189.

213. Harner RN, Katz RI. Electroencephalography in metabolic coma. In: Rémond A, ed. *Handbook of electroencephalography and clinical neurophysiology*, Vol 12. Amsterdam: Elsevier Science, 1975:47–62.

214. Harner RN, Simsarian JP. Triphasic waves in metabolic encephalopathy. *Electroencephalogr Clin Neurophysiol* 1974;36:222(abst).

215. Hawkes CH, Bryan-Smyth L. The electroencephalogram in the "locked in" syndrome. *Neurology* 1974;24:1015–1018.

216. Henchey R, Cibula J, Helveston W, et al. Electroencephalographic findings in Hashimoto's encephalopathy. *Neurology* 1995;45:977–981.

217. Henry CE, Scoville WB. Suppression-burst activity from isolated cerebral cortex in man. *Electroencephalogr Clin Neurophysiol* 1952;4:1–22.

218. Héraut L-A, Lombard C, Cathala H-P. Coma profond à fréquence alpha après pendaison non suivie de mort immédiate: à propos de deux observations. *Rev Electroencephalogr Neurophysiol Clin* 1980;10:21–32.

219. Herkes GK, Wszolek ZK, Westmoreland BF, et al. Effects of midazolam on electroencephalograms of seriously ill patients. *Mayo Clin Proc* 1992;67:334–338.

220. Hess R. Sleep and sleep disturbances in the electroencephalogram. *Prog Brain Res* 1965;18: 127–139.

221. Hess R. Brain tumors and other space occupying processes. In: Rémond A, ed. *Handbook of electroencephalography and clinical neurophysiology*, Vol 14, Part C. Amsterdam: Elsevier Science, 1975:5–10.

222. Hirose G, Kitagawa Y, Chujo T, et al. Acute effects of phenytoin on brainstem auditory evoked potentials: clinical and experimental study. *Neurology* 1986;36:1521–1524.

223. Hockaday JM, Potts F, Epstein E, et al. Electroencephalographic changes in acute cerebral anoxia from cardiac or respiratory arrest. *Electroencephalogr Clin Neurophysiol* 1965;18: 575–586.

224. Holzman BH, Curless RG, Sfakianakis GN, et al. Radionuclide cerebral perfusion scintigraphy in determination of brain death in children. *Neurology* 1983;33:1027–1031.

225. Homan RW, Jones JG. Alpha-pattern coma in a 2-month-old child. *Ann Neurol* 1981;9:611–613.

226. Hormes JT, Benarroch EE, Rodriguez M, et al. Periodic sharp waves in baclofen-induced encephalopathy. *Arch Neurol* 1988;45:814–815.

227. Houlden DA, Li C, Schwartz ML, et al. Median nerve somatosensory evoked potentials and the Glasgow Coma Scale as predictors of outcome in comatose patients with head injuries. *Neurosurgery* 1990;27:701–708.

228. Hrachovy RA, Mizrahi EM, Kellaway P. Electroencephalography of the newborn. In: Daly DD, Pedley TA, eds. *Current practice of clinical electroencephalography*, 2nd ed. New York: Raven Press, 1990:201–242.

229. Hughes JR, Boshes B, Leestma J. Electro-clinical and pathological correlations in comatose patients. *Clin Electroencephalogr* 1976;7:13–30.

230. Hughes JR, Cayaffa J, Leestma J, et al. Alternating "waking" and "sleep" EEG patterns in a deeply comatose patient. *Clin Electroencephalogr* 1972;3:86–93.

231. Hulihan JFJ, Syna DR. Electroencephalographic sleep patterns in post-anoxic stupor and coma. *Neurology* 1994;44:758–760.

232. Hume AL, Cant BR. Conduction time in central somatosensory pathways in man. *Electroencephalogr Clin Neurophysiol* 1978;46:361–375.

233. Hume AL, Cant BR. Central somatosensory conduction after head injury. *Ann Neurol* 1981; 10:411–419.

234. Hume AL, Cant BR, Shaw NA. Central somatosensory conduction time in comatose patients. *Ann Neurol* 1979;5:379–384.

235. Husain AM, Mebust KA, Radtke RA. Generalized periodic epileptiform discharges: etiologies, relationship to status epilepticus, and prognosis. *J Clin Neurophysiol* 1999;16:51–58.

236. Hutchinson DO, Frith RW, Shaw NA, et al. A comparison between electroencephalography and somatosensory evoked potentials for outcome predictions following severe head injury. *Electroencephalogr Clin Neurophysiol* 1991;78:228–233.

237. Illievich UM, Petricek W, Schramm W, et al. Electroencephalographic burst suppression by propofol infusion in humans: hemodynamic consequences. *Anesth Analg* 1993;77: 155–160.

238. Ingvar DH. EEG and cerebral circulation in the apallic syndrome and akinetic mutism. *Electroencephalogr Clin Neurophysiol* 1971;30:272–273.

239. Ingvar DH, Brun A, Johansson L, et al. Survival after severe cerebral anoxia with destruction of the cerebral cortex: the apallic syndrome. *Ann N Y Acad Sci* 1978;315:184–214.

240. Ingvar DH, Häggendal E, Nilsson NJ, et al. Cerebral circulation and metabolism in a comatose patient. *Arch Neurol* 1964;11:13–21.

241. Ingvar DH, Sourander P. Destruction of the reticular core of the brainstem. *Arch Neurol* 1970; 23:1–8.

242. Iragui VJ, McCutchen C. Physiologic and prognostic significance of 'alpha coma'. *J Neurol Neurosurg Psychiatry* 1983;46:632–638.

243. Jacome DE, Morilla-Pastor D. Unreactive EEG: pattern in locked-in syndrome. *Clin Electroencephalogr* 1990;21:31–36.

244. Janati A, Erba G. Electroencephalographic correlates of near-drowning encephalopathy in children. *Electroencephalogr Clin Neurophysiol* 1982;53:182–191.

245. Jasper H, Van Buren J. Interrelationship between cortex and subcortical structures: clinical electroencephalographic studies. *Electroencephalogr Clin Neurophysiol Suppl* 1953;4: 168–202.

246. Jasper HH. The ten-twenty electrode system of the International Federation. *Electroencephalogr Clin Neurophysiol* 1958;10:371–375.

247. Jellinger K, Gerstenbrand F, Pateisky K. Die protrahierte Form der posttraumatischen Enzephalopathie. *Nervenarzt* 1963;34:145–163.

248. Jellish WS, Thalji Z, Fluter E, et al. Etomidate and thiopental-based anesthetic induction: comparisons between different titrated levels of electrophysiologic cortical depression and response to laryngoscopy. *J Clin Anesth* 1977;1997:36–41.

249. Jennett B. Vegetative state: causes, management, ethical dilemmas. *Curr Anaesth Crit Care* 1991;2:57–61.

250. Jennett B, Bond M. Assessment of outcome after severe brain damage. *Lancet* 1975;1: 480–484.

251. Jennett B, Plum F. Persistent vegetative state after brain damage: a syndrome in search of a name. *Lancet* 1972;1:734–737.

252. Jørgensen EO. EEG during severe barbiturate intoxication. *Acta Neurol Scand Suppl* 1970;43: 281.

253. Jørgensen EO, Malchow-Møller A. Natural history of global and critical brain ischaemia. Part I: EEG and neurological signs during the first year after cardiopulmonary resuscitation in patients subsequently regaining consciousness. *Resuscitation* 1981;9:133–153.

254. Jørgensen EO, Malchow-Møller A. Natural history of global and critical brain ischaemia. Part II: EEG and neurological signs in patients remaining unconscious after cardiopulmonary resuscitation. *Resuscitation* 1981;9:155–174.

255. Jouvet M, Pellin B, Mounier D. Etude polygraphique des différentes phases du sommeil au cours des troubles de conscience chroniques (comas prolongés). *Rev Neurol* 1961;105: 181–186.

256. Judson JA, Cant BR, Shaw NA. Early prediction of outcome from cerebral trauma by somatosensory evoked potentials. *Crit Care Med* 1990;18:363–368.

257. Jumao-as A, Brenner RP. Myoclonic status epilepticus: a clinical and electroencephalographic study. *Neurology* 1990;40:1199–1202.

258. Kaada BR, Harkmark W, Stokke O. Deep coma associated with desynchronization in EEG. *Electroencephalogr Clin Neurophysiol* 1961;13:785–789.

259. Kaga K, Takamory A, Mizutani T, et al. The auditory pathology of brain death as revealed by auditory evoked potentials. *Ann Neurol* 1985;18:360–364.

260. Kaji R, McCormick F, Kameyama M, et al. Brainstem auditory evoked potentials in early diagnosis of basilar artery occlusion. *Neurology* 1985;35:240–243.

261. Kane NM, Curry SH, Butler SR, et al. Electrophysiological indicator of awakening from coma. *Lancet* 1993;341:688.

262. Kane NM, Curry SH, Rowlands CA, et al. Event-related potentials—neurophysiological tools for predicting emergence and early outcome from traumatic coma. *Intensive Care Med* 1996; 22:39–46.

263. Kane NM, Moss TH, Curry SH, et al. Quantitative electroencephalographic evaluation of non-fatal and fatal traumatic coma. *Electroencephalogr Clin Neurophysiol* 1998;106: 244–250.

264. Kaplan PW, Genoud D, Ho TW, et al. Etiology, neurologic correlations, and prognosis in alpha coma. *Clin Neurophysiol* 1999;110:205–213.

265. Kaplan PW, Genoud D, Ho TW, et al. Clinical correlates and prognosis in early spindle coma. *Clin Neurophysiol* 2000;111:584–590.

265a. Kaplan PW. Absent cortical somatosensory evoked potentials do not predict persistent vegetative state (PVS) or death. *J Clin Neurophysiol* 2000; 17:529–530.

266. Karnaze DS, Bickford RG. Triphasic waves: a reassessment of their significance. *Electroencephalogr Clin Neurophysiol* 1984;57:193–198.

267. Karnaze DS, Weiner JM, Marshall LG. Auditory evoked potentials in coma after closed head injury: a clinical-neurophysiologic coma scale for predicting outcome. *Neurology* 1985;35: 1122–1126.

268. Karp JS, Hurtig HI. "Locked-in" state with bilateral mid-brain infarct. *Arch Neurol* 1974;30: 176–178.

269. Kifune A, Kubota F, Shibata N, et al. Valproic acid-induced hyperammonemic encephalopathy with triphasic waves. *Epilepsia* 2000;41:909–912.

270. Kim YW, Krieble KK, Kim CB, et al. Differentiation of alpha coma from awake alpha by nonlinear dynamics of electroencephalography. *Electroencephalogr Clin Neurophysiol* 1996;98:35–41.

271. Kimura J, Gerber HW, McCormick WF. The isoelectric electroencephalogram: significance in establishing death in patients maintained on mechanical respirators. *Arch Intern Med* 1968; 121:511–517.

272. Kinney HC, Korein J, Panigrahy A, et al. Neuropathological findings in the brain of Karen Ann Quinlan: the role of the thalamus in the persistent vegetative state. *N Engl J Med* 1994;330: 1469–1475.

273. Klem G, Henry CE. Deterioration within a single tracing from alpha coma to suppression-burst to electrocerebral silence. *Electroencephalogr Clin Neurophysiol* 1976;40:314(abst).

274. Klug N, Csécsei G. Brainstem acoustic evoked potentials in the acute midbrain syndrome and in central death. In: Morocutti C, Rizzo PA, eds. *Evoked potentials: neurophysiological and clinical aspects.* Amsterdam: Elsevier Science, 1985:203–210.

275. Korein J, ed. *Brain death: interrelated medical and social issues.* New York: New York Academy of Sciences, 1978.

276. Kotagal S, Rolfe U, Schwarz KB, et al. Locked-in state following Reye's syndrome. *Ann Neurol* 1984;15:599–601.

277. Kretschmer E. Das apallische syndrom. *Z Gesamte Neurol Psychiatr* 1940;169:576–579.

278. Krieger DW. Commentary: evoked potentials not just to confirm hopelessness in anoxic injury. *Lancet* 1998;352:1796–1797.

279. Kubicki S, Rieger H, Barckow D. The EEG in fatal and near-fatal poisoning with soporific drugs. II. Clinical significance. *Clin Electroencephalogr* 1970;1:14–21.

280. Kubicki S, Rieger H, Busse G. The EEG in fatal and near-fatal poisoning with soporific drugs. I. Typical EEG patterns. *Clin Electroencephalogr* 1970;1:5–13.

281. Kuroiwa Y, Celesia GG. Clinical significance of periodic EEG patterns. *Arch Neurol* 1980;37: 15–20.

282. Kuroiwa Y, Furukawa T. EEG prognostication in drug-related alpha coma [Letter]. *Arch Neurol* 1981;38:200.

283. Kurtz D. The EEG in acute and chronic drug intoxication. In: Rémond A, ed. *Handbook of electroencephalography and clinical neurophysiology*, Vol 15, Part C. Amsterdam: Elsevier Science, 1976:88–107.

284. Lancman ME, Marks S, Mahmood K, et al. Atypical triphasic waves associated with the use of pentobarbital. *Electroencephalogr Clin Neurophysiol* 1997;102:175–177(abst).

285. Leestma JE, Hughes JR, Diamond ER. Temporal correlates in brain death: EEG and clinical relationships to the respirator brain. *Arch Neurol* 1984;41:147–152.

286. Lemmi H, Hubbert CH, Faris AA. The electroencephalogram after resuscitation of cardiocirculatory arrest. *J Neurol Neurosurg Psychiatry* 1973;36:997–1002.

287. Lepetit JM, Vallat JN, Mathieu S, et al. Étude du nycthémère dans un état comateux prolongé: étude électroclinique. *Rev Neurol* 1966;115:526–529.

288. Lersch DR, Kaplan AM. Alpha-pattern coma in childhood and adolescence. *Arch Neurol* 1984; 41:68–70.

289. Levin HS, Saydjari C, Eisenberg HM, et al. Vegetative state after closed-head injury. *Arch Neurol* 1991;48:580–585.

290. Levy DE, Bates D, Caronna JJ, et al. Prognosis in nontraumatic coma. *Arch Intern Med* 1981; 94:293–301.

291. Levy SR, Chiappa KH, Burke CJ, et al. Early evolution and incidence of electroencephalographic abnormalities in Creutzfeldt-Jakob disease. *J Clin Neurophysiol* 1986;3:1–21.

292. Levy SR, Knill-Jones RP, Plum F. The vegetative state and its prognosis following non-traumatic coma. *Ann N Y Acad Sci* 1978;315:293–306.

293. Li C-L, Jasper H, Henderson L Jr. The effect of arousal mechanisms on various forms of abnormality in the electroencephalogram. *Electroencephalogr Clin Neurophysiol* 1952;4:513–526.

294. Lindsay K, Pasaoglu A, Hirst D, et al. Somatosensory and auditory brain-stem conduction after head injury: a comparison with clinical features in prediction of outcome. *Neurosurgery* 1990; 26:278–285.

295. Lindsay KW, Carlin J, Kennedy I, et al. Evoked potentials in severe head injury: analysis and relation to outcome. *J Neurol Neurosurg Psychiatry* 1981;44:796–802.

296. Loeb C, Poggio G. Electroencephalograms in a case with pontomesencephalic hemorrhage. *Electroencephalogr Clin Neurophysiol* 1953;5:295–296.

297. Loeb C, Rosadini G, Poggio GF. Electroencephalograms during coma: normal and borderline records in 5 patients. *Neurology* 1959;9:610–618.

298. Lorenzoni E. Das EEG in posttraumatischen Koma. *Fortschr Neurol Psychiatr* 1975;43: 155–191.

299. Lowenstein DH, Aminoff MJ. Clinical and EEG features of status epilepticus in comatose patients. *Neurology* 1992;42:100–104.

300. Lücking GH, Müllner E, Pateisky K, et al. Electroencephalographic findings in the apallic syndrome. In: Dalle Ore G, Gerstenbrand F, Lücking CH, et al, eds. *The apallic syndrome*. Berlin: Springer-Verlag, 1977:144–154.

301. Luecking C. Sleep-like patterns and abnormal arousal reactions in brain stem lesions. *Electroencephalogr Clin Neurophysiol* 1970;28:214(abst).

302. Lundervold A. Electroencephalographic changes in a case of acute cerebral anoxia unconscious for about three years. *Electroencephalogr Clin Neurophysiol* 1954;6:311–315.

303. Lundervold A, Hauge T, Loken AC. Unusual EEG in unconscious patient with brain stem atrophy. *Electroencephalogr Clin Neurophysiol* 1956;8:665–670.

304. Lütschg J, Pfenninger J, Lundin HP, et al. Brainstem auditory and early somatosensory evoked potentials in neurointensively treated comatose children. *Am J Dis Child* 1983;137:421–426.

305. Maccario M, Messis CP, Vastola EF. Focal seizures as a manifestation of hyperglycemia without ketoacidosis. *Neurology* 1965;15:195–206.

306. MacGillivray BB. The EEG in liver disease. In: Rémond A, ed. *Handbook of electroencephalography and clinical neurophysiology*, Vol 15, Part C. Amsterdam: Elsevier Science, 1976:26–50.

307. MacGillivray BB, Kennedy JK. "The triphasic waves" of hepatic encephalopathy. *Electroencephalogr Clin Neurophysiol* 1970;28:428(abst).

308. Madison D, Niedermeyer E. Epileptic seizures resulting from acute cerebral anoxia. *J Neurol Neurosurg Psychiatry* 1970;33:381–386.

309. Madl C, Grimm G, Kramer L. Early prediction of individual outcome after cardiopulmonary resuscitation. *Lancet* 1993;341:855–858.

310. Madl C, Grimm G, Yeganehfar W, et al. Detection of nontraumatic comatose patients with no benefit of intensive care treatment by recording of sensory evoked potentials. *Arch Neurol* 1996;53:512–516.

311. Mantz JM, Kurtz D, Otteni JC, et al. EEG aspects of six cases of severe barbiturate coma. *Electroencephalogr Clin Neurophysiol* 1965;18:426(abst).

312. Markand ON. Electroencephalogram in "locked in" syndrome. *Electroencephalogr Clin Neurophysiol* 1976;40:529–534.

313. Markand ON, Daly DD. Pseudoperiodic lateralized paroxysmal discharges in electroencephalogram. *Neurology* 1971;21:975–981.

314. Markand ON, Dyken ML. Sleep abnormalities in patients with brain stem lesions. *Neurology* 1976;26:769–776.

315. Markand ON, Lee BI, Warren C, et al. Effects of hypothermia on BAEPs in humans. *Ann Neurol* 1987;22:507–513.

316. Marquardsen J, Harvald B. The electroencephalogram in acute vascular lesions of the brain stem and the cerebellum. *Acta Neurol Scand* 1964;40:58–68.

317. Martin JT, Faulconer A Jr, Bickford RG. Electroencephalography in anesthesiology. *Anesthesiology* 1959;20:359–376.

318. Matsuo F. EEG features of the apallic syndrome resulting from cerebral anoxia. *Electroencephalogr Clin Neurophysiol* 1985;61:113–121.

319. Mauguière F, García-Larrea L, Bertrand O. Utility and uncertainties of evoked potentials monitoring in the ICU. In: Grundy L, Vitali M, eds. *Evoked potentials in ICU and surgical monitoring*. Berlin: Springer-Verlag, 1988:153–167.

320. Mauguière F, García-Larrea L, Murray NMF, et al. Evoked potential diagnostic strategies: EPs in coma. In: Osselton JW, ed. *Clinical neurophysiology. Vol. 1. EMG, nerve conduction, and evoked potentials*. Oxford, England: Butterworth-Heinemann, 1995:482–522.

321. Mauguière F, Grand C, Fisher C, et al. Aspects des potentiels évoqués auditifs et somesthésiques précoces dans les comas neurologiques et la mort cérébrale. *Rev Electroencephalogr Neurophysiol Clin* 1982;12:280–286.

322. Maurri S, Lambruschini P, Barontini F. Total mesencephalic "locked-in" syndrome: a case report and review of the literature. *Riv Neurol* 1989;59:211–216.

323. Mavroudakis N, Brunko E, Nogueira MC, et al. Acute effects of diphenylhydantoin on peripheral and central somatosensory conduction. *Electroencephalogr Clin Neurophysiol* 1991;78: 263–266.

324. May WW. Creutzfeldt-Jakob disease. I. Survey of the literature and clinical diagnosis. *Acta Neurol Scand* 1968;44:1–32.

325. McKeown MJ, Young GB. Comparison between the alpha pattern in normal subjects and in alpha pattern coma. *J Clin Neurophysiol* 1997;14:414–418.

326. Meija RE, Pollack MM. Variability in brain death determination practices in children. *JAMA* 1995;274:550–553.

327. Mellerio F. *L'électroencéphalographie dans les intoxications aigües*. Paris: Masson, 1964.

328. Mellerio F. L'EEG dans le prognostic des comas toxiques: réfléxions à propos de quelques données inhabituelles. *Rev Electroencephalogr Neurophysiol Clin* 1982;12:325–331.

329. Merlo A, Weder B, Ketz E, et al. Locked-in state in Borrelia burgdorferi meningitis. *J Neurol* 1989;236:305–306.

330. Miller JW, Klass DW, Mokri B, et al. Triphasic waves in cerebral carcinomatosis: another non-metabolic cause. *Arch Neurol* 1986;43:1191–1193.

331. Ministère des Affaires Sociales. Circulaire No. 67 du 24 avril 1968 relative à l'application du décret n° 47-2057 du 20 octobre 1947 relatif aux autopsies et prélèvements. *J Officiel République Française* 1968;S.P./18, 12.262:1–3.

332. Ministère des Affaires Sociales et de la Solidarité. Ministère de la Santé. Circulaire n° 03 du 21 janvier 1991 relative à l'application du décret n° 90-844 du 24 septembre 1990 modifiant le décret n° 78-501 du 31 mars 1978 pour l'application de la loi n° 76-1181 du 22 décembre 1976 relative aux prélèvements d'organes. II—La réglementation en viguer sur les critères du constat de la mort cérébrale. 1991:3–4.

333. Mizrahi EM, Pollack MA, Kellaway P. Neocortical death in infants: behavioral, neurologic, and electroencephalographic characteristics. *Pediatr Neurol* 1986;1:302–305.

334. Mjøen S, Nordby HK, Torvik A. Auditory evoked brainstem responses (ABR) in coma due to severe head trauma. *Acta Otolaryngol* 1983;95:131–138.

335. Møller M. "Alpha-pattern coma" and survival after cardiac arrest. *Electroencephalogr Clin Neurophysiol* 1978;44:518–522.

336. Molofsky WJ. Alpha coma in a child [Letter]. *J Neurol Neurosurg Psychiatry* 1982;45:95.

337. Moruzzi G. The sleep-waking cycle. *Ergebn Physiol* 1972;64:1–165.

338. Moseley JI, Molinari GF, Walker AE. Respirator brain: report of a survey and review of current concepts. *Arch Pathol Lab Med* 1976;100:61–64.

339. Moshé SL. Usefulness of EEG in the evaluation of brain death in children: the pros. *J Clin Neurophysiol* 1989;73:272–275.

340. The Multi-Society Task Force on PVS. Medical aspects of the persistent vegetative state (1). *N Engl J Med* 1994;330:1499–1508.

341. The Multi-Society Task Force on PVS. Medical aspects of the persistent vegetative state (2). *N Engl J Med* 1994;330:1572–1579.

342. Murphy MJ, Brenton DW, Aschenbrener CA, et al. Locked-in syndrome caused by a solitary pontine abscess. *J Neurol Neurosurg Psychiatry* 1979;42:1062–1065.

343. Mutschler V, Chaumeil CG, Marcoux L, et al. Etude du P300 auditif chez des sujets en coma post-anoxique: données préliminaires. *Neurophysiol Clin* 1996;26:158–163.

344. Naquet R, Vigouroux RP, Choux M, et al. Étude électroencéphalographique des traumatismes crâniens récents dans un service de réanimation. *Rev Neurol* 1967;117:512–513.

345. Narayan RK, Greenberg RP, Miller JD, et al. Improved confidence of outcome prediction in severe head injury: a comparative analysis of the clinical examination, multimodality evoked potentials, CT scanning, and intracranial pressure. *J Neurosurg* 1981;54:751–762.

346. Neufeld MY. Periodic triphasic waves in levodopa-induced encephalopathy. *Neurology* 1992; 42:444–446.

347. Neufeld MY, Vishnevskaya S, Treves TA, et al. Periodic lateralized epileptiform discharges (PLEDs) following stroke are associated with metabolic abnormalities. *Electroencephalogr Clin Neurophysiol* 1997;102:295–298.

348. Newlon PG, Greenberg RP, Enas GG, et al. Effects of therapeutic pentobarbital coma on multimodality evoked potentials recorded from severely head-injured patients. *Neurosurgery* 1983; 12:613–619.

349. Newlon PG, Greenberg RP, Hyatt MS, et al. The dynamics of neuronal dysfunction and recovery following severe head injury assessed by serial multimodality evoked potentials. *J Neurosurg* 1982;57:168–177.

350. Noachtar S, Binnie C, Ebersole J, et al. A glossary of terms most commonly used by clinical electroencephalographers and proposal for the report form for the EEG findings. *Electroencephalogr Clin Neurophysiol Suppl* 1999;52:21–41.

351. Nöel P, Desmedt JE. Somatosensory cerebral evoked potentials after vascular lesions of the brain stem and diencephalon. *Brain* 1975;98:113–128.

352. Nordgren RE, Markesbery WR, Fukuda K, et al. Seven cases of cerebromedullospinal disconnection: the "locked-in" syndrome. *Neurology* 1971;21:1140–1148.

353. Nowack WJ, King JA. Triphasic waves and spike wave stupor. *Clin Electroencephalogr* 1992; 23:100–104.

354. Nuwer MR. Fundamentals of evoked potentials and common clinical applications today. *Electroencephalogr Clin Neurophysiol* 1998;106:142–148.

355. Obeso JA, Iragui MI, Marti-Masso JG, et al. Neurophysiological assessment of alpha pattern coma. *J Neurol Neurosurg Psychiatry* 1980;43:63–67.

356. Obrador S, Reinoso-Suarez F, Carbonell J, et al. Comatose state maintained during eight years following a vascular ponto-mesencephalic lesion. *Electroencephalogr Clin Neurophysiol* 1975;38:21–26.

357. Ogunyemi A. Triphasic waves during post-ictal stupor. *Can J Neurol Sci* 1996;23:208–212.

358. Oksenberg A, Soroker N, Solzi P, et al. Polysomnography in locked-in syndrome. *Electroencephalogr Clin Neurophysiol* 1991;78:314–317.

359. Onofrj M, Thomas A, Paci C, et al. Event related potentials recorded in patients with locked-in syndrome. *J Neurol Neurosurg Psychiatry* 1997;63:759–764.

360. Ottaviani F, Almadori G, Calderazzo AB, et al. Auditory brain stem (ABRs) and middle latency auditory responses (MLRs) in the prognosis of severely head-injured patients. *Electroencephalogr Clin Neurophysiol* 1986;65:196–202.

361. Pagni CA, Courjon J. Electroencephalographic modifications induced by moderate and deep hypothermia in man. *Acta Neurochir Suppl (Wien)* 1964;13:35–49.

362. Pallis C. ABC of brainstem death: the arguments about the EEG. *Br Med J* 1983;286:284–287.

363. Pallis C. Brainstem death. In: Braskman R, ed. *Handbook of clinical neurology, Vol 13. Head injury*. Amsterdam: Elsevier Science, 1990:441–496.

364. Pallis C, Harley DH. *ABC of brainstem death*, 2nd ed. London: British Medical Journal, 1996.

365. Pampiglione G, Harden A. Resuscitation after cardiocirculatory arrest: prognostic evaluation of early electroencephalographic findings. *Lancet* 1968;1:1261–1264.

366. Papanicolaou AC, Loring DW, Eisenberg HM, et al. Auditory brain stem evoked responses in comatose head-injured patients. *Neurosurgery* 1986;18:173–175.

367. Patterson JR, Grabois M. Locked-in syndrome: a review of 139 cases. *Stroke* 1986;17:758–764.

368. Petty GW, Mohr JP, Pedley TA, et al. The role of transcranial Doppler in confirming brain death: sensitivity, specificity, and suggestions for performance and interpretation. *Neurology* 1990;40:300–303.

369. Pfürtscheller G, Schwartz G, Gravenstein N. Clinical relevance of long-latency SEPs and VEPs during coma. *Electroencephalogr Clin Neurophysiol* 1983;62:88–98.

370. Plum F, Posner JB. *The diagnosis of stupor and coma*. Philadelphia: FA Davis Co, 1966.

371. Pohlmann-Eden B, Hoch DB, Cochius JI, et al. Periodic lateralized epileptiform discharges: a critical review. *J Clin Neurophysiol* 1996;13:519–530.

372. Pollack MA, Kellaway P. Cortical death with preservation of brainstem function: correlation of clinical, electrophysiologic, and CT scan findings in 3 infants and 2 adults with prolonged survival. *Trans Am Neurol Assoc* 1978;103:36–38.

373. Portenoy RK, Kurtzberg D, Arezzo JC, et al. Return to alertness after brain-stem hemorrhage: a case with evoked potential and roentgenographic evidence of bilateral tegmental damage. *Arch Neurol* 1985;42:85–88.

374. Poser CM. Electroencephalographic changes and hyperammonemia. *Electroencephalogr Clin Neurophysiol* 1958;10:51–62.

375. Pratt H, Brodsky G, Goldsher M, et al. Auditory brain-stem evoked potentials in patients undergoing dialysis. *Electroencephalogr Clin Neurophysiol* 1986;63:18–24.

376. Primavera A, Traverso F. Triphasic waves in Alzheimer's disease. *Acta Neurol Belg* 1990;90: 274–281.

377. Prior P. *The EEG in acute cerebral anoxia*. Amsterdam: Excerpta Medica, 1973.

378. Pulst SM, Lombroso CT. External ophthalmoplegia, alpha and spindle coma in imipramine overdose: case report and review of the literature. *Ann Neurol* 1983;14:587–590.

379. Rae-Grant AD, Barbour PJ, Reed J. Development of a novel EEG rating scale for head injury using dichotomous variables. *Electroencephalogr Clin Neurophysiol* 1991;79:349–357.

380. Rae-Grant AD, Eckert N, Barbour PJ, et al. Outcome of severe brain injury: a multimodality neurophysiologic study. *J Trauma* 1996;40:401–407.

381. Rampil IJ, Lockhart SH, Eger EI 2nd, et al. The electroencephalographic effects of desflurane in humans. *Anesthesiology* 1991;74:434–439.

382. Rappaport M, Hall K, Hopkins HK, et al. Evoked brain potentials and disability in brain-damaged patients. *Arch Phys Med Rehabil* 1977;58:333–338.

383. Rappaport M, Hopkins HK, Hall K, et al. Evoked potentials and head injury. 2. Clinical applications. *Clin Electroencephalogr* 1981;12:167–176.

384. Reeves AL, Westmoreland B, Klass DW. Clinical accompaniments of the burst-suppression EEG pattern. *J Clin Neurophysiol* 1997;14:150–153.

385. Reiher J. The electroencephalogram in the investigation of metabolic comas. *Electroencephalogr Clin Neurophysiol* 1970;28:104(abst).

386. Reilly EL, Kondo C, Brunberg JA, et al. Visual evoked potentials during hypothermia and prolonged circulatory arrest. *Electroencephalogr Clin Neurophysiol* 1978;45:100–106.

387. Report of Special Task Force for the Determination of Brain Death in Children. Guidelines for the determination of brain death in children. *Pediatrics* 1987;80:298–300.

388. Report of the Medical Consultants on the Diagnosis of Death to the President's Commission for the Study of Ethical Problems in Medicine and Behavioral Research. Guidelines for the determination of death. *JAMA* 1981;246:2184–2186.

389. Report of the Quality Standards Subcommittee of the American Academy of Neurology. Practice parameters for determining brain death in adults (Summary Statement). *Neurology* 1995; 45:1012–1014.

390. Reutens DC, Dunne JW, Gubbay SS. Triphasic waves in accidental hypothermia. *Electroencephalogr Clin Neurophysiol* 1990;76:370–372.

391. River Y, Zelig O. Triphasic waves in myxedema coma. *Clin Electroencephalogr* 1993;24: 146–150.

392. Rodin E, Tahir S, Austin D, et al. Brainstem death. *Clin Electroencephalogr* 1985;16:63–71.

393. Rosenberg C, Wogensen K, Starr A. Auditory brainstem and middle- and long-latency evoked potentials in coma. *Arch Neurol* 1984;41:835–838.

394. Rossini PM, Pirchio M, Treviso M, et al. Checkerboard reversal pattern and flash VEPs in dialysed and non-dialysed subjects. *Electroencephalogr Clin Neurophysiol* 1981;52: 435–444.

395. Rothstein TL, Austin E, Sumi SM. Evoked responses in neocortical death. *Electroencephalogr Clin Neurophysiol* 1983;56:S162(abst).

396. Rothstein TL, Thomas EM, Sumi SM. Predicting outcome in hypoxic-ischemic coma: a prospective clinical and electrophysiologic study. *Electroencephalogr Clin Neurophysiol* 1991; 79:101–107.

396a. Rothstein TL. The role of evoked potentials in anoxic-ischemic coma and severe brain trauma. *J Clin Neurophysiol* 2000; 17:486–497.

397. Rumpl E. Craniocerebral trauma. In: Niedermeyer E, Lopes da Silva F, eds. *Electroencephalography*. Baltimore: Urban & Schwarzenberg, 1987:347–367.

398. Rumpl E, Lorenzi E, Hackl JM, et al. The EEG at different stages of acute secondary traumatic midbrain and bulbar brain syndromes. *Electroencephalogr Clin Neurophysiol* 1979;46: 487–497.

399. Rumpl E, Prugger M, Bauer G, et al. Incidence and prognostic value of spindles in post-traumatic coma. *Electroencephalogr Clin Neurophysiol* 1983;56:420–429.

400. Rumpl E, Prugger M, Gerstenbrand F, et al. Central somatosensory conduction time and short latency somatosensory evoked potentials in post-traumatic coma. *Electroencephalogr Clin Neurophysiol* 1983;56:583–596.

401. Rumpl E, Prugger M, Gerstenbrand F, et al. Central somatosensory conduction time and acoustic brainstem transmission time in post-traumatic coma. *J Clin Neurophysiol* 1988;5: 237–260.

402. Russ W, Kling D, Loesevitz A, et al. Effect of hypothermia on visual evoked potentials (VEP) in humans. *Anesthesiology* 1984;61:207–210.

403. Schaul N. The fundamental neural mechanisms of electroencephalography. *Electroencephalogr Clin Neurophysiol* 1998;106:101–107.

404. Schneider S. Usefulness of EEG in the evaluation of brain death in children: the cons. *Electroencephalogr Clin Neurophysiol* 1989;73:276–278.

405. Scollo-Lavizzari G, Bassetti C. Prognostic value in EEG in post-anoxic coma after cardiac arrest. *Eur Neurol* 1987;26:161–170.

406. Seales DM, Rossiter VS, Weinstein ME. Brainstem auditory evoked responses in patients comatose as a result of blunt head trauma. *J Trauma* 1979;19:347–352.

407. Seales DM, Torkelson RD, Shuman RM, et al. Abnormal brainstem auditory evoked potentials and neuropathology in "locked-in" syndrome. *Neurology* 1981;31:893–896.

408. Setzer NA, McPherson RW, Johnson RM, et al. Evoked potential determinations in children with brain death. *Anesthesiology* 1983;59:A130.

409. Shafey S, Scheinblum A, Scheinblum P, et al. The ventral pontine syndrome. *Trans Am Neurol Assoc* 1968;93:21–24.

410. Shewmon DA. Commentary on guidelines for the determination of brain death in children. *Ann Neurol* 1988;24:789–791.

410a. Shewmon DA. Coma prognosis in children. Part II: Clinical application. *J Clin Neurophysiol* 2000;17:467–472.

411. Shuttleworth E. Recovery to social and economic independence from prolonged postanoxic vegetative state. *Neurology* 1983;33:372–374.

412. Signorino B, D'Acuto S, Angeleri F, et al. Eliciting P300 in comatose patients. *Lancet* 1995; 345:255–256.

413. Silverman D. Some observations on the EEG in hepatic coma. *Electroencephalogr Clin Neurophysiol* 1962;14:53–59.

414. Silverman D. Retrospective study of the EEG in coma. *Electroencephalogr Clin Neurophysiol* 1963;15:486–503.

415. Silverman D. The electroencephalogram in anoxic coma. In: Rémond A, ed. *Handbook of electroencephalography and clinical neurophysiology, Vol 12. Altered states of consciousness, coma and cerebral death*. Amsterdam: Elsevier Science, 1975:81–94.

416. Silverman D, Saunders MG, Schwab RS, et al. Cerebral death and the electroencephalogram: report of the Ad Hoc Committee of the American Electroencephalographic Society on EEG Criteria for Determination of Cerebral Death. *JAMA* 1969;209:1505–1510.

417. Simon RP, Aminoff MJ. Electrographic status epilepticus in fatal anoxic coma. *Ann Neurol* 1986;20:351–355.

418. Simsarian JP, Harner RN. Diagnosis of metabolic encephalopathy: significance of triphasic waves in the electroencephalogram. *Neurology* 1972;22:456(abst).

419. Smith SH, Kocen RS. A Creutzfeldt-Jakob like syndrome due to lithium toxicity. *J Neurol Neurosurg Psychiatry* 1988;51:120–123.

420. Sohmer H, Gafni M, Chisin R. Auditory nerve and brain stem responses: comparison in awake and unconscious subjects. *Arch Neurol* 1978;35:228–230.

421. Solomon L, Moshé SL, Alvarez LA. Diagnosis of brain death in children. *J Clin Neurophysiol* 1986;3:234–249.

422. Sonnet ML, Perrot D, Floret D, et al. Les potentiels évoqués somesthésiques (PESp) et auditifs (PEAp) précoces dans les comas anoxiques: valeur prognostique. *Neurophysiol Clin* 1993; 23:227–236.

423. Sørensen K, Thomassen A, Wernberg M. Prognostic significance of alpha frequency EEG rhythm in coma after cardiac arrest. *J Neurol Neurosurg Psychiatry* 1978;41:840–842.

424. Soustiel JF, Hafner H, Guilburd JN, et al. A physiological coma scale: grading of coma by combined use of brain-stem trigeminal and auditory evoked potentials and the Glasgow Coma Scale. *Electroencephalogr Clin Neurophysiol* 1993;87:277–283.

425. Speight TM, Avery GS. Pancuronium bromide: a review of its pharmacological properties and clinical application. *Drugs* 1972;4:163.

426. Squires KC, Chu N-S, Starr A. Auditory brainstem potentials with alcohol. *Electroencephalogr Clin Neurophysiol* 1978;45:577–584.

427. Starr A. Auditory brain stem responses in brain death. *Brain* 1976;99:543–554.
428. Starr A, Achor LJ. Auditory brainstem responses in neurological disease. *Arch Neurol* 1975; 32:761–768.
429. Statement issued by the honorary secretary of the Conference of Royal Colleges and Faculties of the United Kingdom on 11 October 1976: diagnosis of brain death. *Br Med J* 1976;2:1187–1188.
430. Steegman AT. The neuropathology of cardiac arrest. In: Minkler J, ed. *Pathology of the nervous system*, Vol 1. New York: McGraw-Hill, 1968:1005–1029.
431. Steinhart CM, Weiss IP. Use of brainstem auditory evoked potentials in pediatric brain death. *Crit Care Med* 1985;13:560–562.
432. Steriade M, Amzica F, Contreras D. Cortical and thalamic cellular correlates of electroencephalographic burst-suppression. *Electroencephalogr Clin Neurophysiol* 1994;90:1–16.
433. Stern BJ, Krumholz A, Weiss HD, et al. Evaluation of brainstem stroke using brainstem auditory evoked responses. *Stroke* 1982;13:705–711.
434. Steudel WI, Krüger J, Grau H. Zur Alpha- und Spindle-Aktivität bei komatösen Patienten nach einer Schädel-Hirn-Verletzung unter besonderer Berücksichtigung der Computer-Tomographie. *EEG EMG* 1979;10:143–147.
435. Stockard JJ, Bickford RG, Aung MH. The electroencephalogram in traumatic brain injury. In: Vinken PJ, Bruyn GW, eds. *Handbook of clinical neurology*, Vol 23. Amsterdam: North-Holland, 1975:317–367.
436. Stockard JJ, Rossiter VS. Clinical and pathologic correlates of brainstem auditory response abnormalities. *Neurology* 1977;27:316.
437. Stockard JJ, Rossiter VS, Jones TA, et al. Effects of centrally acting drugs on brain stem auditory responses. *Electroencephalogr Clin Neurophysiol* 1977;43:550–551.
438. Stockard JJ, Rossiter VS, Wiederholt WC, et al. Brain stem auditory-evoked responses in suspected central pontine myelinolysis. *Arch Neurol* 1976;33:726–728.
439. Stockard JJ, Sharbrough FW. Unique contribution of short-latency auditory and somatosensory evoked potentials to neurologic diagnosis. *Prog Clin Neurophysiol* 1980;7:231–263.
440. Stockard JJ, Stockard JE, Sharbrough FW. Nonpathologic factors influencing brainstem auditory evoked potentials. *Am J EEG Technol* 1978;18:177–209.
441. Stockard JJ, Stockard JE, Sharbrough FW. Brainstem auditory evoked potentials in neurology: methodology, interpretation, clinical application. In: Aminoff J, ed. *Electrodiagnosis in clinical neurology*. New York: Churchill Livingstone, 1980:370–413.
442. Stockard-Pope JE, Werner SS, Bickford RG, et al. *Atlas of neonatal electroencephalography*, 2nd ed. New York: Raven Press, 1992.
443. Strich SJ. Diffuse degeneration of the cerebral white matter in severe dementia following head injury. *J Neurol Neurosurg Psychiatry* 1956;19:163–185.
444. Strich SJ. Shearing of nerve fibres as a cause of brain injury: a pathological study of twenty cases. *Lancet* 1961;2:443–448.
445. Strickbine-Van Reet P, Glaze DG, Hrachovy RA. A preliminary prospective neurophysiologic study of coma in children. *Am J Dis Child* 1984;138:492–495.
446. Sundaram MB, Blume WT. Triphasic waves revisited. *Electroencephalogr Clin Neurophysiol* 1984;58:51P(abst).
447. Sundaram MBM, Blume WT. Triphasic waves: clinical correlates and morphology. *Can J Neurol Sci* 1987;14:136–140.
448. Suter C. Theta coma. *Neurology* 1973;23:445(abst).
449. Suter C. Clinical advances in the evaluation of deep coma. *MCVQ* 1974;10:152–162.
450. Suter C, Brush J. Clinical problems of brain death and coma in intensive care units. *Ann N Y Acad Sci* 1978;315:398.
451. Sutton LN, Frewen T, Marsh R, et al. The effects of deep barbiturate coma on multimodality evoked potentials. *J Neurosurg* 1982;57:178–185.
452. Swash M, Rowan AJ. Electroencephalographic criteria of hypocalcemia and hypercalcemia. *Arch Neurol* 1972;26:218–228.
453. Synek VM. Prognostically important EEG coma patterns in diffuse anoxic and traumatic encephalopathies in adults. *J Clin Neurophysiol* 1988;5:161–174.
454. Synek VM. Value of revised EEG coma scale for prognosis after cerebral anoxia and diffuse head injury. *Clin Electroencephalogr* 1990;21:25–30.
455. Synek VM, Glasgow GL. Recovery from alpha coma after decompression sickness complicated by spinal cord lesions at cervical and midthoracic levels. *Electroencephalogr Clin Neurophysiol* 1985;60:417–419.
456. Tapie P, Feblot P, Tuillas M, et al. Potentiels évoqués auditifs précoces du tronc cérébral dans la mort cérébrale. *Rev Electroencephalogr Neurophysiol Clin* 1985;14:329–332.
457. Taylor MJ, Houston BD, Lowry NJ. Recovery of auditory brainstem responses after a severe hypoxic ischemic insult. *N Engl J Med* 1983;309:1169–1170.
458. Thatcher RW, Cantor DS, McAlaster R, et al. Comprehensive predictions of outcome in closed head-injured patients: the development of prognostic equations. *Ann N Y Acad Sci* 1991;620: 82–101.
459. Thompson JR, Ashwal S, Schneider S, et al. Comparison of cerebral blood flow measurements by xenon computed tomography and dynamic brain scintigraphy in clinically brain dead children. *Acta Radiol Suppl* 1986;369:675–679.
460. Toffol GJ, Lansky LL, Hughes JR, et al. Pitfalls in diagnosing brain death in infancy. *J Child Neurol* 1987;2:134–138.
461. Tomassen W, Kamphuisen HAC. Alpha coma. *J Neurol Sci* 1986;76:1–11.
462. Tomberg C, Desmedt JE, Ozaki I. Right or left ear reference changes the voltage of frontal and parietal somatosensory evoked potentials. *Electroencephalogr Clin Neurophysiol* 1991;80: 504–512.
463. Towle VL, Babikian V, Maselli R, et al. A comparison of multimodality evoked potentials, computed tomography findings and clinical data in brainstem vascular infarcts. In: Morocutti C, Rizzo PA, eds. *Evoked potentials: neurophysiological and clinical aspects*. Amsterdam: Elsevier Science, 1985:383–390.
464. Traub RD, Pedley TA. Virus-induced electronic coupling: hypothesis on the mechanism of periodic EEG discharges in Creutzfeldt-Jakob disease. *Ann Neurol* 1981;10:405–410.
465. Trojaborg W, Jørgensen EO. Evoked cortical potentials in patients with "isoelectric" EEGs. *Electroencephalogr Clin Neurophysiol* 1973;35:301–309.
466. Tsubokawa T, Nishimoto H, Yamamoto T, et al. Assessment of brainstem damage by the auditory brainstem response in acute severe head injury. *J Neurol Neurosurg Psychiatry* 1980;43: 1005–1011.
467. Tsubokawa T, Yamamoto T, Katayama Y. Prediction of outcome of prolonged coma caused by brain damage. *Brain Inj* 1990;4:329–337.
468. Uldry PA, Despland PA, Regli F. Alpha-coma: présentation rétrospective de 20 cas. *Neurophysiol Clin* 1991;21:85–94.
469. Uziel A, Benezech J. Auditory brainstem responses in comatose patients: relationship with brainstem reflexes and levels of coma. *Electroencephalogr Clin Neurophysiol* 1978;45:515–524.
470. Uziel A, Benezech J, Baldy Moulinier M, et al. Étude des potentiels évoqués du tronc cérébral dans les comas traumatiques: intérêt pour la détermination des niveaux de dysfonctionnement du tronc cérébral. *Rev Electroencephalogr Neurophysiol Clin* 1979;9:202–206.
471. Uziel A, Benezech J, Lorenzo S, et al. Clinical applications of brainstem auditory evoked potentials in comatose patients. In: Courjon J, Mauguière F, Revol M, eds. *Clinical applications of evoked potentials in neurology*. New York: Raven Press, 1982:195.
472. Van Zandycke M, Orban LC, Vandereecken HW. Occurrence of triphasic waves in two cases of thyrotoxic crisis. *Acta Neurol Belg* 1977;77:115–120.
473. Verma A, Bedlack RS, Radtke RA, et al. Succinylcholine induced hyperkalemia and cardiac arrest: death related to an EEG study. *J Clin Neurophysiol* 1999;16:46–50.
474. Vignaendra V, Wilkus RJ, Copass MK, et al. Electroencephalographic rhythms of alpha frequency in comatose patients after cardiopulmonary arrest. *Neurology* 1974;24:582–588.
475. Vigouroux R, Naquet R, Baurand C, et al. Évolution électro-radio-clinique de comas graves prolongés post-traumatiques. *Rev Neurol* 1964;110:72–81.
476. Volpe JJ. Brain death determination in the newborn: commentary. *Pediatrics* 1987;80: 293–297.

477. Wagner W. SEP testing in deeply comatose and brain dead patients: the role of nasopharyngeal, scalp and earlobe derivations in recording the P14 potential. *Electroencephalogr Clin Neurophysiol* 1991;80:352–363.

478. Walker AE. Cerebral death. In: Tower DB, ed. *The nervous system*, Vol 2. New York: Raven Press, 1975:75–87.

479. Walker AE. *Cerebral death*. Dallas: Professional Information Library, 1977.

480. Walker AE. *Cerebral death*, 3rd ed. Baltimore: Urban & Schwarzenberg, 1985.

481. Walker AE, Diamond EL, Moseley JI. The neuropathological findings in irreversible coma: a critique of the "respirator brain." *J Neuropathol Exp Neurol* 1975;34:295–323.

482. Walker AE, Molinari GF. Sedative drug surveys in coma: how reliable are they? *Postgrad Med J* 1977;61:105–109.

483. Walser H, Isler H. Frontal intermittent rhythmic delta activity, impairment of consciousness and migraine. *Headache* 1982;22:74–80.

484. Walser H, Kriss A, Cunningham K, et al. Multimodality evoked potential assessment of uremia. In: Noder RH, Barber C, eds. *Evoked potentials II*. Boston: Butterworth-Heinemann, 1984:643–649.

485. Walser H, Mattle H, Keller HM, et al. Early cortical median nerve somatosensory evoked potentials: prognostic value in anoxic coma. *Arch Neurol* 1985;42:32–38.

486. Walter ST, Arfel G. Réponses aux stimulations visuelles dans les états de coma aigu et de coma chronique. *Electroencephalogr Clin Neurophysiol* 1972;32:27–41.

487. Watson CW, Adams RD. The electroencephalogram in its relation to consciousness and responsiveness in destructive lesions of the brain stem: a clinical pathological EEG study of brain stem disease particularly basilar artery occlusion. *Electroencephalogr Clin Neurophysiol* 1951;3:371.

488. Watson CW, Flynn RE, Sullivan JF. A distinctive electroencephalographic change associated with subdural hematoma resembling changes which occur with hepatic encephalopathy. *Electroencephalogr Clin Neurophysiol* 1958;10:780(abst).

489. Weissenborn K, Wilkens H, Hausmann E, et al. Burst suppression EEG with baclofen overdose. *Clin Neurol Neurosurg* 1991;93:77–80.

490. Westmoreland BF, Klass DW, Sharbrough FW, et al. "Alpha coma": EEG clinical, pathologic, and etiologic correlations. *Electroencephalogr Clin Neurophysiol* 1974;37:202(abst).

491. Westmoreland BF, Klass DW, Sharbrough FW, et al. Alpha-coma: electroencephalographic, clinical, pathologic, and etiologic correlations. *Arch Neurol* 1975;32:713–718.

492. Wijdicks EFM. Determining brain death in adults. *Neurology* 1995;45:1003–1011.

493. Wijdicks EFM. Brain death. In: Wijdicks EFM, ed. *The clinical practice of critical care neurology*. Philadelphia: Lippincott–Raven, 1997:320–333.

494. Wijdicks EFM. Diagnostic procedures. In: Wijdicks EFM, ed. *The clinical practice of critical care neurology*. Philadelphia: Lippincott–Raven, 1997:102–131.

495. Wijdicks EFM, Parisi JE, Sharbrough FW. Prognostic value of myoclonus status on comatose survivors of cardiac arrest. *Ann Neurol* 1994;40:1199–1202.

496. Wilkus RJ, Chatrian GE, Lettich E. The electroretinogram during terminal anoxia in humans. *Electroencephalogr Clin Neurophysiol* 1971;31:537–546.

497. Wilkus RJ, Harvey F, Ojemann LM, et al. Electroencephalogram and sensory evoked potentials: findings in an unresponsive patient with pontine infarct. *Arch Neurol* 1971;24:538–544(abst).

498. Woodgate C, Scott DF. Triphasic waves with particular emphasis on phase shift. *Electroencephalogr Clin Neurophysiol* 1983;55:39(abst).

499. Working Group convened by the Royal College of Physicians and endorsed by the Conference of Medical Royal Colleges and their Faculties in the United Kingdom. Criteria for the diagnosis of brain stem death. *J R Coll Physicians Lond* 1995;29:381–382.

500. *Working Party report on the diagnosis of brain stem death in children*. London: British Paediatric Association, 1991.

501. Wytrzes LM, Chatrian G-E, Shaw C-M, et al. Acute failure of forebrain with sparing of brain stem function: electroencephalographic, multimodality evoked potentials, and pathologic findings. *Arch Neurol* 1989;46:93–97.

502. Yagi T, Baba S. Evaluation of the brain stem function by the auditory brain stem response and the caloric vestibular reaction in comatose patient. *Arch Otorhinolaryngol* 1983;238:33–43.

503. Yamada T, Stevland N, Kimura J. Alpha-pattern coma in a 2-year-old child. *Arch Neurol* 1979;36:225–227.

504. Yamashita S, Morinaga T, Ohgo S, et al. Prognostic value of electroencephalogram (EEG) in anoxic encephalopathy after cardiopulmonary resuscitation: relationship among anoxic period, EEG grading and outcome. *Intern Med* 1995;34:71–76.

505. Yang S-S, Chu N-S, Liaw Y-F. Somatosensory evoked potentials in hepatic encephalopathy. *Gastroenterology* 1985;89:625–630.

506. Ying Z, Schmid UD, Schmid J, et al. Motor and somatosensory evoked potentials in coma: analysis and relation to clinical status and outcome. *J Neurol Neurosurg Psychiatry* 1992;55:470–474.

507. Yingling CD, Hosobuchi Y, Harrington M. P300 as a predictor of recovery from coma [Letter]. *Lancet* 1990;336:873.

508. Yli-Hankala A, Jantti V. EEG burst-suppression pattern correlates with the instantaneous heart rate under isoflurane anaesthesia. *Acta Anaesthesiol Scand* 1990;34:665–668.

509. Young GB, Baustin TW, Bolton CF, et al. The electroencephalogram in sepsis-associated encephalopathy. *J Clin Neurophysiol* 1992;9:145–152.

510. Young GB, Blume WT, Campbell VM, et al. Alpha, theta and alpha-theta coma: a clinical outcome study utilizing serial recordings. *Electroencephalogr Clin Neurophysiol* 1994;91:93–99.

511. Young GB, DeRubeis DA. Metabolic encephalopathies. In: Young GB, Ropper AH, Bolton CF, eds. *Coma and impaired consciousness: a clinical perspective*. New York: McGraw-Hill, 1998:307–392.

512. Young GB, Gilbert JJ, Zochodne DW. The significance of myoclonic status epilepticus in postanoxic coma. *Neurology* 1990;40:1843–1848.

513. Young GB, McLachlan RS, Kreeft JH, et al. An electroencephalographic classification for coma. *Can J Neurol Sci* 1997;24:320–325.

513a.Young GB, Kreeft JH, McLachlan RS, Demelo J. EEG and clinical associations with mortality in comatose patients in a general intensive care unit. *J Clin Neurophysiol* 1999;16:354–360.

513b.Young GB. The EEG in coma. *J Clin Neurophysiol* 2000;17:473–485.

514. Zandbergen EGJ, de Haan RJ, Stoutenbeek CP, et al. Systematic review of early prediction of poor outcome in anoxic-ischaemic coma. *Lancet* 1998;352:1808–1812.

514a.Zandbergen EGJ, de Haan RJ, Koelman JHTM, Hijdra A. Prediction of poor outcome in anoxic-ischemic coma. *J Clin Neurophysiol* 2000;17:498–501.

515. Zaret BS. Prognostic and neurophysiological implications of concurrent burst suppression and alpha patterns in the EEG of post-anoxic coma. *Electroencephalogr Clin Neurophysiol* 1985;61:199–209.

516. Zentner J, Rohde V. The prognostic value of somatosensory and motor evoked potentials in comatose patients. *Neurosurgery* 1992;31:429–434.

517. Zentner J, Rohde V. SEP and MEP in comatose patients. *Neurol Res* 1994;16:89–92.

Chapter 15

Drug Effects and Toxic Encephalopathies

Anne C. Van Cott and Richard P. Brenner

The literature addressing the effects of drugs and toxins on electroencephalographic (EEG) activity is abundant and rapidly expanding. Because it is not possible to summarize all the available information, the goal of this chapter is to review the commonly encountered and clinically relevant EEG patterns associated with some drugs and toxins. Reports of the effect of drugs on EEG activity are contradictory; this may result in part from the variety of methods used in analysis of EEG data. Although quantitative EEG analysis has provided a wealth of information, the authors choose to emphasize the changes seen on visual inspection, because this most closely approximates clinical EEG interpretation. A large percentage of patients undergoing EEG are taking one or more medications. Both the EEG technician and interpreter must be aware of changes that may be induced by medications.

A drug or toxin's effect on the EEG is dependent on numerous factors not limited only to its chemical composition. The dose administered and the duration of exposure are critical. Alterations of EEG activity may also reflect systemic effects of a medication: for example, generalized slowing may be secondary to central nervous system hypoperfusion caused by hypotension. Individual patient characteristics, including preexisting brain disease and EEG abnormalities, can influence the impact of drugs and toxins

on background EEG activity. The EEG changes vary considerably from patient to patient, and thus a drug effect cannot be predicted in an individual. The withdrawal of a drug may also greatly influence central nervous system function as reflected by the EEG.

Although changes in EEG activity may indicate central nervous system dysfunction, they are not specific. Diffuse slowing of background EEG activity is the most commonly encountered drug effect, but it does not implicate a particular agent. The presence of superimposed generalized fast activity on an EEG should arouse suspicion of drug toxicity, particularly of medications that are recognized to increase beta activity, such as barbiturates or benzodiazepines. In general, focal slowing or asymmetry of EEG activity is not encountered in toxic encephalopathies; it suggests instead an underlying localized abnormality. Drugs may influence epileptiform discharges. Certain medications, such as clozapine (*Clozaril*) and metronizamide, can activate ictal and interictal epileptiform discharges, which indicates that they reduce seizure threshold. Other medications, including antiepileptic drugs (AEDs), can suppress epileptiform activity, which reflects their anticonvulsant effect. As discussed later, more unique patterns have been associated with certain agents. Generalized, bisynchronous sharp complexes, at times periodic and often with a triphasic configuration, have been associated with a variety of medications, including baclofen, lithium, levodopa, and metrizamide (69,106,110,119,141,145,167,171). Drug intoxications and anesthetic agents can result in seemingly ominous EEG patterns, including alpha-pattern coma, spindle-pattern coma, burst-suppression pattern, and electrocerebral silence.

ANTIEPILEPTIC DRUGS

EEG is an invaluable tool in the management of patients with epilepsy. EEG findings can play a critical role in a variety of decisions, including initiation and withdrawal of antiepileptic drug therapy. In certain situations, the EEG may be used to determine whether AEDs are therapeutic. AEDs have been found to affect both background EEG activity and interictal epileptiform activity. All of the older AEDs may result in increases in slow activity and slowing of the dominant posterior rhythm (28). Each of these issues is addressed for the established AEDs.

Rhythmic fast activity increases with therapeutic doses of both benzodiazepines and barbiturates. With benzodiazepines, rhythmic beta activity increases and is most prominent during drowsiness (17) (Fig. 15.1). A decrease in the voltage of the alpha frequency may also be present (156). These changes depend on the patient's age; they are more marked in younger individuals. In addition, the presence of fast activity is also dependent on duration of treatment; it is more pronounced after the acute administration of benzodiazepines. As the level of the benzodiazepine rises and intoxication occurs, faster frequencies become higher in voltage and are more sustained (5). Eventually, with increasing levels, there is more prominent generalized slowing, which is correlated with the depressed level of consciousness (28).

Rhythmic fast activity associated with barbiturates is usually 18 to 25 Hz and is more prominent in the frontal head regions (121). As the patient becomes increasingly intoxicated with a marked decrease in level of consciousness, background EEG activity can reveal prominent delta activity with superimposed spindle-like activity (12). In deep coma caused by barbiturates, the EEG may show a burst-suppression pattern or even electrocerebral silence (143). A burst-suppression pattern is the therapeutic goal in patients treated for status epilepticus or increased intracranial pressure with intravenous pentobarbital.

At therapeutic levels, phenytoin has no visually discernible effect on background EEG activity. In quantitative EEG analysis, phenytoin, alone or in combination with other drugs, has been reported to decrease background frequency, in comparison with other AEDs (64). With increasing levels (greater than 20 µg per milliliter), there can be slowing of the mean alpha frequency. With clinical neurotoxicity, increased generalized theta activity and intermittent delta activity are present (Fig. 15.2). With severe toxicity, high-voltage delta slowing may be present (128). EEG changes reported with carbamazepine therapy are not consistent and are of no recognized clinical significance. Both mild slowing of the mean alpha frequency and intermittent random generalized theta activity have been reported with therapeutic carbamazepine levels (48,123,126). These changes can be more pronounced with toxic drug levels. Carbamazepine discontinuation has been associated with an increase in the frequency of the dominant rhythm and reduction of slow activity (29). At therapeutic levels, valproic acid has not been found to have an effect on background EEG activity (64), whereas valproate intoxication has been associated with diffuse slowing (1).

Less information about the effect of the newer AEDs on EEG activity is available. Lamotrigine has not been found to slow background activity in normal volunteers or epileptic patients (45,101). In one study (78), patients with partial epilepsy receiving tiagabine had no new EEG abnormalities. Several studies have reported no change in background EEG activity with vigabatrin treatment (58,102).

In general, the reported effects of AEDs on interictal epileptiform activity are variable and inconsistent (5). Most important clinically, for seizures other than absence, the amount of interictal epileptiform activity is often not related to seizure frequency (8,28). Abrupt withdrawal of AEDs has been reported to increase interictal epileptiform discharges (94,100), although later reports found no increase of interictal epileptiform abnormalities after withdrawal of AEDs (54). With regard to seizure activity, reduction of AED dosage can increase seizure frequency and the likelihood that seizures will secondarily generalize. However, So and Gotman (146) found no difference in the electrographic ictal morphological appearance of seizures with dose reduction. With high or low drug levels, there were no changes in the onset of the electrographic seizure, time to contralateral spread, or coherence between discharges in patients.

Ictal and interictal epileptiform activity can be suppressed acutely by benzodiazepine therapy administered intravenously or rectally, but the effects of long-term oral therapy with these agents is less defined (28). Huang and Shen (71) reported that an abnormal EEG pattern that responded positively to intravenous diazepam is a good prognostic indicator of future seizure control with AEDs. Phenobarbital and primidone have been shown to decrease interictal epileptiform abnormalities in patients with controlled seizures (18,80).

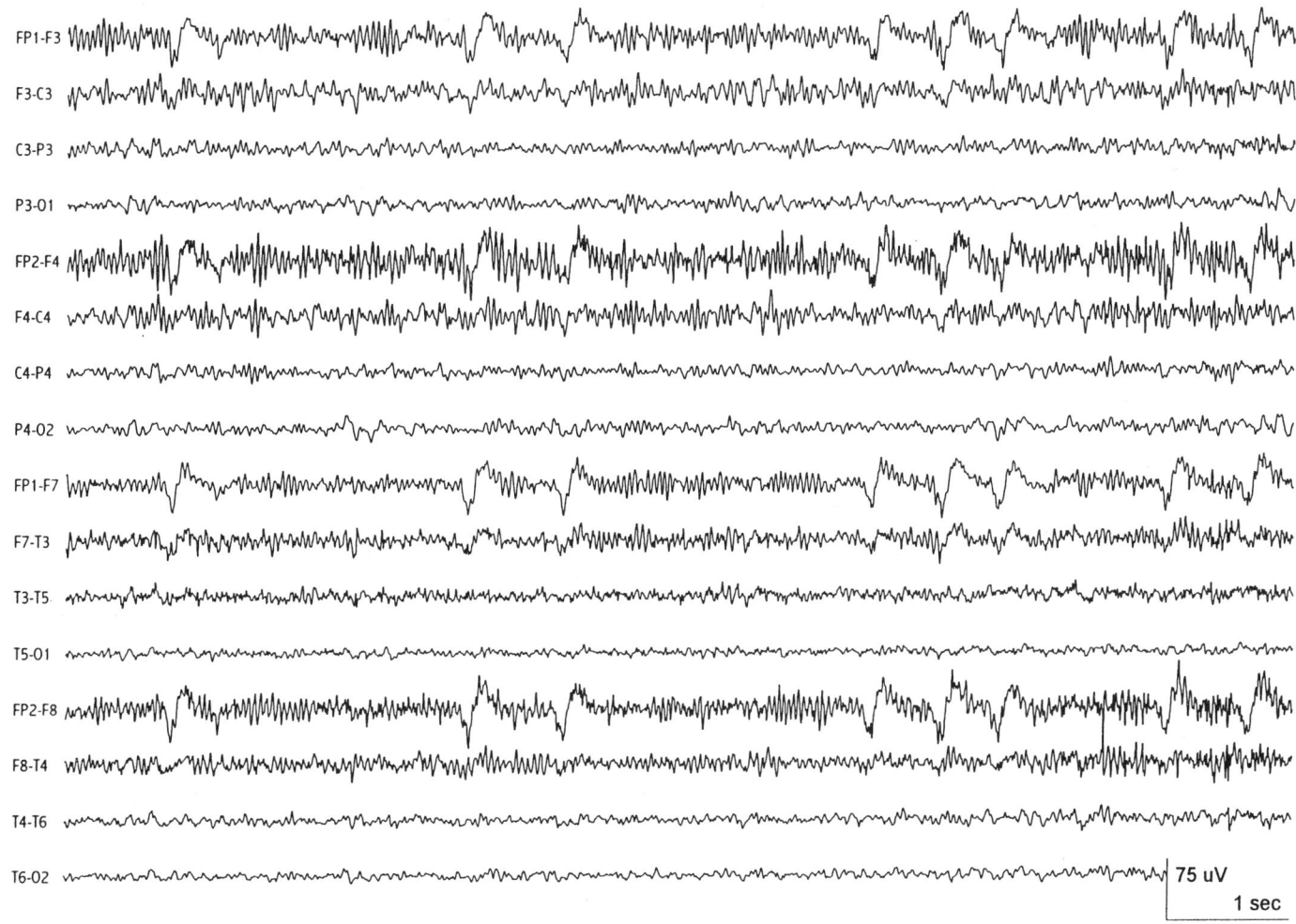

FIG. 15.1. Faster frequencies are prominent in the EEG of an 18-year-old man with a psychotic disorder who was medicated with lorazepam.

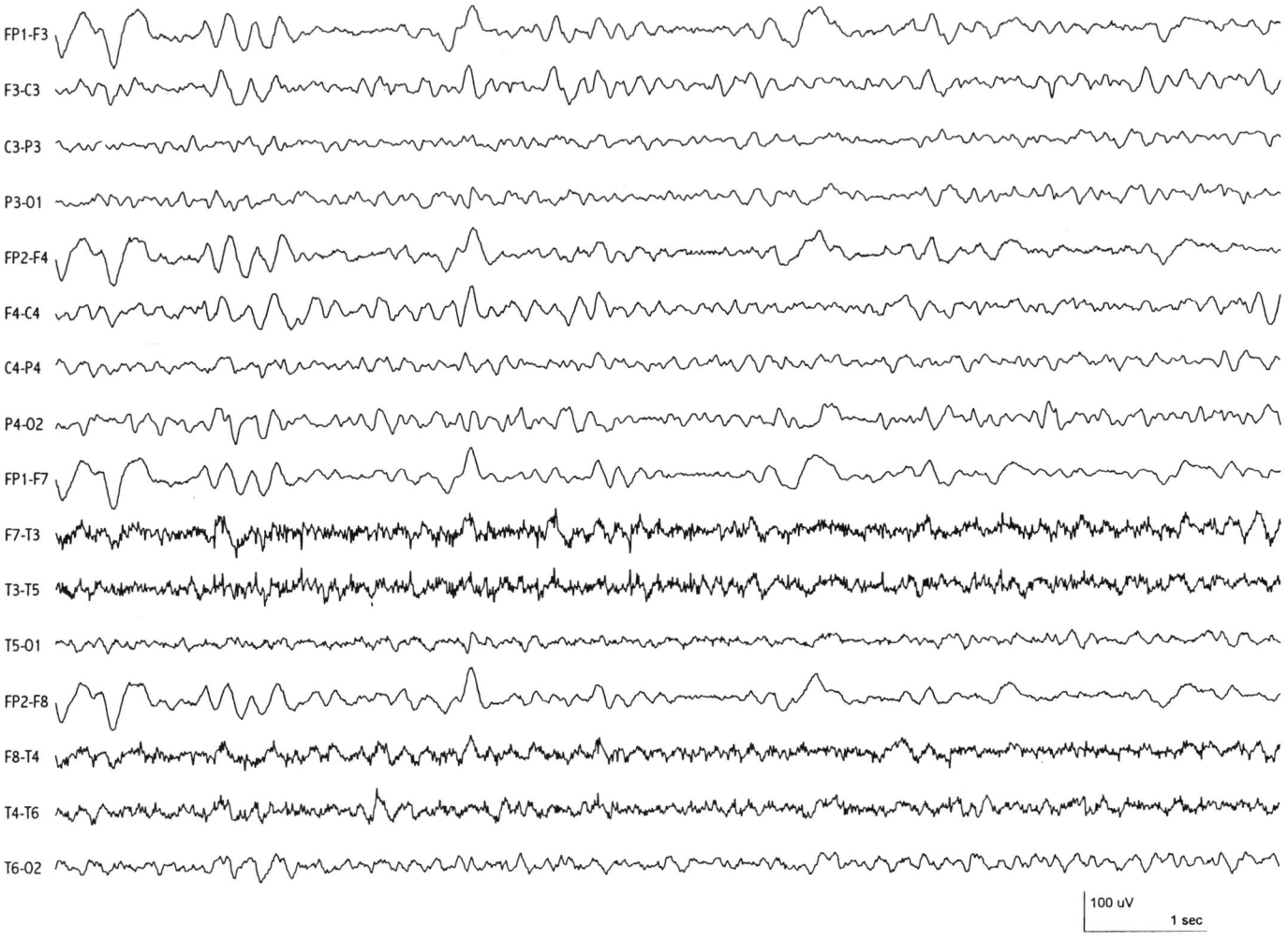

FIG. 15.2. Generalized slowing of the background EEG activity is present in this tracing from a 20-year-old woman with a phenytoin level of 34 µg per milliliter.

Both benzodiazepines and barbiturates can play a useful role in localization of epileptogenic foci. Intravenous diazepam and clonazepam have been shown to suppress spread of electrographic seizures to the contralateral hemisphere (16,89). This may be useful in resolving issues of secondary bilateral synchrony. In a similar manner, barbiturates (intravenous thiopental) have been administered to patients with generalized seizures and bilateral spike-and-wave discharges to allow identification of a focal EEG abnormality (93). Conversely, in patients with partial epilepsy, withdrawal of barbiturates can precipitate generalized epileptiform activity or, less commonly, new or additional foci of seizure onset (148). Barbiturate withdrawal in drug-addicted patients may produce epileptiform discharges consisting of high-voltage bisynchronous spike-and-wave abnormalities superimposed on generalized slowing of background EEG activity (37).

There are contradictory data regarding the effect of phenytoin on interictal epileptiform discharges. Most reports found no effect on interictal epileptiform discharges with phenytoin treatment (5). Phenytoin withdrawal has been reported to falsely localize ictal onset (35). The data about the effect of carbamazepine on interictal discharges is also conflicting. Increased interictal epileptiform activity reported with carbamazepine treatment was not correlated with worse seizure control (75,132,169). Carbamazepine has also been reported to have no effect on interictal abnormalities (123). The frequency of interictal abnormalities was found to be related to seizure activity and not to AED withdrawal (54). Marciani et al. (97) proposed that changes in interictal epileptiform abnormalities may be related to seizure occurrence and not to the direct action of carbamazepine on spike activity.

The effect on valproate therapy on epileptiform activity depends on the epilepsy type. Valproic acid can reduce or abolish generalized spike-and-wave discharges but has little or no effect on focal interictal epileptiform activity (5). The ability of valproic acid to abort or suppress 3-Hz spike-and-wave discharges in patients with absence epilepsy can help gauge therapeutic efficacy (162). Valproate also suppresses photoparoxysmal responses (59). The suppression of generalized epileptiform discharges by valproate may continue for up to 3 months after discontinuation of the medication (59,129). Ethosuximide, like valproate, can reduce generalized spike-and-wave discharges (136).

The effect of the newer AEDs on epileptiform abnormalities in humans is not completely understood. Binnie et al. (9) found that lamotrigine has been reported to decrease spontaneous and light-induced generalized spike-and-wave discharges. Vigabatrin has not been shown to have any consistent effect on interictal spikes (7,99). AEDs may activate epileptiform discharges. Generalized spikes, at times accompanied by myoclonic jerks or absence seizures, have been reported in patients receiving vigabatrin (98,103). In addition, two epileptic patients receiving tiagabine developed nonconvulsive status epilepticus with electroclinical features consistent with atypical absence seizures (32).

EEG can assist in making decisions about the discontinuation of AED therapy in patients who are seizure free. In adult patients who have been seizure free for 2 years or more, EEG abnormalities increase the risk of seizure recurrence after AED withdrawal (20). Some reports refute this finding, stating that only an increase in interictal epileptiform abnormalities during withdrawal of AEDs is associated with a higher seizure relapse rate (49). In children, EEG abnormalities that are present before withdrawal of medications portend a very poor prognosis and are considered a major risk factor for seizure recurrence after discontinuation of medications (140).

Treatment of epileptic patients with AEDs may result in a paradoxical reaction and induction of seizures. Identified clinical risk factors that may predispose a patient to such a reaction include youth, mental retardation, polytherapy, high seizure frequency, and prominent epileptiform abnormalities in EEG before treatment (4). Syndromes in which seizure exacerbation has been attributed to AED therapy include Lennox-Gastaut syndrome and West's syndrome (4). Carbamazepine has been reported to exacerbate a variety of seizures, including absence, atonic, and myoclonic seizures (133, 152). EEGs may reveal bursts of diffuse and bilaterally synchronous spike-and-wave discharges (116).

Increased seizure frequency and an encephalopathy can occur with valproate therapy. This most frequently occurs in patients early (first week to nine months) during a first-time exposure. Valproate levels are frequently within normal limits, and the EEG reveals generalized slowing with an increased number of generalized spike discharges. This has raised the issue about whether the encephalopathy truly represents nonconvulsive status epilepticus. However, no change in the background EEG activity or clinical state after treatment with intravenous benzodiazepines has been reported. Valproate therapy withdrawal is recommended in patients with suspected encephalopathy (4).

NEUROPSYCHIATRIC DRUGS

As a group, the conventional neuroleptic agents, including phenothiazines, butyrophenones, and thioxanthenes, produce similar changes in background EEG activity. Visual analysis of the EEG shows little or no change at therapeutic drug levels, although there are some reports of slowing of the alpha rhythm, reduction of beta activity, and increased amplitude of theta transients (3). Slowing, both focal and generalized, that is present on pretreatment EEGs may be accentuated by phenothiazine administration (92). With acute intoxication, generalized slowing of background EEG activity may be accompanied by generalized paroxysmal activity (72). The neuroleptic agents have been reported to lower seizure threshold in patients with chronic epilepsy (113). Seizure occurrence is usually, but not always, dose dependent, and nonconvulsive status epilepticus has been described (159). Of the newer antipsychotic agents, risperidone has not been associated with seizures and does not produce EEG changes in the awake record (23). However, another novel antipsychotic agent, clozapine, has marked effects on background EEG activity and seizure threshold, both of great clinical significance.

Clozapine selectively blocks cortical and limbic dopamine receptors and is used in the treatment of refractory schizophrenia and schizoaffective disorders. It produces minimal extrapyramidal side effects and has proved beneficial in the treatment of psychosis induced by dopaminomimetic agents in patients with Parkinson's disease. In addition to agranulocytosis and autonomic instability, a serious potential adverse effect of clozapine is seizures.

Clozapine can produce generalized tonic-clonic seizures and myoclonus (135). Myoclonus may manifest as jerking movements of the face, head, fingers, toes, or trunk and can proceed to generalized convulsive seizures (57) (Fig. 15.3). Large-scale studies have previously reported generalized seizure rates of 1.9% to 10% (26,114,170). The risk of seizures is higher during the initial treatment phase than in the maintenance treatment period. Rapid titration of clozapine may be a risk factor in the development of seizures during the initiation of treatment (114). Seizures have been reported with a wide range of dosages, but they seem more likely to occur at higher doses (56,135). Clozapine-associated seizures have been treated with dosage reduction and/or the addition of an antiepileptic agent, most commonly valproic acid or phenytoin.

A wide spectrum of EEG changes can occur in patients treated with clozapine. A high percentage–estimates of 16% to 74%–of patients receiving clozapine have abnormal EEGs; the most prevalent finding is generalized slowing (56,60,96,147). Interictal epileptiform activity indicating a seizure tendency may be present but is less prevalent than slowing of the background EEG activity (Fig. 15.4). Malow et al. (96) described the spectrum of EEG abnormalities in ten patients being treated with clozapine. Interictal epileptiform abnormalities were described as bilateral spike-and-wave discharges predominating in the anterior parasagittal head region and becoming more frequent during drowsiness. Activation by hyperventilation and photic stimulation was present in a few patients. Decreasing the clozapine dosage and/or adding valproic acid therapy diminished epileptiform discharges but did not change background slowing.

Abnormal EEGs have been found to be more common in patients receiving high dosages (56) and with high serum levels of clozapine (47). Even at low dosages in the treatment of delusions and psychotic behavior in parkinsonian patients, clozapine may cause EEG changes, including increased generalized or focal slowing (107). Interestingly, there may be a positive association between clozapine-induced EEG abnormalities and clinical improvement in certain patient populations (118,124,157).

In a retrospective study of 680 EEGs in 593 patients receiving psychopharmaceutical agents, the proportion of abnormal EEGs was found to be highest in patients receiving clozapine (59%), and next highest in those receiving lithium (50%) (147). Lithium is a mood-stabilizing agent with antimanic properties that is used in the treatment of bipolar mood disorders. After a single dose of lithium in an adult, little or no EEG change is observed visually. With ongoing treatment, EEG changes may include slowing of background EEG activity. Frontal intermittent rhythmic delta activity (FIRDA) may be present and accentuated by hyperventilation. EEG abnormalities present before treatment may become more pronounced (144). EEG abnormalities increase with higher serum plasma levels but can occur at therapeutic levels (63). With lithium intoxication, the EEG may show diffuse slowing, paroxysmal abnormalities, and triphasic waves (10) (Fig. 15.5). The electrical abnormalities lessen in parallel with improvement in the patient's clinical state but can persist despite normalization of serum levels (3).

Lithium can enhance preexisting sharp waves and spikes in patients with epilepsy (52,144). However, lithium's actual epileptogenicity remains unclear. According to some reports, lithium treatment has increased seizure frequency in patients with epilepsy and induced seizures in patients without a seizure disorder; according to other reports (36,51), seizure frequency has decreased in epileptic patients receiving lithium. Julius and Brenner (76) reported on two patients who, soon after starting lithium therapy, developed generalized tonic-clonic seizures followed by myoclonic seizures associated with repetitive sharp waves on EEG, which resolved after lithium discontinuation. Smith and Kocen (145) described two cases of a Creutzfeldt-Jakob–like picture accompanied by typical EEG changes (generalized slowing with synchronous periodic complexes) with lithium toxicity that

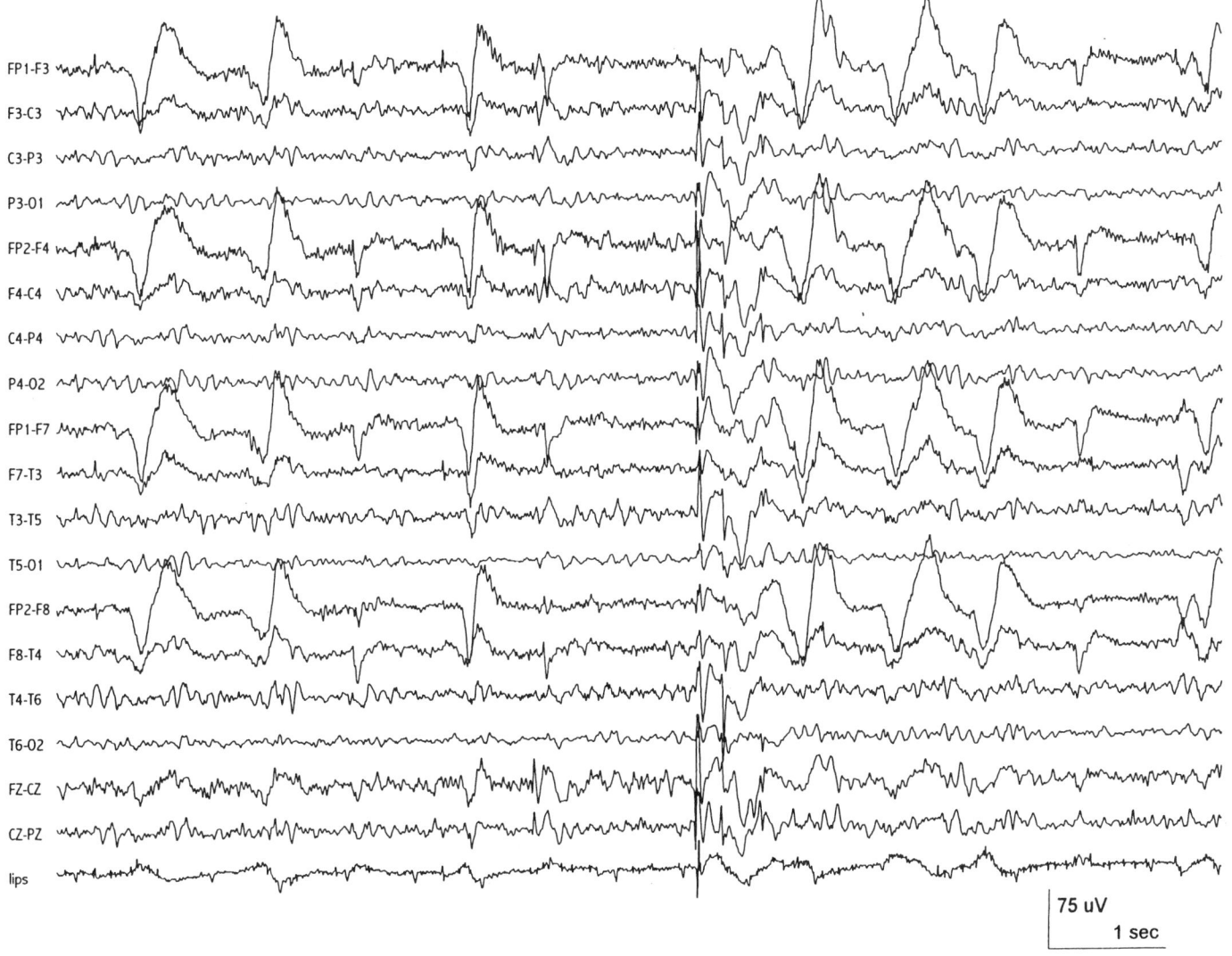

FIG. 15.3. Polyspike discharge in a 32-year-old man taking clozapine (*Clozaril*) therapy for schizophrenia associated with myoclonic movements, including those of the face (lip channel).

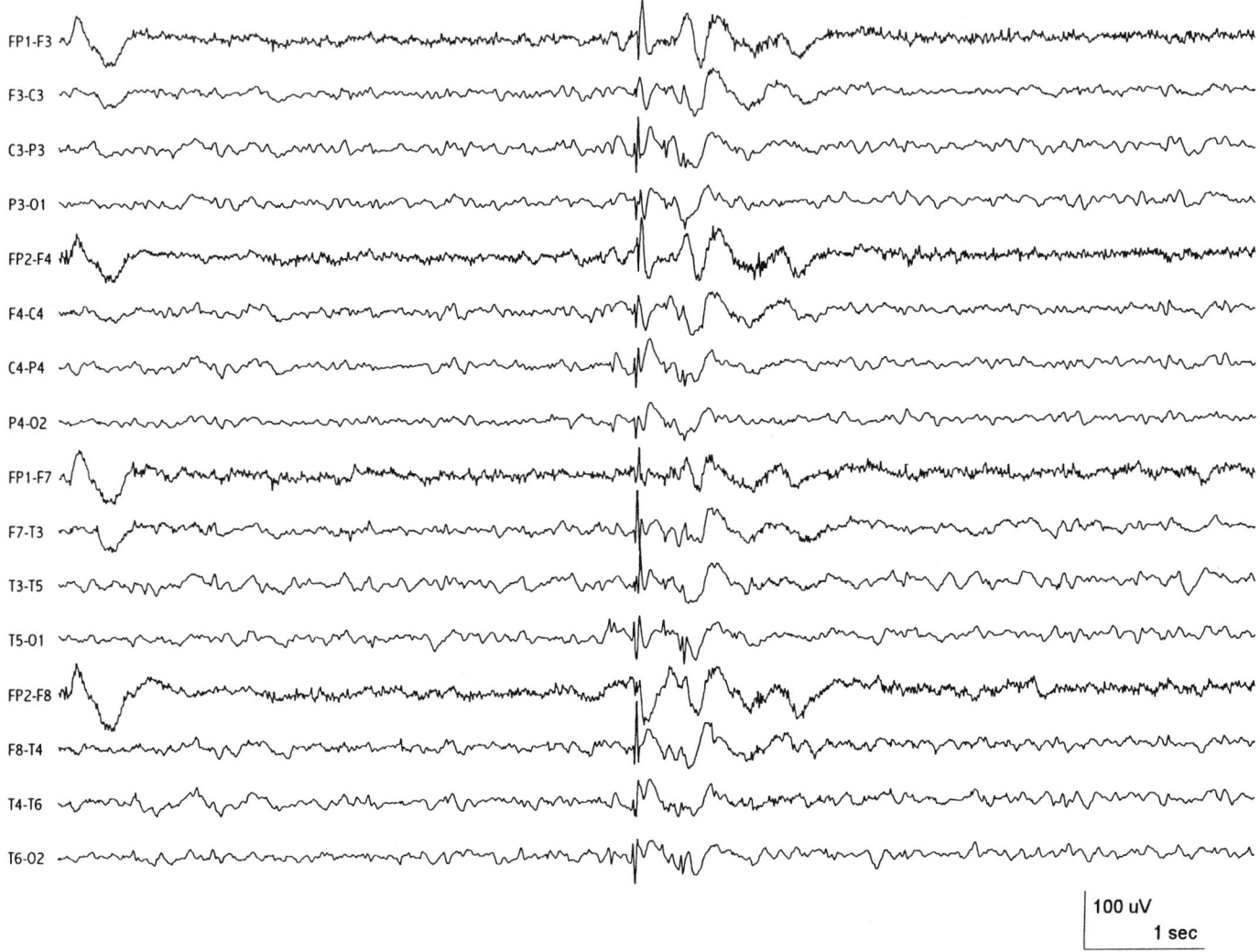

FIG. 15.4. Generalized polyspike discharge accompanied by myoclonic jerks in a 34-year-old woman with bipolar disorder and psychotic symptoms who was taking clozapine (*Clozaril*).

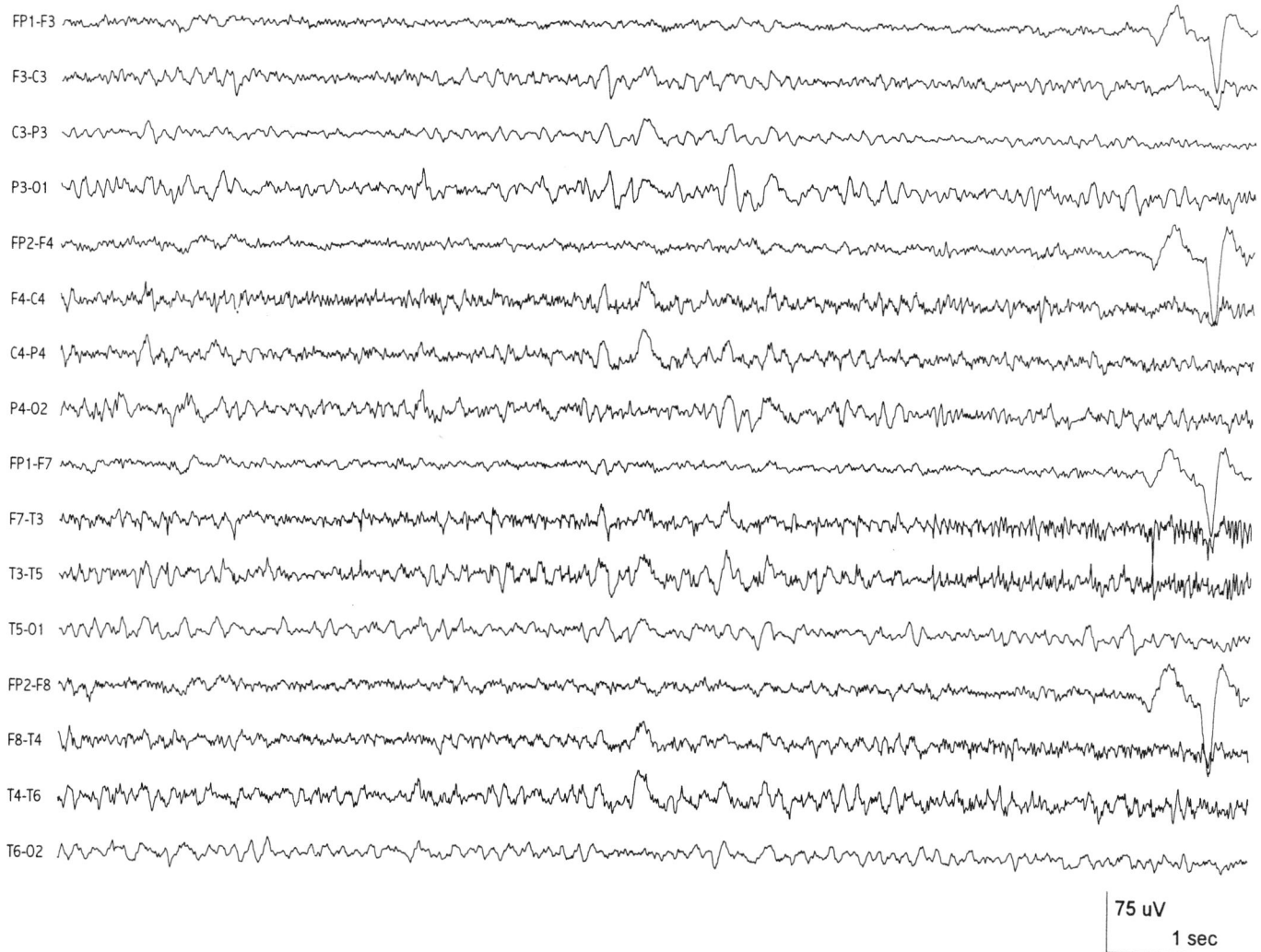

FIG. 15.5. EEG shows generalized slowing in a 50-year-old woman receiving lithium for psychotic depression.

resolved with discontinuation of the medication. Additional cases of Creutzfeldt-Jakob—like syndrome during lithium use, alone or in combination with other medications (including levodopa and tricyclic agents), were reported later (39).

The pharmacological agents available for the treating depression have become more numerous and less toxic since the early 1970s. The first generation of antidepressants included the monoamine oxidase inhibitors (MAOIs) and the tricyclic antidepressants (TCAs). Amoxapine and maprotiline, two TCAs, are pharmacologically similar but differ in chemical structure. Although highly effective, these agents had serious and potentially fatal side effects, particularly if taken in overdose. The first serotonin selective reuptake inhibitor (SSRI), fluoxetine, was introduced in the mid-1980s and provided a much higher therapeutic index. The SSRIs (fluoxetine, sertraline, paroxetine, fluvoxamine, and citalopram) and a heterogeneous group of atypical antidepressants (mirtazapine, nefazodone, and venlafaxine) have largely replaced the TCAs and MAOIs as first-line treatments for depression (46).

Tricyclic drugs, at therapeutic levels, produce only subtle changes on background EEG activity (68). Tricyclic drugs may increase the amount of both fast and slow activities (in the beta and theta frequencies), along with a slowing of the alpha rhythm (40,41). Acute intoxication from overdosage may result in cardiac arrhythmias and is life-threatening. Along with seizures, the clinical picture can include hyperpyrexia, hypertension, and coma (22). During acute intoxication, background EEG activity reveals generalized slowing and paroxysmal activity, including interictal spikes (87) (Fig. 15.6).

Tricyclic agents can lower seizure threshold to a variable degree (142). Seizure frequency may increase in patients with epilepsy after initiation of tricyclic drug therapy. Intravenous administration of imipramine (81) and amitriptyline (24) increased the number of epileptiform discharges in epileptic patients. Although these drugs are rarely a *de novo* cause of seizures, single and multiple seizures have been reported in nonepileptic patients, especially those receiving high doses (32). Itil and Soldatos (73) classified imipramine, along with the MAOIs, as having a slight or no tendency to potentiate epileptiform discharges.

The newer antidepressants offer safer treatment options. Serious adverse events occur rarely; few deaths have resulted from overdose. According to visual analysis, EEG activity exhibits subtle changes in background frequency (3). Maprotiline and bupropion have been reported to have a higher propensity to cause seizures than do the SSRIs trazodone, nefazodone, and mirtazapine (46).

Sleep disturbances, including hypersomnia and insomnia, are an integral feature of the depressive disorders. Polysomnography may document abnormal sleep patterns, including decreased amounts of slow-wave sleep, early onset of first episode of rapid-eye-movement (REM) sleep, and increased amounts of phasic REM sleep (154). Both the tricyclics and MAOIs tend to suppress REM sleep. Paroxetine and fluvoxamine, both SSRIs, showed effects on polysomnographic testing in depressed patients similar to those of amitriptyline; all decreased the amount of REM sleep. However, the SSRIs exhibited an alerting effect on sleep (86,149).

Benzodiazepines, a large class of medications that include diazepam, midazolam, clonazepam, and flurazepam, bind at the γ-aminobutyric acid A (GABA-A) receptor chloride ionophore (50). As already discussed, these drugs can be used as anticonvulsant agents. In addition to being potent anxiolytic agents, benzodiazepines can produce muscle relaxation. As anesthetic agents, they produce hypnotic and amnestic states. As previously indicated, these agents increase beta activity and may cause mild generalized slowing of background EEG activity. Fast activity may persist for up to 2 weeks after drug ingestion. Benzodiazepine-induced fast activity can be reduced at the site of a focal cerebral lesion (53). In addition to producing seizures, psychosis, and delirium, benzodiazepine withdrawal can produce a delirium with catatonic features accompanied by generalized slowing of the background activity without epileptiform discharges (61). Acute withdrawal contributes to *de novo* absence status epilepticus of late onset (155).

Midazolam, frequently used as a sedative or treatment for status epilepticus in the critical care setting, has EEG effects similar to those of other benzodiazepines (65). Side effects, including respiratory depression, hypnosis, and incoordination, may be reversed by a specific benzodiazepine antagonist, flumazenil. In normal controls, flumazenil has no significant effect on EEG activity (13). Although benzodiazepine antagonists have been shown to improve background EEG activity and symptoms of encephalopathy in patients with hepatic failure, several studies have not supported a major therapeutic benefit of flumazenil in most patients with hepatic encephalopathy (2,19,55,158).

Buspirone offers an alternative to diazepam in treatment for patients with generalized anxiety disorders but may lack efficacy in patients with previous exposure to benzodiazepine (88,112). Unlike diazepam, buspirone has little or no effect on background EEG activity (11).

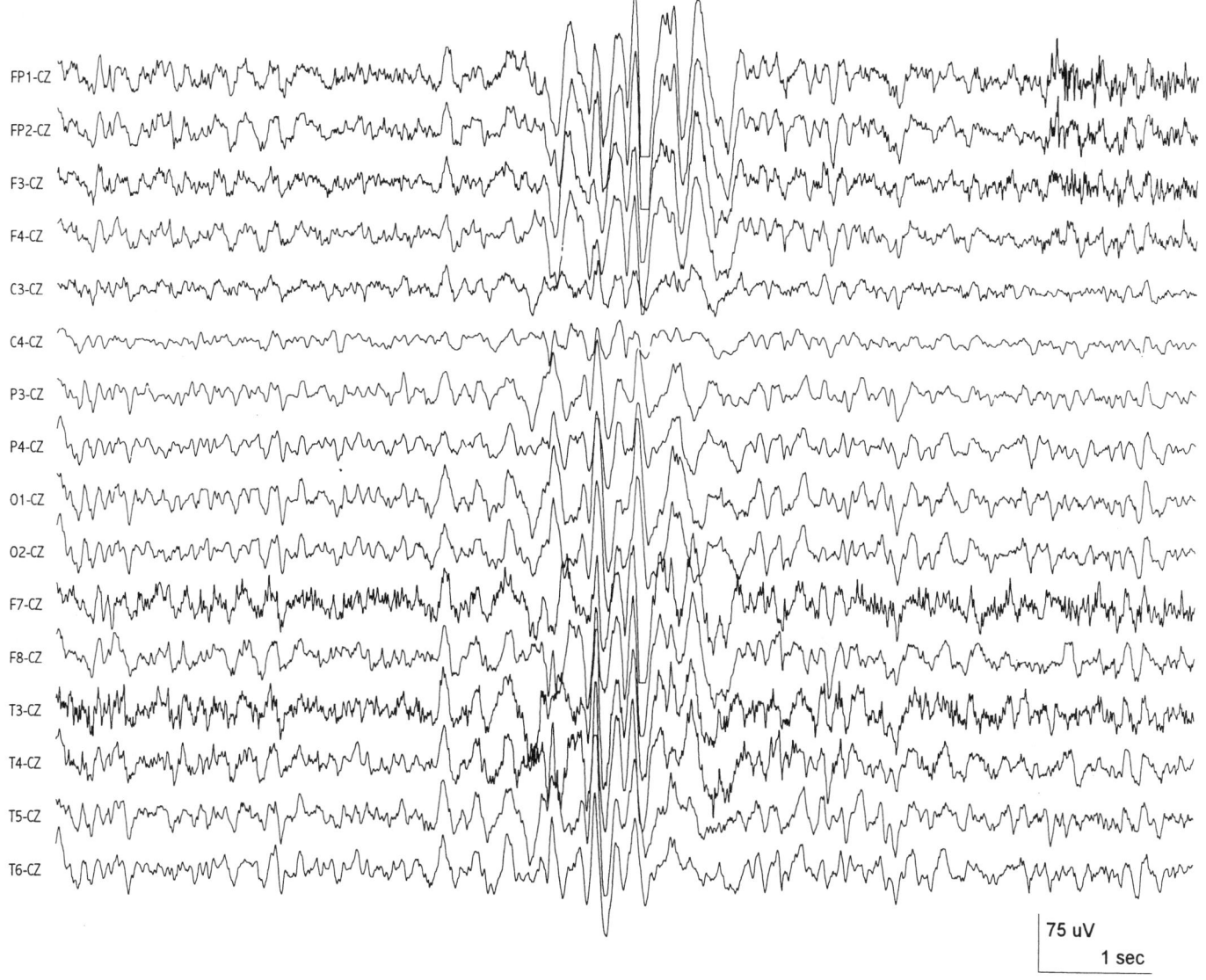

FIG. 15.6. Generalized burst of high-amplitude sharp activity in a 48-year-old woman with toxic levels of amitriptyline and nortriptyline.

ANESTHETICS AND ANALGESICS

The effect of anesthetic agents on the EEG is reviewed elsewhere in this textbook (Chapters 21, especially, but also 25, and 31). The associated EEG patterns depend on several factors, including the type and quantity of the drug used. To complicate the issue, it is common for multiple anesthetic agents to be used in the operative setting. A combination of anesthetics produces an EEG pattern that reflects the impact of the blend of these medications (95).

In selecting anesthetic drugs, in conjunction with EEG recording, the clinician must consider the goal of monitoring. For example, the most common monitoring application is for the detection of focal ischemia intraoperatively. The halogenated inhalation anesthetics, which induce background EEG activity of moderate amplitude and frequency, allow for rapid detection of decreased amplitude and frequency that are associated with reduced blood flow (139). On the other hand, etomidate, which increases epileptiform activity in patients with seizure disorders (30), may be used to enhance spike activity during electrocorticography. In contrast, agents such as barbiturates, which are cortical depressants and can produce electrocerebral silence, have been used to lower cerebral metabolism and oxygen demand.

Most anesthetic agents produce similar changes in the EEG. Barbiturates and most of the nonbarbiturate anesthesia-induction agents (etomidate, propofol) initially cause an increase in faster frequencies (beta) with a loss of the alpha rhythm. As the anesthetic dose is titrated, the frequency of EEG activity decreases and the amplitude increases, accompanied clinically by a loss of consciousness. At high doses, a burst-suppression pattern occurs (Fig. 15.7), and if the dose is titrated further, electrocerebral silence may be present. Surgical stimulation may alter this pattern, opposing the frequency slowing caused by higher doses (95).

Propofol is an ultra–short-acting intravenous agent that is used for both induction and maintenance of anesthesia. Used at doses appropriate for maintenance, propofol induces a regular, frontally dominant delta rhythm with superimposed faster frequencies (Fig. 15.8). Propofol has been reported to have different effects on epileptiform activity (27,31). At lower doses (0.5 mg per kilogram), epileptiform discharges were present in epileptic (40%) and nonepileptic patients (33%). At higher doses (1.5 mg per kilogram), this activating effect was increased to 67% and 73%, respectively. When additional doses were administered, the spike discharges disappeared (166). Propofol at high doses (maintenance infusions of 2 to 4 mg per kilogram per hour) controls refractory status epilepticus more rapidly than high doses of barbiturates (150). Recurrent seizures were common when propofol infusions were abruptly discontinued and may be related to the proconvulsant effects of this medication at lower doses.

Ketamine, which is structurally related to phencyclidine (also known as PCP and angel dust), is useful for anesthesia induction. Initially, a loss of the alpha rhythm and a decrease in background amplitude is present. Increasing the dose further produces frontally dominant rhythmic theta activity. Higher doses produce high-amplitude theta activity accompanied by an increase in beta activity (95).

In general, the halogenated inhalation anesthetics (desflurane, enflurane, halothane, isoflurane, and sevoflurane) produce EEG changes similar to those produced by the barbiturates. With the exception of desflurane, induction with these agents produces alpha frequencies in the anterior head region that may resemble sleep spindles. At higher concentrations, sufficient to produce anesthesia, there is a reduction in the amplitude and frequency of background EEG activity. Unlike isoflurane and desflurane, halothane does not produce a burst-suppression pattern or electrocerebral silence at clinically relevant doses (143). Enflurane may produce interictal epileptiform abnormalities in patients with or without a history of a seizure disorder (44,105). Isoflurane, in comparison with enflurane, has been found to decrease the frequency of spikes on the electrocorticogram of patients with intractable epilepsy who undergo temporal lobectomy (74). Fiol et al. (42) refuted this, reporting that isoflurane in combination with nitrous oxide had no significant effect on spike activity on the electrocorticogram during epilepsy surgery. Enhancement of the EEG activity by enflurane has been considered a disadvantage during neurosurgical procedures, in which increased cerebral metabolic activity is undesirable (143).

A nonhalogenated inhalation anesthetic, nitrous oxide, possesses analgesic and amnestic properties and is used in combination with other agents to achieve surgical anesthesia. In concentrations sufficient to produce analgesia and depressed consciousness, fast (>30 Hz) oscillatory activity is often present (95). The effect of nitrous oxide on the EEG depends on what agents it is combined with, and it has been reported to have both proconvulsant and anticonvulsant properties (143). Hosain et al. (70) found no difference in spike rate during electrocorticography in patients undergoing epilepsy surgery with or without nitrous oxide; this suggests that it may be used without concerns about suppression of epileptiform activity.

The effect of the short-acting synthetic opiates including fentanyl, sufentanil, and alfentanil, on EEG activity can be described on the basis of dosage. At low concentrations, loss of beta activity and slowing of alpha activity occur. With moderate doses, the amplitude increases, whereas the

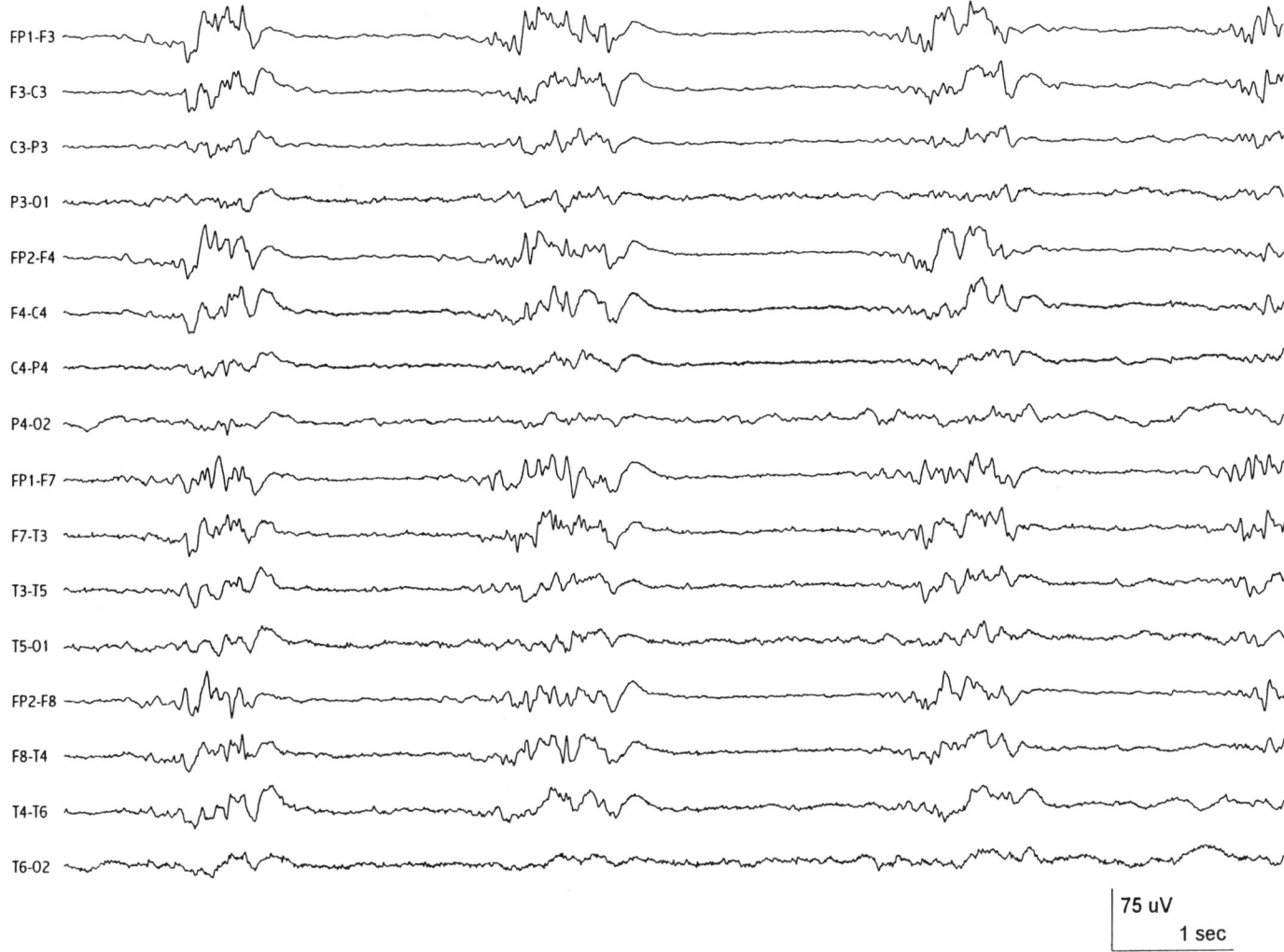

FIG. 15.7. A burst-suppression pattern in a 65-year-old man after an intravenous thiopental sodium (*Pentothal*) bolus during a carotid endarterectomy.

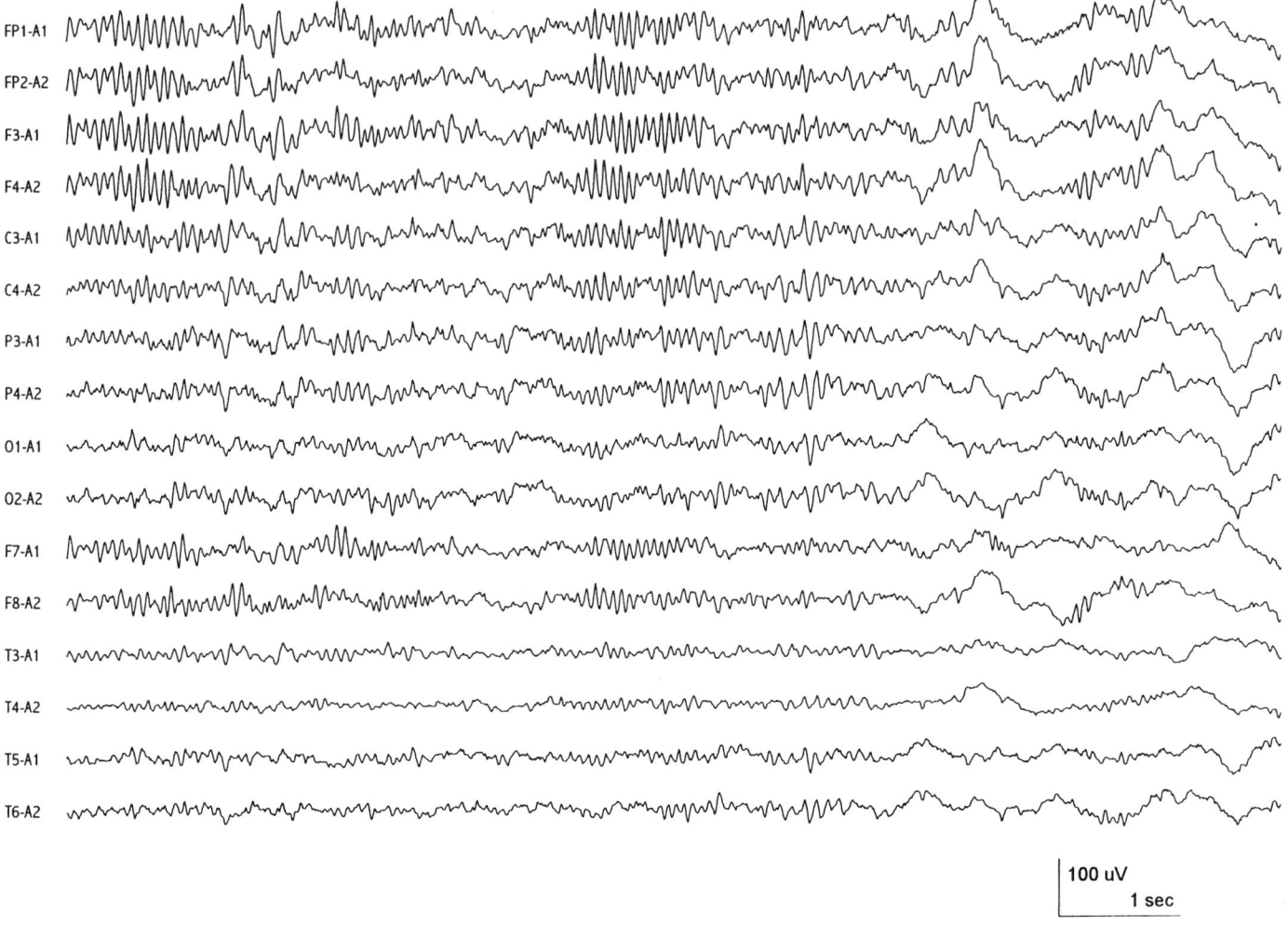

FIG. 15.8. Spindle coma in a 33-year-old woman sedated with propofol after arteriography.

frequency (diffuse theta with some delta activity) decreases. At high concentrations, delta activity, often synchronized and of high amplitude, predominates. Burst-suppression or electrocerebral silence is not present at higher doses (95). Opioid agents are frequently cited as being epileptogenic. Kearse et al. (79) reported that 19 of 20 patients undergoing coronary artery revascularization developed epileptiform activity characterized as low- to moderate-voltage, generalized single-phasic and multiphasic spike discharges "similar in appearance to benign epileptiform transients of sleep." Because of the predominance of slower frequencies at higher doses, opioid agents may reduce the ability to detect changes indicative of ischemia (143).

Benzodiazepines may be used to premedicate or supplement general anesthesia. As reviewed in the AED section, these drugs may produce frontal beta activity with slowing of the alpha rhythm at lower doses. At higher anesthetic doses, benzodiazepines cause generalized slowing (theta and delta activity) without producing a burst-suppression pattern. Because of their potent anticonvulsant properties, they are not used during electrocorticography.

DRUGS OF ABUSE

EEGs are frequently requested for patients who abuse alcohol. In certain patient populations, as many as 15% of EEG referrals are obtained for patients who have a history of chronic alcoholism (85). As with many of the medications already reviewed, alcohol may produce certain characteristic EEG changes, but none are pathognomonic of use or abuse. Patients with a history of alcohol abuse may have EEG abnormalities related to intoxication (both acute and chronic) or withdrawal. Alcohol abusers are prone to a variety of central nervous system diseases and systemic illnesses that may produce additional EEG changes, including focal and interictal epileptiform changes.

During acute alcohol intoxication, mild slowing of the alpha rhythm occurs. Quantitative EEG reveals spectral density shifts to lower frequency ranges (33). The effect of rising concentrations of alcohol is generalized reduction in frequency of EEG activity. With severe intoxication, marked generalized slowing may be present. EEG slowing during intoxication diminishes as tolerance develops (168). EEGs in alcohol abusers are normal or demonstrate only minor degrees of diffuse slowing (85). Patients with a history of chronic alcohol abuse have been reported to have higher incidence (56%) of low-voltage (defined as less than 25-μV) records. Caution is necessary during interpretation because low-voltage background EEG activity in isolation is not considered abnormal, being present in 14% of nonalcoholic adults (84).

Signs of alcohol withdrawal in chronic abusers usually begin within 24 hours after diminished consumption. Mild background EEG slowing may be associated with physiologic artifact (muscle, movement, and sweat) (134). Abstinence may result in alcohol-related seizures, the majority being generalized tonic-clonic, 8 to 72 hours after discontinuation of alcohol (161). Generalized epileptiform discharges during alcohol-related seizures have been described (168). Interictally, patients with seizures associated with withdrawal rarely (2% to 12%) have epileptiform discharges (85).

Withdrawal seizures typically precede delirium tremens, during which time background EEG activity is low voltage with a poorly developed dominant posterior rhythm (138). Most patients with delirium caused by a toxic metabolic encephalopathy have diffuse slowing of background rhythms with theta and delta activity. Thus, an EEG in a delirious patient, which shows generalized low-voltage activity with minimal slowing, should make the interpreter consider that the patient is in a withdrawal state (not limited to alcohol, inasmuch as barbiturate withdrawal may produce similar findings). Niedermyer et al. (109) described periodic lateralized epileptiform discharges (PLEDs) in the rare withdrawal syndrome termed *subacute alcoholic encephalopathy.*

An interesting EEG occurrence described in patients during alcohol withdrawal is photosensitivity, manifested by photomyogenic and photoconvulsive responses during stimulation. Early reports of these phenomena in unmedicated patients led to a hypothesis that they represented a hyperexcitable state of the neuromuscular system and possibly of the central nervous system. Later studies have refuted these findings (62,165), raising the issue that treatment of alcohol withdrawal with benzodiazepines and aggressive medical management of electrolyte abnormalities reduces photosensitivity (43).

Patients with a history of alcohol use are at risk for a variety of medical conditions that may produce abnormalities of the EEG. Focal EEG abnormalities and seizures may result from head injury. The Wernicke-Korsakoff syndrome is caused by thiamine deficiency in chronic alcoholism. It may precipitate an acute psychosis associated with moderate to severe diffuse slowing of EEG activity. In the chronic phase of this illness, EEG slowing is less prominent. Hepatic encephalopathy resulting from alcoholic cirrhosis produces an EEG typical of a metabolic encephalopathy, with generalized slowing and triphasic waves.

Central nervous system stimulants (amphetamines, cocaine, and methylphenidate) potentiate dopamine activity in the brain. These drugs increase faster activity in the beta and alpha ranges and reduce voltage and the amount of slower frequencies (3). Herning et al. (67) examined the effect of various doses of cocaine administered intravenously and orally. Using quantitative EEG techniques, they found an increase in the beta power at all doses and that it occurred earlier in subjects receiving intravenous cocaine. At toxic levels, cocaine produces a nonspecific pattern of generalized slowing with theta and delta activity (68). Quantitative EEG analysis of cocaine-dependent men abstaining from drug use suggests that beta activity may be a neurophysiological sign of withdrawal (66). Cocaine can provoke seizures in nonepileptic patients and can exacerbate seizures in patients with a history of seizures (115). Other cocaine-induced neurological conditions also include vascular insults, including subarachnoid and intracerebral hemorrhages, which can produce focal abnormalities on the EEG, alerting the clinician to other problems besides intoxication.

Information regarding the effects of cannabis on EEG activity is conflicting. Inhalation of both hashish and marijuana produces little or no effect on EEG activity according to visual analysis (25,125). However, the active component of cannabis, delta-9 tetrahydrocannabinol, produces an increase in alpha activity with a decrease in beta and theta frequencies (163). Lysergic acid diethylamide (LSD) and mescaline, both potent hallucinogenic agents, can produce nonspecific changes with reduction in EEG voltage and slower frequencies during the psychotic state (15,41). Phencyclidine, which was introduced as an intravenous veterinarian anesthetic, is structurally related to ketamine. Acute phencyclidine intoxication produces an unusual pattern of rhythmic, nonreactive theta activity interrupted by periodic bursts of delta activity that is highly suggestive of the diagnosis (38,151).

MISCELLANEOUS DRUGS AND TOXINS

It is not possible to review all EEG changes caused by exposure to drugs and toxins. This section summarizes some additional medications and inorganic compounds that can produce distinctive EEG patterns.

Baclofen is a GABA-B receptor agonist used in the treatment of spasticity. Despite its mechanism of action and proepileptic effect in animal models (104), therapeutic levels of this medication do not increase seizure frequency in epileptic patients (153). An encephalopathy associated with periodic sharp waves (similar to the EEG pattern with lithium toxicity) has been reported in a patient receiving low-dose therapy. However, Zak et al. (171) believed that this pattern was ictal, representing nonconvulsive status epilepticus. The encephalopathy and EEG pattern cleared after discontinuation of baclofen (69). Intrathecal baclofen administration by means of an implanted drug delivery system has been used to maximize therapy in the treatment of spinal and supraspinal spasticity. Kofler et al. (82) reported that of 39 of patients, without a prior history of convulsions, who underwent this treatment for "supraspinal" spasticity, four (10.3%) experienced epileptic seizures. All four patients had traumatic brain injuries, and seizure activity was associated with sudden alterations in baclofen levels.

Metrizamide, the first water-soluble contrast medium with mild subarachnoid neurotoxic effects, was used during myelography and cisternography. EEG changes associated with these procedures included slow activity and epileptogenic discharges in 16% to 35% of patients. In the prospective study of Ropper et al. (127), 34% of patients (21 of 62) developed EEG abnormalities, including paroxysmal slow-wave bursts, triphasic waves, spike discharges, and spike-wave discharges. Non-convulsive status epilepticus after metrizamide myelography has been described as either generalized (111,122, 164) or complex partial (34,131). This discrepancy in seizure type may reflect the difficulty in distinguishing these EEG patterns. Iohexol, a second-generation nonionic monomeric contrast media, greatly reduces the risk of neurotoxic side effects (including seizures and mental status changes), but it has been associated with acute encephalopathy, accompanied by diffuse slowing of the background EEG activity, in three patients (21).

Chemotherapeutic and immunosuppressive agents have been associated with slowing of background EEG activity. In pediatric patients, both methotrexate and ifosfamide have been associated with unusual EEG changes. Methotrexate can cause focal polymorphic delta activity, in addition to generalized slowing of background activity (83). Ifosfamide can lead to generalized slowing and high-voltage rhythmic delta activity (120). Ifosfamide can also produce a generalized periodic pattern with bisynchronous sharp complexes, possibly representing nonconvulsive status epilepticus (141,167). L-asparaginase can increase theta and delta activity (90). An encephalopathy related to infusion rate of hepsulfam in patients with hematological malignancies was accompanied by slowing of the alpha rhythm (91). Cyclosporine is associated with diffuse and focal slowing in addition to epileptiform discharges (130).

Antimicrobial agents may lower seizure threshold. An overdose of isoniazid can produce seizures. The interictal EEG shows bilateral sharp waves and generalized paroxysmal and diffuse slowing. Topical application of penicillin is used in experimental models of epilepsy. In humans, intrathecal administration and very high (40 to 80 million units per day) parenteral doses may produce ictal phenomena (3,52).

In animal models, atropine produces slowing of EEG activity, which suggesting a disturbance in cholinergic input to the cortex (137). Atropine is used in military medicine as an antidote after exposure to cholinesterase-inhibiting nerve agents. Quantitative EEG analyses show an increase in delta and theta power with a decrease alpha and beta activity in healthy male volunteers (117). Cholinergic deficits in patients with senile dementia of the Alzheimer type may play a role in memory impairment. In an age-matched normal control population, intravenous scopolamine produced statistically significant changes in quantitative EEG delta activity that was not present in patients with Alzheimer's disease (108).

Bromide salts were the first anticonvulsant agents and were widely used as sedatives. Dose-related toxicity has been related to chloride ion replacement. Advanced forms of bromide encephalopathy are associated with diffuse slowing of background EEG activity (160). Mercury neurotoxicity is most commonly associated with industrial exposure. The EEG changes may include generalized slowing and epileptiform discharges. The severity of the EEG abnormalities and the patient's clinical condition may be correlated with age (14). Lead toxicity may result from ingestion or inhalation of lead-containing compounds (such as paint) and can produce seizures. The EEG shows diffuse slowing in subacute and severe forms of lead poisoning. Diffuse and focal paroxysmal discharges may be present. In chronic lead encephalopathy, the EEG is low voltage with a poorly developed alpha rhythm (6,77).

CONCLUSION

Although the EEG is sensitive to the effects of drugs and toxins on the central nervous system, changes in background activity are not specific. AEDs may reduce ictal phenomena and affect background EEG activity, but most do not suppress interictal abnormalities. Medications used in the treatment of psychiatric disorders may reduce seizure threshold and produce interictal epileptiform activity. Anesthetics and analgesics produce dose-related effects. Drugs may induce EEG changes that include electrocerebral silence and status epilepticus. Drug toxicity should be considered in any comatose patient, especially if background EEG activity includes increased fast activity. As with any neurodiagnostic test, the EEG is a tool that is an adjunct to the clinical evaluation of the patient's history and physical examination.

REFERENCES

1. Adams DJ, Luders H, Pippenger CH. Sodium valproate in the treatment of intractable seizure disorders: a clinical and electroencephalographic study. *Neurology* 1978;28:152–157.
2. Barbaro G, Di Lorenzo G, Soldini M, et al. Flumazenil for hepatic encephalopathy grade III and IVa in patients with cirrhosis: an Italian multicenter double-blind, placebo-controlled, cross-over study. *Hepatology* 1998;28:374–378.
3. Bauer G, Bauer R. EEG, drug effects, and central nervous system poisoning. In: Niedermeyer E, Lopes da Silva FH, eds. *Electroencephalography: basic principles, clinical applications, and related fields,* 4th ed. Baltimore: Williams & Wilkins, 1999:671–691.
4. Bauer J. Seizure-inducing effects of antiepileptic drugs: a review. *Acta Neurol Scand* 1996;94: 367–377.
5. Bazil CW, Pedley TA. General principles. Neurophysiological effects of antiepileptic drugs. In: Levy RH, Mattson RH, Meldrum BS, Perucca E, eds. *Antiepileptic drugs,* 5th ed. New York: Lippincott Williams & Wilkins, 2002:23–35.
6. Benignus VA, Otto DA, Muller KE, et al. Effects of age and body lead burden on CNS functions in young children. II. EEG spectra. *Electroencephalogr Clin Neurophysiol* 1981;52: 240–248.
7. Ben-Menachem E, Treiman DM. Effects of gamma-vinyl GABA on interictal spikes and sharp waves in patients with intractable complex partial seizures. *Epilepsia* 1989;30:79–83.
8. Binnie CD. EEG and blood levels of antiepileptic drugs. *Electroencephalogr Clin Neurophysiol* 1982;36:504–512.
9. Binnie CD, van Emde Boas W, Kastelejn-Nolste-Trenite DG. Acute effects of lamotrigine (BW 430C) in persons with epilepsy. *Epilepsia* 1986;27:248–254.
10. Blatt I, Brenner RP. Triphasic waves in a psychiatric population: a retrospective study. *J Clin Neurophysiol* 1995;13:324–329.
11. Bond AJ, Lader MH. Comparative effects of diazepam and buspirone on subjective feelings, psychological tests and the EEG. *Int Pharmacopsychiat* 1981;16:212–20.
12. Brazier MAB. The effect of drugs on the electroencephalogram of man. *Clin Pharmacol Ther* 1964;5:102–116.
13. Breimer LTM, Hennis PJ, Burm AGL, et al. Pharmacokinetics and EEG effects of flumazenil in volunteers. *Clin Pharmacokinet* 1991;20:491–496.
14. Brenner RP, Snyder RD. Late EEG findings and clinical status after organic mercury poisoning. *Arch Neurol* 1980;37:282–284.
15. Browne BB. Subjective and EEG responses to LSD in visualizer and non-visualizer subjects. *Electroencephalogr Clin Neurophysiol* 1968;25:372–379.
16. Browne TR. Clonazepam—a review of a new anticonvulsant drug. *Arch Neurol* 1976;33: 326–332.
17. Browne TR, Penry JK. Benzodiazepines in the treatment of epilepsy. *Epilepsia* 1973;14: 277–310.
18. Buchtal F, Svensmark O, Simonsen H. Relation of EEG and seizures to phenobarbital in serum. *Arch Neurol* 1968;19:567–572.
19. Cadranel JF, el Younsi M, Pidoux B, et al. Flumazenil therapy for hepatic encephalopathy in cirrhotic patients: a double-blind pragmatic randomized, placebo study. *Eur J Gastroenterol Hepatol* 1995;7:325–329.
20. Callaghan N, Garrett A, Goggin T. Withdrawal of anticonvulsant drugs in patients free of seizures for two years. A prospective study. *N Engl J Med* 1988;318:942–946.
21. Ceylan S, Baykal S, Kuzeyli K, et al. A case of acute encephalopathy after iohexol lumbar myelography. *Clin Neurol Neurosurg* 1993;95:45–47.
22. Chang SS, Davis JM. Toxicity of psychotherapeutic agents (antipsychotics, tricyclic antidepressants, MAO inhibitors and disulfiram). In: Vinken PJ, Bruyn GW, eds. *Handbook of clinical neurology,* vol. 37. Amsterdam: North Holland, 1979:299–327.
23. Cunningham Owens DG. Adverse effects of antipsychotic agents. *Drugs* 1996;51:895–930.
24. Davidson K. EEG activation after intravenous amitriptyline. *Electroencephalogr Clin Neurophysiol* 1965;19:298–300.
25. Deliyannaki SE, Panagopoulos C, Huott AD. The influence of hashish on human EEG. *Clin Electroencephalogr* 1970;1:128–140.
26. Devinsky O, Honigfeld G, Patin J. Clozapine-related seizures. *Neurology* 1991;41:369–371.

27. Drummond JC, Iragui-Madoz VJ, Alksne JF, et al. Masking of epileptiform activity by propofol during seizure surgery. *Anesthesiology* 1992;76:652–654.
28. Duncan JS. Antiepileptic drugs and the electroencephalogram. *Epilepsia* 1987;28:259–266.
29. Duncan JS, Smith SJ, Forster A, et al. Effects of the removal of phenytoin, carbamazepine, and valproate on the electroencephalogram. *Epilepsia* 1989;30:590–596.
30. Ebrahim ZY, DeBoer GE, Luders H, et al. Effect of etomidate on the electroencephalogram of patients with epilepsy. *Anesth Analg* 1986;65:1004–1006.
31. Ebrahim ZY, Schubert A, Van Ness P, et al. The effect of propofol on the electroencephalogram of patients with epilepsy. *Anesth Analg* 1994;78:275–279.
32. Eckardt KM, Steinhoff BJ. Nonconvulsive status epilepticus in two patients receiving tiagabine treatment. *Epilepsia* 1998;39:671–674.
33. Ehlers CL, Wall TL, Schuckit MA. EEG spectral characteristics following ethanol administration in young men. *Electroencephalogr Clin Neurophysiol* 1989;73:179–187.
34. Elian M, Fenwick P. Metrizamide and the EEG: three case reports and a review. *J Neurol* 1985;232:341–345.
35. Engel J, Crandall PH. Falsely localizing ictal onsets with depth EEG telemetry during anticonvulsant withdrawal. *Epilepsia* 1983;24:344–345.
36. Erwin CW, Gerber CJ, Morrison SD, et al. Lithium carbonate and convulsive disorders. *Arch Gen Psychiat* 1973;28:646–648.
37. Essig CF, Fraser HF. Electroencephalographic changes in man during use and withdrawal of barbiturates in moderate dosage. *Electroencephalogr Clin Neurophysiol* 1958;10:649–656.
38. Fariello RG, Black JA. Pseudoperiodic bilateral EEG paroxysms in a case of phencyclidine intoxication. *J Clin Psychiat* 1978;39:579–581.
39. Finelli PF. Drug-induced Creutzfeldt-Jakob like syndrome. *J Psychiatr Neurosci* 1992;17:103–105.
40. Fink M. EEG classification of psychoactive compounds in man: a review and theory of behavioral associations. In: Effron DH, ed. *Psychopharmacology: a review of progress 1957–1967.* U.S. Public Health Service Publication No. 1836. Washington, DC: U.S. Government Printing Office, 1968:497–507.
41. Fink M. EEG and human psychopharmacology. *Annu Rev Pharmacol* 1969;9:241–258.
42. Fiol ME, Boening JA, Cruz-Rodriguez R, et al. Effect of isoflurane (Forane) on intraoperative electrocorticogram. *Epilepsia* 1993;34:897–900.
43. Fisch BJ, Hauser WA, Brust JCM, et al. The EEG response to diffuse and patterned photic stimulation during acute untreated alcohol withdrawal. *Neurology* 1989;39:434–436.
44. Flemming DC, Fitzpatrick J, Fariello RG, et al. Diagnostic activation of epileptogenic foci by enflurane. *Anesthesiology* 1980;52:431–433.
45. Foletti G, Volanschi D. Influence of lamotrigine addition on computerized background EEG parameters in severe epileptogenic encephalopathies. *Eur Neurol* 1994(Suppl 1):S87–S89.
46. Frazer A. Pharmacology of antidepressants. *J Clin Pharmacol* 1997;17(Suppl 1):S1–S18.
47. Freudenreich O, Weiner RD, McEvoy JP. Clozapine-induced electroencephalogram changes as a function of clozapine serum levels. *Biol Psychiatry* 1997;42:132–137.
48. Frost JD, Hrachovy RA, Glaze DG, et al. Alpha rhythm slowing during initiation of carbamazepine therapy: implications for future cognitive performance. *J Clin Neurophysiol* 1995;12:57–63.
49. Galimberti CA, Manni R, Parietti L, et al. Drug withdrawal in patients with epilepsy: prognostic value of the EEG. *Seizure* 1993;2:213–220.
50. Gardner CR, Tully RW, Hedgecock JR. The rapidly expanding range of neuronal benzodiazepine receptor ligands. *Progr Neurobiol* 1993;40:1–61.
51. Gershon S. Use of lithium salts in psychiatric disorders. *Dis Nerv Syst* 1968;29:51–55.
52. Glaze DA. Drug effects. In: Daly DD, Pedley TA, eds. *Current practice of clinical electroencephalography,* 2nd ed. New York: Raven Press, 1990.
53. Gotman J, Gloor P, Quesney LF, et al. Correlations between EEG changes induced by diazepam and the localization of epileptic spikes and seizures. *Electroencephalogr Clin Neurophysiol* 1982;54:614–621.
54. Gotman J, Marciani MG. Electroencephalographic spiking activity, drug levels and seizure occurrence in epileptic patients. *Ann Neurol* 1985;17:597–603.
55. Groeneweg M, Gyr K, Amrein R, et al. Effects of flumazenil on the electroencephalogram of patients with portosystemic encephalopathy. Results of a double blind, randomised, placebo-controlled multicentre trial. *Electroencephalogr Clin Neurophysiol* 1996;98:29–34.
56. Gunther W, Baghai T, Naber D, et al. EEG alterations and seizures during treatment with clozapine: a retrospective study of 283 patients. *Pharmacopsychiatry* 1993;26:69–74.
57. Hallet M, Chadwick D, Marsden CD. Cortical reflex myoclonus. *Neurology* 1979;29:1107–1125.
58. Hammond EJ, Wilder BJ. Effects of gamma-vinyl-GABA on the human electroencephalogram. *Neuropharmacology* 1985;24:975–984.
59. Harding GFA, Herrick CE, Jeavons PM. A controlled study of the effect of sodium valproate on photosensitive epilepsy and its prognosis. *Epilepsia* 1978;19:555–565.
60. Haring C, Neudorfer C, Schwitzer J, et al. EEG alterations in patients treated with clozapine in relation to plasma levels. *Psychopharmacology* 1994;114:97–100.
61. Hauser P, Devinsky O, DeBellis M, et al. Benzodiazepine withdrawal delirium with catatonic features. Occurrence in patients with partial seizure disorders. *Arch Neurol* 1989;46:696–699.
62. Hauser WA, Rich S, Nicolosi A, et al. Electroencephalographic findings in patients with ethanol withdrawal seizures. *Electroencephalogr Clin Neurophysiol* 1982;52:64.
63. Helmchen H, Kanowski S. EEG changes under lithium (Li) treatment. *Electroencephalogr Clin Neurophysiol* 1971;30:269.
64. Herkes GK, Lagerlund TD, Sharbrough FW, et al. Effects of antiepileptic drug treatment on the background frequency of EEGs in epileptic patients. *J Clin Neurophysiol* 1993;10:210–216.
65. Herkes GK, Wszolek ZK, Westmoreland BF, et al. Effects of midazolam on electroencephalograms of seriously ill patients. *Mayo Clin Proc* 1992;67:334–338.
66. Herning RI, Guo X, Better WE, et al. Neurophysiological signs of cocaine dependence: increased electroencephalogram beta during withdrawal. *Biol Psychiat* 1997;41:1087–1094.
67. Herning RI, Jones RT, Hooker WD, et al. Cocaine increases EEG beta: a replication and extension of Hans Berger's historic experiments. *Electroencephalogr Clin Neurophysiol* 1985;60:470–477.
68. Holmes GL, Korteling F. Drug effects on the human EEG. *Am J EEG Technol* 1993;33:1–26.
69. Hormes JT, Benarroch EE, Rodriguez M, et al. Periodic sharp waves in baclofen-induced encephalopathy. *Arch Neurol* 1988;45:814–815.
70. Hosain S, Nagarajan L, Fraser R, et al. Effects of nitrous oxide on electrocorticography during epilepsy surgery. *Electroencephalogr Clin Neurophysiol* 1997;102:340–342.
71. Huang ZC, Shen DL. The prognostic significance of diazepam-induced EEG changes in epilepsy: a follow-up study. *Clin Electroencephalogr* 1993;24:179–187.
72. Itil TM. Convulsive and anticonvulsive properties of neuro-psycho-pharmaca. In: Niedermeyer E, ed. *Epilepsy. Modern problems in pharmacopsychiatry,* vol. 4. New York: S. Karger AG, 1970:270–305.
73. Itil TM, Soldatos C. Epileptogenic effects of psychotropic drugs: practical recommendations. *JAMA* 1980;244:1460–1463.
74. Ito BM, Sato S, Kufta LV, et al. Effect of isoflurane and enflurane on the electrocorticogram of III and IVa in patients with cirrhosis: an Italian multicenter double-blind, placebo-controlled, cross-over study. *Hepatology* 1998;28:374–378.
75. Jongmans JWM. Report of the antiepileptic action of Tegretol. *Epilepsia* 1964;5:74–82.
76. Julius SC, Brenner RP. Myoclonic seizures with lithium. *Biol Psychiat* 1987;22:1184–1190.
77. Kalaidjiev D. Electroencephalographic changes in workers resulting from prolonged exposure to lead. [Abstract]. *Electroencephalogr Clin Neurophysiol* 1983;55:25P.
78. Kalviainen R, Aikia M, Mervaala E, et al. Long-term cognitive and EEG effects of tiagabine in drug-resistant partial epilepsy. *Epilepsy Res* 1996;25:291–297.

79. Kearse LA Jr, Koski G, Husain MV, et al. Epileptiform activity during opioid anesthesia. *Electroencephalogr Clin Neurophysiol* 1993;87:374–379.

80. Kellaway P, Frost JD, Hrachovy RA. Relationship between clinical state, ictal and interictal EEG discharges and serum drug levels. *Ann Neurol* 1978;4:197.

81. Kiloh LG, Davison K, Osselton JW. An electroencephalographic study of the analeptic effects of imipramine. *Electroencephalogr Clin Neurophysiol* 1961;13:216–223.

82. Kofler M, Kroenberg MF, Rifici C, et al. Epileptic seizures associated with intrathecal baclofen application. *Neurology* 1994;44:25–27.

83. Kovnar E, Ward J. EEG manifestations of metabolic, toxic, degenerative and infectious diseases. In: Holmes GL, Moshe SL, eds. *Pediatric clinical neurophysiology.* Norwalk, CT: Appleton & Lange, 1992.

84. Krauss GL, Fisher RS. Alcohol and the EEG. *Am J EEG Technol* 1992;32:118–126.

85. Krauss GL, Niedermeyer E. Electroencephalogram and seizures in chronic alcoholism. *Electroencephalogr Clin Neurophys* 1991;78:97–104.

86. Kupfer DJ, Perel JM, Pollock BG, et al. Fluvoxamine versus desipramine: comparative polysomnographic effects. *Biol Psychiat* 1991;29:23–40.

87. Kurtz D. Section VII. The EEG in acute and chronic drug intoxications. In: Glasser GH, ed. *Handbook of electroencephalography and clinical neurophysiology. Volume 15C—metabolic, endocrine and toxic diseases.* Amsterdam: Elsevier Scientific, 1976:15C-88–15C-104.

88. Lader M. Psychological effects of buspirone. *J Clin Psychiat* 1982;43:62–68.

89. Laguna JF, Korein J. Diagnostic value of diazepam in electroencephalography. *Arch Neurol* 1972;26:265–271.

90. Land VL, Sutow WW, Fernbach DJ, et al. Toxicity of L-asparaginase in children with advanced leukemia. *Cancer* 1972;30:339–347.

91. Larson RA, Geller RB, Janisch L, et al. Encephalopathy is the dose-limiting toxicity of intravenous hepsulfam: results of a phase I trial in patients with advanced hematological malignancies. *Cancer Chemother Pharmacol* 1995;36:204–210.

92. Logothetis J. Spontaneous epileptic seizures and electroencephalographic changes in the course of phenothiazine therapy. *Neurology* 1967;17:869–877.

93. Lombroso CT, Erba G. Primary and secondary bilateral synchrony in epilepsy. *Arch Neurol* 1970;22:321–334.

94. Ludwig BI, Ajmone Marsan C. EEG changes after withdrawal of medication in epileptic patients. *Electroencephalogr Clin Neurophysiol* 1975;39:173–181.

95. Mahla ME. Anesthetic effects on the electroencephalogram. *Neuro Sci Monitor* 1992;3:2–7.

96. Malow BA, Reese KB, Sato S, et al. Spectrum of EEG abnormalities during clozapine treatment. *Electroencephalogr Clin Neurophysiol* 1994;91:205–211.

97. Marciani MG, Gigle GL, Stefanini F, et al. Effect of carbamazepine on EEG background activity and on interictal epileptiform abnormalities in focal epilepsy. *Int J Neurosci* 1993;70:107–116.

98. Marciani MG, Maschio M, Spanedda F, et al. Development of myoclonus in patients with partial epilepsy during treatment with vigabatrin: an electroencephalographic study. *Acta Neurol Scand* 1995;91:1–5.

99. Marciani MG, Stantione P, Maschio M, et al. EEG changes induced by vigabatrin monotherapy in focal epilepsy. *Acta Neurol Scand* 1997;95:115–120.

100. Marossero F, Cabrini GP, Sironi VA, et al. Correlations of anticonvulsant plasma levels with depth EEG recordings in epileptic patients. *Electroencephalogr Clin Neurophysiol* 1977;43:527.

101. Mervaala E, Koivisto K, Hanninen T. Electrophysiological and neuropsychological profiles of lamotrigine in young and age-associated memory impairment (AAMI) subjects. *Neurology* 1995;46(Suppl 4):S259.

102. Mervaala E, Partanen J, Nousiainen U, et al. Electrophysiologic effects of gamma-vinyl GABA and carbamazepine. *Epilepsy* 1989;30:189–193.

103. Michelucci R, Tassinari CA. Response to vigabatrin in relation to seizure type. *Br J Clin Pharmacol* 1989;27:119–124.

104. Mott DD, Bragdon AC, Lewis DV, et al. Baclofen has a proepileptic effect in the rat dentate gyrus. *J Pharmacol Exp Ther* 1989;249:721–725.

105. Neigh JL, Garman JK, Harp JR. The electroencephalographic pattern during anesthesia with enflurane. *Anesthesiology* 1971;35:482–487.

106. Neufeld MY. Periodic triphasic waves in levodopa-induced encephalopathy. *Neurology* 1992;42:444–446.

107. Neufeld MY, Rabey JM, Orlov E, et al. Electroencephalographic findings with low-dose clozapine treatment in psychotic parkinsonian patients. *Clin Neuropharmacol* 1996;19:81–86.

108. Neufeld MY, Rabey JM, Parmet Y, et al. Effects of a single intravenous dose of scopolamine on the quantitative EEG in Alzheimer's disease patients and age-matched controls. *Electroencephalogr Clin Neurophysiol* 1994;91:407–412.

109. Niedermeyer E, Freund G, Krumholz A. Subacute encephalopathy with seizures in alcoholics: a clinical electroencephalographic study. *Clin Electroencephalogr* 1981;12:113–129.

110. Nowack WJ, King JA. Triphasic waves and spike wave stupor. *Clin Electroencephalogr* 1992;23:100–104.

111. Obeid T, Yaqub B, Panayiotopoulos C, et al. Absence status epilepticus with computed tomographic brain changes following metrizamide myelography. *Ann Neurol* 1988;24:582–584.

112. Olajide D, Lader M. A comparison of buspirone, diazepam, and placebo in patients with chronic anxiety states. *J Clin Psychopharmacol* 1987;7:148–152.

113. Oliver AP, Luchius DJ, Wyatt RJ. Neuroleptic-induced seizures. *Arch Gen Psychiat* 1982;39:206–209.

114. Pacia SV, Devinsky O. Clozapine-related seizures: experience with 5,629 patients. *Neurology* 1994;44:2247–2249.

115. Pascual-Leone A, Dhuna A, Altafullah I, et al. Cocaine-induced seizures. *Neurology* 1990;40:404–407.

116. Perucca E, Gram L, Avanzini G, et al. Antiepileptic drugs as a cause of worsening seizures. *Epilepsia* 1998;39:5–17.

117. Pickworth WB, Herning RI, Koeppl B, et al. Dose-dependent atropine-induced changes in spontaneous electroencephalogram in human volunteers. *Mil Med* 1990;155:166–170.

118. Pillay SS, Stoll AL, Weiss MK, et al. EEG abnormalities before clozapine therapy predict a good clinical response to clozapine. *Ann Clin Psychiat* 1996;8:1–5.

119. Potts KM. Seizures and encephalopathies following metrizamide myelography and cisternography. *Am J EEG Technol* 1990;30:45–57.

120. Pratt CB, Green AA, Horowitz ME, et al. Central nervous system toxicity following the treatment of pediatric patients with ifosfamide/mesna. *J Clin Oncol* 1986;4:1253–1261.

121. Prichard JW. Barbiturates: physiological effects I. In: Glaser GH, Perry JK, Woodbury DM, eds. *Antiepileptic drugs: mechanism of action.* New York: Raven Press, 1980:505–522.

122. Pritchard PB, O'Neal DB. Nonconvulsive status epilepticus following metrizamide myelography. *Ann Neurol* 1984;16:252–254.

123. Pryse-Phillips WEM, Jeavons PM. Effect of carbamazepine (Tegretol) on the electroencephalograph and ward behaviour of patients with chronic epilepsy. *Epilepsia* 1970;11:236–273.

124. Risby ED, Epstein CM, Jewart RD, et al. Clozapine-induced EEG abnormalities and clinical response to clozapine. *J Neuropsychiat Clin Neurosci* 1995;7:466–470.

125. Rodin EA, Domino EF. Effects of acute marijuana smoking on the EEG. *Electroencephalogr Clin Neurophysiol* 1970;29:321.

126. Rodin EA, Rim CD, Rennick PM. The effects of carbamazepine on patients with psychomotor epilepsy: results of a double-blind study. *Epilepsia* 1974;15:547–561.

127. Ropper AH, Chiappa KH, Young RR. The effect of metrizamide on the electroencephalogram: a prospective study in 61 patients. *Ann Neurol* 1979;6:222–226.

128. Roseman E. Dilantin toxicity: a clinical and electroencephalographic study. *Neurology* 1961; 11:912–921.

129. Rowan AJ, Binnie CD, Aarfield CA, et al. The delayed effect of sodium valproate on the photoconvulsive response in man. *Epilepsia* 1979;20:61–68.

130. Rubin AM, Kang H. Cerebral blindness and encephalopathy with cyclosporin A toxicity. *Neurology* 1987;37:1072–1076.

131. Russell D, Anke IM, Nyberg-Hansen R, et al. Complex partial status epilepticus following myelography with metrizamide. *Ann Neurol* 1980;8:325–327.

132. Sachdeo R, Chokroverty S. Increasing epileptiform activities in EEG in presence of decreasing clinical seizures after carbamazepine. [Abstract]. *Epilepsia* 1985;26:522.

133. Sachdeo R, Chokroverty S. Enhancement of absence with Tegretol. *Epilepsia* 1985;26:534.

134. Sainio K, Leins T, Huttunen MO, et al. Electroencephalographic changes during experimental hangover. *Electroencephalogr Clin Neurophysiol* 1976;40:535–538.

135. Sajatovic M, Meltzer HY. Clozapine-induced myoclonus and generalized seizures. *Biol Psychiat* 1996;39:367–370.

136. Sato S, White BG, Penry JK, et al. Valproic acid versus ethosuximide in the treatment of absence seizures. *Neurology* 1982;32:157–163.

137. Schaul N, Gloor P, Ball G, et al. The electromicrophysiology of delta waves induced by systemic atropine. *Brain Res* 1978;143:475–486.

138. Schear HE. The EEG pattern in delirium tremens. *Clin Electroencephalogr* 1985;16:30–32.

139. Sharbrough FA. Cerebral function monitoring. In: Daube JR, ed. *Clinical neurophysiology.* Philadelphia: FA Davis, 1996:443–450.

140. Shinnar S, Vining EPG, Mellits ED, et al. Discontinuing antiepileptic medications in children with epilepsy after two years without seizures: a prospective study. *N Engl J Med* 1985;313: 976–980.

141. Simonian NA, Gilliam FG, Chiappa KH. Ifosfamide causes a diazepam-sensitive encephalopathy. *Neurology* 1993;43:2700–2702.

142. Skowron DM, Stimmel GL. Antidepressants and the risk of seizures. *Pharmacotherapy* 1992;12:18–22.

143. Sloan TB. Anesthetic effects on electrophysiologic recordings. *J Clin Neurophysiol* 1998;15: 217–226.

144. Small JG. EEG and lithium CNS toxicity. *Am J EEG Technol* 1986;26:225–239.

145. Smith SJM, Kocen RS. A Creutzfeldt-Jakob like syndrome due to lithium toxicity. *J Neurol Neurosurg Psychiat* 1988;51:120–123.

146. So N, Gotman J. Changes in seizure activity following anticonvulsant drug withdrawal. *Neurology* 1990;40:407–413.

147. Spatz R, Kugler J. Abnormal EEG activities induced by psychotropic drugs. *Electroencephalogr Clin Neurophysiol* 1982;36:549–558.

148. Spencer SS, Spencer DD, Williamson PD, et al. Ictal effects of anticonvulsant medication withdrawal in epileptic patients. *Epilepsia* 1981;22:297–307.

149. Staner L, Kerkhofs M, Detroux D, et al. Acute, subchronic and withdrawal sleep EEG changes during treatment with paroxetine and amitriptyline: a double-blind randomized trial in major depression. *Sleep* 1995;18:470–477.

150. Stecker MM, Kramer TH, Raps EC, et al. Treatment of refractory status epilepticus with propofol: clinical and pharmacokinetic findings. *Epilepsia* 1998;39:18–26.

151. Stockard JJ, Werner SS, Aalbers JA, et al. Electroencephalographic findings in phencyclidine intoxication. *Arch Neurol* 1976;33:200–203.

152. Talwar D, Abora MS, Sher PK. EEG changes and seizure exacerbation in young children treated with carbamazepine. *Epilepsia* 1994;35:1154–1159.

153. Terrence CF, Fromm GH, Roussan MS. Baclofen. Its effect on seizure frequency. *Arch Neurol* 1983;40:28–29.

154. Thase ME. Depression, sleep, and antidepressants. *J Clin Psychiat* 1998;59:55–65.

155. Thomas P, Beaumanoir A, Genton P, et al. *"De novo"* absence status of late onset: report of 11 cases. *Neurology* 1992;42:104–110.

156. Towler ML. The clinical use of diazepam in anxiety states and depressions. *J Neuropsychiat* 1962;3:68–72.

157. Treves IA, Neufeld MY. EEG abnormalities in clozapine-treated schizophrenic patients. *Eur Neuropsychopharmacol* 1996;6:93–94.

158. Van der Rijt CC, Schalm SW, Meulstee J, et al. Flumazenil therapy for hepatic encephalopathy. A double-blind cross over study. *Gastroenterol Clin Biol* 1995;19:572–580.

159. Van Sweden B. Neuroleptic neurotoxicity, electro-clinical aspects. *Acta Neurol Scand* 1984;69:137–146.

160. Van Sweden B, Niedermeyer E. Toxic encephalopathies. In: Niedermeyer E, Lopes da Silva FH, eds. *Electroencephalography: basic principles, clinical applications, and related fields,* 4th ed. Baltimore: Williams & Wilkins, 1999:692–701.

161. Victor M, Brausch C. The role of alcohol in the production of seizures. In: Niedermeyer E, ed. *Epilepsy: recent views on theory, diagnosis, and therapy of epilepsy.* New York: S. Karger AG, 1970:185–199.

162. Villarreal HJ, Wilder BJ, Wilmore LJ, et al. Effects of valproic acid on spike and wave discharges in patients with absence seizures. *Neurology* 1978;28:886–891.

163. Volavka J, Zaks A, Roubicek J, et al. Acute EEG effects of heroin and naloxone. *Electroencephalogr Clin Neurophysiol* 1971;30:165.

164. Vollmer ME, Weiss H, Beanland C, et al. Prolonged confusion to absence status following metrizamide myelography. *Arch Neurol* 1985;42:1005–1008.

165. Vossler DG, Browne TR. Absence of EEG photoparoxysmal responses in alcohol withdrawal seizure patients treated with benzodiazepines. [Abstract]. *Neurology* 1988;38:404.

166. Wang B, Bai Q, Jiao X, et al. Effect of sedative and hypnotic doses of propofol on the EEG activity of patients with or without a history of seizure disorders. *J Neurosurg Anesthesiol* 1997;9:335–340.

167. Wengs WJ, Talwar D, Bernard J. Ifosfamide-induced nonconvulsive status epilepticus. *Arch Neurol* 1993;50:1104–1105.

168. Wikler A, Pescor FT, Fraser HF, et al. Electroencephalographic changes associated with chronic alcohol intoxication and the alcohol abstinence syndrome. *Am J Psychiat* 1956;113: 106–114.

169. Wilkus RJ, Dodrill CB, Troupin AS. Carbamazepine and the electroencephalogram of epileptics: a double-blind study in comparison to phenytoin. *Epilepsia* 1978;19:283–291.

170. Wilson WH, Claussen AM. Seizures associated with clozapine treatment in a state hospital. *J Clin Psychiat* 1994;55:184–188.

171. Zak R, Solomon G, Petito F, et al. Baclofen-induced generalized nonconvulsive status epilepticus. *Ann Neurol* 1994;36:113–114.

Chapter 16

Progressive Pediatric Neurological Syndromes

Douglas R. Nordli, Jr., Linda D. Leary, and Darryl C. De Vivo

Electroencephalography (EEG) is one of the most readily available and well-studied tools for measuring cerebral cortical activity. It is a highly reliable measure of physiological activity, capable of detecting even minor degrees of diffuse cortical dysfunction. It may be useful in the evaluation of the patient with a suspected encephalopathy to confirm the presence of diffuse cerebral dysfunction, suggest a specific etiology, or both. In contrast to the findings in patients with static encephalopathies, for which the EEG is often a sensitive but etiologically nonspecific indicator of dysfunction, the findings in patients with progressive encephalopathies may be very informative. There are more than 11,000 well-recognized and well-characterized inherited disorders in humans, many of which can affect the central nervous system function either directly or indirectly. Published information on the EEG findings in the majority of these disorders is scant, and the EEG results are unlikely to contribute significantly to the clinical decision making. In a subset of nearly 200 disorders, there are associated seizures and epilepsy. The EEG findings in these conditions, whose pathophysiological processes must have some impact on cortical grey function, have been studied in greater detail; in some, very specific EEG findings have been noted. This chapter consequently focuses on the progressive disorders that are associated with seizures or that are characterized by distinctive EEG findings. In addition to progressive encephalopathies, brief mention is made of disorders that manifest with static encephalopathies and prominent seizures, particularly disorders that manifest in childhood or early adolescence.

It is a challenge to organize this wealth of material. In practice, the authors have found it clinically useful to separate diseases by the typical age at manifestation. Accordingly, the conditions are categorized into those commonly manifesting in the neonatal period, those appearing in early and late infancy, and those appearing during childhood. The age of the patient is one piece of clinical information that should always be available to electroencephalographers. This approach has value, but also limitations. Diseases manifest in a biological spectrum, often as a continuum across several age brackets and seldom exclusively at any given age. Diseases categorized within a certain age group may certainly manifest outside that age group. With this caveat in mind, the clinician has at least a starting point for consideration of a differential diagnosis, which may be refined by specific EEG, clinical, or laboratory features.

For each condition, there is a brief description of the clinical manifestation, a concise review of the most recent genetic information available at the time of this writing, and a description of the relevant neuropathological processes. These data will assist the electroencephalographer to be aware of the appropriate clinical context and to integrate EEG and clinical findings. After a discussion of the various entities, we consider an approach to obtaining an EEG in a child with a suspected progressive disorder.

METABOLIC DISORDERS IN THE NEWBORN

In a number of metabolic disorders manifesting in the first month of life, seizures may be a clinical feature. Although the following section cannot be a comprehensive list of all the disorders that should be considered in this age group, it contains those in which seizures are a prominent feature.

Nonketotic Hyperglycinemia

In this inborn error of amino acid metabolism, large amounts of glycine accumulate in the body fluids because of a defect in the multienzyme complex for glycine cleavage. The enzyme system is confined to the mitochondria and is composed of four protein components. A gene localized to 9p24-p23 encodes one component: glycine decarboxylase. The pathophysiological processes have not been fully elucidated, but the elevated glycine level is believed to affect the central nervous system through its roles as an inhibitory transmitter in the brainstem and spinal cord and as an excitatory transmitter in the cortex (62). Cortical malformations or corpus callosum defects may be present. The majority of cases manifest within the first 48 hours after birth, with lethargy, respiratory difficulties, and seizures that are often myoclonic or characterized as infantile spasms. EEG findings may reveal a characteristic burst-suppression pattern or hypsarrhythmia (18). This disorder has been identified as one of the most important metabolic derangements responsible for Ohtahara's syndrome, in which patients present with tonic spasms and a burst-suppression pattern. Similar clinical and electrographic patterns can also be seen with early myoclonic epilepsy, as described by Jean Aicardi. This can lead to diagnostic uncertainty in the differentiation of these two early infantile epilepsy syndromes (48). As patients with these disorders mature, infantile spasms may persist, and the EEG often reveals hypsarrhythmia.

Of note, a transient form of nonketotic hyperglycinemia exists with similar early clinical and biochemical findings. In this condition, however, glycine concentrations normalize between 2 and 8 weeks after birth, and the prognosis is favorable.

Pyridoxine Dependency

In this condition, refractory seizures typically develop within the first several days after birth; they are characterized by infantile spasms or a variety of partial, myoclonic, and atonic seizures. The disorder results from a defect on the binding site of glutamic acid decarboxylase (GAD). Pyridoxine is a key cofactor for this enzyme, and the insufficient γ-aminobutyric acid formation seen in this disorder can be corrected by high doses of pyri-

doxine. Two different genes code for GAD in mammalian brains: GAD1 (gene locus, 2q31) and GAD2 (gene locus, 10p11.23) (10,11).

The EEG is characterized by generalized bursts of high-voltage delta with intermixed spike-and-sharp waves and periods of asynchronous attenuation (Fig. 16.1*A*). Treatment with high doses (100 to 200 mg intravenously) of pyridoxine can result in cession of seizures, conversion of the EEG to a burst-suppression pattern, and later normalization of the EEG with subsequent doses (128) (see Fig. 16.1*B*). The onset of this disease may occur after

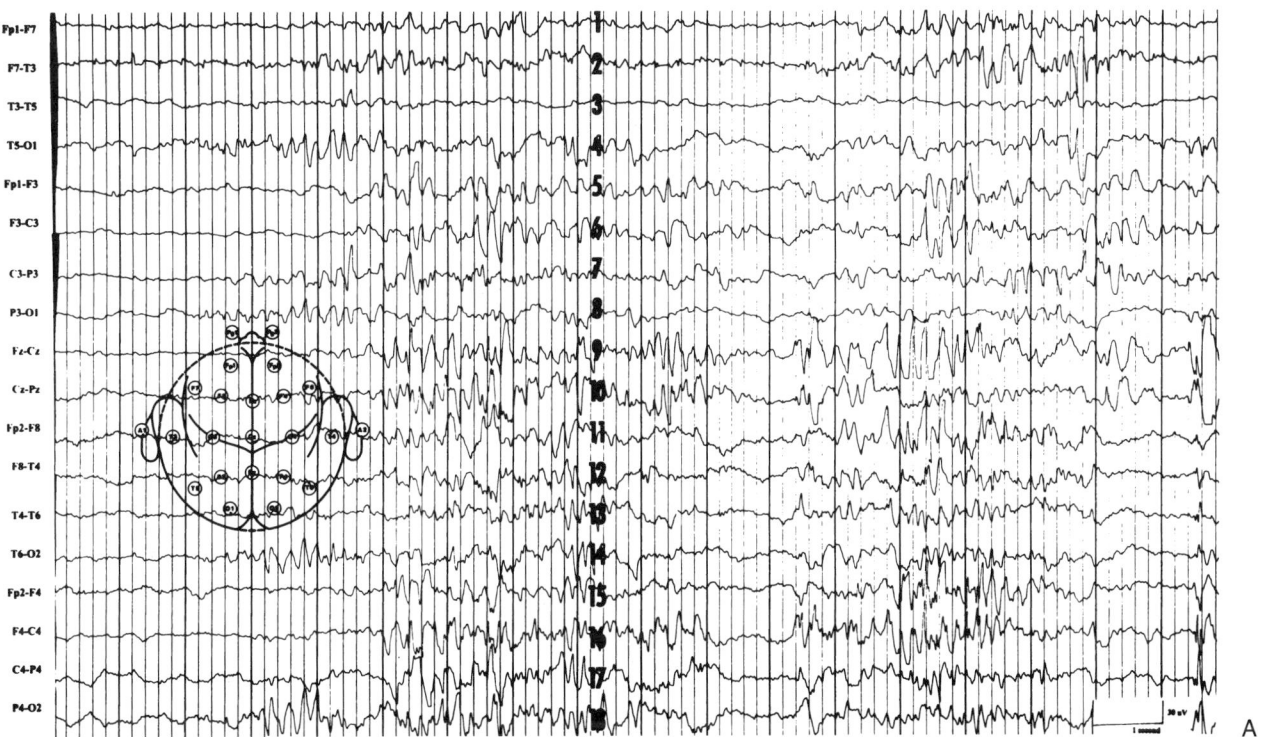

FIG. 16.1. Pyridoxine dependency. **A:** EEG of a 4-week-old child with intractable neonatal seizures. There are bursts of high voltage delta with intermixed spikes and sharp waves and asynchronous epochs of attenuation. *(Figure continues.)*

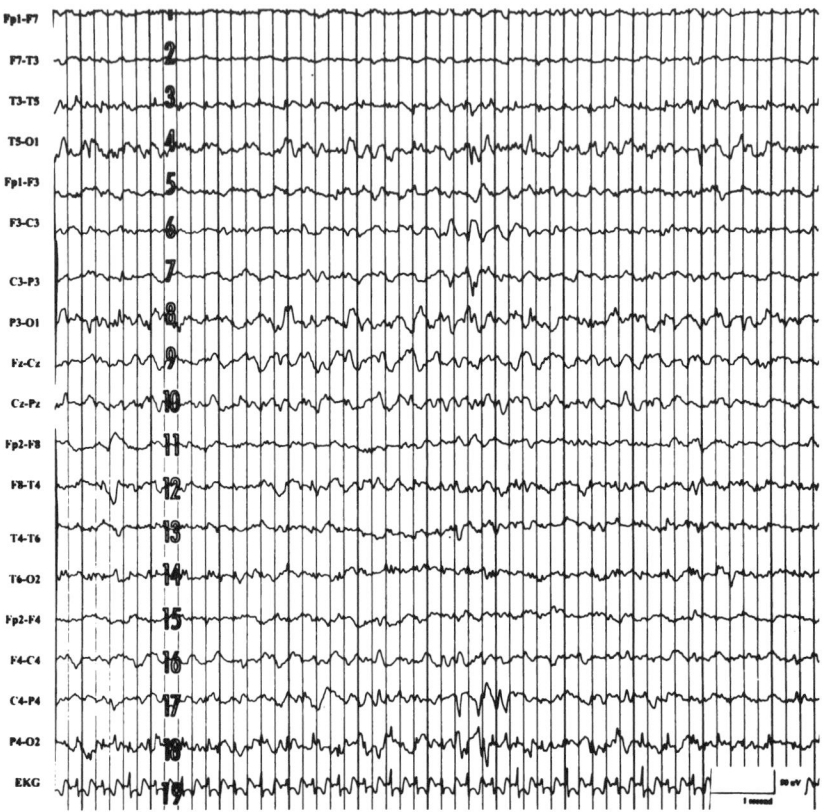

FIG. 16.1. *Continued.* **B:** EEG of the same child after pyridoxine treatment. The tracing is now continuous, and only occasional epileptiform discharges persist. (Courtesy of C. Stack, M.D., and L. Laux, M.D., Children's Memorial Hospital, Chicago, Illinois.)

the newborn period, which makes this disorder a consideration in older infants with refractory seizures as well (14,38).

Molybdenum Cofactor Deficiency and Sulfite Oxidase Deficiency

These rare conditions manifest shortly after birth. Affected neonates develop a progressive encephalopathy, feeding difficulties, hypotonia, and refractory partial, myoclonic, or apparently generalized seizures. Dysmorphic features, lens dislocation, and hepatomegaly are characteristic (46). Neu-roimaging may show poor differentiation between the gray and white matter, severe cerebral and cerebellar atrophy, and multiple cystic cavities in the white matter. The relatively more common molybdenum cofactor deficiency results from an absence of the hepatic cofactor, which leads to a combined enzyme deficiency of the three molybdenum-dependent enzymes: sulfite oxidase, xanthine dehydrogenase, and aldehyde oxidase (99). This may be caused by mutations in the gene (MOCS1; gene locus, 6p21.3) that encodes the two enzymes for synthesis of a precursor. Mutations in molybdopterin synthase (MOCS2; gene locus, 5q11), which converts the precursor into the organic moiety, are responsible for the other form of the disorder (88).

Multifocal paroxysms and a burst-suppression pattern on the EEG have been described (56).

Peroxisomal Disorders

Disorders of the peroxisome have been divided into three categories: disorders of peroxisomal biogenesis (Zellweger's syndrome, neonatal adrenoleukodystrophy [NALD], infantile Refsum's disease], disorders of a single peroxisomal enzyme (X-linked adrenoleukodystrophy, acyl–coenzyme A [CoA] oxidase deficiency AOXD]), and disorders with deficiencies of multiple peroxisomal enzymes (rhizomelic chondrodysplasia punctata. This discussion will be limited to Zellweger's syndrome, AOXD, and NALD.

Zellweger's Syndrome

Zellweger syndrome is the most frequent peroxisomal disorder in early infancy; its incidence is estimated to be 1 in 50,000 to 1 in 100,000. The phenotype in Zellweger's syndrome is caused by mutations in any of several genes involved in peroxisome biogenesis, including peroxin-5 (chromosome 12), peroxin-2 (chromosome 8), peroxin-6 (chromosome 6), and peroxin-12. In addition to these, a locus for Zellweger's syndrome on 7q11 is suspected on the basis of chromosomal aberrations. Mutations in the PEX1 gene, which maps to 7q21-q22, were identified in cases of Zellweger's syndrome, complementation group 1 (70).

Dysmorphic features may be noted shortly after birth. Within the first week, the affected child develops a severe encephalopathy, hypotonia, and hyporeflexia. Eighty percent of patients experience partial, generalized tonic-clonic (rare), and myoclonic seizures and atypical flexor spasms. Multisystem abnormalities of the brain, kidneys, liver, skeletal system, and eyes may be present. Eye abnormalities include cataracts, glaucoma, corneal clouding, optic nerve hypoplasia, pigmentary retinal degeneration, and Brushfield spots. The presence of the latter, along with hypotonia and a mongoloid appearance, may cause the clinician to confuse Zellweger's syndrome with Down's syndrome. Findings on neuroimaging and pathological examination are distinctive, with pachygyria or polymicrogyria localized to the opercular region and with cerebellar heterotopias.

Patients with Zellweger's syndrome have partial motor seizures originating in the arms or legs or corners of the mouth. Their seizures do not culminate in generalized seizures and are easily controlled by antiepileptic drugs (AEDs). Interictal EEGs of the patients with Zellweger's syndrome showed infrequent bilateral independent multifocal spikes, predominantly in the frontal motor cortex and its surrounding regions (113). Less frequently, hypsarrhythmia is observed.

Neonatal Adrenoleukodystrophy

NALD, an autosomal recessive disorder with pathological and biochemical findings resembling those of X-linked adrenoleukodystrophy, bears some similarity to Zellweger's syndrome. Distinguishing features include absent or minimal facial dysmorphisms, later onset of seizures, absent or minimal cerebral malformations, and longer life span. There is evidence that this disorder may be caused by a number of different gene defects, including a mutation in the C-terminal peroxisomal targeting signal (PTS1) receptor gene, PXR1 (25). Frequent, often intractable seizures that may be tonic, clonic, myoclonic, or epileptic spasms occur (122). No characteristic EEG pattern has been defined, but descriptions have included high-voltage slowing, polymorphic delta activity, multifocal paroxysmal discharges, burst-suppression, and hypsarrhythmia.

Acyl-Coenzyme A Oxidase Deficiency

AOXD was initially described in two siblings by Poll-The et al. (86). Clinical features include hypotonia, pigmentary retinopathy, hearing loss, developmental delay, adrenocortical insufficiency, absence of dysmorphic features, and onset of seizures shortly after birth. A deficiency in acyl-CoA oxidase, resulting from a deletion in its coding gene, was identified. Serum levels of very long chain fatty acids are elevated, with normal levels of pipecolic acid. Cortical malformations are generally absent, and the interictal EEG may show continuous, diffuse, high-voltage theta activity.

Urea Cycle Disorders

There are six enzymes in the urea cycle that convert ammonia to urea; five of these may have defects that cause neonatal seizures. The associated diseases and their incidences are as follows: carbamoylphosphate synthetase deficiency, 1 in 800,000; ornithine transcarbamylase deficiency, 1 in 80,000; argininosuccinate synthetase deficiency, 1 in 250,000; argininosuccinate lyase deficiency, 1 in 70,000; and N-acetylglutamate synthetase deficiency, with only a few cases reported. The clinical disorder resulting from a deficiency in the sixth enzyme, arginase, manifests later in infancy. All of these disorders are autosomal recessive except for ornithine transcarbamylase deficiency, which is X-linked dominant.

The clinical manifestations are similar and result, at least in part, from ammonia elevations. Typically, affected newborns exhibit poor feeding, emesis, hyperventilation, lethargy, or convulsions 1 to 5 days after birth. These signs give way to deepening coma with decorticate and decerebrate posturing and progressive loss of brainstem function. Brain imaging and pathological studies reveal cerebral edema with pronounced astrocytic swelling. Ammonium is taken up by the astrocytes and rapidly converted to glutamine in an energy-dependent process. The edema is associated with glutamine accumulation and energy depletion. In experimental models, blocking glutamine synthesis has prevented cerebral edema associated with hyperammonemia (131).

The EEG shows a low-voltage pattern with diffuse slowing and multifocal epileptiform discharges (33) (Fig. 16.2*A*). Two patients studied by Verma et al. in 1984 (121) demonstrated episodes of sustained monorhythmic theta activity (see Fig. 16.2*B*). In acute neonatal citrullinemia, a burst-suppression pattern has been described (74).

Maple Syrup Urine Disease

This disease, resulting from a defect in the branched chain α-keto acid dehydrogenase complex, was first reported by Menkes et al. in 1954 (67). The enzyme defect leads to accumulation of the branched-chain amino acids—valine, leucine, isoleucine—and their keto acids in the body tissues and fluids. The gene locus is 19q13.1-13.2 (29). Pathological studies have revealed diffuse myelin loss and increased total brain lipid content. Cystic degeneration of the white matter associated with gliosis is seen. Disordered neuronal migration may occur with heterotopias and disrupted cortical lamination.

Feeding difficulties and lethargy are observed during the first to second weeks after birth. If left untreated, symptoms may progress to stupor, apnea,

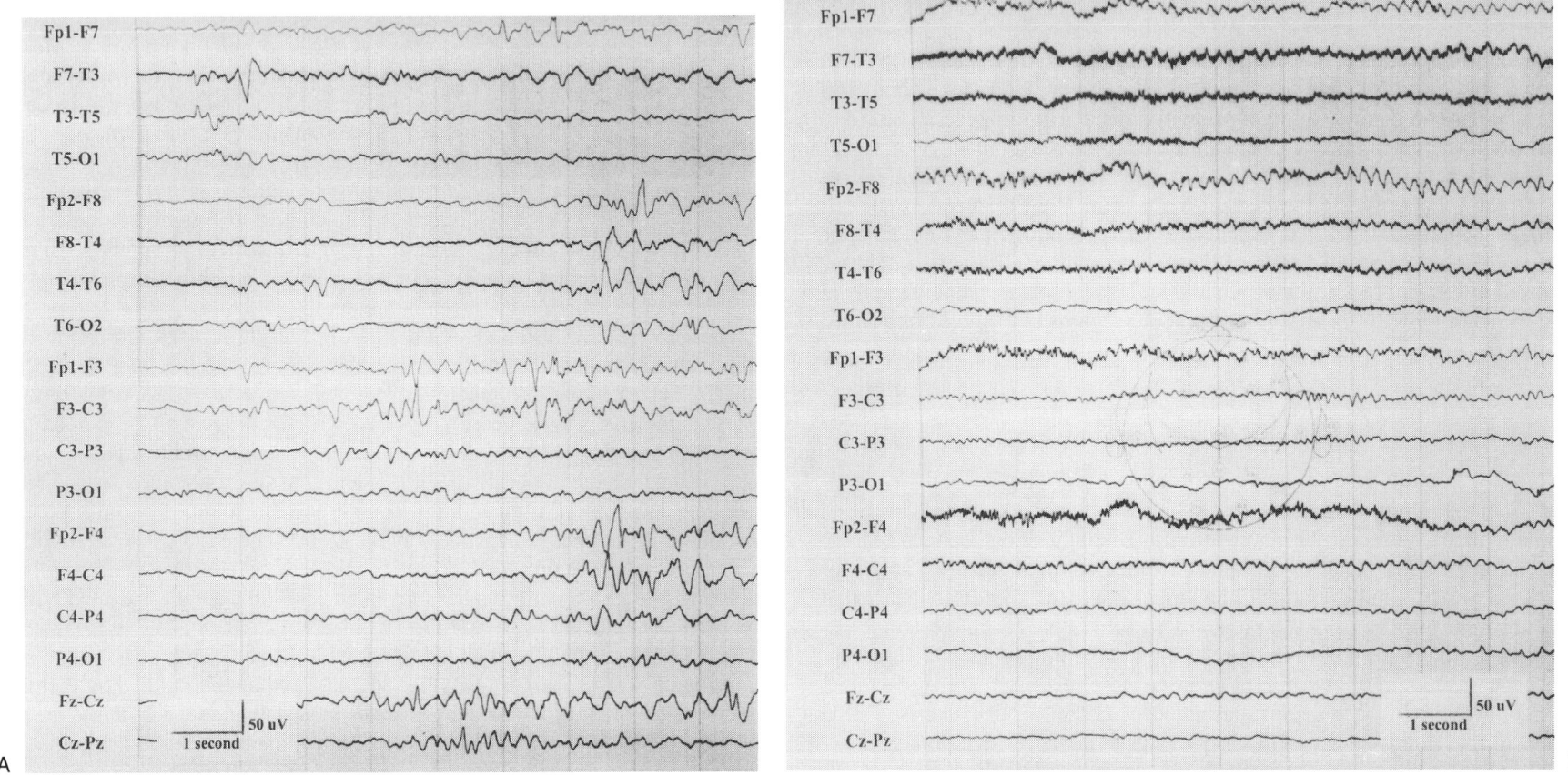

FIG. 16.2. EEGs of a 2-week-old child with ornithine transcarbamylase deficiency. **A:** There is marked attenuation and disorganization of the background with multifocal spikes. **B:** Sustained monorhythmic theta activity is present in the frontal regions. (Courtesy of C. Stack, M.D., and L. Laux, M.D., Children's Memorial Hospital, Chicago, Illinois.)

opisthotonus, myoclonic jerks, and partial and generalized seizures. A characteristic odor can be detected in urine and cerumen, but this may not be detectable until several weeks after birth.

The EEG shows diffuse slowing and a loss of reactivity to auditory stimuli. The comb-like rhythm characteristic of this disease was initially described by Trottier et al. in 1975 when bursts of a central mu-like rhythm were observed in four affected patients (116). Tharp also described this pattern in an infant who developed bursts of primarily monophasic negative 5- to 7-Hz activity in the central and parasagittal regions, which resolved with dietary therapy (115).

Organic Acidurias

The disorders of organic acid metabolism comprise a large number of inborn errors, including isovaleric aciduria and several ketotic hyperglycinemic syndromes (propionic acidemia, methylmalonic acidemia and β-ketothiolase deficiency).

Symptoms of isovaleric aciduria (gene locus, 15q14-q15), which develop during the neonatal period in half of affected children (54), include poor feeding, vomiting, dehydration, and a progressive encephalopathy manifested by lethargy, tremors, seizures, and coma. Platelet and leukocyte counts may be depressed, and the odor of the urine has been described as similar to that of sweaty feet (100). Cerebral edema is present, and seizures are most often partial motor or generalized tonic. The EEG shows dysmature features during sleep.

The symptoms of propionic acidemia also appear during the neonatal period, and in 20% of affected newborns, seizures are the first symptom. Characteristic features include vomiting, lethargy, ketosis, neutropenia, periodic thrombocytopenia, hypogammaglobulinemia, developmental retardation, and intolerance to protein. Patients may have very puffy cheeks and an exaggerated Cupid's bow–shaped upper lip. The gene locus is 13q32 (49). Convulsions are the rule, although more limited partial seizures have also been reported. The EEG shows background disorganization with marked frontotemporal and occipital slow wave activity (109). In 40% of affected children, myoclonic seizures develop in later infancy, and older children may have atypical absence seizures.

Methylmalonic acidemia is the metabolic signature of seven biochemically distinct entities, all of which show decreased activity of methylmalonyl-CoA mutase. Stomatitis, glossitis, developmental delay, failure to thrive, and seizures are the major features. Lesions of the globus pallidus, visible on computed tomography or magnetic resonance images, are characteristic. Diffuse tonic seizures and partial seizures with secondary generalization are the most frequent seizure types. Seizures may also be characterized by eyelid clonus with simultaneous upward deviation of the eyes. In a review of 22 affected patients, Stigsby et al. described abnormalities in seven. These consist of multifocal spike discharges and depressed background activity in two, excessive generalized slowing in two, and mild background slowing with lack of sleep spindles in three (29,109).

Pyruvate Dehydrogenase Deficiency, Pyruvate Carboxylase Deficiency, and Leigh's Syndrome

The pyruvate dehydrogenase complex is composed of multiple copies of three enzymes: pyruvate decarboxylase (E_1), dihydrolipoyl transacetylase (E_2), and dihydrolipoyl dehydrogenase (E_3). The core of the complex is formed by sixty E_2 subunits, and the other enzymes are attached to the surface. The E_1 enzyme is itself a complex structure, a heterotetramer of two α and two β subunits. The E_1-α subunit is particularly important inasmuch as it contains the E_1 active site; its gene locus is Xp22.2-p22.1.

There are various clinical manifestations of pyruvate dehydrogenase deficiency, ranging from acute lactic acidosis in infancy with severe neurological impairment to a slowly progressive neurodegenerative disorder (9). It is one of the most common defined genetic defects of mitochondrial energy metabolism. Structural abnormalities, such as agenesis of the corpus callosum, can be visible on neuroimaging. Seizures frequently occur and may take the form of infantile spasms and myoclonic seizures (80). Electrographic findings include multifocal slow spike-and-wave discharges.

Pyruvate carboxylase deficiency has two predominant clinical forms. The neonatal type manifests with severe lactic acidemia and death in the first few months of life. The juvenile type begins in the first 6 months of life with episodes of lactic acidemia precipitated by an infection. Seizures are related to the hypoglycemia that occurs secondary to dysfunction of the Kreb's cycle. Developmental delay, failure to thrive, hypotonia, and seizures, including infantile spasms with hypsarrhythmia, may be seen. In milder forms, diffuse 1.5- to 3-Hz slowing has been observed (29,109).

Leigh's syndrome (subacute necrotizing encephalomyelopathy) may be related to various metabolic defects, including cytochrome c oxidase deficiency, and defects in other enzymes involved in energy metabolism. Mutations in the mitochondrial deoxyribonucleic acid (DNA)–encoded ATP6 subunit of adenosine triphosphate (ATP) synthase (complex V) and any of the three catalytic subunits (E_1, E_2, or E_3) of the pyruvate dehydrogenase complex may result in the same phenotype described by Leigh in 1951 (23,60). The syndrome may also be caused by isolated deficiency of mitochondrial complex I (reduced nicotinamide adenine dinucleotide (NADH):ubiquinone oxidoreductase) and complex II. In addition, rare causes of Leigh's syndrome include myoclonus epilepsy with ragged red fibers (MERRF), mitochondrial encephalomyopathy with lactic acidosis and stroke-like symptoms (MELAS), and mitochondrial DNA depletion (22). Within the first year of life, classic features include failure to thrive, lactic acidosis, and developmental delay. As the disease progresses, infants develop spasticity, abnormalities of eye movements, and central respiratory failure. Various seizures, including focal and generalized seizures, have been described (24). Cases of infantile spasms and hypsarrhythmia are reported with Leigh's syndrome (47,117). In addition, there have been several cases of epilepsia partialis continua (27). EEG abnormalities, although present, do not appear to be distinctive enough to contribute to the clinical diagnosis of Leigh's syndrome (119).

Disorders of Biotin Metabolism

Early-Onset Multiple Carboxylase Deficiency (Holocarboxylase Synthetase Deficiency)

This rare disorder manifests in the first week after birth with lethargy, respiratory abnormalities, irritability, poor feeding, and emesis. A rash is present in more than 50% of patients. Generalized tonic convulsions, partial motor seizures, and multifocal myoclonic jerks develop in 25% to 50% of cases. A deficiency in the enzyme holocarboxylase synthetase leads to a decrease in holocarboxylase (110). Because this enzyme links biotin to four carboxylases in the mitochondrial and one in the cytosol, an inactivity of all carboxylases results. Electrographically, either multifocal spikes or a burst-suppression pattern is seen.

METABOLIC DISORDERS OF EARLY INFANCY

Lysosomal Disorders

Tay-Sachs Disease

GM_2 gangliosidosis is a lysosomal disorder that invariably includes seizures as a prominent feature. The infantile form of GM_2 gangliosidosis includes Tay-Sachs disease, caused by deficiency of hexosaminidase A, and Sandhoff's disease, caused by deficiency of hexosaminidases A and B.

Tay-Sachs disease, an autosomal recessive disorder localized to chromosome 15 (15q23-q24) (75), is found in the Ashkenazi Jewish population of Eastern or Central European descent. The enzymatic defect leads to intraneuronal accumulation of GM_2 ganglioside. Development is normal until the age of 4 to 6 months, when hypotonia and a loss of motor skills occur. Within the next 1 to 2 years, spasticity, blindness, and macrocephaly develop. The classic cherry-red spot is present in the ocular fundi of more than 90% of patients. At this stage, seizures become prominent with frequent partial motor, complex partial, and atypical absence seizures that respond poorly to medications. Myoclonic jerks are frequent and are often triggered by the exaggerated startle response to noise. The EEG is normal early in the course of the disease. Gradually, background activity slows with bursts of high-voltage delta waves and very fast central spikes (15). Diffuse spike-and-sharp-wave activity can be abundant, and acoustically induced myoclonic seizures appear. As the disease progresses, EEG voltage declines, and background activity becomes undifferentiated.

Krabbe's Disease (Globoid Cell Leukodystrophy)

Another lysosomal disorder occurring at this age is globoid-cell leukodystrophy (Krabbe's disease). This disorder, linked to chromosome 14q31, is caused by a deficient activity of galactosylceramidase. There are four forms of galactosylceramidase: infantile, with onset before the age of 6 months; late infantile, with onset between the ages of 6 months and 3 years; juvenile, with onset between the ages of 3 and 7 years; and adult, with onset after the age of 7 years (132). The majority of cases begin within 3 to 6 months of life with irritability, poor feeding, emesis, and rigidity. Muscular spasms induced by stimulation are prominent. Blindness and optic atrophy ensue. Initially, tendon reflexes are increased; then they gradual diminish as breakdown of peripheral myelin occurs. Partial or generalized clonic or tonic seizures and infantile spasms are seen; they may be difficult to distinguish from muscular spasms (6,40). In contrast to what is observed in many classic white-matter diseases, seizures occur early in the course of 50% to 75% of infants with Krabbe's disease. EEG characteristics include a hypsarrhythmia-like pattern with irregular slow activity and multifocal discharges of lower amplitude than that typically seen with West's syndrome (51). In a study of seven infants by Kliemann et al. in 1969, six children had prominent beta activity independently occurring in the posterior temporal regions and vertex that was superimposed over slower, high amplitude waves. This activity was observed to be state dependent and to occur in long runs without any observed clinical manifestations (51). In the terminal stages of the disease, little electrical activity is detected.

GM₁ Gangliosidosis, Type I and Type II

The infantile form of this disorder, type I, has been localized to chromosome 3 (3p21.33). A deficiency of β-galactosidase leads to the accumulation of GM₁ ganglioside and degradation products in nerve cells and other tissues. Regression of development begins at 3 to 6 months of age with rapid neurological deterioration. Seizures develop by the age of 2 years. Clinical features may include coarse facial features, hepatomegaly, bone deformities (dysostosis multiplex), visual abnormalities, hypotonia, progressive microcephaly, and hematological abnormalities. Examination of the ocular fundi reveals a macular cherry-red spot.

Neurological deterioration in the juvenile form (GM₁ gangliosidosis, type II) is generally slower than in type I. Cerebral manifestations with regression of developmental milestones and visual symptoms typically manifest by the ages of 2 to 4 years. EEG features of both forms include background slowing with increasing, irregular slow activity as the disease progresses (42). In type II, a fluctuating 4- to 5-Hz temporal rhythmic discharge has been observed.

Disorders of Vitamin Metabolism

Biotinidase Deficiency

Disorders of vitamin metabolism with symptoms that appear in early infancy include biotinidase deficiency and disorders of folic acid. As described previously, biotinidase deficiency produces multiple carboxylase deficiency. Seizures occur in 50% to 75% of patients and are the presenting clinical symptoms in one-third of cases. Generalized clonic or tonic-clonic convulsions, infantile spasms, and myoclonic seizures are seen. EEG findings may include a burst-suppression pattern, absence of physiological sleep patterns, poorly organized and slow waking background activity, and frequent spike and spike-and-slow-wave discharges.

Methylene Tetrahydrofolate Reductase Deficiency

Methylene tetrahydrofolate reductase deficiency (gene locus, 1p36.3) (39) is the most common inborn error of folate metabolism. The metabolic defect results from insufficient production of 5-methyltetrahydrofolate, which is needed for the remethylation of homocysteine to methionine, because of a deficiency of methylenetetrahydrofolate reductase. In affected patients, a progressive neurological syndrome develops in infancy. Children with this disorder have acquired microcephaly and seizures, characterized by intractable infantile spasms, generalized atonic and myoclonic seizures, and partial motor features. EEG findings vary from diffuse slowing of background activity to continuous spike-and-wave complexes or multifocal spikes.

Defects in methionine biosynthesis are also associated with seizures. Convulsions are frequent and are predominantly generalized, although myoclonic seizures with hypsarrhythmia have been reported.

Late-Onset Multiple Carboxylase Deficiency (Biotinidase Deficiency)

Seizures are a prominent feature of late-onset multiple carboxylase deficiency, occurring in approximately 75% of affected children. The gene locus is 3p25 (16). Onset of the disease process begins at the age of 3 to 6 months with hypotonia and psychomotor delay. Seborrheic or atopic dermatitis and alopecia are common. As the disease progresses, intermittent ataxia, optic atrophy, and sensorineural hearing loss develop. Seizure types, including generalized tonic-clonic, partial, myoclonic, or infantile spasms, are the presenting symptom in 38% of patients. The EEG may be normal, contain epileptiform discharges, or show diffuse slowing (92).

Glucose Transporter 1 Deficiency Syndrome

The glucose transporter 1 (GLUT-1) deficiency syndrome, previously referred to as the glucose transporter protein deficiency syndrome, was first described in 1991 (20). Affected infants become encephalopathic with seizures and delays of motor and mental development (19). Seizures typically begin after the second month of life and are initially characterized by subtle behavioral alterations consistent with infantile partial seizures. GLUT-1 mutations have been described in several patients (96). The initial EEG may be normal or may show interictal epileptiform discharges in the posterior quadrants. As the child matures, more generalized seizures occur, manifested by nonconvulsive events, myoclonic jerks, or atypical absence seizures. Some patients exhibit 3-Hz spike-and-wave discharges indistinguishable from those seen in childhood absence epilepsy (pyknolepsy). Bursts of generalized spike-and-wave discharges are seen in one-third of older children.

Organic Acidurias

Seizures in early infancy may be the presenting symptom of branched-chain organic acidurias. These include isovaleric aciduria, 3-methylcrotonyl CoA carboxylase deficiency, 3-methylglutaconic aciduria with normal 3-methylglutaconyl-CoA hydratase, and 3-hydroxy-3-methylglutaric aciduria. Seizures, including convulsions and infantile spasms, tend to be prominent in 3-methylcrotonyl CoA carboxylase deficiency.

Severe developmental delay, progressive encephalopathy, and seizures are the most common features of 3-methylglutaconic aciduria with normal 3-methylglutaconyl-CoA hydratase (35). Seizures occur in one-third of cases, and infantile spasms have been reported early on. In another study, eight patients with this disorder were studied, and the most typical finding was mild to moderate slowing of the EEG background. One patient had multifocal sharp-wave discharges as well (109).

Seizures are the presenting symptom in 10% of patients with 3-hydroxy-3-methylglutaric aciduria, a disorder caused by a deficiency of the lyase enzyme that mediates the final step of leucine degradation and plays a pivotal role in hepatic ketone body production. This disorder is one of an increasing list of inborn errors of metabolism that clinically present as Reye's syndrome or nonketotic hypoglycemia. The odor of the urine may resemble that of a cat. The chromosome location for this disorder is 1pter-p33 (129). In many affected patients, EEGs are normal between crises. EEGs in one girl with progressive encephalopathy showed multifocal spikes and intermittent episodes of background attenuation between crises, and focal epileptiform activity during an episode of clinical deterioration (109).

Infantile spasms have been reported in patients with 3-hydroxybutyric aciduria. Facial dysmorphism and brain dysgenesis are prominent manifestations. The enzyme deficiency causing this condition is unknown.

Type I glutaric acidemia is a more common autosomal recessive disorder of lysine metabolism that is caused by a deficiency of glutaryl-CoA dehydrogenase (gene locus, 19p13.2). Seizures are often the first clinical signs of metabolic decompensation after a febrile illness. EEGs are initially normal, but slight background slowing may develop during times of seizure exacerbation (109).

Aminoacidurias

Phenylketonuria and Hyperphenylalaninemias

One of the most frequent inborn errors of metabolism, occurring in 1 in 10,000 to 15,000 live births, phenylketonuria is caused by a deficiency of hepatic phenylalanine hydroxylase (gene locus, 21q24.1) (78). As a consequence of the metabolic defect, toxic levels of the essential amino acid phenylalanine accumulate. If these toxic levels are left untreated, severe mental retardation, behavioral disturbances, psychosis, and acquired microcephaly can result. Seizures are present in 25% of affected children. The majority of children with phenylketonuria (80% to 95%) are found to have abnormalities on EEG. An age-related distribution of EEG findings and seizure types has been observed. Low et al. (61) described characteristic features in 1957. Infantile spasms and hypsarrhythmia predominate in the young affected infant. As the children mature, tonic-clonic and myoclonic seizures become more frequent, and the EEG pattern evolves to mild diffuse background slowing, focal sharp waves, and irregular generalized spike-and-slow waves (84,111). An increase in delta activity has been seen as levels increased during phenylalanine loading (26).

Tyrosinemia, Type III

An inborn error of tyrosine metabolism, type III tyrosinemia (4-hydroxyphenylpyruvate dioxygenase deficiency), has been reported in a newborn with intractable seizures and in children who later developed infantile spasms (98). The EEG pattern has been described as low voltage with spike and polyspike discharges in the parietal-occipital regions.

Menkes' Disease (Kinky Hair Disease)

This X-linked (gene locus, Xq12-q13) disorder of copper absorption was first described by Menkes et al. in 1962 (66). A feature of this disorder is the "kinky hair" of the head and eyebrows. A characteristic twisting of the hair shaft is noted on microscopic examination of these poorly pigmented hairs. Affected boys may be premature, may have neonatal hyperbilirubinemia, or may have hypothermia. Progressive neurological deterioration with spasticity manifests by the age of 3 months, and affected children may have associated bone and urinary tract abnormalities as well. The disease has a rapidly fatal course.

Godwin-Austen et al. (37) described a disorder clinically reminiscent of Wilson's disease but without Kayser-Fleischer rings. Symptoms began at the age of 12 years, and defective copper absorption from the distal intestine, with high copper levels in rectal mucosa, was demonstrated. There is also phenotypic overlap between Menkes' disease and occipital horn syndrome. The topic has been thoroughly reviewed (118).

Seizures, in the form of intractable generalized or focal convulsions, are a prominent feature in Menkes' disease. Stimulation-induced myoclonic jerks are also present. Multifocal spike-and-slow-wave activity can be seen on EEG, sometimes resembling hypsarrhythmia (112).

Progressive Encephalopathy with Edema, Hypsarrhythmia, and Optic Atrophy (PEHO Syndrome)

PEHO syndrome, described by R. Salonen and colleagues in 1991, is characterized by infantile spasms, arrest of psychomotor development, hypotonia, hypsarrhythmia, edema, and visual failure with optic atrophy (105). Characteristic features include epicanthal folds, midfacial hypoplasia, protruding ears, gingival hypertrophy, micrognathia, and tapering fingers. Edema develops over the limbs and face. The progressive decline seen with this disease is suggestive of a metabolic defect, although no biochemical marker has been identified. It is presumed to be an autosomal recessive disorder by its pattern of inheritance. Neuroimaging shows progressive brain atrophy and abnormal myelination. Hypoplasia of the corpus callosum has been reported. Seizures generally begin as infantile spasms with associated hypsarrhythmia on the EEG. Later, other seizure types may be seen, including tonic, tonic-clonic, and absence seizures. The EEG pattern may evolve to a slow spike-and-wave pattern.

METABOLIC DISORDERS OF LATE INFANCY

Metachromatic Leukodystrophy

Metachromatic leukodystrophy is the result of a deficiency of arylsulfatase A (gene locus, 22q13.31-qter) (94). Hypotonia, weakness, and unsteady gait suggestive of a neuropathy or myopathy are the most common presenting symptoms. These are followed by a progressive decline in mental and motor skills. It has become apparent that in some genetic situations, there may be remarkable phenotypic heterogeneity (2). Partial seizures develop late in the clinical course in 25% of patients with the late-infantile form of metachromatic leukodystrophy and in 50% to 60% of patients with the juvenile-onset form (1,32). EEG findings include diffuse high-voltage slowing, which may be asymmetrical, and occasional bursts of spikes.

Schindler's Disease

Schindler's disease results from a deficiency of (α-N-acetylgalactosaminidase (gene locus, 22q11) (50,94,127). Affected patients appear normal at birth, but progressive neurological decline becomes evident in the second year. Manifestations include spasticity, cerebellar signs, and extrapyramidal dysfunction. Generalized tonic-clonic seizures and myoclonic jerks are common. EEG abnormalities include multifocal spikes and spike-and-wave complexes. In older children, Schindler's disease can have the clinical and pathological findings of neuroatonal dystrophy (p. 496).

Mucopolysaccharidoses

The mucopolysaccharidoses are a family of lysosomal storage disorders caused by the deficiency of several enzymes involved in the degradation of glycosaminoglycans. The various mucopolysaccharidoses share many clinical features, including a progressive course, multisystem involvement, organ enlargement, dysostosis multiplex, and abnormal facial features. The most common mucopolysaccharidosis is Sanfilippo's syndrome (mucopolysaccharidosis, type III), in which only heparitin sulfate is excreted in the urine; four different subtypes have been described, each associated with a different enzymatic defect (64). The gene locus is 17q25.3 (95). Generalized seizures develop in about 40% of patients with Sanfilippo's syndrome, but these are often easily controlled by antiepileptic drugs. Progressive dementia and severe behavioral disorders are other features. In a careful study of one patient, the EEG showed lack of normal sleep staging, absence of vertex waves and sleep spindles, and an unusual alteration of low-amplitude fast activity (12 to 15 Hz) with generalized slowing (55).

Neuronal Ceroid Lipofuscinoses

The neuronal ceroid lipofuscinoses (NCLs) are a group of diseases that result in storage of lipopigments in the brain and other tissues. At least five clinical subtypes and rare, atypical forms have been reported, and most are transmitted as autosomal recessive traits.

The infantile form of NCL (type I) is predominantly found in Finland, where the incidence is 1 per 20,000. The majority of affected patients are homozygous for a missense mutation at 1p32 (69). This disorder typically manifests at the age of 12 to 18 months with developmental regression, myoclonus, ataxia, and visual failure. Other features include incoordination of limb movements, acquired microcephaly, and optic atrophy. Seizures, in the forms of myoclonic jerks and astatic, atonic, or generalized seizures, are prominent. EEG features, which include an early, progressive loss of electrocortical activity and attenuation of the background (93), aid in the diagnosis.

Type II NCL shares many clinical features with the infantile form. In contrast to type I NCL, no ethnic predilection for type II NCL exists. The gene responsible for most cases has been mapped to the locus 11p15 (103). Early development is normal or may be mildly delayed. By the age of 2 to 4 years, insomnia, an early clinical sign, and intractable seizures develop. Multiple seizure types develop with staring spells and generalized tonic-clonic, myoclonic, and atonic components. As the disease progresses, irregular myoclonic jerks evoked by proprioceptive stimuli, voluntary movement, or emotional fluctuations become prominent. Cognitive decline, ataxia, and visual failure with optic atrophy and abnormal electroretinographic findings are all common (43). A characteristic EEG pattern of occipital spikes on low-frequency photic stimulation is observed (81). Giant visual evoked responses and somatosensory evoked potentials are also seen.

Alpers' Syndrome (Progressive Infantile Poliodystrophy)

This syndrome of unknown cause probably represents a number of familial disorders that are manifested by a rapidly progressive encephalopathy with intractable seizures and diffuse neuronal degeneration. In the Alpers-Huttenlocher subgroup, liver involvement is present and an autosomal recessive pattern of transmission is suggested. A diagnosis of Alpers' syndrome should be made only in the absence of known metabolic disease or an antecedent event. Along with clinical features suggestive of Alpers' syndrome, neuroimaging should exclude other diagnostic possibilities and should show progressive brain atrophy on successive studies with relative sparing of the white matter. Seizure types include myoclonic, focal, and generalized tonic-clonic convulsions. Brick et al. (8) described continuous anterior high-voltage 1- to 3-per-second spike-and-wave–like activity that persisted despite intermittent focal seizures (Fig. 16.3A). Brick et al. also noted progressive slowing of background activity as the disease progressed. Epilepsia partialis continua and convulsive status epilepticus have been observed in these patients (126). Diffuse slowing with admixed polyspikes has also been described in this disease (see Fig. 16.3B) (7).

Carbohydrate-Deficient Glycoprotein Syndrome

Carbohydrate-deficient glycoprotein syndrome (CDGS) is a multisystemic disease that is characterized by a carbohydrate defect in glycoproteins. Orlean (79) reviewed the congenital disorders of glycosylation caused by defects in the addition of mannose during oligosaccharide assembly. CDGS can be divided into two types, depending on whether they impair lipid-

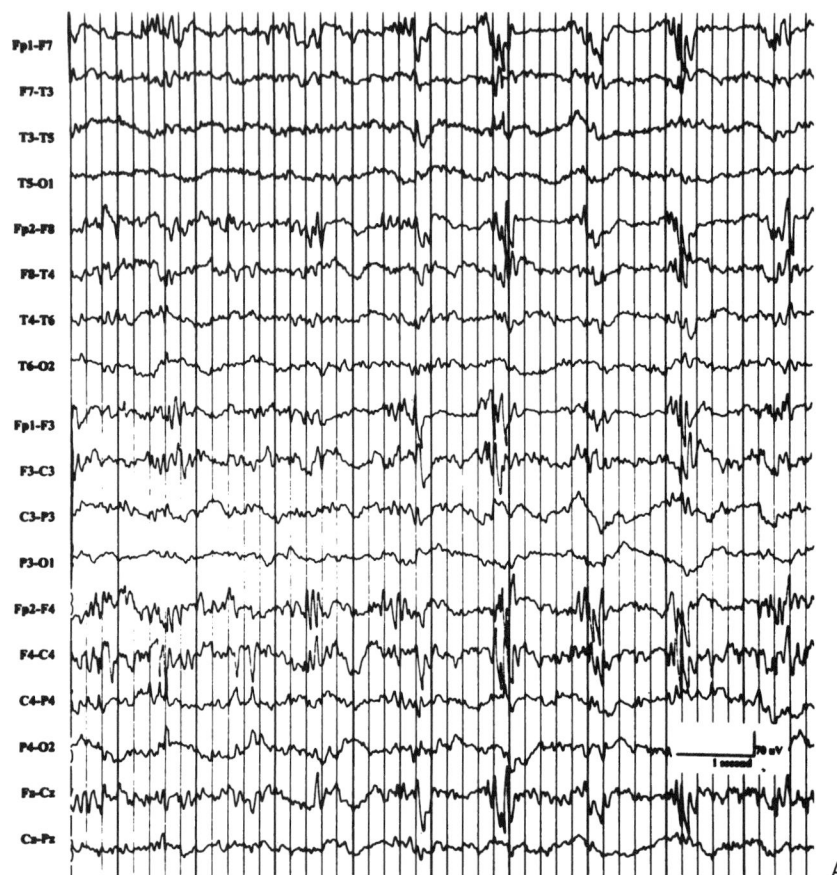

FIG. 16.3. Alpers' syndrome. **A:** EEG of a 10-year-old boy with Alpers' syndrome. Nearly periodic bursts of frontally dominant epileptiform discharges are recorded. (*Figure continues.*)

linked oligosaccharide assembly and transfer (CDGS I) or alter trimming of the protein-bound oligosaccharide or the addition of sugars to it (CDGS II). Participants at the First International Workshop on CDGS in Leuven, Belgium, in November 1999 proposed new nomenclature for CDGS (79). Type Ia CDGS, phosphomannomutase-2 deficiency, is the best characterized and most common of these syndromes (gene locus, 16p13.3-p13.2) (45,65). During infancy, internal organ symptoms are the predominant feature and

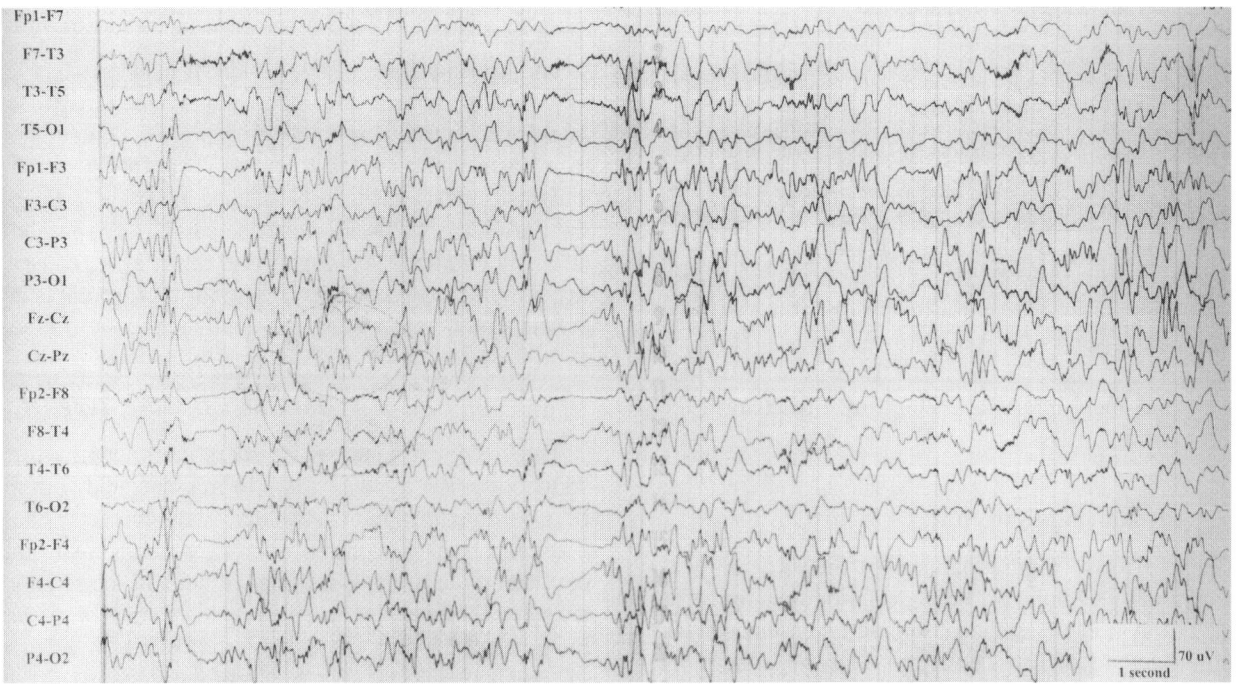

FIG. 16.3. *Continued.* **B:** EEG of a 3-year-old girl with Alpers' syndrome. Bursts of high-voltage slowing with intermixed epileptiform activity punctuated by brief epochs of attenuation were seen. (Courtesy of C. Stack, M.D., and L. Laux, M.D., Children's Memorial Hospital, Chicago, Illinois.)

may be life-threatening. In later childhood, mental deficiency, ataxia, progressive neuropathy involving the legs, retinal degeneration, and skeletal deformities are most common. Subcutaneous tissue changes with an odd distribution of fat, retracted nipples, and odd facies, including almond-shaped eyes, have been described. Imaging studies reveal cerebellar hypoplasia (83). There is a unique pattern of coagulation changes associated with the syndrome, including depression of factor XI, antithrombin III, protein C, and, to a lesser extent, protein S and heparin cofactor II. These changes may account for the stroke-like episodes observed in affected children (120). Clinical neurophysiological studies have demonstrated interictal epileptiform discharges and giant somatosensory evoked potentials (114).

Each of the other subtypes has been found in several patients (41). Type III CDGS was first described by Stibler et al. in 1993 (108). Two patients had severe visual, motor, and mental problems and developed infantile spasms with hypsarrhythmia. Interestingly, these patients had patchy skin changes, similar to those of incontinentia pigmenti (108). The absence of polyneuropathy, pigmentary retinopathy, and cerebellar hypoplasia were thought to differentiate this disorder from the previously described CDGSs. Neuroimaging showed dysmyelination and brain atrophy. A defect in glycosylation of transferrin was identified in both patients. A third child was reported in 1999 by Stibler et al. (107) with similar clinical and biochemical features. EEG findings in this child also showed hypsarrhythmia.

METABOLIC DISORDERS OF CHILDHOOD AND ADOLESCENCE

Homocystinuria

Disorders of transsulfuration include cystathionine β-synthase deficiency, the most frequent cause of homocystinuria. The gene locus is 21q22.3 (72). Some patients respond to pyridoxine administration. Mental retardation, behavioral disturbances, and seizures are manifestations of nervous system involvement; ectopia lentis, osteoporosis, and scoliosis are other common clinical findings (34,71). Generalized seizures occur in about 20% of patients with pyridoxine-nonresponsive homocystinuria and in 16% of patients with the pyridoxine-responsive form. EEG features are relatively nonspecific, with slowing and focal interictal epileptiform discharges that may be ameliorated with treatment (21).

Adrenoleukodystrophy

Symptoms of the X-linked form of adrenoleukodystrophy (gene locus, Xq28) classically appear in early childhood. Parietal motor seizures, often with secondary generalization and generalized tonic-clonic seizures, are common in the peroxisomal disorder. Status epilepticus has been the initial presenting symptom, and epilepsia partialis continua has also been reported. The EEG is characteristic, with high-voltage polymorphic delta activity and loss of faster frequencies over the posterior regions (63).

Lysosomal Disorders

Sialidosis, Type I: Cherry-Red Spot–Myoclonus Syndrome

This autosomal recessive disorder, which appears in late childhood to adolescence, is characterized by progressive visual loss, polymyoclonus, and seizures. The myoclonus can be debilitating and is provoked by voluntary movement, sensory stimulation, or excitement. Reports of increased myoclonus with cigarette smoking and menstruation have been noted. As the disease progresses, cognitive decline, cerebellar ataxia, and blindness with optic atrophy occur. Dysmorphic features, bone abnormalities, and hepatosplenomegaly are absent in contrast to type II and mucopolysaccharidosis. Neuroimaging shows diffuse cerebral and cerebellar atrophy. The EEG contains rhythmical spiking over the vertex with a positive polarity overlying a low-voltage background (28).

Sialidosis, Type II/Galactosialidosis

The juvenile form of this group of disorders has features similar to those of type I sialidosis. Distinguishing characteristics are the less prominent myoclonic activity and the presence of coarse facies, corneal clouding, dysostosis multiplex, and hearing loss. Inheritance is autosomal recessive, and this form has a higher incidence in Japan. In the majority of cases, a partial deficiency of β-galactosidase can be seen in addition to neuraminidase deficiency (galactosialidosis), and this may be caused by a defect in protective protein; the gene locus coding for this protein is 20q13.1 (130). The EEG contains moderate-voltage, generalized four- to six-spike/second paroxysms.

Gaucher's Disease, Type III

Three types of Gaucher's disease are known: type I, a chronic form with adulthood onset; type II, a rare form associated with infantile death; and type III, a chronic form with neurological involvement. These disorders result from a deficiency of glucocerebrosidase, which leads to the accumulation of glucosylceramide in the lysosomes of cells in the reticuloendothelial system. In the type III form, hepatosplenomegaly may be present from birth or early infancy, which may cause it to be confused with the more common type I form of Gaucher's disease. When neurological symptoms develop in childhood to early adulthood, it can be clearly distinguished from type I because cerebral features are absent. Frequent myoclonic jerks and tonic-clonic seizures ultimately develop. A supranuclear palsy of horizontal gaze is present in the majority of cases and is an important diagnostic sign. Generalized rigidity, progressive cognitive decline, and facial grimacing may be present. Paroxysmal EEG abnormalities may be seen before the onset of convulsions with worsening as the disease progresses, and diffuse polyspikes and spike-wave discharges are present. The most characteristic EEG findings are rhythmical trains of spikes or sharp waves at a rate of six to ten per second (77).

Neuroaxonal Dystrophies

Neuroaxonal dystrophies include infantile and juvenile forms of neuroaxonal dystrophy, Hallervorden-Spatz syndrome, and one type of Schindler's disease.

Infantile neuroaxonal dystrophy is an autosomal recessive disorder affecting both the central and peripheral nervous systems. It was first described by Seitelberger in 1952 (97). Characteristic pathological features of axonal spheroids within the peripheral and central nervous system are seen. Clinical manifestations begin between the ages of 1 and 2 years with psychomotor regression, hypotonia, and development of a progressive sensorimotor neuropathy. Seizures occur in one-third of patients with this disease, onset after the age of 3 years. The electrographic finding of high-voltage fast activity (16 to 24 Hz) that is unaltered by eye opening or closure is characteristic of all children with this disorder, regardless of the occurrence of seizures. During sleep, the fast activity may persist, and K complexes are typically absent (30). Seizure types described with infantile neuroaxonal dystrophy include myoclonic and tonic (13,125). In a video EEG case report, Wakai et al. (124) described tonic spasms and an electrographic correlate of a diffuse, 1-second, high-voltage slow complex followed by desynchronization suggestive of infantile spasms. A juvenile form of the disorder presenting with clinical and EEG features of progressive myoclonic epilepsy has been described (26A). The pathological features are identical to those of one infantile type.

Schindler's disease in older children can present as a neuroaxonal dystrophy. It is due to a deficiency of the lysosomal enzyme, α-N-acetylgalactosaminidase, coded on chromosome 22 (50). Tonic seizures and myoclonus are also seen in patients with this disorder. The EEG pattern has been described as diffuse and multifocal paroxysmal discharges with slowing that is maximal over the centroparietal-occipital regions.

Neuronal Ceroid Lipofuscinosis, Type III (Spielmeyer-Vogt Disease or Late-Onset Batten's Disease)

This syndrome with onset in early childhood begins between the ages of 5 and 10 years with visual failure, slow intellectual deterioration, and seizures. A diffuse rigidity later ensues. An autosomal recessive inheritance pattern with localization to 16q12.1 is seen with a worldwide distribution of the disorder. EEG changes are nonspecific. In contrast to the Bielschowsky form of NCL, low-frequency photic does not evoke occipital spikes.

Progressive Myoclonus Epilepsies

Progressive myoclonus epilepsies are a collection of rare disorders characterized by the triad of myoclonic seizures, tonic-clonic seizures, and progressive neurological dysfunction, which often manifests as dementia and ataxia. Onset generally occurs in late childhood to adolescence. If myoclonic features are not prominent, children with this syndrome may be erroneously diagnosed with Lennox-Gastaut syndrome (4). For this reason,

a careful history for myoclonic features is important in children with intellectual deterioration and frequent seizures.

Lafora's Disease

Although the biochemical error remains unknown, the autosomal recessively inherited defect that causes this disease has been localized to 6p23-25. The mean age at onset is 14 years, but symptoms may begin in adulthood. Seizures may precede other clinical signs by months to years; multiple seizure types may occur in a previously normal person. Cognitive decline and personality changes are prominent features. Seizure types include tonic-clonic, myoclonic, and polymyoclonus. Occipital seizures with visual phenomena have been reported in 30% to 50% of cases. Cerebellar ataxia, hypertonia, dyskinesias, and exaggerated tendon reflexes may develop later. Generalized bursts of spikes and polyspikes superimposed on a normal background may be seen initially on EEG. The presence of spikes over the posterior regions is a distinguishing feature that may alert the electroencephalographer to the diagnosis in the appropriate clinical setting (87). Spike-and-wave discharges are uncommon. As the disease progresses, the EEG pattern becomes increasingly disorganized. A photoconvulsive response can be seen with photic stimulation (74). On neuroimaging, cerebellar atrophy is occasionally observed.

Unverricht-Lundborg Progressive Familial Myoclonic Epilepsy (Baltic Myoclonus)

This familial form of progressive encephalopathy is characterized by relentless myoclonus and generalized seizures. The gene locus is 21q22.3 (59). Onset occurs in childhood or adolescence with seizures that are predominantly myoclonic and frequently occur after awakening. Absence and atonic seizures are also observed. Although the familial pattern can initially suggest an idiopathic form of epilepsy, the severity of the myoclonus soon suggests a form of progressive myoclonic epilepsy. Myoclonus can become quite disabling, interfering with speech and swallowing, and is often provoked by voluntary movement and excitement. Cognition is generally retained, although a mild decline may be observed later in the course of the disease. Cerebellar ataxia, hyporeflexia, wasting of the distal musculature, and signs of chronic denervation on electromyograms may be seen. The EEG reveals progressive slowing with generalized spike-and-wave–like bursts at a rate of three to five per second that are frontally predominant. Paroxysmal flicker responses and generalized spikes and polyspikes with photic stimulation are also seen (5,53).

Myoclonic Epilepsy with Ragged Red Fibers (MERFF) and Mitochondrial Encephalomyopathy with Lactic Acidosis and Stroke-Like Episodes (MELAS)

In MERRF, disease onset occurs before the age of 20 years with ataxia and seizures that are predominantly myoclonic. The inheritance pattern is compatible with maternal transmission. In the majority of cases, a point mutation at position 8344 of the mitochondrial gene for transfer ribonucleic acid (tRNA)–lysine has been identified. Affected patients may have short stature, neurosensory hearing loss, optic atrophy, myopathy, or encephalopathy. EEG findings include background slowing, focal epileptiform discharges, and atypical spike- or sharp-and-slow-wave discharges that have a variable association with the myoclonic jerks (104). Suppression of these discharges during sleep is characteristic. As with many of the progressive myoclonic epilepsies, giant somatosensory evoked potentials are observed.

Classically, MELAS manifests during childhood with the sudden onset of stroke-like episodes (Fig. 16.4). Migraine-like headaches, progressive deafness, seizures, cognitive decline, and myopathic features may accompany these symptoms. In an evaluation of 12 patients with MELAS by Berkovic et al. (3), epilepsia partialis continua was frequently seen, and seizures often evolved into partial or generalized status epilepticus. Fujimoto et al. (31) reviewed 79 EEGs in six patients with MELAS and two of their relatives with mitochondrial myopathy, encephalopathy, and lactic acidosis, without stroke-like episodes. In the acute stage after a stroke-like episode, 10 of 11 EEGs showed focal high-voltage delta waves with polyspikes. These discharges were interpreted as ictal phenomena. Later, focal spikes or sharp waves and 14- and 6-Hz positive bursts were frequently recorded (31). The observed seizures were characterized by focal clonic and myoclonic movements with migrainous headache. Four point mutations are predominantly seen with MELAS. Three of these (3243, 3250, 3271) affect the mitochondrial DNA gene of tRNA-leucine. The other mutation involves a coding region of complex I of the respiratory chain. An overlap between clinical characteristics of MERRF and MELAS can be seen with myoclonic features in both syndromes.

Dentatorubral-Pallidoluysian Atrophy

This rare autosomal dominant disease is seen predominantly in the Japanese population. The disorder is related to a trinucleotide (CAG) expansion at

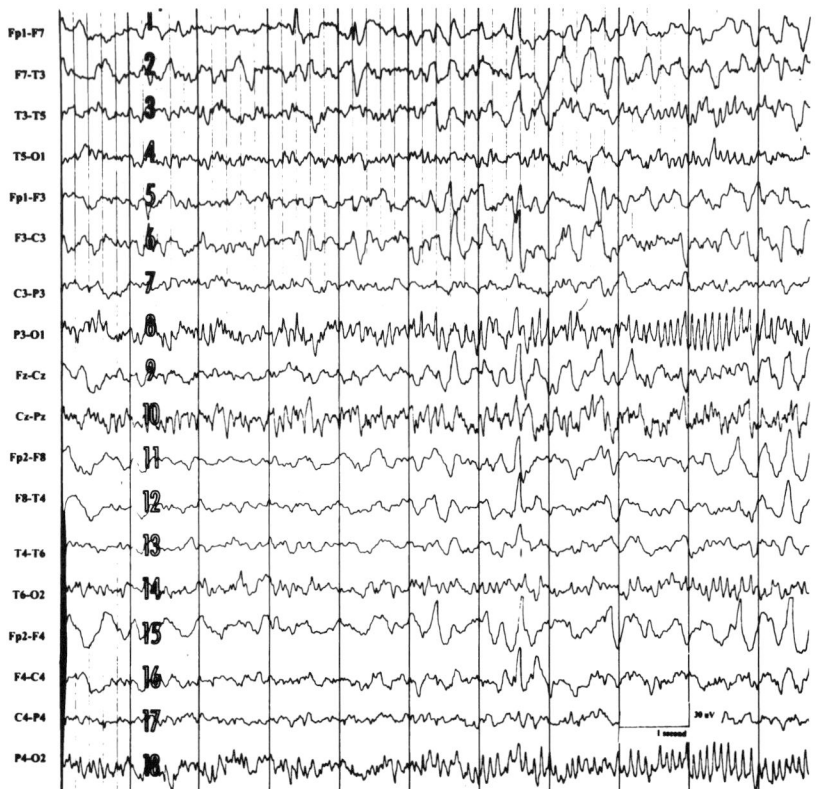

FIG. 16.4. EEG of a 10-year-old boy with mitochondrial encephalomyopathy with lactic acidosis and stroke-like symptoms (MELAS). This tracing was obtained shortly after an acute stroke-like episode. A focal seizure arising from the left posterior quadrant is seen. (Courtesy of C. Stack, M.D., and L. Laux, M.D., Children's Memorial Hospital, Chicago, Illinois.)

12p13.31 (57). Clinical manifestations are dependent on the length of the unstable trinucleotide repeats and vary from a juvenile-onset progressive myoclonic epilepsy to an adult-onset syndrome with ataxia, dementia, and choreoathetosis (44). The juvenile form can also be variable in its manifestation. In general, symptoms begin in infancy to early childhood with myoclonus, ataxia, dementia, opsoclonus, or seizures that can be generalized tonic-clonic, atypical absence, or atonic (91). Pathological features are striking, with neuronal loss and gliosis in the dentatorubral and pallidoluysian structures. EEG characteristically shows bursts of slowing, irregular spike-and-wave discharges, and multifocal paroxysmal discharges. A photoparoxysmal response is seen, and myoclonic seizures can often be triggered by photic stimulation.

OTHER ENCEPHALOPATHIES MANIFESTING IN INFANCY, CHILDHOOD, AND ADOLESCENCE

Fragile X Syndrome

The clinical features of this condition are often characterized by moderate mental retardation; large ears; macroorchidism; large chin; hyperkinesias; jocular, high pitched speech; and associated speech and language disorders. The inheritance pattern of this X-linked condition has been explained by maternal imprinting, with loss of gene deactivation after transmission to offspring of the opposite sex. EEGs in affected boys may show a characteristic pattern of centrotemporal spikes indistinguishable from or very similar to those seen in children with benign epilepsy with centrotemporal spikes. The features of these centrotemporal interictal epileptiform discharges include a stereotyped, diphasic morphological appearance with an apparent horizontal dipole, enhanced by drowsiness and sleep. Musumeci et al. (73) studied 192 boys with fragile X syndrome and found that 18.2% had seizures. The onset occurred exclusively between the ages of 2 and 9 years. The majority of affected boys demonstrated interictal centrotemporal spikes. Interestingly, Singh et al. (102) reported focal spikes similar to those in benign rolandic epilepsy in three related female patients with fragile X syndrome. Two sisters of a boy with fragile X syndrome showed mild developmental delay, but their grandmother was of normal intelligence, and all were carriers of the fragile X chromosome. In a smaller study, Kluger et al. (52) found that the interictal epileptiform discharges were detected in boys between 4 and 8 years of age and were not seen in children younger than 4 years or older than 8 years.

Angelman Syndrome

Children with this disorder exhibit developmental delay, craniofacial abnormalities, ataxia, paroxysmal laughter, and seizures. Children may have atypical absence seizures, partial seizures, and myoclonus. Characteristic EEG findings are diffuse, bilaterally frontal dominant, high-amplitude (1- to 3-Hz) notched or triphasic slow waves (68) (Fig. 16.5). These appear as slow-sharp-wave complexes with a notch of epileptiform activity appearing on the

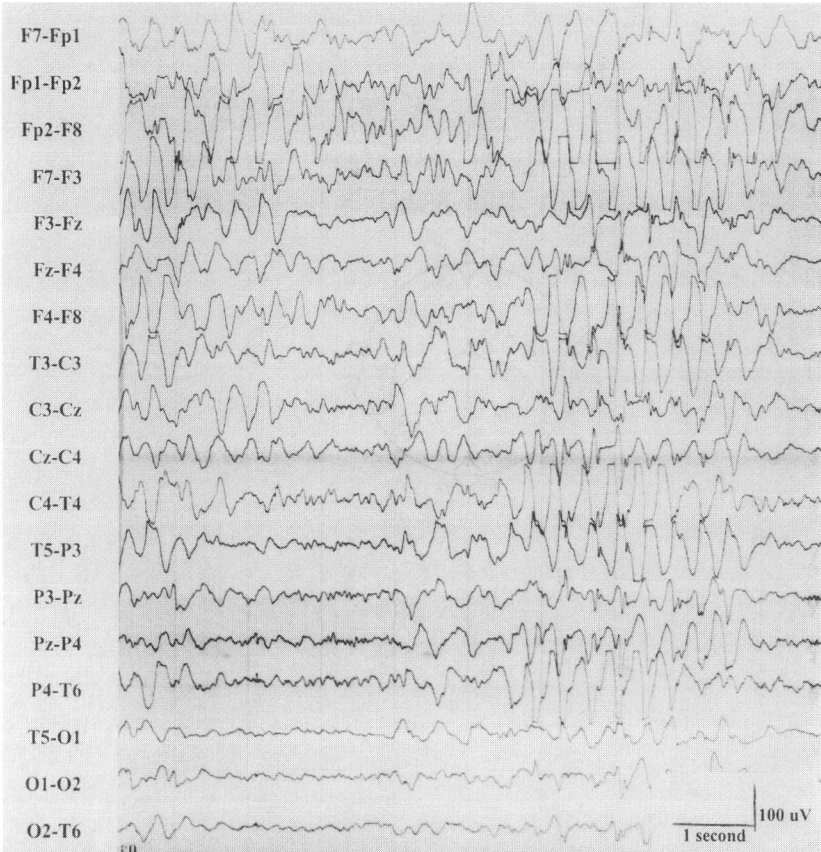

FIG. 16.5. EEG of a 5-year-old with Angelman syndrome. Characteristic high-amplitude 1- to 3-Hz notched slow-sharp-wave complexes are present. (Courtesy of C. Stack, M.D., and L. Laux, M.D., Children's Memorial Hospital, Chicago, Illinois.)

descending portion of the slow wave. Similar discharges have been reported in the occipital region and were facilitated by eye closure (90). In a report on 20 patients with Angelman syndrome, Minassian et al. (68) noted more severe epilepsy in those with maternally inherited 15q11-13 deletions than in patients with loss-of-function UBE3A mutations, uniparental disomy, or methylation imprint abnormalities (68). Angelman syndrome is the probable diagnosis

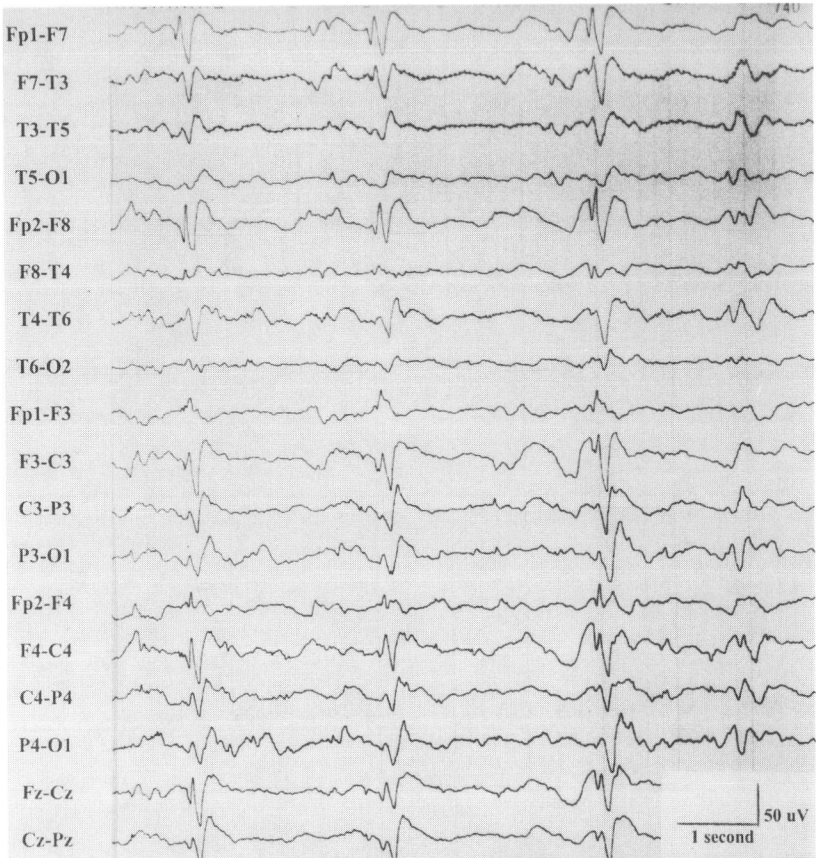

FIG. 16.6. EEG of a 15-year-old girl with Rett syndrome. Characteristic fronto-central needle-like spikes are present. (Courtesy of C. Stack, M.D., and L. Laux, M.D., Children's Memorial Hospital, Chicago, Illinois.)

when the characteristic clinical and electrographic features are present, but it must also be considered in children with severe epilepsy and mental retardation, even when typical EEG features are not present (12).

Rett Syndrome

Rett syndrome is observed only in girls. It is characterized by early psychomotor regression with autistic features, loss of purposeful hand function, ataxia, and acquired microcephaly. The onset of the disease occurs between the ages of 6 months and 3 years, most often before 18 months. Affected girls next experience a rapid decline in function with irritability and loss of purposeful hand use. In the third stage, between the ages of 2 and 10 years, seizures and neurological signs develop. At this stage, the EEG shows interictal epileptiform discharges and a progressive slowing and deterioration of the background in 75% of patients (17,36,89). Characteristic EEG findings include needle-like central spikes, activated by contralateral passive finger pulp palpation (Fig. 16.6). In addition, an unusual and prominent rhythmic theta rhythm (four to five waves per second or five to six waves per second) in the waking state has been noted at the central vertex region and vicinity. This activity blocks with active or passive movements and suggests a slowed equivalent of the mu rhythm (76). These findings can be reliably distinguished from those noted in Angelman syndrome (58).

Down's Syndrome

Children with Down's syndrome are at increased risk for infantile spasms, accompanied by hypsarrhythmia, which is symmetrical and rapidly clears after intravenous administration of diazepam (85,101). Older children may exhibit a variety of seizure types and EEG findings. Overall, epilepsy occurs in 5% to 6% of patients (106). In adulthood, deterioration of the alpha rhythm and changes in its reactivity appears at the onset of dementia in patients with Down's syndrome (82,123).

THE ROLE OF THE EEG IN A CHILD WITH A SUSPECTED PROGRESSIVE ENCEPHALOPATHY

When confronted with a child who is not meeting expected developmental milestones or who exhibits cognitive difficulties, one of the first questions that may arise is whether the patient has a diffuse encephalopathy. The most important parts of the evaluation are the complete medical history and the results of a comprehensive neurological examination. The EEG may help to confirm an encephalopathy by demonstrating diffuse background slowing. The degree of tolerable slowing varies as a function of age and state of the child. In very young children, unrecognized drowsiness can produce abundant intermixed slowing and prolonged bursts of diffuse or posteriorly dominant rhythmic slowing during transition states. In these circumstances, other characteristics of the EEG can be helpful in evaluation, including the frequency of the posterior dominant rhythm, voltage and frequency organization of the background, and sleep architecture.

If an encephalopathy is confirmed, than it should be determined whether it is progressive or static. Progressive encephalopathies are suggestive of a neurodegenerative process, an inborn error of metabolism, or some other type of progressive etiology. Progressive encephalopathy, a family history of relatives with similar unexplained neurological illnesses, and unexplained paroxysmal bouts of obtundation, ataxia, or other neurological phenomena are all indicators of inborn errors of metabolism and merit further investigation. The EEG may help to confirm the presence of a progressive encephalopathy, particularly if serial studies are performed. Deterioration of the background organization, progressive slowing of the dominant rhythm, attenuation of the background, or loss of the usual signposts of maturation are reliable indicators of progressive disease.

The EEG can help to localize the pathological process, thereby limiting the differential diagnosis. Epileptiform discharges indicate the presence of a potentially epileptogenic encephalopathy and implicate at least some degree of gray matter involvement (as in Tay-Sachs disease, NCL, and Alper's syndrome). Conversely, slowing without epileptiform activity indicates dysfunction in the thalamocortical projections and is consistent with white matter involvement (as in NALD, metachromatic leukodystrophy, and Krabbe's disease).

In rare circumstances, the EEG findings are so distinctive that they limit the differential diagnosis. Examples (Table 16.1) include a burst-suppression pattern in nonketotic hyperglycinemia, phenylketonuria, maple syrup urine disease, molybdenum cofactor deficiency, and sulfite oxidase deficiency, in addition to other disorders. A comb-like rhythm with 7- to 9-Hz central activity is present in maple syrup urine disease and propionic academia; vertex positive polyspikes are present in type I sialidosis; biooccipital polymorphic delta activity is present in X-linked adrenoleukodystrophy; and 16- to 24-Hz invariant activity is present with infantile neuroaxonal dystro-

TABLE 16.1. *EEG patterns and their associated disorders*

EEG pattern	Disorder
Comb-like rhythm	Maple syrup urine disease
	Propionic acidemia
Fast central spikes	Tay-Sachs disease
Rhythmic vertex positive spikes	Sialidosis type I
Vanishing EEG	Infantile NCL (type I)
High-voltage 16- to 24-Hz activity	Infantile neuroaxonal dystrophy
Diminished spikes during sleep	PME
Giant somatosensory evoked potentials	
Marked photosensitivity	PME and NCL, particularly type II
Burst-suppression pattern	Neonatal citrullinemia
	Nonketotic hyperglycinemia
	Propionic acidemia
	Leigh's syndrome
	D-glycine acidemia
	Molybdenum cofactor deficiency
	Menkes' disease
	Holocarboxylase synthetase deficiency
	Neonatal adrenoleukodystrophy
Hypsarrhythmia	Zellweger's syndrome
	Neonatal adrenoleukodystrophy
	Neuroaxonal dystrophy
	Nonketotic hyperglycinemia
	Phenylketonuria
	Carbohydrate-deficient glycoprotein syndrome type III

NCL, neuronal ceroid lipofuscinosis; PME, progressive myoclonus epilepsy.

phy. Some static encephalopathies have unusual and distinctive EEG patterns: for example, centrotemporal spikes in fragile X syndrome; needle-like central spikes in Rett's syndrome; and frontally dominant, rhythmic slow-sharp complexes in Angelman syndrome.

Finally, patients with inborn errors of metabolism resulting in epileptogenic encephalopathies may initially appear to have cryptogenic epilepsy. The patterns of clinical presentation and the EEG findings can be organized by epilepsy syndromes in order to facilitate recognition of the more common diagnoses (Table 16.2).

TABLE 16.2. *Metabolic diseases masquerading as epilepsy syndromes*

Neonatal seizures (ILAE 3.1)

1. Urea cycle defects: argininosuccinic acidemia, ornithine transcarbamylase, carbamylphosphate synthetase
2. Organic acidurias: maple syrup urine disease
3. Disorders of biotin metabolism: early-onset multiple carboxylase deficiency (holocarboxylase synthetase deficiency)
4. Peroxisomal disorders: Zellweger's syndrome, acyl-coenzyme A oxidase deficiency
5. Other: molybdenum cofactor deficiency, sulfite oxidase deficiency, disorders of fructose metabolism, pyridoxine dependency

Early myoclonic encephalopathy and early infantile epiletogenic encephalopathy (ILAE 2.3.1)

1. Nonketotic hyperglycinemia
2. Propionic aciduria
3. *D*-glycine acidemia
4. Leigh's disease

Cryptogenic myoclonic epilepsies (ILAE 2.2), other than infantile spasms or Lennox-Gastaut syndrome

1. GM_2 gangliosidoses
2. GM_1 gangliosidosis
3. Infantile neuroaxonal dystrophy
4. Neuronal ceroid lipofuscinosis
5. Glucose transporter 1 deficiency
6. Late-onset multiple carboxylase deficiency
7. Disorders of folate metabolism, methylenetetrahydrofolate reductase deficiency
8. Arginase deficiency (urea cycle defect)
9. Tetrahydrobiopterin deficiency (aminoaciduria)
10. Tyrosinemia type III (case report)

West's syndrome, generalized (ILAE 2.2)

1. Phenylketonuria, hyperphenylalaninemias
2. Pyruvate dehydrogenase
3. Pyruvate carboxylase
4. Carbohydrate-deficient glycoprotein syndrome, type III
5. Organic acidurias
6. Aminoacidurias

Lennox-Gastaut syndrome (ILAE 2.2)

1. Neuronal ceroid lipofuscinosis
2. Sialidoses

Progressive myoclonic epilepsy (ILAE 2.2)

1. Lafora's disease
2. Unverricht-Lundborg disease
3. Myoclonic epilepsy with ragged red fibers and mitochondrial encephalomyopathy with lactic acidosis and stroke-like symptoms
4. Dentatorubral-pallidoluysian atrophy
5. Neuronal ceroid lipofuscinosis
6. Sialidoses
7. Gaucher's disease

ILAE, International League Against Epilepsy.

REFERENCES

1. Balslev T, Cortez MA, Blaser SI, et al. Recurrent seizures in metachromatic leukodystrophy. *Pediatr Neurol* 1997;17:150–154.

2. Berger J, Gmach M, Mayr U, et al. Coincidence of two novel arylsulfatase A alleles and mutation 459A within a family with metachromatic leukodystrophy: molecular basis of phenotypic heterogeneity. *Hum Mutat* 1999;13:61–68.

3. Berkovic SF, Andermann F, Karpati G, et al. The epileptic syndromes associated with mitochondrial disease. [Abstract]. *Electroencephalogr Clin Neurophyiol* 1988;69:50P.

4. Berkovic SF, Cochius J, Andermann E, et al. Progressive myoclonus epilepsies: clinical and genetic aspects. *Epilepsia* 1993;34(suppl 3):S19–S30.

5. Berkovic SF, So NK, Andermann F. Progressive myoclonus epilepsies: clinical and neurophysiological diagnosis. *J Clin Neurophysiol* 1991;8:261–274.

6. Blom S, Hagberg B. EEG findings in late infantile metachromatic and globoid cell leucodystrophy. *Electroencephalogr Clin Neurophys* 1967;22:253–259.

7. Boyd SG, Harden A, Egger J, et al. Progressive neuronal degeneration of childhood with liver disease ("Alpers' disease"): characteristic neurophysiological features. *Neuropediatrics* 1986;17(2):75–80.

8. Brick JF, Westmoreland BF, Gomez MR. The electroencephalogram in Alpers' disease. [Abstract]. *Electroencephalogr Clin Neurophysiol* 58:31P.

9. Brown, GK, Otero LJ, LeGris M, et al. Pyruvate dehydrogenase deficiency. *J Med Genet* 1994;31:875–879.

10. Bu D-F, Erlander MG, Hitz BC, et al. Two human glutamate decarboxylases, 65-kDa GAD and 67-kDa GAD, are each encoded by a single gene. *Proc Natl Acad Sci U S A* 89:2115–2119, 1992.

11. Bu D-F, Tobin AJ. The exon-intron organization of the genes (GAD1 and GAD2) encoding two human glutamate decarboxylases (GAD-67 and GAD-65) suggests that they derive from a common ancestral GAD. *Genomics* 1994;21:222–228.

12. Buoni S, Grosso S, Pucci L, et al. Diagnosis of Angelman syndrome: clinical and EEG criteria. *Brain Dev* 1999;21(5):296–302.

13. Butzer JF, Schochet SS Jr, Bell WE. Infantile neuroaxonal dystrophy: an electron microscopic study of a case clinically resembling neuronal ceroid-lipofuscinosis. *Acta Neuropathol (Berl)* 1975;31:35–43.

14. Chou ML, Wang HS, Hung PC, et al. Late-onset pyridoxine-dependent seizures: report of two cases. *Zhonghua Min Guo Xiao Er Ke Yi Xue Hui Za Zhi* 1995;36:434–437.

15. Cobb W, Martin F, Pampiglione G. Cerebral lipidosis: an electroencephalographic study. *Brain* 1952;75:343–357.

16. Cole H, Weremowicz S, Morton CC, et al. Localization of serum biotinidase (BTD) to human chromosome 3 in band p25. *Genomics* 1994;22:662–663.

17. Cooper RA, Kerr AM, Amos PM. Rett syndrome: critical examination of clinical features, serial EEG and video-monitoring in understanding and management. *Eur J Paediatr Neurol* 1998;2:127–135.

18. Dalla Bernardina B, Aicardi J, Goutieres F, et al. Glycine encephalopathy. *Neuropadiatrie* 1979;10:209–225.

19. De Vivo DC, Garcia-Alvarez M, Ronen G, et al. Glucose transporter protein deficiency: an emerging syndrome with therapeutic implications. *Int Pediatr* 1995;10:51–56.

20. De Vivo DC, Trifiletti RR, Jacobson RI, et al. Defective glucose transporter across the blood-brain barrier as a cause of persistent hypoglycorrhachia, seizures and developmental delay. *N Engl J Med* 1991;325:703–709.

21. Del Giudice E, Striano S, Andria G. Electroencephalographic abnormalities in homocystinuria due to cystathionine synthase deficiency. *Clin Neurol Neurosurg* 1983;85:165–168.

22. DiMauro S, Bonilla E, De Vivo DC. Does the patient have a mitochondrial encephalomyopathy? *J Child Neurol* 1999;14(Suppl 1):S23–S35.

23. DiMauro S; De Vivo DC. Genetic heterogeneity in Leigh syndrome. [Letter]. *Ann Neurol* 1996;40:5–7.

24. DiMauro S, Ricci E, Hirano M, et al. Epilepsy in mitochondrial encephalomyopathies. *Epilepsy Res Suppl* 1991;4:173–180.

25. Dodt G, Braverman N, Wong C, et al. Mutations in the PTS1 receptor gene, PXR1, define complementation group 2 of the peroxisome biogenesis disorders. *Nat Genet* 1995;9:115–125.

26. Donker DNJ, Reits D, Van Sprang FJ, et al. Computer analysis of the EEG as an aid in the evaluation of dietary treatment in phenylketonuria. *Electroencephalogr Clin Neurophys* 1979;46:205–213.

26a. Dorfman LJ, Pedley TA, Tharp BR, Scheitauer BW. Juvenile neuroaxonal dystrophy: clinical electrophysiological and neuropathological features. *Ann Neurol* 1978;3:419–428.

27. Elia M, Musumeci SA, Ferri R, et al. Leigh syndrome and partial deficit of cytochrome c oxidase associated with epilepsia partialis continua. *Brain Dev* 1996;18:207–211.

28. Engel J Jr, Rapin I, Giblin DR. Electrophysiological studies in two patients with cherry red spot–myoclonus syndrome. *Epilepsia* 1977;18:73–87.

29. Fekete G, Plattner R, Crabb DW, et al. Localization of the human gene for the E_1-alpha subunit of branched chain keto acid dehydrogenase (BCKDHA) to chromosome 19q13.1-q13.2. *Cytogenet Cell Genet* 1989;50:236–237.

30. Ferriss GS, Happel L, Duncan MC. Cerebral cortical isolation in infantile neuroaxonal dystrophy. *Electroencephalogr Clin Neurophysiol* 1977;43:168–182.

31. Fujimoto S, Mizuno K, Shibata H, et al. Serial electroencephalographic findings in patients with MELAS. *Pediatr Neurol* 1999;20:43–48.

32. Fukumizu M, Matsui K, Hanaoka S, et al. Partial seizures in two cases of metachromatic leukodystrophy: electrophysiologic and neuroradiologic findings. *J Child Neurol* 1992;7:381–386.

33. Garcia-Alvarez M, Nordli DR, De Vivo DC: Inherited metabolic disorders. In: Engel J Jr, Pedley TA, eds. *Epilepsy: a comprehensive textbook*. Philadelphia: Lippincott-Raven, 1997: 2547–2562.

34. Gerritsen T, Vaughn JG, Waisman HA. The identification of homocystine in the urine. *Biochem Biophys Res Commun* 1962;9:493–496.

35. Gibson KM, Wappner RS, Jooste S, et al. Variable clinical presentation in three patients with 3-methylglutaconyl–coenzyme A hydratase deficiency. *J Inherit Metab Dis* 1998;21:631–638.

36. Glaze DG, Erost JD, Zoghbi HY, et al. Rett's syndrome: correlation of electroencephalographic characteristics with clinical staging. *Arch Neurol* 1987;44:1053–1056.

37. Godwin-Austen RB, Robinson A, Evans K, et al. An unusual neurological disorder of copper metabolism clinically resembling Wilson's disease but biochemically a distinct entity. *J Neurol Sci* 1978;39:85–98.

38. Goutieres F, Aicardi J. Atypical presentations of pyridoxine-dependent seizures: a treatable cause of intractable epilepsy in infants. *Ann Neurol* 1985;17:117–120.

39. Goyette P, Pai A, Milos R, et al. Gene structure of human and mouse methylenetetrahydrofolate reductase (MTHFR). *Mamm Genome* 1998;9:652–656.

40. Hagberg B. Krabbe's disease: clinical presentation of neurological variants. *Neuropediatrics* 1984;15(Suppl):1–15.

41. Hagberg BA, Blennow G, Kristiansson B, et al. Carbohydrate-deficient glycoprotein syndromes: peculiar group of new disorders. *Pediat Neurol* 1993;9:255–262.

42. Harden A, Martinovic Z, Pampiglione G. Neurophysiological studies in GM_1 gangliosidosis. *Ital J Neurol Sci* 1982;3:201–206.

43. Harden A, Pampiglione G, Picton-Robinson N. Electroretinogram and visual evoked response in a form of "neuronal lipidosis" with diagnostic EEG features. *J Neurol Neurosurg Psychiat* 1973;36:61–67.

44. Hattori H, Higuchi Y, Okuno T, et al. Early-childhood progressive myoclonus epilepsy presenting as partial seizures in dentatorubral-pallidoluysian atrophy. *Epilepsia* 1997;38:271–274.

45. Jaeken J, Stibler H, Hagberg B. The carbohydrate-deficient glycoprotein syndrome: a new

inherited multisystemic disease with severe nervous system involvement. *Acta Paediat Scand Suppl* 1991;375:1–71.

46. Johnson JL, Waud WR, Rajagopalan KV, et al. Inborn errors of molybdenum metabolism: combined deficiencies of sulfite oxidase and xanthine dehydrogenase in a patient lacking the molybdenum cofactor. *Proc Natl Acad Sci U S A* 1980;77:3715–3719.

47. Kamoshita S, Mizutani I, Fukuyama Y. Leigh's subacute necrotizing encephalomyelopathy in a child with infantile spasms and hypsarhythmia. *Dev Med Child Neurol* 1970;12:430–435.

48. Kelley KR, Shinnar S, Moshe SL. A 5-month-old with intractable epilepsy. *Semin Pediatr Neurol* 1999;6:138–144.

49. Kennerknecht I, Klett C, Hameister H. Assignment of the human gene propionyl coenzyme A carboxylase, alpha-chain, (PCCA) to chromosome 13q32 by *in situ* hybridization. *Genomics* 1992;14:550–551.

50. Keuleman JL, Reuser AJ, Kroos MA, et al. Human alpha-*N*-acetylgalactosaminidase (alpha-NAGA) deficiency: new mutations and the paradox between genotype and phenotype. *J Med Genet* 1996;33:458–464.

51. Kliemann FAD, Harden A, Pampiglione G. Some EEG observations in patients with Krabbe's disease. *Dev Med Child Neurol* 1969;11:475–484.

52. Kluger G, Bohm I, Laub MC, et al. Epilepsy and fragile X gene mutations. *Pediatr Neurol* 1996;15:358–360.

53. Koskiniemi M, Toivakka E, Donner M. Progressive myoclonus epilepsy: electroencephalographic findings. *Acta Neurol Scand* 1974;50:333–359.

54. Kraus JP, Matsubara Y, Barton D, et al. Isolation of cDNA clones coding for rat isovaleryl-CoA dehydrogenase and assignment of the gene to human chromosome 15. *Genomics* 1987;1: 264–269.

55. Kriel RL, Hauser WA, Sung JH, et al. Neuroanatomical and electroencephalographic correlations in Sanfilippo syndrome, type A. *Arch Neurol* 1978;35:838–843.

56. Kurlemann G, Schuierer G. EEG in diagnosis of other disease pictures than epilepsy. *Klin Padiatr* 1994;206:100–107.

57. Kuwano A, Morimoto Y, Nagai T, et al. Precise chromosomal locations of the genes for dentatorubral-pallidoluysian atrophy (DRPLA), von Willebrand factor (F8vWF) and parathyroid hormone-like hormone (PTHLH) in human chromosome 12p by deletion mapping. *Hum Genet* 1996;97:95–98.

58. Laan LA, Brouwer OF, Begeer CH, et al. The diagnostic value of the EEG in Angelman and Rett syndrome at a young age. *Electroencephalogr Clin Neurophysiol* 1998;106:404–408.

59. Lehesjoki AE, Eldridge R, Eldridge J, et al. Progressive myoclonus epilepsy of Unverricht-Lundborg type: a clinical and molecular genetic study of a family from the United States with four affected sibs. *Neurology* 1993;43:2384–2386.

60. Leigh D. Subacute necrotizing encephalomyelopathy in an infant. *J Neurol Neurosurg Psychiat* 1951;14:216–221.

61. Low NL, Bosma JF, Armstrong MD. Studies on phenylketonuria: VI. EEG studies on phenylketonuria. *AMA Arch Neurol Psychiat* 1957;77:359–365.

62. Lyon G, Adams RD, Kolodny EH. In: Hefta J, Navrozov M, eds. *Neurology of hereditary metabolic diseases of children*, 2nd ed. New York: McGraw-Hill, 1996.

63. Mamoli B, Graf M, Toifl K. EEG, pattern-evoked potentials and nerve conduction velocity in a family with adrenoleucodystrophy. *Electroencephalogr Clin Neurophysiol* 1979;47:411–419.

64. Maroteaux P, Frezal J, Tahbaz-Zadeh NI, et al. Une observation familiale d'oligophrenie polydystrophique. *J Genet Hum* 1966;15:93–102.

65. Matthijs G, Schollen E, Pardon E, et al. Mutations in PMM2, a phosphomannomutase gene on chromosome 16p13, in carbohydrate-deficient glycoprotein type I syndrome (Jaeken syndrome). *Nature Genet* 1997;16:88–92.

66. Menkes JH, Alter M, Steigleder GK, et al. A sex-linked recessive disorder with retardation of growth, peculiar hair and focal cerebral and cerebellar degeneration. *Pediatrics* 1962;29: 764–779.

67. Menkes JH, Hurst PL, Craig JM. A new syndrome: progressive familial infantile cerebral dysfunction associated with unusual urinary substance. *Pediatrics* 1954;14:462–467.

68. Minassian BA, DeLorey TM, Olsen RW, et al. Angelman syndrome: correlations between epilepsy phenotypes and genotypes. *Ann Neurol* 1998;43:485–493.

69. Mole SE. Batten disease: four genes and still counting. *Neurobiol Dis* 1998;5:287–303.

70. Moser AB, Rasmussen M, Naidu S, et al. Phenotype of patients with peroxisomal disorders subdivided into sixteen complementation groups. *J Pediatr* 1995;127:13–22.

71. Mudd SH, Skovby F, Levy, HL, et al. The natural history of homocystinuria due to cystathionine beta-synthase deficiency. *Am J Hum Genet* 1985;37:1–31.

72. Munke M, Kraus J, Watkins P, et al. Homocystinuria gene on human chromosome 21 mapped with cloned cystathionine beta-synthase probe and *in situ* hybridization of other chromosome 21 probes. [Abstract]. *Cytogenet Cell Genet* 1985;40:706–707.

73. Musumeci SA, Hagerman RJ, Ferri R, et al. Epilepsy and EEG findings in males with fragile X syndrome. *Epilepsia* 1999;40:1092–1099.

74. Naidu S, Niedermeyer E: Degenerative disorders of the central nervous system. In Niedermeyer E, Lopes da Silva F, eds. *Electroencephalography: basic principles, clinical applications, and related fields*, 4th ed. pp. 360-382. Baltimore: Williams & Wilkins, 1999:360–382.

75. Nakai H, Byers MG, Nowak NJ, et al. Assignment of beta-hexosaminidase A alpha-subunit to human chromosomal region 15q23-q24. *Cytogenet Cell Genet* 1991;56:164.

76. Niedermeyer E, Naidu SB, Plate C. Unusual EEG theta rhythms over central region in Rett syndrome: considerations of the underlying dysfunction. *Clin Electroencephalogr* 1997;28:36–43.

77. Nishimura R, Omos-Lau N, Ajmone-Marsan C, et al. Electrographic findings in Gaucher disease. *Neurology* 1980;30:152–159.

78. O'Connell P, Leppert M, Hoff M, et al. A linkage map for human chromosome 12. [Abstract]. *Am J Hum Genet* 1985;37:A169.

79. Orlean P. Congenital disorders of glycosylation caused by defects in mannose addition during N-linked oligosaccharide assembly. *J Clin Invest* 2000;105:131–132.

80. Otero LJ, Brown GK, Silver K, et al. Association of cerebral dysgenesis and lactic acidemia with X-linked PDH E_1 alpha subunit mutations in females. *Pediatr Neurol* 1995;13:327–332.

81. Pampiglione G, Harden A. Neurophysiological identification of a late infantile form of "neuronal lipidosis." *J Neurol Neurosurg Psychiat* 1973;36:68–74.

82. Partanen J, Soininen H, Kononen M, et al. EEG reactivity correlates with neuropsychological test scores in Down's syndrome. *Acta Neurol Scand* 1996;94:242–246.

83. Petersen MB, Brostrom K, Stibler H, et al. Early manifestations of the carbohydrate-deficient glycoprotein syndrome. *J Pediatr* 1993;122:66–70.

84. Pietz J, Schmidt E, Matthis P, et al. EEGs in phenylketonuria. I: Follow-up to adulthood; II: Short-term diet-related changes in EEGs and cognitive function. *Dev Med Child Neurol* 1993; 35:54–64.

85. Pollack MA, Golden GS, Schmidt R, et al. Infantile spasms in Down syndrome: a report of 5 cases and review of the literature. *Ann Neurol* 1978;3:406–408.

86. Poll-The BT, Roels F, Ogier H, et al. A new peroxisomal disorder with enlarged peroxisomes and a specific deficiency of acyl-CoA oxidase (pseudo-neonatal adrenoleukodystrophy). *Am J Hum Genet* 1988;42:422–434.

87. Ponsford S, Pye IF, Elliot EJ. Posterior paroxysmal discharge: an aid to early diagnosis in Lafora disease. *J R Soc Med* 1993;86:597–599.

88. Reiss J, Dorche B, Stallmeyer B, et al. Human molybdopterin synthase gene: genomic structure and mutations in molybdenum cofactor deficiency type B. *Am J Hum Genet* 1999;64:706–711.

89. Robb SA, Harden A, Boyd SG. Rett syndrome: an EEG study in 52 girls. *Neuropediatrics* 1989;20:192–195.

90. Rubin DI, Patterson MC, Westmoreland BF, et al. Angelman's syndrome: clinical and electroencephalographic findings. *Electroencephalogr Clin Neurophysiol* 1997;102:299–302.

91. Saitoh S, Momoi M, Yamagata T, et al. Clinical and electroencephalographic findings in juvenile type DRPLA. *Pediatr Neurol* 1998;18:265–268.

92. Salbert BA, Pellock JM, Wolf B. Characterization of seizures associated with biotinidase deficiency. *Neurology* 1993;43:1351–1355.
93. Santavouri P. Neuronal ceroid lipofuscinosis in childhood. *Brain Dev* 1988;4:80–83.
94. Schindler D, Bishop DF, Wallace S, et al. Characterization of alpha-*N*-acetylgalactosaminidase deficiency: a new neurodegenerative lysosomal disease. [Abstract]. *Pediatr Res* 1988;23:333A.
95. Scott HS, Blanch L, Guo XH, et al. Cloning of the sulphamidase gene and identification of mutations in Sanfilippo A syndrome. *Nature Genet* 1995;11:465–467.
96. Seidner G, Garcia-Alvarez M, Yeh J-I, et al. GLUT-1 deficiency syndrome caused by haploinsufficiency of the blood-brain barrier hexose carrier. *Nat Genet* 1998;18:188–191.
97. Seitelberger F. Eine unbekannte form von infantiler lipoid-speicher krankheit des gehirns. In: *Proceedings of the 1st International Congress of Neuropathology, Rome, September 8–13, 1952.* Turin: Rosenberg and Sellier, 1954:323–333.
98. Seshia SS, Perry TL, Dakshinamurti K, et al. Tyrosinemia and intractable seizures. *Epilepsia* 1984;25:457–463.
99. Shalata A, Mandel H, Reiss J, et al. Localization of a gene for molybdenum cofactor deficiency, on the short arm of chromosome 6, by homozygosity mapping. *Am J Hum Genet* 1998; 63:148–154.
100. Sidbury JB Jr, Smith EK, Harlan W. An inborn error of short-chain fatty acid metabolism: the odor-of-sweaty-feet syndrome. *J Pediatr* 1967;70:8–15.
101. Silva ML, Cieuta C, Guerrini R, et al. Early clinical and EEG features of infantile spasms in Down syndrome. *Epilepsia* 1996;37:977–982.
102. Singh R, Sutherland GR, Manson J. Partial seizures with focal epileptogenic electroencephalographic patterns in three related female patients with fragile-X syndrome. *J Child Neurol* 1999;14:108–112.
103. Sleat DE, Donnelly RJ, Lackland H, et al. Associations of mutations in a lysosomal protein with classical late infantile neuronal ceroid lipofuscinosis. *Science* 1997;277:1802–1805.
104. So N, Kuzniecky R, Berkovic S, et al. Electrophysiological studies in myoclonus epilepsy with ragged-red fibers (MERRF). [Abstract]. *Electroencephalogr Clin Neurophysiol* 1988;69:50P.
105. Somer M, Sainio K. Epilepsy and the electroencephalogram in progressive encephalopathy with edema, hypsarrhythmia, and optic atrophy (the PEHO syndrome). *Epilepsia* 1993;34:727–731.
106. Stafstrom CE, Patxot OF, Gilmore HE, et al. Seizures in children with Down syndrome: etiology, characteristics and outcome. *Dev Med Child Neurol* 1991;33:191–200.
107. Stibler H, Gylje H, Uller A. A neurodystrophic syndrome resembling carbohydrate-deficient glycoprotein syndrome type III. *Neuropediatrics* 1999;30:90–92.
108. Stibler H, Westerberg B, Hanefield F, et al. Carbohydrate-deficient glycoprotein (CDG) syndrome: a new variant, type III. *Neuropediatrics* 1993;24:51–52.
109. Stigsby B, Yarworth SM, Rahbeeni Z, et al. Neurophysiologic correlates of organic acidemias: a survey of 107 patients. *Brain Dev* 1994;16(Suppl):125–144.
110. Suzuki Y, Aoki Y, Ishida Y, et al. Isolation and characterization of mutations in the human holocarboxylase synthetase cDNA. *Nature Genet* 1994;8:122–128.
111. Swaiman KF: Aminoacidopathies and organic acidemias resulting from deficiency of enzyme activity and transport abnormalities. In: Swaiman KF, Ashwal S, eds. *Pediatric neurology: principles and practice,* 3rd ed. St. Louis: Mosby, 1996:377–410.
112. Sztriha L, Janaky M, Kiss J, et al. Electrophysiological and 99mTc-HMPAO-SPECT studies in Menkes disease. *Brain Dev* 1994;16:224–228.
113. Takahasi Y, Suzuki Y, Kamazaki K, et al. Epilepsy in peroxisomal diseases. *Epilepsia* 1997; 38:182–188.
114. Tayama M, Hashimoto T, Miyazaki M, et al. [Pathophysiology of carbohydrate-deficient glycoprotein syndrome—neuroradiological and neurophysiological study]. [In Japanese]. *No To Hattatsu* 1993;25:537–542.
115. Tharp BR. Unique EEG pattern (comb-like rhythm) in neonatal maple syrup urine disease. *Pediatr Neurol* 1992;8:65–68.
116. Trottier A, Metrakos K, Geoffroy G, et al. A characteristic EEG finding in newborns with maple syrup urine disease (branched-chain keto aciduria). *Electroencephalogr Clin Neurophysiol* 1975;38:108.
117. Tsao CY, Luquette M, Rusin JA, et al. Leigh syndrome, cytochrome c oxidase deficiency and hypsarrhythmia with infantile spasms. *Clin Electroencephalogr* 1997;28:214–217.
118. Tumer Z, Horn N. Menkes disease: recent advances and new aspects. *J Med Genet* 1997;34: 265–274.
119. Van Erven PM, Colon EJ, Gabreels FJ, et al. Neurophysiological studies in the Leigh syndrome. *Brain Dev* 1986;8:590–595.
120. Van Geet C, Jaeken J. A unique pattern of coagulation abnormalities in carbohydrate-deficient glycoprotein syndrome. *Pediatr Res* 1993;33:540–541.
121. Verma NP, Hart ZH, Kooi KA. Electroencephalographic findings in urea-cycle disorders. *Electroencephalogr Clin Neurophys* 1984;57:105–112.
122. Verma NP, Hart ZH, Nigro M. Electrophysiologic studies in neonatal adrenoleukodystrophy. *Electroencephalogr Clin Neurophysiol* 1985;60:7–15.
123. Visser FE, Kuilman M, Oosting J, et al. Use of electroencephalography to detect Alzheimer's disease in Down's syndrome. *Acta Neurol Scand* 1996;94:97–103.
124. Wakai S, Asanuma H, Hayasaka H, et al. Ictal video-EEG analysis of infantile neuroaxonal dystrophy. *Epilepsia* 1994;35:823–826.
125. Wakai S, Asanuma H, Tachi N, et al. Infantile neuroaxonal dystrophy: axonal changes in biopsied muscle tissue. *Pediatr Neurol* 1993;9:309–311.
126. Walton A. A case study of Alper's disease in siblings. *Am J EEG Technol* 1996;36:18–27.
127. Wang AM, Bishop DF, Desnick RJ. Human alpha-*N*-acetylgalactosaminidase-molecular cloning, nucleotide sequence, and expression of a full-length cDNA. Homology with human alpha-galactosidase A suggests evolution from a common ancestral gene. *J Biol Chem* 1990; 265:21859–21866.
128. Wang PJ, Lee WT, Hwu WL, et al. The controversy regarding diagnostic criteria for early myoclonic encephalopathy. *Brain Dev* 1998;20:530–535.
129. Wang S, Nadeau JH, Duncan A, et al. 3-Hydroxy-3-methylglutaryl coenzyme A lyase (HL): cloning and characterization of a mouse liver HL cDNA and subchromosomal mapping of the human and mouse HL genes. *Mamm Genome* 1993;4:382–387.
130. Wiegant J, Galjart NJ, Rapp AK, et al. The gene encoding human protective protein (PPBG) is on chromosome 20. *Genomics* 1991;10:345–349.
131. Willard-Mack CL, Koehler RC, Hirata T, et al. Inhibition of glutamine synthetase reduces ammonia-induced astrocyte swelling in rat. *Neuroscience* 1996;71:589–599.
132. Zafeiriou DI, Anastasiou AL, Michelakaki EM, et al. Early infantile Krabbe disease: deceptively normal magnetic resonance imaging and serial neurophysiological studies. *Brain Dev* 1997;19:488–491.

Chapter 17

Seizures and Epilepsy

Timothy A. Pedley, Anil Mendiratta, and Thaddeus S. Walczak

In spite of the many remarkable advances in the variety and sensitivity of diagnostic techniques since the mid-1970s, electroencephalography (EEG) continues to play a central role in the diagnosis and management of patients with epilepsy. Epilepsy is a disorder of cortical excitability, and the interictal EEG remains the most convenient and least expensive way to demonstrate the physiological manifestations of this. Although the electrocerebral potentials indicating epileptogenic excitability have not changed, clinicians'

ability to interpret these patterns has grown in tandem with the expanding understanding of the manifestations and natural history of different types of epilepsy. In the past, there was considerable controversy about the relationship between interictal epileptiform discharges and the clinical diagnosis of epilepsy. This was often viewed primarily as a problem of sensitivity and specificity, and this issue remains problematic for some authors (112,221). As it became clear that some forms of epilepsy could be identified as rela-

TABLE 17.1. *Uses of electroencephalography in diagnosis and management of epilepsy*

Diagnosis
1. Is a paroxysmal event an epileptic seizure?
2. Is seizure onset focal or generalized?
3. Are seizures a manifestation of an epilepsy syndrome?

Management
1. What is the probability of recurrence after a single, unprovoked seizure?
2. What types of antiseizure drugs are likely to be most effective in this patient?
3. Is the patient a candidate for epilepsy surgery? Can the area of seizure onset be identified?
4. Why has the patient's cognitive function deteriorated?
5. Is the patient's change in behavior caused by non-convulsive status epilepticus?
6. What is the likelihood of recurrent seizures after discontinuation of antiseizure drugs?

tively unique epilepsy syndromes, EEG findings in patients and close family members became one of the key components of syndromic diagnosis. It has also become clear that EEG is more than a diagnostic tool; it can be very helpful in management decisions that commonly face clinicians treating patients with epilepsy. Thus, even in the era of high-resolution anatomical and functional brain imaging, the information provided by routine EEG is as important as ever, if not more so.

This chapter reviews the use of EEG in addressing several basic questions regularly encountered in clinical practice: (a) Does the patient have epilepsy? (b) Are seizures focal or generalized at their onset? (c) Does the patient have a particular epilepsy syndrome (Table 17.1)? This chapter also reviews how EEG can be used to aid in management of patients with epilepsy by using a few common situations as examples.

ELECTROENCEPHALOGRAPHY IN THE DIAGNOSIS OF EPILEPSY

Epilepsy can have protean clinical manifestations, and some of these can be easily confused with those of other medical conditions. Thus, the first question the physician must address is whether the patient's symptoms rep-

resent epileptic seizures or some other disorder. Although the diagnosis of epilepsy remains a clinical judgment, EEG findings, interpreted in the context of other clinical data, are often pivotal in reaching an answer. However, it is important to recognize that different EEG findings have different degrees of association with epilepsy. This basic observation explains, in part, much of the confusion regarding the sensitivity and specificity of interictal EEG. Clinicians may encounter any of the following abnormalities when evaluating a patient with possible seizures: interictal epileptiform discharges (IEDs), focal slowing, periodic lateralized epileptiform discharges (PLEDs), generalized periodic epileptiform discharges (GPEDs), diffuse slowing, and several nonspecific paroxysmal abnormalities (e.g., frontal intermittent rhythmic delta activity) (Fig. 17.1). Among all of these, *only* IEDs and perhaps PLEDs are associated with epilepsy at rates sufficiently high to be clinically useful. The remaining patterns are much less useful in supporting the diagnosis of epilepsy, although they may provide very important information regarding the underlying conditions associated with seizures or epilepsy.

Sensitivity of Interictal Epileptiform Discharges

The sensitivity of IEDs in identifying patients with epilepsy is an important measure of their clinical utility. Sensitivity is determined by asking how often IEDs are seen in people with epilepsy. Many factors influence the appearance of IEDs, and available studies have not usually standardized or controlled for these. Duration and number of EEG studies are probably the most important variables, because IEDs are intermittent phenomena and thus more likely to be detected with more samples and longer sampling times. Other methodological difficulties further limit most studies. In some, diagnostic criteria for epilepsy are not specified or are unclear. Epilepsy is most often a history-based diagnosis, and this diagnosis may be inaccurate, even when made by experienced clinicians. The possibility that the interictal EEG findings themselves influenced the diagnosis of epilepsy is difficult to exclude in many studies, and this could obviously introduce substantial bias. Furthermore, much of the existing data come from epilepsy centers, which tend to see patients with more refractory and complex cases. Finally, different interpreters have used different criteria for visual detection of IEDs. In view of these difficulties, it is reassuring that the results among different studies are reasonably consistent.

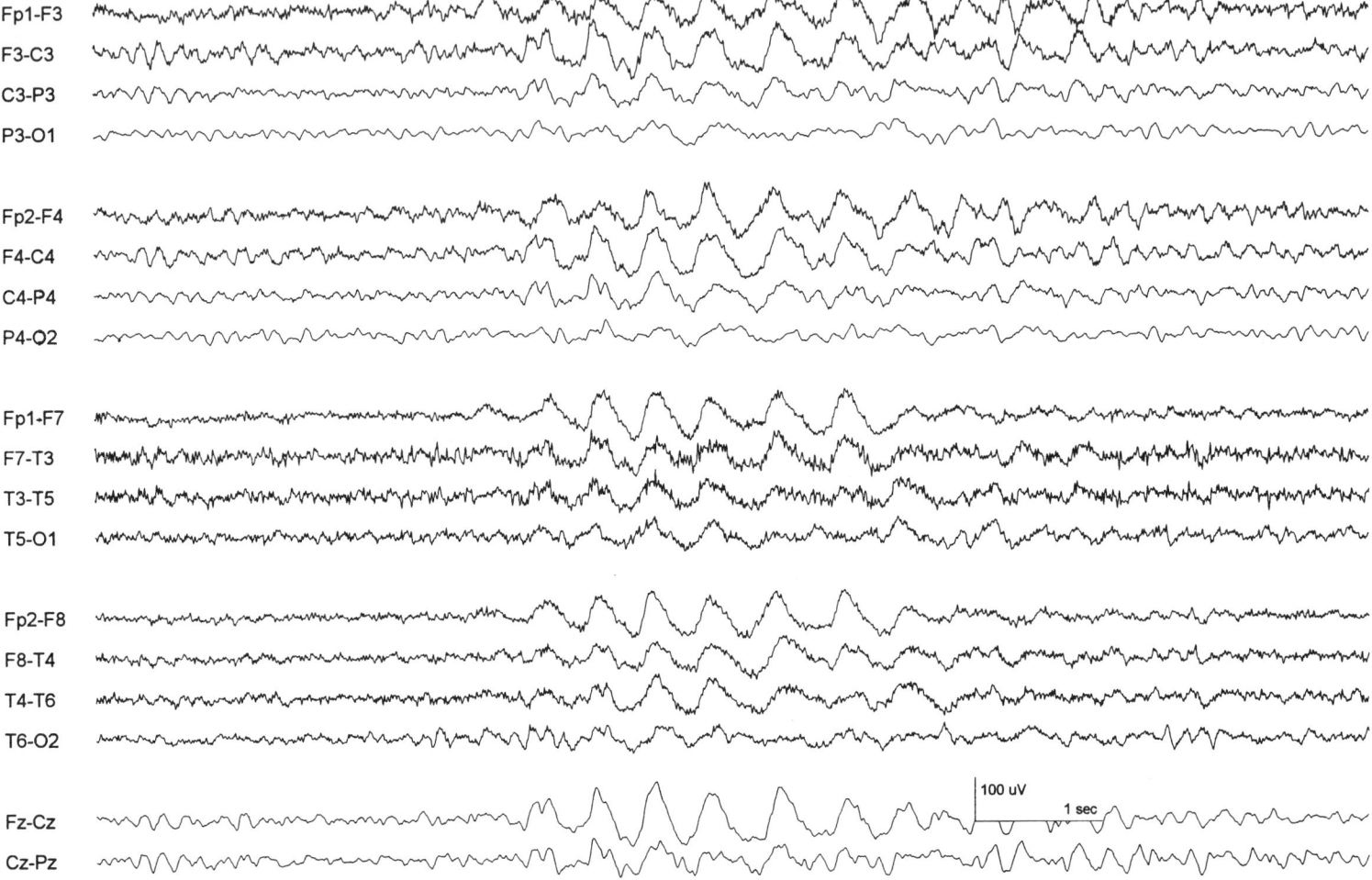

FIG. 17.1. EEG of a 46-year-old man with uremic encephalopathy. The EEG shows 2-Hz frontal intermittent rhythmic delta activity (FIRDA). TC, 0.1 second; HFF, 70 Hz.

In three large studies, mainly of adult patients evaluated at epilepsy centers, initial EEGs detected IEDs in 29% to 55% of patients (117,188,248). Repeated EEGs over varying intervals ultimately demonstrated IEDs in 80% to 90% (188,248). IEDs, if present, were detected by the fourth EEG in 90% of patients (188,248). If the first EEG contained only nonspecific abnormalities (no IEDs), subsequent EEGs were more likely to demonstrate IEDs (248). In another approach (292), adult patients undergoing video-EEG monitoring were screened continuously for IEDs with standard IED detection software. Because the analysis was confined to patients with recorded seizures, the diagnosis was not influenced by the presence of IEDs. Of patients with seizures (average recording duration, 6.9 days), 19% did not have IEDs.

Studies of patients who have experienced only one seizure or of patients for whom antiepileptic drugs were being withdrawn provide information about the prevalence of IEDs in patients with infrequent seizures. Although such studies have less selection bias, the diagnosis of epilepsy was often less secure. In addition, those studies were not designed to evaluate EEGs, and so fewer details are available. What is known is that 12% to 50% of such patients had IEDs recorded during the initial EEG (Table 17.2). Nonepileptiform abnormalities occurred in 6% to 45%, and EEGs were normal in 32% to 74% (see Table 17.2). In two studies (161,285), mainly of adult patients with single seizures, researchers examined the yield of repeated EEGs.

EEGs were repeated if no IEDs were found on the first recording, and these subsequent EEGs captured IEDs in an additional 14% to 18% of such cases. This increased the total yield after two EEGs to 26% in the first study (285) and 61% in the second (161). The wide variability reported in detecting IEDs in patients with infrequent seizures may result from differences in study populations, from different criteria used for classifying or detecting IEDs, and from the many intrinsic and extrinsic factors that affect the occurrence of IEDs.

Several factors influence the likelihood of recording IEDs in patients with epilepsy. These factors were not controlled for in studies in which the sensitivity of IED was evaluated; as a result, they probably account for much of the variability in the findings. IEDs are recorded more frequently in children than in adults, and IEDs are more frequent when epilepsy begins earlier in life (188). Epilepsy syndrome diagnosis also plays a role. For example, IEDs are almost invariably present in children with untreated infantile spasms, Landau-Kleffner syndrome, and benign rolandic epilepsy. Sleep, sleep deprivation, and use of additional recording electrodes also improve detection of IEDs (see Chapter 8), and these were not used consistently in the different studies. In one study, researchers found that greater seizure frequency was associated with an increased likelihood of recording IEDs (188), but in another, researchers obtained opposite results (292). This discrepancy probably arose because the first series included many children, whereas the sec-

TABLE 17.2. *Yield of initial EEG in patients with infrequent seizures*

	Number of patients	Age	Percentage with IED	Percentage with non-IED (abnormal)	Percentage normal
Patients with first unprovoked seizure					
Hopkins et al. (136)	408	Adult	26.8%	26.8%	46.4%
FIRST Group (232)	397	Mixed	50%	6%	44%
Van Donselaar et al. (285)	157	Adult	12%	45%	43%
King et al. (161)	300	Mixed	43%	25%	32%
Shinnar et al. (258)	283	Pediatric	28%	10%	63%
Patients being withdrawn from antiseizure drugs					
Callaghan et al. (44)	92	Mixed	—	—	74%
Shinnar et al. (260)	88	Pediatric	18%	—	49%
Emerson et al. (85)	68	Pediatric	—	—	50%

IED, interictal epileptiform discharge.

ond was performed only in adults. Proximity of the EEG recording to clinical seizure activity seems also to be important, as results of other studies of patients with intractable epilepsy report that IEDs occur more frequently immediately after a seizure (118). In patients who had experienced only one seizure, IEDs were also found more often when the EEG was obtained within 24 hours of the seizure (51%) than when the EEG was obtained later (34%) (161).

In some situations, antiepileptic drugs can affect the likelihood of recording IEDs. The studies just cited did not distinguish among effects caused by the patient's state or by the antiepileptic drug regimen. Furthermore, these studies emphasized findings in patients with frequent IEDs, because effects are easier to demonstrate with a higher baseline IED rate. The effects of antiepileptic drugs on IED are briefly summarized as follows (further details are available in Chapter 15 and in other reviews [12,254]). Benzodiazepines and barbiturates consistently decrease the occurrence of IEDs after acute administration, but this effect wanes with chronic therapy. Acute barbiturate withdrawal may provoke generalized epileptiform discharges or trigger focal discharges in areas from which the habitual epileptogenic abnormality does not originate. Neither chronic phenytoin nor carbamazepine treatment seems to affect either the occurrence or distribution of IEDs in any consistent way. Valproate suppresses generalized spike-wave discharges. In one study (40,286), generalized IEDs were decreased in frequency in 76% of patients ten weeks after valproate treatment began. One year later, discharges remained less frequent in 57% of the patients. Similarly, photoparoxysmal responses were eliminated in 25% of patients ten weeks after they started taking valproate; after 1 year of treatment, photosensitivity was absent in 75% of the patients. Valproate-induced suppression of the photoparoxysmal response persists even after the drug is no longer detectable in the plasma. Although treatment with benzodiazepines, barbiturates, and valproate clearly decreases the amount of recordable IEDs, it is not usually necessary to discontinue these drugs for routine EEGs obtained for diagnostic purposes. In contrast, medication withdrawal is often necessary to facilitate recording of seizures during continuous video-EEG monitoring.

Even after all these factors are considered, EEGs of some patients with epilepsy still lack IEDs. The persistent lack of IED in a minority of patients with an unambiguous diagnosis of epilepsy continues to trouble many physicians. Several explanations can be offered. IEDs may be very infrequent and therefore are not detected even with lengthy recordings. IEDs may be present but not detectable by conventional scalp recordings and montages (1).

The relatively small area of cortex involved in generating the epileptiform activity and the resistive properties of the overlying dura and scalp are partly responsible for this inability to detect IEDs. Furthermore, some areas of cortex, such as the opercular, subfrontal, interhemispheric, and medial temporal areas, are not directly accessible to scalp recording techniques. Therefore, IEDs originating in these areas may not be detected with standard scalp electrodes. Finally, some people with epilepsy apparently lack IEDs, inasmuch as IEDs are not detectable even when intracranial electrodes are used, although such patients are rare. Further study of the pathogenesis of IEDs and of epileptic patients without IEDs should help define characteristics of such patients and explain why this unusual circumstance occurs.

Specificity of Interictal Epileptiform Discharges

How specific IEDs are for epilepsy is another measure of their clinical utility. Specificity is determined by asking how often IEDs occur in normal subjects in comparison with patients with epilepsy. Studies of this issue have all reported that IEDs are rare in EEGs of persons without a history of seizures. Persons with IEDs but without epilepsy at the time of EEG recording seem to have a greater likelihood of developing epilepsy in the future. Occurrence of IEDs in nonepileptic subjects is influenced by the subject's age, the subject's general medical condition, and the circumstances of EEG recording. Only one study was community based (49); some degree of patient selection bias was present in the remainder.

Table 17.3 summarizes available data, and several trends are evident. Among healthy subjects without epilepsy, IEDs are more common in children (1.9 to 3.5%) than in adults (0.5%). Seizures are more likely to develop if IEDs are encountered in a healthy child than if they are encountered in a healthy adult (see also Thorn [277]). In hospitalized adults without neurological or psychiatric disease, the prevalence of IEDs is similar to that found in healthy people (20). As might be expected, the prevalence of IEDs is higher in hospitalized patients with neurological illness but without epilepsy than in adults hospitalized with other conditions (313), probably because the neurologically ill patients included those with cerebral neoplasms, stroke, and craniotomies. Similarly, IED prevalence among psychiatric outpatients is higher than among other hospitalized adults (38), perhaps because anorexia and barbiturate withdrawal are more common in this population.

The types of IEDs seen in nonepileptic subjects differ from those seen in large series of patients with epilepsy. Central-midtemporal discharges, gen-

TABLE 17.3. *Prevalence of interictal epileptiform discharge in subjects without epilepsy*

	Number	Age	General condition	Number with IEDs	Number with IEDs developing seizures
Eeg-Olofson et al. (80)	743	1–15	Highly screened	14 (1.9%)	Not reported
Cavazzuti et al. (49)	3,716	6–13	Screened community-based	131 (3.5%)	7/131 (5.3%)
Bennet (20)	424	Adult	Healthy flight personnel	2 (0.5%)	0/1 (0%)
Gregory et al. (122)	13,658	17–25	Healthy flight personnel	69 (0.51%)	1/38 (2.6%)
Bennet (20)	908	Adult	Hospitalized patients, no neurological illness	6 (0.6%)	0/1 (0%)
Zivin et al. (313)	6,497	1–74	Hospitalized patients, including neurological illness	142 (2.2%)	20/142 (14.1%)
Bridgers (38)	3,143	11–85	Psychiatric inpatients	81 (2.6%)	Not reported

IED, interictal epileptiform discharge.

eralized spike-wave discharges, and photoparoxysmal responses account for the great majority of IEDs, especially in children (20,49,80,122). In contrast, focal (especially temporal) or multifocal IEDs predominate in series of patients with epilepsy (142,158,188). The three types of IEDs observed most often in nonepileptic subjects probably have a lower association with epilepsy than do other types of IEDs. Both central-midtemporal IEDs (132) and generalized IEDs (194) can be seen as asymptomatic manifestations of genetic traits, and so their presence may merely be indicative of epilepsy in siblings or other family members. In an EEG laboratory population, only 40% of children whose EEGs contained central-midtemporal spikes had epileptic seizures (158). Patients who have only photoparoxysmal responses develop seizures infrequently (122,257,266).

Sharp transients are frequent in normal newborns. They occur during all states in the preterm neonate, are present mainly during quiet sleep at term, and gradually disappear over the first 6 to 8 weeks of life. Sharp waves are abnormal in full-term newborns if they are numerous, repetitive, persistently focal, or of positive polarity. Only one study has compared features of sharp waves in normal newborns with those occurring in neonates with epilepsy (57). Epileptiform transients were more abundant, more often spikes, more repetitive, and more persistently focal in newborns with epilepsy (57). It is unlikely, however, that these features alone are sufficient to distinguish between neonates with seizures and those with cerebral abnormalities but no seizures. (For more complete discussion, see Chapter 6).

In infants and older children, the association of IEDs with epilepsy seems to vary with location, distribution, and morphological appearance of the IEDs. Multifocal IEDs and IEDs occurring over the midline, frontal, and anterior temporal regions are highly correlated with clinical seizures: 75%

to 95% of patients with these IEDs have epilepsy (82,158). In contrast, only about 40% of patients with central-midtemporal spikes and 50% with occipital spikes had seizures in one study (158). Blindness occurring in infancy may be associated with occipital spikes and, in the study of Smith and Kellaway (263), accounted for 15% of occipital IEDs. Finally, IEDs that occur in both normal (49) and ill (158,176) children tend to disappear over time, but this is less common in adults (142).

Such observations lead to the conclusion that interictal sharp transients, even those of frankly epileptiform configuration, largely reflect unique responses of the immature brain. They can occur as normal findings, especially in preterm infants, or as an indication of cerebral dysfunction that may or may not be associated with seizures. The occurrence and epileptogenic significance of such discharges change with brain maturation. As a result, sharp transients and IEDs are associated with epilepsy less frequently in children. The age at which the degree of association between IEDs and epilepsy reaches that found in adults is unclear. In infants and children, even more so than in adults, it is essential to consider critically the clinical context for which the EEG recording was obtained before concluding that the presence of IEDs supports a diagnosis of epilepsy.

The association between IEDs and epilepsy is much stronger in adults. However, IEDs without a history of clinical seizures may also be found under certain circumstances. EEGs recorded during periods of metabolic disarray may occasionally reveal IEDs. Triphasic waves, seen in various metabolic encephalopathies, can sometimes be difficult to distinguish from generalized epileptiform activity. Focal spikes, multifocal spikes, and diffuse spikes or sharp waves can occur with the dialysis dementia syndrome, uremic encephalopathy, and hypocalcemia (55,205,284). However, seizures are not regularly observed in the majority of patients with these conditions. IEDs can be recorded in nonepileptic patients treated with chlorpromazine, lithium, or clozapine, especially at high doses (133,144). Some, but by no means all, of such patients develop seizures. IEDs disappear when drug dosages are decreased. EEGs obtained in nonepileptic patients during withdrawal of short-acting barbiturates sometimes demonstrate generalized IEDs or prolonged photoparoxysmal responses (300,309). This is less common with longer acting barbiturates (309). Meperidine, especially when used for a long time, can unmask epileptiform discharges, probably because of an excitatory metabolite interacting with a receptive brain substrate (157; personal observation). Finally, IEDs without a history of clinical seizures are occasionally seen in patients with cerebral mass lesions who do not have a history of seizures. These IEDs are most likely to be seen with cerebral abscesses and slow-growing neoplasms such as astrocytomas and oligodendrogliomas. IEDs in these situations presumably indicate a higher risk of seizures, but studies demonstrating this are not available.

Positive Predictive Value of Interictal Epileptiform Discharges

Although general considerations of sensitivity and specificity are important and useful, clinicians are usually most often interested in knowing the likelihood that an individual patient with IEDs has epilepsy. This probability is termed the *positive predictive value* (PPV) of IEDs. The PPV of IEDs for epilepsy is the ratio of the number of subjects with epilepsy who have IEDs to the number of all subjects (those with epilepsy and those without epilepsy) with IEDs. The PPV is dependent on the sensitivity and specificity of the EEG. However, the prevalence of epilepsy in the population under study may be an even more important determinant of the PPV (116). The following examples illustrate how the PPV varies in accordance with the likelihood of encountering epilepsy in the population being studied. Assume that the prevalence of IEDs in the first EEG of a subject with epilepsy is 55%, and that the prevalence of IEDs in the first EEG of a subject without epilepsy is 4% under similar conditions. When studying a random sample of unselected patients drawn from a defined geographic area, assume an epilepsy prevalence rate of 0.5%. Such a sample of 1,000 patients would therefore be expected to include five persons with epilepsy, three of whom would have IED, and 40 people without epilepsy but whose EEGs show IEDs. In this particular situation, the PPV of IEDs for epilepsy would be only 3/43, or 7%. As a second example,

consider a group commonly used for EEG studies: the referral population of a clinical EEG laboratory. In this setting, the likelihood of encountering epilepsy is much higher because of selection. Assume that 50% of patients referred to a hospital's EEG laboratory have epilepsy. Among 1,000 patients with EEGs recorded in this laboratory, 500 would have epilepsy, and 275 of these would have IEDs. Of the 500 patients who would not have epilepsy, 20 would have IEDs. In this setting, the PPV for IED would be very high: 275/295, or 93%.

The PPV can be calculated more generally in terms of the prevalence of epilepsy in a population, the prevalence of IEDs in the epilepsy patients, and the prevalence of IED in the nonepileptic population, as follows:

$$PPV = \frac{(E)\,(IED_E)}{(E)\,(IED_E) + (1-E)\,(IED_{NE})}$$

where E is the prevalence of epilepsy in a population, IED_E is the prevalence of IEDs in epilepsy patients, and IED_{NE} is the prevalence of IEDs in the nonepileptic subjects (116). This equation allows determination of the PPV of the IEDs for epilepsy on the basis of conditions encountered in different populations.

Interictal Epileptiform Discharges

IEDs (Fig. 17.2) are difficult to describe with meaningful accuracy. To be designated IEDs, discharges should meet at least the following criteria (50,224): (a) They must be paroxysmal; that is, they must be clearly set apart from ongoing background activity and not simply a sharply contoured component of a sequence of waves. (b) They must include an abrupt change in polarity occurring over several milliseconds; this results in the sharp contour or "spikiness" of IED. (c) The duration of each transient should be less than 200 milliseconds. The Committee on Terminology distinguishes between "spikes," which have a duration of less than 70 milliseconds, and "sharp waves," whose duration is between 70 and 200 milliseconds. However, the clinical utility of this distinction has not been demonstrated. Whether an epileptiform discharge has the morphological appearance of a "spike" or "sharp wave" depends on many factors, including the synchrony of the epileptic neuronal aggregate, the proximity of the epileptogenic cortical area to the recording electrodes, and extent of spread of the IED within complex polysynaptic pathways before it is detected at the scalp. (d) The discharge must have a physiological field. This generally means that the discharges are recorded from more than one

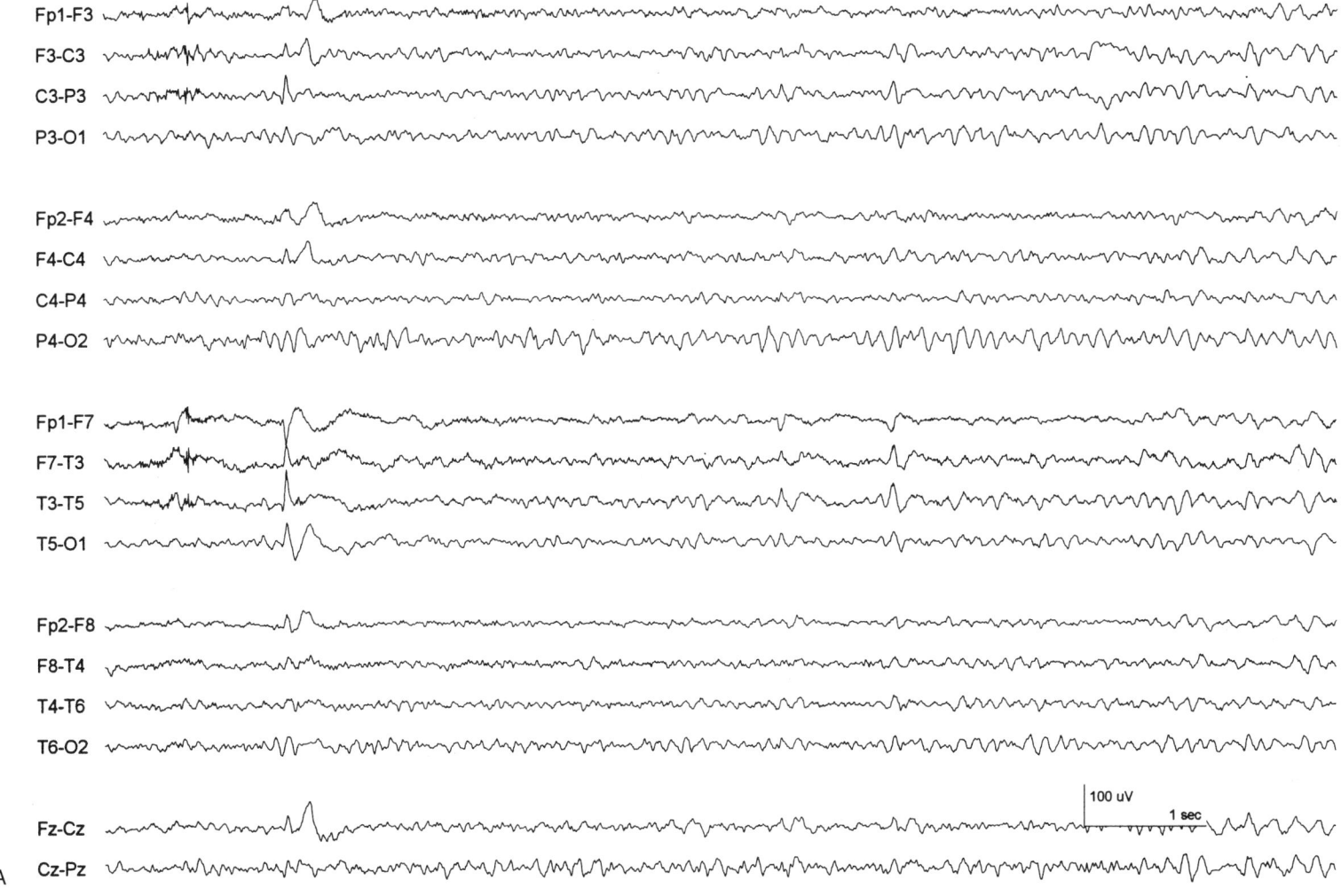

Fp1-F3

F3-C3

C3-P3

P3-O1

Fp2-F4

F4-C4

C4-P4

P4-O2

Fp1-F7

F7-T3

T3-T5

T5-O1

Fp2-F8

F8-T4

T4-T6

T6-O2

100 uV

1 sec

Fz-Cz

Cz-Pz

A

FIG. 17.2. A: EEG of a 22-year-old man with complex partial seizures. The EEG shows mild intermittent left temporal theta activity and anterior temporal epileptiform discharges, which phase reversal at F7. TC, 0.1 second; HFF, 70 Hz. *(Figure continues.)*

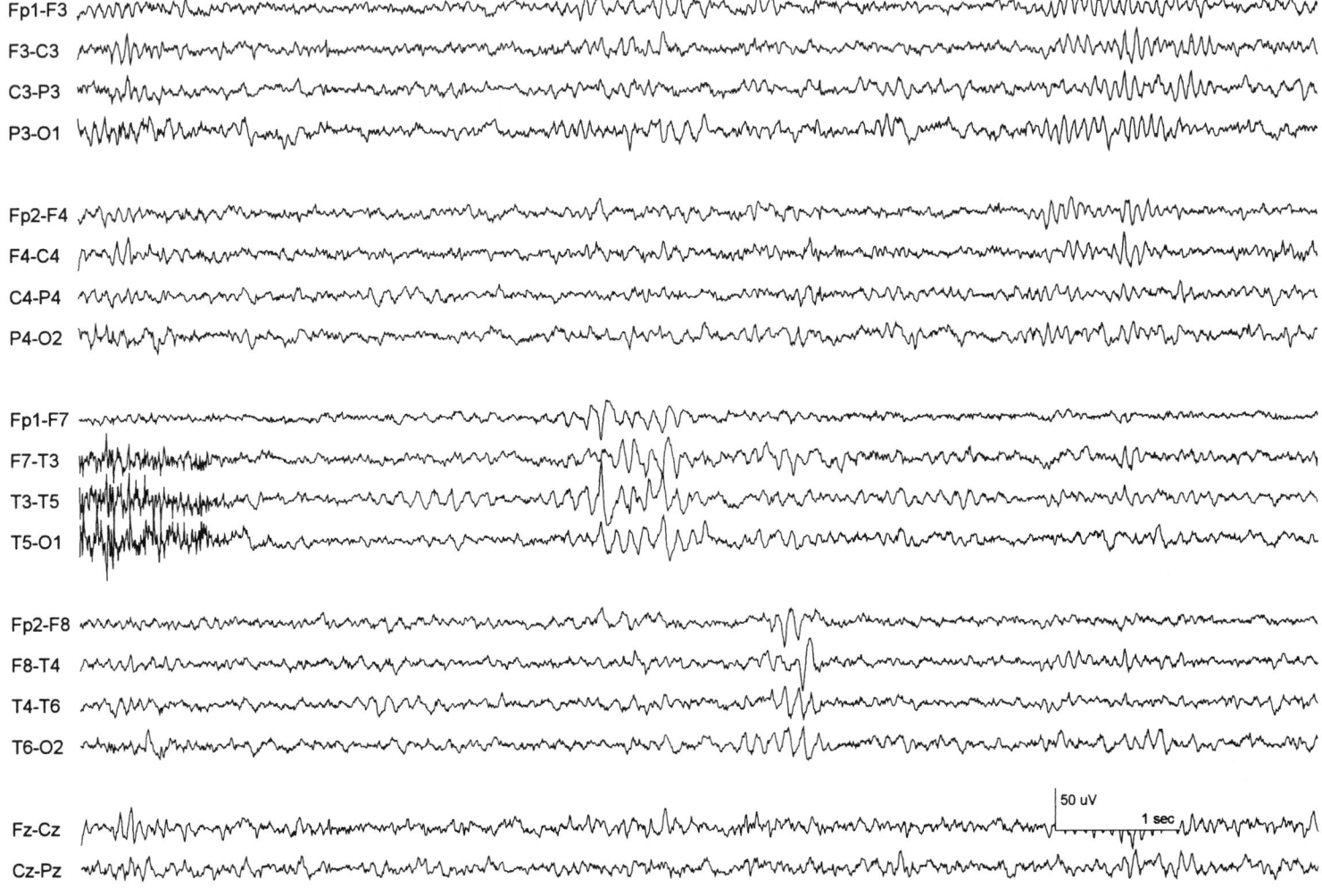

FIG. 17.2. *Continued.* **B:** EEG of a 27-year-old man with no neurological abnormalities. The EEG shows "wicket spikes," a normal variant. Although the waveform is sharply configured, this is not an epileptogenic pattern. (See Chapter 7.) TC, 0.1 second; HFF, 70 Hz.

electrode and typically have a voltage gradient across a region of the scalp. This criterion is particularly useful in distinguishing IEDs from electrode or other artifacts. On occasion, IEDs have very restricted fields, as, for example, in neonates or in children with benign rolandic epilepsy. Additional electrodes can help distinguish IEDs from noncerebral potentials in these situations. In addition to these necessary criteria, the great majority of IEDs are of negative polarity at the scalp, and the majority of IEDs are followed by a slow wave in the range of 2 to 4 Hz. These two features, although not inevitable, are present with sufficient frequency that they are extremely helpful in distinguishing IEDs from other types of paroxysmal activity. Furthermore, they relate closely to the underlying physiological epileptogenic phenomena occurring at the cellular level (see Chapter 1). Within the limitations noted further on, IEDs defined in this manner are highly correlated with epilepsy and are rare in samples of the normal population.

Periodic Lateralized Epileptiform Discharges and Other Periodic Epileptiform Discharges

PLEDs occur most often with acute, usually relatively large, destructive lesions caused by hemorrhagic cerebral infarction or a rapidly growing cerebral malignancy (52,187). The EEG abnormality consists of persistent sharp waves that occur with a nearly regular repetition rate of 0.5 to 2 Hz (Fig. 17.3). PLEDS typically involve a large area of one hemisphere and frequently reflect to homologous regions of the opposite side. They are not sharply focal; hence, the adjective *lateralized.* PLEDs are a transient phenomenon, rarely persisting for more than a few weeks (256), but they are strongly correlated with acute drug-resistant focal seizures during this time. In patients with PLEDs, acute symptomatic seizures occur in about 70% of cases (265). About 20% of patients with PLEDs have preexisting epilepsy (265). Of those without a history of epilepsy, 3% to 66% develop epilepsy after recovering from the acute cerebral injury (255,293,312). In children, PLEDs are more often seen in the setting of seizures and various chronic diffuse encephalopathies (223). De La Paz and Brenner (65) described bilateral independent PLEDs (BiPLEDs). These occur most often with acute infections of the nervous system (especially herpes simplex encephalitis), anoxic encephalopathy, and severe chronic epilepsy. Seizures occur in 55% of affected patients, but 22% have preexisting epilepsy (65). Because the mortality rate is high among patients with BiPLEDs, there is no information on how often epilepsy develops in survivors. Generalized rather than focal seizures predominate in this group. GPEDs are sometimes recorded in patients with severe bilateral brain damage, especially when caused by anoxia, Creutzfeldt-Jakob disease, and refractory status epilepticus. To what extent GPEDs are correlated with the seizures that are common to these conditions is not known. Additional information about periodic epileptiform discharges can be found in Chapters 11 and 14.

Nonepileptiform Electroencephalographic Findings in Epilepsy

Focal slow-wave activity and generalized slowing of background rhythms are common findings in patients with partial seizures and symptomatic epilepsies. However, such findings are also frequent in patients with other neurological disorders, especially focal structural lesions, regardless of whether there are associated seizures. Thus, their specificity and positive predictive value for epilepsy are relatively low. For example, a structural lesion is present in two-thirds of adults with continuous focal polymorphic delta activity, but seizures occur in only about 20% (110). Of patients with continuous focal polymorphic delta activity and no evidence of a structural lesion, seizures occur in more than 50% (110,189). Focal structural lesions are found in only half of children with focal polymorphic delta activity, and only 23% of those without structural abnormalities have epilepsy (192). Transient focal slowing is common after partial and secondarily generalized seizures (156,291), but it is also a frequent interictal finding that localizes to the epileptogenic brain area. Focal interictal slow activity can reflect inhibition evoked by undetected epileptiform discharges occurring deep in the brain (1,63,99) or pathological changes—such as neuronal loss and gliosis, abnormalities of dendrites, axonal spouting, and changes in neurotransmitters—that are common in chronic epileptogenic foci (for review, see Farrell and Vinters [90]).

A particular form of focal slowing that is more specific and predictive of temporal lobe epilepsy is temporal intermittent *rhythmic* delta activity (TIRDA) (Fig. 17.4). TIRDA is distinct from the more common *polymorphic* delta activity, in which frequencies and amplitudes are more variable. TIRDA is found in only 0.3% of all recordings obtained in a general EEG laboratory (206) but in as many as 28% of patients being evaluated for temporal lobe resection (107). TIRDA is often associated with temporal IEDs, and it has a high PPV for temporal lobe epilepsy (107,206,241).

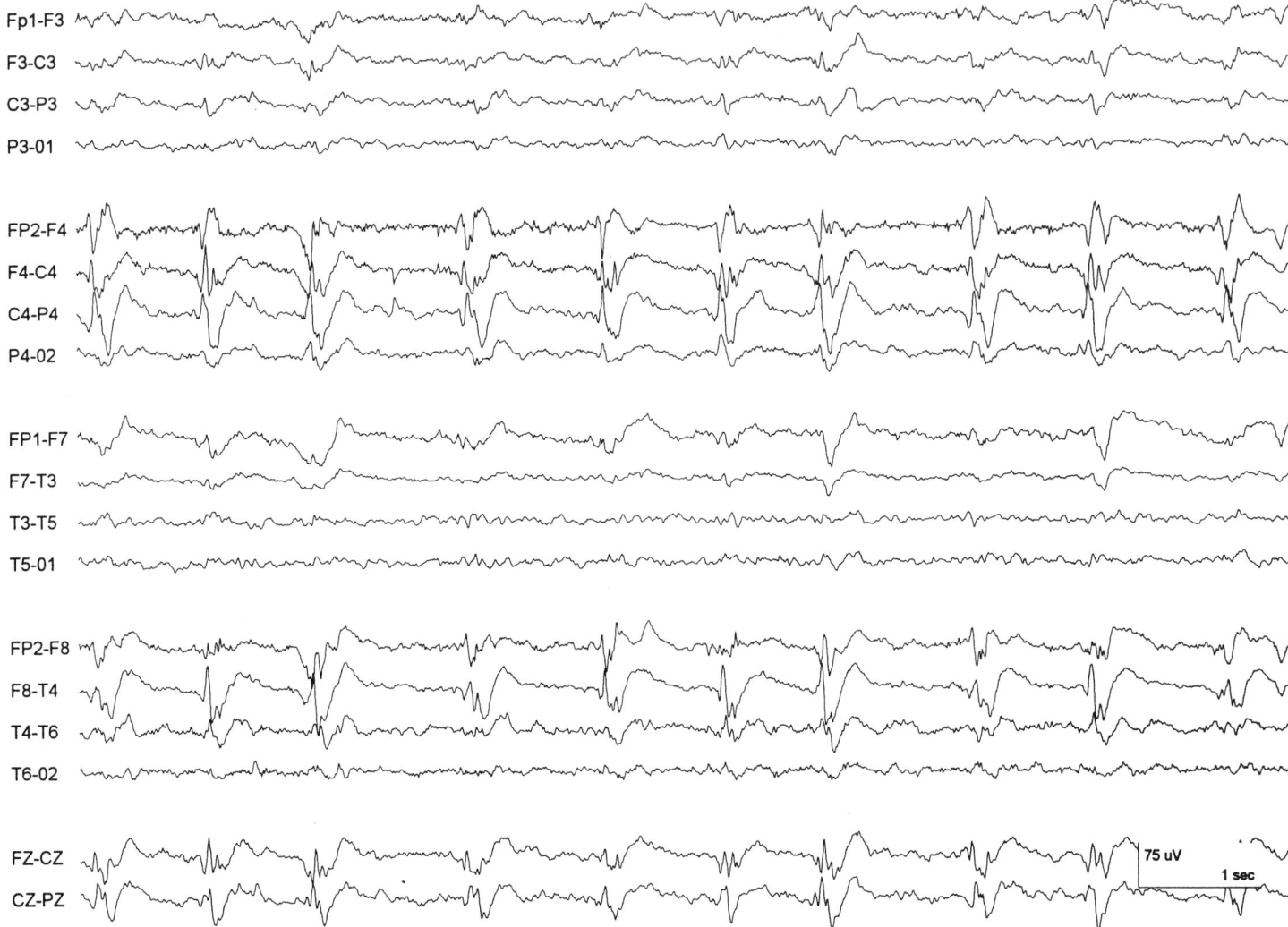

FIG. 17.3. Periodic lateralized epileptiform discharges (PLEDs). EEG of a 78-year-old woman with generalized convulsive seizures after acute infarction of the right middle cerebral artery territory. There are broadly distributed right hemisphere spikes and sharp waves, occurring repetitively at about 1 Hz (PLEDs). TC, 0.1 second; HFF, 70 Hz.

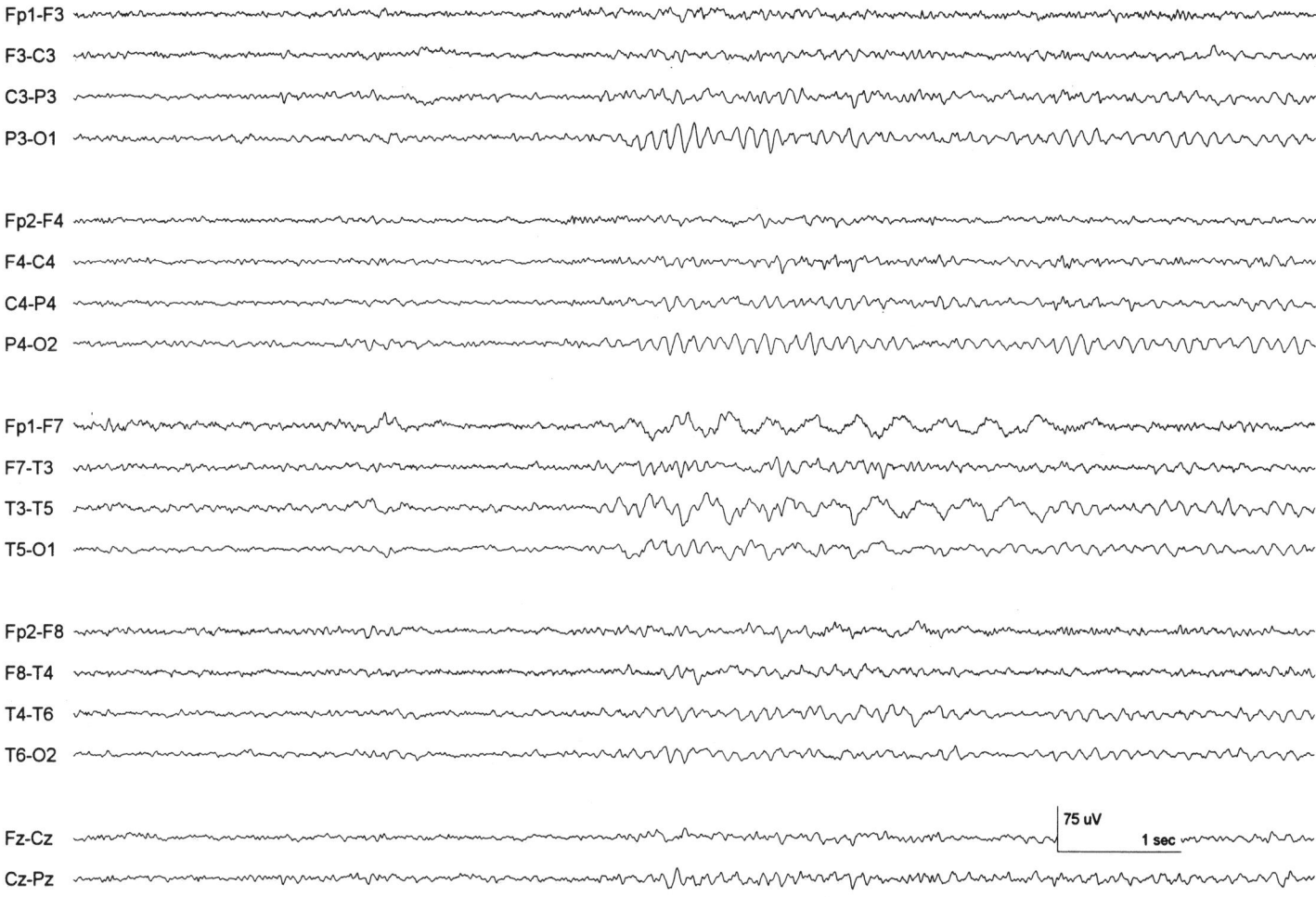

Fp1-F3

F3-C3

C3-P3

P3-O1

Fp2-F4

F4-C4

C4-P4

P4-O2

Fp1-F7

F7-T3

T3-T5

T5-O1

Fp2-F8

F8-T4

T4-T6

T6-O2

Fz-Cz

Cz-Pz

75 uV

1 sec

FIG. 17.4. EEG of a 75-year-old man with complex partial seizures. Previous EEGs had shown left temporal spikes. This EEG demonstrates 2.5-Hz left temporal intermittent rhythmic delta activity (TIRDA). TC, 0.1 second; HFF, 70 Hz.

EPILEPSY SYNDROMES

Identifying the type of epilepsy or "epilepsy syndrome" is important for optimal management and for advising patients and families about prognosis. After the medical history, EEG findings provide the most important information necessary for syndromic diagnosis. The Classification of Epilepsy Syndromes (228) includes more than 24 entities, some of which have engendered controversy. More detailed descriptions (245) have entailed the use of specific features of EEG abnormalities to define syndromes. Because EEG findings are an integral part of syndrome classification, critical analysis of sensitivity, specificity, and predictive value of different EEG features is not possible. Nonetheless, EEG remains very useful in prompting consideration of a particular type of epilepsy and in distinguishing among several possible syndromes in complicated or confusing clinical situations.

Characteristics of the Major Categories of Epilepsy Syndromes

The Classification of Epilepsy Syndromes is based on two distinctions: first, between localization-related and generalized epilepsies and, second, between idiopathic and symptomatic epilepsies. EEG findings assist in making these distinctions. Focal IEDs are seen in localization-related epilepsies, whereas generalized IEDs indicate one of the generalized epilepsies. In the localization-related epilepsies, the location of IEDs usually corresponds approximately to the area of seizure onset, but there are exceptions (described later). Normal or near-normal background activity is most characteristic of idiopathic epilepsy syndromes; focal, multifocal, or diffuse abnormalities of background activity are most suggestive of the symptomatic epilepsies. Persistent focal voltage attenuation, especially of faster frequencies, or polymorphic delta activity is correlated strongly with a structural lesion as the cause of symptomatic epilepsy. These general guidelines help focus initial clinical impressions and prompt a search for the more specific EEG findings associated with the particular epilepsy syndromes.

Specific Epilepsy Syndromes

Childhood and Juvenile Absence Epilepsy

Clinical Features

The International Classification of Epilepsy Syndromes distinguishes between childhood and juvenile onset forms of absence epilepsy. Childhood absence epilepsy (CAE) manifests between the ages of 3 and 12 years. Absence seizures are frequent, often occurring in clusters, a phenomenon known as *pyknolepsy*. In contrast, generalized tonic-clonic seizures are infrequent, and remission by late adolescence is the rule (179). Juvenile absence epilepsy (JAE) manifests at the ages of 10 to 12 years (or later). Absence seizures are less frequent, and generalized tonic-clonic seizures more frequent, than in CAE. Remission is less likely to occur, and seizures often persist into adulthood (307). Such distinctions, although generally applicable to large numbers of patients, are not always clear in individual patients. In addition, the clinical features of JAE overlap with those of two other syndromes: tonic clonic seizures upon awakening and juvenile myoclonic epilepsy. EEG features of CAE and JAE are also broadly similar. Minor differences, however, can sometimes be diagnostically useful.

Electroencephalographic Findings

The classic EEG finding in CAE is the 3-Hz spike-and-slow-wave discharge (Fig. 17.5). Historically, this pattern has been described as consisting of a bisynchronous and symmetrical surface-negative spike that is of maximal voltage in the frontal-central regions. The spike is followed by a surface-negative slow wave. However, careful visual and computerized analyses demonstrate a more complex situation. Depending on electrode location, the duration of the spike-wave paroxysm, and whether a bipolar or referential montage is used, up to three spikes of varying polarity are recorded before the negative slow wave (243,297). The less obvious spike components are of lower voltage and best visualized laterally with the use of referential montages. Consequently, a longitudinal bipolar montage that emphasizes parasagittal regions leaves the impression of a single negative spike and wave. Inspection of the complex through oscillographic or other high-resolution displays reveal that the 3-Hz spike-wave discharge is not truly bisynchronous; rather, spike onset in one hemisphere randomly precedes that of the other by a few milliseconds (243). (Distinguishing primary generalized epileptiform activity from secondary bilateral synchrony is discussed further on p. 570.) Finally, a prolonged surface-negative change in the direct current (DC) potential begins at the onset of each burst and reaches maximal voltage in about 1.5 seconds (53). These observations suggest multiple discrete, albeit linked, sites of cortical onset. Such findings must be accounted for by any theory seeking to explain the origin of the 3-Hz spike-wave discharge. Studies in which magnetoencephalographic imaging and functional magnetic resonance imaging were used have confirmed that several cortical areas are activated during 3-Hz spike-wave bursts (244,294).

Spike-wave frequency varies during the discharge, averaging 3.4 to 4.5 Hz at onset and gradually slowing to an average of 2.5 to 2.8 Hz by the end of the paroxysm (64,218). Eye opening and alerting may terminate the bursts (127). Non–rapid-eye-movement (NREM) sleep increases the number of spike-wave bursts but typically changes their morphological appearance, often dramatically (Fig. 17.6). During sleep, spike-wave discharges are of briefer duration and become fragmented and irregular (250). The repetition rate is usually slower than in the waking state, and polyspike components are common (250). During rapid-eye-movement (REM) sleep, the frequency and morphological appearance of the spike-wave complexes are similar to those of wakefulness, but the duration and number of bursts are somewhat less (246,250). Hyperventilation increases 3-Hz spike-wave bursts in 50% to 80% of patients with CAE, especially if occipital intermittent rhythmic delta activity (OIRDA) is present (64,251). Photic stimulation increases spike-wave bursts in about 18% of cases (307). Valproic acid and ethosuximide typically decrease the number of spike-wave bursts; these bursts cease completely in one-third to one-half of patients treated with either drug (40,252). Both medications also eliminate or greatly attenuate activation by photic stimulation (129).

The distinction between an interictal burst of generalized spike-wave activity and an absence seizure has important clinical implications, but it remains confusing to many. Several studies reported that clinically overt absence seizures averaged 12 seconds in duration (64,179,218) and rarely exceeded 40 seconds and that the spike-wave frequency slowed as the ictal discharge progressed. However, the practical questions are (a) how often cognitive impairment occurs during spike-wave bursts not associated with an obvious absence seizure and (b) whether impairment is related to the duration of the burst of spike-wave activity. Several investigators have carefully analyzed auditory reaction times and demonstrated that about 50% of responses were delayed at the onset of a generalized spike-wave burst. In 80% of responses, the delay occurred within 2 seconds of onset. The degree of responsiveness improved during the remainder of the spike-wave burst, but no more than half of response times were normal at any point. Responsiveness returned abruptly to normal when the burst ended (39,227). A particularly important finding was that responsiveness was equally likely to be impaired in shorter (<3-second) and longer (>3-second) spike-wave paroxysms (39). These data indicate that spike-wave bursts can impair responsiveness regardless of their duration,

depending on the sensitivity of the test used. The therapeutic implication of such findings is that treatment should aim at controlling all spike-wave bursts as much as possible. Duration of bursts also remains important, because longer bursts imply longer periods of altered responsiveness, and duration of impairment is often clinically important. Because valproic acid and ethosuximide decrease the number and duration of generalized spike-wave activity, longer EEG recordings can be used to gauge the efficacy of treatment.

Interictal background activity is usually normal in both CAE and JAE, although minor degrees of slowing have been reported in heterogeneous groups of children (135,251). High-voltage OIRDA is a frequent interictal finding, occurring in 15% to 38% of all patients with absence epilepsy (64,135) (Fig. 17.7). However, the occurrence of OIRDA is strongly age-related: it is found in more than 70% of children between 6 and 10 years of age, and it is rare in persons older than 15 years (64). It is also rare in children with atypical absence seizures (135). Thus, OIRDA is more strongly associated with CAE than with JAE. OIRDA is predictive of activation of generalized spike-wave activity by hyperventilation. OIRDA is distinguished from posterior slow waves of youth by its high-voltage, prominent rhythmicity, persistence, and disruption of the alpha rhythm. However, both OIRDA and posterior slow waves of youth attenuate with eye opening and increase with hyperventilation (59,64).

Ictal EEG recordings during generalized tonic-clonic seizures have shown that the first visually detectable change is usually the appearance of generalized low-voltage beta activity that decreases in frequency (often to 10 Hz or so) as it assumes an increasingly "spiky" configuration and increases in voltage. This electrographic pattern is typically associated with the tonic portion of the seizure. Slower frequencies then appear, developing into repetitive complexes of polyspike and wave activity, which are associated with the clonic portion of the seizure. Immediately after the seizure, EEG voltage is markedly and symmetrically attenuated, but low-voltage polymorphic slow frequencies gradually appear, followed by higher voltage faster and more rhythmic activity as the patient recovers. Normal background activity may not be observed for 30 minutes to 24 hours.

As already noted, EEG findings in CAE and JAE are similar. Background activity is usually normal in both types. OIRDA is uncommon in JAE. The repetition rate of generalized spike-wave bursts is faster at onset in JAE than in CAE, and polyspikes are seen more often in JAE (218). Hyperventilation activates spike-wave activity with equal frequency in CAE and JAE, but photic stimulation is less activating in JAE than in CAE (308).

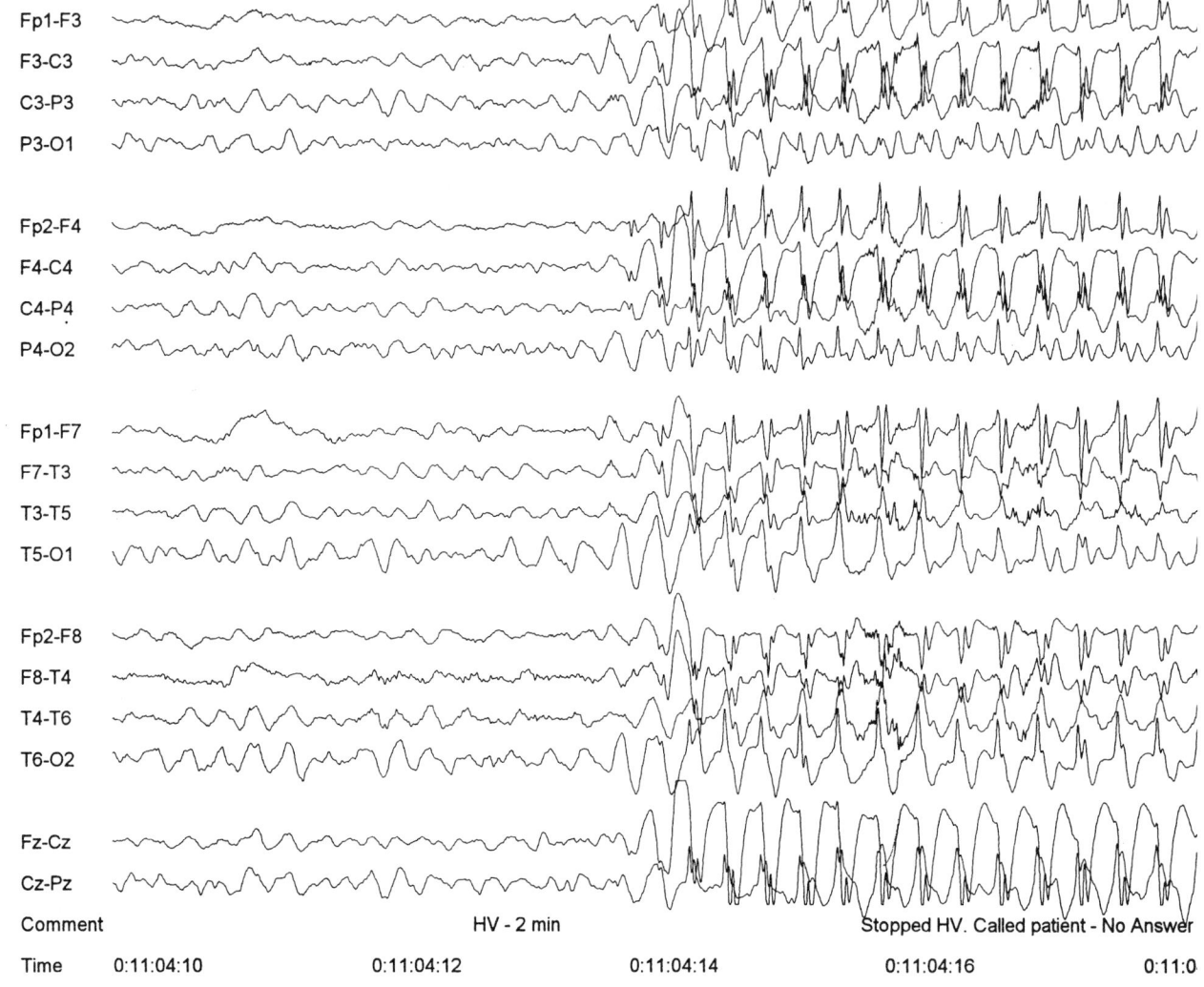

Fp1-F3

F3-C3

C3-P3

P3-O1

Fp2-F4

F4-C4

C4-P4

P4-O2

Fp1-F7

F7-T3

T3-T5

T5-O1

Fp2-F8

F8-T4

T4-T6

T6-O2

Fz-Cz

Cz-Pz

Comment   HV - 2 min   Stopped HV. Called patient - No Answer

A   Time   0:11:04:10   0:11:04:12   0:11:04:14   0:11:04:16   0:11:0

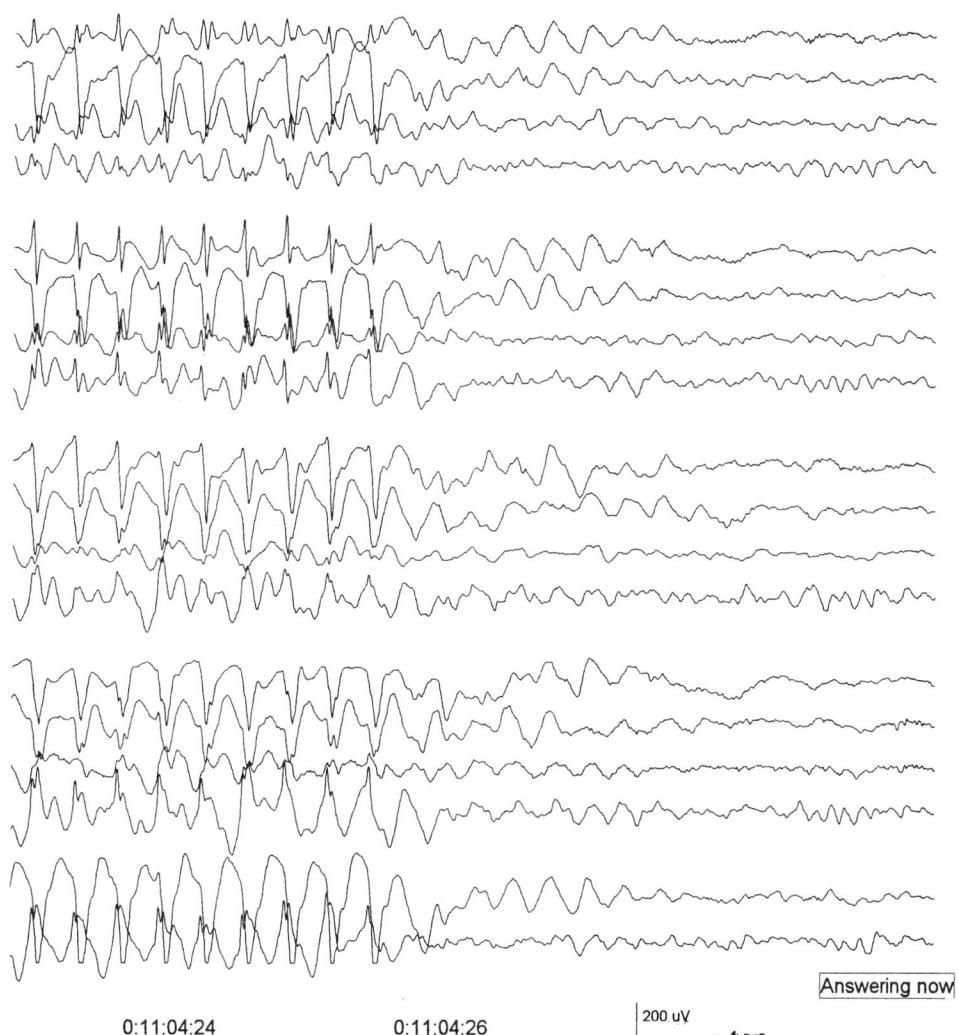

0:11:04:24   0:11:04:26

Answering now

200 uV

1 sec

FIG. 17.5. EEG of a 6-year-old girl with absence seizures. After 2 minutes of hyperventilation, she had a typical absence seizure. The EEG shows the abrupt onset of bilateral synchronous 3-Hz spike-wave discharges lasting 12 seconds (note 5-second break in EEG recording). She began responding normally as soon as the discharge ended. **A:** Longitudinal bipolar montage. TC, 0.1 second; HFF, 70 Hz. *(Figure continues.)*

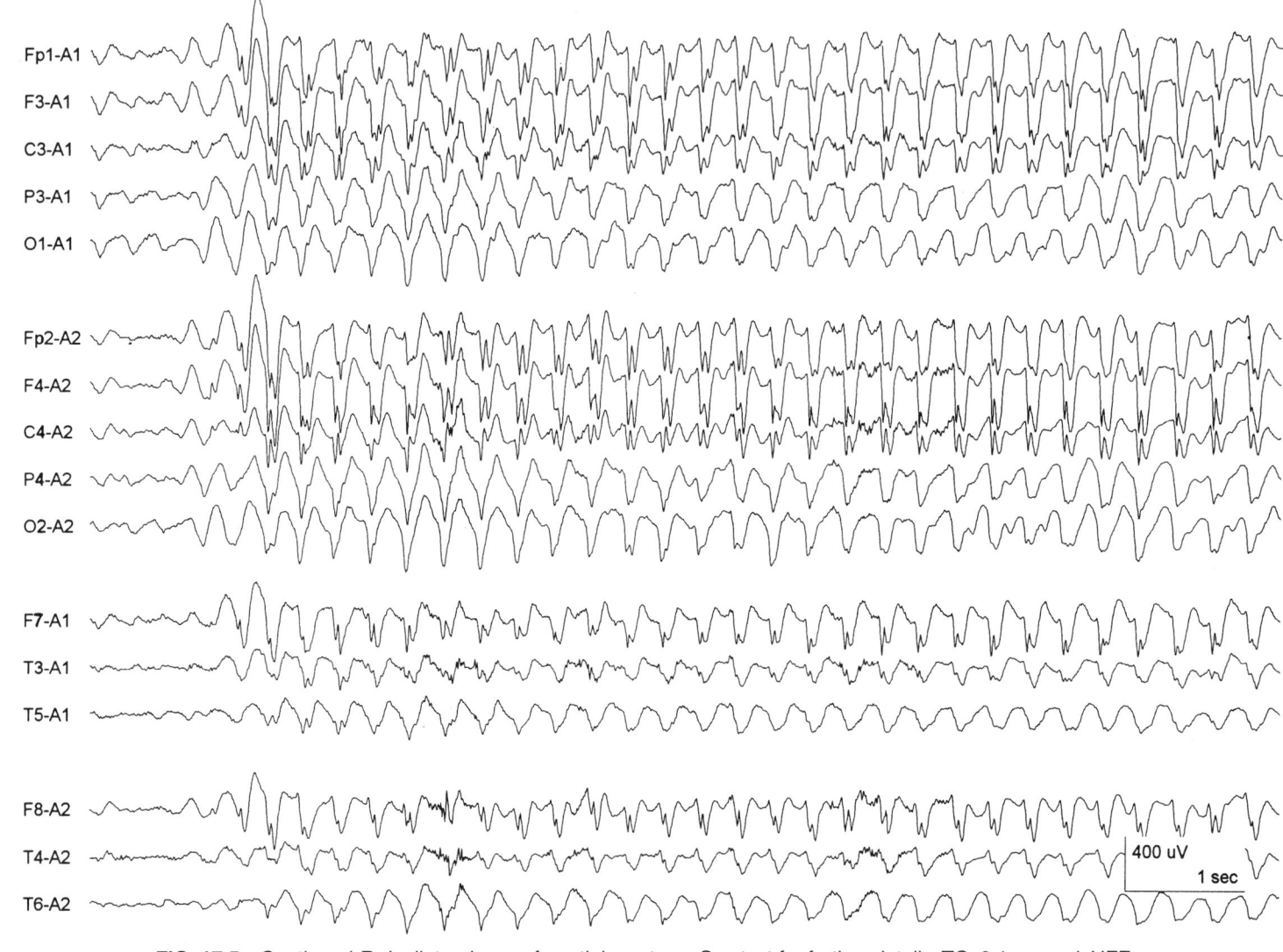

FIG. 17.5. *Continued.* **B:** Ipsilateral ear referential montage. See text for further details. TC, 0.1 second. HFF, 70 Hz.

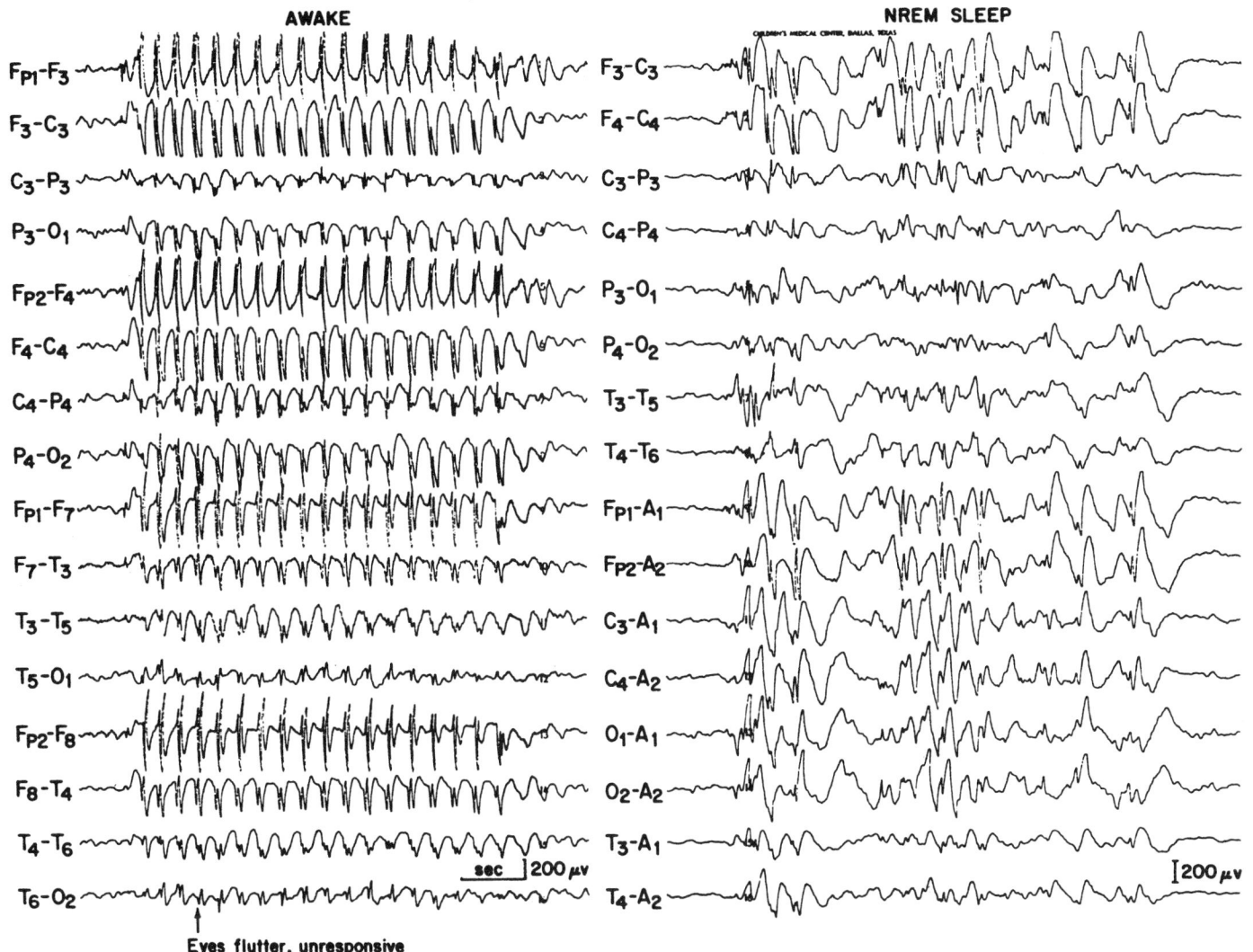

FIG. 17.6 Three-hertz (3Hz) spike-wave complexes in a 7-year-old girl with typical absence seizures. **Left:** While awake, the child had a spontaneous absence seizure. Her eyes fluttered, she did not respond to a test phrase, and she was unaware that she had had a seizure. **Right:** Generalized spike-wave discharges during NREM sleep. Note change in spike-wave morphological appearance during sleep (see text for discussion).

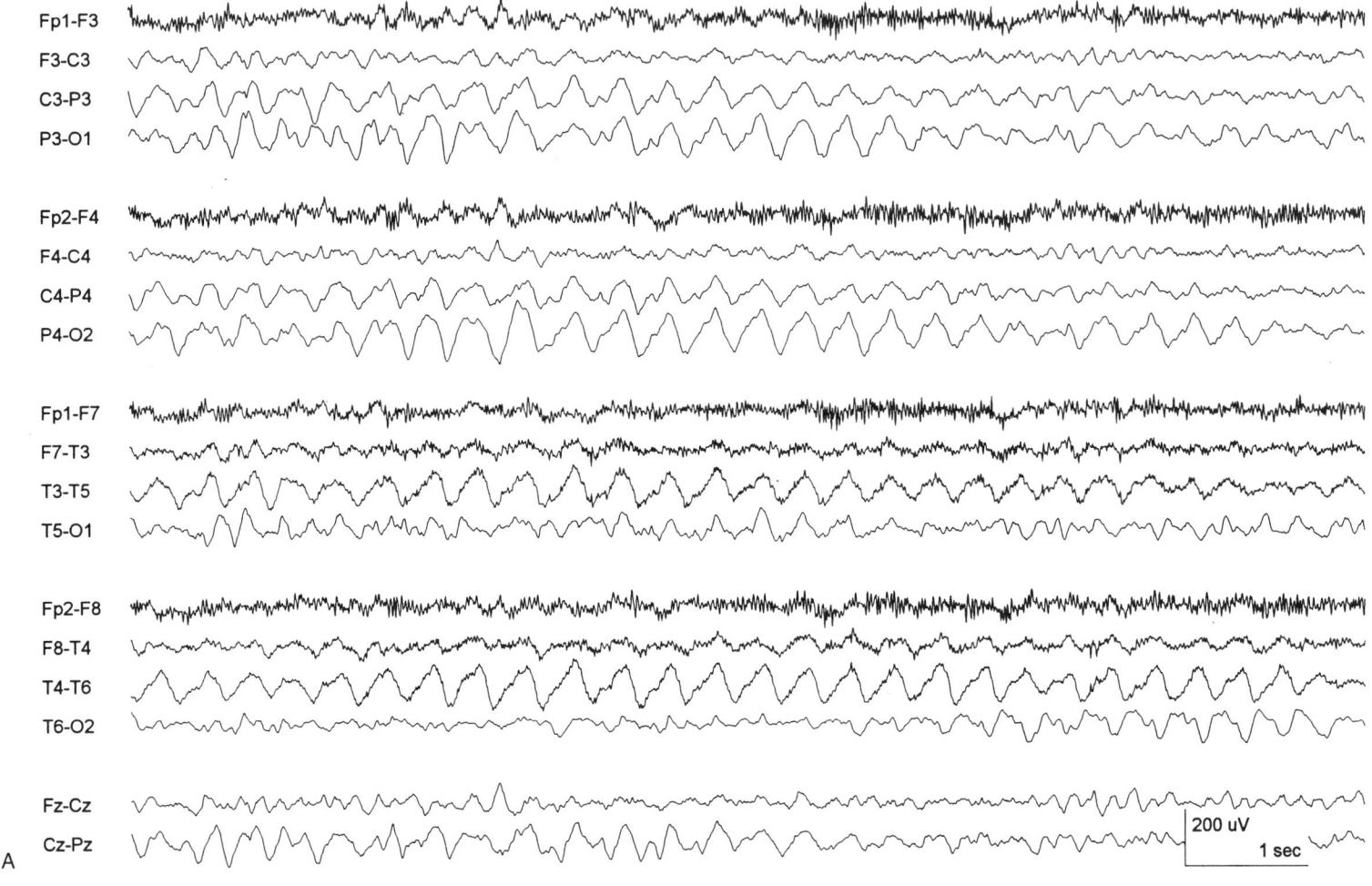

FIG. 17.7 EEG of a 9-year-old girl with childhood absence epilepsy. **A:** The EEG shows runs of 3-Hz bilateral synchronous occipital intermittent rhythmic delta activity (OIRDA). TC, 0.1 second; HFF, 70 Hz. *(Figure continues.)*

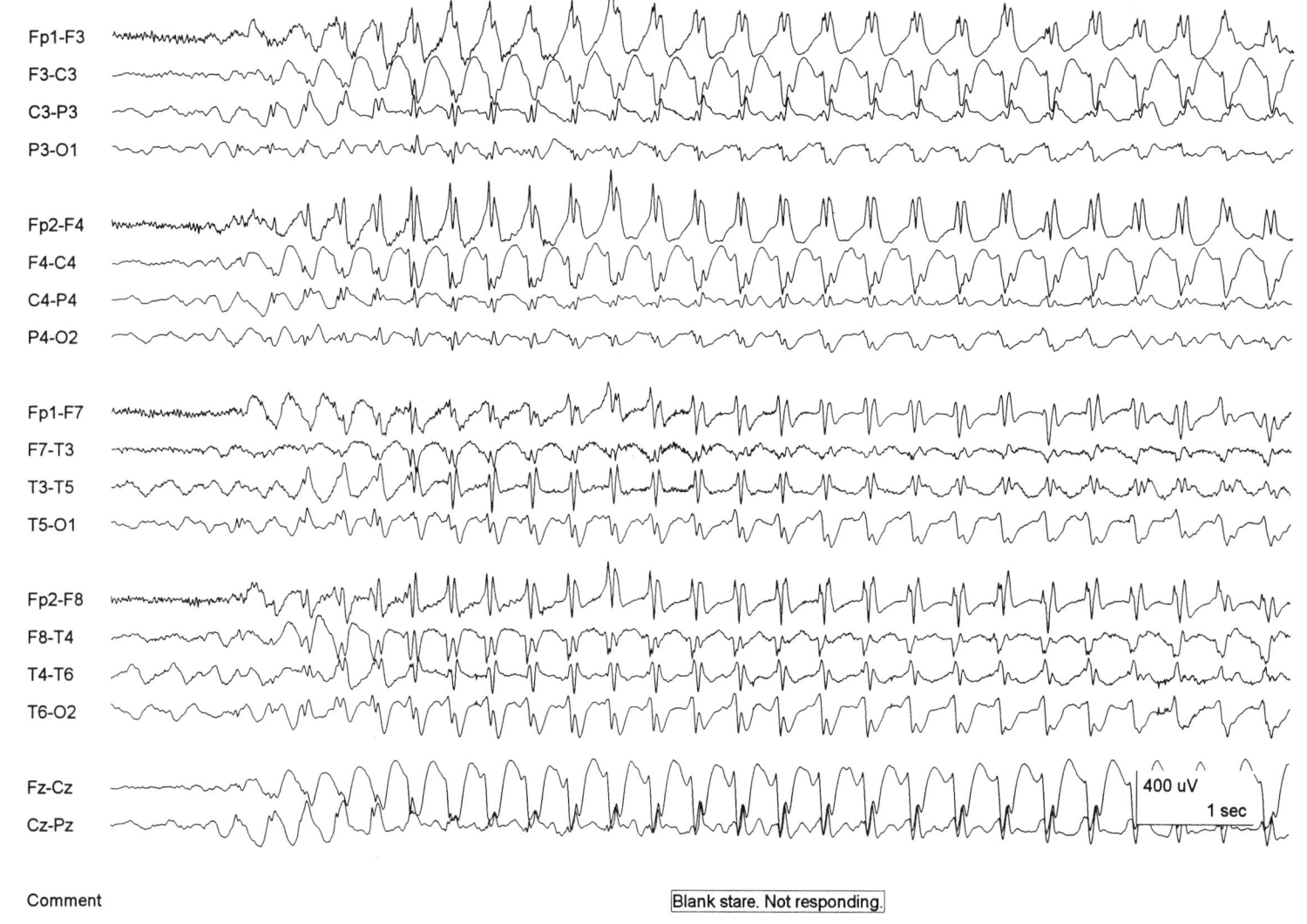

Fp1-F3

F3-C3

C3-P3

P3-O1

Fp2-F4

F4-C4

C4-P4

P4-O2

Fp1-F7

F7-T3

T3-T5

T5-O1

Fp2-F8

F8-T4

T4-T6

T6-O2

Fz-Cz

Cz-Pz

400 uV

1 sec

B   Comment   Blank stare. Not responding.

FIG. 17.7. *Continued.* **B:** Later in the same EEG recording, the patient had a typical absence seizure associated with generalized 3-Hz spike-wave activity. TC, 0.1 second; HFF, 70 Hz.

Benign Epilepsy of Childhood with Central-Midtemporal Spikes

Clinical Features

Benign epilepsy of childhood with central-midtemporal spikes (BECTS) is an idiopathic, localization-related epilepsy syndrome (228). It is also commonly referred to as *benign rolandic epilepsy*. It is one of the most common forms of childhood epilepsy, occurring in 16% to 24% of children with epilepsy (48,131).

BECTS is characterized by two defining features, one clinical and one electrographic:

1. Stereotyped partial seizures consisting of unilateral paresthesias of the tongue, lips, inner cheeks, and gums, accompanied by unilateral tonic or clonic activity of the facial and pharyngeal/laryngeal muscles, speech arrest (anarthria), and excessive salivation. Nocturnal secondarily generalized seizures are common and are often the first manifestation of the disorder. Seizures remit spontaneously during adolescence.
2. Interictal EEG demonstrating central-midtemporal spikes and otherwise normal background activity.

Onset of seizures usually occurs between the ages of 4 and 10 years, although the syndrome can occur as early as the age of 2 years and, rarely, begin as late as 13 years. In the majority of patients, nearly 80% in some series, seizures occur exclusively during sleep (174,180). In about 20%, seizures occur during both sleep and wakefulness. Seizures that occur solely during the waking state are least common (174,180). Seizures are usually infrequent, and 13% to 21% of patients have only a single seizure (174,180). Frequent seizures or seizure clusters are present in only 20% to 25% of cases (174,180). Early onset seems to be predictive of a longer active phase of seizures before remission (180). Partial status epilepticus is rare (61,91).

Electroencephalographic Findings

Interictal EEG. The interictal EEG demonstrates the characteristic central-midtemporal epileptiform discharges (Fig. 17.8). These are stereotyped, diphasic or sometimes triphasic sharp waves, usually followed by an aftergoing slow wave. The sharp waves average 100 to 300 μV in voltage. In bipolar recordings, the discharges most often show maximal voltage in the central (C3-C4) and midtemporal (T3-T4) areas. On occasion, the maximal voltage is displaced posteriorly, to P3-P4 or T4-T6. Discharges are usually seen simultaneously in both central and temporal regions, although they may be of higher voltage in one or the other of these. On occasion, they are confined to either the central or the temporal area. They occur bilaterally and independently in homologous areas of both hemispheres, but in a single recording, they may predominate on one side (see later discussion). The sharp waves occur either as isolated discharges or as runs of repetitive spikes. The latter is especially common during sleep. The frequency of spiking does not correlate with the frequency or severity of seizures. The EEG abnormality typically persists for some time after remission of clinical seizures. The EEG discharge also eventually disappears, almost always by late adolescence; in rare cases, they can be detected in subjects in their early 20s (4,174).

Legarda et al. (170) analyzed the spatial distribution of central-midtemporal spikes in detail, using additional "low central" electrodes (C5, C6) placed equidistant between C3-C4 and between T3-T4. When only standard electrode placements were used, 21 of 33 patients had discharges that were of maximal voltage at C3 and C4. In the rest, discharges were of highest voltage in the midtemporal region. However, when "low central" electrodes were included, all of the apparent T3-T4 loci, and half of the C3-C4 loci were actually of highest voltage at the C5-C6 sites. These data suggest that the term *central-midtemporal* may be a misnomer, because all such discharges actually localize to either high (30%) or low (70%) central regions. This observation is not surprising, inasmuch as the T3 and T4 electrodes actually overlie the junction of the rolandic and sylvian fissures.

Gregory and Wong (121) used digital spike averaging and computerized topographic mapping to analyze the spatial and temporal characteristics of central-midtemporal spikes in 10 children. All of the discharges had stereotyped waveforms that displayed a characteristic tangential dipole over the rolandic region: peak negativity was located over the central or midtemporal area with a lower voltage peak of positivity seen bilaterally over the frontal regions but maximal ipsilaterally. On the basis of these findings, Gregory and Wong postulated a single spike generator in the lower rolandic-sylvian area that was oriented tangentially to the cortical surface.

In many patients, epileptiform discharges occur unilaterally, in the same hemisphere on multiple EEG recordings. In other patients, spikes occur bilaterally and independently, either in a single EEG recording or in consecutive EEG recordings (19,32,174,173). When spikes are present bilaterally, the maximal voltage of the discharges is always in homologous areas (e.g., C3 and C4) (170).

Sleep enhances central-midtemporal discharges, often dramatically. In up to one-third of patients, spikes are seen only during sleep (31,181). This activation occurs in all stages of sleep, including the REM stage, but the effect is most pronounced in slow-wave sleep (27,58). Clemens and Majoros (58) found that the spike discharge rate was highest in stages 3 and 4, lower in

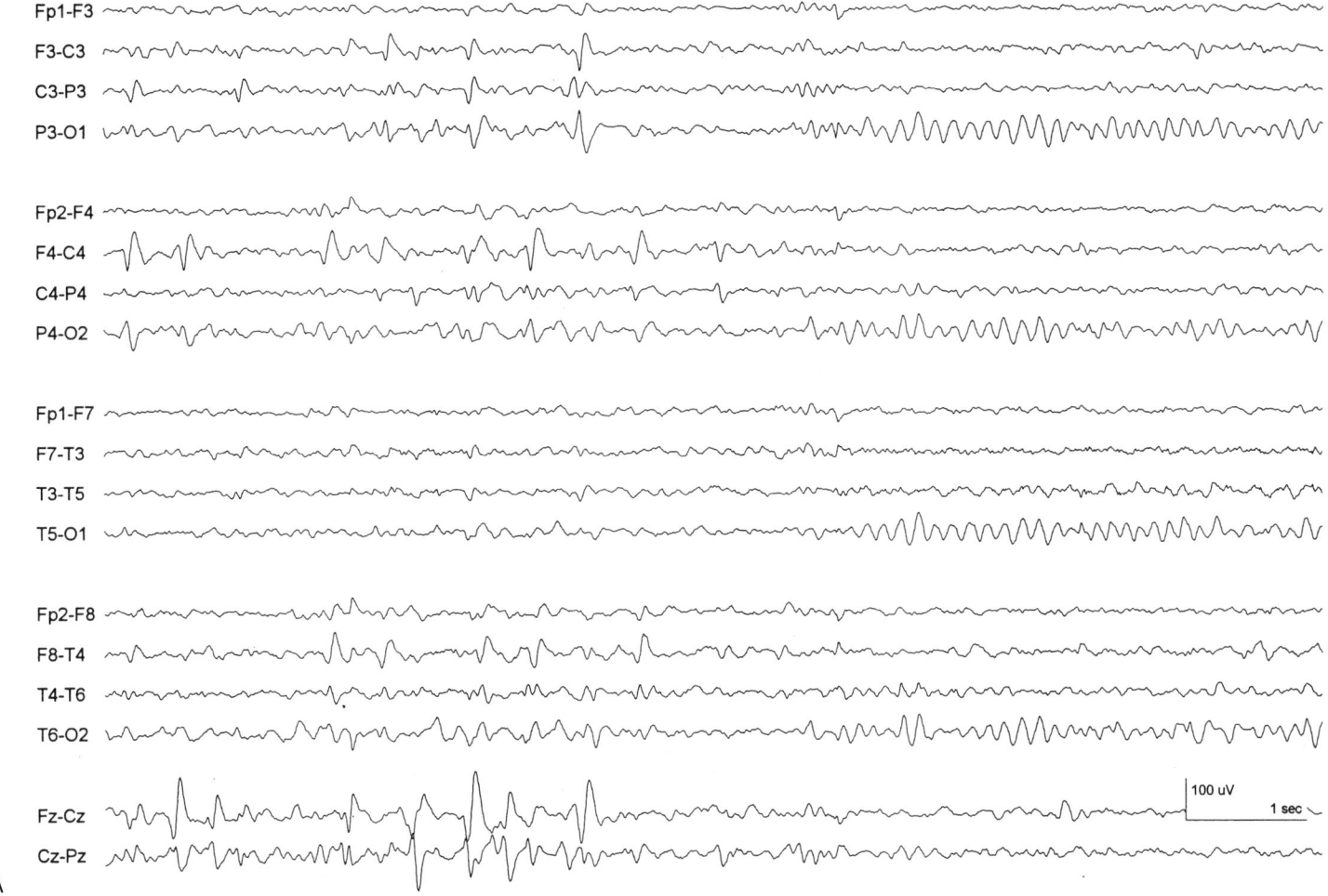

FIG. 17.8. A: EEG of a 6-year-old girl with benign epilepsy of childhood with central-midtemporal spikes (BECTS). She had infrequent seizures consisting of right face and arm clonus with drooling but without loss of consciousness. During drowsiness, the EEG shows frequent, stereotyped sharp waves occurring independently over the left (C3) and right (C4) central regions. Some of the right hemisphere discharges have a more extensive field that includes the temporal region (T4). Note that the vertex sharp transients are clearly distinct with phase reversals at Cz. After arousal, the discharges attenuated completely. TC, 0.1 second; HFF, 70 Hz. *(Figure continues.)*

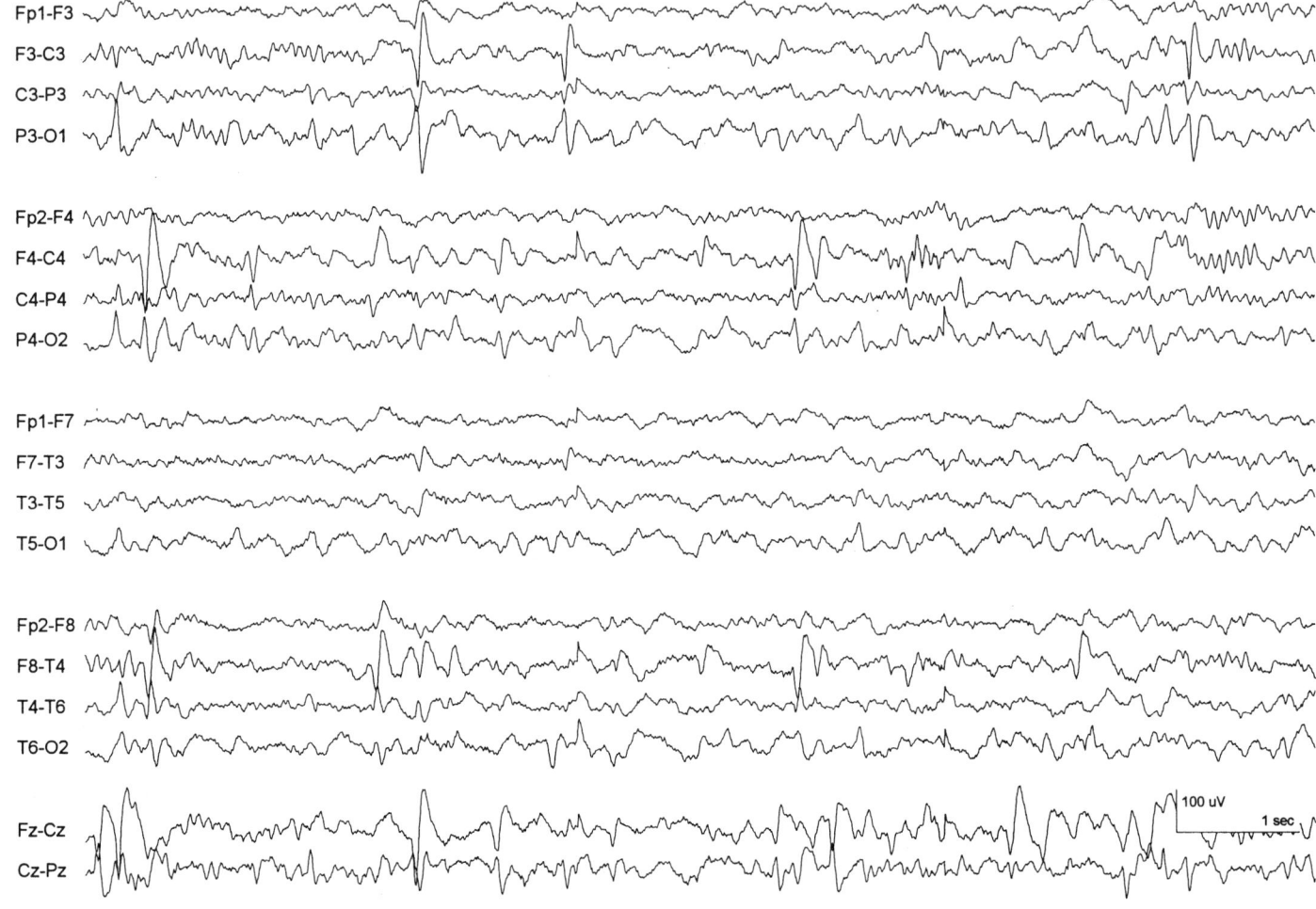

FIG. 17.8. *Continued.* **B:** Stage 2 sleep in the same patient. The discharges occurred more frequently and were more broadly distributed. TC, 0.1 second; HFF, 70 Hz. *(Figure continues.)*

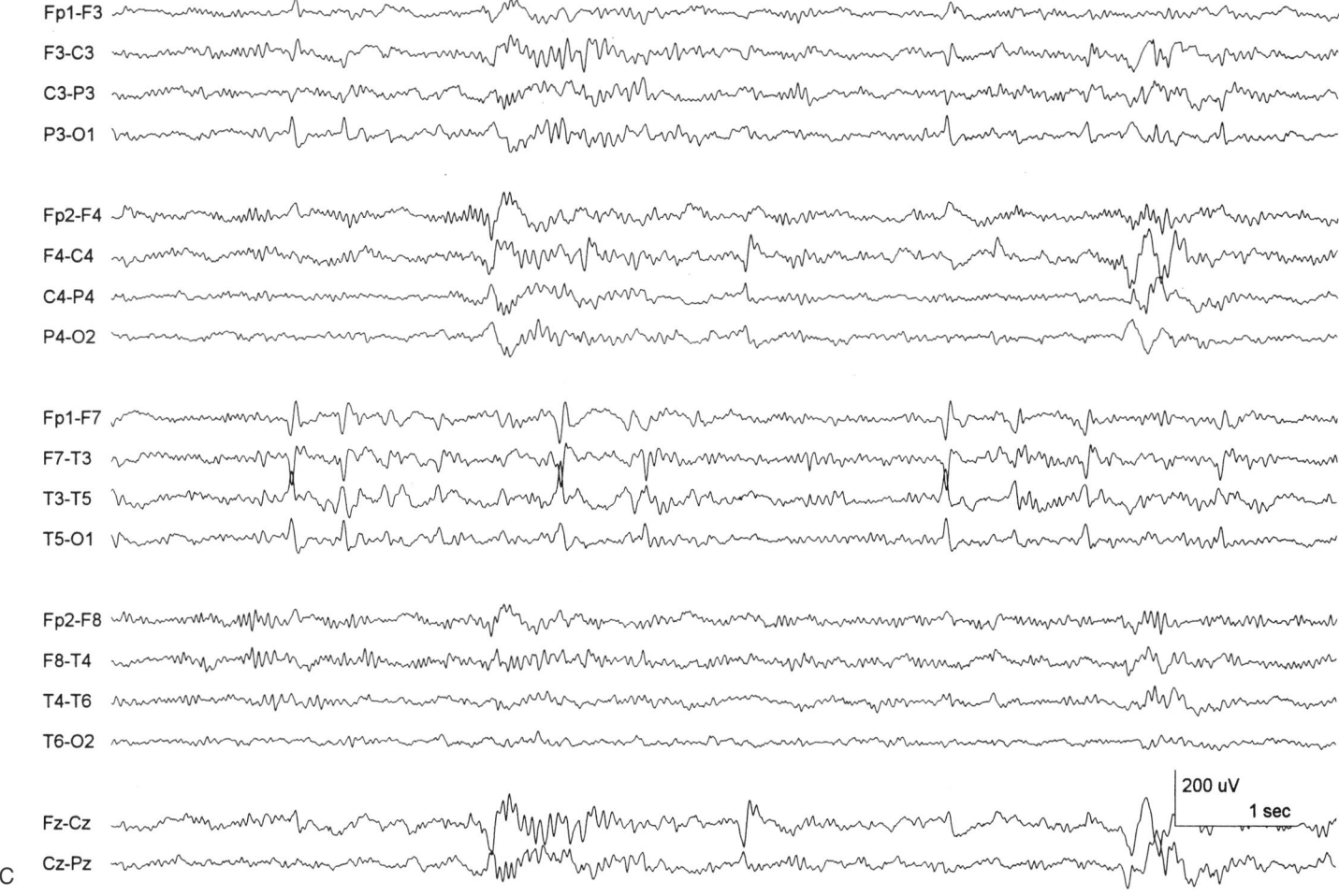

Fp1-F3

F3-C3

C3-P3

P3-O1

Fp2-F4

F4-C4

C4-P4

P4-O2

Fp1-F7

F7-T3

T3-T5

T5-O1

Fp2-F8

F8-T4

T4-T6

T6-O2

200 uV

1 sec

Fz-Cz

Cz-Pz

C

FIG. 17.8. *Continued.* **C:** EEG of a 9-year-old boy with BECTS. In this child, the discharges are predominantly left-sided and mainly temporal in their distribution (see text). TC, 0.1 second; HFF, 70 Hz. *(Figure continues.)*

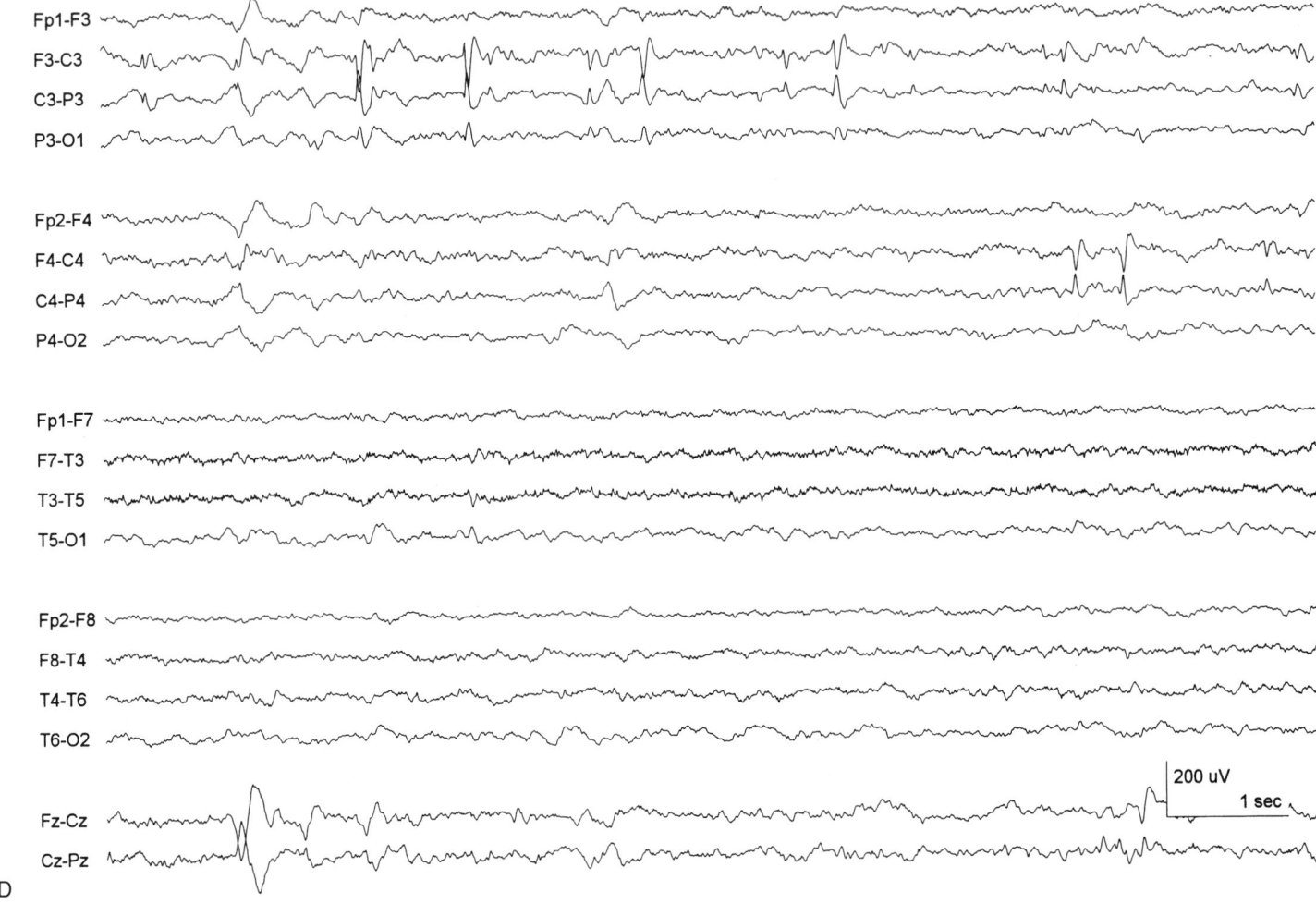

FIG. 17.8. *Continued.* **D:** EEG of a 5-year-old boy with BECTS. There are independent left and right discharges localized to C3 and C4 without significant involvement of temporal electrodes. TC, 0.1 second. HFF, 70 Hz.

stages 1 and 2, even lower in REM sleep, and lowest in the waking state. Epileptiform discharges are also of higher voltage and have more extensive fields during sleep (17,170,195). Spikes that are unilateral during wakefulness often become bilateral during sleep (27). Although there is agreement that central-midtemporal discharges are most apt to be recorded during sleep, the actual sensitivity of this state-dependent effect has not been rigorously examined. Thus, single EEGs, even including sleep, can be normal in children whose clinical presentation is consistent with BECTS.

Hyperventilation and photic stimulation have no consistent effect on central-midtemporal epileptiform discharges (19,29).

In general, EEG background activity is normal in children with BECTS. However, when the discharges are frequent and repetitive, focal slowing can occur in the same distribution as the spikes as a result of summation of aftergoing slow waves.

Other electrographic abnormalities are present in a minority of patients. The most common of these are generalized, bisynchronous 3- to 4-Hz spike-wave discharges. These occur in about 7% of routine EEGs from patients with BECTS (19,174), but the incidence is much higher (up to 70%) with overnight or longer recordings (17,27). Unlike central-midtemporal spikes, the generalized spike-wave complexes can be activated by hyperventilation and, to a lesser extent, photic stimulation (32,195). Other focal spike discharges also occur, most often in the occipital and frontal areas (19), and multiple independent spike foci have also been reported (29). In such cases, the morphological appearance of these other focal spikes is often similar to that of the central-midtemporal discharges.

Ictal EEG. Ictal EEG recordings from patients with BECTS have been reported infrequently. Lerman (173) described the EEG correlate of a diurnal seizure as beginning with a focal decremental pattern followed by dense spikes in the central-midtemporal region during the tonic phase and then by spike-waves in the clonic phase. The ictal discharge remained localized, lasted less than 1 minute, and was not followed by postictal slowing. Bernardina and Tassinari (28) recorded a seizure during stage 2 sleep. The ictal event began with low-voltage (20- to 30-μV) 12-Hz activity over the central and temporal regions on one side, which increased in voltage (to 50 to 100 μV) with an enlarging field before becoming generalized with widespread 8- to 10-Hz rhythmic spike activity. The ictal pattern ended abruptly, and there was no postictal slowing. Interictal spiking was suppressed for 1 minute after the seizure.

Familial Occurrence

Bray and Wiser (36) were among the first to record central-midtemporal discharges in nonepileptic relatives of patients with BECTS. In a study of 40 patients with BECTS, 30% had at least one close relative with central-midtemporal discharges. Siblings and children were more likely to be affected (36%) than were parents (19%). Heijbel et al. (132) found central-midtemporal spikes in 34% of siblings, more than half of these (56%) did not have seizures. In a study of persons whose EEGs contained central-midtemporal spikes (not all of whom had epilepsy), Degen and Degen (66) found that a higher proportion of siblings had generalized epileptiform discharges (31.9%) than central-midtemporal discharges (4.3%). These findings are suggestive of a strong genetic component to the development of BECTS, perhaps a single autosomal dominant gene with age-dependent penetrance.

Differential Diagnosis

Not all patients with central-midtemporal discharges on EEG, however, have BECTS, inasmuch as typical discharges may be seen in several circumstances other than BECTS. The occurrence of central-midtemporal spikes in neurologically normal patients without epilepsy is well recognized (19,27,29,174,195). Cavazutti et al. (49) performed EEGs on 3,726 neurologically normal children 6 to 13 years of age who had no history of epilepsy. They found "rolandic or parietal" or "midtemporal" epileptiform discharges in 2.3% of the children. In a series of 386 neurologically normal children whose EEGs showed central discharges and normal background activity, Kellaway (158) found that only 57% had seizures. In another large series of 315 patients with centrotemporal discharges, Beaussart (19) found that 16% did not have epilepsy.

Central-midtemporal discharges have been recorded in patients with symptomatic forms of epilepsy. In Kellaway's (158) series of 335 patients with central discharges and seizures, only 66% had BECTS; the other 34% were classified as "lesional": that is, having a history of early brain insult or neurological impairment. Central-midtemporal discharges have also been described in patients with a variety of neurological abnormalities, including perinatal hypoxia, agenesis of the corpus callosum, callosal lipoma, congenital toxoplasmosis, Rett's syndrome, fragile X syndrome, cortical dysplasia, and cerebral tumor (74,163,164,201,203). In such cases, the association with BECTS may have several explanations:

1. The occurrence of BECTS is coincidental.
2. The associated neurological insult allowed emergence of rolandic seizures by further lowering seizure threshold in a patient genetically predisposed to BECTS.
3. The neurological lesion resulted in epileptiform discharges and/or seizures similar to those seen in BECTS. In these cases, careful analysis of the clinical features and EEG background may reveal atypical fea-

tures that bring the diagnosis of BECTS into question. In particularly difficult cases, careful topographic analysis of the epileptiform activity, as described by Gregory and Wong (121), may provide useful distinguishing features, such as the characteristic dipole seen in BECTS.

Despite the occurrence of central-midtemporal discharges in the foregoing situations, the characteristic EEG findings, in the absence of atypical features, are quite specific for BECTS.

Childhood Epilepsy with Occipital Paroxysms

Clinical Features

Gastaut (101) was the first to clearly delineate childhood epilepsy with occipital paroxysms (CEOP) as a distinct electroclinical syndrome. The 1989 International League Against Epilepsy (ILAE) Commission on Classification groups this syndrome among the idiopathic localization-related epilepsies (228). Since publication of the initial description, it has become evident that CEOP encompasses a heterogeneous group of patients whose disease is one of two subtypes: an early-onset variant, now termed the *Panayiotopoulos's syndrome,* and a late-onset variant that corresponds to the syndrome initially described by Gastaut (215).

Although there are no epidemiological studies of the incidence of CEOP, several case series indicate that it is two to three times less common that BECTS (46,207,212). The early-onset variant accounts for most cases (46, 207,212).

In addition to the EEG findings (see later discussion), the two variants of CEOP share several features. Children are neurologically normal and have normal computed tomographic and magnetic resonance imaging scans (104,212,213,228). Boys and girls are equally affected in both early- and late-onset variants (92,101,104). As in BECTS, genetic factors are clearly involved, although the pattern of inheritance has not been elucidated. A family history of epilepsy is evident in 37% to 44% of cases (104,273), and occipital spikes have been reported in 26% of nonepileptic relatives (165).

In the late-onset CEOP variant, seizures begin between the ages of 15 months and 17 years; the peak age at onset is between 7 and 9 years (104,215, 273). Seizures nearly always begin with visual symptoms (amaurosis, phosphenes, illusions, or hallucinations) and are typically brief, lasting only seconds, without alteration in consciousness (104,228). In the immediate postictal period, about one-third of patients develop a severe diffuse headache, often with associated nausea and vomiting (104). Seizures tend to occur frequently,

but response to medication is usually good (104,273). Although details of prognosis remain unresolved, the long-term outcome of the late-onset variant CEOP is generally less favorable than that of BECTS.

In the early-onset variant, the peak age at onset is between 3 and 5 years (92,214). In contrast to the late-onset variant, seizures lack the characteristic visual phenomena. Rather, stereotyped seizures consist of lateral gaze deviation and ictal vomiting, with a varying degree of alteration in consciousness (92,214). Seizures are exclusively nocturnal in about two-thirds of cases and are typically prolonged (5 to 10 minutes or longer in duration) (92,214). Partial status epilepticus occurs in nearly half the patients (92, 214). Despite the long duration of seizures and the high incidence of status epilepticus, prognosis in the early-onset variant is universally excellent. Up to 30% of patients experience only a single seizure, and in the remainder, seizures occur infrequently. Ferrie et al. (92) found that the median number of seizures was two, and no more than 15 occurred in any patient. Duration of the disease is typically 1 to 2 years, and nearly all patients become seizure free by age 12 (92). In rare cases, atypical seizures, either generalized or rolandic, recur after remission (92).

Electroencephalographic Findings

Interictal EEG. EEG findings are indistinguishable in the two CEOP variants. The interictal EEG demonstrates normal background activity and occipital epileptiform discharges that are morphologically stereotyped (92,101,104). The characteristic discharge consists of a diphasic spike or sharp wave with a high-voltage (200- to 300-μV) surface-negative peak, followed by a low-voltage surface-positive peak and an aftergoing surface-negative slow wave (104,213) (Fig. 17.9). Although maximal in the occipital derivations, the discharges at times extend into the posterior temporal areas (104). In about 20% of discharges, the principal sharp component has a duration longer than 70 milliseconds. In a similar percentage of discharges, spikes occur without aftergoing slow waves (92).

Gastaut and Zifkin (104) reported that the epileptiform discharges disappeared promptly with eye opening in 94% of cases and returned within 1 to 20 seconds after the eyes closed. Ferrie et al. (92) found less impressive responses to eye opening: The discharges disappeared completely in 54% of instances. Partial attenuation occurred in 15%, and there was no effect in 19%. Panayiotopoulos (211) demonstrated that reactivity of the epileptiform discharges to eye opening and closure is actually determined by central visual fixation. When patients were recorded in darkness, the occipital discharges per-

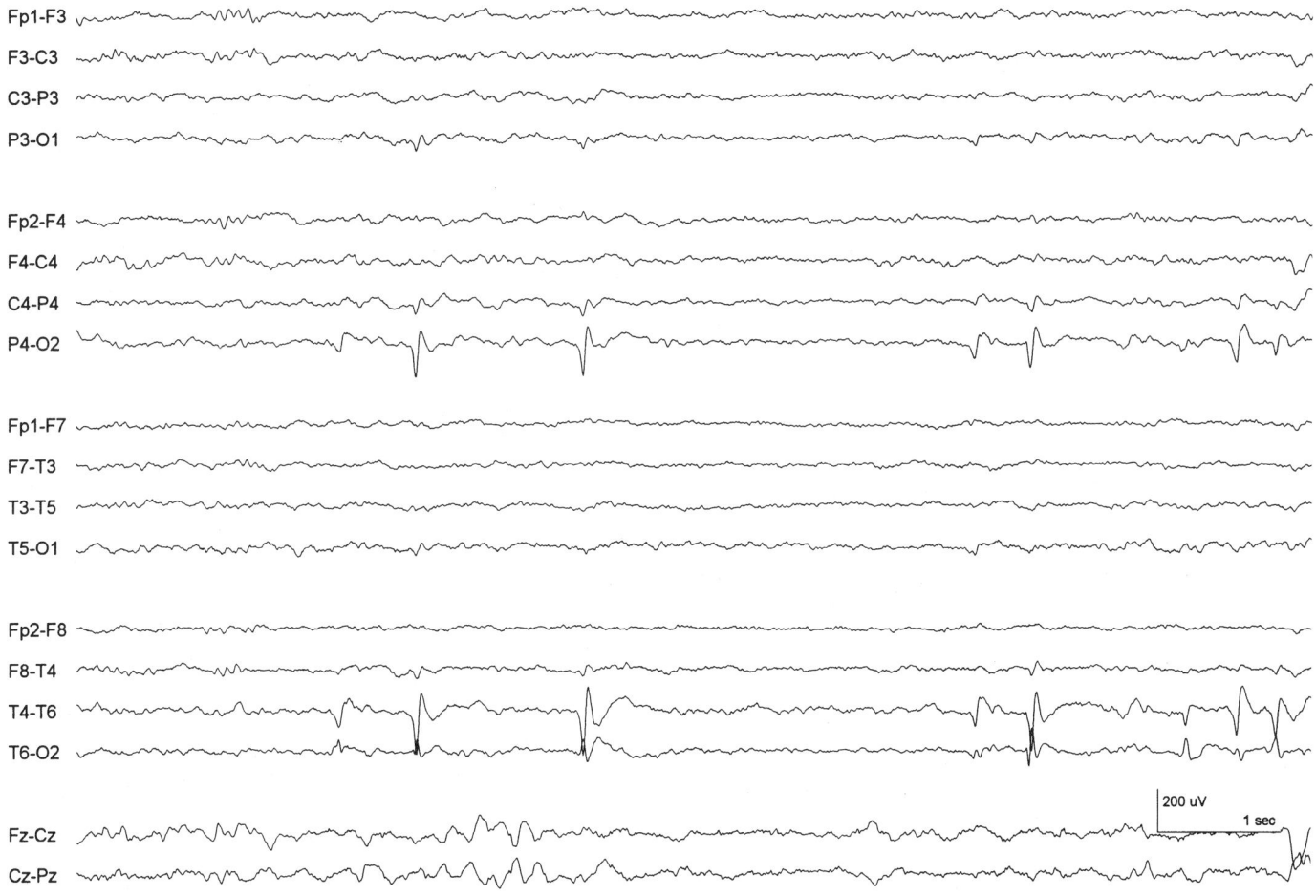

FIG. 17.9. EEG of a 10-year-old girl with childhood epilepsy with occipital paroxysms (CEOP). Her seizures consisted of lateral gaze deviation and vomiting with subtle impairment in awareness. The EEG shows normal background activity and high-amplitude occipital (T6/O2) spikes that have a stereotyped waveform. TC, 0.1 second; HFF, 70 Hz.

sisted, independently of whether the eyes were open or closed. When a small red light was used as a target for visual fixation in an otherwise dark environment, epileptiform activity attenuated promptly. This phenomenon of dependence on central visual fixation has been referred to as *fixation-off sensitivity* or *scotosensitivity*. These findings were confirmed later by Lugaresi et al. (185).

Occipital spikes can occur as isolated discharges, but they are seen most often as 1- to 3-Hz repetitive, semirhythmic paroxysms. At times, such discharges occur nearly continuously (101,104). Spikes may be unilateral or bilateral. When they are bilateral, the discharges on the two sides can be either synchronous or asynchronous (104). Bisynchronous discharges often differ in voltage, which raises the possibility of a single generator located within the medial surface of one occipital lobe with rapid propagation to the homotopic contralateral area.

Hyperventilation usually has no effect on epileptiform activity (104), although a few authors have reported activation (175,273). Similarly, in most patients, photic stimulation has no effect on epileptiform activity (92,104). In a few, however, however, photic stimulation can either activate epileptiform discharges (104,213) or inhibit them (212,213). The inhibition effect seems to occur mainly with high flash rates.

Occipital discharges are activated by NREM sleep and inhibited by REM sleep (92,175) In a minority of cases, occipital discharges may be evident only during sleep (104).

Occipital discharges are not invariably present in CEOP. In 5% to 6% of cases, rhythmic slow waves occur in the occipital regions in the absence of any spike or sharp-wave components (92,104). Interictal epileptiform abnormalities are especially likely to be absent at the beginning of the early-onset variant. For example, Guerrini et al. (125) described four children with early-onset CEOP who did not manifest epileptiform activity until several months after the first seizure.

In many patients—more than half in one series (92)—interictal epileptiform discharges persist after clinical remission of seizures, sometimes for several years.

As in BECTS, some patients have other epileptiform abnormalities as well. Gastaut and Zifkin (104) found generalized spike-wave or central-midtemporal discharges in 38% of their patients. Ferrie et al. (92) made similar observations: 25% of their patients had central-midtemporal spikes, 12% had generalized spike-wave discharges, and 7% had frontal discharges.

Ictal EEG. Ictal EEG recordings have demonstrated a rhythmic spike pattern, initially localized to one occipital region, which evolves into a rhythmic theta or delta frequency discharge. The ictal discharge spreads both anteriorly on the same side and into the contralateral occipital area, but it usually remains best defined and most prominent in the occipital regions. Beaumanoir (14) described the EEG activity recorded during a nocturnal seizure. Interictal occipital spikes disappeared just before seizure onset, replaced by 10-Hz spikes in one occipital region. The rhythmic spike discharged evolved into rhythmic theta activity that was maximal posteriorly. Vigevano and Ricci (287) recorded an EEG during a seizure typical of the early-onset variant. There were unilateral, high-voltage, sharply contoured, rhythmic 1- to 2-Hz waves intermixed with spikes over the occipital-posterior temporal region.

Differential Diagnosis

Occipital spikes by themselves do not indicate a diagnosis of CEOP. Occipital discharges typical of the condition, including scotosensitivity, can be seen in other circumstances as well. Occipital spikes can occur in normal children as the asymptomatic expression of a genetic trait. In a small case series, Kuzniecky and Rosenblatt (165) found occipital spikes in 26% of nonepileptic relatives of patients with CEOP. In a study of 100 children with epileptiform EEGs but no history of seizures, Lerman and Kivity-Ephraim (176) found that 19% had occipital spikes. Kellaway (158) studied children with congenital or acquired amblyopia and found that many of them had occipital spikes and otherwise normal or nearly normal background activity. Such spikes can be very fast and extremely sharp ("needle spikes"). Occipital spikes also occur in patients with idiopathic photosensitive occipital lobe epilepsy. These patients have light-induced seizures and photoparoxysmal EEG responses (126). Occipital spikes can be seen in patients with symptomatic localization-related epilepsy (62) (Fig. 17.10). The best examples of such patients are those with celiac disease, who have occipital seizures, reactive occipital spikes on the EEG, and calcifications in the occipital lobes (114,115). The initial course of seizures in these patients appears benign, but many patients subsequently develop progressively severe epilepsy. Occipital epileptiform discharges have also been reported in hyperglycemia (128) and mitochondrial diseases (6).

Juvenile Myoclonic Epilepsy

Clinical Features

Juvenile myoclonic epilepsy (JME) is the most common syndrome among the idiopathic generalized epilepsies: it comprises 4% to 6% of all types of

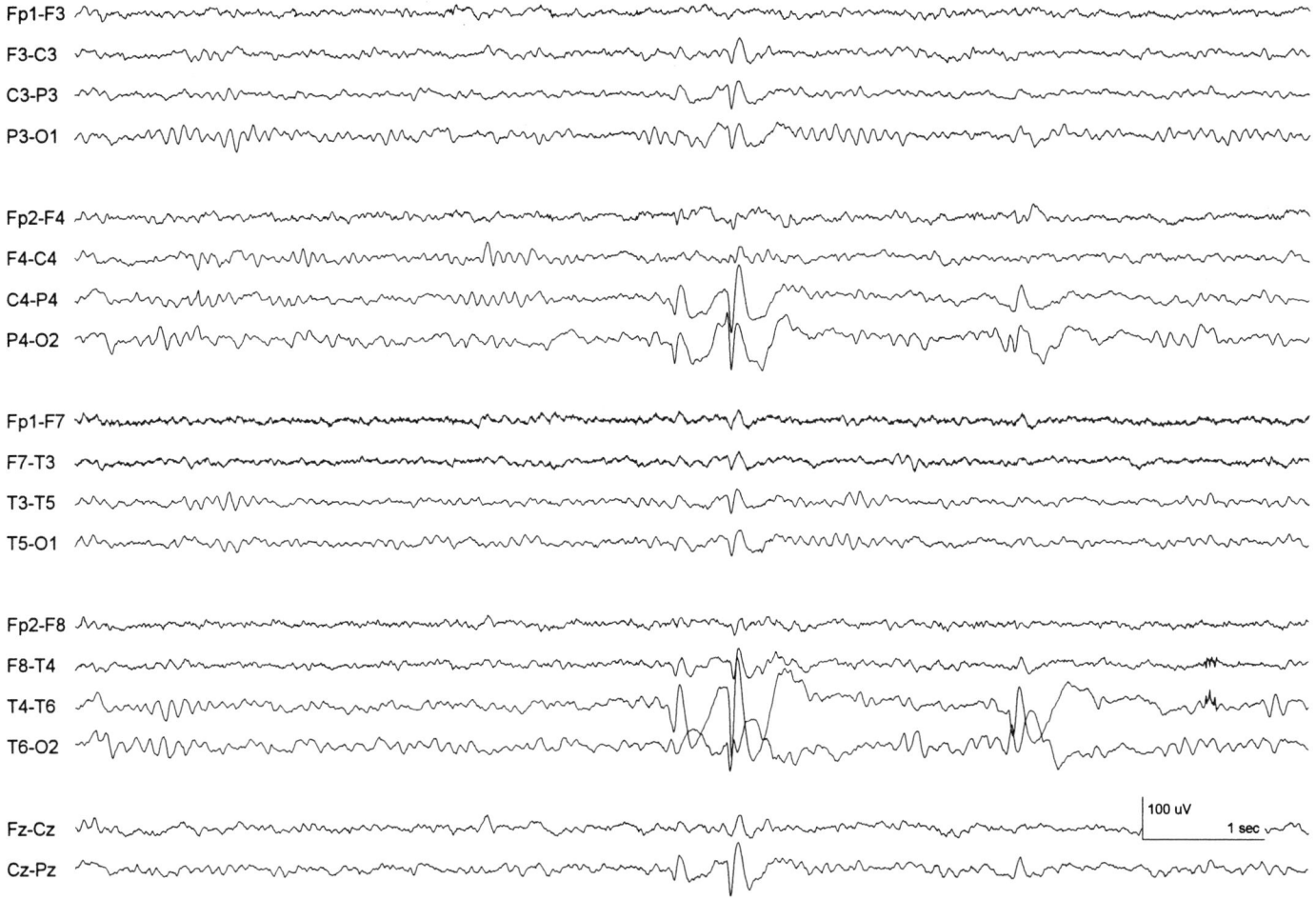

FIG. 17.10. EEG of a 13-year-old boy with intractable epilepsy resulting from heterotopic gray matter in the right temporal-occipital region. Note that the alpha rhythm is less persistent and poorly regulated on the right, and there is associated focal slowing of theta and delta frequencies. Note the similarity of the spike discharges in this example to those shown in Fig. 17.9.

epilepsy (8,148,200). Hereditary factors are clearly evident, and 40% to 50% of patients have a family history of epilepsy (8,67). Boys and girls are affected in equal numbers (67,150,216). Several groups of investigators have reported linkage to chromosome 6p (120), although this has been disputed by others (84,299). No single causative gene has been found, and polygenic factors are likely to be involved (76).

As its name indicates, this epilepsy syndrome usually begins in adolescence. Myoclonic seizures are present in 100% of cases as they are required for diagnosis. They may be the only type of seizure in 2% to 10% of cases (67,216,225). Typically, myoclonic jerks appear 2 to 3 years before the first generalized tonic-clonic seizure, although it is almost always the latter that brings the patient to medical attention. Generalized tonic-clonic seizures occur in more than 90% of patients. Both myoclonic and generalized tonic-clonic seizures occur most often within 1 to 2 hours after awakening. Myoclonus is especially marked in the setting of fatigue and sleep deprivation (216). Sometimes a crescendo of repeated myoclonic jerks terminates in a generalized tonic-clonic seizure (67). Absence seizures occur in about 35% of patients with JME (67,216,225). Sometimes, they may be the first manifestation of the disorder, even preceding the development of myoclonic jerks (8,217,216). Absence seizures in JME are typically less frequent and less intrusive than those seen in childhood absence epilepsy (pyknolepsy) and frequently go unnoticed (218,217).

Electroencephalographic Findings

Interictal EEG: Waking State. As in other idiopathic generalized epilepsy syndromes, the interictal EEG in JME is characterized by two main features:

1. Normal or near-normal background activity, with a well-modulated alpha rhythm (8,67,149).
2. Spontaneous bursts of generalized, bisynchronous epileptiform discharges.

Polyspikes and polyspike-wave discharges are characteristic of JME, although they are not pathognomonic, as initially believed by Janz and Christian (149). Such discharges are also common in other idiopathic generalized epilepsies. However, when polyspikes are abundant and are the predominant form of epileptiform activity, it is more likely that the patient has JME than another idiopathic generalized syndrome. The epileptiform discharge consists of a burst of generalized bisynchronous, symmetrical multiple spikes (polyspikes) that are of maximal voltage in the frontal and central regions, followed by high-voltage, irregular 2- to 5-Hz slow waves with intermixed spikes (148,149) (Fig. 17.11). The polyspike component is often evident only at the beginning of the epileptiform paroxysm. The number of repetitive spikes may be as high as 20; two to four spikes are more usual (148,149). Epileptiform activity can occur either as isolated polyspike-wave bursts or as prolonged paroxysms lasting up to 20 seconds (2). Spike-wave complexes and polyspikes without associated slow waves are also frequent and may sometimes be the only epileptiform abnormality (8).

The spike-wave and polyspike-wave discharges seen in JME are usually "fast"; that is, the repetition rate is higher than the 3-Hz spike-wave pattern seen in childhood absence epilepsy. The most common frequencies are 3.5 to 6 Hz, and the range is between 2 and 10 Hz (67,149,216). "Typical," stereotyped 2.5- to 3-Hz spike-wave discharges, indistinguishable from those seen in childhood absence epilepsy, are present in up to 25% of patients (67).

The sensitivity of the EEG for demonstrating epileptiform activity in patients with JME is widely accepted as being very high, but the actual data from different studies vary considerably in the percentage of "positive" EEG. For example, Delgado-Escueta and Enrile-Bacsal (67) reported epileptiform activity in 100% of patients, Janz and Christian (149) in 92%, Panayiotopoulos et al. (216) in 79%, and Aliberti et al. (2) in 73%. Although much of this variability may result from differences in recording methods, especially the length of the EEG and whether samples of both waking and sleep activity were obtained, antiepileptic drugs may also play a role. Jain et al. (147) found that the probability of detecting epileptiform activity was much greater in untreated (100%) than in treated (63%) JME patients.

Hyperventilation generally activates epileptiform activity (148,216), although there have been no quantitative studies of this effect. In a minority of patients, epileptiform activity is seen only during hyperventilation (2).

A relatively high percentage of patients, 27% to 41%, demonstrate photosensitivity (2,8,124,216,308). Photosensitivity is two to three times more common among girls with JME than among boys with JME (225,308). Like hyperventilation, photic stimulation may be the only way to elicit epileptiform activity in some patients (8). In a minority of patients, epileptiform activity is triggered by eye closure (8,216).

Other EEG abnormalities, including excessive amounts of theta activity and slower than expected alpha rhythms, have been reported in a minority of patients with JME (216). In the study by Panayiotopoulos et al. (216), seizures were uncontrolled at the time of study. Thus, the degree to which slowing of background EEG patterns reflected poorly controlled seizures or other factors is unknown.

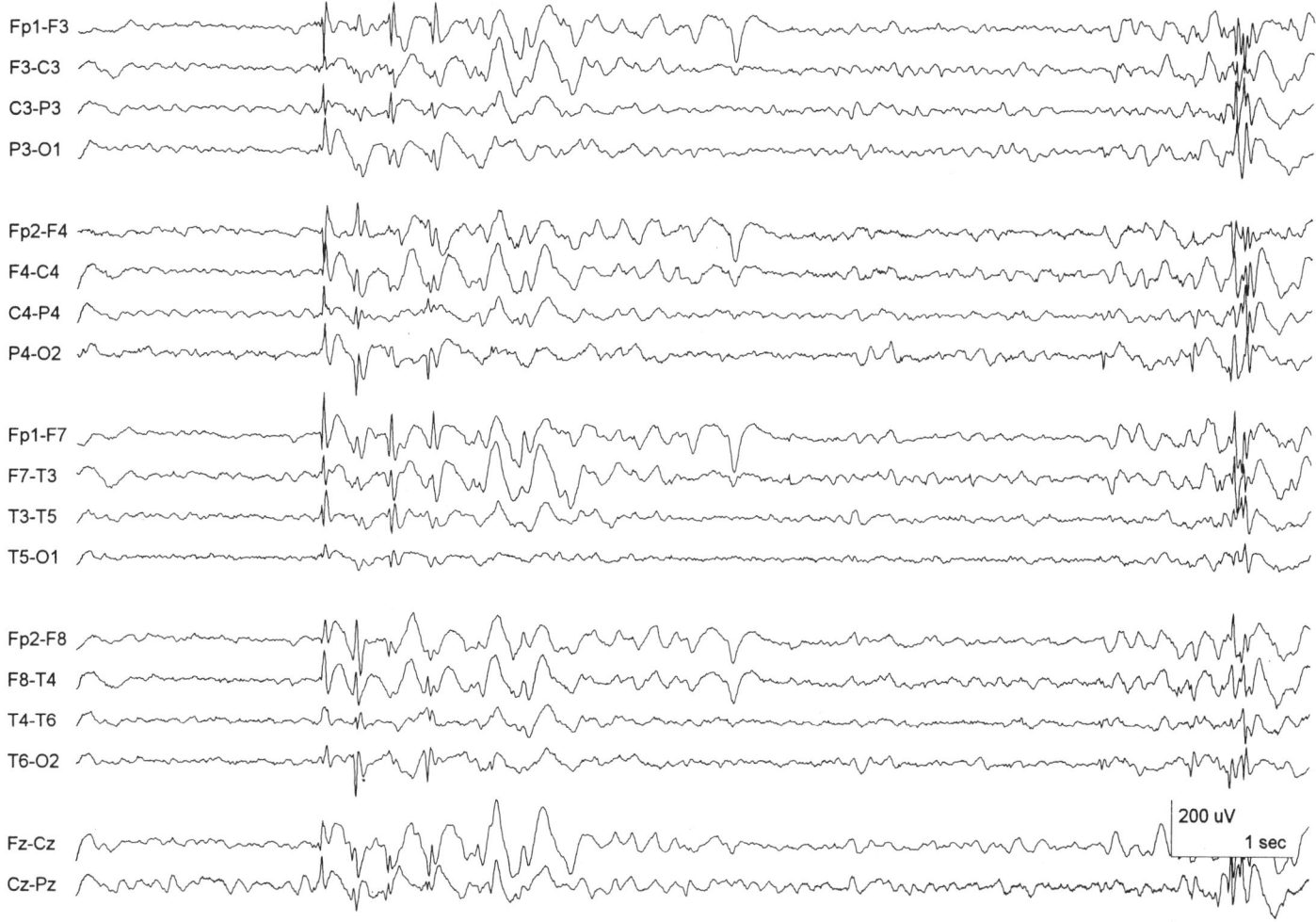

FIG. 17.11. EEG of an 18-year-old woman with juvenile myoclonic epilepsy (JME). The interictal EEG demonstrates generalized spike-wave and polyspike-wave discharges. TC, 0.1 second; HFF, 70 Hz.

Focal EEG abnormalities have been found in 16% to 54% of patients (2, 124,166,219,216). Although details are often lacking, inference of focal regions has usually depended on demonstrating asymmetrical spike-wave discharges, unilateral or focal spike-wave discharges, or unilateral or focal slowing. However, these were often described as inconsistent and shifting in laterality over time. The authors' experience suggests that a detailed analysis would demonstrate that the majority of these "focal discharges" represent limited or fragmentary expression of a generalized abnormality (Fig. 17.12). This conclusion is reasonable when the "focal" discharges have a waveform that mirrors that of the generalized spike-wave discharges, are of maximal

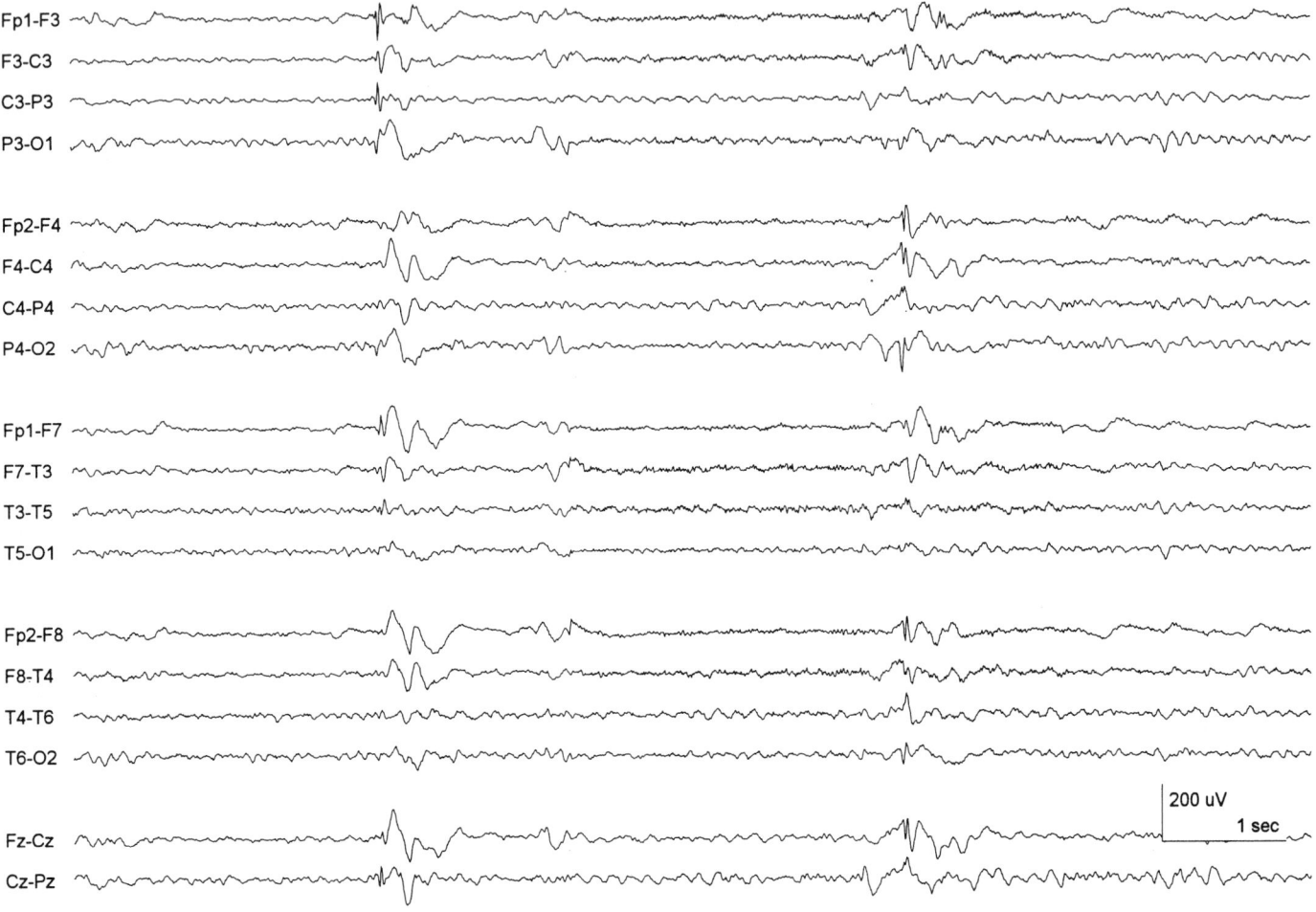

FIG. 17.12. EEG of an 18-year-old patient with juvenile myoclonic epilepsy (JME). Spike-wave discharges seem to shift from side to side during the recording. These asymmetrical fragments are often mistaken for evidence of a localization-related epilepsy syndrome (see text). TC, 0.1 second; HFF, 70 Hz.

voltage over the frontal and frontal-central regions, and lack associated focal slowing of background activity (see section on primary versus secondary bilateral synchrony).

Interictal EEG: Effects of Sleep. In polygraphic EEG studies of 33 patients with JME, Touchon (278) demonstrated that in stage 2 NREM sleep, epilepti-form discharges were suppressed, in contrast to the activation seen with most other types of epilepsy. Discharge rates were equivalent during wakefulness and drowsiness, dropped significantly during REM sleep (although not nearly to the rate seen in NREM sleep), and increased markedly after awakening, especially when the arousal was externally provoked. Epileptiform activity was most abundant after nocturnal and morning awakenings that followed sleepless nights. Sleep deprivation had similar effects and, in some patients, was necessary to elicit epileptiform discharges (8,124).

Ictal EEG. Myoclonic seizures are always associated with polyspike or polyspike-wave bursts (208) that are generally indistinguishable from those that are not accompanied by clinically detectable jerks. Sometimes the num-

ber of multiple spikes is higher (10 to 16 Hz) with ictal discharges, and the voltage may increase from the first spike to the last. The intensity of the myoclonic jerks correlates with a higher number of repetitive spikes (148, 149). The polyspikes are of medium to high voltage, maximally expressed over the frontal regions, and followed by high-voltage, 1- to 3-Hz rhythmic slow waves (67) (Fig. 17.13). While the jerk itself is extremely brief ("light-

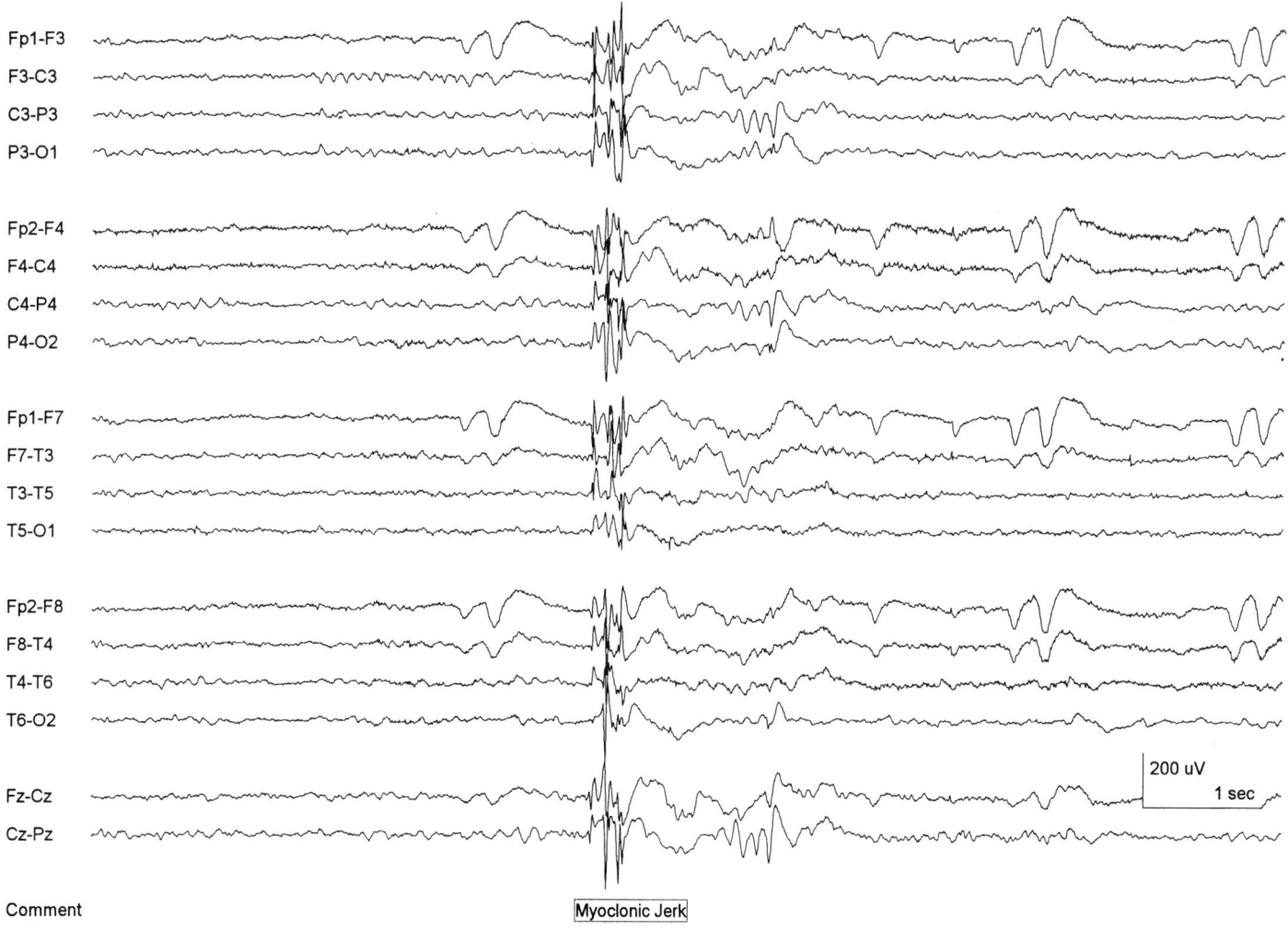

FIG. 17.13. EEG of an 18-year-old patient with juvenile myoclonic epilepsy (JME). A myoclonic jerk of the arms accompanies this burst of bilateral synchronous polyspikes. TC, 0.1 second; HFF, 70 Hz.

ning-like"), the associated EEG discharge is typically 1 to 2 seconds in duration and may last as long as 4 seconds (208).

Absence seizures in JME are associated with generalized, somewhat irregular 2.5- to 4-Hz spike and polyspike-waves that last several seconds and may be interrupted with discontinuities lasting 1 second or less. The repetition rate of the spike-wave and polyspike-wave discharges can range from 2 to 7 Hz. A classical 3-Hz spike-wave pattern is uncommon (217,218).

West's Syndrome

Clinical Features

West's syndrome is named for Dr. W.J. West, who first described the clinical features of infantile spasms in 1841, on the basis of observations of his own son (298). The syndrome consists of the triad of infantile spasms, arrest of psychomotor development, and a grossly abnormal EEG pattern termed *hypsarrhythmia*. Onset nearly always occurs in the first year of life, usually between the ages of 4 and 7 months (153,160,182). Nearly 90% of cases are associated with neurological abnormalities arising from a diverse array of structural, metabolic, and genetic disorders. Only 10% to 15% of cases are cryptogenic/idiopathic (140,159,190).

Electroencephalographic Findings

Interictal EEG. In 1952, Gibbs and Gibbs (108) described the classical EEG pattern associated with infantile spasms. They coined the term hypsarrhythmia, and their description cannot be improved upon:

> "It consists of random high voltage slow waves and spikes. These spikes vary from moment to moment, in both duration and location. At times they appear to be focal, and a few seconds later they seem to originate from multiple foci. Occasionally the spike discharge becomes generalized, but it never appears as a rhythmically repetitive and highly organized pattern....The abnormality is almost continuous...."

The chaotic, high-voltage, and asynchronous features of this abnormality, combined with an absence of virtually all normal activity, give the appearance of near-total disorganization of cortical voltage regulation (Fig. 17.14). This prototypic pattern, however, is usually seen in only the early stages of infantile spasms and most often in younger infants (159). Over time, the degree of abnormality seems to lessen, in that the EEG pattern becomes more organized, decreases in voltage, and shows greater interhemispheric synchrony and symmetry (159).

Hrachovy et al. (140) described five variations of the classical pattern. Each of these variants retained some of the major characteristics of prototypic hypsarrhythmia, and each had the same clinical and electrographic ictal features:

1. Hypsarrhythmia with increased interhemispheric synchronization, which appears as bursts of generalized spike-wave activity or as increased synchronization of the background theta and alpha frequency activities. This variation can evolve from classical hypsarrhythmia over weeks to months. These features sometimes appear only intermittently with frank hypsarrhythmia present at other times (Fig. 17.15*A*).
2. Asymmetrical hypsarrhythmia, in which there are consistent voltage asymmetries, either regionally or affecting an entire hemisphere. This pattern is seen most often when there are large cystic or atrophic defects of one cerebral hemisphere, such as porencephaly or encephalomalacia (see Fig. 17.15*B*).
3. Hypsarrhythmia with a consistent focus of abnormal discharge. In these cases, there is a persistent localized area of spike or sharp wave activity, in addition to the typical multifocal discharges. Focal electrographic ictal discharges can occur in the same region, but the background pattern of hypsarrhythmia is not affected by the focal seizure. Such localized abnormalities can persist after the hypsarrhythmia disappears (see Fig. 17.15*C*).
4. Hypsarrhythmia with episodes of generalized, regional, or lateralized voltage attenuation. These periods of attenuation last 2 to 10 seconds and sometimes occur in a periodic pattern (see Fig. 17.15*D*).
5. Hypsarrhythmia composed primarily of high-voltage, bilaterally asynchronous slow wave activity with relatively little epileptiform activity (see Fig. 17.15*E*).

More than one of these variations may be present at the same time in a given patient.

Hrachovy et al. (140) considered the foregoing variations to be examples of "modified hypsarrhythmia," a term that had been used over the years by many authors to describe any deviation from what, in their view, represents "true" hypsarrhythmia. In fact, the boundaries of what constitutes hypsarrhythmia are not clearly defined, and experienced electroencephalographers have differing opinions about "how abnormal" an EEG must be, and with what constellation of features, before it can be classified accurately as hypsarrhythmia. The authors believe that it is more meaningful to consider hypsarrhythmia as a group of severe abnormalities that share many of the same

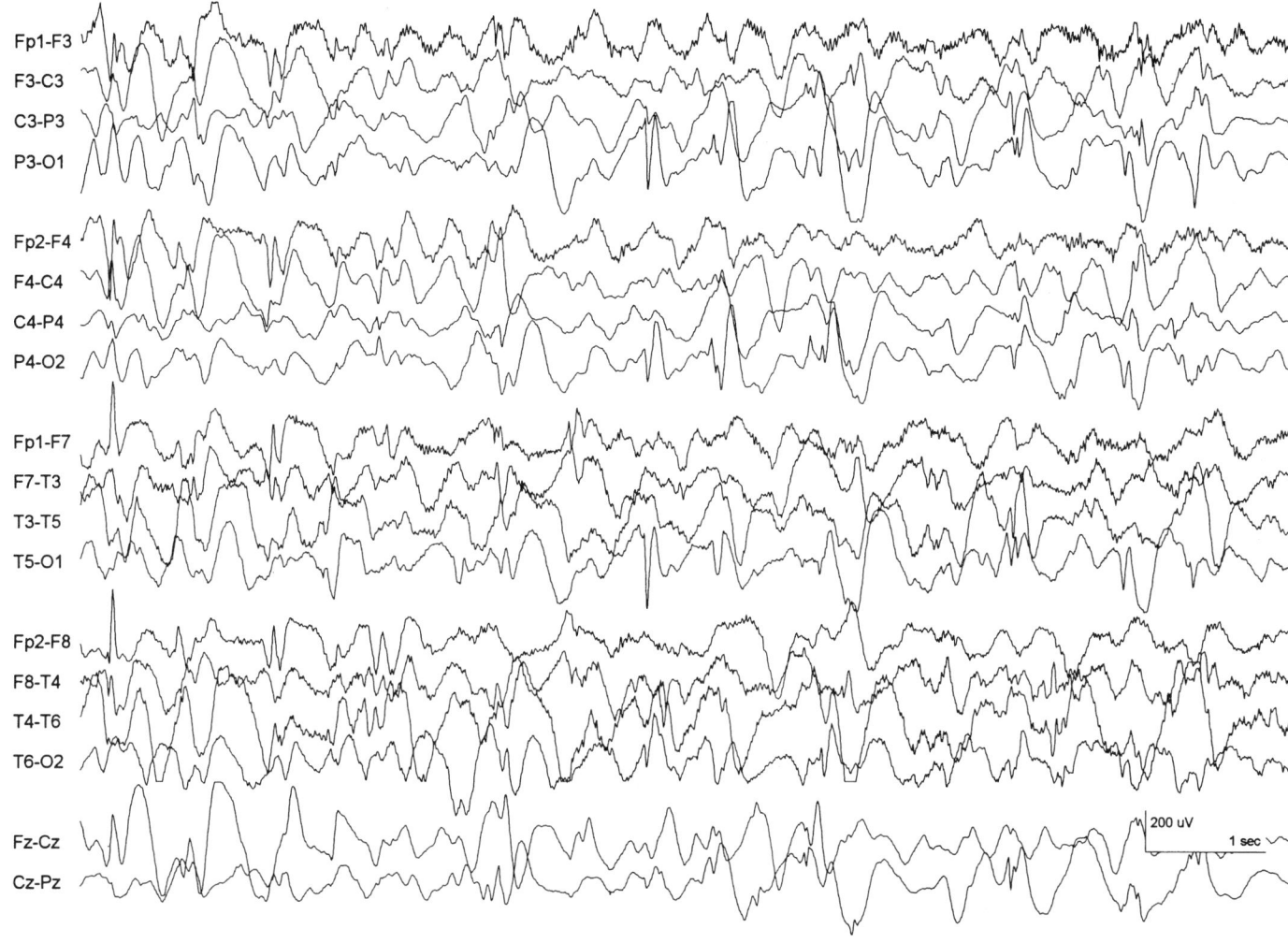

A

FIG. 17.14. A: EEG of an 8-month-old boy with infantile spasms and severe developmental delay. EEG during the waking state shows typical hypsarrhythmia. Note the high voltage, absence of spatial organization, and the multifocal spikes (F4, C3, P3, O1). TC, 0.3 second; HFF, 70 Hz. *(Figure continues.)*

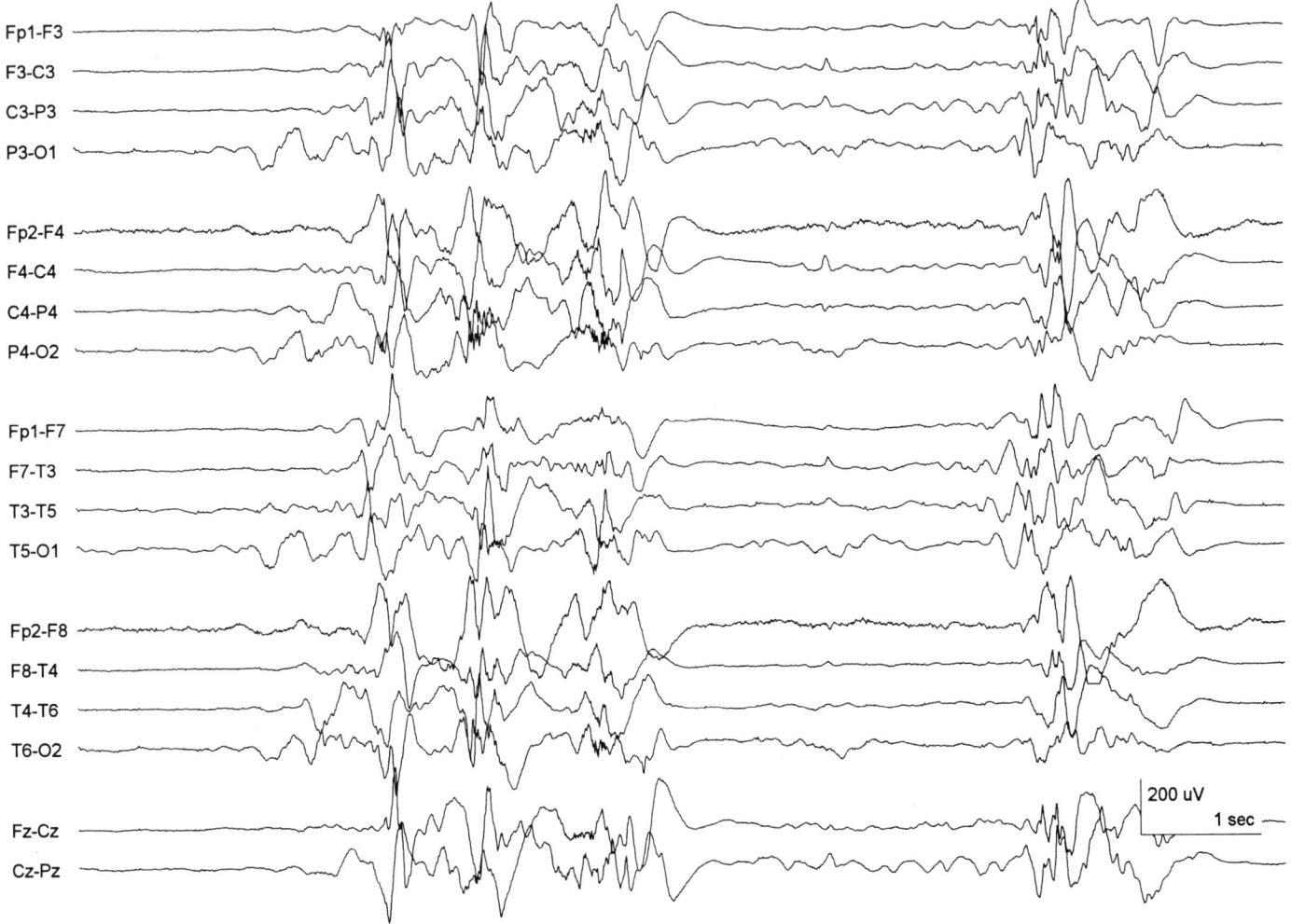

B

FIG. 17.14. *Continued.* **B:** EEG of a 3-month-old boy, also with West's syndrome. The EEG recorded during sleep demonstrates an episodic (burst-suppression) type of hypsarrhythmia pattern. TC, 0.3 second; HFF, 70 Hz.

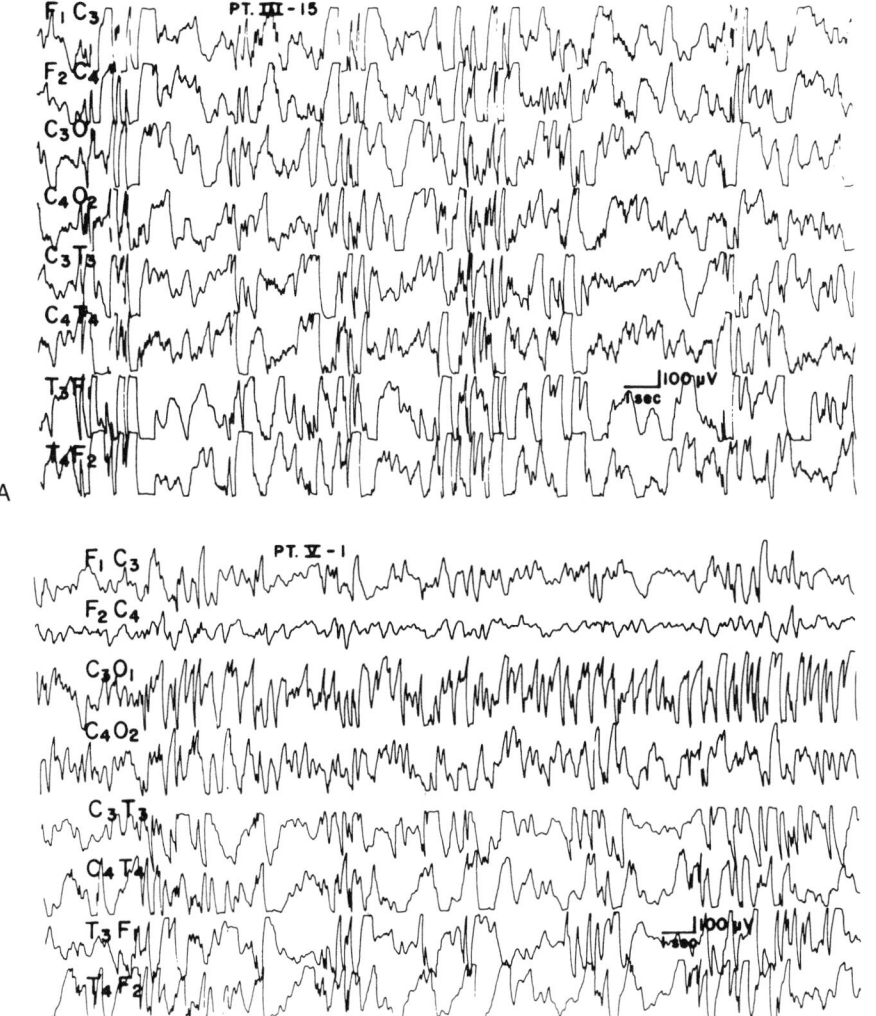

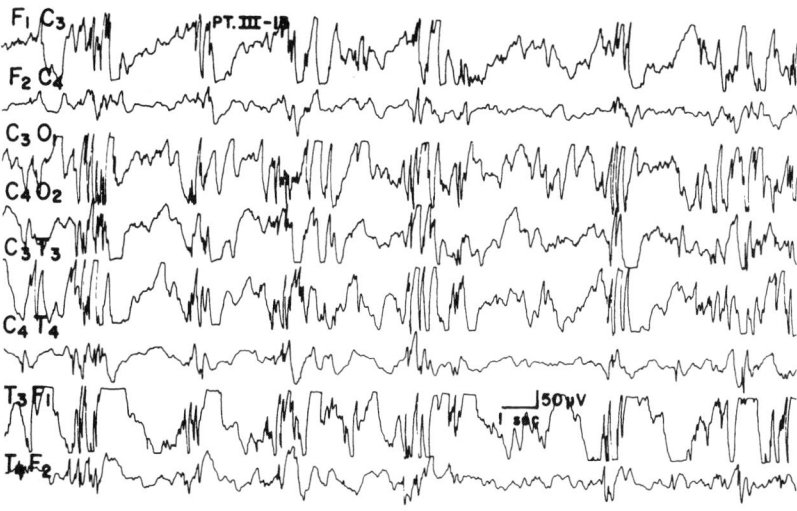

FIG. 17.15 A: EEG of an 8-month-old infant, showing hypsarrhythmia characterized by the presence of synchronous and symmetrical frontal-dominant spike and slow-wave and sharp-and-slow-wave activity. **B:** EEG of a 6-month-old infant, showing asymmetrical hypsarrhythmia. A head computed tomogram revealed a porencephalic defect in the right hemisphere. **C:** EEG of a 3-month-old infant, showing hypsarrhythmia with an identifiable focus of irregular spike and slow-wave and sharp-and-slow-wave activity in the left occipital region. *(Figure continues.)*

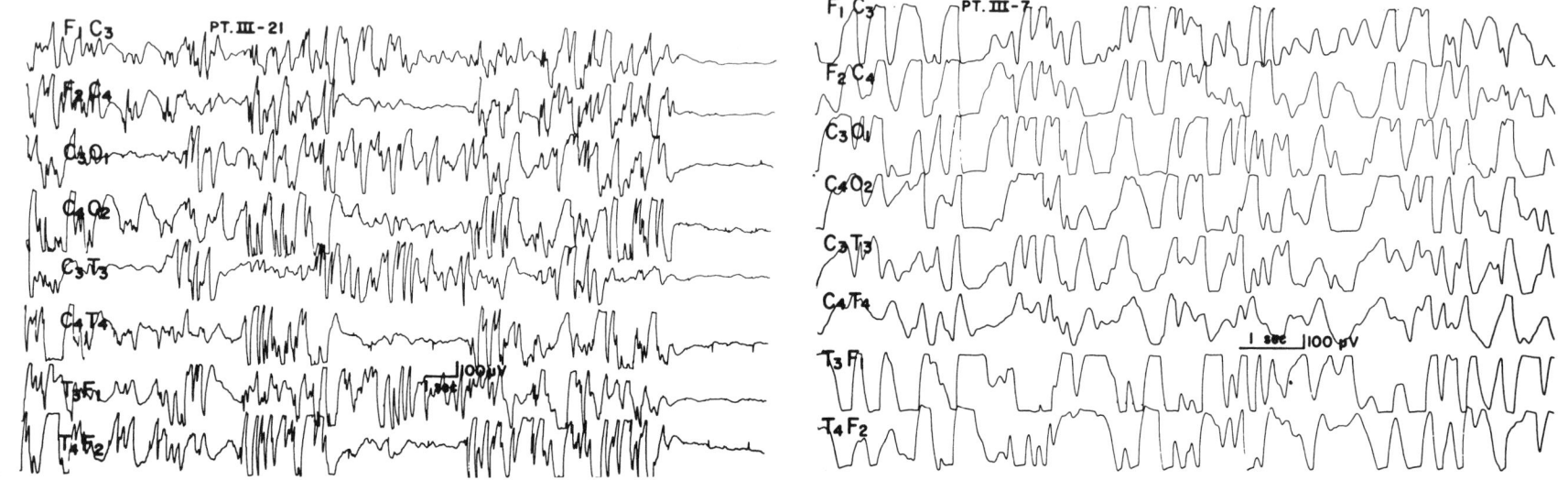

FIG. 17.15. *Continued.* **D:** EEG of a 9-month-old infant, showing hypsarrhythmia with episodes of lateralized and generalized voltage attenuation. **E:** EEG of a 13-month-old infant, showing hypsarrhythmia characterized by the presence of high-voltage, primarily asynchronous slow-wave activity with little spike or sharp wave activity. (From Hrachovy RA, Frost JD Jr, Kellaway P. Hypsarrhythmia: variations on the theme. *Epilepsia* 1984;25:317–325.)

features and exist at one extreme of a spectrum of age-dependent, abnormal EEG findings seen in infants and very young children with severe epileptic encephalopathies. It is not an entity per se, nor does it reflect any common underlying condition or pathological process. It is therefore understandable that physicians encounter considerable variability, including the variations just listed, at one time or another not only among patients but also over time in the same patient. In the authors' view, variations such as those listed are not "modified hypsarrhythmia"; they are simply different manifestations of the hypsarrhythmic type of abnormality.

Although it is characteristic, hypsarrhythmia is not seen in all patients with infantile spasms. *Aicardi's syndrome,* which consists of infantile spasms, agenesis of the corpus callosum, and chorioretinal lacunae, is associated with a distinctive EEG pattern. The interictal EEG is characterized by a background of burst-suppression activity that is completely asynchronous between the two hemispheres. The periods of EEG activity

contain medium-voltage, very irregular theta and delta waves intermixed with multifocal spikes and sharp waves. There is complete absence of any semblance of normal sleep architecture (89). In a longitudinal study of patients with Aicardi's syndrome, Ohtsuka et al. (209) described similar EEG findings but also noted that this pattern may in turn evolve into hypsarrhythmia during the course of the disease. At the same time, not every infant whose EEG demonstrates hypsarrhythmia has infantile spasms. Hypsarrhythmia is sometimes seen in with other types of severe infantile epileptic encephalopathy (96).

In their initial description of hypsarrhythmia, Gibbs and Gibbs (108) described the abnormality as "...almost continuous, and in most cases [evident] as clearly in the waking as in the sleeping record." This description has had to be modified in light of more recent studies. Although the EEG pattern is indeed unreactive to photic or tactile stimulation, hypsarrhythmia commonly varies with changes in state. In a study of 82 children with clinical spasms, Watanabe et al. (295) found that 99% had hypsarrhythmia during stages 2 and 3 NREM sleep, 86% during stage 1 sleep, and only 64% during waking periods. This finding emphasizes the importance of recording adequate samples of sleep to maximize the yield of "positive" EEGs. In slow-wave sleep, background activity voltage and the number of epileptiform discharges typically increase. In addition, background activity often becomes more periodic with intervals of diffuse voltage attenuation (138,140) (see Fig. 17.14*B*). In contrast, the hypsarrhythmia pattern tends to disappear during REM sleep (138,295). Immediately after arousal from either NREM or REM sleep, the EEG may transiently "normalize" before hypsarrhythmia reappears (140). Total sleep time and percentage of REM sleep time are significantly reduced in patients with West's syndrome (138). Of interest is that sleep spindles are commonly preserved even with otherwise profound disturbances in background activity and virtual absence of other normal sleep (138).

The natural evolution of hypsarrhythmia is known mainly from studies performed before 1958, when adrenocorticotropic hormone (ACTH) was introduced (268); treatment with either ACTH or corticosteroids subsequently became widespread. There is gradual modification of the abnormalities over time, with increasing organization and greater interhemispheric synchrony (159). Without treatment, about 25% of patients have spontaneous cessation of spasms with disappearance of hypsarrhythmia within 1 year of onset of the disorder (141). Livingston et al. (178), who studied 531 cases of infantile spasms with hypsarrhythmia, none of whom received corticosteroids, found that only 6% retained a hypsarrhythmic EEG after age 5, and in no case did the abnormality persist after the age of 7. Fewer than half the original patients continued to have spasms after the age of 3 (152); it is extremely rare for spasms to persist after the age of 5 (178).

Until the introduction of vigabatrin, most infants with West's syndrome were treated with ACTH. ACTH usually leads to rapid normalization of the EEG, with response rates ranging from 67% (139) to 97% (264) (Fig. 17.16). Resolution of clinical spasms usually parallels disappearance of hypsarrhythmia, but the two can be dissociated. Improvement in EEG activity is usually long lasting, but a substantial portion (31% to 47%) of patients develop recurrent spasms after being free of seizures for several months (139,264). Longer term follow-up studies have demonstrated that about half the patients develop a normal EEG background (153,154,178). About 35% to 40% develop persistent focal or bilateral abnormalities, and most of these are epileptogenic (153,154).

There is, unfortunately, little evidence that early resolution of spasms and hypsarrhythmia results in lasting, long-term neurological improvement (141). It is therefore important to emphasize that normalization of EEG activity is not necessarily correlated with neurological status and that nearly 90% of patients remain disabled by epilepsy and other neurological abnormalities, including severe mental impairment.

Ictal EEG. Although not all spasms are associated with hypsarrhythmia, spasms are, by definition, present in all cases of West's syndrome. In a video-EEG study, Kellaway et al. (160) reviewed the clinical and electrographic features of 5,042 infantile spasms in 24 infants. The most common electrographic pattern, seen in 37.9% of spasms, consisted of a high-voltage, frontally dominant, generalized slow wave transient, followed by diffuse voltage attenuation (electrodecremental event) (Fig. 17.17). They also noted ten other distinct electrographic ictal patterns:

Generalized sharp-and-slow-wave complexes (17.4%)
Generalized sharp-and-slow-wave discharge followed by a period of attenuation (13.2%)
Period of attenuation only (11.9%)
Generalized slow-wave transients (10.9%)
Attenuation with superimposed fast activity (6.9%)
Generalized slow wave followed by attenuation with superimposed fast activity (1.3%)
Attenuation with rhythmic slow activity (0.2%)
Fast activity only (0.2%)
Sharp-and-slow-wave complex followed by attenuation and superimposed fast activity (0.06%)
Attenuation with superimposed fast activity followed by rhythmic slow activity (0.06%)

The electrodecremental event was the most consistent electrographic feature; it was seen as a part of the ictal discharge in 71.7% of spasms. The duration of the ictal discharge was quite variable, ranging from 0.5 to 106 seconds.

In another video-EEG study, Fusco and Vigevano (98) found less variability in the ictal EEG patterns. All clinical spasms were accompanied by a medium- to high-voltage, positive slow wave that was maximal at the central and vertex regions. Very-low-voltage fast activity was often superimposed. These workers also noted that 70% of spasms were associated with an electrodecremental event but observed that this was a postictal, not an ictal, feature.

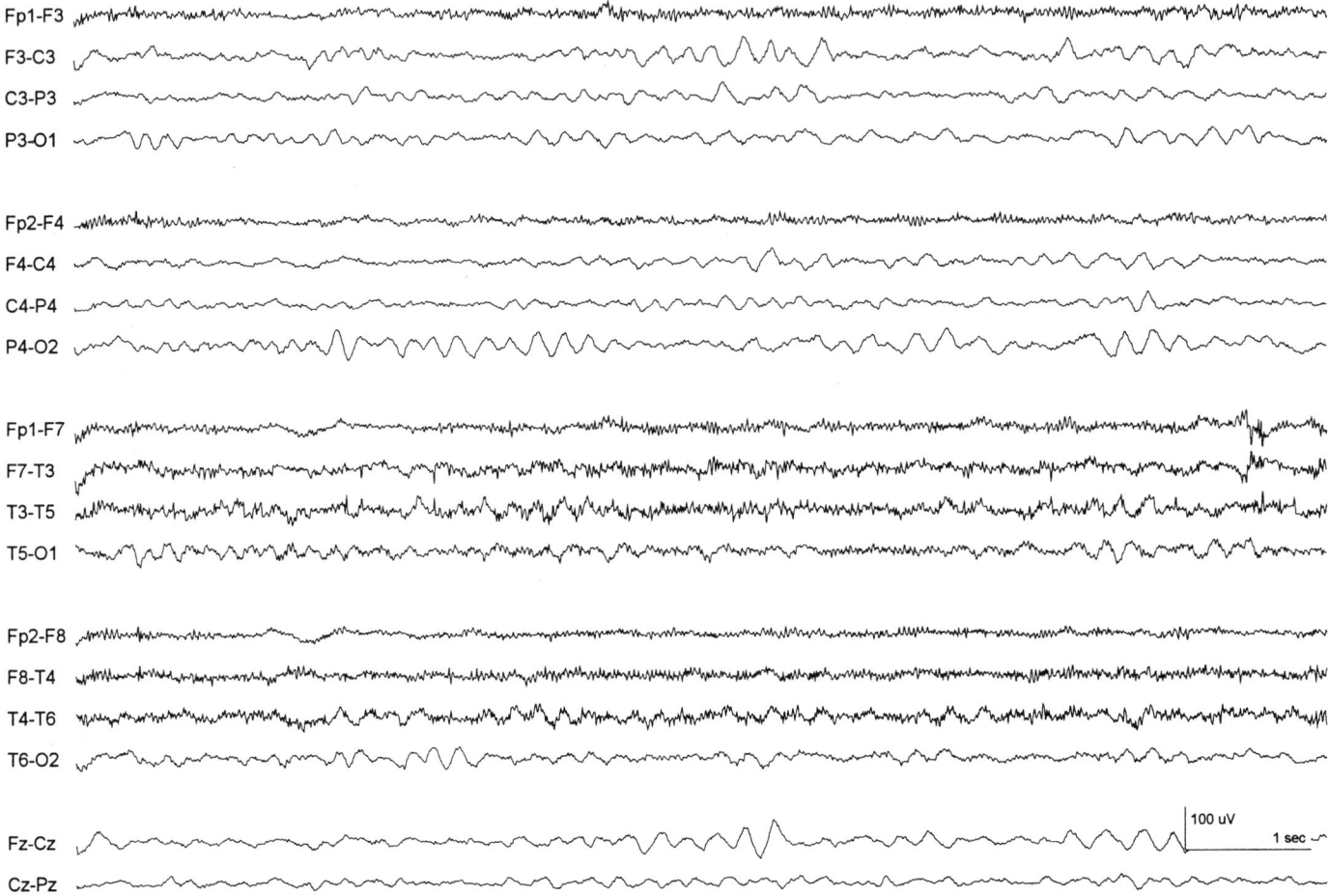

Fp1-F3

F3-C3

C3-P3

P3-O1

Fp2-F4

F4-C4

C4-P4

P4-O2

Fp1-F7

F7-T3

T3-T5

T5-O1

Fp2-F8

F8-T4

T4-T6

T6-O2

Fz-Cz

Cz-Pz

100 uV

1 sec

FIG. 17.16. EEG from the same 8 month-old child as in Fig. 17.14*A* obtained 1 month after treatment with adrenocorticotropic hormone (ACTH). Despite the resolution of both hypsarrhythmia and infantile spasms, the child remained severely impaired neurologically. TC, 0.1 second; HFF, 70 Hz.

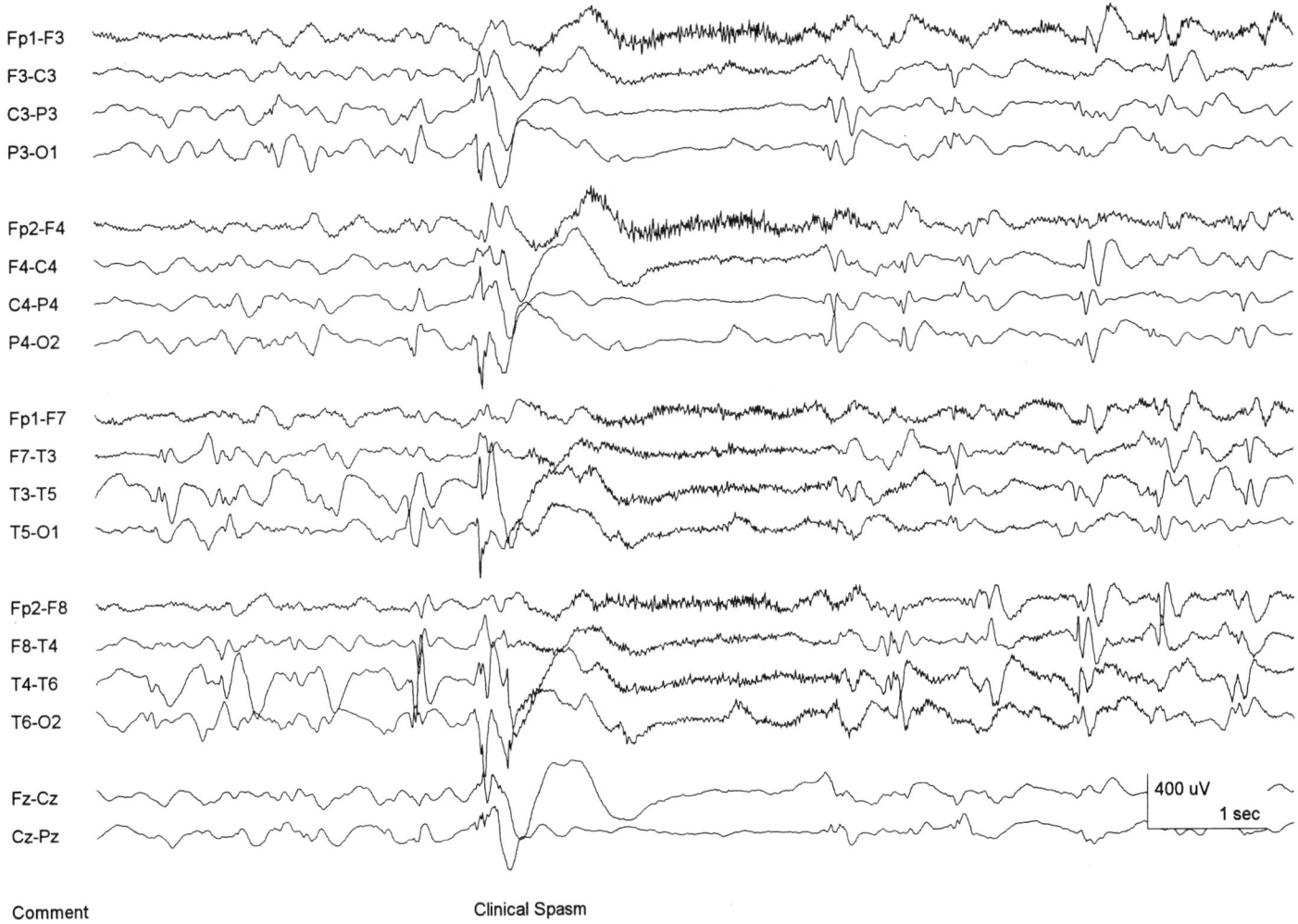

Fp1-F3
F3-C3
C3-P3
P3-O1

Fp2-F4
F4-C4
C4-P4
P4-O2

Fp1-F7
F7-T3
T3-T5
T5-O1

Fp2-F8
F8-T4
T4-T6
T6-O2

Fz-Cz
Cz-Pz

400 uV
1 sec

Comment

Clinical Spasm

FIG. 17.17. Electrodecremental pattern associated with a typical spasm. There is a high-voltage slow wave followed by 3 seconds of greatly attenuated EEG activity. TC, 0.3 second; HFF, 70 Hz.

Lennox-Gastaut Syndrome

Clinical Features

William G. Lennox and, later, Henri Gastaut described the clinical and electrographic features of this disorder. The Lennox-Gastaut syndrome (LGS) encompasses a characteristic triad of severe generalized epilepsy, mental retardation, and an EEG pattern of slow-spike-and-wave discharges (103,171,172). Age at onset is usually between 1 and 8 years; most cases begin between the ages of 2 and 5 years. Onset after 10 years of age is rare (13,18,186).

The ILAE Classification of Epilepsies and Epileptic Syndromes (228) includes LGS among the generalized cryptogenic or symptomatic epilepsies. It is defined by the following criteria:

1. High seizure frequency; tonic, atonic, and atypical absence seizures are the most common. Myoclonic, generalized tonic-clonic, and partial seizures may also be present. As a rule, patients with LGS have multiple seizure types, and at least one episode of status epilepticus occurs in the majority (13).
2. Mental retardation, in general. More recently, some authors have argued that behavioral disorders, not accompanied by cognitive impairment, should be sufficient for diagnosis (105).
3. EEG demonstrating abnormal background activity with diffuse sharp-slow waves that have a repetition rate of less than 3 Hz. There are often multifocal spikes or sharp waves and, during sleep, frequent bursts of 10 Hz and faster frequencies.

LGS accounts for about 10% of all childhood epilepsies (3,102), although the actual prevalence may be much lower if rigorous criteria are used (13,18). Tonic, atonic, and myoclonic seizures can all result in the characteristic "drop attacks" seen in LGS, and differentiating among these on the basis of clinical features alone is often difficult. Moreover, there is significant overlap among the ictal patterns (see later discussion). Despite the consistent electroclinical triad, LGS cannot be attributed to a single cause or common pathological substrate. Diverse prenatal, perinatal, and postnatal disorders have been implicated. About two-thirds of cases are considered symptomatic, because a preexisting neurological condition can be identified. One-third of cases are classified as cryptogenic (54,103,186).

Electroencephalographic Findings

Interictal EEG: Slow-Spike-and-Wave Pattern. Gibbs et al. (109) were the first to describe the characteristic slow-spike-and-wave abnormality, a pattern they called "petit mal variant" to distinguish it from the stereotyped 3-Hz spike-wave discharge of childhood absence epilepsy. The slow-spike-and-wave discharge is more accurately described as a slow-sharp-and-wave (SSW) complex, because it consists predominantly of biphasic or triphasic surface-negative sharp waves of 150 to 200 milliseconds' duration followed by high-voltage (300- to 400-μV) negative slow waves, each lasting about 350 milliseconds (34,103,186). The SSW complexes are bilateral, synchronous, and symmetrical and of highest voltage over the frontal-central regions. These discharges occur repetitively in bursts or extended runs at frequencies of 1.5 to 2.5 Hz (103,186) (Fig. 17.18*A*). It is important to recognize, however, that there are many variations on this general theme. For example, SSW discharges can vary, both between and within individual bursts, in morphological appearance, distribution, voltage, and frequency. The repetition rate of SSW discharges can be quite erratic, with frequencies ranging from 1 to 4 Hz. The extended runs of SSW discharges commonly lack discrete onsets or terminations; sometimes they are nearly continuous during the greater part of an entire recording. Most SSW discharges are not accompanied by obvious clinical manifestations (34,103,186). Although usually symmetrical, SSW complexes sometimes show shifting asymmetries. Persistent focal or lateralized asymmetries of SSW discharges usually occur in symptomatic cases with focal neurological abnormalities (34,186). Asymmetries of SSW discharges usually include associated asymmetries in background activity (186).

Some authors have reported that hyperventilation increases the occurrence and duration of SSW bursts in more than 50% of patients (35,186), but this is disputed by others (34,103). Photic stimulation typically has no effect on SSW activity (18,34,103,186).

NREM sleep dramatically enhances SSW discharges in the great majority of patients (34,103,186). This effect is not universal, however, and in some patients, the discharges may actually decrease in both NREM and REM sleep (35,137). On occasion, SSW discharges are prominent during sleep even when they are infrequent during wakefulness, which underscores the importance of obtaining an adequate sleep recording (186). Polyspike-wave discharges may emerge during sleep (34,51,137). In a minority of patients, sleep causes fragmentation of SSW bursts and a pseudoperiodic or burst-suppression appearance, with 2- to 3-second paroxysms of SSW alternating with diffuse voltage attenuation of background activity (186).

Interictal EEG: Paroxysmal Fast Activity. Paroxysmal fast activity (PFA), the second defining electrographic feature of LGS, is present mainly or exclusively during sleep in nearly all patients (13). PFA consists of diffuse, bilaterally synchronous bursts of 15- to 20-Hz activity that last several seconds. It is of highest voltage in the frontal areas (51) (Fig. 17.19). The frequency of PFA

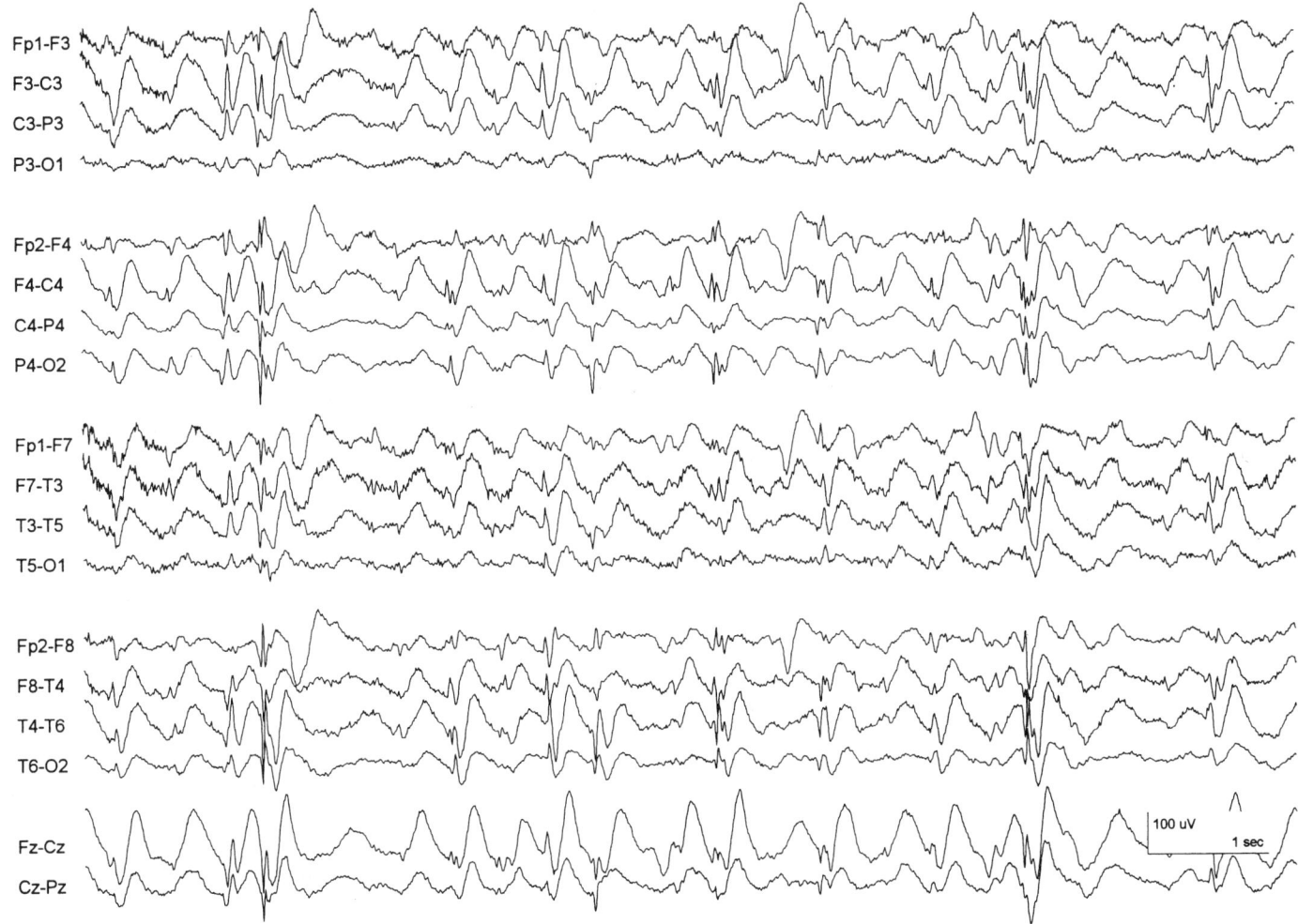

A

FIG. 17.18. EEG of a 29-year-old woman who had had Lennox-Gastaut syndrome (LGS) since early child-hood. **A:** Interictal EEG recording demonstrating diffuse background delta frequency slowing and nearly con-tinuous 1.5- to 2.0-Hz bilateral synchronous slow-spike-and-wave (SSW) discharges. During this time, the patient was attentive and interactive. TC, 0.1 second; HFF, 70 Hz. *(Figure continues.)*

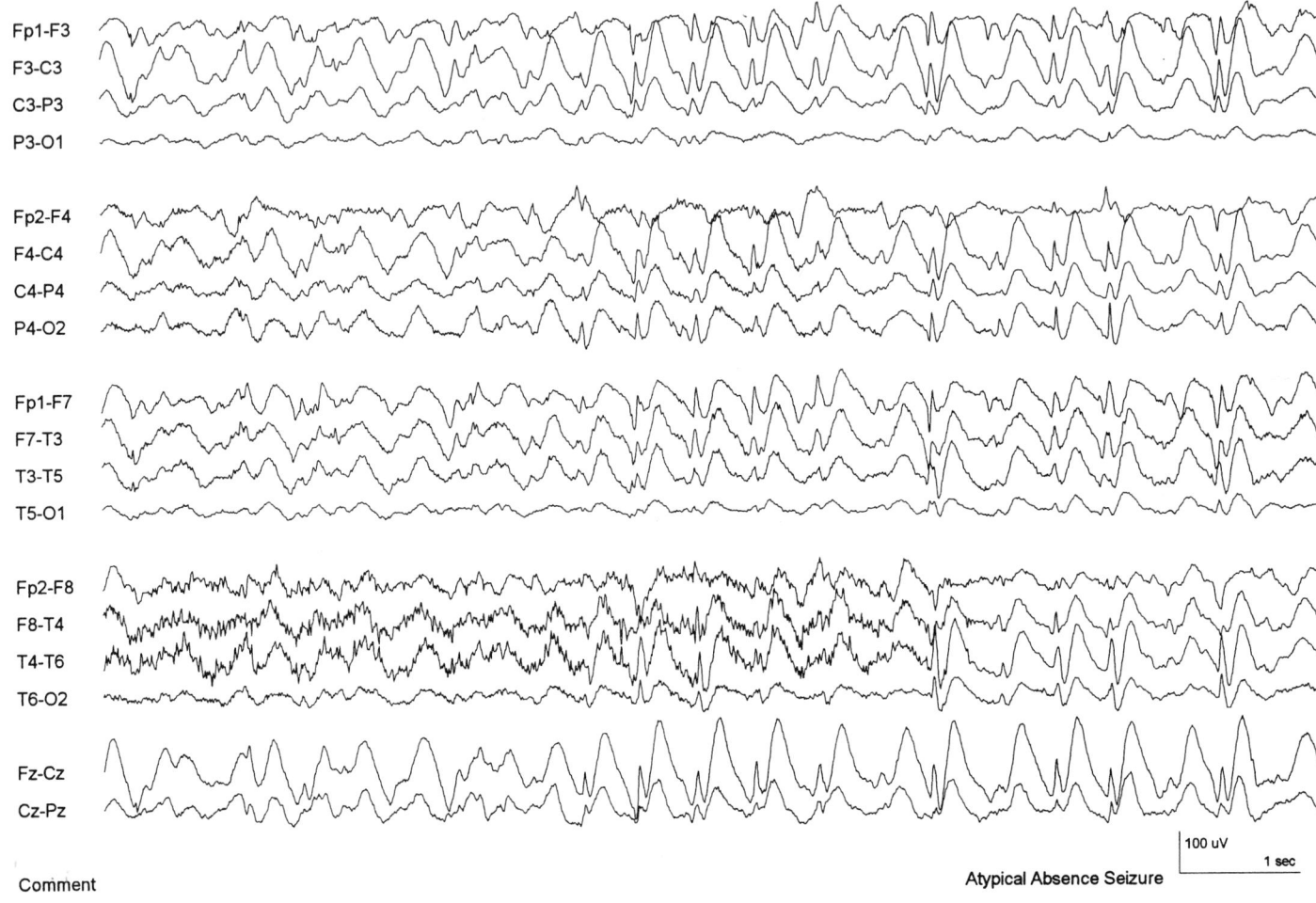

B   Comment

Atypical Absence Seizure

FIG. 17.18. *Continued.* **B:** Atypical absence seizure characterized by decreased responsiveness and gaze deviation to the right. Although very similar to the interictal recording shown in part *A,* the SSW discharges appear more organized and sustained at a consistent 2-Hz frequency. TC, 0.1 second; HFF, 70 Hz.

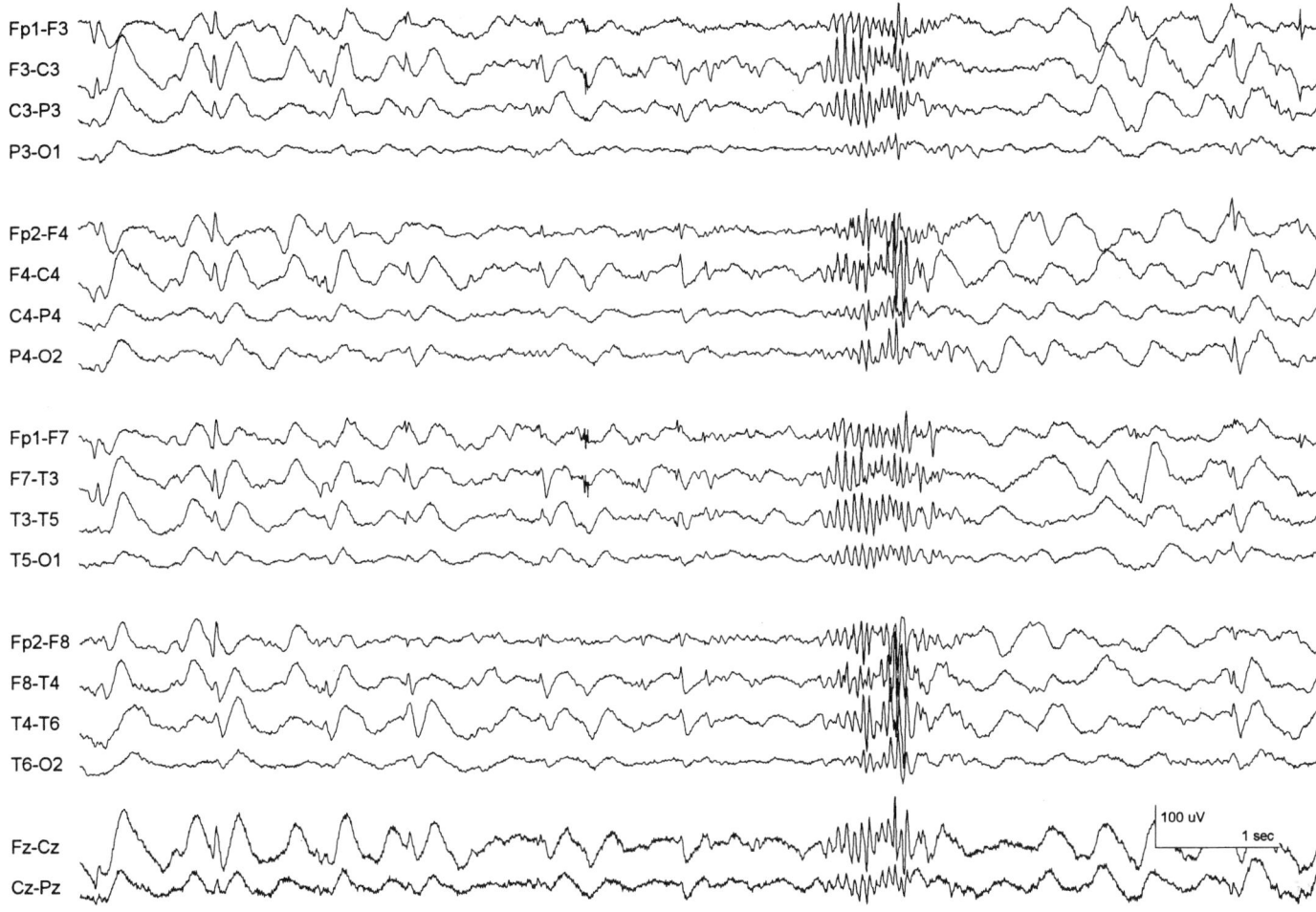

FIG. 17.19. Sleep EEG of a patient with Lennox-Gastaut syndrome (LGS). There are frequent bursts of diffuse 16- to 20-Hz paroxysmal fast activity (PFA) without any visually detectable clinical changes. TC, 0.1 second; HFF, off.

can vary from 7 to 30 Hz, and the voltage may vary from 25 to 250 μV. The duration of PFA bursts ranges from 2 to 12 seconds (51). Bursts of PFA occur up to hundreds of times each night, but only in NREM sleep; they are absent during REM (51).

Although indistinguishable from the ictal pattern associated with tonic seizures (see later discussion), the majority of PFA discharges are not accompanied by any visually discernible clinical changes. Chatrian et al. (51) reported absence of clinical manifestations, even from submental electromyographic electrodes, in 77% of 1,432 discharges. However, electrodes placed over the paraspinous muscles demonstrate subclinical tonic muscle activity that is correlated with bursts of PFA in a higher percentage of patients. Duration of PFA may be one important variable associated with clinical manifestations. Brenner and Atkinson (37) studied 20 patients with LGS and found that bursts of PFA lasting more than 6 seconds usually produced clinical changes, whereas those lasting less than 6 seconds were typically clinically asymptomatic. Autonomic changes, including tachycardia and apnea, can occur in association with PFA, even when motor manifestations are absent (51,137) Thus, it can be argued that PFA is not, strictly speaking, an interictal finding, although the ictal manifestations may be subtle and not visually detectable.

In addition to the characteristic SSW complexes, focal or multifocal epileptiform discharges occur in 14% to 18% of patients (35,186). Additional focal or lateralized abnormalities are present in 23% to 50% of LGS patients (10,186). Diffuse abnormalities of background activity occur in up to 90% of patients with LGS (10,54,103,186). In two-thirds of cases, background slowing is moderate to severe and is generally correlated with the degree of cognitive impairment (186).

Many patients have abnormal sleep architecture. In comparison to normal age-matched controls, REM sleep time in patients with LGS is nearly always reduced and can be absent completely (5,137). In extreme cases, there is complete lack of identifiable sleep stages, and only an undifferentiated pattern of NREM sleep is seen (51). Other patients develop such severe disorganization of background activity during sleep that a quasi-hypsarrhythmic pattern emerges (186).

In most patients with LGS, mental impairment and severe epilepsy persist throughout life. The characteristic electroclinical triad persists into adulthood in 75% of patients (10,13,177).

Ictal EEG. The electrographic correlate of a tonic seizure is the PFA pattern (Fig. 17.20). The discharge is usually of maximal voltage shortly after onset but fluctuates subsequently (51). Diffuse voltage attenuation or a burst of SSW discharges may precede the PFA discharge. After the seizure, baseline EEG activity returns rapidly (51).

Egli et al. (81) described a slightly different type of tonic seizure that they termed *pure axial spasm.* The spasm consists of a high-velocity muscle contraction lasting 0.5 to 0.8 seconds that produces prominent flexion of the neck, trunk, and hips. Consciousness is not impaired, and usually no change in EEG activity is recordable from scalp electrodes.

Atypical absence seizures have been reported in 32% (103), 79% (13), and 100% (310) of patients with LGS. The rising percentage most likely reflects the introduction of continuous video-EEG monitoring and recognition of the more subtle manifestations of these seizures. Although the distinction between typical and atypical absence seizures is not always clearcut (135), several features tend to characterize the majority of atypical absences. First, impairment of consciousness is incomplete, and some purposeful activity may continue. Second, onset and termination are gradual, often making the seizures difficult to recognize, especially when there is marked cognitive impairment. Third, excessive salivation, eyelid or mouth myoclonus, changes in postural tone, and automatisms are common.

Several ictal EEG patterns have been associated with atypical absence seizures. Most often, there is diffuse, bisynchronous, high-amplitude, 1- to 2.5-Hz SSW activity, which may be difficult to distinguish from the interictal EEG pattern. However, ictal paroxysms tend to be more regular, more widely distributed, and of longer duration than interictal bursts (186) (see Fig. 17.18) . Less often, two other patterns are seen: (a) diffuse, bisynchronous, 7-Hz spike-wave discharge or (b) diffuse bursts of 10- to 20-Hz rhythmic activity similar to PFA (35,310).

Ictal EEG recordings during atonic seizures are also variable. Most often, there is a diffuse, high-voltage, bisynchronous burst of polyspikes or polyspike-waves similar to the discharge seen with myoclonic seizures. Less often, the EEG shows diffuse spike-wave, SSW, or generalized fast-frequency activity.

Association of Lennox-Gastaut Syndrome with Other Epileptic Encephalopathies

Blume (33) described a syndrome that is related clinically to LGS with mental retardation and severe generalized epilepsy, but with multiple independent spike foci on EEG. Unlike West's syndrome and LGS, however, this syndrome is not age-specific, and about one-third of patients are mentally normal.

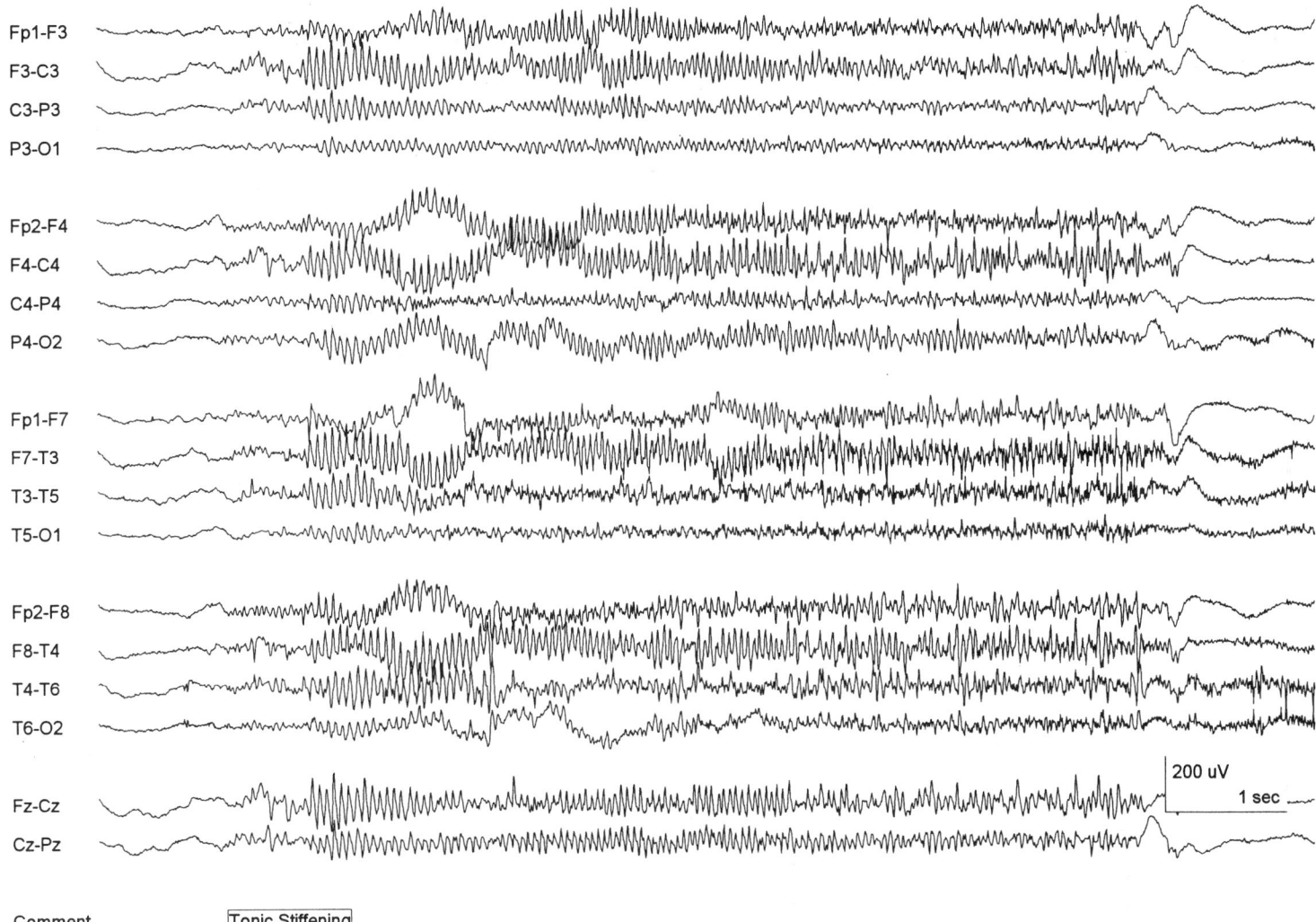

FIG. 17.20. Tonic seizure in Lennox-Gastaut syndrome (LGS). During sleep, the child exhibited abrupt onset of arm and neck stiffening, which lasted several seconds. The EEG shows an 8-second run of bilateral synchronous 16- to 20-Hz activity, which is the ictal discharge. TC, 0.1 second; HFF, off.

There are many associations among infantile spasms, LGS, and multiple independent spike foci. A history of infantile spasms with hypsarrhythmia can be obtained in 17% (13) to 20% (186) of children with LGS. In a few patients, different EEG patterns coexist. For example, in Markand's series (186), some patients showed multiple independent spike foci while awake but SSW during sleep, and nearly one-fourth of patients with SSW in the waking state had hypsarrhythmia during sleep.

Because none of these syndromes is specific with regard to either cause or pathological process, it is likely that the particular manifestations of severe epileptic encephalopathies reflect complex interactions of brain immaturity, developmental mechanisms, timing of brain injury, and pathological processes. When certain sets of clinical and EEG features occur together as the predominant abnormalities, individual clinical-electrographic syndromes can be identified. These groupings, however, show considerable overlap in clinical features and EEG findings, which indicates that although they may be clinically useful, they are fundamentally artificial.

Landau-Kleffner Syndrome and the Syndrome of Continuous Spikes and Waves during Slow Sleep

The Landau-Kleffner syndrome (LKS) and the syndrome of continuous spikes and waves during slow sleep (CSWS) are two rare electroclinical syndromes that have considerable overlap in both clinical and electrographic features.

Landau-Kleffner Syndrome

Clinical Features. This syndrome, first described by Landau and Kleffner (167), is characterized by acquired aphasia associated with epileptiform activity on EEG ("epileptic aphasia"). Although the nature of this syndrome is controversial, it is probably not fundamentally an epileptic disorder. It occurs in previously healthy children between the ages of 3 and 9 years (peak incidence, 5 to 7 years) (15,42,134). The first indication of aphasia is verbal auditory agnosia (234), but language function continues to deteriorate. Some children become mute and do not respond even to nonverbal sounds (15,71). Hyperactivity and personality changes appear as the aphasia worsens (15). Seizures occur in about 70% of patients; they tend to be relatively infrequent, although status epilepticus has been reported. Partial motor, atypical absence, generalized tonic-clonic, and atonic seizures have all been reported (15,134). More subtle seizures, such as eyelid myoclonia, ocular deviation, and head drops also occur (198). Type and frequency of

seizures are not correlated with outcome (16,198). Similarly, treatment with antiseizure drugs does not clearly affect aphasia, EEG findings, or prognosis. Although subpial transection (Morrell's procedure) has recently been used to eliminate epileptiform activity surgically (198), there are no controlled studies to show that this affects the natural history of the disorder. About two-thirds of children have residual language impairment; cognitive and behavioral abnormalities are less frequent consequences.

Electroencephalographic Findings. A paroxysmal EEG is one of the defining features of LKS, and epileptiform discharges are thus invariably present. Epileptiform activity is extremely variable in both location and amount. High-voltage multifocal spikes and spike-wave discharges occur both singly and repetitively (15). Discharges occur over the posterior temporal regions preferentially but are not limited to these areas (Fig. 17.21). Epileptiform activity can be unilateral or bilateral. When bilateral, the discharges can be diffuse and bisynchronous and either symmetrical or asymmetrical (15,134,198). In the early stages of the disorder, epileptiform activity may be limited to sleep. The EEG abnormalities vary considerably over time, so that the distribution, abundance, and topography may change from one tracing to the next (69).

Morrell et al. (198) used a variety of specialized techniques, including the methohexital suppression test, intracarotid injection of amobarbital, and electrocorticography to show that some patients with LKS had a single epileptogenic focus in the perisylvian region. They proposed that bilateral discharges resulted from spread from this one epileptogenic area rather than being manifestations of generalized or independent abnormalities. This argument became the basis for using multiple subpial transections to suppress the perisylvian focus. Although Morrell et al. (198) reported dramatic and clinical improvement after surgery, a controlled study is necessary to confirm these data.

NREM sleep activates epileptiform activity, often to a marked degree. Epileptiform discharges exhibit larger fields, tend to become generalized, and occur repetitively at frequencies of 1.5 to 3 Hz (134). During REM sleep, the slow spike-wave pattern fragments and focal or multifocal discharges appear in a pattern similar to that seen in the waking state (30). Sometimes there is continuous (occupying more than 85% of sleep time) spike-wave activity that is similar to that seen in the syndrome of CSWS (134,220). In a study of five patients with LKS, Hirsch et al. (134) found that all of them showed continuous spike-waves during sleep at some point in their course. Similar findings by other researchers (69,198,220) indicate that this pattern is underrecognized and that perhaps most, if not all, patients with LKS demonstrate this pattern with extended polygraphic sleep recordings.

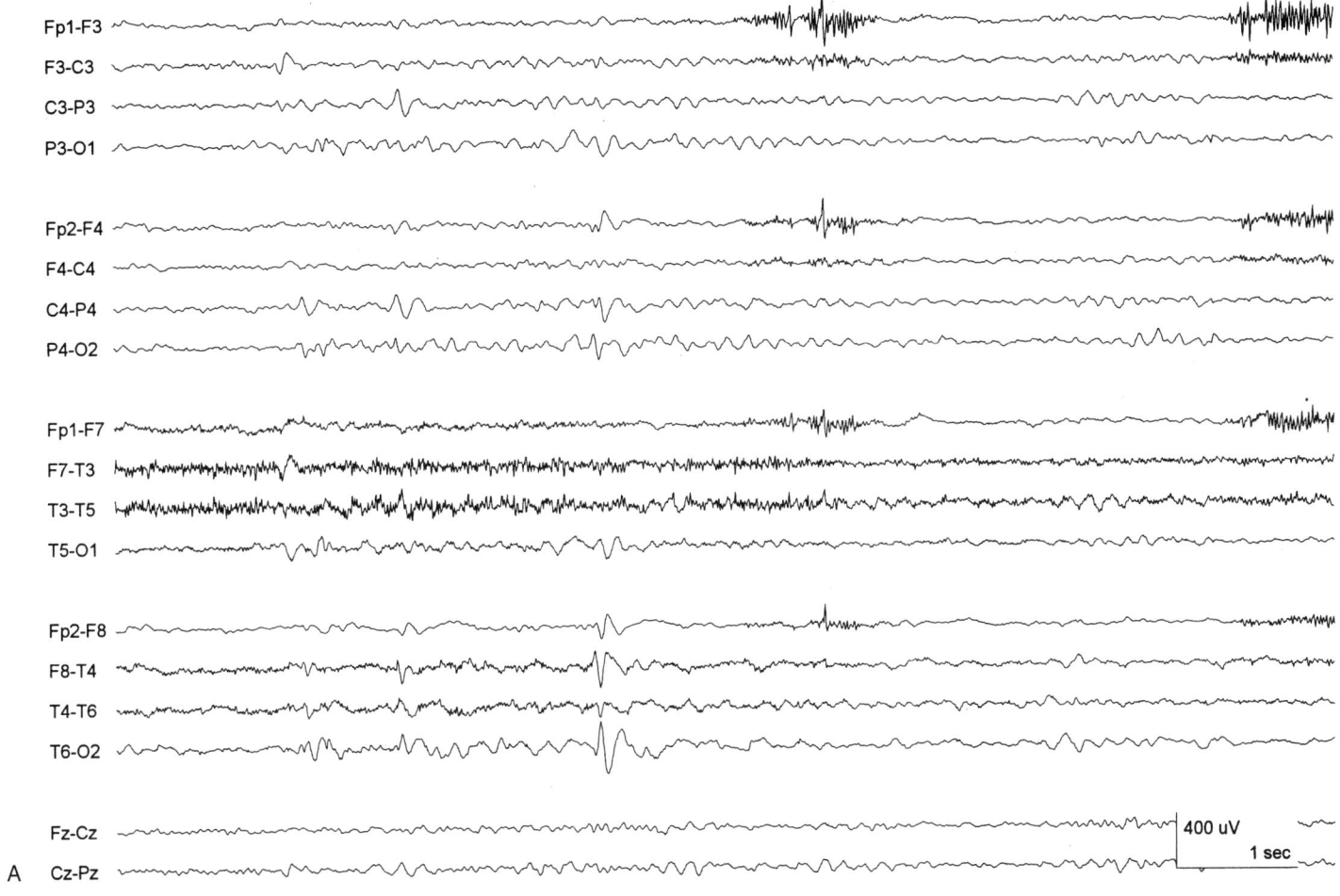

FIG. 17.21. EEG of a 6-year-old boy with Landau-Kleffner syndrome (LKS). He had been neurologically normal until 9 months previously, when he developed rapidly progressive loss of language skills. He had only three seizures, all generalized convulsions. Results of brain imaging, cerebrospinal fluid studies, and metabolic evaluation were normal. **A:** EEG in the waking state demonstrates mild slowing of background activity and infrequent right midtemporal spikes. TC, 0.1 second; HFF, 70 Hz. *(Figure continues.)*

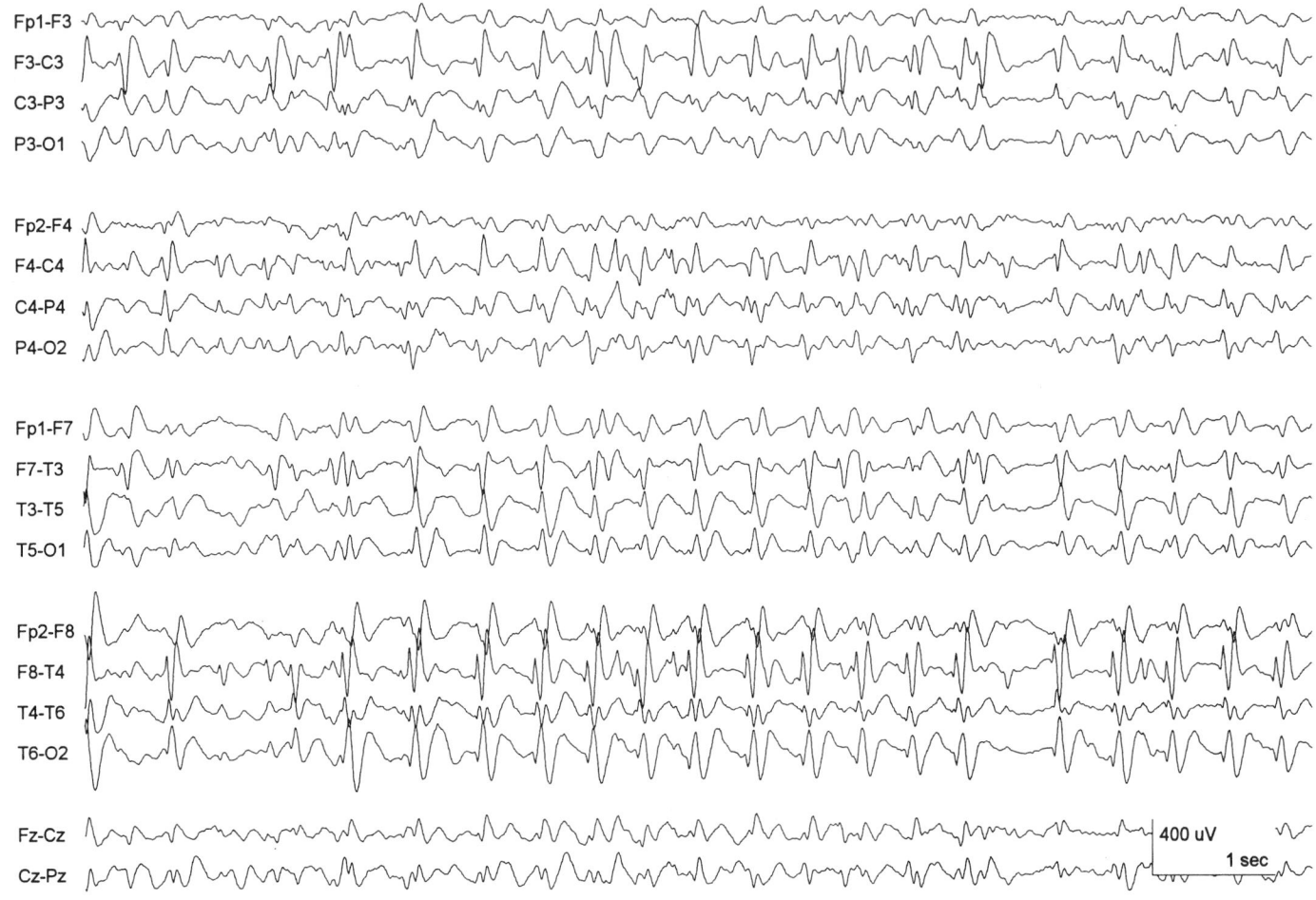

FIG. 17.21. *Continued.* **B:** EEG during non–rapid-eye-movement sleep shows nearly continuous spike-and-wave discharges. Although broadly distributed bilaterally, they are maximal over the right temporal region. TC, 0.1 second; HFF, 70 Hz.

Seizure remit and the EEG normalizes in nearly all patients by the end of adolescence (15,70), but some degree of language dysfunction persists in the majority (15,70,75). Most patients show improvement, but the degree of recovery is variable and unpredictable; some patients remain profoundly impaired.

Continuous Spikes and Waves during Slow Sleep

Clinical Features. This syndrome was first described by Patry et al. (222) as "subclinical electrical status epilepticus induced by sleep." It was later renamed because of the lack of typical clinical features associated with status epilepticus. The ILAE Commission on Classification (228) accepted the proposed name, continuous spike-waves during slow sleep, and described the syndrome as follows:

> "Epilepsy with continuous spike-waves during slow sleep results from the association of various seizure types, partial and generalized, occurring during sleep, and atypical absences when awake. Tonic seizures do not occur. The characteristic EEG pattern consists of continuous diffuse spike-waves during slow-wave sleep, which is noted after the onset of seizures. Duration varies from months to years. Despite the usual benign evolution of seizures, prognosis is guarded because of the appearance of neuropsychologic disorders."

The syndrome of CSWS is a rare condition, accounting for fewer than 0.5% of cases of childhood epilepsies (197). Age at onset ranges from 1 to 12 years, but onset peaks between the ages of 5 and 7 years. Twenty percent of cases begin between the ages of 9 and 12 years (42). Two-thirds of patients are neurologically normal before onset of the syndrome (42,272).

In nearly all patients, seizures appear 1 to 2 years before the EEG abnormality of this syndrome (41,272). Simple partial motor and generalized tonic-clonic seizures predominate. Later, with appearance of the syndrome of CSWS, other seizure types emerge, including atypical absence seizures associated with atonia and falls (42,272). Most patients have frequent seizures, often multiple times in a week or even in a single day (272). Tonic seizures do not occur (30,41,196,272). With development of the syndrome, nearly all patients have a significant decline in IQ with deterioration in language, temporospatial disorientation, impaired memory, and reduced attention span. Behavioral changes such as aggressiveness or, rarely, psychosis also occur (30,41,272).

Electroencephalographic Findings. When seizures first appear, EEG findings are nonspecific. Background activity can be normal or abnormal. Occasional epileptiform discharges occur, and these become more frequent during sleep (41,272). Epileptiform activity consists of generalized spike-wave discharges, occurring singly or in bursts, and focal or multifocal spikes or sharp waves that are best developed over the frontal-central regions. Both focal and generalized discharges often occur in the same patient (41,272).

When the CSWS pattern appears, epileptiform activity in the waking state increases. Diffuse 2- to 3-Hz spike-wave discharges predominate, often occurring in runs (222,272). The CSWS pattern itself consists of continuous, generalized, 1.5- to 2.5-Hz slow spike-wave activity that is maximal frontally (222,272) (Fig. 17.22). Discharges of 3 to 5 Hz also occur in some patients (41). Spike-wave discharges can be asymmetrical, especially in patients with focal cerebral lesions (30,41,196). The continuous spike-wave pattern persists throughout NREM sleep, typically occupying more than 85% of the total NREM sleep recording (spike-wave index) (41,222,272). Beaumanoir (16) observed a subgroup of patients with the syndrome of CSWS who had spike-wave indices between 50% and 85%. In these patients, focal discharges continued to be seen during sleep (16). During REM sleep, the continuous spike-wave activity fragments and occupies only about 5% of REM sleep time, often disappearing completely (16,271,272). Occasional generalized spike-waves or focal spikes are seen in REM sleep (271,272).

The CSWS patterns persist for long periods, ranging from 1 to 3 years in most patients and up to 6 years in some cases (16,41,272). The electrographic pattern gradually resolves in all children, although focal abnormalities may remain somewhat longer. Long-term follow-up demonstrates normalization of the EEG, including sleep architecture, in the majority of patients (272).

Seizures also remit spontaneously in all patients, regardless of their severity and frequency (41,196,272). EEG normalization and remission of seizures do not always occur simultaneously. In some cases, seizures cease while the CSWS pattern is still present, whereas in others, seizures persist after the CSWS pattern has disappeared (272).

Neuropsychological outcome is not as benign. All patients show neurological and behavioral improvement after the CSWS pattern remits, but recovery is slow and often incomplete (41,272). About half of the patients remain profoundly impaired (41,272).

Progressive Myoclonus Epilepsies

Clinical Features

The progressive myoclonus epilepsies (PMEs) are rare syndromes characterized by myoclonic seizures and progressive neurological abnormalities, especially ataxia and dementia. Five entities account for most of the PMEs: myoclonic epilepsy with ragged red fibers (MERRF), Unverricht-Lundborg disease, Lafora's disease, neuronal ceroid lipofuscinosis in its various age-

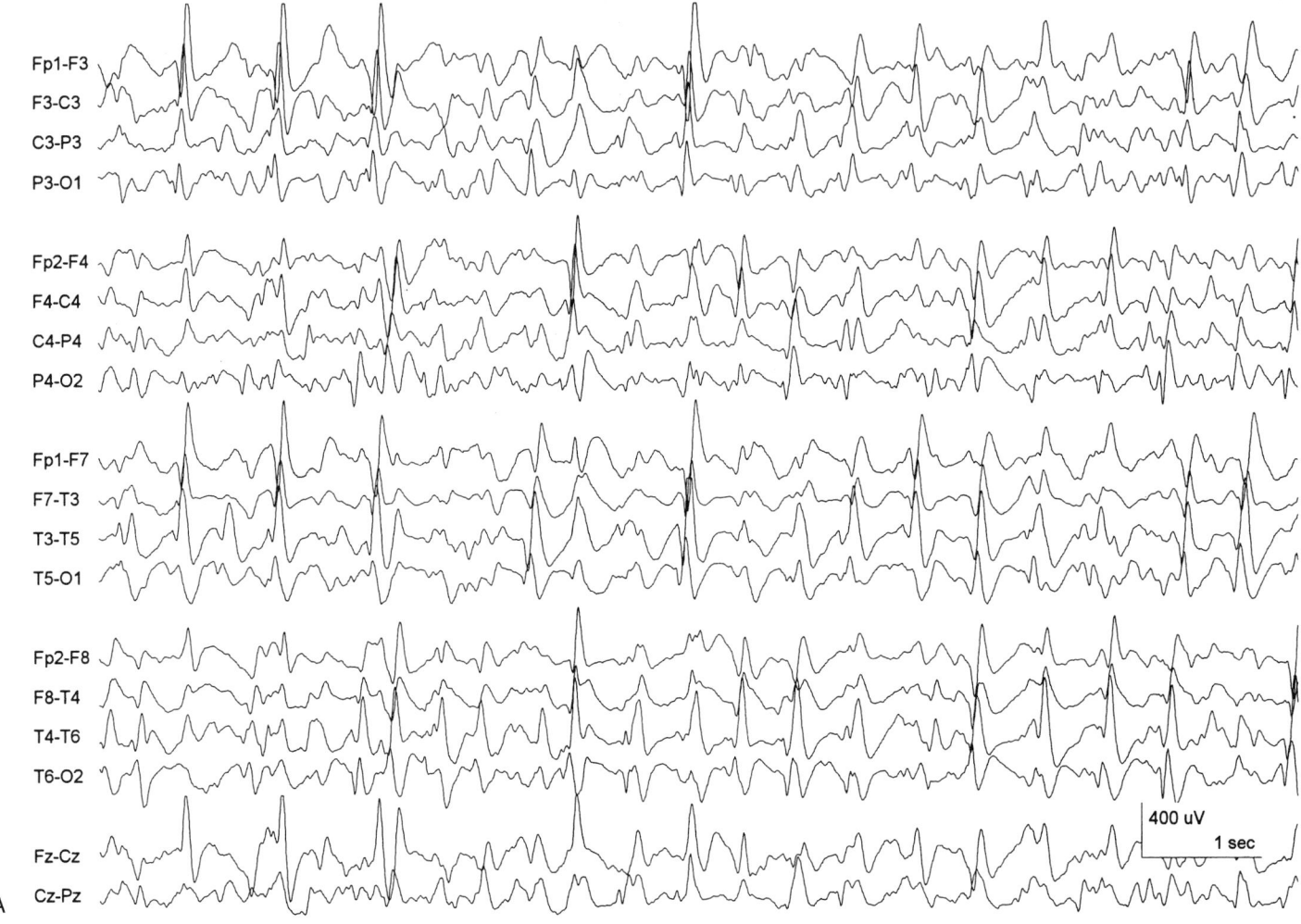

FIG. 17.22. The syndrome of continuous spikes and waves during slow sleep. EEG of an 11-year-old boy with global cognitive decline and seizures. **A:** During sleep, there was continuous sharp-and-slow-wave activity, which shows shifting laterality for waveform definition and voltage. TC, 0.1 second; HFF, 70 Hz. *(Figure continues.)*

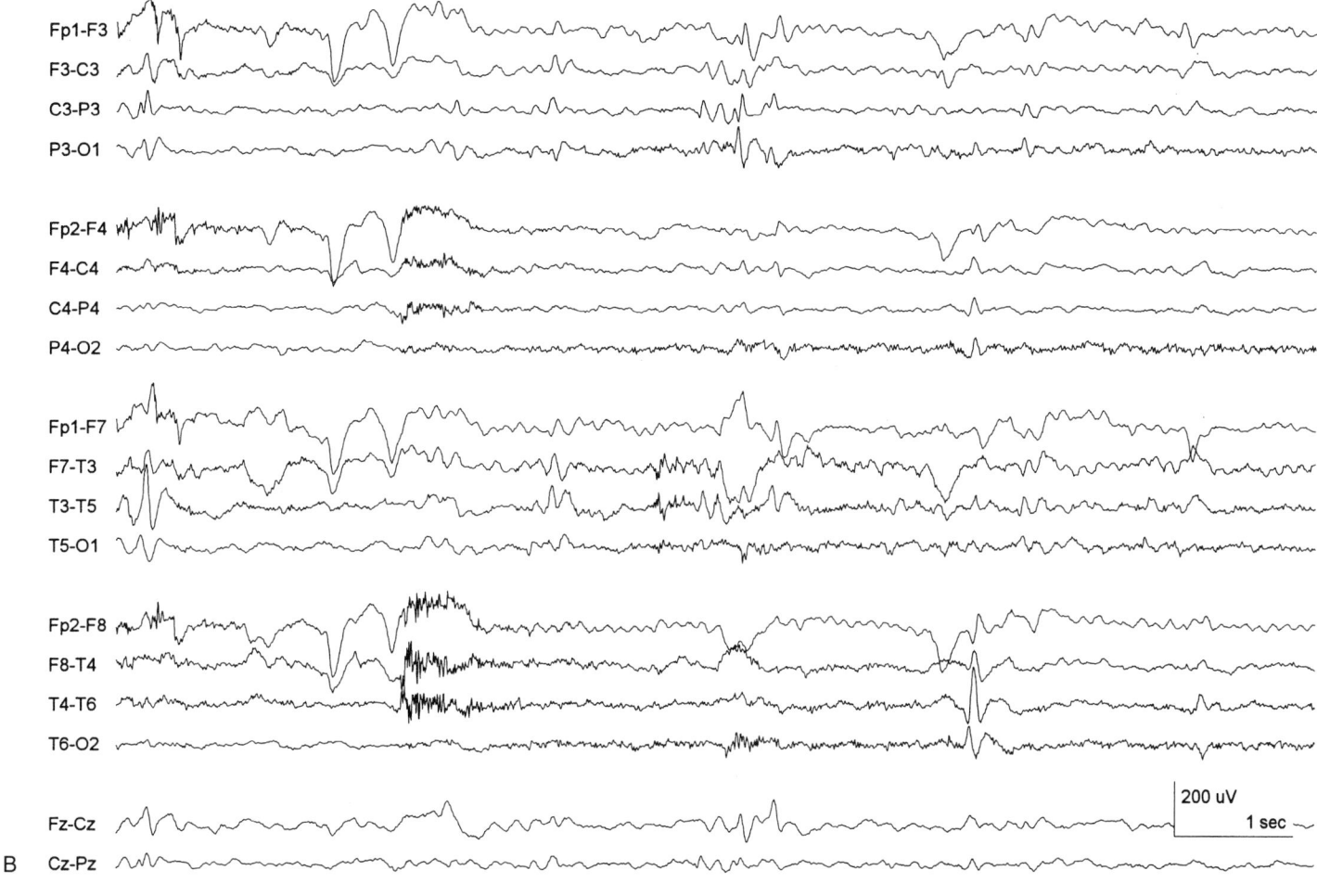

FIG. 17.22. *Continued.* **B:** The EEG in the waking state is strikingly different. Background activity is mildly attenuated with reduced complexity and occasional multifocal sharp waves (T6, P3, F7). TC, 0.1 second; HFF, 70 Hz.

related forms, and sialidoses (24). The clinical forms of each are characteristic. It is often possible to make specific diagnoses from careful review of clinical features, family history, biopsy of skin or muscle, and increasingly, genetic analysis (25). EEG and evoked potential studies help support a clinical diagnosis of PME and distinguish PME from other generalized epilepsies. However, only a few electrophysiological findings are sufficiently specific to indicate a particular syndrome.

Electroencephalographic Findings

EEG findings in PME were reviewed by Berkovic et al. (26). Background activity may be normal initially but inevitably slows as dementia develops. EEG features that distinguish the various sleep stages disappear. In all forms of PME, the predominant epileptiform abnormality consists of generalized spike, spike-wave, and polyspike-wave discharges, most often at a rate of 3 to 6 Hz. Occipital spikes and seizures occurring independently from both hemispheres are seen in all major forms of PME except the sialidoses; these are especially common in Lafora's disease. Photosensitivity and high-voltage, exaggerated somatosensory evoked potentials are also common in most of the PMEs (162,193). Visual and brainstem evoked potentials are usually normal. Prolonged central conduction times occur in late stages of Lafora's disease and MERFF (162,267).

Myoclonic jerks in PME can be generalized, fragmentary, and multifocal in the same patient. Action, or reflex, myoclonus (especially in response to light) is common. Polygraphic studies demonstrate that some, but not all, jerks are accompanied by epileptiform activity (23). Back-averaging techniques may demonstrate EEG potentials preceding muscle jerks that are not obvious with routine recordings. In view of the abundant evidence of cortical hyperexcitability in the PMEs, it is likely that most, if not all, myoclonus in these disorders is of cortical origin, although this has not been demonstrated in careful studies.

A few EEG findings suggest a specific PME syndrome. In the sialidoses, generalized spike-wave activity is infrequent or absent altogether. Instead, myoclonus is associated with characteristic trains of 10- to 20-Hz, low-voltage, positive spikes at the vertex (87,233). Runs of these vertex spikes also occur without myoclonus and are especially frequent during deep sleep. In late infantile and adult neuronal ceroid lipofuscinosis, single light flashes evoke giant potentials over the occipital and posterior scalp regions. Paradoxically, the electroretinographic pattern is greatly attenuated or altogether absent in late infantile and juvenile neuronal ceroid lipofuscinosis (233).

Temporal Lobe Epilepsy

The ILAE Classification of Epilepsy Syndromes (228) distinguishes between medial temporal lobe epilepsy and neocortical temporal lobe epilepsy. Both syndromes can be treated effectively by surgical resection, although the extent of the presurgical evaluation in each is substantially different. Thus, clinical and EEG criteria for distinguishing the two are increasingly important.

Medial Temporal Lobe Epilepsy

Clinical Features. Medial temporal lobe epilepsy (MTLE) is the most common form of localization-related epilepsy occurring in adults. A consistent clinical syndrome has been defined by careful analysis of surgical series (88,95). Onset occurs at the end of the first decade or during adolescence in most cases. Over 80% of patients have a history of at least one convulsive seizure in early childhood; the great majority of these are febrile seizures. Complex partial seizures are the predominant seizure type, with secondarily generalized seizures relatively infrequent or controlled with antiepileptic drugs. Auras, especially epigastric ones, are common. MTLE is highly associated with medial temporal sclerosis, which can be detected reliably by magnetic resonance imaging using appropriate anatomical orientation and imaging sequences (47,145). Anteromedial temporal lobe resection results in freedom from seizure in more than 80% of such patients.

Electroencephalographic Findings. Interictal EEG. Interictal EEG findings in MTLE are also consistent: anterior temporal sharp waves associated with intermittent temporal slowing (Fig. 17.23). Findings are summarized in Table 17.4. Voltage of the IEDs is usually maximal in temporal basal electrodes, such as sphenoidal or "true" anterior (T1/2) temporal electrodes. Because of this, the typical IEDs of MTLE are sometimes referred to as temporal-sphenoidal discharges. IEDs that are of maximal voltage over the lateral temporal area also occur in patients with MTLE, but these are exceptional (93,303). Topographic voltage analysis has demonstrated that most IEDs in MTLE show a relatively discrete region of electronegativity over the ipsilateral inferior temporal scalp that is accompanied by a more diffuse area of positivity over the contralateral central-parietal scalp (78). One-third of patients have bilateral IEDs that occur independently on the two sides (56,86,303). Independent bilateral temporal IEDs often appear during non-REM sleep. IEDs recorded during wakefulness and REM sleep are more often lateralized and closely associated with the area of seizure onset (249).

Ictal EEG. The characteristic ictal EEG pattern associated with complex partial seizures of MTLE is a unilateral, 5-Hz (or faster) temporal discharge

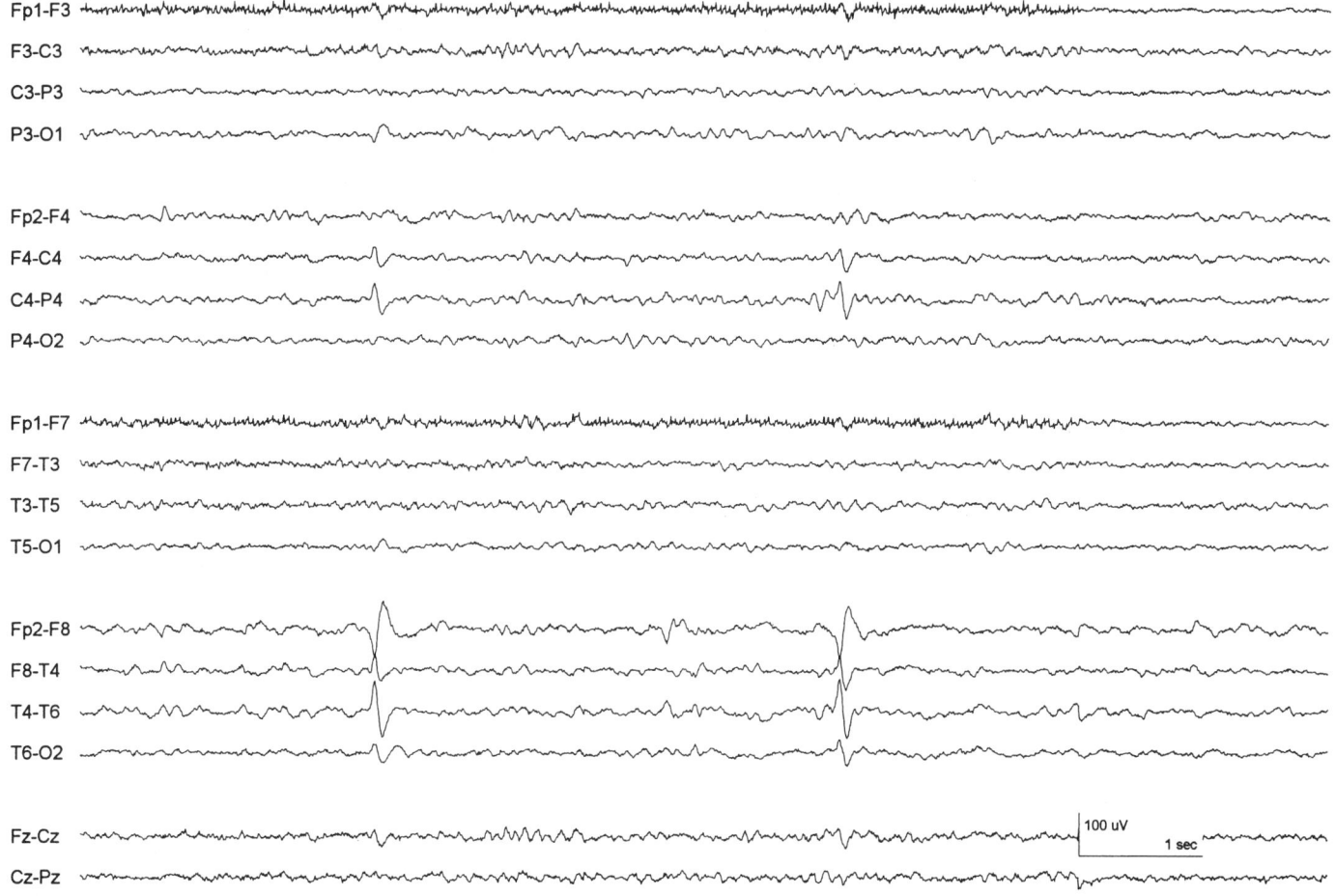

FIG. 17.23. EEG of a 33-year-old woman with complex partial seizures characterized by a rising epigastric sensation, oral automatisms, and impaired responsiveness. Brain magnetic resonance image showed right mesial temporal sclerosis. The interictal EEG shows right temporal polymorphic theta and delta frequency slowing and epileptiform sharp waves which phase reverse at F8. TC, 0.1 second; HFF, 70 Hz.

TABLE 17.4. *Patients with medial temporal lobe epilepsy: scalp*
EEG interictal paroxysmal activity

Total number of patients	67
Present	64
Absent	3
Strictly unilateral	35
Concordant	33
Discordant	2
Anterior temporal	32
Midtemporal	1
Posterior temporal	2
Bilateral independent/anterior temporal predominant	28
Equal	7
Lateralized preponderance	21
Concordant	15
Discordant	6
Bilateral synchronous predominant	1

From Williamson PD, French JA, Thadani VM, et al. Characteristics of medial temporal lobe epilepsy: II. Interictal and ictal scalp electroencephalography, neuropsychological testing, neuroimaging, surgical results, and pathology. *Ann Neurol* 1993;34:781–787.

that appears in anterior and inferior temporal scalp electrodes within 30 seconds or so after onset of clinical symptoms and signs (93,111,242,291) (Fig. 17.24). This finding occurs in 82% to 94% of patients with MTLE (242,291) and lateralizes seizure onset correctly in more than 95% (242,269,291). Table 17.5 summarizes the main ictal scalp findings. Ictal EEG changes are only rarely seen in scalp electrodes when clinical symptoms first appear. The ictal temporal-sphenoidal discharge has less lateralizing value in patients with bilateral temporal IEDs (269,290). Although quite sensitive, temporal-sphenoidal ictal discharges are probably less specific for MTLE than are the interictal discharges, which are also seen in temporal neocortical epilepsy (77,111) and, occasionally, in extratemporal epilepsy. Propagation of the ictal discharge from extratemporal to temporal areas presumably

accounts for the latter observation. Focal slowing or attenuation, usually on the side of seizure onset, occurs postictally in about 70% of patients with MTLE (156,291). Postictal focal EEG findings are more common after partial seizures in MTLE than after partial seizures originating outside the temporal lobe (156,290).

Neocortical Temporal Lobe Epilepsy

Clinical Features. Neocortical temporal lobe epilepsy (NTLE) has been more difficult to characterize because it is less common that MTLE and also because demonstrating a lateral temporal onset requires excluding a medial temporal onset, which can be a difficult challenge. Making the distinction often requires placement of intracranial electrodes. Descriptions of NTLE emphasize absence of features present in MTLE; there are few positive distinctive characteristics (93,111,288). Epigastric auras occur more often in MTLE, but they can also occur with NTLE, probably caused by medial spread of the ictal discharge (79,253). Early oroalimentary automatisms and asymmetrical limb behaviors (contralateral dystonic posture and ipsilateral automatisms) are infrequent in NTLE (111,253).

Electroencephalographic Findings

Interictal EEG. EEG features of NTLE are also less consistent and specific than those of MTLE. IEDs localize to the temporal region but tend to be more broadly distributed than in MTLE. Some researchers have found that IEDs of NTLE are less likely to be of maximal voltage in sphenoidal electrodes (93,226), but this difference has not been found by others (43). Topographic voltage analysis indicates that most IEDs seen in patients with NTLE have a relatively broad negative region over the ipsilateral temporal scalp and lack the contralateral central-parietal scalp positivity seen in MTLE (77). Focal slowing and independent bilaterally temporal IEDs appear to be equally prevalent in the two syndromes (43).

FIG. 17.24. EEG of a 31-year-old man with complex partial seizures consisting of impaired responsiveness, oral automatisms, dystonic posturing of the right hand, and postictal aphasia. Brain magnetic resonance image showed left mesial temporal sclerosis. The interictal EEG demonstrated left temporal slowing and epileptiform discharges. In this example, the ictal discharge appeared 9 seconds after onset of clinical symptoms. There is rhythmic delta activity (maximal at F7-F9), followed by repetitive sharp waves (maximal at F7-F9-T9) and evolution to rhythmic 6-Hz activity that was maximal in the inferior temporal electrode chain (F9-T9). TC, 0.1 second; HFF, 70 Hz.

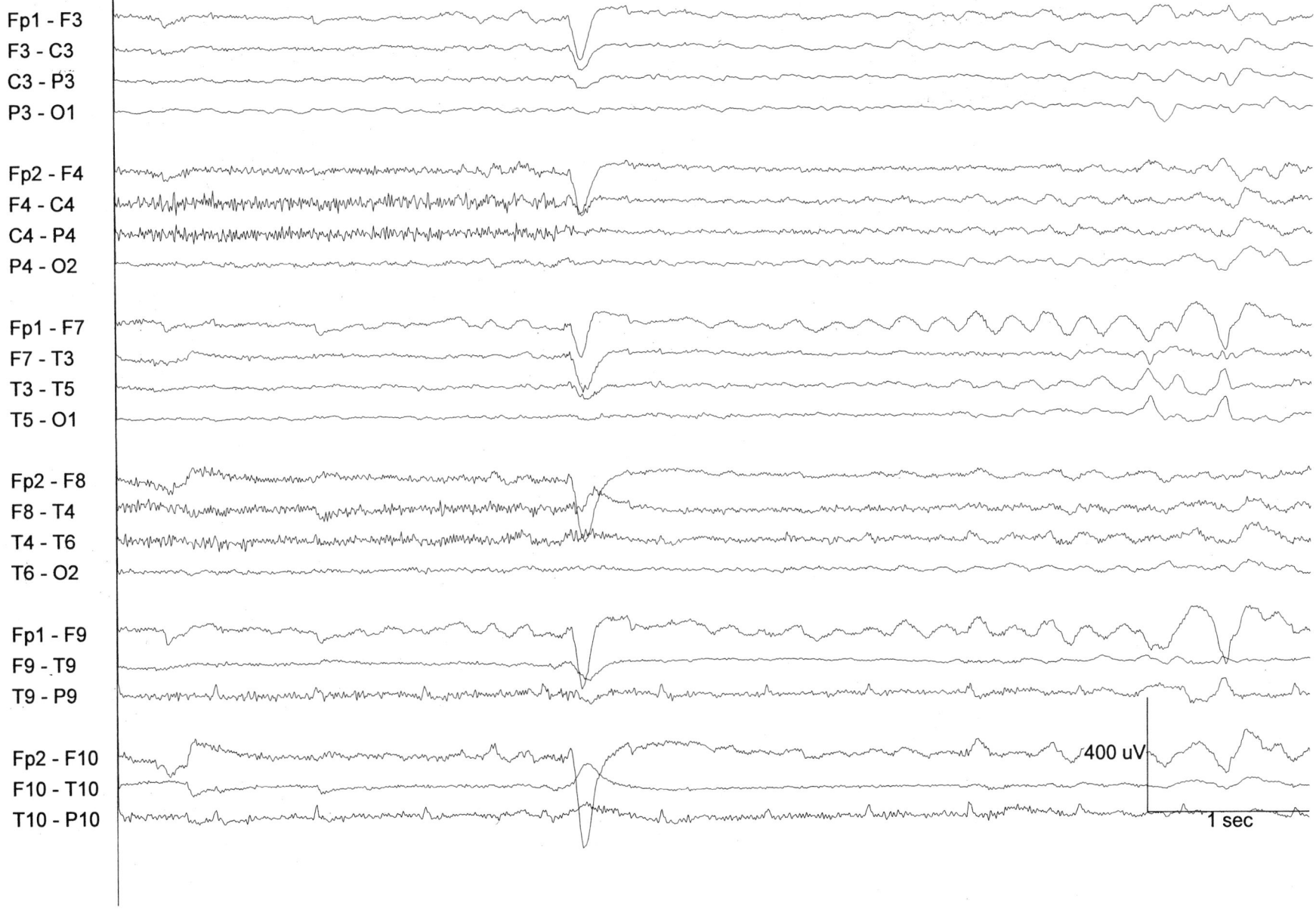

Fp1 - F3
F3 - C3
C3 - P3
P3 - O1

Fp2 - F4
F4 - C4
C4 - P4
P4 - O2

Fp1 - F7
F7 - T3
T3 - T5
T5 - O1

Fp2 - F8
F8 - T4
T4 - T6
T6 - O2

Fp1 - F9
F9 - T9
T9 - P9

Fp2 - F10
F10 - T10
T10 - P10

400 uV

1 sec

1

(Figure continues.)

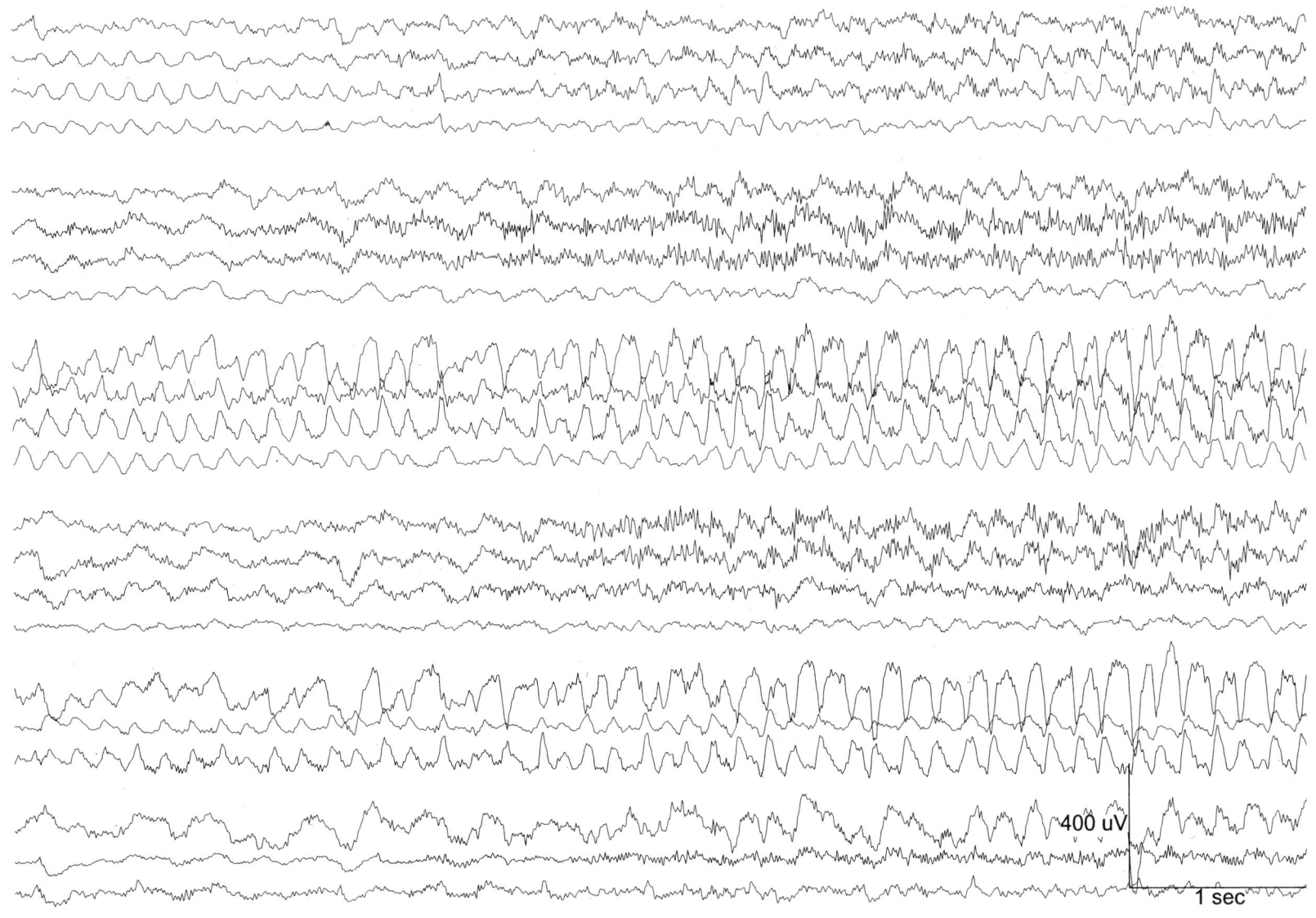

2

FIG. 17.24. *Continued.*

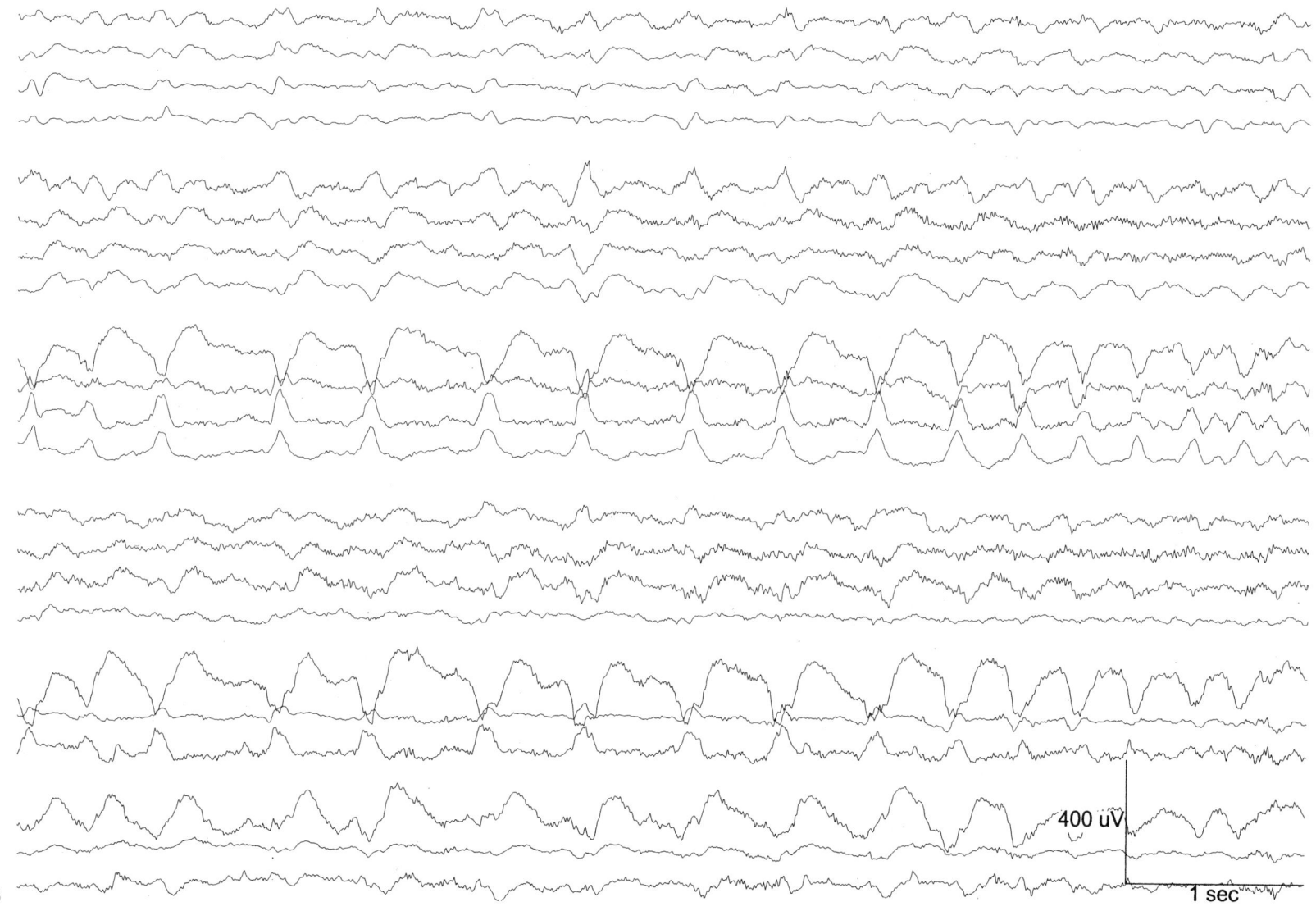

FIG. 17.24. *Continued.*

TABLE 17.5. *Patients with medial temporal lobe epilepsy: scalp EEG ictal changes*

Total number of patients	67
Bilateral ictal changes	13
Lateralized ictal onset	4
Concordant	4
Lateralized buildup (including four with lateralized onset)	54
Concordant	47
Discordant	5
Alternating bilateral	2
Lateralized postictal slowing	45
Concordant	45

From Williamson PD, French JA, Thadani VM, et al. Characteristics of medial temporal lobe epilepsy: II. Interictal and ictal scalp electroencephalography, neuropsychological testing, neuroimaging, surgical results, and pathology. *Ann Neurol* 1993;34:781–787.

Ictal EEG. The temporal-sphenoidal pattern so common in MTLE appears less often in NTLE (93,111,289). Widely distributed, often hemispheric ictal discharges are much more common in NTLE. Other differences are (a) generally slower frequency, (b) less stability of frequency and voltage, and (c) appearance later in the evolution of the seizure (77,93). In two studies, researchers found that parasagittal spread, either ipsilateral or contralateral to the epileptogenic temporal lobe, was seen only in NTLE (93,289), but another report described this in MTLE (77). Absence of a scalp ictal discharge was much more common in NTLE than in MTLE (77).

The overlap in EEG findings between MTLE and NTLE precludes confident distinction of the two syndromes by ictal EEG alone.

Frontal Lobe Epilepsy

Clinical Features

Although neither the incidence nor prevalence of frontal lobe epilepsy (FLE) is known with certainty, large surgical series indicate that it is the second most common localization-related epilepsy, accounting for about 20% of patients undergoing epilepsy surgery (230,237,301). Unlike MTLE, seizure symptoms are heterogeneous, reflecting both the large size of the frontal lobe with its many functional and anatomical divisions, as well as the different pathways of propagation from different areas of the frontal lobe. As a result, several syndromes have been described as types of FLE referable to specific anatomical areas of presumed seizure onset within the frontal lobe. Although

the ictal manifestations of frontal lobe seizures suggest particular localizations, no features are definitive for any. Recognizing significant overlap among the regions, the ILAE Commission (228) classified the frontal lobe epilepsies by anatomical areas that produce relatively characteristic seizure symptoms: supplementary motor, cingulate, anterior frontopolar, orbitofrontal, dorsolateral, opercular, and motor cortex.

All frontal lobe seizures share a number of features: (a) early and prominent motor manifestations, including clonic activity, asymmetrical tonic posturing, or complex semipurposeful, repetitive movements that often involve the legs (e.g., bicycling); (b) short duration with minimal or no postictal confusion; (c) occurrence in clusters; (d) frequent secondary generalization; and (e) predilection for occurring at night (304). Three manifestations are especially correlated with frontal lobe epilepsy:

1. Supplementary motor area seizures manifested by sudden asymmetrical tonic posturing of the limbs, usually with one arm extended upward, and contralateral head and eye deviation; consciousness may or may not be impaired.
2. Complex partial seizures with prominent motor activity, such as vigorous rocking, bicycling, circling, or vocalization; minimal or no impairment in consciousness; and no postictal confusion. Because of their frequently bizarre manifestations, nonepileptic psychogenic seizures are often first suspected. Although such seizures are typical of the medial frontal or orbital frontal areas, they may arise anywhere within the frontal lobe.
3. Simple partial motor clonic seizures, arising from regions within or adjacent to the primary motor cortex.

Electroencephalographic Findings

Interictal EEG. Diagnosis of FLE rests largely on clinical features, inasmuch as the EEG is often normal or nondiagnostic. This is largely because much of the frontal lobe, including the orbital-frontal cortex, interhemispheric convexity and cingulum, and the sulcal depths are relatively inaccessible to scalp EEG recording (229). Consequently, small epileptogenic foci may be missed entirely; conversely, epileptiform abnormalities may appear widespread because of the often large distances and intervening cortex between the epileptogenic area and scalp electrodes. Furthermore, functional networks permit rapid propagation within and outside the frontal lobes, which results in the appearance of diffuse (secondary bilateral synchrony), multifocal, or falsely localizing epileptiform abnormalities (229). In contrast to temporal lobe epilepsy, the placement of additional, closely spaced scalp electrodes does not usually improve the localizing value of scalp EEG in FLE (123).

Interictal EEGs in FLE can demonstrate one of several patterns:

1. For the reasons just listed, epileptiform discharges are not identified on scalp EEG recordings in up to one-third of patients (199,247,305). This is most commonly seen in patients with medial frontal epilepsy (11,204,296).
2. Secondary bilaterally synchronous discharges may be seen in up to two-thirds of patients with FLE (235); these discharges are especially frequent with medial frontal foci. Tükel and Jasper (283) first used the term *secondary bilateral synchrony* in describing the bilateral discharges seen in patients with parasagittal epileptogenic lesions. Secondary bilateral synchrony is discussed in detail later in this chapter.
3. Focal epileptiform discharges occurring over one frontal lobe are seen in 42% to 63% of cases of FLE (169,235,247). When these arise from epileptogenic cortex in the medial frontal lobe, the discharges are of highest voltage at or adjacent to the vertex.
4. High-voltage (up to 300-μV), sharply contoured slow waves that are broadly distributed over the frontal regions but maximal at F3-F4 and Fp1-Fp2 are characteristic of orbital frontal foci. These discharges are almost always seen bilaterally to some extent, but they show voltage and field asymmetries that accurately indicate the epileptogenic hemisphere (184,275).

Ictal EEG. The ictal EEG is nonlocalizing in more than half the patients with FLE (169,199,247). Often, there is no electrographic correlate to be seen in scalp electrodes. Equally problematic, however, is that the early and prominent motor activity of many frontal lobe seizures produces large amounts of muscle and movement artifact that obscures EEG activity. False localization, particularly to the temporal lobe, also occurs as a result of frontal-limbic connections.

Although supplementary motor area seizures can be associated with a focal rhythmic discharge localized or adjacent to the vertex (199), most other seizures of medial frontal origin are not accompanied by a lateralized discharge; EEGs sometimes show only diffuse, bilateral frontal voltage attenuation (11,97,296) followed by bilateral frontal or diffuse rhythmic theta or delta activity (11,305) (Fig. 17.25). Although diffuse, bilateral frontal voltage attenuation is frequently correlated with onset of orbital frontal seizures, focal rhythmic alpha or beta frequency activity is sometimes seen in the frontopolar electrodes (184,275). Seizures of dorsolateral frontal origin are usually associated with a localizing ictal discharge. Bautista et al. (11) reported that focal and lateralizing rhythmic fast activity was associated with seizure onset in 80% of patients with dorsolateral frontal lobe seizures.

Parietal Lobe Epilepsy

Parietal lobe epilepsy is much less common than temporal or frontal lobe epilepsy; it accounts for about 6% of patients who undergo epilepsy surgery (236). As with FLE, scalp EEG is most often nonlocalizing and is sometimes falsely localizing. In a review of 11 patients with parietal lobe epilepsy, 10 of whom had undergone successful surgery, Williamson et al. (302) reported that scalp EEG correctly localized the seizure onset zone in only one patient. Interictal parietal epileptiform discharges were present in four patients (36%), and additional epileptiform abnormalities were noted in three of these. Five patients (45%) without focal parietal epileptiform discharges had other, falsely localizing abnormalities, including temporal and bisynchronous frontal spikes. Scalp ictal EEG was lateralizing in only three patients. There is little doubt that conventional scalp EEG is of limited utility for parietal lobe epilepsy.

Occipital Lobe Epilepsy

Discharges associated with occipital lobe epilepsy have been described in detail in the earlier section on childhood epilepsy with occipital paroxysms.

Focal Cortical Dysplasia

Magnetic resonance imaging, when used as a routine diagnostic procedure, has revealed that focal cortical dysplasia is a relatively common cause of intractable epilepsy, and it enables more thorough study of associated EEG findings, especially in patients being evaluated for epilepsy surgery. Barkovich et al. (9) proposed a useful classification.

EEG abnormalities are related to the extent and location of the lesions. Small lesions often do not disrupt normal background activity. Larger lesions result in ipsilateral or bilateral slowing of the alpha rhythm as well as focal slowing over the involved cortical area. Epileptiform discharges, usual focal, are present in more than 80% of patients (100,239). Generalized epileptiform activity can be seen with multifocal or more diffuse developmental malformations. Focal, bilateral, or generalized discharges can be seen with subependymal heterotopia (240). Epileptiform activity is frequently abundant; discharges occur in repetitive or near-continuous trains, especially during sleep (100,239) (Fig. 17.26). Such findings are especially

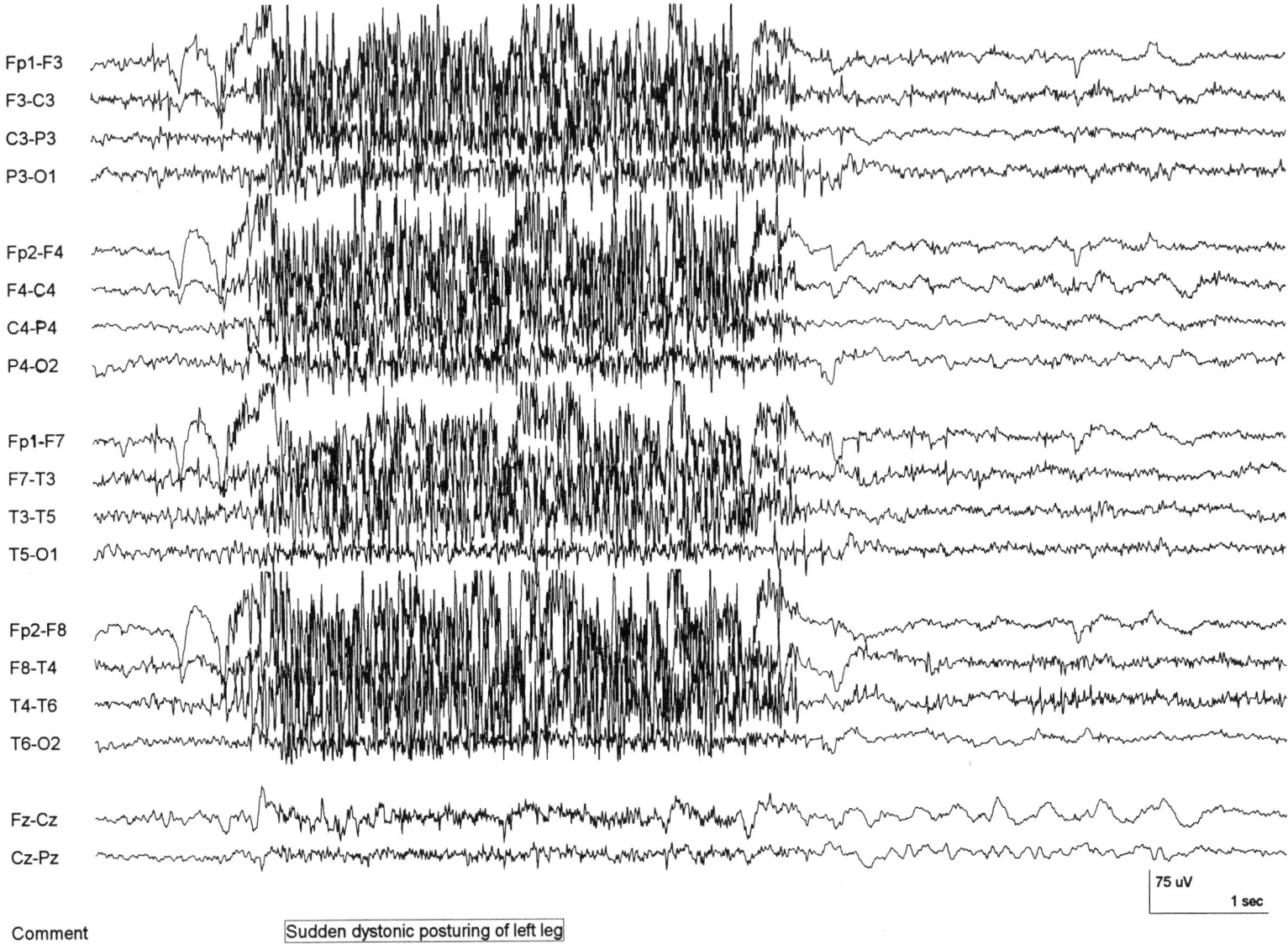

Comment

Sudden dystonic posturing of left leg

75 uV

1 sec

FIG. 17.25. EEG of a 27-year-old man with frontal lobe epilepsy. Seizures consisted of sudden dystonic posturing of the left leg followed by several seconds of large-amplitude clonic activity without loss of consciousness. In the immediate postictal period, there was subtle left leg weakness. The EEG is initially obscured by muscle artifact, but rhythmic 3-Hz delta activity is later seen over the right frontal (F4) and central (C4) regions. TC, 0.1 second; HFF, 35 Hz.

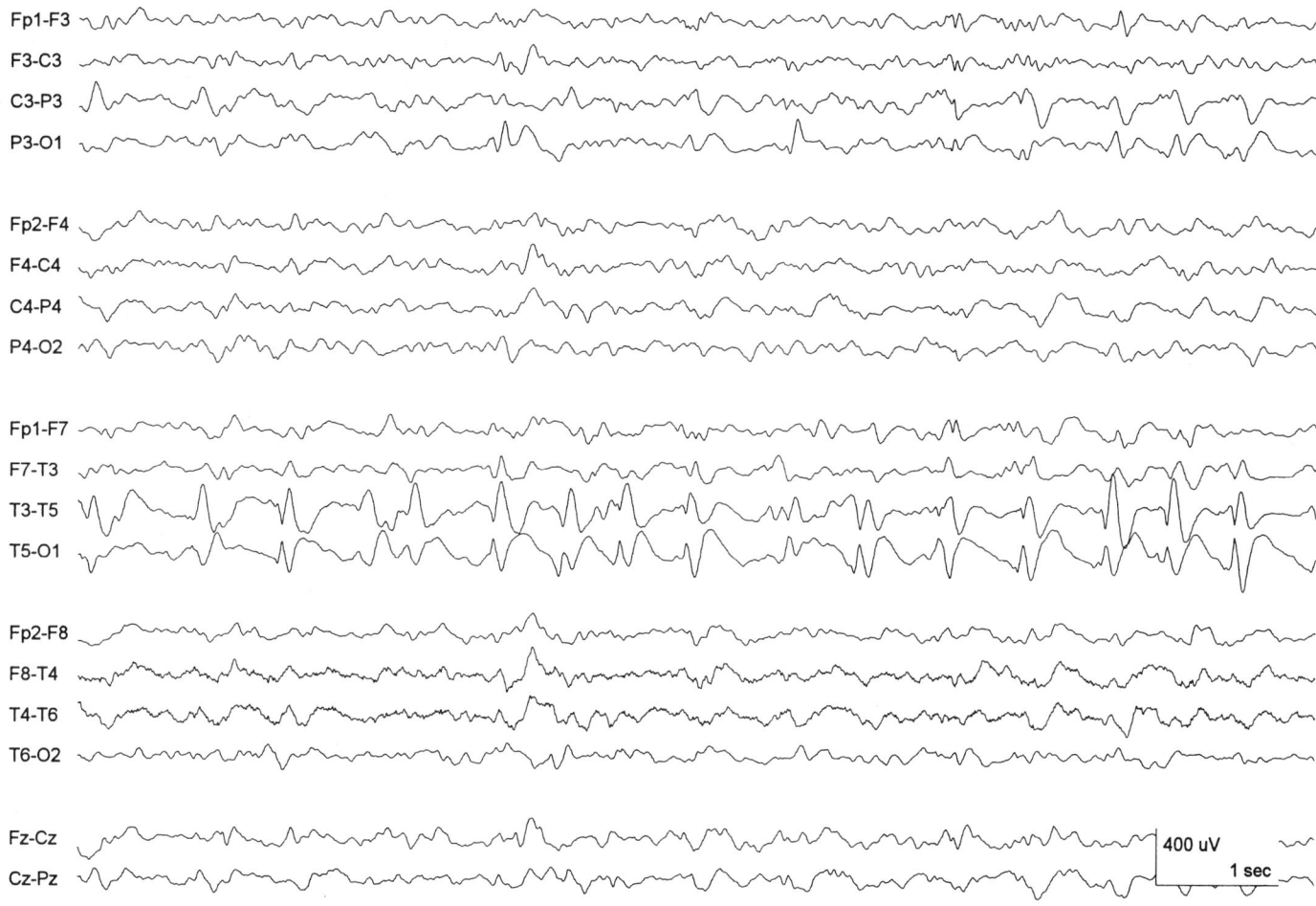

FIG. 17.26. EEG of an 8-year-old girl with intractable epilepsy. During infancy, she had spasms and hypsar-rhythmia. Seizures at the time this EEG was obtained consisted of repetitive flexion of the right shoulder and neck, with speech disruption and decreased attentiveness. Brain magnetic resonance image showed signal abnormalities consistent with a large region of cortical dysplasia in the left posterior hemisphere. The EEG recorded during sleep demonstrates nearly continuous high-voltage epileptiform discharges at T5 (note calibration). These discharges persisted throughout sleep, but there were no visible clinical changes. TC, 0.1 second; HFF, 70 Hz.

characteristic of large neocortical areas of malformation (238) and are strongly suggestive of cortical dysplasia rather than other structural lesions (100). Electrocorticographic recordings in such patients demonstrate continuous rhythmic spiking or repetitive electrographic seizures (210). These patterns, too, are uncommon with other types of lesions and have been considered evidence of the intrinsic epileptogenicity of dysplastic cortex (146). There is often relatively sharp demarcation between epileptogenic and normal cortex, which thus providing a useful guide in determining the extent of surgical resection (210).

EXAMPLES OF USES OF ELECTROENCEPHALOGRAPHY TO AID IN CLINICAL DIAGNOSIS

Seizures with Quiet Staring

Seizures characterized by quiet staring with amnesia but without obvious automatisms are common, especially during childhood, and can occur with such diverse disorders as childhood absence epilepsy, LGS, and temporal lobe epilepsy. EEG findings can provide critical information that aids in diagnosis and management. Generalized 3-Hz spike-wave activity accompanied by staring is pathognomonic of idiopathic absence epilepsy. Generalized sharp-slow wave discharges at a frequency of less than 2.5 Hz and diffusely slow background activity are characteristic of the atypical absence seizures of LGS. Focal IEDs over the anterior temporal region are suggestive of complex partial seizures caused by temporal lobe epilepsy.

Primary Generalized Versus Secondarily Generalized Tonic-Clonic Seizures

Many patients with epilepsy are unaware of the nature of their condition or do not seek medical attention until they have a generalized tonic-clonic seizure. The first manifestations of a seizure are often not witnessed and, even if observed, are not remembered, because the experience of observing a generalized tonic-clonic seizure is often accompanied by panic, fright, and a sense of helplessness. Therefore, it is frequently impossible for the physician to determine whether the convulsion was a symptom of primary generalized epilepsy or of localization-related epilepsy in which rapid secondary generalization occurred. Clinical features such age at onset, history of previous absence or complex partial seizures, and family history are helpful, but not always reliable, in distinguishing the two. In

such circumstances, EEG provides critical additional diagnostic information. Generalized IEDs indicate primary generalized epilepsy, and specific features of the generalized discharges can point to a specific epilepsy syndrome. Focal IEDs or focal slowing, in contrast, are most consistent with localization-related epilepsy. Because treatment and prognosis are usually different for these two groups of syndromes, accurate diagnosis is essential for optimal management.

Primary Versus Secondary Bilateral Synchrony

It is sometimes difficult to distinguish between spike-wave activity that is generalized from the outset and spike-wave activity that reflects rapid generalization from one or multiple foci (*secondary bilateral synchrony*) (Fig. 17.27). The first pattern indicates primary generalized epilepsy, whereas the second implies localization-related epilepsy and raises the possibility of a structural lesion. Sometimes generalized spike-wave activity is expressed incompletely or asymmetrically (see Fig. 17.27). This occurs most often over the frontal regions and during sleep. In such cases, these "focal" aspects are transient and have a morphological pattern that is very similar to that of more typical widespread bursts. Because the IEDs of primary generalized epilepsy are not always perfectly synchronous and symmetrical, subtle asymmetries should be interpreted conservatively and not interpreted as secondary bilateral synchrony. It is useful to remember that the overall appearance of the epileptiform activity in such cases is typical of primary generalized epilepsy. The following criteria for secondary bilateral synchrony helps avoid errors of overinterpretation: (a) Focal IEDs, when present, occur persistently in one area; (b) the morphological pattern of the focal IED is more variable and differs from that of the generalized IEDs; and (c) focal IEDs clearly and consistently precede and initiate most or all of the bursts of generalized IEDs. Simple EEG procedures, such as increasing paper speed or time base, also help distinguish primary from secondary bilateral synchrony. Subtle time differences between IEDs in different regions can be resolved or clarified by the use of special montage designs, such as reference subtraction (151). At one time, the differential effect of intracarotid injections of amobarbital on the spike-wave bursts of each hemisphere was used to recognize secondary bilateral synchrony (113,183). Anesthesia of the dependent hemisphere did not affect contralateral epileptiform activity, whereas anesthesia of the epileptogenic hemisphere suppressed discharges bilaterally. This technique is only rarely used today.

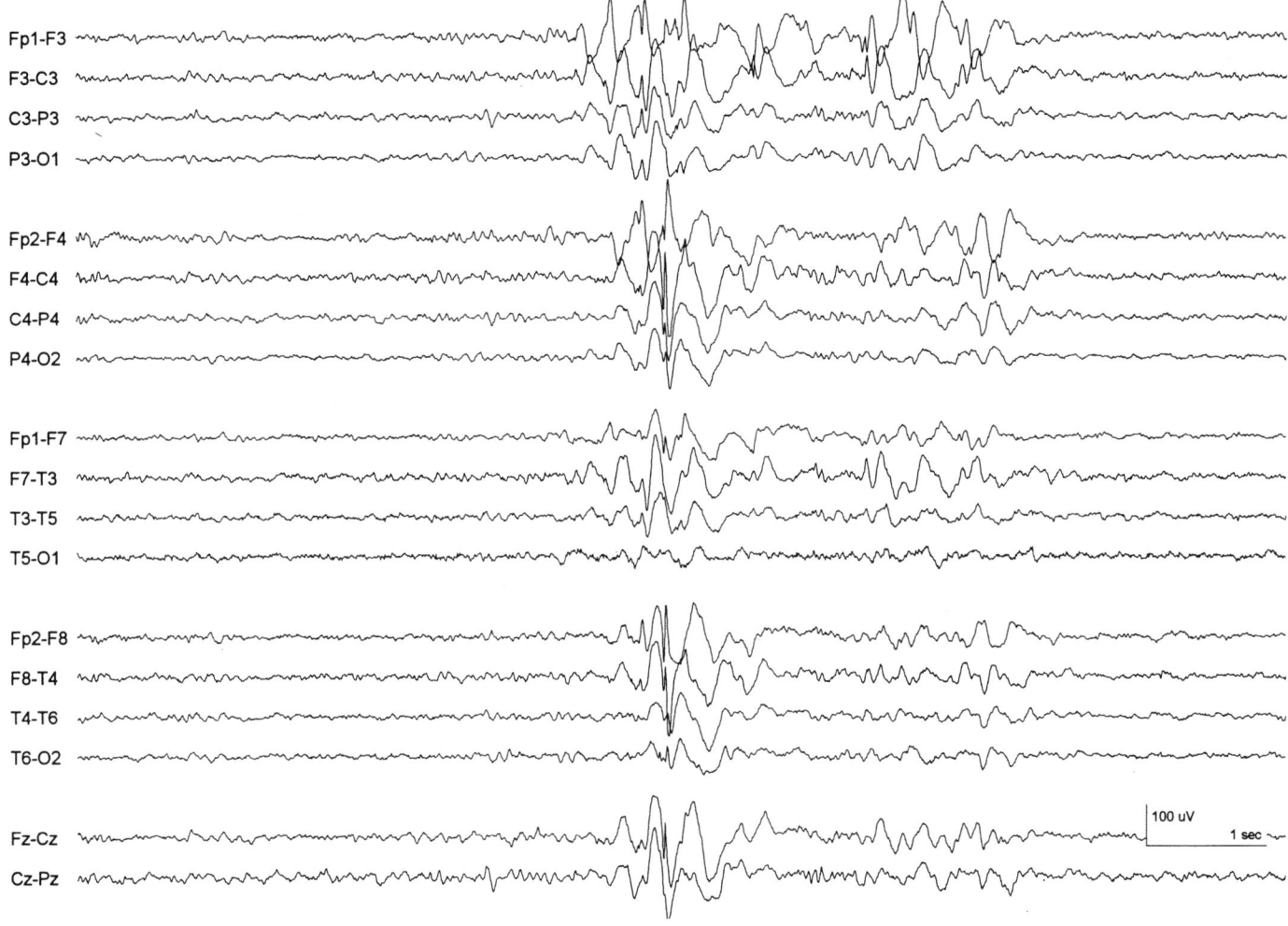

FIG. 17.27. EEG of a 41-year-old woman with nocturnal generalized convulsive seizures. Seizures began with right arm dystonia and forced head deviation to the right with rapid secondary generalization. **A:** Interictal EEG shows frontally predominant bilateral synchronous spike-wave activity that consistently has a left frontal (F3) lead-in, which is consistent with secondary bilateral synchrony. TC, 0.1 second; HFF, 70 Hz. *(Figure continues.)*

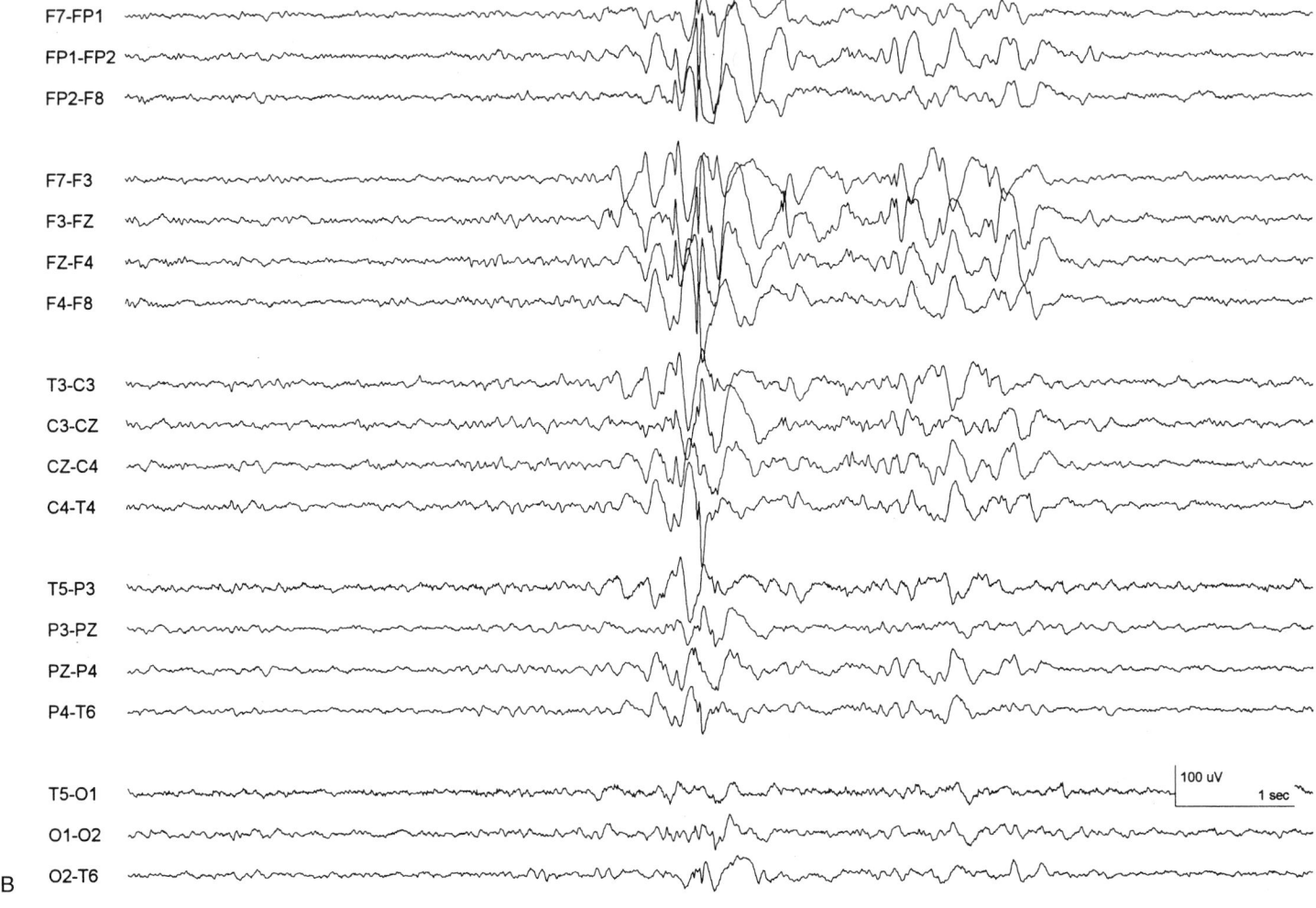

FIG. 17.27. *Continued.* **B:** The F3 lead-in is even clearer in a coronal bipolar montage (compare with part *A*). TC, 0.1 second; HFF, 70 Hz. *(Figure continues.)*

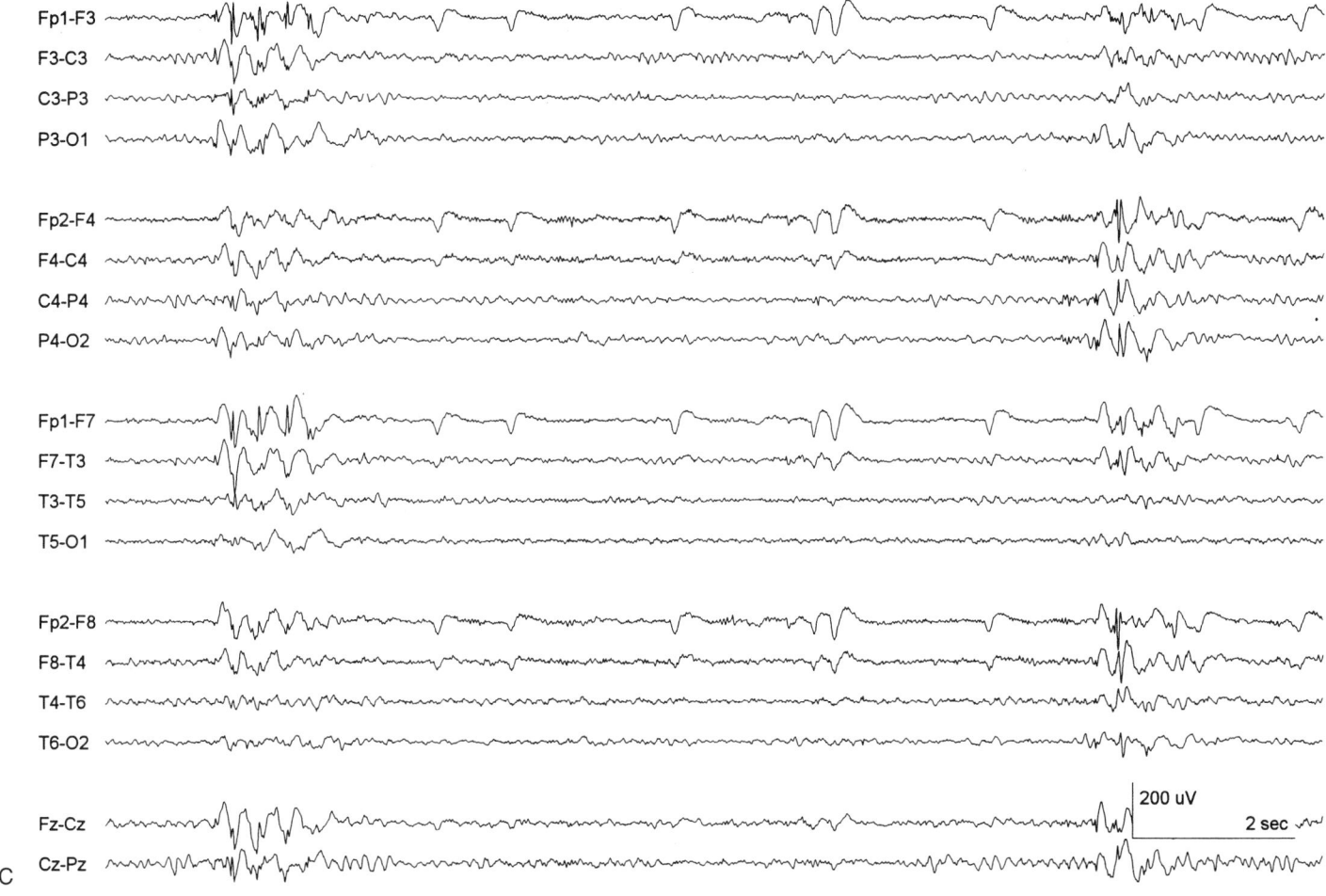

FIG. 17.27. *Continued.* **C:** EEG of a 21-year-old woman with juvenile myoclonic epilepsy. The EEG shows fragments of primary generalized spike-wave discharges that shift in laterality over the course of a recording, rather than demonstrating a consistent focal onset. TC, 0.1 second; HFF, 70 Hz.

Nocturnal Drooling Attacks in Children

Physicians are sometimes asked to see children with a history of night-time drooling and facial twitching with or without unresponsiveness. Diagnostic possibilities include the rolandic seizures of benign focal epilepsy with central-midtemporal spikes and either simple or complex partial seizures that are a manifestation of symptomatic localization-related epilepsy. Although the clinical symptoms of the two types of seizure are quite different, historical details may be incomplete or ambiguous because of the child's age and because the seizures occur during sleep. The EEG can provide definitive information. A central-midtemporal spike discharge supports a diagnosis of benign rolandic epilepsy, whereas an anterior temporal location is indicative of temporal lobe epilepsy. In this case, however, the distinction may not always be straightforward, because not all patients with central-temporal spikes have benign rolandic epilepsy (74,132,158,191). How often central-temporal spikes are associated with symptomatic localization-related epilepsy is not known.

Differentiating Benign Rolandic Spikes from Other Spikes Occurring in the Same Areas

Differences in several EEG features help distinguish discharges of benign rolandic epilepsy from those of perirolandic symptomatic localization-related epilepsy. In the rolandic form of benign focal epilepsy, the IED dipole is oriented tangentially to the cortical surface, with the negative pole near the junction of the rolandic and sylvian fissures and the positive pole more broadly distributed over the frontal regions bilaterally (121,132,181). In symptomatic perirolandic epilepsy, IEDs have a radial distribution (121). In benign rolandic epilepsy, the topographic distribution of the IEDs is typically stereotyped, whereas the distribution of IEDs in symptomatic perirolandic epilepsy is more variable. Focal slowing is absent in benign rolandic epilepsy (except when discharges are so frequent that the aftergoing slow waves summate), but it is often present in symptomatic perirolandic epilepsy. These electrographic differences interpreted within the particular clinical context usually allow firm distinction between two very different types of epilepsy.

Distinction between anterior temporal and centrotemporal spikes usually poses little difficulty. However, distinguishing between benign centrotemporal discharges and midtemporal IEDs that have some suprasylvian representation can be more difficult. The T3/4 electrode placements of the international 10-20 system actually lie near the junction of the sylvian and rolandic fissures, and the short interelectrode distances used in routine longitudinal and bipolar montages do not facilitate assessment of voltage differences in this region. Placement of additional electrodes is frequently very helpful. Recording to an inactive reference and use of the expanded 10-20 system invariably demonstrates that the voltage of IEDs that is characteristic of benign rolandic epilepsy is maximal over C3/4 or C5/6 rather than T3/T4 (170). Similarly, in patients with midtemporal symptomatic epilepsy, the IEDs are of highest voltage when recorded from electrodes below the standard temporal 10-20 placements.

NON-CONVULSIVE STATUS EPILEPTICUS

Non-convulsive status epilepticus is often difficult to diagnose clinically, and it may be confused with dementia, metabolic or toxic encephalopathy, or a psychiatric syndrome. EEG is often the only method for making an accurate diagnosis. The literature has traditionally distinguished between complex partial status epilepticus with lateralized seizure activity occurring continuously or in cycles and generalized non-convulsive status epilepticus with predominantly symmetrical, bilateral synchronous IEDs. However, studies have emphasized practical difficulties in making these distinctions, especially if EEG and clinical findings are followed longitudinally. Consequently, investigators have advanced classifications based on syndromic and etiologic (261), as well as EEG, criteria.

Epilepsia partialis continua is most often characterized by unremitting motor seizures involving part or all of one side of the body. Although the seizures are of cortical origin, correlations between clinical manifestations and EEG changes are inconsistent. One series reported focal discharges in only 22% of affected patients (60). In another, with more aggressive sampling, researchers found focal discharges in 71% of patients, usually in the form of irregular spikes and sharp waves (276). In that series, PLEDs occurred in 14% of patients. More comprehensive neurophysiological investigations demonstrated a relationship between scalp-recorded discharges and muscle jerks in 37% to 45% of patients (60,276). Completely normal EEGs occur in fewer than 10% of cases of epilepsia partialis continua, but focal epileptiform discharges can be demonstrated by electrocorticography (276). In such EEG-negative cases, the discharging cortical region is presumably either oriented unfavorably with regard to scalp electrodes or too small to allow detection at the scalp. PLEDs have been found in 8% to 14% of cases of epilepsia partialis continua (52,256,276), and in these patients, a diagnosis of partial status epilepticus is justified. Most authorities, however, do not believe that PLEDs, by themselves, are a form of non-convulsive status epilepticus. Although mental status is often impaired in patients with PLEDs, this can usually be attributed adequately to the acute structural or metabolic disturbance causing PLEDs, rather than to the PLEDs themselves. PLEDs that occur in the absence of structural lesions or metabolic disturbances may be associated with recurrent episodes of confusion that respond to carbamazepine (274). This unusual situation probably represents a peculiar form of non-convulsive status epilepticus in the elderly.

Initial descriptions of complex partial status epilepticus emphasized recurring periods of automatic activity attributed to partial seizures. These intermittent automatisms with "concomitant cycling of the EEG patterns" were said to be present even in the most advanced stages (279). In one analysis of a large series of EEGs in partial status epilepticus, researchers did, in fact, find that EEG changes remained focal throughout the course of the status epilepticus episode (119). However, in most patients with frontal lobe complex partial status epilepticus, scalp EEGs eventually showed bilateral sharp-slow activity (306). Furthermore, most patients who develop non-convulsive status epilepticus in later life have generalized spike-wave or polyspike-wave discharges during most of the course of the episode (83,168) (Fig. 17.28). The majority of these patients do not have a history of absence seizures, and focal, not generalized, IEDs are recorded subsequently. In these patients, generalized discharges stop altogether or become focal after treatment with phenytoin, and phenytoin also prevents subsequent episodes of status epilepticus (83,168). Such observations provide strong support for the view that non-convulsive status epilepticus occurring later in life and associated with generalized ictal discharges is a localization-related seizure disorder. When confusional episodes in adults are accompanied by generalized ictal discharges, careful inquiry should be made regarding manifestations of primary generalized epilepsy earlier in life. If such history is lacking, brain imaging is mandatory, and treatment with drugs that are effective against partial seizures is reasonable.

Serial EEGs during and after convulsive status epilepticus have demonstrated a wide variety of patterns. It is important to recognize these, because only one of them may be seen during a single EEG study. Treiman et al. (280) proposed that EEG changes occur in a progressive sequence during convulsive status. Seizures occur (a) discretely at first and then (b) gradually merge with waxing and waning voltage and frequency. This is followed by (c) a period of continuous rhythmic ictal discharge. Subsequently, (d) a continuous monorhythmic discharge is punctuated by periods of attenuation. Finally, (e) GPEDs are seen against a severely attenu-ated background (Fig. 17.29). It is not clear where clinical convulsive activity ends in this sequence and what effect treatment has on these patterns. It is also unclear which of these patterns are related to electrographic seizures rather than to the results of cortical injury, whether from the seizures themselves or from the underlying cause of the seizures. Subsequent studies have reported that non-convulsive status (patterns a through d proposed by Treiman et al. [280]) occurred in approximately one-third of patients after convulsive seizure activity had ceased (68). Each of the patterns of Treiman et al. occurred in some patients, but many patients exhibited only a few of the patterns, often out of the sequence proposed (68,202). Non-convulsive status epilepticus accompanied by any of these patterns was associated with a higher rate of mortality, even after investigators accounted for the effects of age and etiology of status epilepticus (68). In contrast, brief electrographic seizures occurring more than 30 minutes after cessation of convulsive activity were not associated with increased rates of mortality (68). GPEDs occurred more often in the elderly and tended to correlate with poorer outcome in one study (202) but not in another (143).

EEGs obtained to rule out non-convulsive status epilepticus sometimes demonstrate a pattern of continuous sharp-slow wave activity or GPEDs. Distinguishing between the more or less continuous sharp-slow wave pattern seen in non-convulsive status epilepticus and the triphasic wave pattern of metabolic or toxic encephalopathies is usually not difficult (see Chapter 12). Distinguishing between GPEDs that occur during or after status epilepticus from those seen in the setting of diffuse anoxia is more problematic. Subtle or overt myoclonus often accompanies GPEDs (155,262,311), and this leads to further confusion. Husain et al. (143) compared GPEDs related to status epilepticus with those caused by other entities. In cases of status epilepticus, GPEDs were of longer duration and of higher but more variable voltage. However, the intergroup variability was too great to formulate clinically useful rules. When status epilepticus is suspected and the EEG shows GPEDs, it is important to review the clinical situation carefully. If the patient has had previous seizures or serial convulsions, vigorous treatment is indicated, because it is possible that the patient has a late stage of status epilepticus. Most experts would probably not use barbiturate anesthesia or a midazolam drip, because it is most likely that the GPEDs represent cerebral aftereffects of the status epilepticus rather than ongoing seizure activity. If the patient has sustained a severe anoxic or other significant cerebral insult, the GPEDs are much more likely to result from the brain injury than from ongoing seizures. In such cases, even aggressive antiepileptic drug treat-

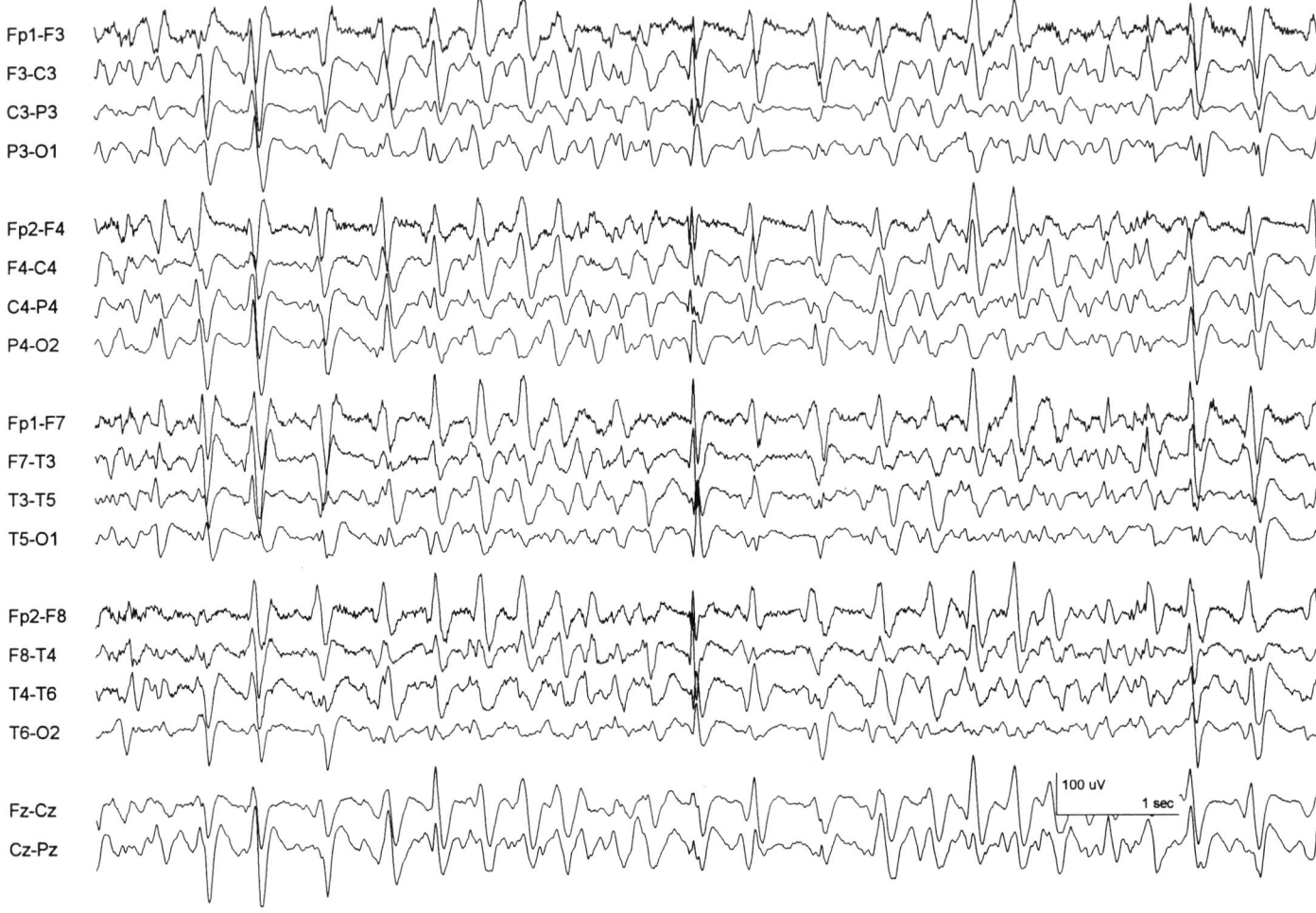

A   Comment

FIG. 17.28. Non-convulsive status epilepticus in a 75-year-old woman with a history of complex partial seizures. On the evening before admission, she had a generalized convulsive seizure. The following morning, she was found staring and poorly interactive. **A:** The EEG shows repetitive bilateral synchronous 2- to 3-Hz spikes and sharp waves. TC, 0.1 second; HFF, 70 Hz. *(Figure continues.)*

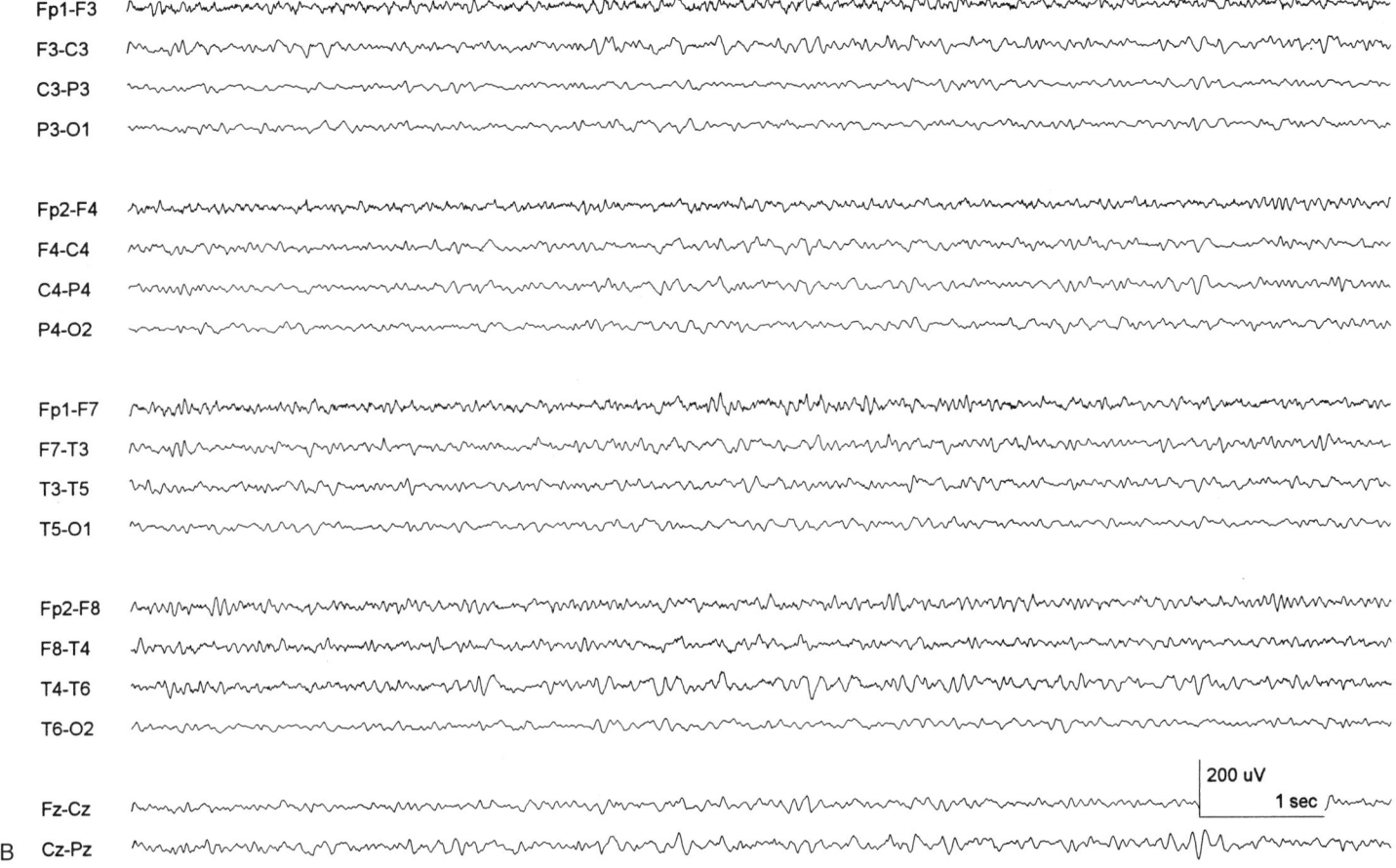

FIG. 17.28. *Continued.* **B:** Fifteen minutes after receiving intravenous lorazepam, she became more responsive, although she remained inattentive. The EEG demonstrates resolution of epileptiform activity and is now notable only for moderate diffuse background slowing. She received a phenytoin loading, and she gradually returned to her baseline neurological status over the next 24 hours. TC, 0.1 second; HFF, 70 Hz.

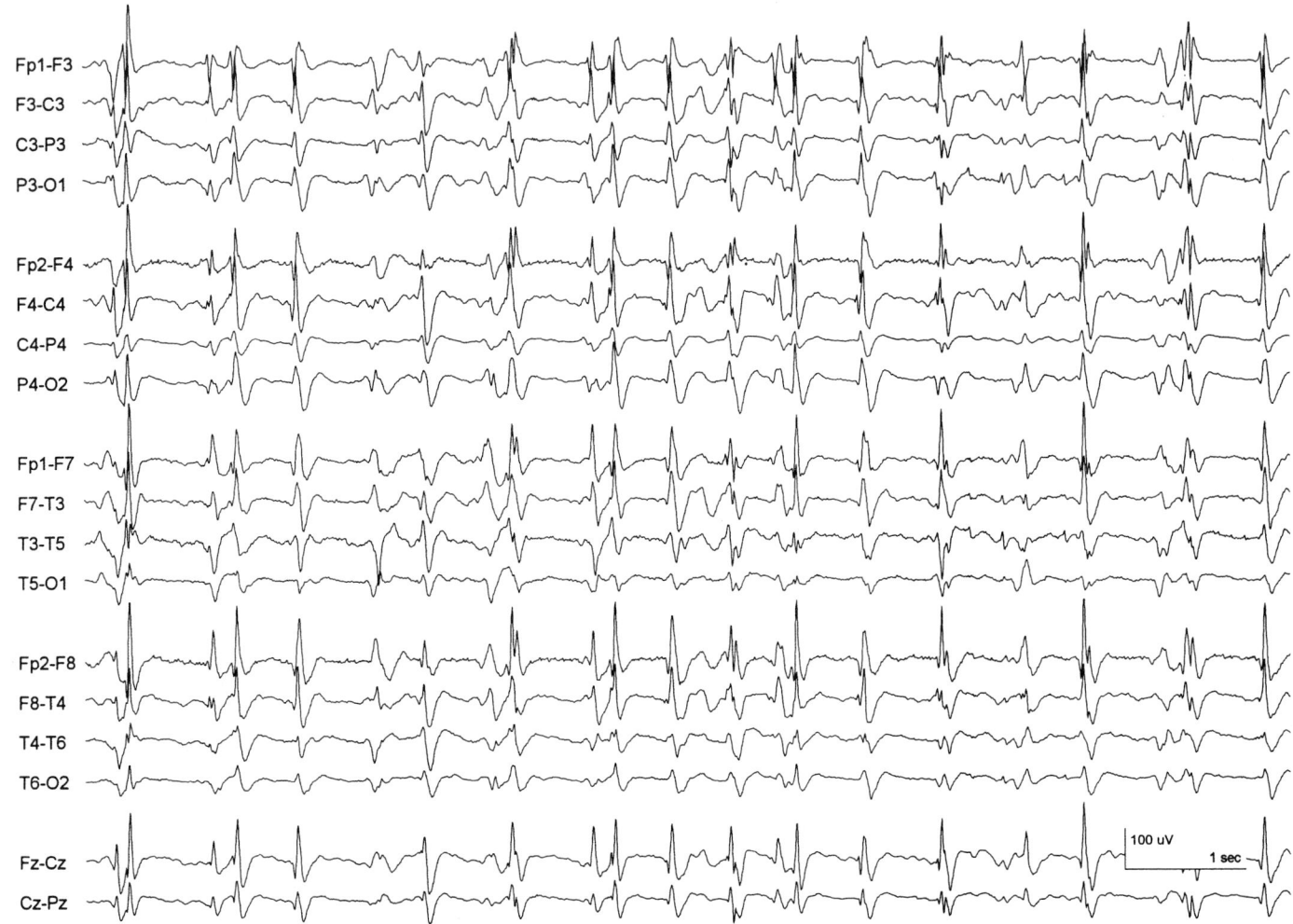

FIG. 17.29. EEG of an 86-year-old woman with refractory non-convulsive status epilepticus after a cardiorespiratory arrest. She remained comatose despite treatment with multiple anticonvulsant medications. She died shortly after the EEG recording shown in *B* was obtained. **A:** EEG demonstrates 1- to 2-Hz generalized periodic epileptiform discharges (GPEDs). Background activity seen between epileptiform discharges is markedly attenuated and undifferentiated. TC, 0.1 second; HFF, 70 Hz. *(Figure continues.)*

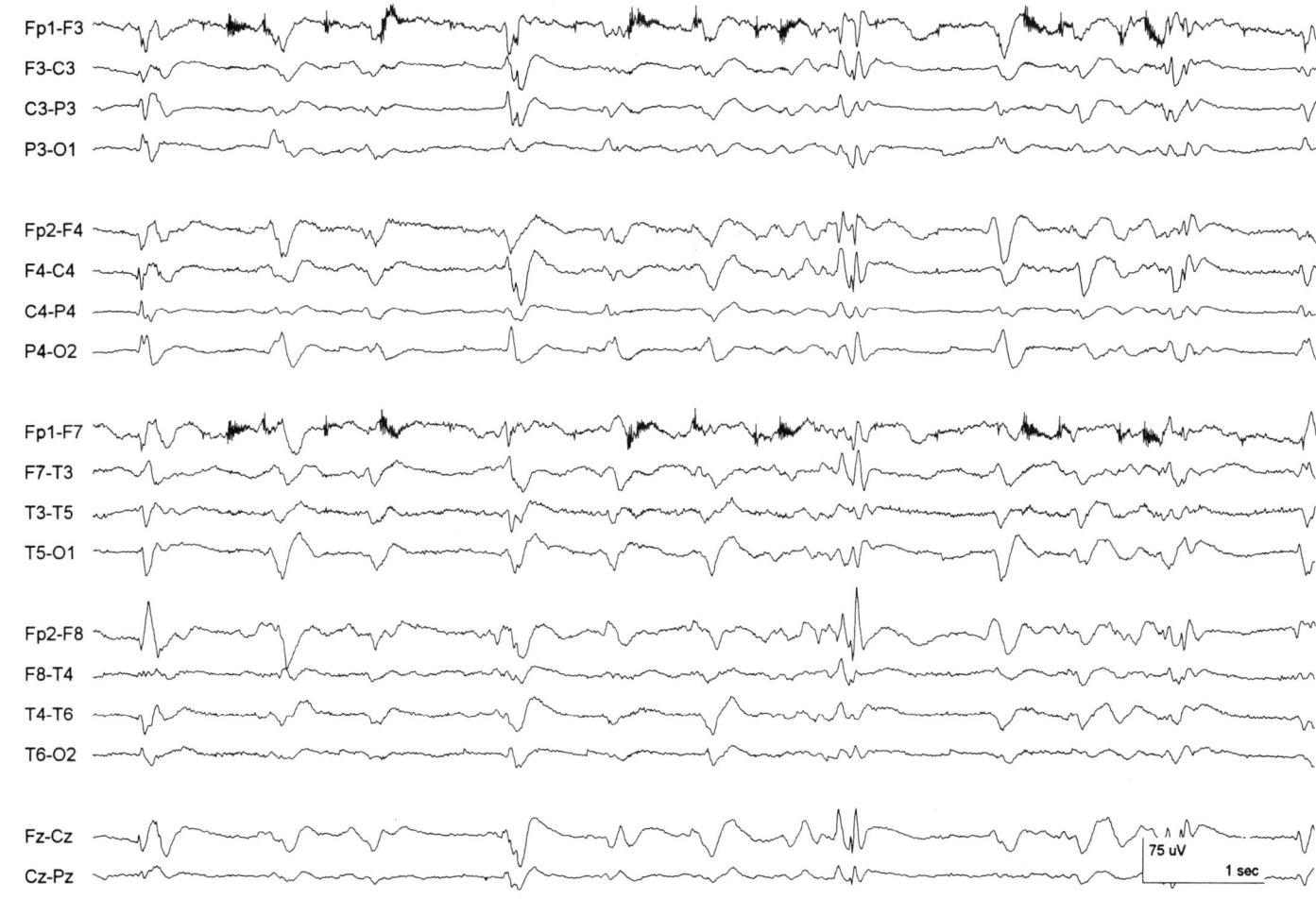

FIG. 17.29. *Continued.* **B:** EEG recorded 1 day later. Background activity remains severely attenuated and undifferentiated. GPEDs have much broader morphological patterns and occur at a slower repetition rate. TC, 0.1 second; HFF, 70 Hz.

ment, including barbiturate anesthesia, is almost always futile, and hypotensive side effects may actually worsen the situation. The prognosis is extremely poor (155,262,311).

EEG interpretation after status epilepticus is sometimes difficult, as indicated in the foregoing section. However, because of the high prevalence of late non-convulsive status epilepticus and the possibility of obtaining useful prognostic information, follow-up EEG should always be obtained after convulsions are controlled, if continuous EEG monitoring is not being used.

ELECTROENCEPHALOGRAPHY AND THE RISK OF SEIZURE RECURRENCE

The likelihood of seizure recurrence is the most important factor in deciding whether to initiate treatment after a first epileptic seizure. EEGs demonstrate IEDs in 10% to 39% of adults after a first seizure and in 32% to 59% of children after a first seizure (45,136,161,259,285). An EEG obtained within 24 hours of the seizure is more likely to yield epileptiform activity (232,285) than is one obtained later, and sleep deprivation increases the yield even further (161,285). Various EEG abnormalities have been associated with increased risk of seizure recurrence (Table 17.6). Three studies found that IEDs were predictive of recurrent seizures (232,130,285). All IEDs were associated with seizure recurrence in two of these studies (232,285), whereas only generalized IEDs were found to increase risk of further seizures in the third (130). A metaanalysis concluded that EEG findings provide useful prognostic information, especially in children, beyond

that already obtained by diagnosis of the epilepsy syndrome, which is itself strongly influenced by EEG results (21).

Febrile seizures represent an exception to the foregoing statements. After a febrile seizure, many children have nonspecific EEG abnormalities, usually generalized slowing that is maximal over the occipital areas, for several days to a week (94,270). Neither slowing nor IEDs have prognostic significance for additional febrile seizures or development of epilepsy (94,277, 282). Serial EEGs obtained for febrile seizures reveal generalized epileptiform discharges in 35% to 45% of children who are older than 2 years, especially between the ages of 3 and 5 years (73,94,281,282). EEG has no role in the evaluation of children with typical febrile seizures.

Determining the probability of seizure relapse also plays a role in deciding whether to discontinue antiepileptic drugs after an appropriate seizure-free period. Most studies have found that an abnormal EEG obtained at the time of drug withdrawal is associated with a greater chance of seizure relapse (relative risk, about 1.5). Results of four of these studies are summarized in Table 17.7. In two of the studies, researchers also examined the value of specific EEG findings. The Medical Research Council (231) found that only generalized IEDs were correlated with recurrent seizures; focal or diffuse abnormalities of background activity were not prognostic. With univariate analysis, Shinnar et al. (258) found that both IEDs and focal or diffuse background abnormalities were associated with a greater chance of recurrence. Using multivariate analysis, they discovered that four of six variables predicting relapse were EEG related: association between age at first seizure and background slowing; presence of IEDs; presence of background slowing; and EEG improvement between seizure diagnosis and antiepileptic drug withdrawal. As is the case with first seizures, epilepsy syndrome also plays an important role in estimating risk of relapse after discontinuation of antiepileptic drugs. For example, benign epilepsy of childhood with central-midtemporal spikes has a uniformly good prognosis (72), whereas in juvenile myoclonic epilepsy, relapse is probable when antiepileptic drugs are stopped (106). It is thus not clear whether the EEG contribution to predictions of seizure relapse exists because EEG findings are a measure of "seizure susceptibility" or an indication of epilepsy syndrome. Berg et al. (22) reported that focal slow wave abnormalities, epilepsy syndrome, and seizure frequency were independent predictors of persistent seizures and lack of response to antiepileptic drugs. This finding supports the conclusion that the utility of EEG in predicting seizure recurrence is greater than its role in diagnosing epilepsy syndromes.

TABLE 17.6. *EEG predictors of recurrence after first unprovoked seizure*

Study	Age	IEDs	Non-IED abnormality	Any abnormality
Annegers et al. (7)	Mixed	NR	NE	+
Hopkins et al. (136)	Adults	0	0	0
Shinnar et al. (258)	Children	0	NR	+
Hauser et al. (130)	Mixed	+	0	0
FIRST Group (232)	Mixed	+	NR	NR
Van Donselaar et al. (285)	Adults	+	+	+

+, factor associated with increased risk; 0, factor not associated with increased risk; IED, interictal epileptiform discharge; NR, effect of factor not reported.

TABLE 17.7. *EEG predictors of relapse after withdrawal of antiseizure drugs*

Study	Population	Definition of abnormality	Relapse risk when abnormality present	Percentage with abnormality suffering relapse
Medical Research Council trial (231)	Mixed	Features analyzed individually	+	NR
Callaghan et al. (44)	Adults	IED, focal slowing	+	70%
Shinnar et al. (260)	Children	Features analyzed individually	+	35%
Emerson et al. (85)	Children	IEDs, focal slowing	+	57%

+, factor associated with increased risk; IED, interictal epileptiform discharge; NR, effect of factor not reported.

CONCLUSIONS

Even in the era of high-resolution anatomical and functional imaging, EEG continues to play a critical role in the evaluation of patients with known or suspected seizures. Because EEG is a physiological test, its results are optimally useful only when considered in the relevant clinical context. This is similar to interpreting findings on neurological examination. Two patients, each with a hemiplegia, may look the same, but if the hemiplegia developed abruptly in one case but evolved slowly over 2 weeks in the other, the diagnostic considerations would be substantially different. The interpretation of epileptiform discharges similarly depends on context. Accurate interpretation and meaningful clinical-electrographic correlations require careful analysis of a spike's voltage distribution on the scalp, the frequency and regularity of its repetition rate, its response to activating procedures, and any alteration that occurs with changes in physiological state. The degree of associated disturbances in EEG background activity must also be taken into account. Finally, when an EEG is "normal," it is important to know whether it was the first EEG or one of several, whether sleep was included in the recording, whether the patient was sleep deprived, and whether appropriate activating procedures were used. Only when these important variables are taken into account is EEG information optimally useful in answering the questions posed in Table 17.1.

REFERENCES

1. Abraham D, Ajmone-Marsan C. Patterns of cortical discharge and their relation to routine scalp EEG. *Electroencephalogr Clin Neurophysiol* 1958;10:447–461.
2. Aliberti V, Grunewald RA, Panayiotopoulos CP, et al. Focal electroencephalographic abnormalities in juvenile myoclonic epilepsy. *Epilepsia* 1994;35:297–301.
3. Alving J. Classification of the epilepsies. An investigation of 402 children. *Acta Neurol Scand* 1979;60:157–163.
4. Ambrosetto G, Tinuper P, Baruzzi A. Relapse of benign partial epilepsy of children in adulthood: report of a case. *J Neurol Neurosurg Psychiat* 1985;48:90.
5. Amir N, Shalev RS, Steinberg A. Sleep patterns in the Lennox-Gastaut syndrome. *Neurology* 1986;36:1224–1226.
6. Andermann F. Occipital epileptic abnormalities in mitochondrial disorders—preferential involvement, illustrations of clinical patterns, current progress in neurobiology, and a hypothesis. In: Andermann F, Beaumanoir A, Mira L, et al., eds. *Occipital seizures and epilepsies in children.* London: John Libbey, 1993:111–120.
7. Annegers JF, Shirts SB, Hauser WA, et al. Risk of recurrence after an initial unprovoked seizure. *Epilepsia* 1986;27:43–50.
8. Asconape J, Penry JK. Some clinical and EEG aspects of benign juvenile myoclonic epilepsy. *Epilepsia* 1984;25:108–114.
9. Barkovich AJ, Kuzniecky RI, Dobyns WB, et al. A classification scheme for malformations of cortical development. *Neuropediatrics* 1996;27:59–63.
10. Bauer G, Aichner F, Saltuari L. Epilepsies with diffuse slow spikes and waves of late onset. *Eur Neurol* 1983;22:344–350.
11. Bautista RE, Spencer DD, Spencer SS. EEG findings in frontal lobe epilepsies. *Neurology* 1998;50:1765–1771.
12. Bazil CW, Pedley TA. Neurophysiological effects of antiepileptic drugs. In: Levy RH, Mattson RH, Meldrum BS, et al., eds. *Antiepileptic drugs,* 5th ed. Philadelphia: Lippincott Williams & Wilkins, 2002.
13. Beaumanoir A. The Lennox-Gastaut syndrome: a personal study. *Electroencephalogr Clin Neurophysiol Suppl* 1982;35:85–99.
14. Beaumanoir A. Infantile epilepsy with occipital focus and good prognosis. *Eur Neurol* 1983; 22:43–52.
15. Beaumanoir A. The Landau-Kleffner syndrome. In: Roger J, Bureau M, Dravet C, et al., eds. *Epileptic syndromes in infancy, childhood, and adolescence.* London: John Libbey, 1992: 231–243.
16. Beaumanoir A. EEG data. In: Beaumanoir A, Bureau M, Deonna T, et al., eds. *Continuous spikes and waves during slow sleepelectrical status epilepticus during slow sleep.* London: John Libbey, 1995:217–223.
17. Beaumanoir A, Ballis T, Varfis G, et al. Benign epilepsy of childhood with rolandic spikes. A clinical, electroencephalographic, and telencephalographic study. *Epilepsia* 1974;15:301–315.
18. Beaumanoir A, Dravet C. The Lennox-Gastaut syndrome. In: Roger J, Bureau M, Dravet C, et al., eds. *Epileptic syndromes in infancy, childhood, and adolescence.* London: John Libbey, 1992:115–132.
19. Beaussart M. Benign epilepsy of children with rolandic (centro-temporal) paroxysmal foci. A clinical entity. Study of 221 cases. *Epilepsia* 1972;13:795–911.
20. Bennet DR. Spike wave complexes in normal flying personnel. *Aerospace Med* 1967;38: 1276–1282.
21. Berg AT, Shinnar S. The risk of seizure recurrence following a first unprovoked seizure: a quantitative review. *Neurology* 1991;41:965–972.

22. Berg AT, Shinnar S, Levy SR, et al. Early development of intractable epilepsy in children: a prospective study. *Neurology* 2001;56:1445–1452.

23. Berkovic S. Progressive myoclonus epilepsies. In: Engel J Jr, Pedley TA, eds. *Epilepsy: a comprehensive textbook.* Philadelphia: Lippincott-Raven, 1997:2455–2468.

24. Berkovic SF, Andermann F, Carpenter S, et al. Progressive myoclonus epilepsies: specific causes and diagnosis. *N Engl J Med* 1986;315:296–305.

25. Berkovic SF, Cochius J, Andermann E, et al. Progressive myoclonus epilepsies: clinical and genetic aspects. *Epilepsia* 1993;34(Suppl 3):S19–S30.

26. Berkovic SF, So NK, Andermann F. Progressive myoclonus epilepsies: clinical and neurophysiological diagnosis. *J Clin Neurophysiol* 1991;8:261–274.

27. Bernardina BD, Beghini G. Rolandic spikes in children with and without epilepsy (20 subjects polygraphically studied during sleep). *Epilepsia* 1976;17:161–167.

28. Bernardina BD, Tassinari CA. EEG of a nocturnal seizure in a patient with "benign epilepsy of childhood with rolandic spikes." *Epilepsia* 1975;16:497–501.

29. Beydoun A, Garofalo EA, Drury I. Generalized spike-waves, multiple loci, and clinical course in children with EEG features of benign epilepsy of childhood with centrotemporal spikes. *Epilepsia* 1992;33:1091–1096.

30. Billard C, Autret A, Laffont F, et al. Electrical status epilepticus during sleep in children: a reappraisal from eight new cases. In: Sterman MB, Shouse MN, Passouant P, eds. *Sleep and epilepsy.* London: Academic Press, 1982:481–494.

31. Blom S, Heijbel J. Benign epilepsy of children with centro-temporal EEG foci. Discharge rate during sleep. *Epilepsia* 1975;16:133–140.

32. Blom S, Heijbel J, Bergfors PG. Benign epilepsy of children with centro-temporal EEG foci. Prevalence and follow-up study of 40 patients. *Epilepsia* 1972;13:609–619.

33. Blume WT. Clinical and electroencephalographic correlates of the multiple independent spike foci pattern in children. *Ann Neurol* 1978;4:541–547.

34. Blume WT. Lennox-Gastaut syndrome. In: Luders H, Lesser RP, eds. *Epilepsy: electroclinical syndromes.* London: Springer-Verlag, 1987:73–92.

35. Blume WT, David RB, Gomez MR. Generalized sharp and slow wave complexes. Associated clinical features and long-term follow-up. *Brain* 1973;96:289–306.

36. Bray PF, Wiser WC. Evidence for a genetic etiology of temporal-central abnormalities in focal epilepsy. *N Engl J Med* 1964;271:926–933.

37. Brenner RP, Atkinson R. Generalized paroxysmal fast activity: electroencephalographic and clinical features. *Ann Neurol* 1982;11:386–390.

38. Bridgers SL. Epileptiform abnormalities discovered on electroencephalographic screening of psychiatric inpatients. *Arch Neurol* 1987;44:312–316.

39. Browne TR, Penry JK, Proter RJ, et al. Responsiveness before, during, and after spike-wave paroxysms. *Neurology* 1974;24:659–665.

40. Bruni J, Wilder BJ, Bauman AW, et al. Clinical efficacy and long-term effects of valproic acid therapy on spike-and-wave discharges. *Neurology* 1980;30:42–46.

41. Bureau M. "Continuous spikes and waves during slow sleep" (CSWS): definition of syndrome. In: Beaumanoir A, Bureau M, Deonna T, et al., eds. *Continuous spikes and waves during slow sleepelectrical status epilepticus during slow sleep.* London: John Libbey, 1995:17–26.

42. Bureau M. Outstanding cases of CSWS and LKS: analysis of the data sheets provided by the participants. In: Beaumanoir A, Bureau M, Deonna T, et al., eds. *Continuous spikes and waves during slow sleepelectrical status epilepticus during slow sleep.* London: John Libbey, 1995:213–216.

43. Burgerman RS, Sperling MR, French JA, et al. Comparison of mesial versus neocortical onset temporal lobe seizures: neurodiagnostic findings and surgical outcome. *Epilepsia* 1995;36:662–670.

44. Callaghan N, Garrett A, Goggin T. Withdrawal of anticonvulsant drugs in patients free of seizures for two years. A prospective study. *N Engl J Med* 1988;318:942–946.

45. Camfield PR, Camfield CS, Dooley JM, et al. Epilepsy after a first unprovoked seizure in childhood. *Neurology* 1985;35:1657–1660.

46. Caraballo R, Cersosimo R, Fejerman N. Idiopathic partial epilepsies with rolandic and occipital spikes appearing in the same children. *J Epilepsy* 1998;11:261–264.

47. Cascino GD, Jack CR, Jr, Parisi JE, et al. Magnetic resonance imaging-based volume studies in temporal lobe epilepsy: pathological correlations. *Ann Neurol* 1991;30:31–36.

48. Cavazzuti GB. Epidemiology of different types of epilepsy in school age children of Modena, Italy. *Epilepsia* 1980;21:57–62.

49. Cavazzuti GB, Cappella L, Nalin A. Longitudinal study of epileptiform EEG patterns in normal children. *Epilepsia* 1980;21:43–55.

50. Chatrian GE. Report of the committee on terminology. The VIIth International Congress of Electroencephalography and Clinical Neurophysiology. *Electroencephalogr Clin Neurophysiol* 1974;35:521–553.

51. Chatrian GE, Lettich E, Wilkus RJ, et al. Polygraphic and clinical observations on tonic-autonomic seizures. *Electroencephalogr Clin Neurophysiol Suppl* 1982:101–124.

52. Chatrian GE, Shaw CM, Lefman H. The significance of periodic lateralizing epileptiform discharges in EEG: an electrographic, clinical, and pathophysiologic study. *Electroencephalogr Clin Neurophysiol* 1964;17.

53. Chatrian GE, Somasundaram M, Tassinari CA. DC changes recorded transcranially during "typical" three per second spike and wave discharges in man. *Epilepsia* 1968;9:185–209.

54. Chevrie JJ, Aicardi J. Childhood epileptic encephalopathy with slow spike-wave. A statistical study of 80 cases. *Epilepsia* 1972;13:259–271.

55. Chokroverty S, Gandhi V. Electroencephalograms in patients with progressive dialytic encephalopathy. *Clin Electroencephalogr* 1982;13:122–127.

56. Chung MY, Walczak TS, Lewis DV, et al. Temporal lobectomy and independent bitemporal interictal activity: what degree of lateralization is sufficient? *Epilepsia* 1991;32:195–201.

57. Clancy RR. Interictal sharp EEG transients in neonatal seizures. *J Child Neurol* 1989;4:30–38.

58. Clemens B, Majoros E. Sleep studies in benign epilepsy of childhood with rolandic spikes. II. Analysis of discharge frequency and its relation to sleep dynamics. *Epilepsia* 1987;28:24–27.

59. Cobb WA, Gordon N, Matthews C, et al. The occipital delta rhythm in petit mal. *Electroencephalogr Clin Neurophysiol* 1961;13:142–143.

60. Cockerell OC, Rothwell J, Thompson PD, et al. Clinical and physiological features of epilepsia partialis continua. Cases ascertained in the UK. *Brain* 1996;119(Pt 2):393–407.

61. Colamaria V, Sgro V, Caraballo R, et al. Status epilepticus in benign rolandic epilepsy manifesting as anterior operculum syndrome. *Epilepsia* 1991;32:329–334.

62. Cooper GW, Lee SI. Reactive occipital epileptiform activity: is it benign? *Epilepsia* 1991;32:63–68.

63. Cooper R, Winter A, Chow HJ, et al. Comparison of subcortical, cortical, and scalp activity using chronically indwelling electrodes in man. *Electroencephalogr Clin Neurophysiol* 1965;18:217–228.

64. Dalby MA. Epilepsy and 3 per second spike and wave rhythms. A clinical, electroencephalographic and prognostic analysis of 346 patients. *Acta Neurol Scand* 1969:Suppl 40:43.

65. de la Paz D, Brenner RP. Bilateral independent periodic lateralized epileptiform discharges. Clinical significance. *Arch Neurol* 1981;38:713–715.

66. Degen R, Degen HE. Some genetic aspects of rolandic epilepsy: waking and sleep EEGs in siblings. *Epilepsia* 1990;31:795–801.

67. Delgado-Escueta AV, Enrile-Bacsal F. Juvenile myoclonic epilepsy of Janz. *Neurology* 1984;34:285–294.

68. DeLorenzo RJ, Waterhouse EJ, Towne AR, et al. Persistent non-convulsive status epilepticus after the control of convulsive status epilepticus. *Epilepsia* 1998;39:833–840.

69. Deonna TW. Acquired epileptiform aphasia in children (Landau-Kleffner syndrome). *J Clin Neurophysiol* 1991;8:288–298.

70. Deonna T, Peter C, Ziegler AL. Adult follow-up of the acquired aphasia-epilepsy syndrome in childhood. Report of 7 cases. *Neuropediatrics* 1989;20:132–138.

71. Deonna T, Roulet E. "Acquired epileptic aphasia" (AEA): definition of the syndrome and cur-

rent problems. In: Beaumanoir A, Bureau M, Deonna T, et al., eds. *Continuous spikes and waves during slow sleepelectrical status epilepticus during slow sleep*. London: John Libbey, 1995:37–46.

72. Dooley J, Gordon K, Camfield P, et al. Discontinuation of anticonvulsant therapy in children free of seizures for 1 year: a prospective study. *Neurology* 1996;46:969–974.

73. Doose H, Ritter K, Volzke E. EEG longitudinal studies in febrile convulsions. Genetic aspects. *Neuropediatrics* 1983;14:81–87.

74. Dravet C. Benign epilepsy with centrotemporal spikes: do we know all about it? In: Wolf P, ed. *Epileptic seizures and syndromes*. London: John Libbey, 1994:231–240.

75. Dugas M, Franc S, Gerard CL, et al. Evolution of acquired aphasia with or without continuous spikes and waves during slow sleep. In: Beaumanoir A, Bureau M, Deonna T, et al., eds. *Continuous spikes and waves during slow sleepelectrical status epilepticus during slow sleep*. London: John Libbey, 1995.

76. Durner M, Sander T, Greenberg DA, et al. Localization of idiopathic generalized epilepsy on chromosome 6p in families of juvenile myoclonic epilepsy patients. *Neurology* 1991;41:1651–1655.

77. Ebersole JS, Pacia SV. Localization of temporal lobe foci by ictal EEG patterns. *Epilepsia* 1996;37:386–399.

78. Ebersole JS, Wade PB. Spike voltage topography identifies two types of frontotemporal epileptic foci. *Neurology* 1991;41:1425–1433.

79. Ebner A. Lateral (neocortical) temporal lobe epilepsy. In: Wolf P, ed. *Epileptic seizures and syndromes*. London: John Libbey, 1994:375–382.

80. Eeg-Olofsson O, Petersen I, Sellden U. The development of the electroencephalogram in normal children from the age of 1 through 15 years. Paroxysmal activity. *Neuropadiatrie* 1971;2:375–404.

81. Egli M, Mothersill I, O'Kane M, et al. The axial spasm—the predominant type of drop seizure in patients with secondary generalized epilepsy. *Epilepsia* 1985;26:401–415.

82. Ehle A, Co S, Jones MG. Clinical correlates of midline spikes. An analysis of 21 patients. *Arch Neurol* 1981;38:355–357.

83. Ellis JM, Lee SI. Acute prolonged confusion in later life as an ictal state. *Epilepsia* 1978;19:119–128.

84. Elmslie FV, Williamson MP, Rees M, et al. Linkage analysis of juvenile myoclonic epilepsy and microsatellite loci spanning 61 cM of human chromosome 6p in 19 nuclear pedigrees provides no evidence for a susceptibility locus in this region. *Am J Hum Genet* 1996;59:653–663.

85. Emerson R, D'Souza BJ, Vining EP, et al. Stopping medication in children with epilepsy: predictors of outcome. *N Engl J Med* 1981;304:1125–1129.

86. Engel J Jr. Recent advances in surgical treatment of temporal lobe epilepsy. *Acta Neurol Scand Suppl* 1992;140:71–80.

87. Engel J Jr, Rapin I, Giblin DR. Electrophysiological studies in two patients with cherry red spot–myoclonus syndrome. *Epilepsia* 1977;18:73–87.

88. Engel J Jr, Williamson PD, Wieser HG. Mesial temporal lobe epilepsy. In: Engel J Jr, Pedley TA, eds. *Epilepsy: a comprehensive textbook*. Philadelphia: Lippincott-Raven, 1997:2417–2426.

89. Fariello RG, Chun RW, Doro JM, et al. EEG recognition of Aicardi's syndrome. *Arch Neurol* 1977;34:563–566.

90. Farrell MA, Vinters HV. General neuropathology of epilepsy. In: Engel J Jr, Pedley TA, eds. *Epilepsy: a comprehensive textbook*. Philadelphia: Lippincott-Raven, 1997:157–175.

91. Fejerman N, Di Blasi AM. Status epilepticus of benign partial epilepsies in children: report of two cases. *Epilepsia* 1987;28:351–355.

92. Ferrie CD, Beaumanoir A, Guerrini R, et al. Early-onset benign occipital seizure susceptibility syndrome. *Epilepsia* 1997;38:285–293.

93. Foldvary N, Lee N, Thwaites G, et al. Clinical and electrographic manifestations of lesional neocortical temporal lobe epilepsy. *Neurology* 1997;49:757–763.

94. Frantzen E, Lennox-Buchthal M, Nygaard A. Longitudinal EEG and clinical study of children with febrile convulsions. *Electroencephalogr Clin Neurophysiol* 1968;24:197–212.

95. French JA, Williamson PD, Thadani VM, et al. Characteristics of medial temporal lobe epilepsy: I. Results of history and physical examination. *Ann Neurol* 1993;34:774–780.

96. Friedman E, Pampiglione G. Prognostic implications of electroencephalographic findings in the first year of life. *BMJ* 1971;4:323–325.

97. Fusco L, Iani C, Faedda MT, et al. Mesial frontal lobe epilepsy: a clinical entity not sufficiently described. *J Epilepsy* 1990;3:123–135.

98. Fusco L, Vigevano F. Ictal clinical electroencephalographic findings of spasms in West syndrome. *Epilepsia* 1993;34:671–678.

99. Gambardella A, Gotman J, Cendes F, et al. Focal intermittent delta activity in patients with mesiotemporal atrophy: a reliable marker of the epileptogenic focus. *Epilepsia* 1995;36:122–129.

100. Gambardella A, Palmini A, Andermann F, et al. Usefulness of focal rhythmic discharges on scalp EEG of patients with focal cortical dysplasia and intractable epilepsy. *Electroencephalogr Clin Neurophysiol* 1996;98:243–249.

101. Gastaut H. A new type of epilepsy: benign partial epilepsy of childhood with occipital spike-waves. *Clin Electroencephalogr* 1982;13:13–22.

102. Gastaut H, Gastaut JL, Goncalves e Silva GE, et al. Relative frequency of different types of epilepsy: a study employing the classification of the International League Against Epilepsy. *Epilepsia* 1975;16:457–461.

103. Gastaut H, Roger J, Soulayrol R, et al. [Epileptic encephalopathy of children with diffuse slow spikes and waves (alias "petit mal variant") or Lennox syndrome]. *Ann Pediatr (Paris)* 1966;13:489–499.

104. Gastaut H, Zifkin BG. Benign epilepsy of childhood with occipital spike and wave complexes. In: Andermann F, Lugaresi E, eds. *Migraine and epilepsy*. Boston: Butterworth, 1987:47–81.

105. Genton P, Dravet C. Lennox-Gastaut syndrome and other childhood epileptic encephalopathies. In: Engel J Jr, Pedley TA, eds. *Epilepsy: a comprehensive textbook*. Philadelphia: Lippincott-Raven, 1997:2355–2366.

106. Gerstle de Pasquet E, Bonnevaux de Toma S, Scaramelli A, et al. Discontinuation of antiepileptic drugs after remission of seizures and risk of relapse: a prospective study. *Adv Epileptol* 1989;17:323–326.

107. Geyer JD, Bilir E, Faught RE, et al. Significance of interictal temporal lobe delta activity for localization of the primary epileptogenic region. *Neurology* 1999;52:202–205.

108. Gibbs FA, Gibbs EL. *Atlas of encephalography*. Cambridge, MA: Addison-Wesley, 1952.

109. Gibbs FA, Gibbs EL, Lennox WG. The influence of the blood sugar level on the wave and spike formation in petit mal epilepsy. *Arch Neurol Psychiat* 1939;41:1111–1116.

110. Gilmore PC, Brenner RP. Correlation of EEG, computerized tomography, and clinical findings. Study of 100 patients with focal delta activity. *Arch Neurol* 1981;38:371–372.

111. Gil-Nagel A, Risinger MW. Ictal semiology in hippocampal versus extrahippocampal temporal lobe epilepsy. *Brain* 1997;120(Pt 1):183–192.

112. Gloor P. The EEG and differential diagnosis of epilepsy. In: Van Duijn H, Donker DN, Van Huffelen AC, eds. *Current concepts in clinical neurophysiology. Didactic lectures of the Ninth International Congress of Electroencephalography and Clinical Neurophysiology*. Amsterdam: NV Drukkerij Trio, 1977:9–21.

113. Gloor P, Rasmussen T, Altuzarra A, et al. Role of the intracarotid amobarbital-pentylenetetrazol EEG test in the diagnosis and surgical treatment of patients with complex seizure problems. *Epilepsia* 1976;17:15–31.

114. Gobbi G, Bouquet F, Greco L, et al. Coeliac disease, epilepsy, and cerebral calcifications. The Italian Working Group on Coeliac Disease and Epilepsy. *Lancet* 1992;340:439–443.

115. Gobbi G, Sorrenti G, Santucci M, et al. Epilepsy with bilateral occipital calcifications: a benign onset with progressive severity. *Neurology* 1988;38:913–920.

116. Goodin DS, Aminoff MJ. Does the interictal EEG have a role in the diagnosis of epilepsy? *Lancet* 1984;1:837–839.

117. Goodin DS, Aminoff MJ, Laxer KD. Detection of epileptiform activity by different noninvasive EEG methods in complex partial epilepsy. *Ann Neurol* 1990;27:330–334.

118. Gotman J, Marciani MG. Electroencephalographic spiking activity, drug levels, and seizure occurrence in epileptic patients. *Ann Neurol* 1985;17:597–603.

119. Grand'Maison F, Reiher J, Leduc CP. Retrospective inventory of EEG abnormalities in partial status epilepticus. *Electroencephalogr Clin Neurophysiol* 1991;79:264–270.

120. Greenberg DA, Delgado-Escueta AV, Widelitz H, et al. Juvenile myoclonic epilepsy (JME) may be linked to the BF and HLA loci on human chromosome 6. *Am J Med Genet* 1988;31:185–192.

121. Gregory DL, Wong PK. Topographical analysis of the centrotemporal discharges in benign rolandic epilepsy of childhood. *Epilepsia* 1984;25:705–711.

122. Gregory RP, Oates T, Merry RT. Electroencephalogram epileptiform abnormalities in candidates for aircrew training. *Electroencephalogr Clin Neurophysiol* 1993;86:75–77.

123. Gross DW, Dubeau F, Quesney LF, et al. EEG telemetry with closely spaced electrodes in frontal lobe epilepsy. *J Clin Neurophysiol* 2000;17:414–418.

124. Grunewald RA, Chroni E, Panayiotopoulos CP. Delayed diagnosis of juvenile myoclonic epilepsy. *J Neurol Neurosurg Psychiatry* 1992;55:497–499.

125. Guerrini R, Belmonte A, Veggiotti P, et al. Delayed appearance of interictal EEG abnormalities in early onset childhood epilepsy with occipital paroxysms. *Brain Dev* 1997;19:343–346.

126. Guerrini R, Dravet C, Genton P, et al. Idiopathic photosensitive occipital lobe epilepsy. *Epilepsia* 1995;36:883–891.

127. Guey J, Bureau M, Dravet C, et al. A study of the rhythm of petit mal absences in children in relation to prevailing situations. The use of EEG telemetry during psychological examinations, school exercises and periods of inactivity. *Epilepsia* 1969;10:441–451.

128. Harden CL, Rosenbaum DH, Daras M. Hyperglycemia presenting with occipital seizures. *Epilepsia* 1991;32:215–220.

129. Harding GF, Herrick CE, Jeavons PM. A controlled study of the effect of sodium valproate on photosensitive epilepsy and its prognosis. *Epilepsia* 1978;19:555–565.

130. Hauser WA, Rich SS, Annegers JF, et al. Seizure recurrence after a 1st unprovoked seizure: an extended follow-up. *Neurology* 1990;40:1163–1170.

131. Heijbel J, Blom S, Bergfors PG. Benign epilepsy of children with centrotemporal EEG foci. A study of incidence rate in outpatient care. *Epilepsia* 1975;16:657–664.

132. Heijbel J, Blom S, Rasmusson M. Benign epilepsy of childhood with centrotemporal EEG foci: a genetic study. *Epilepsia* 1975;16:285–293.

133. Helmchen H, Kanowski S. EEG changes under lithium (Li) treatment. *Electroencephalogr Clin Neurophysiol* 1971;30:269.

134. Hirsch E, Marescaux C, Maquet P, et al. Landau-Kleffner syndrome: a clinical and EEG study of five cases. *Epilepsia* 1990;31:756–767.

135. Holmes GL, McKeever M, Adamson M. Absence seizures in children: clinical and electroencephalographic features. *Ann Neurol* 1987;21:268–273.

136. Hopkins A, Garman A, Clarke C. The first seizure in adult life. Value of clinical features, electroencephalography, and computerised tomographic scanning in prediction of seizure recurrence. *Lancet* 1988;1:721–726.

137. Horita H, Kumagai K, Maekawa K. Overnight polygraphic study of Lennox-Gastaut syndrome. *Brain Dev* 1987;9:627–635.

138. Hrachovy RA, Frost JD Jr, Kellaway P. Sleep characteristics in infantile spasms. *Neurology* 1981;31:688–693.

139. Hrachovy RA, Frost JD Jr, Kellaway P, et al. Double-blind study of ACTH vs prednisone therapy in infantile spasms. *J Pediatr* 1983;103:641–645.

140. Hrachovy RA, Frost JD Jr, Kellaway P. Hypsarrhythmia: variations on the theme. *Epilepsia* 1984;25:317–325.

141. Hrachovy RA, Glaze DG, Frost JD Jr. A retrospective study of spontaneous remission and long-term outcome in patients with infantile spasms. *Epilepsia* 1991;32:212–214.

142. Hughes JR. Long-term clinical and EEG changes in patients with epilepsy. *Arch Neurol* 1985;42:213–223.

143. Husain AM, Mebust KA, Radtke RA. Generalized periodic epileptiform discharges: etiologies, relationship to status epilepticus, and prognosis. *J Clin Neurophysiol* 1999;16:51–58.

144. Itil TM, Soldatos C. Epileptogenic side effects of psychotropic drugs. Practical recommendations. *JAMA* 1980;244:1460–1463.

145. Jackson GD, Berkovic SF, Tress BM, et al. Hippocampal sclerosis can be reliably detected by magnetic resonance imaging. *Neurology* 1990;40:1869–1875.

146. Jacobs KM, Kharazia VN, Prince DA. Mechanisms underlying epileptogenesis in cortical malformations. *Epilepsy Res* 1999;36:165–188.

147. Jain S, Padma MV, Puri A, et al. Juvenile myoclonic epilepsy: disease expression among Indian families. *Acta Neurol Scand* 1998;97:1–7.

148. Janz D. Epilepsy with impulsive petit mal (juvenile myoclonic epilepsy). *Acta Neurol Scand* 1985;72:449–459.

149. Janz D, Christian W. Impulsiv-petit mal. *Dtsch Z Nervenheilk* 1957;176:346–386.

150. Janz D, Durner M. Juvenile myoclonic epilepsy. In: Engel J Jr, Pedley TA, eds. *Epilepsy: a comprehensive textbook*. Philadelphia: Lippincott-Raven, 1997:2389–2400.

151. Jayakar P, Duchowny MS, Resnick TJ, et al. Localization of epileptogenic foci using a simple reference-subtraction montage to document small interchannel time differences. *J Clin Neurophysiol* 1991;8:212–215.

152. Jeavons PM, Bower BD. The natural history of infantile spasms. *Arch Dis Child* 1961;36:17.

153. Jeavons PM, Bower BD, Dimitrakoudi M. Long-term prognosis of 150 cases of "West syndrome." *Epilepsia* 1973;14:153–164.

154. Jeavons PM, Harper JR, Bower BD. Long-term prognosis in infantile spasms: a follow-up report on 112 cases. *Dev Med Child Neurol* 1970;12:413–421.

155. Jumao-as A, Brenner RP. Myoclonic status epilepticus: a clinical and electroencephalographic study. *Neurology* 1990;40:1199–1202.

156. Kaibara M, Blume WT. The postictal electroencephalogram. *Electroencephalogr Clin Neurophysiol* 1988;70:99–104.

157. Kaiko RF, Foley KM, Grabinski PY, et al. Central nervous system excitatory effects of meperidine in cancer patients. *Ann Neurol* 1983;13:180–185.

158. Kellaway P. The incidence, significance, and natural history of spike foci in children. In: Henry CE, ed. *Current clinical neurophysiology: update on EEG and evoked potentials*. Amsterdam: Elsevier, 1981:151–175.

159. Kellaway P, Frost JD Jr, Hrachovy RA. Infantile spasms. In: Morselli PD, Pippinger KF, Penry JK, eds. *Antiepileptic drug therapy in pediatrics*. New York: Raven Press, 1983:115–136.

160. Kellaway P, Hrachovy RA, Frost JD Jr, et al. Precise characterization and quantification of infantile spasms. *Ann Neurol* 1979;6:214–218.

161. King MA, Newton MR, Jackson GD, et al. Epileptology of the first-seizure presentation: a clinical, electroencephalographic, and magnetic resonance imaging study of 300 consecutive patients. *Lancet* 1998;352:1007–1011.

162. Kobayashi K, Iyoda K, Ohtsuka Y, et al. Longitudinal clinicoelectrophysiologic study of a case of Lafora disease proven by skin biopsy. *Epilepsia* 1990;31:194–201.

163. Kraschnitz W, Scheer P, Korner K, et al. Rolandic spikes as an electroencephalographic manifestation of an oligodendroglioma. *Pediatr Padol* 1988;23:313–319.

164. Kuznicky R, Berkovic S, Andermann F, et al. Focal cortical myoclonus and rolandic cortical dysplasia: clarification by magnetic resonance imaging. *Ann Neurol* 1988;23:317–325.

165. Kuznicky R, Rosenblatt B. Benign occipital epilepsy: a family study. *Epilepsia* 1987;28:346–350.

166. Lancman ME, Asconape JJ, Penry JK. Clinical and EEG asymmetries in juvenile myoclonic epilepsy. *Epilepsia* 1994;35:302–306.

167. Landau WM, Kleffner FR. Syndrome of acquired aphasia with convulsive disorder in children. *Neurology* 1957;7:523–530.

168. Lee SI. Non-convulsive status epilepticus. Ictal confusion in later life. *Arch Neurol* 1985;42:778–781.

169. Lee SK, Kim JY, Hong KS, et al. The clinical usefulness of ictal surface EEG in neocortical epilepsy. *Epilepsia* 2000;41:1450–1455.
170. Legarda S, Jayakar P, Duchowny M, et al. Benign rolandic epilepsy: high central and low central subgroups. *Epilepsia* 1994;35:1125–1129.
171. Lennox WG. The petit mal epilepsies; their treatment with tridione. *JAMA* 1945;129:1069–1074.
172. Lennox WG, Davis JP. Clinical correlates of the fast and slow spike-wave electroencephalogram. *Pediatrics* 1950;5:626–644.
173. Lerman P. Benign partial epilepsy with centro-temporal spikes. In: Roger J, Bureau M, Dravet C, et al., eds. *Epileptic syndromes in infancy, childhood, and adolescence.* London: John Libbey, 1992:189–200.
174. Lerman P, Kivity S. Benign focal epilepsy of childhood. A follow-up study of 100 recovered patients. *Arch Neurol* 1975;32:261–264.
175. Lerman P, Kivity S. The benign partial nonrolandic epilepsies. *J Clin Neurophysiol* 1991;8:275–287.
176. Lerman P, Kivity-Ephraim S. Focal epileptic EEG discharges in children not suffering from clinical epilepsy: etiology, clinical significance, and management. *Epilepsia* 1981;22:551–558.
177. Lipinski CG. Epilepsies with astatic seizures of late onset. *Epilepsia* 1977;18:13–20.
178. Livingston S, Eisner V, Pauli L. Minor motor epilepsy: diagnosis, treatment, and prognosis. *Pediatrics* 1958;21:916.
179. Loiseau P. Childhood absence epilepsies. In: Roger J, Dravet C, Bureau M, et al., eds. *Epileptic syndromes in infancy, childhood, and adolescence.* London: John Libbey, 1985:106–120.
180. Loiseau P, Duche B, Cordova S, et al. Prognosis of benign childhood epilepsy with centrotemporal spikes: a follow-up study of 168 patients. *Epilepsia* 1988;29:229–235.
181. Lombroso CT. Sylvian seizures and midtemporal spike foci in children. *Arch Neurol* 1967;17:52–59.
182. Lombroso CT. A prospective study of infantile spasms: clinical and therapeutic correlations. *Epilepsia* 1983;24:135–158.
183. Lombroso CT, Erba G. Primary and secondary bilateral synchrony in epilepsy; a clinical and electroencephalographic study. *Arch Neurol* 1970;22:321–334.
184. Ludwig B, Marsan CA, Van Buren J. Cerebral seizures of probable orbitofrontal origin. *Epilepsia* 1975;16:141–158.
185. Lugaresi E, Cirignotta F, Montagna P. Occipital lobe epilepsy with scotosensitive seizures: the role of central vision. *Epilepsia* 1984;25:115–120.
186. Markand ON. Slow spike-wave activity in EEG and associated clinical features: often called "Lennox" or "Lennox-Gastaut" syndrome. *Neurology* 1977;27:746–757.
187. Markand ON, Daly DD. Pseudoperiodic lateralized paroxysmal discharges in electroencephalogram. *Neurology* 1971;21:975–981.
188. Marsan CA, Zivin LS. Factors related to the occurrence of typical paroxysmal abnormalities in the EEG records of epileptic patients. *Epilepsia* 1970;11:361–381.
189. Marshall DW, Brey RL, Morse MW. Focal and/or lateralized polymorphic delta activity. Association with either "normal" or "nonfocal" computed tomographic scans. *Arch Neurol* 1988;45:33–35.
190. Matsumoto A, Watanabe K, Negoro T, et al. Long-term prognosis after infantile spasms: a statistical study of prognostic factors in 200 cases. *Dev Med Child Neurol* 1981;23:51–65.
191. Mauguiere F, Courjon J. Somatosensory epilepsy. A review of 127 cases. *Brain* 1978;101:307–332.
192. Maytal J, Novak GP, Knobler SB, et al. Neuroradiological manifestations of focal polymorphic delta activity in children. *Arch Neurol* 1993;50:181–184.
193. Mervaala E, Partanen JV, Keranen T, et al. Prolonged cortical somatosensory evoked potential latencies in progressive myoclonus epilepsy. *J Neurol Sci* 1984;64:131–135.
194. Metrakos JD, Metrakos K. Genetic factors in the epilepsies. In: Alter M, Hauser WA, eds. *The epidemiology of epilepsy: a workshop.* National Institute of Neurological Diseases and Stroke Monograph No. 14. Washington, DC: U.S. Government Printing Office, 1972:97–102.
195. Morikawa T, Osawa T, Ishihara O, et al. A reappraisal of "benign epilepsy of children with centro-temporal EEG foci." *Brain Dev* 1979;1:257–265.
196. Morikawa T, Seino M, Osawa T, et al. Five children with continuous spike-wave discharges during sleep. In: Roger J, Dravet C, Bureau M, et al., eds. *Epileptic syndromes in infancy, childhood, and adolescence.* London: John Libbey, 1985:205–212.
197. Morikawa T, Seino M, Watanabe Y, et al. Clinical relevance of continuous spike-waves during slow wave sleep. In: Manelis S, Bental E, Loeber JN, et al., eds. *Advances in epileptology.* New York: Raven Press, 1989:359–363.
198. Morrell F, Whisler WW, Smith MC, et al. Landau-Kleffner syndrome. Treatment with subpial intracortical transection. *Brain* 1995;118(Pt 6):1529–1546.
199. Morris HH 3rd, Dinner DS, Luders H, et al. Supplementary motor seizures: clinical and electroencephalographic findings. *Neurology* 1988;38:1075–1082.
200. Murthy JM, Yangala R, Srinivas M. The syndromic classification of the International League Against Epilepsy: a hospital-based study from South India. *Epilepsia* 1998;39:48–54.
201. Musumeci SA, Colognola RM, Ferri R, et al. Fragile-X syndrome: a particular epileptogenic EEG pattern. *Epilepsia* 1988;29:41–47.
202. Nei M, Lee JM, Shanker VL, et al. The EEG and prognosis in status epilepticus. *Epilepsia* 1999;40:157–163.
203. Niedermeyer E, Naidu S. Further EEG observations in children with the Rett syndrome. *Brain Dev* 1990;12:53–54.
204. Niedermeyer E, Walker AE. Mesio-frontal epilepsy. *Electroencephalogr Clin Neurophysiol* 1971;31:104–105.
205. Noriega-Sanchez A, Martinez-Maldonado M, Haiffe RM. Clinical and electroencephalographic changes in progressive uremic encephalopathy. *Neurology* 1978;28:667–669.
206. Normand MM, Wszolek ZK, Klass DW. Temporal intermittent rhythmic delta activity in electroencephalograms. *J Clin Neurophysiol* 1995;12:280–284.
207. Oguni H, Hayashi K, Imai K, et al. Study on the early-onset variant of benign childhood epilepsy with occipital paroxysms otherwise described as early-onset benign occipital seizure susceptibility syndrome. *Epilepsia* 1999;40:1020–1030.
208. Oguni H, Mukahira K, Oguni M, et al. Video-polygraphic analysis of myoclonic seizures in juvenile myoclonic epilepsy. *Epilepsia* 1994;35:307–316.
209. Ohtsuka Y, Oka E, Terasaki T, et al. Aicardi syndrome: a longitudinal clinical and electroencephalographic study. *Epilepsia* 1993;34:627–634.
210. Palmini A, Gambardella A, Andermann F, et al. Intrinsic epileptogenicity of human dysplastic cortex as suggested by corticography and surgical results. *Ann Neurol* 1995;37:476–487.
211. Panayiotopoulos CP. Inhibitory effect of central vision on occipital lobe seizures. *Neurology* 1981;31:1330–1333.
212. Panayiotopoulos CP. Benign childhood epilepsy with occipital paroxysms: a 15-year prospective study. *Ann Neurol* 1989;26:51–56.
213. Panayiotopoulos CP. Benign nocturnal childhood occipital epilepsy: a new syndrome with nocturnal seizures, tonic deviation of the eyes, and vomiting. *J Child Neurol* 1989;4:43–49.
214. Panayiotopoulos CP. Early-onset benign childhood occipital seizure susceptibility syndrome: a syndrome to recognize. *Epilepsia* 1999;40:621–630.
215. Panayiotopoulos CP. Benign childhood epileptic syndromes with occipital spikes: new classification proposed by the International League Against Epilepsy. *J Child Neurol* 2000;15:548–552.
216. Panayiotopoulos CP, Obeid T, Tahan AR. Juvenile myoclonic epilepsy: a 5-year prospective study. *Epilepsia* 1994;35:285–296.
217. Panayiotopoulos CP, Obeid T, Waheed G. Absences in juvenile myoclonic epilepsy: a clinical and video-electroencephalographic study. *Ann Neurol* 1989;25:391–397.
218. Panayiotopoulos CP, Obeid T, Waheed G. Differentiation of typical absence seizures in epileptic syndromes. A video EEG study of 224 seizures in 20 patients. *Brain* 1989;112(Pt 4):1039–1056.
219. Panayiotopoulos CP, Tahan R, Obeid T. Juvenile myoclonic epilepsy: factors of error involved in the diagnosis and treatment. *Epilepsia* 1991;32:672–676.

220. Paquier PF, Van Dongen HR, Loonen CB. The Landau-Kleffner syndrome or "acquired aphasia with convulsive disorder." Long-term follow-up of six children and a review of the recent literature. *Arch Neurol* 1992;49:354–359.
221. Parsonage MJ, Exley KA. Use and abuse of electroencephalography. *Lancet* 1964;2:753.
222. Patry G, Lyagoubi S, Tassinari CA. Subclinical "electrical status epilepticus" induced by sleep in children. A clinical and electroencephalographic study of six cases. *Arch Neurol* 1971;24:242–252.
223. PeBenito R, Cracco JB. Periodic lateralized epileptiform discharges in infants and children. *Ann Neurol* 1979;6:47–50.
224. Pedley TA. Interictal epileptiform discharges: discriminating characteristics and clinical correlations. *Am J EEG Technol* 1980;20:101–119.
225. Penry JK, Dean JC, Riela AR. Juvenile myoclonic epilepsy: long-term response to therapy. *Epilepsia* 1989;30(Suppl 4):S19–S23; discussion, S24–S17.
226. Pfander M, Arnold S, Henkel A, et al. Clinical features and EEG findings differentiating mesial from neocortical temporal lobe epilepsy. *Epilepsia,* submitted.
227. Porter RJ, Penry JK. Responsiveness at the onset of spike-wave bursts. *Electroencephalogr Clin Neurophysiol* 1973;34:239–245.
228. Proposal for revised classification of epilepsies and epileptic syndromes. Commission on Classification and Terminology of the International League Against Epilepsy. *Epilepsia* 1989;30:389–399.
229. Quesney LF. Preoperative electroencephalographic investigation in frontal lobe epilepsy: electroencephalographic and electrocorticographic recordings. *Can J Neurol Sci* 1991;18:559–563.
230. Quesney LF. Extratemporal epilepsy: clinical presentation, pre-operative EEG localization and surgical outcome. *Acta Neurol Scand Suppl* 1992;140:81–94.
231. Randomised study of antiepileptic drug withdrawal in patients in remission. Medical Research Council Antiepileptic Drug Withdrawal Study Group. *Lancet* 1991;337:1175–1180.
232. Randomized clinical trial on the efficacy of antiepileptic drugs in reducing the risk of relapse after a first unprovoked tonic-clonic seizure. First Seizure Trial Group (FIR.S.T. Group). *Neurology* 1993;43:478–483.
233. Rapin I. Myoclonus in neuronal storage and Lafora diseases. *Adv Neurol* 1986;43:65–85.
234. Rapin I, Mattis S, Rowan AJ, et al. Verbal auditory agnosia in children. *Dev Med Child Neurol* 1977;19:197–207.
235. Rasmussen T. Characteristics of a pure culture of frontal lobe epilepsy. *Epilepsia* 1983;24:482–493.
236. Rasmussen T. Tailoring of cortical excisions for frontal lobe epilepsy. *Can J Neurol Sci* 1991;18:606–610.
237. Rasmussen T. Surgery for central, parietal and occipital epilepsy. *Can J Neurol Sci* 1991;18:611–616.
238. Raymond AA, Fish DR. EEG features of focal malformations of cortical development. *J Clin Neurophysiol* 1996;13:495–506.
239. Raymond AA, Fish DR, Sisodiya SM, et al. Abnormalities of gyration, heterotopias, tuberous sclerosis, focal cortical dysplasia, microdysgenesis, dysembryoplastic neuroepithelial tumour and dysgenesis of the archicortex in epilepsy. Clinical, EEG and neuroimaging features in 100 adult patients. *Brain* 1995;118(Pt 3):629–660.
240. Raymond AA, Fish DR, Stevens JM, et al. Subependymal heterotopia: a distinct neuronal migration disorder associated with epilepsy. *J Neurol Neurosurg Psychiat* 1994;57:1195–1202.
241. Reiher J, Beaudry M, Leduc CP. Temporal intermittent rhythmic delta activity (TIRDA) in the diagnosis of complex partial epilepsy: sensitivity, specificity and predictive value. *Can J Neurol Sci* 1989;16:398–401.
242. Risinger MW, Engel J Jr, Van Ness PC, et al. Ictal localization of temporal lobe seizures with scalp/sphenoidal recordings. *Neurology* 1989;39:1288–1293.
243. Rodin E, Ancheta O. Cerebral electrical fields during petit mal absences. *Electroencephalogr Clin Neurophysiol* 1987;66:457–466.
244. Rodin M, Thompson M. Reassessment of the generalized spike-wave complex. [Abstract]. *Epilepsia* 1995;36(Suppl 3):75.
245. Roger J, Bureau M, Dravet C, et al., eds. *Epileptic syndromes in infancy, childhood, and adolescence.* London: John Libbey, 1992.
246. Ross JJ, Johnson LC, Walter RD. Spike and wave discharges during stages of sleep. *Arch Neurol* 1966;14:399–407.
247. Salanova V, Morris HH 3rd, Van Ness PC, et al. Comparison of scalp electroencephalogram with subdural electrocorticogram recordings and functional mapping in frontal lobe epilepsy. *Arch Neurol* 1993;50:294–299.
248. Salinsky M, Kanter R, Dasheiff RM. Effectiveness of multiple EEGs in supporting the diagnosis of epilepsy: an operational curve. *Epilepsia* 1987;28:331–334.
249. Sammaritano M, Gigli GL, Gotman J. Interictal spiking during wakefulness and sleep and the localization of foci in temporal lobe epilepsy. *Neurology* 1991;41:290–297.
250. Sato S, Dreifuss FE, Penry JK. The effect of sleep on spike-wave discharges in absence seizures. *Neurology* 1973;23:1335–1345.
251. Sato S, Dreifuss FE, Penry JK, et al. Long-term follow-up of absence seizures. *Neurology* 1983;33:1590–1595.
252. Sato S, White BG, Penry JK, et al. Valproic acid versus ethosuximide in the treatment of absence seizures. *Neurology* 1982;32:157–163.
253. Saygi S, Spencer SS, Scheyer R, et al. Differentiation of temporal lobe ictal behavior associated with hippocampal sclerosis and tumors of temporal lobe. *Epilepsia* 1994;35:737–742.
254. Schmidt D. The influence of antiepileptic drugs on the electroencephalogram: a review of controlled clinical studies. *Electroencephalogr Clin Neurophysiol Suppl* 1982;36:453–466.
255. Schraeder PL, Singh N. Seizure disorders following periodic lateralized epileptiform discharges. *Epilepsia* 1980;21:647–653.
256. Schwartz MS, Prior PF, Scott DF. The occurrence and evolution in the EEG of a lateralized periodic phenomenon. *Brain* 1973;96:613–622.
257. Scollo-Lavizzari C. Prognostic significance of epileptiform discharges in the EEG of non-epileptic subjects during photic stimulation. [Abstract]. *Electroencephalogr Clin Neurophysiol* 1971;31:174.
258. Shinnar S, Berg AT, Moshe SL, et al. Risk of seizure recurrence following a first unprovoked seizure in childhood: a prospective study. *Pediatrics* 1990;85:1076–1085.
259. Shinnar S, Berg AT, Moshe SL, et al. The risk of seizure recurrence after a first unprovoked afebrile seizure in childhood: an extended follow-up. *Pediatrics* 1996;98:216–225.
260. Shinnar S, Vining EP, Mellits ED, et al. Discontinuing antiepileptic medication in children with epilepsy after two years without seizures. A prospective study. *N Engl J Med* 1985;313:976–980.
261. Shorvon SD. Definition, classification, and frequency of status epilepticus. In: *Status epilepticus: its clinical features and treatment in children and adults.* Cambridge, UK: Cambridge University Press, 1994:21–33.
262. Simon RP, Aminoff MJ. Electrographic status epilepticus in fatal anoxic coma. *Ann Neurol* 1986;20:351–355.
263. Smith JMB, Kellaway P. The natural history and clinical correlates of occipital foci in children. In: Kellaway P, Petersen I, eds. *Neurological and correlative EEG studies in infancy.* New York: Grune & Stratton, 1964:230–249.
264. Snead OC 3rd, Benton JW, Myers GJ. ACTH and prednisone in childhood seizure disorders. *Neurology* 1983;33:966–970.
265. Snodgrass SM, Tsuburaya K, Ajmone-Marsan C. Clinical significance of periodic lateralized epileptiform discharges: relationship with status epilepticus. *J Clin Neurophysiol* 1989;6:159–172.
266. So EL, Ruggles KH, Ahmann PA, et al. Prognosis of photoparoxysmal response in nonepileptic patients. *Neurology* 1993;43:1719–1722.
267. So N, Berkovic S, Andermann F, et al. Myoclonus epilepsy and ragged-red fibres (MERRF). 2. Electrophysiological studies and comparison with other progressive myoclonus epilepsies. *Brain* 1989;112(Pt 5):1261–1276.
268. Sorel L, Dusaucy-Bauloye A. A propos de cas d'hyposarythmia de Gibbs: son traitement spectulaire par l'ACTH. *Acta Neurol Belg* 1958;58.

269. Steinhoff BJ, So NK, Lim S, et al. Ictal scalp EEG in temporal lobe epilepsy with unitemporal versus bitemporal interictal epileptiform discharges. *Neurology* 1995;45:889–896.

270. Stores G. When does an EEG contribute to the management of febrile seizures? *Arch Dis Child* 1991;66:554–557.

271. Tassinari CA, Bureau M, Dravet C, et al. Electrical status epilepticus during sleep in children (ESES). In: Sterman MB, Shouse MN, Passouant P, eds. *Sleep and epilepsy.* London: Academic Press, 1982:465–479.

272. Tassinari CA, Bureau M, Dravet C, et al. Epilepsy with continuous spikes and waves during slow sleep—otherwise described as ESES (epilepsy with electrical status epilepticus during slow sleep). In: Roger J, Bureau M, Dravet C, et al., eds. *Epileptic syndromes in infancy, childhood, and adolescence.* London: John Libbey, 1992:245–256.

273. Terasaki T, Yamatogi Y, Ohtahara S. Electroclinical delineation of occipital lobe epilepsy in childhood. In: Andermann F, Lugaresi E, eds. *Migraine and epilepsy.* Boston: Butterworth, 1987:125–137.

274. Terzano MG, Parrino L, Mazzucchi A, et al. Confusional states with periodic lateralized epileptiform discharges (PLEDs): a peculiar epileptic syndrome in the elderly. *Epilepsia* 1986; 27:446–457.

275. Tharp BR. Orbital frontal seizures. An unique electroencephalographic and clinical syndrome. *Epilepsia* 1972;13:627–642.

276. Thomas JE, Reagan TJ, Klass DW. Epilepsia partialis continua. A review of 32 cases. *Arch Neurol* 1977;34:266–275.

277. Thorn I. The significance of electroencephalography in febrile convulsions. In: Akimoto H, Kazamatsuri H, Sein M, et al., eds. *Advances in epileptology: the XIIIth Epilepsy International Symposium.* New York: Raven Press, 1982:93–95.

278. Touchon J. Effect of awakening on epileptic activity in primary generalized myoclonic epilepsy. In: Sterman MB, Shouse MN, Passouant P, eds. *Sleep and epilepsy.* London: Academic Press, 1982:239–248.

279. Treiman DM, Delgado-Escueta AV. Complex partial status epilepticus. *Adv Neurol* 1983;34: 69–81.

280. Treiman DM, Walton NY, Kendrick C. A progressive sequence of electroencephalographic changes during generalized convulsive status epilepticus. *Epilepsy Res* 1990;5:49–60.

281. Tsuboi T. Genetic aspects of febrile convulsions. *Hum Genet* 1977;38:169–173.

282. Tsuboi T, Endo S. Febrile convulsions followed by nonfebrile convulsions. A clinical, electroencephalographic and follow-up study. *Neuropadiatrie* 1977;8:209–223.

283. Tükel K, Jasper H. The electroencephalogram in parasagittal lesions. *Electroencephalogr Clin Neurophysiol* 1952;4:481–494.

284. Tyler HR. Neurological complications of dialysis, transplantation, and other forms of treatment in chronic uremia. *Neurology* 1965;15:1081–1088.

285. van Donselaar CA, Schimsheimer RJ, Geerts AT, et al. Value of the electroencephalogram in adult patients with untreated idiopathic first seizures. *Arch Neurol* 1992;49:231–237.

286. Villarreal HJ, Wilder BJ, Willmore LJ, et al. Effect of valproic acid on spike and wave discharges in patients with absence seizures. *Neurology* 1978;28:886–891.

287. Vigevano F, Ricci S. Benign occipital epilepsy in childhood with prolonged seizures and autonomic symptoms. In: Andermann F, Beaumanoir A, Mira L, et al., eds. *Occipital seizures and epilepsies in children.* London: John Libbey, 1993:133–140.

288. Walczak TS. Neocortical temporal lobe epilepsy: characterizing the syndrome. *Epilepsia* 1995; 36:633–635.

289. Walczak TS, Bazil C, Lee N, et al. Scalp ictal EEG differs in temporal neocortical and hippocampal seizures. [Abstract]. *Epilepsia* 1994;35(Suppl 8):134,.

290. Walczak TS, Lewis DV, Radtke R. Scalp EEG differs in temporal and extratemporal complex partial seizures. *J Epilepsy* 1991;4:25–28.

291. Walczak TS, Radtke RA, Lewis DV. Accuracy and interobserver reliability of scalp ictal EEG. *Neurology* 1992;42:2279–2285.

292. Walczak TS, Scheuer ML, Resor S, et al. Prevalence and features of epilepsy without interictal epileptiform discharges. [Abstract]. *Neurology* 1993;43(Suppl 2):287–288.

293. Walsh JM, Brenner RP. Periodic lateralized epileptiform discharges—long-term outcome in adults. *Epilepsia* 1987;28:533–536.

294. Warach S, Ives JR, Schlaug G, et al. EEG-triggered echo-planar functional MRI in epilepsy. *Neurology* 1996;47:89–93.

295. Watanabe K, Negoro T, Aso K, et al. Reappraisal of interictal electroencephalograms in infantile spasms. *Epilepsia* 1993;34:679–685.

296. Waterman K, Purves SJ, Kosaka B, et al. An epileptic syndrome caused by mesial frontal lobe seizure foci. *Neurology* 1987;37:577–582.

297. Weir B. The morphology of the spike-wave complex. *Electroencephalogr Clin Neurophysiol* 1965;19:284–290.

298. West WJ. On a particular form of infantile convulsions. *Lancet* 1841;1:724–725.

299. Whitehouse WP, Rees M, Curtis D, et al. Linkage analysis of idiopathic generalized epilepsy (IGE) and marker loci on chromosome 6p in families of patients with juvenile myoclonic epilepsy: no evidence for an epilepsy locus in the HLA region. *Am J Hum Genet* 1993;53: 652–662.

300. Wikler A, Fraser HF, Isbell H, et al. Electroencephalogram during cycles of addiction to barbiturates in man. *Electroencephalogr Clin Neurophysiol* 1955;7:1–14.

301. Williamson PD. Frontal lobe seizures. Problems of diagnosis and classification. *Adv Neurol* 1992;57:289–309.

302. Williamson PD, Boon PA, Thadani VM, et al. Parietal lobe epilepsy: diagnostic considerations and results of surgery. *Ann Neurol* 1992;31:193–201.

303. Williamson PD, French JA, Thadani VM, et al. Characteristics of medial temporal lobe epilepsy: II. Interictal and ictal scalp electroencephalography, neuropsychological testing, neuroimaging, surgical results, and pathology. *Ann Neurol* 1993;34:781–787.

304. Williamson PD, Jobst BC. Frontal lobe epilepsy. In: Williamson PD, Siegel AM, Roberts DW, et al., eds. *Neocortical epilepsies.* Philadelphia: Lippincott Williams & Wilkins, 2000:215–242.

305. Williamson PD, Spencer DD, Spencer SS, et al. Complex partial seizures of frontal lobe origin. *Ann Neurol* 1985;18:497–504.

306. Williamson PD, Spencer DD, Spencer SS, et al. Complex partial status epilepticus: a depth-electrode study. *Ann Neurol* 1985;18:647–654.

307. Wolf P. Juvenile absence epilepsy. In: Roger J, Bureau M, Dravet C, et al., eds. *Epileptic syndromes in infancy, childhood, and adolescence.* London: John Libbey, 1992:307–312.

308. Wolf P, Goosses R. Relation of photosensitivity to epileptic syndromes. *J Neurol Neurosurg Psychiat* 1986;49:1386–1391.

309. Wuft MH. The barbiturate withdrawal syndrome. A clinical and electroencephalographic study. *Electroencephalogr Clin Neurophysiol* 1959;14(Suppl):1–173.

310. Yaqub BA. Electroclinical seizures in Lennox-Gastaut syndrome. *Epilepsia* 1993;34:120–127.

311. Young GB, Gilbert JJ, Zochodne DW. The significance of myoclonic status epilepticus in postanoxic coma. *Neurology* 1990;40:1843–1848.

312. Young GB, Goodenough P, Jacono V, et al. Periodic lateralized epileptiform discharges (PLEDs): electrographic and clinical features. *Am J EEG Technol* 1987;28:1–13.

313. Zivin L, Marsan CA. Incidence and prognostic significance of "epileptiform" activity in the EEG of non-epileptic subjects. *Brain* 1968;91:751–778.

Chapter 18

Video-Electroencephalographic Monitoring

Eli M. Mizrahi and Ronald P. Lesser

Video-electroencephalographic (video-EEG) monitoring is a valuable tool in the diagnosis and management of those patients suspected of having seizures, from the neonate (71) to the elderly (18). Basic techniques, strategies of recording, and interpretations of findings of video-EEG monitoring are similar for all patients, regardless of age and suspected etiology of the underlying disorder. However, there are also critical differences in the monitoring of certain patients, and the recognition and understanding of these differences will ensure that these studies have a high probability of yielding clinically relevant and valid information.

Technical similarities include EEG and video instrumentation, the requirement for time synchronization of EEG and video, the need for a rel-

atively controlled monitoring environment, the critical role technologists play in recording, and the necessity to prospectively individualize the plans and objectives of each monitoring session. Technical differences relate to requirements, especially in certain pediatric patients, for additional recording sensors; age-dependent instrumentation adaptations; alterations in the recording environment to meet the needs of certain patients, especially young children; and the development of age-dependent strategies for monitoring newborns, infants, and children. Also critical in the monitoring of pediatric patients is the understanding by technologists, referring physicians, and neurophysiologists of the various paroxysmal clinical events that may occur in young patients, in order to determine their significance if or when they are recorded. Finally, it should be emphasized that accurate interpretation of the EEG is the cornerstone of all such studies.

In other reviews and reports, various terminology has been used to describe the simultaneous recording of EEG and video: long-term monitoring, closed-circuit television monitoring, telemetry, and EEG–polygraphic–video monitoring. Here, these techniques are all referred to as "monitoring"—additional information about the specific techniques is provided as needed.

INSTRUMENTATION AND RECORDING

The basic components of monitoring are the electroencephalograph, the polygraph, video recording instruments, and a device to synchronize and display the data. Although these various components have undergone development over the past several years based on contemporary technology, their basic configuration and purposes have not changed. The components are arranged for the simultaneous recording of EEG and clinical events to determine their temporal relationships and to characterize and classify them. Each clinical laboratory may configure instrumentation differently; the physical plant, instrumentation vendor, resources of individual institutions, or preferences of the interpreting neurophysiologist may dictate this. Whatever the configuration, policies and procedures are typically in place to achieve the same clinical objectives: capture clinical events and determine their significance for individual patients. Specific technical guidelines for long-term monitoring have been developed by the American Clinical Neurophysiology Society (formerly the American Electroencephalographic Society) (1).

The Electroencephalograph

Digital units are rapidly replacing analog units in most laboratories, and this is particularly the case for video-EEG monitoring. Critical to the application of either type of EEG recording device are the ability to be synchronized to video; the ability to record a full compliment of EEG channels, at times with several channels of polygraphic data (see below); and the ability to display all channels in a manner that can be visually resolved for analysis. A large number of channels may be needed in particular situations. For example, 128 channels are often needed in patients with implanted subdural electrodes.

Various pediatric age groups pose special challenges in the interpretation of their EEGs (70). Age-dependent features of the EEG exist for premature infants, adolescents, and young adults (41,44; see Chapter 5), including the character of the background of the waking and sleep recordings, the significance of interictal sharp transients, and the characteristics of electrical seizure discharges. For example, not all interictal sharp-wave transients are considered epileptiform in the neonate and young infant. In addition, other transients, including those sometimes called normal variants, may be confused with interictal epileptiform activity, when, in fact, they are variations of normal, sometimes occurring in specific age groups (67). Similarly, other rhythmic activity in adults may be benign and not epileptic activity (97). Therefore, these findings should be interpreted with caution.

The EEG signal can be transmitted to the recording instrument by radio transmission or by hardwired connections. There are strengths and limitations to each technique. Radio transmission allows more freedom of movement for patients, but there is an increased likelihood of movement outside the video camera range, and there is the potential for interference with other radio signals in the vicinity of the EEG recording location. Also, hardwiring will limit patient activities; this may be a concern during long-term monitoring of older children and adults, but is less of a concern for neonates and young infants. However, there may be greater fidelity of signal transmission with the technique. Many laboratories, including our own, prefer hardwired transmission (43,60).

On-line EEG montage and recording variable (filter settings, paper speed, instrumentation sensitivity) selection may be an important consideration in recording, depending on the instrument used. Analog recording instruments and some digital-based instruments require prerecording of montage selection and recording parameters. Many instruments that digitally record EEG allow for initial on-line referential recording and off-line remontaging of the EEG during analysis. If the instrumentation used requires on-line montage selection, it is often best that a single montage be selected for neonates and young infants, to record all wake–sleep states with the same "view" of the electrical activity of the brain (2). It is important that digital devices allow montaging and remontaging to occur in a simple way. There should be a simple way to share montage information between machines—for example, between the instrument used to acquire the EEG data and that used for later review.

Electrode Type and Placement

Although the international 10-20 system remains the benchmark for electrode placement during EEG monitoring, placement of additional electrodes, often using the so-called 10% system (85), can frequently add important information in this setting. These additional electrodes are interpolated between the standard 10-20 electrodes and also placed lower on the scalp, so as to record from the base of the cerebral cortex. Sphenoid electrodes, or the somewhat more invasive foramen ovale electrodes, also can be used (100). Although various electrodes and electrode placements have their proponents, the important question is not which electrode is superior but rather which combination of electrodes is best able to resolve a particular clinical problem. Additional electrodes can help verify a finding that might otherwise occur at only one electrode, can help to record a signal of as high an amplitude as possible, and can aid in determining the field of projection of the discharge, which can in turn help determine its underlying source (15,22,23).

"10%" Electrodes

Electrodes placed between and below the standard positions of the routine EEG electrodes can help to more precisely localize regions of seizure origin. This is particularly important in the case of events originating from the cortical base, because these signals are poorly detected and may not be recorded at all from standard electrodes (64). In one study (75), amplitudes of epileptiform activity were maximal at the standard electrodes 27% of the time and at the "extra" electrodes 61% of the time. Such extra electrodes include zygomatic (cheek) or periorbital electrodes.

Semi-invasive Electrodes

Nasopharyngeal electrodes were widely used at one time to evaluate complex partial seizures arising from the inferior or mesial temporal regions or from the orbitofrontal cortex, but are now used infrequently if at all (29,91). Sphenoid electrodes are more commonly employed. These are thin, flexible wires placed via a needle near the lateral angle of the jaw and directed to the region of the foramen ovale, near the greater wing of the sphenoid bone (78,87). Anterior placements are close to the amygdala and posterior placements close to the hippocampus. However, in practice, there are no clear differences in actual recordings that appear to distinguish various placements. This suggests that the major advantages of the use of sphenoid electrodes are their basal position and subdermal placement. The use of so-called mini-sphenoidal electrodes has been described, and they have been found to provide data similar to that obtained from tra-

ditional sphenoidal electrodes, although recorded waveforms are lower in amplitude (54).

Invasive Electrodes

Invasive electrodes include depth electrodes and subdural electrodes in arrays of strips and grids. They are placed in patients thought to be candidates for seizure surgery and are discussed below in the section on "Epilepsy Surgery."

Polygraphic Variables

Polygraph measures displayed as waveforms or alpha-numeric values in synchronized fashion with an EEG can assist in differentiating epileptic from nonepileptic paroxysmal events and in characterizing these events fully, whatever their pathophysiology. For example, in neonates, paroxysmal changes in heart rate or blood pressure may be investigated during monitoring to determine whether they are part of epileptic seizures or of nonepileptic, yet abnormal, events. In addition, parameters required for sleep staging are recorded in order to characterize events that may be associated with normal sleep or may be abnormal events best categorized as sleep disorders. In older children and adults, heart rate monitoring may detect syncope, and oxygen saturation and respiration measures may detect and characterize apneic episodes. Physiological parameters may be displayed as waveforms along with the EEG or may be displayed on the video screen numerically. The selection of the physiological parameters to be recorded depends on the clinical questions to be addressed during monitoring.

Electrocardiogram

The electrocardiogram is recorded with electrodes placed on the chest. Changes in rate or rhythm, which may occur in isolation or in association with other motor, autonomic nervous system, or behavioral changes, may provide critical data for diagnosis. For example, cardiac syncope may be detected and differentiated from syncope resulting from respiratory arrest in infants and children (65). In addition, syncope resulting from cardiac arrhythmias, alterations in blood pressure, or metabolic changes may occur both in children and in adults and requires differentiation from loss of consciousness associated with epilepsy.

Electro-oculogram

The electro-oculogram (EOG) is recorded to assist in the staging of sleep states and to help in the differentiation of EEG transients recorded by scalp electrodes from electrical potentials generated by eye movements. The EOG electrodes must be placed in order to detect both horizontal and vertical eye movements. This can be done by placing electrodes at both the inner and outer canthi, and both above and below an eye. Alternatively, one electrode can be lateral to and above one eye and the other electrode lateral to and below the other eye.

Respirations

The characterization of respirations is often a critical finding during monitoring studies—particularly those performed in younger infants or those patients suspected of having abnormal events during sleep. Respiratory effort is recorded in a number of complimentary ways: It may be measured by an impedance pneumograph attached to the chest with standard EEG electrodes or by a strain gauge placed around the chest. Abdominal movements associated with respiration are recorded with a strain gauge placed around the abdomen. Airway flow is measured by a thermistor or a thermocouple device placed at the mouth or nares. With these measurements—chest movements, abdominal movements, and airway flow—changes in respiration and the effectiveness of respiratory effort can be determined. Other respiratory parameters that may be recorded include systemic oxygenation and end-tidal carbon dioxide measurements recorded by pulse oximetry from nasal sensors. Regardless of the measurements taken, they must be recorded and displayed synchronously to each other, to the EEG, to other polygraphic parameters, and to the video in order to be clinically useful.

Electromyogram and Triaxial Accelerometry

The movements of selected muscle groups may be documented by using surface electrodes placed over the designated areas with the resultant electromyogram (EMG) recorded and displayed synchronously with other parameters, the video, and the EEG. To assist in identifying sleep stages, a submental EMG is typically recorded. EMGs of other muscle groups may be recorded if these muscle groups are thought to be involved in abnormal clinical events and the correlation of their movements is needed to determine their precise relationship to EEG activity. However, reliance on EMG electrodes to detect limb movement may be limiting because the movement of interest may not require the muscle group that the EMG electrodes are monitoring. Another sensor device, the triaxial accelerometer, can overcome this limitation (26). This compact sensor can be placed on a limb to detect movement in any plane; changes in movement can be represented by a deflection on a polygraph channel.

Systemic Blood Pressure

Continuous recording of systemic arterial blood pressure (SABP) during monitoring is not often performed—it is technically difficult and the clinical relevance of its interpretations is often not clear. However, continuous recording of SABP with other parameters, often including both video and EEG, can address specific clinical questions in the intensive care unit (ICU) setting, such as whether paroxysmal elevations in blood pressure are associated with EEG seizure activity. This parameter usually is measured when an intra-arterial pressure transducer already has been placed for clinical purposes. Values from this transducer can be displayed in parallel with the clinical bedside ICU monitors as a polygraphic analog tracing, or numerically in the video image, simultaneously with other parameters.

Video Recording

The equipment—including cameras, lens, camera mounts, remote control devices, videocassette recorders (or digital video storage media), and lighting—the recording formats, and the method of utilization all can affect the quality of the recorded data and, in turn, the validity of interpretation of the findings. The cameras may record in color or black and white. It may be more difficult to maintain a stable color image over time, and details of the video image may not be as crisp as with black-and-white recording. However, a color image provides clinical information that black-and-white images may not, including, obviously, changes in color of the patient—pallor, flushing, cyanosis, and vasomotor changes. Black-and-white recording is most effective in low-light areas or during nocturnal studies with standard lights out and with the use of infrared or ultraviolet light. The considerations may change with rapidly evolving technology, including the development of cameras that automatically select color or black-and-white recording modes, depending on lighting conditions. The type of questions to be answered will dictate the number of cameras used. A full compliment may include up to four cameras: two color cameras may be used for recording in daylight and two black-and-white cameras for recording in the dark, with one of each pair of cameras used for a full view of the entire body and the other used for a close-up of the face. However, recordings of good quality can be performed using a single camera, carefully adjusted by staff. Lights remain on in the patient's room at night to facilitate continuous color recording.

As with any camera, the lens will determine whether the patient's entire body is on the film (when considered with respect to the distance between camera and patient), whether there is any distortion of the body, and whether there is a capability to obtain close-up views of the face or body parts. Most camera and lens units have the capability for autofocus and automatic monitoring and maintenance of stable color; however, these features must be confirmed for each unit.

Remote control of camera movement and focus is critical in the conduct of accurate monitoring. Many patients, in particular infants and children, move frequently during monitoring. Adults may change locations, such as from bed to chair. Many patients move dramatically during seizures. It is essential that the patient remain on camera at all times in order to capture clinical seizures. Remote control of camera movement, using pan-and-tilt devices, and of camera focus helps ensure this. This control must be accomplished by a technologist assigned to conduct the monitoring; automated sensing devices, placed on the patient and designed to have the camera follow the patient, have not been satisfactory thus far.

For adults, cameras are mounted toward the top of the wall of the monitoring room and directed down toward the bed. This camera placement is appropriate for adults because most of their time is spent in bed or in a chair, often watching a television mounted next to the camera. Care must be taken in camera placement so that visitors cannot block the recording; because they may first greet the patient by standing at the front of the bed, visitors' heads may obscuring the full camera view of the patient. Although high-wall mounting may be appropriate for some children, it may be inadequate for others. Infants and young children may sit in bed and play or interact with family. A camera mounted near the ceiling of the monitoring suite will provide a continuous view of the top of the child's head but not the facial features, which may be crucial in the characterization of a seizure. Thus, for monitoring some children in a laboratory, camera mounting ideally should be flexible to meet specific needs of patients. Bedside monitoring poses different challenges in camera mounting. This type of monitoring is often performed on newborns and infants in neonatal or pediatric ICUs. Mounting the camera directly over the infant, rather than to the side or at a diagonal, allows the most accurate view of the infant without distortion or obscuration

of face, limbs, hands, or feet. Other challenges in this setting include securing the camera so that movement near it does not cause the camera to jitter, and placing the camera so that staff or family will not obscure a view of the patient. Regardless of age of the patient or camera placement, visitors and staff must be educated to stay clear of the camera line of site, particularly during a seizure.

The particular videocassette recorder utilized is often dictated by the vendor of the system(s) installed, but it is often a standard, commercially available unit. Most recently, devices have become available with the capacity to store video images on computer hard drives or compact disks, although this currently requires a significant amount of disk recording space. To accommodate this problem, some configurations allow for simultaneous recording on videotape and hard drive—a complete study is recorded on videotape and significant clinical events are saved on disk. For recording on videotape, the modes of recording (standard vs. extended play) will affect the duration of time it may take to review the video during analysis and may also determine overall quality of the video image if segments are duplicated for teaching. Use of extended-play mode will allow a longer amount of recording on a single videotape and quicker review of the entire video during "fast forward" surveys of the tape compared with recordings made in standard-play mode. However, duplication of video segments obtained during extended-play mode will result in more degraded images than with those obtained during standard play. Fluid, full-motion, digital video, recorded onto computer disk simultaneously with digital EEG, may eliminate these concerns once the recording technology and data storage methods are perfected.

Lighting should be installed in EEG laboratories in order to avoid shadows, particularly on the patient's face and around the eyes. Portable supplemental lighting can be helpful, particularly when recording infants, but may also generate some heat, in addition to shadows, and may cause the patient to sweat, thus compromising EEG recording. Such lighting also can impede movement around the bedside.

Synchronization and Data Display

Synchronization devices are critical to monitoring, providing the basis for the temporal correlation of electrical changes with any clinical events that may be recorded. Time–date generators may be freestanding instruments used in an assembly of analog EEG instrumentation and video equipment or may be embedded within the computer of a digital monitoring unit. The manner of data display will also determine the validity of the interpretation of monitoring. Time–date data must be displayed both on the video image and on the EEG–polygraph. It is often also helpful to display selected channels of EEG on the video image. Digital video can be superimposed on the digital EEG. This has both limitations and strengths. In viewing a small image, subtle movements may be overlooked; however, some instruments have the capacity to expand the image to full screen for more detailed analysis. It can be helpful to see the EEG and video simultaneously on a single screen, although, in interpreting the data, one generally looks at one piece of information at a time and then correlates the two.

With the development and increasing popularity of digital recording devices, the quality of data display, including resolution of waveforms, interchannel distances, and number of displayable channels, has become a significant issue. Because of the limitations of computer monitors, on-screen waveform resolution of EEG is not equal to that available with analog recordings onto paper. Interchannel distances may be too narrow for adequate analysis when utilizing enough channels to record EEG and polygraphic data. For example, the amplitude of the EEGs of children recorded at the scalp may be higher than that of adults, and the number of polygraphic channels recorded may be greater. The display on a monitor may become visually crowded, and greater care may be needed in analysis, particularly among those neurophysiologists who are making the transition from analog to digital recordings. Digital EEG instruments usually can print onto paper using laser or ink-jet printers. The best devices produce very sharp and accurate images, without the problems of pen misalignment occurring with analog machines.

MONITORING ENVIRONMENT

Monitoring suites, often called epilepsy monitoring units, can be located in the clinical neurophysiology laboratory, away from an inpatient hospital unit, or may be placed within an inpatient hospital setting. Regardless of its location or designation, the monitoring facility should be appropriately equipped and staffed.

Children in the laboratory setting have special needs in terms of care, recreation, education, visitation, general activities, and medical attention. Each child must be assessed individually so that the environment is conducive to optimal monitoring. Some laboratories modify cribs with transparent sides in order to record video at a level perpendicular to a sitting or standing infant (21). Other accommodations may include a playroom with video recording capabilities, which will allow the child to roam freely and be more active during monitoring. Although this is an engaging notion for the family of the patient and may be less frustrating for the child, it also increases the chances that the child may be off camera or have critical body parts obscured during a seizure. In such instances, additional events must be recorded for accurate analysis. Thus what may seem an enlightened amenity for children may lead to unnecessarily prolonged monitoring studies in some cases. Monitoring in a more restrictive environment may provide the basis for a more focused and efficient study, but also presents its own sets of challenges in terms of child care.

Bedside monitoring poses different challenges. This technique has been successfully utilized in the monitoring of neonates and children (8,10,71, 83,84) and adults. Bedside recordings are typically requested for newborns and infants who are too ill to be transported to the laboratory. Recording techniques must be adapted to the current status of the individual patient. At times, bedside monitoring is relatively brief in duration compared to epilepsy monitoring unit studies, in part because of limitations of resources, personnel, and instrumentations and in part because the abnormal paroxysmal clinical events that are of most concern in young patients tend to occur more frequently or may be provoked by stimulation of the patient. Thus the yield of brief ICU monitoring in a sick neonate or infant is relatively high compared with a similar study in older patients. Longer studies occur when there is concern that patients may be experiencing unrecognized events, or when the EEG pattern is to be monitored for response to therapy. In the ICU, all the essential instrumental components for monitoring are transported to the bedside. Monitoring is initiated and conducted with the understanding that the clinical care of the patient must continue unimpeded.

ROLE OF TECHNICAL PERSONNEL IN MONITORING

With emerging automated technology, the financial pressures imposed on neurophysiology laboratories, and efforts to "cross-train" hospital personnel, there is a current, and unwelcome, trend to diminish the role of the technologist in monitoring. This role, however, is critical and irreplaceable. The technologist is trained in EEG monitoring, has particular expertise in the recording of EEGs, and is frequently registered by the American Society of Electrodiagnostic Technologists (ASET). The technologist's tasks may include assisting in the planning of the monitoring study; selecting appropriate EEG montages and polygraphic parameters; discussion of the monitoring study with family and other caregivers; conducting a premonitoring visit for the family and, depending on the age of the patient, orienting the patient and family once in the monitoring suite; obtaining historical data; applying electrodes and appropriate sensors for EEG and other polygraphic measurements; initiating and conducting the monitoring study; completing the study; and ending the recordings and removing the electrodes after the study has been completed.

Patient observation, interaction, and testing are important tasks of the technologist. The technologist assures that the patient is constantly on camera and that the EEG and polygraphic measurements are being recorded adequately. (For example, pediatric patients can move quickly off camera and can be very effective and efficient at dislodging recording electrodes.) Adults may suddenly turn and reach for a ringing telephone or, impulsively, try to get out of bed to go to the bathroom. In addition, clinical events can be documented and characterized on a log maintained by the technologist.

Also, during long-term monitoring, patients will require assistance with activities of daily living and, depending on medical necessity, will need recording of vital signs, medication administration, and medical assessments. Technologists may perform some of these tasks; nursing staff must perform others. Policies and procedures should be developed in advance of monitoring studies that delineate the roles of the technologist and nurse in patient care. When children are subject to prolonged monitoring, child-life specialists are helpful in developing age-appropriate activities, education, and recreation.

For bedside monitoring in the ICU, technologists must be available to initiate and conduct studies around the clock, weekdays and weekends, in order to maximize the yield of studies. Studies performed in a timely fashion have a greater likelihood of providing useful clinical information. It is also essential that trained technologists staff the epilepsy monitoring unit whenever patients are monitored.

The purpose of monitoring is to record transient, fleeting clinical events. The malfunction of instrumentation, even for a short time, may cause such events to go unrecorded and thus unnecessarily prolong monitoring. Therefore, dedicated biomedical engineering and computer specialist staffs are critical to the successful operation of a monitoring unit. Regular maintenance is, of course, needed. However, less obvious is the need for on-call biomedical engineering personnel in order to keep monitoring equipment operational around the clock. With new computer-based instrumentation, it is essential that adequate technical support be available to resolve problems rapidly.

The so-called economy of reducing support personnel for monitoring is problematic and, most often, shifts the cost of the study to the patient. Studies conducted with no technologist present, with cameras mounted on the wall with no means of remotely following patients, with little supervision of the patient by knowledgeable personnel, or with the burden of event identification shifted to parents or other caregivers only serve to prolong monitoring unnecessarily, because clinical events may be missed and the patient must be monitored for additional time.

The clinical neurophysiologist is responsible for directing all aspects of the monitoring study and its interpretation. Often, medical issues complicate monitoring, including alteration of antiepileptic drugs (AEDs), intercurrent illnesses, and the management of seizures. There are number of strategies for dealing with these issues. Usually a number of physicians are involved with the patient during an inpatient stay, and comprise an ad hoc team for medical management of these patients. Monitoring, whether within a monitoring unit, in the neurophysiology laboratory, or at the bedside, will require around-the-clock availability of the attending clinical neurophysiologist. In instances in which several physicians are involved in the care of a monitored patient, delineation of responsibilities before recording is important—particularly in regard to management of acute seizures. There is also a tendency for physicians on rounds to review interesting portions of recordings. However, without benefit of the interpretation of the complete study by the neurophysiologist, the specific implications of the study for each patient cannot be determined. Discussion of segments of a study may provide premature information to the patient and may be at odds with the final reported findings.

STRATEGIES OF MONITORING

The strategy of monitoring for each patient is typically individualized and determined prior to monitoring. The type, character, and timing of the clinical events suspected of being abnormal will determine the best strategies for monitoring. This plan may change once monitoring is underway and initial findings are analyzed. The monitoring protocol is devised after consultation with the ordering physician. EEG montages, physiological sensors, and environment should be selected so as to provide for an efficient study and for the highest diagnostic yield during the study. The goal is to conduct a monitoring study that answers the clinical question in the least amount of time, with the least inconvenience and expense.

In addition, the timing of the suspected clinical events may suggest special strategies of timing. For patients with nocturnal events, monitoring must occur at night; monitoring during daytime napping typically cannot be substituted. Some seizure types may occur on arousal from sleep; for example, infantile spasms may occur in a cluster on arousing. Thus monitoring should include recording of a wake–sleep cycle. In addition, specific provocative agents, activities, stressors, or events may trigger a clinical seizure or behavior; these should be included during monitoring.

Sleep and Sleep Deprivation

Sleep activates the occurrence of seizure discharges in about one-third of patients with epilepsy (24). Sleep deprivation also has long been used to activate the occurrence of seizure discharges in patients with suspected seizure disorders (7,82). The technique is effective 30%–70% of the time and can increase the diagnostic yield even if sleep itself does not occur (25). Deprivation can be complete (e.g., no sleep in 24 hours) or partial (e.g., 2–4 hours of sleep the previous night).

Hyperventilation

Hyperventilation commonly produces EEG slowing as a result of hypocapnia and ensuing vasoconstriction and, in some patients, can activate both seizure discharges and actual seizures. This is particularly the case in patients with absence epilepsy but also can occur in patients with complex partial seizures. Hyperventilation is commonly used during routine EEG recordings but also can be useful during video-EEG monitoring. Only generalized or focal spikes on the EEG during hyperventilation should be considered epileptiform (see Chapter 5).

Photic and Other Methods of Sensory Stimulation

In selected patients, photic stimulation can activate epileptiform activity (81), or even seizures, when other modalities will not. However, generalized seizure discharges can occur at times during withdrawal of alcohol, illicit drugs, or medications, including AEDs. Standard flash equipment and flash frequencies are usually used, but special photic devices or activation methods are helpful in some cases (28).

Auditory, cutaneous, and behavioral stimuli can be used in the rare cases in which they are identified as causing seizures to occur (99,108). Startle can activate events in some cases, as can certain games, mental activities, or even eating (17).

Induction of Psychogenic Seizures

From the perspective of video-EEG monitoring, the finding of a normal EEG during a period of unresponsiveness is indicative of a seizure disorder of emotional origin (34,49,52,107). However, certain caveats must be kept in mind. First, seizure activity restricted to very localized areas of the cortex, particularly in adults, may not be reflected at the scalp (but essentially never produces episodes of loss of consciousness). Second, on occasion epileptic seizures can occur during attempts to induce psychogenic seizures immediately following epileptic events (16,59).

Many find it helpful to induce psychogenic seizures under controlled laboratory conditions (6,95). When this is done, the patient is told that a particular technique (e.g., infusion of intravenous saline, an applied tuning fork vibration) will induce a seizure. It has been suggested that hypnotism may be utilized to induce nonepileptic events (4). It is often helpful to review the videotape with the patient and family to ensure that the episode recorded is representative of those occurring spontaneously. If activating techniques are used, they should be employed in a respectful manner. Similarly, when a diagnosis of psychogenic seizures is made, findings must be discussed tactfully with the patient and family. Some patients with psychogenic seizures also have epilepsy (53). If the combination is suspected, it is important to try to make a positive diagnosis of each, so that treatment can be based on an empirically documented disease.

DATA ANALYSIS AND MANAGEMENT

Studies that are short in duration are interpreted by visual analysis. Studies conducted over a long period of time will generate large amounts of data. Typically, these data are also analyzed visually. However, there is a trend to utilize automated EEG spike-and-seizure detection programs. These computer programs have been useful in the analysis of EEGs of older children and adults (30,32,33), and have been applied to neonates and young infants with varied success (30,31,51). The application of spike detection computer programs is confounded by the fact that detection programs can miss seizures. Furthermore, there may be a high number of false positives resulting from detection of artifact or of normal variant patterns; an example of the latter is spike-and-sharp-wave complexes in the neonate, which may not be considered epileptiform (31). Because of these concerns, computer analysis and detection should be followed by human validation of the detected and analyzed data, with the understanding that some interictal and, perhaps, ictal events may be missed.

OVERALL CONSIDERATIONS FOR SYSTEM DEVELOPMENT AND IMPLEMENTATION

Among the principles the user should consider when planning and purchasing a monitoring system are the following (63). The system should be flexible and expandable so that more or fewer channels can be used to assess a given patient or a given problem. Second, breakdowns occur in monitoring equipment; redundancy should be planned into the system so as to account for this, at least some of the time. Third, the system should use standard and interchangeable parts so as to facilitate the flexibility and redundancy already mentioned. Fourth, the system should be modular, enabling separation of data acquisition, analysis, and storage. This facilitates maintenance of the system and allows evaluation of patient data to take place while new data are acquired. Communication between these modular parts should take place using standard methods and protocols. There should be methods of data analysis, data storage, and data reduction that are simple for the average end user.

ROLE OF MONITORING IN CLINICAL MANAGEMENT

The most effective application of monitoring is when it is conducted to answer a specific clinical question for an individual patient (55). Often the goal is to quantify seizures and various aspects of epilepsy (43,58,63,66,69). Applications may be age specific, because a greater variety and range of clinical events may occur in younger patients, events not seen when patients are older. Thus an important aspect of the analysis of pediatric monitoring is the anticipation of the type of clinical events that may occur at various ages.

Neonatal Seizures

Monitoring of neonates is most effectively and most often performed at the bedside (73). Instrumentation that synchronizes EEG, polygraphic para-meters, and video is brought to the nursery for monitoring and used without disrupting the care of the neonate. The differential diagnosis of abnormal clinical paroxysmal events includes normal movements of the waking preterm or full-term infant, normal movements of sleep, nonepileptic apnea and bradycardia, obstructive or central apnea, gastroesophageal reflux, abnormal nonepileptic events such as jitteriness, and epileptic and nonepileptic seizures. The clinical events may occur spontaneously, may be provoked, or both. Thus, in order to characterize any of these events, the full range of polygraphic–physiological sensors is typically applied and recorded with video and EEG. In addition, the duration of recording should be sufficient to include complete wakefulness–sleep cycles and to allow adequate time to capture clinical events, including periods in which maneuvers are performed to provoke them.

The accurate interpretation of the neonatal EEG will allow a more comprehensive understanding of the pathophysiology of the clinical events recorded and, in the absence of any such recorded events, may still provide important information concerning the degree and distribution of brain function (73). The character of the background EEG is conceptional age specific. The findings of serial EEGs, rather than those of a recording from a single point in time, will give the most accurate information concerning prognosis.

Interictal sharp waves are typically not considered epileptiform. Electrical seizure activity may be unifocal or multifocal. It may be confined to one region of the brain (Fig. 18.1), may migrate gradually, or may suddenly change location (Fig. 18.2). When the seizures are multifocal, they may occur simultaneously, but asynchronously in the two hemispheres. The amplitude, frequency, and morphology of the electrical seizures themselves may vary within a single seizure and from seizure to seizure. Electrical seizures may occur in association with clinical events ("electroclinical seizures") or they may occur with no clinical accompaniment ("subclinical seizures"). The latter seizures may occur in infants with significant brain injury and are characterized as seizure discharges of the depressed brain (41) and as alpha seizure discharges (50,96,101). In addition, electrical seizures may occur in the absence of clinical seizures following the treatment of electroclinical seizures with AEDs. In this situation, the clinical seizures are controlled while the electrographic seizures persist, a situation known as "decoupling" (71,72) (Fig. 18.3). Electrical seizures may also occur in the absence of clinical events when the infant is pharmacologically paralyzed for respiratory care.

A number of systems for characterization and classification of neonatal seizures have been proposed and updated (71,73,93,94) (Table 18.1). Clinical

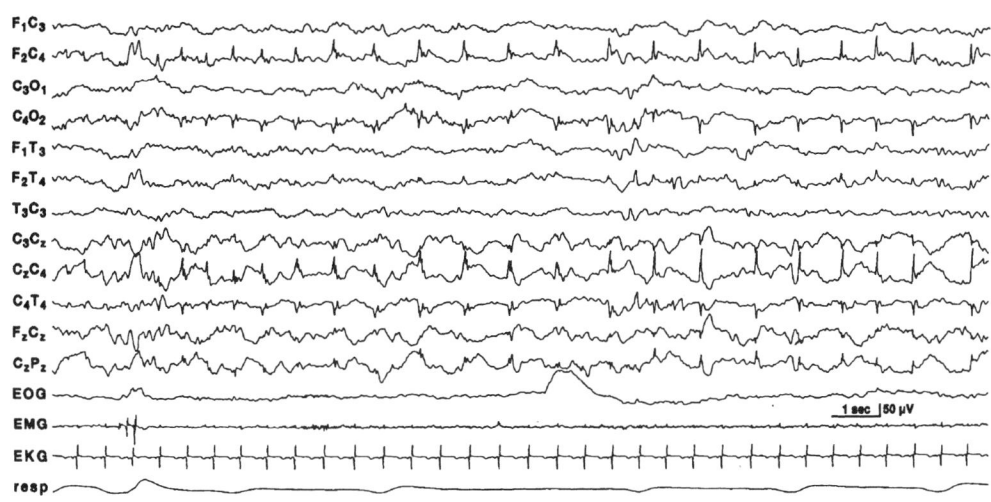

FIG. 18.1. Highly localized neonatal electrical seizure. Seizure discharges arising from the right central region of a 7-day-old, 40-week gestational age female infant with the diagnosis of group B streptococcal meningitis and cerebral infarction of the right temporal-occipital region, demonstrated by contract-enhanced computed tomography. Rhythmic focal clonic activity of the left foot occurred in close association with each seizure discharge. (From Mizrahi EM, Kellaway P. Neonatal electroencephalography. In *Diagnosis and management of neonatal seizures.* New York: Lippincott–Raven Publishers, 1998:99–143, with permission.)

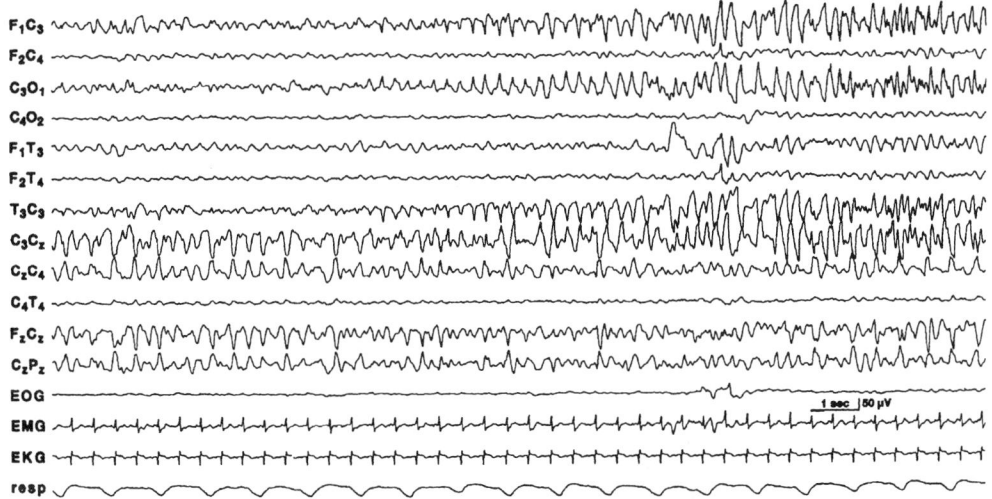

FIG. 18.2. Spread of electrical seizure activity in the neonate. Electrical seizure activity begins in the midline central region, then shifts to the left central region. As the electrical discharge spreads, the midline region becomes uninvolved, just as the left central region was uninvolved at seizure onset. No clinical seizures were associated with this electrical seizure discharge. This recording was obtained from a 4-day-old, 40-week gestational age female infant with hypoxic-ischemic encephalopathy. (From Mizrahi EM, Kellaway P. Neonatal electroencephalography. In *Diagnosis and management of neonatal seizures.* New York: Lippincott–Raven Publishers, 1998:99–143, with permission.)

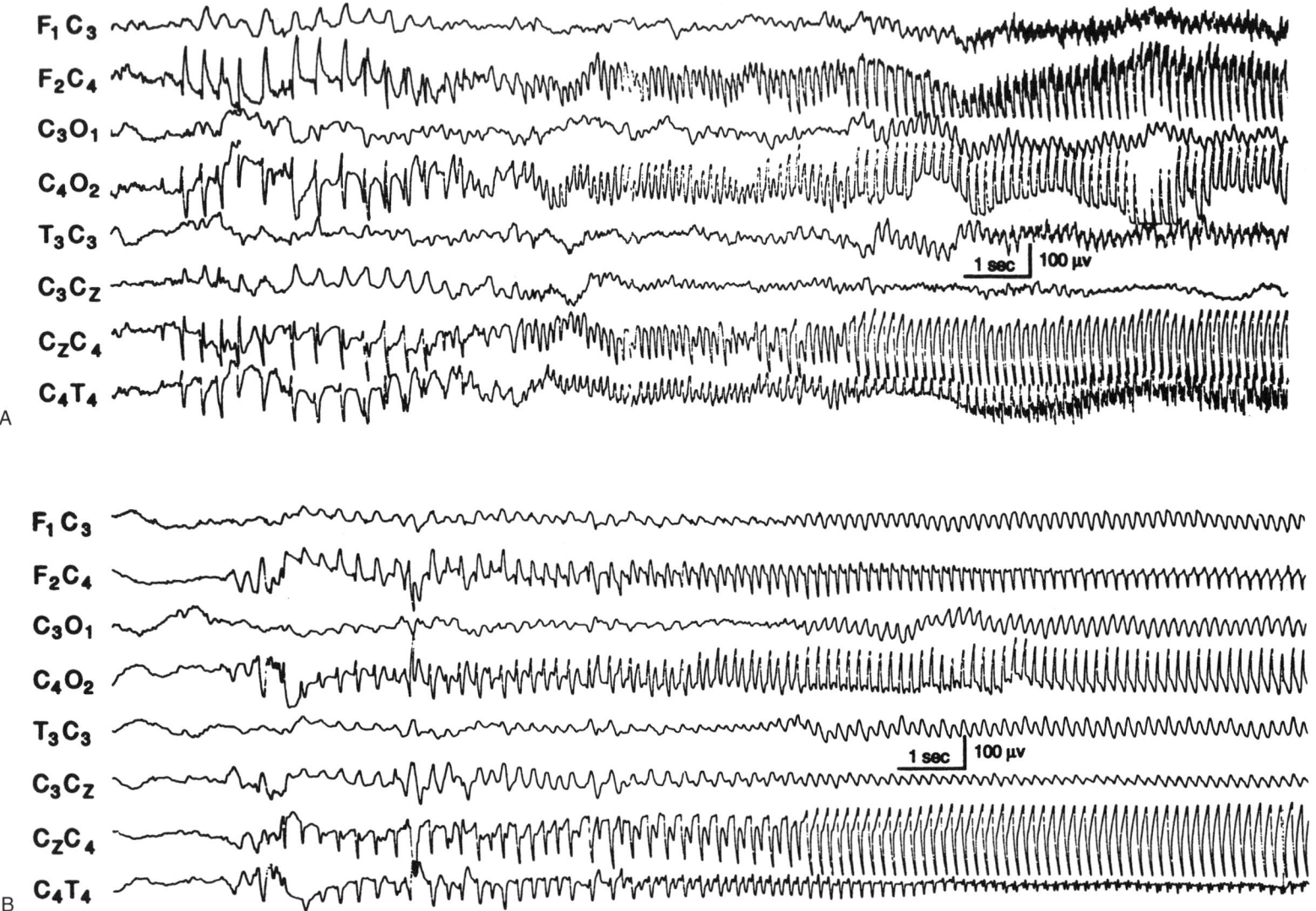

FIG. 18.3. Response to AED therapy in the neonate. **A:** Electrical seizure activity arises in the right central region, clinically associated with focal clonic seizures of the extremities on the left. Recording was obtained prior to AED therapy in this 1-day-old, 40-week gestational age female infant with focal cortical dysplasia in the right central region. **B:** Following administration of a loading dose of phenobarbital (20 mg per kilogram intravenously), no clinical seizures were present, although electrical seizures recurred in the same region as that prior to AED therapy. Thus the clinical seizures had been "decoupled" from the electrical seizures. Both figure parts show selected channels from a 12-channel EEG recording. (From Hrachovy RA, Mizrahi EM, Kellaway P. Electroencephalography of the newborn. In: Daly D, Pedley TA, eds. *Current practice of clinical electroencephalography*, 2nd ed. New York: Raven Press, 1990:201–242, with permission.)

TABLE 18.1. *Clinical characteristics, classification, and presumed pathophysiology of neonatal seizures*

Classification	Characterization
Focal clonic	Repetitive, rhythmic contractions of muscle groups of the limbs, face, or trunk
	May be unifocal or multifocal
	May occur synchronously or asynchronously in muscle groups on one side of the body
	May occur simultaneously but asynchronously on both sides
	Cannot be provoked by stimulation or suppressed by restraint
	Pathophysiology: Epileptic
Focal tonic	Sustained posturing of single limbs
	Sustained asymmetrical posturing of the trunk
	Sustained eye deviation
	Cannot be provoked by stimulation or suppressed by restraint
	Pathophysiology: Epileptic
Generalized tonic	Sustained symmetrical posturing of limbs, trunk, and neck
	May be flexor, extensor, or mixed extensor–flexor
	May be provoked or intensified by stimulation
	May be suppressed by restraint or repositioning
	Presumed Pathophysiology: Nonepileptic
Myoclonic	Random, single, rapid contractions of muscle groups of the limbs, face, or trunk
	Typically not repetitive or may recur at a slow rate
	May be generalized, focal, or fragmentary
	May be provoked by stimulation
	Presumed Pathophysiology: May be epileptic or nonepileptic
Spasms	May be flexor, extensor, or mixed extensor–flexor
	May occur in clusters
	Cannot be provoked by stimulation or suppressed by restraint
	Pathophysiology: Epileptic
Motor automatisms	
Ocular signs	Random and roving eye movements or nystagmus (distinct from tonic eye deviation)
	May be provoked or intensified by tactile stimulation
	Presumed Pathophysiology: Nonepileptic
Oral–buccal–lingual movements	Sucking, chewing, tongue protrusions
	May be provoked or intensified by stimulation
	Presumed Pathophysiology: Nonepileptic
Progression movements	Rowing or swimming movements
	Pedalling or bicycling movements of the legs
	May be provoked or intensified by stimulation
	May be suppressed by restraint or repositioning
	Presumed Pathophysiology: Nonepileptic
Complex purposeless movements	Sudden arousal with transient increased random activity of limbs
	May be provoked or intensified by stimulation
	Presumed Pathophysiology: Nonepileptic

seizures are characterized as clonic (focal or multifocal), tonic (focal or generalized), myoclonic (fragmentary, focal, or generalized), spasm, and motor automatisms (movements of progression, oral–buccal–lingual movements, ocular signs, and paroxysmal purposeless movements) (71). Some of these clinical events have a clear and consistent association with electrical seizure activity, and can best be described as neonatal seizures of epileptic origin. Typically, these are clonic, focal tonic, and some types of myoclonic events. Other clinical seizure types occur without electrographic seizure activity, and the clinical events can also be provoked by tactile stimulation and arrested by restraint. In addition, these types of clinical events have other features that also suggest that they are based in reflex physiology and are best referred to as "brainstem release phenomena" or nonepileptic neonatal seizures (47,71).

Thus the monitoring of neonates for suspected seizures should include a log of suspected clinical events that is well maintained by the technologist, efforts to provoke suspected events by stimulation of the infant, and, when clinical events do occur, efforts to stop them by restraint. These responses are considered in visual analysis of monitoring. In addition, the relationship of clinical and electrical events is given close scrutiny. Because so-called nonepileptic seizures may occur in infants who have also had subclinical electrical seizures unassociated with clinical events, the simple reporting of the occurrence of a clinical event in such a monitored infant may falsely identify that event as epileptic in origin.

The response of electroclinical seizures to treatment with AEDs has been discussed above. However, decoupled, subclinical electrographic seizures in the neonate may be very resistant even to vigorous AED treatment, and, even if eliminated, the discharges may recur. Thus new strategies for treatment and for continued EEG surveillance are needed. Typically, first- and second-line AEDs (phenobarbital and phenytoin) are given in dosages to attain high therapeutic serum levels, with additional dosages of benzodiazepines given. Further AED treatment is often not pursued because it can be associated with adverse effects such as hypotension, bradycardia, apnea, and central nervous system depression (79).

Other needs for new strategies of management concern methods of EEG surveillance for electrical seizures in AED-treated infants, in infants at risk for electrical seizures unassociated with clinical seizures, and in those pharmacologically paralyzed for respiratory care. The latter setting may be ideal for the application of computer-assisted, automated seizure detection systems. In these instances, the infants are relatively immobile and the chance of the occurrence of intrusive movement-induced artifact is minimized.

Infantile Spasms

Monitoring has been successfully utilized to characterize and classify infantile spasms and to assess the efficacy of various therapies (27,38–40, 48). The clinical spasms may be extensor, flexor, or mixed extensor–flexor. Electrographically, a generalized-voltage, slow–sharp transient or an episode of generalized voltage attenuation with low-voltage fast activity superimposed may accompany them (36) (Fig. 18.4). The occurrence of infantile spasms typically has been associated with the interictal EEG finding of hypsarrhythmia background activity, although modified hypsarrhythmic patterns, other abnormal types of EEG background activity, and even normal EEG background activity may occur in infants with spasms (36,37).

Monitoring is effective in establishing the diagnosis of infantile spasms. The duration of monitoring needed for diagnosis is variable, although prolonged recordings are not often needed, particularly in an infant with hypsarrhythmia or a modified pattern. However, additional information may be gained from monitoring these infants because they may also experience other seizure types (77). Thus a child with infantile spasms may also experience recurrent simple or complex partial seizures. Monitoring is critical in the documentation of the various seizure types an infant may have because therapies for each vary and are type specific.

Monitoring is also essential in children with infantile spasms in order to determine the effectiveness of therapy—traditional hormonal treatment with adrenocorticotropic hormone or prednisone, and more recently, new AEDs. Monitoring is more effective in this regard than is parental observation (36). Parents often underestimate spasm frequency or the presence of spasms. A comparison of parental observation with 24-hour monitoring of patients with infantile spasms demonstrated that the infants were actually experiencing several (often unrecognized) events per day. In addition, some parents may report that spasms are occurring when monitoring fails to reveal such events.

Seizures in Infancy

The concerns associated with the monitoring of neonates are also associated with the monitoring of infants suspected of having seizures in the first year of life—seizure types with similar underlying pathophysiology persist, but at relatively different frequencies (67,68). In addition, other seizure types emerge within the first year of life and become more prominent. These include

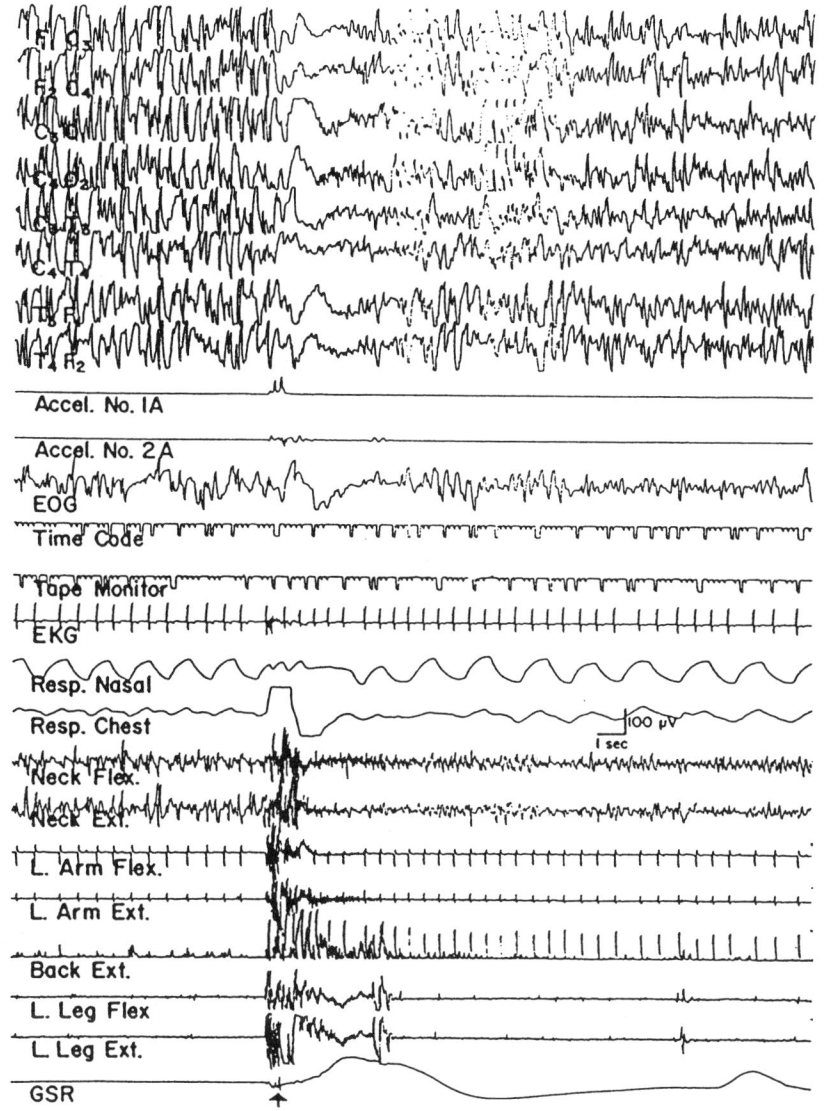

FIG. 18.4. Ictal and interictal recording of infantile spasms. Twenty-four channel EEG and polygraphic recording of an infant with clinical spasms. The preictal EEG background activity demonstrates hypsarrhythmia; the postictal EEG demonstrates relative normalization, which may occur follow electroclinical spasms. The clinical spasm is flexor–extensor, occurring in association with an ictal generalized, high-voltage slow-wave transient, followed by superimposed generalized fast activity. Polygraphic channels that record EMG, accelerometry, and respiration characterize the clinical event and its precise relationship to EEG. Video, capturing the clinical event, was also recorded, and synchronized to the EEG–polygraph with the time code channel.

infantile spasms and other generalized myoclonic events, complex partial seizures, and generalized tonic, generalized tonic–clonic, and generalized clonic seizures (19,76). It should be noted that this period may be characterized by the emergence of generalized epileptic seizures; however, the precise age at which they consistently appear is unknown and may extend beyond the first year of life.

Problems in semiology similar to those with neonatal seizures have led some investigators to develop an additional classification system of seizure for infants, utilizing monitoring (76). Some seizure categories were retained: clonic, tonic, spasms, and myoclonic events. Others added were not part of the seizure classification of older children or adults (11,12). *Astatic seizures* are described as sudden loss of muscle tone of one or more muscle groups or the entire body. *Behavioral seizures* consist of an abrupt change in behavior without other overt features, sometimes with a sudden cessation of movement. *Versive seizures* consist of version of the eyes only—without head or limb turning.

Complex partial seizures in infancy represent an important clinical problem (19). Their characterization and classification by monitoring is the first step in diagnosis and management. Partial epilepsy that presents in infancy and early childhood is considered by some investigators to be a catastrophic disorder that may eventually be associated with profound neurological deterioration (86) and, without effective therapy, a poor prognosis for mental or motor development (9). The diagnosis of complex partial seizures in infants may be difficult, and, because of its association with a poorer prognosis and perhaps the need for more aggressive initial AED therapy, monitoring may be a valuable tool in the management of these patients.

Childhood Epilepsy

The differential diagnosis of suspected seizures in older children may include movement disorders (tics, dystonia, ballismus); sleep disorders (apnea, paroxysmal leg movements, sleep myoclonus, night terrors, other parasomnias) (102); behavioral disorders; pseudoseizures; childhood migraine; cardiac or vagal syncope; esophageal reflux; reflex behaviors; and normal, although, perhaps, unusual behaviors. In addition, childhood seizures themselves can more easily be classified according to the international classification of seizures and, with additional information, epileptic syndromes (11,12). Thus monitoring can provide the basis for the diagnosis of a wide range of paroxysmal clinical events, some caused by epilepsy and some not, and for the classification of epileptic seizures (70).

Prolonged monitoring in childhood also allows for the quantification of epilepsy in the assessment of therapy. Certainly, capture of clinical or electrical seizure activity during monitoring may indicate that AED therapy is not effective. The quantification of EEG interictal generalized spike-and-wave activity during prolonged, overnight recordings in children with generalized seizures has been shown to predict future seizures effectively (45,46,48). In serial monitoring studies, the abundance of generalized spike-and-wave activity has been quantified during 12-hour epochs of EEG before and after therapy with ethosuximide in children with epilepsy characterized by absence seizures and concurrent atonic, myoclonic, or tonic–clonic seizures and 3-Hz generalized spike-and-wave activity. There was a direct relationship between the occurrence of seizures and the amount of interictal spike-and-wave activity. Reduction of the spike-and-wave abundance by AEDs predicted reduced seizure occurrence. At serum levels at which spike-and-wave activity during wakefulness or rapid-eye-movement sleep was

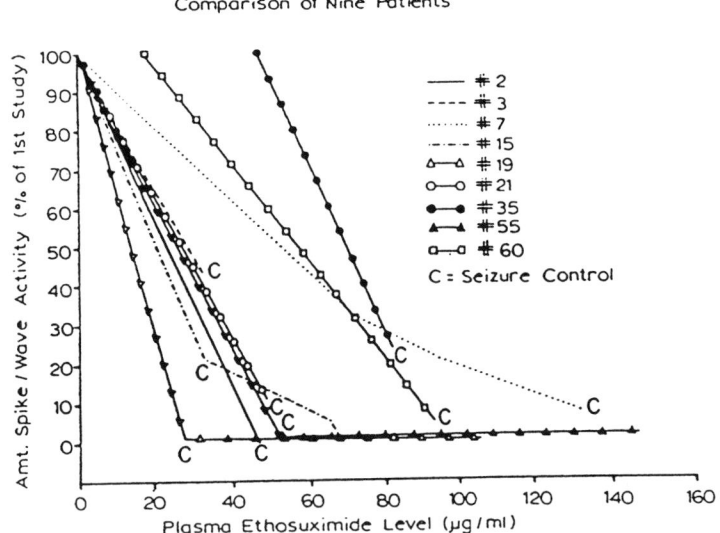

FIG. 18.5. Relationship of interictal generalized spike-and-wave activity, AED serum levels, and clinical control of absence seizures. Control of childhood absence epilepsy associated with 3-Hz spike-and-wave activity is attained with reduction of the amount of spike-and-wave activity during a 24-hour video-EEG monitoring period, compared to a baseline recording. See text for details.

abolished, the seizure types of absence, myoclonic, or atonic did not recur. However, if any spike-and-wave activity was present in a prolonged EEG sample (12–24 hours), the potential persisted for generalized tonic–clonic seizures to recur. Thus prolonged EEG monitoring of patients undergoing AED treatment for some generalized childhood epilepsies may be helpful in the early prediction of eventual seizure control at specific serum levels of AEDs (Fig. 18.5).

Epilepsy Surgery

Prolonged monitoring is an important part of the presurgical evaluation of patients with medically intractable seizures (3,5,20,35,42,56,74,89,105,106). The general principles of monitoring for nonsurgical candidates apply: maintenance of quality recordings, investment in support staff, time synchronization of all recording modalities, and observation for age-specific clinical seizure types.

There are two principle types of invasive leads: depth electrodes and subdural electrodes. The former are thin cylinders with multiple contacts along their length. They can be placed anywhere but are primarily used to record from mesial temporal structures such as the hippocampus and amygdala and from the mesial frontal lobe. They may be surgically placed in a posterior-to-anterior orientation or a lateral-to-mesial (orthogonal) orientation (90). Subdural electrodes are metal disks embedded in plastic. They can be linear "strips" of several electrodes, or larger arrays, often called grids, with several rows of evenly spaced disks. Some strips may be placed through bur holes, whereas other strips and grids require craniotomies. Both stainless steel and platinum–iridium electrodes are used. Depth electrodes (88) are particularly useful when the goal is to determine in which hemisphere seizures of likely mesial temporal lobe origin originate (Fig. 18.6). Subdural strips can be selectively placed: below the basal temporal and frontal lobes (103,104) or over specific cortical regions (Fig. 18.7). Subdural grids can be used to determine the extent of the epileptogenic region over an area of interest and to perform functional localization studies: evoked potential studies or cortical stimulation used to localize cortical regions subsuming motor, sensory, language, or other functions (57,62,64,92). Intracranial electrode utilization is considered safe, with potential benefits outweighing

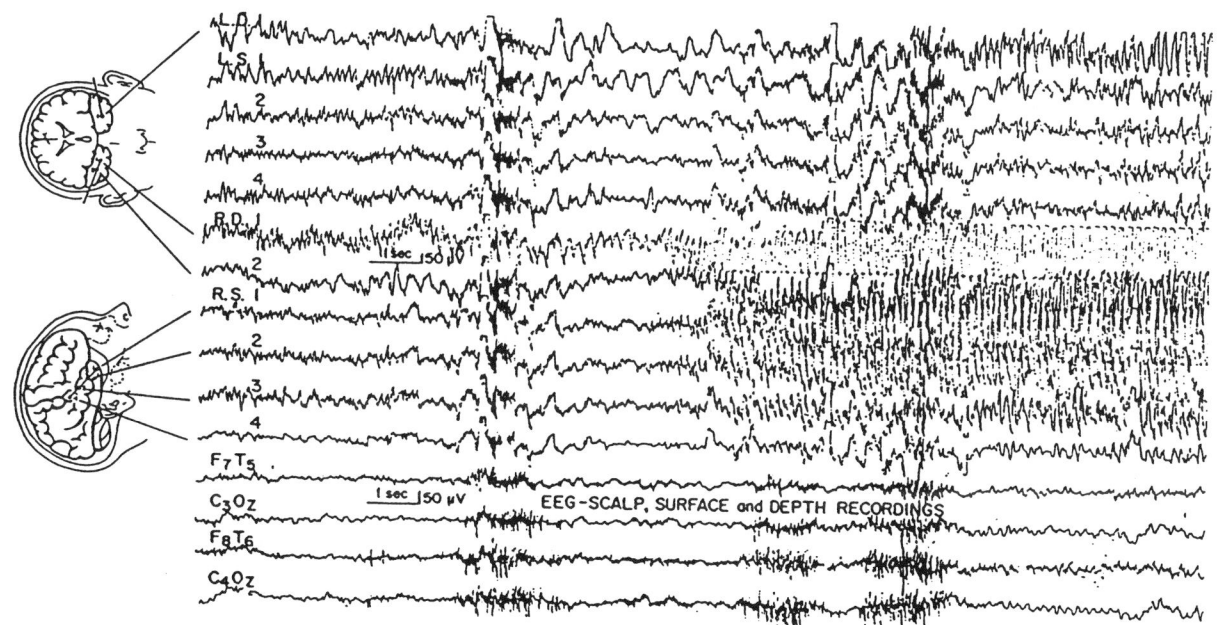

FIG. 18.6. Ictal depth recording in a 35-year-old man with complex partial seizures. Depth electrodes were implanted orthogonally, in lateral-to-medial orientation, into the left and right temporal lobes. Through the same bur hole, additional electrodes were situated over the posterior surface of the temporal lobes in anterior-to-posterior orientation. Electrical seizure activity arises in the depth of the right temporal lobe (*R.D.*) with eventual spread to the right temporal surface (*R.S.*) and finally to the left temporal region (*L.D.*), but there is no representation from the left temporal surface (*L.S.*). Selected EEG channels from scalp electrodes demonstrate no initial focal or lateralizing features. Following right anterior temporal lobectomy, pathology examination demonstrated mesial temporal sclerosis. (From Mizrahi EM, Kellaway P, Grossman RG, et al. Anterior temporal lobectomy and medically refractory temporal lobe epilepsy of childhood. *Epilepsia* 1990;31:302–312, with permission.)

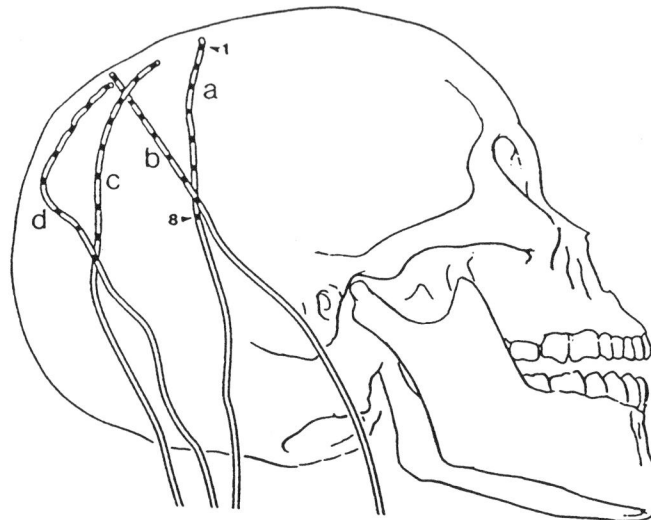

A

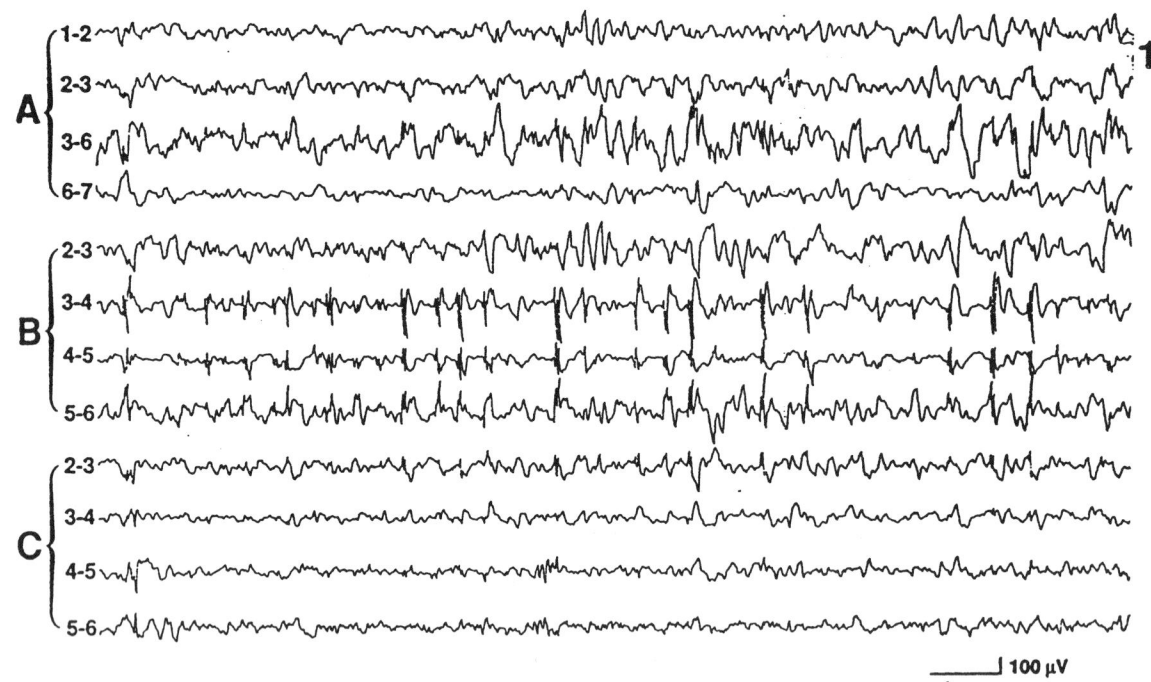

B

FIG. 18.7. Subdural strip electrode recordings. Four electrode strips, in this case arrays originally designed as depth electrodes, were inserted through two bur holes over a cortical region suspected of being the epileptogenic zone in an 11-year-old boy with recurrent, brief partial seizures characterized by initial sensory disturbance of the dorsum of the left hand, followed by transient tonic posturing of the left shoulder and arm, then focal clonic activity of the left arm and hand. **A:** Schematic of skull radiograph indicating location and numbering of electrodes. Electrodes were inserted through two bur holes at the sites of the crossing of each pair of electrodes. The recordings are sequential (labeled 1–5); capital letters on the recordings correspond to lower-case letters on the electrode diagram; and electrode contacts are labeled numerically. **B:** Segment 1. Interictal discharges localize to electrode B5 (calibration: 1 second; 10 μV per millimeter). *(Figure continues.)*

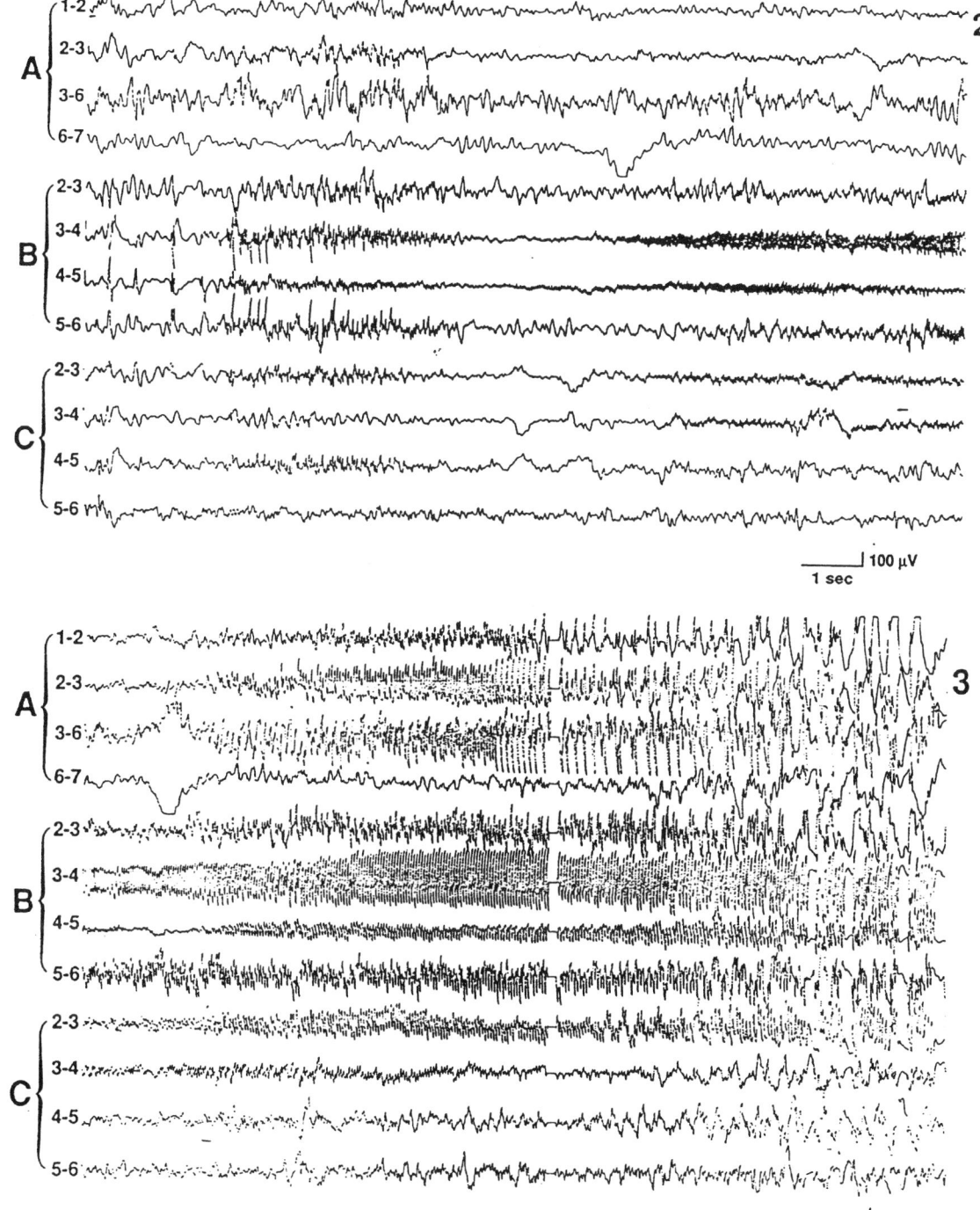

FIG. 18.7. *Continued.* **C:** Segment 2. High-frequency, low-amplitude seizure discharge arises from electrode B5 with involvement of B4 (calibration: 1 second; 10 μV per millimeter). **D:** Segment 3. Electrical seizure activity evolves in morphology and spreads (instrumentation sensitivity is changed, over halfway through this segment, from 10 to 15 μV per millimeter, marked by 0.2-second interruption in recording).*(Figure continues.)*

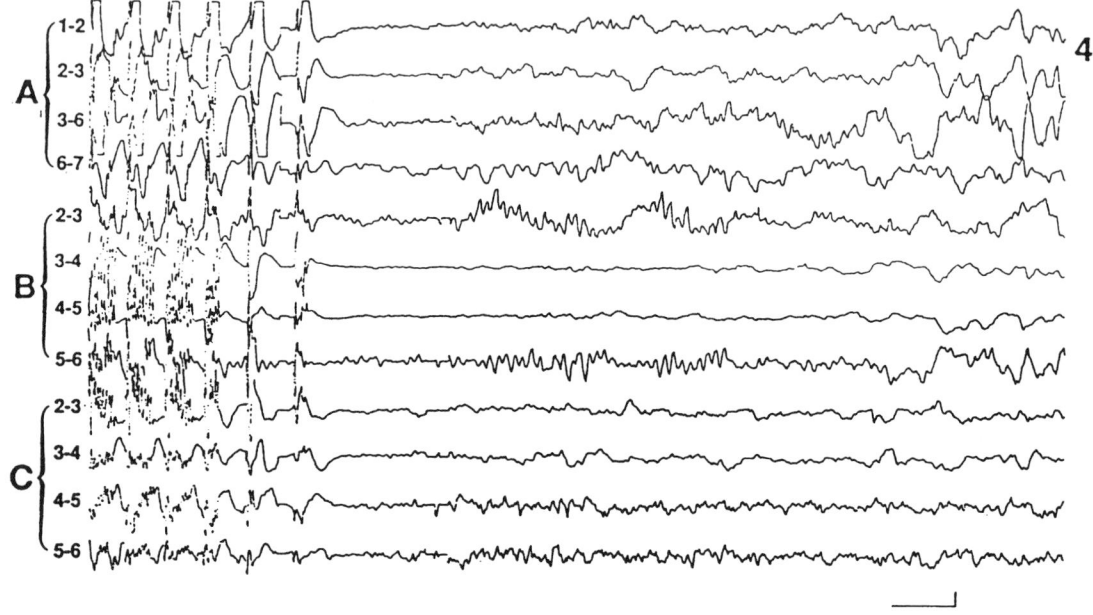

E

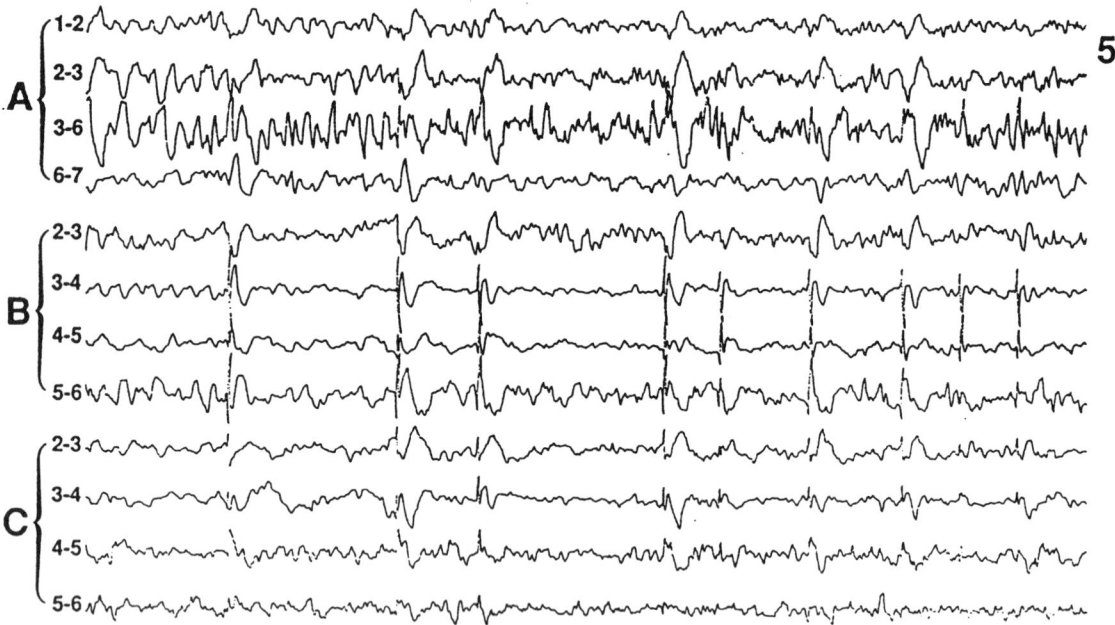

F

FIG. 18.7. *Continued.* **E:** Segment 4. Termination of the electrical seizure, followed by focal postictal depression (calibration: 1 second; 15 μV per millimeter). **F:** Segment 5. Resumption of interictal spike discharges (calibration: 1 second; 15 μV per millimeter). The cortical resection, guided by these recordings and intraoperative electrocorticography, was confined to a small region. Pathology examination demonstrated focal cortical dysplasia characterized by microdysgenesis.

potential risks. However, there have been reports of complications, including infection (98).

In the monitoring unit, cortical stimulation should be optimized at each stimulation site; actual currents used can vary from electrode to electrode and from day to day (61). If this is not done, false negatives can occur from stimulating at too low a current. Conversely, afterdischarges can be produced, and these can confuse the interpretation of any findings produced by stimulation. In addition to cortical stimulation, evoked potentials can be obtained. Somatosensory evoked potentials—to identify the rolandic fissure—have been the most frequently utilized, but visual and auditory evoked potentials also can be obtained, and event-related modalities show great promise for the future (13,14).

REFERENCES

1. American Electroencephalographic Society. Guideline twelve: guidelines for long-term monitoring for epilepsy. *J Clin Neurophysiol* 1994;11:88–110.
2. American Electroencephalographic Society. Guideline two: minimum technical standards for pediatric electroencephalography. *J Clin Neurophysiol* 1994;11:6–9.
3. Arroyo S, Lesser RP, Awad IA, et al. Subdural and epidural grids and strips. In: Pedley J Jr, ed. *Surgical treatment of the epilepsies*, 2nd ed. New York: Raven Press, 1993:377–386.
4. Barry JJ, Atzman O, Morrell MJ. Discriminating between epileptic and nonepileptic events: the utility of hypnotic seizure induction. *Epilepsia* 2000;41:81–84.
5. Bautista RE, Cobbs MA, Spencer DD, et al. Prediction of surgical outcome by interictal epileptiform abnormalities during intracranial EEG monitoring in patients with extrahippocampal seizures. *Epilepsia* 1999;40:880–90.
6. Bazil CW, Kothari M, Luciano D, et al. Provocation of nonepileptic seizures by suggestion in a general seizure population. *Epilepsia* 1994;35:768–770.
7. Bazil CW, Walczak TS. Effects of sleep and sleep stage on epileptic and nonepileptic seizures. *Epilepsia* 1997;38:56–62.
8. Bye AM, Cunningham CA, Chee KY, et al. Outcome of neonates with electrographically identified seizures, or at risk of seizures. *Pediatr Neurol* 1997;16:225–231.
9. Chevrie JJ, Aicardi J. Convulsive disorders in the first year of life: persistence of epileptic seizures. *Epilepsia* 1979;20:643–649.
10. Clancy RR, Legido A, Lewis D. Occult neonatal seizures. *Epilepsia* 1988;29:256–261.
11. Commission on Classification and Terminology of the International League Against Epilepsy. Proposal for revised clinical and electrographic classification of epileptic seizures. *Epilepsia* 1981;22:489–501.
12. Commission on Classification and Terminology of the International League Against Epilepsy. Proposal for revised classification of epilepsies and epileptic syndromes. *Epilepsia* 1989;30:389–399.
13. Crone NE, Mighoretti DL, Gordon B, et al. Functional mapping of human sensorimotor cortex with electrocorticographic spectral analysis. I. Alpha and beta event-related desynchronization. *Brain* 1998;121:2271–2299.
14. Crone NE, Mighoretti DL, Gordon B, et al. Functional mapping of human sensorimotor cortex with electrocorticographic spectral analysis. II. Event-related synchronization in the gamma band. *Brain* 1998;121:2301–2315.
15. Da Silva AM, Cunha JP, de Oliveira PG. Scalp EEG recording: interictal/ictal location and spreading of epileptiform events. *Acta Neurol Scand Suppl* 1994;152:17–19.
16. Devinsky O, Gordon E. Epileptic seizures progressing into nonepileptic conversion seizures. *Neurology* 1998;51:1293–1296.
17. Dreifuss FE. Classification of reflex epilepsies and reflex seizures. *Adv Neurol* 1998;75:5–13.
18. Drury I, Selwa LM, Schuh LA, et al. Value of inpatient diagnostic CCTV-EEG monitoring in the elderly. *Epilepsia* 1999;40:1100–1102.
19. Duchowny M. The syndrome of partial seizures in infancy. *J Child Neurol* 1992;7:66–69.
20. Duchowny M, Jayakar P, Resnick T, et al. Epilepsy surgery in the first three years of life. *Epilepsia* 1998;39:737–743.
21. Duchowny MS, Shewmon DA, Wyllie E, et al. Special considerations for preoperative evaluation in childhood. In: Engel J Jr, ed. *Surgical treatment of the epilepsies*, 2nd ed. New York: Raven Press, 1993:415–27.
22. Ebersole JS. Defining epileptogenic foci: past, present, future. *J Clin Neurophysiol* 1997;14:470–483.
23. Ebersole JS, Pacia SV. Localization of temporal lobe foci by ictal EEG patterns. *Epilepsia* 1996;37:386–399.
24. Ellingson RJ, Wilken K, Bennett DR. Efficacy of sleep deprivation as an activation procedure in epilepsy patients. *J Clin Neurophysiol* 1984;1:83–101.
25. Fountain NB, Kim JS, Lee SI. Sleep deprivation activates epileptiform discharges independent of the activating effects of sleep. *J Clin Neurophysiol* 1998;15:69–75.
26. Frost JD Jr. Triaxial vector accelerometry: a method for quantifying tremor and ataxia. *IEEE Trans Biomed Eng* 1978;25:17–27.
27. Frost JD Jr, Hrachovy RA, Kellaway P, et al. Quantitative analysis and characterization of infantile spasms. *Epilepsia* 1978;19:273–282.
28. Fylan F, Edson AS, Harding GF. Clinical significance of EEG abnormalities during photic stimulation in patients with photosensitive epilepsy. *Epilepsia* 1999;40:370–372.
29. Goodin DS, Aminoff MJ, Laxer KD. Detection of epileptiform activity by different noninvasive EEG methods in complex partial epilepsy. *Ann Neurol* 1990;27:330–334.
30. Gotman J. Automatic recognition of interictal spikes. *Electroencephalogr Clin Neurophysiol Suppl* 1985;37:93–114.
31. Gotman J, Flanagan D, Rosenblatt B, et al. Evaluation of an automatic seizure detection method for newborn EEG. *Electroencephalogr Clin Neurophysiol* 1997;103:363–369.
32. Gotman J, Wang LY. State-dependent spike detection: concepts and preliminary results. *Electroencephalogr Clin Neurophysiol* 1991;79:11–19.
33. Gotman J, Wang LY. State-dependent spike detection: validation. *Electroencephalogr Clin Neurophysiol* 1992;83:12–18.
34. Henry TR, Drury I. Non-epileptic seizures in temporal lobectomy candidates with medically refractory seizures. *Neurology* 1997;48:1374–1382.
35. Henry TR, Ross DA, Schuh LA, et al. Indications and outcome of ictal recording with intracerebral and subdural electrodes in refractory complex partial seizures. *J Clin Neurophysiol* 1999;16:426–438.
36. Hrachovy RA, Frost JD Jr. Severe encephalopathic epilepsy in infants: infantile spasms. In: Dodson WE, Pellock JM, eds. *Pediatric epilepsy: diagnosis and therapy*. New York: Demos Publications, 1993:135–145.
37. Hrachovy RA, Frost JD Jr, Kellaway P. Hypsarrhythmia: variations on the theme. *Epilepsia* 1984;25:317–325.
38. Hrachovy RA, Frost JD Jr, Kellaway P, et al. A controlled study of prednisone therapy in infantile spasms. *Epilepsia* 1979;20:403–407.
39. Hrachovy RA, Frost JD JR, Kellaway P, et al. A controlled study of ACTH therapy in infantile spasms. *Epilepsia* 1980;21:631–636.
40. Hrachovy RA, Frost JD Jr, Kellaway P, et al. Double-blind study of ACTH vs prednisone therapy in infantile spasms. *J Pediatr* 1983;103:641–645.
41. Hrachovy RA, Mizrahi EM, Kellaway P. Electroencephalography of the newborn. In: Daly D,

Pedley TA, eds. *Current practice of clinical electroencephalography*, 2nd ed. New York: Raven Press, 1990:201–242.

42. Jayakar P. Invasive EEG monitoring in children: when, where, and what? *J Clin Neurophysiol* 1999;16:408–418.

43. Kellaway P. Childhood seizures. *Electroencephalogr Clin Neurophysiol Suppl* 1985;37:267–283.

44. Kellaway P. An orderly approach to visual analysis: characteristics of the normal EEG of adults and children. In Daly DD, Pedley TA, eds. *Current practice of clinical electroencephalography*, 2nd ed. New York: Raven Press, 1990:139–199.

45. Kellaway P, Frost JD Jr. Biorhythmic modulation of epileptic events. In: Pedley TA, Meldrum BS, eds. *Recent advances in epilepsy*. Edinburgh: Churchill Livingstone, 1983:139–154.

46. Kellaway P, Frost JD Jr, Crawley JW. Time modulation of spike-and-wave activity in generalized epilepsy. *Ann Neurol* 1980;8:491–500.

47. Kellaway P, Hrachovy RA. Status epilepticus in newborns: a perspective on neonatal seizures. *Adv Neurol* 1983;34:93–99.

48. Kellaway P, Hrachovy RA, Frost JD Jr, et al. Precise characterization and quantification of infantile spasms. *Ann Neurol* 1979;6:214–218.

49. King DW, Gallagher BB, Murvin AJ, et al. Pseudoseizures: diagnostic evaluation. *Neurology* 1982;32:18–23.

50. Knauss TA, Carlson CB. Neonatal paroxysmal monorhythmic alpha activity. *Arch Neurol* 1978;35:104–107.

51. Ko C-W, Chung H-W. Automatic spike detection via an artificial neural network using raw EEG data: effects of data preparation and implications in the limitations of online recognition. *Clin Neurophysiol* 2000;111:477–481.

52. Krumholz A. Nonepileptic seizures: diagnosis and management. *Neurology* 1999;53:576–583.

53. Krumholz A, Niedermeyer E. Psychogenic seizure: a clinical study with follow-up data. *Neurology* 1983;33:498–502.

54. Laxer KD. Mini-sphenoidal electrodes in the investigation of seizures. *Electroencephalogr Clin Neurophysiol* 1984;58:127–129.

55. Lesser RP. The role of epilepsy centers in delivering care to patients with intractable epilepsy. *Neurology* 1994;44:1347–1352.

56. Lesser RP, Fisher RS, Kaplan P. The evaluation of patients with intractable complex partial seizures [Review]. *Electroencephalogr Clin Neurophysiol* 1989;73:381–388.

57. Lesser RP, Gordon B, Fisher R, et al. Subdural grid electrodes in surgery of epilepsy. In Luders H, ed. *Epilepsy surgery*. New York, Raven Press, 1991:399–408.

58. Lesser RP, Kaplan PW. Long-term monitoring with digital technology for epilepsy [Review]. *J Child Neurol* 1994;9:564–70.

59. Lesser RP, Luders H, Conomy JP, et al. Sensory seizure mimicking a psychogenic seizure. *Neurology* 1983;33:800–802.

60. Lesser RP, Luders H, Dinner DS, et al. An introduction to the basic concepts of polarity and localization. *J Clin Neurophysiol* 1985;2:45–61.

61. Lesser RP, Luders H, Klem G, et al. Cortical afterdischarge and functional response thresholds: results of extraoperative testing. *Epilepsia* 1984;25:615–621.

62. Lesser RP, Luders H, Klem G, et al. Extraoperative cortical functional localization in patients with epilepsy. *J Clin Neurophysiol* 1987;4:27–53.

63. Lesser RP, Webber WR, Fisher RS. Design principles for computerized EEG monitoring. *Electroencephalogr Clin Neurophysiol* 1992;82:239–247.

64. Luders H, Hahn J, Lesser RP, et al. Basal temporal subdural electrodes in the evaluation of patients with intractable epilepsy. *Epilepsia* 1989;30:131–142.

65. Maulsby R, Kellaway P. Transient hypoxic crises in children. In: Kellaway P, Petersen I, eds. *Neurological and electroencephalographic correlative studies in infancy*. New York: Grune & Stratton, 1964:349–360.

66. Mizrahi EM. Electroencephalographic/polygraphic/video monitoring in childhood epilepsy. *J Pediatr* 1984;105:1–9.

67. Mizrahi EM. Pathophysiology of seizures in infancy. *Epilepsia* 1991a;32[Suppl 3]:71–72.

68. Mizrahi EM. Seizures in the first year of life. *Pediatr Res* 1991b;29:362A.

69. Mizrahi EM. Electroencephalographic-video monitoring in neonates, infants, and children. *J Child Neurol* 1994;9[Suppl]:S46–S56.

70. Mizrahi EM. Avoiding the pitfalls of EEG interpretation in childhood epilepsy. *Epilepsia* 1996;37[Suppl 1]:S41–S51.

71. Mizrahi EM, Kellaway P. Characterization and classification of neonatal seizures. *Neurology* 1987;37:1837–1844.

72. Mizrahi EM, Kellaway P. The response of electroclinical neonatal seizures to antiepileptic drug therapy. *Epilepsia* 1992;33[Suppl 3]:S114.

73. Mizrahi EM, Kellaway P. Neonatal electroencephalography. In *Diagnosis and management of neonatal seizures*. New York: Lippincott–Raven Publishers, 1998:99–143.

74. Mizrahi EM, Kellaway P, Grossman RG, et al. Anterior temporal lobectomy and medically refractory temporal lobe epilepsy of childhood. *Epilepsia* 1990;31:302–312.

75. Morris HH, Luders H, Lesser RP, et al. The value of closely spaced scalp electrodes in the localization of epileptiform foci: a study of 26 patients with complex partial seizures. *Electroencephalogr Clin Neurophysiol* 1986;63:107–111.

76. Nordli DR Jr, Bazil CW, Scheuer ML, et al. Recognition and classification of seizures in infants. *Epilepsia* 1997;38:553–560.

77. Ohtsuka Y. Symposium II: West syndrome and its related epileptic syndromes. *Epilepsia* 1998;39[Suppl 5]:30–37.

78. Pacia SV, Jung WJ, Devinsky O. Localization of mesial temporal lobe seizures with sphenoidal electrodes. *J Clin Neurophysiol* 1998;15:256–261.

79. Painter MJ, Scher MS, Stein AD, et al. Phenobarbital compared with phenytoin for the treatment of neonatal seizures. *N Engl J Med* 1999;12:485–489.

80. Prats A, Altman N, Birchansky S, et al. Epilepsy surgery in the first three years of life. *Epilepsia* 1998;39:737–743.

81. Quirk JA, Fish DR, Smith SJ, et al. Incidence of photosensitive epilepsy: a prospective national study. *Electroencephalogr Clin Neurophysiol* 1995;95:260–267.

82. Rowan AJ, Veldhuisen RJ, Nagelkerke NJ. Comparative evaluation of sleep deprivation and sedated sleep EEGs as diagnostic aids in epilepsy. *Electroencephalogr Clin Neurophysiol* 1982;54:357–364.

83. Scher MS, Aso K, Beggarly M, et al. Electrographic seizures in preterm and full-term neonates: clinical correlates, associated brain lesions, and risk for neurologic sequelae. *Pediatrics* 1993;91:128–134.

84. Scher MS, Hamid MY, Steppe DA, et al. Ictal and interictal electrographic seizure durations in preterm and term neonates. *Epilepsia* 1993;34:284–288.

85. Sharbrough FW. Scalp-recorded ictal patterns in focal epilepsy. *J Clin Neurophysiol* 1993;10:262–267.

86. Shields WD, Peacock WJ, Roper SN. Surgery for epilepsy: special pediatric considerations. *Neurosurg Clin North Am* 1993;4:301–310.

87. Sirven JI, Liporace JD, French JA, et al. Seizures in temporal lobe epilepsy: I. Reliability of scalp/sphenoidal ictal recording. *Neurology* 1997;48:1041–1046.

88. Spencer SS. Depth electroencephalography in selection of refractory epilepsy for surgery. *Ann Neurol* 1981;9:207–214.

89. Spencer SS, So NK, Engel J Jr, et al. Depth electrodes. In: Pedley J Jr, ed. *Surgical treatment of the epilepsies*, 2nd ed. New York: Raven Press, 1993:359–376.

90. Spencer SS, Sperling MR, Shewmon DA. Intracranial electrodes. In Engel J Jr, Pedley TA, eds. *Epilepsy: a comprehensive textbook*. Lippincott–Raven Publishers, Philadelphia, 1997:1719–1747.

91. Sperling MR, Mendius JR, Engel J Jr. Mesial temporal spikes: a simultaneous comparison of sphenoidal, nasopharyngeal, and ear electrodes. *Epilepsia* 1986;27:81–86.

92. Uematsu S, Lesser RP, Gordon B. Localization of sensorimotor cortex: the influence of Sherrington and Cushing on the modern concept. *Neurosurgery* 1992;30:904–912.

93. Volpe JJ. Neonatal seizures. *N Engl J Med* 1973;289:413–416.

94. Volpe JJ. Neonatal seizures. In: *Neurology of the newborn*. Philadelphia: WB Sanders, 1995:172–207.

95. Walczak TS, Williams DT, Berten W. Utility and reliability of placebo infusion in the evaluation of patients with seizures. *Neurology* 1994;44:394–399.

96. Watanabe K, Hara K, Miyazaki S, et al. Apneic seizures in the newborn. *Am J Dis Child* 1982;136:980–984.

97. Westmoreland BF. Benign EEG variant and patterns of uncertain clinical significance. In Daly DD, Pedley TA, eds. *Current practice of clinical electroencephalography*, New York: Raven Press, 1990:243–252.

98. Wiggins GC, Elisevich K, Smith BJ. Morbidity and infection in combined subdural grid and strip electrode investigation for intractable epilepsy. *Epilepsy Res* 1999;37:73–80.

99. Wieser HG. Seizure induction in reflex seizures and reflex epilepsy. *Adv Neurol* 1998;75:69–85.

100. Wieser HG, Elger CE, Stodieck SR. The foramen ovale electrode': a new recording method for the preoperative evaluation of patients suffering from mesio-basal temporal lobe epilepsy. *Electroencephalogr Clin Neurophysiol* 1985;61:314–322.

101. Willis J, Gould JB. Periodic alpha seizures with apnea in a newborn. *Dev Med Child Neurol* 1980;22:214–222.

102. Wise MS. Parasomnias in children. *Pediatr Ann* 1997;26:427–433.

103. Wyler AR, Ojemann GA, Lettich E, et al. Subdural strip electrodes for localizing epileptogenic foci. *J Neurosurg* 1984;60:1195–1200.

104. Wyler AR, Walker G, Richey ET, et al. Chronic subdural strip recordings for difficult epileptic problems. *J Epilepsy* 1988;1:71–78.

105. Wyler AR, Wilkus RJ, Blume WT. Strip electrodes. In: Pedley J Jr, ed. *Surgical treatment of the epilepsies*, 2nd ed. New York: Raven Press, 1993:387–97.

106. Wyllie E, Comair YG, Kotagal P, et al. Epilepsy surgery in infants. *Epilepsia* 1996;37:625–637.

107. Wyllie E, Friedman D, Rothner AD, et al. Psychogenic seizures in children and adolescents: outcome after diagnosis by ictal video and electroencephalographic recording. *Pediatrics* 1990;85:480–484.

108. Zifkin BG. Some considerations in the intensive electroencephalographic investigation of reflex epilepsy. *Adv Neurol* 1998;75:93–97.

Chapter 19

Ambulatory EEG Monitoring

John S. Ebersole, Donald L. Schomer, and John R. Ives

Ambulatory EEG was developed to fill the diagnostic gap that exists between routine electroencephalography (EEG) and intensive inpatient monitoring in the evaluation of paroxysmal disorders. The brief EEG provided by standard laboratory studies is not well suited to the identification of abnormalities that are infrequent, such as interictal spikes and, in particular, seizures. Prior research indicated that a single 30-minute EEG without sleep deprivation identifies abnormalities in about 50% of patients with epilepsy (1). Sleep deprivation, pharmacological sleep induction, and repeated EEG studies may increase the sensitivity to 70%–85% (1). The remaining patients with unexplained clinical events will not have abnormalities on EEG to support a clinical diagnosis. For this reason, inpatient epilepsy monitoring units evolved to provide long-term EEG recording. Despite widespread acclaim for this form of evaluation, there remain the inherent disadvantages of hospitalization, restricted patient mobility, insufficient availability, and expense. The need continues for a more convenient, mobile, readily available, and less expensive means of obtaining long-term EEG data.

HISTORICAL PERSPECTIVE

The concept of prolonged monitoring of physiological data on mobile patients by means of a portable tape recorder was first introduced by Holter (51) in the electrocardiographic (ECG) evaluation of arrhythmias. This scheme was not immediately applicable to EEG, because the early recorders were limited to one channel, the EEG signals required considerable additional amplification, and there was no efficient method for analyzing the data once recorded. When a four-channel miniature cassette recorder became available (77), Ives and Wood showed that recording EEG on it was feasible (61). Development of a solid-state, on-head preamplifier chip solved the second problem (88), and the introduction of a rapid video–audio playback device solved the last (105). Complete four-channel ambulatory cassette systems were commercially available by 1979. Four-channel cassette recorders were standard analog devices utilizing four recording heads. Tape speed was reduced to approximately 2 mm per second so that a standard C120 cassette could record at least 24 hours of continuous EEG. Recorders weighed approximately 1.5 pounds and were easily worn by belt or strap on most patients, including small children. Paginated rapid video playback was the conceptual breakthrough that made efficient analysis of long-term ambulatory cassette tape recordings practical. The first playback units incorporated a video display of data at selectable page lengths and speeds of replay, plus a simultaneous audio reproduction of the EEG data. At the fastest replay speed, 60 times real time, 24 hours of recording could be reviewed in 24 minutes.

In 1983, a cassette system capable of recording eight channels of continuous EEG, as well as digital real time and event markers, came on the market (26,96). A new recording method called "blocked analog" was developed in order to record eight channels of physiological data plus real digital time and events on 1/8th-inch tape. The size of the early eight-channel recorders was only slightly larger than the four-channel version. The eight-channel playback units provided not only a means of displaying additional physiological data, but also a number of improved operational features.

In 1988, a personal computer (PC)–based replay system made its debut, and 16-channel continuous EEG recordings became possible by electronically linking two cassette recorders. The development in 1996 of a 17-channel continuous recorder was made possible with the use of large-capacity removable hard drives originally designed for notebook computers. With this new recorder, 16 channels of EEG and 1 channel of ECG could be recorded for 24 hours (at a 200-Hz sampling rate). Montage reformatting was possible during replay. EEG analysis could be performed by rapid video review, audio transformation of signals from selected channels (up to 120 times real time), or off-line, computer-assisted spike-and-seizure detection.

Several different 24- to 32-channel continuous recorders have since been introduced that use either miniature hard drives or flash memory technology. Various schemes have been devised for analyzing the data. Most systems use off-line spike-and-seizure detection software. Direct, on-line patient monitoring is now also possible with some systems. Isolation electronics built into the replay unit allow the ongoing EEGs of patients who are attached to recorders to be displayed on the replay screen as scrolling waveforms. Alternatively, an optional laptop computer has also been configured to serve as a display of ongoing EEG. Several systems also have the capability of displaying, editing, and analyzing (either manually or automatically) polysomnographic data, including oximetry.

Ambulatory EEG also developed along another line, namely the discontinuous or epoch recorder. The original concept in this evolution was that more channels could be recorded at a higher sampling rate if only discrete epochs of EEG were recorded rather than continuous data. Ives introduced the first such recorder in 1982 (53). The recorder was like a commercial Walkman and used standard tape speed in order to achieve the frequency response necessary to record faithfully 16 multiplexed channels. The recording was done in selectable periodic epochs, such as 15 seconds every 10 minutes over 24 hours, or the recorder could be turned on by a push button that the patient activated when he or she experienced a spell. An electronic buffer memory allowed recording of the EEG prior to the button push. Approximately 45 minutes of EEG could be recorded on a tape. Both the amplifiers and the multiplexing device were incorporated into one small box that was usually worn on the patient's head and secured by a gauze turban. The 16-channel epoch recorder did not use a video playback device; instead the recorded epochs were transcribed onto paper in real time. Analysis was like that of standard EEG.

Many of the deficiencies of intermittent and push-button EEG sampling were overcome by linking the epoch recorder to a portable computer (54). This device monitored the ongoing EEG and used spike-and-seizure detection programs to identify segments of abnormal EEG that were stored to its hard drive. Although these computers were portable, they were not truly ambulatory because they required mains power. They were appropriate for use in a setting where the patient moved only a limited distance, such as from bed to chair.

Presently, the most common discontinuous system records 16 channels of EEG and 2 channels of other physiological parameters, such as ECG, electromyography (EMG), and electro-oculography (EOG). Up to 15 hours of data can be recorded on the attached portable computer. This includes push-button actuations (with 2 minutes recorded before and after the button push), periodic sampling, and spike-and-seizure detections. The EEG is recorded in one of three bipolar montages, including a standard "double banana" montage. These systems can also be configured with more polygraphic channels, in lieu of EEG channels, in order to record polysomnographic data. Data are routinely printed out on a laser printer and reviewed like standard EEG or burned on a compact disk for review with EEG display software on any PC. An enhanced version of this 18-channel recorder has

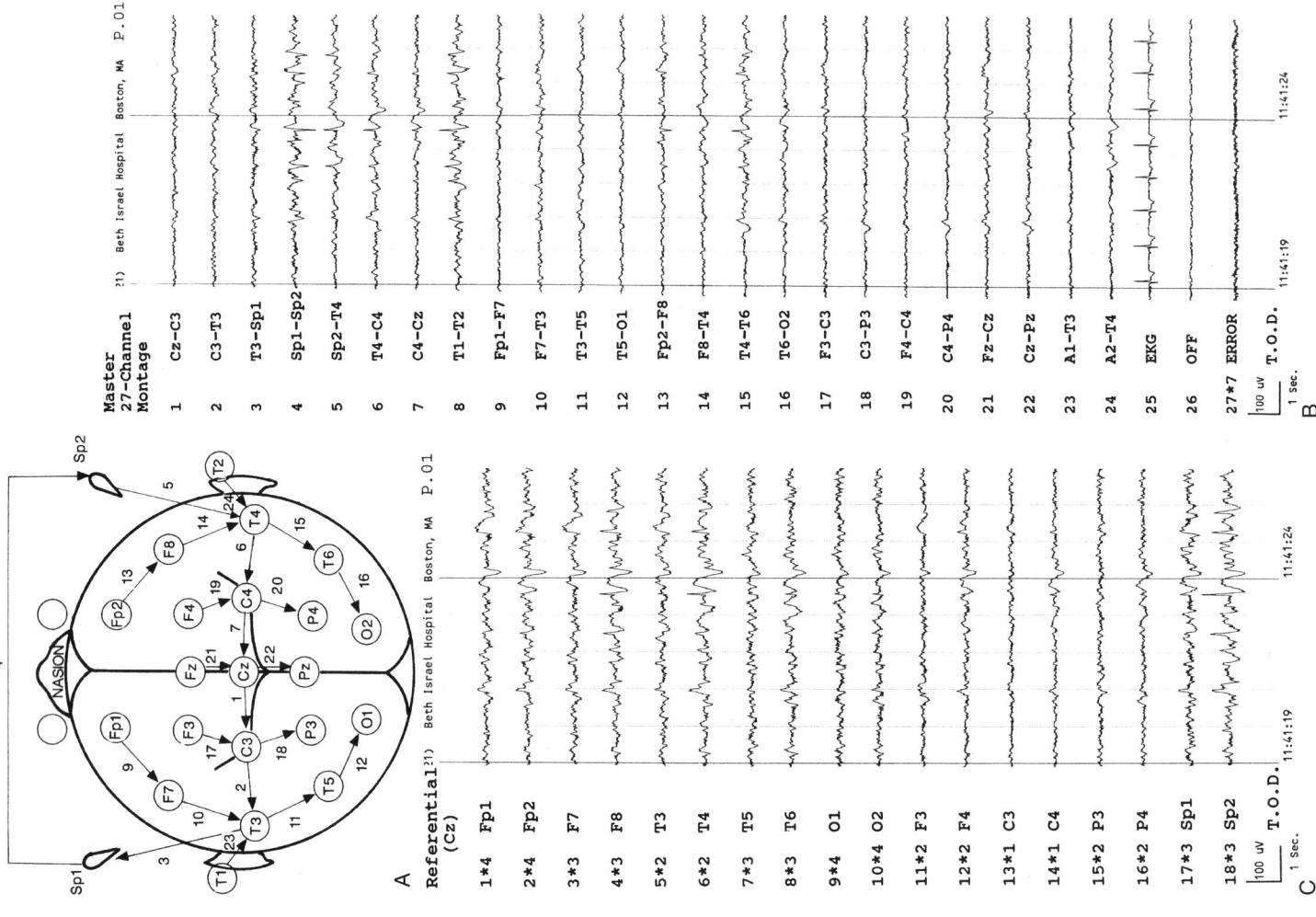

**Master
27-Channel
Montage**

1   Cz–C3
2   C3–T3
3   T3–Sp1
4   Sp1–Sp2
5   Sp2–T4
6   T4–C4
7   C4–Cz
8   T1–T2
9   Fp1–F7
10 F7–T3
11 T3–T5
12 T5–O1
13 Fp2–F8
14 F8–T4
15 T4–T6
16 T6–O2
17 F3–C3
18 C3–P3
19 F4–C4
20 C4–P4
21 Fz–Cz
22 Cz–Pz
23 A1–T3
24 A2–T4
25 EKG
26 OFF
27*7 ERROR

B

11:41:24   11:41:19

?1)   Beth Israel Hospital   Boston, MA   P.01

100 uV   1 Sec.   T.O.D.

A

Referential?1)   Beth Israel Hospital   Boston, MA   P.01
(Cz)

1*4 Fp1
2*4 Fp2
3*3 F7
4*3 F8
5*2 T3
6*2 T4
7*3 T5
8*3 T6
9*4 O1
10*4 O2
11*2 F3
12*2 F4
13*1 C3
14*1 C4
15*2 P3
16*2 P4
17*3 Sp1
18*3 Sp2

C

T.O.D.   11:41:19   11:41:24

100 uV   1 Sec.

been developed that contains within the waist-worn recorder sufficient computing power to perform the spike-and-seizure detection. It is no longer necessary to attach the recorder to a portable computer in order to obtain online EEG analysis. Discontinuous recorders of 27 and 32 channels have also been developed. They offer the possibility of remontaging the output using referential reconstruction from bipolar recordings (Fig. 19.1) (57). The 27- and 32-channel systems include all of the standard electrodes in the 10-20 system plus two basal temporal electrodes (55,58–60). Built-in, on-line spike-and-seizure detection is currently being implemented in these recorders also. Most recently, a digital video recording system with a wide-angle lens has been added to this line of discontinuous recorders. It is synchronized to the recorder to provide on-line monitoring of behavior just as with inpatient monitoring.

It is clear that these two lines of ambulatory recording technology are converging. Given recent increases in the capacity of digital storage devices and decreases in their size and power consumption, continuous recording of 24 or more hours of 24–32 channels of EEG is now reality. A similar evolution of central processing units soon will allow simultaneous on-line spike-and-seizure detection to be done routinely within the confines of a small, truly ambulatory recorder. With these future devices, both detections and their continuous EEG record will be available at the end of a recording session, as is currently the case with inpatient monitoring units. At this point there will be essentially no difference between inpatient and outpatient monitoring technology for EEG. Only greater channel numbers (e.g., 64–128 channels) will differentiate the two.

TECHNICAL ASPECTS OF AMBULATORY RECORDINGS

One of the advantages of ambulatory EEG is that long-term recordings can be obtained without the need for continuous supervision by technical personnel. However, this also means that electrode problems or mechanical failures can go undetected until after the monitoring session. For this reason, proper application of electrodes and faithful maintenance of recorders are of critical importance in minimizing the number of technically inadequate recordings (18).

Application of disk electrodes by collodion technique is currently the only method that will ensure stable long-term recordings. For emergency recordings of several hours' duration on nonambulatory inpatients, self-adhering "stick-on" electrodes, such as those commonly used for nerve conduction studies or pediatric ECG recordings, have been shown to be useful when employed in a subhairline montage (13,29); however, these electrodes are not secure enough for ambulatory outpatients. For outpatients, as well as for most inpatients, it is both convenient and worthwhile to continue the recording for at least 24 hours, including an overnight sleep period. For continuous recorders, battery and/or tape changes are usually needed every 24 hours. Discontinuous recorders commonly run unattended for 48–72 hours.

FIG. 19.1. A: The montage wiring diagram for the master 27-channel system. All of the 10-20–based electrodes are incorporated into a remontageable bipolar array. The Sp1-Sp2 contacts are for additional basal electrode recording and can use any of the standard electrodes employed for that purpose. Channel 8 is dedicated to the monitoring of horizontal eye movements. Channel 25, likewise, is for the monitoring of the cardiac rhythm. Channel 26 is shown as shorted but can be wired for additional noncerebral recordings such as the blood oxygen saturation levels (SPO_2). **B:** Playback of an 8-second epoch of EEG displaying all 27 channels. The time of day (*T.O.D.*) is shown along the bottom margin of the paper along with the 1-second marker and the voltage display. **C:** This remontaged display shows 18 channels of EEG for the same 8-second epoch. Each channel is mathematically recalculated so that it is referenced to the Cz electrode. (From Shomer DL, Ives JR, Schachter SC. The role of ambulatory EEG in the evaluation of patients for epilepsy surgery. *J Clin Neurophysiol* 1999;16:116–129, with permission.)

In hospitals, the conveniences of ambulatory EEG recording can be combined with portable video recording to create a mobile intensive monitoring system. Combined ambulatory EEG and video recording of outpatients can similarly be accomplished in physician's offices, in hotel rooms, or at home, so that the inconvenience and expense of hospitalization can be avoided. The only technical necessity is that the EEG and video recordings must be synchronized so that temporal correlations can be made. This is most easily accomplished by adding the same time code to each recording. Both continuous and discontinuous ambulatory recording systems now offer this option.

The design of the recording montage was particularly important with four- and eight-channel ambulatory systems. Montages had to maximize the likelihood of detecting abnormal EEG features and to display the data in a pattern that was conducive to perception of these abnormalities on rapid video playback. Standard EEG montages are commonly used with recorders of 16 or more channels, particularly those with remontaging capability. An increased number of recording channels improved the localization and characterization of interictal and ictal features more than it did detection probability. Figures 19.2 through 19.5 illustrate the same EEG abnormalities viewed with ambulatory EEG montages of 3, 8, 16, and 26 channels.

Discontinuous ambulatory EEGs are sometimes printed out on paper. Such printouts do not have the same flexibility as EEGs reviewed on a computer screen because gain, filters, and montages cannot be changed to assist in interpretation. Most computer-based EEG replay units offer a variable display gain, simulating sensitivities that are comparable to those of routine EEG. Sensitivity should be varied during playback as required to view ongoing activity clearly. This means using a lower gain during active wakefulness and deep sleep to reduce the visual clutter of high-amplitude artifacts and sleep complexes, respectively, and using a more normal gain during quiet wakefulness and light or rapid-eye-movement (REM) sleep. A rapid review speed of 40–120 times real time may be used in scanning for ictal events. Such high rates of review are not recommended for detecting isolated interictal discharges. Slower scanning rates of 10–40 times real time are more appropriate for perceiving isolated and focal events.

Listening to an audio transformation of ongoing EEG channels can be very useful for detecting abnormalities (24). Seizures, interictal discharges, and various normal transients and artifacts all have characteristic sounds that can be used for event detection and differentiation. Stereo aural monitoring of the EEG from the left versus the right hemisphere further enhances detections. When deriving an audio output with a channel mixer, one should include only every other channel of a linked montage in order to avoid audio cancellation of phase-reversed activity coming principally from one electrode.

Analysis of ambulatory EEG during active wakefulness should be aimed principally at the detection of seizures (see Fig. 19.4). Individual epileptiform transients, even if present, are difficult to recognize or differentiate during periods when activity artifacts are common. The exception may be prominent generalized interictal discharges. Stages 1–3 of sleep, when artifacts are minimal, are the most reliable and productive periods to identify interictal epileptiform abnormalities. Both discontinuous and continuous recording systems have become increasingly dependent on spike-and-seizure detection software, developed originally for long-term monitoring to screen the massive amount of accumulated EEG data for epileptiform abnormalities. Most systems employ variations of the algorithms developed by Gotman and colleagues (43,45–47). More recent investigations have shown that a properly prepared neural network can identify seizures better than standard software detectors, but not as well as traditional video–audio review of the data (41,42).

INDICATIONS FOR AMBULATORY EEG

Generalized Epilepsies

Ambulatory EEG has been most useful in the evaluation of seizure disorders (22,23,25,28). Many of the early investigative efforts were directed at the generalized epilepsies because the electrographic patterns of the abnormalities were distinctive and thus easily recognized even with a reduced number of channels (see Fig. 19.2*A*). Furthermore, in the case of absence seizures, the behavioral manifestations of the seizures were so minimal that ambulatory recordings provided a very convenient way of identifying and quantifying the discharges over a long period. Baseline seizure frequency, circadian or intraday patterns, effects of environmental factors, and changes in medications could be documented in a way far more accurate than by counting clinical seizures.

Numerous clinical reports began appearing in the literature soon after ambulatory EEG equipment became available. Most attested to the usefulness of ambulatory EEG in the differential diagnosis of epilepsy (16,20,49,56,86,92,93,104,111), particularly 3-Hz spike-and-wave or generalized tonic–clonic ictal episodes (90). Objective measurement of drug efficacy in reducing the frequency of interictal and ictal discharges was also

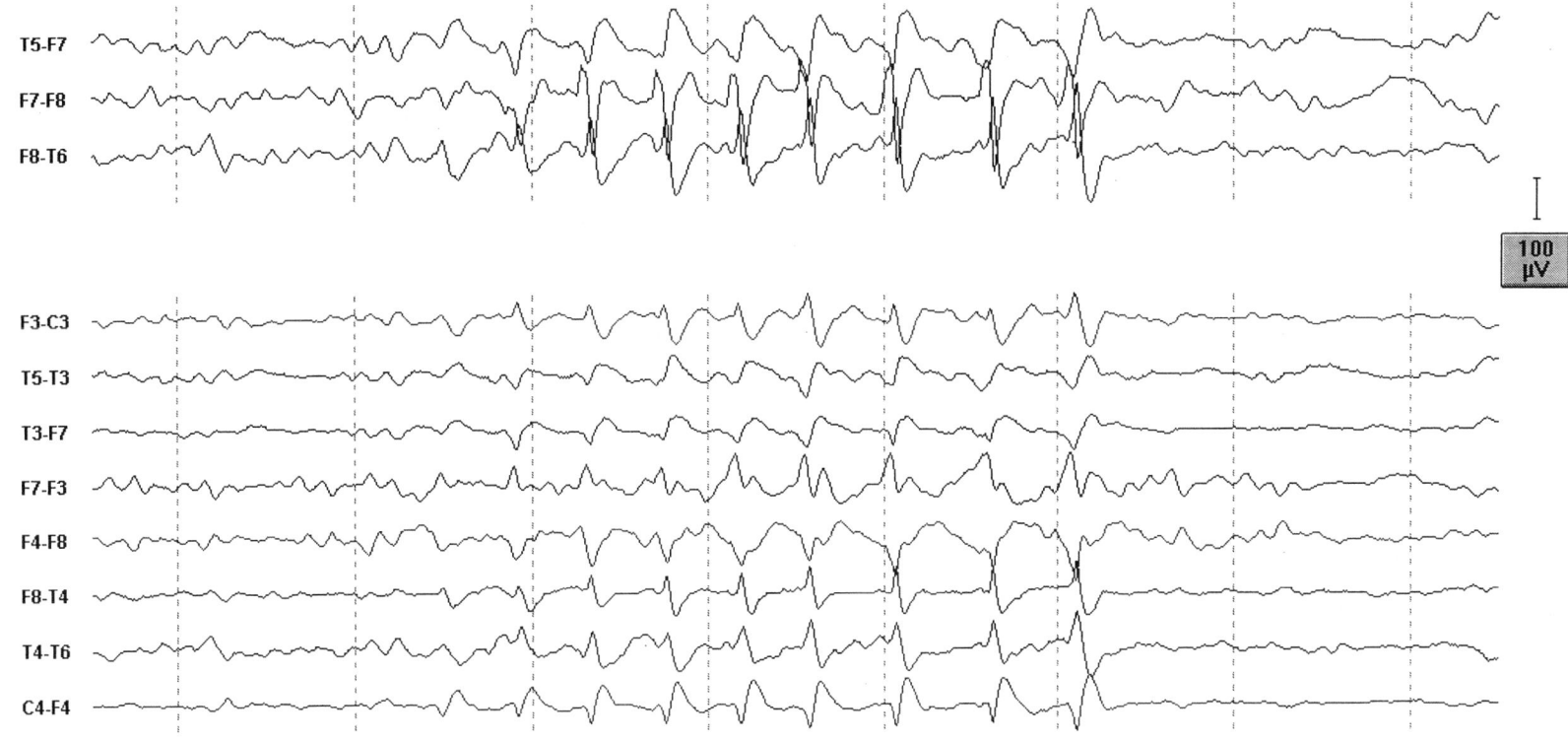

FIG. 19.2. Two-hertz bifrontal spike-and-wave discharges are depicted in 3-channel and 8-channel ambulatory EEG montages **(A)** as well as in 16-channel longitudinal bipolar **(B)** and 26-channel average reference **(C)** montages. Reduced channel number prevents accurate localization of frontopolar spike maxima in ambulatory EEG montages, but identification of the abnormality is easily accomplished with all montages. *(Figure continues.)*

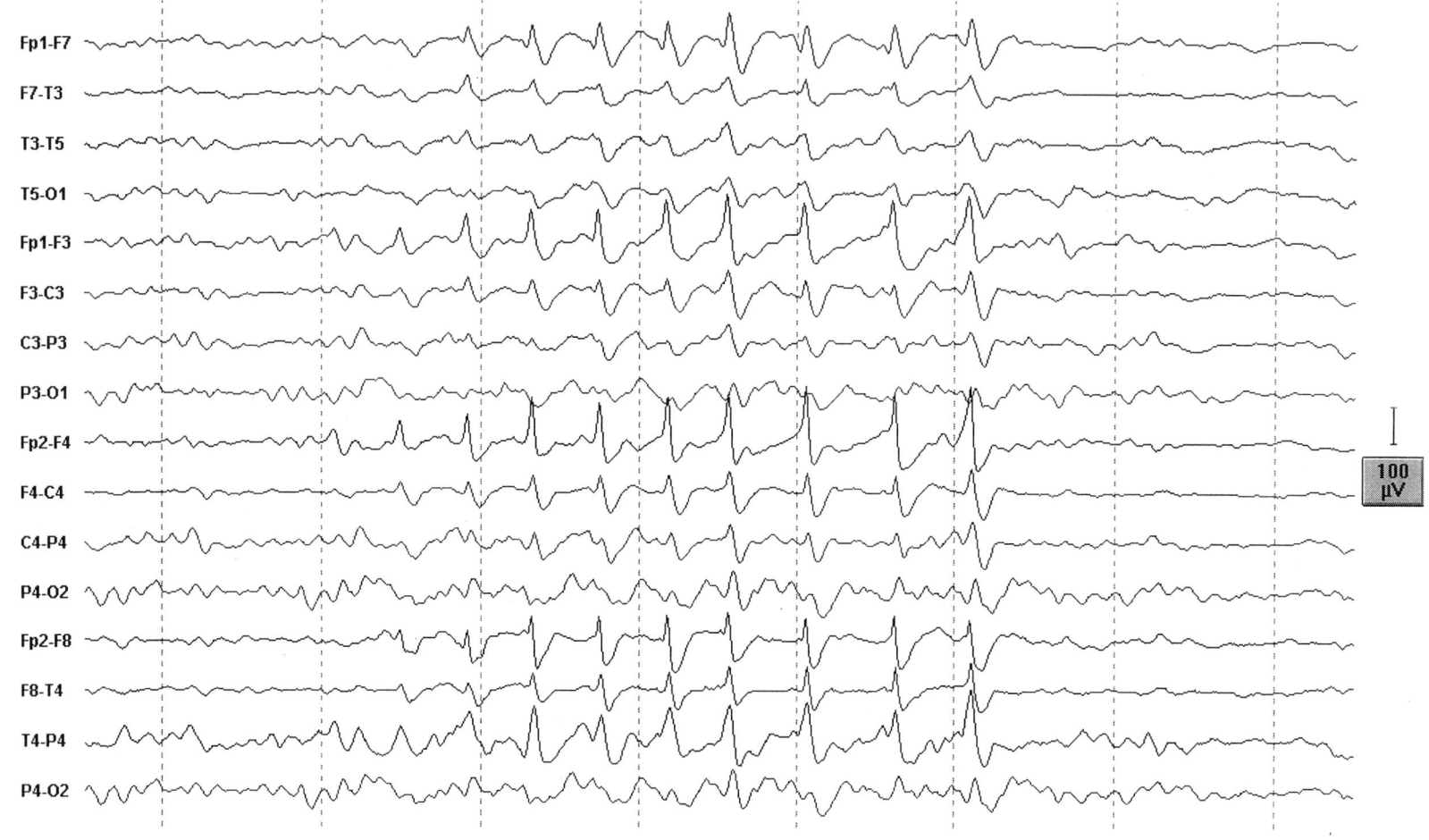

B

FIG. 19.2. *Continued.*

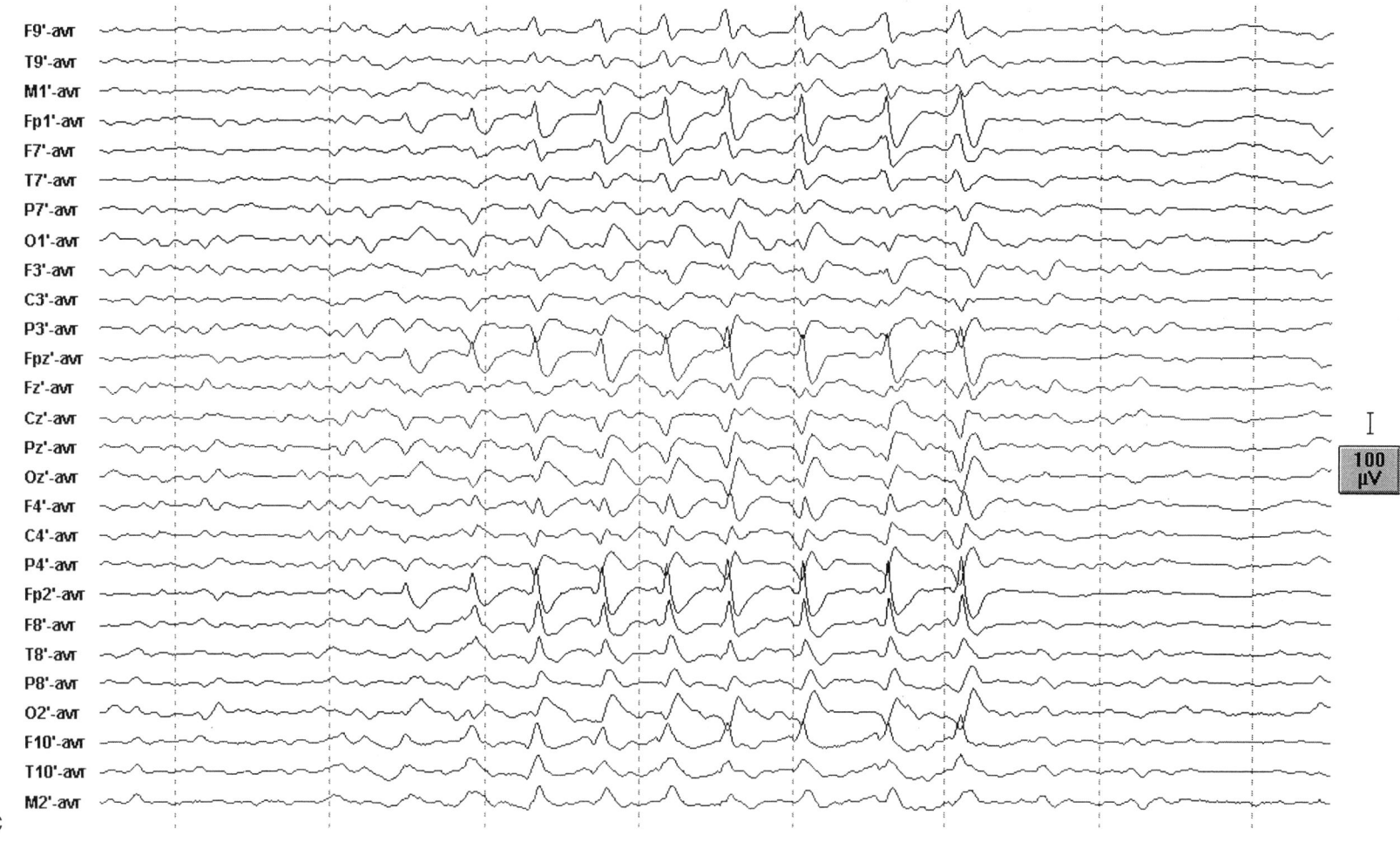

C

FIG. 19.2. *Continued.*

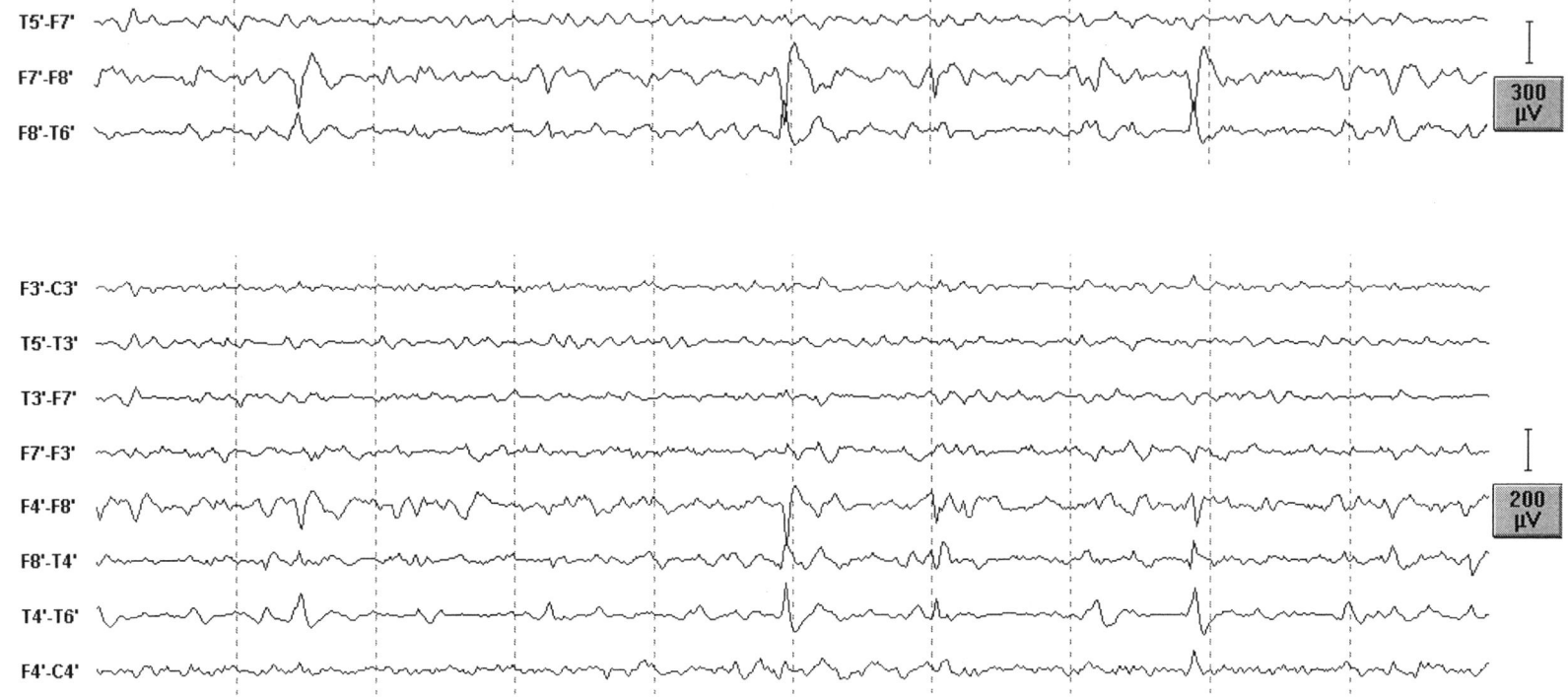

A

FIG. 19.3. Right anterior temporal spikes are depicted in 3-channel and 8-channel ambulatory EEG montages **(A)** as well as in 16-channel longitudinal bipolar **(B)** and 26-channel average reference **(C)** montages. F8 phase reversals in all the bipolar montages, including the 3- and 8-channel ambulatory arrays, easily identify the abnormality. The 26-channel common average reference montage reveals that the spike negative maximum is more inferior and includes electrodes F10 and T10. *(Figure continues.)*

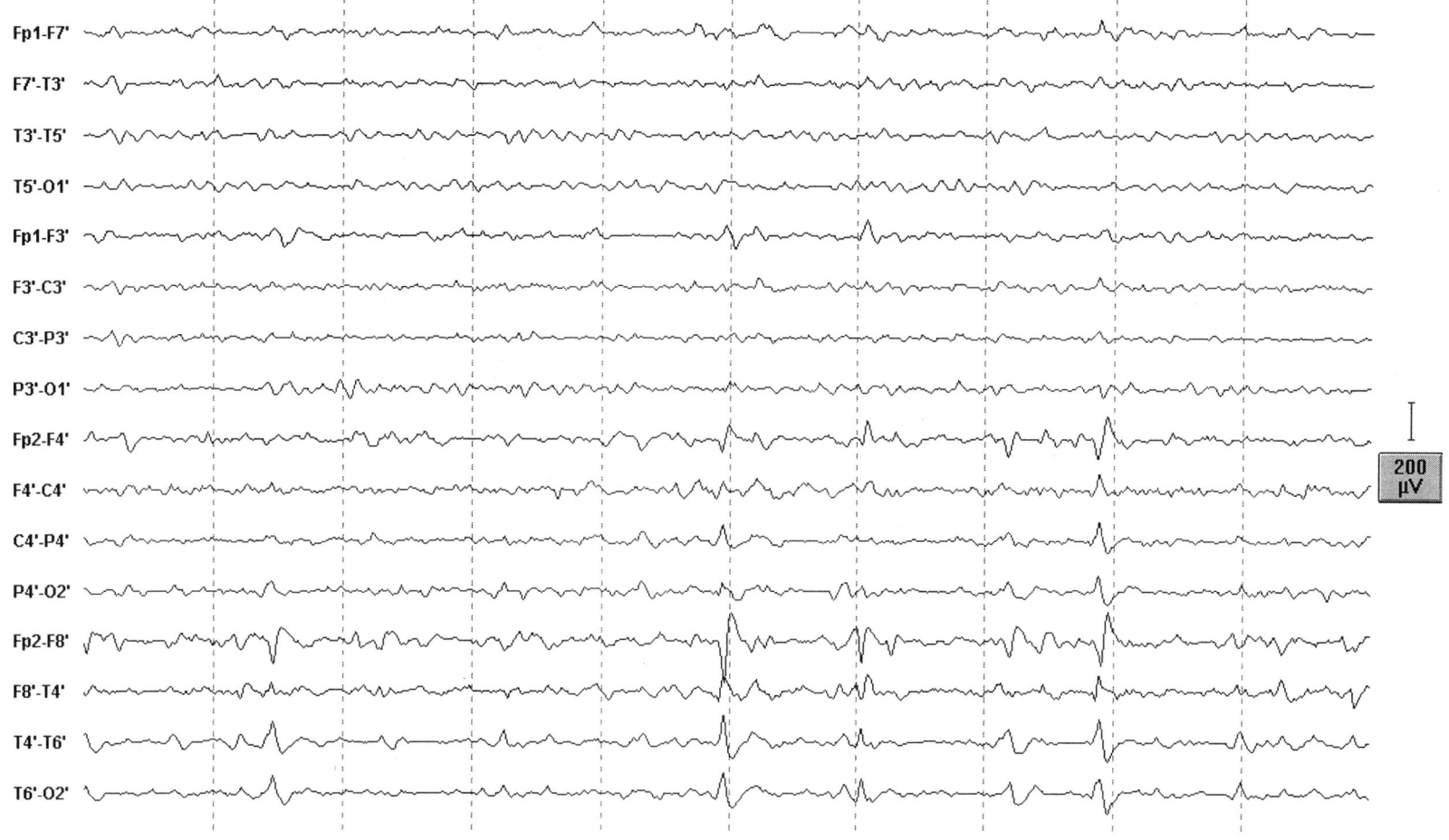

B

FIG. 19.3. *Continued.*

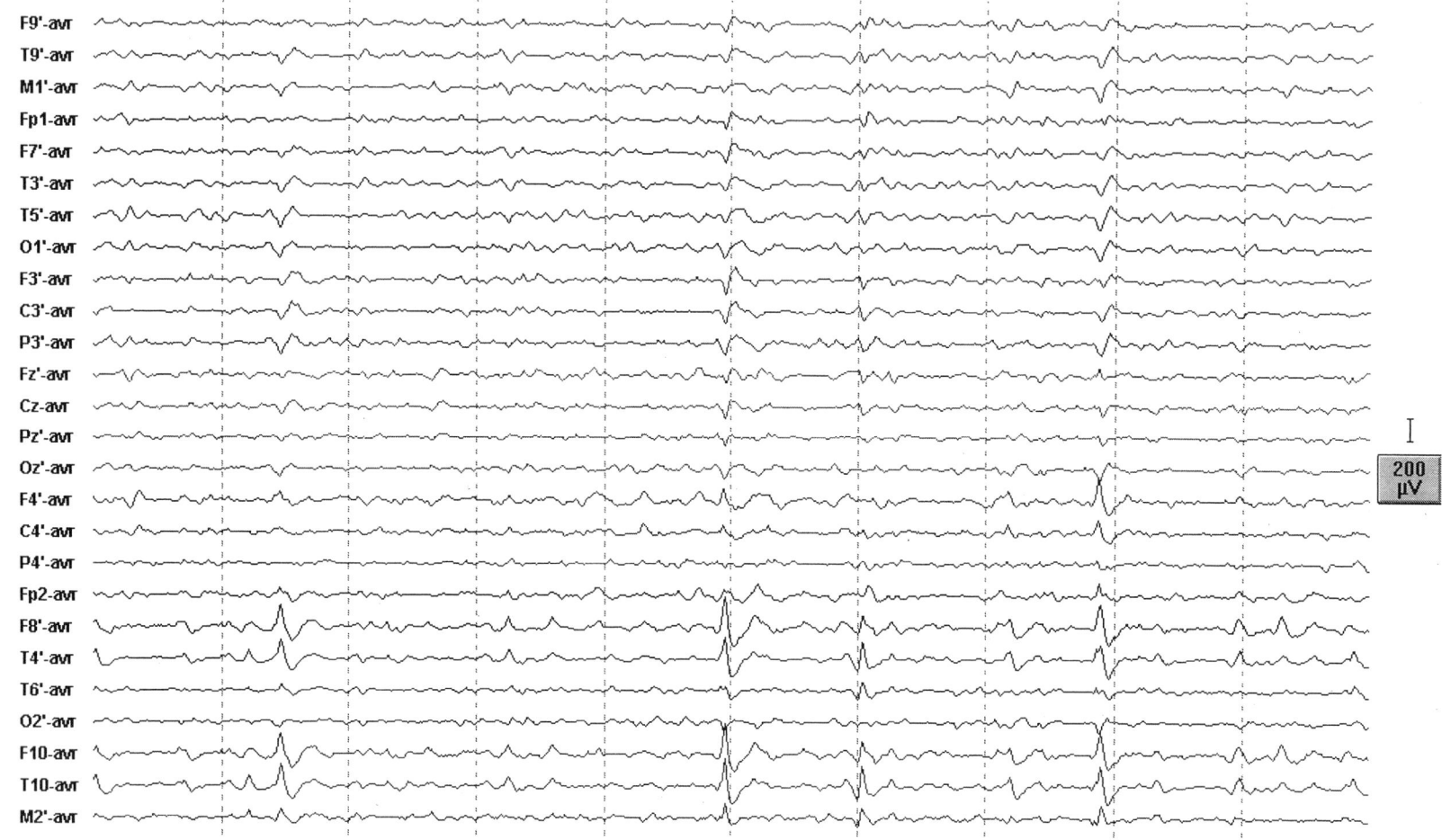

FIG. 19.3. *Continued.*

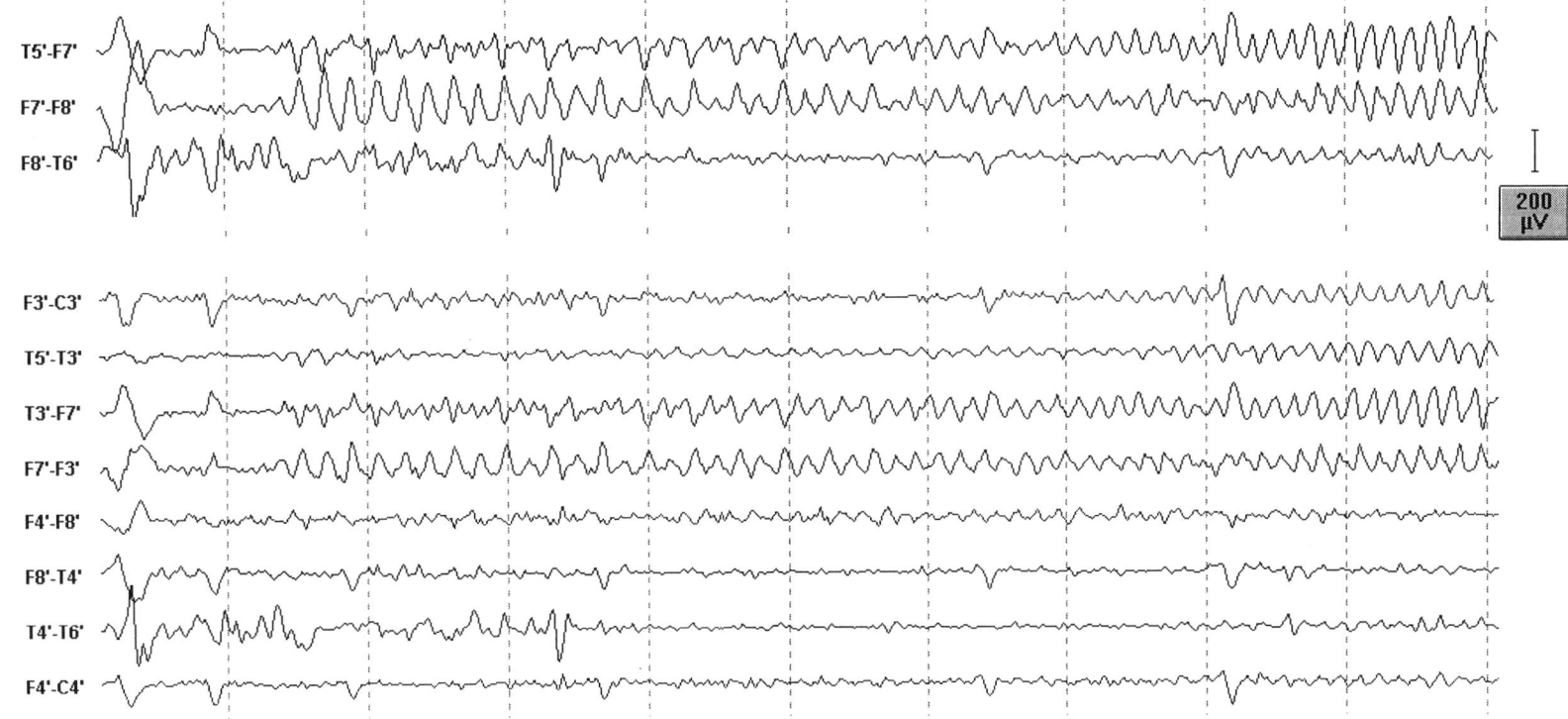

FIG. 19.4. A left anterior temporal seizure is depicted in 3-channel and 8-channel ambulatory EEG montages **(A)** as well as in 16-channel longitudinal bipolar **(B)** and 26-channel average reference 1 **(C)** montages. Anterior temporal location of the seizure is identifiable with all montages. Broad-field ictal discharge makes phase reversals less distinct at seizure onset with bipolar montages that have standard interelectrode distances (8 and 16 channels). Phase differences among temporal channels in these bipolar montages produce a "sham" 11-Hz frequency rhythm that is not apparent in the 26-channel common average reference display. *(Figure continues.)*

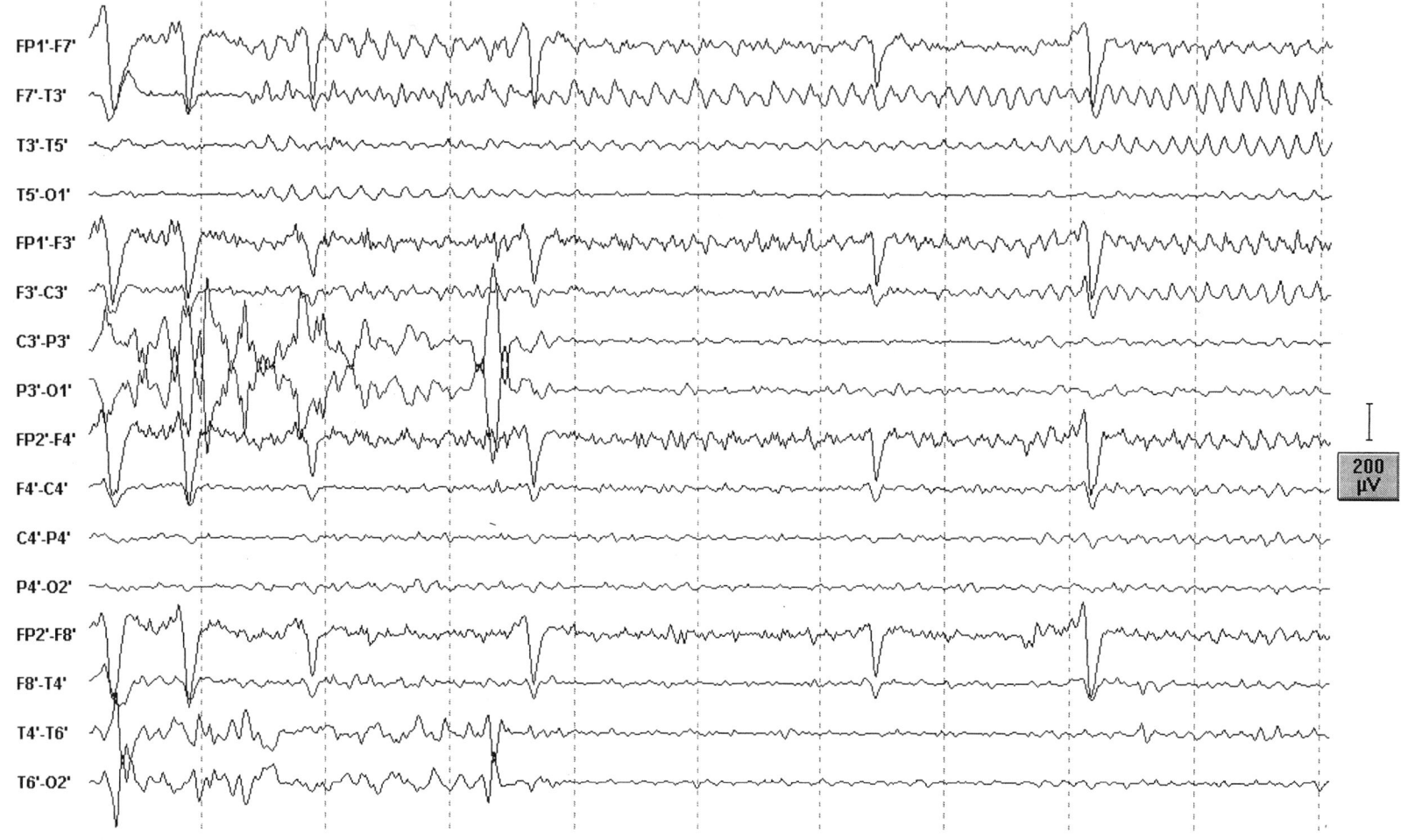

FIG. 19.4. *Continued.*

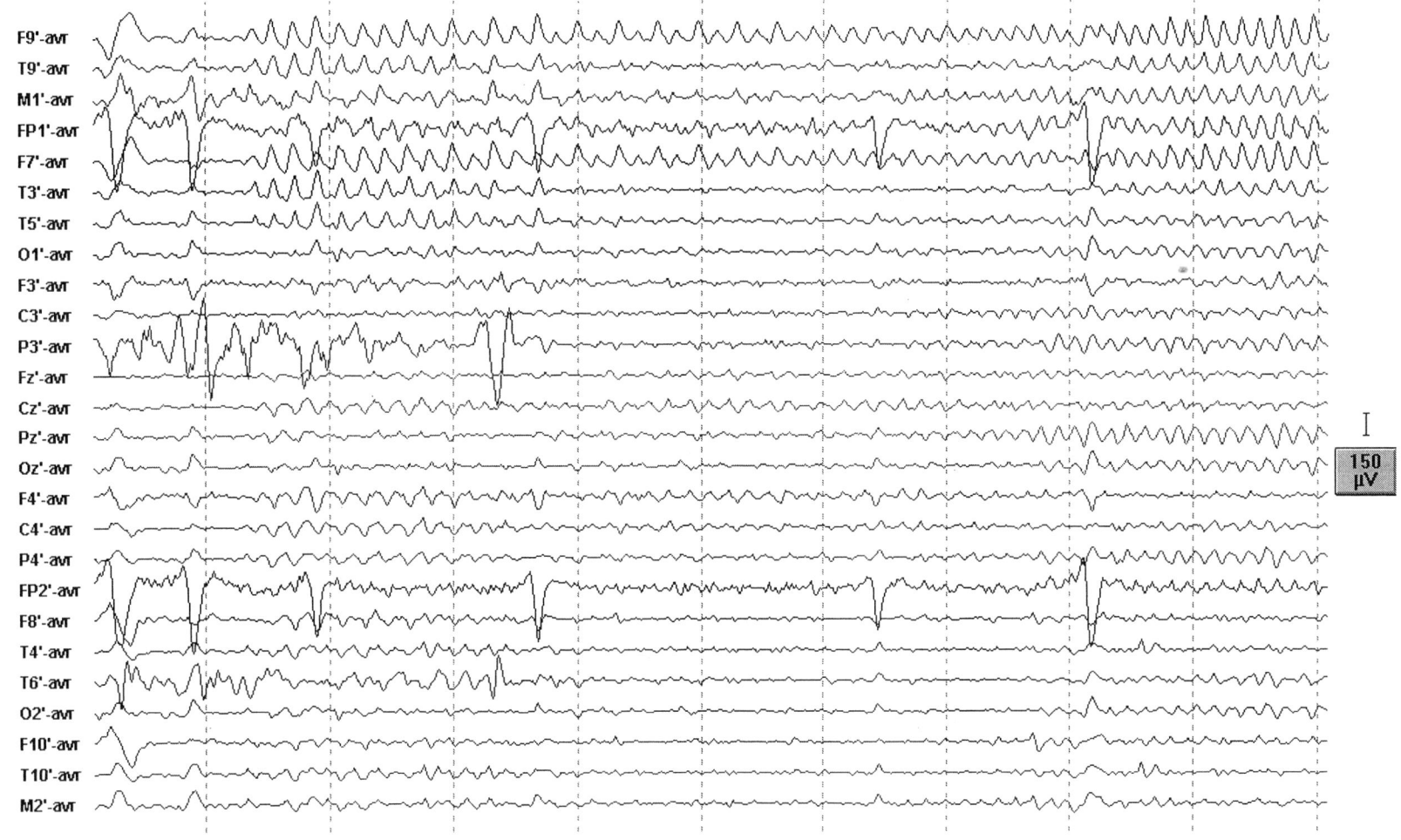

FIG. 19.4. *Continued.*

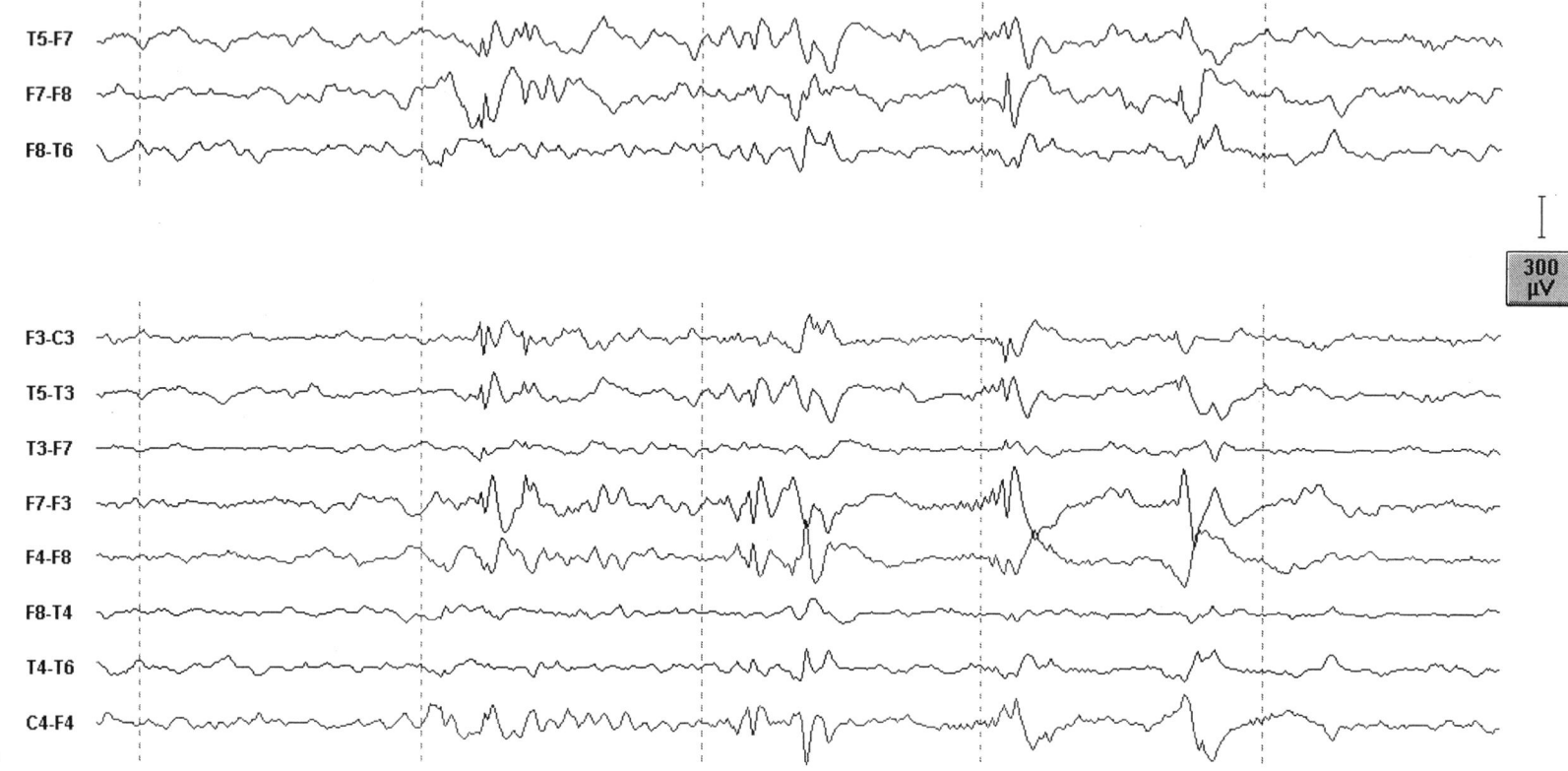

FIG. 19.5. Right frontocentral spikes are depicted in 3-channel and 8-channel ambulatory EEG montages **(A)** as well as in 16-channel longitudinal bipolar **(B)** and 26-channel average reference **(C)** montages. These spikes are not well defined with the 3-channel montage, and localization is difficult with the 8-channel montage. The variability of spike maximum is easiest to appreciate in the 26-channel common average reference montage. Complex phase reversals make this more difficult with the 16-channel bipolar montage. *(Figure continues.)*

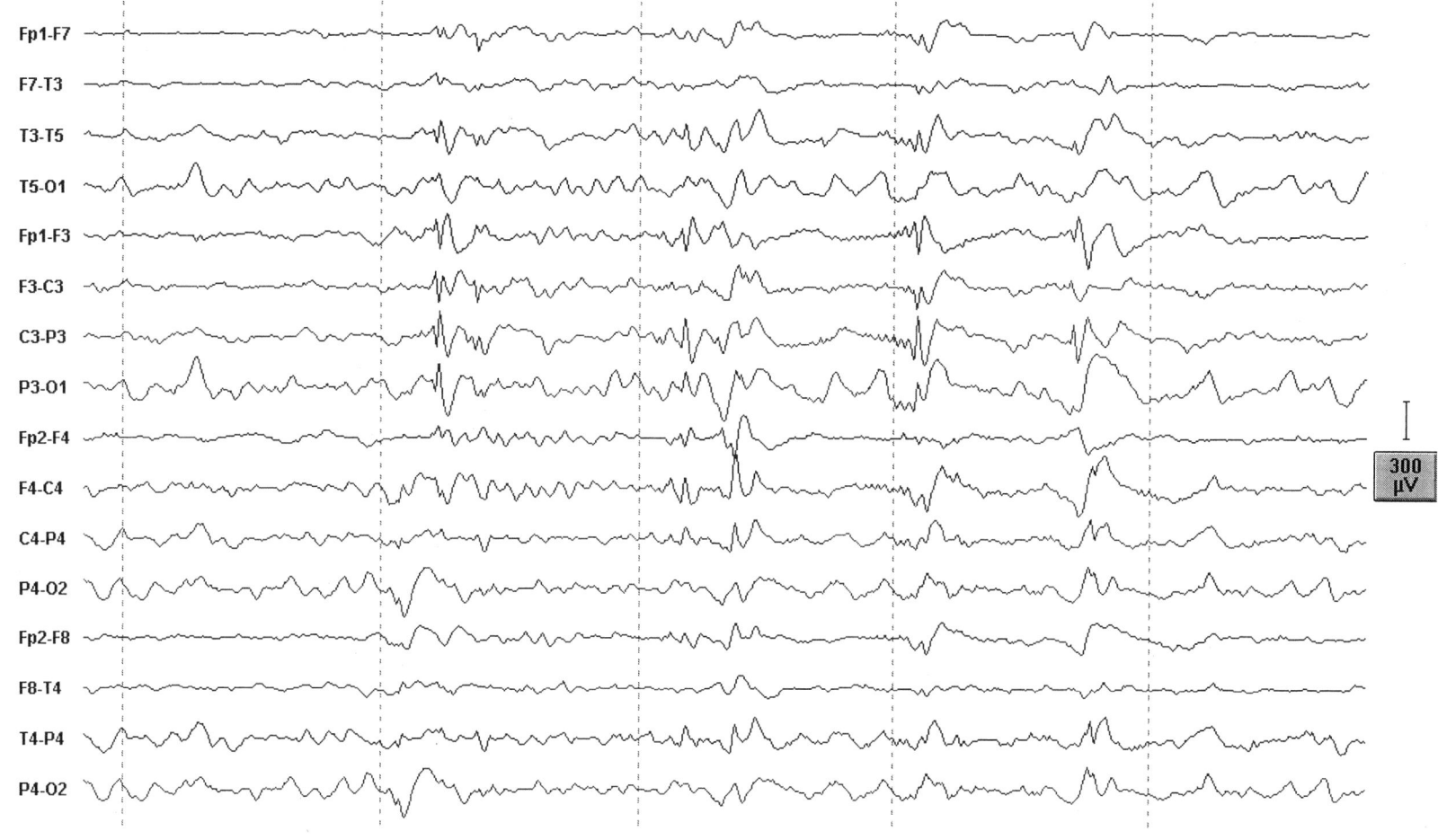

FIG. 19.5. *Continued.*

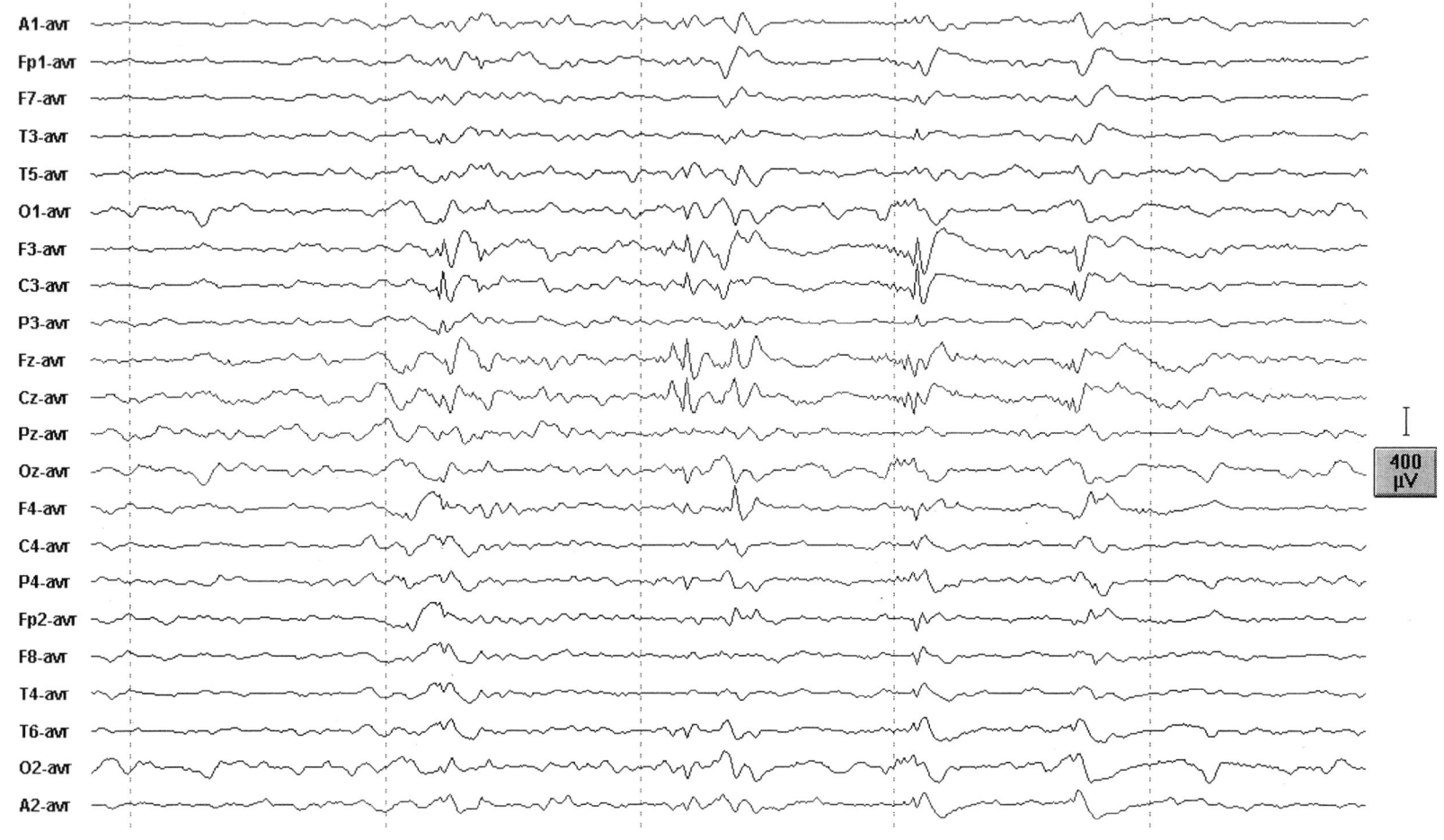

FIG. 19.5. *Continued.*

shown to be feasible (81,102). In nearly all the above studies, improved diagnostic yield over routine EEG recordings was reported. The regular and rhythmic patterns of the generalized epilepsies were also the most promising place to attempt to develop automated means of analyzing recorded data. Generalized spike-and-wave discharges are to date the most common epileptiform features that have been identified and quantitated by automated means (Fig. 19.6) (7,15,44,69,89,107,109,110).

Partial Epilepsies

Many of the patients who would logically be referred for ambulatory EEG because they possess an atypical history and a normal or equivocal routine EEG are likely to have complex partial seizures. Ives and Woods

demonstrated with only four EEG channels the feasibility of cassette monitoring for the lateralized ictal discharges of partial seizures (62). Ebersole and Leroy (30,31,72) later developed ambulatory EEG montages that were designed specifically to maximize the detection of the most common focal, as well as generalized, epileptiform features. They demonstrated that 24 hours of ambulatory EEG could provide identification of most focal (79%) and all generalized interictal abnormalities that were noted on simultaneous eight-channel long-term monitoring, which was the norm at that time. When performed before 4 days of long-term monitoring, 24 hours of ambulatory EEG identified 83% of interictal and ictal abnormalities later found by inpatient EEG recording (12). This diagnostic yield was 2.5 times that of previous routine EEG. The greatest advantage of intensive inpatient monitoring over ambulatory EEG was not its EEG

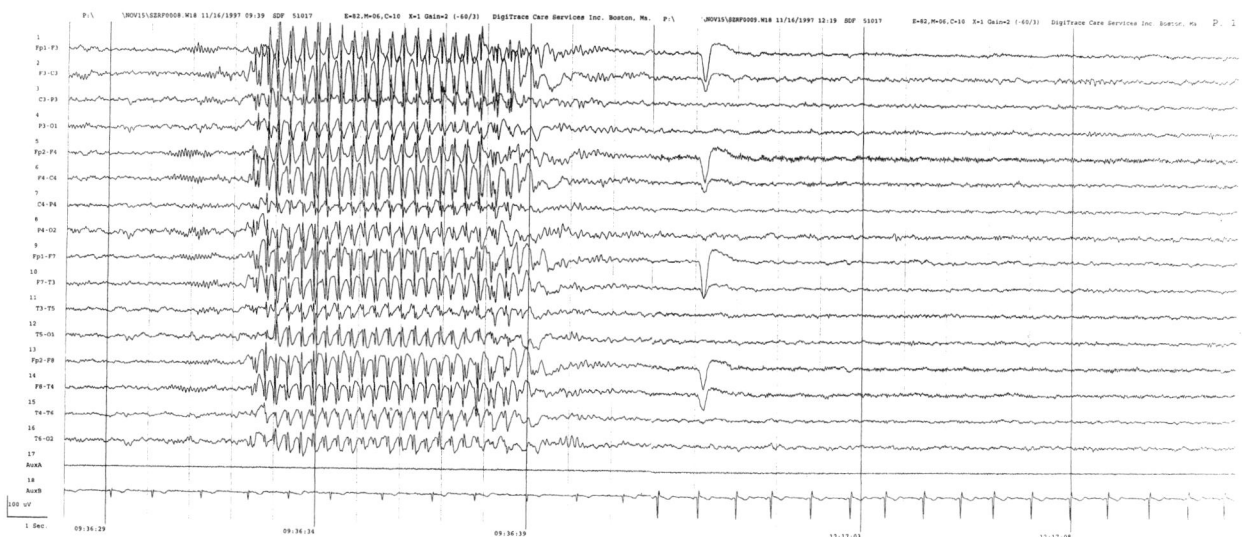

FIG. 19.6. This SZRF***.W18 file represents an automatic seizure detection. In this case, the patient suffered from juvenile absence epilepsy. She had recently experienced a recurrence of events and had undergone a medication change. At the time of this recording, she had rare clinical seizures but was having difficulty with school performance. The tracing did capture silent seizures such as the one shown here. However, extremely few events were detected and no clinically symptomatic events were recorded. This led the treating physician to conclude that the experienced educational difficulty was not secondary to frequent absences. (Tracing and clinical history courtesy of James J. Riviello, M.D., Children's Hospital, Boston, MA. Reprinted from Shomer DL, Ives JR, Schachter SC. The role of ambulatory EEG in the evaluation of patients for epilepsy surgery. *J Clin Neurophysiol* 1999;16:116–129, with permission.)

superiority, but the additional information obtained through video monitoring of behavior and the ability to withdraw antiepileptic medications under medical observation.

The evaluation of partial epilepsies benefited from the introduction of eight-channel ambulatory EEG systems. Compared to simultaneous 16-channel cable telemetry records, both 3- and 8-channel ambulatory EEG reviews correctly identified 93% of the records as either normal or epileptiform (27). Lateralization of abnormalities was equally good with either cassette system, but more detailed characterization was achieved with eight-channel ambulatory EEG. Although 100% of seizures were detected on both systems, there were more false-positive errors when only three data channels were available.

Neonatal and Childhood Seizure Disorders

Ambulatory EEG is particularly useful in pediatric practice because epilepsy is a common neurological affliction of childhood, and these small patients do not tolerate well traditional EEG or especially inpatient long-term monitoring (103). The small size of ambulatory recorders, the resultant mobility, and the outpatient setting make this technique well suited to the pediatric patient. The utility of this method in children, particularly those with absence and other generalized epilepsies, was demonstrated early in the development of the technique (50,52,104,106). Its usefulness in documenting the nature of "spells" of uncertain etiology in children has also been shown (2,6).

Compact recording systems designed for ambulatory outpatients also offer a means of obtaining extended EEG recording in the neonatal intensive care unit with minimal disruption to nursing functions and no limitations of access to the patient being recorded (35). The utility of cassette EEG for seizure detection in neonates has been assessed in several studies (36,38). Extended cassette EEG recording, even when restricted to three EEG channels, can result in substantially increased detection of seizures over routine recordings. Ambulatory EEG can also provide a means of monitoring brain activity in neonates pharmacologically paralyzed in order to improve ventilatory support (37). Given the variable and sometimes localized distribution of neonatal seizure activity, as well as the need for correlative monitoring of other physiological variables, it is likely that newer recorders with multiple polygraph channels will receive greater application in this area.

Presurgical Evaluation

Epilepsy can be diagnosed and its type classified by ambulatory EEG with limited channel numbers. This is not the case with the evaluation of surgical candidates (Table 19.1). Detailed EEG characterization and localization of spikes and seizures are essential. At least 16 and preferably 24–32 scalp EEG channels sampled at a standard 200 Hz are required (see Figs. 19.3 through 19.5). Off-line data manipulations such as remontaging and filtering, as well as more sophisticated analyses such as voltage mapping or source modeling, are often very useful. Video recording of ictal behavior is also considered mandatory at most epilepsy surgery centers. Fortunately, the newest generation of ambulatory recording systems has all these capabilities. In fact, at several epilepsy centers the same recording equipment is used for both inpatient and outpatient monitoring (Figs. 19.7 and 19.8) (97). In the hospital setting, the "ambulatory" recorders are linked to fixed video recording systems, whereas in the outpatient setting they are linked to portable digital video recorders. With responsible patients, sphenoidal electrodes can also be used in home recordings. Withdrawal of antiepileptic medication is perhaps the only part of the normal inpatient scalp EEG evaluation that cannot be performed as an outpatient procedure. For patients with frequent seizures this is not a major consideration.

Sleep Disorders

The capability of recording multiple channels of electrophysiological data over long periods of time also lends itself to the diagnosis or evaluation of sleep-associated disturbances. Sleep staging is easily accomplished using combined video–audio analysis of recorded data (94). Computer programs have been developed that produce sleep statistics and hypnograms from data entered by the reader during such rapid review (32,33). Automated sleep analysis of data from ambulatory recorders has also been introduced and is being progressively refined (19,34,68,75,78).

TABLE 19.1. *Ambulatory EEG usefulness by channel number*

Channels	Use
3–8	Diagnosis, classification, rough localization
16–18	As above plus better localization
24–32	As above plus presurgical localizatio

The physiological parameters other than EEG that are most commonly used for sleep studies with ambulatory recorders are the ECG, EOG, EMG, and partial pressure of oxygen (PO_2). These are used to define disturbances of sleep architecture such as those seen, for example, in the hypersomnias (14). The EMG and movement data from the extremities can be used to identify nocturnal periodic movements and myoclonus (5,91). Measures of res-

piration by means of strain gauges, impedance pneumography, or thermistors, as well as PO_2, may be added in order to investigate paroxysmal disorders of breathing, such as sleep apnea (3,5), sudden infant death syndrome, and neonatal apnea. Monitoring all these sleep parameters in an inpatient setting is now commonplace, but their full utilization in ambulatory cassette recording is just evolving (4,79,80,83,95,108). Being able to monitor

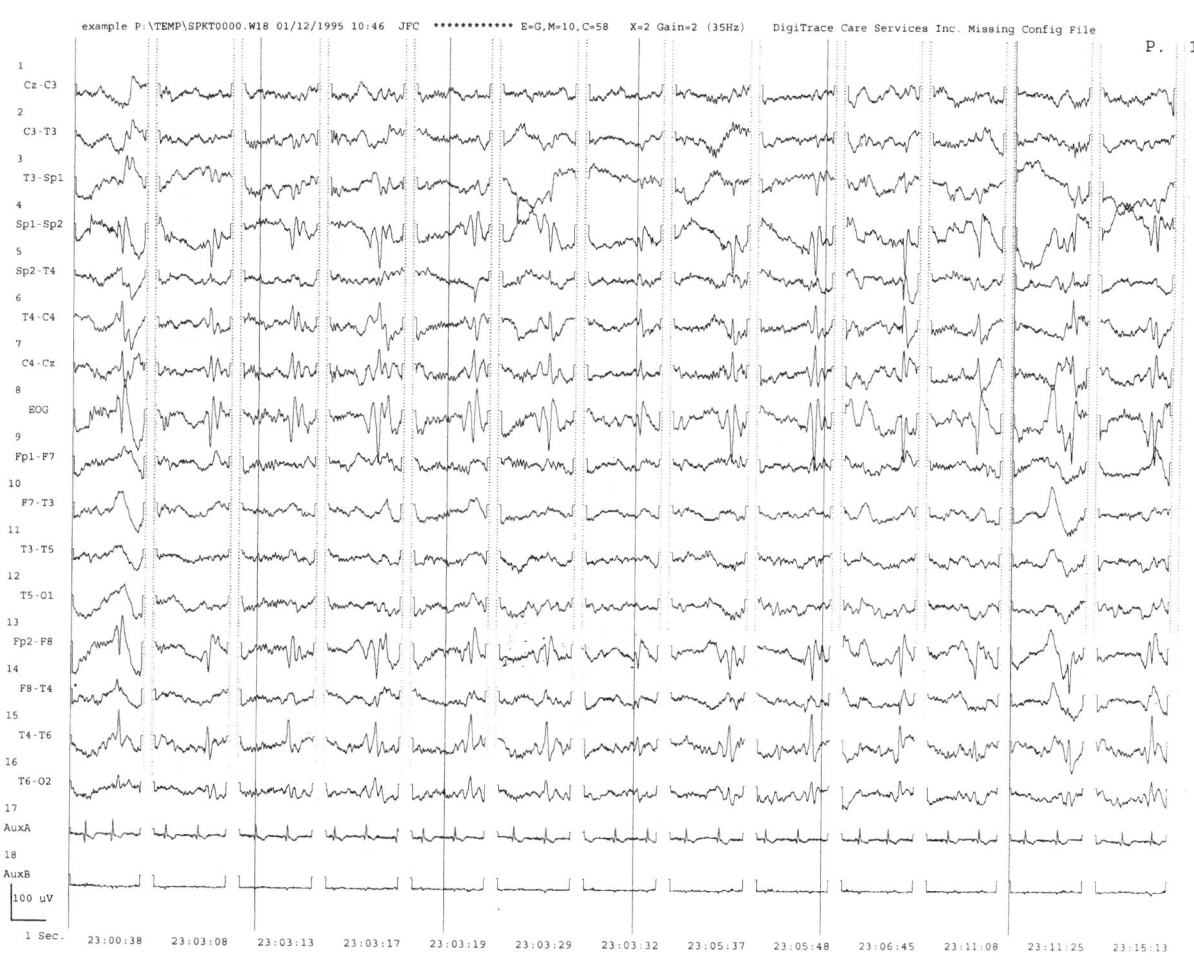

FIG. 19.7. A: The file demonstrated here shows interictal epileptiform discharges detected by an automated spike detection algorithm. The discharges were increased by sleep. All of the discharges were from the right temporal lobe, where phase reversals were noted in the right sphenoidal lead, suggesting that the origin was from the more inferior temporal region. *(Figure continues.)*

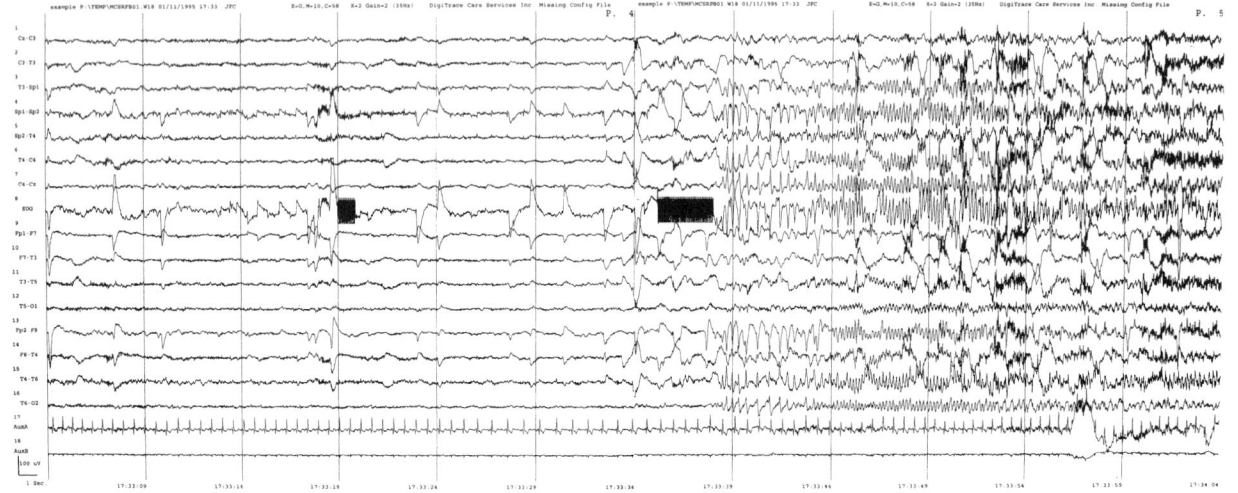

FIG. 19.7. *Continued.* **B:** The PB***.W18 file presented here is a recording made during a typical seizure. The origin appears also to be from the right inferior temporal lobe region, as noted with the interictal files shown above. The time of onset was determined to be 17:33:09 when this file was expanded and enlarged. (From Shomer DL, Ives JR, Schachter SC. The role of ambulatory EEG in the evaluation of patients for epilepsy surgery. *J Clin Neurophysiol* 1999; 16:116–129, with permission.)

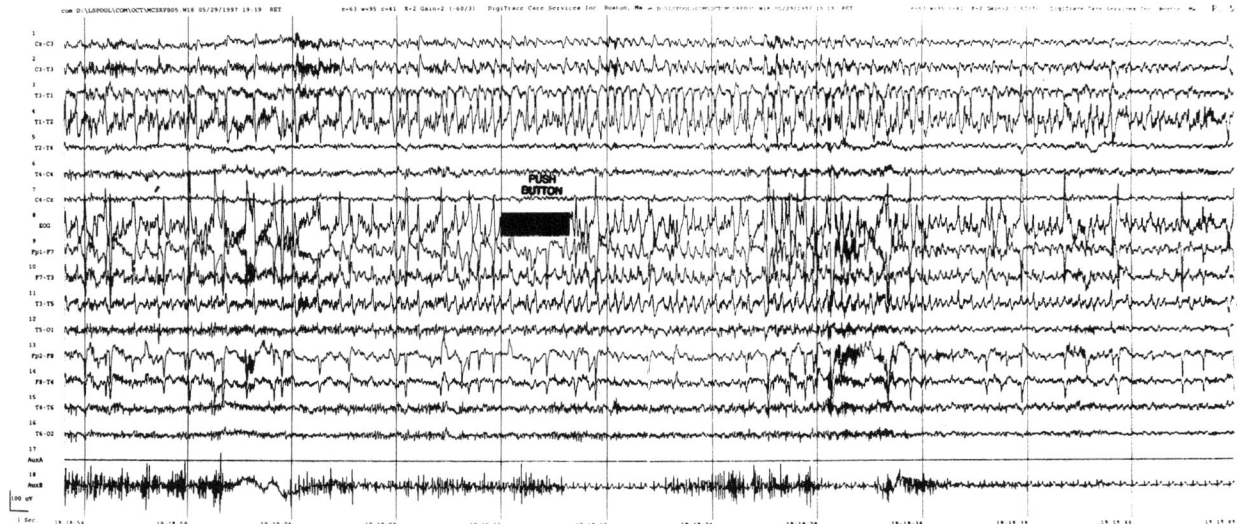

FIG. 19.8. Demonstration of the recording of an "event." The McSR***.W18 file name at the top of the recording identifies it as a waist-worn file of a "push-button" –based recording. In this specific case, the patient had been experiencing episodes of dizziness and aphasia. Channel 8 shows the superimposed artifact for the push-button marking of the time at which the patient felt symptomatic. There is a clear sustained seizure discharge present broadly over the left inferior and lateral temporal area, associated with the symptoms. Previous EEG recording demonstrated only slow-wave activity from the left temporal region. Subsequent to this recording and as a result of the finding of frequent focal left temporal seizures, the patient had repeat magnetic resonance imaging that demonstrated a newly defined left temporal structure that proved to be a glioma. (Case courtesy of Bruce H. Price, M.D., McClean Hospital, Belmont, MA. Reprinted from Shomer DL, Ives JR, Schachter SC. The role of ambulatory EEG in the evaluation of patients for epilepsy surgery. *J Clin Neurophysiol* 1999;16:116–129, with permission.)

patients in their own homes not only is convenient, but also avoids the necessity of habituating the patient to a new environment. Sleep apnea (84,98) may also be associated with behavior that is confused with an ictal event (21,63,70). The new 16- to 32-channel systems are obviously better suited to multiparameter studies (Figs. 19.9 and 19.10). Ambulatory monitoring shows great promise in facilitating the evaluation of all forms of sleep-related disorders.

Syncope and Dizziness

Paroxysmal loss of consciousness or spells of dizziness are common diagnostic problems for neurologists. Ambulatory recordings provide a convenient way to monitor both the ECG and the EEG for a long enough period of time to be likely to record an episode. Several studies have shown that this form of combined monitoring can be useful in clarifying an etiology (8,17,48,66,67,71). Cardiac-related events are the most likely, given the relative infrequency with which epilepsy is uncovered in patients presenting with syncope (80). One study showed that only 1.5% of ambulatory recordings from patients complaining of syncope or dizziness contained epileptiform abnormalities (10,11). Although there continues to be a concern that an increased incidence of sudden death among people with seizure disorders may be related to cardiac arrhythmias, a combined ambulatory EEG and ECG study showed no increase in cardiac rhythm disturbances among known epileptics when compared to nonepileptics (64,65,67). ECG abnormalities may indeed accompany seizures (9,64). In most instances these consist of ictal tachycardia and at times abrupt changes in rate, rather than dangerous rhythm disturbances. Cardiac arrhythmias may, however, masquerade as seizures (Fig. 19.11) (40,66,71).

Nonepileptic Seizures and Psychiatric Disorders

The role of ambulatory EEG in the differential diagnosis of behavioral episodes has also been investigated. Its utility in adults and children has been acclaimed, particularly in documenting those attacks that were seizures rather than spells of psychiatric origin (39,85,99–101). Observing no electrographic changes on recordings made during episodes of apparent total loss of consciousness or major motor convulsions can provide support for a diagnosis of pseudoseizures. A lack of ambulatory EEG findings during reported episodes of only altered consciousness or behav-ior is less diagnostic. It lends some support to the possibility that the spells are functional, but these negative data cannot rule out the possibility of simple partial seizures, for which there may be no surface EEG manifestations. In the evaluation of pseudoseizures, observation of behavior is essential. Ambulatory EEG monitoring can be combined with video recording to provide the objective documentation necessary for these differential diagnoses (73).

In the case of psychiatric disorders that have no paroxysmal features, the yield for detecting underlying epilepsy has been very low, and in one investigation was zero (11). Ambulatory EEG monitoring may, however, be useful in identifying and quantitating disturbances in sleep architecture, particularly REM onset latency, that purportedly are observed in patients with depression and that resolve with drug treatment (76).

OVERALL CLINICAL YIELD

The usefulness of ambulatory EEG in general practice is dependent on the appropriateness of the question being asked and the likelihood of answering the question, even if appropriate. Rates for recording the attacks or spells by means of ambulatory EEG vary dramatically with the clinical frequency of these episodes, as would be expected. A 77% success rate was achieved in patients with one or more seizures daily (20), whereas only 16% of unselected patients had spells recorded (8). A 50% capture rate could be attained in patients who had only one attack per week by allowing at least 3 days for monitoring each of them (87).

Similarly, the yield for documenting epileptiform abnormalities is quite variable in the literature and is most likely due to differences in patient populations. Early reports of continuous four-channel recordings in unselected patients showed a positive yield of evidence to support a diagnosis in the range of 10%–15% (49,92). Of attacks recorded in several series, the proportion that was identifiable as seizures has ranged from 23% to 73% (16,56). In a series of 500 consecutive patients ages 2 months to 82 years who were undergoing eight-channel ambulatory EEG for the first time (11), seizures, interictal epileptiform abnormalities, or both were detected in 17.4%. This represented a 64% increase in the yield of interictal epileptiform abnormalities and a 21-fold increase in seizure recording as compared to a preceding laboratory EEG. A particularly high yield (34.9%) of epileptiform abnormalities was identified in recordings from patients diagnosed as epileptic. The positive yield was 15.3% in patients referred with a wide vari-

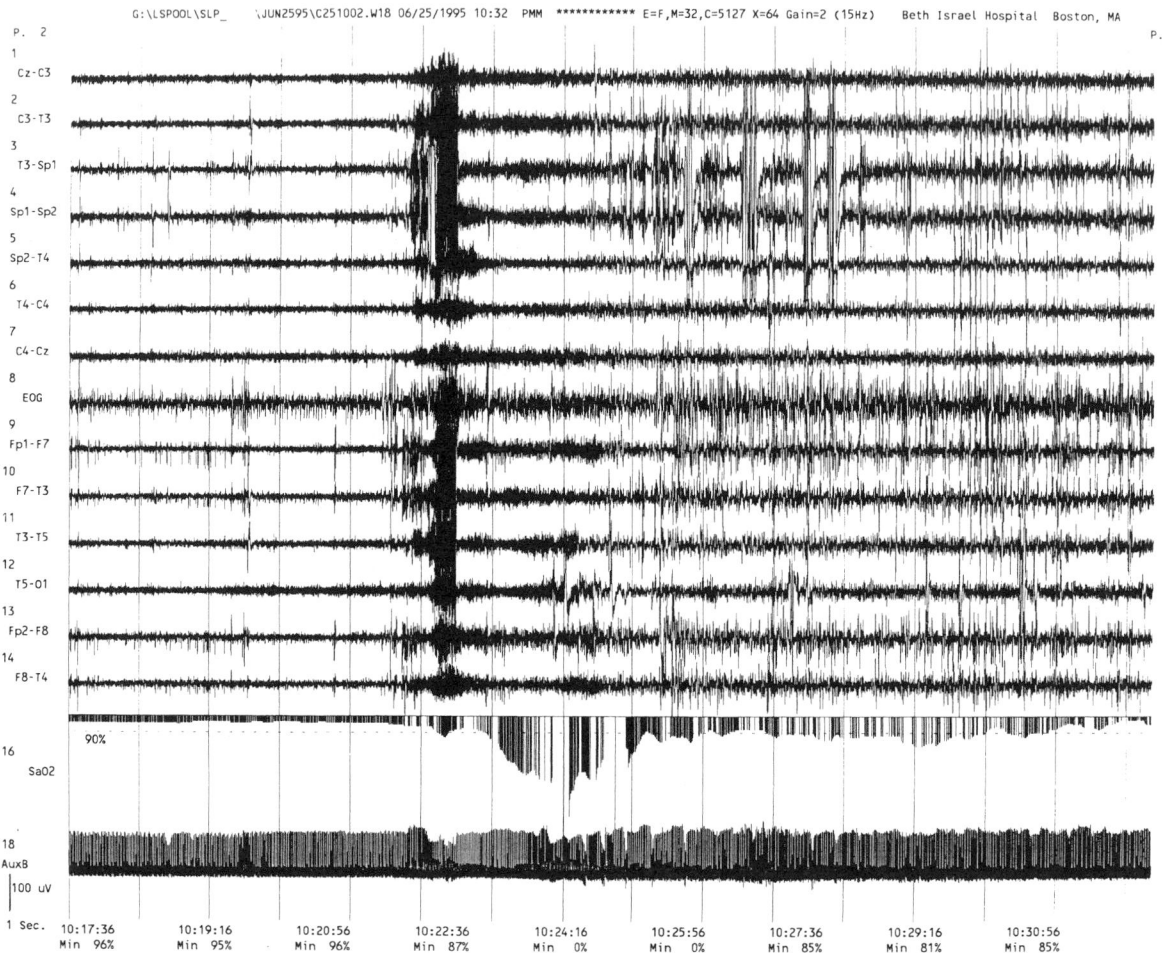

FIG. 19.9. This tracing represents part of a continuous recording done with additional equipment to monitor blood oxygenation levels (SPO₂) on the index finger. This file is compressed for better display of the SPO₂ data. The page shown here represents approximately 15 minutes of recording. From other files, we know that this patient experienced the sensation of a partial seizure at about 10:22:36. He never lost consciousness with this event but, as demonstrated by the SPO₂ monitor, there was a significant drop in his blood oxygen saturation for many minutes. Review of the video recording taken around this event shows that the SPO₂ pulse oximeter was intact. The *dotted line* represents the 90% saturation level. Before the seizure, the patient's oxygen levels were normal, in the 95%+ range. After this simple partial event, the levels dropped approximately to the 70% range. The patient was seemingly unaware of this drop. It took several minutes for the patient to reset his respiratory drive to return his levels to the normal range. (From Shomer DL, Ives JR, Schachter SC. The role of ambulatory EEG in the evaluation of patients for epilepsy surgery. *J Clin Neurophysiol* 1999;16:116–129, with permission.)

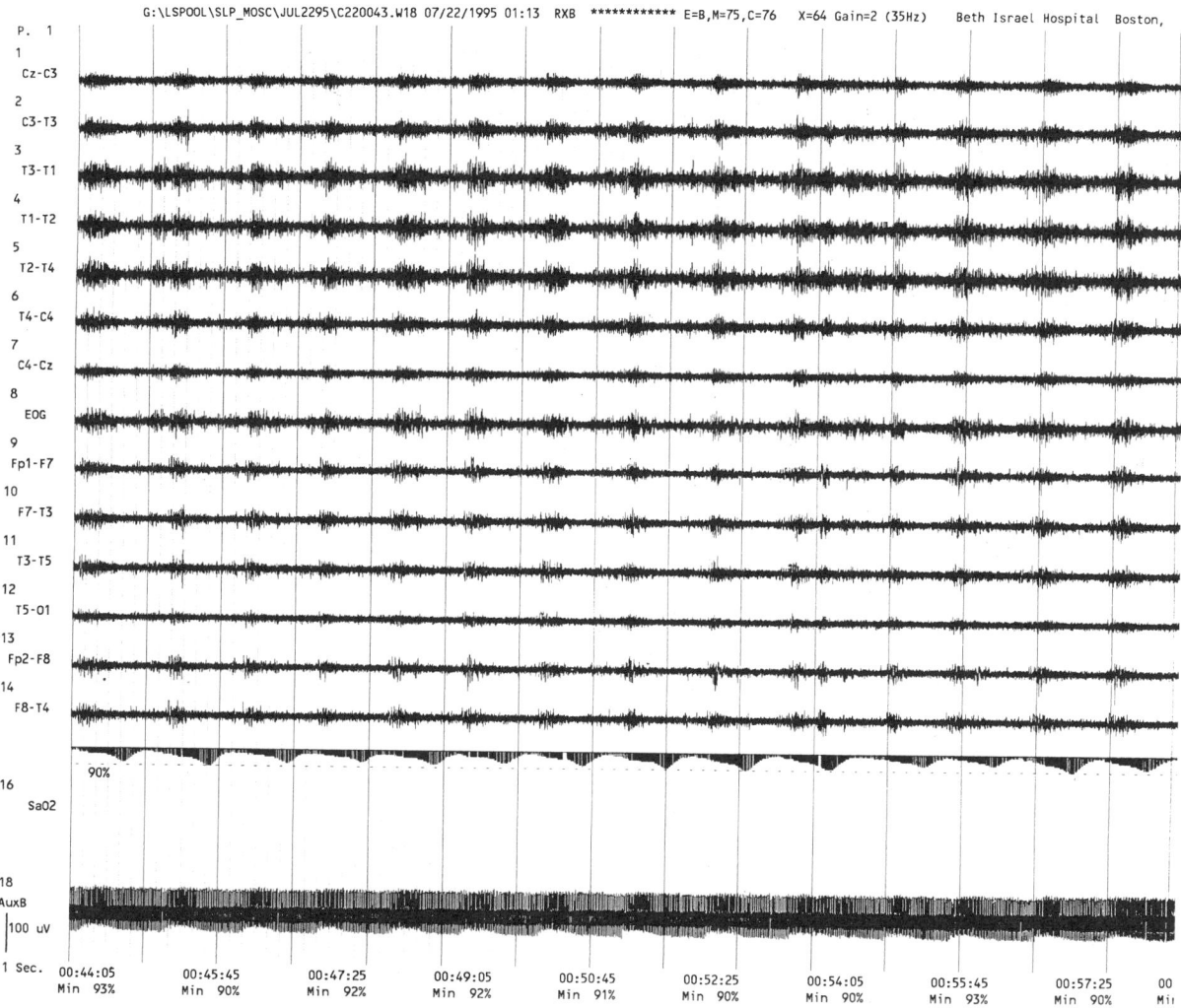

FIG. 19.10. As with the previous tracing, this playback is from a continuous recording with the addition of SPO₂ monitoring. This tracing came from an elderly woman with a history of rare epileptic events. She had experienced a subacute decline in mental status, and the referring physician was concerned that she was having unrecognized seizures, perhaps while asleep. The tracing failed to detect any electrical evidence for such seizures, but it did demonstrate the presence of this Cheyne-Stokes respiratory pattern. The regularly recurring fluctuation in the SPO₂ with about 90-second intervals is classic. The treating physician used this finding to reassess the patient. He found her to be in mild and previously unrecognized cardiac failure. Treatment was instituted and there was a significant improvement in her mental status. (From Shomer DL, Ives JR, Schachter SC. The role of ambulatory EEG in the evaluation of patients for epilepsy surgery. *J Clin Neurophysiol* 1999;16:116–129, with permission.)

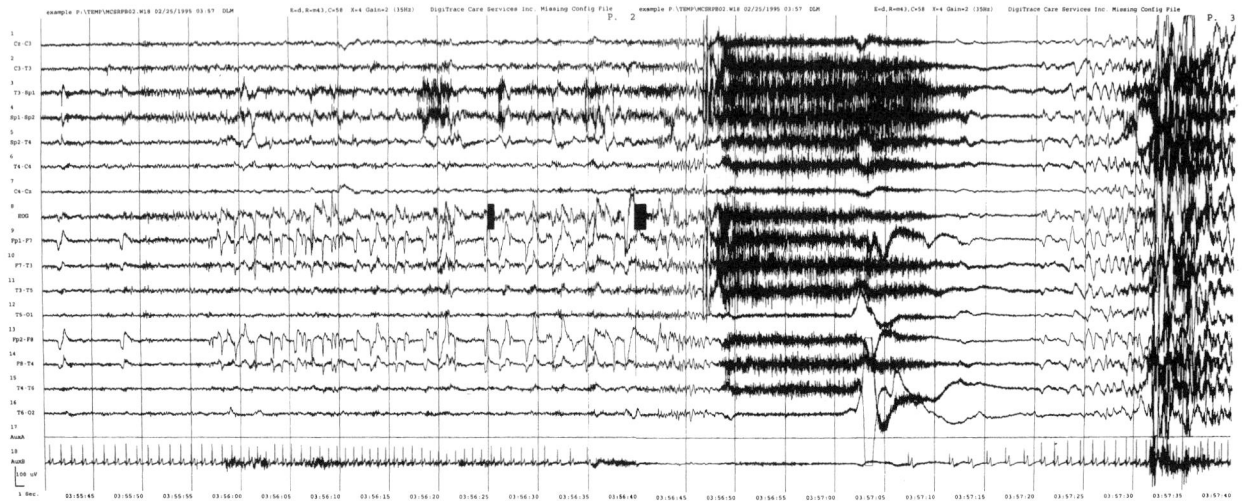

FIG. 19.11. G.H. was a 45-year-old man with a long-standing history of partial epilepsy. He was now having events during his sleep. His wife described being awakened once a week by his abnormal movements, of which he was completely unaware. He had not had any daytime seizures for many months. His recordings revealed the presence of a brief left temporal lobe electrical seizure associated with a profound bradycardia. He was without a pulse for 36 seconds. A cardiology consultant believed that a pacemaker was indicated. This was implanted, but additionally his anticonvulsant regimen was altered because this was believed to be a seizure-driven asystole. (From Shomer DL, Ives JR, Schachter SC. The role of ambulatory EEG in the evaluation of patients for epilepsy surgery. *J Clin Neurophysiol* 1999;16:116–129, with permission.)

ety of episodic alterations of behavior, perception, sensation, or motor function thought possibly to represent seizures. To the contrary, EEG yield was very low in patients with syncope, dizziness, and particularly nonepisodic behavioral alterations without a history consistent with seizure (10,11). These results underscore the need for appropriate clinical judgment in the application of ambulatory EEG.

In 1994, Morris et al. completed a study of the clinical usefulness of 16-channel discontinuous, but computer-assisted, ambulatory EEG recording (82). A total of 344 patients were recorded for an average of 1.4 days using a 16-channel bipolar montage. Push-button events plus spike-and-seizure detections and periodic samples were recorded on a portable computer attached to the recorder. Epileptiform abnormalities (seizures or spikes) were identified in 38% of patients (26% by computer only) and in 25% of patients with previously normal EEGs. Seizures were identified in 12% of patients. The higher overall yield in this study versus previous eight-channel studies may be related to improved detection of EEG abnormalities with the additional channels or to differences in patient population. It is noteworthy that computer assistance is very important in identifying interictal abnormalities with a discontinuous recording system. A full two-thirds of patients had abnormalities identified only by on-line spike-and-seizure detection analysis and not by push-button events or intermittent time samples. Push-button events without associated EEG changes were recorded in 36% of patients. The authors reported "an overall clinical usefulness of 74%" by adding the two yields together.

More recently, Liporace et al. (74) compared the utility of computer-assisted 16-channel, 24-hour ambulatory EEG to routine 30- to 60-minute sleep-deprived EEG in 46 patients using similar recording equipment. Electroencephalographers who were unaware of clinical information on the patients reviewed records independently. Epileptiform abnormalities were found in 33% of ambulatory EEGs and 24% of sleep-deprived EEGs. Statistically significant, however, was the fact that seizures were recorded in 15% of ambulatory EEGs but in none of the routine EEGs.

THE ROLE OF AMBULATORY EEG

What, then, is the current role for ambulatory EEG in the diagnostic spectrum from routine laboratory EEG to inpatient long-term monitoring? In the past the answer to this question was technologically constrained, but this is no longer the case. Ambulatory and fixed EEG monitoring systems have nearly the same capabilities. Cost effectiveness is currently a major factor. Elective hospital admissions for diagnostic purposes are increasingly difficult to justify to insurers despite the fact that, in most situations, inpatient monitoring will provide better quality data. This has mostly to do with the controlled monitoring environment where electrode integrity is maintained and the patient is being watched and carefully recorded on videotape, and where antiepileptic medications can be more safely withdrawn to induce seizures. Conversely, there are few diagnostic situations in which outpatient ambulatory EEG cannot be considered a perfectly reasonable and potentially cost-efficient initial procedure. At present there are few controlled clinical comparisons of ambulatory versus inpatient monitoring. Numerous studies have shown that ambulatory EEG is clearly superior to routine EEG, particularly when seizure recording is essential. Although there are no official guidelines for ambulatory EEG, clinical experience would support the diagnostic flow charts in Tables 19.1 and 19.2.

REFERENCES

1. Ajmone-Marsan C, Zivin LS. Factors related to the occurrence of typical paroxysmal abnormalities in the EEG records of epileptic patients. *Epilepsia* 1970;11:361–381.
2. Aminoff MJ, Goodin DS, Berg BO, et al. Ambulatory EEG recordings in epileptic and nonepileptic children. *Neurology*, 1988;38:558.
3. Ancoli-Israel S. Ambulatory cassette recording of sleep apnea. In: Ebersole JS, ed. *Ambulatory EEG monitoring*. New York: Raven Press, 1988:299.
4. Ancoli-Israel S, Kripke DF, Mason W, et al. Comparisons of home sleep recordings and polysomnograms in older adults with sleep disorders. *Sleep* 1981;4:283.
5. Ancoli-Israel S, Kripke DF, Mason W, et al. Sleep apnea and periodic movements in an aging sample. *J Gerontol* 1985;40:419.
6. Bachman DS. 24 hour ambulatory electroencephalographic monitoring in pediatrics. *Clin Electroencephalogr* 1984;15:164.
7. Bailey C. Evaluation of a spike and wave processor for use in long-term ambulatory EEG monitoring. In: Stott FD, et al, eds. *ISAM 1981: proceedings of the Fourth International Symposium on Ambulatory Monitoring*. London: Academic Press, 1982:203.
8. Blumhardt LD, Oozeer R. Simultaneous ambulatory monitoring of the EEG and ECG in patients with unexplained transient disturbances of consciousness. In: Stott FD, et al, eds. *ISAM 1981: proceedings of the Fourth International Symposium on Ambulatory Monitoring*. London: Academic Press, 1982:171.
9. Blumhardt LD, Smith PEM, Owen L. Electroencephalographic accompaniments of temporal lobe epileptic seizures. *Lancet* 1986;1:1051.
10. Bridgers SL. Evaluation of episodes of altered awareness or behavior. In: Ebersole JS, ed. *Ambulatory EEG monitoring*. New York: Raven Press, 1987:217.
11. Bridgers SL, Ebersole JS. Ambulatory cassette EEG in clinical practice: experience with 500 patients. *Neurology* 1985;35:1767.
12. Bridgers SL, Ebersole JS. The clinical utility of ambulatory cassette EEG. *Neurology* 1985;35:166–173.
13. Bridgers SL, Ebersole JS. EEG outside the hairline: detection of epileptiform abnormalities. *Neurology* 1988;38:146.
14. Broughton RJ. Ambulatory sleep-wake monitoring in the hypersomnias. In: Ebersole JS, ed. *Ambulatory EEG monitoring*. New York: Raven Press, 1988:277.
15. Burr W, Stefan H, Penin H. Spike-wave analysis in 24-hour EEG: comparison between conventional and computerized methods. In: Dam M, Gram L, Penry JK, eds. *Advances in epileptology: XIIth Epilepsy International Symposium*. New York: Raven Press, 1981:275.
16. Callaghan N, McCarthy N. Twenty-four hour EEG monitoring in patients with normal, routine EEG findings. In: Dam M, Gram L, Penry JK, eds. *Advances in epileptology: XIIth Epilepsy International Symposium*. New York: Raven Press, 1981:357.
17. Callaghan N, McCarthy N. Ambulatory EEG monitoring in fainting attacks with normal routine and sleep EEG records. In: Stefan H, Burr W, eds. *Mobile long-term EEG monitoring: proceedings of the MLE Symposium*. New York: Gustav Fischer, 1982:61.
18. Clenney SL. Techniques of cassette EEG recording. In: Ebersole JS, ed. *Ambulatory EEG monitoring*. New York: Raven Press, 1988:27.
19. Crawford C. Evaluation of the Oxford Medilog sleep stager. In: Palu C, Pessina AC, eds. *Proceedings of the Fifth International Symposium on Ambulatory Monitoring*. Padua: Cleup, 1986:697.

TABLE 19.2. *Scalp EEG evaluation of patients with seizure-like spells*

Step 1: Routine laboratory EEG
Step 2: Sleep-deprived EEG or ambulatory EEG
Step 3: Ambulatory outpatient EEG
Step 4: Ambulatory outpatient EEG with video
Step 5: Long-term inpatient monitoring

Patient	Recording montage
New patient with no previous EEGs	Start at Step 1
Referred patient with previous normal or equivocal EEGs	Start at Step 2
Seizure classification/characterization needed	Start at Step 3
Presurgical workup	Start at Step 4

20. Davidson DLW, Fleming AMM, Kettles A. Use of ambulatory EEG monitoring in a neurological service. In: Dam M, Gram L, Penry JK, eds. *Advances in epileptology: XIIth Epilepsy International Symposium*. New York: Raven Press, 1981:319.

21. Devinsky O, Ehrenberg B, Barthlen GM, et al. Epilepsy and sleep apnea syndrome. *Neurology* 1994;44:2060–2064.

22. Ebersole JS. Ambulatory cassette EEG. *J Clin Neurophysiol* 1985;2:397–418.

23. Ebersole JS. Ambulatory EEG: telemetered and cassette recorded. In: Bumnit R, ed. *Intensive neurodiagnostic monitoring*. New York: Raven Press, 1986:139.

24. Ebersole JS. Audio-visual analysis of cassette EEG. In: Ebersole JS, ed. *Ambulatory EEG monitoring*. New York: Raven Press, 1988:69.

25. Ebersole JS. Clinical utility of cassette EEG in adult seizure disorders. In Ebersole JS, ed. *Ambulatory EEG monitoring*. New York: Raven Press, 1988:111.

26. Ebersole JS, Bridgers SL. Performance evaluation of an 8-channel ambulatory cassette EEG system. In: *Abstracts of the XVth Epilepsy International Symposium*, Washington, DC, 1983.

27. Ebersole JS, Bridgers SL. Direct comparison of 3- and 8-channel ambulatory cassette EEG with intensive inpatient monitoring. *Neurology* 1985;35:846–854.

28. Ebersole JS, Bridgers SL. Ambulatory EEG monitoring. In: Pedley TA, Meldrum BS, eds. *Recent advances in epilepsy III*. Edinburgh: Churchill Livingstone, 1986:111.

29. Ebersole JS, Bridgers SL. Cassette EEG monitoring in the emergency room and intensive care unit. In: Ebersole JS, ed. *Ambulatory EEG monitoring*. New York: Raven Press, 1988:231.

30. Ebersole JS, Leroy RF. An evaluation of ambulatory, cassette EEG monitoring: II. Detection accuracy compared to intensive inpatient EEG monitoring. *Neurology* 1983;33:8.

31. Ebersole JS, Leroy RF. Evaluation of ambulatory cassette EEG monitoring: III. Diagnostic accuracy compared to intensive impatient EEG monitoring. *Neurology* 1983;33:853–860.

32. Erwin CW, Ebersole JS. Data reduction of cassette-recorded polysomnographic measures. In: Ebersole JS, ed. *Ambulatory EEG monitoring*. New York: Raven Press, 1988:257.

33. Erwin CW, Ebersole JS, Marsh GR. Combined auditory-visual scoring of polysomnographic data at 60 times real time. *J Clin Neurophysiol* 1987;214:214.

34. Erwin CW, Hartwell JW. Sleep staging in ambulatory tape-recorded polysomnographic data: what a difference an epoch makes. *J Clin Neurophysiol* 1987;4:215.

35. Eyre J. Clinical utility of cassette EEG in neonatal seizure disorders. In: Ebersole JS, ed. *Ambulatory EEG monitoring*. New York: Raven Press, 1982:141.

36. Eyre J, Crawford C. Prolonged electroencephalographic recording in neonates. In: Stott FD, et al, eds. *ISAM 1981: proceedings of the Fourth International Symposium on Ambulatory Monitoring*. London: Academic Press, 1982:143.

37. Eyre JA, Oozeer RC, Wilkinson AR. Diagnosis of neonatal seizures by continuous recording and rapid analysis of the electroencephalogram. *Arch Dis Child* 1983;58:49.

38. Fenichel GM, Ritzpatrick JE. Difficulty in clinical identification of neonatal seizures: an EEG monitor study. *Electroencephalogr Clin Neurophysiol* 1986;58:33P.

39. Forrest GC, Crawford C. Ambulatory monitoring and child psychiatry. In: Stott FD, et al, eds. *ISAM 1981: proceedings of the Fourth International Symposium on Ambulatory Monitoring*. London: Academic Press, 1982:157.

40. Frysinger RC, Harper RM. Cardiac and respiratory correlations with unit discharges in human amygdala and hippocampus. *Electroencephalogr Clin Neurophysiol* 1989;72:463–470.

41. Gabor AJ. Seizure detection using a self-organizing neural network: validation and comparison with other detection strategies. *Electroencephalogr Clin Neurophysiol* 1998;107:27.

42. Gabor AJ, Leach RR, Dowla FU. Automated seizure detection using a self-organizing neural network. *Electroencephalogr Clin Neurophysiol* 1996;99:257.

43. Gotman J. Automatic recognition of epileptic seizures in the EEG. *Electroencephalogr Clin Neurophysiol* 1982;54:530–540.

44. Gotman J. Automated analysis of ambulatory EEG recordings. In: Ebersole JS, ed. *Ambulatory EEG monitoring*. New York: Raven Press, 1988:97.

45. Gotman J. Automatic seizure detection: improvements and evaluation. *Electroencephalogr Clin Neurophysiol* 1990;76:317–324.

46. Gotman J, Gloor P. Automatic recognition and quantification of interictal epileptic activity in the human scalp EEG. *Electroencephalogr Clin Neurophysiol* 1976;41:513–529.

47. Gotman J, Ives JR, Gloor P. Automatic recognition of interictal epileptic activity in prolonged EEG recordings. *Electroencephalogr Clin Neurophysiol* 1979;45:510–520.

48. Graf M, Brunner G, Weber H, et al. Simultaneous long-term recording of EEG and ECG in "syncope" patients. In: Stefan H, Burr W, eds. *Mobile long-term EEG monitoring: proceedings of the MLE Symposium*. New York: Gustav Fischer, 1982:67.

49. Green J, Scales D, Nealis J, et al. Clinical utility of ambulatory EEG monitoring. *Clin Electroencephalogr* 1980;11:173.

50. Hall DMB. Experience with ambulatory monitoring in children. In: Stott FD, et al, eds. *Proceedings of the Fourth International Symposium on Ambulatory Monitoring*. London: Academic Press, 1982:151.

51. Holter NJ. New method for heart studies. *Science* 1961;134:1214–1220.

52. Horwitz SJ, Burgess RC, Kijewski KN. Twenty-four hour, four channel EEG recording in children using a miniature tape recorder and computer analysis. *Am J EEG Technol* 1978;18:133.

53. Ives JR. A completely ambulatory 16-channel recording system. In: Stefan H, Burr W, eds. *Mobile long-term EEG monitoring: proceedings of the MLE Symposium*. New York: Gustav Fischer, 1982:205–217.

54. Ives JR. Evolution of ambulatory cassette EEG. In: Ebersole JS, ed. *Ambulatory EEG monitoring*. New York: Raven Press, 1988:1.

55. Ives JR, Gloor P. New sphenoidal electrode assembly to permit long-term monitoring of the patient's ictal and interictal EEG. *Electroencephalogr Clin Neurophysiol* 1977;42:575–580.

56. Ives JR, Hausser C, Woods JF, et al. Contributions of 4-channel cassette EEG monitoring to differential diagnosis of paroxysmal attacks. In: Dam M, Gram L, Penry JK, eds. *Advances in epileptology: XIIth Epilepsy International Symposium*. New York: Raven Press, 1981:329.

57. Ives JR, Ichihashi K, Gruber LJ, et al. New topographic mapping of temporal lobe seizures. *Epilepsia* 1993;34:890.

58. Ives JR, Schomer DL. Preliminary technical experience using a portable computer (PCAT) for online data analysis of epileptic spike activity on 16 channels of telemetric EEG data. *Epilepsia* 1986;27:626.

59. Ives JR, Schomer DL. Recent technical advances in longterm ambulatory outpatient monitoring. *Electroencephalogr Clin Neurophysiol* 1986;64:37P.

60. Ives JR, Schomer DL. The significance of using chronic sphenoidal electrodes during the recording of spontaneous ictal events in patients suspected of having temporal lobe seizures. *Electroencephalogr Clin Neurophysiol* 1986;64:23P.

61. Ives JR, Woods JF. 4-channel 24 hour cassette recorder for long-term EEG monitoring of ambulatory patients. *Electroencephalogr Clin Neurophysiol* 1975;39:88–92.

62. Ives JR, Woods JF. A study of 100 patients with focal epilepsy using a 4-channel ambulatory cassette recorder. In: Stott FD, Raftery EB, Goulding L, eds. *ISAM 1979: proceedings of the Third International Symposium of Ambulatory Monitoring*. London: Academic Press, 1980:383–392.

63. Kaada BR, Jasper HH. Respiratory responses to stimulation of temporal pole, insula and hippocampal and limbic gyri in man. *Arch Neurol Psychiatry* 1952;68:609–619.

64. Kapoor WN, Karpf M, Wieand S, et al. A prospective evaluation and follow-up of patients with syncope. *N Engl J Med* 1983;309:197.

65. Keilson MJ, Hauser WA, Magrill JP, et al. ECG abnormalities in patients with epilepsy. *Neurology* 1987;37:1624.

66. Keilson MJ, Magrill JP. Simultaneous ambulatory cassette EEG/ECG monitoring. In: Ebersole JS, ed. *Ambulatory EEG monitoring.* New York: Raven Press, 1988:171–193.

67. Keilson MJ, Magrill JP, Hauser WA, et al. Electrocardiographic abnormalities in patients with epilepsy. *Epilepsia* 1984;25:645.

68. Koerner E, Ladurner G, Flooh E, et al. Basic criteria for automatic analysis of mobile long-term EEG. In: Stefan H, Burr W, eds. *Mobile long-term EEG monitoring: proceedings of the MLE Symposium.* New York: Gustav Fischer, 1982:227.

69. Koffler D, Gotman J. Automatic detection of spike and wave bursts in ambulatory EEG recordings. *Electroencephalogr Clin Neurophysiol* 1985;61:165–180.

70. Krieger JR. Obstructive sleep apnea: clinical manifestations and pathophysiology. In: Thorpy MJ, ed. *Handbook of sleep disorders.* New York: Marcel Dekker, 1990:259–284.

71. Lai CW, Ziegler DK. Syncope problem solved by continuous ambulatory simultaneous EEG/ECG. *Neurology* 1981;31:1152–1154.

72. Leroy RF, Ebersole JS. An evaluation of ambulatory, cassette EEG monitoring: I. Montage design. *Neurology* 1983;33:1–7.

73. Leroy RF, Rao KK, Voth BJ. Intensive neurodiagnostic monitoring in epilepsy using ambulatory cassette EEG with simultaneous video recording. In: Ebersole JS, ed. *Ambulatory EEG monitoring.* New York: Raven Press, 1988:157.

74. Liporace J, Tatum W, Morris GL, et al. Clinical utility of sleep-deprived versus computer-assisted ambulatory 16-channel EEG in epilepsy patients: a multi-center study. *Epilepsy Res* 1998;32:357–362.

75. Marsh G, Erwin CW. The Oxford sleep stager: assessment of variability. *J Clin Neurophysiol* 1987;4:291.

76. Marsh GR, McCall WV. Sleep disturbances in psychiatric disease. In: Ebersole JS, ed. *Ambulatory EEG monitoring.* New York: Raven Press, 1988:331.

77. Marson GB, McKinnon JB. A miniature tape recorder for many applications. *Control Instrumentation* 1972;4:46–47.

78. Martens WLJ, Decleck AC, Kums GJTM, et al. Considerations on a computerized analysis of long-term polygraphic recordings. In: Stefan H, Burr W, eds. *Mobile long-term EEG monitoring: proceedings of the MLE Symposium.* New York: Gustav Fischer, 1982:265.

79. Mason WJ, Kripke DF, Messin S, et al. The application and utilization of an ambulatory recording system for the screening of sleep disorders. *Am J EEG Technol* 1986;26:145.

80. McCall WV, Edinger JD, Erwin CW. Clinical utility of cassette polysomnography in sleep and sleep-related disorders. In: Ebersole JS, ed. *Ambulatory EEG monitoring.* New York: Raven Press, 1988:267.

81. Milligan N, Richens A. Ambulatory monitoring of the EEG in the assessment of anti-epileptic drugs. In: Stott FD, et al, eds. *ISAM 1981: proceedings of the Fourth International Symposium on Ambulatory Monitoring.* London: Academic Press, 1982: 224.

82. Morris GL, Galezowshka J, Leroy R, et al. The results of computer-assisted ambulatory 16-channel EEG. *Electroencephalogr Clin Neurophysiol* 1994;91:229.

83. Mounaimne MW, Riley TL. Twenty-four-hour ambulatory recording for diagnosis of narcolepsy. *Electroencephalogr Clin Neurophysiol* 1982;53:37P.

84. Nashef L, Walker F, Sander JWAS, et al. Apnea and bradycardia during epileptic seizures: relation to sudden deaths in epilepsy. *Neurology* 1995;45:938S.

85. Oxley J, Roberts M. The role of prolonged ambulatory monitoring in the diagnosis of nonepileptic fits in a population of patients with epilepsy. In: Stott FD, et al, eds. *ISAM 1981:*

proceedings of the Fourth International Symposium on Ambulatory Monitoring. London: Academic Press, 1982:195.

86. Oxley J, Roberts M, Dana-Haeri J, et al. Evaluation of prolonged 4-channel EEG-taped recordings and serum prolactin levels in the diagnosis of epileptic and nonepileptic seizures. In: Dam M, Gram L, Penry JK, eds. *Advances in epileptology: XIIth Epilepsy International Symposium.* New York: Raven Press, 1981:343.

87. Powell TE, Harding GFA, Jeavons PM. Ambulatory EEG monitoring: a preliminary follow-up study. In: Ross E, Chadwick D, Crawford R, eds. *Epilepsy in young people.* London: John Wiley & Sons, 1987:131.

88. Quy RJ. A miniature preamplifier for ambulatory monitoring of the electroencephalogram. *J Physiol (Lond)* 1978;284:23–24.

89. Quy RJ, Fitch P, Willison RG. High-speed automatic analysis of EEG spike and wave activity using an analogue detection and microcomputer plotting system. *Electroencephalogr Clin Neurophysiol* 1980;49:187.

90. Quy RJ, Fitch P, Willison RG, et al. Electroencephalographic monitoring in patients with absence seizures. In: Wada JA, Penry JK, eds. *Advances in epileptology: The Xth Epilepsy International Symposium.* New York: Raven Press, 1980:69–72.

91. Radtke RA, Hoelscher TJ, Bragdon AC. Ambulatory evaluation of periodic movements of sleep. In: Ebersole JS, ed. *Ambulatory EEG monitoring.* New York: Raven Press, 1988:299.

92. Ramsay RE. Clinical usefulness of ambulatory EEG monitoring of the neurological patient. In: Stott FD, et al, eds. *ISAM 1981: proceedings of the Fourth International Symposium on Ambulatory Monitoring.* London: Academic Press, 1982:234.

93. Ramsay RE, Herskowitz A. 24-hour ambulatory EEG: a clinical appraisal. *Electroencephalogr Clin Neurophysiol* 1981;51:20.

94. Reitman M. Techniques of cassette polysomnography. In: Ebersole JS, ed. *Ambulatory EEG monitoring.* New York: Raven Press, 1988:243.

95. Riley TL, Peterson H, Mounaimne M. Sleep studies in the subject's home. *Electroencephalogr Clin Neurophysiol* 1982;53:37P.

96. Sams MW. Recording and playback instrumentation for ambulatory monitoring. In: Ebersole JS, ed. *Ambulatory EEG monitoring.* New York: Raven Press, 1988:13.

97. Schomer DL, Ives JR, Schachter SC. The role of ambulatory EEG in the evaluation of patients for epilepsy surgery. *J Clin Neurophysiol* 1999;16:116–129.

98. Singh B, Shahwan SAA, Deeb SMA. Partial seizures presenting as life-threatening apnea. *Epilepsia* 1993;34:901–903.

99. Smith EBO. The value of prolonged EEG monitoring to the clinician in a psychiatric liaison service. In: Stott FD, et al, eds. *ISAM 1981: proceedings of the Fourth International Symposium on Ambulatory Monitoring.* London: Academic Press, 1982:162.

100. Stores G. Ambulatory EEG monitoring in neuropsychiatric patients using the Oxford Medilog 4-24 recorder with visual play-back display. In: Stott FD, Raftery EB, Goulding L, eds. *ISAM 1979: proceedings of the Third International Symposium on Ambulatory Monitoring.* London: Academic Press, 1980:399.

101. Stores G. Differential diagnosis of seizures: psychiatric aspects. In: Dam M, Gram L, Penry JK, eds. *Advances in epileptology: XIIth Epilepsy International Symposium.* New York: Raven Press, 1981:259.

102. Stores G. Patterns of occurrence of seizure discharge. In: Stefan H, Burr W, eds. *Mobile long-term EEG monitoring: proceedings of the MLE Symposium.* New York: Gustav Fischer, 1982:115.

103. Stores G, Bergel N. Clinical utility of cassette EEG in childhood seizure disorders. In: Ebersole JS, ed. *Ambulatory EEG monitoring.* New York: Raven Press, 1988:129.

104. Stores G, Brankin P, Crawford C. Aspects of differential diagnosis using ambulatory EEG

monitoring. In: Stefan H, Burr W, eds. *Mobile long-term EEG monitoring: proceedings of the MLE Symposium*. New York: Gustav Fischer, 1982:55.

105. Stores G, Hennion T, Quy RJ. EEG ambulatory monitoring system with visual playback display. In: Woods JA, Penry JK, eds. *Advances in epileptology: Xth Epilepsy International Symposium*. New York: Raven Press, 1989:89–94.

106. Stores G, Lwin R. Precipitating factors and seizure activity. In: Stott FD, et al, eds. *ISAM 1981: proceedings of the Fourth International Symposium on Ambulatory Monitoring*. London: Academic Press, 1982:183.

107. Von Albert HH. Efficacy of non-computerized spike-wave analysis in long-term EEG. In: Stefan H, Burr W, eds. *Mobile long-term EEG monitoring: proceedings of the MLE Symposium*. New York: Gustav Fischer, 1982:237.

108. Wilkinson RT, Mullaney D. Electroencephalogram recording of sleep in the home. *Postgrad Med J* 1976;52:92.

109. Zetterlund B. Quantification of spike and wave episodes in 24-hour tape recordings of EEG. In: Stefan H, Burr W, eds. *Mobile long-term EEG monitoring: proceedings of the MLE Symposium*. New York: Gustav Fischer, 1982:237.

110. Zetterlund B, Bromster O. A system for quantification of spike and wave episodes in 24-hour tape recordings of EEG. In: Dam M, Gram L, Penry JK, eds. *Advances in epileptology: XIIth Epilepsy International Symposium*. New York: Raven Press, 1981:361.

111. Zschoske ST, Hunger J, Alexopoulos T. Gain of information using mobile EEG long-term monitoring. In: Stefan H, Burr W, eds. *Mobile long-term EEG monitoring: proceedings of the MLE Symposium*. New York: Gustav Fischer, 1982:19.

Chapter 20

Intracranial Electroencephalography

Michael R. Sperling

Although easily recorded from scalp electrodes, recording the electroencephalogram (EEG) directly from the cerebral cortex, termed *electrocorticography*, sometimes offers critical advantages (21). Cortical EEG recording is now mainly used for two reasons, planning epilepsy surgery and assessing the brain's electrical activity during cortical mapping sessions (Table 20.1). Planning epilepsy surgery accounts for most cortical recordings by far, although the proportion of surgical patients who require this technique has steadily decreased as noninvasive evaluation methods, such as magnetic resonance imaging (MRI), single-photon emission computed tomography, and positron emission tomography have improved. Monitoring of cortical function during electrical stimulation of the brain is the other major indication for cortical EEG recording. Cortical EEG

recording is used to verify that the stimulus remains local and that after-discharges are not provoked.

This chapter reviews the intracranial EEG, its benefits, and its pitfalls. In many respects, it resembles the extracranial EEG. Some dilemmas posed by extracranial EEG are eliminated with cortical recording, though new difficulties are introduced. The usual waveforms are readily visible, only more so. The intracranial EEG is not filtered by the scalp and skull, and, consequently, ordinary rhythms look different from usual. Normal rhythms sometimes appear sharper and less benign, and waveforms that are not seen in the scalp EEG are sometimes discernible. Definitive answers to clinical questions are not always gained, and, at times, the data are overwhelming. Nonetheless, the intracranial EEG can be immensely rewarding for the

TABLE 20.1. *Intracranial EEG recording objectives*

Define interictal abnormalities
    Epileptiform
    Nonepileptiform
Define ictal onset zone
    Demonstrate site of onset of different seizure types
    Establish reliability of seizure onset pattern
    Demonstrate routes of seizure propagation
Monitor EEG during mapping of cortical function
    Establish lack of afterdischarge during electrical stimulation

patient who derives benefit from its use, and intellectually stimulating to the neurophysiologist who employs it.

WHEN IS INTRACRANIAL EEG INDICATED?

The intracranial EEG may be recorded for a brief time during a neurosurgical procedure or for a longer time in a monitoring suite after electrode insertion in the operating room. Acute intraoperative EEG recording can be done quickly with a minimum of inconvenience and risk. Chronic recording is more complex, expensive, and riskier, and requires greater justification.

Chronic Intracranial EEG Recording

Two requirements must be satisfied before chronically indwelling intracranial electrodes should be used when evaluating someone for epilepsy surgery. First, localization should not be possible through safer noninvasive means or with acute recording during a neurosurgical procedure. The major objective of the presurgical evaluation process is to establish whether a single epileptogenic structural lesion exists that can be safely excised or transected. The widespread adoption of MRI and other ancillary techniques, including positron emission tomography and magnetic source imaging, permits most patients to have surgery without intracranial electrodes. Only when these noninvasive methods yield conflicting data or are insufficiently localizing should intracranial electrodes be employed (17,21,22,25). Second, before placing intracranial electrodes, one must have a reasonable hypothesis regarding the location of the epileptogenic zone; intracranial electrodes should not be placed in the absence of a clear idea of where seizures most likely originate.

The indications and rationale for performing intracranial EEG in epilepsy can be concisely summarized. Intracranial EEG helps establish whether there are one or more well-localized epileptogenic zones, helps demarcate the boundaries of a single zone, and establishes the function of the tissue within and adjacent to that zone. In practice, this means (a) determining the laterality of the focus, (b) localizing the focus to a specific lobe, and (c) defining its location within that lobe. It is also necessary to (a) determine whether there are multifocal epileptogenic areas (which might militate against surgery); (b) confirm that seizures are partial rather than generalized (occasionally, a frontal focus may appear as a generalized spike-and-wave discharge in the scalp EEG); and (c) confirm the diagnosis of epilepsy and define a focus for excision in those rare patients in whom the scalp EEG is negative.

Indwelling intracranial electrodes also provide a unique research opportunity. The electrodes can be utilized for experimental purposes to explore normal and abnormal brain physiology. EEG, evoked potentials, and single neuronal recordings can all be obtained in a passive state or under active experimental conditions, yielding new insights in brain function.

Rarely, chronic indwelling intracranial electrodes are placed for the sole purpose of mapping cortical function. This is generally done in complex cases in which the mapping procedure is expected to last so long that it would not be safe or tolerable to do it in the operating room. For example, most children and some adults cannot remain awake during surgery, so electrodes are inserted and electrical stimulation is performed over the next day or two outside the operating room (30,31). The electrodes are removed after cortical mapping is completed.

Acute Intraoperative Recording

Acute intraoperative electrocorticography is used for identical purposes, to reveal abnormal discharges and to monitor the EEG if electrical stimulation is performed (6,9,14,28,29) (see also Chapter 21 for a more detailed discussion). However, the surgeon must have identified the area for excision with reasonable certainty prior to surgery, and the intraoperative corticogram serves merely to refine the excision margins about a known lesion. Because the recording time is limited, expectations are different and quick decisions must be made.

The same types of electrodes, recording techniques, montage design, and methods of interpretation apply in the operating theater as in chronic recording; therefore, the discussion below is applicable to both acute and chronic recording. The only differences lie in duration of recording, types of artifacts, and potential confounding effects of anesthetic agents during the two types of recording session. Operating suites contain electronic and mechanical equipment that may introduce artifacts in the EEG. Several measures must often be taken to eliminate or reduce extraneous artifacts, ranging from disconnecting some pieces of equipment to conducting a thorough electrical engineering evaluation of the building's grounding cables with appropriate later engineering modifications. Many anesthetics, such as isoflurane and related compounds, propofol, benzodiazepines, and barbiturates, can either provoke or suppress interictal spikes and seizures. These agents are best avoided during intraoperative electrocorticography. Most neurophysiologists prefer to rely on a combination of narcotic medication, such as fentanyl, and nitrous oxide if general anesthesia is used. Local anesthesia provides perhaps the ideal combination of pain control and lack of EEG effect, but is neither suitable nor desirable for all patients.

ELECTRODES

Different types of electrodes can record the intracranial EEG (Table 20.2), including depth electrodes, subdural electrodes, epidural electrodes, and foramen ovale electrodes. Each electrode type has unique advantages and disadvantages, and their use depends on the question being posed in an intracranial evaluation. Often, multiple electrode types are used simultaneously to maximize the yield of an intracranial EEG recording session.

Depth electrodes are constructed as wires or catheters, and pierce the substance of the brain (Fig. 20.1) (13,21). Contacts are placed at regular intervals along the wire. Because depth electrodes penetrate the brain, their contacts lie within the cortex, in contrast to the other types of intracranial electrodes,

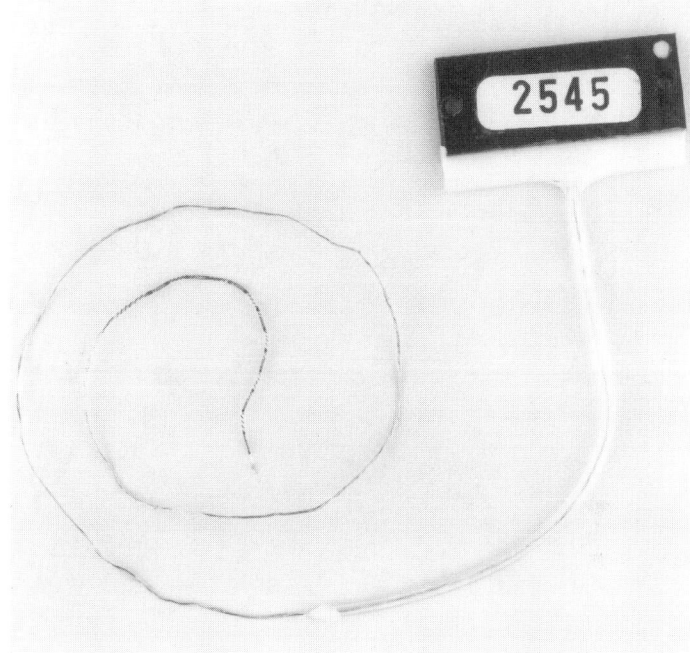

FIG. 20.1. This flexible depth electrode contains eight contacts, spaced every 5 mm beginning at the electrode tip. It is inserted while attached to a trocar insertion device that is removed after the electrode is placed.

which record from the pial or dural surface. Depth electrodes are ideally suited to record from buried, otherwise inaccessible nuclei such as the amygdala, hippocampus, and sulcal depths. At times, they are used to record from the orbitofrontal cortex, though this area can easily be reached by subdural electrodes as well. Limited numbers of these electrodes are used in any one patient to avoid excessive brain punctures; consequently, sampling is limited. They have also been utilized to record from diencephalic nuclei during surgery for Parkinson's disease or tremor.

Subdural electrodes are constructed as thin plastic (Silastic) sheets with embedded electrode contacts (Figs. 20.2 and 20.3). The contacts can be arranged in any pattern, spaced at any interval. The most common electrode types are referred to as strips and grids. Subdural strips have a single or double row of contacts placed in a straight line. Subdural grids are rectangular or square arrays of contacts spaced at regular intervals. Subdural electrodes are placed directly on the pia mater and are not inserted into the brain. They record

TABLE 20.2. *Intracranial electrodes*

Electrode type	Recording characteristics
Depth electrodes	Record from buried cortex (e.g., amygdala, hippocampus), although may be used for superficial or basal cortex; provide limited sampling
Subdural electrodes	Record from superficial, interhemispheric, or basal cortex; ideal for broad sampling
Epidural electrodes	Record from superficial or basal cortex; have dura interposed between electrode and cortex
Foramen ovale electrodes	Record from mesial temporal cortex; extradural location

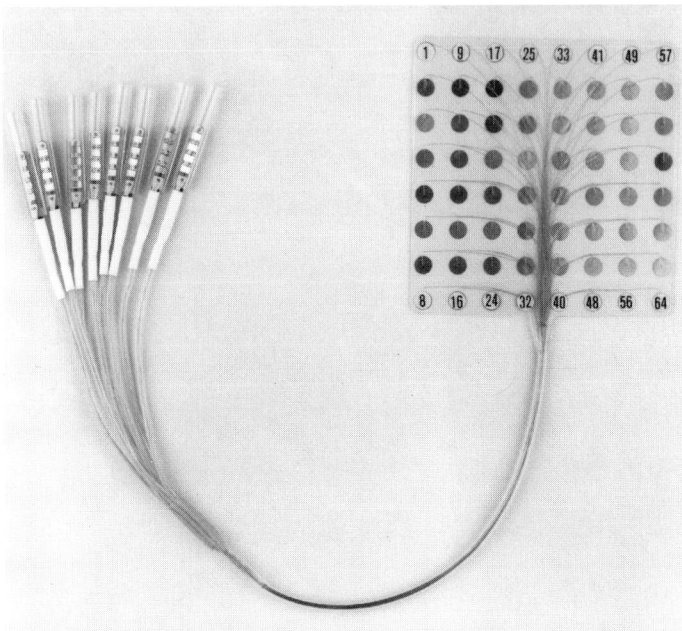

FIG. 20.2. In a subdural grid electrode, the contacts are spaced at 1-cm intervals in an 8-cm by 8-cm array. This electrode requires a craniotomy for placement and is placed in the subdural or epidural space.

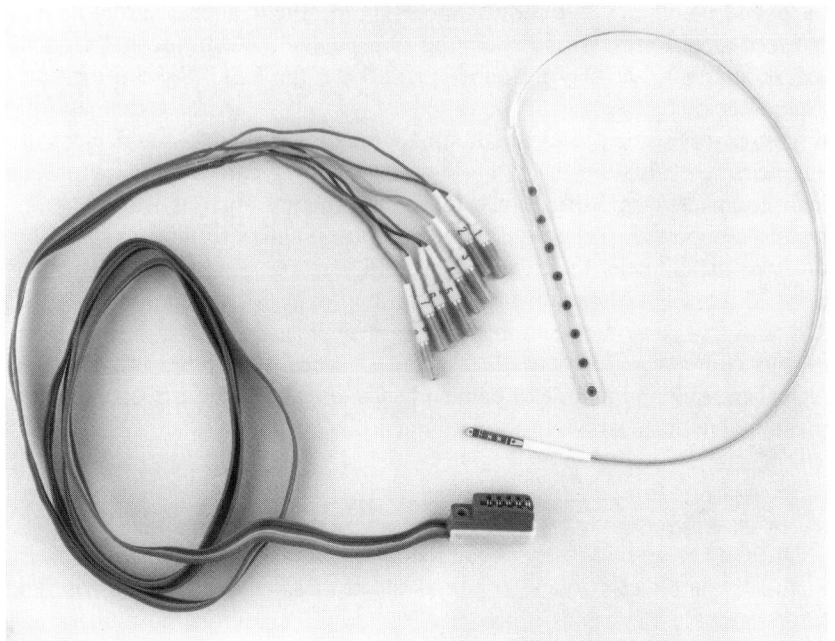

FIG. 20.3. This strip electrode has eight contacts spaced at 1-cm intervals, and can be inserted through a burr hole in the subdural or epidural space.

from the gyral surface and can be placed extensively over cortex to sample widely from one or more lobes (64,70). The same electrodes are used for epidural recording as for subdural recording, but they are placed over rather than under the dura. Epidural EEG recording is less precise than subdural recording, and is mainly reserved for patients who have dural scarring that prevents subdural electrode placement. However, some neurosurgeons prefer an epidural electrode location even in the absence of scarring, and the choice of technique must ultimately rest with the responsible physician.

Foramen ovale electrodes consist of wires with multiple contacts and are similar to depth electrodes (27,68,69). They are inserted via the cheek through the foramen ovale to rest in the epidural space adjacent to the mesial temporal lobe. They were developed as a substitute for depth electrodes. It is not clear that they carry a lower morbidity, though the insertion technique is simpler and less expensive.

ADVANTAGES AND DISADVANTAGES OF INTRACRANIAL ELECTRODES

Intracranial electrodes have several advantages over scalp electrodes (44). They lie in direct proximity to the cortex, so the EEG signal is neither attenuated nor altered by overlying skull or scalp tissue. The scalp and skull act as a frequency-dependent filter, and preferentially pass lower frequencies more readily than higher frequencies (21). Practically speaking, this means that beta and gamma frequencies are attenuated more than delta or theta frequencies, and that the fast components of interictal and ictal spikes are more greatly attenuated. In addition, the EEG signal cannot be obscured by electromyographic artifact when using intracranial electrodes; this is often an insurmountable problem when recording seizures with scalp electrodes. Intracranial electrodes record signals from small pools of neurons that do not generate a sufficiently strong signal for scalp electrode detection. Consequently, intracranial electrodes detect seizures earlier and more often than scalp or sphenoidal electrodes, and hippocampal seizures are usually detected earlier with depth electrodes than subdural electrodes (8,56). Interictal spikes are detected in greater number and in more locations with intracranial electrodes than scalp electrodes. Focal disruptions of normal rhythms are more readily apparent with intracranial electrodes too, because the spatial averaging properties of the scalp are eliminated.

However, these advantages are accompanied by some disadvantages. Only a limited amount of cortex can be sampled by intracranial electrodes, and clinically important signals that are generated at a distance from the electrode may not be detected (21). Because the amplitude of any EEG signal is proportional to the solid angle of the dipole of any potential, potentials with a tangential orientation might not be detected. However, this limitation applies to scalp EEG as well. Signals that derive from the depths of sulci are typically not recorded by intracranial electrodes either, because the usual placement is over the superficial gyral surface. Finally, because the skull and/or dura must be breached to place intracranial electrodes, patients are exposed to risk and significant discomfort. Although the risk of a major complication such as hemorrhage, infection, or herniation is small, the potential for short- and long-term adverse consequences restricts the use of intracranial electrodes.

TECHNICAL CONSIDERATIONS

Depth Electrodes

Depth electrodes may have a variety of designs (see Fig. 20.1). They may be flexible or rigid, have a varying number of contacts, be constructed from different metals, be inserted from different approaches, and be used chronically or acutely in the operating room. The electrodes have blunt tips to avoid severing neural tissue during insertion. Most surgeons prefer to use flexible electrodes because they are safer than rigid electrodes. Flexible electrodes are inserted with a semirigid stylet or introducer placed in a hollow core of a cannula-type electrode or alongside a wire. These electrodes can deviate through natural tissue planes around structures such as arteries, which on occasion leads to less precise placement but a reduced chance of hemorrhage. Once the electrode is placed, the stylet or introducer is removed, leaving the flexible electrode behind. It is possible that removal of the introducer could displace the wire, but this rarely poses a significant problem. With flexible electrodes, a blow to the head cannot cause movement of the electrode through brain tissue with resultant injury. The electrodes are easily removed at the bedside with little discomfort

when they are no longer needed. Rigid electrodes are placed somewhat more precisely in the targeted cortical region. However, caution must be taken to avoid any trauma to the exposed portion of the electrodes so as to avoid movement of the electrodes in the brain.

Commercially produced electrodes typically have multiple contacts placed at regular intervals, either 5 or 10 mm along the course of the electrode, to allow for sampling along the entire course of the electrode. Electrodes can also be fabricated to any desired specification for customized contact spacing. Contacts are usually several square millimeters in area, though size can be varied according to the neurophysiologist's preference. Contacts are typically made of nickel–chromium alloys (nichrome) or, less often, platinum–iridium alloys because these are nonmagnetic and compatible with MRI. In the past, stainless steel, gold–chromium alloy, and other metals were used, but these create more artifact in the MRI scan than does nichrome. Silver and copper cannot be used because of an adverse brain reaction to these substances (12). A separate insulated wire runs from each contact to the proximal end of the electrode, where it inserts into a connector that can be plugged into a cable that connects to the amplifiers of an EEG recording machine.

Subdural and Epidural Electrodes

Subdural and epidural electrodes usually share a common design, irrespective of manufacturer (see Figs. 20.2 and 20.3). They consist of a flexible Silastic matrix, generally less than 0.6 mm thick, with embedded electrode contacts. As with depth electrodes, a separate insulated wire runs from each contact to a connector plug at the end of the electrode. The contacts are made of stainless steel or platinum, the latter producing less artifact in the MRI, and the exposed metal usually has a 2- to 3-mm diameter. Commercial manufacturers usually space the electrode contacts at 5- to 10-mm intervals, though any pattern can be fabricated. Strip electrodes usually have one or two rows of contacts arranged in a straight line, with between four and eight contacts per line. Grid electrodes come in a variety of sizes, and commonly range between four-by-four arrays and eight-by-eight arrays. Subdural strips and grids can be trimmed by the surgeon in the operating room to irregular shapes as needed to accommodate the craniotomy. Subdural strips can be removed at the bedside; an injection of intravenous narcotic prior to removal eases the brief discomfort sometimes experienced by patients. Subdural grid electrodes must be removed in the operating room because of the craniotomy, and the therapeutic surgical procedure is usually performed at the same time.

Another type of epidural electrode is the epidural peg electrode, which is a single contact attached to the skull through a twist drill hole (2). Epidural peg electrodes can be scattered over the skull to sample from different lobes of the brain. Because they are subject to limited spatial sampling, they are more useful for negative information—that is, demonstrating lack of involvement of underlying cortex—than for localizing an epileptogenic zone.

Foramen Ovale Electrodes

These electrodes, which are similar to depth electrodes, are commercially manufactured. They typically contain four to six contacts and have a flexible construction. In contrast to other electrode types, foramen ovale electrodes are inserted under fluoroscopic guidance in the radiology suite or the operating room under local anesthesia, and can be removed at the bedside (27,68,69).

Electrode Insertion

Depth, subdural, and epidural electrodes are inserted under general anesthesia in the operating room. If intraoperative electrocorticography is to be performed, then anesthesia should be restricted to nitrous oxide and narcotics, though propofol can be used briefly at the start of the procedure because it has a short half-life. If intraoperative electrocorticography is not planned, then any anesthetic agent can be used. Depth electrodes are inserted through a twist drill hole or bur hole, and subdural strip electrodes are placed through a bur hole. Subdural grid electrodes typically require a craniotomy, the extent of which depends on the size of the electrode. Depth electrodes are placed with either stereotactic frames or a frameless stereotactic technique, and subdural electrodes are placed freehand. Electrode location is tailored to the clinical picture, and can be modified in the operating room by using acute intraoperative electrocorticography to help define areas of interest for chronic electrode placement. The operative procedure generally takes 2–5 hours depending on the number and type of electrodes placed and whether electrocorticography is done. MRI obtained after implantation of electrodes verifies their location (Fig. 20.4).

Postoperative Course

Patients usually spend the first 24 hours after electrode implantation in the intensive care unit, and may then be transferred to specialized epilepsy units or remain in the intensive care unit for continuous video-EEG monitoring. There is no theoretical limit to how long intracranial electrodes may remain in the brain; the duration of monitoring depends on clinical needs and typically ranges between 1 and 3 weeks.

EEG Acquisition and Playback

The methods used to record and review the intracranial EEG are generally identical to those used for scalp EEG, with a few minor exceptions. The same amplifiers are used for scalp and intracranial EEG. Signals are usually digitized by commercial equipment at a rate of 200 Hz, which allows for adequate display of virtually all clinically relevant EEG signals. Some commercial equipment permits higher sampling rates; these are necessary to record signals greater than 100 Hz. The number of channels required depends on the number of electrode contacts used and the cortical regions that need to be sampled. Most commercial equipment is sufficiently flexible to permit simultaneous recording from at least 128 channels, though fewer channels are usually adequate. The same filter settings are used for depth EEG as scalp EEG (low filter, 1 Hz; high filter, 70 Hz), though high-frequency cutoff limitations do not necessarily apply. Indeed, very-high-frequency activity, up to 500 Hz, has been recorded in the intracranial EEG with depth electrodes using appropriate sampling rates (2,20). Because signal amplitudes are considerably higher, typically three- to eightfold, in the depth EEG than the scalp EEG, amplifier gains must be adjusted accordingly.

The intracranial EEG can be reviewed on a computer screen or on EEG paper; the method depends on the preference of the electroencephalographer. It is often helpful to view an extended period of time when examining a seizure. This is most easily accomplished with paper review, because 1 or more minutes can be laid out for simultaneous review. In addition, low-amplitude beta frequencies are sometimes more difficult to see on a computer screen than in a large paper format. Computer review, however, allows greater flexibility when reviewing data and, in many circumstances, is adequate for clinical purposes. EEG data are most efficiently stored in a digital format on a computer medium such as a compact disk.

Intracranial EEG montages are designed using the same principles as are employed in scalp EEG, although the specifics vary depending on the number of electrodes used and their location. Referential or bipolar montages can be created, and there are often advantages to reviewing data in more than one montage because of in-phase cancellation or active reference contacts. EEG channels are generally best displayed in a logical framework, with lin-

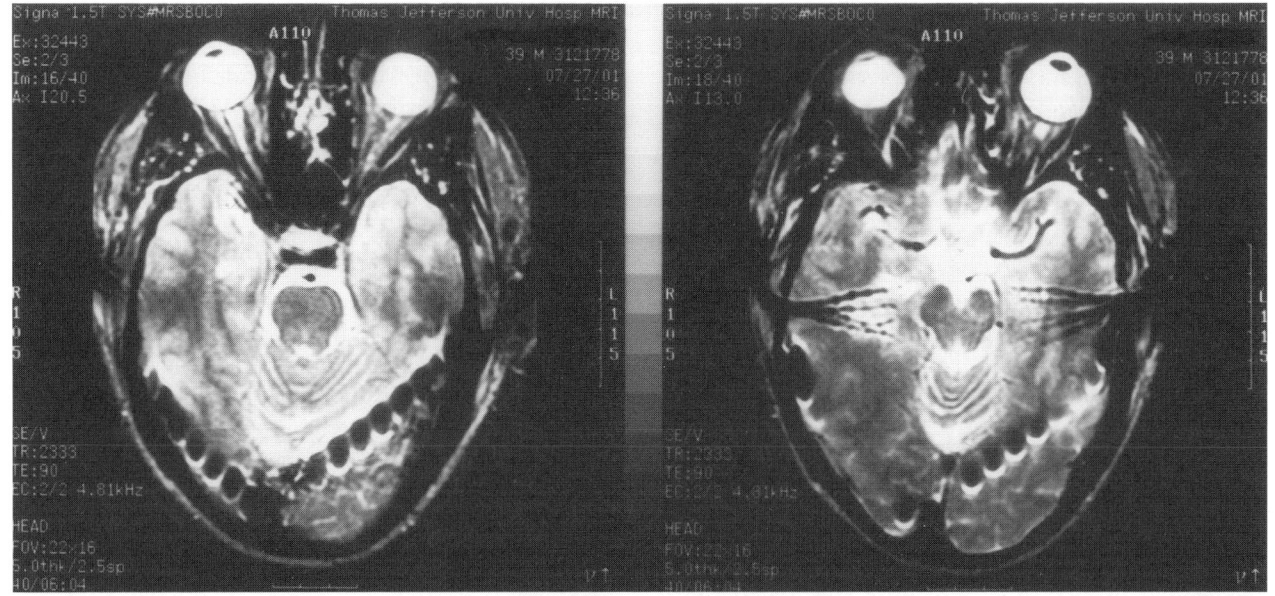

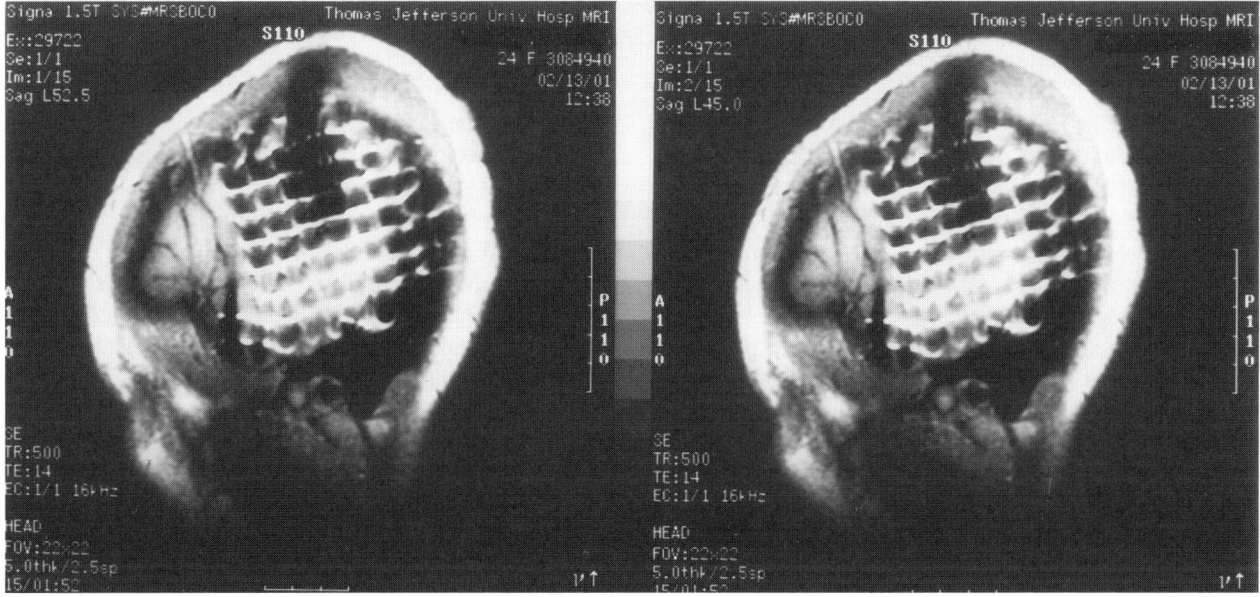

FIG. 20.4. **A:** MRI axial section showing depth and subdural electrodes. The depth electrodes are seen entering the lateral temporal cortex and crossing to the mesial cortex. Subdural electrodes are shown running posteriorly. **B:** MRI sagittal view showing subdural grid electrode contacts overlying the left hemisphere.

ear sequences (e.g., anterior to posterior, superior to inferior) and channels grouped by lobar location. For example, deep temporal lobe contacts may be grouped together in a series of channels, followed then by grouping lateral neocortical temporal contacts in the next series of channels, and so forth. This is shown in the EEG illustrations below. If a referential montage is used, either an extracranial or intracranial contact can be used. It is important to choose a reference contact that has as little artifact as possible and is uninvolved in the discharge of interest. Interpretation of intracranial EEG is often made difficult by the large number of channels needed to display information from all contacts. It is not uncommon to collect 64–128 channels of data, which must then be simultaneously reviewed.

ELECTRODE LOCATION

The majority of refractory patients who come for surgical evaluation have mesial temporal lobe epilepsy (18), which is characterized by seizures originating in the hippocampus or, less often, the amygdala. Depth electrodes are ideally suited to study patients with this condition because they directly record the EEG from limbic structures. In contrast, subdural, epidural, and foramen ovale electrodes are placed at a distance from the hippocampus and amygdala, which limits their sensitivity (this problem is further discussed later in this chapter). Temporal lobe depth electrodes are most often inserted via a lateral approach from the middle temporal gyrus to the desired mesial temporal targets, which include the amygdala, hippocampus, and parahippocampal gyrus. This is a relatively avascular route, which minimizes the risk of producing an intracerebral hematoma. Adequate sampling of mesial temporal structures requires placement of between three and six electrodes when a lateral approach is used. An alternative strategy, used less often, targets the hippocampus from a posterior approach through the occipital lobe. This technique permits placement of multiple contacts within mesial temporal structures with one electrode, though two electrodes are usually placed to ensure adequate sampling. The posterior approach puts the electrode through more brain tissue than the lateral approach, and objections have been raised because this method skewers the hippocampus, theoretically posing greater risk. In practice, however, no clinically significant problems have been reported using the posterior approach. Depth electrodes are generally placed in both mesial temporal lobes because of the possibility of bilateral independent seizure onsets, and to measure the interhemispheric propagation time (35). Unfortunately, temporal lobe neocortex is not well sampled by depth electrodes in either approach, so a combination of temporal lobe subdural strips and depth elec-

trodes is employed to allow for detection of either limbic or extralimbic temporal lobe seizure origin (3,8,42,52,56).

Subdural electrodes are best suited to record from other regions of the brain outside mesial temporal limbic structures, although depth electrodes were used in past years to sample the other lobes of the brain. Advances in subdural electrode technology and increases in the number of recording channels in EEG monitoring equipment have largely rendered the use of extratemporal depth electrodes unnecessary in most cases. Subdural electrodes offer superior sampling of virtually all other neocortical regions at lower risk. Consequently, depth electrodes are now used sparingly outside the temporal lobe in most institutions, and are reserved for situations in which technical considerations prevent adequate sampling with subdural electrodes; the exception is the orbitofrontal cortex, for which some neurophysiologists still use depth electrodes. Finally, depth electrodes have been used in some patients with epilepsy and movement disorders to record from subcortical nuclei, such as the thalamus and basal ganglia (66).

RISKS AND COMPLICATIONS

Intracranial electrodes have a relatively low chance of producing a permanent serious complication. Literature reports suggest that chronic intracranial EEG recording has a serious morbidity and mortality ranging between 1% and 4%, and the low end of that range seems most applicable in recent years (43,59,65,71). Technical advances in electrode fabrication and modern neurosurgical techniques have made intracranial electrode implantation reasonably safe, and there appears to be no safety advantage of one electrode type over another; morbidity and mortality rates appear similar. Even foramen ovale electrodes, introduced as a theoretically safer method, appear to pose risks that do not differ in magnitude from those associated with subdural or depth electrodes. Acute intraoperative recording with subdural or epidural electrodes has virtually no added risk other than that imposed by the added time needed for general anesthesia. If depth electrodes are used for acute intraoperative recording, the main risk consists of hemorrhage, with incidence similar to that when depth electrodes are placed for chronic recording. However, the surgeon has a better capability of treating an acute hemorrhagic complication that occurs during an acute intraoperative procedure, because he or she has already performed the craniotomy and the patient is anesthetized.

Hemorrhage—mainly intracerebral hematoma with depth electrodes, subdural hematoma with subdural electrodes, and epidural hemorrhage with epidural electrodes—is the most feared complication. The incidence of life-threatening hemorrhage has been reduced by using preoperative angiography to define vascular anatomy, directly visualizing cortex through use of a craniectomy rather than a bur hole for insertion, and using relatively avascular routes of electrode insertion in the case of depth electrode placement. In the authors' experience, major hemorrhages requiring therapy are rare, occurring in less than 0.3% of patients. The chance of hemorrhage can be reduced by preoperative evaluation of coagulation and clotting parameters, and counseling patients to avoid drugs that inhibit platelet function in the week before surgery. Because each puncture of the brain poses risk of hemorrhage, limiting the number of depth electrodes to the necessary minimum also reduces risk.

Another major risk is infection, though this is quite infrequent. In addition to the ordinary perioperative risks of any neurosurgical procedure, there is an ongoing risk of developing infection while the electrodes reside in the brain. The wire leading from the intracerebral contacts to the jack box provides a route for organisms to gain entry to the brain and meninges. The risk of infection is minimized by use of a technique whereby the wire is tunneled under scalp tissue for several centimeters before exiting the scalp through a separate stab wound. Tissues can then form a reasonably tight seal around the wire to block infection. Administering antibiotics during the perioperative period also helps prevent infection. Infections usually cause symptoms of meningitis, with fever, headache, photophobia, and stiff neck, and have always cleared with antibiotic use in the author's experience. The vast majority of patients with meningeal symptoms have a chemical meningitis rather than a bacterial infection, but examination and culture of cerebrospinal fluid is needed to clarify the diagnosis. In these circumstances, it is sensible to treat with broad-spectrum antibiotics until cerebrospinal fluid culture results are known. In our experience, infections readily respond to treatment. Antibiotic therapy should treat ordinarily benign skin organisms that may be inadvertently introduced during or after surgery. Although we have not observed brain abscesses following depth electrode placement, these are possible.

Infections sometimes pose a dilemma. Intracranial electrodes are foreign bodies that provide a direct link between the brain and the outside world of pathogenic organisms. Ordinarily, the best course of action when infection occurs is to promptly remove the foreign body and initiate antibiotic therapy. Even if a suboptimal number of seizures have been recorded, this is usually the wisest course of action. However, if seizures have not yet occurred, premature removal of the depth electrodes means that electrodes will need to be reinserted in the future, which exposes the patient to additional risks. If insufficient data have been recorded to make a diagnosis, the authors have elected to leave intracranial electrodes in place, prescribe antibiotics, and aggressively taper medication to record some seizures. The electrodes are removed once enough data are obtained to make a diagnosis; ideally, this is accomplished within a few days, and should be done at once, irrespective of the EEG findings, should any deterioration occur.

The other major risk pertains to subdural grid electrodes. On rare occasions, particularly with older, thicker electrode designs, brain swelling and edema could occur beneath the grid electrode. Herniation has been reported, usually in the first few days after electrode placement, though the incidence of this complication is well under 1% with modern electrodes. Because of this potential complication, careful neurological assessments are required, and emergent grid removal might be necessary.

Histopathological examination of resected tissue usually reveals evidence of the needle track, with reactive gliosis and inflammatory cells, in patients who have had depth electrodes inserted. Mild inflammation is also occasionally seen in tissue that lay beneath subdural electrodes. Because surgery is performed shortly after the electrodes are removed, this probably reflects a temporary alteration resulting from surgical trauma. These pathological findings are believed to be clinically insignificant. Although there is a theoretical risk of electrodes causing permanent brain injury, there is no published evidence suggesting permanent cognitive injury from depth electrodes except in the setting of hemorrhage. The electrodes are believed to be sufficiently small in diameter so that significant interruption of brain function is not seen. Because electrodes are fabricated from biologically inert materials, no toxic tissue reactions occur.

On balance, the decision to use an invasive EEG technique must be made weighing the anticipated benefits against the risks. There are two expected benefits: (i) to gain sufficient knowledge to perform a therapeutic procedure that otherwise could not be done, or could not be done nearly as well or as safely; or (ii) to avoid doing a procedure that would not help—for example, learning that seizures are multifocal and that surgery should not be performed. Although the use of intracranial electrodes carries some risk, it is small, and the benefits to be gained substantially outweigh those risks in carefully chosen patients.

EEG DATA

As detailed above, the intracranial EEG must be cautiously interpreted. When sampling a limited area of brain, one risks recording from cortex that is irrelevant or only marginally relevant to the epileptic process. The electrodes might be in the wrong place, perhaps even in the wrong hemisphere, and all data could be misleading. Only potentials that are near the electrode contacts are detected, and these potentials might consist of propagated activity that has spread from a primary epileptogenic zone. The significance of abnormal interictal paroxysmal and nonparoxysmal discharges is not fully understood. How to interpret seizures is also a subject of debate, and how different seizure types should be weighed is not certain.

Most chronic intracranial EEG recording sessions aim to record and evaluate interictal and ictal data (see Table 20.1). The interictal abnormalities may be epileptiform or nonepileptiform. The ictal onset zone, where seizures begin, should be delineated. The remainder of this section reviews interictal and ictal EEG findings recorded with intracranial electrodes.

Interictal EEG

Normal Findings

All of the EEG rhythms seen in the scalp EEG can be seen in the intracranial EEG. Provided electrodes are placed over the appropriate lobe of the cortical area, any rhythm can be detected. For example, one can record the alpha rhythm, beta activity, mu rhythm, sleep spindles, and any other activity. These are illustrated in Figures 20.5 through 20.9.

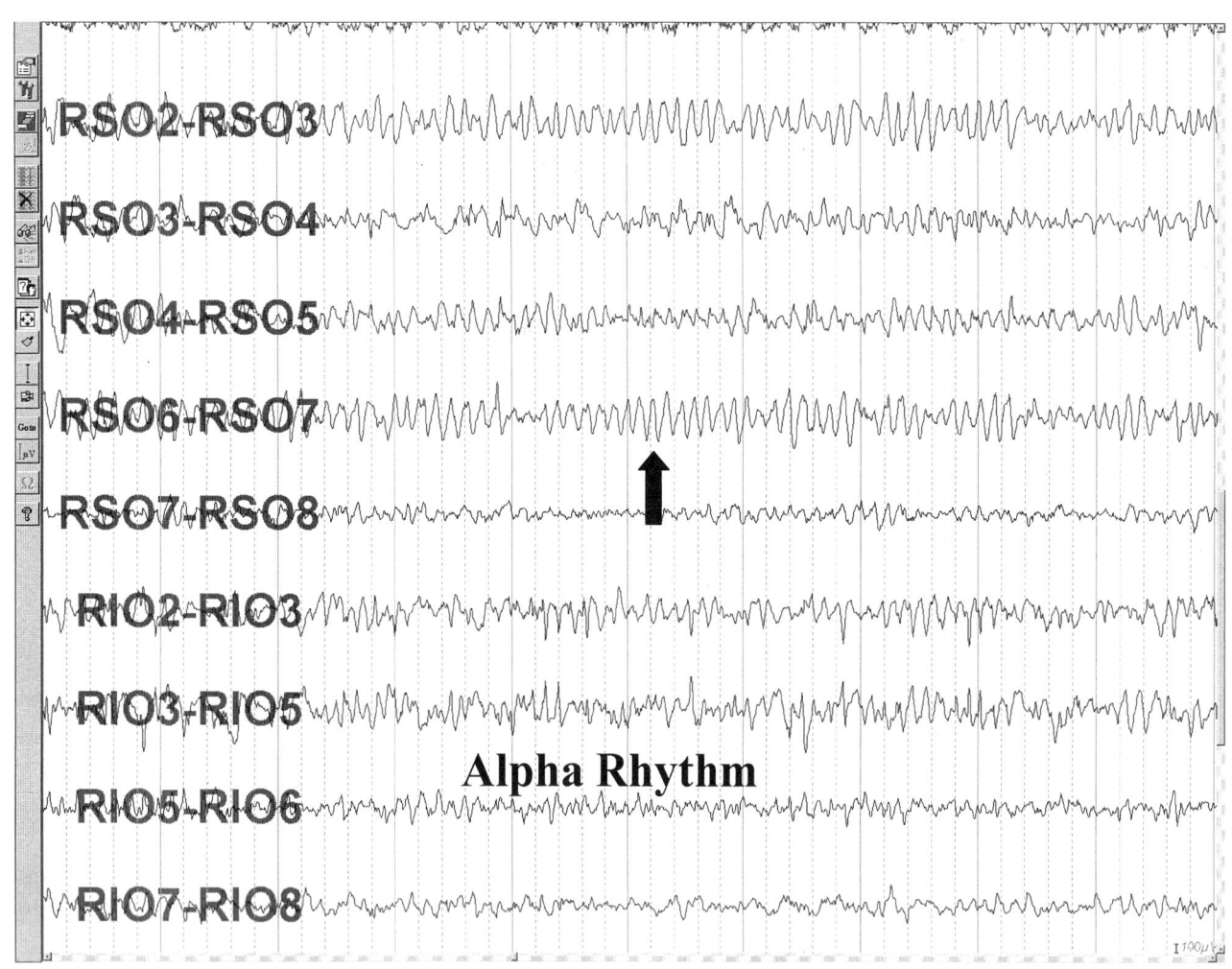

FIG. 20.5. Subdural recording showing the alpha rhythm (*arrow*) in the right occipital lobe.

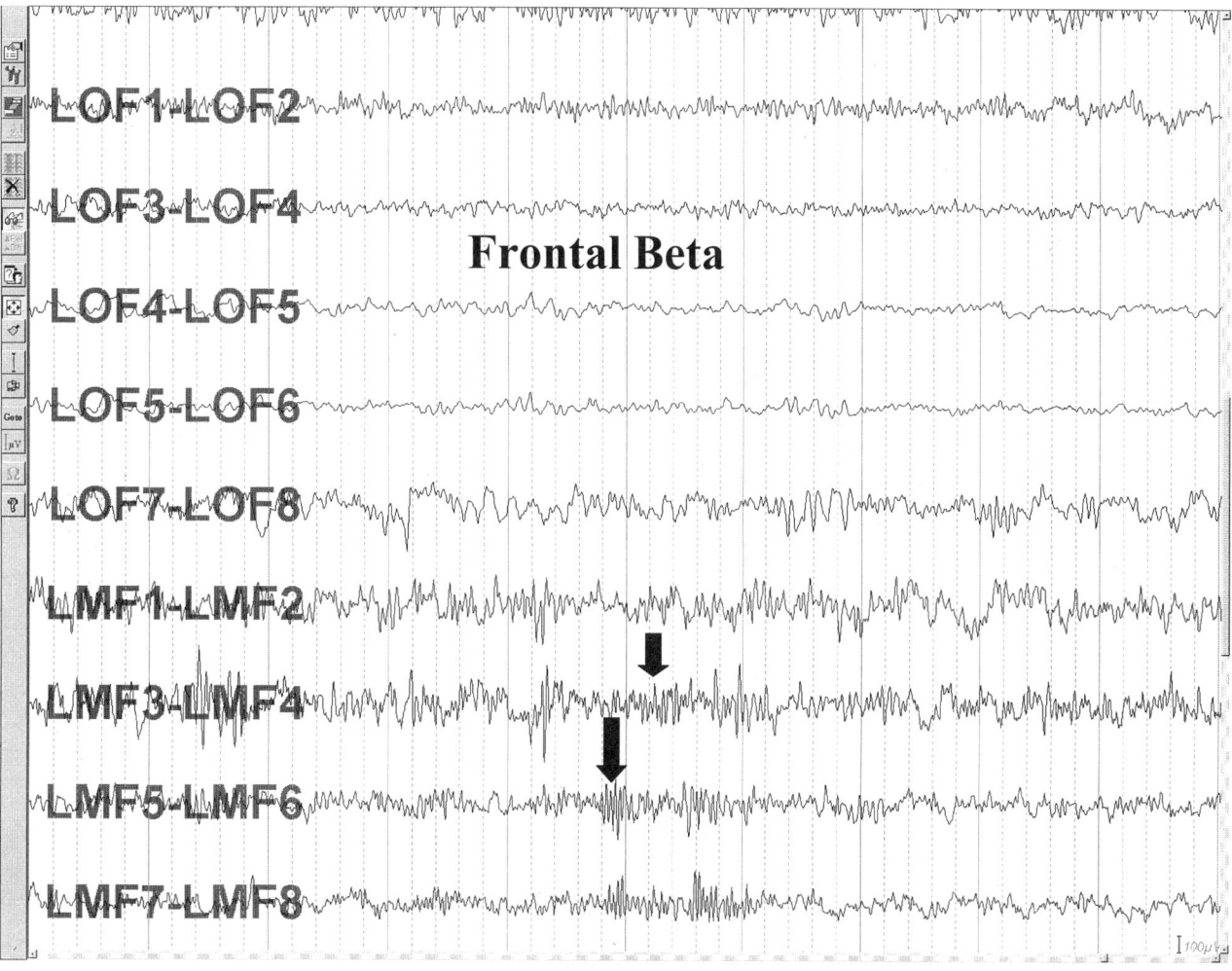

FIG. 20.6. Subdural recording showing normal frontal beta activity, most prominent in the mesial frontal cortex (LMF contacts) (*arrows*). Less beta activity is present in the orbitofrontal cortex (LOF contacts). Note the high frequency of the beta rhythm and its inherent sharpness.

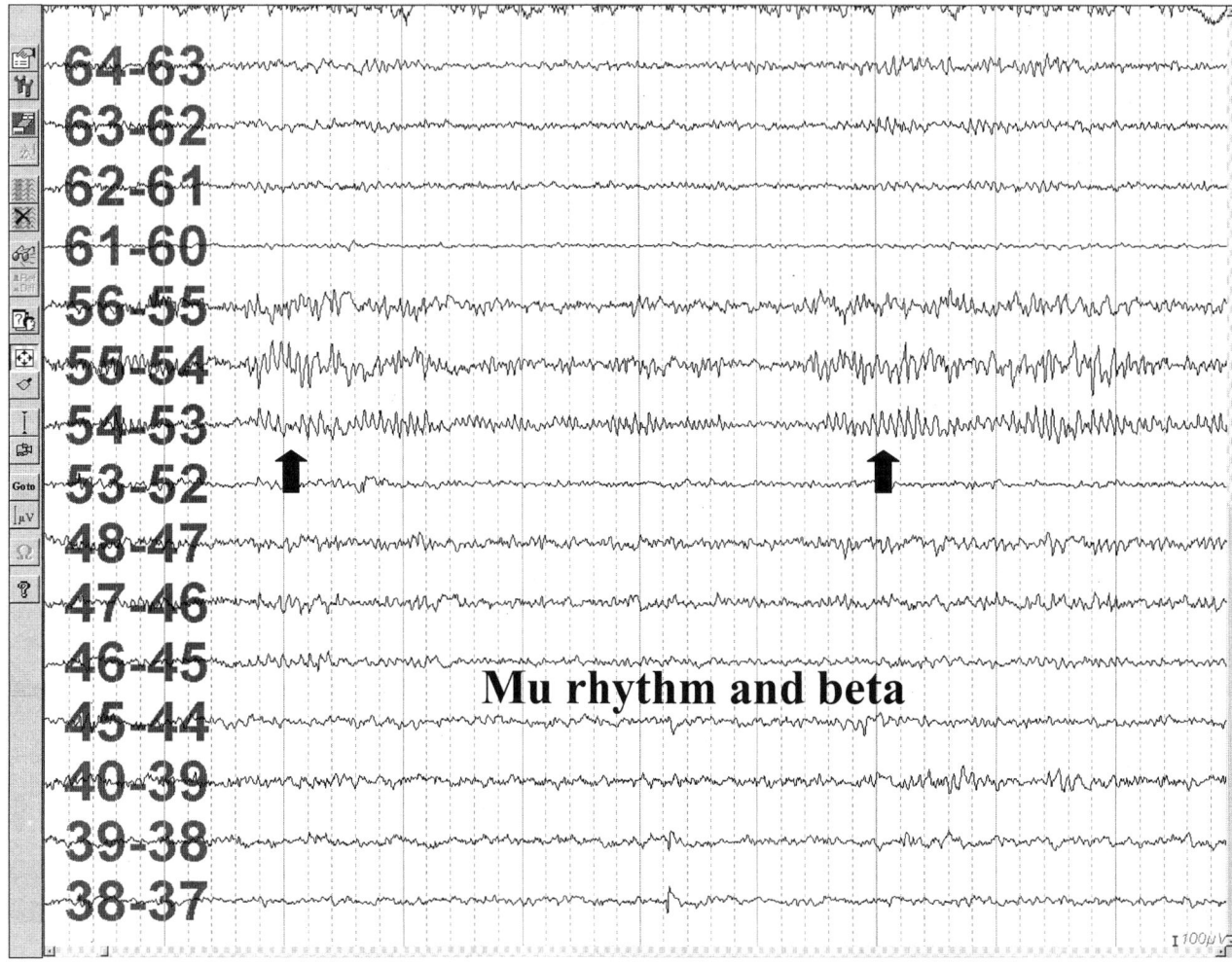

FIG. 20.7. Subdural grid recording showing mu rhythm (*arrows*) and beta activity in the frontal lobe.

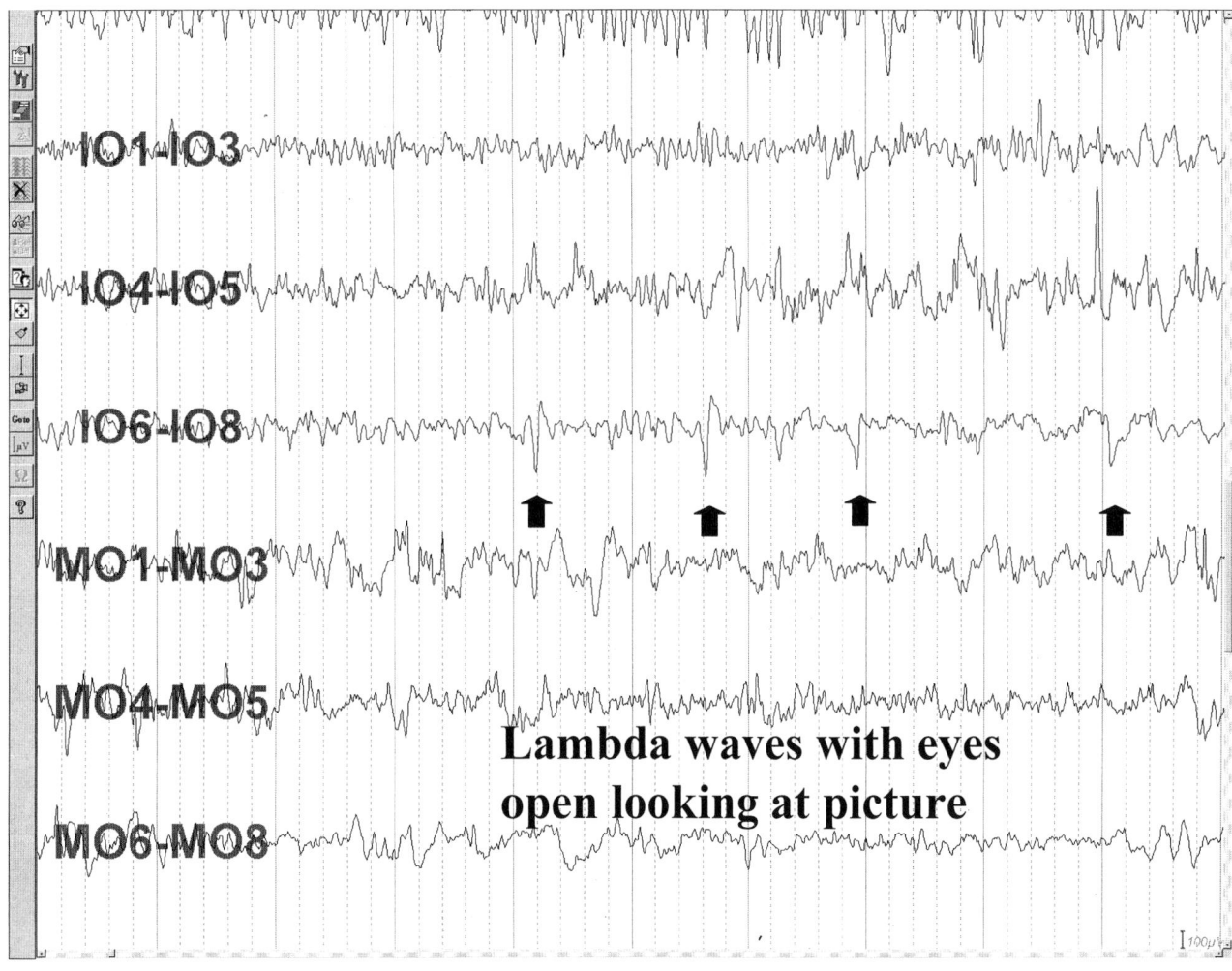

FIG. 20.8. Subdural recording showing lambda waves (*arrows*) while visually scanning a picture. These should not be mistaken for pathological sharp waves, and are abolished by looking at a blank sheet or towel.

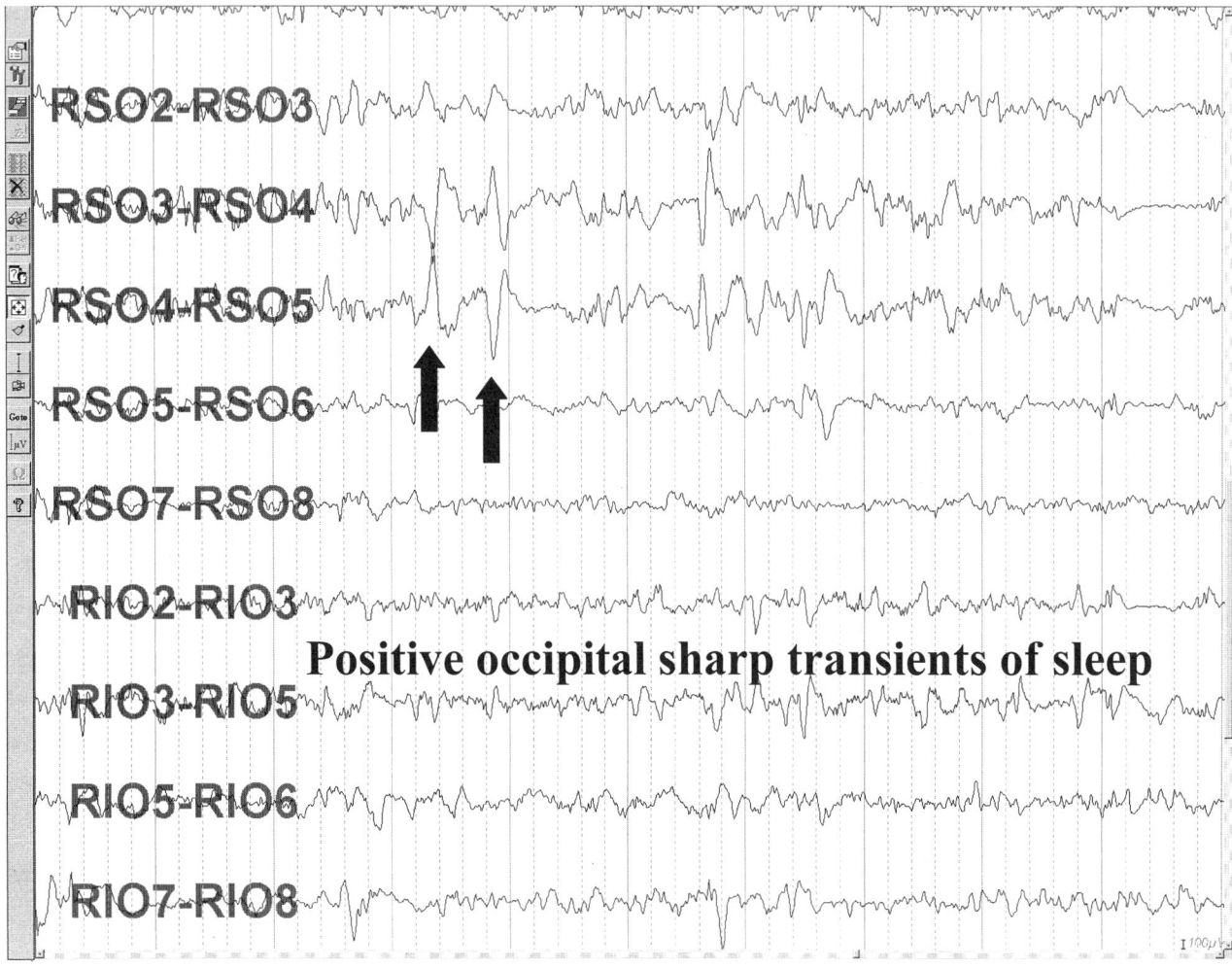

FIG. 20.9. Subdural recording showing positive occipital sharp transients of sleep (POSTS) (*arrows*). Note the varying magnitude of negative and positive components.

Nonepileptiform Abnormalities

The interictal EEG shows a number of focal nonepileptiform abnormalities (Table 20.3) (see also Chapter 17). It is worth reemphasizing that the faster frequencies are not attenuated by scalp and skull, so the electroencephalographer must avoid overinterpreting the EEG. Many normal rhythms, such as normal beta activity, rhythmic temporal theta activity of drowsiness, wicket rhythms, the mu rhythm, positive sharp transients of sleep, and even the alpha rhythm may look quite spiky in the intracranial EEG. These should not be misinterpreted as pathological spikes or sharp waves.

Focal disturbances in the EEG background correlate with the presence of either hippocampal atrophy or neocortical gliosis (11). The following types of nonepileptiform interictal abnormalities have been described:

1. *Focal slowing:* Focal slow waves may appear in the delta- or theta-frequency bands in one or more cortical regions (Fig. 20.10). Because many kinds of artifact can masquerade as focal slowing, diagnosing focal slowing requires comparison of the frequencies in the suspect area with rhythms in homologous contralateral cortex, with rhythms from surrounding cortex in the same lobe, and with an EEG recorded from the same region in other individuals. Transient slowing of frequencies from electrode placement, perhaps related to temporary edema, may be of no clinical consequence, and artifactual sources such as venous pulsation must be excluded as causes (1). Focal slowing may indicate that a structural lesion is present, and but it is reliable only when other abnormalities are present in the same area, as described below. Although focal slowing may indicate the presence of a structural lesion, it does not suggest that the lesion is epileptogenic, and seizures may emanate from a different region of the brain.

2. *Focal attenuation of alpha or beta frequencies:* A localized attenuation of fast frequencies suggests underlying cortical gliosis (see Fig. 20.10). When seen in combination with focal slowing of background frequencies, focal loss of faster frequencies strongly suggests the presence of an underlying structural lesion, such as gliosis or tumor.

3. *Focal attenuation of normal sleep rhythms:* Normal sleep rhythms seen in the scalp EEG are also seen in the depth EEG. During slow-wave sleep, sleep spindles can appear in the frontal, parietal, and temporal cortex. Spindles may even appear in the hippocampus. A focal attenuation of sleep spindles suggests that a lesion is present, such as gliosis.

4. *Focal burst-suppression:* A focal burst-suppression pattern may appear the depth EEG, usually in sleep, suggesting the presence of gliosis (Fig. 20.11).

5. *Lack of full beta induction with pharmacological activation:* Intravenous injection of thiopental or diazepam increases the amount and amplitude of beta activity in the scalp and depth EEG (16). Lack of or reduction in beta induction in one region suggests the presence of gliosis or tumor. Similarly, development of a focal burst-suppression pattern after thiopental injection suggests gliosis (54).

Epileptiform Abnormalities

Interictal spikes look somewhat different in the depth EEG than in the scalp EEG (Chapter 17) because of the lack of filtering by scalp and skull. They are shorter in duration and higher in amplitude, may be either positive or negative, and more often are polyphasic (Figs. 20.12 through 20.15). Some intracranial spikes have a highly restricted field and might appear in a single electrode contact. Other spikes may be quite widespread, involving part or all of a single lobe or more than one lobe in a hemisphere (see Fig. 20.12), or be generalized and synchronous in both hemispheres. Dipoles are more often evident in the intracranial EEG, and both positive and negative phase reversals might be seen along the course of a multicontact depth electrode or in a chain of subdural contacts. However, the usual cautions apply when interpreting spikes. Potential fields must make anatomical and physiological sense. Because spikes are sharper in the intracranial EEG, caution should be exercised when interpreting sharp waves. These may represent distant, temporally spread potentials that have propagated from a distant site or simply be normal sharply contoured activity. One should exercise great caution in interpreting sharp waves in the intracranial EEG as indicative of immediately underlying pathology.

TABLE 20.3. *Interictal EEG abnormalities*

Nonepileptiform
Focal slow waves
Focal loss of fast frequencies
Focal loss of normal sleep rhythms
Focal burst-suppression
Focal attenuation of response to pharmacological activation
Epileptiform
Spikes, sharp waves
   Focal or regional
   Negative or positive
   Synchronous or asynchronous
   Acute or chronic recording

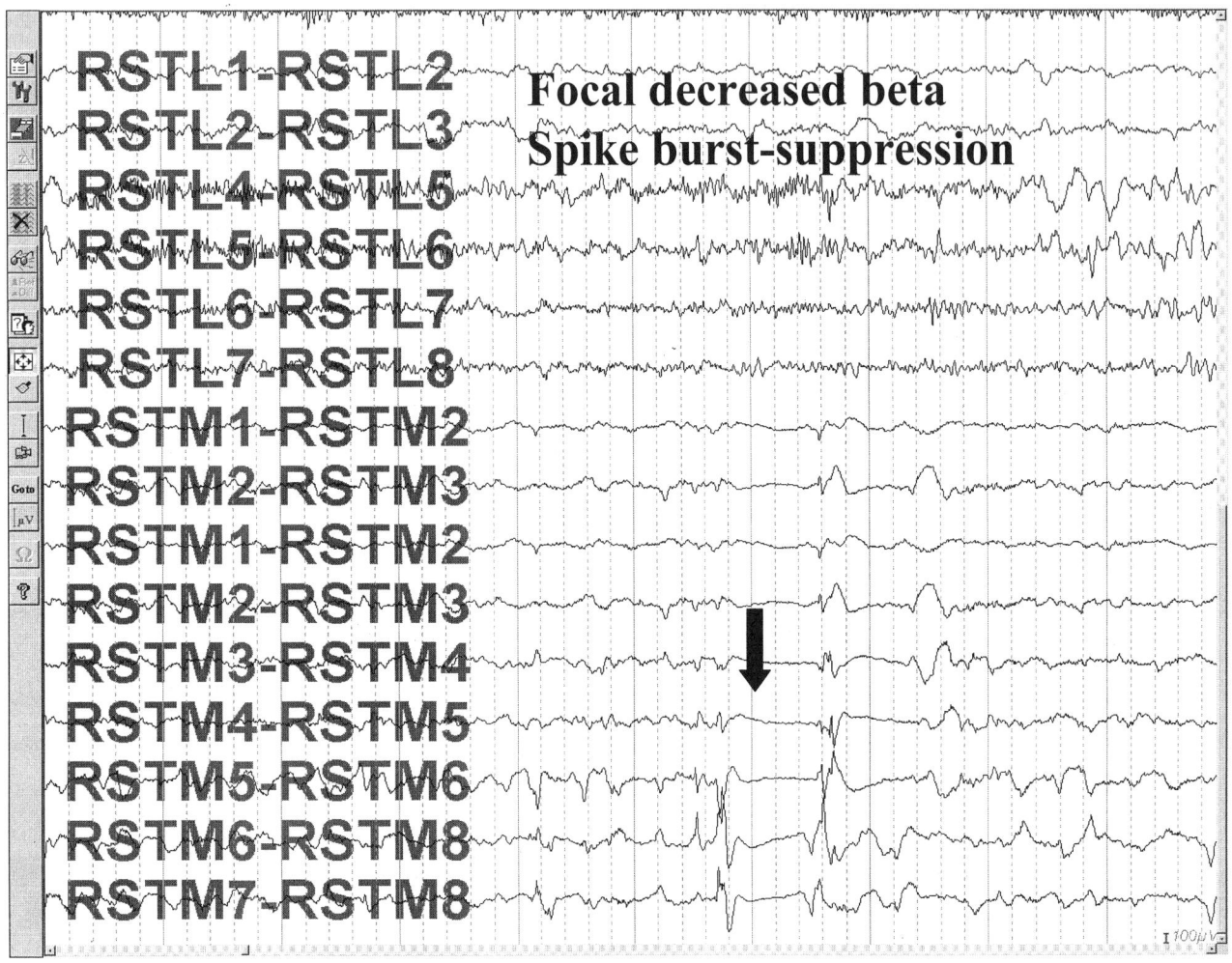

FIG. 20.10. EEG showing focal increase in theta and delta activity, and diminution of beta activity in basomedial right temporal lobe (*RSTM*) compared with basolateral right temporal lobe subdural contacts. In addition, focal spike burst-suppression is seen in the basomedial contacts (*arrow*).

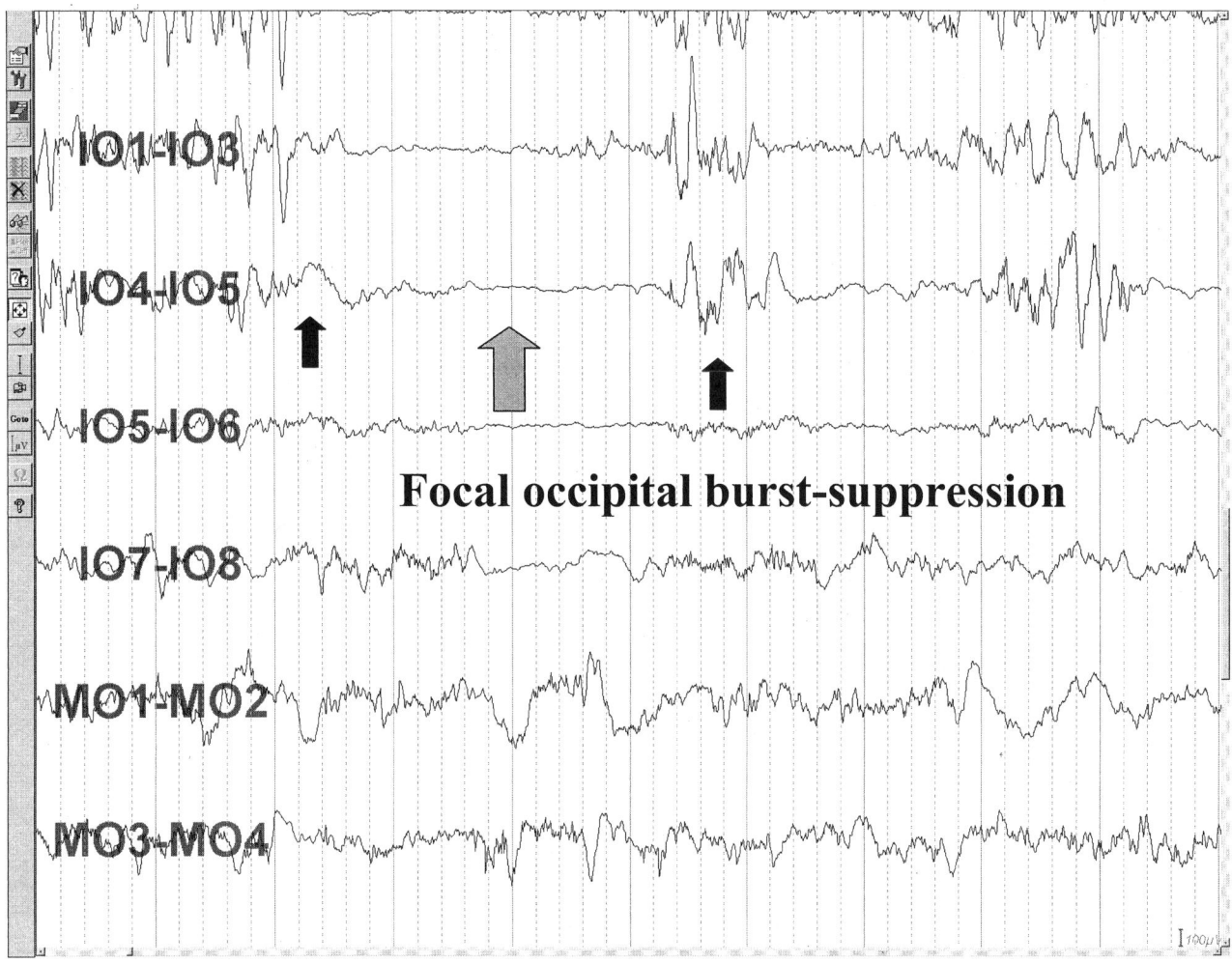

FIG. 20.11. EEG recording showing focal burst-suppression (arrows) in the inferior occipital subdural strip electrode (IO) but not the middle occipital subdural strip electrode (MO) during sleep.

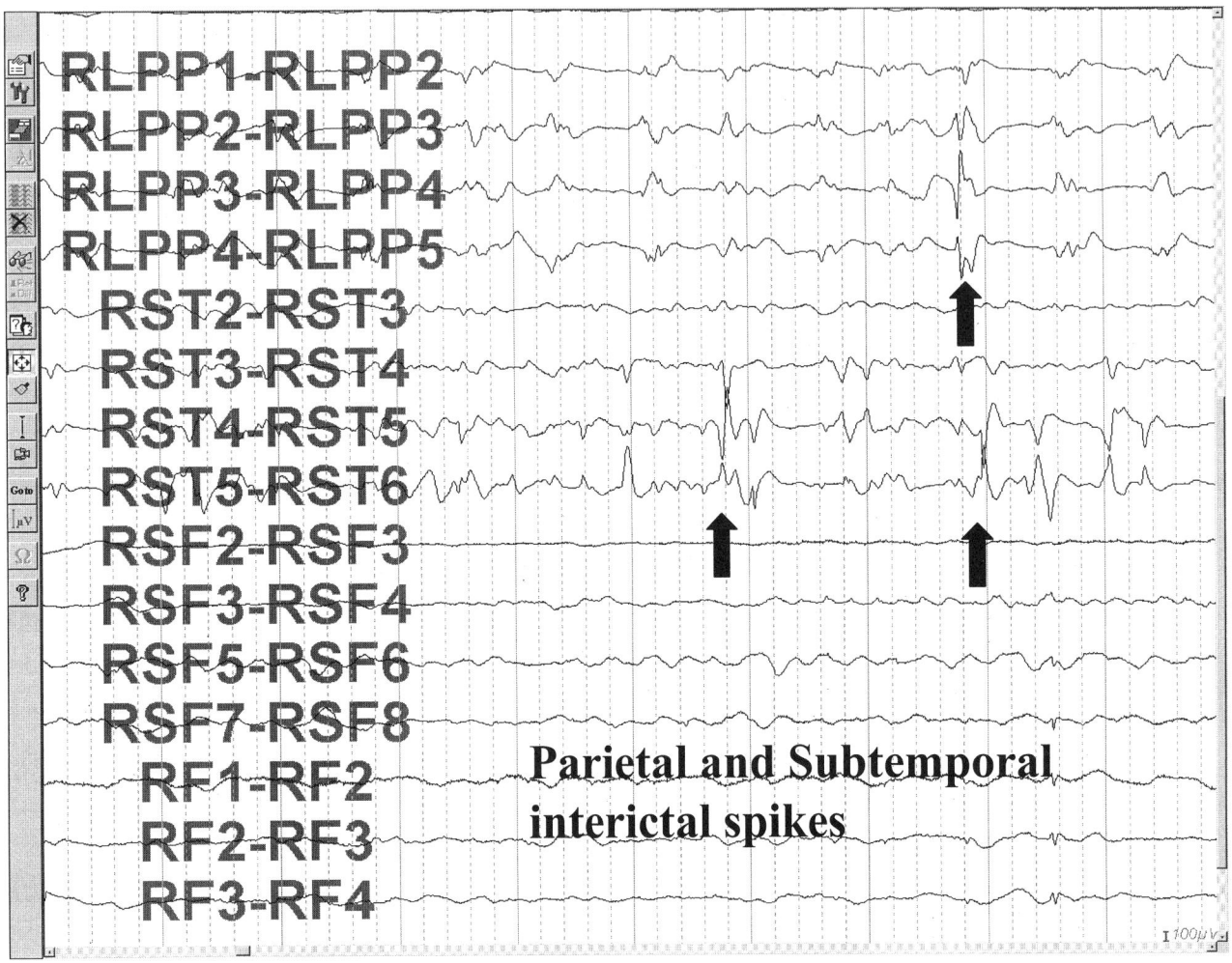

FIG. 20.12. EEG recording showing independent interictal spikes (*arrow*) in the right parietal (*RLPP*) and right temporal subdural (*RST*) electrodes. No spikes are seen in the right frontal lobe electrodes (*RSF, RF*).

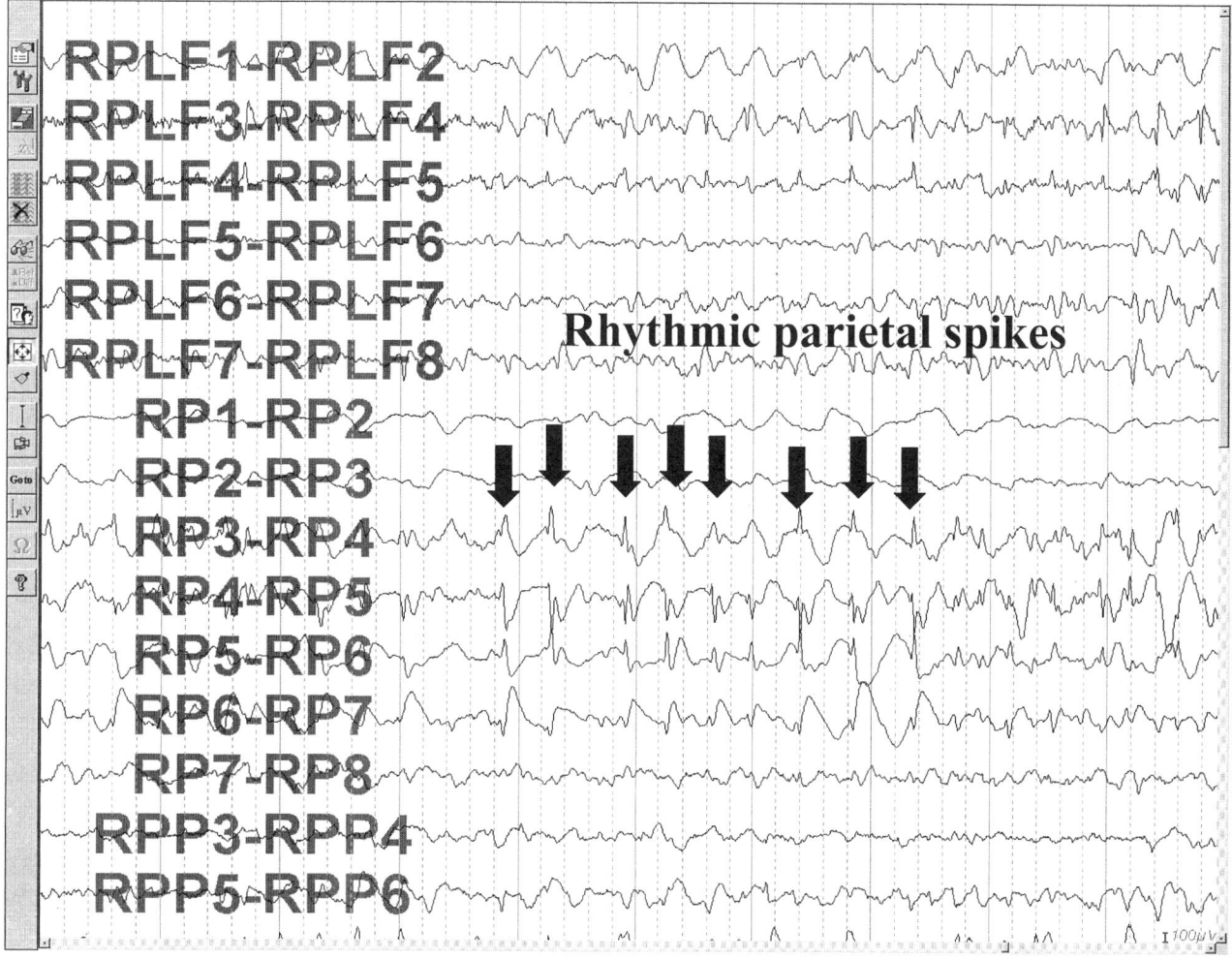

FIG. 20.13. EEG recording showing rhythmic spiking in the right parietal subdural contacts (*arrows*).

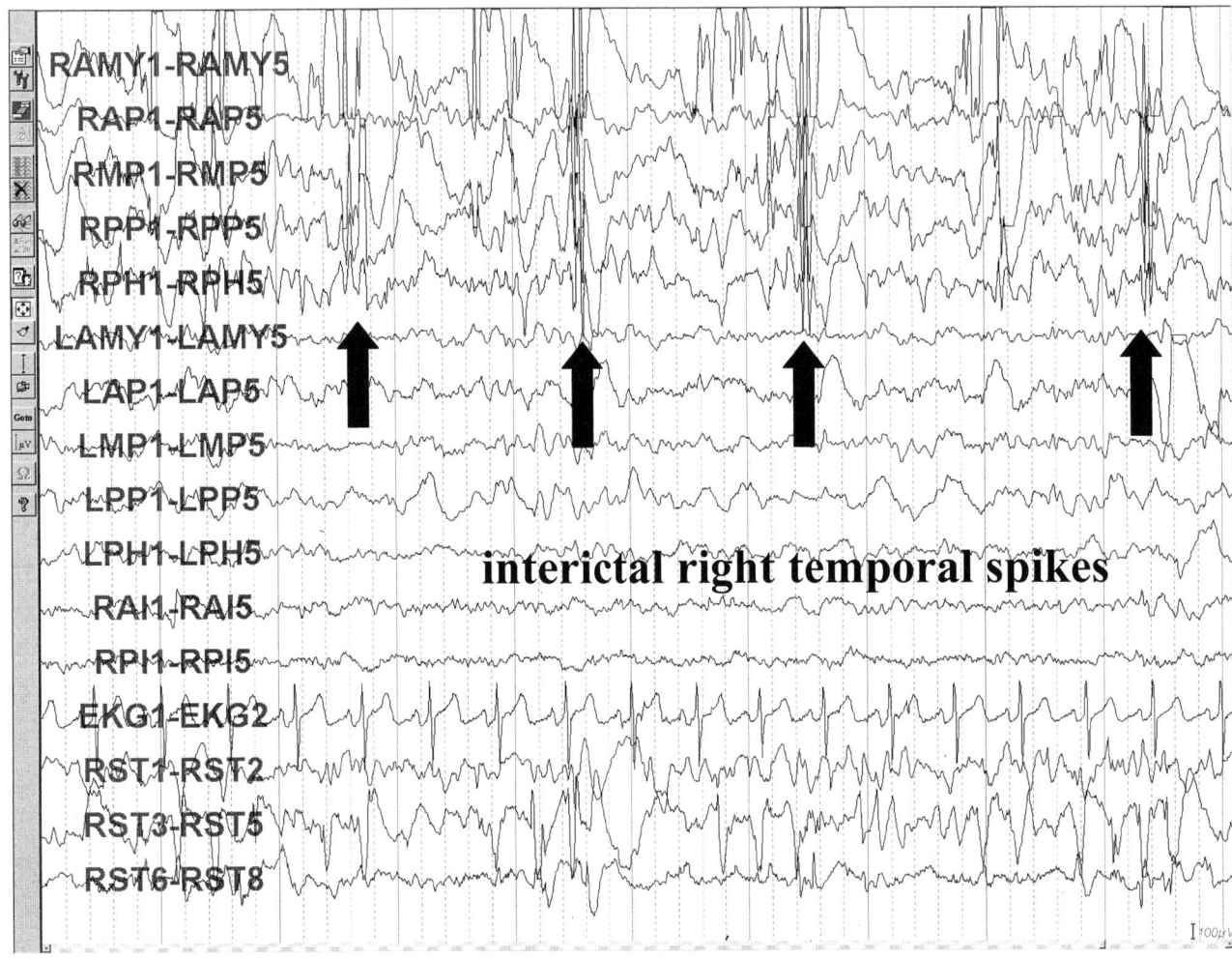

FIG. 20.14. EEG recording showing frequent interictal spikes and polyspikes (*arrows*) in the right mesial depth electrode contacts (*RAMY, RAP, RMP, RPP, RPH*) and occasional low-amplitude spikes in the subtemporal subdural strip electrode (*RST*). No spikes are present in the left mesial temporal depth electrodes (*LAMY, LAP, LMP, LPP, LPH*).

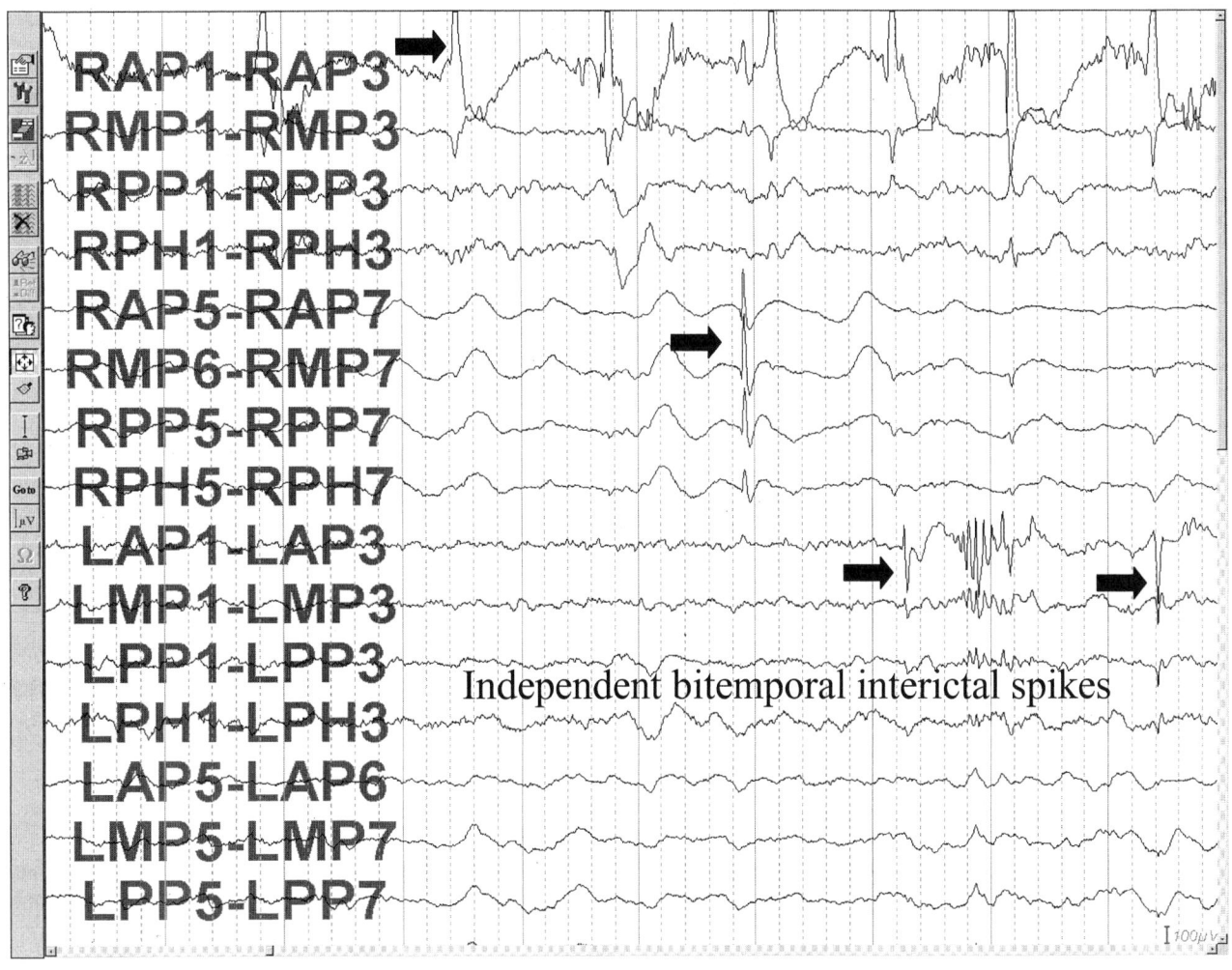

FIG. 20.15. Interictal EEG showing independent asynchronous interictal spikes in right (*R*) mesial and neocortical temporal contacts and left (*L*) mesial temporal depth electrode contacts (*arrows*).

In temporal lobe epilepsy, all patients have interictal spikes on intracranial EEG recording (see Fig. 20.14). Spikes commonly appear bilaterally and independently in the hippocampus, amygdala, and parahippocampal gyrus, and in temporal lobe neocortex (see Fig. 20.15). Negative spikes recorded in the hippocampus are usually not detected by sphenoidal or scalp electrodes (38,55,58). Scalp, nasopharyngeal, and sphenoidal electrodes record from basal temporal neocortex, not from the hippocampus. When a negative spike is seen in the surface EEG, hippocampal electrodes may show no activity, or may show a simultaneous negative or positive component. In the amygdala, a characteristic broad, triangular positive spike is often seen; this is not common in the hippocampus (58). Hippocampal spikes are nearly always asynchronous in mesial temporal lobe epilepsy. The occurrence of synchronous hippocampal spikes is associated with a poor prognosis after temporal lobectomy and suggests a strong possibility of a distant focus (37). In mesial temporal lobe epilepsy, multifocal spikes occur within the hippocampus and amygdala; independent spikes are commonly observed in the amygdala, anterior hippocampus, and posterior hippocampus, along with other widespread "regional" spikes that involve all mesial temporal limbic structures in one hemisphere. In addition, it is common to see interictal spikes occurring independently in other lobes of the brain in patients with temporal lobe epilepsy, especially in the orbitofrontal and cingulate cortex.

Interictal spikes nearly always occur in patients with frontal, parietal, and occipital epilepsies as well (see Figs. 20.12 and 20.13). Both positive and negative spikes and polyspikes can be seen, and their distribution varies from one patient to the next. Multifocal patterns are common, and, even though a structural epileptogenic lesion may be present in one lobe, interictal spikes can be widespread in one or both hemispheres. Interictal spikes are commonly activated by slow-wave sleep and have a reduced rate of occurrence in REM sleep and wakefulness.

Because spikes recorded with intracranial EEG may emanate from a minuscule amount of cortex, a general consensus is lacking with regard to their clinical relevance. It is unclear which types of spike signify the presence of pathological tissue that should be excised. For example, many investigators believe that pseudoperiodic lateralized epileptiform discharge (PLED)-like spikes and spike burst-suppression correlate strongly with the presence of underlying pathological cortex and an epileptogenic zone than do other types of spikes, but few empirical data exist to support this notion. The medical literature does not lend credence to any one interpretation (4,19,39,46,61–63). Fiol and colleagues (19) noted more spikes in the postexcision electrocorticogram in temporal lobectomy patients with recurrent seizures than in those whose seizures stopped. In contrast, Tran et al. (61) and Schwartz et al. (46) found no relation between presence of residual spikes and surgical success. However, no investigators have categorized spikes in a way that might distinguish between different types of discharges (PLED-like, isolated rare spikes, etc.). Lieb et al. (36,37) suggested that some characteristics of hippocampal spikes predict outcome. Spikes with greater autonomy, that is, with less dependence on sleep state and less interspike interval variability, more often indicated the epileptogenic zone than spikes that were less autonomous. The frequency with which spikes occur is a poor predictor of the site of seizure origin or surgical outcome. Lange et al. (33) noted alterations in the spatial organization of limbic spikes shortly before seizures begin, but no interictal spike patterns are yet proven to reliably identify when seizures might occur or their source of origin.

Consequently, most authorities are reluctant to rely on interictal spikes alone for planning surgery. For example, multifocal spikes may be present in patients with well-localized mesial temporal lobe epilepsy who respond to surgery, and interictal spikes may not be present in a location from which seizures arise (26). Hence interictal spikes are probably most useful when considered in conjunction with ictal EEG findings. If most interictal spikes arise from the same area as seizures and other interictal nonepileptiform disturbances, this is *probably* a favorable prognostic sign.

Ictal EEG: Seizures

In the epilepsy surgery patient, intracranial electrodes are mainly placed to record seizures and determine where they begin for purposes of mapping the epileptogenic brain area for resection. Seizures observed with intracranial EEG differ considerably from those recorded with scalp electrodes. A seizure typically only appears in the scalp EEG after it has spread considerably. A larger volume of cortex has been recruited into the seizure, and distant areas, perhaps even in the contralateral hemisphere, may show ictal discharges. Because of lack of filtering by scalp and skull and absence of spatial averaging, discharges with restricted spatial extent, limited voltage, and higher frequencies can be seen, though they were unapparent with scalp electrodes. In

TABLE 20.4. *Seizure characteristics*

Frequency at start of seizure
Location of seizure onset: focal, regional, multilobar, nonlocalized
Propagation routes (pattern and location of spread of ictal discharges)
Latency of spread to other lobes within hemisphere of onset
Latency of spread to contralateral hemisphere
Consistency of localization of seizure onset
Pattern of seizure termination
Location of postictal suppression

many patients, intracranial electrodes show focal seizure onset when extracranial electrodes have not done so. The cortex from which seizures originate often (though not always) harbors pathological changes when examined under the microscope, and excision of this region often results in seizure relief. However, a localized seizure onset in the intracranial EEG does not guarantee a successful surgical result, and a lack of consistently localized seizure onset does not preclude a satisfactory surgical outcome (26,47).

Seizures exhibit diverse features, so much so that one seizure may differ from the next within any particular person (Table 20.4; Figs. 20.16 through 20.25) (1,15,16,24,38,53,58). The electrical pattern usually provides a clear

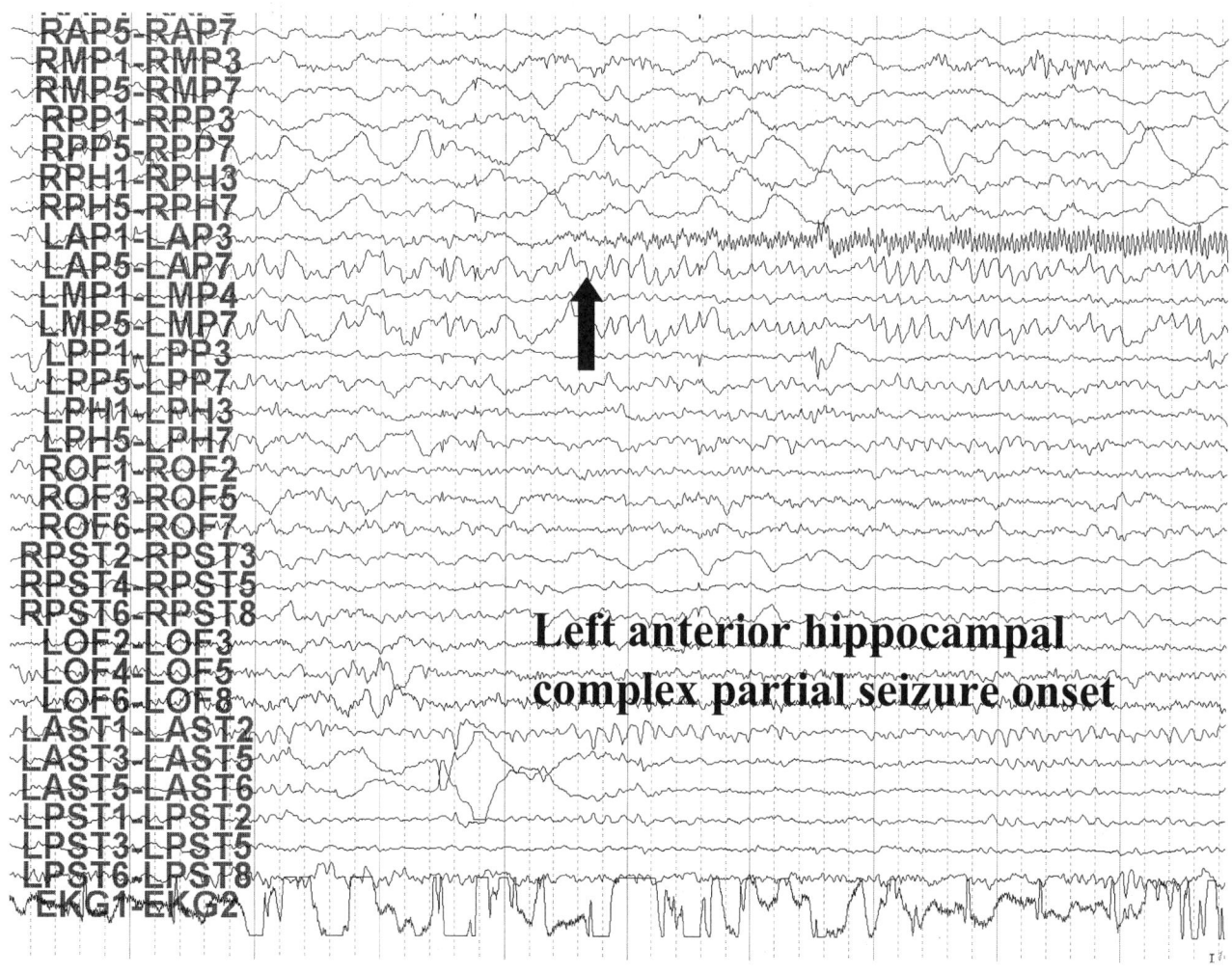

FIG. 20.16. EEG showing focal complex partial seizure onset (*arrow*) in the left anterior hippocampal depth electrode (*LAP*). Note how focal the onset appears, with no involvement of adjacent depth electrode contacts in the middle and posterior hippocampus (*LMP, LPP*) or parahippocampal gyrus (*LPH*), or of left temporal subdural strip electrodes (*LAST, LPST*). Right-sided contacts (all beginning with *R*) are similarly uninvolved.

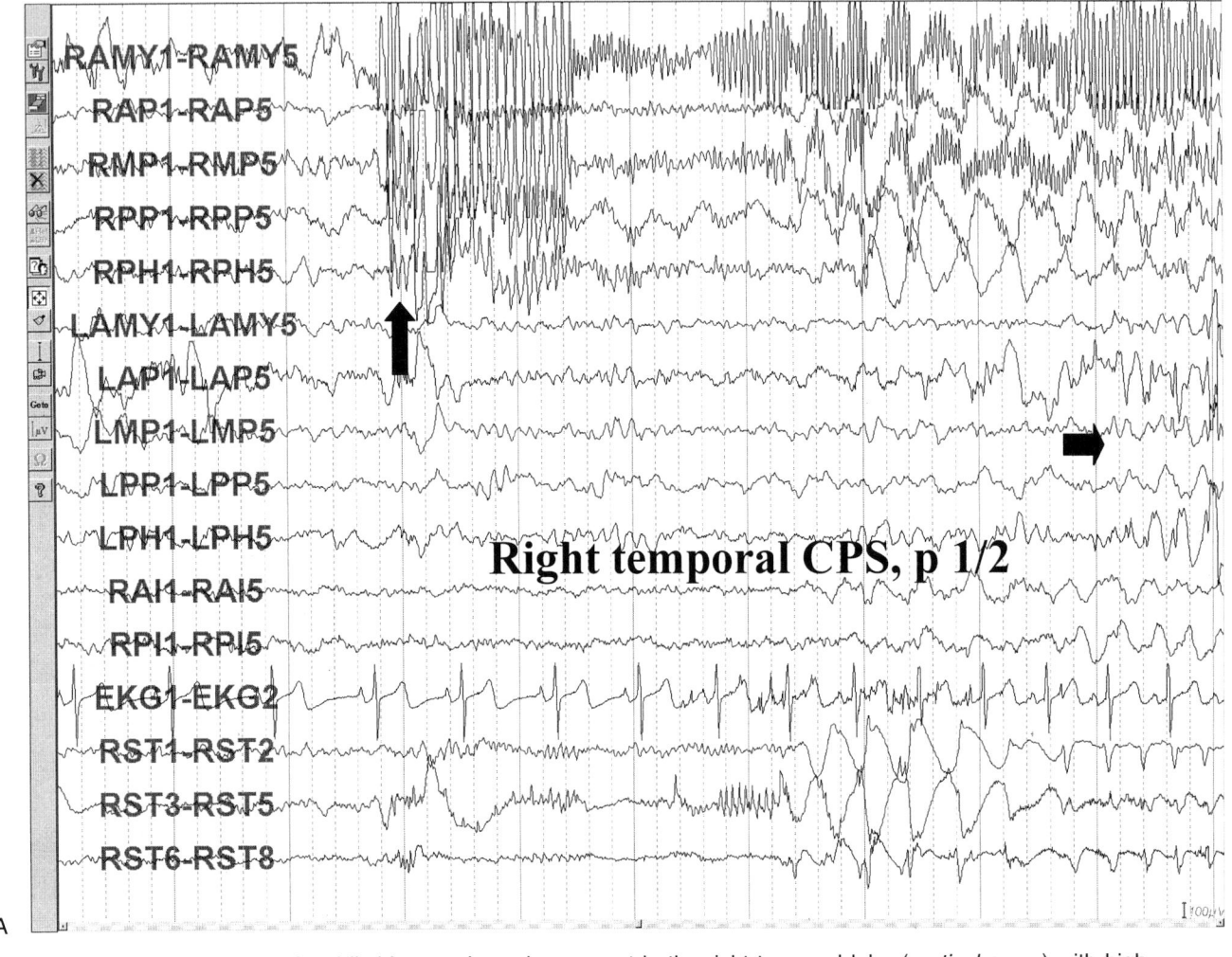

FIG. 20.17. A: Regional limbic complex seizure onset in the right temporal lobe (*vertical arrow*) with high-amplitude fast activity in the amygdala, hippocampus, and parahippocampal gyrus (*RAMY, RAP, RMP, RPP, RPH*) contacts. The subdural contacts beneath the right temporal lobe (*RST*) show the seizure onset nicely as well. The seizure spreads to the left temporal lobe (*horizontal arrow*, right side of figure) approximately 6 seconds after onset, with irregular theta- and alpha-frequency activity. Note the tachycardia that develops in the early seconds of the seizure. *(Figure continues.)*

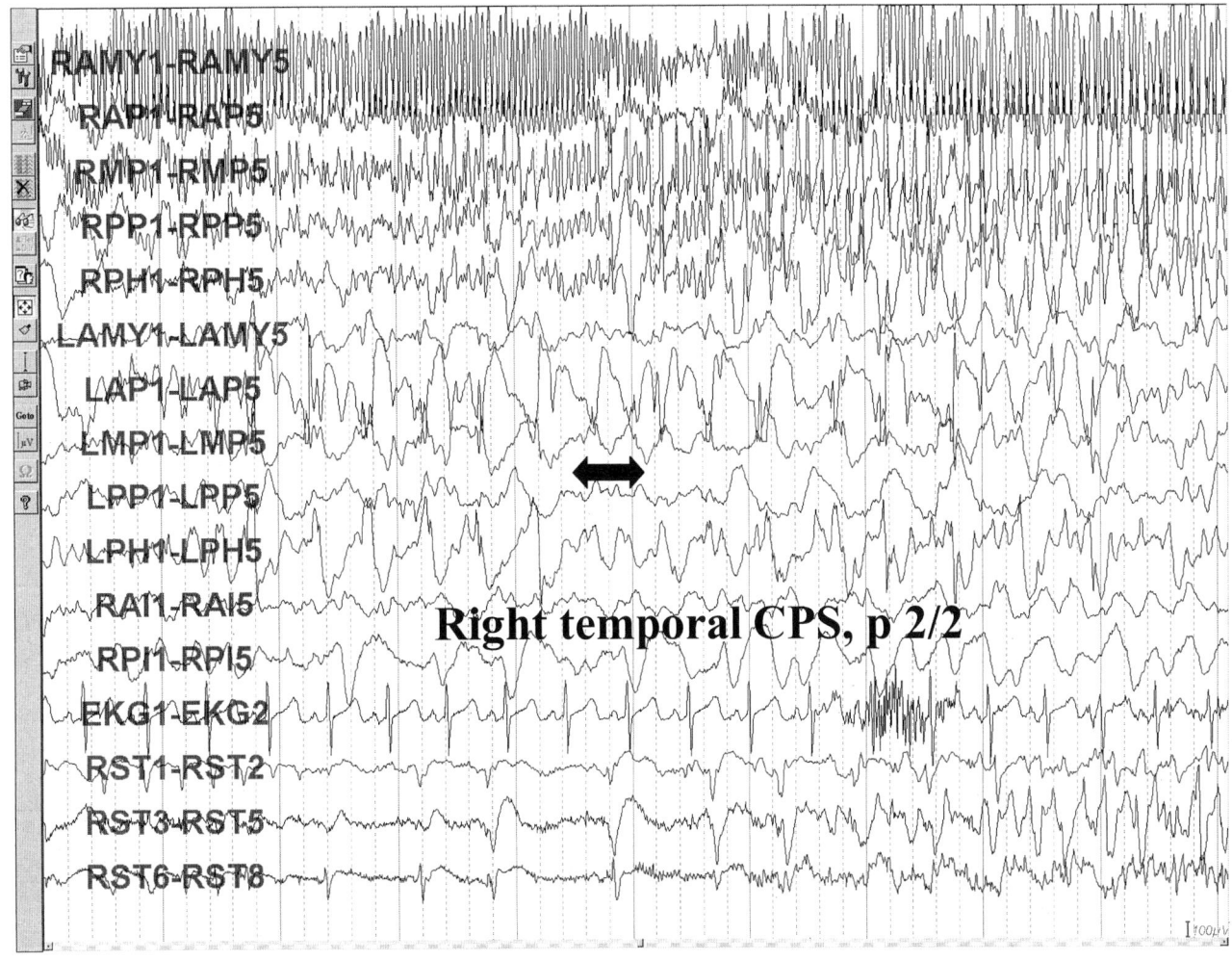

B

FIG. 20.17. *Continued.* **B:** On the second page of the complex partial seizure recording, note that the right and left temporal lobes are seizing independently with different ictal discharge frequencies. The *arrow* highlights the slow discharge frequency in the left temporal contacts.

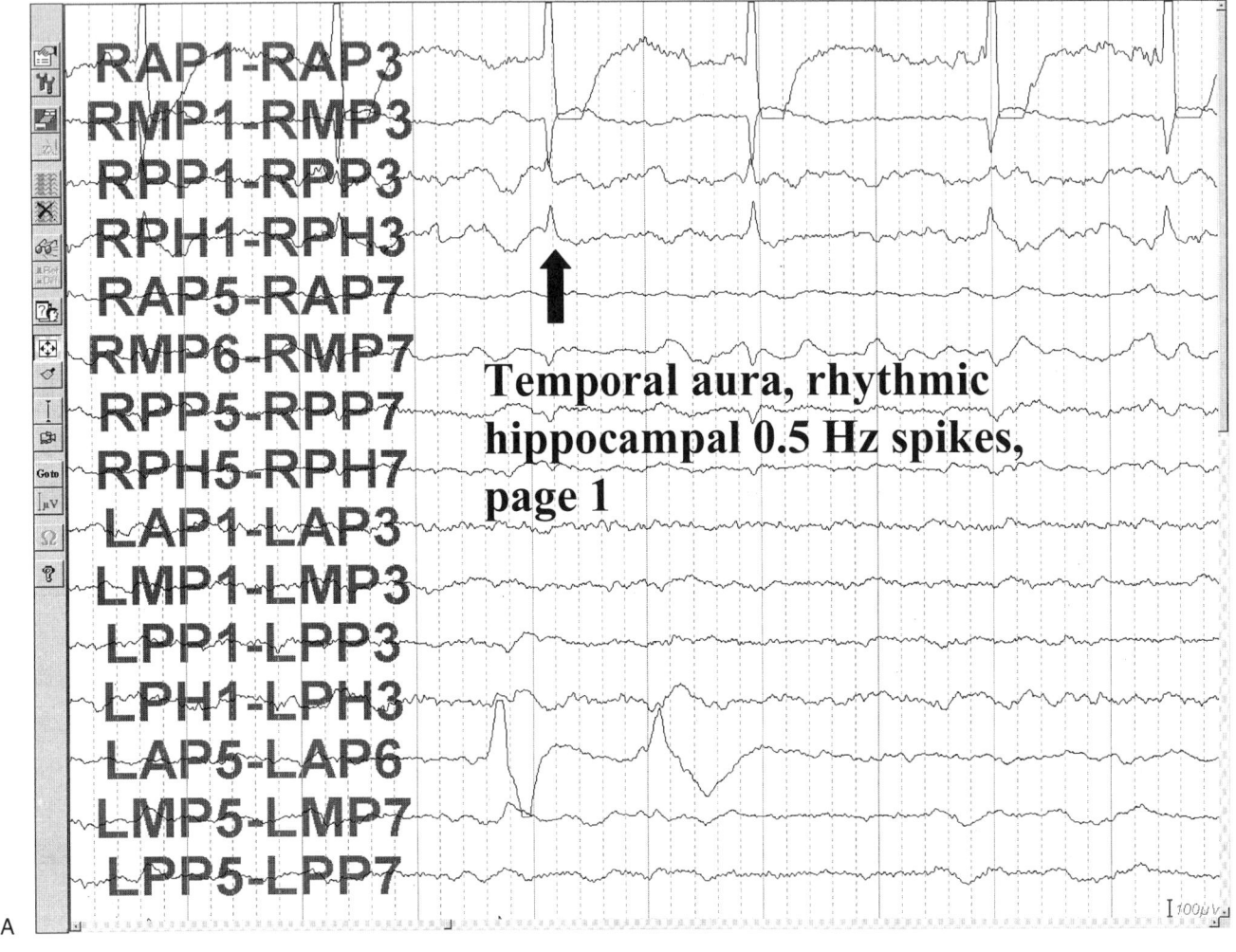

FIG. 20.18. A: EEG showing the beginning of an aura (simple partial seizure) in the right mesial temporal lobe with regional spikes (*arrow*) recurring at a rate of approximately 0.5 Hz. *RAP, RMP, RPP, RPH*, right anterior pes, middle pes, posterior pes hippocampus, and parahippocampal gyrus, respectively. Only the deep contacts of the depth electrode (1–3) are involved in the ictal discharge; the lateral superficial contacts (5–7) are uninvolved. The left-sided electrodes show no ictal activity. The rhythmic spiking was not present prior to the onset of symptoms, and can be considered an ictal pattern in this circumstance because it accompanies a behavioral change and progresses to more obvious ictal activity. *(Figure continues.)*

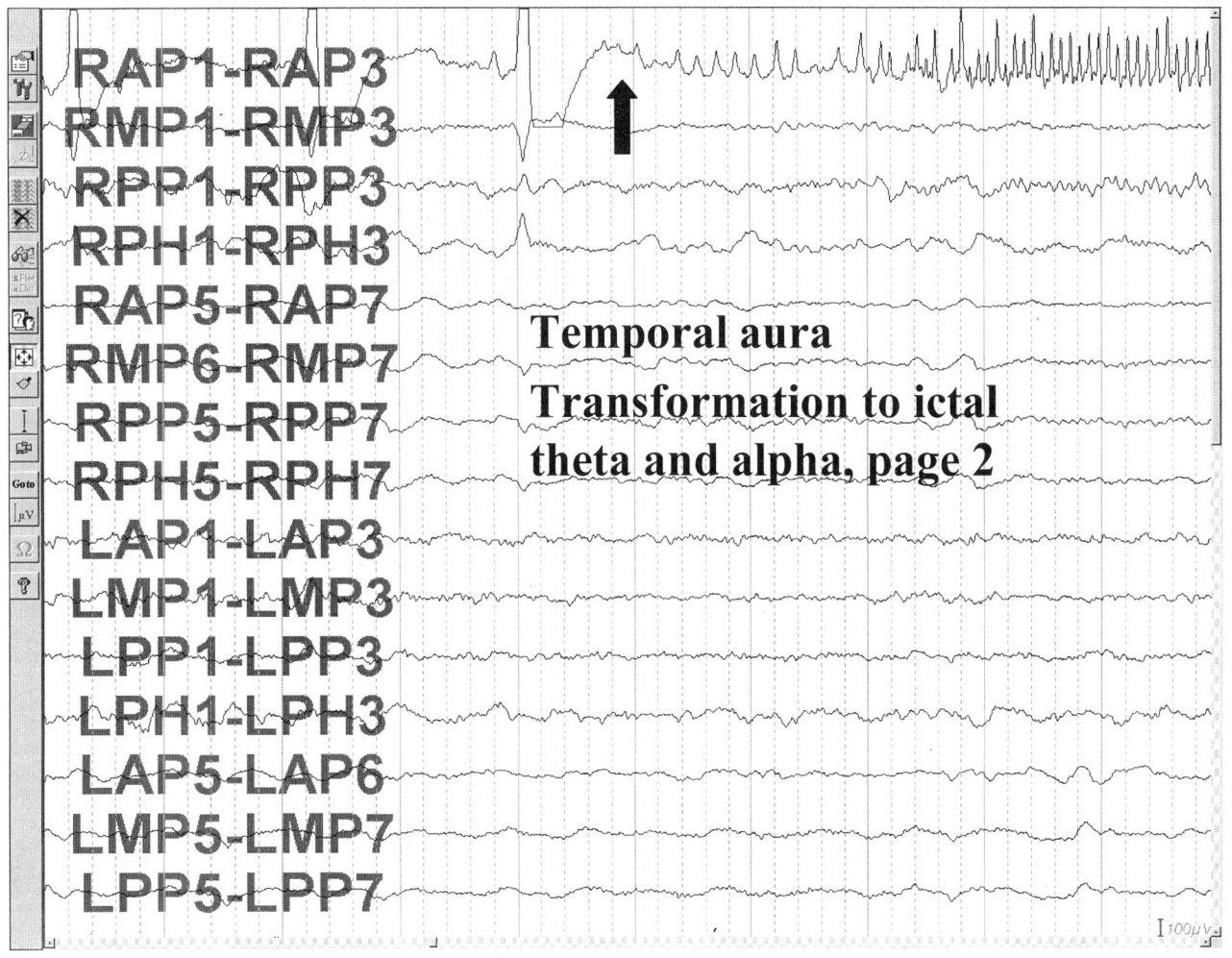

B

FIG. 20.18. *Continued.* **B:** This second page of the seizure recording shows the transformation from rhythmic spiking to rhythmic theta and alpha activity as the seizure progresses.

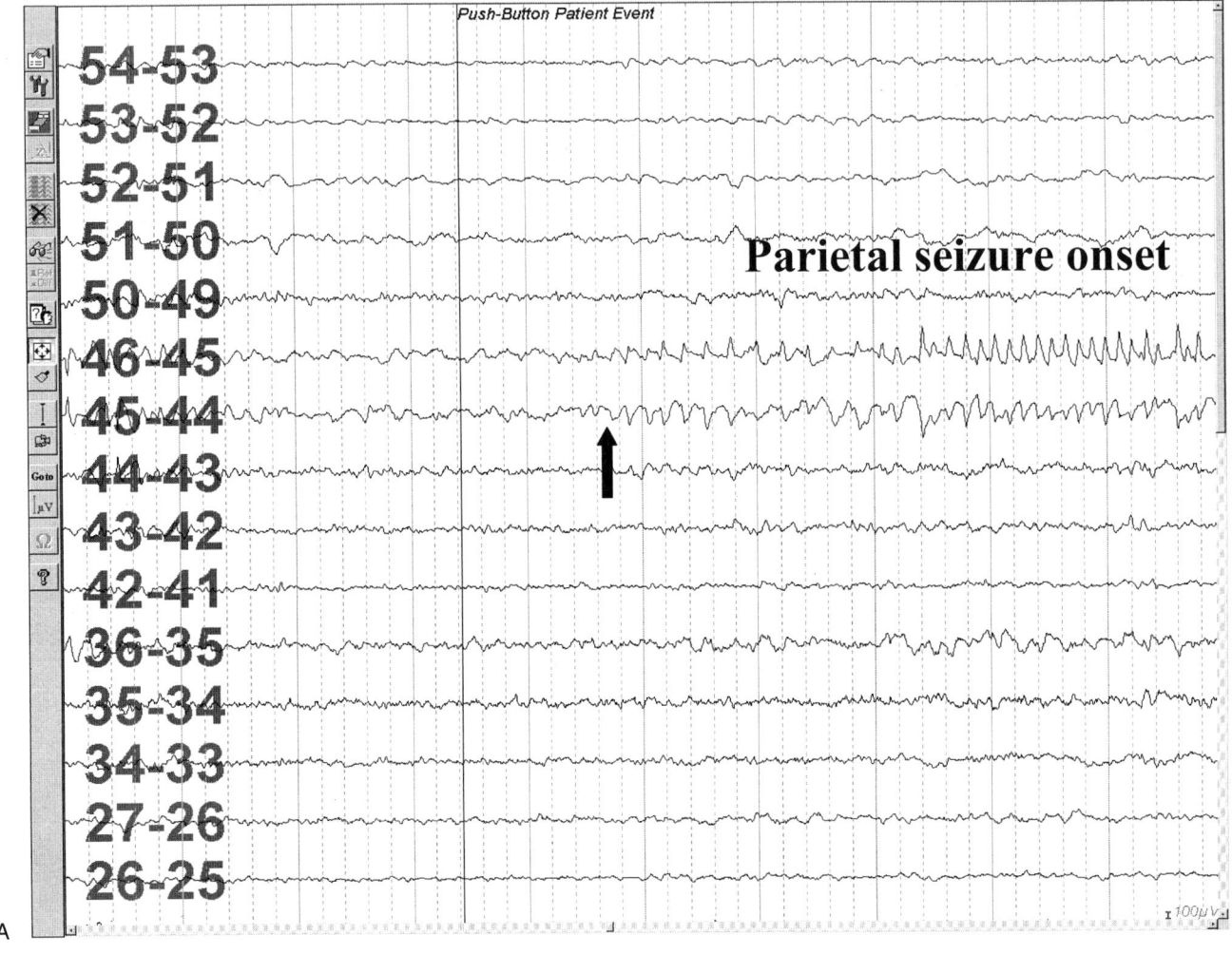

FIG. 20.19. A: EEG showing a parietal seizure beginning in a subdural grid with rhythmic theta-frequency activity (5–6 Hz) (*arrow*) that progressively increases in frequency to 9 Hz. *(Figure continues.)*

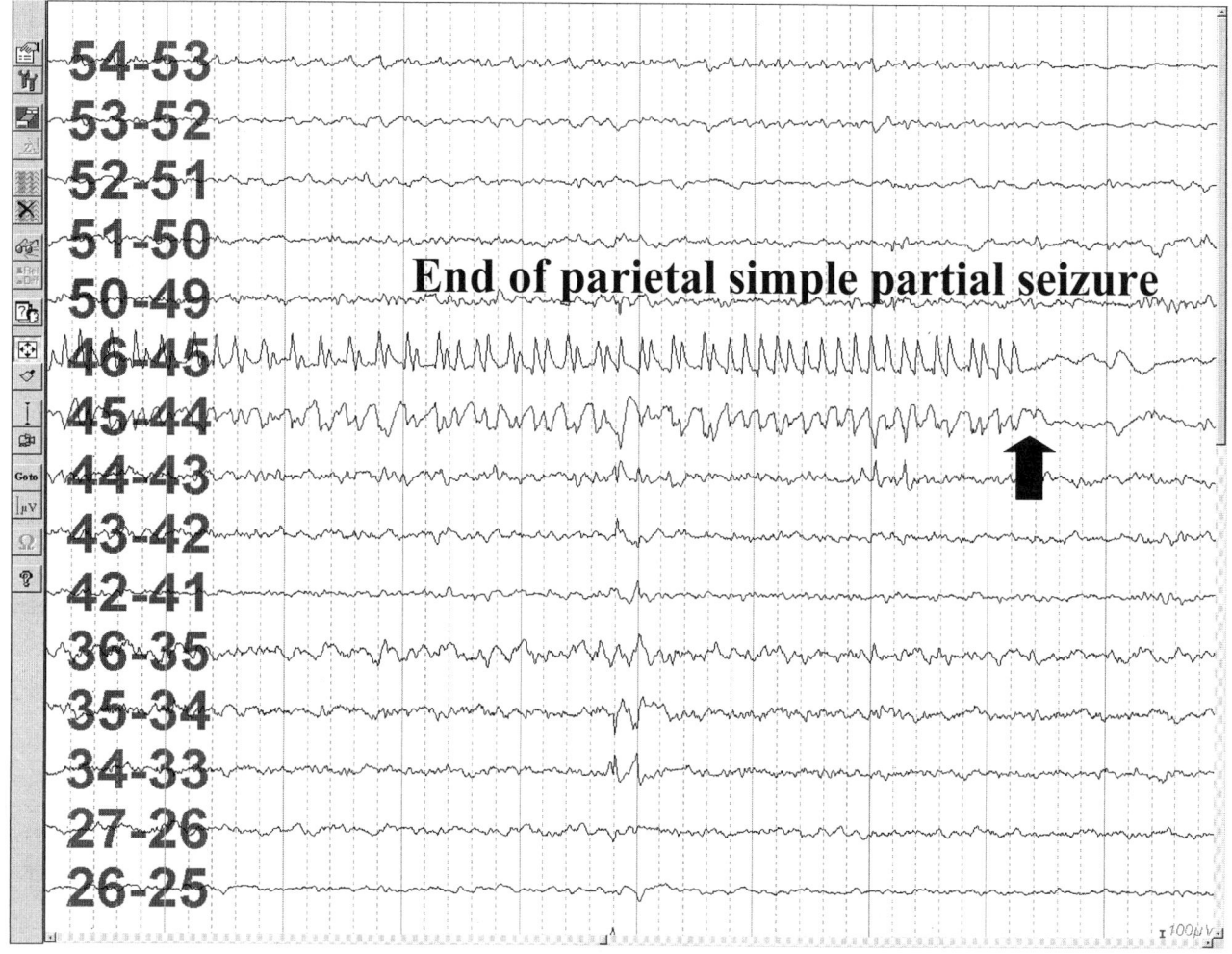

FIG. 20.19. *Continued.* **B:** Second and final 10-second page of the parietal seizure recording shows a slowing and then an increase in ictal frequency prior to seizure termination (*arrow*).

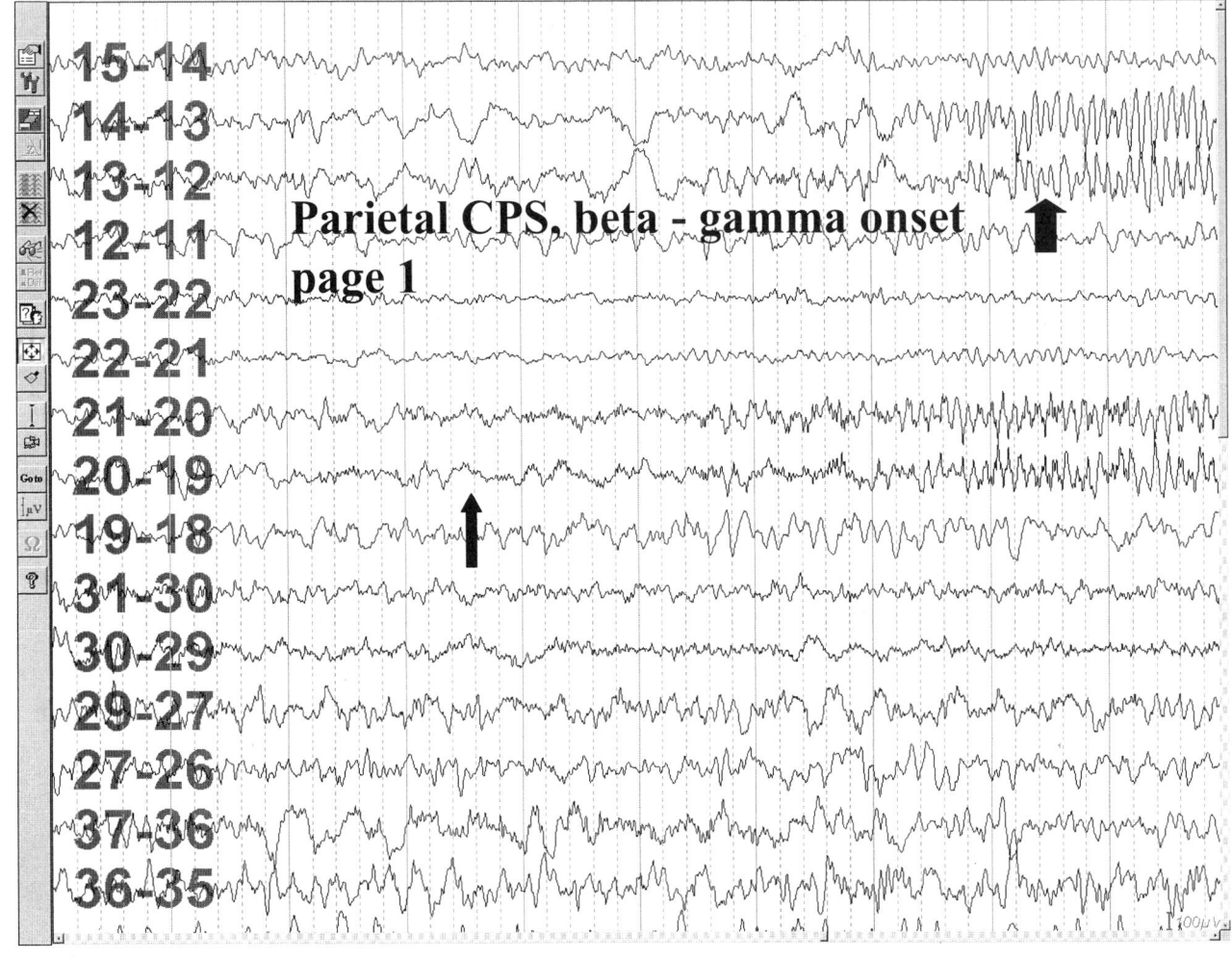

FIG. 20.20. A: This parietal complex partial seizure begins focally with low-amplitude gamma-frequency activity (*thin arrow* on left) in the subdural grid. The seizure slowly spreads through the parietal lobe as it evolves in amplitude and frequency. The pattern, a progressive increase in amplitude and simultaneous decrease in frequency (*thick arrow* on right), is characteristic of many seizures. *(Figure continues.)*

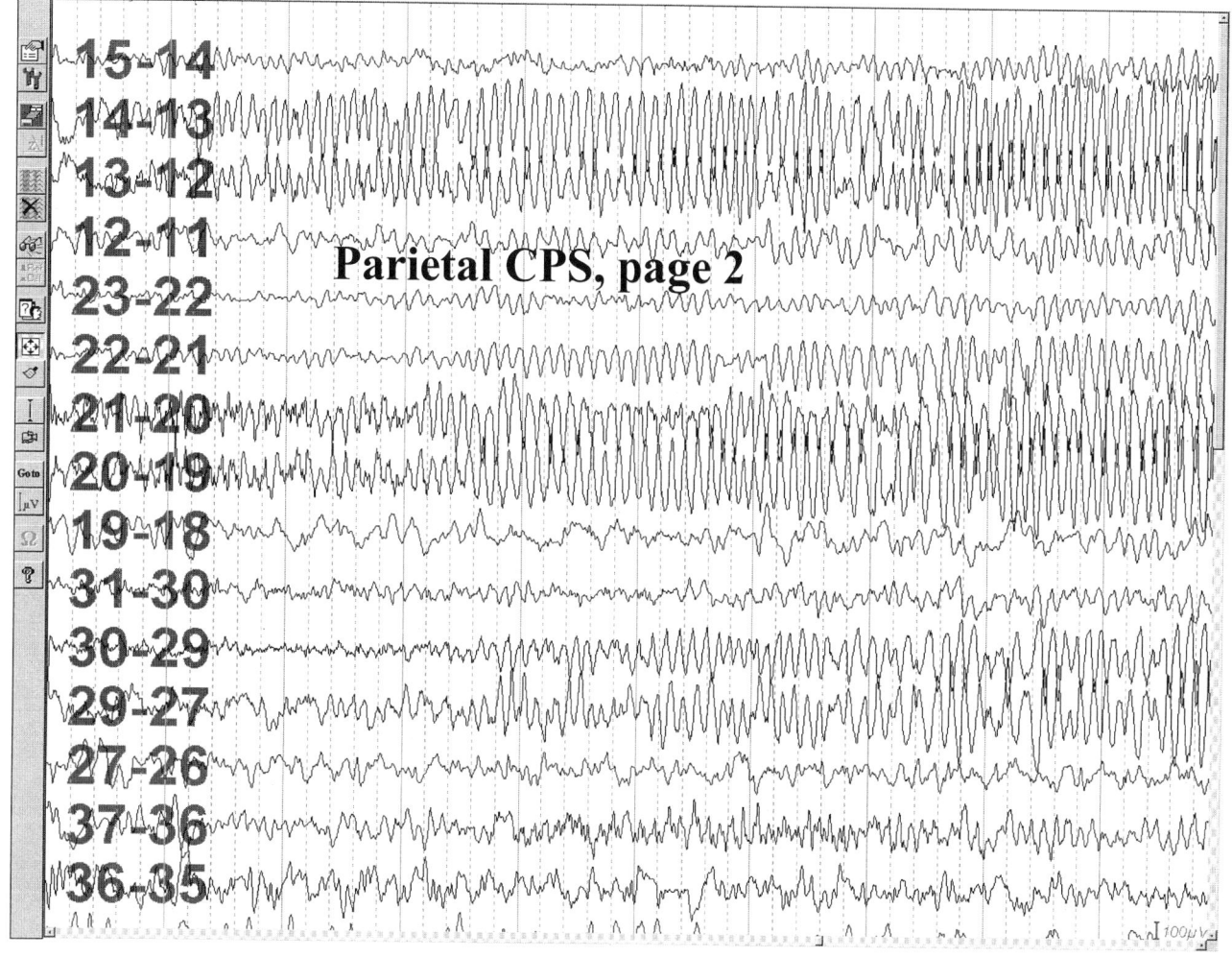

FIG. 20.20. *Continued.* **B:** In the next 10-second epoch during the parietal seizure, note the continuing evolution of amplitude and frequency and the spread of the discharge. *(Figure continues.)*

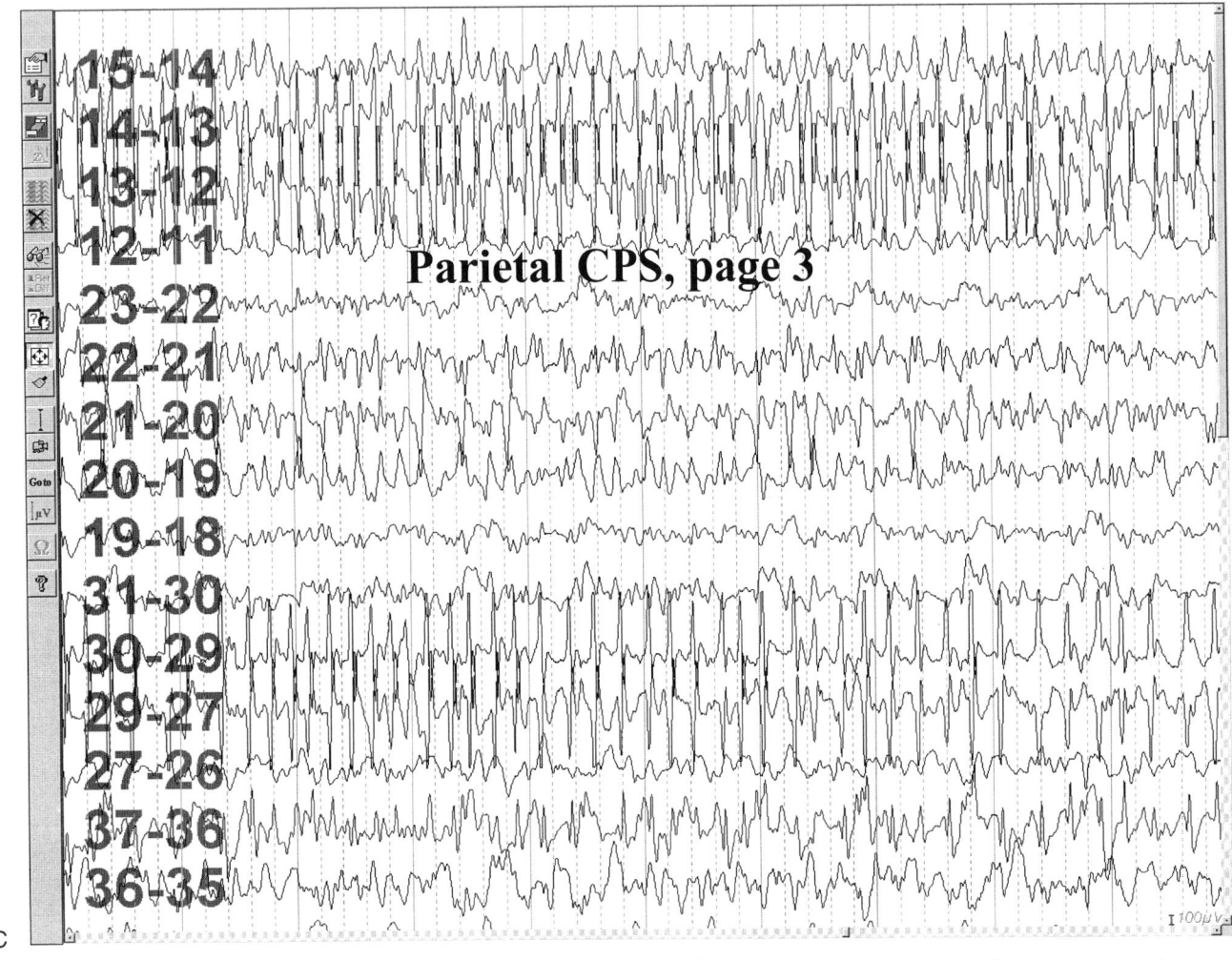

FIG. 20.20. *Continued.* **C:** The seizure continues, changing in electrographic character with less sinusoidal activity and more spike-like activity. *(Figure continues.)*

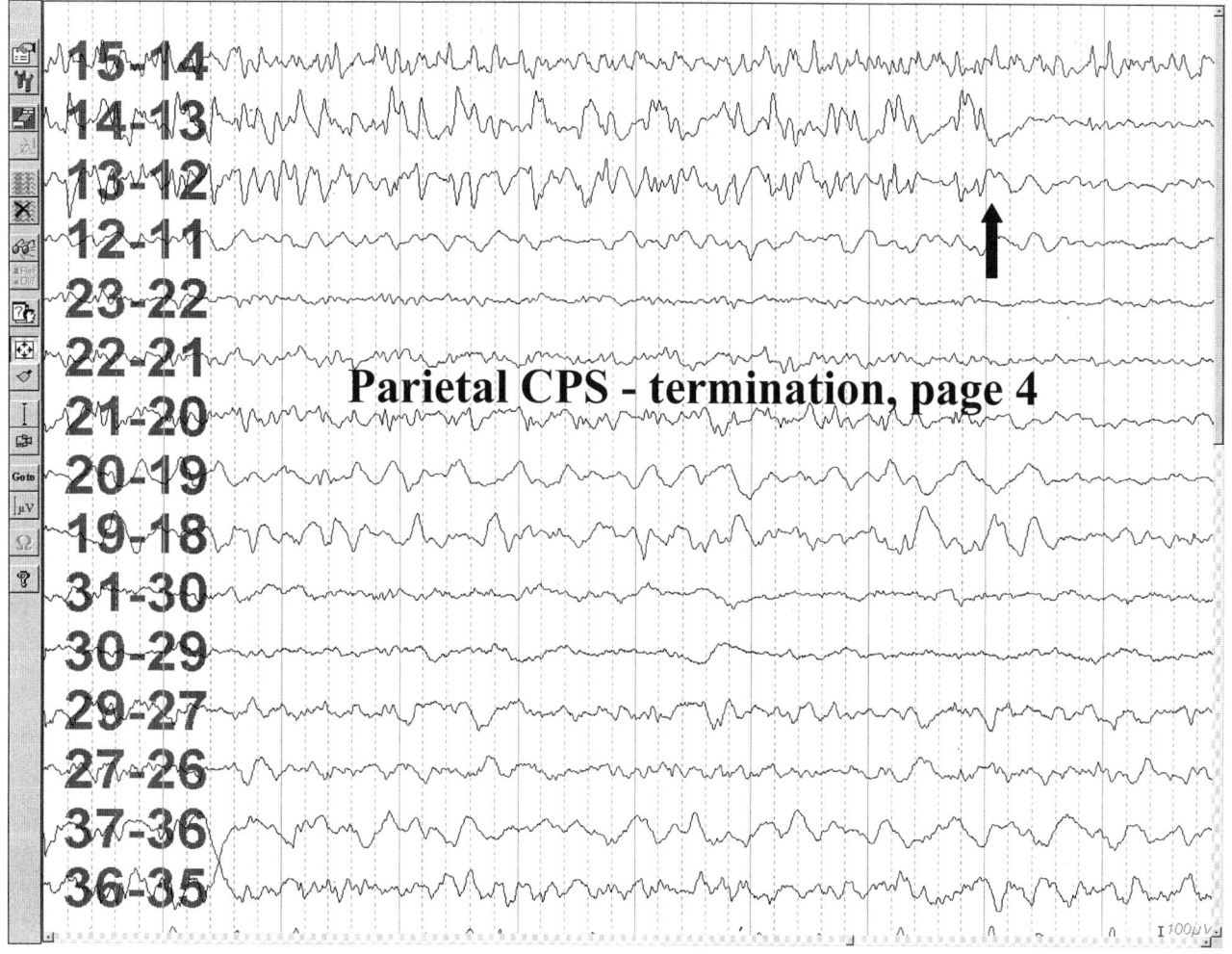

FIG. 20.20. *Continued.* **D:** The seizure gradually slows in frequency of the ictal discharge, and the amplitudes diminish as well. The seizure ends abruptly (*arrow*), terminating focally in contact 13 of the subdural grid.

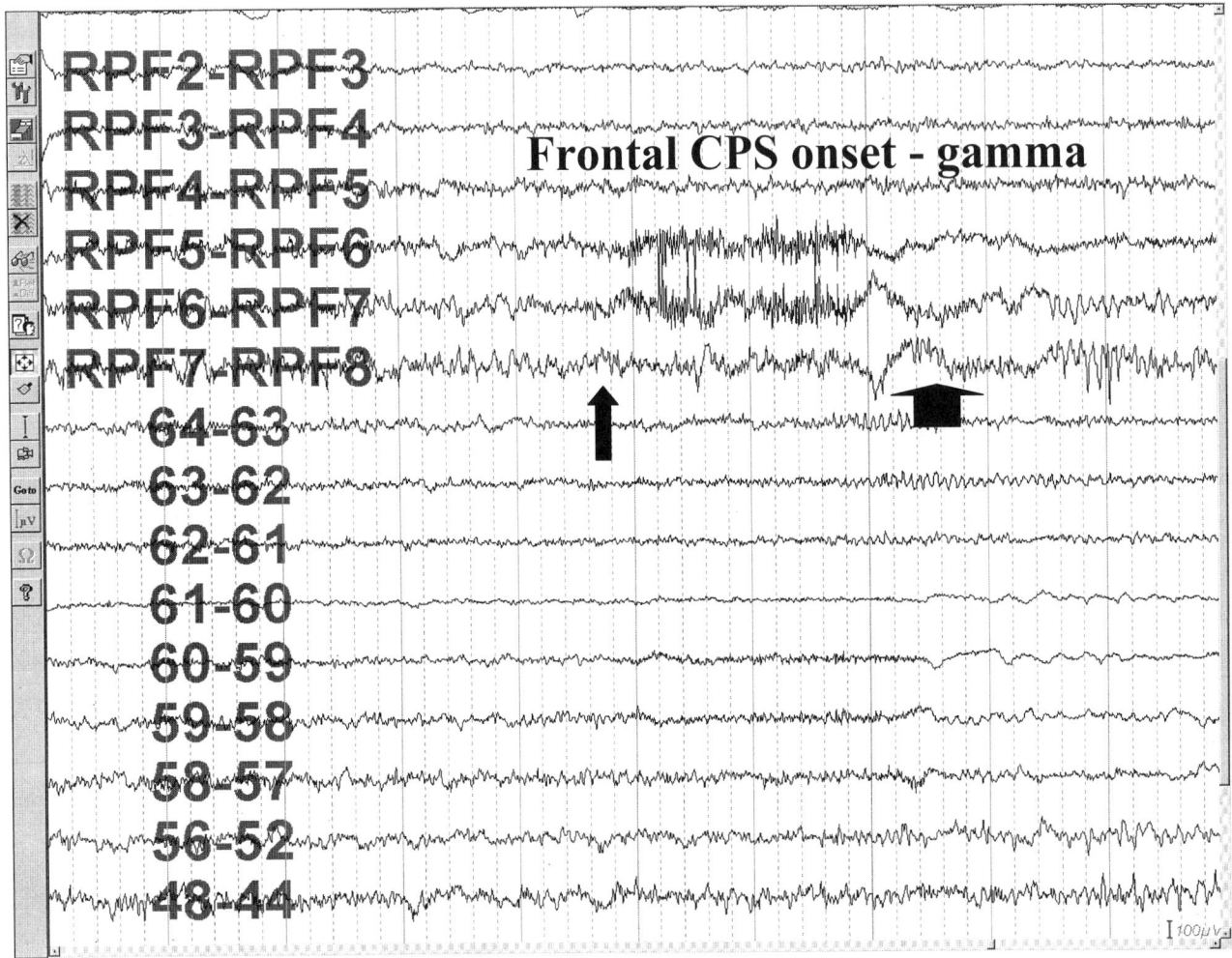

FIG. 20.21. This frontal complex partial seizure begins focally in the right posterior frontal subdural strip electrode (*RPF*) with high-amplitude gamma activity (*left arrow*), with some attenuation of amplitude several seconds after seizure onset (*thick arrow* on right).

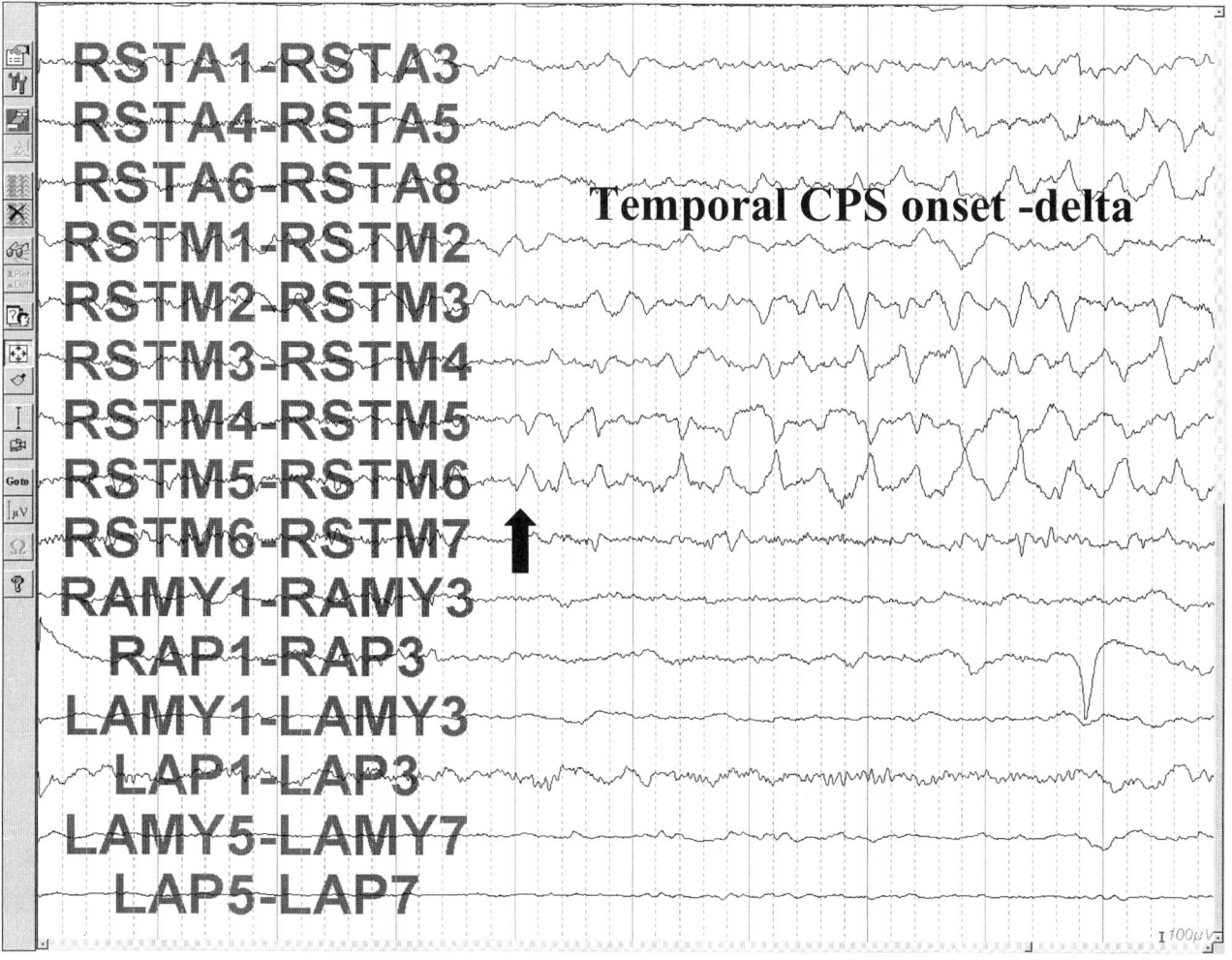

FIG. 20.22. This neocortical temporal lobe seizure begins with focal delta activity (*arrow*) in the middle subtemporal subdural strip contact 5 (*RSTM*), with semirhythmic delta-frequency activity. It spreads to other contacts in the same strip and the adjacent anterior temporal strip (*RSTA*) over the next few seconds. There is no spread to left-sided temporal lobe electrode contacts (beginning with *L*).

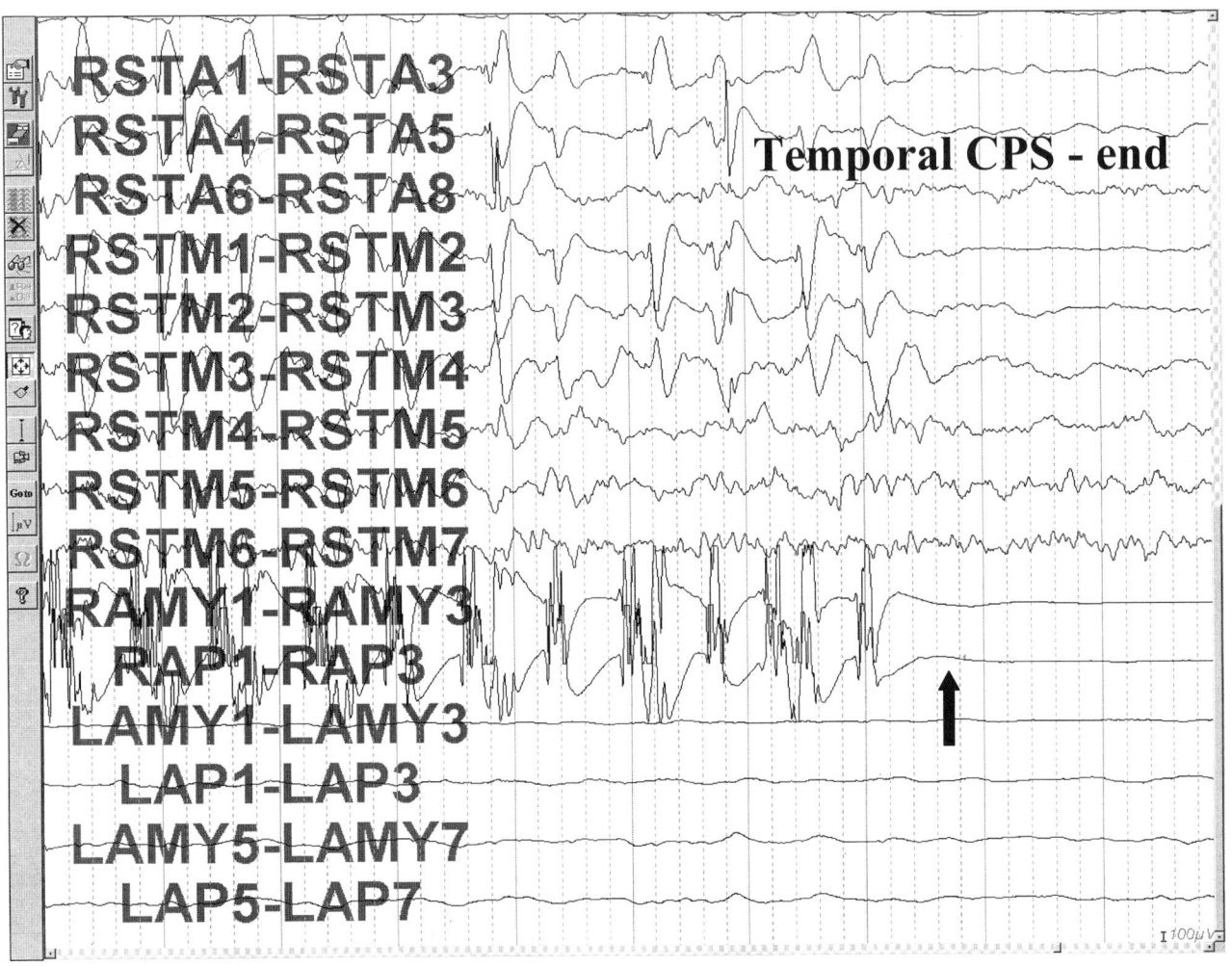

FIG. 20.23. Termination (arrow) of a temporal lobe complex partial seizure with focal suppression of activity in the right amygdala and hippocampus (*RAMY, RAP*) contacts. Other right temporal subdural contacts (*RSTA, RSTM*) show prominent slow waves but not the degree of suppression present in limbic structures. Left-sided temporal lobe depth electrode contacts (beginning with *L*) also register marked attenuation of background activity. This suppression usually lasts for 10 seconds to several minutes.

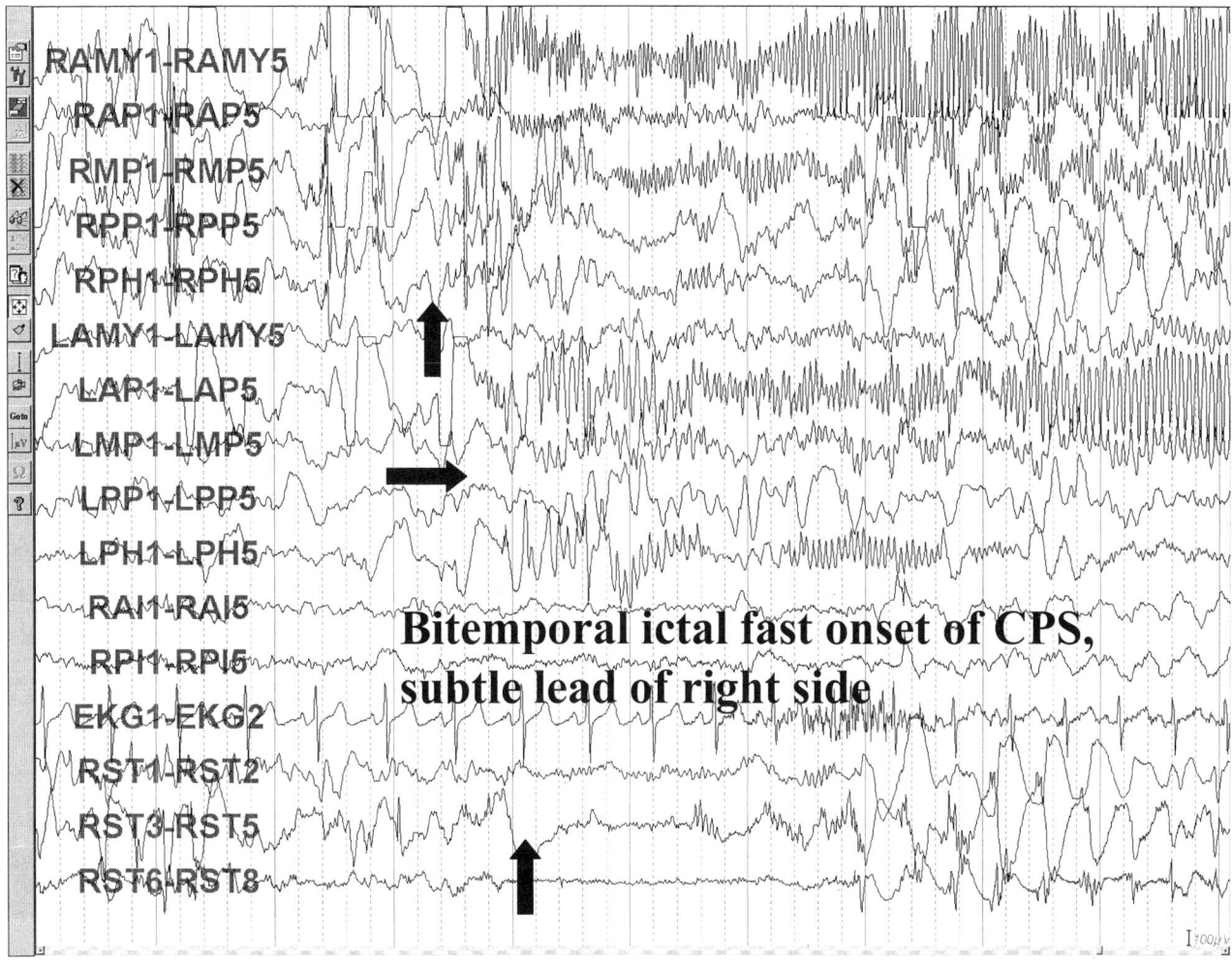

FIG. 20.24. EEG showing nearly synchronous complex partial seizure onset in both temporal lobes. The right temporal lobe depth electrodes show the earliest activity (*upper vertical arrow*), but ictal fast activity appears within 1 second in the left temporal lobe depth electrode contacts (*horizontal arrow*). The right temporal subdural strip contacts show seizure onset slightly later (*bottom arrow*) than the right-sided depth electrodes. This patient had some seizures with a 6- to 9-second interhemispheric propagation delay, and others with rapid spread as shown here. A right temporal lobectomy was performed. Although much reduced in frequency, the seizures have continued.

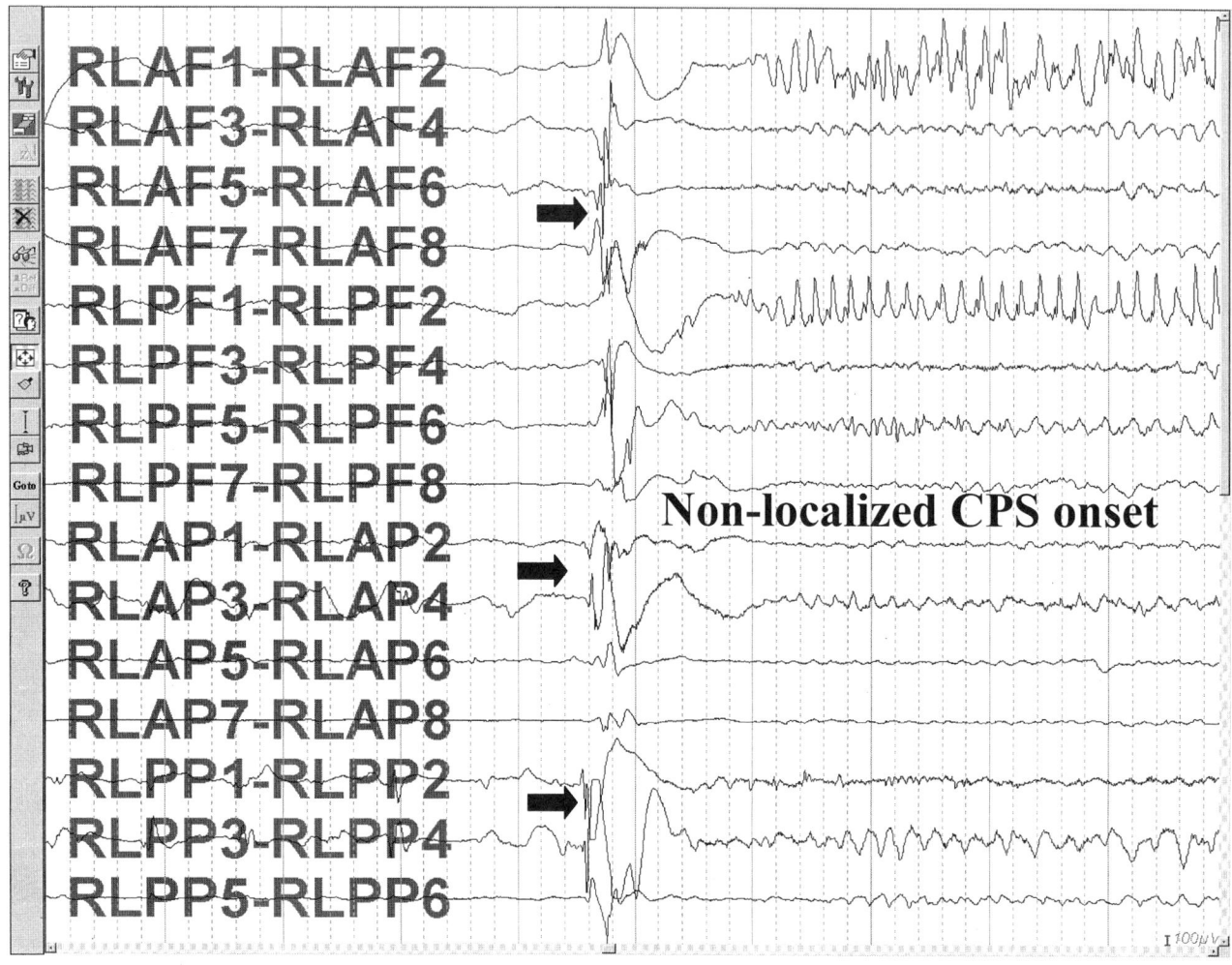

FIG. 20.25. Multilobar nonlocalized complex partial seizure onset in a patient with Rasmussen's encephalitis. Nearly simultaneous seizure onset is seen in the right frontal (*RLAF, RLPF*) and parietal (*RLAP, RLPP*) lobes (*arrows*). Although this seizure appears to start perhaps 20 milliseconds earlier than elsewhere in the posterior parietal subdural strip electrode (*RLPP*), other seizures appeared slightly earlier in the other strips. There was no clear predominant site of earliest seizure onset.

sign that the seizure is partial and not generalized. Partial seizures may begin at any frequency (delta, theta, alpha, beta, or gamma), sometimes preceded by an increase or decrease in the interictal spike rate, whereas generalized seizures begin with a generalized spike-and-wave, polyspike-and-wave, sharp-wave, slow-wave, or diffuse desynchronization pattern (see Figs. 20.16 through 20.22). Nearly all data are derived from patients with partial seizures, because intracranial electrode implantation is appropriately restricted to patients who are potential surgical candidates. The typical EEG pattern is one of varying ictal frequency that evolves during the course of the seizure (see Figs. 20.17 through 20.20), subtle or prominent lateralized amplitude maxima during different portions of the seizure, and postictal slowing or suppression of background frequencies (see Figs. 20.19*B*, 20.20*D*, and 20.23). At times, the beginning or the end of the seizure is not clearly delineated. Subtle changes may develop in the EEG over several seconds or more, and the precise moment of seizure onset or offset cannot be established. Sometimes, seizures appear to start and then stop 5–30 seconds later, only to resume a few seconds later in the same region or elsewhere.

Hippocampal seizures can begin in many ways (see Figs. 20.16 through 20.18) (20,32,40,41,45,48,49,53,60). They often commence with a burst of spikes followed by paroxysmal alpha- or beta-frequency activity of either high or low amplitude. It has been suggested that mesial temporal lobe seizures more often begin with 10- to 16-Hz frequencies, whereas neocortical seizures combine slower (4–10 Hz) and faster (40–50 Hz) frequencies (48). However, seizures of any type arising in any location can begin with any frequency; low-frequency onsets are seen in the hippocampus, and neocortical seizures can begin with frequencies up to 200 Hz (20). It is uncertain whether the frequency of the initial ictal discharge correlates with underlying pathology (48,49,60).

Neocortical seizures usually start with a low-voltage, high-frequency discharge, which may be accompanied by a focal or more widespread electrodecremental response (see Figs. 20.19 through 20.22) (32,40). There is sometimes a localized increase in power at frequencies above 40 Hz hidden within a more broadly distributed electrodecremental response; this localized area may indicate the site of seizure origin (20). However, many neocortical seizures start with slower frequency discharges or focal repetitive spiking that may or may not be well localized. The surface EEG pattern in neocortical seizures, similar to that of hippocampal seizures, reflects propagation and buildup of the ictal discharge rather than seizure onset (40).

Many partial seizures have an obvious focal onset in the intracranial EEG, but this is not a constant feature (see Figs. 20.24 and 20.25). Some partial seizures spread so rapidly that conventional EEG recording methods cannot reliably detect the localized ictal onset. In these cases, the earliest observed ictal changes may appear in more than one lobe of the brain, or in both hemispheres. Seizures recorded from the hippocampus may begin focally in just the anterior hippocampus, or regionally within the entire hippocampus and amygdala (13,16,21,22,35,48,53,58). Seizures that start in the neocortex display varying spatial extent at onset. They may begin in a restricted area of cortex and spread slowly or rapidly, or appear at once in more than one lobe of the brain.

Seizures commonly spread to other regions of the brain, and the extent of propagation determines the clinical behavior exhibited during a seizure. Some seizures remain confined to the cortex in which they begin and produce no symptoms (57). Other seizures may propagate within a single lobe or hemisphere; with unilateral spread, consciousness is generally preserved. When seizures propagate to the contralateral hemisphere, consciousness is nearly always impaired; the rare exception consists of mesial frontal or parietal seizures that remain restricted to the mesial cortex. Secondary generalization occurs as a consequence not only of widespread activation of cortex in both hemispheres and substantial subcortical activation, in both the diencephalon and midbrain.

Intracranial electrodes may be used to study propagation patterns, which relate to prognosis (51). Seizures can be assessed visually or with computer analysis (23,35). Most mesial temporal lobe seizures first propagate to ipsilateral temporal or orbitofrontal cortex, and thence to the contralateral hemisphere, presumably via the corpus callosum. Other propagation patterns occur; for example, some hippocampal seizures spread to the other hemisphere via the hippocampal commissure. Long interhemispheric propagation times predict a better prognosis after anterior temporal lobectomy, whereas short interhemispheric propagation times, particularly those less than 5 seconds, are associated with postoperative seizure recurrence (10, 34,35). Some seizures spread explosively throughout both hemispheres and cannot be localized. The patterns with which seizures stop are of interest, but there is no agreement as to whether they correlate with prognosis after surgery (7,50).

Depth electrodes have a particular advantage when recording hippocampal seizures. They are positioned to detect seizure onset earlier than other electrode types (see Fig. 20.16). Hippocampal electrodes detect seizure onset 30 seconds earlier on average than subdural electrodes in patients with mesial temporal lobe epilepsy (8,56). Because some seizures propagate rapidly throughout both hemispheres once they leave the hippocampus, using depth electrodes offers a major advantage. Several investigators have reported that, because of rapid seizure spread, depth electrodes were needed to identify that seizures began in one hippocampus; had only subdural electrodes been used, localization would not have been possible (5,8,40,56). In several patients, spread of ictal activity from one hippocampus to the contralateral temporal lobe neocortex led to the conclusion that seizure onset would have been incorrectly localized by subdural electrodes (8,56,58). It should be emphasized that subdural and depth electrodes usually lead to the same diagnosis in patients with mesial temporal lobe epilepsy (see Fig. 20.17*A*). Nonetheless, because of the potential for inaccurate localization, the literature supports investigating patients suspected of having temporal lobe epilepsy with both depth and subdural electrodes to maximize the chances of making a correct diagnosis.

When planning to study patients with neocortical epilepsy, whether from the temporal lobe or elsewhere, subdural electrodes offer more comprehensive and versatile recording characteristics. Depth electrodes are not well suited to neocortical seizures. Because of limited sampling, they are more likely to detect propagated ictal discharges. Subdural electrodes also are better suited to electrical stimulation, a task sometimes required prior to epilepsy surgery.

INTRACRANIAL EEG INTERPRETATION

Intracranial EEG recording has been demonstrated to be worthwhile in two ways. First, intracranial EEG reveals epileptogenic cortex that is not apparent by any other testing, permitting surgery that otherwise could not be offered. Second, information gleaned during an intracranial EEG recording session can make it clear that an operation should be avoided, thereby sparing some patients unnecessary resection of brain tissue.

How is the intracranial EEG used to make a surgical decision? In the optimal surgical candidate, the intracranial EEG shows seizures that consistently arise in one location and concordant interictal EEG disturbances. If seizures cannot be localized or are multifocal, then surgery might be inadvisable. However, an ambiguous intracranial EEG evaluation sometimes still leads to a good surgical result. For example, some patients with bitemporal seizures stop having seizures after temporal lobectomy, and excising a structural lesion appears to be the major factor that predicts success (9,10,26,47).

Much must be learned to more effectively employ the intracranial EEG. How many and what types of seizures should be recorded? How should the different aspects of the interictal and ictal EEG be weighed to make the best clinical decision? Most epileptologists try to record at least several typical seizures, but clinical practice varies, and practical considerations (limited monitoring time) may prevent the gathering of all desired data. As discussed above, the interictal abnormalities are even more problematic. Human intuition and insight have triumphed in spite of these deficiencies, but the deficiencies still need remedy.

To assess the usefulness of a technique, one must also assess its yield. Unfortunately, the yield of intracranial EEG is difficult to determine. This depends largely on patient selection, which itself relies on referral patterns, physician judgment and experience, and the availability and sophistication of noninvasive testing methods. Because noninvasive methods provide sufficient information to offer surgery without intracranial electrodes in most individuals (10,17), intracranial EEG is used only in complicated patients with reduced chances of a successful outcome. Despite these biases, most intracranial EEG evaluations lead to a therapeutic procedure, although success rates are somewhat lower than in patients offered surgery on the basis of noninvasive testing alone (10).

A remaining challenge is to integrate intracranial EEG data with other clinical information. Interictal and ictal EEG findings must be interpreted in light of functional deficits (alteration of metabolism, blood flow, cognitive changes), structural lesions, and the clinical symptoms. The intracranial EEG does not proffer better information than noninvasive methods, it merely offers additional information that can be put to better use.

REFERENCES

1. Ajmone-Marsan C. Chronic intracranial recording and electrocorticography. In: Daly DD, Pedley TA, eds. *Current practice of clinical electroencephalograpy*. New York: Raven Press, 1990: 535–560.
2. Barnett GH, Burgess RC, Awad IA, et al. Epidural peg electrodes for the presurgical evaluation of intractable epilepsy. *Neurosurgery* 1990;27:113–115.
3. Barry EE, Bergey GK, Wolf AZ. Simultaneous subdural grid and depth electrode recordings of patients with refractory complex partial seizures. *Epilepsia* 1989;30:695.
4. Bautista RED, Cobbs MA, Spencer DD, et al. Prediction of surgical outcome by interictal epileptiform abnormalities during intracranial EEG monitoring in patients with extrahippocampal seizures. *Epilepsia* 1999;40:880–890.
5. Binnie CD, Elwes RD, Polkey CE, et al. Utility of stereoelectroencephalography in preoperative assessment of temporal lobe epilepsy. *J Neurol Neurosurg Psychiatry* 1994;57:58–65.
6. Binnie CD, McBride MC, Polkey CE, et al. Electrocorticography and stimulation. *Acta Neurol Scand Suppl* 1994;152:74–82.
7. Brekelmans GJ, Demetrios NV, van Veelen CWM, et al. Intracranial EEG seizure-offset termination patterns: relation to outcome of epilepsy surgery in temporal lobe epilepsy. *Epilepsia* 1998;39:259–266.
8. Brekelmans GJ, van Emde Boas W, Velis DN, et al. Comparison of combined versus subdural or intracerebral electrodes alone in presurgical focus localization. *Epilepsia* 1998;39:1290–1301.
9. Cascino GD, Trenerry MR, Jack CR Jr, et al. Electrocorticography and temporal lobe epilepsy: relationship to quantitative MRI and operative outcome. *Epilepsia* 1995;36:692–696.

10. Cascino GD, Trenerry MR, Sharbrough FW, et al. Depth electrode studies in temporal lobe epilepsy: relation to quantitative magnetic resonance imaging and operative outcome. *Epilepsia* 1995;36:230–235.

11. Cendes F, Dubeau F, Andermann F, et al. Significance of mesial temporal atrophy in relation to intracranial ictal and interictal stereo EEG abnormalities. *Brain* 1996;119:1317–1326.

12. Cooper R, Crow JH. Toxic effects of intracerebral electrodes. *Med Biol Eng* 1966;4:575–581.

13. Crandall PH, Walter RD, Rand RW. Clinical applications of studies on stereotactically implanted electrodes in temporal-lobe epilepsy. *J Neurosurg* 1963;20:827–840.

14. Devinsky O, Canevine MP, Sato S, et al. Quantitative electrocorticography in patients undergoing temporal lobectomy. *J Epilepsy* 1992;5:178–185.

15. Devinsky O, Sato S, Kufta CV, et al. Electroencephalographic studies of simple partial seizures with subdural electrode recordings. *Neurology* 1989;38:527–533.

16. Engel J Jr, Crandall PH. Intensive neurodiagnostic monitoring with intracranial electrodes. *Adv Neurol* 1986;46:85–106.

17. Engel J Jr, Henry TR, Risinger MW, et al. Presurgical evaluation for partial epilepsy: relative contributions of chronic depth-electrode recordings versus FDG-PET and scalp-sphenoidal ictal EEG. *Neurology* 1990;40:1670–1677.

18. Engel J Jr, Van Ness PC, Rasmussen TB, et al. Outcome with respect to epileptic seizures. In: Engel J Jr, ed. *Surgical treatment of the epilepsies*, 2nd ed. New York: Raven Press, 1993:609–621.

19. Fiol M, Gates JR, Torres F, et al. The prognostic value of residual spikes in the postexcision electrocorticogram after temporal lobectomy. *Neurology* 1991;41:512–516.

20. Fisher RS, Webber WR, Lesser RP, et al. High-frequency EEG activity at the start of seizures. *J Clin Neurophysiol* 1992;9:441–449.

21. Gloor P. Contributions of electroencephalography and electrocorticography to the neurosurgical treatment of the epilepsies. In: Purpura DP, Penry JK, Walter RD, eds. *Neurosurgical management of the epilepsies*, Vol 8. New York: Raven Press, 1975:59–106.

22. Gloor P. Preoperative electroencephalographic investigation in temporal lobe epilepsy: extracranial and intracranial recordings. *Can J Neurol Sci* 1991;18:554–558.

23. Gotman J. Interhemispheric interactions in seizure of focal onset: data from human intracranial recordings. *Electroencephalogr Clin Neurophysiol* 1987;67:120–133.

24. Havidan M, Katz A, Tran T, et al. Frequency characteristics of neocortical and hippocampal onset seizures. *Epilepsia* 1992;33[Suppl 3]:58.

25. Henry TR, Ross DA, Schuh LA, et al. Indications and outcome of ictal recording with intracerebral and subdural electrodes in refractory complex partial seizures. *J Clin Neurophysiol* 1999;16:426–438.

26. Hirsch LJ, Spencer SS, Williamson PD, et al. Comparison of bitemporal and unitemporal epilepsy defined by depth EEG. *Ann Neurol* 1991;30:340–346.

27. Holthausen H, Noachtar S, Pannek H, et al. Foramen ovale and epidural peg electrodes. *Acta Neurol Scand Suppl* 1994;152:39–43.

28. Jasper H. Electrocorticography. In: Penfield W, Jasper H, eds. *Epilepsy and the functional anatomy of the human brain*. Boston: Little, Brown and Company, 1954:692–738.

29. Jasper HH, Pertuisset B, Flanigin H. EEG and cortical electrocorticograms in patients with temporal lobe seizures. *Arch Neurol Psychiatry* 1951;65:272–299.

30. Jayakar P. Physiological principles of electrical stimulation. *Adv Neurol* 1993;63:17–27.

31. Jayakar P, Alvarez LA, Duchowny MS, et al. A safe and effective paradigm to functionally map the cortex in childhood. *J Clin Neurophysiol* 1992;9:288–293.

32. Jung WY, Pacia SV, Devinsky O. Neocortical temporal lobe epilepsy: intracranial EEG features and surgical outcome. *J Clin Neurophysiol* 1999;16:419–425.

33. Lange HH, Lieb JP, Engel J Jr, et al. Temporo-spatial patterns of preictal spike activity in human temporal lobe epilepsy. *Electroencephalogr Clin Neurophysiol* 1983;56:543–555.

34. Lieb JP, Babb TL. Interhemispheric propagation time of human hippocampal seizures: II. Relationship to pathology and cell density. *Epilepsia* 1986;27:294–300.

35. Lieb JP, Engel J Jr, Babb TL. Interhemispheric propagation time of human hippocampal seizures: I. Relationship to surgical outcome. *Epilepsia* 1986;27:286–293.

36. Lieb JP, Joseph JP, Engel J Jr, et al. Sleep state and seizure foci related to depth spike activity in patients with temporal lobe epilepsy. *Electroencephalogr Clin Neurophysiol* 1980;49:538–557.

37. Lieb JP, Woods SC, Siccardi A, et al. Quantitative analysis of depth spiking in relation to seizure foci in patients with temporal lobe epilepsy. *Electroencephalogr Clin Neurophysiol* 1978; 44: 641–663.

38. Marks DA, Katz A, Booke J, et al. Correlation of surface and sphenoidal electrodes with simultaneous intracranial recording: an interictal study. *Electroencephalogr Clin Neurophysiol* 1992;82:23–29.

39. McBride MC, Binnie CD, Janota I, et al. Predictive value of intraoperative electrocorticograms in resective epilepsy surgery. *Ann Neurol* 1991;30:526–532.

40. Pacia SV, Ebersole JS. Intracranial EEG substrates of scalp ictal patterns from temporal lobe foci. *Epilepsia* 1997;38:642–654.

41. Park YD, Murro AM, King DW, et al. The significance of ictal depth EEG patterns in patients with temporal lobe epilepsy. *Electroencephalogr Clin Neurophysiol* 1996;99:412–415.

42. Privitera MD, Quinlan JG, Yeh H. Interictal spike detection comparing subdural and depth electrodes during electrocorticography. *Electroencephalogr Clin Neurophysiol* 1990;76:379–387.

43. Ross DA, Brunberg JA, Drury I, et al. Intracerebral depth electrode monitoring in partial epilepsy: the morbidity and efficacy of placement using magnetic resonance image-guided stereotactic surgery. *Neurosurgery* 1996;39:327–333.

44. Salanova V, Morris HH, Van Ness PL, et al. Comparison of scalp electroencephalogram with subdural electrocorticogram recordings and functional mapping in frontal lobe epilepsy. *Arch Neurol* 1993;50:294–299.

45. Schiller Y, Cascino GD, Sharbrough FW. Chronic intracranial EEG monitoring for localizing the epileptogenic zone: an electro-clinical correlation. *Epilepsia* 1998;39:1302–1308.

46. Schwartz TH, Bazil CW, Walczak RS, et al. The predictive value of intraoperative electrocorticography in resections for limbic epilepsy associated with mesial temporal sclerosis. *Neurosurgery* 1997;40:302–309.

47. Sirven JI, Malamut BL, Liporace JD, et al. Outcome after temporal lobectomy in bilateral temporal lobe epilepsy. *Ann Neurol* 1997;42:873–878.

48. Spencer SS, Guimaraes P, Katz A, et al. Morphological patterns of seizures recorded intracranially. *Epilepsia* 1992;33:537–545.

49. Spencer SS, Spencer DD. Entorhinal-hippocampal interaction in medial temporal lobe epilepsy. *Epilepsia* 1994;35:721–727.

50. Spencer SS, Spencer DD. Implications of seizure termination localization in temporal lobe epilepsy. *Epilepsia* 1996;37:455–458.

51. Spencer SS, Williamson PD, Spencer DD, et al. Human hippocampal seizure spread studied by depth and subdural recording: the hippocampal commissure. *Epilepsia* 1987;28:479–489.

52. Spencer SS, Williamson PD, Spencer DD, et al. Combined depth and subdural electrode investigation in uncontrolled epilepsy. *Neurology* 1990;40:74–79.

53. Sperling MR. *Atlas of electroencephalography, Vol 3: Intracranial electroencephalography*. Amsterdam, Elsevier Science, 1993.

54. Sperling MR, Brown WJ, Crandall PH. Focal burst-suppression induced by thiopental. *Electroencephalogr Clin Neurophysiol* 1986;63:203–208.

55. Sperling MR, Engel J Jr. Sphenoidal electrodes. *J Clin Neurophysiol* 1986;3:67–73.

56. Sperling MR, O'Connor MJ. Comparison of depth and subdural electrodes in recording temporal lobe seizures. *Neurology* 1989;39:1497–1504.

57. Sperling, MR, O'Connor MJ. Auras and subclinical seizures: characteristics and prognostic significance. *Ann Neurol* 1990;28:320–328.

58. Sperling MR, O'Connor MJ. Electrographic correlates of spontaneous seizures. *Clin Neurosci* 1994;2:17–46.

59. Swartz BE, Rich JR, Dwan PS, et al. The safety and efficacy of chronically implanted subdural electrodes: a prospective study. *Surg Neurol* 1996;46:87–93.

60. Townsend JB, Engel J Jr. Clinicopathological correlations of low voltage fast and high amplitude spike and wave mesial temporal SEEG ictal onsets. *Epilepsia* 1991;32:21(abst).

61. Tran TA, Spencer SS, Marks D, et al. Significance of spikes recorded on electrocorticography in nonlesional medial temporal lobe epilepsy. *Ann Neurol* 1995;38:763–770.

62. Tsai M-L, Chatrian G-E, Pauri F, et al. Electrocorticography in patients with medically intractable temporal lobe seizures: I. Quantification of epileptiform discharges prior to resective surgery. *Electroencephalogr Clin Neurophysiol* 1993;87:10–24.

63. Tsai M-L, Chatrian G-E, Temkin NR, et al. Electrocorticography in patients with medically intractable temporal lobe seizures: II. Quantification of epileptiform discharges following successive stages of resective surgery. *Electroencephalogr Clin Neurophysiol* 1993;87:25–37.

64. Uematsu S, Lesser R, Fisher R, et al. Resection of the epileptogenic area in critical cortex with the aid of a subdural electrode grid. *Stereotact Funct Neurosurg* 1990;54/55:34–45.

65. Van Buren JM. Complications of surgical procedures in the diagnosis and treatment of epilepsy. In: Engel J Jr, ed. *Surgical treatment of the epilepsies*. New York: Raven Press, 1987:465–475.

66. Velasco M, Velasco F, Velasco AL, et al. Electrocortical and behavioral responses produced by acute electrical stimulation of the human centromedian thalamic nucleus. *Electroencephalogr Clin Neurophysiol* 1997;102:461–471.

67. Veznedaroglu E, Sperling M, O'Connor M, et al. Evaluation of intrahippocampal and subdural strip electrodes for seizure localization. *Epilepsia* 1999;40[Suppl 7]:76.

68. Wieser HG, Elger CE, Stodieck SRG. The "foramen ovale electrode": a new recording method for the preoperative evaluation of patients suffering from mesio-basal temporal lobe epilepsy. *Electroencephalogr Clin Neurophysiol* 1985;61:314–322.

69. Wieser HG, Siegel AM. Analysis of foramen ovale electrode-recorded seizures and correlation with outcome following amygdalohippocampectomy. *Epilepsia* 1991;32:838–850.

70. Wyler AR, Ojemann GA, Lettich E, et al. Subdural strip electrodes for localizing epileptogenic foci. *J Neurosurg* 1984;60:1195–1200.

71. Wyler AR, Walker G, Somes G. The morbidity of long-term seizure monitoring using subdural strip electrodes. *J Neurosurg* 1991;74:734–737.

Chapter 21

Intraoperative Electrocorticography

Gian-Emilio Chatrian

Electrocorticography (ECoG), the method of recording electrical potentials directly from the cerebral cortex, was pioneered in humans by Hans Berger, who endeavored to validate the cerebral origin of the scalp electroencephalogram (EEG) by demonstrating that this activity could also be recorded over skull defects (25) as well as with a needle inserted through the cortex and underlying white matter in a patient with a distant brain tumor (26). Subsequent studies confirmed Berger's findings and found that brain tumors caused alterations of electrocerebral activity that contributed to their localization (3,23,96,269,271,320). During the 1940s and 1950s, direct brain recordings became established primarily as aids in the diagnosis and surgery of chronic, medically intractable partial (focal, localization-related) (60) epilepsies (6,124,142,143,148,160,210,234,314).

However, the preeminence of intraoperative ECoG in localizing epileptogenic brain tissue and guiding its removal was soon challenged by increasing sophistication of preoperative electrophysiological studies using noninvasive as well as variously invasive electrodes (20,248,294,297,332). The introduction of prolonged video-EEG monitoring (172) with computer-assisted seizure detection (120) allowed detailed analysis of spontaneous electrographic and clinical seizure patterns only rarely apparent in intraoperative recordings. In most centers, invasive recordings of ictal events and mapping of functionally important cortex by electrical stimulation (151) became the cornerstone of the preoperative examination of most patients suffering from medically intractable partial epilepsies. Neuropsychological (225,261) and intracarotid amobarbital testing (153) complemented these studies. During the 1990s, rapid progress in structural and functional neuroimaging, especially high-resolution magnetic resonance imaging (MRI) (41,131), added a new dimension to the localization of partial epilepsies by revealing previously elusive structural lesions associated with local epileptogenesis. This progress diminished the need for both invasive preoperative studies and the intraoperative ECoG. This chapter reappraises traditional technical and interpretive principles of intraoperative ECoG and highlights controversial aspects and promising developments of this method in the context of current diverse approaches to the surgical treatment of chronic, medically intractable epilepsies.

TECHNIQUE

Electrodes

ECoG electrodes (7) must be capable of detecting the electrical activity of cerebral cortex exposed by the craniotomy as well as that of remote cortical and subcortical areas within the hemisphere undergoing surgery. Until recently, electrode-holder assemblies, or "ECoG sets," have been used (Fig. 21.1); these sets typically incorporate insulated, malleable silver wires whose distal ends terminate with a carbon ball (266) that makes contact with the exposed cortex. The proximal ends of the wires are connected by coiled springs to thin stainless steel rods, which are mounted on the universal ball joints of a holder clamped to the bone edge of the craniotomy. A cable from these joints leads to the inputs of the recording system. The surgeon applies the ECoG electrodes on the exposed cortex, which provides flexibility of electrode placement, ease of identification of individual electrode locations, and clear observation and photography of the operative field, where sites of special interest are marked by small lettered or numbered tags (7). However, these electrodes are limited in number, difficult to align in straight arrays at strictly equal distances as required by mapping studies, and unsuitable for surveying inferior and medial hemispheric surfaces.

An alternative technique that is most often used today utilizes variously shaped assemblies of 4–64 or more small platinum–iridium or stainless steel disk electrodes embedded usually 10 or 15 mm apart in soft, flexible, clear silicone plastic (Silastic) sheets (337). These "strips" or "grids" can be laid over the exposed cortex or introduced from the edges of the craniotomy over or under lateral, inferior, and medial cortical regions, and can be directly stimulated. Grids containing large numbers of equally spaced electrodes are ideally suited for detailed computer-aided mapping of epileptiform discharges and evoked potentials. However, they limit surgical manipulation as well as visual appreciation of the relationships of individual electrodes to the underlying gyri, especially when they are weighted down with cotton strips imbued with saline solution to assure good electrode contacts. Thus, during cortical resections, it is sometimes necessary practice to use both holder-supported electrodes to record from the exposed cortex and strip and grid electrodes to explore more remote cortical areas (307,308). During some surgeries, single- or multicontact "depth" needle electrodes are also introduced into otherwise inaccessible brain regions (75,108,123,148,160,239,298).

Reference leads used for intraoperative brain recordings include two interconnected electrodes on both sides of the neck (307,308), an EEG electrode over the spinous process of the C7 vertebra (108) or on the bone flap distant from the active area (229), or an alligator clip attached to a muscle near the edge of the craniotomy. Grounding of the patient is commonly provided by a metal clamp attached to the post of the electrode holder or the bone edge of the craniotomy. ECoG electrode sets require cleaning and appropriate sterilization after each surgery to prevent transmission of agents highly resistant to decontamination, whereas commercial plastic-embedded and some depth electrodes are disposable.

Instrumentation and Physical Arrangement

ECoGs are now generally recorded with digital instruments, and the electrical activity is displayed on screen, paper, or both. Ideally, both the EEG instrument and the clinical neurophysiologist should be located in a gallery adjacent to but separate from the operating room (142). A large glass window and an intercom system enable the clinical neurophysiologist to view the operating field and to communicate with the neurosurgeon. Photographs of the operating field can be taken through a tilted mirror. A recording system bandpass of 0.5–70 Hz (−3 dB) ensures appreciation of both epileptiform

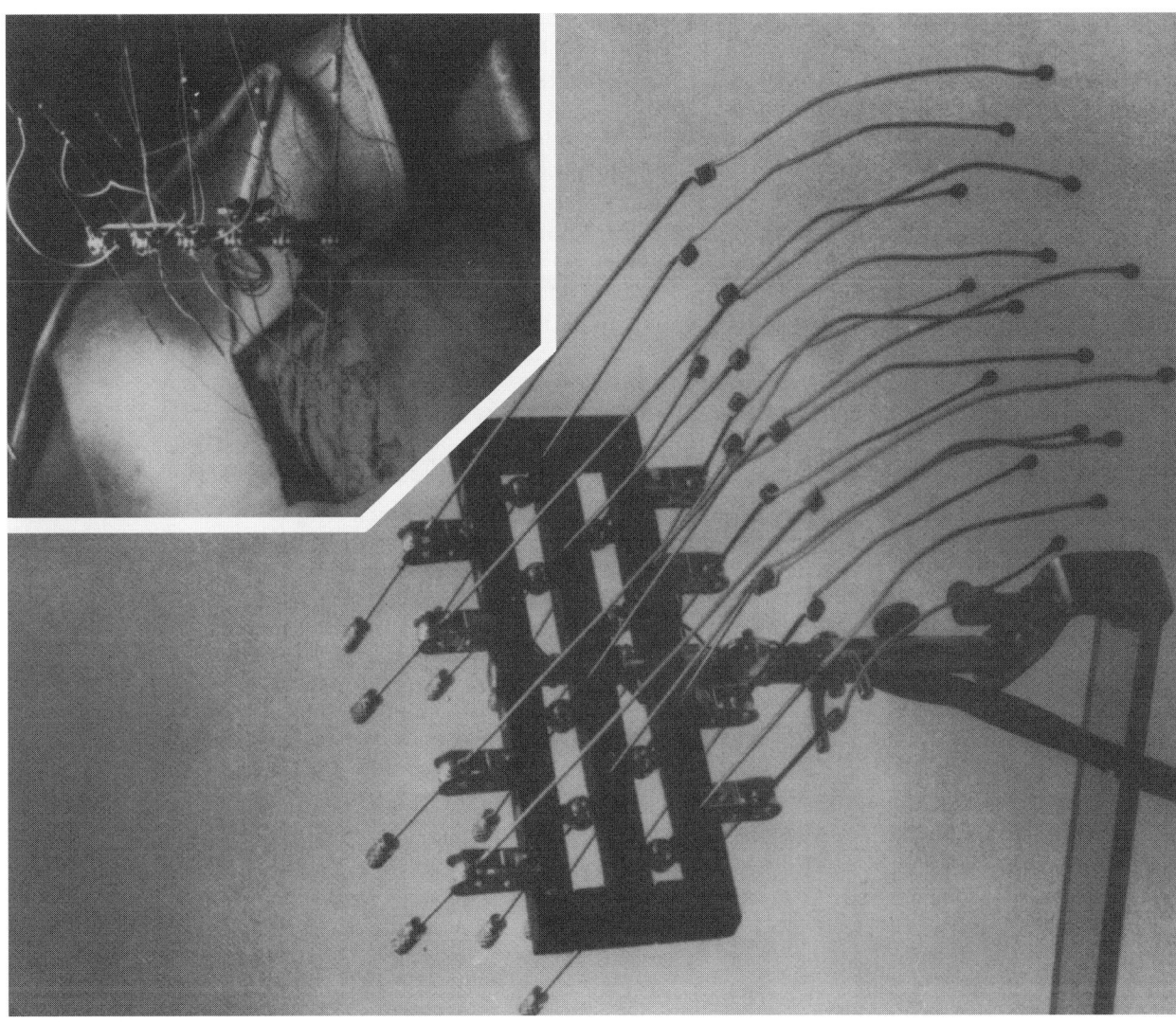

FIG. 21.1. Sixteen-electrode ECoG set used at the University of Miami and at the National Institute of Neurological and Communicative Disorders and Stroke, modified from an original design of the Montreal Neurological Institute. **Inset:** ECoG set in place, with holder clamped to the bone edge of the craniotomy and electrodes in contact with the exposed cortex. (From Ajmone-Marsan C. Chronic intracranial recording and electrocorticography. In: Engel J Jr, Pedley TA, eds. *Epilepsy: a comprehensive textbook*, Vol 2. New York: Lippincott–Raven, 1997:1877–1890, with permission.)

discharges and background activities. During electrical stimulation, a low-frequency cutoff of 1.6 or even 5.0 Hz (−3 dB) helps diminish the duration of amplifier blocking following discontinuation of the stimulus. Because activities recorded directly from the cortical surface are about 2–60 times larger than those detected on the scalp (1), instrumental sensitivities of 10–50 µV per millimeter are most commonly used.

The use of digital recording devices make it possible to survey simultaneously as many as 64–128 brain sites, thus eliminating the need for several successive electrode placements and recordings, while providing detailed topographic assessment of interictal epileptiform discharges, other ECoG patterns, and evoked potentials. These systems also provide the opportunity to supplement the visual appraisal of the ECoG with computer analyses that in the future may increase the localizing power of this method. In addition, developments in the field of neuroimaging have made it possible to generate three-dimensional anatomical maps on which various functional images, such as those from functional MRI, positron emission tomography, single-photon emission computed tomography, magnetoencephalography, EEG, evoked potentials, and the ECoG can be superimposed (165). Frameless stereotactic systems interactively guided by these multimodal images promise to improve the precision of epilepsy surgery (222).

Methods

Preresection ECoGs must survey, in a systematic order, cortical regions within and outside the area of exposure and, whenever appropriate, pertinent subcortical structures. In patients undergoing temporal lobectomy, recordings should include thorough exploration of the infratemporal cortex, hippocampus and parahippocampal gyrus, uncus, and amygdala in addition to the orbital frontal and suprasylvian cortices (307). The hippocampus and amygdala can be surveyed via needle electrodes introduced either manually or stereotactically before resection (32,75,108,123,148,149,160,193,220,231,239,298). Alternatively or additionally, strip or other electrodes can be applied over the ventricular surface of the hippocampus following incision of the lateral temporal cortex or anterolateral temporal lobectomy (32,148,156,193,204,214,239,308). This last approach entails at least partial resection of the amygdala, which precludes the assessment of this structure. Acute deafferentation also may alter hippocampal and parahippocampal functions.

Postresection ECoGs should examine the cortices surrounding the ablation as well as more distant regions. After anteromedial temporal lobectomy, these should include, whenever possible, the remnants of the hippocampus and parahippocampal gyrus, the insula, and neighboring extratemporal cortices. When resection is carried out in stages, at least 10 minutes of technically adequate recording should be obtained following each resection. Total duration of intraoperative ECoG, excluding functional mapping, is generally 1 hour or longer.

Bipolar ECoG recordings are hampered by errors inherent in comparing the voltages of spikes detected by closely and often unequally spaced electrode pairs; difficulties in distinguishing low-voltage records caused by equipotentiality of adjacent electrodes from truly diminished activity related to other causes (7); the long time required to demonstrate instrumental phase reversals between electrode arrays at right angles to each other (108); and inability to readily demonstrate genuine, as opposed to instrumental phase, reversals (32,187,193,239,308). Provided an appropriate reference is chosen, referential montages are unhindered by these difficulties and permit rapid and reliable visual comparison of amplitudes and other features of spikes appearing in multiple channels. In addition, because the voltages of cortical potentials are large compared to those detected by reference electrodes commonly used in ECoG, the activity of the reference is not or is minimally apparent, and generally poses no interpretive problem. Thus displaying ECoGs in the form of referential montages expedites intraoperative interpretation and improves its accuracy. Current computer-based digital recorders offer the advantage that the ECoG, typically obtained referentially, can be displayed in the form of referential, bipolar, or mixed montages depending on circumstances and individual preferences.

Electrical Stimulation

Localized electrical stimulation of the brain is performed during surgery to elicit "afterdischarges" (see "Increased Susceptibility of Epileptic Tissue to Electrical Stimulation: The Afterdischarge" below) (Fig. 21.2), reproduce clinical manifestations of the patients' customary seizures, and map the functions of exposed cortices. In general, the stimulus is applied between two stainless steel ball electrodes that terminate a pencil-shaped probe held by the surgeon (7). Stimulus parameters and technique vary among centers (215), but most commonly individual stimulations consist of a train of diphasic pulses 0.3–1 millisecond in duration delivered at 60 or 50 Hz over 3–5 seconds via electrodes with an exposed surface of about 4 mm^2 and a separation of 5 mm (215). Strategies intended to minimize the chances of thermal (162) or electrolytic (242) damage to tissues that may not be included in the resection have been described (4,108), and a special stimulus paradigm has been suggested to overcome the problems posed by direct cortical stimulation in children, especially infants (150).

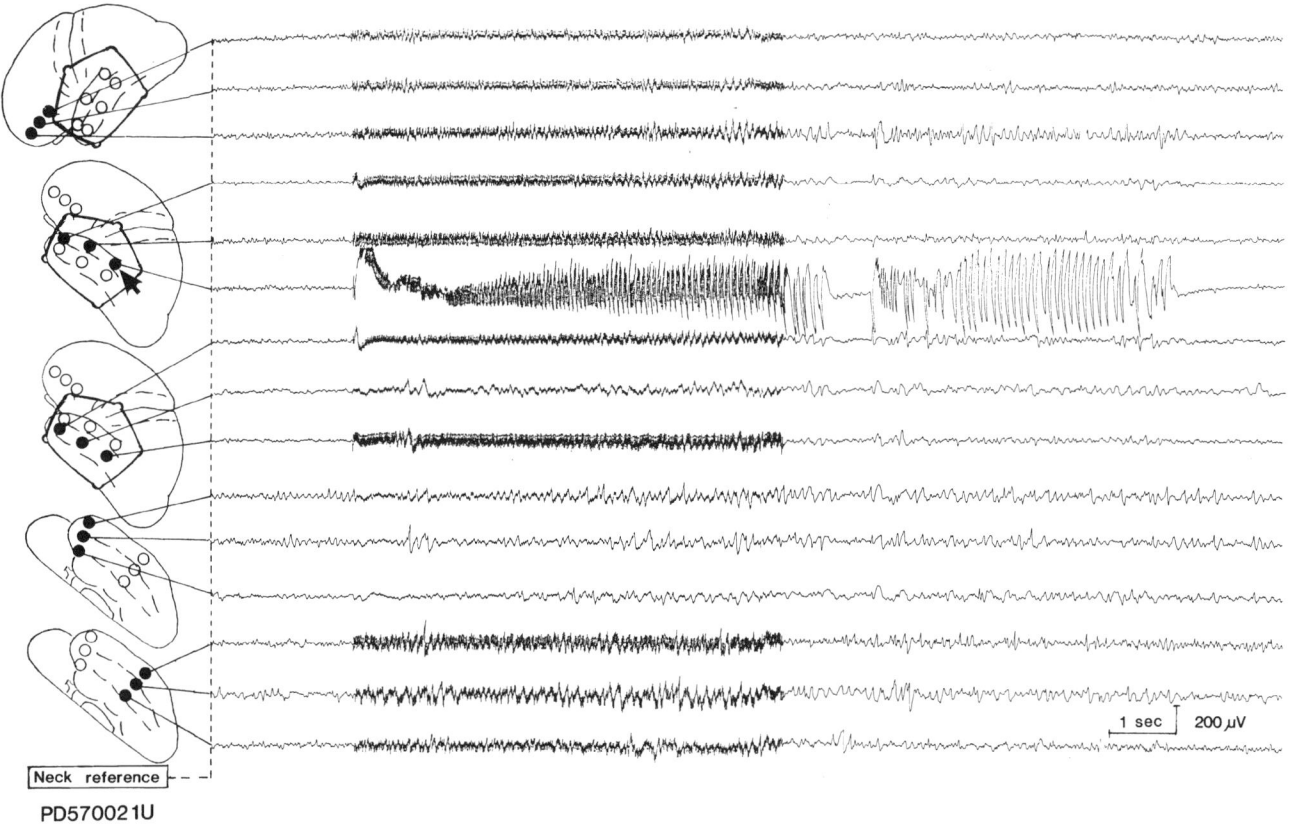

PD570021U

FIG. 21.2. Brief, localized afterdischarge (channel 6) unaccompanied by clinical changes is elicited by electrical stimulation of the posterior portion of the left superior temporal gyrus (rectangular diphasic pulses, 0.3 milliseconds, 60 Hz, 4 mA, 6.5 seconds) in a patient with medial temporal lobe seizures. (From Chatrian GE, Quesney LF. Intraoperative electrocorticography. In: Engel J Jr, Pedley TA, eds. *Epilepsy: a comprehensive textbook*, Vol 2. New York: Lippincott–Raven, 1997:1749–1765, with permission.)

As distinct from stimulation of discrete cortical areas at intensities designed to elicit afterdischarges and reproduce clinical manifestations of the patient's attacks, repetitive electrical excitation at intensities subliminal for afterdischarge is widely used at present to map cortical functions under ECoG control. These stimulations are intended to identify in waking patients motor and sensory cortices often not clearly recognized by visual inspection, and to map regions involved in speech and memory functions that vary remarkably among subjects (218). Delineation of these areas makes it possible to exclude them from resection, thus decreasing the likelihood of functional deficits (218). EEG monitoring allows exclusions of trials in which an afterdischarge is detected. Careful mapping of the earliest cortical components of somatosensory evoked potentials to electrical stimulation of the median or posterior tibial nerves allows localization of motor and sensory cortices during surgery but may be time consuming and is sometimes difficult to interpret. Identification of the central sulcus by this method is most useful in patients undergoing epilepsy surgery under general anesthesia (182,336) and in children (125).

ECOG PATTERNS

The intraoperative ECoG has peculiarities that distinguish it from the scalp EEG. In the absence of gross structural pathology, the same normal rhythms that characterize scalp recordings can be detected from the cortical surface. However, these potentials usually are much larger in amplitude and more sharply demarcated on the cortex than on the scalp (1,7,108,143). Alpha activity predominates over occipital and parietal cortices, and beta activity and, less frequently, a mu rhythm are prominently represented over the central areas. In the temporal region, the alpha rhythm is less abundant, less regular, and variously intermixed with potentials in the theta and delta ranges (7). Because higher frequencies are attenuated to a greater extent than slower frequencies in the transmission of cortical potentials to the scalp (236), most rhythms tend to have a sharper appearance in ECoG than in scalp recordings, and, in general, the ECoG contains more prominent and abundant beta potentials than the scalp EEG (7). The presence of sharp-appearing alpha and mu rhythms over the central cortex (52,147), of occasional sharp potentials over the temporal areas (263), and of prominent beta waves induced by antiepileptic medications sometimes makes it difficult even for experienced interpreters to distinguish individual components of these activities from spike discharges (56).

Among the abnormal patterns recorded in the ECoG, spikes often have larger amplitudes (as much as 0.5–1 mV or more) and shorter durations (as little as 10–20 milliseconds) than in scalp recordings (7). Directly recorded spikes also tend to be more abundant in ECoGs than in scalp EEGs and to involve multiple, often noncontiguous cortical areas, a finding generally not clearly apparent in ordinary extracranial recordings (56,307). Special difficulties may be posed by the interpretation of areas of low-amplitude activity, which may due to equipotentiality of electrodes linked in bipolar derivations, the shunting effect of pooling of saline solution, or structural pathology in the underlying cortex (7). Similarly, in the absence of visually apparent structural alterations, it may be difficult to determine whether areas of arrhythmic delta activity apparent in preresection recordings are related to surgical trauma, such as is caused by division of adhesions, or to preexisting pathology (5,229). Less ambiguous is the finding in postresection ECoGs of similar alterations at and close to the margins of the resection (7). In contrast, a burst-suppression pattern occasionally observed at or near the margins of the excision (71,130) is sometimes difficult to distinguish from bursts of multiple spikes.

Spontaneous seizures are generally not recorded during relatively short-lasting intraoperative ECoGs except when surgery is performed on patients with localized cortical dysplasias (228), or in status epilepticus or by chance. Thus the ECoG examination of patients undergoing epilepsy surgery relies almost exclusively on the detection of interictal spikes.

Because ECoG recordings require instant, unhesitant interpretation that may influence the conduct of surgery, they must be interpreted by a trained and experienced clinical neurophysiologist (5) working in intimate collaboration with a neurosurgeon familiar with the implications of electrophysiological findings.

ACTIVATION AND SUPPRESSION OF ECoG SPIKES

In some patients the ECoG recorded during surgery disappointingly shows no (324) or rare spikes insufficient to define the spiking area. Attempts to elicit or enhance spiking in the intraoperative ECoG include the withdrawal of antiepileptic drugs prior to surgery and the use of physiological as well as pharmacological "activation" procedures. Pharmacological "suppression" of interictal spiking is also used by some to differentiate between primary and secondary spikes.

Withdrawal of Antiepileptic Drugs

In some centers, the patients' antiepileptic medications are discontinued or substantially diminished over a period preceding surgery. However, drug withdrawal is not associated with significant short-term increase of interictal spiking except after the manifestation of clinical seizures (122). Following withdrawal seizures, spikes tend to be more widespread and may even occur contralateral to the side of seizure onset (121). Also, withdrawal seizures may be particularly severe and are sometimes associated with life-threatening complications (283). Because of these drawbacks, several centers prefer to keep antiepileptic medications unchanged in the immediate preoperative period (218).

Physiological and Pharmacological Effects

ECoG spiking can be elicited or enhanced during surgery by activation techniques routinely used in scalp EEG studies, such as hyperventilation and drowsiness or sleep. However, activation of spikes has been achieved more commonly by the administration of pharmacological agents.

Effects of Pentylenetetrazol and Bemegride

In early studies, localized intracortical (14,314) or intravenous (126,148, 314) injection of pentylenetetrazol, a convulsant drug, was used with the intent of promoting ictal discharges in presumably epileptogenic cortex. Because of limited localizing reliability of topical application, and difficulty in preventing the occurrence of generalized seizures with systemic administration (7,108,314), the use of this drug in intraoperative ECoG was abandoned. Another intravenously injected convulsant, bemegride (184,329), had similar shortcomings and fate.

Effects of General Anesthetics, Local Anesthetics, and Opioid Analgesics

General anesthetics, including thiopental, methohexital, etomidate, and propofol, have complex, dose-related effects on the ECoG (40,167).

Methohexital, an ultra-short-acting barbiturate, has been most widely used as an activating agent. Before resection, injection of a 25- to 100-mg bolus of this drug enhanced interictal ECoG spikes in 87% of patients (338) but also promoted expansion of the spiking area in 30% of patients and appearance of new spikes, partly or entirely outside the subsequent resection line, in 43% (92). In other instances, as time elapsed after the injection, the spikes again became restricted to the area involved before activation (Fig. 21.3). Methohexital injection after resection also caused the appearance of new areas of spiking at the margins of the excision or at a distance from it in 35% of patients (92). Additional alterations caused by this drug included induction of slow-wave activity (135,338) (Fig. 21.3) and reduction of beta potentials in the spiking area (135). The expansion of the spiking area under the influence of this, as well as other, agents can be deceptive. Even more

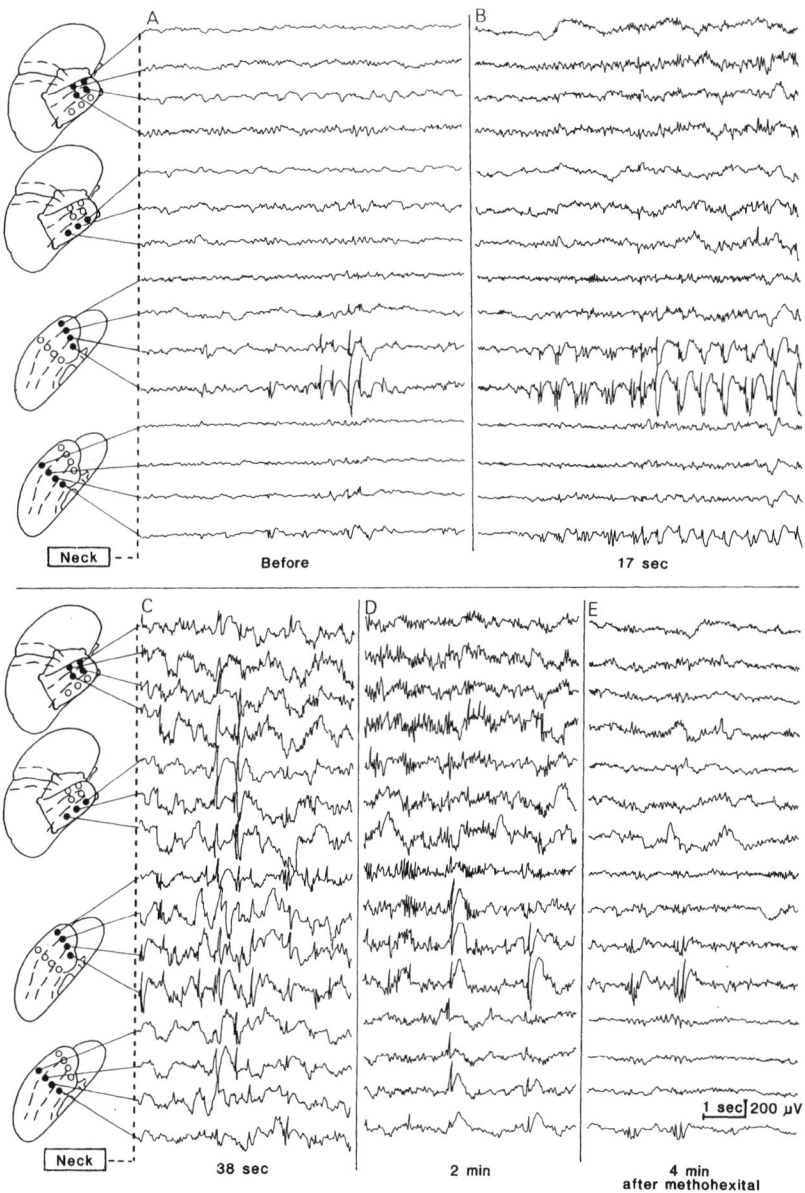

FIG. 21.3. A 23-year-old man experienced episodes of feeling weightless followed by loss of awareness and complex automatisms. **A:** Before activation, intraoperative preresection ECoG shows brief bursts of spike-and-slow-wave activity over the right inferomedial cortex with a maximum on the uncus. **B–E:** After rapid intravenous injection of 100 mg of methohexital, the recording successively demonstrates repetitive spike-and-slow-wave activity of higher voltage at the same location as in **A (B)**; spikes and delta waves occurring diffusely or multifocally throughout the temporal cortex **(C)**; spike-and-slow-wave activity again confined to the anterior infratemporal surface **(D)**; and spikes restricted to the areas involved before activation **(E)**. Beta activity was especially prominent in **D**. The patient fell asleep, and no ictal manifestations accompanied these ECoG changes. His hippocampus showed minor anterior herniation and slight nonspecific sclerosis. (From Chatrian GE, Quesney LF. Intraoperative electrocorticography. In: Engel J Jr, Pedley TA, eds. *Epilepsy: a comprehensive textbook*, Vol 2. New York: Lippincott–Raven, 1997:1749–1765, with permission.)

vexing is the unresolved issue of the significance of those spikes that appear during activation in noncontiguous locations previously free of epileptiform activity. No established criteria allow us to distinguish drug-induced spikes that reveal the existence of epileptogenic tissue to be excised from spikes representing spurious drug effects that can be safely neglected (56,92). Because of these interpretive ambiguities, activation with methohexital or other anesthetic agents is discouraged.

General anesthetic agents such as methohexital may influence epileptiform activity not only when injected as a bolus in small doses to activate interictal spiking but also when used in relatively stable concentrations to produce anesthesia during surgery (97). Various alterations of interictal spiking are also produced by volatile anesthetics, including halothane (108), etomidate (224), enflurane (81,95), and combinations of enflurane and nitrous oxide (138). In contrast, isoflurane (89) and nitrous oxide (134) in commonly used concentrations were found not to alter significantly ECoG spiking.

Other drugs commonly used during surgery that may have epileptogenic effects include intravenously injected local anesthetics such as lidocaine (64) and opioid analgesics such as fentanyl (303) and ultra-short-acting alfentanil (40) and remifentanil (88). These medications enhance interictal spikes and may precipitate electrographic and, sometimes, clinical seizures, mostly in medial temporal structures of patients with temporal lobe epilepsy. However, the combined administration of isoflurane and fentanyl reduces the area and the mean frequency of interictal ECoG spiking (138).

Because many anesthetic drugs variously alter interictal spiking, whenever intraoperative ECoG is to be performed under general anesthesia in children, uncooperative adults, and individuals undergoing special procedures such as corpus callosotomy or medial frontal resections (119,221, 253), the anesthetic agent to be used should be carefully chosen. In some centers, combined short-lasting propofol anesthesia and local anesthetic field block has proved satisfactory in providing comfort to patients undergoing craniotomy while awake (215,274), without substantially altering interictal epileptiform activity (132).

Large doses of intravenously injected anesthetics have been used to suppress rather than activate interictal spiking in the ECoG. The "methohexital sodium suppression test" (198,199) is based on the contention that, because the spikes that characterize primary, autonomous epileptogenic zones are extraordinarily resistant to anesthesia, they tend to persist following methohexital injection even at doses that suppress the background ECoG, and tend to reappear first after the injection. In contrast, secondary, dependent spiking (see "Surgery of Dual Pathology" below), which is more vulnerable to anesthesia, would tend to be obliterated earlier, together with the background ECoG, and to reappear later after the injection. The proponents of this test reported using it successfully during chronic as well as acute ECoGs (135,198,199,280). Further investigation of this method is needed.

TRADITIONAL GOALS AND LIMITATIONS OF INTRAOPERATIVE ECoG

Prior to the introduction of preoperative video-EEG monitoring of spontaneous ictal patterns with noninvasive and variously invasive electrodes and the advent of highly informative structural and functional neuroimaging techniques, ECoG was performed intraoperatively in many centers following clinical and scalp EEG studies that had identified an epileptogenic process within the hemisphere targeted for surgery and established at least its broad location. In this context, intraoperative ECoG was intended to aid in (a) localizing the epileptogenic zone, (b) establishing the limits of the resection, and (c) assessing the completeness of the excision.

Localization of the Epileptogenic Zone

Traditionally, localizing the epileptogenic zone by intraoperative ECoG relied on the identification of an area of brain that (a) displayed interictal spikes,[1] (b) showed greater susceptibility than other regions to repetitive electrical stimulation, and (c) gave rise to the initial or all manifestations of the patient's habitual seizures when electrically stimulated.

Because no seizures are generally recorded during intraoperative ECoG, the utility of this method depends on the correctness of two assumptions: (i) that interictal spikes are reliable markers of the site of origin of the patient's seizures, and (ii) that they provide dependable information on the extent of epileptogenic tissue that must be removed to control the seizures.

Interictal Spikes as Markers of Local Epileptogenicity

Following the demonstration that spikes occurred interictally over limited areas of the scalp and brain of patients suffering from partial seizures

---

[1]For the sake of brevity, interictal epileptiform discharges (i.e., spikes, sharp waves, and their variants) are referred to in this chapter as "interictal spikes" without implying that they are functionally identical, and the full extent of neural tissue displaying spikes is designated the "interictal spiking area." This term is a better descriptor than its frequently used equivalent, the "irritative area."

(140,233), the notion that a close topographic and functional relationship existed between interictal events and ictal discharges became gradually established, although limitations of this concept were recognized (141–143,314), and dissenting opinions were voiced (195). This conjecture found strong support in elegant studies of penicillin-induced epileptic foci in animals. These investigations defined the nature of the cellular events associated with the cortically detected interictal spike (192) and documented the direct transition from interictal into ictal activity within the same neuronal aggregate (250) and even the same neuron (191). However, in patients afflicted by chronic partial epilepsies, the epileptogenic process often by far exceeds in complexity the epileptic focus produced by topical application of convulsants to a discrete cortical area in animals with otherwise normal brains. A manifestation of this complexity is that it is exceedingly difficult to distinguish interictal spikes generated by epileptogenic tissue at the site of recording from spikes neuronally propagated (or volume conducted) from a remote epileptogenic trigger (108,109,143,148,180) and to determine whether or not a secondary epileptogenic zone is capable of independent seizure generation (see "Surgery of Dual Pathology" below). In addition, studies utilizing depth, subdural, and epidural electrodes (20, 180,211,301,326) have demonstrated that, in individuals afflicted with these disorders, seizures sometimes arise outside the ECoG-identified interictal spiking area.

Increased Susceptibility of Epileptic Tissue to Electrical Stimulation: The Afterdischarge

Repetitive electrical stimulation of the brain of sufficient intensity elicits an "afterdischarge" (2,265). Afterdischarges consist of self-sustained rhythmic activity of variable form and frequency, including rhythmic oscillations of alpha or theta frequency and rhythmically repeating spikes, sharp waves, and multiple spikes often evolving into each other (4) (see Fig. 21.2). These electrically elicited seizures vary widely in duration from less than 1 second to 90 seconds or longer (4). They may remain restricted to the area stimulated or spread to wider cortical regions, to subcortical structures, and, sometimes, to distant or contralateral cortices (4,143). Afterdischarges are frequently followed by localized postictal voltage depression, which lasts several seconds and is in turn succeeded by slow activity of variable duration, often most marked at the site of stimulation (4).

Early investigators speculated that human epileptogenic tissues might display increased susceptibility to electrical stimulation in the form of after-discharges of lower threshold, longer duration, or both, compared to non-epileptogenic tissue. They hypothesized that these findings might have special localizing value when associated with prominent, spontaneous interictal spiking or with the initial manifestations of the patients' habitual seizures (142,234,314,317). However, their observations and those of other researchers did not confirm these conjectures (4,108,143,174,181,218,234, 314,317,318). Afterdischarge thresholds also proved unhelpful in determining the presence and location of structural lesions (75), and stimulations of the brain via depth electrodes demonstrated lack of consistent relations between these thresholds and sites of spontaneous ictal onset (29).

Reproduction of Manifestations of the Patients' Habitual Seizures

Penfield and his associates (84,108,145,149,231,232,234,235,252,259) made extensive use of localized electrical stimulation of the brain to reproduce in waking patients undergoing surgery the initial, or all, manifestations of their habitual seizures. The utility of this technique was based on the assumptions that (a) the initial manifestations of partial seizures (i.e., the "aura"), indicated the site of the brain from which the seizures developed, and (b) the reproduction of these manifestations by electrical stimulation of a restricted area of the brain confirmed this localization.

Attempts to reproduce intraoperatively or extraoperatively the initial symptoms and signs of partial seizures by electrically stimulating various brain structures via cortical or depth electrodes provided evidence that these phenomena often did not reflect an ictal discharge arising at the site of stimulation but resulted from spread of the seizure at a distance from this location (20,75,127,145,180,314,329). One study (94) reported that stimulation of numerous frontal and temporal sites evoked in 85% of patients a broad range of clinical phenomena most of which also occurred during the patient's spontaneous attacks. However, similar responses occurred in the presence of an afterdischarge restricted to the site of stimulation or demonstrating only incipient spread from this location, or even the absence of afterdischarge. In addition, the same auras could be elicited from multiple and, sometimes, bilateral sites. These authors concluded that the electrically elicited initial manifestations of the patient's habitual seizures lacked localizing and even lateralizing value, and at best indicated the most likely lobar origin of the patient's spontaneous attacks. Clinical manifestations occurring later during spread of the afterdischarge presumably reflected the involvement of cerebral areas other than that stimulated (94).

Determination of the Limits of Resection

Careful observations have determined that the interictal spiking area defined by intraoperative ECoG often substantially exceeds the extent of brain the excision of which is necessary and sufficient to achieve control of the patient's seizures (254). Removal of the entire interictal spiking area is unnecessary and would increase the likelihood of postoperative neurological deficits (56,72,178,254). That the extent of the "surgically relevant epileptogenic area" (56) remains elusive even when the interictal spiking area has been clearly delineated is not surprising. It is likely that subtle gradations in epileptogenicity exist within the epileptogenic zone, ranging from a maximum (the ictal onset area) to a minimum (the periphery of the interictal spiking area.) Thus it would be unreasonable to expect visual analysis to detect an electrophysiologically sharp demarcation between tissues with sufficiently high epileptogenicity to mandate removal and tissues with sufficiently low epileptogenicity to warrant preservation (56). The frequent finding of multiple spiking areas, especially in the ECoGs of patients with medically intractable temporal lobe seizures (308), is an additional factor of complexity.

Whether or not ECoG recording aids in assessing the completeness of resection and predicting its effectiveness is best determined in the context of each individual operative procedure.

ECOG IN RESECTIVE SURGERIES

Surgery of Medial Temporal Lobe Epilepsy

The majority (about 70%) of patients undergoing surgery for chronic, medically intractable temporal lobe seizures suffer from "medial temporal lobe epilepsy" ("amygdalohippocampal," "mesiobasal limbic," or "rhinencephalic" epilepsy) (60). The electrographic and clinical features of this syndrome; its relations to early risk factors, MRI findings, and neuropsychological profile; and its frequently poor response to medical treatment have been studied in detail (74,76,98,330).

Depth recordings have long established that, in most patients with chronic, medically intractable temporal lobe epilepsy, seizures generally arise at one or multiple sites within a system of closely interconnected structures that include the hippocampus, amygdala, entorhinal cortex (uncus), and parahippocampal gyrus, and may variably propagate to the ipsilateral temporal or frontal neocortex and contralateral hippocampus (8,13,20,55, 62,72,84,111–113,163,177,243,284,290,291,296,310,319,327).

In the majority of patients, a close relationship exists between the medial temporal origin of the seizures and the histological demonstration of "medial temporal sclerosis." This pathology typically consists of a distinct lesion, "hippocampal sclerosis," that is characterized by marked (50% or greater) neuronal loss and gliosis most prominent in the CA1 and CA4 regions (16,80,188) and mossy fiber synaptic reorganization (299). High-resolution MRI reveals hippocampal atrophy and increased T2 signal in over 90% of patients with this pathology (28,42,139,169,170,300). A minority of patients with medial temporal sclerosis display mild, nonspecific hippocampal gliosis without neuronal loss. Variable degrees of sclerosis are also often observed in the amygdala, entorhinal cortex (uncus), and parahippocampal gyrus (48,112). Less frequent lesions include small benign structural lesions such as hamartomas, angiomas, low-grade gliomas, and cysts encroaching on the amygdalohippocampal region (78,190).

At present, surgeries for medically intractable medial temporal lobe epilepsy mostly consist of (a) anteromedial temporal lobectomies designed to remove medial temporal structures and anterior portions of temporal neocortex, and (b) selective removals of medial temporal structures. Anteromedial temporal lobectomy can be anatomically standardized (77,79,210) or individually tailored to ECoG spiking and functional mapping (214).

Temporal Lobe Resection

Preresection ECoG Findings

Intraoperative ECoG findings described in patients undergoing temporal lobe resection reflect the marked prevalence of medial temporal sclerosis among these individuals. However, most surgical series also include some patients with other medial temporal lesions, neocortical temporal lesions (see "Surgery of Neocortical Epilepsies" below), or no demonstrable pathology (see "Surgery of Cryptogenic [Nonlesional] Epilepsies" below).

In a remarkable early study, Jasper et al. (148) reported that the ECoGs of 93% of patients undergoing surgery for chronic, medically intractable temporal lobe seizures showed interictal spikes that involved most commonly the temporal tip, the uncus, the anterior portion of the hippocampus, the parahippocampal and fusiform gyri, and, occasionally, the insula. Subsequent investigators substantially confirmed these findings (6,8,31,32,50,54, 56,66,75,103,123,156,160,193,196,239,247,256,298,307,309,316).

Preresection spikes vary in extent all the way from individual restricted to widespread, often multiple areas (123,160,193,247,298,307) (Figs. 21.4,

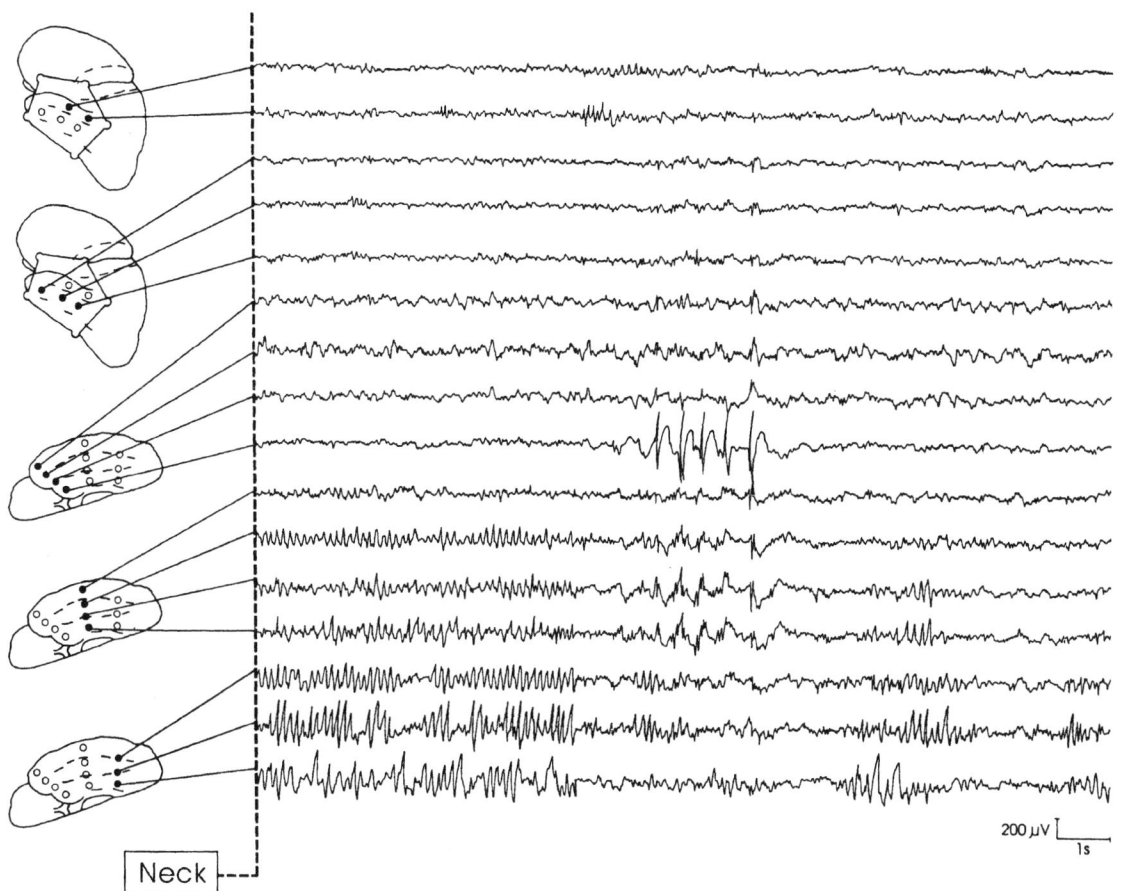

Neck

200 µV
1s

FIG. 21.4. Intraoperative preresection ECoG of a 24-year-old woman with attacks of stomachache, looking to the right, blinking, lip smacking, facial twitching, and impaired awareness. Bursts of spike-and-slow-wave activity occur over the left uncus with minor involvement of adjacent areas. (From Tsai ML, Chatrian GE, Pauri F, et al. Electrocorticography in patients with medically intractable temporal lobe seizures: I. Quantification of epileptiform discharges prior to resective surgery. *Electroencephalogr Clin Neurophysiol* 1993; 87:10–24, with permission.)

21.5, and 21.6*A*). In one series, 81% of all spikes recorded before exposing the hippocampus involved the infratemporal surface, 18% the lateral temporal, and 1% the orbital frontal regions (307). In this group of patients as a whole, the spikes were distributed in an orderly pattern, with the uncus/anterior parahippocampal gyrus and the inferomedial surface of the temporal tip displaying the highest and the lateral temporal and posterior infratemporal cortices showing the lowest propensity for the generation of spikes. Individual patients variously departed from this pattern (307).

In most subjects, electrodes introduced at surgery into the hippocampus through a lateral temporal incision (32) or laid over the ventricular surface of the hippocampus following anterolateral temporal lobectomy (307) demonstrate spikes that occur over the hippocampus and the parahippocampal gyrus apparently simultaneously but with opposite polarities. Commonly, the main component of these discharges is positive on the hippocampus and negative on the parahippocampal gyrus (32,239,307) (Fig. 21.6*B*). However, more complex temporal and polarity relationships between these structures are also frequently evident, suggesting that spikes can be generated at different locations and cortical depths within the hippocampus, the parahippocampal gyrus, or both (307). Hippocampal-parahippocampal spikes are the single most common finding in patients undergoing temporal lobectomy for medial temporal

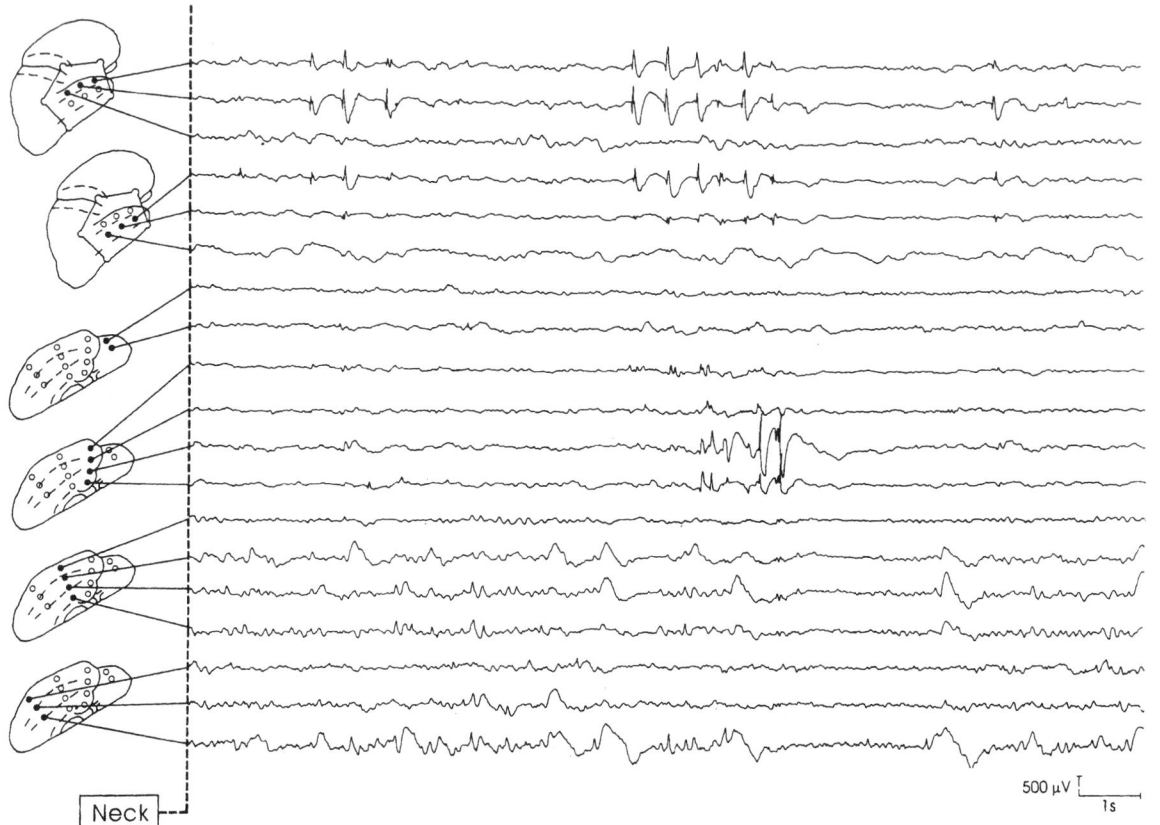

FIG. 21.5. A 31-year-old man had episodes of sour taste, swallowing, chewing, blinking, automatisms of the hands, and unresponsiveness followed by confusion and agitation. Intraoperative preresection ECoG displays spike-and-slow-wave activity that involves the lateral surface and the anterior portion of the inferomedial surface of the right hemisphere independently. (From Tsai ML, Chatrian GE, Pauri F, et al. Electrocorticography in patients with medically intractable temporal lobe seizures: I. Quantification of epileptiform discharges prior to resective surgery. *Electroencephalogr Clin Neurophysiol* 1993;87:10–24, with permission.)

lobe epilepsy. However, electrodes implanted intraoperatively into the amygdala also commonly detect spikes (324). Because these medial temporal discharges frequently fail to appear in recordings from the lateral temporal surface, direct recordings from inferomedial temporal lobe structures are essential to demonstrate them (54,56,307).

In some individuals undergoing temporal lobectomy (as well as other surgeries), no spikes are detected in any location during intraoperative ECoG, however thorough. This negative result is a major drawback if ECoG guides surgery. In a study of selected patients with chronic, medically intractable temporal lobe epilepsy who had undergone both preoperative chronic depth electrode recordings and intraoperative ECoGs (324), those individuals who displayed spikes during the operation had

shown spikes in the same regions preoperatively. However, those patients whose ECoGs failed to show any spiking at surgery had also demonstrated spikes in medial or medial and lateral temporal lobe locations preoperatively (324). This discrepancy strongly contradicts the notion that temporal lobe structures free of interictal epileptiform activity during surgery can be assumed to be functionally intact and should be exempted from resection (158,204).

Preresection Spikes as Indicators of Pathology and Guides to Type of Resection. There is widespread agreement that no dependable relationships exist between the presence or absence as well as the rate, form, location, and polarity of interictal spikes in neocortical and medial temporal structures and the presence or absence and nature of pathology in or outside medial

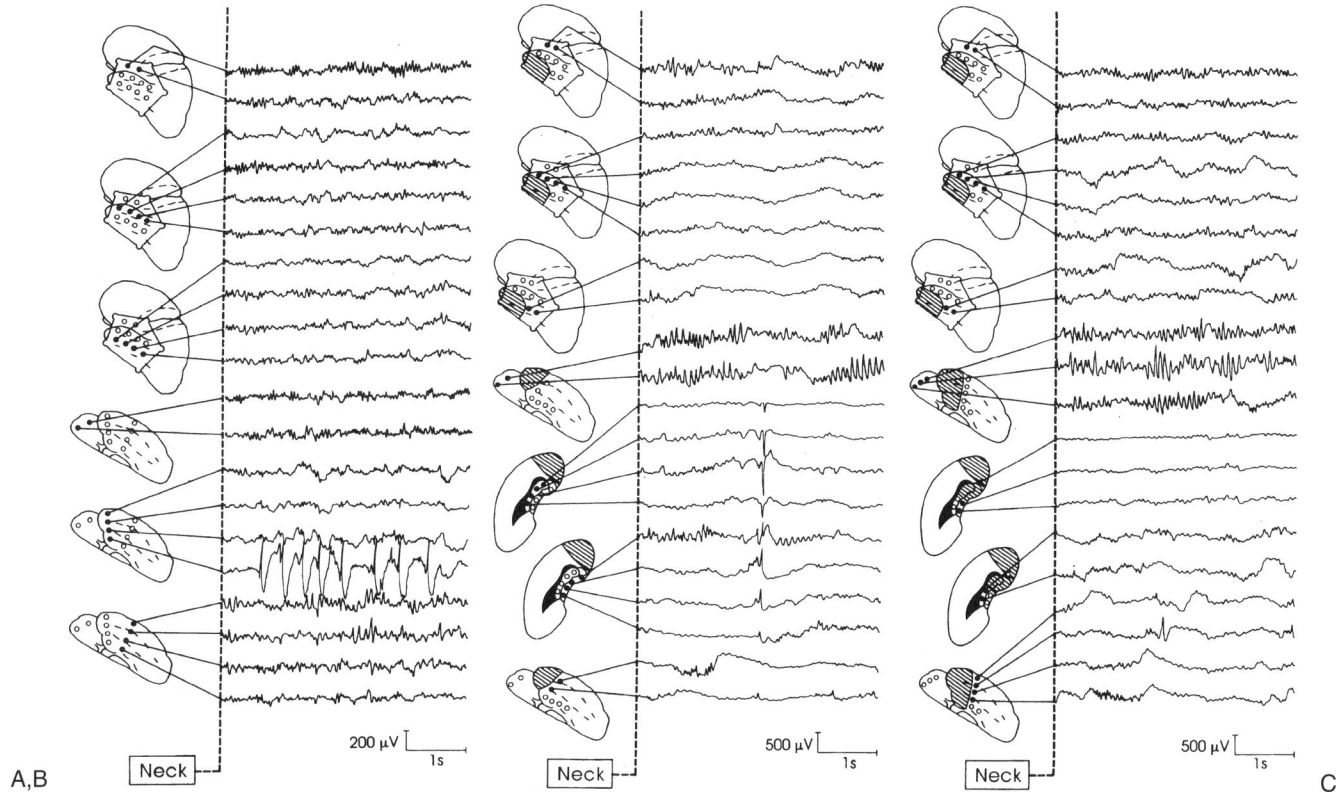

FIG. 21.6. A 33-year-old man had episodes of feeling strange, automatisms of the hands, loss of awareness, and occasional tonic–clonic generalization. **A:** Intraoperative preresection ECoG shows spike-and-slow-wave activity on the anterior hippocampus. **B:** After anterolateral resection, spikes occur simultaneously and with opposite polarities on the hippocampus (channels 11–14) and parahippocampal gyrus (channels 15–18). **C:** Following final ablation, including 2.5 cm of parahippocampal gyrus and hippocampus, infrequent discharges are detected posterior to the inferomedial margin of the excision. (From Tsai ML, Chatrian GE, Temkin N, et al. Electrocorticography in patients with medically intractable temporal lobe seizures: II. Quantification of epileptiform discharges following successive stages of resective surgery. *Electroencephalogr Clin Neurophysiol* 1993;87:25–37, with permission.)

temporal lobe structures (20,32,45,54,75,193,196,197,204,246,308,324). Discrepancies have even been reported between site(s) of seizure onset in neocortical and medial temporal areas and location of pathology (216). It follows that intraoperative ECoG provides no guidance in choosing between temporal lobectomy and amygdalohippocampectomy (32,239).

Preresection Spikes as Guides in Determining the Limits of Resection. Over the past five decades, numerous authors have variously expressed the belief that, in patients suffering from chronic, medically intractable temporal lobe epilepsies of various etiologies, the topography of intraoperative preresection spikes provided guidance in determining the extent of resection (6,24,27,123,148,152,217,234,237,241,251,298,315). Other investigators disagreed with this view (9,61,72,79,282,288,302,318), and some successfully performed "anatomically standardized" temporal lobectomies without ECoG monitoring or consideration of ECoG findings (77,79).

Recognizing that removal of all spiking tissues would be unnecessarily extensive and could cause unacceptable deficits (56,72,75,178,256), those surgeons who perform "ECoG-guided" temporal lobe resections generally exempt from resection one or more of the following:

1. Spiking cortices involved in speech, memory, motor, and sensory functions demonstrated by intraoperative mapping (214)
2. Other cortices located outside anatomically safe boundaries, such as the insula (6,252,275)
3. Posterior temporal extrahippocampal areas
4. Part of the hippocampus when concerns about possible postoperative memory deficits are raised by the preoperative evaluation
5. Cortex displaying comparatively low levels of epileptiform activity
5. Spiking tissues remote from the dominant spiking area

The extent of excision determined by these criteria variably, and sometimes substantially, differs from the limits of the ECoG-defined spiking area (54,56). The presence of spikes outside the limits of the planned resection, whether individually tailored or anatomically standardized, does not detract from the postoperative outcome (66,193) provided that the ablation includes the site(s) from which the seizures arise, those to which the seizures most immediately propagate, and adjacent tissue displaying the most frequent and prominent spiking. Visual assessment of spikes cannot dependably identify these sites, but there is hope that computer analysis of the intraoperative ECoG will facilitate this task in the future (9,31,70,136).

Preresection Spikes as Predictors of Postoperative Seizure Outcome. No measures of preresection spiking, including topography, voltage, rate, and range of rates, reliably distinguish seizure outcomes (30,31,45,86,157,193, 306). Exceptions reported in the literature include maximal spike voltages over posterior temporal and extratemporal areas (31) and very low spike rates (30,31,86,157,193) significantly associated with adverse outcomes, and relatively high discharge rates (24 or more spikes per minute) associated with favorable results (31). A recent comprehensive quantitative study in our center did not confirm any of these relationships (54).

Postresection ECoG Findings

When temporal lobectomy is carried out in stages, following each excision, spikes subside, persist, or newly appear in cortex bordering or neighboring the excision, often varying remarkably in distribution from one ablation to the next (308). After the last of several resections, or after a single lobar resection, the ECoGs of a variable proportion of patients (22%–85%) still display interictal spikes (6,38,54,66,91,116,183,194,306,308) (Figs. 21.6C and 21.7C). Postresection spikes commonly involve multiple cortical areas bordering or neighboring the excision and extend variably into adjacent regions (308). With some exceptions, they are variably diminished in number compared to preresection recordings over the remnants of the hippocampus and parahippocampal gyrus, and other infratemporal cortices, whereas they show no consistent changes in lateral temporal regions (308). In addition, postresection spiking areas are frequently less numerous and less extensive, and attain smaller maximal voltages than did spiking regions before resection (308). Increased spiking is sometimes observed in locations adjacent to the areas most active before resection or at a distance from them (143).

Postresection Spikes as Predictors of Postoperative Seizure Outcome. Whether or not postresection ECoGs contain information of prognostic value has long been the subject of controversy. Early work suggested that persistent or novel spiking following resection was frequently associated with poor postoperative seizure control and warranted additional ablation within neurologically safe boundaries until a normal or clearly improved recording was obtained (143,148,234). Subsequent studies confirmed the existence of a relationship between presence or absence of ECoG spiking after temporal lobectomy and unfavorable or favorable seizure outcome, directly or indirectly advocating the excision of as much epileptogenic tissue as was compatible with avoidance of functional deficits (5,7,24,38,91,108,116,144,146,159, 164,173,193,219,287,298,306,311). No such relationship was found by other investigators (32,45,53,66,68,72,77,107,123,193,256,273,282,305,309,339).

A few studies found that individual measures of postresection spiking were significantly related to postoperative seizure outcome. These included reports of statistically significant associations between low spike rates (five or fewer spikes per minute) and better seizure control (66), and between reductions of postresection spiking to less than 50% of preresection levels and adverse results (32,193). In a somewhat different vein, significant differences in outcome were reported between ECoGs demonstrating simultaneous compared to independent spiking areas and residual compared to increased postresection spiking (183). No such relations were demonstrated

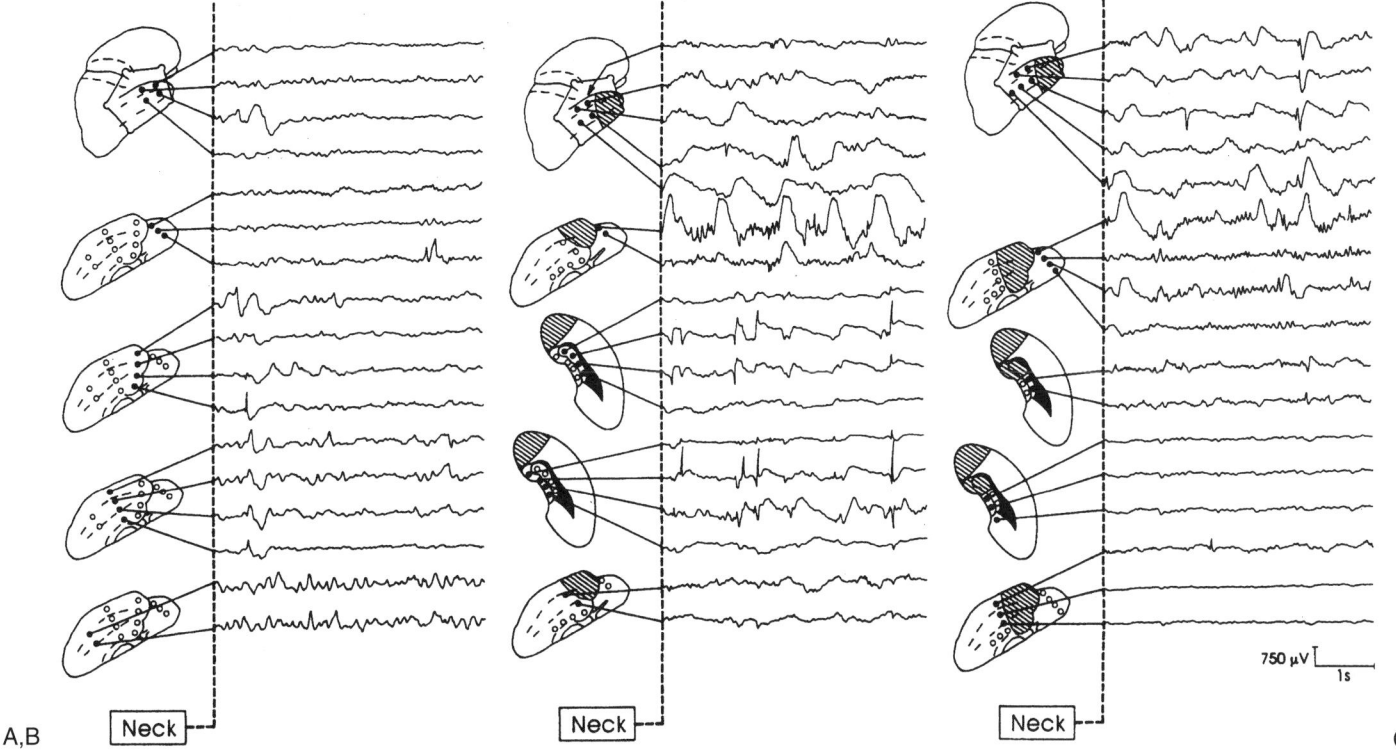

A,B

Neck

Neck

Neck

750 µV
1 s

C

FIG. 21.7. A 20-year-old woman experienced attacks of feeling strange, hot flashes, orofacial automatisms, variably impaired responsiveness, and infrequent tonic–clonic generalization. **A:** ECoG preceding resection displays spike-and-slow-wave activity over the left uncus. **B:** After anterolateral resection, spikes are detected on the hippocampus and parahippocampal gyrus with variable temporal and polarity relationships, and rare lower voltage spikes occur on the right temporal surface posterior to the excision. **C:** Following medial extension of the resection, spikes are recorded posterior to the excision, especially over the lateral temporal areas, and rare low-voltage spikes are noted on the orbital frontal cortex and the residual hippocampus. (From Tsai ML, Chatrian GE, Temkin N, et al. Electrocorticography in patients with medically intractable temporal lobe seizures: II. Quantification of epileptiform discharges following successive stages of resective surgery. *Electroencephalogr Clin Neurophysiol* 1993;87:25–37, with permission.)

by other studies (91), including one by Schwartz et al. (273), who found no statistically significant associations between frequency and voltage of postresection spikes and seizure outcome in a fairly homogeneous group of patients with temporal lobe seizures and preoperatively diagnosed and histologically confirmed mesial temporal sclerosis.

Some investigations focused on the spikes detected postoperatively in individual areas of the temporal lobe. A recent comprehensive quantitative study in our center found no statistically significant relationships between postoperative seizure outcome and any of a number of measures of level (rate and voltage), or change in level, of interictal spiking recorded before and after tailored temporal lobectomy on the hippocampus; the parahippocampal gyrus; the anterior and posterior halves of either of these structures; other infratemporal, lateral temporal, and orbital frontal areas; and all these regions combined (54). A subsequent publication confirmed that the presence or absence of residual spikes in temporal neocortex and the parahippocampal gyrus was not predictive of seizure outcome (194). In contrast, those patients in whom hippocampal resection was pursued until a spike-free hippocampal recording was obtained ($N = 119$) had significantly more favorable results than did individuals in whom spiking persisted on the residual hippocampus, irrespective of the extent of resection ($N = 21$). The latter group included patients in whom hippocampal excision was limited because of concerns about postoperative memory function raised by preoperative intracarotid amobarbital and intraoperative mapping studies ($n = 7$), individuals with bilateral seizure onsets predominantly ipsilateral to the resection ($n = 2$), and individuals with contralateral mesial temporal MRI abnormalities ($n = 1$). The findings of this study were interpreted as strong evidence that ECoG monitoring predicted the extent of hippocampus that should be removed to achieve seizure-free outcome (194), although dissimilarities existed between the two groups compared.

Contradictory findings have been published on the prognostic significance of the frequency of postresection spikes on the insula (157,275). However, there is general agreement that persistent spikes on this cortex do not justify hazardous insulectomy (275).

That ECoG spiking following temporal lobectomy does not reliably predict seizure outcome is not surprising. Postresection spiking may indicate either persistent epileptogenicity resulting from incomplete removal, or inadequate disconnection, of epileptogenic tissue, or may represent new events, most likely caused by the trauma of excision (6,272). It is likely that both mechanisms play a role in the manifestation of spikes after resection, and distinguishing them is a difficult task.

Evolving Role of ECoG in Temporal Lobe Resections

The literature reviewed so far in this chapter suggests that, in patients with chronic, medically intractable medial temporal lobe epilepsy, the presence or absence, topography, and individual measures of interictal spiking detected in medial and lateral temporal locations before as well as after temporal lobectomy are of very limited assistance in the conduct of surgery. These features play no substantial role in establishing the site of onset of the patients' seizures; differentiating between primary and secondary spiking areas; determining the epileptogenic potency of the latter regions; choosing between anteromedial, lateral, and selective medial temporal resections; and predicting postoperative seizure outcome (56). These limitations and the progress of neuroimaging have reduced the dependence of resective temporal lobe surgery on ECoG recordings of interictal spikes, which is increasingly regarded as of primary academic interest. However, when functional mapping is required, ECoG monitoring is essential to determine afterdischarge thresholds and document the subliminal nature of the stimulus.

Reoperation after Unsuccessful Temporal Lobectomy

Failure of surgery following temporal lobectomy is most commonly due to incomplete removal of medial temporal structures. Reoperation with completion of this removal is often successful (106,238) but is usually performed without electrophysiological monitoring.

Selective Medial Temporal Resections and Stereotactic Lesions

Recognition that functional and structural pathologies of medial temporal structures play a central role in medial temporal lobe epilepsy (21,47,73,80, 82,83,104,114,220,326) has inspired a number of selective medial temporal surgeries. These were designed to resect or destroy stereotactically the hippocampus, the amygdala, or both in selected individuals with seizures of established medial temporal lobe onset (36,37,55,85,118,158,161,204, 212,220,230,258,328,333). Remarkably, all these procedures achieved similar good seizure outcomes, suggesting that medial temporal lobe seizures primarily result from concurrent epileptogenesis of closely interconnected medial temporal lobe structures, including the hippocampus and amygdala.

Following resective amygdalohippocampectomy, ECoG-detected interictal spikes (212) increase markedly in frequency, with intervening periods of low voltage or slow activity most evident over the anterior temporal cortex (50,212,323) (Figs. 21.8 and 21.9.) In some patients, a burst-suppression pat-

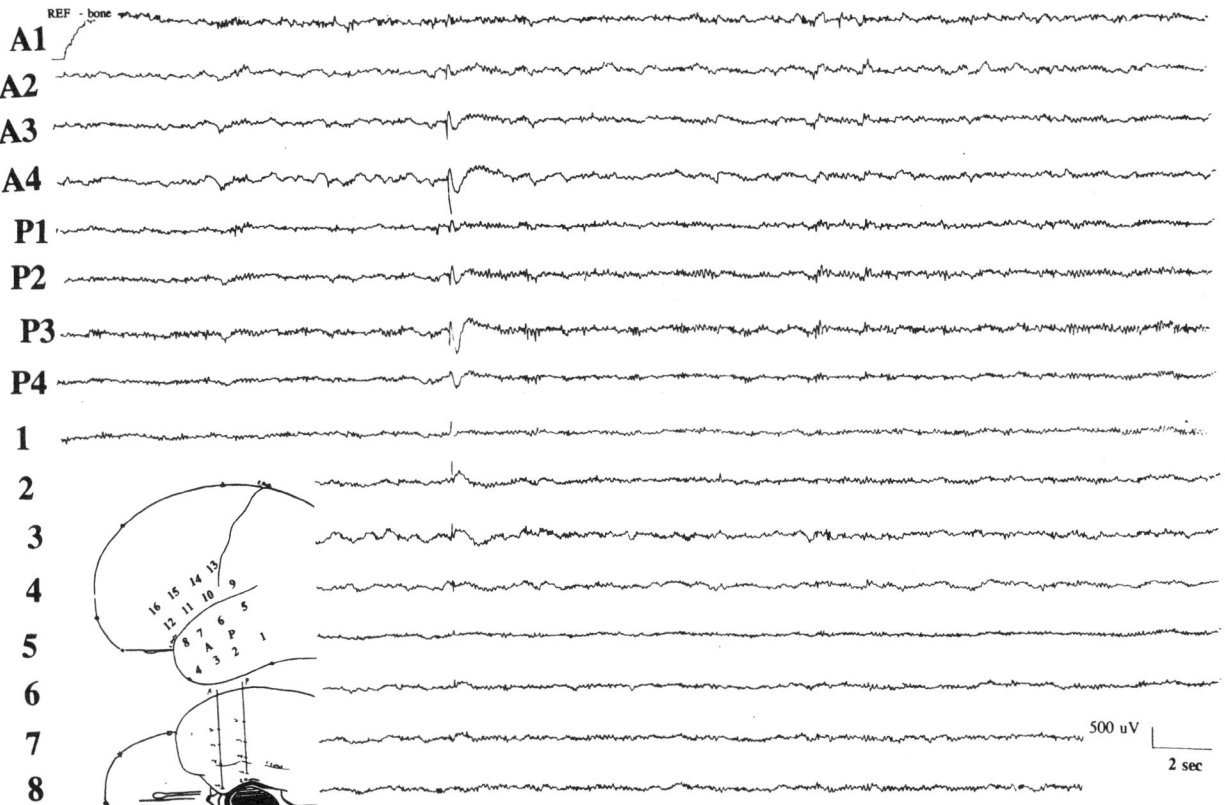

FIG. 21.8. A 36-year-old-man with temporal lobe seizures showed left temporal spikes in his EEG, and MRI demonstrated left amygdalar and hippocampal atrophy. Intraoperative preresection ECoG displays infrequent spikes involving most prominently the left inferior temporal gyrus, the amygdala, and the hippocampus, apparently simultaneously. A1-A4 and P1-P4 are progressively deeper contacts along anterior and posterior depth electrodes inserted manually through the midtemporal gyrus and aimed at the amygdala and the anterior hippocampus, respectively. (From Cendes F, Dubeau F, Olivier A, et al. Increased neocortical spiking and surgical outcome after selective amygdalo-hippocampectomy. *Epilepsy Res* 1993;16:195–206, with permission.)

tern becomes apparent in a similar distribution (323) that may be difficult to differentiate from epileptic activity. This exacerbation of interictal spiking subsides in few days, as indicated by postoperative scalp EEGs (212), and does not presage unfavorable seizure outcome. In contrast to transcortical amygdalohippocampectomies that entail excision of the entorhinal cortex surrounding the amygdala (the uncus), stereotactic amygdalohippocampectomies substantially sparing this cortex are followed by unchanged or decreased spiking in the acute ECoG (36,37,230). Because the entorhinal cortex (the uncus) projects extensively to cortical association areas (112), acute widespread cortical deafferentation incident to ablation of the entorhinal cortex may play a

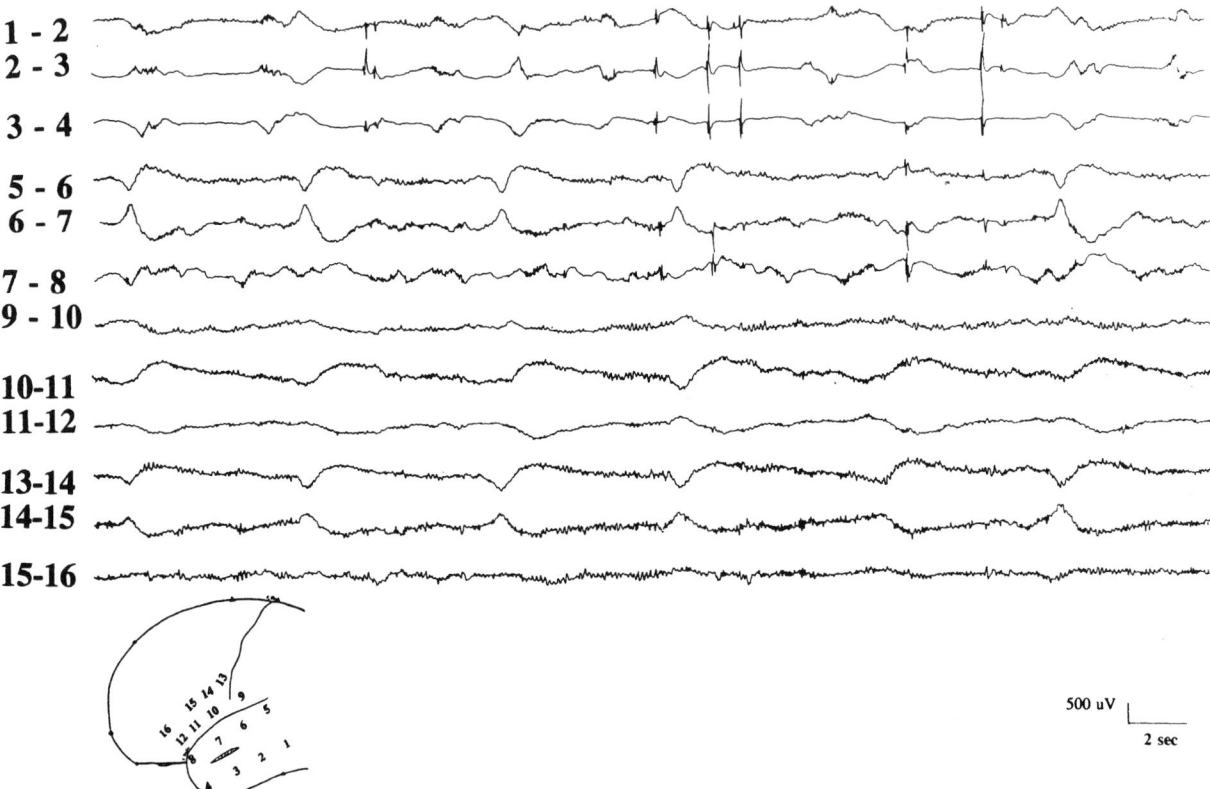

FIG. 21.9. Same patient as in Figure 21.8. After transcortical amygdalohippocampectomy, the ECoG shows frequent spikes over the lateral temporal cortex, with intervening periods of voltage depression and slow waves. (From Cendes F, Dubeau F, Olivier A, et al. Increased neocortical spiking and surgical outcome after selective amygdalo-hippocampectomy. *Epilepsy Res* 1993;16:195–206, with permission.)

major role in the dramatic but transient increase of cortical spiking that follows immediately after amygdalohippocampal resection (230).

In some of the preceding studies, the hippocampus, the amygdala, or both were spared from resection when their intraoperative recordings were free of spikes (158,204). The belief that lack of interictal spiking during a brief intraoperative recording guarantees the functional integrity of any brain area is contrary to basic interpretive EEG criteria and is impugned by the obser-

vation that no spikes were detected intraoperatively in some patients whose earlier preoperative recordings had demonstrated spikes in medial or medial and lateral temporal lobe structures (324) (see "Preresection ECoG Findings" under "Temporal Lobectomy" above). Also, favorable seizure control was achieved by the reoperation of individuals whose seizures had not been relieved by an earlier resection that spared mostly spike-free medial temporal structures (106).

Surgery of Neocortical Epilepsies

Lobar Origin of Neocortical Epilepsies and Factors Hindering Localization

Partial epilepsies symptomatic of structural lesions other than medial temporal sclerosis (and other less frequent medial temporal lesions) are grouped under the term *neocortical* epilepsies (60). The most common lesions include slow-growing tumors, localized cortical dysplasias, vascular malformations, encephalomalacia from previous stroke, and posttraumatic scars.

A major feature of seizures arising in the neocortex is that, because of extensive connecting pathways, they tend to spread rapidly to other areas within and outside the lobe in which they originate. Clinical manifestations of spread to other regions often predominate and tend to obscure the manifestations of the initial localized discharge, thus providing inadequate or even deceptive localizing information. This is evident in neocortical temporal lobe epilepsy, in which ictal activity developing from the temporal neocortex spreads rapidly to medial temporal areas, thus often making it exceedingly difficult to differentiate clinically between seizures of lateral and of medial temporal onset (334). Similarly, seizure spread from functionally distinct areas of the lateral, orbital, or medial frontal lobe surfaces (19) to other regions of the same and adjacent lobes causes clinical manifestations that often provide no precise or even misleading localization (334,335). Major clinical features of seizures originating in the parietal and occipital cortices also reflect spread to other lobes.

Localization of seizure onset and extent of the epileptogenic zone by extracranial as well as intracranial EEG recordings is often difficult, especially in patients undergoing surgery for frontal lobe epilepsy. Biophysical and physiological factors concur to prevent the detection or to hinder the recognition of restricted interictal as well as ictal neocortical discharges while favoring the manifestation of extensive lobar, multilobar, or even widespread discharges. Spikes generated in discrete areas of the depths of cortical sulci often are not detected even by overlying subdural electrodes (109,143,245), and discharges occurring in medial or inferior hemispheric surfaces or in the insula often fail to appear in recordings from the lateral surface while giving rise to secondary widespread discharges. Seizures and interictal spikes rapidly propagating from small cortical sites to other areas of the same and other lobes frequently mimic large spiking areas (245,246). Depth recordings are limited by poor spatial resolution of depth electrodes at the cortical level (129,245,246). The inadequacies of direct cortical recordings were evident in a series of patients with frontal lobe epilepsy only 15% of whom displayed unilateral focal or regional frontal lobe spiking, whereas 32% had lobar and 25% multilobar spikes (244). In harmony with these findings, 75% of patients who underwent frontal lobe resections demonstrated spikes outside the limits of the excision (32) (Fig. 21.10). Despite these limitations, some statistically significant associations have been reported between postoperative seizure outcome and the presence or absence of spikes or individual measures of preresection (193) or postresection (38,193,222,249,268, 321) ECoG spiking.

Lesionectomy for Epileptogenic Slow-Growing Tumors, Vascular Malformations, Encephalomalacia, and Posttraumatic Scars

The relationship between a lesion demonstrated by neuroimaging and the epileptogenic zone varies depending on the pathological substrate. Neocortical lesions such as slow-growing tumors (most commonly low-grade astrocytomas, oligodendrogliomas, gangliogliomas, and dysembryoplastic neuroepithelial tumors), vascular malformations, encephalomalacia from previous stroke, and posttraumatic scars are not intrinsically epileptogenic but often cause interictal spiking whether limited to adjacent tissues or more widespread (15,110,234). Removal of the lesion while sparing "potentially epileptogenic" bordering tissues, or "strict lesionectomy," has given variable results, with seizure-free outcomes being reported in 30%–75% of patients (44,205,289). Resection of potentially epileptogenic adjacent tissues while sparing the lesion has proved unsuccessful (93). In contrast, up to 80%–90% of patients are rendered seizure free or nearly seizure free by excision of both the lesion and a generous margin of potentially epileptogenic bordering tissue, or "extended lesionectomy" (15,27,38,67,101,152,237,251,341). Even partial resection of the lesion met with appreciable success provided all potentially epileptogenic cortex had also been removed (34,100,216).

In principle, intraoperative ECoG appears to be better suited than other methods to identify the potential epileptogenicity of neural tissues bordering the lesion. However, the frequently broad distribution of ECoG spiking may invite unnecessarily large excisions (99,154,295,305). Thus some centers have chosen other approaches to the determination of the margins of the resection that are based on visual inspection, MRI signal abnormalities, histopathological analysis of frozen sections, or combinations of these methods (101). Functional mapping by electrical stimulation may be needed as well to exempt indispensable cortical areas from resection.

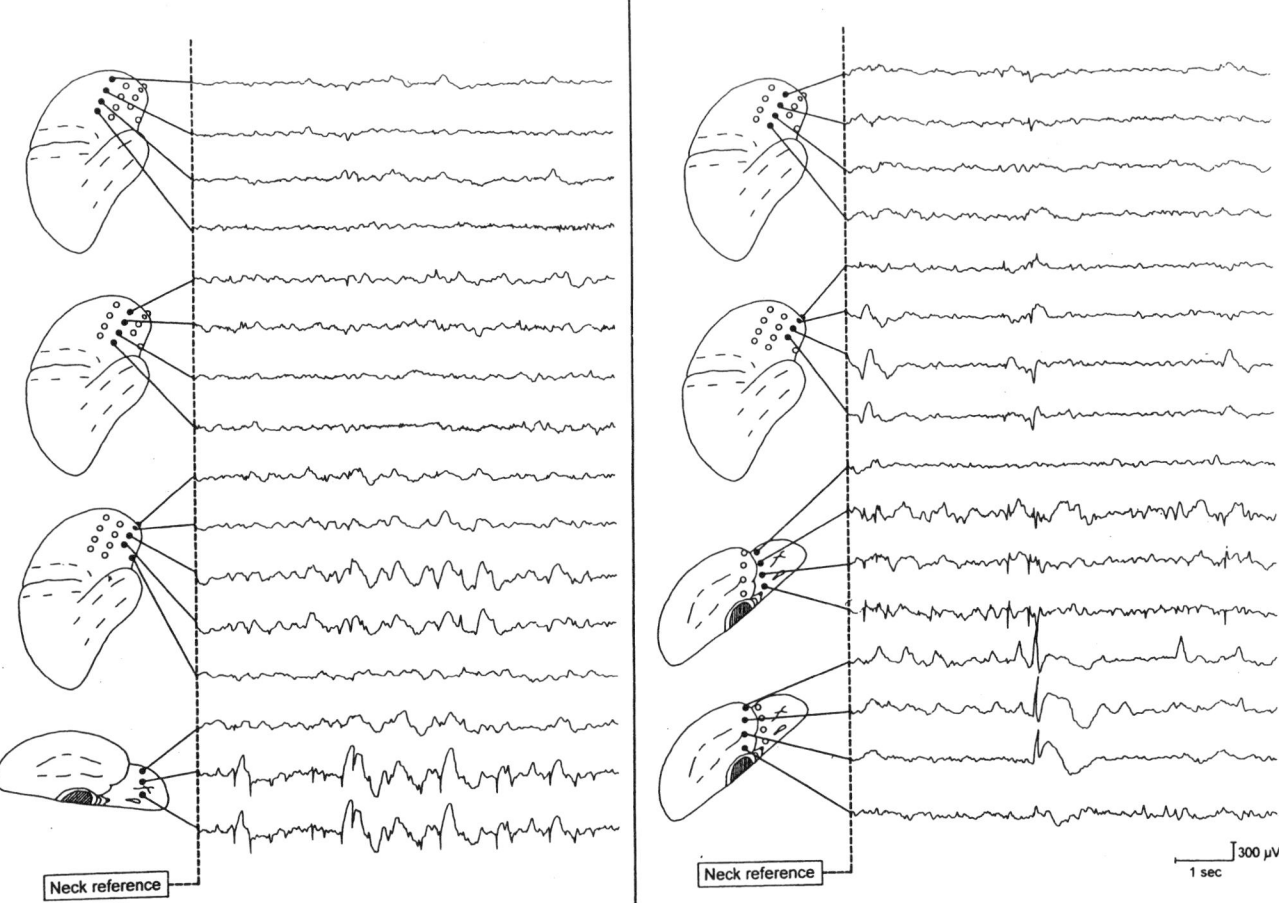

FIG. 21.10. A 31-year-old-man had seizures characterized by body numbness and tingling, a queasy feeling in the stomach, frightened expression and vocalizations, flailing movements of the arms and legs, and infrequent minor automatisms, followed by prompt recovery of responsiveness and denial of having lost consciousness. Occasionally, seizures were followed by tonic–clonic generalization. Intraoperative ECoG shows frequent spikes and sharp waves over the right orbital frontal and inferior frontal cortices, with complex polarity and temporal relationships, and spike-and-slow-wave activity occurring independently over the right infratemporal surface. Two years after surgery, the patient was seizure free. (From Chatrian GE, Quesney LF. Intraoperative electrocorticography. In: Engel J Jr, Pedley TA, eds. *Epilepsy: a comprehensive textbook*, Vol 2. New York: Lippincott–Raven, 1997:1749–1765, with permission.)

Surgery of Localized Cortical Dysplasias

Cortical developmental malformations identified by high-resolution MRI are increasingly recognized as causes of medically intractable neocortical epilepsy. Subdural electrodes overlying these lesions frequently detect seizures, interictal spikes, delta waves, and decreased thiopental-induced beta activity (59,223). The manifestation of seizures that consist of bursts of repetitive spikes mostly restricted to the dysplastic lesion attests to intense intrinsic epileptogenicity that distinguishes dysplastic cortex from most other cerebral lesions (69,228,262) (Fig. 21.11). Sporadic spikes have a more widespread distribution (69,228,262). Remarkably, in a group of patients with frontal lobe epilepsy, seizure activity had 94% sensitivity to and 75% specificity for localized cortical dysplasias, whereas sporadic spikes showed no significant association with type of pathology (87). The detection of intrinsic localized seizures allows the ECoG to complement the MRI delimitation of these lesions, thus contributing to ensure the completeness of resection (222). Abolition of ECoG-detected seizures is significantly associated with favorable seizure outcome, whereas persistent sporadic spikes show no such relationship (87). The use of the ECoG in the resection of localized cortical dysplasias is a promising development that deserves further study.

Surgery of Dual Pathology

In a substantial proportion of patients in whom resection of indolent tumors, arteriovenous malformations, or localized cortical dysplasias involving lateral temporal, posterior temporal (93), or occipital (227) cortices fails to achieve seizure relief, acute and chronic depth recordings demonstrate interictal spikes in the ipsilateral hippocampus (49,93,267,340) and seizures that mostly arise in medial temporal structures, including the hippocampus (189). The finding of this "dual pathophysiology" is mirrored by the intraoperative demonstration of interictal spikes that widely involve the temporal neocortex in patients with epileptogenic tumors confined to the medial temporal structures (128,197). These observations suggest that intense, protracted firing of neocortical epileptic neurons can incite the development of interictal as well as ictal discharges in previously normal, anatomically remote but synap-

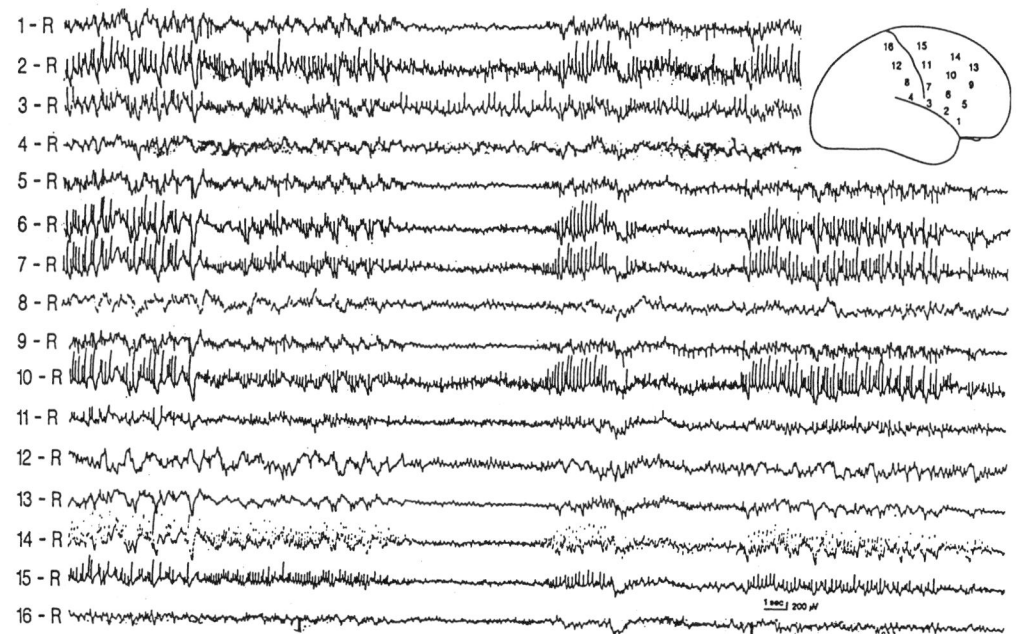

FIG. 21.11. A 7-year-old girl had a right frontocentral cortical dysplasia demonstrated by MRI. Her intraoperative ECoG showed numerous seizures consisting of bursts of high-amplitude spikes over the right frontocentral cortex as in this figure. (From Palmini A, Gambardella A, Andermann F, et al. Intrinsic epileptogenicity of human dysplastic cortex as suggested by corticography and surgical results. *Ann Neurol* 1995;37:476–487, with permission.)

tically connected medial temporal neurons, and that the reverse can also be true. An analogy has been recognized by some between these findings and those characterizing the animal model of secondary epileptogenesis by kindling (39,115,133,313). That interictal spikes can be secondarily elicited in humans at a distance from an epileptogenic zone has long been known (108,143). However, despite suggestive evidence (200,203), it has not been adequately demonstrated that secondary spiking areas can become independently epileptogenic in humans as in animals, that is, capable of spontaneously generating seizures after removal of the primary epileptogenic zone (179). Unfortunately, visual analysis of interictal ECoG spikes occurring independently in distant areas of the temporal lobe can neither differentiate between primary and secondary discharges nor determine the epileptogenic potency of the neural tissues generating them.

Many patients with cortical neuronal migration disorders and porencephalic cysts and a few individuals with slow-growing tumors and vascular malformations also show various degrees of hippocampal neuronal loss and sclerosis (16,51,102,175,289) or MRI-defined hippocampal atrophy (43, 49)—evidence of "dual pathology." In some centers, awareness of the frequency of dual functional and structural pathologies has influenced the surgical approach to extrahippocampal epileptogenic lesions, which currently consists of complete removal of both the extrahippocampal lesion and medial temporal structures to the extent that it is functionally possible. There is no agreement on whether electrophysiological monitoring is useful (51, 164,176,216,340) or unnecessary (43,99) during these resections.

Surgery of Cryptogenic (Nonlesional) Epilepsies

Localization-related epilepsies without a lesion demonstrated by current neuroimaging methods are referred to as "cryptogenic" or, less appropriately, "nonlesional" epilepsies (60). Microdysgenesis and microscopic gray matter heterotopias are frequent findings in resected specimens, suggesting that developmental alterations more discrete and diffuse than those characterizing (lesional) neocortical epilepsies may be the substrate of some cryptogenic epilepsies (171). Such pathology could account for the poor seizure control (15%–30% seizure-free outcome) achieved by localized resections for cryptogenic, as opposed to lesional, epilepsies (46,270,278).

The belief is widely held that most seizures of partial cryptogenic epilepsy arise in the neocortex. Thus several authors include them in the category of neocortical epilepsies, which they subdivide into lesional and nonlesional. However, recent observations suggest that a substantial number of seizures of cryptogenic temporal lobe epilepsy involve at the onset medial temporal structures or both medial temporal and neocortical (temporal or extratemporal) areas (216). The localization of cryptogenic (nonlesional) epilepsies requires careful preoperative studies of ictal patterns with intracranial electrodes. Whether the intraoperative ECoG can contribute additional useful information is unclear at present.

Resection of Large Hemispheric Lesions: Functional Hemispherectomy, Hemidecortication, and Multilobar Removals

Extensive resections such as hemispherectomy, hemidecortication, or multilobar removals are sometimes necessary to alleviate medically refractory seizures in patients displaying profound, lateralized neurological deficits caused by long-standing hemispheric lesions. These include sequelae of prenatal, perinatal, and postnatal insults; extensive cortical dysplasias; hemimegalencephaly; dysplastic gangliocytomas; tuberous sclerosis; Sturge-Weber syndrome; and chronic progressive Rasmussen's encephalitis (11,285). ECoG findings are best known in "functional hemispherectomy," which, unlike complete or "anatomical hemispherectomy," removes the temporal lobe and the central cortex, leaving in place disconnected, vascularized frontal and parieto-occipital cortices (255). Prominent multilobar spikes are commonly demonstrated in the ECoG before this procedure (281,286,322, 325). These discharges often persist or increase, and a burst-suppression pattern may develop over the isolated frontal and parieto-occipital cortices (281,286,322,325) without any relation to seizure outcome (281,312,322). Best seizure control is achieved by carrying out as complete a removal of obviously damaged cortex as can be safely done, irrespective of ECoG findings (257,312). However, in some patients with Rasmussen's encephalitis in whom a more limited resection had been planned preoperatively, the distribution of spiking may suggest the need for additional insulectomy or hemispherectomy (312). Also, the demonstration of spikes in contralateral parasagittal cortex by electrodes applied against the falx has been said to portend poor seizure outcome (312).

ECoG IN CORTICAL DISCONNECTION SURGERIES

Multiple Intracortical Subpial Transections

Morrell and his colleagues (202,207,279) have devised a procedure consisting of multiple intracortical subpial transections designed to selectively interrupt horizontal intracortical connections while largely preserving vertical columnar organization and connections, and blood supply. This alteration of local cortical connectivity is intended to minimize the opportunities for neuronal synchronization and horizontal spread of excitation, thus diminishing epileptogenicity without impairing function. Multiple subpial transections are used, mostly in combination with resection of adjacent dispensable cortex, to relieve partial seizures caused by epileptogenic processes encroaching on nonresectable regions such as precentral, postcentral, Broca's, and Wernicke's areas (137,202,206,207,279). This operation offers an at least temporary alternative to hemispherectomy in conditions that include focal cortical dysplasias and heterotopias, chronic progressive Rasmussen's encephalitis, and epilepsia partialis continua (202,207,279). According to their proponents, transections are followed immediately by marked decrease in voltage of all ECoG activities, followed by recovery of background rhythms but not of spikes (202,207,279). ECoG recordings would be essential to determine the extent of cortex to be transected and to verify the effectiveness of the procedure. However, other investigators have described more variable effects of multiple subpial transections that ranged all the way from complete abolition to 200% increase of ECoG spiking, without demonstrable relation to either seizure outcome or completeness of transection (30,32).

Corpus Callosotomy

EEGs have been monitored during total or partial section of the corpus callosum (264) performed with the intent of mitigating medically intractable drop attacks associated with severe diffuse epileptogenic encephalopathies such as Lennox-Gastaut syndrome (12,35), as well as unilateral seizures with frequent generalization that commonly occur in Rasmussen's encephalitis (10,260,293) and other hemiplegic syndromes, including Sturge-Weber disease, hemimegalencephaly, and cerebral cortical dysgenesis. Evidence was published that increasing disruption of bilaterally synchronous epileptiform discharges occurs in the scalp EEG as callosal section progresses (105,186). Also, combined EEG and ECoG monitoring suggested that sections limited to the most anterior part of the corpus callosum were sufficient to interrupt the bilateral synchrony (185,240). However, synchrony often resumed and generalized seizures variably persisted or returned after callosotomy (35,105,186). Most authors agree that intraoperative loss of bilateral synchrony of epileptiform activity neither reliably determines the extent of corpus callosotomy

to be performed (90) nor dependably predicts the success of this palliative surgery (292). Moreover, it is unclear whether ECoG recording offers appreciable advantages over surface EEGs in monitoring the effects of callosotomy (32).

ECoG IN THE SURGERY OF OTHER EPILEPTIC DISORDERS

Epilepsia Partialis Continua

Occasionally the electrophysiologist is called on to perform an ECoG during surgery for epilepsia partialis continua (166), a particular form of status epilepticus characterized by localized, virtually incessant clonic jerks sometimes associated with intermittent, spreading partial somatomotor seizures. Most commonly, this disorder occurs in patients with (a) a variety of acute or chronic unilateral lesions in or near the motor cortex; (b) more extensive, primarily cortical, unilateral or strongly lateralized inflammatory alterations such as those characterizing Rasmussen's chronic encephalitis; (c) certain systemic metabolic derangements unaccompanied by detectable structural lesions such as nonketotic hyperglycemia; and (d) no demonstrable etiology (18,33,260,276,286,304). In keeping with the variable nature and extent of pathological and scalp EEG alterations, when present (17,57,58,168,286, 304), ECoGs from the hemisphere contralateral to the jerking reveal in some patients spiking and sometimes seizures that may be confined to a small portion of the precentral gyrus or may involve multifocally larger cortical areas, and may or may not be temporally related to the muscular jerks (286,304). These events may be absent in scalp EEGs. In other individuals, no discharges can be demonstrated even by meticulously surveying the cortical surface in the presence of ongoing clonic activity (286,304). Lack of epileptiform activity in the ECoG, the EEG, or both is likely related to the small spatial extent of the cortical area producing the jerks (109,117); the possible location of the discharging neurons in the depths of sulci (109,304); the asynchronous firing of multiple, small groups of neurons within the area involved (304); or a combination of these factors. Results of recordings and electrical stimulations with stereotactically implanted electrodes (18,331) have discredited the alternative interpretation that the electrophysiological and clinical manifestations of epilepsia partialis continua may have a subcortical substrate (155,208).

Limited ECoG-guided corticectomies have succeeded in abolishing epilepsia partialis continua in a few patients, especially in the absence of widespread pathology (63,168). However, in most individuals, particularly those suffering from Rasmussen's encephalitis, spikes persist in cortices spared by limited excisions, and clinical epileptic manifestations show no or little improvement (213,286,304). In these instances, multiple subpial resections with ECoG monitoring have provided at least temporary relief (208) before resorting to multilobar resections or hemispherectomy (213).

Landau-Kleffner Syndrome

The ECoG has contributed to the understanding of the mechanisms underlying the Landau-Kleffner syndrome, or acquired epileptic aphasia. This puzzling disorder characterizes children who have developed age-appropriate speech, lose speech capacity acutely or gradually, and typically manifest various types of epileptic seizures and behavioral deterioration. Although long-term prognosis for seizures is good, serious neuropsychological sequelae are reported in the majority of patients (277).

A peculiarity of most patients with Landau-Kleffner syndrome is that, during non–rapid-eye-movement sleep, their EEGs show virtually continuous bilateral and widespread spike-and-slow-wave activity most prominent over the temporal areas (22,65,277). Methohexital suppression and intracarotid amobarbital tests have demonstrated that the bilateral spike-and-slow-wave activity is dependent on discharges emanating from one hemisphere (201,209), and dipole mapping and magnetic source imaging studies have shown that they originate in the dorsal surface of the superior temporal gyrus (201,226). In a few selected individuals, intraoperative ECoGs have detected spikes that are confined to a small patch of cortex located within the sylvian fissure on or close to Heschl's gyrus, that is, in cortex involved in acoustic processing (201,226). ECoG-guided multiple subpial transections of the intrasylvian source and of surrounding tissues resulted in cessation of seizures, normalization of the EEG, and gradual recovery of speech in the majority of these patients (209) (Fig. 21.12). However, because no localized structural lesion is demonstrated in most cases and the seizure disorder tends to resolve with advancing age (22,277), there are no clear indications at present for the surgical treatment of patients with Landau-Kleffner syndrome.

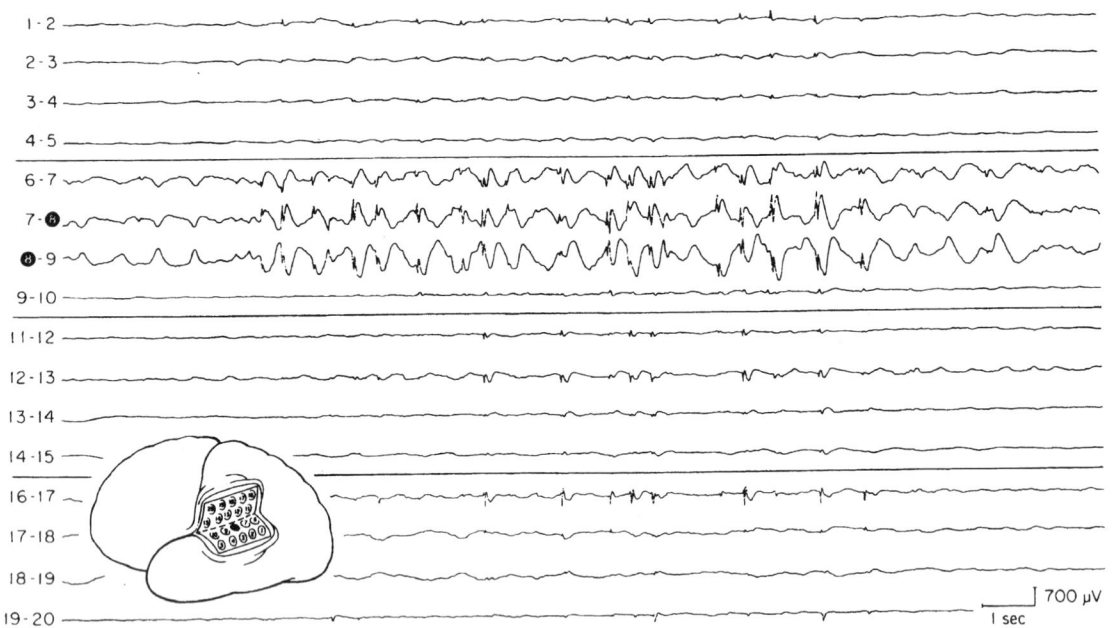

FIG. 21.12. Recordings from a subdural electrode plate inserted between the lips of the Sylvian fissure opened at surgery. Prominent spike-and-slow-wave activity is detected at electrode 8 and to a lesser extent electrode 7, located on the dorsal surface of the superior temporal gyrus immediately posterior to Heschl's gyrus. (From Morrell F. Electrophysiology of CSWS in Landau-Kleffner syndrome. In: Beaumanoir A, Bureau M, Deonna T, et al, eds. *Continuous spikes and waves during slow sleep: electrical status epilepticus during slow sleep*. London: John Libbey, 1995:77–90, with permission.)

CONCLUSIONS

Critical review of traditional principles of intraoperative ECoG reveals that this method has major limitations. Generally, localized interictal spikes directly recorded from the brain are not reliable markers of local epileptogenicity defined as the capacity for active, independent seizure generation. Afterdischarge thresholds and the reproduction of the initial, or all, manifestations of the patient's habitual seizures do not dependably identify the site of origin of the patient's spontaneous seizures. In addition, because interictal spikes often variably exceed the extent of tissue that must be removed to achieve seizure control, their distribution provides no reliable guidance in determining the margins of the resection.

In patients with chronic, medically intractable medial temporal lobe epilepsy, the presence or absence, topography, and individual measures of interictal spiking detected in medial and lateral temporal locations before as well as after temporal lobectomy generally are of little assistance in the conduct of surgery. These features play no substantial role in establishing the site of onset of the patients' seizures; differentiating between primary and secondary spiking areas; determining the epileptogenic potency of the latter regions; choosing between anteromedial, lateral, and selective medial temporal resections; and predicting postoperative seizure outcome. Recognition of these limitations and the progress of neuroimaging have decreased the dependence of resective temporal lobe surgery on intraoperative interictal ECoG (as well as preoperative invasive recordings). Direct recording of interictal spikes during temporal lobectomy is increasingly regarded as of primarily academic interest. However, whenever functional mapping of indispensable cortex is performed, ECoG monitoring is essential to determine afterdischarge thresholds and document the subliminal nature of the stimulus.

Transcortical amygdalohippocampectomy is commonly followed by marked, transient, clinically insignificant increase in interictal spiking in the temporal neocortex. Thus, ECoG monitoring during this surgery serves no practical purpose and may prove misleading.

In neocortical epilepsies symptomatic of lesions such as slow-growing tumors, vascular malformations, encephalomalacia, and posttraumatic scars, whether temporal or extratemporal, excision of the lesion and of a generous margin of potentially epileptogenic bordering tissue is commonly performed. Although, in principle, electrophysiological recordings appear to be eminently suited to identify potential epileptogenicity of surrounding tissues, the frequently extensive distribution of interictal ECoG discharges limits the use of this method in the surgery of these lesions.

Some patients who have undergone unsuccessful excision of epileptogenic lesions involving the lateral temporal, posterior temporal, and occipital cortices but sparing medial temporal structures manifest interictal spikes and seizures that mostly arise from ipsilateral medial temporal structures, especially the hippocampus. In a proportion of cases, medial temporal sclerosis and hippocampal atrophy are demonstrated. Such dual functional and structural pathologies are treated in most centers with resections of both the extrahippocampal lesion and medial temporal structures. However, there is no agreement on the need for ECoG during these surgeries.

There is no indication that ECoG is helpful in performing multilobar resections and functional hemispherectomies, and that direct recordings are more valuable than scalp EEGs in assessing the acute effects and long-term results of corpus callosotomy. Also, it is not clearly established that this method dependably monitors the effects of multiple intracortical subpial transections.

The utility of ECoG in the surgery of epilepsia partialis continua varies depending on factors that include the nature and extent of the underlying pathology. In a few cases, direct cortical recordings during surgery have contributed to clarification of the pathophysiology of Landau-Kleffner syndrome. However, there are no clear indications at present for the surgical treatment of this condition.

REFERENCES

1. Abraham K, Ajmone-Marsan C. Patterns of cortical discharges and their relation to routine scalp electroencephalography. *Electroencephalogr Clin Neurophysiol* 1958;10:447–461.
2. Adrian ED. The spread of activity in the cerebral cortex. *J Physiol (Lond)* 1936;88:127–161.
3. Adrian ED, Matthews BHC. The Berger rhythm: potentials changes from the occipital lobes in man. *Brain* 1934;57:355–385.
4. Ajmone-Marsan C. Focal electrical stimulation. In: Purpura DP, Penry JK, Tower DB, et al, eds. *Experimental models of epilepsy: a manual for the laboratory worker*. New York: Raven Press, 1972:147–172.
5. Ajmone-Marsan C. Chronic intracranial recording and electrocorticography. In: Daly DD, Pedley TA, eds. *Current practice of clinical electroencephalography*, 2nd ed. New York: Raven Press, 1990:535–560.
6. Ajmone-Marsan C, Baldwin M. Electrocorticography. In: Baldwin M, Bailey P, eds. *Temporal lobe epilepsy*. Springfield, IL: Charles C Thomas Publisher, 1958:368–395.
7. Ajmone-Marsan C, O'Connor M. Electrocorticography. In: Ajmone-Marsan C, ed. *Handbook of electroencephalography and clinical neurophysiology*, Vol 10, Part C. Amsterdam: Elsevier Science, 1973:3–49.
8. Ajmone-Marsan C, Van Buren JM. Epileptiform activity in cortical and subcortical structures in the temporal lobe of man. In: Baldwin M, Bailey P, eds. *Temporal lobe epilepsy*. Springfield, IL: Charles C Thomas Publisher, 1958:78–108.
9. Alarcon G, Garcia Seoane JJ, Binnie CD, et al. Origin and propagation of interictal discharges in the acute electrocorticogram: implications for pathophysiology and surgical treatment of temporal lobe epilepsy. *Brain* 1997;120:2259–2282.

10. Andermann F. *Chronic encephalitis and epilepsy: Rasmussen's syndrome.* Boston: Butterworth-Heinemann, 1991.

11. Andermann F, Freeman JM, Vigevano F, et al. Surgically remediable diffuse hemispheric syndromes. In: Engel J Jr, ed. *Surgical treatment of the epilepsies,* 2nd ed. New York: Raven Press, 1993:87–101.

12. Andermann F, Olivier A, Gotman J, et al. Callosotomy for the treatment of patients with intractable epilepsy and the Lennox-Gastaut syndrome. In: Niedermeyer E, Degen R, eds. *The Lennox-Gastaut syndrome.* New York: Alan R. Liss, 1988:361–376.

13. Angeleri F, Ferro-Milone F, Parigi S. Electrical activity and reactivity of the rhinencephalic, pararhinencephalic and thalamic structures: prolonged implantation of electrodes in man. *Electroencephalogr Clin Neurophysiol* 1964;16:100–129.

14. Arseni C, Cinca I, Christian C, et al. Electrocorticography in neurosurgical treatment of epilepsy (method, application and interpretation). *Neurologia* 1963;8:409–428.

15. Awad IA, Rosenfeld J, Ahl J, et al. Intractable epilepsy and structural lesions of the brain: mapping, resection strategies and seizure outcome. *Epilepsia* 1991;32:179–186.

16. Babb TL, Brown, WJ. Pathological findings in epilepsy. In: Engel J Jr, ed. *Surgical treatment of the epilepsies.* New York: Raven Press, 1987:511–540.

17. Bancaud J, Bonis A, Talairach J, et al. Syndrôme de Kojevnikow et accès somatomoteurs (étude clinique, E.E.G. et S.E.E.G.). *Encéphale* 1970;5:391–438.

18. Bancaud J, Bonis A, Trottier S, et al. L'épilepsie partielle continue: syndrôme et maladie. *Rev Neurol (Paris)* 1982;138:802–814.

19. Bancaud J, Talairach J. Clinical semiology of frontal lobe seizures. *Adv Neurol* 1992;57:3–58.

20. Bancaud J, Talairach J, Bonis A, et al. *La stéréo-électroencéphalographie dans l'épilepsie: informations neurophysiopathologiques apportées par l'investigation fonctionnelle stéréotaxique.* Paris: Masson & Cie, 1965.

21. Bancaud J, Talairach J, Morel P, et al. La corne d'Ammon et le noyau amygdalien: effects cliniques et électriques de leur stimulation chez l'homme. *Rev Neurol (Paris)* 1966;115:329–352.

22. Beaumanoir A. The Landau-Kleffner syndrome. In: Roger J, Bureau M, Dravet C, et al, eds. *Epileptic syndromes in infancy, childhood and adolescence,* 2nd ed. London: John Libbey, 1992:231–243.

23. Bechtereva NP. Electrocorticography in supratentorial tumors of the brain. In: Bekhtereva NP, ed. *Biopotentials of cerebral hemispheres in brain tumors.* New York: Consultants Bureau, 1962:115–136.

24. Bengzon ARA, Rasmussen T, Gloor P, et al. Prognostic factors in the surgical treatment of temporal lobe epileptics. *Neurology* 1968;18:717–731.

25. Berger H. Über das Elektrenkephalogramm des Menschen. *Arch Psychiatr Nervenkr* 1929;87:527–520. (Translated by Gloor P. *Electroencephalogr Clin Neurophysiol Suppl* 1969;28:1937–1973.)

26. Berger H. Über das Elektrenkephalogramm des Menschen. *Arch Psychiatr Nervenkr* 1931;94:16–60. (Translated by Gloor P. *Electroencephalogr Clin Neurophysiol Suppl* 1969;28:1995–1132.)

27. Berger MS, Ghatan S, Haglund MM, et al. Low-grade gliomas associated with intractable epilepsy: seizure outcome utilizing electrocorticography during tumor resection. *J Neurosurg* 1993;79:62–69.

28. Berkovic SF, Andermann F, Olivier A, et al. Hippocampal sclerosis in temporal lobe epilepsy demonstrated by magnetic resonance imaging. *Ann Neurol* 1991;29:175–182.

29. Bernier GP, Richer F, Giard N, et al. Electrical stimulation of the human brain in epilepsy. *Epilepsia* 1990;31:513–520.

30. Binnie CD. Unresolved issues in electrocorticography. *Epilepsia* 1995;36[Suppl 3]:S269(abst).

31. Binnie CD, Alarcon G, Elwes RDC, et al. Role of ECoG in 'en bloc' temporal lobe resection: the Maudsley experience. *Electroencephalogr Clin Neurophysiol Suppl* 1998;48:17–23.

32. Binnie CD, McBride MC, Polkey CE, et al. Electrocorticography and stimulation. *Acta Neurol Scand Suppl* 1994;89:74–82.

33. Biraben A, Chauvel P. Epilepsia partialis continua. In: Engel J Jr, Pedley TA, eds. *Epilepsy: a comprehensive textbook,* Vol 3. Philadelphia: Lippincott–Raven, 1997:2447–2453.

34. Blume WT, Aicardi J, Dreifuss FE. Syndromes not amenable to resective surgery. In: Engel J Jr, ed. *Surgical treatment of the epilepsies,* 2nd ed. New York: Raven Press, 1993:103–118.

35. Blume WT, Girvin J, Kaufmann J. Childhood brain tumors presenting as chronic uncontrolled focal seizure disorders. *Ann Neurol* 1982;12:538–541.

36. Blume WT, Parrent AG. Intraventricular recording during and after stereotactic amygdalohippocampotomy. *Epilepsia* 1995;36[Suppl 3]:S169(abst).

37. Blume WT, Parrent AG, Kaibara M. Stereotactic amygdalohippocampotomy and mesial temporal spikes. *Epilepsia* 1997;38:930–936.

38. Britton JW, Cascino GD, Sharbrough FW, et al. Low-grade glial neoplasms and intractable partial epilepsy: efficacy of surgical treatment. *Epilepsia* 1994;35:1130–1135.

39. Cain DP. Kindling and amygdala. In: Aggleton JP, ed. *The amygdala: neurobiological aspects of emotion, memory, and mental dysfunction.* New York: Wiley–Liss, 1992:539–560.

40. Cascino GD. Pharmacological activation. *Electroencephalogr Clin Neurophysiol Suppl* 1998;48:70–76.

41. Cascino GD. Advances in neuroimaging: surgical localization. *Epilepsia* 2001;42:3–12.

42. Cascino GD, Jack CR, Parisi JE, et al. Magnetic resonance imaging-based volumetric studies in temporal lobe epilepsy: pathologic correlations. *Ann Neurol* 1991;30:31–36.

43. Cascino GD, Jack CR Jr, Sharbrough FW, et al. Operative strategy in patients with MRI-identified dual pathology and temporal lobe epilepsy. *Epilepsy Res* 1993;14:175–182.

44. Cascino GD, Kelly PJ, Sharbrough FW, et al. Long-term follow-up of stereotactic lesionectomy in partial epilepsy. *Epilepsia* 1992;33:639–644.

45. Cascino GD, Trenerry MR, Jack CR Jr, et al. Electrocorticography and temporal lobe epilepsy: relationship to quantitative MRI and operative outcome. *Epilepsia* 1995;36:692–696.

46. Cascino GD, Trenerry MR, Sharbrough FW, et al. Depth electrode studies in temporal lobe epilepsy: relations to quantitative magnetic resonance imaging and operative outcome. *Epilepsia* 1995;36:230–235.

47. Cendes F, Andermann F, Gloor P, et al. Atrophy of mesial structures in patients with temporal lobe epilepsy: cause or consequence of repeated seizures? *Ann Neurol* 1993;34:795–801.

48. Cendes F, Andermann F, Gloor P, et al. MRI volumetric measurement of amygdala and hippocampus in temporal lobe epilepsy. *Neurology* 1993;43:719–725.

49. Cendes F, Cook MJ, Watson C, et al. Frequency and characteristics of dual pathology in patients with lesional epilepsy. *Neurology* 1995;45:2058–2064.

50. Cendes F, Dubeau F, Olivier A, et al. Increased neocortical spiking and surgical outcome after selective amygdalo-hippocampectomy. *Epilepsy Res* 1993;16:195–206.

51. Cendes F, Li LM, Andermann F, et al. Dual pathology and its clinical relevance. *Adv Neurol* 1999;81:153–164.

52. Chatrian GE. The mu rhythm. In: Chatrian GE, Lairy GC, eds. *Handbook of electroencephalography and clinical neurophysiology, Vol 6, Part A. The EEG of the waking adult.* Amsterdam: Elsevier Science, 1976:46–69.

53. Chatrian GE. Role of electrocorticography in focal epilepsy. *Epilepsia* 1995;36[Suppl 3]:S269–S270(abst).

54. Chatrian GE. Role of ECoG in tailored temporal lobe resections: the University of Washington experience. *Electroencephalogr Clin Neurophysiol Suppl* 1998;48:24–43.

55. Chatrian GE, Chapman WP. Electrographic study of the amygdaloid region with implanted electrodes in patients with temporal lobe epilepsy. In: Ramey ER, O'Doherty DS, eds. *Electrical studies of the unanesthetized brain.* New York: Hoeber, 1960:351–368.

56. Chatrian GE, Quesney LF. Intraoperative electrocorticography. In: Engel J Jr, Pedley TA, eds. *Epilepsy: a comprehensive textbook,* Vol 2. New York: Lippincott–Raven, 1997:1749–1765.

57. Chatrian GE, Shaw CM, Leffman H. The significance of periodic lateralized epileptiform discharges in EEG: an electrographic, clinical and pathological study. *Electroencephalogr Clin Neurophysiol* 1964;17:177–193.

58. Chatrian GE, Shaw CM, Plum F. Focal periodic slow transients in epilepsia partialis continua:

clinical and pathological correlations in two cases. *Electroencephalogr Clin Neurophysiol* 1964;16:387–393.

59. Chugani HT, Shewmon DA, Shields WD, et al. Surgery for intractable infantile spasms: neuroimaging perspectives. *Epilepsia* 1993;34:764–771.

60. Commission on Classification and Terminology of the International League Against Epilepsy. Proposal for revised classification of epilepsies and epileptic syndromes. *Epilepsia* 1989;30:389–399.

61. Crandall PH. Postoperative management and criteria for evaluation. *Adv Neurol* 1987;8:265–279.

62. Crandall PH, Walter RD, Rand RW. Clinical applications of studies on stereotactically implanted electrodes in temporal-lobe epilepsy. *J Neurosurg* 1963;20:827–840.

63. Dechaume J, Courjon J. L'épilepsie partielle continue: contrôles opératoire et électrocorticographique. *Rev Neurol (Paris)* 1955;93:107–114.

64. DeJong RH, Walts LF. Lidocaine-induced psychomotor seizures in man. *Acta Anaesthesiol Scand Suppl* 1966;23:598–604.

65. Deonna T, Roulet E. Acquired epileptic aphasia (AEA): definition of the syndrome and current problems. In: Beaumanoir A, Bureau M, Deonna T, et al, eds. *Continuous spikes and waves during slow sleep: electrical status epilepticus during slow sleep*. London: John Libbey, 1995;37–45.

66. Devinsky O, Canevini P, Sato S, et al. Quantitative electrocorticography in patients undergoing temporal lobectomy. *J Epilepsy* 1992;5:178–185.

67. Dodick D, Cascino GD, Meyer FB. Vascular malformations and intractable epilepsy: outcome after surgical treatment. *Mayo Clin Proc* 1994;69:741–745.

68. Drake J, Hoffmann HJ, Kobayashi J, et al. Surgical management of children with temporal lobe epilepsy and mass lesions. *Neurosurgery* 1987;21:792–796.

69. Dubeau F, Palmini A, Fish D, et al. The significance of electrocorticographic findings in focal cortical dysplasia: a review of their clinical, electrophysiological and neurochemical characteristics. *Electroencephalogr Clin Neurophysiol Suppl* 1998;48:77–96.

70. Eberhard F, Stefan H. Computerized analysis of the spiking region in temporal lobe epilepsy. *Epilepsia* 1995;36[Suppl 3]:S270(abst).

71. Echlin FA, Arnett V, Zoll J. Paroxysmal high voltage discharges from isolated and partially isolated human and animal cerebral cortex. *Electroencephalogr Clin Neurophysiol* 1952;4:147–164.

72. Engel J Jr. Approaches to the localization of the epileptogenic lesion. In: Engel J Jr, ed. *Surgical treatment of the epilepsies*. New York: Raven Press, 1987:75–100.

73. Engel J Jr. *Seizures and epilepsy*. Philadelphia: FA Davis Co, 1989.

74. Engel J Jr. Recent advances in surgical treatment of temporal lobe epilepsy. *Acta Neurol Scand Suppl* 1992;86:71–80.

75. Engel J Jr, Driver MV, Falconer MA. Electrophysiological correlates of pathology and surgical results in temporal lobe epilepsy. *Brain* 1975;98:129–156.

76. Engel J Jr, Williamson PD, Wieser HG. Mesial temporal lobe epilepsy. In: Engel J Jr, Pedley TA, eds. *Epilepsy: a comprehensive textbook*. Philadelphia: Lippincott–Raven, 1997:2417–2426.

77. Falconer MA. Discussion. In: Baldwin M, Bailey P, eds. *Temporal lobe epilepsy*. Springfield, IL: Charles C Thomas Publisher, 1958:483–499.

78. Falconer MA, Hill D, Meyer A, et al. Treatment of temporal-lobe epilepsy by temporal lobectomy: a survey of findings and results. *Lancet* 1955;268:827–835.

79. Falconer MA, Hill D, Meyer A, et al. Clinical, radiological and EEG correlations with pathological changes in temporal lobe epilepsy and their significance in surgical treatment. In: Baldwin M, Bailey P, eds. *Temporal lobe epilepsy*. Springfield, IL: Charles C Thomas Publisher, 1958:396–410.

80. Falconer MA, Serafetinides EA, Corsellis JAN. Etiology and pathogenesis of temporal lobe epilepsy. *Arch Neurol* 1964;10:233–248.

81. Fariello RO. Epileptogenic properties of enflurane and their clinical interpretation. *Electroencephalogr Clin Neurophysiol* 1980;48:595–598.

82. Feindel W. Temporal lobe seizures. In: Vinken PJ, Bruyn GW, Magnus O, et al, eds. *Handbook of clinical neurology. Vol 15. The epilepsies*. Amsterdam: North Holland, 1974:87–106.

83. Feindel W. Role of brain science in the evolution of epilepsy surgery. *MJM* 1995;1:160–174.

84. Feindel W, Penfield W. Localization of discharge in temporal lobe automatism. *Arch Neurol Psychiatry* 1954;72:605–630.

85. Feindel W, Rasmussen T. Temporal lobectomy with amygdalectomy and minimal hippocampal resection: review of 100 cases. *Can J Neurol Sci* 1991;18:603–605.

86. Fenyes I, Zoltan I, Fenyes G. Temporal lobe epilepsies with deep seated epileptogenic foci. *Arch Neurol* 1961;4:103–105.

87. Ferrier CH, Alarcon G, Engelsman J, et al. Relevance of residual histologic and electrocorticographic abnormalities for surgical outcome in frontal lobe epilepsy. *Epilepsia* 2001; 42:363–371.

88. Fessler AJ, Cascino GD, Thomas Wass C, et al. Remifentanil-induced epileptiform activity in patients undergoing anterior temporal lobectomy. *Epilepsia*, 2000;41[Suppl 7]:228(abst).

89. Fiol ME, Boening JA, Cruz-Rodriguez R, et al. Effect of isoflurane (Forane) on intraoperative electrocorticogram. *Epilepsia* 1993;34:897–900.

90. Fiol ME, Gates JR, Mireles R, et al. Value of intraoperative EEG changes during corpus callosotomy in predicting surgical results. *Epilepsia* 1993;34:74–78.

91. Fiol ME, Gates JR, Torres F, et al. The prognostic value of residual spikes in the postexcision electrocorticogram after temporal lobectomy. *Neurology* 1991;41:512–516.

92. Fiol ME, Torres F, Gates JR, et al. Methohexital (Brevital) effect on electrocorticogram may be misleading. *Epilepsia* 1990;31:524–528.

93. Fish D, Andermann F, Olivier A. Complex partial seizures and small posterior temporal or extratemporal structural lesions: surgical management. *Neurology* 1991;41:1781–1784.

94. Fish DR, Gloor P, Quesney FL, et al. Clinical responses to electrical brain stimulation of the temporal and frontal lobes in patients with epilepsy: pathophysiological implications. *Brain* 1993;116:397–414.

95. Flemming DC, Fitzpatrick J, Fariello RG, et al. Diagnostic activation of epileptic foci by enflurane. *Anesthesiology* 1980;52:431–433.

96. Foerster O, Altenburger H. Elektrobiologische Vorgänge an der menschlichen Hirninde. *Dtsch Z Nervenheilkd* 1935;135:277–288.

97. Ford EW, Morrell F, Whisler WW. Methohexital effect on electrocorticogram may be misleading. *Anesth Analg* 1982;61:997–1001.

98. French JA, Williamson PD, Thadani VM, et al. Characteristics of medial temporal lobe epilepsy: I. Results of history and physical examination. *Ann Neurol* 1993;34:774–780.

99. Fried I. Management of low-grade gliomas: results of resections without electrocorticography. *Clin Neurosurg* 1995;42:453–463.

100. Fried I, Cascino G. Lesional surgery. In: Engel J Jr, ed. *Surgical treatment of the epilepsies*. New York: Raven Press, 1993:501–509.

101. Fried I, Cascino GD. Lesionectomy. In: Engel J Jr, Pedley TA, eds. *Epilepsy: a comprehensive textbook*, Vol 2. Philadelphia: Lippincott–Raven, 1997:1841–1850.

102. Fried I, Kim JH, Spencer DD. Hippocampal pathology in patients with intractable seizures and temporal lobe masses. *J Neurosurg* 1992;76:735–740.

103. Gastaut H, Naquet R, Vigouroux R, et al. Etude électrographique chez l'homme et chez l'animal des décharges épileptiques dites "psychomotrices." *Rev Neurol (Paris)* 1953;88: 310–354.

104. Gastaut H, Vigouroux M, Fischer-Williams M. Partial epilepsies with localized expression (still called "Jacksonian") and those with diffuse expression (still called "psychomotor"). In: Baldwin M, Bailey P, eds. *Temporal lobe epilepsy*. Springfield, IL: Charles C Thomas Publisher, 1958:13–22.

105. Gates JR, Maxwell R, Leppik IE, et al. Electroencephalographic and clinical effects of total corpus callosotomy. In: Reeves AG, ed. *Epilepsy and the corpus callosum*. New York: Plenum Publishing, 1985:315–328.

106. Germano IM, Poulin A, Olivier A. Reoperation for recurrent temporal lobe epilepsy. *J Neurosurg* 1994;81:31–36.

107. Gibbs FA, Amador L, Rich C. Electroencephalographic findings and therapeutic results in sur-

gical treatment of psychomotor epilepsy. In: Baldwin M, Bailey P, eds. *Temporal lobe epilepsy*. Springfield, IL: Charles C Thomas Publisher, 1958:358–367.

108. Gloor P. Contributions of electroencephalography and electrocorticography to the neurosurgical treatment of the epilepsies. *Adv Neurol* 1975;8:59–105.

109. Gloor P. Neuronal generators and the problem of localization in electroencephalography: application of volume conductor theory to electroencephalography. *J Clin Neurophysiol* 1985;2:327–354.

110. Gloor P. Commentary: Approaches to localization of epileptogenic lesion. In: Engel J Jr, ed. *Surgical treatment of the epilepsies*. New York: Raven Press, 1987:97–100.

111. Gloor P. Role of the amygdala in temporal lobe epilepsy. In: Aggleton JP, ed. *The amygdala: neurobiological aspects of emotion, memory, and mental dysfunction*. New York: Wiley–Liss, 1992:508–538.

112. Gloor P. *The temporal lobe and limbic system*. New York: Oxford University Press, 1997.

113. Gloor P, Olivier A, Ives J. Prolonged seizure monitoring with stereotaxically implanted depth electrodes in patients with bilateral interictal temporal epileptic foci: how bilateral is bitemporal epilepsy? In: Wada JA, Penry JK, eds. *Advances in epileptology: 10th Epilepsy International Symposium*. New York: Raven Press, 1980:83–88.

114. Gloor P, Olivier A, Quesney LF, et al. The role of the limbic system in experiential phenomena of temporal lobe epilepsy. *Ann Neurol* 1982;12:129–144.

115. Goddard GV, McIntyre DC, Leech CK. A permanent change in brain function resulting from daily electrical stimulation. *Exp Neurol* 1969;25:295–330.

116. Godoy J, Lüders H, Dinner DS, et al. Significance of sharp waves in routine EEGs after epilepsy surgery. *Epilepsia* 1992;33:285–288.

117. Goldensohn ES. Initiation and propagation of epileptogenic foci. *Adv Neurol* 1975;11:141–162.

118. Goldring S, Edwards I, Harding GW, et al. Results of anterior temporal lobectomy that spares the amygdala in patients with complex partial seizures. *J Neurosurg* 1992;77:185–193.

119. Goldring S, Gregorie EM. Surgical treatment of epilepsy during childhood and adolescence. *Neurosurgery* 1984;60:457–466.

120. Gotman J, Ives J. Computer-assisted data collection and analysis. In: Engel J Jr, Pedley TA, eds. *Epilepsy: a comprehensive textbook*, Vol 1. Philadelphia: Lippincott–Raven, 1997:1029–1044.

121. Gotman J, Koffler DJ. Interictal spiking increases after seizures but does not after decrease in medication. *Electroencephalogr Clin Neurophysiol* 1989;72:7–15.

122. Gotman J, Marciani M. Electroencephalographic spiking activity, drug levels, and seizure occurrence in epileptic patients. *Ann Neurol* 1985;17:597–603.

123. Graf M, Niedermeyer E, Schiemann J, et al. Electrocorticography: information derived from intraoperative recordings during seizure surgery. *Clin Electroencephalogr* 1984;15:83–91.

124. Green JR, Duisberg REH, McGrath WB. Electrocorticography in psychomotor epilepsy. *Electroencephalogr Clin Neurophysiol* 1951;3:293–299.

125. Gregorie EM, Goldring S. Localization of function in the excision of lesions from the sensorimotor region. *J Neurosurg* 1984;61:1047–1054.

126. Guillaume J, Mazars G, Mazars Y. Repérage corticographique préopératoire des foyers épileptogènes et contrôle de l'étendue de l'excision nécessaire. *Rev Neurol (Paris)* 1950;82:497–501.

127. Halgren E, Walter RD, Cherlow DG, et al. Mental phenomena evoked by electrical stimulation of the human hippocampal formation and amygdala. *Brain* 1978;101:83–117.

128. Hamer HM, Najm I, Mohamed A, et al. Interictal epileptiform discharges in temporal lobe epilepsy due to hippocampal sclerosis versus mesial temporal tumors. *Epilepsia* 1999;40:1261–1268.

129. Harner RN, Riggio S, Halgren E, et al. Interictal EEG topography of frontal lobe epilepsy. In: Chauvel P, Delgado-Escueta AV, eds. *Frontal lobe seizures and epilepsies*. New York: Raven Press, 1992:331–338.

130. Henry CE, Scoville WB. Suppression-burst activity from isolated cerebral cortex in man. *Electroencephalogr Clin Neurophysiol* 1952;4:1–22.

131. Henry TR, Duncan JS, Berkovic SF, eds. Functional imaging in the epilepsies. *Adv Neurol* 2000;83.

132. Hewitt PB, Chu DL, Polkey CE, et al. Effect of propofol on the electrocorticogram in epileptic patients undergoing cortical resection. *Br J Anaesth* 1999;82:199–202.

133. Hiyoshi T, Seino M, Kakegawa N, et al. Evidence of secondary epileptogenesis in amygdaloid over-kindled cats: electroclinical documentation of spontaneous seizures. *Epilepsia* 1993;34:325–334.

134. Hosain S, Nagarajan L, Fraser R, et al. Effects of nitrous oxide on electrocorticography during epilepsy surgery. *Electroencephalogr Clin Neurophysiol* 1997;102:340–342.

135. Hufnagel A, Burr W, Elger CE, et al. Localization of the epileptic focus during methohexital-induced anesthesia. *Epilepsia* 1992;33:271–284.

136. Hufnagel A, Dümpellmann M, Zentner J, et al. Clinical relevance of quantified intracranial interictal spike activity in presurgical evaluation of epilepsy. *Epilepsia* 2000;41:467–478.

137. Hufnagel A, Zentner J, Fernandez G, et al. Multiple subpial transection for control of epileptic seizures: effectiveness and safety. *Epilepsia* 1997;38:678–688.

138. Ito B, Sato S, Kufka G, et al. The effect of isoflurane and enflurane on the electrocorticogram of epileptic patients. *Neurology* 1988;38:924–928.

139. Jack CR Jr, Sharbrough FW, Twomey AR, et al. Temporal lobe seizures: lateralization with MR volume measurements of the hippocampal formation. *Radiology* 1990;175:423–429.

140. Jasper HH. Electroencephalography. In: Penfield W, Erickson TC, eds. *Epilepsy and cerebral localization*. Springfield, IL: Charles C Thomas Publisher, 1941:380–454.

141. Jasper HH. Electrical signs of epileptic discharge. *Electroencephalogr Clin Neurophysiol* 1949;1:11–18.

142. Jasper HH. Electrocorticograms in man. *Electroencephalogr Clin Neurophysiol Suppl* 1949;2:16–29.

143. Jasper HH. Electrocorticography. In: Penfield W, Jasper H, eds. *Epilepsy and the functional anatomy of the human brain*. Boston: Little, Brown and Company, 1954:692–738.

144. Jasper HH. Discussion. In: Baldwin M, Bailey P, eds. *Temporal lobe epilepsy*. Springfield, IL: Charles C Thomas Publisher, 1958:488–490.

145. Jasper HH. Functional subdivisions of the temporal region in relation to seizure patterns and subcortical connections. In: Baldwin M, Bailey P, eds. *Temporal lobe epilepsy*. Springfield, IL: Charles C Thomas Publisher, 1958:40–57.

146. Jasper HH, Arfel-Capdeville G, Rasmussen T. Evaluation of EEG and cortical electrographic studies for prognosis of seizures following surgical excision of epileptogenic lesions. *Epilepsia* 1961;2:130–137.

147. Jasper HH, Penfield W. Electrocorticograms in man: effect of voluntary movement upon the electrical activity of the precentral gyrus. *Arch Psychiatr Nervenkr* 1949;183:163–174.

148. Jasper HH, Pertuisset B, Flanigin H. EEG and cortical electrocorticograms in patients with temporal lobe seizures. *Arch Neurol Psychiatry* 1951;65:272–299.

149. Jasper HH, Rasmussen T. Studies of clinical and electrical responses to deep temporal stimulation in man with some considerations of functional anatomy. *Res Publ Assoc Res Nerv Ment Dis* 1958;36:316–334.

150. Jayakar P, Alvarez LA, Duchowny MS, et al. A safe and effective paradigm to functionally map the cortex in childhood. *J Clin Neurophysiol* 1992;9:288–293.

151. Jayakar P, Lesser RP. Extraoperative methods. In: Engel J Jr, Pedley TA, eds. *Epilepsy: a comprehensive textbook*, Vol 2. Philadelphia: Lippincott–Raven Press, 1997:1785–1793.

152. Jennum P, Dhuna A, Davies K, et al. Outcome of resective surgery for intractable partial epilepsy guided by subdural electrode arrays. *Acta Neurol Scand* 1993;87:434–437.

153. Jones-Gotman M, Smith ML, Wieser H-G. Intra-arterial amobarbital procedures. In: Engel J Jr, Pedley TA, eds. *Epilepsy: a comprehensive textbook*, Vol 2. Philadelphia: Lippincott–Raven, 1997:1767–1775.

154. Jooma R, Hwa-Shain Y, Privitera MD, et al. Lesionectomy versus electrophysiologically guided resection for temporal lobe tumors manifesting with complex partial seizures. *J Neurosurg* 1995;83:231–236.

155. Juul-Jensen P, Denny-Brown D. Epilepsia partialis continua. *Arch Neurol* 1966;15:563–578.
156. Kajtor F, Hullay J, Farago L, et al. Electrical activity of the hippocampus of patients with temporal lobe epilepsy. *AMA Arch Neurol Psychiatry* 1958;80:25–38.
157. Kanazawa O, Blume WT, Girvin JP. Significance of spikes at temporal lobe electrocorticography. *Epilepsia* 1996;37:50–55.
158. Kanner AM, Kaydanova Y, de Toledo-Morrell L, et al. Tailored anterior temporal lobectomy: relation between extent of resection of mesial temporal structures and postsurgical seizure outcome. *Arch Neurol* 1995;52:173–178.
159. Kaydanova Y, Kanner AM, Morrell F, et al. Comparative value of postresection ECOG and 10-day postoperative EEGs in predicting seizure outcome in patients with anterotemporal seizure foci. *Epilepsia* 1992;33[Suppl 3]:88–89(abst).
160. Kendrick JF, Gibbs FA. Origin, spread and neurosurgical treatment of the psychomotor type of seizure discharge. *J Neurosurg* 1957;14:270–284.
161. Kim HI, Olivier A, Jones-Gotman M, et al. Corticoamygdalectomy in memory-impaired patients. *Stereotact Funct Neurosurg* 1992;58:162–167.
162. Kim Y, Webster JG, Tomkins WJ. Simulated and experimental studies of temperature elevation around electrosurgical dispersive electrodes. *IEEE Trans Biomed Eng* 1984;31:681–692.
163. King D, Spencer S. Invasive electroencephalography in mesial temporal lobe epilepsy. *J Clin Neurophysiol* 1995;12:32–45.
164. Kirkpatrick PJ, Honavar M, Janota I, et al. Control of temporal lobe epilepsy following en bloc resection of low grade tumors. *J Neurosurg* 1993;78:19–25.
165. Knowlton RC, Wong STC, Woods RP, et al. Coregistration. In: Engel J Jr, Pedley TA, eds. *Epilepsy: a comprehensive textbook*, Vol 1. Philadelphia: Lippincott, 1997:1081–1097.
166. Kojewnikow L. Eine besondere Form von corticaler Epilepsie. *Neurol Zentralbl* 1895;14:47–48.
167. Kraemer DL, Spencer DD. Anesthesia in epilepsy surgery. In: Engel J Jr, ed. *Surgical treatment of the epilepsies*, 2nd ed. New York: Raven Press, 1993:527–538.
168. Kugelberg E, Widén L. Epilepsia partialis continua. *Electroencephalogr Clin Neurophysiol* 1954;6:503–506.
169. Kuzniecky R, Burgard S, Faught E, et al. Predictive value of magnetic resonance imaging in temporal lobe epilepsy surgery. *Arch Neurol* 1993;50:65–69.
170. Kuzniecky RI, Cascino GD, Palmini A, et al. Structural neuroimaging. In: Engel J Jr, ed. *Surgical treatment of the epilepsies*, 2nd ed. New York: Raven Press, 1993:197–209.
171. Lee S, Vives K, Westerveld M, et al. Quantitative temporal lobe volumetrics in the surgical management of nonlesional frontal and temporal neocortical epilepsies. *Adv Neurol* 2000;84:577–593.
172. Legatt AD, Ebersole JS. Options for long-term monitoring. In: Engel J Jr, Pedley TA, eds. *Epilepsy: a comprehensive textbook*, Vol 1. Philadelphia: Lippincott–Raven, 1997:1001–1010.
173. Lehman R, Andermann F, Olivier A, et al. Seizures with onset in the sensorimotor face area: clinical patterns and results of surgical treatment in 20 patients. *Epilepsia* 1994;35:1117–1124.
174. Lesser RP, Lüders H, Klem G, et al. Cortical afterdischarge and functional response thresholds: results and extraoperative testing. *Epilepsia* 1984;25:615–621.
175. Lévesque MF, Nakasato N. Epileptogenicity of structural lesions and the zone of seizure origin: surgical implications. *Epilepsia* 1991;32[Suppl 3]:27.
176. Li LM, Cendes F, Andermann F, et al. Surgical outcome in patients with epilepsy and dual pathology. *Brain* 1999;122:799–805.
177. Lieb JP, Walsh GO, Babb TL, et al. A comparison of EEG seizure patterns recorded with surface and depth electrodes in patients with temporal lobe epilepsy. *Epilepsia* 1976;17:137–160.
178. Lüders HO. Comparison of acute electrocorticography and chronic subdural recordings. *Epilepsia* 1995;36[Suppl 3]:S271.
179. Lüders HO. Clinical evidence for secondary epileptogenesis. *Int Rev Neurobiol* 2001;45:469–480.
180. Lüders HO, Engel J Jr, Munari C. General principles. In: Engel J Jr, ed. *Surgical treatment of the epilepsies*, 2nd ed. New York: Raven Press, 1993:137–153.
181. Lüders HO, Lesser RP, Dinner DS, et al. Commentary: chronic intracranial recording and stimulation with subdural electrodes. In: Engel J Jr, ed. *Surgical treatment of the epilepsies*. New York: Raven Press, 1987:297–321.
182. Lueders HO, Lesser RP, Hahn J, et al. Cortical somatosensory evoked potentials in response to hand stimulation. *J Neurosurg* 1983;58:885–894.
183. MacDonald DB, Pillay N. Intraoperative electrocorticography in temporal lobe epilepsy surgery. *Can J Neurol Sci* 2000;27[Suppl 1]:S85–S91.
184. Magnus P, De Vet AC, Van der Marel A, et al. Electrocorticography during operations for partial epilepsy. *Dev Med Child Neurol* 1962;4:35–48.
185. Marino R Jr, Radvany J, Huck FR, et al. Selected electroencephalograph-guided microsurgical callosotomy for refractory generalized epilepsy. *Surg Neurol* 1990;34:219–228.
186. Marino RJ, Ragazzo PC. Selective criteria and results of selective partial callosotomy. In: Reeves AG, ed. *Epilepsy and the corpus callosum*. New York: Plenum Press, 1985:281–301.
187. Marks DA, Katz A, Booke J, et al. Comparison and correlation of surface and sphenoidal electrodes with simultaneous intracranial recording: an interictal study. *Electroencephalogr Clin Neurophysiol* 1992;82:23–29.
188. Mathern GW, Babb TL, Armstrong DL. Hippocampal sclerosis. In: Engel J Jr, Pedley TA, eds. *Epilepsy: a comprehensive textbook*, Vol 1. Philadelphia: Lippincott–Raven, 1997:133–155.
189. Mathern GW, Babb TL, Pretorius JK, et al. The clinical-pathogenic mechanisms of hippocampal neuron loss and surgical outcomes in temporal lobe epilepsy. *Brain* 1995;118:105–113.
190. Mathieson G. Pathology of temporal lobe foci. *Adv Neurol* 1975;11:163–181.
191. Matsumoto H, Ajmone-Marsan C. Cortical cellular phenomena in experimental epilepsy: ictal manifestations. *Exp Neurol* 1964;9:305–326.
192. Matsumoto H, Ajmone-Marsan C. Cortical cellular phenomena in experimental epilepsy: interictal manifestations. *Exp Neurol* 1964;9:286–304.
193. McBride MC, Binnie CD, Janota I, et al. Predictive value of intraoperative electrocorticograms in resective epilepsy surgery. *Ann Neurol* 1991;30:526–532.
194. McKhann GM, Schoenfeld-McNeill J, Born DE, et al. Intraoperative hippocampal electrocorticography to predict the extent of hippocampal resection in temporal lobe epilepsy surgery. *J Neurosurg* 2000;93:44–52.
195. Meyers R, Knott JR, Hayne RA, et al. The surgery of epilepsy: limitations of the concept of the corticoelectrographic "spike" as an index of the epileptogenic focus. *J Neurosurg* 1950;4:337–346.
196. Mizrahi EM, Kellaway P, Rutecki PA, et al. Electrocorticography during anterior temporal lobectomy in patients with complex partial seizures. *Epilepsia* 1985;26:542(abst).
197. Mizrahi EM, Kellaway P, Rutecki PA, et al. Relationship of electrocorticography to temporal lobe pathology. *Epilepsia* 1986;27:636(abst).
198. Morrell F. Aspects of experimental epilepsy. In: Wada JA, ed. *Modern perspectives in epilepsy*. Montreal: Eden Press, 1978:24–75.
199. Morrell F. Varieties of human secondary epileptogenesis. *J Clin Neurophysiol* 1989;6:227–275.
200. Morrell F. The role of secondary epileptogenesis in human epilepsy. *Ann Neurol* 1991;48:1221–1224.
201. Morrell F. Electrophysiology of CSWS in Landau-Kleffner syndrome. In: Beaumanoir A, Bureau M, Deonna T, et al, eds. *Continuous spikes and waves during slow sleep: electrical status epilepticus during slow sleep*. London: John Libbey, 1995:77–90.
202. Morrell F. Multiple subpial transections and other interventions. In: Engel J Jr, Pedley TA, eds. *Epilepsy: a comprehensive textbook*, Vol 2. Philadelphia: Lippincott–Raven, 1997:1877–1890.
203. Morrell F, deToledo-Morrell L. From mirror focus to secondary epileptogenesis in man: an historical review. *Adv Neurol* 1999;81:11–23.
204. Morrell F, deToledo-Morrell L, Sullivan MP, et al. Direct intraoperative recordings from the hippocampal formation: relation with quantitative volumetric MRI. *Electroencephalogr Clin Neurophysiol Suppl* 1998;48:112–122.
205. Morrell F, Wada J, Engel J Jr. Potential relevance of kindling and secondary epileptogenesis to

the consideration of surgical treatment for epilepsy. In: Engel J Jr, ed. *Surgical treatment of the epilepsies*. New York: Raven Press, 1987:701–707.

206. Morrell F, Whistler W. Multiple subpial transections for epilepsy eliminates seizures without destroying the function of the transected zone. *Epilepsia* 1982;23:440(abst).

207. Morrell F, Whisler WW, Bleck TP. Multiple subpial transection: a new approach to the surgical treatment of focal epilepsy. *J Neurosurg* 1989;70:231–239.

208. Morrell F, Whisler WW, Smith MC. Multiple subpial transection in Rasmussen's encephalitis. In: Andermann F, ed. *Chronic encephalitis and epilepsy: Rasmussen's syndrome*. Boston: Butterworth-Heinemann, 1991:219–233.

209. Morrell F, Whisler WW, Smith MC, et al. Landau-Kleffner syndrome: treatment with subpial intracortical transection. *Brain* 1995;118:1529–1546.

210. Morris AA. Temporal lobectomy with removal of uncus, hippocampus, and amygdala. *Arch Neurol Psychiatry* 1956;76:479–496.

211. Munari C, Hoffman D, Francione S, et al. Stereo-electroencephalography methodology: advantages and limits. *Acta Neurol Scand Suppl* 1994;152:56–67.

212. Niemeyer P. The transventricular amygdala-hippocampectomy in temporal lobe epilepsy. In: Baldwin M, Bailey M, eds. *Temporal lobe epilepsy*. Springfield, IL: Charles C Thomas Publisher, 1958:461–482.

213. Oguni H, Andermann F, Rasmussen TB. The syndrome of chronic encephalitis and epilepsy: a study based on the MNI series of 48 cases. *Adv Neurol* 1992;57:419–433.

214. Ojemann GA. Intraoperative electrocorticography and functional mapping. In: Wyler AR, Hermann BP, eds. *The surgical management of epilepsy*. Boston: Butterworth-Heinemann, 1994:189–196.

215. Ojemann GA. Intraoperative methods. In: Engel J Jr, Pedley TA, eds. *Epilepsy: a comprehensive textbook*, Vol 2. Philadelphia: Lippincott–Raven, 1997:1777–1783.

216. Ojemann GA. Interplay between "neocortical" and "limbic" temporal lobe epilepsy. *Adv Neurol* 2000;84:615–619.

217. Ojemann GA, Engel J Jr. Acute and chronic intracranial recording and stimulation. In: Engel J Jr, ed. *Surgical treatment of the epilepsies*. New York: Raven Press, 1987:263–321.

218. Ojemann GA, Sutherling WW, Lesser RP, et al. Cortical stimulation. In: Engel J Jr, ed. *Surgical treatment of the epilepsies*, 2nd ed. New York: Raven Press, 1993:399–414.

219. Olivier A. Commentary: Cortical resections. In: Engel J Jr, ed. *Surgical treatment of the epilepsies*. New York: Raven Press, 1987:405–416.

220. Olivier A. Relevance of removal of limbic structures in surgery for temporal lobe epilepsy. *Can J Neurol Sci* 1991;18[Suppl 4]:628–635.

221. Olivier A. Surgery of frontal lobe epilepsy. In: Jasper HH, Riggio S, Goldman-Rakic PS, eds. *Epilepsy and the functional anatomy of the frontal lobe*. New York: Raven Press, 1995: 321–352.

222. Olivier A, Boling W Jr. Surgery of parietal and occipital lobe epilepsy. *Adv Neurol* 2000;84: 533–575.

223. Olson DM, Chugani HT, Shewmon DA, et al. Electrocorticographic confirmation of focal positron emission tomographic abnormalities in children with intractable epilepsy. *Epilepsia* 1990;31:731–739.

224. Opitz A, Marshall M, Degen R, et al. General anesthesia in patients with epilepsy and status epilepticus. *Adv Neurol* 1983;34:43–47.

225. Oxbury S. Neuropsychological evaluation—children. In: Engel J Jr, Pedley TA, eds. *Epilepsy: a comprehensive textbook*, Vol 1. Philadelphia: Lippincott–Raven, 1997:989–999.

226. Paetau R, Kajola, M, Korkman M, et al. Landau-Kleffner syndrome: epileptic activity in the auditory cortex. *J Clin Neurophysiol* 1994;11:231–241.

227. Palmini A, Andermann F, Dubeau F, et al. Occipitotemporal relations: evidence for secondary epileptogenesis. *Adv Neurol* 1999;81:115–129.

228. Palmini A, Gambardella A, Andermann F, et al. Intrinsic epileptogenicity of human dysplastic cortex as suggested by corticography and surgical results. *Ann Neurol* 1995;37:476–487.

229. Panet-Raymond D, Gotman J. Can slow waves in the electrocorticogram (ECoG) help localize epileptic foci? *Electroencephalogr Clin Neurophysiol* 1990;75:464–473.

230. Parrent AG, Blume WT. Treatment of mesial temporal lobe seizures by stereotaxic amygdalo-hippocampotomy. *Epilepsia* 1995;36[Suppl 3]:S169(abst).

231. Penfield W, Baldwin M. Temporal lobe seizures and the technique of sub-total temporal lobectomy. *Ann Surg* 1952;136:625–634.

232. Penfield W, Flanigin H. Surgical therapy of temporal lobe seizures. *Arch Neurol Psychiatry* 1950;64:491–500.

233. Penfield W, Jasper H. Electroencephalography in focal epilepsy. *Trans Am Neurol Assoc* 1940;66:209–211.

234. Penfield W, Jasper H, eds. *Epilepsy and the functional anatomy of the human brain*. Boston: Little, Brown, 1954.

235. Penfield W, Kristiansen K. *Epileptic seizure patterns*. Springfield, IL: Charles C Thomas Publisher, 1951.

236. Pfürtscheller G, Cooper R. Frequency dependence of the transmission of the EEG from cortex to scalp. *Electroencephalogr Clin Neurophysiol* 1975;38:93–96.

237. Pilcher WH, Silbergeld DL, Berger MS, et al. Intraoperative electrocorticography during tumor resection: impact on seizure outcome in patients with gangliogliomas. *J Neurosurg* 1993;78:891–902.

238. Polkey CE. Reoperation. In: Engel J Jr, Pedley TA, eds. *Epilepsy: a comprehensive textbook*, Vol 2. Philadelphia: Lippincott–Raven, 1997:1859–1865.

239. Polkey CE, Binnie CD, Janota I. Acute hippocampal recording and pathology at temporal lobe resection and amygdalo-hippocampectomy for epilepsy. *J Neurol Neurosurg Psychiatry* 1989;52:1050–1057.

240. Pressler RM, Binnie CD, Elwes RD, et al. Return of generalized seizures and discharges after callosotomy. *Adv Neurol* 1999;81:171–182.

241. Primrose DC, Ojemann, GA. Outcome of resective surgery for temporal lobe epilepsy. In: Lüders H, ed. *Epilepsy surgery*. New York: Raven Press, 1992:601–611.

242. Pudenz RH, Bullara LA, Jacques S, et al. Electrical stimulation of the brain. III. The neural damage model. *Surg Neurol* 1975;4:389–400.

243. Quesney LF. Clinical and EEG features of complex partial seizures of temporal lobe origin. *Epilepsia* 1986;27[Suppl 2]:S27–S45.

244. Quesney LF. Preoperative electroencephalographic investigation in frontal lobe epilepsy: electroencephalographic and electrocorticographic recordings. *Can J Neurol Sci* 1991;18[Suppl 4]:559–563.

245. Quesney LF. Intracranial EEG investigation in neocortical epilepsy. *Adv Neurol* 2000;84: 253–274.

246. Quesney LF, Gloor P. Localization of epileptic foci. *Electroencephalogr Clin Neurophysiol Suppl* 1985;37:165–200.

247. Quesney LF, Niedermeyer E. Electrocorticography. In: Niedermeyer E, Lopes da Silva F, eds. *Electroencephalography: basic principles, clinical applications, and related fields*, 3rd ed. Baltimore: Williams & Wilkins, 1993:695–699.

248. Quesney LF, Risinger MW, Shewmon DA. Extracranial EEG evaluation. In: Engel J Jr, ed. *Surgical treatment of the epilepsies*, 2nd ed. New York: Raven Press, 1993:173–195.

249. Quesney LF, Wennberg R, Olivier A, et al. ECoG findings in extratemporal epilepsy: the MNI experience. *Electroencephalogr Clin Neurophysiol Suppl* 1998;48:44–57.

250. Ralston BL. The mechanism of transition of interictal spiking foci into ictal seizure discharges. *Electroencephalogr Clin Neurophysiol* 1958;10:217–232.

251. Rasmussen T. Cortical resection in the treatment of focal epilepsy. *Adv Neurol* 1975;8:139–154.

252. Rasmussen T. Surgical treatment of patients with complex partial seizures. *Adv Neurol* 1975; 11:415–449.

253. Rasmussen T. Surgical aspects. In: Wise G, ed. *Topics in child neurology*. Englewood Cliffs, NJ: Spectrum Publications, 1977:143–153.

254. Rasmussen T. Characteristics of a pure culture of frontal lobe epilepsy. *Epilepsia* 1983;24: 482–493.

255. Rasmussen T. Hemispherectomy for seizures revisited. *Can J Neurol Sci* 1983;23:415–449.

256. Rasmussen T. Surgical treatment of complex partial seizures: results, lessons and problems. *Epilepsia* 1983;24:S65–S75.

257. Rasmussen T. Commentary: Extratemporal temporal excisions and hemispherectomy. In: Engel J Jr, ed. *Surgical treatment of the epilepsies.* New York: Raven Press, 1987:417–424.

258. Rasmussen T, Feindel W. Temporal lobectomy: review of 100 cases with major hippocampectomy. *Can J Neurol Sci* 1991;18:601–602.

259. Rasmussen T, Jasper HH. Temporal lobe epilepsy: indications for operation and surgical technique. In: Baldwin M, Bailey P, eds. *Temporal lobe epilepsy.* Springfield, IL: Charles C Thomas Publisher, 1958:440–460.

260. Rasmussen T, Olszewski J, Lloyd-Smith D. Focal seizures due to chronic localized encephalitis. *Neurology* 1958;8:435–445.

261. Rausch R, Le MT, Langfitt JT. Neuropsychological evaluation—adults. In: Engel J Jr, Pedley TA, eds. *Epilepsy: a comprehensive textbook*, Vol 1. Philadelphia: Lippincott–Raven, 1997:977–987.

262. Raymond AA, Fish DR. EEG features of focal malformations of cortical development. *J Clin Neurophysiol* 1996;13:495–506.

263. Reiher J, Lebel M. Wicket spikes: clinical correlates of a previously undescribed EEG pattern. *Can J Neurol Sci* 1977;4:39–47.

264. Roberts DW. Corpus callosotomy. In: Engel J Jr, Pedley TA, eds. *Epilepsy: a comprehensive textbook*, Vol 2. Philadelphia: Lippincott–Raven, 1997:1851–1858.

265. Rosenblueth A, Cannon WP. Cortical responses to electrical stimulation. *Am J Physiol* 1941–1942;135:690–741.

266. Roth JG, MacPherson CH, Milstein V. The use of carbon electrodes for chronic cortical recordings. *Electroencephalogr Clin Neurophysiol* 1966;21:611–615.

267. Rush E, Morrell MJ. Cortical dysplasia with mesiotemporal sclerosis: evidence for kindling in humans. *Epilepsia* 1993;34[Suppl 6]:609–615.

268. Salanova V, Quesney LF, Rasmussen T, et al. Reevaluation of surgical failures and the role of reoperation in 39 patients with frontal lobe epilepsy. *Epilepsia* 1994;35:70–80.

269. Scarff JE, Rahm WE. The human electro-corticogram: a report of spontaneous electrical potentials obtained from the exposed human brain. *J Neurophysiol* 1941;4:418–426.

270. Schiller Y, Cascino GD, Sharbrough FW. Chronic intracranial EEG monitoring for localization of the epileptogenic zone: an electroclinical correlation. *Epilepsia* 1998;39:1302–1308.

271. Schwartz HG, Kerr AS. Electrical activity of the exposed human brain: description of technique and report of cases. *Arch Neurol Psychiatry* 1940;43:457–559.

272. Schwartz TH, Bazil CW, Forgione M, et al. Do reactive post-resection "injury" spikes exist? *Epilepsia* 2000;41:1463–1468.

273. Schwartz TH, Bazil CW, Walczak TS, et al. The predictive value of intraoperative electrocorticography in resections for limbic epilepsy associated with mesial temporal sclerosis. *Neurosurgery* 1997;40:302–311.

274. Silbergeld DL, Mueller WM, Colley PS, et al. Use of propofol (Diprivan) for awake craniotomies: technical note. *Surg Neurol* 1992;38:271–272.

275. Silfvenius H, Gloor P, Rasmussen T. Evaluation of insular ablation in surgical treatment of temporal lobe epilepsy. *Epilepsia* 1964;5:307–320.

276. Singh BM, Strobos RJ. Epilepsia partialis continua associated with nonketotic hyperglycemia: clinical and biochemical profile of 21 patients. *Ann Neurol* 1980;8:155–160.

277. Smith CM. Landau-Kleffner syndrome and continuous spikes and waves during slow sleep. In: Engel J Jr, Pedley TA, eds. *Epilepsy: a comprehensive textbook*, Vol 3. Philadelphia: Lippincott–Raven, 1997:2367–2377.

278. Smith JR, Lee MR, King DW, et al. Results of lesional vs. nonlesional frontal lobe epilepsy surgery. *Stereotact Funct Neurosurg* 1997;69:202–209.

279. Smith MC, Byrne R. Multiple subpial transection in neocortical epilepsy: Part I. *Adv Neurol* 2000;84:621–634.

280. Smith MC, Whisler WW, Morrell F. Neurosurgery of epilepsy. *Semin Neurol* 1989;9:231–248.

281. Smith S, Andermann F, Villemure J-G, et al. Functional hemispherectomy: EEG findings, spiking from isolated brain postoperatively, and prediction of outcome. *Neurology* 1991;41:1790–1794.

282. So EL. Electrocorticography in modified standard temporal lobectomy for nonlesional intractable epilepsy. *Epilepsia* 1995;36[Suppl 3]:S275(abst).

283. So EL, Fisch BJ. Drug withdrawal and other activating techniques. In: Engel J Jr, Pedley TA, eds. *Epilepsy: a comprehensive textbook*, Vol 2. Philadelphia: Lippincott–Raven, 1997:1021–1027.

284. So NK. Depth electrode studies in mesial temporal epilepsy. In: Lüders HO, ed. *Epilepsy surgery.* New York: Raven Press, 1992:371–384.

285. So NK, Andermann F. Rasmussen's syndrome. In: Engel J Jr, Pedley TA, eds. *Epilepsy: a comprehensive textbook*, Vol 3. Philadelphia: Lippincott–Raven, 1997:2379–2388.

286. So NK, Gloor P. Electroencephalographic and electrocorticographic findings in chronic encephalitis of the Rasmussen type. In: Andermann F, ed. *Chronic encephalitis and epilepsy: Rasmussen's syndrome.* Boston: Butterworth-Heinemann, 1991:37–45.

287. So NK, Olivier A, Anderman F, et al. Results of surgical treatment in patients with bitemporal epileptiform abnormalities. *Ann Neurol* 1989;25:432–439.

288. Spencer DD, Inserni J. Temporal lobectomy. In: Lüders HO, ed. *Epilepsy surgery.* New York: Raven Press, 1992:533–545.

289. Spencer DD, Spencer SS, Mattson RH, et al. Intracerebral masses in patients with intractable partial epilepsy. *Neurology* 1984;34:432–436.

290. Spencer SS. Depth electrography in selection of refractory epilepsy for surgery. *Ann Neurol* 1981;9:207–214.

291. Spencer SS. Substrates of localization-related epilepsies: biologic implications of localizing findings in humans. *Epilepsia* 1998;39:114–123.

292. Spencer SS, Gates JR, Reeves AP, et al. Corpus callosum section. In: Engel J Jr, ed. *Surgical treatment of the epilepsies.* New York: Raven Press, 1987:425–444.

293. Spencer SS, Spencer DD. Corpus callosotomy in chronic encephalitis. In: Andermann F, ed. *Chronic encephalitis and epilepsy: Rasmussen's syndrome.* New York: Raven Press, 1991: 213–218.

294. Spencer SS, Sperling MR, Shewmon DA. Intracranial electrodes. In: Engel J Jr, Pedley TA, eds. *Epilepsy: a comprehensive textbook*, Vol 2. Philadelphia: Lippincott–Raven, 1997:1719–1747.

295. Spencer SS, Tran T, Spencer DD. Electrocorticography in lesional epilepsy. *Epilepsia* 1995; 36[Suppl 3]:S270(abst).

296. Sperling MR, O'Connor MJ. Comparison of depth and subdural electrodes in recording temporal lobe seizures. *Neurology* 1989;39:1497–1504.

297. Sperling MR, Shewmon DA. General principles for presurgical evaluation. In: Engel J Jr, Pedley TA, eds. *Epilepsy: a comprehensive textbook*, Vol 2. Philadelphia: Lippincott–Raven, 1997:1697–1705.

298. Stefan H, Quesney LF, Abou-Khalil B, et al. Electrocorticography in temporal lobe epilepsy surgery. *Acta Neurol Scand* 1991;83:65–72.

299. Sutula T, Cascino G, Cavazos J, et al. Mossy fiber synaptic reorganization in the epileptic human temporal lobe. *Ann Neurol* 1989;26:321–330.

300. Swartz BE, Tomiyasu U, Delgado-Escueta AV, et al. Neuroimaging in temporal lobe epilepsy: test sensitivity and relationship to pathology and postoperative outcome. *Epilepsia* 1992;33: 624–634.

301. Talairach J, Bancaud J. Lesion, irritative zone and epileptogenic focus. *Confin Neurol* 1966; 27:91–94.

302. Talairach J, Bancaud J, Bonis JA, et al. Approche nouvelle de la neurochirurgie de l'épilepsie: méthodologie stéréotaxique et résultats thérapeutiques. *Neurochirurgie* 1974;20[Suppl 1].

303. Tempelhoff R, Modica PA, Bernardo KL, et al. Fentanyl-induced electrocorticographic seizures in patients with complex partial epilepsy. *J Neurosurg* 1992;77:201–208.

304. Thomas J, Regan J, Klass D. Epilepsia partialis continua: a review of 32 cases. *Arch Neurol* 1977;34:266–275.

305. Tran TA, Spencer SS, Javidan M, et al. Significance of spikes recorded on intraoperative electrocorticography in patients with brain tumor and epilepsy. *Epilepsia* 1997;38:1132–1139.

306. Tran TA, Spencer SS, Marks D, et al. Significance of spikes recorded on electrocorticography in nonlesional medial temporal lobe epilepsy. *Ann Neurol* 1995;38:763–770.

307. Tsai ML, Chatrian GE, Pauri F, et al. Electrocorticography in patients with medically intractable temporal lobe seizures: I. Quantification of epileptiform discharges prior to resective surgery. *Electroencephalogr Clin Neurophysiol* 1993;87:10–24.

308. Tsai ML, Chatrian GE, Temkin N, et al. Eletrocorticography in patients with medically intractable temporal lobe seizures: II. Quantification of epileptiform discharges following successive stages of resective surgery. *Electroencephalogr Clin Neurophysiol* 1993;87:25–37.

309. Tuunainen A, Nousiainen U, Mervaala E, et al. Postoperative EEG and electrocorticography: relation to clinical outcome in patients with temporal lobe surgery. *Epilepsia* 1994;35:1165–1173.

310. Van Buren JM, Ajmone-Marsan C, Mutsuga N. Temporal-lobe seizures with additional foci treated by resection. *J Neurosurg* 1975;43:596–607.

311. Van Buren JM, Ajmone-Marsan C, Mutsuga N, et al. Surgery of temporal lobe epilepsy. *Adv Neurol* 1975;8:155–196.

312. Villemure J-G, Andermann F, Rasmussen TB. Hemispherectomy for the treatment of epilepsy due to chronic encephalitis. In: Andermann F, ed. *Chronic encephalitis and epilepsy: Rasmussen's syndrome.* Boston: Butterworth-Heinemann, 1991:235–241.

313. Wada JA. The clinical relevance of kindling: species, brain sites and seizure susceptibility. In: Livingston KE, Hornykiewicz H, eds. *Limbic mechanisms: the continuing evolution of the limbic system concept.* New York: Plenum Publishing, 1978:369–388.

314. Walker AE. Electrocorticography in epilepsy: a surgeon's appraisal. *Electroencephalogr Clin Neurophysiol Suppl* 1949;2:30–37.

315. Walker AE. Temporal lobectomy. *J Neurosurg* 1967;26:642–649.

316. Walker AE. Surgery for epilepsy. In: Magnus O, Lorentz de Haas AM, eds. *Handbook of clinical neurology. Vol 15. The epilepsies.* Amsterdam: Elsevier, 1974:739–757.

317. Walker AE, Johnson HC. Normal and pathological after discharge from frontal cortex. *Res Publ Assoc Res Nerv Ment Dis* 1948;27:460–475.

318. Walker AE, Lichtenstein RS, Marshall C. A critical analysis of electrocorticography in temporal lobe epilepsy. *Arch Neurol* 1960;2:172–182.

319. Walter R. Tactical considerations leading to surgical treatment of limbic epilepsy. In: Brazier MAB, ed. *Epilepsy: its phenomena in man.* New York: Academic Press, 1973:99–119.

320. Walter WG. The location of cerebral tumours by electroencephalography. *Lancet* 1936;2:305–308.

321. Wennberg R, Quesney LF, Olivier A, et al. Post-excision residual spiking after frontal lobe removal: outcome. *Electroencephalogr Clin Neurophysiol Suppl* 1998;48:97–104.

322. Wennberg R, Quesney LF, Villemure JG. ECoG findings in hemispherectomy. *Electroencephalogr Clin Neurophysiol Suppl* 1998;48:132–139.

323. Wennberg RA, Quesney LF, Dubeau F, et al. Increased neocortical spiking and surgical outcome after selective amygdalo-hippocampectomy. *Electroencephalogr Clin Neurophysiol Suppl* 1998;48:105–111.

324. Wennberg RA, Quesney LF, Olivier A. Correlation between mesial temporal and temporal neocortical interictal spiking in acute ECoG and chronic depth electrode recordings. *Electroencephalogr Clin Neurophysiol Suppl* 1998;48:123–131.

325. Wennberg RA, Quesney LF, Villemure JG. Epileptiform and non-epileptiform paroxysmal activity from isolated cortex after functional hemispherectomy. *Electroencephalogr Clin Neurophysiol* 1997;102:437–442.

326. Wieser HG. *Electroclinical features of the psychomotor seizure: a stereoelectroencephalographic study of ictal symptoms and chronotopographical seizure patterns including clinical effects of intracerebral stimulation.* Stuttgart: Gustav Fischer, 1983.

327. Wieser HG. Psychomotor seizures of hippocampal-amygdalar origin. In: Pedley TA, Meldrum BS, eds. *Recent advances in epilepsy.* Edinburgh: Churchill Livingstone, 1986:57–79.

328. Wieser HG. Selective amygdalohippocampectomy: indications and follow-up. *Can J Neurol Sci* 1991;18:617–627.

329. Wieser HG, Bancaud J, Talairach J, et al. Comparative value of spontaneous and chemically and electrically induced seizures in establishing the lateralization of temporal lobe seizures. *Epilepsia* 1979;20:47–59.

330. Wieser HG, Engel J Jr, Williamson PD, et al. Surgically remediable temporal lobe syndromes. In: Engel J Jr, ed. *Surgical treatment of the epilepsies,* 2nd ed. New York: Raven Press, 1993:49–63.

331. Wieser HG, Graf HP, Bernoulli C, et al. Quantitative analysis of intracerebral recordings in epilepsia partialis continua. *Electroencephalogr Clin Neurophysiol* 1978;44:14–22.

332. Wieser HG, Morris HI. Foramen ovale and peg electrodes. In: Engel J Jr, Pedley TA, eds. *Epilepsy: a comprehensive textbook,* Vol 2. Philadelphia: Lippincott–Raven, 1997:1707–1717.

333. Wieser HG, Yasargil MG. Selective amygdalohippocampectomy as a surgical treatment of mediobasal limbic epilepsy. *Surg Neurol* 1982;17:445–457.

334. Williamson PD, Engel J Jr, Munari C. Anatomic classification of localization-related epilepsies. In: Engel J Jr, Pedley TA, eds. *Epilepsy: a comprehensive textbook,* Vol 3. Philadelphia: Lippincott–Raven, 1997:2405–2416.

335. Williamson PD, Jobst BC. Frontal lobe epilepsy. *Adv Neurol* 2000;84:215–242.

336. Wood CC, Spencer DD, Allison D, et al. Localization of human sensorimotor cortex during surgery by cortical surface recordings of somatosensory evoked potentials. *J Neurosurg* 1988;68:99–111.

337. Wyler AR, Ojemann GA, Lettich E, et al. Subdural strip electrodes for localizing epileptogenic foci. *J Neurosurg* 1984;60:1195–1200.

338. Wyler AR, Richey ET, Atkinson RA, et al. Methohexital activation of epileptogenic foci during acute electroencephalography. *Epilepsia* 1987;28:490–494.

339. Wyllie E, Lüders H, Morris HH, et al. Clinical outcome after complete or partial cortical resection for intractable epilepsy. *Neurology* 1987;37:1634–1641.

340. Yeh HS, Tew JM Jr, Gartner M. Seizure control after surgery on cerebral arteriovenous malformations. *J Neurosurg* 1993;78:12–18.

341. Zentner J, Hufnagel A, Wolf HK, et al. Surgical treatment of neoplasms associated with medically intractable epilepsy. *Neurosurgery* 1997;41:378–387.

Chapter 22

Automatic Detection and Analysis of Seizures and Spikes

Jean Gotman

When evaluating epileptic patients, it is often important to obtain thorough documentation of ictal and interictal electroencephalographic (EEG) patterns, in conjunction with behavioral patterns if possible. This is critical to help in the differential diagnosis of epilepsy, to determine seizure type for adequate medical treatment, in various situations in the intensive care unit, and of course when considering surgical treatment. This information can be obtained with long-term monitoring, during which the EEG and the patient's behavior are observed and recorded continuously. Thus all spikes and seizures are recorded, the observer may interact with the patient during seizures, and electroclinical correlations may be performed fully. In order to properly characterize a complicated seizure problem that can involve multiple seizure types, or to measure the effect of antiepileptic medication, it may be necessary to monitor a patient for 1–3 weeks. The EEG may include scalp or intracranial electrodes, typically 32–64 chan-

nels. Continuous observation and recording of the EEG and of behavior over a period of several days or weeks is an immense and expensive task, requiring considerable personnel for observation and equipment for recording. If sufficient personnel are not available for constant observation and recording, the following questions arise: Should a complete recording be made on magnetic medium? Should this complete recording be reviewed (also a very time-consuming task), or should a selective review be performed? If a selective review is performed, how is the selection to be made? Or should the recording itself be selective, including only the events of interest?

It has become clear in the last several years that computers can be extremely helpful in making the procedure of long-term epilepsy monitoring less tedious and less expensive. They can also assist in the review and analysis of the EEGs of epileptic patients, and they are used for data archiving. In a more recent development, behavioral video recording can be performed with the assistance of computers as well. The first part of this chapter discusses how computer-based recordings, particularly automatic spike-and-seizure detection methods, can facilitate long-term epilepsy monitoring in the hospital and at home. The second part discusses how spikes and seizures can be further analyzed by computer methods.

COMPUTER-ASSISTED LONG-TERM EEG MONITORING

Whereas it was cumbersome to perform a continuous 24-hour recording on a paper-based machine, the present size of computer disks and the resolution of computer screens are such that it is simple to perform a continuous 24-hour recording on a standard computer. A computer-based recording has the advantages over paper of a flexible review procedure, with immediate access to any part of the recording, and the availability of numerous methods of data manipulation and analysis.

Storing a recording on a computer makes use of its memory capacity, but its computing power also offers the opportunity of attempting to identify the events specific to epilepsy. In most 24-hour recordings, 95%–99% of the recording offers little information of value in the evaluation of the epileptic disorder. Computer analysis methods can help in marking the 1%–5% of the recording that is important, thus greatly facilitating review. The detection of *seizures* and of *interictal spikes* is discussed separately in this section.

Recording Seizures

What Is a Seizure?

In the context of epilepsy monitoring, it is necessary define what is meant by "seizure." We can define first a "behavioral seizure" as the behavioral manifestations of an epileptic seizure, as perceived by the patient, seen by an observer, or recorded on videotape. We can then define the "electrographic seizure" (or "EEG seizure") as an abnormal paroxysmal EEG pattern. In a large fraction of cases, behavioral and electrographic seizures can be observed simultaneously, which is why we have been able to identify the EEG changes specific to seizures. In many cases, however, there is dissociation between behavior and the EEG. Two types of dissociation are possible: a behavioral seizure in the absence of EEG evidence of a seizure, and an electrographic seizure without behavioral manifestations.

When a behavioral seizure is present in the absence of EEG changes, if we assume that the seizure is indeed epileptic (this chapter does not discuss the means of differentiating epileptic from nonepileptic seizures), then abnormal EEG activity is present *somewhere in the brain*. It is simply not available to the particular method of observation being used, that is, to the particular arrangement and location of electrodes. The discharge may, for instance, be limited to the mesial frontal regions, and the patient is being monitored with only scalp electrodes, or only intracerebral electrodes in the temporal lobes. In the context of epilepsy monitoring, it must be clear that such a seizure will be missed by observation, review, or computer analysis of the EEG alone.

An EEG seizure that is present in the absence of a behavioral seizure is commonly referred to as a "pure electrographic seizure" or "subclinical seizure." If the absence of an EEG discharge accompanying a behavioral seizure is a pitfall of the method of measurement (the discharge was present but not visible to the electrodes), the absence of a behavioral manifestation of an EEG seizure may be a pitfall of the method of observation. If a patient is lying in bed watching television, unresponsiveness, inability to speak or to understand, minor automatisms, or loss of muscle tone cannot be observed unless active questioning is performed. Even correct responses to many questions do not exclude clinical signs: Seizures involving only memory have been observed (63). In other words, the presence of clinical signs is a function of the method of questioning or observation, hence the importance of recording all seizures, with and without overt clinical signs, and observing them as precisely as possible. The importance of "subclinical" seizures has been discussed with respect to evaluation for epilepsy surgery (76). Automatic seizure detection and seizure warning systems can be helpful in this situation (see "Limitations and Future Developments" below).

Recording and Review Strategies to Obtain Seizures

All types of seizures, with or without clinical and EEG manifestations, should ideally be recorded. As indicated above, it is possible to perform a continuous recording on a computer disk for a period of 24 hours. This represents a large amount of EEG to be reviewed, but computer review on a high-resolution screen can be quite fast: 32 channels of EEG can be presented 10–20 times faster than real time, resulting in a review lasting 1–2 hours. Such a fast review can result in small seizures being missed, particularly when more than 12–16 channels are utilized (64). The 1–2 hours also do not include the time required for the analysis of seizures or other potentially interesting events. Thus the full review of a 24-hour recording is quite time consuming and strenuous.

Alternative strategies have been developed by many institutions. These strategies consist mainly in a partial review, with an attempt to select the most relevant sections. The most important sections are of course those when a behavioral seizure was noted by the patient or an observer. In addition, randomly selected sections are often reviewed as well. This strategy entails the significant risk that seizures of which the patient is unaware and that are not observed will be almost systematically missed. This may be an acceptable compromise if the patient is under close observation, but could be quite dangerous otherwise.

Methods of Automatic Detection of Seizure Patterns

Some methods of seizure detection are based on behavioral manifestations of seizures; for example, mechanical sensors under a mattress can detect the strong rhythmic movements of generalized tonic–clonic seizures. The limitations of this kind of detection method are obvious—many seizures do not include such strong movements. This discussion instead concentrates on seizure detection methods based on EEG analysis. Because some seizures do not have EEG changes, EEG-based methods cannot be expected to detect them. There are also seizures that have mild or *nonspecific* changes, such as brief desynchronization or groups of theta or delta waves (1), making their differentiation from commonly seen patterns difficult. Thus there are also limitations to seizure detection by EEG, but these are not too restrictive because the vast majority of seizures have clear and relatively specific EEG changes.

The problem of seizure detection is inherently difficult because seizure activity can consist of a variety of morphologies. Unlike spikes, which have a relatively well-defined morphology, seizures can include patterns such as low-amplitude desynchronization, polyspike activity, rhythmic waves at a wide variety of frequencies and amplitudes, and spike-and-wave activity (6). In extracranial recordings, electromyographic (EMG) movement and eye blink artifacts often obscure seizures. From the point of view of pattern recognition, the problem is therefore complex.

Prior et al. (68) described the use of their cerebral function monitor to identify generalized tonic–clonic seizures; these could be recognized on the tracing as a large increase followed by a clear decrease in EEG amplitude (the postictal depression) and by large EMG activity. Such large seizures with major changes could also be identified in monkeys with experimental epilepsy by a characteristic pattern on slow paper tracings (56). Ives et al. (48) described a method in which 16 channels of EEG were added, bandpass filtered, and subjected to amplitude discrimination. This technique could detect large seizure discharges but was quite insensitive. Babb et al. (4) implemented an electronic circuit for the detection of seizures in recordings from intracerebral electrodes. A seizure was recognized when a rapid succession of large-amplitude spikes, lasting at least 5 seconds, was found. Murro et al. (61) described a method based on spectral parameters and discriminant analysis.

Gotman (23,24) presented a computer detection method that attempted to recognize a wide variety of seizure patterns. This method identified patterns that might represent seizure activity, marking them for later examination by traditional visual inspection. The method was therefore designed to be as sensitive as possible. False detections, as long as they were not extremely frequent, were not detrimental because all detections had to be visually reviewed. Observation of numerous seizures with this method led to the conclusion that most seizures, at some time during their development, would include activity that is *paroxysmal* compared to the background (the paroxysm could consist of increased amplitude or increased frequency); such activity would also be *rhythmic* (with frequencies varying from 3 to 20 cycles per second), and relatively *sustained* in duration (lasting several seconds).

Measurements of these characteristics were obtained by breaking down the EEG into half-waves and measuring, for every 2-second epoch, the average amplitude of the half-waves relative to that of the background (indicating whether an epoch was paroxysmal), the average duration of the half-waves (indicating frequency), and the coefficient of variation of half-wave duration (indicating the regularity of duration, or the rhythmicity). The background was constantly updated and included EEG sections recorded before and after the active epoch. Comparing the amplitude, frequency, and rhythmicity measurements of the background to those of the active epoch allowed the development of a decision tree for the detection of seizure activity. Detections may be triggered by rhythmic activity of moderate amplitude (Fig. 22.1) or by a sudden increase in frequency. It is not necessary to detect the *onset* of a seizure because the purpose of detection is to mark the recording. The interpreter will start at the mark and look for the onset. This method of seizure detection has been made available commercially and is in widespread use throughout the world. It has also been used to monitor experimental animals (60).

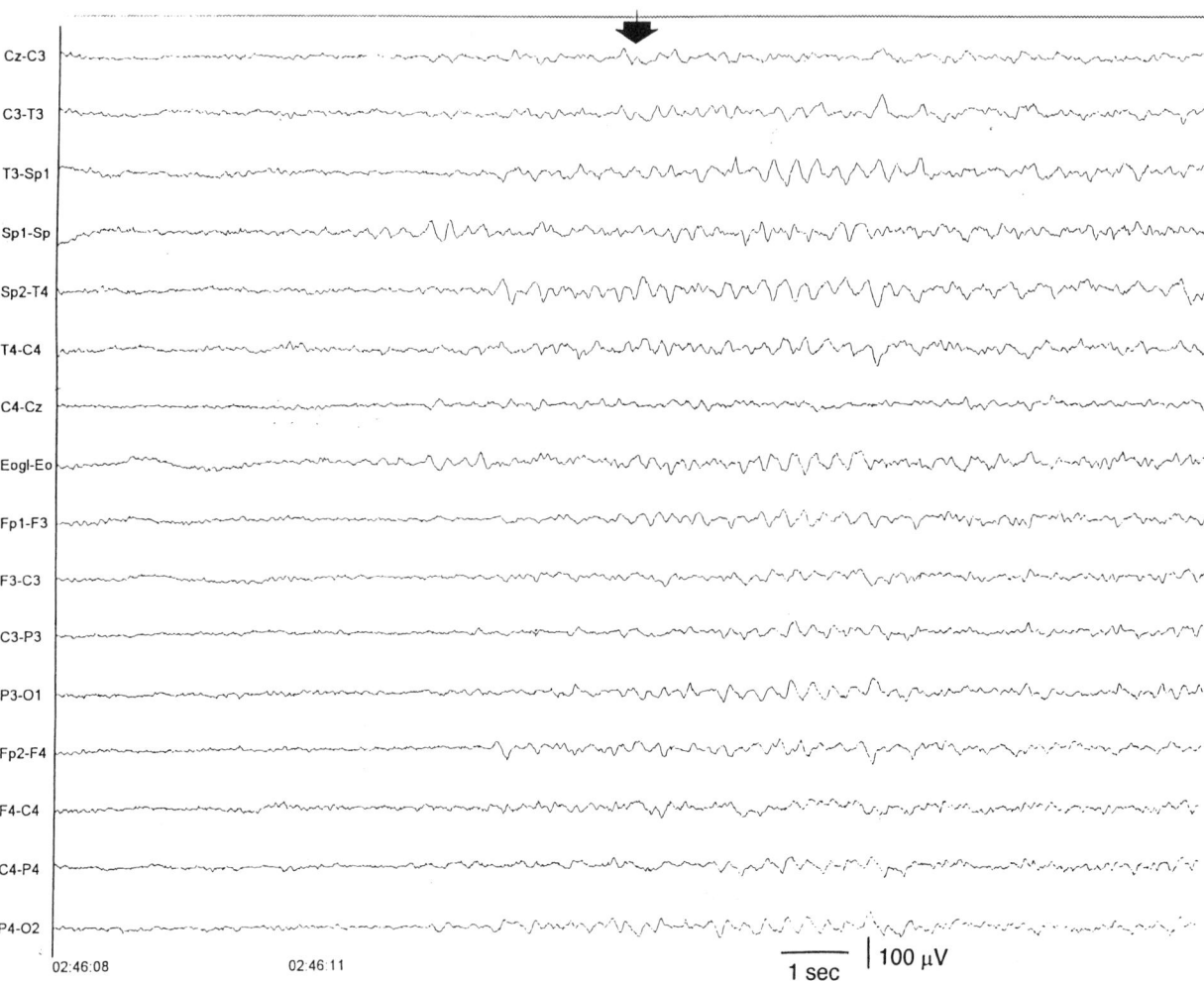

FIG. 22.1. Example of a seizure automatically detected because of a widespread rhythmic discharge (later followed by faster activity and generalized spike-and-wave activity, not shown). The *vertical arrow* marks the time of detection. Note that detection took place even though the rhythmic activity was not very prominent. The push button was not pressed by the patient or an observer.

Harding (43) presented a method specifically for intracerebral recordings, based on the detection of a repetitive spiking pattern, as well as possible flattening at seizure onset. This method was implemented on line and was subjected to an extensive evaluation (see " Clinical Validation of Seizure Detection Methods" below).

The detection of seizures in neonates is quite different from that in adults: discharges are often much slower (down to 0.5 Hz); seizure onset can be very gradual and seizures can last several minutes; and waveforms of seizures and of interictal background show a high level of variability (see

also Chapter 18). Liu et al. (55) presented a method for seizure detection in neonates based on the autocorrelation function for the detection of rhythmic slow patterns of any morphology. Gotman et al. (31) also presented a method specifically for neonates, but based on a combination of spectral analysis and mimetic analysis, aimed at detecting a wide variety of slow rhythms as well as irregular bursts of spikes (Fig. 22.2).

Recent developments in automatic detection have emphasized that performance can be improved significantly by incorporating in detection algorithms a wide context. Rather than defining the event only locally (i.e., com-

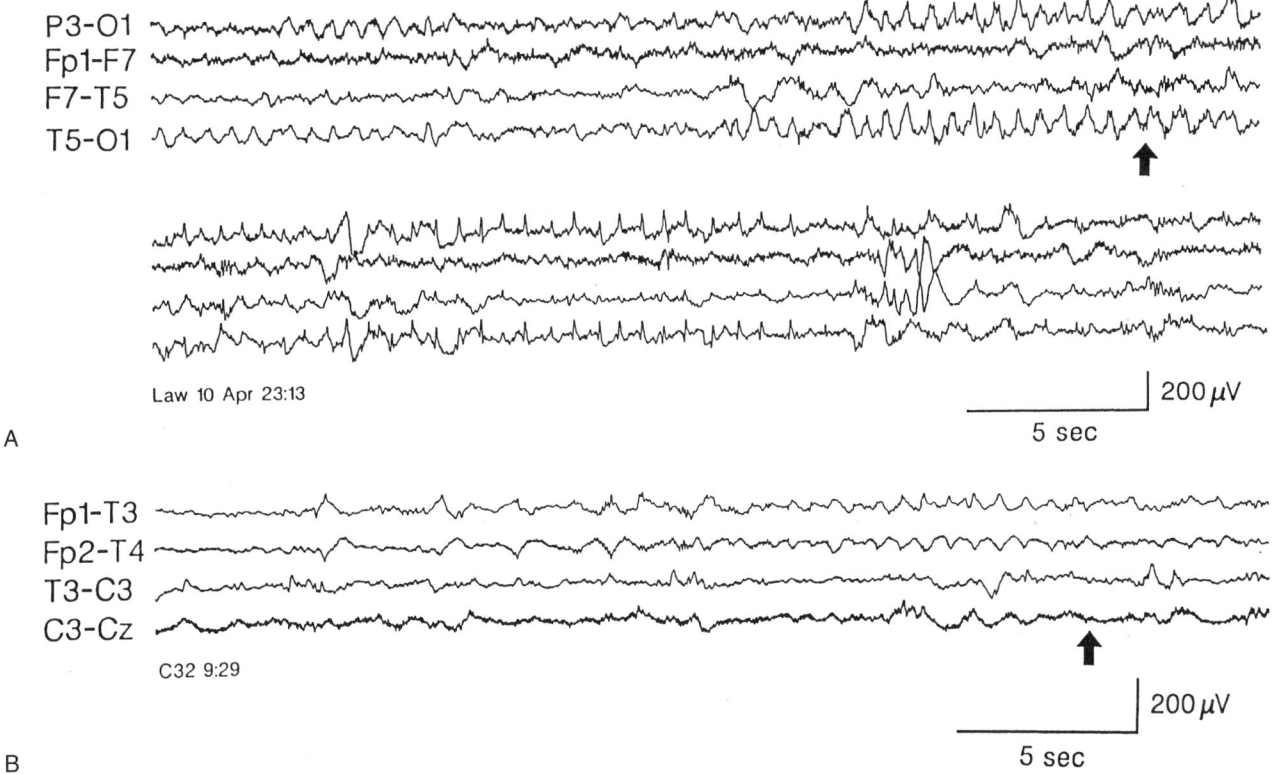

FIG. 22.2. Example of automatically detected seizures in a newborn infant. Only a subset of recorded channels is shown (channels not shown had no seizure activity). The discharges are very slow (note the time scale) and would not be detected by standard methods developed for adults. **A:** Seizure present only in one occipital electrode. **B:** Short seizure in the frontopolar regions. The *arrow* marks the time of detection. (From Gotman J, Flanagan D, Rosenblatt B, et al. Evaluation of an automatic seizure detection method for the newborn EEG. *Electroencephalogr Clin Neurophysiol* 1997;103:363–369, with permission.)

paring the characteristics of a 5-second epoch in one channel to the 30 seconds that precede it), it is important to include measurements of the spatial context (activity in other channels) and the temporal context (state of the subject: awake, stages of sleep, previously recorded events). Using this philosophy, it was possible to greatly reduce the number of false seizure detections by allowing the program to remember the patterns that caused frequent false detections in a particular subject (71). Klatchko et al. (51) presented a method for enhancing seizure detection by clustering in space and time elementary detections made on individual channels, thus obtaining a more global representation of seizures.

Artificial neural networks (ANNs) have found broad applications in many areas of pattern recognition, including seizure detection. Gabor et al. (19) and Webber et al. (77) presented methods of seizure detection based on ANNs, in which the ANN is trained by a large number of sample seizures. This class of method is very powerful because it is not necessary to obtain a formal description of the patterns to be detected; they simply have to be presented to the ANN in sufficiently large number. A large number of "nonseizure" patterns must also be presented, and the ANN learns to separate the two groups optimally. It is still necessary, however, to determine which features must be computed as representing a seizure on the EEG (mean frequency, rhythmicity, relative amplitude, etc.). If the features that really represent the characteristic aspects of seizures are not selected correctly, it will be impossible for the ANN to learn how to detect them. The ANN determines from its learning process which *combination* of features is characteristic of seizures.

Clinical Validation of Seizure Detection Methods

Evaluating the performance of automatic detection methods is difficult because results may depend as much on the selection of EEGs included in the evaluation set as on the detection method itself; for instance, a method may perform well if only very clear seizure patterns are included, but much less well with uncertain patterns, or with a recording having many artifacts. To give a fair impression of performance, what type of EEG should be included in the evaluation? The person selecting the EEG is often subjective, and this can bias strongly the results.

In evaluating the seizure detection method developed at the Montreal Neurological Institute, we made every effort to avoid bias in data selection (24). EEGs were recorded from 293 *consecutive* monitoring sessions from 49 patients. All EEGs were included, independently of EEG patterns and technical quality. Monitoring was performed in the absence of an EEG technologist; electrode problems and other technical difficulties were frequent but all EEGs were retained. Patients were over 10 years old, and the average recording duration was 18.1 hours, for a total of 5,303 hours of EEG.

In 241 of the 293 recordings (44 of 49 patients), scalp and sphenoidal electrodes were used; in the remaining 52 recordings (5 patients), intracerebral and epidural electrodes were used. Twenty-four percent of the 244 seizures were recorded by the push button alone (seizures were missed by the computer, but the patient or an observer pressed the button). In 35% of seizures, both the computer and the push button triggered the recording. In the remaining 41%, only the computer detected the seizures. Pauri et al. (64) performed an independent evaluation of the same method and came to very similar conclusions. In a third evaluation, Salinsky (73) concluded that the use of automatic seizure detection allowed clinicians to catch a large number of seizures missed by the patient and observers, and to reduce significantly the length of hospital stay. As in the above study, approximately 20% of seizures were not detected by the computer but were detected by the patient or an observer.

Thus it is clear that one cannot rely exclusively on human observation (the push button), nor can one rely exclusively on automatic detection. Using both considerably increases the yield of long-term monitoring. In addition, the average detection rates given above poorly reflect the reality of individual patients. Among the five patients with intracerebral electrodes, we had two cases that illustrated the extremes. In one patient 16 clinical seizures were recorded by the push button (with or without computer detection), with only 3 being detected by the computer alone. The computer operated continuously for 2 weeks and yielded little additional information. In another patient, however, 21 seizures were detected by the computer alone and 1 seizure by the computer and the push button. All were clinical seizures consisting of long but quiet automatisms, during which the patient stayed in bed and made no noise; such seizures went unnoticed because the patient was lying in bed, but they were very disruptive in his active life. In this case, the computer was particularly helpful.

We have not given details of false-positive detections. In the majority of cases, false detections are small enough in number not to be disruptive: false detections only cause the EEG to be marked unnecessarily, and can simply be discarded during visual inspection. Rates are usually around one to two false detections per hour of monitoring (24,64).

Harding (43) also performed a thorough evaluation of his method of seizure detection for intracerebral recordings by using large amount of *unselected* data: almost 1,600 hours from 40 patients. He obtained few false negatives and a very acceptable level of false positives. However, the results are difficult to compare directly to other methods because detection parameters were altered slightly in each patient according to results after the first seizure was recorded. Gabor (18) validated his seizure detection method on 4,500 hours of recording from 65 patients with scalp electrodes. He found that 92.8% of seizures were detected and the false alarm rate averaged 1.35 per hour. He also found that fast replay of the EEG to transform it in the audio range allowed the detection of almost all seizures (98.3%).

Gotman et al. (32) evaluated their newborn seizure detection method in a large set of data (from 55 newborns) obtained from three hospitals. Results showed seizure detection rates similar to those of adults (around 70%) and false detection rates of approximately 2 per hour. This study illustrated how it can be difficult to extrapolate results from one patient group to another: the performance varied considerably among the data sets of the three hospitals, reflecting the variability of recording conditions, technical quality, and types of pathology.

Limitations and Future Developments

Current seizure detection programs are not perfect and could use significant improvement. It would be extremely difficult, however, to detect all seizures because some seizures have almost no EEG accompaniment and the discharge morphology is often nonspecific (1). The suggestion is sometimes made that performance could be improved by fine tuning the detection program to each patient's seizure, after the first seizures are detected by the computer or by an observer. However, this would result in the introduction of an unacceptable bias in detection performance, toward seizures of the type recorded early in the monitoring session; in many cases the purpose of monitoring is to document all types of seizures and particularly to see if there are also seizures *different* from those recorded early. Tailoring the detection to a particular seizure type is only acceptable if one is interested in assessing the occurrence of that particular seizure type and is less concerned with other seizures.

The ways in which seizure detection can reduce the load of EEG interpretation during long-term monitoring were discussed above. Seizure detection could also be used to warn the patient or relatives that a seizure is starting. This would allow close clinical observation early in the seizure, and permit necessary precautions in some cases. It could also be useful to increase the applicability of ictal single-photon emission computed tomography (5). One can even conceive of rapid intervention, in the form of electrical stimulation or drug injection with an implanted device to abort the seizure. Unlike *seizure monitoring* as discussed above, this *seizure warning* application requires a very low rate of false alarms and detection very early in the seizure. This places very stringent requirements on the method. Promising results were obtained by the seizure warning system of Qu and Gotman (69,70), which used a first recorded seizure as a template to train the detection system (Fig. 22.3). Such a method can provide a warning only when a seizure similar to the template is taking place. It cannot warn of a new and different type of seizure, and is thus not useful for seizure monitoring. Osorio et al. (62) described a complex method based on time–frequency analysis for seizure warning. They reported perfect performance, although they did not indicate how quickly after the EEG onset the method was able to give a warning.

Recording Interictal Activity

The interictal activity that is specific to epilepsy consists mainly of spikes, sharp waves, and bursts of spike-and-wave activity. This paroxysmal activity occurs unpredictably and sometimes infrequently. In order to obtain a full documentation of the different types of abnormalities, the traditional short EEG recording may not be sufficient. Long-term monitoring may be required, including periods of the different stages of sleep, which most often activate and can modify interictal patterns (74). The reduction of antiepileptic medication, often done during long-term monitoring to precipitate seizures, also results, indirectly, in increased spiking: It has been shown that spikes are more frequent after seizures (28,36,40). It is clear that continuous day-and-night recording is an awkward method to document interictal activity; automatic detection methods can be very helpful.

Past Methods

Numerous publications, particularly in the 1970s and early 1980s, have dealt with automatic spike detection. The usual approach consisted of (a)

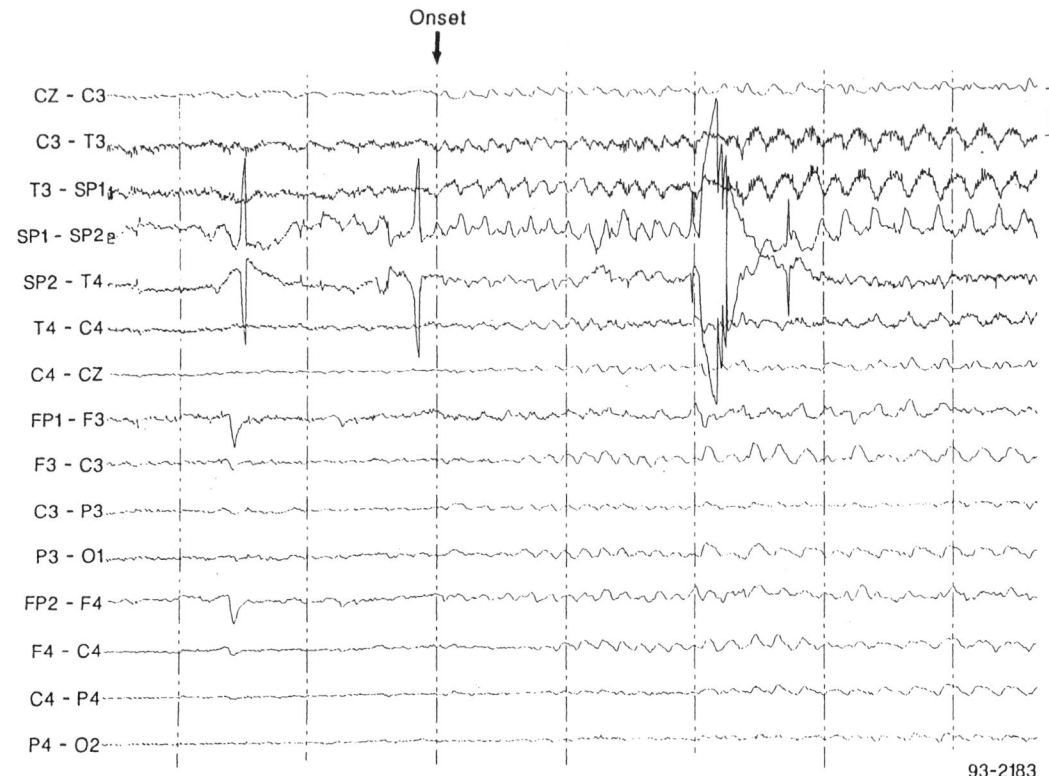

FIG. 22.3. Illustration of seizure warning method. **A:** Template seizure given to the program for training. *(Figure continues.)*

selecting EEG sections lasting 1 or 2 minutes that were free of artifacts and included a sufficient number of spikes, (b) devising a method for their detection, and (c) comparing results of automatic detection to what qualified electroencephalographers considered "true" spikes. Details of the various detection methods have been reviewed extensively (30) and are not repeated here. These methods relied generally on two approaches. In the first, the EEG is broken down into elementary waves and the method attempts to identify the waves having morphological characteristics normally associated with spikes (amplitude, duration, sharpness). In the second, the EEG is analyzed in order to find statistically improbable events of short duration.

For most methods, good performance was obtained, usually with 80%–90% of "true" spikes detected and a low rate of false-positive detection. Many publications ended with statements such as: "As computers become more powerful and less expensive, practical implementation will be simple." In fact, computers became more powerful and less expensive faster than expected but most methods did not reach practical implementation. The major reason is that the detection problem became much more complex when longer sections were analyzed; artifacts and normal transients had to be included, and they caused numerous false detections. In addition, there is little use for spike detection in 10-minute recordings when human inspection is perfect.

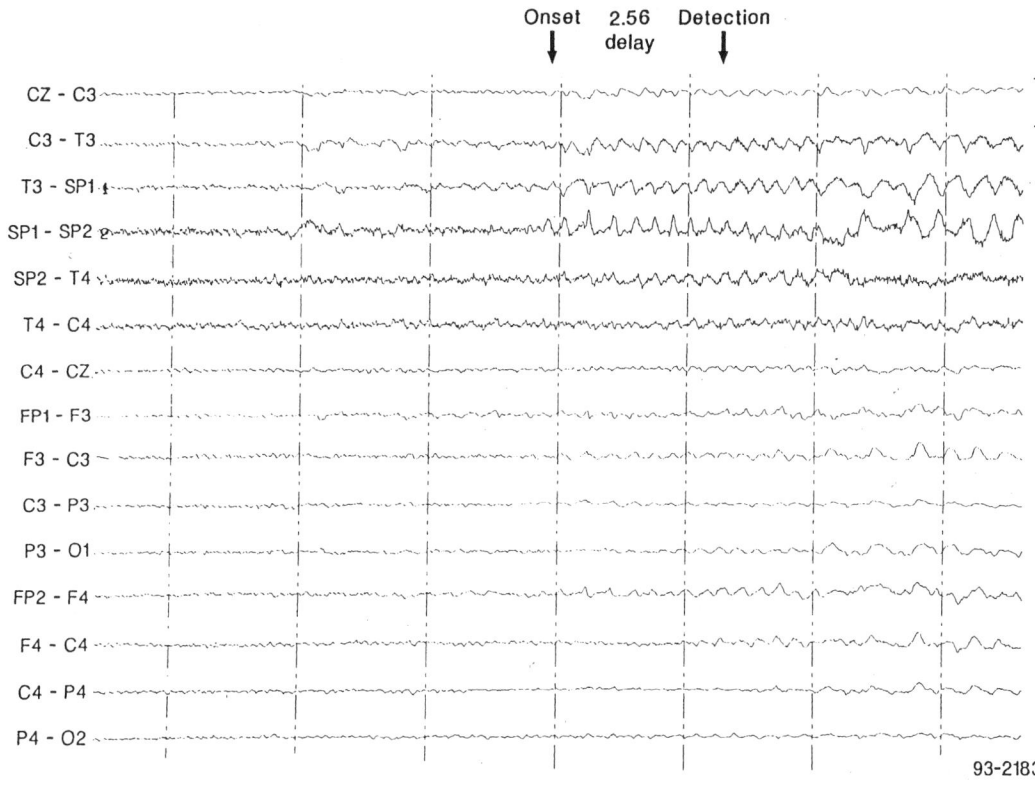

FIG. 22.3. *Continued.* **B:** Seizure occurring at a later time that was detected by the warning system 2.5 seconds after its onset. (From Qu H, Gotman J. A patient-specific algorithm for the detection of seizure onset in long-term EEG monitoring: possible use as a warning device. *IEEE Trans Biomed Eng* 1997;44:115–122, with permission.)

Difficulties of Detection

Spike recognition methods have relied on a definition of a spike adapted from Chatrian et al. (10), quoted in many publications: "a sharp transient, easily distinguishable from the background, having a duration of less than 70 ms for a spike and 70 to 200 ms for a sharp wave." This definition is extremely incomplete because it lacks features differentiating transients that have the same local morphology but that are not spikes, such as eye blinks, vertex sharp waves, isolated alpha or spindle waves, electrode artifacts, and movement artifacts. Such transients are common during long-term monitoring, when automatic spike detection is particularly useful. Figure 22.4 shows a typical example of results from a standard spike detection method: genuine spikes are mixed with false detections resulting from nonepileptiform transients.

Which characteristics allow a human interpreter to separate an epileptiform sharp wave from an eye blink, even though the waves themselves may have the same morphology and emerge from a similar background? These characteristics relate to the overall context in which the waves appear, where "context" covers much wider space and time than "background." When interpreting a wave having the morphology of a spike, the human observer takes into account what happens in other channels (spatial context), what happens in earlier and later parts of the recording (temporal context), and

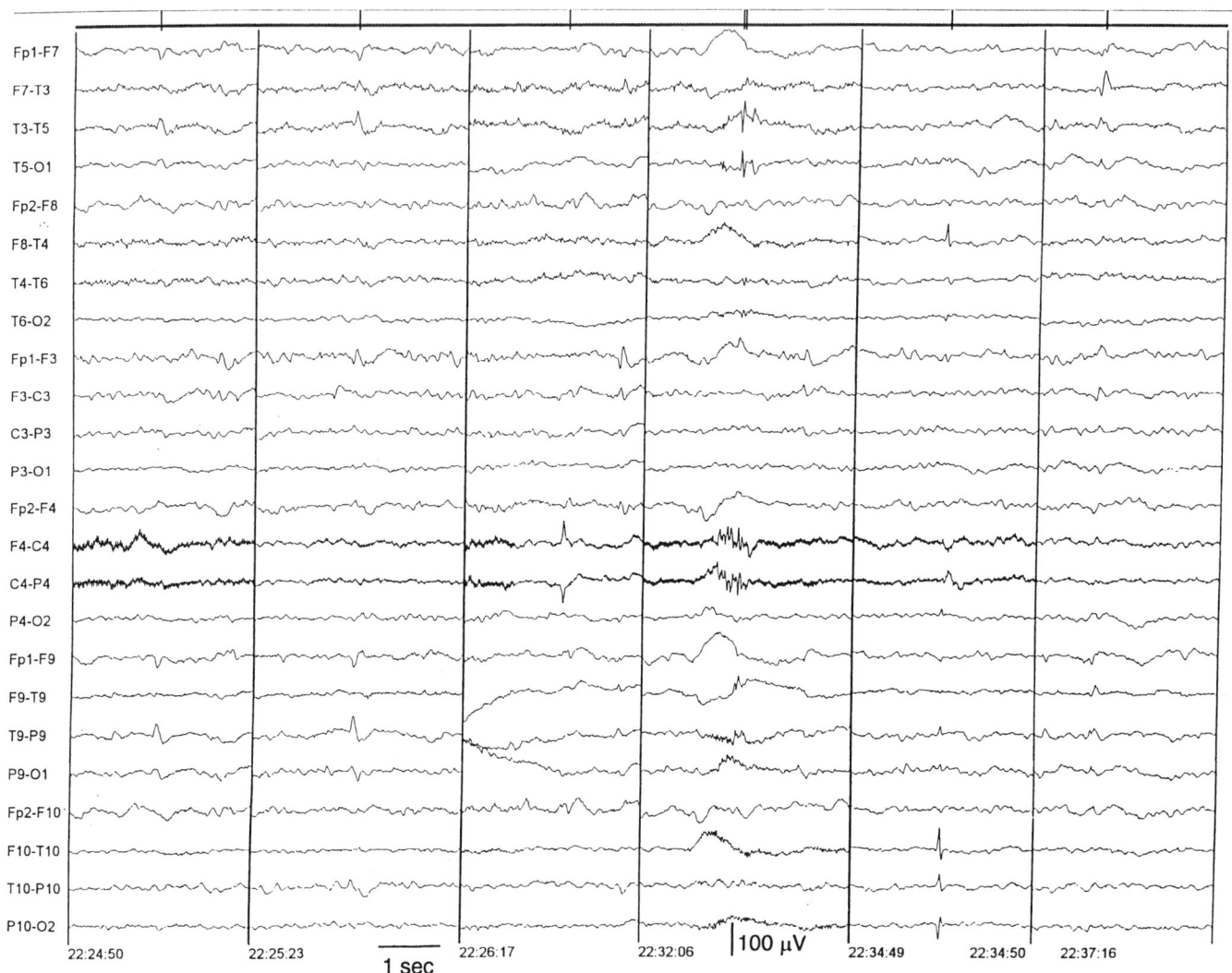

FIG. 22.4. EEG sections marked because of automatic spike detection (method of Gotman et al. [33]). *Vertical lines* represent discontinuities. Sections shown here represent some of the automatically marked events during a 15-minute segment of a 24-hour monitoring session (see time at the beginning of each section, at bottom of page). The intervening EEG is not shown. The method is able to detect clear spikes (section 5) and genuine sharp waves that are not very prominent (sections 1, 2, and 6), mixed with nonepileptiform transients (sections 3 and 4). Even though there are false detections, the method provides valuable data reduction.

even non-EEG information such as the age or clinical state of the subject. Optimism about early detection methods originated in the failure to appreciate how much spike identification relies on this context. In addition, human interpreters have a low level of interrater agreement when asked to mark every spike in a recording (78,81). Although such marking is important in evaluating detection methods or in training detection systems, it is not a task that is normally performed by human interpreters, who look at a record globally and not at each waveform.

The problems discussed above do not affect the ability to detect most epileptiform spikes, but they result in a large number of false-positive detections. For this reason, it is possible to make practical use of an automatic spike detection method, as long as it is conceived as a method to detect a high proportion of the spikes along with a possibly large number of nonepileptiform transients, rather than as a method to detect *only* spikes. Such a practical implementation was made with the spike detection algorithms developed at the Montreal Neurological Institute (24,33). The method has been in use for many years and operates in many other institutions. It runs on line and marks the detected events on the recording; these are subsequently reviewed and the electroencephalographer decides which are true and which are false. Despite false-positive detections, the system allows marking of a large fraction of the spikes and can speed up EEG review considerably. It can be combined with automatic seizure detection and form a system for automatic extraction of epileptiform activity, ictal and interictal, during long-term monitoring. Such a system results in the marking of only 5%–10% of a 24-hour recording, including spikes, seizures, and false detections.

Pietilä et al. (65) presented a system including automatic segmentation of the EEG followed by feature extraction. In comparison to the system of Gotman, their system showed a higher sensitivity but a lower specificity. The system of Gotman was also validated by Hostetler et al. (44), who stated that "the computer system, while not as specific as an EEGer, can be as sensitive and can be a reliable screening editor for large amounts of monitoring data. On balance, it is more effective than an EEGer for this limited purpose." Spatt et al. (75) also confirmed the clinical utility of this method when used as a screening device.

New Approaches

ANNs, a new tool for seizure detection, are also used for spike detection. The process requires a large number of sample patterns for training, including spikes and nonspikes. This method was used by Gabor and Seyal (20), who obtained good performance but evaluated their method on a very small sample. Webber et al. (79), also using a relatively small data set for evaluation, compared the use of the raw EEG to that of preprocessed variables as the input to the ANN and concluded that the raw EEG was not optimal. ANNs have also been used for detecting bursts of spike-and-wave activity in experimental models of epilepsy (49). Wavelet analysis, a new method of signal processing, has also been used to detect spikes (12), but only very preliminary results have been published.

Another approach to improving detection performance is to make automatic methods operate more like humans, that is, to allow them to use information from a wide context, as discussed above. This is conceptually simple but difficult to implement because the context encompasses a large amount of information, and one must decide which part of that information is relevant to spike detection. It is this very selection that humans do so well. Glover et al. (22) described a context-based system aimed largely at reducing false spike detections by making use of *spatial* context: information from all EEG channels, as well as from EMG, electro-oculography, and electrocardiography channels, was used to assess whether a transient in a particular channel was likely to be epileptiform.

Gotman and Wang have proposed an approach in which a wide *temporal and spatial* context is used to decide on the nature of a sharp event (41,42). We labeled the method "state-dependent spike detection" because criteria for spike detection are rendered dependent on the state of the EEG. We defined five states in which spike detection should operate differently: active wakefulness, quiet wakefulness, desynchronized EEG, phasic EEG, and slow-wave EEG. In these different states, the events that cause false detections have to be handled by different means. In active wakefulness, for instance, one must be particularly aware of symmetrical frontal sharp waves that may be due to eye blinks, whereas there is no such concern in the phasic EEG state; in that state, sharp waves maximal at the vertex are a problem (Fig. 22.5). The method was evaluated in 20 patients, each having close to 2 hours of EEG recording covering all states; it showed a reduction in false detection of 65% and an increased sensitivity of 35%, compared to the original method.

Whether using neural nets or more traditional methods, it is unlikely that local wave morphology is sufficient to differentiate epileptiform transients from other transients. Some form of context sensitivity appears necessary.

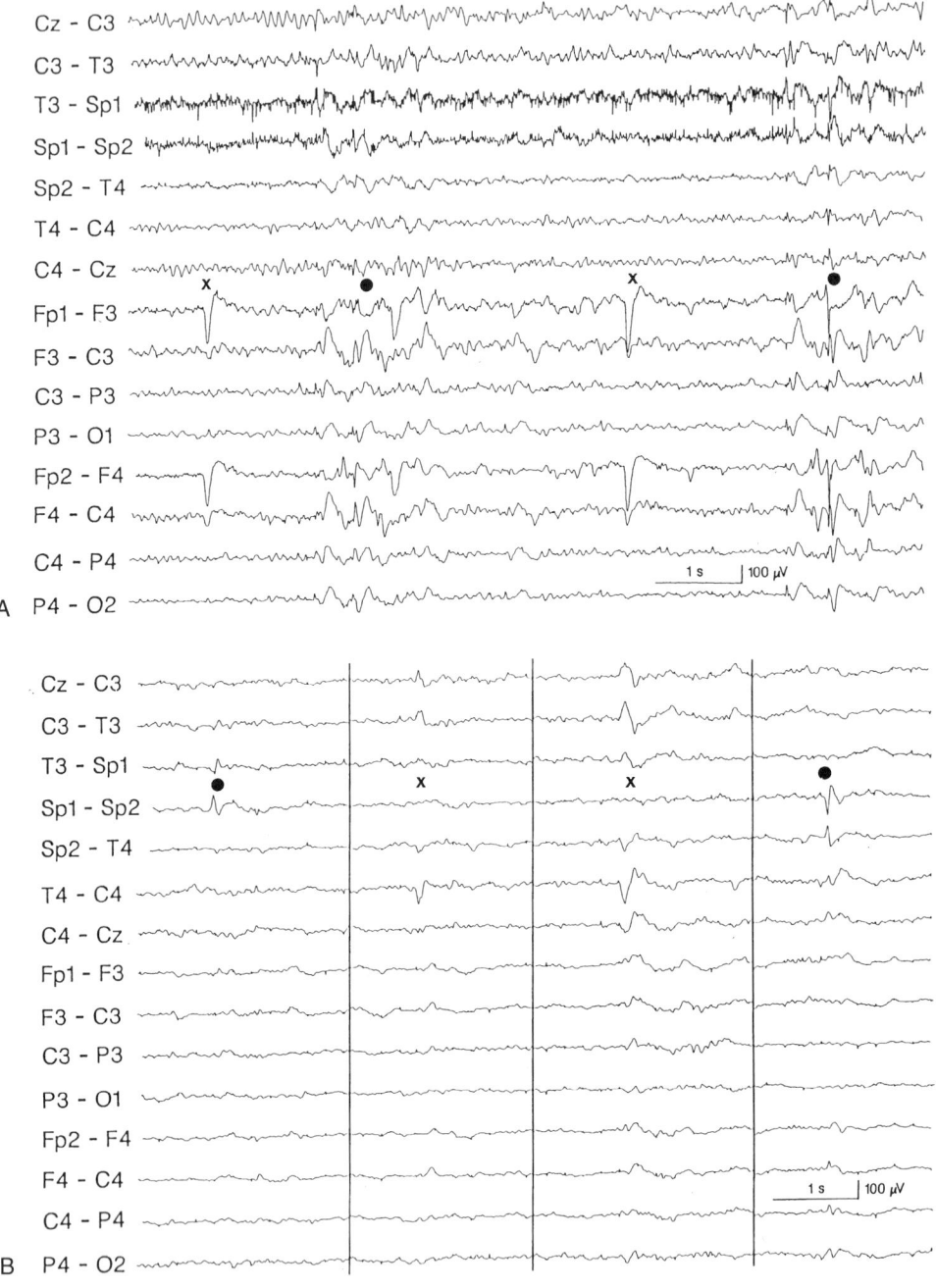

FIG. 22.5. Example of use of spatial and temporal context in spike detection. Nonepileptiform transients are selectively rejected (rejected events are marked with x). **A:** During active wakefulness, as determined by automatic state classification, waves having the morphology and distribution of eye blinks are eliminated. **B:** During phasic sleep, sharp waves having a maximum at the vertex are eliminated. (From Gotman J, Wang L-Y. State-dependent spike detection: concepts and preliminary results. *Electroencephalogr Clin Neurophysiol* 1991;79:11–19, with permission.)

Recording Behavior

The analysis of behavioral manifestations of seizures is obviously a critical element. It can be performed by an observer or by video recording, or often by both. Video recording is simple, most often making use of standard camera and videocassette recorder (VCR) technology. Recent developments in computer technology may, however, have a significant impact. One such development is of minor importance: some VCRs can be controlled by computers, so that the tedious task of finding the right time on the tape is facilitated by use of a direct command from the computer.

A second development will have a much greater impact: it is now possible to record a video image directly in the computer, rather than on videotape (72). This presents important advantages: one has immediate random access to any part of the recording; and behavior and EEG recordings can be replayed simultaneously at many speeds and archived together. However, one problem remains with practical implementation of this technology: The disk space required for storing a 24-hour video recording is still difficult to manage for most computers, even when using powerful image compression techniques (unless one is prepared to accept a lower image quality and a lower frame rate). It is almost certain that this situation will improve rapidly and that computer-based video recording will become standard. Until that time, the difficulty can be overcome by recording the digital video signal selectively, around the times at which the push button is pressed or automatic seizure detections take place.

POSTDETECTION ANALYSIS

The benefits derived from computers are found not only in detecting epileptiform events during long-term monitoring, but also in displaying, manipulating, and analyzing the EEG. Various methods have become standard in the review of digitally recorded EEGs. This section presents some analysis methods specific to epileptic activity.

Analysis of Seizure Activity

One can go beyond visual interpretation and analyze seizures in order to extract information of diagnostic or scientific interest. For instance, digital filtering makes it possible to remove most of the EMG artifact that obscures many seizures recorded from the scalp (34), as well as decrease the effect of electrode movement artifact (Fig. 22.6*A* and *B*). Spectral analysis of the signal contaminated by EMG artifact can sometimes help interpret the result of filtering (Fig. 22.6*C*). One has to be careful in interpreting the filtered signal, however, because there can sometimes be rhythmic low-frequency contraction of scalp muscles (34). The graphic representation of seizures and quantitative measurements of their features can improve EEG interpretation (2,9,11,37,38). It is also possible to develop measures that are able to compare multichannel seizure patterns as one entity. They break down seizures into sections having uniform patterns (low-amplitude fast activity, high-frequency spikes, spike-and-wave activity, etc.), and then determine the similarity between two seizures, taking into account the succession of patterns over multiple channels (80,82).

The ability to analyze the propagation pattern of seizures or the possible influence of one region over another has been the focus of attention of many investigators. The study of interactions between brain regions during seizures was pioneered by Brazier (8). She used the coherence function to measure the strength of interaction between seizure discharges in two locations, and the phase spectrum to measure time differences of a few milliseconds. Thus rapid propagation of seizures could theoretically be followed. The reliability of this method was improved by Gotman (26,27), who included in the measurement a range of frequencies rather than a single frequency. Its validity was established in experimental and human epilepsy, in cases where the location of the focus was known. This method allowed the study of interhemispheric interactions during widespread spike-and-wave activity (26,52) and during temporal lobe seizures (25,39,54). Figure 22.7*A* shows a small seizure recorded with intracerebral electrodes from the hippocampus and amygdala in one patient. The coherence and phase spectra in Figure 22.7*B* show that the discharge in the hippocampus leads that in the amygdala by 25 milliseconds. One should be cautious in interpreting this result; it does not prove that the discharge originates in the hippocampus and propagates to the amygdala. However, if one has to choose between amygdala and hippocampus as the most likely origin of the discharge, results favor the hippocampus.

There are other methods to measure interactions during seizures. The average amount of mutual information (AAMI) has a theoretical advantage over coherence because coherence can only detect *linear* (in the mathematical sense) relationships, whereas AAMI can also detect more complex relationships. However, coherence and AAMI most often give similar results. AAMI and other nonlinear methods have been described by Lopes da Silva and Mars (58). Fernandes de Lima et al. (15) compared a linear and a nonlinear regression coefficient in the study of interhemispheric interactions during hippocampal seizures in rats; they found that the nonlinear measure

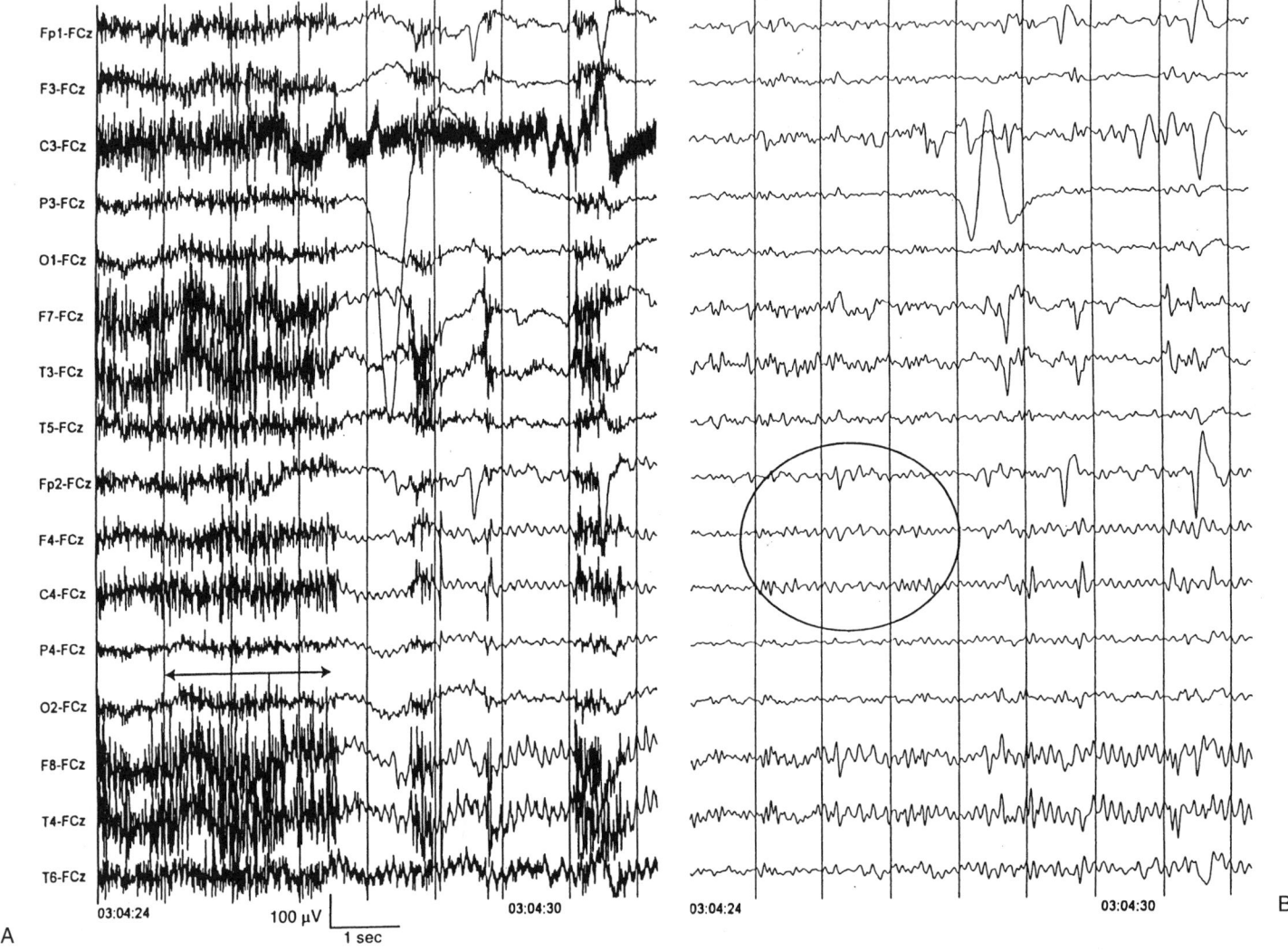

FIG. 22.6. Digital filtering of seizure. **A:** Section of a seizure recording in which one portion is completely obscured by EMG artifact and the following portion shows cerebral seizure activity in the right hemisphere. There is also a large electrode artifact at the P3 electrode. **B:** The same EEG section, but digitally filtered (low-pass finite impulse response filter at 15 Hz and high-pass infinite impulse response filter at 1.5 Hz). The high-pass 1.5-Hz filter reduces the impact of the electrode artifact. The low-pass filter at 15 Hz reveals that rhythmic activity was present under the EMG activity, particularly at C4 and P4; it is more difficult to assess whether cerebral rhythmic activity is also present in F8 and T4 because it appears that there could be some remnants of EMG activity.

(Figure continues.)

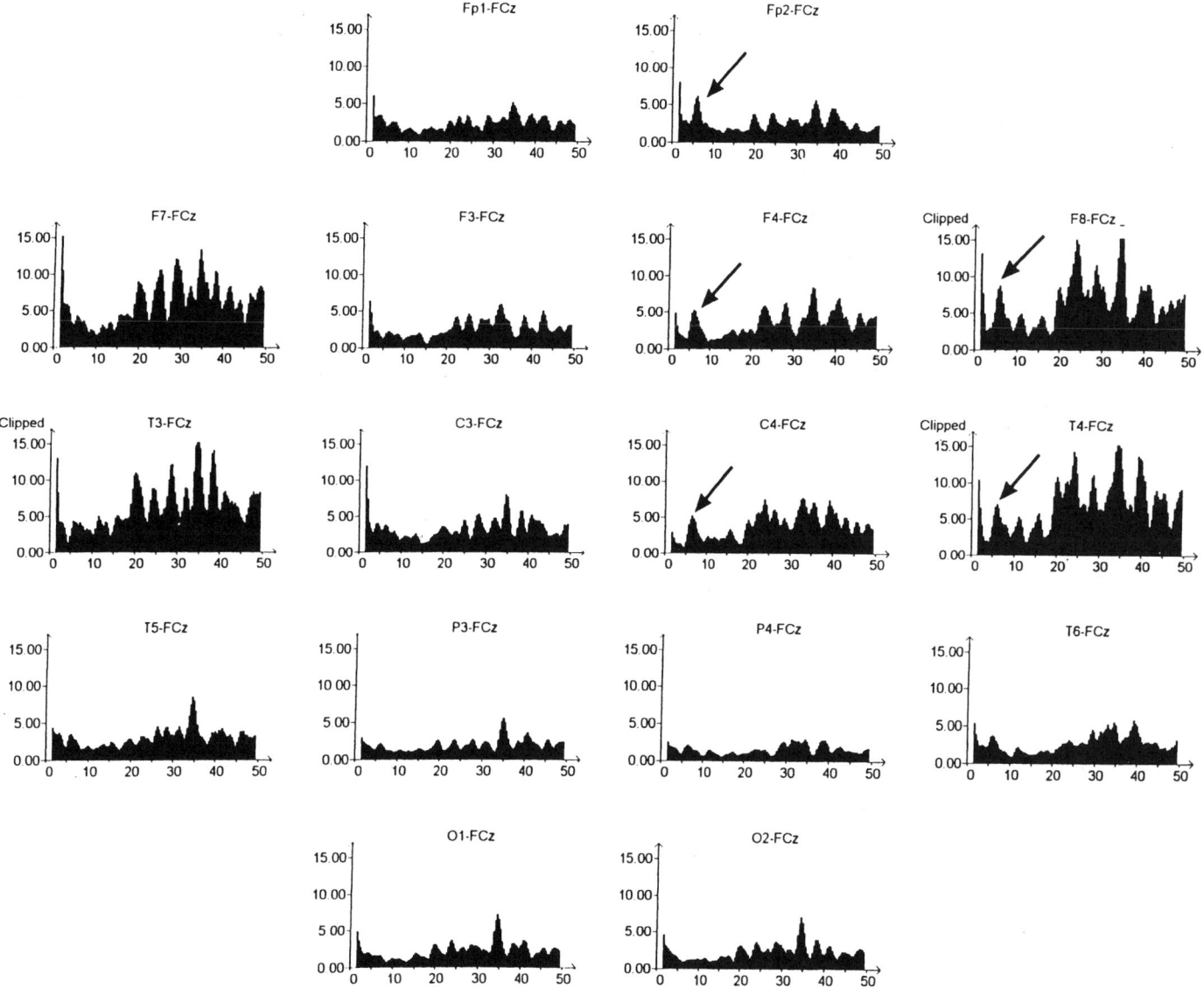

FIG. 22.6. *Continued.* **C:** Frequency spectra of the 2.5-second section marked in **A**. Many peaks are visible at high frequencies, as is always the case with EMG artifact. It is very rare, however, to see rhythmic activity of muscle origin at low frequencies. The peak at 6 Hz, marked by *arrows*, is present in the right hemisphere but not in the left. This is the same frequency as the activity seen after the EMG artifact stops. It therefore clearly represents activity of cerebral origin.

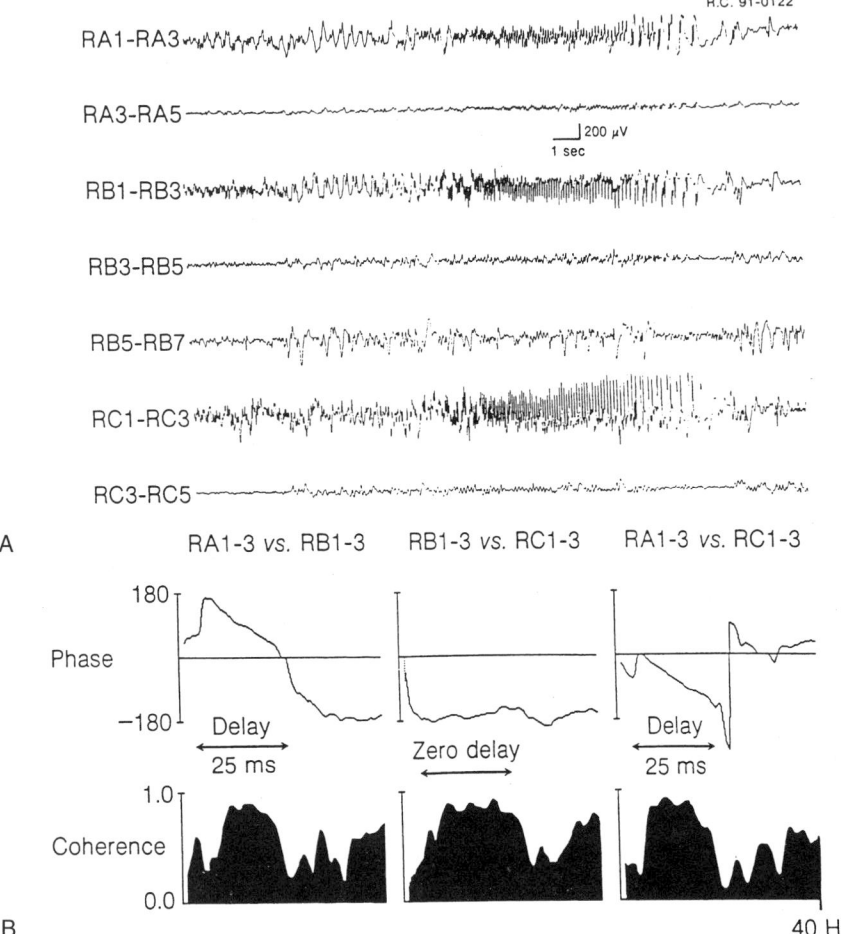

FIG. 22.7. Seizure propagation measured by coherence and phase. **A:** Short seizure localized to deep structures of the temporal lobe; electrodes are in the horizontal plane with contacts 5 mm apart, contact 1 being deepest; RA is aimed at the amygdala, RB at the anterior hippocampus, and RC at the middle hippocampus. **B:** Phase and coherence spectra between the three pairs of deepest channels; phase is linear over the frequency range where coherence is high (*horizontal arrow*); a time delay measurement is therefore possible, indicating a lead from RB1-3 to RA1-3 of 25 milliseconds, a lead from RC1-3 to RA1-3 also of 25 milliseconds, and no time difference between RB1-3 and RC1-3. The discharge in the hippocampus therefore leads the discharge in the amygdala, as was most often the case in seizures limited to mesial temporal structures. (From Gotman J, Levtova V. Amygdala-hippocampus relationships in temporal lobe seizures: a phase-coherence study. *Epilepsy Res* 1996;25:51–57, with permission.)

was more robust and could show interactions when the linear measure was at noise level. One important factor is not often discussed when comparing these methods: The size of the recording electrodes probably influences the type of relationship. Discharges from very small electrodes, which may record multiple-unit activity, are more likely to have nonlinear relationships than discharges from macroelectrodes, which record from large populations of neurons.

Another method of analysis of seizure propagation is that of the directed transfer function, indicating the direction of flow of information. It has been shown in a few seizures that, even when a discharge is widespread, the region in which the seizure originated appears to remain that from which the information flows (16,17). The relationship between the directed transfer function and the coherence/phase method described above has not been established.

Source analysis methods, usually based on dipole modeling, have been used extensively for interictal spikes, but a few studies have also shown their applicability to seizure analysis (3,7).

Concepts of nonlinear dynamics have been used in the study of seizures: Could seizures result from chaotic systems? Some of the complex issues related to the estimation of the correlation dimension, the most commonly used measure, are discussed by Pijn et al. (66) and Lopes da Silva (57). Iasemidis et al. (47) and Pijn et al. (67) showed that, during the seizure, the region of the epileptic focus most often corresponded to an area of low dimensionality. Iasemidis and Sackellares (46) and Iasemidis et al. (45) showed that the Lyapunov exponent (related to the dimensionality of the system) could gradually become synchronous in several channels prior to a seizure (a phenomenon they term *entrainment*). Elger and Lehnertz (13) also indicated that the dimensionality of the EEG may decrease several minutes prior to seizures. A similar finding was also obtained by Martinerie et al. (59), using a multichannel nonlinear measure. These studies raise the interesting possibility that seizures might be predictable.

Analysis of Interictal Activity

Automatic spike detection was described above mainly in the context of data reduction, but it also offers the benefit of quantification. It is possible to edit out the false spike detections interactively on the computer screen so that only valid detections remain. Quantification of spike activity during several days of monitoring has proven invaluable in the study of factors that might affect the rate and localization of spikes. It was found that the rate of focal spiking does not change (increase or decrease) before seizures (40,50).

In contrast, there is a large increase in spiking in the days that follow most secondarily generalized seizures and many partial seizures; surprisingly, spiking rates appear unaffected by changes in antiepileptic drug levels (36,40). The postictal increase in spiking and the absence of decrease in spiking with high antiepileptic drug levels were replicated in the kindling model of epilepsy (21,29,53). Thus quantification of spiking rates has established that spiking does *not* change (increasing before seizures, decreasing with high drug levels), as was intuitively believed.

Spikes were also quantified during the different stages of sleep in patients evaluated for epilepsy surgery with noninvasive recordings. Results indicate that spiking is more focal during rapid-eye-movement (REM) sleep than during slow-wave sleep. The localization obtained from REM sleep spiking correlates better with other tests of localization (e.g., seizure onset, radiological findings) than does the localization obtained during slow-wave sleep or wakefulness (74).

The question of whether spike activity propagates between brain regions has also been studied. Emerson et al. (14) used spike-triggered averaging to measure the propagation between temporal and frontopolar regions and concluded that it was possible to see relationships not visible by visual inspection. Spatiotemporal dipole modeling has also been used to see whether spikes could be represented by one or several dipoles, in an attempt to localize the source of spike activity. This is discussed extensively in Chapter 23.

CONCLUSION

Computers play an important role in assisting in the recording and analysis of the EEGs of epileptic patients. During long-term monitoring, computer assistance is almost indispensable for the detection of epileptic events. There is no single economical method that ensures the detection of all seizures and spikes in every patient: All available help must be used, including staff and patient reporting and computer detection. In some patients, one method will prove more useful than others, but this is not known in advance of the monitoring sessions.

We have seen that spike and seizure detection is not a simple task, as researchers in this area originally thought. The human who reads an EEG uses clues from a wide spatial and temporal context, clues that are difficult to encode in computer programs. Most methods analyze the EEG at a very local level (looking at 10–30 seconds of EEG at a time, often one channel at a time). It would therefore be naive to expect high reliability from such automatic methods. Nevertheless, they can be extremely useful if implemented in the context of human validation. Recent methods incorporate knowledge of a wider context, as does the state-dependent spike detection method mentioned above. This will in all likelihood result in much better performance, but it is very unlikely that we will reach a stage where human validation is not required.

The technological context in which automatic detection methods are implemented is changing rapidly. Detection programs can readily operate in real time in personal computers. Several computers may be connected via a local area network so that review of a recording can take place while the recording is in process. EEGs may be reviewed on several review stations in different locations within a hospital. Given the data reduction ability of detection programs, it is feasible to archive the EEGs from a 3-week monitoring session, including interictal and ictal epileptiform activity, on a single disk.

Finally, computer analysis of seizures and spikes may provide information that is not readily available from traditional visual examination. This is primarily due to the possibility of quantifying the EEG and of making mathematical analyses that can be related to brain function.

ACKNOWLEDGMENT

This work was supported in part by grant MT-10189 of the Medical Research Council of Canada.

REFERENCES

1. Ajmone-Marsan C. Electroencephalographic studies in seizure disorders: additional considerations. *J Clin Neurophysiol* 1984;1:143–157.
2. Alarcon G, Binnie CD, Elwes RDC, et al. Power spectrum and intracranial EEG patterns at seizure onset in partial epilepsy. *Electroencephalogr Clin Neurophysiol* 1995;94:326–337.
3. Assaf BA, Ebersole JS. Continuous source imaging of scalp ictal rhythms in temporal lobe epilepsy. *Epilepsia* 1997;38:1114–1123.
4. Babb TL, Mariani E, Crandall PH. An electronic circuit for detection of EEG seizures recorded with implanted electrodes. *Electroencephalogr Clin Neurophysiol* 1974;37:305–308.
5. Berkovic SF, Newton MR, Chiron C, et al. Single photon emission tomography. In: Engel J Jr, ed. *Surgical treatment of the epilepsies.* New York: Raven Press, 1993:233–244.
6. Blume WT, Young GB, Lemieux JF. EEG morphology of partial epileptic seizures. *Electroencephalogr Clin Neurophysiol* 1984;57:295–302.
7. Boon P, D'Have M. Interictal and ictal dipole modelling in patients with refractory partial epilepsy. *Acta Neurol Scand* 1995;92:7–18.
8. Brazier MAB. Spread of seizure discharges in epilepsy: anatomical and electrophysiological considerations. *Exp Neurol* 1972;36:263–272.
9. Bullmore ET, Brammer MJ, Bourlon P, et al. Fractal analysis of electroencephalographic signals intracerebrally recorded during 35 epileptic seizures: evaluation of a new method for synoptic visualization of ictal events. *Electroencephalogr Clin Neurophysiol* 1994;91:337–345.
10. Chatrian G-E, Bergamini L, Dondey M, et al. A glossary of terms most commonly used by clinical electroencephalographers. *Electroencephalogr Clin Neurophysiol* 1974;37:538–548.
11. Darcey TM, Williamson PD. Spatio-temporal EEG measures and their application to human

intracranially recorded epileptic seizures. *Electroencephalogr Clin Neurophysiol* 1985;61:573–587.

12. D'Attelis CE, Isaacson SI, Sirne RO. Detection of epileptic events in electroencephalograms using wavelet analysis. *Ann Biomed Eng* 1997;25:286–293.

13. Elger CE, Lehnertz K. Seizure prediction by non-linear time series analysis of brain electrical activity. *Eur J Neurosci* 1998;10:786–789.

14. Emerson RG, Turner CA, Pedley TA, et al. Propagation patterns of temporal spikes. *Electroencephalogr Clin Neurophysiol* 1995;94:338–348.

15. Fernandes de Lima VM, Pijn JP, Nunes Filipe C, et al. The role of hippocampal commissures in the interhemispheric transfer of epileptiform after discharges in the rat: a study using linear and non-linear regression analysis. *Electroencephalogr Clin Neurophysiol* 1990;76:520–539.

16. Franaszczuk PJ, Bergey GK. Application of the directed transfer function method to mesial and lateral onset temporal lobe seizures. *Brain Topogr* 1998;11:13–21.

17. Franaszczuk PJ, Bergey GK, Kaminski MJ. Analysis of mesial temporal seizure onset and propagation using the directed transfer function method. *Electroencephalogr Clin Neurophysiol* 1994;91:413–427.

18. Gabor AJ. Seizure detection using a self-organizing neural network: validation and comparison with other detection strategies. *Electroencephalogr Clin Neurophysiol* 1998;107:27–32.

19. Gabor AJ, Leach RR, Dowla FU. Automated seizure detection using a self-organising neural network. *Electroencephalogr Clin Neurophysiol* 1996;99:257–266.

20. Gabor AJ, Seyal M. Automated interictal EEG spike detection using artificial neural networks. *Electroencephalogr Clin Neurophysiol* 1992;83:271–280.

21. Gigli GL, Gotman J. Effects of seizures and carbamazepine on interictal spiking in amygdala kindled cats. *Epilepsy Res* 1991;8:204–212.

22. Glover JR, Raghavan N, Ktonas PY, et al. Context-based automated detection of epileptogenic sharp transients in the EEG: elimination of false positives. *IEEE Trans Biomed Eng* 1989;36:519–527.

23. Gotman J. Interhemispheric relations during bilateral spike-and-wave activity. *Epilepsia* 1981;22:453–466.

24. Gotman J. Automatic recognition of epileptic seizures in the EEG. *Electroencephalogr Clin Neurophysiol* 1982;54:530–540.

25. Gotman J. Measurement of small time differences between EEG channels: method and application to epileptic seizure propagation. *Electroencephalogr Clin Neurophysiol* 1983;56:501–514.

26. Gotman J. Relationships between triggered seizures, spontaneous seizures and interictal spiking in the kindling model of epilepsy. *Exp Neurol* 1984;84:259–273.

27. Gotman J. Interhemispheric interactions in seizures of focal onset: data from human intracranial recordings. *Electroencephalogr Clin Neurophysiol* 1987;67:120–133.

28. Gotman J. Automatic seizure detection: improvements and evaluation. *Electroencephalogr Clin Neurophysiol* 1990;76:317–324.

29. Gotman J. Relationships between interictal spiking and seizures: human and experimental evidence. *Can J Neurol Sci* 1991;18:573–576.

30. Gotman J, Burgess RC, Darcey TM, et al. Computer applications. In: Engel J Jr, ed. *Surgical treatment of the epilepsies.* New York: Raven Press, 1993:429–444.

31. Gotman J, Flanagan D, Rosenblatt B, et al. Evaluation of an automatic seizure detection method for the newborn EEG. *Electroencephalogr Clin Neurophysiol* 1997;103:363–369.

32. Gotman J, Flanagan D, Zhang J, et al. Automatic seizure detection in the newborn: methods and initial evaluation. *Electroencephalogr Clin Neurophysiol* 1997;103:356–362.

33. Gotman J, Ives JR, Gloor P. Automatic recognition of interictal epileptic activity in prolonged EEG recordings. *Electroencephalogr Clin Neurophysiol* 1979;46:510–520.

34. Gotman J, Ives JR, Gloor P. Frequency content of EEG and EMG at seizure onset: possibility of removal of EMG artefact by digital filtering. *Electroencephalogr Clin Neurophysiol* 1981;52:626–639.

35. Gotman J, Ives JR, Gloor P, et al. Long-term monitoring at the Montreal Neurological Institute.

In: Gotman J, Ives JR, Gloor P, eds. *Long-term monitoring in epilepsy.* Amsterdam: Elsevier Science, 1985:327–340.

36. Gotman J, Koffler DJ. Interictal spiking increases after seizures but does not after decrease in medication. *Electroencephalogr Clin Neurophysiol* 1989;72:7–15.

37. Gotman J, Levtova V. Amygdala-hippocampus relationships in temporal lobe seizures: a phase-coherence study. *Epilepsy Res* 1996;25:51–57.

38. Gotman J, Levtova V, Farine B. Graphic representation of the EEG during epileptic seizures. *Electroencephalogr Clin Neurophysiol* 1993;87:206–214.

39. Gotman J, Levtova V, Olivier A. Frequency of the electroencephalographic discharge in seizures of focal and widespread onset in intracerebral recordings. *Epilepsia* 1995;36:697–703.

40. Gotman J, Marciani MG. Electroencephalographic spiking activity, drug levels and seizure occurrence in epileptic patients. *Ann Neurol* 1985;17:597–603.

41. Gotman J, Wang L-Y. State-dependent spike detection: concepts and preliminary results. *Electroencephalogr Clin Neurophysiol* 1991;79:11–19.

42. Gotman J, Wang L-Y. State-dependent spike detection: validation. *Electroencephalogr Clin Neurophysiol* 1992;83:12–18.

43. Harding GW. An automated seizure monitoring system for patients with indwelling recording electrodes. *Electroencephalogr Clin Neurophysiol* 1993;86:428–437.

44. Hostetler WE, Doller HJ, Homan RW. Assessment of a computer program to detect epileptiform spikes. *Electroencephalogr Clin Neurophysiol* 1992;83:1–11.

45. Iasemidis LD, Principe JC, Czaplewski JM, et al. Spatiotemporal transition to epileptic seizures: a nonlinear dynamical analysis of scalp and intracranial EEG recordings. In: Silva FL, Principe JC, Almeida LB, eds. *Spatiotemporal models in biological and artificial systems.* Amsterdam: IOS Press, 1997:81–88.

46. Iasemidis LD, Sackellares JC. The evolution with time of the spatial distribution of the largest Lyapunov exponent of the human epileptic cortex. In: Duke D, Pritchard W, eds. *Measuring chaos in the human brain.* River Edge, NJ: World Scientific Publishing, 1991:49–82.

47. Iasemidis LD, Sackellares JC, Zaveri HP, et al. Phase space topography and the Lyapunov exponent of electrocorticograms in partial seizures. *Brain Topogr* 1990;2:187–201.

48. Ives JR, Thompson CJ, Gloor P, et al. The on-line computer detection and recording of spontaneous temporal lobe epileptic seizures from patients with implanted depth electrodes via a radio telemetry link. *Electroencephalogr Clin Neurophysiol* 1974;37:205.

49. Jandó G, Siegel RM, Horváth Z, et al. Pattern recognition of the electroencephalogram by artificial neural networks. *Electroencephalogr Clin Neurophysiol* 1993;86:100–109.

50. Katz A, Spencer SS. Spatial and temporal relations of interictal spikes and seizures. *Epilepsia* 1989;5:664–664.

51. Klatchko A, Raviv G, Webber WRS, et al. Enhancing the detection of seizures with a clustering algorithm. *Electroencephalogr Clin Neurophysiol* 1998;106:52–63.

52. Kobayashi K, Ohtsuka Y, Oka E, et al. Primary and secondary bilateral synchrony in epilepsy: differentiation by estimation of interhemispheric small time differences during short spike-wave activity. *Electroencephalogr Clin Neurophysiol* 1992;83:93–103.

53. Leung LS. Spontaneous hippocampal interictal spikes following local kindling: time-course of change and relation to behavioral seizures. *Brain Res* 1990;513:308–314.

54. Lieb JP, Hoque K, Skomer CE, et al. Inter-hemispheric propagation of human mesial temporal lobe seizures: a coherence/phase analysis. *Electroencephalogr Clin Neurophysiol* 1987;67:101–119.

55. Liu A, Hahn JS, Heldt GP, et al. Detection of neonatal seizures through computerized EEG analysis. *Electroencephalogr Clin Neurophysiol* 1992;82:30–37.

56. Lockard JS, Congdon WC, Ducharme C, et al. Slow-speed EEG for chronic monitoring of clinical seizures in monkey model. *Epilepsia* 1980;21:325–334.

57. Lopes da Silva F. Dynamics of electrical activity of the brain, local networks, and modulating systems. In: Nunez PL, ed. *Neocortical dynamics and human EEG rhythms.* New York: Oxford University Press, 1995:249–271.

58. Lopes da Silva FH, Mars NJI. Parametric methods in EEG analysis. In: Gevins AS, Rémond A,

eds. *Handbook Of electroencephalography and clinical neurophysiology. Vol. 1. Methods of analysis of brain electrical and magnetic signals.* Amsterdam: Elsevier Science, 1987:243–260.

59. Martinerie J, Adam C, Le Van Quyen M, et al. Epileptic seizures can be anticipated by non-linear analysis. *Nat Med* 1998;4:1173–1176.

60. Mascott C, Gotman J, Beaudet A. Automated EEG monitoring in defining a chronic epilepsy model. *Epilepsia* 1994;35:895–902.

61. Murro AM, King DW, Smith JR, et al. Computerized seizure detection of complex partial seizures (short communication). *Electroencephalogr Clin Neurophysiol* 1991;79:330.

62. Osorio I, Frei, MG, Wilkinson SB. Real-time automated detection and quantitative analysis of seizures and short-term prediction of clinical onset. *Epilepsia* 1998;39:615–627.

63. Palmini A, Gloor P, Jones-Gotman M. Pure amnestic seizures in temporal lobe epilepsy: definition, clinical symptomatology and functional anatomical considerations. *Brain* 1992;115:749–769.

64. Pauri F, Pierelli F, Chatrian G-E, et al. Long-term EEG-video-audio monitoring: computer detection of focal EEG seizure patterns. *Electroencephalogr Clin Neurophysiol* 1992;82:1–9.

65. Pietilä T, Vapaakoski S, Nousiainen U, et al. Evaluation of a computerized system for recognition of epileptic activity during long-term EEG recording. *Electroencephalogr Clin Neurophysiol* 1994;90:438–443.

66. Pijn JPM, van Neerven J, Noest A, et al. Chaos or noise in EEG signals: dependence on state and brain site. *Electroencephalogr Clin Neurophysiol* 1991;79:371–381.

67. Pijn JPM, Velis DN, van der Heyden MJ, et al. Nonlinear dynamics of epileptic seizures on basis of intracranial EEG recordings. *Brain Topogr* 1997;9:249–270.

68. Prior PF, Virden RSM, Maynard DE. An EEG device for monitoring seizure discharges. *Epilepsia* 1973;14:367–372.

69. Qu H, Gotman J. Improvement in seizure detection performance by automatic adaptation to the EEG of each patient. *Electroencephalogr Clin Neurophysiol* 1993;86:79–87.

70. Qu H, Gotman J. A seizure warning system for long-term epilepsy monitoring. *Neurology* 1995;45:2250–2254.

71. Qu H, Gotman J. A patient-specific algorithm for the detection of seizure onset in long-term EEG monitoring: possible use as a warning device. *IEEE Trans Biomed Eng* 1997;44:115–122.

72. Rector D, Burk P, Harper RM. A data acquisition system for long-term monitoring of physiological and video signals. *Electroencephalogr Clin Neurophysiol* 1993;87:380–384.

73. Salinsky MC. A practical analysis of computer based seizure detection during continuous video EEG monitoring. *Electroencephalogr Clin Neurophysiol* 1997;103:445–449.

74. Sammaritano M, Gigli GL, Gotman J. Interictal spiking during wakefulness and sleep and the localization of foci in temporal lobe epilepsy. *Neurology* 1991;41:290–297.

75. Spatt J, Pelzl G, Mamoli B. Reliability of automatic and visual analysis of interictal spikes in lateralising an epileptic focus during video-EEG monitoring. *Electroencephalogr Clin Neurophysiol* 1997;103:421–425.

76. Sperling MR, O'Connor MJ. Auras and subclinical seizures: characteristics and prognostic significance. *Ann Neurol* 1990;28:320–328.

77. Webber WRS, Lesser RP, Richardson RT, et al. An approach to seizure detection using an artificial neural network. *Electroencephalogr Clin Neurophysiol* 1996;98:250–272.

78. Webber WRS, Litt B, Lesser RP, et al. Automatic EEG spike detection: what should the computer imitate? *Electroencephalogr Clin Neurophysiol* 1993;87:364–373.

79. Webber WRS, Litt B, Wilson K, et al. Practical detection of epileptiform discharges (EDs) in the EEG using an artifical neural network: a comparison of raw and parameterized EEG data. *Electroencephalogr Clin Neurophysiol* 1994;91:194–204.

80. Wendling F, Badier JM, Chauvel P, et al. A method to quantify invariant information in depth-recorded epileptic seizures. *Electroencephalogr Clin Neurophysiol* 1997;102:472–485.

81. Wilson SB, Harner RN, Duffy FH, et al. Spike detection. I. Correlation and reliability of human experts. *Electroencephalogr Clin Neurophysiol* 1996;98:186–198.

82. Wu L, Gotman J. Segmentation and classification of EEG during epileptic seizures. *Electroencephalogr Clin Neurophysiol* 1998;106:344–356.

Chapter 23

EEG Voltage Topography and Dipole Source Modeling of Epileptiform Potentials

John S. Ebersole

The ultimate goal of electroencephalography (EEG) is to gain an understanding of brain activity at the time of the recording. Not only is it important to determine if the brain's function is abnormal, but often it is imperative to localize the abnormality. Localization by EEG is a time-honored skill that, for most of its 70-year history, has involved interpreting patterns of EEG traces. Chief among the techniques has been the use of bipolar montages and the identification of phase reversals in bipolar chains, which signify the crossing of a negative field maximum. This method is typically used to localize epileptiform spikes, and it is based on the assumption that the spike generator necessarily lay under the electrode recording maximum negativity. It has been demonstrated in Chapter 2 that this assumption is often not correct.

Although scalp EEG voltage fields of interictal spikes approximate those that would be produced by a dipole, as discussed in Chapters 1 and 2, cerebral sources of EEG are in reality sizable areas of cortex that often encompass 6–20

cm^2. Viewed at a distance, however, as with scalp electrodes, the summed activity of countless aligned pyramidal cells in such a cortical area produces a field that looks dipolar. A particularly useful aspect of this likeness is that there are mathematical techniques for approximating the location and orientation of dipoles in a volume conductor or, in our case, an EEG source within the brain.

PRINCIPLES OF DIPOLE SOURCE MODELING

In the mid-nineteenth century, Helmholtz (24) developed the electromagnetic principles of volume conduction. Nearly 100 years later, Wilson and Bayley (48) developed a method for calculating the voltage field that would appear on the surface of a spherical volume conductor from any given dipole source within it. For a source of specified location, orientation, and magnitude, there can be only one potential field distribution on the surface of the conductor. This answer is called the *forward solution*, and it is unique. Our problem in EEG analysis is the opposite, however—namely trying to characterize an intracerebral source having measured the topography of a scalp potential. The answer to this problem is called the *inverse solution*, and, unfortunately for any given voltage field either on a theoretical spherical volume conductor or on a real head, there is no single answer, but rather multiple possibilities because fields from any number or combination of sources can sum linearly to produce the resultant surface field. This is the principle of *superposition*, and because of it attempts to identify source character (number, location, amplitude, and magnitude) always yield ambiguous results.

Certain assumptions are also usually made to make this inverse problem mathematically tractable and to apply these principles to EEG. The brain is usually modeled as a sphere of uniform conducting material (9), and concentric shells are added around this sphere to imitate the different conductivities of the skull and scalp (12,26,37,45). For ease of modeling, the source of the scalp EEG field is considered to be a theoretical point-like dipole. Although the real generators of EEG potentials are areas of cortex that extend over several square centimeters, the activity of such a region may be modeled effectively by a single dipole, because the field that would be produced by this "equivalent dipole" is very similar to that of a real source. In general, such an equivalent dipole source must reside close to the geometrical center of the actual generator area and have an orientation similar to the net orientation of this cortex. Usually, however, the equivalent dipole must be located deep to the generator cortex in order for it, as a point-like source, to simulate the field produced by an extended cortical region.

The instantaneous, single-dipole, inverse solution is the most common form of source model. This technique defines a single equivalent dipole source for the scalp voltage field at one moment in time (12,25,26,44,45). An iterative minimization technique with a directed search pattern is usually employed. Such dipole modeling programs calculate the forward solution for a given source location/orientation and compare this to the measured voltage field. A difference measure is obtained, and the program repeats the calculations for another source location/orientation multiple times until the one having the minimal difference with respect to the measured field is identified. This is the best equivalent dipole solution for the scalp voltage field at that point in time. Regardless of the complexity or number of real cerebral generators underlying the scalp field, the single-dipole model finds the best single-source explanation.

For some EEG potentials, the voltage field maxima rise and fall as the potential evolves, but the maxima do not move or change shape substantially. Single-dipole models are appropriate for such voltage fields that are spatially stable over time. Repeated dipole solutions over the time course of this type of potential are consistent and vary only in magnitude, not substantially in position or orientation. Such dipole models are consistent with either a single cerebral source or several nearby synchronously activated sources with no propagation of activity (Fig. 23.1).

When the maxima of EEG voltage fields substantially move in location or change shape during the course of the potential, the single-dipole model is inappropriate. The temporal evolution of a changing voltage field can be described, however, by a series of sequential single dipoles (14,19). This "moving dipole" model may usefully reflect characteristics of a propagating source, as commonly seen with spikes or seizures, if the propagation is simple and unidirectional and terminates before the original source repolarizes (Fig. 23.2). Moving dipole models that spiral in a loop or make sudden turns in direction or position are usually the result of fields created by the superposition of several sources with temporally overlapping activity. One-dipole solutions in these instances can be misleading. Moving dipole trajectories should therefore be interpreted with caution. If several cortical areas are active simultaneously, a different technique is needed to identify each of them.

Spatiotemporal dipole modeling is a technique that takes into consideration an overlap of activity from multiple generators (38–40,42). Dipoles are fixed in location and orientation, but they can vary over time in strength and polarity. This technique attempts to determine the fewest number of equivalent sources that can explain the EEG field over time. Not only are the dipole positions given, but the assumed and necessary activity of each dipole over time is estimated in the form of a source potential. This is akin to what an intracerebral electrode would record from the source (see Fig. 23.2).

When dealing with more than a single equivalent dipole, there is no unique solution to the inverse problem. Modeling strategies must be used to constrain the solutions to those that are most realistic. Strategies based on sequential temporal activation of generators or those based on a priori knowledge of the orientation of likely cortical sources are the ones most commonly used. Implicit in the temporal strategy is the idea that early latencies of an EEG potential are more likely to be the result of a single source than are later latencies. Accordingly, one should first model the early evolution of the voltage field with a single dipole, rather than that at the potential peak. Additional dipoles are used for any residual field left unexplained by preceding dipoles. If the initial dipole explains, both in spatial and temporal terms, the entire voltage field evolution, the cortical generator is simple in

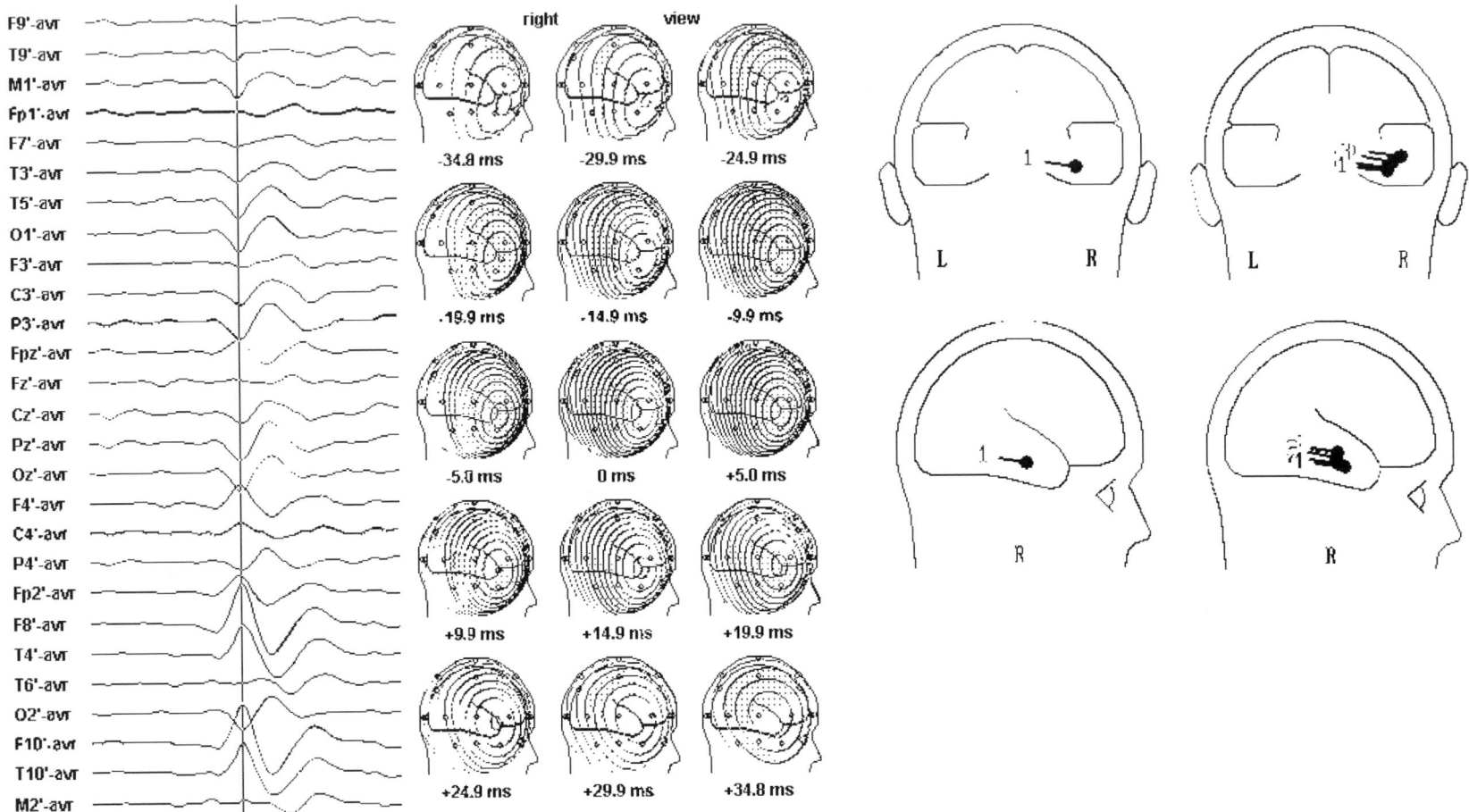

FIG. 23.1. Left: EEG traces (common average reference) of a right, type 2 temporal spike. Cursor denotes 0-millisecond latency. **Middle:** Sequential voltage topography of the spike. Note stable shape of the voltage fields over 70 milliseconds. **Right:** Instantaneous single-dipole model of the spike (at cursor) and moving dipole model of the spike over its duration. Note that voltage field stability and the tight cluster of similar dipoles in a moving model suggest a simple source well modeled by a single, instantaneous dipole. Horizontal, radial orientation is consistent with a lateral temporal cortex source. (From Ebersole J. Noninvasive localization of epileptogenic foci by EEG source modeling. *Epilepsia* 1999;41[Suppl 1]:24–33, with permission.)

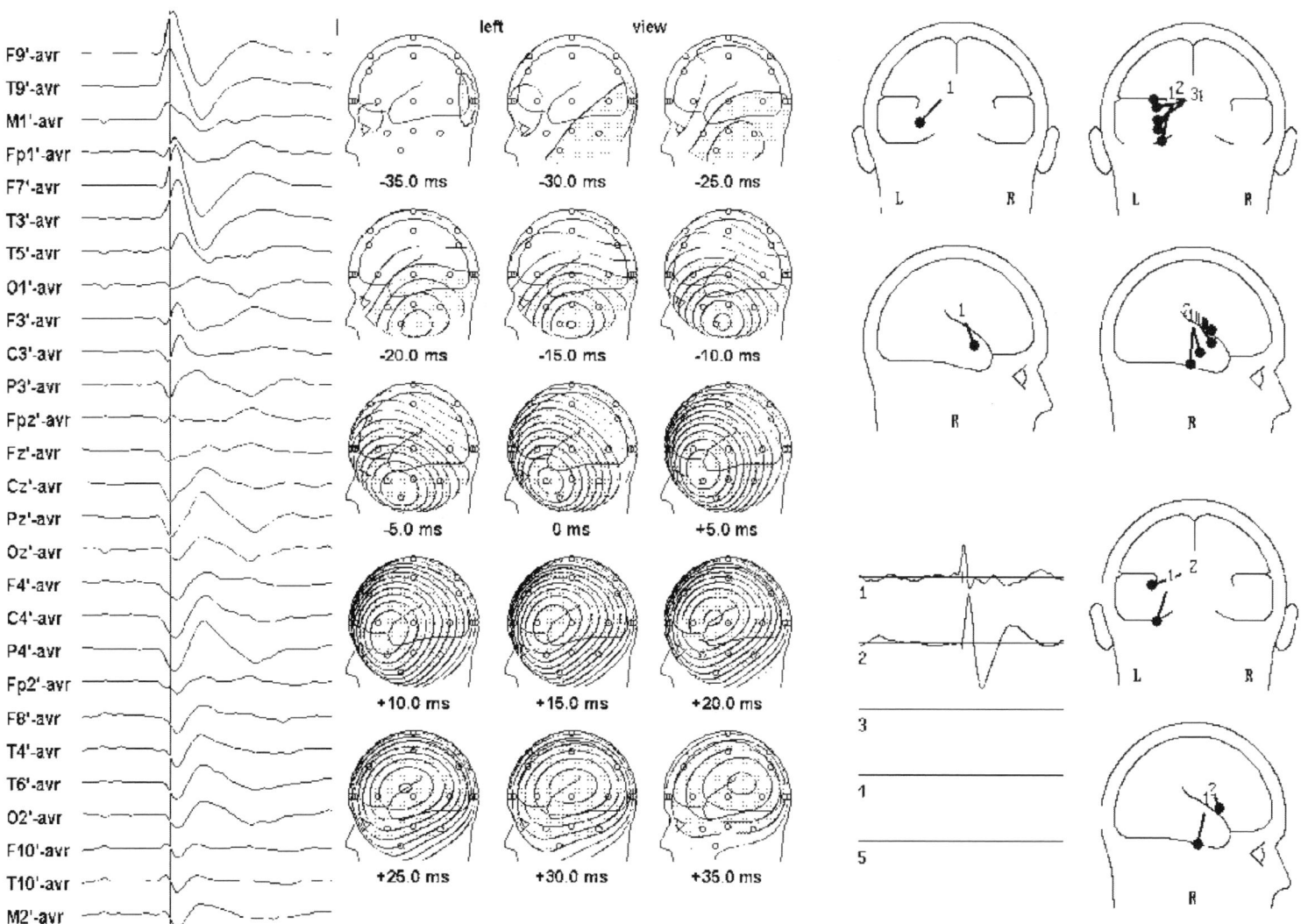

FIG. 23.2. Left: EEG traces (common average reference) of a left, type 1 temporal spike. Cursor denotes 0-millisecond latency. **Middle:** Sequential voltage topography of the spike. Note progressive change in shape of the voltage fields over 70 milliseconds, in particular movement of maxima. **Top right:** Instantaneous single-dipole model of the spike (at cursor) and moving dipole model of spike propagation. **Bottom right:** Spatiotemporal, two-dipole model of the spike. Note that spike field evolution can be explained with as few as two fixed dipoles, if the activity of dipole 1 precedes that of dipole 2. Vertical, tangential orientation of the earliest moving dipole and earlier spatiotemporal dipole is consistent with temporal base source. Later dipoles suggest spike propagation to the lateral temporal cortex. (From Ebersole J. Noninvasive localization of epileptogenic foci by EEG source modeling. *Epilepsia* 1999;41[Suppl 1]:24–33, with permission.)

character. Commonly, however, two or three dipoles may be needed to explain a temporally and spatially changing voltage field, such as that of a propagating spike.

Proper interpretation of equivalent dipoles requires an appreciation for the weaknesses in source modeling assumptions and for the complexity of real cortical source geometry and physiology. Dipole models seldom reflect precisely the location of actual cortical generators. Dipole localization techniques are least accurate in depth determinations because the actual size of the cerebral source is quite variable and always much larger than a point dipole. Activation of a large area of cortex, as is common with epileptic spikes, produces a broad scalp voltage field that will be modeled by a dipole that is deeper than the actual source.

Dipole orientation is often more useful than is dipole location/depth in determining which area of cortex in a given lobe is the likely generator of a scalp field. Because cortical sources of scalp-recordable EEG are large in area, both sides of sulci are commonly active. The tangential fields of opposite polarity generated from opposing sulcal walls tend to cancel one another, however. For this reason, activity in individual sulci tends to contribute less to scalp EEG fields than do gyral crowns. A reasonable simplification for interpreting dipole models of spontaneous potentials, such as epileptiform spikes, is to consider only the overall shape of the brain lobes and not the individual convolutions. Radial scalp EEG fields will come from gyri of convexity cortex, while tangential fields will most likely come from major fissures (interhemispheric and Sylvian) or from basal cortical surfaces (Fig. 23.3).

EEG VOLTAGE TOPOGRAPHY IN TEMPORAL LOBE EPILEPSY

Ebersole and Wade (14,20) first noted that the voltage topography of temporal spikes was not consistent, even among those with a similar frontotemporal negative field maximum. They showed that the corresponding positive field maximum varied in location from near the vertex to the contralateral temporal region. They called the former distribution, with vertex positivity, a type 1 spike field, and the latter pattern, with contralateral temporal positivity, a type 2 spike field (Figs. 23.4 and 23.5). Patients with predominantly type 1 spikes tended to have unilateral hippocampal atrophy, intracranial EEG seizures that began in mesial temporal structures, and an increased likelihood of seizure elimination following standard anteromedial temporal resection. Those patients with type 2 spikes were less likely to have hippocampal atrophy, commonly had seizures originating from non–mesial temporal structures on intracranial EEG, and were less likely to be surgical successes. Subsequent investigation demonstrated that a rigid categorization of spike topography into types 1 and 2 was overly simplistic (15). Although voltage fields may be stable for the duration of the spike, particularly in a type 2 pattern (see Fig. 23.1), voltage fields also commonly evolve, which usually signifies a propagating spike source (see Fig. 23.2). A type 1 pattern may evolve into a type 2 pattern and vice versa. Maxima locations may also shift without a change of spike type.

The location and in particular the orientation of the discharging cortical area determines the resultant spike voltage topography. Type 1 spikes, with an inferior temporal negative maximum and a vertex positive maximum, are generated

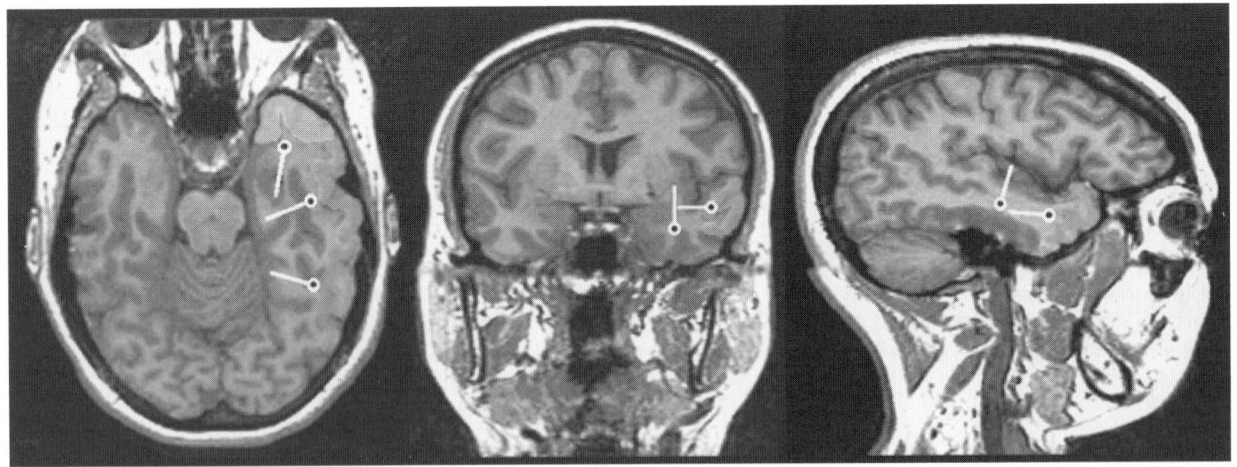

FIG. 23.3. Single dipoles of appropriate location and orientation can effectively model most temporal lobe surfaces. Vertical, tangential dipoles (*middle, right*) model the basal temporal cortex. Horizontal, tangential dipoles (*left, right*) model the temporal pole cortex. Horizontal, radial dipoles (*left, middle*) model the anterior and posterior lateral temporal cortex. (From Assaf BA, Ebersole JS. Continuous source imaging of scalp ictal rhythms in temporal lobe epilepsy. *Epilepsy* 1997;38:1114–1123, with permission.)

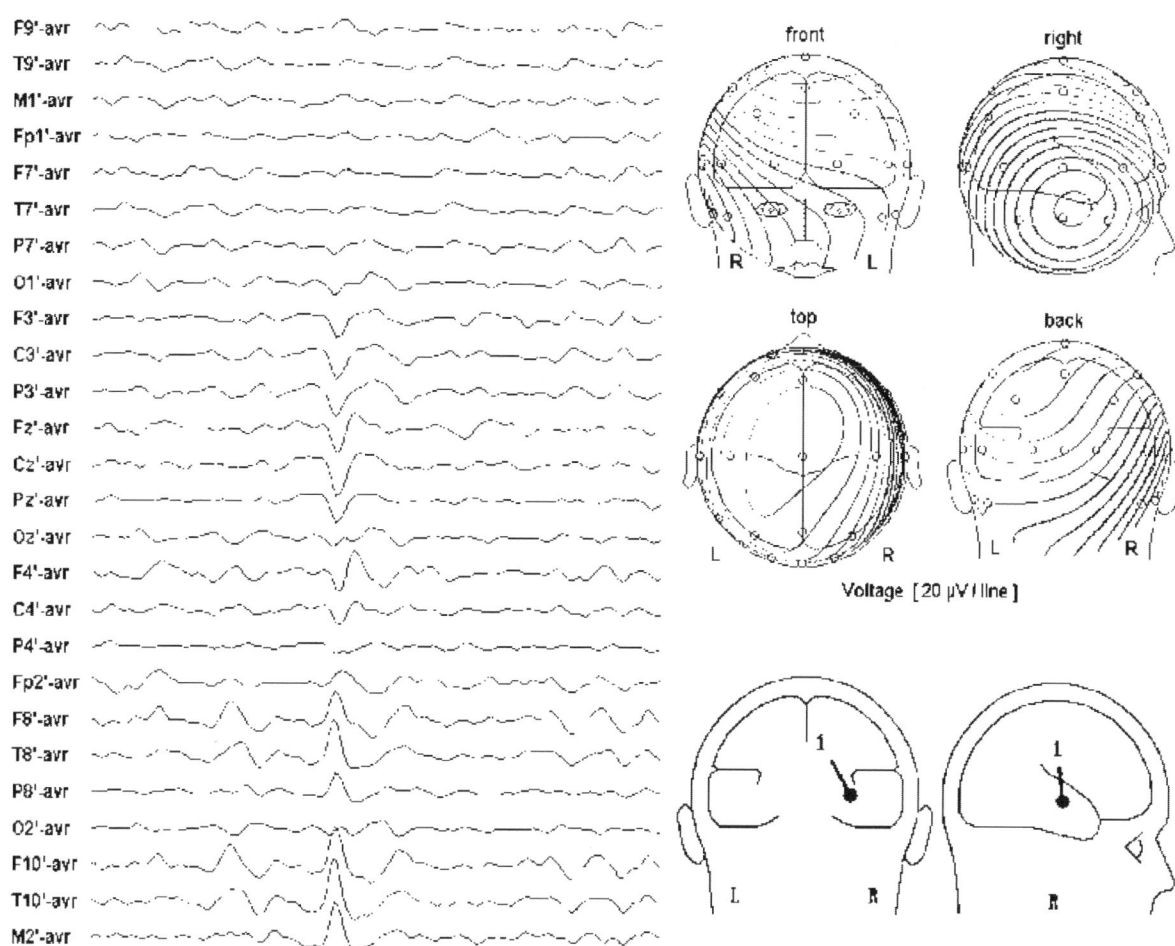

FIG. 23.4. Left: Right temporal type 1 spike. In this and subsequent figures, the EEG is depicted in a common average reference montage. **Top right:** Voltage topography of the spike at the cursor. In this and subsequent figures, the scalp voltage fields are illustrated by isopotential lines; the negative field is speckled. **Bottom right:** Single-dipole model of the spike field at the cursor and in the voltage map. Dot denotes location; vector denotes source orientation. Note the subtemporal negative field maximum and vertex positive field maximum, which are characteristic of type 1 spikes. The dipole model has an elevated orientation. Both the field and the dipole suggest a temporal basal cortex source. (From Ebersole JS. Sublobar localization of temporal epileptogenic foci by EEG source modeling. In: Williamson PD, Siegel AM, Roberts DW, et al, eds. *Neocortical epilepsies*. Philadelphia: Lippincott Williams & Wilkins, 2000:353–364, with permission.)

principally by basal and inferolateral cortex. Only these areas of temporal lobe cortex have a net orientation that could produce such a field. The type 1 spike field does not directly reflect hippocampal or amygdalar activity. Spikes confined to these structures do not generate scalp-recordable voltage fields because of the small source area and curved source shape, which favor voltage cancellation. Rather, it is the common and preferred propagation of this epileptiform activity from mesial structures into the entorhinal, fusiform, and other basal cortex that results in a generator of sufficient area to produce scalp EEG potentials (16,18,34). In general, some degree of propagation commonly occurs before either spike or seizure potentials are recordable at the scalp. Because voltage fields are orthogonal to the net orientation of their source cortex, a temporal lobe base spike is seen as subtemporal negativity and vertex positivity.

Spikes that originate in basal temporal cortex may produce a similar voltage field. Alternatively, these spikes frequently propagate into temporal tip cortex by the time sufficient cortex is activated to produce a scalp EEG field. Temporal tip cortex has a net anterior-facing orientation. Accordingly, spike sources in this cortex result in a voltage field with a frontotemporal-to-frontopolar negative maximum and a posterior positive

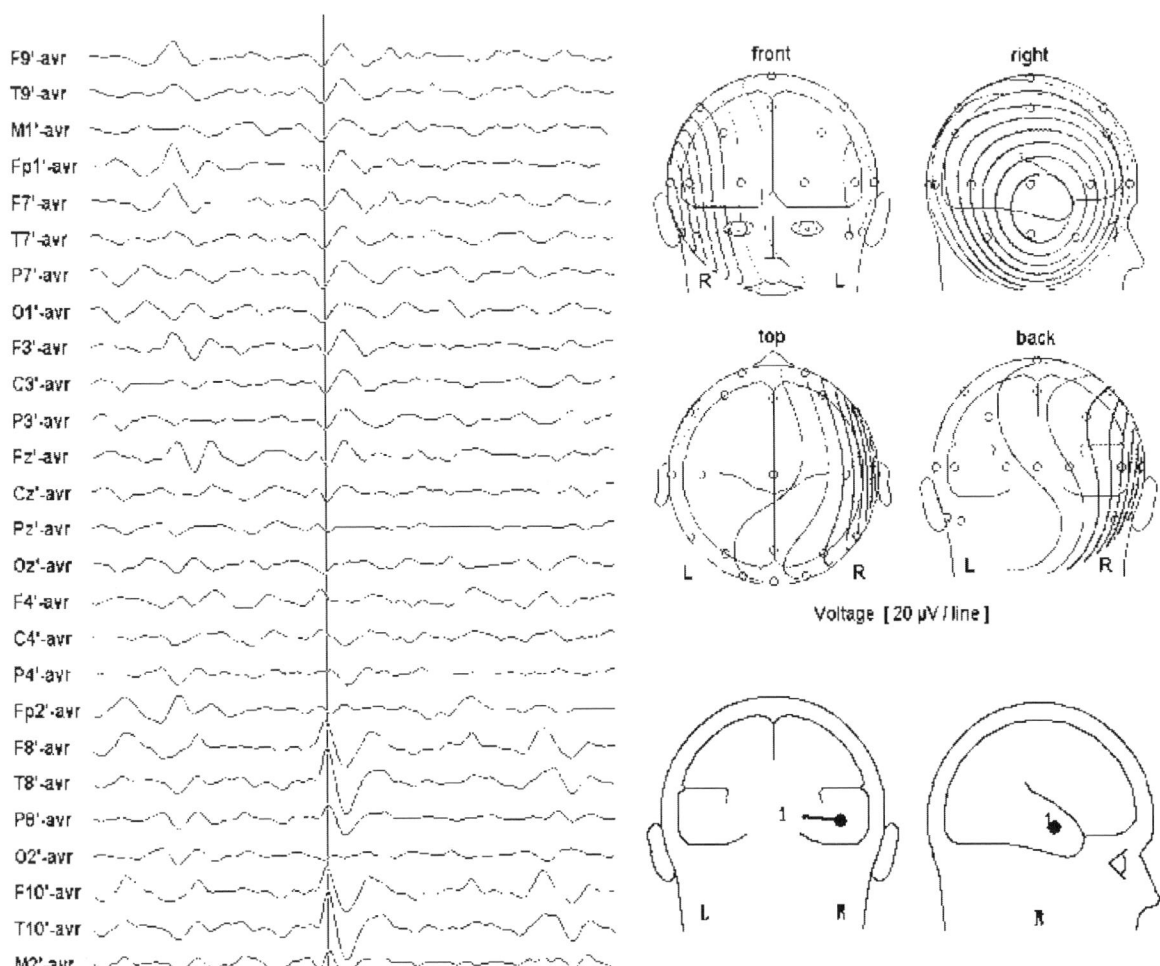

Voltage [20 µV / line]

FIG. 23.5. Left: Right temporal type 2 spike. **Top right:** Voltage topography of the spike at the cursor. **Bottom right:** Single-dipole model of the spike field at the cursor and in the voltage map. Note the lateral temporal negative field maximum and contralateral positive field maximum, which are characteristic of type 2 spikes. The dipole model has a horizontal and radial orientation. Both the field and the dipole suggest a lateral temporal cortex source. (From Ebersole JS. Sublobar localization of temporal epileptogenic foci by EEG source modeling. In: Williamson PD, Siegel AM, Roberts DW, et al, eds. *Neocortical epilepsies.* Philadelphia: Lippincott Williams & Wilkins, 2000: 353–364, with permission.)

maximum (16,47) (Fig. 23.6). That the source of such a field is temporal tip in origin rather than frontal pole can be appreciated by the negative and positive field voltage gradients, which are nearly equal, suggesting that the source lays near the zero isopotential line, which overlays the temporal lobe, rather than beneath the negative maximum over the frontal lobe.

Type 2 spikes are generated by lateral temporal cortex. These spikes commonly propagate in an anterior–posterior (AP) direction along the lateral convexity. The net vertical orientation of this temporal cortex results in a lateral negative maximum and a positive maximum over the contralateral

temporal area. Occasionally lateral temporal spikes will propagate medially into the basal cortex, which causes the later portions of its voltage field to change. It is therefore always important to consider the evolution of each spike voltage field. Because propagation is common, one cannot conclude that the voltage field of the spike peak best represents the character of the spike source. This is only true if the contours of the voltage field do not change over the course of the spike potential. Otherwise, the voltage topography and dipole model of the earliest portion of the spike potential should be regarded as being most closely associated with the spike origin (15,16).

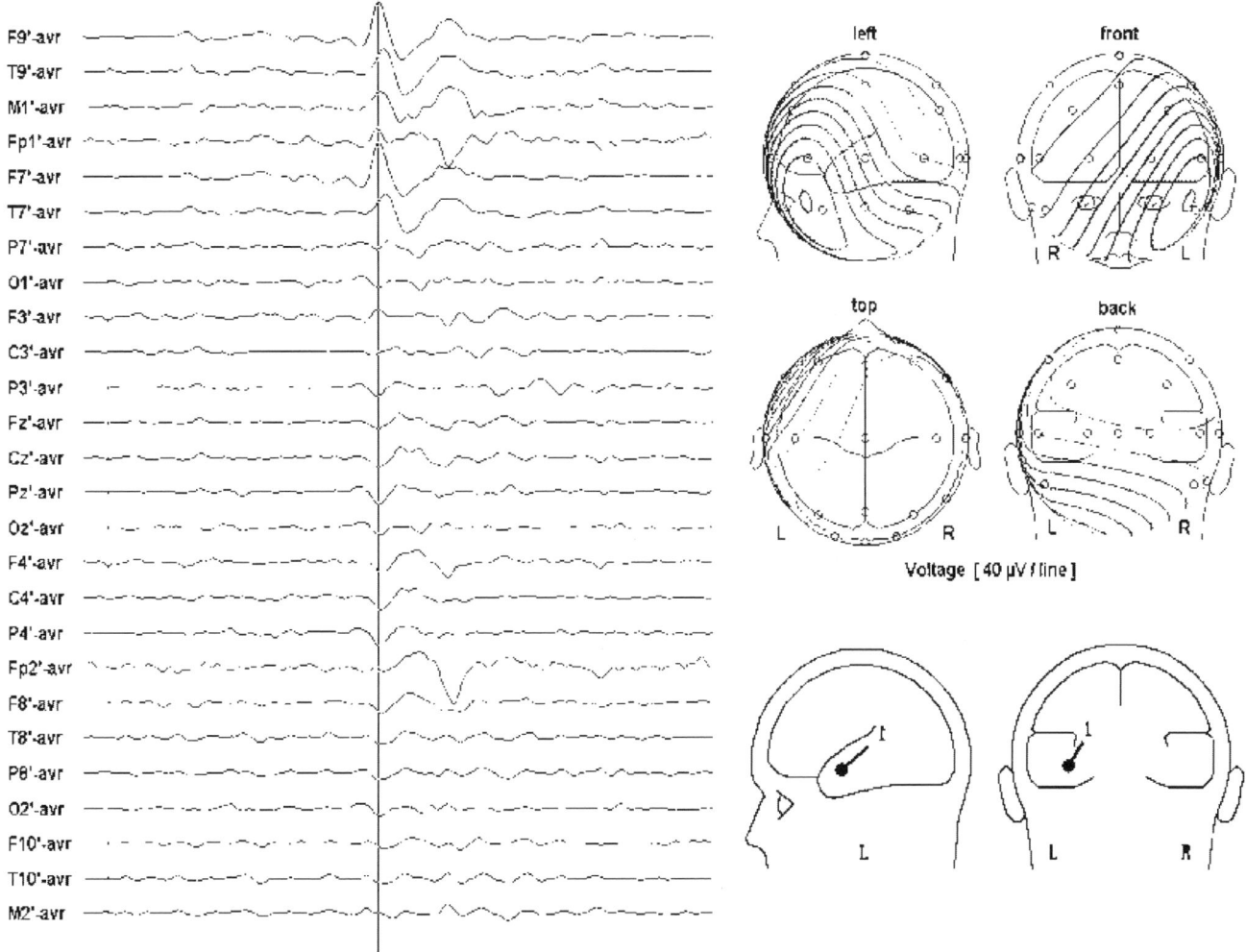

FIG. 23.6. Left: Left temporal tip spike. **Top right:** Voltage topography of the spike at the cursor. **Bottom right:** Single-dipole model of the spike field at the cursor and in the voltage map. Note the inferior frontotemporal negative field maximum and the contralateral posterior positive field maximum, which are characteristic of temporal tip spikes. The dipole model has mostly a horizontal and AP orientation. Both field and dipole suggest a temporal tip cortex source. (From Ebersole JS. Sublobar localization of temporal epileptogenic foci by EEG source modeling. In: Williamson PD, Siegel AM, Roberts DW, et al, eds. *Neocortical epilepsies*. Philadelphia: Lippincott Williams & Wilkins, 2000:353–364, with permission.)

DIPOLE MODELING IN TEMPORAL LOBE EPILEPSY

Single-Dipole Modeling

When single, instantaneous dipole modeling was performed on type 1 versus type 2 spike voltage topography, only dipole orientation (elevation) was significantly different between the two (13,14,19). In a group of 24 patients with anterior temporal discharges, models of type 1 spikes had a mean dipole elevation of 42 degrees (SD 5.0), whereas models of type 2 spikes had a mean dipole elevation of only 2 degrees (SD 10.0). Thus equivalent dipoles for type 2 spikes tend to have an orientation that is radial to the lateral skull convexity (see Fig. 23.5), whereas type 1 spike dipoles have a vertical or oblique orientation (see Fig. 23.4).

For some spikes, repeated single-dipole solutions are very consistent during the course of the spike. Their voltage fields rise and fall in magnitude but change little in position or orientation (see Fig. 23.1). As noted before, a single-dipole model fits these data well and suggests a focal cerebral generator. For other spikes, sequential solutions over the spike time course show progressive drift in dipole location and rotation of vector orientation (see Fig. 23.2). Such behavior is consistent with spike propagation or asynchronous activation of different cortical areas (13,14,19). A single moving dipole model may be misleading in an attempt to explain a complex field, which may be a composite from several generators.

Spatiotemporal Multiple-Dipole Modeling

Several different patterns of multiple-dipole models have emerged when applying this technique to the spikes of patients with temporal lobe epilepsy (13–16). Spikes with type 1 voltage topography usually require two or more dipoles to be modeled adequately (see Fig. 23.2). One of these dipoles typically has an orientation that is vertical and tangential to the lateral skull convexity, whereas the other is horizontal and radial. The tangential dipole is usually deeper than the radial one. Type 1 spike topography is the result of the superposition of fields from both sources when their activity overlaps in time. Source analysis of type 1 spikes from different patients has shown tangential source activity leading, lagging, or being synchronous with radial source activity. The pattern of voltage field evolution for a particular spike is thus dependent on the temporal relationships of its various source components. Information about the direction of spike propagation is conveyed by the sequence in which dipole sources become active. Simultaneous intracranial and scalp EEG recordings have validated previous assumptions that the vertical tangential dipole models activity from the basal temporal lobe cortex and the horizontal radial dipole models activity from the lateral temporal cortex (18,34). Basal-to-lateral cortex propagation and vice versa, suggested by timing differences in dipole source components, have also been confirmed.

The majority of spikes with type 2 topography require only one horizontal radial dipole to be modeled (see Figs. 23.2 and 23.5). In approximately one-third of patients, however, two or more dipoles are needed. In these cases, the dipoles usually differ in azimuth orientation and AP position, yet continue to be predominantly radial. Differences in timing between these sources can suggest anterior-to-posterior or, less commonly, posterior-to-anterior propagation along the lateral temporal convexity.

More recently, a third major cortical source contributing to temporal spike fields has been identified by dipole modeling (17,21,46,47). Synchronous activity of anterior temporal tip cortex results in a field with a negative maximum recorded from frontopolar and frontotemporal electrodes because of its net forward-facing orientation. Dipoles modeling this activity are horizontal, but have a distinct AP direction (see Fig. 23.6). Occasionally, spikes have just this dipole solution, but usually the tip component is present in combination with other temporal source components in more complex spikes exhibiting propagation.

Spatiotemporal modeling strategies using anatomical constraints can also be useful. Unconstrained inverse solutions consider any position within the spherical head model and any orientation of dipole vector to be equally likely as a source. This is obviously not true biologically. Spikes arise from cortex that has limited and definable locations and orientations. Of the two, it is more useful to specify the orientation of possible equivalent sources. As noted previously, it is reasonable to consider for purposes of modeling only the orientations of major lobar surfaces. For the temporal lobes, these dipole orientations are horizontal radial for the lateral convexity cortex, vertical tangential for the basal cortex and superior temporal plane, and AP horizontal tangential for the temporal tip. One approach in using this strategy for the temporal lobes is to create a priori a multiple spatiotemporal dipole model of major lobar surfaces and note from the source potentials of this model to what extent each constituent dipole contributes to explaining the scalp EEG voltage fields over time (1,2,41,46). This technique can be used to review continuous EEG in so-called source montages. Spikes or seizures, along with background rhythms, are decomposed into the source potential contributions of a fixed number of dipoles. For an EEG transient to appear in a particular source channel, it must have a voltage field that is appropriate for the dipole whose source potential that channel is displaying (see Figs. 23.11 through 23.13).

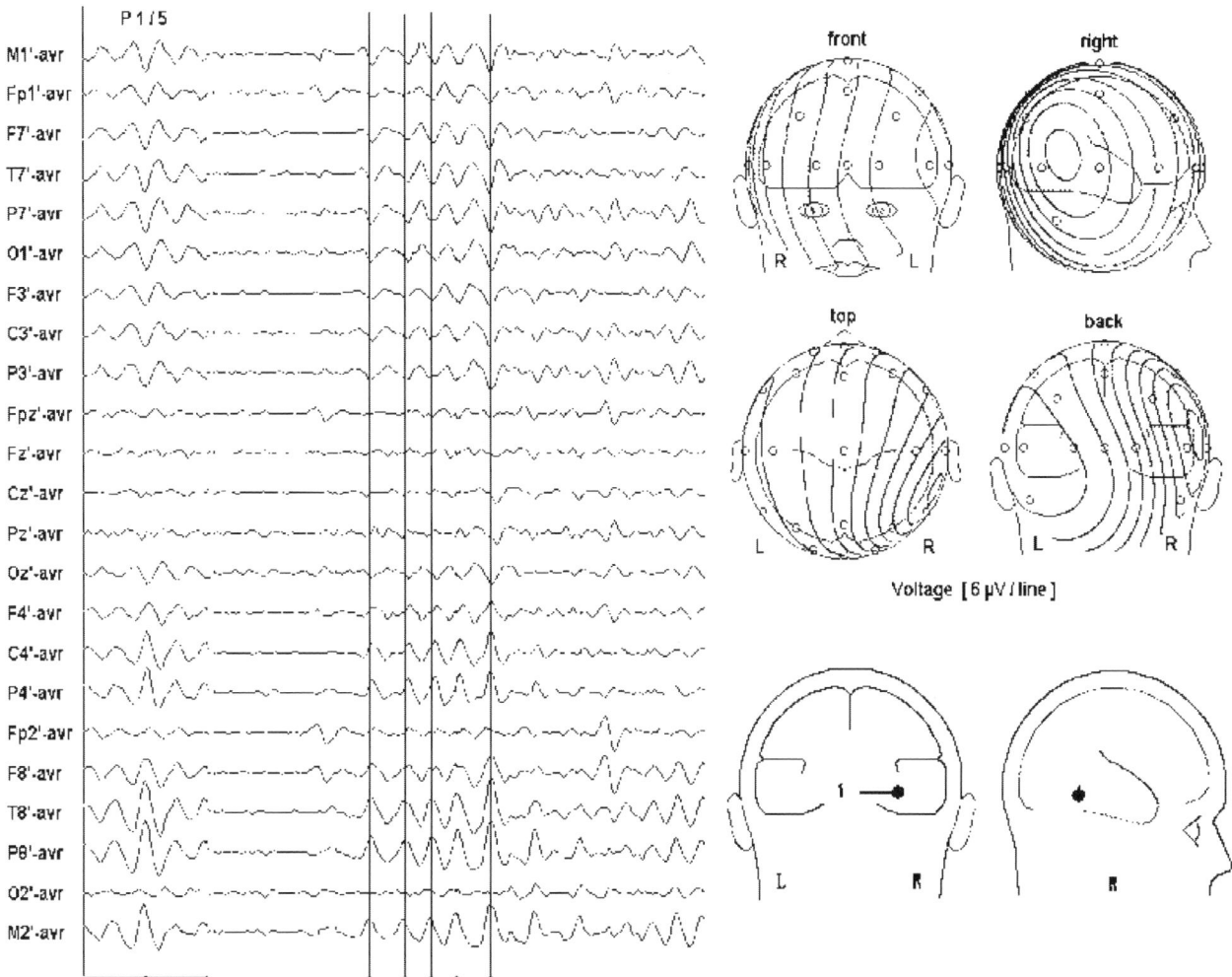

FIG. 23.7. Left: Right temporal type 2 seizure onset pattern. Cursors mark ictal potentials that were averaged to improve the signal-to-noise ratio. The averaged ictal waveform is at the far left. **Top right:** Voltage topography of the averaged ictal waveform at the cursor. **Bottom right:** Single-dipole model of the ictal field at the cursor and in the voltage map. Note the lateral, midposterior negative field maximum and the contralateral positive field maximum, which are characteristic of type 2 seizures. The dipole model has a horizontal and radial orientation. Both the field and the dipole suggest a lateral temporal cortex source. (From Ebersole JS. Sublobar localization of temporal epileptogenic foci by EEG source modeling. In: Williamson PD, Siegel AM, Roberts DW, et al, eds. *Neocortical epilepsies.* Philadelphia: Lippincott Williams & Wilkins, 2000:353–364, with permission.)

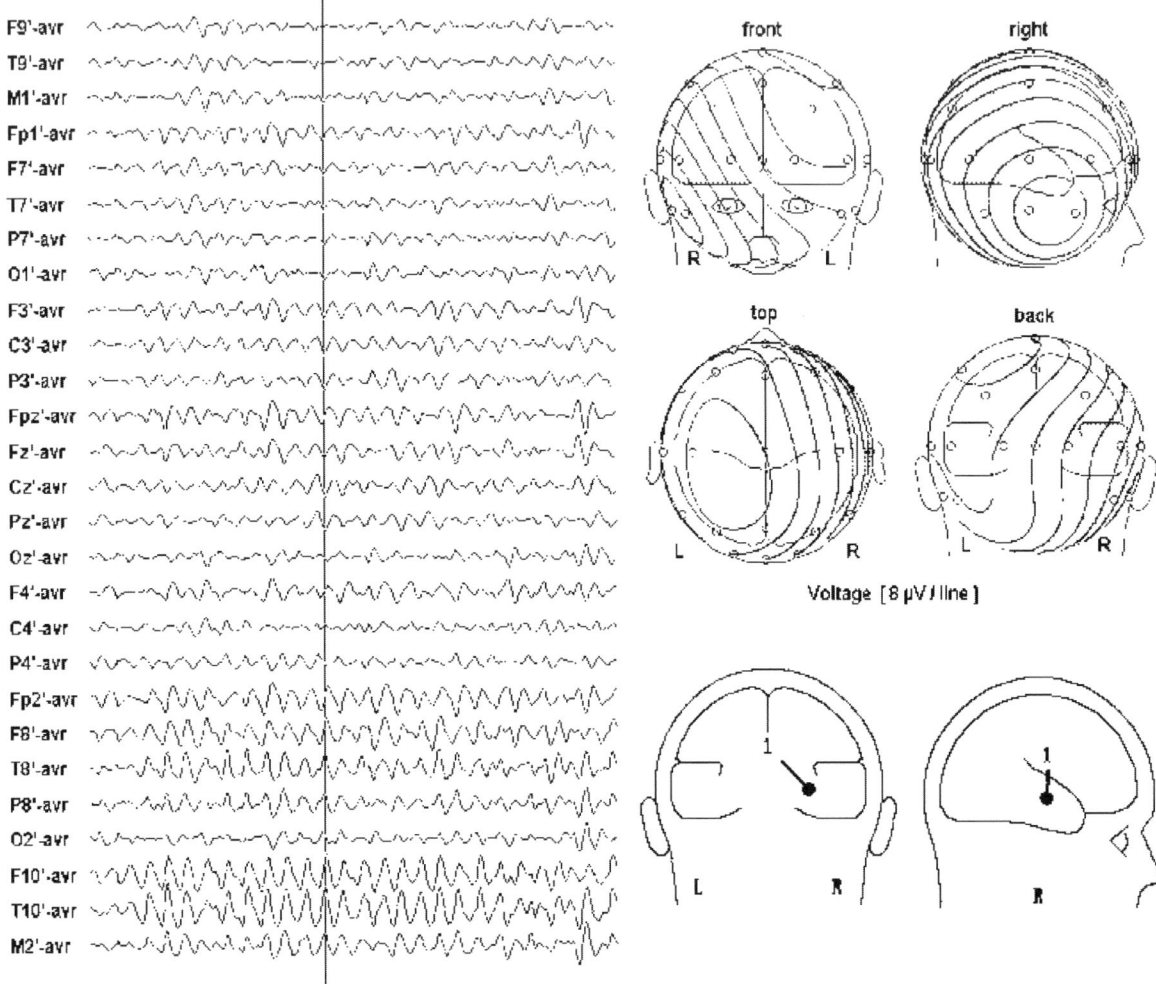

FIG. 23.8. **Left:** Right temporal type 1 seizure onset pattern. **Top right:** Voltage topography of the ictal waveform at the cursor. **Bottom right:** Single-dipole model of the ictal field at the cursor and in the voltage map. Note the anterior subtemporal field maximum and the vertex positive field maximum, which are characteristic of type 1 seizures. The dipole model has an elevated orientation. Both the field and the dipole suggest a temporal basal cortex source. (From Ebersole JS. Sublobar localization of temporal epileptogenic foci by EEG source modeling. In: Williamson PD, Siegel AM, Roberts DW, et al, eds. *Neocortical epilepsies.* Philadelphia: Lippincott Williams & Wilkins, 2000:353–364, with permission.)

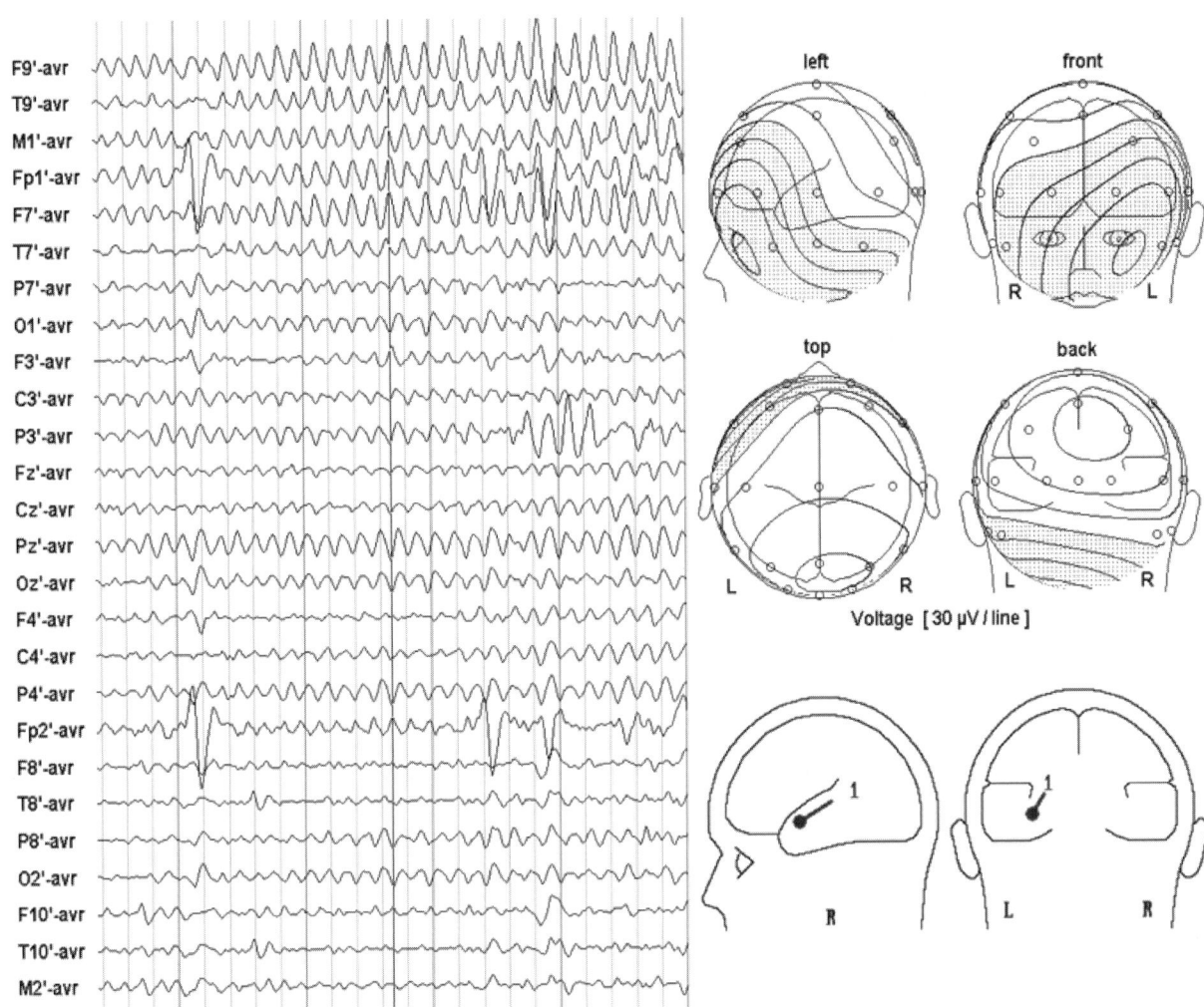

FIG. 23.9. Left: Left temporal tip seizure onset pattern. **Top right:** Voltage topography of the ictal waveform at the cursor. **Bottom right:** Single-dipole model of the ictal field at the cursor and in the voltage map. Note the inferior frontal negative field maximum and the posterior positive field maximum, which are characteristic of temporal tip seizures. The dipole model has mostly a horizontal and AP orientation. Both the field and the dipole suggest a temporal tip cortex source. (From Ebersole JS. Sublobar localization of temporal epileptogenic foci by EEG source modeling. In: Williamson PD, Siegel AM, Roberts DW, et al, eds. *Neocortical epilepsies.* Philadelphia: Lippincott Williams & Wilkins, 2000:353–364, with permission.)

DIPOLE MODELING OF TEMPORAL LOBE SEIZURES

Dipole modeling can also be applied to seizure rhythms with some modifications in the protocol used for spikes (4–7,15,17). The earliest recognizable seizure potentials should be preferentially modeled because they are more likely to reflect the seizure origin than are later rhythms, which usually evolve only after significant propagation. Because ictal-onset rhythms are typically of low amplitude and commonly are confounded with movement and muscle artifact, averaging successive potentials may be necessary to increase the signal-to-noise ratio. The key is to average seizure waveforms with similar voltage topographies (Fig. 23.7); only these reflect the same source configuration. Ictal EEG voltage fields are usually spatially stable for only a few seconds, however. Tight bandpass filtering is also useful in ictal dipole modeling. Most temporal lobe seizure frequencies are less than 12 Hz. A high-frequency filter of 13–20 Hz is therefore reasonable to reduce muscle artifact. Similarly, a low linear filter of 1–2 Hz will minimize low-frequency artifact secondary to movement of the patient or electrode leads.

The orientation of dipole models of ictal waveforms carries the same significance as those of spikes, in that it is most useful in identifying sublobar temporal lobe sources (1,2,4–7,15,17,46). Temporal lobe seizures modeled by dipoles with dominant horizontal radial, vertical tangential, or AP horizontal tangential orientations are most likely associated with lateral temporal, hippocampal/basal, or temporal tip seizures, respectively (Figs. 23.7 through 23.9). Additionally, many temporal lobe seizures are modeled best by dipoles having an anterior oblique orientation, that is, a combination of all three of the previous orientations (Fig. 23.10). In this case, the ictally active cortical region includes inferior, tip, and lateral temporal cortex. Multiple fixed dipole models also can be used to identify the contribution of various sublobar cortical

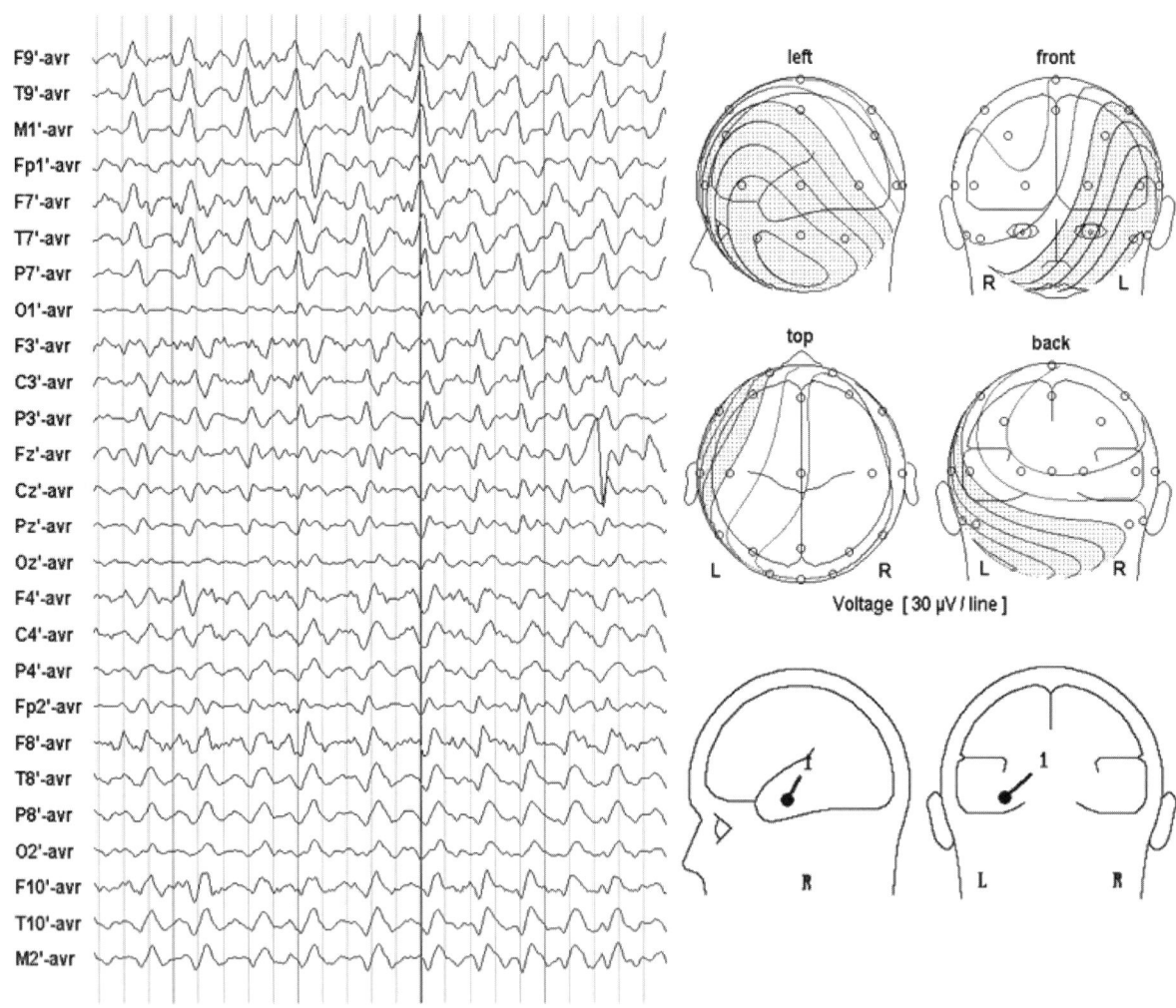

FIG. 23.10. Left: Left temporal, "oblique dipole" seizure onset pattern. **Top right:** Voltage topography of the ictal waveform at the cursor. **Bottom right:** Single-dipole model of the ictal field at the cursor and in the voltage map. Note the anterior subtemporal negative field maximum and the posterior vertex positive field maximum, which are characteristic of these temporal seizures. The dipole model has an anterior oblique orientation. Both the field and the dipole suggest a temporal source involving the anterior basal tip and inferolateral cortex. (From Ebersole JS. Sublobar localization of temporal epileptogenic foci by EEG source modeling. In: Williamson PD, Siegel AM, Roberts DW, et al, eds. *Neocortical epilepsies.* Philadelphia: Lippincott Williams & Wilkins, 2000:353–364, with permission.)

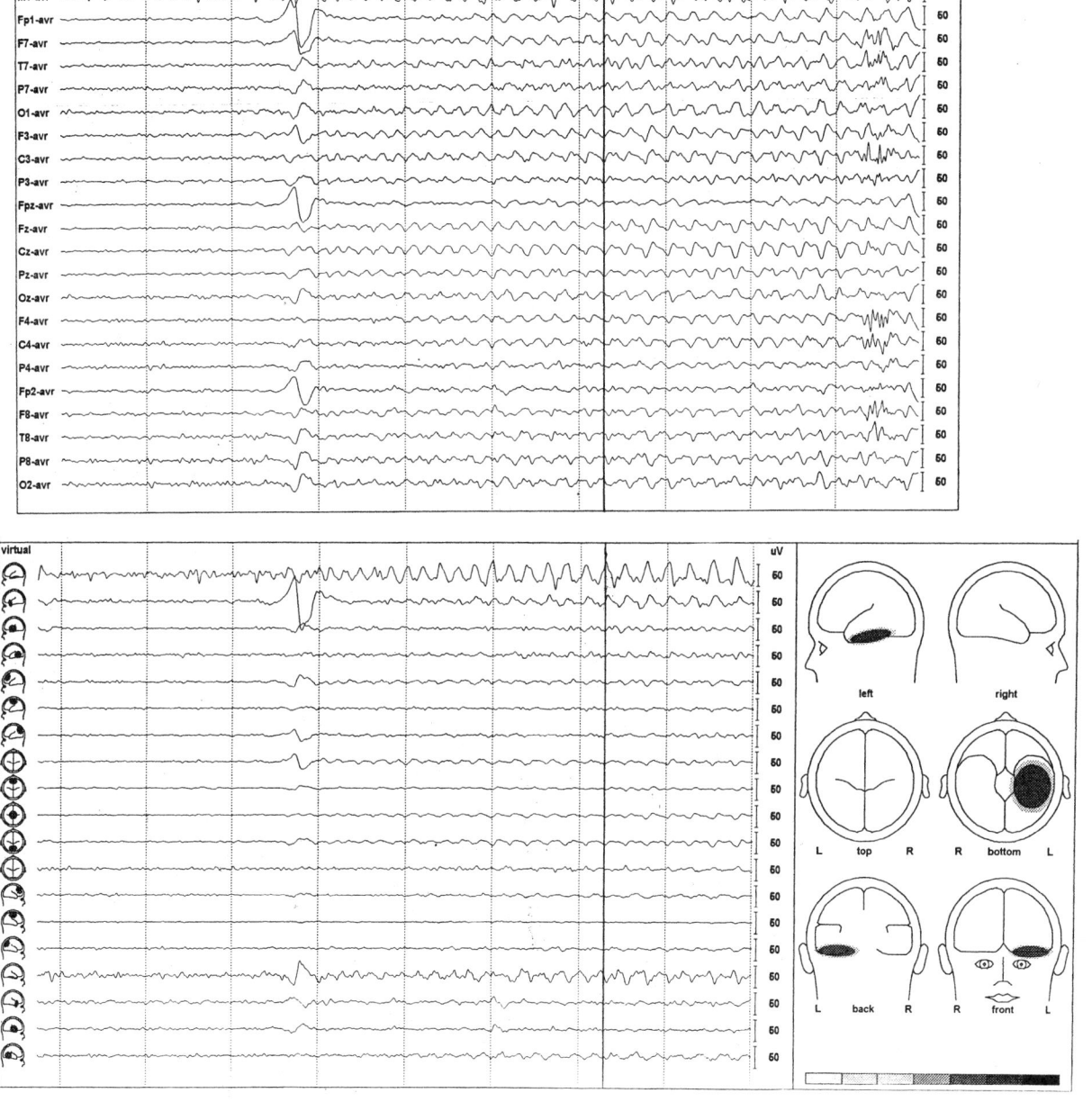

FIG. 23.11. Top: Traditional EEG depiction of a hippocampal-onset seizure, which produces an ictal rhythm with a widespread scalp distribution. **Bottom:** Same seizure displayed in a continuous source imaging montage (Focus 1.1), which decomposes the EEG into the activity of 19 dipolar sources modeling selected cortical surfaces, four of which are in each temporal lobe. The prominent left basal temporal source component (*top trace*) accounts for most of the ictal rhythm. The source image (*right*) displays the most active cortical region at the time of the cursor. In this and in Figures 23.12 and 23.13, the top EEG is displayed in a common average reference with 2- to 20-Hz bandpass filtering. Calibration markers: 60 μV, 1 second. (From Assaf BA, Ebersole JS. Continuous source imaging of scalp ictal rhythms in temporal lobe epilepsy. *Epilepsy* 1997;38: 1114–1123, with permission.)

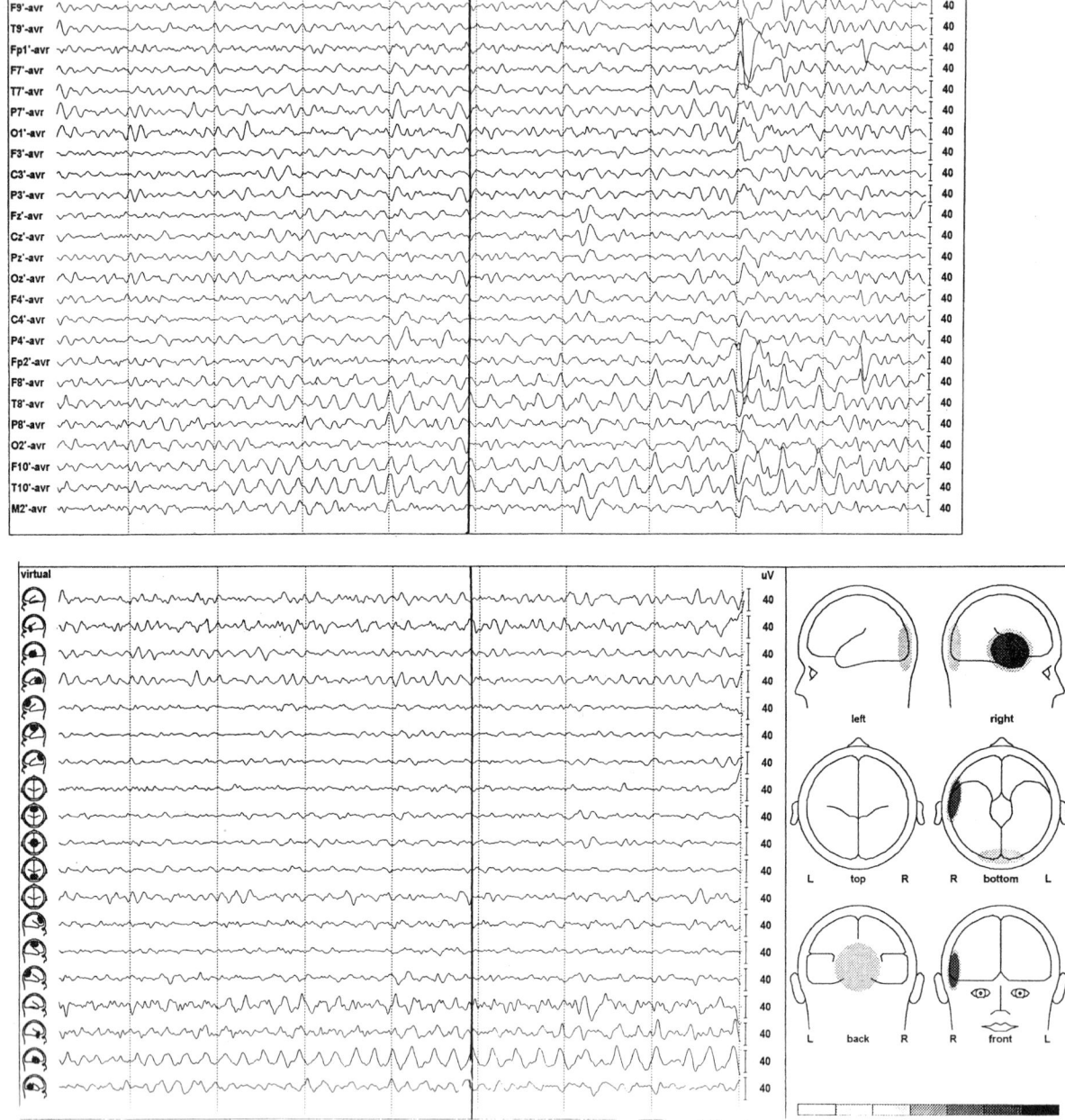

FIG. 23.12. Top: Scalp EEG of a right temporal seizure of lateral neocortical origin. **Bottom:** A prominent anterolateral temporal source component (next to last trace) is evident when the same seizure is displayed in the source imaging montage. **Right:** The most active cortical region at the time of the cursor. Calibration markers: 40 μV, 1 second. (From Assaf BA, Ebersole JS. Continuous source imaging of scalp ictal rhythms in temporal lobe epilepsy. *Epilepsy* 1997;38: 1114–1123, with permission.)

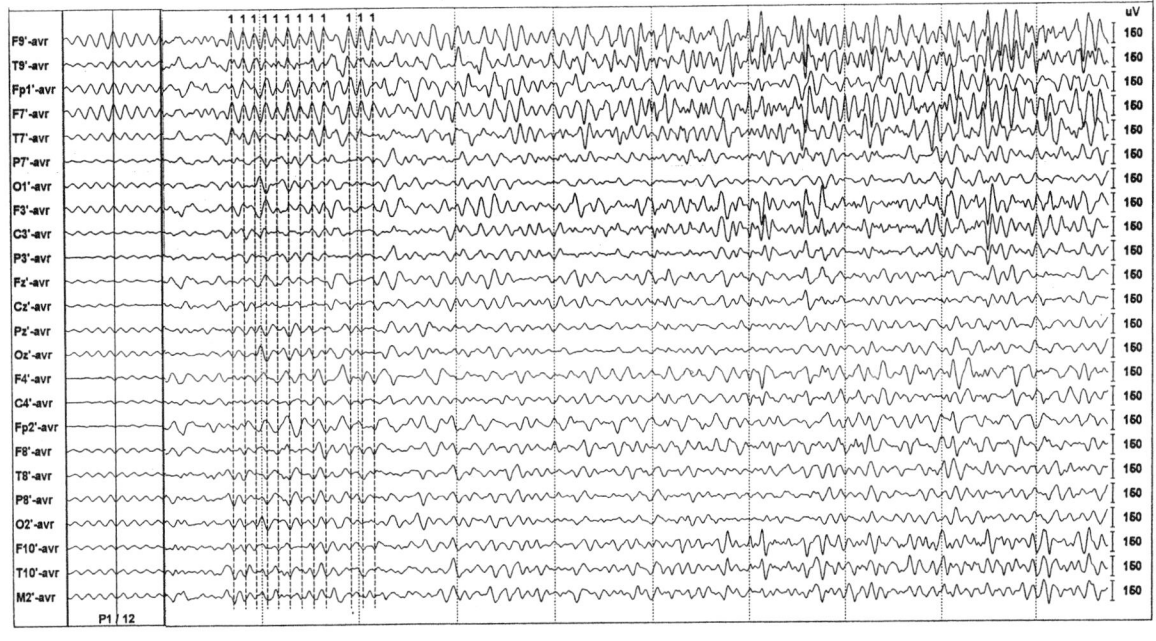

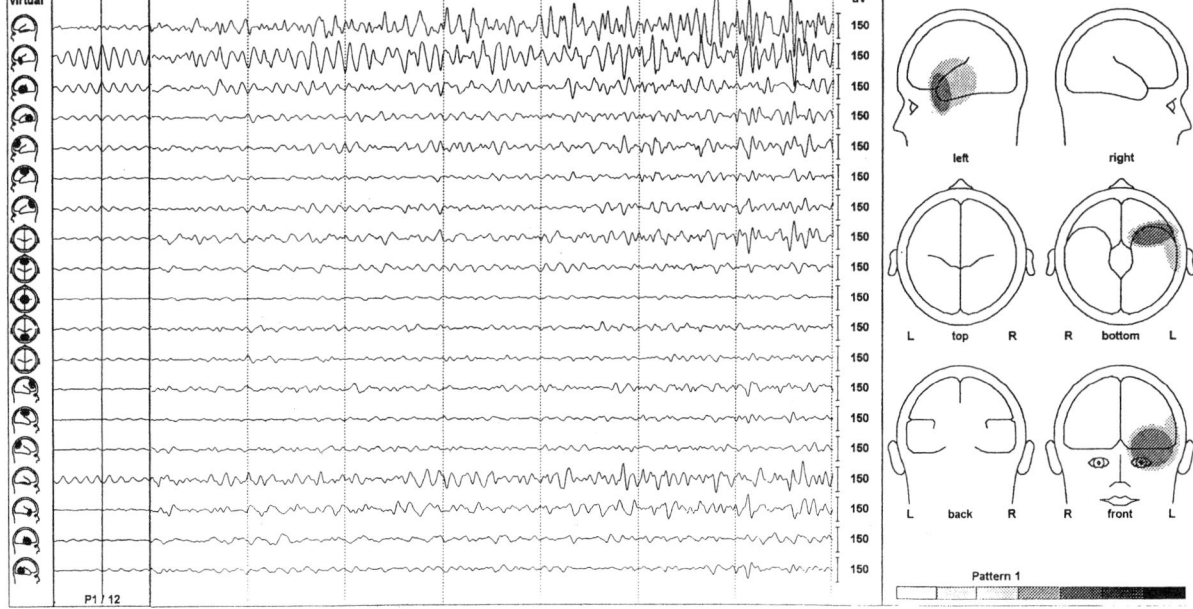

FIG. 23.13. Top: Scalp EEG of a left temporal seizure of entorhinal cortex origin. Cursors "1" mark the 12 waveforms of the ictal rhythm that were averaged to improve the signal-to-noise ratio. **Top Left:** Resultant averaged ictal EEG. **Bottom:** A prominent temporal tip source component is evident when the same seizure is displayed in the source imaging montage. This is better appreciated in the averaged ictal data shown at left. **Bottm Right:** The most active cortical region at the time of the cursor. Calibration markers: 150 μV, 1 second. (From Assaf BA, Ebersole JS. Continuous source imaging of scalp ictal rhythms in temporal lobe epilepsy. *Epilepsy* 1997;38:1114–1123, with permission.)

areas to seizure potentials (Figs. 23.11 through 23.13). This technique has been used to determine temporal lobe seizure origins and to predict surgical outcome following standard temporal lobectomy (1,2,17,41,46).

Ictal EEG dipole models have been correlated with intracranial EEG and surgical outcome (1,2,4–7,15,46). The results are similar to those found with spike dipole modeling. Patients with seizures modeled by horizontal radial dipoles, which suggest a lateral cortex origin, do less well following a standard anteromesial resection and should be considered candidates for invasive monitoring and possibly tailored temporal lobe resections. Patients whose seizures are modeled best by dipoles with a vertical, horizontal AP, or anterior oblique orientation have seizures originating probably in mesial structures: basil, entorhinal, or temporal tip cortex, respectively. All of these patients do well following surgery because these cortices are customarily removed in the standard temporal lobe resection.

Other laboratories have confirmed the utility of EEG dipole modeling in the evaluation of patients with focal epilepsy (3,27–31). There is a consensus that most spikes (and seizures) can be modeled usefully by equivalent dipoles and that activated regions of cortex, rather than mesial structures in the temporal lobe, are the sources. These investigators have also found that dipole orientation more clearly differentiates basomesial from lateral temporal epilepsy than does dipole location. Similarly, change in dipole orientation over time is a better marker of spike propagation than the trajectory of the dipole locus.

CO-REGISTERING EEG DATA WITH MAGNETIC RESONANCE IMAGING AND REALISTIC HEAD MODELS

With the advent of computed tomography and more recently magnetic resonance imaging (MRI), detailed anatomical information about an individual's head and brain are readily available. Only very recently, however, have these data been combined with EEG to provide "functional imaging" of the brain's electrical activity. One of the earliest EEG-related observations using three-dimensional (3-D) MRI reconstructions was the geometrical relationship between standard scalp electrode positions and the underlying brain. As illustrated in Figure 23.14, the standard international 10-20 temporal electrode chain passes across the superior aspect of the temporal lobe. Supplementary inferior temporal electrodes are necessary for properly recording the negative field of basal frontal, temporal, and occipital spikes/seizures. By digitizing the scalp electrode locations and certain head landmark fiducials, such as the nasion and preauricular points in 3-D space, the topography of the scalp EEG fields could be co-registered with and superimposed on a 3-D MRI reconstruction of the patient's head or brain. In similar fashion, calculated dipole models could be co-registered with the same 3-D brain image (16,23,40) (Fig. 23.15).

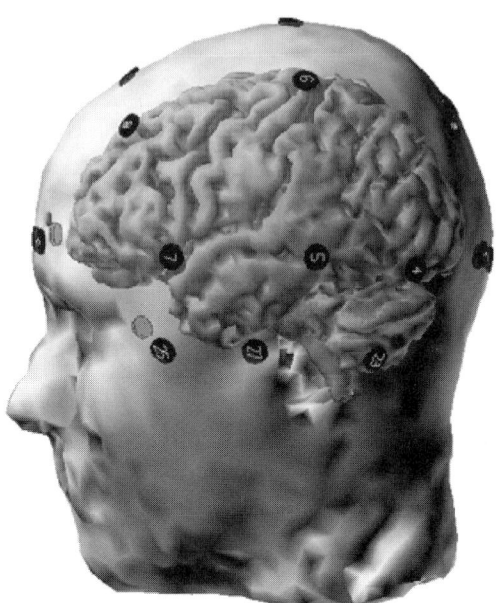

FIG. 23.14. Standard international 10-20 and supplementary subtemporal scalp electrode positions superimposed on transparent three-dimensional reconstructions of the head and brain. Note that the standard longitudinal temporal chain of electrodes passes over the superior aspect of the temporal lobe. Only subtemporal electrodes effectively record from the inferolateral and basal temporal cortex. (From Ebersole JS. Defining epileptogenic foci: past, present, and future. *J Clin Neurophysiol* 1997;14:470–483, with permission.)

It has been appreciated for some time that the spherical head model commonly used to calculate EEG dipoles was a convenient approximation, but an approximation nonetheless. Systematic errors in dipole location introduced by spherical head models have been identified (10,11,43). Roth and colleagues (35,36) first simulated and more recently studied real EEG sources in the temporal and frontal lobes to compare the effects of spherical versus realistic head models on dipole solutions. They noted location errors in the spherical models of 1–3 cm that were worse in the vertical or Z direction. Yvert et al. (49,50) and Fuchs et al. (21,22) simulated EEG dipoles sources throughout the brain and found that spherical head modeling errors were worse for basal regions and in the Z direction. These results were also confirmed using temporal lobe spike and seizure foci as the source and validating the true location of these foci with intracranial EEG (16). Segmented volumetric MRI data were used to calculate a realistic head model by the boundary element method (Fig. 23.16). Dipoles

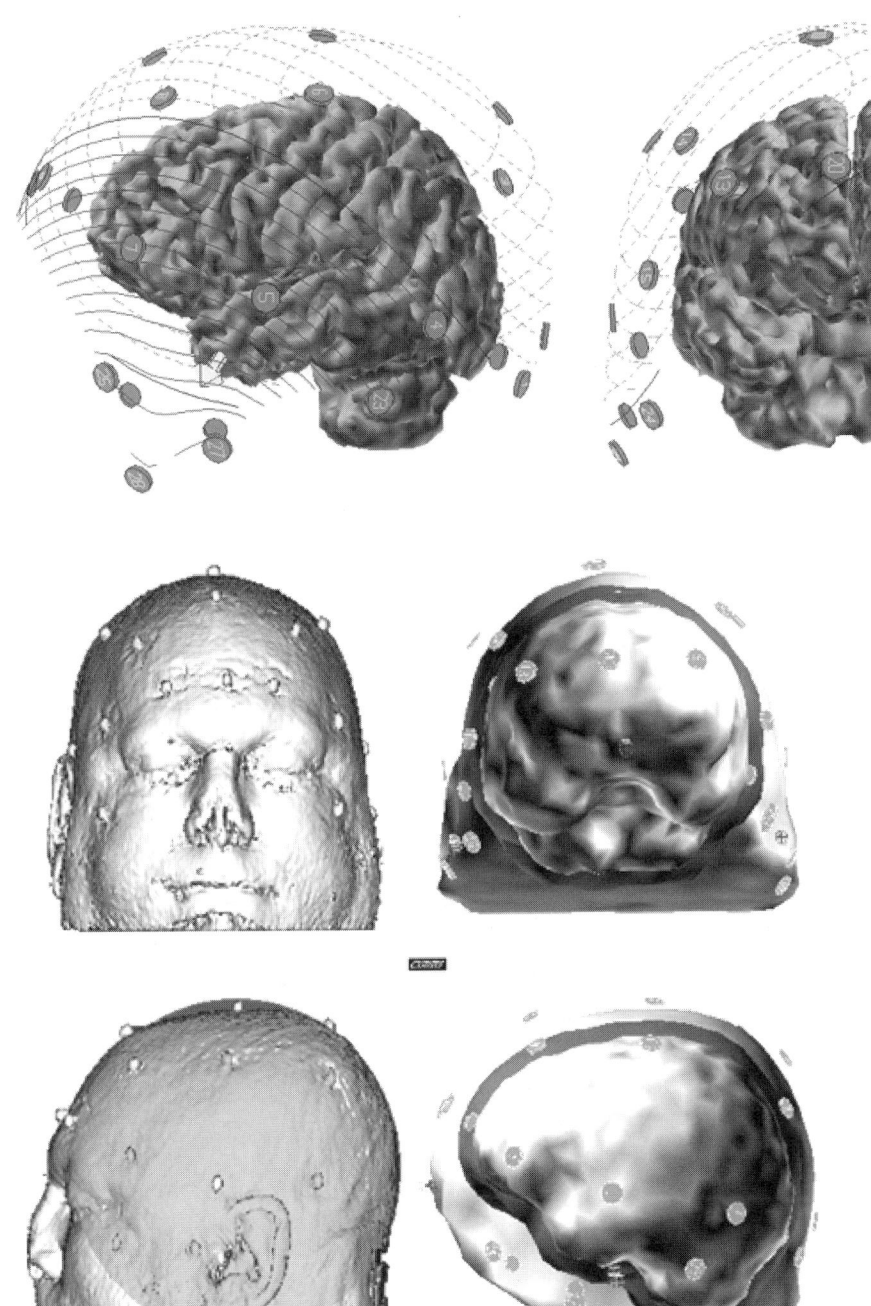

FIG. 23.15. Scalp voltage isopotential field lines of a left temporal spike and recording electrode positions are superimposed on a three-dimensional reconstruction of the patient's brain. Dipole model of the spike source is depicted as an *arrow* emerging from the temporal tip.

FIG. 23.16. Right: Realistic boundary element method (BEM) head model (inner and outer surfaces of skull and scalp) derived from three-dimensional MRI reconstructions. **Left:** *Shaded circle* on patient's head depicts the shape of typical spherical head models. Note divergence of the brain and skull base from this spherical shape. (From Ebersole JS. Defining epileptogenic foci: past, present, and future. *J Clin Neurophysiol* 1997;14:470–483, with permission.)

calculated with spherical head models were misplaced on average 2–3 cm upward from their true temporal lobe source (Figs. 23.17 and 23.18). In several patients, this gave the false impression that the spike/seizure sources were of frontal rather than temporal lobe origin. It would appear that realistic head models should be used whenever dipoles are co-registered with MRI for interpretation. This is particularly so for basal frontal, temporal, and occipital sources, where brain cortex and skull depart most from a spherical shape.

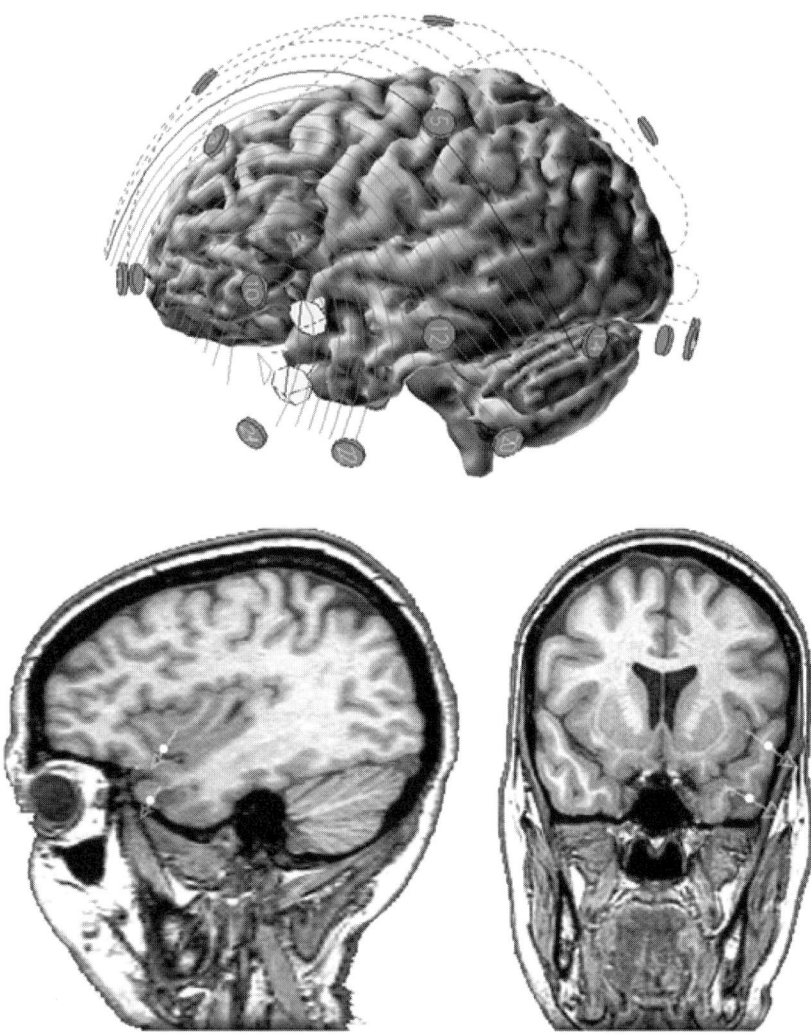

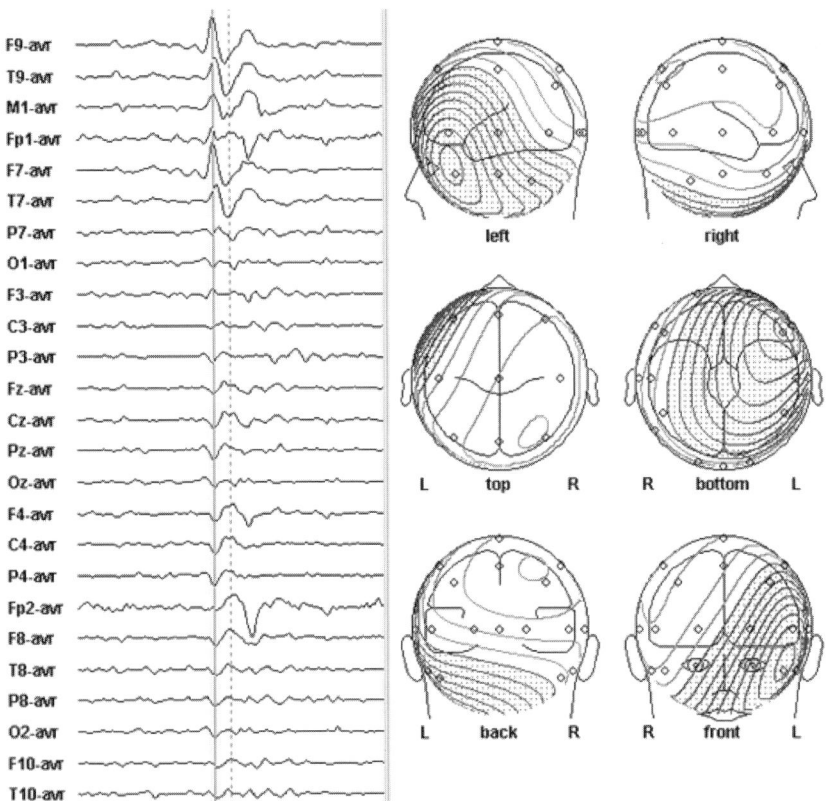

FIG. 23.17. **Left:** Common average reference EEG of a left anterior inferior temporal spike. **Right:** Voltage topography of the same spike at the cursor.

FIG. 23.18. Dipole models of the spike in Figure 23.17, calculated with spherical and realistic BEM head models, are co-registered with three-dimensional (*top*) and two-dimensional MRI sections of the patient's brain. The dipole model derived from a spherical head model is displaced approximately 2.5 cm above that obtained with a realistic head model. The actual spike source is the cortex surrounding the cystic lesion adjacent to the lower dipole.

EXTENDED SOURCE MODELS

Though very useful as a model of EEG sources, the dipole model is unrealistic. Actual brain sources of EEG potentials are extended areas of activated cortex. A number of "extended" or "distributed" models have been employed to simulate more accurately the character of cerebral epileptogenic sources (23,32,34). Some of these use brain anatomy as a powerful reconstruction parameter to restrict the search space to the cortical surface (23). Algorithms have been devised that can calculate discrete approximations of the current density distribution on a defined surface. This current source density estimate is an ill-posed problem, however, if many local sources are to be calculated from measurements at relatively few electrode locations. Regularization is necessary to proceed in these circumstances. This represents a compromise between the demands to explain the measured data and to meet certain source or boundary conditions. One such boundary condition is the minimum norm criterion, in which the source constellation of lowest electrical power is calculated. Variations include the L2 or L1 norms (23) or the minimum spatial Laplacian (34).

Although these methods can produce seductive images of "activated" cortex, much the same as functional MRI, considerable research is needed to validate the accuracy of the results.

REFERENCES

1. Assaf BA, Ebersole JS. Continuous source imaging of scalp ictal rhythms in temporal lobe epilepsy. *Epilepsia* 1997;38:1114–1123.
2. Assaf BA, Ebersole JS. Visual and quantitative ictal EEG predictors of outcome after temporal lobectomy. *Epilepsia* 1999;40:52–61.
3. Baumgartner C, Lindinger G, Ebner A, et al. Propagation of interictal epileptic activity in temporal lobe epilepsy. *Neurology* 1995;45:118–122.
4. Boon P, D'Have M. Interictal and ictal dipole modeling in patients with refractory partial epilepsy. *Acta Neurol Scand* 1995;92:7–18.
5. Boon P, D'Have M, Adam C, et al. Dipole modeling in epilepsy surgery candidates. *Epilepsia* 1997;38:208–218.
6. Boon P, D'Have M, Vanderkerckhove T, et al. Dipole modeling and intracranial EEG recording: correlation between dipole and ictal onset zone. *Acta Neurochir (Wien)* 1997;139:643–652.
7. Boon P, D'Have M, Van Hoey G, et al. Source localization in refractory partial epilepsy. *Rev Neurol* 1999;155:499–508.
8. Brody DA, Terry FH, Ideker RE. Eccentric dipole in spherical medium: generalized expression for surface potentials. *IEEE Trans Biomed Eng* 1973;20:141–143.
9. Cooper R, Winter AL, Crow HJ, et al. Comparison of subcortical, cortical and scalp activity using chronically indwelling electrodes in man. *Electroencephalogr Clin Neurophysiol* 1965;18:217–228.
10. Cuffin BN. Effects of head shape on EEG's and MEG's. *IEEE Trans Biomed Eng* 1990;37:44–52.
11. Cuffin BN. EEG localization accuracy improvements using realistically shaped head models. *IEEE Trans Biomed Eng* 1996;43:299–303.
12. Darcey TM, Ary JP, Fender DH. Methods for the localization of electrical sources in the human brain. *Prog Brain Res* 1980;54:128–134.
13. Ebersole JS. Equivalent dipole modeling: a new EEG method for epileptogenic focus localization. In: Pedley TA, Meldrum BS, eds. *Recent Advances in Epilepsy*, Vol 5. Edinburgh: Churchill Livingstone, 1991:51–72.
14. Ebersole JS. EEG dipole modeling in complex partial epilepsy. *Brain Topogr* 1991;4:113–123.
15. Ebersole JS. Noninvasive localization of the epileptogenic focus by EEG dipole modeling. *Acta Neurol Scand Suppl* 1994;152:20–28.
16. Ebersole JS. Defining epileptogenic foci: past, present, and future. *J Clin Neurophysiol* 1997;14:470–483.
17. Ebersole JS. Sublobar localization of temporal neocortical epileptogenic foci by EEG source modeling. In: Williamson PD, Siegel AM, Roberts DW, et al, eds. *Neocortical epilepsies*. Philadelphia: Lippincott Williams & Wilkins, 2000:353–364.
18. Ebersole JS, Hawes S, Scherg M. Intracranial EEG validation of spike propagation predicted by dipole models. *Electroencephalogr Clin Neurophysiol* 1995;95:18.
19. Ebersole JS, Wade PB. Spike voltage topography and equivalent dipole localization in complex partial epilepsy. *Brain Topogr* 1990;3:21–34.
20. Ebersole JS, Wade PB. Spike voltage topography identifies two types of fronto-temporal epileptic foci. *Neurology* 1991;41:1425–1433.
21. Fuchs M, Drenckhahn R, Wischmann H-A, et al. An improved boundary element method for realistic volume-conductor modeling. *IEEE Trans Biomed Eng* 1998;45:980–997.
22. Fuchs M, Wagner M, Kastner J. Boundary element method volume conductor models for EEG source reconstruction. *Clin Neurophysiol* 2001;112:1400–1407.
23. Fuchs M, Wagner M, Kohler T, et al. Linear and nonlinear current density reconstructions. *J Clin Neurophysiol* 1999;16:267–295.
24. Helmholtz H. Uber einige Gesetze der Vertheilung elektrischer Strome in korperlichen Leitern, mit Anwendung auf die thierischelekrischen Versuche. *Ann Phys Chem* 1853;29:211–233, 353–377.
25. Henderson CJ, Butler SR, Glass A. The localization of equivalent dipoles of EEG sources by the application of electrical field theory. *Electroencephalogr Clin Neurophysiol* 1975;39:117–130.
26. Kavanagh RN, Darcey TM, Lehmann D, et al. Evaluation of methods for three-dimensional localization of electrical sources in the human brain. *IEEE Trans Biomed Eng* 1978;25:421–429.
27. Lantz G, Holub M, Ryding E, et al. Simultaneous intracranial and extracranial recording of interictal epileptiform activity in patients with drug resistant partial epilepsy: patterns of conduction and results from dipole reconstructions. *Electroencephalogr Clin Neurophysiol* 1996;99:69–78.
28. Lantz G, Ryding E, Rosen I. Three-dimensional localization of interictal epileptiform activity with dipole analysis: comparison with intracranial recordings and SPECT findings. *J Epilepsy* 1994;7:117–129.
29. Merlet I, Garcia-Larrea L, Gregoire MC, et al. Source propagation of interictal spikes in temporal lobe epilepsy. *Brain* 1996;119:377–392.
30. Merlet I, Gotman J. Reliability of dipole models of epileptic spikes. *Clin Neurophysiol* 1999;110:1013–1028.
31. Merlet I, Gotman J. Dipole modeling of scalp EEG epileptic discharges: correlation with intracerebral fields. *Clin Neurophysiol* 2001;112:414–430.
32. Michel CM, Grave de Peralta R, Lantz G, et al. Spatiotemporal EEG analysis and distributed source estimation in presurgical epilepsy evaluation. *J Clin Neurophysiol* 1999;16:239–266.
33. Pacia SV, Ebersole JS. Intracranial EEG substrates of scalp ictal patterns from temporal lobe foci. *Epilepsia* 1997;38:642–653.
34. Pasqual-Marqui RD, Michel CM, Lehmann D. Low resolution electromagnetic tomography: a new method for localizing electrical activity in the brain. *Int J Psychophysiol* 1994;18:49–65.

35. Roth BJ, Balish M, Gorbach A, et al. How well does a three-sphere model predict positions of dipoles in a realistically shaped head? *Electroencephalogr Clin Neurophysiol* 1993;87:175–184.
36. Roth BJ, Ko D, von Albertini-Carletti IR, et al. Dipole localization in patient with epilepsy using the realistically shaped head model. *Electroencephalogr Clin Neurophysiol* 1997;102:159–160.
37. Rush S, Driscoll DA. Current distribution in the brain from surface electrodes. *Anaesth Analg Curr Res* 1968;47:717–723.
38. Scherg M. Fundamentals of dipole source potential analysis. In: Grandori F, Hoke M, Romani GL, eds. *Advances in audiology: auditory evoked magnetic fields and potentials*. Basel: Karger, 1990:40–69.
39. Scherg M. Functional imaging and localization of electromagnetic brain activity. *Brain Topogr* 1992;5:103–112.
40. Scherg M, Bast T, Berg P. Multiple source analysis of interictal spikes: goals, requirements, and clinical value. *J Clin Neurophysiol* 1999;16:214–224.
41. Scherg M, Ebersole JS. Brain source imaging of focal and multifocal epileptiform EEG activity. *Neurophysiol Clin* 1994;24:51–60.
42. Scherg M, VonCramon D. A new interpretation of the generators of BAEP waves I–V: results of a spatio-temporal dipole model. *Electroencephalogr Clin Neurophysiol* 1985;62:290–299.
43. Schlitt HA, Heller L, Aaron R, et al. Evaluation of boundary element methods for the EEG forward problem: effect of linear interpolation. *IEEE Trans Biomed Eng* 1995;42:52–58.
44. Schneider MR. A multistage process for computing virtual dipolar sources of EEG discharges from surface information. *IEEE Trans Biomed Eng* 1972;19:1–12.
45. Sidman RD, Giambalvo V, Allison T, et al. A method for localization of sources of human cerebral potentials evoked by sensory stimuli. *Sensory Proc* 1978;2:116–129.
46. Thompson JL, Assaf BA, Ebersole JS. Multiple fixed dipole analysis of scalp-recorded interictal spikes and seizures in temporal lobe epilepsy. *Epilepsia* 1996;37[Suppl 5]:89.
47. Thompson JL, Ebersole JS. Dipole modeling of scalp-recorded interictal EEG spikes in mesial vs. nonmesial temporal lobe epilepsy. *J Clin Neurophysiol* 1995;12:501.
48. Wilson FN, Bayley RH. The electric field of an eccentric dipole in a homogeneous spherical conducting medium. *Circulation* 1950;1:84–92.
49. Yvert B, Bertrand O, Echallier JF, et al. Improved forward EEG calculations using local mesh refinement of realistic head geometries. *Electroencephalogr Clin Neurophysiol* 1995;95:381–392.
50. Yvert B, Bertrand O, Echallier JF, et al. Improved dipoles localization using mesh refinement of realistic head geometries: an EEG simulation study. *Electroencephalogr Clin Neurophysiol* 1996;99:79–89.

Chapter 24

Quantitative Electroencephalography

Marc R. Nuwer

Quantitative methods for analyzing electroencephalograms (EEGs) provide new ways to view data that are different from traditional visual analysis. Sometimes these quantitative techniques can offer new and interesting, even clinically valuable, insights into the EEG. Many types of analysis have been proposed.

The rapid adoption of digital EEG techniques has opened the door for easy application of quantitative analysis. Once EEG data are stored in digital format, applications of various algorithms can become available as simple extensions of the reading process. Although quantitative techniques have been available for 50 years, for much of that time their use was hampered by difficulties accessing these technologies from traditional analog recordings. Digital analysis techniques, however, are accompanied by considerable difficulty in routine use. They still defy attempts to make them easy, user friendly, and free from sources of potential error.

Applications of quantified techniques are discussed in other chapters in this book. Over time, these various techniques imperceptibly will become a standard part of the field of EEG. Successful techniques will be separated from less successful earlier attempts at defining clinically useful analysis. At that point, we shall stop considering quantitative techniques separately from routine EEG. Currently, however, it is still useful to identify separately some of the techniques, inherent problems, and literature in this field. The reader is referred to Chapters 2, 3, 4, 22, 23, and 25 for further discussion.

NOMENCLATURE

A variety of terms are used in the field of quantitative analysis. The terms *digital EEG*, *paperless EEG*, and *quantitative EEG* (qEEG) as well

TABLE 24.1. *Nomenclature used to describe qEEG techniques*

Digital EEG
Quantitative EEG (qEEG)
Signal analysis
   Automated event detection
   Monitoring and trending
   Source analysis
   Frequency analysis
Topographic displays ("brain maps")
Statistical analysis
   Comparisons to normal values
   Diagnostic discriminant analysis

From Nuwer MR. Assessment of digital EEG, quantitative EEG, and EEG brain mapping: report of the American Academy of Neurology and the American Clinical Neurophysiology Society. *Neurology* 1997;49:277–292, with permission.

as *EEG brain mapping* are used to describe certain aspects of these methods. Table 24.1 shows the organization of some of this nomenclature.

Digital EEG

Digital EEG refers to EEG recording on a digital medium, typically a small desktop computer. Recording and display are consistent with existing American Clinical Neurophysiology Society (ACNS; formerly the American Electroencephalographic Society) and International Federation of Clinical Neurophysiology (IFCN) standards for clinical EEG recordings (1–4,19,36,37). Displays are produced on a routine monitor screen, typically of average or larger screen size. Such digital recording allows for subsequent replay with changes and filters, display scales, reformatted montages, remote network access, and larger numbers of recording channels. These topics are reviewed in more detail in Chapters 3 and 4.

Quantitative EEG

Quantitative EEG is a general term for analysis of the EEG, generally with mathematical formulas or statistical comparisons. The EEG data are transformed in ways that highlight certain features that may be difficult to assess by visual inspection of the raw EEG. Numerical results, statistical tables, or transformed datagraphs are produced.

Signal Analysis

Signal analysis refers to techniques to transform the EEG into its frequency components, or to identify or localize possible epileptic spikes, or to determine trends in EEG features over time for monitoring. Several common types of signal analysis are used.

Automated event detection is the process of identifying specific segments of EEG that contain particular events of interest (see Chapter 22 for more detailed discussion). Most often these are epileptic spikes or seizures, which can be flagged during extended recordings. A common application is identification of subclinical or nonconvulsive seizures for patients on long-term epilepsy video-EEG monitoring units. Another common clinical use is automated scoring of sleep architecture in digital polysomnogram recordings (see also Chapter 26). In both instances, the computer flags or scores possible events or states, with varying degrees of success. For many spike or seizure detectors, frequent false-positive identification of artifacts or nonepileptic transients occurs. Expert screening of flagged events or states clarifies these false-positive events. Overall, automated event detection facilitates human review of the data by flagging or prescoring, allowing the expert to scan through or audit data much more rapidly.

Monitoring and trending the EEG is useful in the operating room (OR) or intensive care unit (ICU). Most often this is an aid to detect gradual changes in the EEG that result from changes in the patient's clinical status. In the OR, this can be a sign of gradually developing cerebral ischemia. In the ICU, changes can be due to lightening of coma or development of new complications. Such complications include ischemia, poor tolerance of raised intracranial pressure, postoperative development of subdural hematoma, or occurrence of nonconvulsive seizures (6,8,22,23,25,34,40,48,51) (see Chapter 25). Monitoring the EEG over hours or days allows for identification of such long-term trends or events in ways difficult to appreciate just from occasional 20-minute-long routine EEG testing.

Source analysis is a technique for deducing the likely generator of brief transients such as epileptic spikes or evoked potentials. Multichannel scalp voltage values are used to estimate a likely three-dimensional location of a generator. Sometimes these are displayed superimposed on magnetic resonance imaging (MRI) sections, a technique known as co-registration. As an example, mesial temporal–generated epileptic spikes can be separated from neocortical temporal epileptic spikes (see Chapter 23).

Frequency analysis transforms the EEG into its frequency components. The magnitude of each frequency or frequency band is calculated. As an example, relative amounts of posterior-dominant alpha rhythm can be quantified. *Coherence analysis* takes this method one step further, assessing the relationships between frequency components at different scalp-recording sites. The results of frequency and coherence analysis can be presented as a table of numbers or a multidimensional graph or in a topographic display.

Topographic EEG Displays

Topographic EEG displays most often are stylized maps of the scalp presenting localized electrical features such as frequency content in a particular band. These stylized maps, often collectively referred to as "EEG brain maps," superficially resemble computed tomography or MRI displays. Figure 24.1 shows some EEG brain maps. Actually, the relationship to neuroimaging displays is very superficial, because EEG brain maps are a stylized representation rather than an anatomically accurate rendering. The term *EEG brain maps* should not be confused with functional cortical brain mapping by direct cortical stimulation or with brain mapping by neuroimaging techniques, which have no direct relationship to EEG brain mapping.

Statistical Analysis

Statistical analysis is a way of comparing between EEG recordings or between the EEG recording of an individual subject and those of a group of normal control subjects. Most often such comparisons are made on the basis of signal analysis features such as frequency analysis, and may be displayed as numerical tables or topographic EEG brain maps.

Comparison to normative values uses group statistics to assess a particular EEG feature from an individual. The feature is compared to the same feature in a group of normal control subjects. These statistical techniques identify when a subject's EEG values differ from the expected values based on the control population. Techniques should be used to adjust these for age, nonnormal statistical distributions, and other factors. The results highlight ways in which a particular EEG sample differs from average or expected values.

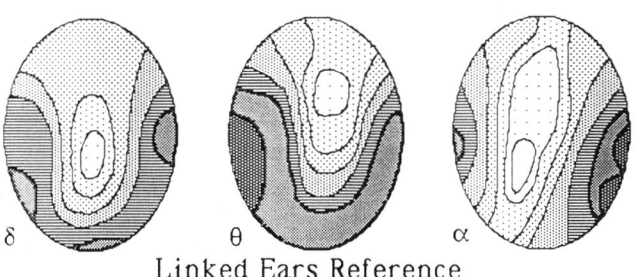

72♂ with an Acute, Small CVA

Linked Ears Reference

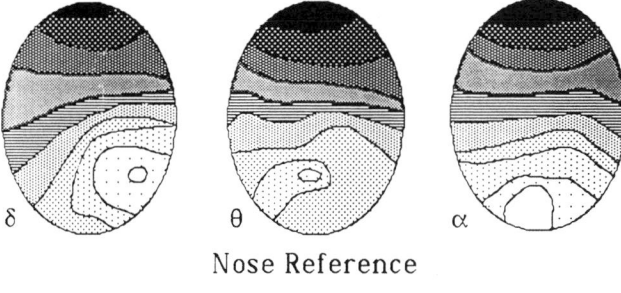

Nose Reference

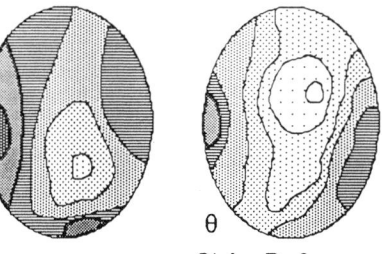

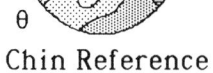

Chin Reference

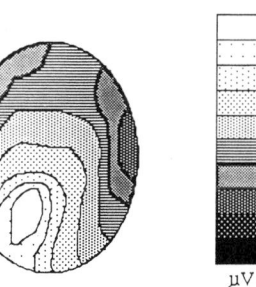

FIG. 24.1. EEG brain maps of the same data compiled using three different references: linked ear, nose, and chin sites. The EEG was recorded on a 72-year-old man who had had a small acute stroke. Right parasagittal slowing is evident as precentral theta and postcentral delta activity. Note how different the maps look depending on the reference chosen. The linked ears reference tends to squeeze the topographic contours toward the sagittal midline. The nose reference tends to flatten the contours and push them toward the occiput. The chin reference is probably the most accurate here. This is an example of the *contaminated reference effect*. (From Nuwer MR. Quantitative EEG: 1. Techniques and problems of frequency analysis and topographic mapping. *J Clin Neurophysiol* 1988;5:1–43, with permission.)

Diagnostic discriminant analysis compares an individual's selected EEG features to a template of features commonly found in a particular disease category. A patient's EEG might be compared with several possible disease categories to see with which the patient's EEG best fits statistically.

PROBLEMS

Various types of problems can interfere with recording of records suitable for qEEG assessments or with their interpretation (31–33).

Artifacts

Artifacts contaminate portions of all EEG records. The sources are many, including eye movements, blinks, electromyograms, electrocardiograms, electrode pops, breathing, nearby electrical equipment, or even intravenous lines. When examining a routine EEG by visual analysis, the expert electroencephalographer is trained to read past these artifacts, seeking the real EEG through or between contaminated regions. In contrast, the computer has great difficulty assessing artifact. Expert human review is needed. Even with such review, many routine clinical EEGs are sufficiently contaminated that finding several minutes of completely artifact-free segments of awake EEG may be challenging or impractical.

"Garbage in, garbage out" is an oft-quoted maxim in the data processing community. This certainly applies to qEEG. Actual qEEG analysis may be contaminated with artifact to some extent. Recognizing and accounting for this is important. One lesson is that the qEEG results cannot be understood unless the raw EEG is visually analyzed by an expert electroencephalographer simultaneously, and referenced back and forth between quantitative results and visual analysis of the EEG tracings. Quantitative results cannot be trusted or interpreted on their own.

"Different" Versus "Diseased"

Statistical analysis can identify ways in which an individual patient's particular EEG segments differ from average or expected values. However, the meaning of this difference can be difficult to interpret, because "different" does not equal "diseased." The fact that a patient's EEG contains features that are different from the ideal average does not imply that this difference is due to a disorder or a disease. Analogously, some people are taller than average and other people are shorter than average, but this height variation does not imply that the differences are due to a pathological cause. Such dif-

ferences should not be considered "abnormal" unless they pass further tests. For example, the difference must represent a type of change that is commonly accepted as indicative of pathology. Artifactual causes also need to be excluded. Other changes may simply reflect the diversity of normal EEG features in the general population, just as the population at large has great diversity in facial or other physical features.

Similarly, the EEG community has long been aware of *"normal variant"* waveforms. Certain features are well known to occur in a minority of patients. Although they may trigger alarm in the uneducated observer, the knowledgeable expert knows to discount these features as nonpathological. Various such features include mu rhythm, rhythmic temporal theta activity (psychomotor variant), and 14- and 6-Hz spikes. These are just some examples of statistical outliers of no clinical significance, but they serve as reminders of how statistical qEEG analysis can yield highly statistically "abnormal" features that are well known to be nonpathological.

Contaminated References

Contaminated references are commonly encountered in EEGs. Many electroencephalographers would concede that there is no optimal montage useful for all patient situations. Digital EEG allows for montage reformatting to help control for this commonplace problem. Yet many qEEG techniques are based on a specific montage, such as using linked ear leads. When either ear lead is contaminated by artifact or normal variant waveforms, the quantitative results can be substantially altered in adverse ways. Even with pathological slowing near one ear lead, the actual location of the slowing may show up at the wrong qEEG scalp sites because of this effect.

Figure 24.1 shows an example of such a problem. One can see how technical differences in processing and displaying can cause major differences in the clinical impression one receives from the brain maps. In these cases, the differences are due simply to changing the reference electrode used. The EEG data themselves are the same. Even an expert electroencephalographer could become confused by such misleading displays.

Alertness

Alertness is assumed for certain qEEG tests, such as comparison to normal controls. Yet all clinicians who routinely read EEGs appreciate how quickly any individual slips into early drowsiness with its concomitant changes in EEG characteristics. The changes in EEG features resulting from drowsiness mimic changes that can be seem with some types of brain damage.

Medication Effects

Medication effects also can cause slowing or other EEG changes. As with drowsiness, these changes may be confused with brain damage by some qEEG analysis techniques. Knowledge of the recent medication history of a patient may be very relevant to understanding the kinds of changes that are seen in any EEG. qEEG worsens the situation when its statistical techniques flag such changes as "abnormal," subverting the usual differential diagnostic process in visual EEG interpretation.

Statistical Problems

Statistical problems are commonplace when assessing large amounts of data with statistical techniques. False-positive "abnormalities" may average about 5% among large numbers of statistical tests run in some applications, but the number can reach 15%–20% in some individual normal control subjects, and even higher numbers may be reached in occasional normal individuals (9). Many statistically generated EEG "abnormalities" are probably clinically meaningless, but flagging them as such can easily mislead an electroencephalographer. Other statistical complexities exist that have yet to be clearly understood, having to do with the lack of independence of EEGs recorded at adjacent sites, the failure of EEG statistics to meet initial tests for a normal distribution, and the use of large numbers of tests simultaneously.

Small Technical Changes

Small technical changes in the collection of EEG data can also cause exaggerated "abnormal" qEEG results. Use of electrode caps can speed conducting the test, but caps sometimes fail to remain adequately in place, becoming slightly tipped or yawed and not ideally accounting for differences in patient head shapes. Sometimes electrodes make poor contact with the scalp or further technical issues intrude. Sometimes filters are set differently from the settings with which the initial normative group of EEGs was run. Each such technical problem can compound itself when processed through qEEG.

Selection of Results

Selection of results is necessary in most qEEG applications. The electroencephalographer must choose among various recorded epochs of EEG. Each epoch may represent 2 seconds of recording. Dozens of such epochs are needed for many qEEG applications. Each must be selected by a knowl-edgeable electroencephalographer so as to exclude artifact, drowsiness, normal variants, and other problems. The skill with which this selection is done is a critical factor in determining the outcome of the test. Furthermore, the selection process can skew results. Intermittent abnormalities truly present in the EEG might be excluded, or certain artifacts might be erroneously included in the epochs chosen. If the electroencephalographer comes to the process with a preconceived bias that a certain result is likely to occur, he or she may bring that bias to the selection process. For example, a record may contain intermittent slowing seen over the left or the right hemisphere at separate times during the recording, but an electroencephalographer seeking just the left-sided slowing could identify those epochs selectively for further processing. In that case the quantitative results will show left-sided slowing. Similarly, frontal slow eye movements of early drowsiness can contaminate the record and produce frontal slow activity in the qEEG. Identification of which epochs are selected for qEEG processing is key for understanding the meaning of the qEEG results. Review of a qEEG test should include review of the concomitantly recorded routine EEG tracings as well as review of the specific epochs chosen.

Some tactics diminish selection bias (10), but, despite such suggestions, commonplace qEEG applications can still be quite problematic. Problems often outweigh the value of specific qEEG tests; however, valuable clinical applications have been found in certain settings, typically when the technique addresses specific quantitative questions, and is used in expert hands with good clinical judgment along with simultaneous visual interpretation of the EEG tracings.

CLINICAL SETTINGS

The American Academy of Neurology (AAN) and the ACNS undertook a joint assessment of the clinical utility of qEEG (35). This evidence-based assessment was conducted through a panel of experts. It widely sought published evidence about qEEG and its potential clinical uses. The panel determined that criteria for assessing the literature should include several ideal elements or concepts (5,7,11–18,20,21,24,26–30,38,39,41–47,49,50). First, the disease study should be clearly defined. Explicit, clear criteria for test abnormality should be defined prospectively. Control groups also should include patient groups with other diseases in the differential diagnosis of the disorder evaluated. Control groups should be different from those originally used to develop the normal limit of the qEEG test. Disease severity should simulate that encountered in the proposed test application. Test–retest reliability should be high. Various validity measures should be calculated and compared to those of other tests already clinically used in that differential diagnosis. Blinded observations are considered more objective. The efficacy or goal of the test (i.e., how will it affect patient care) should be clear. Incremental changes to existing accepted tests require less proof, whereas novel techniques require a greater degree of demonstrated validity and utility. Publications by authors with a potential conflict of interest should preferably be replicated by others. Various gold standards should be taken into account, depending on the clinical question for which a test is being evaluated.

In the end, these societies accepted a series of recommendations about digital EEG, qEEG, and EEG brain mapping. The following is a summary of those recommendations:

A. Digital EEG is an established substitute for recording, reviewing, and storing a paper EEG record. It is a clear technical advance over previous paper methods. It is highly recommended (see Chapter 3).

B. EEG brain mapping and other advanced qEEG techniques should be used only by physicians highly skilled in clinical EEG, and only as an adjunct to and in conjunction with traditional EEG interpretation. These tests may be clinically useful only for patients who have been well selected on the basis of their clinical presentation.

C. Certain qEEG techniques are considered established as an addition to digital EEG in

C.1. Epilepsy—for screening for possible epileptic spikes or seizures in long-term EEG monitoring or ambulatory recording to facilitate subsequent expert visual EEG interpretation (see Chapter 22).

C.2. OR and ICU monitoring—for continuous EEG monitoring by frequency trending to detect early, acute intracranial complications in the OR or ICU, and for screening for possible epileptic seizures in high-risk ICU patients (see Chapter 25).

D. Certain quantitative EEG techniques are considered possibly useful practice options as an addition to digital EEG in

D.1. Epilepsy—qEEG may be useful for topographic voltage and dipole analysis in presurgical evaluations (see Chapter 23).

D.2. Cerebrovascular disease—based on class II and III evidence, qEEG in expert hands may be useful in evaluating certain patients with symptoms of cerebrovascular disease whose neuroimaging and routine EEG studies are not conclusive.

D.3. Dementia—routine EEG has long been an established test in evaluation of dementia and encephalopathy when the diagnosis

remains unresolved after initial clinical evaluation. In occasional clinical evaluation, qEEG frequency analysis may be a useful adjunct to interpretation of the routine EEG when used in expert hands (see Chapter 13).

E. On the basis of current clinical literature, opinions of most experts, and proposed rationales for its use, qEEG remains investigational for clinical use in postconcussion syndrome, mild or moderate head injury, learning disability, attention disorders, schizophrenia, depression, alcoholism, and drug abuse.

F. On the basis of clinical and scientific evidence, opinions of most experts, and the technical and methodological shortcomings, qEEG is not recommended for use in civil or criminal judicial proceedings.

G. Because of the very substantial risk of erroneous interpretations, it is unacceptable for any EEG brain mapping or other qEEG techniques to be used clinically by those who are not physicians highly skilled in clinical EEG interpretation.

CONDITIONS FOR CLINICAL USE

Even within the confines of those clinical circumstances in which qEEG testing is considered established or promising, certain caveats need to be recognized before embarking on test interpretation. First and foremost, quantitative results cannot be interpreted on their own. They can be understood only by referring back and forth between any quantitative tables, charts, graphs, and the like and the visual interpretation of the EEG tracings from which those analyses were made. The individual epochs used should be identified. For multiple-day monitoring or long-term epilepsy EEG monitoring, selected portions are reviewed and interpreted at times when suspicious activity is automatically flagged or at randomly audited other times.

The technical quality of these EEG recordings must be satisfactory for clinical interpretation. The standard guidelines for EEG recordings should be followed (e.g., those from the ACNS and IFCN) (1–7). There is no clinical application for qEEG analysis apart from interpretations by physicians with appropriate skills, training, knowledge, and ability in routine EEG analysis, as well as additional knowledge and experience with the relevant additional technical problems, artifacts, normal variants, and statistical issues encountered in qEEG.

qEEG can be a useful adjunct to traditional visual EEG analysis, in the sense that it acts as a "ruler" that measures certain features more carefully and searches for subtle features of interest. However, qEEG can often be misleading, especially in the hands of practitioners with limited skills in routine EEG interpretation.

As this field gradually develops, a careful evaluation of proposed new applications is needed to separate those that actually work and add clinical value from those that do not. With careful progress, qEEG may come to be a commonly used adjunct to EEG interpretation. Such tools may give us further insights into the pathophysiology of disease as well as further sensitive methods for measuring and diagnosing neurological and psychiatric disorders.

REFERENCES

1. American Electroencephalographic Society. Guidelines for recording clinical EEG on digital media. *J Clin Neurophysiol* 1994;11:114–115.
2. American Electroencephalographic Society. Minimum technical requirements for performing clinical electroencephalography. *J Clin Neurophysiol* 1994;11:2–5.
3. American Electroencephalographic Society. Minimum technical standards for pediatric electroencephalography. *J Clin Neurophysiol* 1994;11:6–9.
4. American Electroencephalographic Society. Standards for practice in clinical electroencephalography. *J Clin Neurophysiol* 1994;11:14–15.
5. Aminoff MJ. Criticism in neurology and medicine. *Neurology* 1994;44:1781–1783.
6. Archibald JE, Drazkowski JF. Clinical applications of compressed spectral analysis (CSA) in OR/ICU settings. *Am J EEG Technol* 1985;25:13–36.
7. Ayres JD. The use and abuse of medical practice guidelines. *J Legal Med* 1994;15:421–443.
8. Cant BR, Shaw NA. Monitoring by compressed spectral array in prolonged coma. *Neurology* 1984;34:35–39.
9. Dolisi C, Suisse G, Delpont E. Quantitative EEG abnormalities and asymmetries in patients with intracranial tumors. *Electroencephalogr Clin Neurophysiol* 1990;76:13–18.
10. Duffy FH, Hughes JR, Miranda F, et al. Status of quantitative EEG (QEEG) in clinical practice, 1994. *Clin Electroencephalogr* 1994;25:vi–xxii.
11. Eddy DM. Principles for making difficult decisions in difficult times. *JAMA* 1994;271:1792–1798.
12. Garber AM. Can technology assessment control health spending? *Health Affairs* 1994 Sum;1:15–126.
13. Guyatt G, Drummond M, Feeny D, et al. Guidelines for the clinical and economic evaluation of health care technologies. *Soc Sci Med* 1986;22:393–408.
14. Guyatt GH, Rennie D, for the Evidence-Based Medicine Working Group. Users' guides to the medical literature. *JAMA* 1993;270:2096–2097.
15. Guyatt GH, Sackett DL, Cook DJ, for the Evidence-Based Medicine Working Group. Users' guides to the medical literature. II. How to use an article about therapy or prevention. A. Are the results of the study valid? *JAMA* 1993;270:2598–2601.
16. Guyatt GH, Sackett DL, Cook DJ, for the Evidence-Based Medicine Working Group. Users' guides to the medical literature. II. How to use an article about therapy or prevention. B. What were the results and will they help me in caring for my patients? *JAMA* 1994;271:59–63.
17. Guyatt GH, Sackett DL, Sinclair JC, et al, for the Evidence-Based Medicine Working Group. Users' guides to the medical literature. IX. A method for grading health care recommendations. *JAMA* 1995;274:1800–1804.
18. Hayward RSA, Wilson MC, Tunis SR, et al, for the Evidence-Based Medicine Working Group. Users' guides to the medical literature. VIII. How to use clinical practice guidelines. A. Are the recommendations valid? *JAMA* 1995;274:570–574.
19. International Federation of Societies for Electroencephalography and Clinical Neurophysiology. *Recommendations for the practice of clinical neurophysiology.* Amsterdam: Elsevier Science, 1983.
20. Jaeschke R, Guyatt GH, Sackett DL, for the Evidence-Based Medicine Working Group. Users' guides to the medical literature. III. How to use an article about a diagnostic test. A. Are the results of the study valid? *JAMA* 1994;271:389–291.
21. Jaeschke R, Guyatt GH, Sackett DL, for the Evidence-Based Medicine Working Group. Users' guides to the medical literature. III. How to use an article about a diagnostic test. B. What are the results and will they help me in caring for my patients? *JAMA* 1994;271:703–707.
22. Jordan KG. Continuous EEG and evoked potential monitoring in the neuroscience intensive care unit. *J Clin Neurophysiol* 1993;10:445–475.
23. Jordan KG. Status epilepticus: a perspective from the neuroscience intensive care unit. *Neurosurg Clin* 1994;5:671–686.
24. Kent DL, Haynor DR, Longstreth WT, et al. The clinical efficacy of magnetic resonance imaging in neuroimaging. *Ann Intern Med* 1994;120:856–871.
25. Labar DR, Fisch BJ, Pedley TA, et al. Quantitative EEG monitoring for patients with subarachnoid hemorrhage. *Electroencephalogr Clin Neurophysiol* 1991;78:325–332.
26. Laupacis A, Wells G, Richardson S, et al, for the Evidence-Based Medicine Working Group. Users' guides to the medical literature. V. How to use an article about prognosis. *JAMA* 1994;272:234–237.
27. Levine M, Walter S, Lee H, et al, for the Evidence-Based Medicine Working Group. Users' guides to the medical literature. IV. How to use an article about harm. *JAMA* 1994;271:1615–1619.
28. Longstreth WT, Koepsell TD, van Belle G. Clinical neuroepidemiology: I. Diagnosis. *Arch Neurol* 1987;44:1091–1099.
29. Longstreth WT, Koepsell TD, van Belle G. Clinical neuroepidemiology: II. Outcomes. *Arch Neurol* 1987;44:1196–1202.
30. McMaster University Health Sciences Centre, Department of Clinical Epidemiology and Biostatistics. How to read clinical journals: 11. To learn about a diagnostic test. *Can Med Assoc J* 1981;124:703–710.
31. Nuwer MR. Quantitative EEG: 1. Techniques and problems of frequency analysis and topographic mapping. *J Clin Neurophysiol* 1988;5:1–43.
32. Nuwer MR. Uses and abuses of brain mapping. *Arch Neurol* 1989;46:1134–1136.
33. Nuwer MR. On the process for evaluating proposed new diagnostic EEG tests. *Brain Topogr* 1992;4:243–247.
34. Nuwer MR. Electroencephalograms and evoked potentials: monitoring cerebral function in the neurosurgical intensive care unit. *Neurosurg Clin* 1994;5:647–659.
35. Nuwer MR. Assessment of digital EEG, quantitative EEG, and EEG brain mapping: report of the American Academy of Neurology and the American Clinical Neurophysiology Society. *Neurology* 1997;49:277–292.
36. Nuwer MR, Comi G, Emerson R, et al. I.F.C.N. standards for digital recording of clinical EEG. *Electroencephalogr Clin Neurophysiol* 1998;106:259–261.
37. Nuwer MR, Lehmann D, Lopes da Silva F, et al. IFCN guidelines for topographic and frequency analysis of EEGs and EPs: report of an IFCN committee. *Electroencephalogr Clin Neurophysiol* 1994;91:1–5.
38. Oxman AD, Cook DJ, Guyatt GH, for the Evidence-Based Medicine Working Group. Users' guides to the medical literature. VI. How to use an overview. *JAMA* 1994;272:1367–1371.
39. Oxman AD, Sackett DL, Guyatt GH, for the Evidence-Based Medicine Working Group. Users' guides to the medical literature. 1. How to get started. *JAMA* 1993;270:2093–2095.
40. Prior PF, Maynard DE. *Monitoring cerebral function.* Amsterdam: Elsevier Science, 1986.
41. Ransohoff DF, Feinstien AR. Problems of spectrum and bias in evaluating the efficacy of diagnostic tests. *N Engl J Med* 1978;299:926–930.

42. Richardson S, Detsky AS, for the Evidence-Based Medicine Working Group. Users' guides to the medical literature. VII. How to use a clinical decision analysis. A. Are the results of the study valid? *JAMA* 1995;273:1292–1295.

43. Richardson S, Detsky AS, for the Evidence-Based Medicine Working Group. Users' guides to the medical literature. VII. How to use a clinical decision analysis. B. What are the results and will they help me in caring for my patients? *JAMA* 1995;273:1610–1613.

44. Sackett DL, Haynes RB, Tugwell P. *Clinical epidemiology: a basic science for clinical medicine.* Boston: Little, Brown and Company, 1985.

45. Sheps SB, Schechter MT. The assessment of diagnostic tests: a survey of current medical research. *JAMA* 1984;252:2418–2422.

46. The Standards of Reporting Trials Group. A proposal for structured reporting of randomized controlled trials. *JAMA* 1994;272:1926–1931.

47. Swets A, Pickett RM, Whitehead SF, et al. Assessment of diagnostic technologies. *Science* 1979; 205:753–759.

48. Vespa PM, Nuwer MR, Juhasz C, et al. Early detection of vasospasm after acute subarachnoid hemorrhage using continuous EEG ICU monitoring. *Electroencephalogr Clin Neurophysiol* 1997; 103:607–615.

49. Wasson JH, Sox HC, Neff RK, et al. Clinical prediction rules: applications and methodological standards. *N Engl J Med* 1985;313:793–799.

50. Wilson MC, Hayward RSA, Tunis SR, et al, for the Evidence-Based Medicine Working Group. Users' guides to the medical literature. VIII. How to use clinical practice guidelines. B. What are the recommendations and will they help you in caring for your patients? *JAMA* 1995;274:1630–1632.

51. Young GB, Jordan KG. Do nonconvulsive seizures damage the brain? *Arch Neurol* 1998;55: 117–119.

Chapter 25

Continuous EEG Monitoring in the Intensive Care Unit

Kenneth G. Jordan and Thomas P. Bleck

THE PROBLEM, ITS HISTORY, AND ITS CONTEXT

Although catheters, transducers, digital readouts, and alarms in the intensive care unit (ICU) enable medical personnel to monitor patients' hearts, lungs, kidneys, blood, and other organs, cerebral function usually remains hidden in the "black box" of the cranial vault, monitored primarily by bedside observations. As treatment options for acute neurological disease have expanded, and as neurologists and neurophysiologists have become more involved in neurological intensive care units (NICU), many clinicians have become uncomfortable relying on the traditional neurological examination for detecting potentially remediable changes in cerebral function. Even in the best circumstances, with expert personnel, intermittent clinical assessment is hampered by discontinuity and subjectivity. In addition, contrary to the goal of a physiological monitor, changes in examination findings occur *after* clinical deterioration. As a result, the intensivist is confronted with the sisyphean task of simultaneously preventing further clinical deterioration while striving to reverse damage that has already occurred. Bedside assessment becomes progressively uninformative when patients are heavily sedated or given neuromuscular junction blocking agents.

Encouraged by the application of the electroencephalogram (EEG) as an intraoperative monitor, neurophysiologists developed methods of employing continuous EEG (CEEG) in the ICU to illuminate the "black box" of cerebral function (14,37,49,84). Traditionally, the raw EEG generated cumbersome amounts of data and was too complex for interpretation by nonexperts. In the 1970s, data compression techniques were introduced in an attempt to simplify EEG interpretation. These techniques entailed the use of quantitative analysis of EEG frequency and amplitude in place of the real-time display of EEG. Examples included compressed spectral array (CSA) (15,21), the cerebral function monitor (73,84), and topographic brain mapping (78,86). In the ICU setting, data reduction—particularly with CSA—was used primarily to predict outcome of patients in a coma (16,20). Until the 1990s, technological limitations and logistical barriers made raw EEG impractical as a real-time physiologic monitor. During that decade, however, digital EEG overcame many of these impediments, making bedside CEEG a clinically relevant tool (51,79,80).

An optimal ICU monitoring system should be:

- More sensitive and specific than clinical observations.
- Noninvasive.
- Simple to operate and interpret by nonexperts.
- Compatible with medical and nursing care of the patients.

Examples of other successful monitors include the bedside electrocardiographic monitor and transcutaneous pulse oximetry. CEEG monitoring in the ICU has not yet reached its potential in simplicity and utility. Advances in digital EEG technology will probably further facilitate its application, online interpretation, and clinical applicability. The early use of CEEG led to the recognition of important and somewhat surprising EEG abnormalities in patients with acute cerebral injuries, including non-convulsive seizures (NCS) and non-convulsive status epilepticus (NCSE) (51). CEEG in the ICU has gradually became more widespread as studies supported its value in providing important and often otherwise unobtainable information (12,19,25,54,80,115). CEEG has more recently been employed in emergency medicine (59,60).

This chapter reviews use of CEEG in the ICU and addresses its scientific basis and the technical and logistical issues of its implementation. It also examines established, emerging, and potential clinical applications; the numerous (often unique) artifacts found in CEEG; and troubleshooting suggestions. Finally, reflecting the maturation of CEEG, we discuss preliminary efforts to assess its cost benefit, cost effectiveness, and impact on patient outcomes.

SCIENTIFIC BASIS FOR CONTINUOUS EEG

Seven major neurobiological and clinical attributes underlie the rationale for CEEG:

1. *The EEG is tightly linked to cerebral metabolism.* A multitude of electrochemical processes produce the extracellular electrical currents that generate the scalp EEG (83; Chapter 1). Measurable activity is generated by the spatial and temporal summation of postsynaptic excitatory and inhibitory potentials in the superficial layers of the cortex. These are modulated by ascending diencephalic input. As a result, the EEG closely reflects cerebral metabolism, becoming abnormal if any of the interdependent components is disrupted.

2. *The EEG is sensitive to two of the most common causes of cerebral injury: ischemia and hypoxia.* Pyramidal neurons in cortical layers 3 and 5 are mainly responsible for EEG generation and are selectively vulnerable to hypoxia and ischemia.

3. *The EEG detects neuronal dysfunction at a reversible stage.* EEG abnormalities arise when cerebral blood flow (CBF) declines to between 25 and 30 mL/100 g/min (5). Progressive changes in EEG morphology, amplitude, and frequency correlate with the severity of cerebral ischemia (92,98) (Fig. 25.1). Synaptic transmission is preserved to 17 mL/100 g/minute, but energy failure and loss of cell membrane integrity (cell death) do not occur until 10 to 12 mL/100 g/minute. This "window of reversibility" between the appearance of EEG abnormalities and neuronal death suggests that appropriate intervention during this time might improve or restore cerebral function (26).

4. *The EEG detects neuronal damage or recovery, whereas the clinical examination cannot.* Two common clinical phenomena illustrate this principle. First, during carotid endarterectomy, EEG changes occur within 60 seconds if clamping of the carotid artery produces significant focal cerebral ischemia. Timely placement of a shunt produces resolution of these EEG abnormalities within minutes (see Fig. 25.1). Because the patient is anesthetized, detection and reversal of cerebral injury would not be possible without EEG monitoring (98). Second, during treatment for refractory status epilepticus, the clinical examination loses much of its value. Seizure activity can persist despite loss of all visible motor activity. When this occurs, only EEG can reveal whether seizure activity has been controlled.

5. *The EEG is the best available method for detecting epileptiform activity.* Acute, observable seizures occur in 10% to 27% of patients with acute brain injuries (38). CEEG has documented a surprisingly high incidence of NCS and NCSE in patients with acute cerebral ischemia, intracranial hemorrhages, head trauma, and convulsive status epilepticus (Fig. 25.2). Conversely, EEG is the only method of confirming absence of EEG seizure activity in NICU patients with motor movements that might be convulsive in origin (50,51,85,101,108).

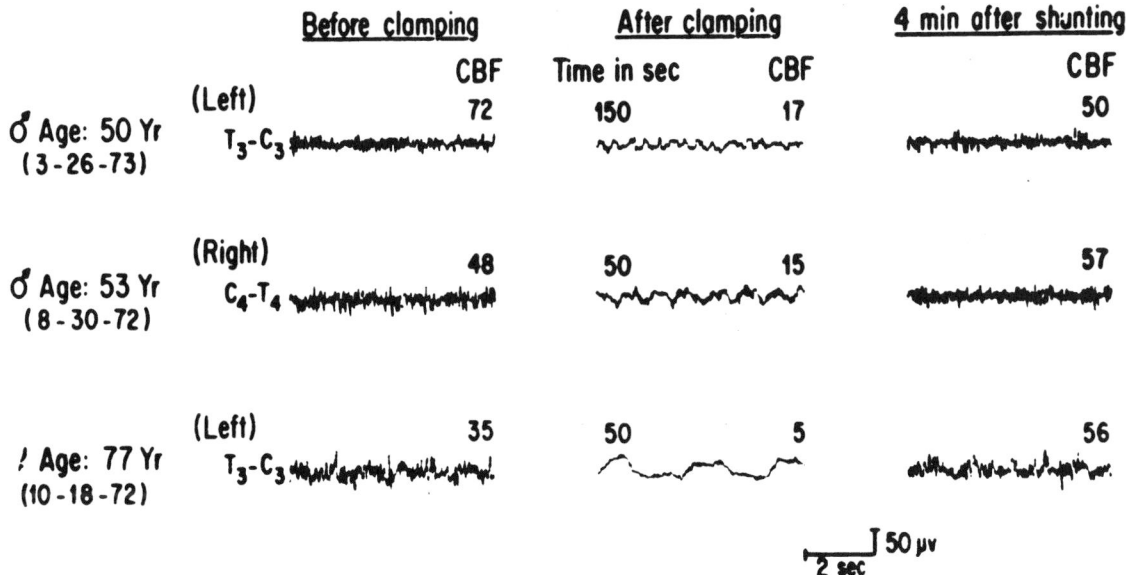

FIG. 25.1 Intraoperative EEG activity in three patients undergoing carotid artery endarterectomy. After carotid clamping, EEG changes correlate with the severity of the drop in cerebral blood flow (CBF). After a shunt is placed and CBF restored, EEG returns rapidly to baseline. (From Sundt TM Jr, Sharbrough FW, Piepgras DG, et al. Correlation of cerebral blood flow and electroencephalographic changes during carotid endarterectomy with results of surgery and hemodynamics of cerebral ischemia. *Mayo Clin Proc* 1981;56:533–543.)

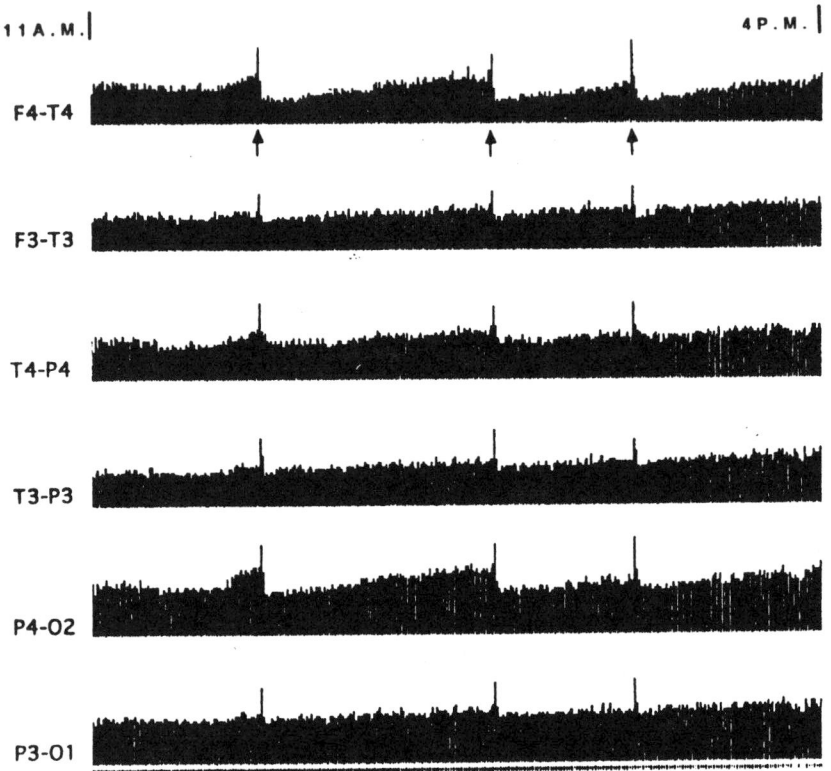

FIG. 25.2. Quantitative EEG detection of non-convulsive seizures. The patient had a hypertensive left thalamic hemorrhage, was comatose, and had no outward signs of seizures. Six EEG channels are displayed, and time is on the horizontal axis. Alpha activity is shown as a percentage of the overall EEG activity from 1 to 30 Hz. Three non-convulsive seizures are characterized by an abrupt jump in percentage of alpha activity *(arrows)* followed by attenuation of alpha activity. Review of the stored raw EEG confirmed that these events were generalized epileptiform discharges. (From Nuwer MR. Electroencephalograms and evoked potentials. Monitoring cerebral function in the neurosurgical intensive care unit. *Neurosurg Clin North Am* 1994;4:647–659.)

6. *CEEG provides dynamic information.* Just as long-term monitoring is necessary to capture spontaneous seizures, the capriciousness and variability of cerebral function in NICU patients necessitate continuous monitoring. Routine bedside EEG provides only a "snapshot" of cerebral activity within a 30- to 45-minute window. Such fragmented testing often misses significant events (Fig. 25.3).

7. *The EEG provides useful information about localization.* The EEG can be used as a bedside tool to approximate localization of cerebral injury to the anterior, posterior, or lateralized head regions. The International

10-20 System of Electrode Placement establishes a consistent relationship between electrode scalp placement and underlying cerebral topography (46). Although this falls short of the anatomical detail provided by modern brain imaging, it can usefully influence the decision to transport a critically ill patient for an imaging study. The transport of critically ill patients out of the ICU for procedures is a logistically intense and potentially hazardous undertaking. Typical adverse events during transport include endotracheal tube mishaps, equipment malfunction, loss of oxygen supply, hypercapnia, and hypotension (103).

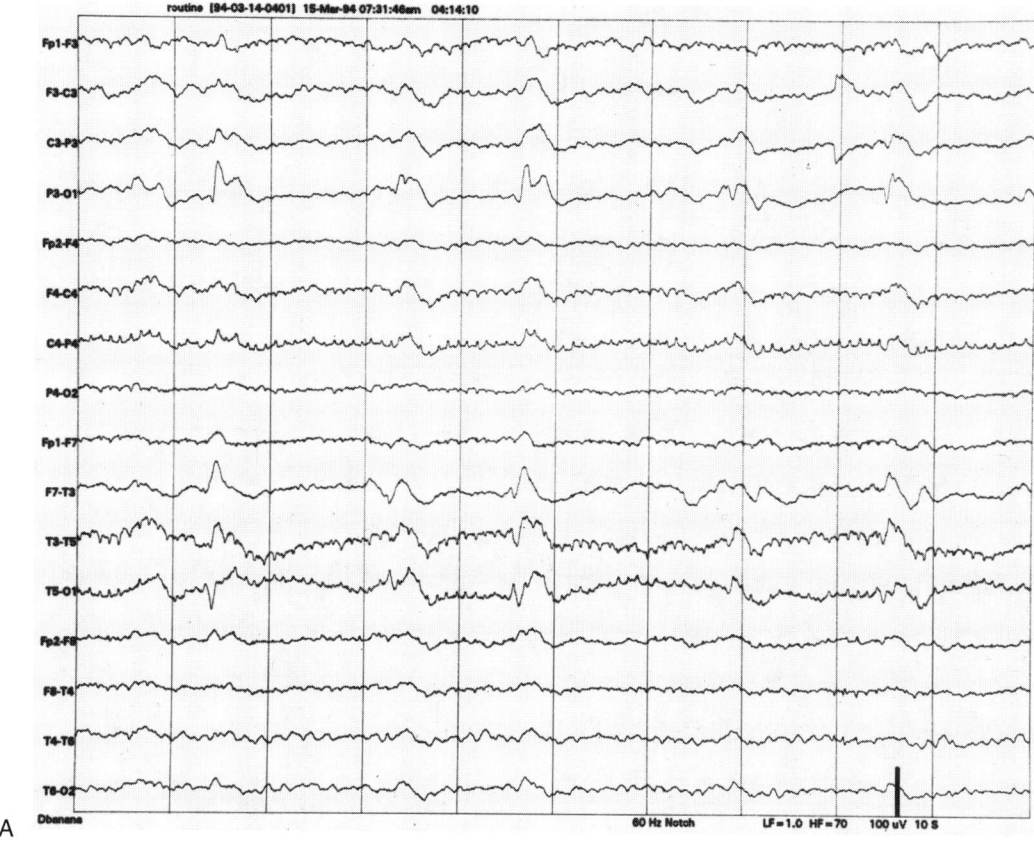

FIG. 25.3. Two samples from continuous EEG recording illustrating why standard EEG might miss significant events. **A:** Periodic lateralized epileptiform discharges (PLEDs) without ictal activity are seen in the left hemisphere. *(Figure continues.)*

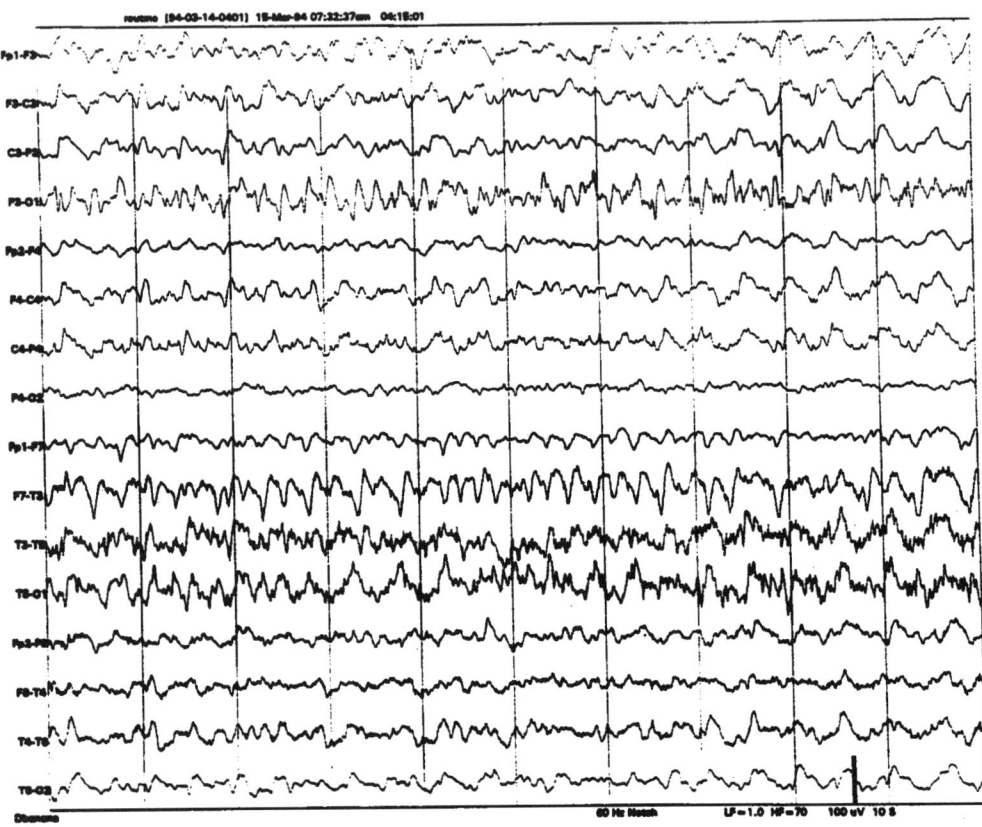

FIG. 25.3. *Continued.* **B:** With continuous monitoring, a prolonged, ictal event is seen arising from the area of PLEDs.

ENVIRONMENTAL AND TECHNICAL CONSIDERATIONS FOR CONTINUOUS EEG

The ICU environment is replete with sources of electrical noise as well as electrical hazards. CEEG is performed on patients who may be restless, agitated, delirious, or combative. Many have altered cranial anatomy, including skull defects, scalp edema, drains, or intracranial catheters. Artifacts of biological, electrical, and environmental sources are seen more frequently, and are more difficult to eliminate, in the ICU than in the EEG laboratory or epilepsy monitoring unit. Duration of monitoring can range from one to many days (the average at the authors' institution is 4.2). During this time, patients require routine medical and nursing care, are often physically manipulated for respiratory and physical therapy, and may be transported out of the ICU for procedures. In this challenging environment, CEEG changes must be identified promptly, accurately interpreted, and correctly correlated with other physiological and clinical data. In comparison with less complex forms of monitoring, such as electrocardiography and pulse oximetry, CEEG generates large amounts of data that require timely review and documentation. Standards for data storage have yet to evolve. Textual notations entered concurrently with patient care maneuvers and any interventions are important for proper interpretation of the EEG data (94).

These challenges can be met with proper equipment, training, and supervision. Digitized real-time EEG (DEEG) is the preferred technological method for CEEG. DEEG allows for on-line or *post hoc* filtering, montage reformatting, and data management. DEEG samples can be saved at preset intervals as well as on an *ad hoc* basis. The record can be annotated, timed, and correlated with other digitized physiological data such as intracranial pressure (ICP) and measurements of cerebral perfusion pressure. Hard copies can be printed and posted for baseline comparisons and documentation, or faxed offsite for expert review. Many commercial systems have automated algorithms for detecting spikes and seizures, although their value in CEEG remains to be determined (51).

A number of commercial DEEG units have programs for quantitative EEG (qEEG). qEEG transforms DEEG signals into frequency and amplitude (or power) measurements using the fast Fourier transformation. The resulting components can be displayed in a variety of formats, including bar graphs, CSA, and topographic scalp maps. Several statistical variables can be analyzed and compared, although the validity of some statistical methods remains to be established (78). The appeal of qEEG resides in its data compression and visual display capabilities, which are perceived as more easily interpretable than raw DEEG data.

The "bispectral index" is one of the more commonly described attempts to process EEG data for the non–EEG-trained user (30). Another approach—automated segmental analysis—holds considerable promise in this regard (3). The expert systems approach may also prove useful (93). qEEG may therefore be easier for non-EEG professionals to identify significant changes. qEEG detects cerebral ischemia earlier than visual analysis, but it remains unclear if these early changes are clinically significant (1).

Vespa et al. (108) analyzed the percentage of alpha-range EEG activity (relative alpha) and found its variability to be a useful tool for detecting cerebral ischemia due to vasospasm. Nuwer (80) used relative alpha to detect NCSE in patients with acute brain injury (see Fig. 25.2). Bleck (12) employed spectral edge frequency and CSA for detecting seizures when sedation or anticonvulsants had suppressed background activity. Another potentially useful area for qEEG is trend analysis of focal slow activity. In patients with baseline encephalopathic slowing, it may be difficult using visual analysis alone to detect progressive regional slowing or further attenuation of background activity. qEEG, such as CSA, may detect these subtle but potentially important changes.

Technical and physiological variables, however, can produce misleading qEEG displays. For this reason, EEGers generally agree that the raw EEG signal must be available for comparison when qEEG is used (78). Sources of potential qEEG misinterpretation include skull asymmetries, scalp edema, and fluctuating states of alertness. Seizures in the delta frequency range, brief seizures, burst-suppression, periodic lateralized epileptiform discharges, and spike discharges may go undetected by qEEG. In addition, a false-negative incidence of up to 10% has been reported, in comparison to raw EEG for the detection of focal abnormalities documented on cerebral imaging studies (81). qEEG has difficulty identifying episodic slowing and variable alertness (personal observation).

ELECTRODES AND MONTAGES

In many patients, including those with head trauma, craniotomies, skull defects, surgical drains, intracranial catheters, fresh suture lines, and head wounds, electrode positions must be modified from those specified by the conventional 10-20 System. Electrode placement should maintain symmetry and be in areas topographically correlated to the cerebral pathological process of interest. Either disk or needle electrodes can be used. Disk electrodes obviate the risk of accidental needle puncture and are more comfortable for conscious patients. However, they produce more artifact on imaging studies than do needle electrodes. Needle electrodes can generally be applied more quickly than disk electrodes, and comfort is not an issue in patients with altered levels of consciousness. Use of collodion to secure the electrodes for long-term recording is mandatory. In the relatively closed environment of the ICU, personnel should be advised of the potentially offensive odor of collodion. Air purifiers, filters, and fans should be used to minimize and disperse the vapors. Reapplication of gel to disk electrodes, at least daily, should be done.

ARTIFACTS AND PITFALLS

When CEEG is used in the ICU, many artifacts are more frequent and may be more difficult to eliminate than those in the EEG laboratory or epilepsy monitoring unit (113). Reasons for this include the following:

- EEG electrodes, wires, and amplifiers are close to electronic devices that generate alternating current fields (automated intravenous pumps, ICU monitors, and ventilator equipment) and to structures that generate static charges (dripping intravenous fluids, condensed water moving in ventilator tubing).
- Long-term recording provides more opportunities for dislodging electrodes and drying of electrode gel, which result in impedance mismatching.
- Patient-generated artifacts are more numerous and also more difficult to control, inasmuch as the patients are critically ill. Artifacts include many of the same body movement and muscle potentials seen in a standard laboratory, but they also include intractable hiccups, myoclonic jerks, palatal myoclonus, nystagmus, asymmetric oculomotor paralysis, and flexor or extensor posturing.
- The scalp and calvaria of patients may be damaged or distorted by trauma, surgery, or disease. Changes include scalp edema, which can be prominent enough to produce artifactual reduction in amplitude either regionally or over an entire hemisphere, mimicking intracranial disease. Skull asymmetries, postcraniotomy defects, or head trauma produce strikingly asymmetrical eye movement, pulse, or electrocardiographic artifacts.

- EEG electrodes and wires can be disturbed by routine nursing activities, including patient turning, manipulation of dressings, suctioning, and placement of nasogastric tubes.

Advances in automated techniques for artifact identification and rejection should greatly increase the utility of CEEG and qEEG in the near future (102).

CLINICAL FACTORS THAT CONFOUND CONTINUOUS EEG IN THE INTENSIVE CARE UNIT

Many clinical variables in ICU patients affect the EEG but do not reflect cerebral abnormalities. For example, most ICU patients receive medications that alter the EEG, including benzodiazepines, barbiturates, narcotics, and neuroleptics. Patients on ventilators may be hyperventilated (intentionally or unintentionally). It is useful for clinicians to know a patient's pH and arterial carbon dioxide tension ($PaCO_2$) when interpreting the EEG. Patients who have been hyperventilated and are being weaned off controlled ventilation may show physiological EEG changes as their hypocapnia normalizes. Most ICU patients have disrupted sleep patterns, or they may lack sleep entirely despite appearing asleep. In patients who are "locked-in," EEG evidence of normal sleep-wake cycling leads to the correct diagnosis.

TECHNICAL ADJUSTMENTS AND SUGGESTIONS FOR TROUBLESHOOTING

It is impossible to avoid the many technical, electrical, mechanical, and physiological sources of artifacts encountered in the ICU. The following suggestions may be valuable:

1. Adjusting the bandpass of the displayed activity can remove some of the bothersome low- and high-frequency transients. With qEEG equipment, the actual data should be stored at wide bandpass. Maintaining the low-frequency filter at 1 Hz usually removes respiratory and other low-frequency artifacts. If epileptiform discharges are superimposed on high-amplitude, low-frequency activity, changing the low-frequency filter setting to 3 or 5 Hz (time constant of 0.03 seconds) attenuates the slow-wave activity and accentuates the sharp signals of interest. Some use a 60-Hz notch filter routinely in the ICU. Reducing the high-frequency

filter to 50 Hz diminishes high-frequency artifacts such as those originating in muscle. Lowering it to 35 Hz risks losing moderate-frequency activity that may have physiological importance. Bipolar montages are usually preferred over referential ones.

2. If generalized or widespread abnormalities appear with atypical waveforms, reference and ground electrode impedances should be checked, as should the preamplified connection to the computer cable.

3. Frequent, simple text notations should be made on the EEG to document nursing and physical therapy treatments, medication administrations, and other variables that can disrupt or affect the EEG record. Without these notations, related EEG changes can easily be misinterpreted as pathological. Developing a standard menu simplifies this task.

4. A database or reference binder with CEEG samples of commonly encountered artifacts is helpful for ICU nurses. As additional or unique examples are identified, these can be added.

TRAINING OF ICU PERSONNEL FOR CONTINUOUS EEG

The word "monitor" is derived from the Latin *monere,* meaning "to warn." CEEG functions much as binoculars do for the lookout on a ship: it provides early warning by extending the viewer's powers of observation. Although impressive technological advances in monitoring devices have improved clinicians' ability to observe physiological and pathophysiological events, the success of a monitoring system depends on a highly trained, skilled, and dedicated team. Like a ship's crew, the monitoring team functions as a feedback loop, consisting of: observation → recognition → communication → analysis → decision making → response → observation, and so forth. Team members must be proficient in use of the equipment, communicate their observations clearly, analyze data thoughtfully, make accurate decisions rapidly, and implement responses appropriately. Key members of the team include the ICU bedside nurse, the EEG technologist, the supervising EEGer, the neurointensivist, and other attending physicians. The team's proper training, continuing education, motivation, compensation, and administrative support require no less commitment than other complex ICU tasks (54).

Our experience of training more than 300 ICU and emergency department nurses in CEEG contradicts the traditional view that the EEG is too complex and visually confusing for non-experts to use. ICU nurses approach EEG already comfortable with waveform recognition from their experience with electrocardiography, pulmonary artery catheters, intraaortic balloon pumps, and ICP monitoring. They consider CEEG a natural extension of physiological monitoring to the brain. Using a structured workshop (51), we have trained a large cadre of ICU nurses to be comfortable with and competent in, recognizing basic CEEG patterns and common artifacts. The workshop

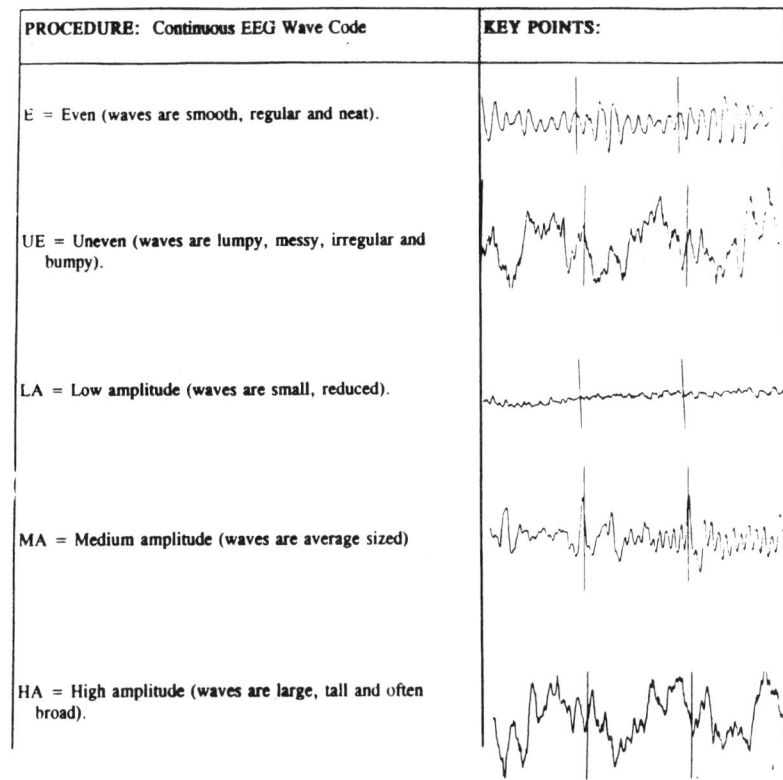

FIG. 25.4. Codes used by nurses to describe CEEG activity. Symbols and respective waveforms from CEEG training manual. (From Jordan KG. Continuous EEG and evoked potential monitoring in the neuroscience intensive care unit. *J Clin Neurophysiol* 1993;10:445.)

includes a training manual, workbooks, a library of CEEG samples with clinical correlations, and hands-on practice with equipment (Fig. 25.4). Neurologists, EEG technologists, and previously trained ICU nurses assume mentoring roles at the bedside. Vespa et al. (106) reported a similar experience. After going through a training program, their nurses achieved 94% accuracy in identifying generalized seizures, burst-suppression, and reduced alpha variability. In a few institutions, CEEG training is a requirement for all ICU nurses, and their competency in this area is regularly assessed. Only nurses who have achieved this competency are assigned to patients requiring CEEG.

SUPERVISION OF CONTINUOUS EEG USING NETWORK TECHNOLOGY

For CEEG to be fully effective and credible, expert supervision must be readily available to ICU nurses and physicians. They may be supervised by a neurointensivist-electroencephalographer or by an EEGer sufficiently experienced in neurological critical care to provide meaningful correlations between EEG and clinical data. In view of its increasing use, CEEG is likely to become part of the curriculum in fellowship programs for clinical neurophysiology and neurointensive care.

Stand-alone bedside EEG units are isolated from expert oversight. Even when CEEG equipment is part of a local ICU network, effective and credible supervision is limited because EEG experts are not in the ICU most of the time. As a computer-based modality, CEEG can be remotely transmitted to experts in an offsite laboratory, office, or home for real-time or *post hoc* interpretation. This makes expert supervision available 24 hours a day. Although speed is a concern because of the voluminous data generated by CEEG, modems at 33.8 or 56 kbps produce a transmission delay of only 10 to 15 seconds for 16 channels of real-time CEEG. Faster and more reliable transmission can be achieved with newer technology.

It is likely that expert supervision via CEEG networking will become increasingly important for at least two reasons. First, management decisions for many acute neurological conditions, such as acute ischemic stroke and status epilepticus, are critically time dependent. With effective treatment now available, it becomes difficult to justify delays in interpretation. Studies have already documented delays in the diagnosis and treatment of NCSE in the emergency department that result in significant

rates of morbidity and mortality (59,60). Second, because there are relatively few certified EEGers to meet the potential demand for CEEG, it may become increasingly important to leverage the limited pool of expertise to an increasing number of patients through a multivenue CEEG network.

CLINICAL APPLICATIONS AND IMPACT OF CONTINUOUS EEG

Table 25.1 lists the diagnoses in 200 patients consecutively monitored in one NICU. Table 25.2 demonstrates the impact of CEEG on the clinical management of these patients, expanding a previously reported experience with 73 patients (51). Jordan (51) examined three specific clinical decisions that commonly arise in the ICU: (a) transporting the patient for cerebral imaging studies; (b) initiating or modifying anticonvulsant drug therapy; and (c) hemodynamic manipulation for cerebral perfusion. Using a retrospective chart review, he categorized the impact of CEEG as "decisive" when the CEEG findings alone led to one or more of these decisions; as "contributing" when CEEG was combined with clinical findings to make one or more decisions; and as "non-contributory" when CEEG data did not assist with any of these decisions. The impact was decisive in 54%, contributing in 32%, and non-contributory in 14% (52). The impact varied somewhat with the specific diagnostic category, as indicated in the Table. Vespa et al. (106) reviewed data from 300 monitored patients to determine

TABLE 25.1. *Indications for continuous EEG in the intensive care unit*

Admitting diagnosis	No. of patients	% of total
Acute cerebral ischemia	57	28
Intracranial hemorrhage	43	22
Uncontrolled seizures	44	22
Metabolic coma	20	10
Brain tumor	16	8
Intracranial infection	13	6
Head trauma	7	4
Total	200	100

K.G. Jordan (unpublished data).

TABLE 25.2. *Impact of continuous EEG in the intensive care unit on clinical management (N = 200)*

Impact	No. of patients	% of total	ACI	HEM	SZ	MC	BT	INF	HT
Decisive	109	54	28	22	36	9	8	4	2
Contributing	64	32	16	16	5	10	5	8	4
None	27	14	13	5	3	1	3	1	1
Total	200	100	57	43	44	20	16	13	7

ACI, acute cerebral ischemia; BT, brain tumor; HEM, intracranial hemorrhage; HT, head trauma; INF, intracranial infection; MC, metabolic coma; SZ, uncontrolled seizures.

the impact of CEEG on clinical decisions in the ICU. They studied 200 patients retrospectively and 100 prospectively. The critical determinations analyzed included decisions to (a) continue aggressive care, (b) send a patient out of the unit for a computerized tomographic (CT) scan, (c) adjust sedation, and (d) determine seizure activity. In more than 90% of their patients, CEEG was used as a daily guide for one of more of these decisions at the bedside.

These data also strongly support the contention that when CEEG is implemented systematically by a well-trained team, it positively influences bedside clinical management decisions (54).

In the following sections, established, emerging, and potential uses of CEEG in patients with status epilepticus, acute focal cerebral ischemia, coma, and acute severe head trauma are reviewed.

CONTINUOUS EEG IN STATUS EPILEPTICUS

Acute seizures, including those of status epilepticus, are common following acute brain injuries. Early convulsive seizures occur in 10% to 27% of patients with various types of acute brain injury (38). More than half of the reported cases of generalized convulsive status epilepticus (GCSE) arise from ischemic trauma, intracranial hemorrhage, cerebral hypoxia, hypoglycemia, drug intoxication, and withdrawal syndromes (33,39,67). Of patients without a history of epilepsy, 59% with status epilepticus have acute brain trauma (7). A new acute brain injury precipitates status epilepticus in about 25% of patients with known epilepsy (8). In other words, various acute brain injuries seen in the ICU and emergency department are commonly associated with status epilepticus. NCSE cannot be reliably

diagnosed by clinical examination, and acute brain injury itself can alter consciousness and behavior, confounding the diagnosis of NCSE. Using CEEG, Jordan (50) found that 34% of 124 NICU patients had nonconvulsive seizures (NCS) and that 76% of these (33 patients) had NCSE. Privitera et al. (85) obtained emergency EEGs from 198 patients with altered consciousness and found that 27% (53 patients) had NCSE. Among their 49 patients with NCS and NCSE, Young et al. (115) found that acute brain injuries were the cause in almost half. Vespa et al. (108) identified seizures in nine (16%) of 56 patients with acute severe head trauma, of whom seven (78%) had NCS. In the Veterans Affairs Cooperative Study of status epilepticus, Treiman et al. (101) found that of patients with overt GCSE who received "adequate" treatment, 20% continued to have NCS and NCSE. Similarly, DeLorenzo et al. (32) found that in 12% of 170 patients with GCSE, NCSE developed after overt convulsive activity stopped. Clinical detection of NCSE could be determined only by CEEG.

In the absence of CEEG, the diagnosis of NCS and NCSE is likely to be delayed or missed. Of 89 ICU patients with NCSE, 77% were not recognized as having seizures at the time of first EEG (34). There was a median delay of 24 hours for the diagnosis of NCSE in those who had had clinical seizures, and a delay of 72 hours for those without clinical seizures. Some of the patients of Young et al. (115) with NCSE were obtunded for hours before an EEG was obtained that led to the correct diagnosis. Conversely, CEEG allows the exclusion of status epilepticus in critically ill patients with unusual movements (88).

Kaplan (60) reported substantial delays in the diagnosis of NCSE in the emergency department. In another study (59), the average time from patients' arrival in the emergency department to the diagnosis of NCSE was 2½ hours, and misdiagnosis of NCSE occurred in 93% (Fig. 25.5). In these

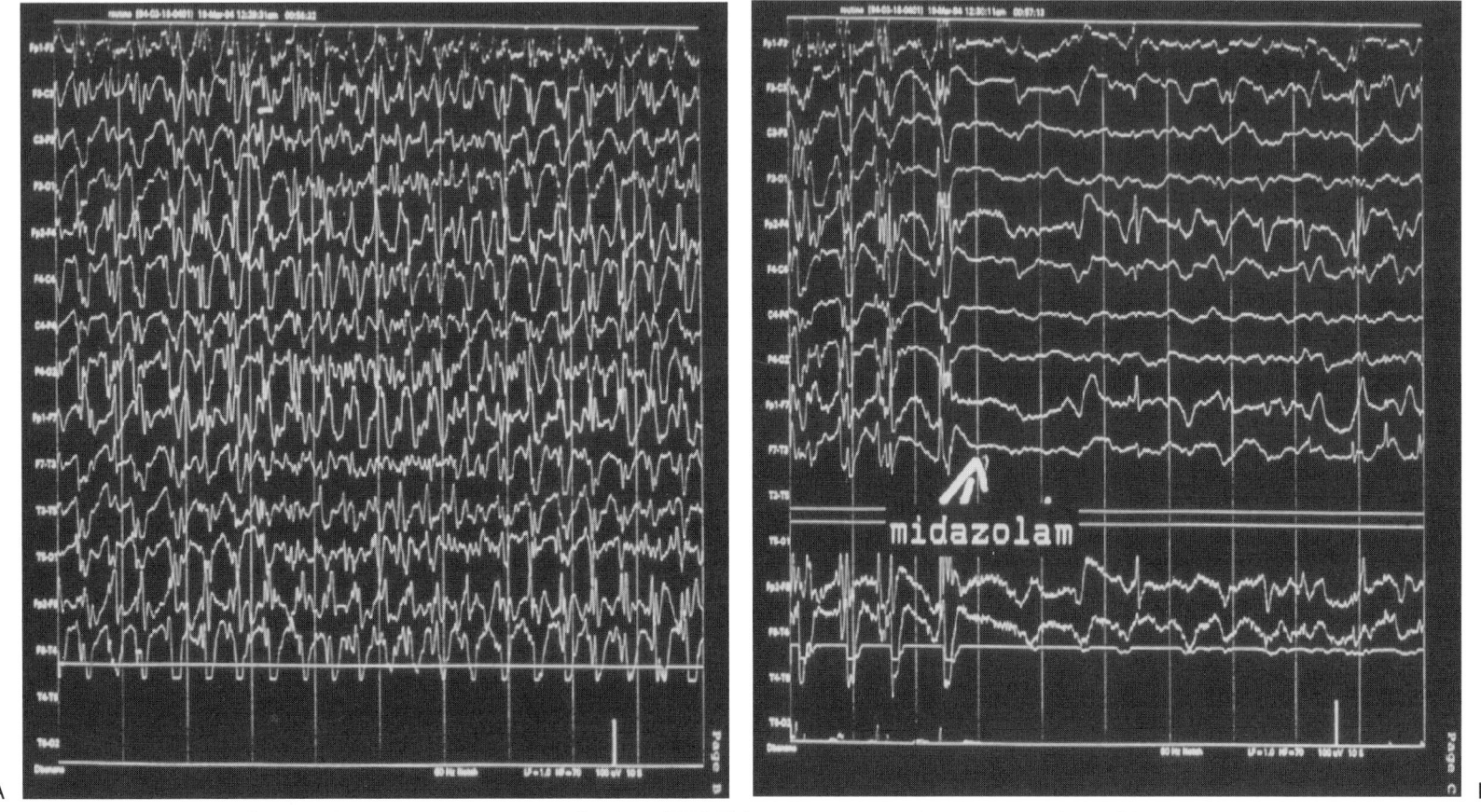

FIG. 25.5. Non-convulsive status epilepticus (NCSE) in an emergency department patient with acute cerebral infarction and theophylline toxicity. The delay from the patient's arrival to diagnosis of NCSE was 210 minutes. **A:** Generalized, highly rhythmic polyspike–slow-wave discharges (channels 15 and 16 turned off). **B:** Once NCSE was identified, intravenous midazolam produced immediate cessation of seizure activity.

two studies from emergency departments, NCSE was often misdiagnosed as postictal state, psychiatric disorder, stroke, or metabolic encephalopathy.

These data lead to the following conclusions:

- GCSE and NCSE are common accompaniments or sequelae of acute brain injury.
- After GCSE convulsions are controlled, NCSE is a common cause of persisting obtundation or behavioral changes.
- Without CEEG, the diagnosis of NCSE is delayed or overlooked.

The longer GCSE or NCSE persists, the more difficult it is to treat, and the higher the rate of mortality. Among patients in whom GCSE lasts more than 1 hour, the mortality rate rises from 3% to 36% (100). After 3 hours, the mortality rate approaches 50% (115). Etiology is an important determinant of progress (67), but multivariate logistic regression analysis has revealed that the variables that most increase the rates of morbidity and mortality in NCSE are seizure duration and delayed diagnosis, independent of etiology (115). Prolonged NCSE is particularly refractory to treatment and carries a higher mortality rate than does GCSE. Of the 30 patients with NCSE in the emergency department study by Jordan et al. (59), only 25% were controlled within 3 hours of treatment, and only 50% were controlled by 5 hours.

In the Veterans Affairs Cooperative Study of status epilepticus, Treiman et al. (101) used definitions somewhat different from those used here. However, many of their cases of "subtle status epilepticus" correspond to NCSE. Their "overt status epilepticus" category includes GCSE and some other forms of status epilepticus as well. Among 518 patients with status epilepticus, the first treatment regimen was successful in 55% with overt status epilepticus but in only 15% with subtle status epilepticus. Mortality rates in those groups were 27% and 65%, respectively.

The concurrence of acute brain injury and status epilepticus appears to compound the risk of morbidity and mortality (57,114). In patients with acute brain injury, GCSE is often resistant to treatment and associated with substantially higher morbidity and mortality rates than is GCSE occurring in non-acute processes (66). In a prospective study, Waterhouse et al. (109) found that when status epilepticus complicated acute ischemic stroke, mortality was three times higher than in stroke without status epilepticus. They also found a highly significant difference in mortality between these two groups that was not attributable to lesion size or to stroke severity. A logistic regression model indicated that the effects of status epilepticus and acute stroke on mortality

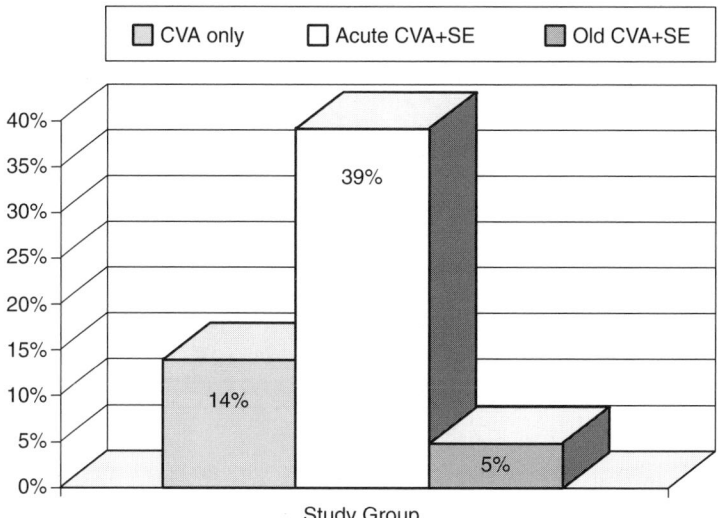

FIG. 25.6. Synergistic effect of status epilepticus and acute ischemic stroke on mortality. The rate of mortality of acute cerebral vascular accident (CVA) with status epilepticus (acute CVA + SE) was significantly higher than that from acute CVA without status epilepticus (CVA only: $p < 0.001$) and also higher than remote CVA with status epilepticus (old CVA + SE; $p < 0.001$). (From Waterhouse EJ, Vaughan JK, Barnes TY, et al. Synergistic effect of status epilepticus and ischemic brain injury on mortality. *Epilepsy Res* 1998;29:175–183.)

rate were synergistic, not simply additive (Fig. 25.6). In the Veterans Affairs Cooperative Study of status epilepticus (101), patients with persistent subtle status epilepticus had a mortality rate twice as high as that of patients with overt status epilepticus (30% versus 16%). In addition, with acute brain injury, subtle status epilepticus was 36% more likely to occur than overt status epilepticus, and more than twice as likely with acute systemic illness. Jordan et al. (59) found a dramatic increase in mortality among patients with acute brain injury associated with prolonged NCSE, with an odds ratio of 23.8 for acute over remote brain injury. In addition, Young et al. (115) found a highly significant difference in mortality between patients with NCSE and acute brain injury and those with remote brain injury (Fig. 25.7). Severe disability or death was seen in 75% of NCSE patients with acute brain injury, in contrast to 38% without acute brain injury (59). There is biochemical evidence sup-

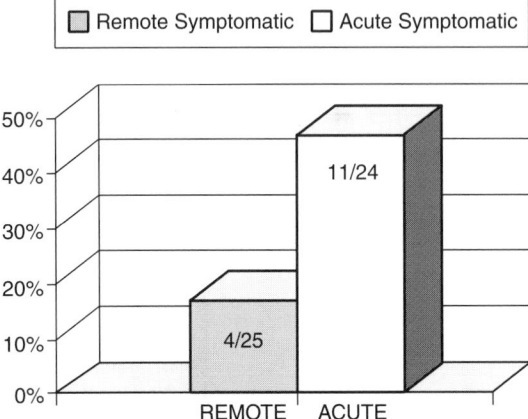

FIG. 25.7. The effect of concurrent acute brain injury and non-convulsive status epilepticus (NCSE) on mortality. In comparison with patients with remote symptomatic etiologies, patients with NCSE and acute symptomatic etiology (called acute brain injury in text) showed a nearly threefold increase in mortality ($p = 0.009$, odds ratio = 6.0). (Based on data from Young GB, Jordan KG, Doig GS. An assessment of nonconvulsive seizures in the intensive care unit using continuous EEG monitoring: an investigation of variables associated with mortality. *Neurology* 1996;47:83–89.)

porting this deleterious synergy. In a study of unselected patients with status epilepticus, DeGiorgio et al. (31) found the highest levels of serum neuron-specific enolase, a marker of neuronal injury, in patients who had both status epilepticus and acute brain injury.

These data are consistent with the accepted concept of secondary neuronal insult described by Miller and Becker (74). Acutely injured neurons are more likely than intact neurons to suffer irreversible injury or death when exposed to comparable levels of ischemic, metabolic, or hypoxic insults. Waterhouse et al. (109) drew an analogy to head injury, in which the combination of two acute injuries produces a worse outcome than either injury alone.

The conclusion from these findings is that in patients with acute brain injury and altered mentation or behavior, an EEG should be obtained promptly to exclude or confirm the diagnosis of NCSE and to guide management. We believe that for patients with acute brain injury and GCSE, it

TABLE 25.3. *Criteria for non-convulsive seizures*

Guideline: To qualify, at least *one* primary criteria *and one or more* secondary criteria, with discharges >10 seconds
Primary criteria
  1. Repetitive generalized or focal spikes, sharp waves, spike-and-wave or sharp-and-slow wave complexes at > three/second
  2. Repetitive generalized or focal spikes, sharp waves, spike-and-wave or sharp-and-slow wave complexes at < three/second *and* secondary criterion 4
  3. Sequential rhythmic waves and secondary criteria 1, 2 *and* 3 with or without 4
Secondary criteria
  1. Incrementally increasing onset: increase in voltage and/or frequency
  2. Decrementally decreasing offset: decrease in voltage and/or frequency
  3. Postdischarge slowing or voltage attenuation
  4. Significant improvement in clinical state or EEG patterns after intravenous antiepileptic drug administration

is urgent to obtain complete control of seizure activity, and control should be confirmed by EEG. Suggested primary and secondary criteria for the EEG diagnosis of NCS are listed in Table 25.3. EEG evolution of NCSE is shown in Figure 25.8.

CEEG provides objective information for physiologically targeted management of both GCSE and NCSE. Without CEEG, the patient may be undertreated, remaining exposed to the effects of unremitting epileptic cerebral activity, or overtreated, subjected to the risk of iatrogenic ventilatory failure, cardiovascular instability, and prolonged coma. After control of status epilepticus, CEEG patterns are useful for prognosis as they are highly correlated with morbidity and mortality, independent of etiology (48). The cumulative published experience from 1995 to 2000 suggests that CEEG is approaching a standard of care in the management of status epilepticus (12,32,77,101).

In cases of refractory GCSE, CEEG is necessary to guide therapy. High-dose pentobarbital has been the agent used most frequently. More recently, midazolam and propofol have been introduced with success and fewer complications (22). Whichever agent is used, CEEG is necessary to guide the intensity and duration of treatment. Different protocols have been recommended, but no optimal regimen has emerged, nor is there consensus about which EEG

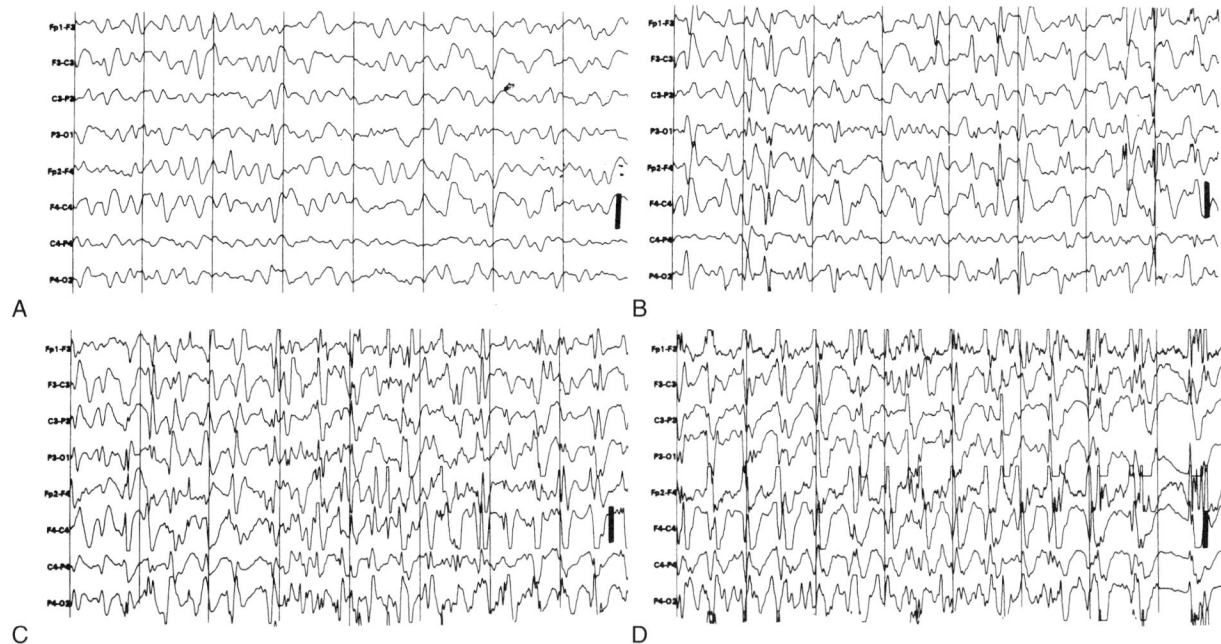

FIG. 25.8. Evolution of generalized non-convulsive status epilepticus (NCSE). **A:** Generalized, low- to medium-voltage theta-delta activity. **B:** Variable but incrementally increasing pattern of generalized spike, spike-wave, and sharp-wave discharges. **C** and **D:** Progressively rhythmic and stereotyped spike, polyspike, and spike-wave generalized discharges. Thick vertical calibration bar is 50 mV. Time interval between vertical dividing lines is 1 second. (From Young GB, Jordan KG, Doig GS. An assessment of nonconvulsive seizures in the intensive care unit using continuous EEG monitoring: an investigation of variables associated with mortality. *Neurology* 1996;47:83–89.)

endpoint is required for treatment to be successful (69,82). Based on our experience, we recommend administering the lowest dose necessary to produce cessation of all EEG epileptiform activity for 12 hours, during which time the patient receives loading doses of maintenance anticonvulsants. After this, the infusion is decreased guided by CEEG (53). As the infusion is decreased by spikes, polyspikes, spike-wave complexes, periodic lateralized epileptiform discharges, and bilateral independent periodic lateralized epileptiform discharges may emerge, which might suggest pending relapse into status epilepticus. However, these "emergent" epileptiform patterns are usually distinct in field distribution and morphological features from the patient's ictal activity, and represent a temporary effect of medication withdrawal. They are not clearly associated with a risk of recurrent seizures. Misconstruing these "medication-emergent" findings can lead to unnecessary, repeated treatment to suppress EEG activity (4) (Fig. 25.9).

Patients in the NICU exhibit a wide variety of non-epileptic involuntary and semipurposeful movements. These can be confused with, and mistakenly treated as, seizures (90). They include struggling movements, tremulousness,

tetanic spasms, septic rigors, neuroleptic-induced rigidity and extrapyramidal movements, myoclonic jerks, tonic head or eye deviations, and decerebrate or decorticate posturing. Routine bedside EEG may capture only a fraction of the movements. CEEG can advantageously identify cerebral activity before, during, and after the movements. In the mechanically ventilated unconscious patient, CEEG during neuromuscular blockade can determine the presence or absence of epileptogenic activity (Fig. 25.10).

Patients with some neurological diseases are at risk for potentially fatal hyperkalemia if given depolarizing neuromuscular junction blocking agents (104). Although this scenario is most commonly encountered in patients with lower motor neuron disorders, nondepolarizing agents are preferable to succinylcholine for this purpose. Vecuronium, 0.1 mg/kg provides adequate blockage for about 20 minutes. Adequate ventilatory support must be provided during this time (e.g., the ventilator mode may require temporary alteration if the patient is receiving pressure support ventilation). Patients with substantial renal dysfunction should receive cisatracurium, 0.1 to 0.2 mg/kg, because vecuronium is renally excreted.

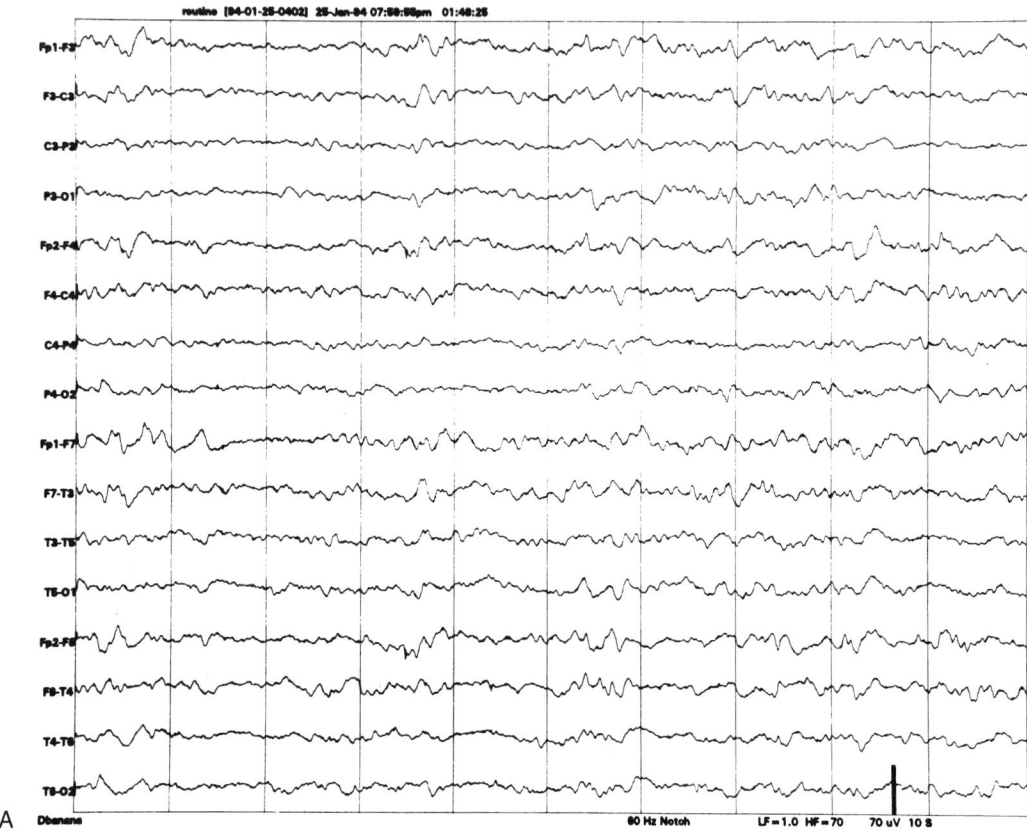

FIG. 25.9. Emergence from pentobarbital-induced cerebral suppression for status epilepticus. **A:** Low-amplitude mixed frequencies with residual burst-suppression. (*Figure continues.*)

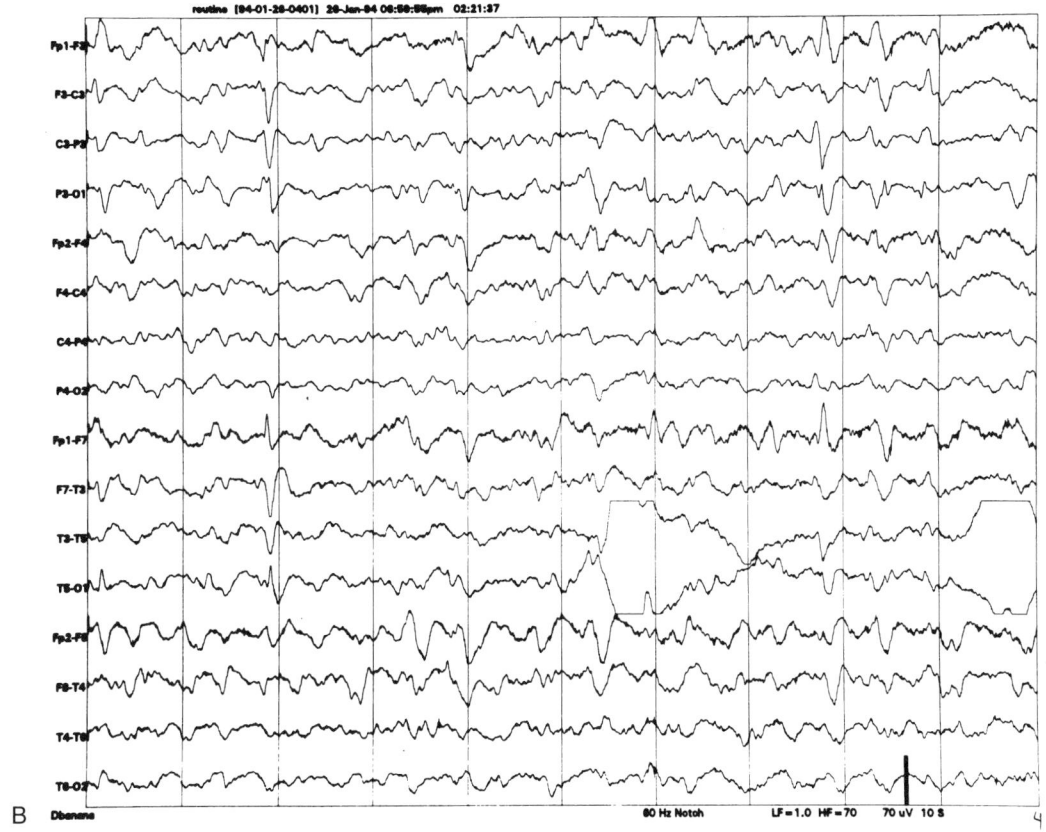

FIG. 25.9. *Continued.* **B:** A variety of epileptiform activity is present, including left hemisphere spikes, right frontal sharp waves, and right frontotemporal triphasic semiperiodic sharp waves. These activities resolved as the patient's coma lightened. (From Jordan KG. Continuous EEG monitoring in the neuroscience intensive care unit and emergency department. *J Clin Neurophysiol* 1999;16:14–39.)

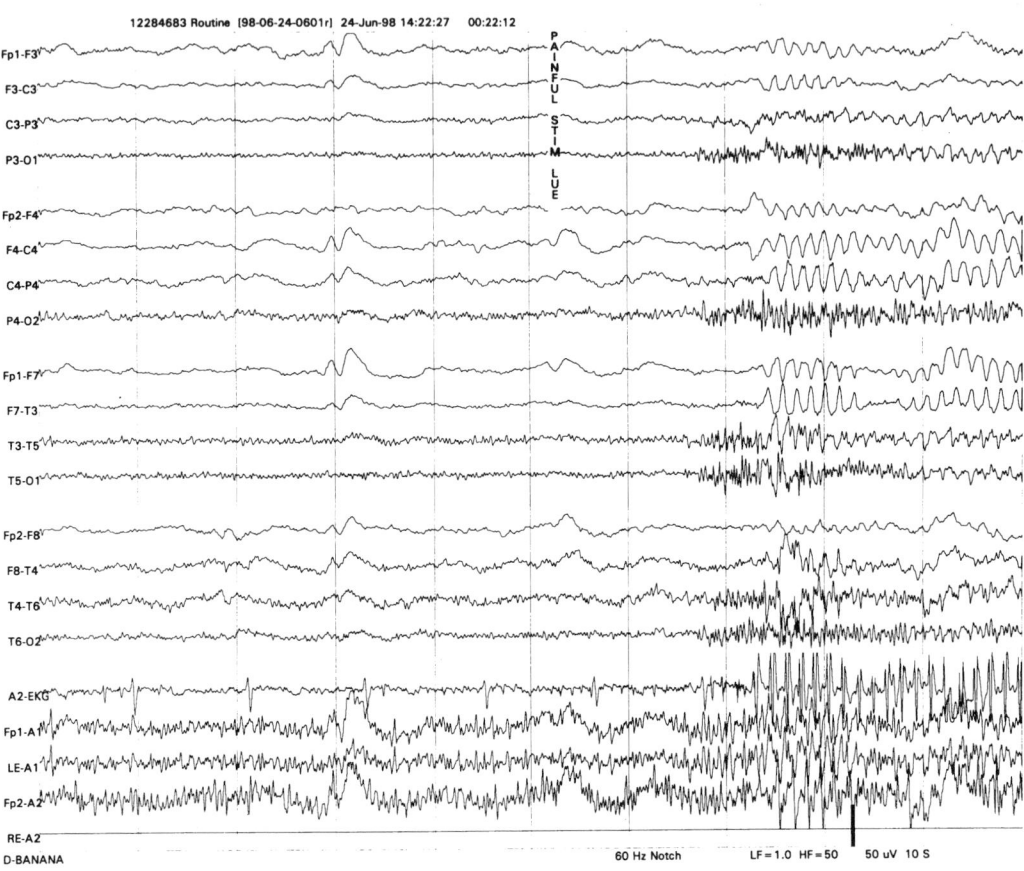

FIG. 25.10. Continuous EEG in a patient with acute severe head trauma and stimulus-induced "seizures." These proved to be non-epileptic. **A** and **B:** Patient stimulation produced incrementally increasing, generalized rhythmic activity. The morphological pattern in the left posterior hemisphere strongly resembles incrementally increasing ictal polyspike activity. (*Figure continues.*)

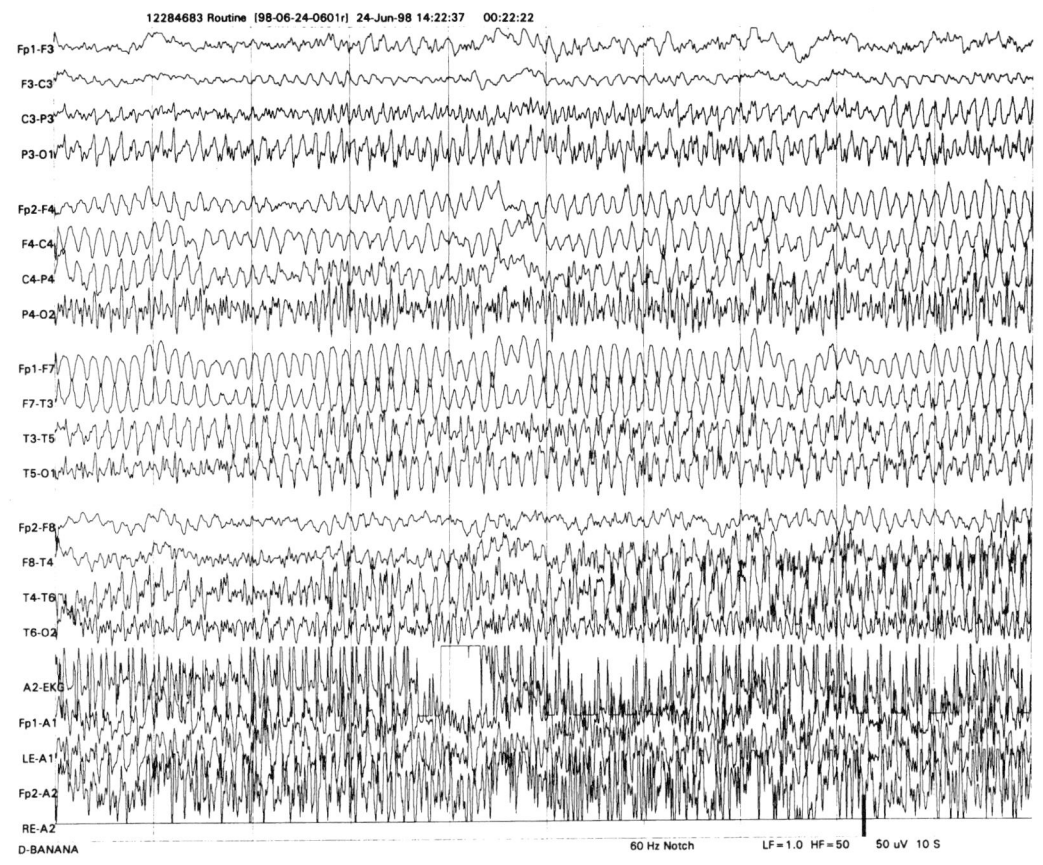

FIG. 25.10. *Continued.*

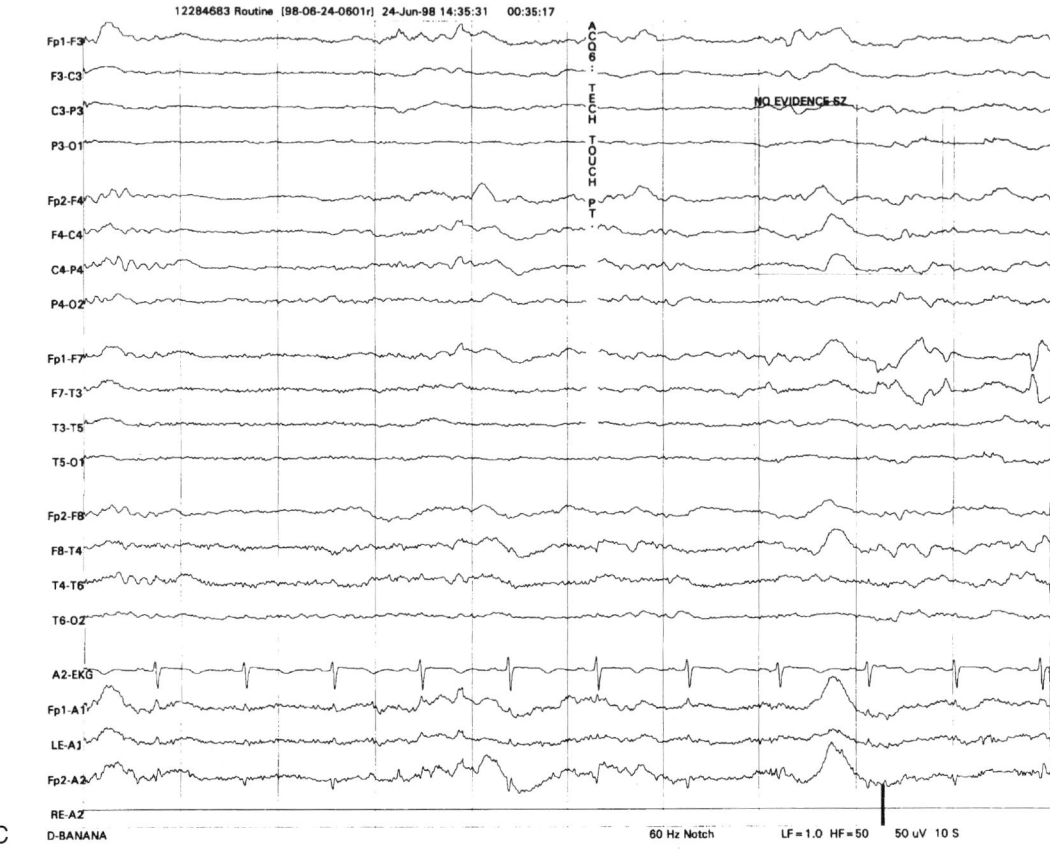

FIG. 25.10. *Continued.* **C:** After administration of a neuromuscular blocking agent, there was no evidence of epileptiform activity, even with stimulation. (From Jordan KG. Continuous EEG monitoring in the neuroscience intensive care unit and emergency department. *J Clin Neurophysiol* 1999;16:14–39.)

The possibility of psychogenic status epilepticus must also be kept in mind. In one specialized epilepsy center, almost 20% of patients in the emergency department with intractable GCS had psychogenic seizures, and several had psychogenic GCSE (38). Psychogenic GCSE can appear genuine even to experts, and CEEG is the only way to determine if the convulsive activity is accompanied by ictal discharges (70). Although convulsive motor activity often obscures the CEEG record, the prompt appearance of a normal alpha rhythm during pauses is strong evidence for psychogenic status epilepticus.

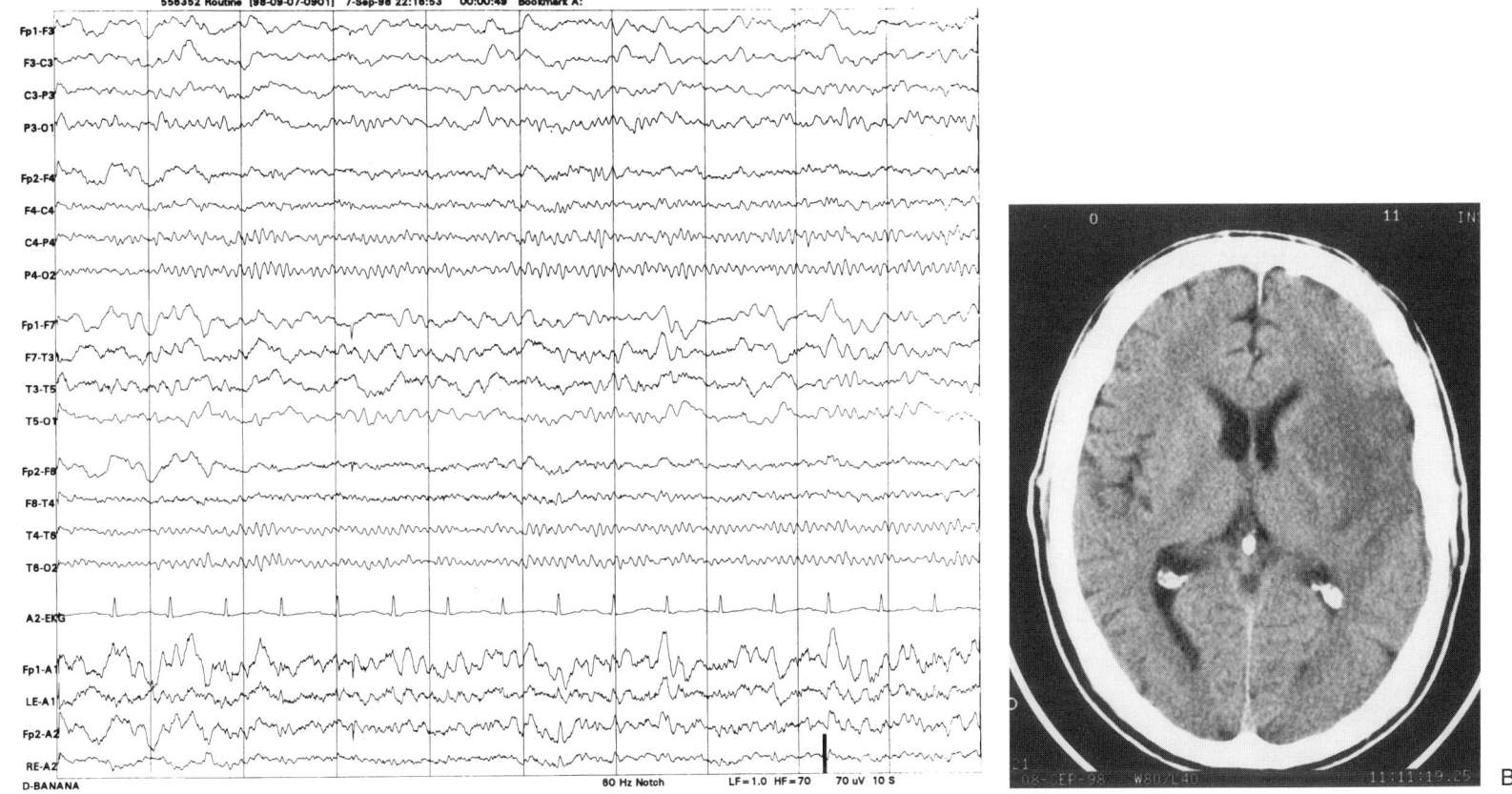

FIG. 25.11. EEG and CT scan in a patient with acute left infarction of the anterior temporal lobe. **A:** Continuous polymorphic delta activity in the left hemisphere, maximal temporally, with well-preserved right hemisphere background activity. **B:** CT scan showing acute left temporal infarction.

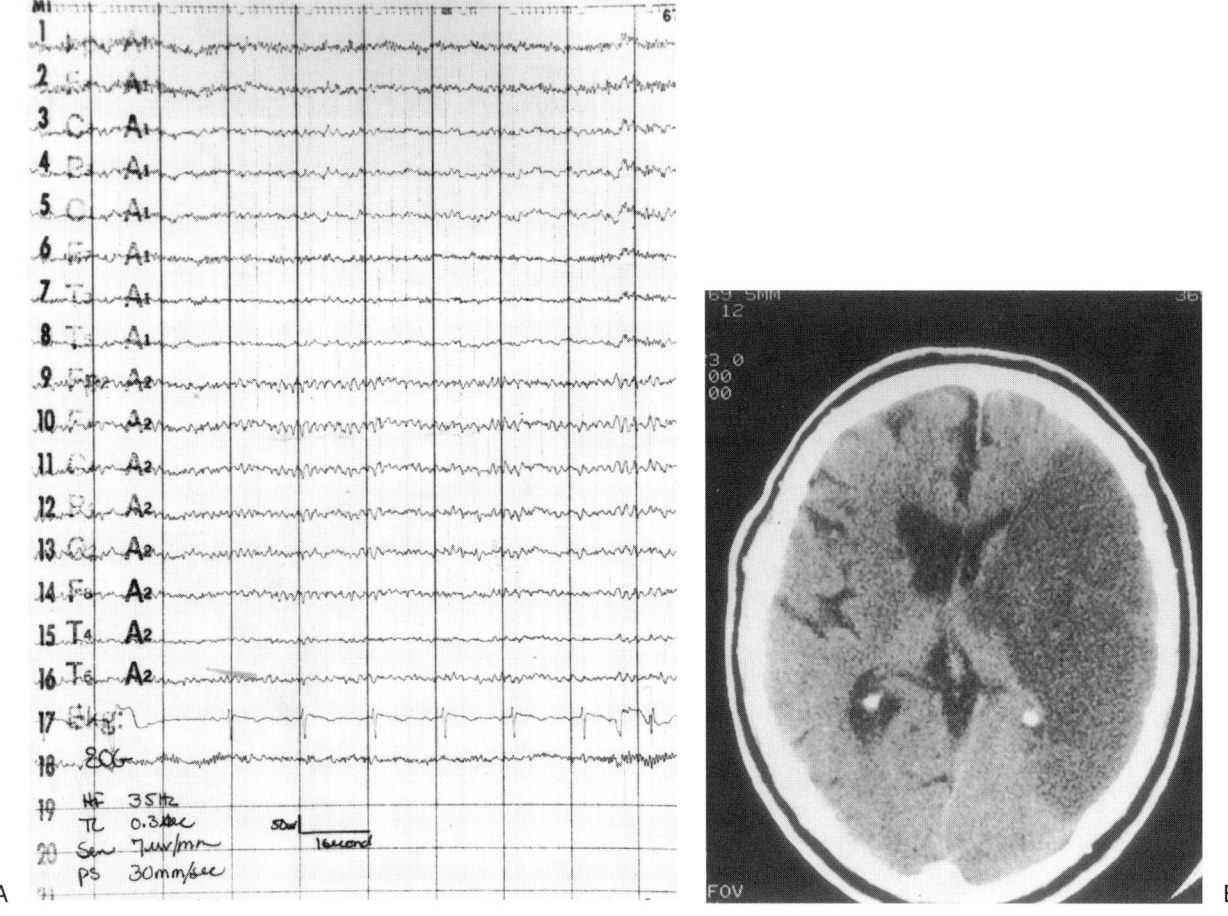

FIG. 25.12. EEG and corresponding CT scan with extensive left hemisphere infarction secondary to middle cerebral artery occlusion. **A:** Referential montage showing marked attenuation of all EEG frequencies over the left hemisphere. **B:** CT showing extensive left hemisphere infarction with mass effect invading the entire middle cerebral artery territory.

CONTINUOUS EEG IN ACUTE FOCAL CEREBRAL ISCHEMIA

EEG abnormalities with large hemispheric infarctions were described as long ago as 1948 (28). In order of increasing severity, these changes include (a) widespread polymorphic delta activity in the involved hemisphere, maximally in the temporal and frontotemporal regions (Fig. 25.11); (b) ipsilateral attenuation or loss of alpha activity, beta activity, and sleep spindles; (c) with extensive hemispheric infarction, marked suppression of all EEG activity (Fig. 25.12); and (d) contralateral frontal delta activity and intermittent projected rhythmic delta activity with mass effect and midline shift. Patients with acute focal ischemia often have precarious cerebral perfusion: in up to 43%, perfusion worsens within the first 24 hours (17). Among patients with subarachnoid hemorrhage vasospasm, 25% to 40% suffer symptomatic ischemia (45). Therefore, a bedside monitor warning of impending deterioration would be helpful. Because of its dependence on CBF, CEEG changes appear within minutes of the onset of ischemia (98). In 45% of 22 such patients, CEEG deterioration was characterized by focal slow activity, appearance of epileptiform discharges, or generalized slowing (49). CEEG abnormalities preceded clinical changes in several patients. The severity of EEG abnormalities in acute focal cerebral ischemia correlates closely with the degree of ischemia measured by xenon CT determination of cerebral blood flow (58). When hypertensive hypervolemic therapy was used to elevate regional CBF above the ischemic threshold, CEEG documented resolution of the focal slow activity. Wood et al. (111) also studied volume expansion therapy and likewise found that CBF and qEEG improved together (111).

In the emergency department, there may be a role for urgent EEG in selected patients with suspected stroke. In one study (65), the rate of stroke misdiagnosis in the emergency department was 13% to 19%; misdiagnosis was caused by conditions that mimicked ischemia (Table 25.4). Another study (40) found that the rate of misdiagnosis by emergency medicine specialists was 9% (16 of 185), and by family physicians 15% (8 of 52). Conversely, a number of stroke syndromes manifest without motor or sensory loss and can be confused with non-stroke conditions, including psychiatric disorders. These include receptive (Wernicke's) aphasia, visual agnosia, Gertsmann's syndrome, alexia with or without agraphia, and right parietal lobe ischemia. In acute stroke, the CT scan is often normal or equivocal early, increasing the likelihood of misdiagnosis. Because the EEG changes within minutes of the onset of ischemia, it provides a strong clue to the presence of ischemia or infarction as the basis of the patient's symptoms. This has obvious implications for the appropriate use of intravenous thrombolytic therapy. The relative roles of CEEG and the newer techniques of diffusion and perfusion magnetic resonance imaging remain to be determined.

The introduction of thrombolytic therapy for stroke has raised both hope and uncertainty within the medical community (21,76). Data support its benefits, but there is also evidence of a low but significant risk of intracranial hemorrhage (27). Jordan (55) studied 49 patients in the emergency department with focal ischemia using acute EEG. Eighteen patients had widespread voltage attenuation of all frequencies without accompanying delta activity, a pattern described by the acronym RAWOD (regional attenuation without delta) (Fig. 25.13A). This is equivalent to the third pattern described by Cohn et al. (28). It is also similar to the EEG pattern seen when clamping of the carotid artery produces cerebral ischemia sufficient to cause infarction (97).

Important clinical, physiological, and anatomic correlations were found with RAWOD: (a) Severe neurological deficits were present in all patients (mean National Institutes of Health Stroke Scale score, 31); (b) regional CBF was decreased to infarction levels in all patients studied (mean regional CBF, 8.6 mL/100 g/min); (c) ipsilateral cortical somatosensory evoked potentials were absent; (d) ipsilateral internal carotid artery and middle cerebral artery transcranial Doppler (TCD) velocities were markedly abnormal; (e) all RAWOD patients had poor outcomes, including a mortality rate of 67% (12 of 18); and, (f) in 56% of RAWOD patients (10 of 18), the ini-

TABLE 25.4. *Early xenon CT cerebral blood flow studies in patients with regional voltage attenuation without delta (RAWOD)*

Patient	MINHSS (NIHSS)	V_i (%)	$mCBF_i$ (mL/100 g/min)	Infarct on initial CT scan
JM	10 (35)	52.9	10.5	+
GN	10 (35)	47	6.8	+
SS	8 (28)	60.6	10.1	−
TP	8 (28)	43.4	10.0	+
HH	10 (35)	53.9	5.7	−
AC	10 (35)	49.8	8.3	−
Mean results	9.3 (33)	51.2 ± 6.6	8.6 ± 2.2	

$mCBF_i$, mean ischemic cerebral blood flow; MINHSS (NIHSS), National Institutes of Health Stroke Scale; V_i, percent volume of ischemic tissue (in affected hemisphere).

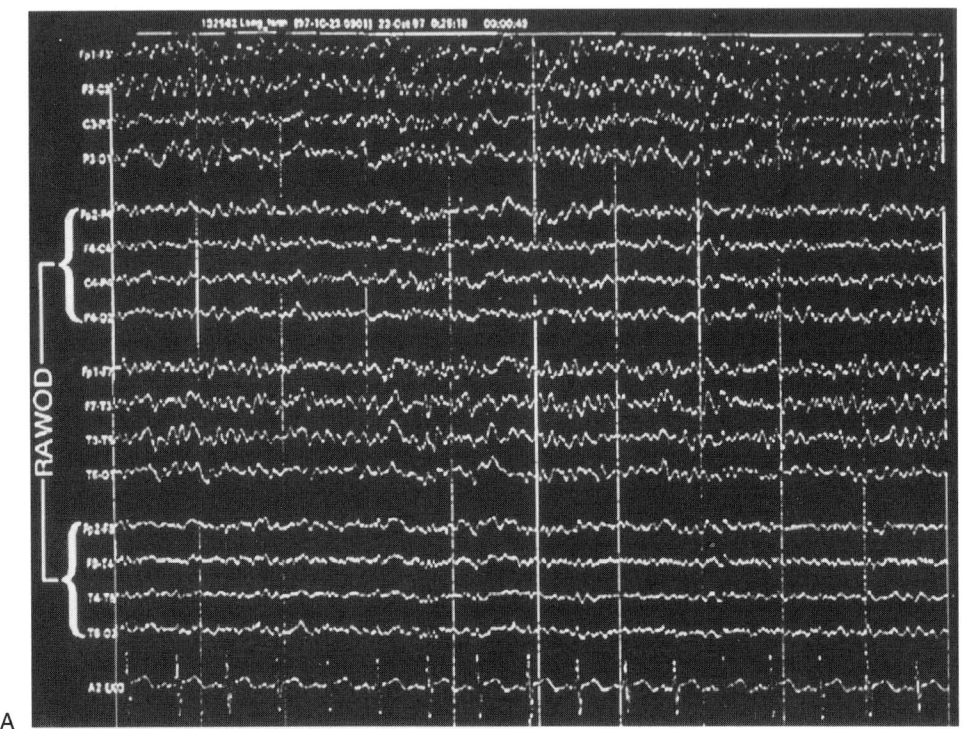

A

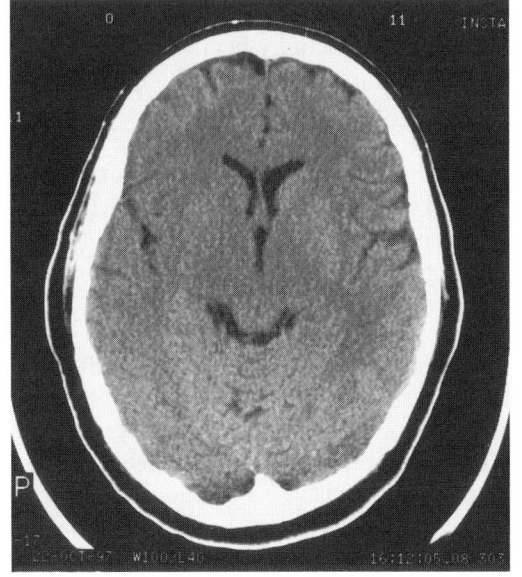

B

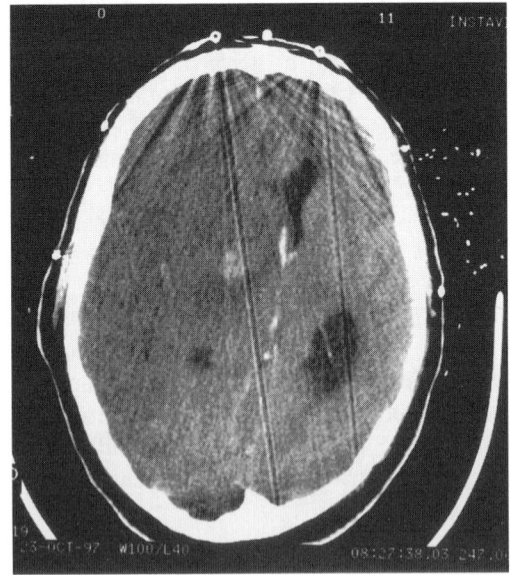

C

FIG. 25.13. Emergency room EEG and CT scans in a patient with massive acute right hemisphere ischemia. **A:** Acute emergency room EEG shows widespread attenuation of all frequencies in the right hemisphere (regional attenuation without delta [RAWOD]). There is diffuse 6-Hz theta slowing and some intermixed delta activity in the left hemisphere. **B:** Initial CT scan taken shortly before emergency room EEG. This scan was interpreted as normal. There may be early cortical edema in the right sylvian fissure. **C:** Repeat CT scan obtained 20 hours after the initial scan. This scan shows massive right hemisphere edema with midline herniation. The streak artifacts are caused by EEG needle electrodes in the patient's scalp.

tial CT showed no new areas of infarction, but on follow-up 48 hours later all 10 showed massive infarctions, often with malignant edema (see Fig. 25.13*B* and *C*). Among 20 patients with clinically severe acute focal cerebral ischemia within the middle cerebral artery territory, xenon CT showed a mean CBF of 10.4 mL/100 g/min in the symptomatic patients who developed severe edema (41). Among those who clinically herniated, mean CBF was 8.6 mL/100 g/min. These values are in the same range measured in the cerebral hemi-

sphere ipsilateral to the RAWOD pattern (personal observation). RAWOD is a distinctive EEG pattern found in extensive and irreversible focal ischemia, and it signifies a high risk of malignant cerebral edema.

Such observations suggest that urgent EEG in the emergency department may be a practical, cost-effective, and objective method for early identification of hemisphere infarctions. If confirmed, this could be a method that contributes to better selection of patients for therapeutic intervention.

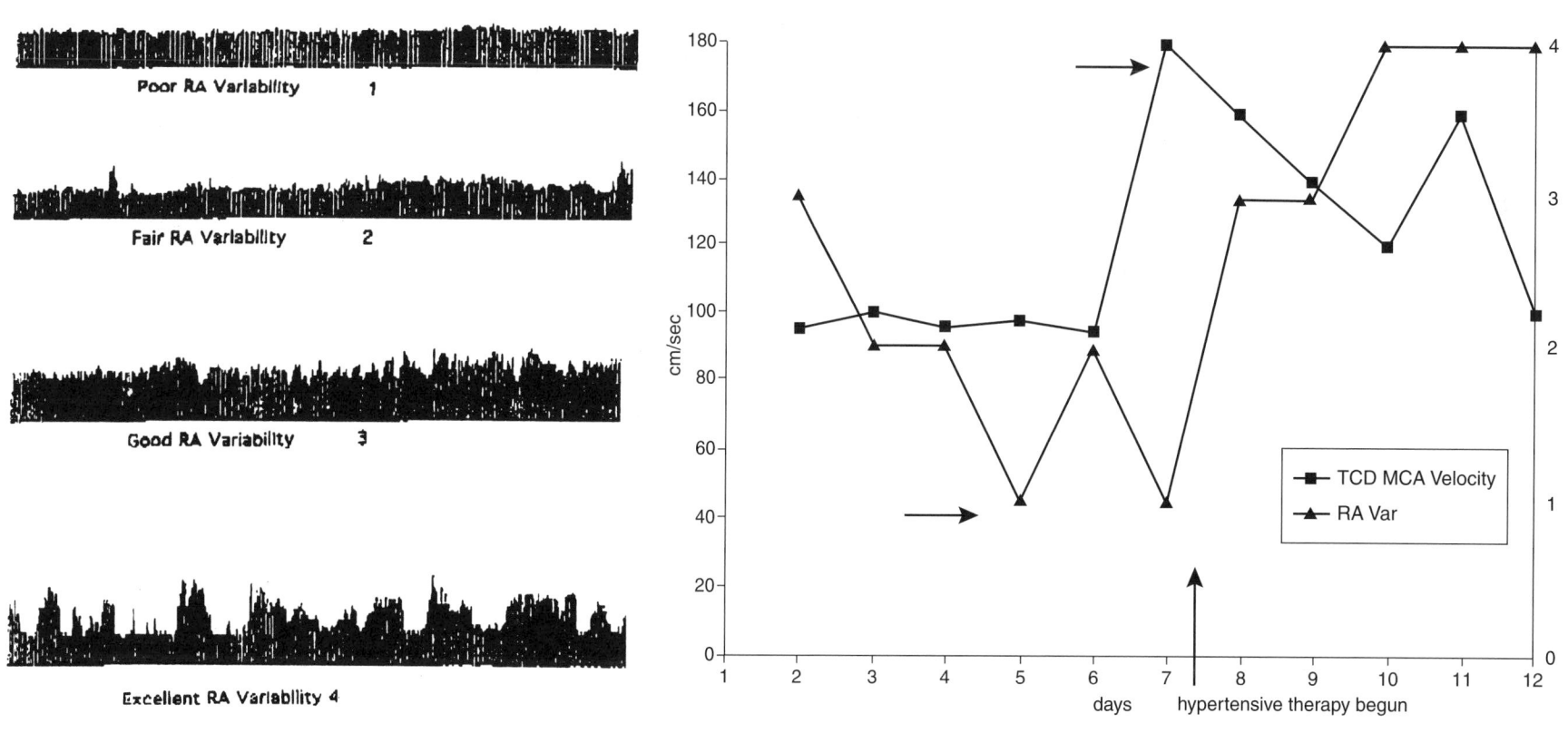

FIG. 25.14. Relative alpha variability on quantitative electroencephalogram (qEEG) correlated with transcranial Doppler (TCD) velocities in subarachnoid hemorrhage vasospasm. **A:** qEEG samples displaying relative alpha variability, graded 1 (abnormal) to 4 (normal). **B:** Graph shows relative alpha variability worsening to grade 1 on day 5. This precedes TCD evidence of vasospasm, detected on day 7. (From Vespa PM, Nuwer MR, Nenov V, et al. Increased incidence and impact of nonconvulsive and convulsive seizures after traumatic brain injury as detected by continuous electroencephalographic monitoring. *J Neurosurg* 1999;91:750–760.)

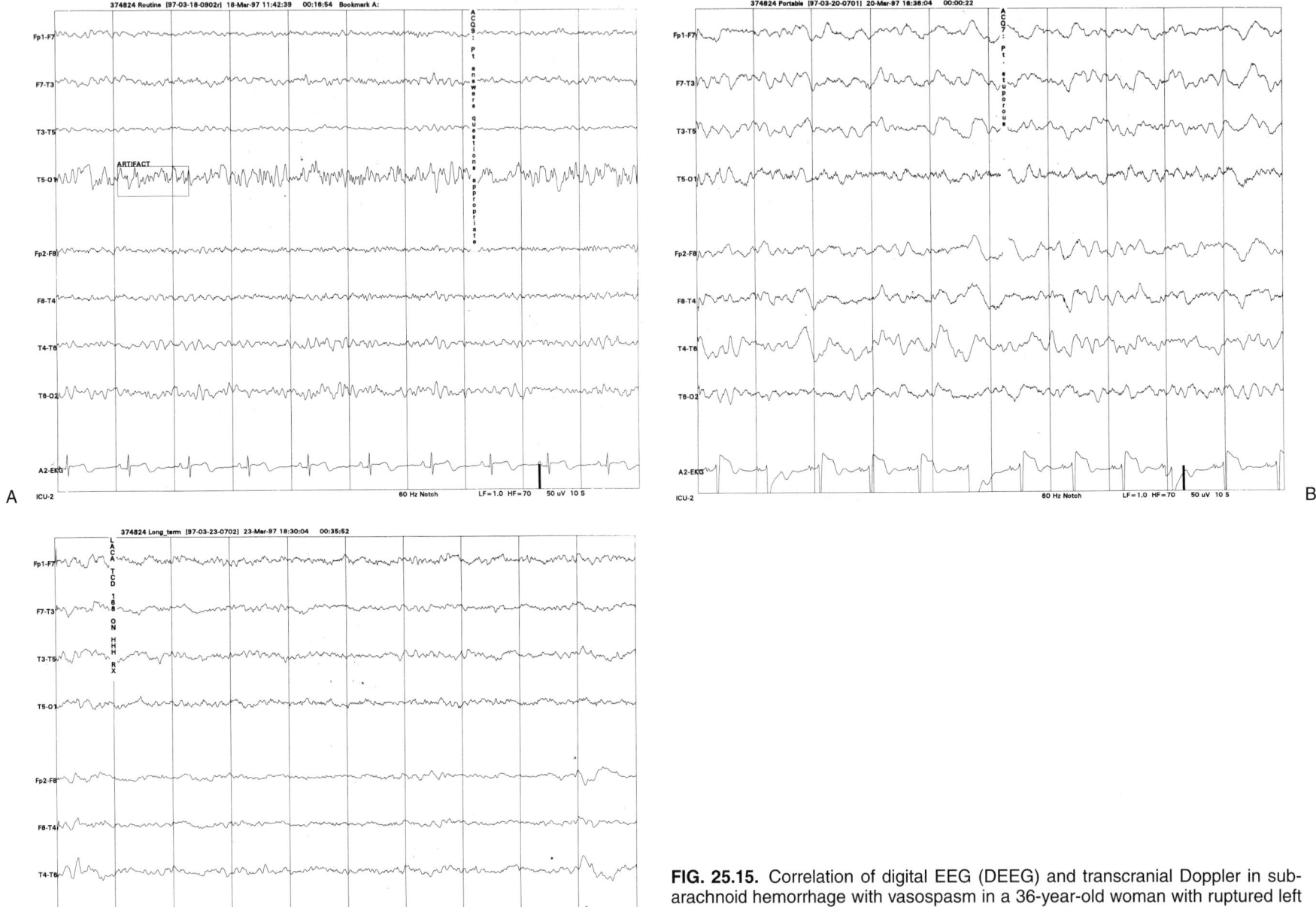

FIG. 25.15. Correlation of digital EEG (DEEG) and transcranial Doppler in subarachnoid hemorrhage with vasospasm in a 36-year-old woman with ruptured left posterior communicating artery aneurysm. **A:** DEEG sample 2 days after the subarachnoid hemorrhage. Mild 7-Hz background slowing is evident. She was drowsy but answered questions appropriately. Artifact is visible at O1 electrode. **B:** DEEG 2 days later. Diffuse, continuous 2-Hz delta with intermixed theta frequencies. Patient's mental status had declined. **C:** Improvement in DEEG activity after hypertensive hypervolemic therapy.

CEEG has been used to monitor patients at risk for vasospasm-induced focal ischemia. Rivierez et al. (87) found that broad, repetitive slow waves were predictive of vasospasm-induced ischemia. Labar et al. (62) reported that qEEG changes preceded clinical evidence of vasospasm in four (36%) of 11 cases. Vespa et al. (107) used qEEG to study 32 consecutive patients with subarachnoid hemorrhage. Data were analyzed blindly and compared with TCD velocities, cerebral angiograms, and CT scans. In 19 (59%) of 32 patients, vasospasm developed. The variability of relative alpha was significantly decreased in all patients with vasospasm, a finding that enabled clinicians to detect vasospasm before TCD studies in over 70%. As vasospasm resolved, baseline relative alpha variability returned (Fig. 25.14).

Raw CEEG data can also help detect vasospasm-induced cerebral dysfunction before TCD findings are diagnostic (Fig. 25.15). In managing vasospasm patients, CEEG may be helpful in targeting therapeutic goals for mean arterial pressure, intravascular volume, and cardiac output (see Fig. 25.15*C*).

CONTINUOUS EEG IN DIAGNOSIS AND PROGNOSIS OF COMA

CEEG assesses the dynamic reactivity, variability, and wake-sleep integrity of the cortex. All of these have prognostic importance in coma. Bricolo et al. (16) reported unfavorable outcomes in 95% of patients with monotonous delta activity, in contrast to 30% of patients with variable or sleep-wake patterns. Other researchers have verified that the presence of physiological sleep-wake cycles suggests a favorable prognosis (9). In a study of posttraumatic coma, Stone et al. (96) found that EEG reactivity was prognostically more useful than the dominant frequency. In their study, reactivity was immediate or delayed and was characterized by desynchronization, attenuation, appearance of new delta or theta activity, or the appearance of sleep spindles. In both traumatic and anoxic-ischemic coma, a poor prognosis is implied by invariant, unreactive alpha activity, burst-suppression patterns, and periodic bursts of epileptiform discharges (99) (see Chapter 14).

In an attempt to provide a systematic approach to EEG in coma, Young et al. (116) developed and validated a grading system that was based on 100 EEGs in comatose patients. Through blinded interpretation by two electroencephalographers, their system achieved a κ score of 0.90, indicating almost perfect agreement. They found that prognosis worsened from grade I to VI but could be further refined by use of "subcategories," including reactivity, generalized or focal distribution, and epileptiform activity.

CEEG may provide clues to the etiology of coma and help exclude competing possibilities. Spindle or alpha coma patterns can be seen in patients with overdoses of tricyclic agents, benzodiazepines, or barbiturates. In the absence of drug overdose, alpha-theta coma is almost always caused by a generalized hypoxic-ischemic insult. Fluctuating, generalized theta-delta activity, especially if accompanied by triphasic wave activity, suggests a metabolic encephalopathy, but the pattern can also be seen in severe hypercapnia, opiate toxicity, and lithium overdose (43). Septic encephalopathy can produce a similar appearance, with the severity of the EEG abnormalities paralleling the degree of mental status impairment, systemic severity of the condition, and correlating with death (112). When severe hydrocephalus produces coma, intermittent bursts of diffuse rhythmic delta activity (FIRDA) can be seen; these may fluctuate dramatically with changes in intraventricular pressure (Fig. 25.16*A* and *B*). Coma caused by structural lesions with mass effect tends to be characterized by attenuated background activity ipsilateral to the lesion, plus bilateral frontal and asymmetric rhythmic delta activity (Fig. 25.20*A* to *D*). Coma can also be a deceptive, nonspecific manifestation of NCSE. Lowenstein and Aminoff (68) reported that of 38 comatose patients with EEG-proved NCS, 10% had no clinical signs of seizures, and 70% had only "subtle motor movements." Corroborating this observation, Jordan (50) reported that of 43 patients with NCS, 37% were comatose without distinguishing clinical motor features (see Fig. 25.17).

In the evaluation of coma, routine bedside EEG can mislead the clinician and result in incorrect conclusions. For example, sleep patterns may not be detected during routine recording times, and prolonged cycles or autonomous activity may not be recognized. In addition, an EEG "snapshot" of a distinctive pattern, such as burst-suppression with epileptiform activity (Fig. 25.18*A*), may lead to management decisions based on the assumption of a hopeless prognosis. The dynamic element of CEEG may, in fact, suggest a more favorable outcome (see Fig. 25.18*B* to *D*). Furthermore, in a comatose patient with NCSE, a nonspecific encephalopathy may be suggested by a routine EEG recorded during an interictal period. Conversely, a number of metabolic encephalopathies can precipitate NCS or NCSE, such as hyperglycemia or hypoglycemia, hypernatremia or hyponatremia, and hepatic encephalopathy (51) (Fig. 25.19).

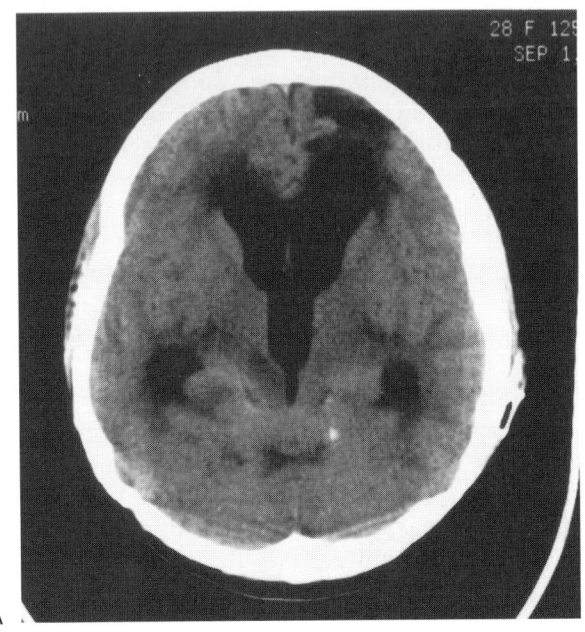

A

FIG. 25.16. CT scan and continuous EEG samples in comatose 28-year-old woman with obstructive hydrocephalus and tuberculous meningitis. **A:** Noncontrast CT scan shows severe dilatation of the supratentorial ventricular system. A right ventriculoperitoneal shunt is not visualized. The left focal encephalomalacia is from prior removal of a tuberculoma. **B:** Semicontinuous delta-theta pattern is punctuated by high-amplitude, generalized, intermittent, rhythmic delta bursts. At the notation "button press," the patient's shunt reservoir is "pumped." **C:** Dramatic improvement in continuous EEG after "pumping" of shunt reservoir.

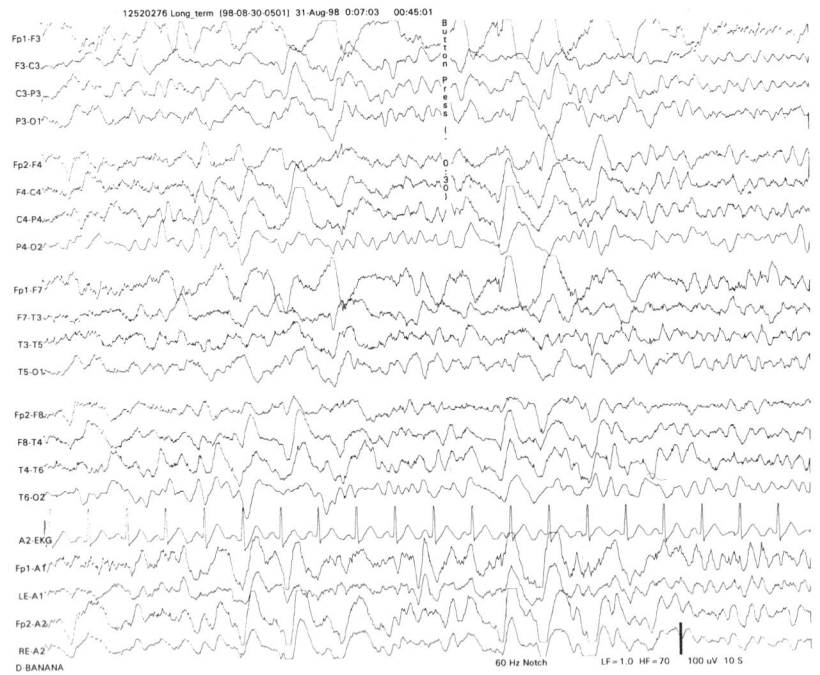

B

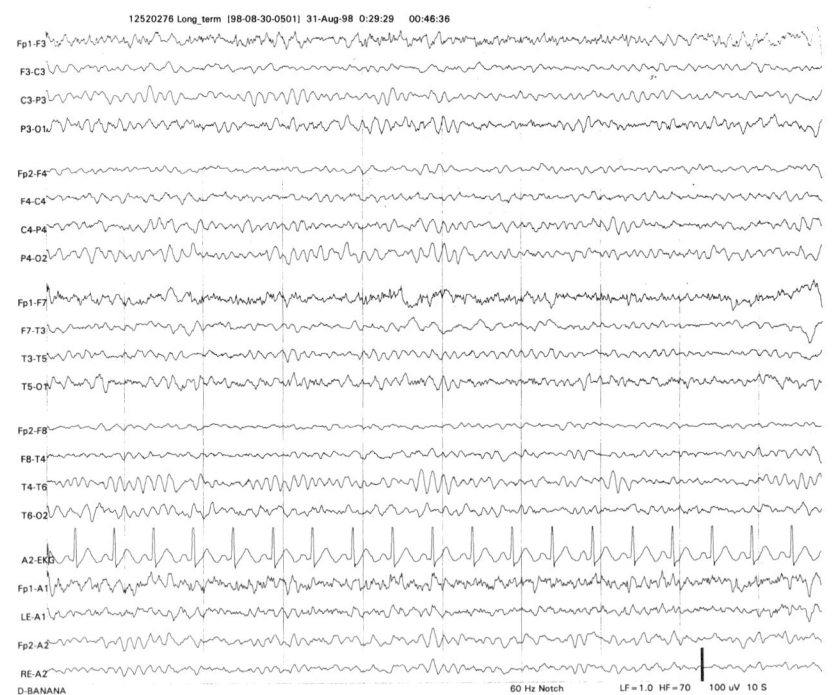

C

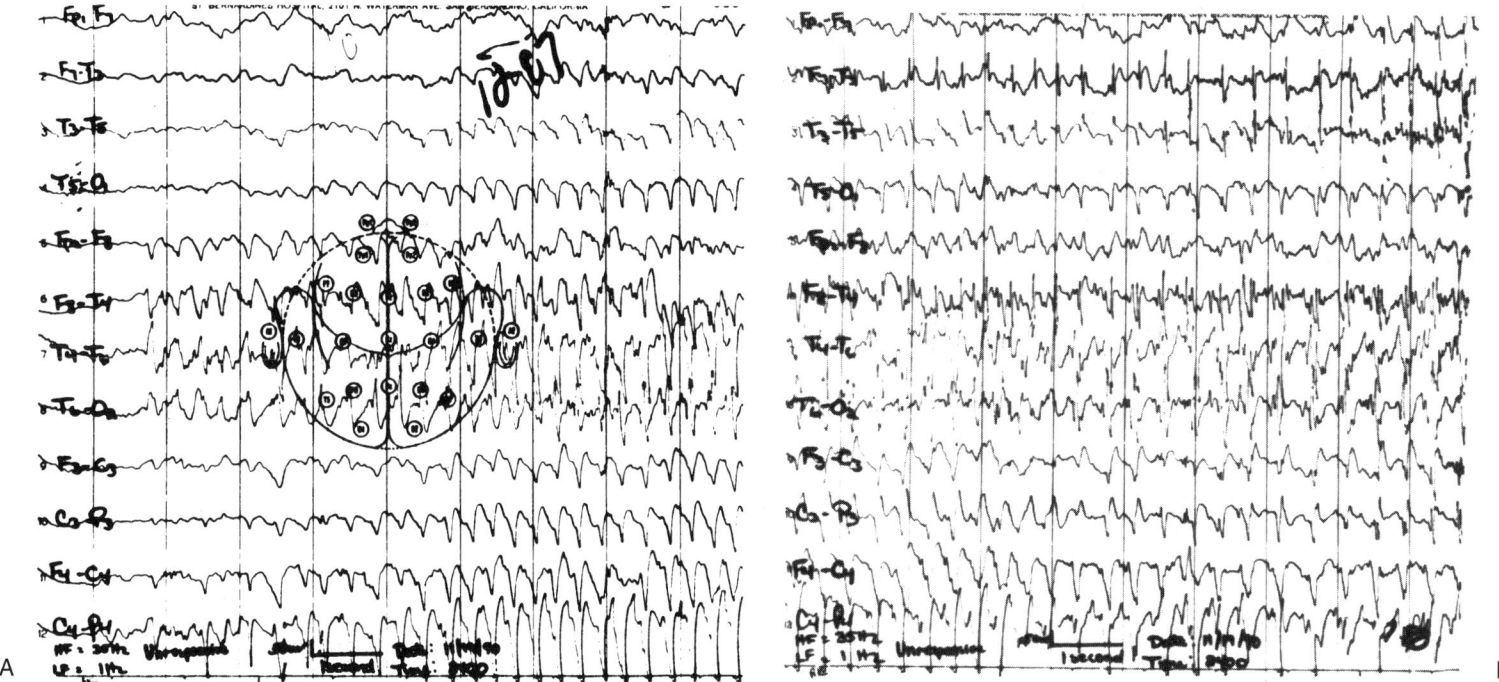

FIG. 25.17. EEG from a comatose patient with small right temporal lobe abscess. The cause of the patient's coma was nonconvulsive status epilepticus (NCSE) arising from the right temporal lobe. No convulsive activity or distinguishing motor features were present. **A:** Focal onset of seizure from the right midtemporal region with beginning secondary generalization. **B:** Generalized seizure activity, during which the patient remained unresponsive without motor activity.

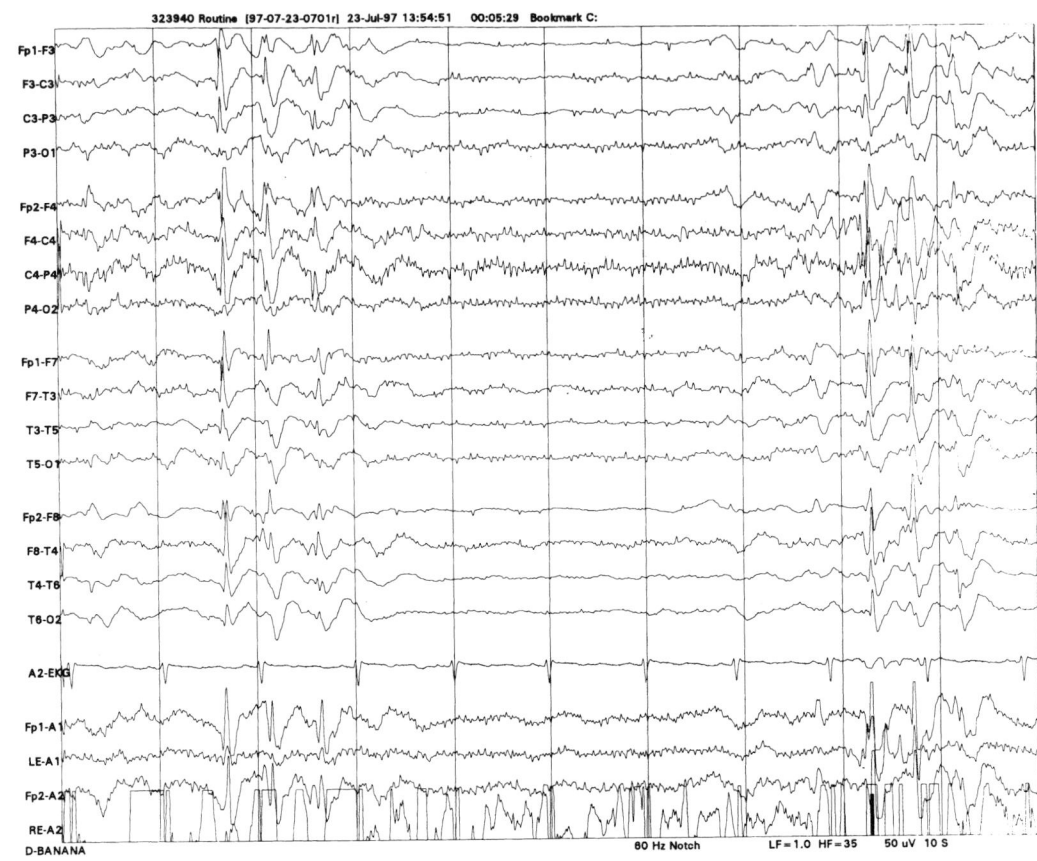

FIG. 25.18. Continuous EEG in a 41-year-old woman with anoxic encephalopathy resulting from generalized convulsive status epilepticus (GCSE). The patient also had elevated ammonia levels in association with chronic valproic acid use. Initial examination revealed deep coma, decerebrate posturing, and bilateral Babinski signs. **A:** Markedly suppressed, unreactive record with bursts of generalized spike discharges. No clinical convulsive activity was seen. (*Figure continues.*)

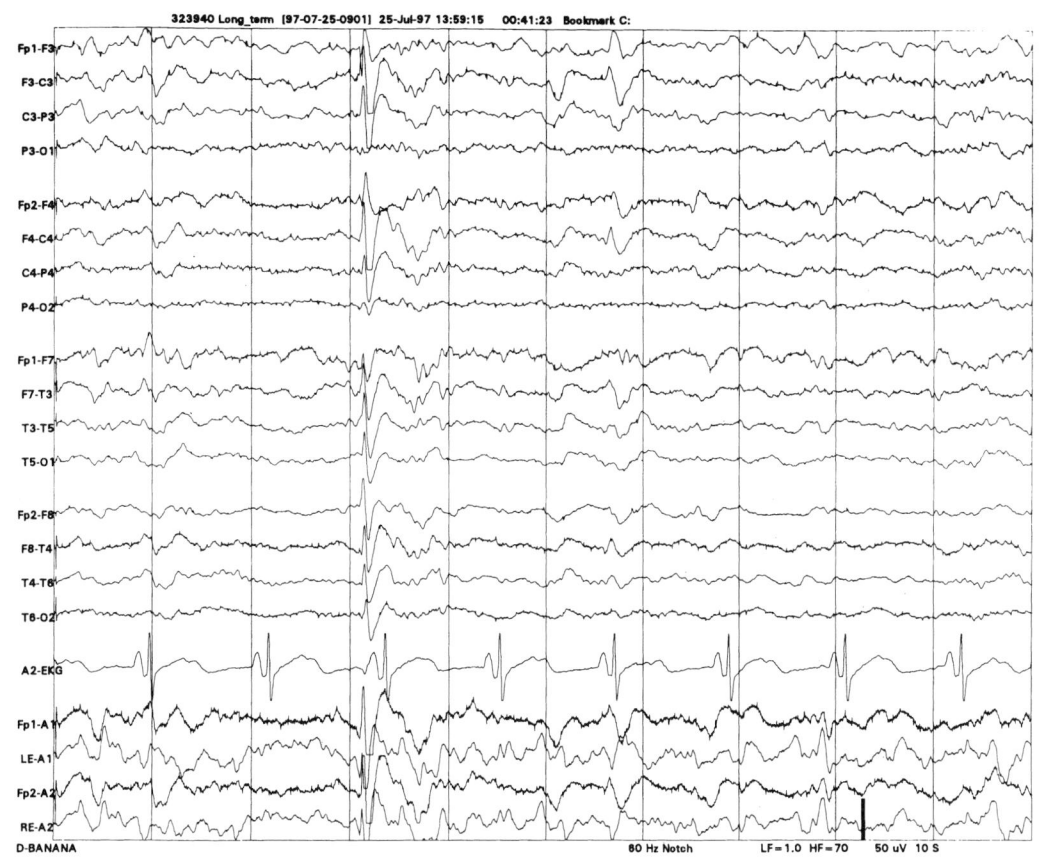

FIG. 25.18. *Continued.* **B:** Two days later, continuous semirhythmic delta activity is present, and occasional generalized spike discharges are still seen. (*Figure continues.*)

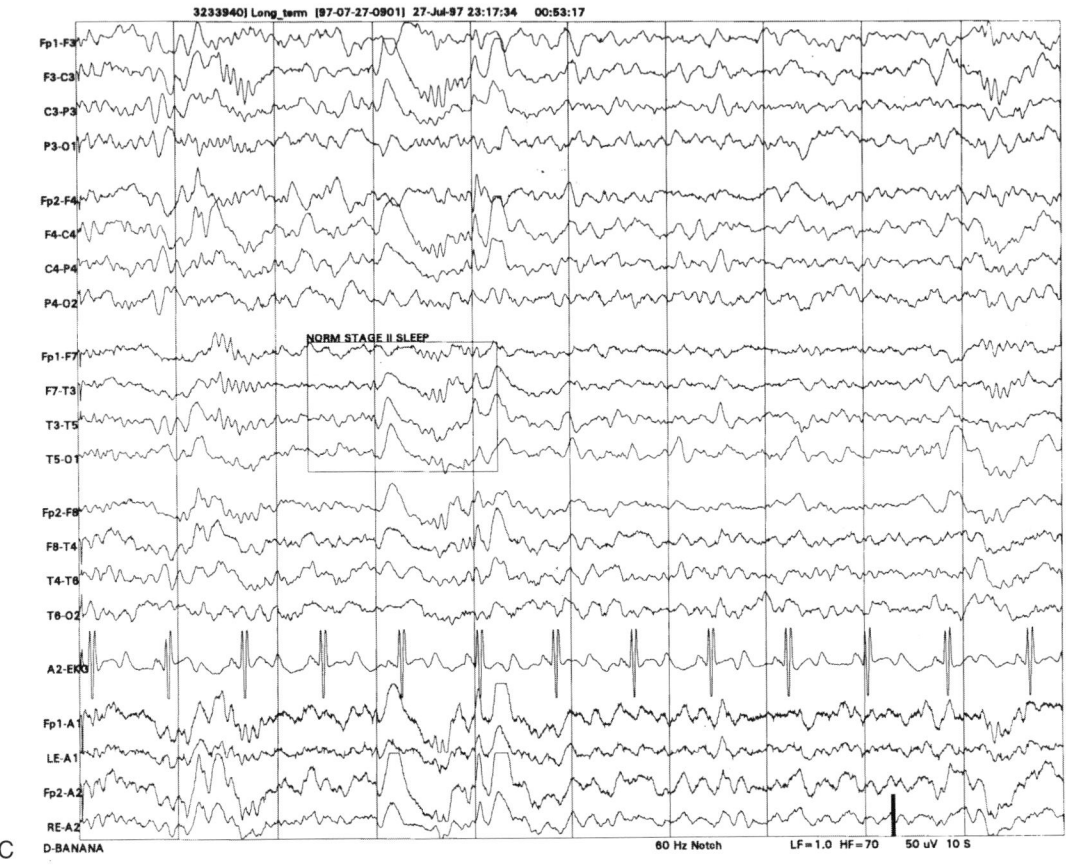

FIG. 25.18. *Continued.* **C:** Two days after the recording in *B.* Generalized theta activity with epochs of physiological stage II sleep patterns is present. (*Figure continues.*)

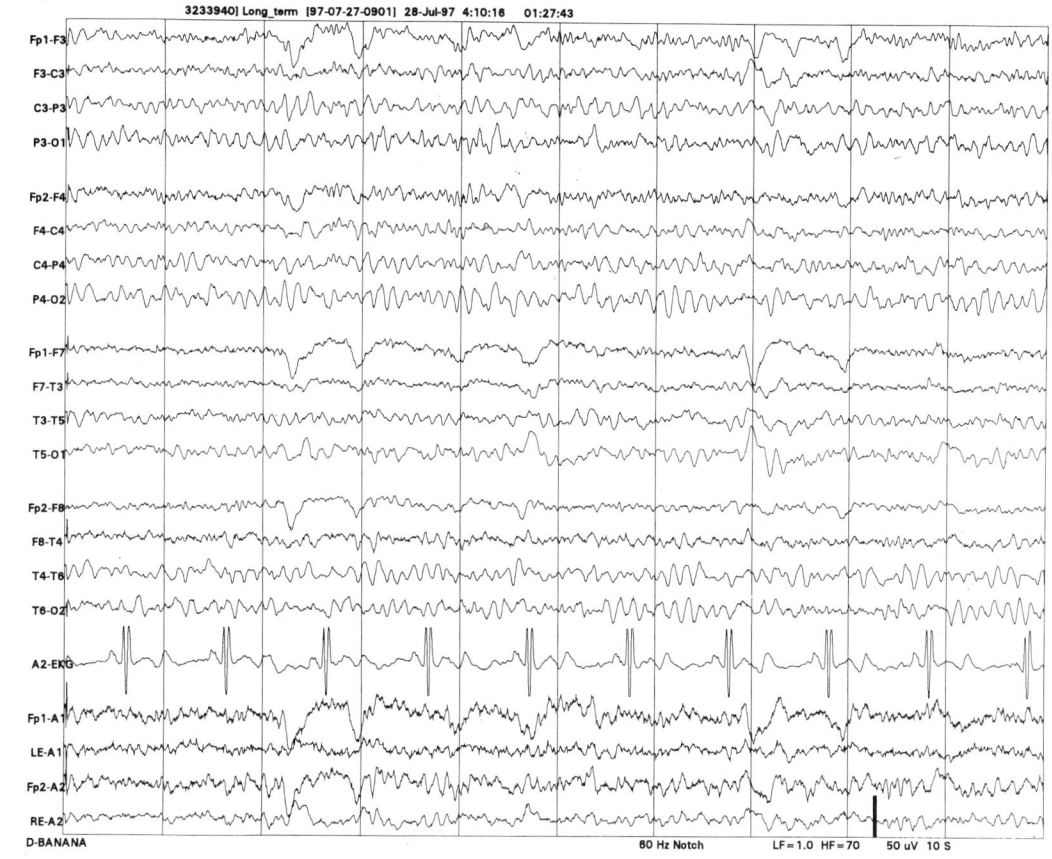

FIG. 25.18. *Continued.* **D:** One day after the recording in part *C.* EEG activity is nearly normal. Only mild posterior background slowing is present. The patient made a complete recovery.

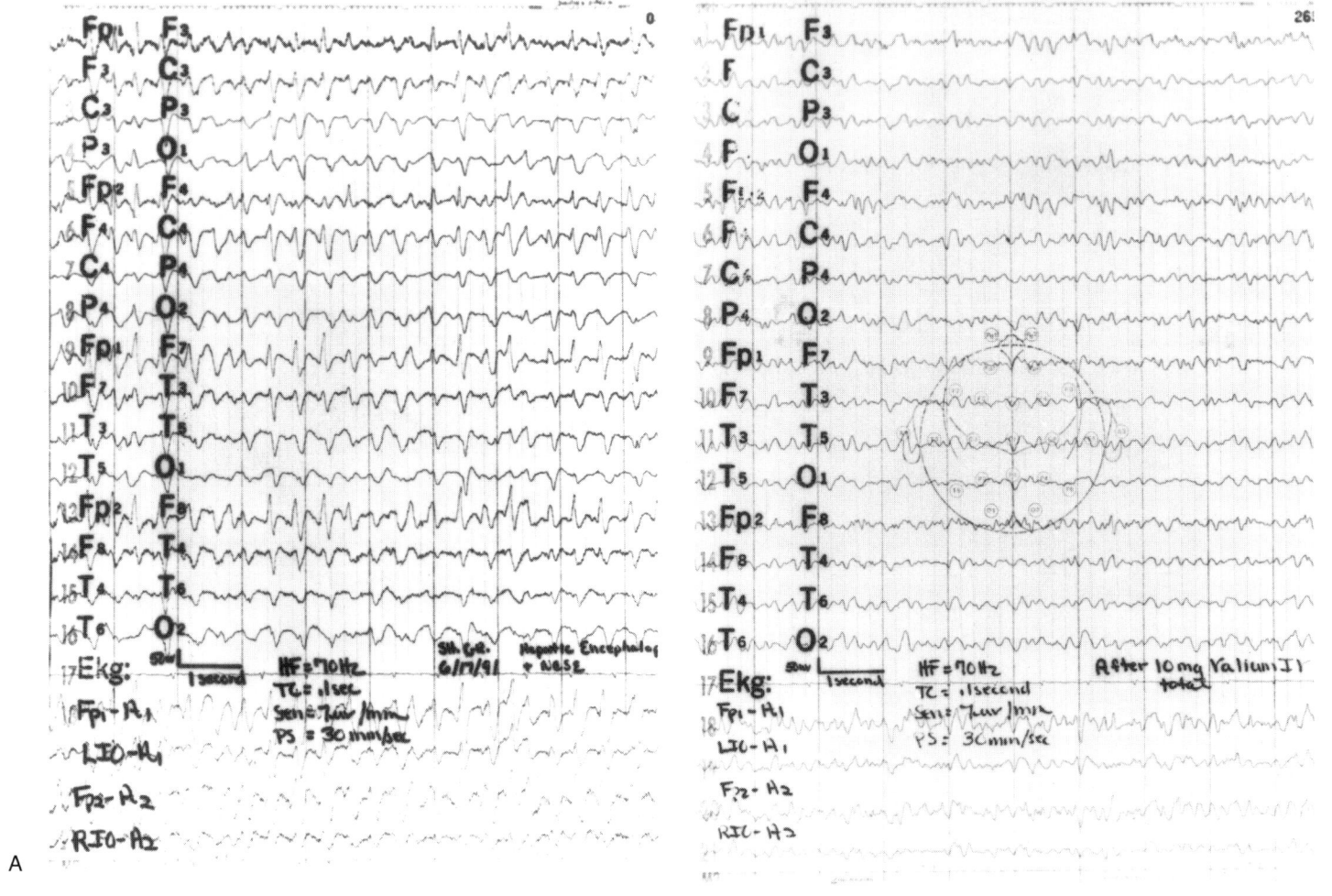

A   B

FIG. 25.19. Continuous EEG of a comatose patient with coexisting NCSE and hepatic encephalopathy. The blood ammonia level was elevated to four times normal. **A:** Continuous 2.5- to 3-Hz spike-wave and triphasic sharp waves. The nurse observed occasional jaw-thrusting movements, suggestive of epileptic automatisms. **B:** After intravenous administration of 10 mg of diazepam, the record rapidly evolved to a generalized rhythmical theta pattern. The patient's level of alertness also improved markedly. (From Jordan KG. Continuous EEG and evoked potential monitoring in the neuroscience intensive care unit. *J Clin Neurophysiol* 1993;10:445.)

Patients with de-efferented ("locked-in") states present a special challenge in the NICU. Their cerebral function is inaccessible by bedside evaluation because motor responses, including facial and bulbar muscles, are absent. In such patients, CEEG reveals normal alertness and responsiveness to various stimuli. Inadequate sedation may leave the paralyzed patient conscious and anxious, whereas excessive sedation may prolong ventilatory dependence, induce coma, or both. CEEG can also reveal superimposed encephalopathic insults, which can be caused by hypercapnia, sepsis, metabolic imbalance, or medication side effects. Some patients are so profoundly de-efferented that clinical findings suggest brain death. In this circumstance, CEEG can confirm normal or near-normal cortical activity, reactivity, and sleep-wake cycles.

The addition of EEG analysis to other systems to predict outcome for ICU patients also improves the utility of these systems (117).

CONTINUOUS EEG IN ACUTE SEVERE HEAD TRAUMA

Since the early 1980s, there have been a number of major breakthroughs in understanding the pathophysiological processes associated with traumatic brain injury. Much of the neurological damage does not occur at the moment of impact. Over the ensuing hours and days, delayed insults cause secondary injury that is apparent biochemically and clinically (23). This discovery spurred renewed interest in neurophysiological monitoring of trauma patients to identify impending secondary brain injury in time to control or reverse it.

In traumatic injury, sequential brain imaging is commonly used to assess structural abnormalities, but, as Sloan (95) pointed out, the functional integrity of the cerebrum and brainstem can be determined only by clinical examination or neurophysiological testing. In many trauma patients, sedative and neuromuscular blockading agents used to control ventilation or agitated behavior render the neurological examination uninformative. In these patients, the functional state of the brain can be determined only by neurophysiological monitoring. The use of CEEG as a management tool in head trauma is in its early stages. Correlative and prospective studies are beginning to appear (10,105,108). Emerging information suggests that CEEG can be beneficial in detecting posttraumatic NCSE, in the management of increased ICP, and in the early detection of cerebral mass effect. From extrapolation of studies in related conditions, CEEG has a potential role in the early detection of posttraumatic vasospasm and, perhaps, injurious levels of hyperventilation.

An important caveat in using EEG in head trauma patients is the common occurrence of skull fractures, surgical defects, edema, and subgaleal hematomas. These extracerebral factors can produce significant abnormalities and asymmetries in the EEG.

Management of Increased Intracranial Pressure

Current guidelines for the management of traumatic brain injury patients (18) suggest ICP monitoring for any patient whose CT scan shows compressed basal cisterns, midline shift, or multiple high- or low-density lesions. When increased ICP does not respond to conventional measures, high-dose barbiturate therapy is effective in lowering it (36). Pentobarbital has been the most widely used barbiturate for this purpose. Neither serum nor cerebrospinal fluid pentobarbital levels correlate with therapeutic efficacy or systemic toxicity (110). CEEG is the most reliable guide to barbiturate dosing, and most experts recommend achieving a burst-suppression pattern, because it correlates with maximal reductions in cerebral oxygen use (as estimated by the cerebral metabolic rate of oxygen [$CMRO_2$]). Increasing the barbiturate dose to induce electrocerebral silence does not diminish $CMRO_2$ further, but it does add to the risk of cardiovascular instability (61). If systemic hypotension complicates barbiturate use, the benefits of the treatment are negated and may be reversed (91).

Non-convulsive Status Epilepticus in Acute Severe Head Trauma

In a small study, Jordan (51), used CEEG to identify NCS in two (29%) of seven patients with head trauma. In a larger, prospective study, Vespa et al. (108) identified seizures in nine (16%) of 56 patients with acute severe head trauma, of whom seven (12.5% of total) had NCS or NCSE. Only one (11%) of the nine patients with seizures had a good outcome, in contrast to 21 (47%) of 45 of the patients without seizures. Bergsneider et al. (10) studied 13 head trauma patients with combined positron emission tomographic (PET) scanning and CEEG. Five of these (38%) showed NCS, and two (15% of the total) had NCSE. PET scans showed that both patients with NCSE had hyperglycolysis in the epileptogenic brain areas.

Armon and Dayes (4) reported NCSE as a complication of acute subdural hematoma. In three cases, the epileptic focus localized to cortex distorted by fresh blood on imaging studies. NCSE was refractory in all patients; two patients required high-dose barbiturates. One patient died, and the two survivors required 65 and 89 days of hospitalization with subsequent custodial care. These observations may relate to an earlier report by Inglis et al. (47), who described glucose hypermetabolism in acute subdural hematoma. The hypermetabolism could be ameliorated by blocking excitatory amino acid receptors, which suggests that it was a manifestation of excitotoxic depolarization, a common substrate for epileptogenic activity. Supporting the observations of Armon and Dayes, Jordan observed a similar association between acute subdural hematoma and NCSE (personal observation). Of four patients with subdural

hematoma, three became alert and interactive after surgical evacuation of the clot. The fourth was in NCSE preoperatively and never regained consciousness after surgery. Within the first two postoperative days, the three alert patients had simple partial seizures. Postoperative CT scans showed successful evacuation of clot with no new abnormalities. Nonetheless, the patients became progressively obtunded and CEEG confirmed NCSE in all three. Aggressive treatment was associated with complete neurological recovery in one patient and good recovery in the other two. These observations suggest the possibility that acute subdural hematoma may impart an excitotoxic vulnerability to status epilepticus and NCSE on the injured cortex.

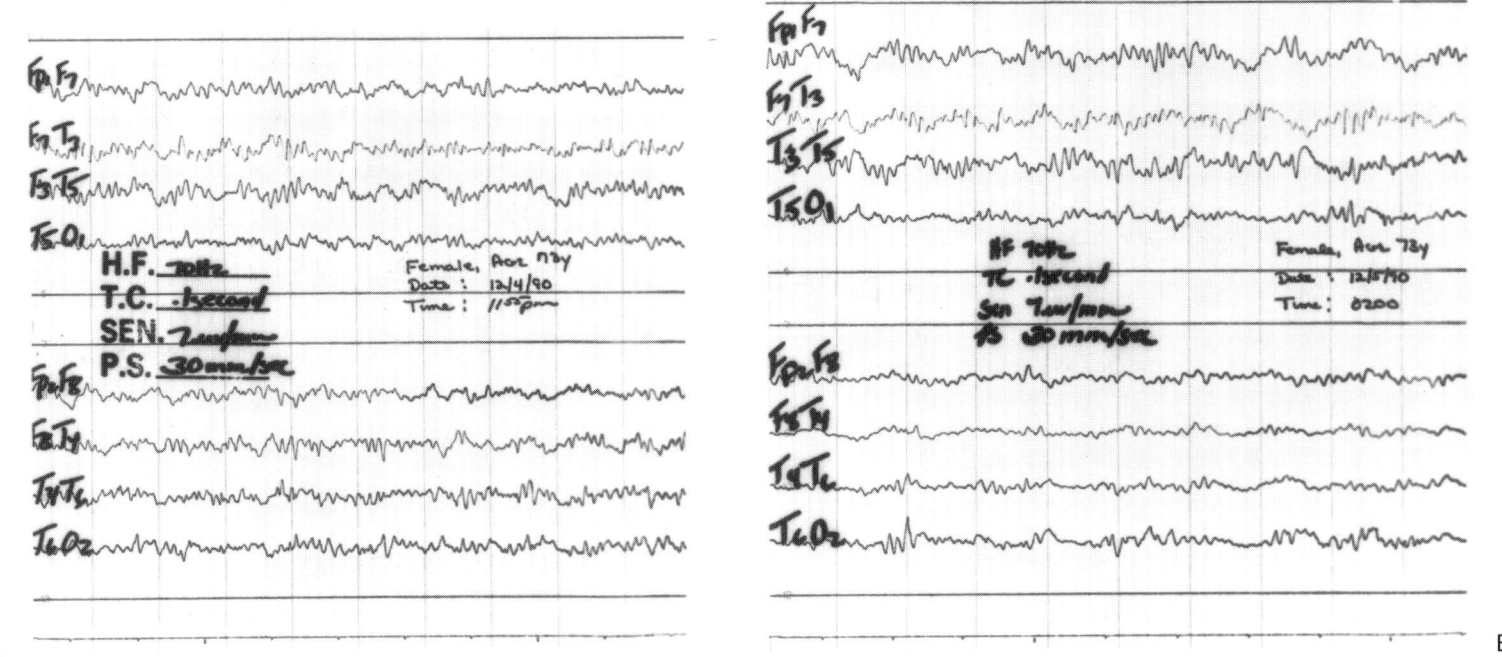

FIG. 25.20. Continuous EEG of a stuporous patient after drainage of right subdural hematoma. **A:** Diffuse spindle-like activity with underlying, continuous 2-Hz delta activity. **B:** Two hours later, right hemisphere activity decreases in amplitude, and left hemisphere delta becomes more prominent. (*Figure continues.*)

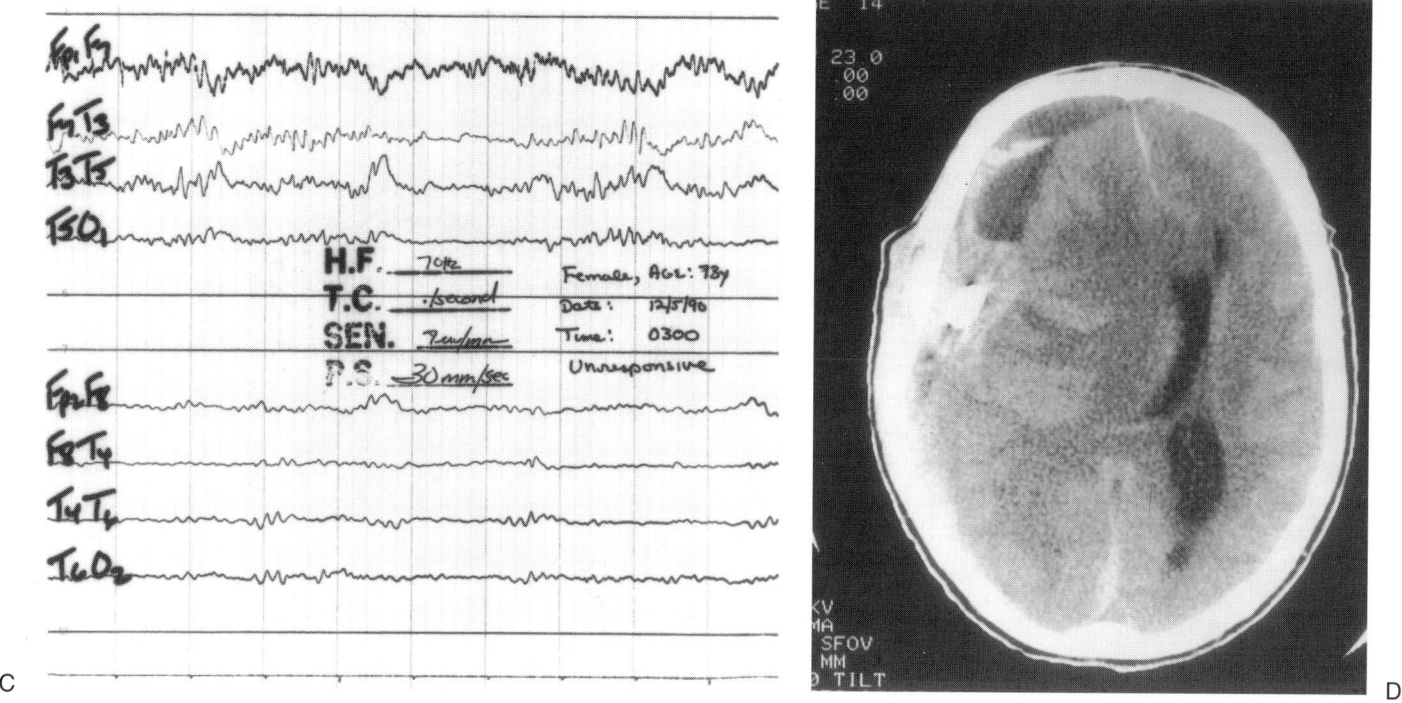

FIG. 25.20. *Continued.* **C:** One hour after the recording in part *B,* the right hemisphere develops a very attenuated burst-suppression pattern. Left hemisphere delta activity is more prominent. **D:** Noncontrast computed tomographic scan taken after the recording in part *C.* There is a fresh hemorrhage below burr hole site with massive right hemisphere edema and transfacial herniation. (From Jordan KG. Continuous EEG and evoked potential monitoring in the neuroscience intensive care unit. *J Clin Neurophysiol* 1993;10:445.)

Detection of New or Increasing Intracranial Masses

Patients with traumatic brain injury may deteriorate as a result of new mass lesions unseen on the initial CT scan, or from rapid enlargement of lesions that initially appeared relatively innocent (23). After the evacuation of large intracranial hemorrhages, the decompression effect can lead to delayed enlargement of contralateral mass lesions. In addition, posttraumatic or postoperative systemic coagulopathies may cause hematomas to enlarge or reaccumulate. Although imaging studies are the best way to identify new or enlarging mass lesions, they require transport of patients out of the ICU. Patients with acute severe head trauma often have multiorgan trauma and cardiovascular instability, which increase the hazard of transport. CEEG can be considered a useful adjunctive tool for suggesting the presence of new or expanding mass lesions (Fig. 25.20), adding objective data to the decision of whether to transport the patient for brain imaging.

Potential Role of Continuous EEG in Traumatic Vasospasm and Therapeutic Hyperventilation

Studies have shown that posttraumatic vasospasm is more common than previously thought (72). CBF measurements have documented the occurrence of severe cerebral ischemia from posttraumatic vasospasm, including cerebral infarctions. Lee et al. (64) demonstrated a close association between posttraumatic vasospasm and poor outcome, which was independent of the admitting Glasgow Coma Scale score. They suggested that early identification of such patients could lead to corrective medical measures similar to those used for treating vasospasm due to subarachnoid hemorrhage vasospasm.

Hyperventilation to a $PaCO_2$ of 25 to 30 mm Hg has been advocated for increased ICP in trauma patients. However, one study suggested that lowering the $PaCO_2$ to about 25 mm Hg may be deleterious in comparison with a $PaCO_2$ in the range of the mid-30s mm Hg (75). Supporting data from CBF, TCD, and $CMRO_2$ studies have led to a consensus that, in severe head trauma, overly vigorous hyperventilation may produce ischemia in vulnerable brain regions (71). Current guidelines therefore no longer recommend hyperventilation as prophylactic therapy. The EEG changes produced by hyperventilation include generalized theta or delta slowing, activation of epileptogenic activity, and accentuation of focal slowing (29). Even moderate hypocapnia ($PaCO_2$ of 35 mm Hg) produces EEG slowing (44).

COST BENEFIT, COST EFFECTIVENESS, AND OUTCOME STUDIES OF CONTINUOUS EEG

Cost benefit and cost effectiveness are complicated and controversial subjects in health care. Their use as analytic tools to examine resource use in ICUs inevitably overlaps with issues of quality of care and medical ethics. In examining a particular variable, cost benefit can be considered as the benefits gained in dollar terms and cost effectiveness as the benefits gained in quality-adjusted life years (63). Therefore, if CEEG provides a *cost benefit* to an institution, the ratio of its setup and operational costs to the sum of the savings that it provides in health care expenditures, plus the monetary value of the increase in lives saved and lives lengthened, will be low. If CEEG is *cost effective*, the ratio of its costs to the sum of the number of lives it saves, years of lives saved, and quality of lives saved will be low.

Vespa et al. (106) calculated the "cost efficiency" for CEEG in the ICU in 100 patients with severe head trauma. They found significant cost effective-

ness and cost benefit for CEEG. Its average cost was $560 per patient, which was 1% of the total hospital cost. Over the 4-year period of study, in which CEEG was part of the standard protocol, hospital costs per patient declined from $88,690 to $49,578, a 44% reduction. Median length of stay declined from 24.3 to 13.6 days, also a 44% reduction. The discharge Glasgow outcome score improved from a mean of 2 to a mean of 3 ($p < 0.01$). Despite the use of needle electrodes, no cases of scalp cellulitis or skin infection were detected. In summary, this study found that inclusion of CEEG in the ICU as standard protocol for management of trauma patients resulted in a cost savings of 44%, a reduction in length of stay by 44%, and relative improvement in outcome of patients by 50%. These preliminary data support the cost benefit and cost effectiveness of CEEG.

The costs of developing a CEEG program include those for personnel, training, continuing education of the monitoring team, purchasing and maintaining equipment, and establishing a computer network. Because CEEG personnel do not dedicate all their time to performing or interpreting CEEG, these costs need to be apportioned accordingly. We estimate that a modest but effective CEEG program can be established at an initial cost of $100,000 to $150,000. As discussed earlier in this chapter, CEEG can have a major impact on the clinical management decisions affecting ICU patients (see Table 25.2). In a retrospective and prospective study of 300 CEEG patients, Vespa et al. (106) found that CEEG was used daily in more than 90% of patients to guide one or more clinical decisions made at the bedside. The impact on care involved both physicians and nurses: nurses increasingly reported suspect EEG ischemia, changes caused by sedative and other drug administration, and EEG patterns contributing to early prognosis. Vespa et al. concluded that "the use of CEEG is cost effective and appears to offer additional quality to intensive care."

CEEG may also help clinicians tailor sedative doses more closely to patient needs, thereby improving efficiency, decreasing costs, and shortening duration of mechanical ventilation. Albrecht et al. (2) demonstrated the utility of a closed-loop control system for sedation that was based on the median frequency of the EEG power spectrum.

It is informative to compare benefit, effectiveness, and outcomes with and without the use of a monitoring device in matched populations. For example, according to historical controls, before electrocardiographic monitoring for acute myocardial infarction was introduced, costs were lower, but there was a significant loss in number of lives saved and in quality-adjusted life years in comparison to similar measures after its introduction. The use of

CEEG in NICU trauma patients improves outcomes, is cost effective, and cost beneficial (106).

Outcome studies examining the role of CEEG in GCSE, NCSE, acute ischemia, and coma remain to be done. The data from reports reviewed for this chapter provide evidence that the rates of morbidity and mortality of GCSE and NCSE can be positively influenced by its use. As the application of CEEG expands in other diagnostic areas, outcome studies should become feasible and informative. It is worth remembering, however, that for outcome studies to have validity and credibility, as Bleck (12) has emphasized, they must carefully define criteria for the competent use of monitoring devices, as well as the management to be followed on the basis of the data obtained. As emphasized earlier, the monitoring device itself has a limited effect on outcome; how the monitoring team extracts information from it and the subsequent clinical decisions and interventions will determine its impact on the patient's course.

SUMMARY

This chapter has placed the current state of CEEG in the ICU in its historical context, reviewed its scientific rationale, presented logistical and technical challenges in its use and implementation, and provided guidelines to meet these challenges. It described major sources of artifacts and methods to reduce them. It presented the rationale and the authors' paradigm for training and supervising ICU bedside nurses in CEEG. It also presented established, emerging, and potential benefits of CEEG emphasizing the clinical importance this monitoring technique brings to the bedside in a variety of NICU and emergency department situations. Increasing numbers of neurointensivists, electroencephalographers, and neurological colleagues are no longer content to rely on bedside examination alone to evaluate cerebral function in critically ill patients. They have thus begun to join with their colleagues in other critical care specialties who have long benefited from physiological monitoring to assess target organs at risk. Network technology and DEEG have made it easier to implement and oversee the use of CEEG in the ICU and emergency department. qEEG is finding a credible role in seizure detection and early identification of cerebral ischemia to complement DEEG. EEG in the emergency department is beginning to carve out a legitimate role in the pre-ICU management of patients with status epilepticus, ischemia, and coma.

Abundant supportive data indicate that in patients with status epilepticus, CEEG may be indispensable for timely and optimally effective management. In this context, it is close to becoming a standard of care. The high incidence of NCS and NCSE in acute brain injury, suggested by early studies, has been confirmed by more recent ones, particularly in patients with GCSE. Without CEEG, the recognition of NCSE is commonly delayed or missed, which likely contributes to the increased rates of morbidity and mortality of NCSE compared to GCSE. As a monitor of the effects of cerebral ischemia, the role of CEEG has expanded to include evaluation of post–subarachnoid hemorrhage vasospasm. CEEG may also be emerging as a valuable tool in focal ischemia. For comatose patients, CEEG can provide otherwise unobtainable prognostic and diagnostic information. Its role in trauma has expanded from monitoring high-dose barbiturate therapy to early detection of NCSE, targeting cerebral perfusion in increased ICP, and providing early detection of progressive mass effect.

One conclusion stands out: In patients with acute brain lesions, unexplained alteration of mental status requires rapid diagnosis and treatment to ensure the best possible outcome. In the clinical settings reviewed in this chapter, this requirement may be impeded without the availability, prompt use, and rapid interpretation of CEEG in the emergency department and NICU. We believe that the timely use of EEG in the emergency department and CEEG will help eliminate diagnostic ambiguity, accurately guide therapy, and prevent potentially harmful delays in treatment.

ACKNOWLEDGMENTS

Kenneth G. Jordan greatly acknowledges the indispensable contributions of the Jordan NeuroScience neurodiagnostic and administrative teams, as well as the excellent and meticulous transcribing and preparation skills of Shirley Smith.

Thomas P. Bleck thanks the staffs of the Neuroscience Intensive Care Unit and the EEG laboratory at the University of Virginia.

REFERENCES

1. Ahn SS, Jordan SE, Nuwer MR, et al. Computed electroencephalographic topographic brain mapping: a new and accurate monitor of cerebral circulation and function for patients having carotid endarterectomy. *J Vasc Surg* 1988;8:247–254.
2. Albrecht S, Frenkel C, Ihursen H, et al. A rational approach to the control of sedation in intensive care unit patients based on closed-loop control. *Eur J Anaesth* 1999;16:678–687.

3. Argarual R, Gotman J, Flanagan D, et al. Automated EEG analysis during long-term monitoring in the ICU. *Electroencephalogr Clin Neurophysiol* 1998;107:44–58.

4. Armon C, Dayes LA. Complex partial status epilepticus in patients with acute, or acute on chronic, subdural hematomas. *J Clin Neurophysiol* 1998;5:274.

5. Astrup J, Simon L, Siesjö BK, et al. Thresholds in cerebral ischemia—the ischemic penumbra. [Editorial]. *Stroke* 1981;12:723–725.

6. Baker NS, Van Ness PC. Evolution of EEG patterns in pharmacologically induced burst-suppression for treatment of status epilepticus. *Neurology* 1998;50:A419.

7. Barry E, Hauser WA. Status epilepticus: The interaction of epilepsy and acute brain disease. *Neurology* 1993;42:1473.

8. Barry E, Hauser WA. Status epilepticus and antiepileptic medication levels. *Neurology* 1994; 44:47.

9. Bergamasco B, Bergamini L, Doriguzzi T, et al. EEG sleep patterns as a prognostic criterion in post-traumatic coma. *Electroencephalogr Clin Neurophysiol* 1968;24:374–377.

10. Bergsneider M, Hovda DA, Shalmon E, et al. Cerebral hyperglycolysis following severe brain injury in humans: a positron emission tomography study. *J Neurosurg* 1997;86:241–251.

11. Bickford RG, Fleming NI, Dillinger TW. Compression of EEG data by isometric power spectral plots. *Electroencephalogr Clin Neurophysiol* 1971;31:632.

12. Bleck TP. Electroencephalographic monitoring in the intensive care unit. In: Tobin MJ, ed. *Principles in practice of intensive care monitoring.* New York: McGraw-Hill, 1997:1035–1045.

13. Bogousslavsky J, Martin R, Regli F, et al. Persistent worsening of stroke sequelae after delayed seizures. *Arch Neurol* 1992;49:385–388.

14. Borel C, Hanley D. Neurological intensive care unit monitoring. In: Rogers MC, Traystman RJ, eds. *Critical care clinics. Symposium on neurological intensive care.* Philadelphia: WB Saunders, 1985;1:223–229.

15. Bricolo A, Turella G, Ore GD, et al. A proposal for the EEG evaluation of acute traumatic coma in neurosurgical practice. *Electroencephalogr Clin Neurophysiol* 1973;34:789.

16. Bricolo A, Turrazzi S, Faccioli F, et al. Clinical application of compressed spectral array in long-term EEG monitoring of comatose patients. *Electroencephalogr Clin Neurophysiol* 1978;45:211–225.

17. Britton M, Roden R. Progression of stroke after arrival at hospital. *Stroke* 1985;16:629–632.

18. Bullock R, Chesnut RM, Clifton G, et al. *Guidelines for the management of severe head injury.* Brain Trauma Foundation 1995;1–29.

19. Buzea CE. Understanding computerized EEG monitoring in the intensive care unit. *J Neurosci Nurse* 1995;27:292–297.

20. Cant BR, Shaw NA. Monitoring by compressed spectral array in prolonged coma. *Neurology* 1984;34:35–39.

21. Caplan LR, Mohr JP, Kissler JP, et al. Should thrombolytic therapy be the first-line treatment for acute stroke? Thrombolysis—not a panacea for ischemic stroke. *N Engl J Med* 1997;337:1309–1310.

22. Chang SWJ, Bleck TP. Status epilepticus. In: Jordan KG, ed. *Neurologic critical care. Neurologic clinics.* Philadelphia: WB Saunders, 1995:529–548.

23. Chesnut RM. Medical management of severe head injury: present and future. *New Horizons* 1995;3:581–593.

24. Chesnut RM. *Bedside brain monitoring: You don't know what you are missing. Point of care testing and bedside brain monitoring.* Medical Association Communications, Yardley, PA 1997. (Excerpted presentation to 7th World Congress of Intensive and Critical Care Medicine, Ottawa, Canada, June 29, 1997:3–4.)

25. Chiappa KH, Hill RA. Evaluation and prognostication in coma. *Electroencephalogr Clin Neurophysiol* 1998;106:149–155.

26. Chiappa KH, Hoch DB. Electrophysiologic monitoring. In: Ropper AH, ed. *Neurological and neurosurgical intensive care,* 3rd ed. New York: Raven Press, 1993:147–165.

27. Chiu D, Krieger D, Villa-Cordova C, et al. Intravenous tissue plasminogen activator for acute ischemic stroke. Feasibility, safety, and efficacy in the first year of clinical practice. *Stroke* 1998;29:18–22.

28. Cohn HR, Raines RG, Mulder DW, et al. Cerebral vascular lesions: electroencephalographic and neuropathologic correlations. *Arch Neurol* 1948;60:163–181.

29. Daly DD. Epilepsy and syncope. In: Daly DD, Pedley TA, eds. *Current practice of clinical encephalography,* 2nd ed. New York: Raven Press, 1990:319–321.

30. De Deyue C, Decruyenaene J, Creupelandt J, et al. Use of continuous bispectral EEG monitoring to assess sedation in ICU patients. *Intensive Care Med* 1998;24:1294–1298.

31. DeGiorgio CM, Correale JD, Gott PS, et al. Serum neuron-specific enolase in human status epilepticus. *Neurology* 1995;45:1134–1137.

32. DeLorenzo RJ, Towne AR, Boggs JG, et al. Nonconvulsive status epilepticus following the clinical control of convulsive status epilepticus. *Neurology* 1997;48:A45.

33. DeLorenzo RJ, Towne AR, Pellock JM, et al. Status epilepticus in children, adults, and the elderly. *Epilepsia* 1992;33(Suppl 4):S15.

34. Drislane FW, Blum AS, Schomer DL. Unsuspected electrographic status epilepticus in intensive care units. *Neurology* 1998;50(Suppl 1):A395–A396.

35. Duarte J, Markus H, Harrison MJG. Changes in cerebral blood flow as monitored by transcranial Doppler during voluntary hyperventilation and their effect on the electroencephalogram. *J Neurol Imaging* 1995;5:209–211.

36. Eisenberg HM, Frankowski RF, Contant CF. High dose barbiturate control of elevated intracranial pressure in patients with severe head injury. *J Neurosurg* 1988;69:15–23.

37. Emmerson RG, Chiappa KH. Electrophysiologic monitoring. In: Ropper AH, Kennedy SK, Zervas NT, eds. *Neurological and neurosurgical intensive care,* 2nd ed. Rockville, MD: Aspen Publishers, 1988:13.

38. Engel J. *Causes of human epilepsy. Seizures and epilepsy.* Philadelphia: FA Davis, 1989:112–134.

39. Epilepsy Foundation of America: Treatment of convulsive status epilepticus: Recommendations of the Epilepsy Foundation of America's Working Group on Status Epilepticus. *JAMA* 1993;270:854.

40. Ferro JM, Pinto AN, Falcao I, et al. Diagnosis of stroke by the nonneurologist. A validation study. *Stroke* 1998;29:1106–1109.

41. Firlik AD, Yonas H, Kaufmann AM, et al. Relationship between cerebral blood flow and the development of swelling and life-threatening herniation in acute ischemic stroke. *J Neurosurg* 1998;89:243–249.

42. Gates JR, Ramani V, Whalen S, et al. Ictal characteristics of pseudoseizures. *Arch Neurol* 1985;42:1183.

43. Glaze DG. Drug effects. In: Daly DD, Pedley TA, eds. *Current practice of clinical electroencephalography,* 2nd ed. New York: Raven Press, 1990;489–512.

44. Gotoh F, Meyer JS, Takagi Y. Cerebral effects of hyperventilation in man. *Arch Neurol* 1965;12:410–423.

45. Hijdra A, Braakman R, Von Gijn J, et al. Aneurysmal subarachnoid hemorrhage. Complications and outcome in a hospital population. *Stroke* 1987;18:1061–1067.

46. Homan RW, Herman J, Purdy P. Cerebral location of International 10-20 System electrode placement. *Electroencephalogr Clin Neurophysiol* 1987;66:376–382.

47. Inglis F, Kuroda Y, Bullock R. Glucose hypermetabolism after acute subdural hematoma is ameliorated by a competitive NMDA antagonist. *J Neurol Trauma* 1992;9:75–84.

48. Jaitly R, Sgro J, Towne AR, et al. Prognostic value of EEG monitoring after status epilepticus: a prospective adult study. *J Clin Neurophysiol* 1997;14:326–334.

49. Jordan KG. Continuous EEG monitoring in the neurological intensive care unit. *Neurology* 1990;40(Suppl 1):180.

50. Jordan KG. Nonconvulsive seizure (NCS) and nonconvulsive status epilepticus (NCSE) detected by continuous EEG monitoring in the neuro ICU. *Neurology* 1992;42(Suppl 1):194.

51. Jordan KG. Continuous EEG and evoked potential monitoring in the neuroscience intensive care unit. *J Clin Neurophysiol* 1993;10:445.

52. Jordan KG. Impact of continuous EEG monitoring in the neuroscience intensive care unit on clinical decision making. *Eur J Neurol* 1994;142:S118.

53. Jordan KG. Status epilepticus. A perspective from the neuroscience intensive care unit. *Neurosurg Clin N Am* 1994;5:671–686.

54. Jordan KG. Neurophysiologic monitoring in the neuroscience intensive care unit. *Neurol Clin* 1995;13:579–626.

55. Jordan KG. Regional attenuation without delta (RAWOD): a distinctive early EEG pattern in severe acute cerebral infarctions (SACI). Implications for thrombolytic therapy. *Neurology* 1998;50:A243.

56. Jordan KG. Continuous EEG monitoring in the neuroscience intensive care unit and emergency department. *J Clin Neurophysiol* 1999;16:14–39.

57. Jordan KG. Nonconvulsive status epilepticus in acute brain injury. *J Clin Neurophysiol* 1999;16:332–340.

58. Jordan KG, Stringer WA. Correlative xenon enhanced CT cerebral blood flow (XeCTCBF) and EEG to functionally stratify acute cerebral infarction. *Neurology* 1991;41(Suppl 1):336.

59. Jordan KG, Young GB, Doig GS. Delays in emergency department (ED) diagnosis and treatment of nonconvulsive status epilepticus (NCSE). *Neurology* 1995;45(Suppl 4):A346.

60. Kaplan PW. Nonconvulsive status epilepticus in the emergency room. *Epilepsia* 1996;37:643–650.

61. Kassel NF, Hitchar PW, Gerk MK, et al. Alterations in cerebral blood flow, oxygen metabolism, and electrical activity produced by high-dose thiopental. *Neurosurgery* 1980;7:598–603.

62. Labar DR, Fish BJ, Pedley TA, et al. Quantitative EEG monitoring for patients with subarachnoid hemorrhage. *Electroencephalogr Clin Neurophysiol* 1991;78:325–332.

63. Lambrinos J, Papadakos PJ. An introduction to the analysis or risks, costs, and benefits in critical care. In: Fine IA, Strosberg MA, eds. *Managing the critical care unit.* Rockville, MD: Aspen Publishers, 1987:358–70.

64. Lee JH, Matin NA, Alsina G, et al. Hemodynamically significant cerebral vasospasm and outcome after head injury: a prospective study. *J Neurosurg* 1997;87:221–233.

65. Libman RB, Wirkowski E, Alvir J, et al. Conditions that mimic stroke in the emergency department. *Arch Neurol* 1995;52:1119–1122.

66. Lowenstein DH. Status epilepticus. Epitomies-neurology. *Arch Neurol* 1998;168:263.

67. Lowenstein DH, Alldredge BK. Status epilepticus at an urban public hospital in the 1980s. *Neurology* 1993;43:483.

68. Lowenstein DH, Aminoff MJ. Clinical and EEG features of status epilepticus in comatose patients. *Neurology* 1992;42:100.

69. Lowenstein DH, Aminoff MJ, Simon RP. Barbiturate anesthesia in the treatment of status epilepticus: Clinical experience in 14 patients. *Neurology* 1988;38:395.

70. Luther JS, McNamara JO, Carwile S, et al. Pseudoepileptic seizures: methods and video analysis to aid diagnosis. *Ann Neurol* 1982;12:458.

71. Marion DW, Firlik A, McLaughlin MR. Hyperventilation therapy for severe traumatic brain injury. *New Horizons* 1995;3:439–447.

72. Martin NA, Doberstein C, Zane C, et al. Post-traumatic cerebral arterial spasm: transcranial Doppler ultrasound, cerebral blood flow, and angiographic findings. *J Neurosurg* 1992;77:575–583.

73. Maynard DE. Development of the CFM: the cerebral function analyzing monitor (CFAM). *Ann Anesthesiol Fr* 1979;3:253–255.

74. Miller JD, Becker DB. Secondary insults to the injured brain. *J R Coll Surg Edinb* 1982;27:292.

75. Muizelaar JP, Marmarou A, Ward JD, et al. Adverse effects of prolonged hyperventilation in patients with severe head injury: a randomized clinical trial. *J Neurosurg* 1991;75:731–739.

76. The National Institute of Neurological Disorders in Stroke r-tPA Stroke Study Group. Tissue plasminogen activator for acute ischemic stroke. *N Engl J Med* 1995;333:1581–1587.

77. Nuwer M. Assessment of digital EEG, quantitative EEG, and EEG brain mapping. Report of the American Academy of Neurology and the American Clinical Neurophysiology Society. *Neurology* 1997;49:277–292.

78. Nuwer MR. Quantitative EEG. I. Techniques and problems of frequency analysis in topographic mapping. *J Clin Neurophysiol* 1988;5:1–43.

79. Nuwer MR. Quantitative EEG. II. Frequency analysis and topographic mapping in clinical settings. *J Clin Neurophysiol* 1988;5:45–85.

80. Nuwer MR. Electroencephalograms and evoked potentials. Monitoring cerebral function in the neurosurgical intensive care unit. *Neurosurg Clin North Am* 1994;4:647–659.

81. Oken BS, Chiappa KH, Selenski M. Computerized EEG frequency analysis: sensitivity and specificity in patients with focal lesions. *Neurology* 1989;39:1281–1287.

82. Osorio I, Reed RC. Treatment of refractory generalized tonic-clonic status epilepticus with pentobarbital anesthesia after high-dose phenytoin. *Epilepsia* 1989;1930:464.

83. Pedley TA, Traub RD. Physiologic basis of the EEG. In: Daly DD, Pedley TA, eds. *Current practice of clinical electroencephalography,* 2nd ed. New York: Raven Press, 1990:107–137.

84. Prior PF, Maynard DE. *Monitoring cerebral function. Long-term monitoring of EEG and evoked potentials.* Amsterdam: Elsevier, 1986:14–140.

85. Privitera M, Hoffman M, Layne Moore J, et al. EEG detection of nontonic-clonic status epilepticus patients with altered consciousness. *Epilepsy Res* 1994;18:155–166.

86. Quinnonez D, Vanoczi W. Computerized EEG topographic brain mapping: noninvasive monitoring in the intensive care unit. *J West Soc Electrodiagn Technol* 1988;29:1–13.

87. Rivierez M, Landau-Ferey J, Grob R, et al. Value of electroencephalogram in prediction and diagnosis of vasospasm after intracranial aneurysm rupture. *Acta Neurochir (Wien)* 1991;110:17–23.

88. Ross C, Blake A, Whitehouse W. Status epilepticus on the paediatric intensive care unit—the role of EEG monitoring. *Seizure* 1999;8:335–338.

89. Rubsamen DS, ed. Mismanagement of status epilepticus. *Professional Liability Newsletter* 1997;27:304.

90. Sander JW, O'Donoghue MF. Epilepsy: getting the diagnosis right. All that convulses is not epilepsy. [Editorial.] *BMJ* 1997;314:158–159.

91. Schwartz, ML, Tator CH, Towed DW, et al. The University of Toronto Head Injury Treatment Study: a prospective randomized comparison of pentobarbital and mannitol. *Can J Neurol Sci* 1980;11:434–440.

92. Sharbrough FW, Messick JM, Sundt TM. Correlation of continuous electroencephalograms with cerebral blood flow measurements during carotid endarterectomy. *Stroke* 1973;4:674–683.

93. Si Y, Gotman J, Flanagan D, et al. An expert system for EEG monitoring in the pediatric intensive care unit. *Electroencephalogr Clin Neurophysiol* 1998;106:488–500.

94. Signorini DF, Piper IR, Jones PA, et al. Importance of textual data in multimodality monitoring. *Crit Care Med* 1997;25:2048–2050.

95. Sloan TB. Electrophysiologic monitoring in head injury. *New Horizons* 1995;3:431–438.

96. Stone JL, Ghaly RF, Hughes JR. Electroencephalography in acute head injury. *J Clin Neurophysiol* 1988;5:124–134.

97. Sundt TM Jr. Correlation of cerebral blood flow measurements and continuous electroencephalography during carotid endarterectomy and risk-benefit ratio of shunting. In: Wood JH, ed. *Cerebral blood flow: physiologic and clinical aspects.* New York: McGraw-Hill, 1987:679–692.

98. Sundt TM Jr, Sharbrough FW, Piepgras DG, et al. Correlation of cerebral blood flow and electroencephalographic changes during carotid endarterectomy with results of surgery and hemodynamics of cerebral ischemia. *Mayo Clin Proc* 1981;56:533–543.

99. Synek VM. Prognostically important EEG coma patterns in diffuse anoxic and traumatic encephalopathies in adults. *J Clin Neurophysiol* 1988;5:164–174.

100. Towne AR, Pellock JM, Ko D, et al. Determinants of mortality in status epilepticus. *Epilepsia* 1994;35:27–34.

101. Treiman DM, Meyers PD, Walton NY, et al. A comparison of four treatments for generalized convulsive status epilepticus. *N Engl J Med* 1998;339:792–798.

102. Van de Velde M, Ghosh I, Clutmans P. Context related artefact detection in prolonged EEG recordings. *Comput Methods Programs Biomed* 1999;60:183–96.

103. Venkataraman SH, Orr RA. Intrahospital transport of critically ill patients. In: Hagman JR, Fetcho S, eds. *Critical care clinics. transport of the critically ill.* Philadelphia: WB Saunders, 1992:535.

104. Verma A, Bedlack R, Erwin C. Succinylcholine induced hyperkalemia and cardiac arrest death related to an EEG study. *J Clin Neurophysiol* 1999;16:46–50.

105. Vespa PM, Bergsneider M, Kelly DF, et al. Effect of early seizures on cerebral metabolism in severe brain trauma. *J Clin Neurophysiol* 1995;12:A104.

106. Vespa PM, Nenov V, Nuwer MR. Continuous EEG monitoring in the intensive care unit: early findings and clinical efficacy. *J Clin Neurophysiol* 1999;16:1–13.

107. Vespa PM, Nuwer MR, Juhasz C, et al. Early detection of vasospasm after acute subarachnoidal hemorrhage using continuous EEG ICU monitoring. *Electroencephalogr Clin Neurophysiol* 1997;103:607–615.

108. Vespa PM, Nuwer MR, Nenov V, et al. Increased incidence and impact of nonconvulsive and convulsive seizures after traumatic brain injury as detected by continuous electroencephalographic monitoring. *J Neurosurg* 1999;91:750–760.

109. Waterhouse EJ, Vaughan JK, Barnes TY, et al. Synergistic effect of status epilepticus and ischemic brain injury on mortality. *Epilepsy Res* 1998;29:175–183.

110. Wilberger JE, Cantella D. High dose barbiturates for intracranial pressure control. *New Horizons* 1995;3:469–473.

111. Wood JH, Polyzoidis KS, Epstein CM, et al. Quantitative EEG alterations after isovolemic hemodilution augmentation of cerebral perfusion in stroke patients. *Neurology* 1984;34:764–768.

112. Young GB, Bolton CF, Archibald YM, et al. The electroencephalogram in sepsis-associated encephalopathy. *J Clin Neurol* 1992;9:145.

113. Young GB, Campbell VC. EEG monitoring in the intensive care unit: pitfalls and caveats. *J Clin Neurophysiol* 1999;16:40–45.

114. Young GB, Jordan KG. Do nonconvulsive seizures cause brain damage? Yes. *Arch Neurol* 1998;55:117–119.

115. Young GB, Jordan KG, Doig GS. An assessment of nonconvulsive seizures in the intensive care unit using continuous EEG monitoring: an investigation of variables associated with mortality. *Neurology* 1996;47:83–89.

116. Young GB, McLachlan RS, Creft JH, et al. An electroencephalographic classification system for coma. *Can J Neurol Sci* 1997;24:320–325.

117. Young GB, McLachlan RS, Demelo J. EEG and clinical association with mortality in comatose patients in a general intensive care unit. *J Clin Neurophysiol* 1999;16:354–360.

Chapter 26

Sleep Disorders: Laboratory Evaluation

Rodney A. Radtke

The rapid growth of sleep disorder medicine in the United States has led to an increasing role for clinical electroencephalographers in the evaluation of sleep and its disorders. However, most clinical neurophysiology training programs still do not incorporate the neurophysiological or clinical aspects of sleep disorders into their curricula. This chapter provides an introductory overview of the sleep laboratory evaluation of sleep disorders that is aimed at the practitioner or trainee in clinical electroencephalography (EEG).

The investigation of sleep and its disorders is a relatively new medical discipline; the greatest development has occurred since 1980. The use of prolonged EEG recording to investigate sleep was pioneered by Kleitman and culminated in his historic discovery (with Aserinsky) of rapid-eye-movement (REM) sleep in 1953 (6). In the 1960s, early investigations described sleep-onset REM periods in narcolepsy (83,102) and defined sleep apnea (39,58). Important progress in standardizing sleep investigation occurred in 1968 when a committee of sleep researchers published a manual for scoring sleep; this system, known by the editors' names, Rechtschaffen and Kales, became the accepted standard that is still used today (82). The Association of Sleep Disorder Centers (ASDA) was formed in 1976 to enhance patient care and standardize the practice of sleep disorders medicine. This group of clinical sleep specialists created an extensive classification system for the diagnosis of sleep and arousal disorders, which was initially published in 1979 (7) and then revised in 1990 (53). The ASDA (which later changed its name to the American Academy of Sleep Medicine) also spearheaded the development of a certification board in sleep medicine, which now functions as the free-standing American Board of Sleep Medicine.

Clinical investigation of sleep disorders relies primarily on two major techniques: the overnight polysomnogram (PSG) and the multiple sleep latency test (MSLT). The overnight PSG allows evaluation of nocturnal sleep and focuses primarily on identification and characterization of respiratory abnormalities in sleep. PSG is also useful in evaluation of movement disorders, parasomnias, and nocturnal sleep disruption. The MSLT offers (a) an objective assessment of daytime sleepiness and (b) a determination of possible early-onset REM sleep. These two study techniques serve as the gold standard of sleep evaluation and are reviewed in detail. A brief overview of the initial assessment of a patient with excessive daytime sleepiness, unusual nocturnal behavior, or insomnia is also presented.

POLYSOMNOGRAPHY: TECHNICAL ASPECTS

Overnight sleep studies are usually performed in a facility dedicated to sleep investigations. Most sleep laboratories have one or more bedrooms in which environmental noise, ambient temperature, lighting, and decor are controlled, thus facilitating the patient's sleep. The technologist and polygraphic equipment are located in a separate room, to minimize any disruption to the patient's sleep. An intercom is used to monitor and communicate with the patient as needed. Most laboratories also videotape the night's sleep so that behavioral or respiratory events that occur can be reviewed. Overnight sleep recordings can be obtained adequately with a standard EEG machine. However, polygraphs that provide several channels with direct current (DC) amplifiers and wider pen excursions offer improved quality of respiratory monitoring and allow simultaneous recording of oxygen saturation directly on the paper record.

The patient is scheduled to arrive for the nocturnal study 60 to 90 minutes before his or her usual bedtime. During electrode application, the technologist reviews the patient's history and offers an explanation of the study procedure. Medical information from the referring physician should be available at the time of the study to ensure that the correct procedure is performed, to assist in decision making during the study, and to complement the interpretation subsequently provided. The usual study duration is 6 to 8 hours, depending on the specific clinical problem. When the patient awakens in the morning, the technologist obtains the patient's impression of the night's sleep and how it may have varied from his or her usual night's rest. This information may be important in the clinical correlation of the sleep study results. Sleep studies are routinely scored by the sleep technologist. The sleep study tracing and scored data are then reviewed by a polysomnographer, who provides the interpretation and clinical correlation.

Digital EEG technology has proved to be an extremely useful tool for PSG studies. It has simplified the handling and storage of large amounts of neurophysiological data. The ability to expand the number of channels also allows a greater EEG sampling, which can then be reviewed at routine EEG paper speed (30 mm per second) to allow better assessment of a possible epileptic event, which can be very difficult to interpret when available only at 10 mm per second (38). The digitalization of the information certainly lends itself to computer analysis. At this time, however, manual scoring of sleep stages according to standard Rechtschaffen and Kales criteria (82) is still the standard, in view of the unreliability of most sleep staging programs (51). Improvement in computer-aided sleep scoring may make sleep study scoring a less laborious task in the future. Computer analysis also has a potential to go beyond the standard (and somewhat arbitrary) epoch-by-epoch scoring of sleep and capture information about the microstructure of sleep that may have important clinical or research implications.

Minimal polygraphic requirements to score sleep adequately include two channels of EEG: one channel for the electro-oculogram (EOG) and one channel for the submental electromyogram (EMG). In routine PSG, additional channels are used to assess respiration, leg movements, oxygenation, and cardiac rhythm. The following is a brief review of "standard" technology involved in PSG recordings. Other reviews of PSG technique may also be helpful to the reader (13,80).

Electroencephalographic Sleep Recording

As with routine EEG, nonpolarizable silver–silver chloride or gold electrodes are standard and are attached with collodion to maintain adequate contact for the 6 to 10 hours required for an overnight study. The International 10-20 System is used for electrode placement (55), but a much more limited EEG montage, described later, is selected. Early sleep investigators were limited by channel availability and could commit only one channel to EEG recording (central EEG lead to contralateral ear; e.g., C4-A1). As a result, the scoring manual of Rechtschaffen and Kales (82) is based on that single lead derivation. However, the poor sampling of waking alpha activity by this montage has led most investigators to add at least one additional channel (occipital lead to more anterior reference; e.g., 01-A2) for better separation of wakefulness from stage 1 (drowsiness). In addition, many laboratories commit at least two additional channels to EEG. A transverse vertex montage (e.g., T3-Cz, Cz-T4) is often preferred because it is sensitive to the identification of sleep spindles and vertex waves. Bilateral central, occipital, and ear electrodes are routinely placed so that in the event of electrode failure, the

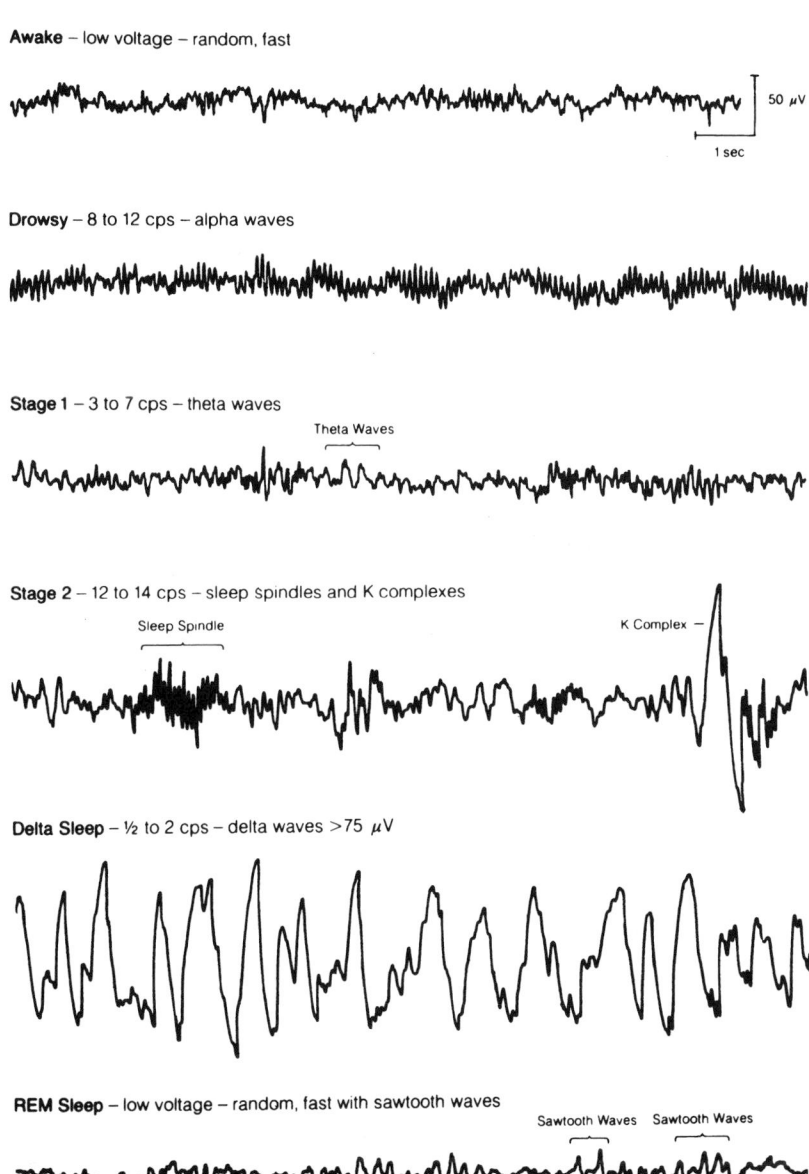

Awake – low voltage – random, fast

50 μV

1 sec

Drowsy – 8 to 12 cps – alpha waves

Stage 1 – 3 to 7 cps – theta waves

Theta Waves

Stage 2 – 12 to 14 cps – sleep spindles and K complexes

Sleep Spindle

K Complex —

Delta Sleep – ½ to 2 cps – delta waves >75 μV

REM Sleep – low voltage – random, fast with sawtooth waves

Sawtooth Waves   Sawtooth Waves

FIG. 26.1. EEG activity characteristic for each of the major sleep stages. The activity is recorded from the usual sleep study derivation (C4-A1) at a paper speed of 10 mm per second. *Delta sleep* is an alternative name for slow-wave sleep. (From Hauri P. *The sleep disorders.* Kalamazoo, MI: Upjohn Co., 1982:5–62.)

homologous contralateral derivation can be used without disturbing the patient. Occasional patients, such as those with possible nocturnal seizures, require a more extensive EEG montage for adequate assessment.

Routine recording or display speed for the PSG is 10 mm per second (82). This is initially disconcerting to the electroencephalographer trained in using a paper speed of 30 mm per second. The slower paper speed was chosen to reduce paper use and to improve visualization of events (e.g., apneas) that occur over a relatively long time. Slow paper speeds still allow clear visualization of alpha rhythm and sleep spindles. In fact, the characteristic appearance of sleep spindles, "sawtooth" waves, and eye movements is more easily recognized at slower paper speeds once the interpreter has adjusted to the altered appearance (Fig. 26.1). The EEG low-frequency filter (LFF) setting is 0.3 Hz, and the high-frequency filter (HFF) setting is 70 Hz. The extended low-frequency band is important for assessing the prominent slow-wave activity seen during deeper stages of non-REM sleep. The amplifier sensitivity setting is usually 5 to 10 μV per millimeter; 7 μV per millimeter is used most commonly. Because voltage of the delta range activity is important in determining sleep stage, any change in EEG channel sensitivity must be clearly flagged to avoid sleep scoring errors.

Electro-oculogram

The EOG is obtained primarily to identify phasic bursts of rapid eye movements, which are the cardinal sign of REM sleep. In addition, these electrodes allow identification of slow lateral eye movements, which are often the first and most dependable manifestation of drowsiness (92). Gold-plated or silver–silver chloride EEG cup electrodes are used to record the EOG, but collodion should be avoided because of possible corneal injury. EEG electrolyte paste with additional sticky tape over the electrodes offers adequate attachment and avoids the risk of eye injury. Two different electrode montages can be used to monitor eye movements. Most commonly (and as recommended in Rechtschaffen and Kales' manual [82]), a referential recording is made from an electrode 1 cm lateral and 1 cm superior to the outer canthus and referred to the ipsilateral ear. A second channel records activity from a location 1 cm lateral and 1 cm inferior to the contralateral outer canthus and referred to the ipsilateral ear. This two-channel derivation shows eye movements as out-of-phase potentials, thus increasing the interpreter's confidence in correctly identifying REMs (Figs. 26.2 and 26.3). Alternatively, eye movements may be recorded from a single bipolar linkage between two electrodes placed near each outer canthus, as described earlier. The advantage of this derivation is that (a) the conjugate eye movements have twice the potential and (b) the EOG

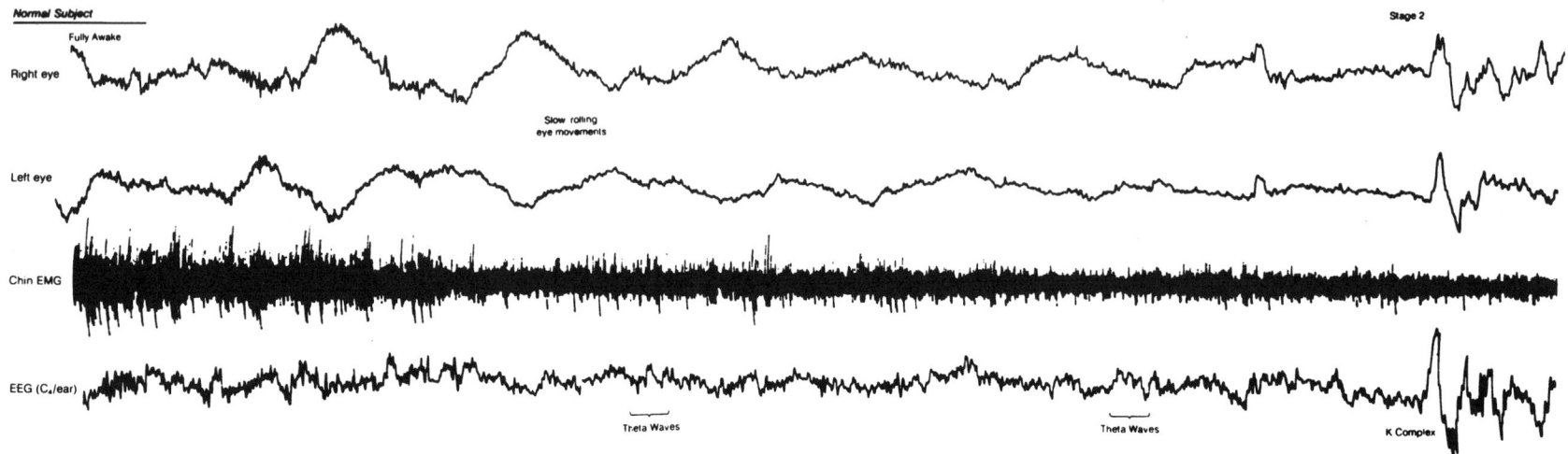

FIG. 26.2. Slow eye movement. Note the slow, rolling eye movements appearing as out-of-phase activity in electro-oculographic (EOG) channels. Slow eye movements accompany the appearance of mixed-frequency theta activity typical for stage 1 sleep. The K complex near the end of the epoch denotes onset of stage 2. The K complex appears as in-phase activity in EOG channels, which reflects its cerebral origin. (From Rechtschaffen A, Kales A, eds. *A manual of standardized terminology, techniques and scoring system for sleep stages of human subjects.* Los Angeles: UCLA Brain Information Service/Brain Research Institute, 1968.)

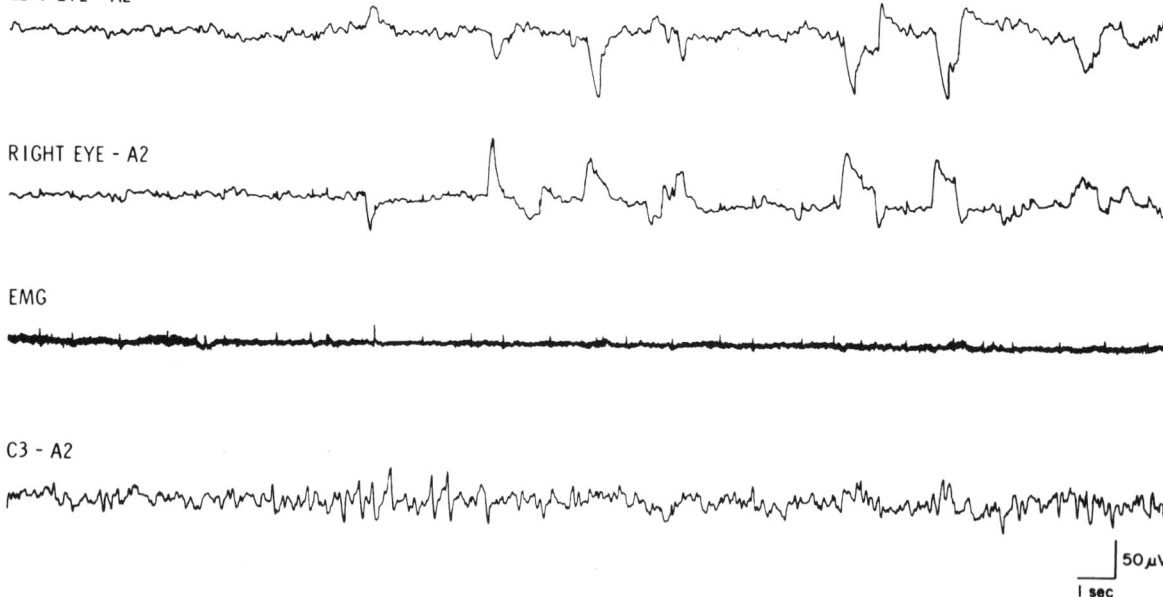

FIG. 26.3. Unambiguous rapid eye movement (REM) sleep with relatively low-voltage, mixed-frequency electroencephalogram, REMs, and tonic electromyogram at lowest level during sleep. Note series of typical "sawtooth waves" at onset of REM activity. (From Rechtschaffen A, Kales A, eds. *A manual of standardized terminology, techniques and scoring system for sleep stages of human subjects.* Los Angeles: UCLA Brain Information Service/Brain Research Institute, 1968.)

occupies only a single polygraph channel. Absence of a phase reversal complicates visual identification of eye movements. Sensitivity and filter settings for the EOG are similar to those used for EEG recording.

There is no standard definition of what constitutes a rapid eye movement as opposed to a slow one. Slow eye movements have a frequency of 0.25 to 0.5 Hz, and the sharpest slope has a duration consistently greater than 0.5 seconds. In comparison, REM waveforms have a sharp slope lasting 50 to 200 milliseconds and a waveform frequency of greater than 1 Hz. Obviously, the rate of return to baseline of any EOG waveform is dependent on the alternating current (AC) filter setting and the superimposition of any additional eye movements. Thus, the abrupt slope of the EOG waveform is the most reliable differentiating feature. A reasonable cutoff is the requirement that the rapid slope of a rapid eye movement be shorter than 300 milliseconds in duration and have an amplitude of at least 20 μV.

Axial Electromyogram

Submental (chin) EMG activity reflects axial muscle tone and is used as one criterion for identifying REM sleep and movement arousals. Submental EMG is recorded by regular EEG electrodes placed over the mylohyoid muscle. One electrode is placed on the tip of the jaw, and the second electrode is placed 3 cm posterior and lateral. This second electrode should be placed bilaterally, functioning as a backup electrode from which to select the most reliable EMG recording.

Tonic EMG activity from axial musculature gradually decreases from wakefulness through stages 1 to 4 of sleep and is usually entirely absent during REM sleep. Sensitivity of the submental EEG channel should be adjusted during drowsiness to reflect moderate activity. Subsequent adjustments should be avoided during the night to permit comparison of EMG activity during different portions of the record. The typical sensitivity setting of the EMG is 2 μV per millimeter, the LFF setting is 5 Hz, and the HFF setting is 70 Hz.

Anterior Tibialis Electromyography

Anterior tibialis EMG activity is monitored to detect periodic leg movements (30,31). Regular EEG electrodes are placed over the anterior tibialis muscle bilaterally. The anterior tibialis muscle can be easily identified on the anterior lower leg by having the patient dorsiflex the foot against resistance. Two electrodes 3 cm apart are placed over each anterior tibialis muscle. A bipolar recording from each anterior tibialis muscle is usually obtained. Sensitivity and filter settings are similar to those described for submental EMG recording. A semistandardized baseline is obtained before the study by asking the patient to dorsiflex a foot gently. Figure 26.4 is an example of periodic leg movements (PLMs) of sleep recorded from the anterior tibialis EMG electrodes.

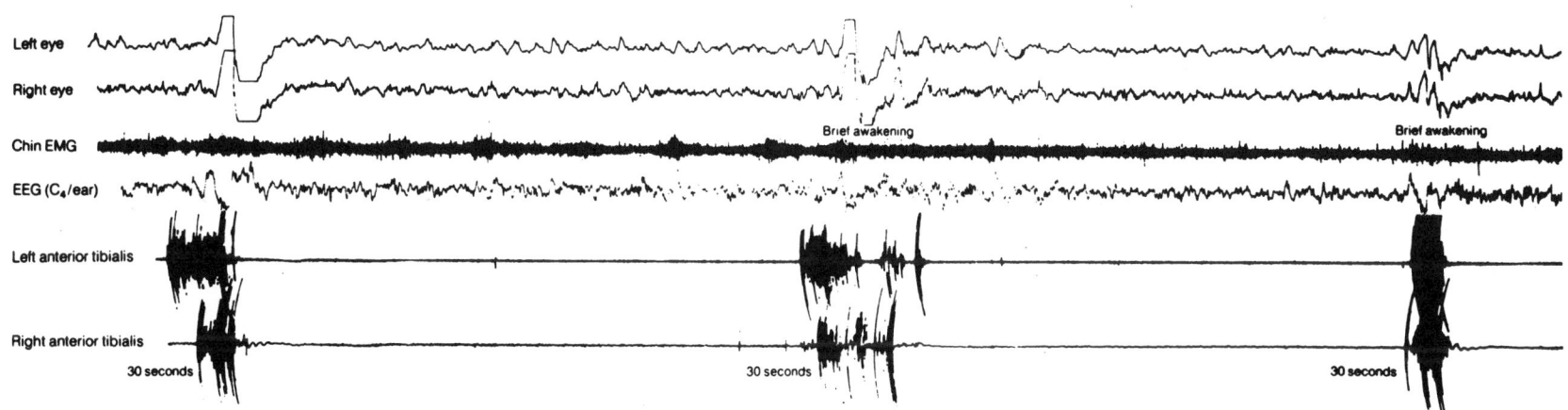

FIG. 26.4. Periodic leg movements (PLMs) of sleep. The anterior tibialis electromyographic (EMG) recording demonstrates bursts of periodic EMG activity associated with electroencephalographic arousals. (From Hauri P. *The sleep disorders.* Kalamazoo, MI: Upjohn Co., 1982:5–62.)

Ventilatory Monitoring

Inasmuch as the suspicion of sleep apnea is the most common indication for overnight PSG, ventilatory monitoring is arguably the most important technical aspect. Although measurements of airflow and ventilatory effort are technically the most difficult of all polygraphic variables to obtain, they are essential for adequate assessment of breathing during sleep. Both airflow and a measure of ventilatory effort must be recorded in order to distinguish among central, mixed, and obstructive apneic events (Fig. 26.5). In central (or nonobstructive) apnea, absence of respiratory drive causes all mechanical efforts to cease, and no airflow occurs at the nose or mouth. In obstructive apnea, ventilatory efforts continue but no airflow occurs; this is because the airway is occluded. A mixed apnea begins as a central apnea (without ventilatory effort or airflow), but then the picture of obstructive apnea develops (ventilatory effort without accompanying airflow). Apneas are arbitrarily defined as cessation of airflow for 10 seconds or longer (1,12). In addition, hypopneas (decreased airflow) may also be clinically significant. Specific scoring criteria for respiratory events are discussed in the section on polysomnographic interpretation.

For all measures of airflow or ventilatory effort, an LFF setting of 0.5 Hz is used. DC amplification is preferred; it is routinely used if a dedicated polygraph machine is available. However, adequate respiratory monitoring is possible with routine EEG AC amplifiers if the lowest LFF available is selected. Polygraph machines have a greater pen excursion, which also aids in assessment of respiratory parameters.

Airflow Monitoring

Thermistors and Thermocouples

Thermistors or thermocouples are the least expensive and most commonly used method of monitoring airflow (1,12,13). Thermistors are small glass beads or wires whose electrical resistance changes as a function of temperature. When they are powered by a 1.5-V battery, the voltage drop across the thermistor varies with temperature. Expired air warms the thermistor and pro-

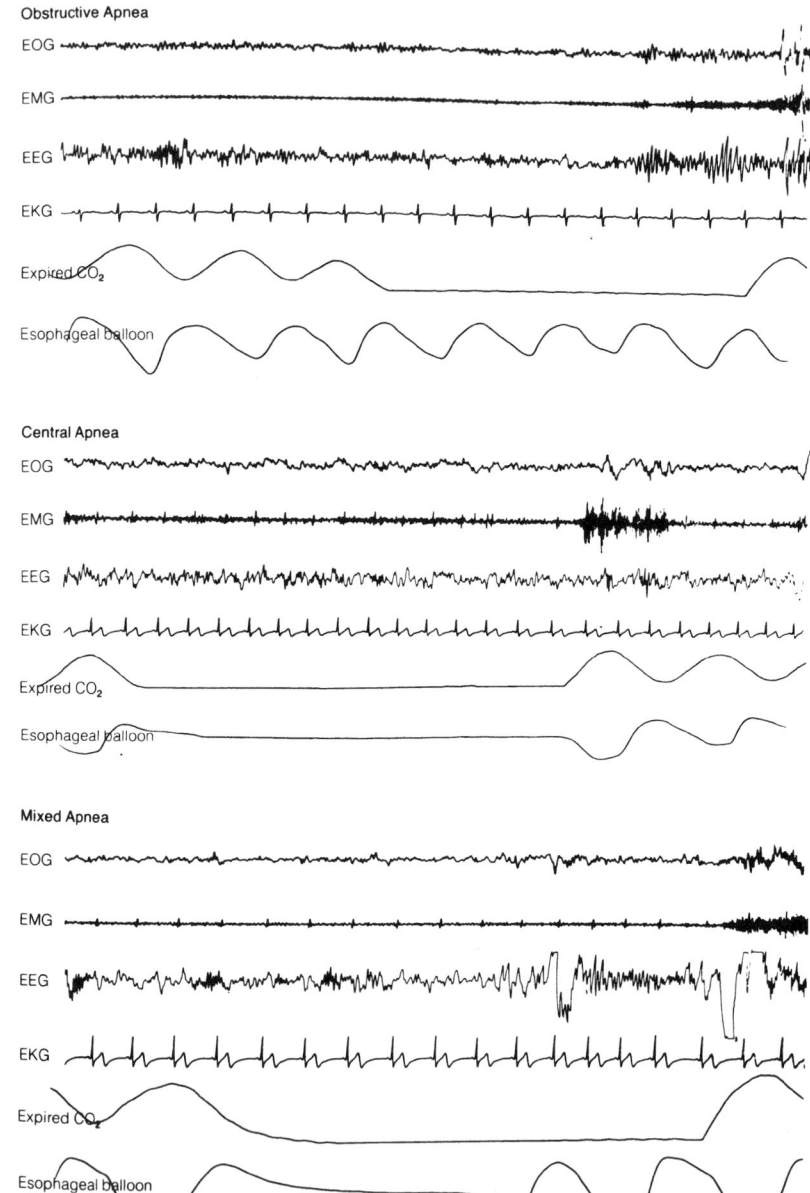

FIG. 26.5. Examples of obstructive, central, and mixed apneas. Compare airflow (measured by CO_2 analysis) and ventilatory effort (measured by intraesophageal balloon). (From Hauri P. *The sleep disorders.* Kalamazoo, MI: Upjohn Co., 1982:5–62.)

duces a signal that can be displayed on a polygraph. A thermocouple consists of two dissimilar metals in electrical contact, which produces a low-voltage signal that varies with the temperature change caused by expired air.

Small, lightweight thermistors (or thermocouples) are taped, under each nostril and in front of the mouth. It is crucial to monitor both nostrils because the airflow path frequently changes during the night as a function of patient position. Activity from the two nasal thermistors can be summed and displayed in a single channel. Patient movement may disturb the position of the thermistors and result in loss of signal. Thus, careful attention needs to be paid to thermistor position throughout the night.

Carbon Dioxide Detectors

Measuring the carbon dioxide (CO_2) of expired air can serve as an alternative method of monitoring airflow (1,76). It is based on the principle that 6% to 7% of exhaled air is CO_2, whereas inhaled air contains negligible amounts of CO_2. In order to sample CO_2 content, a cannula is inserted just inside the nostril and is connected to an infrared or mass spectroscopy analyzer. For routine clinical PSG, the small increase in sensitivity for detecting air movement by using CO_2 detectors does not usually warrant the added expense and technical demands. However, end-tidal carbon dioxide tension (PCO_2) monitoring is an essential component of assessing sleep-disordered breathing in children. The clinical importance of PCO_2 monitoring in pediatric sleep apnea has led to its wide application in pediatric sleep laboratories. Because of the technical difficulties in maintaining adequate end-tidal PCO_2 measurement, transcutaneous CO_2 may be used to complement the end-tidal PCO_2 measurement (76).

Nasal Cannula/Pressure Transducer

Reports have described the successful application of a simple, noninvasive pneumotachygraph consisting of a standard nasal cannula connected to a 2-cm water pressure transducer (52,75,77). These initial reports identified sensitivity to airflow changes comparable with that of thermistor/thermocouples (in identifying hypopneas) and greater sensitivity in recognizing additional events (characterized only by flow limitations) that may be helpful in identifying the respiration-related arousals that are a significant part of the upper airway resistance syndrome (45) (Fig. 26.6). Commercial products are now available, and their use is becoming more widespread. Greater experience is necessary to determine how readily the apparent benefits of this technology can be extended to routine PSG.

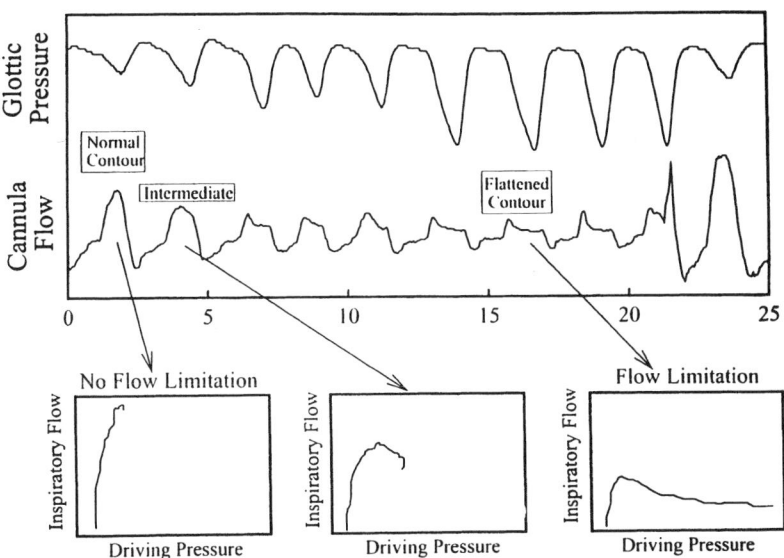

FIG. 26.6. Pressure/flow relationships from nasal cannula/pressure transducer during a single respiratory event. The x-axis shows time in seconds. Breaths with normal, intermediate, and flattened flow contours are labeled, and a plot of the driving pressure/flow relationship is shown. The flattened flow/time contour shows a nonlinear flow/pressure relationship characteristic of flow limitation. (From Hosselet JJ, Norman RG, Ayappa T, et al. Detection of flow limitations with a nasal cannula/pressure transducer system. *Am J Respir Crit Care Med* 1998;157:1461–1467.)

Pneumotachography

Pneumotachography is the only method that allows direct quantification of ventilation during sleep. However, the technique involves an uncomfortable tight-fitting mask and a flow-to-pressure transducer that offers considerable resistance to respiration. Although it is technically superior to the other methods of monitoring airflow, the sleep disruption and increased respiratory resistance preclude the routine use of pneumotachography in PSG (101).

Ventilatory Effort Monitoring

Esophageal Pressure Monitors. An esophageal pressure monitor can be either a catheter-tip or balloon transducer that is placed through the nose into the distal esophagus (72). The output signal of the pressure/voltage transducer shows absolute pressure (with a DC amplifier) or variations in pressure (with an AC amplifier) on the polygraphic record. Esophageal pressure monitors measure pleural pressure swings and are the most accurate devices for assessing ventilatory effort. However, because of their invasive placement and the inability of many patients to tolerate them, esophageal monitors are less than ideal for routine PSG. Nonetheless, in difficult cases, intraesophageal pressure measurement can accurately resolve ambiguities as to the nature of the apnea.

Piezoelectric Belts. This device incorporates a piezo crystal element transducer in an elastic belt. When stretched, the piezo crystal element provides a voltage signal proportional to the stress applied. It requires no power and connects simply to the electrode board or input cable. It incorporates good sensitivity to ventilatory effort with simple and reliable technical application.

Impedence Pneumography. When a high-frequency electrical signal is applied to the chest wall through two electrodes, the electrical impedance

between the two electrodes varies, depending on the position of the chest wall. In practice, an AC carrier signal is applied directly to the chest (or abdominal) wall. The voltage drop across the body wall varies with chest wall movement and modulates the amplitude of the carrier signal. A demodulator system then converts the signal variation into a form that can be displayed on a standard AC or DC polygraph channel.

Impedance pneumography has proved to be a reasonable technique for qualitatively monitoring ventilatory effort (78). The simplicity of the commercially available devices and the stability of this method are significant advantages. The two input electrodes are placed over the point of greatest excursion of the chest wall or abdomen. As with strain gauges, placement on both chest and abdomen increases sensitivity to ventilatory effort and makes identification of paradoxical respirations possible (Fig. 26.7).

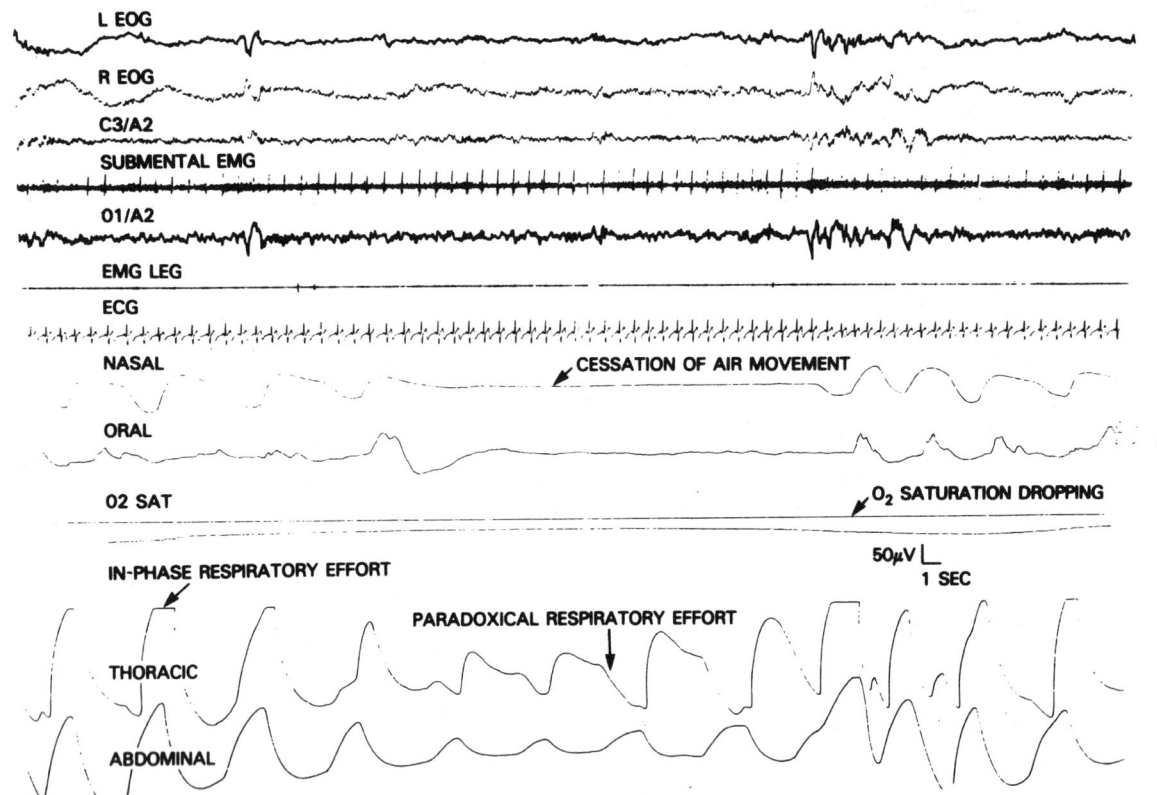

FIG. 26.7. Obstructive apnea. Note the development of out-of-phase or paradoxical movement of thoracic and abdominal monitors during period of obstructive apnea. (From Mendelson WB. *Human sleep.* New York: Plenum Press, 1987:159.)

Inductive Plethysmography. In inductive plethysmography, a conductive wire is sewn into an elastic band or mesh that encircles the chest or abdomen. With expansion of the body wall, the circle of wire enlarges and the inductance of the loop is changed. When an AC current is applied to this wire, the variable inductance can be displayed on an AC or DC polygraph channel. This technique is much more powerful than the methods already described, inasmuch as it provides a quantitative measure of airflow. This method also permits more accurate determination of lung expansion, regardless of patient position (16,27). The instrument is carefully calibrated so that the sum of the chest and abdominal signals is proportional to the volume of airflow. If the airway is obstructed, no air is exchanged; any change in chest volume is associated with an opposite change in abdominal volume (paradoxical respiration), and the sum of the two is zero (representing no airflow). Theoretically, complete ventilatory monitoring can be accomplished with two bands around the chest. The three output channels are rib-cage movement, abdominal movement, and total volume. Obstructive apneas are recorded as continued respiratory movement of both thorax and abdomen but with no significant change in total volume signal (Fig. 26.8). In central apneas, all three signals are suppressed. Mixed apneas, as expected, show a central pattern followed by an obstructive picture. Hypopneas may also be quantified by this technique. Theoretically, an independent measure of airflow (thermistor) is unnecessary. However, because of difficulties in calibration (especially in obese patients) and slippage of coils, this technique usually requires an additional monitor of airflow. Although it increases cost and is more technically demanding, inductive plethysmography offers significant advantages over other methods.

Strain Gauge. Strain gauges are among the most convenient methods of qualitatively recording respiratory effort. Most strain gauges consist of a distensible tube filled with mercury. The electrical resistance of the mercury column varies directly with its length and inversely with its cross-sectional area. The strain gauge tube is strapped to the chest or abdominal wall in the area identified as having the greatest expansion with inspiration, and it is then connected to a battery. Each inspiration stretches the tube, decreasing its diameter and increasing its resistance. The voltage change across this varying resistance can be displayed on the polygraph record. Separate strain gauges should be placed over both the thoracic and abdominal walls. This provides a more sensitive measure of inspiratory effort and also helps identify paradoxical ventilatory effort (e.g., increase in thoracic circumference with decrease in abdominal circumference) seen with obstructive apnea (96). Although convenient and inexpensive, strain gauges depend greatly on stable positioning and are sensitive to artifact created by even small amounts of patient movement.

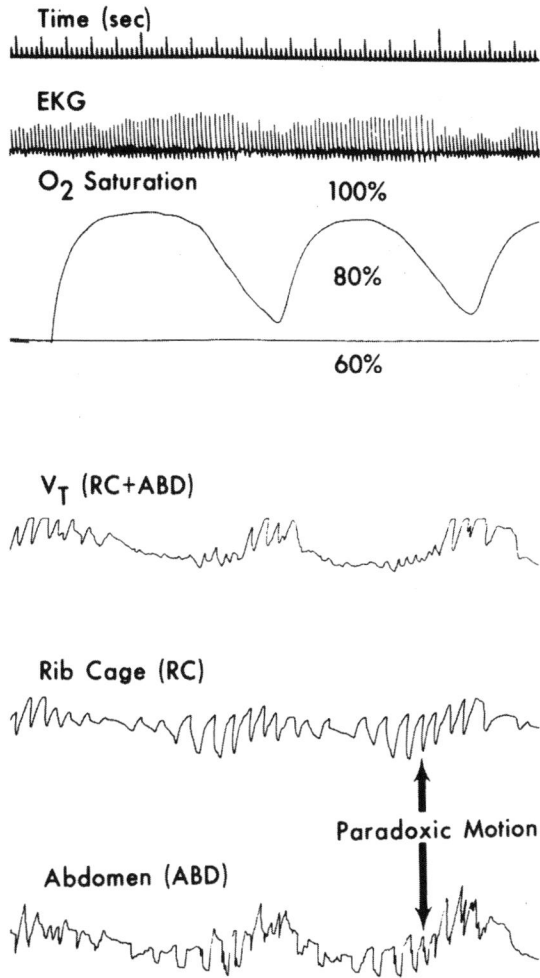

FIG. 26.8. Inductive plethysmography demonstrating paradoxical motion of ribcage and abdominal signals along with absence of significant volume signal (V_T[RC + ABD]), indicating decreased or absent airflow. Note accompanying oxygen desaturation. (From Cohn M. Respiratory monitoring during sleep: respiratory inductive plethysmography. In: Guilleminault C, ed. *Sleeping and waking disorders: indications and techniques.* Menlo Park, CA: Addison-Wesley, 1982:213–223.)

Intercostal Electromyography. Intercostal EMG can be recorded by surface electrodes placed over the intercostal space. This technique identifies thoracic ventilatory movements, but it is frequently inadequate in obese patients. Thus, although sometimes useful as a complementary technique, intercostal EMG alone is not an adequate index of ventilatory effort.

Arterial Oxygen Assessment

Determination of arterial oxygen desaturation is an important adjunct in assessing the severity of apneic episodes (23,34,100). Finger pulse oximetry is the technique that is most commonly used. It measures oxygen saturation by light transmission through the fingernail bed. Oxygen saturation (SaO_2) values obtained from pulse oximetry are continuously recorded, usually through a DC polygraphic channel. The accuracy of pulse oximetry is compromised by the presence of carbon monoxide, hyperbilirubinemia, oxygen saturations of less than 50%, dark skin pigmentation, or significant hypotension. It is important to note that the change in SaO_2 associated with a respiratory event appears 20 to 40 seconds after the actual event. Incorporated in the delay is partial circulation time to the finger and machine measurement delay.

Electrocardiogram

The ECG is monitored during sleep studies to detect arrhythmias that may be associated with sleep-disordered breathing events. Documentation of an associated cardiac arrhythmia can affect treatment decisions in a patient with sleep apnea. In PSG, the ECG is usually derived from two electrodes placed over the anterior chest wall. This placement avoids much of the movement artifact seen with the use of limb leads alone. It is adequate for monitoring heart rate, extrasystoles, and other arrhythmias. However, the differences in recording display, along with the limited derivation, do not allow adequate assessment of P wave and QRS abnormalities. If the precise rhythm disturbance cannot be determined from the PSG alone, then independent evaluation with a Holter monitor or another dedicated ECG recording device is required. The routine LFF setting for ECG is 1 Hz, and the routine HFF setting is 70 Hz; the sensitivity setting is approximately 50 μV per millimeter.

Nocturnal Penile Tumescence

Nocturnal penile tumescence is frequently measured to help differentiate organic from psychogenic causes of impotence. Normal REM sleep-related erections usually persist in the presence of psychogenic causes but are absent with organic causes. Strain gauges are placed on the penis, one at the base and the other just below the glans. Several sizes are commercially available and are selected to fit snugly on the flaccid penis. These devices are very similar to the strain gauges described for monitoring ventilatory effort. Before the study, amplifier signals are carefully calibrated, and the output of each strain gauge is recorded on a DC polygraph channel.

In addition to measuring tumescence, nocturnal penile tumescence studies also record EEG, EOG, and submental EMG. It is important to evaluate sleep continuity and architecture to ensure the validity of the REM-related tumescence observations. Nocturnal penile tumescence studies also include some evaluation of penile rigidity. Karacan (63) gave a description of nocturnal penile tumescence techniques and their clinical interpretation.

Recording Montage

PSG montages are selected in accordance with the clinical question. For screening studies of patients with possible sleep apnea, PSG variables should include EEG, EOG, axial EMG, anterior tibialis EMG, airflow, ventilatory effort, and SaO_2. A representative montage for a 16-channel machine is given in Table 26.1. If there is a more specific clinical question, the montage can be adjusted accordingly. For example, if the primary con-

TABLE 26.1. Screening polysomnographic montage

Channel	Sensitivity (μV/mm)	Filters (LFF/HFF) (Hz)
1. C4-A1	7	0.3/70
2. O1-A2	7	0.3/70
3. T3-Cz	7	0.3/70
4. Cz-T4	7	0.3/70
5. Left outer canthus-A1	7	0.3/70
6. Right outer canthus-A2	7	0.3/70
7. Submental electromyogram (EMG)	2	5/70
8. Electrocardiogram	70	1/70
9. Left anterior tibialis EMG	3–7	5/70
10. Right anterior tibialis EMG	3–7	5/70
11. Snore monitor		
12. Nasal thermistor	—	0.1/15
13. Oral thermistor	—	0.1/15
14. Thoracic movement	—	0.1/15
15. Abdominal movement	—	0.1/15
16. SaO_2 (oximetry)	—	DC/70

HFF, high-frequency filter; LFF, low-frequency filter; SaO_2, oxygen saturation.

cern is involuntary motor activity during sleep, arm and leg EMG monitors can be added. For patients with possible seizures, additional EEG channels are needed (38). The newer digital machines with expanded channel capabilities (e.g., 32 channels) allow greater flexibility in recording all physiological variables and a choice of variables on which to focus in review. In general, assessment for nocturnal seizures is best performed with dedicated video-EEG monitoring designed for recording seizures. If sleep laboratory equipment is used for such a purpose, additional channels of EEG accompanied by simultaneous time-locked video are required and should be able to be reviewed at a 30-mm-per-second display.

Alternatives/Screening Techniques

The laboratory PSG represents the gold standard for the evaluation of patients with sleep disorders. Because of its cost, cumbersome nature, and limited access, alternative approaches have been presented in the literature. Daytime nap studies have been shown to be inappropriate for most noninfant patients. Nap studies have the potential to disrupt sleep or produce an erroneous estimation of apnea severity (4,40).

Nocturnal oximetry has been proposed as a screening tool for patients in whom sleep apnea is suspected. Obviously, this may totally miss the upper airway resistance syndrome or brief apneas without significant oxygen desaturation. In one large study, the sensitivity of nocturnal oximetry was 90%, and specificity was 75% (111). The researchers concluded that, even when used by the most experienced clinicians, nocturnal oximetry has significant limitations that preclude its routine use as a screening tool at this time. In addition, it is totally inadequate in evaluating any other cause of excessive daytime sleepiness (EDS), such as narcolepsy or periodic movements (80,100).

Ambulatory recording of EEG or other physiological recorders have been used extensively in evaluation of patients with EDS (81). Most techniques suffer from limitation of data acquisition (fail to record either adequate EEG or respiratory data), which precludes routine application. Those that do provide comparable physiological sampling to attended PSG still retain some technical limitations and have only minor cost savings. In 1994, the Standards of Practice Committee of the ASDA published practice parameters for the use of portable recording of obstructive sleep apnea (97). The consensus presented is that portable recordings currently have a very limited role (e.g., follow-up studies after diagnosis established with in-laboratory studies). With further technological advances and cost reduction, ambulatory PSG may assume an increasing role but will require careful validation studies.

POLYSOMNOGRAPHY: INTERPRETATION

The clinical interpretation of polysomnographic sleep studies is based primarily on the analysis of three main variables: EEG-related variables (i.e., sleep stage, arousals), respiration-related variables (i.e., apneas or hypopneas), and movement-related variables (i.e., periodic leg movements). This discussion focuses on the guidelines for the scoring of these variables and the subsequent assignment of clinical significance. Both of these areas continue to evolve, and any statement may be outdated within a few years. Because of inconsistency in technique and variability in interpretative guidelines (i.e., criteria for hypopnea [41,108]), it is difficult to compare sleep study results across laboratories (1,5). However, there has been progress (i.e., definition of arousals [11]) that makes sleep scoring today more of a science than it was as practiced during the 1980s.

In contrast, because of the large amount of data demonstrating the presence of apneic or movement events in asymptomatic persons, the assignment of clinical significance today is even more problematic than it was years ago (9,10,19,66,68,112). Previously, a study result was considered abnormal and diagnostic of sleep apnea if the patient had more than five apneic episodes per hour of sleep (46). Today, an apnea index of 5 to 10, particularly in an older patient, is probably best considered normal. The exact limit for attaching clinical significance remains unclear. Guidelines in this area that are based on the author's own standard of practice are provided here, but with the understanding that other experienced practitioners may have different opinions and that these standards are continually evolving.

Electroencephalography-Related Variables

Basic Sleep Scoring

Normal sleep has a clearly defined architecture that is relatively stable from childhood through senescence (86). Sleep onset begins with a transition from wakefulness to stage 1. Stage 1 is normally brief and is followed by stage 2. Slow-wave sleep comes next and is usually sustained, especially in children and young adults. Sleep then briefly lightens to stage 2 before an initial brief REM period. This REM period occurs approximately 90 minute after sleep onset and completes the first sleep cycle. This complete cycle is then repeated three to five times during the night, but the amount of slow-wave sleep diminishes during ensuing cycles, whereas the amount of REM increases. Histograms are useful for visually displaying the ultradian cycle within a night's sleep (Fig. 26.9) (61). Predictable changes in sleep architecture occur with age. Beginning in middle age, slow-wave sleep becomes less prominent, the number of awakenings increase, and sleep efficiency decreases (109). Published information on

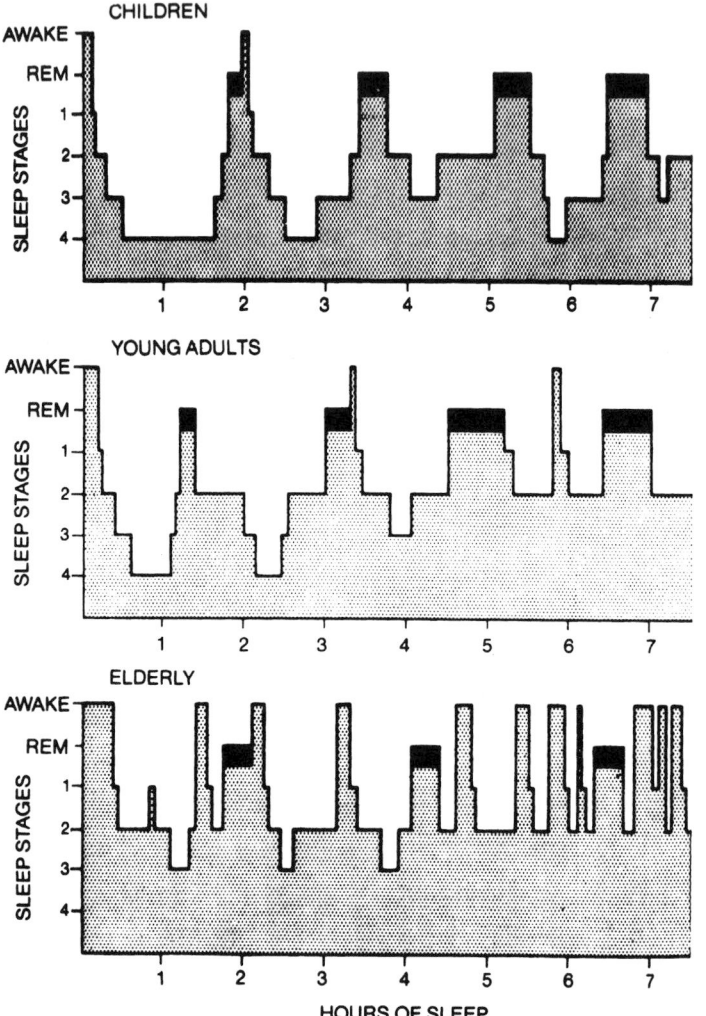

FIG. 26.9. Histograms representing normal sleep cycles for age. Rapid-eye-movement (REM) sleep (darkened area) occurs cyclically throughout the night at intervals of approximately 90 minutes. REM sleep shows little variation in the different age groups, whereas stages 3 and 4 sleep can be seen to decrease with age. Note also the frequent awakenings and increase in total awake time seen in the elderly. (From Kales A, Kales J. Recent findings in the diagnosis and treatment of disturbed sleep. *N Engl J Med* 1974;209:487–499.)

TABLE 26.2. *Average values for men of different ages*

Index	Age (years)		
	20–29	40–49	60–69
Time in bed (TIB) (min)	442	429	451
Total sleep time (TST) (min)	419	389	407
Sleep efficiency (TST/TIB)	95%	91%	90%
Wake (after sleep onset)	1%	6%	8%
Stage 1	4%	8%	10%
Stage 2	46%	55%	57%
SWS	21%	8%	2%
REM sleep	28%	23%	23%
Sleep latency (min)	15	10	8

REM, rapid eye movement; SWS, slow-wave sleep.
(From Williams RI, Karacan I, Hursch CJ. *Electroencephalography (EEG) of human sleep: clinical applications.* New York: John Wiley and Sons, 1974.)

normal sleep can serve as an outline for normal values in PSG (Table 26.2), but each laboratory must study control subjects to identify any significant effects on sleep that result from differences in technique or environment.

Scoring is usually done on an epoch-by-epoch basis, with epoch lengths varying from 20 to 60 seconds. Thirty-second epochs are used as a standard by most laboratories. Epochs are scored according to the guidelines of Rechtschaffen and Kales (82); each epoch is scored as the stage that occupies more than 50% of that epoch (see Fig. 26.1). The following is an abbreviated summary of sleep scoring:

Stage W corresponds to the waking stage and is characterized by alpha activity or low-voltage, mixed-frequency EEG activity. REMs, eye blinks, and tonic EMG activity are usually present.
Stage 1 is scored when more than 50% of an epoch is low-voltage, 2- to 7-Hz activity. Vertex waves may occur in late stage 1. Slow rolling eye movements lasting several seconds are routinely seen early in stage 1, but K complexes and sleep spindles are absent by definition. Tonic EMG activity is usually less than that of relaxed wakefulness.
Stage 2 requires the presence of sleep spindles or K complexes, and less than 20% of the epoch contains delta activity. Sleep spindles bursts must last at least 0.5 second before they can be scored. K complexes are defined as biphasic vertex sharp waves with a total duration of greater than 0.5 second.
Stage 3 is scored when 20% to 50% of an epoch consists of delta activity that is 2 Hz or slower and is greater than 75 µV in amplitude. Sleep spindles may or may not be present.

Stage 4 is scored when more than 50% of an epoch consists of delta activity that is 2 Hz or slower and is more than 75 μV in amplitude. Reliable differentiation of stages 3 and 4 sleep is difficult by visual inspection, and most laboratories combine stages 3 and 4 into a single determination of slow-wave sleep.

Stage REM is characterized by relatively low-voltage, mixed-frequency EEG activity with episodic REMs and absent or markedly reduced axial EMG activity. Phasic EMG activity may occur, but tonic activity must be at a level that is as low as, or lower than, that during any other time in the study. Sleep spindles and K complexes are absent. Series of 2- to 5-Hz vertex-negative "sawtooth waves" occur, particularly just before phasic REM activity. The requirements to score sleep as REM are REMs, low or absent axial EMG, and the typical mixed-frequency EEG recording that does not preclude the scoring of REM (i.e., no sleep spindles can be seen).

Movement time is scored when more than 50% of an epoch is obscured by movement artifact. Movement time must be preceded or followed by sleep and is thus distinguished from movement occurring during wakefulness. If more than 50% of an epoch can be scored as sleep, it is assigned the stage that best describes the majority of the interpretable portion.

Additional sleep values are determined from each sleep study and contribute to the clinical interpretation of the study. These additional variables include the following:

1. Recording time is the time elapsed between "light outs" and "lights on" at end of study.
2. Total sleep time is the total time occupied by stage 1, stage 2, slow-wave sleep, and REM sleep.
3. Sleep efficiency is defined as total sleep time divided by recording time and is expressed as a percentage.
4. Sleep latency is the time from "lights out" to the first epoch scored as sleep. Some authors prefer to use the first epoch of stage 2 in order to be more confident about identifying the onset of sustained sleep. However, when sleep is very disrupted, there may be an extended period of time from recognition of stage 1 until an epoch than can be scored as stage 2.
5. REM latency is the time from sleep onset (as described earlier) to the first epoch scored as REM, minus any intervening epochs scored as wakefulness.
6. Sleep stage percentages (percentages spent in stage 1, stage 2, slow-wave sleep, and REM) are determined by dividing time recorded in each sleep stage by total sleep time.
7. Wake after sleep onset is time spent awake after sleep onset.

The scoring principles of Rechtschaffen and Kales (82) function well when applied to sustained sleep. However, the frequent arousals and movement artifacts seen in a patient with severe sleep apnea can preclude scoring of a study by conventional criteria. Bornstein (12) suggested modified sleep scoring rules to help "smooth over" many of the arousals and sleep stage transitions seen in patients with extremely disrupted sleep.

Arousals and Awakenings

Traditionally, there had been no reasonable consensus about the scoring of arousals from sleep. In Rechtschaffen and Kales' system (82), an awakening was defined as a return of the patient's waking background for at least 30 seconds. An arousal, by Rechtschaffen and Kales' criteria, was scored when a patient's waking alpha activity returned for more than 3 seconds but less than 30 seconds. However, most arousals from sleep are more subtle than that just described, and there previously existed no exact requirements to define these. Standard sleep stage scoring systems are intended to identify sleep stage and not transient interruptions in that stage. The transient nature of these arousals caused them to be overlooked in the standard 30-second-epoch sleep scoring system. These brief arousals are usually characterized on a standard polysomnogram by an abrupt change in EEG frequency with or without brief increase in EMG amplitude. With the increasing recognition that arousals result in fragmented sleep, which in turn leads to increased daytime sleepiness, the need for specific and reliable criteria for the identification of arousals became sorely evident (99). The Sleep Disorders Atlas Task Force of the American Sleep Disorders Association has published a preliminary guide with illustrations (11). These recommendations are summarized as follows.

An EEG arousal is an abrupt shift in EEG frequency, which may include theta waves, alpha waves, and/or frequencies greater than 16 Hz but not spindles, subject to the following rules and conditions:

1. Subjects must be asleep, defined as 10 continuous seconds or more of any stage of sleep, before an EEG arousal can be scored. Arousal scoring is independent of the Rechtschaffen and Kales' (82) epoch scoring (i.e., an arousal can be scored in an epoch of recording that would be classified as wakefulness by Rechtschaffen and Kales' criteria).
2. A minimum of 10 continuous seconds of intervening sleep is necessary to score a second arousal.
3. The EEG frequency shift must be 3 seconds or longer in duration to be scored as an arousal (Fig. 26.10).

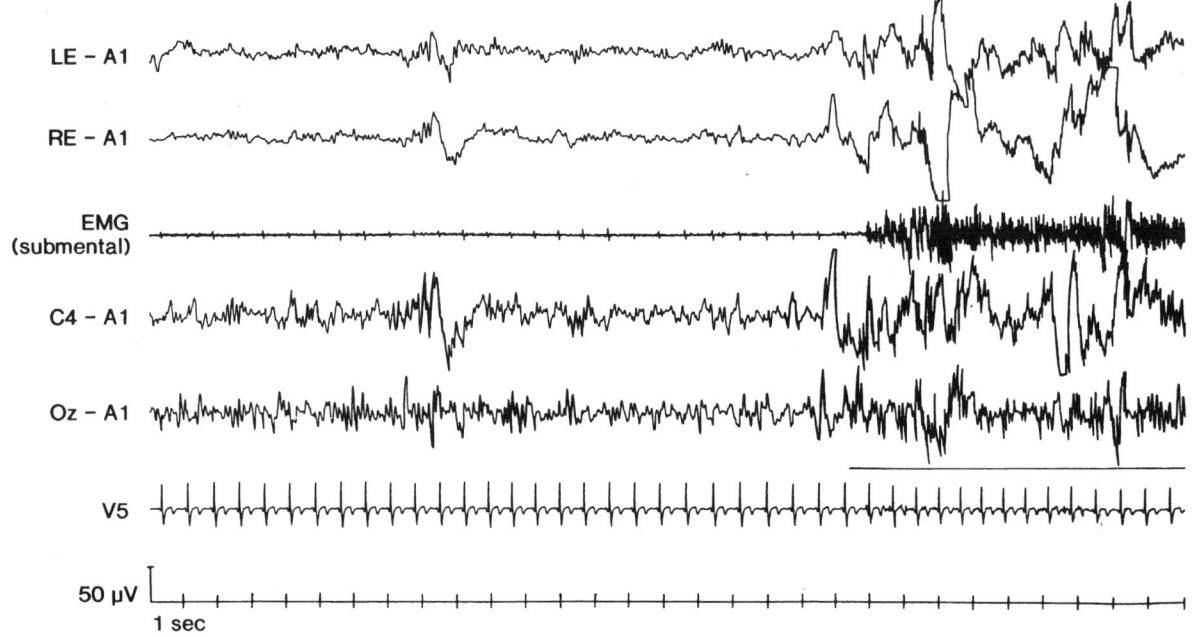

FIG. 26.10. This is a greater-than-3-second electroencephalographic (EEG) change with frequencies higher than 16 Hz and alpha activity. This EEG arousal also has increased electromyographic amplitude. There are more than 10 seconds of sleep preceding this event, and it is scored as an arousal. (From Bonnet M, Carley D, Carskadon M, et al. EEG arousals: scoring rules and examples. *Sleep* 1992;15: 173–184.)

4. Arousals in non-REM sleep may occur without concurrent increases in submental EMG amplitude (Fig. 26.11).
5. Arousals are scored in REM sleep only when accompanied by concurrent increases in submental EMG amplitude (Figs. 26.12 and 26.13).
6. Arousals cannot be scored on the basis of changes in submental EMG amplitude alone.
7. Artifacts, K complexes, and delta waves are not scored as arousals unless accompanied by an EEG frequency shift (as previously defined) in at least one derivation. If such activity precedes an EEG frequency shift, it is not included in reaching the 3-second duration criteria. When occurring within the EEG frequency shift, artifacts or delta wave activity are included in meeting duration criteria.
8. The occurrence of pen-blocking artifact should be considered an arousal only if an EEG arousal pattern is contiguous. The pen-blocking event can be included in reaching duration criteria.
9. Nonconcurrent but contiguous EEG and EMG changes, which were individually less than 3 seconds but together more than 3 seconds in duration, are not scored as arousals.

10. Intrusion of alpha activity of less than 3 seconds' duration into non-REM sleep at a rate higher than one burst per 10 seconds is not scored as an EEG arousal. Three seconds of alpha sleep is not scored as an arousal unless a 10-second alpha-free episode precedes.
11. Transitions from one stage of sleep to another are not sufficient by themselves to scored as EEG arousals unless they meet the criteria just indicated.

These EEG arousal criteria are based on EEG changes alone with one exception: An increase in submental EMG is required for demonstration of arousal from REM sleep. The criteria of defining arousal as being 3 seconds or greater in duration is simply a methodological one and is of uncertain physiological significance. It was simply chosen to increase the reliability between observers for scoring arousals.

In the author's opinion, these current EEG arousal scoring rules underestimate the frequency of arousals. Specifically, rhythmic delta activity or a series of vertex waves is ignored as an arousal (Fig. 26.14). These events, particularly when accompanied by another change in the polysomnogram

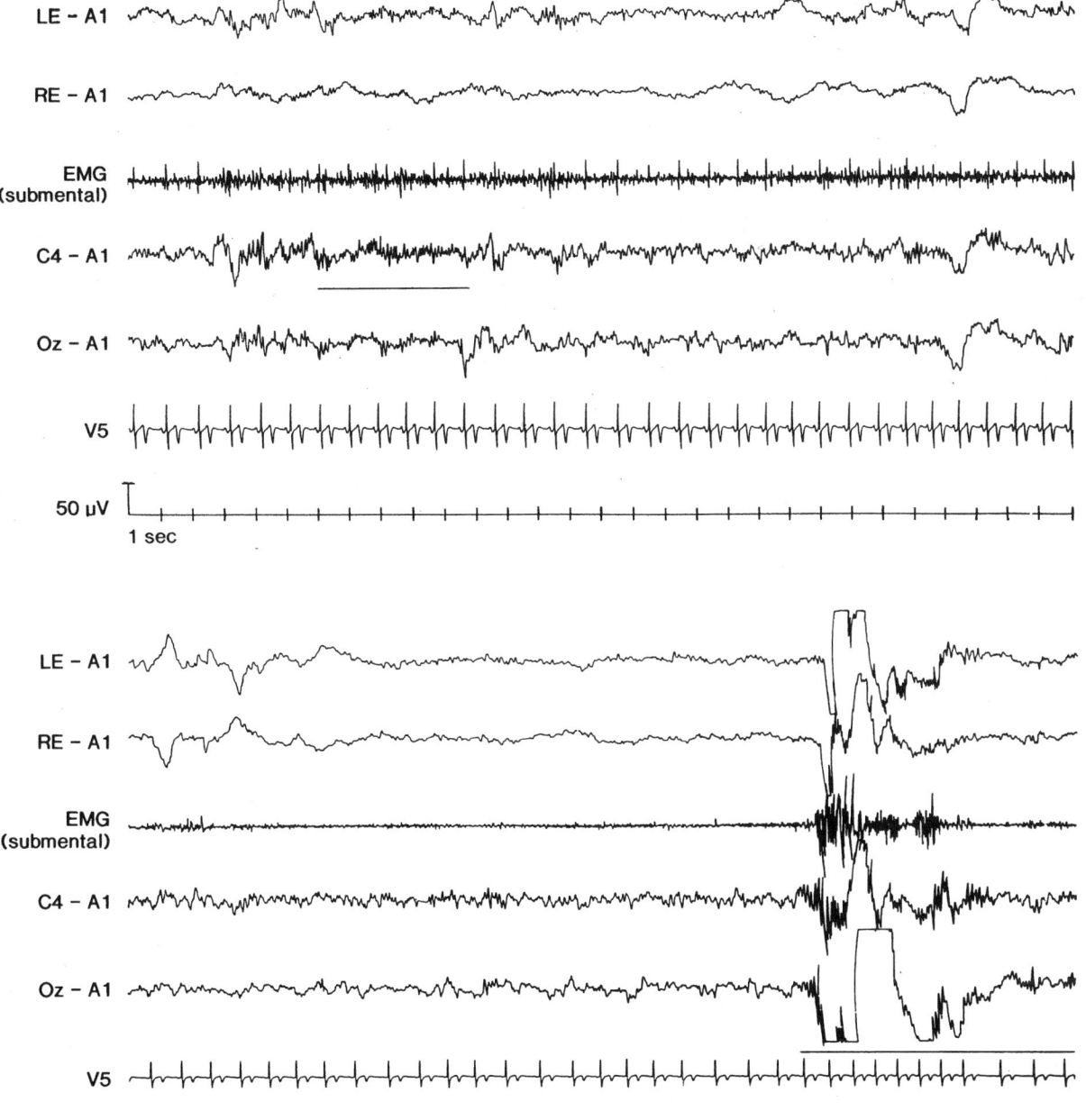

FIG. 26.11. The EEG frequency change in this epoch of non–rapid-eye-movement sleep is scored as an arousal despite the absence of an electromyographic amplitude increase. (From Bonnet M, Carley D, Carskadon M, et al. EEG arousals: scoring rules and examples. *Sleep* 1992;15:173–184.)

FIG. 26.12. The EEG frequency change in this epoch of rapid-eye-movement sleep is scored as an arousal because there are both an electromyographic amplitude increase and an EEG change of more than 3 seconds' duration. (From Bonnet M, Carley D, Carskadon M, et al. EEG arousals: scoring rules and examples. *Sleep* 1992;15:173–184.)

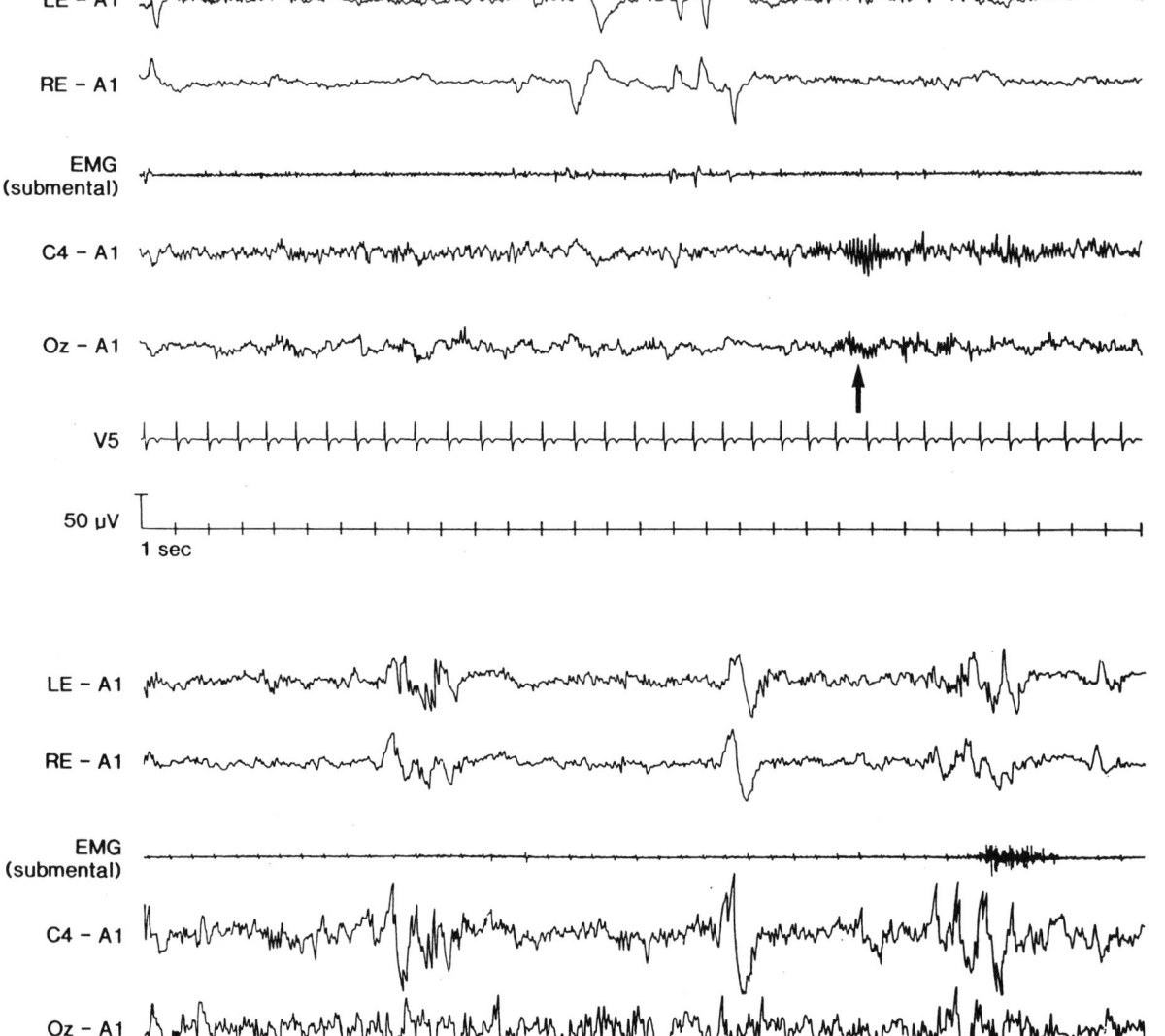

FIG. 26.13. The EEG frequency change on this epoch of rapid-eye-movement sleep *(arrow)* is not accompanied by an increase in electromyographic amplitude and thus is not scored as an arousal. (From Bonnet M, Carley D, Carskadon M, et al. EEG arousals: scoring rules and examples. *Sleep* 1992;15:173–184.)

FIG. 26.14. The delta burst of this example *(arrow)* is not scored as an arousal because there is no arousal-type EEG pattern, although there is an electromyographic amplitude increase. (From Bonnet M, Carley D, Carskadon M, et al. EEG arousals: scoring rules and examples. *Sleep* 1992;15:173–184.)

(i.e., increase in submental EMG or return of ventilation) almost assuredly represent a comparable physiological arousal. In any case, the current availability of rules defining EEG arousals is a major advance in standardizing the scoring of sleep studies.

Respiration-Related Variables

Other than the duration (10 seconds), there is no consensus about the decrement in airflow required for scoring respiratory events as apneas or hypopneas. This ambiguity is further complicated by (a) the variable techniques used in different laboratories, (b) the qualitative nature of airflow measurement by any technique, and (c) the effects of position change on measured airflow and respiratory effort. Many events without complete cessation of airflow are associated with oxygen desaturation and arousal. As a result, most laboratories score both apneas (cessation of airflow) and hypopneas (significant decrease in airflow) as contributing to a respiratory disturbance index (RDI): apneas plus hypopneas, divided by hours of sleep (1,12).

An apnea episode is defined as a cessation (or greater than 90% decrease) of baseline airflow from nasal and mouth thermistors that persists for 10 seconds or more (1,12) (see Fig. 26.5). Baseline airflow is defined by the airflow before and after the respiratory event in question. The event is scored as an obstructive apnea if there is evidence on chest and abdominal monitors of continued respiratory effort throughout the period of apnea. The event is scored as a mixed apnea if there is no apparent ventilatory effort for more than 6 seconds at onset of the apnea, followed by return of ventilatory effort. Central apnea is scored if no respiratory effort can be detected throughout the entire period of apnea. An apparent central apnea that is consistently terminated by a loud snort should be reviewed carefully to confirm the presence or absence of any obstructive component. It should be emphasized that obstructive apneas with feeble accompanying inspiratory efforts may be incorrectly interpreted as purely central apneas by all commonly used techniques for assessing ventilatory effort except for esophageal pressure monitoring (95).

Physiological apneas occur in nearly every study. These are brief (10- to 20-second) central apneas that occur during the transition from wakefulness to sleep or during bursts of phasic REM activity during REM sleep. These events are scored and contribute to the calculation of the respiratory disturbance index. Brief hypopneic periods during REM sleep not associated with arousal or oxygen desaturation are usually ignored.

There is no universal agreement about the polysomnographic criteria necessary to score a hypopnea. The author's criteria has been a more than 50% decrease in airflow at the nasal and oral thermistors associated with an arousal, an awakening, or more than a 3% decrease in oxygen saturation. Whyte et al. (108) demonstrated that hypopneas could be more accurately scored by using the criteria of a 50% decrease in thoracoabdominal movement lasting at least 10 seconds. They used inductive plethysmography as the ventilatory monitoring technique. The same research group had previously demonstrated (41) that examining thoracoabdominal movement was a more sensitive indicator of hypopnea than was airflow monitoring alone. However, the usual standard of practice is currently to use a definition of some noticeable decrement in airflow at the nasal and oral airflow monitors associated with oxygen desaturation or an arousal (1).

Regardless of the definition of an episode of hypopnea, there are frequently other events, presumed to be respiratory in character, that cannot be scored according to the criteria described earlier. These are recurrent episodes of loud snoring and apparent increases in ventilatory effort associated with a brief arousal. However, they do not meet the criteria for a decrease in airflow or an accompanying oxygen desaturation. In view of the lack of objective criteria, these events are usually not scored as respiratory events, although they are most likely part of a continuum that includes apneas and hypopneas. Investigators using an esophageal balloon have demonstrated a similar increase in negative intrathoracic pressure; these events reflect a pathophysiological mechanism similar to that of obstructive apneas and hypopneas. A task force of the American Academy of Sleep Medicine (AASM) labeled these events *respiratory event–related arousals* (RERAs). Such events contribute significantly to sleep disruption and subsequent daytime symptoms. Guilleminault et al. (44) coined the term *upper airway resistance syndrome* to encompass patients who have clinical manifestations of sleep apnea in the absence of respiratory events that can be scored. However, the AASM task force proposed the inclusion of the RERAs as part of the quantification of breathing abnormalities in obstructive sleep apnea. In view of the similar pathophysiological processes, they proposed using the frequency of apneas, hypopneas, and RERAs to define disease severity (1). However, at this time the inclusion of RERAs in assigning obstructive sleep apnea severity is not widely practiced.

In patients who have recurrent hypopneas, no attempt is made to characterize these events as central or obstructive, inasmuch as there are no reliable criteria with current technology. Similarly, it must be recognized that there may be a significant overestimation of central apneas, because of the limitations of routinely used monitoring devices. When a patient has predominantly central apneas, consideration should be given to the use of intraesophageal pressure monitoring to confidently rule out an obstructive component to the patient's respiratory dysrhythmia.

Monitoring of oxygen saturation via pulse oximeter is part of a standard polysomnogram. However, the exact manner in which the results of oxygen saturation monitoring are reported is variable. Several measures of oxygen desaturation have been employed. Most sleep report programs are able to generate a convenient graphic format of the cumulative oxygen saturation histogram (Fig. 26.15). In the histogram, the total percentage of sleep time spent at or below each saturation is demonstrated. From this format, a number of parameters can be derived, such as the percentage of sleep time spent below 90%, 80%, or another identified level of oxygen

saturation. In addition, an oxygen desaturation index is frequently determined, such as the number of oxygen desaturations (greater than 3%) per hour of sleep. This desaturation index can complement the RDI in determining disease severity. Of note is the greater importance of the oxygen desaturation index in pediatric patients as episodes that can be scored as apneas are rare in that population.

Diagnosis of Sleep Apnea

The diagnosis of sleep apnea has traditionally been based on recording five or more respiratory events (apneas and hypopneas) per hour of sleep

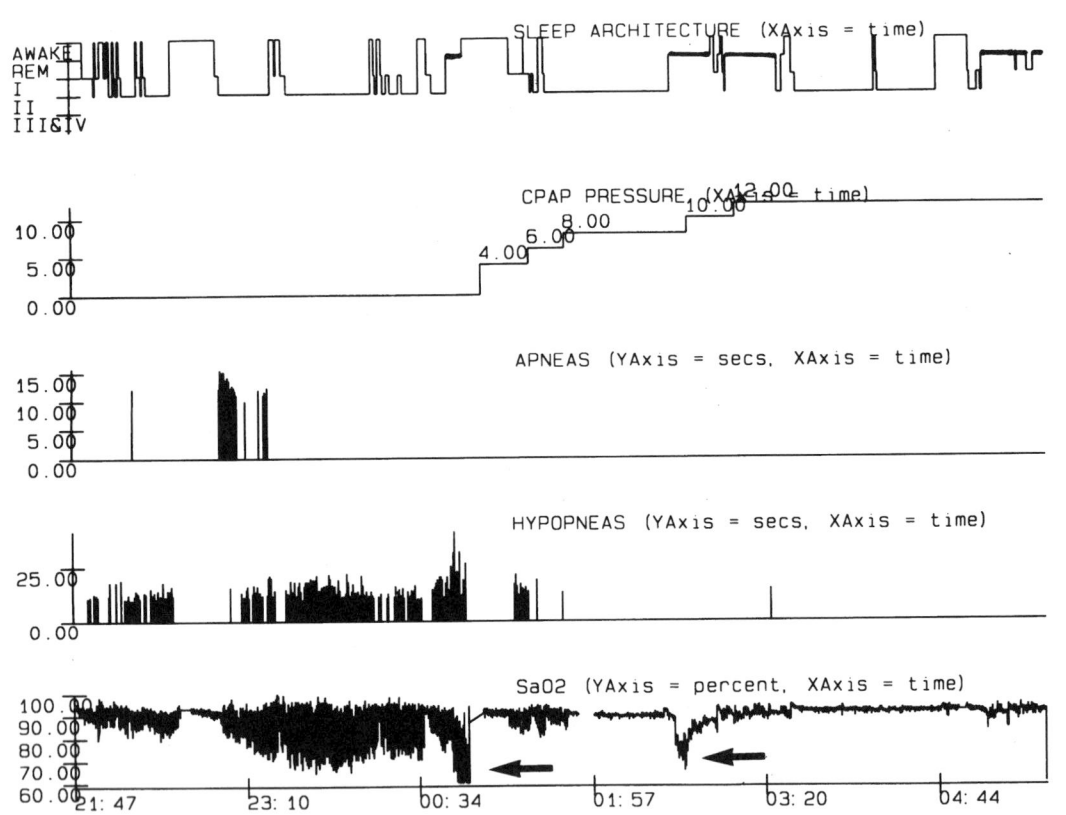

FIG. 26.15. Sleep histogram, continuous positive airway pressure (CPAP), apneas, hypopneas, and oxygen desaturation displayed for overnight polysomnography. Note prominent oxygen desaturations associated with recurrent hypopneas. More severe desaturations (*arrows*) are noted during rapid-eye-movement (REM) sleep (*darkened line*). Marked improvement in respiratory events and oxygen desaturations are noted with CPAP pressure of 8 cm H_2O and above. Slightly higher CPAP pressures were necessary to control desaturations in REM sleep.

(RDI > 5) (46). This standard derived from investigation of a small population of middle-aged control subjects free of sleep complaints. More recent studies, however, indicated that a significant percentage (approximately 40%) of normal subjects older than 60 years have sleep apnea according to that criterion (9,19,66). Knight et al. (64) reported a subtle increase in daytime sleepiness in this "apneic" population, but otherwise these persons have no neuropsychological or general medical complications. Therefore, the rigid use of the RDI of more than 5 as diagnostic of sleep apnea will lead to the overdiagnosis of the sleep apnea syndrome, particularly in an elderly population (9). A more reasonable RDI criterion may be 10 in middle-aged patients and 15 in patients older than 60 years. In the author's experience, this is the minimal degree of sleep apnea that is associated with daytime complaints. Data in the literature have documented that patients with an apnea index exceeding 20 have a significant increase in subsequent mortality during long-term follow-up (49).

Multiple factors must be analyzed in determining the severity of sleep apnea. Certainly the RDI is of great importance, but apnea duration, degree of oxygen desaturation, and associated cardiac dysrhythmias must be incorporated into the decision-making process. The positional nature needs to be assessed, because many patients have severe apnea when lying supine but with little or no apnea when lying on their side. The exact factors that contribute to long-term morbidity or mortality from sleep apnea have not been identified. Surprisingly, the degree of sleepiness is not closely correlated to the RDI or to degree of oxygen desaturation. Rather, sleepiness is more closely correlated to the degree of sleep fragmentation, as reflected by an increase in awakenings, arousals, and percentage of time in stage 1 sleep with an accompanying decrease in percentages of time in stage 3 and 4 sleep (29,43,89). Table 26.3 provides a guide for characterizing disease severity in apneic patients. The AASM task force published their own categorization for obstructive sleep apnea severity but emphasized that there are currently no adequate prospective studies to validate these criteria (1).

Sleep-Disordered Breathing in Pediatric Patients

In the preceding discussion, the emphasis is obviously on adult patients. The diagnosis and sleep laboratory evaluation of pediatric patients for obstructive sleep apnea is much more problematic. Clinically, the patients usually come to medical attention with witnessed snoring and struggling nocturnal respiration. They are much less likely to be sleepy during the day or to have accompanying obesity. The abnormalities identified on polysomnography in pediatric patients are much less profound, and a greater degree of clinical judgment is necessary for evaluation.

The polysomnographic evaluation of normal children indicates that apneas are much less frequent in children than in adults. In 50 normal children studied by Marcus et al. (69), the mean apneic index was 0.1. The mean number of desaturations greater than 4% per hour of sleep was 0.3. Only nine children (18%) had *any* obstructive apnea identified, and only two children (4%) had apnea lasting 10 seconds. Only one child had more than two episodes of obstructive apnea in a night's sleep. From these data, Marcus et al. recommended a "normal value" of less than one for an apnea index in a child. In addition, the mean minimum SaO_2 was 96%, and in only one child did the oxygen saturation ever fall below 90%. Marcus et al. recommended a value of 92% as the minimum SaO_2 in children. The recommended normal value for the number of desaturations greater than or equal to 4% per hour of sleep was less than 1.4.

In an additional study, Rosen et al. (87) examined polysomnographic data from 20 children who had clinical evidence of upper airway obstruction dur-

TABLE 26.3. *Characteristics of sleep apnea by severity*

Degree of apnea	RDI	Apnea duration (sec)	Oxygen saturation (%)	Electrocardiographic findings
Mild	<20	<20	>85	Mild bradytachyarrhythmia
Moderate	20–40	20–40	75–85	Brief asystole (<3 seconds) or prominent bradytachyarrhythmia
Severe	>40	>40	<75	Asystole (>3 seconds) or ventricular tachycardia

RDI, respiratory disturbance index [(apneas + hypopneas)/hours of sleep].

ing sleep (loud snoring and labored breathing) and who had accompanying oxygen desaturations during sleep. The condition of these children was confidently thought to represent a clinical syndrome of obstructive sleep apnea in children. Remarkably, the mean apnea index was only 2 in this population. This was despite the fact they experienced an average of 175 oxygen desaturations greater than 5% each night and with an average minimum SaO_2 of 66%. Rosen et al. concluded from this study that episodes of complete obstructive apnea are generally rare in children, even in the setting of serious sleep-related upper airway obstruction, and that the adult criteria for obstructive sleep apnea fail to identify apnea in the majority of children with serious upper airway obstruction. Although widely accepted normative data in the pediatric population do not currently exist, it is clear that the mere extrapolation of adult values is inappropriate. The presence of any obstructive apneas lasting 10 seconds in a child should be met with suspicion of indicating significant airway compromise. Similarly, greater attention needs to be paid to episodes of oxygen desaturation.

In view of the lack of overt apneas and the possible lack of sensitivity of O_2 changes, additional markers of sleep-disordered breathing have been sought in pediatric patients. The most useful measure identified to date is the end-tidal CO_2. Several defined guidelines have been provided, but the most useful appears to be defining the persistence of an end-tidal PCO_2 equal to or greater than 50 mm of mercury for more than 8% to 10% of the total sleep time. Investigators believe this value to reliably distinguish snoring from clinically significant obstructive hypoventilation (17).

Movement-Related Variables

Periodic leg movements (PLMs) (also called periodic movements of sleep) are repetitive, stereotyped movements of the lower extremities that occur during sleep (28,68,81). They were previously called nocturnal myoclonus, but the movements are not truly myoclonic, and also there might otherwise be confusion with other true myoclonic events that can occur during sleep. PLMs are characterized by tonic extension of the great toe, with occasional superimposed clonic activity, variably accompanied by ankle dorsiflexion and knee flexion. Lower extremity movements are scored as PLMs when anterior tibialis EMG activity lasts 0.5 to 5 seconds and at least five movements occur in a cluster with an intermovement interval of 5 to 90 seconds. The most common intermovement interval is 20 to 40 sec (see Fig. 26.4). Although many authors also require EMG amplitudes to be at least

50% of those of baseline foot dorsiflexion EMG recordings, movements with much smaller amplitudes are frequently associated with an arousal and are potentially significant. Thus, it seems unwise to apply an absolute amplitude requirement for scoring PLMs.

Movement-associated arousals (also termed PLM-associated arousals) are routinely scored with each PLM if there is no associated respiratory dysrhythmia and if the EEG arousal follows the movement within a few seconds. Oftentimes, EEG arousal varies in its relation to anterior tibialis EMG activity. It may occur just before, synchronously with, or just after EMG activity (65). As a result, some authors score arousals occurring 2 to 4 seconds before or after a PLM as being a PLM-associated arousal. Obviously, care must be taken to ensure that there is no other cause (e.g., recurrent hypopneas) for these recurrent arousals. Although arousals that immediately precede the leg movements may not seem to be movement-associated, Lugaresi et al. (68) postulated an internal "pacemaker" that gives rise to both the arousal and leg movement. As such, the leg movement and EEG arousal occur frequently in a mildly asynchronous manner.

Scored PLMs events are counted and divided by hours of sleep to yield a movement index or a PLM index. The number of movement-associated arousals is also divided by the hours of sleep to yield a movement arousal index (or a PLM arousal index). The movement arousal index is believed to be the most clinically relevant measure for assessing the significance of PLMs (28,88).

The basis for diagnosing periodic limb movement disorder was originally determined to be five movements per hour of sleep (31). However, it soon became apparent that there was a large population of asymptomatic persons who had more than five movements per hour (28). Bixler et al. (10) demonstrated an 11% incidence of PLMs (using a movement index greater than 5) in normal subjects and noted a marked increase in incidence with age. However, none of these subjects had more than five arousals per hour related to these leg movements. Other studies have shown that in patients with hypersomnolence, the degree of sleep disruption is correlated with the severity of EDS (46,98). Therefore, the emphasis in PLMs has subsequent been placed on the movement arousal index as a measure of sleep disruption that more closely correlates with clinical symptoms.

PLMs that are associated with few arousals (movement arousal index < 5) are considered clinically insignificant, and patients are classified as having an asymptomatic parasomnia. Even if a movement arousal index of more than 5 is used, there is a large population of asymptomatic individuals who have "significant" periodic limb movement disorder (28,68). As with the RDI, a cutoff of l5 for the movement arousal index appears reasonable, especially in evaluation of an elderly population. The author emphasizes that PLMs are present in a broad range of sleep disorders, and their pathophysiological processes and exact clinical significance remain poorly understood (30,68).

The ASDA Atlas Task Force published standardized rules for scoring, which have not gained wide application to date, at least partly because of the nonintuitive nature of the scoring system and the difficulty in immediately extracting a value comparable to the currently used movement arousal index. The complex guidelines are not repeated here.

MULTIPLE SLEEP LATENCY TEST (MSLT)

The multiple sleep latency test (MSLT) is a multiple-nap trial designed to quantify the patient's sleepiness and assess the presence of sleep-onset REM (SOREM) periods (3,21). It serves as the gold standard for the assessment of EDS, but it clearly has significant limitations. Other measures of sleepiness (pupillometry [95], the Epworth Sleepiness Scale [24,56]) are either too technically cumbersome or too subjective to warrant widespread clinical use. The MSLT provides an objective quantification of "sleepiness" and is useful in the clinical determination of hypersomnolence. Opportunities to nap are given at 2-hour intervals throughout the day, thereby allowing the investigators to obtain a sampling of the diurnal variation of the patient's sleep tendency.

Multiple Sleep Latency Test Procedure

1. The patient obtains a usual night's rest before the study. Most investigators require that the preceding night's sleep be documented by PSG to ensure adequate sleep and exclude sleep disruption (e.g., sleep apnea, PLMs) as a contributing cause of EDS.

2. The patient arrives at the laboratory in time to allow application of electrodes. At a minimum, electrodes are placed to monitor central and occipital EEG, submental EMG, EOG, and ECG. A sample montage is displayed in Table 26.4. The first nap trial is initiated 1.5 to 3 hours after the patient has awakened from nocturnal sleep. Four or five nap times are scheduled during the day (e.g., 9:30 a.m., 11:30 a.m., 1:30 p.m., 3:30 p.m., and 5:30 p.m.). For each scheduled nap time, the patient lies down in street clothes and assumes a comfortable sleep position. In order to standardize physical activity, a 15-minute quiet period immediately precedes each scheduled nap time. The sleep room should be quiet, dark, and free of environmental noise. As the nap time is about to begin, the technician instructs the patient to "close your eyes and attempt to sleep," turns off the lights, exits the room, and begins recording.

3. The MSLT is routinely scored in 30-second epochs. Sleep onset is usually defined as the first 30-second epoch scored as stage 1 or deeper sleep. However, there is some confusion in the literature and some laboratories use the first of three consecutive epochs scored as sleep to define sleep onset. Sleep offset (awakening) is defined as two consecutive epochs of wakefulness after sleep onset. All scoring is done according to the criteria of Rechtschaffen and Kales (82).

4. Each nap is reviewed for evidence of REM sleep (Fig. 26.16). REM sleep is scored as per Rechtschaffen and Kales' criteria (82) and its onset is determined by the first epoch scored as REM sleep. REM latency (latency to REM onset after sleep onset) is usually determined, but the most important observation is the presence or absence of REM during each nap trial.

5. Each nap is terminated (a) 20 minutes after the nap time started if no sleep has occurred, (b) after 15 minutes of continuous sleep as long as sleep onset criteria are met before the end of 20 minutes, or (c) after 20 minutes if the patient awakens, even if the patients has been asleep less than 15 minutes.

6. The patient is instructed to maintain wakefulness (and is observed if at all possible) between nap periods.

TABLE 26.4. *Montage*

Channel	Sensitivity (μV/mm)	Filters (LFF/HFF) (Hz)
1. C4-A1	7	0.3/70
2. O1-A2	7	0.3/70
3. T3-Cz	7	0.3/70
4. Cz-T4	7	0.3/70
5. Left eye-A1	7	0.3/70
6. Right eye-A2	7	0.3/70
7. Submental electromyogram	2	5/70
8. Electrocardiogram	75	1/15

HFF, high-frequency filter; LFF, low-frequency filter.

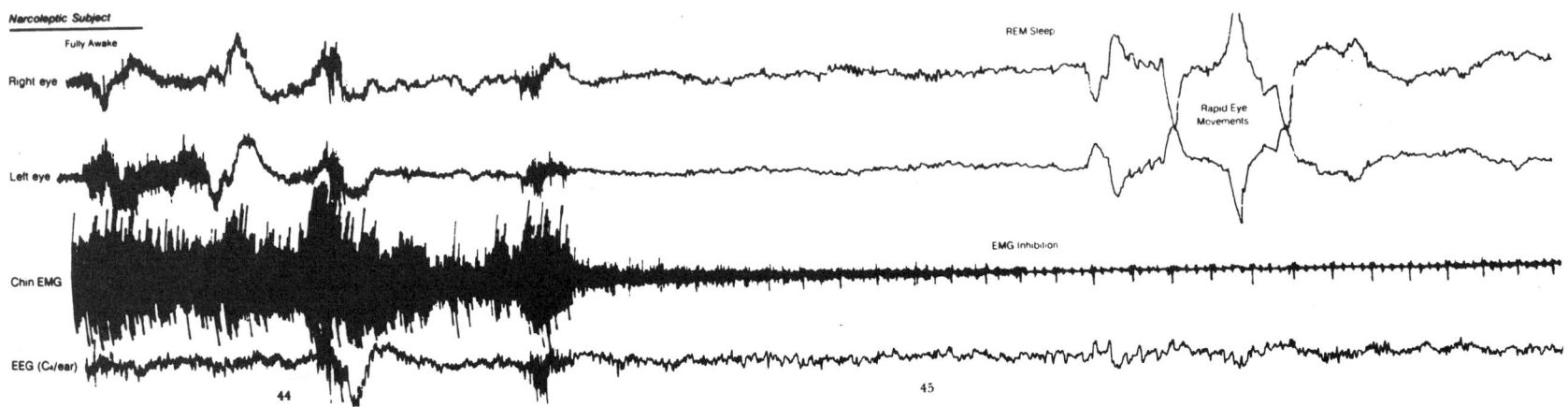

FIG. 26.16. Sleep-onset rapid-eye-movement (REM) period. Polysomnographic record demonstrates the appearance of a low-voltage, mixed-frequency electroencephalogram, accompanied by the abrupt loss of tonic electromyographic activity and the appearance of REM activity. (From Hauri P. *The sleep disorders.* Kalamazoo, MI: Upjohn Co., 1982:5–62.)

Multiple Sleep Latency Test Interpretation

The interpreter determines the latency to sleep onset and the presence or absence of REM sleep for each nap trial. Sleep onset is usually interpreted as the first 30-second epoch of stage 1 sleep or deeper sleep stage. A 30-second epoch is scored as wakefulness if the majority of the 30-second period demonstrates a waking pattern. Stage 1 is determined if the majority of the 30-second epoch is stage 1 sleep. Thus, a brief return of alpha activity for 5 to 10 seconds does not result in an awakening, nor does it necessarily prevent the scoring of an epoch as sleep.

As mentioned previously, there has been some confusion and inconsistencies in the MSLT literature regarding the determination of sleep onset. Richardson et al. (85) used three consecutive epochs scored as stage 1 sleep to determine sleep onset. The most commonly cited "normative data" come from that approach (see Table 26.6). However, starting in 1986 (21) with the publication of the MSLT practice guidelines, many laboratories have begun using the one-epoch criterion, and it is the most widely used definition of sleep onset.

Benbadis et al. (8) examined the various criteria for determining sleep onset and their impact on the MSLT results. Requiring only one epoch of stage 1 sleep resulted in a mean sleep latency of 6.2 minutes, as opposed to 7.5 minutes for the three-epoch criterion. Use of the briefer sleep onset criterion resulted in a change in category (e.g., normal to moderate EDS) in 16 of 100 studies.

Difficulties occasionally occur in determining the exact time of sleep onset or in the interpretation of an ambiguous REM event. Each laboratory needs to develop rules or define approaches to these problems. The most common approach is to require that sleep onset be unambiguous (i.e., cessation of alpha activity and onset of slow eye movements) and not score a decrease in alpha amplitude or frequency as adequate for sleep onset. In the absence of a well-defined posterior alpha rhythm, evidence of increased theta activity (particularly centrally) accompanied by slow eye movements or a vertex wave is usually necessary to score sleep confidently. Similar ambiguities surrounding REM onset sometimes occur. Again, adhering to a strict interpretation for scoring REM sleep is probably the best approach. However, as is evident throughout sleep study interpretation, much has been left to the judgment of the individual polysomnographer.

Individual sleep latencies are then averaged to determine mean sleep latency (MSL). MSLT results from different populations are shown in Table 26.5. A MSL of less than 5 minutes is considered indicative of

TABLE 26.5. *Mean sleep latency test (five nap trials)*

Group	Mean sleep latency (minutes)	Number of REM-sleep episodes (% of group)		
		None	One	Two or more
Narcoleptics (*n* = 49)	2.9 (±2.7)	2	2	96
Nonnarcoleptic, non–sleep apneic EDS (*n* = 63)	8.7 (±4.9)	92	8	0
Controls (*n* = 13)	13.4 (±4.3)	100	0	0

EDS, excessive daytime sleepiness; REM, rapid eye movement.

pathological hypersomnolence. It is a direct indication of the individual's vulnerability to falling asleep in a low-stimulus situation and is associated with performance decrements and unintentional episodes of sleep. A MSL of more than 10 minutes is considered normal and does not reflect significant sleepiness. A MSL between 5 and 10 minutes is the "gray zone" into which some normal persons and some hypersomnolent patients fall. There is no consensus as to the clinical significance that should be applied to results in this range. Labeling a MSL in this range as suggestive but not diagnostic of pathological hypersomnolence is probably the most reasonable approach. Some authors suggest that if a single cut-off value is used, 8 minutes is a rational dividing point between normal (>8 minutes) and abnormal (<8 minutes) (91).

Nonpathological factors affect the MSLT in important ways. MSL is related to the amount of sleep on one or several preceding nights, age, continuity of sleep, time of day, and drug use (18,20,22,33,90). It is therefore necessary to review carefully, preferably with a sleep diary, the patient's sleep pattern over the 7 to 10 days before the study. This need to ensure adequate nocturnal sleep for accurate MSLT results has led most sleep clinicians to require overnight PSG the night before the MSLT. However, sleep deprivation occurring only the night before the study must usually result in less than 4 to 5 hours of total sleep to prominently affect mean sleep latency (18). Drugs also affect sleep latency (sedatives and hypnotics, antihistamines, and stimulants) or REM latency (tricyclic antidepressants, monoamine oxidase inhibitors, and stimulants) (73). Therefore, withdrawal from these medications is necessary before the MSLT is performed. A 2-week period of drug abstinence is empirically required, although there are no good data on the exact time course of medication withdrawal effects. If surreptitious drug use is of concern, a urine drug screen is appropriate on the day of the study.

Somewhat surprisingly, the MSLT has not been an effective measure of treatment response in most patients with narcolepsy. Treated narcoleptic patients do not have a significant change in MSL even though they report improved alertness. Mitler (74) and other researchers (47), in an attempt to be more sensitive to this improvement, devised a "maintenance of wakefulness" test. The main difference from MSLT is that the subjects are instructed to remain awake during each trial. This results in some increased sensitivity to treatment effects, but the test is not widely used clinically.

Premature onset of REM sleep in narcoleptic patients was first noted by Vogel (105) and linked to narcolepsy by Rechtschaffen et al. (83). A single daytime nap to detect early-onset REM was used initially, but it proved to be less than ideal because of its insensitivity in identifying REM sleep pathological processes. The MSLT was developed to allow repeated sampling of sleep and to increase the sensitivity to SOREM periods. When first described by the Stanford University sleep group, each nap allowed a 10-minute period of sustained sleep, and two of five naps had to demonstrate REM sleep onset in order to be diagnostic of narcolepsy. More recently, the recommended protocol for the MSLT was changed to allow the patient a 15-minute period of sustained sleep (21). Because SOREM periods are extremely rare in normal rested persons, some clinicians interpret a single REM-onset nap as adequate for the diagnosis of narcolepsy. However, just as there are many factors that affect MSL, there are circumstances other than narcolepsy that may result in SOREM periods (15,89). Medications, sleep deprivation, time of day, and even subject position have all been described to affect the incidence of SOREMs (73). Nonetheless, a single SOREM period, with documentation of adequate and uninterrupted sleep the night before the study, is certainly abnormal but must be assessed in view of the clinical history or other diagnostic studies. Two REM-onset naps are clearly abnormal and consistent with abnormal REM pressure. Most commonly, this is caused by narcolepsy but also has been described in sleep apnea, drug withdrawal, severe depression, and myotonic dystrophy (27,73,79).

CLINICAL EVALUATION OF SLEEP DISORDERS

The most common sleep-related complaints seen in a sleep center are EDS, disturbed nocturnal breathing, unusual nocturnal behavior (parasomnia), and difficulty with initiating or sustaining sleep (insomnia) (71). The clinical approach to evaluating patients presenting with these common complaints is briefly described in this section. Comprehensive reviews that include discussion of pathophysiological processes and treatment of these disorders are available elsewhere (26,37,67).

Evaluation of Excessive Daytime Sleepiness

A wide range of diagnoses must be entertained in the evaluation of EDS. Table 26.6 lists the final diagnoses in a multicenter report on patients with the complaint of EDS (32). As in nearly every series, sleep apnea, narcolepsy, and idiopathic hypersomnia were the most frequent diagnoses. Figure 26.17 presents a diagnostic algorithm, as proposed by an ASDA task force, that can be applied to the clinical assessment of the "sleepy" patient (4).

The initial evaluation of a hypersomnolent patient focuses on the patient's history. The patient's complaint of EDS must be judged as inappropriate and undesired sleep, as opposed to lethargy, fatigue, or tiredness, which can be reported in a large number of psychiatric and medical conditions. In patients with moderate to severe sleepiness, the history should include episodes of actual inappropriate sleep (e.g., falling asleep at a stoplight). Although the

TABLE 26.6. *Disorders of excessive somnolence (N = 1983)*

Diagnostic category	Total %	Range/center (%)
Sleep apnea	43.2	23.9–81.2
Narcolepsy	25.0	7.7–32.2
Idiopathic hypersomnia	8.8	0.0–26.9
No hypersomnolence disorder	5.4	0.0–16.4
Other hypersomnias	6.1	1.9–7.9
Psychiatric disorders	3.7	0.0–25.3
PLM/RLS	3.5	0.0–13.7
Medical, toxic, environmental	2.7	0.0–5.1
Drug/alcohol dependency	1.5	0.0–4.4

PLM, periodic leg movement; RLS, restless legs syndrome.
Adapted from Coleman RM, Pollak C, Weitzman ED. Periodic movements in sleep (nocturnal myoclonus): relation to sleep-wake disorders. *Ann Neurol* 1980;8:416–421.

character of the patient's sleepiness often varies among these disorders, there is significant overlap that prevents a confident diagnosis based on the character of the patient's sleepiness alone. An observer history is required to corroborate the reports of sleepiness and also to report on the possible presence of loud snoring, witnessed apneic episodes, or excessive motor activity in sleep. Patients frequently deny or underestimate the degree of sleepiness present and are usually unaware of any snoring or nocturnal apneas.

The presence of cataplexy is essentially a pathognomonic feature of narcolepsy. Cataplexy is the sudden development of muscle weakness affecting the head, neck, or entire body. It is usually precipitated by strong emotion (e.g., laughter, anger) and is not associated with impairment of consciousness. The muscular weakness lasts from seconds to minutes and then resolves. A history of unambiguous cataplexy in combination with EDS is sufficient for diagnosing narcolepsy, and further sleep study evaluation is not necessarily indicated. However, the possible coexistence of other sleep disorders (sleep apnea, periodic movements) that may also be clinically significant must not be overlooked. Sleep paralysis and hypnagogic hallucinations are the other auxiliary symptoms of narcolepsy, but they are less specific to narcolepsy and do not serve as pathognomonic markers of the disease.

The initial assessment of a patient's sleep-wake complaint is usually aided by the completion of sleep diaries for 1 to 2 weeks before the appointment. These are particularly helpful in identifying sleep restriction or sleep cycle abnormalities that may be contributing to the patient's complaints.

Routine medical evaluation is appropriate for all patients with EDS. Screening for general medical concerns (e.g., hypothyroidism) is appropriate before sleep center evaluation. Attention to possible psychiatric symptoms is also appropriate. Many patients with EDS present with a picture that resembles depression, and therefore the differentiation is sometimes quite difficult. However, if no overt medical problem is identified and the patient has a history clearly suggestive of pathological sleepiness, sleep laboratory evaluation is appropriate.

The usual recommendation is for overnight PSG and possibly MSLT. If there is a strong clinical suspicion of obstructive sleep apnea, PSG alone is usually adequate. If on the overnight PSG an adequate explanation for the patient's EDS is documented, MSLT is not usually performed. Some sleep laboratories perform the MSLT in all patients in order to quantify sleepiness, which may subsequently influence treatment decisions. However, the associated expense and effort seem unnecessary for patients in whom severe obstructive sleep apnea is demonstrated, in that treatment is

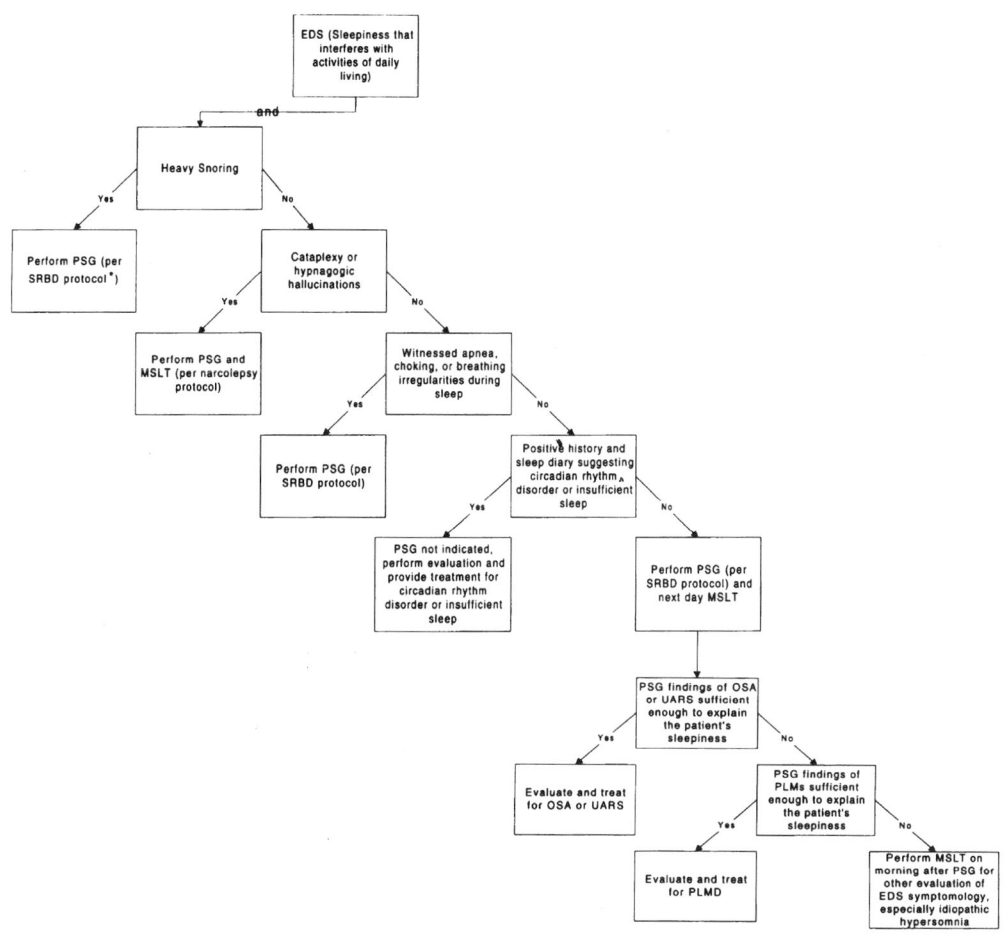

FIG. 26.17. Algorithm for evaluation of patient with a chief complaint of excessive daytime sleepiness. EDS, excessive daytime sleepiness; MSLT, multiple sleep latency test; PLMD, periodic limb movement disorder; PLMs, periodic limb movements; PSG, polysomnography; SRBD, sleep-related breathing disorder; UARS, upper-airway resistance syndrome. (From American Sleep Disorders Association Polysomnography Task Force. Practice parameters for the indications for polysomnography and related procedures. *Sleep* 1997;20:406–422.)

focused on the severity of the PSG abnormality in combination with the patient's subjective complaints.

If the PSG does not demonstrate an obvious cause of EDS, then MSLT is performed the following day to quantify the degree of sleepiness. An overnight PSG before the MSLT is usually required for adequate interpretation of the MSLT to ensure that sleep deprivation or sleep disruption has not artifactually contributed to an abnormal MSLT result. If MSLT is performed without proceeding to PSG, careful historical assessment (e.g., with a sleep diary) of the preceding night's sleep is required at the time of testing.

MSLT results can be used to confirm the diagnosis of narcolepsy and idiopathic hypersomnolence or to refute the complaint of hypersomnolence (21). If the patient has a MSL of less than 5 minutes and at least two REM-onset nap periods, a diagnosis of narcolepsy can be made. It is important to emphasize that the diagnosis of narcolepsy requires both EDS and documentation of REM abnormality. The REM disorder can be represented by cataplexy or by SOREM periods on the MSLT. If a single SOREM period is documented, a diagnosis of possible narcolepsy can be made, and consideration can be given to repeating the MSLT in an attempt to find additional confirmatory evidence of REM pathology. If the MSLT documents hypersomnolence but no REM abnormality, the diagnosis is idiopathic hypersomnia (previously called idiopathic central nervous system hypersomnolence). This is an unfortunate but necessary "wastebasket" category at present. Some of these patients have narcolepsy, but the REM fragmentation has not yet become clinically evident. Other patients appear to have a syndrome characterized by EDS that can be resisted more successfully, resulting in fewer episodes of daytime sleep (42). These patients are not refreshed by daytime naps and respond poorly to stimulant medications. Many also have headaches, syncope, and peripheral vascular complaints, which raises the possibility of accompanying autonomic nervous system dysfunction.

More problematic is what to do for the patient in the "gray zone" with a mean sleep latency of between 5 and 10 minutes. Clinical judgment is needed to assess the appropriateness of stimulant drugs in this setting. Repeating the MSLT may yield more definitive information. A MSL of more than 10 minutes does not support the diagnosis of EDS, and treatment is not generally warranted. In the patient with a convincing clinical complaint of EDS but in whom hypersomnolence is not documented, the clinician must consider syndromes producing episodic hypersomnolence and the possible need to repeat the MSLT.

Approach to Nocturnal Behavioral Events (Parasomnias)

By virtue of their intermittent nature, the parasomnias are less easily investigated with PSG studies. Historical information therefore assumes greater importance. The differential diagnosis in a patient suffering from unusual nocturnal behaviors includes somnambulism, night terrors, confusional arousals, seizures, REM behavior disorder, and nightmares. Table 26.7 lists characteristics that can be useful in differentiating these nocturnal events. If the nocturnal events are ambiguous or occur with predictable frequency, PSG with closed-circuit television recording usually enables diagnosis.

Somnambulism and night terrors are disorders of arousal and classically occur during the first part of the night; the EEG demonstrates a normal awake or paroxysmal slow-wave pattern during the event (54,60,62,103). Night ter-

TABLE 26.7. *Differential diagnosis of common parasomnias*

Type of parasomnia	Usual age at onset	Time of night	Sleep stage	Type of behavior	Postictal confusion	Effect of stimulation	Recall of event	Duration
Somnambulism	Childhood	First half	NREM	Clumsy, trance-like	Absent	Stops episode	Minimal	Seconds to minutes
Night terrors	Childhood	First third	NREM	Intense terror, vocalization autonomic changes	Absent	Variable	Minimal	Seconds to minutes
Nightmares	Variable	Variable	REM	Terror in response to dream content, limited autonomic changes	Absent	Stops episode	Dream content	Seconds to minutes
REM behavior disorder	Elderly	Last third (most common)	REM	Acting out of dream content, frequently aggressive	Absent	Stops episode	Dream content	Seconds to minutes
Confusional arousal	Variable (usually childhood)	First third	NREM	Confusion, incomplete responsiveness, automatic behavior, rarely aggressive	Present	Variable	Minimal	Seconds to minutes
Epileptic seizure	Variable	Variable	Variable	Stereotyped, variable complexity	Present (often agitation)	No effect	Minimal	Seconds to minutes

NREM, non–rapid eye movement; REM, rapid eye movement.

rors resemble nightmares, but the child has intense autonomic arousal, is subsequently amnestic for the event, and cannot recall any precipitating dream content. Nightmares are seen in patients of all ages and are manifested by emotional upset from disturbing dream content with only limited autonomic arousal. Confusional arousals (also called nocturnal sleep drunkenness) arise in patients of all ages who are frequently considered "deep sleepers"; these occurrences are thought to be caused by an inability to rouse from non-REM sleep. During these events, the patient may manifest several minutes of bizarre confused behavior, for which he or she is subsequently amnestic (14). Violent or aggressive behavior is much less common with confusional arousals than that seen with the REM behavior disorder.

REM behavior disorder is believed to arise from the loss of the usual muscle atonia of REM sleep, which results in the acting out of dream content (93,94). This disorder may be a human analogue (50) of an animal model described by Jouvet and Delorme in 1965 (57). These authors observed complex motor activity in cats during REM sleep after they received pontine tegmental lesions. However, only a few humans have had identifiable brainstem disease. Patients with this disorder are most commonly men older than 60 years with no other underlying neurological or psychiatric illness. These patients present with wild dream enactment behaviors that are frequently violent and result in injury to themselves or their bed partners. PSG with video analysis demonstrates that the motor activity is restricted to REM sleep and may allow confirmation of the diagnosis.

Epileptic seizures are almost always accompanied by an ictal discharge on scalp EEG, followed by postictal slowing. However, the limited EEG montage and slow paper speed used in PSG impairs identification of ictal and interictal epileptic activity. Use of expanded EEG montages and a paper speed of 30 mm per second are necessary in order to evaluate possible epileptic events properly (Fig. 26.18). Even with these adjustments, however, some epileptic events have ambiguous scalp correlates or have no scalp correlates whatsoever (14,38,106,107,110). Absence of an EEG correlate during behavioral events has led to symptomatic description of patients in whom the pathophysiological basis of their nocturnal attacks is uncertain. However, most authors believe that syndromes such as hypnagogic paroxysmal dystonia are caused by frontal lobe epilepsy, despite the lack of a consistent electrographic seizure correlate. If nocturnal seizures are likely to occur, evaluation is better carried out in an epilepsy monitoring unit more suited to extended EEG and video analysis.

Hysterical dissociative reactions, including fugue states, are demonstrated by an alert patient (with normal waking EEG) who manifests complex pur-

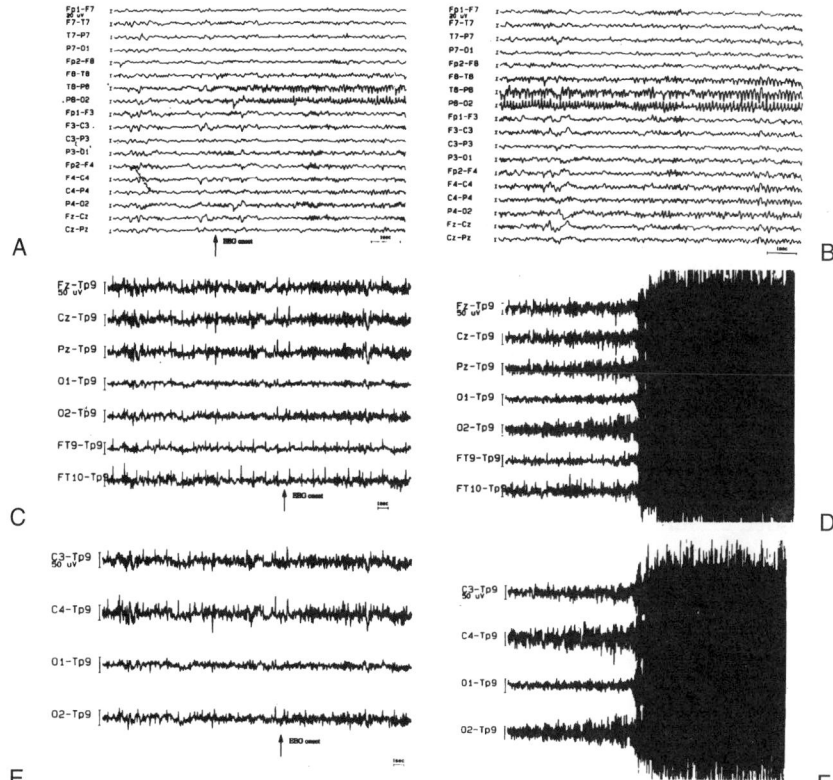

FIG. 26.18. Right temporal lobe seizure in a patient with epilepsy. The electroencephalographic onset (*arrow*) consisted of rhythmic alpha activity in the right temporal region that preceded the clinical onset by 26 seconds, as shown in consecutive 10-second epochs on the 18-channel anteroposterior bipolar montage (**A** and **B**). The evolution of rhythmic activity in the right temporal region (FT10) can be appreciated with difficulty on the seven-channel montage at a paper speed of 10 mm per second but would be extremely difficult to interpret in isolation (**C** and **D**). The pattern is not clearly evident on the four-channel montage (**E** and **F**). (From Foldvary N, Caruso AC, Maschaa E, et al. Identifying montages that best detect EEG seizure activity during polysomnography. *Sleep* 2000;23:221–229.)

poseful behaviors during apparent "sleep" that can last for hours or even days (62). Activity resembling sleepwalking or night terrors in an elderly patient is frequently associated with underlying organic intellectual impairment and is simply an episode of confusion resulting in nocturnal wandering (36).

Approach to the Patient with Insomnia

PSG plays a more limited role in the clinical evaluation of patients complaining of difficulties in initiating or maintaining sleep. The differential diagnosis, as outlined in Table 26.8, includes a wide range of psychiatric and psychological problems that do not routinely necessitate PSG evaluation. However, sleep apnea and periodic movements of sleep (with or without restless leg syndrome) has been identified in 5% to 29% of patients with insomnia (32,59,113).

The author's experience with 100 consecutive chronic insomniac patients evaluated with ambulatory cassette PSG revealed that 34% of the studies provided useful information that was not otherwise available and that sometimes contradicted historical evidence (35). Twenty-five patients had PLMs (mean movement index, 48; mean movement arousal index, 23). Three patients had significant obstructive sleep apnea (mean RDI = 22), subsequently confirmed with laboratory PSG. Six patients had only subjective insomnia because PSG sleep time was five times greater than the amount they had self-reported; four of these patients reported no sleep during the study night even though their total sleep time ranged from 190 to 401 minutes! Age was an important factor in identifying a population more likely to

benefit from PSG. Forty-five percent of patients older than 40 years had sleep apnea, PLM, or subjective insomnia identified on PSG, in contrast to 15% of patients younger than 40.

Although there is disagreement among sleep specialists regarding the necessity of PSG evaluations in patients with insomnia, the author's data argue for at least selective use of PSG. Certainly, patients with difficulties in initiating and maintaining sleep who have clinical evidence of possible sleep apnea or PLM should be evaluated by a PSG. In other such patients, the decision to conduct PSG should be individualized, depending on the chronicity and severity of the sleep problem as well as the age of the patient. In most patients with insomnia, it is reasonable for the sleep clinician to formulate a diagnosis on the basis of clinical judgment and to proceed with initial treatment. For patients failing to respond to treatment efforts, PSG could then be offered in order to provide a more comprehensive diagnostic picture (2,84).

TABLE 26.8. *Disorders of initiating and maintaining sleep*

Diagnostic category	% (N = 1,214)	Range/center %
Psychiatric disorder	34.9	3.9–66.8
Psychophysiological	15.3	1.0–32.9
Drug/alcohol dependency	12.4	2.9–25.2
PLM/RLS	12.2	2.8–26.3
No insomnia abnormality	9.2	0.0–28.7
Sleep apnea	6.2	0.0–18.4
Medical/toxic	3.8	0.0–12.6
Other	5.9	0.0–12.6

PLM, periodic leg movement; RLS, restless legs syndrome.
Adapted from Coleman RM, Pollak C, Weitzman ED. Periodic movements in sleep (nocturnal myoclonus): relation to sleep-wake disorders. *Ann Neurol* 1980;8:416–421.

REFERENCES

1. American Academy of Sleep Medicine Task Force. Sleep-related breathing disorder in adults. *Sleep* 1999;22:667–689.
2. American Sleep Apnea Association Standards of Practice Committee. Practice parameters for the use of polysomnography in the evaluation of insomnia. *Sleep* 1995;18:55–77.
3. American Sleep Disorders Association. The clinical use of the Multiple Sleep Latency Test. *Sleep* 1992;15:268–276.
4. American Sleep Disorders Association Polysomnography Task Force. Practice parameters for the indications for polysomnography and related procedures. *Sleep* 1997;20:406–422.
5. American Thoracic Society. Indications and standards for cardiopulmonary sleep studies. *Am Rev Respir Dis* 1989;139:559–568.
6. Aserinsky E, Kleitman N. Regularly occurring periods of eye motility, and concomitant phenomena, during sleep. *Science* 1953;118:273–274.
7. Association of Sleep Disorders Centers. Diagnostic classification of sleep and arousal disorders, 1st ed. Prepared by the Sleep Disorders Classification Committee, H.P. Roffwarg, chairman. *Sleep* 1979;2:1–137.
8. Benbadis SR, Perry MC, Walgamuth BR, et al. The MSLT: comparison of sleep onset criteria. *Sleep* 1996;19:632–636.
9. Berry DT, Webb WB, Block AJ. Sleep apnea syndrome: a critical review of the apnea index as a diagnostic criterion. *Chest* 1984;86:529–531.
10. Bixler EO, Kales A, Vela-Bueno A, et al. Nocturnal myoclonus and nocturnal myoclonic activity in a normal population. *Res Commun Chem Pathol Pharmacol* 1982;36:129–140.
11. Bonnet M, Carley D, Carskadon M, et al. EEG arousals: scoring rules and examples. *Sleep* 1992;15:173–184.
12. Bornstein SK. Respiratory monitoring during sleep: polysomnography. In: Guilleminault C, ed. *Sleeping and waking disorders: indications and techniques*. Menlo Park, CA: Addison-Wesley, 1982:183–212.
13. Broughton R. Polysomnography: principles and applications in sleep and arousal disorders. In: Niedemeyer E, Lopes da Silva F, eds. *Electroencephalography*. Baltimore: Urban & Schwarzenberg, 1993:765–802.
14. Broughton RJ. NREM arousal parasomnias. In: Kryger MH, Roth T, Dement WC, eds. *Principles and practice of sleep medicine*. Philadelphia: WB Saunders, 2000:693–706.

15. Browman CP, Gujavarty KS, Sampson MG, et al. REM sleep episodes during the maintenance of wakefulness test in patients with sleep apnea syndrome and patients with narcolepsy. *Sleep* 1983;6:23–28.

16. Cantineau JD, Escourrou P, Sartene R, et al. Accuracy of respiratory inductive plethysmography during wakefulness and sleep in patients with obstructive sleep apnea. *Chest* 1991;102:1145–1151.

17. Carroll JL, Loughlan JM. Obstructive sleep apnea syndrome in infants and children: diagnosis and management. In: Ferber R, Kryger MH, eds. *Principles and practices of sleep medicine in the child.* Philadelphia: WB Saunders, 1995:193–216.

18. Carskadon MA, Dement WC. Cumulative effects of sleep restriction on daytime sleepiness. *Psychophysiology* 1981;18:107–113.

19. Carskadon MA, Dement WC. Respiration during sleep in the aged human. *J Gerontol* 1981;36:420–423.

20. Carskadon MA, Dement WC. Sleep loss in elderly volunteers. *Sleep* 1985;8:207–221.

21. Carskadon MA, Dement WC, Milter MM, et al. Guidelines for the MSLT: a standard measure of sleepiness. *Sleep* 1986;9:519–524.

22. Carskadon MA, vander Hoed J, Dement WC. Sleep and daytime sleepiness in the elderly. *J Geriatr Psychiat* 1980;13:135–151.

23. Chaudhary BA, Burki NK. Ear oximetry in clinical practice. *Am Rev Respir Dis* 1978;117:173–175.

24. Chervin R, Aldrich MS. ESS may not reflect objective measures of sleepiness or sleep apnea. *Neurology* 1999;52(1):125–131.

25. Chervin RD, Aldrich MS. Sleep onset REM periods during MSLT in patients evaluated for sleep apnea. *Am J Respir Care Med* 2000;161:426–431.

26. Chokroverty S, ed. *Sleep disorders medicine,* 2nd ed. Boston: Butterworth-Heinemann, 1999.

27. Cohn M. Respiratory monitoring during sleep: respiratory inductive plethysmography. In: Guilleminault C, ed. *Sleeping and waking disorders: indications and techniques.* Menlo Park, CA: Addison-Wesley, 1982:213–223.

28. Coleman RM. Periodic movements in sleep (nocturnal myoclonus) and the restless legs syndrome. In: Guilleminault C, ed. *Sleeping and waking disorders: indications and techniques.* Menlo Park, CA: Addison-Wesley, 1982:265–295.

29. Coleman RM, Bliwise DL, Sajben N, et al. Daytime sleepiness in patients with periodic movements of sleep. *Sleep* 1982;5:S191–S202.

30. Coleman RM, Bliwise DL, Sajben N, et al. Epidemiology of periodic movements during sleep. In: Guilleminault C, Lugares E, eds. *Sleepwake disorders.* New York: Raven Press, 1983:217–229.

31. Coleman RM, Pollak C, Weitzman ED. Periodic movements in sleep (nocturnal myoclonus): relation to sleep-wake disorders. *Ann Neurol* 1980;8:416–421.

32. Coleman RM, Roffwarg HP, Kennedy SJ, et al. Sleep-wake disorders based on a polysomnographic diagnosis: a national cooperative study. *JAMA* 1982;247:997–1003.

33. Dement WC, Seidel W, Carskadon M. Daytime alertness and benzodiazepines. *Sleep* 1982;5:528–545.

34. Douglas NJ, Brash HM, Wraith PK, et al. Accuracy, sensitivity to carboxyhemoglobin, and speed of response of the Hewlett-Packard 47201A ear oximeter. *Am Rev Respir Dis* 1979;119:311–313.

35. Edinger J, Hoelscher TJ, Webb MD, et al. Polysomnographic assessment of DIMS: empirical evaluation of its diagnostic value. *Sleep* 1989;12:315–322.

36. Feinberg I. Sleep in organic brain conditions. In Kales A, ed. *Sleep: physiology and pathology.* Philadelphia: JB Lippincott, 1969:131–147.

37. Ferber R, Kryger MH, eds. *Principles and practice of sleep medicine in the child.* Philadelphia: WB Saunders, 1995.

38. Foldvary N, Caruso AC, Maschaa E, et al. Identifying montages that best detect EEG seizure activity during polysomnography. *Sleep* 2000;23:221–229.

39. Gastaut H, Tassinari C, Duron B. Etude polygraphique des manifestations épisodiques (hypniques et respiratoires) du syndrome de Pickwick. *Rev Neurol* 1965;112:568–579.

40. Goode GB, Slyter HM. Daytime PSG diagnosis of sleep disorders. *J Neurol Neurosurg Psychiat* 1983;46:159–161.

41. Gould GA, Whyte KF, Rhind GB, et al. The sleep hypopnea syndrome. *Am Rev Respir Dis* 1988;137:895–898.

42. Guilleminault C, Faull KF. Sleepiness in non-narcoleptic, non-sleep apneic EDS patients: the idiopathic CNS hypersomnolence. *Sleep* 1982;5:S175–S181.

43. Guilleminault C, Partinen M, Quera-Salva MA, et al. Determinants of daytime sleepiness in obstructive sleep apnea. *Chest* 1988;94:32–37.

44. Guilleminault C, Stoohs R, Clerk A, et al. From obstructive sleep apnea syndrome to upper airway resistance syndrome: consistency of daytime sleepiness. *Sleep* 1992;15:S13–S16.

45. Guilleminault C, Stoohs R, Clerk A, et al. A cause of excessive daytime sleepiness: the upper airway resistance syndrome. *Chest* 1993;104:781–787.

46. Guilleminault C, van den Hoed J, Milter M. Clinical overview of the sleep apnea syndromes. In: Guilleminault C, Dement W, eds. *Sleep apnea syndromes.* New York: Alan R. Liss, 1978:1–12.

47. Hartse KM, Roth T, Zorick FJ. Daytime sleepiness and daytime wakefulness: the effect of instruction. *Sleep* 1982;5(Suppl 2):107–118.

48. Hauri P. *The sleep disorders.* Kalamazoo, MI: Upjohn Co., 1982:5–62.

49. He J, Dryger MH, Zorick FJ, et al. Mortality and apnea index in obstructive sleep apnea. *Chest* 1988;94:9–14.

50. Henley K, Morrison AR. A re-evaluation of the effects of lesions of the pontine tegmentum and locus coeruleus on phenomena of paradoxical sleep in the cat. *Acta Neurobiol Exp* 1974;34:215–232.

51. Hirshkowitz M, Moore CA. Issues in computerized polysomnography. *Sleep* 1994;17(2):105–112.

52. Hosselet JJ, Norman RG, Ayappa T, et al. Detection of flow limitations with a nasal cannula/pressure transducer system. *Am J Respir Crit Care Med* 1998;157:1461–1467.

53. *International classification of sleep disorders: diagnostic and coding manual.* [Diagnostic Classification Steering Committee, Thorpy MJ, Chairman]. Rochester, MN: American Sleep Disorders Association, 1990.

54. Jacobson A, Kales A, Lehmann D, et al. Somnambulism: all night electroencephalographic studies. *Science* 1965;148:975–977.

55. Jasper HH. Ten-Twenty Electrode System of the International Federation. *Electroencephalogr Clin Neurophysiol* 1958;10:371–375.

56. Johns MV. A new method of measuring daytime sleepiness: The Epworth Sleepiness Scale. *Sleep* 1991;14:540–547.

57. Jouyet M, Delorme F. Locus coeruleus et sommeil paradoxal. *C R Soc Biol (Paris)* 1965;159:895–899.

58. Jung R, Kuhlo W. Neurophysiological studies of abnormal night sleep and the pickwickian syndrome. *Prog Brain Res* 1965;18:140–159.

59. Kales A, Bixler EO, Soldatos CR, et al. Biopsychobehavioral correlates in insomnia, part 1: role of sleep apnea and nocturnal myoclonus. *Psychosomatics* 1982;23:589–600.

60. Kales A, Jacobson A, Paulson MJ, et al. Somnambulism: psychophysiological correlates. *Arch Gen Psychiat* 1966;14:586–594.

61. Kales A, Kales J. Recent findings in the diagnosis and treatment of disturbed sleep. *N Engl J Med* 1974;209:487–499.

62. Kales A, Soldatos CR, Kales JD. Sleep disorders: insomnia, sleep-walking, night terrors, nightmares, and enuresis. *Ann Intern Med* 1987;106:582–592.

63. Karacan I. Evaluation of nocturnal penile tumescence and impotence. In: Guilleminault C, ed. *Sleep and waking disorders: indications and techniques.* Menlo Park, CA: Addison-Wesley, 1982:343–372.

64. Knight H, Millman RP, Gur RC, et al. Clinical significance of sleep apnea in the elderly. *Am Rev Respir Dis* 1987;136:845–850.

65. Kotagal P, Ferber RA, Mograss M. Relationship of EEG changes to periodic leg movements. *Sleep Res* 1990;19:224.

66. Krieger J, Turlot J, Mangen P, et al. Breathing during sleep in normal young and elderly subjects: hypopneas, apneas and correlated factors. *Sleep* 1983;6:108–120.

67. Kryger MH, Roth T, Dement WC. *Principles and practice of sleep medicine,* 3rd ed. Philadelphia: WB Saunders, 2000.

68. Lugaresi E, Cirginotta F, Coccagna G, et al. Nocturnal myoclonus and restless legs syndrome. In: Fahn S, Marsden CD, Van Woert M, eds. *Advances in neurology, vol. 43: Myoclonus.* New York: Raven Press, 1986:295–307.

69. Marcus CL, Omlin KJ, Basinki DJ, et al. Normal polysomnographic values for children and adolescents. *Am Rev Respir Dis* 1992;146:1235–1239.

70. Mendelson WB. *Human sleep.* New York: Plenum Press, 1987:159.

71. Mendelson WB. The experience of a sleep disorder center. *Ann Clin Psychiat* 1990;2:277–283.

72. Milic-Emili J, Mead J, Turner JM, et al. Improved technique for estimating pleural pressure from esophageal balloons. *J Appl Physiol* 1984;19:207–211.

73. Mitler MM. The Multiple Sleep Latency Test as an evaluation for excessive somnolence. In: Guilleminault C, ed. *Sleeping and waking disorders: indications and techniques.* Menlo Park, CA: Addison-Wesley, 1982:145–155.

74. Mitler MM, Gujavarty S, Browman CP. Maintenance of wakefulness test: a polysomnographic technique for evaluating treatment efficacy in patients with excessive somnolence. *EEG Clin Neurophys* 1982;53:658–661.

75. Montserrat JM, Farre R, Ballester E, et al. Evaluation of nasal prongs for estimating nasal flow. *Am J Respir Crit Care Med* 1997;155:211–215.

76. Morielli A, Desjardins D, Brouillette RT. To assess hypoventilation during pediatric polysomnography, both transcutaneous and end-tidal CO_2 should be measured. *Am Rev Respir Dis* 1993;148:1599–1604.

77. Norman R, Muhammed A, Walsleben J, et al. Detection of respiratory events during NPSG: nasal cannula/pressure sensor versus thermistor. *Sleep* 1997;20(12):1175–1184.

78. Pacela A. Impedance pneumography—a survey of instrumentation techniques. *Med Biol Eng* 1981;4:1–15.

79. Park YD, Radtke RA. Hypersomnolence in myotonic dystrophy. *J Neurol Neurosurg Psychiat* 1995;58:512–513.

80. Phillips BA, Anstead MI, Gottlieb DJ. Monitoring sleep and breathing: methodology. Part I: monitoring breathing. *Clin Chest Med* 1998;19:203–212.

81. Radtke RA, Hoelscher TJ, Bragdon AC. Ambulatory evaluation of periodic movements of sleep. In: Ebersole J, ed. *Ambulatory EEG.* New York: Raven Press, 1989:317–330.

82. Rechtschaffen A, Kales A, eds. *A manual of standardized terminology, techniques and scoring system for sleep stages of human subjects.* Los Angeles: UCLA Brain Information Service/Brain Research Institute,1968.

83. Rechtschaffen A, Wolpert EA, Dement WC, et al. Nocturnal sleep of narcoleptics. *Electroencephalogr Clin Neurophysiol* 1963;15:599–609.

84. Reite N, Buysse D, Reynolds C, et al. Use of PSG in the evaluation of insomnia. *Sleep* 1995;18(1):58–70.

85. Richardson G, Carskadon MA, Flagg W, et al. Excessive daytime sleepiness in man: multiple sleep latency measurement in narcoleptic and control subjects. *Electroencephalogr Clin Neurophysiol* 1978;45:621–627.

86. Roffwarg HP, Muzio JN, Dement WC. Ontogenetic development of the human sleep-dream cycle. *Science* 1966;152:604–619.

87. Rosen CL, D'Andrea L, Haddad GG. Adult criteria for obstructive sleep apnea do not identify children with serious obstruction. *Am Rev Respir Dis* 1992;146:1231–1234.

88. Rosenthal L, Roehrs T, Sicklesteel J, et al. Periodic movements during sleep, sleep fragmentation, and sleep-wake complaints. *Sleep* 1984;7:326–330.

89. Roth T, Harstse KM, Zorick F, et al. Multiple naps and the evaluation of daytime sleepiness in patients with upper airway sleep apnea. *Sleep* 1980;3:425–439.

90. Roth T, Roehrs T, Koshhorek G, et al. Central effects of antihistamines *Sleep Res* 1986;15:43.

91. Roth T, Roehrs TA, Rosenthal IL. Measurement of sleepiness and alertness: MSLT. In: Chokroverty S, ed. *Sleep disorders medicine,* 2nd ed. Boston: Butterworth-Heinemann, 1999: 133–139.

92. Santamaria J, Chiappa KH. *The EEG of drowsiness.* New York: Demos Publishing, 1987:16–20.

93. Schenck CH, Bundlie SR, Ettinger MG, et al. Chronic behavioral disorders of human REM sleep. A new category of parasomnia. *Sleep* 1986;9:293–308.

94. Schenck CH, Bundlie SR, Patterson AL, et al. REM sleep behavior disorder. *JAMA* 1985;257:1786–1789.

95. Schmidt HA. Pupillometric assessment of disorders of arousal. *Sleep* 1982;5(Suppl 2):157–164.

96. Staats BA, Bonekat HW, Harris CD, et al. Chest wall motion in sleep apnea. *Am Rev Respir Dis* 1984;130:59–63.

97. Standards of Practice Committee of the American Sleep Disorders Association. Practice parameters for the use of portable recording in the assessment of obstructive sleep apnea. *Sleep* 1994;17(4):372–377.

98. Stepanski E, Lamphere J, Badia P, et al. Sleep fragmentation and daytime sleepiness. *Sleep* 1984;7:18–26.

99. Stepanski E, Lamphere J, Roehrs T, et al. Experimental sleep fragmentation in normal subjects. *Int J Neurosci* 1987;33:207–214.

100. Stradling JR, Davies RJ, Atson DJ. New approaches to monitoring sleep-related breathing disorders. *Sleep* 1996;19(Suppl):77–84.

101. Sullivan WJ, Petters GM, Enright PL. Pneumotachographs: theory and clinical applications. *Respir Care* 1984;29:736–749.

102. Takahashi Y, Jimbo M. Polygraphic study of narcoleptic syndrome with special reference to hypnagogic hallucinations and cataplexy. *Folia Psychiat Neurol Jpn [Suppl]* 1963;7:343.

103. Tassinari CA, Mancia D, Bernardina BD, et al. Pavor nocturnus of non-epileptic nature in epileptic children. *Electroencephalogr Clin Neurophysiol* 1972;33:603–607.

104. The Atlas Task Force. Recording and scoring leg movements. *Sleep* 1993;16(8):749–759.

105. Vogel G. Studies in the psychophysiology of dreams. III. The dreams of narcolepsy. *Arch Gen Psychiat* 1960;8:421–428.

106. Walczak TS, Radtke RA, Lewis DV. Accuracy and interobserver reliability of scalp ictal EEG. *Neurology* 1992;42:2279–2285.

107. Waterman K, Purves SJ, Kosaka B, et al. An epileptic syndrome caused by mesial frontal lobe seizure foci. *Neurology* 1987;27:577–582.

108. Whyte KF, Allen MB, Fitzpatrick MF, et al. Accuracy and significance of scoring hypopneas. *Sleep* 1992;15:257–260.

109. Williams RI, Karacan I, Hursch CJ. *Electroencephalography (EEG) of human sleep: clinical applications.* New York: John Wiley and Sons, 1974.

110. Williamson PD, Spencer DD, Spencer SS, et al. Complex partial seizures of frontal lobe origin. *Ann Neurol* 1985;18:497–504.

111. Yamashiro Y, Dryger MH. Nocturnal oximetry: is it a screening tool for sleep disorders? *Sleep* 1995;18(3):167–171.

112. Young T, Palta M, Dempsey J, et al. The occurrence of sleep-disordered breathing among middle-aged adults. *N Engl J Med* 1993;328:1230–1235.

113. Zorick FJ, Roth T, Hartze KM, et al. Evaluation and diagnosis of persistent insomnia. *Am J Psychiat* 1981;138:769–773.

Chapter 27

Visual Evoked Potentials

Charles M. Epstein

The visual evoked potential (VEP) is the largest evoked potential in common use, the easiest to record in cooperative subjects, and, it has been argued, the most sensitive to alteration by neurological disease. However, its deceptively simple waveform is affected by many variables, including nature of the stimulus, choice of recording techniques, and idiosyncrasies of subjects to be tested. There is correspondingly large variation in clinical practice; at times, different authorities appear to give conflicting recommendations. Specific implementations improve the utility of VEPs for some applications but reduce it for others. Two central goals of this chapter are to explain the bases for different techniques and to provide rational criteria for selecting among them. Because the VEP reflects the organization of the human visual system, relevant aspects of visual anatomy and physiology are reviewed.

ANATOMY AND PHYSIOLOGY OF THE HUMAN VISUAL SYSTEM

Retina and Optic Nerve

Light entering the eye crosses behind the lens; thus, images from the temporal field are formed on the nasal portion of the retina, and those from the nasal field appear on the temporal retina (Fig. 27.1). Superior and inferior fields are inverted in a similar manner. Within the human retina, photoreceptor cells classified as rods and cones hyperpolarize in response to light. Rods are more sensitive than cones but function only in dim light and are found predominantly in the peripheral retina. Cones detect color and function in brighter light; they are concentrated especially in the macular region.

After adaptation to a dark environment, the physiological state of the retina is referred to as *scotopic:* rod function predominates. In bright light, in which cone function dominates, the physiological state is *photopic.* Cones sensitive to red light waves are most prominent in the macular region, whereas those sensitive to blue light waves lie almost exclusively outside it.

The output of rods and cones projects to bipolar cells and then to ganglion cells, whose axons form the retinal nerve fiber layer and the optic nerve. Developmentally and physiologically, the retina is part of the central nervous system, and the optic nerve is invested with central myelin. An extensive network of amacrine and horizontal cells mediates lateral interactions between adjacent parts of the retina. These interneurons appear to use a large variety of neurotransmitters, including dopamine.

The macular area at the posterior pole of the retina is specialized for high-acuity vision. The foveal pit, a 1.5-mm depression in the center of the macula, contains only slender cones that are packed densely for maximum resolution. This high-resolution region corresponds to the central 3 degrees of the visual field. The layer of myelinated axons emerging from the fovea is denser than that from other portions of the retina and courses directly to the optic nerve head in the papillomacular bundle. In the optic nerve and cortex, the percentage of fibers devoted to the macula is magnified far out of proportion to the actual size of the macula (see Fig. 27.1). The much larger peripheral retina projects to a proportionally smaller fraction of the visual cortex; it serves predominantly to detect patterns of light and movement and to direct the high acuity of central vision toward appropriate targets. In persons with normalvision, the output of these different retinal areas is integrated so well that people are generally unaware of their different functions.

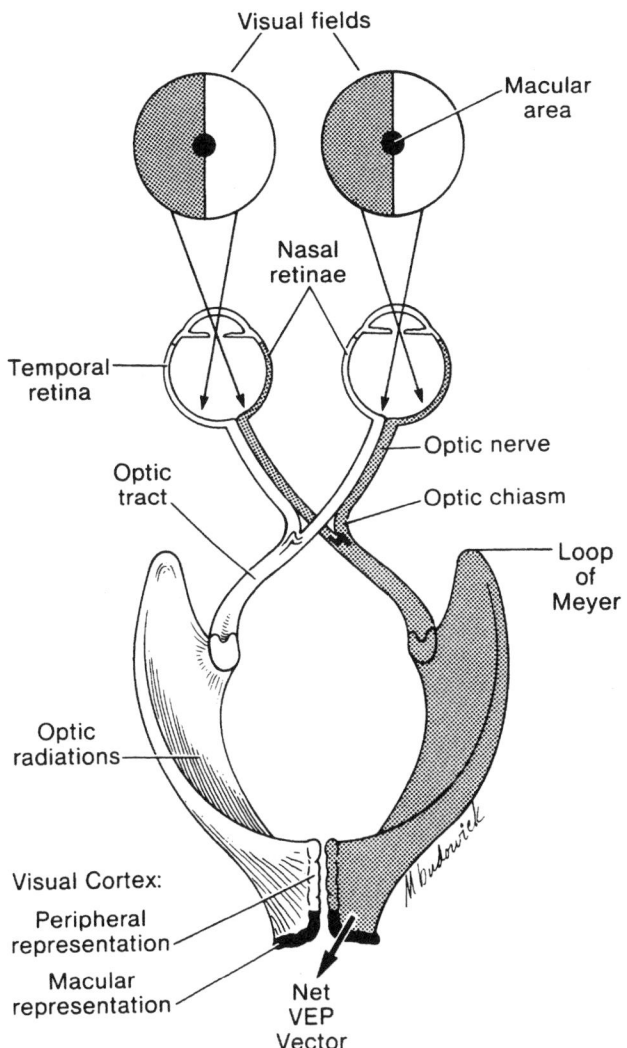

FIG. 27.1. The primary visual pathways, illustrating (i) the crossing of nasal fibers in the optic chiasm, (ii) the macular and peripheral retinal projections to the striate cortex, and (iii) the magnification of the macular area in the visual cortex (shown in black.) The *large arrow* shows the usual direction of the net visual evoked potential vector from hemifield stimulation, which slants obliquely back across the opposite hemisphere.

Each retinal neuron responds to a limited field of photoreceptor cells. For the simplest bipolar and ganglion cells, this receptive field is circular, consisting of a center area and a larger surrounding area. The center and the surrounding area produce opposite responses to light. "Center-on" retinal ganglion cells depolarize and produce more action potentials when light strikes the center of their receptive fields, whereas the firing rate falls when light hits the surrounding area. "Center-off" neurons reduce their firing rate with illumination of the center and increase firing when more light reaches the surrounding area. In the fovea, the center receptive field of a retinal ganglion cell is confined to the width of a single slender cone (1.0 to 1.5 μm), but receptive fields enlarge progressively in the parafoveal and peripheral retina, in which they include multiple photoreceptor cells. Because their input is divided into inhibitory and excitatory fields, retinal neurons are much more sensitive to borders and contrast than to diffuse illumination. This sensitivity to contrasting edges continues with increasing sophistication through the later stages of visual processing (82). Because the primary visual system is arranged to emphasize detection of boundaries and movement, sensitivity to contrasting patterns is a more appropriate way to describe visual function than is simple light detection or even conventional visual acuity.

Overall retinal function is assessed neurophysiologically by the electroretinogram (ERG), which shows the mass response to a bright flash of diffuse or patterned light (Fig. 27.2). Because the peripheral retina is many times larger than the fovea, its response dominates the ERG. The ERG "a" wave represents an early light response from photoreceptors. The ERG "b" wave, peaking at about 50 milliseconds, reflects activity of deeper cell layers; it probably originates in glia rather than in neurons. Retinal processing is relatively slow in comparison with that of other sensory receptors: Direct measurements in humans suggest that the response to a flash of light appears in the optic nerve with a latency of about 40 milliseconds (113).

Optic Tract, Optic Radiations, and Visual Cortex

At the optic chiasm, fibers from the temporal portion of the retina pass ipsilaterally into the optic tract, whereas those from the nasal half of the retina decussate to travel in the contralateral optic tract toward the thalamus (see Fig. 27.1). In primates, there is a small but important exception: For the few degrees around the nasal half of the fovea, a dense ring of ganglion cells also projects ipsilaterally (98). Some crossing fibers for the superior temporal field are said to swing forward into the contralateral optic nerve before turning back in the optic tract. (This bulge is known as Wilbrand's knee,

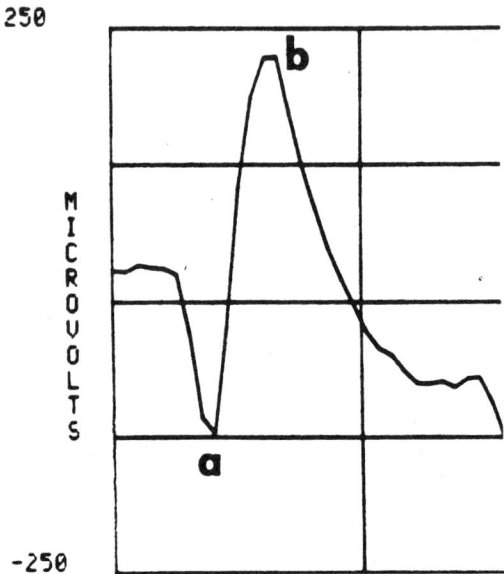

FIG. 27.2. White-flash electroretinogram under scotopic conditions, showing normal "a" and "b" waves from the retina.

although doubts have been raised about its existence in primates (81)). Within the optic tract proper, fibers representing corresponding portions of the visual field are not fully congruous. Thus, lesions at this level produce visual field defects that are nonhomonymous (i.e., they are different in the two eyes). Optic tract fibers from each eye enter alternating layers of the lateral geniculate nucleus.

Myelinated axons projecting from the lateral geniculate nucleus to the cortex form the optic radiations, which swing superiorly and laterally around the lateral ventricle in the temporal and parietal lobes. One portion of the radiations tends to loop especially far forward towards the tip of the temporal horn; known as the loop of Meyer, it contains fibers representing the superior visual field from the contralateral side (see Fig. 27.1). As the radiations near the visual cortex, homologous fibers from the two eyes come closer together; therefore, lesions at a parieto-occipital level produce homonymous field defects. Visual sensory fibers enter the primary visual cortex in Brodmann's area 17. Here, layer IV is markedly thickened and forms a visible stripe in the calcarine fissure, known as the band of Gennari. Its presence has led to the designation of the primary visual area as *striate cortex.*

As a result of foveal magnification, approximately one-third of the primary visual cortex is devoted to the 3 degrees of central vision. The macular projection area occupies the posterior portion of the calcarine cortex, extending in the medial portion of the hemisphere approximately to the occipital pole (see Fig. 27.1). There is considerable anatomical variability in the gross configuration of the occipital lobes, and there is equally wide variability in the representation of macular vision over the occipital pole and medial occipital cortex (162).

LUMINANCE AND CONTRAST SENSITIVITY

The brightness of a light source is commonly measured in candelas; the luminance of a two-dimensional surface is expressed in candelas per square foot, candelas per square meter, or foot-lamberts (1 f-L = 3.426 cd/m^2). The contrast between two adjoining areas has been described in several ways, but in the most common formula, contrast is expressed as a percentage, where *Lmax* is the luminance of the brighter area and *Lmin* represents the dimmer one:

$$\text{contrast} = 100 * \frac{L_{max} - L_{min}}{L_{max} + L_{min}}$$

Contrast sensitivity is the eye's ability to detect small differences in illumination between adjacent areas and is measured with the use of striped patterns or gratings of different sizes. The level of contrast between light and dark stripes is varied to determine the threshold for detection of the pattern. A contrast sensitivity curve can be generated by plotting the size of the grating against the visual threshold for pattern detection (Fig. 27.3). For central vision, peak sensitivity to contrast between light and dark stripes is 3 to 4 cycles per degree (75); the width of individual stripes is 7-10 minutes of arc. At a distance of 1 m, this corresponds to a line 2 to 3 mm wide. Outside the fovea, peak sensitivity is for larger patterns, approaching 1 cycle per degree.

Video-based VEP systems can produce a large variety of stimulus patterns, including solid bars that have uniform luminance within the light and dark areas (Fig. 27.4*A*) and stripes whose luminance varies according to a sine wave function (see Fig. 27.4*B*). Although solid bars may appear to represent the simpler pattern, their optical effects are more complex. The sinusoidal stripes can be represented, through Fourier analysis, by a single fundamental spatial frequency, which is usually given as the number of light-dark cycles in 1 degree of arc. In contrast, Fourier analysis of uniform

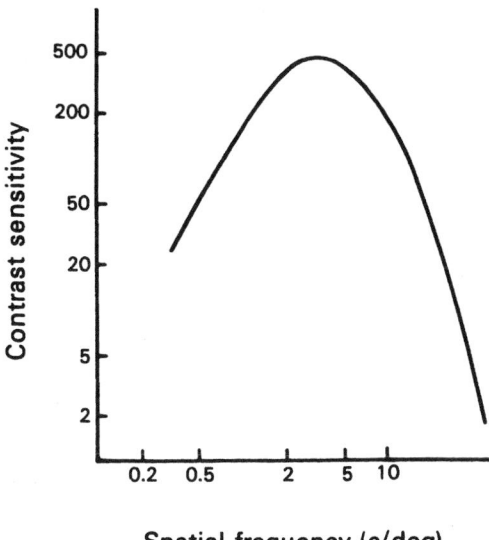

FIG. 27.3. Idealized contrast sensitivity curve, indicating that the human eye is most sensitive to spatial dimensions around three to four cycles per degree. (Modified from Kelly D. Pattern detection and the two-dimensional Fourier transform: flickering checkerboards and chromatic mechanisms. *Vision Res* 1975;16:277–287.)

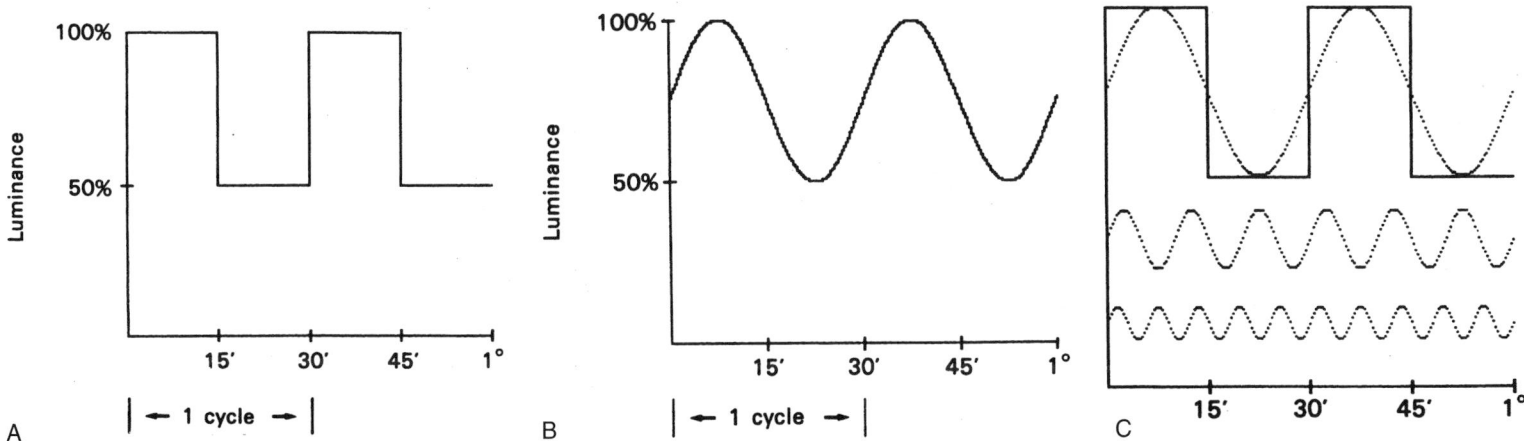

FIG. 27.4. A: Luminance profile for a pattern of solid bars, in which the light elements have twice the brightness of the dark ones and one full cycle is equal to 30 minutes of arc. Individual elements are 15 minutes wide, and the spatial frequency is 2 cycles per degree. **B:** Luminance profile for a sinusoidal grating. Contrast is $100 \times (100 - 50)/(100 + 50) = 33\%$. **C:** A pattern of solid bars shown with the first three sine-wave harmonics of the equivalent Fourier series (*dotted curves*).

bars reveals a whole series of spatial frequencies. The fundamental frequency is still the width of one full light-dark cycle, but there is also an infinite series of weaker harmonics whose frequencies are an odd multiple of the fundamental (see Fig. 27.4C). Thus, a simple-appearing pattern of solid bars may actually stimulate the visual system at many spatial frequencies.

Frequency analysis of a conventional checkerboard pattern yields results that are even more surprising and seem counterintuitive: a two-dimensional Fourier transform shows only components along the diagonals rather than along the edges of the individual checks (75). Thus, if the visual system responds to the underlying frequency components of the pattern, a checkerboard pattern actually stimulates the retina at the oblique angles of 45 and 135 degrees. Data consistent with this hypothesis have been found at both low (87) and high (159) contrast levels with checkerboard stimuli.

Some investigators have argued that the choice of VEP pattern stimuli should be based on these physiological observations: that is, stripes should be used in preference to checks, the luminance profile of the stripes should be sinusoidal rather than uniform, and their size should be near the peak of the contrast sensitivity curve at 3 to 4 cycles per degree. It is further argued that the brightness of the pattern stimulus must be balanced very precisely so that the VEP is not contaminated with any trace of conflicting input in the form of changing luminance. These points are obviously important for research applications in which specifying the exact nature of the stimulus is crucial to understanding the corresponding output. They are less compelling for clinical practice, in which the most important criteria of VEP utility are stable and robust responses, sensitivity, and specificity for certain types of visual dysfunction rather than others. In medical applications, stimuli with the "ideal" characteristics preferred by researchers turn out to have a number of potential drawbacks that are discussed later in this chapter.

SOURCE AND TOPOGRAPHY OF THE FULL-FIELD PATTERN VISUAL EVOKED POTENTIAL

As shown in Fig. 27.1, stimuli confined to half the visual field activate the primary visual cortex of only one hemisphere. Under typical test conditions, checkerboard pattern reversal in one hemifield produces a net pattern VEP (PVEP) vector that points diagonally back across the opposite occipital lobe and is represented by the large arrow in Fig. 27.1 (19,96,152). This net vector reflects almost entirely activity in macular and paramacular areas of the visual cortex (119). The macular area of visual cortex is closer to scalp recording electrodes, and is more responsive than peripheral areas to pat-

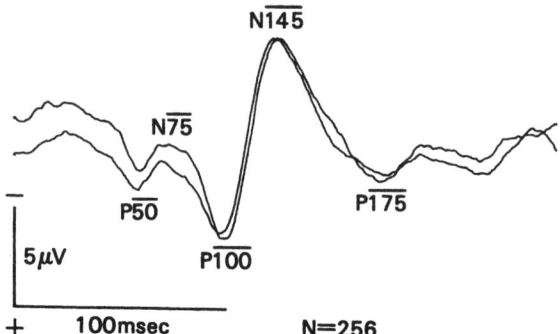

FIG. 27.5. The normal midline pattern visual evoked potential, recorded in an Oz-Cz derivation from an average of 256 responses. Light-emitting diode stimulator with checks measuring 40 minutes of arc, in a 4 × 4 degree pattern; passband is 1.0 to 100 Hz. The major positive and negative peaks are labeled according to their mean latency in normal subjects.

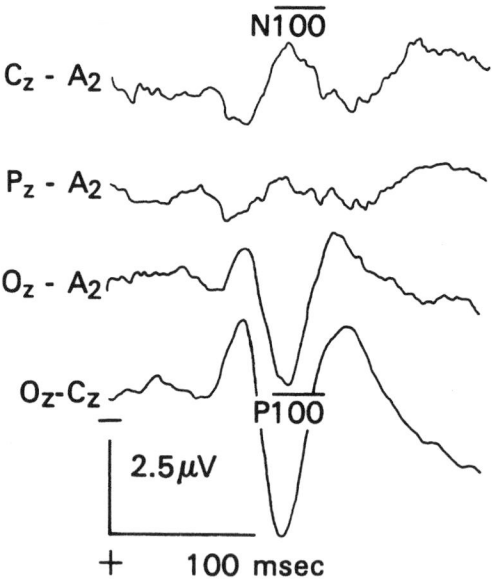

FIG. 27.6. A normal pattern visual evoked potential recorded from a chain of sagittal derivations, showing the occipital $\overline{P100}$, the frontocentral $\overline{N100}$, and their summation in the Oz-Cz derivation.

terns of the sizes most commonly used. When the full visual field is stimulated, vectors from the two hemispheres sum to produce a PVEP maximum at the occipital midline. This full-field PVEP usually has a negative-positive-negative configuration between 70 and 140 milliseconds; maximal positivity occurs at around 100 milliseconds (Figs. 27.5 to 27.7). The most commonly accepted convention is to display relative positivity at the occiput by a downward deflection. Peaks are labeled with nominal latency values derived from the average in normal subjects: $N\overline{75}$, $P\overline{100}$, and $N\overline{145}$ (see Fig. 27.5). In this system, the bar over the numeral means that this number represents an average (*not* a normal limit.) Depending on test conditions, a smaller positive peak may be recorded between 50 and 60 milliseconds and is usually designated either $P\overline{50}$ or $P\overline{60}$.

Electrodes placed more anteriorly along the midline often show a negative wave in the frontocentral region, which occurs at about the same time as the $P\overline{100}$ (see Fig. 27.6, top channel). If a recording derivation interconnects the area of this $N\overline{100}$ and the occiput (e.g., Fz-Oz), then the $P\overline{100}$ and $N\overline{100}$ sum to give a larger and better-defined PVEP (see Fig. 27.6, bottom channel).

All portions of the PVEP are probably of cortical origin and are classified as middle-latency evoked potentials. However, the exact sources of different PVEP components are unresolved. The earliest definable wave, $P\overline{50}$, begins within 50 milliseconds after pattern reversal. This is barely 10 milliseconds after the earliest flash responses that can be recorded directly from the optic nerve and indicates that the "conduction time" in optic nerve, tract, and radiations is only a small fraction of the total latency from pattern-shift to the peak of $P\overline{100}$. Findings from animal studies with flash stimuli have been interpreted to suggest that $N\overline{75}$ may represent the initial excitation associated with the arrival of visual signals at layer IV of the calcarine cortex (91). Kraut et al. (91) proposed that $P\overline{100}$, the most stable and most commonly measured VEP component, arises from a secondary wave of inhibition at pyramidal cells, mediated by γ-aminobutyric acid (GABA). Experiments using several types of stimuli in anesthetized cats demonstrated that the GABA antagonist bicuculline substantially alters the VEP (183). In similar preparations, anticholinesterases reduced VEP amplitudes (88). However, in human studies, γ-vinyl GABA, which increases GABA levels, did not alter $P\overline{100}$ (73). Experiments with magnetic interference over the occipital cortex indicate that the interval from 80 to 100 milliseconds after a retinal stimulus is critical to visual perception. This time frame corresponds fairly well to $P\overline{100}$ and suggests that the latter does in some way reflect active processing of visual information (2).

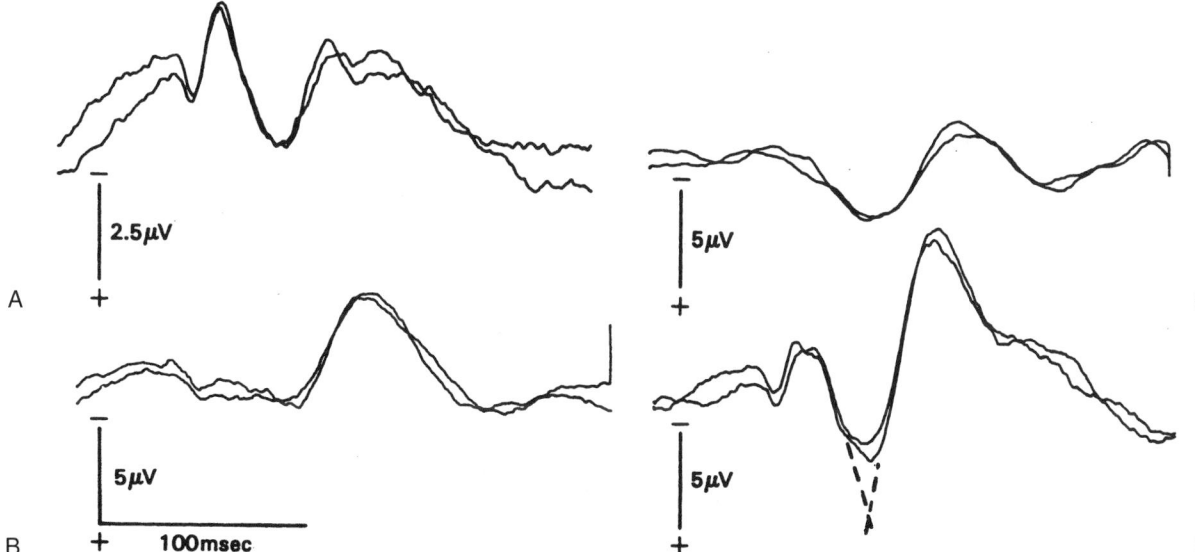

FIG. 27.7. Normal waveform variability of the pattern visual evoked potential in four subjects, all recorded from Oz-Cz as in Fig. 27.5. $N\overline{75}$ may be the largest peak **(A),** or it may be entirely absent **(B).** $P\overline{50}$ is seen in *A, B,* and *D* but not in *C.* $P\overline{100}$ is consistently present at about 100 milliseconds. *Dashed lines* in *D* show one technique for estimating the latency of $P\overline{100}$ when the center is ambiguous.

TRANSIENT AND STEADY-STATE VISUAL EVOKED POTENTIALS

When the interval between visual stimuli is greater than the duration of the VEP and responses are averaged individually, the result is termed a *transient VEP*. This is the type generally used in clinical studies and emphasized in this chapter. At stimulus rates faster than about four per second, sequential VEPs begin to run together and form trains of rhythmic activity. Such trains, seen by electroencephalographers in the form of photic driving, are called *steady-state VEPs*. With increasing stimulus rates, the steady-state VEP resembles a series of sine waves; individual components and individual latencies related to a specific stimulus become difficult to define. However, the much faster stimulus rates that are possible with steady-state VEPs allow presentation of multiple stimuli in a much shorter time. They also enable direct application of special techniques such as phase-locked amplifiers and Fourier analysis (54,120). Although steady-state VEPs sacrifice direct measurement of latency and wave shape, they provide extremely sensitive estimates of evoked potential amplitude and allow distinction among simultaneous responses at closely adjacent frequencies.

Steady-state VEPs have been used most often in attempts to measure visual acuity objectively, as discussed later in this chapter. Alternatively, frequency analysis allows simultaneous stimulation of multiple sectors in the visual field.

INTERPRETATION OF FULL-FIELD PATTERN VISUAL EVOKED POTENTIALS

$P\overline{100}$ latency at the occipital midline is the central measurement for PVEP interpretation. This choice is not attributable to any special physiological significance of $P\overline{100}$; it is neither the earliest component nor even necessarily the largest. In view of the wide range of PVEP variability, it is simply the one that is most stable and most consistently identified in all normal subjects (see Fig. 27.7). $P\overline{50}$, $N\overline{75}$, or $P\overline{175}$ may be absent in some normal persons, and $N\overline{145}$ may be too poorly defined for accurate measurement. Thus, these latter components are difficult to use in distinguishing normal PVEPs from abnormal ones.

$P\overline{100}$ Latency Measurement

$P\overline{100}$ may be narrow or broad, and it may be symmetrical or asymmetrical in shape. A broad $P\overline{100}$ may appear intuitively suspicious and, in fact, has been interpreted as a sign of temporal dispersion in the visual signal. However, there are currently no simple and precise criteria by which $P\overline{100}$ width can be used as an index of disease. In a narrow, symmetrically shaped PVEP, measurement of peak latency is unequivocal. When the response is noisy or asymmetrical, the choice of "peak latency" is more ambiguous. If $N\overline{75}$ is absent (see Fig. 27.7*B*), $P\overline{100}$ should be considered the beginning of the upstroke to $N\overline{145}$. A bifid $P\overline{100}$ should be approached as described later in this chapter. Otherwise, different laboratories deal with ill-defined peaks in different ways. One technique is to extrapolate the downward slopes from $N\overline{75}$ and $N\overline{145}$, taking the $P\overline{100}$ latency as the point of their intersection (see Fig. 27.7*D*). Another is to estimate, simply by gestalt, the center of the entire complex from $N\overline{75}$ to $N\overline{145}$. Whichever criterion is used, it must be applied consistently in collecting normative data, in interpreting clinical studies, and in comparing latencies from the two eyes. Sometimes, $P\overline{100}$ cannot be estimated to better than 2 or 3 milliseconds, and the result lies close to the upper limits of normal. This situation should be described as borderline. The interpretation should not be forced into an "either/or" category beyond the precision allowed by the data.

PVEP latencies have a gaussian distribution in normal subjects, and so conventional parametric statistics may be used to calculate normal limits. Recordings from both eyes in 20 normal subjects are considered the minimum data base for establishing normal values of $P\overline{100}$ latency. There is no clinical interest in recognizing unusually short PVEP latencies, and so one-tailed statistics are appropriate for establishing an upper limit of normal (3). This boundary is commonly set at the 99% tolerance limit, 2.5 standard deviations (SD), or 3.0 SD. For 20 to 30 subjects, the mean plus 2.5 SD and the 99% tolerance limit are similar. These statistics result in classifying about 1% of normal subjects as "abnormal." A one-tailed limit of 2.0 SD results in classifying 5% of normal subjects as abnormal and in an excess number of false-positive findings.

$P\overline{100}$ latency may change appreciably in serial studies of normal volunteers. Oken et al. (127) reported an average absolute latency change of 2.9 milliseconds in controls, with a maximum of 11 milliseconds in one subject. However, Hammond et al. (74) and Stockard et al. (163) found less prominent variability.

Inter-eye latency differences are more sensitive than absolute latency to the presence of subtle disease. They show a less gaussian distribution but also vary far less than absolute latency among different laboratories. Inter-eye differences are also less affected by age than are absolute latency measurements (163). In published normal series, upper limits for interocular latency difference usually lie between 6 and 8 milliseconds. However, patients are generally more likely than controls to have small differences between the two eyes that result from refractive error, changes in pupillary size, retinal disease, cataracts, or other opacities. Patients' PVEPs are less likely to be exquisitely well defined. Thus, a more conservative limit of 10 milliseconds or more is appropriate for defining an abnormal inter-eye latency asymmetry. Mild asymmetries in this range should be considered pathological only when the whole VEP envelope, including N75 and N145—not just the tip of P100—is asymmetrical. On serial studies, inter-eye latency differences have changed by an average of 2.5 milliseconds, with individual shifts of up to 9 milliseconds (127).

P100 Amplitude Measurement

PVEP amplitude is considerably more variable than latency; consequently, it is more difficult to use in identifying neurological disease. Different laboratories measure amplitude from the peak of N75 to P100, from P100 to N145, as the sum of the two, or as whichever is best defined in a given subject. P100 amplitude distribution in normal individuals is non-gaussian; consequently, attempts to calculate normative data by parametric statistics such as mean, standard deviation, and tolerance limits can be inaccurate and misleading. The lower limit of normal for N75 to P100 amplitude is zero (3). Normal limits for P100 to N145 are best determined by nonparametric techniques. In simple terms, this means collecting PVEPs from 100 or so normal persons, measuring the amplitudes, and defining "abnormal" as a value smaller than 99% of these amplitudes.

Comparison of relative PVEP amplitude between the two eyes is somewhat easier than assessment of absolute amplitude. Even here, however, the distribution of raw data and possible data transformations should be evaluated by a trained statistician before "normal limits" are calculated. In various series, amplitude ratios greater than 2:1 or 2.5:1 are considered "abnormal." Such statistical amplitude abnormalities may result from a wide variety of nonneurological factors and should be assessed very carefully before they are interpreted as evidence of neurological disease. Serial studies in normal volunteers have shown amplitude changes of 2:1 for the same eye (127).

Other Statistical Considerations

An important and often-neglected aspect of calculating normal limits is that probability thresholds should be adjusted according to the number of independent parameters that are considered. For example, P100 latency may be measured with three different orientations of the pattern (28). If the laten-

cies under each condition are independent variables (which is, after all, the underlying assumption when they are measured separately) and if the normal limits for each condition include 95% of controls, then three separate statistical tests may produce false-positive results in almost 15% of the normal population!

A large fraction of the VEP literature consists of demonstrating that adding new test conditions and measurements results in a larger number of abnormal VEPs. This is a normal consequence of performing more tests, and without statistical adjustments, the number of false-positive results may rise faster than the number of true abnormalities (62). In testing for disorders such as multiple sclerosis, most clinicians consider that misclassifying a normal subject as diseased is far more deleterious than temporarily missing the diagnosis in a patient with mild illness. To avoid such errors, measurement of increasing numbers of VEP parameters should be accompanied by increasingly conservative statistics, to the level of 3 SD or beyond.

Aberrant Waveforms and Normal Variants

If average background noise is acceptably low (1 μV or less), a nonreproducible PVEP should be considered absent. In cooperative subjects, its absence should be confirmed by additional recordings at Pz and the inion (see Fig. 27.10*B*). A reproducible waveform is "aberrant" if an unequivocal P100 cannot be determined. Many of these aberrant responses appear to contain too many peaks rather than too few, and the origin of each peak must be analyzed individually. Morphological variants that include a prominent P50 should not be confused with aberrant waveforms (see Fig. 27.7).

Apparently bifid, or "W," potentials may be recorded in normal subjects when the frontal N100 and occipital P100 components are asynchronous (161,163). The apparent double peak is seen only with the use of a frontal or central reference. In such cases, P100 latency can be identified easily in simultaneous ear-reference recording (Fig. 27.8). When small check sizes are used, true bifid potentials that fail to resolve with a change of reference are rare in normal persons; many authors consider them pathological. True bifid potentials are best analyzed with hemifield stimulation (85); see later discussion.

Background entrainment is familiar to electroencephalographers as the photic driving response that is seen routinely in conventional EEG. On occasion, the photic response contains higher harmonics at two or more times the actual stimulus rate. This phenomenon, termed *frequency doubling* (134), is seen commonly in steady-state VEPs and more rarely in transient VEPs.

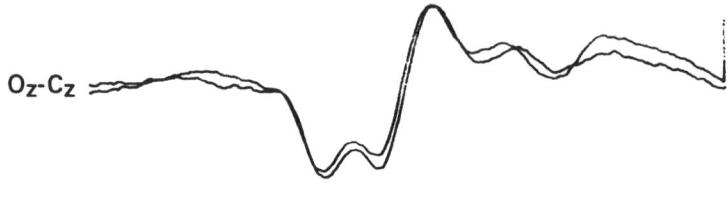

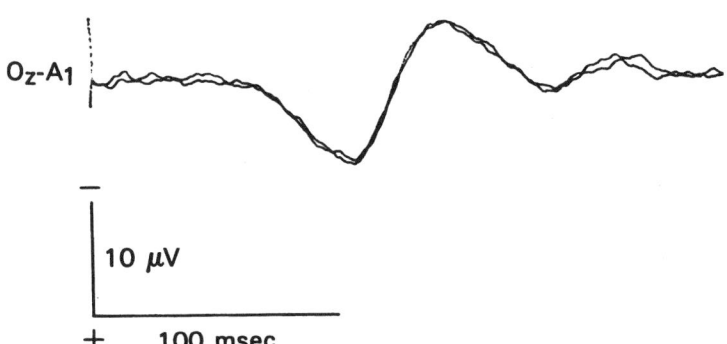

FIG. 27.8. Bifid P$\overline{100}$ with a vertex reference (*top*) resolved to a single peak with a simultaneous ear reference (*bottom*). The W-shape of the P$\overline{100}$ is caused by an asynchronous N$\overline{100}$ picked up by the vertex electrode.

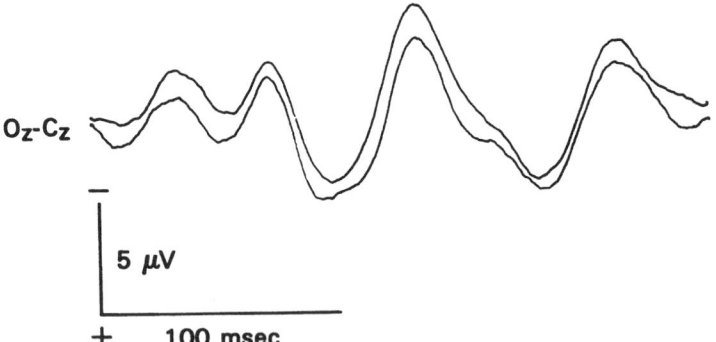

FIG. 27.9. Background entrainment with frequency doubling at 3.7 reversals per second. The very early peaks falling sooner than P$\overline{50}$, as well as the exaggerated P$\overline{175}$, result from driving of harmonics above the actual reversal rate.

PVEPs with frequency doubling appear to contain an excessive number of independent peaks. Usually, P$\overline{175}$ is very large, and there are reproducible components shorter in latency than P$\overline{50}$ (Fig. 27.9). These very early waves can be interpreted only as a late but synchronous response to the penultimate stimulus. Frequency doubling tends to occur at stimulus rates higher than two per second. It can usually be diminished by reducing the reversal frequency and avoiding exact fractions of the original rate.

STIMULI FOR ELICITING PATTERN VISUAL EVOKED POTENTIALS

Pattern Reversal

The most commonly used stimulus for PVEP recording is a pattern of light and dark checks, bars, or stripes that is repeatedly reversed: that is, the light portions of the pattern abruptly become dark, and the dark portions become light. Most clinical laboratories use black-and-white checkerboard patterns.

In the earliest pattern reversal systems, moving mirrors were used to deflect the position of a slide projected on a screen. Such mechanical devices could produce rapid pattern shifts (5 milliseconds) but were clumsy, fragile, and lacking in flexibility. They have been supplanted almost entirely by video pattern generators, which are considerably more versatile. However, pattern reversal is actually slower with conventional video systems than with any other technique. Standard television monitors use an "interlace" mode, which generates only 30 new frames per second (25 in Europe); thus, fully replacing one picture with another requires more than 30 milliseconds. (Faster "noninterlace" modes used in some sophisticated systems require 15 milliseconds or less.) The video sweep generator may be synchronized to the power line, to minimize picture distortion. Synchronizing pattern reversal to sweep onset can then produce excess 60-cycle noise in the VEP. However, desynchronizing the moment of reversal from the sweep generator means that each new pattern begins on a different part of the screen, leading to further uncertainty in timing. This temporal smearing of video images affects the resulting PVEPs. The early, relatively narrow P$\overline{50}$ is less likely to be seen with video pattern generators than with other techniques, and there is a small effect on P$\overline{100}$ latency.

Pattern reversal can also be performed with grids of light-emitting diodes (LEDs), which turn on and off in a few microseconds (53). The luminance of LEDs is precisely controlled by the input current. LED stimulators are small, rugged, and portable, making them suitable for mounting above a supine patient or for the operating room. However, the size of the elements is fixed, and the total stimulus field is small.

Pattern Onset

A complex pattern may be rapidly flashed on and off with the use of LEDs, a tachistoscopic projector, or a computer-controlled video display. Although it is possible to hold luminance constant throughout (141), pattern onset commonly combines both pattern and luminance stimuli and is used less widely than pattern reversal. However, pattern onset produces more robust responses (4,141,149). Aminoff and Ochs (4) reported that this type of stimulus produced a higher yield of diagnostic abnormalities in patients with multiple sclerosis. In the operating room, goggles incorporating small grids of flashing red LEDs are used by some centers to monitor visual function during surgical procedures.

PATTERN VISUAL EVOKED POTENTIAL STIMULUS PARAMETERS

Check Size

As noted previously, the contrast sensitivity function of the fovea suggests that checks with a diagonal around 4 cycles per degree represent an optimal stimulus to central vision. Other considerations, however, mitigate against use of a pattern this fine for routine clinical testing. Many patients referred for PVEP testing have less than 20/20 acuity because of refractive errors, presbyopia, or cataracts; some arrive at the laboratory without their glasses or with the lingering effects of mydriatics that paralyze accommodation. With very small checks or gratings, latency of the PVEP is inordinately sensitive to many factors: blurring of the pattern by poor acuity (159); age (160); ophthalmological disorders such as central serous retinopathy, which can mimic optic neuritis (90,151); and nonvisual disorders such as Parkinson's disease (171). To the neurologist interested in searching for disease of the optic nerve or posterior visual pathways, latency prolongation produced by any of these factors is misleading and reduces the utility of the test. On the other hand, checks larger than 1 degree approach the size of the entire fovea, with increased stimulation of parafoveal and peripheral portions of the retina. As a compromise, the Evoked Potential Guidelines of the American Electroencephalographic Society (now the American Clinical Neurophysiology Society [ACNS]) recommend a check size in the range of 24 to 32 minutes of arc (3). At this size, effects of visual blurring are reduced, and foveal sensitivity remains high. In practice, checks up to 50 minutes of arc in size have proved to be clinically useful for full-field stimulation and are preferred in many laboratories specifically to avoid the confounding factors noted earlier. Checks between 50 and 90 minutes of arc in size are recommended when PVEPs are used for testing visual fields.

Check size also affects PVEP morphological pattern; smaller checks produce a relatively larger $N\overline{75}$, a more sharply defined $P\overline{100}$, and a reduced likelihood of recording a W-shaped $P\overline{100}$.

A simple formula for determining the visual angle of individual checks in a checkerboard pattern is

$$A = 57.3 * W/D$$

where A is the visual angle in degrees, W is the width of the check in millimeters, and D is the distance to the eye in millimeters.

Field Size

Checkerboard patterns used in PVEP testing have ranged in width from 3.0 (33) or 3.8 degrees (23) up to 48 degrees of arc (102). For full-field testing of central vision, a 4×4 degree pattern covers the macula and yields entirely adequate results. Larger fields produce only a small increase in PVEP amplitude. Some researchers suggest that smaller fields increase sensitivity of the PVEP to optic nerve demyelination, perhaps because the response of a large parafoveal area can "swamp" the latency delay produced by a small central scotoma (78). However, larger fields allow the patient's eye to wander more easily during testing. Field size significantly affects the direction of the PVEP net vector from hemifield stimulation. With large stimulus fields, the contribution of the peripheral retina directs the net vector obliquely through the contralateral hemisphere (see Fig. 27.1). With patterns whose size is only a few degrees across, the net vector tends to point straight back, so that the contribution from each hemisphere may be maximal ipsilaterally. In the past, this effect of field size on the PVEP vector led to conflicting experimental results. For hemifield stimulation, the ACNS Guidelines (3) recommend that the total field width subtend at least 16 degrees of arc.

Patient Distance

An eye-to-pattern distance between 0.7 and 1.5 m is generally satisfactory. With longer distances, blurring may result from severe uncorrected myopia or in reduced attention by uncooperative patients. With shorter distances, presbyopia may cause difficulty.

Contrast

PVEP amplitude increases with increasing pattern contrast up to the range of 20% to 40%. Beyond this, the effects of contrast saturate, and there is no further change. In most clinical laboratories, regardless of stimulator type, contrast is well above saturation level.

Luminance

In normal subjects, average latency of P$\overline{100}$ falls by about 12 milliseconds per logarithmic increase in luminance (29); that is, every time the brightness of the pattern is increased tenfold, latency decreases 12 milliseconds. A luminance difference of 100 times produces, on average, a P$\overline{100}$ latency difference of 24 milliseconds. The dependence of PVEP normal values on luminance, and the difficulties in standardizing the brightness of video monitors, are the most important reasons that VEP laboratories must collect their own normative data rather than relying on published results.

The effect of luminance on latency is greater in patients with optic nerve disease, and use of lower luminance has been suggested as a method for increasing PVEP sensitivity (29). Unfortunately (from the neurologist's perspective), lower luminance may also increase sensitivity to other conditions such as retinal disease (151), poor visual acuity, and age (148).

The possibility of *inadvertent* luminance changes is critically important in the VEP laboratory, especially with television pattern generators. Luminance of the television screen is strongly affected by both brightness and contrast controls, and it may be altered by aging of the picture tube. Laboratories collecting normal data sometimes neglect to measure luminance of the screen at the outset or to mark the settings of the controls. At any future time, visitors to the laboratory may randomly twirl knobs, altering the range of normal values and opening the possibility of major errors in interpretation. Control settings should be clearly labeled, and the screen luminance should be checked periodically with a light meter.

PVEP testing should be performed in a moderately well-illuminated room similar to the patient's ordinary environment. This produces a photopic state in which vision is dominated by retinal cones and in which uniform test conditions are relatively simple to attain. In a dark-adapted scotopic test situation, the acuity, color sensitivity, and integrating functions of the retina are different and, of more importance, harder to control. Scotopic adaptation takes 30 minutes, and it is then altered unpredictably by the brightness of the pattern itself.

Color

Retinal cones sensitive to red light are largely confined to the foveal area, and red desaturation is a sensitive clinical sign of paracentral scotomata. On this basis, red/black patterns have been suggested as a means for increasing the sensitivity of the PVEP to central or paracentral lesions (118). In general, the use of different colors produces minor changes in PVEP amplitude and latency, but colored patterns have not been widely adopted for clinical testing.

Reversal Frequency

At "transient" PVEP testing rates, ranging between 0.5 and 4 reversals per second, the average latency of P$\overline{100}$ rises by a few milliseconds with higher reversal frequency (163). Conventional television patterns begin to degrade at approximately two per second, and ACNS Guidelines recommend using patterns of less than four per second for routine clinical studies (3). With patterns of more than four per second, at the faster rates used in steady-state recording, the net VEP vector from pattern reversal swings posteriorly and is seen over the ipsilateral, rather than the contralateral, hemisphere (128). This effect is similar to that of reducing the stimulus field size, and it implies that visual field defects are more likely to be identified as slower reversal rates.

Note that reversal frequency and cycles per second are not the same thing; one full cycle equals two reversals.

PATTERN VISUAL EVOKED POTENTIAL RECORDING PARAMETERS

Passband

The ACNS Guidelines (3) recommend a low filter (high-pass) setting of 1.0 Hz and a high filter (low-pass) setting of 100 Hz. However, the literature includes some studies done with a tighter passband, occasionally as low as 70 Hz (85,141). Waveform distortion may be noticeable at this point.

Sixty-Hertz Filters

The frequency of some VEP components is close enough to 60 Hz that these filters should be avoided in VEP testing.

Sampling Rate

The analog data sampling rate should be fast enough to produce a new data point in each channel every millisecond or less. Thus, the minimum sampling rate for one channel is 1,000 per second; for eight channels, it is

8,000 per second. The inverse of the sampling rate is sometimes called the *dwell time*. At 8,000 samples per second, the dwell time is 0.125 milliseconds per sample.

Sweep Duration

Sampling should continue for at least 250 milliseconds after each stimulus.

Sensitivity

An optimal input range for the analog-to-digital converter is usually 50 to 100 μV. Lower values may lead to excessive distortion or rejection of normal brain activity; higher values may produce inadequate data resolution.

Number of Responses Averaged

Typically, 60 to 250 artifact-free samples are necessary to produce a good signal-to-noise ratio in the final average.

Replications

At least two averages should be taken in each test condition—more if responses are poorly reproduced. Well-reproduced responses should contain a $\overline{P100}$ latency difference of no more than 2.5 milliseconds and an amplitude difference of no more than 15%.

Recording Derivations

All VEP montages must include a midoccipital (MO) electrode. The popularly recommended "Queen Square" technique is to use an MO position 5 cm above the inion (3), which is meant to occupy the average topographic center of $\overline{P100}$. The International 10-20 System's location Oz lies about 1.4 cm below this. Neither MO nor Oz can be considered a fully reliable location in all subjects, however, because the center of $\overline{P100}$ may lie as high as Pz or as low as the inion in normal persons (Fig. 27.10*B*).

The most commonly used reference for PVEPs is Fz (or the Queen Square MF, which is 12 cm above the nasion). Some laboratories place a vertex reference at Cz, where electromyographic activity is usually less prominent. There is no consistent advantage in choosing one of these references over the others. All anterior midline reference sites record the anterior negativity, $\overline{N100}$, that accompanies $\overline{P100}$. This has the consequent advantage of maximizing apparent $\overline{P100}$ amplitude while minimizing noise (see Fig. 27.6), but it has the disadvantage that the contributions of $\overline{N100}$ and $\overline{P100}$ to an aberrant waveform may be impossible to separate. A large $\overline{N100}$ can mask an ectopic or small $\overline{P100}$ or its absence; asynchrony of these two components may lead to an apparently bifid or ambiguous $\overline{P100}$ (161). The easiest way to recognize and resolve such aberrant waveforms is to record routinely from midocciput to one or both ears in a second channel. The ears are relatively uninvolved by the PVEP, and they can be considered inactive for full-field recording. (They are not, however, inactive for hemifield studies.) The ear-reference channel serves as a constant check on the validity of the midline recording and helps identify normal variants that otherwise might lead to serious misinterpretation (see Fig. 27.10*A* and *B*).

For full-field testing, many laboratories use additional electrodes situated lateral to the midline. The International 10-20 System's locations 01 and 02 are generally considered too close together, and so the ACNS (3) recommends left occipital (LO) and right occipital (RO) positions 5 cm to each side of MO (see Fig. 27.10*A*). These additional derivations are most useful in screening for unsuspected field defects, which can then be better defined by subsequent hemifield recording. However, the sensitivity of full-field testing to such defects is limited (13,94,139), and the range of normal variation between LO and RO is large. Even $\overline{P100}$ amplitude asymmetries of greater than 2.5:1 should not be considered definitely abnormal in the absence of corroboration by hemifield studies.

In the author's and some other laboratories (161), an ear reference is considered even more essential than lateral occipital leads for full-field testing. Although the latter prevent a few false-negative results, the former avoids false-positive diagnoses, which are considerably more deleterious for the patients who receive them.

PATIENT FACTORS

Preparation

Ordinarily, each eye is tested individually, while the other eye is occluded by a patch. Binocular testing is occasionally helpful in patients who cooperate poorly, but it is much less sensitive to unilateral optic nerve disease. If possible, patients should not be tested within 24 hours of receiving mydri-

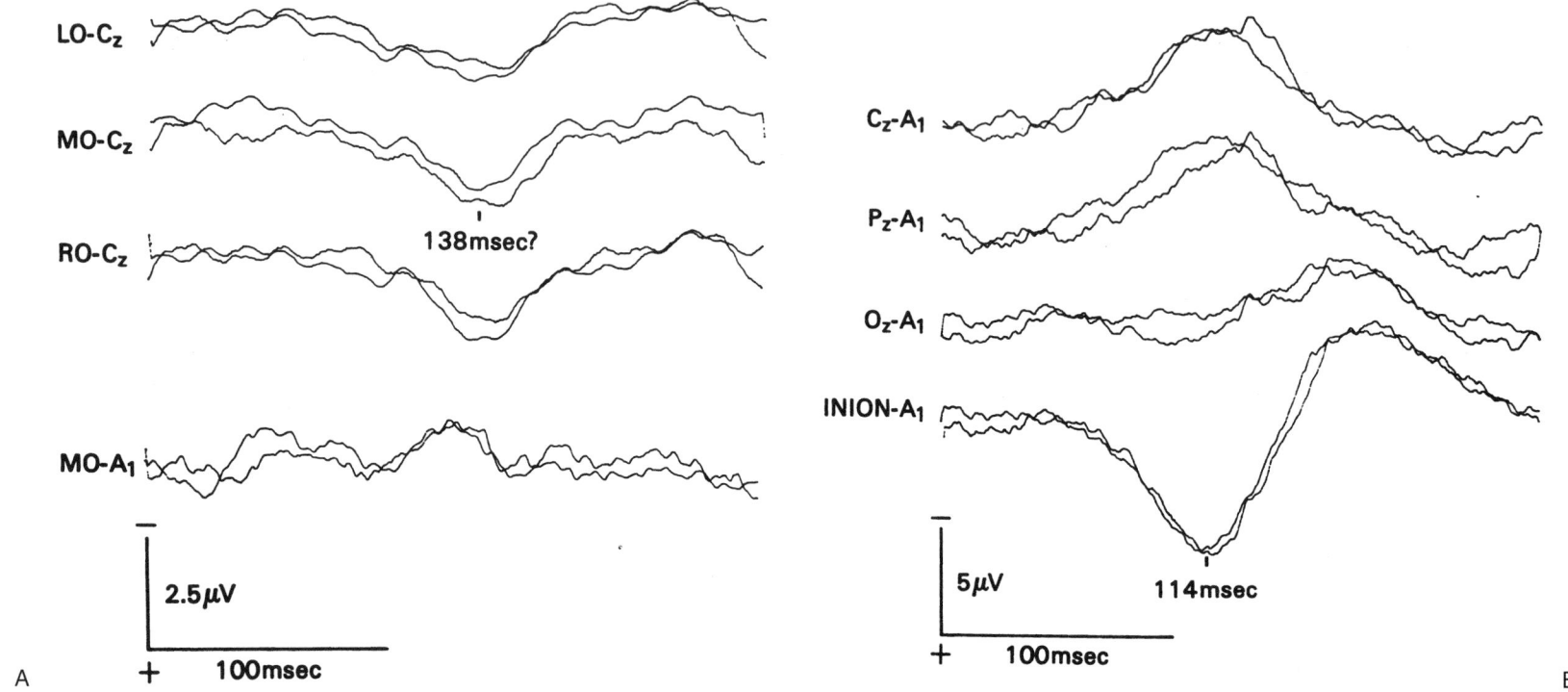

FIG. 27.10. A: Apparently small-amplitude, delayed pattern visual evoked potential to full-field stimulation. However, the response from MO-A1 is discrepant, which suggests an atypical distribution of the electric field. **B:** The same subject as in part *A* recorded 1 day later with a sagittal montage. P$\overline{100}$ is located caudally at the level of the inion, and its latency is normal for this laboratory. The transition zone between P$\overline{100}$ and N$\overline{100}$ is located near MO and Oz, producing small and aberrant waveforms at those sites.

atic agents. Patients who use glasses should try viewing the pattern with and without them and should be tested under the condition in which the image is clearest.

Attention

A PVEP will not be recorded unless the subject is awake and concentrating on the stimulus. Amplitude and latency can be altered substantially if the subject's gaze is allowed to wander around the room, if there is excessive blinking, or if various extracerebral artifacts are generated (178). Unfortu-

nately, other patient variables, more difficult to monitor, may also have an appreciable effect on PVEP amplitude and latency. The difference between relaxed and highly alert states can produce latency differences as large as 11 milliseconds in one eye in the same subject (44). Volunteers using maneuvers such as meditation (Fig. 27.11) and convergence with one eye covered (Fig. 27.12) have been able to abolish the PVEP or alter its latency by up to 15 milliseconds without detection by an attentive technician (27). Similar volitional changes have been demonstrated with different types of pattern stimuli in other laboratories (115,169). These effects may be reduced by the use of larger stimulus fields, larger checks, and binocular testing (169).

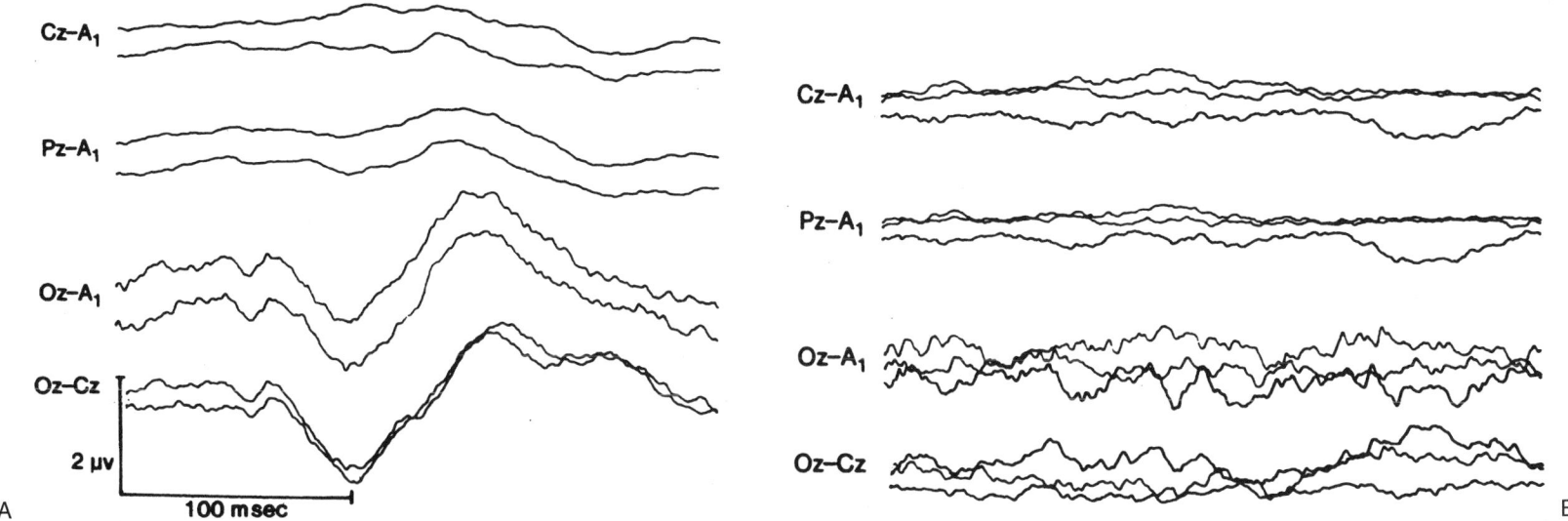

FIG. 27.11. A: Normal pattern visual evoked potential (PVEP) when the subject is attending to the stimulus, which is a light-emitting diode pattern generator with checks measuring 50 minutes of arc, 5-degree field, and maximum luminance of 100 cd per square meter. **B:** Apparently absent PVEP with the same subject performing transcendental meditation under otherwise identical conditions. Cooperation appeared good to the technician. (From Bumgartner J, Epstein C. Voluntary alteration of visual evoked potentials. *Ann Neurol* 1982;12:475–478.)

Only a minority of volunteers have been able to alter their PVEPs surreptitiously without special coaching. However, the PVEP is commonly used to evaluate patients suspected of hysterical visual loss or malingering. Such patients often exhibit unusual difficulty in maintaining fixation on the pattern and repeatedly allow the eye to close unless it is held open by the technician. How many are capable of more sophisticated manipulation is impossible to determine. In general, low-amplitude, absent, or even mildly delayed responses in this setting should be interpreted with caution.

Gender

In large series, women consistently show average latencies that are a few milliseconds shorter than those of men (43,163). In some studies, women have, on average, higher-amplitude PVEPs (43,45). This difference is greater with checks smaller than 30 minutes of arc (52).

Age

It can be difficult to test PVEPs in children until they are a few years old, although with checks of 30 minutes of arc or larger, latencies appear to reach adult values by the age of 20 weeks (158). Latencies for all check sizes are at adult values by the age of 5 years (45,158) and show no significant change from then until about age 40. Many normative studies have yielded conflicting results concerning the nature and degree of latency changes in healthy middle-aged and elderly persons. Some of these discrepant results have been clarified with the discovery that aging effects are dependent on both check size and luminance. Latency rises most rapidly with age with the use of smaller checks (37,159) and decreased luminance (148); these effects appear to be unrelated to pupil size (37,159). They can be minimized by the use of checks of 30 minutes of arc or larger and a luminance of 50 cd per square meter or greater. Otherwise, normative data should be calculated separately for older subjects.

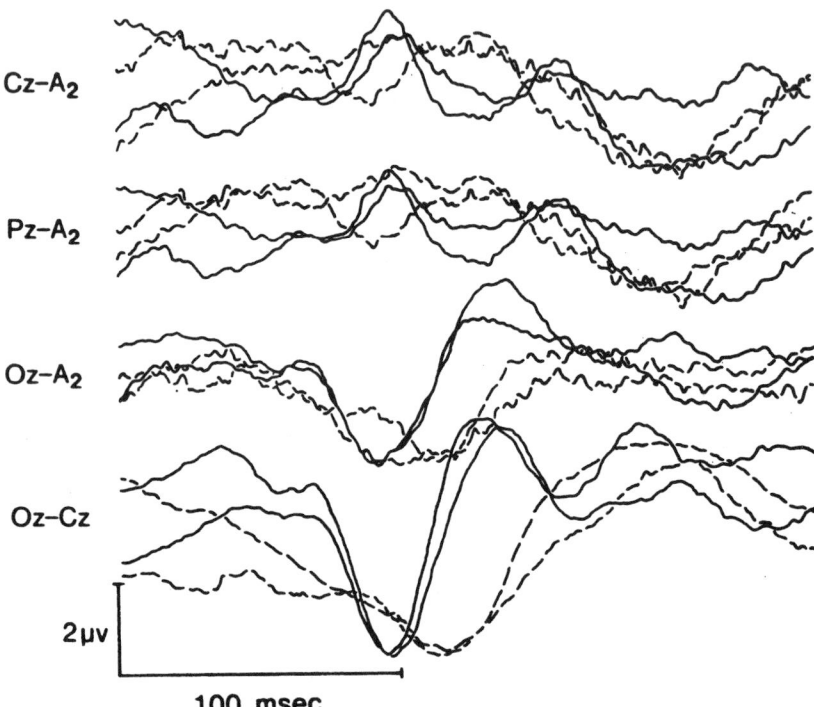

FIG. 27.12. *Solid lines:* normal PVEP with the subject attending to the stimulus, which is a video pattern generator with 21' checks, 10° field. *Dashed lines:* same eye, same subject performing forced convergence with one eye covered. The apparent latency difference is 15 msec. The maneuver was inapparent to the technician. (From Bumgartner J, Epstein C. Voluntary alteration of visual evoked potentials. *Ann Neurol* 1982;12:475–478.)

Pupils

Large pupillary asymmetries can change the amount of light reaching the two retinae by one logarithmic unit or more, and they can alter PVEP latencies by more than 10 milliseconds. Meiotics and cataracts can have similar effects. Pupil size should be noted by the technician and should be considered in evaluating small latency asymmetries.

NEUROLOGICAL APPLICATIONS OF VISUAL EVOKED POTENTIALS

The neurological utility of PVEPs is dependent on two properties: (a) their exquisite sensitivity to subtle lesions of the visual pathways, especially the optic nerve and chiasm, and (b) their relative *insensitivity* to alterations in visual acuity from ophthalmological disorders. Many studies have demonstrated that prolonged $P\overline{100}$ latencies occur without detectable alteration in acuity (71,72), contrast sensitivity (23,117,146), pupillary reactivity, color desaturation, funduscopy, or perimetry (26). Conversely, it is extremely rare for clinical examination to show *any* abnormality of the anterior visual pathways when the PVEP is normal (26). If visual acuity is decreased but the PVEP is normal, a lesion of the optic nerve or chiasm is very unlikely to be the etiology. Figures 27.13 to 27.15 illustrate mild, moderate, and marked latency increases, respectively, for $P\overline{100}$ after full-field monocular stimulation. Although neither these nor any other PVEP abnor-

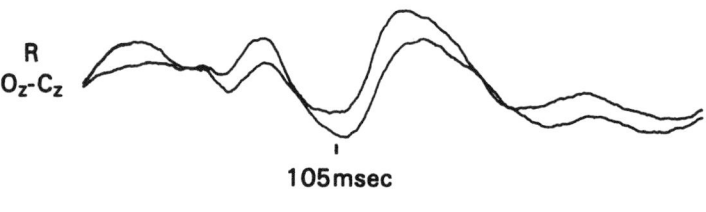

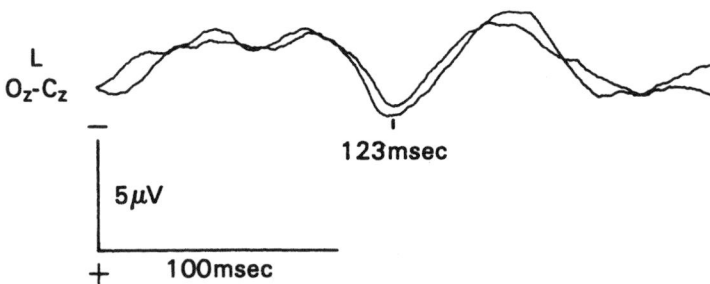

FIG. 27.13. Normal pattern visual evoked potential from right eye, and mild absolute latency prolongation from left eye, recorded as in Fig. 27.5 (99% tolerance limit, 120 milliseconds). In contrast to absolute latency, the interocular latency difference is markedly abnormal.

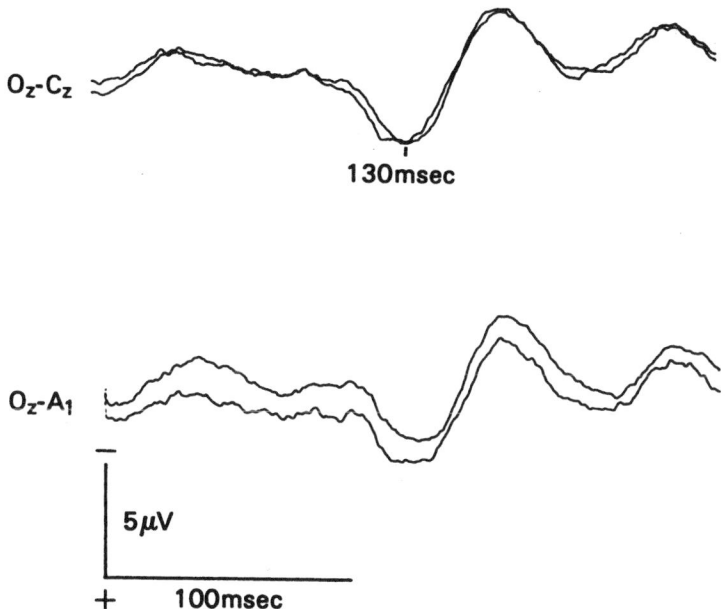

FIG. 27.14. Moderate midline latency prolongation in vertex and ear-reference derivations.

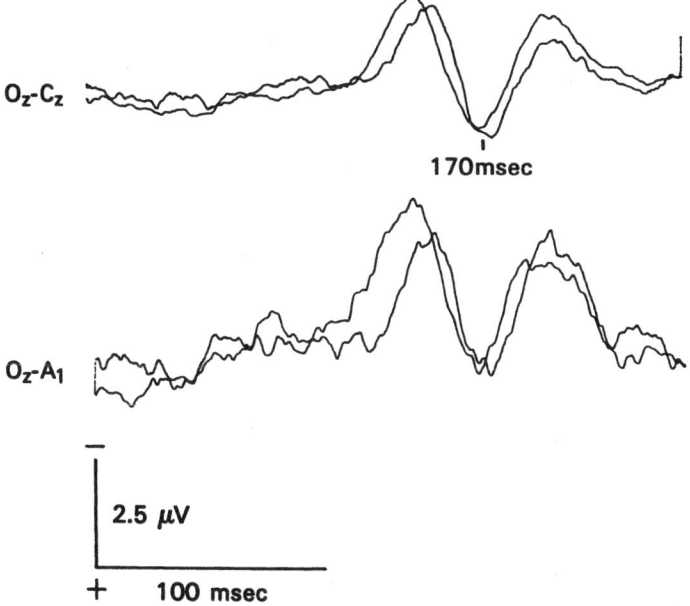

FIG. 27.15. Marked midline latency prolongation.

malities are pathognomonic for one disorder, marked latency prolongation with preservation of $\overline{\text{P100}}$ amplitude is most characteristic of optic nerve demyelination.

Optic Neuritis and Multiple Sclerosis

Screening for asymptomatic lesions in multiple sclerosis is the most common clinical indication for PVEPs. A prolonged PVEP latency is the electrical equivalent of a pale optic disk with a Marcus Gunn pupil, and this helps to document the dissemination in space that is necessary for a diagnosis.

Across many studies on several continents, approximately 90% of patients with an unequivocal history of optic neuritis have abnormalities of the PVEP (8,29,41,71). During an acute attack, the proportion of patients with unobtainable PVEPs or prolonged $\overline{\text{P100}}$ latencies approaches 100%. In most, latency abnormalities persist for many years, even after recovery of normal acuity.

In 1983, Chiappa (41) reviewed 26 clinical series involving nearly 2,000 patients with possible, probable, or definite multiple sclerosis. Overall, PVEP abnormalities were present in 37%, 58%, and 85%, respectively. Among 774 patients without clinical or historical evidence of optic neuritis, 54% had abnormal PVEPs, the majority of which were latency prolongations. Later series (55,84,112,121,126) documented a similar yield and a superior detection rate for asymptomatic lesions, in comparison with those found for somatosensory evoked potentials (SEPs) and brainstem auditory evoked potentials (BAEPs) (55,84). The classic PVEP pattern in multiple sclerosis is a unilateral, marked prolongation of $\overline{\text{P100}}$ with relative preservation of amplitude (see Fig. 27.15). Such striking latency prolongations are unlikely to occur in other disorders; however, multiple sclerosis can commonly produce mildly prolonged PVEPs and their absence as well.

Many modifications have been proposed to increase the yield of PVEP abnormalities in demyelinating disorders. These include hyperventilation (47), decreased field size (32,78,118), smaller checks (121,126), LEDs (6), decreased luminance (29), red/black patterns (118), pattern onset stimulus

(4), hemifield stimulation (121,144), multiple orientations of gratings (28), and Fourier analysis (35). Hyperthermia has been tried as a provocative test; it usually decreases PVEP amplitudes both in normal subjects and in patients with multiple sclerosis but has no effect on latency (104,181). Addition of pattern ERG may help in clarifying the pathophysiological processes of abnormal PVEPs in multiple sclerosis but does not much affect the yield (36).

It is not possible to use all of these additional techniques simultaneously or sequentially in every patient. Some techniques, such as small check or field size and hemifield stimulation, are mutually exclusive. Patient tolerance and the need for multiple additional control studies also limit the number of variations that can be tried in a single subject before PVEPs deteriorate (155). A general screen for patients of varying age, acuity, and cooperation might incorporate full-field testing with checks 50 minutes of arc across and high luminance (at least 50 cd per square meter). For these conditions, a series of 20 to 30 normal controls is adequate. A higher sensitivity approach to cooperative patients with good acuity could involve a full-field pattern with low luminance (less than 40 cd per square meter) (29), small field size, and small checks, followed by hemifield testing. The latter approach would generate a higher yield of VEP abnormalities. It would also be expected to produce a higher percentage of false-positive results and to require a much larger control group compensated for age.

The widespread availability of magnetic resonance imaging (MRI) has modified the indications for evoked potentials (55,60,130). However, in one series (55), six of 11 patients with suspected multiple sclerosis and normal MRIs had abnormal PVEPs, and four of those six had cerebrospinal fluid immunoglobulin abnormalities. Conventional MRI is relatively insensitive to lesions of the optic nerve. Even with special techniques, MRI is less sensitive and less cost effective than PVEPs for detecting optic nerve lesions (111). Thus, the PVEP remains useful as an index of disease progression or improvement in clinical trials for treatment of multiple sclerosis (50,61,124).

Evoked potentials and especially MRI have influenced the criteria for diagnosis of multiple sclerosis, which include dissemination in time as well as in space. Multiple central nervous system lesions at the time of presentation increase the likelihood of progression to multiple sclerosis. However, the presence of other lesions accompanying optic neuritis may be a consequence of acute disseminated leukoencephalitis (130), vasculitis, or other multifocal disorders. A specific diagnosis will still depend on changes over time and on clinical judgment as well as on high technology. With the large number of neurophysiological, radiological, and immunological techniques now available to assist in the diagnosis of multiple sclerosis, clinical skills remain important in choosing and interpreting procedures efficiently and effectively.

Other Neurological Disorders

Diseases of the Optic Nerve

Anterior ischemic optic neuropathy is a common disorder of later life, often associated with temporal arteritis and other forms of vasculitis, tertiary syphilis and other infections, arteriosclerosis, or migraine. Thompson et al. (173) found that the PVEP was abnormal in all cases of ischemic optic neuropathy studied within 2 weeks of onset, as well as in 10 of 12 eyes studied more than 2 months later. Although the $P\overline{100}$ often appeared bifid or delayed, these investigators reported that detailed partial-field analysis showed the true pathophysiological process to be an alteration in PVEP topography resulting from macular field defects. PVEPs are absent or show mild latency increases in almost all cases of Leber's hereditary optic atrophy, but only subtle changes are found in presumed asymptomatic carriers (33).

Optic atrophy occasionally accompanies peripheral neuropathies, and PVEP latency prolongations have been reported in Charcot-Marie-Tooth disease (107,167), giant axonal neuropathy (101), and neuropathy associated with macroglobulinemia (10).

Increased intracranial pressure can produce papilledema and visual loss, and so it is not surprising that $P\overline{100}$ latency changes have been reported with hydrocephalus (49,150) and pseudotumor cerebri (164), although such abnormalities are not particularly frequent.

Sarcoidosis has multiple central nervous system and ocular manifestations, including optic neuropathy. Streletz et al. (166) studied PVEPs in 50 patients with systemic sarcoidosis. Abnormalities of latency and amplitude were found in all four patients with clinical brain involvement, as well as in seven of 29 who had no clinical evidence of ocular or neurological disease.

A variety of toxins may produce clinical or subclinical effects on the optic nerve. PVEPs have been used to monitor therapy with ethambutol (182), cisplatin (99), and deferoxamine (172). Latency prolongations have been described with quinine toxicity (59) and nitrous oxide toxicity (79). $P\overline{100}$ delays are reported in patients with chronic alcoholism (39). PVEPs are uniformly absent or delayed in patients with tobacco-alcohol amblyopia (92). In most of these conditions, improvement has occurred after discontinuation of therapy or after abstinence; no significant $P\overline{100}$ latency prolongation was found in a carefully studied group of abstinent alcoholics (51) One patient who was transiently blind as a result of quinine toxicity had prolonged latencies after recovery (59).

Tumors

Most patients with extrinsic compression of the optic nerve or chiasm have abnormal PVEPs (63,70,80,128). In general, such lesions are expressed by a decrease in amplitude and by relatively modest prolongations in latency. In cases of pituitary adenoma, PVEPs may improve the serial assessment of visual function (80).

Leukodystrophies and Spinocerebellar Disorders

PVEPs are usually abnormal in central nervous system disorders that involve central myelin. Adrenoleukodystrophy, Pelizaeus-Merzbacher disease, and metachromatic leukodystrophy prolong PVEP latency (7,31,102, 103) and may produce abnormalities in presymptomatic affected children (102). The site of the responsible lesion is not clear, given the predilection of these disorders for the cerebral hemispheres. Prolonged latencies have been found in various proportions of patients with Friedreich's and other inherited ataxias (15,32,123,131), familial spastic paraparesis (15,75,131), tropical spastic paraparesis (8), subacute combined degeneration (vitamin B_{12} deficiency) (93), and vitamin E deficiency (86,109). Latency prolongation in this group of disorders is usually symmetrical. Abnormalities resulting from vitamin E and B_{12} deficiency may improve with treatment (86,93,109). Except for the early childhood leukodystrophies, all of these conditions share clinical features with multiple sclerosis, and abnormal evoked potentials should not be overinterpreted as proof of a specific disorder.

Miscellaneous Central Nervous System Disorders

PVEPs are delayed and "desynchronized" in cerebrotendinous xanthomatosis, and they improve after treatment with chenodiol (114). PVEP latencies were prolonged in a patient who suffered decompensation of phenylketonuria in adulthood (105).

PVEP abnormalities have also been found in central nervous system disorders whose major clinical and pathological features lie *outside* the sensory pathways. $P\overline{100}$ latency was delayed in three of eight patients with neurological involvement from Wilson's disease (42), as well as in patients with

idiopathic Parkinson's disease (24). The changes in Parkinson's disease have been correlated with abnormalities of the ERG and have been ascribed to involvement of dopaminergic amacrine cells in the retina (64). However, the nature and existence of PVEP abnormalities in Parkinson's disease have been disputed by several other laboratories. Tartaglione et al. (171) reported that they occurred with sine-wave gratings of 2 cycles per degree but not with checks of 55 minutes of arc. In contrast, Bhaskar et al. (14) found that prolonged latencies occurred with both gratings and checks but that improvement after L-dopa treatment occurred only with checks. Because PVEPs have little practical application in the diagnosis of Parkinson's disease, prudent interpreters might choose to select test conditions that are *less* likely to be affected by it.

As with SEPs and conventional photic stimulation, PVEPs of unusually high amplitude occur in familial myoclonic epilepsies (69,142). Although otherwise nonspecific, this trait has proved to be useful within a large pedigree in screening for mild or asymptomatic mitochondrial encephalomyopathy (Fig. 27.16). VEP latency increases are also described in photosensitive epilepsies (108).

Both flash and pattern VEPs have been studied in patients with Alzheimer's disease and other dementias, with varying results. Changes in $P\overline{100}$ latency seem to be minimal (83) or nonexistent (76). In comparison

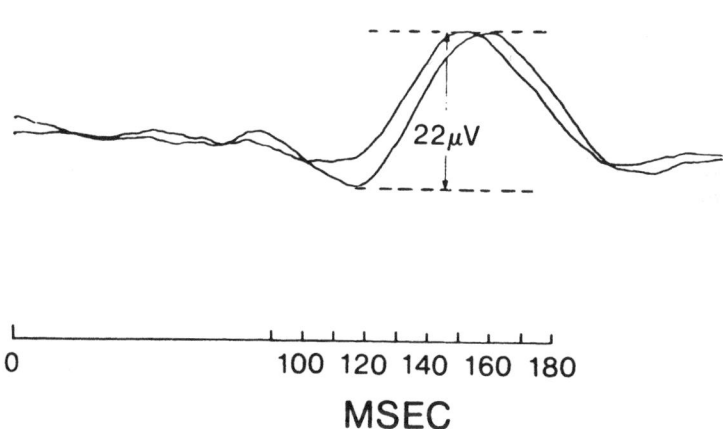

FIG. 27.16. Very high amplitude N$\overline{145}$ and waveform variability in an asymptomatic carrier of mitochondrial encephalomyopathy. (From Rosing H, Hopkins L, Wallace D, et al. Maternally inherited mitochondrial myopathy and myoclonic epilepsy. *Ann Neurol* 1985;17:228–237.)

with appropriate-aged controls, demented subjects have been reported to show latency prolongation in the late components of the PVEP ($\overline{N145}$ and after) (83), as well as in some components of the flash VEP (FVEP) (76). Similar changes have been described with anticholinergics in normal subjects (9,138). Group differences were shown in Alzheimer's patients with the use of steady-state stimulation and Fourier analysis of frequencies from 15 to 30 Hz (174). These changes are not a consequence of diminished attention (83). However, because the affected components of the VEP are present less reliably than $\overline{P100}$ and are more variable, the applicability of VEPs to individual cases of dementia is uncertain.

Migraine has been accompanied by increased high-frequency photic following on EEG (125,154), by increased oscillatory wave amplitude of the PVEP 250 to 500 milliseconds after a flash or pattern stimulus (see Fig. 27.5) (116), and by hemifield changes that are said to match the visual aura (168). However, the specificity and clinical utility of these changes have been disputed (179,180).

Visual Evoked Potentials in Coma

VEPs have been used in conjunction with SEPs and BAEPs to assess disability and attempt prognosis in prolonged coma, usually after closed-head trauma. In most published studies, the stimulus has been a stroboscopic flash, and the ERG has been monitored to verify retinal function. In some series, the FVEPs have been graded by overall configuration rather than by latencies and amplitudes (65), making comparisons among reports difficult. Anderson et al. (5) found that severely abnormal VEPs were accurately predictive of an unfavorable outcome after closed-head trauma. However, normal VEPs did not reliably predict a favorable result, and VEPs did not improve prognostic accuracy beyond that obtained with SEPs alone. Rappaport et al. (135,136) reported that in patients with head injury, the FVEP had a correlation of only 0.24 with disability ratings performed 1 year later. Pfurtscheller et al. (132) had difficulty making any correlation between VEPs and outcome. Gupta et al. (66) studied patients 6 to 24 months after head injury, when they had recovered consciousness and were able to cooperate for PVEPs. Abnormal PVEPs were present in one-third of all patients, as well as in half of those with severe residual cognitive impairment.

In most series, absence of the FVEP (with preserved ERG) appeared to be an accurate predictor of severe disability or death after closed-head trauma. However, a robust flash response is not predictive of recovery.

Visual Evoked Potentials in the Operating Room

Because the PVEP is sensitive to lesions of the optic nerve and chiasm, it has been employed intraoperatively to monitor surgical procedures that might endanger these structures. Unfortunately, the middle-latency PVEP is much more affected by level of consciousness, anesthesia (40,147,153, 177), and hypothermia (140,145) than are short-latency SEPs and BAEPs. Because of the difficulty in presenting true pattern reversal stimuli to the eyes of anesthetized patients, the typical stimulus is a flash from a strobe or from red LEDs mounted in small goggles, delivered through closed eyelids. The resulting evoked potentials are extremely labile, with a high incidence of false-positive changes that detracts from their utility (34,137). Harding et al. found that a combination of enflurane and nitrous oxide had minimal effect on VEPs and that disappearance of a previously normal VEP for more than 4 minutes correlated significantly with postoperative visual loss. Intraoperative evoked potentials are discussed more extensively in Chapter 31.

OPHTHALMOLOGICAL APPLICATIONS OF VISUAL EVOKED POTENTIALS

Visual Acuity

The most common applications of VEPs are chosen largely for their *lack* of correlation with visual acuity and ophthalmological disease. However, checkerboard patterns or gratings with sufficiently small elements can be used to estimate acuity comparable to the Snellen eye chart. Psychophysiological studies in adults indicate that reasonably accurate estimates can be made by plotting PVEP amplitude against spatial frequency for patterns of several different sizes. Amplitudes are then extrapolated to zero, which corresponds approximately to threshold for detection of the pattern (120,156). Sokol (156) used transient PVEPs from checkerboard patterns to determine visual acuity in infancy. He estimated acuities of 20/150 at 2 months of age, improving to 20/20 by age 6 months.

Much more rapid estimates of PVEP amplitude can be obtained with steady-state stimuli (i.e., rapid pattern reversal at 10 to 20 Hz) and signal analysis techniques such as the Fourier transform (54,170) (Fig. 27.17). Using a total test duration of 10 seconds, Norcia and Tyler (120) estimated an acuity of 4.5 cycles per degree in the first month of life; adult values of 20 cycles per degree were reached by the age of 8 months.

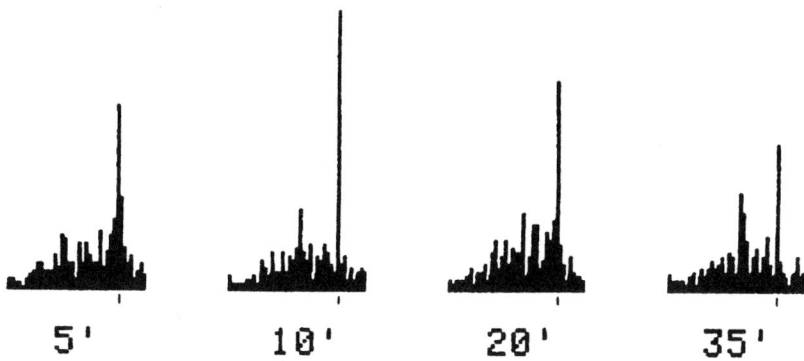

5'   10'   20'   35'

FIG. 27.17. Magnitude spectra obtained from Fourier transforms of steady-state visual evoked potentials, using four consecutive sets of patterns reversing at 15 per second with checks of the indicated dimensions. The histograms cover the range from 0.45 to 18.75 Hz, and the prominent 15-Hz peaks are indicated with tick marks at the bottom of each histogram. The patient, a 6-year-old boy, had normal acuity, and the checks measuring 10 minutes of arc are near the peak of his contrast sensitivity curve. Total recording time was 8.5 seconds. (From Epstein C, Gammon A, Gemmill M, et al. Visual evoked potential pattern generation, recording, and data analysis with a single microcomputer. *Electroencephalogr Clin Neurophysiol* 1984;56:691–693.)

Hysteria and Malingering

Hysterical visual loss or exaggeration of a mild impairment are common problems in neuro-ophthalmology and are frequent sources of referral to the VEP laboratory. Although good cooperation may be difficult to obtain in these patients, technically adequate PVEPs allow some useful conclusions. A normal P$\overline{100}$ latency makes lesions of the optic nerve or anterior chiasm very unlikely as the cause of subjective visual loss. A well-defined response to checks of 10 minutes of arc indicates essentially normal acuity, and a good response to checks of 45 minutes of arc or smaller indicates vision of 20/200 or better (41). Long-latency PVEPs have also been used to document responses to stimuli that patients say they are unable to see (176). However, normal PVEPs do *not* rule out retrochiasmatic visual field defects, especially with full-field stimulation and recording at the occipital midline. Very rare patients with complete cortical blindness have recordable PVEPs when an island of striate cortex is spared by extensive parieto-occipital lesions (21). In general, such cases are easily identified by neurological and radiological evaluation.

As discussed in the section on patient factors, abolition of the PVEP (and even mild degrees of latency prolongation) may be accomplished volitionally by some subjects despite apparently good cooperation (27). In suspect situations, such findings should be assessed with caution before they are interpreted as proof of organic disease.

Amblyopia

With small checks or gratings, amblyopia ex anopsia in children is characterized by decreased amplitude and, occasionally, increased latency of PVEPs. Friendly et al. (57) used reversing checks of 15 minutes of arc on edge and were able to identify the amblyopic eye correctly in 22 of 27 children. They also misclassified one of four normal subjects as amblyopic. Sokol et al. (157) found that PVEPs with checks of 15 minutes of arc had a sensitivity of 96% when the acuity difference between eyes was three lines or more on a Snellen chart. However, sensitivity fell to 50% with a two-line acuity difference, and with a one-line difference, it was only 30%. The magnitude of amplitude asymmetry in amblyopic subjects correlated poorly with the asymmetry in acuity on the Snellen chart.

Glaucoma

PVEP latencies were abnormal at the occipital midline in a little over half of all eyes with glaucomatous field defects (30,175), but in less than one-quarter of those with ocular hypertension (175). Surprisingly, latency prolongation was most likely to be found with checks of 48 minutes of arc rather than with smaller checks of 12 minutes. Transient PVEPs were less sensitive than steady-state PVEPs at 7.5 alternations per second. Increased PVEP latency was associated with visible cupping and pallor of the optic disk.

Retinopathies

Central serous retinopathy is important in the differential diagnosis of optic neuritis. It often produces similar symptoms of central scotoma and decreased acuity, and it commonly produces PVEP delays. Papakostopoulos et al. (129) reported that in six patients with central serous retinopathy, PVEP latencies averaged 7 milliseconds longer in the affected eye. Sherman et al. (151) found significantly increased latencies in nine of ten involved eyes. In comparison with the normal eye, the mean delay was 10.6 milliseconds with checks of 56 minutes of arc and 21 milliseconds with checks of

14 minutes. One subject showed a latency difference of 43 milliseconds. Amplitudes were affected less than latencies, further mimicking PVEP changes seen in demyelinating disorders. Kraushar and Miller (90) reported on three patients in whom ophthalmologists mistook central serous retinopathy for evidence of multiple sclerosis. The retinal disorder most often improves spontaneously, and, in contrast to the usual outcome in optic neuritis, PVEP abnormalities generally remit with it.

PVEP delays have been reported with a variety of other acute and chronic retinal disorders (22,97). Because similar latency delays can be produced by retinal diseases and by optic neuritis, complete ophthalmological examination is *mandatory* in patients with symptomatic, nonhomonymous visual loss, regardless of PVEP findings.

PARTIAL-FIELD STIMULATION

The VEP after full-field pattern stimulation represents the sum of multiple components arising from both hemispheres and from both upper and lower quadrants (Fig. 27.18A). Its apparent simplicity is deceptive: The true complexity of the PVEP can be appreciated—and clinically used—only when portions of the visual field are stimulated selectively.

As previously noted, wide-angle pattern stimulation of either hemifield produces a net VEP vector that tends to point obliquely back through the opposite hemisphere. Thus, as implied by the direction of the arrow in Fig. 27.1, P$\overline{100}$ is most often maximal ipsilateral to the stimulus rather than contralaterally over the active occipital lobe (20,95,152). In addition to occipital electrodes LO and RO, hemifield studies require more lateral recording sites in the form of left and right temporal electrodes LT and RT, placed 5 cm lateral to LO and RO (3). With a circumferential array of five posterior electrodes referenced to a frontal site, normal subjects show an asymmetrical response across the temporal-occipital scalp. P$\overline{100}$ is recorded at the ipsilateral occipital lead, and a nearly simultaneous negative wave, N$\overline{105}$, appears at the contralateral temporal area (Fig. 27.18B) (11,16,67). N$\overline{105}$ is independent of the occipital P$\overline{100}$ and more variable; it arises from projections of the peripheral visual field rather than from the area of the macula (17,18,20,67). In about 50% of normal subjects, the lateral N$\overline{105}$ forms part of a full "PNP" complex, with surrounding P$\overline{75}$ and P$\overline{135}$ waves that roughly mirror the more familiar "NPN" waveform of the full-field response (67) (see Fig. 27.18B). The transition from NPN to PNP complexes usually occurs near the contralateral occipital lead.

If the peripheral retina is stimulated while central vision is occluded by a central scotoma, the contralateral N$\overline{105}$-P$\overline{135}$ complex is enhanced, whereas the ipsilateral P$\overline{100}$ is attenuated (Fig. 27.19) (17,18). The P$\overline{100}$ may disappear entirely with scotomata of 5 to 10 degrees. Under these circumstances, the enhanced N$\overline{105}$-P$\overline{135}$ complex may extend into midline and even ipsilateral leads, and it may be confused with a delayed P$\overline{100}$. If the absence of the true P$\overline{100}$ is not recognized, the preserved P$\overline{135}$ component will be misinterpreted as a latency prolongation. This is probably the mechanism for some apparent P$\overline{100}$ delays reported with macular disease (58) and partial central-field defects (173). In addition, the presence of a prominent P$\overline{75}$ component with the exaggerated P$\overline{135}$ may lead to a W-shaped waveform on full-field testing; this can then be misinterpreted as a bifid P$\overline{100}$ (85). Absence of a true P$\overline{100}$ can be confirmed directly by selective stimulation of the central field with a small field size (2 to 4 degrees) and small checks of 30 minutes of arc or less. Retinal disease—and, occasionally, central lesions—may delay one half-field response in comparison with the other in the same eye. (This is yet another explanation for some W-shaped responses seen on full-field testing.) Such cases can be resolved by testing each half-field separately.

The temporal-occipital asymmetries after hemifield stimulation are most reliably demonstrated with larger field sizes and larger checks than those that may be used for routine full-field testing. Small fields and checks emphasize contributions to the PVEP from the macular region, whereas they minimize input from peripheral elements that produce the N$\overline{105}$. Thus, hemifield testing is best performed with a relatively large stimulus field, extending at least 10 to 16 degrees from the midline, and with check sizes of at least 50 minutes of arc.

Accurate fixation and a consistent level of attention by the subject are even more crucial for partial-field recording than for full-field PVEPs. Partial-field studies produce the clearest results if visual fixation is maintained 1 to 2 degrees outside the edge of the reversing pattern, thereby preventing activation of uncrossed fiber systems in the fovea (98). If patterns occupying the right and left hemifields are reversed sequentially rather than together, the associated PVEPs can be sampled during a single average (143). This modification controls for changes in attention, and often improves the quality of hemifield recording (3).

Applications

Hemifield studies are more successful than full-field PVEPs for evaluating postchiasmatic visual field defects (19,68,94,100,128,139,165). A complete homonymous hemianopia characteristically results in decreased amplitude or complete loss of the response from the affected field (Fig. 27.20) (68,94,128), rather than increased latency (144). Because of the consider-

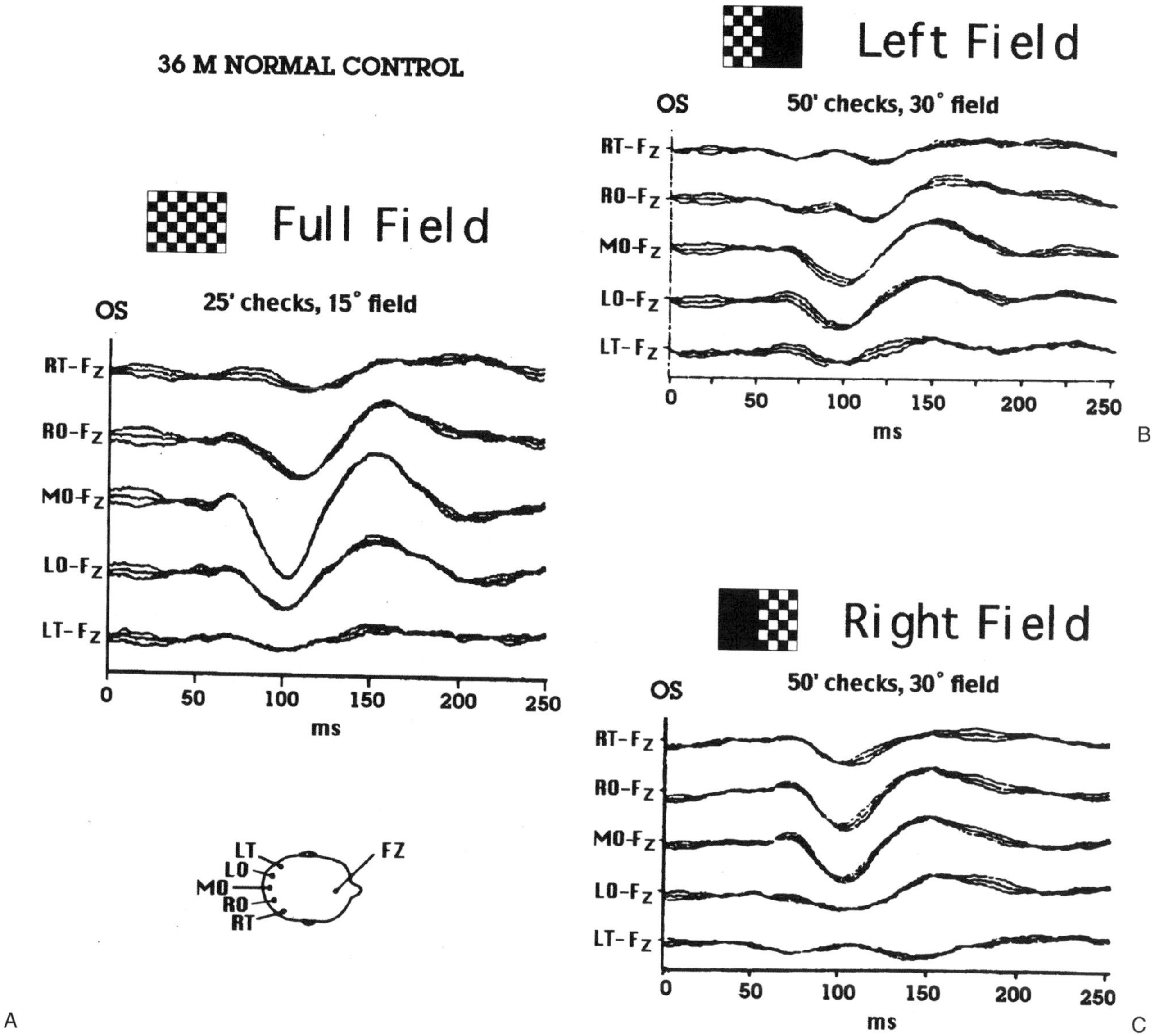

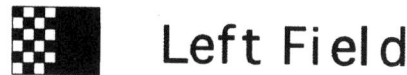

Left Field

OS 50' checks, 30° field

RT–F$_Z$
RO–F$_Z$
MO–F$_Z$
LO–F$_Z$
LT–F$_Z$

0   50   100   150   200   250
ms

B

Full Field

OS 25' checks, 15° field

RT–F$_Z$
RO–F$_Z$
MO–F$_Z$
LO–F$_Z$
LT–F$_Z$

0   50   100   150   200   250
ms

LT
LO
MO
RO
RT
FZ

Right Field

OS 50' checks, 30° field

RT–F$_Z$
RO–F$_Z$
MO–F$_Z$
LO–F$_Z$
LT–F$_Z$

0   50   100   150   200   250
ms

C

A

FIG. 27.18. Normal pattern visual evoked potentials from full-field and hemifield stimulation in a healthy control subject. **A:** The response to full-field stimulation is maximal at the midoccipital electrode and is symmetrical across the posterior temporal-occipital region. **B:** The response to stimulation of the left hemifield shows maximal positivity of P$\overline{100}$ at the midline and the ipsilateral occipital area (LO). The contralateral occipital (RO) and temporal (RT) electrodes register an almost synchronous negativity, N$\overline{105}$, surrounded by positive waves, P$\overline{75}$ and P$\overline{135}$. **C:** A complementary asymmetry is seen on right hemifield stimulation, although N$\overline{105}$ is visible only from the LT electrode. (Figure courtesy of T. A. Pedley.)

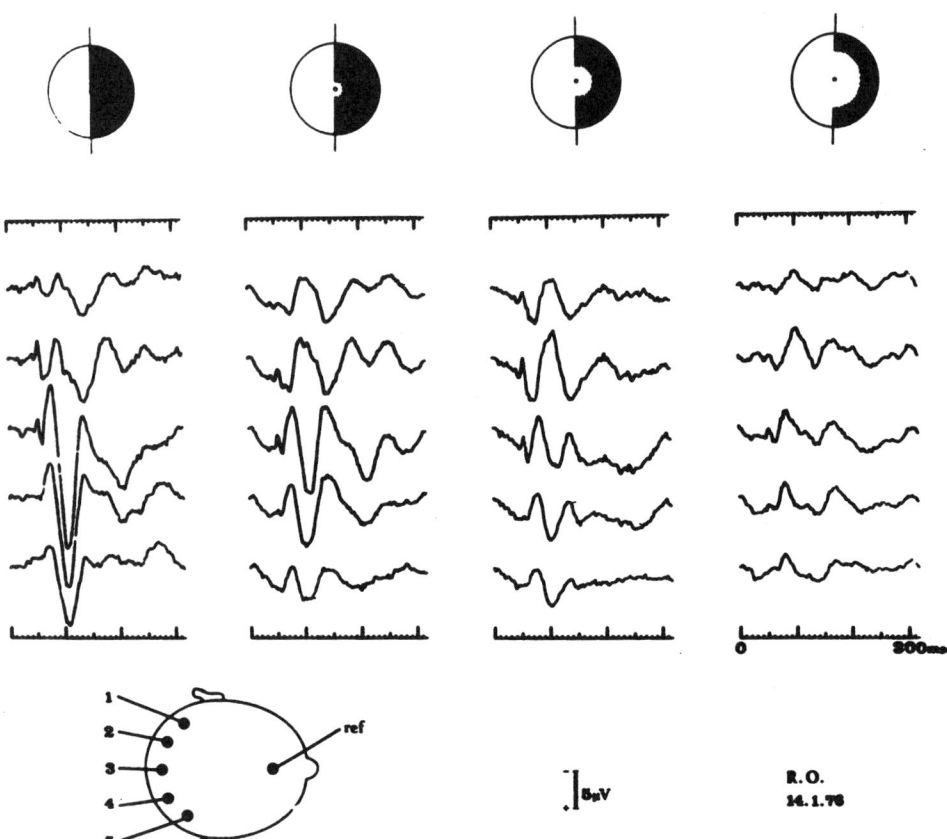

FIG. 27.19. The effect produced by a series of artificial central "scotomata" of increasing radii on the right half-field response in a single subject. The P100 is progressively attenuated, whereas the contralateral N105 is initially enhanced. Tracings from left to right show the complete half-field response, followed by responses with artificial scotomata of 2.5, 5.0, and 10.0 degrees in the central field. (From Blumhardt L, Barrett G, Halliday A, et al. The effect of experimental "scotomata" on the ipsilateral and contralateral responses to pattern-reversal in one half-field. *Electroencephalogr Clin Neurophysiol* 1978;45:376–392.)

able amplitude variability of hemifield responses in normal persons, it is best to interpret amplitude asymmetries conservatively. In laboratories with limited experience in recording half-field PVEPs, an abnormality should be identified only when the hemifield response is absent (68). In laboratories that have developed an adequate series of normative studies and recording experience, clinicians can interpret P100 amplitude asymmetries at the ipsilateral occipital electrode of greater than 3:1 as usually abnormal.

Hemifield latency asymmetries were rare in the reports of Blumhardt et al. (19) and Haimovic and Pedley (68), whose patients had destructive hemisphere lesions resulting from tumor, stroke, trauma, and surgery. Others (85,121,144), however, have reported more frequent half-field latency abnor-

malities in patients suspected of having multiple sclerosis or compressive lesions of the optic chiasm (25). In the latter studies, hemifield recording was also reported to increase the yield of abnormalities or improve analysis of aberrant PVEP waveforms; however, neurophysiological abnormalities were generally not correlated with visual field defects on conventional perimetry.

Unlike PVEPs from lateral hemifields, those from upper and lower fields are generally not symmetrical in normal persons and do not form mirror images above and below a midoccipital electrode. Instead, the full-field response reflects predominantly that from the lower field (96,110). Altitudinal PVEPs have not been widely used. Thus, although complete hemianopia can usually be identified, it has not been possible with partial-field PVEPs to

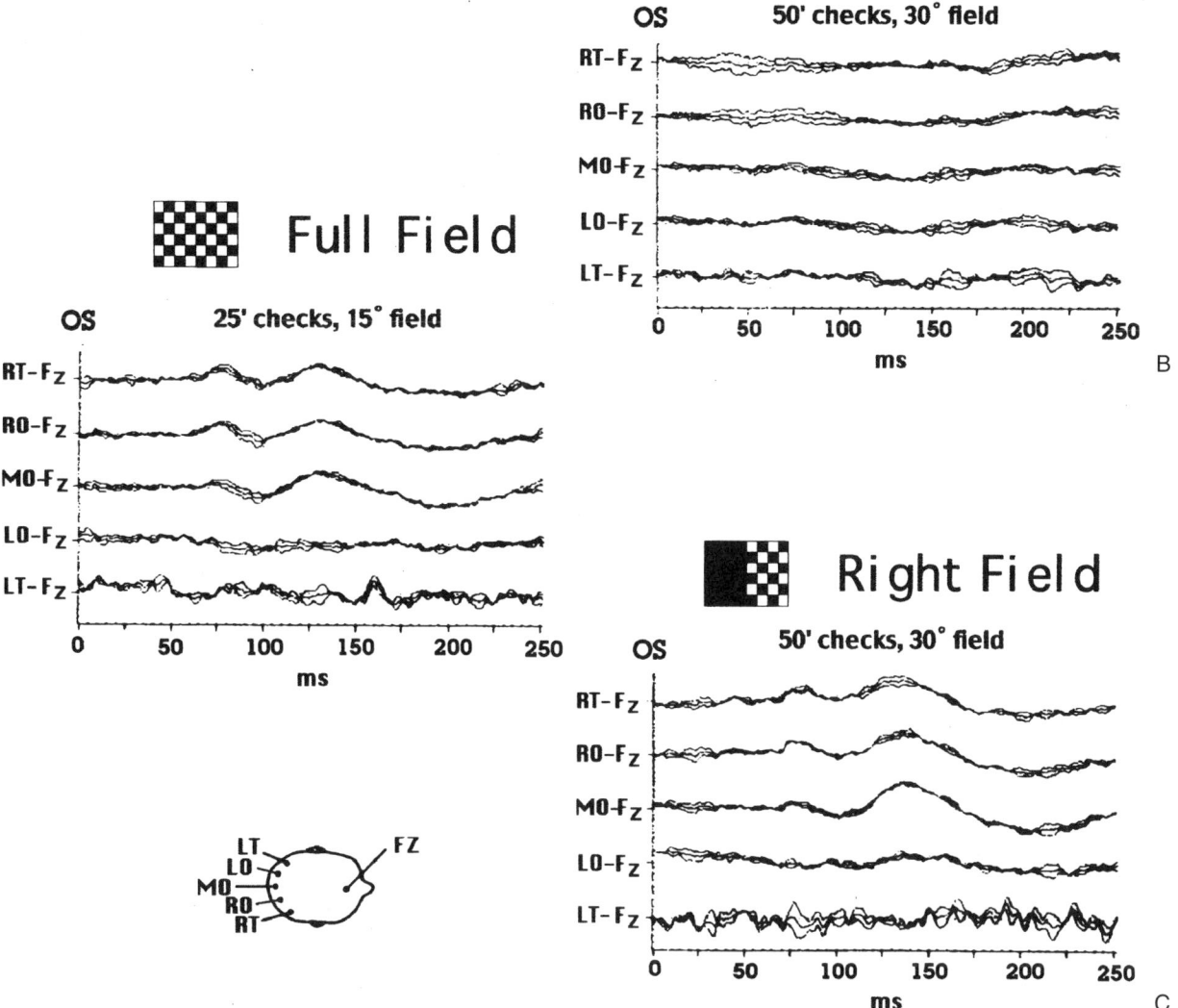

FIG. 27.20. Abnormal pattern visual evoked potentials (PVEPs) in a patient with complete left homonymous hemianopia after a right occipital lobe hemorrhage from an arteriovenous malformation. **A:** The full-field response demonstrates a "paradoxical" asymmetry with the P100 lateralized to the right of midline. **B:** Selective stimulation of the left hemifield elicits no discernible response. **C:** Stimulation of the intact right hemifield elicits a normal response, which is virtually identical to the PVEP after full-field stimulation. (Figure courtesy of T. A. Pedley.)

achieve the precise localization routinely obtained with skilled perimetry and neuro-ophthalmologic examination. Conventional PVEPs do not reliably detect changes involving much less than one hemifield or identify anatomical landmarks such as partial incongruity, Wilbrand's knee, and the loop of Meyer.

Steady-state VEP perimetry has been applied in the visual evoked spectral array (12,38), which delivers stimuli to all quadrants of the retina at slightly different frequencies. Unfortunately, the accuracy of testing with the visual evoked spectral array is restricted by the same factors that confound attempts at perimetry with transient VEPs. In cooperative and communicative patients, it cannot replace conventional visual field testing. In patients who cannot cooperate, results have limited clinical value.

FLASH VISUAL EVOKED POTENTIALS

FVEPs are familiar to electroencephalographers as the photic following (or "driving") response. Averaged FVEPs were studied for many years before evoked potentials came into use as a common clinical test. However, the anatomy, physiological features, and applications of FVEPs are quite different from those of the pattern-shift techniques that have largely superseded them.

The cortical response to flash stimuli is much more widespread, complex, and variable than that resulting from pattern shift. Comprehensive rules for interpretation have been difficult to formulate despite extensive studies (1,89), and none are offered here. The greater topographic complexity of FVEPs may be attributable, in part, to the effects of activating additional cortical projection systems. Before reaching the thalamus, one group of retinal axons leaves the optic tract and courses to the midbrain, synapsing in the pretectal area and superior colliculus. These fibers mediate the pupillary response to light, and they also generate an independent retinotopic field in the superior colliculus. Axons from the superior colliculus project to the pulvinar, which in turn projects to nonstriate areas of the occipital and parietal lobes. "Far-field" VEPs arising from the subcortical pathways have been much more difficult to record than the corresponding short-latency potentials for auditory and somatosensory systems. However, a few investigators using flash stimuli have identified an early oscillatory potential that appears to arise subcortically (46,133).

The great variability of FVEPs limits their utility, because it complicates the task of separating normal responses from abnormal ones. An apparently robust FVEP may occur even with cortical blindness (56). Thus, the ACNS Guidelines (3) advise that only the total absence of a flash response can be considered definitely abnormal. Although some authorities consider this recommendation excessively conservative, the difficulty in interpreting

FVEPs generally confines their clinical use to situations in which pattern stimulation is not feasible.

Applications

The FVEP can be recorded easily through closed eyelids and through all but the most dense ocular opacities (Fig. 27.21). It is unaffected by refractive errors. These properties make it useful in assessing function of the optic

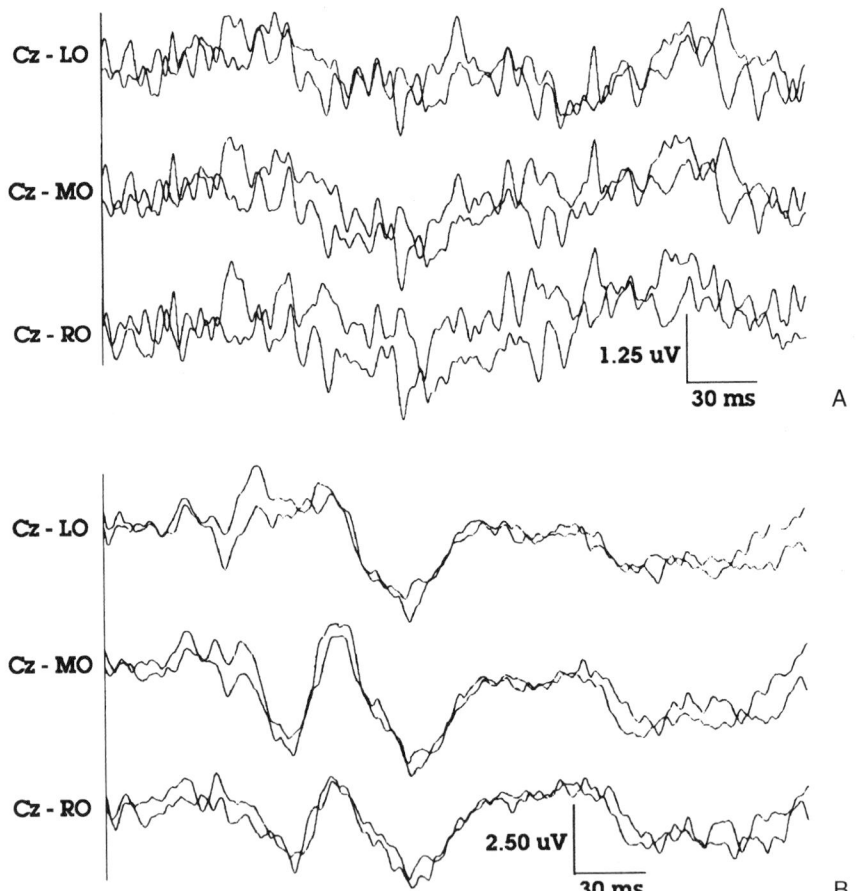

FIG. 27.21. Pattern visual evoked potential (PVEP) in a 68-year-old woman with dense cataracts. **A:** The PVEP is essentially absent, even with 1-degree checks. **B:** The flash visual evoked potential is robust and complex.

nerve and central visual pathways in patients with ocular scarring or hemorrhage. Preservation of a well-defined FVEP in these situations suggests that the visual pathways are at least partially intact, whereas its absence usually indicates that no useful visual function can be salvaged. Note, however, that stroboscopic flash units often produce an audible click with each flash; to prevent auditory evoked potentials from contaminating the FVEP, the subject may have to wear earphones that provide sound attenuation or white noise.

The wide topographic distribution of FVEPs has led to their use with computerized "brain mapping" systems, in which they are preferred over the spatially restricted PVEP. Topographic evoked potential analysis depends primarily on asymmetries between hemispheres, and such asymmetries have been shown to occur at the sites of brain tumors and other structural lesions (48). Amplitudes of FVEPs are increased focally in some children with benign rolandic epilepsy (48). Appropriately localized abnormalities were reported in almost 50% of patients with intractable focal seizures (122). However, such sophisticated computer analyses require at least as much skill as conventional EEG and evoked potentials; they have not gained wide acceptance in clinical medicine.

PATHOPHYSIOLOGY OF LATENCY PROLONGATION IN VISUAL EVOKED POTENTIALS

Because VEPs are sensitive to disorders of myelin, and because damage to the myelin sheath produces slowing of transmission, a decrease in optic nerve conduction velocity is commonly invoked as the cause of VEP latency prolongation in neurological disease. Quantitative calculations support the plausibility of this explanation (106). However, as noted previously, conduction through the optic nerve accounts for only a small fraction of the latency from stimulus onset to the peak of $\overline{P100}$; therefore, other possible mechanisms of latency prolongation must be considered as well. A fall in luminance increases the interpeak interval from $\overline{P50}$ to $\overline{P100}$, although both peaks appear to arise from the cortex (29). Simple refractive errors produce substantial delays with small pattern elements (159), presumably at a retinal level. The retinal response to pattern reversal may be delayed through damage to dopaminergic systems (24,64). Paracentral scotomata may displace the lateral PNP complex into the occipital midline, where $\overline{P135}$ has the appearance of a delayed $\overline{P100}$ (58,173). Retrochiasmatic demyelination may produce true half-field delays (144), although this mechanism has been more difficult to document rigorously. Thus, an apparent latency prolongation may occur at several different sites along the visual pathways. There remains a strong empirical correlation between optic nerve disease and a delayed $\overline{P100}$, but the interpreter must consider the localization, mechanism, and cause of VEP abnormalities separately in every case.

SUMMARY

Full-field PVEPs are exquisitely sensitive to lesions of the optic nerve and anterior chiasm. However, they may also be affected by a wide variety of other ophthalmological and neurological disorders, by patient factors, and by the choice of test conditions. The major benchmark of PVEP interpretation is the latency of $\overline{P100}$ at the occipital midline; normal values for this and other measurements must generally be established independently by each laboratory. Although check sizes of less than 30 minutes of arc may increase the sensitivity of the PVEP in some situations, a size between 30 and 50 minutes lessens the influence of confounding factors and simplifies the collection of normative data.

Retrochiasmatic lesions of the visual system are often not detected by full-field PVEP testing. Hemifield techniques increase the sensitivity of PVEPs to retrochiasmatic lesions, but their interpretation is more difficult and their precision does not match that of conventional visual field assessment.

REFERENCES

1. Allison T, Matsumiya Y, Goff G, et al. The scalp topography of human visual evoked potentials. *Electroencephalogr Clin Neurophysiol* 1977;42:185–197.
2. Amassian VE, Cracco RQ, Maccabee PJ, et al. Suppression of visual perception by magnetic coil stimulation of human occipital cortex. *Electroencephalogr Clin Neurophysiol* 1989;74:458–462.
3. American Electroencephalographic Society. Guidelines on evoked potentials. *J Clin Neurophysiol* 1994;11:40–73.
4. Aminoff M, Ochs A. Pattern-onset visual evoked potentials in suspected multiple sclerosis. *J Neurol Neurosurg Psychiat* 1981;44:608–614.
5. Anderson D, Bundlie S, Rockswold G. Multimodality evoked potentials in closed head trauma. *Arch Neurol* 1984;41:369–379.
6. Andersson T, Siden A. Comparison of visual evoked potentials elicited by light-emitting diodes and TV monitor stimulation in patients with multiple sclerosis and potentially related conditions. *Electroencephalogr Clin Neurophysiol* 1994;92:473–479.
7. Apkarian P, Koetsveld-Baart JC, Barth PG. Visual evoked potential characteristics and early diagnosis of Pelizaeus-Merzbacher disease. *Arch Neurol* 1993;50:981–985.
8. Asselman P, Chadwick D, Marsden C. Visual evoked responses in the diagnosis and management of patients suspected of multiple sclerosis. *Brain* 1975;98:261–282.
9. Bajalan AA, Wright CE, van der Vliet VJ. Changes in the human visual evoked potential caused by the anticholinergic agent hyoscine hydrobromide: comparison with results in Alzheimer's disease. *J Neurol Neurosurg Psychiat* 1986;49:175–182.
10. Barbieri S, Nobile-Orazio E, Baldini L, et al. Visual evoked potentials in patients with neuropathy and macroglobulinemia. *Ann Neurol* 1987;22:663–666.
11. Barrett G, Blumhardt L, Halliday A, et al. A paradox in the lateralisation of the visual evoked response. *Nature* 1976;261:253–255.

12. Baseler HA, Sutter EE, Klein SA, et al. The topography of visual evoked response properties across the visual field. *Electroencephalogr Clin Neurophysiol* 1994;90:65–81.

13. Benbadis SR, Lancman ME, Wolgamuth BR, et al. Value of full-field visual evoked potentials for retrochiasmal lesions. *J Clin Neurophysiol* 1996;13:507–510.

14. Bhaskar P, Vanchilingam S, Bhaskar E, et al. Effect of L-dopa on visual evoked potential in patients with Parkinson's disease. *Neurology* 36:119–121, 1986.

15. Bird T, Crill W. Pattern-reversal visual evoked potentials in the hereditary ataxias and spinal degenerations. *Ann Neurol* 1981;9:243–250.

16. Blumhardt L, Barrett G, Halliday A. The asymmetrical visual evoked potential to pattern-reversal in one half-field and its significance for the analysis of visual field defects. *Br J Ophthalmol* 1977;61:454–461.

17. Blumhardt L, Barrett G, Halliday A, et al. The contralateral negativity of the half-field response and its association with central scotomata. *Electroencephalogr Clin Neurophysiol* 1977;43:286P.

18. Blumhardt L, Barrett G, Halliday A, et al. The effect of experimental "scotomata" on the ipsilateral and contralateral responses to pattern-reversal in one half-field. *Electroencephalogr Clin Neurophysiol* 1978;45:376–392.

19. Blumhardt L, Barrett G, Kriss A, et al. The pattern-evoked potential in lesions of the posterior visual pathways. *Ann N Y Acad Sci* 1982;388:264–289.

20. Blumhardt L, Halliday A. Hemisphere contributions to the composition of the pattern-evoked potential waveform. *Exp Brain Res* 1979;36:53–69.

21. Bodis-Wollner I, Atkin A, Raab E, et al. Visual association cortex and vision in man: pattern-evoked potentials in a blind boy. *Science* 1977;198:629–631.

22. Bodis-Wollner I, Feldman R. Old perimacular pathology causes VEP delays in man. *Electroencephalogr Clin Neurophysiol* 1982;53:38P, 1982.

23. Bodis-Wollner I, Henley C, Mylin L, et al. Visual evoked potentials and the visuogram in multiple sclerosis. *Ann Neurol* 1979;5:40–47.

24. Bodis-Wollner I, Yahr M. Measurements of visual evoked potentials in Parkinson's disease. *Brain* 1978;101:661–671.

25. Brecelj J. A VEP study of the visual pathway function in compressive lesions of the optic chiasm. Full-field versus half-field stimulation. *Electroencephalogr Clin Neurophysiol* 1992;84:209–218.

26. Brooks E, Chiappa K. A comparison of clinical neuroopthalmological findings and pattern shift visual evoked potentials in multiple sclerosis. In: Courjon J, Mauguiere F, Revol M, eds. *Clinical applications of evoked responses in neurology.* New York: Raven Press, 1982:453–458.

27. Bumgartner J, Epstein C. Voluntary alteration of visual evoked potentials. *Ann Neurol* 1982;12:475–478.

28. Camisa J, Mylin L, Bodis-Wollner I. The effect of stimulus orientation on the visual evoked potential in multiple sclerosis. *Ann Neurol* 1981;10:532–539.

29. Cant B, Hume A, Shaw N. Effects of luminance on the pattern visual evoked potential in multiple sclerosis. *Electroencephalogr Clin Neurophysiol* 1978;45:496–504.

30. Cappin J, Nissim S. Pattern visual evoked response in the detection of field defects in glaucoma. *Arch Opthalmol* 1975;93:9–18.

31. Carlin L, Roach E, Riela A, et al. Juvenile metachromatic leukodystrophy: evoked potentials and computed tomography. *Ann Neurol* 1983;13:105–106.

32. Carroll W, Kriss A, Baraitser M, et al. The incidence and nature of visual pathway involvement in Friedreich's ataxia. *Brain* 1980;103:413–434.

33. Carroll W, Mastaglia S. Leber's optic neuropathy. A clinical and visual evoked potential study of affected asymptomatic members of a six generation family. *Brain* 1979;102:559–580.

34. Cedzich C, Schramm J, Fahlbusch R. Are flash-evoked potentials useful for intraoperative monitoring of visual pathway function? *Neurosurgery* 1987;21:709–715.

35. Celesia G, Brigell M, Gunnink R, et al. Spatial frequency evoked visuograms in multiple sclerosis. *Neurology* 1992;42:1067–1070.

36. Celesia G, Kaufman D, Cone S. Simultaneous recording of pattern electroretinography and visual evoked potentials in multiple sclerosis. *Arch Neurol* 1986;43:1247–1252.

37. Celesia G, Kaufman D, Cone S. Effects of age and sex on pattern electroretinograms and visual evoked potentials. *Electroencephalogr Clin Neurophysiol* 1978;68:161–171.

38. Celesia G, Meredith J, Pluff K. Perimetry, visual evoked potentials and visual evoked spectrum array in homonymous hemianopia. *Electroencephalogr Clin Neurophysiol* 1983;56:16–30.

39. Chan Y, McLeod J, Tuck R, et al. Visual evoked responses in chronic alcoholics. *J Neurol Neurosurg Psychiat* 1986;49:945–950.

40. Chi O, McCoy C, Field C. Effects of fentanyl anesthesia on visual evoked potentials in humans. *Anesthesiology* 1987;67:827–830.

41. Chiappa K. *Evoked potentials in clinical medicine,* 3rd ed. Philadelphia: Lippincott-Raven, 1997.

42. Chu N-S. Sensory evoked potentials in Wilson's disease. *Brain* 1986;109:491–507.

43. Chu N-S. Pattern-reversal visual evoked potentials: latency changes with gender and age. *Clin Electroencephalogr* 1987;18:159–162.

44. Cohen S, Syndulko K, Tourtellotte W, et al. Volitional manipulation of visual evoked potential latency. *Neurology* 1982;32:A209.

45. Cohn N, Kircher J, Emmerson R, et al. Pattern reversal evoked potentials: age, sex, and hemisphere asymmetry. *Electroencephalogr Clin Neurophysiol* 1985;62:399–405.

46. Cracco R, Cracco J. Visual evoked potential in man: Early oscillatory potentials. *Electroencephalogr Clin Neurophysiol* 1978;45:731–739.

47. Davies H, Carroll W, Mastaglia F. Effects of hyperventilation on pattern-reversal visual evoked potentials in patients with demyelination. *J Neurol Neurosurg Psychiat* 1986;49:1392–1396.

48. Duffy F. Topographic display of evoked potentials—clinical applications of brain electrical activity mapping (BEAM). *Ann N Y Acad Sci* 1982;388:183–196.

49. Ehle A, Sklar F. Visual evoked potentials in infants with hydrocephalus. *Neurology* 1979;29:1541–1544.

50. Emerson RG. Evoked potentials in clinical trials for multiple sclerosis. *J Clin Neurophysiol* 1998;15:109–116.

51. Emmerson RY, Dustman RE, Shearer DE, et al. EEG, visually evoked and event related potentials in young abstinent alcoholics. *Alcohol* 4:241–248, 1987.

52. Emmerson RY, Dustman RE, Shearer DE, et al. PREP amplitude of older women as a function of check size: visual system responsivity. *Electroencephalogr Clin Neurophysiol* 1987;69:88P.

53. Epstein C. True checkerboard pattern reversal with light-emitting diodes. *Electroencephalogr Clin Neurophysiol* 1979;47:611–613.

54. Epstein C, Gammon A, Gemmill M, et al. Visual evoked potential pattern generation, recording, and data analysis with a single microcomputer. *Electroencephalogr Clin Neurophysiol* 1984;56:691–693.

55. Farlow M, Markand O, Edwards M, et al. Multiple sclerosis: magnetic resonance imaging, evoked responses, and spinal fluid electrophoresis. *Neurology* 1986;36:828–831.

56. Frank Y, Torres F. Visual evoked potentials in the evaluation of "cortical blindness" in children. *Ann Neurol* 1979;6:126–129.

57. Friendly D, Weiss I, Barnet A, et al. Pattern-reversal visual-evoked potentials in the diagnosis of amblyopia in children. *Am J Ophthalmol* 1986;102:329–339.

58. Fukui R, Kato M, Kuroiwa Y. Effect of central scotomata on pattern reversal visual evoked potentials in patients with maculopathy and healthy subjects. *Electroencephalogr Clin Neurophysiol* 1986;63:317–326.

59. Gangitano J, Keltner J. Abnormalities of the pupil and visual-evoked potential in quinine amblyopia. *Am J Ophthalmol* 1980;89:425–430.

60. Giesser B, Kurtzberg D, Vaughan GJ, et al. Trimodal evoked potentials compared with magnetic resonance imaging in the diagnosis of multiple sclerosis. *Arch Neurol* 1987;44:281–84.

61. Gilmore RL, Kasarskis EJ, McAllister RG. Verapamil-induced changes in central conduction in patients with multiple sclerosis. *J Neurol Neurosurg Psychiat* 1985;48:1140–1146.

62. Godfrey K. Comparing the means of several groups. *N Engl J Med* 1985;313:1450–1456.

63. Gott P, Weiss M, Apuzzo M, et al. Checkerboard visual evoked potentials in evaluation and management of pituitary tumors. *Neurosurgery* 1979;5:553–558.

64. Gottlub I, Schneider E, Heider W, et al. Alteration of visual evoked potentials and electroretinograms in Parkinson's disease. *Electroencephalogr Clin Neurophysiol* 1987;66:349–57.

65. Greenberg R, Becker D, Miller J, et al. Evaluation of brain function in severe human head trauma with multimodality evoked potentials. Part 2: localization of brain dysfunction with posttraumatic neurological conditions. *J Neurosurg* 1977;47:163–177.

66. Gupta N, Verma N, Guidice M, et al. Visual evoked response in head trauma: pattern-shift stimulus. *Neurology* 1986;36:578–581.

67. Haimovic I, Pedley T. Hemi-field pattern reversal visual evoked potentials. I. Normal subjects. *Electroencephalogr Clin Neurophysiol* 1982;54:111–120.

68. Haimovic I, Pedley T. Hemi-field pattern reversal visual evoked potentials. II. Lesions of the chiasm and posterior visual pathways. *Electroencephalogr Clin Neurophysiol* 1982;54: 121–131.

69. Halliday A, Halliday E. Photosensitive epilepsy: the electroretinogram and visual evoked response. *Arch Neurol* 1969;20:191–198.

70. Halliday A, Halliday E, Kriss A, et al. The pattern-evoked potential in compression of the anterior visual pathways. *Brain* 1976;99:357–374.

71. Halliday A, McDonald W, Mushin J. Delayed pattern-evoked responses in optic neuritis in relation to visual acuity. *Trans Opthalmol Soc U K* 1973;93:315–324.

72. Halliday A, McDonald W, Mushin J. The visual evoked response in the diagnosis of multiple sclerosis. *BMJ* 1973;4:661–664.

73. Hammond E, Wilder B. Effect of gamma-vinyl GABA on human pattern evoked visual potentials. *Neurology* 1985;35:1801–1803.

74. Hammond S, MacCallum S, Yiannikas C, et al. Variability on serial testing of pattern reversal visual evoked potential latencies from full-field, half-field, and foveal stimulation in control subjects. *Electroencephalogr Clin Neurophysiol* 1987;66:401–408.

75. Happel L, Rothschild H, Garcia C. Visual evoked potentials in two forms of hereditary spastic paraplegia. *Electroencephalogr Clin Neurophysiol* 1980;48:233–236.

76. Harding G, Wright C, Orwin A. Primary presenile dementia: The use of the visual evoked potential as a diagnostic indicator. *Br J Psychiat* 1985;147:532–539.

77. Harding GF, Bland JD, Smith VH. Visual evoked potential monitoring of optic nerve function during surgery. *J Neurol Neurosurg Psychiat* 1990;53:890–895.

78. Hennerici M, Wenzel D, Freund H-J. The comparison of small-size rectangle and checkerboard stimulation for the evaluation of delayed visual evoked responses in patients suspected of multiple sclerosis. *Brain* 1977;100:119–136.

79. Heyer EJ, Simpson DM, Bodis-Wollner I, et al. Nitrous oxide: clinical and electrophysiologic investigation of neurologic complications. *Neurology* 1986;36:1618–1622.

80. Holder GE, Bullock PR. Visual evoked potentials in the assessment of patients with non-functioning chromophobe adenomas. *J Neurol Neurosurg Psychiat* 1989;52:31–37.

81. Horton JC. Wilbrand's knee of the primate optic chiasm is an artefact of monocular enucleation. *Trans Am Ophthalmol Soc* 1997;95:579–609.

82. Hubel D, Wiesel T. Receptive fields and functional architecture of monkey striate cortex. *J Physiol* 1968;195:215–243.

83. Huisman U, Posthuma J, Visser S, et al. The influence of attention on visual evoked potentials in normal adults and dementias. *Clin Neurol Neurosurg* 1987;89:151–156.

84. Javidan M, McLean D, Warren K. Cerebral evoked potentials in multiple sclerosis. *Can J Neurol Sci* 1986;13:240–244.

85. Jones D, Blume W. Aberrant waveforms to pattern reversal stimulation: Clinical significance and electrographic "solutions." *Electroencephalogr Clin Neurophysiol* 1985;61:472–481.

86. Kaplan P, Rawal K, Erwin C, et al. Visual and somatosensory evoked potentials in vitamin E deficiency with cystic fibrosis. *Electroencephalogr Clin Neurophysiol* 1988;71:226–272.

87. Kelly D. Pattern detection and the two-dimensional Fourier transform: flickering checkerboards and chromatic mechanisms. *Vision Res* 1975;16:277–287.

88. Kirby A, Wiley R, Harding T. Cholinergic effects on the visual evoked potential. In Cracco RQ, Bodis-Wollner I, eds. *Evoked potentials.* New York: Alan R. Liss, 1986:296–306.

89. Kooi K. *Visual evoked potentials in central disorders of the visual system.* Hagerstown, MD: Harper & Row, 1979.

90. Kraushar M, Miller E. Central serous choroidopathy misdiagnosed as a manifestation of multiple sclerosis. *Ann Ophthalmol* 1982;4:215–218.

91. Kraut M, Arezzo J, Vaughan HJ. Intracortical generators of the flash VEP in monkeys. *Electroencephalogr Clin Neurophysiol* 1985;62:300–312.

92. Kriss A, Carroll W, Blumhardt L, et al. Pattern and flash-evoked potential changes in toxic (nutritional) optic neuropathy. In Courjon J, Mauguiere F, Revol M, eds. *Clinical applications of evoked responses in neurology.* New York: Raven Press, 1982:11–19.

93. Krumholz A, Weiss H, Goldstein P, et al. Evoked responses in vitamin B12 deficiency. *Ann Neurol* 1981;9:407–409.

94. Kuroiwa Y, Celesia G. Visual evoked potentials with hemifield pattern stimulation: their use in the diagnosis of retrochiasmatic lesions. *Arch Neurol* 1981;38:86–90.

95. Lehmann D, Darcey T, Skrandies W. Intracerebral and scalp fields evoked by hemiretinal checkerboard reversal, and modelling of their dipole generators. In Courjon J, Mauguiere F, Revol M, eds. *Clinical applications of evoked responses in neurology.* New York: Raven Press, 1982:41–48.

96. Lehmann D, Meles H, Mir Z. Average multichannel EEG potential fields evoked from upper and lower hemi-retina: latency differences. *Electroencephalogr Clin Neurophysiol* 1977;43:725–731.

97. Lennerstrand G. Delayed visual evoked cortical potentials in retinal disease. *Acta Ophthalmol* 1982;60:497–504.

98. Leventhal A, Ault S, Vitek D. The nasotemporal division in primate retina: the neural bases of macular sparing and splitting. *Science* 1988;240:66–67.

99. Maiese K, Walker RW, Gargan R, et al. Intra-arterial cisplatin-associated optic and otic toxicity. *Arch Neurol* 1992;49:83–86.

100. Maitland C, Aminoff M, Kennard C, et al. Evoked potentials in the evaluation of visual field defects due to chiasmal or retrochiasmal lesions. *Neurology* 1982;32:986–991.

101. Majnemer A, Rosenblatt B, Watters G, et al. Giant axonal neuropathy: central abnormalities demonstrated by evoked potentials. *Ann Neurol* 1986;19:394–396.

102. Mamoli P, Graf M, Toifl K. EEG, pattern-evoked potentials and nerve conduction velocity in a family with adrenoleucodystrophy. *Electroencephalogr Clin Neurophysiol* 1979;47:411–419.

103. Markand O, DeMeyer W, Worth R, et al. Multimodality evoked responses in leukodystrophies. In Courjon J, Mauguiere F, Revol M, eds. *Clinical applications of evoked responses in neurology.* New York: Raven Press, 1982:409–415.

104. Matthews W, Read D, Pountney E. Effect of raising body temperature on visual and somatosensory evoked potentials in patients with multiple sclerosis. *J Neurol Neurosurg Psychiat* 1978;42:250–255.

105. McCombe PA, McLaughlin DB, Chalk JB, et al. Spasticity and white matter abnormalities in adult phenylketonuria. *J Neurol Neurosurg Psychiat* 1992;55:359–361.

106. McDonald W. Pathophysiology of conduction in central nerve fibres. In: Desmedt JE, ed. *Visual evoked potentials in man: new developments.* Oxford, UK: Clarendon Press, 1977:427–437.

107. McLeod J, Low P, Morgan J. Charcot-Marie-Tooth disease with Leber optic atrophy. *Neurology* 1978;28:179–184.

108. Mervaala E, Keranen T, Penttila M, et al. Pattern-reversal VEP and cortical SEP latency prolongations in epilepsy. *Epilepsia* 1985;26:441–445.

109. Messenheimer J, Greenwood R, Tennison M, et al. Reversible visual evoked potential abnormalities in vitamin E deficiency. *Ann Neurol* 1984;15:499–501.

110. Michael W, Halliday A. Differences between the occipital distribution of upper and lower field pattern-evoked responses in man. *Brain Res* 1971;32:311–324.

111. Miller D, Newton M, Van der Poel J, et al. Magnetic resonance imaging of the optic nerve in optic neuritis. *Neurology* 1988;38:175–179.
112. Miller J, Burke A, Bever C. Occurrence of oligoclonal bands in multiple sclerosis and other CNS diseases. *Ann Neurol* 1983;13:53–58.
113. Moller A, Burgess J, Sekhar L. Recording compound action potentials from the optic nerve in man and monkeys. *Electroencephalogr Clin Neurophysiol* 1987;67:549–555.
114. Mondelli M, Rossi A, Scarpini C, et al. Evoked potentials in cerebrotendinous xanthomatosis and effect induced by chenodeoxycholic acid. *Arch Neurol* 1992;49:469–475.
115. Morgan R, Nugent B, Harrison J, et al. Voluntary alteration of pattern visual evoked responses. *Ophthalmology* 1985;92:1356–1363.
116. Mortimer M, Good P, Marsters J, et al. Visual evoked responses in children with migraine: a diagnostic test. *Lancet* 1990;1:75–77.
117. Neima D, Regan D. Pattern visual evoked potentials and spatial vision in retrobulbar neuritis and multiple sclerosis. *Arch Neurol* 1984;41:198–201.
118. Nilsson B. Visual evoked responses in multiple sclerosis: comparison of two methods for pattern reversal. *J Neurol Neurosurg Psychiat* 1978;41:499–504.
119. Noachtar S, Hashimoto T, Luders H. Pattern visual evoked potentials recorded from human occipital cortex with chronic subdural electrodes. *Electroencephalogr Clin Neurophysiol* 1993;88:435–446.
120. Norcia A, Tyler C. Spatial frequency sweep VEP: Visual acuity during the first year of life. *Vision Res* 1985;25:1399–1408.
121. Novak G, Wiznitzer M, Kurtzberg D, et al. The utility of visual evoked potentials using hemifield stimulation and several check sizes in the evaluation of suspected multiple sclerosis. *Electroencephalogr Clin Neurophysiol* 1988;71:1–9.
122. Nuwer M. Frequency analysis and topographic mapping of EEG and evoked potentials in epilepsy. *Electroencephalogr Clin Neurophysiol* 1988;69:118–126.
123. Nuwer M, Perlman S, Packwood J, et al. Evoked potential abnormalities in the various inherited ataxias. *Ann Neurol* 1983;13:20–27.
124. Nuwer MR, Packwood JW, Myers LW, et al. Evoked potentials predict the clinical changes in a multiple sclerosis drug study. *Neurology* 1987;37:1754–1761.
125. Nyrke T, Kangasniemi P, Lang AH. Difference of steady-state visual evoked potentials in classic and common migraine. *Electroencephalogr Clin Neurophysiol* 1989;73:285–294.
126. Oishi M, Yamada T, Dickens Q, et al. Visual evoked potentials by different check sizes in patients with multiple sclerosis. *Neurology* 1985;35:1461–1465.
127. Oken BS, Chiappa KH, Gill E. Normal temporal variability of the P100. *Electroencephalogr Clin Neurophysiol* 1987;68:153–156.
128. Onofrj M, Bodis-Wollner I, Mylin L. Visual evoked potential diagnosis of field defects in patients with chiasmatic and retrochiasmatic lesions. *J Neurol Neurosurg Psychiat* 1982;45:294–302.
129. Papakostopoulos D, Hart C, Cooper R, et al. Combined electrophysiological assessment of the visual system in central serous retinopathy. *Electroencephalogr Clin Neurophysiol* 1984;59:77–80.
130. Paty D, Oger J, Kastrukoff L, et al. MRI in the diagnosis of MS: a prospective study with comparison of clinical evaluation, evoked potentials, oligoclonal banding and CT. *Neurology* 1988;38:180–185.
131. Pedersen L, Trojaborg W. Visual, auditory, and somatosensory pathway involvement in hereditary cerebellar ataxia, Friedreich's ataxia and familial spastic paraplegia. *Electroencephalogr Clin Neurophysiol* 1981;52:283–297.
132. Pfurtscheller G, Schwartz G, Gravenstein N. Clinical relevance of long-latency SEPs and VEPs during coma and emergence from coma. *Electroencephalogr Clin Neurophysiol* 1985;62:88–98.
133. Pratt H, Bleich N, Berliner E. Short latency visual evoked potentials in man. *Electroencephalogr Clin Neurophysiol* 1982;54:55–62.
134. Previc F. Origins and implications of frequency-doubling in the visual evoked potential. *Am J Optom Physiol Opt* 1987;64:664–674.
135. Rappaport M, Hall K, Hopkins K, et al. Evoked brain potentials and disability in brain-damaged patients. *Arch Phys Med Rehabil* 1977;58:333–345.
136. Rappaport M, Hopkins H, Hall K, et al. Evoked potentials and head injury. Clinical applications. *Clin Electroencephalogr* 1981;12:167–176.
137. Raudzens P. Intraoperative monitoring of evoked potentials. *Ann N Y Acad Sci* 1982;388:308–326.
138. Ray PG, Meador KJ, Loring DW, et al. Effects of scopolamine on visual evoked potentials in aging and dementia. *Electroencephalogr Clin Neurophysiol* 1991;80:347–351.
139. Regan D, Milner B. Objective perimetry by evoked potential recording: limitations. *Electroencephalogr Clin Neurophysiol* 1978;44:393–397.
140. Reilly E, Kondo C, Brunberg J, et al. Visual evoked potentials during hypothermia and prolonged circulatory arrest. *Electroencephalogr Clin Neurophysiol* 1978;45:100–106.
141. Riemslag F, Spekreijse H, Van Wessem T. Responses to paired onset stimuli: implications for the delayed evoked potentials in multiple sclerosis. *Electroencephalogr Clin Neurophysiol* 1985;62:155–166.
142. Rosing H, Hopkins L, Wallace D, et al. Maternally inherited mitochondrial myopathy and myoclonic epilepsy. *Ann Neurol* 1985;17:228–237.
143. Rowe M. A sequential technique for half-field pattern visual evoked potential testing. *Electroencephalogr Clin Neurophysiol* 1981;51:463–469.
144. Rowe M. The clinical utility of half-field pattern reversal visual evoked potential testing. *Electroencephalogr Clin Neurophysiol* 1982;53:73–77.
145. Russ W, Kling D, Loesevitz A, et al. Effect of hypothermia on visual evoked potentials (VEP) in humans. *Anesthesiology* 1984;61:207–210.
146. Sanders E, Volkers A, Van der Poel J, et al. Visual function and pattern visual evoked response in optic neuritis. *Br J Ophthalmol* 1987;71:602–608.
147. Sebel P, Flynn P, Ingram D. Effect of nitrous oxide on visual, auditory and somatosensory evoked potentials. *Br J Anaesth* 1984;56:1403–1407.
148. Shaw N, Cant B. Age-dependent changes in the latency of the pattern visual evoked potential. *Electroencephalogr Clin Neurophysiol* 1980;48:237–241.
149. Shearer D, Creel D, Dustman R. Efficacy of evoked potential stimulus parameters in the detection of visual system pathology. *Am J EEG Technol* 1983;23:137–146.
150. Shearer D, Dustman R, Emmerson R. Hydrocephalus: electrophysiological correlates. *Am J EEG Technol* 1987;27:199–212.
151. Sherman J, Bass S, Noble K, et al. Visual evoked potential (VEP) delays in central serous choroidopathy. *Invest Ophthalmol Vis Sci* 1986;27:214–221.
152. Sidman R, Smith D, Henke J, et al. Localization of neural generators in the visual evoked responses. *Electroencephalogr Clin Neurophysiol* 1982;53:35P.
153. Silva I, Wang A, Symon L. The application of flash visual evoked potentials during operations on the anterior visual pathways. *Neurol Res* 1985;7:11–16.
154. Simon R, Zimmerman A, Sanderson P, et al. EEG markers of migraine in children and adults. *Headache* 1983;23:21–25.
155. Skuse NF, Burke D. Sequence-dependent deterioration in the visual evoked potential in the absence of drowsiness. *Electroencephalogr Clin Neurophysiol* 1992;84:20–25.
156. Sokol S. Measurement of infant visual acuity from pattern reversal evoked potentials. *Vision Res* 1978;18:33–39.
157. Sokol S, Hansen V, Moskowitz A, et al. Evoked potential and preferential looking estimates of visual acuity in pediatric patients. *Ophthalmology* 1983;90:552–562.
158. Sokol S, Jones K. Implicit time of pattern evoked potentials in infants: an index of maturation of spatial vision. *Vision Res* 1979;19:747–755.
159. Sokol S, Moskowitz A. Effects of retinal blur on the peak latency of the pattern evoked potential. *Vision Res* 1981;21:1279–1286.

160. Sokol S, Moskowitz A, Towle V. Age-related changes in the latency of the visual evoked potential: influence of check size. *Electroencephalogr Clin Neurophysiol* 1981;51:559–562.

161. Spitz M, Emerson R, Pedley T. Dissociation of frontal N100 from occipital P100 in pattern reversal visual evoked potentials. *Electroencephalogr Clin Neurophysiol* 1986;65:161–168.

162. Stensaas S, Eddington D, Dobelle W. The topography and variability of the primary visual cortex in man. *J Neurosurg* 1974;40:747–755.

163. Stockard J, Hughes J, Sharbrough F. Visually evoked potentials to electronic pattern reversal: latency variations with gender, age, and technical factors. *Am J EEG Technol* 1979;19:171–204.

164. Stockard J, Iragui V. Clinically useful applications of evoked potentials in adult neurology. *J Clin Neurophysiol* 1984;1:159–202.

165. Streletz L, Bae S, Roeshman R, et al. Visual evoked potentials in occipital lobe lesions. *Arch Neurol* 1981;38:80–85.

166. Streletz L, Chambers R, Bae S, et al. Visual evoked potentials in sarcoidosis. *Neurology* 1981;31:1545–1549.

167. Tackmann W, Radu E. Pattern shift visual evoked potentials in Charcot-Marie-Tooth disease, HMSN type I. *J Neurol* 1980;224:71–74.

168. Tagliati M, Sabbadini M, Bernardi G, et al. Multichannel visual evoked potentials in migraine. *Electroencephalogr Clin Neurophysiol* 1995;96:1–5.

169. Tan C, Murray N, Sawyers D, et al. Deliberate alteration of the visual evoked potential. *J Neurol Neurosurg Psychiat* 1984;47:518–523.

170. Tang Y, Norcia AM. Improved processing of the steady-state evoked potential. *Electroencephalogr Clin Neurophysiol* 1993;88:323–334.

171. Tartaglione A, Pizio N, Bino G, et al. VEP changes in Parkinson's disease are stimulus dependent. *J Neurol Neurosurg Psychiat* 1984;47:305–307.

172. Taylor M, Keenan N, Gallant T, et al. Subclinical VEP abnormalities in patients on chronic deferoxamine therapy: longitudinal studies. *Electroencephalogr Clin Neurophysiol* 1986;68:81–87.

173. Thompson P, Mastaglia F, Carroll W. Anterior ischemic optic neuropathy. A correlative clinical and visual evoked potential study of 18 patients. *J Neurol Neurosurg Psychiat* 1986;49:128–135.

174. Tobimatsu S, Hamada T, Okayama M, et al. Temporal frequency deficit in patients with senile dementia of the Alzheimer type: a visual evoked potential study. *Neurology* 1994;44:1260–1263.

175. Towle V, Moskowitz A, Sokol S, et al. The visual evoked potential in glaucoma and ocular hypertension: effects of check size, field size, and stimulation rate. *Invest Ophthalmol Vis Sci* 1983;24:175–183.

176. Towle V, Sutcliffe E, Sokol S. Diagnosing functional visual deficits with the P300 component of the visual evoked potential. *Arch Ophthalmol* 1985;103:47–50.

177. Uhl R, Squires K, Bruce D, et al. Effect of halothane anesthesia on the human cortical visual evoked response. *J Anesthesiol* 1980;53:273–276.

178. Uren S, Stewart P, Crosby P. Subject cooperation and the visual evoked response. *Invest Ophthalmol Vis Sci* 1979;18:648–652.

179. van Dijk JG, Dorresteijn M, Haan J, et al. No confirmation of visual evoked potential diagnostic test for migraine. *Lancet* 1991;337:517–518.

180. van Dijk JG, Dorresteijn M, Haan J, et al. Visual evoked potentials and background EEG activity in migraine. *Headache* 1991;31:392–395.

181. Wildberger H, Hofmann H, Siegfried J. Fluctuations of visual evoked potential amplitudes and of contrast sensitivity in Uhthoff's symptom. *Doc Ophthalmol* 1987;65:357–365.

182. Yiannikas C, Walsh J. The use of visual evoked potentials in the detection of subclinical optic toxicity secondary to ethambutol. *Neurology* 1982;32:A205.

183. Zemon V, Kaplan E, Ratliff F. The role of GABA-mediated intracortical inhibition in the generation of visual evoked potentials. In Cracco RQ, Bodis-Wollner I, eds. *Evoked potentials.* New York: Alan R Liss, 1986:287–295.

Chapter 28

Brainstem Auditory Evoked Potentials

C. William Erwin and Aatif M. Husain

Potentials elicited from stimulation of the auditory system are called auditory evoked potentials. They are categorized by their latency from stimulus onset and their neural origin. The short-latency auditory evoked potentials are those arising within the first 15 milliseconds after appropriate acoustic stimulation in normal subjects. By neural origin, short-latency auditory evoked potentials are subdivided into the electrocochleogram and the brainstem auditory evoked potentials (BAEPs). BAEPs are widely used in clinical neurology, in contrast to middle-latency auditory evoked potentials and long-latency auditory evoked potentials. The latter two responses are not yet widely used for diagnostic or monitoring applications.

Clinical applications of BAEPs for hearing assessments are particularly useful for patients who are unable to cooperate sufficiently for typical audiological assessment techniques. BAEP testing is common in infants and cognitively impaired older patients. Although usually the domain of audiology, hearing deficits caused by either abnormalities of sound conduction to the inner ear or neurosensory abnormalities of the cochlea and/or acoustic nerve may alter potentials generated in the brainstem. Because of the interpretative problems caused by auditory impairments, this chapter also touches on the effects of audiological deficits on BAEPs and electrophysiological methods of assessing such impairments.

BAEP techniques are useful partly because they are sensitive to the degree that the brainstem auditory pathway can be grossly abnormal without detectable clinical manifestations. This is true both of disorders within the brainstem, such as demyelination, and of extrinsic pathological processes, such as some tumors.

BRAINSTEM AUDITORY EVOKED POTENTIALS

Acoustic Stimulation

Stimulus Types and Applications

The stimulus type selected is determined by the diagnostic application.

Sine Waves

Pure tone audiometry involves the use of sine waves of a specific frequency and relies on behavioral criteria of stimulus detection. The tones last approximately 1 second. There is an interaction between sound intensity and duration for threshold detection. Sine waves are not used to elicit BAEPs.

Clicks

BAEPs are elicited by brief acoustic stimuli that sound like clicks. The acoustic click is usually generated by a 100-microsecond rectangular pulse delivered to a headphone, resulting in an initial deflection of the headphone diaphragm, followed by several rapidly decaying oscillations lasting a few milliseconds. The frequencies of the oscillations are dependent on damping, the natural resonant frequency of the particular headphone, and its housing, and they differ markedly between different makes of headphones. Frequency analysis of oscillations produced by the rectangular wave input reveals a spectrum of frequencies ranging from 500 to 6,000 Hz; the major power is approximately 3,000 Hz (238). The term *broad-band-click* is used to describe BAEP stimuli.

For longer latency auditory evoked potentials, tone pips, which are a series of sine waves of constant frequency lasting approximately 1 second, are used for stimulation. Onset and offset of a tone pip would also generate a click if it were not for a gradual onset and offset (ramp) each lasting approximately 25% of the steady sine-wave duration.

Stimulus Delivery Methods

In animal studies of auditory evoked potentials, researchers often use loudspeakers with open-field stimulation. In adult human clinical studies, open-field stimulation has few applications because of the usual need to assess left- and right-sided responses separately. Neonatal acoustic perception evaluations have been done with open-field stimulation.

Clinical diagnostic BAEP studies are often conducted with audiological grade transducers housed in headphones to provided shielding from environmental noise. Currents flowing in the coils of the transducer generate magnetic fields that cut across the ear electrode and attached lead, which functions like the secondary winding of a transformer. Thus, there is induction of currents into the recording electrodes. The artifact is directly related to the power delivered to the headphones. A linear increase in decibels (dB) requires a logarithmic increase in power (wattage) because 1 dB is 10 times the logarithm of the before-and-after power ratio (1 dB = 10 log P1/P2). Thus, boosting the sound level by 10 dB requires increased power by a factor of 10; boosting sound by 20 dB requires a power factor increase of 100; and a 30-dB increase requires a power factor increase of 1,000. Artifacts from clicks at 70 decibels above hearing level (dBHL) may be acceptable, but at 90 dBHL, the response may be unacceptably distorted when monophasic clicks are used.

More recently, ear insert devices for sound stimulation have come into common use. There are ear inserts that contain the transducer coil. Although they provide less mechanical interference during surgery than do audiological acoustically shielded headphones, they do produce similar amounts of stimulus artifact with no stimulus delay. Ear insert devices that produce little or no artifact are those with a remote transducer connected by a standard length of tubing to the ear canal. The transducer is usually near the clavicle with flexible tubing connecting the source of sound generation to the ear cannel. The usual length of tubing produces a delay of approximately 0.9 milliseconds. Occlusion of the tube from fluids or crimping can be an obscure cause of improper stimulation.

Sound Intensity Methods

In pure tone audiometry, calibrated sine waves of specific frequency are used, with the intensity of sound measured in decibels. Behaviorally, 0 dB is the average threshold of perception for humans with normal hearing. This has been defined to an objective standard of a force of 40 μPa per square centimeter. An "artificial ear" (calibration system) is used to assess an audiometric headphone by measuring the decibel sound pressure level (dBSPL) output of a headphone in response to a sustained sine wave input. Because sound perception requires both physiological and psychological functions, normal thresholds range from −10 to 20 dBSPL at frequencies between 0.5 and 8 kHz.

The calibration of broad-band clicks is different from sustained sine waves because the duration of the click is too short for the electronics of an artificial ear to respond. Behavioral thresholds are often used. The term *decibel sensation level* (dBSL) is used when the zero thresholds have been determined for the person being tested. Thus, if a person has a threshold of 10 dB for the left ear and 20 dB for the right ear, both ears could be tested at 70 dBSL with machine settings of 80 and 90 dB, respectively.

The term *decibel hearing level* is used when the zero thresholds has been determined from a group of persons with normal pure tone audiometry. This level is often 5 to 10 dB higher in a neurophysiology laboratory than in a sound-attenuated audiometric chamber because of masking by low-frequency building noises. Thus, if the mean perceptual threshold were 5 dB, subjects would be tested at 70 dBHL with machine settings of 75 dB. The terms *decibel hearing level* and *decibel normal hearing level* are interchangeable.

Although widely used, both dBHL and dBSL are subjective measures. Audiological applications may require a more objective measure such as decibel peak equivalent sound pressure level (dBpeSPL). With this technique, the amplitude of the initial component of a headphone's acoustic response to the electrical input is displayed and measured on an oscilloscope. The amplitude is matched to a steady sine wave of known decibel intensity and the term *peak equivalent* is used. Although the sine wave and the transient click are of the same amplitude, they evoked different behavioral responses because of their different duration. The measure dBpeSPL is approximately 30 dB higher than dBSL or dBHL.

Stimulus Polarity

When the initial movement of the transducer diaphragm is toward the tympanic membrane, the click acoustic polarity is called *condensation*. When the initial movement is away from the tympanic membrane, the click acoustic polarity is called *rarefaction*. When successive clicks are of opposite polarity, they are called *alternating* (used for stimulus artifact suppression). The electrical impulse delivered to the transducer can be only negative or positive, but there is no industry standard about which electrical polarity should produce which acoustic click polarity. Subjectively, rarefaction and condensation clicks sound identical, and test devices are required to determine click polarity. As noted later in this chapter, there are replicable differences in BAEP responses produced by different click polarities.

Masking

Stimuli from monaural stimulation strike not only the ipsilateral tympanic membrane but continue through the cranium to reach the contralateral cochlea. Transcranial attenuation is approximately 30 to 40 dB. Therefore, if 90-dBHL clicks are delivered to a totally nonfunctional cochlea, about 50- to 60-dBHL clicks pass through the skull and brain to stimulate the opposite cochlea, which if normal will produce normal BAEP responses. This produces confusing responses that can be avoided by delivering noise (e.g., white, pink) to the opposite, nonstimulated ear. The *American Electroencephalographic Society Guidelines in Electroencephalography, Evoked Potentials, and Polysomnography* (6) (referred to henceforth as the *Guidelines*) recommend masking at 60 dBpeSPL.

Recording Strategies

Patient Variables and Recording Strategies

Two important subject or patient variables for the recording of high-quality studies are arousal level and body position. One of the most common impediments to obtaining acceptable BAEP recordings is low-level tonic electromyographic (EMG) activity, found in 30% to 50% of subjects. Sleep, whether spontaneous or induced by medication, greatly reduces such tonic EMG contaminants. Benzodiazepines are frequently used for their combined anxiolytic, myorelaxant, and hypnotic effects with no measurable effects on BAEP latency, amplitude, or morphological pattern. High-amplitude, phasic events are excluded from the average by automatic artifact rejection features found on all modern instruments.

A comfortable bed or reclining chair promotes the likelihood of sleep while relaxing the cervical extensor muscles, which contribute to the postauricular myogenic response. This artifact develops between 10 and 15 milliseconds after presentation of a stimulus.

Electrode Placement

Three recording electrodes are typically used: one at the vertex and one at each of the mastoid/ear locations. The later BAEP components (waves II to VII) are of brainstem, far-field origin and have a widespread distribution over the vertex. Indeed, a Cz-Fz derivation would be expected to be virtually isopotential because of in-phase cancellation. Wave I is both near-field (negative near the ear) and far-field (positive projections to the opposite ear and vertex). On occasion, particularly in neonates, a noncephalic reference is useful because in-phase cancellation can markedly attenuate some components of the BAEP response. All BAEP components can be recorded from both ear electrode locations. With noncephalic recording, it is possible to show all waveforms of the BAEP with different topographies at the three electrode recording sites, and apparent absence of responses from standard bipolar montages can be seen. Distant bone locations such as the patella or medial malleolus are suitable as sites for a noncephalic reference (Fig. 28.1). An increased (often double) number of stimuli are needed to reduce the increased artifact.

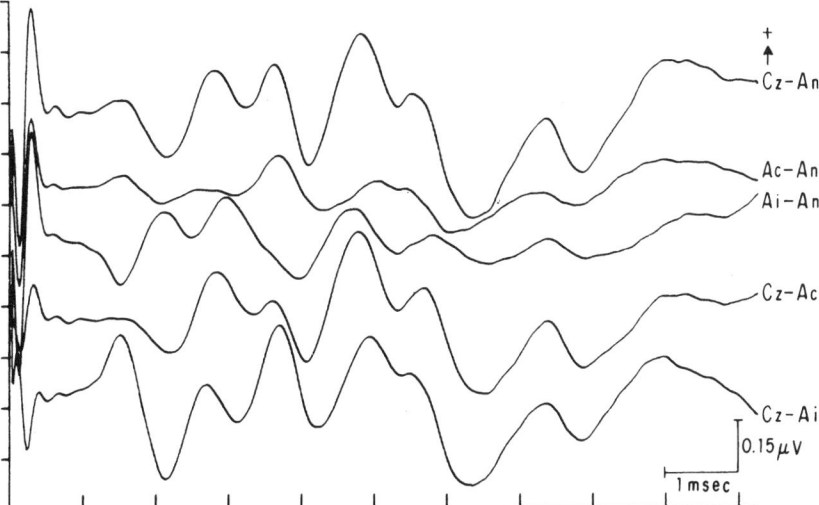

FIG. 28.1. Group BAEP data from five normal subjects (responses from independent stimulation of both ears) is presented. All subject's responses were normal with presence of waves I through V. Stimulation produced by standard TDL 49 audiometric headphones. The bottom two traces are standard bipolar derivations with Cz (vertex) to Ai (ipsilateral ear lobe) and Ac (contralateral ear lobe). This montage caused a positive event at the first named electrode to have an upward deflection. Conversely, a positive event at the second named electrode caused a downward deflection. The top three channels show Cz, Ac, and Ai referenced to An (medial malleolus of the ankle) to provide a distant, relatively uninvolved reference. These three derivations show the unique contributions of responses at each electrode site to the bipolar derivations. There are deflections at each of the three sites for all of the major BAEP components, with the exception of an absent wave III at Ai. (Unless noted otherwise, in Figs. 28.1 to 28.9*B*, BAEP data was recorded with the following stimulation and recording parameters: rate, 11.1 per second; masking of the nonstimulated ear with white noise at 20 dB less than the click level to the stimulated ear; horizontal resolution of 10 microseconds between samples; low-frequency setting, 150 Hz; high-frequency setting, 3,000 Hz; ear insert transducers causing a 0.9-millisecond delay.)

Because BAEP components have different topographies at Ai, Ac, and Cz, this leads to varying degrees of potentiation, attenuation, and apparent latency shift of the individual waves. Wave identification can proceed logically through an understanding of the topographic differences between the ipsilateral and contralateral channels. See the section on waveform identification.

Polarity Conventions

Polarity conventions for electroencephalography (EEG), visual evoked potentials, and somatosensory evoked potentials are the same; a negative event at the first named electrode of a derivation causes an upward deflection. BAEP polarity convention is the opposite. Wave I has a near-field negative field and a far-field positive field with broad projections to Ac and Cz. The near-field, negative component of wave I, when recorded by an Ai electrode connected to negative input, causes an upward deflection. The positive, far-field component, when recorded by the Cz electrode connected to positive input, also causes an upward defection. Thus, all BAEP components are displayed upward, but wave I is negative at the ear and positive at the Cz, whereas waves II to VII are primarily positive at Cz.

Naming of Brainstem Auditory Evoked Potential Components

The up-going, positive peaks of major BAEP components recorded in the ipsilateral Cz-Ai derivation are named waves I, II, III, IV, V, VI, and VII. The down-going negative valleys recorded in this derivation were named I_N, II_N, III_N, IV_N, V_N, VI_N, and VII_N by Stockard et al. (217). The up-going, positive waves recorded in the contralateral (Cz-Ac) derivation are called I_C, II_C, III_C, IV_C, V_C, VI_C, and VII_C; and the down-going negative valleys are called I_{NC}, II_{NC}, III_{NC}, IV_{NC}, V_{NC}, VI_{NC}, and VII_{NC} (Fig. 28.2).

Stimulus Rate and Polarity

Use of stimulus rates of 5 to 90 Hz (and higher) have been reported. A rate of approximately 10 Hz is most common, but many clinical laboratories use approximately 50 Hz for an initial rate. To avoid time locking to 60-Hz artifact, exact multiples of 60 are avoided. Rates faster than 10 per second cause a progressive reduction of amplitude, a broadening of all waves, and a lengthening of all interpeak latencies. Because of this latter factor, sepa-

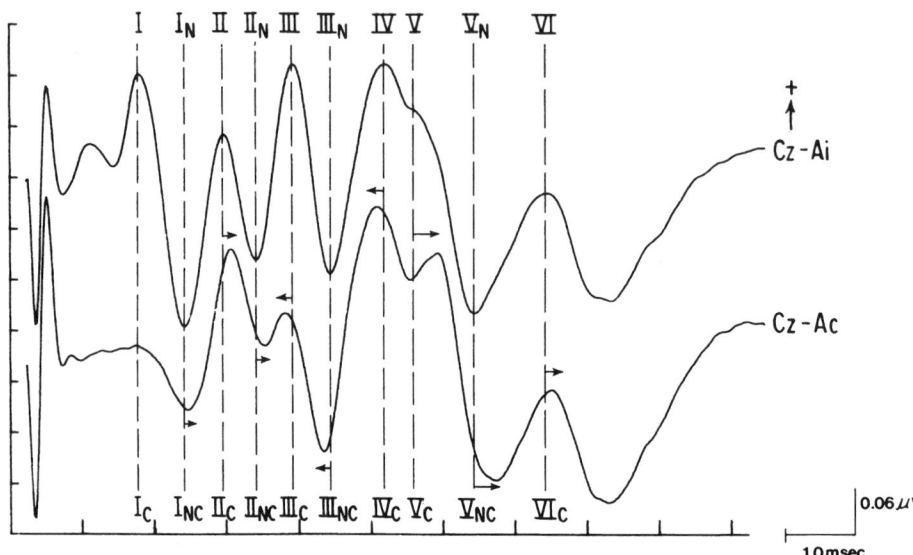

FIG. 28.2. Group BAEP data as in Fig. 28.1, a component-naming method, and apparent latency differences of various peaks as recorded in standard derivations. These latency shifts are useful in waveform identification, particularly when there are missing or redundant peaks or valleys. In the Cz-Ai (ipsilateral) derivation, the up-going peaks are labeled with Roman numerals I through VI. The down-going valleys of this derivation are labeled with Roman numerals followed by a subscripted "N" because they have a negative polarity, with the exception of wave I_N. In the Cz-Ac (contralateral) derivation, the up-going peaks are labeled with Roman numerals followed by a subscripted "C," and the downgoing valleys are labeled with Roman numerals followed by a subscripted "NC." (See legend for Fig. 28.1 for stimulation and recording parameters.)

rate normative values are needed for interpretation of data elicited by different rates of stimulation.

Filtering

Recommended filter settings for BAEPs in adults are 10 to 3000 Hz (6). In the past, the majority of clinical studies were done with low-filter settings of 150 Hz. Lowering the passband has surprisingly little impact on data acquisition (no increase in artifact rejection rate) but produces obvious changes in the morphological pattern of the response. Separate normative data for such filter settings are required for both latency and amplitude criteria of abnormality.

Averaging: Artifact Suppression and Horizontal and Vertical Resolution

The number of responses required to produce relatively artifact-free responses varies between values of 1,000 and 4,000, depending on the signal-to-noise ratio. When responses are large (greater than 0.2 μV) and noise is relatively low in amplitude, fewer responses are required. When low-amplitude responses are present (common in pathological conditions) and/or noise components are relatively high in amplitude, there may be significant

residual noise despite 4,000 or more responses. Increasing the intensity of stimulation increases the amplitude of the response, particularly wave I. Attention to electrode impedance and adequate sedation can significantly reduce environmental artifact and EMG (Fig. 28.3).

Horizontal resolution depends on sweep time and the amount of memory allocated to data. Current commercial systems have adequate horizontal resolution, and responses are usually oversampled. When a 15-millisecond sweep is used with 512 horizontal data points, the intersample interval, or dwell time, is 0.03 millisecond for an effective sampling rate of 33 kHz. This well exceeds the Nyquist number and samples the fastest waveforms adequately (3 kHz is the recommended setting of the high-frequency analog filter).

Vertical resolution is a function of the size of the analog-to-digital (AD) converter, the amplifier sensitivity, and the number of sweeps (stimuli). Even with a minimal 8-bit AD converter. there is overkill of vertical resolution with sweep values as low as 500. Whether such a relatively low number of sweeps is sufficient to adequately reduce noise is a separate issue, but with a full-scale sensitivity of 20 μV, the vertical resolution is 0.00016 μV (20 μV/256/500). Most AD converters are 12-bit, which with full scale sensitivity of 20 μV and 2,000 stimuli produces a vertical resolution of 0.000002 μV (20 μV/4,096/2,000).

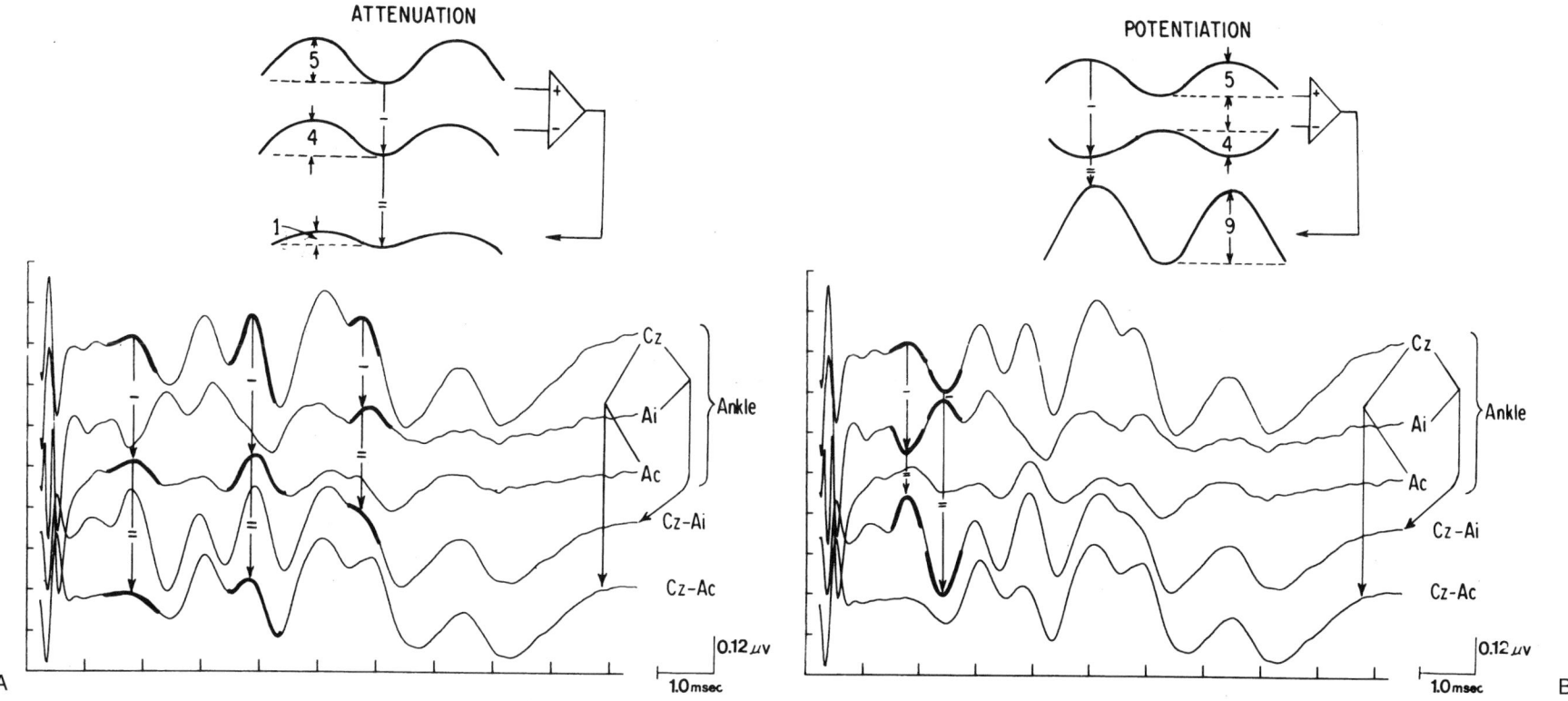

FIG. 28.3. A: Potentiation of waves I and I_N in the Cz-Ai derivation. Wave I is negative as recorded from Ai and projects as a positive event (dipole) at both Cz and Ai (usually larger at Cz). Opposite polarities, when connected to a deferential amplifier, cause additive (potentiating) effects. **B:** Relative attenuation of waves I and III in the Cz-Ac derivation and wave V in the Cz-Ai derivation. It is an example of in-phase cancellation. (See legend for Fig. 28.1 for stimulation and recording parameters.)

Conducting a Brainstem Auditory Evoked Potential Study

Medical History

Before performing the BAEP test, the technologist should obtain a relevant medical history, which may help with interpretation. A directed history should include the symptoms for which the test is being performed, their duration, and coexisting medical conditions. Neurological examination findings, especially those pertaining to cranial nerves, should be noted. Results of prior neuroimaging and audiological tests are particularly helpful.

This historical information is used by the interpreter to suggest clinical relevance to the BAEP findings.

Explanation of the Test to the Patient

Patients undergoing central nervous system evaluations are often understandably anxious. Successful attempts to allay fears about the pending study allow the patient to relax, producing a shorter study with higher quality data. Explanations should be as simple as possible, tailored to the patient's level of medical sophistication. It is better to err on the side of using too simple a language than too complex. The laboratory director, to ensure consistency of the message, should review a written outline of the explanation content.

Sedation

Good-quality BAEPs can be obtained in approximately 60% of unsedated, awake adults (authors' unpublished experience). In patients with varying degrees of anxiety or pain, which causes increased tonic EMG, recording may be more difficult. The authors routinely sedate all adults with orally administered diazepam (usually 10 mg) at the beginning of a BAEP study because it has combined anxiolytic, myorelaxant, and hypnotic qualities. Spectral analysis of scalp surface potentials with an analog passband of 150 to 3,000 Hz taken in an awake state and a sleep state reveals a band of activity from 200 to 500 Hz that is suppressed during sleep (authors' unpublished data). The suppression of this activity probably explains the improvement in data recorded when the patient is sedated.

Electrode Applications

Surface electrodes are preferred because of lower noise characteristics in comparison with needle electrodes. One electrode is placed at the vertex (Cz), and one electrode is placed at each of the two ears (A1 and A2). The ear electrodes are usually designated as Ai and Ac, which indicates the ear ipsilateral and the ear contralateral to stimulation. One study (217) showed a higher amplitude wave I when the ear electrode is placed on the mesial surface of the ear lobe. Comparisons were made between this location and the mastoid or lateral pinna locations. A fourth electrode is required for grounding purposes and can be placed anywhere on the body. A frontal scalp location is commonly used because of the ease of application; however, such a practice could lead to a "ground recording."

Determination of Hearing Threshold for Click Perception

As described in a previous section, determination of the hearing threshold for click perception is needed when dBSL stimulus descriptors are used. To stimulate at 70 dBSL, 70 dB is added to the perception threshold for the person's left and right ears. This technique is used infrequently for two reasons. First, it is inappropriate for a significant number of subjects because of their inability to cooperate (as a result of age, cognitive level, coma, anesthesia); and second, for persons with frequency-specific deficits, the frequency of the broad-band click that is useful for testing hearing may not be the same frequency that elicits various components of the BAEP response.

Usual Parameters for Obtaining Brainstem Auditory Evoked Potential Recordings

The usual parameters for BAEP recording technique (see Guidelines [6]) differ to some degree with the age of the subject and the setting of the study. Thus, a 10-millisecond sweep time is common for diagnostic studies in adults, whereas a 15-millisecond sweep time is common for infants and during intraoperative monitoring because of the distinct possibility that wave V will occur or move later than 10 milliseconds.

Other parameters are common to all studies. Amplifier sensitivity is set to produce an artifact rejection rate of about 15%, which usually translates to a full-scale sensitivity of 10 to 20 μV. Two replications are superimposed, each containing 1,500 to 4,000 responses. The most common is 2,000, but more may be needed when there is a high noise level or when response amplitude is lower than usual. A stimulus level of 60 to 70 dBHL is used initially and adjusted upward to 100 dBHL if no wave I is recorded. The adjustment is in 10-dB increments. Higher intensities shorten the absolute latency of all components of the response but do not affect interpeak latencies (see the Guidelines [6]). Masking of the nonstimulated ear at a level 60 dBSPL reduces the likelihood of significant stimulation of the ear contralateral to stimulation.

Troubleshooting

The four most common technical causes of recording no response and methods of troubleshooting are as follows:

1. Inadequate stimulation, which the technologist can detect by putting on the headset or ear inserts and listening for the presence of adequately loud clicks.
2. A defective amplifier, AD converter, or their connections, which the technologist may detect by viewing the data input rather than the average. Input data is best viewed by extending the sweep to 1 second, decreasing the sensitivity, and touching one or more electrodes, producing an obvious artifact.

3. Improper filters, as from a previous visual evoked potential (1 to 100 Hz) that will essentially eliminate all BAEP responses. The technologist can detect this condition by inspecting the filter controls or settings files.

4. Improper triggering, which prevents averaging of a response. The technologist can detect this condition by slowing the stimulation rate to one per second, viewing the input, and visually confirming that a sweep initiates with each click.

The Normal Brainstem Auditory Evoked Potential

Anatomy and Physiology of the Auditory Pathways

Auditory pathways start in the cochlea. The cochlea coils two and a half times and tapers toward its termination, known as the apex. Two membranes, the vestibular and basilar membranes, separate this coil into three cavities: the scala vestibuli, scala media, and scala tympani. All three are fluid filled; the scala vestibuli and tympani contain perilymph, which communicates with cerebrospinal fluid, and the scala media contains endolymph. The auditory transducer is known as the organ of Corti, which is attached to the basilar membrane throughout its length and lies within the scala media. It contains four rows of hair cells and is stimulated by changes in the hydrostatic pressure of the endolymph. Hydrostatic pressure changes are a result of sound waves that are transmitted to the cochlea through the outer and middle ears. The frequency of the acoustic stimulus determines the precise location on the basilar membrane where the organ of Corti is stimulated; low frequencies stimulate the apex, and high frequencies stimulate the base of the cochlea.

Hair cells of the organ of Corti communicate with processes of bipolar cells, also known as first-order auditory neurons. Bipolar cells have cell bodies located within the cochlea and form the cochlear part of the vestibulocochlear nerve. The vestibulocochlear nerve, after traveling through the petrous bone and the subarachnoid space, enters the brainstem at the pontomedullary junction. Fibers of the cochlear part of the vestibulocochlear nerve terminate in either the ventral or dorsal cochlear nucleus. These nuclei are located along the lateral aspect of the rostrum of the medulla.

The remainder of the auditory pathway from the cochlear nuclei to the auditory cortex is not clearly understood. Although numerous pathways of impulse transmission probably exist, only the one best known and relevant to the discussion of auditory evoked potentials is described here. The cochlear nuclei give rise to second-order auditory neurons, most of which cross to the contralateral side; the ones arising from the ventral cochlear nucleus form the trapezoid body. Most second-order auditory neurons synapse in the superior olivary nucleus, either contralaterally or ipsilaterally. Third-order auditory neurons arise from the superior olivary nuclei and ascend in the lateral lemniscus in the tegmentum of the pons and midbrain to terminate in the inferior colliculus. From the inferior colliculus arise fourth-order auditory neurons that ascend through the inferior brachium to the medial geniculate body of the thalamus. Fifth-order auditory neurons arise in the thalamus and terminate in Heschl's gyri. Auditory perception takes place in Heschl's gyri. Thus, unilateral auditory input is perceived bilaterally.

Generators of Waveforms

BAEPs usually consist of five waveforms, labeled waves I to V (see Fig. 28.2). In addition, two additional waves (VI and VII) are sometimes identified in many, but not all, normal adult humans. Much of the work on waveform generators has been done with animals; the human auditory system is significantly more complex (102), and transspecies correlations require caution.

Results of initial experiments with implanted macroelectrodes in cats suggested discrete synaptic generators for the various BAEP waveforms (96). Wave I was thought to arise from the acoustic nerve, wave II from the cochlear nucleus, wave III from the superior olivary complex, wave IV from the lateral lemniscus, and wave V from the inferior colliculus. Other investigators studied the auditory pathway with different techniques and arrived at comparable results (83,211).

However, other experiments have revealed conflicting findings regarding presumed waveform generators. Whereas there is general agreement that wave I arises in the part of the cochlear nerve closest to the cochlea (35,51,68), there is considerable debate about the generator of wave II. Data have suggested that, instead of arising from the cochlear nucleus, wave II probably originates from the proximal vestibulocochlear nerve (63,140). Additional support for this assertion is provided by studies that demonstrate presence of both waves I and II in patients with brain death, which suggests that these waves arise from the cochlear nerve (68,218). There have been disagreements about the generator of wave III as well. Chiappa (26) suggested that the superior olivary complex generates wave III, whereas other researchers believe that the cochlear nucleus is responsible for this waveform (138,140,194).

The generators of waves IV and V are even more ambiguous. In rat auditory pathway ablation experiments, researchers noted that lesions of the lateral lemniscus had inconsistent effects on waves IV and V, and lesions of the inferior colliculus had no significant effects on these waveforms (25). There is some agreement among many investigators that wave IV arises from the area of the superior olivary nucleus (83,135–137). However, there is much disagreement as to whether the waveform is generated ipsilateral or contralateral to the side of stimulation. Ponton et al. (172) and Moore et al. (142) suggested that wave IV arises from contralateral auditory fibers that do not synapse in the superior olivary complex but run near it. Curio and Oppel (41) suggested that the ipsilateral superior olivary complex produces wave IV with some contribution from contralateral nonsynaptic cochleocollicular fibers. Clinical human data has suggested that lesions in the middle and upper pons cause ipsilateral loss of waves IV and V (15,20,201,211). The exact generator of wave V remains equally uncertain. The contralateral superior olivary complex (41, 142,172,236,237), the contralateral lateral lemniscus (115,137,139,140), and the contralateral inferior colliculus (47,83) have all been proposed as possible generators for wave V. Waves VI and VII are thought to arise from the medial geniculate body and auditory radiations, respectively (28). However, because these waveforms are extremely variable, they are unreliable and are not used in clinical interpretation.

Since the initial attempts at identification of specific neural generators for BAEP waveforms, most investigators have come to believe that each of the waveforms have multiple generators and the various structures along the auditory pathway contribute to more than one peak (2,19,181). Malhotra (119) concluded that waves I and II originate from the acoustic nerve and waves III, IV, and V have multiple generators in the auditory pathway up to the lemniscal level. Chiappa (28) summarized by suggesting that wave I is generated by the distal vestibulocochlear nerve; wave II, by the proximal vestibulocochlear nerve or cochlear nucleus; wave III, by the lower pons (possibly superior olivary complex); wave IV, by the middle or upper pons (possibly lateral lemniscus); and wave V, by the upper pons or inferior colliculus. Although a majority of fibers of the auditory pathway ascend contralaterally, waves I to IV are probably generated ipsilaterally, whereas wave V may be generated contralaterally (28). Markand et al. (121) noted that in patients with unilateral brainstem pathology seen on magnetic resonance imaging (MRI), BAEP abnormalities are elicited from stimulation of the ear ipsilateral to the side of disease. Either the BAEPs elicited by contralateral ear stimulation are normal or the abnormality is not as marked as the ipsilateral abnormality. Markand et al. noted, however, that mesencephalic lesions are more likely to produce bilateral abnormalities.

Variability of Brainstem Auditory Evoked Potentials from Nonpathological Factors: Patient Variables

Age

The effects of age on BAEP are most remarkable in premature infants and neonates. Normal premature infants younger than 30 weeks of conceptional age may not have recordable BAEPs (226). BAEPs recorded in premature infants and neonates are often of higher amplitude than those seen in adults (217); this is presumably because of smaller head size, thinner skull bones, and greater proximity of electrodes to the neural generators of the waveforms. The wave I amplitude is larger than that seen in adults; therefore, the ratio of wave V amplitude to wave I amplitude is smaller (187). Waves II and IV are often difficult to identify in this age group (110). Stimulation rates of ten per second worsened the morphological appearance of waveforms in comparison with a rate of five per second (188) and cause prolongation of wave V (59,112). Waveforms comparable with those seen in adults can be identified by the age of 3 to 6 months (88,132).

Absolute and interpeak latencies undergo remarkable changes as premature infants and neonates mature. The interpeak latency (IPL) from wave I to wave V (I-V IPL) changes at a rate of 0.45 milliseconds per week between the ages of 32 and 34 weeks of conceptional age; the change slows to 0.1 milliseconds per week closer to term (39,162). The change in wave V absolute latency is about 0.2 milliseconds per week between the ages of 26 and 40 weeks of conceptional age (88,189,209). At term, the I-V IPL is 0.8 to 1 millisecond longer than that of adults. Adult values are reached at the ages of about 1 to 2 years (60,132,155). BAEP changes in the early weeks of life have been thought to result from progressive myelination, increase in fiber diameter, and increased synaptic efficiency (86,209). Because of the remarkable latency changes in premature and young infants, Chiappa (28) recommended that age-specific norms be obtained for every 2-week age change before term, at birth, at 3 weeks, at 6 weeks, at 3 months, at 6 months and at 1 year. Of importance, however, is that BAEPs are not affected by prematurity; maturation follows the conceptional age rather than legal age (48).

Beyond childhood, age has variable effects on the BAEP. Although some investigators have noted increases in absolute and interpeak latencies of the waveforms (106,182,185,225), others have found no such effect (12). Malhotra (119) noted that, whereas the latency of wave I does not change with age, the amplitude does. He noted that mean amplitude was 0.21 μV in subjects younger than 40 years and 0.13 μV in those older than 40. Similarly, whereas some researchers have found these latency changes in both genders (182,185), others have found them to be significant in boys and men only (106,119). Chiappa (28) summarized these findings and noted that these latency differences are too small to have an impact in clinical interpretation.

Gender

Girls and women have shorter BAEP absolute and interpeak latencies (3,5,12,95,106,119,128,131,155,225). The wave V latency has been noted to be 0.12 to 0.3 millisecond shorter in girls and women (107,128,168,220). These gender-based differences were seen in children as young as 8 years of age (155). It has been postulated that these shorter latencies resulted from smaller head size (3,8). Mitchell et al. (131) found a correlation between head diameter and the latency of wave V and the I-V IPL. However, Trune et al. (229) controlled for head size and found that girls and women consistently had shorter peak latencies, which thus suggests that factors other than brain size were responsible for the gender differences. Some investigators (128) have attributed shorter waveform latencies in girls and women to hormonal effects. Elevation in progesterone level has been thought to be the cause of these differences (42). Picton et al. (167) noted I-V IPL variability in the menstrual cycle, being a mean of 3.81 milliseconds between days 12 and 26 of the cycle (when the levels of progesterone are the highest) and 3.92 milliseconds on other days. These investigators, as well as others (210), have concluded that shorter latencies in girls and women are caused by their higher core body temperatures.

Temperature

Temperature changes have an effect on both absolute and interpeak latencies; these increase with decreases in body temperature (72,219). Temperature correction factors range from 0.17 to 0.20 millisecond prolongation in wave V latency per degree centigrade below 37 degrees (75,167). Below 27 degrees, centigrade waveforms disappear (43,98). Although decreases in temperature can have significant effect on BAEP absolute and interpeak latencies, most patients undergoing routine BAEP studies do not need their temperatures checked (75). Rather, those at greatest risk for hypothermia (i.e., those acutely ill or with severe head trauma) benefit from temperature determination and latency adjustments (40,75,78). The effects of hyperthermia have been less clearly studied. Hall (75) found a decrease of 0.50 to 0.60 msec in the I-V IPL

in patients with temperatures ranging from 38° to 42°C. He suggested a 0.15-millisecond-per-degree correction for patients who are hyperthermic.

Sleep

Numerous investigators have noted the lack of effects of sleep on BAEP waveform latency and amplitude (5,157,167,202). BAEP waveforms also do not appear to be affected by the level of attention during testing (111,116,165,166,196). Certain pathological states that produce sleep and sedation, such as narcolepsy and metabolic coma, also do not have significant effects on BAEPs (76,89,207,221). The lack of effects of sleep on BAEPs is of particular importance because sleep deprivation and sedation is often employed so that the patient is more relaxed during the procedure. This, in turn, serves to decrease electromyographic artifact that can otherwise degrade the quality of the study.

Drug Effects

BAEP waveforms are not affected by central nervous system depressants in therapeutic doses. This property makes BAEPs a robust evoked potential modality to monitor in operative procedures. Phenobarbital, diazepam, and chloral hydrate do not affect BAEP waveforms in therapeutic doses (134,161,212). However, overdose with phenobarbital and nitrazepam can cause minor BAEP IPL changes (186).

Numerous anesthetics, including thiopental, pentobarbital, etomidate, ketamine, halothane, isoflurane, fentanyl, and nitrous oxide, have minimal to no significant effects on BAEPs (38,73,75,123,191,213). A number of other agents, however, do affect BAEP waveform latencies and morphological features. Methohexital prolongs wave V latency without affecting waves I and III; therefore, it can cause a prolongation of IPLs (75). Thiopental in very high doses has been shown to cause prolongation of IPL and decrease in amplitude (44,67). Enflurane causes a linear increase in IPLs as a function of concentration (45,227).

The effects of alcohol on BAEPs have been extensively studied. Acute intoxication with alcohol has been shown to cause latency prolongations of absolute and interpeak latencies without significant change in amplitude (32,33,173,204,205). Whereas some authorities have contended that these effects result from hypothermia induced by the alcohol (97,215), others have maintained that these changes are temperature independent (204). Lee et al. (113) suggested that the changes depend on how fast the alcohol concentration in blood rises. With chronic use, the latencies remain prolonged (13,32). With discontinuation of alcohol use, there is disagreement as to the changes in BAEP waveforms. Some authorities have argued that during withdrawal, latencies are shorter than usual with higher amplitudes (32), whereas others have argued that even with discontinuation, the latencies remain prolonged, possibly because of demyelination or edema (13).

Aminoglycoside antibiotics are an important class of drugs that may have significant effects on BAEPs because of their ototoxicity. The incidence of ototoxicity ranges between 3% and 25% (46,148,231). Rapid intravenous infusion has been found to result in reduced amplitudes of the waveforms and prolongation of wave I latency; after continued infusion, these effects gradually return to baseline (71,197). Oral administration of these agents results in the same effects, although of smaller magnitude; the effects resolve with discontinuation of medication. Aminoglycosides are proposed to produce these effects on BAEPs by causing destruction of the organ of Corti and loss of microvasculature in the basilar membrane (9).

Other drugs such as salicylates have similar effects on the BAEP, presumably because they too have ototoxic properties. Platinum-containing antineoplastic agents, such as cisplatin and carboplatin, cause a delay in absolute latencies of all waveforms and increase the threshold at which BAEPs are elicited (104,159,222). Depolarizing and nondepolarizing neuromuscular blocking agents have not been found to alter BAEP waveform morphological features and latency (74,82,103,200). The antiepileptic drugs phenytoin and carbamazepine cause a prolongation of absolute and interpeak latencies (24,70,94,163,212,245). In contrast, similar effects have not been noted with valproic acid (245). Electrically induced seizures (electroconvulsive therapy) do not affect BAEPs (239).

Hearing Disorders

Hearing disorders can result from problems with the external or middle ear (conductive hearing loss), the cochlea or vestibulocochlear nerve (sensorineural hearing loss), or a mixture of these (mixed hearing loss). All types of hearing loss cause prolongation of the absolute latencies of the BAEP waveforms (75); however, this does not preclude accurate interpretation relevant to central conduction. Numerous investigators have established that IPLs remain normal in conductive, sensorineural, and mixed types of hearing loss (29,31,50,129,183,203). Some studies have suggested that the prolongation of wave V in sensorineural hearing loss is not as great as that of

wave I; hence, the I-V IPL is shorter than would be expected (36,37) (Fig. 28.4). Keith and Greville (101) found similar shortening of the I-V IPL in patients with conductive hearing loss.

The effects of hearing loss on the latency/intensity series and the behavioral audiogram are more remarkable. Hecox and Galambos (88) discussed these changes in detail. In patients with conductive hearing loss, the curve of the latency/intensity series has the same slope as that of normal persons but is displaced to a higher hearing intensity. Patients with sensorineural hearing loss, on the other hand, have peak latencies that are comparable with those of normal persons at high stimulation intensities. At lower intensities, however, the latencies are significantly prolonged. This is an electrophysiological correlate of the behavioral phenomenon of recruitment typically present in patients with sensorineural hearing losses.

The Abnormal Brainstem Auditory Evoked Potential

Statistical Considerations of Brainstem Auditory Evoked Potential Abnormality

To consider a given finding abnormal, the finding must be shown to occur rarely if ever in a normal person, and it must be seen in persons with recognizable disease conditions (pathological correlates).

The criteria (latency or amplitude) values, above or below which abnormality is implied, are determined by studying a population sample that can be independently determined to be normal according to history and examination. From these data, statistics of central tendency (mean) and dispersion characteristics (standard deviation) are computed. A criterion value is then selected, usually by adding some fixed multiple of standard deviations (SD) to the mean. The expression "X + 3 SD" is a shorthand notation to indicate that three times the standard deviation has been added to the mean. Statistical theory predicts that X ± 3 SD will include values from 99.72% of the population. There is no fixed rule that 3 SD must be added to the mean; the literature contains examples in which 2 or 2.5 SD were added. The amounts of the population contained would be 95.46% and 98.75%, respectively.

The mean BAEP I-V IPL is usually close to 4.0 milliseconds, and the standard deviation of the mean is approximately 0.2 milliseconds. A decision to make the mean plus 2.5 SD the upper limit of normal would yield an upper limit of 4.5 milliseconds. Using 3 SD increases the upper limit to 4.6 milliseconds. The test becomes more specific but less sensitive with 3

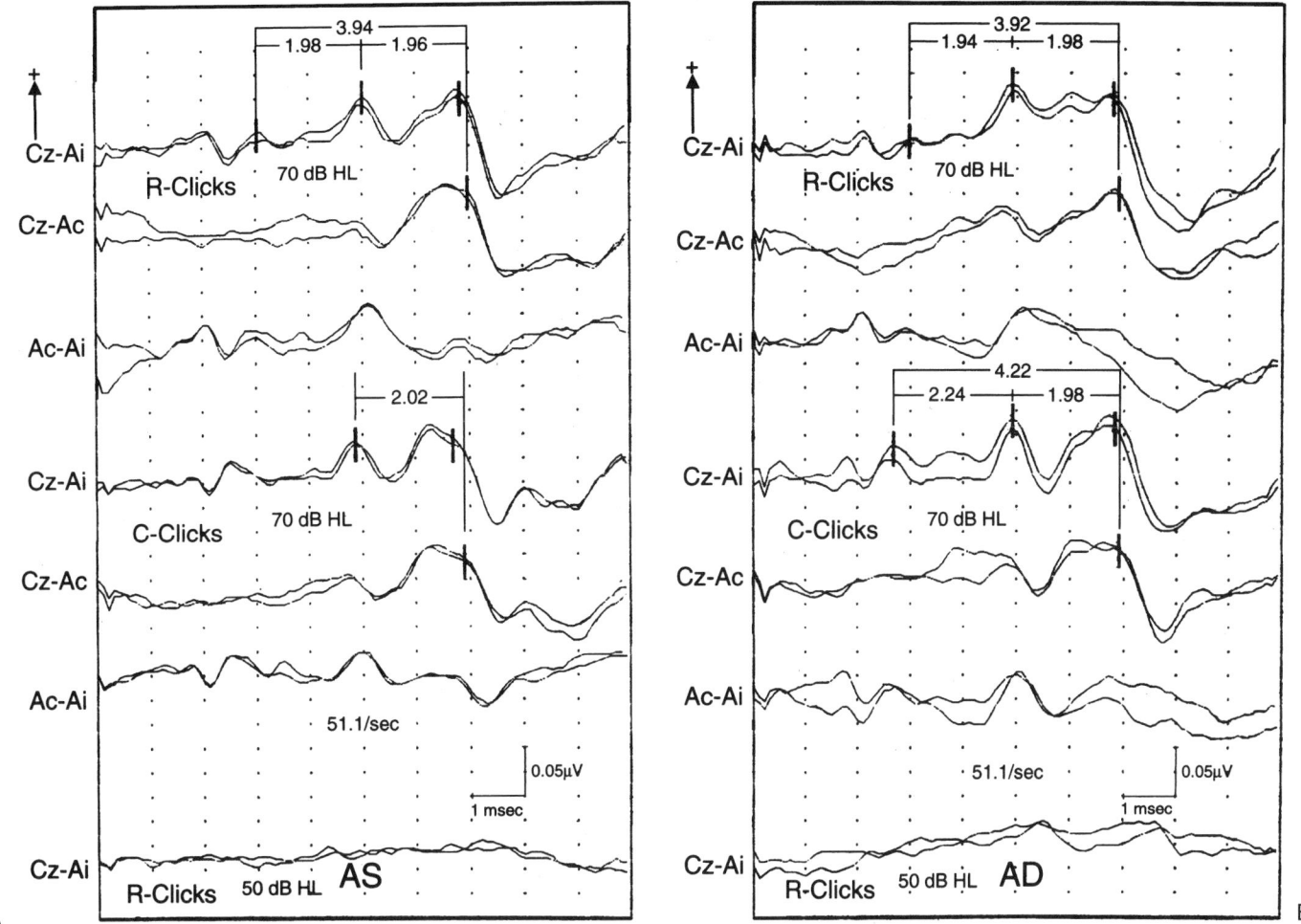

FIG. 28.4. A&**B:** BAEP in an 83-year-old man with worsening hearing loss. The BAEP shows changes related to a neurosensory, high-frequency auditory loss, which resulted in a late and absent to low-amplitude wave I, shortened I-V IPLs, and abnormal latency/intensity testing. It also highlights potential problems in identification of wave I. In this study, waves I are identified as occurring at a delayed absolute latency of ±3.0 milliseconds (0.9-millisecond delay for ear-insert transducers). An up-going event occurs at 2.07 milliseconds, preceding the identified wave I. There are two reasons why this larger event is a cochlear microphonic (CM) rather than a wave I: First, it is too early to be a valid wave I. Subtracting for the ear-insert delay, its absolute latency would be 1.17 milliseconds, which is appropriate for a CM. Second, the polarity of the event reverses when click polarity is changed from rarefaction to condensation clicks, which is to be expected for a CM but not for a wave I. Persons with normal audition have recordable waves V at 30-dBHL (decibel hearing level) of stimulation. In this patient, responses are essentially lost at 50 dBHL. The stimulation rate of 51.1 per second would be expected to produce an average interpeak latency (IPL) from wave I to wave V of 4.2 msec. The shortened IPLs seen in this study are the result of the differential effects of high frequency loss on wave I (smaller and later) and minimal to no change to wave V. (See legend for Fig. 28.1 for stimulation and recording parameters.)

SD added to the mean; there are fewer false-positive results but more false-negative interpretations. Using 2.5 SD does the opposite; the test is less specific but more sensitive, with more false-positive results and fewer false-negative interpretations.

Tolerance Limits

The Guidelines (6) correctly state that addition of a specific number of standard deviations to the mean is not the most appropriate statistical method. The Guidelines (6) indicate that such an application may be correct for dealing with the question "What is the likelihood that two samples were drawn from the same population?"—that is, whether they are different. A more specific example of this type of question is whether a patient group is different from a normal group. Standard deviations were not designed to answer the question of whether a specific value (latency of a person's evoked potential study) is normal or abnormal. To answer this different question, the tolerance limit statistic is suggested. The reader is referred to the Guidelines (6) for a complete discussion of the subtle differences between these two different statistical techniques.

The ultimate goal of the statistical applications is to maximize sensitivity and specificity (in view of the inverse relationship of these concepts), so as to make a clinically relevant interpretation. A BAEP diagnostic study should not be expected to lead to an etiologically specific diagnosis. The BAEP procedure evaluates the physiological integrity of some aspects of the auditory system. Etiologically disparate disorders can produce identical physiological disturbances and identical BAEP abnormalities. The physiological disturbance identified by BAEP abnormality may or may not disturb clinical function. Indeed, a major strength of the study is its ability to demonstrate subclinical disturbance.

Interpretative Criteria of Brainstem Auditory Evoked Potential Abnormality

Obligate Wave Absence

Obligate waves are those that are present in essentially all audiologically and neurologically normal control subjects. The obligate BAEP waves are I, III, and V. Waves II, IV, VI, and VII are known to be absent in some normal subjects, and therefore pathological processes should not be thought to account for their absence. Absence or virtual absence is an amplitude criterion. Absence of any obligate wave indicates abnormality (Fig. 28.5). The obligate wave most commonly absent is wave I, usually as a result of end-organ (cochlear) or conductive deficits; however, retrocochlear (acoustic nerve) dysfunction can also lead to absence of wave I.

Absolute Latency

Prolongation of absolute latency beyond upper limits is a reliable criterion of abnormality. It is common in conductive and neurosensory disturbances. When audiological evaluation indicates no hearing loss, retrocochlear involvement should be considered. Malfunctioning stimulators, transducers, and displaced transducers can indicate absolute latency prolongations.

Interpeak Latency

The I-V IPL is a measure of central brainstem conduction time from the generators of these two waves, generally held to be the distal acoustic nerve to caudal midbrain. Three laboratories independently collecting normative data found remarkable consistency for the I-V IPL when similar ages, genders, stimulation rates, and filter settings were held relatively constant (185). Any IPL can be measured and evaluated, but excessive reliance on IPL is inappropriate on statistical grounds and may lead to excessive false-positive test results. The I-V IPL recorded from stimulation of each ear is usually compared to the upper limits derived from study of normal controls (in the range of 4.6 milliseconds). In addition, a side-to-side comparison is made, whereby asymmetries exceeding 0.4 milliseconds in the interaural I-V IPL are considered abnormal. When the two waves I are relatively symmetrical and the asymmetry is caused by the waves V, the abnormality is that of central conduction. When the waves V are relatively symmetrical and waves I are not, the abnormality is usually caused by a peripheral disturbance. Once an abnormality has been identified, other IPLs (I-III and III-V) may be considered to assess what region of the brainstem may show the major disturbance (Figs. 28.6 and 28.7).

No neuropathological process leads to a shortening of absolute or interpeak latencies. A high-frequency audiological disturbance can shorten I-V IPL by selectively lengthening wave I, which is generated primarily by the high-frequency components of the broad-band click stimuli, and leave the wave V at a normal absolute latency.

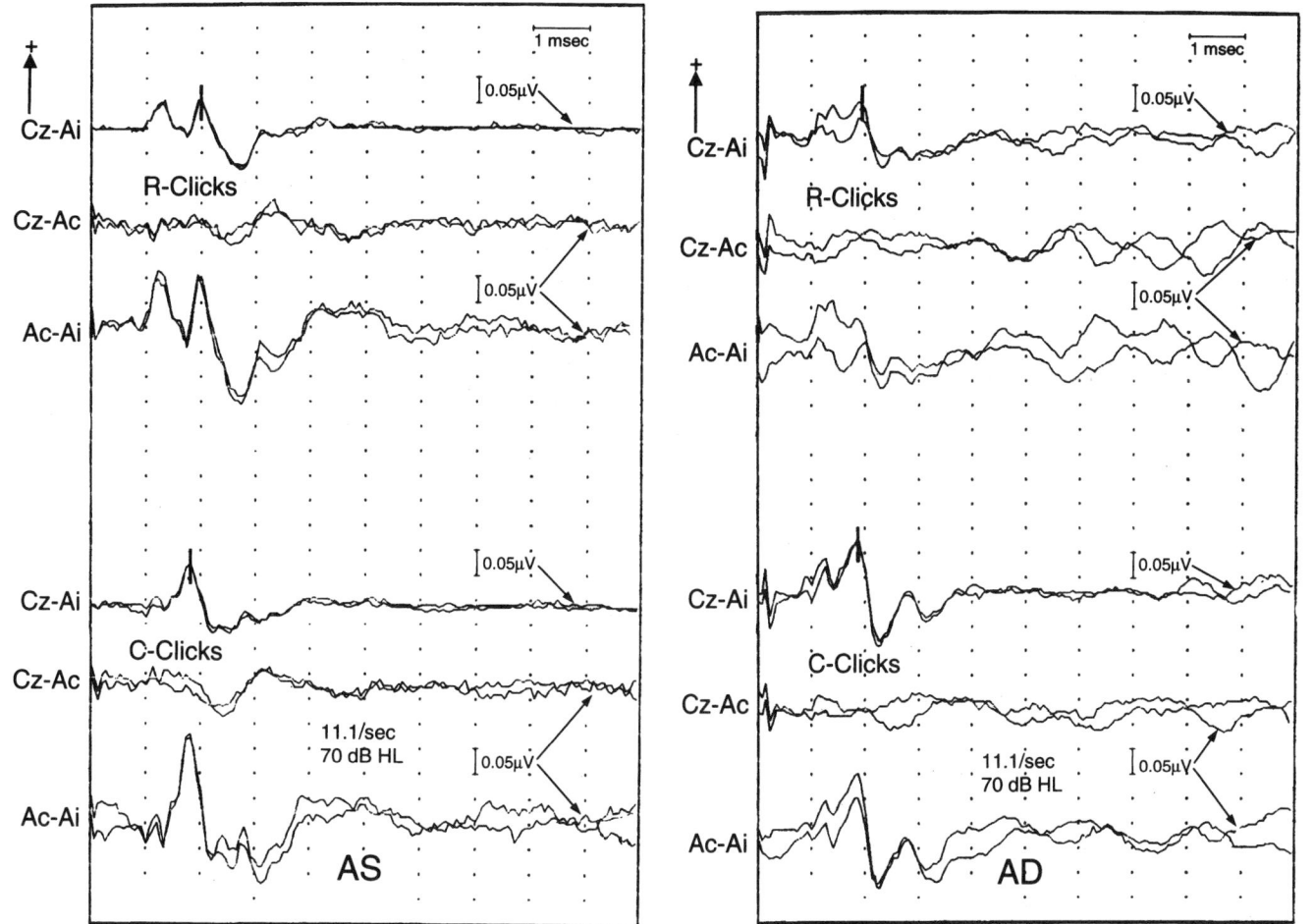

FIG. 28.5. A&**B:** Magnetic resonance imaging shows extensive white matter changes in the cerebral hemispheres and the brainstem of a 1-year-old girl with Krabbe's disease. The BAEP is very abnormal as a result of virtual absence of all waves after wave I_N. This finding indicates severe dysfunction of brainstem structures rostral to the acoustic nerve and is etiologically nonspecific. Whether this represents a block in conduction or marked temporal dispersion cannot be determined from the BAEP data. There is a small stimulus artifact at the beginning of the traces caused by the magnetic fields generated by the transducer near the clavicle. A cochlear microphonic is the first prominent up-going peak, followed by waves I and I_N. There is virtually no activity in the Cz-Ac channels because of in-phase cancellation. (See legend for Fig. 28.1 for stimulation and recording parameters.)

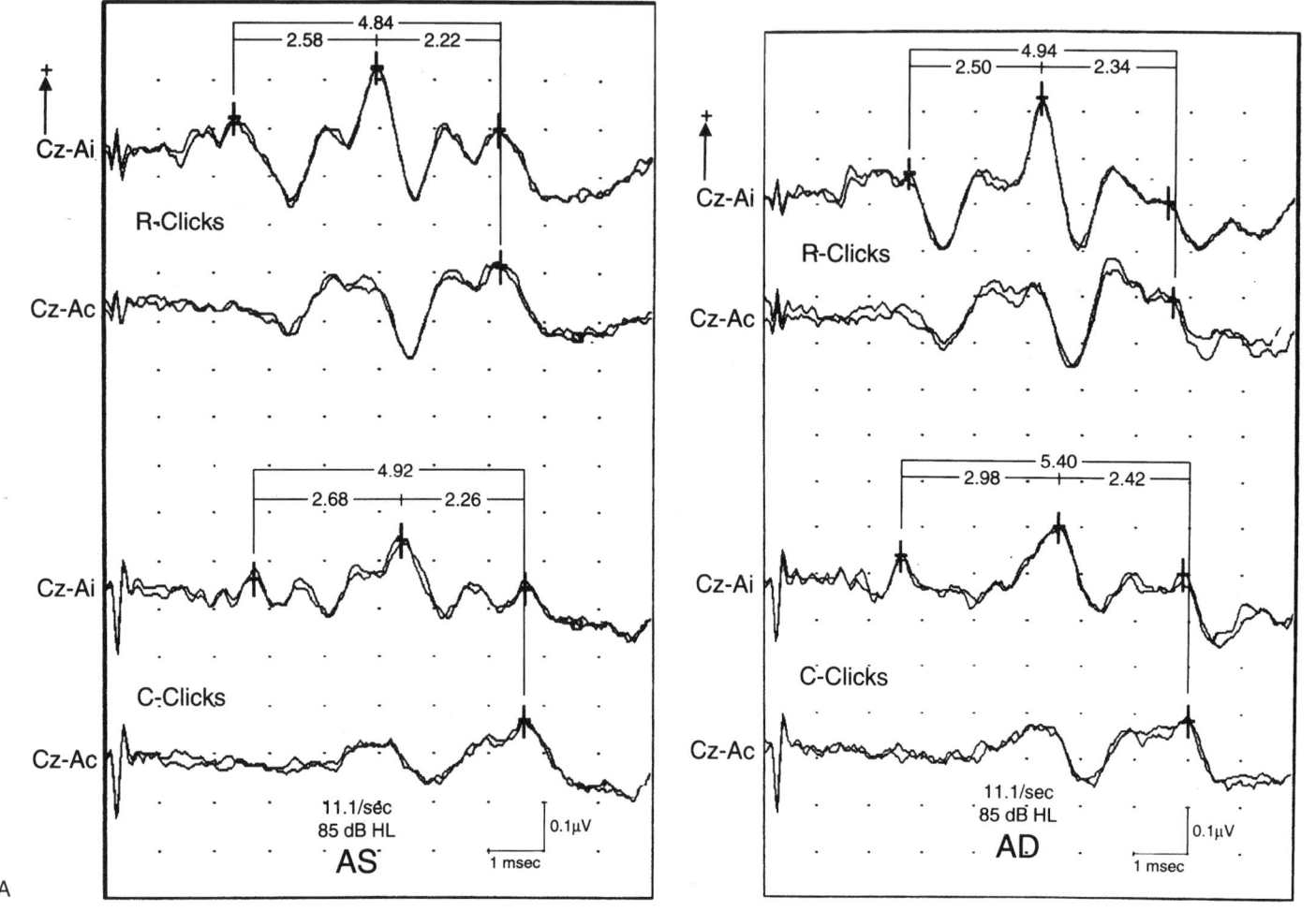

FIG. 28.6. A&B: Magnetic resonance imaging shows T2 hyperintensity in the medulla of an 80-year-old woman with progressive ataxia. The BAEP shows bilaterally prolonged interpeak latencies (IPLs) from wave I to wave V_C to both rarefaction (R) and condensation (C) clicks. The interpeak latency (IPL) from wave I to wave III shows greater bilateral prolongation than the IPL from wave III to wave V, which suggests a greater involvement of the pontine portions of the brainstem. Right ear C clicks produce IPLs from wave I to wave V_C that are 0.46 millisecond longer than those of R clicks because wave I is 0.14 millisecond earlier and wave V is 0.32 millisecond later than those produced by R clicks. Such click polarity discrepancies are often due to cochlear disturbances of neurosensory function, as revealed in the audiogram. (See legend for Fig. 28.1 for stimulation and recording parameters.)

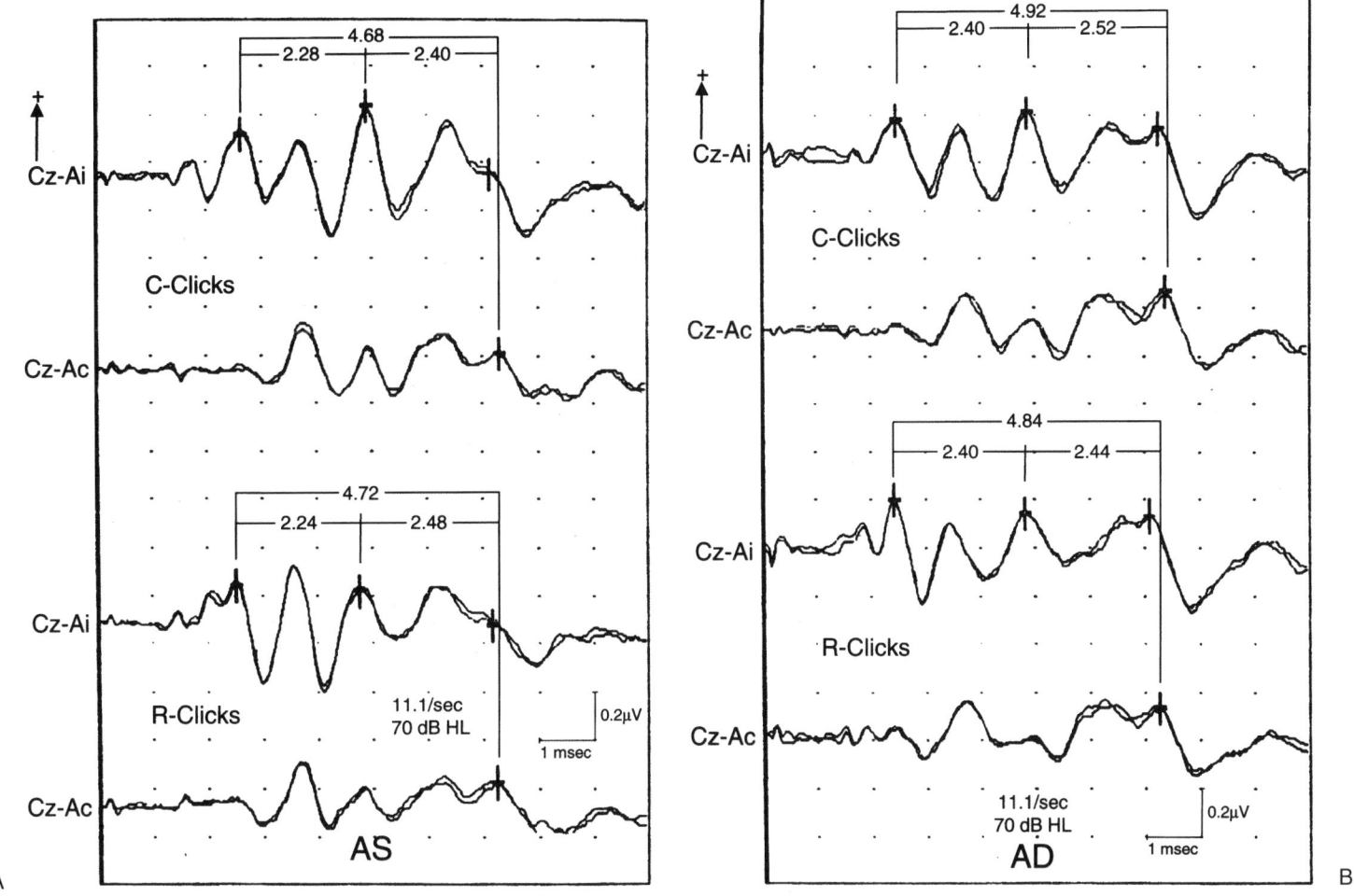

FIG. 28.7. A&B: Magnetic resonance imaging revealed hamartomas in the globus pallidi and upper pons bilaterally in a 10-year-old boy with neurofibromatosis I. The BAEP shows interpeak latencies (IPLs) from wave I to wave V that are well above the upper limits of normal for the laboratory (4.6 milliseconds, rate and age adjusted) bilaterally. The IPL from wave III to wave V shows a greater prolongation than the IPL from wave I to wave III, which is suggestive of greater involvement in the pontomesenphalic region of the brainstem. (See legend for Fig. 28.1 for stimulation and recording parameters.)

Amplitude

The most extreme amplitude abnormality is absence of an obligate wave (see Fig. 28.5). Because of the wide range of amplitudes encountered in the normal population, lesser degrees of absolute low amplitude cannot be assessed; this would lead to excessive variance. Comparing the amplitude of a wave in reference to another wave can partially avoid such problems. When the amplitude ratio of waves IV and V to wave I is less than 0.5, wave V is abnormally small. This criterion is relatively specific because audiological disturbances cause a lowering of wave I amplitude, which in turn cause the amplitude ratio of waves IV and V to wave I to be greater. This ratio, like all ratios, is not normally distributed and must be transformed (usually a by logarithmic transform) before statistics are computed (127).

Latency/Intensity Functions

See Hearing Disorders section (p. 874).

Clinical Correlations

Cerebellopontine Angle Tumors

Acoustic neuromas and meningiomas are the most frequent types of tumors found in the cerebellopontine angle (CPA). These tumors most often produce hearing loss by compression of the vestibulocochlear nerve. About 75% of the nerve fibers need to be involved before pure tone hearing thresholds are affected (195). Acoustic neuromas, by virtue of their attachment to the vestibulocochlear nerve, produce hearing deficits earlier than do other CPA tumors.

The following are the abnormalities noted most often in CPA tumors ipsilaterally (141,164,247):

1. Absence of all waveforms.
2. Absence of all waveforms after wave I.
3. Absence of all waveforms after waves I and II.
4. Absence of all waveforms after waves I, II, and III.
5. Absence of wave I and prolongation of wave V latency.
6. Prolongation of I-III IPL.7. Prolongation of III-V IPL.
7. Prolongation of I-V IPL.

Because many patients with CPA tumors have associated hearing loss, Selters and Brackmann (199) recommended that a correction factor be used if wave I could not be identified and wave V was prolonged. They proposed to use the factor to correct wave V latency for the hearing loss before concluding that the delay in latency was caused by a CPA tumor by subtracting 0.1 millisecond for every 10 dB or fraction thereof of loss of 4-kHz pure-tone threshold over 50 dB. Hyde and Blair (92) recommended subtracting 0.1 millisecond per 5 dB of hearing loss over 55 dB. Because of these problems with absolute latencies, numerous investigators have noted that IPLs are a better measure of abnormality because they are not affected by hearing loss (49,164,190,246). However, even though IPLs are a more definite indicator of abnormality, wave I in many patients with CPA tumors is not recordable by conventional methods (92). For these patients, additional effort should be expended to determine the presence and location of wave I by increasing the stimulation level to the maximum output necessary to elicit wave I. In addition, ear canal electrodes may be used to advantage in recording wave I. These extra efforts may reveal the wave I, making determination of IPLs possible (30,35,51).

CPA tumors can also produce contralateral BAEP abnormalities by distortion and cross-compression of brainstem structures (133,199,213,246). The abnormality most often seen is prolongation of ipsilateral or contralateral III-V IPL (17,133,147); however, investigators have noted I-III IPL prolongation; absence of all waves except wave I; absence of all waves except waves I and II; and absence of all waves except waves I, II, and III (164,199,240). These abnormalities regress with tumor removal (164).

Although large CPA tumors have a higher likelihood of causing contralateral BAEP abnormalities (17,147), severity of ipsilateral abnormalities is related to factors other than size. In their series of 61 tumors, all nearly the same size, Musiek et al. (146) demonstrated that abnormalities ranged from absence of all waves to presence of all waves. Acoustic neuromas limited to the internal acoustic canal produce symptoms early and tend to cause more destructive effects on the vestibulocochlear nerve and to produce abnormalities of the ipsilateral BAEP earlier; they usually do not affect contralateral BAEPs. In contrast, CPA tumors more proximal to the brainstem often produce symptoms later. When they are large enough to affect the ipsilateral vestibulocochlear nerve, they often cause brainstem and contralateral BAEP abnormalities. Malhotra (119) proposed that the following processes may be responsible for producing BAEP abnormalities in patients with CPA tumors: (a) pressure on the vestibulocochlear nerve, which causes asynchrony in neuronal firing; (b) tumors in the CPA, which can cause pressure effects on contiguous brainstem areas; and (c) compression of blood supply to the cochlea, which causes cochlear ischemia.

The sensitivity of BAEPs in detecting CPA tumors has ranged from 93% to 100% in some studies (10,11,34,66) and has been as low as 75% to 76% in others (17,65,232). Faster rates of stimulation have been shown to increase the sensitivity of BAEPs in detecting CPA tumors (223). In comparison to computed tomographic scanning, BAEPs were more sensitive (11,66,164). Before the availability of MRI, BAEPs became the screening study of choice for evaluating for CPA tumors. However, MRI has been shown more recently to be more sensitive than BAEP in evaluation of small tumors (56,149). Wilson et al. (241) demonstrated that BAEP detected only five of 15 small intracanalicular tumors, whereas MRI detected all 15. Because of the significantly higher expense of MRI, Chiappa (28), however, recommended that if the BAEP I-III IPL is normal and there is no other strong evidence of acoustic neuromas, no further testing needs to be performed.

Other Brain Tumors

The results of BAEPs in patients with a variety of intrinsic brainstem tumors have been reported. Brainstem gliomas (20,26,150), fourth ventricle ependymomas (216), cerebellar tumors (117,216), pinealomas, thalamic gliomas (69), and brainstem metastatic tumors (150,156) produce prolongations of absolute and interpeak latencies (Fig. 28.8; see Fig. 28.5). It is widely believed that virtually all intrinsic brainstem tumors produce BAEP abnormalities.

Coma and Brain Death

BAEP is used to evaluate the auditory pathways in the brainstem between the lower pons and the midbrain. Thus, if the cause of coma does not directly affect these pathways, the BAEPs are normal. Coma caused by metabolic dysfunction has little effect on the BAEPs (208,211). Similarly, central nervous system depressant medications do not affect the BAEP significantly (186,218). Support of this observation also comes from studies on patients in persistent vegetative state; these patients have been found to have normal BAEPs (81,99,208), presumably because the site of primary involvement is rostral to the thalamus (233). However, if supratentorial causes of coma cause distortion or pressure on the brainstem, BAEP abnormalities are noted

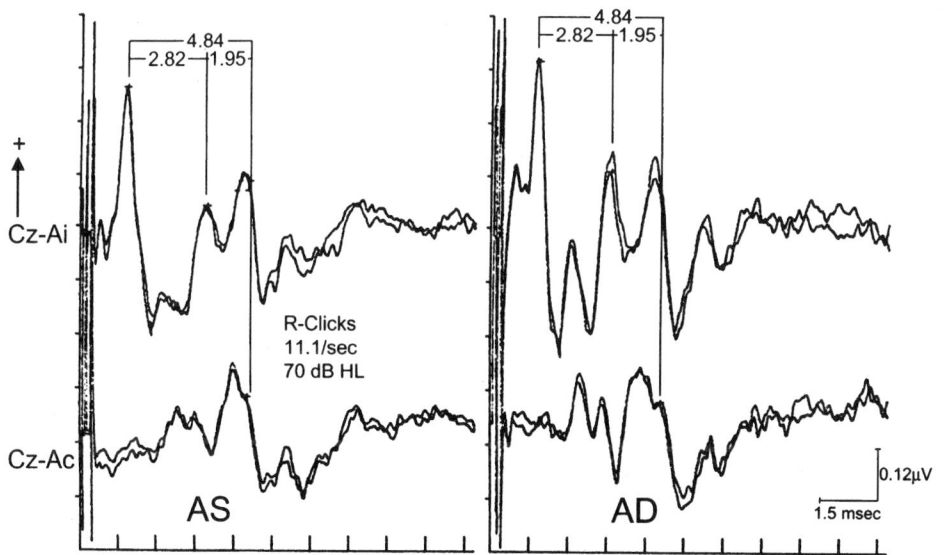

FIG. 28.8. Lower pontine glioma in a 63-year-old man. Brainstem auditory evoked potentials demonstrated prolongedinterpeak latencies from wave I to wave V$_C$ and from wave I to wave III, which are consistent with the lower brainstem lesion. (See legend for Fig. 28.1 for stimulation and recording parameters.)

(28). BAEP abnormalities have also been noted with herniation syndromes and lessen with clinical improvement (55,68,108,207). In such cases, there is gradual disappearance of waves V to II, in a rostrocaudal manner (108,207). Abnormal BAEPs after head injury have been correlated with poor prognosis (99,198).

BAEPs have been shown to be useful for prognosis of patients in coma (7,77,158,192). Elwany (52) correlated BAEPs with neurological outcome. The presence of only wave I or absence of all waves was correlated with a poor outcome. In contrast, 60% of patients with normal BAEPs had a favorable outcome. Presence of wave V, even on only one side, is suggestive of a good outcome (1). BAEPs are most useful prognostically if wave I is completely absent or only wave I is present; this finding is suggestive of a poor outcome. Similar results have been found in children with traumatic coma, in whom absence of BAEPs is suggestive of a poor outcome (16,21).

In patients with brain death, BAEPs are remarkably abnormal; either all waves are completely absent or only wave I is present (68,108). Barbiturates in anesthetic doses sufficient to cause an isoelectric EEG do not affect the BAEP (191,212,218). Thus, BAEPs are useful in confirming brain death in patients being treated with high doses of barbiturates or anesthetics. Before concluding that absence of BAEP waveforms is consistent with brain death, the clinician must rule out preexisting hearing loss and technical problems that may be precluding appropriate stimulation or recording.

Vascular Diseases

Vascular lesions of the brainstem produce BAEP abnormalities only if the auditory pathways are involved. If lesions are below the level of the pontomedullary junction, the BAEP is usually normal (20). This has been demonstrated by the presence of normal BAEPs in patients with locked-in syndrome caused by lesions in the medulla (20,79,228). Various stroke syndromes with lesions above the pontomedullary junction result in BAEP abnormalities (145,156,178,211). There is disagreement about the effect of transient ischemic attacks on BAEPs. Whereas some authors have demonstrated that even brainstem transient ischemic attacks result in BAEP abnormalities (54,184), others have not found this to be the case (105). Rao and Libman (179) noted abnormal BAEPs in patients with isolated vertigo that later progressed to an anterior inferior cerebellar artery stroke. They recommended using BAEPs to differentiate vertigo caused by labyrinthine disease from that caused by vertebrobasilar ischemia.

Brainstem hemorrhages much like ischemic lesions (20,26,55,80). Stockard and Rossiter (211) noted that lower pontine lesions affect wave III and the I-III IPL, whereas higher lesions leave wave III intact. BAEPs have also been shown to be helpful in prognosticating outcome after infratentorial hemorrhages and primary subarachnoid hemorrhages; normal evoked potentials imply good prognosis, whereas absence of waveforms implies poor outcome (84,85). Faster stimulation rates (beyond 50 Hz) have been shown to demonstrate abnormalities more often in patients with vascular brainstem dysfunction (14,58). This is thought to occur because the sites most vulnerable to increased rates of stimulation, the synapses, are the same sites that are most vulnerable to ischemia (176).

Multiple Sclerosis

BAEPs, like other modalities of evoked potentials, are useful in the evaluation of multiple sclerosis. Abnormalities are seen in declining incidence in patients grouped as having definite, probable, and possible multiple sclerosis. BAEP abnormalities have been noted in 39% to 90% of patients with definite multiple sclerosis (160,174,175); 33% to 77% of patients with probable multiple sclerosis (57,100,118,153,174,175,180,216); and 19% to 67% of patient with possible multiple sclerosis (118,174,175) (Fig. 28.9). Chiappa (28) reviewed a number of studies that included all classes of patients with multiple sclerosis. Of the 1,006 patients in these studies, 466 (46%) had abnormal BAEPs. When divided into different classes, 67% of patients with definite multiple sclerosis, 41% with probable multiple sclerosis, and 30% with possible multiple sclerosis had BAEP abnormalities. Most important, 38% of patients without brainstem symptoms or signs had BAEP abnormalities.

The BAEP abnormalities seen most commonly in multiple sclerosis include delay in wave V latency, wave V amplitude abnormalities, and III-V IPL prolongation (29,100,174,175). I-III IPL abnormalities are less common. Fast rates of stimulation have been noted to increase the frequency with which abnormalities are detected.

Other demyelinating and dysmyelinating conditions have been associated with abnormal BAEPs. In leukodystrophy (64,114,120,122,154) and Alpers' syndrome (124), IPL prolongations and absence of waves after wave I have been demonstrated (Fig. 28.10; see Fig. 28.5).

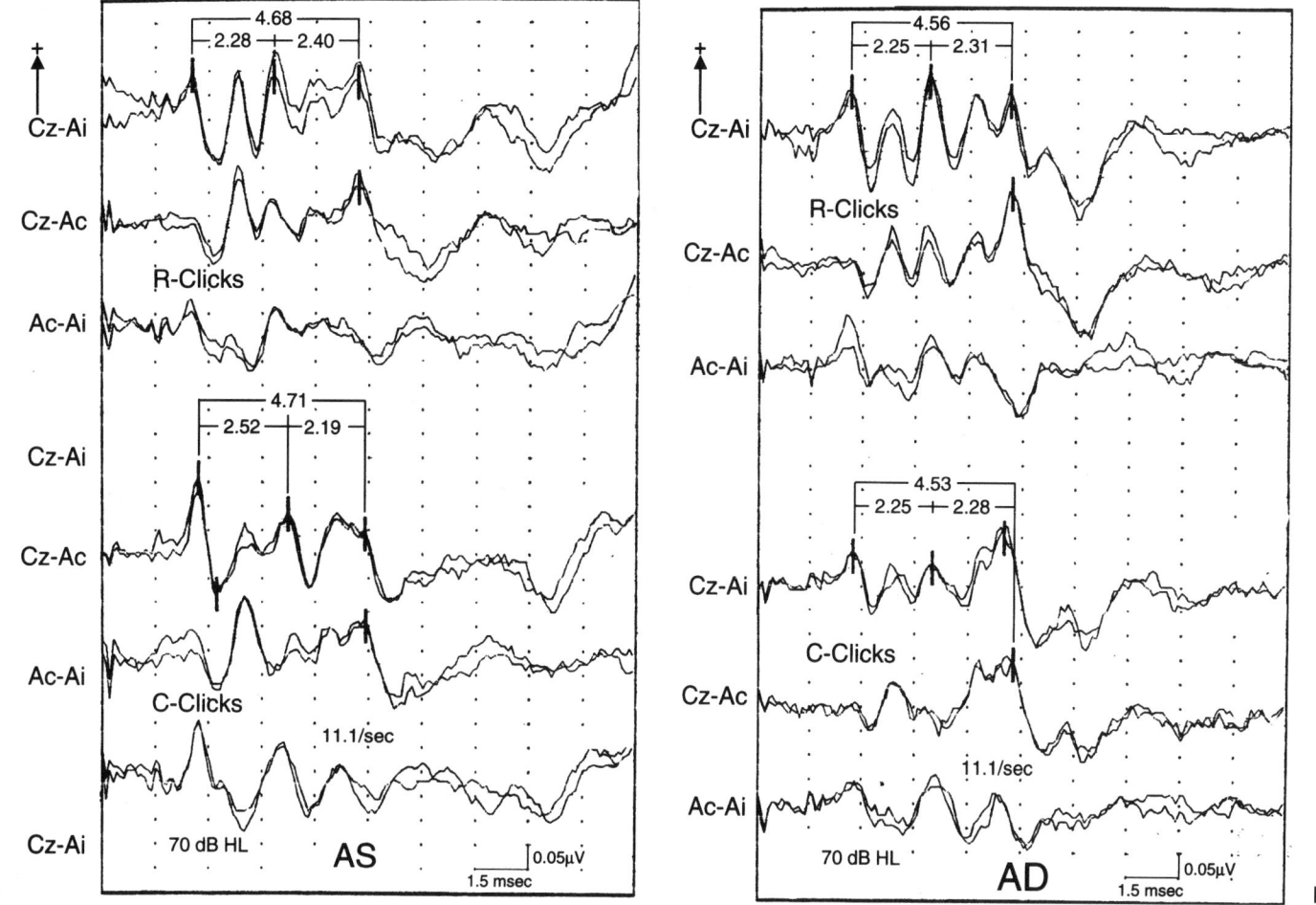

FIG. 28.9. A&**B:** Magnetic resonance imaging (MRI) of the brain of a 50-year-old man with a 5-year history of left lower extremity weakness revealed multiple white matter plaques in the cerebral hemispheres but none in the brainstem. The BAEP revealed prolonged interpeak latencies from wave I to wave V after left ear stimulation that exceed 4.60 milliseconds. The responses from right ear stimulation are just below 4.6 milliseconds. Neither the wave I–wave III nor wave III–wave V segment is prolonged, which suggests that the disturbance is diffuse, from the pontomedullary junction to the caudal midbrain with greater physiological disturbance on the left. This study supports the diagnosis of multiple sclerosis by suggesting yet another site of possible demyelination in the brain stem not seen by MRI. (See legend for Fig. 28.1 for stimulation and recording parameters.)

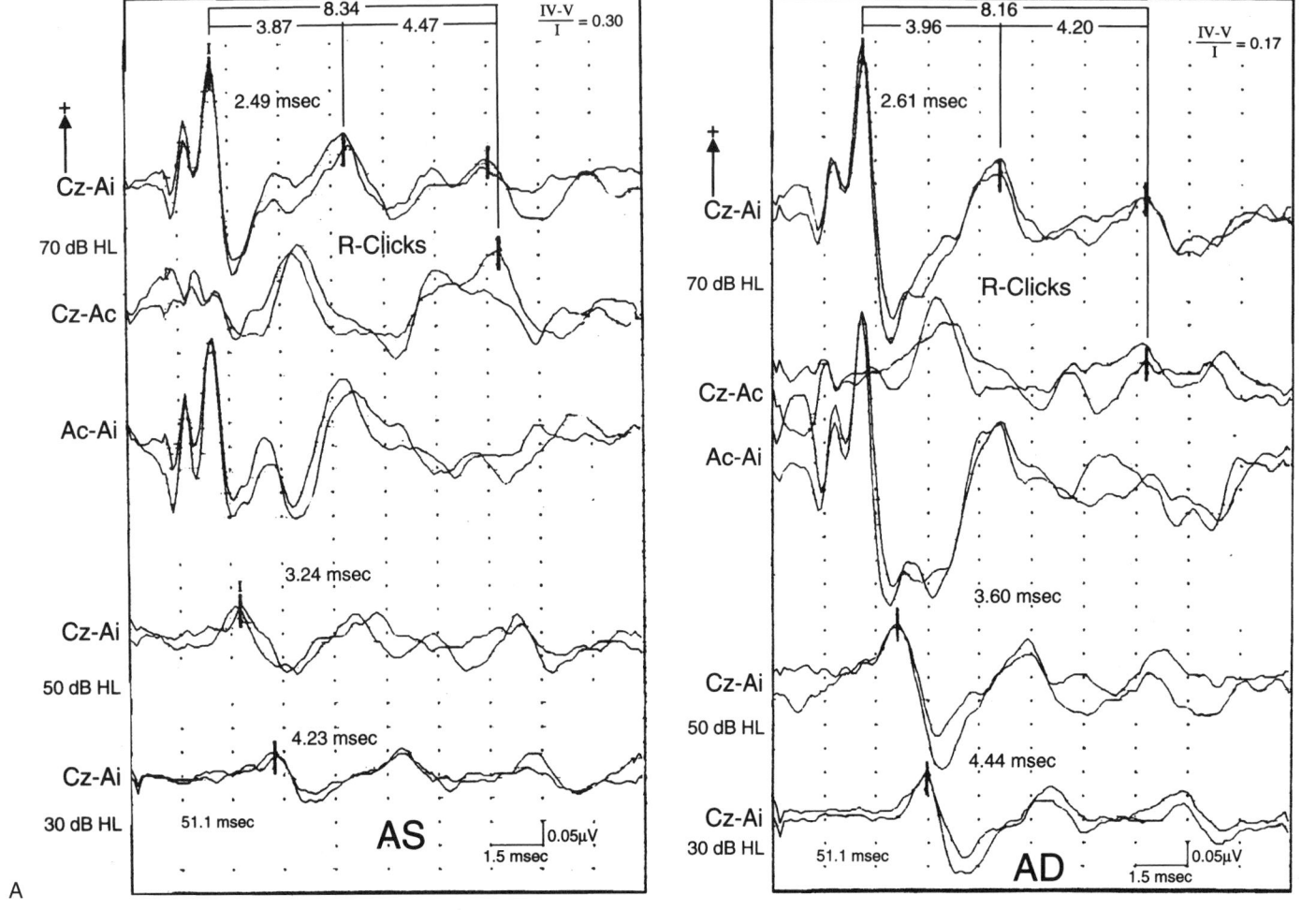

FIG. 28.10 A&**B:** Magnetic resonance imaging revealed diffuse T2 hyperintensity in the subcortical white matter and brainstem of a 5-month-old girl with Krabbe's disease. The BAEP showed markedly prolonged interpeak latencies from wave I to wave V_C of 8.34 milliseconds AS and 8.16 milliseconds AD. The ear insert transducers produce essentially no stimulus artifact and delay the stimulus onset by 0.9 millisecond, producing wave I responses of 2.49 and 2.61 milliseconds after left and right ear stimulation, respectively. Wave I is preceded by a cochlear microphonic response that is more prominent than usual. Waves V and V_C are both prolonged and attenuated, as evidenced by the low amplitude ratios of wave IV or wave V to wave I bilaterally. The latency/intensity series with stimulation at 70, 50, and 30 dBHL (decibel hearing level) shows appropriate time displacements for wave I. Wave V is usually more robust at lower levels of stimulation, but in this instance, wave I is the more robust, confirming the pathological attenuation of wave V at 70 dBHL.

Miscellaneous Disorders

Myelomeningocele and Arnold-Chiari Malformation

BAEPs have been shown to be useful in predicting which patients with myelomeningocele will ultimately have brainstem dysfunction. Children without brainstem symptoms at birth or shortly thereafter and abnormal BAEPs are more likely to become symptomatic than are those with normal BAEPs (224,242). The most common abnormality in this group of children was fusion of waves III, IV, and V, caused in part by the absence of wave III_N (242). The average I-V IPL was also greater in those that later developed symptoms. Others have noted that in natural progression of Arnold-Chiari malformation there is gradual shortening of the III-V IPL and prolongation of I-III IPL (143,151) (Fig. 28.11). Those authors postulate that this is caused by gradual myelination of the brainstem with age. On the other hand, stretching and prolongation of the abnormally placed lower cranial nerves with growth leads to prolongation of the I-III IPL.

Alcoholism

Acute intoxication causes a prolongation in the I-V IPL (204,205,215); these changes do not disappear with discontinuation of alcohol (13).

BAEP abnormalities have also been reported in Wernicke-Korsakoff syndrome (23).

Sleep Disorders

As may be expected, patients with central sleep apnea have been noted to have BAEP abnormalities (214); however, patients with obstructive and mixed apneas often have normal findings (144,214,235). The exception to this observation came from Kotterba and Rasche (109), who found prolongation of IPLs in 12 of 20 patients with obstructive sleep apnea; interestingly, nine of these patients had demonstrable brainstem lesions. In narcolepsy, although a site of pathophysiological abnormality is thought to be the brainstem, BAEPs are normal (89,125).

Neurodegenerative and Other Progressive Neurological Disorders

Although many neurodegenerative disorders have been studied with BAEPs, the number of patients in each group has been small, and the results are thus inconclusive. This is demonstrated by the variability of findings reported in Friedreich's ataxia. Patients with this condition have been reported to exhibit BAEPs with central conduction abnormalities (87,93), only periph-

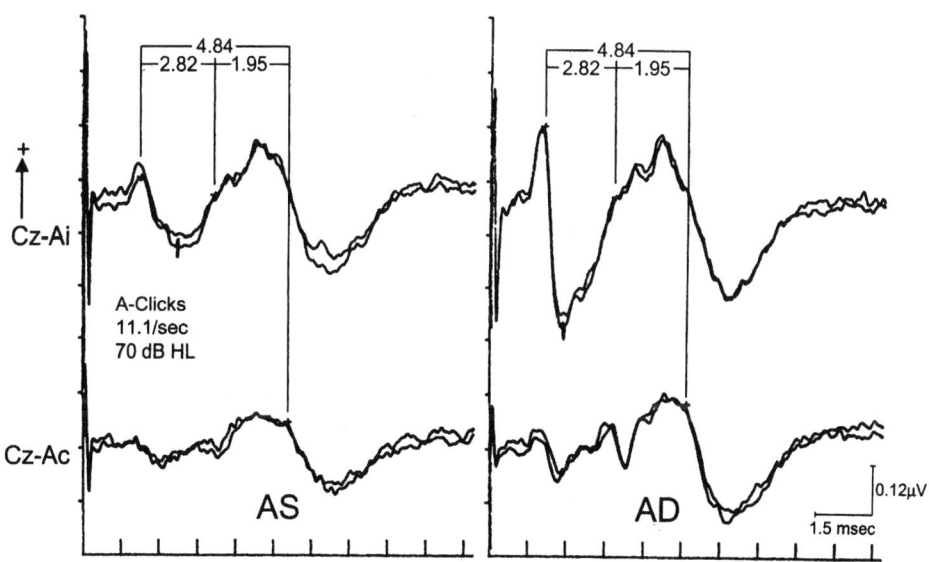

FIG. 28.11. Chiari malformation in a 4-year-old girl. The BAEP showed prolongation of the interpeak latencies from wave I to wave V_C and from wave I to wave III bilaterally, which suggests lower brainstem dysfunction. In addition, fusion of waves III, IV, and V is present bilaterally, forming the typical mitten-shaped waveform.

eral conduction abnormalities (193), and normal findings (152). In numerous other neurodegenerative conditions, including Parkinson's disease (230), Huntington's disease (170), and amyotrophic lateral sclerosis (22), normal BAEPs have been demonstrated. In Creutzfeldt-Jakob disease, there is progressive deterioration of the BAEPs as disease severity increases (171).

REFERENCES

1. Abd al-Hady MR, Shehata O, el-Mously M, et al. Audiological findings following head trauma. *J Laryngol Otol* 1990;104:927–936.
2. Achor LJ, Starr A. Auditory brain stem responses in the cat. II. Effects of lesions. *Electroencephalogr Clin Neurophysiol* 1980;48:174–190.
3. Allison T, Hume AL, Wood CC, et al. Development and aging changes in somatosensory, auditory, and visual evoked potentials. *Electroencephalogr Clin Neurophysiol* 1984;58:14–24.
4. Allison T, Wood CC, Goff WR. Brainstem auditory, pattern-reversal visual and short-latency somatosensory evoked potentials: latencies in relation to age, sex, and brain and body size. *Electroencephalogr Clin Neurophysiol* 1983;55:619–636.
5. Amadeo M, Shagass C. Brief latency click-evoked potentials during waking and sleep in man. *Psychophysiology* 1973;10:244–250.
6. American Electroencephalographic Society Guidelines in Electroencephalography, Evoked Potentials, and Polysomnography. *J Clin Neurophysiol* 1994;11:1–147.
7. Anderson DC, Bundlie S, Rockswold GL. Multimodality EPs in closed head trauma. *Arch Neurol* 1984;41:369–374.
8. Antonelli AR, Bonfioli F, Cappiello J, et al. Auditory evoked potentials test battery related to magnetic resonance imaging for multiple sclerosis patients. *Scand Audiol Suppl* 1988;30: 191–196.
9. Backus RM, De Groot JC, Tange RA, et al. Pathological findings in the human auditory system following long-standing gentamicin ototoxicity. *Arch Otorhinolaryngol* 1987;244:69–73.
10. Baguley DM, Beynon GJ, Grey PL, et al. Audio-vestibular findings in meningioma of the cerebello-pontine angle: a retrospective review. *J Laryngol Otol* 1997;111:1022–1026.
11. Barrs DM, Brackmann DE, Olson JE, et al. Changing concepts of acoustic neuroma diagnosis. *Arch Otolaryngol* 1985;111:17–21.
12. Beagley HA, Sheldrake JB. Differences in brainstem response latency with age and sex. *Br J Audiol* 1978;12:69–77.
13. Begleiter H, Porjesz B, Chou CL. Auditory brainstem potentials in chronic alcoholics. *Science* 1981;211:1064–1066.
14. Ben-David Y, Pratt H, Landman L, et al. A comparison of auditory brain stem evoked potentials in hyperlipidemics and normolipemic subjects. *Laryngoscope* 1986;96:186–189.
15. Boller F, Jacobson GP. Unilateral gunshot wound on the pons. Clinical, electrophysiological and neuroradiological correlates. *Arch Neurol* 1980;37:278–281.
16. Bosch Blancafort J, Olesti Marco M, Poch Puig JM, et al. Predictive value of brain-stem auditory evoked potentials in children with post-traumatic coma produced by diffuse brain injury. *Childs Nerv Syst* 1995;11:400–405.
17. Brackmann DE, Forquer BD. Evaluation of the auditory system: an update. *Ann Otol Rhinol Laryngol* 1983;92:651–656.
18. Brackmann DE, Selters WA. Sensorineural hearing impairment: clinical differentiation. *Otolaryngol Clin North Am* 1978;11:195–199.
19. Britt RH, Rossi GT. Neural generators of brainstem auditory evoked responses. Part I: lesion studies. *Soc Neurosci Abst* 1980;6:594.
20. Brown RH, Chiappa KH, Brooks EB. Brainstem auditory evoked responses in 22 patients with intrinsic brainstem lesions: implications for clinical interpretations. *Electroencephalogr Clin Neurophysiol* 1981;50:38P.
21. Butinar D, Gostisa A. Brainstem auditory evoked potentials and somatosensory evoked potentials in prediction of posttraumatic coma in children. *Pflugers Arch* 1996;431:R289–R290.
22. Cascino GD, Ring SR, King PJL, et al. Evoked potentials in motor system diseases. *Neurology* 1988;38:231–238.
23. Chan YW, McLeod JG, Tuck RR, et al. Brain stem auditory evoked responses in chronic alcoholics. *J Neurol Neurosurg Psychiat* 1985;48:1107–1112.
24. Chan YW, Woo E, Yu YL. Chronic effects of phenytoin on brain-stem auditory evoked potentials in man. *Electroencephalogr Clin Neurophysiol* 1990;77:119–126.
25. Chen TJ, Chen SS. Generator study of brainstem auditory evoked potentials by a radiofrequency lesion method in rats. *Exp Brain Res* 1991;85:537–542.
26. Chiappa KH. Physiologic localization using evoked responses: pattern shift visual, brainstem auditory and short latency somatosensory. In: Thompson RA, Green JR, eds. *New perspectives in cerebral localization.* New York: Raven Press, 1982:63–114.
27. Chiappa KH. *Utility of lowering click intensity in neurologic applications of brainstem auditory evoked potentials.* Presented at Conference on Standards in Clinical BAEP Testing, Laguna Beach, CA, February 1982.
28. Chiappa KH. *Evoked potentials in clinical medicine,* 3rd ed. Philadelphia: Lippincott-Raven, 1997.
29. Chiappa KH, Harrison JL, Brooks EB, et al. Brainstem auditory evoked responses in 200 patients with multiple sclerosis. *Ann Neurol* 1980;7:135–143.
30. Chiappa KH, Parker SW. A simple needle electrode technique for improved registration of wave I in brainstem auditory evoked potentials. In: Starr A, Rosenberg C, Don M, et al., eds. *Sensory evoked potentials, 1. An international conference on standards in auditory brainstem response testing.* Milan: Centro Ricerche e Studi Amplifo, 1984:137–139.
31. Chisin R, Gafni M, Sohmer H. Patterns of auditory nerve and brainstem-evoked responses (ABR) in different types of peripheral hearing loss. *Arch Otorhinolaryngol* 1983;237:165–173.
32. Chu NS, Squires KC, Stan A. Auditory brainstem potentials in chronic alcohol intoxication and alcohol withdrawal. *Arch Neurol* 1978;35:596–602.
33. Church MW, Williams HL, Holloway JA. Dose- and time-dependent effects of ethanol on brain stem auditory evoked responses in young adult males. *Electroencephalogr Clin Neurophysiol* 1982;54:161–174.
34. Clemis JD, McGee T. Brain stem electric response audiometry in the differential diagnosis of acoustic tumors. *Laryngoscope* 1979;89:31–42.
35. Coats AC. On electrocochleographic electrode design. *J Acoust Soc* 1974;56:707–711.
36. Coats AC. Human auditory nerve action potentials and brainstem evoked responses. Latency-intensity function in detection of cochlear and retrocochlear abnormalities. *Arch Otolaryngol* 1978;104:709–717.
37. Coats AC. Martin JL. Human auditory nerve action potentials and brain stem evoked responses. Effects of audiogram shape and lesion location. *Arch Otolaryngol* 1977;103:605–622.
38. Cohen MS, Britt RH. Effects of sodium pentobarbital, ketamine, halothane, and chloralose on brainstem auditory evoked responses. *Anesth Analg* 1982;61:338–343.
39. Cox C, Hack M, Mertz D. Brainstem evoked response audiometry: normative data from the preterm infant. *Audiology* 1981;20:53–64.
40. Cox LC. Infant assessment: developmental and age-related considerations. In: Jacobson JT, ed. *The auditory brainstem response.* San Diego, CA: College Hill Press, 1985:297–316.
41. Curio G, Oppel F. Intraparenchymatous ponto-mesencephalic field distribution of brain-stem auditory evoked potentials in man. *Electroencephalogr Clin Neurophysiol* 1988;69:259–265.
42. Dehan CP, Jerger J. Analysis of gender differences in the auditory brainstem response. *Laryngoscope* 1990;100:18–24.
43. Dorfman LJ, Britt RH, Silverberg GD. Human brainstem auditory evoked potentials during controlled hypothermia and total circulatory arrest. *Neurology* 1981;31:88–89.

44. Drummond JC, Todd MM, Sang H. The effect of high dose sodium thiopental on brain stem auditory and median nerve somatosensory evoked responses in humans. *Anesthesiology* 1985;63:249–254.

45. Dubois M, Sato S, Chassy J, et al. Effect of enflurane on brain stem auditory evoked response (BAER). *Electroencephalogr Clin Neurophysiol* 1982;53:36P.

46. Dumas G, Bessard G, Gavend M, et al. Risk of deafness following ototopical administration of aminoglycoside antibiotic. *Therapie* 1980;35:357–363.

47. Durrant JD, Martin WH, Hirsch B, et al. 3CLT ABR analyses in a human subject with unilateral extirpation of the inferior colliculus. *Hear Res* 1994;72:99–107.

48. Eggermont JJ. Development of auditory evoked potentials. *Acta Otolaryngol* 1992;112:197–200.

49. Eggermont JJ, Don M. Mechanisms of central conduction time prolongation in brain-stem auditory evoked potentials. *Arch Neurol* 1986;43:116–120.

50. Eggermont JJ, Don M, Brackmann DE. Electrocochleography and auditory brainstem electric responses in patients with angle tumors. *Ann Otol Rhinol Laryngol Suppl* 1980;89:1–19.

51. Elberling C. Compound impulse response for the brain stem derived through combinations of cochlear and brainstem recordings. *Scand Audiol* 1978;7:147–157.

52. Elwany S. Auditory brain stem responses (ABR) in patients with acute severe closed head injuries. The use of a grading system. *J Laryngol Otol* 1988;102:755–759.

53. Erwin CW, Cahill WT, Griffiths MF. A mathematical model to explain derivation-specific latency shifts in BAEP studies. *Neurology* 1986;36:30.

54. Factor SA, Dentinger MP. Early brain-stem auditory evoked responses in vertebrobasilar transient ischemic attacks. *Arch Neurol* 1987;44:544–547.

55. Ferbert A, Buchner H, Bruckmann H. Brainstem auditory evoked potentials and somatosensory evoked potentials in pontine hemorrhage. Correlations with clinical and CT findings. *Brain* 1990;113:49–63.

56. Ferguson MA, Smith PA, Lutman ME, et al. Efficiency of tests used to screen for cerebellopontine angle tumours: a prospective study. *Br J Audiol* 1996;30:159–176.

57. Fischer C, Blanc A, Mauguiere F, et al. Diagnostic value of brainstem auditory evoked potentials. *Rev Neurol* 1981;137:229–240.

58. Fradis M, Pdoshin L, Ben-David J, et al. Brainstem auditory evoked potentials with increased stimulus rate in patients suffering from systemic lupus erythematosus. *Laryngoscope* 1989;99:325–329.

59. Fujikawa SM, Weber BA. Effects of increased stimulus rate on brainstem electric response (BER) audiometry as a function of age. *J Am Aud Soc* 1977;3:147–150.

60. Gafni M, Sohmer H, Gross S, et al. Analysis of auditory nerve–brainstem responses (ABR) in neonates and very young infants. *Arch Otorhinolaryngol* 1980;229:167–174.

61. Galambos R, Hecox KE. Clinical applications of the brain stem auditory evoked potentials. *Prog Clin Neurophysiol* 1977;2:1–19.

62. Galambos R, Hecox KE. Clinical applications of the auditory brain stem response. *Otolaryngol Clin North Am* 1978;11:709–722.

63. Garg BP, Markand ON, Bustion PF. Brainstem auditory evoked responses in hereditary motor-sensory neuropathy: site of origin of wave II. *Neurology* 1982;32:1017–1019.

64. Garg BP, Markand ON, DeMyer WE, et al. Evoked response studies in patients with adrenoleukodystrophy and heterozygous relatives. *Arch Neurol* 1983;40:356–359.

65. Gilain L, Bouccara D, Jacquier I, et al. Diagnostic strategy of acoustic neuroma. Evaluation of efficacy of auditory evoked potentials. Apropos of a series of 50 neuroma cases. *Ann Otolaryngol Chir Cervicofac* 1991;108:257–260.

66. Glasscock ME 3rd, Jackson CG, Josey AF, et al. Brain stem evoked response audiometry in clinical practice. *Laryngoscope* 1979;89:1021–1035.

67. Goff GD, Matsumiya Y, Allison T, et al. The scalp topography of human somatosensory and auditory evoked potentials. *Electroencephalogr Clin Neurophysiol* 1977;42:57–76.

68. Goldie WD, Chiappa KH, Young RR, et al. Brainstem auditory and short-latency somatosensory evoked responses in brain death. *Neurology* 1981;31:248–256.

69. Green JB, McLeod S. Short latency somatosensory evoked potentials in patients with neurological lesions. *Arch Neurol* 1979;36:846–851.

70. Green JB, Walcoff M, Lucke JF. Phenytoin prolongs far-field somatosensory and auditory evoked potentials interpeak latencies. *Neurology* 1982;32:85–88.

71. Guerit JM, Mahieru P, Houben-Giurgea S, et al. The influence of ototoxic drugs on brainstem auditory evoked potentials in man. *Arch Otorhinolaryngol* 1981;233:189–199.

72. Hall JW III. Auditory brainstem response audiometry. In: Jerger JF, ed. *Hearing disorders in adults.* San Diego, CA: College Hill Press 1984:1–55.

73. Hall JW III. Effects of high-dose barbiturates on the acoustic reflex and auditory evoked responses: two case reports. *Acta Otolaryngol* 1985;100:387–398.

74. Hall JW III. Auditory evoked responses in the management of acutely brain-injured children and adults. *Am J Otol* 1988;9:36–46.

75. Hall JW III. *Handbook of auditory evoked responses.* Boston: Allyn & Bacon, 1992.

76. Hall JW III, Hargadine JR. Auditory evoked responses in severe head injury. *Semin Hear* 1984;5:313–336.

77. Hall JW, Huangfu M, Gennarelli TA, et al. Auditory evoked responses, impedance measures, and diagnostic speech audiometry in severe head injury. *Otolaryngol Head Neck Surg* 1983;91:50–60.

78. Hall JW III, Tucker DA. Sensory evoked responses in the intensive care unit. *Ear Hear* 1986;7:220–232.

79. Hammond EJ, Wilder BJ. Short latency auditory and somatosensory evoked potentials in a patient with "locked-in" syndrome. *Clin Electroencephalogr* 1982;13:54–56.

80. Hammond EJ, Wilder BJ, Goodman IJ, et al. Auditory brain-stem potentials with unilateral pontine hemorrhage. *Arch Neurol* 1985;42:767–768.

81. Hansotia PL. Persistent vegetative state. Review and report of electrodiagnostic studies in eight cases. *Arch Neurol* 1985;42:1048–1052.

82. Harker LA, Hosick E, Voots RJ, et al. Influence of succinylcholine on middle component auditory evoked potentials. *Arch Otolaryngol* 1977;103:133–137.

83. Hashimoto I, Ishiyama Y, Yoshimoto T, et al. Brain-stem auditory-evoked potentials recorded directly from human brain-stem and thalamus. *Brain* 1981;104:841–859.

84. Haupt WF, Hojer C, Pawlik G. Prognostic value of evoked potentials and clinical grading in primary subarachnoid haemorrhage. *Acta Neurochir* 1995;137:146–150.

85. Haupt WF, Pawlik G. Contribution of initial median-nerve somatosensory evoked potentials and brainstem auditory evoked potentials to prediction of clinical outcome in cerebrovascular critical care patients: a statistical evaluation. *J Clin Neurophysiol* 1998;15:154–158.

86. Hecox K. Electrophysiological correlates of human auditory development. In: Cohen LB, Salapatek P, eds. *Infant perception: from sensation to cognition, vol II: Perception of space, speech and sound.* New York: Academic Press, 1975:151–191.

87. Hecox KE, Cone B, Blaw ME. Brainstem auditory evoked response in the diagnosis of pediatric neurologic disease. *Neurology* 1981;31:832–840.

88. Hecox KE, Galambos R. Brain stem auditory evoked responses in human infants and adults. *Arch Otolaryngol* 1974;99:30–33.

89. Hellekson C, Allen A, Greeley H, et al. Comparison of interwave latencies of brain stem auditory evoked responses in narcoleptics, primary insomniacs and normal controls. *Electroencephalogr Clin Neurophysiol* 1979;47:742–744.

90. Hood LJ, Berlin CI. *Auditory evoked potentials.* Austin, TX: PRO-ED Inc., 1986.

91. Hooks RG, Weber BA. Auditory brain stem responses of premature infants to bone-conducted stimuli: a feasibility study. *Ear Hear* 1984;5:42–46.

92. Hyde ML, Blair RL. The auditory brainstem response in neuro-otology: perspectives and problems. *J Otolaryngol* 1981;10:117–125.

93. Jabbari B, Schwartz DM, MacNeil DM, et al. Early abnormalities of brainstem auditory evoked potentials in Friedreich's ataxia: evidence of primary brainstem dysfunction. *Neurology* 1983;33:1071–1074.

94. Japaridze G, Kvernadze D, Geladze T, et al. Effects of carbamazepine on auditory brainstem response, middle-latency response, and slow cortical potential in epileptic patients. *Epilepsia* 1993;34:1105–1109.

95. Jerger J, Hall J. Effects of age and sex on auditory brainstem response. *Arch Otolaryngol* 1980;106:387–391.

96. Jewett DL. Volume-conducted potentials in response to auditory stimuli as detected by averaging in the cat. *Electroencephalogr Clin Neurophysiol* 1970;28:609–618.

97. Jones TA, Stockard JJ, Weidner WJ. The effects of temperature and acute alcohol intoxication on brain stem auditory evoked potentials in the cat. *Electroencephalogr Clin Neurophysiol* 1980;49:23–30.

98. Kaga K, Kitazumi E, Kodama K. Auditory brainstem responses of kernicterus infants. *Int J Pediatr Otolaryngol* 1979;1:255–264.

99. Karnaze DS, Marshall LF, McCarthy CS, et al. Localizing and prognostic value of auditory evoked responses in coma after closed head injury. *Neurology* 1982;32:299–302.

100. Kayamori R, Dickins QS, Yamada T, et al. Brainstem auditory evoked potential and blink reflex in multiple sclerosis. *Neurology* 1984;34:1318–1323.

101. Keith WJ, Greville KA. Effects of audiometric configuration on the auditory brainstem response. *Ear Hear* 1987;8:49–55.

102. Kiang NY. A survey of recent developments in the study of auditory physiology. *Ann Otol Rhinol Laryngol* 1968;77:656–675.

103. Kileny PR, Dodson D, Gelfand E. Middle latency auditory evoked responses during open-heart surgery with hypothermia. *Electroencephalogr Clin Neurophysiol* 1983;55:268–276.

104. Kingston JE, Abramovich S, Billings RJ, et al. Assessment of the effect of chemotherapy and radiotherapy on the auditory function of children with cancer. *Clin Otolaryngol Allied Sci* 1986;11:403–409.

105. Kjaer M. Localizing brain stem lesions with brain stem auditory evoked potentials. *Acta Neurol Scand* 1980;61:265–274.

106. Kjaer M. Recognizability of brain stem auditory evoked potential components. *Acta Neurol Scand* 1980;62:20–33.

107. Kjaer M. Variations of brain stem auditory evoked potentials correlated to duration and severity of multiple sclerosis. *Acta Neurol Scand* 1980;61:157–166.

108. Klug N, Csecsei G. Brainstem acoustic evoked potentials in the acute midbrain syndrome and in central death. In: Morocutti C, Rizzo PA, eds. *Evoked potentials. Neurophysiological and clinical aspects.* Amsterdam: Elsevier, 1985:203–210.

109. Kotterba S, Rasche K. Acoustic evoked potentials (AEP) in obstructive sleep apnea syndrome. *Pneumologie* 1996;50:924–926.

110. Krumholz A, Feliz JK, Goldstein PJ, et al. Maturation of the brain-stem auditory evoked potential in premature infants. *Electroencephalogr Clin Neurophysiol* 1985;62:124–134.

111. Kuk FK, Abbas PJ. Effects of attention on the auditory evoked potentials recorded from the vertex (ABR) and the promontory (CAP) of human listeners. *Br J Audiol* 1989;27:665–673.

112. Lasky RE. A developmental study on the effects of stimulus rate on the auditory evoked brainstem response. *Electroencephalogr Clin Neurophysiol* 1984;47:607–610.

113. Lee JA, Schoener EP, Nielsen DW, et al. Alcohol and the auditory brain-stem response, brain temperature, and blood alcohol curves: explanation of a paradox. *Electroencephalogr Clin Neurophysiol* 1990;77:362–375.

114. Leombruni S, Vaula G, Coletti Moja M, et al. Neurophysiological study in an Italian family with autosomal dominant late-onset leukodystrophy. *Electromyogr Clin Neurophysiol* 1998;38:131–135.

115. Levine RA, Gardner JC, Fullerton BC, et al. Effects of multiple sclerosis brainstem lesions on sound lateralization and brainstem auditory evoked potentials. *Hear Res* 1993;68:73–88.

116. Lukas JH. The role of efferent inhibition in human auditory attention: an examination of the auditory brainstem potentials. *Int J Neurosci* 1981;12:137–145.

117. Lynn GE, Gilroy J, Taylor PC, et al. Binaural masking-level differences in neurological disorders. *Arch Otolaryngol* 1981;107:357–362.

118. Lynn GE, Taylor PC, Gilroy J. AEP abnormalities in multiple sclerosis. *Electroencephalogr Clin Neurophysiol* 1980;50:167P.

119. Malhotra A. *Auditory evoked responses in clinical practice.* New Delhi: Springer-Verlag, 1997.

120. Markand ON, DeMyer WE, Worth RM, et al. Multimodality evoked responses in leukodystrophies. *Adv Neurol* 1982;32:409–416.

121. Markand ON, Farlow MR, Stevens JC, et al. Brain-stem auditory evoked potential abnormalities with unilateral brain-stem lesions demonstrated by magnetic resonance imaging. *Arch Neurol* 1989;46:295–299.

122. Markand ON, Garg BP, DeMyer WE, et al. Brain stem auditory, visual and somatosensory evoked potentials in leukodystrophies. *Electroencephalogr Clin Neurophysiol* 1982;54:39–48.

123. Marsh RR, Frewen TC, Sutton LN, et al. Resistance of the auditory brain stem response to high barbiturate levels. *Otolaryngol Head Neck Surg* 1984;92:685–688.

124. Martinez-Mena JM, Manquillo A, Saez J, et al. Neurophysiological study in Alpers syndrome. *Rev Neurol* 1998;26:70–74.

125. Marx JJ, Urban PP, Hopf HC, et al. Electrophysiological brain stem investigations in idiopathic narcolepsy. *J Neurol* 1998;245:537–541.

126. Maudlin I, Jerger J. Auditory brain stem evoked response to bone-conducted signals. *Arch Otolaryngol* 1979;105:656–661.

127. McCall WV, Erwin CW, Edinger JD, et al. Ambulatory polysomnography: technical aspects and normative values. *J Clin Neurophysiol* 1992;9:68–77.

128. McClelland RJ, McCrea RS. Intersubject variability of the early auditory-evoked brain stem potentials. *Audiologie* 1979;18:462–471.

129. McGee TJ, Clemis JD. Effects of conductive hearing loss on auditory brainstem response. *Ann Otol Rhinol Laryngol* 1982;91:304–309.

130. Misulis KE. *Spehlmann's evoked potential primer.* Boston: Butterworth-Heinemann, 1994.

131. Mitchell C, Phillips DS, Trune DR. Variables affecting the auditory brainstem response: Audiogram, age, gender and head size. *Hear Res* 1989;40:75–86.

132. Mochizuki Y, Go T, Ohkubo H, et al. Developmental changes of brainstem auditory evoked potentials (BAEPs) in normal human subjects from infants to young adults. *Brain Dev* 1982;4:127–136.

133. Moffat DA, Baguley DM, Hardy DG, et al. Contralateral auditory brainstem response abnormalities in acoustic neuroma. *J Laryngol Otol* 1989;103:835–838.

134. Mokotoff B, Schulman-Galambos C, Galambos R. Brain stem auditory evoked responses in children. *Arch Otolaryngol* 1977;103:38–43.

135. Moller AR. Neural generators of auditory evoked potentials. In: Jacobson JT, ed. *Principles and applications in auditory evoked potentials.* Boston: Allyn & Bacon, 1994:23–46.

136. Moller AR, Jannetta PJ. Auditory evoked potentials recorded intracranially from the brain stem in man. *Exp Neurol* 1982;78:144–157.

137. Moller AR, Jannetta PJ. Evoked potentials from the inferior colliculus in man. *Electroencephalogr Clin Neurophysiol* 1982;53:612–620.

138. Moller AR, Jannetta PJ. Auditory evoked potentials recorded from the cochlear nucleus and its vicinity in man. *J Neurosurg* 1983;59:1013–1018.

139. Moller AR, Jannetta PJ. Interpretation of brainstem auditory evoked potentials: results from the intracranial recordings in humans. *Scand Audiol* 1983;12:125–133.

140. Moller AR, Jannetta PJ, Jho HD. Click-evoked responses from the cochlear nucleus: a study in human. *Electroencephalogr Clin Neurophysiol* 1994;92:215–224.

141. Moller MB, Moller AR. Brainstem auditory evoked potentials in patients with cerebellopontine angle tumors. *Ann Otol Rhinol Laryngol* 1983;92:645–650.

142. Moore JK, Ponton CW, Eggermont JJ, et al. Perinatal maturation of the auditory brain stem response: changes in path length and conduction velocity. *Ear Hear* 1996;17:411–418.

143. Mori K, Nishimura T. Electrophysiological studies on brainstem function in patients with myelomeningocele. *Pediatr Neurosurg* 1995;22:120–131.

144. Mosko SS, Pierce S, Holowach J, et al. Normal brain stem auditory evoked potentials recorded in sleep apneics during waking and as a function of arterial oxygen saturation during sleep. *Electroencephalogr Clin Neurophysiol* 1981;51:477–482.

145. Musiek FE, Geurkink NA, Spiegel P. Audiologic and other clinical findings in a case of basilar artery aneurysm. *Arch Otolaryngol Head Neck Surg* 1987;113:772–776.

146. Musiek FE, Josey AF, Glasscock ME 3d. Auditory brain-stem response in patients with acoustic neuromas. Wave presence and absence. *Arch Otolaryngol Head Neck Surg* 1986;112:186–189.

147. Musiek FE, Kibbe K. Auditory brain stem response wave IV-V abnormalities from the ear opposite large cerebellopontine lesions. *Am J Otol* 1986;7:253–257.

148. Myers RM. Ototoxic effects of gentamicin. *Arch Otolaryngol* 1970;92:160–162.

149. Naessens B, Gordts F, Clement PA, et al. Re-evaluation of the ABR in the diagnosis of CPA tumors in the MRI-era. *Acta Otorhinolaryngol Belg* 1996;50:99–102.

150. Ni D, Li F, Peng P. The analysis of abnormal auditory brainstem response. *Zhonghua Er Bi Yan Hou Ke Za Zhi* 1996;31:36–38.

151. Nishimura T, Mori K, Uchida Y, et al. Brain stem auditory-evoked potentials in myelomeningocele. Natural history of Chiari II malformations. *Childs Nerv Syst* 1991;7:316–326.

152. Nuwer MR, Perlman SL, Packwood JW, et al. Evoked potential abnormalities in the various inherited ataxias. *Ann Neurol* 1983;13:20–27.

153. Oberascher G, Kofler B, Pommer B. Otoneurologic findings in multiple sclerosis. Stapedius reflex, vestibular evaluation, early acoustic evoked potentials. *HNO* 1985;33:23–25.

154. Ochs R, Markand ON, DeMyer WE. Brainstem auditory evoked responses in leukodystrophies. *Neurology* 1979;29:1089–1093.

155. O'Donovan CA, Beagley HA, Shaw M. Latency of brainstem response in children. *Br J Audiol* 1980;14:23–29.

156. Oh SJ, Kuba T, Soyer A, et al. Lateralization of brainstem lesions by brainstem auditory evoked potentials. *Neurology* 1981;46:14–18.

157. Osterhammel PA, Shallop JK, Terkilesen K. The effect of sleep on the auditory brainstem response (ABR) and the middle latency response (MLR). *Scand Audiol* 1985;14:47–50.

158. Ottaviani F, Almadori G, Calderazzo AB, et al. Auditory brain-stem (ABRs) and middle latency auditory responses (MLRs) in the prognosis of severely head-injured patients. *Electroencephalogr Clin Neurophysiol* 1986;65:196–202.

159. Otto WC, Brown RD, Gage-White L, et al. Effects of cisplatin and thiosulfate upon auditory brainstem responses of guinea pigs. *Hear Res* 1988;35:79–85.

160. Pakalnis A, Drake ME Jr, Dadmehr N, et al. Evoked potentials and EEG in multiple sclerosis. *Electroencephalogr Clin Neurophysiol* 1987;67:333–336.

161. Palaskas CW, Wilson MJ, Dobie RA. Electrophysiologic assessment of low-frequency hearing: sedation effects. *Otolaryngol Head Neck Surg* 1989;101:434–441.

162. Paludetti G, Maurizi M, Ottaviani F, et al. Reference values and characteristics of brain stem audiometry in neonates and children. *Scand Audiol* 1981;10:177–186.

163. Panjwani U, Singh SH, sel Vamurthy W, et al. Brainstem auditory evoked potentials in epileptics on different anti-epileptic drugs. *Indian J Physiol Pharmacol* 1996;40:29–34.

164. Parker SW, Chiappa KH, Brooks EB. Brainstem auditory evoked responses in patients with acoustic neuromas and cerebello-pontine angle meningiomas. *Neurology* 1980;30:413–414.

165. Picton TW, Hillyard SA. Human auditory evoked potentials. II. Effects of attention. *Electroencephalogr Clin Neurophysiol* 1974;36:191–199.

166. Picton TW, Hillyard SA, Galambos R, et al. Human auditory attention: a central or peripheral process? *Science* 1971;173:351–353.

167. Picton TW, Hillyard SA, Krausz HI, et al. Human auditory evoked potentials. I. Evaluation of components. *Electroencephalogr Clin Neurophysiol* 1974;36:179–190.

168. Picton TW, Stapells DR, Campbell KB. Auditory evoked potentials from the human cochlea and brainstem. *J Otolaryngol Suppl* 1981;9:1–41.

169. Picton TW, Woods DL, Baribeau-Braun J, et al. Evoked potential audiometry. *J Otolaryngol* 1977;6:90–119.

170. Pierelli F, Pozzessere G, Bianco F, et al. Brainstem auditory evoked potentials in neurodegenerative diseases. In: Morocutti C, Rizzo PA, eds. *Evoked potentials. Neurophysiological and clinical aspects.* Amsterdam: Elsevier, 1985:157–168.

171. Pollak L, Klein C, Giladi R, et al. Progressive deterioration of brainstem auditory evoked potentials in Creutzfeldt-Jakob disease: clinical and electroencephalographic correlation. *Clin Electroencephalogr* 1996;27:95–99.

172. Ponton CW, Moore JK, Eggermont JJ. Auditory brain stem response generation by parallel pathways: differential maturation of axonal conduction time and synaptic transmission. *Ear Hear* 1996;17:402–410.

173. Porjesz B, Begleiter H. Human evoked brain potentials and alcohol. *Alcohol Clin Exp Res* 1981;5:304–317.

174. Prasher DK, Gibson WP. Brain stem auditory evoked potentials: significant latency differences between ipsilateral and contralateral stimulation. *Electroencephalogr Clin Neurophysiol* 1980;50:240–246.

175. Prasher DK, Gibson WP. Brain stem auditory evoked potentials: a comparative study of monaural versus binaural stimulation in the detection of multiple sclerosis. *Electroencephalogr Clin Neurophysiol* 1980;50:247–253.

176. Pratt H, Ben-David Y, Peled R, et al. Auditory brain stem evoked potentials: clinical promise of increasing stimulus rate. *Electroencephalogr Clin Neurophysiol* 1981;51:80–90.

177. Prosser S, Arslan E. Prediction of auditory brainstem wave V latency as a diagnostic tool of sensorineural hearing loss. *Audiology* 1987;26:179–187.

178. Radhakrishnan K, Malhotra AK, Shridharan R, et al. Ataxic hemiparesis: clinical, electrophysiologic, radiologic and pathologic observations. *Clin Neurol Neurosurg* 1982;84:91–100.

179. Rao TH, Libman RB. When is isolated vertigo a harbinger of stroke? *Ear Nose Throat J* 1995;74:33–36.

180. Ricchieri G, Bartolomei L, Pellegrini A, et al. Instrumental diagnosis of multiple sclerosis: correlation between electrophysiologic and cerebrospinal fluid findings. *Rev Neurol* 1984;54:347–357.

181. Robinson K, Rudge P. Wave form analysis of the brain stem auditory evoked potential. *Electroencephalogr Clin Neurophysiol* 1981;52:583–594.

182. Rosenhamer HJ, Lindstrom B, Lundborg T. On the use of click-evoked electric brainstem response in audiologic diagnosis. II. The influence of sex and age upon the normal response. *Scand Audiol* 1980;9:93–100.

183. Rosenhamer HJ, Lindstrom B, Lundborg T. On the use of click-evoked electric brainstem responses in audiological diagnosis. III. Latencies in cochlear hearing loss. *Scand Audiol* 1981;10:3–11.

184. Rossi L, Amantini A, Bindi A, et al. Electrophysiological investigations of the brainstem in the vertebrobasilar reversible attacks. *Eur Neurol* 1983;22:371–379.

185. Rowe MJ III. Normal variability of the brain-stem auditory evoked response in young and old adult subjects. *Electroencephalogr Clin Neurophysiol* 1978;44:459–470.

186. Rumpl E, Prugger M, Battista HJ, et al. Short latency somatosensory evoked potentials and brain-stem auditory evoked potentials in coma due to CNS depressant drug poisoning. Preliminary observations. *Electroencephalogr Clin Neurophysiol* 1988;70:482–489.

187. Salamy A. Maturation of the auditory brainstem response from birth through early childhood. *J Clin Neurophysiol* 1984;1:293–329.

188. Salamy A, McKean CM, Buda FB. Maturational changes in auditory transmission as reflected in human brain stem potentials. *Brain Res* 1975;96:361–366.

189. Salamy A, Mendelson T, Tooley WH. Developmental profiles for the brainstem auditory evoked potential. *Early Hum Dev* 1982;6:331–339.

190. Salomon G, Elberling C, Tos M. Combined use of electrocochleography and brainstem recording in the diagnosis of acoustic neuromas. *Rev Laryngol Otol Rhinol* 1979;100: 697–707.

191. Sanders RA, Duncan PG, McCullough DW, et al. Clinical experience with brain stem audiometry performed under general anesthesia. *J Otolaryngol* 1979;8:24–31.

192. Sanders RA, Smriga DJ, McCullough DW, et al. Auditory brainstem responses in patients with global cerebral insults. *J Neurosurg* 1981;55:227–236.

193. Satya-Murti S, Cacace A, Hanson P. Auditory dysfunction in Friedreich ataxia: Result of spiral ganglion degeneration. *Neurology* 1980;30:1047–1053.

194. Scherg M, von Cramon D. A new interpretation of the generators of BAEP waves I-V: results of a spatio-temporal dipole model. *Electroencephalogr Clin Neurophysiol* 1985;62:290–299.

195. Schuknecht HF. *Otosclerosis.* London: J&A Churchill Ltd., 1962.

196. Schulman-Galambos C, Galambos R. Brain stem auditory-evoked responses in premature infants. *J Speech Hear Res* 1975;18:456–465.

197. Schwent VL, Williston JS, Jewett D. The effects of ototoxicity on the auditory brain stem response and the scalp-recorded cochlear microphonic in guinea pigs. *Laryngoscope* 1980;90:1350–1359.

198. Seales DM, Rossiter VS, Weinstein ME. Brainstem auditory evoked responses in patients comatose as a result of blunt head trauma. *J Trauma* 1979;19:347–352.

199. Selters WA, Brackmann DE. Acoustic tumor detection with brain stem electric response audiometry. *Arch Otolaryngol* 1977;103:181–187.

200. Smith DI, Kraus N. Effects of chloral hydrate, pentobarbital, ketamine, and curare on the auditory middle latency response. *Am J Otolaryngol* 1987;8:241–248.

201. Sohmer H, Feinmesser M, Szabo G. Sources of electrocochleographic responses as studied in patients with brain damage. *Electroencephalogr Clin Neurophysiol* 1974;37:663–669.

202. Sohmer H, Gafni M, Chisin R. Auditory nerve and brain stem responses: comparison in awake and unconscious subjects. *Arch Neurol* 1978;35:228–230.

203. Sohmer H, Kinarti R, Gafni M. The latency of auditory nerve–brainstem responses in sensorineural hearing loss. *Arch Otorhinolaryngol* 1981;230:189–199.

204. Squires KC, Chu N-S, Starr A. Acute effects of alcohol on auditory brainstem potentials in humans. *Science* 1978;201:174–176.

205. Squires KC, Chu N-S, Starr A. Auditory brainstem potentials with alcohol. *Electroencephalogr Clin Neurophysiol* 1978;45:577–584.

206. Stapells DR, Picton TW, Perez-Abalo M, et al. Frequency specificity in evoked potential audiometry. In: Jacobson JT, ed. *The auditory brainstem response.* San Diego, CA: College Hill Press, 1985:147–177.

207. Starr A. Auditory brainstem response in brain death. *Brain* 1976;99:543–554.

208. Starr A. Clinical relevance of brain stem auditory evoked potentials in brain stem disorders in man. *Prog Clin Neurophysiol* 1977;2:45–57.

209. Starr A, Amlie RN, Martin WH, et al. Development of auditory function in newborn infants revealed by auditory brainstem potentials. *Pediatrics* 1977;60:831–839.

210. Stockard JJ, Hughes JF, Sharbrough FW. Visually evoked potentials to electronic pattern reversal: latency variations with gender, age and technical factors. *Am J EEG Technol* 1979;19: 171–204.

211. Stockard JJ, Rossiter VS. Clinical and pathologic correlates of brain stem auditory response abnormalities. *Neurology* 1977;27:316–325.

212. Stockard JJ, Rossiter VS, Jones TA, et al. Effects of centrally acting drugs on brainstem auditory responses. *Electroencephalogr Clin Neurophysiol* 1977;43:550–551.

213. Stockard JJ, Sharbrough FW. Unique contributions of short-latency somatosensory evoked potentials in patients with neurological lesions. *Prog Clin Neurophysiol* 1980;7:231–263.

214. Stockard JJ, Sharbrough FW, Staats BA, et al. Brain stem auditory evoked potentials (BAEPs) in sleep apnea. *Electroencephalogr Clin Neurophysiol* 1980;50:167P.

215. Stockard JJ, Sharbrough FW, Tinker JA. Effects of hypothermia on the human brainstem auditory response. *Ann Neurol* 1978;3:368–370.

216. Stockard JJ, Stockard JE, Sharbrough FW. Detection and localization of occult lesions with brainstem auditory responses. *Mayo Clin Proc* 1977;52:761–769.

217. Stockard JJ, Stockard JE, Sharbrough FW. Nonpathologic factors influencing brainstem auditory evoked potentials. *Am J EEG Technol* 1978;18:177–209.

218. Stockard JJ, Stockard JE, Sharbrough FW. Brainstem auditory evoked potentials in neurology: methodology, interpretation, clinical application. In: Aminoff MJ, ed. *Electrodiagnosis in clinical neurology.* New York: Churchill Livingstone, 1980:370–413.

219. Stockard JE, Westmoreland BF. Technical considerations in the recording and interpretation of the brainstem auditory evoked potential for neonatal neurologic diagnosis. *Am J EEG Technol* 1981;21:31–54.

220. Sturzebecher E, Werbs M. Effects of age and sex on auditory brain stem response. A new aspect. *Scand Audiol* 1987;16:153–157.

221. Sutton LN, Frewen T, Marsh RR, et al. The effects of deep barbiturate coma on multimodality evoked potentials. *J Neurosurg* 1982;57:177–185.

222. Takeno S, Wake M, Mount RJ, et al. Degeneration of spiral ganglion cells in the chinchilla after inner hair cell loss induced by carboplatin. *Audiol Neurootol* 1998;3:281–290.

223. Tanaka H, Komatsuzaki A, Hentona H. Usefulness of auditory brainstem responses at high stimulus rates in the diagnosis of acoustic neuroma. *ORL J Otorhinolaryngol Relat Spec* 1996;58:224–228.

224. Taylor MJ, Boor R, Keenan NK, et al. Brainstem auditory and visual evoked potentials in infants with myelomeningocele. *Brain Dev* 1996;18:99–104.

225. Thivierge J, Cote R. Brain-stem auditory evoked response (BAER): normative study in children and adults. *Electroencephalogr Clin Neurophysiol* 1987;68:479–485.

226. Thivierge J, Cote R. Brainstem auditory evoked responses: normative values in children. *Electroencephalogr Clin Neurophysiol* 1990;77:309–313.

227. Thornton C, Catley DM, Jordan C, et al. Enflurane increases the latency of early components of the auditory evoked response in man. *Br J Anaesth* 1981;53:1102–1103.

228. Towle VL, Babikian V, Maselli R, et al. A comparison of multimodality evoked potentials, computed tomography findings and clinical data in brainstem vascular infarcts. In: Morocutti C, Rizzo PA, eds. *Evoked potentials. Neurophysiological and clinical aspects.* Amsterdam: Elsevier, 1985:383–390.

229. Trune DR, Mitchell C, Phillips DS. The relative importance of head size, gender and age on the auditory brainstem response. *Hear Res* 1988;32:165–174.

230. Tsuji S, Muraoka S, Kuroiwa Y, et al. Auditory brain evoked response (ABSR) of Parkinson-dementia complex and amyotrophic lateral sclerosis in Guam and Japan. *Rinsho Shinkeigaku* 1981;21:37–41.

231. Tucci DL, Rubel EW. Physiologic status of regenerated hair cells in the avian inner ear following aminoglycoside ototoxicity. *Otolaryngol Head Neck Surg* 1990;103:443–450.

232. Turner JS Jr, Saunders AZ. False positive stapedial reflexes and brain stem evoked response findings in patients with suspected retrocochlear lesions. *Laryngoscope* 1984;94:901–903.

233. Uziel A, Benezech J. Auditory brainstem responses in comatose patients: Relationship with brain-stem reflexes and levels of coma. *Electroencephalogr Clin Neurophysiol* 1978;45:515–524.

234. Van der Drift JFC, Brocaar MP, van Zanten GA. Brainstem response audiometry. I. Its use in distinguishing between conductive and cochlear hearing loss. *Audiology* 1988;27:260–270.

235. Verma NP, Kapen S, King SD, et al. Bimodality electrophysiologic evaluation of brainstem in sleep apnea syndrome. *Neurology* 1987;37:1036–1039.

236. Voordecker P, Brunko E, de Beyl Z. Selective unilateral absence or attenuation of wave V of brain-stem auditory evoked potentials with intrinsic brain-stem lesions. *Arch Neurol* 1988;45:1272–1276.

237. Waring MD. Refractory properties of auditory brain-stem responses evoked by electrical stimulation of human cochlear nucleus: evidence of neural generators. *Electroencephalogr Clin Neurophysiol* 1998;108:331–344.

238. Weber BA, Seitz MR, McCutcheon MJ. Quantifying click stimuli in auditory brainstem response audiometry. *Ear Hear* 1981;2:15–19.

239. Weiner RD, Erwin CW, Weber BA. Acute effects of electroconvulsive therapy on brain stem auditory-evoked potentials. *Electroencephalogr Clin Neurophysiol* 1981;52:202–204.

240. Wielaard R, Kemp B. Auditory brainstem evoked responses in brainstem compression due to posterior fossa tumors. *Clin Neurol Neurosurg* 1979;81:185–193.

241. Wilson DF, Hodgson RS, Gustafson MF, et al. The sensitivity of auditory brainstem response testing in small acoustic neuromas. *Laryngoscope* 1992;102:961–964.

242. Worley G, Erwin CW, Schuster JM, et al. BAEPs in infants with myelomeningocele and later development of Chiari II malformation-related brainstem dysfunction. *Dev Med Child Neurol* 1994;36:707–715.

243. Yamada O, Kodera K, Yagi T. Cochlear processes affecting wave V latency of the auditory evoked brain stem response. *Scand Audiol* 1979;8:67–70.

244. Yamada O, Yagi T, Yamane H, et al. Clinical evaluation of the auditory evoked brain stem response. *Auris Nasus Larynx* 1975;2:97–105.

245. Yuksel A, Senocak D, Sozuer D, et al. Effects of carbamazepine and valproate on brainstem auditory evoked potentials in epileptic children. *Childs Nerv Syst* 1995;11:474–477.

246. Zappulla RA, Karmel BA, Greenblatt E. Prediction of cerebellopontine angle tumors based on discriminant analysis of brain stem auditory evoked responses. *Neurosurgery* 1981;9:542–547.

247. Zileli M, Idiman F, Hicdonmez T, et al. A comparative study of brain-stem auditory evoked potentials and blink reflexes in posterior fossa tumor patients. *J Neurosurg* 1988;69:660–668.

Chapter 29

Somatosensory Evoked Potentials

Ronald G. Emerson and Timothy A. Pedley

Stimulation of peripheral nerves results in generation of electrical signals that are recordable over the spine and scalp. Potentials evoked in this manner reflect activity within the large fiber sensory systems. Abnormalities of somatosensory evoked potentials (SSEPs) occur in a wide variety of pathological conditions:

Focal lesion affecting the somatosensory pathways: tumors, strokes, and spinal cord compression (16,21,39,107)
Demyelinating diseases: multiple sclerosis (15), adrenoleukodystrophy and adrenomyeloneuropathy (26,48,71,146), metachromatic leukodystrophy (140,160), and Pelizaeus-Merzbacher disease (97)

In adrenoleukodystrophy and adrenomyeloneuropathy, even asymptomatic heterozygotes manifest SSEP abnormalities (48,146).
Diseases that affect the nervous system diffusely: hereditary system degenerations (110), subacute combined degeneration (65), vitamin E deficiency (12, 70), human immunodeficiency virus encephalopathy (61,106), amyotrophic lateral sclerosis (49,167), myotonic dystrophy (55,142), diabetes (44,95)
Brain death (54)

Lesions generally alter SSEPs by prolonging interpeak latencies, reflecting delayed conduction, or attenuating or abolishing component waveforms, indicating conduction block or dysfunction of the responsible generator(s). An exception is cortical reflex myoclonus, in which high-voltage SSEPs reflect enhanced excitability of sensory cortex (57,68).

SSEPs are best utilized as an extension of the neurological examination. They help to document lesions of the nervous system and often suggest their location. SSEPs are therefore most useful when they detect clinically occult abnormalities that might otherwise be unrecognized. They also often assist in resolving clinically vague symptoms or ambiguous sensory findings on examination. Increasing, SSEPs are being used intraoperatively, both to identify specific structures and to detect injury to neural structures while it is still reversible.

ORIGINS OF SURFACE-RECORDED SSEPS

Although Dawson (24) first recorded SSEPs over 40 years ago, there is still considerable uncertainty about their neural generators. The present level of understanding provides an adequate basis for many clinical purposes; however, improved interpretation of complex abnormalities, as well as precise localization of lesions, requires additional detailed knowledge of generator sources.

An appreciation of the basis for uncertainties about the origins of SSEPs can be gained by considering the criteria that must be met to establish a causal relation between activity in a neural structure and a scalp-recorded potential (2):

1. The neural event and the surface potential must occur simultaneously.
2. There must be evidence that the neural event produces a signal that can be recorded beyond the bounds of the active structure.
3. No other simultaneous neural activity must exist that could explain or substantially contribute to the scalp recording.

These criteria are virtually impossible to fulfill in humans. On a few occasions, temporal coincidence has been demonstrated between (a) neural activity occurring at likely generator sites and (b) surface recordings. However, even when intracranial or spinal recordings are made, it is almost never possible to track a potential from its origin to the surface, which makes it difficult to prove a direct relation (2,4). Therefore, the present conclusions about the origins of SSEP components are derived largely from indirect evidence, including (a) analysis of surface distributions of waveforms; (b) inferences about probable anatomical sites from calculations measured in peripheral nerves with adjustment for fiber size, tract length, and synaptic delays; and (c) the effects of lesions.

At least two distinct classes of neural events contribute to brain electrical activity recorded at the scalp: (i) synaptic potentials arising in gray matter and (ii) propagated action potentials generated in white matter fiber tracts. The following discussion reflects our own beliefs and prejudices; nonetheless, we believe it is a reasonable synthesis based on the current evidence.

Contributions from White Matter Structures

White matter fiber tracts generate propagated compounded action potentials. An overlying electrode records these as triphasic, positive–negative–positive waveforms representing, respectively, outward current flow in advance of the active region of depolarization, inward current flow in the actively depolarized area, and then outward current flow as a depolarization passes and repolarization occurs (Fig. 29.1) (11). Such signals can be recorded ordinarily only in the vicinity of the fiber tract itself and have been termed *near-field potentials* (NFPs). Because current density gradients are steep in the vicinity of a localized area of depolarization, the voltage of NFPs is highly dependent on the position of the recording electrode. Small changes in electrode position produce large changes in voltage. Another important characteristic of NFPs is that, when recorded from an array of electrodes along the course of a fiber tract, NFPs increase in latency at recording sites progressively more distant from the point of stimulation.

White matter fiber tracts also generate another class of signals, known as *far-field potentials* (FFPs). These are unlike NFPs in that they are widely distributed and their latency is independent of electrode position (i.e., they are stationary). Their amplitude and morphology also remain relatively constant despite substantial changes in position of the recording electrode (10,62). FFPs are generated when a propagated action potential reaches or traverses certain fixed points along the course of a nerve or fiber tract. In classical neurophysiology, FFPs were recognized only as positive signals that reflected the moving front of an approaching volley recorded from a point beyond the termination of active fibers (159). A theoretical model involving an exploring electrode situated at a distance from an active neural element in a uniform volume conductor supports this view, as does an experimental model in which a recording electrode was placed beyond the crushed end of a nerve in a saline bath (91,159).

More recently, investigators recognized that FFPs also are generated under other conditions (40,75,76,92,108). Kimura and colleagues (72,73,75, 164) demonstrated in humans that FFPs are generated at specific sites along a peripheral nerve where physical boundaries are crossed. These potentials, which Kimura et al. labeled "junctional" or "intercompartmental" potentials, are typically diphasic but may appear predominantly either negative or positive. Far-field signals also may be generated at points where nerve trunks bend or branch (34).

Nakanishi (108,109) presented an experimental model that showed that FFPs could be generated at points along the course of a nerve where the impedance of the surrounding tissue changed abruptly. He passed a nerve through a series of chambers separated by slotted partitions sealed with petroleum jelly. Each chamber was filled with Ringer's solution and contained a recording electrode so as to become a fluid electrode surrounding the portion of the nerve coursing through it. The sealed partitions constituted high-impedance boundaries between fluid electrode chambers. Nakanishi recorded a potential between two adjacent chambers at the moment the volley reached the separating partition and the recorded potential reversed polarity as the volley crossed the partition (Fig. 29.2.). Recordings across multiple partitions produced a multipeaked waveform, with the number of peaks equaling the number of partitions crossed by the nerve (Fig. 29.3).

Generation of junctional FFPs seems to depend on a change in current density in tissues surrounding a nerve, caused by abrupt alteration in either their geometry (75,76) or conductive properties (93,108; see also ref. 121). Kimura et al. (72) hypothesized that tissue on either side of a boundary approximates a volume conductor acting as a lead connecting all points within an anatomical compartment to the voltage source at the boundary. This is consistent with Nakanishi's model (108) and suggests that there may be no inactive site on the body for junctional FFPs.

Other factors may influence the distribution of a FFP within a compartment, including the direction of the volley crossing the partition (33,69). A model based on a moving quadrupole in a cylindrical volume conductor, in which FFPs result from asymmetries between leading and trailing dipoles, has been proposed (34).

Figure 29.4 illustrates the generation of junctional FFPs (N$\overline{3}$, N$\overline{6}$, and N$\overline{9}$) as the median nerve afferent volley crosses borders between anatomically distinct compartments. This figure also illustrates the use of bipolar and referential derivations to emphasize near-field and far-field components selectively. Sequential bipolar recordings from a chain of electrodes overlying the course of the median nerve depict only the propagated near-field volley. Referential recordings from the same electrodes also detect the more widely distributed far-field stationary signals that are generated as the volley enters the brachioradialis muscle, enters the distal end of the deltoid, and crosses the boundary between arm and body. These far-field signals in phase cancel in the bipolar recordings (164).

Yamada et al. (164) further demonstrated that the N$\overline{3}$, N$\overline{6}$, and N$\overline{9}$ potentials could be recorded from distant electrodes and were therefore, by definition, FFPs. Three subjects were electrically connected at the forearm. Fol-

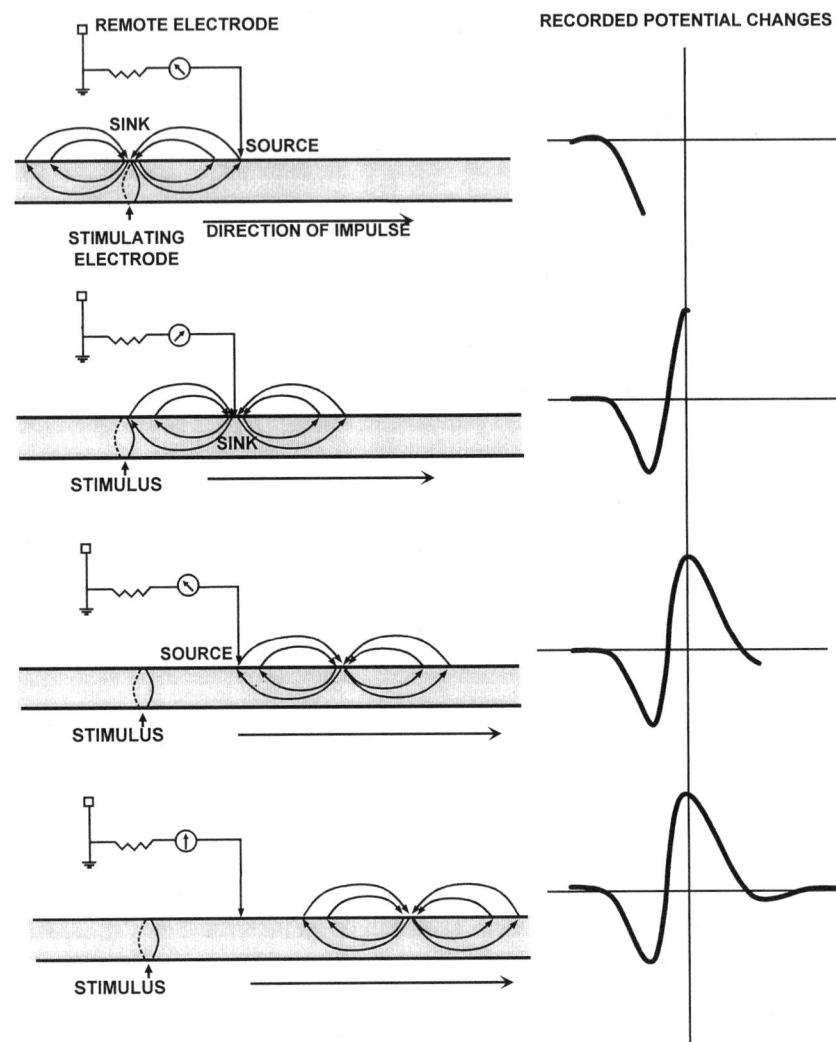

FIG. 29.1. Generation of the classical triphasic, positive–negative–positive signal by a propagated action potential. (From Brazier MAB. *Electrical activity of the nervous system.* Baltimore: Williams & Wilkins, 1977:68, with permission.)

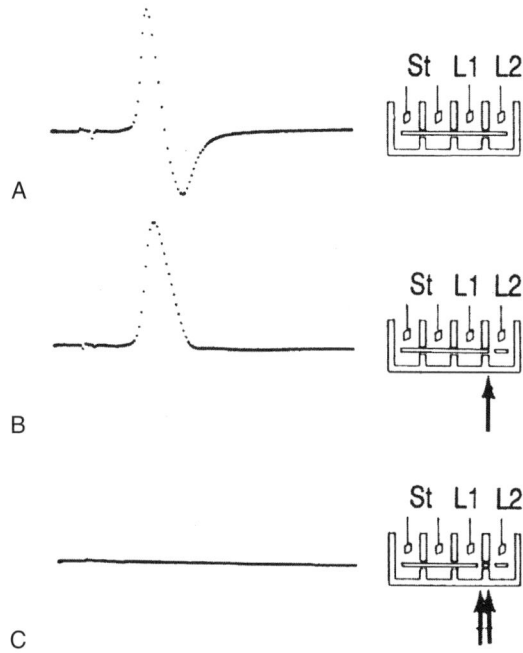

FIG. 29.2. Action potential recorded differentially between adjacent fluid electrodes, L1 and L2, following stimulation at electrode S1. **A:** With the nerve intact, a biphasic signal is recorded. **B:** When the nerve is severed at its point of exit from the partition between L1 and L2, only a monophasic signal is recorded. **C:** When the nerve is cut prior to entering the partition, no signal is recorded. (From Nakanishi T, Tamaki M, Arasaki K, et al. Origins of the scalp-recorded far field potentials in man and cat. *Electroencephalogr Clin Neurophysiol Suppl* 1982;36:336–348, with permission.)

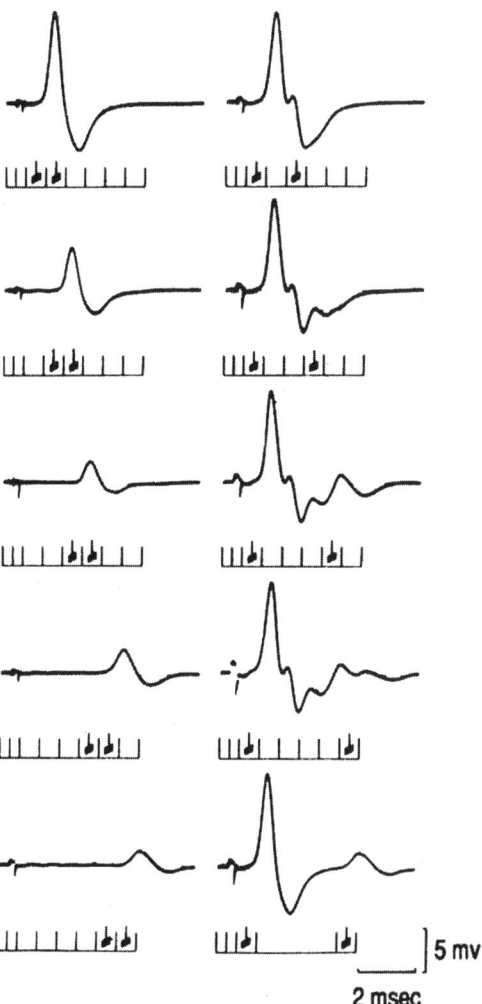

FIG. 29.3. Action potentials recorded differentially between fluid electrodes separated by a variable number of partitions. (From Nakanishi T. Action potentials recorded by fluid electrodes. *Electroencephalogr Clin Neurophysiol* 1982;53: 343–346, with permission.)

lowing stimulation of the median nerve of the middle subject, this series of negativities, recordable as stationary potentials over the stimulated forearm, was conducted to the nonstimulated subject on either side. Yamada et al. (164) observed that the $N\overline{9}$ stationary potential was precisely coincident with the scalp-recorded $P\overline{9}$ FFP, and found evidence that N6 had a positive counterpart over the lower third of the body. Although unable to identify a corresponding positivity for $N\overline{3}$, they suggested that a negative stationary potential may be necessary for the occurrence of the familiar positive FFP. It is now clear, however, that junctional FFPs can be recorded as either predominantly negative or positive, or as diphasic potentials.

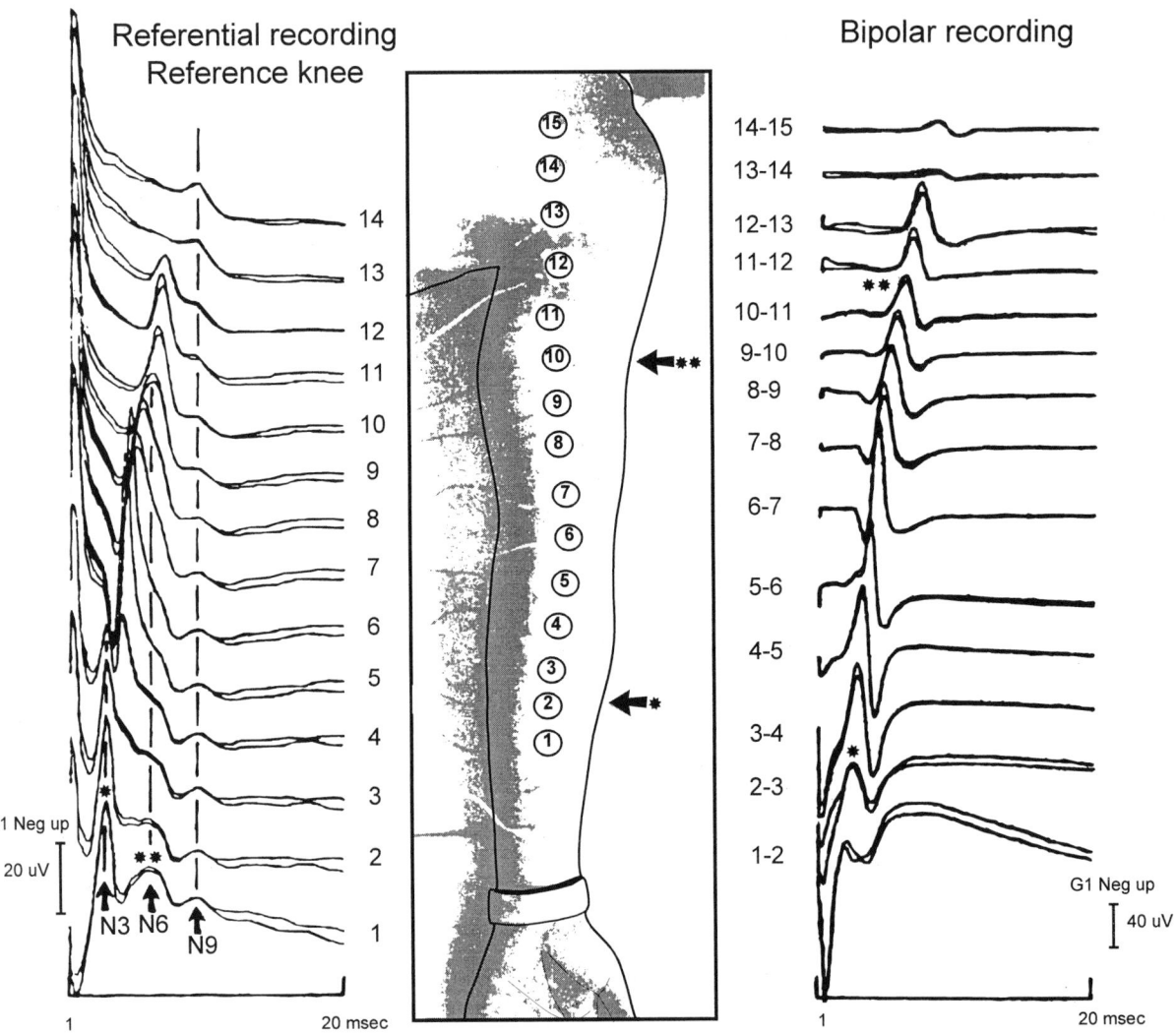

FIG. 29.4. Near-field and far-field potentials generated in the arm and shoulder following stimulation of the median nerve at the wrist. *Right:* A series of bipolar recordings from sequential pairs of electrodes over the course of the median nerve show near-field signals corresponding to the afferent volley. *Left:* Referential recordings from the same electrodes to a knee reference show both near-field (propagated) and far-field (stationary) signals. Far-field signals are generated when the afferent volley enters the brachioradialis (*) and deltoid (**) muscles, and crosses the boundary between the arm and the trunk. (Modified from Yamada T, Machida M, Oishi M, et al. Stationary negative potentials near the source vs. positive far-field potentials at a distance. *Electroencephalogr Clin Neurophysiol* 1985;60:509–524.)

Contributions from Gray Matter Structures

Graded postsynaptic potentials (PSPs) generated in gray matter structures also contribute to surface-recorded evoked potentials. The scalp-recorded electroencephalogram primarily reflects extracellular current flow resulting from summated excitatory and inhibitory PSPs generated in the parallel, vertically oriented pyramidal cells and their dendrites (35,78,147,164). Similar postsynaptic activity is probably responsible for the primary and subsequent cortical components of median nerve and posterior tibial nerve (PTN) SSEPs.

Although many subcortical nuclei are considered "closed-field" systems because their internal geometries are not conducive to producing current flow much beyond their boundaries (6,78,90), some subcortical nuclear structures do generate surface-recordable evoked potentials ("open-field" system). Examples include (a) central gray matter of the cervical (29,40,93) and lumbar spinal cord (125) and (b) the cochlear nuclear complex (85).

The terms *near field* and *far field* are also used to classify evoked potentials generated predominantly by PSPs. However, the distinction between the two is not always clear in this setting, and, in fact, a continuum probably exists. Furthermore, when applied to synaptically generated potentials, the terms do not necessarily imply a difference in generator mechanisms—in contrast to their use with potentials reflecting propagated volleys in white matter. Close to the region of depolarization, current gradients are steep, causing the voltage to vary substantially with changes in electrode position; evoked potentials recorded close to their generators appear as near-field potentials. In contrast, evoked potential signals recorded far from their generators are much less affected by alterations in electrode position, and hence appear as far-field signals (10).

COMPONENTS OF THE MEDIAN NERVE SSEP

For 18 milliseconds following electrical stimulation of the median nerve at the wrist, electrodes distributed widely over the scalp record similar waveforms (Fig. 29.5). Using an elbow reference, these consist of an initial positivity occurring at approximately 9 milliseconds (P$\overline{9}$), followed first by a

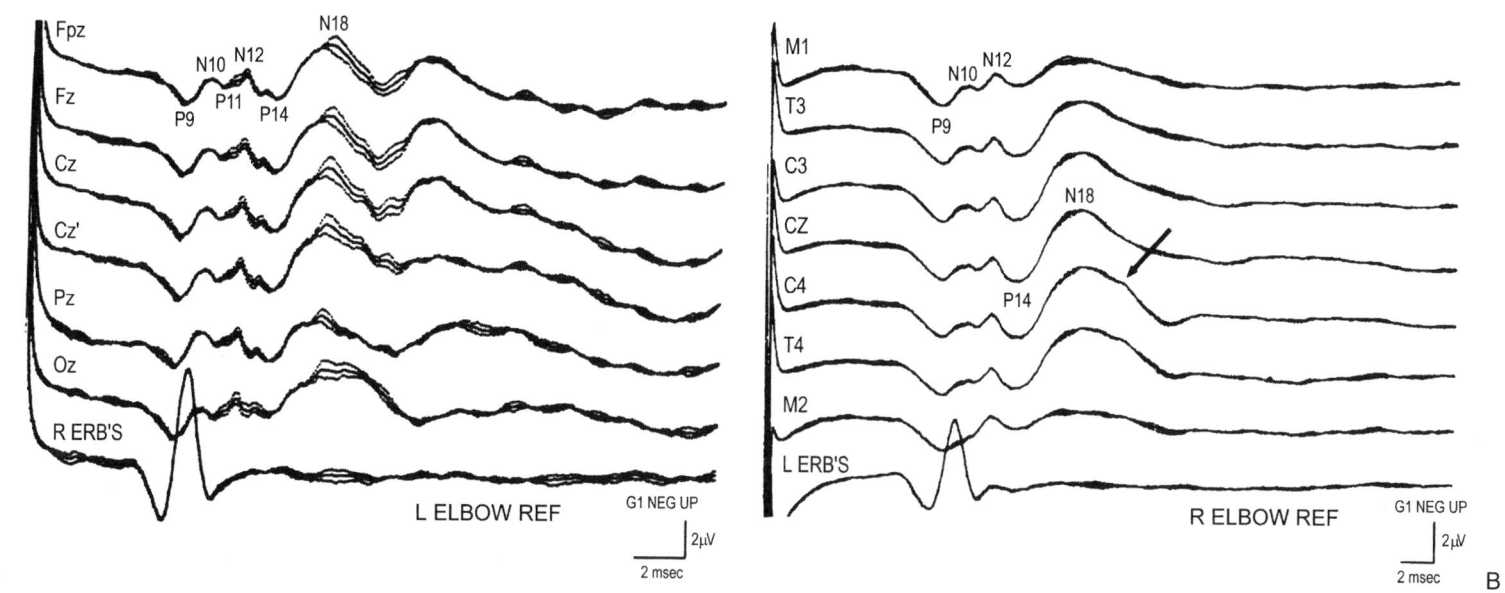

FIG. 29.5. Median-nerve SSEPs recorded in midsagittal (**A**) and coronal (**B**) planes using elbow references in two different normal individuals. In this and subsequent figures, amplifier passband settings are 30–3,000 Hz (−6 dB) unless noted. Upward deflections correspond to a relative negative voltage at the noninverting amplifier input.

series of small oscillations and then by a large-amplitude negative deflection of relatively long duration. The homogeneity of the recordings from virtually all scalp locations suggests that these components correspond to FFPs generated by relatively remote subcortical structures. After 18 milliseconds, differences appear in recordings from different scalp regions that reflect localized near-field activity (arrow, Fig. 29.5B).

Scalp-recorded activity following P$\overline{9}$ is customarily described as a series of two or more positive waves (5,6,19,20,28–30,64,79,93,99,109,148,157, 163). This view is consistent with, and may have been influenced by, the traditional concept that FFPs "should" be positive. It is clear from the foregoing section, however, that mechanisms of FFP generation are complex and that FFPs can appear either positive or negative.

Electrodes placed over the neck allow identification of signals corresponding to passage of the afferent volley through the proximal brachial plexus and the cuneate tract of the cervical spinal cord. Comparison of these measurements with simultaneous scalp recording provides important clues to the origins of the scalp-recorded FFPs. In addition to activity in ascending long tracts, neck electrodes register a distinct, localized stationary potential most likely generated in the gray matter of the cervical cord.

Brachial Plexus Volley

The scalp P$\overline{9}$ potential corresponds to the afferent volley in the brachial plexus (93,99,109,148,157,163) and occurs after the onset of afferent depolarization at the axilla but prior to arrival of the volley at Erb's point (28,163). The exact latency of P$\overline{9}$ can be influenced by changes in shoulder position (33).

Activity in Proximal Brachial Plexus and Cervical Roots

A vertical array of electrodes placed laterally over the anterior border of the sternocleidomastoid muscle, ipsilateral to the stimulated nerve, records a propagating wave that begins immediately after the afferent volley passes beneath Erb's point. No similar wave occurs contralaterally. The timing and topography of this potential indicate that it must represent activity in the brachial plexus or cervical spinal roots proximal to Erb's point. As illustrated in Fig. 29.6, the N$\overline{10}$ scalp FFP coincides with passage of this proximal plexus volley (PPV) through the neck. Although N$\overline{10}$ is widely distributed over the scalp, it is not identical at all electrode sites. It is maximal at the auricular electrode ipsilateral to the stimulus and is of significantly lower voltage contralaterally (Fig. 29.6). The exact point along the brachial plexus at which the N$\overline{10}$ FFP is generated is not known. There is considerable inter-

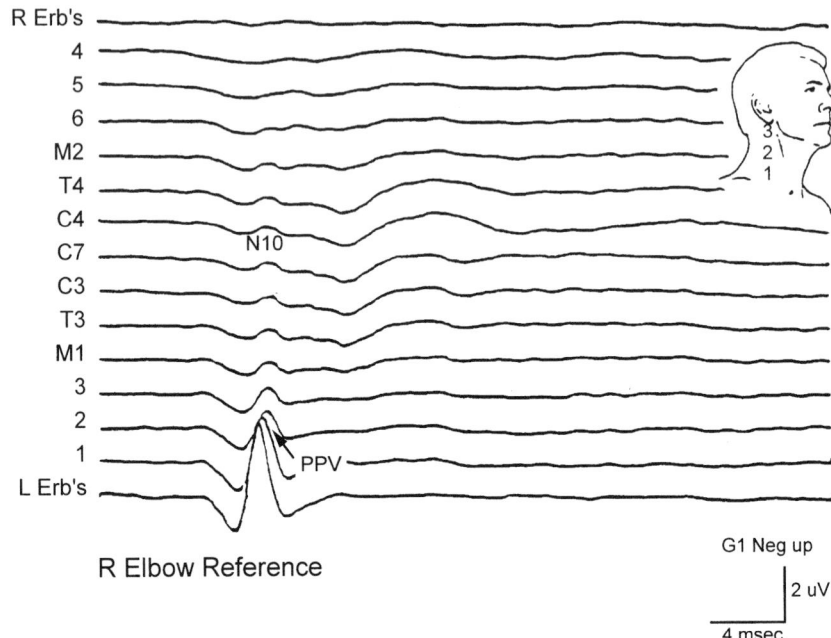

FIG. 29.6. Scalp topography of the N$\overline{10}$ potential in the coronal plane following left median nerve stimulation. Amplifier passband is 1–3,000 Hz.

subject variation in the position over the lateral neck where the negative peak of PPV becomes coincident with the scalp N$\overline{10}$ potential. It is likely that the relation of activity in the brachial plexus both to the propagating wave recorded over the neck and to its far-field counterpart on the scalp is determined by individual considerations of neck geometry and the electrical properties of intervening structures.

Dorsal Column Volley

Approximately 2 milliseconds after N$\overline{10}$, a second negative deflection, N$\overline{12}$, appears at scalp electrodes (see Fig. 29.5). This corresponds to another propagated volley that can be recorded directly from an ascending series of electrodes placed over the dorsal aspect of the neck (Fig. 29.7). Its characteristics are compatible with the sensory signal ascending the cuneate tract, and we have accordingly designated this the "dorsal column volley" (DCV). The scalp N$\overline{12}$ FFP occurs simultaneously with arrival of the DCV at the first cer-

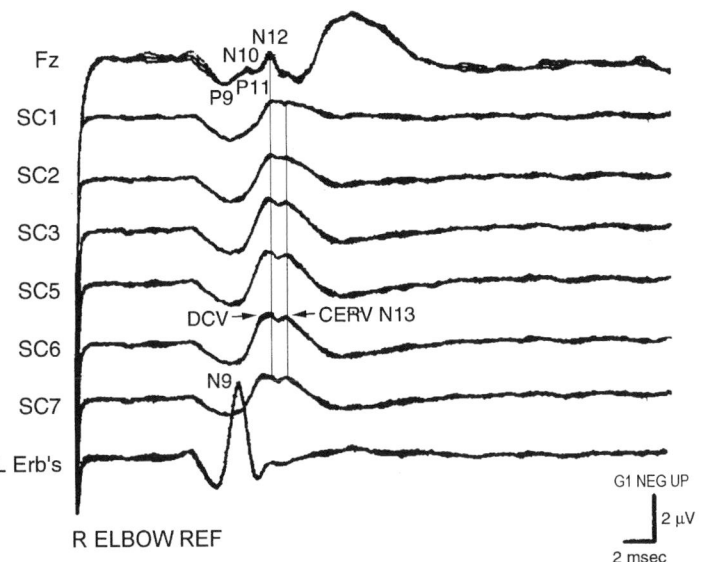

FIG. 29.7. Median nerve SSEPs recorded from a series of ascending cervical electrodes and from FZ using a noncephalic common reference.

vical level, SC1 (Fig. 29.7). This relationship suggests that the $N\overline{12}$ potential is generated at or before termination of the cuneate tract at the cuneate nucleus, perhaps because of changes in current density occurring as the afferent volley passes the boundary between spinal and cranial compartments.

Postsynaptic Activity in the Cervical Cord

Desmedt and Cheron (30) and Lueders et al. (93) provided evidence for a fixed generator of NFPs in the cervical spinal cord. Figure 29.7 demonstrates that a negativity (Cerv $N\overline{13}$) follows the DCV over the posterior neck. The Cerv $N\overline{13}$ potential is stationary in time (i.e., its latency does not change with rostral–caudal movement of the recording electrode), and its voltage is maximal over the low to middle cervical region. Desmedt and Cheron (30) used electrodes placed within the esophagus to identify a stationary positivity that was synchronous with the simultaneously recorded fixed dorsal negativity. We confirmed this observation using a ring of electrodes around the neck at the level of the fifth cervical spine (SC5) posteriorly and the superior border of the thyroid cartilage anteriorly (40). As illus-

trated in Figure 29.8, this stationary cervical potential attenuates laterally, passes through a null point, and becomes positive over the anterolateral neck, reaching maximal positivity in the anterior midline (Cerv $P\overline{13}$). It is not uncommon for the Cerv $N\overline{13}$ potential to mask the DCV. In these subjects, placement of lateral neck electrodes, where the stationary potential is near its null point, permits separation of the DCV from the Cerv $N\overline{13}$ potential.

It is most probable that the Cerv $N\overline{13}/P\overline{13}$ complex reflects postsynaptic activity in the central gray matter of the cervical spinal cord generated in response to input from axon collaterals. This conclusion is supported by direct intramedullary recordings in cats (7,17,43) and monkeys (7,8) that demonstrated potentials that reversed polarity between dorsal and ventral horns of the spinal cord gray matter. A contribution to Cerv $N\overline{13}$ from the cuneate nucleus has also been proposed (127).

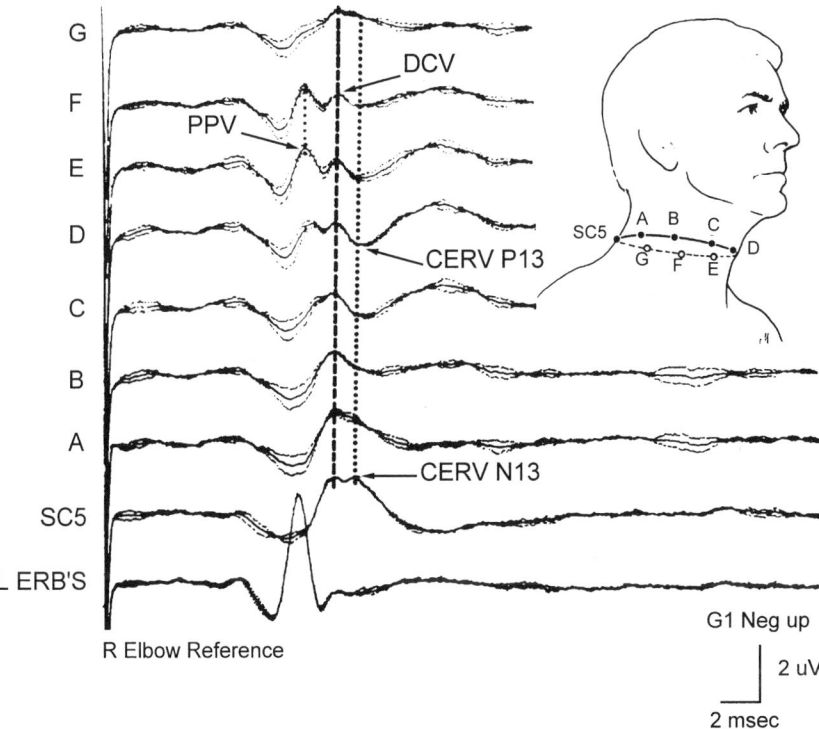

FIG. 29.8. Median nerve SSEPs recorded from a ring of electrodes about the neck using a noncephalic site.

Between N$\overline{10}$ and N$\overline{12}$, a downward deflection is present that has been designated P$\overline{11}$ (see Fig. 29.5). Desmedt and Cheron (28) concluded, by extrapolating from measurements of the velocity of the approaching volley in peripheral nerve, that P$\overline{11}$ onset coincided with the spinal entry of the afferent signal. Similarly, Lueders et al. (93) observed intraoperatively that the peak latency of the afferent volley at the C6 posterior rootlet corresponded to P$\overline{11}$ latency.

The P$\overline{14}$ Complex

Following N$\overline{12}$, a clearly demarcated positive deflection, P$\overline{14}$, is seen at all scalp electrodes (see Fig. 29.5). P$\overline{14}$ often appears as a single positive wave (see Fig. 29.5B), although frequently one or more inflections appear superimposed on it (see Fig. 29.5A) (6,28,38,60,93,163).

Although the exact origin of the P$\overline{14}$ potential is debated, based on observations in normal subjects (28–30), patients (100,143,161), and experimental animals (2,6), it is generally agreed that P$\overline{14}$ reflects activity in the medial lemniscus in the caudal brainstem. A presynaptic contribu-

tion from the upper cervical cord has also been suggested (66,119,120). Figure 29.9 is the median nerve SSEP of a 70-year-old woman with locked-in syndrome secondary to basilar artery occlusion. She had sudden onset of quadriparesis and a right hemisensory deficit that included the face. Pupillary reflexes and vertical eye movements were intact, but horizontal eye movements were absent. Although an autopsy was not permitted, the clinical picture indicated a bilateral lesion affecting the ventral portion of the midpons. Additionally, the right hemisensory deficit suggested that the lesion had sufficient dorsal extension to affect lemniscal fibers in the left pontine tegmentum. The SSEP in response to right median nerve stimulation revealed a normal P$\overline{14}$ complex, but N$\overline{18}$ was absent (see below). Preservation of P$\overline{14}$ in this patient is consistent with a generator site in the caudal medial lemniscus, below the midpons. A patient with a right pontine arteriovenous malformation showed similar findings (Fig. 29.10). Additionally, intraoperative recordings have demonstrated activity in the caudal medulla that is coincident with the scalp-recorded P$\overline{14}$ complex (Fig. 29.11).

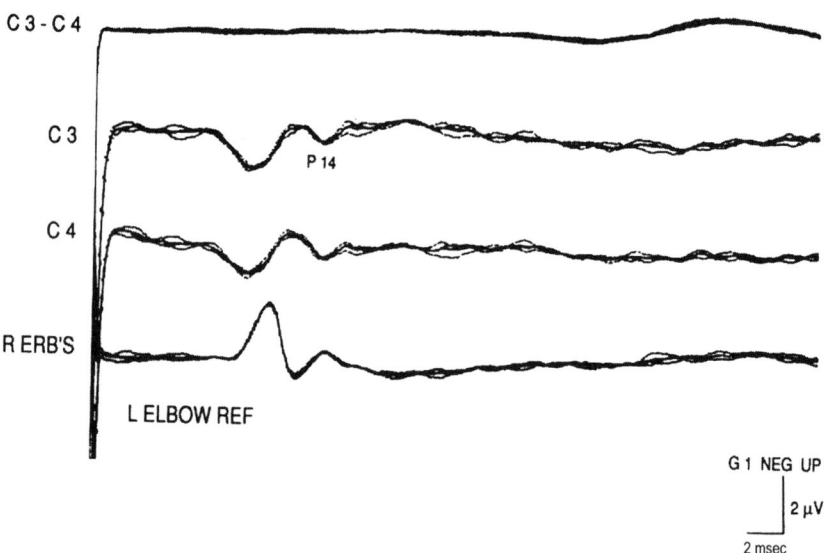

FIG. 29.9. Median nerve SSEP of a patient with locked-in syndrome as a result of basilar artery occlusion. P$\overline{14}$ is preserved, but subsequent short-latency potentials are lost.

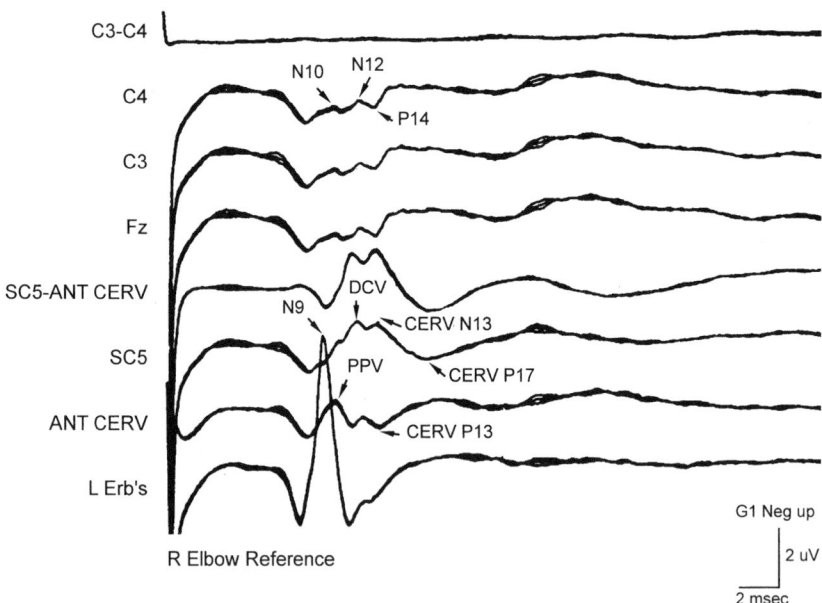

FIG. 29.10. Loss of potentials following P$\overline{14}$ in a patient with a pontine arteriovenous malformation.

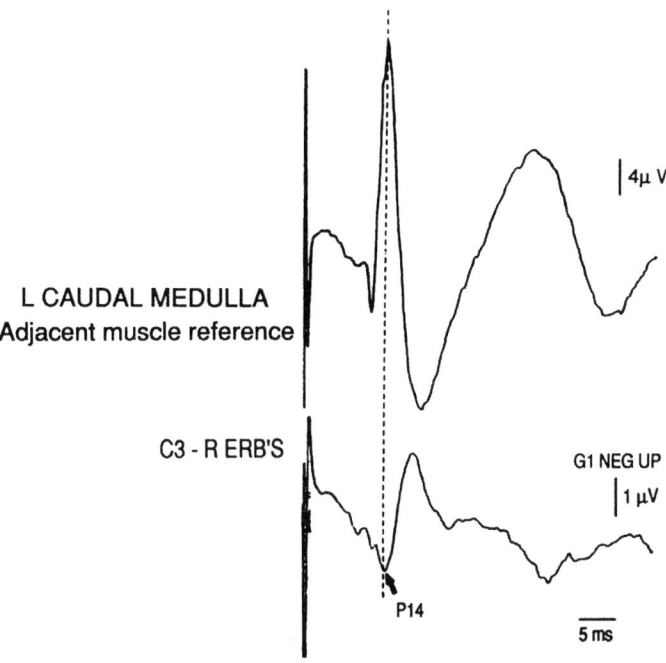

FIG. 29.11. Intraoperative recording demonstrating coincidence of the scalp-recorded P14 potential with activity in the caudal medulla.

The morphology of P14 varies considerably among individuals, although it is remarkably stable for individual subjects on repeat testing (134). Among 62 normal subjects, Sonoo et al. observed that P14 consisted of one, two, and three distinct peaks in 22, 35, and 5 subjects, respectively. Based on the timing of these peaks with respect to the onset of P14, they proposed that P14 is a composite of three components (P14a, P14b, and P14c[1] Figure 29.12), that are variably expressed among normal subjects (134,136).

Sonoo suggested that, whereas components P14a and P14b are most likely generated in the caudal medial lemniscus, P14c may originate more rostrally (134). Figure 29.13 illustrates the unilateral loss of P14c (and N20), but preservation of P14a and P14b, in a patient with a midpontine tumor. In contrast to the symmetrically distributed P14a and P14b, P14c is of greatest voltage over the central scalp region opposite the stimulated median nerve.

<hr>

[1]P14a, P14b, and P14c, in this discussion, correspond to Sonoo's P13, P14a, and P14b (134).

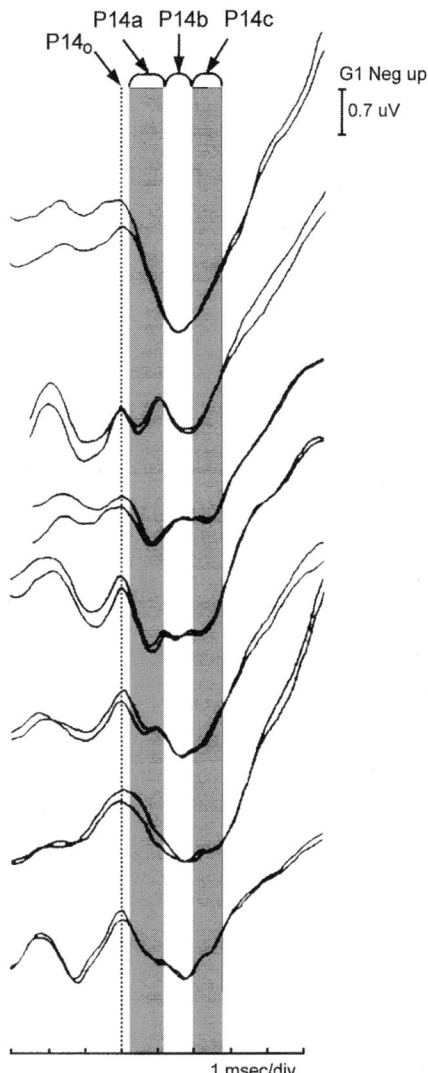

FIG. 29.12. Scalp-to-noncephalic recording following median nerve stimulation in seven normal subjects, illustrating the range of normal variability of the P14 complex. Tracings are aligned at the onset of P14 (P14o), and subcomponents P14a, P14b, and P14c are identified. (Modified from Sonoo M, Kobayashi M, Genba-Shimizu K, et al. Detailed analysis of the latencies of median nerve somatosensory evoked potential components, 1: selection of the best standard parameters and the establishment of normal values. *Electroencephalogr Clin Neurophysiol* 1996;100:319–331.)

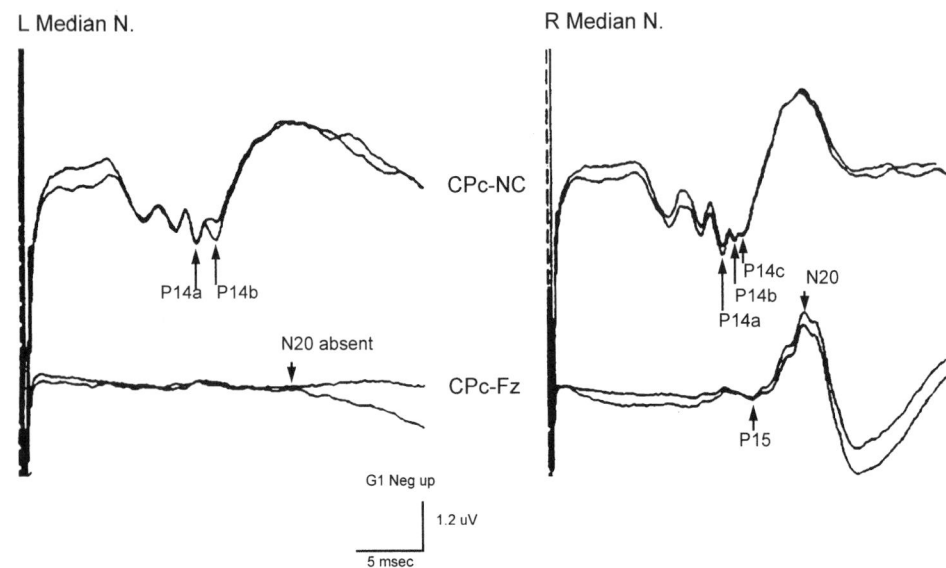

FIG. 29.13. Median nerve SSEP recorded in a patient with a low-grade astrocytoma in the midpons, in the vicinity of the right medial lemniscus. The right median nerve SSEP is normal, and components P14a, P14b, and P14c are identified. The left median nerve SSEP is abnormal, with loss of both N20 and P14c; P14a and P14b are preserved. (From Sonoo M, Kobayashi M, Genba-Shimizu K, et al. Detailed analysis of the latencies of median nerve somatosensory evoked potential components, 1: selection of the best standard parameters and the establishment of normal values. *Electroencephalogr Clin Neurophysiol* 1996; 100:319–331, with permission.)

P14c may be lost in patients with lesions of the brainstem and thalamus, and with long-standing lesions of cerebral cortex. For these reasons, Sonoo et al. suggested that P14c may originate in the thalamocortical radiations (134). Intracranial recording in monkeys have also shown that the third of three positive far-field signals, which together appear to correspond to the human P14 complex, originates in the thalamocortical radiations (6). Because of asymmetry of its scalp distribution, P14c most likely corresponds to the small positivity that is sometimes detectable prior to the onset of N20 on bipolar scalp derivations (41).

Many clinical laboratories routinely utilize a recording montage that combines Cerv N13 with the scalp P14 FFP (e.g., SC5-Fpz). In contrast to this practice, we cannot overemphasize the importance of employing montages that preserve the distinct identities of the Cerv N13 and scalp P14 FFPs (39,105). As shown in Figure 29.14, a compressive cervical myelopathy produced a marked dissociation between these normally near-simultaneous components. Two distinct upward deflections are present in the SC5-Fpz derivation, but it is not possible to identify each. Separate referential recordings from SC5 and Fpz demonstrated that the first inflection is a normal-latency Cerv N13 potential; the second is a markedly prolonged P14 complex. In Figure 29.15, from a patient with syringomyelia (152), there is no Cerv N13, but P14 is normal. In both of these cases, use of a SC5-Fpz derivation would have obscured the abnormality.

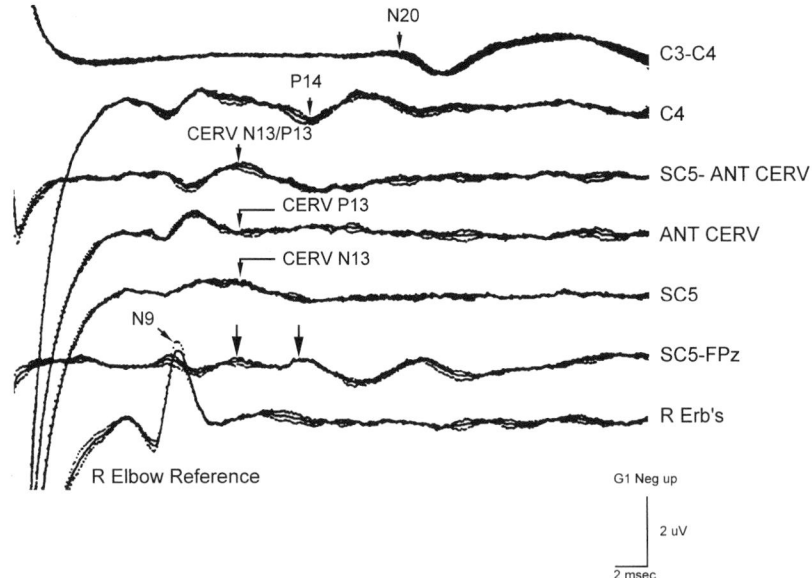

FIG. 29.14. Right median nerve SSEP in a patient with a compressive cervical myelopathy. Cerv N13 occurs at normal latency, but P14 is delayed. The potentials may be properly identified on separate referential derivations from SC5 and Fpz but not in the bipolar SC5-Fpz derivation.

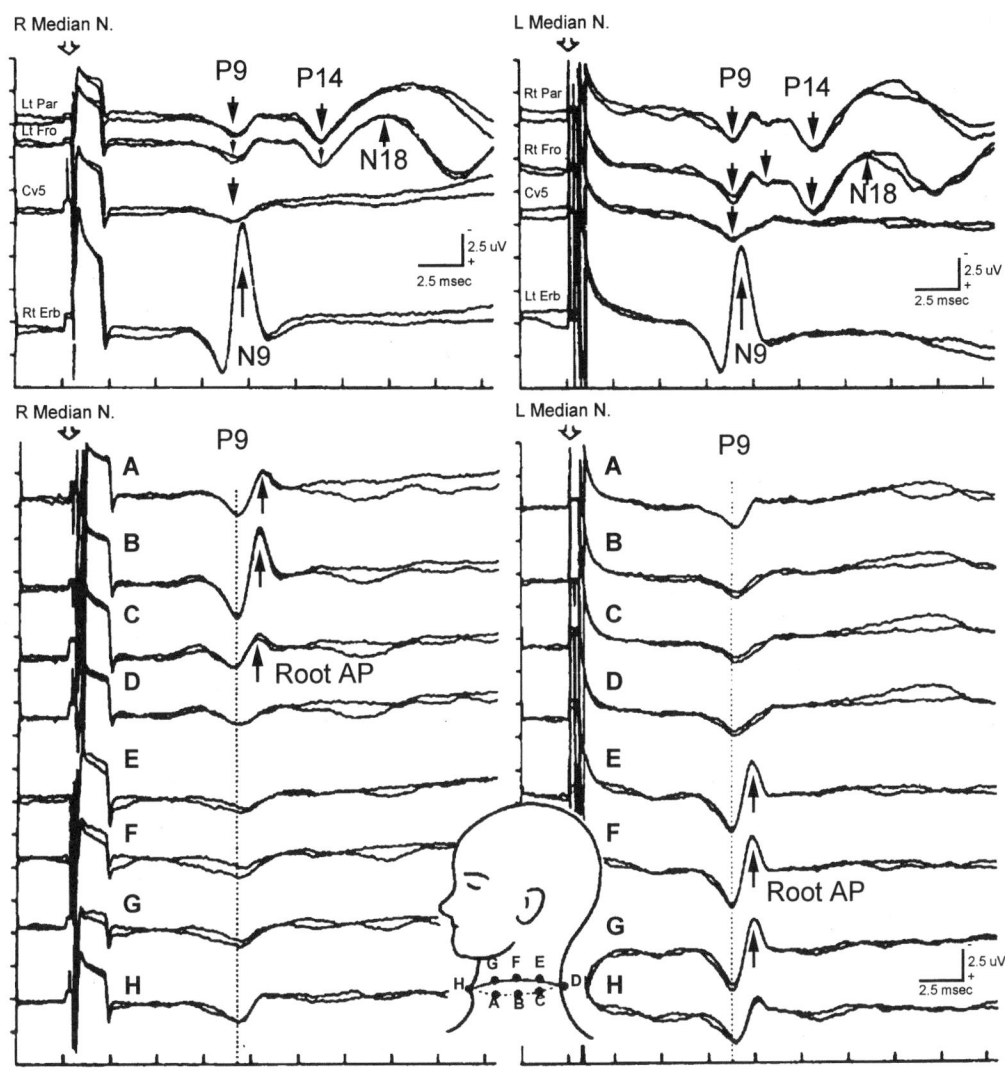

FIG. 29.15. Median nerve SSEPs in a patient with syringomyelia extending from C1 to T11. In all recordings, the reference electrode was at Erb's point on the side opposite the stimulated arm. Scalp-recorded components are preserved, but the cervical N13/P13 complex is abolished. (From Urasaki E, Wada S, Kadoya C, et al. Absence of spinal N13-P13 and normal scalp far-field P14 in a patient with syringomyelia. *Electroencephalogr Clin Neurophysiol* 1988;71:400–404, with permission.)

The N18 Potential

Following P14, a prolonged negative potential, N18, is recorded from all scalp electrodes. The distribution of N18 is illustrated in Figure 29.5. The initial part of the deflection is symmetrical, but a notch (arrow, Fig. 29.5B) at the contralateral parietal area indicates an additional negative component restricted to this region. Desmedt and Cheron (29) have carefully defined the characteristics of these two waves and designated them, respectively, N18 and N20. N20 may be separated from the underlying N18 potential by subtracting recordings made simultaneously from the ipsilateral and contralateral parietal electrodes (Fig. 29.16; see also "The N20 and Other Short-Latency Cortical Potentials" below).

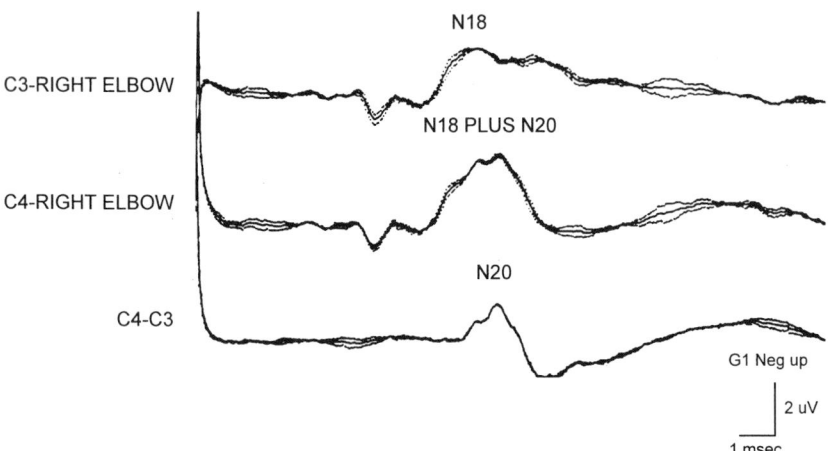

FIG. 29.16. Separation of N$\overline{20}$ from the underlying N$\overline{18}$. The lower channel was computed by subtracting the upper channel from the middle channel.

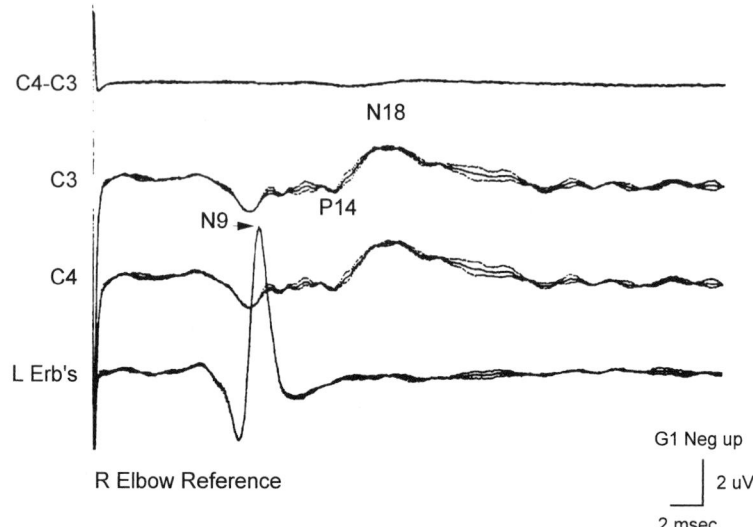

FIG. 29.17. Preservation of N$\overline{18}$ with loss of N$\overline{20}$ in a patient with a bilateral thalamic astrocytoma.

The widespread distribution of N$\overline{18}$ is characteristic of a FFP and suggests a subcortical origin. Desmedt and Cheron (29) originally proposed that N$\overline{18}$ reflected delayed activity within the thalamus or caudal portions of thalamocortical projection fibers. However, it was subsequently demonstrated that N$\overline{18}$ is preserved with destructive lesions of the thalamus that cause the loss of later components of the median nerve SSEP (104) (Fig. 29.17). Although postsynaptically generated signals, coincident with the scalp N$\overline{18}$, have been recorded from the Vim nucleus of the thalamus, they have been confined to that structure, demonstrating high-voltage gradients that are characteristic of closed-field systems (153). In contrast, direct brainstem recording from within the forth ventricle demonstrates a stationary peak, with shallow spatial voltage gradients, coincident with the scalp-recorded N$\overline{18}$ potential, beginning above the level of the midpons (153). This observation is consistent with the view that N$\overline{18}$ reflects postsynaptic activity in the upper brainstem gray matter structures, especially tectal and pretectal nuclei, that receive axon collaterals from the medial lemniscus (101,151,153,154). The organization of the tectum is compatible with an open-field system that could generate scalp-recordable far-field evoked potentials (101). Loss of N$\overline{18}$ amplitude has been observed in patients with lesions of the pons and midbrain (154) (see Fig. 29.10). Conversely, reports of patients with largely intact N$\overline{18}$ despite pontine and rostral medullary lesions suggest that postsynaptic activity in the cuneate nuclei may contribute to the N$\overline{18}$ potential (118,135).

N$\overline{18}$ has a long duration (up to 19 milliseconds), which supports postsynaptic (rather than axonal) activity as a major contributor to scalp-recorded FFPs (104). Careful inspection of the N$\overline{18}$ potential often reveals small, superimposed inflections that persist even when hemispherectomy has removed the possibility of cortical near-field contamination (2,101) (Fig. 29.18). These inflections plus its long duration suggest that N$\overline{18}$ is a complex wave with multiple, possibly sequentially activated, brainstem generators (101).

The N$\overline{20}$ and Other Short-Latency Cortical Potentials

The earliest localized scalp potential is the N$\overline{20}$ potential. It is recorded only over parietal regions contralateral to the stimulated side, where it is superimposed on N$\overline{18}$ and represents the initial cortical response to the sensory volley (1,2,29,60,103). Loss of the N$\overline{20}$ potential, with preservation of the underlying N$\overline{18}$ potential, can be seen in patients with small lesions of the parietal cortex that produce severe astereognosis and loss of graphesthesia but do not disturb perception of intact touch, pain, temperature, position, and vibration. Like earlier components, N$\overline{20}$ often has several small inflections superimposed on it (see Figs. 29.16 and 29.23), suggesting that it may result from activity within multiple generators (1,2,29,60,103,104). The view of N$\overline{20}$ as a

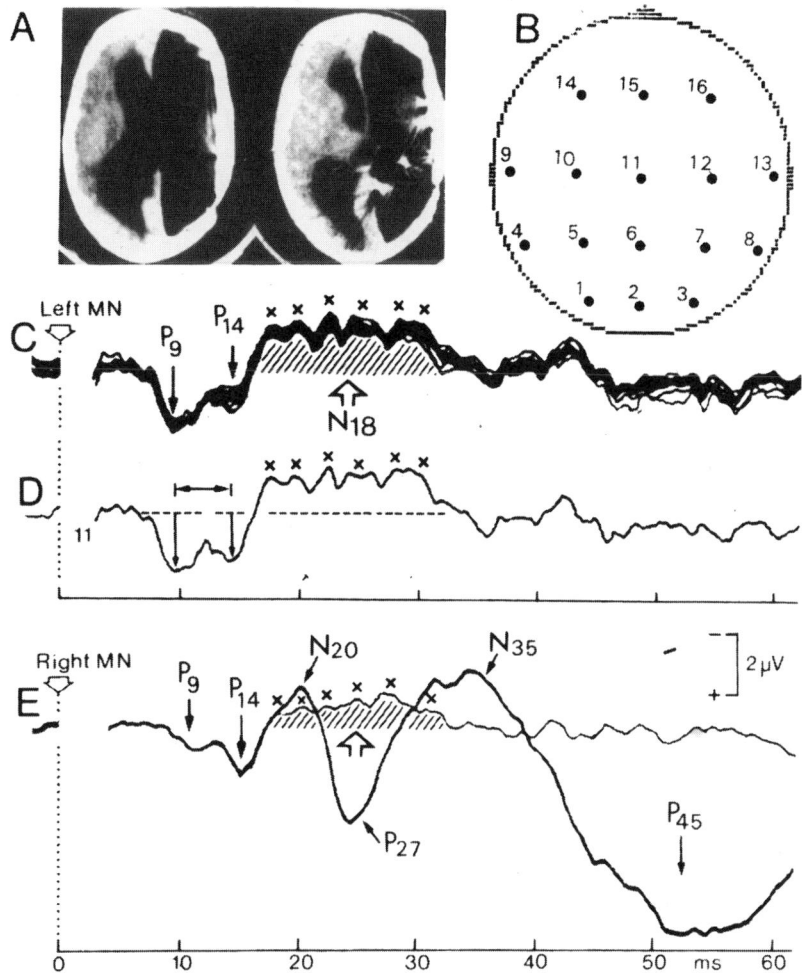

FIG. 29.18. Median SEPs recorded from a patient with a long-standing right hemispherectomy performed for intractable epilepsy. **A:** Computed tomography scans. **B:** Electrode placements. For all recordings, the reference electrode was on the shoulder opposite the stimulated arm. **C:** Left median nerve SSEP, with all 16 channels superimposed. Responses are essentially identical in all channels. **D:** Left median nerve SSEP, recorded from electrode 11. **E:** Right median nerve SSEP, showing superimposed recordings from electrodes 5 (thicker line) and 7. In **B** and **D**, N$\overline{18}$ is shown as the *hatched area*. (From Mauguière F, Desmedt JE. Bilateral somatosensory evoked potentials in four patients with long-standing surgical hemispherectomy. *Ann Neurol* 1989;26: 724–731, with permission.)

composite waveform is supported by (a) recordings from subdural electrodes (92); (b) studies of state-dependent effects (42,162); and (c) changes in N$\overline{20}$ topography produced by selective stimulation of muscle and cutaneous afferents in the median nerve using intrafascicular microelectrodes (45).

Recorded from a subdural strip electrode perpendicular to the central fissure, the earliest cortical response is a negativity beginning at approximately 18 milliseconds and peaking at about 20 milliseconds following median nerve stimulation (93). This signal, which corresponds to the scalp-recorded N$\overline{20}$ potential, is maximal in voltage just posterior to the central fissure, and is accompanied by a simultaneous, nearly mirror-image positivity occurring anterior to the central sulcus (Fig. 29.19). This postcentral negativity and the corresponding precentral positivity are thought be volume conducted from a tangentially oriented "dipole" in the posterior wall of the central sulcus, generated by activation of area 3b, with possible contributions from area 3a (Fig. 29.20.) (6,92,115,155).

In scalp recordings, the parietal N$\overline{20}$ potential is accompanied by a frontal positivity, the P$\overline{22}$ potential, which usually peaks slightly later. P$\overline{22}$ is generated separately from N$\overline{20}$. It does not share a common generator with N$\overline{20}$ in the posterior wall of the central sulcus, as was previously thought (1,13). N$\overline{20}$ and P$\overline{22}$ have different peak and onset latencies (25,28,32,122). They respond differently to changes in stimulation rate, to anesthetic drugs, and to ischemia (122). They can be affected separately by focal internal capsular lesions (Figs. 29.21 and 29.22) (81,85). Anatomical and physiological studies have previously established independent thalamocortical projections to the crown of the postcentral gyrus and to anterior and posterior banks of the central sulcus (63,98,112). Mauguière and Desmedt suggested that, whereas activation of the posterior bank of the central sulcus following input from VPL$_c$ is responsible for generation of the N$\overline{20}$ potential, depolarization of motor area 4 on the opposing anterior bank, in response to independent input from VPL$_o$, results in generation of the P$\overline{22}$ potential (102).

Over the central-parietal scalp, N$\overline{20}$ is followed by a positivity, P$\overline{27}$, that likely reflects activation of area 1 on the crown of the postcentral gyrus (102). Over the frontal scalp, P$\overline{22}$ is followed by a negativity, N$\overline{30}$, thought to be generated by supplementary motor and premotor cortex (102). Although the electrical fields of P$\overline{22}$ and N$\overline{30}$ extend bilaterally, recordings following hemispherectomy indicate that these signal are generated only by the hemisphere opposite the stimulated side (101).

Most studies of SSEPs in humans have been conducted with subjects or patients relaxed and often asleep, frequently with the aid of sedative drugs. By recording median nerve SSEPs with subjects both fully alert and in stage 2 sleep, we demonstrated that the multiple inflections superimposed on the

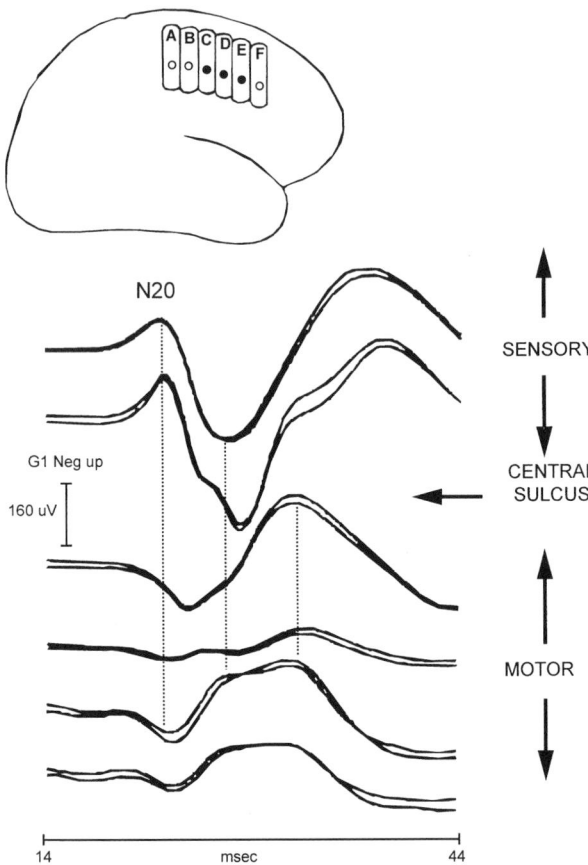

FIG. 29.19. Cortical surface recordings of a median nerve SSEP made from a subdural electrode grid crossing the central sulcus. Motor potentials were elicited by electrical stimulation at electrode locations shown as *black circles*. (Modified from Lueders H, Lesser RP, Hahn J, et al. Cortical somatosensory evoked potentials in response to hand stimulation. *J Neurosurg* 1983;58:885–894.)

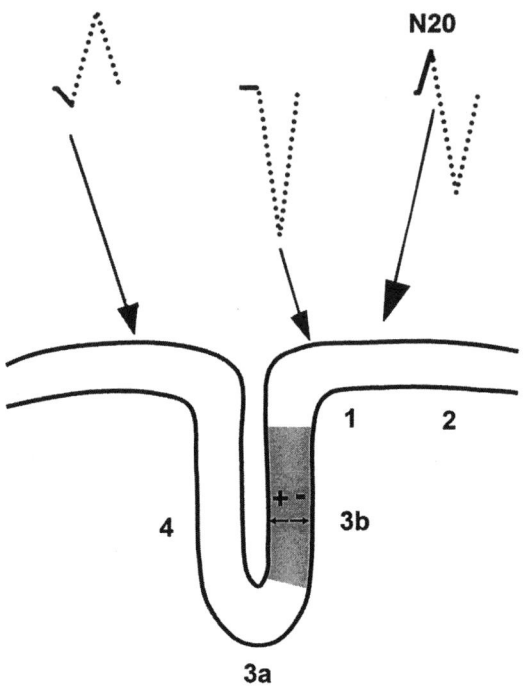

FIG. 29.20. Model proposed to explain the generation of N$\overline{20}$. Waveforms corresponding to the median nerve SSEP in immediate pre- and postcentral regions are illustrated. Depolarization of area 3b is responsible for the solid portion of the waveform. Subsequent depolarization of adjacent cortical regions contributes to subsequent dotted portions of the waveform. (Modified from Lueders H, Lesser RP, Hahn J, et al. Cortical somatosensory evoked potentials in response to hand stimulation. *J Neurosurg* 1983;58:885–894.)

initial upstroke of the N$\overline{20}$ potential are state dependent: They are prominent during wakefulness but attenuate or disappear during sleep (42). Yamada et al. (162) have confirmed this. Stage 2 sleep also prolongs N$\overline{20}$ peak latency by 0.2–0.9 millisecond (mean 0.6 millisecond) (Fig. 29.23) (42,130). We have speculated that loss of the inflections, along with the associated shift in N$\overline{20}$ peak latency, reflects selective downward modulation (during sleep) of

specific thalamocortical projection systems that contribute to the composite N$\overline{20}$ waveform (42,46,47,138).

In fully alert subjects, N$\overline{20}$ is often preceded by a small positivity (mean latency 15.4 milliseconds; $n = 10$), P$\overline{15}$, which has a similar scalp topography (see Fig. 29.23) (41). P$\overline{15}$, recorded using a bipolar scalp derivation, is nearly coincident with P$\overline{14}$c on referential scalp derivations, and is most likely generated in the thalamocortical radiations (134).

Although the caudal–rostral organization of the large-fiber sensory system might suggest serial processing of sensory signals, examples of selective loss of subcortical SSEP components with preservation of the cortical

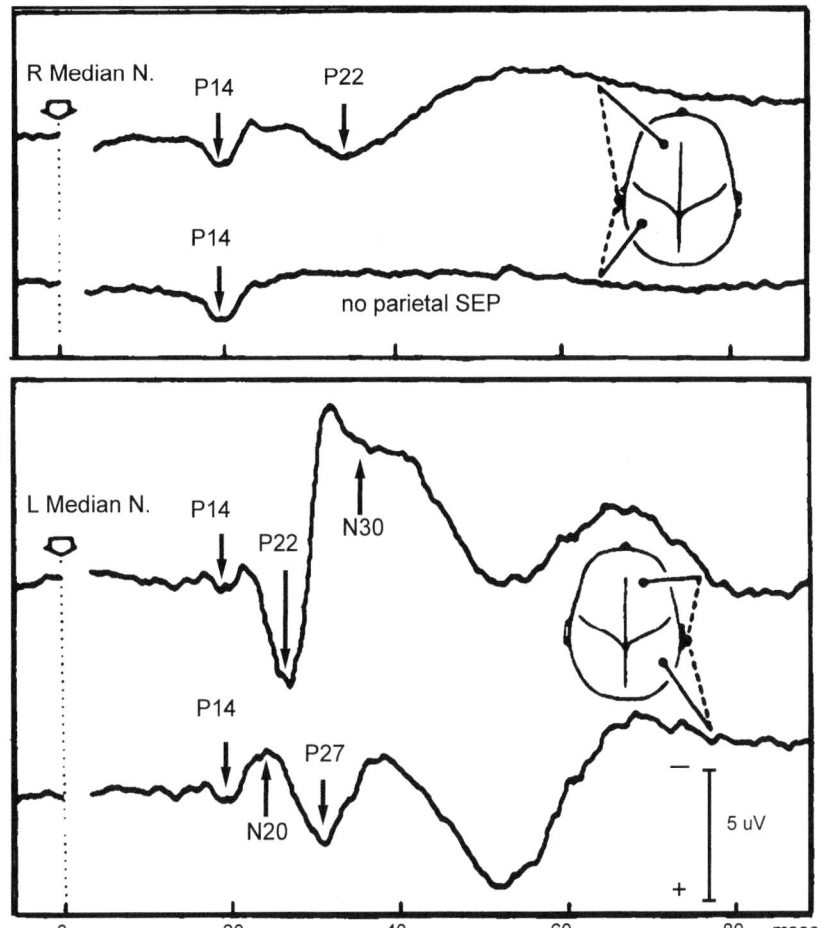

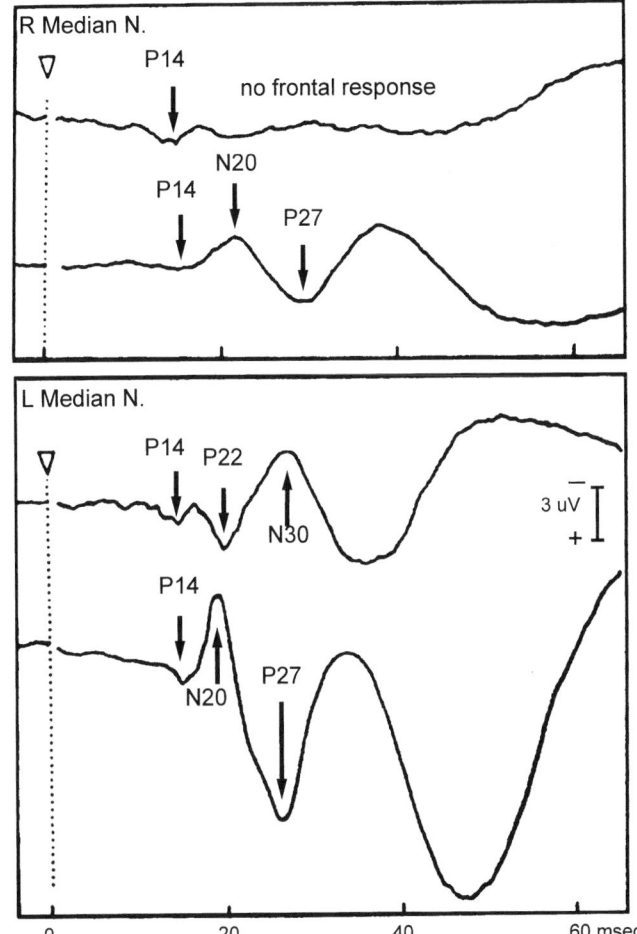

FIG. 29.21. Median nerve SSEPs from a patient with a small left internal capsular hematoma, presenting with severe right-sided motor and sensory deficits. The right median SSEP shows complete absence of the N$\overline{20}$ potential, and the P$\overline{22}$ potential, although present, is delayed and of lower voltage when compared with the normal response obtained to left-sided stimulation. (From Mauguière F, Desmedt JE. Focal capsular vascular lesions can selectively deafferent the prerolandic of the parietal cortex: somatosensory evoked potentials evidence. *Ann Neurol* 1991;30:71–75, with permission.)

FIG. 29.22. Median nerve SSEPs from a patient with a left internal capsular hematoma, presenting with right hemiplegia and partially preserved touch, point position, pain, and temperature sensation on the right. The right median nerve SSEP shows loss of the frontal P$\overline{22}$ potential. The parietal N$\overline{20}$ potential is present, but delayed and lower in voltage than that obtained following stimulation of the normal left side. (From Mauguière F, Desmedt JE. Focal capsular vascular lesions can selectively deafferent the prerolandic of the parietal cortex: somatosensory evoked potentials evidence. *Ann Neurol* 1991;30:71–75, with permission.)

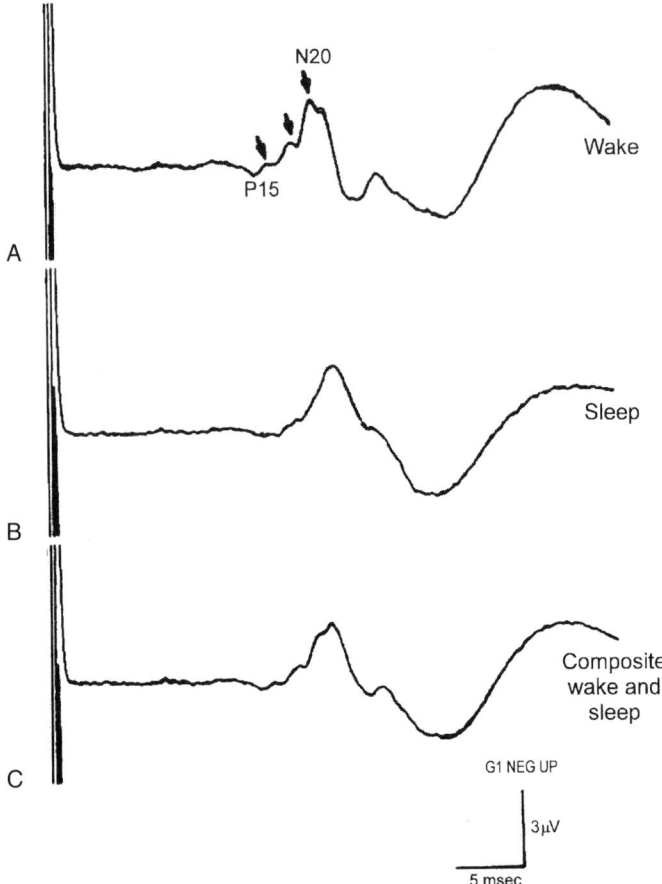

FIG. 29.23. State-dependent changes in N$\overline{20}$. **A:** Changes in N$\overline{20}$ during transition from wakefulness to sleep are depicted using a two-dimensional filtering technique. Each line represents the average of 32 sequential trials; sequential sets are stacked vertically. (**A** from Sgro JA, Emerson RG, Pedley TA. Real-time reconstruction of evoked potentials using a new two dimensional filter method. *Electroencephalogr Clin Neurophysiol* 1985;62:372–380, with permission.) **B:** N$\overline{20}$ recorded with the subject awake. **C:** N$\overline{20}$ recorded with the subject asleep after oral diazepam. **D:** "Composite" N$\overline{20}$ including responses obtained during wakefulness, drowsiness, and sleep. Note that both morphology and peak latency are intermediate between waking and sleep N$\overline{20}$ potentials. (**B–D** from Emerson RG, Sgro JA, Pedley TA, et al. State-dependent changes in the N20 component of the median nerve somatosensory evoked potential. *Neurology* 1988;38:64–68, with permission.)

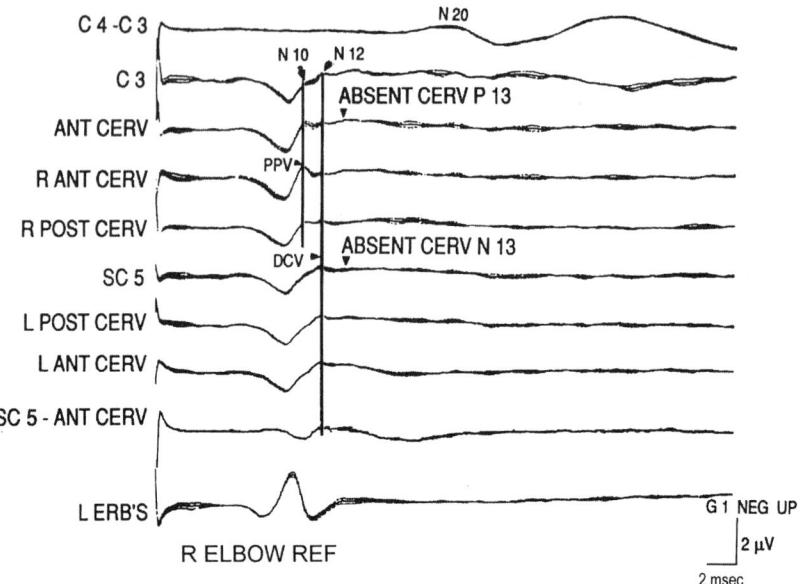

FIG. 29.24. Left median nerve SSEP record from a patient with multiple sclerosis, demonstrating loss of Cerv N$\overline{13}$/P$\overline{13}$, P$\overline{14}$, and N$\overline{18}$ with preservation of a normal N$\overline{20}$ potential.

response are occasionally encountered (15,133). Figure 29.24 depicts the left median nerve SSEP recorded in a patient with multiple sclerosis. Although Cerv N$\overline{13}$/P$\overline{13}$, P$\overline{14}$, and N$\overline{18}$ are absent, N$\overline{20}$ is normal. The relative independence of subcortical and cortical SSEPs may be explained either by nonserial linkage of at least some component generators or by central amplification of abnormally weak input signals (36,39).

COMPONENTS OF THE PTN SSEP

SSEPs recorded following PTN stimulation are, in part, analogous to responses evoked by median nerve stimulation. The afferent signals that produce the PTN SSEP traverse the dorsal columns (23,53), although signals mediated by other pathways, (e.g., the dorsolateral funiculus) may also play a role (14,50,139). Some laboratories routinely use common peroneal nerve stimulation for lower-limb SSEPs. However, common peroneal nerve SSEPs show a greater degree of intersubject variability than PTN SSEPs (113), and the latter are therefore preferred for routine clinical use.

Following PTN stimulation, electrodes over the lumbar spine record both a propagated volley and a stationary potential that are analogs of the DCV and Cerv N$\overline{13}$ potentials seen after median nerve stimulation. Scalp electrodes initially record widely distributed potentials reflecting subcortical activity, and then register lateralized activity that represents the early cortical response.

Spinal Components

Electrodes positioned over the lower spine record two distinct components (Fig. 29.25) (125). The potential labeled N$\overline{22}$ is of maximal amplitude between T10 and L1 (37) and has properties identical to the Cerv N$\overline{13}$ potential. Its amplitude attenuates, but its latency remains fixed, in elec-

trodes rostral and caudal to the point of maximal voltage. It reverses phase from dorsal to ventral, and electrodes over the abdominal wall record a positivity, P$\overline{22}$ (Fig. 29.26). The N$\overline{22}$/P$\overline{22}$ complex most likely represents postsynaptic activity in the lumbar enlargement of the spinal cord.

Electrodes over the lumbosacral spine record a second waveform that occurs just before the N$\overline{22}$ potential. The latency of this potential increases at progressively more rostral electrode sites (see Fig. 29.25). This potential arises from the propagated volley (PV), occurring first in the spinal roots of the cauda equina and subsequently in the gracile tract. Because its latency changes depending on recording electrode position, its timing in relation to N$\overline{22}$ is variable. Thus PV precedes N$\overline{22}$ over the lumbosacral spine but occurs with, or just following, N$\overline{22}$ over the thoracic spine.

As already mentioned, N$\overline{22}$ is normally of maximum voltage over the lower thoracic spine, at the level of the spinal cord's lumbar enlargement just

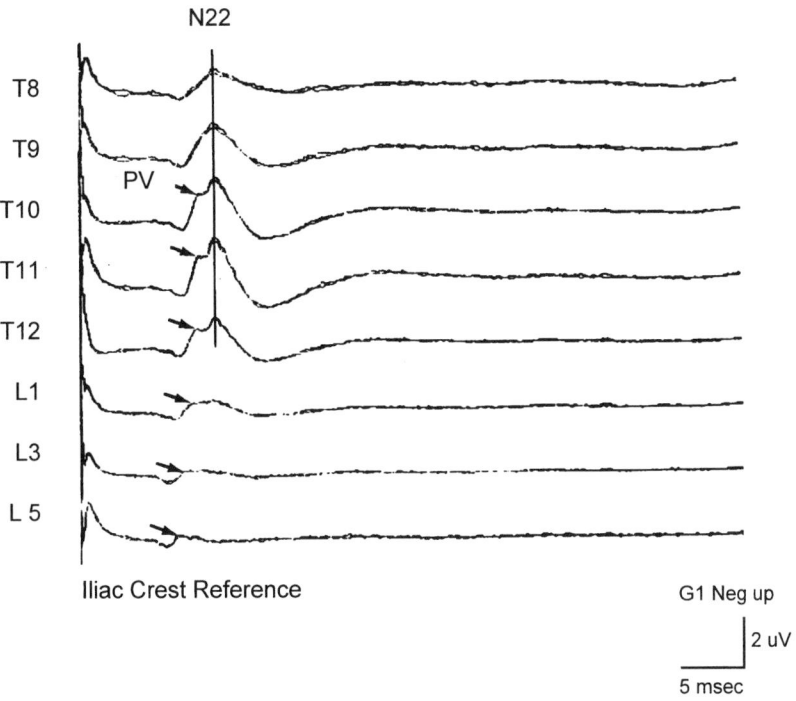

FIG. 29.25. Left PTN SSEP recorded over the lower thoracic and lumbar spine using a reference electrode on the right iliac crest. The thoracolumbar response consists of two distinct signals: a propagated volley (PV) that increases in latency at more rostral electrodes, and a stationary potential (N$\overline{22}$) whose voltage is maximal between T10 and L1.

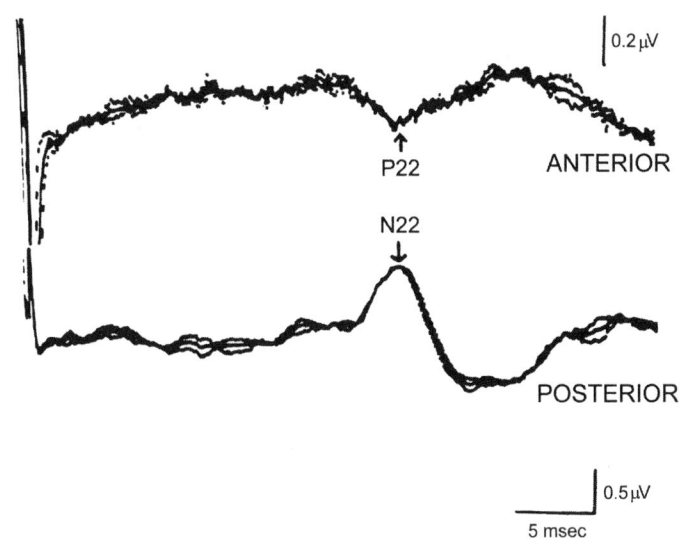

FIG. 29.26. PTN SSEP recorded simultaneously from a lumbar electrode 10 cm rostral to the L4 spinous process (*lower tracing*) and an electrode over the abdomen at the same level (*upper tracing*). The reference electrode was on the elbow opposite the site of stimulation. (From Seyal M, Gabor AJ. The human posterior tibial somatosensory evoked potential: synapse dependent and synapse independent spinal components. *Electroencephalogr Clin Neurophysiol* 1985;62: 323–331, with permission.)

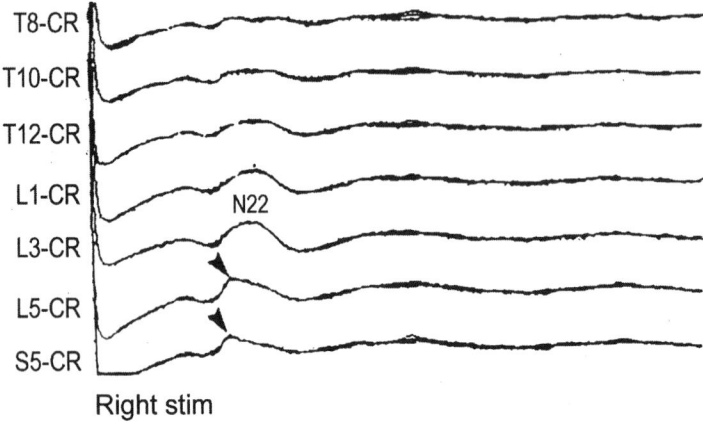

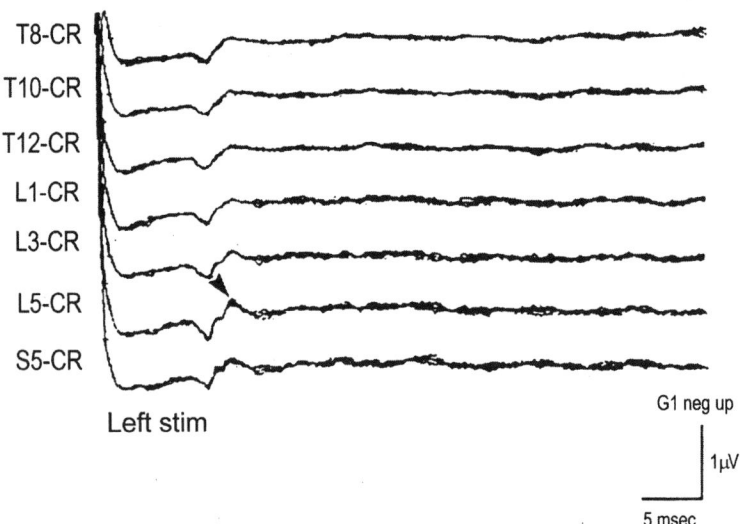

FIG. 29.27. PTN SSEP recorded in a 7-year-old boy with a lumbosacral lipoma and tethering of the spinal cord. Reference electrode was on the contralateral iliac crest. **Upper panel:** Right PTN stimulation reveals caudal displacement of N$\overline{22}$. **Lower panel:** Following left PTN stimulation, N$\overline{22}$ is absent, and only the PV (*arrowhead*) component of the lumbar response is seen.

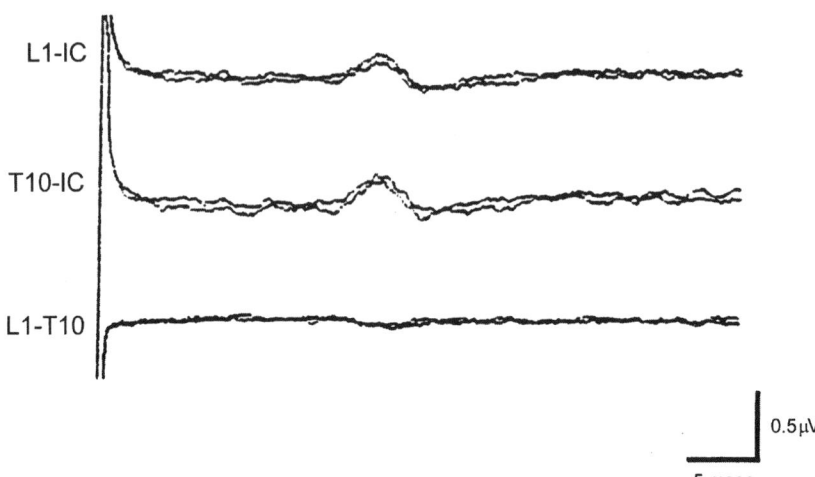

FIG. 29.28. Comparison of bipolar and referential techniques for recording the lumbar response to PTN stimulation. N$\overline{22}$ is well delineated using the iliac crest (IC) reference, but it is virtually absent on the L1-T10 bipolar derivation because of in-phase cancellation.

rostral to the termination of the conus medullaris at L1 or L2 (8). In patients with tethered cord syndrome, the N$\overline{22}$ potential, if preserved, is displaced caudally, corresponding to the abnormally low position of the terminal spinal cord (Fig. 29.27) (37).

The most prominent evoked potential component recorded over the lower thoracic and upper lumbar spine following PTN stimulation is N$\overline{22}$, not the afferent volley. Indeed, in many recordings, N$\overline{22}$ is the only spinal component identifiable. Because N$\overline{22}$ is widely distributed over the lower spine, bipolar spinal recordings frequently result in in-phase cancellation. Referential recording (e.g., T12 to iliac crest) (Fig. 29.28) allows clear characterization of N$\overline{22}$ and also allows distinction between N$\overline{22}$ and the more variable PV (87). Over the upper cervical spine, a second low-amplitude stationary potential can be recorded following PTN stimulation, which may reflect postsynaptic activity in the gracile nucleus (126).

Subcortical Components

Scalp recordings using a non

cephalic reference (shoulder or lower cervical spine) initially demonstrate a series of widespread waves representing FFPs arising at subcortical sites. The most consistent of these are a small positive deflection, P$\overline{31}$, and a following negative potential of larger amplitude and longer duration, N$\overline{34}$ (Fig. 29.29). Sometimes another positive component, P$\overline{28}$, precedes P$\overline{31}$. At sites away from the vertex, N$\overline{34}$ shows a gradual return to baseline approximately 40 milliseconds after the stimulus (124).

The best information about the origin of the subcortical components of the PTN SSEP comes from analogies to the more extensively studied median nerve SSEP (74,150). P$\overline{31}$ is strikingly similar to P$\overline{14}$ recorded after median

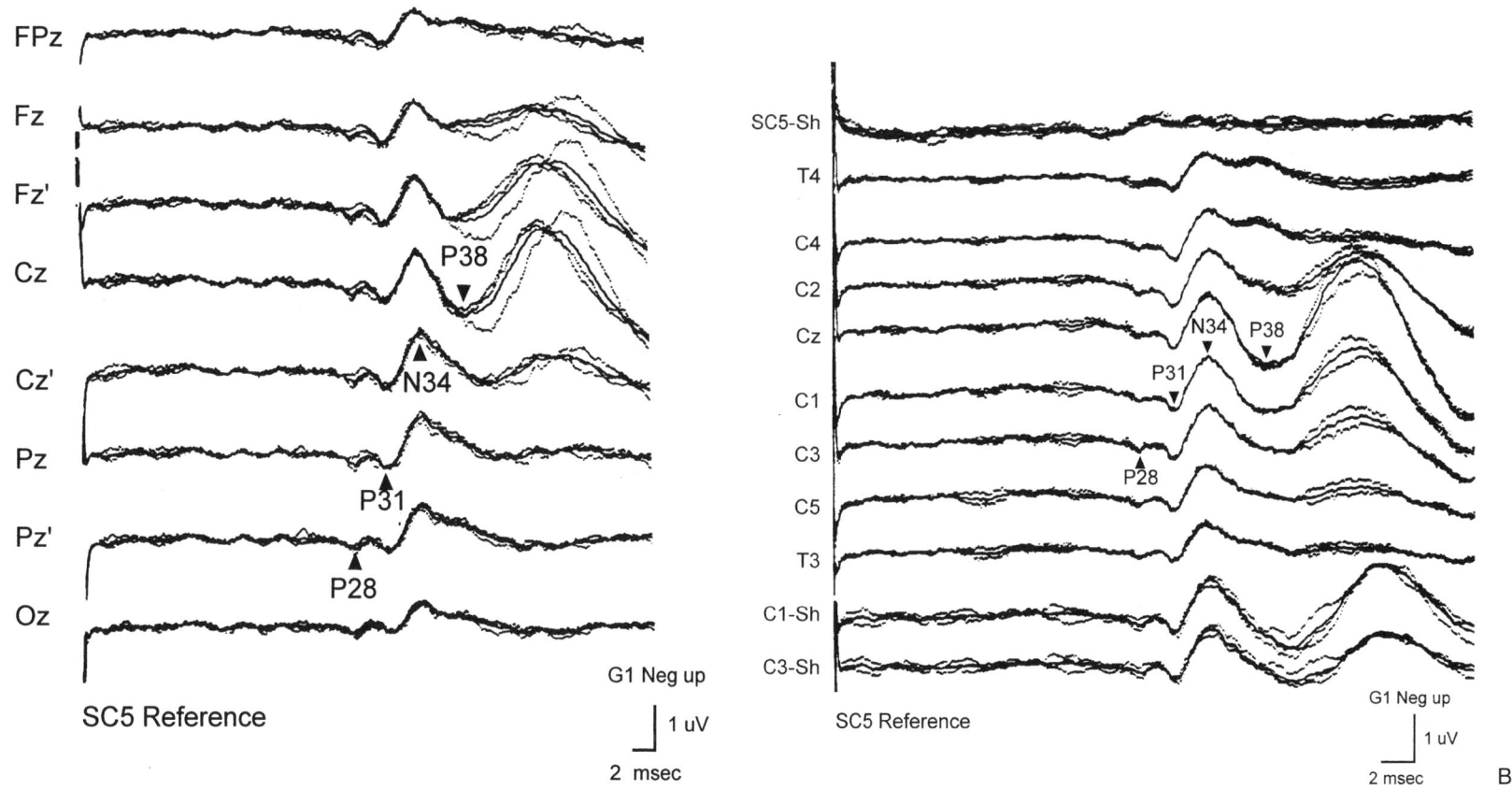

FIG. 29.29. A: Left PTN SSEP recorded in the coronal plane through Cz, with electrodes in channels 2–9 referred to an electrode on the spinous process of the fifth cervical vertebra (SC5). Responses are nearly identical if a contralateral shoulder reference (sh) is used for comparison (*bottom two tracings*). There is no detectable response in the SC5-sh derivation confirming the relative inactivity of SC5. **B:** Left PTN SSEP recorded in the midsagittal plane using a SC5 reference. Note that Fpz is relatively inactive for events occurring after the N$\overline{34}$ potential.

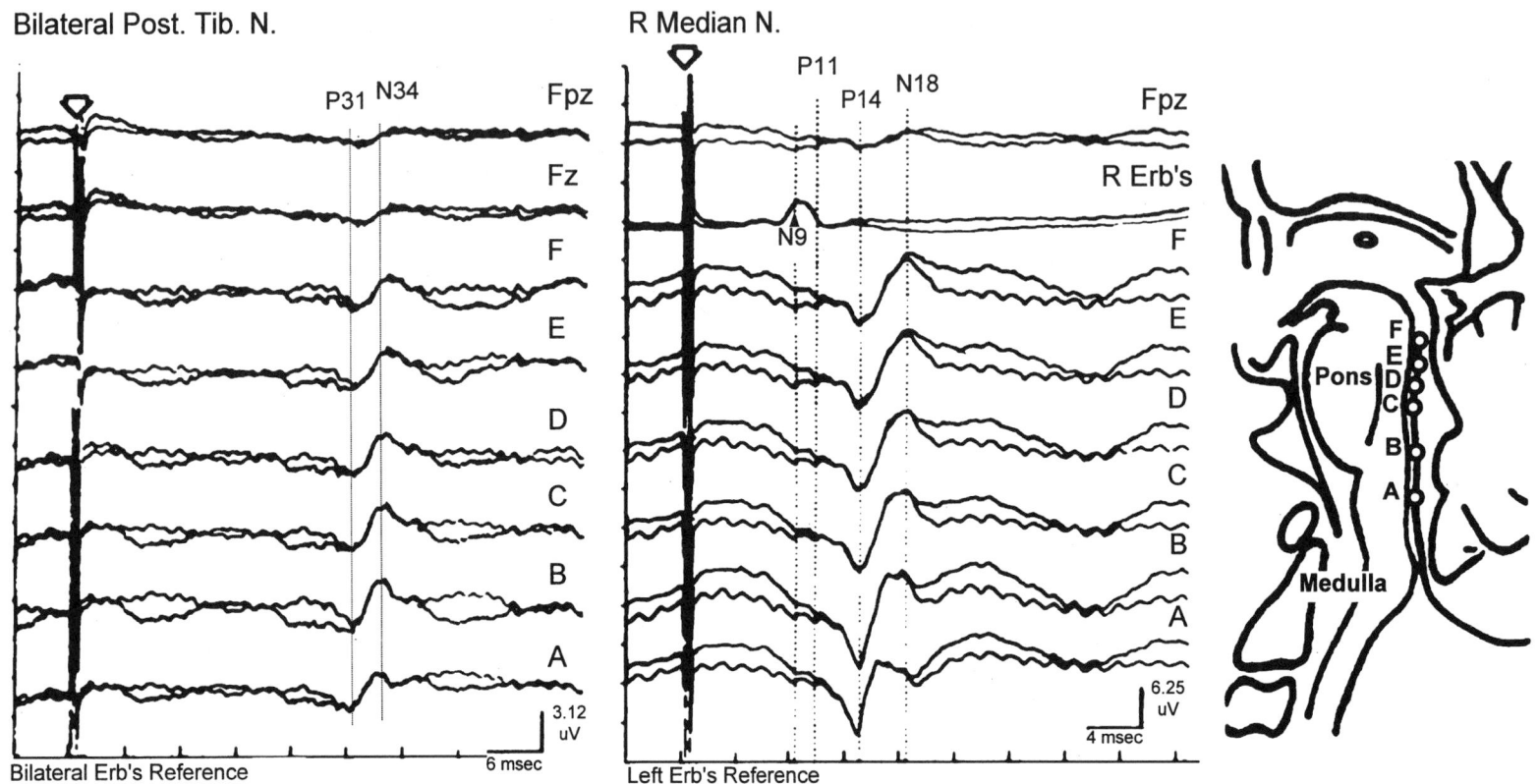

FIG. 29.30. PTN and median nerve SSEPs recorded referentially from both scalp and intracranial electrodes. Electrode positions are illustrated in the accompanying diagram. The analogy of the P$\overline{31}$ and N34 following PTN stimulation to P$\overline{14}$ and N$\overline{18}$ following median nerve stimulation is clear. (From Urasaki E, Tokimura T, Yasukouchi H, et al. P$\overline{30}$ and N$\overline{33}$ of posterior tibial nerve SSEPs are analogous to P$\overline{14}$ and N$\overline{18}$ of median nerve SSEPs. *Electroencephalogr Clin Neurophysiology* 1993;88:525–529, with permission.)

nerve stimulation in terms of polarity, distribution, and morphology, and N$\overline{34}$ closely resembles N$\overline{18}$. These similarities are illustrated in Figure 29.30, which shows PTN and median nerve SSEPs recorded referentially both from Fpz and from within the fourth ventricle. Electrodes along the dorsal surface of the medulla and pons record stationary positivities that coincide with scalp-recorded P$\overline{14}$ and P$\overline{31}$, and electrodes over the mid- and upper pons record stationary negativities that correspond to N$\overline{18}$ and

N$\overline{14}$ (150). Accordingly, P$\overline{31}$ most likely is generated in the medial lemniscus, and N$\overline{34}$ probably arises from multiple brainstem nuclear generators (29,104,150).

The effects of clinical lesions on the subcortical components of both PTN and median nerve SSEPs also support this relationship. For example, Figure 29.31 illustrates absent upper and lower extremity far-field SSEPs that returned following removal of a cervical chondrosarcoma (143).

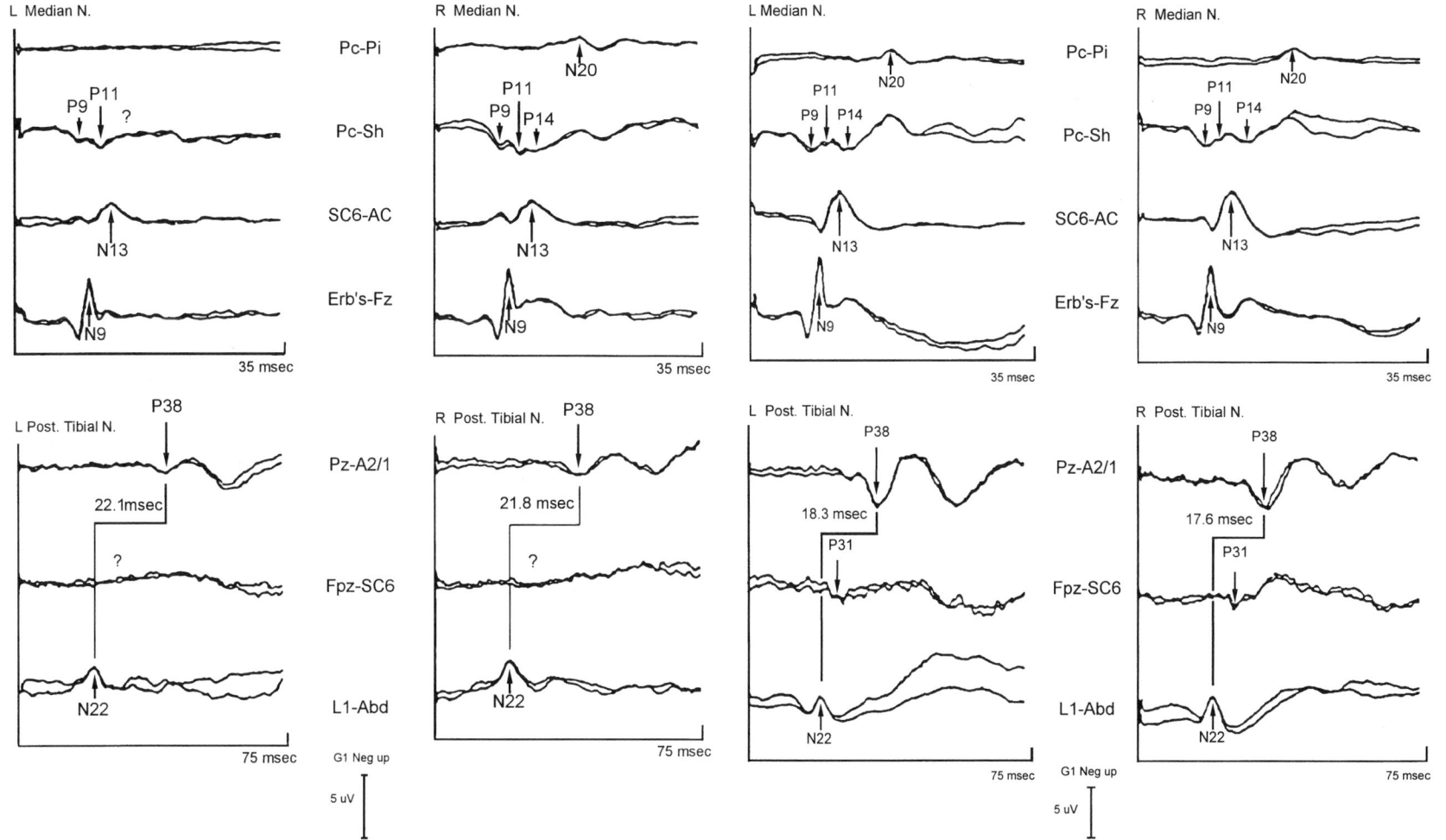

FIG. 29.31. Pre- and postoperative SSEPs in a patient with a C2-C4 chondrosarcoma. **A:** Preoperative median nerve SSEPs demonstrate loss of P14 and subsequent waves in response to left-sided stimulation and attenuation of P14 in response to right-sided stimulation. PTN SSEPs show delay of the P38 potential and loss of subcortical P31 and N38 signal bilaterally. **B:** Seven months postoperatively, both median nerve and PTN SSEPs are normal. Note that a bipolar SC6–anterior cervical electrode derivation is used to record the stationary cervical N13 potential, and similarly an L1-abdominal electrode derivation is used to record N22. (From Tinazzi M, Zanette G, Bonato C, et al. Neural generators of tibial nerve P30 somatosensory evoked potential studied in patients with a focal lesion of the cervicomedullary junction. *Muscle Nerve* 1996;19:1538–1548, with permission.)

The P$\overline{38}$ Potential

At Cz and adjacent scalp areas ipsilateral to the stimulus, the N$\overline{34}$ deflection terminates with the onset of a large positive wave, P$\overline{38}$ (see Fig. 29.29). Unlike earlier far-field subcortical components, P$\overline{38}$ has a restricted field involving mainly the central parasagittal region. Because Fpz is virtually inactive with respect to potentials occurring after 34 milliseconds, it is a useful reference electrode for selectively recording P$\overline{38}$ and other localized scalp activity. Figure 29.32A shows the nearly complete in-phase cancellation of the widespread early potentials in scalp Fpz recordings, with preservation of localized activity near Cz.

P$\overline{38}$ is the first localized wave in the scalp-recorded PTN SSEP. It is asymmetrically distributed about Cz with consistently greater involvement of areas ipsilateral to the stimulated PTN. P$\overline{38}$ topography is somewhat variable from subject to subject, and the maximal positivity can occur either at Cz or in the lateral parasagittal region ipsilateral to the stimulated leg (compare Fig. 29.32A with Fig. 29.32B). In the midsagittal plane, P$\overline{38}$ is of greatest voltage just posterior to Cz. In most subjects, an approximately simultaneous signal, N$\overline{38}$, can be recorded over the contralateral frontocentral scalp (144). N$\overline{38}$ amplitude is usually lower than that of P$\overline{38}$, although in some subjects the two components are of nearly equal voltage (22,67,124,144).

The apparently "paradoxical" localization of P$\overline{38}$ to scalp areas ipsilateral to the stimulated leg is best explained by considering the location of the primary sensory areas for the leg and foot on the mesial aspect of the postcentral gyrus within the interhemispheric fissure. PTN stimulation

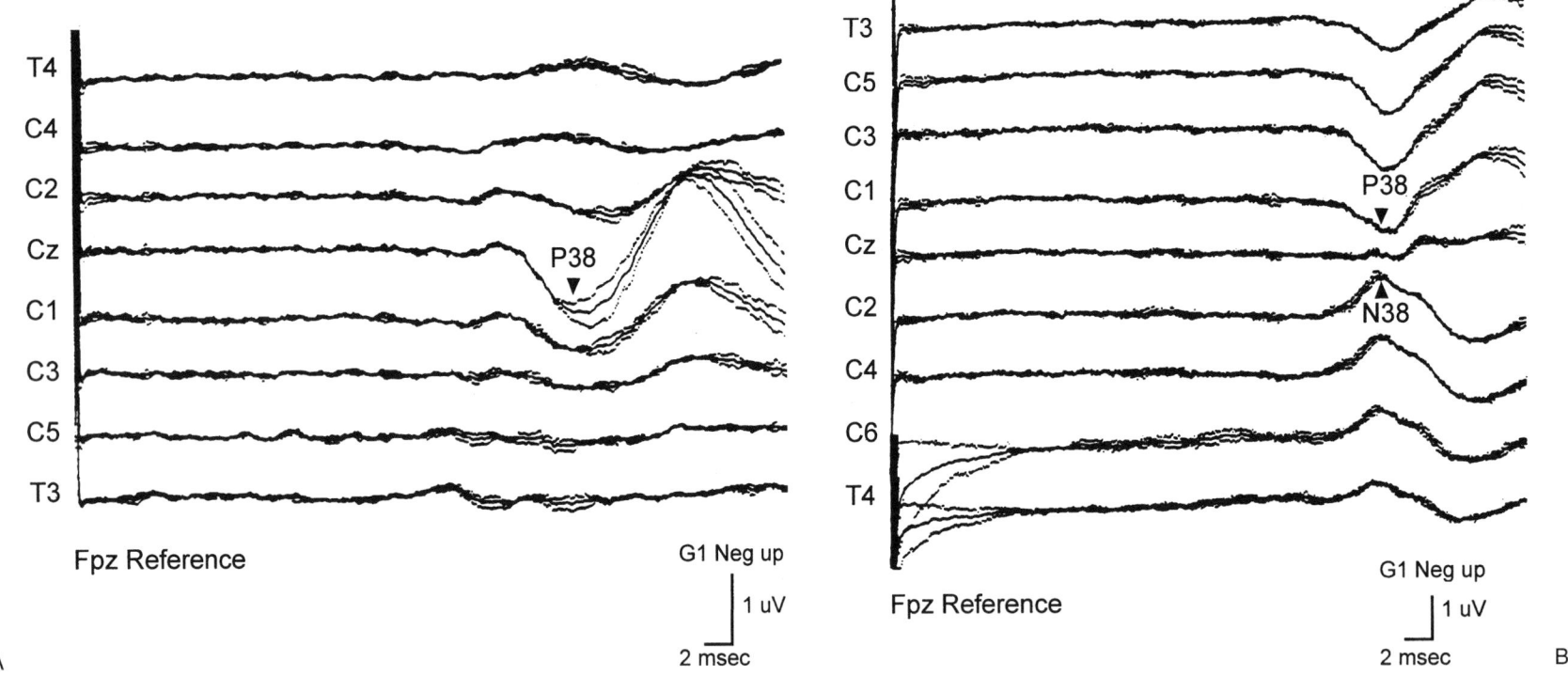

FIG. 29.32. Left PTN SSEPs recorded in two different subjects (**A** and **B**), illustrating the wide range of normal variability in scalp topography of the responses.

results in depolarization of layer IV pyramidal cells of the cortical receiving area, with a corresponding passive source located at the cortical surface (52). The cortical surface positivity projects ipsilateral to the simulated side, and the negative end of this "dipole" projects contralaterally (22,89,124). Intraoperative cortical surface recordings have supported this explanation by demonstrating a localized positivity on the contralateral mesial cortical surface coincident with the contralateral N$\overline{38}$ and the ipsilateral P$\overline{38}$ scalp-recorded signals (89).

Although this model for producing P$\overline{38}$ based on a single dipole located within sensory cortex is appealing, it is an oversimplification. In many normal subjects, the P$\overline{38}$ peak occurs following, rather than simultaneous with, the peak of N38. Furthermore, P$\overline{38}$ is selectively sensitive to increases in stimulus rate and active and passive foot movement during stimulation (144,145). These observations are inconsistent with the single cortical generator model, and it is likely that there are contributions from multiple sources that modify the distribution and latency of the scalp-recorded response (67,89,103). As with the median nerve N$\overline{20}$, the P$\overline{38}$/N$\overline{38}$ complex probably reflects nearly simultaneous activation of several regions within the primary sensory receiving areas for the lower extremity.

Intersubject differences in P$\overline{38}$/N$\overline{38}$ scalp topography probably reflect known anatomical variability in location of primary sensory cortex subserving the lower extremity (114). Location of the leg area near the superior edge of the interhemispheric fissure would cause vertical orientation of P$\overline{38}$'s cortical generator and result in scalp positivity that is maximal at or close to the midline. In contrast, location of the foot area deep within the interhemispheric fissure would cause the cortical generator to have a more horizontal orientation, with the P$\overline{38}$ potential projecting to lateral parasagittal scalp leads (22,89,124). Consistent with this view and reflecting representation of the proximal leg close to the upper edge of the interhemispheric fissure or over the lateral convexity, Yamada et al. have shown that stimulation of the lateral femoral cutaneous nerve of the thigh produces a positivity with greater interindividual variability than the response to PTN, but generally lateralized to the hemisphere *contralateral* to stimulation (165).

Latencies of P$\overline{38}$ and N$\overline{38}$ are affected by alterations in a subject's level of arousal. In normal adults, stage 2 sleep can prolong P$\overline{38}$ latency by more than 2 milliseconds and can prolong N38 latency by over 4 milliseconds (Fig. 29.33) (131). We speculate that P$\overline{38}$ and N$\overline{38}$, like N$\overline{20}$, are composite waveforms reflecting activity from multiple cortical generators, and that, during sleep, downward modulation of selective components results in the observed latency shifts.

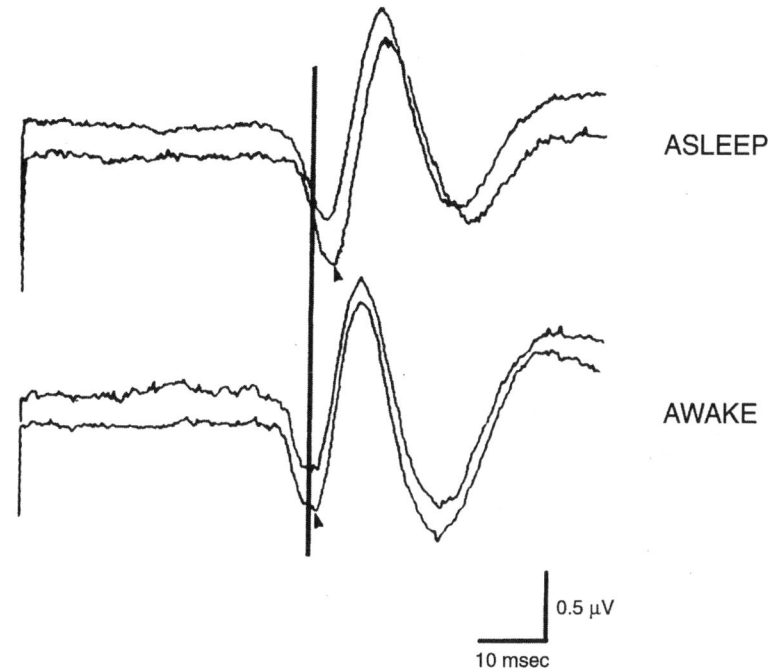

FIG. 29.33. PTN SSEP recorded from Cz-Fpz in a subject asleep (*upper tracing*) and immediately following arousal (*lower tracing*).

MATURATIONAL DEVELOPMENT OF SSEPS

There is less information available about SSEPs in children than in adults. Much of the available literature consists of studies performed using only limited scalp-to-scalp and neck-to-scalp bipolar derivations that, for reasons discussed in previous sections, are not adequate for detailed analysis of recorded potentials. Nonetheless, median nerve and PTN SSEPs may be recorded from earliest infancy. They are similar to responses obtained from adults in many ways, although important differences exist that largely reflect the degree of nervous system maturation.

Term neonates reliably demonstrate subcortical components following median nerve stimulation. The N$\overline{20}$ potential (recorded from parietal scalp referred to a midfrontal electrode) is almost always present by 2 months of age, although some authors have observed it to be absent in as many as one-third of newborns (84,96,158).

Maturation of the median nerve SSEP is nonlinear. Central conduction time decreases dramatically prior to 40 weeks' postconceptional age (9) (Fig. 29.34), continues to fall rapidly during the first year, and declines more slowly thereafter, reaching adult values by 6–8 years of age (Fig. 29.35) (27,59,82,83,141). In children, as in adults, the N20 response is partially dependent on level of arousal (31,84,96), and the effect is most pronounced in infants and younger children. This state dependence may contribute to the apparent absence of N20 in many normal term babies.

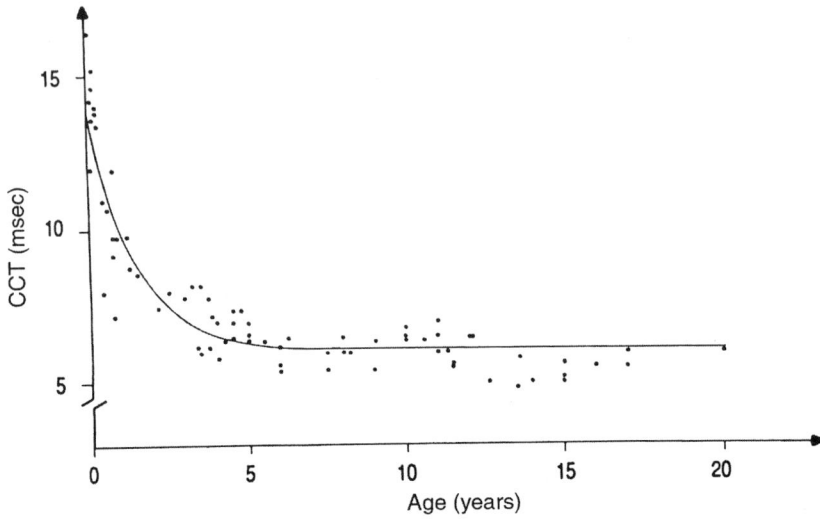

FIG. 29.35. Central conduction time (CTT) as a function of age. In this study, CTT was defined as the interpeak latency difference between N20 (recorded from C3 or C4 to Fz) and N14 (recorded from SC2 to Fz). (From Lauffer H, Wenzel D. Maturation of central somatosensory conduction time in infancy and childhood. *Neuropadiatrie* 1986;71:72–74, with permission.)

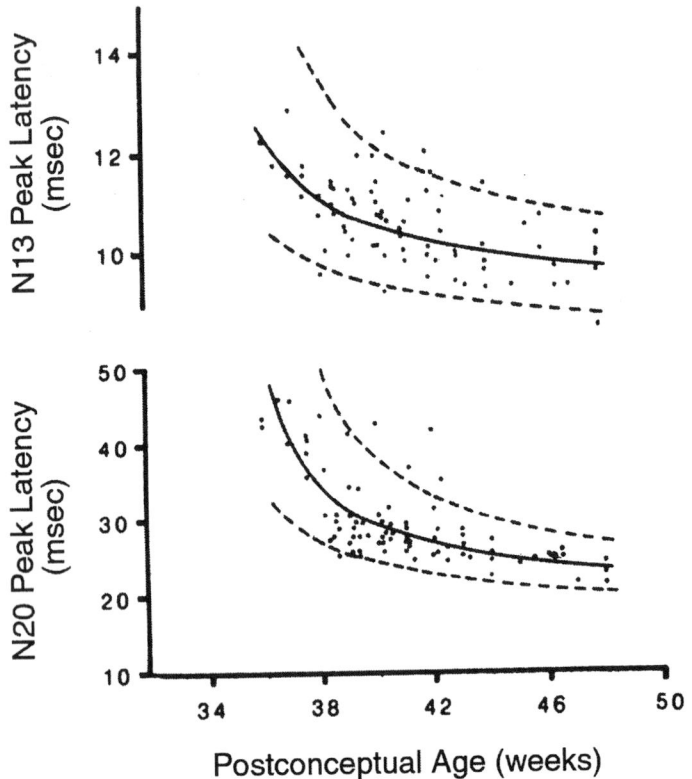

FIG. 29.34. Maturation of the median SSEP in the neonate. Between 36 and 48 weeks' postconceptional age, the N20 latency decreases dramatically compared with a more modest decrease in the N13 latency, producing a dramatic decrease in central conduction time. The N13 latency was measured using a bipolar SC2-Fpz derivation. (From Bongers-Schokking JJ, Colon EJ, Hoogland RA, et al. Somatosensory evoked potentials in term and preterm infants in relation to postconceptional age and birth weight. *Neuropediatrics* 1989;21:32–36, with permission.)

Spinal and subcortical components are readily recorded following PTN stimulation in infants and young children (18,51,59). Spinal conduction velocity increases from birth until about 5–7 years of age, when it reaches adult values (18,51,59). The P38 cortical response is reliably present in awake infants older than 1 year of age (18,51,59). Like N20, the P38 potential appears to be much more susceptible to the effects of level of arousal in infants and children. Indeed, by recording selectively during active sleep, Pike et al. were able to obtain reproducible cortical responses to PTN stimulation in each of 67 premature infants studied, ranging from 27 to 37 weeks' postconceptional age (mean 31 weeks) (116).

RECORDING TECHNIQUES AND INTERPRETIVE CONSIDERATIONS

Stimulation

Peripheral nerves are usually stimulated transcutaneously using electrodes placed on the skin over the selected nerve. Subdermal needle electrodes also may be used, however. The cathode electrode should be placed 2–3 cm proximal to the anode to avoid anodal block. Either constant-voltage or constant-current stimulators can be used. Typical stimulus parameters include a pulse width of 100–300 microseconds, a stimulation rate of 3–5 per second (79,117,132), and a stimulus intensity adequate to produce a consistent, but comfortable muscle twitch. Lesser et al. (88) found that median nerve stimulation at the motor threshold produced SSEPs of submaximal amplitude, and that optimal responses required a stimulus intensity of motor plus sensory threshold. Tsuji et al. (149) recommended an intensity level three times the sensory threshold for PTN SSEPs.

Amplifier and Averager Settings

Most laboratories use a passband of approximately 30–3,000 Hz (–6 dB per octave), which is consistent with American Electroencephalographic Society guidelines (4). Although a wider passband—extending down to 1 Hz, for example—may be advantageous in recording long-duration signals (104), the additional low-frequency noise requires averaging a larger number of responses. Use of a 1- or 2-Hz high-pass filter setting has been reported to facilitate the recording of cortical SSEPs in young infants (9,116). More restrictive passbands are sometimes useful for examining selected SSEP components (36,94,162). When recording with restricted passbands, linear phase-shift digital filtering should be used to avoid distortions produced by analog filters (56).

Recording Montage

A minimum of four channels is necessary to record either median nerve or PTN SSEPs. For median nerve SSEPs, a minimal montage is as follows:

Channel 1: Erb's point–noncephalic (e.g., contralateral elbow or shoulder)
Channel 2: SC5-noncephalic
Channel 3: CPi-noncephalic
Channel 4: CPc-CPi

Channel 1 registers the afferent volley passing Erb's point. Channel 2 records activity in the cervical cord, principally CERV $N\overline{13}$. Channel 3 displays subcortical activity as FFPs, including $P\overline{14}$ and $N\overline{18}$. Channel 4 selectively records $N\overline{20}$.

If additional channels are available, other bipolar scalp derivations are useful (e.g., Pc-Pi) because of normal variation in the location of the maximal $N\overline{20}$ response (86). In cases of possible cervical spinal lesions, it is desirable to utilize an expanded montage including a ring about the neck (as in Figs. 29.8 and 29.15) to delineate cervical components optimally. Bipolar derivations using posterior and anterior cervical electrodes, or lumbar and abdominal electrodes, can be used to enhance cervical $N\overline{13}/P\overline{13}$ and lumbar $N\overline{22}/P\overline{22}$ potentials (see Fig. 29.31).

For PTN SSEPs, a minimal montage is as follows[2]:

Channel 1: T12–iliac crest
Channel 2: Fpz-SC5
Channel 3: CPi-Fpz
Channel 4: CPz-Fpz

Channel 1 records the stationary lumbar potential, and a relatively inactive distant reference should be used. Bipolar recordings using closely spaced lumbar electrodes are ill advised because of in-phase cancellation of the stationary lumbar response. Channel 2 records subcortical far-field activity ($P\overline{31}$ and $N\overline{34}$). SC5 is a reasonably inactive reference site and, in our experience, is usually subject to less artifactual contamination than shoulder or elbow placements. Channels 3 and 4 each record the $P\overline{38}$ cortical responses selectively by causing in-phase cancellation of widely distributed far-field activity. Reliable detection of $P\overline{38}$ requires use of at least two channels because of the normal interindividual variability in $P\overline{38}$ scalp topography (see Fig. 29.32).

Availability of additional channels permits recording of the afferent volley at the level of the popliteal fossa and the $N\overline{38}$ cortical response (CPi-Fpz). In additional, the topography of the lumbar stationary potential can be defined; this is useful in cases of spinal dysraphism.

Criteria of Abnormality

Clinical interpretation of SSEP recordings is based largely on identifying abnormal latency or absence of waveforms that are consistently present in normal individuals. Each laboratory should study at least 20 neurologically normal subjects who have no family history of neurological disease and should ensure that measurements in this control group are comparable to published values. Patient conduction times that are beyond 2.5 or 3 standard deviations from the mean for this control group are regarded as abnormal.

---

[2]The letters *i* and *c* denote, respectively, locations ipsilateral and contralateral to the stimulated limb. The designated CP locations are midway between standard central and parietal international 10-20 electrode placement locations. Similarly, CPz refers to scalp locations midway between Cz and Pz.

Statistical considerations and limitations of this approach are discussed in the American Electroencephalographic Society guidelines (4).

Interpeak latency measurements are used to minimize the effects of (a) peripheral conduction times and (b) differences in arm and leg lengths, and to evaluate segments of central sensory pathways separately. For median nerve SSEPs, the Erb's point–to-$\overline{P14}$ and the $\overline{P14}$-to-$\overline{N20}$ interwave latencies provide measures of conduction between the brachial plexus and lower brainstem, and between lower brainstem and primary sensory cortex. For PTN SSEPs, similar information is provided by calculating the $\overline{N22}$-to-$\overline{P31}$ and $\overline{P31}$-to-$\overline{P38}$ latencies. Because amplitude of SSEP waveforms shows considerable normal variability, amplitude criteria alone generally are not used to interpret a response as abnormal. During intraoperative monitoring, however, when an amplitude baseline is established for each patient, a significant decrease in SSEP waveform amplitude is often the principal indicator of injury.

The $\overline{P14}$-to-$\overline{N20}$ and $\overline{P31}$-to-$\overline{P38}$ interpeak latencies are often regarded as measures of "central conduction time" (60) between the lower brainstem and sensory cortex. Although it is clinically useful, one must remember that this concept is an approximation. In all likelihood, each of these waveforms has more than a single, anatomically discrete generator (36,42,162). The latencies of peak amplitudes, therefore, do not correspond to occurrence of unitary physiological events, but rather to the maxima or minima of summated signals from several simultaneously active neural generators. For example, the model depicted in Figure 29.20 implies that, whereas the rising phase of $\overline{N20}$ is generated by depolarization of area 3b, the peak latency of $\overline{N20}$ is influenced by onset of subsequent positivity arising from activation of adjacent cortical areas. Although technically demanding, more accurate measures of central conduction time may be obtained using inter-onset rather than interpeak latency differences (111).

It has been generally assumed that short-latency evoked potentials are stable in a given individual, reproducible between testing sessions, and independent of effects of state or level of arousal (42,131,162). As already indicated, the peak latencies of $\overline{N20}$ and $\overline{P38}$ do, in fact, vary depending on the subject's level of arousal (42,131,162). This state effect is especially prominent for the $\overline{P38}$ potential, whose latency may change by 2 milliseconds or more between the fully alert state and stage 2 sleep. Thus normative data for clinical testing should control for state. In the absence of such data, clinical interpretation of minor latency "abnormalities" should be appropriately cautious.

An evoked potential signal should only be reported as abnormal or absent if the technical quality of the recording is sufficient to permit that signal to have been adequately recorded. In some normal unsedated subjects, cortical SSEPs, recorded using scalp-to-scalp derivations, may be reliably recorded, whereas subcortical signals, recorded using noncephalic reference derivations, may be obscured by movement and muscle-related noise. For that reason, we favor the use of sedation for routine clinical SSEP testing.

STIMULATION OF OTHER PERIPHERAL NERVES

We have focused on SSEPs elicited by median nerve and PTN stimulation, because these nerves are used most commonly in clinical situations. However, stimulation of virtually any peripheral mixed or sensory nerve, including radial, ulnar, peroneal, sural, lateral femoral cutaneous, trigeminal, and pudendal nerves, gives rise to an SSEP (3,58,77,123,128,129,137, 156,165,166). To assess dorsal root integrity in patients with lumbar radiculopathy, Seyal et al. (129) compared stationary lumbar potentials evoked by stimulating saphenous, superficial peroneal, and sural nerves. Specific characteristics of the SSEP will vary, of course, depending on which nerve is stimulated. Allison et al. used SSEPs to stimulate median, posterior tibial, pudendal, and trigeminal nerves to map primary sensory and supplementary motor and sensory regions on the mesial cortex in patients undergoing evaluation for surgical treatment of epilepsy (3). Responses are influenced not only by the somatotropic representation of the structure(s) innervated by a nerve but also by the sensory elements within the nerve itself (e.g., relative amount of muscle and cutaneous afferents) (14,80,113).

REFERENCES

1. Allison T, Goff WR, Williamson PD, et al. On the neural origin of early components of the human somatosensory evoked potential. In: Desmedt JE, ed. *Clinical uses of cerebral, brainstem and spinal somatosensory evoked potentials*. Basel: Karger, 1980:51–68.
2. Allison T, Hume AL. A comparative analysis of short-latency somatosensory evoked potentials in man, monkey, cat and rat. *Exp Neurol* 1981;72:592–611.
3. Allison T, McCarthy G, Luby M, et al. Localization of functional regions of human mesial cortex by somatosensory evoked potential recording and by cortical stimulation. *Electroencephalogr Clin Neurophysiol* 1996;100:126–140.
4. American Electroencephalographic Society. Guideline nine: guidelines on evoked potentials. *J Clin Neurophysiol* 1994;11:40–73.
5. Anziska BJ, Cracco RQ. Short latency SEPs to median nerve stimulation: comparison of recording methods and origins of components. *Electroencephalogr Clin Neurophysiol* 1981; 52:531–539.
6. Arezzo J, Legatt AD, Vaughn HG. Topography and intracranial sources of somatosensory evoked potentials in the monkey. I. Early components. *Electroencephalogr Clin Neurophysiol* 1979;46:155–172.
7. Austin GM, McCouch GP. Presynaptic components of intermedullary cord potential. *J Neurophysiol* 1955;18:441–451.

8. Beall JE, Applebaum AE, Foreman RD, et al. Spinal cord potentials evoked by cutaneous afferents in the monkey. *J Neurophysiol* 1977;40:199–211.

9. Bongers-Schokking JJ, Colon EJ, Hoogland RA, et al. Somatosensory evoked potentials in term and preterm infants in relation to postconceptional age and birth weight. *Neuropediatrics* 1989;21:32–36.

10. Brazier MAB. A study of the electrical field at the surface of the head. *Electroencephalogr Clin Neurophysiol Suppl* 1949;2:38–52.

11. Brazier MAB. *Electrical activity of the nervous system*. Baltimore: Williams & Wilkins, 1977.

12. Brin MF, Pedley TA, Lovelace RE, et al. Electrophysiological features of abetalipoproteinemia: functional consequences of vitamin E deficiency. *Neurology* 1986;36:669–673.

13. Broughton RJ. Discussion. In: Donchin E, Lindsley DB, eds. *Average evoked potentials*. Washington, DC: National Aeronautics and Space Administration, 1969:79–84.

14. Burke D, Gandevia SC. Muscle afferent contribution to the cerebral potentials of human subjects. In: Cracco RQ, Bodis-Wollner I, eds. *Evoked potentials*. New York: Alan R. Liss, 1986:262–268.

15. Chiappa KH. Pattern shift visual, brainstem auditory and short latency somatosensory evoked potentials in multiple sclerosis. *Neurology* 1980;30:110–123.

16. Chiappa KH, Choi SK, Young RR. Short-latency somatosensory evoked potentials following median nerve stimulation in patients with neurological lesions. In: Desmedt JE, ed. *Clinical uses of cerebral, brainstem and spinal somatosensory evoked potentials*. Basel: Karger, 1980:254–281.

17. Coombs JS, Curtis DR, Laudren S. Spinal cord potentials generated by impulses in muscle and cutaneous afferent fibers. *J Neurophysiol* 1956;19:452–457.

18. Cracco JB, Cracco R, Stolove R. Spinal evoked potentials in man: a maturational study. *Electroencephalogr Clin Neurophysiol* 1979;46:48–84.

19. Cracco RQ. Scalp-recorded potentials evoked by median nerve stimulation: subcortical potentials, traveling waves, and somatomotor potentials. In: Desmedt JE, ed. *Clinical uses of cerebral, brainstem and spinal somatosensory evoked potentials*. Basel: Karger, 1980:1–14.

20. Cracco RQ, Cracco JB. Somatosensory evoked potentials in man: far-field potentials. *Electroencephalogr Clin Neurophysiol* 1976;41:460–466.

21. Cracco RQ, Evans B. Spinal evoked potentials in the cat: effects of asphyxia, strychnine, cord section and compression. *Electroencephalogr Clin Neurophysiol* 1978;44:187–201.

22. Cruse R, Klem G, Lesser RP, et al. Paradoxical lateralization of the cortical potentials evoked by stimulus of the posterior tibial nerve. *Arch Neurol* 1982;39:222–225.

23. Cusick JF, Myklebust JB, Larson SJ, et al. Spinal cord evaluation by cortical evoked responses. *Arch Neurol* 1979;36:140–143.

24. Dawson GD. Cerebral responses to electrical stimulation of peripheral nerve in man. *J Neurol Neurosurg Psychiatry* 1947;10:137–140.

25. Deiber MP, Giard MH, Mauguière F. Separate generators with distinct orientations for N20 and P22 somatosensory evoked potentials to finger stimulation. *Electroencephalogr Clin Neurophysiol* 1986;65:321–324.

26. DeMeirleir LJ, Taylor MJ, Logan WJ. Multimodal evoked potential studies in leukodystrophies of children. *Can J Neurol Sci* 1988;15:26–31.

27. Desmedt JE, Brunko E, Debecker J. Maturation of the somatosensory evoked potentials in normal infants and children, with special reference to the early N1 component. *Electroencephalogr Clin Neurophysiol* 1976;40:43–58.

28. Desmedt JE, Cheron G. Central somatosensory conduction in man: neural generators and interpeak latencies of the far-field components recorded from neck and right or left scalp and earlobes. *Electroencephalogr Clin Neurophysiol* 1980;50:382–403.

29. Desmedt JE, Cheron G. Non-cephalic reference recording of early somatosensory potentials to finger stimulation in adult or aging normal man: differentiation of widespread N18 and contralateral N20 from prerolandic P22 and N30 components. *Electroencephalogr Clin Neurophysiol* 1981;52:553–570.

30. Desmedt JE, Cheron G. Prevertebral (esophageal) recording of subcortical somatosensory evoked potentials in man: the spinal P13 component and the dual nature of the spinal generators. *Electroencephalogr Clin Neurophysiol* 1981;52:257–275.

31. Desmedt JE, Manil J. Somatosensory evoked potentials of the normal human neonate in REM sleep, in slow wave sleep and in waking. *Electroencephalogr Clin Neurophysiol* 1970;29:113–126.

32. Desmedt JE, Nguyen TH, Bourguet M. Bit-mapped color imaging of human evoked potentials with reference to the N20, P22, P27 and N30 somatosensory responses. *Electroencephalogr Clin Neurophysiol* 1987;68:1–19.

33. Desmedt JE, Nguyen TH, Carmeliet J. Unexpected latency shift of the stationary P9 somatosensory evoked potential far field with changes in shoulder position. *Electroencephalogr Clin Neurophysiol* 1983;56:628–634.

34. Dumitru D, King JC. Far-field potentials produced by quadrupole generators in cylindrical volume conductors. *Electroencephalogr Clin Neurophysiol* 1993;88:421–431.

35. Eccles JC. Interpretation of action potentials evoked in the cerebral cortex. *Electroencephalogr Clin Neurophysiol* 1951;3:449–464.

36. Eisen A, Roberts K, Low M, et al. Questions regarding the sequential neural generator theory of the somatosensory evoked potential raised by digital filtering. *Electroencephalogr Clin Neurophysiol* 1984;59:388–395.

37. Emerson RG. The anatomic and physiologic bases of posterior tibial nerve somatosensory evoked potentials. *Neurol Clin North Am* 1988;6:735–749.

38. Emerson RG, Pedley TA. Generator sources of median somatosensory evoked potentials. *J Clin Neurophysiol* 1984;2:203–218.

39. Emerson RG, Pedley TA. Effect of cervical spinal cord lesions on early components of the median nerve somatosensory evoked potential. *Neurology* 1986;36:20–26.

40. Emerson RG, Seyal M, Pedley TA. Somatosensory evoked potentials following median nerve stimulation. I. The cervical components. *Brain* 1984;107:169–182.

41. Emerson RG, Sgro JA, Pedley TA. Identification of a state-dependent Pre-N20 "near-field" positivity in the human median nerve SEP. *Neurology* 1987;37[Suppl 1]:359.

42. Emerson RG, Sgro JA, Pedley TA, et al. State-dependent changes in the N20 component of the median nerve somatosensory evoked potential. *Neurology* 1988;38:64–68.

43. Fernandez de Molinda A, Gray JAB. Activity in the dorsal spinal grey matter after stimulation of cutaneous nerves. *J Physiol (Lond)* 1957;137:126–140.

44. Fierro B, Meli F, Brighina F, et al. Somatosensory and visual evoked potentials in young insulin-dependent diabetic patients. *Electromyogr Clin Neurophysiol* 1996;36:481–486.

45. Gandevia SC, Burke D, McKeon B. The projection of muscle afferents from the hand to cerebral cortex. *Brain* 1984;107:1–13.

46. Gandolfo G, Arnaud C, Gottesmann C. Transmission processes in the ventrobasal complex of rat during the sleep-waking cycle. *Brain Res Bull* 1980;5:553–562.

47. Gandolfo G, Gottesmann C. Transmission in the ventrobasal complex of thalamus during rapid sleep and wakefullness in the homolaterally neodecorticated rat. *Acta Neurobiol Exp* 1982;42:443–455.

48. Garg BP, Markand ON, DeMyer WE, et al. Evoked response studies in patients with adrenoleukodystrophy and heterozygous relatives. *Arch Neurol* 1983;40:356–359.

49. Georgesco M, Salerno A, Camu W. Somatosensory evoked potentials elicited by stimulation of lower-limb nerves in amyotrophic lateral sclerosis. *Electroencephalogr Clin Neurophysiol* 1997;104:333–342.

50. Giblin D. Somatosensory evoked potentials in healthy subjects and in patients with lesions of the nervous system. *Ann N Y Acad Sci* 1964;112:93–142.

51. Gilmore RL, Bass NH, Wright EA. Developmental assessment of spinal cord and cortical evoked potentials after tibial nerve stimulation: effects of age and stature on normative data during development. *Electroencephalogr Clin Neurophysiol* 1985;62:241–251.

52. Goff WR, Allison T, Vaughn HG. Functional neuroanatomy of event-related potentials. In:

Callaway E, Tueting P, Koslow SH, eds. *Event related potentials in man*. New York: Academic Press, 1978:1–79.

53. Goldie WD, Chiappa KH, Young RR, et al. Brainstem auditory and short latency somatosensory evoked responses in brain death. *Neurology* 1981;31:248–256.

54. Goldie WD, Chiappa KH, Young RR, et al. Brainstem auditory and short latency somatosensory evoked potentials in brain death. *Neurology* 1981;31:248–256.

55. Gott PS, Karnaze DS. Short-latency somatosensory evoked potentials in myotonic dystrophy: evidence for a conduction disturbance. *Electroencephalogr Clin Neurophysiol* 1985;62:455–458.

56. Green JB, Nelson AV, Michael D. Digital zero-phase shift filtering of short-latency somatosensory evoked potentials. *Electroencephalogr Clin Neurophysiol* 1986;63:384–388.

57. Hallett M, Chadwick D, Marsden CD. Cortical reflex myoclonus. *Neurology* 1979;29:1107–1125.

58. Hashimoto I. Trigeminal evoked potentials following brief air puff: enhanced signal to noise ratio. *Ann Neurol* 1988;23:332–338.

59. Hashimoto T, Tayama M, Hiura K, et al. Short latency somatosensory evoked potentials in children. *Brain Dev* 1983;5:390–396.

60. Hume AL, Cant BR. Conduction time in central somatosensory pathways in man. *Electroencephalogr Clin Neurophysiol* 1978;45:361–375.

61. Iragui VJ, Kalmijn J, Thal LJ, et al. Neurological dysfunction in asymptomatic HIV-1 infected men: evidence from evoked potentials. *Electroencephalogr Clin Neurophysiol* 1994;92:1–10.

62. Jewett DL, Williston JS. Auditory-evoked far fields averaged from the scalp of humans. *Brain* 1971;94:681–696.

63. Jones EG, Powell TPS. Connexions of the somatic sensory cortex of the rhesus monkey. *Brain* 1970;93:37–56.

64. Jones SJ. Short latency potentials recorded from the neck and scalp in man. *Electroencephalogr Clin Neurophysiol* 1977;43:853–863.

65. Jones SJ, Yu YL, Rudge P, et al. Central and peripheral SEP defects in neurologically symptomatic and asymptomatic subjects with low vitamin B12 levels. *J Neurol Sci* 1987;82:55–65.

66. Kaji R, Sumner AJ. Vector short-latency somatosensory evoked potentials after median nerve stimulation. *Muscle Nerve* 1990;13:1174–1182.

68. Kakigi R, Shibasaki H. Generator mechanisms of giant somatosensory evoked potentials in cortical reflex myoclonus. *Brain* 1987;110:1359–1373.

67. Kakigi R, Shibasaki H. Scalp topography of the short latency somatosensory evoked potential following posterior tibial nerve stimulation in man. *Electroencephalogr Clin Neurophysiol* 1983;56:430–437.

69. Kameyama S, Yamada T, Matsuoka H, et al. Stationary potentials after median nerve stimulation: changes with arm position. *Electroencephalogr Clin Neurophysiol* 1988;71:348–356.

70. Kaplan PW, Rawal K, Erwin CW, et al. Visual and somatosensory evoked potentials in vitamin E deficiency with cystic fibrosis. *Electroencephalogr Clin Neurophysiol* 1988;71:266–272.

71. Kaplan PW, Tusa RJ, Rignani J, et al. Somatosensory evoked potentials in adrenomyelopathy. *Neurology* 1997;48:1662–1667.

72. Kimura J, Ishida T, Suzuki S, et al. Far field recording of the junctional potential generated by median nerve volleys at the wrist. *Neurology*, 1986:36:1451–1457.

73. Kimura J, Kimura A, Ishida T, et al. What determines the latency and amplitude of stationary peaks in far-field recordings. *Ann Neurol* 1986;19:479–486.

74. Kimura J, Kimura A, Machida M, et al. Model for far-field recordings of SEP. In: Cracco RQ, Bodis-Wollner I, eds. *Evoked potentials*. New York: Alan R. Liss, 1986:246–261.

75. Kimura J, Mitsudome A, Beck DO, et al. Field distribution of antidromically activated digital nerve potentials: model for far field recording. *Neurology* 1983;33:1164–1169.

76. Kimura J, Mitsudome A, Yamada T, et al. Stationary peaks from a moving source in far-field recording. *Electroencephalogr Clin Neurophysiol* 1984;58:351–361.

77. Kirkeby HJ, Poulsen EU, Petersen T, et al. Erectile dysfunction in multiple sclerosis. *Neurology* 1988;38:1366–1371.

78. Klee M, Rall W. Computed potentials of cortically arranged populations of neurons. *J Neurophysiol* 1977;40:647–666.

79. Kritchevsky M, Widerhold WC. Short-latency somatosensory evoked potentials. *Arch Neurol* 1978;35:706–711.

80. Kunesch E, Knecht S, Schnitzler A, et al. Somatosensory evoked potentials elicited by intraneural microstimulation of afferent nerve fibers. *J Clin Neurophysiol* 1995;12:476–487.

81. Labar DR, Petty GW, Emerson RG, et al. Abnormal somatosensory evoked potentials in patients with motor deficits due to lacunar strokes. *Electroencephalogr Clin Neurophysiol* 1988;69:91P.

82. Lafreniere L, Laureau E, Vanasse M, et al. Maturation of short latency somatosensory evoked potentials by median nerve stimulation: a cross sectional study in a large group of children. *Electroencephalogr Clin Neurophysiol Suppl* 1990;41:236–242.

83. Lauffer H, Wenzel D. Maturation of central somatosensory conduction time in infancy and childhood. *Neuropadiatrie* 1986;71:72–74.

84. Laureau E, Majnemer A, Rosenblatt B, et al. A longitudinal study of short latency somatosensory evoked responses in healthy newborns and infants. *Electroencephalogr Clin Neurophysiol* 1988;71:100–108.

85. Legatt AD, Arezzo JC, Vaughan HG. Anatomic and physiologic bases of brain stem auditory evoked potentials. In: Gilmore R, ed. *Evoked potentials*. Philadelphia: WB Saunders, 1988:681–704.

86. Legatt AD, Emerson RG, Labar DR, et al. Surface near-field mapping of the median nerve SEP N20 component. *Neurology* 1987;37[Suppl 1]:366.

87. Legatt AD, Emerson RG, Pedley TA. Use of the stationary lumbar potential increases the diagnostic yield of posterior tibial nerve somatosensory evoked potentials. *Electroencephalogr Clin Neurophysiol* 1986;64:72P.

88. Lesser RP, Koehle R, Lueders H. Effect of stimulus intensity of short latency somatosensory evoked potentials. *Electroencephalogr Clin Neurophysiol* 1979;47:377–382.

89. Lesser RP, Luders H, Dinner DS, et al. The source of 'paradoxical lateralization' of cortical evoked potentials to posterior tibial nerve stimulation. *Neurology* 1987;37:82–88.

90. Lorente de No RA. Action potentials of motorneurons of the hypoglossus nucleus. *J Cell Comp Physiol* 1947;29:207–287.

91. Lorente de No RA. A study of nerve physiology. *Stud Rockefeller Inst* 1947;132:384–477.

92. Lueders H, Lesser RP, Hahn J, et al. Cortical somatosensory evoked potentials in response to hand stimulation. *J Neurosurg* 1983;58:885–894.

93. Lueders H, Lesser R, Hahn J, et al. Subcortical sensory evoked potentials to median nerve stimulation. *Brain* 1983;106:341–372.

94. Maccabee PJ, Pickhasov EI, Cracco RQ. Short latency somatosensory evoked potentials to median nerve stimulation: effect of low frequency filter. *Electroencephalogr Clin Neurophysiol* 1983;55:34–44.

95. Maetzu C, Villoslada C, Cruz Martinez A. Somatosensory evoked potentials and central motor pathway conduction after magnetic stimulation of the brain in diabetes. *Electromyogr Clin Neurophysiol* 1995;35:443–448.

96. Majnemer A, Rosenblatt B, Willis D, et al. The effects of gestational age at birth on somatosensory-evoked potentials performed at term. *J Child Neurol* 1990;5:329–335.

97. Markand ON, Garg BP, DeMyer WE, et al. Brain stem auditory, visual and somatosensory evoked potentials in leukodystrophies. *Electroencephalogr Clin Neurophysiol* 1982;54:39–48.

98. Marshall WH, Woolsey CN, Bard P. Observations on cortical somatic sensory mechanisms in cat and monkey. *J Neurophysiol* 1941;4:1–24.

99. Matthews WB, Beauchamp M, Small DG. Cervical somatosensory evoked potentials in man. *Nature* 1947;252:230–232.

100. Mauguière F, Courjon J. The origins of short-latency somatosensory evoked potentials in humans. *Ann Neurol* 1981;9:607–611.

101. Mauguière F, Desmedt JE. Bilateral somatosensory evoked potentials in four patients with long-standing surgical hemispherectomy. *Ann Neurol* 1989;26:724–731.

102. Mauguière F, Desmedt JE. Focal capsular vascular lesions can selectively deafferent the pre-rolandic of the parietal cortex: somatosensory evoked potentials evidence. *Ann Neurol* 1991; 30:71–75.

103. Mauguière F, Desmedt JE, Courjon J. Astereognosis and dissociated loss of frontal or parietal components of somatosensory evoked potentials in hemispheric lesions. *Brain* 1983;106: 271–311.

104. Mauguière F, Desmedt JE, Courjon J. Neural generators of N18 and P14 far-field somatosensory evoked potentials studied in patients with lesions of thalamus or thalamo-cortical radiations. *Electroencephalogr Clin Neurophysiol* 1983;56:283–292.

105. Mauguière F, Ibanez V. The dissociation of early SEP components in lesions of the cervico-medullary junction. *Electroencephalogr Clin Neurophysiol* 1985;56:283–292.

106. McAllister RH, Herns MV, Harrison MJ, et al. Neurological and neuropsychological performance in HIV seropositive men without symptoms. *J Neurol Neurosurg Psychiatry* 1992;55: 143–148.

107. Nagle KJ, Emerson RG, Adams DC, et al. Intraoperative motor and somatosensory evoked potential monitoring: a review of 116 cases. *Neurology* 1996;47:999–1004.

108. Nakanishi T. Action potentials recorded by fluid electrodes. *Electroencephalogr Clin Neurophysiol* 1982;53:343–346.

109. Nakanishi T, Tamaki M, Arasaki K, et al. Origins of the scalp-recorded far field potentials in man and cat. *Electroencephalogr Clin Neurophysiol Suppl* 1982;36:336–348.

110. Nuwer MR, Perlman SL, Packwood JW, et al. Evoked potential abnormalities in the various inherited ataxias. *Ann Neurol* 1983;13:20–27.

111. Ozaki I, Takada H, Shimamura H, et al. Central conduction in somatosensory evoked potentials. *Neurology* 1996;47:1299–1304.

112. Paul RL, Merzenich M, Goodman H. Representation of slowly and randomly adapting cutaneous mechanoreceptors of the hand in Brodmann's areas 3 and 1 of Macaca mulatta. *Brain Res* 1972;36:229–249.

113. Pelosi L, Cracco JB, Cracco RQ, et al. Comparison of scalp distribution of short latency somatosensory evoked potentials (SSEPs) to stimulation of different nerves in the lower extremity. *Electroencephalogr Clin Neurophysiol* 1988;71:422–428.

114. Penfield W, Rasmussen T. *The cerebral cortex of man: a clinical study of localization of function.* New York: Macmillan, 1950.

115. Peterson NN, Schroeder CE, Arezzo JC. Neural generators of early cortical somatosensory evoked potentials in the awake monkey. *Electroencephalogr Clin Neurophysiol* 1995;96: 248–260.

116. Pike A, Marlow N, Dawson C. Posterior tibial somatosensory evoked potentials in very preterm infants. *Early Hum Dev* 1997;47:71–84.

117. Pratt H, Politoske D, Starr A. Mechanically and electrically evoked somatosensory potentials in humans: effects of stimulus presentation rate. *Electroencephalogr Clin Neurophysiol* 1980; 49:240–249.

118. Raroque HG Jr, Batjer H, White C, et al. Lower brain-stem origin of the median nerve N18 potential. *Electroencephalogr Clin Neurophysiol* 1994;90:170–172.

119. Restucci D, Di Lazzaro V, Valeriani M, et al. Scalp, nasopharyngeal and neck recording in healthy subjects and in patients with cervical and cervico-medullary lesions. *Electroencephalogr Clin Neurophysiol* 1995;96:371–384.

120. Restuccia D, Di Lazzaro V, Valeriani M, et al. Brain-stem somatosensory dysfunction in a case of long-standing left hemispherectomy with removal of the left thalamus: a nasopharyngeal and scalp study. *Electroencephalogr Clin Neurophysiol* 1996;100:184–188.

121. Robinson BW, Bryan JS, Rosvold HE. Locating brain structures: extensions to the impedance method. *Arch Neurol* 1965;13:477–486.

122. Rossini PM, Gigli GL, Marciani MG, et al. Non-invasive evaluation of input-output characteristics of sensorimotor cerebral areas in healthy humans. *Electroencephalogr Clin Neurophysiol* 1987;68:88–100.

123. Seyal M, Browne JK. Short latency somatosensory evoked potentials following mechanical taps to the face: scalp recordings with a non-cephalic reference. *Electroencephalogr Clin Neurophysiol* 1989;74:271–276.

124. Seyal M, Emerson RG, Pedley TA. Spinal and early scalp-recorded components of the somatosensory evoked potential following stimulation of the posterior tibial nerve. *Electroencephalogr Clin Neurophysiol* 1983;55:320–330.

125. Seyal M, Gabor AJ. The human posterior tibial somatosensory evoked potential: synapse dependent and synapse independent spinal components. *Electroencephalogr Clin Neurophysiol* 1985;62:323–331.

126. Seyal M, Kraft LW, Gabor AJ. Cervical synapse-dependent somatosensory evoked potentials following posterior tibial nerve stimulation. *Neurology* 1987;37:1417–1421.

127. Seyal M, Ortstadt JL, Kraft LW, et al. Effects of movement on human spinal and subcortical potentials. *Neurology* 1987;37:650–655.

128. Seyal M, Palma GA, Sandhu LS, et al. Spinal somatosensory evoked potentials following segmental sensory stimulation: a direct measure of dorsal root function. *Electroencephalogr Clin Neurophysiol* 1988;69:390–393.

129. Seyal M, Sandhu LS, Mack YP. Spinal segmental somatosensory evoked potentials in lumbosacral radiculopathies. *Neurology* 1989;39:801–805.

130. Sgro JA, Emerson RG, Pedley TA. Real-time reconstruction of evoked potentials using a new two dimensional filter method. *Electroencephalogr Clin Neurophysiol* 1985;62:372–380.

131. Sgro JA, Emerson RG, Pedley TA. State dependent non-stationarity of the P38 cortical response following posterior tibial nerve stimulation. *Electroencephalogr Clin Neurophysiol* 1988;69:77P.

132. Shaw NA. Effects of stimulus rate on the cortical somatosensory evoked potential in cat. *Electroencephalogr Clin Neurophysiol* 1987;27:235–241.

133. Small DG, Beauchamp M, Matthews WB. Subcortical somatosensory evoked potentials in normal man and in patients with central nervous system lesions. In: Desmedt JE, ed. *Clinical uses of cerebral, brainstem and spinal somatosensory evoked potentials.* Basel: Karger, 1980:190–204.

134. Sonoo M, Genba-Shimizu K, Mannen T, et al. Detailed analysis of the latencies of median nerve somatosensory evoked potential components, 2: analysis of subcomponents of P13/14 and N20 potentials. *Electroencephalogr Clin Neurophysiol* 1997;104:296–311.

135. Sonoo M, Hagiwara H, Motoyoshi Y, et al. Preserved widespread N18 and progressive loss of P13/P14 of median nerve SEPs in a patient with unilateral medial medullary syndrome. *Electroencephalogr Clin Neurophysiol* 1996;100:488–492.

136. Sonoo M, Kobayashi M, Genba-Shimizu K, et al. Detailed analysis of the latencies of median nerve somatosensory evoked potential components, 1: selection of the best standard parameters and the establishment of normal values. *Electroencephalogr Clin Neurophysiol* 1996;100: 319–331.

137. Soustiel JF, Chistyakov AV, Hafner H, et al. Intracranial recording from the brain-stem and trigeminal nerve following upper lip stimulation. *Electroencephalogr Clin Neurophysiol* 1996;100:51–54.

138. Steriade M, Iosif G, Apostol V. Responsiveness of thalamic and cortical motor relays during arousal and various stages of sleep. *J Neurophysiol* 1969;32:251–265.

139. Synder BGE, Holliday TA. Responsiveness of thalamic and cortical motor relays during arousal and various stages of sleep. *J Neurophysiol* 1984;32:251–265.

140. Takakura H, Nakano C, Kasagi S, et al. Multimodality evoked potentials in progression of metachromatic leukodystrophy. *Brain Dev* 1985;7:424–430.

141. Taylor MJ, Fagan ER. SEPs to median nerve stimulation: normative data for pediatrics. *Electroencephalogr Clin Neurophysiol* 1988;71:323–330.

142. Thompson DS, Woodward JB, Ringel SP, et al. Evoked potential abnormalities in myotonic dystrophy. *Electroencephalogr Clin Neurophysiol* 1983;56:453–456.

143. Tinazzi M, Zanette G, Bonato C, et al. Neural generators of tibial nerve P30 somatosensory evoked potential studied in patients with a focal lesion of the cervicomedullary junction. *Muscle Nerve* 1996;19:1538–1548.

144. Tinazzi M, Zanette G, Fiaschi A, et al. Effects of stimulus rate on the cortical posterior tibial nerve SEPs: a topographic study. *Electroencephalogr Clin Neurophysiol* 1996;100:210–219.

145. Tinazzi M, Zanette G, La Porta F, et al. Selective gating of lower limb cortical somatosensory evoked potentials (SEPs) during passive and active foot movements. *Electroencephalogr Clin Neurophysiol* 1997;104:312–321.

146. Tobimatsu S, Fukui R, Kato M, et al. Multimodality evoked potentials in patients and carriers with adrenoleukodystrophy and adrenomyeloneuropathy. *Electroencephalogr Clin Neurophysiol* 1985;62:18–24.

147. Towe AL. On the nature of the primary evoked response. *Exp Neurol* 1966;15:113–139.

148. Trojaborg W, Jorgensen EO. Evoked cortical potentials in patients with "isoelectric" EEGs. *Electroencephalogr Clin Neurophysiol* 1973;35:301–309.

149. Tsuji S, Luders H, Dinner DS, et al. Effect of stimulus intensity of subcortical and cortical somatosensory evoked potentials by posterior tibial nerve stimulation. *Electroencephalogr Clin Neurophysiol* 1984;59:229–237.

150. Urasaki E, Tokimura T, Yasukouchi H, et al. P30 and N33 of posterior tibial nerve SSEPs are analogous to P14 and N18 of median nerve SSEPs. *Electroencephalogr Clin Neurophysiology* 1993;88:525–529.

151. Urasaki E, Uematsu S, Lesser RP. Short latency somatosensory evoked potentials around the human upper brain-stem. *Electroencephalogr Clin Neurophysiol* 1993;88:92–104.

152. Urasaki E, Wada S, Kadoya C, et al. Absence of spinal N13-P13 and normal scalp far-field P14 in a patient with syringomyelia. *Electroencephalogr Clin Neurophysiol* 1988;71:400–404.

153. Urasaki E, Wada S, Kadoya C, et al. Origin of the scalp far-field N18 of SSEPs in response to median nerve stimulation. *Electroencephalogr Clin Neurophysiol* 1990;77:39–51.

154. Urasaki E, Wada S, Kadoya C, et al. Amplitude abnormalities in the scalp far-field N18 of SSEPs to median nerve stimulation in patients with midbrain-pontine lesion. *Electroencephalogr Clin Neurophysiol* 1992;84:232–242.

155. Valeriani M, Restuccia D, Di Lazzaro V, et al. Giant central N20-P22 with normal area 3B N20-P20: an argument in favour of an area 3a generator of early median nerve cortical SEPs. *Electroencephalogr Clin Neurophysiol* 1997;104:60–67.

156. Veilleux M, Daube JR. The value of ulnar somatosensory evoked potential in infants. *Electroencephalogr Clin Neurophysiol* 1987;68:415–423.

157. Wiederholt WC. Early components of the somatosensory evoked potential in man, cat and rat. In: Desmedt JE, ed. *Clinical uses of cerebral, brainstem and spinal somatosensory evoked potentials*. Basel: Karger, 1980:105–117.

158. Willis J, Seales D, Frazier E. Short latency somatosensory evoked potentials in infants. *Electroencephalogr Clin Neurophysiol* 1984;59:366–373.

159. Woodbury WJ. Potentials in a volume conductor. In: Ruch TC, Patton HD, Woodbury JW, et al, eds. *Neurophysiology*. Philadelphia: WB Saunders, 1965:85–91.

160. Wulff CH, Trojaborg W. Adult metachromatic leukodystrophy: neurophysiologic findings. *Neurology* 1985;35:1776–1778.

161. Yamada T, Ishida T, Kudo Y, et al. Clinical correlates of abnormal P14 in median SEPs. *Neurology* 1986;36:765–771.

162. Yamada T, Kameyama S, Fuchigami Y, et al. Changes of short latency somatosensory evoked potential during sleep. *Electroencephalogr Clin Neurophysiol* 1988;70:126–136.

163. Yamada T, Kimura J, Nitz DM. Short latency somatosensory potentials following median nerve stimulation in man. *Electroencephalogr Clin Neurophysiol* 1980;48:367–376.

164. Yamada T, Machida M, Oishi M, et al. Stationary negative potentials near the source vs. positive far-field potentials at a distance. *Electroencephalogr Clin Neurophysiol* 1985;60:509–524.

165. Yamada T, Matsubara M, Shiraishi G, et al. Topographic analyses of somatosensory evoked potentials following stimulation of tibial, sural and lateral femoral cutaneous nerves. *Electroencephalogr Clin Neurophysiol* 1996;100:33–43.

166. Yiannikas C, Shahani BT, Young RR. Short-latency somatosensory evoked potentials from radial, median, ulnar and peroneal nerve stimulation in the assessment of cervical spondylosis. *Arch Neurol* 1986;43:1264–1271.

167. Zanette G, Tinazzi M, Polo A, et al. Motor neuron disease with pyramidal tract dysfunction involves the cortical generators of the early somatosensory evoked potentials to tibial nerve stimulation. *Neurology* 1996;47:932–938.

Chapter 30

Long-Latency Event-Related Potentials

Douglas S. Goodin

Event-Related Potentials	**Other Uses of the ERP**
Effects of Age and Other Factors on the ERP	**References**
Clinical Utility of the ERP	

External stimuli produce changes of electrical potential within the nervous system that can be recorded using the technique of signal averaging (9). The nature of these so-called evoked potentials (EPs) depends, to a large extent, on the physical nature of the stimulus that is used to elicit them, and such potentials are commonly referred to as "exogenous" or "stimulus-related." These exogenous EPs include the brainstem auditory evoked potentials (BAEPs), the short-latency somatosensory evoked potentials (SSEPs), and visual evoked potentials (VEPs), all of which are in widespread clinical use. They also include the motor evoked potentials that are produced following transcranial electrical or magnetic stimulation of the brain. In general, these potentials do not depend on the subject's level of attention or interest in the task, and they often can be recorded when the subject is asleep or unconscious.

However, there is another type of EP, the so-called endogenous or event-related potential (ERP). Like exogenous EPs, these ERPs also can be recorded in response to an external stimulus (14,46,47,75,83,102). However, unlike exogenous EPs, these potential changes occur only when the subject is selectively attentive to the stimulus train and are elicited only when a subject is able to distinguish one stimulus or event (the target) from another group of stimuli (the nontargets). In addition, these potentials can be recorded in the circumstance (the event) where an anticipated stimulus is unexpectedly omitted (66, 92,96,103). ERPs are thus relatively independent of the physical nature of the stimulus, depending more importantly on the setting in which the target stimulus or event actually occurs.

As a result of experimental observations such as these, ERPs have been linked to a variety of cognitive processes thought to be associated with the task of distinguishing a target from a nontarget stimulus. Thus attempts even have been made to link different components of the ERP to particular stages of information processing, such as stimulus detection, stimulus classification, or response selection. The successful completion of these stages is often held to be a necessary prerequisite for a subject to respond selectively and accurately to a target stimulus (15,27,30,32,34,35,47,51,57,59,81,84,85, 106). As a result of this presumed relationship between these basic cognitive processes and the ERP, there has been considerable interest in the potential clinical role that the recording of these potentials might have in the evaluation of patients with impaired cognitive function.

EVENT-RELATED POTENTIALS

The usual experimental design used to elicit the ERP is the so-called odd-ball paradigm. In this design, a subject attends to a sequence of two different stimuli. One of these stimuli occurs quite often (the frequent stimulus) and thus is anticipated by the subject. The other stimulus occurs much less frequently (the rare stimulus), and it is this stimulus that evokes the endogenous components of the ERP. In order to ensure that the subject pays attention to the sequence of stimuli, he or she is typically required to count mentally or otherwise respond to one stimulus or the other.

The cerebral responses to the different stimuli are then recorded and averaged separately. The cerebral response to frequent stimuli consists of a series of waves that relate, to a large extent, to the sensory modality involved. Thus, following an auditory stimulus, this response has been divided into three sequential time periods. The early-latency response (occurring within the first 10 milliseconds after the stimulus) is the BAEP, and this reflects neural activity in auditory nerve and brainstem auditory structures such as the choclear nucleus, the superior olive, the lateral lemniscus, and the inferior colliculus (67). The midlatency response (10–50 milliseconds after the stimulus) is thought to reflect both reflex muscle activity and neural activity possibly arising in the thalamocortical radiations, the primary auditory cortex, and the early auditory association cortex (67). The long-latency response to the frequent stimulus (occurring more than 50 milliseconds after the stimulus) consists of a negative ($N\overline{1}$)–positive ($P\overline{2}$) complex that has been referred to as the vertex potential because it is of maximal amplitude in this scalp region (13). The neural basis for long-latency responses (including the vertex potential) is less well defined than it is for the earlier responses. Nevertheless, dipole localization methods using magnetoencephalography have generally localized the vertex potential to the superior temporal lobe (18,44,60,82,91). This vertex potential represents an obligate response of the nervous system to the external stimulus and can be recorded even when a subject is asleep (66). Therefore, like the early- and midlatency components, the vertex potential is an exogenous response.

In contrast to the long-latency response to the frequent tone, the response to the rare auditory stimulus consists not only of a negative ($N\overline{1}$)–positive (apparent $P\overline{2}$) complex but also of a following negative ($N\overline{2}$)–positive ($P\overline{3}$) complex (Fig. 30.1). The first positive wave in this sequence (apparent $P\overline{2}$) reflects the sum of the stimulus-related $P\overline{2}$ and the

event-related $P\overline{165}$ (37). The amplitude and latency of this response are quite consistent for the same subject performing the same task (18,48,93). Although several other ERP components have been described in the literature (e.g., 22,37,43,50,58,75,100–102), most of the components other than this $N\overline{2}$-$P\overline{3}$ complex have not been studied widely in clinical contexts or are only elicited in special experimental circumstances. This $P\overline{3}$ response is a large wave of positive polarity that peaks in the midline central-parietal scalp approximately 300 milliseconds after an unexpected stimulus or event. An EP component with a scalp distribution similar to $P\overline{3}$ can be recorded in response to a stimulus of any sensory modality and, as mentioned earlier, can be recorded (in the absence of an associated vertex potential) even when an anticipated stimulus is unexpectedly omitted (66,68,92,96,103). The neural generators of this $P\overline{3}$ response are largely unknown, although a mesial cortical or subcortical location has been suggested by some authors (12,42,89,95,108,109).

The amplitude and latency of ERPs can be affected by several experimental manipulations that have little appreciable affect on exogenous EPs, and, conversely, other variables affect exogenous EPs without appreciable affect on ERPs. Thus the $P\overline{3}$ response is markedly influenced by the ease or difficulty with which targets are distinguished from nontargets (Fig. 30.2) (16,39), by the expectancy of the stimulus (21,73), or by the attention of the subject (see Fig. 30.1), whereas exogenous EPs are not (14,15,46,47, 66,67,75,83,102). By contrast, a change in the intensity of stimulation has relatively little effect on the $P\overline{3}$ component but a major influence on the associated exogenous EPs (14,46,47,66,67,75,83,102).

In order to record ERPs in a clinical setting, it is necessary to have a stimulator that is capable of delivering rare and frequent stimuli and recording the averaged EP in response to each stimulus separately. The stimuli need to be easily distinguished from each other in order to maximize the likelihood of eliciting robust ERPs. When two auditory stimuli are used (as is common in clinical practice), each stimulus is delivered binaurally. Typically, the stimuli used are 1000- and 2000-Hz tones (50–100 milliseconds in duration) delivered at an intensity of 65–75 decibels sensation level (dBSL). Because of the relatively long refractory period of the vertex potential, the interstimulus interval is usually more than 1 second. The amplitude of the $P\overline{3}$ response is typically 50–100 times the amplitude of the BAEP and, therefore, an average of only a few cerebral responses to rare tones is generally adequate to improve the signal-to-noise ratio to the point where the $P\overline{3}$ response can be seen easily (8). In fact, the $P\overline{3}$ amplitude is often large enough that this component often

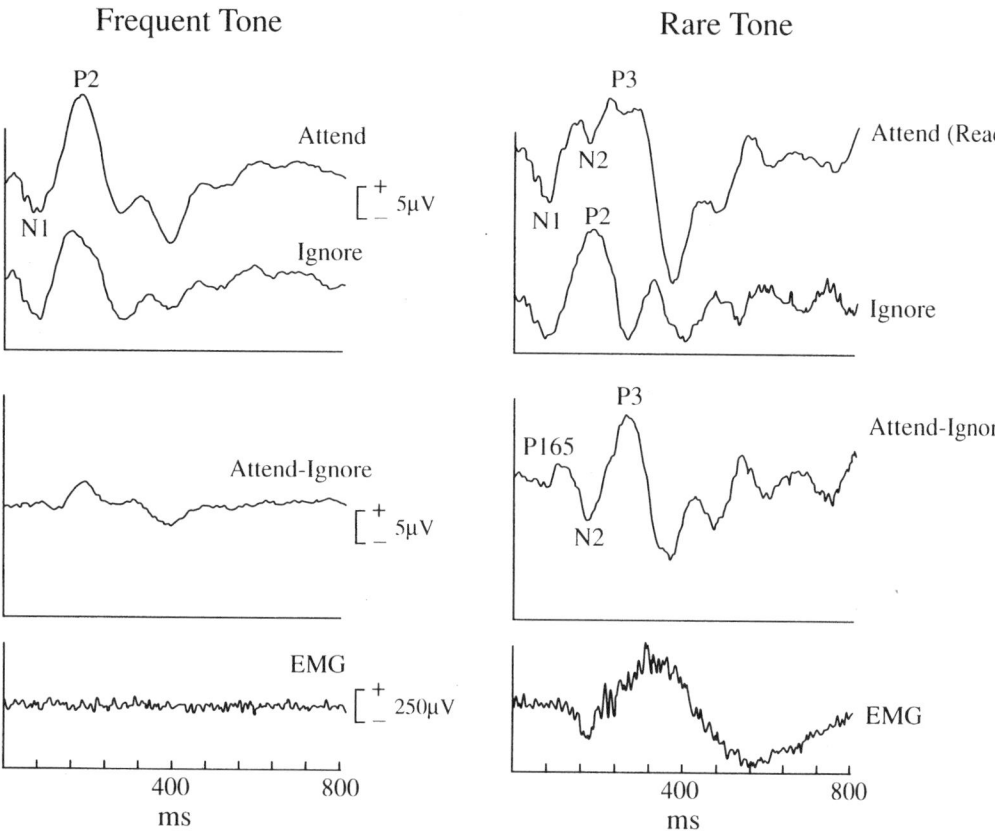

FIG. 30.1. Long-latency ERPs recorded from the vertex in a normal subject. Responses to the frequent stimulus are shown on the left and responses to the rare stimulus are shown on the right. Waveforms in the top row (react) were recorded when the subject listened to the stimuli and responded to each rare stimulus by extension of the right middle finger. Waveforms in the second row (ignore) are those recorded when the subject ignored the stimuli and read a book. Waveforms in the third row (react-ignore) represent difference waveforms obtained by digital subtraction of the ignore waveforms from the react waveforms. Compound muscle action potentials (CMAPs) from the right extensor digitorum communis muscle in the react condition are shown in the bottom row. (Modified from Goodin DS, Aminoff MJ. The relationship between the evoked potential and brain events in sensory discrimination and motor response. *Brain* 1984;107:241–251.)

can be identified in the response to a single stimulus. The ratio of rare to frequent tones is generally set at 20:80 or less. This allows approximately 50 responses to the rare tone per trial to be averaged in 10 minutes. At least two trials should be done to ensure that the responses are replicable.

Responses are recorded from Fz, Cz, and Pz electrode placements on the scalp (international 10-20 system) referenced to a common site such as linked mastoids. Eye movements should also be monitored to ensure that eye movement artifact has not contaminated the recordings, although it is possible with some recording systems either to reject contaminated trials automatically or to remove such artifacts from the recordings mathemati-

cally (54). Most of the electrical power present in ERPs is in the frequency band of less than 10 Hz, so that a high-frequency filter of 40 or 50 Hz is appropriate. The best low-frequency filter is controversial (17,31) because much of the power in ERP recordings is in the 1- to 4-Hz frequency band, and a marked distortion of the P$\overline{3}$ amplitude begins to occur when low-frequency filters greater than this are used (31). As a result, high-pass filters of more than 1 Hz should be avoided. In addition, because high-pass analog filters will shift responses to earlier latencies, even at very low filter settings (31), it is important to ensure that both normal controls and clinical patients are recorded at an identical bandpass.

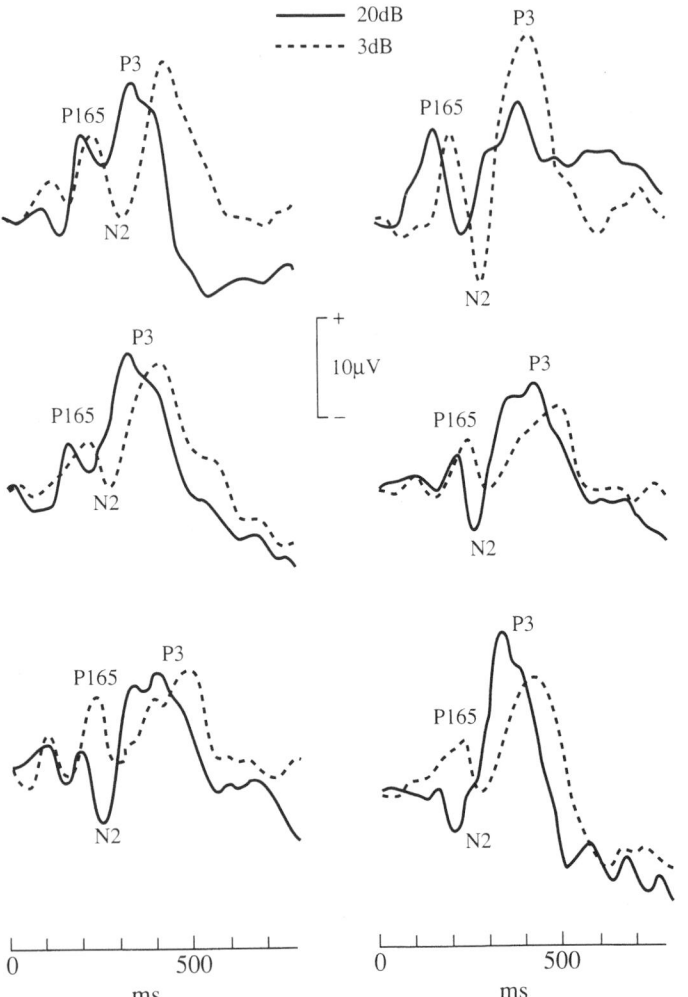

FIG. 30.2. Difference waveforms showing the ERPs in six subjects engaged in tasks of two different levels of difficulty. In the easy condition (*solid lines*), the frequent tone had an intensity of 40 decibels hearing level (dBHL), whereas the rare tone had an intensity of 60 dBHL. In the difficult condition (*dashed lines*), the rare tone was the same but the frequent tone had an intensity of 57 dBHL. The peak latencies of the ERP components are consistently longer in the difficult task compared to the easy one. (Modified from Goodin DS, Squires KC, Starr A. Variations in early and late event-related components of the auditory evoked potential with task difficulty. *Electroencephalogr Clin Neurophysiol* 1983;55:680–686.)

EFFECTS OF AGE AND OTHER FACTORS ON THE ERP

The long-latency ERP is strongly influenced by age (Fig. 30.3; Table 30.1). The exogenous $N\overline{1}$ and $P\overline{2}$ components seem to reach their adult latencies at the latest by the age of 5 or 6 years (10,36). By contrast, the $N\overline{2}$ and $P\overline{3}$ components are quite prolonged in young children and decrease in latency until reaching adult values in the mid- to late teenage years (10,36). Following this, the latency of both the stimulus-related ($P\overline{2}$) and event-related ($N\overline{2}$ and $P\overline{3}$) components increases linearly with age (Fig. 30.3; Table 30.1). These findings have, in general, been confirmed by several studies (Table 30.2), although there has been some variation in the rate of change among reports (2,3,7,20, 36,41,63,68–70,76,80). A few groups have reported that the age–latency relationship for $P\overline{3}$ is curvilinear, with an increased slope in elderly subjects compared to young controls (7,41). Picton and colleagues, however, specifically investigated this possibility and found no nonlinear trends on either trend analysis or formal testing for curvilinearity (68). As a result of these discrepancies, it is unclear whether nonlinear factors are important determinants of the $P\overline{3}$ latency–age function. However, in two of the larger studies that have reported significant curvilinear effects (2,41), the incorporation of these effects into the model increased the explained variance by only a small amount, so that, from a practical standpoint, a linear approximation can be used to establish normal values for clinical purposes. In addition, because the changes in $P\overline{3}$ latency that occur with maturation are so marked, separate normative data are necessary in children (10,36).

In addition to an increase in latency with age, there is also a decrease in the amplitude of both the stimulus-related and event-related components of the long-latency ERP (see Tables 30.1 and 30.2). Unlike the generally small intersubject variability of latency measurements, this variability of amplitude is large. Thus a single standard error around the regression line at age 60 years usually represents 60%–80% of the predicted amplitude of $P\overline{3}$ (Table 30.2). This marked intersubject variability limits the clinical usefulness of measuring amplitude.

Medications can also affect the ERP. For example, metabolic encephalopathies (as might be caused by an overdose of many drugs) are known to affect the ERP (40). Of particular interest in the context of clinical ERP recordings are the medications used to treat depression or other psychiatric conditions, because these illnesses are often confused with dementia (24,49,107). The effect of these drugs taken in therapeutic dosages, however, has not been studied extensively. Baribeau-Braun and co-workers reported no difference in either $P\overline{3}$ latency or amplitude between schizophrenic patients treated with high- and low-dose phenothiazines (4). In another

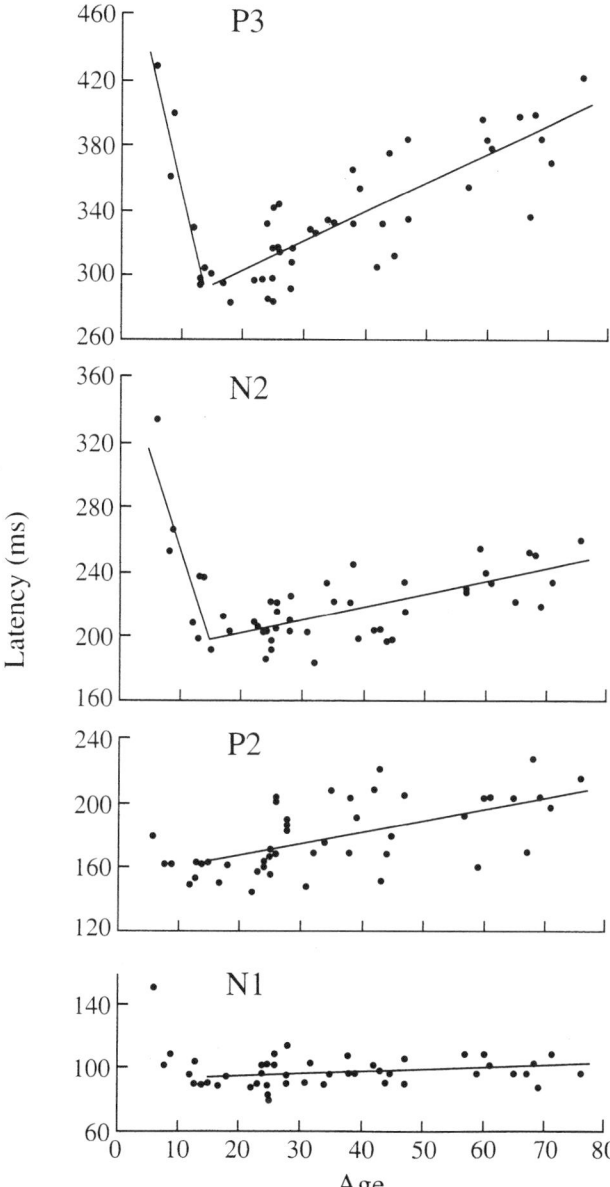

FIG. 30.3. Age–latency regression lines for the different long-latency ERP components. During maturation (age 6–15 years), the peak latency of the later N$\overline{2}$ and P$\overline{3}$ components becomes progressively shorter, reaching its shortest latency at approximately 15 years. Following this, each component increases in latency with age, although the rate of this change is faster for components that occur later in the sequence. (Modified from Goodin DS, Squires KC, Henderson BH, et al. Age-related variations in evoked potentials to auditory stimuli in normal human subjects. *Electroencephalogr Clin Neurophysiol* 1978;44:447–458.)

study, Pfefferbaum and co-workers (65) studied 20 schizophrenic patients and found no difference in the P$\overline{3}$ response between treated and untreated patients. In depressed patients, by contrast, they found a P$\overline{3}$ amplitude reduction, but no latency difference, in the drug-free depressed patients compared with those receiving antidepressant medication. Therefore, from the available evidence, it seems that these psychiatric medications, at least when taken in therapeutic doses, do not have major effects on the ERP.

Certain other variables, such as how recently food has been consumed, body temperature, fitness, sleep deprivation, or time of day, also have been reported to affect the P$\overline{3}$ response (23,71). These findings still need to be confirmed, although, because the magnitude of the changes reported tends to be small, the relevance of these effects to clinical recordings is unclear.

Table 30.1. *Variation in the amplitude and latency of the auditory ERPs with age*

	Slope	SE[a]	Value at age 15 yr	Significance[b]
Latency				
N$\overline{1}$ component	0.1 msec/yr	8 msec	94 msec	NS
P$\overline{2}$ component	0.7 msec/yr	19 msec	168 msec	$p < 0.001$
N$\overline{2}$ component	0.8 msec/yr	15 msec	199 msec	$p < 0.001$
P$\overline{3}$ component	1.6 msec/yr	21 msec	310 msec	$pp < 0.001$
Amplitude				
N$\overline{1}$-P$\overline{2}$	0.2 µV/yr	5.6 µV	15.6 µV	$p < 0.01$
N$\overline{2}$-P$\overline{3}$	0.2 µV/yr	7.9 µV	17.7 µV	$p < 0.05$

[a]Standard error of the estimate around the regression line.
[b]NS indicates that the regression slope is not significantly different from zero.
Data from Goodin DS, Squires KC, Henderson BH, et al. Age-related variations in evoked potentials to auditory stimuli in normal human subjects *Electroencephalogr Clin Neurophysiol* 1978;44:447–458.

Table 30.2. *Comparison of age-related changes in the auditory P3 amplitude and latency in different studies*

	Latency			Amplitude		
	Slope (msec/yr)	Intercept (msec)	SE (msec)	Slope (μV/yr)	Intercept (μV)	SE (μV)
Goodin et al. (36)	+1.64	285	21	−0.18	17.6	5.6
Picton et al. (68)	+1.71	294	25	−0.15	16.6	4.0
Syndulko et al. (104)	+1.07	297	22	*	*	*
Brown et al. (7)	+1.12	272	28	−0.15	*	*
Pfefferbaum et al. (63)	+0.94	*	51	−0.13	*	*
Emmerson et al. (20)	+1.46	*	*	*	*	*
Gordon et al. (41)	+0.91	*	31	*	*	*
Puce et al. (80)	+1.34	281	*	−0.28	23.0	*
Polich (69)	+0.92	304	32	*	*	*
Anderer et al. (2)	+0.92	327	33	−0.12	19.2	6.3

Asterisks indicate data are not included in the reports.

ERPs also may be difficult to interpret in certain situations. For example, unlike the interpretation of many clinically used EPs such as the BAEP, the VEP, and the SSEP, the complete absence of a P3 response should not be considered as an abnormality. On occasion, the P3 response may absent in alert, attentive, and cooperative nondemented subjects who are engaged in the task. Conversely, such a finding might simply reflect a subject's inattention to the task. Another difficulty is that occasionally the P3 peak consists of two distinct subcomponents, the so-called P3a and P3b, as initially described by Squires and co-workers (98). These authors found the P3a sub-component in the averaged response to rare tones regardless of the subject's attention, whereas the P3b subcomponent was present only when subjects attended to the stimulus train. They therefore concluded that it was the P3b subcomponent that was sensitive to task requirements. Some authors have recommended separate measurement of these two subcomponents in order to improve the sensitivity of the test (72). In practice, however, the P3a and P3b subcomponents often are fused and cannot be identified separately. Even so, measuring a single P3 latency generally results in both small standard errors and high sensitivities (Tables 30.2 and 30.3).

Table 30.3. *Clinical experience with P3 latency in neurological and psychiatric patients[a]*

Study	Demented	Psychiatric	Nondemented
Squires et al. (97)	74% (58)	3% (33)	4% (51)
Brown et al. (6)	61% (18)	0% (7)	
Pfefferbaum et al. (65)	30% (37)	19% (54)	
Leppler and Greenberg (52)	73% (15)	0% (15)	
Slaets and Fortgens (94)	38% (8)	17% (6)	
St. Clair et al. (99)	7% (14)		
Gordon et al. (41)	80% (19)	12% (32)	
Polich et al. (74)	28% (39)		
Goodin and Aminoff (28)	61% (36)		
Patterson et al. (62)	13% (15)	0% (8)	

[a]Percentages of patients with abnormally prolonged P3 latencies in each of the three categories: demented and nondemented patients with neurological illnesses and psychiatric patients with either depression or schizophrenia. Numbers in parentheses represent the total number of patients studied in each category.

CLINICAL UTILITY OF THE ERP

The clinical syndrome of dementia describes a deterioration of intellect simultaneously involving several different areas of cognitive function, such as memory, orientation, judgment, and abstraction. Senile dementia of the Alzheimer's type (SDAT) is, at present, the most common (albeit untreatable) cause of dementia, particularly in the elderly, among whom this diagnosis accounts for considerably more than 50% of demented patients in most series (24,49,107). However, other causes of dementia, if recognized early enough, can be successfully treated. As a result, it is necessary to exclude other treatable causes of dementia in all patients. This is particularly important for patients with an apparent deterioration in intellect resulting from a "pseudodementia" caused by depression or other psychiatric illness. These patients cannot be distinguished from those with SDAT by commonly used radiological and laboratory tests, and yet they have an eminently treatable condition. The recording of ERPs has been used most widely in this clinical circumstance.

Several groups have reported that the P$\overline{3}$ component is prolonged in latency and reduced in amplitude in demented patients compared to age-matched controls (Fig. 30.4; Table 30.3) (6,28,38,52,62,65,74,76,94,97,99,104). Squires and co-workers (97) found that 74% of their demented patients had a P$\overline{3}$ latency that was more than 2 standard errors above the normal age–latency regression line (Fig. 30.5). The P$\overline{3}$ amplitude was also reduced significantly in the patients with dementia (38). By contrast, only 3.5% of their nondemented patients with other neurological and psychiatric conditions had a similar prolongation of their P$\overline{3}$ latency (Fig. 30.5). These findings, again, were similar in all diagnostic categories, including depressive illness (Table 30.4). The finding of 74% sensitivity and 96.5% specificity suggests that recording the

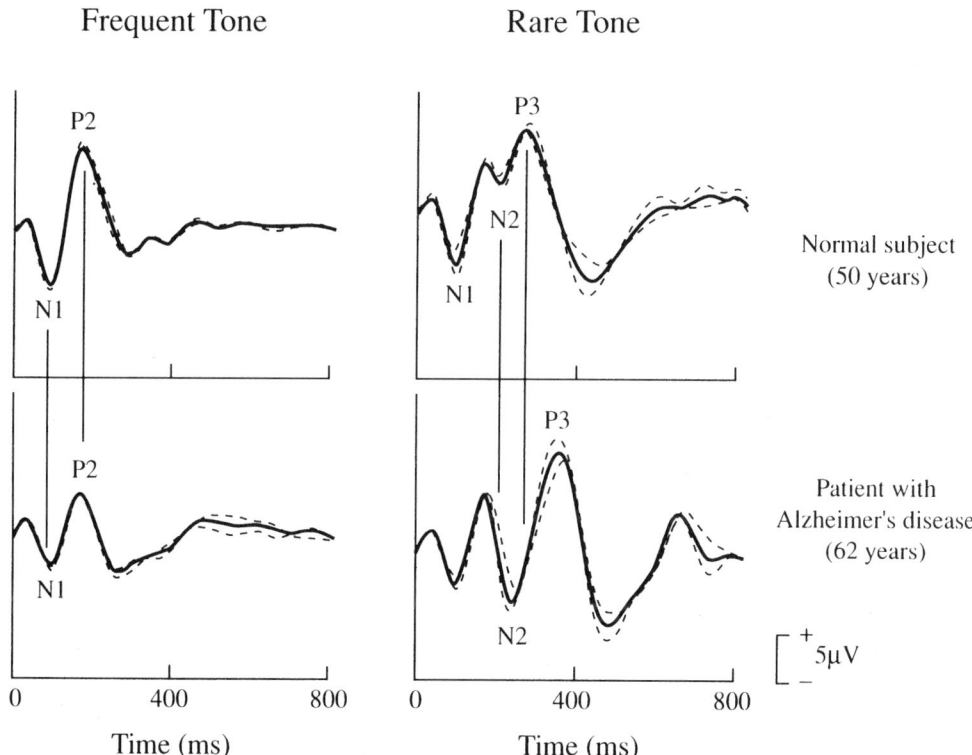

FIG. 30.4. Long-latency ERPs recorded from the vertex in a demented and a nondemented subject of similar age. **Top:** Responses from the nondemented subject. **Bottom:** Responses from the demented subject. Responses to the frequent tone are on the left and those to the rare tone are on the right. The N$\overline{1}$ and P$\overline{2}$ components are similar in the two subjects, whereas the later event-related components (N$\overline{2}$ and P$\overline{3}$) are delayed in the demented subject relative to the nondemented subject. (Modified from Goodin DS, Aminoff MJ. Electrophysiological differences between subtypes of dementia. *Brain* 1986;109:1103–1113.)

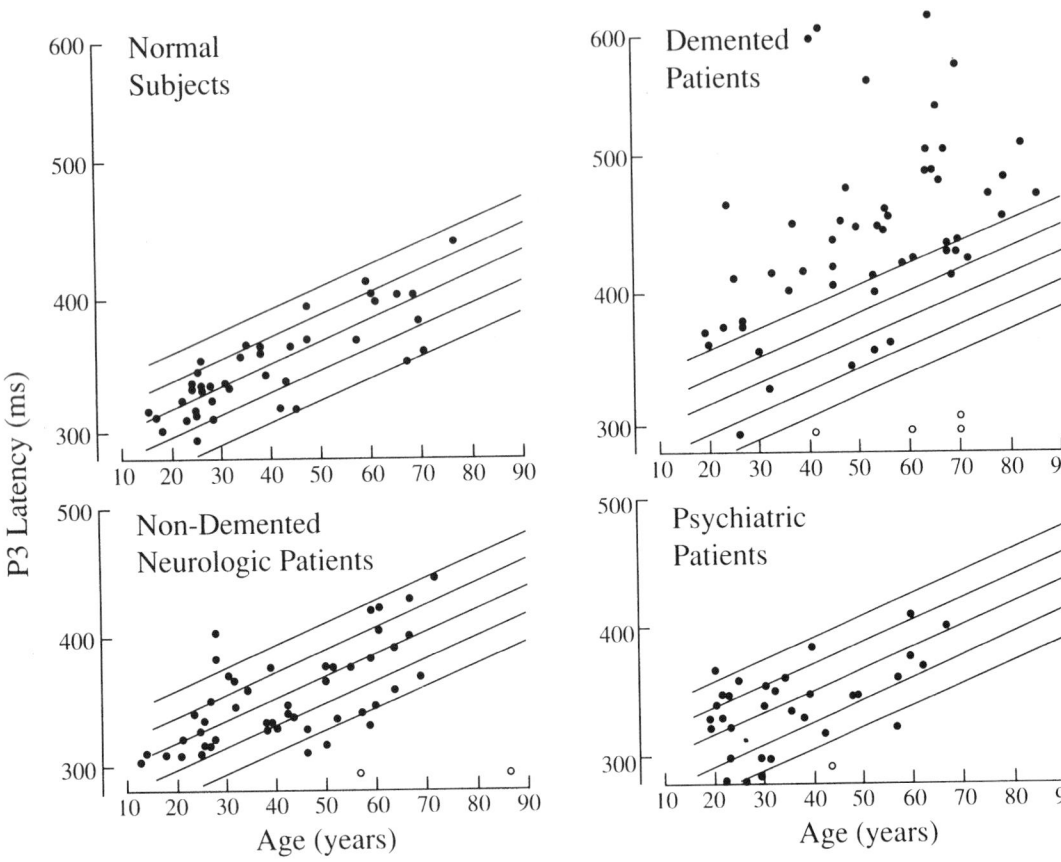

FIG. 30.5. The relationship between P$\bar{3}$ latency and age in three patient groups and in normal subjects. *Open circles* represent persons without an identifiable P$\bar{3}$ response. The normal age–latency regression line (in addition to the 1 and 2 standard error lines) is superimposed on each plot. (Modified from Squires KC, Chippendale TJ, Wrege KS, et al. Electrophysiological assessment of mental function in aging and dementia. In: Poon LW, ed. *Aging in the 1980s.* Washington, DC: American Psychological Association, 1980:125–134.)

P$\bar{3}$ could be quite helpful in the evaluation of demented patients. For example, if the diagnoses of dementia and pseudodementia were thought (on clinical impression) to be equally likely, the finding of a prolonged P$\bar{3}$ latency would effectively establish the diagnosis of dementia beyond reasonable doubt (25). A normal P$\bar{3}$ latency in this circumstance, by contrast, would suggest (but not establish) the diagnosis of pseudodementia.

Most published studies have confirmed these general findings, although the sensitivity of the P$\bar{3}$ latency has varied among reports (see Table 30.3). In addition, although the specificity of the test also has varied among reports, no study has shown a significant prolongation in the P$\bar{3}$ latency of depressed patients or patients with other psychiatric conditions. Thus the sensitivity and

specificity of the test, both in the more favorable reports as well as in the average experience, make it useful in the proper clinical setting (25) and give it an important role in the evaluation of selected patients with cognitive impairment.

ERPs also have been studied (33) in patients infected with human immunodeficiency virus (HIV), some of whom were asymptomatic from their infection and others of whom were demented and met other diagnostic criteria for the acquired immunodeficiency syndrome (AIDS). As in other subcortical dementias (see below), patients with the AIDS-dementia complex have a prolongation of the early components of the ERP, particularly of the N$\bar{1}$ component, in addition to the prolongation of later N$\bar{2}$ and P$\bar{3}$ components that occurs in other dementing disorders (see Table 30.4). Almost a

Table 30.4. $\overline{P3}$ *latency in neurological and psychiatric illnesses*

	Number	P3 Latency (SE)[a]
Diagnoses of Demented Patients		
Alzheimer's type	13	2.79
Uncertain cause	12	3.17
Toxic-metabolic	11	4.09
Vascular disease	8	4.98
Hydrocephalus	7	2.84
Brain tumor	4	4.20
Multiple sclerosis	2	8.19
Herpes simplex encephalitis	1	0.29
Total	*58*	*3.61*
Diagnoses of Psychiatric Patients		
Depression	12	−0.22
Paranoid schizophrenia	11	−0.30
Manic-depression	6	0.16
Acute schizophrenia	4	−0.23
Total	*33*	*−0.18*
Diagnoses of Nondemented Patients		
Miscellaneous	17	0.20
Brain tumor	8	−0.52
Vascular disease	7	−0.41
Multiple sclerosis	6	−0.42
Parkinsonism	5	0.50
Hydrocephalus	5	0.87
Trauma	3	0.41
Total	*51*	*−0.30*

[a]Indicates the average number of standard errors away from the normal age–latency regression line in each group of patients.

Data from Goodin DS, Squires KC, Starr A. Long latency event-related components of the auditory evoked potential in dementia. *Brain* 1978;101:635–648.

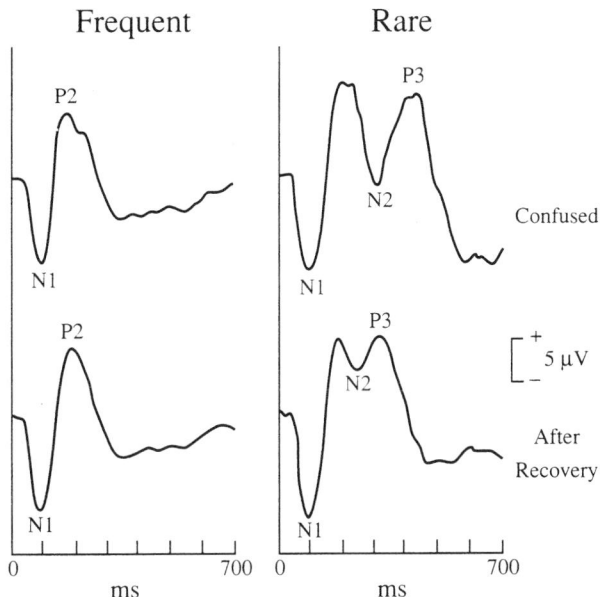

FIG. 30.6. Long-latency ERPs recorded in a man of age 60 who was initially comatose from hyponatremia. Responses to the frequent tone are shown on the left and responses to the rare tone are shown on the right. **Top:** Waveforms recorded while the patient was awake but mentally slow from his metabolic encephalopathy. **Bottom:** Waveforms recorded after he had recovered fully. The stimulus-related N1 and P2 components were unchanged between recordings. The latencies of the N2 and P3 components of the ERP, by contrast, were considerably shorter after the patient had returned to normal mental functioning. (Modified from Goodin DS, Starr A, Chippendale T, et al. Sequential changes in the P3 component of the auditory evoked potential in confusional states and dementing illnesses. *Neurology* 1983;33:1215–1218.)

third of asymptomatic HIV patients in this study had ERP changes similar to those that occurred in patients with dementia. These results suggest that ERPs may be used to identify a subgroup of asymptomatic patients who have a particularly high risk of developing future cognitive difficulties, perhaps thereby identifying patients who require more aggressive treatment.

Because ERPs are known to fluctuate with clinical state (40), they can be used to study the same individual over time in order to provide an objective measure of the changes that occur in cognitive function (Fig. 30.6). This clinical role for ERPs may increase as the therapeutic options for dementia become more prevalent.

The use of the ERP in diseases other than dementia has not been clearly defined. Several authors have reported P3 amplitude to be reduced in schizophrenia (4,5,53,61,65,86,87,90), and some have reported a latency prolongation as well (4,55,65). Similarly, the ERP has been studied in both acute alcohol intoxication and chronic alcohol abuse. In general, the P3 amplitude is reduced in both settings (19,45,64,77–79,88), although, again, latency differences occasionally are reported (64). In addition, some studies have reported that subjects with a family history of alcoholism (and therefore at increased risk of becoming alcoholics) had large-amplitude decrements in recorded ERPs, unlike subjects without such a history (19,45). As discussed previously, however, such a large normal variation in amplitude exists that the actual clinical utility of these findings in individual patients is uncertain, even though such results may have considerable theoretical importance to our understanding of schizophrenia and of alcoholism.

OTHER USES OF THE ERP

The recording of ERPs also may provide insight into other clinical or theoretical controversies. For example, there has been debate about whether a distinction can be made between the dementia syndrome produced by neocortical diseases such as Alzheimer's disease and that produced by subcortical diseases such as Huntington's or Parkinson's disease (1,11,56). By recording ERPs in patients with these different illnesses, however, Goodin and Aminoff were able to demonstrate differences in the ERP not only between the cortical and subcortical dementias but also within the subcortical group (28,29). Other groups also have investigated the electrophysiological changes that occur in Parkinson's, Huntington's, and Alzheimer's diseases (see ref. 26 for a review), and the reported changes generally have paralleled each other. In this circumstance, ERPs are able to provide direct evidence that, in fact, different subtypes of dementia exist.

Suggestions also have been made in the literature that SDAT represents an acceleration of the normal aging process (e.g., ref. 105). By recording of the ERP, however, it can be demonstrated (e.g., ref. 38) that patients with SDAT have markedly prolonged (i.e., age-inappropriate) P$\bar{3}$ latencies but normal (i.e., age-appropriate) P$\bar{2}$ latencies (see Fig. 30.5). The finding of such a selective effect of dementia on the ERP indicates that the aging process has not simply been accelerated in these patients.

ERPs also have been used to study the central organization utilized by the brain to detect and identify different stimuli, discriminate among them, and select appropriate motor responses to each. As mentioned earlier, many authors have attempted to link different ERP components to the so-called stages of information processing (e.g., stimulus detection, stimulus classification, and response selection) that are presumed to take place during the performance of a discrimination task such as the oddball task used to elicit the P$\bar{3}$ response (15,27,30,32,34,35,43,57–59,81,83,85). Many of these authors assume (either explicitly or implicitly) that the various stages of information processing proceed in a serial manner, with the completion of one stage being a necessary prerequisite for the beginning of the next. However, whether such processing occurs serially or in parallel is controversial.

Several experimental observations bear on this issue. First, not only is the timing of the ERP dependent on the difficulty of the discrimination task (see Fig. 30.2), but the coupling of the motor response to the ERP also varies with task difficulty (Fig. 30.7) and with the response strategy adopted by the subject (30,32,34,35,59). In fact, with particularly easy tasks (18), the entire ERP

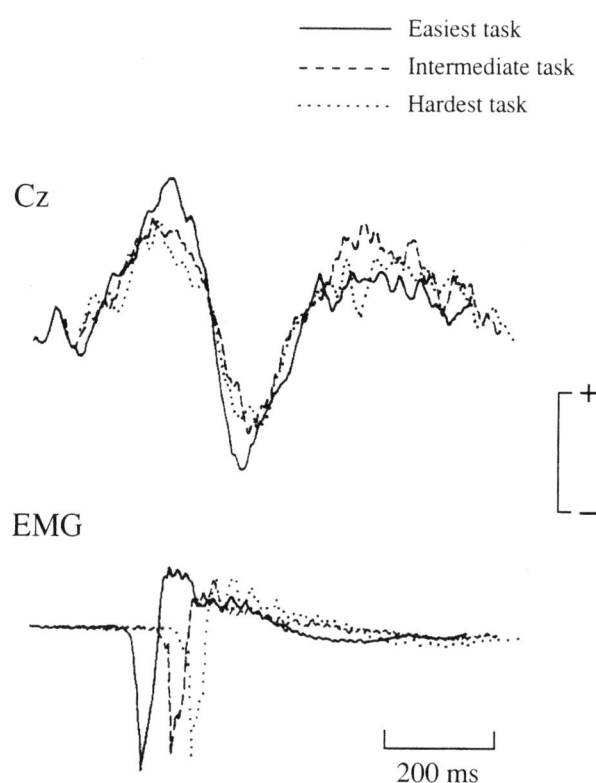

FIG. 30.7. Long-latency response-synchronized ERPs recorded from the vertex when subjects were engaged in tasks of varying difficulty (easiest task: *solid line*; intermediate task: *dashed line*; hardest task: *dotted line*). **Top:** The cerebral responses, which have been aligned with each other. **Bottom:** CMAPs recorded from the responding muscle as described in Figure 30.1. As can be seen, there is a progressive delay between the ERP and the onset of the CMAP as the tasks become harder. (Modified from Goodin DS, Aminoff MJ, Mantle MM. Sensory, discrimination and its relationship to cerebral processing of infrequent stimuli. *Can J Neurol Sci* 1987;14:642–648.)

may actually follow the motor response (see Fig. 30.1). Conversely, when a subject correctly anticipates a future event, the correct motor response may be initiated prior to the onset of the stimulus (35,59). The importance of these observations is that no ERP component can be linked consistently to any specific cerebral process related to the making of such a sensory discrimination (30,32,34,35,59). Moreover, based on comparisons between response-synchronized and stimulus-synchronized averages, the $\overline{N1}$ and $\overline{P2}$ components of the ERP seem to be on a separate (i.e., parallel) branch of the stimulus processing sequence from the $\overline{P165}$-$\overline{N2}$-$\overline{P3}$ complex, and errors seem to arise when a response is inappropriately generated from the wrong branch (30). Thus ERPs seem to reflect neural activity in substantially parallel networks and, thereby, provide physiological evidence of parallel processing. Indeed, as a result of considerations such as these, the discrimination and response systems appear to be so intertwined that even the notion of discrete stages of information processing seems somewhat implausible.

REFERENCES

1. Albers ML, Feldman RG, Willis AL. The subcortical dementia of supranuclear palsy. *J Neurol Neurosurg Psychiatry* 1974;37:121–130.
2. Anderer P, Semlitsch HV, Saletu B. Multichannel auditory event-related brain potentials: effects of normal aging on the scalp distribution of N1, P2, N2, and P300 latencies and amplitudes. *Electroencephalogr Clin Neurophysiol* 1996;99:458–472.
3. Ball SS, Marsh JT, Schubarth G, et al. Longitudinal P300 latency changes in Alzheimer's disease. *J Gerontol* 1989;44:M195–M200.
4. Baribeau-Braun J, Picton TW, Gosselin JY. Schizophrenia: a neurophysiological evaluation of abnormal information processing. *Science* 1983;219:874–876.
5. Brecher M, Begleiter H. Event-related brain potentials to high incentive stimuli in unmedicated schizophrenics. *Biol Psychiatry* 1983;18:661–674.
6. Brown WS, Marsh JT, LaRue A. Event-related potentials in psychiatry: differentiating depression and dementia in the elderly. *Bull Los Angeles Neurol Soc* 1982;47:91–107.
7. Brown WS, Marsh JT, LaRue A. Exponential electrophysiological aging: P3 latency. *Electroencephalogr Clin Neurophysiol* 1983;55:277–285.
8. Cohen J, Polich J. On the number of trials needed for P300. *Int J Psychophysiol* 1997;25: 249–255.
9. Cooper R, Ossilton JW, Shaw JC. *EEG technology*, 3rd ed. London: Butterworth-Heinemann, 1980.
10. Courchesne E. Neurophysiological correlates of cognitive development: changes in long-latency event-related potentials from childhood to adulthood. *Electroencephalogr Clin Neurophysiol* 1978;45:468–482.
11. Cummings JL, Benson DF. Subcortical dementia: review of an emerging concept. *Arch Neurol* 1984;41:874–879.
12. Daruna JH, Nelson AV, Green JB. Unilateral temporal lobe lesions alter P300 scalp topography. *Int J Neurosci* 1989;46:243–247.
13. Davis H, Zerlin S. Acoustic relations of the human vertex potential. *J Acoust Soc Am* 1966;39:109–116.
14. Donchin E, Ritter W, McCallum WC. Cognitive psychophysiology: the endogenous components of the ERP. In: Callaway E, Tueting P, Koslow S, eds. *Brain event-related potentials in man*. San Diego: Academic Press, 1978:349–411.
15. Duncan-Johnson CC. P300 latency: a new metric of information processing. *Psychophysiology* 1981;18:207–215.
16. Duncan-Johnson CC, Donchin E. On quantifying surprise: the variation of event-related potentials with subjective probability. *Psychophysiology* 1977;14:456–467.
17. Ebmeier KP, Potter DD, Cochrane RHB, et al. Lower-bandpass filter frequency in P3 experiments: a possible cause for divergent results in schizophrenia research. *Biol Psychiatry* 1990;27:667–670.
18. Elberling C, Bak C, Kofoed B, et al. Magnetic auditory responses from the human brain: a peliminary report. *Scand Audiol* 1980;9:185–190.
19. Elmasian B, Neville H, Woods D, et al. Event-related brain potentials are different in individuals at high risk and low risk for developing alcoholism. *Proc Natl Acad Sci U S A* 1982;79:7900–7903.
20. Emmerson RY, Dustman RE, Shearer DE, et al. P3 latency and symbol digit performance correlations in aging. *Exp Aging Res* 1989;151:151–159.
21. Fitzgerald PG, Picton TW. The effects of probability and discriminability on the evoked potentials to unpredictable stimuli. *Ann N Y Acad Sci* 1984;425:199–203.
22. Ford JM, Roth WT, Dirks SJ, et al. Evoked potential correlates of signal recognition between and within modalities. *Science* 1973;181:465–466.
23. Geisler MW, Polich J. P300 and time of day circadian rhythms, food intake, and body temperature. *Biol Psychol* 1990;31:117–136.
24. Goodin DS. Electrophysioiogic evaluation of dementia. *Neurol Clin* 1985;3:633–647.
25. Goodin DS. Clinical utility of long latency 'cognitive' event-related potentials (P3): the pros. *Electroencephalogr Clin Neurophysiol* 1990;76:2–5.
26. Goodin DS: Electrophysiological correlates of dementia in Parkinson's disease. In: Huber SJ, Cummings JL, eds. *Neurobehavior of Parkinson's disease*. New York: Oxford University Press, 1992:199–213.
27. Goodin DS, Aminoff MJ. The relationship between the evoked potential and brain events in sensory discrimination and motor response. *Brain* 1984;107:241–251.
28. Goodin DS, Aminoff MJ. Electrophysiological differences between subtypes of dementia. *Brain* 1986;109:1103–1113.
29. Goodin DS, Aminoff MJ. Electrophysiological differences between demented and non-demented patients with Parkinson's disease. *Ann Neurol* 1987;21:90–94.
30. Goodin DS, Aminoff MJ. Event-related potentials and their relationship to discrimination and response in simple and choice reaction tasks. *J Clin Neurophysiol* 1998;15:34–43.
31. Goodin DS, Aminoff MJ, Chequer RS. The effect of different high-pass filters on the long latency event-related potentials in normal subjects and individuals infected with human immunodeficiency virus. *J Clin Neurophysiol* 1992;9:97–104.
32. Goodin DS, Aminoff MJ, Chequer RS, et al. Response compatibility and the relationship between event-related potentials and the timing of a motor response *J Neurophysiol* 1996; 76:3705–3713.
33. Goodin DS, Aminoff MJ, Chernoff DN, et al. Long latency event-related potentials in patients infected with human immunodeficiency virus. *Ann Neurol* 1990;27:414–419.
34. Goodin DS, Aminoff MJ, Mantle MM. Sensory discrimination and its relationship to cerebral processing of infrequent stimuli. *Can J Neurol Sci* 1987;14:642–648.
35. Goodin DS, Aminoff MJ, Shefrin SL. The organization of sensory discrimination and response selection in choice and nonchoice conditions: a study using cerebral evoked potentials. *J Neurophysiol* 1990;64:1270–1281.
36. Goodin DS, Squires KC, Henderson BH, et al. Age-related variations in evoked potentials to auditory stimuli in normal human subjects. *Electroencephalogr Clin Neurophysiol* 1978;44: 447–458.
37. Goodin DS, Squires KC, Henderson BH, et al. An early event-related cortical potential. *Psychophysiology* 1978;15:360–365.

38. Goodin DS, Squires KC, Starr A. Long latency event-related components of the auditory evoked potential in dementia. *Brain* 1978;101:635–648.

39. Goodin DS, Squires KC, Starr A. Variations in early and late event-related components of the auditory evoked potential with task difficulty. *Electroencephalogr Clin Neurophysiol* 1983;55:680–686.

40. Goodin DS, Starr A, Chippendale T, et al. Sequential changes in the P3 component of the auditory evoked potential in confusional states and dementing illnesses. *Neurology* 1983;33:1215–1218.

41. Gordon E, Kraiuhin C, Harris A, et al. The differential diagnosis of dementia using P300 latency. *Biol Psychiatry* 1986;21:1123–1132.

42. Halgren E, Squires NK, Wilson CL, et al. Endogenous potentials generated in the human hippocampal formation amygdala by infrequent events. *Science* 1980;210:803–805.

43. Hansen JC, Hillyard SA. Endogenous brain potentials associated with selective auditory attention. *Electroencephalogr Clin Neurophysiol* 1980;49:277–290.

44. Hari R, Aittoniemi K, Jarvinen ML, et al. Auditory evoked transient and sustained magnetic fields of the human brain. *Exp Brain Res* 1980;40:237–240.

45. Hill SY, Steinhauer S, Park J, et al. Event-related potential characteristics in children of alcoholics from high density families. *Alcohol Clin Exp Res* 1990;14:6–16.

46. Hillyard SA, Kutas M. Electrophysiology of cognitive processing. *Annu Rev Psychol* 1983;34:33–61.

47. Hillyard SA, Wood DL. Electrophysiological analysis of human brain function. In: Gazzaniga MS, ed. *Handbook of behavioral neurobiology*. New York: Plenum Publishing, 1979:345–377.

48. Karniski W, Blair RC. Topographical and temporal stability of the P300. *Electroencephalogr Clin Neurophysiol* 1989;72:373–383.

49. Kiloh LG. The investigation of dementia: results in 200 consecutive admissions. *Lancet* 1981;1:824–827.

50. Kutas M, Hillyard SA. Reading senseless sentences: brain potentials reflect semantic incongruity. *Science* 1980;207:203–205.

51. Kutas M, McCarthy G, Donchin E. Augmenting mental chronometry: the P300 as a measure of stimulus evaluation time. *Science* 1977;197:792–795.

52. Leppler JG, Greenberg HJ. The P3 potential and its clinical usefulness in the objective classification of dementia. *Cortex* 1984;20:427–433.

53. Levit RA, Sutton S, Zubin J. Evoked potential correlates of information processing in psychiatric patients. *Psychol Med* 1973;3:487–494.

54. Lins OG, Picton TW, Berg P, et al. Ocular artifacts in recording EEG and event-related potentials. II: source dipoles and source components. *Brain Topogr* 1993;6:65–78.

55. Louza MR, Maurer K: Differences between paranoid and non-paranoid schizophrenic patients on the somatosensory P300 event-related potential. *Neuropsychobiology* 1989;21:59–66.

56. Mayeux R, Stern Y, Rosen J, et al. Is "subcortical dementia" a recognizable clinical entity? *Ann Neurol* 1983;14:278–283.

57. McCarthy G, Donchin E. A metric for thought: a comparison of P300 latency and reaction time. *Science* 1981;211:77–80.

58. Naatanen R, Michie PT. Early selective attention effects on the evoked potential: a critical review and reinterpretation. *Biol Psychol* 1979;8:81–136.

59. Ortiz TA, Goodin DS, Aminoff MJ. Neural processing in a three-choice reaction time task: a study using cerebral evoked potentials and single trial analysis. *J Neurophysiol* 1993;69:1499–1512.

60. Papanicolaou AC, Baumann SB, Rogers RL, et al. Localization of auditory response sources using magnetoencephalography and magnetic resonance imaging. *Arch Neurol* 1990;47:33–37.

61. Pass HL, Korman R, Salzman LF, et al. The late positive component of the evoked response in acute schizophrenics during a test of sustained attention. *Biol Psychiatry* 1980;15:9–20.

62. Patterson JV, Michalewski JH, Starr A. Latency variability of the components of auditory event-related potentials to infrequent stimuli in aging, Alzheimer-type dementia, and depression. *Electroencephalogr Clin Neurophysiol* 1988;71:450–460.

63. Pfefferbaum A, Ford JM, Wenegrat BG, et al. Clinical applications of the P3 component of event-related potentials: I. Normal aging. *Electroencephalogr Clin Neurophysiol* 1984;59:85–103.

64. Pfefferbaum A, Horvath TB, Roth WT, et al. Event-related potential changes in chronic alcoholics. *Electroencephalogr Clin Neurophysiol* 1979;47:637–647.

65. Pfefferbaum A, Wenegrat BG, Ford JM, et al. Clinical application of the P3 component of event-related potentials: II, Dementia, depression and schizophrenia. *Electroencephalogr Clin Neurophysiol* 1984;59:104–124.

66. Picton TW, Hillyard SA. Human auditory evoked potentials: II. Effects of attention. *Electroencephalogr Clin Neurophysiol* 1974;36:191–199.

67. Picton TW, Hillyard SA, Krausz HL, et al. Human auditory evoked potentials: I. Evaluation of components. *Electroencephalogr Clin Neurophysiol* 1974;36:179–190.

68. Picton TW, Stuss DT, Champagne SC, Nelson RF. The effects of age on the human event-related potential. *Psychophysiology* 1984;21:312–326.

69. Polich J. Meta-analysis of P300 normative aging studies. *Psychophysiol* 1996;33:334–353.

70. Polich J. EEG and ERP assessment of normal aging. *Electroencephalogr Clin Neurophysiol* 1997;104:244–256.

71. Polich J. On the relationship between EEG and P300: individual differences, aging, and ultradian rhythms. *Int J Psychophysiol* 1997;26:299–317.

72. Polich J. P300 clinical utility and control of variability. *J Clin Neurophysiol* 1998;15:14–33.

73. Polich J, Bondurant T. P300 sequence effects, probability, and interstimulus interval. *Physiol Behav* 1997;61:843–849.

74. Polich J, Ehlers CL, Otis S, et al. P300 latency reflects the degree of cognitive decline in dementing illness. *Electroencephalogr Clin Neurophysiol* 1986;63:138–144.

75. Polich J, Kok A. Cognitive and biological determinants of P300: an integrative review. *Biol Psychol* 1995;41:103–146.

76. Polich J, Starr A. Evoked potentials in aging. In: Albert ML, ed. *Clinical neurology of aging*. New York: Oxford University Press, 1984:149–177.

77. Porjesz B, Begleiter H. Human evoked brain potentials and alcohol. *Alcohol Clin Exp Res* 1981;5:304–317.

78. Porjesz B, Begleiter H. Genetic basis of the event-related potentials and their relationship to alcoholism and alcohol use. *J Clin Neurophysiol* 1998;15:44–57.

79. Porjesz B, Begleiter H, Samuelly I. Cognitive deficits in chronic alcoholics and elderly subjects assessed by evoked brain potentials. *Acta Psychiatr Scand Suppl* 1980;286:15–29.

80. Puce A, Donnan GA, Bladin PF. Comparative effects of age on the limbic and scalp P3. *Electroencephalogr Clin Neurophysiol* 1989;74:385–393.

81. Renault B, Ragot R, Lesevre N, et al. Onset and offset of brain events as indices of mental chronometry. *Science* 1982;215:1413–1415.

82. Rif J, Hari R, Hamalainen MS, et al. Auditory attention affects two different areas in the human supratemporal cortex. *Electroencephalogr Clin Neuroplysiol* 1991;79:464–472.

83. Ritter W, Ford JM, Gaillard AWK, et al. Cognition and event-related potentials: I. The relation of negative potentials and cognitive processes. *Ann N Y Acad Sci* 1984;425:24–38.

84. Ritter W, Simson R, Vaughan HG Jr, et al. A brain event related to the making of a sensory discrimination. *Science* 1979;203:1358–1361.

85. Ritter W, Simson R, Vaughan HG Jr, et al. Manipulation of event-related potential manifestations of information processing stages. *Science* 1982;218:909–911.

86. Roth WT, Cannon EH. Some features of the auditory evoked response in schizophrenics. *Arch Gen Psychiatry* 1972;27:466–471.

87. Roth WT, Pfefferbaum A, Horvath TB, et al. P3 reduction in auditory evoked potentials of schizophrenics. *Electroencephalogr Clin Neurophysiol* 1980;49:497–505.

88. Roth WT, Tinklenberg JR, Kopell BS. Ethanol and marihuana effects on event-related potentials in a memory retrieval paradigm. *Electroencephalogr Clin Neurophysiol* 1977;42:381–388.

89. Rugg MD, Roberts RC, Potter DD, et al. Endogenous event-related potentials from sphenoidal electrodes. *Electroencephalogr Clin Neurophysiol* 1990;76:331–338.

90. Shagass C, Roemar RK, Struamanis JJ, et al. Evoked potential correlates of psychosis. *Biol Psychiatry* 1978;13:163–184.

91. Siedenberg R, Goodin DS, Aminoff MJ, et al. Comparison of late components in the simultaneously recorded event-related electrical potentials and event-related magnetic fields. *Electroencephalogr Clin Neurophysiol* 1996;96:191–197.

92. Simson R, Vaughan HG Jr, Ritter W. The scalp topography of potentials associated with missing visual and auditory stimuli. *Electroencephalogr Clin Neurophysiol* 1976;40:33–42.

93. Sklare DA, Lynn GE. Latency of the P3 event-related potential: normative aspects and within subject variability. *Electroencephalogr Clin Neuroplysiol* 1984;59:420–424.

94. Slaets JPJ, Fortgens C. On the value of P300 event-related potentials in the differential diagnosis of dementia. *Br J Psychiatry* 1984;145:652–656.

95. Smith ME, Halgren E, Sokolik M, et al. The intracrainal topography of the P3 event-related potential elicited during auditory oddball. *Electroencephalogr Clin Neurophysiol* 1990;76:235–248.

96. Snyder E, Hillyard SA, Galambos R. Similarities and differences among the P3 waves to detected signals in three modalities. *Psychophysiology* 1980;17:112–122.

97. Squires KC, Chippendale TJ, Wrege KS, et al. Electrophysiological assessment of mental function in aging and dementia. In: Poon LW, ed. *Aging in the 1980s*. Washington, DC: American Psychological Association, 1980:125–134.

98. Squires NK, Squires KC, Hillyard SA. Two varieties of long-latency positive waves evoked by unpredictable auditory stimuli in man. *Electroencephalogr Clin Neurophysiol* 1975;38: 387–401.

99. St. Clair DM, Blackwood DHR, Christie JE. P3 and other long latency auditory evoked potentials in presenile dementia Alzheimer type and alcoholic Korsakoff syndrome. *Br J Psychiatry* 1985;147:702–706.

100. Stuss DT, Picton TW. Neurophysiological correlates of human concept formation. *Behav Biol* 1978;23:135–162.

101. Sutton S, Braren M, Zubin J, et al. Evoked potential correlates of stimulus uncertainty. *Science* 1965;150:1187–1188.

102. Sutton S, Ruchkin DS. The late positive complex: advances and new problems. *Ann N Y Acad Sci* 1984;425:1–23.

103. Sutton S, Tueting P, Zubin J, et al. Information delivery and the sensory evoked potential. *Science* 1967;155:1436–1439.

104. Syndulko K, Hansch EC, Cohen SN, et al. Long latency event-related potentials in normal aging and dementia. In: Courjon J, Mauguiere F, Revol M, eds. *Clinical application of evoked potentials in neurology*. New York: Raven Press, 1982:279–285.

105. Terry R. Dementia: a brief and selected review. *Arch Neurol* 1976;33:1–4.

106. Verleger R. On the utility of P3 latency as an index of mental chronometry. *Psychophysiology* 1997;34:131–156.

107. Wells CE. Diagnostic evaluation and treatment in dementia. In: Wells CE, ed. *Contemporary neurology series. Vol 15. Dementia*. Philadelphia: FA Davis Co, 1978:247–276.

108. Wood CC, Allison T, Goff WR, et al. On the neural origins of P300 in man. *Prog Brain Res* 1980;54:51–56.

109. Yingling CD, Hosobuchi Y. Subcortical correlate of P300 in man. *Electroencephalogr Clin Neurophysiol* 1984;59:72–76.

Chapter 31

Intraoperative Monitoring

Ronald G. Emerson and David C. Adams

Neurophysiological techniques have traditionally been used to detect relatively static structural or functional disturbances of the nervous system: for example, demyelinative and mass lesions, encephalopathies, and epileptic disorders. Even when employed in connection with evolving disease processes, electroencephalograms (EEGs) and evoked potentials (Eps) were classically recorded at infrequent intervals, providing only "snapshot" measurements. However, in contrast to other, imaging-based technologies, electrophysiological measures are uniquely well suited to providing almost real-time measures of nervous system function. For this reason, continuous neurophysiological monitoring is now routinely employed intraoperatively during surgical procedures, which entail risk of nervous system injury. For example, intraoperative monitoring is now considered a standard of care during carotid endarterectomy, correction of scoliosis, and resection of acoustic nerve tumors.

Monitoring can reduce the risk of intraoperative neurological damage in two ways: First, monitoring enables detection of neurological injury at a time when it can be reversed or minimized. During scoliosis surgery, for example, deteriorating long tract function can be detected by somatosensory evoked potential (SEP) and motor evoked potential (MEP) monitoring early enough to avert permanent spinal cord damage. Second, neurophysiological techniques can distinguish vital neural structures that may otherwise be difficult to distinguish from surrounding tissue. For example, the rolandic fissure is commonly identified through SEP monitoring during surgery involving cortical resection.

The evolution of intraoperative neurophysiological monitoring strategies has resulted from the collaborative efforts of neurophysiologists, anesthesiologists, and surgeons. Neurophysiologists have modified existing techniques and developed new methods and interpretative strategies for use in the operating room. Anesthesiologists have developed anesthetic techniques that facilitate neurophysiological monitoring. Surgeons have learned how to best incorporate and appropriately respond to neurophysiological information in a real-time surgical context.

Intraoperative neurophysiological monitoring continues to evolve with a seemingly continuous stream of literature describing innovative and imaginative approaches to various clinical circumstances. This chapter illustrates how standard diagnostic laboratory techniques have been extended to the intraoperative setting. It serves as an introduction to intraoperative monitoring as it is currently employed rather than as an instruction manual or exhaustive reference.

MONITORING SPINAL CORD FUNCTION

Intraoperative EP monitoring of long tract function is commonly employed during procedures such as spine surgery, neuroradiological procedures, brainstem surgery, and aortic surgery, in which motor and sensory tracts are placed at risk (13,26,32,69,84,89,114,128). There are early reports of the failure of EP monitoring to detect neurological injury (58,34,75). However, at least some of these failures are traceable to human errors, such as monitoring an inappropriate EP, not monitoring for a long enough period, and not recognizing artifact, rather than to inherent limitations of EP monitoring.

In the past, the "wake-up" test (124) was used to verify spinal cord integrity during surgery. However, EP monitoring offers important advantages over the wake-up test. A review of 1,168 scoliosis operations at The Royal Orthopedic Hospital concluded that EP monitoring was more sensitive than the wake-up test (32). In contrast to EP monitoring, the wake-up test provides only a single snapshot of spinal cord integrity and exposes the patient to additional risks, including dislodgment of instrumentation, laminar fractures, venous air embolism, and accidental extubation (9).

Although SEPs are direct measures of posterior column function and MEPs depend on the integrity of descending motor pathways, each modality alone serves as a good measure of spinal cord integrity. Graded changes in both MEPs and SEPs accompany spinal cord injury produced by ischemia, compression, and blunt trauma (8,20,21,24,28,31,59,60,64,65,68,90,105,112). Intraoperative spinal cord compression generally results in degradation of both MEP and SEP signals (82). Concurrent MEP and SEP recording provides an added level of security, inasmuch as, if technical difficulties compromise one monitoring modality, the other is likely to continue functioning. In this manner, SEPs and MEPs are complementary, and optimal monitoring of long tract function ideally entails concurrent recording of both.

However, because SEPs and MEPs are mediated by distinct anatomical pathways, surgical injury to either the motor or sensory system can occur independently (10,11,25,120,131). Their relatively tenuous vascular supply, provided by the anterior spinal artery with large watershed regions along its length, makes the motor tracts particularly vulnerable to ischemia resulting from hypotension, potentially producing loss of motor function without altered SEPs (119,122,131). Monitoring both MEPs and SEPs allows detection of the occasional insult that selectively affects either motor or sensory long tracts separately.

Somatosensory Evoked Potential Monitoring

Although it is similar to techniques employed in the diagnostic laboratory, certain features of intraoperative SEP recording are unique. For example, although many anesthetic agents can attenuate cortical SEP components, making them difficult to record, the use of neuromuscular blocking agents facilitates the recording of subcortical components.

The montages used for recording SEPs in the diagnostic laboratory and in the operating room are determined by the relatively restricted distribution of the primary cortical components and the widespread topography of the subcortical SEP components. Because the primary cortical response for median nerve SEPs, the $N\overline{20}$ response, is confined to the centroparietal scalp opposite the stimulated arm, a bipolar "scalp-to-scalp" recording, between symmetrical centroparietal electrodes, detects it in isolation. However, because the subcortical $P\overline{14}$ and $N\overline{18}$ median nerve responses are widely and symmetrically distributed, a referential "scalp-to-noncephalic" recording, by a scalp electrode ipsilateral to the stimulated median nerve, detects mainly subcortical far-field potentials (see Chapter 29, Figs. 29.5 and 29.29). The posterior tibial nerve SEP has a more complex topography. Although the primary cortical $P\overline{38}$ response is present at the vertex but lateralized to the scalp *ipsilateral* to the stimulated leg, there is considerable individual variation in the "normal" $P\overline{38}$ scalp topography. Thus, it is suggested that two channels, such as Cz-Fpz and C3/4$_{ipsilateral}$-Fpz, be used to reliably record $P\overline{38}$ in all patients. A referential Fpz-to-noncephalic derivation detects the subcortical $P\overline{31}$ and $P\overline{34}$ components in isolation (5).

In general, the cortical $N\overline{20}$ and $P\overline{38}$ responses are easily recorded in awake or lightly sedated patients in the diagnostic laboratory. However, changes in the cortical SEP amplitude and latency are often observed while patients are under general anesthesia. This effect typically is most pronounced in infants and young children (42), in lower extremity SEP recordings, and when halogenated inhalational agents, such as isoflurane and halothane, are used (12,38,94,110). Similar but less prominent effects are also seen with most other anesthetic agents, including narcotics, benzodiazepines, and barbiturates (54,72,94). For these reasons, cortical SEPs are sometimes difficult to record intraoperatively and are insufficiently stable to use for monitoring. Subcortical far-field signals (P$\overline{14}$, P$\overline{31}$), in contrast, are much less affected by anesthetic agents and are often preferred as indicators of spinal cord function (110) (Fig. 31.1).

In the diagnostic laboratory, subcortical far-field potentials can be very difficult to record. Noncephalic referential recordings are often contaminated by movement and muscle related artifacts, particularly in awake patients. In the operating room, the recording of far-field potentials is facilitated by the use of neuromuscular blocking agents, which significantly reduce muscle-related noise (Fig. 31.2).

On occasion, particularly in patients with preexisting neurological deficits, only cortical SEP signals may be recordable, despite the use of neuromuscular blocking agents. In these cases, it is important to limit the use of

anesthetic agents that attenuate cortical components. Small variations in the doses of anesthetic drugs, particularly halogenated inhalational agents, can produce changes in SEP amplitude that mimic surgical injury. Etomidate, an intravenous anesthetic agent that increases the amplitude of cortical SEP components, has occasionally been used to augment the cortical response (Fig. 31.3; however, there is a possibility that etomidate could mask intraoperative SEP changes (72).

Surgical spinal cord injury typically results in loss of EP amplitude and degradation in the morphological appearance of the signal. Prolonged latencies tend to be less prominent and consistent findings (32,86). Thus, strategies for intraoperative SEP interpretation differ from those used in standard testing, which rely primarily on response latencies (5). Furthermore, intraoperative SEPs are compared primarily with the patient's baseline values, rather than with those of normative controls. Two general approaches have been developed for intraoperative interpretation of SEP recordings. One is to adopt predefined, somewhat arbitrary limits (typically a 50% decrement

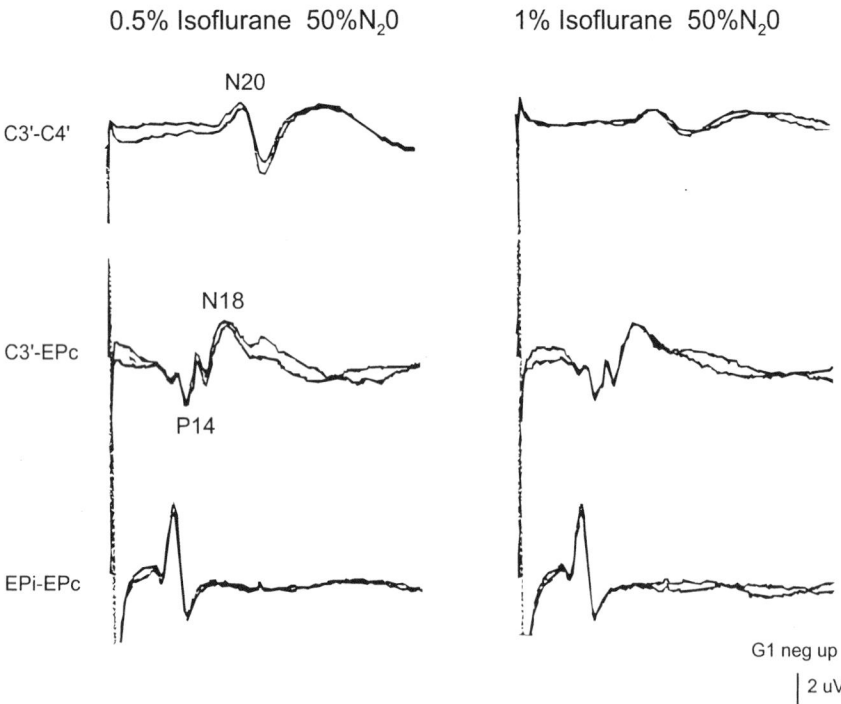

FIG. 31.1. Median SSEP recorded in a patient receiving isoflurane and nitrous oxide. Increasing the concentration of isoflurane from 0.5% to 1% causes attenuation of the N$\overline{20}$ cortical response but does not alter the subcortical N$\overline{18}$ potential. In this and subsequent figures, EPi and EPc refer to electrode locations over Erb's points, ipsilateral and contralateral to the stimulated nerve. C3' and C4' designate electrode locations halfway between C3 and P3 and halfway between C4 and P4, respectively.

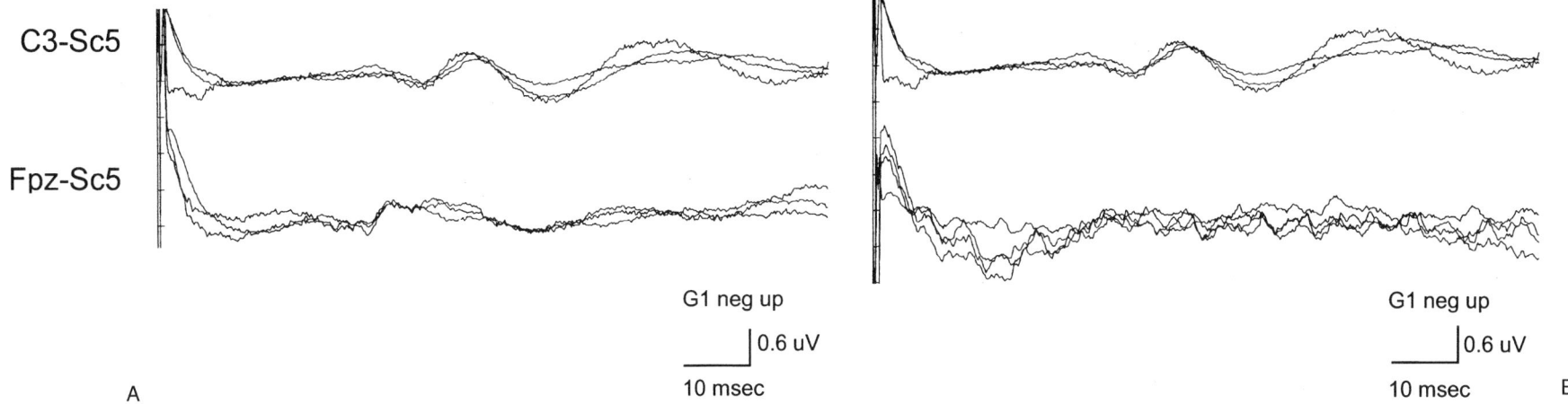

C3-Sc5

Fpz-Sc5

G1 neg up

0.6 uV

10 msec

A

G1 neg up

0.6 uV

10 msec

B

FIG. 31.2. Posterior tibial SSEP recorded during nitrous oxide/fentanyl anesthesia with **(A)** and without **(B)** neuromuscular blockade. In panel *A,* a vecuronium infusion eliminates muscle-related artifact and improves the quality of the subcortical recording (Fpz-SC5). SC5 denotes an recording site over the fifth cervical vertebra.

in amplitude or a 10% increase in latency), beyond which there is considered to be substantial risk of neurological insult, and to inform the surgeon when those limits are surpassed. An alternative approach is to inform the surgeon of changes, even if small, in SEP amplitude, latency, and morphology, that exceed the baseline variability in the patient's recordings. Because this approach enables the surgeon to better identify the cause of these changes and to use that information to decide whether to take a wait-and-see approach or to act immediately (78), the authors favor its use.

The implications of SEP deterioration depend on the type of surgery being performed. For example, in the absence of corrective intervention, loss of SEP amplitude during correction of spinal deformities is ominous and carries a high risk of serious neurological injury (32). On the other hand, loss of SEP amplitude during intramedullary surgery is predictive of neurological deficits in the immediate postoperative period but is less predictive of the ultimate outcome (52,126). It may be that, in these cases, surgical manipulation of the spinal cord produces transient conduction block without producing permanent axonal injury (126). Furthermore, although the stability of SEPs during intramedullary surgery provides reassurance that neurological injury has not occurred, sudden loss of SEPs does not necessarily indicate permanent injury (52).

Motor Evoked Potential Monitoring

It has long been recognized that the motor cortex can be activated by electrical stimulation (93), but the application of motor system stimulation to intraoperative monitoring is a relatively recent development. Currently, intraoperative MEP monitoring is routine at some centers (44,82,115), although the techniques employed are not yet uniform. Either electrical or magnetic transcranial stimulation or electrical spinal cord stimulation can be used to elicit the MEP response. The "motor" response may be a compound nerve action potential recorded over the spinal cord (13,36) or over peripheral nerve (88), or it may be a compound muscle action potential (CMAP) recorded over an appropriate distal muscle (2).

Transcranial stimulation allows relatively selective activation of spinal motor pathways because intervening synapses prevent retrograde firing of sensory tracts. Direct spinal stimulation, in contrast, activates sensory as well as motor pathways. Furthermore, transcranial techniques permit stimulating electrodes to remain outside of the surgical field. Transcranial stimulation may either fire pyramidal neurons directly or activate cortical interneurons, which then fire pyramidal cells. Direct pyramidal stimulation produces the earlier,

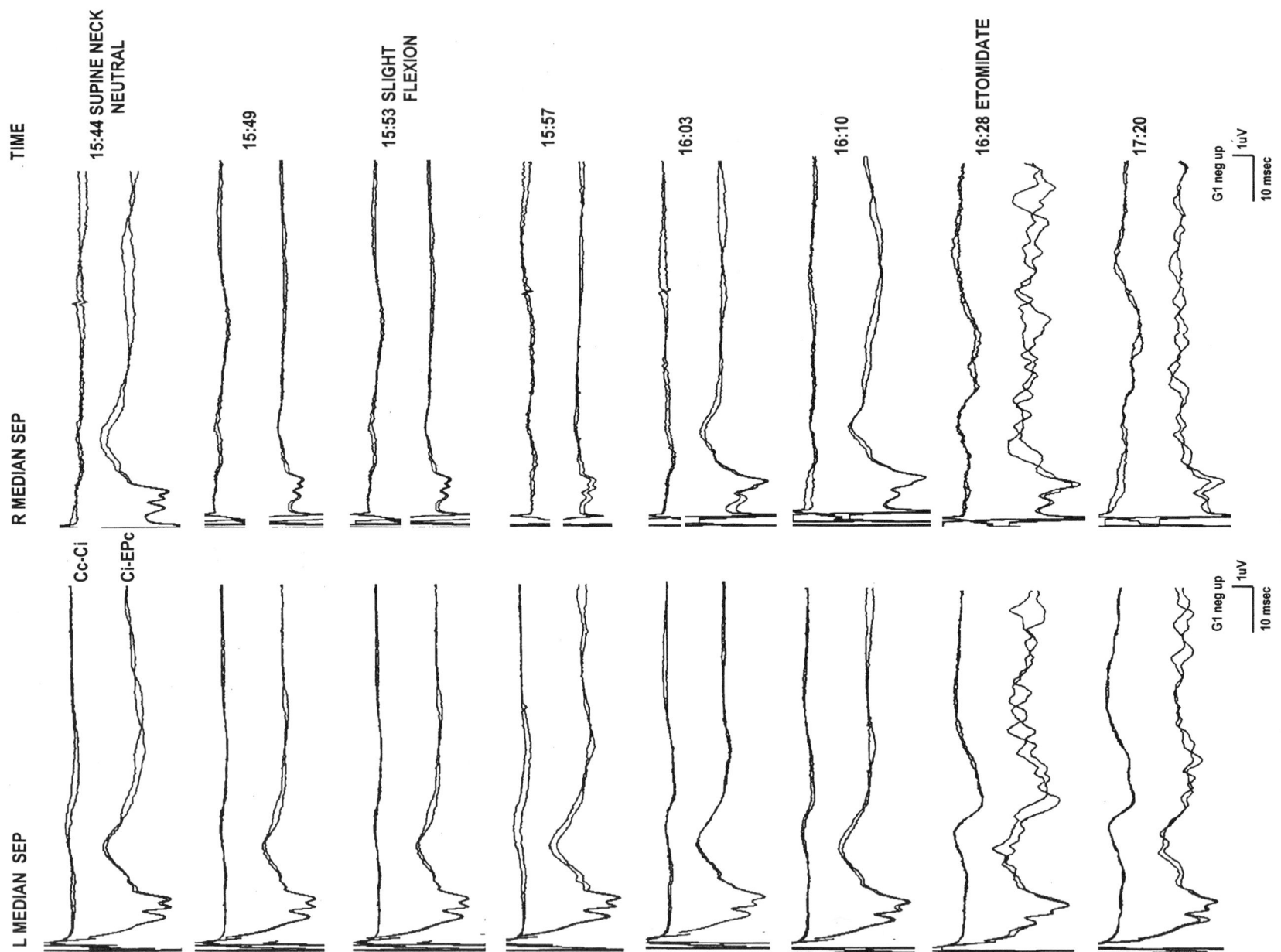

more stable components of the MEP known as D waves, whereas indirect pyramidal activation results in the longer latency, less stable I waves (4,107). Whereas transcranial electrical stimulation results in both D and I waves, magnetic stimulation generally elicits only I waves (73).

Magnetically elicited transcranial motor evoked potentials (tcm-MEPs) are of limited use for intraoperative monitoring because they are significantly attenuated by most commonly used anesthetics (33,48,50) and vary widely with minor alterations in coil position (Fig. 31.4) (1). Although advances in magnetic coil design and stimulus parameters, such as the use of paired or trains of stimuli, may improve the reliability of tcm-MEPs (123), tcm-MEPs are currently not sufficiently reliable for intraoperative use. Transcranial magnetic stimulation, in contrast, is easily accomplished in awake subjects and it may have a role in the preoperative assessment of patients with spinal cord lesions.

Transcranial electrical motor evoked potentials (tce-MEPs) are also substantially attenuated by the commonly used inhalational anesthetics (39,49,130), generally necessitating the use of intravenous anesthetic techniques (91). Although special high-voltage stimulators have been developed for transcranial stimulation (13,46,129), a method allowing standard SEP stimulators to be used for transcranial stimulation under general anesthesia has been introduced. Rather than a single high-voltage pulse, a series of lower voltage pulses are rapidly delivered (47,91). There is a marked increase in amplitude and a reduction in latency of the tce-MEP at interstimulus intervals of 1 to 3 milliseconds, which presumably reflect temporal summation at cortical or spinal levels (91) (Fig. 31.5).

An alternative MEP technique, suitable for cases in which the region at risk is at or below the upper thoracic cord, entails electrical stimulation of the spinal cord with CMAPs monitored over appropriate muscles. For stimulation, needle electrodes are positioned, either transcutaneously or through the surgical exposure, near the ligamentum flavum at two adjacent vertebral levels (Fig. 31.6). Partial neuromuscular blockade produced by an infusion

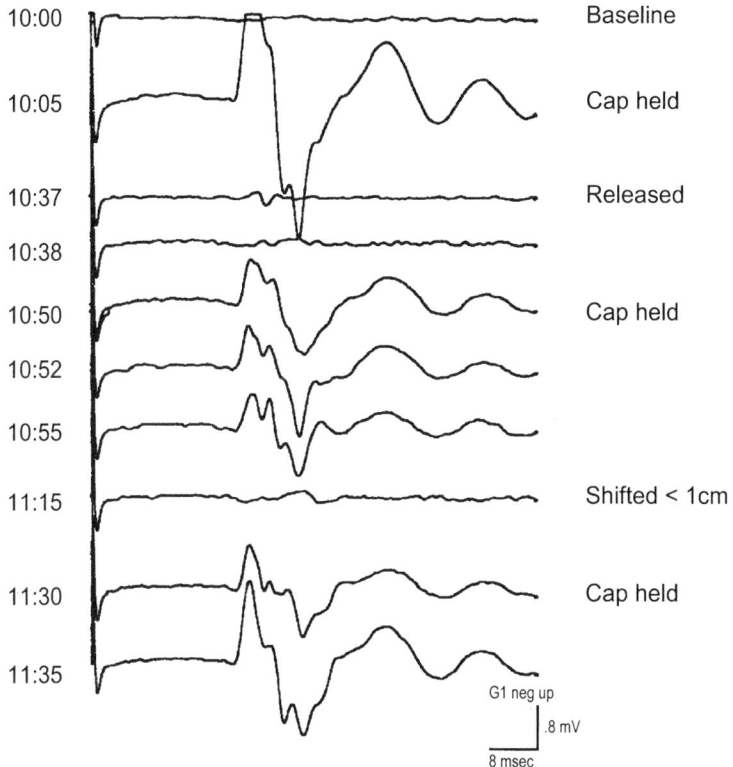

FIG. 31.4. Small movements of the stimulating "skull cap" coil produce large changes in transcranial motor evoked potentials recorded from quadriceps during nitrous oxide/fentanyl anesthesia.

FIG. 31.3. A series of median SSEPs recorded during myringotomy in preparation for cleft palate repair in a 3-year-old child with achondroplasia. Halothane was administered by mask. Baseline recordings showed an intact subcortical response (Ci-Epc) bilaterally. The very low voltage N20 cortical response (Cc-Ci) is a normal finding in a young child receiving a halogenated anesthetic agent. On the right, N18 was lost after slight neck flexion and returned when the head was moved to the neutral position. The cleft palate repair was deferred, and during the remainder of the procedure, etomidate was used to facilitate monitoring of the cortical N20. The patient awoke with no neurological deficits.

Double pulses 300V

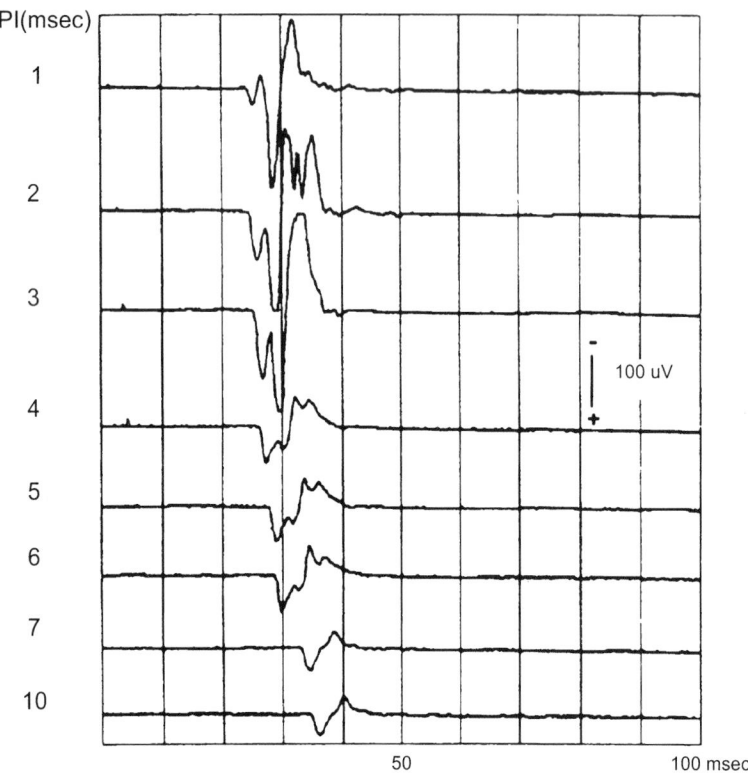

FIG. 31.5. Effect of interpulse interval (IPI) on transcranial electrical motor evoked potentials (MEPs) recorded from abductor digit minimi using paired pulses. Interpeak intervals of less than 2 milliseconds produced the highest amplitude and shortest latency MEPs. (From Jones et al, 1966, with permission).

of non-depolarizing muscle relaxant eliminates movements that would interfere with surgery but allows CMAPs to be easily recorded, even when the patient has been given potent inhalational anesthetic drugs (2). Stimulation is achieved with single pulses, 10 to 40 mA and 0.1 to 0.3 milliseconds in duration, or with brief trains of similar pulses (2,74). Typically, 2 to 20 such stimuli delivered at 0.5 Hz are averaged, producing an updated MEP every few seconds. As with transcranial electrical stimulation, several pulses delivered in rapid succession may produce higher amplitude MEPs and help

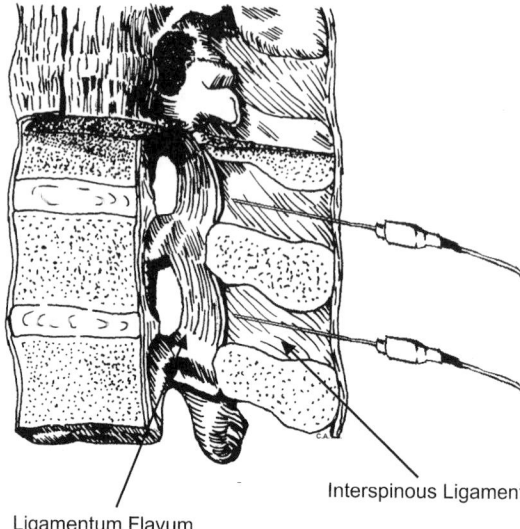

FIG. 31.6. For spinal cord stimulation, electrode tips lie close to the ligamentum flavum at two adjacent vertebral levels.

overcome the effects of anesthetic agents (74). Although it is possible to record "neurogenic motor evoked potentials" over mixed nerve or spinal cord, these recordings represent a composite of both orthodromic motor signals and antidromic sensory signals (88). It has been suggested that, under certain circumstances, antidromic sensory volleys produced by direct stimulation for spinal cord monitoring could activate motor neurons in the ventral horn (95,116). In cats anesthetized with ketamine, Mochida et al. (74) demonstrated that dorsal column stimulation could abolish CMAPs to single pulse spinal cord stimulation. However, they observed that paired pulses produced much larger CMAPs that were not affected by dorsal column section, and they concluded that these were mediated by spinal motor pathways. Furthermore, potent inhalational agents known to suppress spinal reflexes (103) would probably diminish any contribution of antidromic sensory volley. An important benefit of recording CMAPs is that they incorporate the ventral gray matter of the spinal cord in the monitored pathway, which is a site of potential operative injury (2,18,60).

Figure 31.7 illustrates a case in which permanent paraplegia was probably prevented by MEP and SEP monitoring during correction of severe

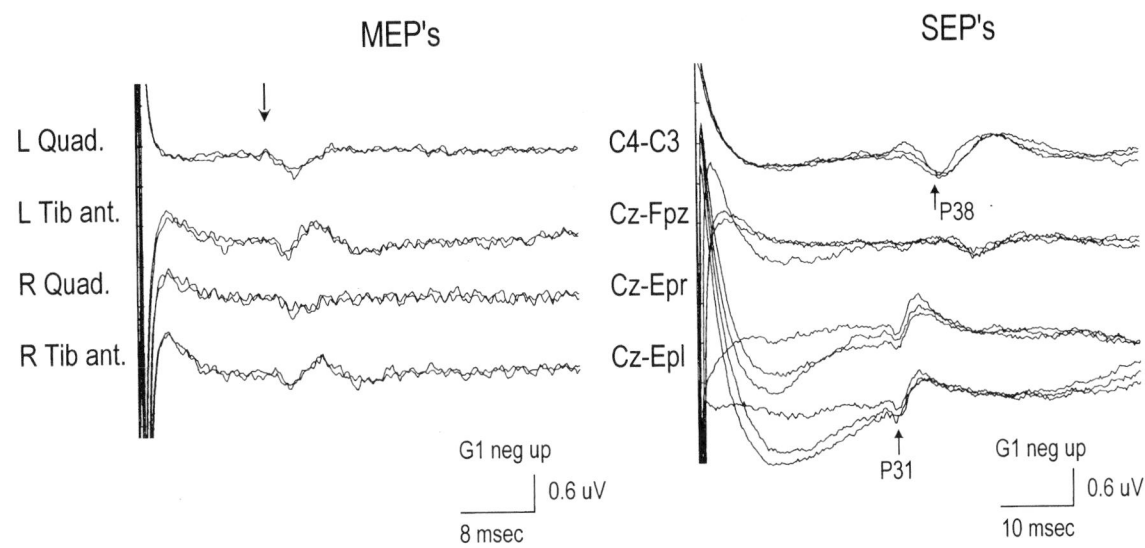

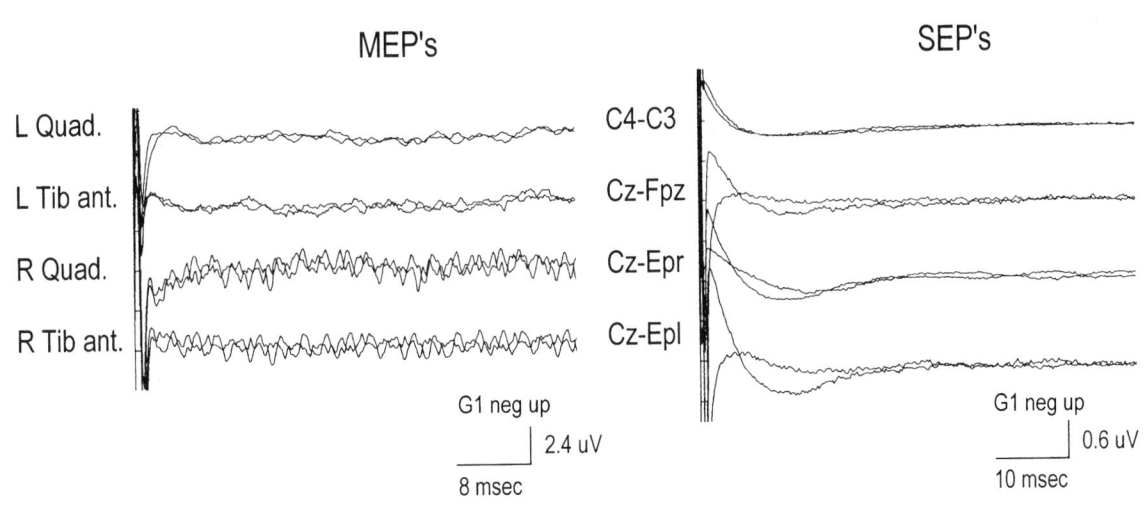

FIG. 31.7. Loss of both motor evoked potentials and SSEPs after distraction in a 14-year-old girl with severe thoracolumbar scoliosis. **A:** Baseline. **B:** After distraction. EPr and EPl denote electrode positions over right and left Erb's points.

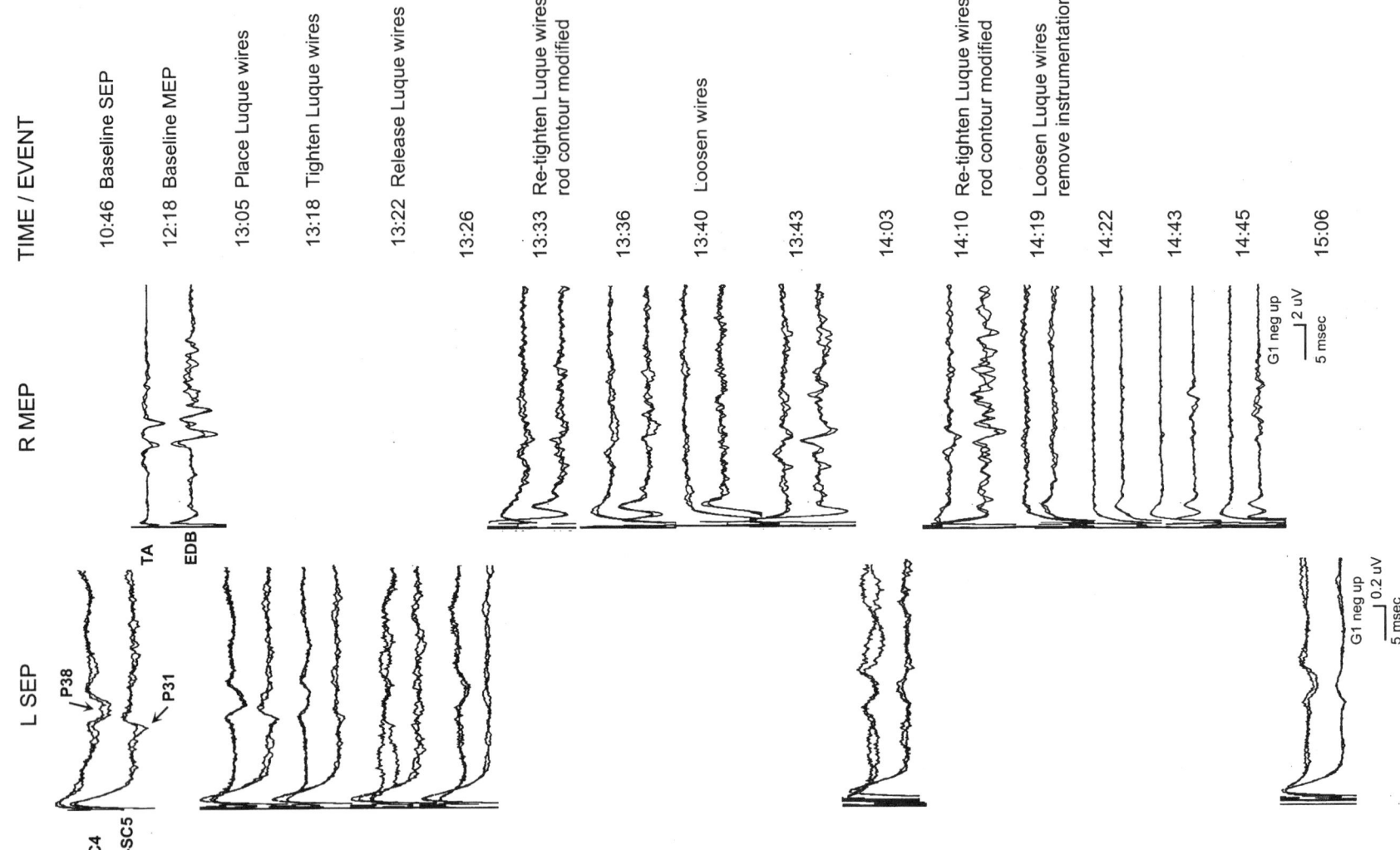

FIG. 31.8. SSEPs and motor evoked potentials monitored in a 17-year-old girl during scoliosis surgery with Luque segmental spinal instrumentation. Each time the wires were tightened, there was reversible loss of monitored potentials. Therefore, the instrumentation was removed, and the patient was treated with a body cast. Although paraplegic immediately postoperatively, the patient recovered to baseline examination levels within 2 weeks and was ambulatory at discharge.

thoracolumbar scoliosis. After multiple osteotomies and spinal distraction, both MEPs and SEPs were lost. Thereafter the distraction was reduced and the spine was stabilized, but the EPs remained absent. Although an emergency computed tomographic myelogram was negative, the patient was paraplegic postoperatively; the injury was attributed to overdistraction. Motor function returned over the ensuing several months, and the patient currently is fully ambulatory.

The authors reported their experience of 116 spine or spinal cord surgical cases monitored with SEPs and MEPs elicited by electrical spinal cord stimulation (82). In eight cases in which MEPs and SEPs deteriorated, and in an additional case in which only MEPs changed, there were corresponding postoperative motor deficits. In four cases, intraoperative MEP deterioration prompted changes in surgical management. In two patients undergoing correction of scoliosis, there was repeated reversible loss of MEPs and SEPs during spinal instrumentation. In both cases, instrumentation was removed, and patients were placed in body casts (Fig. 31.8). In another patient with severe kyphoscoliosis and spinal stenosis, MEP and SEP signals were lost during anterior decompression, prompting early termination of the surgery and delaying a planned second operation. In the fourth case, a vessel supplying a spinal cord arteriovenous malformation was spared after temporary occlusion was found to produce reversible loss of MEPs. One of these four patients died of a concurrent illness; the other three had good neurological recoveries. Because intraoperative SEP and MEP monitoring does not add any substantial risk to the patient, the only cost is monetary (22). The costs associated with a single avoidable case of neurological injury could well dwarf the expense of monitoring several hundred cases.

CRANIAL NERVE AND SPINAL ROOT MONITORING

Intraoperative neurophysiological monitoring both facilitates identification of cranial nerves and spinal roots and allows continuous assessment of their functional integrity. The facial nerve is monitored during resection of acoustic neuromas and other cerebellopontine angle surgeries, during which it may be injured or accidentally severed. These risks are increased with large tumors, which may either engulf the facial nerve or distort its appearance. Reduced rates of morbidity after acoustic neuroma surgery performed with facial nerve monitoring have been confirmed by several studies (40,57,83). At the Mayo Clinic, 91 monitored acoustic neuroma operations were compared with unmonitored controls matched for patient age, tumor size, and year of surgery; results demonstrated a threefold reduction in the rate of facial paralysis in the monitored cases (40).

In a similar manner, cranial nerves III, IV, and VI may be monitored during cavernous sinus surgery (111), and the lower cranial nerves may be monitored during skull base surgery (76). During surgery that places the spinal roots at risk (such as spinal cord untethering, placement of pedicle screws for instrumentation, and certain types of tumor resection), spinal root monitoring may be indicated (30,44,45,55).

Compound Muscle Action Potentials

Monitoring of CMAPs over appropriate muscles can be used to identify cranial nerves or spinal roots when scarring or anatomical distortion makes visual identification difficult. In contrast to the clinical laboratory setting in which constant-current stimulators are preferred, constant-voltage stimulators are often more suitable for intraoperative use. In stimulating within the operative site, constant voltage stimulators are better able to compensate for variable shunting of current through ambient fluid and to deliver a constant depolarizing current to a nerve (77,127).

Either surface or intramuscular electrodes may be used to record CMAPs. A monopolar probe is directed by the surgeon. Initially, nerve roots are located through the use of relatively high stimulation intensities. Then the intensity is decreased to selectively stimulate only the target root in order to confirm its identity and establish its stimulation threshold. In general, stimulation thresholds are 0.03 to 0.1 mA for cranial nerves and slightly higher for nerve roots. Higher stimulation intensities (about three times threshold) are used to confirm that an intended area of resection does not contain nerve, and lower stimulation intensity (near threshold) is used to confirm identity of the nerve. Elevation of the stimulus threshold may reflect nerve injury and an increased likelihood of postoperative deficit (51). Stimulation near a nerve may fail to produce a CMAP if the nerve has been injured, causing conduction block, or has been transected proximal to the site of stimulation.

The close relationship of the many muscles of the face can lead to ambiguity in recordings. Electrodes in muscles innervated by cranial nerve VII may also record signals generated the masseter and temporalis muscles, innervated by cranial nerve V. However, latencies of these responses differ and can be used to distinguish them. For example, after intracranial stimulation, cranial nerve VII has an onset latency of about 6 milliseconds, whereas cranial nerve Vm has a latency of only 3 milliseconds. Similarly, activation of lateral rectus muscle from cranial nerve VI stimulation is observed in the orbicularis oculi channel but can be properly identified by its latency (127) (Fig. 31.9).

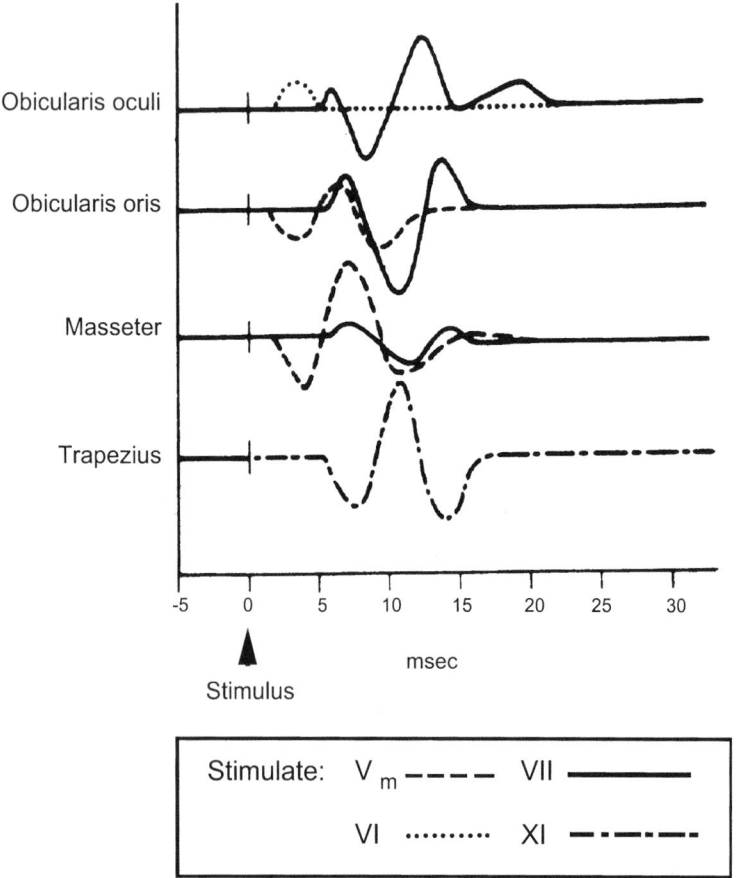

FIG. 31.9. The proximity of various cranial muscles results in "cross-talk" between recording sites. Characteristic latency differences help distinguish among responses to stimulation of cranial nerves Vm, VII, VI, and XI. (Reproduced from Yingling CD, Gardi JN. Intraoperative monitoring of facial and cochlear nerves during acoustic neuroma surgery. *Otolaryngol Clin North Am* 1992;25:413–448.)

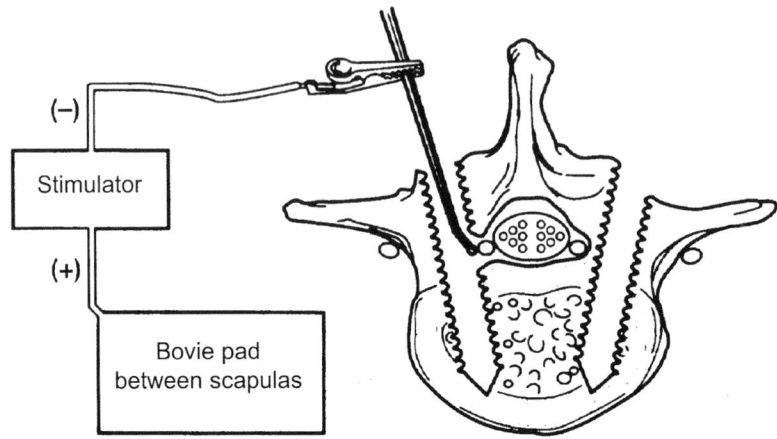

FIG. 31.10. Method for testing of lumbar pedicle screw hole integrity before screw placement. (From Calancie B, Madsen P, Lebwohl N. Stimulus-evoked EMG monitoring during transpedicular lumbosacral instrumentation. *Spine* 1994;19:2780–2786.)

CMAP thresholds are employed to test the placement of metal screws used for transpedicular spinal fixation. Postoperative radiculopathy may result from inadvertent penetration of the pedicle cortex with a screw. Either the wall of the intended screw hole or the screw itself is stimulated (Fig. 31.10), and the threshold for stimulation is measured by recording over the corresponding muscles (Fig. 31.11). Intact bone surrounding the screw provides insulation between it and the adjacent root. If the bone is perforated, a low-impedance path is created, lowering the stimulation threshold. Thresholds below 6 to 11 mA are suggestive of pedicle wall breakthrough (14,17,66).

Neurotonic Discharges

Mechanical nerve stimulation can produce neurotonic electromyographic discharges. In contrast to CMAPs, which can be recorded with surface electrodes, these discharges are best recorded with intramuscular electrodes (23). Although partial neuromuscular blockade allows monitoring of CMAPs, its use precludes reliable recording of neurotonic discharges (51). Instead, higher concentrations of inhaled anesthetics are

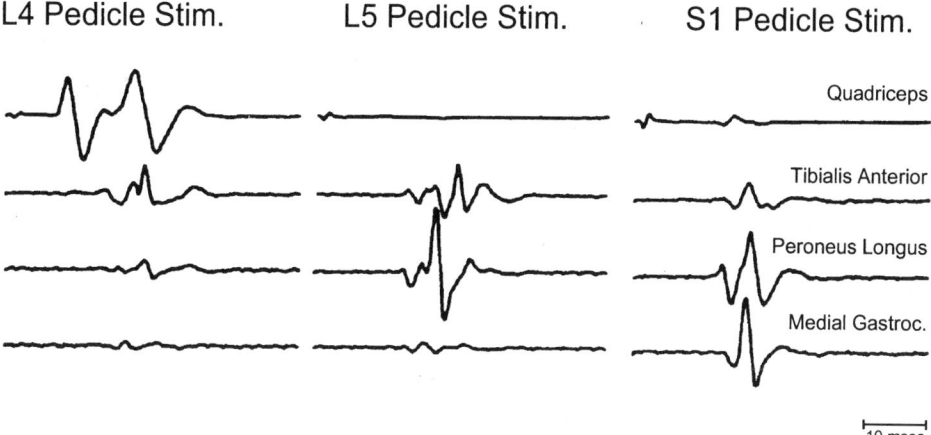

L4 Pedicle Stim.   **L5 Pedicle Stim.**   **S1 Pedicle Stim.**

Quadriceps

Tibialis Anterior

Peroneus Longus

Medial Gastroc.

10 msec

FIG. 31.11. Compound muscle action potentials from lower extremity muscles after stimulation of L4, L5, and S1 pedicle screws at 1 to 2 mA above threshold. (Reproduced from Calancie B, Madsen P, Lebwohl N. Stimulus-evoked EMG monitoring during transpedicular lumbosacral instrumentation. *Spine* 1994;19:2780–2786.)

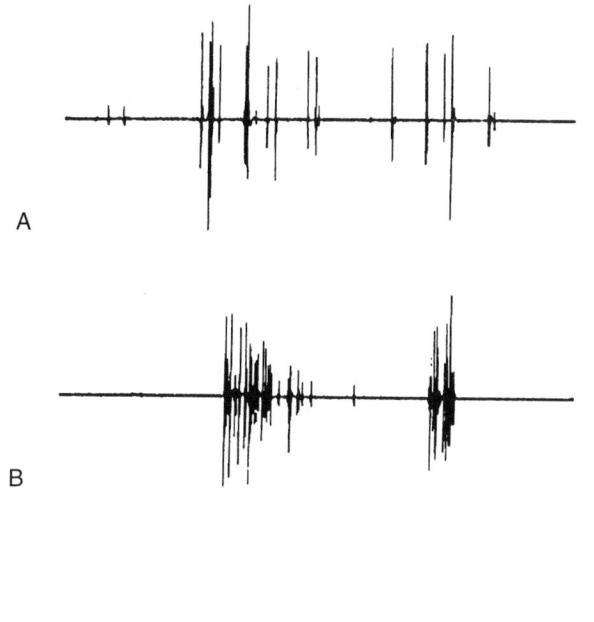

A

B

500 msec

FIG. 31.12. Brief burst electromyographic response recorded with blunt dissection **(A)** and after a rapid squirt with Ringer's lactate solution **(B)** during acoustic neuroma surgery. (From Prass RL, Luders H. Acoustic (loudspeaker) facial electromyographic monitoring: part 1. Evoked electromyographic activity during acoustic neuroma resection. *Neurosurgery* 1986;19:392–400.)

typically used to achieve relaxation when neurotonic discharges are recorded.

Mechanical stimulation—for example, from dissecting instruments and irrigation—produces brief (<1-second) bursts of motor unit potentials that occur with the mechanical stimulus and fatigue on repeat stimulation (Fig. 31.12). Easily elicited, relatively synchronous bursts indicate functional integrity of the nerve distal to the stimulated site. Loss of this response may signal nerve injury (97). However, because injured nerves may not be sensitive to mechanical stimulation, and because severing a nerve may produce only a minimal electromyographic response (51), mechanically elicited discharges should be supplemented with periodic electrical stimulation.

Prolonged asynchronous "train" discharges lasting up to several seconds or minutes signal nerve damage. These may result from ischemia, heating, or prolonged mechanical deformation, and their onset may be delayed seconds to minutes after the insult (Fig. 31.13). On the basis of their sounds when monitored on a loudspeaker, two types of tonic discharges, 50- to -100-Hz "bomber" discharges or 1- to 50-Hz "popcorn" discharges have been described (97). Both have been associated with postoperative neurological deficits (23,98). The frequent association of train discharges with lateral-to-medial facial nerve traction during acoustic neuroma surgery led Prass and Luders (98) to identify that manipulation as a likely source of nerve injury and to modify their dissection strategy to minimize it.

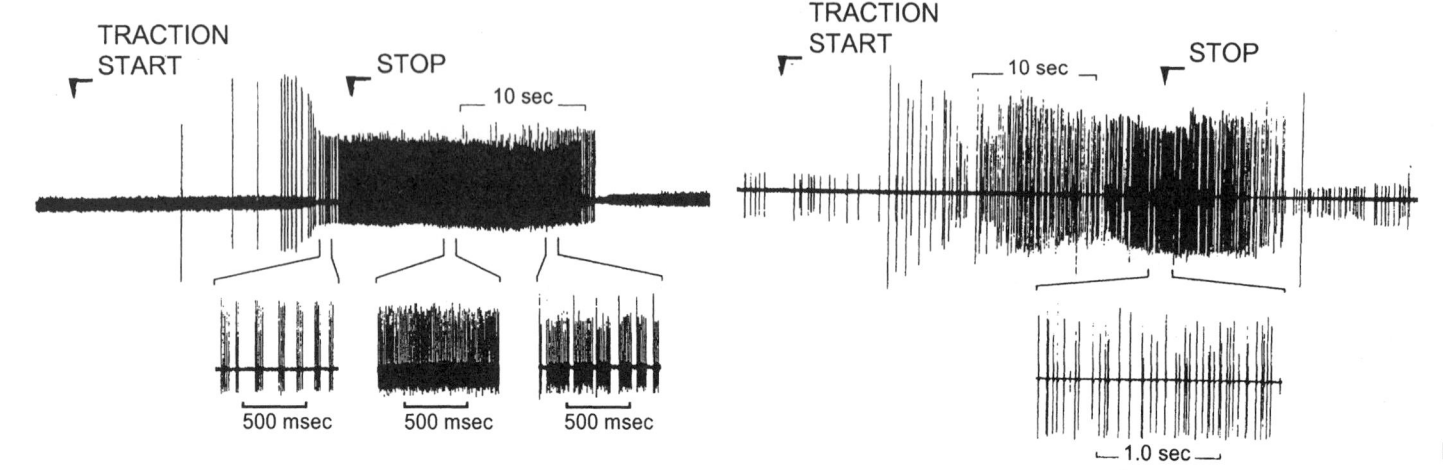

FIG. 31.13. Prolonged "bomber" **(A)** and "popcorn" **(B)** train discharges produced by lateral to medial facial nerve traction. (From Prass RL, Luders H. Acoustic (loudspeaker) facial electromyographic monitoring: part 1. Evoked electromyographic activity during acoustic neuroma resection. *Neurosurgery* 1986;19:392–400.)

ACOUSTIC NERVE AND BRAINSTEM AUDITORY EVOKED POTENTIAL MONITORING

Brainstem auditory evoked potentials (BAEPs) reflect the functional integrity of the cochlea, auditory nerve, and brainstem auditory pathways. Accordingly, BAEPs are monitored during cerebellopontine angle surgery to help preserve auditory nerve function. They may be recorded intraoperatively to assess brainstem function. Clinically relevant components of the BAEP are wave I, generated by the acoustic nerve; wave III, generated in the lower pons and wave V, generated in the lower midbrain.

Intraoperatively, BAEPs are recorded in a manner similar to that employed in the clinical laboratory, except that bulky headphones are replaced either with small earphones that can be inserted or with molded earplugs. In the operating room, a faster stimulation rate, typically 30 Hz rather than 10 Hz, is often used. Although this results in a small reduction in signal amplitude, it allows more rapid signal acquisition. BAEPs are largely unaffected by general anesthetic drugs, although potent inhalational agents may produce small increases in wave V latency (27,61,67). Similarly, decreases in core temperature, as well as local cooling at the surgical site, increase wave V latency approximately 0.2 millisecond per degree Celsius (127).

The utility of monitoring BAEPs to preserve hearing was demonstrated by a study in which the outcomes of 70 microvascular decompressions for trigeminal neuralgia or hemifacial spasm monitored with BAEP were compared to those of 152 historical control procedures performed without monitoring (99). The incidence of profound hearing loss was 0% in the monitored group, in comparison with 6.6% in the unmonitored group (99). Similarly, the efficacy of BAEP monitoring to reduce the risk of hearing loss during acoustic neuroma surgery is well documented (41,53,81,113, 125). In another study, 90 consecutive monitored acoustic neuroma resections were compared with 90 unmonitored historical controls; hearing was preserved in 79% of the monitored patients but in only 42% of the unmonitored patients for tumors smaller than 1.1 cm in diameter (98). BAEP monitoring in patients with tumors larger than 2 cm is unlikely to be of significant benefit because preservation of hearing is unlikely in such patients (41).

In general, a 50% or greater loss of wave V amplitude or a 0.5-millisecond or greater increase in wave V latency is recognized as a potentially important alteration in the BAEP waveform (15,41,99). Surgical maneuvers most likely to cause deterioration of BAEPs include electrocautery near the auditory nerve, pulling of the tumor-nerve bundle, drilling of the internal auditory canal, and direct manipulation of the auditory nerve (19,71). Because BAEP monitoring is capable of providing feedback to the surgeon at approximately 1- to 2-minute intervals, it is suggested that the most dangerous maneuvers be performed in incremental steps, in order to use BAEP feedback to guide the resection. Simply pausing may allow the deteriorated BAEP signals to recover (71,96).

Modified recording techniques, such as recording directly from the cochlear nerve (19,106) or from near the brainstem (70,79), have been introduced to provide more rapid feedback to the surgeon. These techniques offer improved signal-to-noise ratios, potentially allowing changes to be detected within seconds rather than minutes.

Although it provides direct surveillance of only the portion of brainstem between the lower pons and the lower midbrain, BAEP monitoring is sensitive to manipulations of the brainstem and may be used to assess its integrity (6). In patients with large cerebellopontine angle tumors, it has been observed that the wave V latencies measured after stimulation of the ear opposite the lesions are more closely related to brainstem manipulation than either the wave V amplitude or other hemodynamic parameters (6).

FUNCTIONAL LOCALIZATION

Intraoperative visual identification of the central sulcus may be difficult; however, it is easily identified functionally through the use of median nerve SEPs recorded from a cortical electrode array. Because activation of area 3b in the posterior bank of the central fissure produces the initial component of $\overline{N20}$, a horizontal dipole—positive precentrally and negative postcentrally—is recorded from a row electrodes traversing the central sulcus (Fig. 31.14). (62,63). Demonstration of this phase reversal is critical for accurate localization of the rolandic fissure, and if the surgical exposure does not permit placement of sufficient cortical electrodes, comparison of cortical SEPs with those recorded simultaneously from scalp electrodes may be helpful (62).

The precentral cortex can also be identified through the use of direct electrical stimulation with 50-Hz trains and observing target muscles for movement. However, electrical cortical stimulation may be difficult in young children, whose motor cortices are difficult to stimulate electrically (37,62,87).

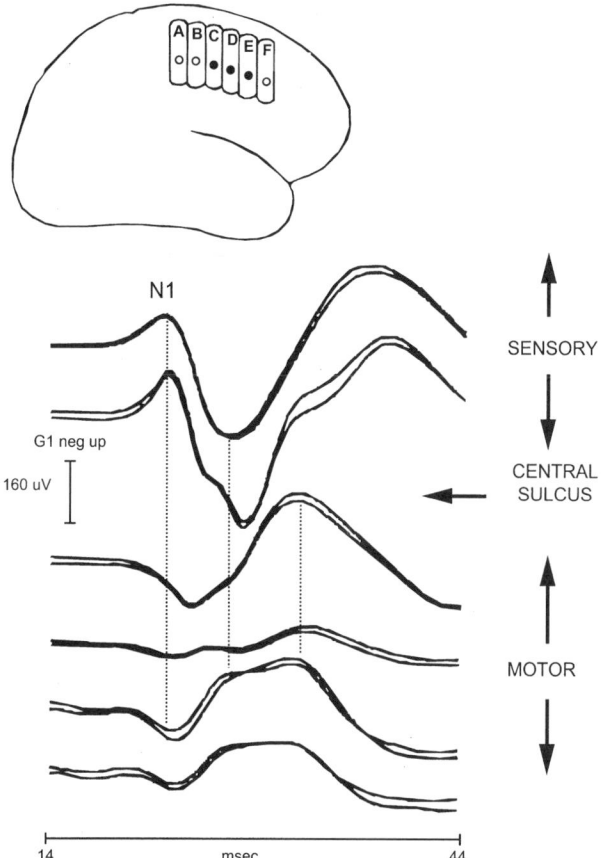

FIG. 31.14. The primary cortical response to median nerve stimulation (labeled N1) demonstrates a characteristic phase reversal when recorded from electrodes on their side of the central sulcus. (From Lueders H, Lesser RP, Hahn J, et al. Cortical somatosensory evoked potentials in response to hand stimulation. *J Neurosurg* 1983;58:885–894.)

DETECTION OF CEREBRAL ISCHEMIA

The rationale for using EEG and EP recording techniques to monitor patients at risk for cerebral ischemia is based on the observation that neuronal activity is measurably altered before cellular integrity is lost (7). Under normal conditions, global cerebral blood flow is approximately 50 mL per 100 g of brain tissue per minute, and oxygen consumption is in the range of 3 to 3.5 mL per 100 g of brain tissue per minute (117). Although influenced by anesthetic drugs and brain temperature, ischemic EEG changes generally occur at a cerebral blood flow of 20 mL per 100 g of brain tissue per minute, and isoelectric EEG changes occur at a cerebral blood flow below 12 mL per 100 g of brain tissue per minute. In the absence of cerebral protective agents, further decline in cerebral blood flow may result in loss of cellular integrity and in permanent neuronal injury (117).

Electroencephalographic Monitoring

Ischemic EEG changes typically consist of a progressive loss of fast frequency activity and an increase in slow frequency activity, followed by loss of amplitude, ultimately leading to electrical silence. In patients undergoing carotid endarterectomy, intraoperative EEG changes are correlated both with changes in regional cerebral blood flow, as measured by intracarotid xenon 133 injection (117), and with postoperative neurological deficits (16,102,117). Nonetheless, the ultimate clinical utility of EEG during carotid surgery has been debated (100). Although selective arterial shunting on the basis of EEG evidence of cerebral ischemia during carotid cross-clamping, rather than universal placement of a temporary shunt, is an inherently attractive notion, there is no conclusive evidence that selective shunting improves outcome after carotid surgery. This may, at least in part, be explained by the relatively low overall incidence of stroke after carotid surgery, along with the observation that cerebral embolism, rather than global ischemia, is the most common cause of cerebral injury after carotid endarterectomy.

In order to facilitate EEG monitoring, techniques have been developed to simplify and condense EEG data. Most commonly, the fast Fourier transform is used to convert EEG to the frequency domain, and methods of display such as the compressed spectral array (CSA) are used to depict the amplitude or power of the EEG in various frequency ranges. Although CSA can function as a useful graphic summary of the EEG background, the CSA or other forms of spectral analysis alone cannot enable the clinician to reliably distinguish between real EEG changes and artifacts from sources such as skeletal muscle activity, cardiac electrical activity, and external electrical devices (85) (Fig. 31.15). For this reason, the American Clinical Neurophysiology Society has indicated that the clinical application of quantitative EEG techniques such as CSA should be "considered to be limited and adjunctive" (5).

Successful intraoperative use of EEG to warn of cerebral ischemia requires that ischemic related alterations in the EEG be distinguished from potentially similar changes resulting from other causes, including effects of anesthetic drugs, surgical stimulation, and changes in temperature and carbon dioxide tension, in addition to artifacts. Failure to recognize this leads to overinterpretation. It is likely that data reduction techniques such as CSA, intended to make the EEG "easier" to read, may in fact make this distinction more difficult. For example, although increases in delta power on EEG power spectra were interpreted as "ischemic" patterns and used as the basis the initiation of "therapeutic interventions" during cardiopulmonary bypass (29), similar increase in delta power were commonly observed in a control population of patients undergoing abdominal surgery (3).

Somatosensory Evoked Potential Monitoring

Intraoperative SEP recording has also been used to detect ischemia during cerebrovascular procedures such as carotid endarterectomy (43), clipping of cerebral aneurysms (43,80,108,118), and various neuroradiological procedures (128). Because the generators of the primary cortical $\overline{N20}$ component of the median nerve SEP lie within the territory of the middle cerebral artery, these have been used to monitor cortical function during carotid enterectomy. The SEP that is being monitored must correspond with the cortical territory at risk. For example, whereas median nerve SEPs are appropriate for surgery involving the internal carotid and middle cerebral arteries, they are not appropriate for surgery involving aneurysms of the anterior circulation. In one series, reversible changes occurred of N20 occurred in approximately 10% and irreversible changes in 0.7% of 994 patients undergoing carotid enterectomy (43). The incidence of SEP abnormalities during carotid cross-clamping correlated with the degree of contralateral carotid stenosis, and all patients with irreversible changes had corresponding postoperative deficits (43).

Although SEP and EEG monitoring have been shown to have similar sensitivities and specificities during carotid enterectomy (56), EEG monitoring appears to have the advantages of being somewhat less complicated, providing continuous real-time feedback, and surveying the function of more widespread cortical regions.

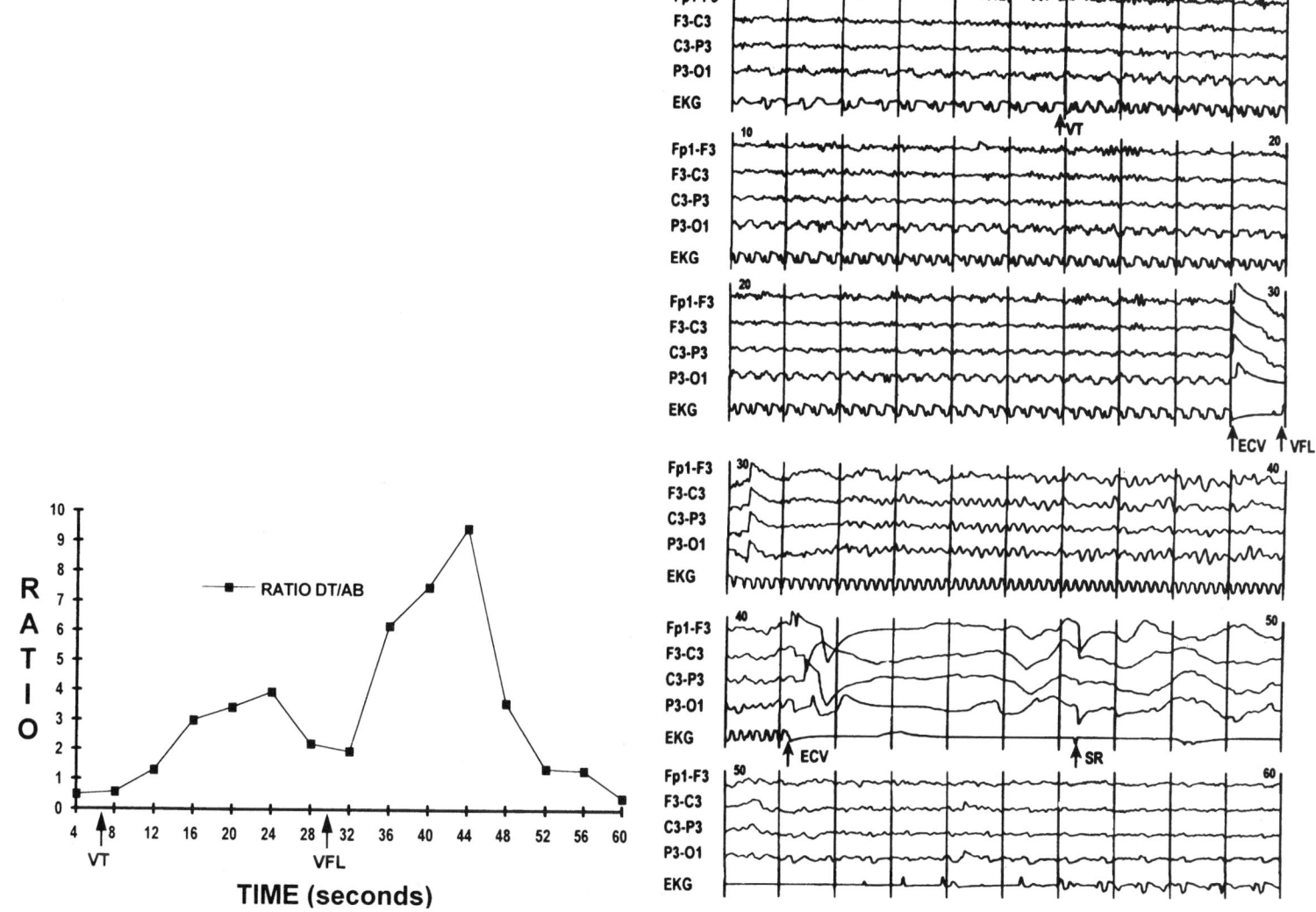

FIG. 31.15. Apparent increase in the delta/theta–to–alpha/beta power ratio during ventricular tachycardia and ventricular flutter **(A).** Careful inspection of the raw electroencephalogram **(B)** reveals that the graph in panel *A* depicts changes in power spectrum of the electrocardiographic artifact. (From Adams DC, Heyer EJ, Emerson RG, et al. The reliability of quantitative electroencephalography as an indicator of cerebral ischemia. *Anesth Analg* 1995;81:80–83.)

MONITORING DEPTH OF ANESTHESIA

The EEG effects of virtually every inhaled and intravenous anesthetic agent have been described (124). Certain measures based on EEG frequency analysis, such as the spectral edge frequency, have been correlated with hemodynamic responses to noxious stimuli during specific anesthetic regimens (104). However, attempts to correlate various EEG parameters over a broad range of anesthetic techniques with clinical measurements of anesthetic depth, such as movement to incision, have not produced uniform results (121). More complex measures, such as the "EEG bispectrum," which incorporates phase relationships of the various frequency components of the EEG along with other EEG descriptors, have been proposed as better measures of anesthetic depth (35,101,109,121).

REFERENCES

1. Adams DC, Emerson RG, Heyer EJ. Intraoperative motor tract monitoring using transcranial magnetic evoked potentials. *Neurology* 1993;43:426.
2. Adams DC, Emerson RG, Heyer EJ, et al. Monitoring of intraoperative motor evoked potentials under conditions of controlled neuromuscular blockade. *Anesth Analg* 1993;77:913–918.
3. Adams DC, Heyer EJ, Emerson RG, et al. The reliability of quantitative electroencephalography as an indicator of cerebral ischemia. *Anesth Analg* 1995;81:80–83.
4. Amassian VE, Stewart M, Quirk GJ, et al. Physiological basis of motor effects of a transient stimulus to cerebral cortex. *Neurosurgery* 1987;20:74–93.
5. American Electroencephalographic Society: Guideline nine: guidelines on evoked potentials. *J Clin Neurophysiol* 1994;11:40–73.
6. Angelo R, Moller AR. Contralateral evoked brainstem auditory potentials as an indicator of intraoperative brainstem manipulation in cerebellopontine angle tumors. *Neurol Res* 1996;18:528–540.
7. Astrup J, Siesjo BK, Symon L. Thresholds in cerebral ischemia—the ischemic penumbra. *Stroke* 1981;12:723–725.
8. Baskin DS, Simpson RK Jr. Corticomotor and somatosensory evoked potential evaluation of acute spinal cord injury in the rat. *Neurosurgery* 1987;20:871–877.
9. Ben-David B. Spinal cord monitoring. *Orthop Clin North Am* 1988;19:427–448.
10. Ben-David B, Haller GS, Taylor PD. Anterior spinal fusion complicated by paraplegia. A case report of a false-negative somatosensory-evoked potential. *Spine* 1987;12:536–539.
11. Ben-David B, Taylor PD, Haller GS. Posterior spinal fusion complicated by posterior column injury. A case report of a false-negative wake up test. *Spine* 1987;12:540–543.
12. Browning JL, Heizer ML, Baskin DS. Variations in corticomotor and somatosensory evoked potentials: effects of temperature, halothane anesthesia, and arterial partial pressure of CO_2. *Anesth Analg* 1992;74:643–648.
13. Burke D, Hicks R, Stephen J, et al. Assessment of corticospinal and somatosensory conduction simultaneously during scoliosis surgery. *Electroencephalogr Clin Neurophysiol* 1992; 85:388–396.
14. Calancie B, Madsen P, Lebwohl N. Stimulus-evoked EMG monitoring during transpedicular lumbosacral instrumentation. *Spine* 1994;19:2780–2786.
15. Cheek JC. Posterior fossa intraoperative monitoring. *J Clin Neurophysiol* 1993;10:412–424.
16. Chiappa KH, Burke SR, Young RR. Results of electroencephalographic monitoring during 367 carotid endarterectomies. Use of a dedicated minicomputer. *Stroke* 1979;10:381–388.
17. Clements DH, Morledge DE, Martin WH, et al. Evoked and spontaneous electromyography to evaluate lumbosacral pedicle screw placement. *Spine* 1996;21:600–604.
18. Coles JG, Wilson GJ, Sima AF, et al. Intraoperative detection of spinal cord ischemia using somatosensory cortical evoked potentials during thoracic aortic occlusion. *Ann Thorac Surg* 1982;34:299–306.
19. Colletti V, Fiorino FG. Vulnerability of hearing function during acoustic neuroma surgery. *Acta Otolaryngol* 1994;114:264–270.
20. Cracco RQ, Evans B. Spinal evoked potentials in the cat: effects of asphyxia, strychnine, cord section and compression. *Electroencephalogr Clin Neurophysiol* 1978;44:187–201.
21. D'Angelo CM, VanGilder JC, Taub A. Evoked cortical potentials in experimental spinal cord trauma. *J Neurosurg* 1973;38:332–336.
22. Daube JR. Intraoperative monitoring by evoked potentials for spinal cord surgery: the pros. *Electroencephalogr Clin Neurophysiol* 1989;73:374–377.
23. Daube JR, Harper CM. Surgical monitoring of cranial and peripheral nerves. In: Desmdet JE, ed. *Neuromonitoring in surgery*. Amsterdam: Elsevier, 1989:115–138.
24. Deecke L, Tator CH. Neurophysiological assessment of afferent and efferent conduction in the injured spinal cord of monkeys. *J Neurosurg* 1973;39:65–74.
25. Dorfman LJ, Perkash I, Bosley TM, et al. Use of cerebral evoked potentials to evaluate spinal somatosensory function in patients with traumatic and surgical myelopathies. *J Neurosurg* 1980;52:654–660.
26. Drenger B, Parker SD, McPherson RW, et al. Spinal cord stimulation evoked potentials during thoracoabdominal aortic aneurysm surgery. *Anesthesiology* 1992;76:689–695.
27. Dubois MY, Sato S, Chassy J, et al. Effects of enflurane on brainstem auditory evoked responses in humans. *Anesth Analg* 1982;61:898–902.
28. Ducker TB, Salcman M, Lucas JT, et al. Experimental spinal cord trauma, II: Blood flow, tissue oxygen, evoked potentials in both paretic and plegic monkeys. *Surg Neurol* 1978;10:64–70.
29. Edmonds HL Jr, Griffiths LK, van der Laken J, et al. Quantitative electroencephalographic monitoring during myocardial revascularization predicts postoperative disorientation and improves outcome. *J Thorac Cardiovasc Surg* 1992;103:555–563.
30. Epstein NE, Danto J, Nardi D. Evaluation of intraoperative somatosensory evoked potential monitoring during 100 cervical operations. *Spine* 1993;18:737–747.
31. Fehlings MG, Tator CH, Linden RD. The relationships among the severity of spinal cord injury, motor and somatosensory evoked potentials and spinal cord blood flow. *Electroencephalogr Clin Neurophysiol* 1989;74:241–259.
32. Forbes HJ, Allen PW, Waller CS, et al. Spinal cord monitoring in scoliosis surgery. *J Bone Joint Surg Br* 1991;73:487–491.
33. Ghaly RF, Stone JL, Levy WJ, et al. The effect of nitrous oxide on transcranial magnetic-induced electromyographic responses in the monkey. *J Neurosurg Anesthesiol* 1990;2:175–181.
34. Ginsburg HH, Shetter AG, Raudzens PA. Postoperative paraplegia with preserved intraoperative somatosensory evoked potentials. Case report. *J Neurosurg* 1985;63:296–300.
35. Glass PS, Bloom M, Kearse L, et al. Bispectral analysis measures sedation and memory effects of propofol, midazolam, isoflurane, and alfentanil in healthy volunteers. *Anesthesiology* 1997;86:836–847.
36. Gokaslan ZL, Samudrala S, Deletis V, et al. Intraoperative monitoring of spinal cord function using motor evoked potentials via transcutaneous epidural electrode during anterior cervical spinal surgery. *J Spinal Disord* 1997;10:299–303.
37. Goldring S, Gregorie EM. Surgical management of epilepsy using epidural recordings to localize the seizure focus. Review of 100 cases. *J Neurosurg* 1984;60:457–466.
38. Gravenstein MA, Sasse F, Hogan K. Effects of stimulus rate and halothane dose on canine far-field somatosensory evoked potentials. *Anesthesiology* 1984;61:A342.
39. Haghighi SS, Green KD, Oro JJ, et al. Suppression of motor evoked potentials by inhalation anesthetics. *J Neurosurg Anesthesiol* 1990;2:73–78.

40. Harner SG, Daube JR, Beatty CW, et al. Intraoperative monitoring of the facial nerve. *Laryngoscope* 1988;98:209–212.
41. Harper CM, Harner SG, Slavit DH, et al. Effect of BAEP monitoring on hearing preservation during acoustic neuroma resection. *Neurology* 1992;42:1551–1553.
42. Harper CM, Nelson KR. Intraoperative electrophysiological monitoring in children. *J Clin Neurophysiol* 1992;9:342–356.
43. Haupt WF, Horsch S. Evoked potential monitoring in carotid surgery. A review of 994 cases. *Neurology* 1992;42:835–838.
44. Herdmann J, Deletis V, Edmonds HL Jr, et al. Spinal cord and nerve root monitoring in spine surgery and related procedures. *Spine* 1996;21:879–885.
45. Hormes JT, Chappuis JL. Monitoring of lumbosacral nerve roots during spinal instrumentation. *Spine* 1993;18:2059–2062.
46. Jellinek D, Jewkes D, Symon L. Noninvasive intraoperative monitoring of motor evoked potentials under propofol anesthesia: effects of spinal surgery on the amplitude and latency of motor evoked potentials. *Neurosurgery* 1991;29:551–557.
47. Jones SJ, Harrison R, Koh KF, et al. Motor evoked potential monitoring during spinal surgery: response of distal limb muscles to transcranial cortical stimulation with pulse trains. *Electroencephalogr Clin Neurophysiol* 1996;100:375–383.
48. Kalkman CJ, Drummond JC, Kennelly NA, et al. Intraoperative monitoring of tibialis anterior muscle motor evoked responses to transcranial electrical stimulation during partial neuromuscular blockade. *Anesth Analg* 1992;73:584–589.
49. Kalkman CJ, Drummond JC, Ribberink AA. Low concentrations of isoflurane abolish motor evoked responses to transcranial electrical stimulation during nitrous oxide/opioid anesthesia in humans. *Anesth Analg* 1991;73:410–415.
50. Kalkman CJ, Drummond JC, Ribberink AA, et al. Effects of propofol, etomidate, midazolam, and fentanyl on motor evoked responses to transcranial electrical or magnetic stimulation in humans. *Anesthesiology* 1992;76:502–509.
51. Kartush JM. Electroneurography and intraoperative facial monitoring in contemporary neurology. *Otolaryngol Head Neck Surg* 1989;101:496–503.
52. Kearse LA, Lopez-Bresnahan M, McPeck K, et al. Loss of intraoperative somatosensory evoked potentials during intramedullary spinal cord injury predicts postoperative neurological deficits in motor function. *J Clin Anesth* 1993;5:392–398.
53. Kemink JL, LaRouere MJ, Kileny PR, et al. Hearing preservation following suboccipital removal of acoustic neuromas. *Laryngoscope* 1990;100:597–602.
54. Koht A, Moss JL. Effects of etomidate, midazolam, and thiopental on median nerve somatosensory evoked potentials and the additive effects of fentanyl and nitrous oxide. *Anesth Analg* 1988;67:435–441.
55. Kothbauer K, Schmid UD, Seiler RW, et al. Intraoperative motor and sensory monitoring of the cauda equina. *Neurosurgery* 1994;34:702–704.
56. Lam AM, Manninen PH, Ferguson GG, et al. Monitoring electrophysiologic function during carotid endarterectomy: a comparison of somatosensory evoked potentials and conventional electroencephalogram. *Anesthesiology* 1991;75:15–21.
57. Leonetti JP, Brackmann DE, Prass RL. Improved preservation of facial nerve function in the infratemporal approach to the skull base. *Otolaryngol Head Neck Surg* 1989;101:74–78.
58. Lesser RP, Raudzens P, Luders H, et al. Postoperative neurological deficits may occur despite unchanged intraoperative somatosensory evoked potentials. *Ann Neurol* 1986;19:22–25.
59. Levy WJ, McCaffrey M, Hagichi S. Motor evoked potential as a predictor of recovery in chronic spinal injury. *Neurosurgery* 1987;20:138–142.
60. Levy WJ, McCaffrey M, York D. Motor evoked potential in cats with acute spinal cord injury. *Neurosurgery* 1986;19:9–19.
61. Loyd-Thomas AR, Cole PV, Prior PF. Quantitative EEG and brainstem auditory potentials: comparison of isoflurane with halothane using cerebral function analysing monitor. *Br J Anaesth* 1990;65:306–312.
62. Lueders H, Dinner DS, Lesser RP, et al. Evoked potentials in cortical localization. *J Clin Neurophysiol* 1986;3:75–84.
63. Lueders H, Lesser RP, Hahn J, et al. Cortical somatosensory evoked potentials in response to hand stimulation. *J Neurosurg* 1983;58:885–894.
64. Machida M, Weinstein SL, Imamura Y, et al. Compound muscle action potentials and spinal evoked potentials in experimental spine maneuver. *Spine* 1989;14:687–691.
65. Machida M, Weinstein SL, Yamada T, et al. Dissociation of muscle action potentials and spinal somatosensory evoked potentials after ischemic damage of spinal cord. *Spine* 1988;13:1119–1124.
66. Maguire J, Wallace S, Madiga R, et al. Evaluation of intrapedicular screw position using intraoperative evoked electromyography. *Spine* 1995;20:1068–1074.
67. Manninen PH, Lam AM, Nicholas JF. The effects of isoflurane and isoflurane-nitrous oxide anesthesia on brainstem auditory evoked potentials in humans. *Anesth Analg* 1985;64:43–47.
68. Martin SH, Bloedel JR. Evaluation of experimental spinal cord injury using cortical potentials. *Neurosurgery* 1973;39:75–81.
69. Matsui Y, Goh K, Shiiya N, et al. Clinical application of evoked spinal cord potentials elicited by direct stimulation of the cord during temporary occlusion of the thoracic aorta. *J Thorac Cardiovasc Surg* 1994;107:1519–1527.
70. Matthies C, Samii M. Direct brainstem recording of auditory evoked potentials during vestibular schwannoma resection: nuclear BAEP recording. *J Neurosurg* 1997;86:1057–1062.
71. Matthies C, Samii M. Management of vestibular schwannomas (acoustic neuromas): the value of neurophysiology for intraoperative monitoring of auditory function in 200 cases. *Neurosurgery* 1997;40:459–468.
72. McPherson RW, Sell B, Traystman RJ. Effects of thiopental, fentanyl and etomidate on upper extremity somatosensory evoked potentials in humans. *Anesthesiology* 1986;65:584–589.
73. Mills KR. Magnetic brain stimulation: a tool to explore the action of the motor cortex on single human motoneurones. *Trends Neurosci* 1991;14:401–405.
74. Mochida K, Shinomiya K, Komori H, et al. A new method of multisegment motor pathway monitoring using muscle potentials after train spinal stimulation. *Spine* 1995;20:2240–2246.
75. Molaie M. False negative intraoperative somatosensory evoked potentials with simultaneous bilateral stimulation. *Clin Electroencephalogr* 1986;17:6–9.
76. Moller AR. *Evoked potentials in intraoperative monitoring.* Baltimore: Williams & Wilkins, 1988.
77. Moller AR. Neuromonitoring in operations in the skull base. *Keio J Med* 1991;40:151–159.
78. Moller AR. Intraoperative neurophysiological monitoring. *Am J Otol* 1992;16:115–117.
79. Moller AR, Jho HD, Janetta PJ. Preservation of hearing in operations on acoustic tumors: an alternative to recording brainstem auditory potentials. *Neurosurgery* 1994;34:688–642.
80. Momma F, Wang AD, Symon L. Effects of temporary arterial occlusion on somatosensory evoked responses in aneurysm surgery. *Surg Neurol* 1987;27:343–352.
81. Morioka T, Tobimatsu S, Fujii K, et al. Direct spinal versus peripheral nerve stimulation as monitoring techniques in epidurally recorded spinal cord potentials. *Acta Neurochir (Wien)* 1991;108:122–127.
82. Nagle K, Emerson RG, Adams DC, et al. Intraoperative monitoring of motor evoked potentials: a review of 116 cases. *Neurology* 1996;47:999–1004.
83. Niparko JK, Kileny PR, Kemink JL, et al. Neurophysiologic intraoperative monitoring: II. Facial nerve function. *Am J Otol* 1989;10:55–61.
84. Noordeen MH, Lee J, Gibbons CE, et al. Spinal cord monitoring in operations for neuromuscular scoliosis. *J Bone Joint Surg Br* 1997;79:53–57.
85. Nuwer MR. Intraoperative electroencephalography. *J Clin Neurophysiol* 1993;10:437–444.
86. O'Brien MF, Lenke LG, Bridwell KH, et al. Evoked potentials monitoring of upper extremities during thoracic and lumbar spinal deformity surgery: a prospective study. *J Spinal Disord* 1994;7:277–284.
87. Ojemann G. Temporal lobectomy tailored to electrocorticography and functional mapping.

In: Spencer SS, Spencer DD, eds. *Surgery for epilepsy.* London: Blackwell Scientific, 1991: 137–149.

88. Owen JH, Laschinger J, Bridwell K, et al. Sensitivity and specificity of somatosensory and neurogenic-motor evoked potentials in animals and humans. *Spine* 1988;13:1111–1118.

89. Padberg AM, Russo MH, Lenke LG, et al. Validity and reliability of spinal cord monitoring in neuromuscular spinal deformity surgery. *J Spinal Deform* 1996;9:150–158.

90. Patil AA, Nagaraj MP, Mehta R. Cortically evoked motor action potential in spinal cord injury research. *Neurosurgery* 1985;16:473–476.

91. Pechstein U, Cedzich C, Nadstawek J, et al. Transcranial high-frequency repetitive electrical stimulation for recording myogenic motor evoked potentials with the patient under general anesthesia. *Neurosurgery* 1996;39:335–344.

92. Pechstein U, Nadstawek J, Zentner J, et al. Isoflurane plus nitrous oxide versus propofol for recording of motor evoked potentials after high frequency repetitive electrical stimulation. *Electroencephalogr Clin Neurophysiol* 1998;108:175–181.

93. Penfield W, Boldrey E. Somatic motor and sensory representation in the cerebral cortex of man as studied by electrical stimulation. *Brain* 1939;60:389–443.

94. Perlik SJ, VanEgeren R, Fisher MA. Somatosensory evoked potential surgical monitoring. Observation during combined isoflurane–nitrous oxide anesthesia. *Spine* 1992;17:273–276.

95. Poncelet L, Michaux C, Balligand M. Motor evoked potentials induced by electrical stimulation of the spine in dogs: which structures are involved? *Electroencephalogr Clin Neurophysiol* 1995;97:179–183.

96. Post KD, Eisenberg MB, Catalano PJ. Hearing preservation in vestibular schwannoma surgery: what factors influence outcome. *J Neurosurg* 1995;83:191–196.

97. Prass RL, Kinney SE, Hardy RW Jr, et al. Acoustic (loudspeaker) facial EMG monitoring: II. Use of evoked EMG activity during acoustic neuroma resection. *Otolaryngol Head Neck Surg* 1987;97:541–551.

98. Prass RL, Luders H. Acoustic (loudspeaker) facial electromyographic monitoring: part 1. Evoked electromyographic activity during acoustic neuroma resection. *Neurosurgery* 1986; 19:392–400.

99. Radke RA, Erwin CW, Wilkins RH. Intraoperative brainstem auditory evoked potentials: significant decrease in postoperative morbidity. *Neurology* 1989;39:187–191.

100. Rampil IJ. Electroencephalogram. In: Albin MS, ed. *Textbook of neuroanesthesia with neurosurgical and neuroscience perspectives.* New York: McGraw-Hill, 1997:193–219.

101. Rampil IJ. A primer for EEG signal processing in anesthesia. *Anesthesiology* 1998;89:980–1002.

102. Rampil IJ, Holzer JA, Quest DO, et al. Prognostic value of computerized EEG analysis during carotid endarterectomy. *Anesth Analg* 1983;62:186–192.

103. Rampil IJ, King BS. Volatile anesthetics depress spinal motor neurons. *Anesthesiology* 1996;85:129–134.

104. Rampil IJ, Matteo RS. Changes in EEG spectral edge frequency correlate with the hemodynamic response to laryngoscopy and intubation. *Anesthesiology* 1987;67:139–142.

105. Reuter DG, Tacker WA Jr, Badylak SF, et al. Correlation of motor-evoked potential response to ischemic spinal cord damage. *J Thorac Cardiovasc Surg* 1992;104:262–272.

106. Roberson J, Senne A, Brackmann D, et al. Direct cochlear nerve action potentials as an aid to hearing preservation in middle fossa acoustic neuroma resection. *Am J Otol* 1996;17:653–657.

107. Rothwell J, Burke D, Hicks R, et al. Transcranial electrical stimulation of the motor cortex in man: further evidence of site of activation. *J Physiol* 1994;481:243–250.

108. Schramm J, Koht A, Schmidt G, et al. Surgical and electrophysiological observations during clipping of 134 aneurysms with evoked potential monitoring. *Neurosurgery* 1990;26: 61–70.

109. Sebel PS, Bowles SM, Saini V, et al. EEG bispectrum predicts movement during thiopental/ isoflurane anesthesia. *J Clin Monit* 1995;11:83–91.

110. Sebel PS, Erwin CW, Neville WK. Effects of halothane and enflurane on far and near-field somatosensory evoked potentials. *Br J Anaesth* 1987;57:1492–1496.

111. Sekhar LN, Moller AR. Operative management of tumors involving the cavernous sinus. *J Neurosurg* 1986;64:879–889.

112. Shiau JS, Zappulla RA, Nieves J. The effect of graded spinal cord injury on the extrapyramidal and pyramidal motor evoked potentials of the rat. *Neurosurgery* 1992;30:76–84.

113. Slavit DH, Harner SG, Harper CM Jr, et al. Auditory monitoring during acoustic neuroma removal. *Arch Otolaryngol Head Neck Surg* 1991;117:1153–1157.

114. Stechison MT. Neurophysiologic monitoring during cranial surgery. *J Neurooncol* 1994;20: 313–325.

115. Stephen JP, Sullivan MR, Hicks RG, et al. Cotrel-Dubousset instrumentation in children using simultaneous motor and somatosensory evoked potential monitoring. *Spine* 1996;21:2450–2457.

116. Su CF, Haghighi SS, Oro JJ, et al. "Backfiring" in spinal cord monitoring. High thoracic spinal cord stimulation evokes sciatic response by antidromic sensory pathway, not motor tract conduction. *Spine* 1992;17:504–508.

117. Sundt TM Jr, Sharbrough FW, Piepgras DG, et al. Correlation of cerebral blood flow and electroencephalographic changes during carotid endarterectomy: with results of surgery and hemodynamics of cerebral ischemia. *Mayo Clin Proc* 1981;56:533–543.

118. Symon L, Momma F, Murota T. Assessment of reversible cerebral ischaemia in man: intraoperative monitoring of the somatosensory response. *Acta Neurochir (Wien)* 1988;(Suppl 42):3–7.

119. Szilagyi D, Hageman JH, Smith RF, et al. Spinal cord damage in surgery of the abdominal aorta. *Surgery* 1978;83:38–56.

120. Takaki O, Okumura F. Application and limitation of somatosensory evoked potential monitoring during thoracic aortic aneurysm surgery. A case report. *Anesthesiology* 1985;63:700–703.

121. Todd MM. EEGs, EEG processing, and the bispectral index. [Editorial; comment]. *Anesthesiology* 1998;89:815–817.

122. Turnbull IM, Brieg A, Hassler O. Blood supply of the cervical spinal cord in man: a microangiographic cadaver study. *J Neurosurg* 1966;24:951–965.

123. Valzania F, Quatrale R, Strafella AP, et al. Pattern of motor evoked response to repetitive transcranial magnetic stimulation. *Electroencephalogr Clin Neurophysiol* 1994;93:312–317.

124. Vauzelle C, Stagnara C, Jouvinroux P. Functional monitoring of spinal cord activity during spinal surgery. *Clin Orthop Rel Res* 1973;93:173–178.

125. Watanabe E, Schramm J, Strauss C, et al. Neurophysiologic monitoring in posterior fossa surgery. II. BAEP—waves I and V and preservation of hearing. *Acta Neurochir (Wien)* 1989;98:118–128.

126. Whittle IR, Johnston IH, Besser M. Recording of spinal somatosensory evoked potentials for intraoperative spinal cord monitoring. *J Neurosurg* 1986;64:601–612.

127. Yingling CD, Gardi JN. Intraoperative monitoring of facial and cochlear nerves during acoustic neuroma surgery. *Otolaryngol Clin North Am* 1992;25:413–448.

128. Young WL, Pile-Spellman J. Anesthetic considerations for interventional neuroradiology. *Anesthesiology* 1994;80:427–456.

129. Zentner J. Motor evoked potential monitoring during neurosurgical operations on the spinal cord. *Neurosurg Rev* 1991;14:29–36.

130. Zentner J, Albrecht T, Heuser D. Influence of halothane, enflurane, and isoflurane on motor evoked potentials. *Neurosurgery* 1992;31:298–305.

131. Zornow MH, Grafe MR, Tybor C, et al. Preservation of evoked potentials in a case of anterior spinal artery syndrome. *Electroencephalogr Clin Neurophysiol* 1990;77:137–139.

Subject Index

Note: Page numbers followed by f indicate figures; page numbers followed by t indicate tables.

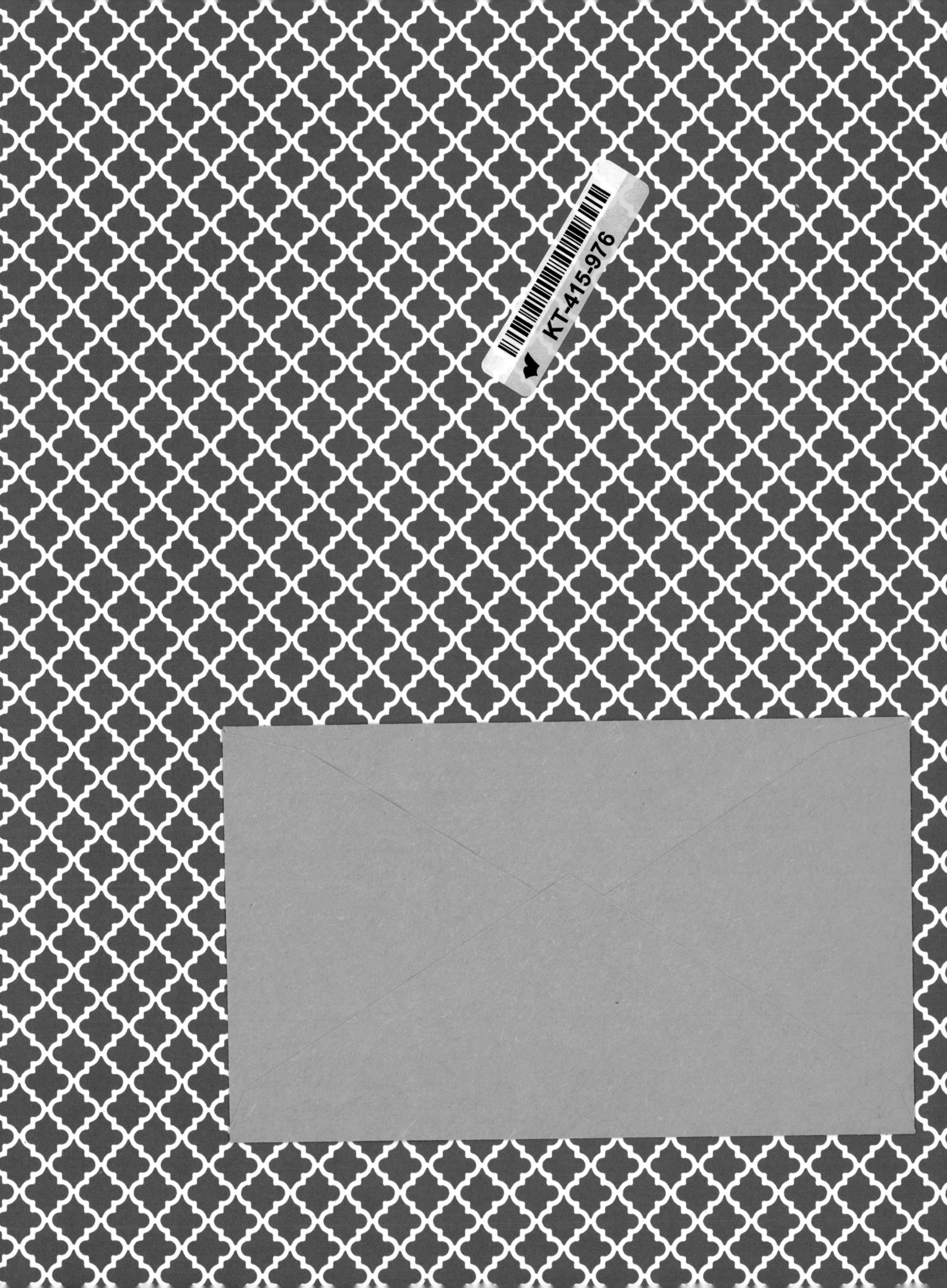

VOLUME 2
Gynecologic Oncology

For Churchill Livingstone

Publisher: Peter Richardson
Project Editor: Elif Fincanci-Smith
Editorial Co-ordination: Editorial Resources Unit
Production Controller: Neil Dickson
Design: Design Resources Unit
Sales Promotion Executive: Louise Johnstone

Contents
Volume 1

PART IV TUMORS OF VAGINA AND CERVIX AND RELATED ABNORMALITIES IN YOUNG FEMALES EXPOSED TO DIETHYLSTILBESTROL (DES)

PART V CARCINOMA OF CERVIX

PART VI

Carcinoma of endometrium and its precursors

VOLUME 2

Gynecologic Oncology
Fundamental Principles and Clinical Practice

Edited by

Malcolm Coppleson MB BS MD(Syd) FRCOG FRACOG
Clinical Professor, University of Sydney; Head, Department of Gynecologic Oncology, King George V Memorial Hospital, Royal Prince Alfred Hospital, Sydney, Australia

Associate Editors

John M. Monaghan MB FRCS(Ed) FRCOG
Director of Gynaecological Oncology Services, Regional Department of Gynaecological Oncology, Queen Elizabeth Hospital, Gateshead, UK

C. Paul Morrow MD
Professor and Director, Division of Gynecologic Oncology, Department of Obstetrics and Gynecology, University of Southern California School of Medicine, Los Angeles, USA

Martin H. N. Tattersall MA MD MSc FRCP FRACP
Professor of Cancer Medicine, University of Sydney; Honorary Physician, Royal Prince Alfred Hospital and King George V Memorial Hospital, Sydney, Australia

SECOND EDITION

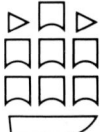

CHURCHILL LIVINGSTONE
EDINBURGH LONDON MELBOURNE NEW YORK AND TOKYO 1992

CHURCHILL LIVINGSTONE
Medical Division of Longman Group UK Limited

Distributed in the United States of America by Churchill
Livingstone Inc., 650 Avenue of the Americas, New York, N.Y.
10011, and by associated companies, branches and
representatives throughout the world.

First edition 1981
Second edition 1992
  Reprinted 1992

ISBN 0-443-04114-8

British Library Cataloguing in Publication Data
A catalogue record for this book is available from the British Library.

Library of Congress Cataloging in Publication Data
Gynecologic oncology / edited by Malcolm Coppleson . . . [et al.]. —
  2nd ed.
      p.   cm.
    Includes bibliographical references.
    Includes index.
    ISBN 0-443-04114-8
    1. Generative organs, Female — Cancer. I. Coppleson, Malcolm.
    [DNLM: 1. Genital Neoplasms, Female. WP 145 G99652]
RC280.G5G896   1992
616.99′465—dc20
DNLM/DLC
for Library of Congress   91–8296
                                                 CIP

The
publisher's
policy is to use
paper manufactured
from sustainable forests

Produced by Longman Group (FE) Ltd
Printed in Hong Kong

Preface

Gynecological neoplasms have shared in that incredible surge of progress in medicine which characterizes the late 20th century. Requirement for a second edition of *Gynecologic Oncology* can therefore come as no surprise, mandated as it was by its share of the many novelties exposed in this book and by rapid advances in both scientific and clinical aspects of the specialty. Amplification and extension of theory and practice have taken their toll of the content of the previous edition such that it became apparent that much of it warranted major change. As an example of this growth the second edition contains an additional 12 chapters.

The sheer compass of the proposed second edition very early in the planning stage made it essential to share the editorial load. To this end three respected colleagues, from various parts of the world, John Monaghan, Paul Morrow and Martin Tattersall, were invited onto a panel as co-editors. This successful arrangement has enhanced the comprehensiveness of the volume. Considerable rearrangement of the author list has occurred from the inevitable attrition involved in the lapse of a decade in time.

The goal for this edition is the same as the first: a comprehensive, indeed encyclopedic account of the current state of the art. The format and organizational concepts are basically unchanged. The structure of the work is that of a textbook, not a series of articles by multiple authors. Each author was given a commission, the precise format being dependent on that section of the book occupied by the chapter. As many contributors could testify, editorial liberty has been ruthlessly taken with the dual purposes of providing cohesiveness and minimizing duplication.

As before, the book is subdivided into several parts. The first chapter of the book discusses *Training of the Gynecologic Oncologist*. There follows discussion of *Epidemiology, Carcinogenesis* including the *Scientific Basis* of the contained disciplines of immunology, pharmacology (chemotherapy), endocrinology and radiation therapy. Authors in these chapters have given a thorough yet concise and easily grasped survey of each topic, maintaining relevance to Gynecologic Oncology. The second section of the book is devoted to *Diagnostic Aids* and includes two new chapters, one on needle biopsy, the other on CT scanning and magnetic resonance imaging. The main bulk of the book deals with the many and varied *Gynecological Malignancies, and their Precursors*, in great detail. On this occasion the structure of this section has been changed so that separation of pathological and clinical matters is consistent throughout. Again our colleagues in pathology have provided a series of valuable chapters which collectively have the effect of veritable provision of a textbook of gynecological oncological pathology within the book. Each of the clinical chapters consists of a detailed comprehensive cover of the subject following a classical format of introduction, clinical features, staging, diagnosis, management and prognosis. In the sections on management authors were asked to review all management options prior to developing their own recommendations concerning therapy. They were asked also not to omit discussion of rarities.

In the section of *Operative Techniques* authors have concentrated on finer points of detail. These chapters have been profusely illustrated. Authors were asked to draw on their experience on discussion of possible errors and risks, how to avoid them and how to correct them if they occur. A review of the literature and detailed results were not requested. Such matters are discussed earlier in the book. The section on *Postoperative Complications* after radical surgery and irradiation has been expanded and a new section devoted to improvement of quality of life by ingenious techniques aimed at the surgical reconstruction of the gynecologic oncology patient has been added. In the final section of the book *After Care*, chapters on the problems of psychological and sexual dysfunction have been amplified and a new chapter on palliative care added.

The Editor of a series of writings by exponents of diverse aspects covered in these volumes is in an unequalled position to sense groundswells of approach which prompt comment in a general synopsis such as a Preface. This is the more especially true in considering that a decade separates the two editions. Undoubtedly the question that recurs in my mind is the abject imbalance between the enormous effort extended in the laboratory and clinic on the cancer problem on the one hand and the quite minor improvements in survival rates on the other. What is the meaning of this profound paradox?

I am well aware of the view of the optimists who can point to considerable advances in therapy of some cancers as a result of rapid progress in chemotherapy more especially in hematological disciplines. My query concerns the great bulk of cancers the subject of these volumes.

Were I to pursue my notions on the nature of the paradox at the philosophical level I could assert that the great majority of our present research is underpinned by an approach that has been dubbed reductionism. If we reduce the problem and its parts to even more refined fragments in pursuit of their understanding, then it will be solely a problem of reassembly of the understood fragments to produce a thorough understanding of the whole. This idea which presently saturates the vast majority of Western scientific thought, particularly in the basic bio- and medical sciences, encompasses the notion that what is then most needed is merely a more intensive prosecution of attempts to understand the reduced parts. It is these more-of-the-same aspects which I ponder most in casting about for an explanation of the paradox. I wonder whether there needs to be a qualitative rather than a quantitative change in the road ahead to the understanding of the cancer problem, a road which takes a new direction rather than a more-of-the-same direction.

If we acknowledge the prospective value of history then it is likely that the smallest hints of this new direction are already with us in the literature but in their obscurity and isolation they bear no banner. Were I bold enough to strain editorial privilege even further and cite at least one of these yet embryonic portents I find myself loitering over the contribution of our colleagues, the physicists. Compared with the chemists their entry to the bioscene at the cell level is rather belated, and by volume of these chemical contributions minor. Rather than an intense concern with the fragments which make up the biosystem, which are of course chemicals, the physicist is more concerned with energy as it permeates amongst these chemicals. The physicist monitors this energy flow through the system as though it were the driver and it will be interesting to note whether the driver has special qualities in the case of cancer tissue. This is not the place to enter details of process of an approach with more claim to be termed holistic but the idea spawns the prospect of a remote control of the biosystem using an entity renowned for its flexibility and its abundance. Such approaches are genuine qualitative breaks with the present scene.

It is a great pleasure to thank my co-editors and all authors and to acknowledge all those who have helped so much in the preparation of this edition. The exercise of superb skills by artists and photographers who have drawn and produced new illustrations and the assistance of my own secretarial force, Jan Hepples, Suzanne Glennon and Christine Young is very much appreciated. A special word of thanks goes to our publisher, Churchill Livingstone, and especially to Andrew Stevenson, Managing Director, Peter Richardson, Publishing Director, Elif Fincanci-Smith, Senior Project Editor, Graham Birnie, Editorial Manager and Alison Crombie, Editorial Assistant, who have been ever helpful from the planning stage to completion of the book.

Malcolm Coppleson

Contributors

Barbara L Andersen PhD
Professor, Departments of Psychology and Obstetrics and Gynecology, The Ohio State University, Columbus, USA

Barrie Anderson MD
Department of Obstetrics and Gynecology, University of Iowa, Iowa City, USA

Diane Anderson BA
Research Analyst, Department of Obstetrics and Gynecology, University of Chicago, Chicago, USA

Bruce Armstrong BMedSc MBBS FRACP D Phil(Oxon)
Commissioner of Health, Health Department of Western Australia, Perth, Australia

Kenneth H Atkinson MBBS FRCOG FRACOG CGO
Gynecologic Surgeon, Department of Gynecologic Oncology, King George V Hospital, Royal Prince Alfred Hospital, Sydney, Australia

Hervy E Averette MD
Professor of Obstetrics and Gynecology and Director, Division of Gynecologic Oncology, University of Miami School of Medicine, Miami, USA

Jan P A Baak MD PhD FRCPath
Professor of Pathology, Institute for Pathology, Free University Hospital, Amsterdam, The Netherlands

Kenneth D Bagshawe CBE MD FRS DSc FRCP FRCOG FRCR
Emeritus Professor of Medical Oncology, Charing Cross Hospital, London, UK

Patricia M Bannatyne MBBS FRCPA
Formerly Senior Histopathologist, Royal Prince Alfred Hospital and King George V Memorial Hospital, Sydney, Australia

Hugh R K Barber MD
Director, Department of Obstetrics and Gynecology, Lenox Hill Hospital, New York City; Professor of Clinical Obstetrics and Gynecology, Cornell University Medical College, New York City, USA

John L Benedet MD FRCS(C)
Professor, Department of Obstetrics and Gynaecology, University of British Columbia and Head, Department of Gynaecology, Vancouver General Hospital, Vancouver, Canada

Jonathan S Berek MD
Director, Division of Gynecologic Oncology; Professor, Department of Obstetrics and Gynecology, UCLA School of Medicine, Jonsson Comprehensive Cancer Center, Los Angeles, USA

Michael L Berman MD
Director, Division of Gynecologic Oncology, Department of Obstetrics and Gynecology, University of California, Irvine Medical Center, Orange, USA

F Xavier Bosch MD MPH
International Agency for Research on Cancer, Lyon, France

Luther W Brady MD
Hylda Cohn/American Cancer Society Professor of Clinical Oncology and Chairman, Department of Radiation Therapy and Nuclear Medicine, The Hahnemann Medical College and Hospital, Philadelphia, USA

William G Brose MD
Assistant Professor and Director of the Pain Management Unit, Stanford University Medical Center, Stanford, USA

C Hilary Buckley MD FRCPath
Senior Lecturer in Gynaecological Pathology, Department of Pathological Sciences, University of Manchester, Manchester; Honorary Consultant Histopathologist, St Mary's Hospital, Manchester, UK

Erich Burghardt MD
Professor and Head, Department of Gynecology and
Obstetrics, University of Graz, Graz, Austria

William Chanen MBBS DGO(Melbourne) FRCSE FRACS
FRCOG FRACOG
Honorary Consulting Surgeon and former Head of the
Gynecologic Oncology and the Dysplasia and
Colposcopy Units, Royal Women's Hospital, Melbourne,
Australia

William M Christopherson MD
Professor of Pathology, University of Louisville School
of Medicine, Louisville, USA

Philip B Clement MD FRCP(C)
Pathologist, Vancouver General Hospital; Clinical
Professor of Pathology, Faculty of Medicine, University
of British Columbia, Vancouver, Canada

Carmel J Cohen MD
Professor of Obstetrics and Gynecology, Director,
Division of Gynecologic Oncology, Chairman,
Department of Obstetrics and Gynecology, The Mount
Sinai School of Medicine of the City University of New
York, New York, USA

Malcolm Coppleson MB BS MD(Syd) FRCOG FRACOG
Clinical Professor, University of Sydney; Head,
Department of Gynecologic Oncology, King George V
Memorial Hospital, Royal Prince Alfred Hospital,
Sydney, Australia

Michael J Cousins MB BS MD(Syd) FFARACS FFARCS
Professor and Head, Department of Anesthesia and Pain
Management, Royal North Shore Hospital, University of
Sydney, Sydney, Australia

Wendy Cozen DO MPH
Research Associate Professor, Department of Preventive
Medicine, University of Southern California School of
Medicine, Los Angeles, USA

William T Creasman MD
Sims-Hester Professor and Chairman, Department of
Obstetrics and Gynecology, Medical University of South
Carolina, Charleston, USA

John L Currie MD
Director, Division of Gynecologic Oncology,
Department of Obstetrics and Gynecology, Johns
Hopkins University School of Medicine, Baltimore, USA

John P Curtin MD
Assistant Professor, Division of Gynecologic Oncology,
Department of Obstetrics and Gynecology, University of
Southern California Medical School, Los Angeles, USA

J Christopher Dalrymple MBBS FRACOG
Staff Specialist, Department of Gynecologic Oncology,
King George V Hospital, Royal Prince Alfred Hospital,
Sydney, Australia

Brian Daunter BSc MSc PhD
Senior Lecturer in Human Reproductive Biology,
Department of Obstetrics and Gynecology, University of
Queensland, Brisbane, Australia

A D DePetrillo MD FRCS(C)
Director, Division Gynecologic Oncology, University of
Toronto; Head, Surgical Oncology, Princess Margaret
Hospital, Toronto, Canada

Sir John Dewhurst FRCOG FRCSE Hon DSc MD FACOG
FRCSI
Formerly Professor of Obstetrics and Gynaecology,
Institute of Obstetrics and Gynaecology, Queen
Charlotte's Maternity Hospital, London, UK

Philip J DiSaia MD
The Dorothy Marsh Chair in Reproductive Biology;
Professor, Department of Obstetrics and Gynecology,
University of California, Irvine, Orange, USA

Janneke van der Does MD
Resident, University Hospital, Leiden, The Netherlands

Daniel M Donato MD
Assistant Professor, Division of Gynecologic Oncology,
Department of Obstetrics and Gynecology, University of
Miami, Miami, USA

James H Dorsey MD
Chairman, Department of Gynecology, Greater Baltimore
Medical Center, Baltimore, USA

Peter M Elliott MD BS DGO FRCOG FACOG FRACOG
FCOG(SL) FAOFOG
Senior Gynecologic Surgeon, Department of Gynecologic
Oncology, King George V Memorial Hospital, Royal
Prince Alfred Hospital, Sydney, Australia

Alex Ferenczy MD
Professor of Pathology, Obstetrics and Gynecology,
McGill University and the Sir Mortimer B Davis Jewish
General Hospital, Montreal, Canada

Sir Rustam Feroze MD FRCS FRCOG FACOG
Formerly Consultant Obstetrician and Gynaecologist,
King's College Hospital, London, UK

Neil J Finkler MD
Division of Gynecologic Oncology, Brigham and
Women's Hospital, Dana Farber Cancer Institute,
Harvard Medical School, Boston, USA

Harold Fox MD FRCPath
Professor of Reproductive Pathology, University of
Manchester, Honorary Consultant Pathologist, United
Manchester Hospitals, Manchester, UK

Yao S Fu MD
Professor of Pathology, Department of Pathology,

UCLA School of Medicine, Jonsson Comprehensive Cancer Center, Los Angeles, USA

William J Garrett AM MD BS DPhil FRCSEd FRACS FRCOG FRACOG HonFRACR
Director, Department of Diagnostic Ultrasound, Royal Hospital for Women, Sydney, Australia

David M Gershenson MD
Professor and Deputy Chairman, Department of Gynecology, The University of Texas, MD Anderson Cancer Center, Houston, USA

Laman A Gray MD
Clinical Professor of Obstetrics and Gynecology, University of Louisville School of Medicine, Louisville, USA

C Thomas Griffiths MD
Gynecologic Oncologist, New England Baptist Hospital, Boston, USA

Neville F Hacker FRACOG FRCOG FACOG FACS
Director, Department of Gynaecological Oncology, School of Obstetrics and Gynaecology, The University of New South Wales and the Royal Hospital for Women, Sydney, Australia

William R Hart MD
Chairman, Department of Pathology; Vice Chairman, Division of Laboratory Medicine, The Cleveland Clinic Foundation, Cleveland, USA

Harald zur Hausen MD DSc (Hon)
Scientific Director, The German Cancer Research Centre, Heidelberg, Germany

Arthur L Herbst MD
Chairman and Joseph Bolivar DeLee Distinguished Service Professor, Department of Obstetrics and Gynecology, University of Chicago, Chicago, USA

Robert V Higgins MD
Assistant Professor, Division of Gynecologic Oncology, University of Kentucky Medical Center, Lexington, USA

Michael K Hohl Prof Dr
Professor and Head of Department of Obstetrics and Gynecology, Kantonsspital, Baden, Switzerland

William J Hoskins MD
Attending Surgeon and Chief, Gynecology Service, Department of Surgery, Memorial Sloan-Kettering Cancer Center, New York, USA

Shirley J Huang MD
Resident, Department of Pathology, UCLA School of Medicine, Los Angeles, USA

Christopher C Hudson MCHIR FRCS FRCOG FRACOG
Physician Accoucheur, St Bartholomew's Hospital, London, UK

Robert P S Jansen BSc(Med) MB BS FRACP FRCOG FRACOG
Visiting Gynaecologist, The Endocrinology Fertility Unit, King George V Memorial Hospital, Royal Prince Alfred Hospital, Sydney, Australia

Joseph A Jordan MD FRCOG
Consultant Gynaecologist, Birmingham and Midland Hospital for Women, Honorary Senior Lecturer, University of Birmingham, Birmingham, UK

Charles A F Joslin MB BS DMRT FRCR MIERE CEng
Professor and Head of University Department of Radiotherapy, Leeds; Honorary Consultant Radiotherapist, Leeds Area Health Authority, UK

Soo Keat Khoo MB BS MD FRCOG FRACOG
Professor, Department of Obstetrics and Gynaecology, University of Queensland, Brisbane, Australia

Carolyn V Kirschner MD
Department of Obstetrics and Gynecology, Rush Medical College, Rush Presbyterian, St Luke's Medical Center, Chicago, USA

Olle Kjellgren MD PhD FIAC(Hon)
Formerly Professor, Department of Gynecologic Oncology, University of Umea, Sweden

Alf Kolbenstvedt MD
Professor, Department of Radiology, Rikshospitalet, The National Hospital, University of Oslo, Oslo, Norway

Per Kolstad MD FRCOG(Hon)
Research Chief Gynecologic Oncology, Norsk Hydro's Institute for Cancer Research, the Norwegian Radium Hospital, Oslo, Norway

Philip J Krupp BS MD
Clinical Professor in Obstetrics and Gynecology, Tulane University; Medical Director, Oncology Center Mercy Hospital; Senior Visiting Surgeon, Charity Hospital at New Orleans, Louisiana, USA

Raymond L Lee MD
Chairman, Division of Gynecologic Surgery, Mayo Clinic and Mayo Foundation; Professor of Obstetrics and Gynecology, Mayo Medical School, Rochester, USA

Richard Lee MBBS FFARACS
Senior Specialist, Intensive Care Unit, St Vincent's Hospital, Sydney, Australia

John L Lewis Jr MD
Chief, Gynecology Service, Memorial Sloan-Kettering Cancer Center, New York, USA

J Norelle Lickiss MD(Syd) FRCP(Edin) FRACP
Director of Palliative Care, Royal Prince Alfred Hospital and King George V Memorial Hospital; Clinical Associate Professor, University of Sydney, Sydney, Australia

Hans H Lien MD
Department of Diagnostic Radiology, The Norwegian
Radium Hospital, Oslo, Norway

Bengt Lindahl MD
Department of Obstetrics and Gynecology, University
Hospital, Lund, Sweden

John R Lurain MD
John and Ruth Brewer Professor of Gynecology and Cancer
Research; Chief, Section of Gynecologic Oncology,
Department of Obstetrics and Gynecology, Northwestern
University of Medical School, Chicago, USA

Thomas M Mack MD MPH
Associate Professor, Department of Family and
Preventive Medicine; Director, Cancer Surveillance
Program, University of Southern California School of
Medicine, Los Angeles, USA

Eric V Mackay MB BS MGO(Melb) FRCSE FRCOG FRACS
FRACOG
Professor Emeritus, Department of Obstetrics and
Gynecology, University of Queensland, Brisbane,
Australia

Don R McNeil PhD FASA
Professor of Statistics, Macquarie University, Sydney,
Australia

Alberto Manetta MD
Associate Professor, Department of Obstetrics and
Gynecology, University of California, Irvine Medical
Center, Orange, USA

Otoniel Martinez-Maza PhD
Assistant Professor, Departments of Obstetrics and
Gynecology, Microbiology and Immunology,
UCLA School of Medicine, Los Angeles, USA

Warwick Middleton
Deputy Director of Psychiatry, Royal Brisbane Hospital;
Senior Lecturer in Psychiatry, University of
Queensland, Brisbane, Australia

Anthony B Miller MB FRCP
Professor, Department of Preventive Medicine and
Biostatistics, Faculty of Medicine, University of
Toronto, Toronto, Canada

Dianne M Miller BSc MD FRCSC
Division of Gynecologic Oncology, Cancer Control
Agency of British Columbia and Assistant Professor,
Department of Obstetrics and Gynecology, Faculty of
Medicine, University of British Columbia, Vancouver,
Canada

John M Monaghan MB FRCS (ED) FRCOG
Director of Gynaecological Oncology Services, Regional
Department of Gynaecological Oncology, Queen
Elizabeth Hospital, Gateshead, UK

Fredrick J Montz MD FACOG FACS
Assistant Professor, Division of Gynecologic Oncology,
UCLA School of Medicine, Los Angeles, USA

George W Morley MD
Associate Chairman and Norman F Miller Professor of
Gynecology, The University of Michigan Medical
School, Ann Arbor, USA

C Paul Morrow MD
Professor and Director, Division of Gynecologic
Oncology, Department of Obstetrics and Gynecology,
University of Southern California School of Medicine,
Los Angeles, USA

Nubia Munoz MD MPH
Chief, Unit of Field and Intervention Studies,
International Agency for Research on Cancer, Lyon,
France

John R van Nagell Jr MD
Director, Division of Gynecologic Oncology, American
Cancer Society Professor of Clinical Oncology,
University of Kentucky Medical Center, Lexington, USA

James H Nelson Jr MD
Professor and Director, Division of Gynecologic
Oncology, New York Medical College, New York, USA

Alan B P Ng MD
Professor of Pathology, Department of Pathology,
University of Sydney and Head, Department of
Anatomic Pathology, Royal Prince Alfred Hospital and
King George V Memorial Hospital, Sydney, Australia

Henry J Norris MD
Director, Department of Gynecologic and Breast
Pathology, Armed Forces Institute of Pathology; Clinical
Professor, Department of Pathology, Uniformed Services
University of the Health Sciences, F Edward Herbert
School of Medicine, Washington DC, USA

Dennis M O'Connor MD COL MC
Assistant Professor, Departments of Obstetrics and
Gynecology and Pathology, Uniformed Services
University of the Health Sciences, F Edward Herbert
School of Medicine; Staff Physician, Department of
Obstetrics and Gynecology, National Naval Medical
Center, Bethesda, USA

Cees Oudejans MD PhD
Research Scientist, Institute for Pathology, Free University
Hospital, Amsterdam, The Netherlands

Fernando J Paradinas FRCPath
Department of Histopathology, Charing Cross and
Westminster Medical School, University of London,
London, UK

Roy T Parker MD
F Bayard Carter Professor, Chairman Emeritus,

Department of Obstetrics and Gynecology, Duke University Medical Center, Durham, USA

William A Peters III MD
Gynecologic Oncologist; Clinical Associate Professor of Obstetrics and Gynecology, University of Washington, Seattle, USA

M Steven Piver MD
Chief, Department of Gynecologic Oncology, Roswell Park Cancer Institute; Clinical Professor and Director of Gynecologic Oncology, State University of New York at Buffalo, Buffalo, USA

Ellis C Pixley MB BS FRCOG FRACOG
Consultant Gynecologist to Health Department of Western Australia, Perth, Australia

Martin C Powell FRCS MRCOG
Senior Registrar, Obstetrics & Gynaecology, City Hospital, Nottingham, UK

Michael A Quinn MBChB MGO MRCP FRACOG CGO
Director, Gynecological Oncology, Royal Women's Hospital, Melbourne; Associate Professor, Department of Obstetrics and Gynaecology, University of Melbourne, Melbourne, Australia

Beverley Raphael MD FRANZCP MRCPsych
Professor and Head, Department of Psychiatry, University of Queensland and Royal Brisbane Hospital, Brisbane, Australia

Bevan L Reid MD(Syd) BVSc DTMH
Formerly Reader, Queen Elizabeth Research Institute, The University of Sydney, Sydney, Australia

Richard Reid MD
Assistant Professor, Wayne State University School of Medicine, Detroit, USA

Ralph M Richart MD
Professor of Pathology, Columbia University College of Physicians and Surgeons; Director, Division of Obstetrical and Gynecologic Pathology and Cytology, The Sloane Hospital for Women, New York City, USA

Stephen C Rubin MD
Gynecology Service, Department of Surgery, Memorial Sloan-Kettering Cancer Center, New York, New York, USA

Peter Russell BSc(Med) MD FRCPA
Senior Histopathologist, Royal Prince Alfred Hospital and King George V Memorial Hospital, Sydney, Australia

Shoichi Sakamoto MD
Professor, Tokyo Women's Medical College, Professor Emeritus and formerly Chairman, Department of

Obstetrics and Gynecology, Faculty of Medicine, University of Tokyo, Tokyo, Japan

Peter Scheidel MD
Professor and Chief Surgeon, Department of Gynecology and Obstetrics, Marienkrankenhaus, University of Hamburg, Hamburg, Germany

Robert E Scully MD
Professor of Pathology, Massachusetts General Hospital, Harvard Medical School, Boston, USA

John H Shepherd FRCS MRCOG
Consultant Gynaecological Surgeon, St Bartholomew's and the Royal Marsden Hospitals, London, UK

John Simes MD MSc FRACP
Director, National Health and Medical Research Council Clinical Trials Center, University of Sydney, Sydney, Australia

Albert Singer PhD DPhil(Oxon) FRCOG
Consultant Gynaecologist, Whittington and Royal Northern Hospitals, London, UK

H John Solomon MB BS(Syd) FRCOG FRACOG CGO
Gynecologic Surgeon, Department of Gynecological Oncology, King George V Memorial Hospital, Royal Prince Alfred Hospital, Sydney, Australia

Adolf Stafl MD PhD
Professor, Department of Obstetrics and Gynecology, Medical College of Wisconsin, Milwaukee, USA

Osamu Sugimoto MD
Professor and Head, Department of Obstetrics and Gynecology, Osaka Medical College, Osaka, Japan

Richard E Symmonds MD
Emeritus Senior Consultant, Department of Obstetrics and Gynecology, Mayo Clinic and Mayo Foundation; Emeritus Professor of Obstetrics and Gynecology, Mayo Medical School, Rochester, USA

E Malcolm Symonds MD FRCOG
Professor and Head of Department of Obstetrics and Gynaecology, University Hospital, Queen's Medical Centre, The University of Nottingham, Nottingham, UK

Martin H N Tattersall MA MD MSc FRCP FRACP
Professor of Cancer Medicine, University of Sydney Honorary Physician, Royal Prince Alfred Hospital and King George V Memorial Hospital, Sydney, Australia

John D Thompson MD
Professor, Department of Gynecology and Obstetrics, Emory University, School of Medicine, Atlanta, USA

Leslee J Thompson RN MScN
Director of Nursing, Toronto — Bayview Regional Cancer Centre; Assistant Professor, Faculty of Nursing, University of Toronto, Toronto, Canada

Duane E Townsend MD
Professor and Vice Chairman, Department of Obstetrics
and Gynecology, University of California, Davis,
Sacramento, USA

Claes Trope MD PhD
Professor and Head, Department of Gynecologic
Oncology, The Norwegian Radium Hospital, Oslo,
Norway

Jan M M Walboomers PhD
Head of Molecular Pathology, Institute for Pathology, Free
University Hospital, Amsterdam, The Netherlands

Peter S Warren MB ChB FRACR
Senior Specialist, Department of Medical Imaging,
Royal Hospital for Women, Sydney, Australia

Maurice J Webb MD
Professor of Obstetrics and Gynecology, Mayo Medical
School; Consultant, Division of Gynecologic Surgery,
Mayo Clinic and Mayo Foundation, Rochester, USA

John C Weed Jr MD
Professor and Director of Gynecologic Oncology,
University of Kansas, Medical Center, Kansas City, USA

Clifford R Wheeless Jr MD
Professor of Gynecology, Director of Gynecologic
Oncology, Emory University School of Medicine,
Atlanta, USA

George D Wilbanks MD
The John M Simpson Professor and Chairman,
Department of Obstetrics and Gynecology, Rush
Medical College, Rush Presbyterian, St Luke's Medical
Center, Chicago, USA

Barbara Winkler MD
Associate Professor of Clinical Pathology, Columbia
University College of Physicians and Surgeons, New
York City, USA

Brian S Worthington BSc MB BS DMRD FRCR
Professor of Diagnostic Radiology, Department of
Radiology, University Hospital, Nottingham, UK

Robert C Wright MB BS FFARACS FRACP
Director of Intensive Care, St Vincent's Hospital,
Sydney, Australia

Robert H Young MD
Associate Professor of Pathology, Massachusetts General
Hospital, Harvard Medical School, Boston, USA

Contents
Volume 2

46. Premalignant lesions of the endometrium: endometrial hyperplasia and adenocarcinoma in situ

W. M. Christopherson   L. A. Gray

INTRODUCTION

The term 'premalignant' is rather imprecise and at times evasive. It has been applied to a variety of lesions that would appear to have varying degrees of potential for the subsequent development of cancer. The degree of risk is known for only a few precancerous lesions, for example xeroderma pigmentosa and familial polyposis. Other less obvious cancer precursors such as solar keratosis and isolated colonic adenomatous polyps have a less well documented premalignant connotation.

In the female genital tract there are several lesions which at one time or another were presumed to be premalignant but have not endured the test of time. One such example is vulvar leukoplakia. At one time it was so highly regarded as to have resulted in what presently would be considered excessive surgery. Leukoplakia currently is not even recognized as a specific pathologic entity and vulvectomy is no longer recommended for these white patches. Other lesions exist which, because of their worrisome histological appearance, would seem likely to be cancer precursors. The association of clear cell carcinoma with vaginal and cervical adenosis resulted in the postulation that adenosis was probably a precursor of clear cell carcinoma. Evidence for this has not materialized.[22] To date only 16 clear cell carcinomas have apparently developed in young women while under surveillance for vaginal adenosis. (See p. 529.)

The association of hyperplasia with adenocarcinoma of the endometrium has been amply documented.[4,8,16,17,40,49,50] Both are associated with estrogen,[5,12,32,34,35,42] however, proof that hyperplasia is a transition stage is more difficult to document (see Chs 3 and 8).

The lack of uniform terminology and the impreciseness of definitions that have existed for over half a century compound the problem of understanding the predestination of endometrial hyperplasia. Prospective studies are difficult to conduct because of the lengthy follow-up required. Another obstacle to long-term surveillance is that hysterectomy is often performed in the interim or the exogenous estrogens withdrawn after hyperplasia is diagnosed. The studies also lack consistency of terminology and definitions previously mentioned.[6,11,23,33] The precise relative risk is thus difficult to determine from past studies. The risk, however, does seem greater for postmenopausal than for premenopausal women.[29,40]

It is now generally agreed that invasive cancer of most, if not all, sites must evolve through an in situ stage. There is convincing biological evidence that such is the case.[46] Logic would compel us to believe that even carcinoma in situ is not likely to develop de novo but rather evolve from precursor lesions. The important point is that the many morphologically disturbing epithelial lesions have not only a wide spectrum of cytologic and morphologic changes, but undoubtedly a wide variety of initiating factors, and for some at least a similar wide spectrum of biologic potential.

There is ample evidence that both endometrial hyperplasia and carcinoma are estrogen-dependent and that either endogenous estrogens in excess or unopposed exogenous estrogen predispose to their development. There appears to be an increased risk for endometrial hyperplasia as well as for carcinoma in women with estrogen-producing tumors[32] and in women with sclerocystic ovaries.[27] The latter are anovulatory and thus would presumably have non-cyclic estrogen stimulation of the endometrium. At the other end of the spectrum women with gonadal dysgenesis rarely develop endometrial hyperplasia or endometrial adenocarcinoma unless they receive estrogen therapy to promote secondary sexual development.[12,42] To complicate the picture, most of the estrogen-treated hypogonadal patients appear not to develop hyperplasia and in one study those that did received a lifetime conjugated estrogen dose of 2500 mg or more for periods longer than 4.2 years.[42]

While it appears to be unlikely that endometrial hyperplasia or adenocarcinoma develops in the absence of estrogens, the precise role of estrogen is poorly understood. The endometrium is perhaps the most dynamic tissue in the body. Its cyclic regeneration, maturation and shedding is dependent on the female sex hormones, notably estrogen and progesterone. In women with anovulation or irregular ovulation the persistent estrogen stimulation can produce a continuous proliferation of the endometrium that could, by pathologic definition, be considered hyperplastic. Recognizing the significance of such changes in a younger woman, most pathologists would prefer to diagnose such samples as being consistent with ovulation failure rather than reporting the change as 'proliferative hyperplasia or simple hyperplasia', which in fact it is, albeit not immediately related to a premalignant change. Atypical endometrial changes are also associated with the presence of chorionic tissue.[2] This is a physiological phenomenon which is totally reversible.

Essentially every author who has written on the subject of endometrial hyperplasia has stressed the need for uniform terminology and for uniform definitions, usually pointing out the difficulties in determining the premalignant potential of a particular pattern due to the inconsistency of definitions. For this reason we have chosen to use the classification adopted by Vellios who wrote the Armed Forces Institute of Pathology (AFIP) fascicle on the uterus (Table 46.1).[51] These authoritative volumes are widely used as standard references by pathologists both in the United States and abroad. We have no other *a priori* reason to select this classification. Since the diagnoses are highly subjective all definitions must be somewhat imprecise within the limits of subjectivity, however, a degree of uniformity is absolutely essential in classification if more precise knowledge of the relative significance of the various degrees of hyperplasia is to be elucidated sometime in the future.

The historical account of the lesions under discussion has been thoroughly covered by numerous authors[17,18,52] so it need not be repeated here. The discussion will be confined to those types of endometrial hyperplasia and carcinoma in situ that may be precursors of adenocarcinoma of the endometrium. (See also Ch. 47.)

Table 46.1 Precursor lesions of invasive endometrial carcinoma[51]

1. Cystic hyperplasia
2. Adenomatous hyperplasia
3. Atypical hyperplasia
4. Carcinoma in situ

PATHOLOGY

Cystic hyperplasia

The least controversial type of hyperplasia is cystic hyperplasia. It must be distinguished histologically from proliferative endometrium with the occasional cystic gland. In patients using sequential contraceptives and in the occasional anovulatory endometrium, the glands may also be dilated.[51] Cystic atrophy can acquire a polypoid configuration and should not be confused with regressing cystic hyperplasia. In cystic atrophy the glandular epithelium is flattened and atrophic and the stroma tends to be reduced in amount and often appears fibrous (Fig. 46.1).

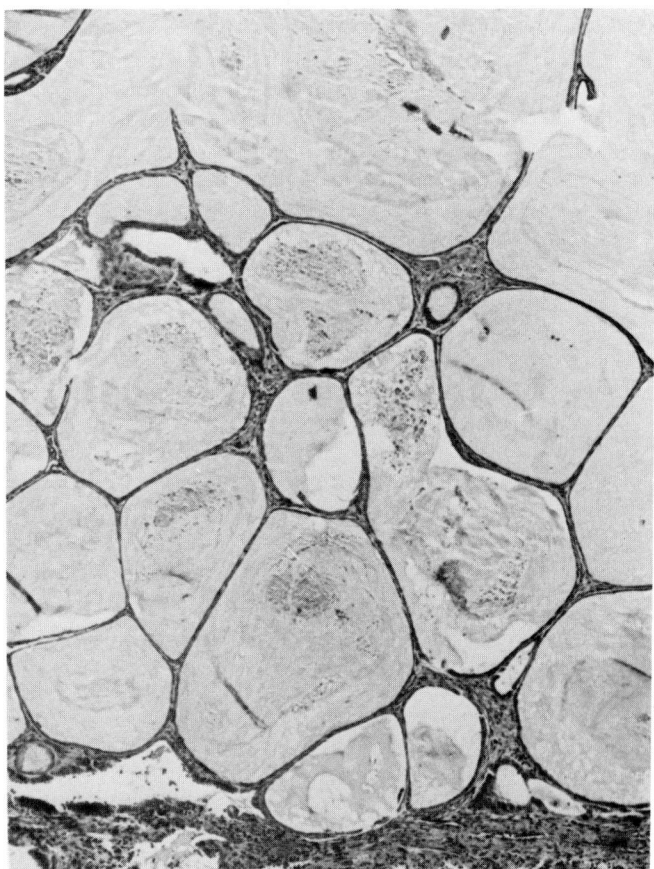

Fig. 46.1 Cystic atrophy of the endometrium (H & E ×79)

On gross examination endometrium in cystic hyperplasia may be increased in thickness and polypoid areas may be present. The amount of material obtained by curettage is usually more abundant than is the case in proliferative phase endometrium. Unlike carcinoma the gross specimen is soft and appears mucoid and glistening.

Under low power magnification it is characterized by dilated cystic glands whose lumens may contain debris and histiocytes. There is no particular crowding of the glands as opposed to the more marked forms of hyperplasia. The stroma often in fact appears to be increased in amount. The morphology had led to the term 'Swiss cheese hyperplasia' (Fig. 46.2).

Under higher magnification the stromal cells are densely packed and their nuclear diameter is larger than the stromal cells in proliferative phase endometrium.[21] Mitoses in both stroma and glands are variable but can usually be found without much difficulty. Atypical mitoses are not encountered. The surface epithelium and the cells lining the gland lumens may be columnar, cuboidal or flattened, largely dependent on the degree of dilatation of the particular gland examined. Pseudostratification, if present, is patchy and minimal. Well formed cilia can be found, usually in large numbers. They are often absent in the very distended glands. The nuclei of the columnar cells are

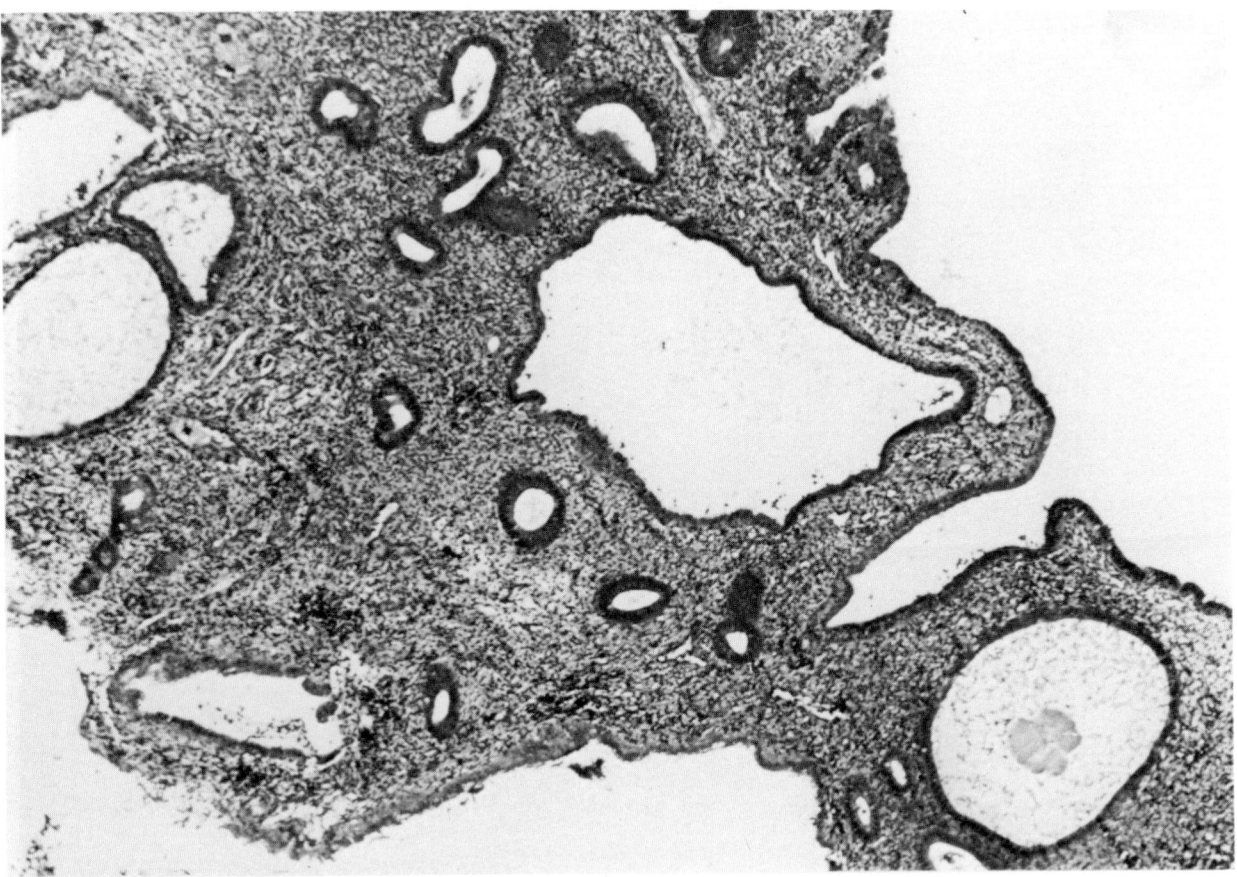

Fig. 46.2 Cystic hyperplasia from curettings. Note the abundant stroma and non-crowding of the glands. (H & E ×79)

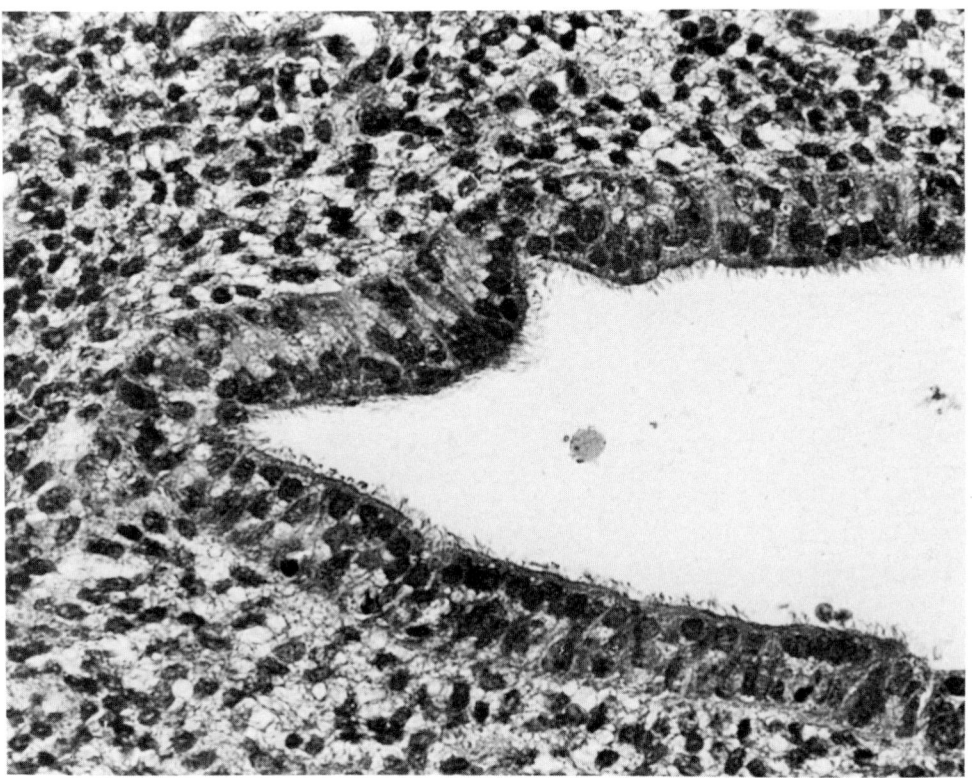

Fig. 46.3 High power of gland in cystic hyperplasia. Note pseudostratification and numerous cilia. (H & E ×500)

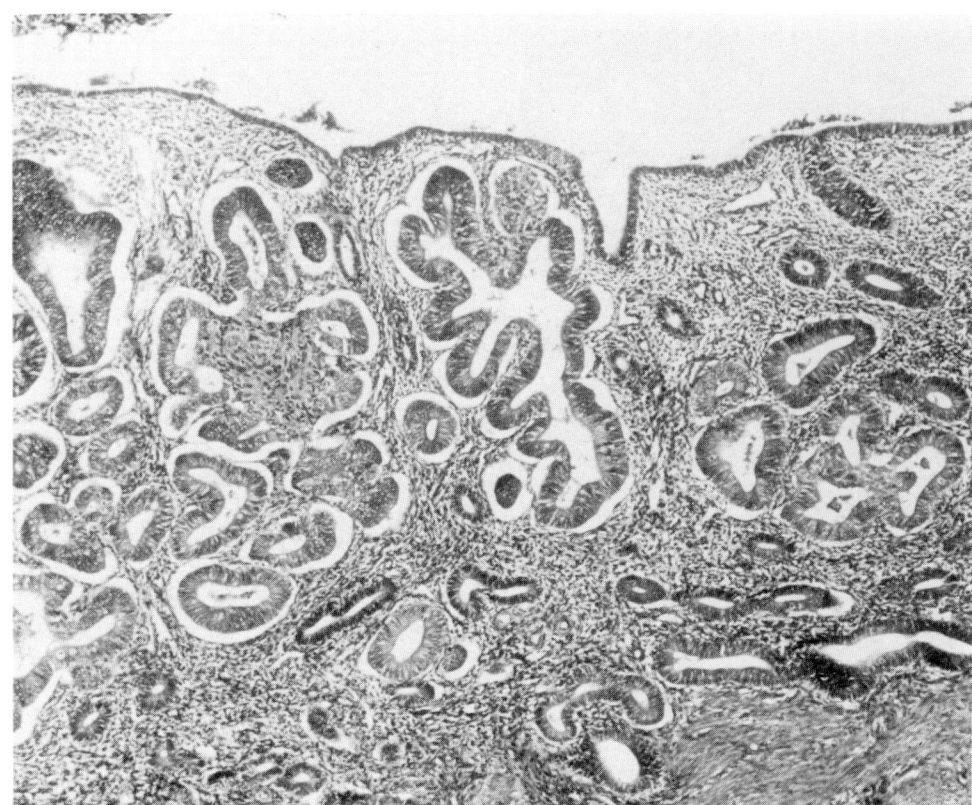

Fig. 46.4 Adenomatous hyperplasia. Note the irregular glands with outpouching and crowding of the adjacent smaller glands. There is a squamous morule to the left. (H & E ×79).

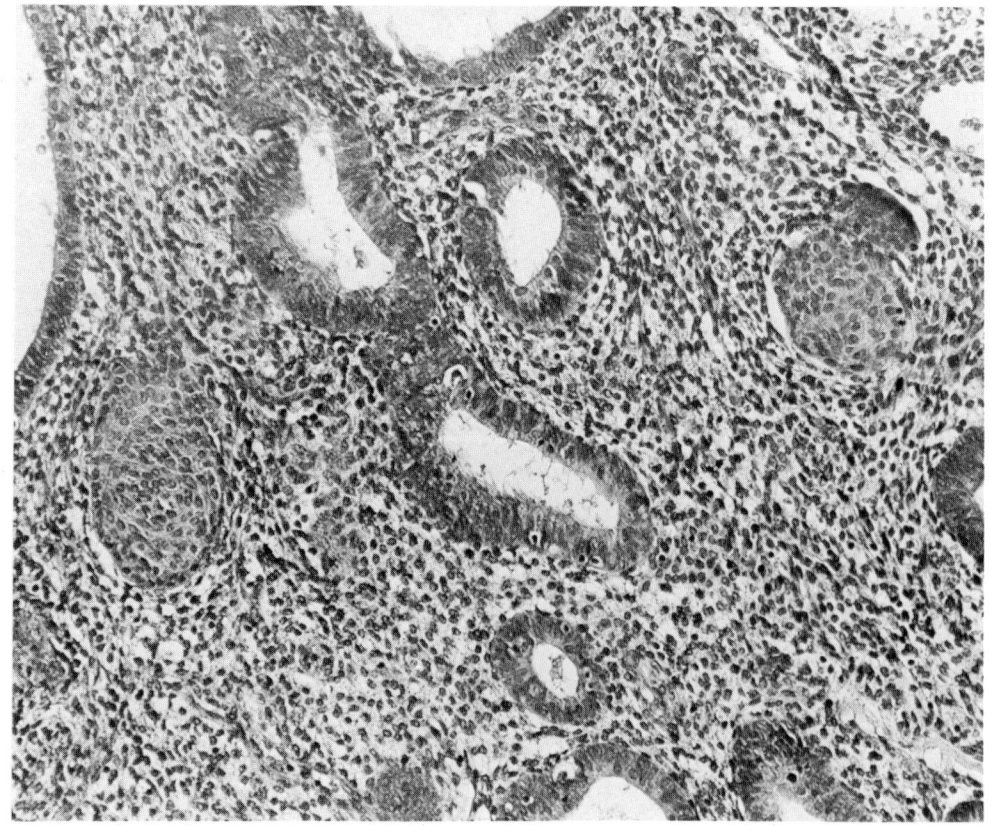

Fig. 46.5 Adenomatous hyperplasia with squamous morules. Same case as Figure 46.4. Note pseudostratification and numerous mitoses in the glands which are much less crowded than in Figure 46.4. (H & E ×197).

elongated, usually vesicular and are oriented perpendicular to the surface. Chromocenters may be distinct but nucleoli are not (Fig. 46.3). Chromosome analysis and microspectrophotometric patterns are said to be identical with those of nuclei of the normal proliferative endometrium.[26,54]

Adenomatous hyperplasia

This category of endometrial hyperplasia is noted by essentially all authors as an area of some confusion and disagreement, due largely to terminology and definitions. The term as used by Gusberg is a comprehensive one which also includes atypical hyperplasia and carcinoma in situ.[18,19,20] It has been modified by subsequent authors to denote more specific histologic changes.[23,51] Since the more recent trend seems to be to attempt to separate adenomatous hyperplasia from lesions which appear morphologically and cytologically more advanced, we will use the more restrictive definition.

Adenomatous hyperplasia produces an increased thickness of the endometrium either in a diffuse pattern or in an irregular fashion with the hyperplasia intermingled with normal endometrium. At times it occurs as a focal change in cystic hyperplasia, and scattered dilated cystic glands are occasionally present in predominantly adenomatous hyperplasia. The low magnification appearance is one of closely packed, irregularly distributed glands. There is glandular outpouching into the endometrial stroma and these evaginations may appear in clusters with a microfollicular pattern adjacent to the larger irregular gland (Fig. 46.4). The appearance is dependent on the plane of section. The epithelium is similar to that of proliferative endometrium. The nuclei are uniform and tend to be oval and are without prominent nucleoli. The degree of pseudostratification is usually minimal and depends largely on the thickness of the section. Mitoses are usually frequent. Squamous morules are occasionally found (Fig. 46.5). The stroma is variable and rarely the stromal cells are fat-laden as they may also be in atypical hyperplasia as well as in endometrial carcinoma. When the term 'adenomatous hyperplasia' is used in this more restrictive sense it is not easily confused with well differentiated adenocarcinoma.

Atypical hyperplasia

Atypical hyperplasia, like the other forms, usually produces a thickened endometrium which may be quite copious in the curettage specimen. It usually occurs in conjunction with one of the lesser forms of hyperplasia and is

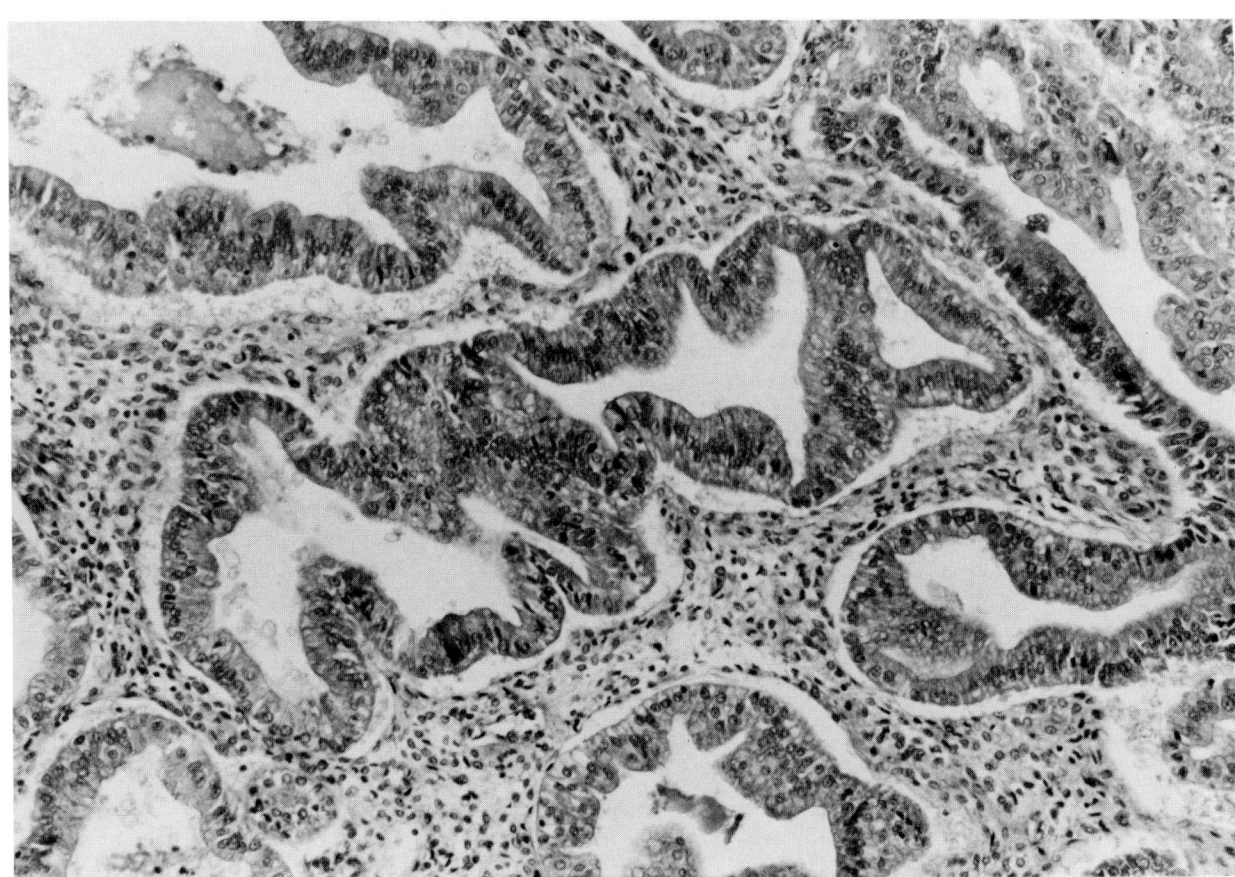

Fig. 46.6 Atypical endometrial hyperplasia. Note the large convoluted glands and decreased stroma. (H & E ×197)

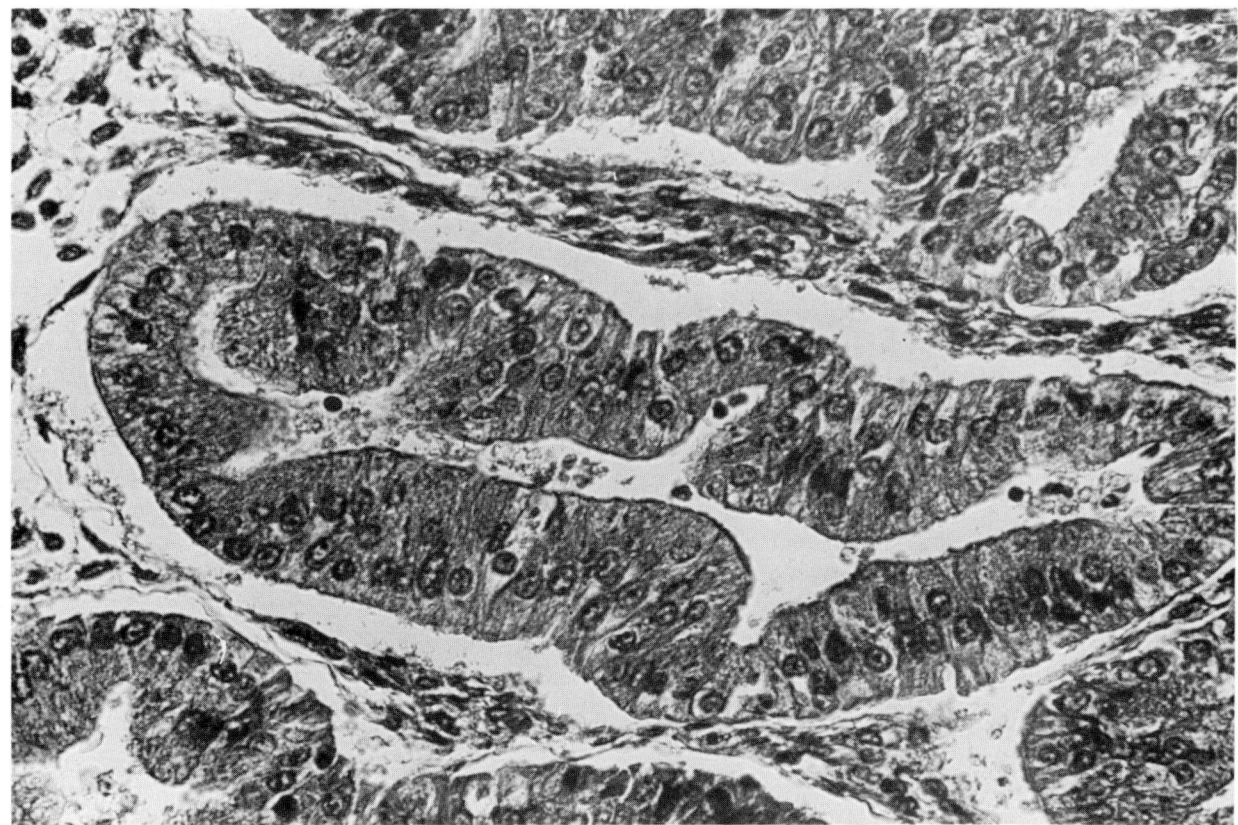

Fig. 46.7 Atypical endometrial hyperplasia. Note the rounding of the nuclei and scanty stroma. (H & E ×500).

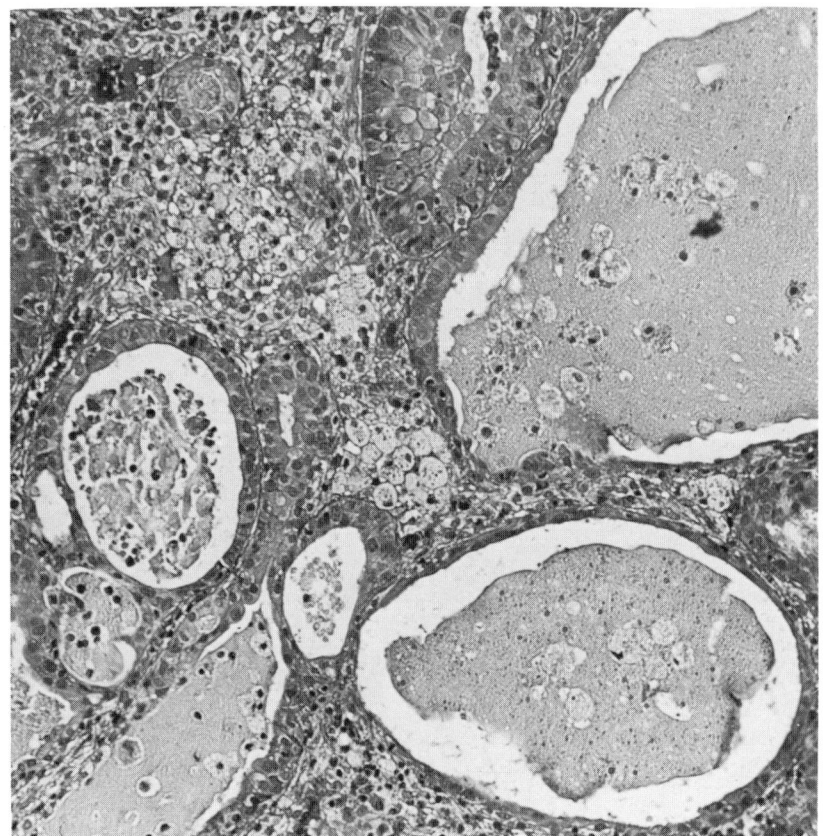

Fig. 46.8 Atypical endometrial hyperplasia to illustrate lipid-laden stromal cells. (H & E ×197)

rarely diffuse throughout the entire endometrium. It is characterized by larger, very irregular glands with a pronounced decrease in the intervening stroma. The process of proliferation produces infolding into the glandular lumen. This at times may be extensive (Fig. 46.6). The definitive diagnosis depends on a critical evaluation of the epithelial cells (Fig. 46.7). The nuclei are large and tend to round out, there is nuclear pleomorphism but distinct nucleoli are not common. When they are present they are not as prominent, as irregular nor as often multiple as they are in carcinoma in situ. In contrast to carcinoma in situ the amount of cytoplasm is not greatly increased and is not eosinophilic. Both squamous morules and fat-laden stromal cells may occasionally be present (Fig. 46.8).

Carcinoma in situ

Carcinoma in situ of the endometrium is perhaps the most controversial lesion under discussion. Some authors do not use the term, preferring to group such cases with adenomatous hyperplasia,[18,19,20] or atypical hyperplasia.[38] The lesion as defined by Hertig and associates[14,24] and later by Buehl et al[7] and by Vellios[52] has a distinctive histologic appearance. Using the criteria of these authors it is possible to delineate a group of endometria that can be dis-

tinguished from adenomatous and atypical hyperplasia as herein described and on the other hand from invasive endometrial carcinoma. Whether this delineation can be correlated with the malignant potential of the various lesions remains to be proven.

In a review Welch & Scully stressed the cytologic features and the limited extent of carcinoma in situ as important criteria for diagnosis.[55] If more than five or six glands are involved those authors designate the lesions as adenocarcinoma with the realization that invasion of the stroma is often impossible to distinguish from the crowding of non-invasive atypical glands. We are in agreement with these authors in that the cytologic features are most important, however, we are less restrictive about the extent of the lesion.

Table 46.2 Criteria for diagnosis of carcinoma in situ of endometrium[7]

Nuclear hyperchromatism
Nuclear irregularity in size and shape
Clumping of nuclear chromatin
Enlarged nucleoli
Eosinophilia of the cytoplasm
Loss of nuclear polarity
Piling up of epithelial cells
Intraglandular epithelial bridges

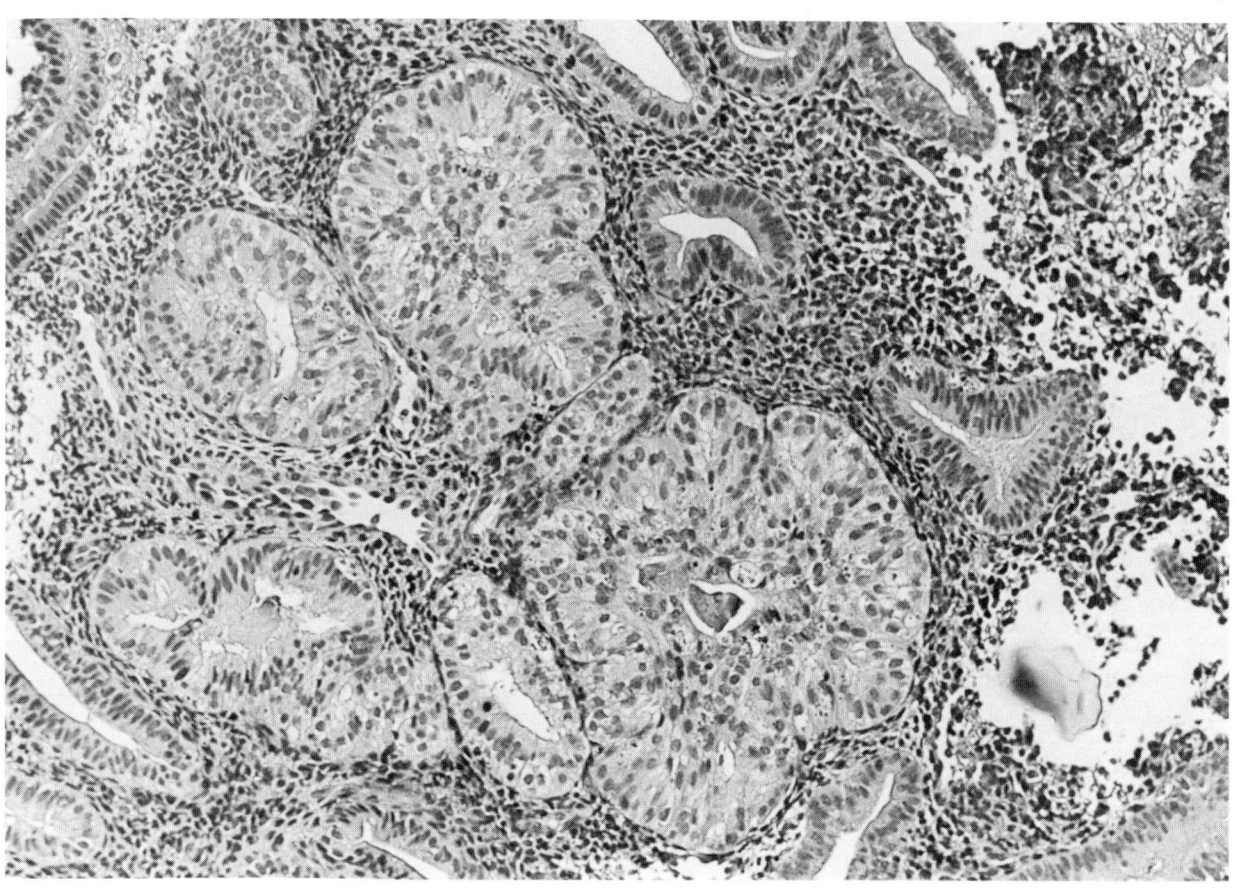

Fig. 46.9 Small focus of carcinoma in situ of endometrium. Only five or six glands were involved. There is no stromal invasion. The remaining endometrium had cystic and adenomatous hyperplasia. (H & E ×192).

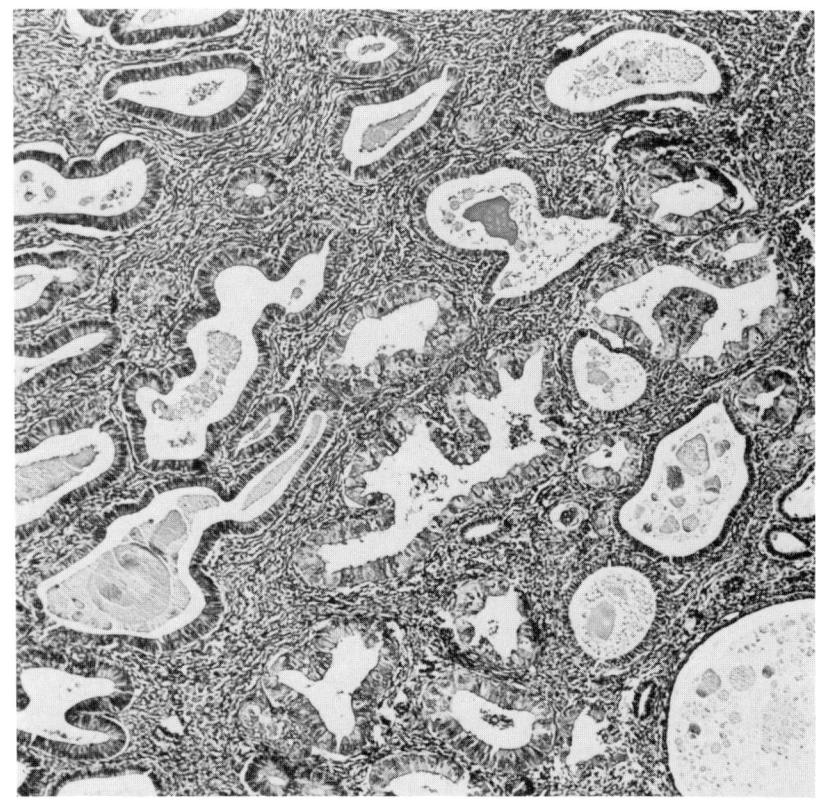

A

Fig. 46.10A Foci of adenocarcinoma in situ arising in an area of adenomatous hyperplasia. This low power magnification shows the focal nature of the carcinoma in situ, which can be identified by the larger pale cells. (H & E ×79).

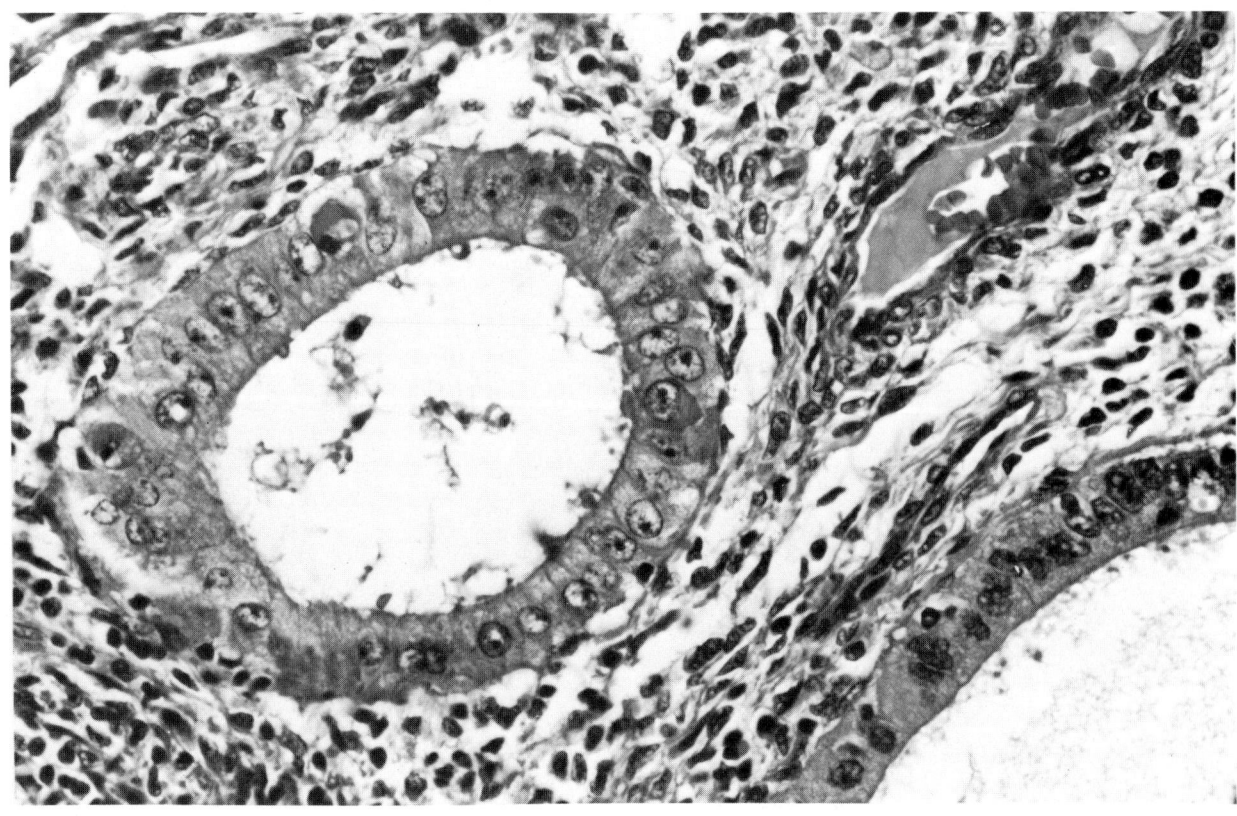

B

Fig. 46.10B Carcinoma in situ. The epithelial cells are large with abundant eosinophilic cytoplasm. The nuclei are large and rounded and have large irregular nucleoli. (H & E ×500).

Endometrial carcinoma in situ has no gross characteristics which distinguish it from other hyperplastic lesions. Histologically the most striking feature is the focal nature of the lesion in combination with hyperplasia. Curiously the change seems to accompany cystic hyperplasia as frequently as it does the more advanced types. The epithelial cells are large and oncocytic in appearance, usually the cytoplasm stains brightly with eosin[24] but the degree of eosinophilia is variable.[7] The nuclear and structural features of the lesion as defined by Buehl, Vellios, et al[7] are shown in Table 46.2 and the lesion illustrated in Figures 46.9 and 46.10A and B. Gore & Hertig found that the more complex the pattern in hyperplasia the more likelihood of future invasive carcinoma. They further state that they have never observed carcinoma to arise from normal endometrium and that only rarely was cystic hyperplasia followed by carcinoma.[15]

The controversy of carcinoma in situ of the endometrium is unlikely to be settled in the near future. A major problem is a better understanding of what constitutes endometrial stromal invasion. It is at this upper end of the spectrum that careful and precise evaluation is of greatest importance. Variations in the interpretation would have a significant effect on the presumed incidence of endometrial carcinoma as well as the prognosis. Stage I Grade 1 endometrial carcinoma has an excellent prognosis, especially in women under age 50.[10] It has been our experience and that of others that there is a tendency to overdiagnosis by as much as 25%.[13,47]

Kurman & Norris[31] studied 204 patients with severe forms of atypical hyperplasia, carcinoma in situ and well differentiated carcinoma in curettings. They compared the results of this review with the findings in the hysterectomy specimens. Stromal invasion was the single most important feature in predicting the likelihood of carcinoma in the hysterectomy specimen. Subsequent studies support this view.[28,31]

Special problems in diagnosis

Secretory changes may be present in endometrial carcinoma, the so-called secretory carcinoma, and in the various forms of hyperplasia as well.[9] This is thought to be the result of superimposed ovulation or progestagen therapy.[55] While we indicate secretory change when it is present, we do not consider the lesion to be a separate category of hyperplasia. In the case illustrated there was atypical hyperplasia and focal carcinoma both with secretory activity but no evidence of secretion in the hysterectomy specimen at a later date even though there was persistent hyperplasia and carcinoma (Fig. 46.11).

There are other changes which must be distinguished

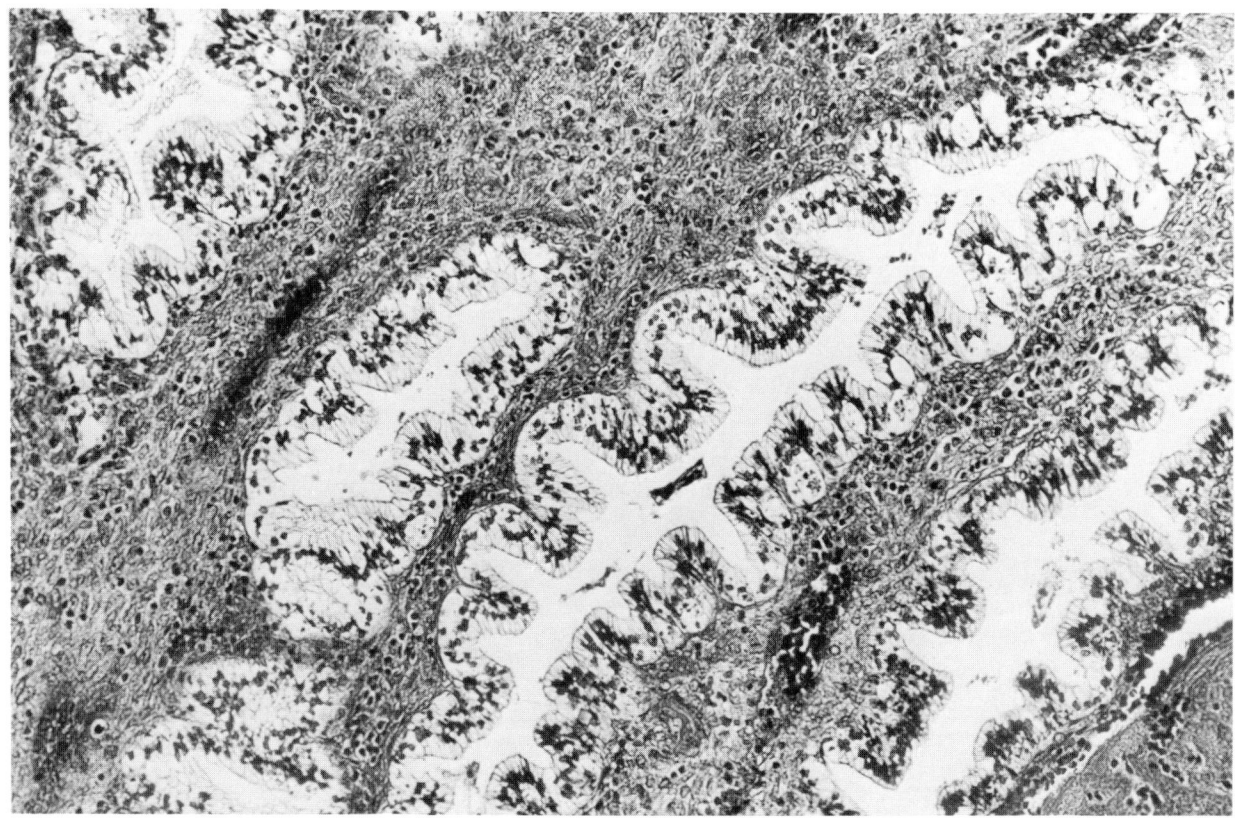

Fig. 46.11 Secretory activity in a patient with atypical hyperplasia and secretory carcinoma. The subsequent hysterectomy about 6 weeks later had both atypical hyperplasia and a focus of early adenocarcinoma which did not invade the myometrium. There was no secretory activity in the latter specimen. (H & E ×197).

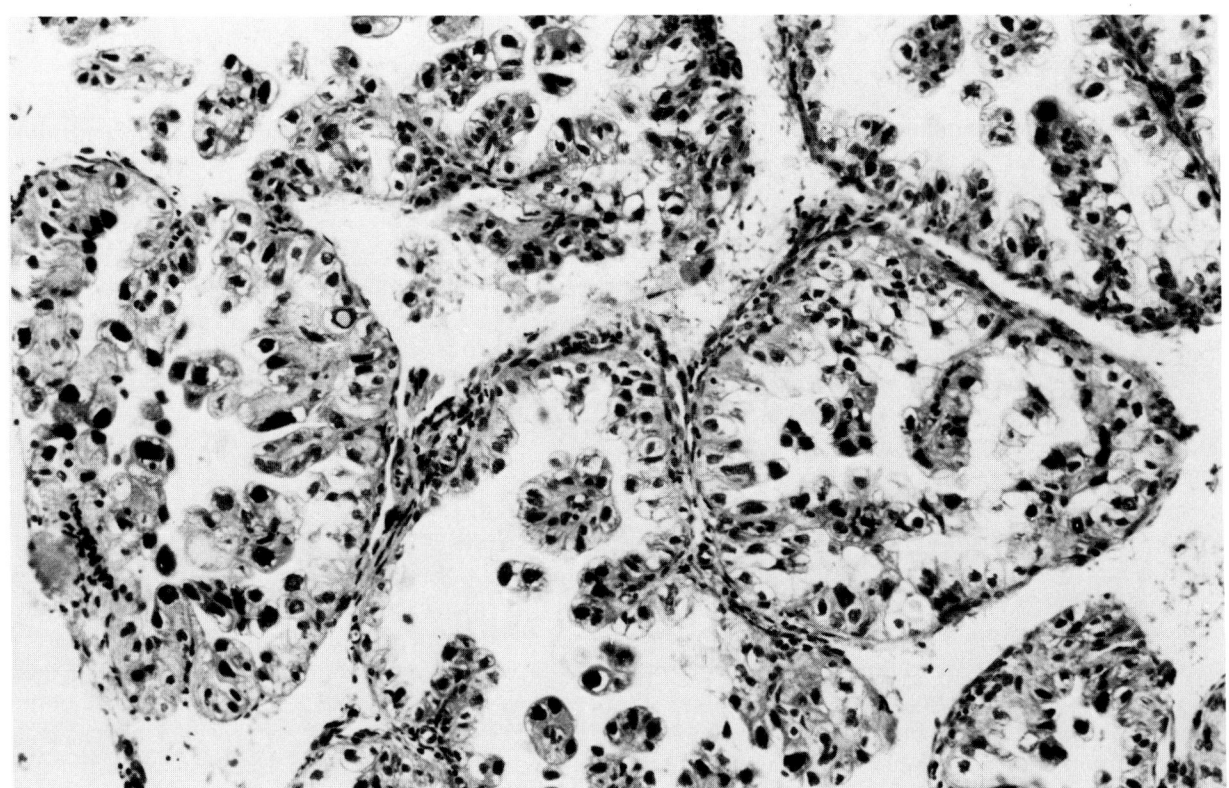

Fig. 46.12   Endometrium showing early pregnancy changes in the glands, Arias-Stella phenomenon. (H & E ×196).

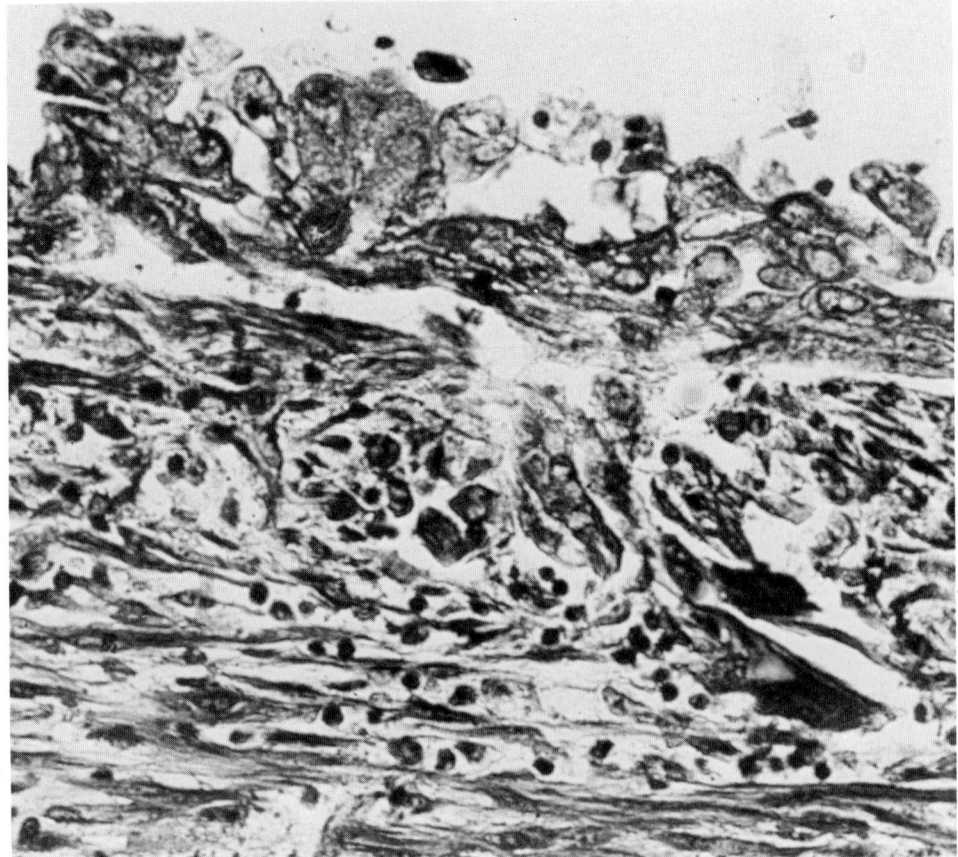

Fig. 46.13   Regenerating epithelium following curettage. Note the piling up of disorganized atypical cells. (H & E ×500).

from carcinoma in situ or atypical hyperplasia. The changes which take place in early pregnancy have already been mentioned (Fig. 46.12). This lesion is quite familiar to all pathologists and should rarely present a problem.

Tubal metaplasia is less widely appreciated and because of the cytoplasmic eosinophilia it may be confused with carcinoma in situ. The ciliated border should be the clue as to the nature of the change since the cells in carcinoma in situ are not ciliated.[24]

Regenerating surface epithelium often displays nuclear atypia and the cells may be quite irregular with numerous mitoses. Such changes can result in errors in the interpretation of endometrial cell studies performed following endometrial biopsy or endometrial curettage (Fig. 46.13). The location of the lesion and the history of prior biopsy assists in recognizing the nature of such changes.[51]

The presence of squamous metaplasia, often in the form of intraglandular morules, is quite frequently associated with adenocarcinoma, the so-called adenoacanthoma. Such changes are also found in adenomatous and atypical hyperplasia and should not be interpreted as evidence of malignancy. There is no evidence that these metaplastic changes alter the behavior of either carcinoma or hyperplasia. Finally, the telescoping effect commonly found in curettage specimens is an artifact without special significance (Fig. 46.14).

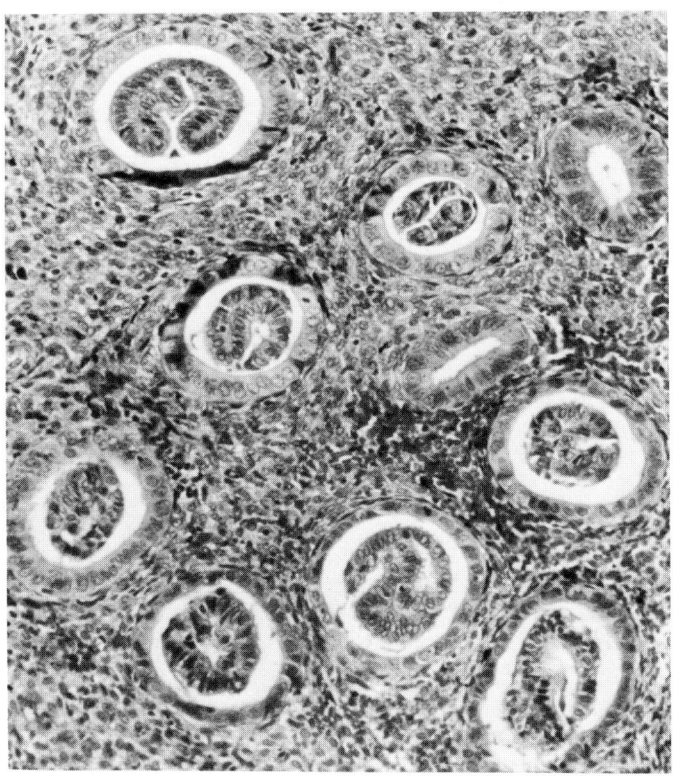

Fig. 46.14 Proliferative endometrium with 'telescoping' of glands. This is a common phenomenon and should not be confused with hyperplasia. (H & E ×79).

Adenomatous polyps

A discussion of premalignant changes in the endometrium would not be complete without the inclusion of adenomatous polyps. While polyps are rather common in uteri containing endometerial carcinoma[17,23] this appears to reflect a common etiology, estrogens.[41] The presence of atypical endometrial hyperplasia in polyps also raises the question of their significance. It has been pointed out, however, that the frequency of such an occurrence is apparently no greater than carcinoma arising in the adjacent non-polypoid endometrium.[15] One study found only four acceptable cases of primary carcinoma arising in a polyp. The study included 1100 polyps for a rate of 0.36%. There were four other cases where the possibility of carcinoma arising in a polyp existed.[41] Other authors cite the figure for carcinoma arising in a polyp of less than 1%.[57] In one report, however, the author believes there is a nine-fold risk. He studied 520 patients with endometrial polyps excised or removed by curettage without hysterectomy. In a follow-up ranging from 3 to 19 years, with a median of 10 years, endometrial cancer developed in 17 patients whereas only 2 could have been expected.[3] When carcinoma is confined to a polyp the prognosis is said to be excellent.[43] From available evidence it would seen wise to remove all polyps and to examine them carefully as well as scrutinize the remaining endometrium.

Polyps are easily recognized grossly if they are removed intact. Except for the base they are covered with epithelium that is smooth and glistening. The surface may be ulcerated, usually at the tip. When the polyps are large they may be infarcted. When fragmented in the curettage specimen they may be identified in that they differ in appearance from the remainder of the specimen. More often than not polyps are non-responsive to cyclic endometrial changes in premenopausal endometrium (Fig. 46.15). They may, however, show secretory changes and may contain any of the various types of hyperplasia or even carcinoma. In the typical polyp the glands appear dilated and a few may be cystic. Sections through the base often reveal a large thick walled nutrient artery. This vessel is thought to be derived from one of the straight arteries that normally supply the basal zone of the endometrium. Since polyps probably develop as localized overgrowths of the basal zone as they increase in size the straight artery continues to enlarge to supply it with blood.[51] Polyps occurring in the lower uterine segment may have areas of endocervical type glands intermixed with non-reactive endometrial glands. The stroma of polyps is usually more fibrous, especially in the larger ones. The stroma thus appears to be less cellular than in endometrial hyperplasia.

Relative frequency of precursor lesions

We know of no published data on the actual incidence rates for the various lesions under discussion. Wentz[56] & Sher-

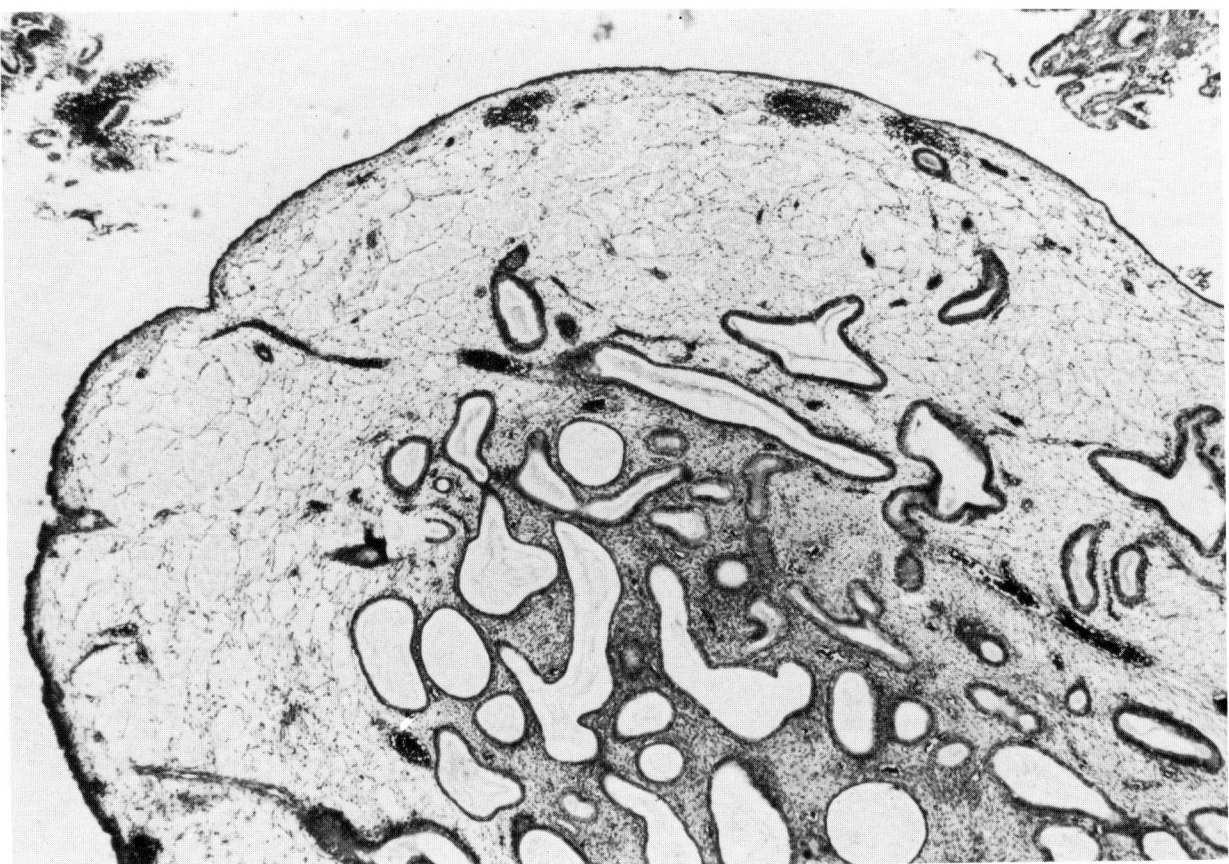

Fig. 46.15 Edematous endometrial polyp found in the curettings of a patient with secretory hyperplasia and secretory carcinoma (see Fig. 46.11). This polyp showed no secretory activity. (H & E ×53).

man[44] have both published relative frequency rates from their institutions. They were compiled on the basis of curettage specimens unrelated to pregnancy. Wentz has two such series, the first on 3888 specimens between 1964 and 1968, and a subsequent series which includes 7106 specimens. Sherman analyzed 12 206 curettage specimens. The relative frequencies found in the two studies are remarkably similar and are shown in Table 46.3. We have incidence data for endometrial carcinoma in situ as diagnosed in our community. We have not reviewed all of the material but a comparison is shown in Table 46.4. Unlike

Table 46.4 Comparison of number of cases and rates for in situ carcinoma of endometrium and of cervix in relation to their invasive counterparts[a]

	No.	Endometrium (Adenocarcinoma only) Age adjusted Rate[a] Rate[b]		No.	Cervix (Squamous carcinoma only) Age adjusted Rate[a] Rate[b]	
Carcinoma	1283	25.0	15.0	1720	33.6	21.6
In situ carcinoma	88	1.7	1.1	2513	49.0	34.4

[a] Based on the female population of Louisville, Kentucky, 20 years old and over, 1953–1976. Rates/100 000 women.
[b] Adjusted to the 1950 US population.

carcinoma in situ of the cervix which is diagnosed more often than is invasive cervix cancer, carcinoma in situ of the endometrium is much less frequently diagnosed than is endometrial carcinoma.

The relative frequency with which a particular lesion is diagnosed is heavily dependent on the diagnostic criteria utilized. Critical pathologic reviews of the slides from two studies of endometrial carcinoma in relationship to replacement estrogen therapy have been published. The review in one study indicated that about 20% of the lesions were benign[47] and in the other study there was a reduction of 8

Table 46.3 Relative frequency of hyperplasia and carcinoma: curettage specimens unrelated to pregnancy.

	Wentz 1964–1968[56] 3888 specimens	Wentz after 1968[56] 7106 specimens	Sherman[44] 12 206 specimens
Cystic hyperplasia	5.6	4.8	—
Adenomatous hyperplasia	2.9	2.4	2.7
Atypical hyperplasia	0.9	1.3	1.2
Carcinoma in situ	0.2	0.1	0.2
Endometrial carcinoma	2.2	2.9	2.6

to 26% dependent on whether only the majority, or all three pathologists agreed. The degree of overestimation in that study was similar in both estrogen takers and in controls.[13] In a review of the situation in King County, Washington, where very high rates of endometrial cancer associated with estrogen replacement therapy had been reported, there has been a striking overall drop in the incidence which accompanied a decrease in prescription rate for replacement estrogens. This striking decrease in carcinoma rates occurred within a 6 month period, and is attributed to the decrease in prescriptions for estrogens that occurred following the original publication.[25] The decrease was so striking and the interval so short that an alternate hypothesis might be that stricter criteria for the diagnosis of endometrial carcinoma are now utilized.

Finally there is the observation that death from disease almost never occurs in women under 40 years of age with well differentiated endometrial adenocarcinoma.[10,45] The consistent feature of all carcinoma is autonomous growth. Could not some of these disturbing histologic changes represent unusually florid estrogen stimulation of the endometrium which in fact lack autonomy of growth and which revert upon estrogen withdrawal?

CLINICAL PRESENTATION

Abnormal vaginal bleeding is by far the most common symptom in patients with the more advanced hyperplasias.[24] Strangely enough, among young women with ovarian dysgenesis treated with estrogen and progestagens none reported abnormal bleeding.[42] Hyperplasia is first diagnosed in some younger women during fertility studies or is found incidentally at time of hysterectomy. Postmenopausal women treated with estrogens for prolonged periods, if they do not bleed, may have the diagnosis made by biopsy performed as a precautionary measure.

Cytology has been used as a surveillance method, but in very few hands has it had any degree of success. The major problem is obtaining a suitable sample. Ng has reported excellent results in detecting precursor lesions by means of endocervical aspiration samples with a positive rate of 71.8% of 163 cases.[36] Unfortunately, few have been able to duplicate this performance. Our own experience with a variety of collection methods has been less than satisfactory. We prefer some type of aspiration tissue biopsy which if skilfully done is highly diagnostic (see Chs 14 and 49).

MALIGNANT POTENTIAL OF PRECURSOR LESIONS

At present there is little, if any, disagreement that the lesions under discussion have some malignant potential. The degree to which they are premalignant, however, is still being debated. The difference in the estimates is

largely due to reasons previously alluded to. Since hyperplasia and endometrial carcinoma share a common factor, estrogen, it is not surprising that both types of epithelial proliferation are frequently found in the same specimen. The magnitude of this association would seem to be dependent on the thoroughness of sampling and the criteria for diagnosis.

Prospective studies provide better evidence but they are becoming progressively more difficult because of the conviction of most gynecologists that hyperplasia does place a woman in a high category for either concurrent or future endometrial cancer. This results in hysterectomy, which abruptly ends the investigation. Within the limitations of classification and definition at that time, a few older prospective studies revealed varying degrees of risk. Essentially all show a greater risk for postmenopausal than for premenopausal women. A 1937 study indicated that 2.4% of premenopausal and 11% of postmenopausal women with hyperplasia developed carcinoma within the time frame of the study.[40] Presumably more would have during their entire life span. Another study found that 1.57% of patients with hyperplasia subsequently developed carcinoma. The authors interpreted the risks for postmenopausal women to be 10-fold that of women without hyperplasia.[9] Yet another study arrives at the figures of a 3% risk for premenopausal and 25% for postmenopausal women.[29]

Data are available from at least two prospective studies. Wentz[56] presents data on patients with adenomatous hyperplasia, atypical hyperplasia and carcinoma in situ using the criteria of Vellios. He gathered patients who had had one of the three lesions on two curettage specimens at least 8 weeks apart. He included only women who did not undergo hysterectomy and had not had hormonal therapy. A significant number of women developed invasive adenocarcinoma of the endometrium during the subsequent period of 2 to 8 years (Table 46.5).

Table 46.5 Persistent endometrial hyperplasia: premalignant potential[56]

| | Developed invasive adenocarcinoma | |
	Number	%
Adenomatous hyperplasia	75	26.7
Atypical hyperplasia	22	81.8
Adenocarcinoma in situ	18	100.0

Sherman reported 204 women with precursor type lesions followed for not less than 2 and for up to 15 years. There was a high rate of subsequent carcinoma (Table 46.6). In only 20% did the endometrium revert to a benign state.[44]

Sherman also reports the results of a retrospective study of 201 patients with endometrial carcinoma. They were all over 60 years of age at the time of diagnosis. All had a curettage specimen within the previous 10 years. The

Table 46.6 Follow-up of women with precursor lesions (1960–70) treated for 2–15 years[44]

	Total no. of patients	Endometrial carcinoma %	Intraepithelial carcinoma %
Adenomatous hyperplasia	106	19.8	49.1
Atypical hyperplasia	91	57.1	87.4
Adenocarcinoma in situ	7	57.1	1[a]
	204	37.7	

[a] one persisted, two treated progestins reverted.

specimens within 2 years were excluded to avoid the problem of a concomitant cancer. 72% had one of the precursor lesions.[44] Avoiding the inclusion of patients with less than a 2-year interval increases the validity of the study since Wentz found 10 of 150 patients with endometrial cancer had the diagnosis of hyperplasia made on the curettage specimen only to find invasive cancer in the hysterectomy.[56] The accuracy of sampling is thus an important consideration in interpreting the results of the reported studies.

In a more recent study Kurman et al examined curettings from 170 patients with all grades of endometrial hyperplasia who did not undergo a hysterectomy for at least one year. Follow-up ranged from 1 to 26.7 years (mean 13.4 yrs). Classification of proliferative lesions based solely on cytologic atypia revealed that atypia was a discriminate factor. Proliferations lacking cytologic atypia were designated hyperplasia and those displaying atypia designated atypical hyperplasia. Only 1.6% with hyperplasia progressed to carcinoma compared to 23% of women with atypical hyperplasia. When architectural abnormalities were considered, the difference between the subgroups suggested a trend, but were not statistically significant.[30]

Although the above classification (Table 46.7) has much to recommend it the one in general use will probably persist for some time to come. (See also p. 747.)

In contrast to the more worrisome hyperplasia, the premalignant potential of cystic hyperplasia would appear to be low. In a frequently quoted study with a follow-up period of up to 24 years, cancer developed in less than 0.4%.[33] Others have found cystic hyperplasia was present in patients who did not subsequently develop cancer while finding that the greater the degree of hyperplasia, the higher was the risk.[6,15,23] The severity of the hyperplasia also increased inversely with the time interval before the diagnosis of cancer.[23]

Chromosomal and DNA studies also support the low malignant potential of cystic hyperplasia (see Ch. 47).[26,54]

Table 46.7 Comparison of follow-up of patients with simple and complex hyperplasia and simple and complex atypical hyperplasia: 170 patients[30]

	No. of patients	Regressed No.	(%)	Persisted No.	(%)	Progressed to carcinoma No.	(%)
Simple hyperplasia	93	74	(80)	18	(19)	1	(1)
Complex hyperplasia	29	23	(80)	5	(17)	1	(3)
Simple atypical hyperplasia	13	9	(69)	3	(23)	1	(8)
Complex atypical hyperplasia	35	20	(57)	5	(14)	10	(29)

(Reproduced from J. B. Lippincott, 1985)

REFERENCES

1. Anderson B, Watring W G, Edinger D D Jr, Small E C, Netland M T, Safaii H 1979 Development of DES-associated clear-cell carcinoma. The importance of regular screening. Obstet Gynecol 53: 293
2. Arias-Stella J 1959 Atypical endometrial changes associated with the presence of chorionic tissue. AMA Arch Pathol 58: 112
3. Armenia C S 1967 Sequential relationship between endometrial polyps and carcinoma of the endometrium. Obstet Gynecol 30: 524
4. Bamforth J 1956 Carcinoma of body of uterus and its relationship to endometrial hyperplasia: histological study. J Obstet Gynaecol Brit Commonw 63: 415
5. Benjamin I, Block R E 1977 Endometrial response to estrogen and progesterone therapy in patients with gonadal dysgenesis. Obstet Gynecol 50: 136
6. Beutler H K, Dockerty M B, Randall L M 1963 Precancerous lesions of the endometrium. Am J Obstet Gynecol 86: 433
7. Buehl I A, Vellios F, Carter J E, Huber C P 1964 Carcinoma in situ of the endometrium. Am J Clin Pathol 42: 594
8. Campbell P E, Barter R A 1961 The significance of atypical endometrial hyperplasia. J Obstet Gynaecol Br Commonw 68: 668
9. Christopherson W M, Alberhasky R C, Connelly P J 1982 Carcinoma of the endometrium. I. A clinicopathological study of clear-cell carcinoma and secretory carcinoma. Cancer 49: 1511
10. Christopherson W M, Connelly P J, Alberhasky R C 1983 Carcinoma of the endometrium V. An analysis of prognosticators in patients with favorable subtypes and Stage I disease. Cancer 51: 1705
11. Corscaden J A, Fertig J W, Gusberg S B 1946 Carcinoma subsequent to the radiotherapeutic menopause. Am J Obstet Gynecol 51: 1
12. Dewhurst C J, DeKoos E B, Haines R M 1975 Replacement hormone therapy in gonadal dysgenesis. Br J Obstet Gynecol 82: 412
13. Gordon J, Reagan J W, Finkle W D, Ziel H K 1977 Estrogen and endometrial carcinoma; an independent pathology review supporting original risk estimate. N Engl J Med 297: 570
14. Gore H, Hertig A T 1962 Premalignant lesions of the endometrium. Clin Obstet Gynecol 5: 1148

15. Gore H, Hertig A T 1966 Carcinoma in situ of endometrium. Am J Obstet Gynecol 94: 134
16. Gray L A, Barnes M L 1964 Histogenesis of endometrial carcinoma. Ann Surg 159: 976
17. Gray L A, Robertson R W Jr, Christopherson W M 1974 Atypical endometrial changes associated with carcinoma. Gynecol Oncol 2: 93
18. Gusberg S B 1947 Precursors of corpus carcinoma: estrogens and adenomatous hyperplasia. Am J Obstet Gynecol 54: 905
19. Gusberg S B, Kaplan A L 1963 Precursors of corpus cancer. IV. Adenomatous hyperplasia as stage 0 carcinoma of the endometrium. Am J Obstet Gynecol 87: 662
20. Gusberg S B, Moore D B, Martin F 1954 Precursors of corpus cancer. A clinical and pathological study of adenomatous hyperplasia. Am J Obstet Gynecol 68: 1472
21. Hanson D J 1959 Studies of the endometrial stroma in cystic glandular hyperplasia. Am J Clin Pathol 32: 1952
22. Herbst A L, Norusis M J, Rosenow P J, Welch W R, Scully R E 1979 An analysis of 346 cases of clear cell adenocarcinoma of the vagina and cervix with emphasis on recurrence and survival. Gynecol Oncol 7: 111
23. Hertig A T, Sommers S C 1949 Genesis of endometrial carcinoma. Study of prior biopsies. Cancer 2: 964
24. Hertig A T, Sommers S C, Bengloff H 1949 Genesis of endometrial carcinoma. Carcinoma in situ. Cancer 2: 946
25. Jick H, Watkins R N, Hunter J R et al 1979 Replacement estrogens and endometrial cancer. N Engl J Med 300: 218
26. Katayama K T, Jones H W 1967 Chromosomes of atypical (adenomatous) hyperplasia and carcinoma of the endometrium. Am J Obstet Gynecol 97: 978
27. Kaufman R H, Abbott J P, Wall J A 1959 The endometrium before and after wedge resection of the ovaries in the Stein-Leventhal syndrome. Am J Obstet Gynecol 77: 1271
28. King A, Seraj I M, Wagner R J 1984 Stromal invasion in endometrial carcinoma. Am J Obstet Gynecol 149: 10
29. Kucera F 1957 The histogenesis of carcinoma of the body of the uterus. Zentralby Gynaekol 79: 345
30. Kurman R J, Kaminski P F, Norris H J 1985 The behavior of endometrial hyperplasia. A long-term study of 'untreated' hyperplasia in 170 patients. Cancer 56: 403
31. Kurman R J, Norris H J 1982 Evaluation of criteria for distinguishing atypical endometrial hyperplasia from well-differentiated carcinoma. Cancer 49: 2547
32. Mansell H, Hertig A T 1955 Granulosa-theca cell tumors and endometrial carcinoma. A study of their relationship and a survey of 80 cases. Obstet Gynecol 6: 385
33. McBride J M 1959 Pre-menopausal cystic hyperplasia and endometrial carcinoma. J Obstet Gynaecol Br Emp 66: 288
34. Meissner W A, Sommers S C, Sherman G 1957 Endometrial hyperplasia, endometrial carcinoma and endometriosis produced experimentally by estrogen. Cancer 10: 500
35. Merriam J C Jr, Easterday C L, McKay D G, Hertig A T 1960 Experimental production of endometrial carcinoma in the rabbit.

36. Ng A B P 1974 The cellular detection of endometrial carcinoma and its precursors. Gynecol Oncol 2: 162
37. Norris H J, Travassoli F A, Kurman R J 1983 Endometrial hyperplasia and carcinoma. Diagnostic considerations. Am J Surg Pathol 7: 839
38. Novak E, Rutledge F 1948 Atypical endometrial hyperplasia simulating adenocarcinoma. Am J Obstet Gynecol 55: 46
39. Novak E, Yui E 1936 Relation of endometrial hyperplasia to adenocarcinoma of the uterus. Am J Obstet Gynecol 32: 674
40. Payne F L 1937 The clinical significance of endometrial hyperplasia. Am J Obstet Gynecol 34: 762
41. Peterson W F, Novak E R 1956 Endometrial polyps. Obstet Gynecol 8: 40
42. Rosenwaks Z, Wentz A C, Jones G S et al 1979 Endometrial pathology and estrogens. Obstet Gynecol 53: 403
43. Salm R 1972 The incidence and significance of early carcinomas in endometrial polyps. J Pathol 108: 47
44. Sherman A I 1978 Precursors of endometrial cancer. Israel J Med Science 14: 370
45. Silverberg S G 1977 The disease in young women. Endometrial Carcinoma and Its Treatment. Thomas, Springfield, p 26
46. Stewart F W 1957 Factors influencing the curability of cancer. Proceedings of the Third National Cancer Conference. Lippincott, Philadelphia, p 62
47. Szekely D R, Weiss N S, Schweid A I 1978 Incidence of endometrial carcinoma in King County, Washington: a standardized histologic review. J Natl Cancer Inst 60: 985
48. Tavassoli F A, Kraus F T 1978 Endometrial lesions in uteri resected for atypical endometrial hyperplasia. Am J Clin Pathol 70: 770
49. Taylor H C Jr, Millen R 1938 The causes of vaginal bleeding and the histology of the endometrium after the menopause. Am J Obstet Gynecol 36: 22
50. TeLinde R W, Jones H W Jr, Galvin G A 1953 What are the earliest endometrial changes to justify diagnosis of endometrial cancer? Am J Obstet Gynecol 66: 953
51. Vellios F 1972 Endometrial hyperplasia, precursors of endometrial carcinoma. Pathology Annual. Appleton-Century-Crofts, New York, p 201
52. Vellios F 1978 Personal communication
53. Wade T R, Kopf A W, Ackerman A B 1979 Bowenoid papulosis of the genitalia. Arch Dermatol 115: 306
54. Wagner D, Richart R M, Terner J Y 1967 Deoxyribonucleic acid content of presumed precursors of endometrial carcinoma. Cancer 20: 2067
55. Welch W R, Scully R E 1977 Precancerous lesions of the endometrium. Hum Pathol 8: 503
56. Wentz W B 1974 Progestin therapy in endometrial hyperplasia. Gynecol Oncol 2: 362
57. Wolfe S A, Mackles A 1962 Malignant lesions arising from benign endometrial polyps. Obstet Gynecol 20: 542

Obstet Gynecol 16: 253

47. Premalignant lesions of the endometrium: clinical features and management

C. Trope   B. Lindahl

CLINICAL PRESENTATION AND DIAGNOSIS

Obesity is a predisposing factor for endometrial hyperplasia because androstenedione is converted in peripheral fatty tissue to estrone and estradiol. Hence obese women should try to lose weight, but weight-loss per se does not prevent the development of all cases of endometrial carcinoma. In adolescence there may be a short anovulatory period after the menarche, associated with endometrial hyperplasia of the simple or complex type, but seldom of the more severe atypical type. The hyperplasia ends with the onset of regular ovulatory cycles. In patients with infertility due to anovulation, hyperplasia is often diagnosed, and the most rational treatment of these patients is to stimulate ovulation. If this is not achieved, the patients should undergo endometrial sampling in order to detect precursors to, or frankly invasive endometrial carcinoma.[19] In climacteric women the quality of life can today be improved by exogenous estrogens, but this will result in an increased risk of endometrial hyperplasia or endometrial cancer. Under careful control and with strict indications for estrogenic substitution therapy combined with gestagens, for example, in a cyclic way, no significant increase in the endometrial carcinoma rate compared to untreated postmenopausal women is found.[10] In the premenopausal woman anovulation is the cause of endometrial hyperplasia. To mimic ovulation intermittent gestagen therapy is given, and then as a rule regular bleeding will occur and at the same time the endometrial hyperplasia disappears.[2] (See also Chs 3 and 8.)

Abnormal vaginal bleeding is the most common reason for endometrial sampling, and consequently the most common symptom of endometrial hyperplasia. However, we all have experience of patients with infertility or uterine fibroids who have shown signs of endometrial hyperplasia. Asymptomatic climacteric women treated with estrogens may have the diagnosis made by screening biopsies. Thus, there probably exists a rather high but unknown frequency of undiagnosed hyperplasia.

The correct diagnosis can only be made by histologic examination of the endometrial tissue. This demands endometrial biopsy or fractional dilatation and curettage (D&C.) This is the most commonly performed gynecologic operative procedure. Office procedures such as endometrial lavage, aspiration, scraping, brushing and biopsy have been carried out in the last 15 years and have been reviewed by Bonte[2] with regard to accuracy, adequacy, feasibility, acceptance and cost. It has been difficult to identify endometrial hyperplasia and to separate it from endometrial polyps and glandular changes by these techniques. Histologic sampling by D&C is considered a more accurate and adequate technique compared with cytologic sampling in detecting precancerous endometrial lesions. Nevertheless, D&C induces more discomfort and complications and is more expensive compared with cytologic sampling. In addition even a D&C at times will not result in a correct diagnosis.[28] (See also Ch. 14.)

A retrospective study of 1383 women submitted to D&C, showed that the current practice of routine D&C for abnormal uterine bleeding resulted in a low yield of cancer diagnosis for women below 60, and that the indications for this procedure should be re-evaluated, and in many cases replaced by simpler methods.[27]

CLASSIFICATION AND BEHAVIOR

As has been stressed elsewhere, the absence of a uniform terminology and the impreciseness of definitions constitutes a problem in understanding the malignant potential of endometrial hyperplasias. Norris et al[22] have summarized the recent advances in our understanding of endometrial hyperplasia with particular emphasis on its relationship to endometrial carcinoma, and it seems clear that atypical cytology and architectural changes are definitely associated with an increased risk of endometrial cancer. The International Society of Gynecological Pathologists, under the auspices of the World Health Organization, has proposed a classification that will provide uniformity in diagnostic terminology. This classification defines three groups: simple hyperplasia, complex hyperplasia (adenomatous hyperplasia without atypia), atypical hyperplasia (adenomatous hyperplasia with atypia). Cytologic abnormalities are primarily taken into account. Proliferations showing no evidence of cytologic atypia are classified as either simple or complex hyperplasia depending on the extent of glandular complexity and crowding whereas those showing cytologic atypia regardless of the architectural pattern are classified as atypical hyperplasia (Table 47.1).[16] Recently, Kurman et al[15] reviewed the histologic pattern of 170 women with all grades of endometrial hyperplasia. In this study the patients were followed for at least one year after the curettage (mean 13.4 years) without hysterectomy. Only 2 (2%) of 122 patients with hyperplasia lacking cytological atypia progressed to carcinoma whereas 11 (23%) of the 48 women with atypical hyperplasia progressed to carcinoma (p < 0.001). Thus, cytologic atypia was the most useful feature in identifying a lesion that may progress to carcinoma. The mean duration of progression of hyperplasia without atypia to carcinoma is nearly 10 years compared to 4 years for atypical hyperplasia.[15] Thus, it seems clear that there is a highly increased risk for patients with atypical hyperplasia to develop endometrial cancer. 17 to 25% of women with atypical hyperplasia in curettings will have a well differentiated carcinoma in the uterus if hysterectomy is performed within 1 month after curettage.[28] Yet, we know that in long-term follow-up studies only 11 to 23% of women with atypical hyperplasia developed a carcinoma.[15] There may be many explanations why untreated patients with atypical hyperplasia have a relatively low percentage of progression to endometrial carcinoma, but one of the most provocative explanations is based on epidemiologic and clinical-pathologic evidence.[14]

Table 47.1 Classification of endometrial hyperplasia*

Simple hyperplasia

Complex hyperplasia (adenomatous hyperplasia without atypia)

Atypical hyperplasia (adenomatous hyperplasia with atypia)

* International Society of Gynecological Pathologists after Kurman[14]

MANAGEMENT OF ENDOMETRIAL HYPERPLASIA

Despite various techniques, no screening method today has sufficient diagnostic accuracy to be used for early detection of endometrial hyperplasia or endometrial carcinoma. This is because cytological interpretation of endo-uterine specimens can be difficult even for experienced cytologists.[24,25] (See also Chs 14 and 49.)

The treatment of endometrial hyperplasia is controversial because of the varying degree and extent of the lesion, the medical condition and desires of the patient, and the lack of uniform recognition of the malignant potential of various lesions. In this chapter a treatment recommendation will be presented using the classification of the International Society of Gynecological Pathologists. The therapeutic approach to the precancerous endometrial lesions can be hormonal or surgical and should be based on age, health and reproductive status. Whether the patient has received exogenous estrogen treatment prior to the diagnosis should also be considered.

After the diagnosis the very first thing to do is to exclude tumors of endocrine origin as the cause of hyperplasia. The patients can be divided into two different categories, namely women of 40 and younger, and women older than 40. In the group <40 efforts should be made to distinguish between endogenous and exogenous caused hyperplasia. In premenopausal women (<40) endometrial hyperplasia is often an innocuous and self-limiting process, and very often these women need no more than a diagnostic curettage.[14]

Women with simple and complex hyperplasia induced by estrogen therapy have an extremely low risk of progression to carcinoma.[14,15,16] These patients should be treated with D&C and withdrawal of the estrogen treatment. If the patient requires estrogen treatment, this could be prescribed again, but only with the addition of gestagen, for example, in a cyclic pattern.[33] In some patients the hyperplasia is caused by endogenously produced hormones. In these patients, there is need for a control curettage and a close follow-up because the condition is prone to reappear if the reason for the endogenous production is not corrected. It must be stressed that the low dose gestagen treatment introduced to prevent the development of endometrial hyperplasias in patients on estrogen therapy may not cure an endometrial hyperplasia. After the hyperplasia has been cured, low dose gestagen treatment might be introduced to control irregular bleeding or to prevent a new hyperplasia.[19]

When anovulation is the cause of simple or complex endometrial hyperplasia in women of child-bearing ages, treatment with megestrol acetate 40 mg orally four times daily for 8 weeks, or intermittent medroxyprogesterone acetate 10 mg per day for 10 days every month or high dose medroxyprogesterone acetate 1000 mg per week for 3 months is often successful. This treatment should be monitored by endometrial biopsy or curettage. In the majority of patients (90%) this treatment results in elimination of simple and complex hyperplasia[19,32] In the more severe atypical hyperplasias a higher dose is needed.[19] Even if the risk of finding frank invasive carcinoma in the uterus after curettage exists, it is relatively low in women younger than 40 years,[13] and therefore a conservative treatment is justified in these women if they desire to bear children. We know that about 30% of young women with atypical hyperplasia will deliver normally. Even if these progress to carcinoma they rarely die of their disease.[14] If no response to the progestin treatment is achieved, a total hysterectomy should be performed. For treatment recommendations see Table 47.2.

Table 47.2 Treatment scheme of endometrial hyperplasia

| | <40 years | 40–50 years | >50 years | |
			Operable	Inoperable
Simple hyperplasia	EC or HDP or OI or TAH	EC or HDP or TAH + BSO	HDP or TAH + BSO	HDP or ICR
Complex hyperplasia	EC or HDP or OI or TAH	EC or HDP or TAH + BSO	HDP or TAH + BSO	HDP or ICR
Atypical hyperplasia	EC or HDP or OI or TAH	HDP or TAH + BSO	TAH + BSO	HDP or ICR

EC	=	Endometrial curettage every 3 months
HDP	=	High dose progestin
OI	=	Ovulation induction
TAH	=	Total abdominal hysterectomy
BSO	=	Bilateral salpingo-oophorectomy
ICR	=	Intracavitary radium

It has been reported that the malignant potential of endometrial hyperplasias is more pronounced in postmenopausal women.[30,31,32] This means that a more aggressive therapy should be considered for women in whom it is difficult to separate severely atypical hyperplasia from well-differentiated endometrial carcinoma ('not carcinoma, but better out'). However, many postmenopausal women with endometrial hyperplasia present with surgical risk factors such as hypertension, diabetes or obesity. This has contributed to the preference in certain cases of hormone therapy as an alternative to surgery. Progestins have been used in the treatment of recurrent endometrial carcinoma for the past 30 years with a response rate of 15 to 30%.[13] From these protocols different treatment schedules have been adapted to the treatment of endometrial hyperplasias (Table 47.3).

High dose medroxyprogesterone acetate or megestrol acetate which creates a medical curettage is adequate in 80% of the patients. Repeated problems with irregular

Table 47.3 Different effective hormonal treatment regimens of endometrial hyperplasias

Type of progestin	Dosage	Duration
Dimethisterone[2]	75 mg/day	6 weeks
Megestrol acetate[30]	160 mg/day	8 weeks
Medroxyprogesterone acetate[17]	100 mg/day	continuous
17α-Hydroxyprogesterone caproate[13]	500 mg/week	12 weeks
Medroxyprogesterone acetate[17]	1000 mg/week	12 weeks
Levo-Norgestrel intrauterine[23]		1 year

bleeding may require hysterectomy. Excellent results, at least for a limited time, have been published.[5,8,12,19,30,31,32]

Kistner[12] stressed that the hyperplasia may be held in a regressive state as long as the progestational agent is administered. Wentz[32] used progestins for only 6 weeks to control endometrial hyperplasia, but that is too short according to Eichner & Abellera[6] who found that the disease progressed or recurred when the progestin therapy was stopped. Gal[8] disproved the theory that intracellular progesterone receptors decreased after a short treatment period and therefore should not be administered as a long-term treatment. He has shown that the progesterone effect was maintained during many years of treatment. Lindahl et al[19] claim that it is only during a short period in the life of women that it is possible to develop a hyperplasia, and if this development is stopped the possibility of developing a new hyperplasia again is low. They propose a high dose gestagen treatment for only 3 months to avoid the negative side effects of gestagen treatment.

For patients with atypical hyperplasias nearly 50 to 60% regress, but since risk of residual undiagnosed carcinoma in the uterus after a curettage increases with age, hysterectomy plus bilateral salpingo-oophorectomy is the recommended treatment for women over 50 years of age.[16] For patients who are judged inoperable, high dose gestagen treatment should be given. Lindahl et al[19] reported a nearly 100% response rate to 1000 mg medroxyprogesterone acetate weekly for 3 months. Similar results were obtained with megestrol acetate 20 to 40 mg 4 times per day for 8 weeks.[32] Prompt response to treatment judged by control curettage specimens is mandatory, and the patient should agree to a long-term follow-up. Patients who are not operable and who do not respond to hormone therapy may be treated with intracavitary irradiation, for example, according to Heyman. For treatment recommendations see Table 47.2.

Another approach to the problem is by anti-estrogenic treatment with tamoxifen or Danazol. In our own experience treatment with tamoxifen in a daily dose of 20 mg results in a response rate of 70% in patients with simple and complex hyperplasia; whereas 4 out of 8 patients with atypical hyperplasia responded to tamoxifen, which is in agreement with the observations of El-Tomi et al.[7] No serious side effects were noted. Although it is too early to say anything about long-term results, tamoxifen is clearly an alternative to progestins in patients in whom progestins are contraindicated. Danazol, an isoxazol derivative of ethinyltestosterone, has a significant anti-proliferative effect on the endometrium in daily doses of 200 mg for 3 months. A very high response rate[3] has been reported (Table 47.4). In a pilot study topical treatment of endometrial hyperplasia by an intrauterine device releasing levonorgestrel has shown very promising results with complete histological regression of the hyperplasia, regardless of pattern.[23] Complete remission of hyperplasia to a normal

Table 47.4 Different anti-estrogenic hormonal treatment regimens of endometrial hyperplasia

Type of anti-estrogen	Dosage	Duration
Tamoxifen[7,19]	10–30 mg/day	6 months
Danazol[3]	200 mg/day	3 months

endometrial pattern was achieved in 87.5% of the patients in this study. This device seems to represent a significant step toward the ideal medical treatment of endometrial hyperplasia (Table 47.3).

THE FUTURE

Although the number of patients with atypical hyperplasia with progression to cancer is rather small, usually patients with this diagnosis are treated with hysterectomy. The absence of diagnostic criteria which can accurately predict the outcome of the disease is the major cause of overtreatment. In addition there is considerable disagreement between pathologists in differentiating between cases of atypical hyperplasia and those of well differentiated carcinoma. There is an increasing interest in the search of additive prognostic factors in order to be able to give patients with endometrial hyperplasia a more individualized therapy. Recently, a classification based on nuclear morphometric features has been described,[1] which can predict the outcome in the majority of patients with atypical hyperplasia. In endometrial carcinomas steroid receptor concentrations[4,11,18] and flow cytometrical DNA-measurements in individual cells[9,18] have been reported as prognostic parameters. In order to investigate if these parameters are also valuable in endometrial hyperplasia, prospective studies are in progress. Preliminary results have been reported regarding steroid receptor concentrations and DNA-measurements.[20,21] The steroid receptor concentrations in 128 endometrial hyperplasias revealed that only the progesterone receptor concentration tended to be higher than that of proliferating histopathologically normal endometria (Table 47.5). The DNA-measurements in 194 patients revealed that about 20% of simple and complex hyperplasia have an aneuploid DNA content compared to 6% in normal endometria and 33% in atypical hyperplasia and well to moderately differentiated cancers (Table 47.6). 122 patients were randomized between control curettage only and treatment with 1000 mg medroxyprogesterone weekly for 3 months. In the control group (64 patients) it was found that at first control curettage 3 months later, 60% of the patients presented with normal endometria regardless whether it was a simple, complex or atypical hyperplasia. Hitherto only a short follow-up time is presented regarding the steroid receptor content, and these results gave no further information. The DNA analyses seem more promising. After 2 years of follow-up for the

Table 47.5 The mean concentrations of steroid receptors in different groups of hyperplasia

Endometrial hyperplasia	N	Estradiol receptors fmol/mg DNA	N	Progesterone receptors fmol/mg DNA
Simple	92	1100	84	7800
Complex	28	1100	28	7400
Atypical	8	1200	8	6400
Secretory phase	140	850	123	3500
Proliferative phase	148	1100	127	5800

There are no significant differences between concentrations of steroid receptors comparing the three diagnoses (multiple range test). After Lindahl et al[20]

Table 47.6 DNA-index in relation to degree of endometrial hyperplasia

Diagnosis at first curettage	Number and percentage	
	Diploidy	Aneuploidy
Simple	109(79%)	33(21%)
Complex	28(80%)	12(20%)
Atypical	8(67%)	4(33%)

After Lindahl et al[17]

64 patients there was an overrepresentation of atypical hyperplasia or endometrial cancer in the group with aneuploidy at the initial curettage compared to the diploid ones (Table 47.7).[21] Due to the small numbers, the differences were not significant. However, the only two carcinomas developed in patients who had aneuploid simple hyperplasia before treatment. All the patients in the treatment arm are still in complete remission after 2 years of observation (see also Ch. 6).

Another prognostic factor which perhaps in the future can help us to define high risk patients is the plasminogen activator. Recent results support the contention that plasminogen activator reflects malignant transformation of endometrial cells and it is suggested that determination of plasminogen activator may facilitate diagnosis and proper treatment of precancerous and cancerous states of endometrium.[26]

Thus, in the future we may well have a test-set including DNA profile,[21] nuclear morphometry,[1] progesterone chal-

Table 47.7 Diagnosis at control curettage 2 years after the initial curettage without further treatment in relation to DNA.

Initial DNA index	N	Simple	Complex	Atypical	Normal	Adeno-carcinoma
Diploidy	48	6	4	4	34(71%)	0
Aneuploidy	14	2	0	3	8(57%)	2

Lindahl et al (Unpublished data)

lenge test[29] and plasminogen activator[26] analysed in a multi-range setup which could give us a prognostic index able to separate the high-risk from the low-risk patients. This is especially important in young patients.

REFERENCES

1. Ausems E W, van der Kamp J K, Baak J P 1985 Nuclear morphometry in the determination of the prognosis of marked atypical endometrial hyperplasia. Int J Gynecol Pathol 4: 180
2. Bonte J 1986 Diagnosis and treatment of precancerous endometrial lesions. In: Schultz (ed) Endometrial Cancer. Int Symp Marburg, p 26
3. Bulletti C, Jasonni V M, Tabanelli S, Balducci M, Fuschini G, Flamigni C 1987 Danazol reverses endometrial hyperplasia to normal endometrium. Acta Eur-Fertil 18: 185
4. Creasman W T, Soper J T, McCarthy Jr K S, Hanshaw W, Clarke-Pearson D L 1985 Influence of cytoplasmic steroid receptor content on prognosis of early stage endometrial carcinoma. Am J Obstet Gynecol 151: 922
5. Dallenbach-Hellweg G, Czernobilsky B, Allemann J 1986 Medroxyprogesteron acetat bei der adenomatosen Hyperplasie des Korpusendometriums. Geburtsh Frauenheilk 46: 601
6. Eichner E, Abeller M 1987 Endometrial hyperplasia treated by progestins. Obstet Gynecol 38: 739
7. El-Tomi N F, Hassan S, Youssef F, Labib N, Ali N, Hathout H 1985 The effect of tamoxifen on endometrial hyperplasia. J Kuveit Med Assoc 19: 175
8. Gal D 1986 Hormonal therapy for lesions of the endometrium. Seminars Oncology 13: 33
9. Geisinger K R, Homesley H D, Morgan T M, Kute T E, Marshall R B 1986 Endometrial adenocarcinoma. A multiparameter clinicopathological analysis including the DNA profile and the sex steroid hormone receptors. Cancer 58: 1518
10. Greenblatt R B, Gambrell R D Jr, Stoddard L D 1982 The protective role of progesterone in the prevention of endometrical cancer. Pathol Res Pract 174: 127
11. Kauppila A, Kujansuu E, Vikko R 1982 Cytosol estrogen and progestin receptors in endometrial carcinoma of patients treated with surgery, radiotherapy and progestin. Cancer 50: 2157
12. Kistner R W 1970 The effects of progestational agents on hyperplasia and carcinoma in situ of the endometrium. Int J Gynecol Obstet 84: 561
13. Kjørstad K E, Welander C, Halvorsen T, Grude T, Onsrud M 1978 Progestogens as primary treatment in pre-malignant changes of the endometrium. In: Bush, King and Taylor (eds) Endometrial Cancer. Bailliere Tindall, London, p 188
14. Kurman R J 1988 Endometrial hyperplasia and its relationship to certain types of carcinoma. In: Surgery in the Treatment of Gynecologic Cancer. Proceedings of the international symposium. University Press, Antwerp, Sept 30–Oct 1 p 11
15. Kurman J R, Karrinski P F, Norris H J 1985 The behavior of endometrial hyperplasia. A long-term study of untreated hyperplasia in 170 patients. Cancer 56: 403
16. Kurman R J, Norris H J 1987 Endometrial carcinoma. In: Kurman R J (ed) Blaustein's Pathology of the Female Genital Tract (3rd edn) Springer Verlag, New York, p 324
17. Lindahl B, Alm P 1991 Flow cytometrical DNA-measurements on endometrial hyperplasias. A prospective follow-up study after curettage only or additional high-dose gestagen treatment. Submitted for publication.
18. Lindahl B, Alm P, Fernö M, Killander D, Långström E, Norgren A, Trope C 1987 Prognostic value of flow cytometrical DNA measurements in stage I–II endometrial carcinoma. Correlations with steroid receptor concentration, tumor myometrial invasion and degree of differentiation. Anticancer Res 7: 791
19. Lindahl B, Alm P, Fernö M, Norgren A 1988 Endometrial hyperplasia II. Endocrine factors. Submitted for publication.
20. Lindahl B, Alm P, Fernö M, Norgren A 1990 Endometrial hyperplasia: A prospective randomized study of histopathology, tissue steroid receptors and plasma steroids after curettage, with or without high dose gestagen treatment. Anticancer Research 10: 725
21. Lindahl B, Willen R 1991 Endometrial hyperplasia. Clinicopathological considerations of a prospective randomized study after curettage only or high dose gestagen treatment. Results of 2 years follow-up of 292 patients. Submitted for publication.
22. Norris H J, Connor M P, Kurman R J 1986 Preinvasive lesions of the endometrium. Clin Obstet Gynecol 13: 725
23. Scarselli G, Tantini C, Colafranceschi M, Taddei G L, Bargelli G, Venturini N, Branconi F 1988 Levo-Norgestrel-Nova T and precancerous lesions of the endometrium. Eur J Gynecol Oncol 9: 284
24. Schneider M L 1985 Möglichkeiten und Grenzen eines zytologischen Frühererkennungsprogramms beim Endometriumkarzinom. Geburtsh u Frauenheilk 45: 831
25. Schneider M L 1986 Die Lokalisation der Endometriehyperplasien und ihre Kernmorphologie. Geburtsh u Frauenheilk 46: 381
26. Soszka T, Olszewski K 1986 Plasminogen activators and their inhibitors in normal, hyperplastic and carcinomatous human endometrium. Thromb Res 42: 835
27. Smith J J, Schulman H 1985 Current dilatation and curettage practice: A need for revision. Obstet Gynecol 65: 516
28. Tavasolli F A, Kraus F T 1978 Endometrial lesions in uteri resected for atypical endometrial hyperplasia. Am J Clin Pathol 70: 770
29. Toppozada M K, Ismail A A, Hamed R S, Ahmed K S, El-Faras A 1988 Progesterone challenge test and estrogen assays in menopausal women with endometrial adenomatous hyperplasia. Int J Gynecol Obstet 26: 115
30. Wentz W B 1964 Effect of a progestational agent on endometrial hyperplasia and endometrial cancer. Obstet Gynecol 24: 370
31. Wentz W B 1974 Progestin therapy in endometrial hyperplasia. Gynecol Oncol 2: 362
32. Wentz W B 1985 Progestin therapy in lesions of the endometrium. Seminar Oncology 12: 23
33. Whitehead M 1987 The effects of estrogens and progestogens on the postmenopausal endometrium. Maturitas 1: 87

48. Pathology of endometrial carcinoma

S. J. Huang J. S. Berek Y. S. Fu

GENERAL CONSIDERATIONS

Endometrial cancer is the most common malignant neoplasm of the female genital tract in American women, although it ranks behind ovarian and cervical cancers in deaths caused by pelvic malignancies.[113] Incidence rates which increased by a third during the 1970s were followed by a near comparable decline during the 1980s.[34] However, overall 5-year survival for cancer of the uterine corpus as reported by the American Cancer Society decreased in 1979–1984 compared to 1974–1976, from 89 to 83% for whites and from 61 to 52% for blacks.[113]

While increased detection through the use of cytologic smears has contributed to the changing frequency of cancer arising in the uterine cervix, there is little evidence to suggest that this has had any direct effect on the increasing frequency of endometrial cancer. The changing incidence does appear to reflect the use of exogenous estrogens during the 1960s.[34] There is a geographic correlation among the frequencies of endometrial, breast, and ovarian cancers, with low rates of these cancers in Asiatic populations and high rates in North Americans; such a correlation is not seen with cancer of the cervix.[36] In recent years, the growing interest in endometrial cancer can be attributed to its increasing frequency, its relationship to the use of estrogen and oral contraceptives, and a better understanding of the factors affecting the ultimate prognosis. An understanding of the pathologic features is essential if optimal results are to be achieved in the management of endometrial cancer.

Changing frequency and nature

In the United States, age-adjusted incidence rates for endometrial carcinoma in white females were essentially unchanged between the late 1940s and 1970, remaining in the range 23.2 to 24.6 per 100 000. The rates increased gradually and peaked during the mid-1970s, with an overall increase of 30% over the decade.[34] This was followed by a gradual decrease in the 1980s, most notably among women aged 25 to 64 years. During the last two decades, a rising incidence of endometrial cancer has also been reported in Norway,[52] Japan,[84] and England.[122]

While increased clinical awareness, improved detection, and changes in the histopathologic criteria used to establish the diagnosis of endometrial carcinoma may have contributed to the increase in its incidence rate, it is unlikely that these totally account for a rise of this magnitude.[101] Conditions leading to excess endogenous estrogens are well known to heighten the risk of developing endometrial cancer[52,112] and the rising frequency of this carcinoma has been attributed to the increased usage of estrogen.[34,100,129] (See also Chs 3 and 8.)

Several studies have demonstrated differences between carcinomas in women exposed or not exposed to estrogen.[9,31,103,117] Silverberg et al[117] found that carcinoma patients who were estrogen non-users had a lower parity, later menopause, obesity, hypertension, and diabetes mellitus, compared to patients who received exogenous estrogens; these features were thought to represent constitutional risk factors for endometrial cancers. Estrogen users tended to have well differentiated, non-invasive cancers. In contrast, the cancers in estrogen non-users tended to be more poorly differentiated, more deeply invasive, less sensitive to progesterone therapy, and of an unfavorable histology or higher grade; they also were associated with a poorer prognosis and greater recurrence rate.[103,117] However, when carcinomas of similar grade were compared, the survival rates in estrogen users and non-users were similar.[103] Early detection of carcinoma in estrogen users has been suggested as a reason for its better prognosis.[103]

Deligdisch and Cohen[31] found that patients with endometrial carcinoma, adenomatous hyperplasia, and hyperestrogenism had more well differentiated and less invasive cancers than patients with carcinomas unassociated with adenomatous hyperplasia. Similar findings were reported by Bokhman,[9] who compared cancer patients with obesity, hyperlipidemia, and signs of hyperestrogenism to those lacking these features; the 5-year survival for the former was 85.6% compared to 58.8% for those lacking endocrine or metabolic disturbances. Thus, two patterns of pathogenesis are suggested by these studies: better differentiated carcinomas sometimes associated with hyperplasia may arise in a background of endogenous or exogenous hyperestrogenism, and cancers of poorer prognosis may arise from normal or atrophic endometrium without increased estrogen.

When compared with past experience, cancers arising in the endometrium are currently detected at an earlier stage in their evolution. The cancers detected in recent years are more likely to be localized, confined to the endometrium or characterized by limited penetration of the myometrium.[114]

DIAGNOSIS

Endometrial cancer may be detected by the use of appropriate cellular samples interpreted by skilled observers. The detection of endometrial carcinoma in cervical smears depends on the exfoliation of malignant cells. In one retrospective review, 58 of 154 patients with endometrial cancer had a prior cervical smear.[79] Smears were more often positive or suspicious when carcinomas were of higher grade, extended over a greater endometrial surface area, involved the endocervix, or were associated with benign or malignant squamous elements. A polypoid pattern of growth and clear cell or papillary histologies, but not myometrial invasion, also correlated with exfoliation.[79] In another retrospective study of 220 endometrial cancer patients, cervical smears were positive in 33%, suspicious in 26%, and negative in 41%; smears were more often positive in high grade and high stage lesions.[109]

While conventional cervical smears have an accuracy of 50 to 75% in the detection of symptomatic endometrial carcinomas, various endometrial sampling techniques for cytologic or histologic examination of the endometrium are being tested and evaluated, such as endometrial aspiration and vacuum curettage, with accuracies ranging from 74 to 97%.[4,43,46,53,96] The benefits of screening tests for treatable diseases are dependent to some extent on test sensitivity and disease prevalence. Through prospective screening of 2586 asymptomatic women over 40 years of age by endometrial sampling technique (Isaacs cannula and Mi-Mark Helix), 16 adenocarcinomas were detected cytologically and two adenocarcinomas were missed.[72] The prevalence rate based on carcinomas detected on or within one year of first screening was 6.96 per 1000.[72]

In many institutions, endometrial curettage is still the traditional method for detecting the presence of endometrial cancer. Kurman and Norris[75] have developed criteria for stromal invasion, applicable to curettage specimens. Stromal invasion is indicated by (1) an infiltrate associated with a desmoplastic response, (2) a confluent glandular, cribriform pattern, (3) an extensive papillary pattern, or (4) replacement of stroma by masses of squamous epithelium; the latter three patterns should involve at least 2.1 mm or half of a 4.2 mm diameter low power field.[75] For neoplasms that met these criteria in endometrial curettings, 50% (58/115) of the subsequent hysterectomy specimens contained carcinoma, and mid to deep myometrial invasion was present in 24% of these. For tumors which did not show stromal invasion by these criteria, residual carcinoma was found in 17% (15/89) of uteri, and invasion in seven was limited to the superficial myometrium.

King et al[71] applied these criteria to endometrial biopsies or curettages from 83 women with Stage I, Grade 1 adenocarcinomas. Of the 40 patients whose lesions fulfilled the definition of stromal invasion, 25, or 67%, had myometrial invasion on subsequent hysterectomy. Seven (16%) of the 43 patients lacking stromal invasion on preliminary sampling had myometrial invasion on hysterectomy.

Among others, Stock and Kanbour[120] have emphasized that endometrial curettage may fail to provide a comprehensive sampling of the endometrium. In 100 consecutive cases of ultimately proven endometrial cancer, the curetted material obtained by 35 different obstetrician-gynecologists was thought to be 'suspicious' in only 45% of the cases. Palmer and Roth[95] similarly found that the gross appearance of the endometrial curettings was often misleading in the presence of endometrial cancer and recommended the use of frozen sections of the endometrial curettings prior to hysterectomy.

With modern equipment, the overall accuracy of frozen section diagnosis in the hands of a skilled surgical pathologist is 95% or more. Considerable skill is required to evaluate the endometrium by frozen section, which has several limitations. In about 20% of cases, the tissue submitted for frozen section may be less than 0.5 ml, a tissue volume small enough to create technical difficulties. The artifacts induced by freezing may make it more difficult to interpret the subsequently processed permanent sections. More importantly, the changes identified in endometrial curettings studied by frozen section may not be representative of lesions in the uterus, which may be more advanced than anticipated or which may include other elements, e.g. adenosquamous cancer or malignant mixed müllerian tumor. Distinguishing between complex hyperplasia with atypia and well differentiated adenocarcinoma is notoriously difficult. The presence of hyperplasia on a frozen section of endometrial curettings does not exclude the presence of cancer in the resected uterus; however, the recognition of cancer has a high degree of validity.

The histologic grade of tumors based on curettings obtained in the office or operating room is at least one grade lower than the grade derived from hysterectomy specimens in 15 to 20% of patients.[29] Intraoperative consultation at the time of hysterectomy, for the evaluation of gross pathology and possibly for frozen section to determine histologic grade and tumor extent, may aid in the selection of appropriate staging procedures.[29]

Although endocervical curettage is performed for FIGO staging of endometrial carcinoma, its accuracy in the determination of cervical involvement has been questioned. Endocervical curettings (ECC) may show tumor in contiguity with endocervical tissue (in 3%), isolated endometrial tumor fragments only (28%), or no tumor (54%), or be insufficient for diagnosis (14%).[45] When endometrial cancer was found in direct contact with identifiable endocervical tissue, 60[45] to 100%[16] of hysterectomy specimens had proven cervical involvement. Not finding cervical disease on hysterectomy can be explained by preoperative radiotherapy, by inadequate cervical sampling for histologic examination, or by prior vigorous curettage, which may completely remove the tumor or cause tumor necrosis.

When only isolated fragments of endometrial cancer are present in endocervical curettings, the probability of cervical involvement in the hysterectomy specimen is 31%.[45] In the majority of cases, this represents free floating endometrial tumor cells in the cervical canal, removed along with normal endocervical epithelium or stroma. In spite of this, Larson et al[77] have found that the presence of endometrial tumor in ECC, in any pattern, with or without demonstrable cervical invasion, is a poor prognostic sign.

When ECC samples are free of tumor, the risk of cervical involvement in hysterectomy specimens is 1[45] to 8%.[16] False negative results can be explained by sampling error or by the inaccessibility of tumor confined to the stroma without mucosal disease. In the series of Frauenhoffer,[45] the predictive value of positive findings in ECC was 35% and of the negative results 99%. Thus, the value of a well performed ECC lies in its ability to exclude rather than to confirm the cervical involvement. When ECCs are inadequate for interpretation, 10% of hysterectomy specimens demonstrate cervical extension.[45]

GROSS MANIFESTATIONS

Endometrial cancer may occur in a localized or a diffuse form. When localized, the neoplasm uncommonly may be confined to a polyp. In postmenopausal women, the yield from endometrial curettage in the presence of cancer may exceed the yield from an atrophic endometrium. The tumor tissue is firm, somewhat dry, and often friable, and has a granular appearance. Necrotic foci may be yellow, white, or red. With associated pyometra, an exudate may be conspicuous. In the presence of uterine cancer, endometrial curettings will not always have the typical gross features of cancer. Hyperplastic endometrium may also be polypoid and abundant, but is more likely to be soft, with a moist or mucoid surface, and to lack necrosis.

The gross identification and evaluation of cancer in the resected uterus is best achieved by employing a standardized method of examination. The uterus should be transversely sectioned at 4 mm intervals down to the level of the internal os. The uterine cervix is removed, pinned out on a cork board, and allowed to fix for a minimum of 2 hours. If warranted by the tumor location and extent, the entire cervix may be embedded for histologic examination by sectioning around the clock, parallel to the axis of the canal.

The endometrium may be focally or diffusely involved. Carcinoma may appear as a localized thickening of the endometrium, but diffuse involvement is more common, particularly in the upper portion of the uterine cavity (Fig. 48.1). The posterior wall is more likely to be involved than the anterior wall. Less frequently, there is involvement of the lower uterine segment. Residual neoplasm is often identified in the cornual areas of the resected uterus, since these are less accessible to curettage. It may be difficult to determine the precise origin of the cancer since considerable tissue may be removed by curettage or destroyed by prior radiation. In the presence of coexistent disease, such as polyps and leiomyomas, cancer may be overlooked (Fig. 48.2).

Comprehensive survey and sampling are needed to provide information about tumor size, gross appearance, and histologic classification. Particularly important is the assessment of the depth of penetration into the myometrium and of involvement of extrauterine sites. Sections for histology should include the full thickness of the uterine wall, where there is deepest tumor invasion. With extended surgical procedures, lymph nodes should be separately embedded and identified as to site of origin.

Anderson et al[3] evaluated two major growth characteristics: exuberance of exophytic growth and diffuseness of origin. Of tumors that were both diffuse, arising from more than one-quarter of the endometrial cavity, and polypoid or shaggy, 61.1% had greater than 30% myometrial penetration. All recurrences occurred in this group. When neither bulky nor diffuse cancer was present, no patient had more than 30% myometrial penetration. Tumors with only one poor prognostic gross feature had intermediate levels of myoinvasion.[3]

TYPES OF NEOPLASM

A variety of neoplasms may originate in the endometrium, including classical adenocarcinoma and its variants, adenocarcinoma with squamous elements, rare squamous cell carcinomas, and rarer small cell carcinomas.

Of 1009 consecutive cancers evaluated at the Institute of Pathology of the University Hospitals of Cleveland, 65% were classified as adenocarcinomas, 19.0% as adenoacanthomas, 13.8% were considered to be adenosquamous cancers, 1.2% were clear cell carcinomas, and 1.0% had

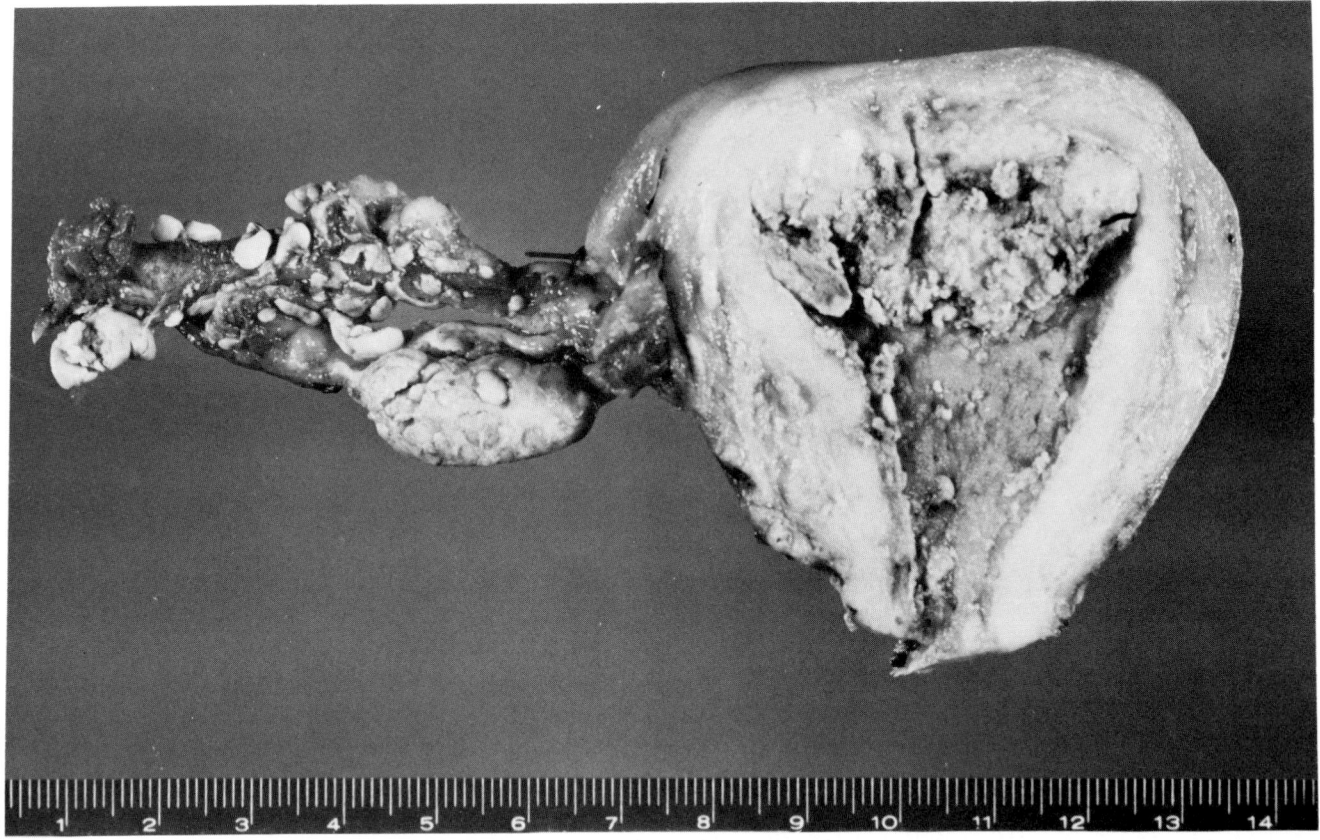

Fig. 48.1 Adenosquamous cancer of endometrium. Residual carcinoma is readily identified in the uterine specimen. Transtubal seeding accounts for the cancer implants observed over the fallopian tube and ovary. The uterine cervix has been removed for comprehensive evaluation.

characteristics of secretory adenocarcinoma.[102] Comparable frequencies were reported by Christopherson et al;[18a] in a review of 989 invasive endometrial cancers, 59.6% were adenocarcinomas, 21.7% adenoacanthomas, 6.9% adenosquamous carcinomas, 5.7% clear cell carcinomas, 4.7% papillary carcinomas, and 1.5% secretory carcinomas.

Among the rare primary cancers of endometrial origin, the most common is squamous cell cancer. According to Fluhmann[44] and Kay,[70] the diagnosis of squamous cell carcinoma of the endometrium is only justified when there is no coexisting endometrial adenocarcinoma and no connection between the neoplasm and squamous abnormalities of the uterine cervix, and when primary origin in the cervix is excluded by careful examination. Direct extension of cervical condyloma, intraepithelial neoplasia, invasive carcinoma, and verrucous carcinoma to the endometrium can occur.[69,123] This event is more common than is primary squamous neoplasm of the endometrium. In a case presentation of a spindle cell variant and a review of 28 previously reported squamous cell carcinomas of the endometrium, Yamashina et al[130] noted that this tumor was associated with pyometra in recent cases less frequently than in the past, that while the average age of patients was 61 years, premenopausal cases did occur rarely, and that squamous

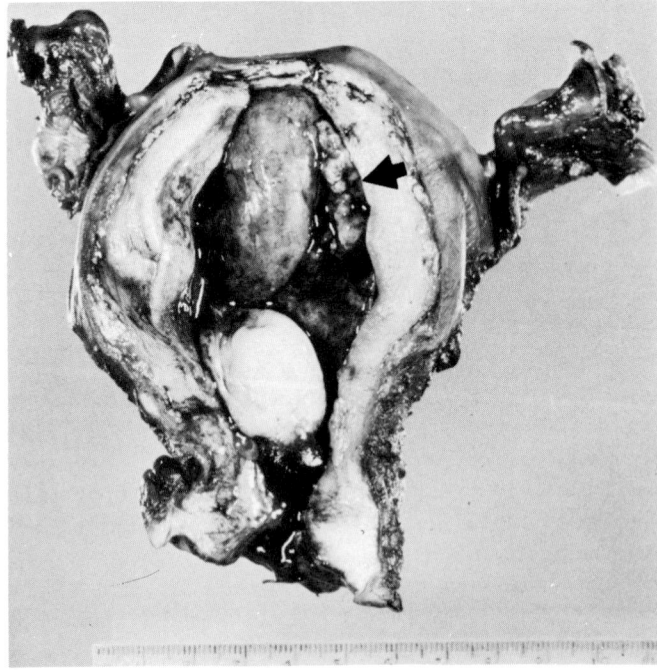

Fig. 48.2 Endometrial adenocarcinoma coexisting with adenomatous polyps of the endometrium and uterine cervix. The cancer, initially detected by cell studies, was not apparent on endometrial biopsy. The neoplasm located in the cornual area was confined to the endometrium.

metaplasia was not always present. Too few cases of squamous cell carcinoma of the endometrium have been reported to evaluate its prognosis. Rare examples of primary verrucous carcinoma of the endometrium have been reported.[106]

Argyrophil cell adenocarcinomas originating in the endometrium have been reported; these may represent counterparts of apudomas (*a*mine *p*recursor *u*ptake and *d*ecarboxylation-oma) seen elsewhere.[124] Argyrophil cells may be found in normal, hyperplastic, and carcinomatous endometria. Such cells are reported in about 26% of endometrial cancers[1] although rare Grimelius positive cells may be found in up to 68% of tumors.[6] At least two types of Grimelius positivity have been described: (1) in cells similar to non-Grimelius positive cells in an apical or diffuse cytoplasmic distribution, or (2) within the cytoplasm of round, oval, or flask-shaped cells similar to the enterochromaffin cells of the gastrointestinal tract. In the former cells, argyrophilia in some cases has been attributed to mucin or glycogen.[1] Chromogranin positivity and APUD type functions have been demonstrated in the latter cell type.[65,124] Positivity for serotonin, somatostatin, and ACTH has also been noted.[1] The presence of these cells has not been associated with any clinical endocrine syndromes. The morphology of the carcinomas containing argyrophil cells is the same as that for usual adenocarcinomas.

In contrast, reports of small cell carcinomas of the endometrium are very rare.[6,74,93,97] These appear morphologically similar to oat cell carcinomas of the lung or small cell carcinomas of the cervix, and contain neurosecretory granules by electronmicroscopy. Three of the four reported cases were argyrophil negative and were associated with aggressive behavior. It is postulated that small cell carcinomas of the endometrium arise either from neuroendocrine-derived argyrophilic cells in the normal endometrium, or from a stem cell precursor capable of either epithelial or neuroendocrine differentiation.

Rare melanin-producing neoplasms of the endometrium have been reported which resemble, in part, the retinal anlage tumors of children.[58,110] Secondary neoplasms involving the endometrium most commonly originate from the cervix, breast, stomach, pancreas, colon and kidney. The endometrium is involved in one-third of the women with ovarian endometrioid cancer according to Scully[111] although this may represent simultaneous neoplastic transformation rather than metastasis.

HISTOLOGIC APPEARANCE

Adenocarcinoma, the most common neoplasm arising in the endometrium, is characterized by glands having an abnormal architectural relationship with one another (Figs 48.3 and 48.4). Recognizable stroma is not identified between the abnormal glands (Fig. 48.4). The size of the glands is

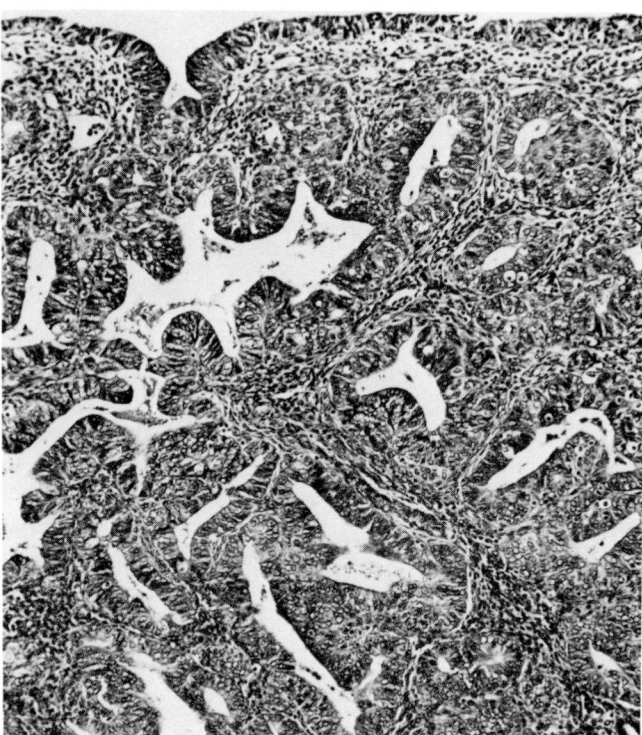

Fig. 48.3 Grade I adenocarcinoma of the endometrium occurring in a 32 year old woman with a history of Oracon (ethinyl estradiol 100 mg, dimethisterone 25 mg) therapy. In some glands there is infolding of the lining epithelium. (×100.)

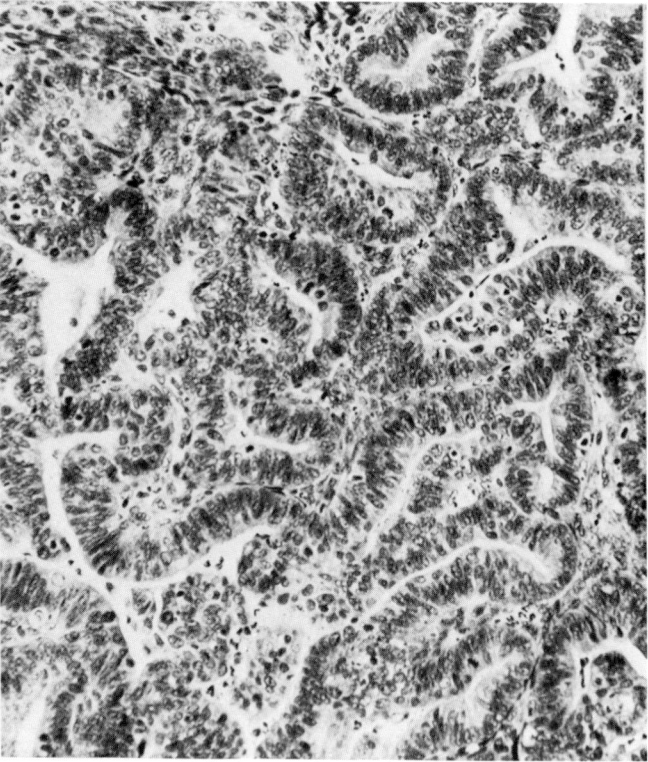

Fig. 48.4 Grade II adenocarcinoma of endometrium. The glands are in close apposition and lined by a pseudostratified columnar epithelium. Nucleoli are more conspicuous than in Grade I cancer and mitoses are more numerous. (×150.)

variable within a given neoplasm and also varies from one cancer to another. There may be infolding of the lining epithelium into the gland lumens or evidence of a papilliferous growth. Rarely, the carcinoma consists of sheets of cells and gland formation is inconspicuous (Fig. 48.5). The constituent cells are increased in size and often pseudostratified, and have enlarged nuclei which occur at varying levels within the epithelium. The nuclear chromatin is clumped and nucleolar enlargement may be observed. Nucleoli tend to be few in number. Mitoses are variable in frequency; occasional abnormal mitotic figures may be observed. Necrosis, hemorrhage and the formation of psammoma bodies may occur.

In the stroma, foam cells or lipid laden macrophages, characterized by abundant, pale, finely vacuolated cytoplasm and small central nuclei, are believed to be of endometrial stromal cell derivation. They may be found in 15% of endometrial cancers.[30] Their presence, although not related to specific clinical or pathologic features, is supportive of origin from the endometrium.[30]

Various metaplastic cells seen in benign endometria may also occur in endometrial malignancy, such as mucinous, ciliated, oxyphilic, squamous, clear, and serous cells. Focal

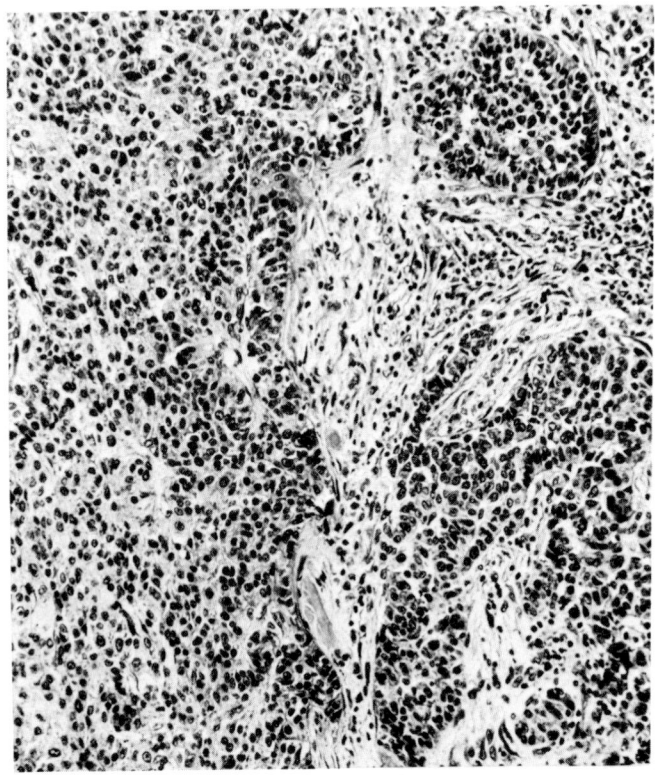

Fig. 48.5 Grade 3 adenocarcinoma of endometrium. The tumor cells are arranged predominantly in solid nests and sheets with rare glandular formations. The nuclei are hyperchromatic and variable in size. (×150.)

mucinous metaplasia, which resembles endocervical mucous cells, occurs in 10[27] to 38%[104] of ordinary endometrial cancers. The cells feature abundant, foamy cytoplasm or discrete basophilic mucous vacuoles. They form a complex villoglandular architecture and usually have only mild to moderate nuclear atypia (Fig. 48.6). When these cells comprise more than 50% of tumor cells, the tumor is designated a *mucinous adenocarcinoma*. Mucinous adenocarcinomas constitute 9% of endometrial adenocarcinomas.[104] The rates of relapse and myometrial invasion for mucinous adenocarcinoma are similar to those for non-mucinous adenocarcinoma. Mucinous adenocarcinoma must be distinguished from benign mucinous metaplasia of the endometrium and from involvement of the endometrium by endocervical, ovarian, or gastrointestinal primaries.

Ciliated cells may be seen in up to one-quarter of endometrial cancers. Such cells may appear singly or in focal clusters, and are more often found in Grade 1 than higher grade tumors.[117] Ten cases of *ciliated carcinoma* have been reported, in which, by definition, more than 75% of the cancerous cells were ciliated.[59] In addition to cilia, granular structures corresponding to ciliary rootlets were seen in the apical cytoplasm. These rare carcinomas accounted for 2.5% of cases in this series. The 10 cases were Grade 1 or 2, some were myoinvasive, and 9 of the 10 were accompanied by unciliated endometrial cancer.[59] Although ciliated cells are more often found in benign conditions, they may infrequently be part of a carcinoma.

Adenocarcinoma may coexist with squamous epithelium. The squamous component may be focal or more commonly multicentric in its distribution, superficially or diffusely distributed, and adjacent to or intermixed with the glandular component. It may demonstrate varying degrees of differentiation and keratinization.[47,92,114] Adenocarcinomas accompanied by benign appearing squamous epithelium are designated adenoacanthomas (Figs 48.7 and 48.8), while adenosquamous cancers by definition have both malignant glandular and malignant squamous components (Figs 48.9 to 48.11).

In *adenoacanthomas*, the squamous cells appear well differentiated and resemble cervical squamous metaplasia; there is minimal nuclear atypia and low mitotic activity. Squamous cells may proliferate within glandular lumens (Fig. 48.7), forming the so-called morules of Dutra,[37] or yield solid nests with smooth pushing borders (Figs 48.7 and 48.8).

The squamous cells in *adenosquamous carcinoma* have moderate to severe nuclear atypia and high mitotic activity, grow in irregular nests and solid sheets (Fig. 48.9), and infiltrate the stroma (Fig. 48.10). Some squamous cells in adenoacanthoma and adenosquamous carcinoma may assume an elongated configuration (Fig. 48.11) or have abundant clear cytoplasm. The Nomenclature and Classification Committee of the International Society of

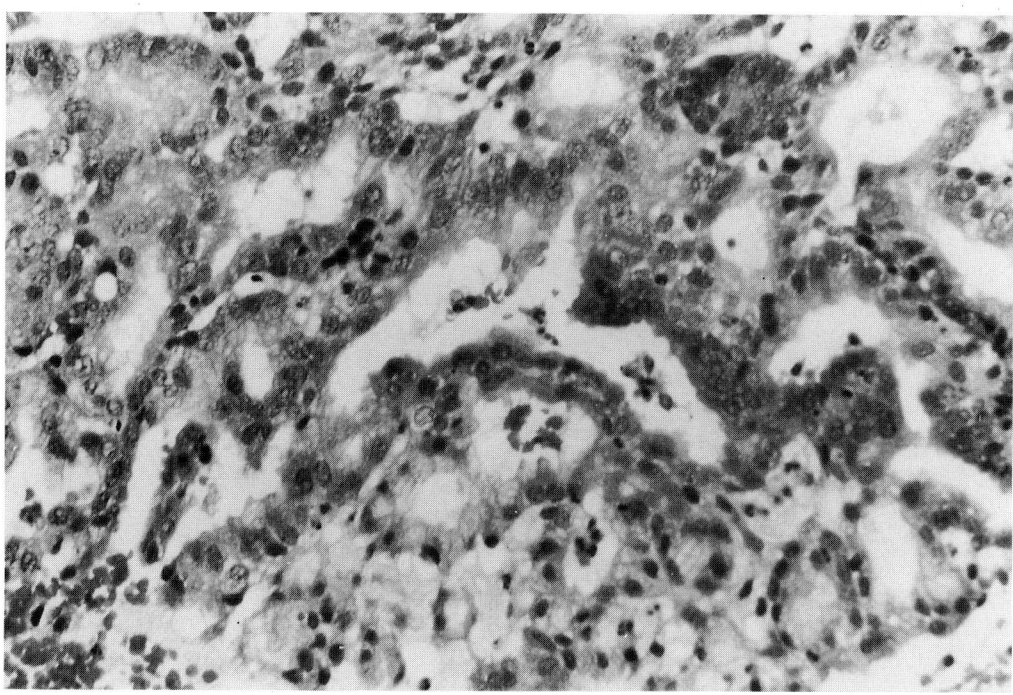

Fig. 48.6 Mucinous metaplasia consists of tall columnar cells with foamy vacuolated cytoplasm. Nuclear atypia is mild. The cells form complex back to back glands. (×255.)

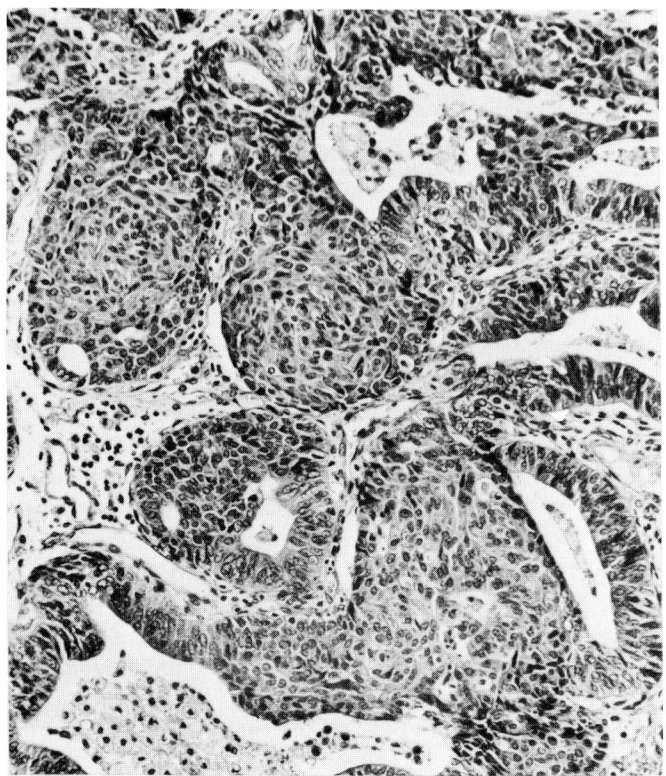

Fig. 48.7 Adenoacanthoma of endometrium. There are multicentric and well circumscribed foci of squamous epithelium. The squamous cells resemble those observed in immature squamous metaplasia. (×150.)

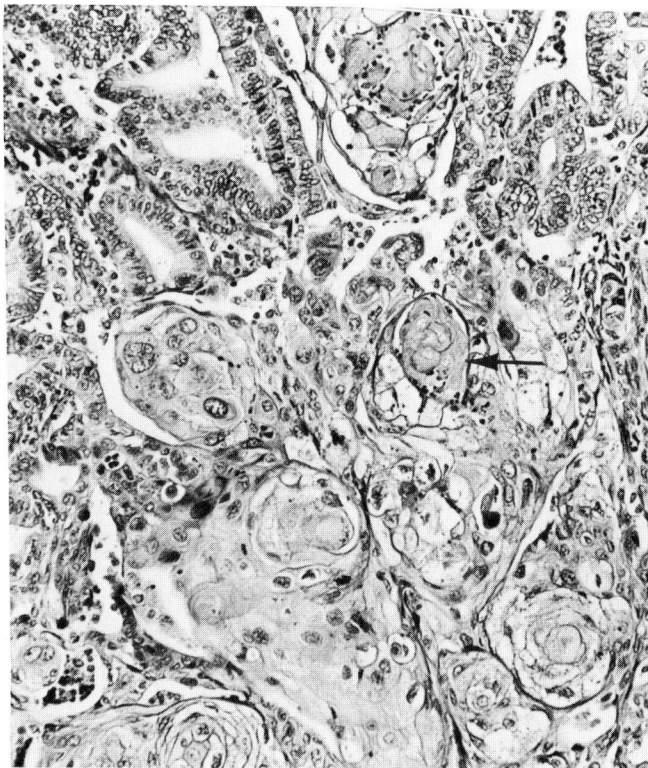

Fig. 48.8 Adenoacanthoma of endometrium. The squamous component is more differentiated than that of Figure 48.5. Focal keratinization is evident (see arrow). There is limited nuclear atypicality in the squamous cells. (×150.)

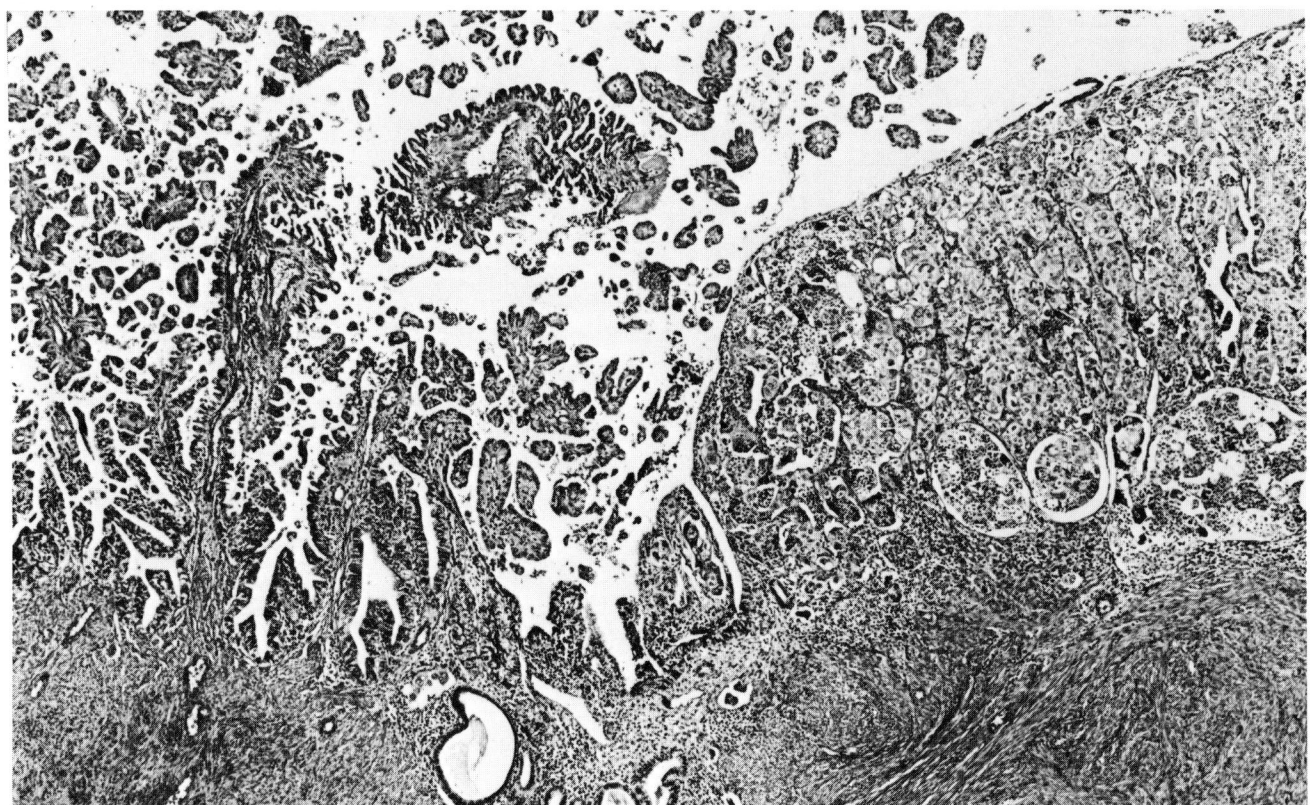

Fig. 48.9 Adenosquamous cancer of endometrium. The glandular and squamous components are in juxtaposition. The cells of the squamous component had the ultrastructural features of squamous cells. Despite the limited myometrial invasion the patient survived only 2 years. (×70.)

Gynecological Pathologists recommends that the cells interpreted as squamous type should meet at least one of the following criteria: (1) recognizable keratinization on H&E slide, (2) presence of intercellular bridges, and (3) presence of three or more of the following features: (a) solid sheets without glands or palisading, (b) sharp cell borders, (c) eosinophilic, thick or glassy cytoplasm, and (d) decreased nuclear/cytoplasmic ratio when compared with other tumor areas. These guidelines may improve consistency among pathologists in the classification of solid foci in adenocarcinoma and adenosquamous carcinoma.

Glassy cell carcinoma has been described by Christopherson et al[19] as a variant of adenosquamous carcinoma. Histologic features include a ground glass cytoplasm, accentuated cell margins, an irregular, opaque, hyperchromatic nucleus, a prominent nucleolus, and numerous mitotic figures. These comprised 7.4% of their cases of adenosquamous carcinoma, and four of the five cases reported behaved more aggressively than adenosquamous carcinomas without glassy cell features.[19]

In addition to the usual endometrial adenocarcinoma, with and without squamous elements, there are several histologic adenocarcinoma subtypes. The growth patterns of these variants may overlap; for example, papillary architec-

ture occurs in usual adenocarcinomas, uterine papillary serous tumors and clear cell carcinomas. Some subtypes may coexist, such as uterine papillary serous tumor and clear cell carcinoma. In most instances, subtypes can be separated from usual endometrial adenocarcinoma by their characteristic cytologic features.

Uterine *papillary serous tumor*, as defined by Hendrickson et al,[61] is morphologically and clinically distinct from the usual endometrial adenocarcinoma. It comprises less than 10% of Stage I endometrial carcinomas. Its appearance resembles that of ovarian papillary serous carcinoma, and is characterized by a complex papillary architecture with a broad fibrovascular framework lined by markedly atypical epithelial cells, occasionally in a hobnail pattern (Fig. 48.12A). The cells are notable for their nuclear pleomorphism and macronucleoli; bizarre nuclei may be seen (Fig. 48.12B). Mitotic figures are frequent, and are often abnormal. When invasive, the tumor tends to form gaping spaces lined by protruding atypical cells. Psammoma bodies are found in 33% of the tumors. The diagnosis of uterine papillary serous carcinoma should be made on the basis of the predominantly papillary architecture and the marked cytologic atypia. An endometrial adenocarcinoma in which less than 50% of the architecture is papillary and which

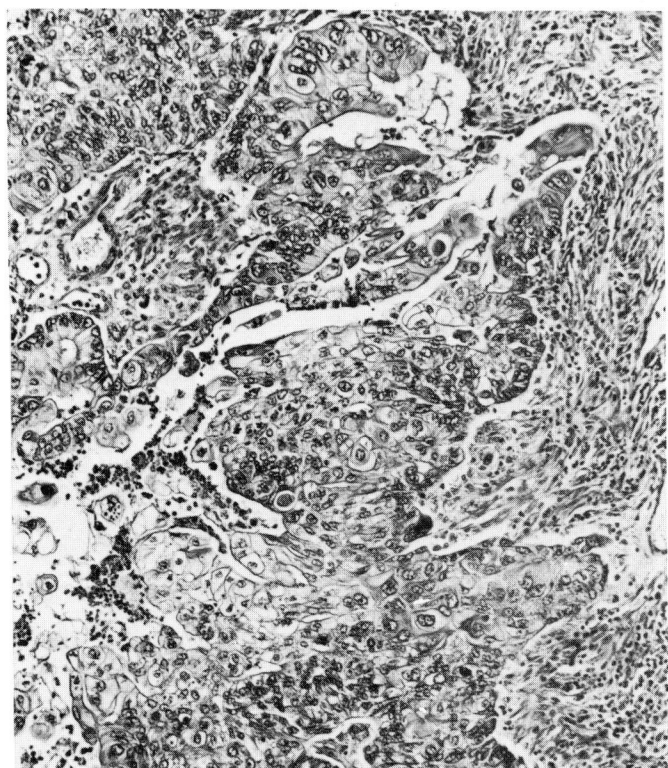

Fig. 48.10 Adenosquamous cancer. In this lesion squamous and glandular components are intermingled. The nuclear changes and the infiltration of the stroma indicated that the squamous component is malignant. (×100.)

Fig. 48.11 Adenosquamous cancer. The glandular and squamous components are intermingled. In this field the squamous component is made up of spindle-shaped cells. (×150.)

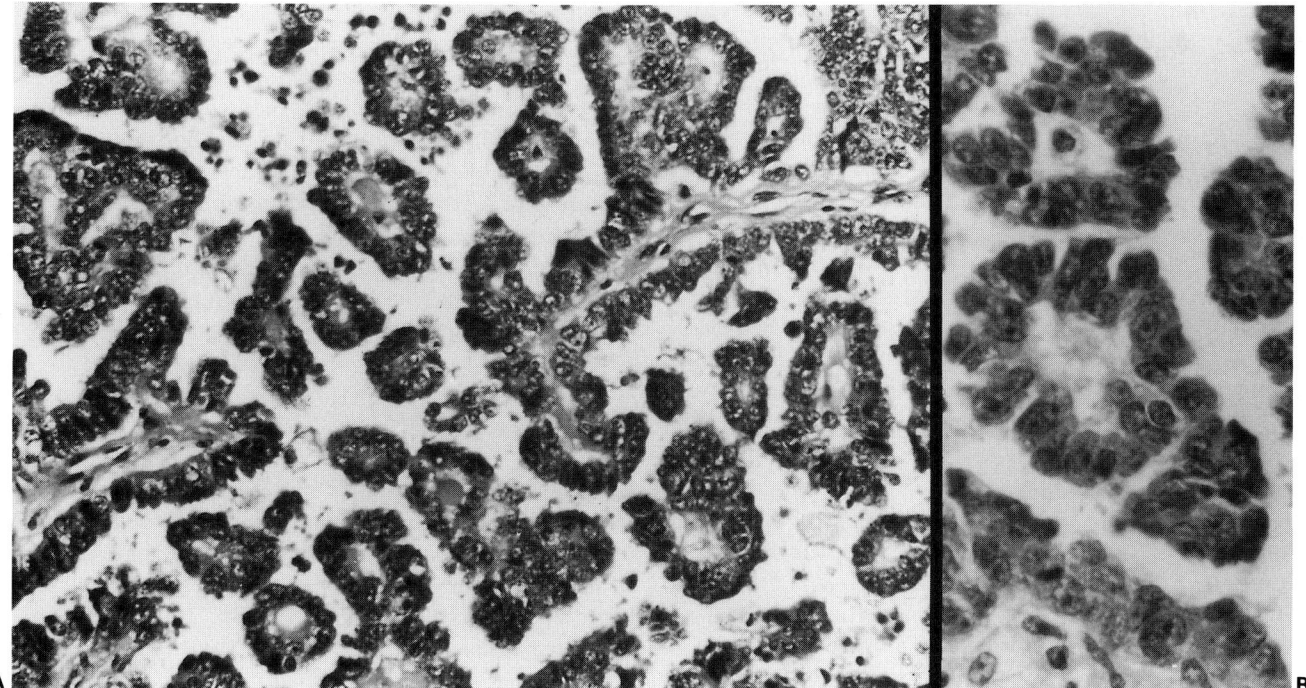

Fig 48.12 A. Papillary serous adenocarcinoma with complex papillary fronds supported by fibrous cores. B. Nuclear enlargement and pleomorphism, prominent nucleoli, and high mitotic activity are common features. (A. ×255, B. ×510.)

displays only mild nuclear atypia should be classified as the ordinary type.

Using these criteria, uterine papillary serous carcinoma is distinctive because of its poor prognosis and high mortality, independent of the depth of tumor invasion. These tumors are frequently clinically understaged, and invasion and spread may be grossly inapparent. They have a propensity for lymphatic invasion. Myometrial invasion is present in 40%, endocervical involvement in about one-third, and extrauterine spread in 50 to 55%.[61,78,126] As in ovarian papillary serous carcinomas, spread over the peritoneal surface may be seen. The overall relapse rate for patients with pathologic Stage I tumors in one series was 50%.[61] Recurrence has been reported in a tumor with less than 1 mm of myometrial invasion.[78] In another study, the combined 5-year survival for cases of surgical Stages I and II was 45%; the 3-year survival for Stages III and IV was 11%.[13] Uterine papillary serous carcinoma is accompanied in slightly over one-third of cases by clear cell carcinoma.[61] However, unlike ovarian serous carcinoma, which may be accompanied by a mucinous component, uterine papillary serous carcinoma has not been associated with mucinous elements.[78]

Neoplasms classified as *clear cell carcinomas* are composed of polygonal, hobnail-shaped, or flattened cells with a clear cytoplasm, according to Kurman and Scully.[76] The cells are arranged in solid masses or in papillary, tubular or cystic patterns (Fig. 48.13). With PAS stains there is evidence of diastase digestible glycogen in the cytoplasm of the neoplastic cells. In 13 of the 21 cases studied, clear cells accounted for more than half the cells; hobnail cells were dominant in only one case. In the remaining seven cases, there was an admixture of the described cell types. In five cases, clear cell carcinoma coexisted with other variants of endometrial cancer: secretory adenocarcinoma in two and endometrial adenocarcinoma associated with benign appearing squamous epithelium in three. Psammoma bodies were evident in three cases. These neoplasms are thought to be of müllerian rather than mesonephric origin. Clear cell carcinomas constitute 5.5% of endometrial carcinomas and are generally seen in women with a mean age of 67 years.[18] The 5-year survival for white patients was 39%.[18] Crum and Fechner[26] found that the 3-and 5-year survivals for clear cell carcinomas were not worse than survival rates for ordinary adenocarcinomas of the same clinical stage, but that clear cell carcinomas in general presented with a higher clinical stage. They also noted that clear cell carcinomas were present in a greater proportion of black women, who had a worse prognosis than white patients, and that it was sometimes associated with a positive syphilis serology or a history of prior radiation exposure.

In *secretory adenocarcinoma*, the neoplastic glands are lined by cells with uniform subnuclear vacuolization, reminiscent of normal immediately postovulatory en-

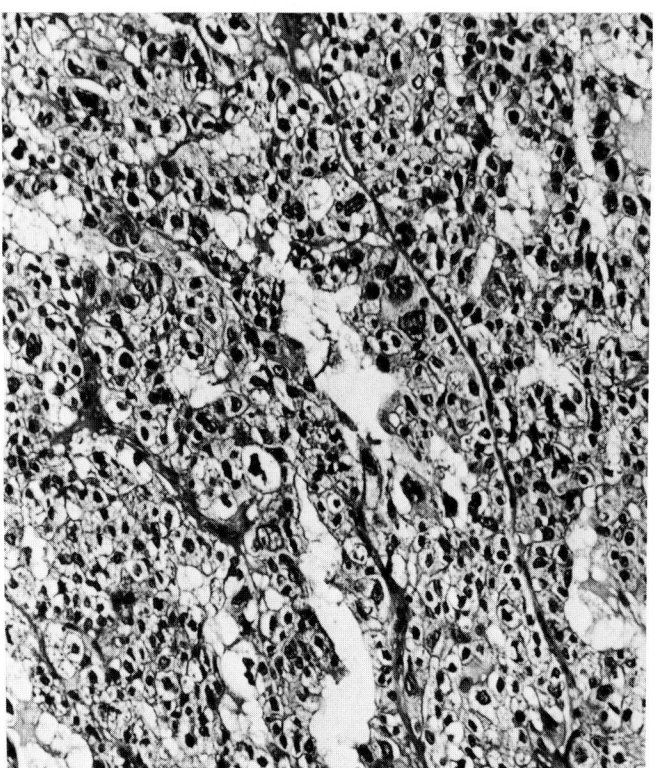

Fig. 48.13 Clear cell carcinoma of endometrium. In this neoplasm the cells are predominantly polygonal in form with clear cytoplasm. There is conspicuous variation in nuclear size and shape. (×150.)

dometrium (Fig. 48.14). In contrast to clear cell carcinoma, secretory carcinoma lacks significant cytologic atypia, its morphology may not be preserved in recurrences or metastases, and its prognosis is no worse than that of the usual endometrial adenocarcinoma.[18] Secretory adenocarcinoma is more often observed in premenopausal than in postmenopausal women, and it may coexist with normal endometrium exhibiting progesterone related changes. In women who have received progesterone therapy prior to biopsy, perinuclear vacuoles may be seen focally or diffusely in otherwise typical well differentiated endometrial adenocarcinomas.

HISTOLOGIC GRADE

Histologic grading of endometrial cancer provides important information about the malignant potential of the neoplasm. In some grading systems there are four grades, while in others, grades 3 and 4 are combined. With the latter approach the three grades are comparable to the FIGO subdivisions* of well differentiated (G1), moderately differentiated with partly solid areas (G2), and predominantly solid or entirely undifferentiated (G3) en-

---

* For new FIGO classification see p. 778

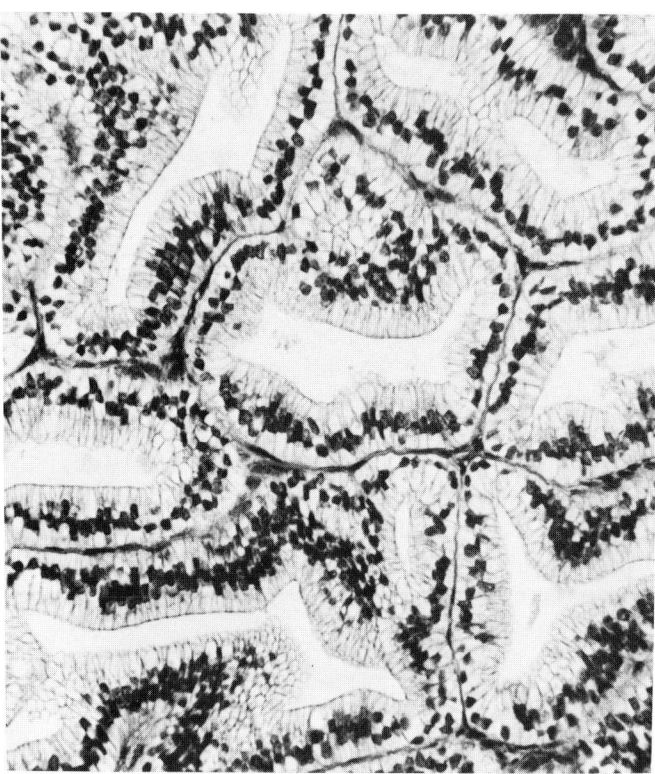

Fig. 48.14 Secretory adenocarcinoma of endometrium. Subnuclear vacuolization is prominent. Elsewhere there was normal secretory endometrium. (Courtesy of Dr William M. Christopherson). (×250.)

dometrial cancers. More specifically, by the FIGO grading method, Grade 1, highly differentiated carcinomas consist of 98% or more glandular or papillary formations; Grade 2, moderately differentiated adenocarcinomas consist of 20 to 50% solid areas; and grade 3 poorly differentiated or undifferentiated carcinomas are more than 50% or entirely solid in pattern.[73] The Pathology Committee of the Gynecologic Oncologic Group (GOG) defines Grade 1 well differentiated tumors as having less than 5% solid, non-glandular foci; Grade 2, moderately differentiated adenocarcinomas have from 5 to 50% solid areas; and Grade 3, poorly differentiated adenocarcinomas are composed architecturally of more than 50% solid sheets of tumor.[54] The World Health Organization[99] and others[18a,47,102] combine both architectural criteria and cytologic features, including mitotic activity and nuclear and nucleolar findings, for final grading. When graded by nuclear morphology alone, tumor cells having oval or elongated nuclei with evenly distributed chromatin, inconspicuous nucleoli, and few mitoses are classified as Grade 1 neoplasms. Tumors composed of cells with enlarged, irregular, rounded nuclei with prominent large, eosinophilic nucleoli and frequent mitoses are designated Grade 3. Grade 2 carcinomas have cytologic features intermediate between those in grades 1 and 3.[18a,20]

In the evaluation of the histologic grade of the glandular component of 615 endometrial cancers, 33.6% were considered Grade 1 (Fig. 48.3), 48.0% were Grade 2 (Fig. 48.4), 15.6% were Grade 3 and 2.8% were Grade 4.[102] In another series of 262 endometrial adenocarcinomas classified by FIGO criteria, 24.5% were Grade 1, 62.7% were Grade 2, and 12.8% were Grade 3.[33] Series including only Stage I endometrial carcinomas show a higher proportion of well differentiated cancers. Of 222 and 140 Stage I endometrial carcinomas from two studies, 41.9 and 46.4% were Grade 1, 39.6 and 35.7% were Grade 2, and 18.5 and 17.9% were Grade 3, respectively, by GOG criteria.[10,22]

IMMUNOHISTOCHEMICAL AND ULTRASTRUCTURAL STUDIES

The distinction between poorly differentiated glandular and squamous neoplasms may be difficult to make on routine histologic examination, because both grow in solid sheets or nests. Electronmicroscopy reveals specialized cell surfaces and cytoplasmic organelles allowing for the separation of different cell types. Cells of well differentiated adenocarcinoma maintain a columnar or cuboidal configuration and an orderly arrangement of the cytoplasmic organelles. More importantly, they form extracellular or intracytoplasmic luminal formations lined by microvilli. Less commonly, cilia and ciliary rootlets may be seen. Junctional complexes and desmosomal junctions are occasionally seen. The cytoplasmic organelles consist of profiles of rough endoplasmic reticulum, well developed Golgi membranes, vacuoles and scattered ribosomes. Mucinous vacuoles are rarely identified. Bundles of intermediate filaments with a thickness of 80–100 Angstroms may be present, but tonofilaments are scant or absent. In poorly differentiated glandular tumors, the cytoplasmic organelles are scant. Intercellular and intracytoplasmic lumens may be small, irregular, and slit-like (Fig. 48.15).

Squamous cells, on the other hand, have abundant tonofilaments and desmosomal junctions between neighboring cells, and lack glandular lumens (Fig. 48.16). In keratinizing cells, tonofilaments form coarse aggregates, sometimes with condensation into keratohyaline granules. Rough endoplasmic reticulum and Golgi apparatus are poorly developed and sparse. Pools of glycogen particles may be seen and usually correspond to the clear cytoplasm seen on light microscopy.

Clear cell adenocarcinoma is characterized by accumulations of glycogen particles and lipid droplets. Rough endoplasmic reticulum and Golgi membranes are abundant. In cells having granular cytoplasm, mitochondria are often more numerous than in the clear cells. Rhomboid, electron-dense, membrane-bound bodies with a crystalline appearance are sometimes observed. Microvilli are short, few in number, and irregularly spaced. These characteristics are unlike those seen in the clear cell variant of

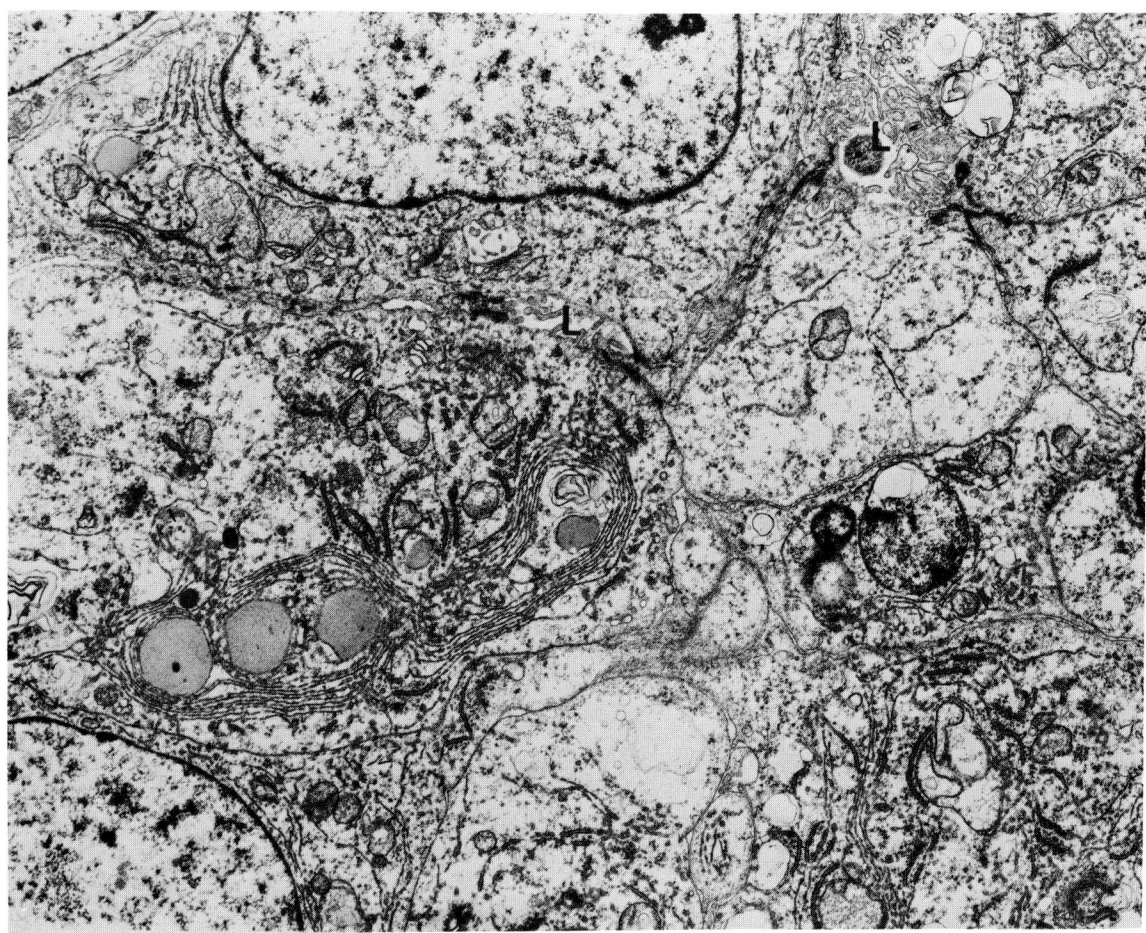

Fig. 48.15 Electronphotomicrograph of a poorly differentiated adenocarcinoma. Small inconspicuous lumens (L) lined by microvilli are seen. The remaining plasma membranes are closely apposed to each other and joined by a few desmosomes. Profiles of rough endoplasmic reticulum, some arranged in concentric whorls, are abundant. Other organelles are disorderly arranged. Tonofilaments are absent. (×7650.)

renal cell carcinoma, in which microvilli are tall and numerous.

Intermediate filaments seen in benign and malignant endometrial cells by electronmicroscopy correspond to vimentin and keratin by immunohistochemical studies. In addition, involucrin, detectable in the suprabasal layers of normal squamous epithelium, is a useful marker of squamous differentiation. It was identified in 57% of adeno-acanthomas and 87% of adenosquamous carcinomas.[127]

The distinction between endocervical and endometrial adenocarcinomas can usually be made by mucicarmine or PAS stains. A positive reaction is limited to the lumens and apical cell borders of endometrial cells, as compared to intracytoplasmic localization in endocervical cells. However, mucinous cells present in both neoplasms react positively with these stains.[48] In an early study by Wahlstrom et al,[125] 80% of endocervical adenocarcinomas and all adenosquamous carcinomas were reported to be positive for CEA. None of 122 endometrial adenocarcinomas, including clear cell adenocarcinomas, were positive for CEA.

In recent studies, although 87 to 100% of endocervical adenocarcinomas contain predominantly cytoplasmic CEA,[21,28] 52 to 72% of endometrial adenocarcinomas also react weakly with CEA; positivity is usually focal and extracellular, for example, at the cell surface and lumen.[21,28] Vimentin immunohistochemistry further aids in this differential diagnosis; whereas 65% of endometrial adenocarcinomas are reactive with anti-vimentin, endocervical adenocarcinomas are consistently nonreactive.[28] These studies suggest that PAS and mucicarmine positivity, CEA localization to cytoplasmic or surface sites, and anti-vimentin reactivity permit identification of the majority of endocervical and endometrial carcinomas.

MODE OF SPREAD

Myometrial invasion

In a study of 222 patients with Stage I endometrial cancer, tumor was confined to the endometrium in 41%, infiltrated

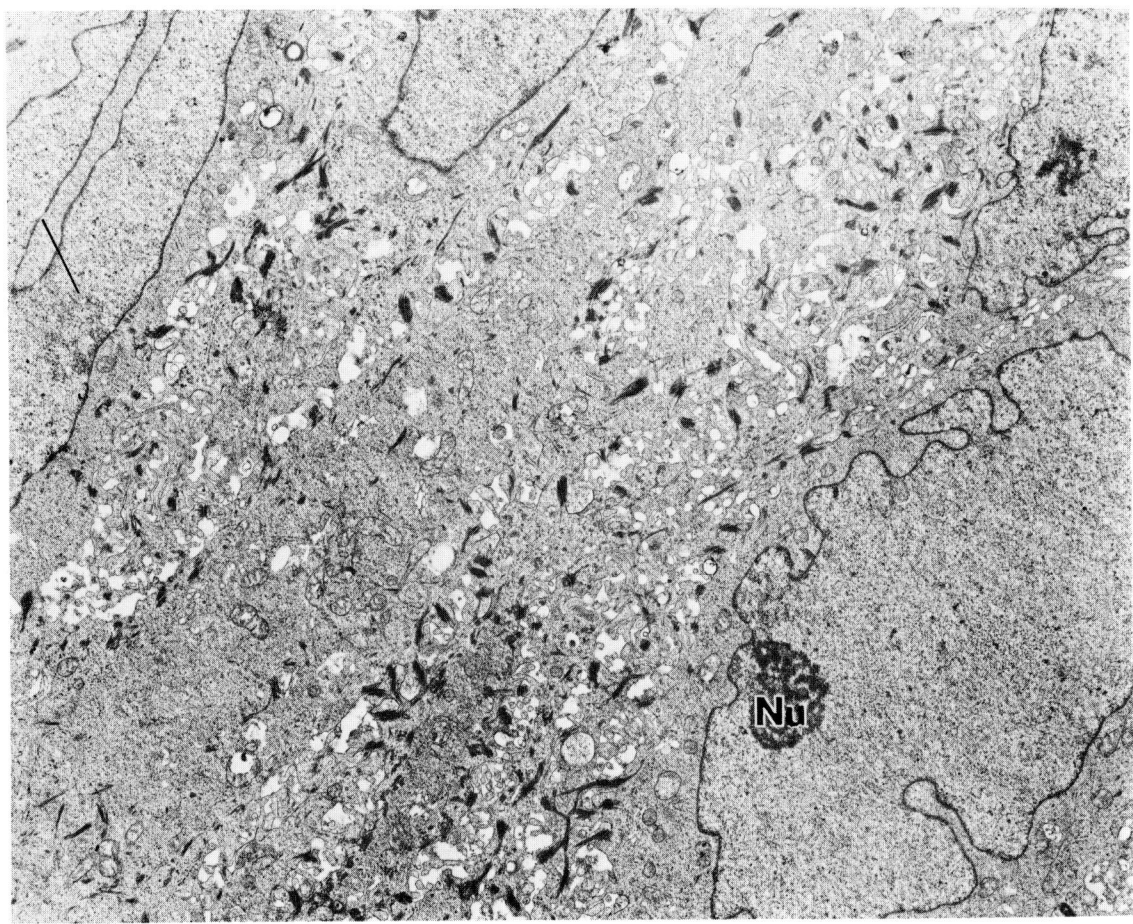

Fig. 48.16 Electronphotomicrograph of squamous component in an adenosquamous carcinoma. This area corresponds to spindle-shaped cells shown in Figure 48.11. The cells are joined by numerous desmosomes. Tonofilaments are abundant. Rough endoplasmic reticulum and Golgi membranes are few in number. Note convoluted nuclear envelope and nucleolus (Nu). (×7650.)

the upper third of the myometrium in 26%, extended into the middle third of the myometrium in 7.7%, and invaded the deeper third in 14.9%.[10] The extent of myometrial invasion correlates with tumor grade by GOG criteria. Of 93 Grade 1 cancers, 62% were confined to the endometrium; 27 or 77% of the remaining 35 invasive tumors were limited to the upper third of the myometrium. Of Grade 2 cancers, 24% (21/88) had infiltrated the middle or deeper thirds of the myometrium. Only 17% (7/41) of the Grade 3 cancers were non-invasive; 51% were myoinvasive beyond the upper third of the myometrium. 16 of the 33 cancers which invaded the outer third of the myometrium were Grade 3 neoplasms.[10]

Adenocarcinomatous invasion into the myometrium must be distinguished from carcinomatous extension into adenomyosis, since the latter finding carries the same prognosis as that of adenocarcinoma confined to the endometrium.[55,62] Carcinomatous foci of adenomyotic extension, which can occur below the upper third of myometrium, retain smooth, circumscribed outer borders.

The presence of residual benign endometrial glands or stroma in the periphery of these foci confirms pre-existing adenomyosis (Fig. 48.17). True myometrial invasion is characterized by irregular, angular borders associated with desmoplasia and chronic inflammation in the stroma (Fig. 48.18).

Lymphatic spread

Of 64 cases of endometrial cancer studied at autopsy, lymph node spread was present in only one of eight clinical Stage I cancers, in 10 of 18 Stage II cancers, and in all of the remaining 38 cases with advanced disease. In a review of the literature dealing with surgically treated cases, pelvic lymph node metastases were present in 10.6% of 369 clinical Stage I endometrial cancers and in 36.5% of 85 cases of clinical Stage II cancers.[10,22] Lymphography revealed node metastases in 8.9% of clinical Stage I, 28.6% of Stage II, 57.1% of Stage III, and 66.6% of Stage IV carcinomas.[91] In studies of Stage I endometrial carcinoma, the

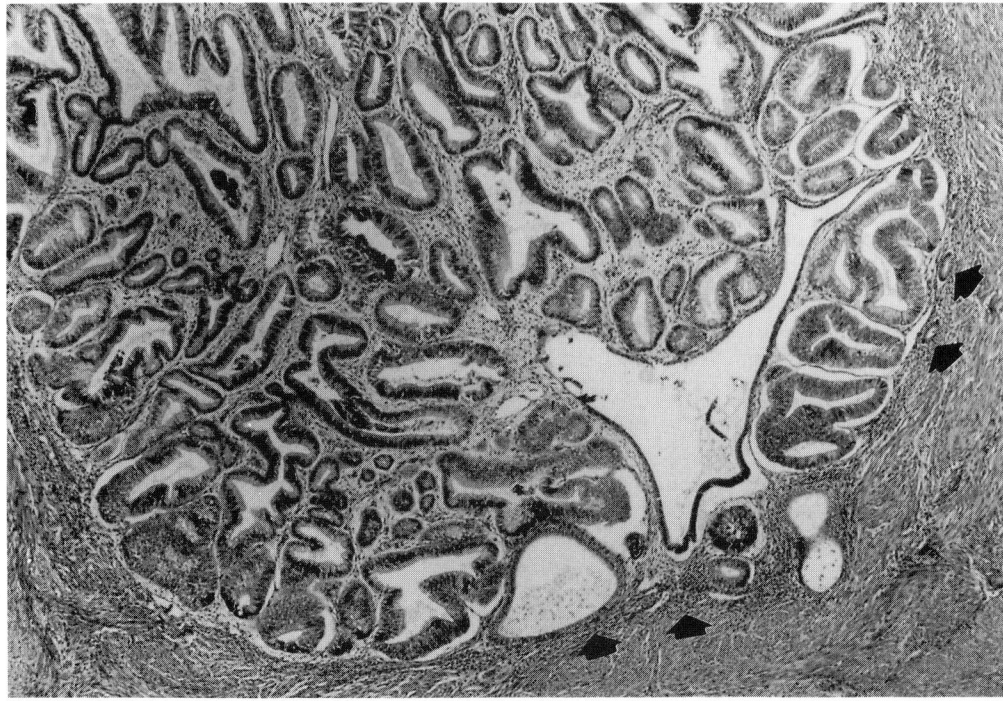

Fig. 48.17 Located in the middle third of myometrium, this represents carcinomatous extension of preexisting adenomyosis rather than myometrial invasion. The borders of this focus are smooth and regular. The normal myometrium shows no evidence of desmoplastic reaction. Benign endometrial glands and stroma (arrows) at the periphery further support this interpretation. (×150.)

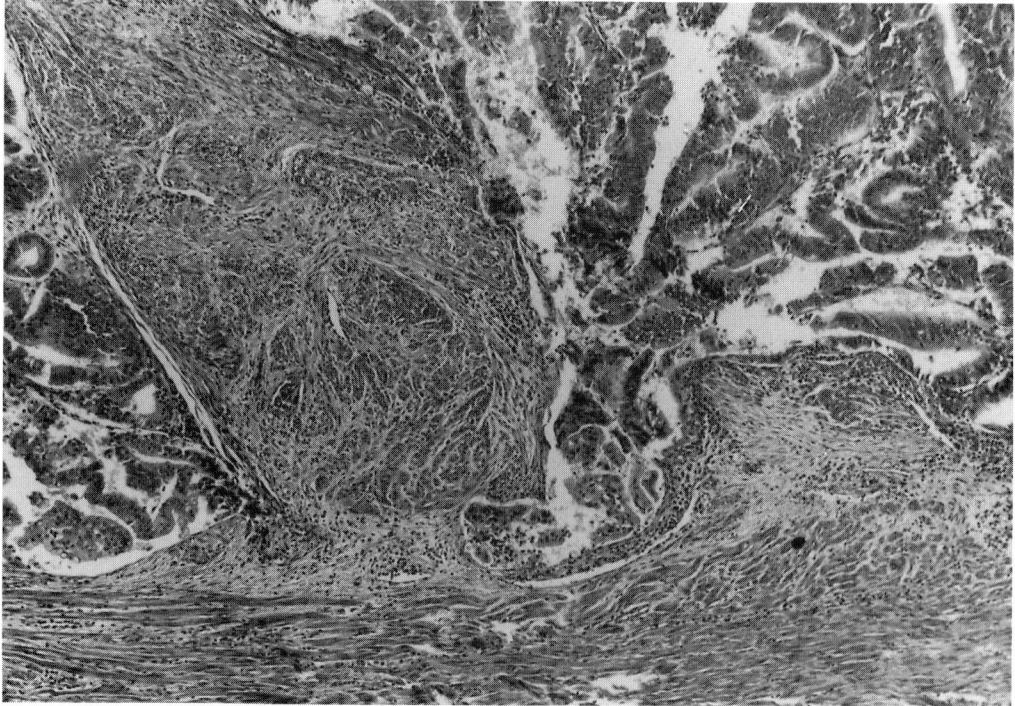

Fig. 48.18 In this true myometrial invasion, irregular, angulated glands are surrounded by a fibrotic, desmoplastic reaction and chronic inflammatory response. (×150).

incidence of positive pelvic nodes ranged from 10.4 to 11.4%, and of positive para-aortic nodes from 8.0 to 14.6%. [10,22,98]

Spread to lymph nodes has been correlated with various pathological features; advanced tumor grade and deeper myometrial invasion appear to be the most consistent indicators of potential lymph node involvement. By GOG grading criteria, pelvic lymph node metastasis was present in 2.2 to 3.1% of Grade 1 tumors, 10 to 11.4% of Grade 2, and 26.8 to 36.0% of Grade 3 tumors. [10,22] Para-aortic node metastasis was present in 0.0 to 1.5% of Grade 1 cancers, 4.0 to 13.6% of Grade 2, and 28.0 to 37.5% of Grade 3 tumors. [10,22,98] In reference to myometrial invasion, pelvic and para-aortic lymph nodes were involved in 3.6 and 1.8% of endometrial adenocarcinomas without myometrial invasion, respectively, and in 11.5 and 9.8% with superficial third, 10.0 and 0.0% with middle third, and 43.0 and 21.0% with outer third myometrial invasion, respectively. [22]

The presence of lymphatic-vascular invasion on histologic sections of the primary cancer was found to correlate with tumor grade and myoinvasion, as well as with tumor recurrence. It was observed in 2% of Grade 1, 25% of Grade 2, and 42% of Grade 3 carcinomas, and in 5% with inner third myometrial involvement, 24% with middle third myometrial invasion, and 70% with outer third invasion. [56] Recurrence of Stage I cancer increased from 2% without vascular invasion to 44% in the presence of this finding. [56]

Metastasis to lymph nodes has also been reported to correlate with tumor involvement of greater than one-third of the endometrial surface area, gross cervical involvement, uterine cavity length, [15] and tumor size greater than 2 cm. [108] Schink et al [108] noted nodal metastases in 9.3% of adenocarcinomas, 8.3% of adenoacanthomas, 28.6% of adenosquamous carcinomas, 35.7% of papillary carcinoma, and 75.0% of clear cell carcinoma.

Cervical involvement

There is considerable variation in the reported frequency of cervical involvement in endometrial cancer. Among 7561 women represented in 17 individual studies cited by Rutledge, [105] 881 or 11.6% had cervical involvement (clinical Stage II endometrial cancer). The frequency of involvement varied from 3 to 24% among the studies, and tended to be somewhat higher in the more recently reported studies as compared with those published in earlier years. While variations in the represented populations may in part explain this difference in frequency, it is more likely due to the lack of a standardized procedure for establishing the presence of cervical involvement. As discussed earlier, fractional curettage may be misleading, unless cancer is identified in continuity with recognizable cervical tissue (Fig. 48.19). Biopsy may confirm the presence of overt

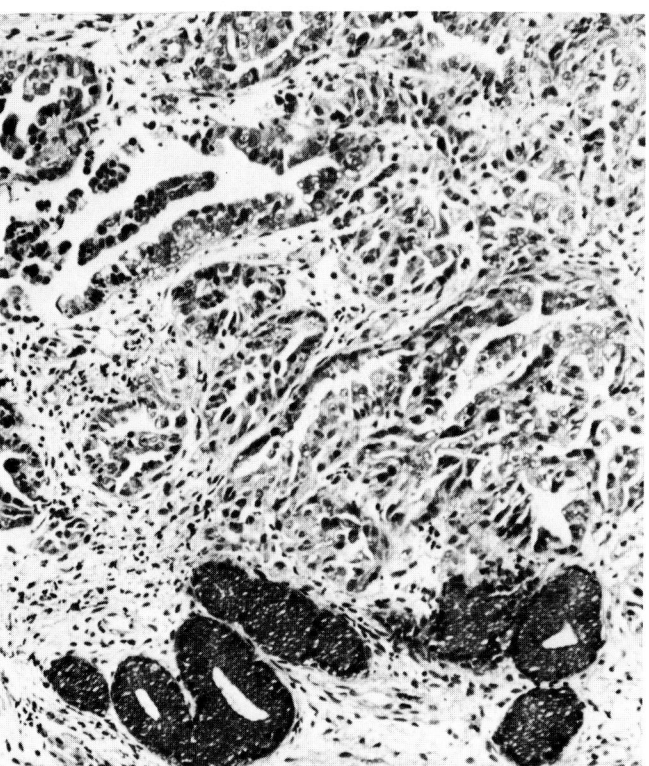

Fig. 48.19 Cervical involvement in endometrial cancer. In this PAS stained section the intracellular mucin contained within a normal endocervical gland appears black. Adjacent to the normal gland there is evidence of adenocarcinoma. (×150).

cancer but is less reliable in identifying occult involvement.

The preponderance of occult cervical spread was demonstrated in a report of 617 patients with endometrial cancer, in which 90 or 14.6% had cervical involvement. [63] Only 27% (24/90) of the cases with cervical involvement were detected prior to surgery. This represents only 3.9% of the patients with endometrial cancer. In the remaining 73% (66/90) of patients, cervical involvement was occult and detected only on histopathologic examination of the resected uterus. Similar results were reported by others. [94,128]

The malignant endometrial cells may reach uterine cervix by direct extension or by embolization via lymphatic vascular spaces. In Stage II tumors, direct extension seems to be the most common pathway. This is supported by the presence of tumor in the cervical mucosa in the majority of hysterectomy specimens, either with (69%) or without (26%) underlying stromal involvement; only 5% showed tumor infiltration of the cervix limited to the stroma. [8,45] On the other hand, Kadar et al [68] found tumor cells limited to the cervical stroma in 65%, in both the mucosa and the stroma in 22%, and in the cervical mucosa in 13% of uteri. A high frequency of cases without mucosal involvement led to the suggestion that tumor cells reach the cervix predominantly by lymphatic vascular spaces. However, radiotherapy administered prior to hysterectomy may have contributed to the lack of mucosal disease in some patients.

The prognostic value of ECC findings is controversial. When isolated endometrial tumor fragments without connection to normal endocervical tissue are found, the prognosis is found to be similar to that of Stage I carcinoma.[68,94] Only when the tumor is contiguous with cervical tissue is there a decrease in 5-year survival to 65%, suggesting that this finding is indicative of true cervical spread.[68] In the study by Larson et al,[77] 5-year survival rates were 65 to 70% for both those with gross cervical disease and for those with fragments of endometrial tumor in ECC with or without contiguity with cervical tissue.

Transtubal spread

Although pathologic involvement of the fallopian tube was found in 5% of Stage I carcinomas,[10] malignant cells were found in 21% (10/47) of tubal aspirates obtained prior to any manipulation of the uterus from women undergoing hysterectomy.[88] This positive finding apparently did not correlate with tumor size, histologic grade, clinical stage or prognosis. Of the four women who had positive peritoneal cytology, only one had concurrent positive tubal cytology. Thus, transtubal passage of tumor cells to peritoneal cavity, although common, does not necessarily result in detectable viable tumor cells in the peritoneal fluid or in abdominal tumor implants.[88] A positive peritoneal cytology, on the other hand, is a poor prognostic indicator in this[88] and other studies.[57,121]

Pelvic spread

Of 222 cases of Stage I endometrial carcinoma, 4.5% had ovarian spread, 0.9% had pelvic implants, 1.8% had extrapelvic implants, and 13.5% had positive or suspicious peritoneal washings.[10] In another study, pelvic implants and positive pelvic washings were reported in 4.3 and 8.5% respectively of 94 endometrial cancers.[15]

Simultaneous involvement of the endometrium and the ovary by carcinoma occurs uncommonly. 16 patients with endometrioid carcinoma in both sites, including one with myometrial invasion in the uterine corpus, were found to have an excellent prognosis. There were no deaths and only one successfully treated vaginal relapse, suggesting that these represented cases of separate primary tumors rather than advanced stage endometrial or ovarian carcinoma.[40]

RELATION OF PATHOLOGIC FINDINGS TO SURVIVAL

Several different factors which can be assessed by the pathologist are known to have a bearing on the survival of women with endometrial cancer (Table 48.1). Of these, the most important is the extent of the disease at the time of detection. In a series of 404 women with endometrial cancer of all stages treated by radiation and surgery the 5-year survival was 82% when the neoplasm was confined to the endometrium, 69% with infiltration of the inner one-half of the myometrium, 31% with involvement of the outer one-half of the myometrium and only 7% with extrauterine involvement.[47] Survival and relapse rates similarly related to the extent of myometrial invasion are reported by others.[10,11,20,33,35,60]

The differentiation of the neoplasm can also be correlated with the 5-year survival. In women treated by radiotherapy and surgery the 5-year survival was 85% for Grade 1 neoplasms, 67% for Grade 2 neoplasms, 24% for Grade 3 cancers and 15% for Grade 4 cancers. If Grades 3 and 4 are combined, the 5-year survival is 23%.[47] Similar findings are reported in other studies.[10,11,20,33,35,81] Christopherson et al[20] and Mittal et al[89] found nuclear grading to be a more accurate prognosticator than either FIGO grading, based on architecture alone, or the grading by architecture and nuclear morphology used by WHO.[99]

Tumor type may also bear an important relationship to

Table 48.1 Prognostic variables in Stage I endometrial carcinoma

	5-year survival (a)	(b)	Recurrences (c)
Grade			
Grade 1	93.2%	98.2%	4.0%
Grade 2	76.2%	95.2%	15.0%
Grade 3	61.5%	79.2%	42.0%
Myoinvasion			
Endometrium only	100.0%	97.2%	8.0%
Superficial third	88.2%	96.4%	13.0%
Middle third	80.0%	90.5%	12.0%
Outer third	60.0%	100.0%	46.0%
Pelvic nodes			
negative			11.0%
positive			57.0%
Para-aortic nodes			
negative			11.0%
positive			59.0%
Histologic type			
Adenocarcinoma	79.8%		
Adenoacanthoma	87.5%		
Adenosquamous carcinoma	53.1%		
Papillary carcinoma	69.7%		
Clear cell carcinoma	44.2%		
Estrogen receptors		(d) 2-year survival	
negative		67.0%	
positive		90.0%	

(a) Christopherson, 1983[20]
(b) DePalo, 1982[33]
(c) DiSaia, 1985[35]
(d) Creasman, 1985[24]

survival. Usually endometrial adenocarcinoma, mucinous carcinoma, and secretory carcinoma have similar prognoses, while poor prognosis variants include papillary serous carcinoma and clear cell carcinoma. Christopherson et al[18a] reported 5-year survival rates of 75.2% for adenocarcinoma, 87% for adenoacanthoma, 47.5% for adenosquamous carcinoma, 51.1% for papillary carcinoma and 35.2% for clear cell carcinoma. Crum and Fechner[26] noted a 53% 5-year survival for clear cell carcinoma compared to 63% for other types. Hendrickson et al[61] emphasized the 50% relapse rate of uterine papillary serous carcinomas, compared to 5% for ordinary Stage I adenocarcinomas.

Several studies have shown a poorer prognosis for adenosquamous carcinoma than for adenocarcinoma or adenoacanthoma. At the University Hospitals of Cleveland the overall 5-year survival for women with endometrial adenocarcinoma was 72%, for women with adenoacanthoma 68%, and for women with adenosquamous cancer 26%.[47] Boutselis[11] reported a 24.3% survival for adenosquamous cancer of the endometrium and in the cases reviewed by Silverberg et al[114] the 5-year survival was 35.3%. Alberhasky et al[2] reported a 5-year survival for adenosquamous carcinoma of 46.7% compared to 87.0% for adenoacanthomas. Demopoulos et al[32] reported 5-year survivals of 54.7% for adenosquamous carcinoma, 70.5% for adenocarcinoma, and 87.4% for adenoacanthoma. Silverberg[114] suggested that the poor prognosis of adenosquamous carcinoma was related to the high grade and poor differentiation of its associated adenocarcinoma. In support of this argument, Salazar et al[107] found no differences in incidence, clinical history, or 5-year survivals for adenoacanthoma, adenocarcinoma or adenosquamous carcinomas of the same grade. Nevertheless, several studies indicate a poorer prognosis for adenosquamous carcinoma independent of tumor grade.[32,47] Other factors that lead to a less favorable prognosis compared to adenocarcinoma include the deeper myometrial invasion, more advanced stage, and more frequent vascular invasion in adenosquamous cancers.[32]

Recurrence rates for carcinomas are dependent on extrauterine spread; 43% recurrence is noted with, and 7% recurrence without, extrauterine spread.[35] Pelvic and para-aortic lymph node involvement reflects a more advanced stage of disease. While 5-year survival for endometrial carcinoma is extremely favorable without lymph node involvement, metastases to lymph nodes portend a poor prognosis.[10,35,85,90] In one study, when pelvic nodes were involved, the tumor recurrence rate was 57%, compared to 11% recurrence when pelvic nodes were uninvolved.[35] Recurrence rates with and without para-aortic node metastases were 59 and 11%.[35]

Pelvic extension also indicates advanced disease. The significance of positive pelvic washings was studied by Szpak et al[121] in 54 women with Stage I endometrial adenocarcinoma. None of the 42 patients with negative washings developed a recurrence after a median disease-free survival of 36 months. Of the 12 patients with malignant cells, four had a high concentration (>1000 cells/100 ml sample) and all four died within 2 years. The remaining eight had lower concentrations; six of these patients had no evidence of disease after 37 to 64 months. Positive pelvic washings were predictive of a higher likelihood of recurrence, and a high cell concentration portended a worse prognosis.

In the study of Harouny et al,[57] malignant pelvic washings were detected in 17, 20, 69, and 86% of women with Stage I, II, III, and IV disease, respectively. Among patients with Stage I disease, malignant cytology was associated with higher grade, deeper myometrial invasion, and adnexal spread. Tumor recurred in 29% (12/41) with positive cytology, but in only 3% (6/207) with negative cytology.

SPECIALIZED TECHNIQUES

Recent studies of endometrial cancers have utilized cytometry for nuclear DNA quantitation and various assays for the measurement of steroid hormone receptor protein levels. These analyses can further improve the prognostic accuracy achieved by regular clinical and pathologic examinations. Of particular promise are the new techniques that make it possible to perform DNA ploidy analysis and steroid hormone receptor assessment in paraffin-embedded tissue. (See also Chs 6 and 8.)

Chromosomal karyotyping and nuclear DNA studies

Previous studies of endometrial cancer by chromosome karyotyping have demonstrated diploid or near-diploid chromosome counts in a majority of the cases.[5,50,119] Less frequently the chromosome number is higher.[5,119] In a review of the literature, 69% of endometrial cancers studied by karyotyping were diploid and 31% aneuploid.[66] A slightly higher frequency of endometrial cancers (73%) is reported to be diploid when ploidy is assessed by flow cytometry on single cells prepared from fresh tissue.[67] This finding is not unexpected, however, because of the difficulty in detecting minor chromosome abnormalities by flow cytometry.

The DNA ploidy patterns correlate with histologic grade. Aneuploid patterns were found in 10, 31, and 78% of Grade 1, 2, and 3 tumors, respectively.[67] There was no relation to clinical stage, depth of myometrial invasion, or patient age. Patients with aneuploid tumors had a higher tumor recurrence rate, shorter disease-free period, and shorter survival compared to those with diploid tumors.[67] In the diploid group, there was 11% (4/38) mortality, as compared to 50% (7/14) in the aneuploid group. Among the patients who died, the length of median survival was 27.5 and 17 months for the diploid and aneuploid groups, respectively.[67] The majority of adenosquamous carcinomas of the endometrium are aneuploid.[5] This is another poor prognostic indicator associated with this neoplasm.

Others have found the sum of the S and G2 phase cells, which represent the proliferating population, to be of prognostic value.[49] A favorable outcome is associated with a low proliferative fraction. Essentially, DNA ploidy analysis by flow or static cytometry identifies a subset of endometrial tumors with aneuploidy, high proliferative activity, and aggressive behavior. It is also suitable for the detection of malignant aneuploid cells in pelvic washings and other specimens.

Steroid hormone receptors

Estrogen and progesterone receptors have been demonstrated in cytosol preparations from normal, hyperplastic, and carcinomatous endometria.[38] Progesterone administration reduces the levels of estrogen and progesterone receptors.[83] This finding may provide an explanation for the anti-proliferative effect of progestins in normal endometrium and in endometrial cancers. By biochemical assay, two-thirds of endometrial carcinomas are estrogen receptor positive, with levels comparable to or lower than those in proliferative endometrium.[23] Many, but not all, authors have found a correlation between hormone receptor levels and tumor grade (see also Ch. 8).[14,39,49,86]

Increased length of survival has been correlated with biochemical estrogen and progesterone receptor positivity, independent of histologic grade and myometrial invasion.[82] Creasman et al[24] reported a 2-year disease-free survival of 90% for estrogen receptor positive and of 67% for estrogen receptor negative patients with endometrial adenocarcinoma. In a biochemical assay study of 175 endometrial carcinomas by Ehrlich et al,[39] progesterone receptor positivity correlated with tumor grade, histology, adenexal spread, age, and recurrence; 7% (4/57) of progesterone receptor positive tumors recurred, compared to 37% (16/43) recurrence in progesterone receptor negative tumors. Progesterone receptor status also correlated significantly with response to progestin therapy and survival. Similarly, estrogen receptor positivity correlated with decreased recurrence; there was 12.7% and 41.2% recurrence with estrogen receptor positive and negative tumors, respectively. No correlation between estrogen receptor status and response to progestin therapy or survival was observed.[39] In another study of 74 patients evaluated for estrogen and progesterone receptors, there was a 92% concordance between their presence and a clinical response to progestin therapy.[23]

Biochemical assay of endometrial tissue for estrogen and progesterone receptors has several drawbacks. The sample may not contain an adequate amount of neoplastic tissue or may be non-representative, because of the presence of normal endometrium and myometrium which also contain receptors. In a review of 100 endometrial specimens submitted for steroid receptor analysis, non-malignant epithelium accounted for the majority of specimens in 20%; 5% of cases contained cancer only.[118] Even within tumors, receptors are heterogeneous in distribution.[131] With the development of monoclonal anti-estrophilin (estrogen receptor) antibodies,[51] immunohistochemical studies can now be performed on fresh or paraffin-embedded tissue. This minimizes the sampling problems mentioned above.

By immunohistochemistry on fresh frozen tissue, decreased epithelial estrogen receptor staining has been reported in Grade 3 tumors compared to Grades 1 and 2.[7] Budwit-Novotny et al[12] found that 92% (34/37) of Grade 1, 62% (23/37) of Grade 2, and 12% (3/26) of Grade 3 cancers were estrogen receptor positive, proportions comparable to estrogen receptor positivity determined by biochemical assay. It is now possible to visualize estrogen receptors in paraffin-embedded tissue sections (Fig. 48.20).[17,64] False positives that may occur in biochemical assays due to inadvertent inclusion of adjacent normal endometrium or myometrium can be avoided, since estrogen receptors can be localized to cancer cells.

ENDOMETRIAL CANCER IN WOMEN UNDER 40 YEARS OF AGE

Endometrial cancer in women under 40 years of age is estimated to account for less than 3% of all endometrial cancers.[116] Patients with polycystic ovaries, obesity, anovulation, or ovarian tumors (functional or nonfunctional) are believed to have a higher risk for developing endometrial cancer.[42,112] Of 137 women under 40 years of age with endometrial cancer reported by Silverberg,[116] 52% were nulliparous, 54% were obese, and 48% had polycystic ovaries. Diabetes and hypertension were uncommon.

Endometrial cancers have been observed in women who are long-term users of oral contraceptive agents or of exogenous estrogen for gonadal dysgenesis.[80,87,115,116] Of 29 long term users of contraceptive agents who developed endometrial carcinoma; 20 were on sequential agents and 9 were on combined agents. Secretory carcinoma occurred more frequently in this group than in the non-contraceptive users.[116] Overall, the prognosis of young women with endometrial carcinoma is excellent. In the majority of the reported cases, there was no residual tumor in the excised uterus or tumor was confined to the endometrium. Myometrial invasion was infrequent. Only a few patients, all among the small group with a poorly differentiated cancer and myometrial invasion, died of the disease.

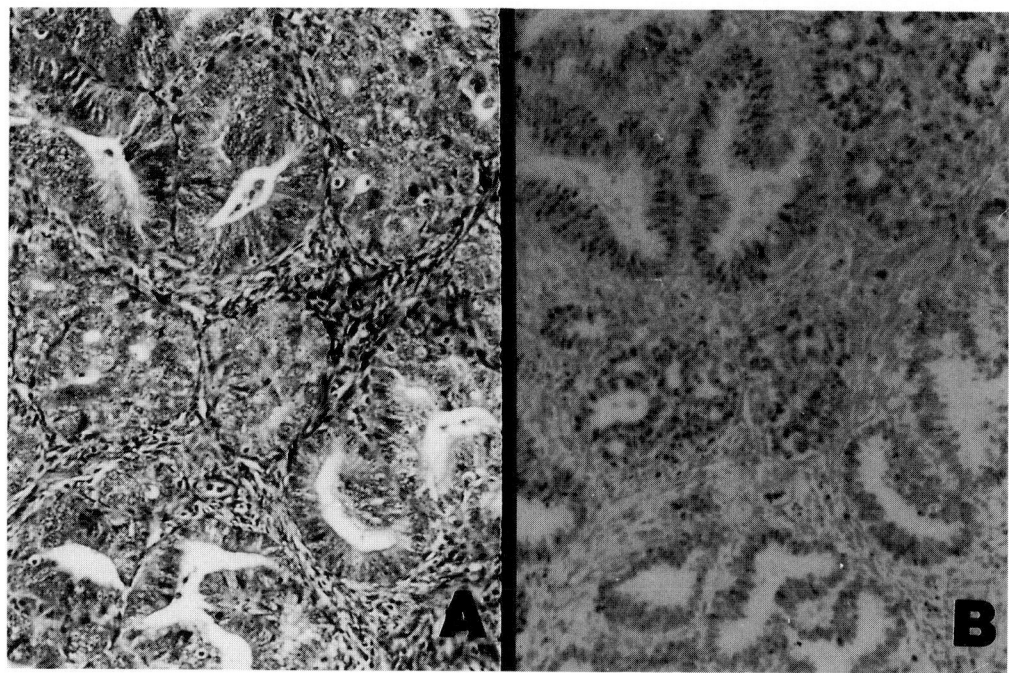

Fig. 48.20 A. Grade 1 adenocarcinoma. B. A parallel section of Figure 48.20A is stained immunohistochemically with a monoclonal antibody for estrogen receptor proteins. Estrogen receptor proteins are localized in the nuclei of epithelial cells but not in the fibroblasts in the stroma. (A. & B. ×150)

Fechner & Kaufman[42] reviewed 47 cases of endometrial cancer in women with Stein-Leventhal syndrome from the literature and added 4 cases of their own. The age of the patients varied from 16 to 40 years. All but four had well-differentiated endometrial cancers. None of the patients with well differentiated tumors developed recurrence or metastasis following hysterectomy. A small number of patients were cured following endometrial curettage, induction of ovulation after wedge resection of the ovaries, or institution of clomiphene therapy. As expected, poorly differentiated carcinomas had a poorer prognosis.[42]

In Crissman et al's series[25] of 32 patients 40 years of age or younger, none had Stein-Leventhal syndrome, none were on sequential oral contraceptives, 37.5% were obese, 37.5% were nulligravid, and 25% were hypertensive. 19% (6/32) had coexisting ovarian malignant neoplasms. A careful adnexal examination at the time of clinical staging was recommended. It was noted that many cases of hyperplasia had been misdiagnosed as carcinoma.[25]

Of 10 women under 25 years of age with endometrial cancer, 7 had the clinical features of Stein-Leventhal syndrome.[41] Nine tumors (6 adenoacanthomas and 3 adenocarcinomas) were well differentiated and confined to the endometrium. The remaining case was a moderately differentiated adenosquamous carcinoma, without myometrial invasion, but with metastatic carcinoma in one ovary and in the pelvic wall. This may have represented multiple synchronous primary tumors. At the time of report, two patients were lost to follow-up; the remaining 8 patients were alive and well 3 months to 10 years following therapy (see also Ch. 8).[41]

REFERENCES

1. Aguirre P, Scully R E, Wolfe H J, DeLellis R A 1984 Endometrial carcinoma with argyrophil cells: a histochemical and immunohistochemical analysis. Hum Pathol 15: 210
2. Alberhasky R C, Connelly P J, Christopherson W M 1982 Carcinoma of the endometrium. IV. Mixed adenosquamous carcinoma. A clinical-pathological study of 68 cases with long-term follow-up. Am J Clin Pathol 77: 655
3. Anderson B, Louis F, Watring W G, Edinger D D 1980 Growth patterns in endometrial carcinoma. Gynecol Oncol 10: 134
4. An-Foraker S H, Kawada C Y, McKinney D 1979 Endometrial aspiration studies on Isaacs cell sampler with cytohistologic correlation. Acta Cytol 23: 303
5. Atkin N B 1976 Prognostic significance of ploidy level in human tumors. I. Carcinoma of the uterus. J Natl Cancer Inst 56: 909
6. Bannatyne P, Russell P, Wills E J 1983 Argyrophilia and endometrial carcinoma. Int J Gynecol Pathol 2: 235
7. Bergeron C, Ferenczy A, Shyamala G 1988 Distribution of estrogen receptors in various cell types of normal, hyperplastic, and neoplastic human endometrial tissues. Lab Invest 58: 338
8. Bigelow B, Vekshtein V, Demopoulos R I 1983 Endometrial carcinoma, Stage II: route and extent of spread to the cervix. Obstet Gynecol 62: 363

9. Bokhman J V 1983 Two pathogenetic types of endometrial carcinoma. Gynecol Oncol 15: 10

10. Boronow R C, Morrow C P, Creasman W T et al 1984 Surgical staging in endometrial cancer: clinical-pathologic findings of a prospective study. Obstet Gynecol 63: 825

11. Boutselis J G 1978 Endometrial carcinoma. Prognostic factors and treatment. Surg Clin N Am 58: 109

12. Budwit-Novotny D A, McCarty Sr K S, Cox E B et al 1986 Immunohistochemical analyses of estrogen receptor in endometrial adenocarcinoma using a monoclonal antibody. Cancer Res 46: 5419

13. Chambers J T, Merino M, Kohorn E I, Peschel R E, Schwartz P E 1987 Uterine papillary serous carcinoma. Obstet Gynecol 69: 109

14. Chambers J T 1988 Sex steroid receptors in endometrial cancer. Yale J Biol and Med 61: 339

15. Chen S S 1985 Extrauterine spread in endometrial carcinoma clinically confined to the uterus. Gynecol Oncol 21: 23

16. Chen S S, Lee L 1986 Reappraisal of endocervical curettage in predicting cervical involvement by endometrial carcinoma. J Reprod Med 31: 50

17. Cheng L, Binder S W, Fu Y S, Lewin K J 1988 Methods in laboratory investigation. Demonstration of estrogen receptors by monoclonal antibody in formalin-fixed breast tumors. Lab Invest 58: 346

18. Christopherson W M, Alberhasky R C, Connelly P J 1982 Carcinoma of the endometrium. I. A clinicopathologic study of clear-cell carcinoma and secretory carcinoma. Cancer 49: 1511

18a. Christopherson W M, Alberhasky R C, Connelly P J 1982 Carcinoma of the endometrium. II. Papillary adenocarcinoma: A clinical pathological study of 46 cases. Am J Clin Pathol 77: 534

19. Christopherson W M, Alberhasky R C, Connelly P J 1982 Glassy cell carcinoma of the endometrium. Hum Pathol 13: 418

20. Christopherson W M, Connelly P J, Alberhasky R C 1983 Carcinoma of the endometrium. V. An analysis of prognosticators in patients with favorable subtypes and Stage I disease. Cancer 51: 1705

21. Cohen C, Shulman G, Budgeon L R 1982 Endocervical and endometrial adenocarcinoma. An immunoperoxidase and histochemical study. Am J Surg Pathol 6: 151

22. Creasman W T, Boronow R C, Morrow C P, DiSaia P J, Blessing J 1976 Adenocarcinoma of the endometrium: its metastatic lymph node potential. A preliminary report. Gynecol Oncol 4: 239

23. Creasman W T, McCarty K S Sr, Barton T K, McCarty K S Jr 1980 Clinical correlates of estrogen- and progesterone-binding proteins in human endometrial adenocarcinoma. Obstet Gynecol 55: 363

24. Creasman W T, Soper J T, McCarty K S Jr, McCarty K S Sr, Hinshaw W, Clarke-Pearson D L 1985 Influence of cytoplasmic steroid receptor content on prognosis of early stage endometrial carcinoma. Am J Obstet Gynecol 151: 922

25. Crissman J D, Azoury R S, Barnes A E, Schellhas H F 1981 Endometrial carcinoma in women 40 years of age or younger. Obstet Gynecol 57: 699

26. Crum C P, Fechner R E 1976 Clear cell adenocarcinoma of the endometrium. A clinicopathologic study of 11 cases. Am J Diag Gynecol Obstet 1: 261

27. Czernobilsky B, Katz Z, Lancet M Gaton J 1980 Endocervical-type epithelium in endometrial carcinoma. Am J Surg Pathol 4: 481

28. Dabbs D J, Geisinger K R, Norris H T 1986 Intermediate filaments in endometrial and endocervical carcinomas. The diagnostic utility of vimentin patterns. Am J Surg Pathol 10: 568

29. Daniel A G, Peters W A III 1988 Accuracy of office and operating room curettage in the grading of endometrial carcinoma. Obstet Gynecol 71: 612

30. Dawagne M P, Silverberg S G 1982 Foam cells in endometrial carcinoma — a clinicopathologic study. Gynecol Oncol 13: 67

31. Deligdisch L, Cohen C J 1985 Histologic correlates and virulence implications of endometrial carcinoma associated with adenomatous hyperplasia. Cancer 56: 1452

32. Demopoulos R I, Dubin N, Noumoff J, Blaustein A, Sommers G M 1986 Prognostic significance of squamous differentiation in Stage I endometrial adenocarcinoma. Obstet Gynecol 68: 245

33. DePalo G, Kenda R, Andreola S, Luciani L, Musumeci R, Rilke F 1982 Endometrial carcinoma: Stage I. A retrospective analysis of 262 patients. Obstet Gynecol 60: 225

34. Devesa S S, Silverman D T, Young J L Jr et al 1987 Cancer incidence and mortality trends among whites in the United States, 1947–84. J Natl Cancer Inst 79: 701

35. DiSaia P J, Creasman W T, Boronow R C, Blessing J A 1985 Risk factors and recurrent patterns in Stage I endometrial cancer. Am J Obstet Gynecol 151: 1009

36. Dunn J E 1974 Geographic considerations of endometrial cancer. Gynecol Oncol 2: 114

37. Dutra F R 1959 Intraglandular morules of the endometrium. Am J Clin Pathol 31: 60

38. Ehrlich C E, Young P C M, Cleary R E 1981 Cytoplasmic progesterone and estradiol receptors in normal, hyperplastic, and carcinomatous endometria: therapeutic implications. Am J Obstet Gynecol 141: 539

39. Ehrlich C E, Young P C M, Stehman F B, Sutton G P, Alford W M 1988 Steroid receptors and clinical outcome in patients with adenocarcinoma of the endometrium. Am J Obstet Gynecol 158: 796

40. Eifel P, Hendrickson M, Ross J, Ballon S, Martinez A, Kempson R 1982 Simultaneous presentation of carcinoma involving the ovary and the uterine corpus. Cancer 50: 163

41. Farhi D C, Nosanchuk J, Silverberg S G 1986 Endometrial adenocarcinoma in women under 25 years of age. Obstet Gynecol 68: 741

42. Fechner R F, Kaufman R H 1974 Endometrial adenocarcinoma in Stein-Leventhal syndrome. Cancer 34: 444

43. Ferenczy A, Gelfand M M 1984 Outpatient endometrial sampling with Endocyte: Comparative study of its effectiveness with endometrial biopsy. Obstet Gynecol 63: 295

44. Fluhmann C F 1928 Squamous epithelium in the endometrium in benign and malignant conditions. Surg Gynecol Obstet 46: 309

45. Frauenhoffer E E, Zaino R J, Wolff T V, Whitney C E 1987 Value of endocervical curettage in the staging of endometrial carcinoma. Int J Gynecol Pathol 6: 195

46. Fu Y S, Ferenczy A, Huang I, Gelfand M M 1988 Digital imaging analysis of normal, hyperplastic and malignant endometrial cells in endometrial brushing samples. Anal Quant Cytol Histol 10: 139

47. Fu Y S, Parks P J, Reagan J W, Wentz W B, Storaasli J P 1979 The ultrastructure and factors relating to survival of endometrial cancers. Am J Diag Gynecol Obstet 1: 55

48. Fu Y S, Reagan J W 1989 Pathology of the Uterine Cervix, Vagina and Vulva. Saunders, Philadelphia

49. Geisinger K R, Homesley H D, Morgan T M, Kute T E, Marshall R B 1986 Endometrial adenocarcinoma. A multiparameter clinicopathologic analysis including the DNA profile and the sex steroid hormone receptors. Cancer 58: 1518

50. Granberg I, Gupta S, Joelsson I, Sprenger E 1974 Chromosome and nuclear DNA study of a uterine adenocarcinoma and its metastases. Acta Pathol Microbiol Scand, [A] 82: 1

51. Greene G L, Nolan C, Engler J P, Jensen E V 1980 Monoclonal antibodies to human estrogen receptor. Proc Natl Acad Sci USA 77: 5115

52. Gusberg S B 1976 The individual at risk for endometrial carcinoma. Am J Obstet Gynecol 126: 535

53. Gusberg S B, Milano C 1981 Detection of endometrial cancer and its precursors. Cancer 47: 1173

54. Gynecologic Oncology Group, Pathology Manual, Philadelphia, Pa

55. Hall J B, Young R H, Nelson J H 1982 The prognostic significance of adenomyosis in endometrial carcinoma. Gynecol Oncol 17: 32

56. Hanson M B, van Nagell J R, Powell D E et al 1985 The prognostic significance of lymph-vascular space invasion in stage I endometrial cancer. Cancer 55: 1753

57. Harouny V R, Sutton G P, Clark S A, Geisler H E, Stehman F B Ehrlich C E 1988 The importance of peritoneal cytology in endometrial carcinoma. Obstet Gynecol 72: 394

58. Hausman D H, Roitman H B 1962 A malignant melanotic tumor of the uterus. Bull Ayer Clin Lab 4: 79

59. Hendrickson M R, Kempson R L 1983 Ciliated carcinoma — a

variant of endometrial adenocarcinoma: a report of 10 cases. Int J Gynecol Pathol 2: 1

60. Hendrickson M, Ross J, Eifel P J, Cox R S, Martinez A, Kempson R 1982 Adenocarcinoma of the endometrium: analysis of 256 cases with carcinoma limited to the uterine corpus. Gynecol Oncol 13: 373

61. Hendrickson M, Ross J, Eifel P, Martinez A, Kempson R 1982 Uterine papillary serous carcinoma. A highly malignant form of endometrial adenocarcinoma. Am J Surg Pathol 6: 93

62. Hernandez E, Woodruff J D 1980 Endometrial adenocarcinoma arising in adenomyosis. Am J Obstet Gynecol 138: 827

63. Homesley H D, Boronow R C, Lewis J L Jr 1977 Stage II endometrial adenocarcinoma. Memorial Hospital for Cancer 1949–1965. Obstet Gynecol 49: 604

64. Huang S J, Cheng L, Lewin K J, Fu Y S 1989 Immunohistochemical estrogen receptor assessment in normal and abnormal formalin fixed endometria. Submitted for publication

65. Inoue M, Ueda G, Yamasaki M et al 1982 Capacity for amine precursor uptake and decarboxylation of argyrophil cell adenocarcinoma of the endometrium. Gynecol Oncol 13: 19

66. Iversen O E, Laerum O D 1985 Ploidy disturbances in endometrial and ovarian carcinomas. A review. Anal Quant Cytol Histol 7: 327

67. Iversen O E 1986 Flow cytometric deoxyribonucleic acid index: A prognostic factor in endometrial carcinoma. Am J Obstet Gynecol 155: 770

68. Kadar N R D, Kohorn E I, LiVolsi V A, Kapp D S 1982 Histologic variants of cervical involvement by endometrial carcinoma. Obstet Gynecol 59: 85

69. Kanbour A I, Stock R J 1978 Squamous cell carcinoma in situ of endometrium and fallopian tube as superficial extension of invasive cervical carcinoma. Cancer 42: 570

70. Kay S 1974 Squamous cell carcinoma of the endometrium. Am J Clin Pathol 61: 264

71. King A, Seraj I M, Wagner R J 1984 Stromal invasion in endometrial adenocarcinoma. Am J Obstet Gynecol 149: 10

72. Koss L G, Schreiber K, Oberlander S G, Moussouris H F, Lesser M 1984 Detection of endometrial carcinoma and hyperplasia in asymptomatic women. Obstet Gynecol 64: 1

73. Kottmeier H L 1967 Annual report on the results of treatment in carcinoma of the uterus, vagina, and ovary. J Int Fed Gynaecol Obstet 15: 4

74. Kumar N B 1984 Small cell carcinoma of the endometrium in a 23-year-old woman: light microscopic and ultrastructural study. Am J Clin Pathol 81: 98

75. Kurman R J, Norris H J 1982 Evaluation of criteria for distinguishing atypical endometrial hyperplasia from well differentiated carcinoma. Cancer 49: 2547

76. Kurman R J, Scully R E 1976 Clear cell carcinoma of the endometrium: an analysis of 21 cases. Cancer 37: 872

77. Larson D M, Copeland L J, Gallager H S et al 1987 Nature of cervical involvement in endometrial carcinoma. Cancer 59: 959

78. Lauchlan S C 1981 Tubal (serous) carcinoma of the endometrium. Arch Pathol Lab Med 105: 615

79. Lozowski M S, Mishriki Y, Solitare G B 1986 Factors determining the degree of endometrial exfoliation and their diagnostic implications in endometrial adenocarcinoma. Acta Cytol 30: 623

80. Lyon F A 1975 The development of adenocarcinoma of the endometrium in young women receiving long-term sequential oral contraception: Report of four cases. Am J Obstet Gynecol 123: 299

81. Malkasian G D, Annegers J F, Fountain K S 1980 Carcinoma of the endometrium: Stage I. Am J Obstet Gynecol 136: 872

82. Martin J D, Hahnel R, McCartney A J, Woodings T L 1983 The effect of estrogen receptor status on survival in patients with endometrial cancer. Am J Obstet Gynecol 147: 322

83. Martin P M, Rolland P H, Gammerre M, Serment H, Toga M 1979 Estradiol and progesterone receptors in normal and neoplastic endometrium: correlations between receptors, histopathological examinations and clinical responses under progestin therapy. Int J Cancer 23: 321

84. Masubuchi K, Nemoto H, Masubuchi S Jr, Fujimoto I, Uchino S 1975 Increasing incidence of endometrial carcinoma in Japan. Gynecol Oncol 3: 335

85. Masubuchi S, Fujimoto I, Masubuchi K 1979 Lymph node metastasis and prognosis of endometrial carcinoma. Gynecol Oncol 7: 36

86. McCarty K S Jr, Barton T K, Fetter B F, Creasman W T, McCarty K S Sr 1979 Correlation of estrogen and progesterone receptors with histologic differentiation in endometrial adenocarcinoma. Am J Pathol 96: 171

87. McCarty K S, Barton T K, Peete C H Jr, Creasman W T 1978 Gonadal dysgenesis with adenocarcinoma of the endometrium: an electron microscopic and steroid receptor analysis with review of the literature. Cancer 42: 512

88. Menczer J, Modan M, Gloor E 1980 The significance of positive tubal cytology in patients with endometrial adenocarcinoma. Gynecol Oncol 10: 249

89. Mittal K R, Schwartz P E, Barwick K W 1988 Architectural (FIGO) grading, nuclear grading, and other prognostic indicators in stage I endometrial adenocarcinoma with identification of high-risk and low-risk groups. Cancer 61: 538

90. Morrow C P, DiSaia P J, Townsend D E 1973 Current management of endometrial carcinoma. Obstet Gynecol 42: 399

91. Musumeci R, DePalo G, Conti U et al 1980 Are retroperitoneal lymph node metastases a major problem in endometrial adenocarcinoma? Cancer 46: 1887

92. Ng A B P, Reagan J W, Storaasli J P, Wentz W B 1973 Mixed adenosquamous carcinoma of the endometrium. Am J Clin Pathol 59: 765

93. Olson N, Twiggs L, Sibley R 1982 Small-cell carcinoma of the endometrium: light microscopic and ultrastructural study of a case. Cancer 50: 760

94. Onsrud M, Aalders J, Abeler V, Taylor P 1982 Endometrial carcinoma with cervical involvement (Stage II): prognostic factors and value of combined radiological-surgical treatment. Gynecol Oncol 13: 76

95. Palmer A L, Roth E 1970 Gross examination of curettings in endometrial carcinoma. Ohio State Med J 66: 44

96. Palermo V G, Glythe J G, Kaufman R H 1985 Cytologic diagnosis of endometrial adenocarcinoma using the Endo-pap sampler. Obstet Gynecol 65: 271

97. Paz R A, Frigerio B, Sundblad A S, Eusebi V 1985 Small-cell (oat cell) carcinoma of the endometrium. Arch Pathol Lab Med 109: 270

98. Piver M S, Lele S B, Barlow J J, Blumenson L 1982 Paraaortic lymph node evaluation in Stage I endometrial carcinoma. Obstet Gynecol 59: 97

99. Poulsen H E, Taylor C W 1975 Histological Typing of Female Genital Tract Tumors. International Histological Classification of Tumors. No 13. World Health Organization, Geneva

100. Quint B C 1975 Changing patterns in endometrial adenocarcinoma: a study of 291 consecutive cases at a large private hospital, 1960–1973. Am J Obstet Gynecol 122: 498

101. Reagan J W 1974 The changing nature of endometrial cancer. Gynecol Oncol 2: 144

102. Reagan J W, Fu Y S 1981 Pathology of endometrial carcinoma. In: Coppleson M (ed) Gynecologic Oncology. Fundamental Principles and Clinical Practice. Churchill Livingstone, London. p 546

103. Robboy S J, Miller A W III, Kurman R J 1982 The pathologic features and behavior of endometrial carcinoma associated with exogenous estrogen administration. Path Res Pract 174: 237

104. Ross J C, Eifel P J, Cox R S, Kempson R L, Hendrickson M R 1983 Primary mucinous adenocarcinoma of the endometrium. A clinicopathologic and histochemical study. Am J Surg Pathol 7: 715

105. Rutledge F 1974 The role of radical hysterectomy in adenocarcinoma of the endometrium. Gynecol Oncol 2: 331

106. Ryder D E 1982 Verrucous carcinoma of the endometrium: a unique neoplasm with long survival. Obstet Gynecol 59: 78s–80s

107. Salazar O M, DePapp E W, Bonfiglio T A, Feldstein M L, Rubin P, Rudolph J H 1977 Adenosquamous carcinoma of the endometrium. An entity with an inherent poor prognosis? Cancer 40: 119

108. Schink J C, Lurain J R, Wallemark C B, Chmiel J S 1987 Tumor size in endometrial cancer: a prognostic factor for lymph node metastasis. Obstet Gynecol 70: 216

109. Schneider M L, Wortmann M, Weigel A 1986 Influence of the histologic and cytologic grade and the clinical and postsurgical stage on the rate of endometrial carcinoma detection by cervical cytology. Acta Cytol 30: 616

110. Schultz D M 1957 A malignant melanotic neoplasm of the uterus resembling the 'retinal anlage' tumors. Am J Clin Pathol 28: 524

111. Scully R E 1975 Recent progress in ovarian cancer. Hum Pathol 1: 73

112. Siiteri P 1978 Steroid hormones and endometrial cancer. Cancer Res 38: 4360

113. Silverberg E, Lubera J A 1988 Cancer statistics, 1988. CA-A Cancer J Clin 38: 14

114. Silverberg S G, Bolin M G, DeGiorgi L S 1972 Adenoacanthoma and mixed adenosquamous carcinoma of the endometrium: A clinicopathologic study. Cancer 30: 1307

115. Silverberg S G, Makowski E I 1975 Endometrial carcinoma in young women taking oral contraceptive agents. Obstet Gynecol 46: 503

116. Silverberg S G, Makowski E L, Roche W D 1977 Endometrial carcinoma in women under 40 years of age. Comparison of cases in oral contraceptive users and non-users. Cancer 39: 592

117. Silverberg S G, Mullen D, Faraci J A et al 1980 Endometrial carcinoma: clinical-pathologic comparison of cases in postmenopausal women receiving and not receiving exogenous estrogens. Cancer 45: 3018

118. Soper J T, McCarty K S Jr, Creasman W T, McCarty K S Sr 1985 Histologic control of biochemical steroid receptor analysis in endometrial carcinomas. Am J Obstet Gynecol 153: 520

119. Stanley M A, Kirkland J W 1968 Cytogenetic studies of endometrial carcinoma. Am J Obstet Gynecol 102: 1070

120. Stock R J, Kanbour A 1975 Prehysterectomy curettage. Obstet Gynecol 45: 537

121. Szpak C A, Creasman W T, Vollmer R T, Johnston W W 1981 Prognostic value of cytologic examination of peritoneal washings in pateints with endometrial carcinoma. Acta Cytol 25: 640

122. Taylor C W 1969 Premalignant changes in endometrium. In: Kellar R J (ed) Modern Trends in Gynecology. Butterworth, London

123. Tiltman A J, Atad J 1982 Verrucous carcinoma of the cervix with endometrial involvement. Int J Gynecol Pathol 1: 221

124. Ueda G, Nishino T, Saito J, Abe Y, Shimizu H, Tanizawa O 1987 Detection of chromogranin in argyrophil cells of endometrial carcinoma. Gynecol Oncol 27: 159

125. Wahlstrom T, Lindgren J, Korhonen M 1979 Distinction between endocervical and endometrial adenocarcinoma with immunoperoxidase staining of carcinoembryonic antigen in routine histologic tissue specimens. Lancet ii: 1159

126. Walker A N, Mills S E 1982 Serous papillary carcinoma of the endometrium. A clinicopathologic study of 11 cases. Diag Gynecol Obstet 4: 261

127. Warhol M J, Rice R H, Pinkus G S, Robboy S J 1984 Evaluation of squamous epithelium in adenoacanthoma and adenosquamous carcinoma of the endometrium: Immunoperoxidase analysis of involucrin and keratin localization. Int J Gynecol Pathol 3: 82

128. Weiner J, Bigelow B, Demopoulos R I, Beckman E M, Weiner I 1980 The value of endocervical sampling in the staging of endometrial carcinoma. Diag Gynecol Obstet 2: 265

129. Weiss N S, Szekely D R, Austin D F 1976 Increasing incidence of endometrial cancer in the United States. New Eng J Med 294: 1259

130. Yamashina M, Kobara T Y 1986 Primary squamous cell carcinoma with its spindle cell variant in the endometrium. Cancer 57: 340

131. Zaino R J, Clarke C L, Mortel R, Satyaswaroop P G 1988 Heterogeneity of progesterone receptor distribution in human endometrial adenocarcinoma. Cancer Res 48: 1889

49. Carcinoma of endometrium (FIGO Stages I and II): clinical features and management

W. T. Creasman   J. C. Weed Jr

INTRODUCTION

In the United States, cancer of the uterine corpus is the most common malignancy in the female pelvis. According to the American Cancer Society, approximately 35 000 women will develop a uterine cancer in 1988[7]. Therefore, this lesion is seen over twice as frequently as carcinoma of the ovary and cervix. Although the Third National Cancer Survey noted no increase in the incidence of adenocarcinoma of the endometrium compared with the Second National Cancer Survey, some authors during the recent past have reported a marked increase in the incidence. In reviewing the predicted incidence for the decade of the 1970s, the American Cancer Society noted a one and a half fold increase in the number of patients with endometrial cancer. It is interesting to note during that time interval the predicted deaths from this malignancy actually decreased slightly.[7,72] When selected areas of the country are evaluated the same trend is apparent. This changing frequency has been discussed earlier (Chs 3 and 48). Greenblatt & Stoddard[23] in 1978 suggested several reasons. (1) Greater availability of medical care: more women are provided medical care; thus more cancers are detected. (2) More women reach the critical age for the development of endometrial cancer. (3) A broadening of criteria for the diagnosis of endometrial cancer by the inclusion of severe dysplasia, atypical adenomatous hyperplasia, carcinoma in situ, and so-called well differentiated endometrial cancers into the cancer registry as adenocarcinoma. (4) A worldwide increase in endometrial cancer, possibly due to environmental and unknown factors. The increased use of estrogen has been implicated; however, Norway and Czechoslovakia reported a 50 to 60% increase in endometrial cancer despite the fact that estrogens are rarely prescribed or are not generally available.[41]

For many years, corpus cancer was considered less malignant than other genital malignancies. Total abdominal hysterectomy and bilateral salpingo-oophorectomy has been the hallmark of therapy and has withstood close scrutiny over the years. Although various forms of radiation therapy have been advocated, many studies in the literature demonstrate that the use of only simple hysterectomy and bilateral salpingo-oophorectomy is as effective as combined therapy at least in certain circumstances. As a result, there appears to be some complacency regarding this so-called 'good' cancer. In this chapter a review of corpus cancer will be given with such areas as important prognostic factors and appropriate therapy discussed in detail.

RISK FACTORS IN ENDOMETRIAL CANCER*

Age

Endometrial carcinoma is a disease which spans the reproductive and menopausal years. The median age of cases of corpus cancer is 61.1 years,[72] and the largest number of cases is found in the age group of 55 to 59 years. The age range extends from the second to the ninth decades yet only approximately 5% of patients with endometrial carcinoma are under 40 years of age. Mattingly reports 20 to 25% of cases are diagnosed before menopause.[54]

Obesity, nulliparity, and late menopause

These variants of normal anatomy or physiology are classically associated with endometrial carcinoma. Studies by Damon[17] demonstrated a 13% increase in the mean body weight of patients with endometrial cancer as compared to control patients of similar height. Wynder, Escher & Mantel[79] showed an increasing risk of developing endometrial cancer in obese women. The risk was 3 times that of the normal weight woman when 21–50 lbs overweight increasing approximately 10 times for greater than 50 lbs overweight. Similar studies in Boston demonstrated 1.8 times the risk for women in the upper one-third of weight

---

* See also Chapters 3 and 8.

775

distribution increasing to 2.4 times the risk for patients in the top 15% of the weight distribution.[50] Unfortunately, screening limited to the obese population would detect only 50% of endometrial cancers.

Nulliparity is commonly associated with endometrial carcinoma. 24 to 31% of patients with endometrial cancer are nulliparous.[50,53] The risk of developing endometrial cancer in the nulligravida is twice as high as the primipara increasing to treble the risk of the quintapara. Masubuchi[53] reports age of first pregnancy is lower in parous patients than in controls. Again, screening the nulliparous population would identify only 48% of the endometrial carcinomas in the population.[50]

Late menopause was reported by Kaplan & Cole[35] to be associated with an increased risk of developing endometrial carcinoma. Women with menopause after age 52 had 2.4-fold risk as women with menopause before age 49. This association was valid retrospectively for women with cancers diagnosed many years postmenopausally. Late occurrence of spontaneous menopause should be differentiated from abnormal bleeding in perimenopausal women.

Associated medical disease

Hypertension and diabetes mellitus are frequently associated with endometrial cancers. Kaplan & Cole report a relative risk of 2.8 for women with a history of diabetes after controlling for age, body weight and socioeconomic status.[35] Frequently, the abnormality of carbohydrate metabolism is diagnosed during the staging evaluation for endometrial carcinoma. Frick and associates[22] reported from 5.3 to 41% of patients with endometrial cancer had abnormal carbohydrate intolerance. Similarly, high blood pressure is prevalent in the elderly, obese population and does not appear to be a significant risk factor by itself, yet 25% of the patients will have hypertension or arteriosclerotic heart disease. There is a slightly higher frequency of arthritis and hypothyroidism in patients with endometrial carcinoma as compared to controls.[35]

Immunodeficiency diseases and immunosuppressive states are highly correlated with the development of malignancy. Husslein and associates[28] reported one patient with endometrial cancer diagnosed 20 months after successful renal transplantation. The patient had had a prior curettage which was normal. Abnormal bleeding in this group of patients cannot be ascribed to anovulation secondary to chronic disease, and increased surveillance with tissue evaluation is required.

Hormone-secreting tumors

It has been known for years that endometrial cancer can occur in patients with hormone-secreting tumors, particularly of the ovary. Many studies have been reported concerning this entity since it was first described by Novak & Yui[62] in 1936 in the American literature. Gusberg & Kardon[24] noted the highest correlation between endometrial cancer and the so-called feminizing ovarian tumors. Of 115 patients 21% were found to have corpus cancer and another 43% were found to have cancer precursors such as endometrial hyperplasia and carcinoma in situ. Despite this association the authors were unable to draw any solid conclusions about the possible carcinogenic role of estrogen in humans. Norris & Taylor[61] evaluated 203 patients with granulosa theca cell tumor at the Armed Forces Institute of Pathology. Only 9% of these patients had adenocarcinoma of the uterus, although the authors do not mention endometrial precursors. Mansell & Hertig[52] reviewed 80 feminizing tumors at the Free Hospital in Boston between 1905 and 1953. Only 11 patients had adenocarcinoma; however 60% of the endometria had changes suggestive of estrogen stimulation. McDonald, Malkasian & Gaffey[49] approached the situation from another viewpoint. Between 1905 and 1975 at the Mayo Clinic there were 44 patients with functional ovarian tumors associated with endometrial cancer. Unfortunately, the authors do not mention the total number of functional ovarian tumors and adenocarcinomas of the endometrium during that time interval. In addition there were 28 patients with polycystic ovarian disease and endometrial cancer. The control group consisted of 523 adenocarcinoma patients who were seen in the years 1952 to 1962. The 72 patients with endometrial cancer associated with functional tumors or polycystic ovaries had a predominance of Stage I, Grade I lesions, less myometrial involvement and better survival compared with the other 523 adenocarcinoma patients. Some authors have qualified the stromal tumors with the word 'feminizing' while others have not used this designation. It is well known that granulosa cell tumors can produce androgens, although fewer than those which produce estrogen. (See Ch. 59.)

Polycystic ovary syndrome

Another situation in which endogenous estrogen might be a contributing factor to the development of endometrial cancer is in patients with the polycystic ovary syndrome. Endometrial cancer has been reported to be as high as 25% in patients with Stein-Leventhal syndrome, although in fact, this number is probably considerably smaller. If the unopposed estrogen can be overcome in this syndrome by wedge resection or clomiphene citrate, the estrogen stimulated endometrium and its possible premalignant changes can be reversed. Kistner[38] has reported that progestogens can cause regression of hyperplasia and carcinoma in situ of the endometrium.

Ovarian dysgenesis

Patients with ovarian dysgenesis (Turner's syndrome) have

also been reported as being at high risk for endometrial cancer because of the long-term supplemental estrogen that is given to these individuals beginning at an early age. Several case reports have appeared recently in the literature, and 14 patients have been reported to date.[48,64]

Exogenous determinants of endometrial cancer

The relationship of endometrial cancer to ionizing radiation, oral contraceptives and exogenous estrogens is discussed in Chapter 3: Epidemiology of cancer of the endometrium, ovary, vulva and vagina.

DIAGNOSIS

Abnormal uterine bleeding is the cardinal symptom of endometrial carcinoma, especially when it occurs in the perimenopausal and postmenopausal age groups. Nevertheless, 20 to 25% of cases of corpus cancer are found in patients before the menopause. There is only a 17 to 63% finding of malignancy as a cause of postmenopausal bleeding in the United States as reviewed by Caspi and associates.[8] Approximately half of the cancers will be endometrial in origin, the remainder will be cervical carcinomas with a few ovarian or other primaries. Other common causes of postmenopausal bleeding which enter the differential diagnosis are estrogen therapy, uterine polyps and atrophic endometritis or cervicitis. An uncommon but important presentation, sometimes overlooked, is a watery discharge. Pain is rarely an early symptom. In the postmenopausal patient the presence of pyometra signals great care in excluding this cancer.

A high index of suspicion is crucial for the early diagnosis of endometrial carcinoma. No attempt at routine screening of the female population has been made although Hofmeister[27] reported that 17% of endometrial carcinomas diagnosed by routine office biopsy occurred in asymptomatic perimenopausal women. Multiple techniques utilizing cytologic and histologic studies are available for office diagnosis[12] and a formal, fractional curettage remains the definitive diagnostic procedure.

Cervico-vaginal cytologic sampling has a diagnostic accuracy of 47 to 67% for invasive endometrial carcinoma. Studies by Ng et al,[59] have revealed that normal endometrial cells found in routine vaginal pool smears of women in the secretory phase of the cycle or in menopause are associated with endometrial carcinomas in 2% and 5.2% respectively. Precursor lesions were noted in 4.9% of women with normal endometrial cells found in the secretory phase and 13.2% after menopause. Their findings indicate a 15% occurrence of precursor cancer lesions when normal endometrial cells are found on smears of postmenopausal women aged 50 to 59 and a 33% occurrence in women over 59 years of age (see also Ch. 14).

A wide variety of mechanical devices has been developed for cytologic sampling of the endometrial cavity. Samples may be obtained by uterine sounds, endometrial brushes, or irrigation instruments. The diagnostic accuracy of cytologic preparations ranges from 57 to 92%. Table 49.1 presents our results at Duke Medical Center in patients referred with a histologic diagnosis of endometrial cancer.[15] No single technique achieved the desired performance of

Table 49.1 Accuracy of multiple diagnostic techniques in uterine cancer

	Number of patients
Total with cancer	21
Pap	14 (67%)
Post sound	12 (57%)
Brush	16 (76%)
Jet wash	17 (81%)
Endometrial biopsy	13 (62%)

detecting all cancers. The results of combining cytologic screening with tissue sampling endometrial biopsy are shown in Table 49.2. With this approach there is greater accuracy than with either technique used alone. Unfortunately, the diagnostic accuracy for precursor lesions is lower than that for carcinoma. Abate, Edwards & Vellios[1] reported the jet wash correctly diagnosed only one of seven endometrial hyperplasias present in material obtained by simultaneous endometrial biopsy.

Biopsy curettage of the endometrial cavity may be performed by using small curettes or suction instruments. The overall accuracy of curette biopsy approaches 90% and vacuum curettage approaches 100%. A reported advantage of the vacuum technique is a high detection rate of precursor lesions. Other techniques are reported for obtaining endometrial samples. The intrauterine sponge technique reported by Chatfield & Bremner[9] had a 97.6% rate of adequate samples and correctly diagnosed 13 of 17 invasive endometrial cancers. Three of the remaining patients had material suspicious for cancer, and one patient was asymptomatic. The Kuper Brush technique, according to

Table 49.2 Accuracy of combination of diagnostic techniques in uterine cancer

Brush + jet wash	19/21 (91%)[a]
Brush + biopsy	19/21 (91%)[b]
Brush + Vabra aspirator	24/27 (89%)
Brush + biopsy	23/27 (85%)[d]

[a] One patient misdiagnosed had a prior curettage; the other patient had adenocarcinoma in situ.
[b] Both patients misdiagnosed had a prior curettage.
[c] All three patients misdiagnosed had a prior curettage.
[d] All three patients misdiagnosed had a prior curettage; and one had a diagnosis of glandular hyperplasia.

Butler, Monahan & Warrell[6], yields material suitable for a histologic sample in approximately 96% of cases. They correctly identified all invasive and one of three precursor lesions. The Milan-Markley technique yields both cytologic and histologic specimens.[55]

The diagnosis of endometrial carcinoma may be made by cytology and biopsy in the office. Endocervical curettage at the same time rules out cervical involvement and obviates the need for fractional curettage. Any cytologic or histologic abnormality short of invasive cancer demands formal, fractional curettage to rule out a small focus of invasive disease. All patients with persistent symptoms despite normal cytology and biopsy should also be submitted to fractional curettage.

STAGING

The International Federation's (FIGO) clinical staging for endometrial carcinoma, in effect until October 1989, is shown in Table 49.3. With this classification, approximately 75% patients present with Stage I disease. The remaining patients are about equally divided between the other stages. However the value of clinical staging as a

Table 49.3 FIGO classification of endometrial carcinoma until September, 1989

Stage I	The carcinoma is confined to the corpus
Stage Ia	The length of the uterine cavity is 8 cm or less
Stage Ib	The length of the uterine cavity is more than 8 cm

Stage I cases should be subgrouped with regard to the histologic type of adenocarcinoma as follows:
G1 Highly differentiated adenomatous carcinomas
G2 Differentiated adenomatous carcinomas with partly solid areas
G3 Predominantly solid or entirely undifferentiated carcinomas

Stage II	The carcinoma involves corpus and cervix
Stage III	The carcinoma extends outside the corpus but not outside the true pelvis (it may involve the vaginal wall or the parametrium but not the bladder or the rectum)
Stage IV	The carcinoma involves the bladder or rectum or extends outside the pelvis

predictor of prognosis is compromised because of the large proportion of Stage I cases. Other prognostic factors, some of which are only available after surgery, assume greater importance. To overcome this problem the Cancer Committee of FIGO recently introduced a surgical-pathological staging system (Table 49.4).

After the tissue diagnosis of endometrial malignancy is established, the patient should have a thorough diagnostic evaluation prior to the initiation of therapy. Endocervical curettage should be performed in any patient who has not had a fractional curettage. The problem of establishing the

Table 49.4 Surgical-pathological staging of endometrial carcinoma* (Adapted from FIGO cancer committee report, Rio de Janiero, October, 1989)

STAGE Ia	(G123)	Tumor limited to endometrium
Ib	(G123)	Invasion to <1/2 myometrium
Ic	(G123)	Invasion >1/2 myometrium
IIa	(G123)	Endocervical glandular involvement only
IIb	(G123)	Cervical stromal invasion
IIIa	(G123)	Tumor invades serosa and/or adnexae and/or positive peritoneal cytology
IIIb	(G123)	Vaginal metastases
IIIc	(G123)	Metastases to pelvic and/or para-aortic lymph nodes
IVa	(G123)	Tumor invasion bladder and/or bowel mucosa
IVb	(G123)	Distant metastases including intra-abdominal and/or inguinal lymph node

* 1. Since corpus cancer is now surgically staged, procedures previously used for differentiation of stages are no longer applicable, such as the finding on D&C to differentiate between Stage I and Stage II.
   a) It is appreciated that there may be a small number of patients with corpus cancer who will be treated primarily with radiation therapy. If that is the case, the clinical staging adopted by FIGO in 1971 would still apply but designation of that staging system would be noted.
2. Ideally, width of the myometrium should be measured along with the width of tumor invasion.
3. Notable nuclear atypia, inappropriate for the architectural grade, raises the grade of a Grade 1 or Grade 2 tumor by 1.
4. In serous adenocarcinomas, clear cell adenocarcinomas, and squamous cell carcinomas, nuclear grading takes precedent.
5. Adenocarcinomas with squamous differentiation are graded according to the nuclear grade of the glandular component.

presence of cervical involvement (Stage II) prior to hysterectomy has already been discussed (Ch. 48). Routine hematologic studies and clotting profiles are obtained in all patients. Completion of the evaluation is carried out with chest X-ray, electrocardiogram, intravenous urogram, and a metabolic profile. Some authorities recommend hysteroscopy (Ch. 17) and hysterography. Sigmoidoscopy and barium enema are reserved for patients with palpable disease outside the uterus or with symptoms of bowel disease. Brain, liver and bone scans are indicated in patients suspected of having extant disease. Kademian, Buchler & Wirtanen[34] recommended the use of bipedal lymphography. Although we appreciate the significance of positive lymphadenopathy, we have been disappointed in the lymphogram's ability to demonstrate pelvic lymph nodes which are involved in a significant percentage of patients with higher grades of tumor.

PROGNOSTIC FACTORS

Pretreatment evaluation of patients with malignant neoplasms coupled with clinicopathological experience should allow the physician to individualize therapy for the best results. Several factors have been identified for endometrial adenocarcinoma which have significant predictive value for these patients (Table 49.5). Factors relative to host resistance and modality of therapy also are important for determining patient outcome. On the basis of clinical experiences, Nolan & Huen[60] developed a mathematical model for evaluating prognosis wherein prognosis is directly proportional to host resistance factors, inversely proportional to tumor virulence factors, and enhanced by treatment factors.

$$\text{Prognosis} \propto \frac{\text{Resistance}}{\text{Virulence}} \times \text{Treatment}$$

The resistance factors are age and general constitutional condition. The virulence factors are stage of disease, grade of tumor, and tumor volume.

Table 49.5 Prognostic factors in endometrial adenocarcinoma

1. Age at diagnosis
2. Stage of tumor
3. Histologic differentiation
4. Myometrial penetration
5. Lymph node metastasis
6. Peritoneal cytology
7. Histologic subtype

Age

The significance of age at the time of diagnosis has been appreciated for years. Frick et al[22] found that patients under age 59 at diagnosis had improved survival as compared to older patients in Stage I disease, even after correcting for deaths from intercurrent disease. The survival rate was greater than 80% for women below age 59 and less than 56% for women over age 60. De Muelenaere[19] noted similar results in his review. Jones[32] points out that the improved survival of younger patients is secondary to the tendency to earlier (smaller), better differentiated lesions without myometrial invasion occurring in those patients. This assumption is borne out by reports of excellent survival in endometrial cancer patients who were using sequential oral contraception or who were pregnant. Other factors such as lack of host immunocompetence may be more active in older patients.

Stage at diagnosis

The pretreatment staging of patients with malignant neoplasia was designed to have prognostic value by determining the size and extent of tumor. Reported figures of stage and survival have been consistent (Table 49.6). The

Table 49.6 5-year survival in endometrial cancer

Stage	Patients
I	7729/10 285 (75.1%)
II	1089/1885 (51.8%)
III	253/844 (30.0%)
IV	48/452 (10.6%)

From Pettersson F (ed) (1985) *Annual report on the results of treatment in gynecological cancer*, vol. 19. FIGO/Stockholm

new FIGO surgical-pathological classification will in time provide more accurate data.

Uterine size has been recognized as a predictor of survival and was incorporated into the subgrouping of Stage I patients into Ia and Ib. Creasman and associates[13] demonstrated a progressive increase in lymph node metastasis to pelvic and para-aortic areas with increase in the size of the uterus. However, Lutz and associates[47] point out that uterine size does not always reflect tumor volume as benign lesions may account for a large corpus. De Muelenaere[19] reports that the uterine cavity of 10 cm is a better discriminator for assessing survival as opposed to the 8 cm limit of the FIGO classification (Table 49.7). The size of the uterus is associated with both grade of tumor and degree of myometrial invasion, both factors which may have more significance for prognosis.

Table 49.7

Depth of uterine cavity	No. of patients	Crude survival	Died of disease
Less than 8 cm	39	28 (71.8%)	3 (7.7%)
Greater than 8 cm	32	26 (81.3%)	4 (12.5%)
Less than 10 cm	55	43 (78.2%)	4 (7.3%)
Greater than 10 cm	16	11 (68.8%)	3 (18.8%)

Adapted from De Muelenaere, G.F.G.O. (1975) Prognostic factors in endometrial carcinoma. *S Afr Med J* **49**: 695

Prognosis for women with cervical involvement (Stage II) is much poorer than for earlier lesions. The importance of establishing endocervical involvement by fractional curettage or endocervical curettage is shown by the overall drop in survival from the 80% to the 50% range. Location of the tumor within the endometrial cavity could be significant, as tumors low in the cavity might involve the cervix earlier than fundal lesions. Data from staging studies of Creasman and associates[13] reveal 92% of clinical Stage I lesions are located in the fundus.

Similarly, Surwit and associates[75] reviewed 117 patients with histologically documented Stage II endometrial cancer. The preoperative endocervical curettage findings were compared with operative findings in the uterus and with survival. Overall survival was 58% at 3 years. However, patients with stromal invasion of the cervix had poorer survival (47%) than those in whom involvement was limited to the endocervical glands or in whom no stroma was present in the endocervical curettage (74%). The key factor seems to be penetration of cervical stroma with its increased propensity for pelvic nodal spread (36%).

Histologic differentiation

The degree of histologic differentiation of endometrial carcinoma has long been accepted as one of the most sensitive indicators of prognosis. Jones' review[32] of the treatment of endometrial carcinomas from 15 reports covering 3990 patients shows progressive fall in survival with decreasing differentiation. Average 5-year survival for Grade 1 (highly differentiated) lesions was 81%; for Grade 2, 74%; and for Grade 3 (undifferentiated), 50%. Some reports indicated very low survivals with Grade 3 lesions. Creasman and associates[13] report a higher percentage of pelvic and para-aortic lymph node involvement with increasing stage and grade, but the largest percentage increase is seen when Grade 3 lesions are compared with Grade 2 (Table 49.8).

Grade of tumor is correlated with other factors of prognosis. Cheon[10] reported an increasing percentage of deep myometrial involvement with increasing grade of tumor. Here again the jump between Grade 1 and 2 and Grade 3 lesions is impressive and reflects the lymph node data from Creasman.[13] The relationship of grade to survival persists regardless of the mode of therapy as reported in the Annual Report of FIGO (Table 49.9) The recently adopted FIGO surgical-pathological staging system (Table 49.4) takes into account nuclear atypia. Thus nuclear atypia that is regarded as inappropriate for the architectural grade raises the grade of a Grade 1 or Grade 2 tumor by one. In serous adenocarcinomas, clear cell adenocarcinomas, and squamous cell carcinomas, nuclear grading takes precedence over the degree of histologic differentiation. Adenocarcinomas with squamous differentiation are graded according to the nuclear grade of the glandular component.

Table 49.8 Grade versus positive pelvic and aortic nodes

Grade		Pelvic	Aortic
G1	(N=180)	5 (3%)	3 (2%)
G2	(N=288)	25 (9%)	14 (5%)
G3	(N=153)	28 (18%)	17 (11%)

Modified from Creasman et al (1987) *Cancer* **60**: 2035

Myometrial penetration

The degree of myometrial penetration is a consistent indicator of tumor virulence. The literature, as reviewed by Jones[32] and Plentyl & Friedman[65] demonstrates a decrease in survival rate as myometrial penetration increases, sur-

vival dropping from 80 to 60%. Lutz and associates[47] determined that the depth of myometrial penetration was not as important as the proximity of the invading tumor to the uterine serosa. Patients whose tumors invaded to within 5 mm of the serosa had 65% 5-year survival compared to 97% survival in patients whose tumors were more than 10 mm from the serosa (see also Ch. 48).

The depth of myometrial invasion is associated with the other poor prognosis factors, poor differentiation and lymph node involvement (Tables 49.8 and 49.10). In the past, it has been difficult to accurately assess myometrial invasion in women who have received preoperative irradiation due to the interval between irradiation and operation. The current approach of primary surgical exploration yields more accurate data.

Several authors recommend routine pretreatment hysterography in an effort to obtain more precise information concerning the size, location, and extent of the endometrial lesions.[2,31,70,78] The discovery of subclinical anomalies or uterine perforations is helpful. Tak and associates[76] correlated the pattern of hysterographic defects

Table 49.9 Survival rate in Stage I carcinoma of the endometrium with regard to grade and treatment

Grade	Survival	
	Surgery only	Combined therapy
1	601/734 (82%)	1314/1540 (85%)
2	253/324 (78%)	716/891 (80%)
3	69/114 (61%)	205/319 (64%)

From Pettersson F (ed.) (1985) *Annual report on the results of treatment in gynecological cancer*, Vol. 19, Stockholm

Table 49.10 Maximal invasion and node metastasis

Maximal invasion	Pelvic	Aortic
Endometrium only (N=87)	1 (1%)	1 (1%)
Superficial muscle (N=279)	15 (5%)	8 (3%)
Intermediate muscle (N=116)	7 (6%)	1 (1%)
Deep muscle (N=139)	35 (25%)	24 (17%)

Modified from Creasman et al (1987) *Cancer* **60**: 2035

with myometrial involvement. Shallow defects were infrequently associated with significant invasion; whereas large defects were found with myometrial penetration. The information obtained from this technique may be useful if preoperative radiation is planned. If a primary surgical approach is the management of choice then this added diagnostic procedure is unnecessary.

Peritoneal cytology

The routine use of cytologic sampling of peritoneal fluids

or washings is common practice as an adjunct to staging in patients who require celiotomy for pelvic malignancies. Creasman & Rutledge[14] reported positive washings in 12% of corpus cancer patients. Creasman and associates[13] routinely obtain peritoneal washings, and note a 15% rate of positive washings in a group of 228 corpus cancer patients. Five of 15 patients with positive washings and no clinical evidence of extrauterine spread sustained intra-abdominal recurrence.

Lymph node involvement

Since total abdominal hysterectomy and bilateral salpingo-oophorectomy has been the hallmark of therapy in endometrial cancer the true incidence of lymph node metastases has been difficult to determine. Although the remote as well as the recent literature has indicated that a significant number of women with endometrial cancer, even Stage I disease, have lymph node involvement, the potential metastatic sites have not been routinely included in the treatment plan.

In 1952, Javert[29] noted that 14 (28%) of 50 patients with endometrial cancer had pelvic node metastasis, although the stage of disease was not recorded. Lymph node metastases occurred more frequently when there was deep invasion of the myometrium. His review of the literature noted that Cullen in 1900 described 27 patients, of whom one had a positive pelvic lymph node.[16] During the first part of the twentieth century, several reports in the literature, as noted by Javert, contained information suggesting that endometrial cancer did metastasize to the pelvic and occasionally to the aortic lymph node areas. He found 30 of 591 patients (5%) with pelvic lymph node metastases and an additional 3 patients with para-aortic disease. Autopsy reports showed a much higher incidence of nodal disease with 54 of 211 patients (25.5%) having metastases in the pelvic areas. Javert observed that 4 of his 14 patients with lymph node metastases survived at least 3 years (28%) compared with 94.4% of the other 36 patients who had negative lymph nodes. He reported subsequently that all the patients with positive nodes eventually died of their disease. Javert believed that it was extremely important to determine the depth of invasion, whether or not metastases to the lymph nodes had occurred, and most importantly the presence or absence of vascular emboli and thrombi in the uterus and perinodal veins. He felt that involvement of the vessels carried extremely poor prognosis.

In 1956, Lefèvre[43] reviewed the literature of the preceding 5 years noting 19% of 217 endometrial cancer patients had positive lymph nodes. He reported another 45 patients whose treatment included lymphadenectomy; seven with positive nodes. Unfortunately, this was an unstaged study, and some of those with positive nodes had recurrence at the time the lymph node metastasis was discovered.

Table 49.11 Endometrial carcinoma: frequency of lymph node metastases

| Author | Year | Patients with positive nodes | | | |
		No.	%	Stage I	Stage II
Randall	1950	4/20	20%	Not stated	Not stated
Brunschwig	1954	10/57	17%		
Liu and Meigs	1955	11/47	23%	4/33 (12%)	7/14 (50%)
Lefèvre	1956	7/45	16%	Not stated	Not stated
Schwartz and Brunschwig	1957	13/96	14%		
Roberts	1961	10/34	29%	5/22 (23%)	2/8 (25%)
Anderson and Stephens	1961	4/52	8%	Not stated	Not stated
Barber et al	1962	12/85	20%		
Davis	1964	7/56	12.5%	Not stated	Not stated
Parsons	1959	4/50	8%		
Hawksworth	1964	8/64	12.5%		6/11 (18.7%)
Winterton	1964	8/76	10%		
Rickford	1968	5/50	10%	2/36	2/9
Lees	1969	13/76	17%	3/56	4/8
Morris	1967	4/21	20%	16	5
Lewis	1970	17/129	13.2%	12/107 (11.2%)	5/22 (23%)
Stallworthy	1973	18/131	14%		11/27 (40%)
Boronow	1984	23/222	(10% pelvic — all Stage I)		
GOG	1986	58/621	(9% pelvic — all Stage I)		

Adapted from Rutledge, F. (1974) *Gynecol Oncol* 2: 331.

Lees[42] in 1969, and Lewis, Stallworthy & Cowdell[44] in 1970, presented their data concerning Stage I endometrial cancer and the incidence of lymph node metastases. Lees noted 3 of 56 cases (5.4%) and Lewis, Stallworthy & Cowdell 12 of 107 cases (11.2%) with pelvic node metastases in Stage I. The incidence of lymph node metastases in Stage II was considerably higher.

Morrow, DiSaia & Townsend[57] in 1973, reviewed the recent literature and noted that in collected series 39 (10.6%) of 369 patients with Stage I carcinoma and 31 (36.5%) of 85 patients with Stage II carcinoma, had pelvic node metastases. The 5-year survival was only 31% in patients with Stage I disease and positive nodes. Most patients had been treated with postoperative radiation.

Rutledge[67] in his excellent review of the role of radical hysterectomy in adenocarcinoma of the endometrium, made an exhaustive review of the literature of the last 25 years, and noted that approximately 10% of patients with Stage I carcinoma from the collective series had metastases to the pelvic nodes. Some of the studies reported a higher incidence, but this was usually explained by the selection of patients (Table 49.11). The incidence of pelvic node metastases was increased when the tumor was more undifferentiated and penetrated further into the myometrium.

The information gained from these pelvic lymphadenectomy studies indicated that a significant number of patients with early stage disease have metastases outside the uterus.

More recently, the Gynecologic Oncology Group reported[13] approximately 11% incidence of pelvic node metastases in Stage I carcinoma of the endometrium and 7 to 10% with para-aortic nodal metastases. Metastases were directly related to the size of the uterus, differentiation of the tumor, depth of myometrial invasion as well as tumor site within the uterus. These data were based on selective lymphadenectomies only, and therefore represent minimal incidence figures. The correlation of pelvic with para-aortic nodal metastases is of prime importance and the first to date so identified. Although Stage II lesions were not evaluated it is assumed, based on pelvic lymph node data in the literature, that pelvic and para-aortic involvement would have been higher than in Stage I disease.

TREATMENT

Historical review

Thomas Cullen, in his book *Cancer of the Uterus* published in 1900, stated that the treatment of choice in patients with endometrial cancer was abdominal hysterectomy with the removal of the adnexae.[16] Although during the first part of the twentieth century radium became available, surgery continued to be the most common therapy applied to this malignancy. Howard Kelly, in 1916, reported a large series

of patients with uterine cancer which had been treated with radium.[36] He felt, however, that the surgical treatment was still an important part of the overall therapy.

Beginning in the 1920s Healy studied the effects of radiation therapy alone and in combination with surgery in the treatment of endometrial cancer. He confirmed that poorly differentiated lesions are more difficult to treat successfully. His report with Brown[25] in 1939 showed no better results in poorly differentiated lesions using radiation therapy than occurring in the early surgical series as noted by Mahle.[51] Although further studies indicated that irradiation plus surgery did not appear to improve survival over surgery alone; it was the strong opinion of these investigators that the combination of radiation followed 3 to 6 weeks later by hysterectomy was the best method to treat cancer of the corpus uteri.[3] Unfortunately, many of these early reports did not correct for important prognostic factors as we now understand them in endometrial cancer. Because of these enthusiastic reports, radiation therapy was applied to a greater degree in the management of adenocarcinoma of the endometrium. Heyman, during the 1930s, developed a technique of packing the uterus with multiple capsules of radium prior to hysterectomy.[26] His results showed approximately a 60% 5-year survival in Stage I carcinoma.

During the 1940s, renewed interest in radical surgery for the treatment of malignancies of the female genital tract became apparent. Javert & Douglas[30] were early proponents for using radical hysterectomy and pelvic lymphadenectomy for endometrial cancer. On the basis of their own study and the literature review, they recommended exploratory laparotomy without irradiation in the operable patient with endometrial cancer. If no metastases were noted on intra-abdominal evaluation, hysterectomy and complete pelvic lymphadenectomy was carried out. With obvious metastases a selective lymphadenectomy was advised since the lymph node data might be important in assessing prognosis. They felt that preoperative radiation added nothing to the surgical procedure. They also maintained that selective lymphadenectomy was worthless from the stand-point of cure when the nodes were positive; however, the use of postoperative external irradiation might be efficacious in patients found to have positive nodes or pelvic extension. No increased morbidity or mortality was attributed to either selective or complete lymphadenectomy.

Radical hysterectomy and pelvic lymphadenectomy has been performed by several other investigators and as mentioned in Rutledge's excellent review[67] the incidence of pelvic node involvement was shown to be in the vicinity of 10 to 12% even in Stage I disease. However, patients treated by such radical surgery had essentially the same 5-year survival as those treated with other modalities. In Rutledge's opinion the frequency of positive nodes in Stage I disease did not justify routine lymphadenectomy. However he conceded 'lymphadenectomy may very well be useful treatment if by selectivity, the patient with a greater risk for nodal metastases can be identified'. Patients with Stage I disease treated by radical hysterectomy had decreased incidence of vaginal recurrence but on its own this finding does not necessarily warrant lymphadenectomy since several studies have shown that radiation either by radium or external therapy, in combination with simple hysterectomy will yield the same low incidence of vaginal recurrence. The number of operative deaths and major postoperative complications was not significantly greater than that found in other reports of treatment utilizing conservative hysterectomy. From Rutledge's review it appears that most authors agree that radical hysterectomy and pelvic lymphadenectomy is not indicated in Stage I carcinoma of the endometrium. However, many authorities recommend the procedure in women with Stage II disease. Those surgeons who did use radical hysterectomy and pelvic lymphadenectomy confirmed, as might be anticipated, that patients with positive nodes had a much poorer survival than those with negative nodes even if postoperative irradiation was given.

Also during the 1940s and the following decades, a continued interest was evident in the use of preoperative irradiation. A miscellany of regimes was used including the packing technique of Heyman, standard uterine tube and vaginal ovoids and, infrequently, external irradiation. Many reports were presented indicating that patients treated with preoperative irradiation had less residual disease in the uterus at the time of hysterectomy, and that this group had much better survival than those who had tumor identified. Reports also indicated that patients treated with preoperative irradiation had less vaginal recurrence than if surgery alone was used. In theory the irradiation should have minimized the viability of cancer cells which might be disseminated at operation and also sterilized any subclinical vaginal metastases. Jones,[32] in his excellent review article, surveyed the extensive literature of the 1950s, 1960s and 1970s and noted that the 5-year survival rate for patients treated with surgery only was essentially the same as that following radiation plus surgery (Table 49.12). Unfortunately, the vast majority of these reports were not evaluated in regards to grade of the tumor or myometrial involvement. It is probable that many patients with poorly differentiated lesions were in the combined group, thus prejudicing the overall survival in this therapy category. Other investigators have suggested that postoperative irradiation also reduced the incidence of vaginal metastases and achieved as good a 5-year survival rate as preoperative irradiation. Some investigators therefore have suggested that postoperative irradiation by intracavitary and/or external techniques should be applied either routinely or to those individuals who, at the time of surgery, were found to have poorly differentiated carcinomas or deep myometrial penetration.[56]

Table 49.12 Comparison of the 5-year survival results using surgery alone and radiation plus surgery in the treatment of endometrial carcinoma

| | Surgery alone | | Combined therapy | |
	No. Pts	5-year survival	No. Pts	5-year survival
		%		%
Webb	43	65	79	71
Graham	103	70	135	64
Boutselis	19	64	130	66
Javert	101	65	209	68
Davis	167	46	238	56
Gusberg	178	66	217	81
Dobbie	236	81	384	79
Carmichael	140	85	193	81
Copenhaver	141	79	43	77
Wade	43	75	156	86
Burr	36	78	112	82
Geisler	22	82	99	86
Nilsen	97	84	262	85
Sall	198	82	46	72
Vongtama	50	76	327	85
Graham	33	64	90	78
Joslin	280	79	230	84
Beiler	68	79	64	90
Moltz	83	72	68	81
Shah	37	63	80	72
Wentham	98	70	119	68
Monson	179	92	322	92
Silverberg	40	70	76	79
Total Patients	2392		3679	
Total Survivors	1794		2886	
Average 5 Year Survival		75		78

Jones, H W, III. 1975 Treatment of adenocarcinoma of the endometrium. Review. *Obstet and Gynecol Survey* 3, No. 3.

More recently, a considerable amount of data has been collected concerning the incidence of vaginal recurrence and survival after either combined therapy with mainly preoperative radium and surgery or surgery alone.[22,77] More importantly, the authors also considered the effect of the grade of tumor (Table 49.13), and in some instances the depth of myometrial involvement (Table 49.14). As a generalization, it appears that patients who had pre- or postoperative irradiation had a lower incidence of vaginal vault recurrence. However, the overall survival did not seem to be greater in the combined therapy group than in those individuals who were treated with surgery only. This was particularly true of those patients with Grade 1 and Grade 2 lesions. Patients with poorly differentiated adenocarcinoma treated with combined therapy had a slightly better survival, although in most studies the differences were not statistically significant.

Onsrud, Kolstad & Norman[63] have evaluated the role of postoperative external pelvic irradiation in Stage I carcinoma of the endometrium in a prospective, randomized trial. This is the only study of this kind. Patients judged to have clinical Stage I carcinoma of the endometrium were all treated by total abdominal hysterectomy and bilateral

Table 49.13 Survival in Stage I carcinoma of the endometrium comparing grade and treatment

	G1		G2		G3	
	S[a]	S+R[a]	S	S+R	S	S+R
Wharam[77]	80/82	14/14	63/69	60/69	5/9	15/26
Frick[22]	78/88	78/86	7/10	25/36	3/5	9/14
Salazar[68a]	10/12	10/11	13/14	38/42	12/17	67/81
Total	168/182	102/111	83/93	123/147	20/31	91/121
	(92.3%)	(91.8%)	(89.2%)	(83.6%)	(64.5%)	(75.2%)

S[a]: Surgery.
R[a]: Radiation therapy.

Table 49.14 Survival in Stage I carcinoma of the endometrium comparing depth of invasion and treatment

Residual	Surgery only	Surgery + Radiation
No tumor	11/12 (91.6%)	27/28 (96.4%)
Endometrium + inner muscle	69/80 (86.2%)	49/64 (76.5%)
Mid or outer muscle	8/11 (72.7%)	36/44 (81.8%)

Adapted from Frick H C, Munnell E W, Richart R M, Berger A D and Lawry M F (1973). Carcinoma of endometrium. *Am J Obstet Gynecol* 115: 663

salpingo-oophorectomy. All patients then received postoperative intravaginal radium application, delivering approximately 60 Gy (6000 rads) to the surface of the vaginal vault. Then, by random number, patients were allocated either into a no-treatment arm or treated with external pelvic irradiation to 40 Gy (4000 rads.) There were 195 patients in the group who received surgery and vaginal radium, and 191 patients in the group that received in addition external irradiation. The 5-year survival was 90% for patients who did not receive the pelvic irradiation and 88% for those who did. The death and recurrence rates in both groups were identical. There was no difference in results of the two treatment groups when the histological grades were considered. The combined death and recurrence rate for histological Grade 1 and 2 tumors was 6.8% when no external irradiation was given, and 6.1% in the group receiving external irradiation. With Grade 3 tumors the respective rates were 15.0% and 17.6%. The death and recurrence rate in patients with involvement in the outer half of the myometrium was lower in the external irradiation group although the differences were not statistically significant. In patients who did not receive external irradiation, recurrences were detected in the vagina in 4.6% of cases and on the pelvic wall in 2.5% whereas, in the patients who received irradiation therapy the percentages were 2.1 and zero respectively. This prospective randomized study suggests that external radiation therapy, although decreasing local recurrence, does not benefit survival except, perhaps, in Grade 3 lesions. The role of vaginal radium in this study may have been of benefit in decreasing vaginal recurrences but certainly would have little or no effect upon pelvic wall recurrences.

Joslin's group[33] reported on the results of postoperative radiotherapy in 256 cases of cancer of the corpus uteri treated between 1967 and 1973. Unfortunately, the stage is not stated. Like so many other clinics the approach of this group had previously been determined on ad hoc grounds. In this study they adopted a more formal approach by subdividing the patients into two groups (a) those with disease limited to the endometrium and (b) those with myometrial involvement. The former group was treated by intravaginal radiation using an obturator of suitable diameter and length whose central catheter is connected to an afterloading device (the Cathetron) capable of delivering a source of high activity [60]Cobalt. Five daily fractions were used to deliver a total of 35 Gy at 0.5 cm from the surface of the obturator. The latter group was treated by a combination of external irradiation and intravaginal therapy. To treat the lymph nodes, supervoltage therapy was given, in 15 fractions over 3 weeks, delivering a dose of 35 Gy. This was followed by intravaginal irradiation of 20 Gy given in 4 daily fractions of 5 Gy each.

The results showed an overall improvement compared with the previous ad hoc approach. Myometrial invasion was shown to be significantly related to histological grading as it was to recurrence rates. The results also substantiated those of other series in showing marked reduction in the incidence of vaginal vault recurrence, in this series only 3 of 256 cases. The addition of external beam therapy significantly improved survival in the group with deep myometrial spread. The commonest immediate reaction to treatment was diarrhea; 7% of patients with intracavitary and 50% of those with external irradiation. This symptom was more prevalent in the older age groups, so that the authors recommended that in women over 55 years of age, the dose of external therapy should not exceed 30 Gy. The most common late reaction was an adhesive vaginitis occurring in approximately 5% of all cases in both treatment groups, more especially in older women not exposed to regular intercourse.

Since radiation therapy may be beneficial only in patients with poor prognostic factors, it would seem prudent to evaluate these factors first and then apply irradiation selectively after surgery. The grade of the tumor can be determined before surgery, but the depth of myometrial invasion is unknown. Some patients with well differentiated lesions will have deep myometrial involvement, and it appears that in this small group the recurrence rate is higher and the survival is lower than a like grade lesion with limited invasion. Conversely, a poorly differentiated lesion limited to the endometrium would not seem to require the same therapy as a more differentiated tumor with significant myometrial invasion. By such post-surgical evaluation, specific therapy can then be applied to the individual patient.

Recommended surgery

Since individualized treatment for endometrial cancer appears to be desirable and since the true extent of the disease cannot be determined preoperatively, it would seem that the best approach is to perform surgery initially. From the foregoing discussion the following prognostic factors are important in Stage I and II endometrial cancer: size of the uterus, differentiation of the tumor, depth of myometrial involvement, subclinical adnexal metastases, tumor location in the uterus, peritoneal cytology, and pelvic and para-aortic lymph node metastases. Since 75% of all endometrial cancer is Stage I, these factors would seem even more pertinent in individualizing management.

In order to evaluate these multiple parameters a proper surgical procedure would be a conservative total abdominal hysterectomy, bilateral salpingo-oophorectomy, and selective pelvic and para-aortic lymphadenectomy (see also Ch. 80). The cervix is not sutured before the hysterectomy. Specimens for cytology should be obtained immediately upon opening the peritoneal cavity either by removing the fluid that is present in the cul-de-sac or irrigating the pelvis with saline. The pelvic lymphadenectomy is selective and not as thorough as in a standard pelvic lymphadenectomy for cervical cancer. The retroperitoneal spaces in the pelvis are entered, the vessels outlined, and any enlarged nodes are removed separately for histologic evaluation. In the absence of node enlargement the lymph-node bearing tissue along the external iliac vessels from the bifurcation of the common iliac vessels to the inguinal ligament is removed. The obturator fossa, anterior to (above) the obturator nerve is cleaned of the lymph node tissue. Any enlarged nodes along the common iliac vessels are also removed. No attempt at exploration behind the vessels is made. The use of hemovac drains in the retroperitoneal space has decreased the incidence of postoperative lymphocysts. The para-aortic node sampling is approached by retracting the small intestines into the upper abdomen, and incising the peritoneum over the upper common iliac artery and lower aorta. The main vessels are outlined and the tissue overlying the vena cava and aorta is removed beginning

at the bifurcation and extending cephalad. The upper limit of the dissection, unless enlarged nodes are noted above this area, is usually at the level of the second and third portion of the duodenum as it crosses the main vessels retroperitoneally. Hemostasis can be easily managed with hemoclips. Using this technique approximately 15 to 20 lymph nodes will be available for evaluation.

In a prospective surgical-pathologic study undertaken by the Gynecologic Oncology Group, 621 patients with clinical Stage I carcinoma of the endometrium were evaluated in regards to these multiple prognostic factors. 346 (56%) of the patients had a Stage Ia lesion, 235 patients had a Stage Ib. 180 (29%) patients had a well differentiated lesion while 158 (25%) had a poorly differentiated carcinoma. In 59%, only the endometrium and superficial myometrium (less than one-third depth invasion) were involved.

The grade of the tumor and the depth of myometrial invasion correlated well as has been previously reported; however, there were notable exceptions in that there were several patients with a Grade 3 lesion in which only the endometrium was involved, while in others a Grade 1 malignancy and deep muscle invasion was noted. 5% of the patients had occult disease present in the adnexa which was not recognized preoperatively. 58 (9.3%) had metastases in one or more pelvic lymph nodes. Some patients had grossly enlarged nodes while in most the metastasis was only recognized on histological examination. In some cases, the disease was in a single node, in others multiple nodes on one side, and there were some individuals who had bilateral positive pelvic nodes. 34 (5.4%) patients had para-aortic node metastases (Table 49.15). There was cor-

Table 49.15 Grade versus positive pelvic and aortic nodes

Grade	Pelvic	Aortic
G1 (N=180)	5 (3%)	3 (2%)
G2 (N=288)	25 (9%)	14 (5%)
G3 (N=153)	28 (18%)	17 (11%)

Modified from Creasman et al (1987) *Cancer* **60**: 2035

relation between pelvic and para-aortic nodal metastases and the size of the uterus (Table 49.16). When the grade of the tumor was correlated with pelvic or para-aortic node metastasis, again, an excellent correlation is noted (Table 49.16). Likewise, when the depth of invasion was correlated with nodal metastasis, the chance of having regional nodal metastases increased with the depth of myometrial invasion (Table 49.10). When the six sub-stages of Stage I carcinoma were evaluated for nodal metastasis, the incidence, both in Stage Ia and Stage Ib, increased as the tumor became less differentiated (Table 49.16). This relationship is also present when the depth of invasion is evaluated within each grade of the tumor, in that, as depth

Table 49.16 Stage and grade versus pelvic and aortic node metastasis

Stage		Pelvic	Aortic
IaG1	(N=101)	2 (2%)	0 (0%)
IaG2	(N=169)	13 (4%)	6 (4%)
IaG3	(N=76)	8 (11%)	5 (7%)
IbG1	(N=79)	3 (4%)	3 (4%)
IbG2	(N=119)	12 (10%)	8 (7%)
IbG3	(N=77)	20 (26%)	12 (16%)

Modified from Creasman et al (1987) *Cancer* **60**: 2035

increased within each grade, the chances of nodal metastasis also increased.

Adjunctive radiotherapy

Radiation therapy techniques in endometrial cancer are almost as varied as the articles appearing in the literature. Some prefer radium application only, others a combination of radium plus external radiation while still others would treat with only external radiation. Newer forms of intracavitary radiation including afterloading techniques and radium substitutes (e.g. [137]cesium or [60]cobalt) have been used. The recommended interval from radiation to hysterectomy varies from immediate to 6 weeks or more. Other investigators give radiation therapy post-hysterectomy either routinely or depending upon pathologic evaluation of the operative specimen. Many advocate primary surgery alone for well differentiated carcinoma in a small uterus but give adjunctive radiation where a high risk is indicated by the pathology. (See also p. 236.)

In view of the previous discussion of the advantages of prior surgery it is proper to describe the postoperative techniques first. In all technical descriptions, pre- and postoperative, which follow, the authority of Fletcher[21] will be recognized. Vaginal ovoids are applied to give 60 to 70 Gy surface dose. If deep myometrial invasion is present without extra-uterine spread, 40 to 45 Gy external radiation to the whole pelvis is given over 4 to 5 weeks. The fields should cover the upper one-third to one-half of the vagina. Vaginal radium is probably unnecessary in this circumstance. When lymph node metastases have been identified, external radiation should be given to the appropriate fields. If only pelvic nodes are involved, 50 Gy over 5 to 6 weeks to the pelvic area can be given. If para-aortic lymph node involvement is present, radiation of this area to the level of T-12 should be added in a dosage of 40 to 45 Gy. When higher doses are given to the para-aortic area, complications mainly referable to the small bowel are appreciable.

In those clinics where preoperative irradiation is in routine use there has been a tendency to individualize the treatment. In the presence of a small uterine cavity, a uterine tandem and vaginal ovoids are inserted to give 3000 to 3500 mg-hrs and 70 Gy surface dose respectively in one application. Hysterectomy follows immediately. With a moderately enlarged uterus and well differentiated tumor, two Heyman-type packings or tandem applications, 2 to 3 weeks apart, each to give 2500 mg-hrs to the uterus, are advocated. Vaginal ovoids are used to give a surface dose of 80 Gy if two applications are used or 70 Gy with a single application. Hysterectomy follows immediately after completion of the second treatment. In both groups of patients postoperative external radiation (approximately 40 Gy) to the whole pelvis may be added if deep myometrial invasion is noted. When the uterus is large or an anaplastic tumor is present, 40 Gy of external radiation to the whole pelvis (15 × 15 cm) is given preoperatively over 4 weeks. This is then followed with a Heyman-type packing or tandem application to the uterus to give 2500 mg-hrs and together with vaginal ovoids to give a surface dose of 40 Gy. The hysterectomy is performed 4 to 6 weeks later.

In the patients who are inoperable for whatever reason, radiotherapy should also be individualized. However, there are today few patients, whether due to age or medical disorder, who should be judged inoperable. The patient with a small or normal size uterine cavity and a well differentiated tumor is treated with two radium applications usually a tandem and vaginal ovoids. Two 72 hour applications give a uterine dose of 5000 to 6000 mg-hrs and a vaginal surface dose of 80 Gy. The implants are inserted 2 to 3 weeks apart. If a patient has a moderately enlarged uterus a similar schedule is recommended. If Heyman packing is used, care must be taken to insert as many capsules as possible so that the uterine wall can be 'thinned' and the radiation source placed as close as possible to the tumor. In the patient with the large uterus or anaplastic tumor the irradiation protocol is similar to that just described for preoperative management of the same conditions except that the external irradiation is followed by two radium applications (Heyman or tandem) to give 3500 to 4000 mg-hrs to the uterus. The surface dose to the vagina from the ovoids should be 40 Gy.

There is a small group of patients who require special consideration. The large GOG study[13] reported positive peritoneal washings for malignant cells in approximately 16% of patients with early corpus cancer. Follow-up of these cases revealed an increased relapse rate. The use of intraperitoneal radiocolloid (^{32}P) or abdominal radiation for patients with positive peritoneal cytology is currently being evaluated.

Adjunctive hormonal and cytotoxic chemotherapy

The use of hormones and cytotoxic agents in the adjunctive therapy of patients with early endometrial cancer has not proved effective. A report of the use of progestational agents in treatment of recurrent disease appeared in 1962. Kelly & Baker[37] reported a response rate up to 37%. The treatment is now popular for both recurrence and advanced disease (see Ch. 50). Progestin therapy, usually administered by intramuscular or oral routes, offers the advantage of therapeutic response with very limited toxicity. In a large, multi-institutional study Lewis and associates[45] prospectively evaluated two groups of patients with endometrial carcinoma limited to the corpus (Stage I). Medroxyprogesterone or placebo was given randomly to 285 and 287 patients respectively over 14 weeks prior to surgery or surgery plus radiotherapy. Survival at 4 years showed no significant improvement in the hormone-treated group.

Decoster, Bonte & Marcq[18] have suggested that intracavitary hormonal therapy may be as effective as intracavitary irradiation preoperatively in patients with Stage I carcinoma of the endometrium. The advantage of the micronized medroxyprogesterone acetate in silastic elastomer is its freedom from the side effects of radiation on neighboring organs. They report their early experience as total destruction of the carcinoma in approximately 60% of patients treated preoperatively with either intracavitary radium or intracavitary medroxyprogesterone acetate. In patients with myometrial infiltration, the number of patients with residual foci of disease was similar in both groups. The hormone group was free of radiation side effects, and additionally there was the theoretical advantage of systemic absorption of hormone.

Cytotoxic chemotherapy as an adjuvant is a recent development. Donovan[20] in 1974 reviewed the scattered reports in the literature concerning the use of various single cytotoxic agents in patients with endometrial carcinoma. The majority of these patients reportedly had advanced disease, and a shortcoming of these reports was failure to define 'regression'. Nevertheless, the overall responders were 27%. Active agents included 5-fluorouracil (25%), cyclophosphamide (28%) and adriamycin (38%).

The Gynecologic Oncology Group initiated a study concerning the effectiveness and tolerance of adjuvant cytotoxic therapy. Adriamycin after surgery and radiotherapy for Stage I patients who had unsuspected disease outside of the uterus, deep myometrial invasion, cervical involvement or nodal disease, was compared to patients not receiving adriamycin. There were 23% recurrences in the adriamycin arm versus 26% in the non-adriamycin arm. The site of recurrence was greater in the abdomen in the adriamycin-treated patients but distant metastases were higher in those not receiving adriamycin. The role of adjunctive therapy in high risk patients with early stage disease has not been found to be effective to date.

CONCLUSIONS

It would appear from the material presented that corpus cancer is a more significant entity than previously regarded. Since approximately 75% of all endometrial cancer is Stage I, prognostic factors assume greater significance in determining therapy on an individual basis. For appropriate evaluation of these factors, one must examine the surgical specimen in critical detail. We feel the best approach is to proceed with a total abdominal hysterectomy and bilateral salpingo-oophorectomy and, particularly for the more anaplastic Grade 2 and Grade 3 lesions, selective pelvic and para-aortic lymphadenectomy. Peritoneal cytology should be obtained immediately upon entering the peritoneal cavity. The histological data may then be reviewed. In many instances, surgery alone will be adequate. If poor prognostic factors such as deep myometrial involvement, adnexal metastases, or lymph node metastases are present, radiation therapy could then be tailored to the specifically involved areas. By following such a protocol, one would hope that optimal individualized therapy would be applied to each patient in some instances saving unnecessary radiation while in others directing radiation to the appropriate areas for improved survival. The role of adjunctive chemotherapy in these high risk patients is currently lacking. Although selected studies have shown a 90% or better survival in Stage I carcinoma of the endometrium, the last report from the International Federation of Gynecologists and Obstetricians notes only a 75% 5-year survival.

Several options are available for the treatment of Stage II carcinoma. The conventional approach consists of external or intracavitary irradiation followed by simple hysterectomy with bilateral salpingo-oophorectomy, as described for Stage I patients with large or anaplastic tumors (see p. 786). We prefer to combine this operation with pelvic and para-aortic lymphadenectomy prior to selected external irradiation. This approach allows the more thorough evaluation of nodal status and the earlier detection of disease which may be outside the portals of conventional teletherapy. We have not recommended the use of the radical Wertheim hysterectomy for Stage II patients as they tend to be elderly, obese and require radiation therapy.

REFERENCES

1. Abate S D, Edwards C L, Vellios F 1972 A comparative study of the endometrial jet-washing technic and endometrial biopsy. Am J Clin Path 58: 118

2. Anderson B, Marchant D J, Munzenrider J E, Moore J P, Mitchell G W Jr 1976 Routine noninvasive hysterography in the evaluation and treatment of endometrial carcinoma. Gynecol Oncol 4: 354

3. Arneson A 1936 Clinical results and histologic changes following

the radiation treatment of cancer of the corpus uteri. Am J Roentgenol 36: 461

4. Boronow R C, Morrow C P, Creasman W T et al 1985 Surgical staging in endometrial cancer. Clinical pathologic findings of prospective study. Obstet Gynecol 63: 825

5. Bruckner H W, Deppe G 1977 Intensive combination chemotherapy of advanced endometrial adenocarcinoma with adriamycin, cyclophosphamide, 5-fluorouracil, and medroxyprogesterone acetate. Obstet Gynecol 50: 10

6. Butler E B, Monahan P B, Warrell D W 1971 Kuper brush in the diagnosis of endometrial lesions. Lancet ii: 1390

7. Cancer Statistics 1988 CA — A Cancer Journal for Clinicians 38: 5

8. Caspi E, Perpinial S, Reif A 1977 Incidence of malignancy in Jewish women with post-menopausal bleeding. Israel J Med Sci 13: 299

9. Chatfield W R, Bremner A D 1972 Intrauterine sponge biopsy. Obstet Gynecol 39: 323

10. Cheon H K 1969 Prognosis of endometrial carcinoma. Obstet Gynecol 34: 680

11. Cohen C J, Deppe G, Bruckner H W 1977 Treatment of advanced adenocarcinoma of the endometrium with melphalan, 5-fluorouracil, and medroxyprogesterone acetate. A preliminary study. Obstet Gynecol 50: 415

12. Cohen C J, Gusberg S B 1975 Screening for endometrial cancer. Clin Obstet Gynecol 18: 27

13. Creasman W T, Morrow C P, Bundy L et al 1987 The surgical pathologic spread pattern of endometrial cancer. A Gynecologic Oncology Group Study. Cancer 60: 2035

14. Creasman W T, Rutledge F N 1971 The prognostic value of peritoneal cytology in gynecologic malignant disease. Am J Obstet Gynecol 110: 773

15. Creasman W T, Weed J C Jr 1976 Screening techniques in endometrial cancer. Cancer 38: 436

16. Cullen T H 1900 Cancer of the Uterus. Saunders, Philadelphia

17. Damon A 1960 Host factors in cancer of the breast and uterine cervix and corpus. J Natl Cancer Inst 24: 483

18. Decoster J M, Bonte J, Marcq A 1977 Medroxyprogesterone acetate release from silastic devices as replacement for local irradiation by radium tubes in preoperative intrauterine packing for endometrial adenocarcinoma. A preliminary study. Gynecol Oncol 5: 189

19. De Muelenaere G F 1975 Prognostic factors in endometrial carcinoma S Afr Med J 49: 1695

20. Donovan J F 1974 Non-hormonal chemotherapy of endometrial adenocarcinoma. Cancer 34: 1587

21. Fletcher G H 1973 Textbook of Radiotherapy. Lea and Febiger, Philadelphia

22. Frick H C, Munnell E W, Richart R M, Berger A P, Lawry M F 1973 Carcinoma of endometrium. Am J Obstet Gynecol 115: 663

23. Greenblatt R B, Stoddard L D 1978 The estrogen — cancer controversy. J Am Geriat Soc 26: 1

24. Gusberg S B, Kardon P 1971 Proliferative endometrial response to theca-granulosa cell tumors. Am J Obstet Gynecol 3: 633

25. Healy W P, Brown R 1939 Experience with surgical radiation therapy in carcinoma of the corpus uteri. Am J Obstet Gynecol 38: 1

26. Heyman J 1935 The so-called Stockholm method and the results of treatment of uterine cancer at Radiumhemmet. Acta Radiol 16: 129

27. Hofmeister F J 1974 Endometrial biopsy. Another look. Am J Obstet Gynecol 118: 773

28. Husslein H, Breitenecker G, Tatra G 1978 Premalignant and malignant uterine changes in immunosuppressed renal transplant recipients. Acta Obstet Gynecol Scand 57: 73

29. Javert C T 1952 The spread of benign and malignant endometrium in the lymphatic system with a note on co-existing vascular involvement. Am J Obstet Gynecol 64: 780

30. Javert C T, Douglas R 1956 Treatment of endometrial carcinoma. Am J Roentgenol 75: 508

31. Johnsson J E, Norman O 1979 Relation between prognosis in early carcinoma of the uterine body and hysterographically assessed localization and the size of tumor. Gynecol Oncol 7: 71

32. Jones H W 1975 Treatment of adenocarcinoma of the endometrium. Obstet Gynecol Surv 30: 147

33. Joslin C A, Vaishamtayan G V, Mallick A 1977 The treatment of early cancer of the corpus uteri. Br J Radiol 50: 38

34. Kademian M T, Buchler D A, Wirtanen G W 1977 Bipedal lymphangiography in malignancies of the uterine corpus. Am J Roentgenol 129: 903

35. Kaplan S D, Cole P 1980 Epidemiology of cancer of the endometrium. In Press

36. Kelly H A 1916 Radium therapy in cancer of the uterus. Transactions American Gynecological Society 41: 532

37. Kelly R M, Baker W H 1961 Progestational agents in the treatment of carcinoma of the endometrium. N Eng J Med 264: 216

38. Kistner R W 1970 The effects of progesteronal agents on hyperplasia and carcinoma in situ of the endometrium. Int J Gynecol Obstet 8: 561

39. Kohorn E I 1976 Gestagens and endometrial carcinoma. Gynecol Oncol 4: 398

40. Kottmeier H, Kolstad P (eds) Annual Report Gynecological Cancer FIGO Vol 16 Stockholm

41. Lauritzen C 1977 Oestrogens and endometrial cancer: a point of view. Clinics Obstet Gynecol 4: 145

42. Lees D H 1969 An evaluation of treatment in carcinoma of the body of the uterus. J Obstet Gynaecol Br Commonw 76: 615

43. Lefèvre H 1956 Node dissection in cancer of the endometrium. Surg Gynecol Obstet 102: 649

44. Lewis B V, Stallworthy J A, Cowdell R 1970 Adenocarcinoma of the body of the uterus. J Obstet Gynaecol Br Commonw 77: 343

45. Lewis G C Jr, Slack N H, Mortel R, Bross I D J 1974 Adjuvant progestogen therapy in the primary definitive treatment of endometrial cancer. Gynecol Oncol 2: 368

46. Lloyd R E, Jones S E, Salmon S E 1975 Southwest oncology group members: 'Phase II trial of adriamycin and cyclophosphamide: A southwest oncology group pilot study'. Proc Am Assoc Cancer Res 16: 265

47. Lutz M H, Underwood P B Jr, Kreutner A Jr, Miller M C 1978 Endometrial carcinoma: a new method of classification of therapeutic and prognostic significance. Gynecol Oncol 6: 83

48. McCarty K S Jr, Barton T K, Peete C H Jr, Creasman W T 1978 Gonadal dysgenesis with adenocarcinoma of the endometrium. An electron-microscopic and steroid receptor analysis with a review of the literature. Cancer 42: 512

49. McDonald T W, Malkasian G D, Gaffey T A 1977 Endometrial cancer associated with feminizing ovarian tumor and polycystic ovarian disease. Obstet Gynecol 49: 654

50. MacMahon B 1974 Risk factors for endometrial cancer. Gynecol Oncol 2: 122

51. Mahle A E 1923 The morphological histology of adenocarcinoma of the body of the uterus in relation to longevity. Surg Gynecol Obstet 36: 385

52. Mansell H, Hertig A T 1955 Granulosa-theca cell tumors and endometrial carcinoma. A study of their relationship and a survey of 80 cases. Obstet Gynecol 6: 385

53. Masubuchi K, Nemoto H 1972 Epidemiologic studies on uterine cancer at Cancer Institute hospital. Tokyo, Japan. Cancer 30: 268

54. Mattingly R F 1977 Malignant tumors of the uterus. TeLinde's Operative Gynecology, 5th Edn. Lippincott, Philadelphia, p 779

55. Milan A R, Markley R L, Fisher R S, Linthicum C M, Witherspoon B, Eidschun A G 1976 Endometrial cytology. Using the Milan-Markley technic. Obstet Gynecol 48: 111

56. Monson R R, MacMahon B, Austin J H 1973 Postoperative irradiation in carcinoma of the endometrium. Cancer 31: 630

57. Morrow C P, DiSaia P J, Townsend D E 1973 Current management of endometrial carcinoma. Obstet Gynecol 42: 399

58. Muggia F M, Perloff M, Chia G A, Juden-Reed L, Escher G C 1974 Adriamycin (NSC123127) in combination with cyclophosphamide (NSC26271): A phase I and II evaluation. Cancer Chemotherapy Rep 58: 919

59. Ng A B, Reagan J W, Hawliczek S, Wentz W B 1974 Significance of endometrial cells in the detection of endometrial carcinoma and its precursors. Acta Cytol 18: 356

60. Nolan J F, Huen A 1976 Prognosis in endometrial cancer. Gynecol Oncol 4: 384

61. Norris H J, Taylor H B 1968 Prognosis of granulosa thecal tumor of the ovary. Cancer 21: 255

62. Novak E, Yui E 1936 Relation of endometrial hyperplasia to adenocarcinoma of the uterus. Am J Obstet Gynecol 32: 674

63. Onsrud M, Kolstad P, Norman T 1976 Postoperative external pelvic irradiation in carcinoma of the corpus Stage I: A controlled clinical trial. Gynecol Oncol 4: 222

64. Ostör A G, Fortune D W, Evans J H, Kneale B L 1978 Endometrial carcinoma in gonadal dysgenesis with and without estrogen therapy. Gynecol Oncol 6: 316

65. Plentyl A A, Friedman E A 1971 Lymphatic System of the Female Genitalia: The Morphologic Basis of Oncologic Diagnosis and Therapy. Saunders, Philadelphia, p 123

66. Rauramo L 1978 Estrogen replacement therapy and endometrial carcinoma. Front Hormone Res 5: 117

67. Rutledge F N 1974 The role of radical hysterectomy in adenocarcinoma of the endometrium. Gynecol Oncol 2: 331

68. Rutledge F N, Tan S K, Fletcher G H 1958 Vaginal metastases from adenocarcinoma of the corpus uteri. Am J Obstet Gynecol 75: 167

68a. Salazar O M, Bonfiglio T A, Patten S F et al 1978 Uterine sarcomas: natural history, treatment and prognosis. Cancer 42: 1152

69. Sall S, Sonnenblick B, Stone M L 1970 Factors affecting survival of patients with endometrial adenocarcinoma. Am J Obstet Gynecol 107: 116

70. Schwartz P E, Kohorn E I, Knowlton A H, Morris J McL 1975 Routine use of hysterography in endometrial carcinoma and postmenopausal bleeding. Obstet Gynecol 45: 378

71. Segaloff A 1975 Steroids and carcinogenesis. J Steroid Biochem 6: 171

72. Silverberg E 1975 Gynecologic cancer: statistical and epidemiological information. American Cancer Society Publication

73. Silverberg E, Holleb A 1971 Cancer Statistics 1971. CA — A Cancer Journal for Clinicians 21: 13

74. Speert H 1949 Carcinoma of the endometrium in young women. Surg Gynecol Obstet 88: 332

75. Surwit E A, Fowler W C Jr, Rogoff E E et al 1979 Stage II carcinoma of the endometrium. Int J Radiation Oncol Biol Phys 5: 323

76. Tak W K, Anderson B, Vardi J R, Beecham J B, Marchant D J 1977 Myometrial invasion and hysterography in endometrial carcinoma. Obstet Gynecol 50: 159

77. Wharam M D, Philips T L, Bagshaw M A 1976 The role of radiation therapy in clinical stage I carcinoma of the endometrium. Int J Radiat Oncol Biol Phys 1: 1081

78. Wolff J R, Goldfarb E, Rumeau-Rouquette C, Breart G 1975 The value of hysterogram for the prognosis of endometrial cancer. Gynecol Oncol 3: 103

79. Wynder E L, Escher G C, Mantel N 1966 An epidemiological investigation of cancer of the endometrium. Cancer 19: 489

50. Advanced (FIGO Stages III and IV) and recurrent carcinoma of the endometrium

C. J. Cohen

GENERAL CONSIDERATIONS

Endometrial carcinoma has traditionally been viewed as a neoplasm with diminished virulence when compared to the other gynecologic cancers. In the past this assumption has invited a complacency among the therapeutic community which, in fact, is unjustified. If one inspects the treatment reports summarized in the Annual Report of the International Federation of Gynecology and Obstetrics,[53] it will be apparent that only 67.7% of women with endometrial cancer are alive and free of disease 5 years after treatment. One may ascribe this failure to three general features: (1) imperfect application of proven therapeutic techniques, (2) understaging or application of therapeutic techniques to inappropriate fields, and (3) aggressive biology of the tumor or diminished host response which combine to resist appropriately applied known therapeutic modalities. For two decades, investigators retrospectively studied the patterns of spread of endometrial carcinoma, including the distribution of invaded lymph nodes and blood vessels. The systematic prospective staging study completed by the Gynecologic Oncology Group[18] has verified the relationship between cell differentiation, depth of myometrial invasion, and presence of cancer in the regional and aortic lymph nodes. From these data, it is clear that poorly differentiated cancers, even in clinically early disease, will have spread beyond conventional treatment fields with greater frequency than has been appreciated. In the last 20 years, there has been an increase in the incidence of endometrial cancer[78] in the United States, and in many therapeutic centers it is the most common gynecologic cancer treated. This observation has variously been ascribed to an increase in the life expectancy of the American female, an increase in the accuracy of diagnostic techniques and their greater application, and improvement in data collection and reporting. However, others have suggested that many of the factors associated with the development of endometrial cancer, such as high percentage of unsaturated fat in the diet, exposure to exogenous estrogen, obesity, diminished parity, and exposure to exogenous carcinogens, are intensified in

the Western world. An interesting and still classic model for this concept is provided by the observation of a changing cancer risk for Japanese females who migrate to the United States. Haenszel & Kurohara[36] report that these women experienced a diminished incidence of cancer of the stomach and cervix compared to their Japanese cohorts; however, their incidence of cancer of the endometrium doubled, approaching the incidence among United States-born Caucasians.

The final consideration in assessing the possibility of having to treat advanced or recurrent endometrial carcinoma is the consideration that more virulent forms of this cancer are emerging. Over a decade ago, Reagan[58] described a rising incidence of adenosquamous carcinoma of the endometrium which comprised almost one-third of the endometrial neoplasms in his institution. He found a sharp diminution in survival among patients with this histologic variant. While this increase was not noted universally in the United States, and while today there is a convention to ignore the squamous element in this histologic variant and assign virulence according to the degree of differentiation of the adenocarcinoma, there does seem to be an increase in the incidence of poorly differentiated lesions. Some have noted these to occur with greater incidence as a function of age; others have suggested that exposure to estrogen alone, while increasing the risk of endometrial cancer, produces a lesion of diminished virulence. Nevertheless there is general agreement that the poorly differentiated lesions are increasing in incidence, are more virulent, spread more rapidly, involve lymph nodes more often, and are less frequently cured.

Thus, since life expectancy in the West among females is increasing and since endometrial carcinoma is rising in incidence and virulence; since adequate staging techniques are being employed more frequently; it is reasonable to expect that more patients will be seen with recognized advanced disease at the time of initial therapy, or that more patients will be seen with residual or recurrent disease after initial therapy. We can expect this therapeutic challenge in more than one out of three of all patients with endometrial

791

cancer. Since more than 90% of all neoplasms of the endometrium are adenocarcinomas, we will confine our discussion to cancers of this histologic designation.

PATTERNS OF SPREAD

If one is to identify endometrial carcinoma in extrauterine sites prior to initial therapy, an understanding of the routes of extension is essential. Contiguous spread from the endometrial surface into the endocervical canal, the fallopian tube, or penetration into the myometrium occurs commonly. Invasion of blood vessels can explain distant metastases to lung, bone, and other sites, and such vascular invasion can be identified in the surgical specimen by careful inspection. Retrograde spill of cancer cells through the fallopian tubes into the peritoneal cavity has been observed. In the recent experience of the Gynecologic Oncology Group, approximately 15% of all patients with Stage I and II endometrial cancers[19] who were examined by staging laparotomy had positive or suspicious peritoneal cytology. The survival in these patients was markedly diminished in spite of their early clinical stage. Others[47] have verified this observation.

Cervical invasion by the tumor, especially when grossly observable, exposes the patient not only to the conventional patterns of spread from the corpus itself but also makes available transport of tumor through the cervical lymphatic network. This observation was suggested by Stallworthy[67] who found that at the time of radical hysterectomy for endometrial carcinoma, patients in FIGO Stage II had positive lymph nodes 41% of the time.

The lymphatics of the uterus have been well described[56] and the importance of selective lymphadenectomy for staging has been explained elsewhere (see Ch. 49). Only by careful application of staging techniques can one identify extrauterine extension of cancer at the time of initial therapy and thus construct a proper therapeutic plan.

PATTERNS OF RECURRENCE

Most recurrences are diagnosed before the completion of the second year following therapy. While recurrences have been noted more than 10 years after therapy, in most series at least 85% of the recurrences have been diagnosed by the fifth year following therapy. Representative series may be inspected in Table 50.1. Less well differentiated tumors tend to recur earlier and tend to be found in the lower vagina or in distant sites. Well differentiated tumors recur later and, more frequently, involve the upper vagina, either as isolated lesions or in combination with pelvic sites of recurrence. In recent years, with wider employment of radiation therapy as an adjuvant to hysterectomy, the incidence of isolated vaginal recurrence has diminished significantly. A summary of the effect of radiation therapy in diminishing vaginal vault recurrence may be inspected in Table 50.2. Thus, the site of recurrence is related not only to the virulence of the tumor but the type of therapy initially employed. For example, Spanos[65] observed that on the basis of staging laparotomy data at the M. D. Anderson Hospital, pelvic lymph node involvement occurred in 11% of patients with early endometrial cancers. When, at this same institution, 431 patients were treated with preoperative radiation therapy followed by conservative hysterectomy, the overall clinical recurrence rate in pelvic nodes was 1%. The recurrence rate in the same series for vaginal sites was 3% and for central pelvic structures was 3%. In a study of Stage I endometrial cancer performed at the Norwegian Radium Hospital,[52] all patients were treated postoperatively with radiation therapy, consisting of a 60 Gy (6000 rads) vaginal surface dose. Patients were then randomized into two groups. One group was given external radiation of 40 Gy (4000 rads) to whole pelvis and the other group received no further therapy. Clinically, the group receiving only vaginal radium experienced a pelvic wall recurrence of 2.5%, whereas when the whole pelvis was treated, there were no pelvic wall recurrences.

More recently, Chambers et al[11] have demonstrated that radiation therapy to the pelvis, whether administered by intracavitary and/or external source, either preoperatively or postoperatively, or both, diminishes the incidence of

Table 50.1 Time from initial treatment to recurrence: cumulative percentage by year

Author	No. of pts.	6 mths %	1 year %	2 years %	3 years %	4 years %	5 years %
Badib[2]	300	10	20	50	70	78	85
Copenhaver[17]	29	—	24	48	58	72	83
Finn[29]	49	40	55	67	67	78	—
[a]Boronow[5]	95	—	41	—	87	—	93
Dede[21]	124	20	30	62	70	—	90

[a] Cumulative percent of those dying of recurrence

Table 50.2 Vaginal recurrences following therapy: hysterectomy alone vs hysterectomy & radiation (modified from Cohen and Gusberg, 1970)[15]

Author	Treatment	Patients No.	Vaginal recurrences
Gusberg	Hysterectomy	191	14.6
	Hysterectomy & Radiation	219	4.5
Boutselis	Hysterectomy	61	14.7
	Hysterectomy & Radiation	208	1.8
Wade	Hysterectomy	43	9.3
	Hysterectomy & Radiation	156	1.9

vaginal vault and pelvic recurrence. However, in poorly differentiated lesions, it does not seem to change survival patterns. The most frequent site of recurrence in such patients is pulmonary and upper abdominal.

Thus, the evolution of new therapeutic plans will alter the patterns of recurrence.

DIAGNOSIS OF RECURRENCE

All patients treated for endometrial cancer require a frequent, careful, and complete physical examination every 3 to 4 months for the first 3 years following treatment and then less frequently until the fifth year, when an annual examination should suffice. During these examinations, periodic cytologic sampling from the vagina should be made. Previous radiation therapy may confuse cytologic findings; however, abnormalities will be detected prior to clinically detectable recurrence and careful, systematic biopsies from the vagina should be made when cytology is abnormal. The value of non-invasive radiographic scanning techniques is controversial because the accuracy is largely dependent on the artistry of the radiologist. We have noted variability in skills within our own institution. A recent analysis of our own data comparing the accuracy of sonography, CT scan, and MRI, by the same group of expert radiologists examining patients with gynecologic cancers demonstrated no advantage for any single technique.[7] Chest X-ray should be performed at least every 6 months for the first 2 years and then annually. CT scan of the chest should be selectively applied, especially in patients who have G2 or G3 lesions. Clinical enlargement of the liver should be clarified by radioisotope scanning and directed biopsy when indicated.

When a mass is identified on physical examination, biopsy should be performed, either by needle aspiration or by excision to verify the diagnosis. If a lesion is noted on chest X-ray, confirmed as a single lesion by radiographic techniques, and if a metastatic investigation reveals no evidence of disease elsewhere, we have no hesitation in recommending surgical excision if the lesion is amenable to segmental resection. At the time of excision of any possible recurrence, tissue should be collected for assay of estrogen and progesterone receptors to assist in predicting possible response to hormone treatment should it be instituted. An increasing number of investigators have studied the value of measuring newly acquired serum proteins in the blood of patients with proven gynecologic cancers. Van Nagell[75] and his colleagues have found that carcinoembryonic antigen (CEA) levels are elevated in 67% of patients with poorly differentiated lesions and when patients have recurrent endometrial cancer, elevations in the serum CEA may be detectable several months prior to clinical diagnosis. Several investigators[26,53,51] have verified Nyloff's first observation that CA125 measurements in patients with endometrial cancer were elevated in 78% of patients with Stage IV or recurrent endometrial carcinoma, but normal in patients with early disease. Patsner found that 90% of 31 patients with surgically staged endometrial adenocarcinoma who were found to have extrauterine disease had elevations of CA125 levels. Duk and his colleagues found that patients with clinically confined disease who had invasion of lymphatic or vascular spaces were more likely to have elevated CA125 levels even though there was no surgical evidence of distant metastasis.

MANAGEMENT

Surgical treatment

Advanced carcinoma (Stages III and IV)

The role of surgery in patients with Stages III or IV endometrial carcinoma is controversial since in most series individualization has been essential. Because surgery will not be curative for most such patients, the reasonableness of a surgical approach has been questioned. If the diagnosis is made at the time of laparotomy, surgery should be accomplished only to improve the patient's candidacy for adjuvant or subsequent combined therapy with other modalities. While the concept of cytoreduction has not been justified in prospective trials, if one extrapolates from the experience with ovarian carcinoma, where cytoreduction is essential for a proven chemosensitive tumor, then for endometrial carcinoma, a somewhat less chemosensitive tumor, cytoreduction would seem even more attractive. Resection of masses, omentum, enlarged lymph nodes, invaded intestine, as well as removal of uterus, tubes and ovaries would seem desirable.

Routine radical hysterectomy would not seem indicated if one inspects the experience of Javert,[39] Brunschwig & Murphy.[9] In these collected series of 110 patients, 27 had positive lymph nodes of whom 6 survived 5 years. The experience of Stallworthy[67] is not appreciably different. Since many patients with adenocarcinoma of the endometrium are aged and obese, we prefer to reduce the tumor burden to microscopic levels surgically and to apply postoperative adjuvant treatment. This can best be accomplished by extrafascial hysterectomy with selective pelvic and aortic lymphadenectomy, and removal of tumor masses rather than routine radical hysterectomy and complete lymphadenectomy.

Recurrent carcinoma

Surgery for recurrent carcinoma requires even more individualization. Patients who have been treated previously with radiation therapy alone and who have recurrent disease in the cervix, uterus or upper vagina may profit from local extirpation. Those patients with central pelvic recurrences of a bulky nature may occasionally be candidates for pelvic exenteration. Barber and Brunschwig reported on 36 patients treated by exenteration.[3] 14 had anterior exenteration of whom two survived for 5 years; 22 had a total exenteration of whom three survived for 5 years. There are doubtless patients for whom an exenterative procedure is indicated; however, such circumstances would appear to be unusual.

Radiotherapy

Advanced carcinoma (Stages III and IV)

When patients are found to have disease outside of the uterus but confined to the pelvis, after initial surgery has been completed, postoperative radiation to the whole pelvis is commonly employed. The aim of laparotomy should be removal of the uterus and adnexa and any bulky disease. Lymph node sampling should be performed and removal of enlarged lymph nodes should be carried out. However, complete lymphadenectomy should be avoided if radiation is to be employed because the complication rate from the combined treatment will be increased. The margins of dissection should be clearly marked with metallic clips and areas from which positive lymph nodes are taken should be identified similarly. Meticulous postoperative description of the distribution of disease will aid in localization for radiation therapy planning. Structures to be included in the radiation fields are identified by verification films with the patient in the precise treatment position, either on a simulator or under the machine. The equipment available for radiation therapy varies among institutions. However, the aim of therapy should be to deliver 40–50 Gy to the whole pelvis either by parallel-opposed or 4-field beam directed techniques over a period of 4 to 5 weeks. When the whole pelvis has been treated to 50 Gy a smaller field should be constructed for additional treatment to known areas of residual disease. For example, an additional 15 Gy can be delivered to one pelvic side wall or to an 8 × 8 cm field

which would include the upper vaginal vault. Another alternative is the introduction of intracavitary radiation by ovoids or colpostats to administer a 40 Gy vaginal surface dose if there is residual disease in the upper vagina and no more than 50 Gy has been administered by external therapy. For lesions which are irregular or which extend deeply beneath the vaginal mucosa, interstitial radiation may be useful.

For patients in whom cytologic washings are the only evidence of extrauterine spread of disease, the administration of intraperitoneal radioisotopes may provide therapeutic benefit. The most frequently employed isotope is ^{32}P and it can be administered postoperatively prior to the patient's discharge with appropriate surveillance after proof of absence of loculation because of postoperative adhesions.

When common iliac or para-aortic lymph nodes are involved, some would treat these regions by radiation therapy. The extended field should include the entire para-aortic lymph node chain with a field up to T12 and 8 cm in width. A dose of 45 to 55 Gy in 4 to $6\frac{1}{2}$ weeks can be delivered at a dose of 8.5 Gy per week. Several individual reports have suggested 5-year survival rates of 40% for patients with microscopic disease but meager survival for patients with gross para-aortic disease.[4,28,57,45]

An alternate radiation therapy plan for patients with disease outside of the pelvis would be treatment to the whole abdomen either with open field or moving strip technique followed by a pelvic boost to 50 Gy.[31]

Because patients with endometrial carcinoma are often obese, aged, and arteriosclerotic, the complications from para-aortic radiation might not be justified in view of the low probability of eradicating disease in this region. Suppression of the bone marrow by total pelvic radiation therapy with extended para-aortic fields will be significant, and this will limit the possibilities for subsequent cytotoxic chemotherapy. Thus, when disease is present outside of the pelvis at the time of laparotomy, we prefer to limit the radiation therapy to smaller volumes where disease control is possible, and to treat the patient systemically, either by hormone therapy, by cytotoxic chemotherapy or by a combination of both depending on the differentiation of the tumor and the presence or absence of hormone receptors.

Recurrent or residual disease outside of the abdomen is often best treated with systemic therapy. An exception, however, is the bone metastasis which frequently is painful or causes significant dysfunction. Radiation therapy of such a lesion can produce rapid amelioration of symptoms. Ideally, the field should be large enough to include the entire area of metastasis, and it is preferable to construct a single field. Parallel-opposed fields may be required if the lesion is extensive or if it is located in the midline of the trunk. A single exposure of 12 Gy, tumor dose, will usually control pain. Small areas of metastasis to the long bones or to selected segments of the spine can be treated well by 20 Gy tumor dose, administered in 1 week. When multiple metastases exist in the skull, they may be treated by the administration of 40 Gy tumor dose, over a period of 4 weeks. We prefer to treat the thorax by radiation therapy only when there is obstruction of vital structures, requiring immediate relief. In this case, a tumor dose of 40 Gy administered through two parallel-opposed fields over a 4-week period will provide palliation. The field size should be kept deliberately small so as not to complicate subsequent therapy with cytotoxic agents.

Finally, when the patient is observed to have Stage III endometrial carcinoma on clinical evaluation and is not a candidate for any surgical exercise, one may treat the whole pelvis with 40 Gy over 4 weeks by external radiation and then add intracavitary treatment to the uterus by a packing technique which delivers 3000 to 4000 mg hours. Vaginal colpostats can be applied to give a surface dose of 40 Gy. Occasionally, the uterine cavity will be so diminished in size after the external radiation therapy that packing is not efficient or valuable. In such cases, a single application of uterine tandem and colpostats for a dose of 3500 to 4000 mg hours will complete the treatment. If it is technically impossible to insert carriers into the uterus either because of irregularities in the cavity, cervical stenosis, distortion of the vagina or other anatomic variance, then the whole pelvis may be treated with up to 55 Gy of external radiation, and a smaller field can be applied to include the uterus, cervix and vagina to complete the radiation.

When the disease extends primarily to the vagina and the patient is not a surgical candidate, whole pelvis radiation should be administered followed by interstitial radiation. After the external radiation is complete, an additional 30–40 Gy tumor dose, can be administered in 3 to 4 days with needles. If the tumor is not thicker than 1.5 cm then a single plane implant will suffice.

Recurrent carcinoma

In patients who have not received radiation therapy as part of their initial treatment, the vaginal vault will be a common site of recurrence. If such is the case, this disease can be treated by local excision, by vaginal radiation from placement of ovoids for a tumor dose of 50–60 Gy or by a combination of external radiation therapy of 40–50 Gy to a 10 × 10 cm pelvic field followed by placement of vaginal intracavitary radiation to deliver an additional 30–40 Gy mucosal dose. On occasion, combinations of surgical reduction of tumor bulk followed by radiation therapy can be highly effective. 5-year survival in patients who are treated for recurrence to the upper vagina approximates 35 to 40% with any of these optimally individualized treatment plans.[1]

When a central pelvic recurrence is diagnosed in patients who have previously not received radiation therapy and in whom there is no requirement for diminishing the dose because of intercurrent ailment, whole pelvis radiation of 55 Gy in 5 weeks may be administered or 40 Gy whole pelvis may be administered with additional radiation therapy to smaller fields where tumor is known to exist in bulk. Addition of intracavitary vaginal radiation sources is indicated only if the tumor is close to the vaginal vault and can receive a significant contribution from the vaginal sources by virtue of proximity. When the cancer occurs outside of the pelvis, it should be treated according to the principles previously outlined in treatment of patients with Stage III and Stage IV disease.

Lower vaginal recurrence usually implies disseminated disease and it is reasonable to treat the whole pelvis while boosting the vaginal dose by either volume interstitial implants or additional external radiation with a field size which includes the vagina. The 5-year survival in patients treated for lower vaginal recurrence is approximately 25%. When the recurrence is confined to a single locus in the pelvis, one may expect a 30% 5-year survival, and if there are multiple areas confined to the pelvis, 20% 5-year survival can be achieved by radiation therapy alone. Distant metastases or a combination of pelvic recurrence with metastases elsewhere respond poorly to radiation therapy alone.

Conclusion

Because adenocarcinoma of the endometrium is radiosensitive, it is reasonable to treat advanced cancer or recurrent disease by radiation therapy. The advantages are obvious: surgery in a population which is frequently unfit can be reduced, applied selectively, or restricted in scope. Palliation can be achieved quickly, often within 2 weeks from the onset of treatment. The treatment time is less than for chemotherapy. Finally, the technique is effective. The disadvantages include combinations of bowel and bladder dysfunction, often of a severe nature in older people; marrow suppression when large fields are employed so that subsequent cytotoxic chemotherapy may be restricted; and limited applicability in patients who have primary disease in the intestinal tract, vascular insufficiency due to atherosclerosis, and history of previous radiation therapy. By careful individualization, radiation therapy can be applied with good benefit.

Hormone therapy

It has long been known that certain endometrial adenocarcinomas are related to estrogen activity.[35] Gusberg[34] cites the following evidence for this inferred relationship: (1) the co-existence of granulosa-theca cell tumors in the ovary and endometrial cancer; (2) increased incidence of endometrial cancer in patients with failure of ovulation; (3) the coincidence of obesity in patients with endometrial cancer.

Other examples include the observed aromatization of estrogen precursors to produce estrogen in body fat, the many case-controlled studies demonstrating an increased risk conferred by long estrogen usage, and, finally, considerable experience in creating animal models which demonstrate the influence of estrogenic stimulation in the production of endometrial cancers.

It is not remarkable, then, that Kelly & Baker,[42] observing the 'profound effect' of progesterone on the normal endometrium, tending to produce maturation, should have applied progestational agents in the treatment of patients with advanced endometrial cancers. In their original series, they treated 21 patients and observed an objective response in six patients, ranging from 9 months to $4\frac{1}{2}$ years.

Since 1960, the literature is replete with reports of treatment of advanced or recurrent endometrial carcinoma with progestins.[30,44,46,64,76,77,79] The drug initially employed for metastatic endometrial carcinoma was 17 alpha-hydroxyprogesterone caproate. Subsequently, medroxyprogesterone was introduced and then megestrol acetate. While other gestagens have been investigated, most are no longer employed and the major experience is with the three drugs cited. Reifenstein[59] analyzed 992 patients treated by 113 investigators with hydroxyprogesterone acetate. He analyzed in detail the records of 314 patients and observed little response in patients who were treated for less than 7 weeks and the longest remissions and best responders were treated for at least 12 weeks initially. There appeared in his analysis to be no relationship between response and patient age when correction is made for tumor differentiation. Others have analyzed large collections by multiple authors,[77] but this total experience varies little in response from the original publication of Kelly & Baker in 1960, i.e. 30%.

The optimum dose for each agent has not been defined with precision. In Kohorn's[44] survey of the prominent centers of gynecologic oncology in the United States, he identified 15 different dose schedules for the use of medroxyprogesterone. Other doses and schedules have been employed for the other agents. The Gynecologic Oncology Group, employing a dose of 50 mg of medroxyprogesterone orally three times daily in a large group of well studied patients, observed a 15% objective response rate.[70] The Group is currently undertaking a two-arm study, measuring the effect of 200 mg vs. 1 gm of oral medroxyprogesterone given daily.

Geisler[30] has demonstrated that a dosage of 160 mg per day of megestrol is superior to either 40 mg per day or 80 mg per day. Podratz studied alpha hydroxyprogesterone caproate, dimethyl-6-dihydroprogesterone, and methyl-dihydroprogesterone acetate in 155 patients and found no advantage for any one drug. It is not clear from his report how many patients had recurrent disease and how many had untreated metastatic disease. However, he observed an objective response rate in 11.2% of his study population.

Oral administration has been demonstrated by Sall and his co-workers[60] to be at least as effective as parenteral administration when treating with medroxyprogesterone.

Since the demonstration by Gurpide[33] that progesterone reduces the number of estrogen receptors available in the endometrium and induces the enzyme 17-beta-hydroxysteroid dehydrogenase, there has been considerable interest in the receptor status of endometrial carcinomas. Several investigators have studied the presence and quantity of hormone receptors in patients with endometrial carcinoma and related such observations to prognosis in their own study populations.[20,41,27] Most investigators agree that the presence of receptors correlates with the degree of differentiation of the cancer. The presence of progesterone receptors was related to improved prognosis in all studies, however, only in Creasman's report was the presence of estrogen receptor similarly favorable prognostically. Mortel[48] cautions against over-reliance on the presence of progesterone receptors in predicting response to progestational therapy. He points out that many tumors are heterogenous and that while receptors may be identified, the cell's capacity to transport it to the nucleus and to have it activate genes and to synthesize RNA for progestin-specific protein elaboration should not be assumed. These considerations may, in fact, explain why many receptor-rich endometrial cancers fail to respond to progestational therapy.

With the availability of tamoxifen, several investigators have employed it in an 'anti-estrogenic' therapeutic effort on the assumption that if estrogen can stimulate endometrial cancer, an anti-estrogen might control it. Swenerton,[68] employing a dose of 10 mg twice daily by mouth on a continuous basis observed an objective response in four of seven patients who had previously failed surgery, radiation therapy, and progestational agents. Carlson demonstrated the capacity of tamoxifen to induce the progesterone receptor in patients with previously untreated endometrial carcinomas. His group then treated patients who had recurrent endometrial carcinoma with tamoxifen followed by progestational treatment. They observed a 33% total objective response rate with the combination hormone therapy which was not superior to that of standard single progestin therapy. Kline[43] and his co-workers were similarly disappointed in their treatment of 20 consecutive patients with recurrent or metastatic poorly differentiated adenocarcinoma. It may well be that Mortel's admonition is justified by the experience of these two investigative groups or that they have not yet found the appropriate dose of progestin.

Hormone treatment of advanced endometrial cancer is rational, is successful from 15 to 30% of the time and is easily administered. We should be mindful that responses may require 12 weeks of therapy, that patients with poorly differentiated cancers will probably not respond and that while the adverse effects are infrequent, fluid retention, occasional phlebitis, and weight gain may be problems in patients who are already obese, diabetic, or suffering from impaired vascularity.

Chemotherapy

Cytotoxic chemotherapy in the treatment of patients with endometrial cancer was unusual prior to 15 years ago. In 1974, Donovan reviewed the literature[25] and identified only 126 patients who had been treated with 16 different agents. An objective response was identified in 34 of 126 patients, or 27%. Definitions of response were highly variable, and there was no minimum duration required in definition of response. Donovan's review may be inspected in Table 50.3.

Table 50.3 Nonhormonal chemotherapy of endometrial cancer (from Donovan, 1974)[25]

Agent	% responding
5-Fluorouracil	25
Cyclophosphamide	28
Chlorambucil	9
Miscellaneous	
12 drugs in 53 patients	28
Total	27 (34/126)

In 1974, Muggia and his co-workers[49] evaluated adriamycin in combination with cyclophosphamide for treatment of patients with recurrent endometrial cancer. In 1979,[50] they published a more complete experience in which 11 patients were treated with adriamycin (37.5 mg per m^2) and cyclophosphamide (500 mg per m^2) given intravenously every 21 days. Three ill patients died within 2 weeks of the first treatment. Of the remaining eight, five had objective responses, of which three were complete. Thus, the combination proved effective against poorly differentiated cancers. The major toxicity in this small group of patients was thromboembolism. Four patients suffered this complication with the onset of treatment and in another three who had previous thrombophlebitis this was exacerbated. Leukopenia was not a problem in this small study.

The Gynecologic Oncology Group studied adriamycin alone in patients with advanced or recurrent endometrial adenocarcinoma at a dose rate of 60 mg per m^2 administered intravenously every 3 weeks with appropriate dose modifications for diminished liver function.[69] 43 patients were evaluated and achieved an objective response of 37.2%. An additional 30.2% of these patients had stable disease and only 32.6% progressed. Performance status was an independent prognostic variable but histologic grade of tumor, site of metastasis, and length of time from initial diagnosis to first recurrence all had no effect on the response rate. The major toxicity was hematologic with half of the patients experiencing some evidence of myelosup-

pression. This occurred most frequently after the second course of drug. Cardiac toxicity occurred in five of 43 patients, and there was one death from cardiotoxicity in a patient who had received more than the recommended maximum cumulative dose of 500 mg per m^2. This study clearly established the value of adriamycin as a single agent in treatment of endometrial cancer; it evaluated the role of several prognostic features and offered a model for the evaluation of other cytotoxic regimens.

Horton and his co-workers from the Eastern Cooperative Oncology Group (ECOG)[38] reported a prospective study testing adriamycin vs. cyclophosphamide in single agent treatment of patients with advanced or recurrent endometrial adenocarcinoma. Adriamycin was administered at a dose rate of 50 mg per m^2 IV every 3 weeks to a maximum dose of 550 mg per m^2. Cytoxan was given at a dose of 660 mg per m^2 IV every 3 weeks. These investigators found a 19% objective response rate in the adriamycin arm and of the 19 patients receiving cyclophosphamide, there were no objective responses. Among the adriamycin patients, there were five (25%) instances of severe or life-threatening hematologic toxicity which the authors attributed to the influence of previous radiation therapy with which all their patients had been treated.

Investigators at the M. D. Anderson Hospital and Tumor Institute treated 26 patients with adriamycin and cyclophosphamide, of whom 13 had recurrent endometrial adenocarcinoma and 13 had untreated disseminated disease. 31% of the patients demonstrated a partial response, however, there were no complete responders. The median duration of remission was 4 months.[62] The Gynecologic Oncology Group tested adriamycin with or without cyclophosphamide in the treatment of advanced or recurrent endometrial carcinoma and found no advantage for the combination over adriamycin alone.[71]

Our own study group demonstrated activity of adriamycin, cyclophosphamide, 5-fluorouracil and medroxyprogesterone acetate in patients with advanced and recurrent adenocarcinoma of the endometrium.[8] In an attempt to avoid the cardiotoxicity of adriamycin, a combination of melphalan and 5-fluorouracil was employed and achieved objective response in six of the first seven patients treated.[14] An expanded experience[22] produced objective responses in 11 of 26 patients, of whom five had complete responses. Of the complete responders, two had no evidence of disease at the time of repeat laparotomy and in the other complete responders, the site of metastasis was not amenable to second-look surgery. Piver[55] treated 13 women with advanced endometrial carcinoma with this same regimen. Of this group, 11 were evaluable for response and there were six objective responders (54.5%).

Based on these preliminary studies, the Gynecologic Oncology Group undertook a prospective randomized study comparing the efficacy of these two combination regimens.[16] 358 patients with advanced (FIGO Stages III and IV) or recurrent endometrial cancer were treated with one of two regimens: (1) melphalan, 7 mg per m^2 per day orally for four days plus 5-fluorouracil 525 mg per m^2 per day i.v. for 4 days, repeated every 28 days; and (2) i.v. administration of adriamycin 40 mg per m^2, cyclophosphamide 400 mg per m^2, and 5-fluorouracil 400 mg per m^2 every 21 days. In both arms, 180 mg of megestrol was administered orally daily for 8 weeks and then discontinued. The megestrol was included since at the time of the investigation, few patients with recurrent endometrial carcinoma were referred to treatment centers without previous prescription for megestrol by their local physicians. A dose modification of 25% was imposed in the first arm early in the study when myelosuppression was noted to be profound in some patients.

The objective response rate in those with measurable disease was 36.8% in both groups and 36.8% of each group had stable disease. 26.4% progressed on treatment. Response was unaffected by site of recurrence, time to first recurrence, or presence or absence of previous treatment by progestational or radiation therapy, or age. While grade of tumor and performance status did affect response, 44 of 57 objective responders had undifferentiated tumors. While this trial did not demonstrate an advantage of these combinations over single agent treatment by adriamycin, it did demonstrate that there is an alternative to adriamycin therapy for patients who have cardiac disease or other contraindications to adriamycin therapy.

Our study group[23] demonstrated the activity of cisplatin in patients with endometrial cancer by treating patients who had failed conventional surgery, radiation therapy, hormonal therapy, and other cytotoxic chemotherapeutic programs, with cisplatin at a dose rate of 100–120 mg per m^2 by 4-hour intravenous infusion. We observed four objective responses in 13 patients where others, employing a dose rate of 50 mg per m^2, observed no activity of the drug. Seski[63] and his colleagues, in treating 26 women with advanced or recurrent endometrial cancer, in a dose-seeking regimen of 50, 70, or 100 mg per m^2 every 4 weeks, observed an objective response rate of 42% with 10 partial responses and one complete response. Of note is the fact that 21 of the 26 patients in Seski's study had not been previously treated with cytotoxic agents. In the experience of the Gynecologic Oncology Group,[72] 23 patients were treated with cisplatin at a dose of 50 mg per m^2 every 3 weeks and only one responded. However, 20 of these 23 patients had previously been treated with adriamycin or an alkylating agent and thus no responses were observed at the conventional dose of 50 mg per m^2. In support of this notion is Trope's[73] report of treating 11 patients who had recurrent endometrial cancer without previous cytotoxic treatment. Four of 11 patients (36%) experienced objective response at a dose rate of 50 mg per m^2.

Others have exploited the observed activity of cisplatin by investigating its use in combination with adriamycin

with or without cyclophosphamide in the treatment of patients with advanced endometrial cancer.[74,61] The range of response to these platinum-based regimens appears to be 33 to 47%. While this figure seems promising, it is not clear that combination therapy offers an advantage over cisplatin or adriamycin as single agent treatment; thus, the Gynecologic Oncology Group has embarked on a study of adriamycin alone at a dose of 60 mg per m^2 intravenously every 3 weeks vs. adriamycin 60 mg per m^2 plus cisplatin 50 mg per m^2, both given intravenously every 3 weeks. Hopefully, the results of this study will help with the formulation of optimal regimens for cytotoxic chemotherapy in patients with endometrial carcinoma.

It is clear that there is a role for non-hormonal cytotoxic chemotherapy in the treatment of patients with advanced or recurrent endometrial carcinoma. Selection of a regimen is dependent on the patient's performance status, whether or not she has been recently or heavily radiated, the adequacy of her hepatic and renal function, and perhaps her age. It is clear, however, that this treatment approach offers advantages of rapid disease control, effectiveness against cancers which are not well treated by other modalities (poorly differentiated cancer which has recurred quickly) and is effective against all sites of recurrence except the central nervous system. These considerations raise the attractive possibility of adjuvant treatment and some trials are already in place. To date, however, there is no clear evidence that adjuvant treatment is effective in this disease.

SPECIAL HISTOLOGIC VARIANTS

Until now, this chapter has addressed the treatment of adenocarcinoma of the endometrium without regard to special histologic subclassifications. However, following the description in 1982 of uterine papillary serous carcinoma (UPSC),[37] a series of reports have appeared uniformly confirming the virulence of this pathologic entity.[10,12,40,66] Between 1960 and 1980, there were several reports of endometrial carcinomas that were observed to have histologic appearances suggestive of serous ovarian carcinoma. These observations included the presence of psammoma bodies, papillary structure, and a high degree of cytologic anaplasia.[13] However, Hendrickson's report affixed the current designation and this stimulated others to search their own material. Important features include the following: (1) There is a papillary histologic pattern which can be diagnosed in the curettings and which is very similar to papillary serous cystadenocarcinoma of the ovary. (2) Approximately half of the patients will have more advanced disease at the time of laparotomy than is appreciated in preoperative clinical staging, imposing a requirement for careful surgical staging as in patients with early ovarian adenocarcinoma. (3) Patients may not present with a long history of intermittent vaginal bleeding nor with the somatotypes or endocrinopathies typical of patients with endometrial adenocarcinoma. (4) The survival is only 20 to 50% of that expected in corresponding stage for patients with endometrial adenocarcinoma. Some investigators report having no survivors. (5) While there are reports of unique survivorship after treatment with abdominal radiation therapy or cisplatin-based chemotherapy or combinations of both, most reports describe failure in spite of aggressive therapy.

There are currently therapeutic trials being undertaken in collaborative groups to identify optimal treatment for this subgroup of virulent disorders. Until such trials are mature, individualized treatment will be necessary but therapists must quickly recognize the diagnosis so that meticulous staging and sufficiently aggressive therapy can be applied.

REFERENCES

1. Badib A O, Kurohara S S, Beitia A A, Webster J H 1969 Recurrent cancer of the corpus uteri: techniques and results of treatment. Am J Roentgenol Radium Ther Nucl Med 105: 596
2. Badib A O, Kurohara S S, Beitia A A, Webster J H 1970 The treatment of recurrent endometrial carcinoma. Prog Clin Cancer 4: 368
3. Barber H R K, Brunschwig A 1968 Treatment and results of recurrent cancer of corpus uteri in patients receiving anterior and total pelvic exenteration (1947–1963). Cancer 22: 949
4. Blythe J G, Hodel K A, Wahl T P, Baglan R J, Lee F A, Zivnuska F R 1986 Para-aortic node biopsy in cervical and endometrial cancers: does it affect survival? Am J Obstet Gynecol 155: 306
5. Boronow R C 1969 Carcinoma of the corpus: treatment at M.D. Anderson Hospital. Cancer of the Uterus and Ovary. Yearbook Medical Publishers, Chicago, p 35
6. Boronow R C, Morrow C P, Creasman W T, DiSaia P J, Silverberg S G, Miller A, Blessing J A 1984 Surgical staging in endometrial cancer: I. Clinical pathologic findings of a prospective study. Obstet Gynecol 63: 825
7. Brodman M, Friedman F Jr, Dottino P, Janus C, Plaxe S, Cohen C 1989 A comparative study of computerized tomography, magnetic resonance imaging, and clinical staging in cervical cancer. Gynecol Oncol. In press
8. Bruckner H W, Deppe G 1977 Combination chemotherapy of advanced endometrial carcinoma with adriamycin, cyclophosphamide, 5-fluorouracil, and medroxyprogesterone acetate. Obstet Gynecol 50: 10
9. Brunschwig A, Murphy A I 1954 The rationale for radical panhysterectomy and pelvic node excision in carcinoma of the corpus uteri. Am J Obstet Gynecol 68: 1482
10. Chambers J T, Merino M, Kohorn E I, Peschel R E, Schwartz, P E 1987 Uterine papillary serous carcinoma. Obstet Gynecol 69: 109
11. Chambers S K, Kapp D S, Peschel R E, Lawrence R, Merino M, Kohorn E I, Schwartz P E 1987 Prognostic factors and sites of failure in FIGO Stage I, Grade 3 endometrial carcinoma. Gynecol Oncol 27: 180
12. Christman J E, Kapp D S, Hendrickson M R, Howes A E, Ballon S C 1985 Therapeutic approaches to uterine papillary serous carcinoma: a preliminary report. Gynecol Oncol 36: 228
13. Christopherson W M, Alberhasky R C, Connelly P J 1982 Carcinoma of the endometrium. II. Papillary adenocarcinoma: a clinical pathologic study of 46 cases. Am J Clin Pathol 77: 534
14. Cohen C J, Deppe G, Bruckner H W 1977 Treatment of advanced adenocarcinoma of the endometrium with melphalan, 5-fluorouracil, and medroxyprogesterone acetate: a preliminary study. Obstet Gynecol 50: 415
15. Cohen C J, Gusberg, S B 1970 Contribution of radiotherapy to the surgical treatment of endometrial cancer. Progress in Gynecology, Vol 5. Grune & Stratton, New York, p 349
16. Cohen C J, Bruckner H W, Blessing J A, Homesley H, Lee J H, Watring W 1984 A randomized study comparing multi-drug chemotherapeutic regimens in the treatment of advanced and recurrent endometrial cancer. A Gynecologic Oncology Group study. Obstet Gynecol 63: 719
17. Copenhaver E H, Nahhas W A 1968 Recurrent endometrial adenocarcinoma. Surg Clin N Am 48: 619
18. Creasman W T, Boronow R C, Morrow C P, DiSaia P J, Blessing J 1976 Adenocarcinoma of the endometrium: its metastatic lymph node potential. Gynecol Oncol 4: 239
19. Creasman W T, DiSaia P J, Blessing J, Wilkinson R H, Johnston W, Weed J C Jr 1981 Prognostic significance of peritoneal cytology in patients with endometrial cancer and preliminary data concerning therapy with intraperitoneal radio-pharmaceuticals. Am J Obstet Gynecol 141: 921
20. Creasman W T, Soper J T, McCarty K S Jr, McCarty K S Sr, Hinshaw W, Clarke-Pearson D L 1985 Influence of cytoplasmic steroid receptor content on prognosis of early stage endometrial carcinoma. Am J Obstet Gynecol 151: 922
21. Dede J A, Plentl A A, Moore J G 1968 Recurrent endometrial carcinoma. Surg Gynecol Obstet 126: 533
22. Deppe G, Bruckner H W, Cohen C J 1980 Combination chemotherapy for advanced endometrial adenocarcinoma. Int J Gynecol Obstet 18: 168
23. Deppe G, Cohen C J, Bruckner H W 1980 Treatment of advanced endometrial carcinoma with cisdiamminedichloroplatinum (II) after intensive prior therapy. Gynecol Oncol 10: 51
24. DiSaia P J, Creasman W T, Boronow R C, Blessing J A 1985 Risk factors and recurrent patterns in stage I endometrial cancer. Am J Obstet Gynecol 151: 1009
25. Donovan J F 1974 Nonhormonal chemotherapy of endometrial carcinoma: a review. Cancer 34: 1587
26. Duk J M, Aalder J G, Fleuren G J, deBruijn H W A 1986 CA125: a useful marker in endometrial carcinoma. Am J Obstet Gynecol 155: 1097
27. Ehrlich C E, Young P C M, Stehman F B, Sutton G P, Alford W M 1988 Steroid receptors and clinical outcome in patients with adenocarcinoma of the endometrium. Am J Obstet Gynecol 158: 796
28. Feuer G A, Calanog A 1987 Endometrial carcinoma: treatment of positive para-aortic nodes. Gynecol Oncol 27: 104
29. Finn W R 1950 Time site and treatment of recurrence of endometrial carcinoma. Am J Obstet Gynecol 60: 773
30. Geisler H E 1973 The use of megestrol acetate in the treatment of advanced malignant lesions of the endometrium. Adv Med Oncol Res Edu 8: 191
31. Genest P, Drouin P, Girard A, Gerig L 1987 Stage III of carcinoma of the endometrium: a review of 41 cases. Gynecol Oncol 26: 77
32. Greer B E, Hamberger A D 1982 Treatment of intraperitoneal metastatic adenocarcinoma of the endometrium by the whole-abdomen moving-strip technique and pelvic boost irradiation. Gynecol Oncol 16: 365
33. Gurpide E, Satyaswaroop P G, Fleming H, Bressler R S 1979 Hormonal aspects of carcinoma of the endometrium. Adv Med Oncol Res Edu 8: 191
34. Gusberg S B 1978 Corscaden's Gynecologic Cancer (5th edn). Williams & Wilkins, Baltimore, Md

35. Gusberg S B 1947 Precursors of corpus carcinoma: estrogens and adenomatous hyperplasia. Am J Obstet Gynecol 54: 905
36. Haenszel W, Kurohara M 1968 Studies of Japanese migrants. J Natl Cancer Inst 40: 43
37. Hendrickson M, Ross J, Eifel P, Martinez A, Kempson R 1982 Uterine papillary serous carcinoma, a highly malignant form of endometrial adenocarcinoma. Am J Surg Pathol 6: 93
38. Horton J, Begg C B, Arseneault J, Bruckner H, Creech R, Han R G 1978 Comparison of adriamycin with cyclophosphamide in patients with advanced endometrial cancer. Cancer Treatment Rep 62: 159
39. Javert C T 1952 The spread of benign and malignant endometrium in the lymphatic system with a note on co-existing vascular involvement. Am J Obstet Gynecol 64: 780
40. Jeffrey J F, Krepart G V, Lotocki R J 1986 Papillary serous adenocarcinoma of the endometrium. Obstet Gynecol 67: 670
41. Kauppilla A, Kujansuv E, Vihko R 1982 Cytosol estrogen and progestin receptors in endometrial carcinoma of patients treated with surgery, radiotherapy and progestin. Cancer 50: 2157
42. Kelly R M, Baker W H 1961 Progestational agents in the treatment of carcinoma of the endometrium. N Eng J Med 264: 216
43. Kline R C, Freedman R S, Jones L A, Atkinson E N 1987 Treatment of recurrent or metastatic poorly differentiated adenocarcinoma of the endometrium with tamoxifen and medroxyprogesterone acetate. CA Treatment Reports 71: 327
44. Kohorn E I 1976 Gestagens and endometrial carcinoma. Gynecol Oncol 4: 398
45. Komaki R, Mattingly R F, Hoffman R G 1983 Irradiation of para-aortic lymph node metastases from carcinoma of the cervix or endometrium. Radiology 147: 245
46. Malkasian G D, Decker D G, Mussey E, Johnson C E 1971 Progestin treatment of recurrent endometrial carcinoma. Am J Obstet Gynecol 110: 15
47. Mazurka J L, Krepart G V, Lotocki R J 1988 Prognostic significance of positive peritoneal cytology in endometrial carcinoma. Am J Obstet Gynecol 158: 303
48. Mortel R, Zaino R, Satyswaroop P G 1984 Sex steroid receptors and hormonal treatment of endometrial cancer. In: Deppe G (ed) Chemotherapy of Gynecologic Cancer. Alan Liss Inc, New York
49. Muggia F M, Perloff M, Chia G A, Juden-Reed L, Escher G C 1974 Adriamycin in combination with cyclophosphamide: a Phase I and II evaluation. Cancer Chemotherapy Rep 58: 919
50. Muggia F M, Chia G A, Reed L J, Romney S L 1979 Doxorubicin-cyclophosphamide: effective therapy for advanced endometrial cancer. Am J Obstet Gynecol 128: 314
51. Niloff J M, Klug T, Schaetzl E, Zurawski R, Knapp R C, Bast R C 1984 Elevation of CA125 in carcinomas of the fallopian tube, endometrium and endocervix. Am J Obstet Gynecol 148: 1057
52. Onsrud M, Kolstad P, Norman T 1976 Postoperative external pelvic irradiation in carcinoma of the corpus, Stage I: a controlled clinical trial. Gynecol Oncol 4: 222
53. Patsner B, Mann W J, Cohen H, Loesch M 1988 Predictive value of preoperative serum CA125 levels in clinically localized and advanced endometrial carcinoma. Am J Obstet Gynecol 158: 399
54. Pettersson F 1978 Annual report of the results of treatment in gynecologic cancer, Vol 19. Int Fed Gynecol Obstet, Stockholm
55. Piver M S, Shashikant L, Barlow J J 1980 Melphalan, 5-fluorouracil, and medroxyprogesterone acetate in metastatic or recurrent endometrial carcinoma. Obstet Gynecol 56: 370
56. Plentl A A, Friedman E A 1971 Lymphatic System of the Female Genitalia: Morphologic Basis of Oncologic Diagnosis and Therapy. Saunders, Philadelphia
57. Potish, R A, Twiggs L B, Adcock L L, Savage J E, Levitt S H, Prem K A 1985 Paraaortic lymph node radiotherapy in cancer of the uterine corpus. Obstet Gynecol 65: 251
58. Reagan J W 1974 The changing nature of endometrial cancer. Gynecol Oncol 2: 144
59. Reifenstein E C Jr 1974 The treatment of advanced endometrial cancer with hydroxyprogesterone caproate. Gynecol Oncol 2: 377
60. Sall S, DiSaia P, Morrow C P, Mortel R, Prem K, Thigpen T, Creasman W 1979 A comparison of medroxyprogesterone serum concentrations by the oral or intramuscular route in patients with persistent or recurrent endometrial carcinoma. Am J Obstet Gynecol 135: 647
61. Seltzer V, Vogl S E, Kaplan B H 1984 Adriamycin and cis-diamminedichloroplatinum in the treatment of metastatic endometrial adenocarcinoma. Gynecol Oncol 19: 308
62. Seski J C, Edwards C L, Gershenson D M, Copeland L J 1981 Doxorubicin and cyclophosphamide chemotherapy for disseminated endometrial cancer. Obstet Gynecol 58: 88
63. Seski J C, Edwards C L, Herson J, Rutledge F N 1982 Cisplatin chemotherapy for disseminated endometrial cancer. Obstet Gynecol 59: 225
64. Smith J P, Rutledge F, Soffar S W 1966 Progestins in the treatment of patients with endometrial adenocarcinoma. Am J Obstet Gynecol 94: 977
65. Spanos W J, Fletcher G H, Wharton J T, Gallager H S 1978 Patterns of pelvic recurrence in endometrial carcinoma. Gynecol Oncol 6: 495
66. Sutton G P, Brill L, Michael H, Stehman F B, Ehrlich C E 1987 Malignant papillary lesions of the endometrium. Gynecol Oncol 27: 294
67. Stallworthy J A 1971 Surgery of endometrial cancer in the Bonney tradition. Ann Roy Coll Surg Eng 48: 293
68. Swenerton K D, White G W, Boyes D A 1979 Treatment of advanced endometrial carcinoma with tamoxifen. N Eng J Med 301: 105
69. Thigpen J T, Buchsbaum H J, Mangan C, Blessing J A 1979 Phase II trial of adriamycin in the treatment of advanced or recurrent endometrial carcinoma: a Gynecologic Oncology Group study. Cancer Treatment Rep 63: 21
70. Thigpen T, Blessing J, DiSaia P, Ehrlich C 1985 Treatment of advanced or recurrent endometrial adenocarcinoma with medroxyprogesterone acetate. Gynecol Oncol 2, 20: 250
71. Thigpen T, Blessing J, DiSaia P, Ehrlich C 1985 A randomized comparison of adriamycin with or without cyclophosphamide in the treatment of advanced or recurrent endometrial carcinoma (Abstract). ASCO, #C-448
72. Thigpen J T, Blessing J A, LaGasse, L D, DiSaia P J, Homesley H D 1984 Phase II trial of cisplatin as second-line chemotherapy in patients with advanced or recurrent endometrial carcinoma. Am J Clin Oncol: Cancer Clinical Trials 7: 253
73. Trope C, Grundsell H, Johnsson J E, Cavallin-Stahl E 1980 A phase II study of cisplatinum for recurrent corpus cancer. Eur J Cancer 16: 1025
74. Turbow M M, Ballon S C, Sikic B I, Koretz M M 1985 Cisplatin, doxorubicin and cyclophosphamide chemotherapy for advanced endometrial carcinoma. Cancer Treat Rep 69: 465
75. van Nagell J R, Donaldson E S, Wood E G, Sharkey R M, Goldenberg D F 1978 The prognostic significance of carcinoembryonic antigen in the plasma and tumors of patients with endometrial adenocarcinoma. Am J Obstet Gynecol 128: 308
76. Varga A, Henriksen E 1961 Clinical and histopathologic evaluation of the effect of 17-alpha-hydroxyprogesterone-17-N-caproate on endometrial carcinoma. Obstet Gynecol 18: 658
77. Wait R B 1973 Megestrol acetate in the management of advanced endometrial carcinoma. Obstet Gynecol 41: 129
78. Weiss N S, Szekely D R, Austin D F 1976 Increasing incidence of endometrial cancer in the United States. N Eng J Med 294: 1259
79. Wentz W B 1964 Effect of a progestational agent on endometrial hyperplasia and endometrial cancer. Obstet Gynecol 24: 370

PART VII

Uterine sarcomas

51. Pathology of uterine sarcomas

P. B. Clement   R. E. Scully

INTRODUCTION

Sarcomas and related neoplasms account for only 3% of uterine cancers in the western world, but are relatively common in populations with a low prevalence of endometrial carcinoma. These tumors present a challenge to the pathologist, who must distinguish them histologically, as well as for the clinician, who must appreciate their varied and occasionally bizarre biologic manifestations. Table 51.1 represents a classification of the non-epithelial, the mixed epithelial non-epithelial, and miscellaneous related tumors of the uterus. Although a complete classification is listed, this chapter will consider only sarcomas and benign mesenchymal tumors that may mimic them on gross or microscopic examination.

Table 51.1 Classification of mesenchymal and related tumors of the uterus*

I. NON-EPITHELIAL TUMORS AND RELATED LESIONS
A. Endometrial stromal tumors
  1. Stromal nodule
  2. Stromal sarcoma
    a) low-grade (endolymphatic stromal myosis)
    b) high-grade

B. Smooth muscle tumors
  1. Leiomyoma
  variants
    a) cellular
    b) epithelioid (leiomyoblastoma;** clear cell)
    c) bizarre (symplastic)
    d) lipoleiomyoma
  2. Smooth muscle tumor of uncertain malignant potential
  3. Leiomyosarcoma
  variants
    a) epithelioid (leiomyoblastoma**)
    b) myxoid
  4. Others
    a) intravenous leiomyomatosis
    b) diffuse leiomyomatosis
    c) disseminated peritoneal leiomyomatosis
    d) benign metastasizing leiomyoma

C. Mixed endometrial stromal and smooth muscle tumors

D. Adenomatoid tumor

E. Other soft tissue tumors (benign and malignant)
  1. Homologous
  2. Heterologous

II. MIXED EPITHELIAL/NON-EPITHELIAL TUMORS
A. Benign
  1. Adenofibroma
  2. Adenomyoma
    variant: atypical polypoid adenomyoma

B. Malignant
  1. Malignant müllerian mixed tumor (malignant mesodermal mixed tumor, carcinosarcoma)
    a) homologous
    b) heterologous
  2. Adenosarcoma
    a) homologous
    b) heterologous
  3. Carcinofibroma

III. MISCELLANEOUS TUMORS AND RELATED LESIONS
A. Sex cord-like tumors

B. Tumors of germ cell type

C. Gliomas

D. Lymphoma and leukemia

E. Others

* The classification represents the current, but not necessarily final, version of the World Health Organization classification of mesenchymal and related tumors of the uterus.
** See page 808.

NON-EPITHELIAL TUMORS

Endometrial stromal tumors

Endometrial stromal sarcomas, which account for approximately 10% of non-epithelial uterine cancers, are composed exclusively or almost exclusively of neoplastic cells that resemble the endometrial stromal cells of a proliferative endometrium.[34,41,44,54,59,63,64,65,66,71,93,98,114,122] Rare stromal tumors with circumscribed borders, so-called stromal nodules, are clinically benign and will not be discussed further.[110] Tumors with infiltrating borders, designated endometrial stromal sarcomas (ESSs), have been subdivided on the basis of mitotic activity and nuclear pleomorphism into low grade ESSs (endolymphatic stromal myosis; endometrial stromatosis) and high grade ESSs. Recently, however, doubt has been cast on the stromal nature of the high grade tumors (see below).[41,66]

ESSs form single or multiple masses that typically protrude into the endometrial cavity. Nodular or diffuse invasion of the myometrium is common, with extension to the serosa in approximately one-half of cases. A rare stromal sarcoma is confined to the myometrium, possibly having arisen from the stroma of adenomyosis, or appears to have originated within the cervix.[2] The neoplastic tissue is typically soft, fleshy and tan to yellow, with a bulging, cut surface. Areas of cystic degeneration, necrosis and hemorrhage may be seen, especially in the high-grade tumors. Worm-like plugs of tumor within myometrial and extra-uterine pelvic vessels may be recognized at the time of operation or on gross examination of the hysterectomy specimen, and are a much more characteristic feature of the low grade tumors (Fig. 51.1).

On microscopic examination, ESSs are typically cellular tumors that involve the endometrium and invade the myometrium in irregular tongues. As noted above, myometrial as well as extra-uterine veins and lymphatics frequently contain extensions of the tumor (Fig. 51.2). The cardinal features of low grade ESSs are a content of uniform, oval to spindle-shaped cells of endometrial stromal type (Fig. 51.3A) and a network of small arteries resembling the spiral arteries of the late secretory endometrium. Low grade ESSs are typically mitotically inactive, with usually three or fewer mitotic figures per 10 high-power-fields (MF/10 HPFs); higher mitotic rates, however, can be encountered occasionally and do not exclude the diagnosis.[34,41,66] Collections of lipid-filled histiocytes and rounded bands of hyalinized collagen are often present. Reticulin stains usually reveal a dense network of fibrils surrounding individual cells or small groups of cells. Foci of epithelial or epithelial-like differentiation occur in up to 25% of the cases in the form of endometrial-type glands or tubules, nests, cords and trabeculae in plexiform arrangements, and cavities resembling Call-Exner bodies, resulting in patterns reminiscent of ovarian sex cord tumors (Fig. 51.4).[27,44,93,96,126] When such elements form the predominant component of a stromal tumor, the designation 'uterine tumor resembling ovarian sex cord tumor' has

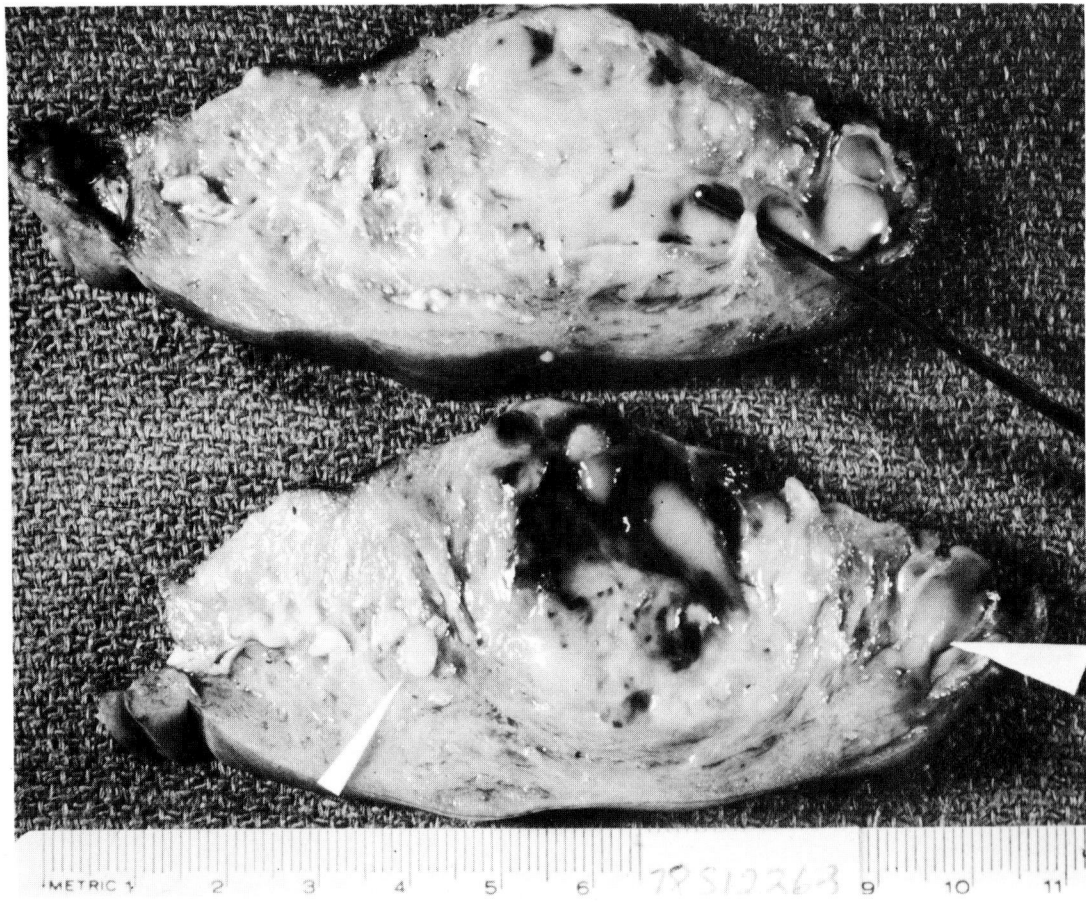

Fig. 51.1 Endometrial stromal sarcoma, low grade. Two sections of myometrium show fleshy, focally hemorrhagic tumor invading the myometrium and myometrial vascular channels (indicated by probe and arrows).

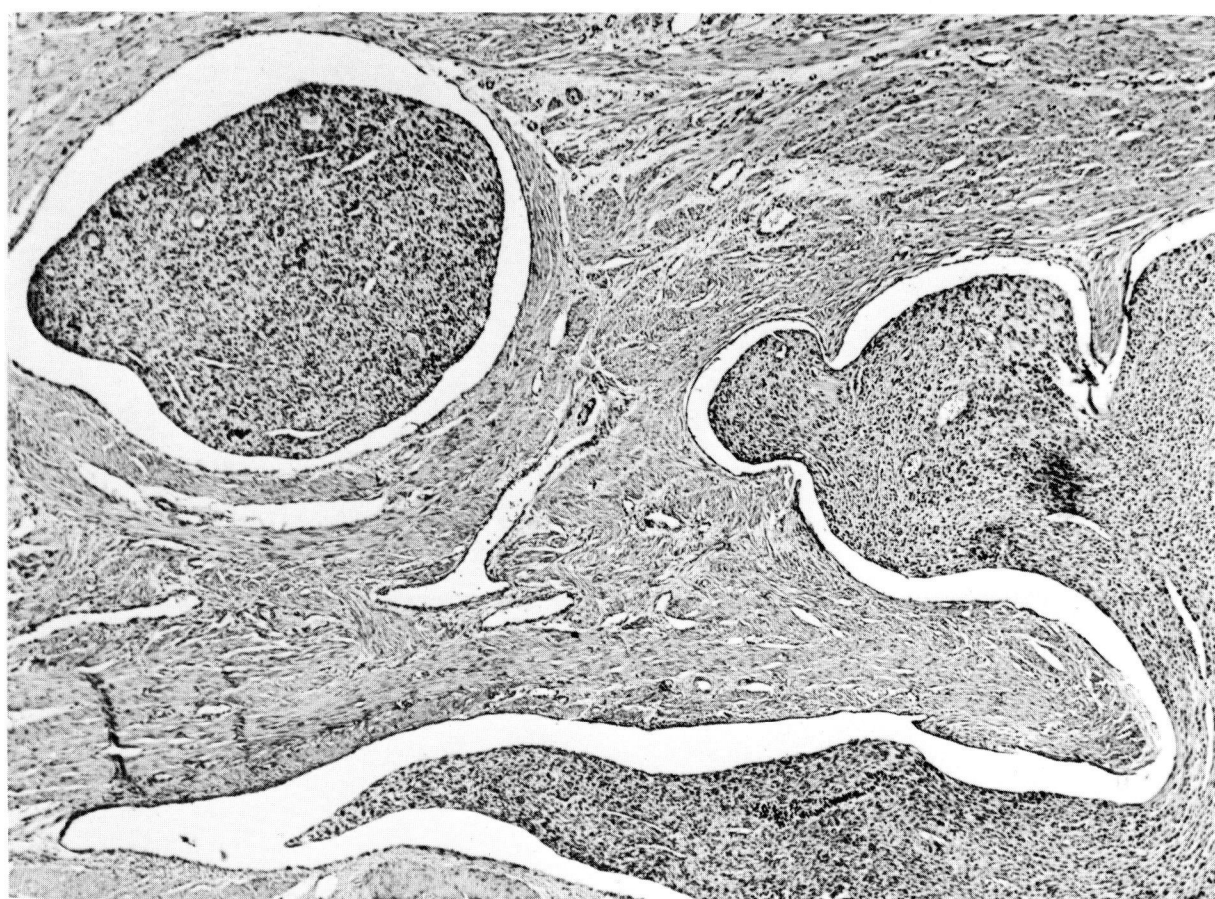

Fig. 51.2 Endometrial stromal sarcoma, low grade. Intravascular growth of tumor is seen in myometrium (×44).

been used (see p. 820). A distinction between an endometrial stromal nodule and low grade ESS can rarely be made on a curettage specimen, since the appearance of the interface of the tumor with the myometrium is the essential criterion in the differential diagnosis.

Most of the tumors that have been previously interpreted as high grade ESSs, in contrast to low grade ESSs, are composed of spindle to polygonal cells with marked degrees of nuclear pleomorphism and mitotic rates greater than 10 MF/10 HPFs, often exceeding 20 or 30 MF/10 HPFs (Fig. 51.3B).[41,66] The distinctive vascular pattern of the low grade tumors is typically absent. As the cells of these tumors bear little or no resemblance to endometrial stromal cells, they are of uncertain and possibly variable nature. 'Poorly differentiated endometrial sarcoma'[41] or 'high grade undifferentiated uterine sarcoma'[66] have recently been proposed as appropriate designations for these tumors. It has been suggested that some of them may be monophasic variants of malignant müllerian mixed tumors.[41]

The distinction between low grade ESSs and high grade endometrial sarcomas has important prognostic and therapeutic implications. Pelvic or abdominal recurrences develop in from one-third to one-half of the patients with the low grade tumors.[93,98] These tumors are typically indolent with a tendency to late recurrence; the interval before recurrence in one series was 3 months to 23 years, with a median interval of 3 years.[98] Distant metastases to the lungs and occasionally bone and other sites, are uncommon. In many cases, recurrent tumor may be successfully treated by resection, radiation therapy or both. Recurrent tumor may also respond to progestin therapy, consistent with the presence of estrogen and progesterone receptors in some tumors.[6,63,75,114] Almost 90% of patients in one study,[98] and 100% of patients in another,[93] survived 10 years. In contrast, high grade endometrial sarcomas are aggressive tumors, with death from local and hematogenous metastases within 3 years after hysterectomy in most of the cases.[41,64,65,66,122]

Smooth muscle tumors: Leiomyosarcomas

Leiomyosarcomas (LMS) account for approximately 45%

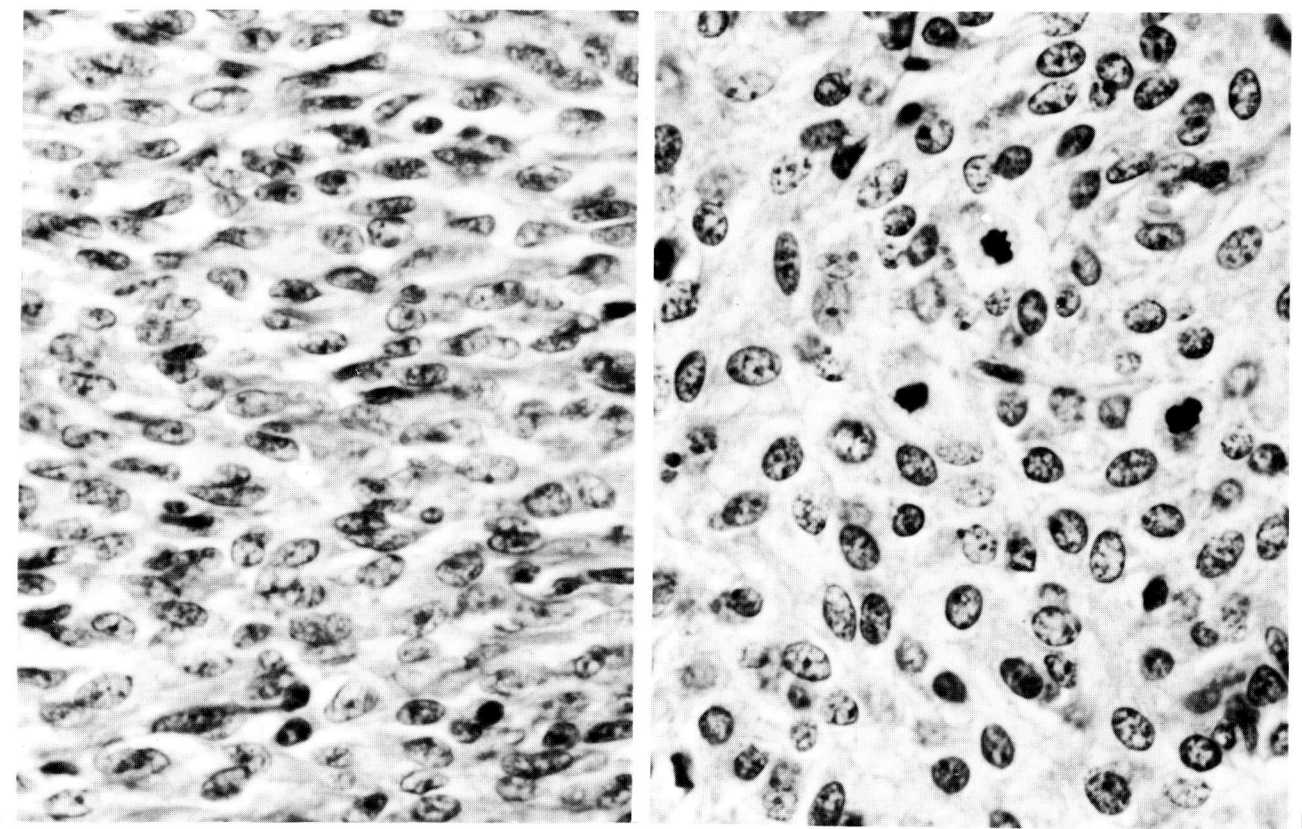

A ... B

Fig. 51.3 Endometrial stromal sarcoma. (A) Low grade endometrial stromal sarcoma: the neoplastic cells resemble the stromal cells of a proliferative endometrium (×840). (B) High grade endometrial sarcoma: the tumor cells show nuclear pleomorphism, a coarse chromatin pattern, and mitotic activity (×840).

of non-epithelial uterine cancers.[9,14,19,42,52,64,65,66,97,112] On gross examination, they are typically solitary masses with a median diameter of 10 cm. Approximately two-thirds of them are intramural, one-fifth submucosal, and one-tenth subserosal. They are almost always less circumscribed than leiomyomas and cannot be shelled out from the adjacent myometrium. The cut surface is typically bulging, soft, fleshy and focally necrotic and hemorrhagic, without the whorled appearance characteristic of a leiomyoma (Fig. 51.5). Gross evidence of vascular invasion is rare. 5% of these tumors originate in the cervix, where they usually form an intramural or an intraluminal mass. Occasional leiomyosarcomas develop in pre-existing leiomyomas.

The single most important microscopic criterion for separation of a LMS from a cellular leiomyoma is the mitotic rate (Fig. 51.6). Zaloudek & Norris,[127] combining the results of eight series of cases,[14,19,47,65,103,106,112] found that three-quarters of cellular smooth muscle tumors with mitotic rates of five or more MFs/10 HPFs were clinically malignant, i.e. leiomyosarcomas, whereas those tumors with four or fewer MFs/10 HPFs were almost invariably benign. Leiomyosarcomas, however, typically have considerably higher mitotic rates (more than 15 MFs/10 HPFs) than benign tumors, as well as a number of other clinical

or pathological features that are useful in differentiating them from the occasional leiomyomas that exhibit unusual degrees of mitotic activity. These include, alone or in combination: predominant occurrence after the menopause, extra-uterine extension at operation, a diameter usually greater than 10 cm, an infiltrating border, necrosis, marked cytologic atypia and atypical mitotic figures. In one study, patients with smooth muscle tumors that lacked these features but had intermediate mitotic counts (5 to 15 MFs/10 HPFs) exhibited a benign clinical course after hysterectomy.[97] The term 'mitotically active leiomyoma' was proposed for such tumors.[97] Rare smooth muscle tumors with some, but not all, of the above features have been referred to as 'smooth muscle tumors of uncertain malignant potential' (UMP);[66,127] the criteria for tumors in the UMP category, however, have varied from one group of investigators to another.

Rare variants of leiomyosarcoma, specifically epithelioid leiomyosarcoma (see below) and myxoid leiomyosarcoma, may lack the high mitotic activity of typical leiomyosarcomas. Myxoid leiomyosarcomas are usually grossly gelatinous and characterized by a sparsely cellular, myxoid appearance on histological examination.[67] Such tumors are almost always clinically malignant despite low

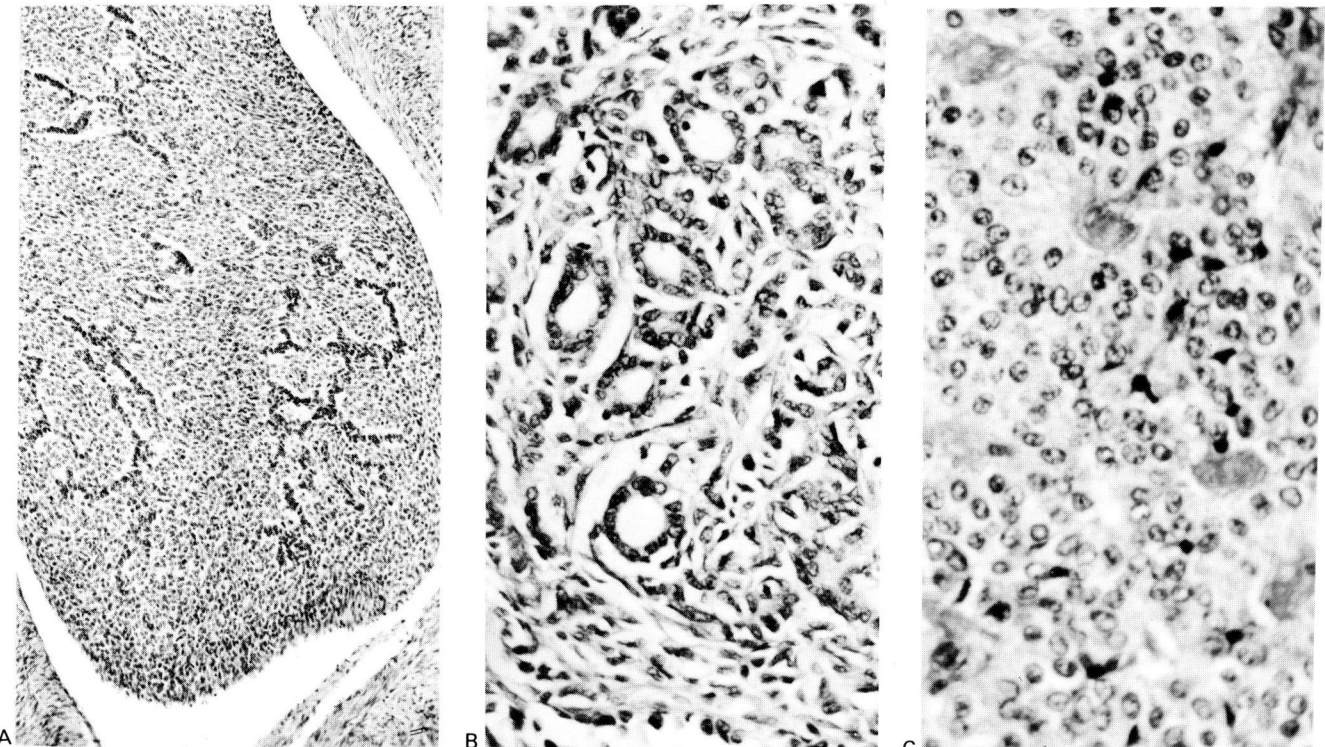

Fig. 51.4 Endometrial stromal sarcoma with sex-cord-like patterns. (A) Tumor within myometrial vascular channel exhibits focal cord-like arrangement of its cells (×70). (B) The tumor cells form small hollow tubules (×27). (C) The tumor cells have round nuclei and enclose Call-Exner-like spaces containing acellular darkly staining material (×390).

mitotic rates (0 to 2 MF/10 HPF) and bland nuclear features; they are diagnosable as sarcomas on the basis of their highly infiltrative borders.

One-third to one-half of the patients with leiomyosarcoma have extra-uterine extension at the time of diagnosis, and the 5-year survival is only 15%. Autopsy almost always reveals pelvic and intra-abdominal spread as well as distant metastasis to the lungs, less often the pleura, liver and bone, and, in half the cases, regional lymph nodes.[112] There has been no consistency among various studies with respect to showing a correlation between survival and age of the patient, mitotic rate, and the presence or absence of necrosis, nuclear pleomorphism, and vascular invasion. One study, however, found a correlation between tumor size and survival: five of eight patients with tumors less than 5 cm in diameter survived, whereas all the patients with tumors greater than 5 cm in diameter died.[42]

The differential diagnosis of leiomyosarcomas on histological examination includes, in addition to the aforementioned mitotically active leiomyomas and smooth muscle tumors of UMP, mitotically inactive tumors containing numerous cells with enlarged, bizarre nuclei (Fig. 51.7).[14,19,43,52,100] Such tumors, synonymously referred to as 'atypical leiomyomas', 'symplastic leiomyomas' or 'leiomyomas with bizarre nuclei' are benign

if mitotic figures are rare and other features suggesting a malignant potential are absent. Another problem in interpreting the malignant potential of smooth muscle tumors is that mitotic counts in otherwise bland leiomyomas may be increased in pregnancy and by oral contraceptive medication.[89,115] Tiltman has shown that the exogenous hormones that induce mitotic activity in leiomyomas are progestins.[115] Focally hemorrhagic or 'apoplectic' leiomyomas have also been described in women who are pregnant or on oral contraceptive medication;[87,89] the patients typically present with abdominal pain. The distinctive features on microscopic examination are stellate zones of recent hemorrhage surrounded by cellular, mitotically active, but otherwise benign-appearing smooth muscle.[87,89]

Distinguishing benign smooth muscle tumors, those of uncertain malignant potential, and leiomyosarcomas can be difficult because of subjectivity in interpreting degrees of mitotic activity, differences in techniques of mitotic counting, problems in interobserver reproducibility of mitotic counting, variations in fixation and staining, and the confusing effects of hormones on the appearance of these tumors. Additional research is essential to solve these problems.

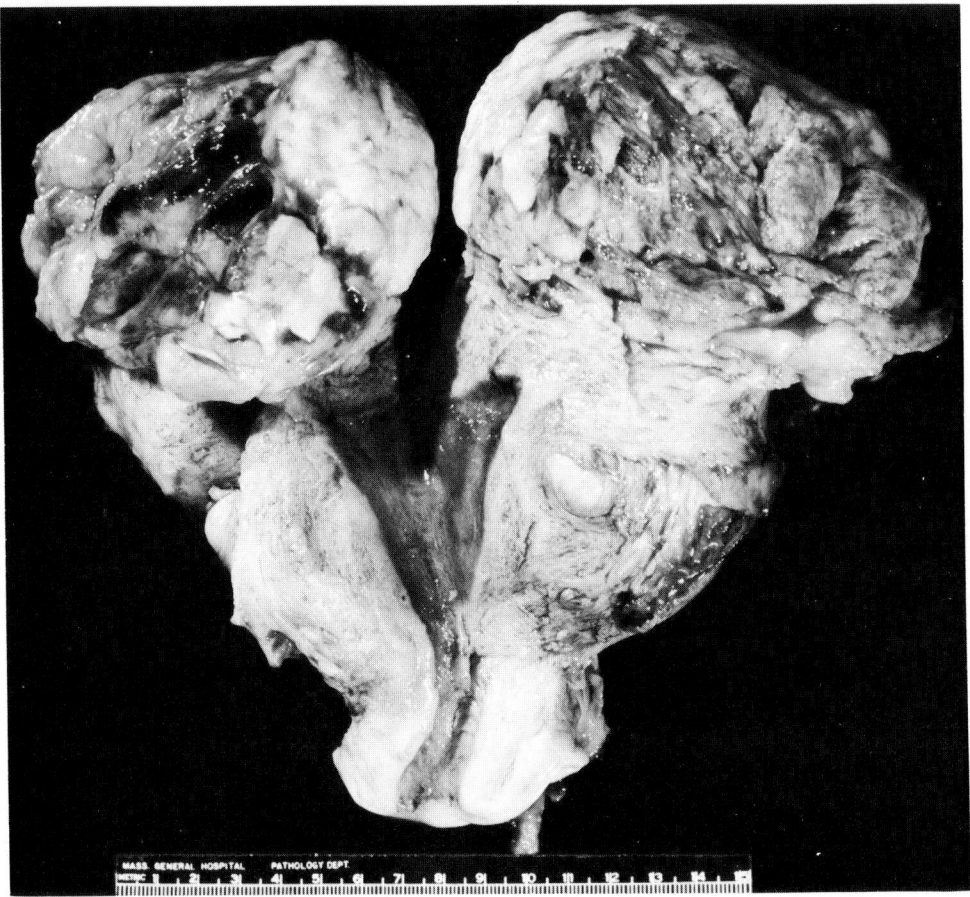

Fig. 51.5 Leiomyosarcoma. The poorly circumscribed mural mass exhibits a fleshy, focally hemorrhagic cut surface.

Epithelioid smooth muscle tumors

Rare smooth muscle tumors, composed predominantly or entirely of epithelial-like cells, have been referred to as epithelioid smooth muscle tumors, leiomyoblastomas, or clear cell smooth muscle tumors.[16,17,60,72,77,102] On gross examination, many of these tumors resemble typical leiomyomas, but some lack a whorled cut surface, are poorly circumscribed, and are more suggestive of leiomyosarcomas. The neoplastic cells grow diffusely, in nests, in long cords, or in a plexiform pattern. The cells are predominantly or exclusively round or polygonal; in one-half of cases, spindle-shaped cells characteristic of typical smooth muscle tumors are present in some areas. The cytoplasm is usually eosinophilic, but may be clear, and in about 25% of the cases the entire tumor is composed of clear cells (Fig. 51.8). Cytoplasmic glycogen is present in one-half of cases, and small amounts of lipid less often. The round or angular nucleus is typically central but may be eccentric, occasionally resulting in a signet-ring appearance. Nuclear pleomorphism is usually minimal, but occasionally moderate to marked. The mitotic rate is generally less than 3 MF/10 HPF. Stromal hyalinization may be slight and focal, or marked and diffuse, particularly

in association with a plexiform pattern. Most of the tumors infiltrate the adjacent myometrium but vascular invasion is rare.

Three of 6 tumors in one series[77] and 3 of 26 in another[72] recurred or metastasized. In the second series, the malignant tumors exhibited one or more of the following features: a component of eosinophilic cells, an infiltrating margin, necrosis, a diameter greater than 6 cm, and the absence of a hyaline stroma.[72] Neither the mitotic rate nor the presence or absence of vascular invasion appeared to be reliable prognostically. Because reliable microscopic criteria for predicting their behavior have not been established, epithelioid smooth muscle tumors should be considered to have a malignant potential unless they are small and well circumscribed, and lack necrosis, mitotic activity, and nuclear pleomorphism.

Other smooth muscle tumors

Intravenous leiomyomatosis is an uncommon uterine tumor characterized by the presence of intravenous proliferations of benign-appearing smooth muscle in the absence of a

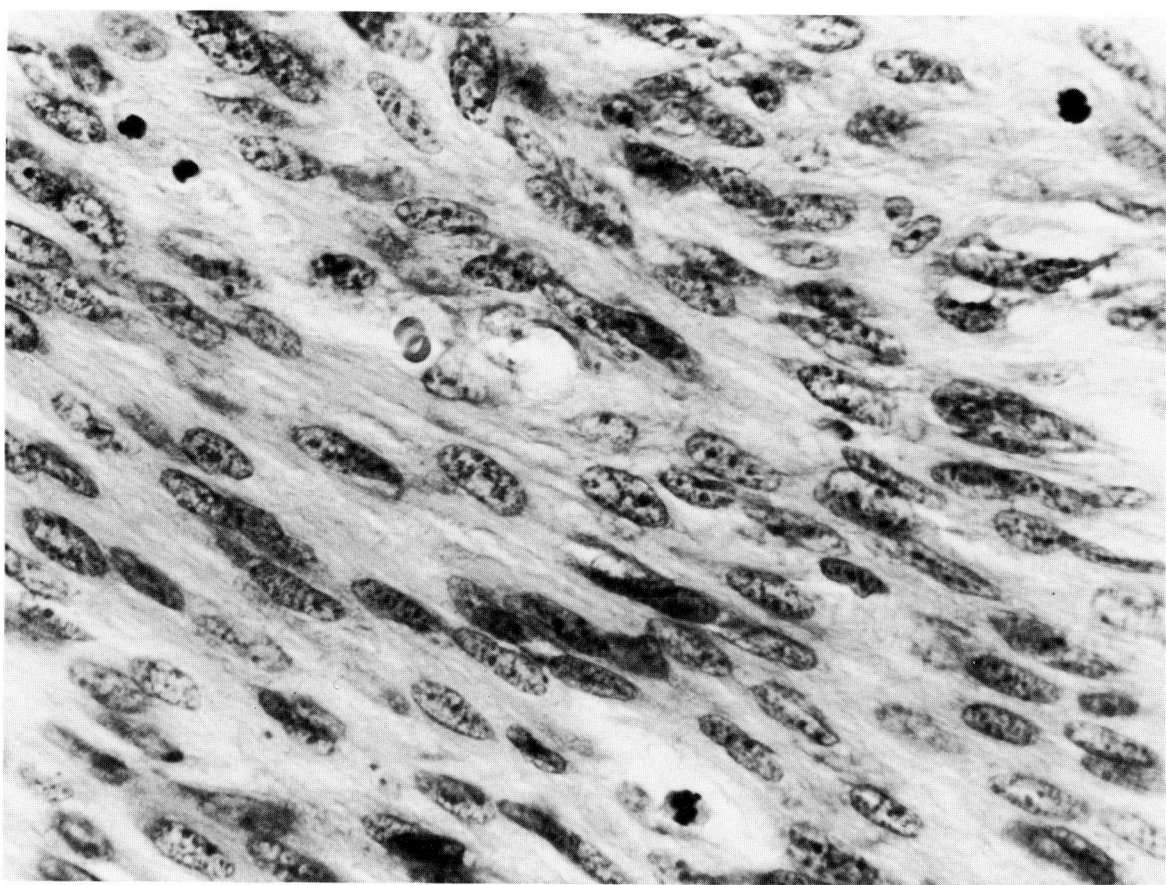

Fig. 51.6 Leiomyosarcoma. Nuclear hyperchromatism and three mitotic figures are evident (×660).

leiomyoma or outside its confines.[24,30,88,90] Extra-uterine extension, particularly within the veins of the broad ligament, and less often in ovarian and vaginal veins, has been reported in 80% of cases.[24] In 40% of cases with extension, the tumor has reached the right side of the heart, sometimes causing the death of the patient. Extra-uterine extension may be diagnosed intraoperatively or on gross examination of the hysterectomy specimen, but in other cases is evident only after the patient has presented with recurrent tumor in the pelvis or heart, in some cases many years after hysterectomy.

The uterus is usually enlarged and bosselated, with thickening of the myometrium by multinodular, rubbery, gray-white masses. Although not always appreciated on initial examination of the hysterectomy specimen, the diagnostic gross feature is the presence of one or more worm-like extensions of tumor within vessels (Fig. 51.9). Leiomyomas are also usually present, but occasionally all discernible tumor is intravascular without a discrete mass.

Microscopic examination reveals endothelium-coated plugs of cytologically benign smooth muscle within myometrial vessels outside one or more leiomyomas. When the vessels contain thrombi, or communicate with large veins,

they can be identified as veins, but other involved vessels may be lymphatics. In areas where the intravenous tumor is attached to a vessel wall, it may merge with, and appear to arise from, a subendothelial smooth muscle proliferation, or it may be continuous with an extravascular leiomyoma. The intravascular growth usually resembles a typical leiomyoma, but rarely has the appearance of one or another variant of uterine leiomyoma, including cellular leiomyoma, epithelioid leiomyoma, leiomyoma with bizarre nuclei, lipoleiomyoma and myxoid leiomyoma.[30] The intravascular tumor is characterized by a clefted or lobulated contour (Fig. 51.10), extensive hydropic change or hyalinization, and a content of numerous thick-walled vessels (angiomatoid pattern). The extravascular tumor may be less well circumscribed than a typical leiomyoma, and often exhibits hydropic degeneration.

Intravenous leiomyomatosis should be distinguished from low grade endometrial stromal sarcoma, which typically lacks thick-walled vessels, lobulation and hydropic degeneration in its intravascular extensions, and usually involves the endometrium as well as the myometrium. Immunohistochemical staining characteristic of smooth muscle may be helpful diagnostically in difficult cases.

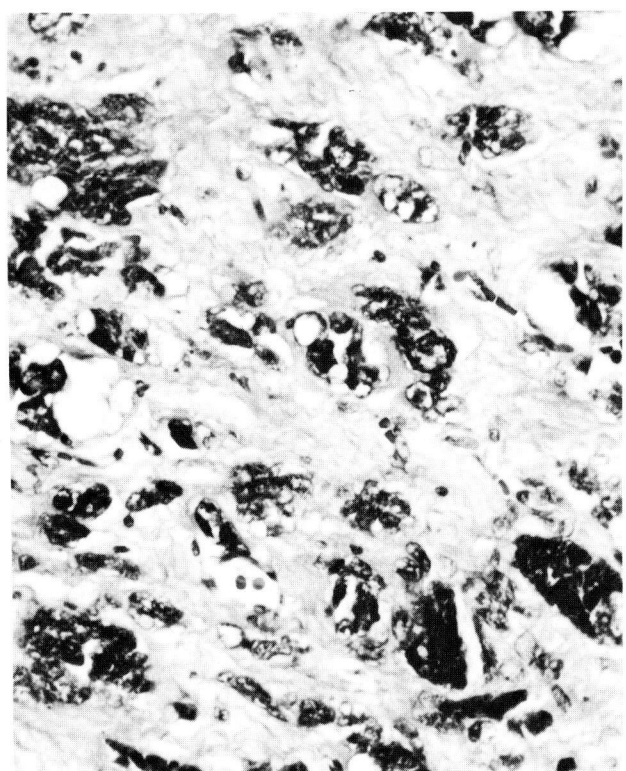

Fig. 51.7   Leiomyoma with bizarre nuclei. Smooth muscle cells contain markedly atypical nuclei with smudged chromatin; no mitotic figures are seen (×256).

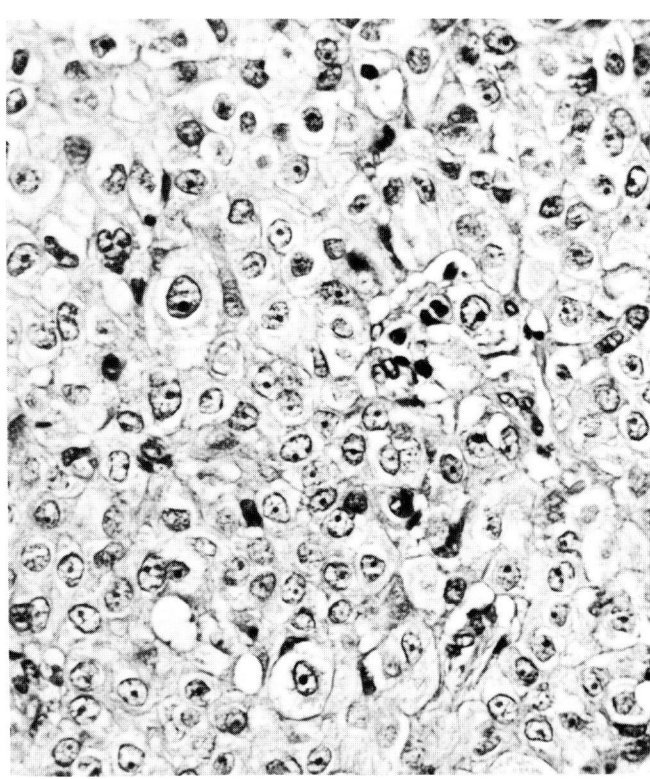

Fig. 51.8   Epithelioid smooth muscle tumor (leiomyoblastoma). Polygonal tumor cells have clear to eosinophilic cytoplasm (×400).

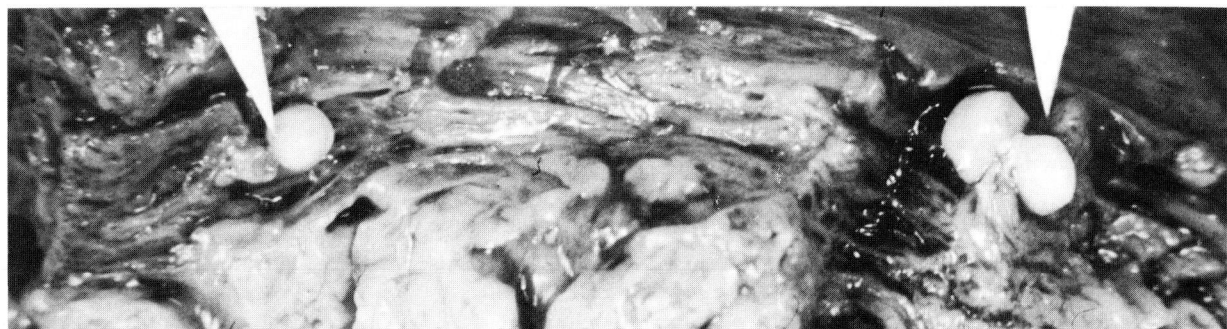

Fig. 51.9   Intravenous leiomyomatosis. Tumor involves myometrial veins (arrows).

Diffuse uterine leiomyomatosis is a rare disorder characterized by symmetrical uterine enlargement due to the presence of countless, confluent, leiomyomatous nodules within the myometrium (Fig. 51.11).[32] Microscopic examination reveals that the nodules, including many not appreciable grossly, consist of cytologically benign, typically cellular, mitotically inactive smooth muscle.

Leiomyomatosis peritonealis disseminata (LPD) is characterized by multiple peritoneal nodules of benign smooth muscle; approximately 60 cases have been reported.[111,117] The patients can be categorized into one of three groups: pregnant or puerperal (43%), oral contraceptive (OC) users (27%), or women who are neither pregnant nor on OCs (30%). A single case has been associated with a

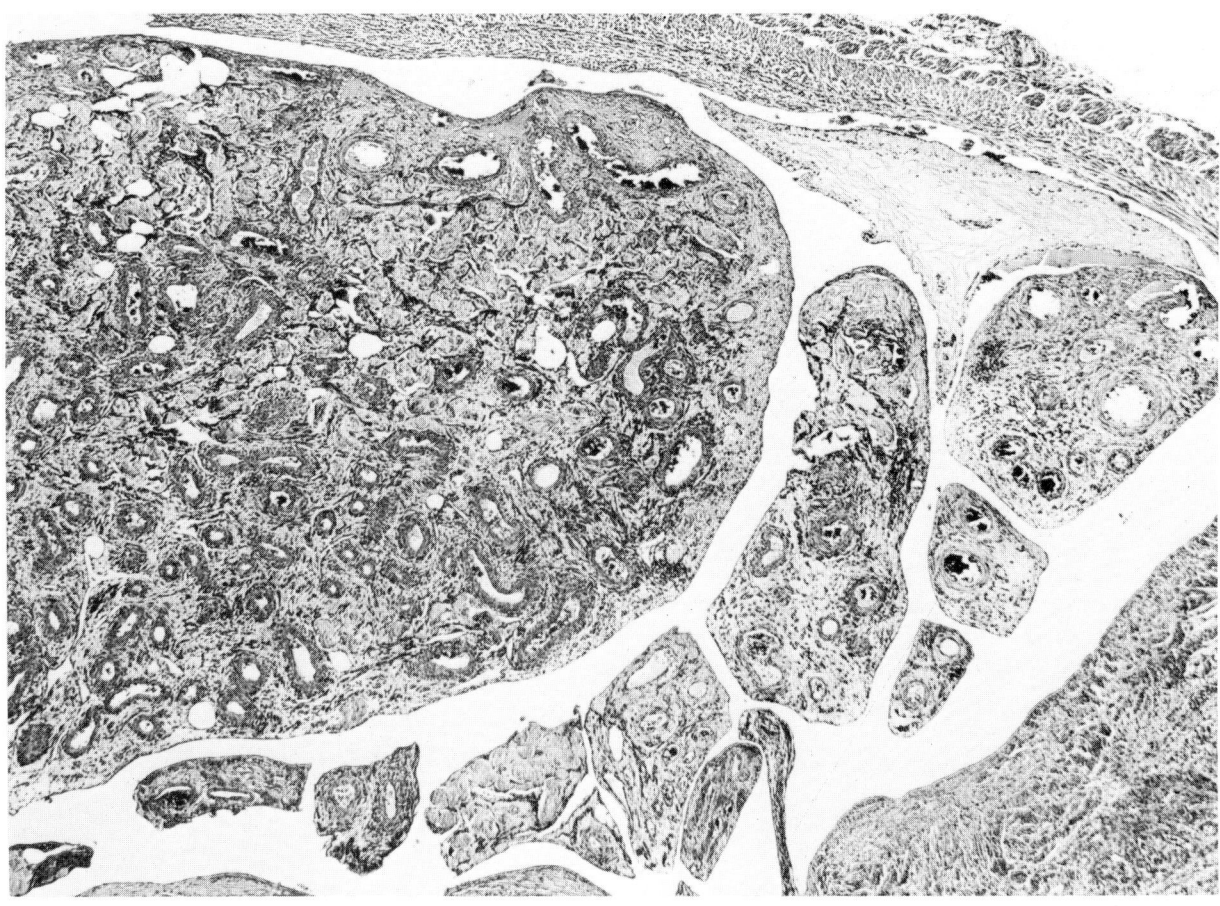

Fig. 51.10 Intravenous leiomyomatosis. The intravascular tumor has a characteristic lobulated appearance and contains numerous thick-walled vessels (×44).

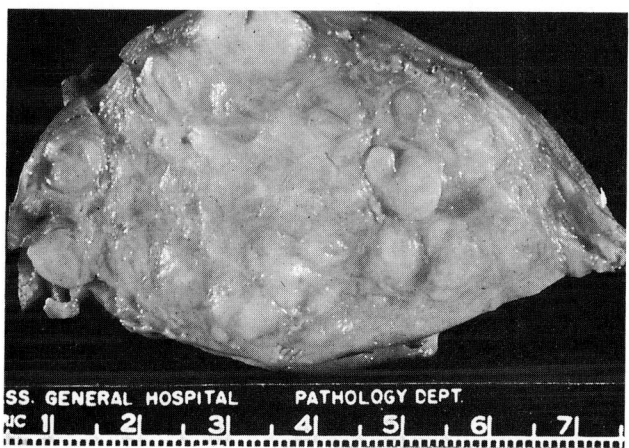

Fig. 51.11 Diffuse leiomyomatosis. The sectioned surface of the myometrium is almost completely replaced by numerous, confluent small leiomyomas.

granulosa cell tumour. In pregnant women, the disorder is usually an incidental finding during the course of a laparos-

copy or laparotomy for cesarean section or postpartum tubal ligation. Symptoms in non-pregnant women or in occasional symptomatic pregnant women are usually related to the coexistence of uterine leiomyomas; in other cases, laparotomy has been prompted by palpable pelvic nodularity.

Several to innumerable firm, discrete, solid, round nodules ranging in size from microscopic to 10 cm in diameter are scattered over the parietal and visceral pelvic peritoneum and omentum, producing a matted nodularity or an ill-defined sheet-like thickening that can simulate a metastatic tumor (Fig. 51.12A). Similar nodules also frequently involve the serosa of the uterus, ovary, bowel and mesentery; the upper abdominal peritoneum may be involved less commonly. Two cases of simultaneous pelvic lymph node involvement have also been reported.[57]

On microscopic examination, the nodules have the appearance of typical leiomyomas, usually with no significant nuclear pleomorphism or mitotic activity (Fig. 51.12B). Occasionally, they are more cellular and may contain up to 3 MF/10 HPF.[111] Decidual cells and cells intermediate in

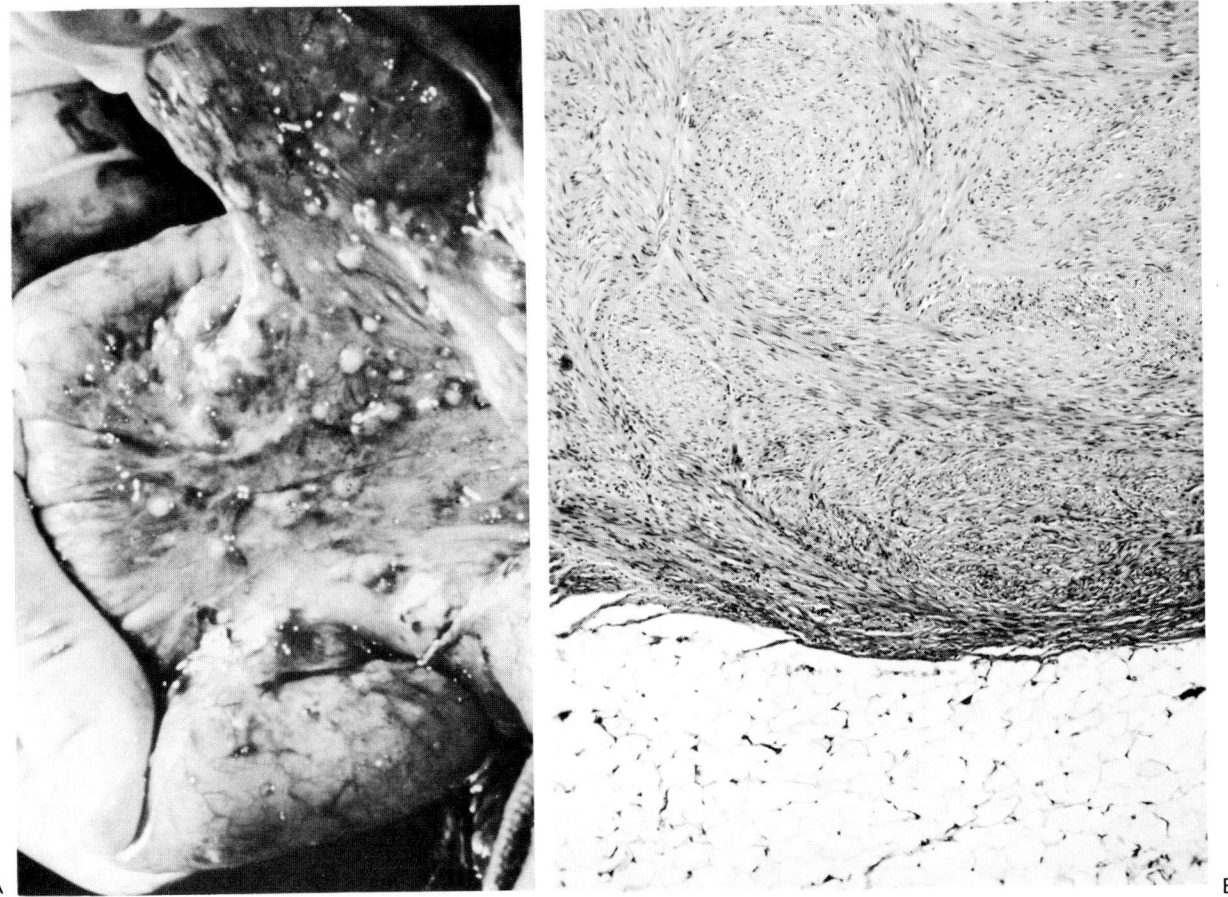

Fig. 51.12 Leiomyomatosis peritonealis disseminata. (A) Mesentery of small bowel is studded with numerous nodules. (B) Peritoneal nodule composed of histologically benign smooth muscle abuts mesenteric fat (×100).

appearance between muscle and decidual cells have been found admixed with the smooth muscle cells in many of the pregnant patients.[111] Foci of endometriosis or endo-salpingiosis have likewise been identified in continuity with the nodules in 10% of cases.

With the exception of one case of leiomyosarcomatous transformation,[101] there have been no reports of progressive disease on follow-up examination, despite incomplete excision. In patients receiving a second-look procedure, the nodules have completely or partially regressed. After frozen section confirmation of the diagnosis, conservative therapy is therefore indicated. The disorder, however, may recur in subsequent pregnancies.

LPD is considered to be a result of metaplastic transformation of subperitoneal mesenchymal cells into proliferating smooth muscle cells. The submesothelial location of the nodules, and the occasional juxtaposition to other forms of metaplasia, such as ectopic decidua, endometriosis and endosalpingiosis, support this interpretation. The association with pregnancy or exogenous hormone use in 70% of cases, the reduction in size of the tumors after pregnancy or surgical castration, and the production in guinea pigs of similar uterine and subperitoneal nodules by the administration of estrogen alone or in combination with progesterone,[79,80] indicate a hormonal background for this disorder in most of the cases.

Benign metastasizing leiomyoma, an exceedingly rare disorder, is characterized by the presence of single or multiple pulmonary nodules composed of benign-appearing smooth muscle in women who have had typical uterine leiomyomas.[5,7,8,12,22,56,62,99,108,113] Spread to the retroperitoneal and mediastinal lymph nodes[10,57] and other sites, such as bone and soft tissue, has been reported less often, with or without associated pulmonary involvement.

The pulmonary tumors, which range up to 10 cm in diameter, are circumscribed, and may be solid or contain cysts filled with fluid. The uterus, which has been removed many years previously in most of the cases, contains typical leiomyomas, which are usually multiple. On microscopic examination, the pulmonary metastases are typically circumscribed; entrapment of bronchio-alveolar epithelium

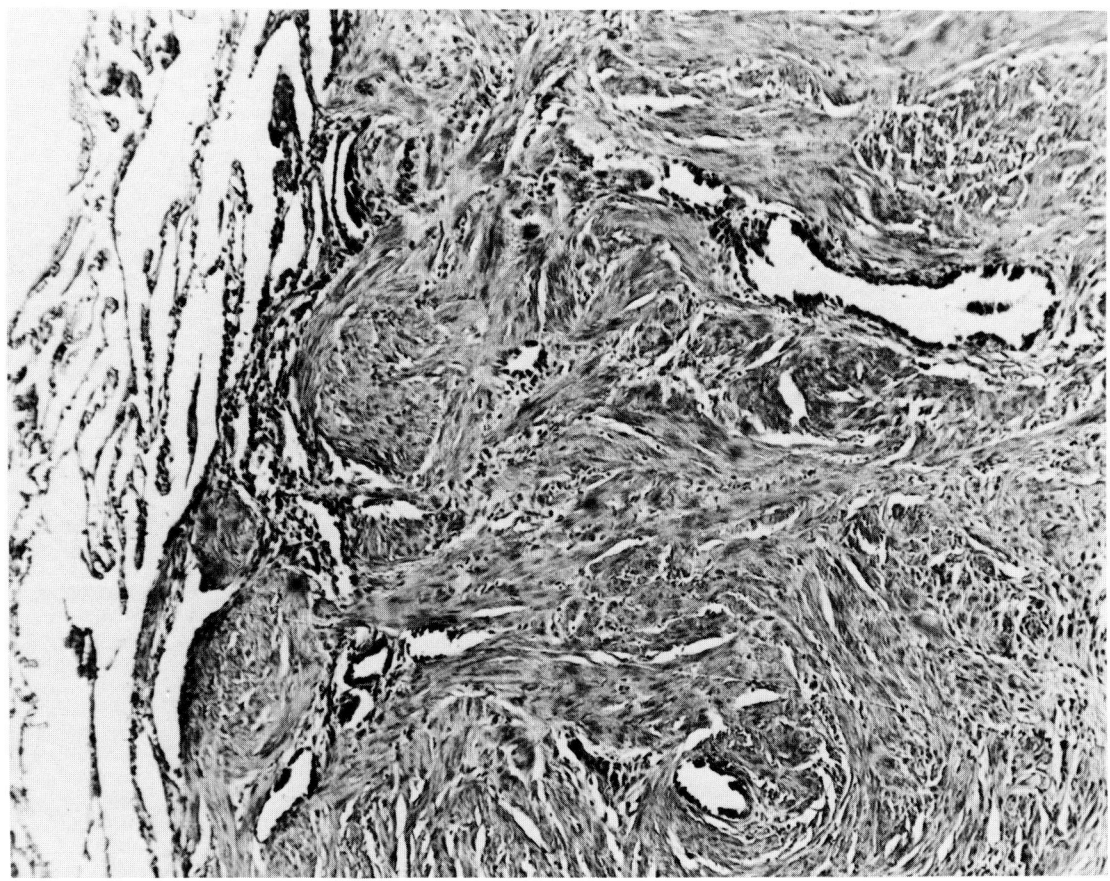

Fig. 51.13 Metastasizing leiomyoma. Pulmonary nodule is composed of smooth muscle, which encloses gland-like spaces; normal pulmonary parenchyma is at left (×97).

can result in the formation of gland-like spaces, which may be cystic and contain mucin (Fig. 51.13). With occasional exceptions, there is no evidence of vascular invasion either within the uterine leiomyomas or the adjacent myometrium, but in many cases it has not been examined extensively.

The metastasizing leiomyoma should be differentiated from the lesions of pulmonary lymphangiomyomatosis[7,33,73] as well as from primary smooth muscle tumors of the lung, which are extremely rare. In pulmonary lymphangiomyomatosis, which is sometimes associated with tuberous sclerosis, proliferating smooth muscle infiltrates the pleura, septa and bronchial and alveolar walls accompanied by honeycombing and bulla formation. Pulmonary vessels, particularly lymphatics, and lymph nodes are also involved in the myoproliferative process. Uterine involvement is rare;[73] more commonly, uterine leiomyomas, which are probably coincidental, are additionally present.

The extreme rarity of primary pulmonary smooth muscle tumors, the association with uterine leiomyomas and the occasional additional involvement of pelvic and abdominal lymph nodes establish the interpretation that the pulmonary nodules encountered in this disorder are metastatic. Additional evidence includes an occasional paradoxical reduction in their size during pregnancy[56] and a cessation in their growth after the menopause, suggesting hormone dependence.

Heterologous sarcomas

Rare uterine sarcomas, composed entirely of heterologous elements, include in order of frequency: rhabdomyosarcoma,[13,37,53,85,116] chondrosarcoma[23,69] osteosarcoma[35,116] and liposarcoma.[116,120]

Heterologous sarcomas typically form large polypoid masses that fill the endometrial cavity, often prolapsing through the external os, and invade the myometrium; rare tumors may be confined to the myometrium. Botryoid forms of rhabdomyosarcoma in the cervix of young women histologically resemble the more common sarcoma botryoides of the vagina of infants and children.[13,37] In contrast to tumors in the latter site, however, the cervical tumors have an excellent prognosis. Some patients have been cured by polypectomy, wide local excision, or cervicectomy.[37]

Rhabdomyosarcomas must be differentiated from polyps containing bizarre cells resembling rhabdomyoblasts (pseudosarcoma botryoides).[15,92] These lesions have been encountered in the cervix as well as the vagina and vulva, particularly in pregnant or recently pregnant women. The stromal cells in these polyps typically have pointed cytoplasmic processes and rarely contain mitotic figures; a cambium layer, immature cells and rhabdomyoblasts are absent.

MIXED EPITHELIAL/NON-EPITHELIAL TUMORS

Tumors in this category are characterized by an intimate admixture of an epithelial and a non-epithelial component, both of which are neoplastic. In the vast majority of the cases, both components are histologically malignant and the tumor is designated a malignant müllerian mixed tumor. Uncommonly, a malignant stromal component occurs with a benign-appearing epithelial component (müllerian adenosarcoma) or, very rarely, the epithelial component is carcinomatous but the stromal component appears benign (carcinofibroma or carcinomesenchymoma).

Malignant müllerian mixed tumors

The terms, malignant müllerian mixed tumor, malignant mesodermal mixed tumor (MMMT) and carcinosarcoma have all been applied to uterine neoplasms composed of a mixture of malignant epithelial and stromal elements.[2,4,11,20,21,28,40,48,68,81,91,94,104,107,118,121] They account for approximately 40% of uterine sarcomas. MMMTs are usually soft, broad-based, polypoid tumors that fill the endometrial cavity (Fig. 51.14) and may protrude through the external os. Rare tumors appear to be multicentric, with two or more separate exophytic masses. The surface of the tumor is characteristically smooth in contrast to the more rough and irregular surface of the typical endometrial carcinoma. The cut surface is usually fleshy, often with areas of hemorrhage, necrosis and cystic degeneration. Gritty or hard areas may be produced by the presence of bone or cartilage; the latter may have a translucent appearance. Myometrial invasion is usually evident. The cervix may be involved by downgrowth of tumor, and rare MMMTs are primary in the endocervix.[2]

Microscopic examination reveals an intimate admixture of malignant epithelial (carcinomatous) and malignant mesenchymal (sarcomatous) components (Fig. 51.15). The carcinoma in over 90% of the cases is an adenocarcinoma, usually endometrioid and less often clear cell, serous, mucinous or undifferentiated, alone or in combination. In occasional tumors, the glandular component focally lacks

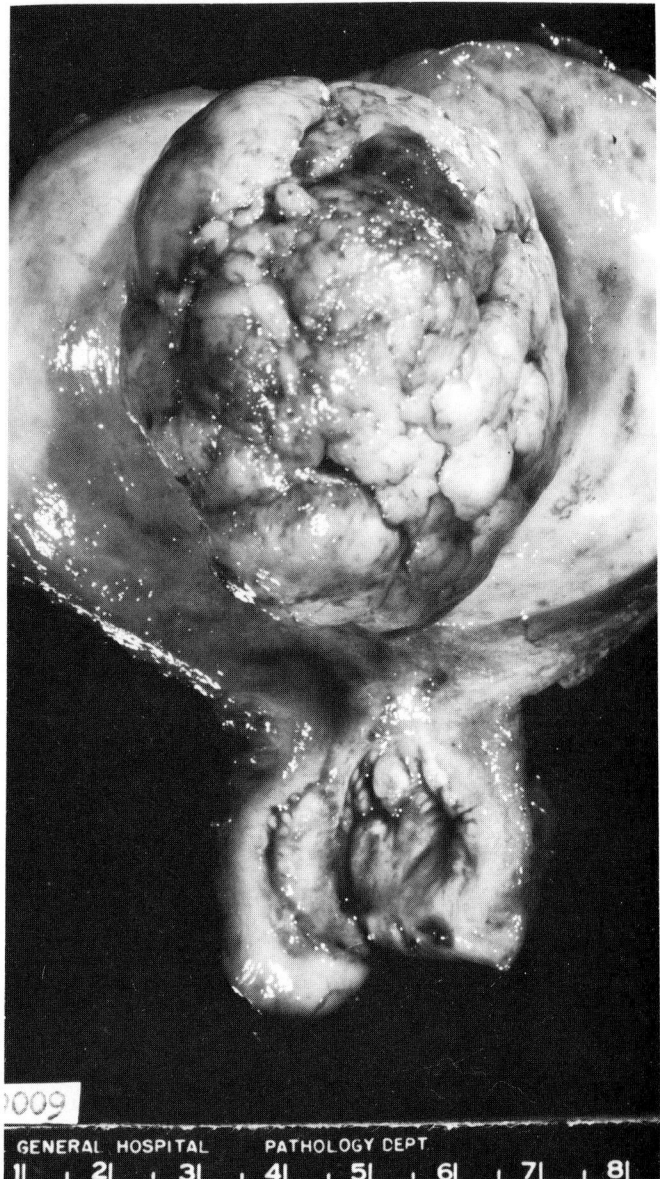

GENERAL HOSPITAL   PATHOLOGY DEPT

Fig. 51.14 Malignant müllerian mixed tumor. Large fleshy polypoid mass with relatively smooth surface fills endometrial cavity.

frankly malignant features, exhibiting a benign or dysplastic appearance. Squamous cell carcinoma alone is found in approximately 5% of cases, but more frequently it is admixed with an adenocarcinoma as an adenosquamous carcinoma.

The sarcomatous component of MMMTs may be homologous or heterologous. Homologous sarcoma typically has the appearance of a spindle cell sarcoma, resembling an endometrial stromal sarcoma, leiomyosarcoma, fibrosarcoma, malignant fibrous histiocytoma, undifferentiated sarcoma, or any combination thereof. Bizarre cells with eosinophilic cytoplasm but no cross striations, which may

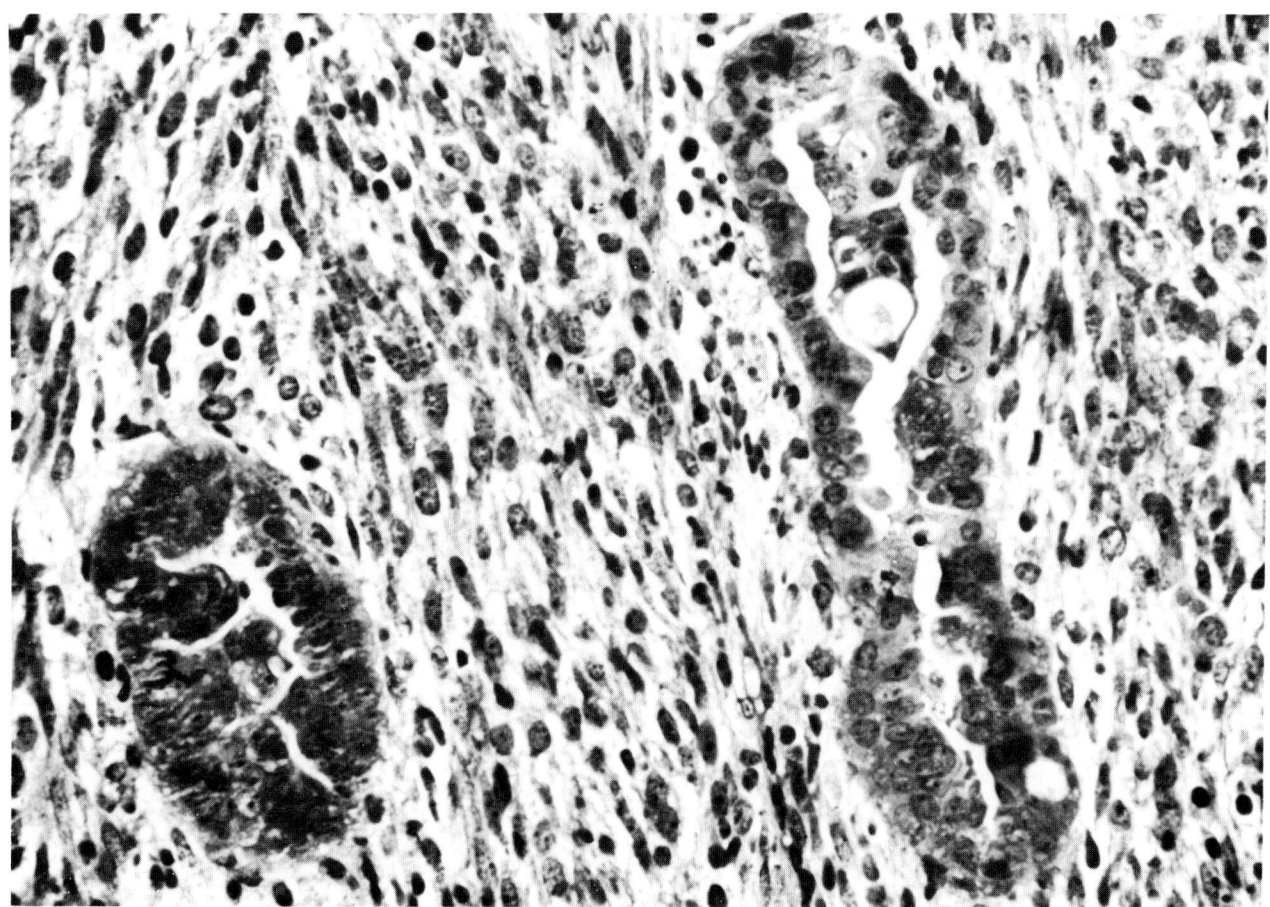

Fig. 51.15 Malignant müllerian mixed tumor, homologous type. Carcinomatous glands are surrounded by a high-grade spindle-cell sarcoma (×660).

be present, should not be considered rhabdomyoblasts on the basis of light-microscopic examination of routinely stained sections alone. Edematous or myxoid areas are common. In the heterologous tumors, the heterologous foci typically merge with, and appear to be derived from, undifferentiated homologous sarcoma. Heterologous tumors contain one or more of the following elements, in descending order of frequency: rhabdomyoblasts (Fig. 51.16B); foci of cartilage that may appear mature or have the features of chondrosarcoma (Fig. 51.16A); osteoid, bone or osteosarcoma; and liposarcoma.

Homologous and heterologous MMMTs have occurred with approximately equal frequency in most studies. Heterologous tumors have predominated, however, in some series of postradiation MMMTs,[118] as well as in other series in which an assiduous search for heterologous elements has been performed.[68] It has been suggested that, because these elements are often sparsely and irregularly distributed, heterologous tumors are probably underdiagnosed and truly homologous tumors may be rare.[68]

Eosinophilic hyaline droplets, 1 to 50 micra in diameter, are commonly present in both uterine and ovarian

MMMTs.[38] They are usually arranged in grape-like clusters within the perinuclear cytoplasm; extracellular droplets, however, are also commonly present. The droplets stain consistently with periodic acid-Schiff after diastase digestion, and are light blue to deep purple with phosphotungstic acid staining. In some tumors they may be inconspicuous, whereas in others large numbers of closely packed droplets may be a striking finding on low power examination. The droplets are most commonly within mesenchymal cells in edematous or myxomatous areas, but in approximately one-half of cases, they are also seen within carcinoma cells.

The rarest type of differentiation in MMMTs is neural or neuroendocrine. Young et al[123] have described an MMMT with focal glial differentiation, and another possible example of such an occurrence has also been reported.[105] Additionally, one MMMT contained foci of small cell carcinoma that stained positively with the Grimelius method and for 'neuron-specific' enolase (NSE).[82]

Immunohistochemical staining may be useful in confirming the presence of both an epithelial component

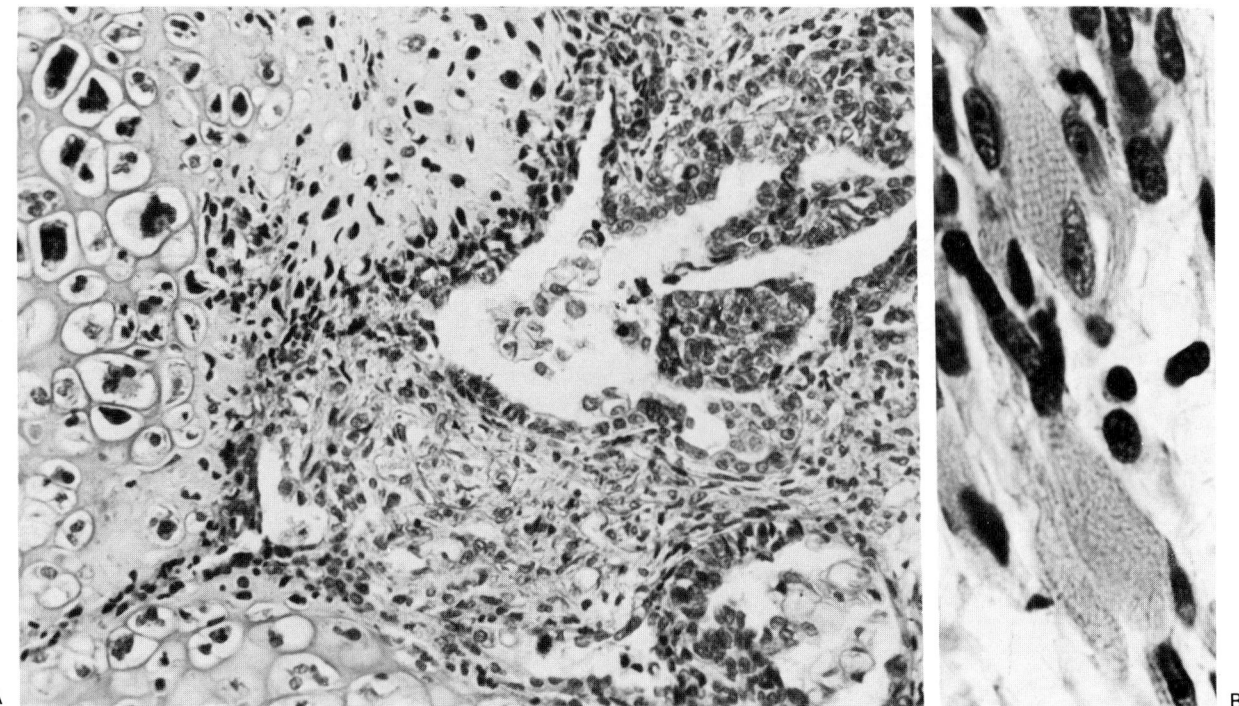

Fig. 51.16 Malignant müllerian mixed tumor, heterologous type. (A) Carcinomatous glands are admixed with nodules of chondrosarcoma (×250). (B) Rhabdomyoblasts exhibit cytoplasmic cross striations (×1250).

(cytokeratin, epithelial membrane antigen) and a mesenchymal component (vimentin, desmin, actin, myosin) in tumors in which one or both of the suspected neoplastic elements are poorly differentiated.[4,21,48] Similarly, staining for myoglobin can be useful in confirming the presence of rhabdomyoblasts. Both epithelial and mesenchymal cells may stain for alpha-1-antitrypsin (AAT) and alpha-1-antichymotrypsin.[83] Hyaline droplets have been shown to be consistently positive for AAT,[38] although it is unclear whether it is a secretory product of the tumor cells or is derived from the serum. Recently, expression of glial fibrillary acidic protein (GFAP) has been demonstrated within otherwise non-specific neoplastic spindle cells in 9 of 13 MMMTs.[78]

80% of MMMTs invade beyond the inner third of the myometrium, and 40% extend into the outer third.[39] Myometrial, lymphatic, and vascular invasion is present in almost all the cases. Rare MMMTs may be confined to an otherwise typical endometrial polyp.

The uninvolved endometrium may be the site of an atypical endometrial hyperplasia or contain pure endometrial carcinoma in as many as one-half of cases.[121] The latter finding, in addition to rare cases in which an apparently pure endometrial carcinoma has recurred or metastasized as an MMMT, suggests that occasional MMMTs may evolve from pure carcinomas.

Histologic grading, mitotic activity, and the presence or absence of heterologous elements have not been consistently useful in predicting the prognosis of patients with MMMTs; the only important prognostic factor appears to be the extent of tumor at the time of treatment. Most survivors have tumors confined to the endometrium and inner myometrium, although some patients with tumor of this extent succumb.[11,65,68] The much poorer survival associated with deeper invasion is related to the high frequency of lymphatic and blood vessel involvement. DiSaia et al found pelvic and para-aortic lymph node metastases in 36% and 14%, respectively, of clinical Stage I cases, but metastases occurred only in those cases in which the neoplasms invaded the outer half of the myometrium.[39] Other studies have shown that approximately 50% of clinical Stage I tumors are associated with extra-uterine spread at the time of operation.[40,81,91] Clinical staging in patients with MMMTs, therefore, is a poor discriminator of outcome and is misleading as a guideline for therapy.

90% of recurrences appear within 2 years.[107] Most patients die as a result of complications of tumor growth within the pelvis and abdomen, although the majority of such patients also have hematogenous spread, most commonly to the lungs, liver, bone and brain.[20,40,91,94,107,121] The recurrent or metastatic tumor may mimic the primary tumor on histological examination, contain only carcinoma or only sarcoma, or be undifferentiated.

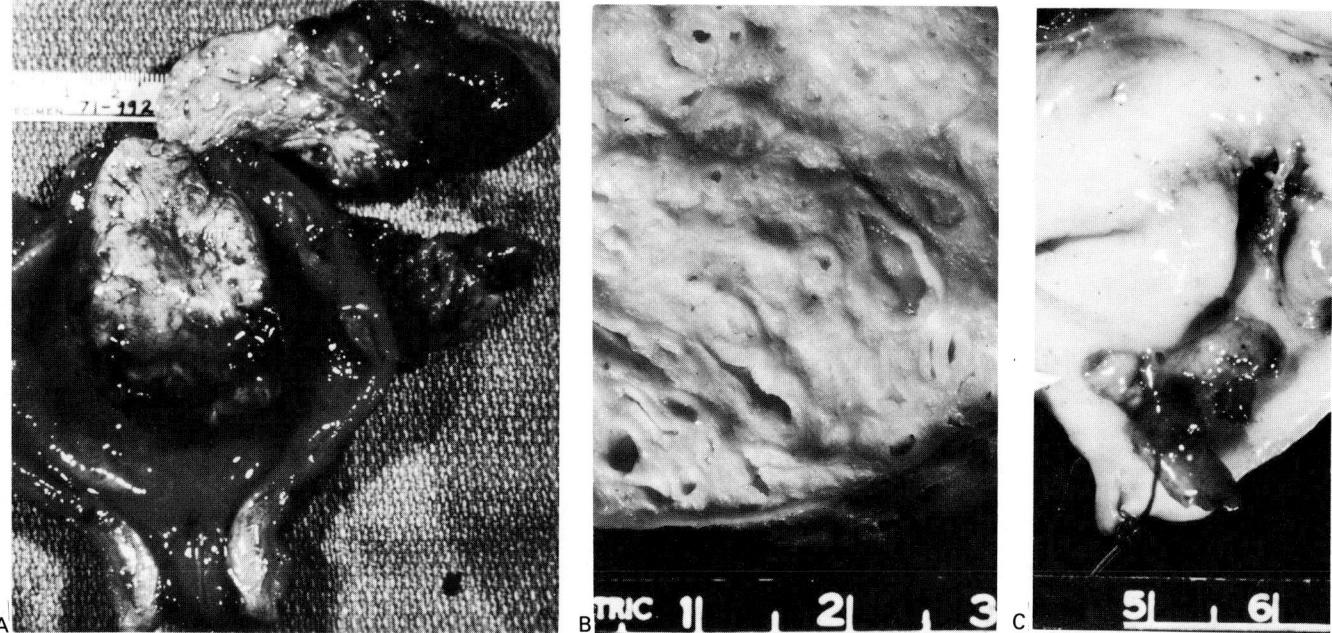

Fig. 51.17 Müllerian adenosarcoma (A) Cross section of fleshy, focally hemorrhagic polypoid tumor fills endometrial cavity. (B) Cut surface of mural tumor shows characteristic sponge-like appearance of cut surface with cystic spaces surrounded by collars of tumor. (C) Polypoid recurrence at vaginal apex, which developed 18 months following hysterectomy.

Müllerian adenosarcoma

Much less common than MMMTs is the müllerian adenosarcoma, which is characterized by a malignant stromal component and an epithelial component that has a benign or atypical appearance.[26,28,36,46,50,95,128] Adenosarcomas usually occur in postmenopausal women with a median age of 62 years, but, in contrast to MMMTs, approximately 30% of adenosarcomas are found in premenopausal patients, including adolescents and young adults. The most common symptom is abnormal vaginal bleeding, often accompanied by lower abdominal or pelvic pain. Pelvic examination typically reveals an enlarged uterus and, in about one-half of cases, tumor protruding through the external os. The diagnosis can frequently be made prior to hysterectomy by biopsy or dilatation and curettage.

Adenosarcomas form typically polypoid, broad-based tumors that frequently fill the endometrial cavity (Fig. 51.17A); prolapse of the tumor through the external os is common. Approximately 10% of the tumors originate in the endocervix and, rarely, the tumor is confined to the myometrium without mucosal involvement.[28] The cut surface is typically spongy, characterized by cystic spaces filled with a watery or mucoid fluid, surrounded by white to tan tissue (Fig. 51.17B). Myometrial invasion, which is present in approximately 25% of adenosarcomas, may be appreciable on gross examination of the hysterectomy specimen.

On microscopic examination, adenosarcomas have an epithelial component characterized by glands that are frequently cystically dilated and are scattered regularly or irregularly throughout the mesenchymal component of the tumor (Fig. 51.18A). Occasional tumors have a villous pattern, with the neoplastic epithelium lining mesenchymal papillae, and only a minor component of glands. The glands may be lined by a variety of benign or atypical müllerian epithelia, most commonly of proliferative endometrial type, although endocervical (mucinous), tubal (ciliated), secretory-endometrial (with subnuclear vacuoles), hobnail, or indifferent epithelia may also be seen. Metaplastic squamous epithelium, typically nonkeratinizing, is often present and may fill the gland lumens. Uncommonly, the glandular epithelium exhibits focal architectural or cytological atypia, rarely creating a resemblance to endometrial adenocarcinoma in situ, but invasive carcinoma, by definition, is absent in these tumors. The stromal component of the adenosarcoma is composed of round to spindle-shaped cells that most commonly resemble those of an endometrial stromal sarcoma (Fig. 51.18B); less often they appear fibrosarcomatous or, rarely, leiomyosarcomatous. The stromal cells exhibit nuclear atypia that is usually mild or moderate, but occasionally marked. Stromal mitotic figures are an almost constant

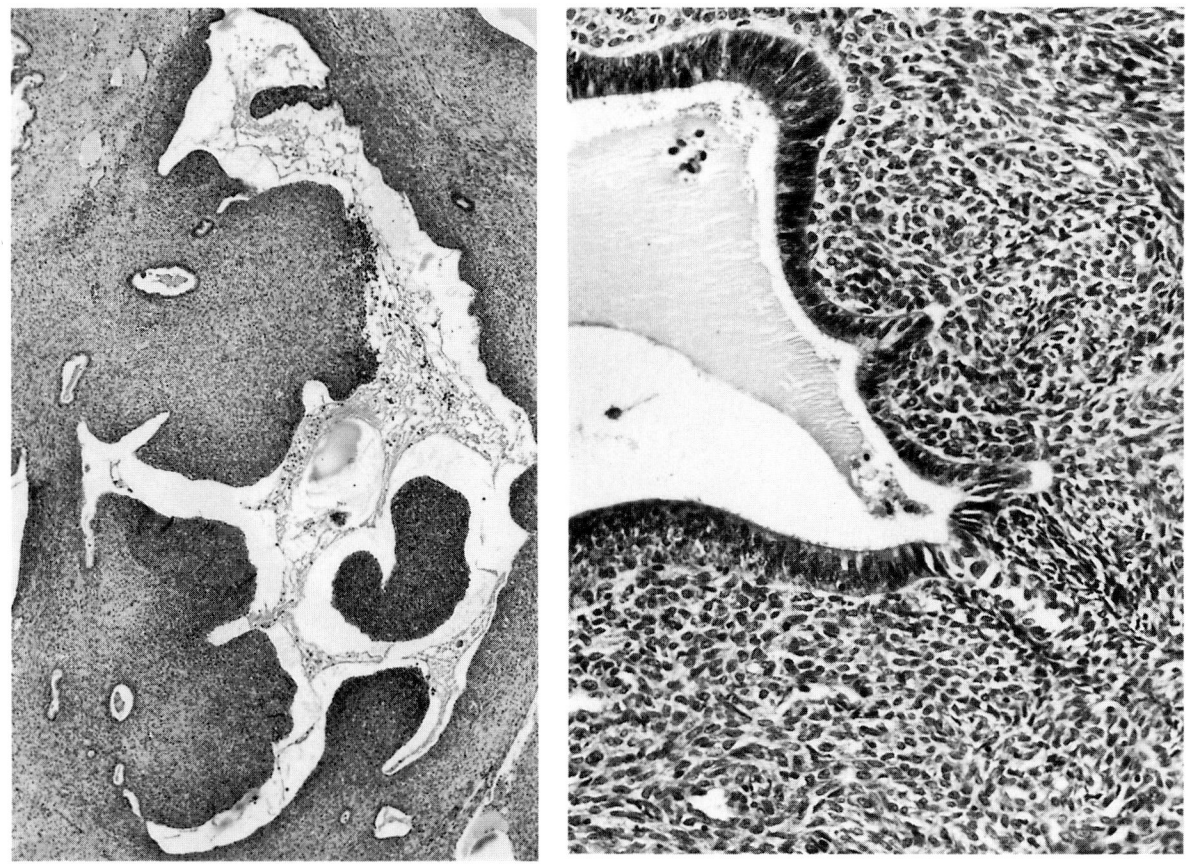

Fig. 51.18 Müllerian adenosarcoma. (A) The tumor is composed of a cellular sarcomatous stroma and benign glands. The sarcomatous component exhibits periglandular condensation and forms intraglandular polypoid projections (×50). (B) The sarcomatous stroma, which resembles low grade endometrial stromal sarcoma, surrounds a benign-appearing gland lined by proliferative-type endometrial epithelium (×270).

finding, with most tumors exhibiting a mitotic rate of four or more per 10 HPF.[28,128] Characteristically, the stroma is more cellular around the glands, creating a cuff-like appearance, and intraluminal polypoid or papillary stromal projections are common (Fig. 51.18B). The stroma at a distance from the glands is often less cellular, and may consist of sparsely cellular or hyalinized fibrous tissue, which can impart a deceptively benign appearance to large areas of the tumor. In rare cases, the stromal cells exhibit differentiation into epithelial type cords or trabeculae, similar to those encountered in occasional endometrial stromal tumors and in the rare uterine tumors with predominant sex cord-like patterns.[29] In 25% of cases of adenosarcoma, heterologous elements are present and may have a benign or malignant appearance on histologic examination.[28] These elements include, in descending order of frequency, skeletal muscle, cartilage, bone or osteoid, and fat. Approximately 25% of adenosarcomas invade the myometrium, usually with a well circumscribed margin; in other cases, the border is more obviously infiltrative.

The histologic dividing line between adenosarcomas and the rarer adenofibroma has not been clearly established. We currently diagnose as adenosarcoma tumors with two or more MF/10 HPF, a mitotic rate that will detect almost all the tumors with a malignant potential.[28] Because rare, essentially amitotic tumors with marked stromal cellularity, stromal atypia or both have recurred after hysterectomy, we also consider tumors with these features low grade adenosarcomas. The diagnosis of adenofibroma is rendered only rarely, and only after the tumor has been extensively sampled to exclude foci exhibiting mitotic activity, marked cellularity, or stromal cell atypia.

Adenosarcomas typically have a low malignant potential, manifested primarily by local vaginal or pelvic recurrence in approximately one-third of the cases, and hematogenous spread in less than 5% of the cases.[28] The only morphologic features that have so far been associated with a high risk of recurrence are deep myometrial invasion[28,128] and the presence of sarcomatous overgrowth.[25] Adenosarcomas frequently have an indolent growth rate, so that recurrences may appear at postoperative intervals of 5 years or more. Long-term clinical follow-up is therefore essential in these patients. Death from tumor occurred in 25% of the series of Zaloudek & Norris, with a median survival time of 7 years.[128] In contrast, adenosarcomas with sarcomatous overgrowth are aggressive tumors with a high risk for recurrence and blood-borne metastases, and a prognosis similar to that of other high grade uterine sarcomas.[25]

Recurrent adenosarcomas, which most commonly appear as a polypoid mass at the vaginal apex (Fig. 51.17C), may mimic the primary tumor in their histologic appearance, with both components present; more commonly, however, they are pure spindle cell sarcomas, often with a greater degree of nuclear pleomorphism and a higher mitotic rate than the sarcomatous component of the primary tumor. Rare recurrent tumors have contained foci of adenocarcinoma or heterologous mesenchymal elements that were not found in the primary tumor.[28] Distant metastases of adenosarcomas are almost always purely sarcomatous.

Atypical polypoid adenomyoma

Approximately 1% of benign polypoid tumors of the endometrium have a stroma composed of smooth muscle,

rather than the endometrial or fibrous stroma of the typical endometrial polyp. When these adenomyomas are bland cytologically, they pose no diagnostic problem. In 1981, however, Mazur focused attention on the presence of atypical features in some adenomyomas that occasionally led to confusion with a malignant tumor.[84] Since then, 35 of these 'atypical polypoid adenomyomas' (APAs) have been reported.[31,84,125]

APAs characteristically occur in premenopausal women, who are usually in their fourth or fifth decade (average age 39 years); rarely, the tumor is encountered after the menopause. Three APAs have been reported in patients with Turner's syndrome, at least two of whom had been on long-term estrogen therapy.[31] The presenting symptom is almost always abnormal vaginal bleeding. Pelvic examination is usually negative, although rare tumors have been visible as polypoid masses projecting through the external os.[31]

APAs typically involve the lower uterine segment and, less commonly, the endocervix or upper corpus. They are usually solitary and less than 2 cm in diameter, although multiple tumors and examples up to 6 cm have been described.[31] The cut surfaces are yellow-tan to gray to

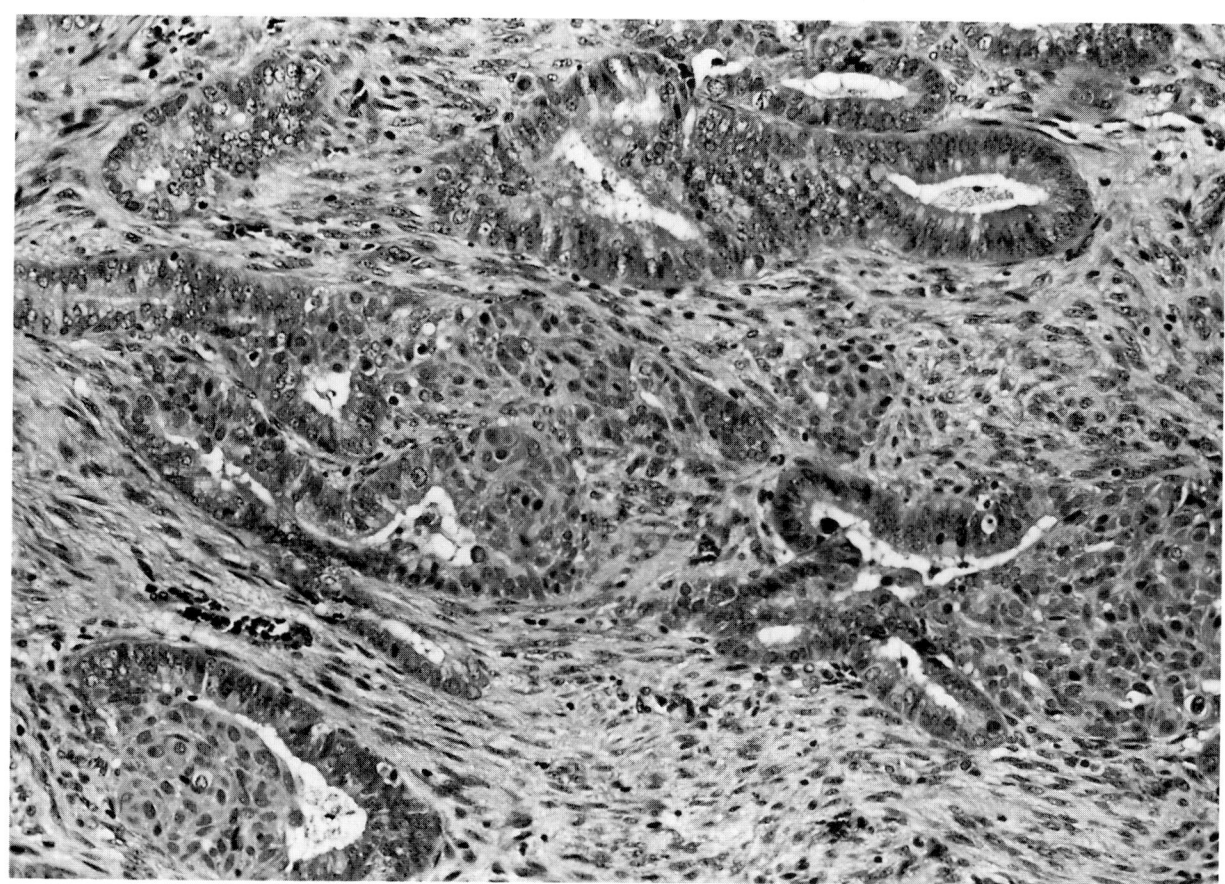

Fig. 51.19 Atypical polypoid adenomyoma. The tumor is composed of an intimate admixture of endometrial-type glands and benign cellular smooth muscle. The glands are lined by atypical columnar cells, and some contain squamous morules (×300).

white, solid, bulging, lobulated or bosselated, and firm or rubbery. The tumors may be pedunculated or sessile and are well demarcated from the underlying myometrium.

On histologic examination, APAs are composed of endometrial glands admixed with smooth muscle that is usually cellular (Fig. 51.19). The glands exhibit varying degrees of architectural and cytological atypia with mitotic activity. In occasional cases, severe cytological atypia with an intraglandular cribriform pattern may warrant a diagnosis of adenocarcinoma in situ. In 90% of the cases, squamous metaplasia is present and may be extensive, obliterating glandular lumens (Fig. 51.19). The stromal component consists of interlacing bundles of smooth muscle cells that appear benign (Fig. 51.19), but exhibit mild to moderate atypia in a minority of cases; occasional mitotic figures are usually present, but the mitotic rate is typically less than 2 MF/10 HPF. In some cases, occasional glands are surrounded by a narrow cuff of cells of endometrial stromal type. In curettage specimens, the diagnostic fragments are usually admixed with normal proliferative or secretory endometrium, although occasionally there may be associated endometrial hyperplasia or even adenocarcinoma, which may also involve and, rarely, originate in adenomyoma. In hysterectomy specimens, APAs usually have a well circumscribed non-invasive border with the adjacent endometrium and underlying myometrium, but rarely invade the myometrium in irregular tongues.

Follow-up of the 35 reported cases treated by curettage or hysterectomy has shown no evidence of a malignant behavior. In most cases, however, the postcurettage follow-up has been short, or hysterectomy was performed soon after diagnosis. The ultimate fate of the conservatively treated lesion is thus uncertain at the present time. In several patients in whom a repeated curettage was performed, the lesion has persisted for as long as 4 years after the initial procedure. In several other cases, a repeated curettage has revealed atypical endometrial hyperplasia, with or without squamous metaplasia, or an adenoacanthoma.

MISCELLANEOUS TUMORS AND RELATED LESIONS

Uterine tumors resembling ovarian sex-cord tumors

We have applied the term 'uterine tumor resembling ovarian sex-cord tumor' to a heterogeneous group of rare neoplasms characterized by pure or predominant histologic patterns that closely resemble those of ovarian sex-cord tumors (granulosa cell and Sertoli cell tumors).[27,28,61,109] Several previously described 'granulosa cell tumors' of the uterus most likely belong in this category.[74,86] The patients, who are in the reproductive and postmenopausal age groups, typically present with abnormal vaginal bleeding, although occasionally they are asymptomatic. An enlarged uterus is usually found on pelvic examination.

On gross examination, these tumors are generally solid, round, well circumscribed myometrial masses that range from 3 to 10 cm in diameter (Fig. 51.20); occasional tumors have been predominantly cystic. The tumors are usually submucosal or intramural, but occasionally subserosal; the submucosal and subserosal tumors may be polypoid. Rare tumors have been located predominantly within the endometrium. The cut surfaces are often yellow, but occasionally grey to tan, and are soft, fleshy and homogeneous without the whorled pattern of a leiomyoma (Fig. 51.20).

Histologic examination usually reveals a well circumscribed, pushing border with the adjacent myometrium. Less commonly, the tumor infiltrates the myometrium, usually to a limited degree, but occasionally more extensively. In such cases, invasion of lymphatics, blood vessels or both have been encountered. The tumor cells typically form solid or hollow tubules, cords and trabeculae often disposed in a plexiform arrangement, and solid nests (Fig. 51.21). The neoplastic cells vary from small, round and regular with scanty cytoplasm, to large with abundant eosinophilic, clear, or foamy cytoplasm that is often lipid-rich. The nuclei are generally small and regular with little pleomorphism and indistinct nucleoli. Nuclear grooves are rare or absent and mitotic figures are typically scarce. The stroma ranges from scanty to abundant, and from moderately cellular to hypocellular and hyalinized. Leydig or theca cell-like differentiation has not been observed, although lipid-laden stromal cells of questionable origin have been present in some cases.

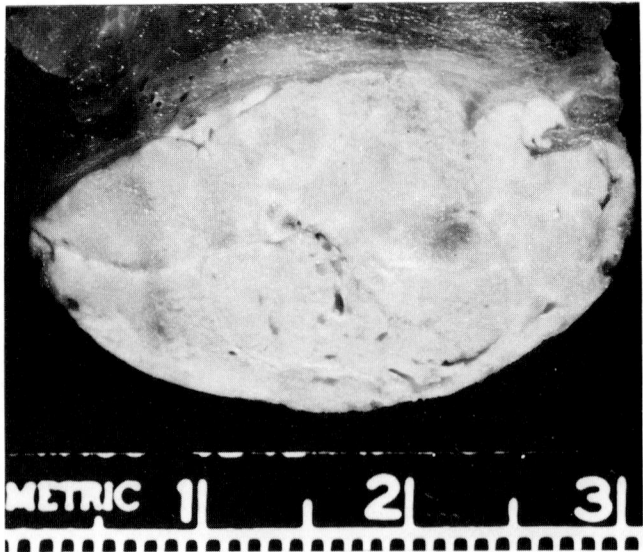

Fig. 51.20 Uterine tumor resembling ovarian sex-cord tumor. Well-circumscribed mural tumor exhibits a faintly lobulated fleshy (yellow) cut surface (tumor was completely surrounded by myometrium, some of which has become detached).

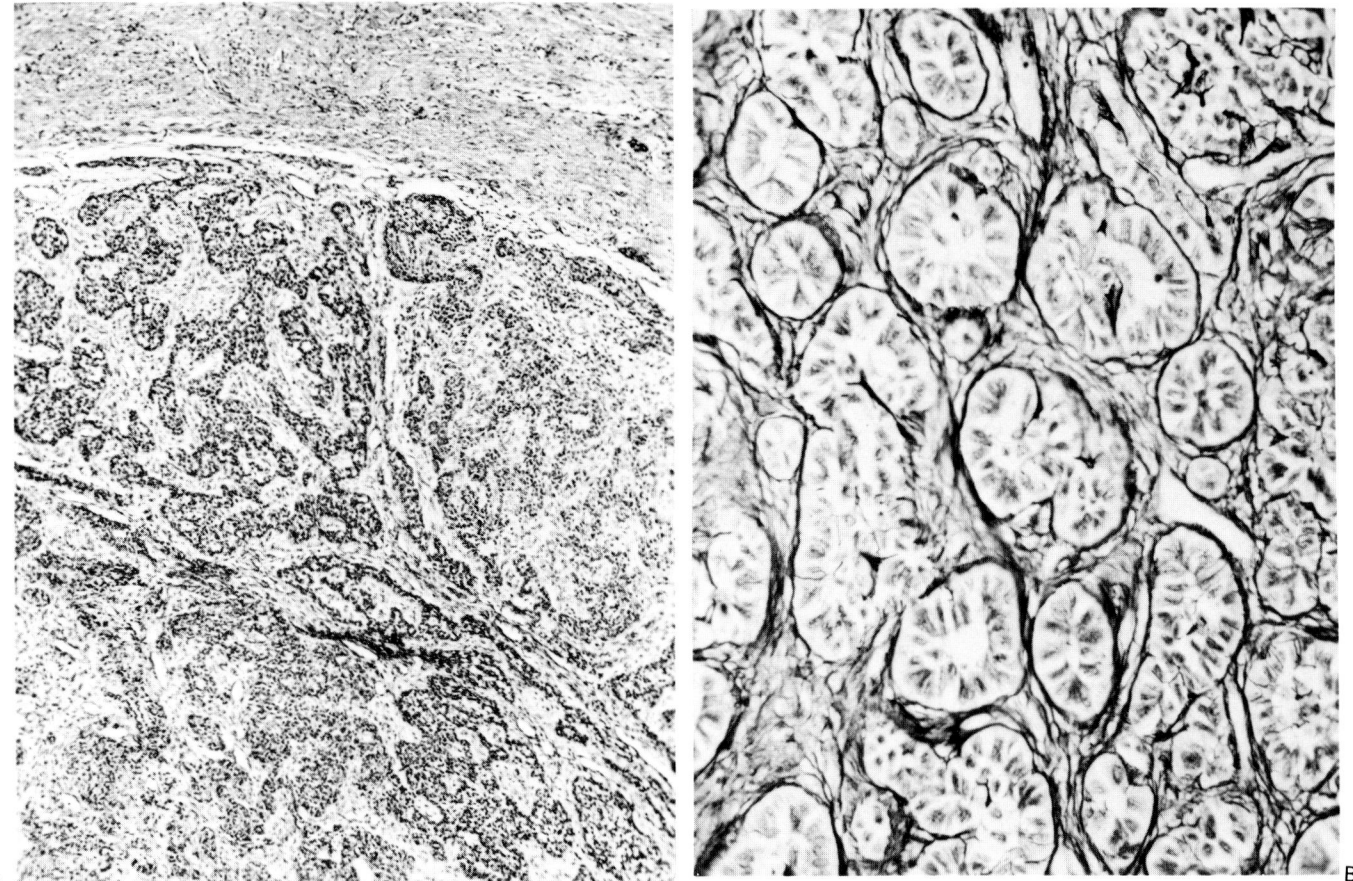

Fig. 51.21 Uterine tumor resembling ovarian sex-cord tumor. (A) Tumor exhibits a trabecular pattern and a pushing border with adjacent myometrium (×70). (B) The tumor cells form hollow tubules and have abundant vacuolated cytoplasm; reticulum is sparse and does not penetrate tubules (×320; reticulum stain).

Because of the close resemblance of these tumors to ovarian sex-cord tumors, a possible origin from displaced ovarian tissue has been considered. However, the neoplastic cells lack the characteristic pale nuclei with grooves and typical Call-Exner body formation of ovarian granulosa cell tumors, and there has been no clinical evidence of endocrine function in the reported cases. In one case, however, structures resembling Charcot-Bottcher filament-bundles, characteristic inclusions of testicular Sertoli cells, were enigmatically present.[61] The histologic heterogeneity of these tumors suggests the possibility of more than a single cell of origin. The similarity of the epithelial patterns to those seen focally in endometrial stromal tumors strongly supports a derivation from endometrial stromal cells in most cases. The plexiform pattern seen in some cases, which may be similar to that seen in some epithelioid smooth muscle tumors and plexiform tumorlets, favors a smooth muscle origin in occasional cases.

Although most of these tumors have had a benign clinical course after hysterectomy, we have encountered several examples that have recurred or metastasized. In two such cases, myometrial lymphatic or blood vessel invasion was observed. Until larger numbers of cases have been studied and criteria for malignancy established, these neoplasms should be regarded as potentially malignant, except when they are small and circumscribed and lack significant nuclear pleomorphism, mitotic activity and angio-invasion.

Lymphoma and leukemia

The uterus is often infiltrated by leukemia or non-Hodgkin's lymphoma as a manifestation of generalized disease. Analysis of one autopsy series of patients with leukemia and lymphoma that was predominantly of the non-Hodgkin's type showed uterine infiltration in 41% of the patients dying with leukemia, and involvement of the corpus in 10% and the cervix in 6% of those dying with lymphoma.[76] The demonstration of Hodgkin's disease in the uterus is much less common,[55,58] with only a 3% frequency in one autopsy series.[55]

Rarely, uterine involvement may be the initial manifestation of a disseminated lymphoma, or the uterus may be the primary site of lymphoma.[18,51,70] The diagnosis of primary uterine lymphoma should be restricted to cases in which the disease is confined to the uterus or has spread only to contiguous areas including regional lymph nodes. Of the approximately 65 such cases in the literature, 90% have originated in the cervix, and the remainder in the corpus. Approximately 85% of these tumors were classified as

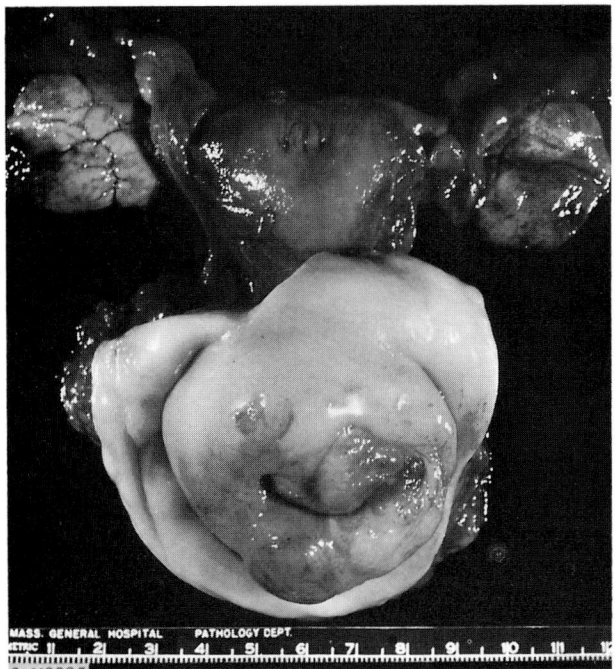

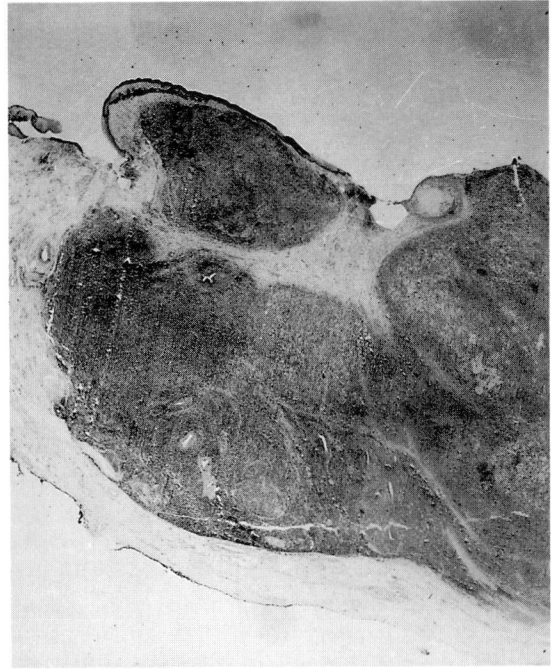

Fig. 51.22 Primary lymphoma of the uterine cervix. (A) The cervix is diffusely enlarged with several areas of nodularity and mucosal congestion. (B) The tumor consists of large solid masses with pushing margins, and penetrates almost to the deep margin of resection (×5; Giemsa stain). (Reproduced from Chung et al (1988),[21] with permission.)

non-Hodgkin's lymphoma, most commonly 'reticulum cell sarcoma', large cell, or 'histiocytic' lymphoma and, rarely, as Hodgkin's disease. A few cases of granulocytic sarcoma of the cervix have been associated with the subsequent development of rapidly progressive leukemia.[1,51]

Involvement by lymphoma or granulocytic sarcoma typically results in diffuse enlargement of the cervix or corpus by homogeneous pale, fish-flesh tissue (Fig. 51.22A). Microscopic examination typically reveals deeply invasive tumor (Fig. 51.22B) with a diffuse or nodular pattern. The neoplastic cells usually surround glands and vessels without destroying them, although infiltration of vessel walls is common. Occasionally, a cord-like pattern of growth simulates that of a carcinoma. One form of cervical lymphoma that is difficult to differentiate from both inflammatory disorders and other malignant neoplasms, including sarcomas, is the sclerosing 'histiocytic' type.[51] In biopsy specimens of such a tumor, the neoplastic cells may be artifactually shrunken and easily confused with benign lymphocytes or the cells of a small cell carcinoma. In larger specimens, the abundant fibrous stroma and the presence of varying numbers of lymphocytes in the tumor may be misleading. Careful examination of areas where the neoplastic cells are numerous and well preserved may be necessary to establish the diagnosis.

Granulocytic sarcomas can be easily confused with non-Hodgkin's lymphomas, but chloroacetate esterase stains and immunoperoxidase stains for lysozyme are sometimes helpful in this distinction. Evaluation of the blood and bone marrow is of obvious additional importance in such cases. Finally, staining of direct smears of the neoplastic tissue may be of great diagnostic aid in cases of leukemia as well as lymphoma.

In the differential diagnosis of granulocytic sarcomas, a variety of lymphoma-like lesions that involve the uterus, most commonly the cervix but also the endometrium, must be considered.[124] These lesions are characterized by an accumulation of inflammatory cells, often including immunoblasts with mitotic activity, but the presence of other cell types, such as plasma cells and polymorphonuclear leukocytes, in the infiltrate is helpful in identifying the lesion as inflammatory. Additional features that aid in the distinction from a lymphoma include absence of a mass, associated ulceration, mucosal involvement, absence of deep invasion and absence of a prominent perivascular distribution.[124] The differential diagnosis of lymphomas also includes rare, otherwise typical uterine leiomyomas with massive lymphoid infiltration,[45] inflammatory pseudotumors of the uterus,[49] and exceptional cases of decidual transformation of the cervical stroma during pregnancy that may mimic a lymphoma.[3] Stage I and occasional higher stage lymphomas are curable with radiotherapy, surgical therapy or both: 14 of 19 patients in one series were alive with no evidence of disease at the time of reporting.[51]

REFERENCES

1. Abeler V, Kjorstad K E, Langholm R, Marton P F 1983 Granulocytic sarcoma (chloroma) of the uterine cervix: report of two cases. Int J Gynecol Pathol 2: 88

2. Abell M R, Ramirez J A 1973 Sarcomas and carcinosarcomas of the uterine cervix. Cancer 31: 1176

3. Armenia C S, Shaver D N, Modisher M W 1964 Decidual transformation of the cervical stroma simulating reticulum cell sarcoma. Am J Obstet Gynecol 89: 808

4. Auerbach H E, LiVolsi V A, Merino M J 1988 Malignant mixed müllerian tumors of the uterus. An immunohistochemical study. Int J Gynecol Pathol 7: 123

5. Bachman D, Wolff M 1976 Pulmonary metastases from benign-appearing smooth muscle tumors of the uterus. Am J Roentgenol 127: 441

6. Baker V V, Walton L A, Fowler W C Jr, Currie J L 1984 Steroid receptors in endolymphatic stromal myosis. Obstet Gynecol 63: 72S

7. Banner A S, Carrington C B, Emory W B et al 1981 Efficacy of oophorectomy in lymphangioleiomyomatosis and benign metastasizing leiomyoma. New Engl J Med 305: 204

8. Barnes H M, Richardson P J 1973 Benign metastasizing fibroleiomyoma. Br J Obstet Gynaecol 80: 569

9. Barter J F, Smith E B, Szpak C A, Hinshaw W, Clarke-Pearson D L, Creasman W T 1985 Leiomyosarcoma of the uterus; clinicopathologic study of 21 cases. Gynecol Oncol 21: 220

10. Barter J F, Szpak C, Creasman W T 1987 Uterine leiomyomas with retroperitoneal lymph node involvement. South Med J 80: 1320

11. Barwick K W, LiVolsi V A 1979 Malignant mixed müllerian tumors of the uterus. A clinicopathologic assessment of 34 cases. Am J Surg Pathol 3: 125

12. Boyce C R, Buddhdev H N 1973 Pregnancy complicated by metastasizing leiomyoma of uterus. Obstet Gynecol 47: 525

13. Brand E, Berek J S, Nieberg R K, Hacker N F 1987 Rhabdomyosarcoma of the uterine cervix. Cancer 60: 1552

14. Burns B, Curry R H, Bell M E A 1979 Morphologic features of prognostic significance in uterine smooth muscle tumors: A review of 84 cases. Am J Obstet Gynecol 135: 1979

15. Burt R L, Prichard R W, Kim B S 1976 Fibroepithelial polyp of the vagina. A report of five cases. Obstet Gynecol 47: 52s

16. Buscema J, Carpenter S E, Rosenshein N B, Woodruff J D 1986 Epithelioid leiomyosarcoma of the uterus. Cancer 57: 1192

17. Chang V, Aikawa M, Druet R 1977 Uterine leiomyoblastoma. Ultrastructural and cytological studies. Cancer 39: 1563

18. Chorlton I, Karnei R F Jr, King F M, Norris H J 1974 Primary malignant reticuloendothelial disease involving the vagina, cervix, and corpus uteri. Obstet Gynecol 44: 735

19. Christopherson W M, Williamson E O, Gray L A 1972 Leiomyosarcoma of the uterus. Cancer 29: 1512

20. Chuang J T, Van Velden J J, Graham J B 1970 Carcinosarcoma and mixed mesodermal tumor of the uterine corpus. Review of 49 cases. Obstet Gynecol 35: 769

21. Chung M, Mukai K, Teshima S, Kishi K, Shimosato Y 1988 Expression of various antigens by different components of uterine mixed müllerian tumors. An immunohistochemical study. Acta Pathol Jpn 38: 35

22. Clark D H, Weed J C 1977 Metastasizing leiomyoma: a case report. Am J Obstet Gynecol 127: 672

23. Clement P B 1978 Chondrosarcoma of the uterus: report of a case and review of the literature. Hum Pathol 9: 726

24. Clement P B 1988 Intravenous leiomyomatosis. Pathology Annual 23 (part 2): 153

25. Clement P B 1989 Müllerian adenosarcoma of the uterus with sarcomatous overgrowth. A clinicopathological analysis of ten cases. Am J Surg Pathol 13: 28

26. Clement P B, Scully R E 1974 Müllerian adenosarcoma of the uterus. A clinicopathologic analysis of ten cases of a distinctive type of müllerian mixed tumor. Cancer 34: 1138

27. Clement P B, Scully R E 1976 Uterine tumors resembling ovarian sex-cord tumors. Am J Clin Pathol 66: 512

28. Clement P B, Scully R E 1988 Uterine tumors with mixed epithelial and mesenchymal elements. Semin Diagn Pathol 5: 199

29. Clement P B, Scully R E 1990 Müllerian adenosarcoma of the uterus with sex cord-like elements. Am J Clin Pathol 91: 664

30. Clement P B, Young R H, Scully R E 1988 Intravenous leiomyomatosis of the uterus: A clinicopathologic analysis of 16 cases with unusual histologic features. Am J Surg Pathol 12: 932

31. Clement P B, Young R H 1987 Atypical polypoid adenomyoma of the uterus associated with Turner's syndrome. Int J Gynecol Pathol 6: 104

32. Clement P B, Young R H 1987 Diffuse leiomyomatosis of the uterus: a report of four cases. Int J Gynecol Pathol 6: 322

33. Corrin B, Liebow A A, Frediman P J 1975 Pulmonary lymphangiomyomatosis. Am J Pathol 79: 348

34. Crabtree T, Kempson R L, Hendrickson M R 1985 Endometrial stromal sarcoma: A clinicopathological study of 56 cases (abstract). Lab Invest 52: 1985

35. Crum C P, Rogers B H, Andersen W 1980 Osteosarcoma of the uterus: case report of review of the literature. Gynecol Oncol 9: 256

36. Czernobilsky B, Hohlweg-Majert P, Dallenbach-Hellweg G 1983 Uterine adenosarcoma: a clinicopathologic study of 11 cases with a reevaluation of histologic criteria. Arch Gynäkol 233: 281

37. Daya D A, Scully R E 1988 Sarcoma botryoides of the uterine cervix in young women: a clinicopathological study of 13 cases. Gynecol Oncol 29: 290

38. Dictor M 1982 Ovarian malignant mixed mesodermal tumor: The occurrence of hyaline droplets containing alpha-1-antitrypsin. Human Pathol 13: 930

39. DiSaia P J, Morrow C P, Boronow R, Creasman W, Mittelstaedt L 1978 Endometrial sarcoma: lymphatic spread pattern. Am J Obstet Gynecol 130: 104

40. Doss L L, Llorens A S, Henriquez E M 1984 Carcinosarcoma of the uterus: a 40-year experience from the state of Missouri. Gynecol Oncol 19: 43

41. Evans H L 1982 Endometrial stromal sarcoma and poorly differentiated endometrial sarcoma. Cancer 50: 2170

42. Evans H L 1988 Smooth muscle neoplasms of the uterus other than ordinary leiomyoma. A study of 46 cases, with emphasis on diagnostic criteria and prognostic factors. Cancer 62: 2239

43. Fechner R E 1968 Atypical leiomyomas and synthetic progestin therapy. Am J Clin Pathol 49: 697

44. Fekete P S, Vellios F 1984 The clinical and histologic spectrum of endometrial stromal neoplasms: a report of 41 cases. Int J Gynecol Pathol 3: 198

45. Ferry J A, Harris N L, Scully R E 1990 Uterine leiomyomas with lymphoid infiltration simulating lymphoma: a report of seven cases. Int J Gynecol Pathol. In press

46. Fox H, Harilal K R, Youell A 1979 Müllerian adenosarcoma of the uterine body: a report of nine cases. Histopathol 3: 167

47. Gallup D G, Cordray D R 1979 Leiomyosarcoma of the uterus: case reports and a review. Obstet Gynecol Surv 34: 300

48. Geisinger K M, Dabbs D J, Marshall R B 1987 Malignant mixed müllerian tumors. An ultrastructural and immunohistochemical analysis with histogenetic considerations. Cancer 59: 1781

49. Gilks G B, Taylor G P, Clement P B 1987 Inflammatory pseudotumor of the uterus. Int J Gynecol Pathol 6: 275

50. Gloor E 1979 Müllerian adenosarcoma of the uterus. Clinicopathologic report of five cases. Am J Surg Pathol 3: 203

51. Harris H L, Scully R E 1984 Malignant lymphoma and granulocytic sarcoma of the uterus and vagina: a clinicopathologic analysis of 27 cases. Cancer 53: 2530

52. Hart W R, Billman J K 1978 A reassessment of uterine neoplasms originally diagnosed as leiomyosarcomas. Cancer 41: 1902

53. Hart W R, Craig J R 1978 Rhabdomyosarcomas of the uterus. Am J Clin Pathol 70: 217

54. Hart W R, Yoonessi M 1977 Endometrial stromatosis of the uterus. Obstet Gynecol 49: 393

55. Hennessey J P 1958 Discussion of paper by Hahn G: Gynecologic considerations in malignant lymphoma. Am J Obstet Gynecol 75: 673

56. Horstmann J P, Pietra G G, Harman J A, Cole N G, Grinspan S

1977 Spontaneous regression of pulmonary leiomyomas during pregnancy. Cancer 39: 314

57. Hsu Y K, Rosenshein N B, Parmley T H, Woodruff J D, Elberfeld H T 1981 Leiomyomatosis in pelvic lymph nodes. Obstet Gynecol 57: 91A

58. Hung L H Y, Kurtz D M 1985 Hodgkin's disease of the endometrium. Arch Pathol Lab Med 109: 952

59. Jensen P A, Dockerty M B, Symmonds R E, Wilson R B 1966 Endometrioid sarcoma ('stromal endometriosis'). Report of 15 cases including 5 with metastases. Am J Obstet Gynecol 95: 79

60. Kaminski P F, Tavassoli F A 1984 Plexiform tumorlet: a clinical and pathological study of 15 cases with ultrastructural observations. Int J Gynecol Pathol 3: 124

61. Kantelip B, Cloup N, Dechelotte P 1986 Uterine tumor resembling ovarian sex cord tumors: report of a case with ultrastructural study. Human Pathol 17: 91

62. Kaplan C, Katoh A, Shamoto M et al 1973 Multiple leiomyomas of the lung: benign or malignant. Am Rev Respir Dis 108: 656

63. Katz L, Merino M J, Sakamoto H, Schwartz P E 1987 Endometrial stromal sarcoma: a clinicopathologic study of 11 cases with determination of estrogen and progestin receptor levels in three tumors. Gynecol Oncol 26: 87

64. Kempson R L 1973 Sarcomas and related neoplasms. The Uterus. Williams and Wilkins, Baltimore

65. Kempson R L, Bari W 1970 Uterine sarcomas. Classification, diagnosis and prognosis. Hum Pathol 1: 331

66. Kempson R L, Hendrickson M R 1988 Pure mesenchymal neoplasms of the uterine corpus: selected problems. Semin Diagn Pathol 5: 172

67. King M E, Dickersin G R, Scully R E 1982 Myxoid leiomyosarcoma of the uterus. A report of six cases. Am J Surg Path 6: 589

68. King M E, Kramer E E 1980 Malignant müllerian mixed tumors of the uterus. Cancer 45: 188

69. Kofinas A D, Suarez J, Calame R J, Chipeco Z 1984 Chondrosarcoma of the uterus. Gynecol Oncol 19: 231

70. Komaki R, Cox J D, Hansen R M, Gunn W G, Greenberg M 1984 Malignant lymphoma of the uterine cervix. Cancer 54: 1699

71. Kriegir P D, Gusberg S B 1973 Endolymphatic stromal myosis — a grade 1 endometrial sarcoma. Gynecol Oncol 1: 299

72. Kurman R J, Norris H J 1976 Mesenchymal tumors of the uterus. VI. Epithelial smooth muscle tumors including leiomyoblastoma and clear-cell leiomyoma. A clinical and pathologic analysis of 26 cases. Cancer 37: 1853

73. Lack E E, Dolan M F, Finisio J, Grover G, Singh M, Triche T J 1986 Pulmonary and extrapulmonary lymphangioleiomyomatosis. Am J Surg Pathol 10: 650

74. Langley F A, Smith J P, Woodcock A S 1953 Debatable uterine tumors. Acta Obstet Gynaecol Scand 32: 143

75. Lantta M, Kahanpaa K, Karkkainen J, Lehtovirta P, Wahlstrom T, Widholm O 1984 Estradiol and progesterone receptors in two cases of endometrial stromal sarcoma. Gynecol Oncol 18: 233

76. Lathrop J C 1967 Malignant pelvic lymphomas. Obstet Gynecol 30: 137

77. Lavin P, Hajdu S I, Foote F W 1972 Gastric and extragastric leiomyoblastomas. Clinicopathologic study of 44 cases. Cancer 29: 305

78. Liao S Y, Choi B H 1986 Expression of glial fibrillary acidic protein by neoplastic cells of müllerian origin. Virchows Arch [Cell Pathol] 52: 185

79. Lipschutz A 1950 Tumorigenic and antitumorigenic actions of steroid hormones and the steroid homeostasis: experimental aspects. In: Steroid Hormones and Tumors. Williams and Wilkins, Baltimore

80. Lipschutz A, Vargas L 1941 Structure and origin of extragenital fibroids induced experimentally in the guinea pig by prolonged administration of estrogen. Cancer Res 1: 236

81. Macasaet M A, Waxman M, Fruchter R G et al 1985 Prognostic factors in malignant mesodermal (müllerian) mixed tumors of the uterus. Gynecol Oncol 20: 32

82. Manivel C, Wick M R, Sibley R K 1986 Neuroendocrine differentiation in müllerian neoplasms. An immunohistochemical study of a 'pure' endometrial small-cell carcinoma and a mixed müllerian tumor containing small cell carcinoma. Am J Clin Pathol 86: 438

83. Marshall R J, Braye S G 1985 Alpha-1-antitrypsin, alpha-1-antichymotrypsin, actin, and myosin in uterine sarcomas. Int J Gynecol Pathol 4: 346

84. Mazur M T 1981 Atypical polypoid adenomyomas of the endometrium. Am J Surg Pathol 5: 473

85. Montag T W, d'Ablaing G, Schlaerth J B, Gaddis O Jr, Morrow C P 1986 Embryonal rhabdomyosarcoma of the uterine corpus and cervix. Gynecol Oncol 25: 171

86. Morehead R P, Bowman M C 1945 Heterologous mesodermal tumors of the uterus. Report of a neoplasm resembling a granulosa cell tumor. Am J Pathol 21: 53

87. Myles J L, Hart W R 1985 Apoplectic leiomyomas of the uterus. Am J Surg Pathol 9: 798

88. Nogales F F, Navarro N, de Victoria J M M et al 1987 Uterine intravascular leiomyomatosis: an update and report of seven cases. Int J Gynecol Pathol 6: 331

89. Norris H J, Hilliard G D, Irey N S 1988 Hemorrhagic cellular leiomyomas ('apoplectic leiomyoma') of the uterus associated with pregnancy and oral contraceptives. Int J Gynecol Pathol 7: 212

90. Norris H J, Parmley T 1975 Mesenchymal tumors of the uterus. V. Intravenous leiomyomatosis. A clinical and pathological study of 14 cases. Cancer 36: 2164

91. Norris H J, Roth E, Taylor H B 1966 Mesenchymal tumors of the uterus. III. A clinical and pathologic study of 31 mixed mesodermal tumors. Obstet Gynecol 28: 57

92. Norris H J, Taylor H B 1966 Polyps of the vagina. A benign lesion resembling sarcoma botryoides. Cancer 19: 227

93. Norris H J, Taylor H B 1966 Mesenchymal tumors of the uterus. I. A clinical and pathologic study of 53 endometrial stromal tumors. Cancer 19: 755

94. Norris H J, Taylor H B 1966 Mesenchymal tumors of the uterus. III. A clinical and pathologic study of 31 carcinosarcomas. Cancer 19: 1459

95. Ostor A G, Fortune D W 1980 Benign and low grade variants of mixed müllerian tumor of the uterus. Histopathol 4: 369

96. Paulsen S M, Nielsen V T, Hansen P, Ferenczy A 1982 Endolymphatic stromal myosis with focal tubular-glandular differentiation (biphasic endometrial stromal sarcoma). Ultrast Pathol 3: 31

97. Perrone T, Dehner L P 1988 Prognostically favorable 'mitotically active' smooth-muscle tumors of the uterus. A clinicopathologic study of ten cases. Am J Surg Pathol 12: 1

98. Piver M S, Rutledge F N, Copeland L, Webster K, Blumenson L, Suh O 1984 Uterine endolymphatic stromal myosis: a collaborative study. Obstet Gynecol 64: 173

99. Pocock E, Craig J R, Bullock W K 1976 Metastatic uterine leiomyomata. A case report. Cancer 38: 2096

100. Prakash S, Scully R E 1964 Sarcoma-like pseudopregnancy changes in uterine leiomyomas. Obstet Gynecol 24: 106

101. Rubin S C, Wheeler J E, Mikuta J J 1986 Malignant leiomyomatosis peritonealis disseminata. Obstet Gynecol 68: 126

102. Rywlin A M, Recher L, Benson J 1964 Clear cell leiomyoma of the uterus. Report of 2 cases of a previously undescribed entity. Cancer 17: 100

103. Saksela E, Lampinen V, Procope B 1974 Malignant mesenchymal tumors of the uterine corpus. Am J Obstet Gynecol 120: 452

104. Schaepman-Van Guens E J 1970 Mixed tumors and carcinosarcomas of the uterus evaluated five years after treatment. Cancer 25: 72

105. Schroder R, Hillejahn A 1920 Uber einen heterologen Kombinationen — tumor des uterus. Zentralbl Gynaekol 44: 1050

106. Silverberg S G 1971 Leiomyosarcoma of the uterus. A clinicopathological study. Cancer 38: 613

107. Spanos W J, Wharton J T, Gomez L, Fletcher G H, Oswald M J 1984 Malignant mixed müllerian tumors of the uterus. Cancer 53: 311

108. Spiro R H, McPeak C J 1966 On the so-called metastasizing leiomyoma. Cancer 19: 544

109. Tang C, Toker C, Ances I G 1979 Stromomyoma of the uterus. Cancer 43: 308

110. Tavassoli F A, Norris H J 1981 Mesenchymal tumours of the uterus. VII. A clinicopathological study of 60 endometrial stromal nodules. Histopathol 5: 1
111. Tavassoli F A, Norris H J 1982 Peritoneal leiomyomatosis (leiomyomatosis peritonealis disseminata): a clinicopathologic study of 20 cases with ultrastructural observations. Int J Gynecol Pathol 1: 59
112. Taylor H B, Norris H J 1966 Mesenchymal tumors of the uterus. IV. Diagnosis and prognosis of leiomyosarcomas. Arch Pathol 82: 40
113. Tench W D, Dail D, Gmelich J T 1978 Benign metastasizing leiomyomas: a review of 21 cases (abstract). Lab Med 38: 37
114. Thatcher S S, Woodruff J D 1982 Uterine stromatosis: a report of 33 cases. Obstet Gynecol 59: 428
115. Tiltman A J 1985 The effect of progestins on the mitotic activity of uterine fibromyomas. Int J Gynecol Pathol 4: 89
116. Vakiani M, Mawad J, Talerman A 1982 Heterologous sarcomas of the uterus. Int J Gynecol Pathol 1: 211
117. Valente P T 1984 Leiomyomatosis peritonealis disseminata. A report of two cases and review of the literature. Arch Pathol Lab Med 108: 669
118. Varela-Duran J, Nochomovitz L E, Prem K A, Dehner L P 1980 Postirradiation mixed müllerian tumors of the uterus: a comparative clinicopathologic study. Cancer 45: 1625
120. Veliath A J, Hannah P, Ratnakar C, Jayanthi K, Aurora A L 1978 Primary liposarcoma of the cervix: a case report. Int J Gynaecol Obstet 16: 75
121. Williamson E O, Christopherson W M 1972 Malignant mixed müllerian tumors of the uterus. Cancer 29: 585
122. Yoonessi M, Hart W R 1977 Endometrial stromal sarcomas. Cancer 40: 898
123. Young R H, Kleinman G M, Scully R E 1981 Glioma of the uterus: report of a case with comments on histogenesis. Am J Surg Pathol 5: 695
124. Young R H, Harris N L, Scully R E 1985 Lymphoma-like lesions of the female genital tract: a report of 16 cases. Int J Gynecol Pathol 4: 289
125. Young R H, Treger T, Scully R E 1986 Atypical polypoid adenomyoma of the endometrium. A report of 27 cases. Am J Clin Pathol 86: 139
126. Yu T J, Iwasaki I, Teratani T, Tanaka T, Aoki M 1986 Circumscribed endometrial stromatosis of the uterus with marked epitheliogenesis. Gynecol Oncol 24: 367
127. Zaloudek C J, Norris H J 1981 Mesenchymal tumors of the uterus. Prog Surg Pathol 3: 1
128. Zaloudek C J, Norris H J 1981 Adenofibroma and adenosarcoma of the uterus. A clinicopathologic study of 35 cases. Cancer 48: 354

52. Uterine sarcomas: clinical features and management

J. R. Lurain   M. S. Piver

INTRODUCTION

Uterine sarcomas are relatively rare tumors of mesodermal origin. They comprise 2 to 6% of uterine malignancies and account for about 1% of all tumors of the female genital tract.[40,52,55,75] They are the most malignant group of uterine tumors and present intriguing problems in regard to diagnosis, clinical behavior, pattern of spread and management.

The three most common histologic variants of uterine sarcoma are endometrial stromal sarcoma (ESS), leiomyosarcoma (LMS), and malignant müllerian mixed tumor of both homologous and heterologous types (MMMT). Other, less common types include pure heterologous sarcomas, blood vessel sarcomas and lymphosarcomas (Table 52.1). Variations in the relative incidences of uterine sarcomas occur in different published series, probably related to the

Table 52.1 Histologic classification of uterine sarcoma

1. Endometrial stromal sarcoma
   Endolymphatic stromal myosis (low grade stromal sarcoma) (ESM)
   Stromal sarcoma (high grade) (ESS)

2. Leiomyosarcoma (LMS)

3. Malignant müllerian mixed tumor (MMMT)
   Homologous type (carcinosarcoma)
   Heterologous type

4. Other

strictness of criteria used to classify smooth muscle and endometrial stromal tumors as sarcomas. In general, LMS and MMMT each make up about 40% of tumors followed by ESS (15%) and other sarcomas (5%), although MMMTs predominate in more recent reports (Table 52.2).

Table 52.2 Incidence of uterine sarcomas by histology

| Authors | No. of patients | Histology | | | |
		LMS	MMMT	ESS	Other
Aaro et al[1]	177	105	52	17	3
Badib et al[5]	147	71	46	30	—
Bartsich et al[11]	125	56	57	12	—
Chuang et al[23]	118	48	49	14	7
Giarratano & Slate[45]	40	15	16	9	—
Kempson & Bari[63]	82	29	36	17	—
Neiminen & Soderlin[84]	117	71	16	17	13
Norris & Taylor[87]	144	50	62	12	20
Saksela et al[106]	66	28	14	21	3
Salazar et al[107]	73	20	44	6	3
Sorbe[118]	87	37	28	19	3
Kahanpaa et al[61]	119	51	45	23	—
Wheelock et al[137]	71	19	47	5	—
Covens et al[27]	74	17	43	7	7
Total	1440	617 (43%)	555 (39%)	199 (14%)	59 (4%)

Staging of uterine sarcomas is based on the International Federation of Gynecology and Obstetrics (FIGO) system for adenocarcinoma of the endometrium (Table 52.3).

Table 52.3 Staging of uterine sarcomas

Stage	Criteria
Stage Ia	Tumor limited to endometrium
Stage Ib	Invasion to $<\frac{1}{2}$ myometrium
Stage Ic	Invasion $>\frac{1}{2}$ myometrium
Stage IIa	Endocervical glandular involvement only
Stage IIb	Cervical stromal invasion
Stage IIIa	Tumor invades serosa and/or adnexa and/or positive peritoneal cytology
Stage IIIb	Vaginal metastases
Stage IIIc	Metastases to pelvic and/or para-aortic lymph nodes
Stage IVa	Tumor invasion of bladder and/or bowel mucosa
Stage IVb	Distant metastases including intra-abdominal and/or inguinal lymph nodes

An increased incidence of uterine sarcomas following radiation therapy to the pelvis for either carcinoma of the cervix or a benign condition is well documented in the literature (Table 52.4). The relative risk of developing uterine sarcoma following pelvic radiotherapy has been estimated to be 5.38.[30] The time interval between radiation therapy and the diagnosis of the uterine malignancy ranges between 18 months and $27\frac{1}{2}$ years, but is usually 10 to 20 years. Most of the sarcomas arising after irradiation are malignant müllerian mixed tumors. The prognosis for these radiation-related sarcomas appears worse than for those with no prior history of pelvic radiotherapy.[78,139]

Table 52.4 Prior pelvic radiotherapy in uterine sarcomas

Authors	No. of patients	Prior pelvic radiotherapy No.	%
AFIP[87]	144	17	12
Badib et al[5]	147	7	5
Bartsich et al[11]	32	12	37
Edwards et al[36]	7	2	29
Masterson & Kremper[76]	25	5	20
Salazar et al[107]	73	4	5
Symmonds & Dockerty[125]	28	9	32
Williamson & Christopherson[139]	48	6	12.5
Total	504	42	8.3

The classification and pathology of uterine sarcomas has been well covered in the preceding chapter. The purpose of this chapter will be to present information on the incidence, criteria for diagnosis, clinical features, patterns of spread, and prognosis of the major types of sarcomas. Management of each type of uterine sarcoma will be

discussed together with the recommended treatment plans for localized as well as advanced disease, including surgery, radiation therapy and chemotherapy.

ENDOMETRIAL STROMAL TUMORS

Endometrial stromal tumors are rare tumors composed purely of cells resembling normal endometrial stroma. They can be divided into three types on the basis of mitotic activity, vascular invasion and observed differences in prognosis. The *endometrial stromal nodule* is a lesion confined to the uterus, with pushing margins, less than 10 MF/10 HPF and no lymphatic or vascular invasion. The second type of endometrial stromal tumor is *endolymphatic stromal myosis* or *endometrial stromatosis*. This lesion infiltrates the myometrium and may extend beyond the uterus and metastasize. Vascular and lymphatic invasion is common. Endolymphatic stromal myosis (ESM) is distinguished from the third type, *endometrial stromal sarcoma* (ESS), mainly on the basis of mitotic activity. Endometrial stromal sarcoma, by definition, has 10 or more MF/10 HPF and a much more aggressive course and poorer prognosis than the more indolent ESM. Flow cytometric analysis has also proven useful in separating ESS with aneuploidy and a high proliferative index from ESM, and in predicting response to therapy.[3]

Stromal tumors occur primarily in the perimenopausal age group, between 45 and 50 years, with about one-third being in postmenopausal women. There is no relationship to parity, associated diseases or prior pelvic radiotherapy. These tumors are rare in blacks. The most frequent symptom is abnormal vaginal bleeding. Abdominal pain and pressure and a pelvic mass are less common, and some patients are asymptomatic. Symptoms are usually of short duration. Pelvic examination usually reveals regular or irregular uterine enlargement, sometimes associated with rubbery parametrial induration. The diagnosis may be made by dilatation and curettage, but the usual preoperative diagnosis is uterine leiomyoma. At surgery, an enlarged uterus filled with soft, gray-white to yellow necrotic and hemorrhagic tumors with bulging surfaces, associated with worm-like elastic extensions into the pelvic veins suggests the diagnosis.

Endometrial stromal nodule

Endometrial stromal nodule is an expansile, non-infiltrating, solitary lesion. Mitotic activity rarely exceeds 3 MF/10 HPF. In a series of 53 endometrial stromal tumors, Norris & Taylor found 18 tumors conforming to this description.[88,126] There were no recurrences or tumor deaths following surgery in this group. They should be considered benign.

Endolymphatic stromal myosis

Endolymphatic stromal myosis is a low grade stromal sarcoma differing from the true endometrial stromal sarcoma only in the mitotic rate. These stromal tumors, with less than 10 MF/10 HPF have a more protracted clinical course, with recurrences typically occurring late and local recurrence being more common than distant metastases.[57,63,68,88,101,129] Although ESM often behaves in a histologically aggressive fashion, it lacks the aneuploid DNA content commonly associated with malignancy.[49]

Endolymphatic stromal myosis has extended beyond the uterus in 40% of cases at the time of diagnosis, but in two-thirds of the cases the extra-uterine spread is confined to the pelvis. Upper abdominal and pulmonary metastases are less common. Recurrence occurs in almost 50% of cases after initial therapy. The interval between initial treatment and the diagnosis of recurrent or metastatic tumor averages about 5 years, but recurrences as late as 25 years have been reported. Prolonged survival and even cure are not uncommon even after the development of recurrent or metastatic disease, as shown by the relatively low incidence of tumor-related deaths in Table 52.5.

Optimum initial therapy for patients with ESM consists of surgical excision of all grossly detectable tumor. Total abdominal hysterectomy and bilateral salpingo-oophorectomy should be performed. All patients treated with local excision (myomectomy) will have recurrence. Supracervical hysterectomy is inadequate since cervical involvement is not uncommon and recurrences following this procedure have been reported. The adnexa should be removed because of the propensity for extension into the parametrium, broad ligament and adnexal structures, as well as the possible stimulating effect on the tumor cells of estrogen from the retained ovaries. Krieger & Gusberg[68] suggested that radical hysterectomy may be the treatment of choice because of the high incidence of parametrial involvement and pelvic recurrences, but there is no clinical data to support this concept. Recurrent or metastatic lesions are also amenable to surgical excision, with many long-term survivors reported living without residual tumor following excision of recurrent pelvic disease or pulmonary metastases.

A beneficial effect of radiation therapy has been reported. Twelve patients with extra-uterine pelvic tumor received radiation therapy in the AFIP series.[88] A description of the effect of radiation on the size of the tumor was available in six cases: five tumors decreased and one remained unchanged. Only three of the 12 patients who received radiation therapy died of their tumor. Koss et al[67] recommend pelvic irradiation for recurrent and inadequately excised pelvic disease.

There is evidence that endolymphatic stromal myosis is also hormone dependent or responsive. Baggish & Woodruff[6] reported a decrease in tumor mass of approximately 50% with oophorectomy alone. They also described the complete disappearance of pulmonary metastases with large parenteral doses of progestins. Piver et al noted an objective response to progestin therapy in six of 13 patients (48%).[101] Effective control of pulmonary and intra-abdominal metastases using progestational agents has been reported in other cases as well.[47,62,69,92] Estrogen and progesterone receptors have been identified in high concentrations in some of these tumors, possibly explaining this sensitivity to progestin therapy.[9,47,62]

Endometrial stromal sarcoma

Endometrial stromal sarcoma can be a highly lethal neoplasm. Only a few series have clearly separated pure stromal sarcomas from endolymphatic stromal myosis (Table 52.6). Norris & Taylor[88] reported that six of their 15 patients with ESS died of tumor from 0.1 to 6.2 years after therapy. Four other patients were living with tumor at last contact, but only one of these patients had been followed for more than 15 months. Thus, the tumor-free 5-year survival was 26%. This study indicated that the prognosis was excellent for patients having sarcomas confined to the uterus at initial treatment and measuring less than 4 cm. Kempson & Bari,[63] however, recorded a 100% mortality in the nine patients with ESS for which they had follow-up data, all dying within 2.5 years. Yoonessi & Hart[141] described seven patients with ESS, five of whom had tumor confined to the uterus at diagnosis; all seven patients died of tumor within 27 months of diagnosis.

Table 52.5 Recurrence and death in endolymphatic stromal myosis

Authors	No of patients	Recurrences (%)	Tumor-related deaths (%)
Krieger & Gusberg [68]★	182	91 (50)	35 (19)
Kempson & Bari[63]	7	0 (0)	0 (0)
Norris & Taylor[88]	19	7 (37)	1 (5)
Hart & Yoonessi[57]	9	7 (78)	2 (22)
Thatcher & Woodruff[129]	33	4 (12)	2 (6)
Total	250	109 (44)	40 (16)

★ Review

Table 52.6 5-year survival in endometrial stromal sarcoma

Authors	No. of patients	Survival (%)
Norris & Taylor[88]	15	8 (55)[a]
Kempson & Bari[63]	9	0 (0)
Yoonessi & Hart[142]	7	0 (0)
Salazar et al[107]	6	2 (33)
Evans[38]	7	1 (14)
Total	44	11 (25)[b]

[a] 4 patients living with tumor; tumor-free 5-year survival = 26%
[b] Tumor-free 5-year survival = 16%

Salazar et al[107] had two of six patients with ESS survive 5 years. Only one of seven patients reported by Evans survived; the lone survivor had tumor limited to the endometrium.[38]

Treatment for ESS should consist of total abdominal hysterectomy and bilateral salpingo-oophorectomy, for the reasons previously discussed in connection with ESM. The dismal therapeutic results obtained in the above series suggest that radiotherapy and/or chemotherapy should be combined with surgery. Suggestive evidence for increased survival by the addition of radiation therapy has been reported by several authors. Progesterone therapy will probably not be as beneficial in these tumors, as demonstrated in some instances of metastatic ESM. No evidence of tumor regression was identified in the three patients treated in the Yoonessi & Hart series.[142]

LEIOMYOSARCOMAS

The incidence of sarcomatous change in uterine leiomyomata is reported to be between 0.13% and 0.81%.[26,39,52,75,80,94,95] Some authors, however, doubt the existence of sarcomatous change in a leiomyoma. In a comparative ultrastructural study, Ferenczy et al[41] could not demonstrate an intermediate form between leiomyoma and leiomyosarcoma, and suggested that the cellular leiomyoma represents a variety of benign leiomyoma. Nevertheless, benign leiomyomata are found associated with leiomyosarcoma in a high proportion of cases.[1,113,122,128] In addition, Silverberg[113] and Spiro & Koss[121] were able to demonstrate evidence of origination of leiomyosarcoma in leiomyomata in 11 of 34 and 14 of 33 cases, respectively.

Clinical features

The median age for women with leiomyosarcoma is somewhat lower than that for other sarcomas, ranging from 43 to 56 years.[11,22,52,75,135] This malignancy has no relationship with parity, as in endometrial carcinoma, and the incidence of associated diseases in patients with leiomyosarcoma is not so high. Silverberg,[113] and Christopherson et al[22] reported a higher incidence and a poorer prognosis in blacks. Although a history of prior pelvic radiotherapy for carcinoma of the cervix or benign conditions occurs in about 4% of patients with leiomyosarcoma,[1,52,80,87,113,121] prior radiotherapy is much more commonly associated with malignant müllerian mixed tumors.

Many series list a significant percentage (47 to 81%) of patients as premenopausal, and report that the survival in these patients is improved.[13,32,52,113,135] Gudgeon reported a 75% 5-year survival in premenopausal patients as opposed to a 37% 5-year survival after menopause.[52] Vardi & Tovell noted a 5-year survival of 63.6% in 11 premenopausal patients compared to only 5.5% in 18 postmenopausal patients.[135] Silverberg found that, of patients available for follow-up, 16 of 18 premenopausal patients were alive at 5 years, whereas only 2 of 13 postmenopausal patients survived.[113] Bartsich,[11] and Hart & Billman[56] both emphasized that the lower average age of patients in some reports and the improved survival in premenopausal patients may be due to the inclusion of cellular myomas in the tumors diagnosed as leiomyosarcoma. Bartsich reclassified 22 of 45 tumors as cellular myomas; 63% were in premenopausal women and there were no tumor-related deaths in this group. Of the remaining 20 patients considered to have true leiomyosarcoma, only 20% were premenopausal and all were dead of disease within $2\frac{1}{2}$ years. Hart & Billman found no difference in survival between pre- and postmenopausal women with leiomyosarcoma. Patients with tumors reclassified as cellular myomas had a median age of 47 years, as compared to a median age of 54 years in the leiomyosarcoma group.

Presenting symptoms are usually of short duration (mean = 6 months) and are not specific for the disease, but resemble those of other benign and malignant conditions of the uterus. The most common symptoms, in order of frequency, are vaginal bleeding, pelvic pain or pressure and awareness of an abdominal-pelvic mass. Pain and a palpable mass are more frequently associated with intramural tumors, while vaginal bleeding occurs more often with submucosal lesions. Other, less common symptoms are weakness, lethargy, weight loss and fever. Occasionally, patients present with symptoms of distant metastases.[1]

The principal physical finding in patients with leiomyosarcoma is the presence of a pelvic mass. The diagnosis should be suspected if rapid uterine growth occurs, especially in a postmenopausal woman. Dilatation and curettage (D&C), although not as useful as in other sarcomas, may establish the diagnosis if the lesion is submucosal. In one reported series where D&C was done prior to laparotomy, a diagnosis of leiomyosarcoma was obtained in 33% of cases.[45] Occasionally, a leiomyosarcoma may form a polypoid mass which protrudes through the cervix and can be biopsied, but this is less common than with malignant müllerian mixed tumors.

Prognosis

Survival of women with leiomyosarcoma ranges from 20 to 63% with a mean of 47%.[15,22,42,52,106,113,128] The pattern of tumor spread is to the myometrium, pelvic blood vessels and lymphatics, contiguous pelvic structures, abdomen, and then distantly, most commonly to the lungs. The number of mitoses in the tumor seems to be the most reliable indicator of malignant behavior (Table 52.7). Taylor and Norris[128] found that none of their 21 patients with tumors having fewer than 10 mitoses (MF) per 10 high power fields (HPF) died of disease, whereas 31 of the 36 patients with tumors having 10 or more MF/10 HPF developed metastatic or recurrent disease. Kempson & Bari,[63] however, reported that all 5 patients whose tumors had a mitotic count of 5 to 9 MF/10 HPF and who had been followed for 5 years, died of tumor or developed metastatic disease. Similarly, Silverberg,[113] and Vardi & Tovell[135] reported that 50% and 82% of patients, respectively, with tumors having mitotic counts between 5 and 9 MF/10 HPF died or developed metastatic disease. Most investigators agree that tumors with less than 5 MF/10 HPF usually behave in a benign fashion, and tumors with 10 or more mitoses are frankly malignant with a poor prognosis. Tumors with 5 to 10 MF/10 HPF are less predictable, and many will recur or metastasize.

Thus, the qualitative estimation of mitotic activity is useful as one of the diagnostic and prognostic criteria but probably should not be used as the sole criterion for distinguishing between benign and malignant smooth muscle tumors and planning treatment. Silverberg[115] presented a reference set of 10 microscopic slides from smooth muscle tumors of the uterus to six different pathologists who were asked to record the number of mitoses per 10 HPF in the most active region of each slide. The diagnosis based on mitotic count alone was unanimous in only 4 of the 10 cases, whereas the diagnosis based on other histologic criteria as well was unanimous in all cases and correlated well with the subsequent clinical evolution of the cases. Other histologic indicators of poor prognosis, besides high mitotic count, are marked anaplasia, necrosis and blood vessel invasion.

The gross presentation of the tumor at the time of surgery is the most important prognostic indicator. Tumors with infiltrating tumor margins or extension beyond the uterus are associated with a poor prognosis, whereas those tumors originating within myomas or with pushing margins are associated with prolonged survival (Table 52.8). When a leiomyosarcoma is confined to a myoma and the diagnosis is not suspected grossly but made histologically only after myomectomy, the prognosis appears to be excellent. Davids[31] found five sarcomas in his series of 1150 myomectomies; none of the patients had further treatment and all were without evidence of disease (NED) after 5 years, including three who subsequently became pregnant. Langstadt & Javert[72] likewise found five unsuspected sarcomas in 690 myomectomies. Four of the five patients subsequently underwent hysterectomy, and no residual sarcoma was found; all five were alive with no evidence of disease at 5 years. Gudgeon[52] treated one patient by myomectomy only, and she survived without evidence of disease at 7 years. Aaro et al[1] reported on two patients in their series who had myomectomy only for leiomyosarcoma. One was alive without evidence of disease $2\frac{1}{2}$ years later, and the other had a hysterectomy 3 years

Table 52.7   Relationship of mitotic activity to 5-year survival in leiomyosarcoma

Authors	1 to 4		5 to 9		≥ 10	
	No.	alive NED	No.	alive NED	No.	alive NED
Silverberg[113]	10	9[a]	8	4[b]	12	4
Kempson & Bari[63]	10	10[c]	6	0[d]	12	1[e]
Taylor & Norris[128]	21	21	—	—	34	3
Christopherson et al[22]	40	40	2	1	29	1[f]
Hart & Billman[56]	13	13[a]	1	0	14	0
Saksela et al[106]	22	22	3	1	28	11
Vardi & Tovell[135]	6	5	11	2	15	1
Dinh & Woodruff[32]	9	8[b]	16	12	5	1
Total	131	128 (98%)	47	20 (42%)	149	22 (15%)

NED no evidence of disease
[a] 1 patient followed only 4 years
[b] 1 other patient living with metastatic disease
[c] 1 patient had metastatic disease removed and is now NED
[d] 1 patient lost to follow-up at 3 years
[e] 2 other patients NED at 3 and 14 months only
[f] 3 patients died at 6, 7 & 28 years; 1 patient living with disease at $9\frac{1}{2}$ years

Table 52.8 Survival in LMS as related to origin within a leiomyoma or encapsulated LMS

Authors	Total no. of patients	Patients dead	% survival
Fenton & Burke[40]	10	2	80
Kimbrough[64]	26	9	65[a]
Laberge[71]	20	1[b]	85[c]
Spiro & Koss[121]	11	4[d]	65
Bass & O'Leary[13]	14	2	85
Silverberg[113]	13	0	100[e]
Dinh & Woodruff[32]	9	0	100[f]
Total	103	17	83

[a] 7 patients followed less than 5 years/5-year survival = 53 %
[b] died of intercurrent disease
[c] 2 patients lost to follow-up
[d] 1 patient died of intercurrent disease
[e] 1 patient followed only 4 years; 1 patient developed metastatic disease
[f] 1 patient alive with recurrent disease 6 years; 4 patients followed less than 5 years

later with no tumor found. Dinh & Woodruff[32] noted only one recurrence in nine patients who underwent myomectomy for infertility with the finding of unsuspected leiomyosarcoma. Thus, it appears that if a leiomyosarcoma is confined to a myoma at the time of surgery and has none of the gross features to lead one to suspect a sarcoma, a myomectomy is usually curative. This may be important in deciding how to treat a young patient who desires to retain her fertility under such circumstances.

Clinico-pathologic variants

There are five other clinico-pathologic variants of leiomyosarcoma that deserve special comment. These are: intravenous leiomyomatosis, metastasizing uterine leiomyoma, leiomyoblastoma, leiomyomatosis peritonealis disseminata, and myxoid leiomyosarcoma.

Intravenous leiomyomatosis is characterized by the growth of histologically benign smooth muscle into venous channels in the broad ligaments, and uterine and iliac veins.[85,110] The intravascular growth takes the form of visible, worm-like projections that extend out from a myomatous uterus into the parametria towards the pelvic sidewalls and may be confused with endolymphatic stromal myosis or leiomyosarcoma (see also p. 809). Tumor involvement is not symmetrical. The tumors may arise from the walls of veins themselves, or may be the result of extensive vascular invasion from a leiomyoma. Symptoms are related to the associated uterine myomas and the presence of a pelvic mass. Most patients are in the late fifth and early sixth decade of life. The prognosis in most cases is excellent, even when tumor is left behind in pelvic vessels. Late local recurrences can occur, however, and

deaths from extension into the inferior vena cava or metastases to the heart have been reported.[7,37] Several authors have noted that tumor left behind after hysterectomy is no longer capable of independent or metastatic growth. There is some evidence to suggest that estrogen stimulates the proliferation of such vascular lesions.[59] Treatment should therefore be total abdominal hysterectomy, and bilateral salpingo-oophorectomy with removal of as much of the tumor as possible.

Benign metastasizing leiomyoma is a rare condition where a histologically benign uterine smooth muscle tumor acts in a somewhat malignant fashion producing benign metastases, usually to the lungs or lymph nodes.[2,10,24,28,102] In most instances, intravenous leiomyomatosis is not demonstrable; the metastasizing myomata are capable of growth at sites distant from the primary focus, whereas the intravenous tumors spread only by direct extension within blood vessels (see also p. 812). There is experimental and clinical data that suggest an estrogen stimulus to such tumors, and that removing that stimulus by castration, withdrawal of exogenous estrogen, or treatment with progestins, tamoxifen or a gonadotropin agonist has an ameliorating effect. Surgical treatment should consist of total abdominal hysterectomy and bilateral salpingo-oophorectomy, combined with segmental resection of pulmonary metastases if possible.

Leiomyoblastoma includes smooth muscle tumors that have been designated as epithelioid leiomyomas, clear cell leiomyomas and plexiform tumorlets (see also p. 808). This group of atypical smooth muscle tumors is distinguished from the usual leiomyoma by the predominance of rounded, rather than spindle-shaped, cells and by a clustered or cord-like pattern.[21,70] In Kurman & Norris' series of 26 cases, only 3 patients developed recurrent disease during the follow-up period. Two patients with recurrent disease 4 and 5 years following hysterectomy are now living without evidence of disease following chemotherapy or additional surgery.[70] These lesions should be regarded as specialized low grade leiomyosarcomas with fewer than 5 MF/10 HPF, and standard treatment should be hysterectomy.

Leiomyomatosis peritonealis disseminata is a rare clinical entity characterized by the finding of smooth muscle subperitoneal nodules scattered throughout the peritoneal cavity.[48,105,123,127] This condition probably arises as a result of metaplasia of subperitoneal mesenchymal stem cells to smooth muscle, fibroblasts, myofibroblasts and decidual cells under the influence of estrogen and progesterone. Less than 30 cases have been reported in the literature (see also p. 810). Most of these have occurred in non-white females in their thirties and forties who are, or have recently been, pregnant, or who have a long history of oral contraceptive use. Intriguing features of this disease are its grossly malignant appearance, benign histology and favorable clinical behavior. Intraoperative diagnosis requires frozen-section examination. Extirpative surgery, including total abdominal hysterectomy, bilateral salpingo-oophorectomy, omentectomy and excision of as much gross disease as possible may be indicated after the reproductive years. Surgical castration may remove an hormonal stimulus for growth of residual tumor, and actual regression of unresected tumor masses has been noted. Almost all patients have done well postoperatively.

Myxoid leiomyosarcoma of the uterus is characterized by a gelatinous appearance and apparent circumscribed border, but microscopically the tumors have a myxomatous stroma and extensively invade adjacent tissue and blood vessels (see also p. 806). Their mitotic activity is low, with mitotic counts of 0 to 2 MF/10 HPF. This belies their aggressive behavior. Four of six patients reported by King et al[65] were dead, and two were living with disease. Patients ranged in age from 47 to 68 and presented with abnormal vaginal bleeding or a pelvic mass. Surgical excision by total abdominal hysterectomy is the mainstay of treatment. The low mitotic rate and abundance of intracellular myxomatous tissue suggest that these tumors might not be responsive to radiotherapy or chemotherapy.

MALIGNANT MÜLLERIAN MIXED TUMORS

Malignant müllerian mixed tumors are histologically composed of a mixture of sarcoma and carcinoma (see also p. 814). The carcinomatous element is usually glandular, while the sarcomatous element may resemble the normal endometrial stroma (homologous) or the so-called carcinosarcoma, or be composed of tissues foreign to the uterus, such as cartilage, bone or striated muscle (heterologous). Malignant müllerian mixed tumors are most likely derived from totipotential endometrial stromal cells having the capacity for glandular and stromal differentiation.

Clinical features

Almost all of these tumors occur after menopause with the median age being about 62 years.[5,12,23,36,76,86,89,96,139] Several studies report a higher incidence in blacks.[33,86,139] Associated clinical conditions, such as obesity, diabetes mellitus and hypertension, are found in a significant percentage of women as in endometrial adenocarcinomas.[12,33,86,103] A history of previous pelvic irradiation for benign conditions or carcinoma of the cervix can be obtained in 7 to 37% of patients.[12,76,86,87,89,96,103,125]

The most frequent presenting symptom is postmenopausal bleeding, occurring in 80 to 90% of cases. Other less common symptoms are vaginal discharge, abdominal-pelvic pain, weight loss and passage of tissue from the vagina. The duration of symptoms is usually only a few months. On physical examination, uterine enlargement is the rule (50 to 95%). A polypoid mass may be seen in up to 50% of cases in the endocervical canal or protruding through the cervical os.[5,23,33,76,86,89,96,139] Diagnosis can usually be made by physical examination and biopsy of an endocervical mass, or by dilatation and curettage. Cytology is negative in up to 45% of cases.[138] Uterine curettings are often misleading in that only one type of tissue may be obtained, i.e. adenocarcinoma or stromal sarcoma, allowing a definitive histologic diagnosis to be made in only 60 to 70% of cases.[19]

Grossly, the tumor grows as a large, soft, polypoid mass filling and distending the uterine cavity, with necrosis and hemorrhage as prominent features. The myometrium is invaded to various degrees in almost all cases. The most frequent areas of spread are the pelvis, lymph nodes, peritoneal cavity, lungs and liver. This metastatic pattern suggests that these neoplasms spread by local extension and regional lymph node metastasis similar to the manner of spread of endometrial adenocarcinomas, but behave more aggressively.[23,33,76,86,103,139]

Prognosis

Evidence from the Armed Forces Institute of Pathology (AFIP) suggests that homologous tumors are confined to the uterus more frequently than are heterologous tumors, and that they therefore have an improved survival.[86,89] Schaepman-van Geuns recorded a 43.7% 5-year survival in patients with homologous tumors, and a 30% 5-year survival in those with heterologous elements.[109] However, other reports have not confirmed this relationship and could find no statistical differences in survival based on histology.[5,23,73,112,120,125,136,139] Reports from the AFIP[86] and Kempson & Bari[63] also record a poor prognosis if the heterologous elements are rhabdomyoblasts or osteoblasts, and an improved prognosis if the tumor contains cartilage as the only heterologous element. Others have not been able to demonstrate such a relationship.[5,23,73,96,112,120,125,136,139]

The most important single factor affecting prognosis is the extent of the tumor at the time of treatment. DiSaia et al[33] noted that survival was directly related to extent of disease. In 94 patients with malignant müllerian mixed tumors, those with tumor confined to the uterine corpus (Stage I) had a 53% 2-year survival, whereas survival dropped to 8.5% when the disease had extended to the cervix, vagina or parametrium (Stages II and III); there were no survivors in those patients with disease outside the pelvis (Stage IV). Unfortunately, disease has clinically already extended outside the uterus in 40 to 60% of cases at the time of diagnosis, indicating the highly malignant nature of this lesion. Even when disease is thought to be confined to the uterus preoperatively and potentially still curable (Stages I and II), surgical-pathologic staging identifies extra-uterine spread of disease in a significant percentage of cases. Macasaet et al[74] reported that, in their series, 55% of women with clinical Stage I disease had a higher surgical-pathologic stage. Only 28% of tumors were actually confined to the uterine corpus, 16% had additionally spread to the cervix and 56% showed extra-uterine spread. DiSaia et al[34] and Geszler et al[44] have also reported a significant occurrence of lymph node metastasis and positive peritoneal cytology, respectively, in early stage müllerian mixed tumors, which influences survival.

Deep myometrial invasion is present in about one-half of Stage I cases and is associated with poor prognosis. In Kempson & Bari's report, all patients whose tumors extended more than one-half the thickness of the myometrium died.[63] Vongtama et al[136] found that the survival in Stage I disease was two times greater when the depth of myometrial invasion was less than one-half the myometrial thickness (58% versus 29%). Peters and colleagues[96] noted that the strongest correlate with survival in patients with disease apparently confined to the uterus was depth of myometrial invasion. All patients with tumor limited to the endometrium survived, while involvement of the outer one-third of the myometrium was almost uniformly fatal.

Patients dying from these tumors also tend to have larger tumors and a higher incidence of lympho-vascular invasion.[74,86,89] Patients with a history of prior pelvic irradiation generally have a poorer prognosis.[78,139] The overall 5-year survival approximates 20 to 30% in most series (Table 52.9).

Adenosarcomas

Adenosarcoma is an uncommon variant of malignant müllerian mixed tumor, first described by Clement & Scully in 1974.[25] It consists of an admixture of benign-appearing neoplastic glands and a sarcomatous stroma. Most patients are white, present with postmenopausal vaginal bleeding, and do not have a history of prior pelvic radiotherapy. The diagnosis is made or suspected by dilatation and curettage. Most adenosarcomas are well-circumscribed and limited to the endometrium, with deep myometrial invasion being very unusual. The treatment is total abdominal hysterectomy and bilateral salpingo-oophorectomy with or without adjuvant radiotherapy. Recurrences have been reported in 5 of 10 cases by Clement & Scully,[25] and in 10 of 25 cases from the AFIP.[143] Most recurrences were local (pelvic or vaginal), causing these authors to recommend adjuvant postoperative intravaginal or pelvic irradiation. More recently, Baker et al[8] noted recurrences in five of six patients and advocated more aggressive treatment of these tumors similar to that given for their müllerian mixed counterpart.

TREATMENT OF UTERINE SARCOMAS AND RESULTS

As noted by Vongtama et al,[136] Salazar et al[108] and Spanos et al,[119] recurrences occur in over one-half of cases of uterine sarcoma even when the disease is localized, and at least 50% of all recurrences occur outside the pelvis. In the series from Roswell Park Memorial Institute, 65% of the 104 cases of Stage I and II uterine sarcoma recurred.[136] Of these 68 patients, 51% had their initial recurrence in the pelvis, and 21% had recurrences in the pelvis plus some distant site. The remaining 28% recurred at distant sites only, most commonly the lungs and abdomen. There were no significant differences in the recurrence patterns among the different histologic types, and 72% of recurrences occurred within 2 years. Salazar et al[108] found that 20 of 41 patients (56%) with Stage I tumors failed treatment, with an average failure time of 32 months. Once corrected for stage, there were no significant differences in failure rates, spread patterns, or survival among the three main histologic variants. Isolated pelvic failures constituted only 4% of all failures. Forty percent of failures occurred both in the pelvis and at distant sites, while distant metastases accounted for 47% of failures. The most common distant failures were in the upper abdomen and lungs. Lung metastases alone were the only site of failure in 16% of cases. Recurrences were seen in 56% of 120 patients with MMMT treated primarily at the M. D. Anderson

Table 52.9 5-year survival in malignant mixed müllerian tumors

Authors	No. of patients	Survival No.	%
AFIP[86,89]	62	14	23
Badib et al[5]	46	14	30
Bartsch et al[12]	32	0	0
Chuang et al[23]	49	6	14
Edwards D L et al[36]	10	3	30
Edwards C L[35]	85	7	8
Giarratano & Slate[45]	12	4	33
Kempson & Bari[63]	36	2	6
Masterson & Kremper[76]	25	4	16
Mortel et al[81,82]	32	9	28
Nieminen & Soderlin[84]	16	6	38
Perez et al[93]	54	17	31
Saksela et al[106]	14	7	50
Salazar et al[107]	44	13	30
Schaepman-van Geuns[109]	61	23	38
Spanos et al[120]	99	38	38
Symmonds & Dockerty[125]	28	6	21
Williamson & Christopherson[139]	48	8	17
White et al[138]	10	3	30
Total	763	184	24

Hospital.[119] The distant metastasis rate was 49% accounting for 84% of first recurrences. The locoregional-only recurrence rate was 10%. The most common sites of recurrence were the lung and abdomen. These reports emphasize that the major limitation to cure of uterine sarcomas is distant spread.

Because of the high distant failure rate in uterine sarcomas presumed to be localized to the uterus despite good local control with surgery and radiotherapy, the Gynecologic Oncology Group (GOG) undertook to study lymph node metastases in these tumors.[34] Extensive sampling of the pelvic and para-aortic lymph nodes was carried out at the time of standard treatment for uterine sarcoma. Ten of 28 patients (35.7%) reported had histologically positive pelvic lymph nodes, and four patients (14.3%) had positive aortic nodes. In two subsequent reports, positive pelvic nodes were found in two of 10 (20%) and two of 15 (13%) patients in whom lymph node sampling was done at the time of surgery for Stage I disease.[27,137] Although the numbers are small, these reports demonstrate that spread of uterine sarcomas via lymphatics to the pelvic and para-aortic nodes occurs in a significant percentage of patients with this disease.

Based on this type of evidence, treatment of Stage I and II uterine sarcomas should include hysterectomy, bilateral salpingo-oophorectomy, and treatment of the pelvic lymphatics by irradiation or surgery. Strong consideration should also be given to the use of adjuvant chemotherapy to decrease the incidence of distant metastases.[99] Stage III uterine sarcomas are probably best treated by an aggressive, combined surgical, radiotherapeutic and chemotherapeutic approach similar to that used to treat childhood rhabdomyosarcomas.[140] Stage IV disease must be treated with combination chemotherapy.[4,50,53,98,117,124,130]

Surgery

The first step in the treatment of early uterine sarcomas (Stages I & II) should be exploratory laparotomy. Since extirpative surgery is the most important aspect of treatment, and knowledge of the extent and spread of the disease is crucial to further management, one should not forego or delay surgery by using radiotherapy first. At the time of surgery, careful exploration of the peritoneal cavity should be made, with special attention given to the pelvic and para-aortic nodes. Total abdominal hysterectomy is the standard procedure, but consideration may be given to radical hysterectomy in Stage II disease. Bilateral salpingo-oophorectomy should also be performed in all patients except premenopausal women with leiomyosarcoma, in whom the presence of retained ovaries seems to improve the prognosis.[1,13,32,122,128] The role of pelvic and para-aortic node sampling at the time of laparotomy for the purpose of determining future therapy needs additional study.

Based on the surgical, as well as the histopathologic, findings, additional therapy with irradiation and/or chemotherapy can then be more rationally planned. Rarely, a patient may be cured by the excision of an isolated single pulmonary metastasis.

Radiotherapy

The role of radiotherapy in the treatment of uterine sarcomas is controversial. Classically, uterine sarcomas have been thought to be radioresistant.[116] Radiation therapy alone is clearly inadequate primary treatment for uterine sarcomas. However, many authors have found adjuvant pre- or postoperative radiation therapy to be of value in terms of increased survival and decreased pelvic recurrence in patients with localized ESS and MMMT, but not LMS. Edwards, in 1969, reported the previous 21 year experience at the M. D. Anderson Hospital with uterine sarcomas.[35] Fifty-two percent of 29 patients with localized uterine sarcoma treated with preoperative irradiation survived, as compared to 30% of 21 patients treated by surgery alone. This improved survival with irradiation was true for all histologic subgroups, except LMS. The amount of tumor remaining in the excised uterus was less in the group receiving preoperative irradiation, demonstrating the ability of irradiation to destroy sarcomatous tissue. Belgrad et al,[14] combining results from four institutions, found that the 2-year survival was improved by pre- and postoperative irradiation in MMMT (35% vs. 20%) and ESS (57% vs. 37%), but not in LMS.

Vongtama et al[136] reported an overall 5-year survival of 53% in 31 patients receiving either pre- or postoperative irradiation, compared to 40% in 61 patients treated by surgery alone and 29% in 12 patients who received only radiotherapy. LMS patients responded better to surgery alone. Also of significance is the fact that local treatment failures, i.e. pelvic recurrences, were less than half for the group receiving combined therapy (26%) than for those having surgery alone (57%). Salazar et al,[107] in 1978, reviewed the literature and included their own cases of uterine sarcoma. They found that the 5-year survival of Stage I patients treated with surgery and irradiation (62%) was not significantly better than for those treated by surgery alone (53%); however, patients treated with irradiation alone had a considerably lower 5-year survival (33%). This study did demonstrate an increase in disease-free interval and a two-fold increase in pelvic disease control by the addition of irradiation to surgery. Vongtama and co-authors also noted that surgery without the addition of supplemental irradiation was ineffective treatment in Stage II disease.[136]

Other studies have confirmed the value of adding pelvic radiotherapy to operation for the treatment of Stage I and II uterine sarcomas. Perez et al[93] noted pelvic recurrences in only three of 17 patients (17%) receiving preoperative pelvic irradiation compared to three of six patients (50%) treated with surgery alone for Stage I müllerian mixed tumors. Covens and colleagues[27] reported that local recurrences decreased in Stage I tumors, from nine of 22 cases in which operation alone was performed to none of 15 cases in which pelvic radiotherapy was added. In a Gynecologic Oncology Group study, those patients who received radiation therapy to the pelvis postoperatively for Stage I and II müllerian mixed tumors had a significant reduction in recurrences within the radiation treatment field.[58] In none of these reports, however, was radiotherapy demonstrated to have any impact on survival or any effect on leiomyosarcomas. Radiotherapy thus seems to have a role in the combined treatment of müllerian mixed tumors and endometrial stromal sarcomas confined to the pelvis by increasing the disease-free progression interval and by increasing pelvic control, thereby probably increasing the overall survival to some degree.

Chemotherapy

There is increasing interest in the role of chemotherapy in the treatment of metastatic, as well as adjuvant treatment of localized, uterine sarcomas. Several chemotherapeutic agents have been found to have activity in sarcomas. Retrospective combined data show that cyclophosphamide and vincristine are active single agents,[17] and they have been employed in combination with actinomycin-D, the so-called VAC regimen, yielding response rates in the range of 24%.[60] Generally, adult sarcomas do not respond as favorably to this combination as do childhood rhabdomyosarcomas. Smith et al[117] reported treating 38 patients with advanced recurrent or metastatic pelvic sarcomas with combined irradiation and VAC chemotherapy. Twenty four uterine sarcomas in the group included 13 malignant müllerian mixed tumors, 8 leiomyosarcomas and 3 endometrial stromal sarcomas. Ten of these patients were alive and well without evidence of disease 10 to 56 months following completion of therapy (3 müllerian mixed tumors and 7 leiomyosarcomas). Complications with this aggressive combined treatment were severe, with five deaths resulting. In 1983, Hannigan summarized the experience at the M. D. Anderson Hospital in treating 74 patients with recurrent or metastatic uterine sarcomas with VAC.[53] The response rate for the 45 patients with measurable disease was 28.9% (13.3% complete responses and 15.6% partial responses). The toxicity was considerable and included an 11% death rate.

In the early 1970s, adriamycin and dimethyl-triazeno-imidazole carboxamide (DTIC) were found to be active agents against sarcomas. The overall response rate for adriamycin in patients with sarcomas of all types is reported to be 26%, ranging in individual studies from 10% to 40%.[17] However, Piver et al reported only a 6% objective response in 17 patients treated with adriamycin for metastatic uterine sarcoma.[97] DTIC produced a 17% response rate in 53 patients studied by the Southwest Oncology Group (SWOG), but only 1.9% were complete responses.[50] Because animal studies suggested a synergism between adriamycin and DTIC, these two agents were combined in nearly full doses of each in a study by SWOG involving 218 patients with sarcomas. A 42% overall response rate, including a 10% complete response rate was observed.[50] A similar, but not statistically increased, response rate was observed in a randomized trial of adriamycin versus adriamycin-DTIC in metastatic uterine sarcomas conducted by the GOG.[91] Thirteen of 80 patients (16%) responded to adriamycin alone, compared to 16 of 66 patients (24%) responding to adriamycin-DTIC. Lung metastases responded much better in patients treated with the combination. In a subsequent randomized study of adriamycin versus adriamycin and cyclophosphamide, the GOG was unable to determine any benefit for the combination regimen, both groups having a 19% response rate.[83] Gottlieb and associates in the SWOG added vincristine to the combination of adriamycin and DTIC (VAD).[50] The observed response rate was no greater than that for the two drug combination, but the percentage of patients with progressive disease fell and there was an increase in the duration of remission. Azizi et al,[4] employing a similar combination (VAD) in six patients with metastatic uterine leiomyosarcoma, obtained complete remissions in three patients and a partial remission in a fourth. There was no serious chemotherapeutic toxicity. The Mayo Clinic could not duplicate the results reported by Gottlieb et al[50] and Azizi et al[4] with VAD, or by Smith et al[117] and Hannigan et al[53] with VAC. Using the VAD combination, an 11% response rate occurred as primary and secondary chemotherapy, whereas using VAC only an 8% overall response rate was obtained. Only two complete responses were achieved in the 69 patients treated with these two drug regimens, one in each category.[29]

With the addition of cyclophosphamide to vincristine, adriamycin and DTIC (CYVADIC), Gottlieb et al were able to increase the complete and overall response rates to 14% and 55%, respectively, in 136 patients with various sarcomas.[50] By the use of CYVADIC at even higher doses in a protected-environment-prophylactic-antibiotic program (PEPA), the M. D. Anderson Hospital obtained a complete remission rate of 33%, versus 15% in the control group, and the PEPA patients survived substantially longer.[18] Other investigators have also reported significant responses of metastatic soft tissue sarcomas to combinations of cyclophosphamide, adriamycin and DTIC, with or without vincristine.[16,140] Piver et al[98] noted a 23% objective response rate (11.5% complete response rate) using the CYVADIC regimen in 26 patients with sarcomas of the female genital tract, most of whom had had extensive prior treatment.

More recently, cisplatin and ifosfamide have been used

to treat advanced or recurrent uterine sarcomas with some success. In a GOG Phase II trial of cisplatin for treatment of metastatic müllerian mixed tumors, five of 28 evaluable patients (18%) had an objective response (2 complete and 3 partial).[130] Gershenson et al[43] reported an overall response rate of 42% in 12 patients with measurable disease treated with cisplatin for metastatic MMMT. Responses have also been noted when cisplatin was used in combination with other agents in treatment of advanced pelvic sarcomas.[51,100,111] Piver et al[100] reported on 20 patients with pelvic sarcomas treated with cisplatin and DTIC; seven (35%) achieved an objective response (4 complete and 3 partial).

Ifosfamide with mesna uroprotection has been demonstrated to have activity in sarcomas. The GOG reported the preliminary results of a phase II trial of ifosfamide in patients with metastatic uterine müllerian mixed tumors. Of 23 evaluable patients, responses were seen in 35% (4 complete and 4 partial).[124] Ifosfamide, when combined with etoposide, has also been shown to be an effective regimen in the treatment of recurrent sarcomas in children and young adults, and deserves study in advanced uterine sarcomas.[79]

Most of the above trials suggest that tumor response in sarcomas is partially a function of histologic type and tumor location. Leiomyosarcomas appear to be more responsive to chemotherapy than MMMT or ESS. Also, pulmonary metastases tend to respond better to chemotherapy than pelvic, intraperitoneal or liver metastases.

Because of the relatively low survival rate in localized uterine sarcomas, and the high incidence of failure due to subsequent distant metastasis, adjuvant treatment programs employing chemotherapy have recently been tested. At Roswell Park Memorial Institute, 19 patients with Stage I uterine sarcomas were prospectively studied, comparing postoperative adjuvant adriamycin (60 to 75 mg/m^2 every 4 weeks for six courses) versus no adjuvant chemotherapy. Nine patients also received postoperative

vaginal radium, but not external pelvic irradiation. Two of eight adriamycin treated patients (25%) developed recurrences compared to seven of 11 women (64%) treated by surgery alone. The median survival time for the surgery alone patients was 38 months versus 68 months for the surgery plus adriamycin group. Because of these encouraging results, together with the apparent improved response to CYVADIC over adriamycin alone for the treatment of advanced sarcomas, the adriamycin trial was terminated and a new adjuvant trial employing CYVADIC after surgery for Stage I uterine sarcomas was initiated. Eleven patients received nine courses of CYVADIC after total abdominal hysterectomy and bilateral salpingo-oophorectomy, and have been followed from 2 to 5 years. No patient received adjuvant radiotherapy. Only two patients (18%) have developed recurrences at 14 and 28 months.[99]

Buchsbaum et al[20] reported on 17 patients with Stages I and II uterine sarcoma who were treated with postoperative VAC chemotherapy. Only 10 of the 17 patients completed treatment, and five patients were alive free of disease after 4 years, a crude survival rate of only 29%. Van Nagell et al[134] similarly treated seven patients with Stage I uterine sarcoma with surgery plus adjuvant VAC chemotherapy. Two patients developed recurrent sarcoma; the remaining five patients were alive and well with no evidence of disease 48 to 73 months after therapy. The GOG conducted a trial of adjuvant adriamycin postoperatively in 131 Stage I and 25 Stage II uterine sarcoma patients. Of the 75 patients randomized to receive adriamycin, 31 (41%) developed a recurrence, compared with 43 of 81 (53%) receiving no adjuvant chemotherapy. These results were not significantly different, and there was no difference in progression-free interval or survival.[90] Other reports have also been unable to demonstrate a clear improvement in survival by the addition of postoperative adjuvant chemotherapy in early uterine sarcoma.[54,66,104,118]

REFERENCES

1. Aaro L A, Symmonds R E, Dockerty M D 1966 Sarcoma of the uterus: a clinical and pathologic study of 177 cases. Am J Obstet Gynecol 94: 101
2. Abell M R, Littler E R 1975 Benign metastasizing uterine leiomyoma: multiple lymph node metastases. Cancer 36: 2206
3. August C Z, Bauer K, Lurain J R, Murad T 1990 Neoplasms of endometrial stroma: histopathologic and flow cytometric analysis with clinical correlation. Hum Pathol. In press
4. Azizi F, Bitran J, Javehari G, Herbst A L 1979 Remission of uterine leiomyosarcomas treated with vincristine, adriamycin, and dimethyl-triazenoimodazole carboximide. Am J Obstet Gynecol 133: 379
5. Badib A O, Vongtama V, Kurohara S S, Webster J H 1969 Radiotherapy in the treatment of sarcomas of the corpus uteri. Cancer 24: 724
6. Baggish M S, Woodruff J D 1972 Uterine stromatosis: clinicopathologic features and hormone dependency. Obstet Gynecol 40: 487
7. Bahary C M, Gorodeski I G, Nilly M, Neri A, Avidor I, Garti I J 1982 Intravascular leiomyomatosis. Obstet Gynecol 59: 73s
8. Baker T R, Piver M S, Lele S B, Tsukada Y 1988 Stage I uterine adenosarcoma: a report of 6 cases. J Surg Oncol 37: 128
9. Baker V V, Walton L A, Fowler W C, Currie J L 1984 Steroid receptors in endolymphatic stromal myosis. Obstet Gynecol 63: 725
10. Banner A S, Carrington C B, Emory W B et al 1981 Efficacy of oophorectomy in lymphangioleiomyomatosis and benign metastasizing leiomyoma. N Engl J Med 305: 204
11. Bartsich E G, Bowe E T, Moore J G 1968 Leiomyosarcoma of the uterus: a 50-year review of 42 cases. Obstet Gynecol 32: 101
12. Bartsich E G, O'Leary J A, Moore J G 1967 Carcinosarcoma of the uterus: A 50-year review of 32 cases (1917–1966). Obstet Gynecol 30: 518
13. Bass J C, O'Leary J A 1970 Leiomyosarcoma of the uterus. South Med J 63: 473
14. Belgrad R, Elbadawi N, Rubin P 1975 Uterine sarcomas. Radiology 114: 181
15. Berchuck A, Rubin S C, Hoskins W J, Saigo P E, Pierce V K,

Lewis J L Jr 1988 Treatment of uterine leiomyosarcoma. Obstet Gynecol 71: 845

16. Blum R H, Carter S K 1974 Adriamycin: a new anticancer drug with significant clinical activity. Ann Int Med 80: 249

17. Blum R H, Corson J M, Wilson R E, Greenberger J S, Canellos G P, Frei E 1980 Successful treatment of metastatic sarcomas with cyclophosphamide, adriamycin, and DTIC (CAD). Cancer 46: 1722

18. Bodey G P, Rodriquez V, Murphy W K, Burgess M A, Benjamin R S 1981 Protected environment-prophylactic antibiotic program for malignant sarcomas. Cancer 47: 2422

19. Boram L H, Erlandson R A, Hajdu S I 1972 Mixed mesodermal tumor of the uterus: a cytologic, histologic, and electron microscopic correlation. Cancer 30: 1295

20. Buchsbaum H J, Lifshitz S, Blythe J G 1979 Prophylactic chemotherapy in Stages I and II uterine sarcoma. Gynecol Oncol 8: 346

21. Buscema J, Carpenter S E, Rosenshein N B, Woodruff J D 1986 Epithelioid leiomyosarcoma of the uterus. Cancer 57: 1192

22. Christopherson W M, Williamson E O, Gray L A 1972 Leiomyosarcoma of the uterus. Cancer 29: 1512

23. Chuang J T, van Velden J J, Graham J B 1970 Carcinosarcoma and mixed mesodermal tumor of the uterine corpus: review of 49 cases. Obstet Gynecol 35: 769

24. Clark D H, Weed J C 1977 Metastasizing leiomyoma: a case report. Am J Obstet Gynecol 127: 672

25. Clement P B, Scully R E 1974 Müllerian adenosarcoma of the uterus. Cancer 34: 1138

26. Corscaden J A, Singh B P 1958 Leiomyosarcoma of the uterus. Am J Obstet Gynecol 75: 149

27. Covens A L, Nisker J A, Chapman W B, Allen H H 1987 Uterine sarcoma: analysis of 74 cases. Am J Obstet Gynecol 156: 370

28. Cramer S F, Meyer J S, Kraner J F, Camel M, Mazur M T, Tanenbaum M S 1980 Metastasizing leiomyoma of the uterus. Cancer 45: 932

29. Creagan E T, Hahn R G, Ahmann D L, Edmonson J H, Bisel J F, Eagan R T 1976 A comparative trial evaluating the combination of adriamycin, DTIC and vincristine, the combination of actinomycin D, cyclophosphamide and vincristine, and a single agent methyl-CCNU, in advanced sarcomas. Cancer Treat Rep 60: 1385

30. Czesnin K, Wronkowski Z 1976 Second malignancies of the irradiated area in patients treated for uterine cervix cancer. Gynecol Oncol 6: 309

31. Davids A M 1952 Myomectomy: surgical technique and results in a series of 1150 cases. Am J Obstet Gynecol 63: 592

32. Dinh T V, Woodruff J D 1982 Leiomyosarcoma of the uterus. Am J Obstet Gynecol 144: 817

33. DiSaia P J, Castro J R, Rutledge F N 1973 Mixed mesodermal sarcoma of the uterus. Am J Roentgenol 117: 632

34. DiSaia P J, Morrow C P, Boronow R, Creasman W, Mittelstaedt L 1978 Endometrial sarcoma: Lymphatic spread pattern. Am J Obstet Gynecol 130: 104

35. Edwards C L 1969 Undifferentiated tumors. In Cancer of the Uterus and Ovary: A collection of papers presented at the 11th Annual Clinical Conference on Cancer at the M.D. Anderson Hospital and Tumor Institute. Year Book Medical Publishers, Inc., Chicago, p 84

36. Edwards D L, Sterling L N, Keller R H, Nolan J F 1963 Mixed heterologous mesenchymal sarcoma (mixed mesodermal sarcomas) of the uterus. Am J Obstet Gynecol 85: 1002

37. Evans A T III, Symmonds R E, Gaffey T A 1981 Recurrent pelvic intravenous leiomyomatosis. Obstet Gynecol 57: 260

38. Evans H L 1982 Endometrial stromal sarcoma and poorly differentiated endometrial sarcoma. Cancer 50: 2170

39. Fehr P E, Prem K A 1974 Malignancy of the uterine corpus following irradiation therapy for squamous cell carcinoma of the cervix. Am J Obstet Gynecol 119: 685

40. Fenton A N, Burke L 1952 Sarcoma of the uterus: a record of 26 cases. Am J Obstet Gynecol 63: 158

41. Ferenczy A, Richart R H, Okagaki T 1971 A comparative

ultrastructural study of leiomyosarcoma, cellular leiomyoma, and leiomyoma of the uterus. Cancer 28: 1004

42. Gallup D G, Cordray D R 1979 Leiomyosarcoma of the uterus: case reports and a review. Obstet Gynecol Surv 34: 300

43. Gershenson D M, Kavanagh J J, Copeland L J, Edwards C L, Stringer C A, Wharton J T 1987 Cisplatin therapy for disseminated mixed mesodermal sarcoma of the uterus. J Clin Oncol 5: 618

44. Geszler G, Szpak C A, Harris R E, Creasman W T, Barter J F, Johnston W W 1986 Prognostic value of peritoneal washings in patients with malignant mixed müllerian tumors of the uterus Am J Obstet Gynecol 155: 83

45. Giarratano R C, Slate T A 1971 Sarcomas of the uterus. Obstet Gynecol 38: 472

46. Gilbert H A, Kagan A R, Lagasse L, Jacobs M R, Tawa K 1974 The value of radiation therapy in uterine sarcoma. Obstet Gynecol 45: 84

47. Gloor E, Schnyder P, Cikes M et al 1982 Endolymphatic stromal myosis: surgical and hormonal treatment of extensive abdominal recurrence 20 years after hysterectomy. Cancer 50: 1888

48. Goldberg M F, Hurt W G, Frable W J 1977 Leiomyomatosis peritonealis disseminata: report of a case and review of the literature. Obstet Gynecol 49: 46s

49. Goldfarb S, Richart R M, Okagaki T 1970 Nuclear DNA content in endolymphatic stromal myosis. Am J Obstet Gynecol 106: 524

50. Gottlieb J A, Baker L H, O'Bryan R M et al 1975 Adriamycin used alone and in combination for soft tissue and bony sarcomas. Cancer Chemother Rep Part 3, 6: 271

51. Grosh W W, Jones H W III, Burnett L S, Greco F A 1986 Malignant mixed mesodermal tumors of the uterus and ovary treated with cisplatin-based combination chemotherapy. Gynecol Oncol 25: 334

52. Gudgeon D H 1968 Leiomyosarcoma of the uterus. Obstet Gynecol 32: 96

53. Hannigan E V, Freedman R S, Elder K W, Rutledge F N 1983 Treatment of advanced uterine sarcoma with vincristine, actinomycin D, and cyclophosphamide. Gynecol Oncol 15: 224

54. Hannigan E V, Freedman R S, Rutledge F N 1983 Adjuvant chemotherapy in early uterine sarcoma. Gynecol Oncol 15: 56

55. Harlow B L, Weiss N S, Lofton S 1986 The epidemiology of sarcomas of the uterus. JNCI 76: 399

56. Hart W R, Billman J K 1978 A reassessment of uterine neoplasms originally diagnosed as leiomyosarcomas. Cancer 41: 1902

57. Hart W R, Yoonessi M 1977 Endometrial stromatosis of the uterus. Obstet Gynecol 49: 393

58. Hornback N B, Omura G, Major F J 1986 Observations on the use of adjuvant radiation therapy in patients with Stage I and II uterine sarcoma. Int J Radiat Oncol Biol Phys 12: 2127

59. Irey N S, Norris H J 1973 Intimal vascular lesions associated with female reproductive steroids. Arch Path 96: 227

60. Jacobs E M 1970 Combination chemotherapy of metastatic testicular germinal cell tumors and soft part sarcomas. Cancer 25: 324

61. Kahanpaa K V, Wahlstrom T, Grohn P, Heinonen E, Neiminen U, Widholm O 1986 Sarcomas of the uterus: a clinicopathologic study of 119 patients. Obstet Gynecol 67: 417

62. Katz L, Merino M J, Sakamoto H, Schwartz P E 1987 Endometrial stromal sarcoma: a clinicopathologic study of 11 cases with determination of estrogen and progestin receptor levels in three tumors. Gynecol Oncol 26: 87

63. Kempson R L, Bari W 1970 Uterine sarcomas: classification, diagnosis and prognosis. Hum Pathol 1: 331

64. Kimbrough R A 1934 Sarcoma of the uterus. Am J Obstet Gynecol 28: 723

65. King M E, Dickersin G R, Scully R E 1982 Myxoid leiomyosarcoma of the uterus. Am J Surg Pathol 6: 589

66. Kohorn E I, Schwartz P E, Chambers J T, Peschel R E, Kapp D S, Merino M 1986 Adjuvant therapy in mixed müllerian tumors of the uterus. Gynecol Oncol 23: 212

67. Koss L G, Spiro R H, Brunschwig A 1965 Endometrial stromal sarcoma. Surg Gynecol Obstet 121: 531

68. Krieger P D, Gusberg S B 1973 Endolymphatic stromal myosis-a grade 1 endometrial sarcoma. Gynecol Oncol 1: 299
69. Krumholz B A, Lobovsky F Y, Halitsky V 1973 Endolymphatic stromal myosis with pulmonary metastases. Remission with progestin therapy: report of a case. J Reprod Med 10: 85
70. Kurman R J, Norris H J 1976 Mesenchymal tumors of the uterus VI. Epithelioid smooth muscle tumors including leiomyoblastoma and clear cell leiomyoma. A clinical and pathologic analysis of 26 cases. Cancer 37: 1833
71. Laberge J L 1962 Prognosis of uterine leiomyosarcomas based on histopathologic criteria. Am J Obstet Gynecol 84: 1833
72. Langstadt J R, Javert C T 1955 Sarcoma and myomectomy. Cancer 8: 1142
73. Lotocki R, Rosenshein N B, Grumbine F, Dillon M, Parmley T, Woodruff J D 1982 Mixed müllerian tumors of the uterus: clinicopathologic correlations. Int J Gynaecol Obstet 20: 237
74. Macasaet M A, Waxman M, Fruchter R G et al 1985 Prognostic factors in malignant mesodermal (müllerian) mixed tumors of the uterus. Gynecol Oncol 20: 32
75. MacFarlane K T 1950 Sarcoma of the uterus: an analysis of 42 cases. Am J Obstet Gynecol 59: 1304
76. Masterson J G, Kremper J 1969 Mixed mesodermal tumors. Am J Obstet Gynecol 104: 693
77. McFarland J 1935 Dysontogenetic and mixed tumors of the urogenital region. Surg Gynecol Obstet 61: 42
78. Meredith R F, Eisert D R, Kaka Z, Hodgson S E, Johnston G A Jr, Boutselis J G 1986 An excess of uterine sarcomas after pelvic irradiation. Cancer 58: 2003
79. Miser J S, Kinsella T J, Triche T J et al 1987 Ifosfamide with mesna uroprotection and etoposide: an effective regimen in the treatment of recurrent sarcomas and other tumors of children and young adults. J Clin Oncol 5: 1191
80. Montague A C W, Swartz D P, Woodruff J D 1965 Sarcoma arising in a leiomyoma of the uterus. Am J Obstet Gynecol 92: 421
81. Mortel R, Koss L G, Lewis J L Jr, D'Urso J R 1974 Mesodermal mixed tumors of the uterine corpus. Obstet Gynecol 43: 248
82. Mortel R, Nedwich A, Lewis G C Jr, Brady L W 1970 Malignant mixed müllerian tumors of the uterine corpus. Obstet Gynecol 35: 468
83. Muss H B, Bundy B, DiSaia P J et al 1985 Treatment of recurrent or advanced uterine sarcoma: a randomized trial of doxorubicin versus doxorubicin and cyclophosphamide. Cancer 55: 1648
84. Nieminen U, Soderlin E 1974 Sarcoma of the corpus uteri: results of the treatment of 117 cases. Strahlentherapie 148: 57
85. Norris H J, Parmley T 1975 Mesenchymal tumors of the uterus V. Intravenous leiomyomatosis: a clinical and pathologic study of 14 cases. Cancer 36: 2164
86. Norris H J, Roth E, Taylor H B 1966 Mesenchymal tumors of the uterus II. A clinical and pathologic study of 31 mixed mesodermal tumors. Obstet Gynecol 28: 57
87. Norris H J, Taylor H B 1965 Postirradiation sarcomas of the uterus. Obstet Gynecol 26: 689
88. Norris H J, Taylor H B 1966 Mesenchymal tumors of the uterus I. A clinical and pathologic study of 53 endometrial stromal tumors. Cancer 19: 755
89. Norris H J, Taylor H B 1966 Mesenchymal tumors of the uterus III. A clinical and pathologic study of 31 carcinosarcomas. Cancer 19: 1459
90. Omura G A, Blessing J A, Major F et al 1985 A randomized clinical trial of adjuvant adriamycin in uterine sarcomas: a Gynecologic Oncology Group Study. J Clin Oncol 3: 1240
91. Omura G A, Major F J, Blessing J A et al 1983 A randomized study of adriamycin with and without triazenoimidazole carboxamide in advanced uterine sarcomas. Cancer 52: 626
92. Pellillo D 1968 Proliferative stromatosis of the uterus with pulmonary metastases. Remission following treatment with a long-acting synthetic progestin: a case report. Obstet Gynecol 31: 33
93. Perez C A, Askin F, Baglan R J et al 1979 Effects of irradiation on mixed müllerian tumors of the uterus. Cancer 43: 1274
94. Persaud V, Arjoon P D 1970 Uterine leiomyoma: incidence of degenerative change and a correlation of associated symptoms. Obstet Gynecol 35: 432
95. Persaud V, Knight L P 1968 Malignant mesenchymal tumors of the corpus uteri. W Indian Med J 17: 96
96. Peters W A III, Kumar N B, Fleming W P, Morley G W 1984 Prognostic features of sarcomas and mixed tumors of the endometrium. Obstet Gynecol 63: 550
97. Piver M S, Barlow J J, Lele S B, Yazigi R 1979 Adriamycin in localized and metastatic uterine sarcomas. J Surg Oncol 12: 263
98. Piver M S, DeEulis T G, Lele S B, Barlow J J 1981 Cyclophosphamide, vincristine, adriamycin, and dimethyltriazenoimidazole carboxamide (CYVADIC) for sarcomas of the female genital tract. Gynecol Oncol 14: 319
99. Piver M S, Lele S B, Marchetti D L, Emrich L J 1988 The effect of adjuvant chemotherapy on time to recurrence and survival of Stage I uterine sarcomas. J Surg Oncol 38: 233
100. Piver M S, Lele S B, Patsner B 1988 cis-diamminedichloroplatinum plus dimethyl-triazenoimidazole carboxamide as second- and third-line chemotherapy for sarcomas of the female pelvis. Gynecol Oncol 23: 371
101. Piver M S, Rutledge F N, Copeland L, Webster K, Blumenson L, Suh O 1984 Uterine endolymphatic stromal myosis: a collaborative study. Obstet Gynecol 64: 173
102. Pocock E, Craig J R, Bullock W K 1976 Metastatic uterine leiomyomata: a case report. Cancer 38: 2096
103. Rachmaninoff N, Climie A R W 1966 Mixed mesodermal tumors of the uterus. Cancer 19: 1705
104. Rose P G, Boutselis J G, Sacks L 1987 Adjuvant therapy for Stage I uterine sarcoma. Am J Obstet Gynecol 156: 660
105. Rubin S C, Wheeler J E, Mikuta J J 1986 Malignant leiomyomatosis peritonealis disseminata. Obstet Gynecol 68: 126
106. Saksela E, Lampinen V, Procope B J 1974 Malignant mesenchymal tumors of the uterine corpus. Am J Obstet Gynecol 120: 452
107. Salazar O M, Bonfiglio T A, Patten S E et al 1978 Uterine sarcomas: natural history, treatment, and prognosis. Cancer 42: 1152
108. Salazar O M, Bonfiglio T A, Patten S F et al 1978 Uterine sarcomas: analysis of failures with special emphasis on the use of adjuvant radiation therapy. Cancer 42: 1161
109. Schaepman-van Geuns E J 1970 Mixed tumors and carcinosarcomas of the uterus evaluated five years after treatment. Cancer 25: 72
110. Scharfenberg J C, Geary W L 1974 Intravenous leiomyomatosis. Obstet Gynecol 43: 909
111. Seltzer V, Kaplan B, Vogel S, Spitzer M 1984 Doxorubicin and cisplatin in the treatment of advanced mixed mesodermal uterine sarcoma. Cancer Chemother Rep 68: 1389
112. Shaw R W, Lynch P F, Wade-Evans T 1983 Müllerian mixed tumor of the uterus corpus: a clinical histopathological review of 28 patients. Br J Obstet Gynaecol 90: 562
113. Silverberg S G 1971 Leiomyosarcoma of the uterus. A clinicopathologic study. Obstet Gynecol 38: 613
114. Silverberg S G 1971 Malignant mixed mesodermal tumor of the uterus: an ultrastructural study. Am J Obstet Gynecol 110: 702
115. Silverberg S G 1976 Reproducibility of the mitosis count in the histologic diagnosis of smooth muscle tumors of the uterus. Hum Pathol 7: 451
116. Smith F R 1941 Sarcoma of the uterus. New York State J Med 41: 681
117. Smith J P, Rutledge F, Delclos L, Sutow W 1975 Combined irradiation and chemotherapy for sarcomas of the pelvis in females. Am J Roentgen Rad Ther Nucl Med 123: 571
118. Sorbe B 1985 Radiotherapy and/or chemotherapy as adjuvant treatment of uterine sarcomas. Gynecol Oncol 20: 281
119. Spanos W J, Peters L J, Oswald M J 1986 Patterns of recurrence in malignant mixed müllerian tumors of the uterus. Cancer 57: 155
120. Spanos W J, Wharton J T, Gomez L, Fletcher G H, Oswald M J

1984 Malignant mixed müllerian tumors of the uterus. Cancer 53: 311

121. Spiro R H, Koss L G 1965 Myosarcoma of the uterus. Cancer 18: 571

122. Stearns H C, Sneeden V D 1966 Leiomyosarcoma of the uterus. Am J Obstet Gynecol 95: 374

123. Sutherland J A, Wilson E A, Edger D E, Powell D 1980 Ultrastructure and steroid-binding studies in leiomyomatosis peritonealis disseminata. Am J Obstet Gynecol 136: 992

124. Sutton G, Blessing J, McGuire W, Photopulos G, Rettenmaier M 1988 Phase II trial of ifosfamide and mesna in patients with recurrent or advanced mixed mesodermal tumors of the uterus. Proc ASCO 7: 137

125. Symmonds R E, Dockerty M B 1955 Sarcoma and sarcoma-like proliferations of the endometrial stroma. Surg Gynecol Obstet 100: 232

126. Tavassoli F A, Norris H J 1981 Mesenchymal tumors of the uterus. VII. A clinicopathologic study of 60 endometrial stromal nodules. Histopathology 5: 1

127. Tavassoli F A, Norris J J 1982 Peritoneal leiomyomatosis (leiomyomatosis peritonealis disseminata): a clinicopathologic study of 20 cases with ultrastructural observations. Int J Gynecol Pathol 1: 59

128. Taylor H B, Norris H J 1966 Mesenchymal tumors of the uterus IV. Diagnosis and prognosis of leiomyosarcomas. Arch Path 82: 40

129. Thatcher S S, Woodruff J D 1982 Uterine stromatosis: A report of 33 cases. Obstet Gynecol 59: 428

130. Thigpen T, Shingleton H, Homesley H, Blessing J 1982 Phase II trial of cis-diaminedichloroplatinum (DDP) in treatment of advanced or recurrent mixed mesodermal sarcoma of the uterus. Proc ASCO 23: 110

131. Thomas W O Jr, Harris H H, Enden J A 1969 Postirradiation malignant neoplasms of the uterine fundus. Am J Obstet Gynecol 104: 209

132. Tseng L, Tseng J K, Mann W J et al 1986 Endocrine aspects of human uterine sarcoma: a preliminary study: Am J Obstet Gynecol 155: 95

133. Tsukamoto N, Kamura T, Matsukuma K et al 1985 Endolymphatic stromal myosis: a case with positive estrogen and progesterone receptors and good response to progestins. Gynecol Oncol 20: 120

134. Van Nagell J R Jr, Hanson M B, Donaldson E S, Gallion H H 1986 Adjuvant vincristine, dactinomycin, and cyclophosphamide therapy in Stage I uterine sarcomas. Cancer 57: 1451

135. Vardi J R, Tovell H M M 1980 Leiomyosarcoma of the uterus: clinicopathologic study. Obstet Gynecol 56: 428

136. Vongtama V, Karlen J R, Piver M S, Tsukada Y, Moore R H 1976 Treatment results and prognostic factors in Stage I and II sarcomas of the corpus uteri. Am J Roentgen Rad Ther Nucl Med 126: 139

137. Wheelock J B, Krebs H-B, Schneider V, Goplerud D R 1985 Uterine sarcoma: analysis of prognostic variables in 71 cases. Am J Obstet Gynecol 151: 1016

138. White T H, Glover J S, Pette C H Jr, Parker R T 1965 A 34-year clinical study of uterine sarcomas, including experience with chemotherapy. Obstet Gynecol 25: 657

139. Williamson E O, Christopherson W M 1972 Malignant mixed müllerian tumors of the uterus. Cancer 29: 585

140. Yap B-S, Baker L H, Sinkovics J G et al 1980 Cyclophosphamide, vincristine, adriamycin and DTIC (CYVADIC) combination chemotherapy for the treatment of advanced sarcomas. Cancer Treat Rep 64: 93

141. Yazigi R, Piver M S, Barlow J J 1979 Stage III uterine sarcoma: case report and literature review. Gynecol Oncol 8: 92

142. Yoonessi M, Hart W R 1977 Endometrial stromal sarcomas. Cancer 40: 898

143. Zaloudek C J, Norris H J 1981 Adenofibroma and adenosarcoma of the uterus: a clinicopathologic study of 35 cases. Cancer 48: 354

PART VIII

Tumors of fallopian tube and broad ligament

53. Pathology of tumors of fallopian tube and broad ligament

R. H. Young   R. E. Scully

INTRODUCTION

Neoplasms of the fallopian tube, which account for only a small minority of female genital tract tumors, may pose diagnostic difficulties both clinically and pathologically. This chapter will describe the pathological features of these tumors, and the non-neoplastic lesions that simulate them; tumors of the broad ligament will also be discussed.

FALLOPIAN TUBE TUMORS

Carcinoma

In most cases, the diagnosis of tubal carcinoma is not suspected preoperatively, and an abnormality of the tube is first appreciated by the gynecologist at the time of operation or by the pathologist on gross or microscopic examination.[15,19,34] In approximately 10% of cases, however, malignant cells are detected in a cytologic smear of the lower genital tract and, if the vagina, uterus and ovaries appear to be free of tumor, the diagnosis of tubal carcinoma may be suspected preoperatively.[4,17,65,72,79] In some cases, fragments of tumor discovered in an endocervical or endometrial curettage specimen obtained during the investigation of abnormal bleeding are the first evidence of the disease.[19]

Tubal carcinoma is bilateral in 10 to 20% of cases.[67,79] At operation, it characteristically appears as a fusiform swelling that may be indistinguishable from a non-neoplastic hydrosalpinx or hematosalpinx. In some cases, however, the tube is not enlarged, or is only minimally enlarged, and a neoplasm is not detected until the structure is opened. The intraluminal tumor may be a soft, friable mass that fills the lumen (Fig. 53.1), a localized solid mucosal nodule (Fig. 53.2) or an ulcerated lesion. Hemorrhage and necrosis are common, and cysts are occasionally seen in large endophytic tumors. Sectioning of the tumor and the

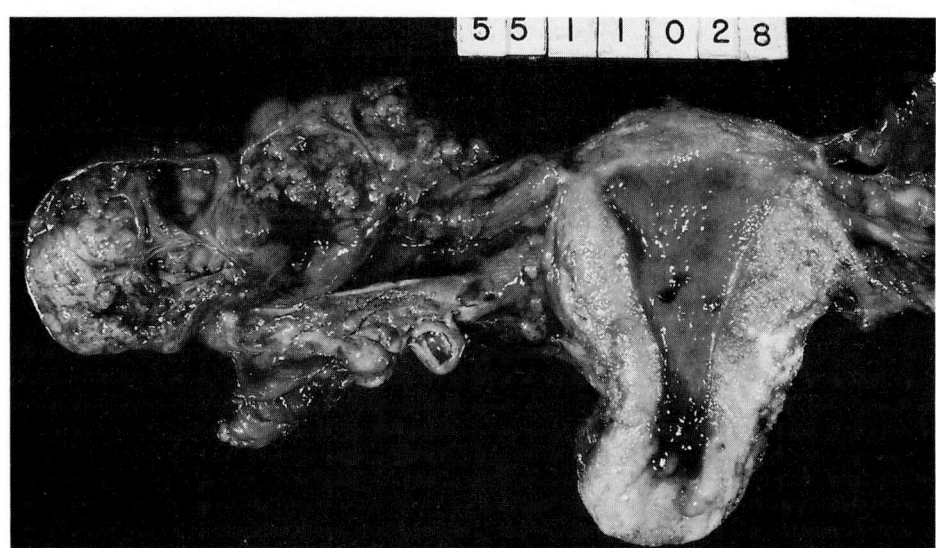

Fig. 53.1 Carcinoma of fallopian tube. A markedly distended tube has been opened to disclose papillary tumor occupying most of the lumen. (Reproduced from Green & Scully (1962),[28] with permission.)

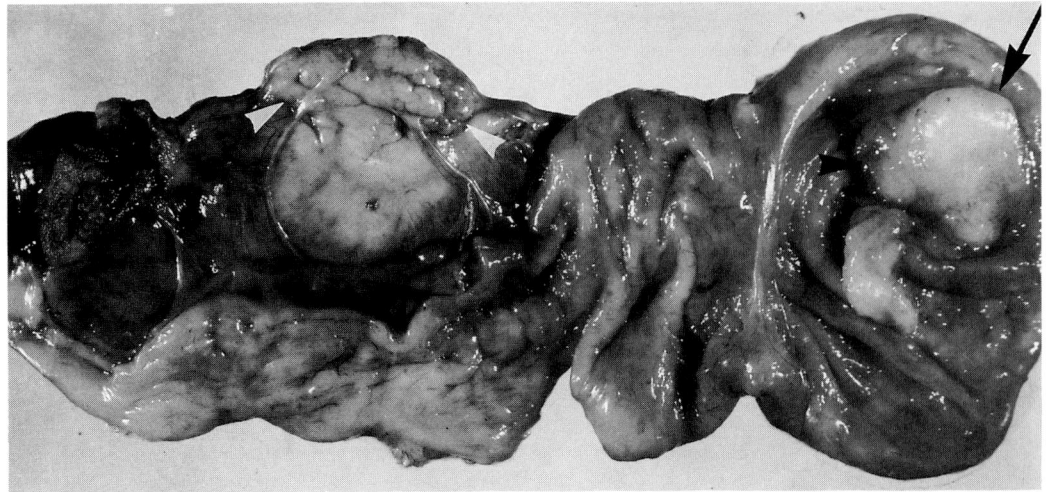

Fig. 53.2 Carcinoma of fallopian tube. Discrete nodule of white tumor tissue (black arrow) is visible on the mucosa. The opened tube occupies the lower portion of the left half of the specimen and the entire right half. The ovary and adjacent fibrous adhesions are visible (white arrow). (Reproduced from Green & Scully (1962),[28] with permission.)

underlying tubal wall may show no invasion, minimal invasion, or extensive infiltration, sometimes associated with involvement of adjacent structures, including the ovary. As tubal carcinoma usually closely resembles ovarian carcinoma on microscopic examination, gross examination is important in determining the primary site whenever both organs are involved.[28] Since ovarian carcinoma is much commoner than tubal carcinoma, the bias should be towards considering the ovary the primary site in doubtful cases. Occasional cases of apparently independent synchronous serous neoplasia of the tube and ovary have been reported[7] and, indeed, it has been suggested that if the tube is serially blocked, microscopic foci of tubal carcinoma may be found in as many as 5 to 10% of cases of serous carcinoma of the ovary.[7]

On microscopic examination, tumors that are primarily endophytic are typically papillary (Fig. 53.3). Some tubal carcinomas, however, particularly those that invade the wall, grow in the form of diffuse sheets, nests with or without focal gland formation (Figs 53.4 and 53.5), clusters, or single cells. Glands resembling those of serous adenocarcinoma of the ovary and psammoma bodies are occasionally seen. Most of the tumors are moderately or poorly differentiated. Endometrioid adenocarcinomas (Fig. 53.6), including some with squamous differentiation,[17,20,34] and squamous cell carcinomas,[46] clear cell carcinomas,[75] transitional cell carcinomas[18] and mucinous carcinoma occur rarely and are similar in their microscopic features to their more common ovarian counterparts. One fallopian tube tumor that was associated with pseudomyxoma peritonei was interpreted as a mucinous tumor of border-

line malignancy,[49] and another tumor that resembled an ovarian serous papillary tumor of borderline malignancy has also been reported.[22]

Occasional cases of carcinoma in situ of the tube have been described.[7,29,60] Such lesions have typically been incidental findings in tubes that have been entirely excised. Therefore, their natural history is unclear. Their recognition has been based on conventional histologic criteria,

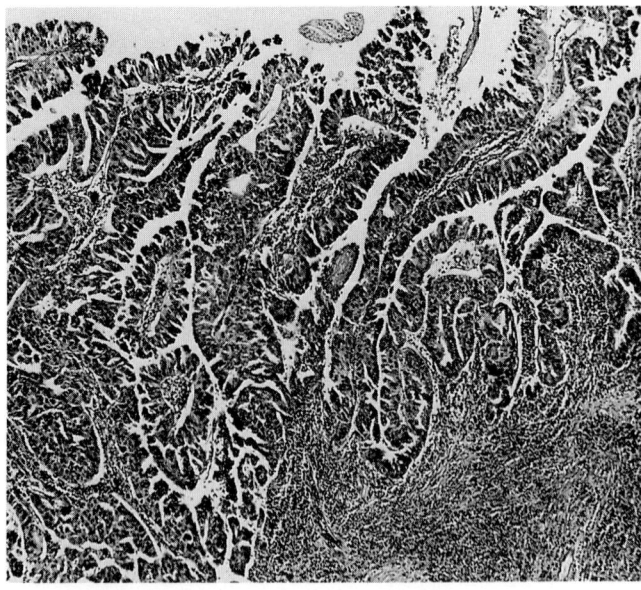

Fig. 53.3 Carcinoma of fallopian tube. A papillary neoplasm projects into the lumen (×50).

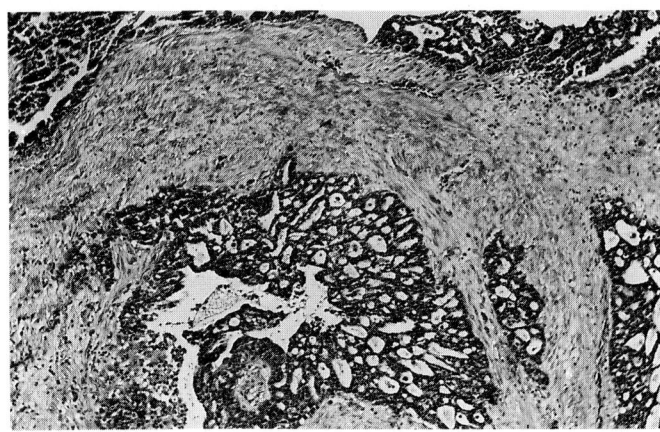

Fig. 53.4 Carcinoma of fallopian tube. Nests of tumor with glandular differentiation are invading the wall. The lumen is present at the top of the illustration (×63).

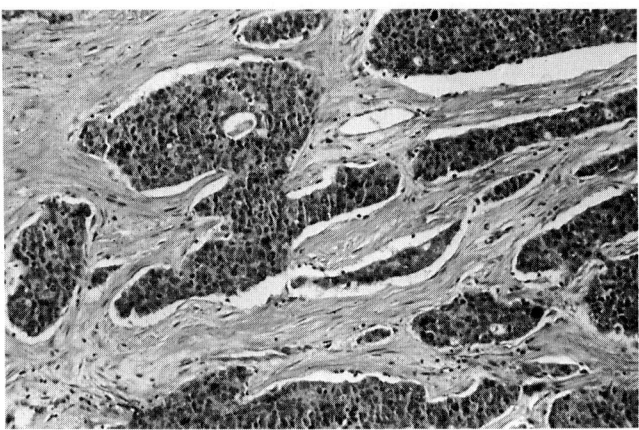

Fig. 53.5 Carcinoma of fallopian tube. Solid nests of tumor are invading the wall of the tube and have elicited a prominent fibrous stromal response (×135).

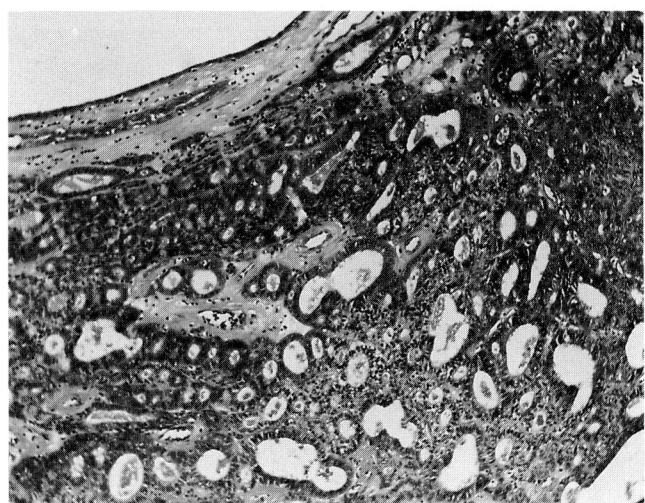

Fig. 53.6 Endometrioid adenocarcinoma of fallopian tube. The tumor is characterized by tubular glands and resembles the typical adenocarcinoma of the endometrium (×63).

and they should be distinguished from the reactive atypias that are usually associated with tubal inflammatory disease. Carcinoma in situ is typically focal (Fig. 53.7),[7] whereas reactive atypias are often widespread. In addition, the degree of nuclear atypia, nucleolar prominence and mitotic activity of carcinoma in situ (Fig. 53.7) is greater than that of reactive atypia.

The most important problem in the differential diagnosis of invasive tubal carcinoma is its distinction from atypical epithelial hyperplasia, which may be seen under a variety of circumstances.[16,51,54,58,70] The most florid examples occur in association with chronic salpingitis, in which the formation of papillae and pseudoglands (Fig. 53.8) and mild to moderate nuclear pleomorphism, nuclear hyperchromatism, and mitotic activity of the epithelial cells may occur.[54] Also, the abnormal epithelium may penetrate into the muscularis of the tube in the form of irregular gland-like structures, simulating invasive adenocarcinoma. Finally, pseudoglandular hyperplasia of the overlying mesothelial cells, which often become entrapped in inflamed fibrous tissue, enhances the resemblance to carcinoma.

It has long been recognized that these pseudocarcinomatous changes are associated with tuberculous salpingitis (Fig. 53.8), but they are also seen with other forms of bacterial salpingitis. A number of differences between carcinomas and pseudocarcinomatous inflammatory lesions aid in their distinction. The great majority of carcinomas are visible grossly, are unassociated with active inflammatory disease and exhibit severe nuclear atypia. The pseudocarcinomatous changes, in contrast, are usually incidental microscopic findings accompanied by overt evidence of active salpingitis. Additionally, carcinoma typically occurs in women who are older than those with a

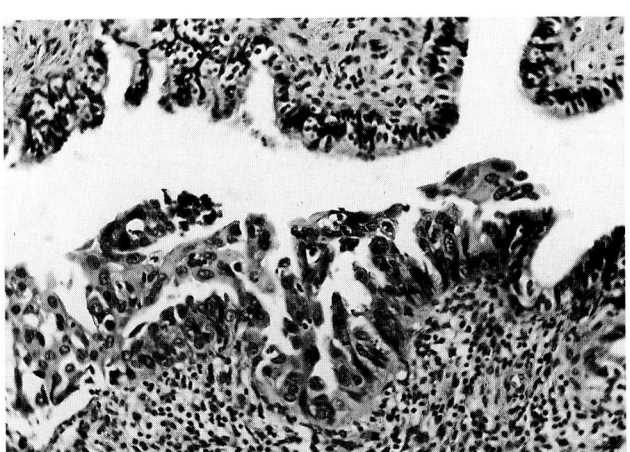

Fig. 53.7 Carcinoma in situ of fallopian tube. Most of the mucosa in the lower portion of the illustration has been replaced by highly atypical stratified epithelial cells. Contrast with normal mucosa in upper portion of illustration (×150).

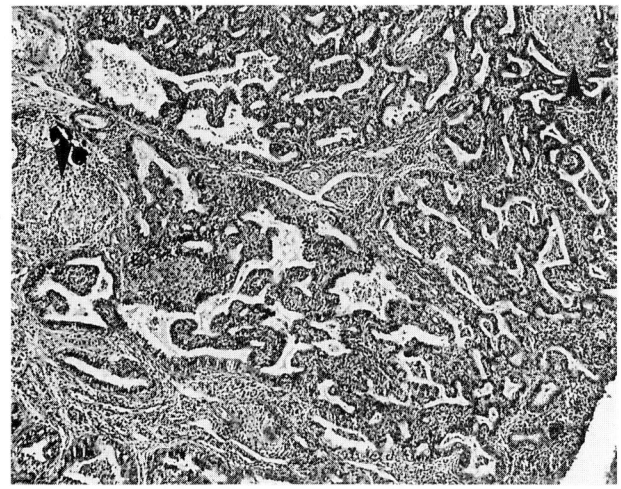

Fig. 53.8 Tuberculous salpingitis. The plicae contain tubercles (arrows) and the associated epithelial hyperplasia simulates adenocarcinoma (×51). (Reproduced from: Pathology of the fallopian tube. In: Hunt R B (ed) (1986) *Atlas of Female Infertility Surgery.* Yearbook Medical Publishers Inc, Chicago, with permission.)

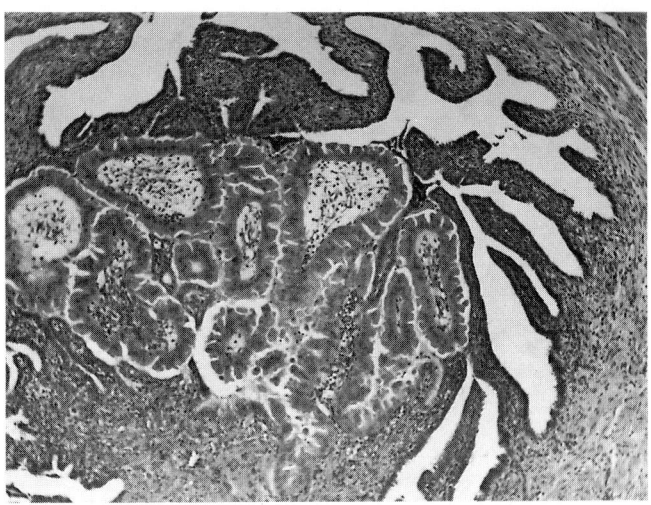

Fig. 53.9 Metaplastic papillary tumor of fallopian tube. A portion of the tubal mucosa has been replaced by cells with abundant cytoplasm that was eosinophilic. There is some papillary tufting off the surfaces of the papillae (×66).

pseudocarcinomatous lesion of inflammatory origin. If atypical mesothelial proliferation is a component of the lesion, the mesothelial cells are typically cuboidal, are often lined up in rows more or less parallel to the serosal surface, and generally exhibit only mild nuclear atypia.

Tubal hyperplasia is occasionally an incidental microscopic finding in a tube that is not the seat of inflammation. One study reported the presence of proliferative epithelial changes with nuclear stratification and atypia in 18.5% of a series of unselected fallopian tubes removed surgically;[16] there was no significant inflammation in half of the cases.

A microscopic appearance characterized by marked cellular stratification and nuclear elongation suggestive of carcinoma very rarely results from prolonged intraoperative cautery or inadvertent heating of the tube after surgical removal.[13] The rare lesion designated metaplastic papillary tumor of the fallopian tube[61] may also be confused with tubal carcinoma. In almost all of the cases, this lesion has been encountered as an incidental microscopic finding in a tubal segment removed from a pregnant or postpartum woman. It involves only part of the circumference of the mucosa (Fig. 53.9) and is characterized by large epithelial cells with abundant, eosinophilic cytoplasm which occasionally contain mucin, and large, oval vesicular nuclei; mitotic figures are rare. The lesion is distinguishable from a primary carcinoma of the tube by its microscopic size, lack of invasion, the bland or only slightly atypical appearance of its nuclei, and its special relation to pregnancy. Whether this lesion is metaplastic or neoplastic is unclear, but it has been associated with an uneventful course in the small number of cases encountered to date.

Malignant müllerian mixed tumor

Malignant müllerian mixed tumors (MMMTs) of the tube are rare, with only 36 cases reported.[11,31,39,47,55] This figure must be viewed in the context of the rarity of tubal malignancies in general; in one series, these tumors accounted for 18% of tubal cancers.[55] The well-documented examples of MMMTs have occurred in patients of 35 to 76 (average 58) years of age.[55] The clinical presentation is similar to that of tubal carcinoma, but at operation more widespread tumor is usually found. These tumors, which are typically large, are characteristically polypoid and may obliterate the tubal lumen (Fig. 53.10). Some of them are uniformly solid

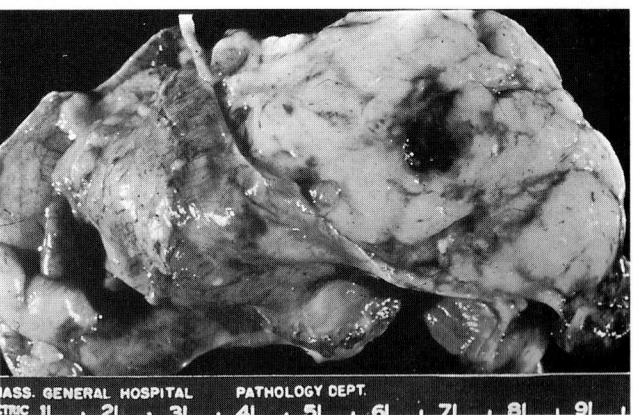

Fig. 53.10 Malignant müllerian mixed tumor. A markedly dilated tube has been opened to disclose a large white mass with focal hemorrhage. (Reproduced from Young R H, Clement P B, Scully R E 1988 The fallopian tube and broad ligament. In: Sternberg S (ed) *Diagnostic Surgical Pathology.* Raven Press, New York, with permission.)

and white to yellow, while others exhibit extensive cystic degeneration, hemorrhage and necrosis. Microscopic examination shows the typical admixture of malignant müllerian epithelial and mesenchymal elements that characterize this neoplasm in other locations. These two components are typically intimately admixed and approximately equal in amount, but in occasional tumors one or the other predominates. In the rare case in which the sarcomatous component is minor, the prognosis may be better; one patient with a tumor of this type was alive and well 10 years postoperatively, at which time the tumor recurred and was fatal after 2 more years.[55]

The epithelial component of the MMMT typically has the appearances of a moderately to poorly differentiated adenocarcinoma, often with focal squamous differentiation. The mesenchymal component may appear non-specific or may resemble a leiomyosarcoma, fibrosarcoma or high grade endometrial stromal sarcoma. Heterologous elements in the form of malignant-appearing cartilage or skeletal muscle, more often the former, are found in 40% of cases. The metastases of these tumors may be epithelial or mesenchymal or both. The prognosis is poor, with survival of only 3 of 19 patients (16%) who have been followed for at least 5 years.[55]

Sarcomas

Primary sarcomas of the tube are exceedingly rare, with only sporadic case reports in the literature.[2,64] Most of the reported tumors have been leiomyosarcomas.

Malignant lymphoma and leukemia

The tube may be involved in women with disseminated lymphoma, as well as those in whom the tumor appears to be confined to or involve predominantly the genital tract. In one large series of lymphomas presenting as ovarian masses, the tube was infiltrated in 26% of the cases,[57] but its involvement was rarely conspicuous on gross inspection. There are no reported cases of lymphoma apparently confined to the tube at the time of presentation, but one such case, a follicular lymphoma, has been seen by us. The gross and microscopic features of lymphoma of the tube are similar to those seen elsewhere. Like lymphomas of the female genital tract in general, tubal lymphomas may exhibit extensive sclerosis. The tube may also be infiltrated in patients with leukemia.[12]

Germ cell tumors

Forty-eight teratomas of the tube have been reported.[36] They are usually attached by a pedicle to the tubal mucosa and have ranged up to 20 cm in diameter. Most have been dermoid cysts, but rare examples have been solid mature teratomas[66] or immature teratomas.[71] One solid mature teratoma contained an area of insular carcinoid;[66] another tubal teratoma was composed entirely of thyroid tissue.[32]

Trophoblastic disease

The great majority of reported examples of trophoblastic disease of the tube have been choriocarcinomas. The 58 neoplasms considered acceptable in an authoritative review arose in patients from 16 to 56 (average 33) years of age.[56] Most of the patients complained of acute abdominal symptoms, which often mimicked those of ectopic pregnancy. The remaining patients usually presented with abdominal swelling. One choriocarcinoma that formed a large mass confined to the mesosalpinx has been reported.[43] Gross examination of the reported choriocarcinomas has typically shown a friable, hemorrhagic mass, which may contain soft, spongy tissue reminiscent of placental tissue. Small neoplasms may be difficult to distinguish on gross examination from an ectopic pregnancy. Microscopic examination shows the typical intimate admixture of cytotrophoblast and syncytiotrophoblast that characterizes choriocarcinoma. The distinction between choriocarcinoma and an ectopic pregnancy is occasionally difficult, because in some cases of ruptured ectopic pregnancy, villi are not present in the material submitted for microscopic examination. In these cases, in which only cytotrophoblast and syncytiotrophoblast are present, the pathologist may erroneously misinterpret the findings as choriocarcinoma. Unless the trophoblast is excessive in amount or significantly atypical, a benign interpretation is more appropriate in this circumstance. Conversely, the presence of villi does not inevitably exclude the diagnosis of choriocarcinoma, as they were present in two of the cases accepted by Ober & Maier[56] in their critical literature review of gestational neoplasms of the fallopian tube.

Ober & Maier[56] also identified in the literature 22 reported cases of hydatidiform mole of the tube. Most of these lesions, however, were reinterpreted by the authors as probable cases of ectopic pregnancy with hydropic change of the villi; only four of the cases were accepted as true mole.[56,77] The distinction between a hydatidiform mole and hydrops is made according to the criteria used for uterine trophoblast lesions (see Ch. 64). One hydatidiform mole of the tube was associated with lung metastases.[27]

Secondary tumors

The commonest secondary carcinoma of the fallopian tube has its origin in the ipsilateral or, occasionally, contralateral ovary. The spread from the ipsilateral ovary is usually direct, and from the contralateral ovary is usually by implantation. The tube is also invaded in occasional cases of advanced uterine cancer. In cases of ovarian and uterine cancer, tumor is often found in the lumen of the tube.

Rarely, a carcinoma of the uterus spreads solely or predominantly along the mucosal surface of the tube. This phenomenon has been seen not only in cases of endometrial carcinoma, but also in cases of squamous cell and mucinous adenocarcinoma of the cervix.[80] Rarely, squamous cell carcinoma in situ of the cervix spreads upward to involve the tubal mucosa.[40]

The tube is the site of metastasis from an extragenital site less often than is the ovary. In one review of 149 cases of metastasis to the genital tract from extragenital sites, there was only one case of tubal metastasis in contrast to 113 cases of ovarian metastasis.[48] In our experience, however, microscopic evidence of tubal metastasis is not as rare as the above figure indicates. In two other studies, 3%[19] and 7%[48] of metastases to the tube had their origin outside the genital tract.

Adenomatoid tumor

Adenomatoid tumor is the most common benign neoplasm of the tube.[26,38,59,62,74,81] It is usually an incidental finding in the myosalpinx but may compress the tubal lumen or project from the serosa; it is typically 2.0 cm or less in diameter, and is circumscribed, firm, and gray, white or yellow (Fig. 53.11); rarely, it is bilateral.[81] The microscopic patterns include irregular, gland-like spaces that range from elongated and slit-like to round and cystically dilated (Fig. 53.12) oval vacuoles, and small cords and clusters of cells in varying proportions. The neoplastic cells range from flattened cells, that are sometimes confused with endothelial cells, to large cells containing abundant eosinophilic cytoplasm. The nuclei appear bland and

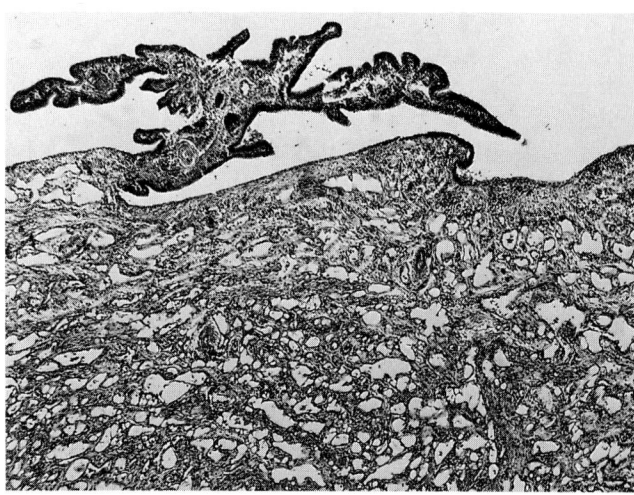

Fig. 53.12 Adenomatoid tumor. Numerous gland-like spaces lie beneath the surface epithelium (×40).

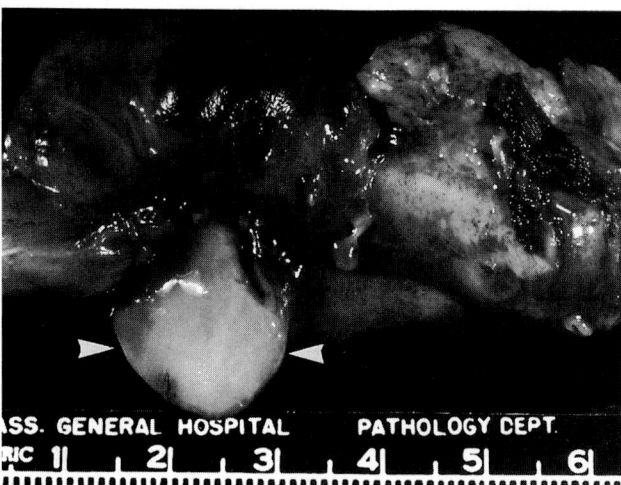

Fig. 53.11 Adenomatoid tumor. The tumor (arrows) has a glistening white sectioned surface. (Reproduced from Young R H, Clement P B, Scully R E 1988 The fallopian tube and broad ligament. In: Sternberg S (ed) *Diagnostic Surgical Pathology.* Raven Press, New York, with permission.)

mitotic figures are rare. The glandular lumens and vacuoles may contain slightly basophilic fluid which is rich in hyaluronic acid. The stroma may be hyalinized and contain smooth muscle and lymphocytes, which occasionally form prominent follicles.

An origin from mesothelium is now supported by most investigators, and continuity with the overlying mesothelium is occasionally seen.[74] The adenomatoid tumor may be confused with other benign tumors, particularly lymphangiomas and leiomyomas. Careful examination of the tumor cells should permit their distinction from endothelial cells and immunoperoxidase stains for cytokeratin and ulex europaeus aid in their distinction in difficult cases.[62] Although smooth muscle may be present in tubal adenomatoid tumors, it is rarely as prominent as it is in uterine adenomatoid tumors, and the characteristic spaces of an adenomatoid tumor are not compatible with the diagnosis of a leiomyoma. Adenomatoid tumors may also be confused with malignant tumors, such as malignant mesotheliomas and adenocarcinomas, but the circumscribed gross appearance, bland cytologic findings, and mitotic inactivity characteristic of adenomatoid tumors are not features of malignant neoplasms.

Benign epithelial and soft tissue tumors

Benign epithelial tumors of the types encountered in the ovary are very rare in the fallopian tube. Serous adenofibromas occur particularly at the fimbriated ends, and are similar to their ovarian counterparts.[68] Rare adenomas, papillomas and adenomyomas have also been reported.[25] Leiomyomas are the most common form of soft tissue tumor of the tube. They are grossly similar to uterine leiomyomas and may undergo similar degenerative changes.

Most tubal leiomyomas are relatively small; they may be submucosal, intramural or subserosal. On microscopic examination, they may exhibit the variety of appearances encountered in their uterine counterparts. Smooth muscle tumors of epithelioid type may cause a particular diagnostic problem, which may be solved by electronmicroscopic demonstration of myofibrils, dense bodies and pinocytosis, or by immunohistochemical demonstration of the intermediate filament, desmin. Other benign soft-tissue tumors also occur rarely in the tube.

BROAD LIGAMENT TUMORS

Paratubal cysts

Cysts of various types are a common finding attached to the fallopian tube or within the leaves of the broad ligament. These are usually small and often microscopic, but on occasion are large and symptomatic. The majority of these cysts are of müllerian origin, but some are derived from the mesothelium and a few result from the cystic dilatation of mesonephric tubules which are commonly present in the broad ligament.[23,63]

Müllerian tumors

Serous cystadenomas and serous cystadenomas of borderline malignancy are the commonest müllerian tumors of the broad ligament.[5,21] The former, which accounted for one-third of broad ligament tumors in one series of cases,[21] are grossly and microscopically identical to their ovarian counterparts. Borderline tumors are more troublesome, in part, because many clinicians and pathologists are not aware of their occurrence in this location. Aslani and his associates[5] recently described 25 serous papillary cystadenomas of borderline malignancy of the broad ligament, arising in patients from 19 to 67 (average 32) years of age. All the tumors were unilateral, confined to the broad ligament and unassociated with ovarian tumors of similar type. They were 1 to 13 cm in diameter, had smooth outer surfaces and contained straw-colored, watery fluid. Their inner linings had one or more papillary areas ranging up to 2.6 cm in greatest extent (Fig. 53.13). Microscopic examination showed the typical features of a serous borderline tumor. Papillae of various sizes projected from the cyst lining and were lined by stratified, moderately atypical cells. Smaller papillae typically budded off the surfaces of larger papillae. There was no invasion of the cyst wall, which was characteristically composed of tissue resembling ovarian stroma, but lacked follicles or their derivatives. Follow-up data were obtained in 23 cases and revealed that all of the patients were alive and free of disease 6 months to 11 years (average 4.5 years) postoperatively. Conservative removal of the cyst was appropriate management in the younger patients.

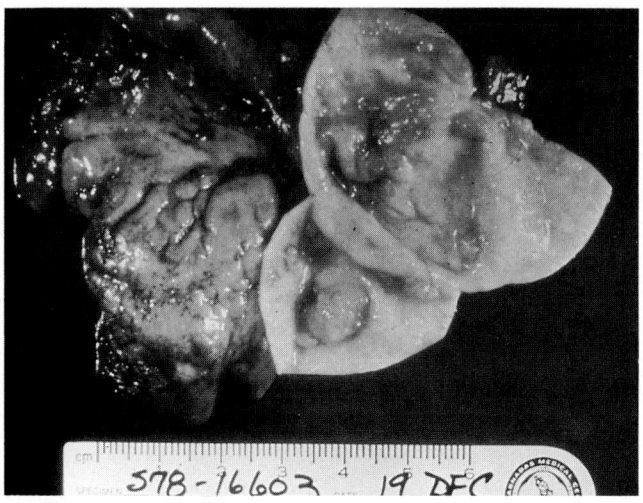

Fig. 53.13 Serous papillary cystadenoma of borderline malignancy of broad ligament. The inner surface of a cystic mass contains focal papillary projections. Note the adjacent unremarkable ovary and fallopian tube. (Reproduced from Aslani et al (1988),[5] with permission.)

Twelve cases of carcinomas of müllerian type arising within the broad ligament have been reported,[6] occurring in patients of 29 to 70 (average 46) years of age. These tumors ranged from 4.5 to 13 cm in diameter and were solid, cystic or both. All of them were unilateral. On microscopic examination, four of the tumors were endometrioid carcinomas, four clear cell carcinomas, one a probable mucinous adenocarcinoma, two papillary adenocarcinomas of undetermined cell types and one a serous papillary cystadenoma of borderline malignancy with microinvasion of its stroma. Endometriosis was reported to have been present in three of the cases and was the likely source of the tumor both in those cases and possibly in some of the others in which its presence was not documented. An endometrioid stromal sarcoma associated with endometriosis and originating in the broad ligament has also been reported.[53] Two of the patients with müllerian carcinomas of the broad ligament, one with an endometrioid carcinoma and one with a clear cell carcinoma, had independent, well-differentiated adenocarcinomas of the endometrium. One of the uterine tumors was non-invasive of the myometrium and the other was only superficially invasive. One of these patients had a distant metastasis in the rib at the time of operation, but was still alive 27 months later. Follow up was available for eight of the remaining patients, all of whom were free of disease 6 months to 7 years postoperatively.

Adnexal tumor of probable wolffian origin

Adnexal tumors of probable wolffian origin have occurred in patients from 18 to 72 (average 47) years of

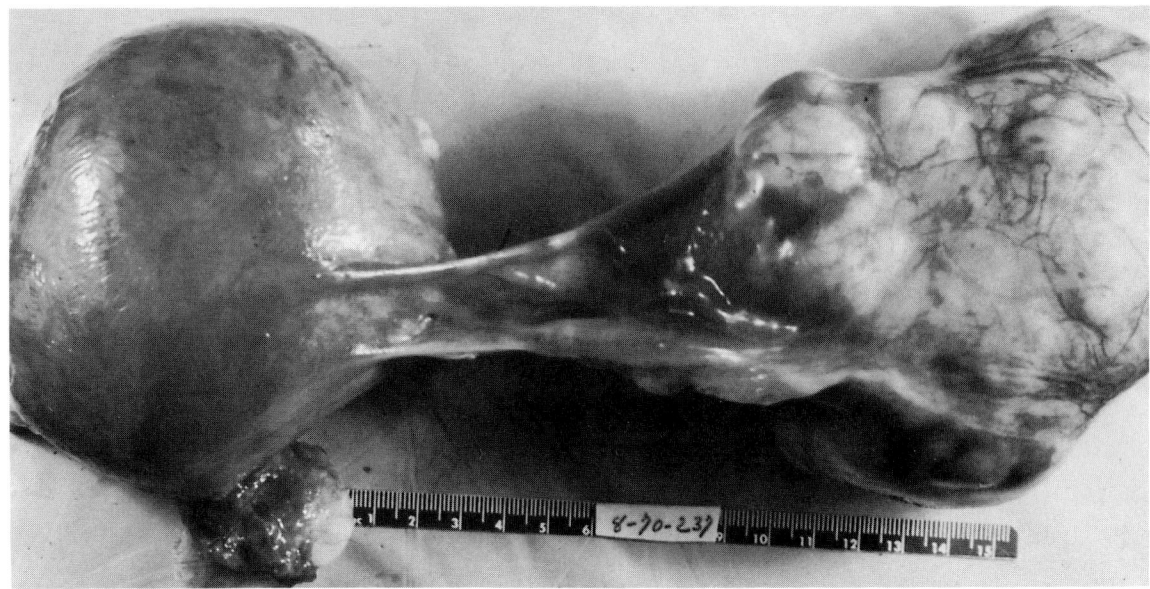

Fig. 53.14   Female adnexal tumor of probable wolffian origin. Posterior view of uterus and tumor within the leaves of the broad ligament. Note the smooth bosselated surface of the tumor. (Reproduced from Kariminejad & Scully (1973),[42] with permission.)

age.[14,41,42,69,73] Some of the patients have been asymptomatic while others have had abdominal pain or swelling; in still other patients, masses have been discovered on physical examination or at operation. The tumors lie within the broad ligament (Fig. 53.14) or hang from it or from the fallopian tube by a pedicle. They are typically large, round to oval masses with bosselated external surfaces (Fig. 53.14) and solid or solid and cystic cut surfaces. The solid tissue varies from gray-white to tan or yellow and is usually firm or rubbery; hemorrhage and necrosis are rare. Microscopical examination reveals dif-

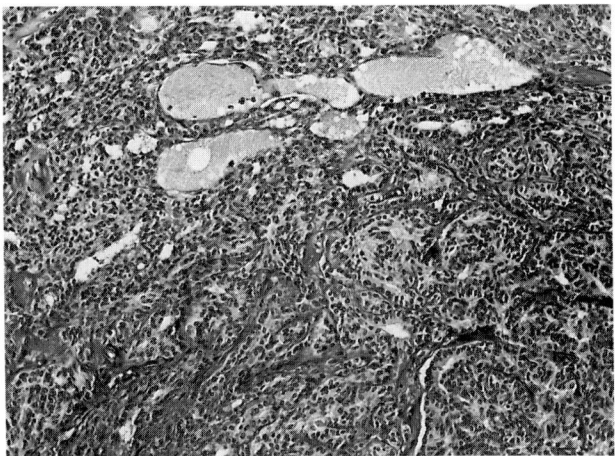

Fig. 53.15   Female adnexal tumor of probable wolffian origin. The tumor has a sieve-like pattern characterized by cyst formation (upper center) and a tubular pattern (lower right) (×94).

fuse, tubular, cystic and sieve-like patterns alone or in combination (Fig. 53.15). The tumor cells are cuboidal, columnar, or spindle-shaped with scanty cytoplasm and generally bland cytologic features. The tumors are considered to be of probable wolffian origin because of their location in areas where wolffian remnants are present in abundance, and because of the striking difference in their microscopic features from those of tumors of müllerian type.

Most of the reported examples of adnexal tumors of probable wolffian origin have been benign, but two tumors exhibiting malignant behavior have been reported.[55,59] Both recurred after 6 years, and one of them was fatal.[73]

Soft tissue tumors

Benign soft tissue tumors occur occasionally in the broad ligament[21] and round ligament.[10] The most common tumor encountered is the leiomyoma, with adenomyomas being relatively frequent, particularly in the round ligament.[10] Other tumors of soft tissue type occasionally occur in this location, and are classified according to criteria utilized elsewhere in the body.

Sarcomas are rare in the broad ligament, with leiomyosarcoma being the most common form.[33] One leiomyosarcoma arose within a pre-existing leiomyoma.[33] It should be remembered that large uterine leiomyosarcomas may grow into, and extensively involve, the broad ligament.[44] Careful gross evaluation is important in determining the primary site in cases in which both the myometrium and broad ligament are involved.

Miscellaneous tumors

Three ependymomas of the broad ligament have been reported in patients of 13, 45 and 47 years of age.[9,30] They were 1.0, 9.5 and 13 cm in largest dimension and had a microscopic appearance similar to that of ependymomas of the central nervous system; immunoperoxidase stains for glial fibrillary acidic protein were positive in all the cases. Intra-abdominal spread was present at presentation in one case, and was detected 11 years later in a second.[9] Various other tumors of miscellaneous types occur very rarely in the broad ligament. Of special interest are various tumors of ovarian type not mentioned above, such as Brenner tumor,[76] yolk sac tumor,[37] immature teratoma (personal observation), 'fibrothecoma',[50] steroid cell tumor (lipid cell tumor),[52] hyperplastic nodules of adrenal rest origin in Nelson's syndrome,[8] and bilateral mesonephric papillary cystadenomas occurring in association with the von Hippel-Lindau syndrome.[24] Rare tumors of other types reported as primary in this location include Ewing's sarcoma[45] and phaeochromocytoma.[3]

REFERENCES

1. Abbot R L, Barlogie B, Schmidt W A 1981 Metastasizing malignant juxtaovarian tumor with terminal hypercalcemia: a case report. Cancer 48: 860
2. Abrams J, Kazal H L, Hobbs R E 1958 Primary sarcoma of the fallopian tube. Am J Obstet Gynecol 75: 180
3. Al-Jafari M S, Panton H M, Gradwell E 1985 Phaeochromocytoma of the broad ligament. Case report. Br J Obstet Gynaecol 92: 649
4. Amendola B E, LaRouere J, Amendola M A, McClatchey K D, Han I H, Morley G W 1983 Adenocarcinoma of the fallopian tube. Surg Gynecol Obstet 157: 223
5. Aslani M, Ahn G-H, Scully R E 1988 Serous papillary cystadenoma of broad ligament: a report of 25 cases. Int J Gynecol Pathol 7: 131
6. Aslani M, Scully R E 1989 Primary carcinoma of the broad ligament: report of four cases and review of the literature. Int J Gynecol Pathol 64: 1540
7. Bannatyne P, Russell P 1981 Early adenocarcinoma of the fallopian tubes. A case for multifocal tumorigenesis. Diag Gynecol Obstet 3: 49
8. Baranetsky N G, Zipser R D, Goebelsmann U, Kurman R J, March C M, Morimoto I, Stanczyk F Z 1979 Adenocorticotropin-dependent virilizing para-ovarian tumors in Nelson's syndrome. J Clin Endocrinol Metab 49: 381
9. Bell D A, Woodruff J M, Scully R E 1984 Ependymoma of the broad ligament. A report of two cases. Am J Surg Pathol 8: 203
10. Breen J L, Neubecker R O 1962 Tumors of the round ligament. A review of the literature and a report of 25 cases. Obstet Gynecol 19: 771
11. Buchino J J, Buchino J J 1987 Malignant mixed müllerian tumor of the fallopian tube. Arch Pathol Lab Med 111: 386
12. Cecalupo A J, Frankel L S, Sullivan M P 1982 Pelvic and ovarian extramedullary leukemic relapse in young girls. A report of four cases and review of the literature. Cancer 50: 587
13. Cornog J L, Currie J L, Rubin A 1970 Heat artifact simulating adenocarcinoma of fallopian tube. JAMA 214: 1118
14. Demopoulos R I, Sitelman A, Flotte T, Bigelow B 1980 Ultrastructural study of a female adnexal tumor of probable Wolffian origin. Cancer 46: 2273
15. Dodson M G, Ford J H, Averette H E 1970 Clinical aspects of fallopian tube carcinoma. Obstet Gynecol 36: 935
16. Dougherty C M, Cotten N M 1964 Proliferative epithelial lesions of the uterine tube. I. Adenomatous hyperplasia. Obstet Gynecol 24: 849
17. Eddy G L, Copeland L J, Gershenson D M, Atkinson E N, Wharton J T, Rutledge F N 1984 Fallopian tube carcinoma. Obstet Gynecol 64: 546
18. Federman Q, Toker C 1973 Primary transitional cell tumor of the uterine adnexa. Am J Obstet Gynecol 115: 863
19. Finn W F, Javert C T 1949 Primary and metastatic cancer of the fallopian tube. Cancer 2: 803
20. Gaffney E F, Cornog J 1978 Endometrioid carcinoma of the fallopian tube arising in endometriosis. Obstet Gynecol 52: 34s
21. Gardner G H, Greene R R, Peckham B 1957 Tumors of the broad ligament. Am J Obstet Gynecol 73: 536
22. Gatto V, Selim M A, Lankerani M 1986 Primary carcinoma of the fallopian tube in an adolescent. J Surg Oncol 33: 212
23. Genadry R, Parmley T, Woodruff J D 1977 The origin and clinical behavior of the paraovarian tumor. Am J Obstet Gynecol 129: 873
24. Gersell D J, King T C 1988 Papillary cystadenoma of the mesosalpinx in von Hippel-Lindau disease. Am J Surg Pathol 12: 145
25. Gisser S D 1986 Obstructing fallopian tube papilloma. Int J Gynecol Pathol 5: 179
26. Golden A, Ash J E 1945 Adenomatoid tumors of the genital tract. Am J Pathol 21: 63
27. Govender N S K, Goldstein D P 1977 Metastatic tubal mole and coexisting intra-uterine pregnancy. Obstet Gynecol 49: 67s
28. Green T H, Scully R E 1962 Tumors of the fallopian tube. Clin Obstet Gynecol 5: 886
29. Greene R R, Gardner G H 1949 A preinvasive carcinoma of the uterine tube. Arch Path 48: 362
30. Grody W W, Nieberg R K, Bhuta S 1985 Ependymoma-like tumor of the mesovarium. Arch Pathol Lab Med 109: 291
31. Hanjani P, Petersen R O, Bonnell S A 1980 Malignant mixed müllerian tumor of the fallopian tube. Report of a case and review of the literature. Gynecol Oncol 9: 381
32. Henricksen E 1955 Struma salpingii. Report of a case. Obstet Gynecol 5: 833
33. Herbold D R, Fu Y S, Silbert S W 1983 Leiomyosarcoma of the broad ligament. A case report and literature review with follow-up. Am J Surg Pathol 7: 285
34. Hershey D W, Fennell R H, Major F J 1981 Primary carcinoma of the fallopian tube. Obstet Gynecol 57: 367
35. Honoré L H 1981 Para-uterine leiomyomas in women: a clinicopathologic study of 22 cases. Europ J Obstet Gynecol Reprod Biol 11: 273
36. Horn T, Jao W, Keh P C 1983 Benign cystic teratoma of the fallopian tube. Arch Pathol Lab Med 107: 48
37. Huntington R W, Bullock W K 1970 Yolk sac tumors of extragonadal origin. Cancer 25: 1368
38. Jackson J R 1958 The histogenesis of the 'adenomatoid' tumor of the genital tract. Cancer 11: 337
39. Kahanpaa K V, Laine R, Saksela E 1983 Malignant mixed müllerian tumor of the fallopian tube: report of a case with 5-year survival. Gynecol Oncol 16: 144
40. Kanbour A I, Stock R J 1978 Squamous cell carcinoma in situ of the endometrium and fallopian tube as superficial extension of invasive cervical carcinoma. Cancer 42: 570
41. Kao G F, Norris H J 1978 Juxtaovarian adnexal tumor — a clinical and pathologic study of 19 cases. Lab Invest 38: 350
42. Kariminejad M H, Scully R E 1973 Female adnexal tumor of probable Wolffian origin. A distinctive pathologic entity. Cancer 31: 671
43. Kay S, Schneider V, Litt J 1983 Choriocarcinoma of the mesosalpinx masquerading as congestive heart failure. Ultrastructural observations of the tumor. Int J Gynecol Pathol 2: 72

44. King M E, Dickersin G R, Scully R E 1982 Myxoid leiomyosarcoma of the uterus: a report of six cases. Am J Surg Pathol 6: 589

45. Longway S R, Lind H M, Haghighi P 1986 Extraskeletal Ewing's sarcoma arising in the broad ligament. Arch Pathol Lab Med 110: 1058

46. Malinak L R, Miller G V, Armstrong J T 1966 Primary squamous cell carcinoma of the fallopian tube. Am J Obstet Gynecol 95: 1167

47. Manes J L, Taylor H B 1976 Carcinosarcoma and mixed müllerian tumors of the fallopian tube. Report of four cases. Cancer 38: 1687

48. Mazur M T, Hsueh S, Gersell D J, 1984 Metastases to the female genital tract. Analysis of 325 cases. Cancer 53: 1978

49. McCarthy J H, Aga R 1988 A fallopian tube lesion of borderline malignancy associated with pseudomyxoma peritonei. Histopathology 13: 223

50. Merino M J, LiVolsi V A, Trepeta R W 1980 Fibrothecoma of the broad ligament. Diagn Gynecol Obstet 2: 51

51. Moore S W, Enterline H T 1975 Significance of proliferative epithelial lesions of the uterine tube. Obstet Gynecol 45: 385

52. Morris J M, Scully R E 1958 Endocrine Pathology of the Ovary. Mosby, St. Louis, p 104

53. Mostoufizadeh M, Scully R E 1980 Malignant tumors arising in endometriosis. Clin Obstet Gynecol 23: 951

54. Mostoufizadeh M, Scully R E 1983 Pseudocarcinomatous lesions of the fallopian tube. Lab Invest 48: 61a

55. Muntz H G, Rutgers J L, Tarraza H M, Fuller A F 1989 Carcinosarcomas and mixed müllerian tumors of the fallopian tube. Report of four cases. Gynecol Oncol 34: 109

56. Ober W, Maier R C 1982 Gestational choriocarcinoma of the fallopian tube. Diagn Gynecol Obstet 3: 213

57. Osborne B M, Robboy S J 1983 Lymphomas or leukemia presenting as ovarian tumors. An analysis of 42 cases. Cancer 52: 1933

58. Pauerstein C J, Woodruff J D 1966 Cellular patterns in proliferative and anaplastic disease of the fallopian tube. Am J Obstet Gynecol 96: 486

59. Pauerstein C J, Woodruff J D, Quinton S W 1968 Developmental patterns in 'adenomatoid lesions' of the fallopian tube. Am J Obstet Gynecol 100: 1000

60. Ryan G M Jr 1962 Carcinoma in situ of the fallopian tube. Am J Obstet Gynecol 84: 198

61. Saffos R O, Rhatigan R M, Scully R E 1980 Metaplastic papillary tumor of the fallopian tube — a distinctive lesion of pregnancy. Am J Clin Pathol 74: 232

62. Salazar H, Kanbour A, Burgess F 1972 Ultrastructure and observations on the histogenesis of mesotheliomas 'adenomatoid tumors' of the female genital tract. Cancer 29: 141

63. Samaha M, Woodruff J D 1985 Paratubal cysts: frequency, histogenesis, and associated clinical features. Obstet Gynecol 65: 691

64. Scheffey L C, Lang W R, Nugent F B 1941 Clinical and pathologic aspects of primary sarcoma of the uterine tube. Am J Obstet Gynecol 52: 904

65. Schenck S B, Mackles A 1961 Primary carcinoma of fallopian tubes with positive smears. Case report. Am J Obstet Gynecol 81: 782

66. Scully R E 1963 Germ cell tumors of the ovary and fallopian tube. In: Progress in Gynecology, Vol. IV. Grune, Stratton, New York, p 335

67. Sedlis A 1961 Primary carcinoma of the fallopian tube. Obstet Gynecol Surv 16: 209

68. Silverman A Y, Artinian B, Sabin M 1978 Serous cystadenofibroma of the fallopian tube: a case report. Am J Obstet Gynecol 130: 593

69. Sivathondan Y, Salm R, Hughesdon P E, Faccini J M 1979 Female adnexal tumour of probable Wolffian origin. J Clin Pathol 32: 616

70. Stern J, Buscema J, Parmley T, Woodruff J D, Rosenshein N B 1981 Atypical epithelial proliferations in the fallopian tube. Am J Obstet Gynecol 140: 309

71. Sweet R L, Selinger H E, McKay D G 1975 Malignant teratoma of the uterine tube. Obstet Gynecol 45: 553

72. Takashina T, Ito E, Kudo R 1985 Cytologic diagnosis of primary tubal cancer. Acta Cytol 29: 367

73. Taxy J B, Battifora H 1976 Female adnexal tumor of probable wolffian origin. Evidence for a low grade malignancy. Cancer 37: 2349

74. Taxy J B, Battifora H, Oyasu R 1974 Adenomatoid tumors: a light microscopic, histochemical, and ultrastructural study. Cancer 34: 306

75. Voet R L, Lifshitz S 1982 Primary clear cell adenocarcinoma of the fallopian tube: light microscopic and ultrastructural findings. Int J Gynecol Pathol 1: 292

76. Wagner I, Bettendorf U 1980 Extra-ovarian Brenner tumor. Case report and review. Arch Gynakol 229: 191

77. Westerhout F C Jr 1964 Ruptured tubal hydatidiform mole. Report of a case. Obstet Gynecol 23: 138

78. Woodruff J D, Julian C G 1969 Multiple malignancy in the upper genital cancer. Am J Obstet Gynecol 103: 810

79. Yoonessi M 1979 Carcinoma of the fallopian tube. Obstet Gynecol Surv 34: 257

80. Young R H, Scully R E 1988 Mucinous ovarian tumors associated with mucinous adenocarcinomas of the cervix. Int J Gynecol Pathol 7: 99

81. Youngs L A, Taylor H B 1967 Adenomatoid tumors of the uterus and fallopian tube. Am J Clin Pathol 48: 537

54. Tumors of fallopian tube: clinical features, staging and management

J. L. Benedet D. M. Miller

INTRODUCTION

Primary tumors of the fallopian tube, both benign and malignant, are rare. Nevertheless, a surprisingly wide variety of benign tumors have been reported as originating in the fallopian tube (see Ch. 53). Such lesions as salpingitis isthmica nodosa, endometriosis, adenomyosis and the hydatid of Morgagni are usually excluded from consideration as benign tubal tumors. The majority of benign tubal tumors are little more than interesting pathologic curiosities and are generally incidental findings at the time of pelvic surgery. Nonetheless, some have important clinical significance. A classification of fallopian tube tumors is presented in Table 54.1.

The most common benign tumor is the adenomatoid tumor, sometimes called an angiomyoma or reticuloendothelioma; it is a small, circumscribed tumor usually confined to the smooth muscle wall of the tube and found incidentally at the time of hysterectomy. Its importance clinically relates to its microscopic picture, which may be confused with a low grade adenocarcinoma. These tumors are not thought to possess malignant potential.

Leiomyomas of the tube, on occasion, may enlarge and undergo torsion and degeneration producing symptoms similar to those of their more common uterine counterparts.

Cystic teratomas of the fallopian tube have been reported to produce clinical findings simulating pelvic inflammatory disease, and they also may undergo rupture with spill of their contents leading to peritoneal irritation. There are no reported cases of malignancy arising within a cystic teratoma of the fallopian tube as has been described for those of the ovary.

The vast majority of malignant lesions involving the fallopian tube are secondary malignancies, generally arising from the adjacent ovary or uterus. Occasionally, the fallopian tube is involved by intraperitoneal dissemination of disease from gastrointestinal tract lesions.

Table 54.1 Classification of tumors of the fallopian tube

I. Benign tumors
1. Adenomatoid tumor
2. Leiomyoma
3. Teratoma
   a) Cystic
   b) Solid
4. Fibroma
5. Fibroadenoma
6. Papilloma
7. Lipoma
8. Hemangioma
9. Lymphangioma
10. Mesothelioma
11. Mesonephroma

II Malignant tumors
A. Primary
   1. Adenocarcinoma
      a) Papillary
      b) Papillary-alveolar
      c) Alveolar-medullary
   2. Sarcoma
   3. Choriocarcinoma
B. Secondary, e.g. ovary, bowel, etc.

PRIMARY ADENOCARCINOMA OF THE FALLOPIAN TUBE

Adenocarcinoma is the most common primary malignancy of the fallopian tube. It is responsible for approximately 0.3% of all gynecologic cancers in most reported series,[11,20,34,38] ranking it with carcinoma of the vagina as the most infrequent gynecological malignancies. A summary of its relative frequency according to literature reports is presented in Table 54.2.[11,13,15,20,28,34,38]

Orthmann is generally credited with the first classic case description of the disease in 1886, although Renaud is said to have made drawings of this tumor in 1847.

Etiology

The etiology of fallopian tube carcinoma is not certain, although earlier reports have suggested chronic tubal inflammation and infertility as possible predisposing

Table 54.2   Relative frequency of fallopian tube cancer

Principal author	Year	Patients with gynecological cancer	Adenocarcinoma of fallopian tube	Relative frequency
Finn[13]	1949	952	5	0.50%
Hu[20]	1950	3878	12	0.31%
Green[15]	1962	3200	2	0.10%
Momtazee[28]	1968	4341	8	0.18%
Sieck[38]	1978	2947	10	0.34%
Roberts[34]	1982	8974	28	0.33%
Eddy[11]	1984	22 200	71	0.36%
Total		44 492	136	0.31%

factors. However, the longstanding infertility in many patients, together with the frequent occurrence of chronic pelvic inflammatory disease in these individuals, suggest that these changes were present long before malignant change developed and that, in themselves, they are not factors in the etiology of this disease. Furthermore, when one contrasts the rarity of tubal carcinoma with the frequency of salpingitis, it would appear that little causal relationship exists. Tuberculous salpingitis has been noted to coexist with tubal carcinoma, and this association has also led some to speculate on whether it is a predisposing factor. Sedlis' review[36] showed that the rate of pelvic tuberculosis was not higher than that of the general population. It is important to distinguish the adenomatous response of tuberculous salpingitis from low grade adenocarcinoma of the tube.

Pathological diagnosis

Finn & Javert[13] have suggested the following criteria for the diagnosis of primary cancer of the fallopian tube.

Gross:
1. The tubes, at least in the distal portion, are grossly abnormal. The fimbriated ends may be dilated and occluded, resembling chronic salpingitis.
2. There is a papillary growth in the endosalpinx.
3. The uterus and ovaries are either grossly normal or affected by a lesion other than cancer.

Microscopic:
1. The epithelium of the endosalpinx is replaced in whole or in part by adenocarcinoma, and the histological character of the cells resembles the epithelium of the endosalpinx.
2. The endometrium and ovaries are normal, or contain a malignant lesion that by its size, distribution and histologic appearance is secondary to a tubal primary.
3. Tuberculosis has been carefully excluded.

The pathology of fallopian tube cancer is described in detail in Chapter 53.

Clinical features

Primary adenocarcinoma of the fallopian tube has been reported in patients ranging in age from 18 to 87 years, although it most often occurs between the ages of 40 and 65. The mean age as derived from numerous reports is 55 years (Table 54.3).[1,2,3,11,23,31,36,44]

Table 54.3   Age range — patient with fallopian tube cancer

Author	Year	Total no. of patients	Age range	Mean age
Eddy[11]	1984	71	36 to 84	54
Brown[3]	1985	21	34 to 82	52
Yoonessi[44]	1979	47	21 to 78	53
Benedet[1]	1977	41	33 to 80	54
Kinzel[23]	1976	26	33 to 80	55
Phelps[31]	1974	15	43 to 87	61
Boutselis[2]	1971	14	44 to 73	56
Sedlis[36]	1961	232	20 to 80	52

Primary carcinoma of the fallopian tube, like ovarian cancer, may be asymptomatic for variable periods of time. In 1916, Latzko[24] called attention to a triad of profuse vaginal discharge, pain and an adnexal mass. This symptom complex of *hydrops tubae profluens*, although said to be pathognomonic for fallopian tube cancer, is uncommon in most of the reported series.[18,23,26,27,33,34] Furthermore, the individual components of this triad are not specific for either cancer in general or fallopian tube carcinoma. The most common presenting complaints are those of abnormal vaginal bleeding and discharge, which are present in 35 to 55% of cases.[1,3,6,11,32,34,44] Next in frequency is abdominal pain, which may be of an intermittent or colicky type. This pain may be a manifestation of increased peristaltic activity as the tube attempts to rid itself of its contents. Pain of a dull, aching nature has also been frequently described and is probably related to distension of the tube.

The most common finding on examination is a pelvic or abdominal mass. Usually, this is thought to be an ovarian tumor and little consideration is given to the possibility of a tubal primary. This is, perhaps, the reason why so few patients are diagnosed preoperatively.[6,11,26,37] Three recent literature reports[11,18,32] with a combined total of 168 patients noted the correct diagnosis in only five cases (3%).

Several studies[18,37] have shown that delay in diagnosis

from the onset of symptoms with fallopian tube carcinoma is common.

The correct preoperative diagnosis may, on occasion, be made as a result of abnormal Pap tests showing malignant gland cells.[11,30,32,39,44] Takashina,[39] in his review of 184 patients who had cytologic assessment, found positive smears in 67 (36%). This, however, should not be relied upon as a diagnostic or screening test for fallopian tube carcinoma. Rarely, patients may present with Pap tests showing abnormal or suspicious, poorly differentiated epithelial or gland cells alternating with apparently negative smears, and results of the usual investigations may be unremarkable. This paradox should suggest the possibility of tubal carcinoma.

Similarly, patients with postmenopausal bleeding or spotting in whom diagnostic curettage is negative should have the diagnosis of fallopian tube carcinoma seriously entertained. Laparoscopy may be of diagnostic value in such individuals.

Hysterosalpingography has been employed in some reports but has not gained popularity as a diagnostic test due to the fear of extruding malignant cells through patent tubal ostia.

Ultrasonography and computerized transaxial tomography scanning are helpful in the preoperative evaluation of patients with suggested fallopian tube carcinoma. This may help to localize the extent of the primary lesion, and also to document possible spread to other intra-abdominal structures or pelvic and para-aortic lymph node areas. Lymphography may also be employed in the preoperative evaluation of patients to exclude obvious disease in the para-aortic and pelvic node areas, although the relative inaccuracy of this technique in the evaluation of metastatic cervical carcinoma makes one hesitant to recommend major changes in treatment policy on the basis of an equivocally abnormal lymphogram. The only tumor marker shown to be helpful in fallopian tube cancer is CA-125.[25,29] Although it does not distinguish this tumor from other more common gynecological malignancies or, indeed, even some benign conditions, it can be useful in assessing response to treatment in patients who have elevated titers initially.

Clinical staging

There is no universally accepted staging system for fallopian tube carcinoma. Most of the recent reports[3,6,18,26,30,32] have used a staging system that parallels that of the FIGO system for ovarian cancer (Fig. 54.1). This has the advantage of familiarity to most gynecologists and oncologists. One of its major disadvantages, however, is that it subdivides the relatively few cases that occur into many subgroups, making analysis of results even more difficult. The fallopian tube, unlike the ovary, is a hollow viscus with a muscular wall, and the mechanics of tumor spread may be different from that in the ovary. Most ovarian car-

Fig. 54.1 Clinical and operative staging for fallopian tube carcinoma (FIGO type)

Stage	Criteria
Stage I	Growth limited to the fallopian tubes
Ia	Growth limited to one fallopian tube; no ascites; no tumor on the external surface; tubal serosa intact
Ib	Growth limited to both fallopian tubes; no ascites; no tumor on external surface; tubal serosa intact
Ic	Tumor is either Stage Ia or Ib, but with tumor on the surface of one or both fallopian tubes; tubal serosa ruptured or with ascites present containing malignant cells, or with positive peritoneal cytology
Stage II	Growth involving one or both tubes with pelvic extension
IIa	Extension or metastases to the uterus and/or ovaries
IIb	Extension to other pelvic tissues
IIc	Tumor either IIa or IIb or with ascites present containing malignant cells, or with positive peritoneal washings
Stage III	Tumor involving one or both fallopian tubes with peritoneal implants outside the pelvis and/or positive retroperitoneal or inguinal nodes; tumor is limited to pelvis but with histologically proven malignant extension to small bowel or omentum
IIIa	Tumor grossly limited to the true pelvis with negative nodes but with histologically confirmed microscopic seeding of the abdominal peritoneal surface
IIIb	Tumor of one or both fallopian tubes with histologically confirmed implants of abdominal peritoneal surfaces, none exceeding 2 cm in diameter; nodes are negative
IIIc	Abdominal implants larger than 2 cm in diameter and/or positive retroperitoneal or inguinal nodes
Stage IV	Growth involving one or both fallopian tubes with distant metastases; if pleural effusion is present, there must be positive cytologic findings to allot the case to Stage IV; parenchymal liver metastases equal Stage IV

cinomas spread by transcelomic means, whereas tubal cancers not infrequently have been found to spread by lymphatic metastasis. Several other staging systems have been proposed taking these factors into account. One such system, similar to that proposed by Erez, Kaplan & Wall in 1967,[12] is shown in Figure 54.2. Schiller & Silverberg[35] used such a system in a review of 76 cases of fallopian tube carcinoma and were able to show the importance of disease confined either to the mucosa or to the lumen of the tube. Once serosal penetration had occurred, survival was exceedingly poor. It is generally accepted that the prognosis for fallopian tube cancer is determined by the anatomic extent of the disease thus the importance of meticulous surgical staging must be emphasized.

Table 54.4 lists the stage at presentation of fallopian tube cancer as derived from several literature series utilizing the

Fig. 54.2 Staging system for fallopian tube carcinoma (modified Erez's classification)

Stage	Criteria
I	Tumor limited to the tube, whether in the mucosa or invading the muscularis.
IIA	Tumor has extended through the serosa but has not invaded the contiguous organs.
IIB	Tumor directly invading surrounding organs, whether in the pelvis or abdomen. This would include metastases to the pelvic organs.
III	True metastatic lesions to organs outside the pelvis but confined to the abdomen.
IV	Metastatic disease outside the abdomen.

Table 54.4 Stage distribution at presentation by various staging system

Stage	FIGO type system No.	%	Modified Erez system No.	%
I	154	34%	64	26%
II	142	32%	59	24%
III	119	27%	70	29%
IV	33	7%	49	20%
Total	448*		242**	

* Reference: 2, 3, 4, 6, 10, 11, 18, 26, 30, 31, 32, 33, 34
** Reference: 1, 12, 19, 23, 28, 35, 37, 44

staging systems described. The FIGO type system[2 to 4, 6,10,11,18,26,30 to 34] shows that approximately two-thirds of patients are Stage I to II at the time of diagnosis, whereas the Erez system[1,12,19,23,28,35,37,44] distributes the cases almost equally between all of the stages.

Mechanism of spread

Although numerous pathways exist for the spread of fallopian tube cancer, it would appear that lymphatic dissemination and transcelomic migration are the two most commonly encountered.

The fallopian tube is richly supplied with a parenchymal lymphatic network with intercommunications throughout the mucosa, muscularis and serosa. The efferent trunks of this network emerge through the mesosalpinx to anastomose with the subovarian lymphatic plexus. The main channels then pass via the infundibulopelvic ligament to terminate in para-aortic lymph nodes at the level of the lower pole of the kidney. Tamimi & Figge[40] noted in their review that spread to the para-aortic area was a major site for metastasis.

Frequently, accessory channels may also pass through the broad ligament to drain into the internal iliac lymph nodes or, rarely, into the superior gluteal lymph nodes. Thus, when one appreciates the rich lymphatic network of the tube, together with its common drainage sites, it is easy to understand how widespread disease can occur once lymphatic dissemination has started. On occasion, metastases to inguinal lymph nodes may be the first manifestation of fallopian tube cancer.

The other major mechanism of spread in patients with fallopian tube cancer appears to be transcelomic migration of malignant cells. This pathway may arise either as spill of tumor cells through an open tubal ostia or by disease penetrating through the wall of the tube and shedding cells from its serosal surface. Once this method of spread is established, the intra-abdominal findings are very similar to those of advanced ovarian carcinoma. Sedlis[36] found the most frequent site of metastasis to be the peritoneum, followed by the ovaries and uterus. These findings led him to state that direct extension through the open tubal ostium was the most common mechanism of spread.

Surgical findings

The lesions are typically unilateral, although in approximately 20% of cases the lesions are bilateral at the time of diagnosis (Table 54.5). The distal or ampullary portion of the tube appears to be involved twice as often as the more proximal isthmic area when the site can be determined. Classically, the tube appears as a purplish, fusiform-like structure which, at times, may be similar in appearance to a hydrosalpinx or a pyosalpinx. Small lesions may produce no discernible gross change apart from some nodularity, present only on palpation, at the site of the primary. More advanced cases may demonstrate serosal penetration by tumor, with papillary growth and seedlings on surrounding structures. In advanced cases, large tumor masses enclosing the ovary and adherent to the pelvic sidewall are frequent, making distinction from an ovarian or uterine malignancy difficult. The fimbriated ends appear to be open or closed in an equal number of cases. On cut section, the lesion usually appears as a friable, granular, gray or yellowish tissue.

Treatment

The optimum method of treatment for fallopian tube carcinoma has not been clearly defined. The establishment of treatment protocols has been hampered by the relative rarity of this disorder, together with a lack of uniformity in staging observed cases.

Surgery

A variety of surgical procedures have been utilized. Cur-

Table 54.5 Site of primary

Principal author	Year	Total no. of patients	Right	Left	Bilateral
Brown[3]	1985	21	8	12	1
Roberts[34]	1982	22	12	8	2
Yoonessi[44]	1979	47	22	19	6
Benedet[1]	1977	37	17	17	3
Kinzel[23]	1976	26	15	9	2
Schiller[35]	1971	78	26	26	16
Dodson[10]	1970	10	3	5	2
Fogh[14]	1969	38	10	13	15
Momtazee[28]	1968	8	5	2	1
Green[15]	1962	18	9	9	0
Sedlis[36]	1961	176	63	67	46
Total		471	190	187	94 (20%)

rently, surgical exploration with peritoneal washings and staging similar to that done for ovarian carcinoma is recommended. The basic primary surgical procedure is total abdominal hysterectomy, bilateral salpingo-oophorectomy and omentectomy, where technically feasible. Certainly, for lesions confined to the tube, this would appear logical and desirable. Furthermore, the high incidence of bilaterality of these tumors and their ability to spread transcelomically as well as their frequent spread to ovary and uterus would support this concept.

Radical surgery does not appear to offer any advantages over simple hysterectomy in spite of the not infrequent spread of this tumor by lymphatic channels, since the extensive lymphatic drainage of the fallopian tube would necessitate complete node dissection of the pelvic and para-aortic areas and, perhaps, the inguinal nodes as well.

Retroperitoneal node sampling is recommended, particularly in patients with early stage disease. In patients with advanced disease, attempts to 'debulk' or optimally reduce the size of the tumor deposits, utilizing principles similar to those for advanced stage ovarian carcinoma, are advocated. Eddy et al,[11] in their review, showed a statistically significant difference in median survival between those patients with no gross residual disease post-surgery compared to those with a tumor diameter greater than 2 cm. The studies of Podratz[32] and those of Peters[30] have also confirmed the importance of residual tumor volume.

Radiotherapy

The role of radiotherapy in the management of carcinoma of the fallopian tube is less clear than that of surgery. Analysis of the literature[1 to 3,10,11,18,19,26,31,32,34] is hampered not only by the lack of uniformity in staging but also by the variability in radiotherapeutic dosage, field size, fractionation and type of radiation employed.

Certain authors,[1 to 3,31] however, have reported series of patients treated with radiotherapy where the results would seem to indicate definite benefit in terms of survival and disease-free intervals. In patients with widespread intra-abdominal disease, radiotherapy has not been shown to have an appreciable benefit. In such cases, the large field size needed, together with the radiosensitivity of small bowel and adjacent organs, makes the application of a useful radiotherapeutic dose virtually impossible.

However, when serosal penetration by disease has occurred and ostial patency is present, postoperative radioactive chromic phosphate may be of merit in patients with no gross residual disease. Radioactive colloidal chromic phosphate, 12 millicuries, is instilled intraperitoneally and has the potential for controlling microscopic deposits of tumor. Significant adhesions within the peritoneal cavity always raise the concern that the isotope will loculate, producing extensive bowel damage from high dose irradiation to fixed loops of small or large bowel. After administration of the drug, the patient should be turned frequently for the first 6 hours to ensure that the isotope distributes adequately throughout the peritoneal cavity, and scans should also be performed to ensure an adequate drug distribution. Alternately, pelvic-abdominal irradiation may be utilized in patients with positive peritoneal cytology and/or no macroscopic residual disease. These patients are treated sequentially, first with 2250 cGy in 10 fractions to a 17 × 17 cm pelvic field, followed by whole abdominal irradiation designed to deliver a mid-plane dose of 2250 cGy in 22 fractions. Shields are used to limit the dose to the kidneys to 1800 cGy.

Until some form of central registry and cooperative type

trials are established, the relative worth of radiotherapy in the treatment of fallopian tube cancer will remain controversial.

Chemotherapy

The similar morphologic appearance of tubal epithelium and certain serous ovarian carcinomas suggests that chemotherapeutic agents effective in the management of epithelial ovarian cancers should be effective for tubal cancer also. Cyclophosphamide, melphalan and thiotepa appear to have been the most widely used drugs as single agents. All appear to have about the same degree of effectiveness. Interpretation of the data is often difficult as many of the literature reports[6,9,16,33,42] regarding the use of these medications are brief, and the patients often receive chemotherapy because of recurrent disease or for palliation. The use of these agents in an adjuvant setting may produce results which are quite different from those produced when used in a palliative setting or for patients with extensive or large residual tumor deposits.

More recently, favorable results have been reported for combination chemotherapy employing cisplatin-containing regimens. These reports have utilized doses and schedules similar to those used in ovarian cancer. Six different literature reports[8,11,21,26,27,33] encompassing experience gained with the use of these medications in 35 patients have shown response rates in excess of 85%. The duration of response has ranged from 6 to 56 months. Unfortunately, however, as has been noted with ovarian carcinoma, in an appreciable number of patients who achieve complete clinical and histological remission, the disease does show a tendency to recur at a later date.

Certainly, patients with residual disease post-surgery warrant a trial with cisplatin containing regimens to see what benefit may accrue. In addition, given the general tendency for this disease to spread, and to extraperitoneal areas, the use of chemotherapy in an adjuvant setting, even in patients with complete resection of disease, would also appear justified. What is less clear, however, is whether or not adjuvant therapy, in patients with early stage disease where complete surgery has been carried out, should take the form of primary chemotherapy or radiotherapy. Also, the role of combined therapy with these modalities and their sequence is not clear. Toxicity can be substantial[9] with combination chemotherapy with cisplatin-based regimens, and difficulty in administering full therapeutic doses of drugs may occur, particularly if whole abdomen and pelvis irradiation has previously taken place. Conversely, optimum doses of radiotherapy are often difficult after multiple cycles of combination chemotherapy.

The role of hormonal therapy has not been fully evaluated but remains attractive, particularly as normal tubal epithelium undergoes cyclic changes in response to hormonal fluctuations during the menstrual cycle. Also, this epithelium embryologically and histologically is derived from the same sources as endometrial tissue and thus may be responsive to the same type of agents. Hormonal receptor studies with tubal carcinoma have been inconclusive and this avenue needs further study. A treatment schema based on risk categories is presented in Figure 54.3.

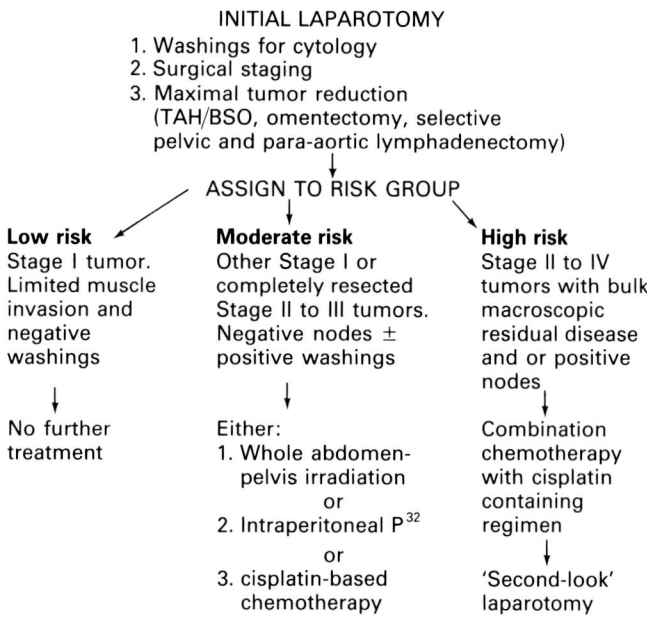

Fig. 54.3 Suggested management for fallopian tube carcinoma

Prognosis

The stage or extent of disease at the time of diagnosis appears to be the most important factor regarding prognosis of fallopian tube carcinoma. Table 54.6 lists the 5-year survival rates by stage for 278 patients collected from recent journal reports[3,6,18,26,30,32] using a FIGO-type staging system. Similarly, 155 patients[1,35,37,44] staged by a modified Erez classification had a 5-year survival rate of 58%. It is apparent that disease confined to the tube, i.e. Stage I, has a 5-year survival rate of approximately 60%, regardless of what staging system is used.

The prognostic significance of the histological degree of differentiation of the tumor is not clear. Hu et al[20] were among the first to correlate grade of tumor with survival, and they felt that a positive relationship existed. Recent reports,[26,27,30,32] however, show little difference between the various histologic grades. In addition, the observation that various patterns can be seen in the same lesion would appear to cast some doubt on the value of histologic differentiation as it relates to survival. There is a tendency for the more poorly differentiated tumors to be more advanced at the time of diagnosis. Therefore, until one is able to

Table 54.6 Survival rate by stage (FIGO) in recent selected series

Principal author	Year	Eligible for assessment	5-Year survival rate			
			Stage I	Stage II	Stage III	Stage IV
Denham[6]	1984	40	68%	39%	21%	0
Brown[3]	1985	17	60%	46%	16%*	—
Podratz[32]	1986	47	64%	60%	18%	25%
McMurray[26]	1986	30	56%	27%	14%	0
Hee[18]	1987	50	65%	13%	—	—
Peters[30]	1988	94	61%	29%	17%	—
Total		278	62%	36%	17%	—

* Stages III and IV combined

collect and analyze a sufficient number of cases of different grades within a given stage, uncertainty will continue to exist.

Green & Scully[15] reported that all five of 18 patients who survived 5 years had ostial closure. This suggests that tubal occlusion may act as a protective barrier against local spill and dissemination.

No firm evidence exists to indicate that the particular site of the lesion within the tube has prognostic significance in itself. However, it may be logical to assume that whereas lesions located in the cornual half of the tube have a tendency to spread to endometrium, those in the distal portion spread to ovaries and para-aortic lymph nodes, which may lead to an earlier widespread dissemination. Recently, the presence of positive cytology indicates that this is also an unfavorable prognostic factor. In general, most patients who relapse or recur do so within the first 2 to 3 years;[37] however, instances of recurrences 7 to 9 years post-treatment have been reported.[3,6] The potential value of DNA flow cytometry in this disease also needs assessment.

SARCOMAS

Sarcomas of the fallopian tube are extremely rare tumors. It has been estimated that the ratio of sarcoma to carcinoma is approximately 1:25.

The most common tumors of this type, malignant mixed müllerian tumors, have less than 35 cases reported to date in the world literature.[17,41,43] These tumors may be subdivided according to their mesenchymal component, which may contain either homologous or heterologous elements, i.e. elements native or foreign to the fallopian tube. It is thought that müllerian mixed tumors arise from the multi-potential mesoderm of the müllerian stroma. This stroma apparently retains a latent capability to differentiate into a variety of cell types. Most of the reported cases[43] to

date have been of the homologous type, with the mean age of the reported cases being 57 years. The routes of spread of this tumor are similar to that of fallopian tube cancer, that is dissemination via intraperitoneal or lymphatic-hematogenous pathways. The adjacent structures, such as the ovaries, uterus, peritoneal surfaces and bowel, are the most common metastatic sites. According to the review by Hanjani et al,[17] distant metastases are rare, and may include liver, lungs and bone. The metastatic lesions may contain either epithelial or stromal elements or both.

The prognosis of patients with these tumors is usually poor. The longest reported survival to date is a patient of Kahanpaa et al[22] who survived more than 5 years. According to the review of Yabushita et al,[43] the mean survival of all reported patients is 18.6 months. Prognosis may be influenced by stage, histologic type and grade, although the rarity of this tumor makes assessment difficult. Primary therapy should be complete surgical removal. In addition, chemotherapy has been used with some success and is advocated by several authors.[7,17,22,43] The role of radiotherapy is less clear, particularly when one considers the relative radio-resistance of malignant mixed müllerian tumours of other sites.

CHORIOCARCINOMA

Choriocarcinomas are exceedingly rare.[5] They arise as a consequence of trophoblastic neoplasia within an ectopic tubal pregnancy, or from transportation of trophoblast from an intra-uterine pregnancy that undergoes malignant transformation. These rare lesions are characterized histologically by the typical appearance of abnormal trophoblastic proliferation. Treatment is by chemotherapy in the same fashion as their uterine counterparts, utilizing hCG monitoring.

REFERENCES

1. Benedet J L, White G W, Fairey R N, Boyes D A 1977 Adenocarcinoma of the fallopian tube. Obstet Gynecol 50: 654
2. Boutselis J G, Thompson J M 1971 Clinical aspects of primary carcinoma of the fallopian tube: a clinical study of 14 cases. Am J Obstet Gynecol 3: 98
3. Brown M D, Kohorn E I, Kapp D S, Schwartz P E, Merino M 1985 Fallopian tube carcinoma. J Radiation Oncol Biol Phys 11: 583
4. Chalmers J A, Marshall A T 1976 Carcinoma of the fallopian tube. Br J Obstet Gynaecol 83: 580
5. Dekel A, Van Iddekinge B, Isaacson C, Dicker D, Feldberg D, Goldman J 1986 Primary choriocarcinoma of the fallopian tube: report of a case with survival and postoperative delivery. Review of the literature. Obstet Gynecol Surv 41: 142
6. Denham J W, MacLennan K A 1984 The management of primary carcinoma of the fallopian tube: experience of 40 cases. Cancer 53: 166
7. Deppe G, Zbella E, Fribert J, Thomas W 1984 Combination chemotherapy for mixed müllerian tumor of the fallopian tube. Cancer 54: 1517
8. Deppe G, Bruckner H W, Cohen C J 1980 Combination chemotherapy for advanced carcinoma of the fallopian tube. Obstet Gynecol 56: 530
9. Diamond S B, Rudolph S H, Lubicz S S, Deppe G, Cohen C J 1982 Cerebral blindness in association with cis-platinum chemotherapy for advanced carcinoma of the fallopian tube. Obstet Gynecol 59: 84S
10. Dodson M G, Ford J H, Averette H E 1970 Clinical aspects of fallopian tube carcinoma. Obstet Gynecol 36: 935
11. Eddy G L, Copeland L J, Gershenson D M, Atkinson E N, Wharton J T, Rutledge F N 1984 Fallopian tube carcinoma. Obstet Gynecol 64: 546
12. Erez S, Kaplan A L, Wall J A 1967 Clinical staging of carcinoma of the uterine tube. Obstet Gynecol 30: 547
13. Finn W F, Javert C T 1949 Primary and metastatic cancer of the fallopian tube. Cancer 2: 803
14. Fogh I 1969 Primary carcinoma of the fallopian tube. Cancer 23: 1332
15. Green T H, Scully R E 1962 Tumors of the fallopian tube. Clin Obstet Gynecol 5: 886
16. Guthrie D, Cohen S 1981 Carcinoma of the fallopian tube treated with a combination of surgery and cytotoxic chemotherapy. Br J Obstet Gynaecol 88: 1051
17. Hanjani P, Petersen R O, Bonnell S A 1980 Malignant mixed müllerian tumor of the fallopian tube: report of a case and review of literature. Gynecol Oncol 9: 381
18. Hee P, Pagel J D 1987 Primary carcinoma of the fallopian tube. Eur J Obstet Gynecol Reprod Biol 25: 131
19. Hershey D W, Fennell R H, Major F J 1981 Primary carcinoma of the fallopian tube. Obstet Gynecol 57: 367
20. Hu C Y, Taymor M L, Hertig A T 1950 Primary carcinoma of the fallopian tube. Am J Obstet Gynecol 50: 58
21. Jacobs A J, McMurray E H, Parham J et al 1986 Treatment of carcinoma of the fallopian tube using cisplatin, doxorubicin, and cyclophosphamide. Am J Clin Oncol 9: 436
22. Kahanpaa K V, Laine R, Saksela E 1983 Malignant mixed müllerian tumor of the fallopian tube: report of a case with 5-year survival. Gynecol Oncol 16: 144
23. Kinzel G E 1976 Primary carcinoma of the fallopian tube. Am J Obstet Gynecol 125: 816
24. Latzko W 1916 Linkseitiges tubenkarzinom rechtseitige karzinomatose tubo-ovarial cyste. Zentralbl Gynakol 40: 599
25. Lootsma-Miklosova E, Aalders J G, Willemse P H B, de Bruijn H W A 1987 Levels of CA 125 in patients with recurrent carcinoma of the fallopian tube: two case histories. Eur J Obstet Gynecol Reprod Biol 24: 231
26. McMurray E H, Jacobs A J, Perez C A, Camel H M, Kao M-S, Galakatos A 1986 Carcinoma of the fallopian tube: management and sites of failure. Cancer 58: 2070
27. Maxson W Z, Stehman F B, Ulbright T M, Sutton G P, Ehrlich C E 1987 Primary carcinoma of the fallopian tube: evidence for activity of cisplatin combination therapy. Gynecol Oncol 26: 305
28. Momtazee S, Kempson R L 1968 Primary adenocarcinoma of the fallopian tube. Obstet Gynecol 32: 649
29. Niloff J M, Klug T L, Schaetzl E, Zurawski V R, Knapp R C, Bast R C 1984 Elevation of serum CA 125 in carcinomas of the fallopian tube, endometrium, and endocervix. Am J Obstet Gynecol 148: 1057
30. Peters W A, Andersen W A, Hopkins M P, Kumar N B, Morley G W 1988 Prognostic features of carcinoma of the fallopian tube. Obstet Gynecol 71: 757
31. Phelps H M, Chapman K E 1974 Role of radiation therapy in treatment of primary carcinoma of the uterine tube. Obstet Gynecol 43: 669
32. Podratz K C, Podczaski E S, Gaffey T A, O'Brien P C, Schray M F, Malkasian G D 1986 Primary carcinoma of the fallopian tube. Am J Obstet Gynecol 154: 1319
33. Raju K S, Wiltshaw E 1981 Primary carcinoma of the fallopian tube: report of 22 cases. Br J Obstet Gynaecol 88: 1124
34. Roberts J A, Lifshitz S 1982 Primary adenocarcinoma of the fallopian tube. Gynecol Oncol 13: 301
35. Schiller H M, Silverberg S G 1971 Staging and prognosis in primary carcinoma of the fallopian tube. Cancer 28: 389
36. Sedlis A 1961 Primary carcinoma of the fallopian tube. Obstet Gynecol Surv 16: 209
37. Semrad N, Watring W, Fu Y-S, Hallatt J, Ryoo M, Lagasse L 1986 Fallopian tube adenocarcinoma: common extraperitoneal recurrence. Gynecol Oncol 24: 230
38. Sieck U V 1978 Primary adenocarcinoma of the fallopian tube. Aust NZ J Obstet Gynaecol 18: 147
39. Takashina T, Ito E, Kudo R 1985 Cytologic diagnosis of primary tubal cancer. Acta Cytol 29: 367
40. Tamimi H K, Figge D C 1981 Adenocarcinoma of the uterine tube: potential for lymph node metastases. Am J Obstet Gynecol 141: 132
41. Viniker D A, Mantell B S, Greenstein R J 1980 Carcinosarcoma of the fallopian tube: a case report and review of the literature. Br J Obstet Gynaecol 87: 530
42. Wong W S F, Tindall V R, Wagstaff J, Bramwell V, Crowther D 1985 Surgery and radiotherapy in the treatment of primary carcinoma of the fallopian tube – report of 18 cases. Aust NZ J Obstet Gynaecol 25: 211
43. Yabushita H, Ogawa A, Hoshina S, Okamoto T, Nakanishi M, Ishihara M 1987 Malignant mixed mesodermal tumour of the fallopian tube: case report. Br J Obstet Gynaecol 94: 179
44. Yoonessi M 1979 Carcinoma of the fallopian tube. Obstet Gynecol Surv 34: 257

PART IX

Tumors of ovary

55. Pathology of malignant and borderline (low malignant potential) epithelial tumors of ovary

W. R. Hart

GENERAL CONSIDERATIONS

The most common neoplasms of the ovary are composed principally of epithelial cells. Epithelial tumors account for at least 50% of all benign ovarian neoplasms, and from 85 to 90% of the primary malignant tumors. The frequency with which they are encountered is age dependent. While epithelial neoplasms comprise over 80% of all primary benign and malignant ovarian tumors in women over 50 years of age, they are infrequent in children and rare prior to puberty.[1,74] In premenarchial girls, practically all epithelial neoplasms are benign. Borderline and malignant epithelial tumors are occasionally discovered in adolescents and young adults. Ovarian carcinoma generally is a disease of perimenopausal and postmenopausal women. The mean age of patients at the time of diagnosis of a malignant ovarian epithelial tumor is about 52 years.[173] Borderline tumors affect women about 4 to 10 years younger.[7,134] Although ovarian carcinomas occur less frequently than do carcinomas of the uterine cervix or endometrium, they cause more deaths than any other group of malignancies of the female genital tract.

Ovarian tumors are notorious for the wide variation in degree of histologic differentiation that can be found in different areas of the same neoplasm. While classification by cell type is based on the most differentiated areas of a tumor, malignant potential is determined by assessment of the least differentiated portion. Consequently, extensive sampling by multiple sections is essential for accurate diagnosis. Special attention should be given to markedly papillary areas, nodular thickenings, roughened portions of a cyst wall, solid areas and regions where hemorrhage or necrosis are conspicuous. As a guideline, a block of tissue should be taken for each 1 to 2 cm of a tumor's maximum dimension.[68] The presence or absence of tumor on the external cortical surface of the ovary should be documented. This is important for staging of the tumor and may influence therapeutic decisions, since entirely intracystic, encapsulated lesions are less likely to produce peritoneal implants than are those which involve the cortical surface.

Accurate staging of ovarian epithelial tumors also requires information on whether the 'capsule' of the tumor is intact or ruptured. The need for a careful, thorough gross description of each ovarian tumor by the pathologist cannot be overemphasized.

HISTOGENESIS

The histogenesis of most common epithelial tumors is linked to the embryonic celomic epithelium. Some tumors may have other origins which are discussed later. Just lateral to each urogenital ridge wherein the gonad is developing, the celomic epithelium invaginates to form the müllerian (paramesonephric) ducts, from which the mucosae of the fallopian tube, endometrium and endocervix are derived. The celomic epithelium also gives rise to a thin layer of mesothelial cells which line the peritoneal cavity and cover the cortical surfaces of the ovaries and serosa of the adjacent pelvic organs. Following puberty, and especially later in life, invaginations of the ovarian surface epithelium, a modified mesothelium, recapitulate the formation of the fetal müllerian ducts. Narrow clefts lined by the infolded surface cells impart a convoluted appearance to the cortical surface. Frequently, the bases of these clefts are pinched-off, resulting in small inclusion cysts. Metaplasia of the mesothelial cells lining the clefts and cysts produces tall epithelial cells which often resemble the epithelium of the endosalpinx or endometrium and, occasionally, that of the endocervix.

In view of the common ancestry and close anatomic relationship of cells of the ovarian surface and the müllerian ducts, it is not surprising that tubal-, endometrial-, and endocervical-like epithelial cells are found in cysts and neoplasms of the ovary. In fact, similar types of metaplasias and neoplasms also arise in extra-ovarian pelvic peritoneum. Lauchlan designated cells capable of differentiation into epithelium similar to or identical with the mucosal lining of the uterus or tubes as forming a secondary müllerian system.[95] The greatest concentration of secondary müllerian epithelium is found on the surface of the ovaries, while the pelvic peritoneum provides the next most fruitful source.[95] Primary peritoneal tumors histologically identical to ovarian tumors may arise from such multipotential mesothelial cells.

Besides müllerian-type epithelium, other types of epithelial cells are also commonly encountered in ovarian and pelvic peritoneal lesions. The potential for metaplasia into transitional epithelial cells simulating the urothelium of the urinary bladder is seen in Walthard nests ('rests'), and is important in the genesis of Brenner and transitional cell tumors. Intestinal differentiation with goblet cells, neuroendocrine cells and even Paneth cells is also a relatively common metaplastic change.

The cause of metaplasia and neoplasia of ovarian surface cells is unknown. Ovulation is believed to play a major role in the production of inclusion cysts in the ovarian cortex[123,179] since they are seen with regularity only after puberty. The absence of ovulation in childhood is an explanation for the rarity of inclusion cysts and epithelial ovarian neoplasms in prepubertal girls. Animal studies support the notion that ovulation contributes to the development of epithelial neoplasms. Subhuman mammals with estrous cycles and infrequent ovulation rarely have epithelial tumors, while in animals with frequent ovulations, such as egglaying domestic fowl, ovarian adenocarcinomas are common.[43,96,173] Moreover, hens caused to ovulate incessantly have an increased frequency of ovarian adenocarcinomas.[43,96,173] The use of combination oral contraceptive medications appears to exert a protective effect against the development of ovarian epithelial cancer in women younger than 60 years.[126] Focal cortical stromal hyperplasia secondary to the effects of an excess of pituitary follicle-stimulating-hormone on the aging ovary,[69] and stimulation due to steroid hormones secreted by subjacent ovarian stromal cells[28] are two other proposed theories for the proliferative activity of ovarian surface cells. The low frequency of epithelial tumors in patients with gonadal dysgenesis, their increased incidence in nuns, and the positive correlation with infertility may also be manifestations of the relationships between ovulation, surface epithelial activity with inclusion cyst formation and the genesis of epithelial neoplasms.[43]

Mesothelial cells of the pelvic and ovarian surfaces are unique in females for reasons other than those related to ovulation and hormone secretion. The entire pelvic peritoneum and its encasements are susceptible both to environmental substances, which may reach them by upward passage through the interconnected lumina of the genital tract organs, and to endogenous fluid and debris regurgitated from the endometrium and fallopian tubes; irritant materials within such substances and secretions may serve as proliferative or carcinogenic agents in some women.[117] (See also Ch. 3.)

CLASSIFICATION OF COMMON EPITHELIAL TUMORS

Numerous classifications of epithelial neoplasms have been proposed over the years. While all schemes have certain defects, the histological classification of the World Health Organization (WHO)[152] published in 1973 has gained widespread acceptance. This scheme has been followed in this chapter, although it has been slightly modified to more closely conform to the topics under discussion. Table 55.1 shows the common epithelial tumors classified according to cell type. As indicated in the table, benign, borderline and overtly malignant tumors are found in each of the five specific cell type categories and in the mixed epithelial tumor group. While carcinosarcomas, malignant mixed mesodermal (müllerian) tumors, adenosarcomas and endometrioid stromal sarcomas have been classified with the endometrioid epithelial tumors in the WHO classification,[149] they are discussed with the ovarian sarcomas (Ch. 61) and are not considered here.

Table 55.1 Classification of primary common epithelial neoplasms of the ovary

I. Serous tumors	
II. Mucinous tumors	A. BENIGN
III. Endometrioid tumors	B. BORDERLINE (low malignant potential)
IV. Clear cell (mesonephroid) tumors	C. MALIGNANT
V. Transitional cell (Brenner) tumors	
VI. Mixed epithelial tumors	
VII. Undifferentiated carcinomas	
VIII. Unclassified and miscellaneous epithelial tumors	

The benign epithelial neoplasms are usually cystadenomas, papillary cystadenomas, adenofibromas, cystadenofibromas or, occasionally, surface papillomas, while the malignant varieties are usually cystadenocarcinomas, papillary cystadenocarcinomas, surface papillary carcinomas, adenocarcinomas or, occasionally, 'malignant adenofibromas' (carcinoma arising in adenofibromas). The relative frequency of malignancy varies considerably in each of the cell type categories. For example, most mucinous and almost all Brenner tumors are benign, while about half the serous, most endometrioid and the overwhelming majority of clear cell tumors are overtly malignant. Most borderline tumors are of either serous or mucinous type. Although the WHO classification has been widely used, some problems in interobserver and intraobserver reproducibility continue to exist.[32,160] While these are troublesome and of some concern, they do not lessen the usefulness of this system.

Epithelial ovarian neoplasms usually are not regarded as functional tumors, since the epithelial cells themselves only rarely elaborate hormonal substances. Production and secretion of sex steroids by reactive ovarian stromal cells adjacent to the epithelial cells, however, are not infrequent. Masculinization may result from secretion of androgens derived from these stromal cells, and hyperestrinism from aromatization of androgens to estrogens. The typical morphologic manifestation of such epithelial tumors with 'functional stroma' is hyperplasia and luteinization of the stromal cells which can be shown to have enzymatic activity and lipidic deposits in their cytoplasm. The lush stromal components of mucinous, endometrioid and Brenner tumors are especially likely to become functional, whilst the typically fibrous stroma of serous and clear cell tumors rarely displays steroidogenic activity (see also Ch. 8).

CONCEPT OF BORDERLINE (LOW MALIGNANT POTENTIAL) TUMORS

About 10 to 20% of the common epithelial tumors are intermediate in their histologic appearance and clinical behavior between the innocuous benign tumors and the clearly malignant carcinomas. In 1961, the International Federation of Gynecology and Obstetrics (FIGO) developed a classification wherein all common epithelial tumors of the ovary were subdivided into three groups:[145]

1. benign cystadenomas
2. cystadenomas with proliferating activity of the epithelial cells and nuclear abnormalities, but with no infiltrative destructive growth (low potential malignancy)
3. cystadenocarcinomas.

The WHO classification designated the intermediate proliferative neoplasms synonymously as 'tumors of borderline malignancy' or 'carcinomas of low malignant potential.' By definition, a borderline tumor is 'one that has some, but not all, of the morphological features of malignancy; those present include in varying combinations: stratification of epithelial cells, apparent detachment of cellular clusters from their sites of origin, and mitotic activity and nuclear abnormalities intermediate between those of clearly benign and unquestionably malignant tumors of a similar cell type; on the other hand, obvious invasion of the adjacent stroma is lacking'.[152] In recent years, these borderline tumors have become popularly designated as tumors of low malignant potential (LMP). They have an excellent prognosis when confined to the ovaries, and an indolent behavior when disseminated. Very few women who die of ovarian epithelial neoplasms within 10 years of diagnosis have a borderline tumor.[113] Diagnosis is based exclusively on histologic examination of the primary ovarian tumor without consideration of whether spread beyond the ovary has taken place.[152] Therefore, a diagnosis of carcinoma is not justified for a histologically borderline (LMP) tumor with peritoneal or omental implants, or even lymph node metastases. In fact, a substantial proportion of borderline serous tumors are Stage II or III at presentation.

Invasion of the ovarian stroma must be absent before a proliferating tumor can qualify for the designation of borderline or LMP. However, assessment of stromal invasion is at times difficult, and pathologists sometimes differ in their criteria for stromal invasion. Generally, tumors exhibiting unequivocal stromal invasion also show unequivocally malignant cytologic features, but the reverse is not always true. Some unquestionably malignant tumors, as well as many carcinomas metastatic to the ovary, do not display an obviously invasive pattern of growth. It is perilous to insist on finding a pattern of infiltrative destructive growth in every carcinoma. Carcinomas may invade the substance of the ovary in a very orderly pattern without evoking any stromal reaction. Moreover, some high grade surface carcinomas are devoid of stromal invasion but are fully capable of producing widespread carcinomatosis and rapid death of the patient by their easy access to the peritoneal cavity. In keeping with the definition of the WHO classification,[152] some proliferative epithelial tumors lacking 'obvious invasion of the adjacent stroma' are best classified as well-differentiated carcinoma when their microscopic features are those of 'unquestionably malignant tumors'.[67,68] This is especially true in mucinous tumors and in proliferating adenofibromatous tumors.

Russell has attempted to address the range of epithelial proliferation and nuclear atypia found in borderline tumors by dividing them into four histologic grades.[134] Grade I proliferating tumors have features only slightly more atypical than benign tumors, while Grade IV proliferating tumors have the microscopic features of well-differentiated adenocarcinomas without recognizable stromal invasion.[135] The relationship of histologic grade to survival has been variable in different studies.[88,138] Advocates of grading borderline tumors have concluded, however, that it is a moot point whether the high grade proliferating tumors should be classified with the invasive carcinomas and managed accordingly.[138]

Because of these differing approaches in the application of the WHO criteria for borderline tumors and the difficulties in recognition of unequivocal stromal invasion, the diagnosis of borderline (LMP) tumors continues to cause problems in evaluation of some high grade proliferating epithelial tumors. More studies are necessary to further refine the criteria for diagnosis of borderline tumors. Whether more objective analytic or morphometric methods will resolve these issues remains to be seen. DNA ploidy analysis of borderline tumors has recently been proposed as an adjunct to diagnosis.[56]

In spite of these recognized problems, a large number

of reported series has substantiated the clinical validity of separating the borderline tumors from the outright carcinomas.[13,21,25,65,68,72,75,81,88,89,111] While most information was initially available only for serous and mucinous borderline (LMP) tumors, clinicopathologic studies of borderline endometrioid, clear cell and transitional (Brenner) tumors have recently been published.

HISTOLOGIC GRADING

One of the most important prognostic factors in patients with ovarian carcinoma is the stage of the disease. The value of histologic grading of the tumors has been less certain. In studies in which the category of borderline (LMP) tumor was not utilized, the highly favorable outcome of patients with low grade tumors could be attributed to the failure to exclude them from the Grade 1 carcinomas.[24,105,106] When borderline (LMP) tumors and undifferentiated carcinomas are excluded, the prognostic importance of histologic grading of the common epithelial carcinomas is somewhat lessened.

Several different grading systems have been used and no single system has been widely embraced by pathologists. To compound matters, problems with both reproducibility and consistency of grading have been documented.[11] Nonetheless, there are highly significant relationships between histologic grade, tumor stage and survival. Poorly differentiated (high grade) carcinomas are most common in the advanced stages while the vast majority of Grade 1 carcinomas are of low stage. Multivariate analyses of patients receiving postoperative radiotherapy and/or chemotherapy have shown histologic grade to be a highly significant independent prognostic factor.[146,162] Grading may be especially valuable in assessing prognosis and selecting treatment for patients with low stage carcinomas. DNA ploidy analysis of tumor tissue by flow cytometry promises to provide additional important prognostic information on ovarian carcinomas[55,85] (see also Ch. 6).

SEROUS TUMORS

The serous tumors are by far the most commonly encountered histologic type, comprising about 40% of all primary ovarian neoplasms.[1] About 50 to 70% are benign. The malignant variants comprise about one-half of all ovarian carcinomas. The outright carcinomas outnumber the borderline (LMP) serous tumors by a two-fold to four-fold margin.[7,81,87,122,145]

Serous carcinomas tend to be large tumors. In one large series, 56.2% were over 15 cm in diameter, 39.9% were from 5 to 15 cm, and only 3.9% were less than 5 cm in diameter.[4] Grossly, the majority are papillary and cystic with multiple friable papillary masses and solid nodules of adenocarcinoma obliterating the cystic cavities and invad-

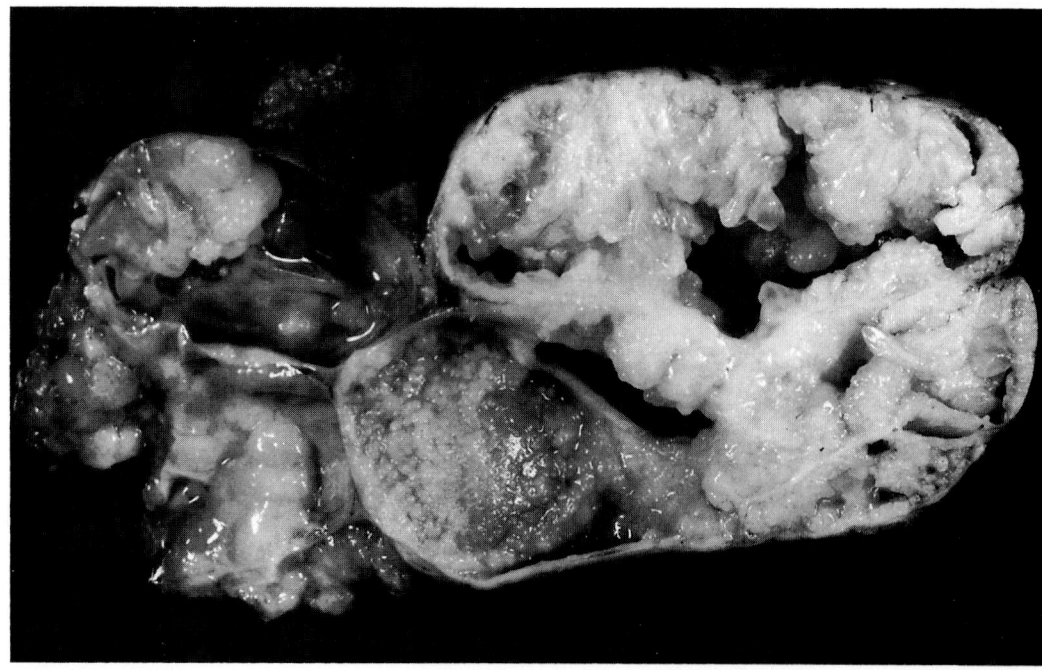

Fig. 55.1 Cut surface of a papillary serous cystadenocarcinoma. Exuberant papillary processes have overgrown cysts and partially obliterated their cavities. (Reproduced from Morrow C P, Hart W R 1975 The ovaries. In: Romney S et al (eds) *Gynecology and Obstetrics: The Health Care of Women.* McGraw-Hill, New York, with permission.)

ing adjacent ovarian parenchyma (Fig. 55.1). The fluid within the cysts tends to be watery and thin or 'serous' in quality. However, in 28% of all benign and malignant serous tumors it is viscid and mucoid.[4] About 8% are solid adenocarcinomas without an appreciable cystic element.[4] Tumor growth on the cortical surface can be seen in almost half of the carcinomas and borderline (LMP) tumors but is observed in less than 10% of benign lesions.[52] An infrequent variant of serous carcinoma is an entirely exophytic tumor that arises directly from the surface epithelium of the ovarian cortex. These surface serous carcinomas are often bilateral and associated with widespread tumor within the peritoneal cavity at presentation.[64,169] When the affected ovaries are only slightly enlarged or appear 'normal' to the gynecologist at operation, such surface serous carcinomas probably represent multicentric tumors of the peritoneum and ovarian surfaces. The least common malignant serous tumor is a carcinoma arising within an adenofibroma ('malignant adenofibroma' or 'adenofibrocarcinoma').

Serous neoplasms are composed of cells that resemble those of the surface epithelium of the ovary or of the fallopian tubal mucosa. At one time, the well-differentiated serous tumors were termed 'endosalpingiomas'.[14] Immunohistologic reactivity of monoclonal antibody OC 125 with the ovarian tumor associated antigen CA 125 is characteristically found in benign, borderline and malignant serous tumors, as well as in some other ovarian and non-ovarian epithelial tumors.[76,77] Amylase activity has also been demonstrated in serous tumors as well as in endosalpingeal epithelium.[22,167] Ultrastructurally, three to five types of cells have been described.[62,87,124] Ciliated cells are prominent in benign and borderline tumors but are rare in carcinomas.[62,87]

The well differentiated (low grade) carcinomas are usually papillary cystadenocarcinomas. They have broad and finely-branched papillations with connective tissue stroma. Overgrowth of epithelial cells results in anastomosing bridges of tumor cells that interconnect adjacent papillae (Fig. 55.2). Stromal invasion is usually obvious but, even in some high grade carcinomas, infiltrative growth into ovarian parenchyma may be minimal or difficult to identify. Nuclei are large, vesicular and have prominent nucleoli. The size and number of nucleoli increase with increasing grades of malignancy.[61,87,164] Moderately and poorly differentiated carcinomas have more alveolar and medullary configurations, with solid sheets of cells surrounding irregular small spaces; cysts and papillae are less conspicuous. The least differentiated and most aggressive variants are predominantly solid adenocarcinomas. They contain undifferentiated cells and large bizarre cells (Fig. 55.3). Multinucleated tumor giant cells, suggesting an attempt at trophoblastic differentiation, may be responsible for hormonal production in the reported instances of gonadotropin-producing ovarian carcinomas.[28,153] Rounded hyaline globules similar to those seen in endodermal sinus tumors and other cancers are often present. Barzilai[14] referred to these extremely high grade tumors as 'sero-anaplastic carcinoma', a term which we have found useful, although some pathologists classify them as undifferentiated carcinoma when a solid pattern becomes the exclusive or almost exclusive feature.[149]

Small, laminated calcospherites, or psammoma bodies, are frequent in papillary serous tumors (Fig. 55.4). They are found in about one-third or more of the carcinomas[9] but also occur in benign cystadenomas and inclusion cysts. They are more often seen in patients with disseminated peritoneal implants than in patients with localized tumors.[9,122] The better prognosis associated with tumors having psammoma bodies[9] probably reflects the fact that they are more copious in the borderline (LMP) tumors and well-differentiated carcinomas than in the poorly differentiated carcinomas. Ultrastructurally, psammoma bodies are composed of microcrystals similar to calcium-phosphate apatite crystals of bone and are produced intracellularly.[49] They are believed to be a consequence of dystrophic calcification associated with cellular degeneration.[49]

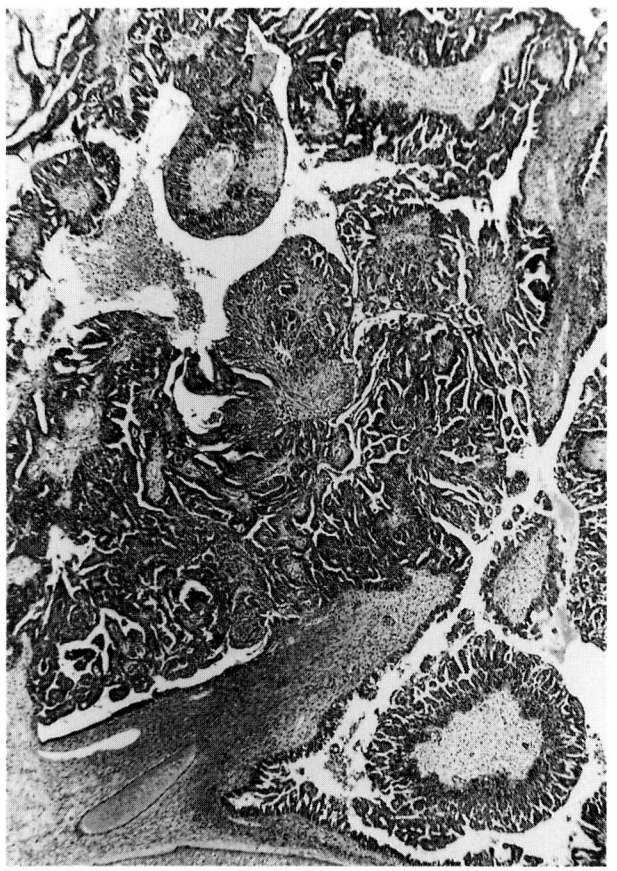

Fig. 55.2 Papillary serous cystadenocarcinoma. Broad and finely branched papillae are interconnected by anastomosing bridges of carcinoma cells.

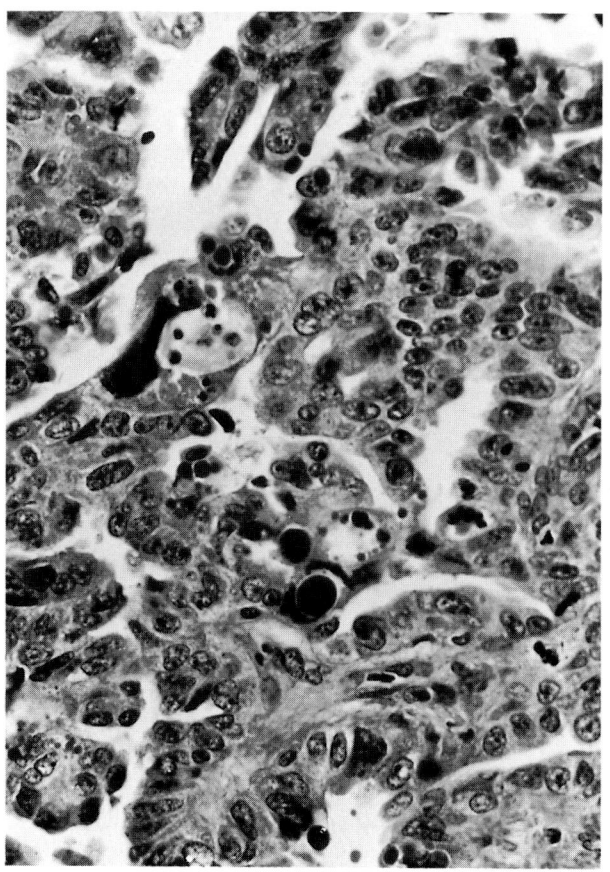

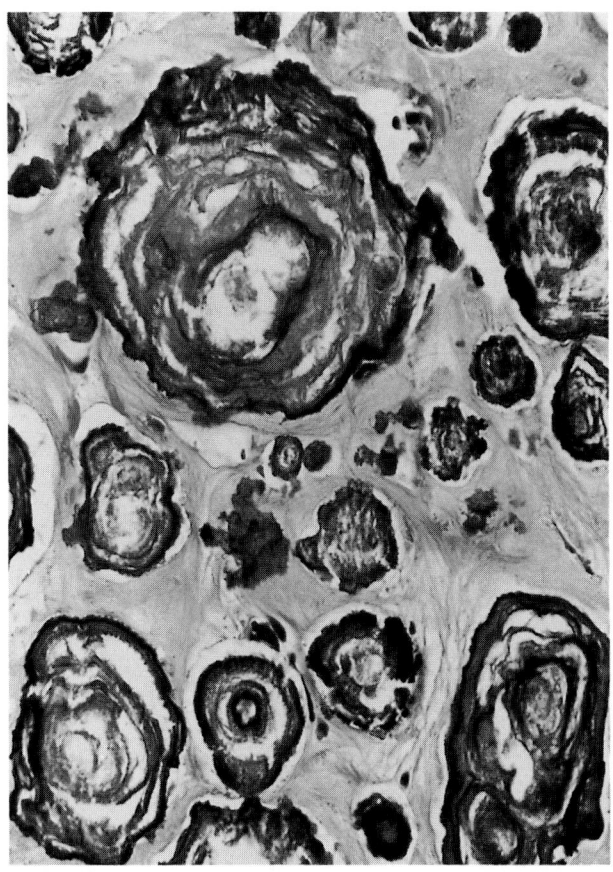

Fig. 55.3 Anaplastic serous ('seroanaplastic') carcinoma. Pleomorphic, poorly differentiated serous carcinoma has cells with anaplastic nuclei and numerous mitotic figures. Amongst the cells are several round hyaline bodies.

Fig. 55.4 Psammoma bodies. Multiple calcospherites with concentric laminations in fibrous tissue from a metastatic serous carcinoma. Epithelial cells are not visible in this field.

Some serous tumors produce mucus. Unlike mucinous cell tumors, however, the mucin is extracellular and appears to be secreted into the cysts from the apical surfaces of the epithelial cells. If mucin droplets are within the cytoplasm, they occupy only a small portion adjacent to the lumen.[61,87] Histochemical studies have shown both neutral and acidic mucins within the cysts of some tumors.[87]

Bilaterality occurs in 35 to 50% of serous carcinomas, but both ovaries may be involved in two-thirds of cases with extensive peritoneal spread.[89] Serous carcinomas spread rapidly throughout the peritoneal cavity, and typically produce marked ascites. Only about 20% of patients have tumors confined to one or both ovaries (Stage I) when the diagnosis is established.[7] The tendency for involvement of the cortical surfaces, either by de novo malignant transformation of surface epithelium or secondary to invasion from underlying carcinoma, is responsible for early intra-abdominal dissemination. It is not surprising that the prognosis is poor in view of the minority of patients that are diagnosed and treated before extra-ovarian spread has occurred. After exclusion of borderline tumors, the overall 5-year survival rate for patients with serous carcinoma is only 15 to 30%.[7,145] The most important prognostic factors are the stage and histologic grade of the tumor.

Borderline (LMP) serous tumors

About 9 to 15% of all serous neoplasms are of borderline or LMP type.[81,122,134] Grossly, most are cystic and papillary and may not be distinguishable from papillary serous cystadenocarcinomas or markedly papillary cystadenomas (Fig. 55.5). Papillary excrescences on the external cortical surface occur in almost one-half of all patients, and in one-quarter to one-third of those with Stage I tumors.[52,75,81] Surface growth of this type does not result from invasion through the cortex, but represents direct origin from surface epithelium. In less than 10% of cases, the entire lesion is an exophytic papillary surface borderline (LMP) tumor unassociated with internal cysts or with only a minor cystic

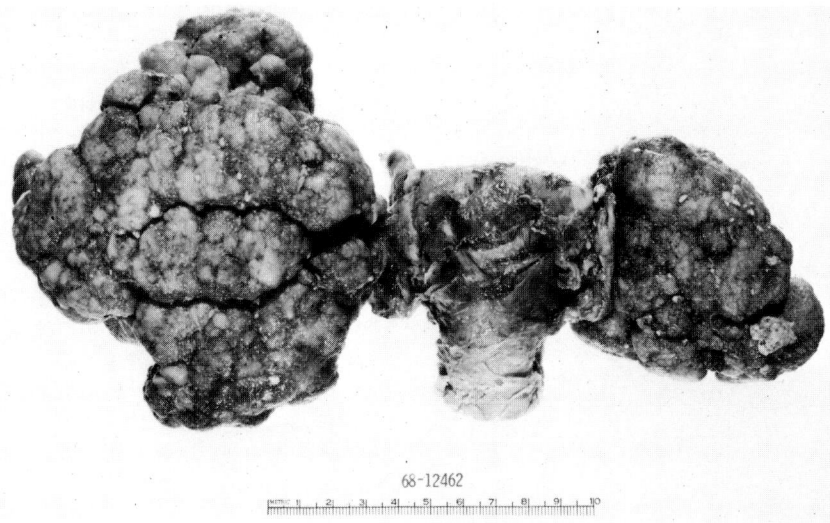

68-12462

Fig. 55.5 Bilateral papillary serous borderline (low malignant potential) tumors. Cortical surfaces of ovaries and serosa of uterus are studded with small papillary excrescences.

component.[81] The least frequent variant is a predominantly solid adenofibromatous or cystadenofibromatous borderline tumor.[79,166]

Histologically, borderline serous tumors are non-invasive, proliferative neoplasms characterized by multiple fibrous papillae with extensive and complex branching (Fig. 55.6). Epithelium covering the papillae is multi-layered forming cellular tufts. Detachment and exfoliation of cells from the papillae is characteristic. Mitotic figures may be present, but they are not found in large numbers. Only about 5% of tumors have more than 4 mitotic figures per 10 high power fields.[21,81] Abnormal mitotic figures are not usually observed.[21] The cells generally show mild to moderate nuclear atypia. Up to 26% have severe atypia,[21,81] and some resemble carcinoma in situ. Many cells display cilia. Some cells assume a rounded shape and resemble mesothelial cells. Psammoma bodies are often numerous, especially in peritoneal implants where they become encased in dense fibrous tissue. On rare occasions, isolated foci of microinvasion are discovered in an otherwise typical borderline tumor. The clinical significance of such 'early' invasion has yet to be determined.

Bilateral ovarian tumors are found in about 14 to 40% of cases.[75,81,122,134] Of greatest concern is the high frequency of extra-ovarian involvement. Extension beyond the ovaries has been found at the time of initial operation in from 20 to 46% of patients.[7,75,81] Multiple superficial implantation metastases are seen on the peritoneum, omentum and serosal surfaces of abdominopelvic organs (Fig. 55.7). Implants often accompany those tumors with prominent involvement of the external ovarian surface,[21,102] but also are found in tumors without a surface component.[8,135] Ascites may be present, and cytologic

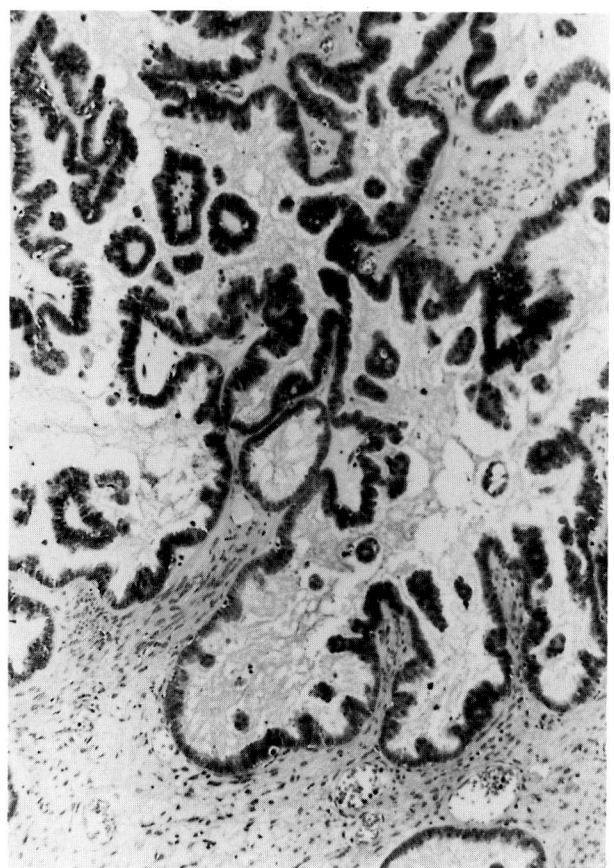

Fig. 55.6 Borderline (low malignant potential) papillary serous tumor. Finely branching papillae are covered by atypical epithelial cells which form small tufts. Stromal invasion is absent. (Reproduced from Hart W R 1977 Ovarian epithelial tumors of borderline malignancy (carcinoma of low malignant potential). *Human Pathol* 8: 541, with permission.)

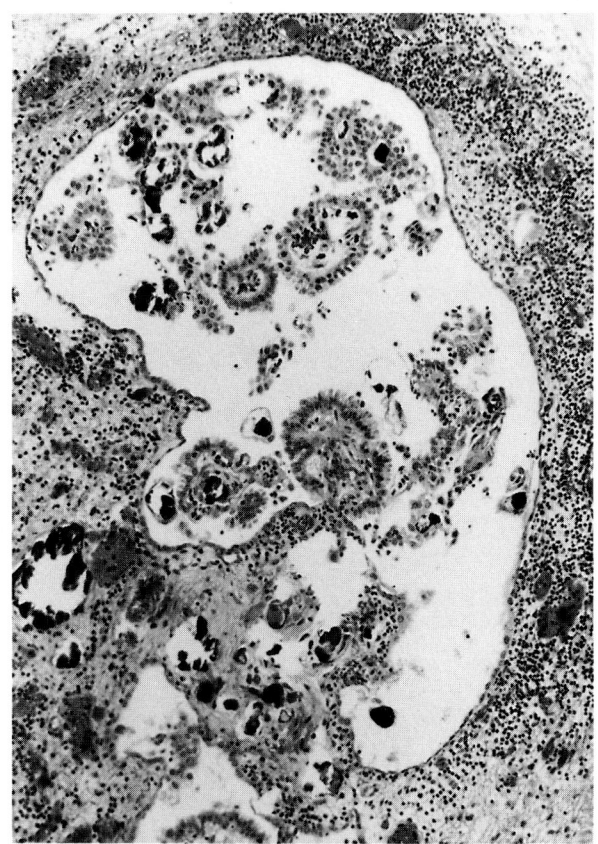

Fig. 55.7 Superficial implant of borderline (low malignant potential) papillary serous tumor. There is no invasion of surrounding connective tissue.

examination of peritoneal fluid may reveal papillary clusters of neoplastic cells.

Prognosis is excellent for patients with limited extent of tumor, and surprisingly good even for those with extensive peritoneal spread. Actuarial survival rates for tumors of all stages have ranged from 92 to 100% at 5 years,[7,75,81,122] and 10-year rates of 75 to over 90% have been recorded.[7,122,145] The survival rate for Stage I tumors has been over 95% at 5 and 10 years and 78% at 20 years.[7] Most deaths due to tumor result from Stage III neoplasms.[81] Attempts at correlating prognosis with the degree of proliferative activity and cytologic atypia of the primary ovarian tumor have not been particularly successful.[21,81]

Recurrent lesions may develop after latent intervals of as long as 20 to 50 years,[75,106] and eventually up to 25% of patients may die from tumor if followed for sufficiently long periods of time.[7] About 15% of patients with conservatively treated unilateral tumors have developed second primary borderline tumors in the preserved contralateral ovary.[21] Recurrences are usually histologically similar to the primary tumors.[67,171] Some peritoneal implants fail to

continue to proliferate, and rare instances of spontaneous regression have been cited.[57,163] Correlations between prognosis and the microscopic features of peritoneal and omental implants have been attempted. In some studies, deeply invasive implants or those with marked nuclear atypia seemed to be more aggressive (Fig. 55.8).[17,102,137] Other studies have not found prognostic significance in the invasiveness or atypia of implants.[21,88,107] Some cases with apparent peritoneal dissemination actually may be examples of multicentric primary peritoneal borderline serous tumors, rather than metastases from the ovarian tumors.[67,135] Occasionally, lymph node metastases develop.[75,106] Hematogenous metastasis is uncommon, as is extension outside the peritoneal cavity, although the author has seen a case in which subcutaneous metastases developed more than 20 years after operation.

Endosalpingiosis and primary peritoneal serous tumors

The pelvic peritoneum is a rich source of cells for the secondary müllerian system.[95] The same histologic spectrum of serous cell metaplasias and neoplasms en-

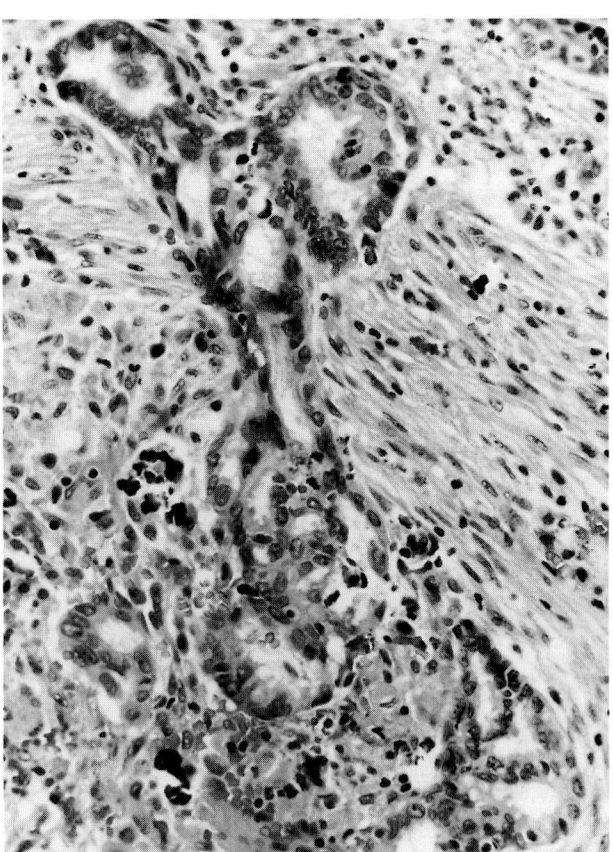

Fig. 55.8 Invasive implant of a borderline (low malignant potential) papillary serous tumor. Desmoplastic stromal reaction surrounds neoplastic glandular epithelium.

countered in the ovary occasionally originate directly from the pelvic peritoneum and serosal coverings of the fallopian tubes, uterus, broad ligament and omentum. Multifocal metaplasia and neoplasia of pelvic peritoneum and ovarian surface epithelium are believed to be manifestations of a 'field effect'.

The most frequent primary peritoneal lesions are small, benign inclusion cysts or tubules of infolded mesothelium that have undergone metaplasia towards tubal or serous epithelium (Fig. 55.9). Small papillary projections and psammoma bodies are sometimes seen. Currently, these benign glandular inclusions are termed endosalpingiosis.[23,63,118,143,147,158] They sometimes coexist and blend with foci of typical endometriosis. Endosalpingiosis may occur alone or in combination with benign, borderline or frankly malignant ovarian serous tumors.[17,31,102,134] They are frequently found at second-look operations during the course of treatment for ovarian epithelial tumors.[30] Identical glandular inclusions occur in the fibrous capsule and trabeculae of pelvic and para-aortic lymph nodes in females.[41,80]

Shedding of tubal epithelium following salpingectomy or

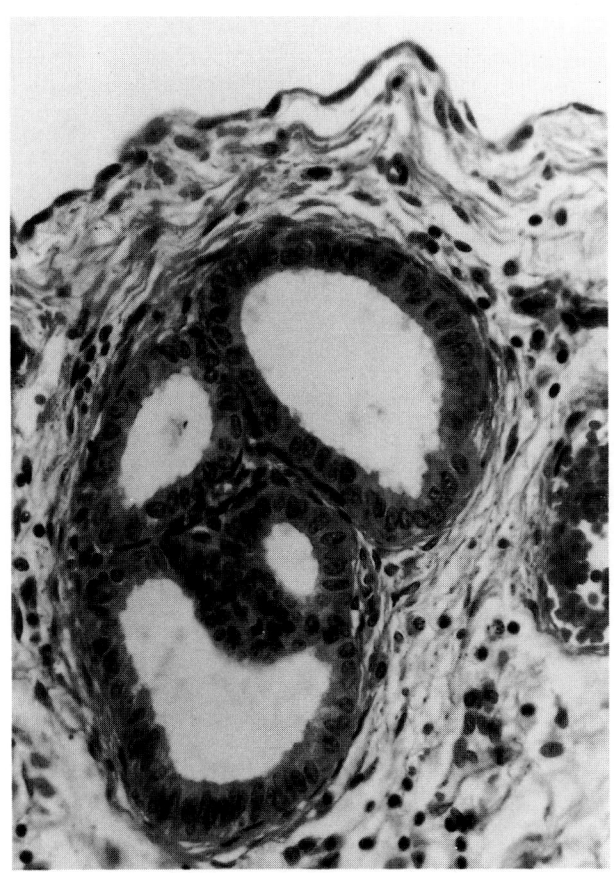

Fig. 55.9 Endosalpingiosis of peritoneum. Cluster of benign tubular glands is just beneath surface mesothelium.

salpingitis has been proposed as an alternative theory of histogenesis of endosalpingiosis.[143,180] However, the metaplastic theory seems more likely. Regardless of histogenesis, the potential for multifocal benign epithelial inclusions to affect pelvic peritoneum, omentum and lymph nodes must be remembered, lest a misdiagnosis of metastatic carcinoma be made. Occasionally, endosalpingiotic proliferations become florid and cytologically atypical.[58,101] In some instances, it may not be possible to distinguish atypical endosalpingiosis from metastases of ovarian borderline (LMP) serous tumors. Furthermore, examples of primary serous borderline (LMP) tumors of the peritoneum without accompanying ovarian tumors also occur.[18,101]

Serous carcinomas sometimes arise from pelvic peritoneum in the absence of ovarian carcinoma, or with only minor involvement of the surfaces of the ovaries.[5,54,78,110] Some of the high grade surface serous carcinomas described above belong to this group of tumors. While origin from modified peritoneal mesothelium is now accepted, these multicentric surface serous carcinomas are histologically different from epithelial mesotheliomas of the peritoneal cavity. True papillary mesotheliomas do occasionally arise in the female pelvis[2,60,101] and may extensively involve the ovarian surfaces. If careful attention is paid to their histologic, cytologic, immunohistologic and ultrastructural features, mesotheliomas can usually be distinguished from ovarian or extra-ovarian serous carcinomas.

MUCINOUS TUMORS

Ovarian cysts lined by mucin-rich epithelial cells form a common variety of benign cystoma. The müllerian nature of most mucinous tumors is generally accepted, since they commonly are composed of endocervical type cells. However, their histogenesis is complicated by the presence of other cellular elements. Often, the tumors contain goblet cells similar to those of gastrointestinal mucosa. Enterochromaffin cells and argyrophil cells can be detected in 20 to 60% of cases, and in over half of the carcinomas and borderline tumors.[3,45,46,53,83,86] A few have Paneth cells.[20] Gastrointestinal enzymes and polypeptides can be found in tumor fluid and tissue,[3,24] and a gastrin-producing mucinous tumor that appeared to produce the Zollinger-Ellison syndrome has been documented.[29] Some of the endocervical-like cells may actually represent mucinous cells of the stomach or Brunner's glands.[3] Dermoid cysts coexist in 4.5% of cases.[24] These features have suggested that some mucinous tumors are monodermal gastrointestinal teratomas of germ cell origin while others are of an endocervical müllerian nature. Ultrastructural studies have supported the contention that all or most mucinous tumors are derived from ovarian surface epithelium,[45,86] but alternate theories of histogenesis cannot be totally dismissed.

From 77 to 87% of all mucinous neoplasms are benign.[4,68,83] Of the remainder, somewhat more than half are borderline (LMP) tumors while the rest are outright carcinomas. Of all primary ovarian carcinomas, mucinous tumors account for 15%. Only about 10% of mucinous carcinomas are bilateral,[4,68,89,172] if cases with extensive spread are excluded to reduce the influence of metastatic spread to the contralateral ovary.

Grossly, mucinous tumors may attain huge proportions (Fig. 55.10). Massive size alone, however, does not indicate malignancy, as several tumors of 200 to 300 pounds have proved to be benign cystadenomas. The carcinomas may range from 5 to over 20 cm in size.[68] In one study, over 80% were 15 cm or more in diameter.[4] Mucinous carcinomas are usually cystic, with 76% being multilocular and 24% unilocular.[68] Solid areas and firm mural nodules are common,[68] and 4% are predominantly or entirely solid.[4] The capsular surface is usually smooth. A few have intracystic or surface papillary excrescences. Cyst fluid is mucoid and tenacious, but one-fourth of the cysts also may contain serous fluid.[4]

Greater variations in degree of differentiation occur in mucinous tumors than in most ovarian epithelial neoplasms. Benign cystadenomas may have small, localized areas of carcinoma which require extensive sampling to identify. Most carcinomas consist of multiple glands and cysts of variable size lined by malignant mucinous cells (Fig. 55.11). Intestinal differentiation with goblet cells may be prominent. Rarely, the majority of the tumor is composed of signet-ring cells with large cytoplasmic vacuoles of mucin; some of these may correspond to so-called primary Krukenberg tumors. Endocervical, enteric and gastric types of mucinous cells are seen with the electron microscope.[92] According to some ultrastructural studies, carcinomas contain only intestinal-type cells, while benign cystadenomas are composed of either endocervical-type cells alone or mixtures of endocervical- and intestinal-type cells; borderline (LMP) tumors have both.[45,46] A few mucinous cystadenomas and cystadenocarcinomas also contain foci of anaplastic carcinoma,[121] sarcoma,[119] or sarcoma-like mural nodules.[120]

Stromal invasion is often difficult to recognize in mucinous tumors because of their complex multilocular patterns, with closely packed glands of various sizes. Consequently, the distinction between borderline (LMP) tumors and carcinomas is more difficult in mucinous than in serous tumors, and the diagnostic criteria used are more controversial. Invasion may take the form of irregular cords and nests of cells haphazardly scattered in the ovarian stroma (Fig. 55.12) or large sheets of glands with a back-to-back arrangement without intervening stroma.[68] Some tumors infiltrate with a pattern of colloid or gelatinous car-

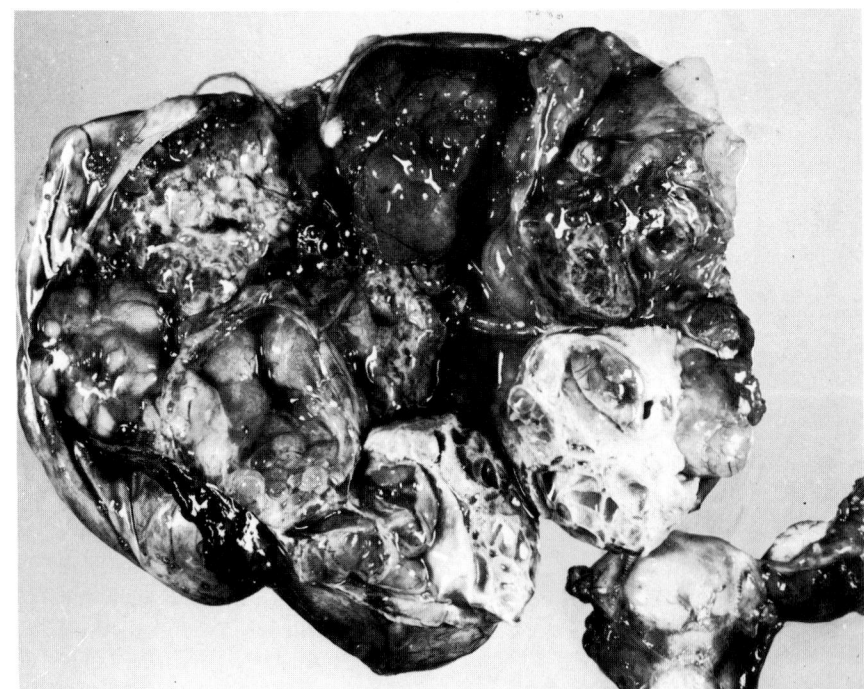

Fig. 55.10 Cut surface of a huge unilateral mucinous cystadenocarcinoma. Solid nodular areas alternate with cysts of various sizes. (Reproduced from: Hart W R, Norris H J 1977 Borderline and malignant mucinous tumors of the ovary: histologic criteria and clinical behavior. Cancer 31: 1031, with permission.)

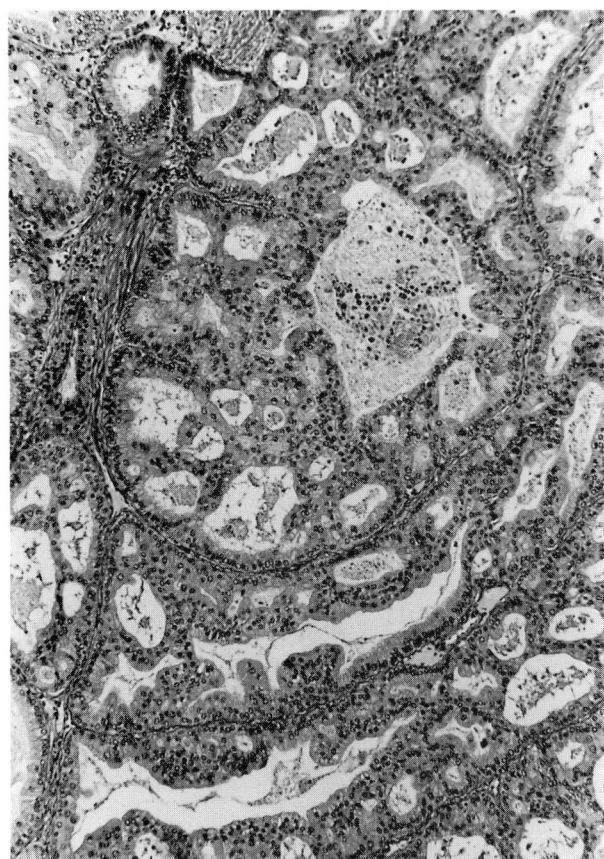

Fig. 55.11 Mucinous cystadenocarcinoma. Large cysts are lined by numerous layers of malignant mucinous epithelial cells. Intraglandular cellular bridges produce a cribriform pattern. Although a destructive infiltrative pattern of stromal invasion is not apparent, these histologic features are indicative of well differentiated mucinous carcinoma.

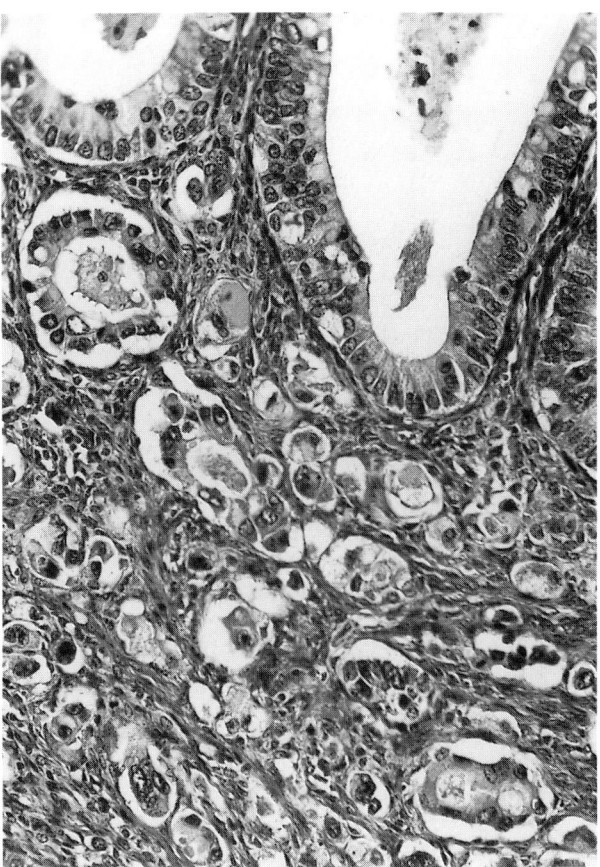

Fig. 55.12 Mucinous cystadenocarcinoma with stromal invasion. Irregular nests and clusters of mucinous carcinoma cells haphazardly infiltrate the ovarian stroma adjacent to small cysts. (Reprinted from Hart W R 1977 Ovarian epithelial tumors of borderline malignancy (carcinoma of low malignant potential). *Human Pathol* 8: 541, with permission.)

cinoma, as seen in colonic and rectal mucinous carcinomas. In tumors without an obviously invasive component, a diagnosis of carcinoma is also warranted whenever the atypical cells lining the cysts are severely anaplastic, stratified into more than three layers, form intraglandular bridges or produce a cribriform pattern.[68] Thus, so-called 'high grade' proliferating mucinous tumors should be classified as well differentiated carcinoma.[161] Patients whose carcinomas have demonstrable stromal invasion have poorer survival and tend to have higher stage tumors.[25,68] With increasing grades of malignancy, the amount of intracytoplasmic mucin diminishes, and recognition of the tumor as a mucinous adenocarcinoma becomes dependent on finding better differentiated areas.[68]

The possibility of a metastatic adenocarcinoma must always be kept in mind when a mucinous ovarian carcinoma is encountered. Mucinous adenocarcinomas from the intestinal tract and the pancreas may closely mimic primary mucinous tumors of the ovary. Bilaterality favors a diagnosis of metastatic adenocarcinoma. Recently, an association between mucinous adenocarcinomas of the ovary and the endocervix has been found.[97,177] Some have occurred in patients with the Peutz-Jeghers syndrome.[177] While most examples are believed to represent separate primary mucinous carcinomas, some of the ovarian tumors result from metastases of the endocervical carcinoma.[177]

Changes in the chemical composition of mucins have been described, including a reduction in the ratio of neutral to acidic mucopolysaccharides, increasing sulfomucins with greater degrees of malignancy,[83,98] and a shift from sulfated mucins to sialomucins with transitions from cystadenoma to carcinoma.[44] Sialomucins are said to correlate well with the presence of carcinoembryonic antigen (CEA), and levels of CEA may be markedly elevated in plasma of patients with mucinous carcinomas.[168] CEA positivity by immunohistologic techniques is demonstrable in most mucinous carcinomas and borderline tumors, as is found in intestinal carcinomas. The pattern of staining is identical in both endocervical and intestinal types of primary mucinous tumors.[26] CA 19–9 immunoreactivity is also common.[26] However, neither tumor marker is specific for any type of ovarian epithelial tumor, primary or metastatic.

When discovered, half of the patients with mucinous carcinoma have Stage I lesions.[7] The absence of surface involvement together with the high proportion of tumors confined to the ovaries at diagnosis are important factors that contribute to the relatively favorable prognosis for patients with mucinous carcinomas. Actuarial survival rates of 66% at 5 years and 59% at 10 years have been recorded for women with Stage I neoplasms,[68] and overall 5-year rates of 40 to 45% can be expected.[7,25,145]

Borderline (LMP) mucinous tumors

Borderline (LMP) mucinous tumors are less common than borderline serous tumors. However, they constitute a large percentage of all non-benign mucinous neoplasms.[68] From 50 to 71% of Stage I mucinous tumors that previously may have been classified as mucinous carcinoma are now regarded as borderline tumors.[25,68] The gross appearance of borderline tumors cannot reliably distinguish them from cystadenomas or cystadenocarcinomas. Typically, they are large cystic masses. Three-fourths are multilocular, and the average diameter is 17 cm.[68] Some have thick cyst walls or intracystic papillations. Growth on the cortical surface is rare.

Mucinous borderline tumors commonly have intestinal as well as endocervical epithelium. Microscopically, they are characterized by complex glandular arrangements (Fig. 55.13). Some have patterns reminiscent of tubular and villous adenomas of the colon or appendix.[68] The cysts are lined by epithelial cells with variable amounts of intracellular mucin that are stratified into two or three layers and display mild to moderate nuclear atypia (Fig. 55.14). 'High grade' proliferating mucinous tumors with microscopic features of adenocarcinoma are usually best diagnosed as well-differentiated carcinoma, even if obvious stromal invasion cannot be demonstrated with certainty.[25,67,68,161]

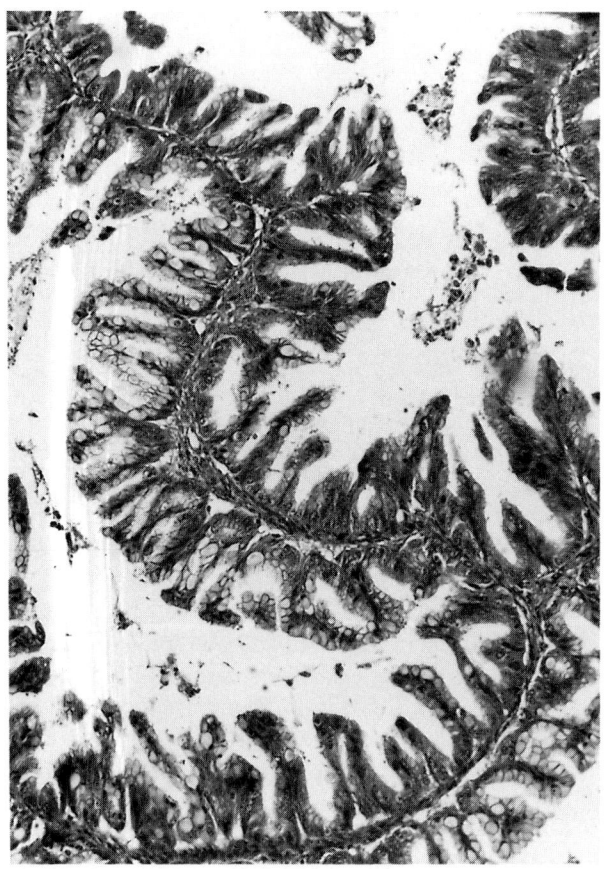

Fig. 55.13   Mucinous borderline (low malignant potential) tumor. Several cysts are lined by proliferating atypical epithelial cells. Delicate micropapillae produce a filagree pattern. (Reproduced from Hart W R 1977 Ovarian epithelial tumors of borderline malignancy (carcinoma of low malignant potential). *Human Pathol* 8: 541, with permission.)

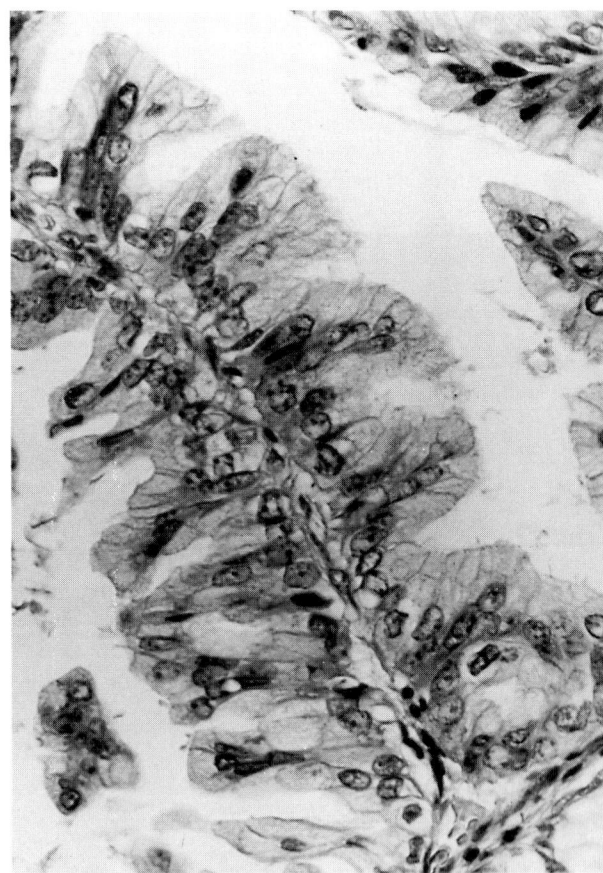

Fig. 55.14   Borderline (low malignant potential) mucinous tumor. Two adjacent cysts are lined by atypical mucinous epithelium of endocervical-type. (Reproduced from Hart W R, Norris H J 1973 Borderline and malignant mucinous tumors of the ovary: histologic criteria and clinical behavior. *Cancer* 31: 103, with permission.)

Secondary cysts and short papillary infoldings are characteristic. Mitotic figures may be plentiful. Small daughter cysts and glandular outpouchings can usually be delineated from stromal invasion if they have an orderly arrangement with smooth contours, are lined by cells similar to those in the larger cysts and are not associated with a reactive desmoplastic stromal proliferation.

About 15% of mucinous borderline tumors have a predominantly papillary gross and microscopic architecture simulating a borderline tumor of serous type. When the epithelium is of endocervical type, this variant has been designated müllerian mucinous borderline tumor (MMBT).[139] There is a surprisingly high association with endometriosis. MMBTs have several features which differ from intestinal-type borderline tumors (IMBTs). MMBTs are devoid of goblet cells and only a few contain argyrophil cells. They are smaller, and usually unilocular or paucilocular rather than multilocular.[139]

Only about 10% or less of borderline mucinous tumors are bilateral,[68] although 40% of MMBTs synchronously involve both ovaries.[139] In some series, about 15% had extended beyond the ovaries at the time of the initial diagnosis.[7,134] Discrete implants and/or lymph node metastases have been found in 20% of MMBTs, while pseudomyxoma peritonei is said to be the characteristic pattern of extra-ovarian spread of IMBTs.[139]

Borderline mucinous tumors have a better prognosis than serous borderline tumors. Corrected actuarial survival rates of 98% and 96% at 5 and 10 years, respectively, were found in a study of patients with Stage I tumors; over half had been treated by unilateral salpingo-oophorectomy alone.[68] A 20-year survival rate of about 85% has been recorded for patients with tumors of all stages.[7]

Pseudomyxoma peritonei

Accumulations of gelatinous mucus within the pelvic and abdominal cavities is termed pseudomyxoma peritonei ('Werth's tumor'). This enigmatic and poorly understood condition is quite rare, occurring in only 0.001% of all women admitted to the obstetric and gynecological service of one hospital during a 5-year period.[144] Most patients are in the age range of 50 to 70 years.[59,116,144,154] Young women are sometimes affected, and rare cases occur in childhood.[100]

At least 10 different mucinous lesions, ranging from benign developmental cysts to invasive adenocarcinomas, have been incriminated in the genesis of pseudomyxoma peritonei.[116] Undoubtedly, spontaneous leakage of mucus and neoplastic epithelial cells from proliferating, borderline or low grade malignant mucinous tumors of the ovary or appendix causes the majority of cases of peritoneal pseudomyxoma. About 3.5 to 12% of all mucinous ovarian neoplasms,[24,154] and from 10.6 to 29% of appendiceal mucoceles and tumors,[70,170] are associated with pseudo-myxoma of limited or diffuse extent. In up to one-third of patients with pseudomyxoma peritonei, both ovarian and appendiceal mucinous tumors are found.[50,154] Colonic adenocarcinomas coexist in many instances.[50,70,170]

When ovarian tumors are found, they are often bilateral, contain areas resembling borderline mucinous tumor and have large pools of mucus dissecting through the parenchyma and covering the cortical surfaces. Small strands of mildly atypical or borderline mucinous epithelium are suspended in the mucus and are often hard to find (Fig. 55.15). Opinions differ about whether this pattern signifies stromal invasion.[25,108,137] Such tumors have often been referred to as 'pseudomyxoma ovarii'.[14,68,134,152] Cogent arguments have been made for diagnosing them as 'ovarian carcinoma with extracellular mucin production'.[108] For treatment and prognostic purposes, they are probably best regarded as a form of low grade mucinous carcinoma. When an appendiceal carcinoma coexists, many of the ovarian tumors are likely to be metastatic rather than primary carcinomas.

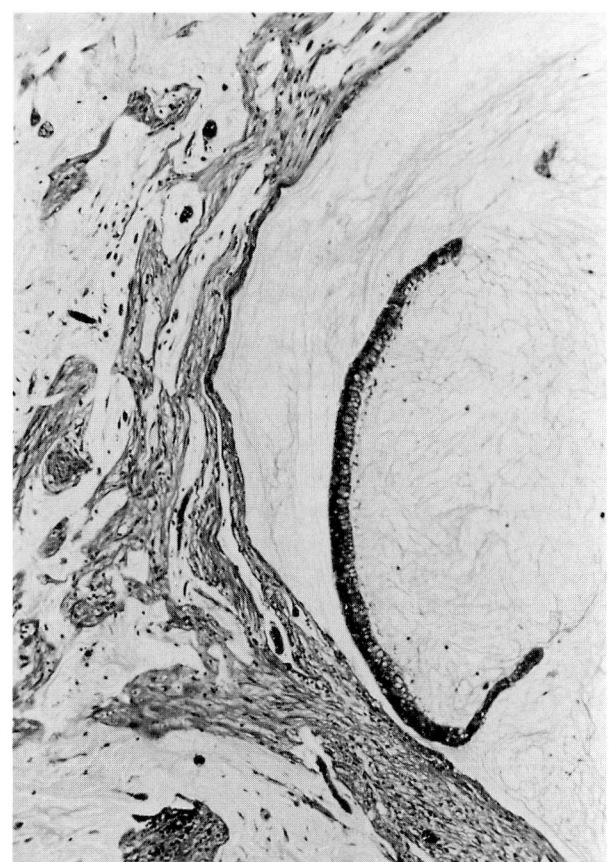

Fig. 55.15 Pseudomyxoma peritonei associated with mucinous ovarian tumor. Pools of mucin with a suspended strand of mildly atypical mucinous epithelium are enmeshed in granulation tissue on ovarian surface.

Several studies have proved that neither intraoperative rupture of a mucinous ovarian tumor, nor evacuation by trocar prior to removal, regularly lead to pseudomyxoma peritonei. None of 11 patients with borderline mucinous tumors that ruptured before or during operation developed pseudomyxoma during follow up intervals of 3 to 19 years, nor did any of five women with ruptured Stage I mucinous carcinomas in the same series.[68]

About 80% of patients with pseudomyxoma peritonei gradually deteriorate and succumb to inanition and infection following repeated bouts of intestinal obstruction.[24] Extra-abdominal spread, or metastases to the liver or lymph nodes are rare. Survival rates of 45 to 54% at 5 years and 18% at 10 years have been reported, with fatalities occurring from 3 months to 24 years after initial diagnosis.[50,100] Pseudomyxoma peritonei associated with ovarian mucinous neoplasms diagnosed as mucinous LMP tumor, IMBT or carcinoma with extracellular mucin production has caused progressive disease and eventual death in most patients.[108,139] It is still argued whether a truly benign form of pseudomyxoma peritonei exists, or whether all cases represent metastatic, low grade, mucus-secreting adenocarcinomas.

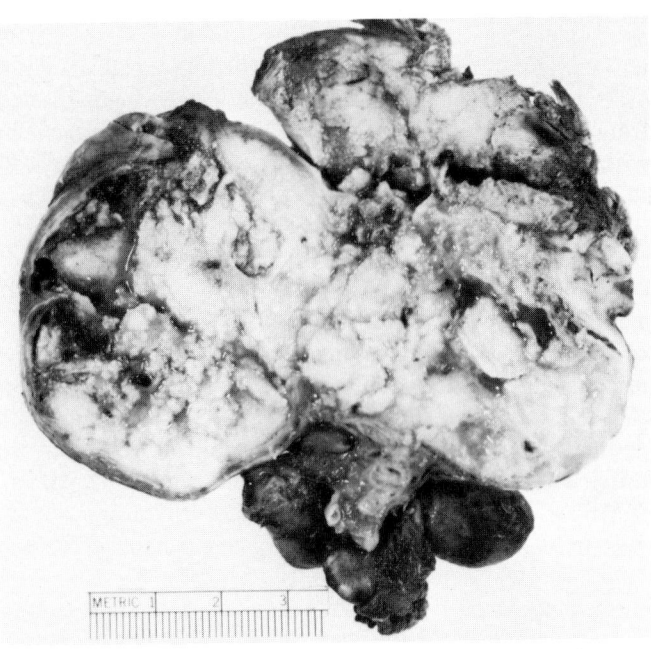

Fig. 55.16 Sectioned surface of an endometrioid carcinoma of ovary in a patient who also had adenocarcinoma of the endometrium. Tumor is predominantly solid and composed of friable, granular tissue.

ENDOMETRIOID TUMORS

Endometrioid tumors have the microscopic features of one or more of the typical forms of endometrial neoplasia.[152] Benign endometrioid tumors are rare, usually appearing as adenofibromas or cystadenomas. Endometriosis is generally excluded from this category since it is not regarded as a neoplasm. Endometrial-like carcinomas of the ovary were first described in 1925 by Sampson.[142] Two modes of histogenesis are possible: from the epithelium of antecedent endometriosis, or from the surface epithelium of the ovary. In 1961, the term 'endometrioid carcinoma' was agreed upon for all primary ovarian carcinomas having microscopic features resembling carcinoma of the uterine corpus, whether or not origin from endometriosis could be demonstrated.[151] Endometrioid carcinomas account for 16 to 30% of all ovarian carcinomas.[37,90,99,134]

Endometrioid carcinomas tend to be less cystic than serous or mucinous carcinomas (Fig. 55.16). Solid nodular areas of yellow-tan to dark red tissue often alternate with cysts, or comprise the bulk of the tumor. Their sizes range from 2 to 35 cm;[37] most are 10 to 20 cm in diameter. Intracystic papillary projections are found in some, but surface papillations are infrequent. Dark hemorrhagic fluid in the cysts should prompt a thorough microscopic search for evidence of origin from an endometriotic cyst.

The diagnostic microscopic features of endometrioid carcinomas were clearly delineated in 1964 by Long & Taylor.[99] The vast majority are relatively well-differentiated adenocarcinomas with tubular or branching glands

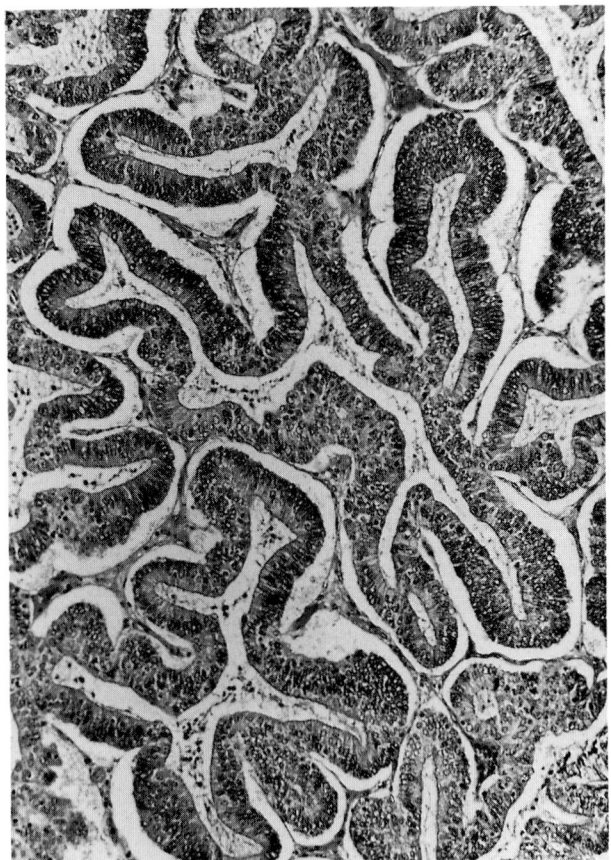

Fig. 55.17 Endometrioid carcinoma. Stellate branching and tubular glands in a back-to-back arrangement resemble well differentiated adenocarcinoma of endometrium.

(Fig. 55.17). However, all the subtypes of endometrial carcinoma may be observed, including poorly differentiated medullary tumors that are difficult to recognize as endometrioid carcinoma. When papillary, the papillae are blunt and broad, in contrast to the finer branching, slender papillations of serous carcinomas. Psammoma bodies are found in less than 10% of the papillary forms.[37] Squamous metaplasia or differentiation is characteristic of endometrioid carcinoma, occurring in one-fourth to one-half of cases.[136,149] Intra-glandular squamoid morules or nests of keratinizing squamous epithelium are frequent elements (Fig. 55.18). Occasionally, most or practically all of the tumor appears as squamous cell carcinoma. Mucin production is sometimes prominent. Typically, the mucin is predominantly extracellular or periapical. Foci of secretory adenocarcinoma with prominent subnuclear and supranuclear vacuoles are sometimes seen. About one-third contain mixtures with other types of müllerian-directed epithelium, with minor components of serous, mucinous or clear cell carcinoma.[37,90] An unusual histologic variant consisting of hollow or solid tubules may be mistaken for a Sertoli cell tumor ('Sertoliform endometrioid carcinoma').[132,174]

Endometrioid carcinomas have ultrastructural features similar to those of well differentiated adenocarcinomas of the endometrium and to normal endometrium.[34,47,84] Bundles of microfilaments adjacent to the nucleus are typically found in the better differentiated tumors.[47] Immunohistologic coexpression of vimentin and cytokeratin intermediate filaments is very common.[38] CEA immunoreactivity is sometimes present,[26,38] especially in the squamous elements, and positivity for CA 125 and CA 19–9 may also be found.[26,76,77]

Ovarian endometriosis is present in about 9 to 17% of cases,[6,37,90] while pelvic endometriosis has been reported in as many as 28% of patients.[134] However, origin from an endometriotic cyst can be demonstrated in only 5 to 10% of cases.[148] Atypical hyperplastic changes within ovarian endometriosis may be precursors of some endometrioid carcinomas.[35,91] Origin from pre-existent cystadenoma or adenofibroma also occurs.

About one-third of endometrioid carcinomas involve both ovaries, but only 13% of Stage I to IIa tumors are bilateral.[89] One of the most important aspects of endometrioid carcinoma is the inordinately high frequency of associated carcinomas and hyperplasias of the endometrium. From 15 to 26% of women with ovarian endometrioid carcinoma also harbor a uterine endometrial carcinoma,[37,84,151] and an additional 12% have endometrial hyperplasia.[37] The endometrial lesions may be synchronous or asynchronous, and they are often microscopically similar. In contrast, only about 4% of ovarian carcinomas of all cell types are associated with carcinoma of the endometrium.[4,157] Available evidence indicates that, in most cases, the ovarian and endometrial neoplasms are separate, independent primary tumors and not metastases from one organ to the other. Endometrial carcinomas that are small, well differentiated, confined to the endometrial mucosa or only superficially invasive of myometrium, and are accompanied by a background of endometrial hyperplasia are almost certain to be separate primary tumors. Even larger and more extensive endometrial carcinomas probably represent independent autochthonous tumors in many instances. Patients whose simultaneous ovarian and uterine carcinomas are of non-endometrioid type (e.g. papillary carcinoma, clear cell carcinoma) and those whose uterine carcinoma deeply invades the myometrium and is widespread, are more likely to have a single primary with metastases.[42]

Approximately 40 to 55% of patients with endometrioid carcinoma survive 5 years.[7,37,84,90,145,157] Survival is best related to the stage of the tumor. Histologic grade is also of importance. Grade 1, Stage I carcinomas have resulted in 10-year survival rates of 100% in some reports.[37,90] Patients with endometrioid carcinoma and an associated endometrial carcinoma have about the same prognosis as

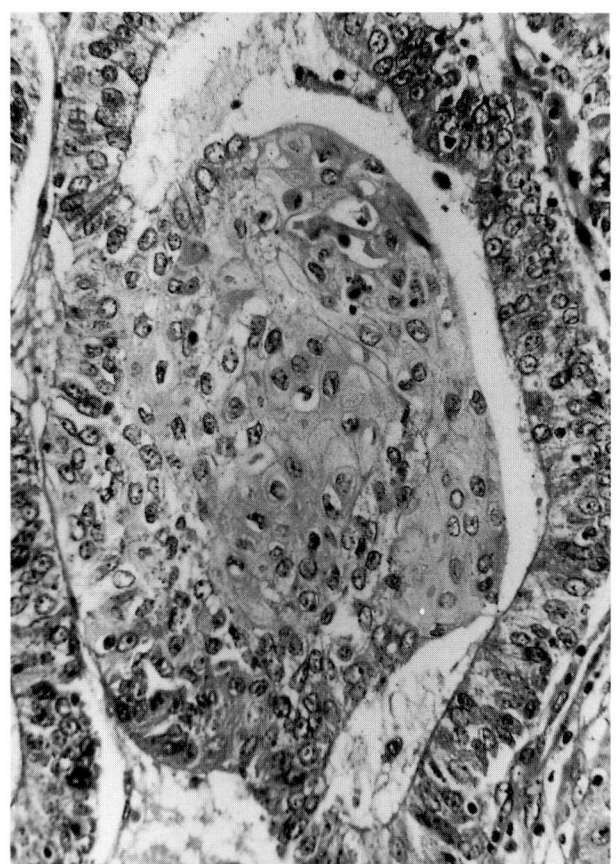

Fig. 55.18 Endometrioid carcinoma. A well differentiated gland contains a nest of squamous epithelium.

those without such a lesion, another factor indicating that the ovarian and uterine carcinomas commonly are separate primary tumors.[37,40,42,89,103,157]

Metastatic adenocarcinoma of the large intestine commonly masquerades as an endometrioid carcinoma of the ovary.[93] Carefully performed light microscopy is required to identify the tell-tale histologic features of metastatic colonic adenocarcinoma. Immunohistochemical staining for carcinoembryonic antigen (CEA) is characteristically present in colonic metastases, but also may be found in some primary ovarian carcinomas.

Borderline (LMP) endometrioid tumors

In recent years, a number of endometrioid tumors have been variously designated as 'atypical', 'proliferating', 'borderline', and 'low malignant potential'.[15,79,129,134,159] Typically, these intermediate tumors have predominantly been adenofibromas and cystadenofibromas with cytologic or architectural atypia of the glandular epithelium. Squamous metaplasia with the formation of adenoacanthomatous nodules is often present. Several investigators have attempted to separate these uncommon tumors into those with no malignant potential and those with low malignant potential, on the basis of either qualitative cytologic features or quantitative assessments of the extent of atypical epithelial proliferation. The low malignant potential tumors have generally been those with apparently non-invasive nests of carcinoma (carcinoma in situ) or those with relatively large confluent areas with microscopic features similar to those of atypical endometrial hyperplasia. In several of the reported LMP tumors, foci of microinvasive carcinoma have also been found.[15,159] The problems in distinguishing borderline endometrioid tumors from low grade adenocarcinoma arising in adenofibromas are essentially the same as those in separating atypical hyperplasias from Grade 1 adenocarcinomas of the endometrium. A consensus on definitive diagnostic criteria has yet to be reached.

CLEAR CELL TUMORS

Clear cell carcinomas account for about 5 to 11% of all ovarian carcinomas.[8,36,51,90,134] While the histogenesis of clear cell tumors of the female genital tract was a contested issue in the past, it is now generally accepted that they are müllerian in nature and are not derived from remnants of the embryologic mesonephric duct system.[150] The close relationship of clear cell carcinoma to endometrioid carcinoma and to endometriosis was established in 1967 by Scully & Barlow.[150] Histologically identical clear cell carcinomas arise in the ovary, cervix, vagina, endometrium and broad ligament. At one time, confusion with endodermal sinus (yolk sac) tumor was disconcertingly common

because of some overlapping microscopic features. This is rarely a problem today.

Clear cell carcinomas of the ovary are found almost exclusively in adult women. The average age at diagnosis is about 48 to 58 years, and practically all are diagnosed after the age of 25 years.[8,36,82,90,112,155] They are curiously infrequent in black women.[36,51,112] A fascinating association with para-endocrine hypercalcemia simulating hyperparathyroidism has been documented.[48,82,153] About 10% of patients with ovarian clear cell carcinoma have hypercalcemia.[82]

The tumors usually exceed 15 cm in diameter and are a mixture of cystic and solid tissues.[51,82] Less than 15 to 20% are predominantly solid with a few small cysts, while more than half are unilocular cysts with solid mural nodules.[36,112] Bilaterality occurs in 3% or less of Stage I tumors.[112,125] Clear cell carcinoma is one of the commonest types of carcinoma to originate from the epithelium of endometriosis. Homolateral ovarian endometriosis has been demonstrated in up to 24% of cases,[6,8] and pelvic endometriosis in one-quarter to one-half of all patients.[36,82,134,150] In contrast, only 3.5 to 6.5% of all types of primary ovarian carcinoma are closely associated with endometriosis.[6,90]

Microscopically, clear cell carcinomas have numerous distinctive architectural and cellular patterns. Cells with abundant clear or vacuolated cytoplasm that contain abundant glycogen are arranged diffusely in solid sheets (Fig. 55.19), line tubular glandular or cystic spaces, or cover papillary projections. Most tumors have a mixture of patterns.[82] Glomerulus-like tufts sometimes protrude into microcysts. Clear cells are typically present but usually are mixed with other cell types. A variant of the clear cell has scanty cytoplasm draped around a prominent protruding nucleus, producing the so-called hobnail cell. Hobnail cells tend to predominate in the tubular and cystic examples (Fig. 55.20) and occasionally are the predominant cell type.[112] Frequently, the carcinoma cells are not vacuolated but have abundant eosinophilic, granular cytoplasm. Tumors with a prominent component of such eosinophilic cells have recently been designated 'oxyphilic clear cell carcinoma'.[175] An important feature is abundant basement-membrane-like hyaline material, especially in papillary areas. Marked nuclear pleomorphism with scattered, large, hyperchromatic, bizarre cells are very common.[82] Calcific deposits are observed in up to 30% of tumors.[112] Intracellular mucin is absent or very scant, but mucinous secretions are often found within tubular lumens. Mixtures with other müllerian cell types, such as endometrioid or serous carcinomas, are said to be frequent. Confusion between endometrioid carcinomas of secretory type and clear cell carcinomas may be partly responsible for the seemingly high frequency of mixtures. Clear cell carcinomas with a marked infiltrate of inflammatory lymphoid cells occasionally are mistaken for dysgerminoma.

Prognosis is similar to that for patients with endo-

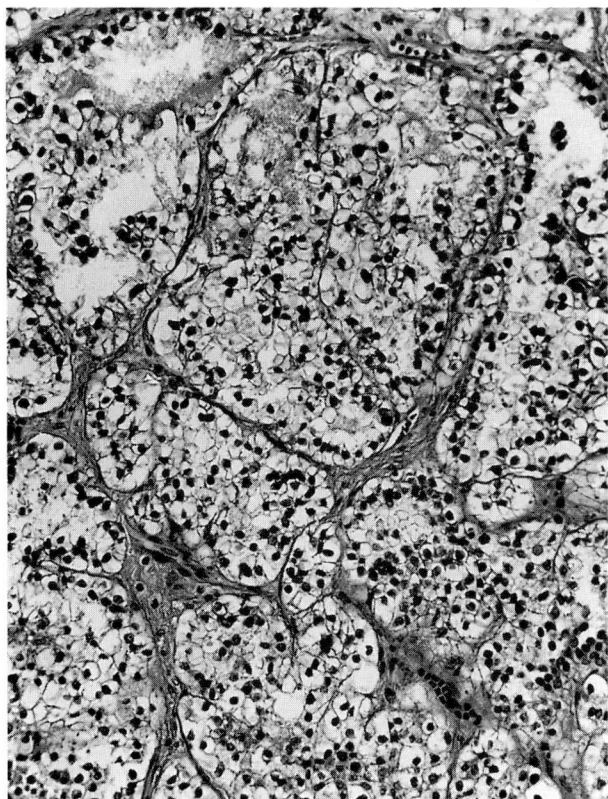

Fig. 55.19 Clear cell carcinoma. Epithelial cells with abundant vacuolated or clear cytoplasm form solid nests and glands.

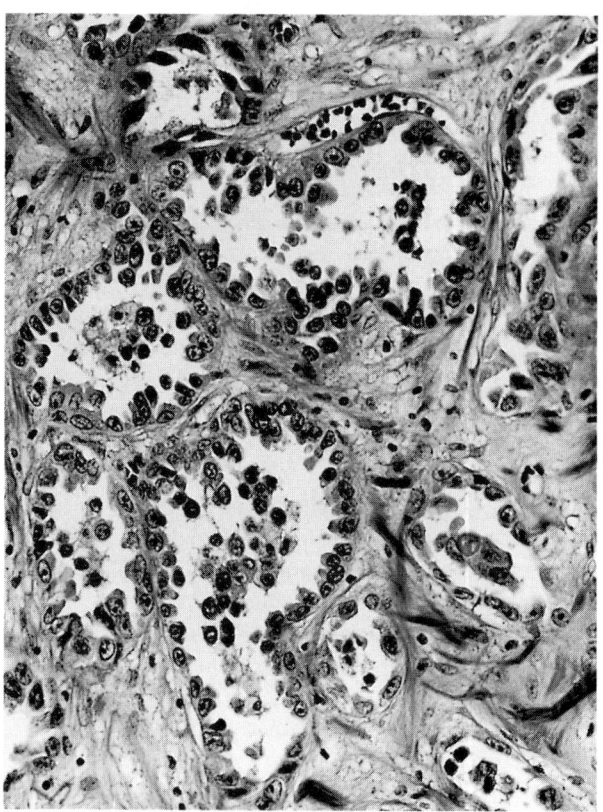

Fig. 55.20 Tubular area of clear cell carcinoma. The tubules are lined by 'hobnail' cells with prominent protruding nuclei and scanty amounts of cytoplasm.

metrioid and mucinous carcinomas, probably because 56 to 68% of tumors are localized to the ovaries at the time of diagnosis.[8,125] In Stage I cases, 5-year survival rates range from 60 to 80% and about 40 to 50% of all patients survive 5 years when all stages are considered.[8,36,82,112,125,155] Attempts to correlate survival with the predominant histologic pattern or percentage of clear cells have yielded inconstant results.[8,82,112,125] Prognosis is unrelated to the presence of endometriosis,[8,82] and histologic grading has not proved reliable.[125,155]

Ultrastructural studies have been of some value in evaluating histogenesis. Consistent differences between primary clear cell carcinoma of the kidney and those of the female genital tract have been demonstrated. Unlike renal tumors, genital clear cell carcinomas do not possess the numerous, long, slender microvilli characteristic of a brush border, abundant lipidic droplets or deep infoldings of the basilar plasma membrane.[114,115,141,156] Distinction from metastatic renal carcinoma is rarely a practical problem, since the ovaries are involved in only 0.3% of patients dying of renal carcinoma.[112] A striking resemblance to the Arias-Stella reaction of gestational endometrium is seen with both the light and electron microscope.[156] No

ultrastructural similarities with fetal mesonephric glomeruli or mesonephric tubules have been identified.

The preponderance of evidence indicates that clear cell carcinomas of the ovary are derived from surface epithelial elements in most cases, and from endometriosis in some patients. Origin from remnants of the mesonephric apparatus remains unproven. No link to intra-uterine stilbestrol exposure has been established. The term 'mesonephroid' carcinoma has been advocated to communicate the historical perspective of these distinctive tumors, and to serve as a practical label for those lesions in which clear cells are in meager numbers or altogether absent.[125] In the WHO classification, clear cell carcinoma and mesonephroid carcinoma are used as synonyms.[152]

Borderline (LMP) clear cell tumors

Clear cell tumors of borderline type are extremely rare and not well defined. Separation of clear cell adenofibromas and some well differentiated clear cell carcinomas from borderline clear cell tumors remains problematic. Adenofibromas with tubules, glands or small nests lined by clear cells or hobnail cells with significant nuclear atypia but without invasion of the stromal component have been regarded as borderline or LMP tumors.[16,131,134] Some tumors without stromal invasion, in which the epithelial cells have nuclear characteristics of high-grade carcinoma have however, been diagnosed as malignant adenofibromas, as have those with foci of microinvasion.[16] It cannot be overemphasized that small or large portions of clear cell carcinoma may have the microscopic features of a benign or borderline clear cell adenofibroma. Hence, extensive sampling to search for areas of clear cell carcinoma must be undertaken before a diagnosis of either benign or borderline clear cell tumor can be safely made.

TRANSITIONAL CELL (BRENNER) TUMORS

About 1.5 to 2.5% of all ovarian neoplasms are composed of nests of benign transitional epithelium resembling urothelium of the urinary bladder surrounded by dense fibrous tissue;[12] they are popularly called Brenner tumors. While their histogenesis has been controversial, an origin from derivatives of the surface epithelium is favored.[94] Some may arise from rete ovarii. Although 5 to 6% are associated with teratomas, a germ cell origin is unlikely. Ultrastructural studies have corroborated the light microscopic impressions that the epithelial nests closely simulate normal urothelium, transitional papillomas of the urinary tract and metaplastic Walthard cell nests of pelvic peritoneum.[33,127] Mucinous cells are often within normal urothelium, and a close relationship exists between mucinous cell and transitional cell ovarian tumors. About 2% of mucinous cystadenomas have a component of Brenner tumor, and up to 25% of Brenner tumors have significant mucinous areas.[134] Examples with prominent mucinous and ciliated cell metaplasia, often with a complex glandular pattern, have been termed 'metaplastic Brenner tumor'.[130] Immunohistologic positivity for CEA and CA 19–9 is common.[26]

Practically all Brenner tumors are benign. Most are less than 5 cm in diameter[12] and are incidental, unsuspected findings identified during operative procedures for unrelated gynecologic conditions, or at the time of routine pathological examination. Benign Brenner tumors are sometimes coincidental lesions adjacent to serous, mucinous and endometrioid carcinomas.[12] Malignant and borderline variants occur, but they are very unusual and criteria for diagnosis are often disputed.

Malignant Brenner tumors resemble urothelial carcinomas of the bladder and lower urinary tract. The potential for confusion with metastatic transitional cell carcinoma is small, since ovarian metastases from primary carcinomas of the urinary bladder are rare (only 1.1% of cases confirmed by autopsy).[109] However, cases of metastatic transitional cell carcinomas of the ovary have, rarely, been reported, as have anecdotal examples of

patients with identical transitional cell carcinomas of the ovary and urinary tract in which the primary site could not be definitely determined.[178]

Primary carcinomas of the ovary resembling transitional cell carcinoma of the urinary tract may originate by two different pathways: malignant transformation of the epithelial component of a pre-existent benign Brenner tumor, or direct malignant transformation of surface epithelial derivatives without an antecedent benign Brenner tumor. Some authorities require the presence of a benign or proliferating Brenner tumor with transition into carcinoma for a diagnosis of malignant Brenner tumor (MBT),[10,109,128] those without an associated Brenner tumor being diagnosed as transitional cell carcinoma (TCC).[10]

MBT and TCC are decidedly rare. Only a few series of cases have been reported.[10,12,66,109,128] They occur in elderly women (mean age 58 to 68 years), are usually unilateral, and grossly are unilocular or multilocular cystic tumors with solid areas. Their maximum dimension ranges from 5 to 30 cm, with an average diameter of about 15 cm. Irrespective of the presence or absence of identifiable benign Brenner tumor, the carcinomas are basically invasive transitional cell carcinomas (Fig. 55.21), often

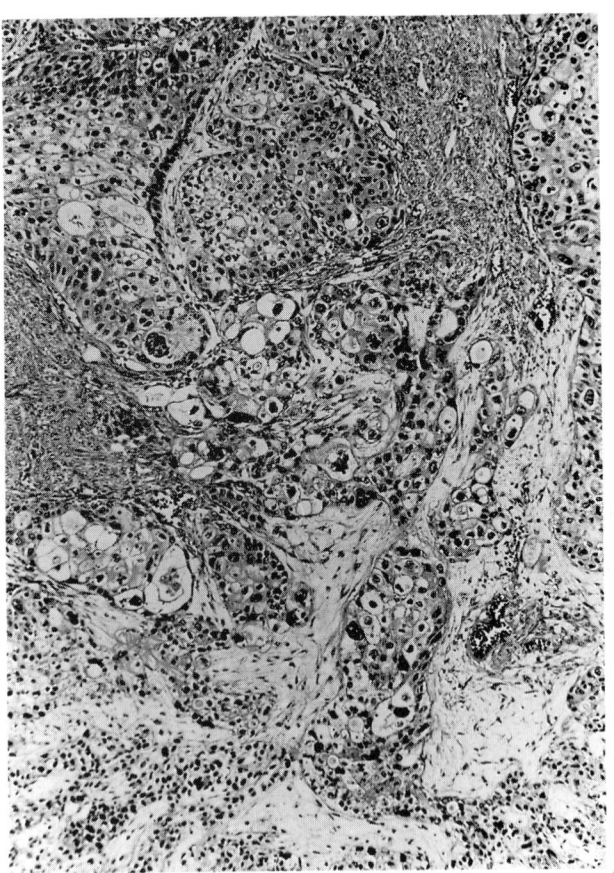

Fig. 55.21 Malignant Brenner tumor. High grade transitional cell carcinoma with pleomorphic nuclei infiltrates ovarian stroma.

with a papillary component. Squamous differentiation is very common, as are minor elements of adenocarcinoma.[10]

The prognosis of these rare tumors is difficult to determine because of the small number of documented cases. Tumors without an associated Brenner tumor (i.e. transitional cell carcinomas) have been reported to be more aggressive.[10] As with other ovarian carcinomas, the stage of the tumors is an important prognostic factor. Well differentiated tumors may have a better prognosis than poorly differentiated tumors;[128] however, most are predominantly Grade 2 or 3 carcinomas.[10]

Borderline (proliferating and LMP) transitional cell (Brenner) tumors

The first description of a tumor intermediate between typical benign and malignant Brenner tumors was the 'proliferating Brenner tumor' reported by Roth & Sternberg in 1971.[133] Subsequently, the proliferating Brenner tumor was included in the WHO classification as a Brenner tumor of borderline malignancy.[152] Recently, this approach has been challenged.[130] Regardless of terms, all

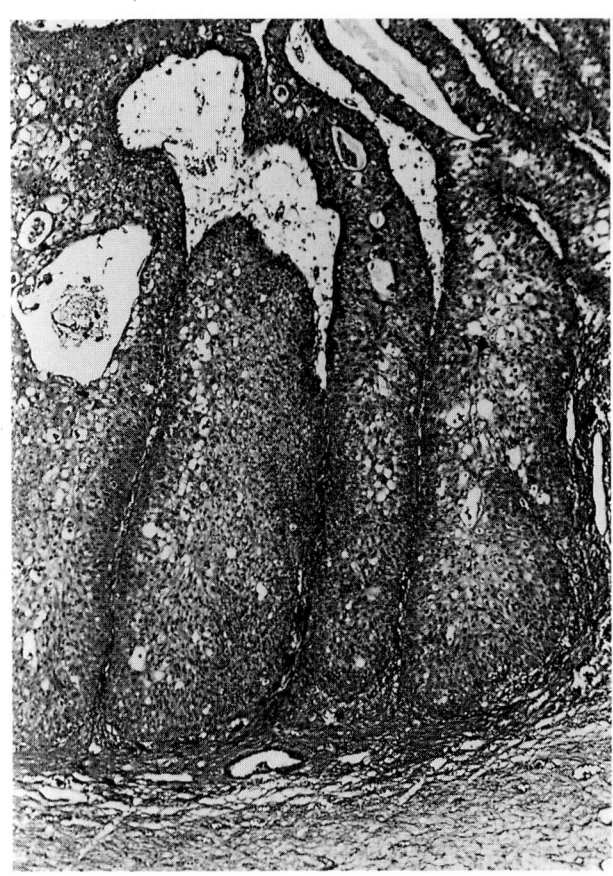

Fig. 55.22 Borderline (proliferating) Brenner tumor. Thick papillary masses of proliferating transitional epithelial cells resting on delicate connective tissue septa protrude into a cyst.

of the microscopic variants of intermediate Brenner tumors are extremely infrequent. The majority occur between the ages of 45 to 75 years and present as large unilateral tumors.[12,130]

Most are larger than 8 to 10 cm in greatest dimension, and some have attained a diameter of 28 to 31 cm.[66,109,130] Typically, the tumors are cystic or semicystic. Polypoid and papillary masses often protrude into the cystic cavities. Microscopically, the epithelial proliferation resembles noninvasive, low grade papillary transitional cell carcinomas of the urinary bladder. Exuberant papillary processes of multilayered transitional epithelial cells resting on delicate fibrovascular stalks protrude into or obliterate the cavities of large cysts (Fig. 55.22). According to Roth et al, only those proliferating Brenner tumors with areas of high grade transitional cell carcinoma in situ or squamous cell carcinoma in situ should be classified as Brenner tumor of low malignant potential.[130] Squamous metaplasia and mucinous cells are common. Large plaques of dystrophic calcific deposits may be numerous, as they are in many benign Brenner tumors. Mucinous cystadenomas coexist in some instances.[133]

The borderline Brenner tumors have been associated with a benign clinical course in practically all reported cases,[130,149] although few women have been followed for 10 or more years. Hence, the utility of separately subdividing borderline Brenner tumors into proliferating and LMP categories has not been satisfactorily determined.

MIXED EPITHELIAL TUMORS

Mixtures of two or more of the five cell types can be found in 10% of the common epithelial tumors, but neoplasms in which each subtype constitutes at least 10% of the total area are found in less than 3% of all benign and malignant epithelial tumors.[134] Such neoplasms are designated as mixed epithelial tumors with each element specified. When only a small quantity of a second or third type of epithelium is present, the tumor should be classified according to the predominant element.[152]

Mixed epithelial tumors may be benign, borderline (LMP) or malignant. The most common mixtures in benign tumors are of transitional (Brenner)-mucinous cells and serous-mucinous cells. Mixed borderline epithelial tumors most often contain mucinous cells in combination with serous or endometrioid epithelium.[140] Amongst malignant epithelial tumors, mixtures of endometrioid carcinoma with clear cell or mucinous carcinomas are most frequent. Problems in distinguishing high grade serous carcinomas from endometrioid carcinomas sometimes arise. Such tumors should not be classified as mixed serous-endometrioid carcinoma unless unequivocally diagnostic features of both cell types are found. Most pathologists interpret poorly differentiated carcinomas consisting of cells with overlapping microscopic characteristics shared by serous and endometrioid epithelium as serous carcinomas. Hence, only relatively well differentiated carcinomas of mixed cell type can be confidently diagnosed.

UNDIFFERENTIATED CARCINOMAS

Primary ovarian carcinomas that are too poorly differentiated to be recognized as belonging to any of the specific common epithelial categories are classified as undifferentiated carcinoma. Rare foci of differentiation, such as gland formation, psammoma bodies or mucin production, do not exclude the diagnosis of undifferentiated carcinoma in the WHO system.[152] Many of these tumors can be identified histologically as extremely poorly differentiated adenocarcinomas. The decision to diagnose a tumor as undifferentiated carcinoma, rather than as poorly differentiated serous or endometrioid adenocarcinoma, is highly subjective. The criteria are sufficiently vague to cause difficulties in uniform application, and problems in reproducibility in the diagnosis of undifferentiated carcinoma have been found in several studies.[32,160] Since classification of any neoplasm is based on recognition of its most differentiated portion, multiple histologic sections may have to be examined before recognizable areas of one of the specific epithelial cell types are identified in an otherwise undifferentiated carcinoma.

Probably no more than 5 to 10% of primary carcinomas belong in the category of undifferentiated carcinoma. Obviously, this is a heterogeneous group of high-grade carcinomas of diverse microscopic appearances. Over half are bilateral, and about 75% have spread beyond the ovaries before diagnosis is accomplished.[7] The prognosis for patients with these aggressive tumors is poor, with overall 5- and 10-year survival rates of only 15% or less.[7] Differential diagnosis includes metastatic carcinoma, and misdiagnosis of an undifferentiated carcinoma as a granulosa cell tumor continues to be a common pitfall.

Small cell carcinoma

A distinctive type of undifferentiated carcinoma of the ovary was designated small cell carcinoma (SCC) by Dickersin et al in 1981.[39] Previously, these tumors had usually been diagnosed as undifferentiated malignant sex-cord or gonadal stromal tumors.[71] SCC typically is a unilateral tumor found in young females (average age, 23 years). About three-quarters of reported tumors are Stage I, and two-thirds of patients have hypercalcemia. It is the most common type of primary ovarian tumor to be associated with para-endocrine hypercalcemia in young females. The tumor consists of sheets and nests of malignant, small, undifferentiated epithelial cells, often with follicle-like structures containing eosinophilic secretions (Figs. 55.23

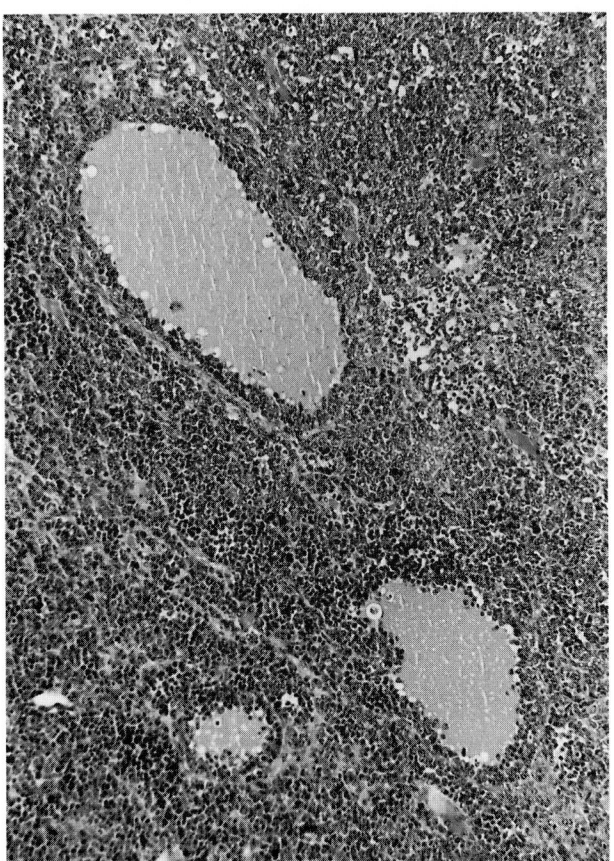

Fig. 55.23 Small cell carcinoma. The tumor consists of sheets and nests of small epithelial cells with occasional follicle-like structures. (Reprinted from McMahon J T, Hart W R 1988 Ultrastructural analysis of small cell carcinomas of the ovary. *Am J Clin Pathol* 90: 523, with permission.)

and 55.24). In about 25% of cases, larger cells with more abundant cytoplasm are found ('large cell variant').[176] Occasional glands lined by mucinous epithelium have been reported in about 9% of cases.[176] Ultrastructurally, the neoplastic cells have epithelial features and consistently contain prominent vesicles composed of dilated cisterns of rough endoplasmic reticulum filled with granular proteinaceous material.[104] SCC is an extremely aggressive neoplasm with a dismal prognosis. Almost 90% of patients have died within 1 year of diagnosis.[176] Ovarian SCC must be distinguished from lymphoma, juvenile granulosa cell tumor and metastatic small cell undifferentiated carcinoma (neuroendocrine carcinoma) from the lung or other anatomic sites.

UNCLASSIFIED AND MISCELLANEOUS EPITHELIAL TUMORS

According to the WHO scheme, the category of unclassified epithelial tumors should be used for those neoplasms

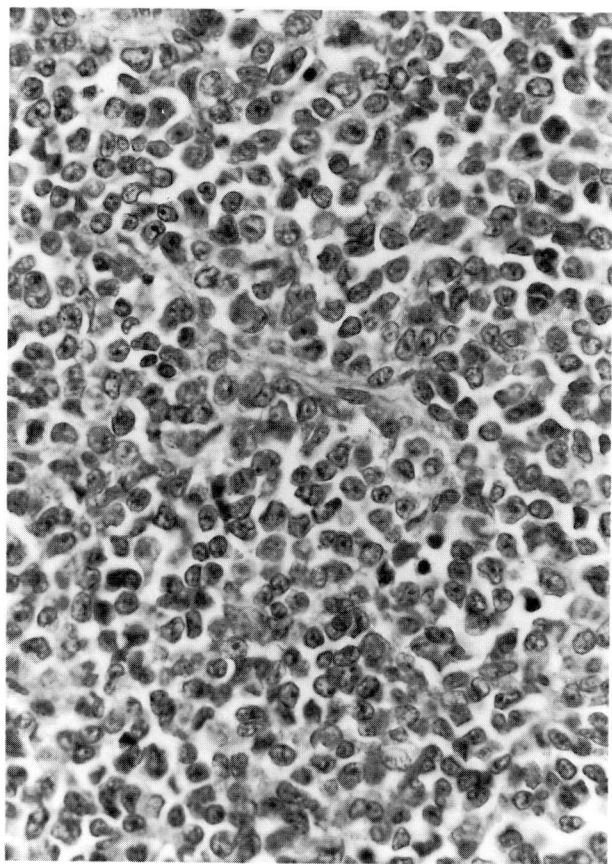

Fig. 55.24 Undifferentiated carcinoma cells of small cell carcinoma have indistinct cytoplasm and relatively uniform vesicular nuclei. (Reprinted from McMahon J T, Hart W R 1988 Ultrastructural analysis of small cell carcinomas of the ovary. *Am J Clin Pathol* 90: 523, with permission.)

of common epithelial type with features intermediate between two or more of the specific cell types.[152] As mentioned above, however, tumors with features intermediate between serous and endometrioid are most often diagnosed as serous tumors. Consequently, most pathologists either do not use this category or reserve it for microscopically unusual tumors of uncertain nature. In such cases, the possibility that the tumor is a metastasis to the ovary, rather than a primary carcinoma, must always be explored.

On rare occasions, carcinomas not generally found as primary ovarian tumors are encountered. Amongst these miscellaneous neoplasms are primary pure squamous cell carcinoma and the newly described 'hepatoid carcinoma'. Primary squamous cell carcinomas are curiosities.[19,165] Exclusion of metastatic spread from a carcinoma of the cervix or elsewhere must be done. A number of primary ovarian tumors may contain a component of squamous cell carcinoma. Endometrioid carcinomas, malignant Brenner tumors and malignant mixed müllerian tumors (carcinosarcomas) often have malignant squamous epithelium as a prominent histologic element. Squamous cell carcinomas also originate from mature cystic teratomas (dermoid cysts) and endometriosis. A case believed to have developed from an ovarian epidermoid cyst has been reported.[27]

'Hepatoid carcinoma' has been recently described as a new type of primary ovarian tumor.[73] The few reported cases have occurred in adult women. Histologically, they resemble hepatocellular carcinoma and immunoreactive alphafetoprotein (AFP) is present. Hepatoid carcinoma must be distinguished from hepatoid yolk sac tumors and from metastases of liver cell carcinomas or hepatoid adenocarcinomas of the stomach.

REFERENCES

1. Abell M R 1966 The nature and classification of ovarian neoplasms. Canad Med Assoc J 94: 1102
2. Addis B J, Fox H 1983 Papillary mesothelioma of ovary. Histopathol 7: 287
3. Aguirre P, Dayal Y, Scully R E, DeLellis R A 1984 Mucinous tumors of the ovary with argyrophil cells. Am J Surg Pathol 8: 345
4. Allen M S, Hertig A T 1949 Carcinoma of the ovary. Am J Obstet Gynecol 58: 640
5. August C Z, Murad T M, Newton M 1985 Multiple focal extraovarian serous carcinoma. Int J Gynecol Pathol 4: 11
6. Aure J C, Hoeg K, Kolstad P 1971 Carcinoma of the ovary and endometriosis. Acta Obstet Gynecol Scandinav 50: 63
7. Aure J C, Hoeg K, Kolstad P 1971 Clinical and histologic studies of ovarian carcinoma: long-term follow-up of 990 cases. Obstet Gynecol 37: 1
8. Aure J C, Hoeg K, Kolstad P 1971 Mesonephroid tumors of the ovary: clinical and histopathologic studies. Obstet Gynecol 37: 860
9. Aure J C, Hoeg K, Kolstad P 1971 Psammoma bodies in serous carcinoma of the ovary: a prognostic study. Am J Obstet Gynecol 109: 113
10. Austin R M, Norris H J 1987 Malignant Brenner tumor and transitional cell carcinoma of the ovary: a comparison. Int J Gynecol Pathol 6: 29

11. Baak J P A, Langley F A, Talerman A, Delemarre J F M 1986 Interpathologist and intrapathologist disagreement in ovarian tumor grading and typing. Analyt Quant Cytol Histol 8: 354
12. Balasa R W, Adcock L L, Prem K A, Dehner L P 1977 The Brenner tumor: a clinicopathologic review. Obstet Gynecol 50: 120
13. Barnhill D, Heller P, Brzozowski P, Advani H, Gallup D, Park R 1985 Epithelial ovarian carcinoma of low malignant potential. Obstet Gynecol 65: 53
14. Barzilai G 1943 Atlas of Ovarian Tumors. Grune & Stratton, New York
15. Bell D A, Scully R E 1985 Atypical and borderline endometrioid adenofibromas of the ovary: a report of 27 cases. Am J Surg Pathol 9: 205
16. Bell D A, Scully R E 1985 Benign and borderline clear cell adenofibromas of the ovary. Cancer 56: 2922
17. Bell D A, Weinstock M A, Scully R E 1988 Peritoneal implants of ovarian serous borderline tumors: Histologic features and prognosis. Cancer 62: 2212
18. Bell D A, Scully R E 1990 Serous borderline tumors of the peritoneum. Am J Surg Pathol 14: 230
19. Ben-Baruch G, Menashe Y, Herczeg E, Menczer J 1988 Pure primary ovarian squamous cell carcinoma. Gynecol Oncol 29: 257
20. Bigelow B, Blaustein A 1978 Paneth cells in a mucinous cystadenoma of the ovary: light and electron microscopic study. Gynecol Oncol 6: 391
21. Bostwick D G, Tazelaar H D, Ballon S C, Hendrickson M R,

Kempson R L 1986 Ovarian epithelial tumors of borderline malignancy: a clinical and pathologic study of 109 cases. Cancer 58: 2052

22. Bruns D E, Mills S E, Savory J 1982 Amylase in fallopian tube and serous ovarian neoplasms. Arch Pathol Lab Med 106: 17

23. Burmeister R E, Fechner R E, Franklin R R 1969 Endosalpingiosis of the peritoneum. Obstet Gynecol 34: 310

24. Cariker M, Dockerty M B 1954 Mucinous cystadenomas and mucinous cystadenocarcinomas of the ovary: a clinical and pathological study of 355 cases. Cancer 7: 302

25. Chaitin B A, Gershenson D M, Evans H L 1985 Mucinous tumors of the ovary: a clinicopathologic study of 70 cases. Cancer 55: 1958

26. Charpin C, Bhan A K, Zurawski U R, Scully R E 1982 Carcinoembyronic antigen (CEA) and carbohydrate determinant 19–9 (CA 19–9) localization in 121 primary and metastatic ovarian tumors. An immunohistochemical study with the use of monoclonal antibodies. Int J Gynecol Pathol 1: 231

27. Chen K T K 1988 Squamous cell carcinoma of the ovary. (Letter to the Editor) Arch Pathol Lab Med 112: 114

28. Civantos F, Rywlin A M 1972 Carcinomas with trophoblastic differentiation and secretion of chorionic gonadotrophins. Cancer 29: 789

29. Cocco A E, Conway S J 1975 Zollinger-Ellison syndrome associated with ovarian mucinous cystadenocarcinoma. N Engl J Med 293: 485

30. Coffin C M, Adcock L L, Dehner L P 1985 The second-look operation for ovarian neoplasms: a study of 85 cases emphasizing cytologic and histologic problems. Int J Gynecol Pathol 4: 97

31. Copeland L J, Silva E G, Gershenson D M, Sneige N, Atkinson E N, Wharton J T 1988 The significance of müllerian inclusions found at second-look laparotomy in patients with epithelial ovarian neoplasms. Obstet Gynecol 71: 763

32. Cramer S F, Roth L M, Ulbright T M et al 1987 Evaluation of the reproducibility of the World Health Organization classification of common ovarian cancers with emphasis on methodology. Arch Pathol Lab Med 111: 819

33. Cummins P A, Fox H, Langley F A 1973 An ultrastructural study of the nature and origin of the Brenner tumor of the ovary. J Pathol 110: 167

34. Cummins P A, Fox H, Langley F A 1974 An electron microscopic study of the endometrioid adenocarcinoma of the ovary and a comparison of its fine structure with that of normal endometrium and of adenocarcinoma of the endometrium. J Pathol 113: 165

35. Czernobilsky B, Morris W J 1979 A histologic study of ovarian endometriosis with emphasis on hyperplastic and atypical changes. Obstet Gynecol 53: 318

36. Czernobilsky B, Silverman B B, Enterline H T 1970 Clear cell carcinoma of the ovary: a clinicopathologic analysis of pure and mixed forms and comparison with endometrioid carcinoma. Cancer 25: 762

37. Czernobilsky B, Silverman B B, Mikuta J J 1970 Endometrioid carcinoma of the ovary: A clinicopathologic study of 75 cases. Cancer 26: 1141

38. Dabbs D J, Geisinger K R 1988 Common epithelial ovarian tumors: immunohistochemical intermediate filament profiles. Cancer 62: 368

39. Dickersin G R, Kline I W, Scully R E 1982 Small cell carcinoma of the ovary with hypercalcemia: a report of eleven cases. Cancer 49: 188

40. Dockerty M B 1954 Primary and secondary ovarian adenoacanthoma. Surg Gynecol Obstet 99: 392

41. Ehrmann R L, Federschneider J M, Knapp R C 1980 Distinguishing lymph node metastases from benign glandular inclusions in low-grade ovarian carcinoma. Am J Obstet Gynecol 136: 737

42. Eifel P, Hendrickson M, Ross J, Ballon S, Martinez A, Kempson R 1982 Simultaneous presentation of carcinoma involving the ovary and the uterine corpus. Cancer 50: 163

43. Fathalla M F 1972 Factors in the causation and incidence of ovarian cancer. Obstet Gynecol Surv 27: 751

44. Fenoglio C M, Contrall G A, Ferenczy A, Richart R M 1976 Mucinous tumors of the ovary: III. Histochemical studies. Gynecol Oncol 4: 151

45. Fenoglio C M, Ferenczy A, Richart R M 1975 Mucinous tumors of the ovary: ultrastructural studies of mucinous cystadenomas with histogenetic considerations. Cancer 36: 1709

46. Fenoglio C M, Ferenczy A, Richart R M 1976 Mucinous tumors of the ovary: II. Ultrastructural features of mucinous cystadenocarcinomas. Am J Obstet Gynecol 125: 990

47. Fenoglio C M, Puri S, Richart R M 1978 The ultrastructure of endometrioid carcinomas of the ovary. Gynecol Oncol 6: 152

48. Ferenczy A, Okagaki T, Richart R M 1971 Para-endocrine hypercalcemia in ovarian neoplasms: Report of mesonephroma with hypercalcemia and review of literature. Cancer 27: 427

49. Ferenczy A, Talens M, Zoghby M, Hussain S S 1977 Ultrastructural studies on the morphogenesis of psammoma bodies in ovarian serous neoplasia. Cancer 39: 2451

50. Fernandez R N, Daly J M 1980 Pseudomyxoma peritonei. Arch Surg 115: 409

51. Fine G, Clarke H D, Horn R C Jr 1973 Mesonephroma of the ovary: a clinical, morphological, and histogenetic appraisal. Cancer 31: 398

52. Fisher E R, Krieger J A, Skirpan P J 1955 Ovarian cystoma: clinicopathological observations. Cancer 8: 437

53. Fox H, Kazzaz B, Langley F A 1964 Argyrophil and argentaffin cells in the female genital tract and in ovarian mucinous cysts. J Pathol Bacteriol 88: 479

54. Foyle A, Al-Jabi M, McCaughey W T E 1981 Papillary peritoneal tumors in women. Am J Surg Pathol 5: 241

55. Friedlander M L, Hedley D W, Taylor I W, Russell P, Coates A S, Tattersall M H N 1984 Influence of cellular DNA content on survival in advanced ovarian cancer. Cancer Res 44: 397

56. Friedlander M L, Russell P, Taylor I W, Hedley D W, Tattersall M H N 1984 Flow cytometric analysis of cellular DNA content as an adjunct to the diagnosis of ovarian tumors of borderline malignancy. Pathol 16: 301

57. Gaudrault G L 1961 Papillary carcinoma of the ovary: report of a case with prolonged dormancy and spontaneous regression of metastases. N Engl J Med 264: 398

58. Genadry R, Poliakoff S, Rotmensch J, Rosenshein N B, Parmley T H, Woodruff J D 1981 Primary papillary peritoneal neoplasia. Obstet Gynecol 58: 730

59. Ghosh B C, Huvos A G, Whiteley H W 1972 Pseudomyxoma peritonei. Dis Col Rect 15: 420

60. Goepel J R 1981 Benign papillary mesothelioma of peritoneum: a histological, histochemical and ultrastructural study of six cases. Histopathol 5: 21

61. Gondos B 1971 Electron microscopic study of papillary serous tumors of the ovary. Cancer 27: 1455

62. Gondos B 1975 Surface epithelium of the developing ovary: possible correlation with ovarian neoplasia. Am J Pathol 81: 303

63. Goodall J R 1943 A Study of Endometriosis, Endosalpingiosis, Endocervicosis, and Peritoneo-Ovarian Sclerosis. A Clinical and Pathologic Study. Lippincott, Philadelphia

64. Gooneratne S, Sassone M, Blaustein A, Talerman A 1982 Serous surface papillary carcinoma of the ovary: a clinicopathologic study of 16 cases. Int J Gynecol Pathol 1: 258

65. Guthrie D, Davy M L J, Phillips P R 1984 A study of 656 patients with 'early' ovarian cancer. Gynecol Oncol 17: 363

66. Hallgrimsson J, Scully R E 1972 Borderline and malignant Brenner tumours of the ovary: a report of 15 cases. Acta Pathol Microbiol Scand, Sect A, 80 (Suppl 233): 56

67. Hart W R 1977 Ovarian epithelial tumors of borderline malignancy (carcinomas of low malignant potential). Human Pathol 8: 541

68. Hart W R, Norris H J 1973 Borderline and malignant mucinous tumors of the ovary: Histologic criteria and clinical behavior. Cancer 31: 1031.

69. Hertig A T, Gore H 1961 Tumors of the ovary and fallopian tube. In: Tumors of the Female Sex Organs. Part 3. Atlas of Tumor Pathology. Sect IX-Fascicle 33. Armed Forces Institute of Pathology, Washington, DC

70. Higa E, Rosai J, Pizzimbono C A, Wise L 1973 Mucosal hyperplasia, mucinous cystadenoma, and mucinous

cystadenocarcinoma of the appendix: a re-evaluation of appendiceal 'mucocele'. Cancer 32: 1525

71. Holtz G, Johnson T R and Schrock M E 1979 Paraneoplastic hypercalcemia in ovarian tumors. Obstet Gynecol 54: 483

72. Hopkins M P, Kumar N B, Morley G W 1987 An assessment of pathologic features and treatment modalities in ovarian tumors of low malignant potential. Obstet Gynecol 70: 923

73. Ishikura H, Scully R E 1987 Hepatoid carcinoma of the ovary: a newly described tumor. Cancer 60: 2775

74. Jensen R D, Norris H J 1972 Epithelial tumors of the ovary: occurrence in children and adolescents less than 20 years of age. Arch Pathol 94: 29

75. Julian C G, Woodruff J D 1973 The biologic behavior of low grade papillary serous carcinoma of the ovary. Obstet Gynecol 40: 860

76. Kabawat S E, Bast R C, Welch W R, Knapp R C, Colvin R B 1983 Immunopathologic characterization of a monoclonal antibody that recognizes common surface antigens of human ovarian tumors of serous, endometrioid and clear cell types. Am J Clin Pathol 79: 98

77. Kabawat S E, Bast Jr R C, Bhan A K, Welch W R, Knapp R C, Colvin R B 1983 Tissue distribution of a coelomic-epithelium-related antigen recognized by the monoclonal antibody OC 125. Int J Gynecol Pathol 2: 275

78. Kannerstein M, Churg J, McCaughey W T E, Hill D P 1977 Papillary tumors of the peritoneum in women: mesothelioma or papillary carcinoma. Am J Obstet Gynecol 127: 306

79. Kao G F, Norris H J 1978 Cystadenofibromas of the ovary with epithelial atypia. Am J Surg Pathol 2: 357

80. Karp L A, Czernobilsky B 1969 Glandular inclusions in pelvic and abdominal para-aortic lymph nodes: a study of autopsy and surgical material in males and females. Am J Clin Pathol 52: 212

81. Katzenstein A A, Mazur M T, Morgan T E, Kao M 1978 Proliferative serous tumors of the ovary: histologic features and prognosis. Am J Surg Pathol 2: 339

82. Kennedy A W, Biscotti C V, Hart W R, Webster K D 1989 Ovarian clear cell adenocarcinoma. Gynecol Oncol 32: 342

83. Klemi P J 1978 Pathology of mucinous ovarian cystadenomas: 1. Argyrophil and argentaffin cells and epithelial mucosubstances. Acta Pathol Microbiol Scand, Sect. A, 86: 465

84. Klemi P J, Gronroos M 1978 Endometrioid carcinoma of the ovary: a clinicopathologic, histochemical, and electron microscopic study. Obstet Gynecol 53: 572

85. Klemi P J, Joensuu H, Kiilholma P, Maenpaa J 1988 Clinical significance of abnormal nuclear DNA content in serous ovarian tumors. Cancer 62: 2005

86. Klemi P J, Nevalainen T J 1978 Pathology of mucinous ovarian cystadenomas: 2. Ultrastructural findings. Acta Pathol Microbiol Scand, Sect. A, 86: 471

87. Klemi P J, Nevalainen T J 1978 Ultrastructural and histochemical observations on serous ovarian cystadenomas. Acta Pathol Microbiol Scand, Sect. A, 86: 303

88. Kliman L, Rome R M, Fortune D W 1986 Low malignant potential tumors of the ovary: a study of 76 cases. Obstet Gynecol 68: 338

89. Kottmeier H L 1968 Surgical management – conservative surgery: Indications according to the type of the tumor. In: Gentil F, Junqueira A C (eds) Ovarian Cancer. UICC Monograph Series, Vol 11. Springer-Verlag, New York, p 157

90. Kurman R J, Craig J M 1972 Endometrioid and clear cell carcinoma of the ovary. Cancer 29: 1653

91. LaGrenade A, Silverberg S G 1988 Ovarian tumors associated with atypical endometriosis. Hum Pathol 19: 1080

92. Langley R A, Cummins P A, Fox H 1972 An ultrastructural study of mucin secreting epithelia in ovarian neoplasms. Acta Pathol Microbiol Scand, Sect A, 80 (Suppl 233): 76

93. Lash R H, Hart W R 1987 Intestinal adenocarcinomas metastatic to the ovaries: a clinicopathologic evaluation of 22 cases. Am J Surg Pathol 11: 114

94. Lauchlan S C 1966 Histogenesis and histogenetic relationships of Brenner tumors. Cancer 19: 1628

95. Lauchlan S C 1972 The secondary Müllerian system. Obstet Gynecol Surv 27: 133

96. Lingeman C H 1974 Etiology of cancer of the human ovary: a review. J Natl Cancer Inst 53: 1603

97. LiVolsi V A, Merino M J, Schwartz P E 1983 Coexistent endocervical adenocarcinoma and mucinous adenocarcinoma of ovary: a clinicopathologic study of four cases. Int J Gynecol Pathol 1: 391

98. Long M E, Sommers S C 1968 Histochemical characterization of epithelial mucins in human ovarian mucinous tumors. J Histochem Cytochem 16: abstract 511

99. Long M E, Taylor H C Jr. 1964 Endometrioid carcinoma of the ovary. Am J Obstet Gynecol 90: 936

100. Long R T L, Spratt J S Jr, Dowling E 1969 Pseudomyxoma peritonei: new concepts in management with a report of seventeen patients. Am J Surg 117: 162

101. McCaughey W T E 1985 Papillary peritoneal neoplasms in females. Pathol Annual 20 (Part 2): 387

102. McCaughey W T E, Kirk M E, Lester W, Dardick I 1984 Peritoneal epithelial lesions associated with proliferative serous tumours of ovary. Histopathol 8: 195

103. Mackillop W J, Pringle J F 1985 Stage III endometrial carcinoma: a review of 90 cases. Cancer 56: 2519

104. McMahon J T, Hart W R 1988 Ultrastructural analysis of small cell carcinomas of the ovary. Am J Clin Pathol 90: 523

105. Malkasian Jr G D, Decker D G, Webb M J 1975 Histology of epithelial tumors of the ovary: clinical usefulness and prognostic significance of the histologic classification and grading. Semin Oncol 2: 191

106. Malloy J J, Dockerty M B, Welch J S, Hunt H B 1965 Papillary ovarian tumors: I. Benign tumors and serous and mucinous cystadenocarcinomas. Am J Obstet Gynecol 93: 867

107. Michael H, Roth L M 1986 Invasive and noninvasive implants in ovarian serous tumors of low malignant potential. Cancer 57: 1240

108. Michael H, Sutton G, Roth L M 1987 Ovarian carcinoma with extracellular mucin production: reassessment of 'pseudomyxoma ovarii et peritonei'. Int J Gynecol Pathol 6: 298

109. Miles P A, Norris H J 1972 Proliferative and malignant Brenner tumors of the ovary. Cancer 30: 174

110. Mills S E, Andersen W A, Fechner R E, Austin M B 1988 Serous surface papillary carcinoma: a clinicopathologic study of 10 cases and comparison with Stage III–IV ovarian serous carcinoma. Am J Surg Pathol 12: 827

111. Nikrui N 1981 Survey of clinical behavior of patients with borderline epithelial tumors of the ovary. Gynecol Oncol 12: 107

112. Norris H J, Robinowitz M 1971 Ovarian adenocarcinoma of mesonephric type. Cancer 28: 1074

113. Obel E B 1976 A comparative study of patients with cancer of the ovary, who have survived more or less than 10 years. Acta Obstet Gynecol Scand 55: 429

114. Ohkawa K, Amasaki H, Terashima Y, Aizawa S, Ishikawa E 1977 Clear cell carcinoma of the ovary: light and electron microscopic studies. Cancer 40: 3019

115. Okagaki T, Richart R M 1970 'Mesonephroma ovarii (hypernephroid carcinoma)': light microscopic and ultrastructural study of a case. Cancer 26: 453

116. Osborn C L 1973 Pseudomyxoma peritonei: a report of seven cases. Gynecol Oncol 1: 195

117. Parmley T, Woodruff J D 1974 The ovarian mesothelioma. Am J Obstet Gynecol 120: 234

118. Powers E G, Hooker O N 1948 Salpingiosis (endosalpingiosis): case report. Texas Med J 44: 457

119. Prat J, Scully R E 1979 Sarcomas in ovarian mucinous tumors: a report of two cases. Cancer 44: 1327

120. Prat J, Scully R E 1979 Ovarian mucinous tumors with sarcoma-like mural nodules: a report of seven cases. Cancer 44: 1332

121. Prat J, Young R H, Scully R E 1982 Ovarian mucinous tumors with foci of anaplastic carcinoma. Cancer 50: 300

122. Purola E 1963 Serous papillary ovarian tumours: a study of 233 cases with special reference to the histological type of tumour and its influence in prognosis. Acta Obstet Gynecol Scand 42 (Suppl 3): 7

123. Radisavljevic S V 1977 The pathogenesis of ovarian inclusion cysts and cystomas. Obstet Gynecol 49: 424

124. Roberts D K, Marshall R B, Wharton J T 1970 Ultrastructure of ovarian tumors: I. Papillary serous cystadenocarcinoma. Cancer 25: 947

125. Rogers L W, Julian C G, Woodruff J D 1972 Mesonephroid carcinoma of the ovary: a study of 95 cases from the Emil·Novak Ovarian Tumor Registry. Gynecol Oncol 1: 76

126. Rosenberg L, Shapiro S, Slone D et al 1982 Epithelial ovarian cancer and combination oral contraceptives. JAMA 247: 3210

127. Roth L M 1974 The Brenner tumor and the Walthard cell nest: an electron microscopic study. Lab Invest 31: 15

128. Roth L M, Czernobilsky B 1985 Ovarian Brenner tumors II. Malignant. Cancer 56: 592

129. Roth L M, Czernobilsky B, Langley F A 1981 Ovarian endometrioid adenofibromatous and cystadenofibromatous tumors: benign, proliferating, and malignant. Cancer 48: 1838

130. Roth L M, Dallenbach-Hellweg G, Czernobilsky B 1985 Ovarian Brenner tumors I. Metaplastic, proliferating, and of low malignant potential. Cancer 56: 582

131. Roth L M, Langley R A, Fox H, Wheeler J E, Czernobilsky B 1984 Ovarian clear cell adenofibromatous tumors: benign, of low malignant potential, and associated with invasive clear cell carcinoma. Cancer 53: 1156

132. Roth L M, Liban E, Czernobilsky B 1982 Ovarian endometrioid tumors mimicking Sertoli and Sertoli-Leydig cell tumors: Sertoliform variant of endometrioid carcinoma. Cancer 50: 1322

133. Roth L M, Sternberg W H 1971 Proliferating Brenner tumors. Cancer 27: 687

134. Russell P 1979 The pathological assessment of ovarian neoplasms. I. Introduction to the common 'epithelial' tumours and analysis of benign 'epithelial' tumours. Pathol 11: 5

135. Russell P 1979 The pathological assessment of ovarian neoplasms. II: The proliferating 'epithelial' tumours. Pathol 11: 251

136. Russell P 1979 The pathological assessment of ovarian neoplasms. III: The malignant 'epithelial' tumours. Pathol 11: 493

137. Russell P 1984 Borderline epithelial tumours of the ovary: a conceptual dilemma. Clin Obstet Gynecol 11: 259

138. Russell P, Merkur H 1979 Proliferating ovarian 'epithelial' tumours: a clinico-pathological analysis of 144 cases. Aust NZ J Obstet Gynaecol 19: 45

139. Rutgers J L, Scully R E 1988 Ovarian müllerian mucinous papillary cystadenomas of borderline malignancy: a clinicopathologic analysis. Cancer 61: 340

140. Rutgers J L, Scully R E 1988 Ovarian mixed-epithelial papillary cystadenomas of borderline malignancy of müllerian type: clinicopathologic analysis. Cancer 61: 546

141. Salazar H, Merkow L P, Walter W S, Pardo M 1974 Human ovarian neoplasms: light and electron microscopic correlations. II. The clear cell tumor. Obstet Gynecol 44: 551

142. Sampson J A 1925 Endometrial carcinoma of ovary arising in endometrial tissue in that organ. Arch Surg 10: 1

143. Sampson J A 1930 Post-salpingectomy endometriosis (endosalpingiosis). Am J Obstet Gynecol 20: 443

144. Sandenbergh H A, Woodruff J D 1977 Histogenesis of pseudomyxoma peritonei: review of 9 cases. Obstet Gynecol 49: 339

145. Santesson L, Kottmeier H L 1968 General classification of ovarian tumors. In: Gentil F, Junqueira A C (eds) Ovarian Cancer. UICC Monograph Series, Vol 11. Springer-Verlag, New York, p 1

146. Schray M, Martinez A, Cox R, Ballon S 1983 Radiotherapy in epithelial ovarian cancer: analysis of prognostic factors based on long-term experience. Obstet Gynecol 62: 373

147. Schuldenfrei R, Janovski N A 1962 Disseminated endosalpingiosis associated with bilateral papillary serous cystadenocarcinomas of the ovaries. Am J Obstet Gynecol 84: 382

148. Scully R E 1977 Ovarian tumors: a review. Am J Pathol 87: 686

149. Scully R E 1979 Tumors of the ovary and maldeveloped gonads. In: Atlas of Tumor Pathology, Second Series, Fascicle 16. Washington D.C., Armed Forces Institute of Pathology

150. Scully R E, Barlow J F 1967 'Mesonephroma' of ovary: tumor of Müllerian nature related to the endometrioid carcinoma. Cancer 20: 1405

151. Scully R E, Richardson G S, Barlow J F 1966 The development of malignancy in endometriosis. Clin Obstet Gynecol 9: 384

152. Serov S F, Scully R E, Sobin L H 1973 International Histologic Classification of Tumours. No. 9. Histological Typing of Ovarian Tumours. World Health Organization, Geneva

153. Shane J M, Naftolin F 1975 Aberrant hormone activity by tumors of gynecologic importance. Am J Obstet Gynecol 121: 133

154. Shanks H G I 1961 Pseudomyxoma peritonei. J Obstet Gynaecol Br Emp 68: 212

155. Shevchuk M M, Winkler-Monsanto B, Fenoglio C M, Richart R M 1981 Clear cell carcinoma of the ovary: a clinicopathologic study with review of the literature. Cancer 47: 1344

156. Silverberg S G 1973 Ultrastructure and histogenesis of clear cell carcinoma of the ovary. Am J Obstet Gynecol 115: 394

157. Silverman B B, O'Neill R T, Mikuta J J 1972 Multiple malignant tumors associated with primary carcinoma of the ovary. Surg Gynecol Obstet 134: 244

158. Sinykin M B 1960 Endosalpingiosis. Minn Med 43: 759

159. Snyder R R, Norris H J, Tavassoli F 1988 Endometrioid proliferative and low malignant potential tumors of the ovary: a clinicopathologic study of 46 cases. Am J Surg Pathol 12: 661

160. Stalsberg H, Abeler V, Blom P, Bostad L, Skarland E, Westgaard G 1988 Observer variation in histologic classification of malignant and borderline ovarian tumors. Hum Pathol 19: 1030

161. Sumithran E, Susil B J, Looi L M 1988 The prognostic significance of grading in borderline mucinous tumors of the ovary. Hum Pathol 19: 15

162. Swenerton K D, Hislop T G, Spinelli J, LeRiche J C, Yang N, Boyes D A 1985 Ovarian carcinoma: a multivariate analysis of prognostic factors. Obstet Gynecol 65: 264

163. Taylor H C Jr, Alsop W E 1932 Spontaneous regression of peritoneal implantations from ovarian papillary cystadenoma. Am J Cancer 16: 1305

164. Taylor H C Jr, Long M E 1955 Problems of cellular and tissue differentiation in papillary adenocarcinoma of the ovary. Am J Obstet Gynecol 70: 753

165. Tetu B, Silva E G, Gershenson D M 1987 Squamous cell carcinoma of the ovary. Arch Pathol Lab Med 111: 864

166. Timonen S, Purola E 1967 Adenofibroma and cystadenofibroma of the ovary. Ann Chir Gynaecol Fenn 56(Suppl 154): 5

167. Van Kley H, Cramer S, Bruns D E 1981 Serous ovarian neoplastic amylase (SONA): a potentially useful marker for serous ovarian tumors. Cancer 48: 1444

168. Van Nagell J R, Donaldson E S, Gay E C, Sharkey R M, Rayburn P, Goldenberg D M 1978 Carcinoembryonic antigen in ovarian epithelial cystadenocarcinomas: the prognostic value of tumor and serial plasma determinations. Cancer 41: 2335

169. White P F, Merino M J, Barwick K W 1985 Serous surface papillary carcinoma of the ovary: a clinical, pathologic, ultrastructural, and immunohistochemical study of 11 cases. Pathol Annual 20 (Part 1): 403

170. Wolff M, Ahmed N 1976 Epithelial neoplasms of the vermiform appendix (exclusive of carcinoid): II. Cystadenocarcinomas, papillary adenomas and adenomatous polyps of the appendix. Cancer 37: 2511

171. Woodruff J D, Julian C G 1970 Histologic grading and morphologic changes of significance in the treatment of semi-malignant and malignant ovarian tumors. Proc Natl Cancer Conf 6: 346

172. Woodruff J D, Perry H, Genadry R, Parmley T 1978 Mucinous cystadenocarcinoma of the ovary. Obstet Gynecol 51: 483

173. Wynder E L, Dodo H, Barber H K 1969 Epidemiology of cancer of the ovary. Cancer 23: 352

174. Young R H, Prat J, Scully R E 1982 Ovarian endometrioid carcinomas resembling sex-cord-stromal tumors: a clinicopathologic analysis of 13 cases. Am J Surg Pathol 6: 513

175. Young R H, Scully R E 1987 Oxyphilic clear cell carcinoma of the ovary: a report of nine cases. Am J Surg Pathol 11: 661

176. Young R H, Scully R E 1987 Sex-cord-stromal, steroid cell, and other ovarian tumors with endocrine, paraendocrine, and paraneoplastic manifestations. In: Kurman R J (ed) Blaustein's Pathology of the Female Genital Tract, 3rd edn. Springer-Verlag, New York, p 647

177. Young R H, Scully R E 1988 Mucinous ovarian tumors

associated with mucinous adenocarcinomas of the cervix. Int J Gynecol Pathol 7: 99

178. Young R H, Scully R E 1988 Urothelial and ovarian carcinomas of identical cell types: problems in interpretation. A report of three cases and review of the literature. Int J Gynecol Pathol 7: 197

179. Zajicek J 1978 Prevention of ovarian cystomas by inhibition of ovulation: a new concept. J Reprod Med 20: 297

180. Zinsser K R, Wheeler J E 1982 Endosalpingiosis in the omentum: a study of autopsy and surgical material. Am J Surg Pathol 6: 109

56. Malignant and borderline epithelial tumors of ovary: clinical features, staging, diagnosis, intraoperative assessment and review of management

C. P. Morrow

INTRODUCTION

Malignancies arising from the ovarian surface epithelium account for 80 to 90% of all ovarian cancers and, as a group, are more malignant than the cancers of stromal origin and less curable than the germ cell malignancies. The majority of cases are found at initial surgery to have spread beyond the ovaries and perhaps half the cases will have gross residual disease at the conclusion of their operative therapy. Even those cases with apparently 'early' disease have a high recurrence rate. Although the overall curability of ovarian carcinoma may have increased somewhat during the past 50 years, progress must be attributed to the cumulative effect of small improvements in diagnosis, surgical management and adjuvant therapy rather than a breakthrough in any of these areas.

Like other visceral malignancies, ovarian carcinoma does not cause early symptoms. Consequently, there is little prospect for improved results by patient education. Nor does frequent pelvic examination appear to have promise as a means of early detection, since the disease often grows rapidly and the methodology is intrinsically inaccurate. Cul de sac cytology has proven to be inaccurate and inapplicable to large scale screening. In recent years, hope for an effective screening method has been revived by the promise of a serum immunodiagnostic test for tumor-associated antigens, but none has yet arrived. The outcome for patients with ovarian malignancy remains, therefore, largely in the hands of fate, the skill of the surgeon, the acumen of the pathologist and the selection of optimal postoperative therapy. In most countries it is an inescapable fact of life that often the most important phase of ovarian cancer management, surgery, is carried out by the least specialized physician who will be involved in the patient's care. The gynecologic oncologist, radiation oncologist or chemotherapist ordinarily are not called upon until after surgery since the diagnosis is not usually made preoperatively. This situation results inevitably in some patients having suboptimal oncoreductive surgery and others being understaged with its attendant risk of undertreatment. To counteract this problem, a number of treatment centers have resorted to laparoscopic or laparotomy re-evaluation so that adjunctive chemo- or radiotherapy will be administered only after optimal surgical management.

The proper place for radiation therapy in ovarian carcinoma has not been established even after 50 years of experience. The appropriate stage of disease, optimal dose, field size and technique remain undecided. Is the pelvic field without abdominal radiation therapeutic in early ovarian cancer? Which is more effective, the moving strip or open field technique for whole abdomen radiation? Are intraperitoneal nuclides curative for any stage of ovarian carcinoma? What is the largest volume of residual abdominal tumor which can be expected to respond favorably to radiation therapy? The situation with respect to chemotherapy is also uncertain. What are the most effective single agents? What are the best combinations? What are their indications? Are they useful as an adjuvant in early ovarian cancer? For how long must they be given? Can they be used in combination with radiation therapy? Is intraperitoneal chemotherapy more effective than intravenous chemotherapy?

Many of these questions can only be answered by large scale, controlled studies. Fortunately, much clinical research has been initiated in ovarian cancer management during the past few years and the results should lead to a more effective plan of treatment. In this chapter these new studies, as well as many of the older reports, are reviewed and collated to present a comprehensive status report on the clinical and therapeutic facets of ovarian carcinoma. Emphasis has been placed on those aspects which the author believes might enhance the quality of patient evaluation and therapy, thus maximizing survival.

CLINICAL FEATURES

Age

The epithelial ovarian malignancies rarely occur before

puberty and are uncommon prior to age 40. Thereafter their incidence rises rapidly until the 7th decade of life when a plateau occurs.

Jensen & Norris,[88] reporting on 353 cases of benign and malignant ovarian neoplasms in females under age 20, found no epithelial malignancies among 54 neoplasms in the 0 to 9 age group, 1 among 82 neoplasms in the 10 to 14 age group, and only 7 among 217 neoplasms in the 15 to 19 year group. Five of the 8 malignant epithelial ovarian tumors were classified as cystadenomas of low malignant potential (borderline malignant tumors). Thus, outspoken epithelial malignancies in children and young women are rare, and such a diagnosis must be viewed with circumspection. Several investigators[13,60,174] have documented that younger women with ovarian carcinoma have a better prognosis than older women. This reflects the higher incidence of borderline tumors and the lower stage at diagnosis that occurs in the younger age groups (Table 56.1). Grönroos

Table 56.1 Age-related frequency of borderline versus true ovarian carcinoma. (From: Grönroos, Lauren, Lehto & Rauramo, 1969)[70]

Age in years	Borderline tumors	True carcinomas	Total cases	Borderline tumors (% of total)
20 to 29	5	1	6	(83)
30 to 39	10	5	15	(67)
40 to 49	17	18	35	(49)
50 to 59	19	35	54	(35)
60 to 69	9	28	37	(24)
>70	1	4	5	(20)
Total	61	91	152	(40)

and associates[70] found the mean age of women with benign cystadenomas, borderline tumors and true cancers to be 45, 49 and 55 years respectively. Aure, Hoeg & Kolstad,[5] reporting on 161 women with borderline tumors and 829 with true carcinomas, found the mean age at diagnosis to be 45.7 ± 13.7 years for the former and 52.5 ± 11.5 years for the latter. According to Vol. 20 of the FIGO Annual Report,[4] the mean age of patients with ovarian carcinoma increases with stage as well as histologic differentiation. The stage distribution for borderline tumors and true carcinomas is presented in Table 56.2. Fifty percent of the less aggressive, borderline ovarian tumors are Stage I at the time of diagnosis, compared with 23.5% of the true carcinomas reported in the same series.

Yancik, Ries & Yates,[203] in an analysis of 11 062 cases of ovarian cancer (National Cancer Institute of the United States SEER program 1973 to 1982), noted that the proportion of advanced cases increased with age, while the survival within stage, especially the more advanced stages, declined (Table 56.3). These differences are in part due to the greater frequency of borderline ovarian tumors in younger women. Others have reported similar findings. For example, Beller et al[13] reported that 39% of their 31 ovarian cancer patients below 40 years of age had borderline tumors, and 55% of the 31 patients were in FIGO Stage I. Smedley & Sikora, in a study of 2305 ovarian cancer patients in the United Kingdom, found that the 5-year survival for women aged 15 to 35 years was approximately 60%, versus 30% for older women.

Symptoms

Ovarian carcinoma does not produce specific symptoms. As the tumor enlarges, its weight and the space it occupies cause urinary urgency or frequency, constipation, a sense of heaviness in the pelvis, occasional sharp twinges, or dyspareunia. With growth beyond 12 to 15 cm in diameter or ascites, abdominal enlargement begins. The patient may interpret the tight fit of her clothes to simple weight gain. If amenorrhea develops in the premenopausal woman, whether due to some endocrine effect of the tumor or coincidental menopause, she may interpret these developments as the symptoms of pregnancy.

Other frequent symptoms are: (1) pelvic or abdominal pain or discomfort. This is often intermittent, vague and seldom severe; (2) bloating, dyspepsia, selective food intolerance, bouts of nausea, vomiting, cramps, diarrhea, dyschezia, epigastric distress or anorexia which often lead the patient to an internist and direct attention away from

Table 56.2 Stage distribution of borderline and true ovarian epithelial carcinomas*

FIGO stage	Borderline tumors		True carcinomas		Total	
	Cases	%	Cases	%	Cases	%
I	265	(50.6)	1838	(23.5)	2103	(25.2)
II	114	(21.7)	1265	(16.1)	1379	(16.5)
III	128	(24.4)	3311	(42.3)	3439	(41.1)
IV	17	(3.2)	1420	(18.1)	1437	(17.2)
Total	524		7834		8358	

* From: Annual Report Gynecologic Cancer FIGO, Vol 20. (1988)[4]

Table 56.3 Stage distribution and survival by age for ovarian cancer in the United States, 1973 to 1982*

| Age group (yr) | Stage I (N=2074) | | Stages III and IV (N=5618) | |
	% in stage	% survived	% in stage	% survived
<45	47	87	47	41
45 to 54	32	84	60	24
55 to 64	23	75	70	16
65 to 74	18	79	75	11
≥75	17	83	74	7

* From: Yancik et al[203]

the pelvis. This is entirely understandable because the symptoms suggest biliary, gastric or intestinal disease. In one series[186] of ovarian cancer cases, 22% of the patients were initially referred to an internist or surgeon because of gastrointestinal complaints. Clinically apparent ascites may mimic primary liver, heart or renal disease or tuberculosis, particularly in the patient with wasting and shortness of breath. This misconception may be reinforced by the presence of edema resulting from retroperitoneal spread of the ovarian carcinoma.

Abnormal uterine bleeding is a relatively frequent symptom in women with ovarian epithelial malignancy although it is more common in the presence of a functional granulosa-theca cell tumor. In the reproductive years the abnormal bleeding is manifested by irregular or excessive uterine bleeding; in the postmenopausal woman by any vaginal spotting or bleeding. The cause of the vaginal bleeding associated with ovarian cancer is due to several factors: production of estrogen by the stromal component of the neoplasm producing endometrial hyperplasia; bleeding from a concomitant primary malignancy of the uterus; and bleeding from metastases to the uterus, cervix or vagina.

Ovarian carcinoma may present as a surgical emergency because of torsion (Figs 56.1a & 56.1b), rupture or intra-abdominal hemorrhage. This is evidently uncommon since few series mention it. Vara & Pankamma[188] noted a 10% incidence of torsion >120° (not necessarily symptomatic) for malignant ovarian tumors compared with 16 to 20% for ovarian benign neoplasms. The highest incidence of torsion was in the under 20 year age group. The greater incidence of adhesions associated with malignant tumors (60%) compared with various benign tumors (15 to 40%) probably contributes to this discrepancy. Rupture of an ovarian tumor prior to surgery is another event which is seldom mentioned in the literature on ovarian cancer. Disruption of the capsule of ovarian malignancies is common, but is nearly always due to destructive growth of the tumor rather than a sudden bursting with acute symptoms. In one series,[188] 6.2% of mucinous cystadenomas and 5% of serous cystadenomas had ruptured spontaneously, but only 1 of 21 (4.8%) mucinous carcinomas and 7 of 47

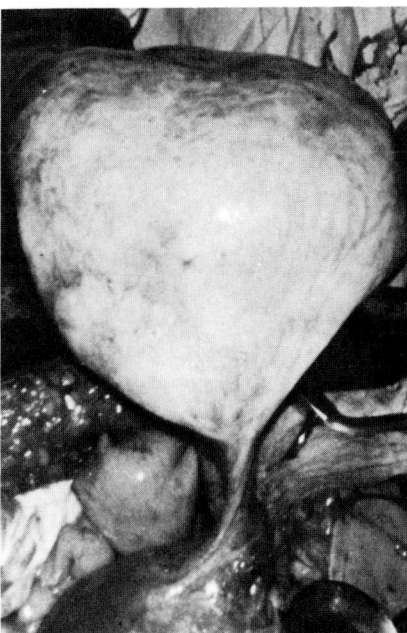

Fig. 56.1a Large, twisted, but not infarcted mucinous cystadenoma of low malignant potential. The patient was 34 years old and presented with intermittent abdominal pain.

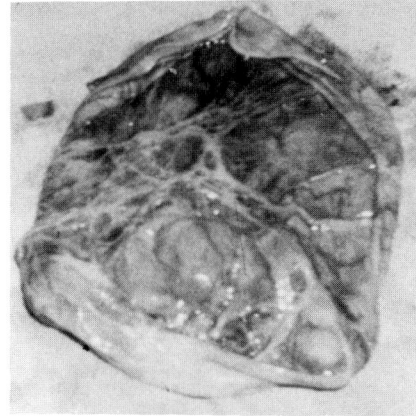

Fig. 56.1b The same neoplasm as in Figure 56.1a after removal and subsequent incision. It has numerous locules with areas of thickening in the septa.

(14.9%) serous malignancies had capsular disruption preoperatively.

Ovarian carcinoma is seldom diagnosed in the asymptomatic patient. MacFarlane, Sturgis & Fetterman[108] discovered only 6 ovarian cancers during 18 753 routine pelvic examinations performed on 1319 women aged 30 to 80 years from 1938 to 1952. Only one of the six was cured of her disease. Uncommon or rare modes of presentation include: hypoglycemia,[130] hypercalcemia (clear cell or endometrial carcinoma),[82] Cushings syndrome,[139] Zollinger-Ellison's syndrome,[34] dermatomyositis,[143] hyperpyrexia,[46] migratory thrombophlebitis,[29] disseminated intravascular coagulation,[171] cerebellar degeneration[74] and distant metastases (skin, peripheral lymph node, lung).[24]

The presenting symptoms and duration of symptoms have a crude prognostic value. Holme[81] reported that 23% of patients with symptoms for less than 6 months at diagnosis survived 5 years compared with 35.5% if symptoms were present 6 to 12 months, and 38% if symptoms were present longer than 1 year. Timm[186] noted certain symptoms augured a better or worse prognosis. Women presenting with abnormal bleeding had a 46.7% 5-year survival (his series includes only epithelial carcinomas). In contrast, constipation and weight loss were attended by a 16.7 and 14.3% 5-year survival respectively. Those patients presenting with abdominal swelling, pain and urinary complaints had a 32 to 35% 5-year survival. Stone & Weingold[183a] also found the best survival among patients presenting with vaginal bleeding (45% at 5 years), while those with pain, gastrointestinal complaints or ascites had a 20, 18 and 9.8% survival respectively.

Davis, Latour & Philpott[39] found no correlation of stage with duration of symptoms, but found anorexia and weight loss were considerably more common with advanced disease. Pearse & Behrman[140] reported the *first* symptom noted in their group of 262 patients with ovarian malignancy: abdominal swelling 41.2%, abdominal pain 22.4% and vaginal bleeding 15.8%. Six of their patients (2%) were asymptomatic at the time of diagnosis, three of whom were dead within 2 years. The duration of symptoms in their study group was <3 months in 35%, <6 months in 60% and <12 months in 86%.

Obel[126] studied prognosis within each stage based on symptoms. Only polyuria in Stage II cases had a statistically significant poorer prognosis. The symptoms of constipation, diarrhea, nausea, vomiting and poor general condition in his study group were bad signs largely because they reflected an advanced stage of disease. For example 29% of Stage III and IV patients had constipation, compared with 11% of Stage I cases and 22% for Stage II. It is interesting to note that the proportion of patients reporting abnormal bleeding decreased with increasing stage.

The symptoms of ovarian cancer relative to stage have also been studied by Flam et al (Table 56.4). Gastrointestinal symptoms, fatigue, fever, dyspnea and back pain are

Table 56.4 Main initial symptoms reported by patients with early and advanced ovarian carcinoma*

Symptom	Stage (N=362)	
	Early (%)	Advanced (%)
Abdominal swelling	26.8	24.3
Abdominal pain	16.9	10.6
Gastrointestinal	14.5	24.2
Vaginal bleeding	12.2	11.6
Dysuria	9.9	4.7
Fatigue/fever	4.1	14.6
Dyspnea/back pain	1.8	7.9
None	10.2	2.1

* From: Flam et al 1988[56]

clearly more common with advanced ovarian cancer. Abdominal swelling was more likely to cause the patient with advanced cancer to seek medical help (27.9% advanced vs 18.0% of early cases) suggesting that the swelling is more severe. Smith & Anderson[176] found no relationship between delay, seriousness of symptoms and stage of disease at diagnosis.

Physical findings

The results of physical examination are not often included in articles on ovarian cancer. From five reports[3,23,61,138,140] it can be concluded that 40 to 75% have a palpable abdominal mass and 20 to 30% have clinically detectable ascites. Only 1 to 2% of cases will have a negative examination. Buka & MacFarlane[23] reported that 66% of their 223 cases had a palpable ovarian mass, 18% had a mass and ascites, 9% had ascites without a palpable mass and 18% had pelvic nodules. They also noted 13% of the patients had a pleural effusion with a similar incidence on both sides. One patient had no clinical findings while six (3%) were diagnosed prior to the appearance of symptoms. In Bernstein's 190 patient study group[17] 2.7% had pleural effusion; Javert[87] reported this finding in only 2 of 127 patients with ovarian serous carcinoma (1.5%).

In the report of Parker, Parker & Wilbanks[138] 14% of the patients with ovarian cancer had a preoperative diagnosis of fibroids (Fig. 56.2) or other 'pelvic pathology'. They also found that of the patients in their study group who had Papanicolaou smears, the test was reported as suspicious or positive in 11%. Pearse & Behrman[140] observed that the abdominal examination was negative in 20% of their 277 cases of ovarian carcinoma; 13% had pelvic nodules without a palpable mass and 4 patients had no findings on physical examination; 2 of these had widespread metastases at surgery. In only 55% of the patients in their series was the diagnosis of ovarian cancer suspected prior to surgery. Distant metastases (skin, inguinal, supraclavicular or

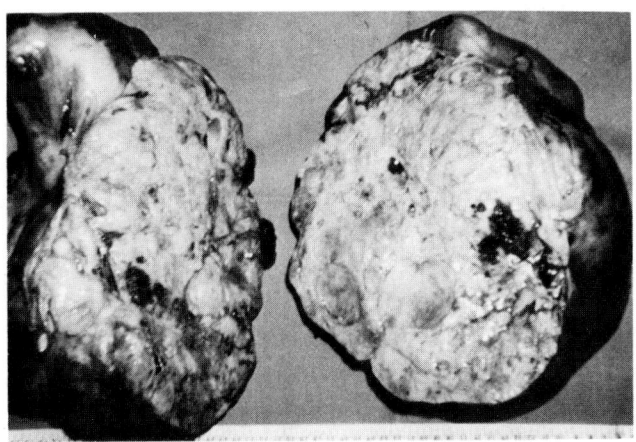

Fig. 56.2 This 25 cm solid ovarian tumor had been present for several years and was believed to be large uterine fibromyomas. The cut section shows areas of hemorrhage. The microscopic pathology revealed predominantly benign fibroadenoma with adenocarcinoma in the hemorrhagic areas.

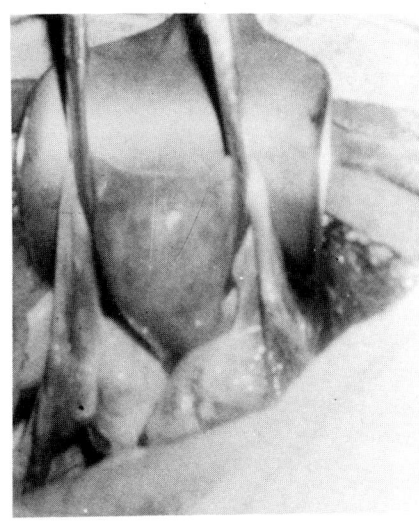

Fig. 56.3 Bilateral ovarian 'tumors' typical of the Stein-Leventhal syndrome. Both ovaries are a little smaller than the uterine fundus. The clinical picture is the key to diagnosis.

axillary lymph nodes) are clinically detectable in about 5% of patients with ovarian carcinoma.[24] The most common mistaken preoperative diagnosis is uterine fibroids. Lynch[107] reported that 2.5% of 1200 patients with a preoperative diagnosis of 'fibroids' had ovarian cancer, a figure which underscores the difficulty of this clinical problem.

When ascites accompanies ovarian carcinoma it augurs a poor outcome because it is usually associated with advanced disease. The caveat propagated by Meigs,[115] however, must not be forgotten. Peritoneal and pleural effusions may be caused by otherwise harmless ovarian tumors (Meigs syndrome). Particularly in the older woman, emaciation may result, and the failure to intervene surgically because of a presumptive diagnosis of advanced ovarian cancer can result in a wrongful death or unnecessary suffering.

The most productive 'test' and the cornerstone for the detection of ovarian neoplasia is the pelvic examination. Patient prerequisites include an empty bladder and rectosigmoid, and relaxed abdominal muscles. An appropriate examining facility is also a necessity. Even under optimal circumstances the patient with symptomatic ovarian cancer may have a negative pelvic examination. If the patient is obese, anxious, in pain, or has a full bladder or rectosigmoid the examination will be even less reliable.

The bimanual rectovaginal palpation of the pelvic organs is essential. It provides the most accurate assessment of the posterior uterine surface, the uterosacral ligaments, the pouch of Douglas and the parametria (cardinal ligaments). Small ovarian tumors and nodularity of the cul de sac, uterosacral ligaments or rectovaginal septum might otherwise be missed. The presence of cul de sac nodularity is

an indication of malignancy and should not be treated as endometriosis without visual confirmation.

The character of the adnexal or pelvic mass is an important indicator of its nature. While it is seldom possible to conclude with absolute confidence whether a tumor is benign or malignant (or even ovarian or non-ovarian), benignancy (Fig. 56.3) is favored if the mass is mobile, smooth, cystic, small (<10 cm), or unilateral. Solid, fixed, irregular, nodular, bilateral and large tumors are more likely to be malignant. Paradoxically, the extremely large ovarian tumors are usually benign mucinous cystadenomas.

Distension of the abdomen is one of the most common physical findings and is usually a sign of ascites, or a large tumor. Distension also may be due to partial bowel obstruction, ileus, masses of intra-abdominal cancer (e.g. omental cake), or various combinations of these. Ascites and a large ovarian cyst may both give a fluid wave; ascites distends the umbilicus, a cyst will not. Another point of differentiation is the location of the tympanitic area of the bowel on percussion: with ascites it is over the central abdomen in the supine patient, while an ovarian cyst will push the bowel laterally. A large omental metastasis is often ballotable and has a solid, irregular feel. Adhesions from prior surgery or pelvic inflammatory disease can obscure an associated adnexal neoplasm or be mistaken itself for a neoplastic mass.

Important positive findings can be elicited by the general physical examination of the patient with ovarian carcinoma. Supraclavicular, inguinal and even axillary nodes may be enlarged by metastases. Pleural effusion most commonly accompanies ascites, but does occur alone. Emaciation, leg edema, skin metastasis and the stigmata of abnormal hormone production should also be noted.

DIAGNOSIS

The diagnosis of ovarian carcinoma ultimately depends upon operative intervention. Much of the preoperative evaluation is directed toward excluding other important causes of a pelvic mass, particularly non-gynecologic (Table 56.5) causes such as colonic carcinoma, diverticular

Table 56.5 Non-gynecologic causes of a pelvic mass in 45 women (from Schnur, Symmonds & Williams, 1969)[163]

		Total cases
Inflammatory		25
Diverticulitis	16	
Regional enteritis	5	
Appendiceal abscess	3	
Ileal volvulus with abscess	1	
Neoplastic		22
Sigmoid carcinoma	9	
Cecal carcinoma	2	
Intestinal leiomyosarcoma	2	
Pancreatic carcinoma	2	
Metastatic sarcoma	2	
Retroperitoneal sarcoma	2	
Gastric carcinoma	1	
Gallbladder cancer	1	

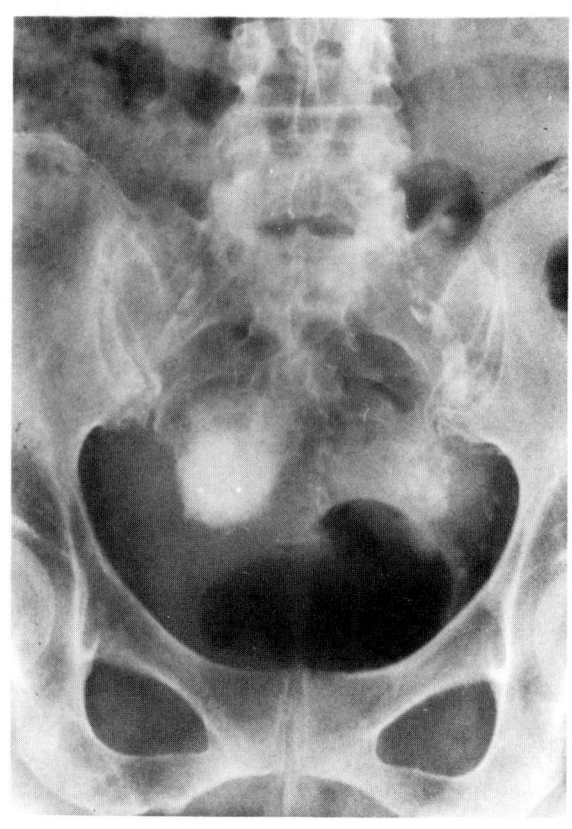

Fig. 56.4 Plain radiograph of abdomen. Patient was 55 years old and thought to have uterine fibromyomata. Bilateral calcified masses proved to be Brenner tumors.

disease, and upper abdominal cancers with ovarian and/or peritoneal involvement. Preoperative diagnostic measures must also be directed toward the genital organs other than the ovary, since uterine and occasionally endocervical carcinoma present with a concomitant ovarian primary or ovarian metastasis.[51,207] Thus, the work up may require cervical cytology, colposcopy, endocervical curettage and endometrial biopsy. Sounding the uterus helps identify a pelvic mass as uterine if the instrument passes into the mass, but this is by no means an entirely reliable test. Stool guaiac, rectal examination, sigmoidoscopy and barium enema are indicated whenever the patient has gastrointestinal symptoms, anemia, weight loss or other than a mobile, unilateral smooth, cystic adnexal mass. A plain roentgenogram of the abdomen is most helpful in diagnosing dermoid cysts.[182] Various patterns of calcification (Fig. 56.4) may suggest a serous ovarian tumor (psammoma bodies) or uterine myomas. Stomach and small bowel radiologic studies are warranted if the patient has ascites or related upper gastrointestinal symptoms, since gastric carcinoma can present with dominant ovarian metastases. The presence of ascites suggests other diseases which must be considered in the differential diagnosis: heart disease with failure, chronic liver disease (cirrhosis), pancreatitis, or tuberculous peritonitis. If no pelvic mass is palpated and the origin of the ascites is unclear, the ascites should be drained (and examined cytologically) to facilitate the pelvic examination. Chest X-ray is routine. Pleural fluid should also be removed and evaluated cytologically. The contrast urogram will identify ureteral anomalies and urinary obstruction which aid in the surgical phase of treatment.

Numerous studies have demonstrated the value of preoperative serum CA-125 measurements in identifying patients with pelvic malignancy.[52,111,126,189] In a series of 182 gynecology patients with a pelvic mass, Vasilev et al found that 77.8% of the 18 patients with malignant tumors (11 primary ovarian, 4 metastatic to ovary and 3 leiomyosarcomas of the uterus) had CA-125 values above 35 U/ml, while 22% of the 164 benign masses had values above 35 U/ml. The specificity was increased by raising the normal value to 65 U/ml (11.5% of benign masses) but the test sensitivity declined. Specificity was also increased if the diagnosis of malignancy was limited to women older than 50 years. Falsely elevated CA-125 values can be associated with pregnancy, endometriosis, adenomyosis, benign ovarian tumors and inflammatory conditions of the peritoneum, inter alia. Mucinous carcinomas are less likely to cause an elevated CA-125 value (see Ch. 24).

There are a number of special diagnostic studies available which can be of assistance. Tumor imaging by computerized tomography,[173,192] which employs ionizing radiation, and ultrasonography[55,78], which does not, are most useful in the patient with suspicious pelvic signs, or persistent symptoms with a normal pelvic examination, or an inadequate pelvic examination due to a muscular abdominal wall, obesity or ascites. These methods can also be helpful in delineating the mass as uterine or adnexal, cystic or solid. Transvaginal and transrectal ultrasonography may be more useful than transabdominal ultrasound for evaluating the pelvis.[103,181] Other promising techniques for ovarian cancer diagnosis and evaluation are magnetic resonance imaging[114] (Mawhennig et al) and radio-imaging with monoclonal antibodies[102] (see also Chs 19 and 20) Other methods of evaluating the pelvis with doubtful findings are laparoscopy (see Ch. 21), pneumogynography and examination under anesthesia. Much interest has developed in thin needle biopsy of internal lesions, but this method cannot be recommended for the usual case of ovarian carcinoma, since surgery is the primary mode of therapy and a preoperative histologic diagnosis is not often helpful (see Ch. 22). It would be contraindicated in the patient with an ovarian mass of any composition which might be intact and unaccompanied by metastases.

There have been several reports[120,137] on the use of lymphography in detecting metastases to retroperitoneal nodes from ovarian malignancy (see Ch. 18). These studies show that the method is capable of identifying metastases, that the incidence in advanced disease is high, and that frequently both pelvic and aortic nodes are involved, but that there is a predominance of pelvic nodal disease (Table 56.6).

Table 56.6 The frequency of retroperitoneal lymph node metastasis by lymphography in ovarian carcinoma*

Stage	Total cases	Cases positive (%)
I	51	4 (8)
II	10	0 (0)
III	90	26 (29)
IV	15	8 (53)
Recurrent	99	46 (46)
Restaging NED**	24	4 (17)

* From: Musumeci, Banfi, Bolis et al (1977)[120]
** Restaging NED = patients re-operated on to determine the status of disease when there is no clinical evidence of cancer after completing therapy.

PROGNOSTIC FEATURES

Stage

The FIGO stage grouping for ovarian carcinoma is presented in Table 56.7. It is apparent that the FIGO Cancer Committee believes that the following features may have an adverse effect on prognosis: malignant cells in the peritoneal cavity, surface excrescences, ruptured capsule,

Table 56.7 Carcinoma of ovary: FIGO staging*

Stage	Criteria
Stage I	Growth limited to the ovaries
Ia	Growth limited to one ovary; no ascites No tumor on the external surfaces; capsule intact
Ib	Growth limited to both ovaries; no ascites No tumor on the external surfaces; capsules intact
Ic**	Tumor either Stage Ia or Ib, but with tumor on surface of one or both ovaries; or with capsule ruptured; or with ascites present containing malignant cells or with positive peritoneal washings
Stage II	Growth involving one or both ovaries with pelvic extension
IIa	Extension and/or metastases to the uterus and/or tubes
IIb	Extension to other pelvic tissues
IIc**	Tumor either Stage IIa or IIb, but with tumor on surface on one or both ovaries; or with capsule(s) ruptured; or with ascites present containing malignant cells or with positive peritoneal washings
Stage III	Tumor involving one or both ovaries with peritoneal implants outside the pelvis and/or positive retroperitoneal or inguinal nodes. Superficial liver metastasis equals Stage III Tumor is limited to the true pelvis but with histologically-proven malignant extension to small bowel or omentum
IIIa	Tumor grossly limited to the true pelvis with negative nodes but with histologically confirmed microscopic seeding of abdominal peritoneal surfaces
IIIb	Tumor involving one or both ovaries with histologically confirmed implants of abdominal peritoneal surfaces none exceeding 2 cm in diameter. Nodes are negative
IIIc	Abdominal implants greater than 2 cm in diameter and/or positive retroperitoneal or inguinal nodes
Stage IV	Growth involving one or both ovaries with distant metastases. If pleural effusion is present there must be positive cytology to allot a case to Stage IV

* From: Annual Report Gynecologic Cancer FIGO, Vol. 20 (1988)[4]
** In order to evaluate the impact on prognosis of the different criteria for allotting cases to Stage Ic or IIc it would be of value to know:
1. If the source of malignant cells detected was a) peritoneal washings or b) ascites
2. If rupture of the capsule was a) spontaneous or b) caused by the surgeon

involvement of both ovaries; involvement of the uterus, tubes or other pelvic structures; abdominal metastases and their size; positive retroperitoneal nodes or extension to the small bowel or omentum (even within the pelvis); distant metastases including parenchymal liver metastases; and pleural effusion with positive cytology. The stage is assigned on the basis of clinical and surgical findings, the final histology, and the cytology of peritoneal fluid. Peritoneal cytology based on washings in the absence of ascites is also part of the standard staging procedure. Once the stage group has been assigned it cannot be changed. When there is doubt, the lower or earlier stage is assigned.

The FIGO Cancer Committee recommends that the clinical staging of ovarian carcinoma be based upon the findings at laparotomy, as well as the usual clinical examination and roentgenological studies. Thus, surgery with resection of the ovarian tumor and hysterectomy with biopsy of all suspicious sites, such as omentum, mesentery, liver, diaphragm, pelvic nodes and aortic nodes, form the basis for staging. The final histologic and cytologic data are to be considered in the staging, as are clinical studies, including chest X-ray and CT scan.

It has been a longstanding practice of many surgeons[118,138,141] to remove the greater omentum as part of the surgical management of ovarian carcinoma. Some have recommended routine appendectomy[118] and, more recently, excision of peritoneal patches, random diaphragmatic biopsy and routine sampling of pelvic and aortic retroperitoneal nodes.[41a] In one report on the results of extended surgical staging, 8 of 49 (15%) of apparent Stage I cases were upstaged and 22 of 51 (43%) of apparent Stage II cases were upstaged.[205] The Gynecology Oncology Group (GOG) ovarian carcinoma staging study found in nearly 100 apparent Stage I cases, that 1% or fewer had a positive random diaphragm biopsy, omentectomy or pelvic node sampling, while 4% had subclinical aortic node involvement and about 15% positive peritoneal cytology. Overall, 9 of 97 cases were upstaged.[21] Thus, the most fruitful studies at surgery that have not been a standard of practice are peritoneal cytology and aortic node biopsies.

A common problem in staging ovarian cancer is that of adhesions. Kottmeier[99] recommended that fixation of small bowel or omentum to the ovarian tumor (whether to the ovary itself or tumor implanted on some other pelvic structure) represents 'tumor adherent to surrounding organs, not primary disease above the pelvis', i.e. Stage IIb. To qualify for Stage III, there must be histologic documentation of tumor involving these organs. Kottmeier also considers a tumor incompletely removed if there are firm adhesions, and microscopic examination shows extracapsular extension of tumor. He could not demonstrate, however, any difference in outcome between the adherent tumor and the free tumor with visible pelvic metastases. Dembo et al[45] found only adherence and grade to be significant adverse features of Stage I ovarian carcinoma.

A systematic visual and palpatory exploration of the abdomen and pelvis is the single most important aspect of surgically defining the extent of disease. The patient with no obvious metastases must be examined most thoroughly. The parietes, the large and small bowel and the omentum are carefully evaluated. Also assessed are the liver, diaphragm, the umbilical recess, the retroperitoneal nodes, pancreas, colon, stomach and biliary structures. If the ovarian lesions are consistent with Krukenberg cancer or mucinous tumors, the gastrointestinal examination is even more crucial. The pelvic culs de sac, the uterus and tubes, both sides of the sigmoid colon, and the round and broad

ligament peritoneum are inspected and palpated. If adhesions are present, they must be lysed to assure the absence of metastases buried by the adherent structures.

In the absence of ascites and obvious tumor spread, washings are taken from the pelvis and abdomen for cytology. Even with apparent metastatic disease, biopsies are needed and frozen section may be helpful. Tuberculous peritonitis, endometriosis, granulomatous disease secondary to a ruptured dermoid cyst or talc, implants of benign ovarian tumors, or suture granulomas are among the many conditions that mimic carcinomatous spread. Biopsy of the diaphragm has been recommended,[41a] but it is not reported whether this is more accurate than cytology or palpation. Certainly, any lesion suspicious of cancer needs to be biopsied when spread is not obvious and extensive.

The therapeutic benefit of partial or total omentectomy is disputed (infra vide). Regardless, it is a common site of metastasis and is resectable with relative impunity. At least partial excision is recommended. The specimen needs careful microscopic examination. The peritoneum can be studied for occult involvement by taking strips or patches from the anterior parietes, the paracolic gutters and the posterior cul de sac. While their value is unknown, this is probably useful in restaging the more advanced cases after chemotherapy. Banfi et al[7] have recommended routine excision of the ovarian vascular pedicle. The high frequency with which ovarian carcinoma involves the retroperitoneal lymphatics suggests lymph node evaluation in apparently early stage disease (FIGO I and II) might be warranted. However, the documented incidence of pelvic node metastasis is very low in apparent Stage I cases (none in 106 cases, combining the GOG data[21] with Burghardt et al[22]) compared to 17% for 47 Stage II cases. Aortic node involvement in the GOG study was 4.2% and 19.5% for apparent Stages I and II respectively. Thus, node sampling is highly productive when there is pelvic spread of cancer. Palpable nodes should be excised for study in all but the most advanced cases.

Grade

Although not part of the stage, the influence histologic grade can have on overall survival in any series of patients treated for ovarian cancer must not be underrated. In the older literature, the majority of survivors in Stages III and IV may be patients with tumors of low malignant potential (Table 56.8). Other authors support the idea that many, if not most, of the patients with advanced ovarian cancer who survive for long periods have tumors of low malignant potential or well differentiated carcinomas. Munnell[117] noted that of 13 patients with FIGO Stage III disease who survived 5 or more years, 7 had a borderline or Grade I tumor. Elahi and colleagues[54] reported twelve 5-year survivors with advanced ovarian carcinoma (10 Stage III, 2 Stage II). Six were Grade 1 ('differentiated tumors with one to several

Table 56.8 Ovarian carcinoma. 5-year survival for borderline[a] and true carcinomas

FIGO Stage	I				II				III and IV			
	Borderline tumors		True carcinomas		Borderline tumors		True carcinomas		Borderline tumors		True carcinomas	
Author	Cases	Alive 5 years (%)	Cases	Alive 5 years (%)	Cases	Alive 5 years (%)	Cases	Alive 5 years (%)	Cases	Alive 5 years (%)	Cases	Alive 5 years (%)
Grönroos[70]	35	(91)	24	(54)	8	(50)	27	(11)	5	(100)	14	(14.0)
Obel[125]	51	(96)	105	(72)	8	(88)	46	(28)	2	(50)	85	(2.4)
Julian[90]	5	(100)	28	(75)	6	(100)	29	(24)	13	(62)	76	(2.6)
Kottmeier[99]	90	(88)	162	(60)	38	(92)	225	(42)	30	(70)	314	(5.4)
Aure[5]	138	(97)	292	(65)	20[c]	(d)	214	(30)	6[c]	(d)	320	(9.4)
Annual report[4]	395	(86)	1838	(70)	50	(76)	1265	(45)	62	(69)	4731	(13.6)
Total	714	(91)	2449	(67)	130	(68)	1806	(42)	112	(71)	5540	(14.4)

[a] Most patients received postoperative radiotherapy. Cause of death not usually given.
[b] 10-year survival.
[c] Deleted from total.
[d] Not specified.

layers of epithelial cells'). This group undoubtedly included borderline cases. Obel,[125] in a detailed study of women in Denmark surviving more than 10 years after the diagnosis of ovarian cancer, found that 57 of the 148 study cases (38.5%) were of low malignant potential. Of the 84 patients with Stage III or IV disease, only 3 were alive at 10 years and one of these had a borderline tumor. Numerous more recent studies continue to document the important influence of grade on survival[110,134,172,180] (see Fig. 56.5). Obviously, the efficacy of any therapy must be assessed in the light of this information.

Age

As discussed on page 889, the prognosis of ovarian carcinoma is related to patient age because younger women are more likely to have lower stage and better differentiated cancers. However, age also seems to have an independent prognostic significance. For example, in a study of women with serous carcinoma, Demopoulos et al[45] found that women less than age 50 had a better survival than older women, after correcting for stage and grade differences. Several authors using multivariate analysis have found advancing age to be associated with a significantly worsening prognosis, although this factor is generally less important than residual disease, grade and stage.[18,43a,164a] Others, however, did not find age to be prognostic by multivariate analysis.[77,183b]

Other prognostic factors

Performance status is frequently reported to be correlated with survival in ovarian cancer patients,[77,183b] as is histologic type, especially clear cell carcinoma which has a poorer prognosis than the more common varieties. The relationship between ovarian carcinoma cytosol estrogen and progestin receptor levels and prognosis is uncertain, although one or both are found in more than half the cases. It appears, however, that the presence of estrogen receptor may have little prognostic significance. Regarding progestin receptor content, Schwartz et al[167] noted that patients with receptor-rich tumors had a more favorable prognosis in early stage disease, but a worse prognosis in advanced stage disease. Kuhnel et al[100] noted that well differentiated endometrioid carcinomas more often contained progestin receptor than poorly differentiated tumors, a situation similar to endometrial carcinoma, and presumably predictive of hormone responsiveness.

Another prognostic parameter of ovarian tumors is DNA content. Friedlander et al[57] studied the nuclear DNA content of ovarian carcinomas and found a significant as-

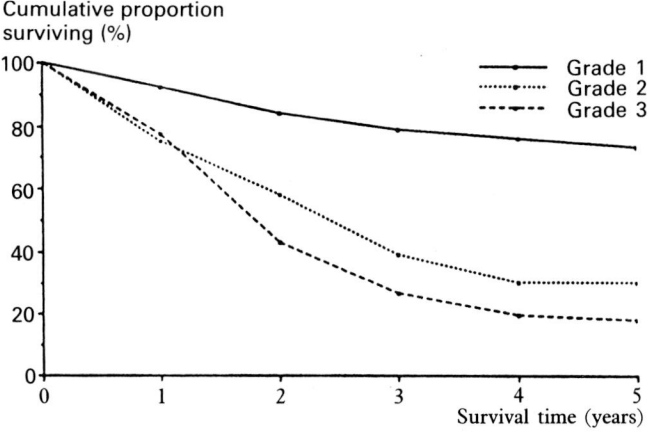

Fig. 56.5 Obviously malignant serous carcinoma of the ovary Stage IIIb, 1979–1981. Life table presentation by histological grade. From Annual Report Vol. 20, p. 125. Reprinted with permission.

sociation of ploidy with stage, but not grade, for obviously malignant tumors. All diploid tumors were early stage, and all late stage (III and IV) tumors were aneuploid. However, 40% of early stage tumors were also aneuploid. In their study, there were only three borderline tumors, all early stage and all diploid. In a study of the DNA content of early stage serous tumors, Erhardt et al[54a] found the DNA content of borderline tumors to be slightly higher, but within the limits of normal proliferating cells. The well differentiated invasive cancers had DNA patterns usually resembling those of the borderline tumors, while the Grade 2 and 3 tumors generally had a high, scattered DNA content. Nevertheless, no clearcut demarcation was possible between borderline and benign or malignant serous tumors (see also Ch. 6).

SURGICAL THERAPY

General principles

The cornerstone of any scheme of management for ovarian malignancy is necessarily surgery. Not only is surgery the most effective treatment, but it plays a primary role in establishing the diagnosis and determining the extent of the malignancy which form the basis upon which adjunctive therapy can most accurately be planned.

The basic principle of surgical therapy for ovarian carcinoma is to remove the primary lesion and all metastases without putting the patient's life in immediate jeopardy. For unilateral ovarian carcinoma the adjacent tube is removed since it may be a site of metastasis. This gives maximum information without compromising the patient's fertility (assuming the other tube is normal). When fertility is not a consideration the opposite adnexa and uterus are also removed. The remaining ovary is excised because (a) it is expendable even if no other treatment is planned; (b) occult metastatic or primary carcinoma is frequently present; (c) there is a relatively high risk of a carcinoma developing eventually in the uninvolved ovary. For these reasons, even though studies have not demonstrated a clear superiority of results with unilateral versus bilateral oophorectomy, the procedure is standard. Removal of the uterus also has its controversial aspects, but is generally recommended as part of the treatment in resectable ovarian cancer because it is a common site for lymphatic metastases, there is often a coexistent endometrial primary, there may be serosal implants, the organ is dispensable when fertility is not a consideration, it can usually be removed with little risk, patients with ovarian cancer have a propensity to develop at a later date other müllerian primaries (endometrium, cervix),★ and it is easier to assess the pelvis on

<hr>

★Obel[125] found that of 103 women with ovarian carcinoma surviving 10 or more years and who had their uterus preserved, 10 developed endometrial carcinoma and 6 cervical carcinoma.

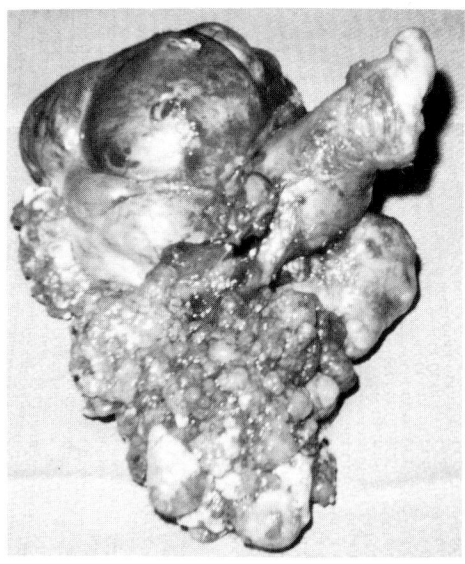

Fig. 56.6 The uterus is encased by a papillary serous carcinoma. The cervix is pointing to the upper right. Even though the patient had numerous abdominal metastases hysterectomy was performed to facilitate removal of the bulk of the neoplastic mass prior to chemotherapy (cytoreductive surgery).

follow-up examinations with the uterus absent. Even in the presence of unresectable abdominal metastases, removal of the uterus may be warranted when removal will contribute significantly to tumor reduction (Fig. 56.6) or the patient has been bleeding from the uterus, or the ovaries are small and there is reason to believe the primary might be endometrial. In cases of advanced ovarian cancer, supracervical hysterectomy is sometimes advisable because of its simplicity and the improbability that excising the cervix will have any therapeutic value.

Cytoreductive surgery

The surgical management of the patient with advanced ovarian carcinoma often requires fine judgement and considerable skill (see Chs 82 and 83). In the early cases, outcome will be more a consequence of adequate surgical staging and postoperative adjuvant therapy, but in cases with more advanced disease the curability is more dependent upon the surgeon's ability to maximally reduce the tumor burden (Table 56.9). Aure et al[5] reporting from the Norwegian Radium Hospital, noted a 5-year survival rate of 55% versus 18% in Stage II, and 30% versus 8% in Stage III resectable and incompletely resected true carcinomas of the ovary employing a variety of radiation therapy (RT) methods. From the same institution, Welander[198] observed in a subsequent study a 24% survival at 5 years for resectable cases versus 7% for incompletely resected cases of Stage III ovarian cancer employing 5000 rads (cGy) whole

Table 56.9 Influence of resectability on ovarian carcinoma survival

| Author | FIGO stage | 5-year survival | | | |
| | | Residual carcinoma | | No residual carcinoma | |
		Total cases	(%)	Total cases	(%)
Barr[10]	IIb	30	(13)	21	(29)
Fuks[58]	IIb	50	(46)	16	(67)
Aure[5]	II	141	(18)	71	(55)
Bush[25]	Ib & II	48	(52)	77	(75)[a]
Delclos[42]	II	6	(33)	18	(72)[b]
Aure[5]	III	191	(8)	34	(30)
Bush[25]	III (asymptomatic)	48	(33)	10	(70)[c]
Delclos[42]	III	24	(8)	20	(25)[b]
Zylberberg[209]	IIb & III	28	(13)	14	(25)
Welander[198]	III	73	(7)	78	(24)
Griffiths[68]	III	26	9.5 months	19	26 months[d]

[a] 4-year follow-up.
[b] Palpable residual vs. non-palpable residual disease.
[c] 3-year follow-up.
[d] Mean survival time.

abdomen irradiation. Delclos & Fletcher[42] at the M. D. Anderson Hospital noted that 72% (13/18) of Stage II cases with non-palpable disease after surgery (serous carcinoma) and 33% (2/6) with palpable disease postoperatively survived 4 years after radiotherapy. For Stage III cases the survival figures were 25% (5/20) and 8.3% (2/24). On the other hand, Parker et al[138] found no statistically significant difference in the 5-year survival of Stage III patients completely resected (1 of 9) versus incompletely resected (7.5% of 136). In a preliminary analysis by Bush et al[25] of a randomized study of treatment for ovarian carcinoma, 52% (25/48) of Stages Ib and II patients were clinically free of disease although they had postsurgical residual tumor, compared with 75% (58/77) of the completely resected group. For asymptomatic patients with Stage III disease, the corresponding figures were 33% (16/48) and 70% (7/10). They found no difference in treatment results of either stage relative to residual disease if the cases were analyzed according to the completeness of the surgery, i.e. whether or not they had a total hysterectomy and bilateral salpingo-oophorectomy. In a randomized trial, the Gynecologic Oncology Group (GOG) compared various combinations of radiation therapy and chemotherapy in Stage III ovarian carcinoma.[19] Among 106 evaluable cases, those with ≤3 cm residual masses had a significantly longer progression free interval and survival time than those with larger disease (respective medians were 11.8 vs 7.3 months and 28.5 vs 15.7 months). Approximately 40% of the cases were considered to have residual disease ≤3 cm in size.

Munnell[118] has championed what he terms the 'maximal surgical effort' based on improved results attributed to this policy. He defines this surgical approach as a 'maximal, tedious, careful, painstaking effort . . . carried out by aggressive, persistent, persevering surgeons'. The implication is clear that he is not necessarily talking about radical surgery, but rather, as in the case of tubovarian abscesses, the experienced, persistent surgeon can often resect the ovarian carcinoma which the dilettante might simply biopsy and close. In a study of 102 patients with Stage II and III ovarian carcinoma, Griffiths employed a multivariate analysis to control potentially confounding variables in order to assess the effect of surgical resection on survival.[67] While survival was significantly related to the size of the largest residual mass, there was no difference in survival among patients with masses greater than 1.5 cm in diameter. The experience of Wharton & Herson[199] is similar. The most aggressive surgery, then, should be reserved for those cases in which all or nearly all of the gross tumor can be excised. It is this group of patients who stand to gain most by extending the surgical procedure to include resection of adjacent viscera, provided there is not an excessive risk of fatal complications (see Chs 82 and 83).

Even in the hands of the best operators, many patients will have unresectable ovarian carcinoma. In this situation, the surgeon's responsibility is to establish the correct diagnosis. Whenever possible, the diagnosis of ovarian cancer should be based upon excision of an entire, involved ovary or biopsy of an involved ovary.

Omentectomy

There can be no disputing that the greater omentum is a common site of metastasis from ovarian carcinoma. For this reason, greater omentectomy has been recommended by some authorities as an important part of the surgical treatment of ovarian cancer.[118,138,141] However, total omentectomy is rarely, if ever, done. Furthermore, the omentum in its entirety is subject to implantation metastasis, as are all peritoneal surfaces. Thus, there is little reason to expect that excising the omentum or any part of it will result in a cure. Table 56.10 presents data from several reports comparing survival of patients having and not having omentectomy. None of them is randomized and no conclusions can be drawn. Omentectomy may be valid for reasons other than a curative benefit. It is a common site of metastases and, therefore, may be a valuable site to 'biopsy' although this was not substantiated for Stage I cases by the GOG study (vide supra). Since it is an expendable organ, this is a feasible reason for excision. Omental removal may facilitate the even distribution of radioactive colloids,[36] an important consideration in their use as therapeutic agents. If the gastrocolic ligament is excised, the lesser sac will be more accessible to the radioactive material. Removal of the omentum with gross metastasis may be important as a therapeutic procedure (tumor reductive surgery) and as a palliative, since an omental 'cake' can be very uncomfortable and contribute significantly to the production of ascites. However, removing the normal appearing omentum in the patient with resectable ovarian cancer and ascites will contribute nothing to eliminate the ascites, since the fluid does not reform if the cancer is resected. The suggestion that omentectomy may increase the risk of postoperative bowel obstruction has not been borne out in clinical practice and is, therefore, either not true or a low risk event.

Rupture

Considering the numerous variables which influence outcome in ovarian cancer, it is not expected that the impact of intraoperative rupture from a retrospective review of individual series would establish any inimical effect unless the event were highly fatal. However, it is illogical to believe that the malignant cells and epithelial fragments which are contained in the fluid of these cystic cancers are incapable of producing implants in vivo when they can be grown in tissue culture. Furthermore, the ability of ovarian carcinoma to grow on the peritoneal surfaces of the pelvis and abdomen is well known. The only reason for the surgeon not to accept the potential harm of rupture is that a vertical (and larger), rather than transverse, incision might be necessary, and that more care is required in performing the surgery. For most patients these are hardly justifications for taking the small but undoubted risk that attends spill. That is not to say that in some circumstances whatever risk there is may not be justified or acceptable to the patient. For example, the extremely large ovarian cystic tumors are usually benign mucinous neoplasms. Controlled tapping of such a tumor might be warranted not only to minimize the incision, but also to avoid uncontrolled rupture and to obtain better operative exposure (Figs 56.7 and 56.8).

Conservative surgery

The minimal treatment for ovarian carcinoma is unilateral ovariectomy. Although in the case of smaller cystadenomas enucleation is possible, this should not be attempted if the lesion has demonstrated any of the signs suggestive of malignancy, such as adhesions, necrosis, solid areas, hemorrhage, ascites, papillary excrescences or a multilocular character. Preservation of the involved ovary is not a reasonable alternative in the presence of carcinoma. Adhesions or rupture are also relative contraindications to surgical conservatism.[193] In general, when fertility is desirable and malignancy is suspected, the ovary and tube are removed for pathologic examination before more

Table 56.10 Survival* in ovarian cancer in patients having omentectomy compared with patients not having omentectomy

Author	FIGO stage	Omentectomy		No omentectomy	
		Total cases	(%) alive	Total cases	(%) alive
Munnell[117]	III and IV	52	(27)	84	(11)
Villasanta[190]	Ib to III	56	(33)	108	(32)
Carter[29]	I	21	(86)	2	(0)
	II	1	(100)	8	(50)
Parker[138]	III and IV	8	(25)	11	(0)
	I	21	(81)	25	(48)
Harris[79]	III	94	(2)	56	(9)
	I (surgery)	5	(80)	26	(61)
	I (surgery)	16	(87)	10	(100)

* Not all survival data 5 years. Some reports included non-epithelial ovarian malignancies.

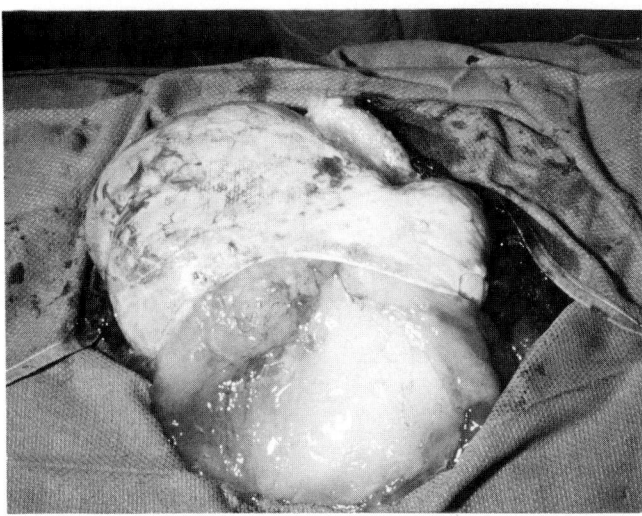

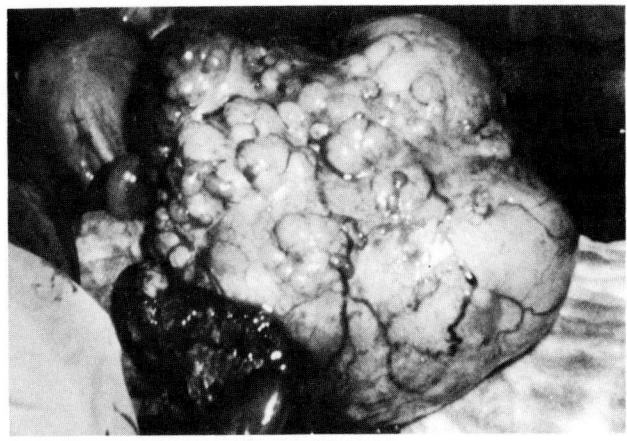

Fig. 56.9 Ovarian neoplasm confined to one ovary, but adherent to the sigmoid colon. The frozen section diagnosis was moderately well differentiated serous carcinoma. Although Stage Ia, all other features were unfavorable for conservative therapy.

Fig. 56.7 Intraoperative rupture of this mucinous cystadenoma resulted from forced delivery through an inadequate incision. Although unilocular, the mass could not have been decompressed because the mucin is too viscous.

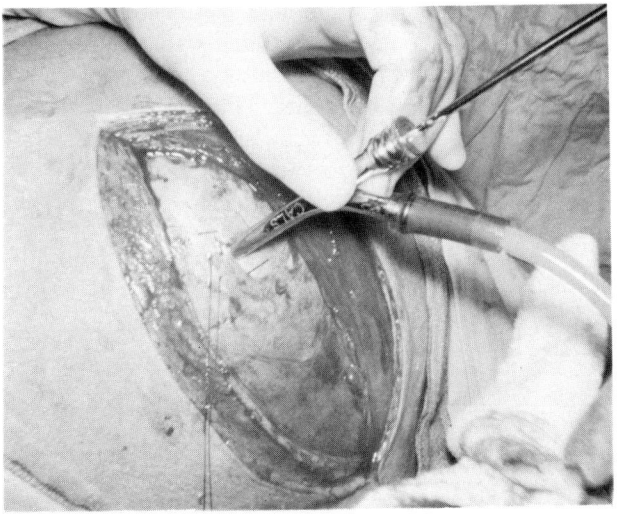

Fig. 56.8 Although this large ovarian neoplasm could have been removed intact by enlarging the vertical incision, the operator elected to aspirate its contents under controlled conditions. Nevertheless, a certain amount of 'spill' is unavoidable.

plasms, cystectomy is the treatment of choice. Partial omentectomy and peritoneal cytology are recommended as part of the staging procedure.

The need for biopsy of the opposite ovary and the risk of leaving it have been debated for years in the gynecologic literature. The propensity for simultaneous occult bilaterality is reasonably well established (Table 56.11). The risk of bilaterality is not, however, as great as suggested by the overall incidence of overt bilaterality among ovarian epithelial tumors. Nor does there seem to be any histologic species exempt from this threat,[201] although the mucinous tumors are generally thought to be a very low risk. The reliability of ovarian biopsy, the optimal means of obtaining the biopsy and the risk to the ovary have not been determined, but there must be some threat of mechanical infertility[195] or ovarian failure.[127] Certainly any abnormality of the contralateral ovary requires histologic evaluation. Because the long term risk for ovarian carcinoma may be significantly higher than that for women in general, it has been recommended that the woman whose fertility has been preserved undergoes sterilization by removal of the residual ovary after her childbearing has been completed.[202] The recommended requirements for conservative

radical surgery is carried out. While the presence of adhesions, rupture and surface tumor (Fig. 56.9) are contraindications to cystectomy, these are factors only if the neoplasm is malignant. Internal papillations strongly suggest the presence of malignancy, although often of a borderline category. If the pathologist is unable to give an unequivocal diagnosis of frank malignancy or borderline histology, conservative surgery is advised until the final pathology review is done. If both ovaries have cystic neo-

Table 56.11 Frequency of occult bilaterality in apparently Stage Ia ovarian carcinoma

Author	Total cases	Occult bilaterality	
		Number	(% of total)
Munnell[119]	134	7	(5)
Williams[201]	54	4*	(7)
Total	188	11	(6)

* Another 5 cases had microscopic benign tumors. Includes only Stage Ia, Grade 1 tumors.

surgical management of epithelial ovarian malignancy are presented in Table 56.12

In attempting to preserve the reproductive potential of young women with early ovarian cancer, an alternative to

Table 56.12 Recommended criteria for conservative surgical therapy in ovarian carcinoma

1. Stage Ia
  a) No ascites
  b) No dense adhesions
  c) No surface excrescences
  d) Unruptured
  e) Unilateral, confined neoplasm

2. Adequate surgical-pathologic evaluation
  a) Borderline or Grade I histology
  b) Negative peritoneal washings
  c) Negative omentum
  d) Negative evaluation of opposite ovary
  e) Negative endometrial biopsy

conservative surgery alone is conservative surgery with adjuvant chemotherapy. This therapy is applicable to Grade 1 cases confined to one ovary, which are ruptured, adherent or extracystic. Adjunctive therapy is also recommended for all unilateral Stage I, Grade 2 or 3 ovarian cancer cases. Therapy should be limited to six cycles in order to minimize the risk of gonadal damage. A second-look procedure is indicated if the initial evaluation was inadequate, but pelvic dissection should be kept to a minimum to avoid causing infertility due to adhesions.

RADIATION THERAPY

Treatment results

Radiation has been employed as an adjuvant to surgery in the management of ovarian carcinoma for over 50 years. At first, it was reserved for the patient with 'inoperable', that is, incompletely resected, cancer. It soon became common practice to administer at least pelvic radiation to patients with resectable disease which was more extensive than Stage Ia or which was ruptured during surgery. Several authors have reviewed the literature over the years[142,157,187,191] to evaluate the efficacy of radiation therapy in ovarian cancer in general, and the epithelial malignancies in particular. In reviewing these papers, there was no obvious survival gradient comparing the earliest reports to later ones. As a number of authors have observed, there is no clear evidence of a therapeutic advantage to the use of radiation therapy in Stages I, III and IV. This may simply reflect the problem of demonstrating in clinical studies the effect of treatment on patients who have a good prognosis without adjuvant therapy (Stage I) or who have a very poor prognosis (Stages III and IV).

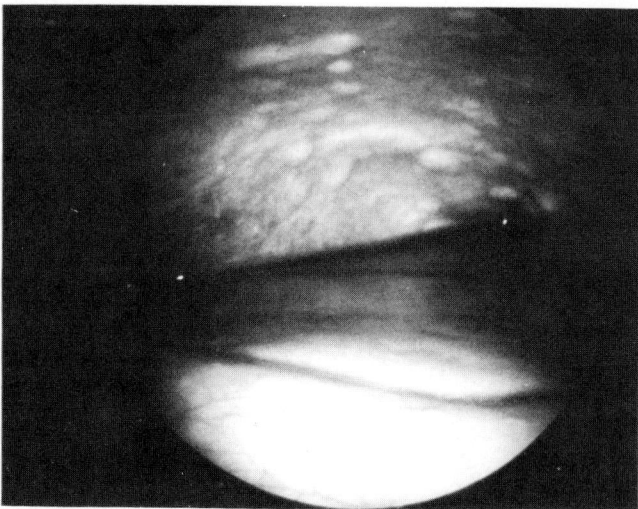

Fig. 56.10 Implants on the diaphragm, as seen in this photograph, and liver surface are common in ovarian carcinoma which has spread to the abdomen. The sensitivity of the liver limits the radiation dose which can be delivered to this important area.

It may also reflect the limitations of abdominal radiation imposed by the radiation sensitivity of the liver and kidneys, especially the liver, since ovarian cancer has a predilection for implanting there (Fig. 56.10).

In the past decade, several randomized clinical trials employing postoperative radiation therapy in ovarian carcinoma have been reported (Table 56.13). These studies

Table 56.13 Ovarian carcinoma: randomized clinical trials employing postoperative radiation therapy

Reference	Postoperative therapy	Recurrent	
		N	(%)
Dembo et al[43b]	No treatment	20	(5)
Stage Ia	Pelvic RT	21	(19)
Hreshychyshyn et al[85]	No treatment	29	(17)
Stages Ia and b	Pelvic RT	23	(23)
	Melphalan	34	(6)
Dembo et al[43b]	Pelvic RT + CHL	51	(22)
Stages I, II, III optimal	WAR strip	50	(45)
Smith et al[178]	WAR strip	70	(37)
Stages I, II, III <3 cm residual	Melphalan	79	(37)
Klaassen et al[94]	WAR strip	107	(38)[b]
Stages I, III[a]	Pelvic RT +	106	(39)[b]
	Melphalan	44	(34)[c]
	Pelvic RT + P[32]		

Abbreviations: RT = radiation therapy; CHL = Chlorambucil; WAR = whole abdomen radiation therapy.
[a] Stage III cases had tumor confined to pelvis
[b] Disease free 5 year survival statistically superior in melphalan arm (P=0.015)
[c] Arm discontinued prematurely because of toxicity.

help to answer some of the questions regarding the contribution of radiation therapy to the treatment of this disease. Both the Gynecologic Oncology Group (GOG) study[85] and the Princess Margaret study[43b] indicate that the results of pelvic radiation therapy after surgery in Stage I ovarian carcinoma are no better, and possibly worse, than those obtained with no further treatment. Combining these studies, 110 of 127 cases were Stage Ia, of which more than half were Grade I. While the overall Stage Ia recurrence rate in the two series was 13.6%, in the Stage Ia, Grade 1 group, only 2 of 51 malignancies (3.9%) recurred. This supports the long-held opinion that these patients need no treatment as an adjunct to surgery. However, the prognosis for the Stage Ia, Grade 2 and 3 cases without postoperative treatment, or with pelvic radiation therapy, was not so favorable; approximately 25% experienced recurrence after 3 to 5 years of follow-up.

Using a multivariate analysis, Dembo et al in a later report from the Princess Margaret Hospital[45], found that only grade and adherence were significantly associated with the risk of relapse in a series of 252 Stage I invasive ovarian carcinomas. There were 6 relapses among 103 Grade 1 cases, compared to 42 of 146 (29%) Grade 2 and 3 cases. Relapse with dense adhesions was twice that for cases with minor or no adhesions, 8 of 23 (35%) versus 32 of 222 (17%). In this study, it is of interest that postoperative treatment did not significantly correlate with the risk of relapse. Nevertheless, these studies identify the Stage Ia cases needing adjuvant therapy: Grades 2 and 3, and cases with densely adherent tumors.

There have been no randomized studies comparing whole abdomen radiation therapy (WAR) to no further treatment, but the Princess Margaret study of favorable Stage II ovarian carcinomas found a statistically superior relapse-free 5-year actuarial survival with strip whole abdomen radiation therapy (79%), compared to pelvic radiation only (51%).[43b,44] Klaassen et al[94], however, reported that melphalan plus pelvic radiation was superior to WAR alone. In another randomized study, Dembo et al (1984) compared strip to open-field whole abdomen radiation therapy.[43a] No statistically significant differences were found for the 5-year actuarial survival in the two treatment groups. Furthermore, while the acute toxicity was similar in the two groups, there were more serious late complications with the strip technique. These data indicate that whole abdomen radiation therapy is superior to pelvic radiation therapy only, for treating ovarian cancer, and the open field technique is preferable to the strip method.

Randomized studies utilizing intraperitoneal radioactive colloidal gold plus pelvic radiation versus pelvic radiation only have been reported from the Norwegian Radium Hospital.[6,97] There were significantly fewer tumor deaths in the Stage I patients receiving intraperitoneal gold than in the pelvic radiation group (Stage I: 15% of 87 cases

versus 24% of 88 cases). For Stage II cases, there were fewer cancer deaths in the gold group, but the difference, which occurred primarily in the residual disease cases, was not statistically significant. Because of a high serious complication rate in the gold plus pelvic radiation therapy cases (23 of 198, 8 deaths), this treatment is not recommended by the authors, despite its apparent therapeutic superiority. Intraperitoneal P[32] is unfortunately also attended by a high serious complication rate[95,145], despite the fact that, unlike gold, it does not have any gamma radiation (Table 56.14). A randomized study of surgically-staged

Table 56.14 Comparison of ^{198}Au and $Cr^{32}PO_4$*

Feature	^{198}Au	$Cr^{32}PO_4$**
Emission	Beta and gamma	Beta
Energy of beta (MeV)	0.331	0.690
Maximum penetration of beta (mm)	3.8	8.0
Average penetration of beta (mm)	0.7	2.5
Beta dose rate (rads/g/Ci)	76	885
Half-life (days)	2.69	14.3
Usual dose (Ci)	150	15

* From: Julian, Inalsingh & Burnett (1978)[91]
** P[32]: Chromic phosphate

early ovarian carcinoma patients was conducted by the GOG and National Cancer Institute (NCI).[204] One hundred and forty-eight patients (Stages I to II, exclusive of Ia and Ib, G1, G2) were randomized to receive either melphalan for 12 cycles or intraperitoneal P[32]. Disease free survival was about 80% in both arms. In the P[32] group, one patient had bacterial peritonitis and four required surgery for bowel obstruction. One patient in the melphalan arm died with preleukemia. Others[150,153] have reported results using P[32] as postoperative adjuvant therapy in ovarian cancer, and concluded that, for properly selected cases, it is effective, safe and inexpensive. Contraindications to its use are macroscopic residual disease, extensive adhesions, prior abdominal or pelvic radiation and the desire to preserve fertility.

The only contemporary study of advanced ovarian cancer comparing surgery to surgery plus radiotherapy is that of Zylberberg et al.[209] The study is not randomized. Most patients had Stage III disease (a few IIb) with either little or no gross residual tumor. The regime was not described in detail, but presumably the radiation encompassed the entire abdomen. If these two groups are comparable it is surprising that the surgery-only group did so well (17% of 35 patients alive at 5 years) and the radiation therapy group did so poorly (19% of 42 patients alive at 5 years).

Site of failure

Site of recurrence or failure following adjuvant radiation therapy has been reported in detail for one large series of patients with ovarian carcinoma (Table 56.15). The failure site in 52 (21.6%) was pelvic only, in 5 (2.1%) there were distant metastases only, and in the remaining 183 (76.2%) the recurrences were abdominal, usually with pelvic and occasionally distant metastases. It is interesting that even in Stage I cases, where microscopic residual tumor is the target of adjuvant therapy, the ratio of pelvic to abdominal failures is similar to that for Stage III cases. Hintz et al[80] found a similar incidence of failures in the abdomen and pelvis with relatively few patients recurring in both sites. Recurrence in the retroperitoneal nodes only is rarely reported.[37]

Table 56.15 Site of recurrence of ovarian cancer (post-radiation therapy)[a]

Site of recurrence	Number of cases by stage and site				
	I	II	III	IV	Total
Pelvic only	4	30	16	2	52
Abdomen only	4	6	13	0	23
Pelvis and abdomen	8	29	92	6	134
Pelvis, abdomen and DM[b]	1	10	8	2	21
DM only	0	3	1	1	5
Abdomen or pelvis plus DM	0	3	1	1	5
Total	17	81	130	12	240

From: Rutledge (1976)[161]
[a] DM = Distant metastases

CHEMOTHERAPY

The treatment of advanced ovarian carcinoma with cytotoxic drugs has been a standard practice for three decades, but only in the past 15 years has this therapy been subjected to intense evaluation. The early results of numerous clinical trials demonstrate a remarkable similarity in the clinical features of patients most likely to have a prolonged, objective benefit from chemotherapy.[47,69,133,194] Studies indicate that patients with bulky disease, or slowly growing malignancies or who are in poor health will be less responsive. In addition, failure after prior radiation therapy or chemotherapy make it less likely that a good effect will be obtained. There is little evidence that tissue type per se among the epithelial tumors has any substantial influence on their sensitivity to chemotherapy. Results of clinical trials must be evaluated in several aspects to make a proper assessment of their worth to the patient. While residual measurable disease defines a population relatively easy to evaluate for response, i.e. tumor regression, this variable does not

necessarily correlate with the patient-oriented objectives of improved function, attenuation of symptoms and prolonged life.

The collective experience of organized clinical trials has recognized the need for standardizing study end points and the means by which they are calculated. Table 56.16

Table 56.16 Objective response criteria for chemotherapy trials in ovarian carcinoma — measurable lesions

Grade of response	Definition
Complete (CR)	Disappearance of all evidence of disease for a minimum of one month.
Partial (PR)	≥50% reduction in the product of the two larger diameters of each tumor mass for at least one month.
Stable (SD)	No change in the measurement of any tumor mass; or a measurable reduction which does not meet the criteria for a partial response; or a measurable increase which does not meet the criteria for progression.
Progression (PD)	≥50% increase in the product of the two larger diameters of any tumor mass, or the appearance of a new lesion.

presents commonly used definitions of the various levels or grades of objective response. Perhaps more important is the measurement of survival as an indicator of benefit to the patient. The general experience that a small percentage of women with advanced ovarian carcinoma can be cured by chemotherapy has led to more aggressive efforts to effectively treat ovarian cancer with drugs. Accompanying this effort has been a corresponding increase in what is considered to be an acceptable risk to the patient. The evolution of cytotoxic therapy has been one of combining effective agents, preferably with divergent modes of action and toxicities, and administering them in sometimes complex schedules in order to produce a larger fractional kill of the tumor cells. The success of drug therapy in advanced ovarian carcinoma has led also to the use of active agents to treat early cases with presumed residual microscopic disease. It thus becomes even more important to determine as reliably as possible the patient benefit. The reported activity of standard and investigational drugs is presented in Table 56.17.

Early ovarian carcinoma

The GOG randomized study of postoperative Stage I ovarian carcinoma indicates that patients who receive melphalan have a better prognosis than those who receive pelvic radiation or no further treatment. The M.D. Anderson Hospital randomized trial[178] found melphalan to be as

Table 56.17 Advanced ovarian carcinoma. Objective response rates in chemotherapy trials with single agents

Reference	Drug	CR + PR	
		Total cases	%
Thigpen[185]	Alkylating agents[a]	1419	45
	Cyclophosphamide[b]	45	80
	Cisplatin	190	32
	Adriamycin (Doxorubicin)	102	33
	Hexamethylmelamine	215	24
	5-Fluorouracil	126	29
	Methotrexate	34	18
	Mitoxantrone	40	25
	Carboplatin	82	24
	Iproplatin	89	36
	Ifosfamide	61	79
	Prednimustine	36	28
	Dihydroxybusulfan	26	27
	Galactitol	39	15
	Mitomycin	49	16
Kuhnle[101]	Etoposide	111	31

CR = Complete clinical response;
PR = Partial clinical response
[a] Melphalan, Cyclophosphamide, Leukeran
[b] "High dose"

effective as, and less toxic than, strip whole abdomen radiation therapy in the postoperative treatment of women with Stage I, II or III optimal (<3 cm residual masses) ovarian carcinoma. The Princess Margaret study of optimal Stage I, II and III cases found strip whole abdomen radiation therapy to be significantly superior to pelvic radiation therapy plus chlorambucil,[43b] while Young et al,[205] in a preliminary report, observed no survival difference (median follow-up, 26 months) among patients with Stage Ia, Grade 1 and 2 ovarian carcinoma treated postoperatively with melphalan or followed without further therapy. Forty percent of their 56 patients, however, had borderline histology. They also reported a study of the 101 higher-risk Stage I, plus Stage II resectable patients who were randomized to receive melphalan or intraperitoneal P[32] with a median follow up of 31 months. The relapse rate in each arm was 12%. Six percent of the P[32] patients experienced severe abdominal complications.

These studies, on balance, point to the superiority of chemotherapy to radiation therapy in the treatment of resectable ovarian carcinoma. The comparative data are limited but, certainly for short-term chemotherapy, the toxicity and expense are less, while the efficacy appears to be similar to that of whole abdomen radiation therapy, with the exception of the Princess Margaret study. The observation of Potish & Twiggs[151] is relevant here. They found that the rate of radiation therapy complications increased sharply with decreasing midplane depth, while the risk of leukemia, which is related to total drug dose, increased with patient weight. Thus, the thin woman may be more suited to chemotherapy and the stout one to radiation therapy.

Advanced ovarian carcinoma

Turning to the more advanced stages of ovarian carcinoma, a profusion of randomized and non-randomized trials have been conducted in the last decade, testing single-agent and multi-agent chemotherapy, usually involving adriamycin (doxorubicin), cyclophosphamide, 5-fluorouracil, hexamethylmelamine, melphalan, and cisplatin.[12,20,28,41b,48,49,71,116,122,128,129,165,186] The introduction of cisplatin has probably had a greater impact on the treatment of ovarian carcinoma in recent years than any other single event. Unfortunately, its gastrointestinal effects, neurotoxicity and nephrotoxicity have seriously limited its usefulness, leading to concerted clinical research seeking means of reducing these adverse effects by manipulating the schedule, using more effective anti-emetics, and developing less toxic platinum salts, such as carboplatin and CHIP. These efforts have been successful to a considerable degree.

The results of the randomized clinical trials of chemotherapy in advanced ovarian carcinoma have established the superiority of combination chemotherapy to single alkylating-agent therapy with respect to inducing complete clinical remission (CR), a response which confers some potential for cure. In the National Cancer Institute (NCI),[206] GOG,[129] and Milan[112] trials, the combination drug arms also had a higher frequency of surgically-confirmed, complete responses. Furthermore, the median duration of survival in the NCI combination drug arm (29 months) was significantly better than that of the melphalan arm (17 months). There was no statistically significant survival difference, however, in either of the GOG studies, despite the better rate of complete response in the combination drug treatment arm and the longer survival of the complete remission patients (the median survival period in months was 21.4, 12.3, 11.5, and 4.2 for the complete remission, partial remission, stable disease and increasing disease categories, respectively).

A few trials have suggested that cyclophosphamide plus cisplatin is as effective as the combination with adriamycin. Not all the evidence is in agreement, but deleting the adriamycin is attractive because of its cardiac toxicity and because of the constant hazard of tissue necrosis accompanying extravasation. There have now been three major studies comparing cyclophosphamide, adriamycin and cisplatin (CAP) to cyclophosphamide and cisplatin (CP) in ovarian cancer, and the results are mixed. In the Italian study, CAP was superior to CP (and P alone) in terms of pathological response rates (complete plus partial) and progression-free survival (PFI), but not complete pathologic response or disease-free survival. However, the CP and P doses were the same as in CAP; thus, the regimens were not equitoxic and the CP dose could, therefore, have been increased. Bertlesen et al[17b] similarly reported an advantage for CAP over CP utilizing the same doses of CP in each regimen. In the 350-patient GOG study, CAP and CP were compared at equitoxic doses.[128] No significant difference was observed in PFI or survival, although the CAP patients did slightly better.

It is conceivable that, for example, patients with endometrioid carcinoma will need adriamycin as part of their therapy, but none of the studies compared results among the histologic subtypes. While CAP should still be considered the standard chemotherapy for ovarian carcinoma, one should not hesitate to delete the adriamycin when there are compelling reasons to do so (heart disease, suboptimal venous access, patient intolerance, etc.). A summary treatment plan for epithelial ovarian carcinoma is presented in Table 56.18, and the recommended chemotherapy regimens are in Table 56.19.

Table 56.18 Treatment plan for epithelial carcinoma of the ovary

Tumor	Treatment plan
Borderline tumors	
Stage I, IIa	USO or TAH-BSO, depending on reproductive status. No adjuvant therapy.
Stage IIb to III	Complete surgery; tumor-reductive surgery. If implants invasive, give chemotherapy (CP). Otherwise monitor for progression.
True carcinomas	
Stage Ia, Grade 1 without dense adhesions	USO or TAH-BSO, depending on reproductive status. No adjuvant therapy.
All other Stage I, IIa, and resectable IIb	1. CAP[a] or CP for 6 to 12 cycles; or 2. Whole abdomen radiation therapy; or 3. Intraperitoneal P[32]
All other cases	CAP or CP for 6 cycles. Second look. Continue chemotherapy for 6 cycles postsurgery if surgical CR or microscopic residual disease occurs.

USO = unilateral salpingo-oophorectomy; TAH-BSO = total abdominal hysterectomy and bilateral salpingo-oophorectomy; CP = cylcophosphamide and cisplatin; CAP = cyclophosphamide, adriamycin, and cisplatin; CR = complete response; PR = partial response.
[a] Some patients are disinclined or medically unsuited to take such toxic chemotherapy. Melphalan should be offered to them.

Table 56.19 Recommended drugs and doses for first line chemotherapy of ovarian carcinoma.

Drug	Dose	
	CAP	CP
Cyclophosphamide (C)	500 mg/m^2	750 to 1000 mg/m^2
Adriamycin (A)	50 mg/m^2	
Cisplatin (P)	50 mg/m^2	50 to 100 mg/m^2
All drugs given IV on day 1 every 21 days as toxicity permits		

Intraperitoneal chemotherapy

The rationale and status of intraperitoneal (IP) chemotherapy of ovarian carcinoma has been reviewed by several authors.[83,113,154] The demonstration that intraperitoneal administration of certain common oncocidal chemicals can produce local concentrations many times greater than can be achieved in the serum, has led to an intense investigation of this mode of therapy during the past decade. The agents which have received the greatest attention are cisplatin alone,[73] cisplatin with various combinations of cytarabine, adriamycin and bleomycin,[84,147] and cisplatin plus etoposide.[83] The mean area under the curve (AVC) ratio for IP cisplatin versus IV cisplatin is 12. The AVC ratios for other agents are: etoposide 65, melphalan 65, 5-FU 367 and bleomycin 7. The usefulness of certain agents (adriamycin, mitomycin C) is seriously limited because of the attendant chemical peritonitis. The success of IP chemotherapy is limited by the tumor volume, because direct tumor penetration by IP drugs is very superficial. Extensive adhesions also militate against success of this regimen.

The specific details of treatment vary considerably but, in general, subjects have been patients with small residual disease at the time of second-look assessment laparotomy. A totally implantable access system is placed at the time of surgery, and chemotherapy begun as soon as feasible postoperatively (the totally implantable device has sharply reduced the infection risk). The treatment course is repeated every 3 to 4 weeks for 6 courses. Response to therapy is measured by peritoneal cytology, peritoneal and serum CA-125 or other markers and, in some cases, repeat laparotomy. In this manner, Howell et al[84] reported a median survival of >49 months for 25 patients with <2 cm residual disease, compared with 8 months for 65 patients with >2 cm disease using a variety of platinum-based regimens. Piver et al[147] observed that all 8 responders in their 31 patient study group (cisplatin plus adriamycin plus bleomycin) had residual disease <1 cm at the onset of IP therapy. They also had previously responded to IV platinum. In 1987, the GOG and SWOG, two US-based national cooperative study groups, initiated a randomized comparison of IV cisplatin plus cyclophosphamide to IP cisplatin plus IV cyclophosphamide in the postoperative primary treatment of Stage III optimal disease ovarian carcinoma patients. This study should determine finally whether or not the IP route of giving cisplatin is superior to the IV route.

MANAGEMENT OF SEROUS EFFUSIONS

Ascites is found in 5 to 10% of patients with Stages I and II, and 30 to 50% of patients with Stages III and IV ovarian carcinoma. While the etiology is not entirely clear, there are two components — increased production and decreased absorption. The protein and electrolyte-rich fluid is derived from the parietal and visceral peritoneum, particularly the omentum and small bowel serosa. Preoperatively, removal of an aliquot of ascitic fluid has been recommended for diagnostic purposes. This is seldom helpful in the patient with a pelvic mass and no evidence of liver or heart disease. Other causes of serous effusions, such as pancreatitis, tuberculosis, salpingitis, Meig's syndrome and endometriosis, must be kept in mind. Even in the presence of intraperitoneal cancer, the peritoneal cytology may be negative (especially if only a small amount of fluid is analyzed). When the peritoneal fluid is positive, the malignant cells are seldom diagnostic of the site of origin. At least two adverse effects relative to the malignancy can result from diagnostic paracentesis: first, the trochar may rupture a large, encapsulated ovarian carcinoma resulting in 'spill'; second, the cancer tends to grow in the tract of the paracentesis needle.

Drainage of the peritoneal fluid has been cited as a reason for preoperative paracentesis, to avoid hypotension from sudden decompression of the abdomen at surgery. If this occurs at all it is an exception.[75] Furthermore, preoperative paracentesis may be deleterious because it is often followed by rapid reaccumulation of ascites. Consequently, when the ascites again must be removed at surgery, plasma volume, serum proteins and electrolytes will be further depleted. Occasionally, ascites will require removal preoperatively because it is causing respiratory distress, pain or gastrointestinal symptoms. Complete removal will not only provide gratifying relief to the patient, but will facilitate the pelvic-abdominal examination. Slow removal of ascites at surgery while the anesthesiologist monitors the patient's cardiovascular response is the preferred management in the relatively asymptomatic patient.

The patient with resectable cancer will not form ascites postoperatively. Although, in theory, the ascites should recur if it is due to decreased absorption because peritoneal and diaphragmatic lymphatics are plugged with tumor, this has not occurred in our experience. On the other hand, patients with ascites and unresectable disease invariably continue to produce ascites postoperatively, sometimes at an increased rate.

The postoperative management of ascites is systemic chemotherapy. Serous effusions are, in fact, one of the most sensitive indicators of tumor response. Control rates of 80% or more are usually reported. The radioactive colloids are also effective in controlling serous effusions in about 50% of the cases,[27] but their effectiveness is less in cases refractory to chemotherapy.

When ascites is forming so rapidly that it must be constantly removed during surgery, and postoperatively the patient's abdomen is quickly distended, hypovolemia, oliguria, respiratory embarrassment and the threat of wound disruption result. Such a profuse production of ascites should prompt the initiation of systemic chemotherapy when the problem is recognized. Response may be observed within a few hours, making the recovery period much smoother. The use of cisplatin, methotrexate and other nephrotoxic agents must be avoided, however.

Ascites which fails to respond to systemic chemotherapy may respond to intraperitoneal radioactive colloids or bleomycin.[135] If these measures fail, repeated paracentesis must be done to alleviate the patient's symptoms. Drainage more than once or twice a week is poorly tolerated and should be viewed as an ominous sign. The use of peritoneal-venous shunts might prove helpful in the patient with refractory ascites.[32]

Pleural effusion often accompanies ovarian carcinoma with ascites. There seems to be a predilection for the right side, presumably because the right hemi-diaphragm has more lymphatic or anatomic connections between the pleural and peritoneal spaces. Thoracentesis must be done for the patient with symptoms, and may be life-saving. If thoracentesis is necessitated more than once, intrapleural therapy should be employed using bleomycin, tetracycline, nitrogen mustard or radioactive colloids.[132,135,208] Effusions refractory to these methods and systemic chemotherapy can be controlled by thoracotomy tube drainage.[86] Pericardial effusion is a rare complication of ovarian carcinoma. The diagnosis may be obscured by a concomitant pleural effusion. Treatment with sclerosing agents such as those used for pleural effusions appears to be better than surgical approaches.[40,177]

SECOND-LOOK PROCEDURES

Indications

There are many reasons for reoperating on the patient with ovarian carcinoma,[158] but the term, second-look, applies specifically to a laparotomy undertaken after 6 to 12 courses of chemotherapy to determine whether the patient with a complete clinical response is surgically and pathologically free of disease. Such an operation is clearly more specific and sensitive than any other method of measuring residual tumor, including CT scan, ultrasound, magnetic resonance imaging, CA-125 ovarian cancer antigen serum levels and clinical examination.[33,124] A second-look laparotomy may also be beneficial in other circumstances (Table 56.20) (see also Ch. 82).

The most cogent argument in favor of the second-look operation is the toxicity of continuing chemotherapy which has already induced a complete remission or which has proved to be ineffective. This permits secondary cytoreductive surgery and a change of therapy, for example to intraperitoneal chemotherapy. Perhaps a greater danger for the former group is the increased risk of acute non-lymphocytic leukemia, a risk which may be as high as 5 to 10% for long-term survivors.[53,66]

Table 56.20 Indications for second-look laparotomy

1. A sustained clinical complete response to chemotherapy.

2. Postoperative non-measurable residual disease exhibiting no evidence of progression on chemotherapy.

3. Stable disease or a partial response to chemotherapy if residual disease might be resectable.

4. Cases other than Stage I, Grade 1, which were not optimally staged at initial surgery.

The role of second-look surgery for patients with early ovarian carcinoma has not been delineated. It appears that the general experience with second-look operation in Stages I and II finds about 15% of patients to be positive after 6 to 12 courses of chemotherapy, intraperitoneal P[32] or whole abdomen radiation therapy. This relatively high rate probably reflects inadequate initial staging and patient selection. It seems appropriate to recommend a second-look procedure to patients with Stage I, Grade 2 or 3 ovarian carcinoma with incomplete initial staging, and all Stage II patients.

In the absence of gross tumor, the second-look laparotomy involves multiple biopsies and cytologies in a concerted effort to detect any residual microscopic disease (Table 56.21). The probability of finding residual car-

Table 56.21 Operative procedure for second-look laparotomy in ovarian carcinoma

1. Methodical, meticulous exploration of the abdomen and pelvis.

2. Peritoneal cytology specimens from the abdomen and pelvis.

3. Biopsy of all target lesions.

4. Removal of residual omentum.

5. Resection of ovarian pedicles with peritoneum.

6. Resection of cul-de-sac peritoneum, bowel adhesions, and peritoneal patches from paracolic gutters.

7. Selective dissection of pelvic and aortic lymph nodes.

8. Appendectomy.

9. Removal of residual uterus, tubes, and ovaries.[a]

10. Resection of residual carcinoma.

11. Obtain hormone receptors on residual tumor.

[a] In some instances, preservation of the uterus and residual adnexa is feasible.

cinoma at second-look surgery is inversely related to the extent and resectability of the disease at the first operation, the histologic grade, the response to chemotherapy, the number of drug courses before second-look and the thoroughness of the second-look staging procedure. Similarly, the relapse rate after a negative second-look pro-

cedure will be influenced to a degree by all of these factors. Collating data from several reported series,[9,14,63,149,175] the probability of having a surgically/pathologically negative second-look in patients with Stage II to IV ovarian carcinoma after 6 to 18 cycles of chemotherapy and no clinical evidence of disease is about 35%. Another 20% of cases will have microscopic disease only, and perhaps one-third to one-half of the remaining cases will be resectable.[35,64,106,166]

Results

Unfortunately, a negative second-look laparotomy is not equivalent to a cure. The reported relapse rate for this group of patients is 25 to 50%. When microscopic residual disease is found, 30 to 60% of patients have relapsed, while those patients whose disease was reduced to microscopic dimensions or who had small residual disease after second-look surgery are reported to have a recurrence rate of 70% or greater after 1 to 5 years of follow-up. Long-term survivors among patients with invasive ovarian cancer and residual tumor >2 cm after second-look surgery are unusual. Factors other than the amount of residual disease at second-look surgery are prognostic. Considering negative second-look cases, Gershenson et al[63] reported that 32% of Grade 3 cases recurred, compared to 17% of Grade 2 and none of Grade 1 cases. They also observed a higher relapse rate (46% versus 19%) in cases with 10 or fewer biopsy specimens, compared to those with more than 10. It has not been clearly demonstrated that the complete clinical response induced by combination drug therapy is more likely to be surgically/pathologically complete, or that treatment for more than six cycles increases the rate of surgically-negative second-looks.

Laparoscopy

Laparoscopy has been both recommended and condemned as a tool for staging, or restaging, selected patients with ovarian carcinoma. For early cases, the major shortcoming is evaluation of the retroperitoneal nodes. But this objection can be partly overcome by the use of lymphography or CT scanning. Certainly, it can be very effective for inspecting the peritoneal surfaces, including the right diaphragm (Fig. 56.10). Target biopsies and peritoneal cytology can also be obtained. Thus, while laparoscopy is not as accurate or thorough as a full laparotomy, it is undoubtedly superior to no second-look, and may be the procedure of choice when laparotomy is rejected or undesirable. The laparoscope can also be employed to identify cases that, on the basis of clinical and previous surgical data, are most likely to have persistent, unresectable disease before proceeding with a laparotomy.[146] Lele & Piver[104] used laparoscopy to evaluate the response to chemotherapy. None of the 11 patients who had a positive biopsy at 6 months had a negative second-look at 12 months. (See also Ch. 21).

Salvage therapy

There is no proven, effective salvage regimen for patients with a positive second-look, although the report of Copeland et al (1985) indicates that the prognosis for cases with only microscopic residual disease is excellent (70% alive at 5 years) if chemotherapy is given postoperatively. Thus, if the patient has had a good response to therapy and the second-look is done after six cycles, it seems reasonable to continue the chemotherapy for another three to six cycles when only microscopic residual disease is present. Intraperitoneal P^{32} or whole abdomen radiation therapy is also appropriate for patients with microscopic residual disease, but there is less supportive evidence for their efficacy.[59,72,144,164b,168,175,179] These treatments are especially applicable to the patient who, because of gastrointestinal effects or neurotoxicity, will not tolerate further chemotherapy. Investigational therapies, such as intraperitoneal chemotherapy (supra vide) or immunotherapy, also may be beneficial to the patient with microscopic or <1 cm macroscopic residual disease.[15,152]

Tumor hormone-receptor measurements should be obtained at second-look surgery, because high-dose progestin or tamoxifen therapy may provide some measure of tumor control, especially in cases of ovarian carcinoma with significant levels of cytosol receptor protein.[1,62,121,169] Although in vitro testing of tumor sensitivity to chemotherapeutic agents remains largely an investigational tool, the clonogenic assay may be useful in excluding drugs for second-line chemotherapy, since there is a high correlation between the in vitro and in vivo results of inactive drugs.[197,200] Although it is unusual today to encounter a patient with recurrent ovarian cancer who has not previously received cisplatin, it is well to remember that cisplatin is the most effective therapy known for alkylating-agent treatment failures.

BORDERLINE EPITHELIAL TUMORS

For many years, the existence of a group of epithelial ovarian tumors that have histologic and biologic features occupying a position between those of the clearly benign and frankly malignant ovarian epithelial neoplasms has been recognized (see Ch. 55). Clinically, these tumors are characterized by a predominantly early stage at diagnosis, infrequent and late recurrence, and long survival with residual or recurrent malignancy. Nearly three-quarters are Stage I at the time of diagnosis. The average age of women with the borderline serous and mucinous tumors is between that of women with frankly malignant ovarian carcinomas and those with benign cystomas.

Characteristics of histologic subtypes

Serous tumors of borderline malignancy

Approximately three-quarters of the serous borderline neoplasms are confined to the ovaries at the time of diagnosis, but 30% of these Stage I cases involve both ovaries. Ascites is unusual, and bilateralism is the rule in more advanced stages. Surface papillations are common, even in Stage I, with occasional tumors composed predominantly of an exophytic growth pattern (surface papilloma). The typical lesion, however, is a unilocular cyst with intracystic, warty growths which cannot be readily distinguished grossly from benign or even some malignant serous tumors. Psammoma bodies are common, and may be extensive. Among 168 Stage I cases from six series,[8,92,93,96,123,159] there were two recurrences, both in the preserved ovary. However, Tazelaar et al[184] observed five recurrences in their series of 42 Stage Ia, borderline serous tumors. Of these five recurrences, three were in a residual ovary 2 to 3 years after the initial surgery. In the same six series cited above, the recurrence or progression rate for Stages II and III was about 30%. However, many of the Stage III patients with recurrence were well, without clinical evidence of cancer. Patients not cured of their malignancy have a mean life expectancy of about 10 years after diagnosis.[93] Discordance between the ovarian primary and peritoneal implants has been reported. Thus, resection of the implants for histologic study is highly desirable for purposes of staging and treatment planning (invasive or benign implants can occur with a borderline ovarian lesion). Spontaneous regression of peritoneal implants from borderline serous tumors has been documented. It is probably uncommon and usually incomplete. Benign glandular inclusions are not infrequent in pelvic and aortic nodes in women. These must not be interpreted as metastases.[50]

Mucinous tumors of borderline malignancy

In Russell & Merkur's[160] series of 144 ovarian neoplasms of borderline malignancy, 36% were mucinous and 49% were serous. Mucinous borderline tumors are three times as common as mucinous carcinomas, and 80 to 90% of these are Stage I at diagnosis. Less than 5% of Stage I cases have bilateral involvement. An entirely benign neoplasm is as common in the contralateral ovary. Ascites is unusual. Characteristically, mucinous borderline tumors are multi-locular.

Mucinous borderline tumors appear to have a greater malignant potential than their serous counterparts. Although only 9 of 234 Stage I patients (8 of 220 Stage Ia) from collected series recurred, all died of disease: four within 2 years and three between 4.5 and 9.5 years. Of 20 Stage III patients, 8 were dead with disease, 7 within 3 years, and 2 were alive with disease less than 2 years after diagnosis. Death usually results from uncontrolled mucinous ascites.[8,31,76,96,123,159,184]

Pseudomyxoma peritonei

Pseudomyxoma peritonei, named and described by Werth in 1884, referred to a complication of ovarian mucinous cysts characterized by a gelatinous material filling the peritoneal cavity, partly attached to the peritoneal surfaces, forming masses contained within a connective tissue membrane.[155] Today, this term is generally used to refer to a more or less chronic state of viscid, mucinous 'ascites' which cannot be drained by paracentesis, thus requiring repeated laparotomy for removal of the material and/or encysted masses because of discomfort, distension or bowel obstruction. Review of the literature, however, fails to provide any consistent perception of this entity other than ascites accompanying a mucinous neoplasm.

Pseudomyxoma peritonei is nearly always associated with a ruptured mucinous tumor of the ovary or appendix, although the defect may be microscopic in dimension. The intraperitoneal mucin contains, or arises from, mucinous epithelium growing on the visceral and parietal peritoneum. While it may be difficult to demonstrate the presence of mucinous cells because of their scarcity, if they are, in fact, absent, removing the ruptured ovarian and/or appendiceal lesion along with the mucin invariably results in a cure. Similarly, if all of the involved peritoneum is excised, cure can be anticipated. On the other hand, if the primary and the peritoneal lesions cannot be removed in toto, the usual history is continued production of mucin with repeated small bowel obstruction eventuating in death.

The reported association of pseudomyxoma peritonei with benign or malignant mucinous tumors varies widely, but the majority probably should be classified as lesions of borderline malignant potential. There are well-documented, histologically benign cases, but these have nevertheless shown evidence of stromal invasion or manifested pools of apparently acellular mucin in the ovarian stroma (pseudomyxoma ovarii). Concomitant ovarian and appendiceal lesions are frequent, the latter potentially occult with a microscopic ovarian tumor. The appendiceal lesions (mucocele) may be a simple retention cyst or a benign or malignant neoplasm.[2] In half of the cases of pseudomyxoma peritonei, both ovaries are involved.

Treatment of pseudomyxoma consists of hysterectomy, bilateral salpingo-oophorectomy, and removal of the mucin and the peritoneal implants along with the appendix when feasible. If the implants cannot be entirely removed, recurrence is probable. Repeat laparotomy with evacuation of the mucin, resection of encysted masses, and relief of bowel obstruction are recommended, as indicated. No other therapy has established value, although systemic chemotherapy,[89] radiation therapy and abdominal lavage

with 5% aqueous dextrose have all been recommended.[65,148] When the mucin is encysted, creation of a mucous fistula may prevent relaparotomy.[109] Reported survival varies in the extreme. Of 15 patients in the combined series of Limber et al[105] and Sandenbergh & Woodruff,[162] 13 were dead. Only four survived for more than 3 years. Of two who survived longer than 5 years, one died of disease at 11 years and the other was alive at 8 years. Campbell et al,[26] however, in a literature review of pseudomyxoma peritonei with ovarian and appendiceal lesions, reported only seven deaths, with a mean survival of 6 years among 26 patients. Survival is probably related to the degree of cellular malignancy and the extent of disease (resectability) at the time of diagnosis.

Endometrioid and clear cell tumors of borderline malignancy

In Russell's series,[159] the endometrioid variety of borderline ovarian malignancy accounted for only 7% of all cases. These tumors are associated with pelvic endometriosis (30%) and endometrial carcinoma. The majority have a predominantly stromal component and are, therefore, properly termed adenofibromas. Histologically, the endometrial-like, glandular epithelium recapitulates the usual variations of endometrial hyperplasia, including atypia and squamous metaplasia. Peritoneal implants are distinguished from endometriosis by the absence of both endometrial stroma and evidence of hemorrhage.

Clear cell tumors of borderline malignancy accounted for 2% of Russell's series. All were cystadenofibromas. Bell & Scully[11] found histologic criteria for classifying 25 clear cell adenofibromas (21.3% of 122 adenofibromas) as benign in 3 cases, borderline in 11 and malignant in 11. All borderline and malignant lesions were Stage I. Ten of the 11 women with borderline tumors were postmenopausal. Bilateralism was observed once. Three of the 25 cases were associated with endometriosis. Three of the tumors classified as malignant were Stage Ia, predominantly borderline tumors with several foci of microinvasion. One of these recurred locally at 3.3 years of follow-up. Roth et al[156] reported one tumor death (after 5.2 years) among two patients with microinvasion.

Treatment of borderline ovarian malignancies

The majority of ovarian neoplasms in the borderline malignant category occur in women of reproductive age and are Stage I at the time of diagnosis. These cases are adequately managed by unilateral salpingo-oophorectomy. For serous tumors, the opposite ovary should be carefully evaluated for evidence of bilateralism. If the patient has no interest in fertility, a hysterectomy with bilateral adnexectomy is recommended. Appendectomy should accompany pelvic surgery for mucinous tumors. In the presence of bilateral ovarian cystic neoplasms or a single ovary, cystectomy is the procedure of choice when fertility is desired by the patient. The value of peritoneal cytology, partial omentectomy, and pelvic and aortic lymph node sampling is not known. In the absence of target lesions and a presumptive diagnosis of a borderline lesion based on the clinical situation and a frozen section, it is unlikely that node sampling will be of value. No postoperative therapy is needed.

In those unusual cases of ovarian borderline malignancy more advanced than Stage I, the cornerstone of therapy is surgery. Whenever feasible, complete excision should be done, recognizing, however, that if the preliminary diagnosis is right, the patient stands to benefit little from life-threatening surgery because these tumors typically have an indolent course. Careful pathologic evaluation of the primary tumor and its 'metastases' is essential, even for serous tumors, to exclude areas of frank invasion. If the tumor has a purely borderline histology, there is scant evidence that postoperative chemotherapy or radiation therapy alters in any beneficial way the course of the disease.[8,38,96,123] In the face of clinical progression, further tumor reductive surgery followed by chemotherapy seems reasonable. The recommended regimen is cisplatin plus cyclophosphamide for six cycles. The leukemia risk of long-term alkylating-agent therapy argues against prolonged treatment.[131] It must be kept in mind, however, that borderline ovarian carcinoma can be a progressive, fatal disease. At least for the serous tumors, the distribution of metastases in fatal cases includes liver, lymphatic, and even bone, similar to that of the frankly malignant tumors.[16] Thus, regional therapy has intrinsic shortcomings, if applied in this situation.

REFERENCES

1. Aabo K, Pedersen A G, Hald I 1982 High-dose medroxyprogesterone acetate (MPA) in advanced chemotherapy-resistant ovarian carcinoma: a phase II study. Cancer Treat Rep 66: 407
2. Aho A J, Heinonen R, Lauren P 1973 Benign and malignant mucocele of the appendix. Am J Obstet Gynecol 139: 392
3. Allan M S, Hertig A T 1949 Carcinoma of the ovary. Am J Obstet Gynecol 58: 640
4. Annual Report Gynecologic Cancer FIGO 1988 Pettersson F (ed) Panorama Press, Stockholm, Vol 20
5. Aure J C, Hoeg K, Kolstad P 1971 Clinical and histologic studies of ovarian carcinoma. Long-term follow-up of 990 cases. Obstet Gynecol 37: 1
6. Aure J C, Hoeg K, Kolstad P 1971 Radioactive colloidal gold in the treatment of ovarian carcinoma. Acta Radiol 10: 399
7. Banfi A, De Palo G M, DeRe F, Lattuada A, Luciani L, Musumeci R, Pizzetti F 1975 The value of radio-surgical-anatomical staging in ovarian epithelial cancer. In: DeWatteville H (ed) Diagnosis and Treatment of Ovarian Neoplastic Alterations. Excerpta Medica, Oxford, p 63
8. Barnhill D, Heller P B, Brzozowski P, Advani H, Gallup D, Park R 1985 Epithelial ovarian carcinoma. Obstet Gynecol 65: 53
9. Barnhill D, Hoskins W J, Heller P B, Park R 1984 The second-look surgical reassessment for epithelial ovarian carcinoma. Gynecol Oncol 19: 148
10. Barr W, Cowell M A, Chatfield W R 1970 The management of ovarian carcinoma. A review of 420 cases. Scot Med J 15: 250
11. Bell D A, Scully R E 1985 Benign and borderline clear cell adenofibromas of the ovary. Cancer 56: 2922
12. Bell D R, Woods R L, Levi J A, Fox R M, Tattersall M H 1982 Advanced ovarian cancer: a prospective randomised trial of chlorambucil versus combined cyclophosphamide and cis-diamminedichloroplatinum. Aust NZ J Med 12: 245
13. Beller U, Bigelow B, Beckman M, Brown B, Demopoulos R 1982 Epithelial carcinoma of the ovary in the reproductive years: clinical and morphological characterization. Gynecol Oncol 15: 422
14. Berek J S, Hacker N F, Lagasse L D, Poth T, Resnick B, Nieberg R K 1984 Second-look laparotomy in Stage III epithelial ovarian cancer: clinical variables associated with disease status. Obstet Gynecol 64: 207
15. Berek J S, Knapp R C, Hacker N F et al 1985 Intraperitoneal immunotherapy with corynebacterium parvum. Am J Obstet Gynecol 152: 1003
16. Bergman F 1966 Carcinoma of the ovary: a clinicopathological study of 86 autopsied cases with special reference to mode of spread. Acta Obstet Gynecol Scand 45: 211
17a. Bernstein P 1936 Tumors of the Ovary. Am J Obstet Gynecol 32: 1023
17b. Bertlesen K, Jakobsen A, Andersen J E et al 1987 A randomized study of cyclophosphamide and cis-platinum with or without doxorubicin in advanced ovarian carcinoma. Gynecol Oncol 28: 161
18. Bjorkhom E, Pettersson F, Einhorn H 1982 Longterm follow-up and prognostic factors in ovarian carcinoma. Acta Radiol Oncol Radiat Phys Biol 21: 413
19. Brady L, Blessing J, Homesley H, Lewis G C 1979 Radiotherapy (RT) chemotherapy (CT) and combined therapy in Stage III epithelial ovarian cancer. Proc Am Ass Cancer Res 20: 218.
20. Brodovsky H S, Bauer M, Horton J, Elson P J 1984 Comparison of melphalan with cyclophosphamide, methotrexate and 5-fluorouracil in patients with ovarian cancer. Cancer 53: 844
21. Buchsbaum H J, Brady M F, Delgado G, Miller A, Hoskins W J, Manetta A, Sutton G 1989 Surgical staging of ovarian carcinoma: Stage I, II and III (optimal). A Gynecologic Oncology Group Study. Surg Gynecol Obstet 169: 226
22. Burghardt E, Pickel H, Lahousen M, Stettner H 1986 Pelvic lymphadenectomy in operative treatment of ovarian cancer. Am J Obstet Gynecol 155: 315
23. Buka N I, Macfarlane K T 1964 Malignant tumors of the ovary. Am J Obstet Gynecol 90: 383
24. Burns B C, Underwood P B, Rutledge F N 1969 A review of carcinoma of the ovary at The University of Texas M.D. Anderson Hospital and Tumor Institute at Houston. Cancer of the Uterus and Ovary. Year Book Med Pub, Chicago
25. Bush R S, Allt W E, Beale F A, Bean H, Pringle J F, Sturgeon J 1977 Treatment of epithelial carcinoma of the ovary: operation, irradiation and chemotherapy. Am J Obstet Gynecol 127: 692
26. Campbell J S, Ferguson P, Krongold I, Kemeny T, Mitton D M, Allan N 1973 Pseudomyxoma peritonei et ovarii with occult neoplasms of appendix. Obstet Gynecol 42: 897
27. Card R Y, Cole D R, Hensche U K 1960 Summary of ten years of the use of radioactive colloids in intracavitary therapy. J Nucl Med 1: 195
28. Carmo-Pereira J, Costa D F, Henriques E, Ricardo J 1981 Advanced ovarian carcinoma: a prospective and randomized clinical trial of cyclophosphamide versus combination cytotoxic chemotherapy (hexa-CAF). Cancer 48: 1947
29. Carter J P 1964 Thrombophlebitis as an early sign of visceral cancer. Angiology 15: 236
30. Carter W F 1964 Primary ovarian malignancy. Am J Obstet Gynecol 90: 951
31. Chaitin B A, Gershenson D M, Evans H L 1985 Mucinous tumors of the ovary. Cancer 55: 1958

32. Cheung D K and Raaf J H 1982 Selection of patients with malignant ascites for a peritoneovenous shunt. Cancer 50: 1204

33. Clarke-Pearson D L, Bandy L C, Dudzinski M, Heaston D, Creasman W T 1986 Computed tomography in evaluation of patients with ovarian carcinoma in complete clinical remission. Correlation with surgical-pathologic findings. JAMA 255: 627

34. Cocco A E, Conway S J 1975 Zollinger-Ellison syndrome associated with ovarian mucinous cystadenocarcinoma. N Engl J Med 293: 485

35. Copeland L J, Gershenson D M, Wharton J T, Atkinson E N, Sneige N, Edwards C L and Rutledge F N 1985 Microscopic disease at second-look laparotomy in advanced ovarian cancer. Cancer 55: 472

36. Covington E, Hilaris B S 1973 P^{32} scans for intracavitary distribution studies. Am J Roentgenol Radium Ther Nucl Med 118: 895

37. Creasman W T, Abu-Ghazaleh S, Schmidt H J 1978 Retroperitoneal metastatic spread of ovarian cancer. Gynecol Oncol 6: 447

38. Creasman W T, Park R, Norris H, DiSaia P J, Morrow C P, Hreshychyshyn M M 1982 Stage I borderline ovarian tumors. Obstet Gynecol 59: 93

39. Davis B A, Latour J P, Philpott N W 1956 Primary carcinoma of the ovary. Surg Gynecol Obstet 102: 565

40. Davis S, Rambotti P, Grignani F 1984 Intrapericardial tetracycline sclerosis in the treatment of malignant pericardial effusion: An analysis of thirty-three cases. J Clin Oncol 2: 631

41a. Day T G, Smith J P 1975 Diagnosis and staging of ovarian carcinoma. Semin Oncol 2: 217

41b. Decker D G, Fleming T R, Malkasian G D, Webb M J, Jefferies J A, Edmonson J H 1982 Cyclophosphamide plus cis-platinum in combination: Treatment program for Stage III or IV ovarian carcinoma. Obstet Gynecol 60: 481

42. Delclos L, Fletcher G H 1969 Postoperative irradiation for ovarian carcinoma with the cobalt-60 moving strip technique. Clin Obstet Gynecol 12: 993

43a. Dembo A J, Bush R S 1982 Choice of postoperative therapy based on prognostic factors. Int J Radiat Oncol Biol Phys 8: 893

43b. Dembo A J, Bush R S, Beale F A, Bean H A, Pringle J F, Sturgeon J F 1979 The Princess Margaret Hospital study of ovarian cancer: Stage I, II and asymptomatic III presentations. Cancer Treat Rep 63: 249

44. Dembo A J, Bush R S, Beale F A, Bean H A, Pringle J F, Sturgeon J, Reid J G 1979 Ovarian carcinoma: improved survival following abdominopelvic irradiation in patients with a completed pelvic operation. Am J Obstet Gynecol 134: 793

45a. Dembo A J, Prefontaine M, Miceli P, Bush R S 1986 Prognostic factors in Stage I epithelial ovarian carcinoma (ECO). Presented at the 17th Annual Meeting of the Society of Gynecologic Oncologists, Palm Springs, Calif., Feb. 2–5, 1986.

45b. Demopoulos R I, Bigelow B, Blaustein A, Chait J, Gutman E, Dubin N 1984 Characterization and survival of patients with serous cystadenocarcinoma of the ovaries. Obstet Gynecol 64: 557

46. Drukker B H, Hodgkinson C P 1971 Ovarian carcinoma: perspective for the 70's. Am J Obstet Gynecol 109: 825

47. Edmonson J H, Fleming T R, Decker D G et al 1979 Different chemotherapeutic sensitivities and host factors affecting prognosis in advanced ovarian carcinoma versus minimal residual disease. Cancer Treat Rep 63: 241

48. Edmonson J H, McCormack G W, Fleming T R et al 1985 Comparison of cyclophosphamide plus cisplatin versus hexamethylmelamine, cyclophosphamide, doxorubicin, and cisplatin in combination as initial chemotherapy for Stage III and IV ovarian carcinomas. Cancer Treat Rep 69: 1243

49. Edwards C L, Herson J, Gershenson D M, Copeland L J, Wharton J T 1983 A prospective randomized clinical trial of melphalan and cis-platinum versus hexamethylmelamine, adriamycin, and cyclophosphamide in advanced ovarian cancer. Gynecol Oncol 15: 261

50. Ehrmann R L, Federschneider J M, Knapp R C 1980 Distinguishing lymph node metastases from benign glandular inclusions in low-grade ovarian carcinoma. Am J Obstet Gynecol 136: 737

51. Eifel P, Hendrickson M, Ross J, Ballon S, Martinez A, Kempson R 1982 Simultaneous presentation of carcinoma involving the ovary and the uterine corpus. Cancer 50: 163

52. Einhorn N, Bast R C, Knapp R C, Tjernberg B, Zurawski V R 1986 Preoperative evaluation of serum CA 125 levels in patients with primary epithelial ovarian cancer. Obstet Gynecol 67: 414

53. Einhorn N, Eklund G, Franze S, Lambert B, Lindsten J, Soderhall S 1982 Late side effects of chemotherapy in ovarian carcinoma: A cytogenetic, hematologic and statistical study. Cancer 49: 2234

54a. Elahi E H, Long M E, Frick H C, Sommers S C 1967 Long-term survival in disseminated ovarian carcinoma. Am J Obstet Gynecol 99: 522

54b. Erhardt K, Auer G, Bjorkholm E et al 1985 Combined morphologic and cytochemical grading of serous ovarian tumors. Am J Obstet Gynecol 151: 356

55. Ferrucci J T 1979 Body ultrasonography. N Engl J Med 300: 538

56. Flam F, Einhorn N, Sjovall K 1988 Symptomatology of ovarian cancer. Eur J Obstet Gynecol Reprod Biol 27: 53

57. Friedlander M L, Hedley D W, Swanson C, Russell P 1988 Prediction of long-term survival by flow cytometric analysis of cellular DNA content in patients with advanced ovarian cancer. J Clin Oncol 6: 282

58. Fuks Z, Bagshaw M 1975 The rationale for curative radiotherapy for ovarian carcinoma. Int J Radiat Oncol Biol Phys 1: 21

59. Fuks Z, Rizel S, Biran S 1988 Chemotherapeutic and surgical induction of pathological complete remission and whole abdominal irradiation for consolidation does not enhance the cure of stage III ovarian carcinoma. Clin Oncol 6: 509

60. Gallup D G, Cody W M, Metheyny W P, Talledo O E 1988 Epithelial tumors of the ovary in women less than 40 years old. S Med J 81: 10

61. Gardiner G A, Slate J 1955 Malignant tumors of the ovary. Am J Obstet Gynecol 70: 554

62. Giesler H E 1983 Megestrol acetate for the palliation of advanced ovarian carcinoma. Obstet Gynecol 61: 95

63. Gershenson D M, Copeland L J, Wharton J T, Atkinson E N, Sneige N, Edwards C L, Rutledge F N 1985 Prognosis of surgically determined complete responders in advanced ovarian cancer. Cancer 55: 1129

64. Greco F A, Julian C G, Richardson R L, Burnett L, Hande K R, Oldham R K 1981 Advanced ovarian cancer: brief intensive combination chemotherapy and second-look operation. Obstet Gynecol 58: 199

65. Green N, Gancedo H, Smith R, Bernett G 1975 Pseudomyxoma peritonei — nonoperative management and biochemical findings: a case report. Cancer 36: 1834

66. Greene M H, Boice J C, Greer B E, Blessing J A, Dembo A J 1982 Acute nonlymphocytic leukemia after therapy with alkylating agents for ovarian cancer: a study of five randomized clinical trials. N Engl J Med 307: 1416

67. Griffiths C T 1974 Surgical resection of tumor bulk in the primary treatment of ovarian carcinoma. In Symposium on Ovarian Carcinoma National Cancer Institute Monograph. 42: 1010

68. Griffiths C T, Grogan R H, Hall T C 1972 Advanced ovarian cancer, primary treatment with surgery, radiotherapy and chemotherapy. Cancer 29: 1

69. Griffiths C T, Parker L M, Fuller A R 1979 Role of cytoreductive surgical treatment in the management of advanced ovarian cancer. Cancer Treat Rep 63: 235

70. Grönroos M, Lauren P, Lehto J, Rauramo L 1969 Ovarian cancer and its treatment. Ann Chir Gynaecol Fenn 58: 83

71. Gruppo Interegionale Cooperativo Oncologico Ginecologia 1987 Randomised comparison of cisplatin with cyclophosphamide/cisplatin and with cyclophosphamide/doxorubicin/cisplatin in advanced ovarian cancer. Lancet ii: 353

72. Hacker N F, Berek J S, Burnison C M, Heintz P M, Juillard J F, Lagasse L D 1985 Whole abdominal radiation as salvage therapy for epithelial ovarian cancer. Obstet Gynecol 65: 60

73. Hacker N F, Berek J S, Pretorius R G, Zuckerman J, Eisenkop S, Lagasse L D 1987 Intraperitoneal cis-platinum as salvage

therapy for refractory epithelial ovarian cancer. Obstet Gynecol 70: 759

74. Hall D J, Dyer M L, Parker J C 1985 Ovarian cancer complicated by cerebellar degeneration: a paraneoplastic syndrome. Gynecol Oncol 21: 240

75. Halpin T F, McCann T O 1971 Dynamics of body fluids following the rapid removal of large volumes of ascites. Am J Obstet Gynecol 110: 1

76. Hart W R, Norris H J 1973 Borderline and malignant mucinous tumors of the ovary. Cancer 31: 1031

77. Heintz A P, Van Oosterom A T, Trimbos J M C, Schaberg A, Van Der Velde E A, Nooy M 1988 The treatment of advanced ovarian carcinoma (1): clinical variables associated with progress. Gynecol Oncol 30: 347

78. Herrmann U J Jr, Locher G W, Goldhirsch A 1987 Sonographic patterns of ovarian tumors: prediction of malignancy. Obstet Gynecol 69: 777

79. Hilaris B S, Clard D G 1971 The value of postoperative intraperitoneal injection of radiocolloids in early cancer of the ovary. Am J Roentgenol Radium Ther Nucl Med 112: 749

80. Hintz B L, Fuks Z, Kempson R L, Eltringham J R, Zaloudek C, Williamson T J, Bagshaw M A 1975 Results of postoperative megavoltage radiotherapy of malignant surface epithelial tumors of the ovary. Radiology 114: 695

81. Holme G M 1963 Prognostic factors in malignant ovarian disease. Acta Unio Internat Contra Cancrum 19: 1135

82. Holtz G 1980 Paraneoplastic hypercalcemia in gynecologic malignancy. Obstet Gynecol Sur 35: 129

83. Howell S B 1988 Intraperitoneal chemotherapy for ovarian carcinoma. J Clin Oncol 6:1673

84. Howell S B, Zimm S, Markman M, Abramson I S, Cleary S, Lucas W E, Weiss R J 1987 Long-term survival of advanced refractory ovarian carcinoma patients with small-volume disease treated with intraperitoneal chemotherapy. J Clin Oncol 5: 1607

85. Hreshychyshyn M W, Park R C, Blessing J A, Norris H J, Levy D, Lagasse L D, Creasman W T 1980 The role of adjuvant therapy in stage I ovarian cancer. Am J Obstet Gynecol 138: 139

86. Izbici R, Weyhing B T, Baker L, Caoili E, Vaitkevicius V 1975 Pleural effusion in cancer patients: a prospective randomized study of pleural drainage with the addition of radioactive phosphorus to the pleural space vs pleural drainage alone. Cancer 36: 1511

87. Javert C T, Roscoe R R 1953 Serous cystadenocarcinoma of the ovary: a review of 127 cases. Surg Clin Nth Am 33: 557

88. Jensen R D, Norris H J 1972 Epithelial tumors of the ovary: occurrence in children and adolescents less than 20 years of age. Arch Pathol 94: 29

89. Jones C M, Homesley H D 1985 Successful treatment of pseudomyxoma peritonei of ovarian origin with cisplatinum, doxorubicin, and cyclophosphamide. Gynecol Oncol 22: 257

90. Julian C G 1974 Germinal epithelial neoplasia of the ovary. Clin Obstet Gynecol 17: 241

91. Julian C G, Inalsingh A, Burnett L S 1978 Radioactive phosphorus and external radiation as an adjuvant to surgery for ovarian carcinoma. Obstet Gynecol 52: 155

92. Julian C G, Woodruff J D 1972 The biologic behavior of low-grade papillary serous carcinoma of the ovary. Obstet Gynecol 40: 860

93. Katzenstein A L, Mazur M T, Morgan T E, Kao M S 1978 Proliferative serous tumors of the ovary. Am J Surg Pathol 2: 339

94. Klaassen D, Shelly W, Starreveld A et al 1988 Early stage ovarian cancer: a randomized clinical trial comparing whole abdominal radiotherapy, melphalan, and intraperitoneal chromic phosphate: a National Cancer Institute of Canada clinical trials group report. Clin Oncol 6: 1254

95. Klaassen D, Starreveld A, Shelly W, Miller A, Boyes D, Gerulath A, Levitt M 1985 External beam pelvic radiotherapy plus intraperitoneal, radioactive chromic phosphate in early stage ovarian cancer: a toxic combination. A National Cancer Institute of Canada clinical trials report. J Radiat Oncol Biol Phys 11: 1801

96. Kliman L, Rome R M, Fortune D W 1986 Low malignant potential (LMP) tumors of the ovary: a clinical and pathological study of 76 cases. Obstet Gynecol 68: 338

97. Kolstad P, Davy M, Hoeg K 1977 Individualized treatment of ovarian cancer. Am J Obstet Gynecol 128: 617

98. Kottmeier H L 1968 Clinical staging in ovarian carcinoma. In: Gentil, F, Junqueira A (eds) UICC Monograph Series No 11 Springer Verlag, New York, p 146

99. Kottmeier H L 1971 Ovarian cancer with special regard to radiotherapy. In: Deeley T J (ed) Modern Radiotherapy and Gynecologic Cancer. Butterworth, London, p 186

100. Kuhnel R, Delemarre F M, Rao B R, Stolk J G 1987 Correlation of multiple steroid receptors with histological type and grade in human ovarian cancer. Int J Gynecol Pathol 6: 248

101. Kuhnle H, Meerpohl H G, Lenaz L et al 1988 Etoposide in cisplatin-refractory ovarian cancer. Proc Am Soc Clin Oncol, Vol 7, p 137, Abstract 527

102. Lastoria S, D'Amico P, Mansi L et al 1988 A prospective imaging study of I-B72.3 monoclonal antibody in patients with epithelial ovarian cancer: preliminary report. Nucl Med Commun 9: 347

103. Leibman A J, Kruse B, McSweeney M B 1988 Transvaginal sonography: comparison with transabdominal sonography in the diagnosis of pelvic masses. AJR 151: 89

104. Lele S B, Piver M S 1986 Interval laparoscopy as predictor of response to chemotherapy in ovarian carcinoma. Obstet Gynecol 68: 345

105. Limber G K, King R E, Silverberg S G 1973 Pseudomyxoma peritonei: a report of ten cases. Ann Surg 178: 587

106. Luesley D M, Chan K K, Fielding J W, Hurlow R, Blackledge G R, Jordan J A 1984 Second-look laparotomy in management of epithelial ovarian carcinoma: an evaluation of fifty cases. Obstet Gynecol 64: 421

107. Lynch F W 1936 A clinical review of 110 cases of ovarian carcinoma. Am J Obstet Gynecol 32: 753

108. MacFarlane C, Sturgis M C, Fetterman F S 1955 Results of an experiment in the control of cancer of the female pelvic organs and report of a fifteen-year research. Am J Obstet Gynecol 69: 294

109. Magell J 1969 Pseudomyxoma peritonei. Lancet ii: 846

110. Malkasian G D, Melton L J, O'Brien P C, Greene M H 1984 Prognostic significance of histologic classification and grading of epithelial malignancies of the ovary. Am J Obstet Gynecol 149: 274

111. Malkasian G D, Podratz K C, Stanhope C R, Ritts R E Jr, Zurawski V R Jr 1986 CA 125 in gynecologic practice. Am J Obstet Gynecol 155: 515

112. Mangioni C, Colombo N, Marsoni S et al 1986 Treatment of advanced ovarian cancer (OC): a randomized trial comparing different platinum (P) combinations. Presented at the 17th Annual Meeting of the Society of Gynecologic Oncologists, Palm Springs, Calif., Feb 2–5, 1986.

113. Markman M, Howell S B 1985 Intraperitoneal chemotherapy for ovarian carcinoma. In: Alberts D S and Surwit E A (eds) Ovarian Cancer. Martinus Nihoff, Boston, p 179

114. Mawhinney R R, Powell M C, Worthington B S, Symonds E M 1988 Magnetic resonance imaging of benign ovarian masses. Br J Radiol 61: 179

115. Meigs J V, Armstrong S H, Hamilton H H 1943 A further contribution to the syndrome of fibroma of the ovary with fluid in the abdomen and chest: Meigs syndrome. Am J Obstet Gynecol 46: 19

116. Miller A B, Klaassen D J, Boyes D A et al 1980 Combination v. sequential therapy with melphalan, 5-fluorouracil and methotrexate for advanced ovarian cancer. CMA J 123: 365

117. Munnell E W 1968 The changing prognosis and treatment in cancer of the ovary. Am J Obstet Gynecol 100: 790

118. Munnell E W 1969 Surgical treatment of ovarian carcinoma. Clin Obstet Gynecol 12: 980

119. Munnell E W 1969 Is conservative therapy ever justified in Stage I (Ia) cancer of the ovary? Am J Obstet Gynecol 103: 641

120. Musumeci R, Banfi A, Bolis G et al 1977 Lymphangiography in patients with ovarian epithelial cancer. An evaluation of 289 consecutive cases. Cancer 40: 1444

121. Myers A M, Moore G E, Major F J 1981 Advanced ovarian carcinoma: response to antiestrogen therapy. Cancer 48: 2368

122. Neijt J P, Bokkel Huinink W W, van der Burg M E L et al 1987 Randomized trial comparing two combination chemotherapy regimens (CHAP-5 v CP) in advanced ovarian carcinoma. J Clin Oncol 5: 1157

123. Nikrui N 1981 Survey of clinical behavior of patients with borderline epithelial tumors of the ovary. Gynecol Oncol 12: 107

124. Niloff J M, Knapp R C, Lavin P T et al 1986 The CA-125 assay as a predictor of clinical recurrence in epithelial ovarian cancer. Am J Obstet Gynecol 155: 56

125. Obel E B 1976 A comparative study of patients with cancer of the ovary, who have survived more or less than 10 years. Acta Obstet Gynecol Scand 55: 429

126. O'Connell G J, Ryan E, Murphy K J, Prefontaine M 1987 Predictive value of CA 125 for ovarian carcinoma in patients presenting with pelvic masses. Obstet Gynecol 70: 930

127. Oelsner G, Menczer J, Insler V, Serr D M 1975 Fertility after ovarian surgery for benign tumor under the age of twenty. Int J Gynaecol Obstet 13: 145

128. Omura G, Blessing J A, Ehrlich C E, Miller A, Yordan E, Creasman W T, Homesley H D 1986 A randomized trial of cyclophosphamide and doxorubicin with or without cisplatin in advanced ovarian carcinoma. Cancer 57: 1725

129. Omura G A, Morrow C P, Blessing J A, Miller A, Buchsbaum H J, Homesley H D, Leone L 1983 A randomized comparison of melphalan versus melphalan plus hexamethylmelamine versus adriamycin plus cyclophosphamide in ovarian carcinoma. Cancer 51: 783

130. O'Neill R T, Mikuta J J 1970 Hypoglycemia associated with serous cystadenocarcinoma of the ovary. Obstet Gynecol 35: 287

131. O'Quinn A G, Hannigan E V 1985 Epithelial ovarian neoplasms of low malignant potential. Gynecol Oncol 21: 177

132. Ostrowski M J, Halsall G M 1982: Intracavitary bleomycin in the management of malignant effusions: a multicenter study. Cancer Treat Rep 66: 1903

133. Ozols R F, Garvin A J, Costa J, Simon R M, Young R C 1979 Histologic grade in advanced ovarian cancer. Cancer Treat Rep 63: 255

134. Ozols R F, Garvin A J, Costa J, Simon R M, Young R C 1980 Advanced ovarian cancer: correlation of histologic grade with response to therapy and survival. Cancer 45: 572

135. Paladine W, Cunningham T J, Sponzo R, Donavan M, Olson K, Horton J 1976 Intracavitary bleomycin in the management of malignant effusions. Cancer 38: 1903

136. Park R C, Blom J, DiSaia P J, Lagasse L D, Blessing J A 1980 Treatment of women with disseminated or recurrent advanced ovarian cancer with melphalan alone, in combination with 5-fluorouracil and dactinomycin or with the combination of cytoxan, 5-fluorouracil and dactinomycin. Cancer 45: 2529

137. Parker B R, Castellino R A, Fuks Z Y, Bagshaw M A 1974 The role of lymphography in patients with ovarian cancer. Cancer 34: 100

138. Parker R T, Parker C H, Wilbanks G D 1970 Cancer of the ovary. Am J Obstet Gynecol 108: 878

139. Parson V, Rigby B 1958 Cushing's syndrome associated with adenocarcinoma of the ovary. Lancet ii: 992

140. Pearse W H, Behrman S J 1954 Carcinoma of the ovary. Obstet Gynecol 3: 32

141. Pemberton F A 1940 Carcinoma of the ovary. Am J Obstet Gynecol 40: 751

142. Perez C A, Bradfield J S 1972 Radiation therapy in the treatment of carcinoma of the ovary. Cancer 29: 1027

143. Peters W A, Andersen W A, Thornton W N 1983 Dermatomyositis and coexistent ovarian cancer: A review of the compounding clinical problems. Gynecol Oncol 15: 440

144. Peters W A, Blasko J C, Bagley C M Jr et al 1986 Salvage therapy with whole-abdominal irradiation in patients with advanced carcinoma of the ovary previously treated by combination chemotherapy. Cancer 58: 880

145. Pezner R D, Stevens K R Jr, Tong D, Allen C V 1978 Limited epithelial carcinoma of the ovary treated with curative intent by the intraperitoneal instillation of radiocolloids. Cancer 42: 2563

146. Piver M S, Lele S B, Barlow J J, Gamarra M 1980 Second-look laparoscopy prior to proposed second-look laparotomy. Obstet Gynecol 55: 571

147. Piver M S, Shashikant B L, Marchetti D L, Baker T R, Emrich L J, Hartman A B 1988 Surgically documented response to intraperitoneal cisplatin, cytarabine, and bleomycin after intravenous cisplatin-based chemotherapy in advanced ovarian adenocarcinoma. J Clin Oncol 6: 1679

148. Piver M S, Lele S B, Patsner B 1984 Pseudomyxoma peritonei: possible prevention of mucinous ascites by peritoneal lavage. Obstet Gynecol 64: 95

149. Podratz K C, Malkasian G D Jr, Hilton J F, Harris E A, Gaffey T A 1985, Second-look laparotomy in ovarian cancer: evaluation of pathologic variables. Am J Obstet Gynecol 152: 230

150. Powell J L, Burrell M O, Kirchner A B 1987 Intraperitoneal radioactive chromic phosphate P-32 in the treatment of ovarian cancer. S Med J 80: 1513

151. Potish R A, Twiggs L B 1986 A decision theory analysis of radiotherapeutic and chemotherapeutic toxicity in the management of ovarian cancer. In: Morrow C P, Smart G E (eds) Gynaecological Oncology (Proceedings of the Second International Conference on Gynaecological Cancer held in Edinburgh in September 1983). Springer-Verlag, New York, p 201

152. Rambaldi A, Introna M, Colotta F, Landolfo S, Colombo N, Mangioni C, Mantovani A 1985 Intraperitoneal administration of interferon B in ovarian cancer patients. Cancer 56: 294

153. Reddy S, Sutton G P, Stehman F B, Hornback N B, Ehrlich C E 1987 Ovarian carcinoma: adjuvant treatment with P-32. Radiology 165: 275

154. Regelson W, Parker G 1986 The routinization of intraperitoneal (intracavitary) chemotherapy and immunotherapy. Cancer Inv 4: 29

155. Ries E 1924 Pseudomyxoma peritonei. Surg Gynecol Obstet 39: 569

156. Roth L M, Langley F A, Fox H, Wheeler J E, Czernobilsky B 1984 Ovarian clear cell adenofibromatous tumors. Cancer 53: 1156

157. Rubin P, Grise J W, Terry R 1962 Has postoperative irradiation proved itself? Am J Roentgenol Radium Ther Nucl Med 88: 849

158. Rubin S C, Lewis J L Jr 1988 Second-look surgery in ovarian cancer. CRC Crit Rev Oncol 8: 75

159. Russell P 1979 The pathological assessment of ovarian neoplasms. II. The proliferating 'epithelial' tumors. Pathology 11: 251

160. Russell P, Merkur H 1979 Proliferating ovarian 'epithelial' tumors: a clinico-pathological analysis of 144 cases. Aust NZ J Obstet Gynaecol 19: 45

161. Rutledge F N 1976 In: Rutledge F N, Boronow R C, Wharton J T (eds) Gynecologic Oncology. Wiley, New York, p 183

162. Sandenbergh H A, Woodruff J D 1977 Histogenesis of pseudomyxoma peritonei. Obstet Gynecol 49: 339

163. Schnur P L, Symmonds R E, Williams T J 1969 Intestinal disorders masquerading as gynecologic problems. Surg Gynecol Obstet 128: 1016

164. Schray M, Martinez A, Cox R 1983 Radiotherapy in epithelial ovarian cancer: analysis of prognostic factors based on long term experience. Obstet Gynecol 62: 373

164b. Schray M F, Martinez A, Howes A E et al 1988 Advanced epithelial ovarian cancer: salvage whole abdominal irradiation for patients with recurrent or persistent disease after combination chemotherapy. J Clin Oncol 6: 1433

165. Schwartz P E, Lawrence R, Katz M 1981 Combination chemotherapy for advanced ovarian cancer: a prospective randomized trial comparing hexamethylmelamine and cyclophosphamide to doxorubicin and cyclophosphamide. Cancer Treat Rep 65: 137

166. Schwartz P E, Smith J P 1980 Second-look operations in ovarian cancer. Am J Obstet Gynecol 138: 1124

167. Schwartz P E, MacLusky N, Merino M J, Livolsi V A, Kohorn E I, Eisenfeld A 1986 Are cytosol estrogen and progestin receptors of prognostic significance in the management of epithelial ovarian cancers? Obstet Gynecol 68: 751

168. Shelley W E, Starreveld A A, Carmichael J A, O'Connell G, Roy M, Swenerton K 1988 Toxicity of abdominopelvic radiation in advanced ovarian carcinoma patients after

cisplatin/cyclophosphamide therapy and second-look laparotomy. Obstet Gynecol 71: 327

169. Shirey D R, Kavanagh J J, Gershenson D M, Freedman R S, Copeland L J, Jones L A 1985 Tamoxifen therapy of epithelial ovarian cancer. Obstet Gynecol 66: 575

170. Siegman-Igra Y, Flatau E, Deligdish L 1977 Chronic diffuse intravascular coagulation (DIC) in nonmetastatic ovarian cancer. Gynecol Oncol 5: 92

171. Sigurdsson K, Alm P, Gullberg B 1983 Prognostic factors in malignant epithelial ovarian tumors. Gynecol Oncol 15: 370

172. Silverberg E 1986 Statistical and epidemiological information on gynecological cancer. American Cancer Society, New York.

173. Simon A, Fields S, Schenker J G, Anteby S O 1986 Computed tomography prior to surgery for ovarian carcinoma. Aust NZ J Obstet Gynaecol 26: 199

174. Smedley H, Sikora K 1985 Age as a prognostic factor in epithelial ovarian carcinoma. Br J Obstet Gynaecol 92: 839

175. Smirz L R, Stehman F B, Ulbright T M, Sutton G P, Ehrlich C E 1985 Second-look laparotomy after chemotherapy in the management of ovarian malignancy. Am J Obstet Gynecol 152: 661

176. Smith E M, Anderson B 1985 The effects of symptoms and delay in seeking diagnosis on stage of disease at diagnosis among women with cancers of the ovary. Cancer 56: 2727

177. Smith F E, Lane M, Hudgins P T 1974 Conservative management of malignant pericardial effusion. Cancer 33: 47

178. Smith J P, Rutledge F N 1975 Random study of hexamethylmelamine, 5-fluorouracil, and melphalan in treatment of advanced carcinoma of the ovary. In: Symposium on Ovarian Cancer. National Cancer Institute Monograph 42, p 169

179. Soper J T, Wilkinson R H, Bandy L C, Clarke-Pearson D L, Creasman W T 1987 Intraperitoneal chromic phosphate P32 as salvage therapy for persistent carcinoma of the ovary after surgical restaging. Am J Obstet Gynecol 156: 1153

180. Sorbe B, Frankendal B, Veress B 1982 Importance of histologic grading in the prognosis of epithelial ovarian carcinoma. Obstet Gynecol 59: 576

181. Squillaci E, Salzani M C, Grandinetti M L, Auffermann W, Marsella A, Maresca G, Colagrande C 1988 Recurrence of ovarian and uterine neoplasms: Diagnosis with transrectal ultrasound. Radiol 169: 355

182. Stern W Z 1979 Radiology of the ovary. Obstet Gynecol Surv 31: 518

183a. Stone M L, Weingold A B 1969 Factors affecting survival of patients with ovarian carcinoma. Clin Obstet Gynecol 12: 1025

183b. Swenerton K D, Hislop T G, Spinelli J, LeRiche J C, Yang N, Boyes D A 1985 Ovarian carcinoma: a multivariate analysis of prognostic factors. Obstet Gynecol 65: 264

184. Tazelaar H D, Bostwick D G, Ballon S C, Hendrickson M R, Kempson R L 1985 Conservative treatment of borderline ovarian tumors. Obstet Gynecol 66: 417

185. Thigpen T, Vance R, Lambuth B et al 1987 Chemotherapy for advanced or recurrent gynecologic cancer. Cancer 60: 2104

186. Timm J, 1973 Ovarian carcinoma: a 10 year series from a provincial hospital. Acta Obstet Gynecol Scand 52: 103

187. Tobias J S, Griffiths C T 1976 Management of ovarian carcinoma. N Engl J Med 294: 818

188. Vara P, Pankamma P 1946 A clinical-statistical investigation of ovarian tumors operated at the Helsinki University Clinic of Gynecology during the years 1900–1944. Acta Obstet Gynecol Scand 26, Suppl 4

189. Vasilev S A, Schlaerth J B, Campeau J, Morrow C P 1988 Serum CA 125 levels in preoperative evaluation of pelvic masses. Obstet Gynecol 71: 751

190. Villasanta U, Bloedorn F G 1968 Operation, external irradiation, radioactive isotopes, and chemotherapy in treatment of metastatic ovarian malignancies. Am J Obstet Gynecol 102: 531

191. Walter R I, Bachman A L, Harris W 1941 The treatment of carcinoma of the ovary: improvement of results with postoperative radiotherapy. Am J Roentgenol Radium Ther Nucl Med 45: 403

192. Warde P, Rideout D F, Herman S et al 1987 Computed tomography in advanced ovarian cancer: an evaluation of diagnostic accuracy. Am J Med Sci 293: 94

193. Webb M J, Decker D G, Mussey E, Williams T J 1973 Factors influencing survival in Stage I ovarian cancer. Am J Obstet Gynecol 116: 222

194. Webb M J, Malkasian G D, Jorgensen E O 1974 Factors influencing ovarian cancer survival after chemotherapy. Obstet Gynecol 44: 564

195. Weinstein D, Polishuk W Z 1975 The role of wedge resection of the ovary as a cause for mechanical sterility. Surg Gynecol Obstet 141: 417

196. Weiss N S, Lyon J L, Liff J M 1981 Incidence of ovarian cancer in relation to the use of oral contraceptives. Int J Cancer 28: 669

197. Welander C E 1985 The human tumor clonogenic assay used to study ovarian cancer. In Alberts D S, Surwit E A (eds) Ovarian Cancer. Martinus Nijhoff, Boston, p 37

198. Welander C, Kjorstad K, Kolstad P 1978 Postoperative irradiation and chemotherapy in patients with advanced ovarian cancer. Acta Obstet Scand 57: 161

199. Wharton J T, Herson J 1981 Surgery for common epithelial tumors of the ovary. Cancer 48: 589

200. Williams C J 1985 The usefulness of the human tumour stem cell assay: In Bleehan N M (ed) Ovarian Cancer. Springer-Verlag, Berlin, p 98

201. Williams T J, Dockerty M B 1976 Status of the contralateral ovary in encapsulated low grade malignant tumors of the ovary. Surg Gynecol Obstet 143: 763

202. Williams T J, Symmonds R E, Litwak O 1973 Management of unilateral and encapsulated ovarian cancer in young women. Gynecol Oncol 1: 143

203. Yancik R, Ries L G, Yates J W 1986 Ovarian cancer in the elderly: an analysis of surveillance, epidemiology and end results program data. Am J Obstet Gynecol 154: 639

204. Young R C 1987 Initial therapy for early ovarian carcinoma. Cancer 60: 2042

205. Young R C, Decker D G, Wharton J T et al 1983 Staging laparotomy in early ovarian cancer. JAMA 250: 3072

206. Young R C, Chabner B A, Hubbard S P et al 1978 Advanced ovarian adenocarcinoma: a prospective clinical trial of melphalan (L-PAM) versus combination chemotherapy. N Engl J Med 299: 1261

207. Young R H, Scully R E 1988 Mucinous ovarian tumors associated with mucinous adenocarcinomas of the cervix. Int J Gynecol Pathol 7: 99

208. Zalonik A J, Oswald M, Langin M 1983 Intrapleural tetracycline in malignant pleural effusions: a randomized study. Cancer 51: 752

209. Zylberberg B, Abbes M, Benoit M et al 1986 Initial therapeutic strategies applied to treatment of common epithelial cancers of the ovary (Stage IIb–III) In: Mathé G (ed) Recent Results in Cancer Research No. 62. Tactics and Strategy in Cancer Treatment. Springer-Verlag, New York, p 181

57. Pathology of malignant germ cell tumors of ovary

H. J. Norris   D. M. O'Connor

INTRODUCTION

One-fifth to a quarter of all ovarian tumors are derived from germ cells. Most are mature cystic teratomas. Less than 5% of all ovarian germ cell tumors are malignant. In the United States Third National Survey of Ovarian Cancer, the three most common malignant germ cell tumors accounted for only 2.4% of ovarian malignancies.[83] The younger a patient is, the more common is the diagnosis of a germ cell tumor and the greater the likelihood that it is malignant. Approximately 60% of ovarian tumors in patients under 20 years of age are germ cell tumors and a quarter of these are malignant in girls younger than 15 years of age.[1,46] In girls less than 10 years old, 84% of germ cell tumors are malignant.[46] In adults, 95% of germ cell tumors are benign mature cystic teratomas, and will not be considered further in this chapter. Thus, children, adolescents, and young women with pelvic and abdominal masses are the main candidates for a malignant germ cell tumor of the ovary.

Table 57.1 Classification of malignant germ cell tumors of the ovary

I Germ cell tumors[a]
A. Dysgerminoma
B. Endodermal sinus tumor
C. Teratomas
   1. Immature (malignant) teratoma
   2. Mature cystic teratoma with malignant transformation
   3. Monodermal or highly specialized
      a) Struma ovarii
      b) Carcinoid and adenocarcinoid
      c) Strumal carcinoid
      d) Others
D. Embryonal carcinoma
E. Choriocarcinoma
F. Combination germ cell tumor

II Mixed germ cell and sex cord stromal tumors
A. Gonadoblastoma
B. Others

III Germ cell tumors arising in dysgenetic gonads

[a] Major types are listed in order of incidence

Because of their rarity, malignant germ cell tumors until recently were little understood. The reported series were small, heterogeneous mixtures of different tumors, the diagnostic criteria were uncertain and treatment met with little success. The situation began to change with the recognition that pure tumors, unlike the combinations and mixtures, had a characteristic behavior,[6] and that combinations of different malignant types were uncommon compared to germ cell tumors of the testis.

A modification of the WHO classification is shown in Table 57.1. An improved classification, together with better staging in recent years, has provided a uniform basis for understanding the behavior of these tumors and for predicting their response in therapy. Clinical interest particularly has been stimulated by effective chemotherapy and the identification of serum tumor markers: alpha-fetoprotein (AFP), lactic acid dehydrogenase (LDH), human placental lactogen (HPL), placental alkaline phosphatase (PLAP), and human chorionic gonadotrophin (hCG). The latter have opened up new possibilities in monitoring treatment (see also Chs 8 and 24).

Based largely on information obtained from the new developments and the experience at the Armed Forces Institute of Pathology with over 300 malignant germ cell tumors, this review emphasizes diagnostic criteria and behavior. Where a histologic type of tumor, like dysgerminoma, is described, this means a histologically proven *pure* tumor. It is not acceptable to bracket various types of mixed malignant germ cell tumors and poorly studied tumors of dubious composition with pure malignant germ cell tumors; to do so only perpetuates the confusion of earlier years. Neoplasms that are combinations are considered separately, as is the rare but clinically important topic of malignant germ cell tumors in intersex states.

DYSGERMINOMA

Incidence

Dysgerminoma is the most common malignant germ cell

tumor of the ovary, representing between 0.9 and 2% of all ovarian malignancies. Three-quarters of patients are between 10 and 30 years old and the median age is about 20 years.[6,25] Few occur under age six or over age 60; only 4% of patients are over 40 years.[6] Dysgerminoma is rare in infants but it is the most common ovarian malignancy of children, adolescents and pregnant women, and the most common associated with gonadoblastoma in dysgenetic gonads. There is a tendency for these tumors to occur in intersex individuals, and in abdominally located gonads associated with a Y chromosome. As many as 17% of dysgerminomas are associated with pregnancy.[31]

Clinical features

The presentation in over half the patients is non-specific, that of a pelvic or abdominal mass with abdominal enlargement and pain. Despite the large size of most dysgerminomas when discovered, the duration of symptoms ranges from 1 month to 2 years,[6] and is under 4 months in one-half of patients. If discovered during pregnancy, the tumor is usually an incidental finding, or it may obstruct labor. Menstrual abnormalities are uncommon in younger women with dysgerminoma. About 10% of patients are asymptomatic.[6] Children may have isosexual precocious puberty or virilization; the former is associated with a positive pregnancy test. About 2% of non-pregnant women have positive pregnancy tests from hCG production by isolated syncytiotrophoblastic cells within the tumor.

Operative findings

Three-quarters of patients have Stage I disease at the time of laparotomy. Dysgerminoma is the only malignant germ cell tumor with a significant incidence of bilaterality. 86% of Stage I tumors are substage Ia (confined to one ovary) and 14% are substage Ib (confined to both ovaries).[6] Although most of the Stage Ib cases are macroscopically obvious at operation, nearly one-third of grossly normal contralateral ovaries harbor microscopic areas of dysgerminoma.

Gross pathology

Typically, dysgerminoma is a solid, fleshy tumor with a smooth lobulated exterior. The cut section appears pink or tan with focal hemorrhage or necrosis (Fig. 57.1). Large, yellowish, sharply demarcated zones of infarction are common. Areas of hemorrhage raise the possibility of focal endodermal sinus tumor or choriocarcinoma. Cystic spaces are uncommon and may represent teratoma. Focal calcification at the periphery suggests gonadoblastoma. Dysgerminoma contains other malignant germ cell elements in up to one-fifth of cases.

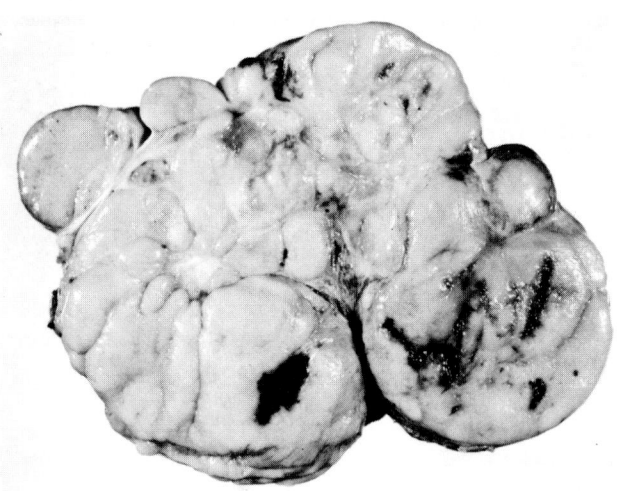

Fig. 57.1 Typical gross appearance of the fleshy cut surface of a dysgerminoma.

Histologic appearance

Dysgerminoma has a distinctive microscopic appearance, identical with that of seminoma arising in testis, mediastinum, sacrococcygeal area and the pineal region. It is composed of cells that resemble primordial germ cells morphologically, histochemically and ultrastructurally,[26,80] but tend to be smaller (Fig. 57.2 and Fig. 57.3). The cells

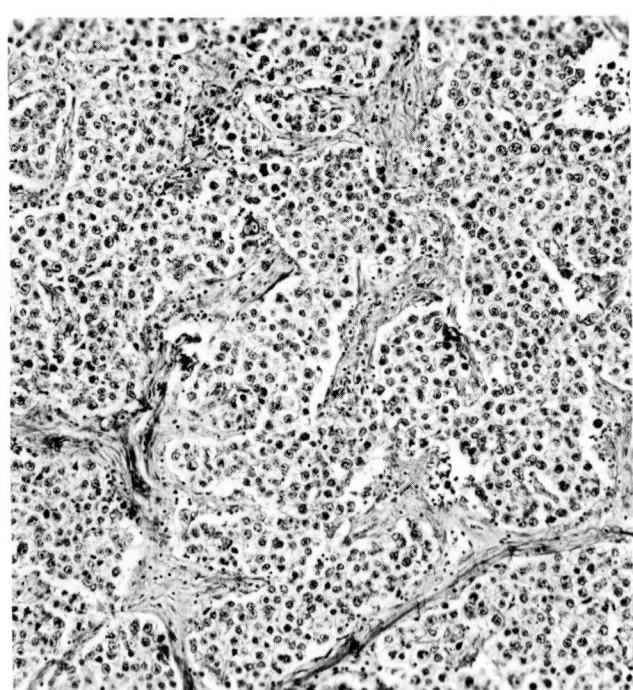

Fig. 57.2 The typical histologic pattern of dysgerminoma. Large polygonal cells are shown interspersed with fibrous trabeculae. (H & E ×150)

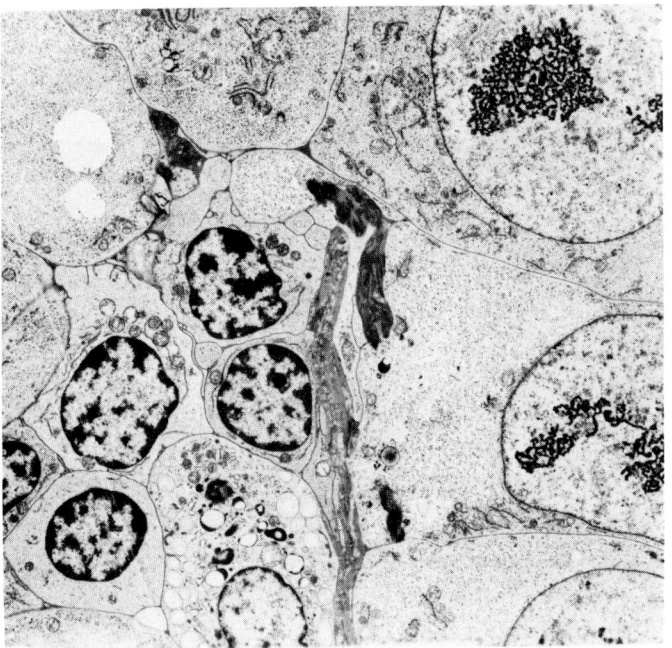

Fig. 57.3 Ultrastructure of an ovarian dysgerminoma. Large electronlucent cells with large nuclei and chromatin spiremes (right field) contrast with lymphoctyes (left center) and macrophage (lower center). (× 2200) (Courtesy of Dr Francisco F Nogales, Seville, Spain.)

are round or polygonal and are about 20 μ in diameter. When the cells are well fixed, they display a prominent vesicular nucleus containing one or more large eosinophilic nucleoli. The cytoplasm is clear or slightly granular, contains glycogen and gives positive periodic acid Schiff and alkaline phosphatase reactions. Most dysgerminomas have a solid pattern with variable amounts of intervening connective tissue and are usually infiltrated with lymphocytes. A vague glandular trend may be evident in some tumors, reflecting differentiation towards embryonal carcinoma. Immunokeratin stains are usually negative. Positive reactivity for alphafetoprotein reflects a trend towards endodermal sinus tumor or embryonal carcinoma. Dysgerminoma cells are negative for AFP and hCG, but positive for placental alkaline phosphatase.

In 2 to 3% of dysgerminomas, rare giant cells resembling syncytiotrophoblast are present. hCG has been demonstrated by immunoperoxidase reaction in these cells.[35,80,87] Even small clusters of syncytiotrophoblasts can produce elevation of serum hCG and luteinization in residual ovarian stroma. The syncytiotrophoblastic cells lack the two-cell population of admixed syncytiotrophoblast and cytotrophoblast found in choriocarcinoma. Thus, by convention, they are not sufficient by themselves for a diagnosis of choriocarcinoma.

About 20% of dysgerminomas contain foreign-body-type giant cells which, like the presence of a diffuse lymphocytic infiltrate, correlate with a better prognosis. Foreign body giant cells and fibrosis may produce a granulomatous appearance.[6]

A rare subtype, the anaplastic dysgerminoma (Fig. 57.4), is analogous with anaplastic seminoma of the testis. It has the overall pattern of a dysgerminoma but with more cellular pleomorphism, multinucleated cells and increased numbers of mitoses. It is unclear whether the prognosis is worse for anaplastic dysgerminoma. DNA studies reveal that most dysgerminomas have an aneuploid or polyploid DNA content. Ploidy does not correlate with stage, recurrence or survival in dysgerminoma, however.[49]

A well preserved dysgerminoma presents little diagnostic difficulty for the pathologist. Poor preservation and fixation artifact, however, can obscure the diagnosis, particularly in metastatic deposits. Granulomatous dysgerminomas, and dysgerminomas with much sclerosis and few cells, may mimic an undifferentiated carcinoma or Hodgkin's disease.

Therapy and prognosis

Therapy for dysgerminoma can be individualized according to the age and childbearing status of the patient. It is based on careful staging of the tumor by radiographic studies and surgery. LDH, PLAP, and CA 125 may be elevated and in some instances can serve as tumor markers. LDH,

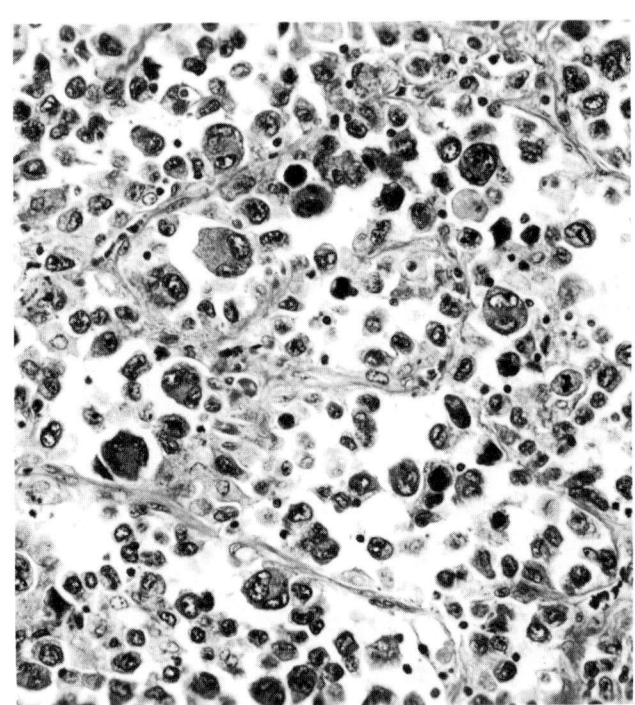

Fig. 57.4 Anaplastic dysgerminoma. Multiple nuclei, cell pleomorphism and unusually numerous mitotic figures identify this rare type of dysgerminoma. (H & E ×330)

in particular, has been successful in predicting recurrence in testicular seminomas and dysgerminomas.[63] Metastasis is primarily via lymphatics rather than peritoneal seeding. Metastasis seldom occurs in small dysgerminomas.

For patients with biopsy-proven Stage Ia disease, the recurrence rate is higher (22%) with unilateral salpingo-oophorectomy than with bilateral salpingo-oophorectomy with or without hysterectomy (9%). However, recurrences can be controlled with radiation or chemotherapy[9,10,18,79] in half of the first group, resulting in a comparable 10-year survival rate of about 85% in both groups (see Ch. 58).[6]

In addition to the presence of metastases, extension beyond the ovary, bilaterality, and large tumor size worsen the prognosis. Most recurrences are evident within 2 years.

The 5-year survival in dysgerminoma drops from 96% to 63% when it has extended beyond the ovaries.[6] Bilateral salpingo-oophorectomy is recommended for patients with dysgenetic gonads or abnormal karyotypes containing a Y chromosome. (See p. 944.)

ENDODERMAL SINUS TUMOR

Incidence

Endodermal sinus tumor (yolk sac carcinoma) is the second most common ovarian malignant germ cell tumor in girls and young women.[46] It represents about 1% of all ovarian malignancies. Originally confused with carcinoma of mesonephroid type (clear cell carcinoma) and embryonal carcinoma, collected series of pure tumors are still infrequent.

Clinical features

The age range of patients is from 14 months to 45 years, but very few cases are reported in persons over 40 years. The median age is 19 years,[33] or younger in some series.

The clinical presentation of endodermal sinus tumor is frequently acute, and half of patients have symptoms for 1 week or less. Three-fourths of the patients have abdominal pain and nearly all have a large abdominal or pelvic mass.[33] Symptoms produced by rupture, torsion or hemorrhage occasionally mimic appendicitis. Patients usually do not have endocrine or menstrual abnormalities and the serum hCG is not elevated. AFP is the characteristic marker for endodermal sinus tumor, either primary or recurrent. Occasional reports of endodermal sinus tumor with hormonal activity probably represent inadequately sampled tumors containing choriocarcinoma or embryonal carcinoma.

Operative findings

About a quarter of tumors are ruptured before or during surgery. As many as 71% are Stage I and all of these are Stage Ia; involvement of the contralateral ovary does not occur in the absence of peritoneal spread (Table 57.2). At least 6% of tumors are Stage II and 23% are Stage III. Few neoplasms are Stage IV.

Table 57.2 Status of contralateral ovary in patients with Stage I germ cell tumors of the ovary

Tumor	Stage Ia patients	Stage Ib patients	Stage I patients with microscopic spread to opposite ovary	
			No. examined	No. positive
Dysgerminoma[6]	71	7	21	4[a]
Endodermal sinus tumor[33]	51	0	24	0
Immature teratoma[47]	40	0	6	0
Embryonal carcinoma[32]	9	0	0	0
Combination germ cell tumors[34]	20	0	5	1[b]

[a] Dysgerminoma developed subsequently in two additional patients in the contralateral ovary which appeared normal at the time of operation.
[b] An identical neoplasm (mixed dysgerminoma and endodermal sinus tumor) developed subsequently in one additional patient in the contralateral ovary which appeared normal at the time of operation.

Gross pathology

Endodermal sinus tumors are unilateral and large, the majority being over 10 cm in diameter. They typically have a smooth, lobulated exterior surface. Usually very soft and predominantly solid, they contain large and small cysts throughout, which give the cut surface a honeycombed appearance (Fig. 57.5). 14% of endodermal sinus tumors coexist with benign cystic teratoma in the same ovary, and 5% with it in the opposite ovary. Visible necrosis and hemorrhage are common, often leading to rupture and spillage at the time of surgery.

Histologic appearance

Endodermal sinus tumors display five basic interrelated growth patterns, described in detail by Teilum.[75,76] The most common is the reticular pattern, composed of a loose meshwork of spaces and channels lined by flattened or cuboidal cells with scanty cytoplasm and indistinct borders. Schiller-Duval bodies ('festoons'), the tufted structures pathognomonic of this neoplasm, are infrequent, but present in most instances. Hyaline bodies are common in the reticular pattern. The typical reticular endodermal sinus pattern is the easiest to identify and it may contain abundant Schiller-Duval bodies. This pattern recapitulates the endodermal sinus of the rodent yolk sac (Fig. 57.6). The

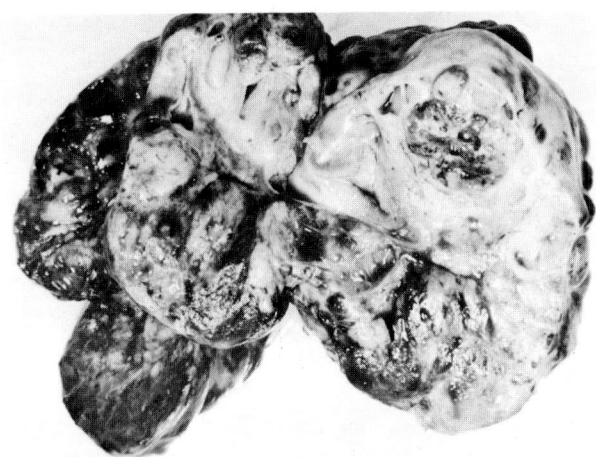

Fig. 57.5 Endodermal sinus tumor, opened to show multiple cysts.

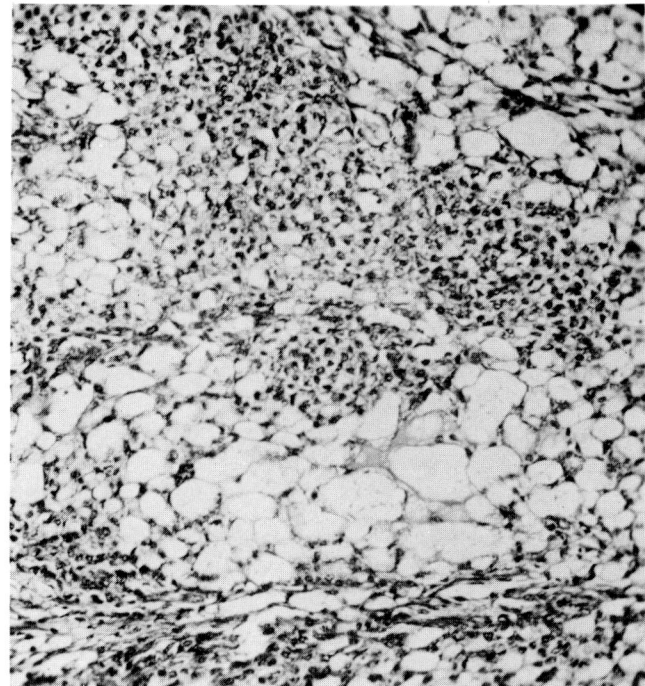

Fig. 57.7 Mixed solid and reticular pattern of endodermal sinus tumor. (H & E ×100)

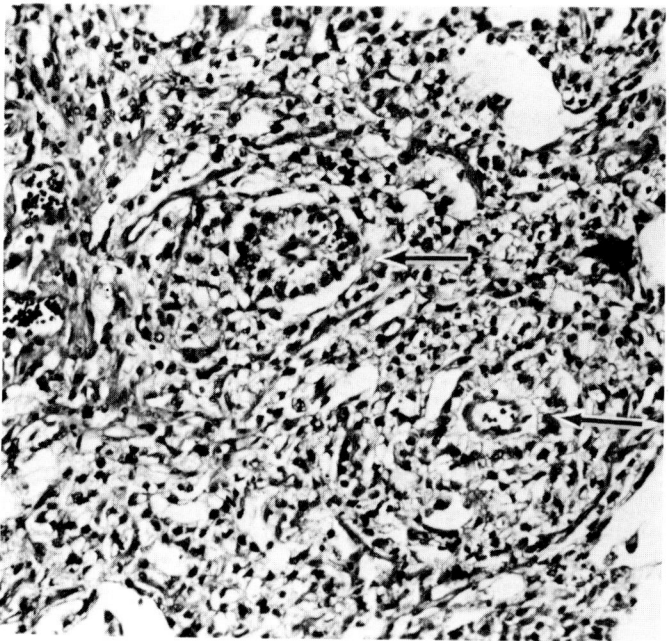

Fig. 57.6 The reticular pattern of endodermal sinus tumor showing typical Schiller-Duval bodies (arrows). (H & E ×150)

bryonal carcinoma. In most cases the growth patterns are mixed (Fig. 57.7). There is no prognostic difference between any of the types. One-fifth of the endodermal sinus tumors contain admixtures with one or more malignant germ cell elements, usually dysgerminoma.

Schiller-Duval bodies, diagnostic of endodermal sinus tumor, are absent in one-fourth of tumors. On the other hand, hyaline droplets, which stain positively with the periodic acid-Schiff reaction are always present.[33] Immunohistochemical studies have established that the droplets represent mainly AFP,[33,35] with alpha anti-trypsin[50] and other proteins also present (Fig. 57.8).

Therapy and prognosis

Endodermal sinus tumors constitute a surgical and therapeutic emergency. The tumor growth rate is probably the fastest of any human malignancy and some patients have had normal pelvic examinations a week before the removal of a large tumor. Any delay in treatment may therefore be fatal.

It is clear that staging procedures for endodermal sinus tumors are inaccurate, since prior to modern chemotherapy 84% of Stage Ia tumors recurred and the mortality rate for all stages combined was 93%.[33] Regardless of the type of surgery or use of adjunctive irradiation, 90% of recurrences appeared within a year of diagnosis and nearly all of these patients were dead within 2 years. Radiation and

polyvesicular vitelline pattern is rarer, being characterized by microcysts with flat or columnar epithelial cells having clear cytoplasm lying in a dense fibroblastic stroma. This pattern has seldom been encountered in pure form. A fourth pattern is the alveolar-glandular type, in which cystic spaces are lined by papillary processes having cuboidal epithelium. A subset of this category is the hepatoid yolk sac tumor, with a cellular pattern reminiscent of hepatocellular carcinoma.[56] The fifth and rarest form is a relatively solid growth of undifferentiated cells resembling em-

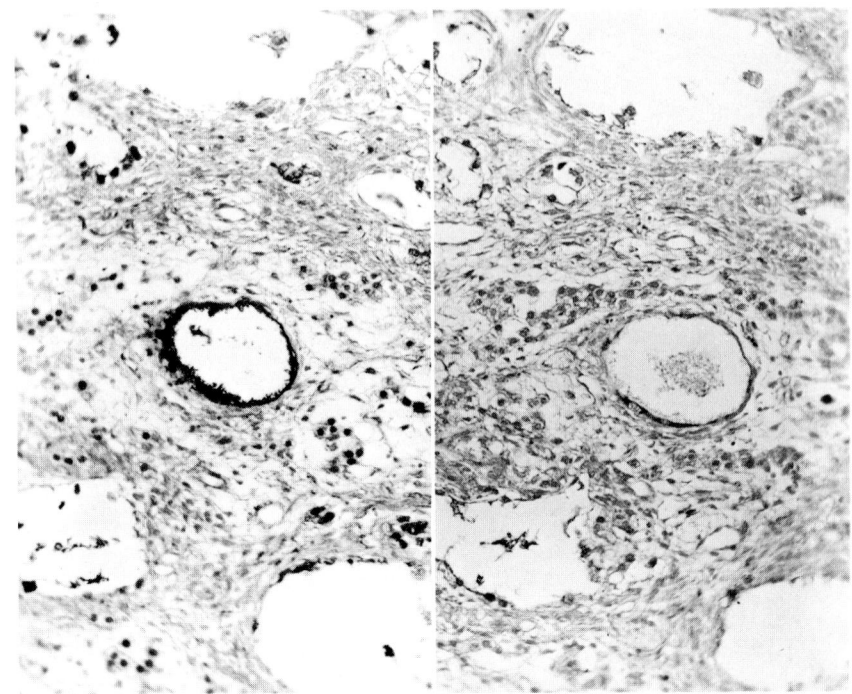

Fig. 57.8 Polyvesicular vitelline pattern of endodermal sinus tumor showing (on left) alphafetoprotein (AFP) in cells lining a cyst. Right field is a control section using normal rabbit serum. (Peroxidase stain × 130)

radical surgery are ineffective. Success has been reported with chemotherapy utilizing combinations of vincristine, actinomycin-D and cyclophosphamide,[33] or methotrexate, actinomycin-D, and chlorambucil. A survival rate of greater than 50% after postoperative intervals of 11 and 63 months (which includes some patients with Stage III disease) has been achieved (see Ch. 58).

TERATOMAS

Many teratomas arise from premeiotic cells, possibly with failure in the first meiotic division. At least some immature teratomas originate from a pre- or post second meiotic division error. More than 90% arise from fertilization of an empty ovum by a haploid sperm, with subsequent duplication without cytokinesis.[28,48] While the majority of teratomas are 46 XX, a small number of tumors demonstrate deviations from the normal karyotype. This finding correlates with tumors of higher grade.[28]

Immature (malignant) teratomas

The term *immature teratoma*, introduced by the World Health Organization classification,[65] is reserved for a pure teratoma that contains a variable amount of immature tissue derived from any of the three germ cell layers. Immaturity in teratomas indicates a potential for recurrence and metastasis which is directly related to the

quantity and grade of immature neuroepithelium present.[45,47,59] Neoplasms arising in otherwise mature and benign teratomas are discussed separately below.

Incidence

Pure immature teratoma is the third most common malignant germ cell tumor of ovary after dysgerminoma and endodermal sinus tumor.[46] Immature teratomas account for only 1% of all ovarian teratomas, but in children younger than 15 years of age they represent nearly one-quarter of all ovarian germ cell tumors.[46]

Clinical features

Children and young women are principally affected. The median age is 17 to 19 years and the oldest patients are about 40 years.[21,47] The symptoms are non-specific and are usually present for only a few weeks; occasionally they are acute. About 80% of patients have a palpable abdominal or pelvic mass, frequently combined with pain or local tenderness. A minority of patients have menstrual irregularities. Characteristically, AFP and hCG levels are not elevated.

Operative findings

Approximately 70% of tumors are Stage Ia. 5% of contralateral ovaries contain a benign cystic teratoma, which

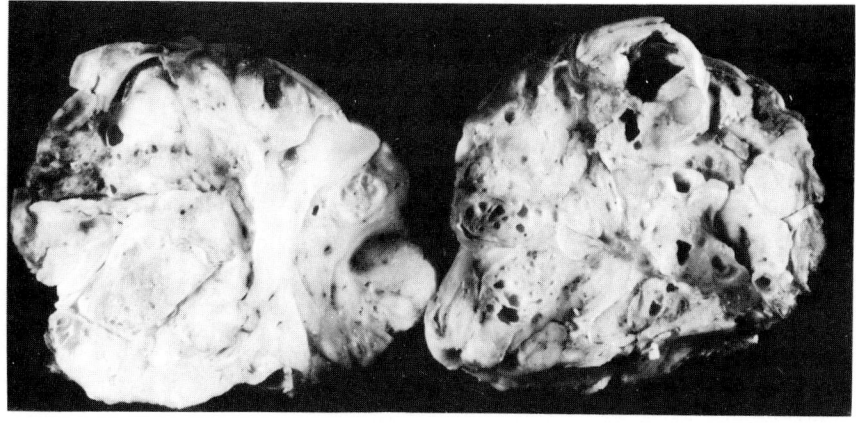

Fig. 57.9 Pure immature (malignant) teratoma. The cut surface shows a basically solid tumor.

was previously often mistaken for a metastasis. In the three largest series, no patient had contralateral involvement without diffuse peritoneal spread.[21,45,47] Thus, Stage Ib has not been reported. Early spread is by direct extension to the adnexa and adjacent pelvic tissues, and by peritoneal implantation. Metastasis via lymphatic invasion is unusual, as is extra-abdominal spread.

Gross pathology

Most immature teratomas are large, unilateral tumors with a median size of 18 cm, and a mean tumor weight of about 2510 g.[45] The external surface is smooth, and the cut surface is soft and fleshy, gray to pink with visible hemorrhage and necrosis. Perforation of the capsule, adhesions and invasion to adjacent structures can occur. Predominantly solid, all contain cysts, with a variegated cut surface. Hair is present in two-fifths of tumors. Teeth are rare, but bone, cartilage or calcification are usually evident macroscopically.

Although mainly solid, immature teratomas always contain some cysts and a third may contain large cysts (Fig. 57.9). The use of the terms 'solid teratoma' and 'cystic teratoma' to imply malignant and benign behavior respectively is misleading, but the principle that solid areas of teratoma may reflect malignancy should prompt the surgeon to request an intraoperative frozen section examination.

Histologic appearance

A variety of tissues with different degrees of immaturity are typically found. Glia comprises most of the ectodermal tissue, but retina, nerve bundles and skin components are also prominent. Mesodermal elements, such as connective tissue, cartilage and smooth muscle are common, but their immaturity has little or no influence on outcome. Endo-

dermal derivatives include respiratory and intestinal epithelium. These may contain AFP.

Immature teratomas must be graded histologically because chemotherapy is used to treat the higher grade tumors. The grade is based on the degree of immaturity of the neural tissue and its quantity (Fig. 57.10). The most common grading system uses the method of Norris, Zirkin & Benson,[47] who proposed a simple quantitative method amplifying that of Robboy & Scully[59]:

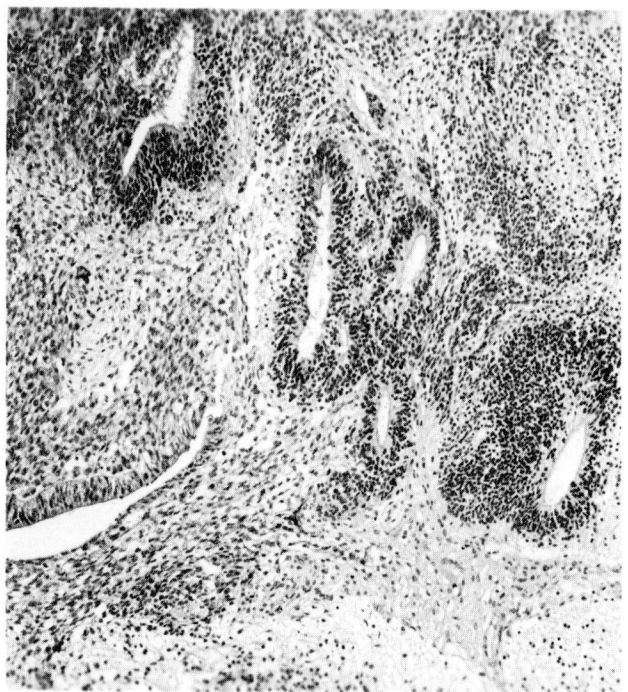

Fig. 57.10 Grade 2 immaturity in malignant teratoma. Neuroepithelium is shown. The technique for grading teratomas is discussed in the text. (H & E ×80)

Grade 0: Wholly mature tissue

Grade 1: Abundant mature tissue but some immaturity, mainly glial, with loose, primitive mesenchyme. Mitoses are present, but neuroepithelium is restricted to one low power field (40×) per slide.

Grade 2: Greater immaturity, with neuroepithelium not exceeding 3 low power fields per slide.

Grade 3: Marked immaturity, with neuroepithelium found in 4 or more low power fields per slide and frequently merging with sarcomatous stroma.

Accurate grading requires adequate sampling. One block of tissue should be taken for every 1 cm of maximum tumor diameter. For neoplasms exceeding 20 cm in diameter, and therefore requiring more than 20 blocks of tissue to evaluate, the quantitative allowance of immaturity for grading may be doubled. It has been proposed that up to 10% of neuroectoderm on one slide be considered Grade 1, between 10 and 33% assigned Grade 2, and greater than 33% identify Grade 3 neoplasms.[68]

Therapy and prognosis

Prognosis is related both to the stage of the tumor (Fig. 57.11) and to its histologic grade (Table 57.3). In view of the rarity or nonexistence of Stage Ib disease (Table 57.2), surgical Stage I disease is treated by unilateral salpingo-oophorectomy. Patients with Grade 2 and 3 Stage I neoplasms and all more advanced stages require adjunctive chemotherapy; it is also probably indicated for all Stage I tumors with rupture.

Table 57.3 Comparison of grade and stage with survival for patients with immature teratoma[a]

| Grade | Stage I | | Stages II and III | | |
	No. of patients	% surviving	No. of patients	% surviving	Total % surviving
1	14	100	8	50	82
2	20	70[b]	4	50	62
3	6	33	4	35	30
Total	40		16		

[a] Results were derived prior to modern chemotherapy.[47]
[b] Includes 3 patients living with tumor.

Once metastasis has occurred, the grade of the metastasis is a major determinant of prognosis. Thorough sampling of deposits is therefore important to determine prognosis and therapy. Grade 0 implants (Fig. 57.12) do not have an adverse effect on survival. Before the advent of effective chemotherapy, Grade 1 or 2 metastasis carried a 40 to 50% survival rate and no patient with Grade 3 metastases survived. Combination chemotherapy with vincristine, actinomycin D and cyclophosphamide will produce an 85% cure rate (see Ch. 58).[21]

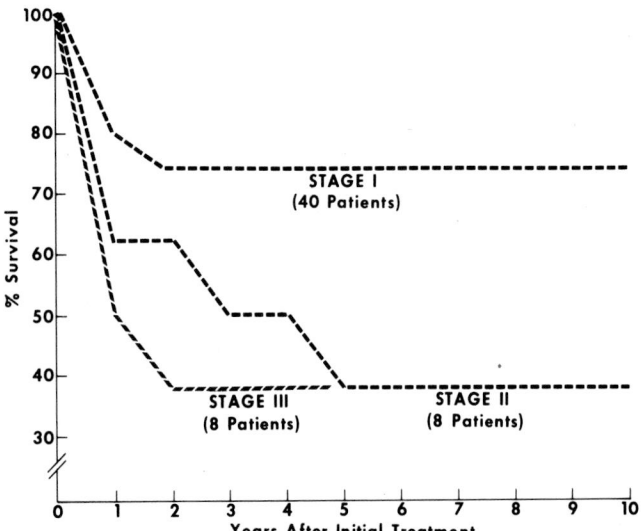

Fig. 57.11 Actuarial survival of 56 patients with malignant teratoma prior to the era of chemotherapy by stage of the neoplasm. Two patients who were lost to follow-up were excluded.[47]

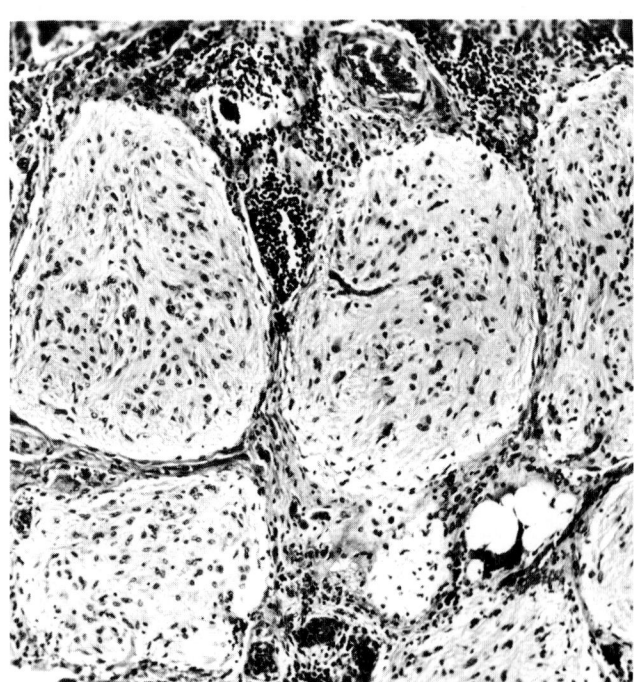

Fig. 57.12 Grade 0 glial implants originating from a Grade 3 malignant teratoma. Grade 0 implants rarely if ever progress, regardless of the degree of immaturity of the primary tumor. (H & E ×110)

Malignant transformation in mature cystic teratoma

Incidence

Between 1 and 2% of benign cystic teratomas undergo malignant transformation.[17,29,40,53] This occurs most frequently in postmenopausal women, who account for only 10% of benign cystic teratomas. A wide variety of neoplasms arise in the mature tissues of otherwise benign teratomas. Of the malignancies arising in teratomas, squamous carcinoma is the most common (83%) with sarcomas accounting for 7%; adenocarcinoma and carcinoid tumors make up most of the others.

Clinical features

The presentation in Stage I disease does not differ from that of benign cystic teratoma, except that ascites is occasionally present. In the more advanced neoplasms, the symptoms are those of epithelial ovarian cancer of the same stage.

Gross pathology

The gross specimen resembles a cystic teratoma with a soft to firm mass invading part of the cyst wall, often with necrosis. The appearance varies with the type of supervening malignancy. Squamous cell carcinoma tends to grow through the teratoma and invade neighboring tissue.[11,29,53] In two-thirds of cases, invasion or metastasis have occurred before diagnosis.[53]

Histologic appearance

Almost any component of a teratoma may undergo malignant change; in up to 80% of cases, it is a squamous cell carcinoma arising from epidermis.[53] The only other malignancies occurring with any regularity are carcinoid tumors and adenocarcinomas, including struma ovarii (described below). Small and single numbers of bronchogenic carcinoma, leiomyosarcoma,[29] osteosarcoma, chondrosarcoma,[11] basal cell carcinoma, melanoma,[37] melanotic 'retinal anlage tumor',[22] sebaceous tumors, nevi[24] and other less acceptable entities have all been reported. Sarcomatous or pseudosarcomatous changes in stroma surrounding areas of carcinoma also occur.[12]

Monodermal and highly specialized teratomas

1. Struma ovarii. The term, struma ovarii, is restricted to teratomas in which thyroid tissue represents more than half of the tumor. Biologically malignant struma ovarii is exceedingly rare. In 5 to 20% of cases, a diagnosis of carcinoma has been made,[16,86] but metastases occurred in only a minority.[52,84,86] The frequency of malignancy is exaggerated because the criteria for carcinoma in struma ovarii are not the same as those in primary thyroid carcinoma. Thyroid tissue within a teratoma is not encapsulated, giving the false impression of invasion, and papillary processes have no proven significance.

Grossly, the thyroid tissue is firm and brownish red, as in the neck. The diagnosis of malignant struma ovarii should only be made when there are the cytologic features of malignancy. Very infrequently peritoneal implants of benign thyroid tissue, termed 'strumosis', occur in struma ovarii and should not be confused with malignancy.

2. Carcinoid. More than 150 primary ovarian carcinoids have been reported.[72] Carcinoid tumor is found in less than 1% of ovarian teratomas.[58] Grossly, it appears as a solid yellow nodule, usually with visible elements of cystic teratoma. It forms insular (midgut) or trabecular (foregut and hindgut) histologic patterns, depending on the type of tissue from which it arises.[58,60] Argentaffin granules are identified in over 80% of the former and two-thirds of the latter type. A few insular carcinoids have given rise to local metastasis, but metastasis from a trabecular carcinoid has been reported only once.[72]

A goblet cell (adenocarcinoid) primary tumor also occurs. This is distinguished from metastatic adenocarcinoid in that it is unilateral and often associated with a cystic teratoma. Metastatic adenocarcinoids are nearly always bilateral and have their primary site in the appendix.[15]

Carcinoid syndrome is only found with the midgut tumors and is present in one-third of them.[58] Since venous blood from the ovary drains to the inferior vena cava, bypassing the portal circulation, a primary ovarian carcinoid can produce carcinoid syndrome without metastases. Patients with primary ovarian carcinoid therefore are symptomatic early, and all have been cured after total excision. Carcinoid syndrome with tricuspid valve involvement secondary to an ovarian carcinoid has been reported.[5] Insulin production by an ovarian carcinoid has also been reported,[43] as has substance 'p'.[69]

In nearly one-quarter of midgut tumors, carcinoid is the sole component and must therefore be distinguished from metastatic carcinoid.[58] Primary carcinoid is unilateral, occurs with other teratomatous components in three-quarters of cases, and has no metastases; urinary 4-hydroxy-indole-acetic acid levels are normal after complete excision.

3. Strumal carcinoid. Occasionally, carcinoid tissue is combined with thyroid tissue as 'strumal carcinoid'. Myoglobin and neuroendocrine granules can occur in the same cell comprising the tumor.[66] Only one malignant example has been documented,[57] and one case caused masculinization.[14]

4. Malignant neuroectodermal tumor. Malignant neuroectodermal tumor is a monodermal germ cell tumor composed entirely of neuroectoderm.[4] It is the equivalent of a Grade 3 immature teratoma and requires combination chemotherapy even in Stage I. Of four patients with a primary ovarian neuroectodermal tumor, only one survived longer than 7 years.[4]

5. Miscellaneous. Sebaceous tumors, melanotic neoplasms resembling a retinal anlage tumor, and some pure mucinous cystadenomas and cystadenocarcinomas of intestinal differentiation are found. These rare neoplasms may contain goblet cells, argentaffin and Paneth cells. Functioning pituitary tissue has been described and chondrosarcoma and other rare sarcomas have also arisen in mature cystic teratoma.

EMBRYONAL CARCINOMA

Incidence

Embryonal carcinoma has only recently been characterized as a separate clinicopathologic entity.[32] It is analogous morphologically with embryonal carcinoma of the adult testis. In the past, it was included with endodermal sinus tumor of the ovary and both terms were used indiscriminately. However, a retrospective study of 85 tumors accessioned at the AFIP as endodermal sinus tumor or embryonal carcinoma showed that 15 could be distinguished on a clinical, histologic and immunochemical basis.[32] Eleven were pure embryonal carcinoma and four contained elements of other germ cell tumors. Thus, pure embryonal carcinoma is rare, accounting for no more than 5% of malignant ovarian germ cell tumors.

Clinical features

The patient age range is 4 to 28 years (median 14 years) with nearly one-half of tumors occurring in prepubertal females.[32] A majority of patients have an abdominal or pelvic mass and half have abdominal pain at presentation. Symptoms tend to be of short duration (mean of 3 weeks) and occasionally mimic appendicitis or ruptured ectopic pregnancy, particularly when the pregnancy test is positive. Unlike patients with endodermal sinus tumor, most patients with embryonal carcinoma have abnormal hormonal manifestations. Signs of precocious puberty are present in almost half of prepubertal girls.[32] Amenorrhea or abnormal vaginal bleeding are found in postmenarchial women. Mild hirsutism and virilization may also occur.

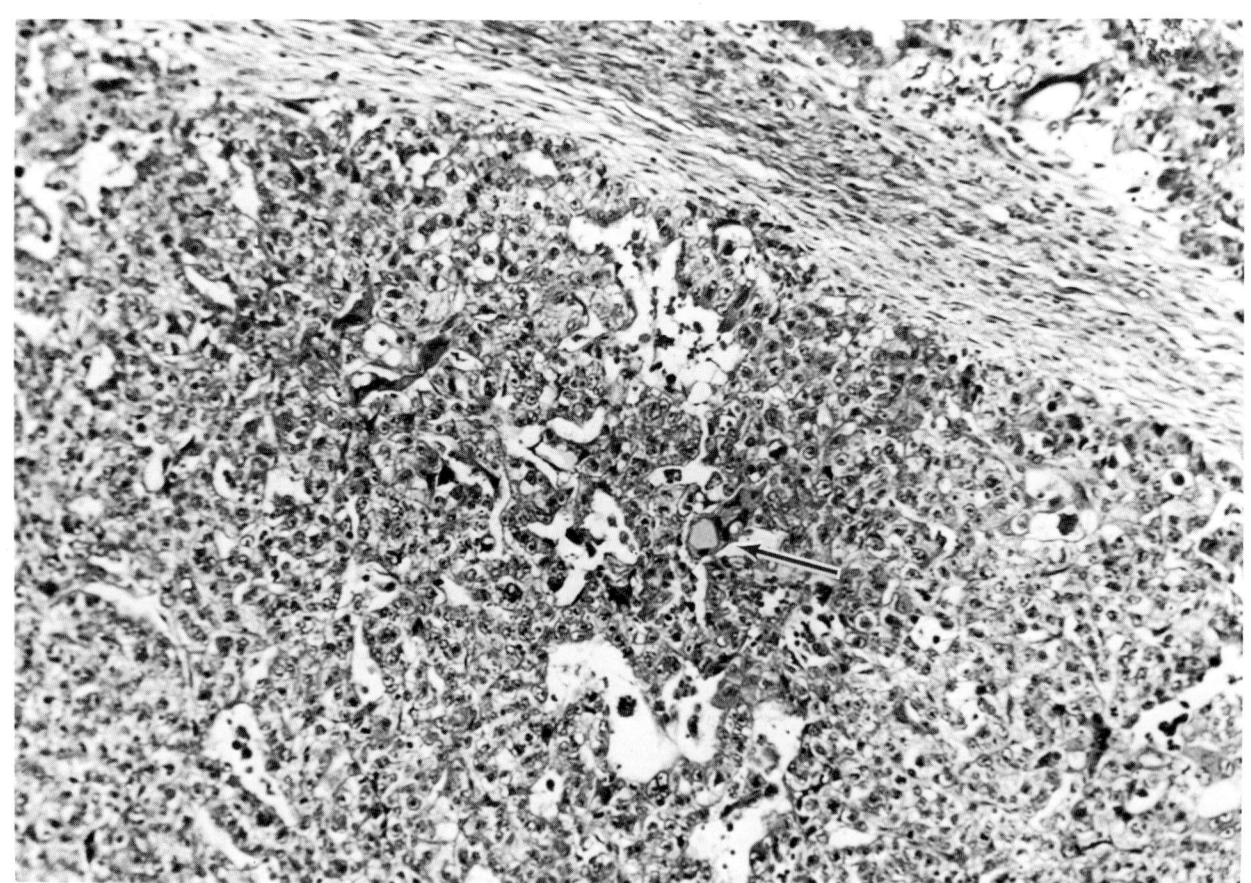

Fig. 57.13 Embryonal carcinoma. Solid sheets of primitive cells are interspersed with occasional gland-like clefts. The large intracellular hyaline droplet (arrow) is characteristic of AFP production. (H & E ×300)

HCG is elaborated by the syncytiotrophoblasts in the tumor.

Operative findings

About 60% of cases are Stage I and, like endodermal sinus tumor and immature teratoma, none are bilateral. The remainder divide equally between Stage II and Stage III. Stage IV disease is rarely encountered. In two of six patients undergoing biopsy, the opposite ovary harbored microscopic foci of dysgerminoma. Both had occult areas of dysgerminoma in the main neoplasm.[32]

Gross pathology

The tumor is typically encapsulated, soft and round. Focal hemorrhage and infarcts are common. The appearance of embryonal carcinoma is not distinctive among the malignant germ cell tumors. The median size is 17 cm. The cut surface is gray-yellow and variegated with cysts common.

Histologic appearance

Microscopically, embryonal carcinoma is composed of solid sheets of large, primitive pleomorphic cells with amphophilic vacuolated cytoplasm and vesicular nuclei with one or more nucleoli (Fig. 57.13). These cells may form gland-like spaces and clusters, but they lack the reticular, polyvesicular vitelline and festoon growth pattern of endodermal sinus tumor. The stroma is variable, being either loose and myxoid or cellular with primitive fibroblastic mesenchymal cells.

All tumors contain isolated clusters of syncytiotrophoblastic cells and mononuclear cells with cytoplasmic hyaline droplets. These droplets have been shown by immunoperoxidase stains, even in paraffin embedded tissue up to 20 years old, to contain hCG, AFP and keratin.[8,32,35] The first two, which are secreted by different cell lines, serve as tumor markers in tissue and serum. The relationship of embryonal carcinoma to endodermal sinus tumor is demonstrated by the fact that both elaborate AFP (Fig. 57.14). In one-half of both tumors mucinous glands are present, and both patterns occur in some neoplasms.

The close relationship of embryonal carcinoma to choriocarcinoma is illustrated by the presence of hCG and syncytiotrophoblastic cells, and the occasional existence of both tumors in combination. Embryonal carcinoma also has a tendency to differentiate towards teratoma, as sug-

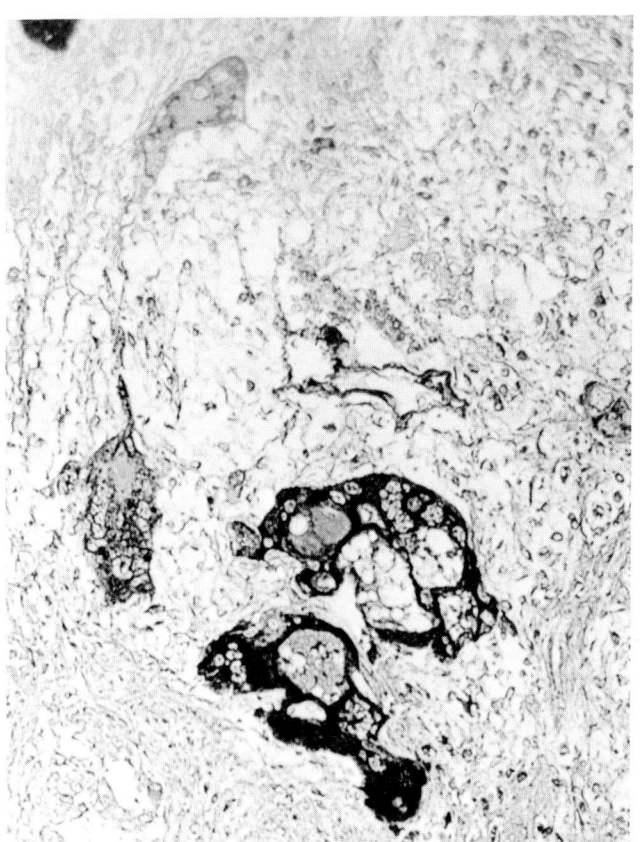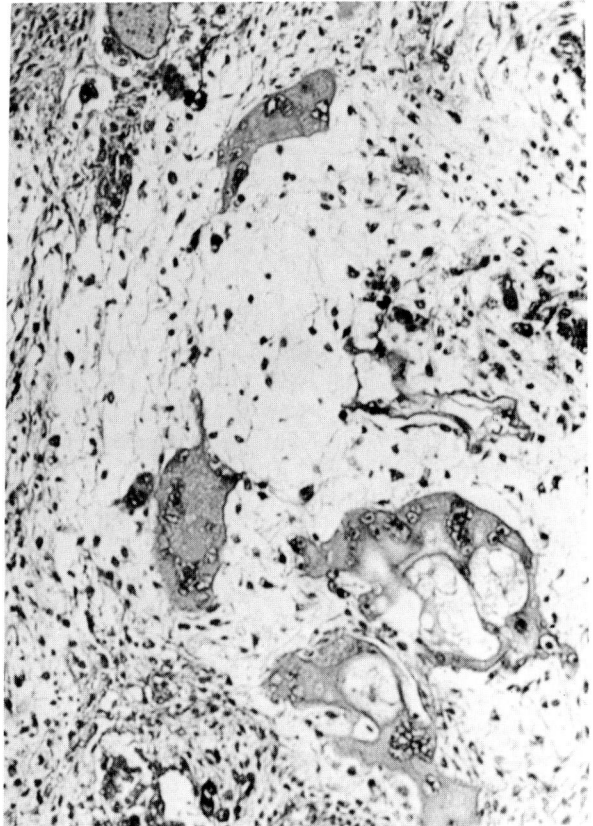

Fig. 57.14 Syncytiotrophoblastic cells in embryonal carcinoma showing (on left) a positive reaction for hCG with indirect immunoperoxidase preparation. Right field shows the same section stained with H & E ×60.

gested by its primitive stroma and by the cartilage and squamous epithelium found in some examples. It is considered a primitive germ cell tumor, intermediate between dysgerminoma and the others, and capable of both embryonic (teratoma) and extra-embryonic (yolk sac carcinoma, choriocarcinoma) differentiation.

Therapy and prognosis

Prior to combination chemotherapy, the 5-year actuarial survival for patients with embryonal carcinoma was 50% in Stage I and 39% for all stages combined (Table 57.4). Patients who developed recurrences following treatment died within 2 years from widespread intra-abdominal metastases. With modern chemotherapy, most patients

Table 57.4 5-year actuarial survival of malignant germ cell tumors[a]

Tumor	No. followed	% survival of Stage I	% survival of all Stages
Dysgerminoma[6]	98	90	86
Endodermal sinus[33]	67	16	13
Immature teratoma[47]	56	75	63
Mixed germ cell[34]	28	50	46
Embryonal carcinoma[32]	14	50	39

[a] Results were derived prior to modern chemotherapy.

should be cured, as in the case of endodermal sinus tumors. Radiation therapy is ineffective (see Ch. 58).

CHORIOCARCINOMA

Ovarian choriocarcinoma may be found as pure choriocarcinoma or, far more commonly, as part of a mixed germ cell tumor. The distinction is important; if pure, it is more likely to be gestational than germ cell in origin. If the origin is gestational, ovarian choriocarcinoma is more likely to be a metastasis from a uterine or tubal primary than a choriocarcinoma resulting from an ovarian pregnancy. This has some practical importance because non-gestational choriocarcinoma may be less sensitive to chemotherapy than gestational choriocarcinoma.

Incidence

To be unequivocally derived from germ cells, pure ovarian choriocarcinoma should be diagnosed in a prepubertal child excluding the possibility of pregnancy. Primary ovarian choriocarcinoma is extremely rare.[7,20,23,51,81] Two probable cases were encountered in the first 5000 ovarian tumors accessioned at the AFIP.

Most non-gestational choriocarcinomas of the ovary occur in combination with immature teratoma, endodermal sinus tumor, embryonal carcinoma or dysgerminoma. Among eight examples of non-gestational ovarian choriocarcinoma in the AFIP files, at least six were mixed with other malignant germ cell elements. Of the first 40 examples of choriocarcinoma cited in the literature, only one-half were pure.[17] Gestational choriocarcinoma is not found in association with other malignant germ cell components. The remainder of this section concerns only the teratomatous form of choriocarcinoma.

Clinical features

In a review of published cases of both pure and combination germ cell tumors with choriocarcinoma, the age range was seven months to 35 years with a mean of about 13 years.[17] About 40% of patients had abdominal pain, half of them with abdominal enlargement. Hemoperitoneum is common. Half the premenarchial girls had signs of isosexual precocious puberty.

Gross pathology

Choriocarcinoma is a solid, soft, hemorrhagic neoplasm with abundant necrosis and little viable tumor at the periphery. Usually unilateral, the purer the tumor, the more hemorrhagic it is. Other gross characteristics depend on the proportions of other germ cell elements.

Histologic appearance

Microscopically, choriocarcinoma is composed of two populations of cells, cytotrophoblast and syncytiotrophoblast, arranged in a characteristic biphasic plexiform pattern. The hCG-producing syncytiotrophoblast is relatively well differentiated, with distinct immunological, histochemical and ultrastructural features. Both elements must be present to identify choriocarcinoma and avoid confusion with embryonal carcinoma. Because of extensive hemorrhage, only a small amount of viable trophoblast may be evident microscopically.

Prognosis and therapy

A highly malignant neoplasm, non-gestational choriocarcinoma of the ovary has not been as amenable to methotrexate-based therapy as gestational choriocarcinoma of the uterus has been, but this may be partly because some cases represented misdiagnosed embryonal carcinoma while others were poorly sampled and may have contained occult areas of other malignant germ cell elements.

Irradiation is of no value in the treatment of choriocarcinoma. Modern treatment depends on surgical excision and a choice of combination chemotherapy based upon thorough histologic evaluation of all elements present.[7,20,81] Serial hCG estimations are of value in monitoring treatment. (See also Ch. 65.)

COMBINATION GERM CELL TUMORS

There remains a group of germ cell tumors which contain a mixture of two or more malignant components. Dysgerminoma and endodermal sinus tumor are the most common combination and, when dysgerminoma is present, the dysgerminoma component may be bilateral (Stage Ib).

Incidence

Combination germ cell tumors represent about 8% of malignant germ cell tumors in the ovary, compared with 60% in the testes.

Clinical factors

The age of patients ranges from 5 to 33 years with a median of 16 years. 40% are prepubertal and one-third of these are children with signs of isosexual precocious puberty. The pregnancy test is positive in 38% of non-pregnant patients, reflecting syncytiotrophoblast in the tumor.[34] The majority of patients present with non-specific signs of an abdominal or pelvic mass; half of them have lower abdominal pain, and one-fifth have fever. A fifth of the patients present with an acute abdomen. The mean duration of symptoms is 4 weeks.

Operative findings

The tumor arises in the right ovary more often than in the left. Two-thirds of patients at laparotomy have Stage I disease, with no macroscopic involvement of the opposite ovary; most of the others have either Stage II or III disease in equal numbers. In advanced stages, the abdominal and pelvic peritoneum and pelvic organs are the principal sites of metastasis. The lungs are involved infrequently and late.

Gross pathology

Like other germ cell tumors, these neoplasms tend to be large, with a mean diameter of 15 cm. The outer surface is smooth, but the appearance of the cut surface depends on the type and quantity of the components. Solid fleshy areas correspond with dysgerminoma, mucoid cystic areas with teratoma, and hemorrhage and necrosis result most frequently from endodermal sinus tumor or choriocarcinoma.

Careful examination of the gross specimen, and selective sampling are essential for accurate histologic diagnosis. Quantitation of the various components is also important for estimating the likely behavior of the tumor. Areas of immature teratoma should be graded histologically.

Histologic appearance

By definition, at least two malignant elements are present. The most common is dysgerminoma, found in 80% of tumors, followed by endodermal sinus tumor in 70%, immature teratoma in 53%, choriocarcinoma in 20% and embryonal carcinoma in 13%.[34]

In two-thirds of tumors, only two malignant components are present. The mixture of dysgerminoma and endodermal sinus tumor is most common and accounts for a third of all combinations (Fig. 57.15). When immature teratoma is present, it is Grade 1 in half the cases. When the opposite ovary is examined microscopically and found to contain a malignancy, it is invariably dysgerminoma (Fig. 57.16). The other components are not known to exist as Stage Ib.

Therapy and prognosis

Prior to modern combination therapy, the overall actuarial survival for mixed germ cell tumors was 46%, and for Stage I tumors 50%.[34] The most important factors in predicting the prognosis in Stage I disease are the size and composition of the neoplasm. If more than one-third of a Stage I tumor is composed of endodermal sinus tumor, choriocarcinoma or Grade 3 teratoma, the tumor is very

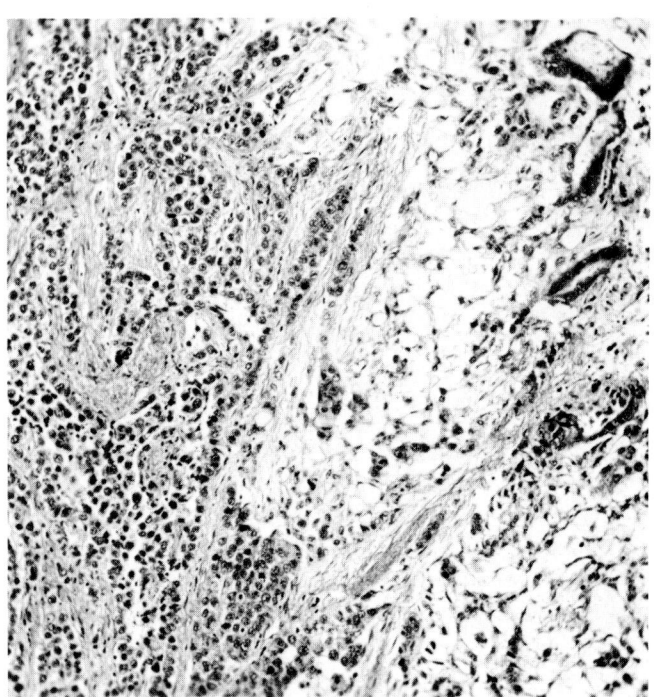

Fig. 57.15 Malignant mixed germ cell tumor with dysgerminoma (left) and endodermal sinus tumor (right). (H & E ×100)

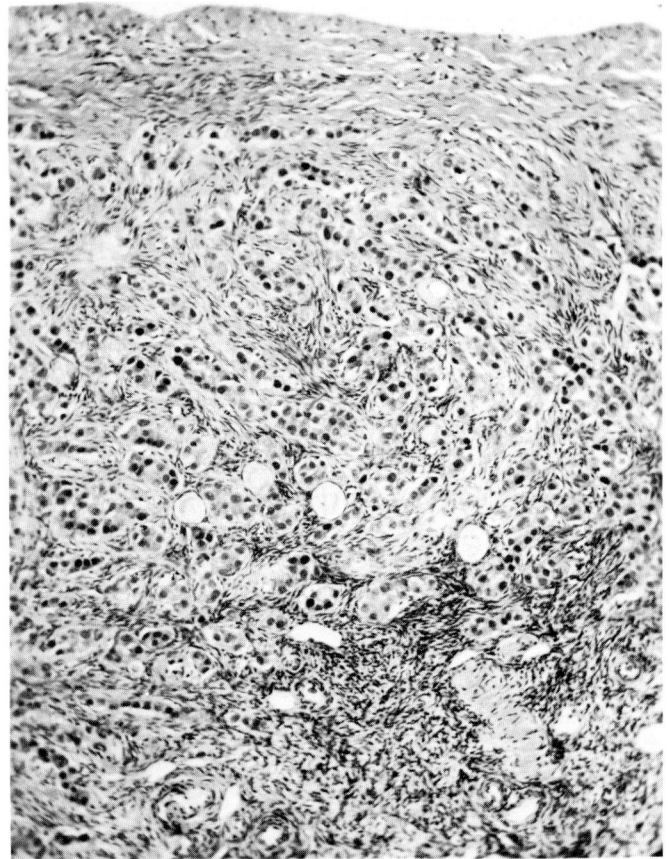

Fig. 57.16 Metastatic dysgerminoma in the ovary opposite a mixed germ cell tumor composed of dysgerminoma and endodermal sinus tumor. (H & E ×60)

aggressive. When these elements comprise less than one-third of the tumor, or it contains combinations of dysgerminoma, embryonal carcinoma or Grade 1 or 2 teratoma, it is less aggressive. Patients with tumors less than 10 cm diameter are more likely to survive, regardless of the composition of the tumor.

POLYEMBRYOMA

Polyembryoma is a rare tumor pattern occurring with other malignant germ cell components, and is best classified as a combination germ cell tumor with embryoid formation rather than a separate entity, since it does not appear in a pure form. Occurring in patients under age 40, most of these tumors have associated teratomatous trophoblastic differentiation. The original description by Peyron[54] was in a testicular teratoma; further cases were reported in the ovaries associated with dysgerminoma, endodermal sinus tumor, embryonal carcinoma and teratoma. Only about nine cases have been described in the ovary, one of which

produced AFP, HPL and hCG. It has never been reported as a pure neoplasm. Embryoids are microscopic structures replicating the features of a presomite embryo. Most resemble the 13 to 15th day of gestational age.[71] Structures resembling the embryonic disc, yolk sac and amniotic cavity can usually be identified (Fig. 57.17). Embryoid types are described as complete, imperfect or amorphous, depending on the degree of organization.[39] Embryoids have been observed in transplanted embryonal carcinoma after germ cells were no longer identifiable. This suggests that they are a stage in the differentiation of embryonal carcinoma or primitive multipotential cells.[55,67] The behavior is as aggressive as with other malignant germ cell tumors.

MIXED GERM CELL AND SEX-CORD STROMAL TUMORS

The category of mixed germ cell and sex-cord stromal tumors includes tumors that contain large numbers of germ cells resembling intermixtures of dysgerminoma cells and neoplastic gonadal stromal cells. The only tumor of numerical significance is the gonadoblastoma. A very small number of other types have been described.[36,74] Their clinical and pathological features justify distinguishing them from gonadoblastoma, but they are very rare.[27]

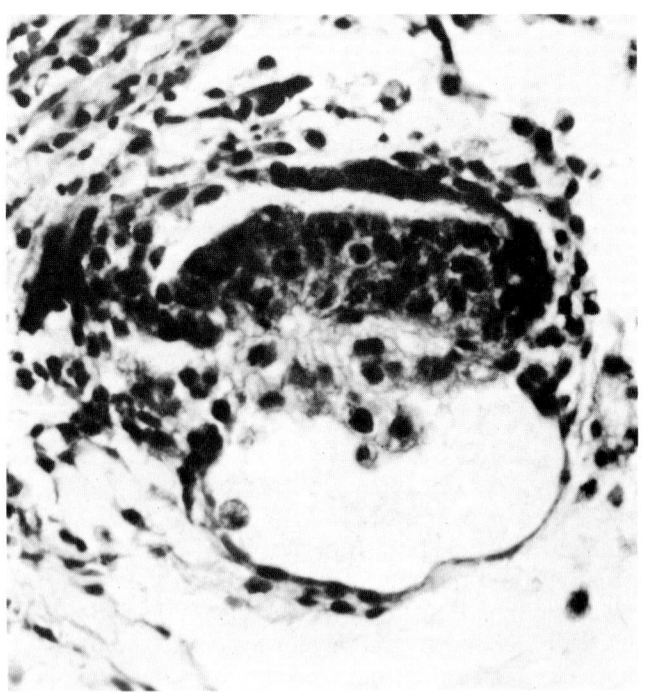

Fig. 57.17 Embryoid body. Top cavity represents the future amniotic cavity, the lower cavity represents the primitive allantoic yolk sac cavity. A germ disc is in the center (H & E ×400)

Gonadoblastoma

Gonadoblastoma is the commonest neoplasm arising in dysgenetic gonads and arises almost exclusively in them. More than 100 have been reported.[74] 22% arise in a streak gonad, 18% in a cryptorchid, dysgenetic testis and the majority in an abnormal gonad of indeterminate type.[64] Over 80% of patients are phenotypic females who are usually virilized, and 90% of all patients have a Y chromosome,[64] although it is not essential to the diagnosis.[19] An abnormal ring type of Y chromosome has been reported.[30] Gonadoblastoma has been reported very rarely in women with a normal 46XX karyotype,[13,41,61] fertile women[13,64] and, very rarely, in true hermaphrodites.[42,70] These patients may be mosaics, as gonadal mosaicism can be difficult to establish reliably. Gonadoblastoma resembles the polyovular follicles found in immature ovaries and stillborns, suggesting origin as a developmental anomaly.

The age range of patients at diagnosis is from 1 to 38 years. The clinical presentation depends on the nature of the underlying gonadal abnormality. Primary amenorrhea with or without signs of virilization is common in the phenotypic females, as is abnormal genitalia among the phenotypic males. Most patients, because of gonadal failure, have high serum and urinary gonadotropin levels.[85]

Grossly, gonadoblastomas vary in size from millimeters to a large solid, soft, firm or gritty mass, depending on the degree of calcification and the contribution of other germ cell elements. Most are only a few centimeters in diameter. Calcification is very common and may be recognized in abdominal X-ray films prior to surgery. Bilaterality is also common, occurring in at least half of the patients.

The essential histologic feature is a mixture of primordial germ cells, similar to those found in dysgerminomas, with cells that resemble granulosa cells. The latter have the same ultrastructural features as ovarian stromal cells or testicular Leydig cells, but do not contain crystals of Reinke (Fig. 57.18). In two-thirds of cases, cells identical with Leydig cells and luteinized stromal cells are present.[64] The granulosa cells form a supporting matrix for the germ cells. At times, seminiferous tubules and Sertoli-like cells are formed. Hyalinization, calcification and overgrowth by malignant germ cells occur to varying degrees.

Approximately half of gonadoblastomas are overgrown by dysgerminoma. 10% are associated with endodermal sinus tumor, embryonal carcinoma or choriocarcinoma.[73] Comprehensive sampling of all elements in these tumors is important, since pure gonadoblastoma does not metastasize. Metastasis of the dysgerminoma component in gonadoblastoma is uncommon, even when the tumor is bilateral and large. In contrast, other malignant combinations have been fatal within 18 months.[73]

Bilateral salpingo-oophorectomy is usually indicated in patients with gonadoblastoma because it tends to be overgrown by malignant elements and because a third of tumors are bilateral. In addition, since most gonadoblastomas develop in patients with gonadal dysgenesis, the contralateral ovary is usually dysgenetic. Subsequent treatment is determined by the histologic nature of any malignant germ cell element present.

Mixed germ cell sex-cord stromal tumors other than gonadoblastoma

To date, mixed germ cell sex-cord stromal tumors other than gonadoblastoma have been benign, with few exceptions.[74] They are unilateral, occur in males and females of all ages and are unassociated with a chromosomal abnormality. These neoplasms are composed of two admixed cellular elements and are differentiated from gonadoblastoma by the absence of calcification, a nest-like pattern, and the paucity of germ cells. Overgrowth by dysgerminoma has not occurred, and the neoplasm is dominated by the stromal proliferation. In one report, a metastasis contained both cellular components.[36] One case has been associated with a dysgerminoma, and one with a gonadoblastoma.[74] Karyotyping is recommended as an adjunct to diagnosis.

MALIGNANT GERM CELL TUMORS AND GONADAL DYSGENESIS

Any patient with gonadal dysgenesis and a Y chromosome

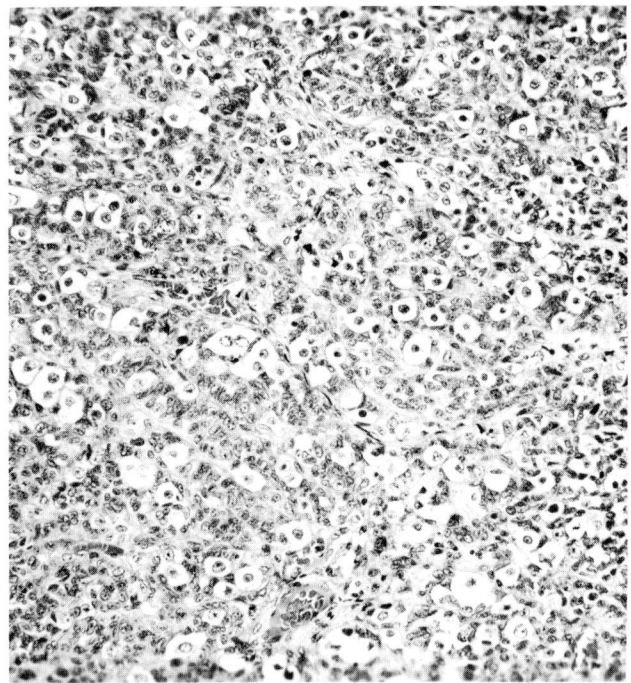

Fig. 57.18 Mixed germ cell and sex cord tumor. Large cells resembling primordial germ cells are interspersed with neoplastic stromal cells resembling granulosa cells. (H & E ×60)

runs a high risk of developing a malignant germ cell tumor, particularly a gonadoblastoma. In one review,[64] at least nine-tenths of gonadoblastomas arose in these patients. Dysgerminoma also appears in some reports to arise de novo, but most of these probably originated in a gonadoblastoma and had overgrown it, obscuring the origin.

A review of several studies showed that the median incidence of malignant germ cell tumors in patients with gonadal dysgenesis and a Y chromosome was 25%.[62] Two papers showed a cumulative incidence of 41%.[3,77]

In assessing the level of risk for malignancy developing in the individual patient, the karyotype, rather than the type of dysgenesis, is decisive. Despite clarification of the histologic sequence in gonadal differentiation, the subject of gonadal dysgenesis is still hampered by imprecise nomenclature and criteria. Individual cases may not fit a particular category,[2] or precise classification may be impossible because tumor has destroyed the original gonadal tissue. In addition, mosaicism may be difficult to exclude because it can be incomplete or limited to the gonads.

Pure gonadal dysgenesis

Patients with pure gonadal dysgenesis have a female phenotype with normal height, but they suffer the effects of prepubertal castration due to bilateral streak gonads. They lack the stigmata of Turner's syndrome. The majority have either a 46XY male karyotype or XY mosaicism. Less commonly, a 46XX karyotype is found.

Gonadal tumors are very rare with the 46XX pattern, but among 15 patients with 46XY karyotype, Teter found three with gonadoblastoma and four with dysgerminoma.[77]

Mixed gonadal dysgenesis

Patients with mixed gonadal dysgenesis are phenotypic females, usually with a streak ovary on one side and a dysgenetic testis on the other. They may be regarded as intermediate between pure gonadal dysgenesis and Turner's syndrome. In most cases, they are chromatin-negative, 45XO/46XY mosaics. Depending on the criteria selected, stigmata suggesting Turner's syndrome are present in about half of patients. In 51 cases of 45XO/46XX mosaicism, of which two-fifths were classified as mixed gonadal dysgenesis, 9 patients (18%) had a neoplasm.[82] The incidence reached 23% among individuals with abnormal external genitalia.

Turner's syndrome

Patients with Turner's syndrome having the typical 45XO karyotype (or, less frequently, 45XO/46XX), without signs of virilization, have a very low incidence of gonadal

malignancy. Teter found none among 21 of his patients[77] and von Camperhout identified only one in the literature.[82] Although germ cells are rarely identified in the gonads of 45XO patients, they do occur and there are reports of individuals having a full term pregnancy.[44] In contrast, among four patients with phenotypes of Turner's syndrome displaying virilization (which is usually associated with a Y chromosome) Teter reported one gonadoblastoma and one interstitial hilar cell tumor.[77,78]

Testicular feminization

Patients with testicular feminization are phenotypic females who have a 46XY karyotype and androgen insensitivity. They commonly present with primary amenorrhea or inguinal hernias. Since they are XY individuals with abdominal or labial testes, a proportion of them have a gonadal tumor that is either classified as a hamartoma or as a Sertoli cell adenoma. The incidence of malignant germ cell tumors is elevated, but the degree of risk is difficult to ascertain since the gonads are usually removed prophylactically at a young age. About a third can expect to develop a gonadal tumor, most commonly dysgerminoma, by the age of 50 years.[38] This finding alone justifies gonadectomy after puberty. Indeed, this precaution is indicated in all intersex individuals with a Y chromosome and abdominal, inguinal or labial testes.

Hermaphroditism

Dysgerminoma has been reported in true hermaphrodites. Gonadoblastoma has been reported both in 46XX and 46XY hermaphrodites.[42] The predisposing factor is the Y chromosome and the abdominal, inguinal or labial position of the gonad.

Summary

It can be seen that the likelihood of a patient with abnormal gonads developing a germ cell tumor depends on the karyotype rather than on classification of the dysgenesis, which is often imprecise. Patients not having scrotal testes with a pure XY karyotype or XY mosaicism have a high incidence of malignancy, regardless of their clinical features. Patients with a normal 46XX karyotype, 45XO karyotype or a mosaic not containing a Y chromosome are at low risk.

Acknowledgements

Figures 57.7, 57.8, 57.11, 57.14, and 57.3 are reproduced by permission of Cancer, Figure 57.5 and Tables 57.2 and

57.4 by permission of *Pathology Annual* and Figures 57.1 and 57.15 by permission of *Obstetrics and Gynecology*.

The opinions or assertions contained herein are the private views of the authors and are not to be construed as official or as reflecting the views of the Departments of the Army or Defense.

REFERENCES

1. Abell M R, Johnson V J, Holtz F 1965 Ovarian neoplasms in childhood and adolescence I — Tumors of germ cell origin. Am J Obstet Gynecol 92: 1059
2. Adashi E, Farber M, Safaii H S, Mitchell G W Jr 1977 Mixed gonadal dysgenesis without virilization. Obstet Gynecol 50: 397
3. Andrews J 1971 Streak gonads and the Y chromosome. J Obstet Gynaecol Brit Commonw 78: 448
4. Aguirre P, Scully R E 1982 Malignant neuroectodermal tumor of the ovary, a distinctive form of monodermal teratoma. Report of 5 cases. Am J Surg Pathol 6: 283
5. Artaze A, Beiner J T, Gonzales H, Aranela I, de Teresa E G, Palpon L A 1985 Carcinoid heart disease: report of a case secondary to pure carcinoid tumor of the ovary. Eur Heart J 6: 800
6. Asadourian L A, Taylor H B 1969 Dysgerminoma. An analysis of 105 cases. Obstet Gynecol 33: 370
7. Axe S R, Klein V R, Woodruff J D 1985 Choriocarcinoma of the ovary. Obstet Gynecol 66: 111
8. Battefora H, Sheibani K, Tubbs R R, Kopinski M I, Sun T 1984 Antikeratin antibodies in tumor diagnosis: distinction between seminoma and embryonal carcinoma. Cancer 54: 843
9. Boyes D A, Pankratz E, Galliford B W, White G W, Fairey R N 1978 Experience with dysgerminomas at the Cancer Control Agency of British Columbia. Gynecol Oncol 6: 123
10. Burkons D M, Hart W R 1978 Ovarian germinomas (dysgerminomas). Obstet Gynecol 51: 221
11. Climie A R W, Heath L P 1968 Malignant degeneration of benign cystic teratomas of the ovary. Cancer 22: 824
12. Czernobilsky B, Rotenstreich L, Lancet M 1972 Ovarian dermoid with squamous carcinoma — pseudosarcoma. Arch Pathol 93: 141
13. de Bacalao E B, Dominguez I 1969 Unilateral gonadoblastoma in a pregnant woman. Am J Obstet Gynecol 105: 1279
14. Dikman S H, Toker C 1971 Strumal carcinoid of the ovary with masculinization. Cancer 27: 925
15. Edmunds P, Marino H J, Livolsi P A, Duray P H 1984 Adenocarcinoids of the appendix. Gastroenterology 86: 302
16. Emge L A 1940 Functional and growth characteristics of struma ovarii. Am J Obstet Gynecol 40: 738
17. Fox H, Langley F A 1976 Tumours of the Ovary. Heinemann, London
18. Freel J H, Cassir J F, Pierce V K, Woodruff J, Lewis J L 1979 Dysgerminoma of the ovary. Cancer 43: 798
19. Garvin A J, Pratt-Thomas H R, Spector M, Spicer S S, Williamson H O 1976 Gonadoblastoma: histologic, ultrastructural and histochemical observations in five cases. Am J Obstet Gynecol 125: 459
20. Gerbie M V, Brewer J I, Tamimi H 1975 Primary choriocarcinoma of the ovary. Obstet Gynecol 46: 720
21. Gershenson D M, Del Junco G, Silva E, Copland L J, Wharton J T, Rutledge F N 1986 Immature teratoma of the ovary. Obstet Gynecol 68: 624
22. Hameed K, Bruslem M R G 1970 A melanotic ovarian neoplasm resembling the retinal 'anlage tumor'. Cancer 25: 564
23. Hay D M, Stewart D B 1969 Primary ovarian choriocarcinoma. J Obstet Gynaecol Br Commonw 76: 941
24. Hermann W J Jr, Humes J J 1976 A compound nevus in a benign cystic teratoma of the ovary. Am J Clin Pathol 66: 54
25. Higuchi K, Kato T 1958 Dysgerminoma of the ovary. J Jap Obstet Gynecol Soc 5:206
26. Hou-Jensen K, Kempson R L 1974 The ultrastructure of gonadoblastoma and dysgerminoma. Human Pathol 5: 79
27. Hughesdon P E, Kumarasamy T 1970 Mixed germ cell tumors (gonadoblastomas) in normal and dysgenetic gonads. Virchows Arch (Pathol Anat) 349: 258
28. Ihara T, Ohama K, Satoh N, Fujii T, Nomura K, Fujiwara A 1984 Histologic grade and karyotype of immature teratoma of the ovary. Cancer 54: 2988
29. Kelley R R, Scully R E 1961 Cancer developing in dermoid cysts of the ovary. Cancer 14: 989
30. Khudr G, Bernirschke K 1973 Y ring chromosome associated with gonadoblastoma in situ. Obstet Gynecol 41: 897
31. Krepart G, Smith J P, Rutledge F, Delclos L 1978 The treatment for dysgerminoma of the ovary. Cancer 41: 897
32. Kurman R J, Norris H J 1976 Embryonal carcinoma of the ovary. A clinicopathologic entity distinct from endodermal sinus tumor resembling embryonal carcinoma of the adult testis. Cancer 38: 2420
33. Kurman R J, Norris H J 1976 Endodermal sinus tumor of the ovary. A clinical and pathologic analysis of 71 cases. Cancer 38: 2404
34. Kurman R J, Norris H J 1976 Malignant mixed germ cell tumors of the ovary. A clinical and pathologic analysis of 30 cases. Obstet Gynecol 48: 579
35. Kurman R J, Scardino P T, McIntire K R, Waldmann T A, Javadpour N, Norris H J 1978 Cellular localization of AFP and hCG in germ cell tumors of the testis and ovary. Scand J Immunol 8 (suppl 8): 127
36. Lacson A G, Gillis D A, Shawwa A 1988 Malignant mixed germ cell-sex cord stromal tumor of the ovary associated with isosexual precocious puberty. Cancer 61: 2122
37. Leo S, Rorat E, Parekh M 1973 Primary malignant melanoma in a dermoid cyst of the ovary. Obstet Gynecol 41: 205
38. Manuel M, Katayama K P, Jones H W Jr 1976 The age of occurrence of gonadal tumors in intersex patients with a Y chromosome. Am J Obstet Gynecol 124: 293
39. Marin-Padilla M 1965 Origin, nature and significance of the 'embryoids' of human teratomas. Virchows Arch (Pathol Anat) 340: 105
40. Matz M H 1961 Benign cystic teratomas of the ovary. Obstet Gynecol Surv 16: 591
41. McDonough P G, Rogers-Byrd J, Freedman M A 1971 Gonadal dysgenesis with ovarian function. Clinical and cytogenetic findings in six patients. Obstet Gynecol 37: 868
42. McDonough P G, Rogers-Byrd J, Tho P T, Otken L 1976 Gonadoblastoma in a true hermaphrodite with a 46XX karyotype. Obstet Gynecol 47: 355
43. Morgello S, Schwartz I, Horwith M, King M E, Gorden P, Alonso D R 1988 Ectopic insulin production by primary ovarian carcinoid. Cancer 61: 800
44. Nakashima I, Robinson A 1971 Fertility in a 45X female. Pediatrics 47: 770
45. Nogales F F, Favara B E, Major F J, Silverberg S G 1976 Immature teratoma of the ovary with a neural component ('solid teratoma'). Hum Pathol 7: 625
46. Norris H J, Jensen R D 1972 Relative frequency of ovarian neoplasms in children and adolescents. Cancer 30: 713
47. Norris H J, Zirkin H J, Benson W L 1976 Immature (malignant) teratoma of the ovary. A clinical and pathologic study of 58 cases. Cancer 37: 2359
48. Ohama K, Nomura F, Okamoto E, Fukuda Y, Ihara T, Fujiwara A 1985 Origin of immature teratoma. Am J Obstet Gynecol 152: 896
49. Oud P S, Soeters R P, Pahlplatz M M, Hermkens P G, Beck H L M, Reubsaet-Veldhuisen J, Vooijs G P 1988 DNA cytometry

of pure dysgerminoma of the ovary. Int J Gynecol Pathol 7: 258

50. Palmer P E, Safaii H, Wolfe H J 1976 Alpha-antitrypsin and alphafetoprotein. Protein markers in endodermal sinus (yolk sac) tumors. Am J Clin Pathol 65: 575

51. Panayaton P P, Vrettos A S, Papatheodorou B, Kadas K 1971 Primary nongestational choriocarcinoma of the ovary. Int Surg 55: 137

52. Pardo-Mindan F J, Vazquez J J 1983 Malignant struma ovarii. Cancer 51: 337

53. Peterson W F 1957 Malignant degeneration of benign cystic teratomas of the ovary: a collective review of the literature. Obstet Gynecol Surv 12: 793

54. Peyron A 1939 Faits nouveaux relatifs a l'origine et à l'histogénése des embryomes. Bull Cancer (Paris) 28: 658

55. Pierce G B, Dixon F J 1959 Testicular teratomas. I. Demonstration of teratogenesis by metamorphosis of multipotential cell. Cancer 12: 573

56. Prat J, Bhan A K, Dickersin G R, Robboy S J, Scully R E 1982 Hepatoid yolk sac tumor of the ovary (endodermal sinus tumor with hepatoid differentiation). Cancer 50: 2355

57. Robboy S J, Scully R E 1980 Strumal carcinoid of the ovary. An analysis of 50 cases of a distinctive tumor composed of thyroid tissue and carcinoid. Cancer 46: 2019

58. Robboy S J, Norris H J, Scully R E 1975 Insular carcinoid primary in the ovary. A clinicopathologic analysis of 48 cases. Cancer 36: 404

59. Robboy S J, Scully R E 1970 Ovarian teratoma with glial implants on the peritoneum. An analysis of 12 cases. Hum Pathol 1: 643

60. Robboy S J, Scully R E, Norris H J 1977 Primary trabecular carcinoid of the ovary. Obstet Gynecol 49: 202

61. Salet J, de Gennes J L, de Grouchy J, Musset R, Pelissier I, Yaneva H, Sebaoun M, Netter A 1970 A propos d'un cas de gonadoblastome 46 XX. Ann Endocrinol (Paris) 31: 927

62. Schellhas H F 1974 Malignant potential of the dysgenetic gonad — I. Obstet Gynecol 44: 302

63. Schwartz P F, Morris J M 1988 Serum lactic dehydrogenase: a tumor marker for dysgerminoma. Obstet Gynecol 72: 511

64. Scully R E 1970 Gonadoblastoma, a review of 74 cases. Cancer 25: 1340

65. Serov S F, Scully R E, Sobin L H 1973 International histological classification of tumors, No 9. WHO: Histological typing of ovarian tumors

66. Snyder R R, Tavassoli F A 1986 Ovarian strumal carcinoid: immunohistochemical, ultrastructural and clinicopathologic observations. Int J Gynecol Pathol 5: 187

67. Stevens L C Jr 1960 Embryonic potency of embryoid bodies derived from a transplantable testicular teratoma of the mouse. Dev Biol 2: 285

68. Steeper T A, Mukai K 1984 Solid ovarian teratomas: an immunocytochemical study of thirteen cases with clinicopathologic correlation. Path Ann 19 (Part I): 81

69. Strodel W E, Vinik A I, Jaffe B M, Eckhauser F F, Thompson N W 1984 Substance P in the localization of carcinoid tumor. J Surg Oncol 27: 106

70. Szokol M, Kondrai G, Papp Z 1977 Gonadal malignancy and 46 XY karyotype in a true hermaphrodite. Obstet Gynecol 49: 358

71. Takeda A, Ishizuka T, Goto T, Ohta M, Tomoda Y, Hushino M 1982 Polyembryoma of ovary producing alphafetoprotein and hCG. Cancer 49: 1878

72. Talerman A 1984 Carcinoid tumors of the ovary. J Cancer Res Clin Oncol 107: 125

73. Talerman A 1974 Gonadoblastoma associated with embryonal carcinoma. Obstet Gynecol 43: 138

74. Talerman A 1980 The pathology of gonadal neoplasms composed of germ cells and sex cord stromal derivatives. Pathol Res Pract 170: 21

75. Teilum G 1959 Endodermal sinus tumors of the ovary and testis. Comparative morphogenesis of the so-called mesonephroma ovarii (Schiller) and extraembryonic (yolk sac-allantoic) structures of the rat's placenta. Cancer 12: 1092

76. Teilum G 1978 The concept of endodermal sinus (yolk sac) tumor. Scand J Immunol 8 (Supp 8): 75

77. Teter J 1969 Rare gonadal tumors occurring in intersexes and their classification. Int J Gynaecol Obstet 7: 183

78. Teter J, Bozkowski K 1967 Occurrence of tumors in dysgenetic gonads. Cancer 20: 1301

79. Thomas G M, Dembo A J, Hacher N F, DePetrillo A D 1987 Current therapy for dysgerminoma of the ovary. Obstet Gynecol 70: 268

80. Ueda G, Hamanaka N, Hayakawa K et al 1972 Clinical, histochemical and biochemical studies of an ovarian dysgerminoma with trophoblasts and Leydig cells. Am J Obstet Gynecol 114: 748

81. Vance R P, Geisenger K R 1985 Pure nongestational choriocarcinoma of the ovary. Report of a case. Cancer 56: 2321

82. von Camperhout J, Lord J, Lanthier A, Berard M 1969 The phenotype and gonadal history in XO/XY mosaic individuals: report of two personal cases. J Obstet Gynaecol Br Commonw 76: 631

83. Weiss N S, Homonchuk T, Young J L 1977 Incidence of the histologic type of ovarian cancer: the US third national cancer survey, 1969–1971. Gynecol Oncol 5: 161

84. Williamse P H, Oosterhuis J W, Aalders J G, Piers D A, Sleijfet D T, Vermey A, Doorenbos H 1987 Malignant struma ovarii treated by ovariectomy, hysterectomy, and ^{131}I administration. Cancer 60: 178

85. Winter J S D, Faiman C 1972 Serum gonadotrophin concentrations in agonadal children and adults. J Clin Endocrinol Metabol 35:561

86. Yannopoulos D, Yannopoulos K, Ossowski R 1976 Malignant struma ovarii. Pathol Ann 11: 403

87. Zaloudek C S, Tavassoli F A, Norris H J 1981 Dysgerminoma with syncytiotrophoblastic giant cells. A histologically distinct subtype of dysgerminoma. Am J Surg Pathol 5: 361

58. Malignant germ cell tumors of ovary: clinical features and management

D. M. Gershenson

INTRODUCTION

Malignant germ cell tumors of the ovary are those neoplasms derived from primitive germ cells of the embryonic gonad. As a group, they account for less than 5% of all ovarian neoplasms.[106] Younger patients with ovarian tumors, however, have a much greater likelihood of having a malignant germ cell tumor.[1,69]

These tumors generally occur in girls and young women, and are highly malignant and rapidly growing. Because of the rarity of these tumors, only recently have we been able to appreciate their biologic behavior and to clarify their terminology. Over the last three decades these aspects have been refined and effective treatment has evolved.

The concept of germ cell tumors as a specific group of ovarian neoplasms is based, as suggested by Teilum,[98] on their common histogenesis, on the presence of histologically different elements within the same neoplasm, on the occurrence of histologically similar neoplasms on extragonadal sites along the line of migration of the primitive germ cells,[42,111] and on homology between specific tumor types in the different sexes.[18,29,96,97]

The World Health Organization (WHO) introduced the currently accepted classification of germ cell tumors of the ovary in 1973. This represented a major advance in terms of standardization of nomenclature and histologic criteria. The present chapter will review the clinical features of each of the malignant germ cell tumors, with emphasis on the clinical management of these rare neoplasms. Details of the pathology of malignant germ cell tumors are given in Chapter 57. A modification of the WHO classification is shown in Table 57.1 (p. 917).

DIAGNOSIS

Once the diagnosis of a malignant germ cell tumor of the ovary is suspected, preoperative evaluation should include routine blood studies, serologic tumor markers (hCG, AFP, LDH, isoenzymes), intravenous pyelography, and chest X-ray. Optional studies, depending on the clinical situation, include barium enema, sonography, lymphangiography, computed tomography and magnetic resonance imaging. In the case of acute abdominal pain, of course, time may not allow the completion of many of these studies in the preoperative period. Selected studies not performed in the preoperative period should be considered in the postoperative period, especially for patients who have undergone inadequate staging procedures at primary surgery.

CLINICAL FEATURES

As noted above, malignant germ cell tumors of the ovary occur principally in girls and young women. In the University of Texas M. D. Anderson Cancer Center (UTMDACC) series, the age of the patients ranged from 6 to 46 years, with a median age of 16 to 20 years, depending upon histologic type. Of course, the age of patients with malignant germ cell tumors reported in the literature have ranged from a few months to the eighth decade.

These tumors are known to be associated with pregnancy in a small percentage of cases. For example, approximately 15 to 20% of all dysgerminomas are diagnosed during pregnancy or in the immediate postpartum period.[52] In our series, pregnancy was noted at the time of diagnosis in nine patients with dysgerminoma, one patient with immature teratoma, three patients with endodermal sinus tumor, and two patients with mixed germ cell tumors.

Signs and symptoms in these patients are rather consistent. Abdominal pain associated with a palpable pelvic-abdominal mass are most commonly noted. In our series, abdominal pain was present in 87% of patients, and a palpable mass was present in 85%. Approximately 10% of patients will present with acute abdominal pain, usually caused by rupture, hemorrhage, or torsion of these tumors. This finding may be somewhat more common in patients with an endodermal sinus tumor or a mixed germ cell tumor, and is frequently misdiagnosed as acute appendicitis. Less common signs and symptoms include abdominal distension (35%), fever (10%). and vaginal bleeding (10%). A few patients will exhibit isosexual precocity, presumably due to hCG production by the tumor (only noted in a few patients with choriocarcinoma, embryonal carcinoma, polyembryoma or mixed germ cell tumors).

Among ovarian neoplasms, many germ cell tumors possess the unique property of producing biologic markers which can be detected in the serum (see also Chs 8 and 24). The development of specific and sensitive radioimmunoassay techniques for measuring hCG and AFP has led to dramatic improvements in the monitoring of patients with these tumors. Serial measurement of these serum markers may aid in the diagnosis of these tumors and, more importantly, may be used in monitoring the response to treatment as well as in detecting subclinical disease recurrence. Table 58.1 illustrates the typical findings in the

Table 58.1 Serum tumor markers in malignant ovarian germ cell tumors

Histology	AFP	hCG
Choriocarcinoma	−	+
Endodermal sinus tumor	+	−
Dysgerminoma	−	±
Immature teratoma	±	−
Mixed germ cell tumor	±	±
Embryonal carcinoma	±	+
Polyembryoma	±	+

AFP = alphafetoprotein; hCG = human chorionic gonadotropin

sera of patients with the various histologic types. Endodermal sinus tumor and choriocarcinoma are the prototypical tumors producing AFP and hCG, respectively. Embryonal carcinoma and polyembryoma are capable of producing both hCG and AFP, more commonly the former. Of course, mixed tumors may produce either, both or none, depending on the type and quantity of elements present. Dysgerminoma is commonly considered to be devoid of any hormonal production, although a small percentage of these tumors do produce low levels of hCG from the multinucleated syncytiotrophoblastic giant cells.[11,102] Likewise, although immature teratomas usually are associated with negative markers, a few do produce AFP.[6,22,92]

A third serologic marker that has recently received increasing attention is the glycolytic enzyme, lactic dehydrogenase (LDH). Certain LDH isoenzymes have been reported to be elevated in patients with testicular cancer[58,59] as well as in ovarian dysgerminomas.[4,28,83,112] Serologic testing of LDH isoenzymes in malignant germ cell tumors of the ovary certainly deserves further attention.

Dysgerminoma, as is true of any malignant germ cell tumor of the ovary, may arise in phenotypic females with gonadal dysgenesis. Most commonly, this condition occurs in a pre-existing precursor lesion, the gonadoblastoma. Gonadoblastoma was first described by Scully.[81] There have been several subsequent reports of malignant germ cell tumors, usually dysgerminomas, arising in dysgenetic gonads.[2,46,78,79,91,94,99,100] The majority of these patients, but not all, have a Y chromosome. Classic examples of this type of patient include testicular feminization (phenotypic female, 46XY karyotype, androgen insensitivity), pure gonadal dysgenesis (phenotypic female, 46XY or XY mosaic karyotype, normal height), hermaphroditism (46XY or 46XX karyotype), mixed gonadal dysgenesis (phenotypic female, 45XO/46XY mosaic karyotype, with or without stigmata of Turner's syndrome), or Turner's syndrome (phenotypic female, 45XO karyotype). The probability of a patient with dysgenetic gonads and a Y chromosome developing a malignant germ cell tumor is 25 to 30% (see Ch. 57). The management of such lesions will be discussed below.

OPERATIVE FINDINGS

Malignant germ cell tumors of the ovary tend to be quite large. In our series, these tumors ranged in size from 7 to 40 cm with a median size of 16 cm. There was also slight predominance of right-sided involvement over left-sided involvement. Bilaterality of tumor involvement, especially true Stage Ib disease, is exceedingly rare, except in the case of dysgerminoma and, perhaps, embryonal carcinoma (see Ch. 57). Bilateral involvement occurs in 10 to 15% of dysgerminoma cases,[3,18,66,76] although it has been reported to be lower in some series[44,62] and higher in one.[93] With the non-dysgerminomatous tumors, bilateral involvement almost always signifies advanced disease with metastatic spread to the contralateral ovary or a mixed germ cell tumor with a dysgerminoma component. Likewise, while contralateral occult ovarian disease may occasionally be seen with dysgerminoma, it is exceedingly rare in the non-dysgerminomatous tumors, except in the case of mixed tumors containing dysgerminoma.[56]

Ascites may be noted in approximately 20% of cases. Rupture of these tumors, either preoperatively or intraoperatively, also occurs in approximately 30% of cases. Endodermal sinus tumor has a somewhat higher predilection for rupture than the other histologic types. Torsion of the ovarian pedicle could be documented in only 5% of patients in our series.

Benign cystic teratoma is associated with malignant germ cell tumors in 5 to 10% of cases. It may occur in the ipsilateral ovary, the contralateral ovary or bilaterally. Likewise, a pre-existing gonadoblastoma may be noted. This occurred in seven of our patients. This situation is generally accompanied by dysgenetic gonads with a Y chromosome.

Malignant germ cell tumors spread by peritoneal surface spread or by lymphatic dissemination. While the relative incidence of these two principal mechanisms is difficult to discern, it is generally accepted that these neoplasms more commonly metastasize to lymph nodes than epithelial tumors. The prevalence of inadequate staging procedures makes the true incidence of lymph node involvement uncertain. It is also our impression that, although still uncommon, malignant germ cell tumors also have a somewhat greater predilection than epithelial tumors to metastasize hematogenously to parenchyma of liver or lung.

The staging of malignant germ cell tumors is identical to that of epithelial tumors. The stage distribution, however, is very different from that of epithelial tumors. In most large series, approximately 60 to 70% of tumors will be Stage I. The next most common Stage is III, accounting for 25 to 30% of tumors. Stages II and IV are relatively uncommon.

CLINICAL MANAGEMENT

Primary surgery

The initial treatment approach for a patient suspected of having a malignant ovarian germ cell tumor is surgery, for diagnosis, appropriate staging and therapy. After an adequate vertical midline incision, a thorough determination of disease extent should be made by inspection and palpation. If the disease seems to be confined to one or both ovaries, it is imperative that proper staging biopsies be performed. Our routine consists of taking one or more peritoneal cytologic specimens (or ascitic fluid if present) and random biopsies of tissue from the omentum, abdominal peritoneum, pelvic peritoneum and retroperitoneal lymph nodes. Most patients undergoing surgery for this condition still do so outside major centers and, for most of them, the staging information available upon referral is inadequate.

The type of primary operative procedure depends upon the surgical findings. Bilateral ovarian involvement with tumor is exceedingly rare except in the case of pure dysgerminoma, wherein the incidence of bilaterality is 10 to 15%.[3,18,66,76] Bilateral involvement may also be found in cases of advanced disease (Stages II to IV) in which there is metastasis from one ovary to the opposite, and in cases of mixed germ cell tumors with a dysgerminoma component. Therefore, unilateral salpingo-oophorectomy with preservation of the contralateral ovary and the uterus can be performed in most patients with a malignant ovarian germ cell tumor, thus preserving the potential for fertility. If the contralateral ovary appears grossly normal on careful inspection, it should be left undisturbed; however, in the case of pure dysgerminoma, biopsy should be considered, because occult or microscopic tumor involvement does occur in a small percentage of patients.[56] If the contralateral ovary appears abnormal or enlarged, a biopsy or ovarian cystectomy should be performed. If frozen section analysis reveals malignant disease or a dysgenetic gonad, then bilateral salpingo-oophorectomy is indicated. If a benign cystic teratoma is found (approximately 5 to 10% of cases), however, then only ovarian cystectomy with preservation of normal ovarian tissue is recommended.

In cases wherein bilateral salpingo-oophorectomy is necessary, experience has dictated that hysterectomy be performed as well. With the advent of in vitro fertilization with donor oocytes, however, preservation of the uterus should be considered in a young patient desirous of future childbearing.

If advanced disease is encountered, it is recommended that the same principles concerning cytoreductive surgery that have been applied in the surgical management of advanced epithelial ovarian cancer be followed, with resection of as much tumor as is technically feasible. There is, however, scant information in the literature to support aggressive cytoreductive surgery. Slayton et al,[86] in a study of the Gynecologic Oncology Group (GOG), found that 15 of 54 (28%) patients with completely resected disease at primary surgery failed chemotherapy with a combination of vincristine, actinomycin-D and cyclophosphamide (VAC), as opposed to 15 of 22 (68%) patients with incompletely resected disease treated with the same regimen. Moreover, a higher percentage of patients with bulky residual disease (82%) failed chemotherapy compared to those with minimal residual disease (55%). Even in the face of extensive metastatic disease, it is not uncommon for the surgeon to be able to preserve a normal contralateral ovary.

Postoperative management of pure dysgerminoma

Early reports indicated a rather poor prognosis for patients with pure dysgerminoma; the overall 5-year survival was 27 to 33%.[23,66] Several factors undoubtedly contributed to these poor results, including suboptimal therapy and the inclusion of patients with advanced disease or those with mixed tumors. Other studies have shown a much improved prognosis and a 5-year survival of 75 to 90%.[3,8,18,44,62,63,101]

Two major factors influence treatment decisions in patients with dysgerminoma – survival and preservation of childbearing capacity. While dysgerminomas are exquisitely radiosensitive, the majority of patients are young and desirous of future childbearing.

Management of Stage Ia

One of the major dilemmas in the management of pure dysgerminoma is deciding whether patients with Stage Ia disease can be safely treated with surgery alone. Following unilateral salpingo-oophorectomy only for Stage Ia disease, reported recurrence rates vary from 17 to 53%.[3,44,62,63,71,101] Higher recurrence rates in many series are probably attributable to inadequate staging and inclusion of mixed tumors. With careful initial disease staging and inclusion of patients with pure dysgerminoma only, the recurrence rate following surgery alone for Stage Ia disease should be 20% or less. Table 58.2 lists the criteria to be considered in selecting patients with pure dysgerminoma for treatment with surgery alone. Some clinicians or patients, however, will choose conservative therapy without meeting all these criteria. The matter of

Table 58.2   Criteria for conservative management of pure dysgerminoma

1. Young patient desirous of future childbearing
2. Patient and family consent, and agreement to close follow-up
3. Unilateral, nonadherent, encapsulated, unruptured tumor (Stage Ia)
4. No evidence of dysgenetic gonads or presence of Y chromosome
5. No ascites or positive cytologic washings
6. No evidence of extra-ovarian tumor on staging biopsies, including lymph nodes and contralateral ovary
7. Negative lymphogram

tumor size is a controversial point. Some investigators[8,27,52] have recommended that only patients with tumors less than 8 to 10 cm in diameter be considered for conservative therapy; they contend that with larger tumors, disease is more likely to recur. The evidence for this recommendation, however, is somewhat lacking, because it is based on only a few cases. Other investigators[3,44,63] have found no statistical difference in survival based on tumor size. Further studies are necessary to clarify this issue.

According to traditional medical practice, all patients who do not meet the criteria for conservative management should be treated with abdominal hysterectomy and bilateral salpingo-oophorectomy followed by radiotherapy. Also, most patients with recurrent disease after treatment with surgery alone have been candidates for radiotherapy. (Details of radiotherapy techniques are discussed below.) For those patients treated with surgery alone who have subsequently developed recurrent disease, reported survival rates in radiotherapy series have varied from 60 to 100%, with an average of approximately 70%.[3,44,52,62,63] These excellent salvage rates make a strong case for adequately staging all patients with pure dysgerminoma, and treating all those with Stage Ia disease by surgery alone. Our preference, however, is to consider adjuvant chemotherapy for all patients with Stage I disease, because salvage therapy is not yet 100% successful. Moreover, most

patients undergoing surgery for dysgerminoma continue to be inadequately staged. In the last few years, we have recommended postoperative chemotherapy consisting of a combination of bleomycin, etoposide, and cisplatin (BEP) to all patients with Stage Ia to c disease. Chemotherapy has been administered for a total of three cycles; thus far, none of the patients treated with this regimen have developed recurrent disease, and no significant toxicity has occurred. More experience, however, will be necessary to prove the efficacy of such an approach. The obvious advantage of chemotherapy over radiotherapy in this situation is preservation of fertility.

Management of Stages II to IV and recurrent disease

The traditional approach for all patients with metastatic dysgerminoma (either primary or recurrent) has been abdominal hysterectomy and bilateral salpingo-oophorectomy followed by radiotherapy. The standard radiotherapy program consists of treatment of the whole abdomen in a dose of approximately 20 Gy either by the moving-strip technique with a ^{60}Co unit, or with the open-field technique employing a 25-MeV photon beam. An additional 15 Gy is delivered to the pelvis. If para-aortic nodal disease is present, as documented at surgery or by lymphangiography, a 10 to 15 Gy boost is administered to the para-aortic field. Following a hiatus of 4 weeks, the mediastinum and supraclavicular areas receive 25 Gy over a 3 week period. These are the radiotherapy procedures employed at UTMDACC.[17] Radiotherapy prescriptions often vary from center to center, however.

Because radiotherapy has produced excellent survival rates in patients with ovarian dysgerminoma, information in the early literature concerning chemotherapy is limited. There has been a growing body of literature documenting the efficacy of chemotherapy in the treatment of advanced or metastatic testicular seminoma.[20,25,60,75,84,90] Similarly, there is an increasing number of reports regarding the sensitivity of ovarian dysgerminoma to chemotherapy. Creasman et al[14] reported sustained remissions in five patients with Stage Ia anaplastic dysgerminoma treated with the combination of methotrexate, actinomycin-D, and cyclophosphamide (MAC). The surgical treatment in four of these patients consisted of unilateral salpingo-oophorectomy alone.

Chemotherapy has also been used as treatment for advanced or recurrent dysgerminoma. Krepart et al[52] reported three cases wherein chemotherapy was administered for recurrent disease. Two of these patients responded to a combination of actinomycin-D, 5-fluorouracil, and cyclophosphamide (ACFUCY). The other patient failed to respond to single-agent cyclophosphamide. Boyes et al[8] treated two patients with recurrent disease with alkylating agents. Both patients experienced a complete remission and were disease-free 7 and 12 years later, respectively. Cohen & Goldsmith[13] reported a prolonged complete remission in one patient with metastatic dysgerminoma who was treated with a combination of vincristine and bleomycin followed by maintenance therapy with vincristine and methotrexate. Weinblatt & Ortega[105] reported a survival of 10 years in a patient with inoperable Stage III dysgerminoma who was treated with 20 cycles of the VAC combination. Newlands et al[68] described three patients with metastatic dysgerminoma who achieved a complete remission with sequential combination therapy including vincristine, methotrexate, bleomycin, cisplatin, etoposide, actinomycin-D, cyclophosphamide, vinblastine, hydroxyurea and chlorambucil. De Palo et al[17] treated two patients with recurrent disease with combination chemotherapy – doxorubicin (adriamycin) and cyclophosphamide in one patient and doxorubicin and vincristine alternating with cyclophosphamide and cisplatin in the other. Both patients experienced a complete remission and were alive and disease-free at 24 and 26 months, respectively, at the time of the report. More recent reports include one by Vriesendorp et al[104] in which a patient with Stage IV dysgerminoma experienced a complete response after treatment with a combination of vinblastine, bleomycin, and cisplatin (VBP). Pinkerton et al[72] also reported a complete response in a patient with Stage IV dysgerminoma treated with the same regimen.

The BEP combination has also been used for patients with dysgerminoma. We reported sustained complete remissions in two patients with metastatic dysgerminoma (one with recurrent and one with Stage III disease) with this combination.[41] Subsequently, we have treated other patients with this regimen for metastatic dysgerminoma with equally favorable results. Smales & Peckham[87] treated four patients with this regimen; all experienced a complete remission and were disease-free from 6 to 62 months after diagnosis.

Therefore, there is ample evidence in the literature that ovarian dysgerminoma is exquisitely chemosensitive as well as radiosensitive. Although postoperative therapy should continue to be individualized, the obvious advantage of choosing chemotherapy over comprehensive radiotherapy after unilateral adnexectomy is the preservation of fertility. The optimal chemotherapy regimen or optimal duration of therapy for dysgerminoma is yet to be established. We prefer the BEP regimen administered for three cycles in Stage I disease and for four to six cycles in Stages II to IV and recurrent disease.

Postoperative management of non-dysgerminomatous tumors

Until the advent of combination chemotherapy in the mid-1960's, the prognosis for patients with non-dysgerminomatous tumors was dismal; virtually all patients with advanced disease died. Even in Stage I disease, only 5 to 20% of patients survived after treatment with surgery alone.[31,36,38,48,49,54,55,70] In the entire series from UTMDACC,[40] 30 of 33 patients treated with initial surgery alone developed recurrent disease. Currently, the only patients in this category who should be considered for treatment with surgery alone are those with a well-documented Stage Ia, Grade 1 pure immature teratoma. In the AFIP Series,[70] 13 of 14 patients with Stage I, Grade 1 immature teratoma treated with surgery alone remained disease-free; the other patient developed a recurrence, but was successfully treated.

Equally dismal survival rates have resulted from postoperative treatment with radioisotopes,[37,54,55,70] radiotherapy,[48,53,54,55,70] or single alkylating agent therapy.[37,48,70] These postoperative therapies are mentioned only to emphasize that there is no role for them in the management of non-dysgerminomatous tumors. Combination chemotherapy is clearly the postoperative treatment of choice.

ACFUCY was one of the earliest regimens administered for malignant germ cell tumors. Although there was modest success with ACFUCY,[24,31,89] its popularity was short-lived, and it was replaced by other combination regimens.

The MAC combination was also used in the early combination chemotherapy era and is still advocated by some today.[14] MAC, or variations thereof, has been particularly applied in cases of non-gestational choriocarcinoma of the ovary, simulating the traditional therapy for gestational trophoblastic disease.[5,32,43] Nevertheless, the MAC regimen has never been widely used for patients with malignant germ cell tumors of the ovary.

The VAC regimen

Beginning in approximately 1970, the VAC combination became the standard therapy for patients with non-dysgerminomatous germ cell tumors. In 1974, Malkasian et al[64] reported sustained remissions in two patients with malignant ovarian teratomas who were treated with VAC. The following year, Smith & Rutledge[89] reported on the experience at UTMDACC with the VAC regimen in the treatment of 20 patients with 'embryonal carcinoma'. Fifteen of those patients were surviving at the time of the report. Subsequent studies[9,15,30,31,35,65,80,85,86] documented the efficiency of VAC in the treatment of patients with malignant germ cell tumors of the ovary.

Initially, the VAC regimen was administered for a total of 2 years (18 to 24 cycles) at UTMDACC. Vincristine was administered weekly for a total of 12 weeks, and actinomycin-D and cyclophosphamide were administered for 5 consecutive days and repeated every 4 to 6 weeks (higher doses and longer intervals were used in the Pediatric Department). Since the late 1970's, the treatment at UTMDACC has been limited to a maximum of 12 cycles (6 cycles in some patients with Stage I disease), and vincristine has been administered on day 1 of each cycle instead of weekly. This current modified regimen is shown in Table 58.3.

Table 58.3 Combination chemotherapy regimens for malignant germ cell tumors of the ovary

Regimen	Drugs	Dosages
VAC	Vincristine	1 to 1.5 mg/m^2 on cycle day 1
	Actinomycin-D	0.5 mg/d on days 1 to 5 every 4 weeks
	Cyclophosphamide	5 to 7 mg/kg/d on days 1 to 5 every 4 weeks
VBP	Vinblastine	0.3 mg/kg in divided doses, days 1 and 2
	Bleomycin	15 mg on days 1 to 5 by continuous infusion
	Cisplatin	100 mg/m^2 on day 1
		Repeat cycles at 3 to 4 week intervals
BEP	Bleomycin	10 to 15 mg/d iv on days 1 to 3 by continuous infusion
	Etoposide	100 mg/m^2/d on days 1 to 3
	Cisplatin	100 mg/m^2 on day 1
		Repeat cycles at 3 to 4 week intervals

The VAC regimen has produced a high proportion of cures for early-stage disease. Table 58.4 presents the sustained remission rates in Stage I malignant germ cell tumors from three of the larger series in the literature. As noted, sustained remission rates varied from 73 to 100%; the overall sustained remission rate from these studies is 82%. The lowest sustained remission rate was noted in the GOG study.[86] When the results from these studies are further analyzed by the four main histologic subtypes, as noted in Table 58.4, the sustained remission rates are good in all subgroups except for those patients with Stage I endodermal sinus tumor in the study of Slayton et al.[86] The reason for the much poorer survival of 50% in the latter group remains unclear, because the drug doses and schedules were similar to those in the other two studies. One possible explanation is that disease was understaged in the GOG study, or treatment was initiated at a suboptimal interval postoperatively.

For patients with advanced disease (Stages II to IV), the results with VAC have been disappointing. Table 58.5 shows sustained remission rates from the three studies mentioned above in patients with advanced disease. As noted, survival is uniformly less than 50%. When analyzed by histologic subtype (Table 58.5) the sustained remission rates are suboptimal in all subgroups except for those patients with pure immature teratoma in the studies from UTMDACC and Yale (only one patient). Based on these results, it has been our distinct impression that patients with advanced immature teratoma respond much better to VAC than do patients with the other common histologic subtypes. Therefore, although VAC seems to provide excellent results for Stage I germ cell tumors of all types, it is inadequate for advanced disease, except the immature teratoma. Consequently, when the use of VAC is contemplated, it is quite important that the patient should have undergone an adequate staging procedure.

The toxicity of the VAC regimen is quite acceptable. Most patients tolerate it in an outpatient setting, and severe myelotoxicity is rare. Of course, ototoxicity, nephrotoxicity and pulmonary toxicity are not of concern with this regimen, as they are with the regimens containing cisplatin and bleomycin.

Although we are currently studying other combination regimens at UTMDACC, VAC remains safe and effective therapy for patients with a Stage I germ cell tumor. The optimal duration of therapy remains unknown. We believe this regimen should be administered for a maximum of 12 cycles, and consideration should be given to limiting it to 6 cycles, especially if serum tumor markers can be monitored or second-look laparotomy is employed in patients with negative markers.

The VBP regimen

In 1977, Einhorn and Donohue[21] reported their preliminary experience with the VBP combination in the treatment of testicular cancer. Subsequent reports[10,16,39,47,50,61,77,80,82,95,103,104,110] have documented the efficacy of the VBP regimen in the treatment of malignant ovarian germ cell tumors. At UTMDACC, we have used a modification of the Einhorn regimen (Table 58.3). We administer cisplatin at a dosage of 100 mg/m^2 on day 1 in-

Table 58.4 VAC chemotherapy for Stage I ovarian germ cell tumors: reported sustained remission rates

Study	Malignant germ cell tumor		Immature teratoma		Mixed germ cell tumor		Endodermal sinus tumor	
	No.	(%)	No.	(%)	No.	(%)	No.	(%)
Gershenson 1985[35]	32/37[a]	(86)	8/9	(89)	9/12	(75)	15/16	(94)
Slayton 1985[86]	32/44	(73)	16/16	(100)	5/6	(83)	11/22	(50)
Schwartz 1984[80]	16/16	(100)	7/7	(100)	2/2	(100)	5/5	(100)

VAC = vincristine, actinomycin-D and cyclophosphamide
[a] Patients in remission/total patients treated

Table 58.5 VAC chemotherapy for Stages II to IV ovarian germ cell tumors: reported sustained remission rates

Study	Malignant germ cell tumors		Immature teratoma		Mixed germ cell tumor		Endodermal sinus tumor	
	No.	(%)	No.	(%)	No.	(%)	No.	(%)
Gershenson 1985[35]	14/29[a]	(48)	7/9	(78)	3/9	(33)	3/10	(30)
Slayton 1985[86]	14/32	(44)	7/12	(58)	2/9	(22)	5/9	(56)
Schwartz 1984[80]	1/3	(33)	1/1	(100)	0/1	(0)	0/1	(0)

VAC = vincristine, actinomycin-D and cyclophosphamide
[a] Patients in remission/total patients treated

stead of 20 mg/m^2 daily for 5 days. We do this in an effort to limit the duration of potentially severe nausea and vomiting. Moreover, bleomycin is administered as a 24-hour continuous infusion over 5 days, rather than as a weekly bolus injection. The rationale for continuous infusion of bleomycin is based on data that indicate that the half-life is short (less than 2 hours), tissue inactivation is rapid, and the drug is cell-cycle specific, acting at the G_2-M interphase.[74] Nevertheless, there is as yet no firm evidence that continuous infusion is definitely superior.

The results of the treatment of Stage I and advanced stage disease with VBP in several series from the literature is presented in Tables 58.6 and 58.7 respectively. A review of the aforementioned data suggests that with the VBP regimen, excellent results can be achieved in Stage I disease, and results are superior to the VAC regimen in advanced disease. Because of the rarity of malignant germ cell tumors, to randomized clinical trials have been conducted to compare the two combinations. The VBP regimen or similar combinations should also be considered as salvage therapy for those patients who have failed VAC chemotherapy. Several reports[10,39,47] have documented remissions with VBP after VAC failure. Although the

precise salvage rate under these circumstances remains unknown, it probably approximates 50%.

The VBP regimen is potentially more toxic than the VAC regimen. With the former, the incidence of severe neutropenia and concurrent sepsis is greater. Although bleomycin pulmonary toxicity and cisplatin nephrotoxicity are rare, the occurrence of either side effect in a young patient with potentially curable disease may be devastating. Drug-related deaths with this regimen have been reported.[95,107] Therefore, for patients who receive VBP, we recommend meticulous monitoring before each cycle with complete blood count and creatinine clearance, as well as tests to determine D_LCO and pulmonary function.

The optimal duration of therapy with VBP remains unclear. The duration of treatment, however, is somewhat restricted by the potential cumulative toxicities of cisplatin and bleomycin. Most patients with Stage I disease require 3 to 4 cycles, whereas the majority of patients with advanced disease are cured with 4 to 6 cycles of therapy.

The BEP regimen

Etoposide (VP-16) was initially shown in 1977 to have

Table 58.6 VBP chemotherapy for Stage I germ cell tumors: reported sustained remissions

Study	Immature teratoma	Mixed germ cell tumor	Endodermal sinus tumor
	No.	No.	No.
Carlson et al 1983[10]	3/3[a]	1/1	1/1
Taylor et al 1984[95]	2/2	—	1/1
Vriesendorp et al 1984[104]	—	—	1/1
Gershenson et al 1986[39]	—	0/1	1/1
Lokey et al 1981[61]	—	—	1/1
Wiltshaw et al 1982[110]	—	—	4/4
Davis et al 1984[16]	—	—	3/3
Sawada et al 1985[77]	—	—	2/2
Sessa et al 1987[82]	—	—	4/4
Total	5/5	1/2	18/18

VBP = vinblastine, bleomycin and cisplatin
[a] Patients in remission/total patients treated

Table 58.7   VBP chemotherapy for Stages II to IV and recurrent germ cell tumors: reported sustained remissions

Study	Immature teratoma No.	Mixed germ cell tumor No.	Endodermal sinus tumor No.
Carlson et al 1983[10]	1/1[a]	1/1	2/2
Taylor et al 1984[95]	3/4	6/6	0/1
Gershenson et al 1986[39]	0/2	7/10	1/1
Vriesendorp et al 1984[104]	1/1	2/2	2/2
Schwartz 1984[80]	—	2/3	1/2
Julian et al 1979[50]	—	—	2/3
Wiltshaw et al 1982[110]	—	—	3/4
Davis et al 1984[16]	—	—	1/1
Sawada et al 1985[77]	—	—	2/3
Sessa et al 1987[82]	—	—	5/9
Total	5/8	18/22	19/28

VBP = vinblastine, bleomycin and cisplatin
[a] Patients in remission/total patients treated

single-agent activity in the treatment of refractory testicular cancer;[67] subsequently, a number of investigators confirmed its usefulness in this disease.[7,12,45,57,109] In a multi-institutional randomized trial, Williams et al[108] reported that, when compared with the VBP combination, BEP showed equal efficacy and less toxicity.

Based on the results of the above studies, it seemed logical for investigators to test the activity of etoposide in malignant ovarian germ cell tumors. Smith et al[88] treated three patients with recurrent germ cell tumors with etoposide-containing combination regimens; all three patients achieved remissions for a duration of 9 to 50 months. Pinkerton et al[72] described a complete response in a patient with Stage III mixed germ cell tumor who was treated with the BEP combination. Smales & Peckham[87] reported sustained remissions of 6 to 62 months in eight of nine patients with malignant ovarian germ cell tumors treated with etoposide, bleomycin, and either cisplatin or carboplatin. At UTMDACC, two patients with metastatic dysgerminoma were treated with BEP. Both patients achieved complete remission and remain disease-free.[41] We have subsequently treated a number of patients with malignant ovarian germ cell tumors with this regimen with excellent success. Our current BEP regimen is outlined in Table 58.3.

Second-look laparotomy

Since the advent of successful combination chemotherapy for malignant non-dysgerminomatous germ cell tumors, management for patients with these lesions has been similar to that for epithelial ovarian cancer. Namely, patients who responded to chemotherapy and remained clinically disease-free underwent second-look laparotomy after a fixed interval of treatment. In a review of the experience with second-look laparotomy at UTMDACC, 52 of 53 patients had negative findings.[34] One patient with negative findings subsequently relapsed and died. Thirteen patients had biopsy-proven evidence of mature teratoma at second-look laparotomy; treatment was discontinued in all patients, and none has had disease recurrence.

Our philosophy concerning second-look laparotomy in this patient population is to limit its use as much as possible. The procedure is not recommended for patients with initially positive serum tumor markers, especially those with early disease, which return to normal. Some patients with advanced disease, particularly those with initially negative serum tumor markers, continue to undergo second-look surgery. Nevertheless, as better therapies are devised, second-look laparotomy will inevitably be discontinued except in unusual situations.

Post-therapy surveillance

Following completion of chemotherapy, patients are examined at monthly intervals for the first year, and less frequently thereafter. If serum tumor markers are initially positive, patients are monitored at monthly intervals during the first year and every 2 to 3 months post-therapy during the second year. Imaging studies are performed as indicated and are used more commonly in those patients with initially negative tumor markers. If disease relapse does occur in this patient population, it is generally within 1 to 2 years after therapy. There are, however, a few reports of patients developing recurrent disease at intervals longer than 2 years.

LONG-TERM SEQUELAE

There is currently a great deal of interest in the long-term effects of chemotherapy in patients cured of malignant ovarian germ cell tumors. Secondary malignancies, especially leukemias, have been reported after treatment for testicular cancer and ovarian germ cell tumors.[34,51,73] The leukemogenic potential of cytotoxic agents, especially alkylating agents, is now well-recognized. More data concerning this subject will undoubtedly be forthcoming in the next few years.

There is also much concern over the long-term effects of chemotherapy on menstrual status, reproductive function and progeny. In a recent analysis of our experience at UTMDACC[33] of 40 patients who had retained a normal contralateral ovary and uterus after successful treatment with combination chemotherapy for malignant ovarian germ cell tumors, 68% maintained regular menses after completion of chemotherapy, and 83% of patients were having regular menses at the time of follow-up. In the same study, we discovered that 12 of 16 patients who had attempted to become pregnant did so. Three of these 12 patients, however, had some difficulty in conceiving, and required infertility consultation. One patient had an elective first-trimester abortion, and the other 11 patients delivered 22 healthy infants, none of whom had a major birth defect. Other reports have also documented cases of successful pregnancies following combination chemotherapy.

FUTURE DIRECTIONS

As has been shown recently, future progress in the treatment for ovarian germ cell tumors will continue to occur on the heels of advances in treatment of the more common testicular cancer. New drug development and methods for limiting both acute and long-term toxicities will most probably originate from studies of male patients. Randomized studies in the near future will clarify such issues as the relative efficacy and toxicity of bleomycin versus non-bleomycin regimens and cisplatin-carboplatin regimens. Cure rates approaching 100% may well be within our grasp during the next decade.

REFERENCES

1. Abell M R, Johnson V J, Holtz F 1965 Ovarian neoplasms in childhood and adolescence. I, Tumors of germ cell origin. Am J Obstet Gynecol 92: 1059

2. Andrews J 1971 Streak gonads and the Y chromosome. J Obstet Gynaecol Br Commonw 78: 448

3. Asadourian L A, Taylor H B 1969 Dysgerminoma: an analysis of 105 cases. Obstet Gynecol 33: 370

4. Awais G M 1983 Dysgerminoma and serum lactic dehydrogenase levels. Obstet Gynecol 62: 99

5. Axe S R, Klein V R, Woodruff J D 1985 Choriocarcinoma of the ovary. Obstet Gynecol 66: 111

6. Bahari C M, Lurio M, Schoenfeld A et al 1980 Ovarian teratoma with peritoneal gliomatosis and elevated serum alphafetoprotein. Am J Clin Pathol 73: 603

7. Bosl G J, Yagoda A, Whitmore W F Jr et al 1984 VP-16-213 and cisplatin in the treatment of patients with refractory germ cell tumors. Am J Clin Oncol 7: 327

8. Boyes D A, Pankratz E, Galliford B W et al 1978 Experience with dysgerminoma at the Cancer Control Agency at British Columbia. Gynecol Oncol 6: 123

9. Cangir A, Smith J, van Eys J 1978 Improved prognosis in children with ovarian cancer following modified VAC chemotherapy. Cancer 42: 1234

10. Carlson R W, Sikic B I, Turbow M M et al 1983 Cisplatin, vinblastine, and bleomycin (PVB) therapy for ovarian germ cell cancers. Proc Am Soc Clin Oncol (Abstract) 2: 156

11. Case records of the Massachusetts General Hospital (Case 11–1972) 1972 N Engl J Med 286: 594

12. Cavalli F, Klepp O, Renard J et al 1981 A phase II study of oral VP-16-213 in non-seminomatous testicular cancer. Eur J Cancer 17: 245

13. Cohen S M, Goldsmith M A 1977 Prolonged chemotherapeutic remission of metastatic ovarian dysgerminoma: Report of a case. Gynecol Oncol 5: 299

14. Creasman W T, Fetter B F, Hammond C B, Parker R T 1979 Germ cell malignancies of the ovary. Obstet Gynecol 53: 226

15. Curry S L, Smith J P, Gallagher H S 1978 Malignant teratoma of the ovary: prognostic factors and treatment. Am J Obstet Gynecol 131: 845

16. Davis T E, Loprinzi C L, Buchler D A 1984 Combination chemotherapy with cisplatin, vinblastine, and bleomycin for endodermal sinus tumor of the ovary. Gynecol Oncol 19: 46

17. Delclos L, Dembo A J 1980 Ovaries. In: Fletcher G H (ed) Textbook of Radiotherapy, 3rd edn. Lea & Febiger, Philadelphia, p 834

18. De Palo G, Pilotti S, Kenda R et al 1982 Natural history of dysgerminoma. Am J Obstet Gynecol 143: 799

19. Dixon F J, Moore R A 1952 Tumors of the male sex organs. Atlas of Tumor Pathology. Section VIII, Fascicles 31b and 32. Armed Forces Institute of Pathology, Washington, D.C.

20. Einhorn L H 1980 Chemotherapy of metastatic seminoma. In Testicular Tumors: Management and Treatment. Masson, New York, p 151

21. Einhorn L H, Donohue J 1977 Cis-diamminedichloroplatinum, vinblastine, and bleomycin combination chemotherapy in disseminated testicular cancer. Ann Intern Med 87: 293

22. Esterhay P J, Shamiro H M, Sutherland J C et al 1973 Serum alpha-fetoprotein concentration and tumor growth disassociation in a patient with ovarian teratocarcinoma. Cancer 31: 835

23. Felmus L B, Pedowitz P 1967 Clinical malignancy of endocrine tumors of the ovary and dysgerminoma. Obstet Gynecol 29: 344

24. Forney J P, DiSaia P J, Morrow P C 1975 Endodermal sinus: A report of two sustained remissions treated postoperatively with a combination of actinomycin-D, 5-fluorouracil and cyclophosphamide. Obstet Gynecol 45: 186

25. Fossa S D, Borge L, Aass N, Johannessen N B, Stenwig A E, Kaalhus O 1987 The treatment of advanced metastatic seminoma: experience in 55 cases. J Clin Oncol 5: 1071.

26. Fox H, Langley F A 1976 Tumors of the ovary. Heinemann, London

27. Freel J H, Cassir J F, Pierce V K et al 1979 Dysgerminoma of the ovary. Cancer 43: 798

28. Friedman M, White R G, Nissenbaum M M, Browde S 1984 Serum lactic dehydrogenase — a possible tumor marker for an ovarian dysgerminoma: a literature review and report of a case. Obstet Gynecol Surv 39: 247

29. Friedman N B, Moore R A 1946 Tumors of the testis: a report of 922 cases. Mil Surgeon 99: 573
30. Gallion H, van Nagell J R Jr, Donaldson E S, Hanson M B, Powell D F 1983 Immature teratoma of the ovary. Am J Obstet Gynecol 146: 361
31. Gallion H, van Nagell J R Jr, Powell D F et al 1979 Therapy of endodermal sinus tumor of the ovary. Am J Obstet Gynecol 135: 447
32. Gerbie M V, Brewer J I, Tamimi H 1975 Primary choriocarcinoma of the ovary. Obstet Gynecol 46: 720
33. Gershenson D M 1988 Menstrual and reproductive function after treatment with combination chemotherapy for malignant ovarian germ cell tumors. J Clin Oncol 6: 270
34. Gershenson D M, Copeland L J, Del Junco G, Edwards C L, Wharton J T, Rutledge F N 1986 Second-look laparotomy in the management of malignant germ cell tumors of the ovary. Obstet Gynecol 67: 789
35. Gershenson D M, Copeland L J, Kavanagh J J et al 1985 Treatment of malignant nondysgerminomatous germ cell tumors of the ovary with vincristine, actinomycin-D, and cyclophosphamide. Cancer 56: 2756
36. Gershenson D M, Del Junco G, Copeland L J, Rutledge F N 1984 Mixed germ cell tumors of the ovary. Obstet Gynecol 64: 200
37. Gershenson D M, Del Junco G, Herson J, Rutledge F N 1983 Endodermal sinus tumor of the ovary: the M.D. Anderson experience. Obstet Gynecol 61: 194
38. Gershenson D M, Del Junco G, Silva E G, Copeland L J, Wharton J T, Rutledge F N 1986 Immature teratoma of the ovary. Obstet Gynecol 68: 624
39. Gershenson D M, Kavanagh J J, Copeland L J et al 1986 Treatment of malignant non-dysgerminomatous germ cell tumors of the ovary with vinblastine, bleomycin, and cisplatin. Cancer 57: 1731
40. Gershenson D M, Wharton J T 1985 Malignant germ cell tumors of the ovary. In: Alberts D S, Surwit E A (eds) Ovarian Cancer. Martinus Nijhoff, Hingham, p 227
41. Gershenson D M, Wharton J T, Kline R C, Larson D M, Kavanagh J J, Rutledge F N 1986 Chemotherapeutic complete remission in patients with metastatic ovarian dysgerminoma. Cancer 58: 2594
42. Gillman J 1948 The development of the gonads in man with consideration of the role of fetal endocrines and the histogenesis of ovarian tumors. Contrib Embryol 32: 83
43. Goldstein D P, Piro A J 1972 Combination chemotherapy in the treatment of germ cell tumors containing choriocarcinoma in males and females. Surg Gynecol Obstet 134: 61
44. Gordon A, Lipton D, Woodruff J D 1981 Dysgerminoma: a review of 158 cases from the Emil Novak ovarian tumor registry. Obstet Gynecol 48: 497
45. Hainsworth J D, Williams S D, Einhorn L H, Birch R, Greco F A 1985 Successful treatment of resistant germinal neoplasms with VP-16 and cisplatin: Results of a Southeastern Cancer Study Group trial. J Clin Oncol 3: 666
46. Hart W R, Burkons D M 1979 Germ cell neoplasms arising in gonadoblastomas. Cancer 43: 669
47. Jacobs A J, Harris M, Deppe G et al 1982 Treatment of recurrent germ cell tumors with cisplatin, vinblastine, and bleomycin. Obstet Gynecol 59: 129
48. Jimerson G K, Woodruff J D 1977 Ovarian extraembryonal teratoma. I. Endodermal sinus tumor. Am J Obstet Gynecol 127: 73
49. Jimerson G K, Woodruff J D 1977 Ovarian extraembryonal teratoma: II. Endodermal sinus tumor mixed with other germ cell tumors. Am J Obstet Gynecol 127: 302
50. Julian C G, Barrett J M, Richardson R L et al 1979 Bleomycin, vinblastine, and cis-platinum in the treatment of advanced endodermal sinus tumor. Obstet Gynecol 56: 396
51. Kaldor J M, Day N E, Band P et al 1986 Second malignancies following testicular cancer, ovarian cancer and Hodgkin's disease: an international collaborative study among cancer registries. Int J Cancer 39: 571
52. Krepart G, Smith J P, Rutledge F, Delclos L 1978 The treatment for dysgerminoma of the ovary. Cancer 41: 986
53. Kurman R J, Norris H J 1976 Embryonal carcinoma of the ovary. A clinico-pathologic entity distinct from endodermal sinus tumor resembling embryonal carcinoma of the adult testis. Cancer 38: 2420
54. Kurman R J, Norris H J 1976 Endodermal sinus tumor of the ovary. A clinical and pathologic analysis of 71 cases. Cancer 38: 2404
55. Kurman R J, Norris H J 1976 Malignant mixed germ cell tumors of the ovary. Obstet Gynecol 48: 579
56. Kurman R J, Norris H J 1977 Malignant germ cell tumors of the ovary. Hum Pathol 8: 551
57. Lederman G S, Garnick M B, Canellos G P et al 1983 Chemotherapy of refractory germ cell cancer with etoposide. J Clin Oncol 1: 706
58. Lippert M C, Javadpour N 1981 Lactic dehydrogenase in the monitoring and prognosis of testicular cancer. Cancer 48: 2274
59. Liu F, Fritsche H A, Trujillo J M, Samuels M L 1982 Serum lactate dehydrogenase isoenzyme I in patients with advanced testicular cancer. Am J Clin Pathol 78: 178
60. Loehrer P J, Birch R, Williams S D, Greco F A, Einhorn L H 1987 Chemotherapy of metastatic seminoma: The Southeastern Cancer Study Group experience. J Clin Oncol 5: 1212
61. Lokey J L, Baker J J, Prince N A et al 1981 Cisplatin, vinblastine, and bleomycin for endodermal sinus tumor of the ovary. Ann Intern Med 94: 56
62. Lucraft H H 1979 A review of thirty-three cases of ovarian dysgerminoma emphasizing the role of radiotherapy. Clin Radiol 30: 585
63. Malkasian G D, Symmonds R E 1964 Treatment of the unilateral encapsulated ovarian dysgerminoma. Am J Obstet Gynecol 90: 379
64. Malkasian G D, Webb M J, Jorgensen E O 1974 Observations on chemotherapy of granulosa cell carcinomas and malignant ovarian teratomas. Obstet Gynecol 44: 885
65. Micha J P, Kucera P R, Berman M L, Romansky S, Flamm M, Reynolds J, DiSaia P J 1985 Malignant ovarian germ cell tumors: a review of thirty-six cases. Am J Obstet Gynecol 152: 842
66. Mueller C W, Topkins P, Lapp W A 1950 Dysgerminoma of the ovary: an analysis of 427 cases. Am J Obstet Gynecol 60: 153
67. Newlands E S, Bagshawe K D 1977 Epipodophyllin derivative (VP-16-213) in malignant teratomas and choriocarcinomas. Lancet ii: 87
68. Newlands E S, Begent R H J, Rustin G J S, Bagshawe K D 1982 Potential for cure in metastatic ovarian teratomas and dysgerminomas. Br J Obstet Gynaecol 89: 55
69. Norris H J, Jensen R D 1972 Relative frequency of ovarian neoplasms in children and adolescents. Cancer 30: 713
70. Norris H J, Zirkin H J, Benson W L 1976 Immature (malignant) teratoma of the ovary. Cancer 37: 2359
71. Pedowitz P, Felmus L B, Grayzel D M 1955 Dysgerminoma of the ovary. Prognosis and treatment. Am J Obstet Gynecol 70: 1284
72. Pinkerton C R, Pritchard J, Spitz L 1986 High complete response rate in children with advanced germ cell tumors using cisplatin-containing combination chemotherapy. J Clin Oncol 4: 194
73. Redman J R, Vugrin D, Arlin Z A et al 1984 Leukemia following treatment of germ cell tumors in men. J Clin Oncol 2: 1080
74. Samuels M L, Johnson D E, Holoye P Y 1975 Continuous intravenous bleomycin therapy with vinblastine in Stage III testicular neoplasia. Cancer Chemother Rep 59: 563
75. Samuels M L, Logothetis D J 1983 Follow-up study of sequential weekly pulse-dose cisplatinum for far-advanced seminoma. Proc Am Soc Clin Oncol 2 (C-535): 137
76. Santesson L 1947 Clinical and pathological survey of ovarian

tumours treated at the Radiumhemmet. I. Dysgerminoma. Acta Radiol (Stockholm) 28: 643

77. Sawada M, Okudaira Y, Matsui Y, Nishiura H, Iwasaki T, Kasamatsu H 1985 Cisplatin, vinblastine, and bleomycin therapy of yolk sac (endodermal sinus) tumor of the ovary. Gynecol Oncol 20: 162

78. Schellhas H H, Trujillo J M, Rutledge F N 1971 Germ cell tumors associated with XY gonadal dysgenesis. Am J Obstet Gynecol 109: 1197

79. Schwartz I S, Cohen C J, Deligdisch L 1980 Dysgerminoma of the ovary associated with true hermaphroditism. Obstet Gynecol 56: 102

80. Schwartz P E 1984 Combination chemotherapy in the management of ovarian germ cell malignancies. Obstet Gynecol 64: 564

81. Scully R E 1953 Gonadoblastoma. A gonadal tumor related to dysgerminoma (seminoma) and capable of sex hormone production. Cancer 6: 445

82. Sessa C, Bonazzi C, Landoni F, Pecorelli S, Sartori E, Mangioni C 1987 Cisplatin, vinblastine, and bleomycin combination chemotherapy in endodermal sinus tumor of the ovary. Obstet Gynecol 70: 220

83. Sheiko M C, Hart W R 1982 Ovarian germinoma (dysgerminoma) with elevated serum lactic dehydrogenase: case report and review of literature. Cancer 49: 994

84. Simon S D, Srougi M, Goes G M 1983 Treatment of advanced seminoma with vinblastine (VBL), actinomycin-D (AcD), cyclophosphamide (CTX), bleomycin (BLEO) and cis-platinum (CPDD). Proc Am Soc Clin Oncol 2 (C-517): 132

85. Slayton R E, Hreshchyshyn M M, Silverberg S G et al 1978 Treatment of malignant ovarian germ cell tumor. Cancer 42: 390

86. Slayton R E, Park R C, Silverberg S G, Shingleton H, Creasman W T, Blessing J A 1985 Vincristine, dactinomycin, and cyclophosphamide in the treatment of malignant germ cell tumors of the ovary: a Gynecologic Oncology Group Study (A final report). Cancer 56: 243

87. Smales E, Peckham M J 1987 Chemotherapy of germ-cell ovarian tumours: first-line treatment with etoposide, bleomycin and cisplatin or carboplatin. Eur J Cancer Clin Oncol 23: 469

88. Smith E B, Clarke-Pearson D L, Creasman W T 1984 A VP16-213- and cisplatin-containing regimen for treatment of refractory ovarian germ cell malignancies. Am J Obstet Gynecol 150: 927

89. Smith J P, Rutledge F N 1975 Advances in chemotherapy for gynecologic cancer. Cancer 36: 669

90. Stanton G F, Bosl G J, Vugrin D et al 1983 Treatment of patients (pts) with advanced seminoma with cyclophosphamide, bleomycin, actinomycin-D, vinblastine, and cisplatin (VAB-6). Proc Am Soc Clin Oncol 2 (C-551): 141

91. Talerman A 1974 Gonadoblastoma associated with embryonal carcinoma. Obstet Gynecol 43: 138

92. Talerman A, Haije W G 1974 Alpha-fetoprotein and germ cell tumors: a possible role of yolk sac tumor in production of alpha-fetoprotein. Cancer 34: 1722

93. Talerman A, Huyzinga W T, Juipers T 1973 Dysgerminoma clinicopathologic study of 22 cases. Obstet Gynecol 41: 137

94. Talerman A, Jarabak J, Amarose A P 1981 Gonadoblastoma and dysgerminoma in a true hermaphrodite with a 46XX karyotype. Am J Obstet Gynecol 140: 475

95. Taylor M H, DePetrillo A D, Turner A R 1984 Vinblastine, bleomycin, and cisplatin in malignant germ cell tumors of the ovary. Cancer 56: 1341

96. Teilum G 1944 Homologous tumours in ovary and testis: contribution to classification of gonadal tumours. Acta Obstet Gynecol Scand 24: 480

97. Teilum G 1946 Gonocytoma: homologous ovarian and testicular tumours. I. with discussion of 'mesonephroma ovarii' (Schiller: Am J Cancer 1939). Acta Pathol Microbiol Scand 23: 242

98. Teilum G 1965 Classifications of endodermal sinus tumour (mesoblastoma vitellinum) and so-called 'embryonal carcinoma' of the ovary. Acta Pathol Microbiol Scand 64: 407

99. Teter J, Bozkowski K 1967 Occurrence of tumors in dysgenetic gonads. Cancer 20: 1301

100. Teter J 1969 Rare gonadal tumors occurring in intersexes and their classification. Int J Gynaecol Obstet 7: 183

101. Thoeny R H, Dockerty M B, Hunt A B, Childs D S Jr 1961 Study of ovarian dysgerminoma with emphasis on the role of radiation therapy. Surg Gynecol Obstet 113: 692

102. Ueda G, Kamanaka N, Hayakawa K et al 1972 Clinical, histochemical, and biochemical studies of an ovarian dysgerminoma with trophoblasts and Leydig cells. Am J Obstet Gynecol 114: 748

103. Vance R P, Geisinger K R 1985 Pure nongestational choriocarcinoma of the ovary. Cancer 56: 2321

104. Vriesendorp R, Aalders J G, Sleijfer D T, Willemse P H B, Bouma J, Mulder N H 1984 Treatment of malignant germ cell tumors of the ovary with cisplatin, vinblastine, and bleomycin (PVB). Cancer Treat Rep 68: 779

105. Weinblatt M E, Ortega J A 1982 Treatment of children with dysgerminoma of the ovary. Cancer 49: 2608

106. Weiss N S, Homonchuk T, Young J L 1977 Incidence of the histologic type of ovarian cancer: the US third national cancer survey, 1969-1971. Gynecol Oncol 5: 161

107. Williams S D, Blessing J, Adcock L, Homesley H 1984 Treatment of ovarian germ cell tumors with cisplatin + vinblastine + bleomycin (PVB). Proc Am Soc Clin Oncol (Abstract) 3: 175

108. Williams S D, Birch R, Einhorn L H, Irwin L, Greco F A, Loehrer P J 1987 Treatment of disseminated germ-cell tumors with cisplatin, bleomycin, and either vinblastine or etoposide. N Engl J Med 316: 1435

109. Williams S D, Einhorn L H, Greco F A et al 1980 VP-16-213 salvage therapy for refractory germinal neoplasms. Cancer 46: 2154

110. Wiltshaw E, Stuart-Harris R, Barker G H et al 1982 Chemotherapy of endodermal sinus tumour (yolk sac tumor) of the ovary: Preliminary communication. J Roy Soc Med 75: 888

111. Witschi E 1948 Migration of the germ cells of human embryos from the yolk sac to the primitive gonadal folds. Contrib Embryol 32: 69

112. Zondag H A 1964 Enzyme activity in dysgerminoma and seminoma: a study of lactic dehydrogenase isoenzymes in malignant diseases (The 1963 Fiske Essay). Rhode Island Med J 47: 273

59. Pathology of malignant gonadal stromal tumors of ovary

H. Fox   C. H. Buckley

INTRODUCTION

The gonadal stromal tumors, perhaps nowadays more commonly referred to as sex cord stromal tumors, of the ovary are formed of cells which are believed to be derived ultimately from the sex cords or mesenchyme of the embryonic gonad. Such neoplasms may contain granulosa cells, Sertoli cells, Leydig cells, thecal cells or fibroblasts of gonadal stromal origin, either singly or in any combination and in any degree of differentiation.[52] Traditionally, the lipid, or steroid cell tumors are also included under the general heading of gonadal stromal neoplasms.

Many gonadal stromal tumors secrete sex steroids, and the clinical picture of patients with these neoplasms is often dominated by the results of their endocrinological activity. It has to be stressed, however, that the individual tumor entities are defined solely in morphological terms, without reference to their ability or otherwise to secrete particular sex hormones.

HISTOGENESIS AND ETIOLOGY

It is widely thought that both granulosa and Sertoli cells differentiate from the sex cords of the developing gonad, which are now thought to originate as downgrowths from the celomic epithelium rather than as a condensation from gonadal mesenchyme.[32,40] There is, however, disagreement as to the eventual fate of the sex cord cells; many believe that these cells differentiate into granulosa cells if the gonad is destined to become an ovary, and into Sertoli cells if development is deflected along a testicular pathway by the presence of H-Y antigen in the germ cells.[40] According to this view, granulosa and Sertoli cells, and the neoplasms derived from these cells, are homologues of each other. This relationship is, however, denied by others who believe that, whilst granulosa cells originate from cortical sex cords, the Sertoli cells derive from medullary cords of mesonephric origin.[32] The possible mesonephric, or Wolffian, origin of Sertoli cell tumors is further suggested by the retiform pattern seen in some of these neoplasms,[72]

whilst the 'Sertoli cell' component in Sertoli-Leydig cell tumors usually contains both vimentin and cytokeratins, unlike the Sertoli cells of the testis which contain only vimentin.[33,34] These findings, together with ultrastructural observations, question the long held belief that Sertoli-Leydig cell tumors recapitulate phases in the development of the male gonad,[63] and have prompted the suggestion that the apparent Sertoli cells in these neoplasms may be more akin to the cells lining the efferent ducts or rete of the testis.[17]

The stromal element of ovarian gonadal stromal tumors may be of an indifferent nature, or may be differentiated into either thecal or Leydig cells. These stromal elements can exist in a pure form or may be admixed with epithelial elements of putative sex cord origin. These latter tumors pose a histogenetic dilemma, for one would have to postulate a dual origin for such entities as granulosa-theca or Sertoli-Leydig cell tumors, with simultaneous neoplastic origin of cells from epithelial and stromal sources. This histogenic problem can be overcome by suggesting that, in such cases, the epithelial component is the only true neoplastic element, the stromal components arising as a result of differentiation in non-neoplastic reactive stroma. It would also have to be postulated that granulosa cell tumors have a particular tendency to induce thecal cell differentiation in reactive stroma, and that Sertoli cells have a similar propensity for inducing Leydig cell differentiation. This does not, however, seem an unlikely hypothesis.

Virtually nothing is known about the etiology of sex cord stromal tumors in the human. Somewhat surprisingly, however, the granulosa cell tumor is the form of ovarian neoplasia most easily and consistently inducible in animals, particularly rodents, under experimental conditions. Such tumors can be induced by a variety of techniques which, however, have three factors in common: firstly, that the tumor only develops after oocyte depletion; secondly, that a tumor will not arise unless the pituitary gland is functioning normally; and thirdly, that tumorigenesis is prevented by the presence of normally sited functional ovarian tissue.[25,31] The sequence of events in experimental granulosa cell tumor induction appears, therefore, to be: oocyte loss, subsequent degeneration of follicular granulosa cells, and a compensatory rise in pituitary gonadotrophins with resulting irregular proliferation, and eventual neoplasia, of the granulosa cells. These experimentally induced tumors thus reflect reasonably accurately the situation occurring in humans, in so far as many granulosa cell tumors occur at, or soon after, the menopause when similar conditions of oocyte depletion and high levels of pituitary gonadotrophins prevail. Nevertheless, these studies shed no light on the etiology of granulosa cell tumors developing during the reproductive years or before menarche, and provide no clues as to the etiology of other types of sex cord stromal tumors.

CLASSIFICATION

The classification of sex cord stromal tumors used here, and shown in Table 59.1, is a slight modification of that introduced by Young & Scully[71,76] and is an expansion of the WHO classification[53] which is now woefully out of date. Not all the neoplasms listed in Table 59.1 are malignant, and those which are invariably benign, such as thecomas, fibromas and sclerosing stromal tumors, will not be considered in this chapter. The pure Leydig cell tumor can be considered as a form of androblastoma, but is more logically regarded as a type of lipid cell tumor.

GRANULOSA–STROMAL CELL TUMORS

Granulosa cell tumors — adult type

Since the delineation of the juvenile granulosa cell tumor,[51] it has become necessary to refer to the conventional form of this neoplasm as the 'adult-type of granulosa cell tumor'. These tumors account for about 1.5% of all ovarian neoplasms. One-third of adult-type granulosa cell tumors develop in women of reproductive age, the bulk of the remainder occurring in patients who have passed the menopause. Approximately 5% of adult-type granulosa cell neoplasms develop in premenarchal girls.

Macroscopic appearances

The tumors are unilateral in 95% of cases, and vary in size from microscopic lesions to masses measuring 40 cm in diameter; the average size, however, is about 12 cm in diameter. Most adult granulosa cell tumors are predominantly solid, with a smooth or bosselated outer surface. On section, they may be hard, rubbery or soft, and their cut surface may be white, brown, yellow, pink or gray: focal hemorrhage or necrosis is common, and any cystic areas may contain watery, serosanguinous or gelatinous fluid. A small proportion of granulosa cell tumors are predominantly cystic and may closely resemble a cystadenoma.

Microscopic features

Histologically, the tumor cells are round, ovoid or angular, with scanty eosinophilic cytoplasm and indistinct cell boundaries. The nuclei are vesicular, round or oval and characteristically, though not invariably, show well marked longitudinal grooving (coffee bean appearance).

The neoplastic granulosa cells may be arranged in a variety of patterns and, although in any individual tumor a particular histological pattern may predominate, there is usually a combination of cellular arrangements in any single neoplasm. The tumor may show an insular, trabecular, diffuse or follicular pattern (Figs 59.1 and 59.2). The follicles are of three types: firstly, microfollicular or rosette-like structures (Call-Exner bodies) which usually contain eosinophilic material and nuclear debris; secondly, macrofollicles which are really areas of liquefaction in islands of granulosa cells; and thirdly, large follicles lined by circumferentially arranged cells which resemble the Graafian follicles of the newborn infant. The insular parts of a granulosa cell tumor are composed of large groups, or islands, of polygonal cells arranged, except at

Table 59.1 Classification of sex cord stromal tumors of the ovary

(A) Granulosa-stromal cell tumors
(1) Granulosa cell tumor
  (i) Adult type
  (ii) Juvenile form
(2) Thecoma-fibroma group of tumors
  (i) Thecoma*
    (a) Typical thecoma
    (b) Luteinized thecoma
    (c) Leydig cell containing thecoma
  (ii) Fibroma-fibrosarcoma
    (a) Fibroma*
    (b) Fibroma with sex cord elements*
    (c) Cellular fibroma
    (d) Fibrosarcoma
  (iii) Fibrothecoma*
(3) Sclerosing stromal tumor*

(B) Sertoli-Leydig cell tumors (androblastomas)
(1) Sertoli cell tumor
(2) Leydig cell tumor**
(3) Sertoli-Leydig cell tumor
  (i) Well differentiated
  (ii) Of intermediate differentiation
  (iii) Poorly differentiated
  (iv) Retiform variant
  (v) With heterologous elements

(C) Gynandroblastoma

(D) Sex cord tumor with annular tubules
(1) Pure form
(2) With granulosa cell overgrowth
(3) With Sertoli cell overgrowth

(E) Unclassified

* Benign tumors not discussed in this chapter
** More logically regarded as lipid cell tumor (see Table 59.2)

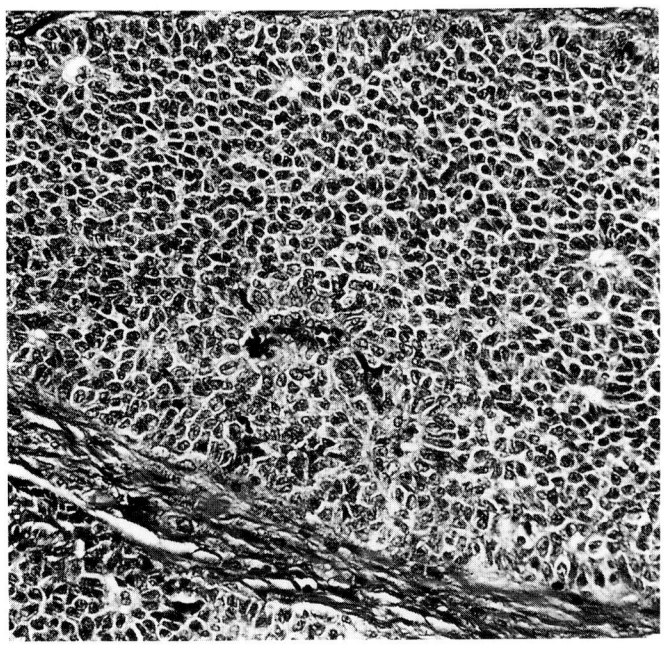

Fig. 59.1 An adult-type granulosa cell tumor. This has an insular pattern and typical Call-Exner bodies are present.

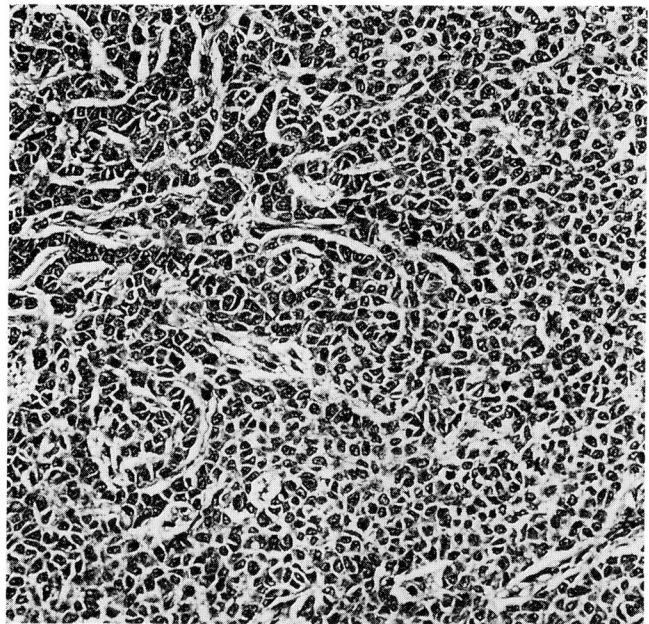

Fig. 59.2 An adult-type granulosa cell tumor showing, in part, a trabecular pattern.

the margin, without polarity and with few microfollicles. In the trabecular regions, the cells are arranged in ribbons, one, two or several layers thick, set in a stromal matrix. The cells adjacent to the stroma tend to be regimented at right angles to the axis of the ribbon with their nuclei arranged antipodally. When the ribbons are narrow and the stroma scanty, the pattern is sometimes described as 'watered silk'. The diffuse form of these neoplasms, often incorrectly called 'sarcomatoid', may be formed by polygonal or spindle-shaped cells. Cystic granulosa cell tumors have a lining which resembles that of a Graafian follicle, but which contains microfollicles (Fig. 59.3).

There is usually little pleomorphism, but about 2% of these tumors contain cells with large, bizarre, hyperchromatic nuclei.[73] Mitotic figures are usually scanty (less than three mitotic figures per 10 high power fields). The stromal component of a granulosa cell tumor is variable in amount and may have a fibromatous or thecomatous appearance.

Prognosis and prognostic features

A proportion of adult-type granulosa cell tumors will recur or metastasize, but this proportion has, in the past, been minimized by an over-reliance on 5-year survival rates.[4,11,13,36] Granulosa cell tumors which pursue a malignant course do so in a leisurely and indolent manner, with one-third of recurrences presenting more than 5 years after initial treatment, and one-fifth after 10 years;[10] indeed, recurrences can develop after as long a period as 25 years.[27] A true estimate of the malignancy of these neoplasms can only be achieved, therefore, by prolonged surveillance, probably lifelong but for at least 20 years. In a number of such studies, the corrected 20-year survival rate for

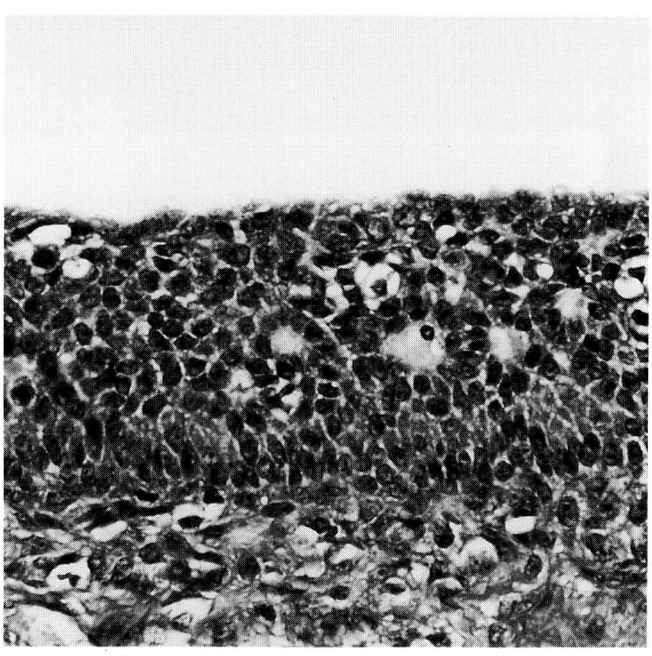

Fig. 59.3 A cystic adult-type granulosa cell tumor.

women with adult-type granulosa cell neoplasms has been in the region of only 50 to 60%,[14,27,39,54,55] though a considerably higher survival rate was noted in one series.[35] It is clear, therefore, that all granulosa cell tumors should be regarded as being at least potentially malignant, and it has to be stressed that no tumor of this type can, on pathological grounds, be unequivocally classed as fully benign. Conversely, the only absolute indication of a poor prognosis is the presence of extra-ovarian spread at the time of initial diagnosis. Other prognostic indicators are more debatable and, although there has been a measure of agreement that the larger the neoplasm the greater is the tendency towards a poor outcome,[14,54,55] it has not been clearly established that this factor is prognostically significant for those tumors confined to the ovary.[6] The type of histological pattern seen in the tumor is not prognostically relevant,[5,6,14,54,55] whilst it has not been proved that a high mitotic count is of strict relevance for those tumors without extra-ovarian spread.[6,14,55] Atypia is not, by itself, indicative of a poor prognosis.[73]

Juvenile granulosa cell tumors

About 85% of granulosa cell neoplasms which occur before puberty have a distinctive histological appearance which has therefore been considered typical of the juvenile granulosa cell tumor.[29,46,51,67,80] Neoplasms showing this pattern are not, however, confined to the prepubertal years, for, whilst 45% occur in the first decade of life and 32% in the second decade, 20% develop in the third decade and 3% present after the age of 30 years.

The tumor usually arises in otherwise normal children, though there is a suggestion of a specific, though weak, association with Ollier's disease and Mafucci's syndrome.[58,60,64,65]

Pathological features

The tumors are usually unilateral and characteristically largely solid, though cystic forms are occasionally encountered.

Histologically (Figs 59.4 and 59.5), there is a nodular or, less commonly, a diffuse pattern of tumor cells set in an edematous, loose stroma. The nodules may be solid, but usually contain a number of sharply etched, rounded or irregular follicles which bear some resemblance to normal developing follicles. These are lined by one or more layers of granulosa cells, and their lumens commonly contain mucinous material. Cystic spaces, often relatively large, may be present and have a multilayered lining of granulosa cells. Thecal cells may lie in the stroma adjacent to the granulosa cell nodules, but the two cell types can be intermingled in a haphazard fashion. Luteinization is often a striking feature of these neoplasms, whilst the granulosa cell nuclei tend to be hyperchromatic and lack the charac-

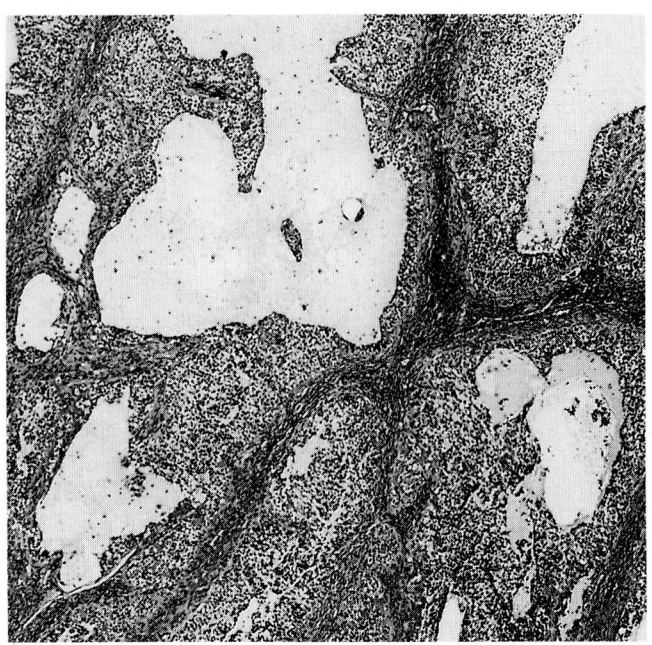

Fig. 59.4 A juvenile-type granulosa cell tumor.

teristic longitudinal grooving of an adult-type granulosa cell tumor. A degree of cytological atypia is not uncommon, and mitotic figures, sometimes of abnormal form, are frequently plentiful.

Prognosis

Approximately 5% of juvenile granulosa cell tumors behave in a malignant fashion; these are usually, but not invariably, those showing the greatest degree of atypia and mitotic activity. The indolent course pursued by malignant adult-type granulosa cell tumors is not, however, mirrored by the malignant juvenile forms, for these tend to recur rapidly and disseminate widely throughout the abdominal cavity within 2 years of initial diagnosis.

Cellular fibromas and fibrosarcomas

The vast majority of ovarian fibromas are clearly benign, but occasional examples are encountered which show an increased cellularity together with a variable degree of pleomorphism and mitotic activity; such neoplasms have been subdivided into cellular fibromas and fibrosarcomas.[42] Cellular fibromas are characterized by mild pleomorphism, increased cellularity and a mitotic count of less than 4 per 10 high power microscopic fields. Fibrosarcomas show a greater degree of pleomorphism and more than 3 mitotic figures per 10 high power fields. The prognosis for patients with a cellular fibroma is generally good, but a minority, perhaps 20%, of these tumors recur, particularly if

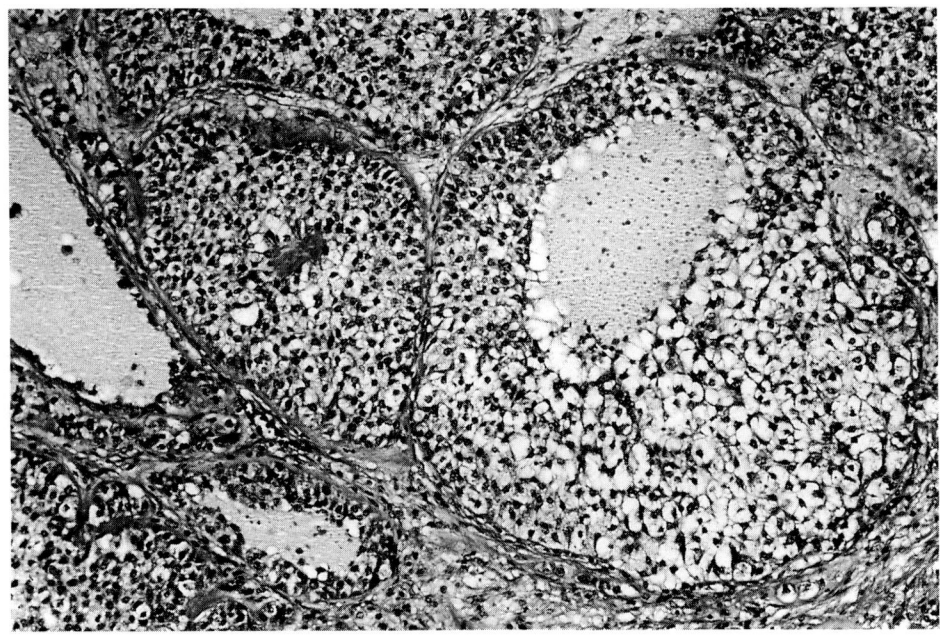

Fig. 59.5 A higher power view of a juvenile-type granulosa cell tumor.

removal has been incomplete. Fibrosarcomas, by contrast, are highly malignant and are associated with an extremely poor prognosis.

SERTOLI AND SERTOLI-LEYDIG CELL TUMORS

Pure Sertoli cell tumors

Pure Sertoli cell tumors are rare and present at an average age of 27 years[75]. Occasional cases have occurred in women with the Peutz-Jeghers syndrome.

Pathology

Pure Sertoli cell tumors are usually intra-ovarian, small (average diameter 9 cm), solid and have an orange or yellow cut surface.

Histologically, Sertoli cell neoplasms have a predominantly tubular pattern (Fig. 59.6), the tubules being either hollow or solid. The hollow tubules are generally uniform, rounded or ovoid, and lined by a single layer of cuboidal or low columnar cells with clear cytoplasm and basal nuclei. The lining cells often have well defined apical margins, but in some instances their apical cytoplasm trails off towards the lumen to form intertwining fibrils. The solid tubules are usually elongated and are sometimes admixed with Sertoli cells arranged in a diffuse pattern. The Sertoli cells commonly contain cytoplasmic lipid droplets, and in a proportion the tumor cells are

markedly distended by fat, a pattern sometimes given the term 'folliculoma lipidique'.[62]

A complex tubular form of Sertoli cell tumor has been described,[61] but this corresponds to the sex cord tumor with annular tubules (see p. 955).

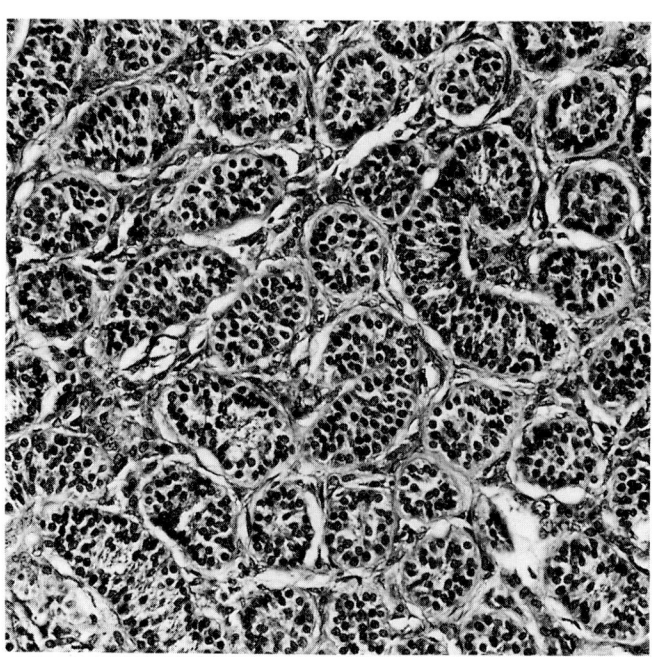

Fig. 59.6 A pure Sertoli cell tumor.

Prognosis

Virtually all Sertoli cell tumors are benign, but one such neoplasm, occurring in a young girl, recurred rapidly and led to death within 5 months.[75] In this particular tumor, there was a typical tubular pattern in some areas but elsewhere there were aggregates of pleomorphic cells showing much mitotic activity.

Sertoli-Leydig cell tumors

Sertoli-Leydig cell tumors are rare, accounting for only about 0.2% of all ovarian neoplasms. They occur most commonly between the ages of 11 and 45 years, the mean age of patients being 25 years. A few familial cases of Sertoli-Leydig cell tumor have been described; these women also had a high incidence of associated thyroid abnormalities, such as goitres and adenomas.[24]

Macroscopic features

Sertoli-Leydig cell tumors are unilateral in 98% of cases and are of variable size, averaging, however, about 10 cm in diameter. The neoplasms have a smooth external surface and are usually solid and firm; the cut surface often has a yellowish tinge. Cystic change is sometimes apparent, but areas of necrosis or hemorrhage are uncommon except in poorly differentiated neoplasms.

Histological appearances

Sertoli-Leydig cell tumors are traditionally, and probably

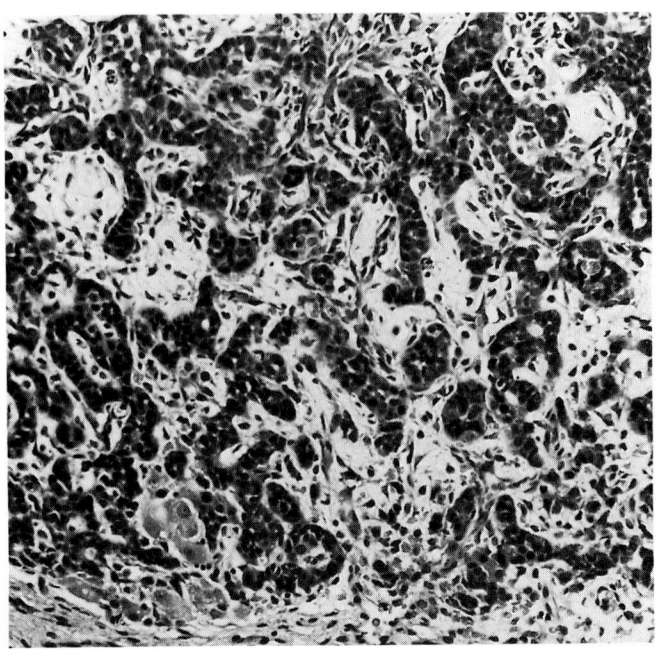

Fig. 59.8 A Sertoli-Leydig cell tumor of intermediate differentiation.

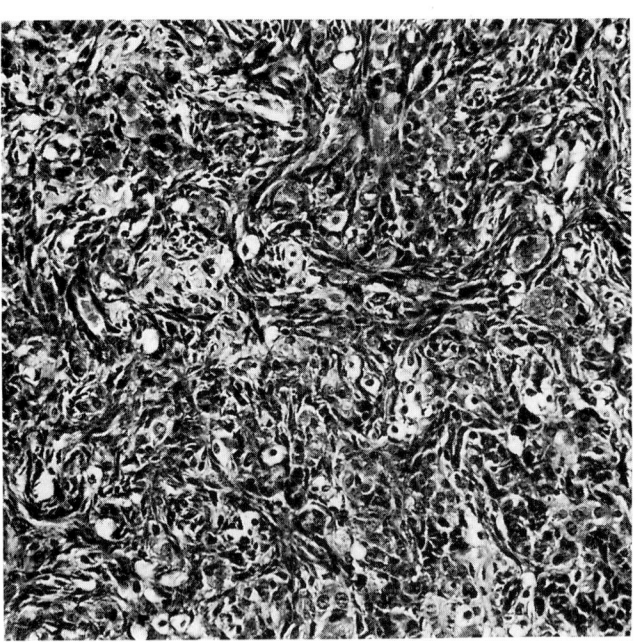

Fig. 59.9 A poorly differentiated Sertoli-Leydig cell tumor.

usefully, categorized according to their degree of differentiation.[15] The well differentiated neoplasms (Fig. 59.7) are formed by clearly defined tubular structures, which may be hollow or solid, lined by Sertoli cells. These tubules are set in a fibrous stroma which contains a variable number

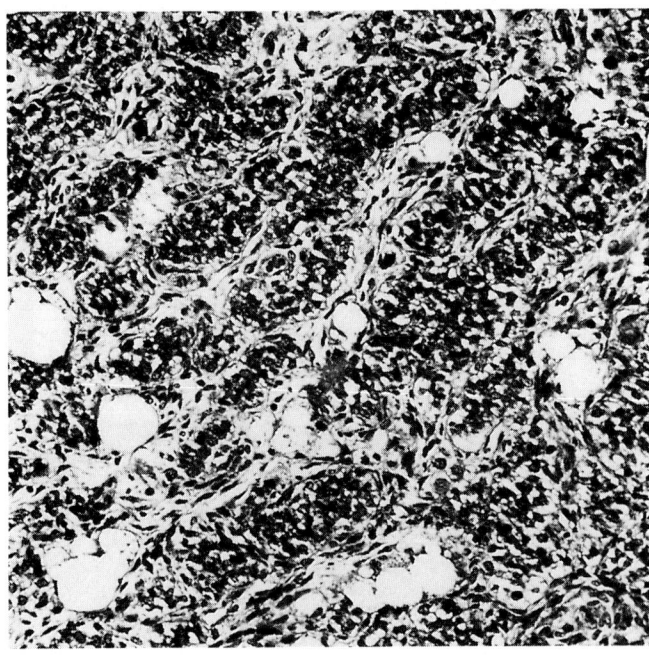

Fig. 59.7 A well differentiated Sertoli-Leydig cell tumor.

of cells resembling Leydig cells; it is unusual, however, for Reinke's crystals to be identifiable in these cells.

Tumors of intermediate differentiation (Fig. 59.8) tend to have a lobular pattern, and contain Sertoli cells arranged in islands, trabeculae, sheets or cords; solid or hollow tubules are occasionally encountered. This Sertoli cell element is set in a fibrous or edematous stroma in which Leydig cells are found singly, in clumps or in sheets. The Leydig cells are seen most conspicuously at the periphery of the cellular lobules and at the margin of the tumor as a whole.

Poorly differentiated Sertoli-Leydig cell tumors (Fig. 59.9) are formed largely of sheets of closely packed, spindle-shaped cells, this tissue bearing a close resemblance to the stroma of the undifferentiated gonad. Set in this undifferentiated sex cord stromal tissue are, however, occasional poorly formed tubules or irregular epithelial cords, and in most cases there are also a few clusters of Leydig cells.

Any Sertoli-Leydig cell tumor may contain foci of cells with bizarre nuclei[73], whilst if these neoplasms are encountered in a pregnant patient they often contain broad sheets of Leydig cells.[68]

Prognosis

The biological behavior, and hence the prognosis, of Sertoli-Leydig cell tumors is still not fully defined, though it is now reasonably clear that well differentiated neoplasms always behave in a benign fashion.[74] The outlook for patients with tumors of intermediate or poor differentiation is, however, less clear.[15,44] In one series of 64 tumors showing intermediate or poor differentiation, the corrected 10-year survival rate was 92%.[81] However, in another large study, the survival rate for patients with neoplasms of intermediate differentiation was 87% but that for women with poorly differentiated tumors only 44%.[77] It is clear, however, that most Sertoli-Leydig cell tumors which behave in a malignant fashion fall into the poorly differentiated category. In those tumors which do pursue a malignant course, metastasis or recurrence is usually apparent within 12 months of initial treatment and most women with malignant tumors are dead within 2 years. Metastases usually occur in the omentum, abdominal lymph nodes or liver, but deposits have been noted in sites such as lung, bone and brain.

Retiform Sertoli-Leydig cell tumors

Approximately 10% of Sertoli-Leydig cell tumors contain, at least in part, areas which show a pattern of growth resembling that of the rete testis.[47,59,72] The retiform areas may be only a minor component of such neoplasms, represent a moderate proportion of the tumor, or be a predominant, even exclusive, feature of a Sertoli-Leydig

cell neoplasm. Tumors with prominent retiform components tend to occur in children and in women who are, on average, younger than are those whose tumors lack a retiform element (average age 17 years).

Retiform neoplasms tend to be larger and more often cystic than more conventional Sertoli-Leydig cell tumors. Histologically, the retiform areas of these tumors are characterized by a network of elongated, irregularly shaped, not uncommonly slit-like, tubules and spaces. The tubules are sometimes dilated and contain eosinophilic material, thus having a slight resemblance to thyroid follicles. Papillary structures are also present in most cases (Fig. 59.10), projecting into the tubules and cysts; these papillae may be short with a hyalinized core, large or polypoid with fibrous or edematous cores, or have a complex branching pattern. The stroma may be fibrous or of a loose mesenchymal nature, and often shows foci of hyalinization. The Sertoli-Leydig cell component of these tumors is invariably of intermediate or poor differentiation.

Retiform Sertoli-Leydig cell tumors appear to have a relatively poor prognosis. In one series of 21 such neoplasms, 5 patients succumbed to their tumors at intervals ranging from 6 months to 17 years after initial therapy.[72]

Sertoli-Leydig cell tumors with heterologous elements

Heterologous elements are present in about 20% of Sertoli-Leydig cell tumors, most commonly gastrointestinal-type epithelium[19,23,37,38,45,66,69] and, less frequently, muscle or cartilage;[26,28,43] very rarely, cells resembling hepatocytes[70] or neuroectodermal elements[7] may be seen. There has been debate as to whether neoplasms of this type are teratomatous in nature[15] or whether the heterologous elements develop by a process of neometaplasia;[52] on balance, the latter view appears the more convincing.

In tumors containing gastrointestinal-type epithelium, the enteric component may be inconspicuous but in some cases predominates, the Sertoli-Leydig cells occurring in the wall of what at first sight appears to be an unexceptional mucinous neoplasm. The mucinous epithelium is usually benign but occasionally shows a pattern of borderline malignancy, whilst, rarely, it may be frankly malignant. The enteric epithelium often contains argyrophil cells, and in such cases small microscopic foci of carcinoid tumor may develop.[69] Heterologous skeletal muscle or cartilage in Sertoli-Leydig cell tumors is always immature, and the muscle component (Fig. 59.11) sometimes develops into a rhabdomyosarcoma.[16]

Sertoli-Leydig cell tumors containing heterologous gastrointestinal epithelium have a good prognosis, and in a study of 31 such neoplasms only two behaved in a malignant fashion and proved fatal.[69] By contrast, neoplasms containing heterologous muscle or cartilage are associated

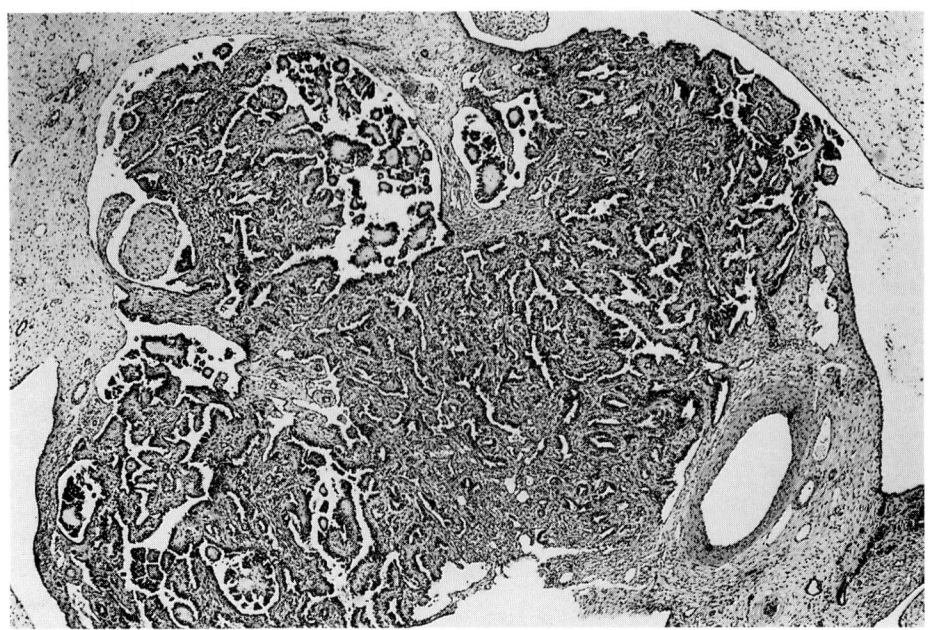

Fig. 59.10 A retiform Sertoli-Leydig cell tumor. In this field, only the retiform pattern is seen but elsewhere there was a transition to a more conventional Sertoli-Leydig cell pattern.

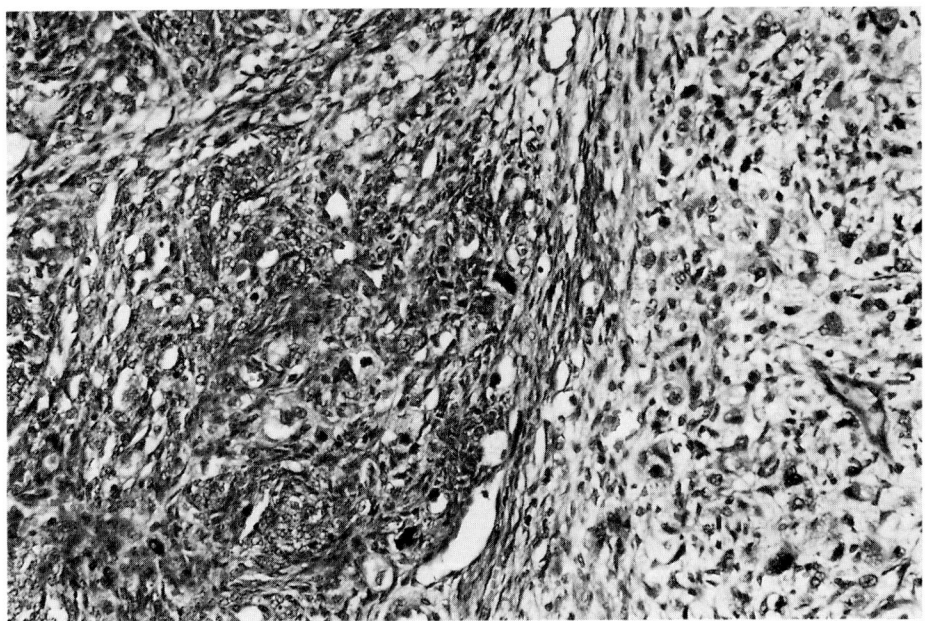

Fig. 59.11 A Sertoli-Leydig cell tumor containing heterologous striated muscle which has developed into a rhabdomyosarcoma (on the right).

with a poor outlook; in a series of 10 patients with such tumors only two survived.[43]

GYNANDROBLASTOMA

The diagnosis of gynandroblastoma has commonly been applied in an indiscriminate manner, but should be restricted to neoplasms in which both Sertoli-Leydig and granulosa-thecal components are present in substantial quantities and in typical and unequivocal form. There must also be a true mingling of the two cell patterns, for there have been instances of a granulosa cell tumor and a Leydig cell neoplasm occurring as separate and discrete entities within the same ovary.[15]

With the application of these precise criteria, only a very small number of acceptable cases of gynandroblastoma have been reported;[3,8] all of these appeared to behave in a benign fashion, but insufficient examples have accumulated for the true biological behavior of these neoplasms to be defined.

SEX CORD TUMOR WITH ANNULAR TUBULES

Sex cord tumors with annular tubules have a very distinctive histological appearance (Fig. 59.12), being formed of sharply circumscribed, rounded or ovoid, nests of epithelial cells set in a fibrous stroma.[1,2,9,18,22,50,79] The epithelial cells have clear or eosinophilic cytoplasm, indistinct margins, and regular, round, occasionally grooved, nuclei. The cell nests contain acidophilic, PAS-positive, hyaline bodies, which may coalesce with each other to form complex networks within the epithelial nests. The hyaline material, which is occasionally so abundant as to obliterate most of the cellular elements in some or even most nests, appears to be basement membrane protein. The epithelial cells are characteristically palisaded around the periphery of the cell nests and around the hyaline bodies, so as to give two basic patterns: there may be a simple, closed, ring-shaped tubule with a central hyaline body, or there may be a network of continuous tubules rotating around numerous single or confluent hyaline bodies. Between the epithelial islands is ovarian-type stroma which may show extensive hyalinization.

There has been considerable debate as to whether the epithelial cells in a sex cord tumor with annular tubules are of granulosa or Sertoli cell type, but they are best regarded as immature cells of sex cord origin which have a potentiality for differentiating into either granulosa or Sertoli cells.

The original descriptions of the sex cord tumor with annular tubules stressed the association between these neoplasms and the Peutz-Jegher's syndrome, but as more cases have accumulated it has become clear that they can also occur in women with no stigmata of this syndrome. Furthermore, it has become apparent that those tumors associated with the Peutz-Jegher's syndrome differ both clinically and pathologically from those arising in otherwise normal women.[79] Thus, sex cord tumors with annular tubules occurring in women with the Peutz-Jegher's syndrome are usually bilateral, commonly only of microscopic size, frequently calcified, not associated with granulosa or Sertoli cell tumoral overgrowth and never behave in a malignant fashion. By contrast, histologically identical tumors developing in women lacking the stigmata of the Peutz-Jegher's syndrome are unilateral, usually large, rarely calcified and are associated not infrequently with an overgrowth of either granulosa (Fig. 59.13) or Sertoli cells, about 15% of these neoplasms behaving in a malignant fashion.[79]

UNCLASSIFIED SEX CORD STROMAL TUMORS

Between 5 and 10% of tumors which are clearly of sex cord stromal type defy any more specific diagnosis. Difficulties

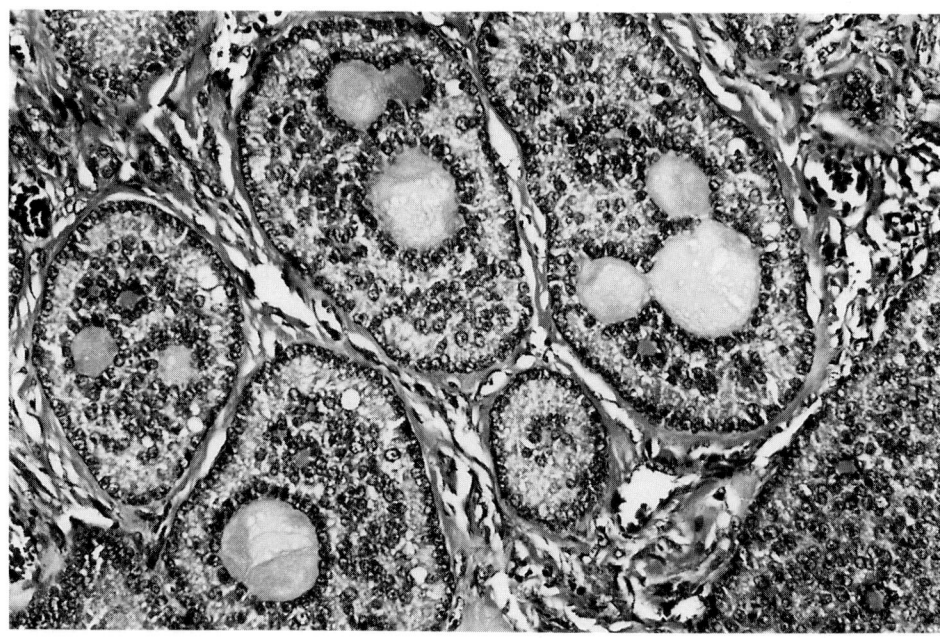

Fig. 59.12 A sex cord tumor with annular tubules.

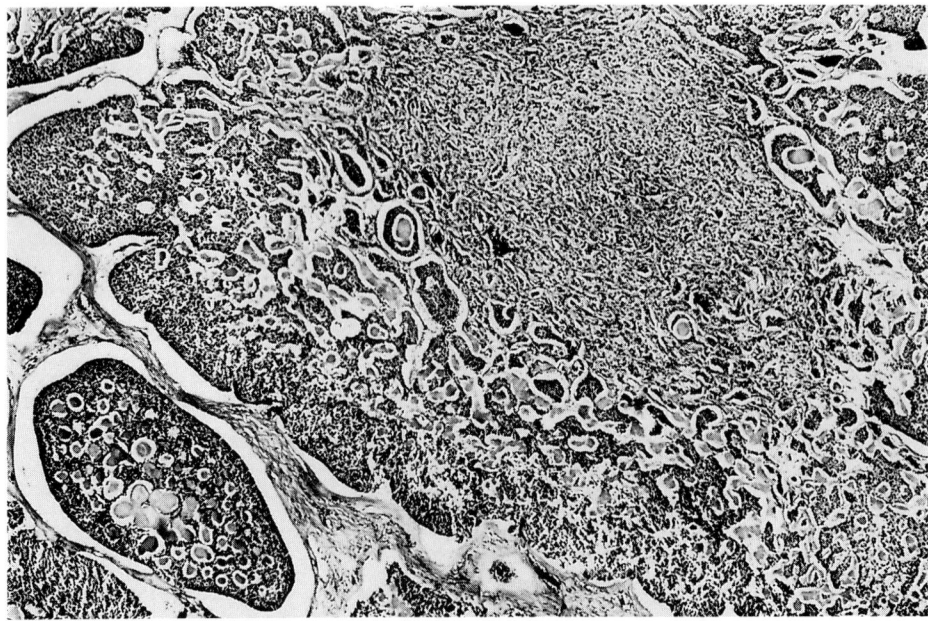

Fig. 59.13 A sex cord tumor with annular tubules which is showing granulosa cell overgrowth.

in precise categorization are particularly likely to arise in sex cord stromal tumors occurring in pregnant women,[68] the combination of edema and luteinization contributing markedly to the diagnostic difficulties.

LIPID CELL (STEROID CELL) TUMORS

The term 'lipid cell tumor' is used to describe a group of neoplasms having an endocrine type architecture and formed of cells resembling luteal, Leydig or adrenocortical cells.[15] Most of these tumors do contain intracellular lipid, but a substantial minority do not, these latter leading to the paradox of 'lipid-free' lipid cell tumors. In order to overcome this incongruity, the term 'steroid cell tumors' has been introduced to describe these neoplasms.[52] Unfortunately, this term could also be applied, with justification, to granulosa and Sertoli cell tumors, and in this account we therefore adhere to the historically entrenched term 'lipid cell neoplasms', whilst recognizing its inadequacy.

The various types of lipid cell tumors are listed in Table 59.2. Central to this classification is the belief that all lipid

Table 59.2 Classification of lipid cell tumors

(A) Stromal luteoma

(B) Leydig cell tumor

(C) Adrenal-like tumor

(D) Lipid cell tumor of indeterminate type

cell tumors are derived from the ovarian stroma, which is presumed to have the capacity to differentiate along a variety of pathways. The Leydig cell tumors present a particular difficulty in classification, for, although some such neoplasms appear to develop from ovarian stromal cells, a majority arise from pre-existing hilar cells;[48,50] the inclusion of Leydig cell tumors in this category of lipid cell tumors is thus a matter of expediency rather than of fact. Adrenal-type tumors do not, as is often thought, arise from ovarian adrenal rests; this concept is difficult to sustain in view of the fact that intra-ovarian rests of this nature have never been demonstrated.[15] Experimental studies have shown that ovarian stromal cells have a facultative ability to differentiate into adrenal cells and this is substantiated by the finding, in a number of cases, of a peripheral transition between tumor and stromal cells.[15] The adrenocortical nature of the cells in these neoplasms has been confirmed by ultrastructural studies and by the fact that some patients with tumors of this type develop many of the features of Cushing's syndrome.[78]

Of the various lipid cell neoplasms, the stromal luteoma is invariably benign[20,49] and will not be further discussed.

Leydig cell tumors

A pure Leydig cell tumor can arise either from pre-existing hilar cells or, much less commonly, from ovarian stromal cells. The neoplasms appear as unilateral, small (usually less than 5 cm in diameter), well circumscribed, solid, brown, orange or yellow, masses; those arising from hilar cells present as nodules within the mesovarian, while those of stromal origin occur within the medullary portion of the ovary. If the tumors are small, a distinction can usually be drawn between hilar and stromal types, but large neoplasms often cannot be specifically categorized in these terms.

Histologically, Leydig cell neoplasms (Fig. 59.14) are formed of uniform, rounded or polygonal cells with abundant granular or vacuolated eosinophilic cytoplasm and large central nuclei. These cells are arranged in nests, sheets and cords, and a characteristic feature is the presence, in some areas, of nuclear 'pooling' or aggregation. There is some controversy as to whether it is permissable to make a diagnosis of a Leydig cell tumor in the absence of Reinke's crystals. The crystals, when present, are very unevenly distributed and are absent from hilar Leydig cells in many adult ovaries, thus making an insistence on their presence as a diagnostic criterion appear too stringent. It would be a reasonable compromise not to insist on the finding of the crystals for those mesovarian tumors which are clearly of hilar cell origin, but to retain this diagnostic requirement for tumors of stromal origin and for those whose large size will not permit their recognition as either hilar or non-hilar.

The vast majority of ovarian Leydig cell tumors are benign, but a small proportion, probably less than 5%, pursue a malignant course and give rise to widespread metastases;[12,57] those which behave in this fashion may or may not show histological features suggestive of malignancy.

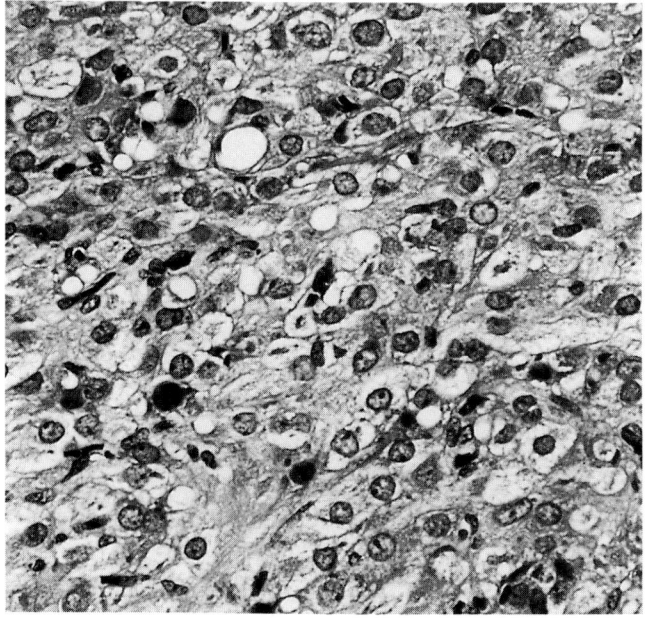

Fig. 59.14 A Leydig cell tumor.

Adrenal-type lipid cell tumors

Adrenal-type lipid cell tumors are commonly small, usually unilateral and are formed of large, polygonal or rounded cells with well defined borders and abundant, usually lipid-containing, clear, vacuolated or foamy cytoplasm which are arranged in nests or columns around a rich capillary network (Fig. 59.15). The histological mimicry by these neoplasms of an adrenocortical adenoma is usually quite striking.[41] Most behave in a benign fashion, but about 5% recur locally in the pelvis or metastasize to lymph nodes, liver or omentum.[30] In some of these latter cases, their malign nature has been recognizable histologically, but others have not shown any features to suggest their aggressive nature.

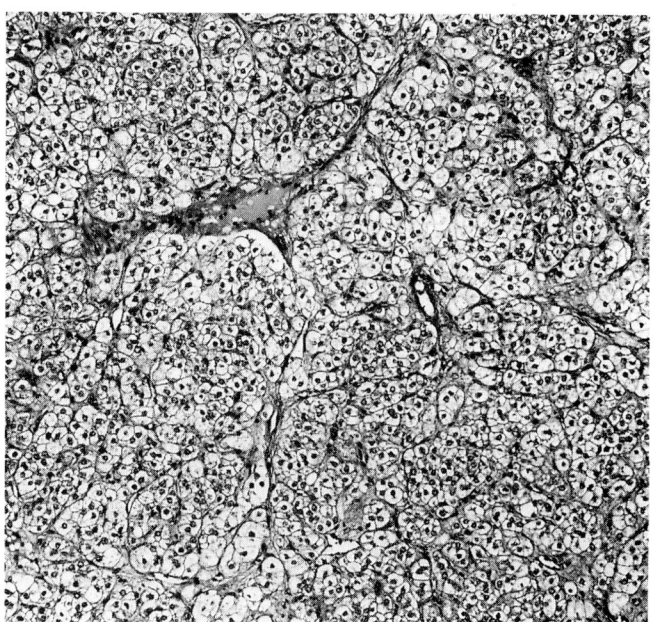

Fig. 59.15 An adrenal-type lipid cell tumor.

Lipid cell tumors of indeterminate type

Lipid cell tumors of indeterminate type are neoplasms which, whilst clearly falling into the lipid cell category, cannot be further categorized in more specific terms.

These neoplasms range in size up to 45 cm in diameter but have an average diameter of 8 to 9 cm. Most are solid with a yellow or orange cut surface but some are reddish or brown. Histologically, polygonal or rounded cells are arranged in nests or columns separated by a rich vascular network. The tumor cells have granular or foamy cytoplasm, sharp-cut cell borders and central nuclei.

About 40% of lipid cell tumors of indeterminate type are clinically malignant and, although the only absolute evidence of malignancy in these neoplasms is the presence of metastases, certain pathological features correlate well with malignant behavior. Thus, nearly 80% of tumors measuring more than 7 cm in diameter are malignant, whilst neoplasms smaller than this appear to be invariably benign; two-thirds of the neoplasms showing marked nuclear atypia, and 80% of those with two or more mitotic figures per 10 high power fields pursue a malignant course.[21]

REFERENCES

1. Ali F 1981 Sex cord tumor with annular tubules. Diag Gynecol Obstet 3: 137
2. Anderson M C, Govan A D T, Langley F A, Woodcock A S, Tayagi S F 1980 Ovarian sex cord tumours with annular tubules. Histopathology 4: 137
3. Anderson M C, Rees D A 1975 Gynandroblastoma of the ovary. Br J Obstet Gynaecol 82: 68
4. Anderson W R, Levine A J, Macmillan D 1971 Granulosa-theca cell tumors: clinical and pathological study. Am J Obstet Gynecol 110: 32
5. Björkholm E, Pettersson F 1980 Granulosa cell and theca cell tumours: the clinical picture and long term outcome for the Radiumhemmet series. Acta Obstet Gynecol Scand 59: 361
6. Björkholm E, Silfverswäld C 1981 Prognostic factors in granulosa cell tumors. Gynecol Oncol 11: 261
7. Chadha S, Honnebier W J, Schaberg A 1987 Raised serum alpha-fetoprotein in Sertoli-Leydig cell tumor (androblastoma) of ovary: report of two cases. Int J Gynecol Pathol 6: 82
8. Chalvardjian A, Derzko C 1982 Gynandroblastoma: its ultrastructure. Cancer 50: 710
9. Crissman J D, Hart W R 1981 Ovarian sex cord tumors with annular tubules: an ultrastructural study of three cases. Am J Clin Pathol 75: 11
10. Diddle A W 1952 Granulosa-theca-cell ovarian tumors: prognosis. Cancer 5: 215
11. Dinnerstein A J, O'Leary J A 1968 Granulosa-theca cell tumors: a clinical review of 102 patients. Obstet Gynecol 31: 654
12. Echt C R, Heald H E 1968 Androgen excretion patterns in a patient with a metastatic hilus cell tumor of the ovary. Am J Obstet Gynecol 100: 1055
13. Felmus L B, Pedowitz P 1967 Clinical malignancy of endocrine tumors of the ovary and dysgerminoma. Obstet Gynecol 29: 344
14. Fox H, Agrawal K, Langley F A 1975 A clinicopathological study of 92 cases of granulosa cell tumor of the ovary with special reference to the factors influencing prognosis. Cancer 35: 231
15. Fox H, Langley F A 1976 Tumours of the Ovary. Heinemann, London
16. Gueraro M J, Ferenczy A, Arguelles M A 1982 Ovarian Sertoli-Leydig cell tumor with rhabdomyosarcoma: an ultrastructural study. Ultrastruc Pathol 3: 347
17. Harris M, Balgobin B 1978 Pure Sertoli cell tumour of the ovary: report of a case with ultrastructural observations. Histopathology 2: 449
18. Hart W R, Kumar N, Crissman J D 1980 Ovarian neoplasms resembling sex cord tumors with annular tubules. Cancer 45: 2352
19. Hayes D M, Hunter R J 1973 Androblastoma of the ovary with heterotopic elements. J Pathol 100: 267
20. Hayes M C, Scully R E 1987 Stromal luteoma of the ovary: a clinicopathological analysis of 25 cases. Int J Gynecol Pathol 6: 313
21. Hayes M C, Scully R E 1987 Ovarian steroid cell tumors, not otherwise specified (lipid cell tumors): a clinicopathological analysis of 63 cases. Am J Surg Pathol 11: 835
22. Hertel B F, Kempson R L 1977 Ovarian sex cord tumor with annular tubules: an ultrastructural study. Am J Surg Pathol 1: 145
23. Hertz P H 1945 Giant cystic arrhenoblastoma of the ovary containing endodermal epithelium and carcinoid. Am J Pathol 21: 1167
24. Jensen R D, Norris H J, Fraumeni J F 1974 Familial arrhenoblastoma and thyroid adenoma. Cancer 33: 218
25. Jull J W 1973 Ovarian tumorigenesis. Meth Cancer Res 7: 131
26. Kawter A E, Klawan A H 1940 Arrhenoblastoma of the ovary. Am J Cancer 40: 474
27. Kolstad P 1986 Clinical Gynecologic Oncology. The Norwegian Experience. Norwegian University Press, Oslo
28. Krock F, Wolferman S J 1941 Arrhenoblastoma of the ovary. Ann Surg 114: 78
29. Lack E E, Perez-Atayzo A R, Murphy A S A, Goldstein D P, Crigler J F, Wawther G F 1981 Granulosa-theca cell tumors in premenarchal girls: a clinical and pathologic study of ten cases. Cancer 48: 1846
30. Lipsett M B, Kirschner M A, Wilson H, Barlow C W 1970 Malignant lipoid cell tumor of the ovary: clinical, biological and etiologic considerations. J Clin Endocrinol 30: 336
31. Marchant J 1980 Animal models for tumours of the ovary. In: Murphy E D and Beamer W C (eds) Biology of Ovarian Neoplasia. International Union Against Cancer, Geneva, p 50
32. McLean J M 1987 Embryology and anatomy of the female genital tract and ovaries. In: Fox H (ed) Haines and Taylor: Obstetrical and Gynaecological Pathology 3rd edn. Churchill-Livingstone, Edinburgh, p 1
33. Miettinen M, Virtanen I, Talerman A 1985 Intermediate filament proteins in human testis and testicular germ cell tumors. Am J Pathol 120: 402
34. Miettinen M, Wahlstrom T, Virtanen I, Talerman A, Astenco-Osuna C 1985 Cellular differentiation in ovarian sex cord stromal and germ cell tumors studied with antibodies to intermediate filament proteins. Am J Surg Pathol 9: 640
35. Norris H J, Taylor T H B 1968 Prognosis of granulosa-theca tumors of the ovary. Cancer 21: 255
36. Novak E R, Kutchmeshgi J, Mudas A S, Woodruff J D 1971 Feminizing gonadal stromal tumors: analysis of the granulosa-theca cell tumors of the Ovarian Tumor Registry. Obstet Gynecol 38: 701
37. Novak E R, Long J H 1965 Arrhenoblastoma of the ovary: a review of the Ovarian Tumor Registry. Am J Obstet Gynecol 92: 1082
38. O'Hern T M, Neubecker R D 1962 Arrhenoblastoma. Obstet Gynecol 19: 758
39. Pankratz E, Boyes D A, White G W, Galliford B W, Fairey R N, Benedet J L 1978 Granulosa cell tumors, a clinical review of 64 cases. Obstet Gynecol 52: 718
40. Parmley T 1987 Embryology of the female genital tract. In Kurman R J (ed) Blaustein's Pathology of the Female Genital Tract 3rd Edn. Springer-Verlag, New York, p 1
41. Pedowitz P, Pomerance W 1962 Adrenal-like tumors of the ovary: review of the literature and report of two new cases. Obstet Gynecol 19: 183
42. Prat J, Scully R E 1981 Cellular fibromas and fibrosarcomas of the ovary: a comparative clinicopathologic analysis of seventeen cases. Cancer 47: 2663
43. Prat J, Young R H, Scully R E 1982 Ovarian Sertoli-Leydig cell tumors with heterologous elements. II. Cartilage and skeletal muscle: a clinicopathologic analysis of twelve cases. Cancer 50: 2465
44. Roth L M, Anderson M C, Govan A D T, Langley F A, Gowing N F C, Woodcock A S 1981 Sertoli-Leydig cell tumors: a clinicopathological study of 34 cases. Cancer 43: 187
45. Roth L M, Cleary R E, Rosenfeld R L 1974 Sertoli-Leydig cell tumor of the ovary with an associated mucinous cystadenoma: an ultrastructural and endocrine study. Lab Invest 31: 648
46. Roth L M, Nicholas T R, Ehrlich C E 1979 Juvenile granulosa cell tumor: a clinicopathologic study of three cases with ultrastructural observations. Cancer 44: 2194
47. Roth L M, Slayton R E, Brady L W, Blessing J A, Johnson G 1985 Retiform differentiation in ovarian Sertoli-Leydig cell tumors: a clinicopathologic study of six cases from a Gynecologic Oncology Group study. Cancer 55: 1093

48. Roth L M, Sternberg W H 1973 Ovarian stromal tumors containing Leydig cells. I. Pure Leydig cell tumor, non-hilar type. Cancer 32: 940
49. Scully R E 1964 Stromal luteoma of the ovary. Cancer 17: 769
50. Scully R E 1970 Sex cord tumor with annular tubules: a distinctive ovarian tumor of the Peutz-Jegher's syndrome. Cancer 25: 1107
51. Scully R E 1977 Ovarian tumors: a review. Am J Pathol 87: 686
52. Scully R E 1979 Tumors of the ovary and maldeveloped gonads. Atlas of Tumor Pathology. Second Series, Fascicle 16. Armed Forces Institute of Pathology, Washington D.C.
53. Serov S F, Scully R E, Sobin L H 1973 International Histological Classification of Tumours. No. 9. Histological Typing of Ovarian Tumours. World Health Organization, Geneva
54. Sjöstedt S, Wahlen T 1961 Prognosis of granulosa cell tumours. Acta Obstet Gynecol Scand 40 (suppl 6): 3
55. Stenwig J T, Hazekamp J T, Beecham J B 1979 Granulosa cell tumors of the ovary: a clinicopathological study of 118 cases with long term follow up. Gynecol Oncol 7: 136
56. Sternberg W H, Dhyrandha H N 1977 Functional ovarian tumors of stromal and sex cord origin. Hum Pathol 56: 565
57. Stewart R S, Woodward D E 1962 Malignant ovarian hilus cell tumor. Arch Pathol 73: 91
58. Takeuchi H, Hamada H, Sodemoto Y, Ushigome S 1983 Juvenile granulosa cell tumor with rapid distant metastases. Acta Pathol Jap 33: 537
59. Talerman A 1987 Ovarian Sertoli-Leydig cell tumor (androblastoma) with retiform pattern: a clinicopathologic study. Cancer 60: 3056
60. Tamini H K, Bolen J 1984 Enchrondomatosis (Ollier's disease) and ovarian juvenile granulosa cell tumor. Cancer 53: 1605
61. Tavassoli F A, Norris H J 1980 Sertoli tumors of the ovary: a clinicopathologic study of 28 cases with ultrastructural observations. Cancer 46: 2281
62. Teilum G 1949 Homologous ovarian and testicular tumors. III. Estrogen-producing Sertoli cell tumors (androblastoma tubulare lipoides) of the human testis and ovary. J Clin Endocrinol 8: 301
63. Teilum G 1971 Special Tumors of the Ovary and Testis. Munksgaard, Copenhagen
64. Vaz R M, Turner C H 1986 Ollier's disease (enchrondomatosis) associated with ovarian juvenile granulosa cell tumor and precocious pseudopuberty. J Paediat 108: 945
65. Velasco-Oses A, Alonso-Alvaro A, Blanco-Pozo A, Nogales F F 1988 Ollier's disease associated with ovarian juvenile granulosa cell tumor. Cancer 62: 222
66. Waxman M, Damsanov I, Alpert L, Sardinsky T 1981 Composite mucinous ovarian neoplasms associated with Sertoli-Leydig and carcinoid tumors. Cancer 47: 2044
67. Young R H, Dickersin G R, Scully R E 1984 Juvenile granulosa cell tumor of the ovary: a clinicopathologic analysis of 125 cases. Am J Surg Pathol 8: 575
68. Young R H, Dudley A G, Scully R E 1984 Granulosa cell, Sertoli-Leydig cell and unclassified sex-cord stromal tumors associated with pregnancy: a clinicopathological analysis of thirty six cases. Gynecol Oncol 18: 181
69. Young R H, Prat J, Scully R E 1982 Ovarian Sertoli-Leydig cell tumors with heterologous elements. I. Gastrointestinal epithelium and carcinoid: a clinicopathologic analysis of thirty six cases. Cancer 50: 2448
70. Young R H, Perez-Ayayde A R, Scully R E 1984 Ovarian Sertoli-Leydig cell tumor with retiform and heterologous elements: report of a case with hepatocytic differentiation and elevated serum alphafetoprotein. Am J Surg Pathol 8: 709
71. Young R H, Scully R E 1982 Ovarian sex cord-stromal tumors: recent progress. Int J Gynecol Pathol 1: 101
72. Young R H, Scully R E 1983 Ovarian Sertoli-Leydig tumors with a retiform pattern: a problem in histopathologic diagnosis: a report of 25 cases. Am J Surg Pathol 7: 755
73. Young R E, Scully R E 1983 Ovarian sex cord-stromal tumors with bizarre nuclei: a clinicopathologic analysis of seventeen cases. Int J Gynecol Pathol 1: 325
74. Young R H, Scully R E 1984 Well differentiated ovarian Sertoli-Leydig cell tumors: a clinicopathological analysis of 23 cases. Int J Gynecol Pathol 3: 277
75. Young R H, Scully R E 1984 Ovarian Sertoli cell tumors: a report of 10 cases. Int J Gynecol Pathol 2: 349
76. Young R H, Scully R E 1984 Ovarian sex cord-stromal tumours; recent advances and current status. Clinics Obstet Gynaecol 11: 93
77. Young R H, Scully R E 1985 Ovarian Sertoli-Leydig cell tumors: a clinicopathological analysis of 207 cases. Am J Surg Pathol 9: 543
78. Young R H, Scully R E 1987 Ovarian steroid cell tumors associated with Cushing's syndrome: a report of three cases. Int J Gynecol Pathol 6: 40
79. Young R H, Welch W R, Dickersin G R, Scully R E 1982 Ovarian sex cord tumor with annular tubules: a review of 74 cases including 27 with Peutz-Jegher's syndrome and 4 with adenoma malignum of the cervix. Cancer 50: 1384
80. Zaloudek C, Norris H J 1982 Granulosa tumors of the ovary in children: a clinical and pathologic study of 32 cases. Am J Surg Pathol 6: 503
81. Zaloudek C, Norris H J 1984 Sertoli-Leydig cell tumors of the ovary: a clinico-pathologic study of 64 intermediate and poorly differentiated neoplasms. Am J Surg Pathol 8: 405

60. Malignant gonadal stromal tumors of ovary: clinical features and management

W. J. Hoskins   S. C. Rubin

INTRODUCTION

Stromal tumors of the ovary are estimated to constitute approximately 7% of ovarian malignancies. In the United States, with about 18 000 new cases per year of ovarian cancer, roughly 1260 women yearly will be diagnosed with stromal tumors of the ovary. The development of our understanding of the natural history and management of these tumors has been limited by their scarcity. Thus, a good deal of the literature on stromal tumors of the ovary consists of retrospective surveys of non-uniform treatment spanning many decades. In some reports, stromal tumor types with different clinical behavior are analyzed together, accurate surgical staging is lacking, histologic review of tissue specimens has not been performed, and long-term follow up is not available. In series where histologic review has been performed, a substantial proportion of cases are rejected. Stenwig[52] reported that of 177 cases originally diagnosed as granulosa tumors, 41 (23%) failed to meet their histologic criteria when reviewed. Similarly, Bjorkholm[5] rejected 80 of 278 (29%) cases on review. More recently, collaborative groups such as the Gynecologic Oncology Group in the United States have attempted to study the management of certain stromal tumors of the ovary in a systematic, prospective manner. These studies have not yet yielded usable information due primarily to slow patient accrual. Despite these problems, we have been able to gain a rudimentary understanding of the behavior of these interesting neoplasms, and to formulate some recommendations for treatment.

The classification and histopathology of the stromal tumors of the ovary have been considered in detail in the preceding chapter. Here, we will review their clinical features and management.

GRANULOSA–STROMAL CELL TUMORS

Granulosa cell tumors — adult type

Epidemiology and clinical features

Perhaps 70% of the ovarian stromal tumors will fall into the category of granulosa tumors. These tumors occur at an average age of about 52 years, according to a compilation of information on over 600 cases (Table 60.1). Hormone production is frequent, as is characteristic of the ovarian stromal tumors, and results in abnormal vaginal bleeding in about two-thirds of the patients. Estrogen production predominates, although there are reports of androgenic granulosa cell tumors as well[37] (see also Ch. 8). As a result, endometrial hyperplasia and even frank carcinoma may be found in a substantial proportion of patients with granulosa cell tumors. The reported incidence of hyperplasia ranges from 24% to above 80%, depending on diagnostic criteria. In Gusberg's[22] series of 69 carefully studied cases, 13% had cystic glandular hyperplasia, 42% had atypical glandular hyperplasia, 5% had adenocarcinoma in situ, and 22% had adenocarcinoma. Most authors have reported adenocarcinoma of the endometrium in about 10% of cases in which the endometrium has been examined. Hormone production by granulosa cell tumors has been documented by changes in serum hormone levels following surgical excision,[33] by direct measurement of hormone concentrations in the tumor,[19] and by the demonstration of the in vitro production of estrone and estradiol by a human ovarian granulosa tumor cell line.[25]

Table 60.1 Age at diagnosis of granulosa cell tumor

Author	Years studied	No. of cases	Mean age
Anikwue[2]	1955 to 76	32	50.2
Evans[15]	1910 to 72	118	51.0
Stenwig[52]	1932 to 70	118	53.7
Bjorkholm[5]	1923 to 72	198	52.6
Goldston[20]	1940 to 71	41	52.7
Fox[16]	1948 to 73	92	52.6
Pankratz[42]	1944 to 74	61	50.1
Total		660	52.2

A large majority of granulosa cell tumors are diagnosed in Stage I, although it must be remembered that accurate and complete surgical staging is not available in most of the published series. In three of the largest series,[5,15,52] the proportion of patients having Stage I tumors ranges from 78 to 91%. In each of these series, patients (some diagnosed as early as 1910) were retrospectively staged. Undoubtedly complete surgical staging as we conceive it today would reveal a somewhat greater incidence of extra-ovarian spread. Bilateral ovarian involvement is unusual. In combined series totalling over 700 patients (Table 60.2), the incidence of bilaterality ranges from 0 to 8%, with a weighted mean of 3.75%. Again, it must be noted that this information was obtained retrospectively, although it is probably more accurate than the information on overall staging. Granulosa cell tumors tend to be of substantial size. In Norris' series,[39] the average diameter of the pure granulosa tumors was 11.9 cm; the average diameter of the granulosa-theca variant was 6.6 cm. Goldston[20] reported that 25 of 41 tumors in his series were greater than 10 cm in diameter. Stage[51] has reported a granulosa-theca tumor as large as 36 cm.

Table 60.2   Frequency of bilateral granulosa cell tumors

Author	No. of cases	No. bilateral
Norris[39]	97	2
Evans[15]	118	0
Stenwig[52]	118	6
Bjorkholm[5]	198	5
Antolic[3]	28	2
Goldston[20]	33	2
Fox[16]	92	7
Pankratz[42]	61	5
Stage[51]	29	0
Total	774	29 (3.75%)

The patterns of spread and recurrence that have been observed in patients with granulosa tumors indicate that the tumor disseminates by the same routes as do the epithelial cancers: exfoliation of clonogenic cells into the peritoneal cavity, direct extension to adjacent organs and lymphatic and hematogenous metastases. It would appear that the latter two routes assume greater importance for the granulosa tumors than for the epithelial tumors. Another interesting feature of granulosa tumors is their propensity for indolent growth and late recurrence. In Stenwig's series,[52] the mean time to recurrence was 8.9 years; Evans[15] reported a 6 year mean interval. Fox,[16] however, found most recurrences were diagnosed within 2 years. These dif-ferences may be due in part to differing durations of patient follow-up. Certainly there are many reports of granulosa tumors recurring 10 to 20 years after diagnosis.

Management

Granulosa tumors, whether or not admixed with theca elements, should be considered low-grade malignancies, similar to the so-called borderline epithelial cancers of the ovaries, and must be managed as such. In the past, a number of authors have sought to distinguish 'benign' from 'malignant' granulosa tumors, based on their clinical behavior and histology. Some have even adopted the curious position that only those granulosa tumors that have metastasized or recurred are malignant, as if finding a cancer prior to the development of spread renders it benign. The waters have been further muddied by the inclusion of pure thecomas along with granulosa tumors. Thecomas are nearly always benign, and must be considered separately.

The diagnosis of granulosa tumor is generally not made until surgery, except for the occasional case where an astute clinician is able to make a tentative diagnosis based on the findings of an adnexal mass in a patient with evidence of hormonal imbalance, usually excess estrogen production. The surgeon may thus be faced with making decisions based on a frozen section diagnosis, which can be a challenge even to experienced gynecologic pathologists. The distinction between a granulosa tumor and other ovarian malignancies of similar histologic appearance (e.g other stromal tumors, carcinoid, undifferentiated carcinoma, lymphoma) can be difficult, and may require the assistance of a consultant pathologist.

If a granulosa tumor is suspected and future reproductive potential is not an issue (as it generally will not be in the age group likely to develop these tumors), total hysterectomy and bilateral salpingo-oophorectomy should be performed. In addition, a complete cancer staging operation should be undertaken. This includes a thorough exploration of the abdominal cavity, ideally through a vertical incision extending from the pubic symphysis to above the umbilicus. Washings for cytologic analysis are taken from multiple sites, and omentectomy is performed. Aortic and pelvic lymph node sampling may be done, with particular attention paid to the nodes on the side of the tumor but its value is unproven. In the occasional younger woman with a granulosa tumor who may wish to preserve reproductive potential, a unilateral salpingo-oophorectomy may be considered if a complete staging operation shows no evidence of tumor spread. Dilatation and curettage to rule out significant endometrial pathology should be considered. Although the incidence of occult bilateral involvement is certainly low, most gynecologic oncologists would recommend a thin-wedge biopsy of the opposite ovary.

The majority of patients with granulosa tumors of the

ovary will have no evidence of spread found at surgery. Our understanding of the role of adjuvant therapy in these patients is hampered by a lack of basic information. The risk of recurrence without treatment, and the efficacy of the various treatment options are largely unknown. Evans[15] reported a 9% risk of recurrence in Stage Ia; Stenwig[52] reported a 91.8% 5-year survival for Stage I patients. The lack of thorough surgical staging in these and other studies, and the indolent nature of the tumor make interpretation of these data difficult. It would appear that patients with Stage I disease based on optimal surgery have a very low risk of recurrence.

In Bjorkholm's retrospective series, there was no observed benefit to adjuvant irradiation in Stage I patients. There have been no reports suggesting a benefit to adjuvant chemotherapy in early granulosa cell tumors. Currently, there is no basis to recommend adjuvant treatment of any sort following surgery for Stage I granulosa cell tumor of the ovary.

There is little information available concerning the use of radiation therapy or chemotherapy in advanced or recurrent granulosa tumors. Many of the reported series include patients treated with irradiation, but the lack of proper staging, standardized treatment programs, and adequate follow-up render the results uninterpretable. A recent report by Neville[38] includes six patients with advanced (Stage IIb to III) granulosa tumors treated with postoperative radiotherapy. All were alive with no evidence of disease, although only one has been followed for longer than 3.5 years. Response to chemotherapy has been reported for a number of regimens. Malkasian[31] reported a partial response in three of 12 patients treated with cyclophosphamide, as well as a secondary response to actinomycin D. Schwartz & Smith[48] reported a partial response in two of 13 patients treated with an alkylating agent, and two of two patients treated with the combination of actinomycin-D, 5-fluorouracil, and cyclophosphamide. More recently, a complete clinical response has been reported in two patients treated with cisplatin and doxorubicin[26] and in a single patient treated with cisplatin, doxorubicin, and cyclophosphamide.[8] Neville[38] has also reported responses to alkylating agents, doxorubicin, and cisplatin-containing combination regimens. In Italy, Colombo et al[12] have reported that of 11 previously untreated cases of recurrent or metastatic granulosa tumors treated with cisplatin, vinblastine and bleomycin, there were six pathological complete responses and three partial responses. In the United States, the Gynecologic Oncology Group used the combination of vincristine, actinomycin-D, and cyclophosphamide in the treatment of advanced or recurrent ovarian granulosa cell tumors. Although some responses were seen, not enough patients were accrued for a definitive analysis.

There is essentially no experience in the use of hormonal manipulation in the treatment of advanced or recurrent

granulosa cell tumors. Receptors for follicle stimulating hormone (FSH) have been demonstrated in granulosa cell tumors, and FSH has been shown to support the growth of granulosa tumors in nude mice.[13] FSH has also been shown to stimulate the metabolic activity of granulosa cell tumors in vitro.[21] These observations lead one to speculate that the elevated levels of FSH seen in hypo-estrogenic women following treatment for a granulosa cell tumor may adversely affect prognosis.

Prognosis

The relationship of the histologic features of granulosa cell tumors to their clinical behavior has been the subject of substantial debate. Perhaps the clearest work on the subject comes from Bjorkholm et al[5] who analyzed 198 cases of granulosa and granulosa-theca tumors diagnosed between 1923 and 1972. Using a multivariate analysis with a minimum of 10 years clinical follow-up, they found that nuclear atypia and in Stages II to IV, mitotic activity, were related to prognosis. Stenwig[52] also found mitotic activity and nuclear atypia related to prognosis in a univariate analysis not corrected for tumor stage. The prognostic value of the various histologic features is detailed in Chapter 59.

The overall survival of patients with granulosa tumors of the ovary is quite good, probably due in large part to the fact that they are generally diagnosed early. The highest reported survival comes from the series of Norris,[39] who found actuarial survival at 5 and 10 years to be 97% and 93% respectively. Others (Table 60.3) have reported lower survivals; techniques for calculation of survival have varied. Although many reports do not stratify patients by stage, those that do, agree that it is an important prognostic factor. Evans[15] found an overall rate of recurrence of 19%, as compared to 9% in Stage Ia tumors. This is particularly significant since, in their series, 20 of 22 patients with recurrence died of tumor. Stenwig[52] & Pankratz[42] also reported a greater survival in Stage I as compared to more advanced stages. Some authors have considered the size of the tumor to be of prognostic import.[39,52] This is certainly due in part to the fact that larger tumors are more likely to have occult metastases that are missed at incomplete surgical staging. Whether tumor size would retain its prognostic significance in thoroughly staged patients is un-

Table 60.3 Survival of patients with granulosa cell tumors

Author	No. of cases	Survival
Norris[39]	97	97% 5-yr; 93% 10-yr
Evans[15]	118	88% 5-yr; 82% 10-yr
Stenwig[52]	118	80% 5-yr; (91.8% Stage I)
Pankratz[42]	61	61% 5-yr; 56% 10-yr (75% Stage I, 5 and 10-yr)

known. The propensity of granulosa cell tumors for indolent growth and late recurrence should be borne in mind. The specific sites of recurrence are not well documented in most series, but 15 of 22 recurrences in Evans' report[15] were apparently within the peritoneal cavity, three were in the lungs, and one involved the liver.

Juvenile granulosa cell tumors

Scully's group[68] has described a variant of granulosa cell tumor that tends to occur in younger women and has distinct histopathologic features, including hyperchromatic granulosa cells with round nuclei, a generally high mitotic rate, and prominent luteinization. About 90% of granulosa tumors occurring in prepubertal girls, and many of those seen in patients under 30 years of age are of this juvenile granulosa cell tumor (JGCT) type. In Scully's series of 125 cases, the clinical features seem similar to those of the adult granulosa tumors. Only 3 cases were bilateral, and only 3 were diagnosed beyond Stage I. With an average of 5 years follow up for 95 patients, 92% were alive and free of disease. Thus, the outlook for these tumors is quite good despite their worrisome histologic appearance. There is no information to suggest that they should be managed any differently from adult granulosa cell tumors. (See also p. 950.)

Theca cell tumors

Epidemiology and clinical features

Theca cell tumors of the ovary are best regarded as benign stromal neoplasms. They generally occur in women in the early postmenopausal years. Many reports have included these tumors among granulosa and granulosa-theca tumors, although there is no clinical justification for doing so. In Bjorkholm's series,[4] which does not mix theca and granulosa tumors, the thecomas occurred at a mean age of 59 years, with an age range of 19 to 81 years. In this report, 62 cases were considered after review to represent theca cell tumors. Only 39 of these cases were originally diag-

nosed as thecomas; 17 had previously been called granulosa-theca tumors, and six had been considered fibromas. As with other stromal tumors, hormonal production is common, with associated abnormal uterine bleeding in approximately 60% of patients (Table 60.4). The reported incidence of concomitant endometrial hyperplasia varies from 25% to above 50%, while from 4.5% to 27% of patients were found to have a concomitant adenocarcinoma of the endometrium.

Thecomas of the ovary are usually of moderate size. In Norris' series,[39] mean tumor diameter was 8.1 cm; in Bjorkholm's report,[4] mean size was 7 cm, with a range of less than 1 to 20 cm. Bilateral involvement occurs in less than 4% of cases (Table 60.5). A number of authors have reported cases of so-called 'malignant thecoma'. In their 1979 review, Waxman et al[62] have analyzed these cases and considered them to be inadequately documented. Most were felt to represent either 'sarcomatoid' granulosa cell tumors, stromal sarcomas, or fibrosarcomas. The authors further state that 'if a thecoma ever becomes malignant, the tumor cells de-differentiate so that they cannot be recognized any longer as thecal cells; instead, they proliferate as a *stromal sarcoma* or *fibrosarcoma*', and propose that the term 'malignant thecoma' not be used. If malignant ovarian tumors derived from thecal cells do exist, they are certainly extremely rare.

Table 60.5 Frequency of bilateral ovarian thecomas

Author	Total cases	No. bilateral
Norris[39]	106	3
Stage[51]	22	1
Antolic[3]	46	4
Bjorkholm[4]	62	2
Evans[15]	81	0
Total	317	10 (3.1%)

Management and outcome

Ovarian thecomas can be managed as any other benign solid tumor of the ovary. Oophorectomy in younger women should be curative. The endometrium must be evaluated, with the disposition of the uterus dependent on the histologic findings and individual patient considerations. If the opposite ovary is to be conserved, it should be carefully inspected for evidence of bilateral involvement.

Sclerosing stromal tumors

Sclerosing stromal tumors are uniformly benign tumors that occur most often in the first three decades of life.[43]

Table 60.4 Abnormal bleeding and endometrial histology in patients with ovarian thecoma

Author	Total	Abnormal bleeding (%)	Endometrium	
			Hyperplasia (%)	Cancer (%)
Norris[39]	106	61	46	7.7
Stage[51]	22	50	64	4.5
Antolic[3]	46	—	25	22
Bjorkholm[4]	62	60	—	21
Evans[15]	81	—	37	27

Tang & Liu[55] reported 10 cases with both menstrual irregularities and infertility and postulated that these tumors may be hormonally active. Gee & Russell[17] also reported indirect evidence of hormonal activity. These tumors should be managed by unilateral salpingo-oophorectomy in young patients and by hysterectomy and bilateral salpingo-oophorectomy in older patients not desiring to preserve fertility.

SERTOLI AND LEYDIG CELL TUMORS

Sertoli-Leydig cell tumors were described by Meyer in 1930 and 1931 as arrhenoblastomas or androblastomas.[34 to 36] The term arrhenoblastoma should not be used as it implies virilization and, while some of these tumors do produce defeminization or virilization, this is by no means true for all tumors of this type. These sex-cord stromal tumors arise from cells exhibiting a testicular differentiation and may imperfectly recapitulate stages in the development of the testis.[50,65] Kurman et al[29] analyzed Sertoli-Leydig tumors for testosterone, estradiol and progesterone by an indirect immunoperoxidase method, and found both testosterone and estradiol in Sertoli cells, Leydig cells and in primitive spindle cells resembling those of the embryonic gonad; they suggested that the latter cell was the precursor for both Sertoli and Leydig cells.

Sertoli-Leydig cell tumors represent 0.2 to 0.5% of ovarian neoplasms.[46,50,57] In an analysis of malignant ovarian tumors in girls under age 15 in the United Kingdom, LaVecchia et al[30] reported nine stromal tumors among 172 cases. Only three of these nine stromal tumors were clearly Sertoli-Leydig tumors. Most occur in young women. Scully[50] has stated that the average age is 28 years, with 5% being seen in prepubertal girls and 10% in women over age 45 years. Bilaterality is reported to occur in only 1 to 3% of cases. Sertoli-Leydig cell tumors can be found as pure Sertoli cell tumors, pure Leydig cell tumors or, most commonly, as mixtures of both cell types. These latter tumors, the Sertoli-Leydig cell group, account for most of those cases in which the tumor behaves in a malignant fashion.

Pure Sertoli cell tumors

Sertoli cell tumors are neoplasms of the gonadal stroma which are composed of Sertoli cells and lack any Leydig cell element. They may demonstrate a variety of histologic appearances depending on the complexity of tubular differentiation, amount of intracellular lipid and extent of hyalinization[57] (see also p. 951). Tavassoli & Norris[57] reported isosexual precocious puberty in three prepubertal females, and in nine other cases there was evidence of estrogenic activity (menometrorrhagia, postmenopausal bleeding and endometrial hyperplasia). However, five of their patients did show virilization or defeminization. In all, 17 of 28 patients reported by these authors had evidence of hormonal activity by the tumor, and 12 of these appeared to produce estrogen. Young & Scully[64] reported that four of 10 pure Sertoli tumors exhibited estrogenic stimulation. Two prepubertal girls showed isosexual precocity and two postmenopausal women had estrogenic stimulation of the endometrium. Korzets et al[28] reported a single case of a 17-year-old girl with a pure Sertoli cell tumor that produced renin. The patient experienced both hypertension and hypokalemia which returned to normal after removal of the tumor.

Although Sertoli cell tumors can be seen at any age, most occur between 15 and 50 years. Tavassoli & Norris[57] reported a median age of 33 years. The tumors in their series were unilateral, more often solid, and ranged in size from 2.5 to 28 cm with a median of 7 cm. In the series reported by Young & Scully,[64] tumors ranged in size from 0.8 to 17 cm in diameter. The usual clinical behavior of Sertoli cell tumors is benign, although Tavassoli & Norris[57] reported recurrence in two of 28 Stage Ia patients, and Young & Scully reported that one of 10 patients in their series had a tumor which behaved in a malignant fashion. Treatment should consist of total abdominal hysterectomy and bilateral salpingo-oohorectomy in the older patient, but Stage Ia tumors in children and in women who desire further childbearing should be managed by unilateral salpingo-oophorectomy. It seems logical to recommend a thorough staging evaluation of the abdomen in all patients, but there are too few cases reported to prove definite benefit from such a procedure. There are too few cases with metastases to dictate therapy for recurrent disease; however, it seems reasonable to utilize the same regimens suggested for Sertoli-Leydig cell tumors.

Pure Leydig cell tumors (hilus cell tumors)

The Leydig cell tumor is composed completely of Leydig cells. Scully[50] states that these cells arise from three areas in the ovary: 1) directly from hilus cells, 2) from the ovarian stroma or 3) as one-sided development of a Sertoli-Leydig cell tumor. The distinguishing histopathologic feature in these tumors are crystals of Reinke, which are found in the cytoplasm of the cells.[43] Scully[50] limits the diagnosis of these tumors to those in which the crystals can be identified with certainty. Although the pure Leydig cell tumor is included herein as a form of androblastoma, others (such as Fox & Buckley in the preceding chapter) have classified them as a type of lipid cell tumor.

The majority of Leydig cell tumors produce virilization, although estrogenic activity has been reported. Occasional tumors appear to be hormonally inactive[6,27,61] (see also Ch. 8). Zhang et al[70] reported four cases, of which one showed virilization, two exhibited estrogenic activity and one was not associated with any endocrinologic activity. Manifestations of other endocrinologic abnormalities, such as hypertension, diabetes and Cushing's syndrome, have been reported.[50]

Leydig cell tumors are most often seen in peri-menopausal and postmenopausal women. Of four cases reported by Zhang et al,[70] the average age was 61 years. Occasionally, these tumors are seen in young women or children.[50] The tumors are usually small, and Casthely et al[9] have reported hormonal activity in a very small tumor.

These tumors rarely behave in a malignant fashion, although metastases have been reported.[14,53] Since most tumors occur in older women, total abdominal hysterectomy and bilateral salpingo-oophorectomy is the usual therapy. In those rare cases which occur in younger females, unilateral salpingo-oophorectomy is adequate treatment.

Sertoli-Leydig cell tumors

Epidemiology and clinical features

Stromal tumors which contain both Sertoli cells and Leydig cells are by far the most common of the Sertoli-Leydig cell group. Not only are these tumors the most numerous, they also account for the majority of those tumors which metastasize and thus behave as malignant tumors. Most authors have divided these tumors into three groups based on their histologic characteristics: well differentiated tumors, tumors of intermediate differentiation and poorly differentiated tumors.[46,50,65,69] The usefulness of this classification is borne out by a rather marked difference in the clinical behavior of these subtypes, although the difference is more marked between the well differentiated variety and the other two types. Many authors have also grouped separately those Sertoli-Leydig cell tumors that are associated with heterologous elements, such as cartilage, skeletal muscle, carcinoid and gastrointestinal epithelium[7,44,66] (see also p. 953).

The mean age of patients with Sertoli-Leydig cell tumors is 25 years, with a range of 2 to 84 years. Patients with well differentiated tumors tend to be somewhat older, with a mean age of 36 years. Table 60.6 shows the age distribution and weighted mean from three large reviews.[46,65,69]

Table 60.6 Age at diagnosis of Sertoli-Leydig cell tumors of the ovary

Sertoli-Leydig cell tumors	Age Mean (yr)	Range (yr)
Well differentiated		
Young & Scully[65]	34.5	18 to 61
Roth et al[46]	41.0	
Weighted mean	36	
Intermediate differentiation		
Young & Scully[65]	25	2 to 75
Zaloudek & Norris[69]	24	3 to 74
Roth et al[46]	23	20 to 79
Weighted mean	25	
Poor differentiation		
Young & Scully[65]	25	4 to 61
Zaloudek & Norris[69]	24	3 to 74
Roth et al[46]	19	9 to 84
Weighted mean	24	

Presenting symptoms include evidence of androgen excess, abdominal pain, pelvic or abdominal mass and menstrual disturbances. A small number of patients present with an acute abdomen due to torsion of the adnexa or rupture of the mass. Menstrual disturbances are one of the most frequent symptoms (Table 60.7). Amenorrhea and oligomenorrhea account for 51% of the menstrual disorders reported.

Clinical evidence of defeminization or masculinization is reported to be present in 25 to 77% of patients[46,69] (see also Ch. 8). Evidence of some hormonal activity as manifested by either clinical virilization or menstrual disturbances is found in over 75% of patients in most series. Virilization is seen less frequently in well differentiated tumors.[14] In those patients in whom endocrine studies have been obtained, elevated testosterone levels, decreased estrogen levels and elevated urinary 17-ketosteroids have been reported. Haruyama et al[24] studied a patient with clinical virilization and an ovarian Sertoli-Leydig cell tumor by selective ovarian vein catheterization, and found levels of testosterone of 40.5 ng/ml on the side with the tumor and 7.1 ng/ml on the normal side. Brumsted et al[7] reported that they were able to inhibit testosterone production by giving a patient with a Sertoli-Leydig cell tumor an oral contraceptive.

Unfortunately, no definite pattern of endocrine abnormalities occurs, and patients with clinical virilization often

Table 60.7 Menstrual disturbances in patients with Sertoli-Leydig cell tumors

Author	Total patients	No. with menstrual disturbance			
		Amenorrhea	Oligomenorrhea	Menometrorrhagia	Postmenopausal bleeding
Zaloudek & Norris[69]	64	10	3	6	4
Roth et al[46]	34	13	2	3	4
Total cases (%)	98	23 (24)	5 (5)	9 (9)	8 (8)

have normal endocrine studies.[46,50,65,69] Kurman et al[29] utilized immunohistological stains and found considerable variation in the staining of cells for testosterone, estradiol and progesterone, even though all the patients whose tumors were studied had clinical evidence of virilization. Recently, several authors[11,32,59] have reported elevated alphafetoprotein (AFP) levels in patients with Sertoli-Leydig cell tumors. Omar & Tabbakh[41] reported elevated levels of immunoreactive beta endorphin in the Leydig cells of patients with Sertoli-Leydig cell tumors.

The size of the tumors found at the time of surgical exploration varies from microscopic foci to over 50 cm. The average size is larger in tumors of intermediate and poor differentiation. Table 60.8 summarizes the size of tumors found in three large series from the literature.[46,65,69] Sertoli-Leydig cell tumors can be mostly solid, or mixed solid and cystic. Roth et al[46] found that the larger tumors were more likely to be partially cystic. Young & Scully[65] reported that tumors of intermediate and poor differentiation were more likely to be partially cystic than well differentiated tumors (67 of 116 intermediate and poorly differentiated tumors were partially cystic versus three of 23 well differentiated tumors).

Table 60.8 Size of Sertoli-Leydig cell tumors found at surgical exploration

Author	Size	
	Range (cm)	Mean (cm)
Roth et al[46]	—	
Well differentiated		6
Intermediate differentiation	Microscopic to 22	7.5
Poor differentiation	—	13.5
Young & Scully[65]		
Well differentiated	1.5 to 10	5.3
Intermediate differentiation	Microscopic to 35	12.5
Poor differentiation	7 to 51	17.5
Zaloudek & Norris[69]		
Intermediate and poor differentiation	3 to 30	14.5

The distribution of cases by stage of disease at the time of diagnosis is shown in Table 60.9. Young & Scully[65] reported that when spread beyond the ovary was found, it was always in patients with tumors of intermediate or poor differentiation. Neither Zaloudek & Norris[69] nor Roth et al[46] found bilateral tumors in their patients. Young & Scully[65] reported bilaterality in 1.5% of their patients. Rupture of the tumors is infrequent, but more likely to occur in larger tumors of intermediate and poor differentiation.

Table 60.9 Stage of disease at the time of diagnosis of Sertoli-Leydig cell tumors

Author	% in each stage		
	I	II	III
Young & Scully[65]	97.5	1.5	1
Roth et al[46]	100*	—	—
Zaloudek & Norris[69]	97	—	3

* Two of 34 tumors had the omentum adherent to the ovary containing the tumor

Management

Treatment of Sertoli-Leydig cell tumors in older women in whom child-bearing is complete is total abdominal hysterectomy, bilateral salpingo-oophorectomy and appropriate staging procedures for ovarian carcinoma. In younger women, unilateral salpingo-oophorectomy and a proper staging evaluation of the entire abdomen is sufficient for Stage Ia neoplasms. More advanced stage disease requires total abdominal hysterectomy and bilateral salpingo-oophorectomy. Recurrence in patients with Stage I neoplasms is unusual. Zaloudek & Norris[69] reported recurrence in three of 62 (5%) patients with Stage I disease of intermediate or poor differentiation. Young & Scully[65] reported recurrence in 20 of 138 (7%) patients with Stage I tumors of intermediate or poor differentiation. None of the 23 well differentiated tumors recurred. Roth et al[46] reported no recurrences in patients with well differentiated tumors and only one of 26 (3%) intermediate and poorly differentiated tumors.

Because of the rarity of these tumors and the infrequent finding of advanced or recurrent disease, there is little experience with chemotherapy or radiation therapy. Isolated reports have indicated that these tumors may respond to radiation therapy or combination chemotherapy, but response rates are low. Roth et al[46] reported one patient with recurrent intra-abdominal disease that failed to respond to chlorambucil, but had a partial response to triosulfan. Zaloudek & Norris[69] reported failure of therapy with thiotepa and 5-fluorouracil in one patient with recurrent disease, but a complete response to vincristine, actinomycin-D and cyclophosphamide (VAC). They also reported two long-term survivors after treatment of persistent or recurrent disease with VAC chemotherapy plus pelvic irradiation. Gershenson et al[18] reported one partial response and one complete response to a regimen of cisplatin, adriamycin and cyclophosphamide (PAC). The complete response occurred in a heavily pretreated patient. Young & Scully[65] reported responses in five of 13 patients using various combinations of radiation and chemotherapy. They reported definite responses to vincristine, actinomycin-D and cyclophosphamide, a combination of methotrexate, cyclophosphamide and cisplatin, as well as actinomycin, cisplatin, vinblastine and bleomycin. Pride et al[45] have reported a complete response in a patient with metastatic Sertoli-Leydig cell tumor with a combination of bleomycin, vincristine, cyclophosphamide, cisplatin and doxorubicin.

Although it is not possible from the above isolated cases to draw definitive conclusions, it is apparent that Sertoli-Leydig tumors may respond to chemotherapy regimens that utilize cisplatin, cyclophosphamide, adriamycin, actinomycin, vinblastine or bleomycin in various combinations. It also appears clear that radiation therapy may be beneficial in patients with small residual disease. There appears to be no place for single alkylating agent therapy. In the absence of definitive evidence of activity of any single regimen in advanced disease, it is not possible to suggest a regimen to be employed for adjuvant therapy, nor is it possible to clearly define a population of patients that might benefit from such therapy.

Sertoli-Leydig cell tumors with a retiform pattern

The variant of the Sertoli-Leydig cell tumor showing a retiform pattern has been reported by Young & Scully,[63] Roth et al,[47] and others.[54,60] Most of these tumors are of intermediate and poor differentiation and should be managed as such. They appear to be important only because they are often mistaken for other ovarian tumors, such as endodermal sinus tumor, ovarian sarcoma and epithelial carcinoma.[47,54]

Sertoli-Leydig cell tumors with heterologous elements

Several authors[44,46,65,66,69] have singled out Sertoli-Leydig cell tumors that contain heterologous elements for special consideration. Gastrointestinal epithelium and carcinoids are the most frequently reported heterologous elements. Tumors with these elements are not more likely to recur or behave in a malignant fashion than non-heterologous tumors of similar differentiation.[66,69] On the other hand, those tumors with heterologous elements of mesenchymal origin, such as skeletal muscle and cartilage, do appear more likely to behave in a malignant fashion. Prat et al[44] reported that eight of 12 cases of Sertoli-Leydig cell tumors with mesenchymal elements (skeletal muscle, nine cases; cartilage, seven cases; neuroblastoma, one case) died of their tumors from 5 months to 7 years after initial diagnosis. Zaloudek & Norris[69] reported metastases in one of two patients with rhabdomyosarcoma. There does not appear to be any difference in the frequency with which tumors containing heterologous elements are hormonally active.

GYNANDROBLASTOMA

The gynandroblastoma is an extremely rare ovarian tumor that contains both female type (granulosa cell) and male type (Sertoli or Leydig cell) tumor elements[43,50] (see also Ch. 8). Scully[50] states that these tumors are of more theoretical than practical interest because of their rarity. Chalvardjian & Derzko[10] have performed electronmicroscopy on one of these tumors, and pointed out the striking similarity of the various sex-cord elements of the tumor on an ultrastructural level. Tavassoli[56] reported a gynandroblastoma that contained epithelial elements as well as granulosa cell and Sertoli cell elements. These tumors behave in a benign fashion and should be treated by unilateral salpingo-oophorectomy in young patients.

SEX CORD TUMORS WITH ANNULAR TUBULES

Sex cord tumors with annular tubules (SCTAT) were described by Scully[49] and have also been called Scully's tumor. They comprise about 10% of all sex-cord stromal tumors and have been reported to be estrogenic, androgenic or endocrinologically inactive.[50] One-third of these tumors are associated with the Peutz-Jegher's syndrome and two-thirds are bilateral.[43] When not associated with the Peutz-Jegher's syndrome, these tumors are usually poorly differentiated and are more likely to behave in a malignant fashion than either granulosa cell or Sertoli-Leydig cell tumors. Young et al[67] found 27 tumors of this type associated with the Peutz-Jegher's syndrome to be typically multifocal, bilateral and very small (the largest tumor was 3 cm). All were benign. On the other hand, they found that 47 tumors not associated with the Peutz-Jegher's syndrome were unilateral and large (28 of 47 were greater than 5 cm in diameter and one was 20 cm in diameter). Seven of the 47 tumors not associated with the Peutz-Jegher's syndrome were malignant (four of them fatal). The mean age of the patients reported by Young et al[67] was 27 years for those with the Peutz-Jegher's syndrome, and 34 years for those without the syndrome. Hart et al[23] reported six patients with sex-cord tumors with annular tubules, none of which were associated with the Peutz-Jegher's syndrome. The mean age of these patients was 34 years and the mean size of the tumor was 10 cm. Two of the six patients had metastatic disease.

Based on the limited numbers of cases reported in the literature to date, it would appear that bilateral salpingo-oophorectomy and hysterectomy is the treatment of choice for this tumor in the older woman who does not desire further childbearing, whether or not the tumor is associated with the Peutz-Jegher's syndrome. In younger women in whom future fertility is important, those tumors associated with the Peutz-Jegher's syndrome will usually be benign and conservatism is justified. In those not associated with the Peutz-Jegher's syndrome, unilateral salpingo-oophorectomy and an ovarian staging operation are indicated if the tumor is confined to one ovary (Stage Ia). It is important to note that both of the patients in the report by Hart et al[23] with metastatic disease had lymph node metastases. Thus, a full staging operation including nodal biopsies appears to be important in this sex-cord stromal tumor variant.

LIPID (LIPOID) CELL TUMORS

Although lipid cell tumors are listed as a separate type of ovarian tumor, they are discussed under the section of sex-cord stromal tumors for convenience. The exact origin of the tumor is unknown, but Scully[50] states that there is no strong evidence to suggest an adrenal rest origin. He feels that they probably develop from hilus cells or Leydig cells and thus ultimately from ovarian stromal cells.

These tumors may be hormonally active and usually produce virilization. Occasionally, they may be estrogenic or endocrinologically inactive. Taylor & Norris[58] reported 30 cases in which none were bilateral. As many as 20% of these tumors may exhibit clinical behavior that is malignant, with either metastases or recurrence.[50]

Treatment should be unilateral salpingo-oophorectomy in the young patient with the tumor confined to one ovary, as these tumors are essentially always unilateral. In older women not desiring to preserve fertility, hysterectomy and bilateral salpingo-oophorectomy is indicated. Too few cases exist to have good information as to the role of chemotherapy or radiation.

CONCLUSION

Because stromal tumors of the ovary occur infrequently, there are few collected series in the literature large enough to provide a clear picture of their clinical behavior. In addition, since most of these tumors are diagnosed in early stages and do not recur or metastasize, even less is known about their response to therapy. Thus, whenever possible, patients with these tumors should be entered into prospective clinical trials so that we may not only document their natural history, but also establish optimal methods of therapy for those few patients who develop recurrent or metastatic disease.

Based on what little information can be gleaned from the literature at present, the following statements can be made:

1. stromal tumors are often hormonally active
2. bilaterality is consistently found in less than 5% of cases
3. when these tumors are confined to one ovary in young women, unilateral salpingo-oophorectomy with complete surgical staging is the treatment of choice
4. for women in whom childbearing is complete, total abdominal hysterectomy, bilateral salpingo-oophorectomy and complete surgical staging should be carried out
5. recurrent or metastatic disease should be treated with multi-drug chemotherapy utilizing a combination of vincristine, actinomycin-D and cyclophosphamide, or cisplatin, bleomycin plus vinblastine or etoposide
6. radiation therapy may be effective, providing the disease is localized or there is microscopic residual disease.

REFERENCES

1. Anderson W R, Levine H J, MacMillan D 1971 Granulosa-theca cell tumors: clinical and pathological study. Am J Obstet Gynecol 110: 32
2. Anikwue C, Dawood Y, Kramer E 1978 Granulosa and theca cell tumors. Obstet Gynecol 51: 214
3. Antolic Z N, Kovacic J, Rainier S 1980 Theca and granulosa cell tumors and endometrial adenocarcinoma. Gynecol Oncol 10: 273
4. Bjorkholm E, Silfversward C 1980 Theca-cell tumors. Acta Radiol 19: 241
5. Bjorkholm E, Silfversward C 1981 Prognostic factors in granulosa-cell tumors. Gynecol Oncol 11: 261
6. Bonaventura L M, Judd H, Roth L M, Cleary R E 1978 Androgen, estrogen and progesterone production by a lipid cell tumor of the ovary. Am J Obstet Gynecol 131: 403
7. Brumsted J R, Chapitis J, Riddick D, Gibson M 1987 Norethindrone inhibition of testosterone secretion by an ovarian Sertoli-Leydig cell tumor. J Clin Endocrinol Metab 65: 194
8. Camlibel F, Caputo T A 1983 Chemotherapy of granulosa cell tumors. Am J Obstet Gynecol 145: 763
9. Casthely S, Diamandis H P, Pierre-Louis R 1977 Hilar cell tumor of the ovary: Diagnostic value of plasma testosterone by selective ovarian vein catheterization. Am J Obstet Gynecol 129: 108
10. Chalvardjian A, Derzko C 1982 Gynandroblastoma. Its ultrastructure. Cancer 50: 710
11. Chumas J C, Rosenwaks Z, Mann W J, Finkel G, Pastore J 1984 Sertoli-Leydig cell tumor of the ovary producing alpha-fetoprotein. Int J Gynecol Pathol 3: 213
12. Colombo N, Sessa C, Landoni F, Sartori E, Pecorelli S, Mangioni C 1986 Cisplatin, vinblastine, and bleomycin combination chemotherapy in metastatic granulosa cell tumor of the ovary. Obstet Gynecol 67: 265
13. Davy M, Torjesen P A, Aakvaag A 1977 Demonstration of an FSH receptor in a functioning granulosa cell tumor. Acta Endocrinol 85: 615
14. Echt C R, Hadd H E 1968 Androgen excretion patterns in a patient with metastatic hilus cell tumor of the ovary. Am J Obstet Gynecol 100: 1055
15. Evans A T, Gaffey T A, Malkasian G D, Annegers J F 1980 Clinicopathologic review of 118 granulosa and 82 theca cell tumors. Obstet Gynecol 55: 231
16. Fox H, Agrawal M B, Langley F A 1975 A clinicopathologic study of 92 cases of granulosa cell tumor of the ovary with special reference to the factors influencing prognosis. Cancer 35: 231
17. Gee D C, Russell P 1979 Sclerosing stromal tumors of the ovary. Histopathology 3: 367
18. Gershenson D M, Copeland L J, Kavanagh J J, Stringer C A, Saul P B, Wharton J T 1987 Treatment of metastatic stromal tumors of the ovary with cisplatin, doxorubicin and cyclophosphamide. Obstet Gynecol 70: 765
19. Givens J R, Anderson R N, Wiser W L, Donelson A J, Coleman

S A 1975 A testosterone-secreting, gonadotrophin-sensitive pure thecoma and polycystic ovarian disease. J Clin Endocrinol Metab 41: 845

20. Goldston W R, Johnston W W, Fetter B F, Parker R T, Wilbanks G D 1972 Clinicopathologic studies in feminizing tumors of the ovary. Am J Obstet Gynecol 112: 422

21. Graves P E, Surwit E A, Davis J R, Stouffer R L 1985 Adenylate cyclase in human ovarian cancers: sensitivity to gonadotrophins and nonhormonal activators. Am J Obstet Gynecol 153: 877

22. Gusberg S B, Kardon P 1971 Proliferative endometrial response to theca-granulosa cell tumors. Am J Obstet Gynecol 111: 633

23. Hart W R, Kumas N, Crissman J D 1980 Ovarian neoplasms resembling sex cord tumors with annular tubules. Cancer 45: 2352

24. Haruyama Y, Miyakawa I, Inoue H, Mori N C 1987 Endocrinological study of Sertoli-Leydig cell tumors. Nippon Sanka Fujinka Gakkai Zasshi 39: 765

25. Ishiwata I, Ishiwata C, Soma M, Kobayashi N, Ishikawa H 1984 Establishment and characterization of an estrogen-producing human ovarian granulosa tumor cell line. JNCI 72: 789

26. Jacobs H J, Deppe G, Cohen C J 1982 Combination chemotherapy of ovarian granulosa cell tumor with cis-platinum and doxorubicin. Gynecol Oncol 14: 294

27. Jeffcoate S L, Prunty F T G 1968 Steroid synthesis in vitro by a hilar cell tumor. Am J Obstet Gynecol 101: 684

28. Korzets A, Nouriel H, Steiner Z et al 1986 Resistant hypertension associated with a renin-producing ovarian Sertoli cell tumor. Am J Clin Pathol 85: 242

29. Kurman R J, Andrade D, Goebelsmann U, Taylor C R 1978 An immunohistological study of steroid localization in Sertoli Leydig tumors of the ovary and testis. Cancer 42: 1772

30. LaVecchia C, Morris H B, Draper G J 1983 Malignant ovarian tumors in childhood in Britain, 1962–78. Br J Cancer 48: 363

31. Malkasian G D, Webb M J, Jorgensen E O 1974 Observations on chemotherapy of granulosa cell carcinomas and malignant ovarian teratomas. Obstet Gynecol 44: 885

32. Mann W J, Chumas J, Rosenwaks Z, Merrill J A, Davenport D 1986 Elevated serum alpha-fetoprotein associated with Sertoli-Leydig cell tumors of the ovary. Obstet Gynecol 67: 141

33. Marsh J M, Savard K, Baggett B 1962 Estrogen synthesis in a feminizing ovarian granulosa tumor. J Clin Endocrinol Metab 22: 1196

34. Meyer R 1930 Tubulare testiculare und solide formen des andreiblastoma ovarii und ihre Beziehnug zur Vermannlichung. Beitr Pathol Anat 84: 485

35. Meyer R 1930 Zur pathologie der zur vermannlichung fuhrenden tumoren des ovarien (arrhenoblastoma ovarii). Vehr Dtsch Ges Pathol 25: 328

36. Meyer R 1931 Pathology of some special ovarian tumors and their relation to sex characteristics. Am J Obstet Gynecol 22: 697

37. Nakashima N, Young R H, Scully R E 1984 Androgenic granulosa cell tumors of the ovary. Arch Pathol Lab Med 108: 786

38. Neville A J, Gilchrist K W, Davis T E 1984 The chemotherapy of granulosa cell tumors of the ovary: experience of the Wisconsin Clinical Cancer Center. Med Ped Oncol 12: 397

39. Norris H J, Taylor H B 1968 Prognosis of granulosa-theca tumors of the ovary. Cancer 21: 255

40. Novak E R, Kutchmeshgi J, Mupas R S, Woodruff J D 1971 Feminizing gonadal stromal tumors. Obstet Gynecol 38: 701

41. Omar R A, Tabbakh G H 1987 Immunoreactive beta endorphin in ovarian sex cord stromal tumors. Arch Pathol Lab Med 111: 436

42. Pankratz E, Boyes D A, White G W, Galliford B W, Fairey R N, Benedet J L 1978 Granulosa cell tumors. Obstet Gynecol 52: 718

43. Piver M S 1986 Non-epithelial tumors. In: Blackledge G, Chan K K (eds) Management of Ovarian Cancer. Butterworths, London, p 143

44. Prat J, Young R H, Scully R E 1982 Ovarian Sertoli-Leydig cell tumors with heterologous elements. II. Cartilage and skeletal muscle: a clinicopathologic analysis of twelve cases. Cancer 50: 2465

45. Pride G L, Pollock W J, Norgard M J 1982 Metastatic Sertoli-Leydig cell tumor of the ovary during pregnancy treated by BV-CAP chemotherapy. Am J Obstet Gynecol 143: 231

46. Roth L M, Anderson M C, Govan A D T, Langley F A, Gowing N F C, Woodcock A S 1981 Sertoli-Leydig cell tumors: a clinicopathologic study of 34 cases. Cancer 48: 187

47. Roth L M, Slayton R E, Brady L W, Blessing J A, Johnson G 1985 Retiform differentiation in ovarian Sertoli-Leydig cell tumors: a clinicopathologic study of six cases from a Gynecologic Oncology Group study. Cancer 55: 1093

48. Schwartz P E, Smith J P 1976 Treatment of ovarian stromal tumors. Am J Obstet Gynecol 125: 402

49. Scully R E 1970 Sex cord tumor with annular tubules: a distinctive ovarian tumor of the Peutz-Jeghers syndrome. Cancer 25: 1107

50. Scully R E 1979 Tumors of the ovary and maldeveloped gonads. In: Atlas of Tumor Pathology, Second series, Fascicle 16. Armed Forces Institute of Pathology, Bethesda, p 190

51. Stage A H, Grafton W D 1977 Thecomas and granulosa-theca cell tumors of the ovary. Obstet Gynecol 50: 21

52. Stenwig J T, Hazekamp J T, Beecham J B 1979 Granulosa cell tumors of the ovary. Gynecol Oncol 7: 136

53. Stewart R S, Woodward D E 1962 Malignant ovarian hilus cell tumor. Arch Pathol 73: 91

54. Talesman A 1987 Ovarian Sertoli-Leydig cell tumor (androblastoma) with retiform pattern: a clinicopathologic study. Cancer 60: 3056

55. Tang M Y, Liu T H 1982 Ovarian sclerosing stromal tumors: clinicopathologic study of 10 cases. Clin Med J 95: 186

56. Tavassoli F A 1983 A combined germ cell-gonadal stromal-epithelial tumor of the ovary. Am J Surg Pathol 7: 73

57. Tavassoli F A, Norris H J 1980 Sertoli tumors of the ovary: a clinicopathologic study of 28 cases with ultrastructural observations. Cancer 46: 2281

58. Taylor H B, Norris H J 1967 Lipid tumors of the ovary. Cancer 29: 1953

59. Tiltman A, Dehaeck K, Soeters R, Goldberg G, Levin W 1986 Ovarian Sertoli-Leydig cell tumor with a raised serum alpha-fetoprotein. A case report. Virchows Arch 410: 107

60. Tokuoka S, Aoki Y, Hayashi Y et al 1985 A mixed germ cell-sex cord stromal tumor of the ovary with retiform tubular structure: a case report. Int J Gynecol Pathol 4: 161

61. Wagner V P, Smale L E 1973 Androgen and estrogen production by a lipid ovarian tumor. Obstet Gynecol 42: 903

62. Waxman M, Vuletin J C, Urcuyo R, Belling C G 1979 Ovarian low grade stromal sarcoma with thecomatous features. Cancer 44: 2206

63. Young R H, Scully R E 1983 Ovarian Sertoli-Leydig cell tumors with a retiform pattern. A problem in histopathologic diagnosis: a report of 25 cases. Am J Surg Pathol 7: 755

64. Young R H, Scully R E 1984 Ovarian Sertoli cell tumors: a report of 10 cases. Int J Gynecol Pathol 2: 349

65. Young R H, Scully R E 1985 Ovarian Sertoli-Leydig cell tumors: a clinicopathological analysis of 207 cases. Am J Surg Pathol 9: 543

66. Young R H, Prat J, Scully R E 1982 Ovarian Sertoli-Leydig cell tumors with heterologous elements. I. Gastrointestinal epithelium and carcinoid: a clinicopathologic analysis of thirty six cases. Cancer 50: 2448

67. Young R H, Welch W R, Dickersin G R, Scully R E 1982 Ovarian sex cord tumor with annular tubules: review of 74 cases including 27 with Peutz-Jeghers syndrome and four with adenoma malignum of the cervix. Cancer 50: 1384

68. Young R H, Dickersin G R, Scully R E 1984 Juvenile granulosa cell tumor of the ovary. Am J Surg Pathol 8: 575

69. Zaloudek C, Norris H J 1984 Sertoli-Leydig tumors of the ovary: a clinicopathologic study of 64 intermediate and poorly differentiated neoplasms. Am J Surg Pathol 8: 409

70. Zhang J, Young R H, Arseneau J, Scully R E 1982 Ovarian stromal tumors containing lutein or Leydig (luteinized thecomas and stromal Leydig cell tumors): a clinicopathological analysis of fifty cases. Int J Gynecol Pathol 1: 270

61. Malignant müllerian and miscellaneous mesenchymal tumors of ovary ('ovarian sarcomas')

P. Russell   P. Bannatyne   H. J. Solomon

INTRODUCTION

Ovarian mesenchymal neoplasms are uncommon and of diverse origin. Tumors of fibrous tissue are considered part of the spectrum of fibrothecomas and, as such, to be of specific gonadal stromal origin. Smooth muscle tumors, based on their homology with tumors occurring more commonly in the uterus, are included in the group of müllerian mesenchymal tumors. Remaining mesenchymal tumors are considered to arise directly from those elements of the ovary not committed to its specific gonadal function, such as connective tissue, vessels, nerves and lymphoid cells.[25,73] Other histogenetic possibilities include monophyletic teratomatous origin (as proposed for struma ovarii and ovarian carcinoids), secondary malignant transformation in benign or mature cystic teratomas[13,25,28,53,55,79,88] or overwhelming predominance of sarcomatous components in mixed müllerian tumors, Sertoli-Leydig cell tumors[25,60,83] or even granulosa cell tumors.[82]

Specific müllerian mesenchymal lesions are characterized by neoplastic stromal or mesenchymal cells exhibiting varying degrees of proliferation and malignant potential as well as many patterns of mesenchymal differentiation. Many, additionally, contain neoplastic epithelial elements which may be benign or malignant. All have more frequently observed homologues elsewhere in the female genital tract (particularly the uterus) and, rarely, beneath the pelvic and abdominal peritoneum or within the omentum (presumably from the same cells which give rise to endometriosis and endosalpingiosis). In view of the diverse nature of these mesenchymal tumors, the ovarian tumors should be sampled extensively by the pathologist for evidence of a specific origin, since this may have a bearing on prognosis. In general, pure sarcomas have a better outlook than those which are components of teratomas or malignant mixed müllerian tumors. Primary pure ovarian sarcomas also seem, from the limited reports available for analysis, to have a better prognosis than the same tumors occurring in extra-ovarian sites; this may relate to the greater ease of local excision of these tumors (oophorec-tomy) compared with that of similar tumors occurring in the deep soft tissues. It is important that the possibility, although rare, that an ovarian sarcoma is metastatic should be investigated clinically.

All types of lymphoma have been reported to occur in the ovaries. Hodgkin's disease presenting as ovarian disease is extremely rare and has been of mixed cellularity,[29,43] or unspecified type.[67] It is uncommonly encountered even in autopsy series, being found in less than 5% of patients compared with approximately 25% of other lymphoma patients.[71] Amongst non-Hodgkin's lymphomas, there is a preponderance of diffuse lymphomas with small cell ('lymphocytic'-Rappaport) lymphomas being more common than the large cell ('histiocytic'-Rappaport) types.[9,51,52,67] Burkitt's lymphoma is relatively well represented because of its propensity for extra-nodal involvement.[37] In fact, bilateral massive ovarian enlargement is a classical manifestation of this disease, and occurs in approximately 50% of patients at some stage.[9,37,83] Involvement of the ovaries by plasma cell dyscrasias is even rarer than the other lymphoproliferative disorders. Infiltration by multiple myeloma has been observed at autopsy, and there are very rare reports of primary plasmacytomas of ovary.[14,33,83]

A comprehensive scheme of classification, modified from that used by Hendrickson & Kempson[34] for uterine mesenchymal tumors, is outlined in Table 61.1.

PURE HOMOLOGOUS (MÜLLERIAN) TUMORS

Leiomyoma and leiomyosarcoma

Although smooth muscle is sometimes seen as a minor component of benign or low grade ovarian müllerian epithelial tumors (particularly endometrioid and mucinous) and, uncommonly, as part of the cellular proliferation in stromal hyperplasia, true leiomyomas in the ovary are rare neoplasms.[23] Reported cases have occurred in women aged 20 to 65 years (85% of cases occurring in premenopausal women) and usually present as an abdominal mass or as an incidental finding at hysterectomy for uterine myomas.

971

Table 61.1 Classification of ovarian mesenchymal tumors.

Benign tumors and tumor-like conditions

Leiomyomas and histological variants
Leiomyomatosis peritonealis disseminata (LPD)
Hemangiomas
Lymphangiomas
Chondromas
Osteomas
Giant cell tumors
Myxomas
Neurofibromas
Neurilemmomas (schwannomas)
Ganglioneuromas
Pheochromocytomas

Malignant tumors

Pure sarcomas
   Homologous (müllerian)
      Leiomyosarcomas
      Low grade endometrioid stromal sarcomas ('endolymphatic
      stromal myosis', 'stromatosis')
      High grade endometrioid stromal sarcomas
   Heterologous
      Hemangioendotheliomas (angiosarcomas)
      Lymphangiosarcomas
      Hemangiopericytomas
      Rhabdomyosarcomas
      Chondrosarcomas
      Osteogenic sarcomas
      Fibrosarcomas (? ovarian stromal sarcoma)
      Neurofibrosarcomas
Mixed sarcomas — homologous or heterologous
Malignant mixed müllerian tumors
   Low grade ('adenosarcomas')
      Homologous
      Heterologous
   High grade
      Homologous ('carcinosarcomas')
      Heterologous ('mixed mesodermal tumors')
Sarcomas, not otherwise differentiated
Malignant lymphomas and leukemias

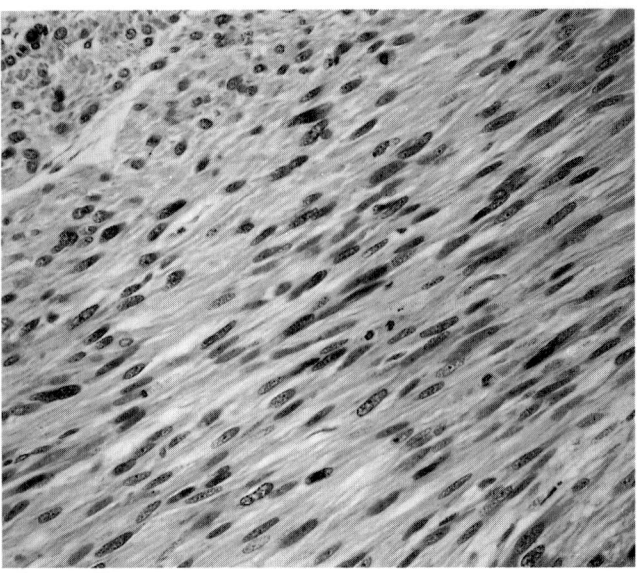

Fig. 61.1 Ovarian leiomyosarcoma. Broad bundles of spindled cells with elongate, blunt-ended nuclei and prominent mitotic activity. (H&E; ×100)

Ascites may accompany the tumor, but pleural effusions have not been recorded.[87] A solitary case has presented with virilization due to associated hilus cell hyperplasia.[54]

Leiomyosarcomas of teratomatous and non-teratomatous origin[1,74] are equally rare, but have been reported in the ovaries in elderly women. Grossly, they are large, soft, pale, fleshy tumors indistinguishable from other ovarian sarcomas on gross examination. Focal cystic degeneration is frequently seen. Histologically, leiomyosarcomas differ from their benign counterparts in being hypercellular (Fig. 61.1) and in exhibiting a markedly increased mitotic rate (greater than 10 per 10 HPF). Cells tend to be uniform and spindled, and organized in whorled, interwoven bundles with pleomorphism prominent only in areas of ischemia. Nuclei are elongate and blunt-ended.

Too few cases of leiomyosarcoma have been reported to test the sophisticated criteria of malignancy which have been applied to uterine smooth muscle neoplasms.[34] Our recommendations are that they be utilized in the interim with the additional proviso that consideration be given to the proclivity for smooth muscle tumors to increase their mitotic activity under conditions of ischemia, such as torsion, which not infrequently complicates ovarian neoplasms and pregnancy.

Peritoneal leiomyomatosis

Clinical features

Peritoneal leiomyomatosis (also known as leiomyomatosis peritonealis disseminata; LPD) is a rare, typically self-limiting tumor-like condition of the peritoneal subcelomic mesenchyme, manifesting as myriad nodules of smooth muscle up to a centimeter or so in diameter. LPD affects the ovaries in about one-quarter of cases.[85] It occurs mostly in young women with a median age of 30 years, and 50% are pregnant or immediately post-partum. Many other women are taking oral contraceptive agents at the time of presentation. Spontaneous regression is the rule, while clinical recurrence may be observed with subsequent pregnancies. A single example of malignant LPD has been reported, but in this case the ovaries were not involved.[68] The significance of this disease entity is principally in its clinical differentiation from peritoneal carcinomatosis at laparotomy.

Pathology

LPD is characterized grossly by tens to hundreds of firm, rounded nodules, seldom exceeding 1 cm in diameter and distributed widely in the omentum and beneath the pelvic peritoneum. Less frequently, they are seen on the serosal surfaces of the ovaries, uterus, fallopian tubes and bowel. Histologically, LPD exhibits small, subperitoneal nodules which cytologically and architecturally resemble small seedling myomas in the uterus. The typical spindled smooth muscle cells, often with prominent eosinophilic cytoplasm, may merge with the surrounding tissue or be sharply demarcated from it. Nuclear atypia is absent but mitoses may be easily found. Decidual cells are prominent in pregnant or immediately post-partum patients. The intimate association of LPD with such cells, as well as with endometriosis[40] and benign serosal inclusions,[8] has led most investigators to favor a subcelomic mesenchymal metaplastic origin for LPD.[85,90]

Low and high grade endometrioid stromal sarcomas

Clinical features

Occasional reports of primary ovarian stromal sarcomas of müllerian or endometrioid type have appeared in the literature, although clear interpretation of instances with synchronous or metachronous involvement of both uterus and ovary is seldom given.[92] Some such lesions are high grade endometrioid stromal sarcomas, whilst most are less frankly malignant tumors and correspond to low grade stromal sarcomas or endolymphatic stromal myosis ('stromatosis').[74] Most of these latter lesions are thought to arise in pre-existing endometriosis, which is found in association with 50% to 85% of cases.[71,77,92] They are often bilateral and widespread within the abdomen at the time of diagnosis, and occur in women in their fifth and sixth decades.

Pathology

Low grade endometrioid stromal sarcoma (endolymphatic stromal myosis) tends to appear as an ill-defined and homogeneous ovarian enlargement with tumor extension into adjacent tissues; rather less commonly, it appears as a multinodular fleshy tumor, although a cystic component may occasionally be prominent. Focal intracystic hemorrhage may be an indication of associated endometriosis. High grade sarcomas are usually discrete, white, fleshy ovarian masses averaging 10 cm in diameter, with prominent necrosis and evidence of local invasion.

Microscopically, endometrioid stromal sarcomas, either low or high grade, show the same spectrum of changes observed in the more common uterine lesions. Most often they are composed of closely packed sheets of small, round to oval cells which often are whorled around a fine meshwork of small arteriolar vessels. Reticulin fibers invest individual cells and highlight the vascularity. Tongues of apparently intravascular tumor growth, as seen in endo-

lymphatic stromal myosis, may also be present (Fig. 61.2). Cytoplasm is scant, and the nuclei are round to oval with inapparent nucleoli (Fig. 61.3).

A second distinct pattern is created by the deposition of intercellular hyaline material, which may be focally prominent (Fig. 61.4) and which separates clusters of small tumor cells. Thick-walled, cleft-like vascular spaces are evident in this variant. Storiform patterns are sometimes seen, as are less cellular areas more closely resembling those of ovarian fibromas.[92]

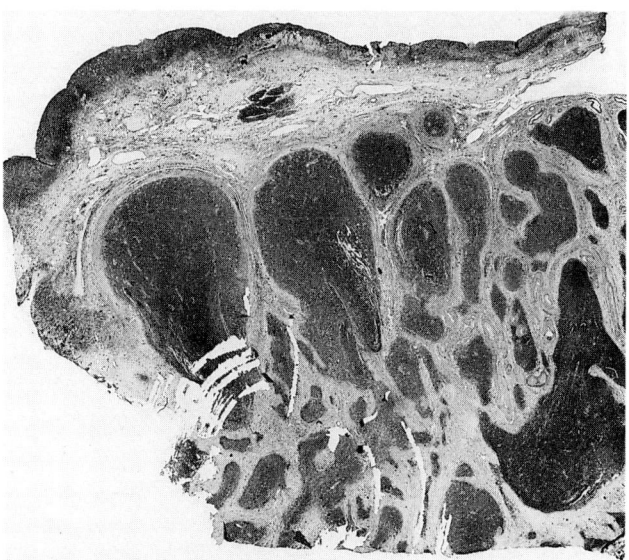

Fig. 61.2 Low grade endometrioid stromal sarcoma. Slug-like processes of hypercellular tumor infiltrate the ovarian medulla. The contralateral ovary was the site of a primary tumor mass 15 cm in diameter. (H&E; ×3)

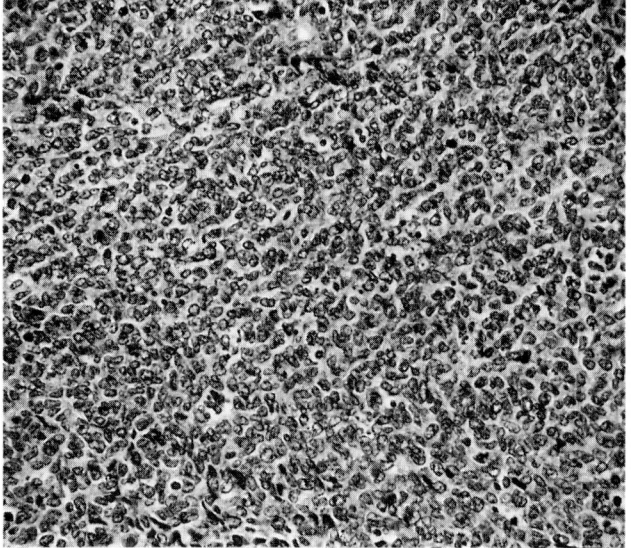

Fig. 61.3 Low grade endometrioid stromal sarcoma. Cells show scant cytoplasm, no appreciable mitotic activity and little nuclear atypia. (H&E; ×100)

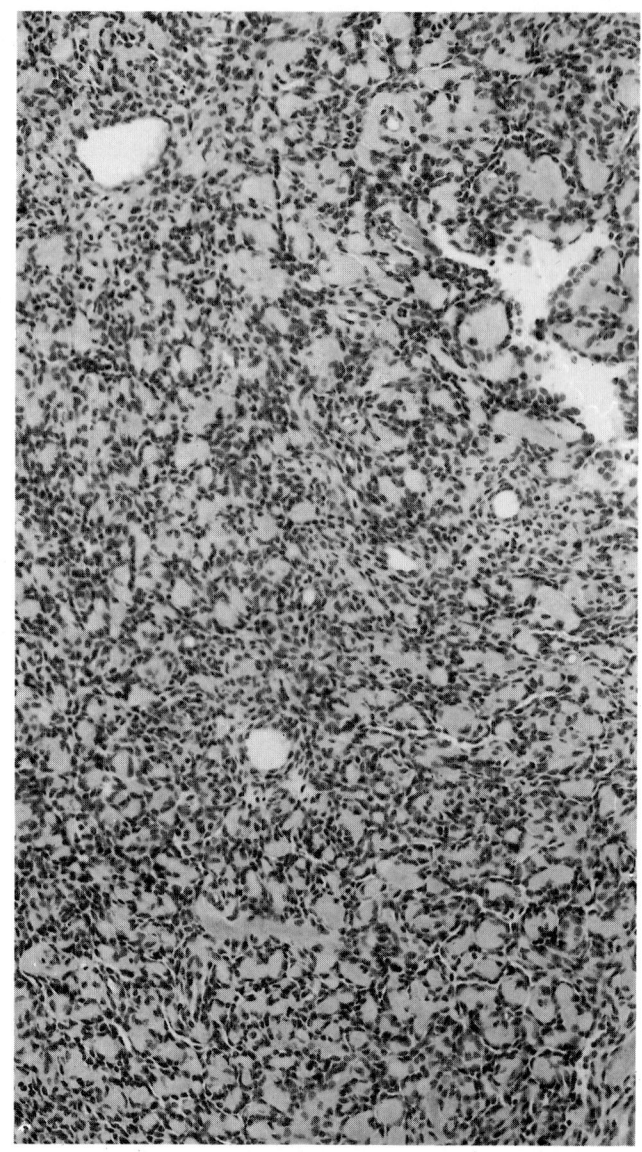

Fig. 61.4 Low grade endometrioid stromal sarcoma. Prominent deposition of intercellular hyaline material. (H&E; ×83)

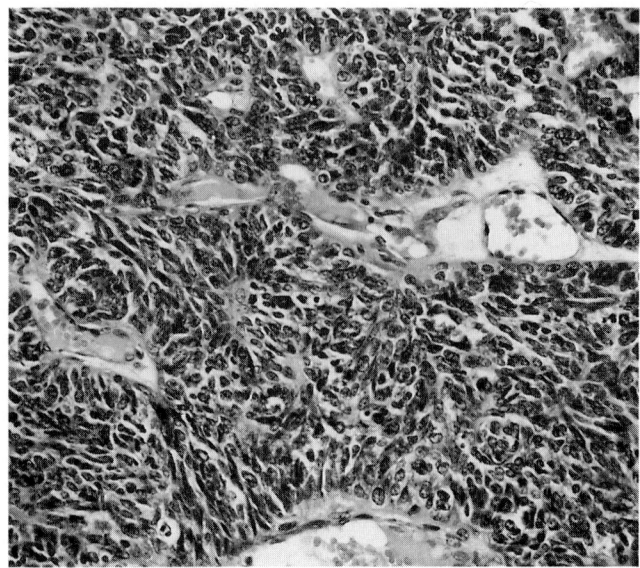

Fig. 61.5 High grade endometrioid stromal sarcoma with larger, more pleomorphic and densely hyperchromatic nuclei (contrast with Fig. 61.3). (H&E; × 100)

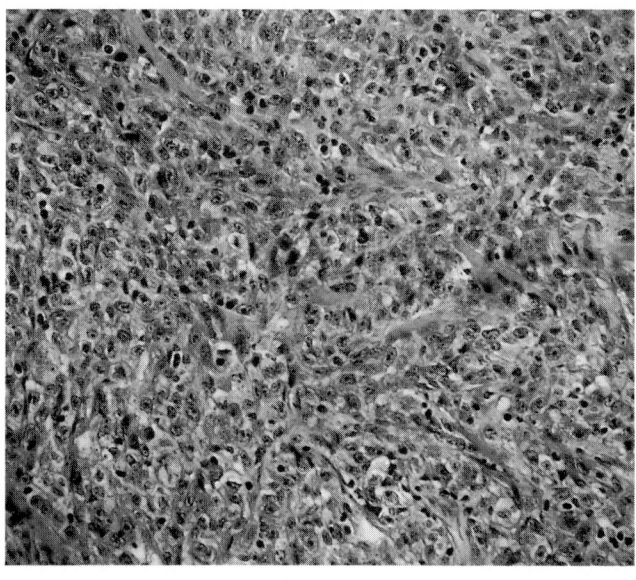

Fig. 61.6 High grade endometrioid stromal sarcoma. Cells exhibit pronounced nuclear pleomorphism and prominent nucleoli. (H&E; × 100)

Nuclei in low grade lesions are bland, and mitoses infrequent (by definition fewer than 10 per 10 HPF) and never atypical. Nuclear atypia is seen in high grade tumors (Figs 61.5 and 61.6) with mitoses numbering over 10 per 10 HPF.

Therapy

Primary treatment is surgical, with hysterectomy and bilateral salpingo-oophorectomy the preferred treatment in all age groups. The tumors tend to invade local structures without necessarily being grossly apparent.[74] Because of their proclivity for bilaterality, or for prior, synchronous or subsequent uterine stromal sarcoma,[92] conservative surgery is associated with a high risk of persistent disease. Progression is largely dependent on tumor grade. Low grade tumors (mitoses fewer than 10 per 10 HPF) have an indolent course, spread of tumor still being compatible with long survival. Only 2 of 19 patients reported by

Young et al[92] died of their disease, whilst 3 of 4 patients with high grade sarcoma (greater mitotic rate than 10 per 10 HPF) died.

Progesterone has been used successfully in low grade endometrioid uterine sarcomas[32,86] and is the treatment of choice for low grade ovarian lesions where residual or recurrent disease is present. Treatment must be prolonged, or recurrence may occur on cessation of therapy. Radiation therapy has been used for residual or recurrent low grade endometrial stromal sarcoma with some success, and is also of benefit in high grade uterine tumors.[57] Its place in the treatment of analogous ovarian tumors is uncertain. We similarly have little knowledge of the efficacy of chemotherapy in this disease. The equivalent uterine tumor has been shown to respond to single agent cyclophosphamide[35] or to multiple agent therapy with vincristine, adriamycin and cyclophosphamide.[42] Treatment along these lines may be appropriate in the management of recurrent or widespread disease.

PURE HETEROLOGOUS TUMORS

Hemangioma and hemangioendothelioma (angiosarcoma)

Benign hemangiomas are the most common of the miscellaneous mesenchymal ovarian tumors, although some controversy exists as to whether they represent malformations, hamartomas or true tumors. About 35 cases have been reported.[25] They occur at any age, but most are found in children or young adults.[20,36] In some cases, there is an association with generalized or abdominopelvic hemangiomatosis, or with hemangiomas elsewhere in the genital tract.[41,83]

Hemangiosarcomas are extremely rare tumors which have been reported only in adults and have presented as abdominal masses. Torsion and rupture are not uncommon complications.[18,25] They pursue a malignant course, with local infiltration, peritoneal seeding and vascular dissemination.[25,83] Hemangiosarcomas are large, soft, friable, spongy masses with areas of hemorrhage and necrosis. The vascular spaces are lined by endothelial cells showing nuclear pleomorphism and mitotic activity which, although sometimes only focal, may be the only features which distinguish these tumors from their benign counterparts. The presence of solid cores of endothelial cells helps to confirm the diagnosis.

Lymphangiosarcoma

The only reported case of lymphangiosarcoma of which we are aware occurred in a 31-year-old woman who died within a year from widespread metastases. The 15 cm tumor was distinguished from a lymphangioma by the presence of focal endothelial proliferation, with some pleomorphism and nuclear hyperchromatism.[66]

Hemangiopericytoma

Ovarian hemangiopericytoma has only recently been reported. The first case[48] was a 48-year-old woman who developed bilateral large (10 cm) ovarian tumors with small subperitoneal metastases in the terminal ileum. The patient was given postoperative chemotherapy, but died from surgical complications and inanition 2 years later, with residual but non-progressive disease. The second case[74] was a 63-year-old woman with a 28 cm tumor associated with adhesions and ascites, who was alive with disease 5 years postoperatively.

Hemangiopericytomas have a complex vascular network composed of gaping, thin-walled channels which often show a staghorn pattern of branching. The tumor cells which surround the vessels are regular ovoid fibroblast-like cells, each surrounded by abundant reticulin fibers. Fibrosis and myxoid change may be present.[21] Electron microscopy confirms the pericytic origin of hemangiopericytomas, showing abundant cytoplasmic fibrils, basal lamina and micropinocytotic vesicles.[5]

Rhabdomyosarcoma

Clinical features

No case of ovarian rhabdomyoma has been reported. By contrast, rhabdomyosarcomas are the most common of the pure heterologous ovarian sarcomas.[60,70,74] Although they possibly arise from undifferentiated ovarian mesenchyme, they may also represent one-sided development of mixed müllerian tumors (in which rhabdomyosarcoma is a relatively frequent component) or Sertoli-Leydig cell tumors. Diagnosis of pure rhabdomyosarcoma requires the examination of multiple blocks in order to exclude other diagnostic possibilities, as indicated at the beginning of this chapter.

The age at presentation ranges from early childhood to old age. In a review of 29 cases, Shakfeh & Woodruff[74] found 32% under the age of 20 years, the youngest being 13 months. The symptomatology is non-specific. Pelvic discomfort, pressure symptoms on the bladder and rectum, or a rapidly enlarging abdominal mass are the commonest modes of presentation. Metastases are often apparent at initial presentation and, until recently, death usually occurred within 1 year.[25,74]

Pathology

The tumors are unilateral and usually more than 10 cm in diameter. The cut surfaces show soft, gray-white tissue with areas of hemorrhage, necrosis and cystic degeneration. The histological subtypes are comparable with extraovarian rhabdomyosarcomas; embryonal and alveolar types are most common in young patients, and pleomorphic in the elderly.

Therapy

Primary treatment is surgical, with hysterectomy, bilateral salpingo-oophorectomy and omentectomy the treatment of choice in the past. With a large percentage of patients in the younger age group, and with current chemotherapy approaches giving encouraging results, fertility-conserving surgical procedures require reassessment.

There are few reports in the literature relating to chemotherapy regimes for ovarian rhabdomyosarcoma. Other sites of genital rhabdomyosarcoma have, however, been more fully assessed. In 1969, Pratt[61] introduced the now commonly used regime of vincristine, actinomycin D and cyclophosphamide (VAC), and this combination regime has been widely used in the treatment of all forms of rhabdomyosarcoma. Until 1970, radical surgery, including exenteration, was widely performed for pelvic rhabdomyosarcoma, and this was followed by radiotherapy with or without chemotherapy. The Intergroup Rhabdomyosarcoma Study Group was formed in 1972 and initially studied the effects of radiotherapy and chemotherapy given after surgery. Their findings confirmed the excellent results of other studies of genital rhabdomyosarcoma treated by combined modalities.[22,64] During the 1970's, chemotherapy and/or radiotherapy were evaluated as primary therapy, so that less radical surgery would then be required subsequently to excise the residual tumor mass. Ortega[50] demonstrated a response rate of 90% to VAC, with survival rates of 60% at 2 to 8 years (median 4.5 years); Flamanat et al,[24] treating eight cases of vaginal rhabdomyosarcoma with primary radiotherapy and chemotherapy, found only one case requiring subsequent surgery.

Drawing on the experience of therapy of rhabdomyosarcomas in other pelvic sites, a rational approach to treatment would involve surgery (conservative in the younger patient) followed by combination chemotherapy. VAC is the combination most commonly used up to this time; however, adriamycin may be introduced into the regime.[63]

Chondroma and chondrosarcoma

Only one case of an ovarian chondroma has been reported.[62] Ovarian tumors with conspicuous benign cartilaginous components are most likely to be fibromas with cartilaginous metaplasia, or teratomas with prominent cartilage formation.[25]

Talerman et al[84] have reported a pure primary ovarian chondrosarcoma. The large tumor occurred in a 61-year-old woman who was free of tumor 4.5 years after total hysterectomy and bilateral salpingo-oophorectomy. Extensive sampling of the tumor revealed no other histological elements, but the authors nonetheless suggested that the tumor probably resulted from malignant transformation of cartilage in a mature cystic teratoma (an example of which

has been documented previously).[13] A subsequent case, briefly described by Shakfeh & Woodruff,[74] died of disease 8 years postoperatively.

Osteogenic sarcomas

The rare reports of ovarian osteomas probably represent examples of osseous metaplasia in fibromas, leiomyomas or non-neoplastic lesions.[25,36,76,83] There are two reports of apparently pure osteogenic sarcomas, that is, with no evidence of associated teratoma or malignant mixed müllerian tumor.[1,74] The tumors developed in women aged 24 and 41 years, both of whom had metastatic disease at the time of initial surgery and died 5 months later. These large tumors had histological features similar to those of skeletal osteogenic sarcomas. Stowe & Watt[81] described an ovarian osteogenic sarcoma which, although associated with a cyst lined by ciliated epithelium, may also have been a pure lesion.

Liposarcoma

There are no well documented cases of pure ovarian lipomas. Lesions which simulate lipomas are benign cystic teratomas with prominent adipose tissue, adherent adipose tissue or auto-amputated infarcted appendices epiploicae, and adipocytic prosoplasia.[25,36,38] No pure primary ovarian liposarcoma has been reported, but liposarcoma may be identified in the ovary as a component of a malignant mixed müllerian tumor or as a metastasis.[83]

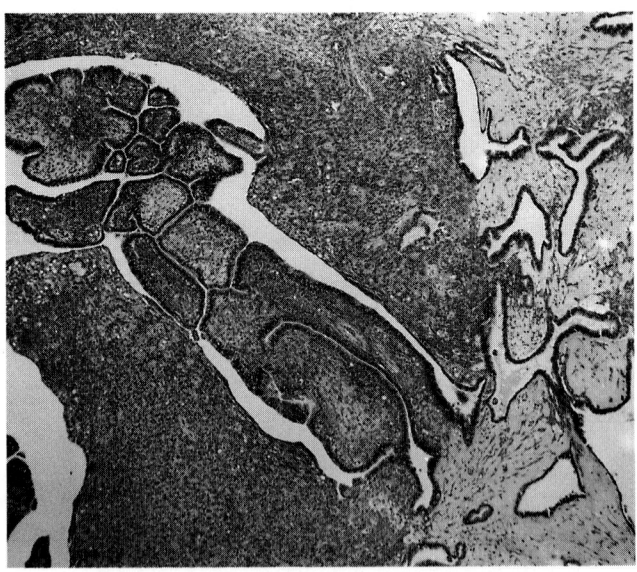

Fig. 61.7 Ovarian adenosarcoma. Low power showing a coarse papillary pattern and hypercellular stroma. (H&E; ×20)

Neural and related tumors

Neural and related tumors are very rare, and their histogenesis is similar to that proposed for other mesenchymal ovarian tumors. Some are associated with von Recklinghausen's disease. Neuroectodermal tumors (ependymomas, neuroblastomas, glioblastomas), even if apparently pure, are considered to be of teratomatous origin and are discussed elsewhere. One case each of neurofibroma and neurofibrosarcoma has been described in association with von Recklinghausen's disease.[19,78] Three cases of neurilemmoma (schwannoma) have been reported, all with symptoms of a pelvic mass and an uneventful postoperative course. The tumors were solid, and histologically similar to non-ovarian neurilemmomas.[83] Two malignant schwannomas have been reported in elderly women who died with metastatic disease 5 to 18 months after initial surgery.[75,80] One presented with episodic hypoglycemia; insulin was extracted from the 12 cm tumor.[75]

MALIGNANT MIXED MÜLLERIAN TUMORS

Low grade (müllerian adenosarcomas)

Low grade malignant mixed müllerian tumors (müllerian adenosarcomas) differ from the sarcomas described above in that a benign epithelial component is also present. They differ from ordinary adenofibromas in that their stroma is hypercellular and often frankly sarcomatous. The term, adenosarcoma, was used first by Clement & Scully[11] to describe such tumors in the uterus, and has since been applied to adnexal neoplasms.[12,36,69] These tumors are unilateral and mostly confined to the ovaries at laparotomy. Their mean age of incidence is about 50 years.

Adenosarcomas measure about 10 cm in average diameter, some with a smooth external surface and others with external papillary or polypoid excrescences. Their cut surface is spongy and multicystic (containing clear or yellowish fluid), with intervening tough fibrous tissue. Focal hemorrhage may be present in larger tumors.

Histologically, adenosarcomas show an epithelial component which is usually endometrial in type and disposed in clefts or cystic spaces. Less often, they exhibit a serous papillary pattern (Figs 61.7 and 61.8). Pseudostratification and nuclear hyperchromatism are sometimes present. The stroma is usually most cellular immediately adjacent to the epithelium, but varies greatly within each tumor. Stromal cell nuclei are more pleomorphic than in benign adenofibromas, and mitoses are increased up to 5 per 10 HPF in tumors subcategorized as 'cellular adenofibromas', and 2 to 25 per 10 HPF in those designated as 'adenosarcoma' by Kao & Norris.[39] Heterologous elements infrequently occur in the stroma of corresponding uterine lesions, for which reason Kao & Norris[39] prefer to designate them as 'benign and low grade variants of mixed mesodermal tumors'.

High grade (carcinosarcomas, mixed mesodermal tumors)

High grade malignant mixed müllerian tumors (car-

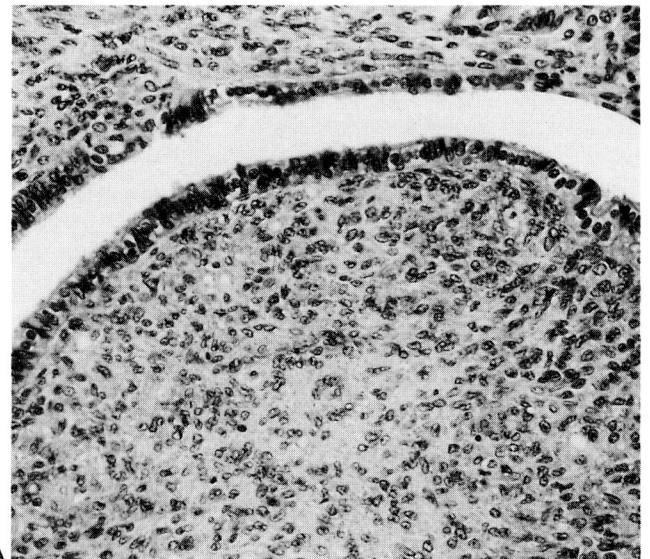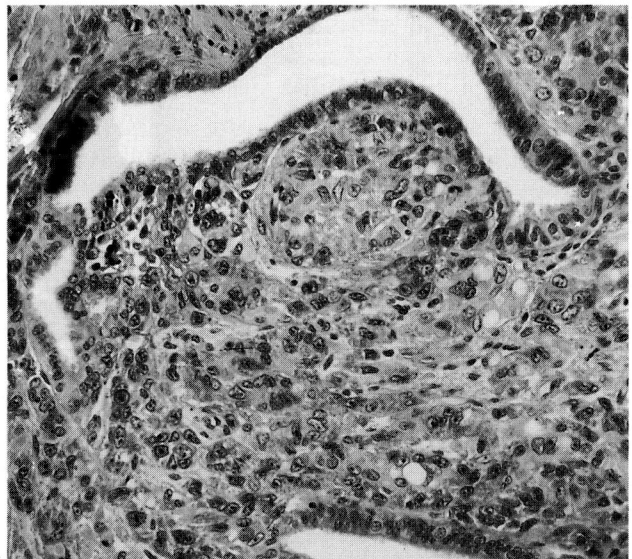

Fig. 61.8 Ovarian adenosarcoma. **A.** benign, ciliated, serous (tubal) type epithelium and atypical, hypercellular stroma. **B.** pelvic metastasis which developed 5 months after initial surgery. Nuclear changes in the stromal cells are more marked, but the epithelium is still cytologically benign. (Reproduced from Russell et al (1979),[69] with permission.) (H&E; ×100)

cinomas, mixed mesodermal tumors) are comparatively rare, and contain epithelial and mesenchymal elements, both of which are histologically malignant. The mesenchymal elements may, on the one hand, differentiate towards tissues 'homologous' to the müllerian tract (endometrial stroma, fibrous tissue, smooth muscle), and such tumors are also termed carcinosarcomas in the WHO classification. On the other hand, they may show 'heterologous' tissues foreign to the müllerian tract (bone, cartilage, fat, skeletal muscle); these tumors are also known as mixed mesodermal tumors. The heterologous elements can be prominent and widespread, or limited to occasional small foci. Of the 200 or so cases in the English literature,[6,17,45] one-third fall into the homologous group. Barwick & LiVolsi[4] point out that all sarcomas (except fibrosarcoma) are heterologous to the ovary, and suggest that there is no justification for this distinction. Although they are closely related neoplasms, there may be merit in separating the homologous from heterologous types, because of the reduced median survival claimed for the latter.[15,17] Rarely, mixed müllerian tumors are seen to arise in ovarian endometriosis.

Clinical features

These tumors account for less than 1% of malignant ovarian neoplasms and are reported almost exclusively in postmenopausal women (often nulliparous) with a mean age of incidence of 60 years. They are bilateral in 10% of cases, and in over 80% of patients the tumor exhibits extra-ovarian abdominal spread at diagnosis. The symptoms, signs and operative findings are identical to those associated with the common epithelial carcinomas; the final differentiation from these tumors is histological.

The progression of these tumors tends to be rapid, and survival has been reported as inferior to that of epithelial tumors. Hanjani[31] reported 23% survival at 12 months, whilst Morrow et al[45] and Dictor[17] reported 30% and 29% survivals for the same period. A more recent report by Moore et al[44] showed a median survival of 21 months for patients treated by combination chemotherapy, bringing the survival more into parity with pure epithelial ovarian tumors.

Early reports suggested that carcinosarcomas had a better prognosis than mixed mesodermal tumors.[15] Hanjani et al,[31] reporting 8 cases and reviewing the published literature of 193 cases, concluded that when age, stage and therapeutic modality were considered there was no significant survival difference. A Gynecologic Oncology Group study[45] found no apparent differences in stage distribution or survival between the two tumor types.

Pathology

Carcinosarcomas and malignant mixed mesodermal tumors

average 15 to 20 cm in diameter, with bosselated outer surfaces showing prominent vessels and focal hemorrhage. The cut surface reveals yellow to brown, friable, fleshy nodules, soft in consistency and showing obvious hemorrhage and necrosis. A variable cystic component usually contains polypoid excrescences and bloodstained fluid. Heterologous (mixed mesodermal) sarcomas and mixed tumors may show cartilage or bone.

Histologically, the epithelial element in high grade malignant mixed müllerian tumors is, in our experience, most commonly serous carcinoma (Fig. 61.9). Less frequently, endometrioid (Fig. 61.10), mucinous, clear cell or

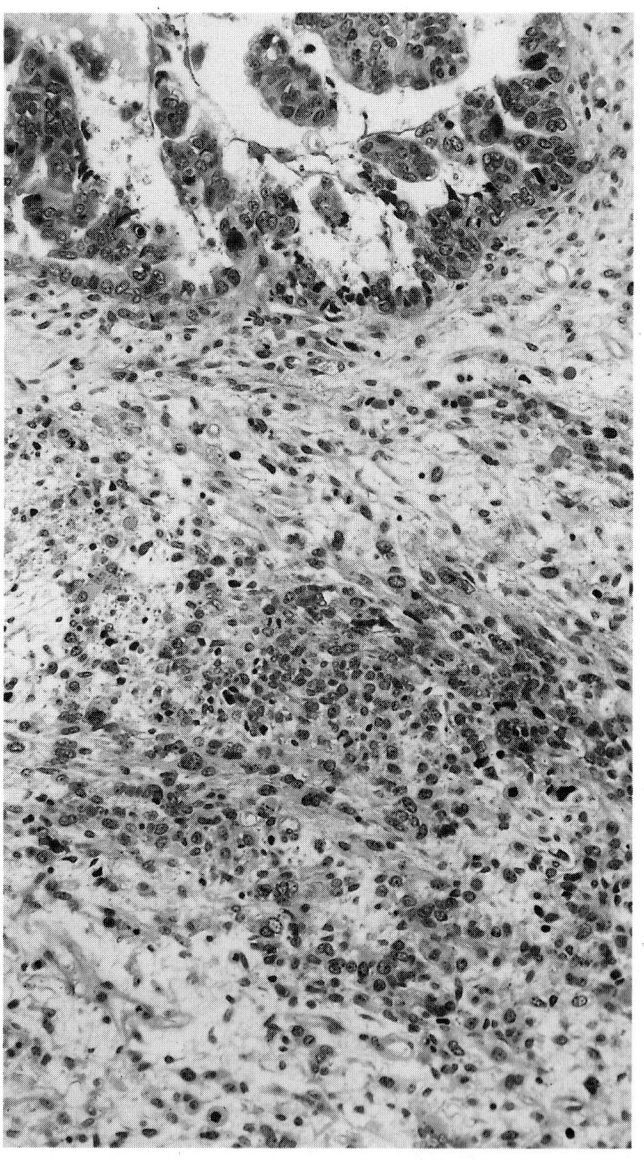

Fig. 61.9 Homologous malignant mixed müllerian tumor with typical high grade serous carcinoma (top) and a malignant stromal component of poorly defined and rather non-descript small cells with marked mitotic activity. (H&E; ×83)

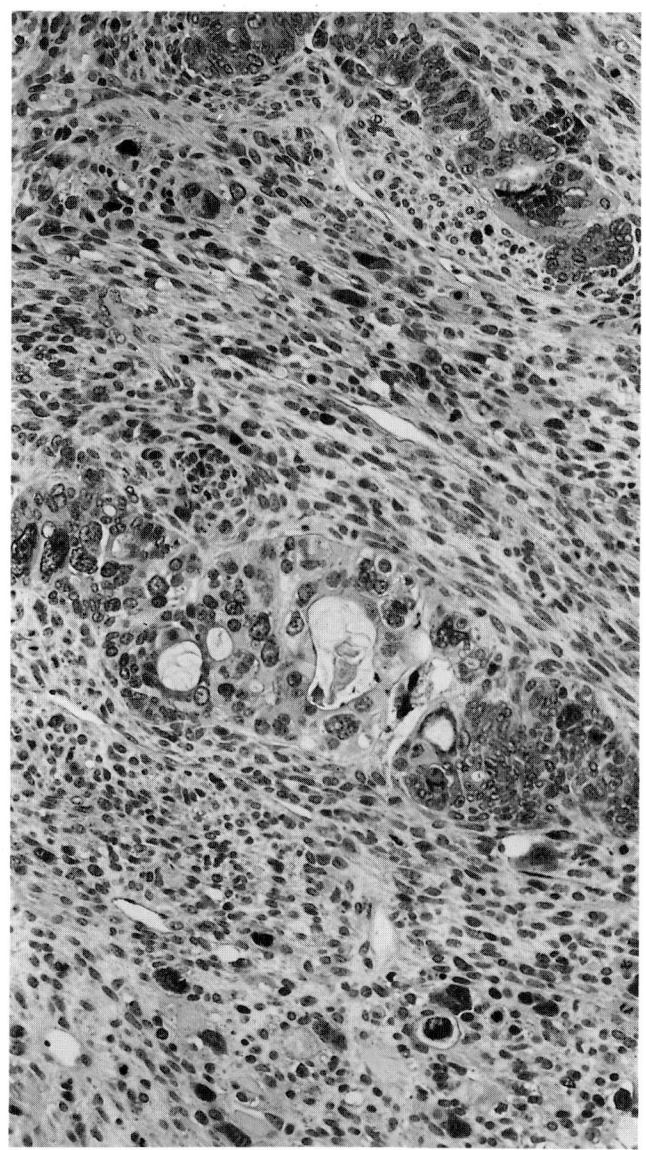

Fig. 61.10 Homologous malignant mixed müllerian tumor with poorly differentiated endometrioid carcinoma admixed with high grade 'spindle-cell' sarcoma. Cellular pleomorphism is prominent in both components. (H&E; × 83)

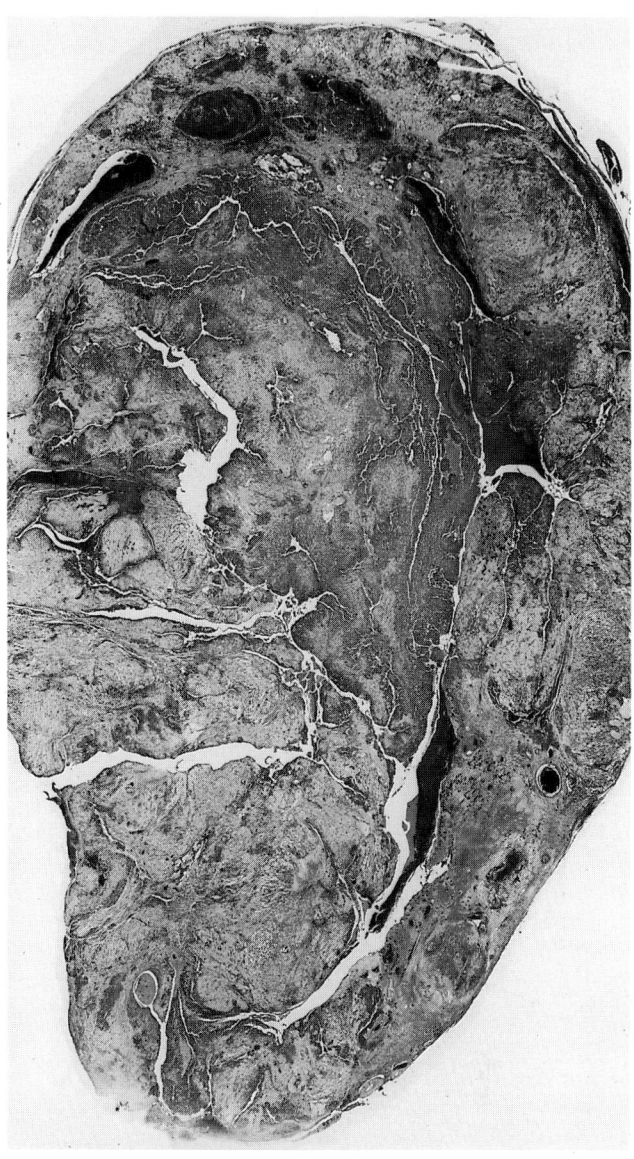

Fig. 61.11 Homologous malignant mixed müllerian tumor showing the variegated appearance occasioned by a complex admixture of epithelial and stromal elements. The fine slit-like spaces (top-center) suggest serous epithelial differentiation. Pale myxoid stroma is noted to the lower left. (H&E; ×2)

squamous elements are noted. Other investigators have found endometrioid differentiation the most common.[45] If the epithelium is mucinous, care should be taken to differentiate such tumors from mucinous lesions with mural nodules.[58,59] The latter nodules may be reactive to invasive carcinoma or truly sarcomatous.

There is generally a complex admixture of epithelial and malignant stromal elements (Fig. 61.11), particularly if the latter is composed of undifferentiated or primitive myxoid mesenchyme; transitions, however, are uncommon.

Reticulin stains and immunoperoxidase stains for epithelial membrane antigen (EMA) and cytokeratins assist in distinguishing sarcomatous areas from undifferentiated carcinoma. Pleomorphic and bizarre epithelial giant cells are common (Fig. 61.12), as are cells with hyaline cytoplasmic droplets.[71] Large fields composed entirely of either carcinoma or sarcoma may be encountered, and in occasional tumors one or other component may predominate. However, the finding of even a small focus of sarcoma in a large tumor justifies the diagnosis of malignant mixed

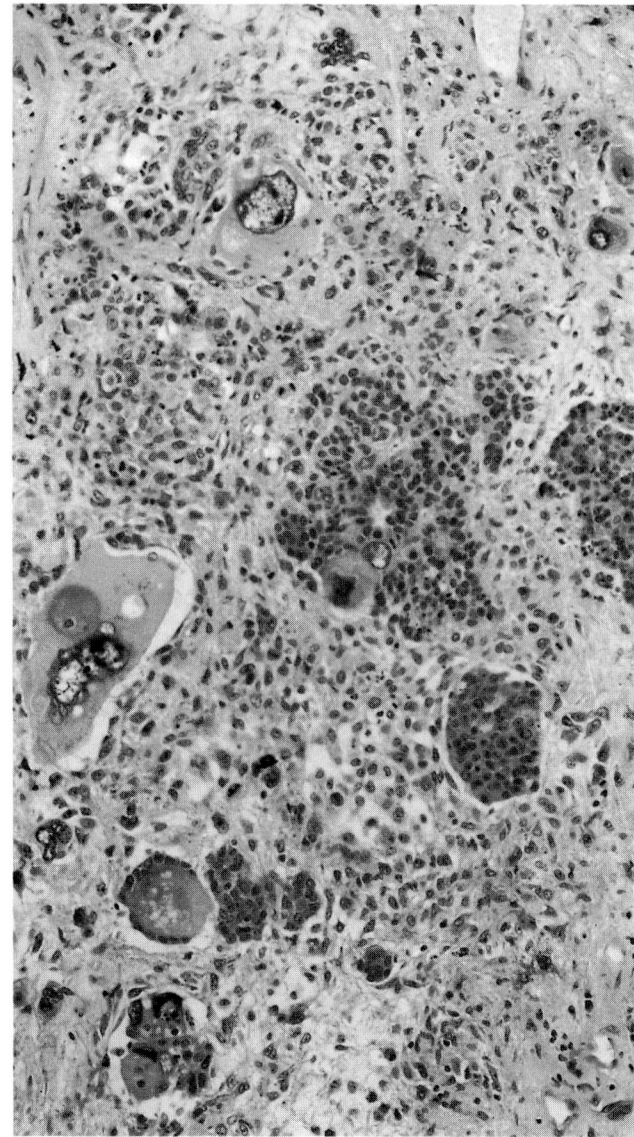

Fig. 61.12 Homologous malignant mixed müllerian tumor with much variability in the epithelial component. Clustered small uniform cells are seen as well as bizarre giant cells, the latter identified only immunohistochemically as epithelial in nature. (H&E; ×83)

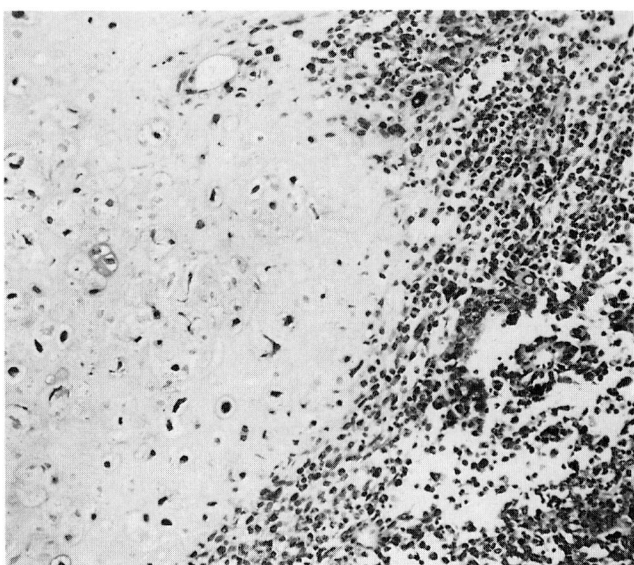

Fig. 61.13 Heterologous malignant mixed müllerian tumor with islands of malignant cartilage. (H&E; ×50)

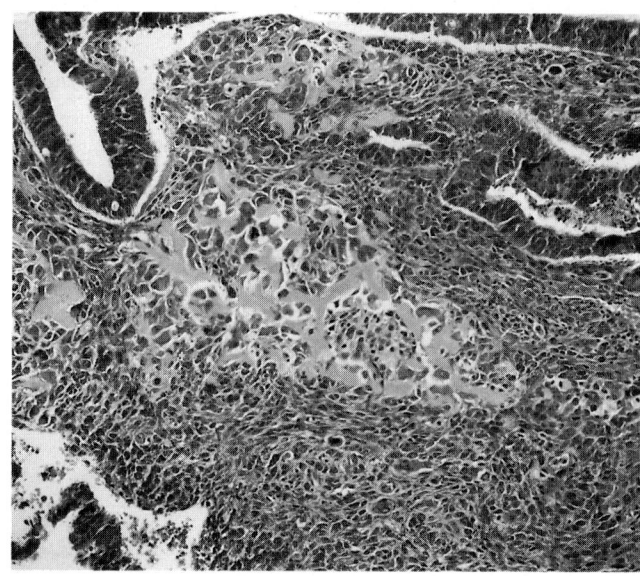

Fig. 61.14 Heterologous malignant mixed müllerian tumor with small discrete foci of malignant osteoid. The nearby epithelium is endometrioid in type. (H&E; ×50)

müllerian tumor, as the behavior of the lesion and its attendant prognosis are significantly and unfavorably altered in such cases.

Sarcomatous elements are predominantly hypercellular sheets of small, hyperchromatic, round to spindle cells with a high mitotic rate and without apparent differentiation. In routine hematoxylin and eosin sections, chondrosarcoma is the most frequently encountered heterologous stromal element (Fig. 61.13); less often, malignant osteoid (Fig. 61.14) and skeletal muscle (Fig. 61.15) are present. Recent use of immunohistochemical techniques to identify myoglobin[46] and desmin suggest that rhabdomyoblasts are more common than has been previously reported.[15] Rarely, bizarre malignant lipoblasts are encountered.[17]

Evidence of pelvic endometriosis is seen more frequently than would be expected by chance, and the tumors may rarely arise within ovarian endometriotic cysts.

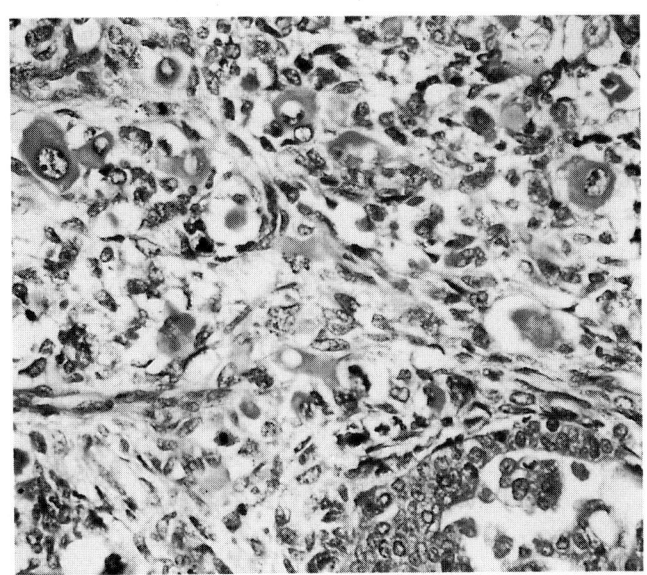

Fig. 61.15 Heterologous malignant mixed müllerian tumor with bizarre mononuclear cells having dense eosinophilic cytoplasm and resembling embryonal rhabdomyoblasts. Immunohistochemical stains for myoglobin or desmin should be positive to confirm skeletal muscle differentiation. (H&E; ×100)

Therapy

The surgical management is as for malignant epithelial ovarian tumors; it comprises full staging procedures followed by total hysterectomy, bilateral salpingo-oophorectomy, total omentectomy and radical debulking of all resectable tumor within the pelvis and abdomen.

In the literature review of 106 cases with adequate follow-up, Hanjani et al[31] found the major prognostic indicator to be stage of disease. Of patients with Stage I disease, 56% were dead at one year, whilst of those with Stages II, III and IV, 80%, 81.5% and 88.8% respectively had died. In the majority of cases, surgery was followed by radiation therapy, or single or combination chemotherapy. VAC was the most commonly used regime.

Carlson et al[6] reported treatment of 20 cases at the M.D. Anderson Hospital and Tumor Institute. Twelve patients were treated postoperatively with radiotherapy (whole pelvis and abdomen strip irradiation) in combination with VAC, with complete disease control achieved in four. The mortality from combined treatment was high, with two deaths related to myelosuppression and sepsis. Subsequently, a reduction in dosage of chemotherapeutic agents was instituted.

Because of the uncommon occurrence of these tumors, most reports deal with small numbers of patients collected over many years, and with differing treatment modalities. In these regimes, adriamycin began to emerge as an active single agent for sarcoma, with response rates of 27 to 40%.[29,91] These results were not, however, corroborated in the treatment of uterine sarcomas. Though Barlow et al[3] demonstrated a partial response in 5 of 7 (71%) patients with metastatic uterine sarcoma, Piver et al[56] could only demonstrate a 6% response rate in 17 similar tumors. The place of adriamycin in the treatment of gynecological sarcomas, therefore, remains in doubt.

Moore et al[44] more recently reported results of treatment of 27 patients from 1968 to 1984. Since 1975, 15 patients with bulky residual disease have been treated with adriamycin-containing combination therapy, either VAC and DTIC (CYVADIC), or cyclophosphamide, adriamycin and cisplatin (CAP). Complete response occurred in 6 of 15 patients (40%), with a median duration of 23 months, and there were three (20%) partial responders (median duration of 10 months). The median survival was 21 months for the chemotherapy treated group (34 months for complete responders), while 10 of 15 patients (67%) were alive at 12 months. The report suggested that CYVADIC or CAP are appropriate first line chemotherapy regimes for mixed müllerian tumors. Further trials with these adriamycin-containing regimes are at present being evaluated.

SARCOMAS NOT OTHERWISE DIFFERENTIATED

Rarely, one may encounter malignant mesenchymal tumors with no apparent specific differentiation or evidence of underlying lesions, known to be associated with, or complicated by, sarcomas. Multiple blocks should be examined closely for evidence of müllerian epithelial components or teratomatous elements. It is worth performing immunohistochemical stains for epithelial markers or electronmicroscopy to exclude undifferentiated carcinoma. The possibility of a metastasis should also be considered; the clinical history and operative findings should be reviewed. If the patient is young with hypercalcemia, primary small cell 'carcinoma' enters the differential diagnosis.[16]

MALIGNANT LYMPHOMA AND LEUKEMIA

Lymphomas

Clinical features

Ovarian involvement by malignant lymphomas is rare, except as a manifestation of disseminated nodal lymphoma. In patients dying of lymphoma, the ovaries are found to be infiltrated in approximately 25% of cases.[10,71] By contrast, only 0.2 to 0.3% of lymphomas present initially as gonadal disease;[10,27] most of these patients probably have occult nodal disease,[51,52,89] and overt generalized disease usually develops within a short time.[26,52,83] The third type of expression of malignant lymphoma in the ovaries is of primary extranodal lymphoma. Fox & Langley[25] proposed the following criteria for the diagnosis of primary ovarian lymphoma:

1. At the time of diagnosis, the lymphoma is clinically confined to the ovary and full investigation fails to reveal evidence of lymphoma elsewhere. A lymphoma can still, however, be considered primary if spread has occurred to immediately adjacent lymph nodes or if there has been direct spread to infiltrate immediately adjacent structures.
2. The peripheral blood and bone marrow should not contain any abnormal cells.
3. If further lymphomatous lesions occur at sites remote from the ovary, then at least several months should have elapsed between the appearance of the ovarian and extra-ovarian lesions.

There has always been scepticism about the existence of primary ovarian lymphoma because of the lack of a physiological lymphocyte population in the gonads,[30,51] and the failure to identify a prelymphomatous hyperimmune stage as has been recognized in sites such as thyroid or small intestine.[51] However, the possibility of true primary extranodal ovarian lymphomas is supported by reports of long survival of patients with ovarian disease after only local ablative therapy.[10,30,52] The report of a diffuse, large cell lymphoma arising within thyroid tissue of a mature cystic teratoma suggests a plausible, but probably rare, histogenesis.[72]

In patients with apparent initial gonadal disease only, or with a dominant ovarian tumor and minor disease elsewhere (e.g. peritoneal) consistent with the pattern of spread expected in primary ovarian neoplasms, staging procedures reveal that in 27 to 64% the disease is more advanced than FIGO Stage I.[10,51,52]

Presentation is similar to that of other ovarian tumors, namely abdominal or pelvic mass, often accompanied by pain. Ascites is not unusual. Less commonly, the tumors are incidental findings at routine pelvic examination or surgery for other indications.[26,51]

The age of patients with malignant lymphoma initially manifest in the ovaries is similar to that of patients with equivalent nodal disease. This varies more in relation to the histological type than the anatomical site affected. Thus, diffuse lymphomas are most common in the 35 to 45 year age group, while nodular lymphomas are more often found in older women. First presentation may occur during pregnancy.[26,37,67] Burkitt's lymphoma (both endemic and sporadic) typically affects children in the 5 to 10 year age group.[9]

A large recent study (40 cases) of lymphoma presenting in the ovaries reported a 5-year survival rate of 35%, with most deaths occurring in the first 2 years. The outlook was better in patients with Stage Ia disease or unilateral tumors of any stage. These authors considered that the relatively poor prognosis of 'primary' ovarian lymphomas compared with other Stage Ie (Ann Arbor) extra-nodal lymphomas could be due in part to the high proportion of diffuse lymphomas.[51] In the analysis of 34 cases by Fox et al,[26] 19 patients died (15 in the first year). Poor prognostic factors were: the rapid onset of abdominal symptoms, presence of systemic symptoms, bilateral tumors, advanced stage, and histological type other than B-cell lymphoma.

Pathology

Malignant lymphomas presenting as ovarian disease are bilateral in 50% of cases, irrespective of stage.[10,51,67,71] Burkitt's lymphoma is almost always bilateral.[9] The ovarian tumors range from 2 to 25 cm in diameter, with most in the range of 8 to 15 cm. In disseminated lymphoma affecting the ovaries, the latter may be of normal size or only slightly enlarged.[83]

The ovaries are usually free of adhesions and show a nodular or bosselated surface. The cut surface shows uniform pale grayish white to tan tissue with a rubbery or fleshy consistency. Gross edema was present in a recent case of Burkitt's lymphoma at our institution (Fig. 61.16). Small foci of necrosis, cystic degeneration and hemorrhage may be present, but they are rarely conspicuous features. Although the ovaries appear to be preferentially infiltrated relative to the remainder of the female genital tract,[67] other organs, especially the adjacent fallopian tubes, may also appear swollen and edematous owing to peritoneal or interstitial infiltration.

Histologically, there is a diffuse monotonous infiltrate of neoplastic lymphoid cells with a superimposed nodularity in selected subtypes (Fig. 61.17). The infiltrate of diffuse lymphomas often forms cords, sometimes only one cell thick. The malignant cells may infiltrate and surround structures, such as pre-existing follicles, corpora lutea and corpora albicantes, without destroying them; blood vessel walls are also invaded in this way. The nodular lymphomas may demonstrate bands of fibrous tissue or even dense sclerotic areas. Microscopic foci of necrosis, in addition to those evident macroscopically, may be seen. In high grade tumors with rapid cell turnover, such as diffuse large cell, lymphoblastic and, especially, Burkitt's lymphoma, the presence of large macrophages dispersed amongst the tumor cells leads to a 'starry-sky' appearance. The cytology of the lymphomatous cells is that of the corresponding lesions in lymph nodes. Lymphoma cells are EMA-negative and leucocyte-common-antigen-(LCA) positive by immunohistochemical techniques — characteristics shared by the leukemias. To distinguish the various subtypes of malignant lymphoma, special stains may be necessary, for example methyl green pyronin and immunohistochemical stains for immunoglobulins, light chains and T- and B-cell markers (some of the latter require frozen sections of fresh tumor tissue). Imprint preparations from fresh tumor tis-

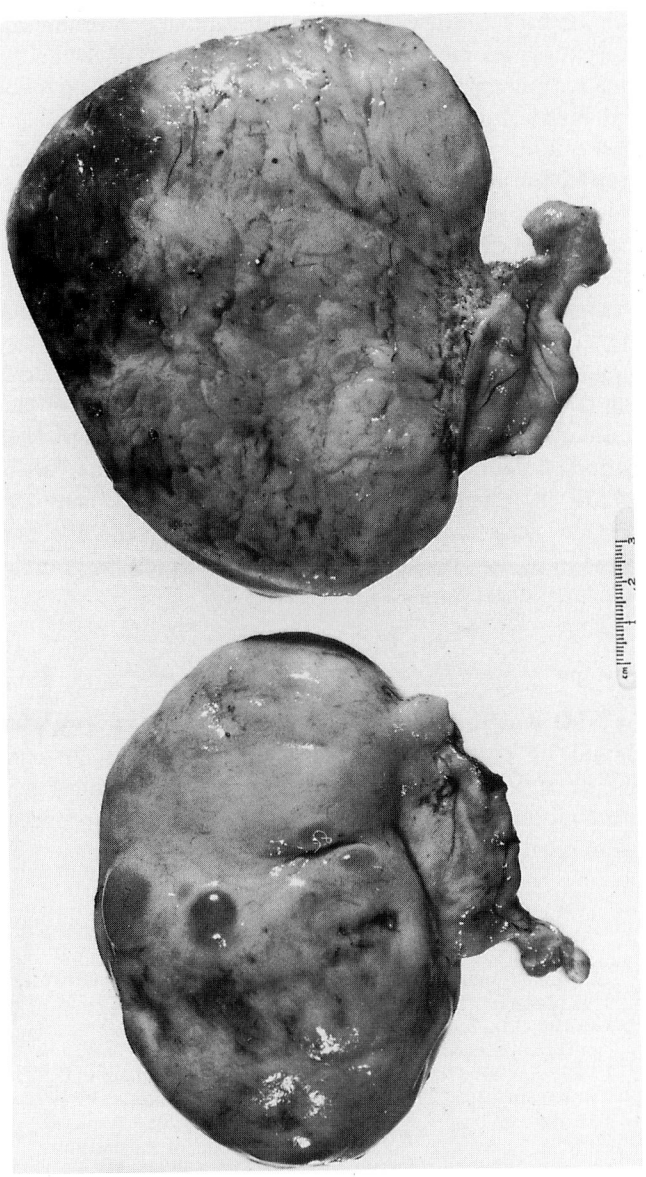

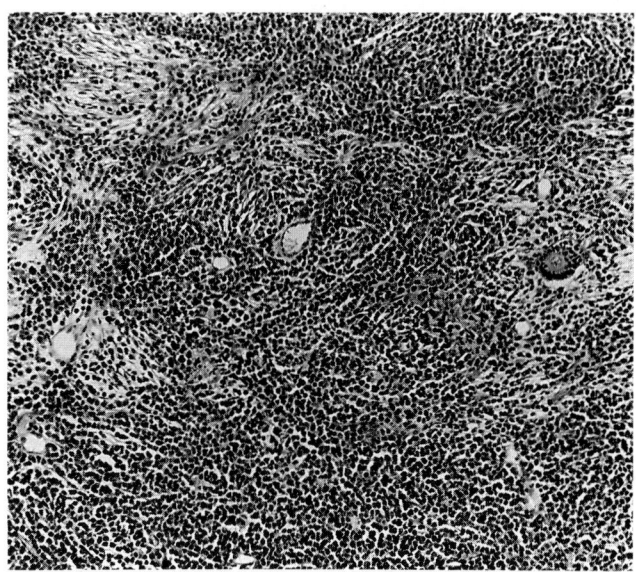

Fig. 61.17 Malignant lymphoma (Burkitt's lymphoma; same patient as in Fig. 61.16). Monotonous infiltrate of uniform lymphoid cells, focally in linear arrangements. A primary follicle is noted at right. (H&E; ×53)

Fig. 61.16 Burkitt's lymphoma presenting as bilateral ovarian masses in a 16-year-old girl. The cut surface (top) shows uniformly edematous fleshy tumor tissue with focal hemorrhage.

sue may be very useful; Romanowsky-stained slides will be helpful in identifying the cytoplasmic lipid vacuoles in Burkitt's lymphoma and also the granules of leukemic cells.

Referral centers have found that the diagnosis of ovarian lymphomas is often missed initially, and that misdiagnosis is frequently the result, in part, of poor histological technique.[51] The non-hematopoietic tumors most commonly confused with lymphomas are granulosa cell tumors and dysgerminomas; others are metastatic carcinomas and primary undifferentiated small cell carcinoma. In children,

embryonal rhabdomyosarcoma and neuroblastoma may also have to be considered.

Therapy

The rarity of ovarian lymphoma as a clinical entity has hindered development of treatment protocols. The most recent treatment data relates to a series of 34 lymphomas presenting as ovarian tumors and submitted to the Ovarian Tumor Panel of the Royal College of Obstetricians and Gynaecologists.[26] Two of 6 patients treated by surgery alone were alive 22 and 3 years later; one of 5 patients receiving surgery plus radiotherapy was alive, whilst 6 of 10 having postoperative chemotherapy were alive. Patients treated by both postoperative radiotherapy and chemotherapy had no survival advantage over those having chemotherapy alone. It is probable, therefore, that surgery plus chemotherapy offers the best prognosis.

Although true primary ovarian lymphomas can rarely occur, lymphoproliferative disorders diagnosed initially in the ovaries should always be considered, for therapeutic purposes, as probable manifestations of systemic disease and treated accordingly.

Leukemias

Clinical features

Ovarian infiltration occurs more commonly in patients

with leukemias than in those with lymphomas, and is more often seen in children than in adults. Ovarian infiltration at autopsy has been found in up to 66% of leukemic patients.[9,65,83] The more recent studies have yielded higher rates, possibly reflecting longer survival times with modern therapeutic regimes. However, any clinical enlargement of the ovaries in leukemic patients is rare. Myeloid leukemias are encountered more frequently than the lymphocytic types.[7,71,83] An ovarian tumor may be the initial presentation of leukemia, or herald a relapse.[7,49,51] Extramedullary tumor-like masses of leukemic cells are called granulocytic sarcomas (formerly called chloromas because of their greenish hue). Hematological investigations usually reveal leukemia but, rarely, a leukemic picture may not develop for some time and even be absent at the time of death, although the bone marrow may reveal infiltration.[10,71] The prognosis of leukemias initially presenting as an ovarian tumor is poor,[51] as it is for other extramedullary lesions, and generalized disease develops within a few months.[47]

Pathology

Leukemic ovaries do not differ from those of lymphomas, although some tumors have a greenish tinge best seen when the tissue is fresh. Bilateral involvement is frequent. The histological features can closely mimic those of ovarian lymphomas. Diffuse monotonous cellular infiltrates are present, sometimes with cord-like formations as in the diffuse lymphomas. Leukemic infiltrates may also surround and invade follicular structures without destroying them. In the autopsy study of Reid et al,[65] most involved ovaries showed preservation of oocytes. The nuclear features are those of the corresponding blast cells in the leukemic bone marrow. The folded nuclei of myeloid leukemic cells may imitate the cleft, or irregularly shaped, nuclei of some lymphomas. In myeloid leukemias, cytoplasmic granulation may be apparent in the hematoxylin- and eosin-stained sections, but identification can be aided by periodic acid-Schiff or Giemsa stains, which will highlight neutrophilic and eosinophilic precursors respectively. Imprints of fresh tumor tissue stained by a Romanowsky technique can be useful in identifying cytoplasmic granules, and also provide very clear nuclear cytological detail. Electron microscopy can be used to search for the sparse granules of poorly differentiated leukemias.

Therapy

As with lymphomas, ovarian manifestations of leukemias should be regarded as local manifestations of systemic disease and treated accordingly. Surgery (by definition, a prerequisite to diagnosis) with postoperative appropriate chemotherapy is the treatment of choice.

REFERENCES

1. Azoury R S, Woodruff J D 1971 Primary ovarian sarcomas. Report of 43 cases from the Emil Novak ovarian tumor registry. Obstet Gynecol 37: 920
2. Bare W W, McCloskey J F 1961 Primary Hodgkin's disease of the ovary. Report of a case. Obstet Gynecol 17: 477
3. Barlow J J, Piver M S, Chuang T T, Cortes E P, Ohnuma T, Holland J F 1973 Adriamycin and bleomycin, alone and in combination in gynecologic cancers. Cancer 32: 735
4. Barwick K W, LiVolsi V A 1980 Malignant mixed mesodermal tumors of the ovary. A clinicopathologic assessment of 12 cases. Am J Surg Pathol 4: 37
5. Battifora H 1973 Hemangiopericytoma: ultrastructural study of five cases. Cancer 31: 1418
6. Carlson J A Jr, Edwards C, Wharton J T, Gallager H S, Delclos L, Rutledge F 1983 Mixed mesodermal sarcoma of the ovary. Treatment with combination radiation therapy and chemotherapy. Cancer 52: 1473
7. Chan E Y C, Glassberg A B, Rosenblum M A 1980 Chloroma. Rare manifestation of acute leukemia. Postgrad Med 67: 125
8. Chen K T K, Hendricks E J, Freeburg B 1982 Benign glandular inclusions of the peritoneum associated with leiomyomatosis peritonealis disseminata. Diag Gynecol Obstet 4: 41
9. Chorlton I 1987 Malignant lymphoma of the female genital tract and ovaries. In: Fox H (ed) Haines and Taylor Obstetrical and Gynaecological Pathology, 3rd edn. Churchill Livingstone, Edinburgh, p 737
10. Chorlton I, Norris H J, King F M 1974 Malignant reticuloendothelial disease involving the ovary as a primary manifestation. A series of 19 lymphomas and 1 granulocytic sarcoma. Cancer 34: 307
11. Clement P B, Scully R E 1974 Müllerian adenosarcoma of the uterus. A clinicopathologic analysis of ten cases of a distinctive type of müllerian mixed tumor. Cancer 34: 1138
12. Clement P B, Scully R E 1978 Extrauterine mesodermal (müllerian) adenosarcoma. Am J Clin Pathol 69: 276
13. Climie A R W, Heath L P 1968 Malignant degeneration of benign cystic teratomas of the ovary; review of the literature and report of a chondrosarcoma and carcinoid tumor. Cancer 22: 824
14. Cook H T, Boylston A W 1988 Plasmacytoma of the ovary. Gynecol Oncol 29: 378
15. Dehner L P, Norris H J, Taylor H B 1971 Carcinosarcomas and mixed mesodermal tumors of the ovary. Cancer 27: 207
16. Dickersin G R, Kline I W, Scully R E 1982 Small cell carcinoma of the ovary with hypercalcemia: a report of eleven cases. Cancer 49: 188
17. Dictor M 1985 Malignant mixed mesodermal tumor of the ovary: a report of 22 cases. Obstet Gynecol 65: 720
18. DiOrio J, Lowe L C 1980 Hemangioma of the ovary in pregnancy. A case report. J Reprod Med 24: 232
19. Dover H 1950 Neurofibrosarcoma of the ovary associated with neurofibromatosis. Can Med Assoc J 63: 488
20. Ebrahimi T, Goldsmith J W, Okagaki T 1971 Hemangioma of the ovary. A case report. Obstet Gynecol 38: 677
21. Enzinger F, Smith B H 1976 Hemangiopericytoma: an analysis of 106 cases. Hum Pathol 7: 61
22. Exelby P R, Ghavimi F, Jereb B 1978 Genitourinary rhabdomyosarcoma in children. J Ped Surg 13: 746
23. Fallahzadeh H, Dockerty M B, Lee R A 1972 Leiomyoma of the ovary: report of five cases and review of the literature. Am J Obstet Gynecol 113: 394
24. Flamanat F, Chassagne D, Cosset J, Gerbaulet A, Lemerle J 1979 Embryonal rhabdomyosarcoma of the vagina in children: conservative treatment with curietherapy and chemotherapy. Euro J Cancer 15: 527

25. Fox H, Langley F A 1976 Tumours of the ovary. Heinemann, London, p 278
26. Fox H, Langley F A, Govan A D T, Hill S A, Bennett M H 1988 Malignant lymphoma presenting as an ovarian tumour: a clinicopathological analysis of 34 cases. Br J Obstet Gynaecol 95: 386
27. Freeman C, Berg J W, Cutler S J 1972 Occurrence and prognosis of extranodal lymphomas. Cancer 29: 252
28. Genadry R, Parmley T, Woodruff J D 1979 Secondary malignancies in benign cystic teratomas. Gynecol Oncol 8: 246
29. Gottlieb J A, Baker L H, O'Bryan R M et al 1975 Adriamycin (NSC-123127) used alone, and in combination for soft tissue and bony sarcomas. Cancer Chemo Rep (Part 3) 6: 271
30. Halpin T F 1975 Gynecologic implications of Burkitt's tumor. Obstet Gynecol Surv 30: 351
31. Hanjani P, Petersen R P, Lipton S E, Nolte S A 1983 Malignant mixed mesodermal tumors and carcinosarcoma of the ovary: report of eight cases and review of literature. Obstet Gynecol Surv 38: 537
32. Hart W R, Yoonessi M 1977 Endometrial stromatosis of the uterus. Obstet Gynecol 49: 393
33. Hautzer N W 1984 Primary plasmacytoma of ovary. Gynecol Oncol 18: 115
34. Hendrickson M R, Kempson R L 1980 Surgical Pathology of the Uterine Corpus. Saunders, Philadelphia, p 389
35. Hoovis M L 1970 Response of endometrial stromal sarcoma to cyclophosphamide. Am J Obstet Gynecol 108: 1117
36. Janovski N A, Paramanandhan T L 1973 Ovarian Tumors. Tumors and Tumor-like Conditions of the Ovaries, Fallopian Tubes and Ligaments of the Uterus. Saunders, Philadelphia, p 46
37. Jones D E D, d'Avignon M B, Lawrence R, Latshaw R F 1980 Burkitt's lymphoma: obstetric and gynecologic aspects. Obstet Gynecol 56: 533
38. Kanter A E, Zummo B P 1956 Lipomas of gynecologic interest. Am J Obstet Gynecol 71: 376
39. Kao G F, Norris H J 1978 Benign and low grade variants of mixed mesodermal tumor (adenosarcoma) of the ovary and adnexal region. Cancer 42: 1314
40. Kuo T-T, London S N, Dinh T V 1980 Endometriosis occurring in leiomyomatosis peritonealis disseminata. Ultrastructural study and histogenetic consideration. Am J Surg Pathol 4: 197
41. Lawhead R A, Copeland L J, Edwards C L 1985 Bilateral ovarian hemangiomas associated with diffuse abdominopelvic hemangiomatosis. Obstet Gynecol 65: 597
42. Lehner L M, Miles P A, Enck R E 1979 Complete remission of widely metastatic endometrial stromal sarcoma following combination chemotherapy. Cancer 43: 1189
43. Long J P, Patchefsky A S 1971 Primary Hodgkin's disease of the ovary. A case report. Obstet Gynecol 38: 680
44. Moore M, Fine S, Sturgeon J 1986 Malignant mixed mesodermal (MMM) tumors of the ovary: the Princess Margaret Hospital (PMH) experience (abstract). Proc Am Soc Clin Oncol 5: 114
45. Morrow C P, d'Ablaing G, Brady L W, Blessing J A, Hreshchyshyn M M 1984 A clinical and pathologic study of 30 cases of malignant mixed müllerian epithelial and mesenchymal ovarian tumors: A Gynecologic Oncology Group study. Gynecol Oncol 18: 278
46. Mukai K, Varela-Duran J, Nochomovitz L E 1980 The rhabdomyoblast in mixed müllerian tumors of the uterus and ovary: an immunohistochemical study of myoglobin in 25 cases. Am J Clin Pathol 74: 101
47. Neiman R S, Barcos M, Berard C et al 1981 Granulocytic sarcoma: a clinicopathologic study of 61 biopsied cases. Cancer 48: 1426
48. Norgaad M, Hansborg N, Fischer-Rasmussen W 1985 Malignant hemangiopericytoma of the ovary. Acta Obstet Gynecol Scand 64: 87
49. Obeid D, Cotter P, Sturdee D W 1979 Acute leukaemia relapse presenting as ovarian tumour. Br J Obstet Gynaecol 86: 578
50. Ortega J 1979 A therapeutic approach to childhood pelvic rhabdomyosarcoma without pelvic exenteration. J Pediat 94: 205
51. Osborne B M, Robboy S J 1983 Lymphomas or leukemia presenting as ovarian tumors. An analysis of 42 cases. Cancer 52: 1933
52. Paladugu R R, Bearman R M, Rappaport H 1980 Malignant lymphoma with primary manifestation in the gonad. A clinicopathologic study of 38 patients. Cancer 45: 561
53. Pantoja E, Rodriguez-Ibanez I, Axtmayer R W, Noy M A, Pelegrina I 1975 Complications of dermoid tumors of the ovary. Obstet Gynecol 45: 89
54. Parish J M, Lufkin E G, Lee R A, Gaffey T A 1984 Ovarian leiomyoma with hilus cell hyperplasia that caused virilization. Mayo Clin Proc 59: 275
55. Peterson W F 1957 Malignant degeneration of benign cystic teratomas of the ovary. A collective review of the literature. Obstet Gynecol Surv 12: 793
56. Piver M S, Barlow J J, Lele S B, Yagazi R 1979 Adriamycin in localized and metastatic uterine sarcomas. J Surg Oncol 12: 263
57. Piver M S, Lurain J R 1981 Uterine sarcomas. Clinical features and management. In: Coppleson M (ed) Gynecologic Oncology. Churchill Livingstone, New York, p 608
58. Prat J, Scully R E 1979a Ovarian mucinous tumors with sarcoma-like mural nodules. A report of seven cases. Cancer 44: 1332
59. Prat J, Scully R E 1979b Sarcomas in ovarian mucinous tumors. A report of two cases. Cancer 44: 1321
60. Prat J, Scully R E 1986 Ovarian sarcomas and related tumors. A clinicopathologic analysis of 98 cases (Abst.). Lab Invest 54: 50a
61. Pratt C B 1969 Response of childhood rhabdomyosarcoma to combination chemotherapy. J Pediat 74: 791
62. Ramos Martinez E, Rodriguez Muguel L, Quijano Narezo M, Santiago Payan H 1983 Condromo primario del ovario. Informe de un caso. Ginecol Obstet Mex 51: 95
63. Raney R B Jr, Crist W M, Maurer H M, Foulkes M A 1983 Prognosis of children with soft tissue sarcoma who relapse after achieving a complete response. A report from the Intergroup Rhabdomyosarcoma Study 1. Cancer 52: 44
64. Rayek A A, Peres C A, Lee F A, Ragab A H, Askin F, Vietti T 1977 Combined treatment modalities of rhabdomyosarcoma in children. Cancer 39: 2415
65. Reid H, Marsden H B 1980 Gonadal infiltration in children with leukaemia and lymphoma. J Clin Pathol 33: 722
66. Rice M, Pearson B, Treadwell W B 1943 Malignant lymphangioma of the ovary. Am J Obstet Gynecol 45: 884
67. Rotmensch J, Woodruff J D 1982 Lymphoma of the ovary: report of twenty new cases and update of previous series. Am J Obstet Gynecol 143: 870
68. Rubin S C, Wheeler J E, Mikuta J J 1986 Malignant leiomyomatosis peritonealis disseminata. Obstet Gynecol 68: 126
69. Russell P, Slavutin L, Laverty C R, Cooper-Booth J 1979 Extrauterine mesodermal (Müllerian) adenosarcoma. A case report. Pathol 11: 557
70. Sandison A T 1955 Rhabdomyosarcoma of the ovary. J Pathol Bacteriol 70: 433
71. Scully R E 1979 Tumors of the Ovary and Maldeveloped Gonads (AFIP Fascicle 16, Second Series). Armed Forces Institute of Pathology, Washington, p 53
72. Seifer D B, Weiss L M, Kempson R L 1986 Malignant lymphoma arising within thyroid tissue in a mature cystic teratoma. Cancer 58: 2459
73. Serov S F, Scully R E, Sobin L H 1973 Histological Typing of Ovarian Tumours (International histological classification of tumours No. 9). World Health Organization, Geneva, p 17
74. Shakfeh S M, Woodruff J D 1987 Primary ovarian sarcomas: report of 46 cases and review of the literature. Obstet Gynecol Surv 42: 331
75. Shetty M R, Boghossian H M, Duffell D, Freel R, Gonzales J C 1982 Tumor-induced hypoglycemia. A result of ectopic insulin production. Cancer 49: 1920
76. Shipton E A, Meares S D 1965 Heterotopic bone formation in the ovary. Aust NZ J Obstet Gynaecol 5: 100
77. Silverberg S G, Fernandez F N 1981 Endolymphatic stromal myosis of the ovary. A report of three cases and literature review. Gynecol Oncol 12: 129

78. Smith F R 1931 Neurofibroma of the ovary associated with von Recklinghausen's disease. Am J Cancer 15: 859

79. Stamp G W H, McConell E M 1983 Malignancy arising in cystic ovarian teratomas. A report of 24 cases. Br J Obstet Gynaecol 90: 671

80. Stone G C, Bell D A, Fuller A, Dickersin G R, Scully R E 1986 Malignant schwannoma of the ovary. Report of a case. Cancer 58: 1575

81. Stowe L M, Watt J Y 1952 Osteogenic sarcoma of the ovary. Am J Obstet Gynecol 64: 422

82. Susil B J, Sumithran E 1987 Sarcomatous change in granulosa cell tumor. Hum Pathol 18: 397

83. Talerman A 1982 Mesenchymal tumors and malignant lymphoma of the ovary. In: Blaustein A (ed) Pathology of the Female Genital Tract, 2nd edn. Springer-Verlag, New York, p 561

84. Talerman A, Auerbach W M, van Meurs A J 1981 Primary chondrosarcoma of the ovary. Histopathol 5: 319

85. Tavassoli F A, Norris H J 1982 Peritoneal leiomyomatosis (leiomyomatosis peritonealis disseminata): a clinicopathologic study of 20 cases with ultrastructural observations. Int J Gynecol Pathol 1: 59

86. Thatcher S S, Woodruff J D 1982 Uterine stromatosis. A report of 33 cases. Obstet Gynecol 59: 428

87. Tsalacopoulos G, Tiltman A J 1981 Leiomyoma of the ovary. A report of 3 cases. S Afric Med J 59: 574

88. Ueda G, Sato Y, Yamasaki M et al 1977 Malignant fibrous histiocytoma arising in a benign cystic teratoma of the ovary. Gynecol Oncol 5: 313

89. Ulbright T M, Roth L M, Stehman F B 1984 Secondary ovarian neoplasia; a clinicopathologic study of 35 cases. Cancer 53: 1164

90. Walley V M 1983 Leiomyomatosis peritonealis disseminata. Int J Gynecol Pathol 2: 222

91. Yap B S, Baker L H, Sinkovics J G et al 1980 Cyclophosphamide, vincristine, adriamycin and DTIC (CYVADIC) combination chemotherapy for the treatment of advanced sarcomas. Cancer Treat Rep 64: 93

92. Young R H, Prat J, Scully R E 1984 Endometrioid stromal sarcomas of the ovary. A clinicopathologic analysis of 23 cases. Cancer 53: 1143

62. Metastatic tumors of ovary

R. T. Parker   J. L. Currie

INTRODUCTION

Malignant neoplasms frequently find the ovary a fertile ground for metastasis, and virtually any cancer can establish secondary growth in the female gonad. Approximately 10 to 30% of reported ovarian cancers are metastatic, and diagnosis and management continue to be a problem.

Despite the importance of this group of cancers, considerable confusion still exists regarding their terminology, classification, and incidence. Entwined in this confusion is the classic eponym 'Krukenberg tumor.' Ironically, Krukenberg's original report[38] in 1896 of six tumors was an accurate description of metastatic gastrointestinal cancer to the ovary, but he considered them to be primary connective tissue tumors and thus his original term fibrosarcoma ovarii mucocellulare (carcinomatodes) was a misnomer. Although Schlagenhaufer in 1902 correctly analyzed Krukenberg's original tumor as being epithelial in origin and metastatic,[52] probably from the gastrointestinal tract, the Krukenberg name became linked in perpetuity with metastatic cancer to the ovary. For many clinicians, any secondary cancer in the ovary is synonymous with the 'Krukenberg tumor.' Woodruff & Novak[69] attempted to clarify this confusion by adhering to the histologic criteria of Krukenberg, that is, the presence of (1) tumor in the ovary, (2) intracellular mucin production with the microscopic picture of the signet ring cells, and (3) diffuse sarcomatoid infiltration of ovarian stroma. These criteria did not require that the primary lesion originate in the gastrointestinal tract, as would be more specifically compatible with the signet ring cell (stomach). This departure from the strict metastatic phenomenon allows the inclusion of the so-called 'primary Krukenberg tumor.' The latter, as a distinct entity, has been reported frequently[16,34,69] and its origin said to be from totipotential müllerian or mesothelial epithelium. To use the eponym, Krukenberg, for the primary mucus producing adenocarcinoma only tends to confuse the clinician. Thus, the term Krukenberg tumor probably should be deleted, unless it is accompanied by a precise description of what it is intended to describe.

The relative incidence of metastatic ovarian cancer is quite difficult to establish accurately, and figures vary greatly from 10 to 30%. Webb, Decker & Mussey[66] found 357 (28%) cancers metastatic to the ovary among 1285 ovarian malignancies from 1950 to 1966 at the Mayo Clinic. Israel, Helsel & Hausman[32] reported that 28% of 87 ovarian neoplasms were secondary, and six patients could not be classified. Woodruff and associates[68] reported 120 metastatic tumors from the files of the Emil Novak Ovarian Tumor Registry; these authors made no effort to establish the frequency of such occurrences and did not include 50 Krukenberg tumors reported earlier from 1700 ovarian cancers in the Registry at that time.[69] In the Duke Medical Center study there were 132 patients with cancer metastatic to the ovary among approximately 1350 ovarian cancer patients treated, a much lower frequency of 10%.[13,50] During the 40 years of this study (1950 to 1989), the occurrence rate has remained in the 10% range for cancers metastatic to the ovary, while the incidence of primary ovarian cancer has doubled due to the referral practice.

Autopsy studies suggest that metastatic cancers in the ovary are more frequent than primary ones.[32,33] Of 1000 autopsied patients dying of epithelial tumors, Abrams[1] found 11% had metastatic disease in the ovaries, while 6.4% had primary ovarian cancers. Karsh[35] reported 72 (0.7%) patients who had cancer metastatic to the ovary among 10 287 consecutive autopsies. Hundley[31] found only 11 cases in 11 200 autopsies. Random autopsy series are apt to find a low incidence of metastatic cancer to the ovary, while autopsy studies on patients dying of cancer report a high frequency of secondary ovarian disease.

Since many ovaries containing metastatic foci are normal in gross appearance, careful microscopic analysis is essential to discover occult metastasis.

OVERVIEW OF CANCER METASTATIC TO OVARY

Site of primary tumor

Approximately three-fourths of patients who have cancer metastatic to the ovaries will have the primary originating

Table 62.1 Cancer metastatic to the ovary: sites of primary tumor

Primary cancers	Webb[66] (1975)	Woodruff[b68] (1970)	Israel[32] (1965)	Parker (1989)
Gastrointestinal	169 (47%)	24 (20%)	12 (36%)	42 (32%)
Breast	109 (31%)	16 (14%)	13 (39%)	28 (21%)
Uterine body[a]	44 (12%)	32 (27%)	5 (15%)	28 (21%)
Other	35 (<10%)	48 (40%)	3 (9%)	34 (26%)
Total (n)	357	120	33	132

[a] Includes uterine sarcomas
[b] Does not include 50 Krukenberg tumors

in the gastrointestinal tract, breast or uterus. Although figures for each of these primary sites vary in large series, the overall proportion of the three is consistent. Table 62.1 shows an occurrence rate in the studies noted, of a low of 20% to a high of 47% for primary lesions in the gastrointestinal tract, 14 to 39% for breast, and 12 to 27% for uterine body. Other primary tumors metastatic to the ovary in the Duke study are: melanoma, 9 patients; lymphoma, 6; squamous carcinoma of cervix, 3; lung, 3; one patient each of kidney, bladder, gallduct, angiosarcoma of heart, carcinoid and choriocarcinoma; and of unknown origin, 7 patients.

Age and parity

Patients with metastatic ovarian cancer from the breast and gastrointestinal tract generally are younger than patients with primary epithelial cancer of the ovary, and significantly younger than patients with metastatic endometrial cancer to the ovaries.[13] When the diagnosis of secondary ovarian cancer is related to menopause, more than 50% of patients will be postmenopausal at the time of diagnosis, with the exception of patients with breast cancer, where it is reported that up to 83% of patients who have metastatic breast cancer in the ovary develop it prior to menopause.[66] In assessing the younger patient with probable ovarian cancer, the possibility of metastatic disease from another primary always must be kept in mind.

There seems to be no relationship between the development of cancer metastatic to the ovaries and parity.

Symptoms

Patients with secondary ovarian cancer may, like those with early primary ovarian cancer, be asymptomatic, or may present with vague and non-specific symptoms. Patients with primary disease in the gastrointestinal tract are more apt to have symptoms of weight loss, pelvic pain, abdominal fullness and bowel complaints. Although most patients with endometrial carcinoma metastatic to the ovaries have abnormal bleeding, this symptom is usually caused by the primary endometrial growth. Patients with breast cancer metastatic to the ovaries are likely to have no pelvic complaints.[13] Occasionally, patients with marked enlargement of the ovaries due to metastatic cancer from the gastrointestinal tract may have symptoms of acute pelvic pain, pelvic heaviness, and the presence of rapidly enlarging ovarian masses. This is thought to be secondary to massive obstruction of lymphatics by tumor emboli with resultant accumulation of edema fluid, and has been termed the 'acute Krukenberg syndrome.'[33]

Interval from primary diagnosis to secondary ovarian cancer

Metastatic cancer to the ovaries of uterine origin is most apt to be recognized at the time of diagnosis of the initial cancer, because removal of the ovaries is standard surgical procedure along with total abdominal hysterectomy. On the other hand, there is often a significant interval between the diagnosis of metastatic ovarian cancer from breast and gastrointestinal primaries and the time of original diagnosis. Approximately 65% of patients with gastrointestinal metastatic disease will have the ovarian metastasis diagnosed at the time of original surgery; the interval for the remaining patients may be quite lengthy, as long as several years. Fully one-fourth of the patients in the Mayo Clinic study had the secondary tumors diagnosed greater than 1 year after the diagnosis of primary.[66] In the Duke Medical Center experience, if the secondary disease was not diagnosed at the time of the primary, the mean interval between the diagnosis of the primary and secondary was 22 months, with the longest interval 51 months. Similarly, unless castration accompanies the original breast operation, the diagnosis of secondary breast disease in the ovaries may be many months after the primary diagnosis. The mean interval to secondary diagnosis of metastatic ovarian cancer from breast primary was 12 months, with a range of 2 to 74 months. Table 62.2 demonstrates the interval from primary diagnosis to diagnosis of secondary ovarian cancer in the Duke study. In the last 10 years since the data were gathered for the first edition of this volume, the mean interval between the diagnosis of the primary cancers and the secondary ovarian cancers has been shortened, an improvement resulting from more frequent use of ultrasound and computerized tomography studies to characterize question-

Table 62.2 Interval from primary diagnosis to diagnosis of secondary ovarian cancer[a]

Primary sites	Metastatic cancer to ovaries diagnosed at the time of primary diagnosis	Mean interval between diagnosis of the primary cancer and secondary ovarian cancer (if not concurrent with primary)
Gastrointestinal	65%	22 months
Breast	27%	12 months
Uterine	90%	5 months
Other	30%	40 months

[a] Duke Medical Center study.

able enlargement of an ovary. The diagnostic feature is the complex ovarian mass (cystic and/or solid), rather than a distinct difference between the image of a primary and a secondary ovarian tumor.[3,10,43,57]

It is apparent that long intervals between the diagnosis of the primary malignancy and the ovarian metastasis are not uncommon, especially with breast and gastrointestinal primaries. Thus, a remote history of cancer of the breast or the gastrointestinal tract should elicit strong suspicion of metastatic disease of the ovary whenever an abnormal pelvic examination or abnormal bleeding are encountered.

Diagnosis

The definitive diagnosis of metastatic cancer to the ovary is a surgical diagnosis. The presence of an adnexal mass on examination, or as suggested by the roentgenographic studies of the large bowel or urinary tract, is almost never a definitive diagnosis for metastatic ovarian cancer, and usually mandates celiotomy. Almost half of the patients with metastatic ovarian cancer will have the diagnosis established at the time of exploratory surgery for an unknown pelvic mass. Approximately one-fourth of the patients who have gastrointestinal primaries will have ovarian metastases found at the time of planned surgery. Almost all patients with ovarian extension of endometrial cancer will have this diagnosis made at the time of the initial operation. Prophylactic oophorectomy is usually the method of diagnosis of metastatic breast cancer to the ovary.[36,41,62] Metastatic ovarian cancer may not be diagnosed until autopsy.

Gross pathology (surgical findings)

The classic picture of metastatic ovarian cancer is that of the Krukenberg tumor with bilateral involvement of the ovaries, with tumor masses that symmetrically enlarge the ovaries, retaining the overall ovarian outline (Fig. 62.1). The capsules are quite friable and easily ruptured.

Three types of gross ovarian pathology may be expected:

(1) patients with asymptomatic microscopic metastases, most likely to be metastatic from breast primary, found at the time of ablative oophorectomy but occasionally seen in endometrial carcinoma; (2) patients with the typical Krukenberg tumor described above, usually recognized months after the gastrointestinal primary; and (3) patients with widespread abdominal carcinomatosis at the time of diagnosis of metastatic ovarian cancer.[13] Approximately one in five patients with metastatic ovarian cancer will have malignant effusion, either pleural or ascitic, at the time of diagnosis. In patients with lymphomatous involvement of the ovary, there is frequently chylous ascites.

Microscopic pathology

Microscopic studies of metastatic ovarian cancer can be a challenge to the pathologist. There can be wide variations in patterns, and often the distortion produced by the small foci of metastasis and the accompanying stromal reaction in the ovary can make comparison with the primary tumor difficult. In general, the presence of intracytoplasmic secretion with compression of the chromatin associated with an infiltrated, edematous, or reactive stroma is indicative of metastatic neoplasm,[68] and this pattern is usually associated with a primary in the gastrointestinal tract (Fig. 62.2).

For patients with an endometrial primary, the characteristic adenocarcinoma of the endometrium with papillations and mucus-secreting epithelium is common. Occasionally, a clear cell pattern is present. When both the primary endometrial carcinoma and the secondary ovarian tumor are well differentiated, the possibility of multicentric primary is raised (Fig. 62.3).

Breast carcinoma varies most in microscopic pattern, with the earliest metastases characterized by cords of tumor cells reminiscent of an arrhenoblastoma. At other times, breast cancers can show a definite adenomatous lesion of the ductal variety or, more unusually, a lymphomatous infiltration with the epithelial elements obscured. The common adenoid patterns show variations but occasionally simulate lobular carcinoma. All of the tumor cell infiltrates can stimulate ovarian stromal proliferation, and this may further confuse the picture (Fig. 62.4).

The typical Krukenberg tumor with signet ring cells and infiltration of the stroma is one of several microscopic presentations of gastrointestinal metastasis (Fig. 62.5). Occasionally, the metastasis is a characteristic primary mucus-secreting tumor, which can be confused with primary mucinous carcinoma of the ovary. Less common features from gastrointestinal primaries are the cord-like patterns typical of breast cancer, occasionally with small acini and a Brenner-like stromal pattern.[68] The similarities between granulosa cell tumors and metastatic carcinoid may make this diagnosis difficult to establish.

Considering metastasis from other sites, it is usual that

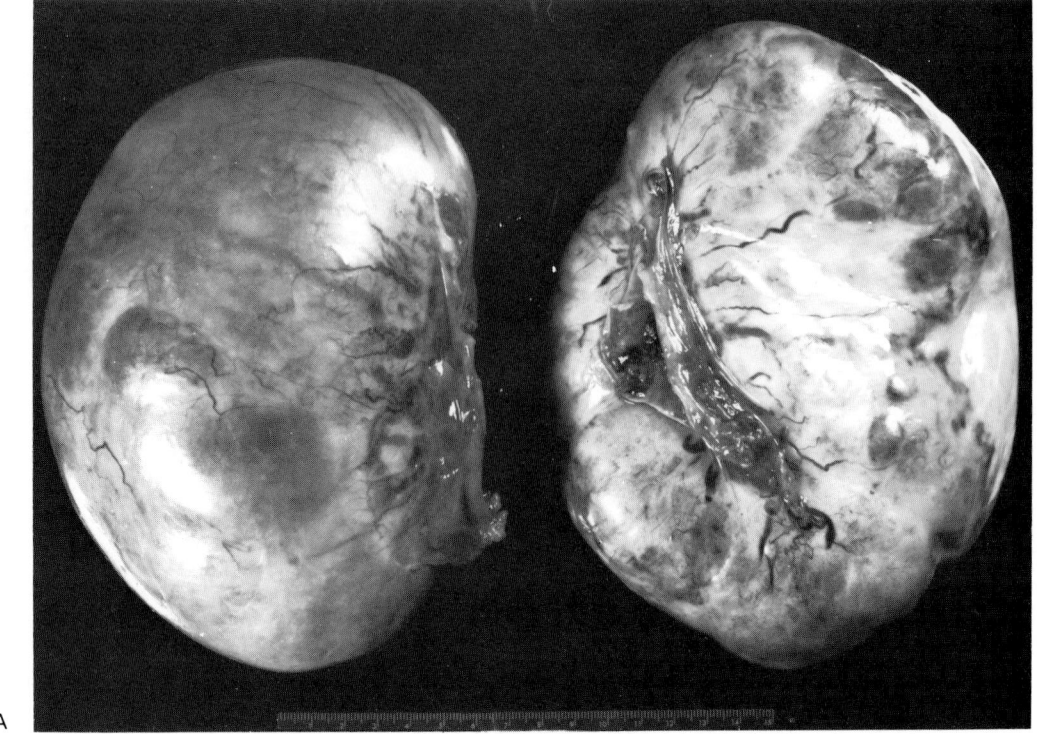

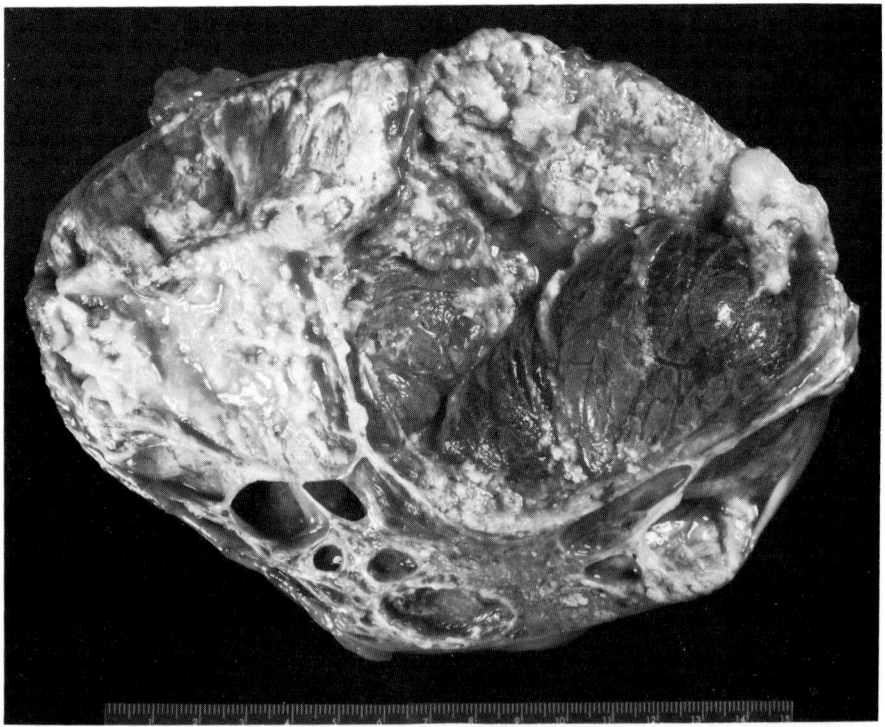

Fig. 62.1 Metastatic ovarian cancer from adenocarcinoma of the sigmoid colon. Metastatic cancers to both ovaries have caused gross enlargement, yet the overall ovarian architecture is preserved (A). The cut surface shows virtual replacement of ovarian tissue with multiloculated cystic and solid masses, with no grossly discernible normal ovarian tissue (B).

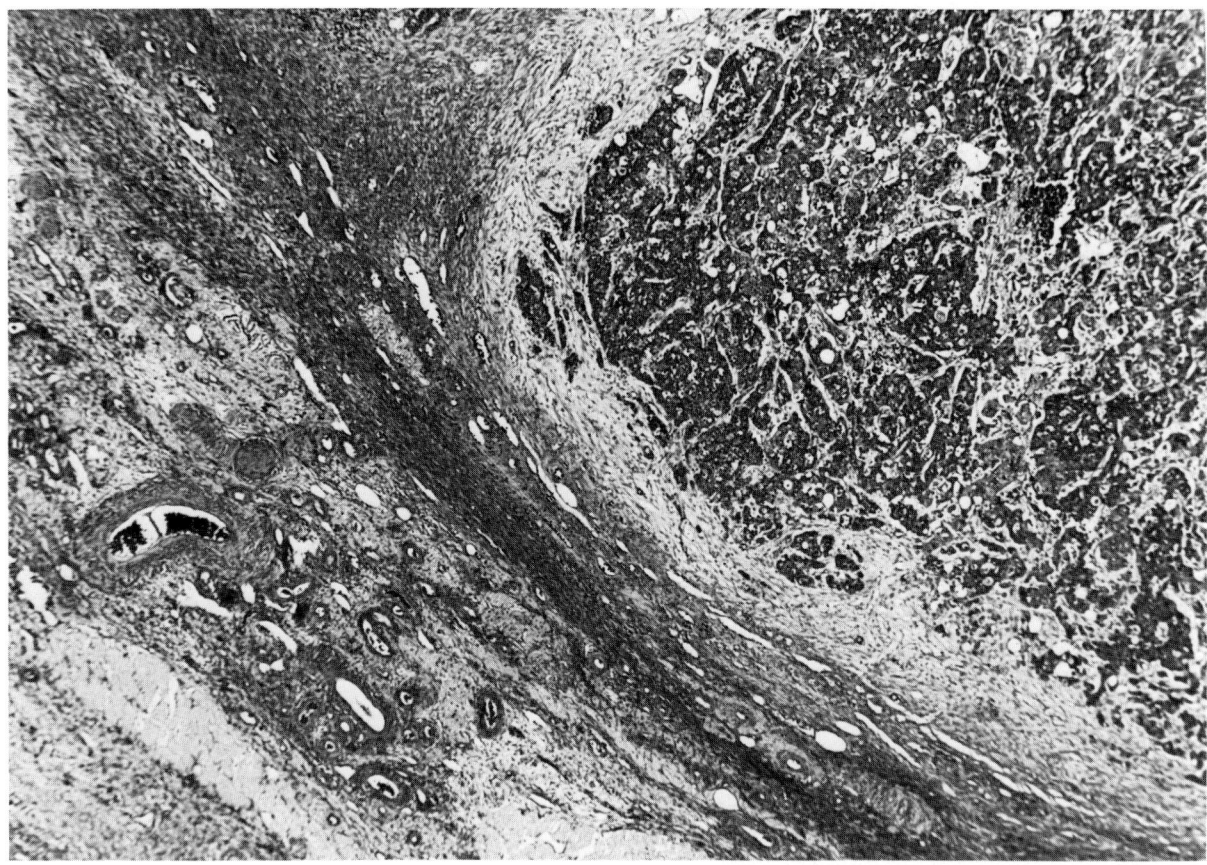

Fig. 62.2 Metastatic adenocarcinoma of unknown origin involving the ovary. The ovarian stroma, with corpus albicans and vasculature, is visible in the lower left portion of the photomicrograph. Although multiple signet ring cells are evident in the poorly differentiated adenocarcinoma, lack of sarcomatoid infiltration of the stroma prevents this from being labelled a Krukenberg tumor. (H & E, original magnification 25×)

the primary tumor microscopic pattern is preserved and easily recognized. For example, in metastatic carcinoma of the cervix, the characteristic epidermoid pattern is usually preserved. All metastatic cancers can simulate the cord-like or tubular arrangement previously described, and when stromal reaction is marked, interpretation may be difficult.

Pathophysiology

It is generally accepted that the ovary is a fertile field for metastasis and, indeed, it may be a privileged site for tumors of certain origin. In considering the pathobiology of metastasis, the rich blood supply of the ovary, especially in the premenopausal ovulatory patient, would suggest that metastasis would have little difficulty establishing sites of growth. In general, a small cluster of circulating tumor cells may initiate the metastatic process, and there is some evidence to suggest that a recognition occurs between the tumor cell and the site of metastasis.[22] After localization, the tumor cell must invade the local capillary walls and create a fibrin matrix. From this point an increase to 10^6 to 10^7 cells can be supported by metabolites and oxygen supplied by diffusion. Further growth requires a vascular supply, and at this point, neovascularization is necessary for future growth.[22] The concept of tumor angiogenesis factor (TAF) and its relationship to ovarian stroma as a privileged site for metastasis requires further elaboration and study. Whether in the ovary or elsewhere, metastases which induce their own blood supply begin early exponential growth resulting in the known proliferative thrust of solid tumors.

Hormonal activity

The ovarian stroma is rich in enzymatic capabilities for hormone production, and secretion of estrogen, progesterone and testosterone is a totipotential capability of specialized stromal cells. The presence of metastatic disease in the ovary stimulates hormone production,[70] and varying clinical manifestations may be present. Signs of hyperestrogenism and ovarian mass suggest a granulosa cell tumor, but a metastatic lesion in the ovary could likewise simulate this pattern. In fact, it has been reported that over half of women who have ovarian tumors, other than granulosa cell and thecal cell tumors, can have an increase in urinary estrogens and pregnanediol.[54]

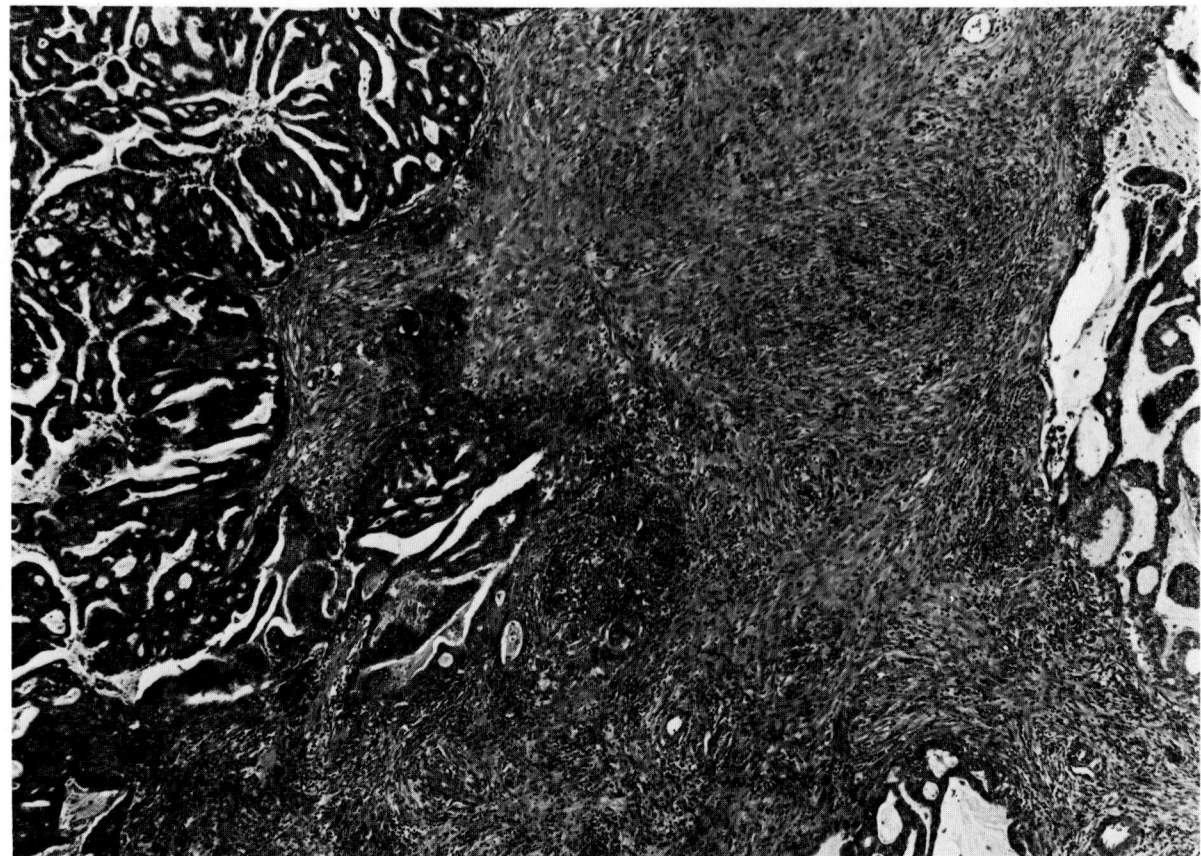

Fig. 62.3 Adenocarcinoma of the endometrium metastatic to the ovary. This moderately differentiated papillary metastatic adenocarcinoma is typical of endometrial carcinoma metastatic to the ovary, but could also represent an endometrioid carcinoma of the ovary. (H & E, original magnification 40×)

Virilization of the fetus due to maternal Krukenberg tumor emphasizes the importance of testosterone secretion.[7] Also, urinary testosterone values have been reported to be high in patients with metastasis from breast carcinoma.[55] Scully states that the phenomenon of tumor growing in an endocrine organ and stimulating it to produce hormones is, among all other endocrine glands, unique in the ovary.[54]

Thus, the presence of unusual hormonal activity and ovarian mass should raise the possibility of metastatic ovarian cancer. While hormonal studies may be helpful, definitive surgical diagnosis is necessary.

Routes of metastasis to the ovaries

In cancer metastatic to the ovaries, there are six possible routes of spread of the primary, and one or more mechanisms may be extant in any circumstance.

1. *Direct extension.* This method of metastasis applies only to those structures in close geographic approximation to the ovaries, such as fallopian tube, uterus and colon. Direct extension of lymphoma can occur from the retroperitoneal lymph node systems, and squamous cell carcinoma from the cervix or vulva could extend directly to the ovaries. Extension of primary bladder tumor to the ovaries has also been reported.

2. *Dissemination through peritoneal fluid.* Any · tumor which primarily or secondarily invades the peritoneal surfaces can exfoliate tumor cells; these are known to be viable and can establish metastatic foci. The surface of the premenopausal ovary is vulnerable to implantation of exfoliated cells in the ostium created by the rupture of the ripe follicle. Likewise, the peritoneal surface of the ovary, through some unknown mechanism, may attract the lodging of exfoliated cells. Although this is certainly a method of metastasis to the ovaries, its exact importance in any individual patient is unknown.

3. *Metastasis through the lumen of the fallopian tube.* Although the usual flow of fluid and particles through the fallopian tube is from the fimbria towards the uterus, certainly the reverse pathway is possible. This mechanism of spread of tumor cells may be the etiology of positive peritoneal cytology in patients who have endometrial or fallopian tube cancer, and may be important in the spread of endometrial cancer to the ovarian surface. Although less likely, cervical cancer and uterine sarcomas could also spread to the ovary in this manner.

4. *Lymphatic metastasis.* The ovaries have a rich network

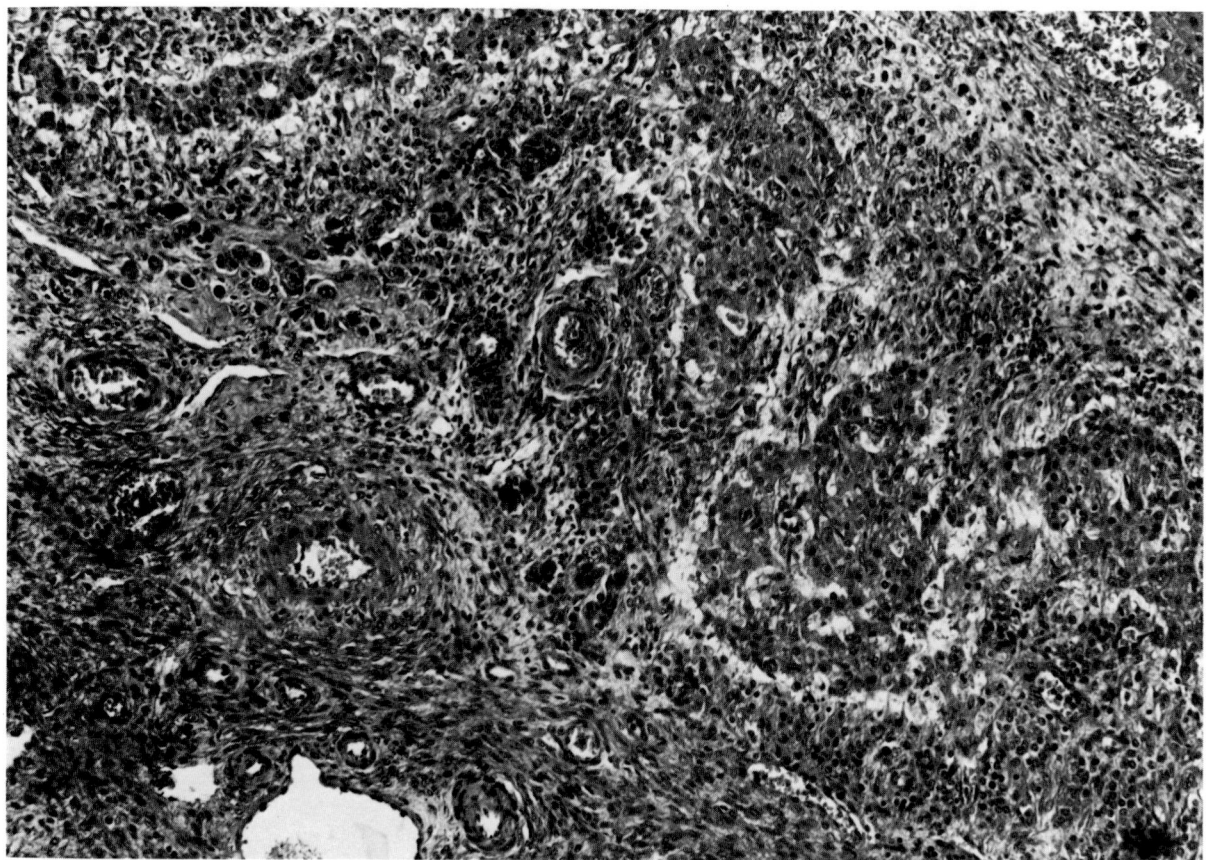

Fig. 62.4 Metastatic breast carcinoma to the ovary. In the central portion of the photomicrograph clumps of malignant cells, metastatic from primary breast carcinoma are visible in ovarian stroma. There is accompanying luteinization of the stroma, and in the upper left portion luteinized stromal cells are associated with a corpus luteum. (H & E, original magnification 100×)

of intra-ovarian and extra-ovarian lymphatics, whose collecting trunks extend upward with the utero-ovarian vessels to the lumbar aortic and lateral caval nodes at the lower pole of the kidneys. This is probably the most important means of spread of cancer from other sites to the ovary. Lymphatics connecting the fallopian tubes, uterus and each ovary with the other have been established, and these provide obvious patterns of spread for genital cancers to the ovary. In addition, the ovary has anastomotic channels with all the pelvic lymphatics, and retrograde flow can occur, especially when the channels are filled with tumor cells. In gastrointestinal cancer, the network of lymphatics from the ovary meeting with those from the mesenteric axis in the aortic pathways could allow for metastasis. This theory is most attractive in the case of very small primary tumors in the gastrointestinal tract whose ovarian metastases are discovered before the primary site can be determined. Likewise, in patients with cancer of unknown primary, lymphatic spread is an attractive theory for establishing ovarian metastasis. Breast cancer may metastasize to the ovaries by lymphatic spread via the internal mammary chain in retrograde flow from that point. Retrograde lymphatic flow is a reasonable explanation for the bilateral ovarian involvement often encountered.

5. *Hematogenous metastasis.* The chances of hematogenous spread are exceedingly good, especially in the highly vascular premenopausal ovary. When tumors metastasize by the cascade phenomenon, the metastases originate from sites of early metastases, invade the blood stream and cascade throughout the body.[64] When the metastasis is present deep in the ovarian stroma near the hilum, one can postulate that the route of spread is via the blood stream.

6. *Iatrogenic metastasis.* Spread of cancer may occur by errant needle biopsies, culdocentesis, paracentesis, or during surgical manipulation. Although theoretically possible, these routes of spread are probably not important clinically.

Treatment

The treatment of choice for metastatic ovarian cancer is bilateral salpingo-oophorectomy, hysterectomy and omentectomy. If there is no gross evidence of intraperitoneal metastasis, pelvic lymph node sampling should be done to determine further evidence of disease. Additionally, debulking of intra-abdominal tumor may be helpful in reducing the tumor mass before chemotherapy. Further management of patients depends upon the site and extent

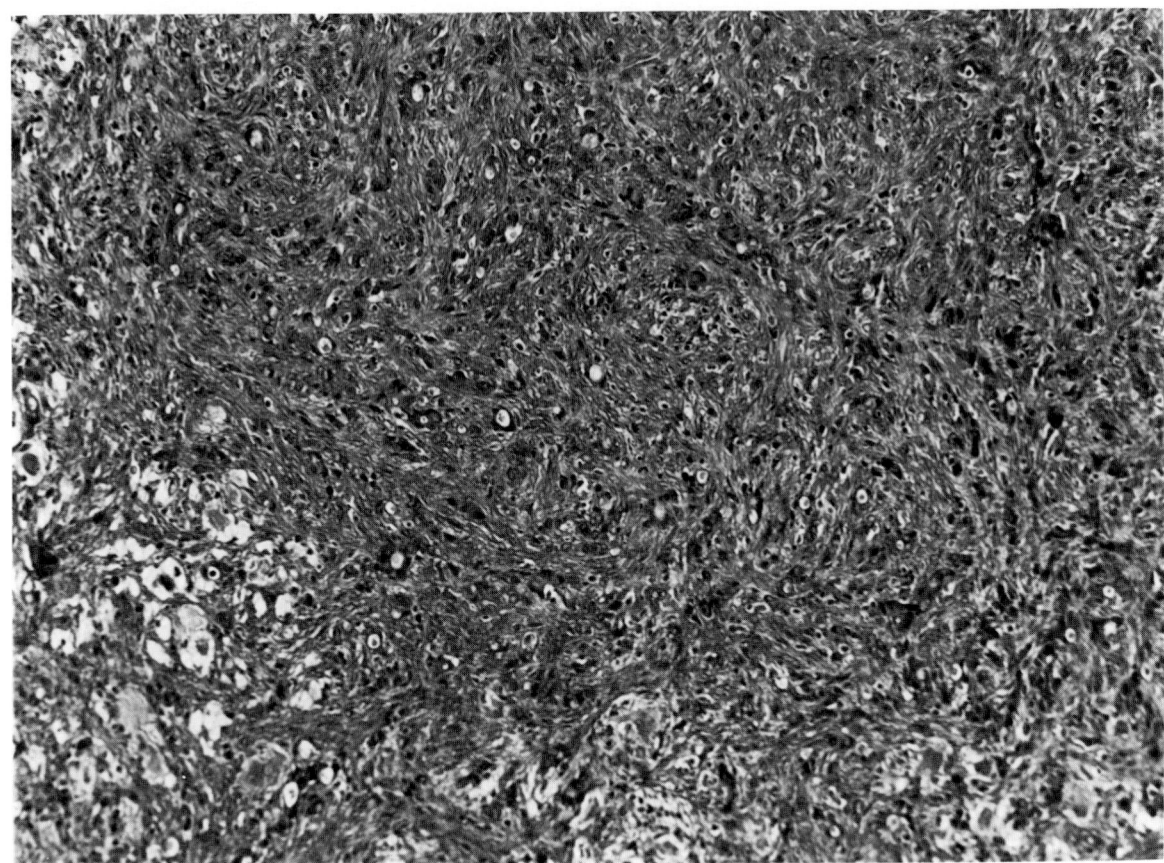

Fig. 62.5 Krukenberg tumor of the ovary. Metastatic cancer from the gastrointestinal tract which shows infiltration of the stroma with malignant cells, giving a sarcoma-like pattern, and frequent signet ring type cells. This histologic pattern is characteristic of true Krukenberg tumors. (H & E, original magnification 100×)

of the primary disease. In most instances, aggressive management is the cornerstone of further therapy.

Prognosis

In general, the survival of patients with metastatic ovarian cancer is poor.[61] In the Mayo Clinic experience, the overall survival at 5 years was 12%, and at 10 years, 7.5%.[66] The most important factor in survival is the extent of tumor at the time of original diagnosis. Morrow & Enker[45] reported that in carcinoma metastatic from the colon the ability to remove all gross disease at the time of oophorectomy was the major determinant of survival. Patients who were operatively free of disease (n=15) lived a mean of 48 months, compared with 9.6 months for patients with localized but unresectable disease (n=9), and 8 months for patients with non-resectable diffuse disease (n=35). In addition, patients with poorly differentiated tumors are less likely to survive as long as patients with well differentiated tumors.[66] Because of the hormonal influence of oophorectomy on selected breast tumors, patients with breast primaries have a significantly longer survival after diagnosis of metastatic

ovarian cancer. Selected patients with microscopic ovarian disease from endometrial cancer, thought to be those patients with lymphatic dissemination of the ovaries rather than direct extension of cancer from the uterus, have minimal disease at the time of the initial operation and thus a reasonable chance for survival. Most patients with gastrointestinal primaries have bulky ovarian tumors or generalized abdominal carcinomatosis, and an expected poor prognosis.

COMMON SITES OF CANCER METASTATIC TO THE OVARY

Gastrointestinal tract

Krukenberg tumors. Although the Krukenberg tumor is diagnosed on strict histologic criteria, the majority of these tumors arise in the gastrointestinal tract, usually in the stomach. Hale found the stomach to be the primary site in 76 of 81 histologically classified Krukenberg tumors,[25] and of the other 5, 2 arose in the sigmoid, 1 in the cecum, and

2 in the breast. Woodruff[69] described 48 Krukenberg tumors, of which 19 (40%) arose in the stomach, 4 in the colon, 1 in the gallbladder, 1 in the breast, 13 from unknown primaries, and 10 were primary in the ovary. All of Diddle's 557 collected cases, of which the origin was known, had the primary site in the gastrointestinal tract, with 80% arising in the stomach and the remainder divided among other gastrointestinal sites, including the small bowel, gallbladder, appendix and pancreas.[14] It is apparent that the capability of producing the microscopic picture of the Krukenberg tumor can be associated with virtually any mucin-producing adenocarcinoma, other examples being the appendix[49,57] and the urinary bladder.[6]

Non-Krukenberg gastrointestinal primary sites. In some reports, the colon and the rectum are much more commonly the sites of the primary tumor than is the stomach.[13,39,45,61,67] These metastases appear to retain the characteristic microscopic picture of the primary tumor, with duplication of the papillary and acinar features of adenocarcinomas of the large intestine.[37,67] As is the case with Krukenberg tumors, these are apt to be bilateral (75%) and may achieve massive size. When such massive enlargement occurs, retention of the ovarian shape is less likely than when a true Krukenberg tumor is present, probably because of the latter's sarcomatoid infiltration of the stroma.

The striking similarity microscopically between secondary ovarian carcinoma metastatic from the colon and primary mucinous cystadenocarcinoma of the ovary may lead to diagnostic confusion and inappropriate management. Even with multiple special staining techniques,[18] microscopic differentiation may be impossible; thus, accurate operative assessment is essential. In patients who have bilateral mucinous tumors, careful inspection and palpation of the bowel is mandatory. The juxtaposition of the ovaries and the pelvic colon likewise may make the diagnosis of which lesion is the primary more difficult. Careful description of the relationships of the tumor masses, both pelvic and mesenteric lymph node evaluations, and the location of other metastases may assist in establishing the site of the primary tumor.

Occasionally, the secondary ovarian tumor may precede the discovery of the primary bowel lesion, usually because of symptoms of a large pelvic mass. Even with careful evaluation of the gastrointestinal tract, the primary lesion may not become manifest until months later.

The incidence of metastasis to the ovaries from gastrointestinal cancer varies, depending upon the source of the patient material. If autopsy data are used, 13 to 15% of patients dying of gastrointestinal carcinoma will be found to have ovarian metastasis. On the other hand, clinical reports suggest a lower incidence, in the range of 3 to 8%.[2,9,37] In young patients with carcinoma of the stomach, the incidence may be as high as 50%.[25,53] This high predilection for ovarian involvement, accompanied by the chance of unsuspected metastasis in normal appearing ovaries, leads many clinicians to advocate prophylactic oophorectomy for patients undergoing surgery for gastrointestinal malignancy.[2,8,9,24,42,45,61,69] In the absence of other demonstrable metastasis, such ablative surgery seems reasonable.

The route of spread of gastrointestinal cancer to the ovaries could be any of the six mechanisms noted. Probably lymphatic spread, direct extension in the case of the pelvic colon, and intraperitoneal seeding are the most important. In a meticulous study of the spread of gastrointestinal tumors, Viadana, Bross & Pickren[65] demonstrated that most metastases from tumors of the digestive system occurred after initial spread to the liver or lungs, via hematogenous mode, i.e. 'the cascade spread.' The ovaries were the exception to this rule, with the chance of ovarian metastasis occurring with or without lung and liver involvement. In 50% of patients, spread to the ovaries seemed to occur directly from the primary tumor, lending further credence to the theory of lymphatic or intraperitoneal extension. Additionally, the infiltration of the stroma, as seen in the microscopic picture of the Krukenberg tumor, would suggest a diffuse lymphatic spread.

The survival of patients with the primary tumor in the gastrointestinal tract is dependent on the extent of disease at the time of diagnosis, the interval between the diagnosis of the primary and secondary tumor, and the presence of ascites. Tunca and colleagues[61] recommended '(1) compulsory colon examination to include colonoscopy prior to surgery for ovarian masses, and (2) prophylactic bilateral salpingo-oophorectomy at the time of colectomy for colon cancer' in an effort to improve long-term survival. Morrow & Enker[45] concurred in performing oophorectomy in curative cases, and emphasized the role of bilateral oophorectomy at the same time as palliative operations for cancer of the colon, since 27% of patients in the Memorial Hospital, New York study required a second palliative operation to remove huge ovarian metastases. In a prospective and controlled study, Graffner, Alm & Oscarson[24] found that 6 of 58 patients (10%) had ovarian metastases (random variation at a confidence level of 95% equals 3.9 to 21.1%), and in 4 of the 6 patients, the ovaries were macroscopically judged to be free of metastatic disease. Their conclusions were that these data, plus the risk of the development of a primary ovarian carcinoma 'favors prophylactic oophorectomy' in the presence of colorectal carcinoma. MacKeigan & Ferguson[42] reported a higher risk of ovarian metastases in younger women, and advocated bilateral salpingo-oophorectomy in this group. It is apparent from the literature of the past 10 years that this aggressive attitude towards removal of ovaries at the time of colorectal surgery for cancer is gaining ground, and we concur in this concept.

Ascites is present in up to 46% of patients with Krukenberg type tumors,[69] and if present, portends a poor prognosis.[13,44] Patients with ascites are unlikely to survive more than 6 months. Isolated metastasis, occurring months after the primary surgical procedure, may not preclude long-term survival. On the other hand, presence of multiple sites of metastasis in addition to the ovaries, especially if ascites is present, would suggest little chance of salvage. The efficacy of chemotherapy for these patients is low, but vigorous treatment of selected patients in carefully controlled circumstances is probably worthwhile.

Breast

There is good evidence indicating that the ovary is a frequent site of metastasis from breast carcinoma. Abrams[1] found that 23% of patients autopsied who died of breast carcinoma had ovarian metastasis. The most frequent source of information for breast metastasis to the ovaries comes from studies of ovaries removed in the treatment of advanced breast disease. Kasilag & Rutledge[36] found that 23 of 91 patients (25%) undergoing oophorectomy for breast carcinoma had metastatic disease in the ovary. Lumb & MacKenzie[41] discovered metastatic foci in 90 of 190 patients (47%) who had ovaries removed because of carcinoma of the breast. Turksoy[62] found metastatic carcinoma in 8 of 26 specimens (31%) of castration material, and in 8 of 19 autopsied patients; the report was subtitled 'A surgical surprise'. Although these figures are higher than those earlier reported, they are remarkably consistent, and approximately one-third of patients may be expected to have breast cancer spread to the ovaries. Because of the increasing frequency of the use of annual mammogram screening in patients beyond 40 years of age in the Duke Medical Center Clinics, and the increasing frequency of early diagnosis of breast cancer ('early' meaning mammogram diagnosis without palpable mass), it is anticipated that the occurrence rate of breast cancer metastatic to ovary will decrease; however, the data in the past 10 years have not reflected a significant change to date.

Ovarian metastasis from breast cancer occurs primarily in premenopausal women. Fifty-six percent of Kasilag & Rutledge's patients were menstruating at the time of discovery of the ovarian metastasis,[36] while the average ages of patients in the Duke series[13] and as reported by Osborne & Pitts[47] were 44 and 45 years, respectively. Almost one-third of the patients from the Emil Novak Registry with breast metastasis to the ovary were 39 years old or younger.[68] Such occurrence is not uncommon in the very young. Premenopausal women who have cancer of the breast should be followed with periodic pelvic ultrasound studies to characterize the ovaries for subtle changes in size, consistency and bilateral involvement, all of which are suggestive of metastasis. Celiotomy and wedge resection of ovaries should be done if there is suspicion.

Oophorectomy for treatment of metastases of breast cancer has been a time honored mode of treatment.[28] Prior to the advent of sensitive measurements of estrogen receptor status, such castration was performed empirically, and 25 to 37% of patients, roughly one-third, could expect objective tumor regression.[58] Utilizing receptor knowledge, between 50 and 60% of receptor-positive patients respond to ablative therapy.[30] If knowledge of receptor status is unknown, a short 'free interval' between mastectomy and recurrence demands castration.[58]

Prophylactic oophorectomy is widely used as adjuvant therapy in premenopausal women.[29] Unfortunately, when all patients are considered, there is no significant overall increase in the mean recurrence-free interval or survival time when castration is done prophylactically.[58] However, if more than four lymph nodes are positive at the time of breast surgery, castration may increase the disease-free interval, but not survival. When metastases are found in the ovary at the time of castration, these patients have a higher remission rate.[58] Attempts to relate this to stromal activation by metastatic disease have been unconvincing.[47] With today's multiple agent chemotherapeutic regimen used in metastatic breast cancer, the influence of castration upon improvement in survival will be difficult to prove. Current practice is to administer anti-estrogen compounds, such as tamoxifen citrate (Novaldex)®, instead of castration in selected patients, and often in conjunction with multiple agent chemotherapy. This practice is reasonable in view of the poor prognosis for patients who have metastatic breast cancer. Tamoxifen citrate may produce a significant palliative response, even in patients who are estrogen receptor negative. Toremifene is another anti-estrogen which is under study in clinical trials, but as yet there are no definitive data.

Metastatic breast cancer is frequently microscopic, and the removed ovaries often appear grossly normal. As is the case for metastasis from the gastrointestinal tract, breast metastases are bilateral in three-fourths of patients. The ovarian architecture is less likely to be preserved in advanced disease, and solid nodules on the surface of the ovary are common and may indicate hematogenous spread. Microscopically, duplication of the primary tumor pattern is often seen, along with a diffuse, infiltrative picture. Woodruff states that patterns may vary within the same patient, and the presence of wide microscopic variations should arouse suspicion that the disease is metastatic.[68]

The capability of metastatic disease in the ovaries to produce autocastration has been hypothesized, but the remarkable reserve of the ovary makes this unlikely, except in the case of massive replacement. Indeed, active ovulation with the formation of corpora lutea was present in all patients who were still ovulating in the M.D. Anderson report.[36] The considered opinion is that autocastration, although a theoretical possibility, rarely occurs.

Endometrial carcinoma

Spread from carcinoma of the endometrium to the adjacent

adnexa is a well-established phenomenon, occurring in approximately 8 to 10% of patients. Retrograde dissemination through the fallopian tubes is virtually unique for this cancer. The rich lymphatic network, both efferent and afferent, between the two structures is an often demonstrated route of extension. Additionally, direct growth through the wall of the uterus into the ovaries is common for advanced disease.

Roughly one out of six metastatic neoplasms in the ovary is of endometrial origin, and this frequency increases if endometrial sarcomas are included.[13] Assigning which organ is the primary may at times be impossible,[19,63] since histologically the pictures of metastatic endometrial cancer and primary endometrioid carcinoma of the ovary can be identical (Fig. 62.3). This is especially true in early, well differentiated tumors. Presenting symptoms, myometrial invasion, differentiation of the tumor, and patterns of intra-abdominal spread may offer clues as to which is the primary site. Occasionally, the theory of double primary tumors must be invoked. Woodruff[68] has for years postulated the multicentric focus of origin of all müllerian tumors, believing them to be of mesothelial origin. Histologically, this theory has merit, but its clinical significance is unknown.

Almost all ovarian metastases from endometrial carcinoma will be diagnosed at the time of definitive surgery for the primary disease. Routine removal of the tubes and ovaries is standard operative treatment when removing the uterus for malignancy. Microscopic spread may be detected despite normal appearing ovaries.

Patients with metastasis from endometrial carcinoma confined to the ovaries have a better prognosis than patients who have other forms of Stage III disease. Bruckman et al[7] divided Stage III patients into two groups depending on limitation of spread to the ovaries and/or fallopian tubes versus spread to other pelvic structures, and found a significantly better relapse-free survival at 5 years for the former group. Others[13,68] have shown a marked increase in survival rate when metastases were limited to the ovaries.

Pelvic irradiation for patients with ovarian involvement from endometrial cancer is accepted treatment. The use of pelvic irradiation for metastatic endometrial cancer to the ovaries is one of the limited circumstances when radiotherapy would be applicable for secondary disease.[66]

Other tumors with secondary ovarian metastasis

Lymphoma and leukemia

Lymphomatous involvement of the gonad may be primary extra-nodal disease, the initial manifestation of clinically occult nodal disease, or a late focus of disseminated lymphoma. When autopsy data are considered, involvement of the ovary with lymphoma is quite common, but occasionally lymphoma presents as its primary manifestation in the ovary.[11,48] Most authorities believe that, despite the presentation of the disease in the ovary, the primary site was in the reticulo-endothelial system. Lymphomas in the gonads are usually non-Hodgkins lymphomas, although all types, even Burkitt's tumor, can be present in the ovary.[26]

Bickers et al[5] point out that acute leukemia, the most common neoplasm of children, spreads to the testes and to the ovaries in about equal frequency (8%) and that disease in the testicle can be palpated, whereas metastasis to the ovary requires sonography to detect early leukemic involvement. Chu and colleagues[12] report a patient who developed a large ovarian tumor due to leukemic infiltration while in bone marrow remission, and recognized that 36% of girls who die of leukemia have ovarian involvement. Zarrouk et al[72] report two additional patients who developed ovarian related relapse after 3 years of chemotherapy and in the presence of negative evaluations of the bone marrow and central nervous system. These data and numerous other reports clearly indicate the gonads as a primary site of extramedullary relapse in acute lymphoblastic leukemia in children, and the need for periodic non-invasive pelvic ultrasound studies as a vital part of the follow-up regimen in females.

The presence of an ovarian mass accompanied by symptoms of fatigue, night sweats and fever, especially if ascites is present, suggests a diagnosis of lymphoma. In those cases, the finding at operation of bilateral solid ovarian tumors is virtually diagnostic, and enlarged nodal chains are usually present. After accurate staging, a combination of surgery, irradiation and chemotherapy is the treatment of choice.[21] (See also Ch. 61.)

Melanoma

Of patients dying with melanoma, as high as 16% are found at autopsy to have metastatic disease in the ovaries. A member of the Duke Cancer Center Faculty is heavily involved in melanoma research and has a large referral practice of patients with malignant melanoma, and this accounts for the high number (9) of patients with melanoma metastatic to the ovaries. Of these nine patients, seven have accrued in the past 10 years and this inordinately high rate is related to the advanced disease of these melanoma patients. Other reports[20,23] indicate the normally expected incidence of this malignancy. Almost all of these patients have bilateral ovarian disease.[27] Occasionally, the primary site will be unknown, and the metastatic disease in the ovary will be the only known site of metastasis.[56] Although a case of peritonitis following rupture of metastatic malignant melanoma has been reported, it is rare that melanoma metastatic to the ovary is sufficiently symptomatic to require surgical excision.[56] Although the ovary does not contain melanin in cells as such, melanoma has been described arising in teratomas, perhaps the only means by which they could arise primarily in the ovary. Complete surgical removal including omentectomy, and chemotherapy and/or immunotherapy are the only hope at present for patients with melanotic neoplasms involving the ovary (see also Ch. 67).

Uterine sarcomas

Ovarian metastasis from the uterine sarcomas is common, and, as ongoing staging studies for sarcomas continue, both lymph node spread and ovarian metastasis are found in increasing numbers. While the route of spread is similar to that of endometrial cancer, the hematogenous route must be considered, especially in the anaplastic tumors. Operation and vigorous adjunctive chemotherapy is presently the only hope of long-term survival in patients with metastatic disease in the ovaries from sarcomas.

Carcinomas from unknown primary

The presence of metastatic disease in the ovaries from unknown primary is a frustrating experience for the clinician. Despite exhaustive radiographic procedures, often the primary site is not disclosed even at autopsy.[46] It is estimated that 3 to 4% of all cancers present with a metastatic lesion from an occult primary tumor.[15]

When the primary manifestation of a carcinoma of unknown origin is in the ovary, the diagnosis is usually made at the time of celiotomy for an undiagnosed pelvic mass. In such patients, the disease will often be beyond the confines of surgical resection at the time of diagnosis.[13] Even with the probabilistic models of micrometastasis formation,[40] it is difficult to assess how a tumor can create a metastasis that is more virulent than that of the primary and thereby elude diagnosis. Still, exhaustive search is necessary since determination of the primary source prior to definitive therapy is essential if choice of proper chemotherapeutic agents is to be effective.[17]

Carcinoid metastatic to the ovary

Metastatic carcinoid occasionally involves the ovary, and Robboy, Scully & Norris[51] recently described 35 cases. In 25 patients, diagnosis was discovered at surgical exploration, and all but 2 patients had tumor in both ovaries. Microscopically, the carcinoid can be confused with a bone tumor or granulosa cell tumor, and the presence of a primary site is needed to exclude primary ovarian carcinoid.[57,71] The latter is usually unilateral and associated with other teratomatous elements.[51] The presence of a pelvic mass and carcinoid syndrome should prompt urinary determinations for 5-hydroxyindole acetic acid, a GI and liver work up and surgical exploration with the presumptive diagnosis of metastatic carcinoid in the ovary.

Less common tumors that metastasize to the ovary

Virtually any malignant neoplasm can establish secondary growth in the ovaries. Usually, these are adenocarcinomas; however, squamous cell carcinoma of the cervix will occasionally directly invade the ovaries and rarely metastasize to the ovaries.[59] Metastasis to the ovary from squamous cell carcinoma of the esophagus[60] and lung[13,71] has been reported. Even more rarely, the ovary may be the site of cancer to cancer metastasis,[30] but this is more a pathological curiosity than of clinical significance.

SUMMARY

Cancer metastatic to the ovary comprises an important part of all ovarian tumors, and this eventuality should be included in the differential diagnosis of pelvic masses. Most commonly, the primary sites are in the gastrointestinal tract, the breast and endometrium, but lymphomas, sarcomas, melanomas and carcinoid, as well as virtually any other tumor can establish a secondary growth in the ovaries. A remote history of breast carcinoma or gastrointestinal malignancy accompanying the presence of a pelvic mass should double the suspicion that the disease is secondary in the ovary. Although most such metastatic tumors are diagnosed at the time of definitive surgery, remote recurrence in the ovary is common. Usually, and especially in the gastrointestinal primaries, the ovary retains its normal shape and resembles an enlarged version of its previous form. Over three-fourths of metastatic ovarian neoplasms are bilateral and may reach tremendous size, and are symptomatic. Histologically, the primary tumor is duplicated frequently, but a specific picture of signet ring cell formation and sarcomatoid infiltration of the stroma prompts a diagnosis of Krukenberg tumor, a term which is purely histologic and not specific in defining the primary site. Although aggressive surgical therapy as well as indicated chemotherapy and radiation are advised, most patients with cancer metastatic to the ovary have a poor prognosis.

REFERENCES

1. Abrams H L, Spiro R, Goldstein N 1950 Metastases in carcinoma. Cancer 3: 74
2. Antoniades K, Spector H B, Hecksher R H 1977 Prophylactic oophorectomy in conjunction with large bowel resection for cancer. Dis Colon Rectum 20: 506
3. Athey P A, Butters H E 1984 Sonographic and CT appearance of Krukenberg tumors. J Clin Ultrasound 12: 205
4. Bell R J M 1977 Fetal virilization due to maternal Krukenberg tumor. Lancet i: 1162
5. Bickers G H, Siebert J J, Anderson J C, Golladay S, Berry D L 1981 Sonography of ovarian involvement in childhood acute lymphocytic leukemia. Am J Radiol 137: 399

6. Bowlby L S, Smith McL 1986 Signet-ring cell carcinoma of the urinary bladder; primary presentation as a Krukenberg tumor. Gynecol Oncol 25: 376

7. Bruckman J E, Bloomer W D, Marck A, Ehrmann R L, Knapp R C 1980 Stage III adenocarcinoma of the endometrium: two prognostic groups. Gynecol Oncol 9: 12

8. Burt C A V 1957 Modern concepts in the surgical management of diseases of the colon and rectum. Am J Surg 93: 77

9. Burt C A V 1951 Prophylactic oophorectomy with resection of the large bowel for cancer. Am J Surg 82: 571

10. Carnovale R L, Samuels B I 1976 Complex ovarian mass on ultrasonography: Primary or metastatic tumor? (Letter) N Engl J Med 294: 446

11. Chorlton I, Norris H J, King F M 1974 Malignant reticuloendothelial disease involving the ovary as a primary manifestation. Cancer 34: 397

12. Chu J Y, Craddock T V, Danis R K, Tennant N E 1981 Ovarian tumor as manifestation of relapse in acute lymphoblastic leukemia. Cancer 48: 377

13. Currie J L, Parker R T 1980 Cancer metastatic to the ovary. Unpublished observations.

14. Diddle A W 1955 Krukenberg tumors: diagnostic problem. Cancer 8: 1026

15. Didolkar M S, Fanous N, Elias E G, Moore R H 1977 Metastatic carcinomas from occult primary tumors. Ann Surg 186: 625

16. Engeler V, Siebenmann R, Schreiner W E 1976 Primary Krukenberg tumor in pregnancy. Arch Gynäekol 220: 293

17. Feleppa V B, Lemon H M 1977 The therapeutic dilemma of carcinomas of unknown origin. J Surg Oncol 9: 453

18. Fenoglio C M, Cottral G A, Ferenczy A, Richart R M 1976 Mucinous tumors of the ovary: III. Histochemical studies: Gynecol Oncol 4: 151

19. Finn W F 1951 The diagnostic confusion of ovarian metastases from endometrial carcinoma with primary ovarian carcinoma. Am J Obstet Gynecol 62: 403

20. Fitzgibbons P L, Martin S E, Simmons T J 1987 Malignant melanoma metastatic to the ovary. Am J Surg Pathol 11: 959

21. Fox H D, Cartnick E N, Shohov P, Zaino E C 1975 Lymphoma of the ovary. A case report and a review of the literature. Gynecol Oncol 3: 347

22. Frei E III 1977 Rationale for combined therapy. Cancer 40: 569

23. Gonzalez M S, Hammond D O 1983 Malignant melanoma in the ovary with ultrastructural confirmation. Am J Obstet Gynecol 147: 722

24. Graffner H O, Alm P O, Oscarson J E 1983 Prophylactic oophorectomy in colorectal carcinoma. Am J Surg 146: 233

25. Hale R W 1968 Krukenberg tumor of the ovaries. Obstet Gynecol 32: 221

26. Halpin T F 1975 Gynecologic implications of Burkitt's tumor. Obstet Gynecol Surv 30: 351

27. Hameed K 1973 Melanotic ovarian neoplasms. Prog Clin Cancer 5: 209

28. Henderson I C, Canellos G P 1980(a) Cancer of the breast. N Engl J Med 302: 17

29. Henderson I C, Canellos G P 1980(b) Cancer of the breast. N Engl J Med 302: 78

30. Hines J R, Gordon R T, Widger C, Kolb T 1976 Cystosarcoma phyllodes metastatic to a Brenner tumor of the ovary. Arch Surg 111: 299

31. Hundley J M 1931 Krukenberg tumors and other secondary ovarian carcinomas. South Med J 24: 579

32. Israel S L, Helsel E V, Hausman D A 1965 The challenge of metastatic ovarian carcinoma. Am J Obstet Gynecol 93: 1094

33. Janovski N A, Paramanandhan T L 1973 Ovarian Tumors. Saunders, Philadelphia

34. Joshi V V 1968 Primary Krukenberg tumor of the ovary. Cancer 22: 1199

35. Karsh J 1951 Secondary malignant disease of the ovaries. Am J Obstet Gynecol 61: 155

36. Kasilag F B, Rutledge F N 1957 Metastatic breast carcinoma in the ovary. Am J Obstet Gynecol 74: 989

37. Knoepp L F, Ray J E, Overby I 1973 Ovarian metastasis from colorectal carcinoma. Dis Colon Rectum 16: 305

38. Krukenberg F E 1896 Ueber das Fibroma Ovarii Mucocellulare (Carcinomatodes). Arch Gynäekol 50: 287

39. Lash R H, Hart W R 1987 Intestinal adenocarcinomas metastatic to the ovaries. Am J Surg Pathol 11: 114

40. Liotta L A, Delisi C, Saidel G, Kleinerman J 1977 Micrometastases formation: a probabilistic model. Cancer Lett 3: 203

41. Lumb G, MacKenzie D H 1959 The incidence of metastases in adrenal glands and ovaries removed for carcinoma of the breast. Cancer 12: 521

42. MacKeigan J M, Ferguson J A 1979 Prophylactic oophorectomy and colorectal cancer in premenopausal patients. Dis Colon Rectum 22: 401

43. Megibow A J, Hulnick D H, Bosniak M A, Balthazar E J 1985 Ovarian metastases: computed tomographic appearances. Radiology 156: 161

44. Metz S A, Karnei R T, Veach S R, Hoskins W J 1980 Krukenberg carcinoma of the ovary with bone marrow involvement. Obstet Gynecol 55: 99

45. Morrow M, Enker W E 1984 Late ovarian metastases in carcinoma of the colon and rectum. Arch Surg 119: 1385

46. Nystrom J S, Weiner J M, Wolf R M, Bateman J R, Viola M V 1979 Identifying the primary site in metastatic cancer of unknown origin. JAMA 241: 381

47. Osborne M P, Pitts R M 1961 Therapeutic oophorectomy for advanced breast cancer. Cancer 14: 126

48. Paladugu R T, Bearman R M. Rappaport H 1980 Malignant lymphoma with primary manifestation in the gonad. Cancer 45: 561

49. Paone J F, Bixler T J II, Imbembo A L 1978 Primary mucinous adenocarcinoma of the appendix with bilateral Krukenberg ovarian tumors. Johns Hopkins Med J 143: 43

50. Parker R T, Parker C H, Wilbanks G D 1970 Cancer of the ovary. Am J Obstet Gynecol 108: 878

51. Robboy S J, Scully R E, Norris H J 1974 Carcinoid metastatic to the ovary. Cancer 33: 397

52. Schlagenhaufer F 1902 Ueber das metastatische Ovarialcarcinom nach Krebs des Magens, Darmes und anderer Bauchorgane. Monatshr f Geburtsh u Gynak 15: 485

53. Schmutzer K J, Zaki A E, Regan J F 1973 Gastric carcinoma in a 22-year-old Negro woman with metastases to ovaries and breast. J Natl Med Assoc 65: 426

54. Scully R E (ed) 1975 Case records of the Massachusetts General Hospital. N Engl J Med 292: 521

55. Secreto G 1977 Urinary testosterone values in patients with ovarian metastases from breast cancer. Tumori 63: 457

56. Silveira E, Palhares F A B, Filho J A O, Alberta O, Alverti V N, Silveira M I G S 1977 Peritonitis following rupture of metastatic malignant melanoma of the ovary. Gynecol Oncol 5: 305

57. Skoane P, Sauer T, Jewe F 1986 Mucinous adenocarcinoma of the appendix presenting as an ovarian cystadenocarcinoma. Eur J Surg Oncol 12: 379

58. Stoll B A (ed) 1972 Endocrine Therapy in Malignant Disease. Saunders, Philadelphia

59. Tabata M, Ichinoe K, Sakuragi N, Shina Y, Yamaguchi T, Mabachi Y 1987 Incidence of ovarian metastasis in patients with cancer of the uterine cervix. Gynecol Oncol 28: 255

60. Takita H, Vincent R G, Caicedo V, Gutierrez A 1977 Squamous cell carcinoma of the esophagus: a study of 153 cases. J Surg Oncol 9: 547

61. Tunca J C, Starling J R, Hafez G R, Buchler D A 1983 Colon carcinoma metastatic to the ovary. J Surg Oncol 23: 269

62. Turksoy N 1960 Ovarian metastasis of breast carcinoma. Obstet Gynecol 15: 573

63. Ulbright T M, Roth L M 1985 Metastatic and independent cancers of the endometrium and ovary: a clinicopathologic study of 34 cases. Human Pathol 16: 28

64. Viadana E, Bross I D J, Pickren J W 1973 An autopsy study of some routes of dissemination of cancer of the breast. Human Pathol 16: 28

65. Viadana E, Bross I D J, Pickren J W 1978 The metastatic spread of cancers of the digestive system in man. Oncology 35: 114

66. Webb M J, Decker D G, Mussey E 1975 Cancer metastatic to the ovary. Obstet Gynecol 45: 391

67. Wheelock M C, Putong P 1959 Ovarian metastases from adenocarcinoma of the colon and rectum. Obstet Gynecol 14: 291

68. Woodruff J D, Murthy Y S, Bhaskar T N, Bordbar F & Tseng S S 1970 Metastatic ovarian tumors. Am J Obstet Gynecol 107: 202

69. Woodruff J D, Novak E R 1960 The Krukenberg tumor. Obstet Gynecol 15: 351

70. Woodruff J D, Williams T F, Goldberg B 1963 Hormone activity of the common ovarian neoplasm. Am J Obstet Gynecol 87: 679

71. Young R H, Scully R E 1985 Ovarian metastases from cancer of the lung: problems in interpretation — a report of seven cases. Gynecol Oncol 21: 337

72. Zarrouk S O, Kim T H, Hargreaves H K, Ragab A H 1982 Leukemic involvement of ovaries in childhood acute lymphocytic leukemia. J Pediat 100: 422

PART X

Presacral tumors

63. Presacral tumors: anatomy, classification, clinical features and management

R. A. Lee

INTRODUCTION

A relatively infrequent and heterogeneous group of tumors with similar clinical presentations may arise in the presacral space. Depending on their origin, size and degree of invasion, the lesions may be asymptomatic and are found only on routine pelvic examination. Occasionally, they are first discovered when they produce pressure on adjacent structures and thus cause urinary frequency or obstruct the bladder or bowel. Computed tomography is capable of depicting the intraosseous and soft tissue extensions of these tumors. Magnetic resonance imaging is valuable for examining musculoskeletal structures because it provides a high-contrast image of soft tissue, in addition to having the unique capacity of imaging in virtually any anatomic plane.

Depending on the location, size and mobility of the tumor, various surgical approaches will prove advantageous. Because of the variety of histologic types of tumors and of their sizes and locations, specific surgical management is individualized and, on occasion, is best accomplished by a combination or team of surgeons. Excellent results with minimal morbidity can be obtained in patients with benign tumors. In patients with very large, complex or malignant tumors, encroachment on contiguous structures results in increased morbidity and limited curability.

GROSS ANATOMY

Teplick and associates[12] defined the gross anatomy of the retrorectal area. It is generally accepted that this is a potential space bounded in front by the posterior wall of the rectum and behind by the ventral surface of the sacrum. The inferior extent is formed by the pelvic floor, composed mainly of the levator ani and coccygeal muscles. Cephalad, the space is limited by the peritoneal reflection at the rectosigmoid junction, adjacent to about the third sacral segment.

The presacral space is contained by two fascial layers — the parietal pelvic fascia (Waldeyer's fascia) covers the anterior sacral surface, and the fascia propria covers the posterior rectum. These layers enclose the retrorectal fat, areolar tissue, lymph nodes and hemorrhoidal vessels. The presacral space contains branches of the sacral and hypogastric nerve plexuses, and the median, sacral and iliolumbar vessels.

EMBRYOLOGY

Laird[4] reviewed the embryologic changes occurring in the caudal end of the embryo during the third to eighth weeks of development. Study of these changes certainly implicates this portion of the embryo as the site of origin for the various neoplasms that invade the presacral area.

Within a few weeks, the neuroenteric canal — the connection from the neural groove — becomes obliterated. The postanal gut, i.e. the portion of the hind gut caudal to the proctodeum, is obliterated as the anus and the rectum form; the notochord, having become segmented, leaves vestiges of the neural canal at its distal tip. It is assumed that any of these pluripotential cells left behind as 'rests' in the developing embryo are capable of later multiplication, with resultant neoplastic capabilities. Ewing[2] suggested that the embryonal structures giving rise to presacral tumors are the fovea coccygeal and coccygeal vestiges of the neural canal, the neuroenteric canal, the postanal gut and the proctodeal membrane.

FREQUENCY

The incidence of retroperitoneal tumors in females is difficult to determine, but it is low. Spencer & Jackman[10] found only three coccygeal cysts (0.014%) during 20 851 proctoscopic examinations done in a single year at the Mayo Clinic. Only 63 presacral tumors in adults were seen over a 30-year period at the Portland Surgical Center.[13] Cody et al[1] described 39 patients with malignant retrorectal tumors managed at the Memorial Sloan-Kettering Center over a 28-year period, and Localio and associates[6] reported the management of 20 patients with presacral tumors at the

1003

New York University Medical Center over a 15-year period.

From 1965 to 1980, 70 female patients with primary presacral or pelvic retroperitoneal tumors underwent operation at the Mayo Clinic.[5] Excluded from this study were patients who had chordomas, who had had previous treatment at another institution, or who had metastasis to the presacral space. The tumors were benign in 70% and malignant in 30% of patients. This is similar to Uhlig & Johnson's[13] finding of 31% as the proportion of malignancy in females. Stewart et al[11] found 50% of the tumors to be malignant in the adults in their series, a finding similar to the 40% reported by Whittaker & Pemberton[14] who also noted a preponderance of males (60%).

CLASSIFICATION

Stewart et al[11] reviewed an amalgamation of reports representing 311 presacral tumors, of which 63% were congenital lesions, 8% were inflammatory, 10% were neurogenic, 7% were osseous and 12% were grouped as miscellaneous. Some series included large numbers of chordomas with few teratomas. Freier et al[3] found no mucous or secretory tumors, but did find numerous chordomas. Histologic review of our female patients has allowed us to use a modification of the classification of Lovelady & Dockerty,[7] which includes congenital, neurogenic, osseous, soft tissue and miscellaneous tumors. This excludes patients with metastatic cancers, chordomas, inflammatory masses, and recurrent tumors who have been operated on at other hospitals, and patients who do not have a tissue diagnosis.

Congenital tumors

Thirty four patients (48% of our series) had congenital tumors. Of these, 30 were benign (teratoma, 24; epidermoid cyst, 5; meningocele, 1) and 4 were malignant teratomas. The patients ranged in age from 13 days to 51 years.

Neurogenic tumors

Sixteen patients, ranging from 18 to 60 years of age, had neurogenic tumors. Six of these tumors were benign (neurofibroma, 4; neurolemmoma, 2) and 10 were malignant (neuroblastoma, 6; ganglioneuroblastoma, 2; ependymoma, 1; neurofibrosarcoma, 1). Low back, sacral and nerve root pain were reported in all of the patients with malignant tumors. Three of the six patients with benign tumors also complained of pain over the sacral and hip areas. Patients in this group ranged from 5 to 47 years of age.

Osseous tumors

Ten patients in this category, ranging in age from 7 to 28 years, accounted for 7% of our series. Six tumors were benign (giant cell tumor, 4; osteoblastoma, 1; aneurysmal bone cyst, 1). The four malignant tumors were Ewing sarcoma in two cases and myeloma in two. All 10 patients had some degree of bone destruction preoperatively. All four patients with giant cell tumors had local recurrence after operation, but remained alive 6 to 19 years after the initial treatment.

Soft tissue tumors

Seven of the 10 soft tissue tumors were benign (leiomyoma, 3; lipoma, 2; fibroma, 2), and all were resected without complication or need for reoperation. The three malignant tumors (hemangiopericytoma, 2; fibrosarcoma, 1) were treated by incomplete resection; two of these patients remain alive, 2 years and 3 years postoperatively. The third lived for 4 years before succumbing to metastatic disease.

CLINICAL PRESENTATION

Retroperitoneal tumors of the pelvis are well concealed lesions with no classic signs or symptoms. Most grow slowly in a functionally 'silent' area, permitting them to achieve sizable proportions without producing obvious symptoms. Because of the vague nature of the symptoms, it is difficult to determine the onset of the condition accurately prior to operation. Twenty percent of our patients had no symptoms, and their tumor was found on incidental pelvic examination. In two patients, the tumor was first recognized when obstruction of labor required cesarean section. Sixteen patients underwent prior exploration with a presumptive diagnosis of uterine fibroids or ovarian tumor (in most of these cases the incision was promptly closed, but in four, a biopsy was performed prior to referral for definitive care).

Many patients complained of multiple symptoms resulting from compression or obstruction of adjacent organs or pressure on pelvic nerves or bone. Thirty-five percent of our patients had bowel symptoms consisting of incomplete emptying, tenesmus, obstipation or rectal pain. Urinary retention, incontinence, or urgency and frequency were ascribed to the tumor mass in 10% of our patients. Pain was most commonly associated with malignant tumors, and was described as steady and located low in the back or over the buttocks or sacral area. All bone tumors were associated with back or sacral pain. Their presence becomes apparent when neurologic deficits occur as a result of invasion or distortion of the nerve roots or of the trunks of the sciatic or pudendal nerves. Motor dysfunction of the lower extremity may be manifested in the gluteal, hamstring, gastrocnemius, or soleus group, with coincidental atrophy and diminished Achilles reflex. In our experience, impairment of the anal or saddle area was not a frequent finding, nor were anal or urinary incontinence or fecal soiling.

Aside from the palpable presacral mass, which can be noted on pelvic examination in more than 90% of the patients and occasionally even felt on abdominal examination, there are other, less-striking findings. These consist of small café-au-lait spots in conjunction with scattered neurofibromas, venous engorgement of the buttocks over the tumor, or distortion of the outer contour of the buttocks. Other suggestive findings noted by review of the history were tender sciatic nerve, positive sciatic stretch test, draining perirectal sinuses, and palpable mass in the buttocks. The gynecologist is so accustomed to palpating for a primary tumor of the bowel or of the structures lying anterior to it (uterus, ovary or pelvic peritoneum) during the rectovaginal and pelvic examinations, that it requires a conscious effort to palpate the presacral region (Fig. 63.1).

DIAGNOSIS

Accurate diagnosis prior to operation is essential for successful management of retroperitoneal tumors. Some tumors can attain remarkable size without associated clinical symptoms. Developmental cysts are usually located in the midline, and are soft and non-tender. Occasionally, a communicating sinus will be associated with one of these and can be detected in the posterior midline of the anal canal, inferior to the dentate line; it may be confused with a fistulous opening. Anterior sacral meningoceles have similar characteristics; however, pressure may elicit a headache or a cough impulse. Sacral chordomas are solid tumors, are fixed to the sacrum, and have a rubbery consistency. Neurogenic tumors lie laterally, on one side or the other but not on both, on the posterior rectal wall; they are firm, smooth, semifixed and non-tender. Bony tumors are often solid and fixed; rarely, they are soft.

Results of sigmoidoscopy, intravenous pyelography, and barium enema examination are either normal or demonstrate only extrinsic compression by the tumor (Fig. 63.2). Plain anterior or posterior and lateral radiographs are useful (some tumors are seen only on the lateral view). Fine calcific deposits are found in patients with benign teratomas. Twenty-nine patients had some lytic bone destruction of the pelvis associated with the presacral

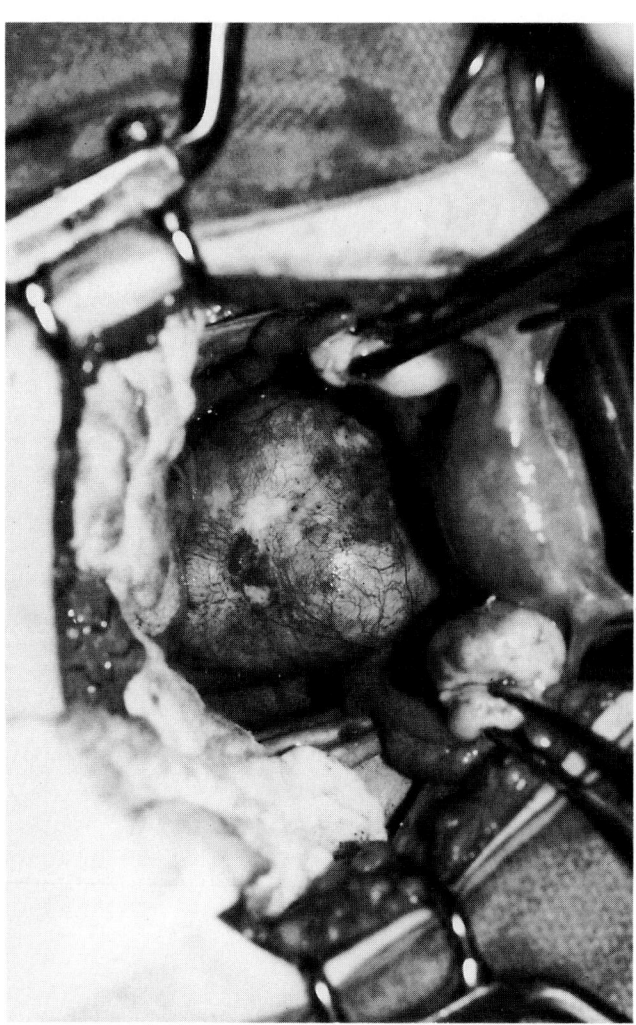

Fig. 63.1 Presacral location of an 11 cm dermoid in an asymptomatic patient.

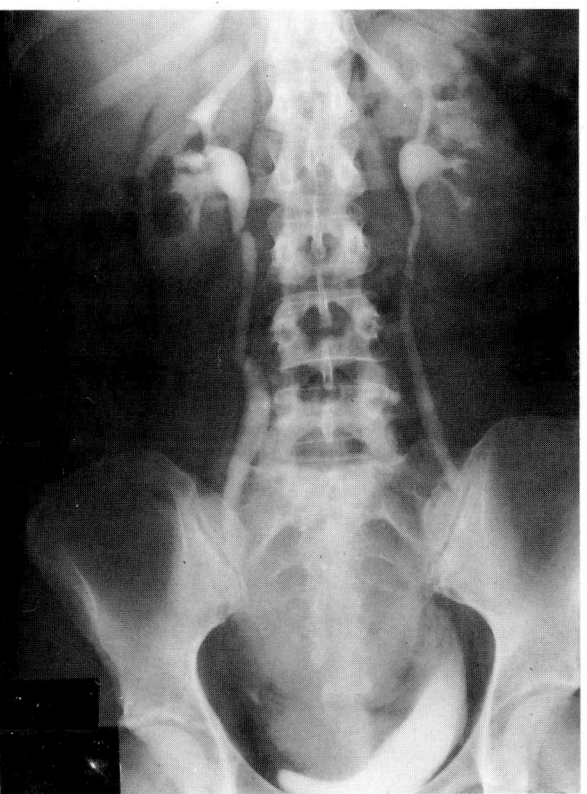

Fig. 63.2 Distortion of the bladder by a neurolemmoma of the right pelvic sidewall.

tumor (80% with malignant tumors and 20% with benign tumors). Recently, computed tomography has proven valuable in the delineation of intraosseous and presacral tumors (Fig. 63.3). The exact degree of tumor invasion can be determined; however, the diagnosis remains non-specific.

The differential diagnosis between anterior sacral meningocele and other presacral cysts is very important. Prior to 1960, the operative mortality with anterior sacral meningocele was more than 40%, chiefly due to misdiagnosis. Oren et al[9] emphasized that aspiration for diagnosis or therapy was worthless because the cyst simply refilled, and it was also dangerous because of ascending meningitis. Transrectal and transvaginal drainage of the cyst is also to be condemned because of the high mortality. Ascending meningitis can also occur from aspiration at the time of laparotomy. A congenital malformation of the sacrum suggests the possibility of an anterior meningocele or a myelomeningocele that presents as a protrusion of the sacral nerves and their covering through an anterior sacral defect associated with spina bifida. On a plain radiograph, a scimitar (short, curved sword with its edge on the convex side) defect of the sacrum and the absence of a coccyx are typical (Fig. 63.4). A myelogram usually shows passage of contrast medium from the caudal sac into the presacral cyst (Fig. 63.5). When operation is undertaken, the neck of the sac is ligated via a trans-sacral approach.

It should be emphasized that needle biopsy has little or no role in the diagnosis of presacral tumors unless the tumor is obviously unresectable or metastatic. Because of the potential complications associated with biopsy, especially of a meningocele, or the potential for seeding of a malignant tumor, it is our recommendation that, whenever possible, the only biopsy of a resectable presacral tumor should be total excision. Trans-sacral or transrectal biopsy of chordomas and other osseous malignancies potentially

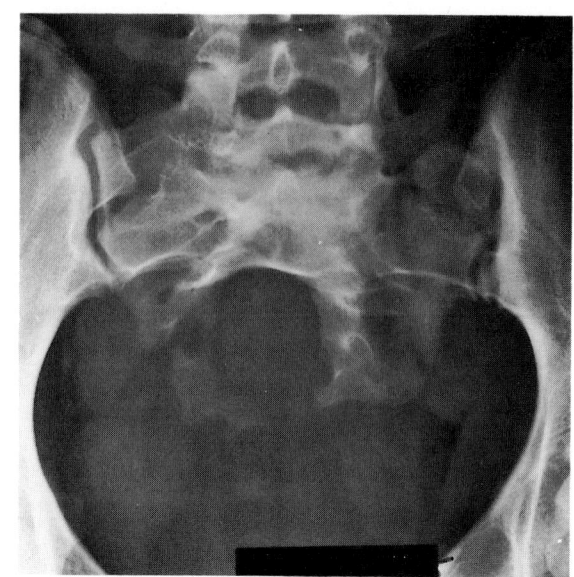

Fig. 63.4 Scimitar defect of the sacrum.

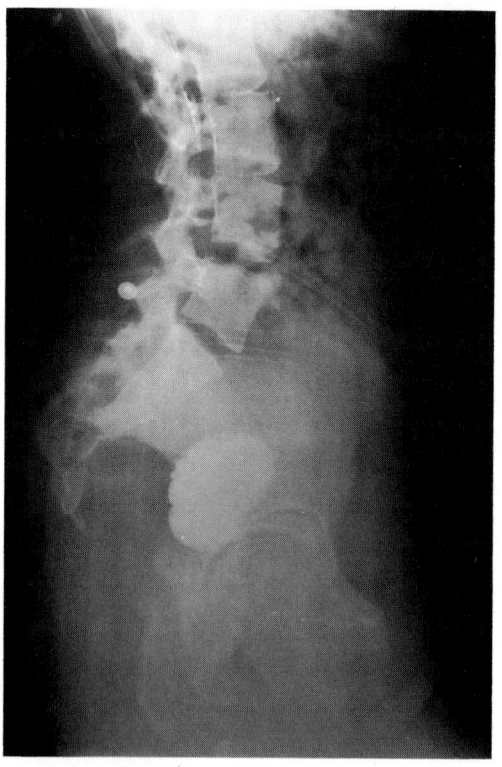

Fig. 63.5 Myelogram (lateral view) from the same patient as Fig. 63.4, showing radiopaque dye in the meningeal sac.

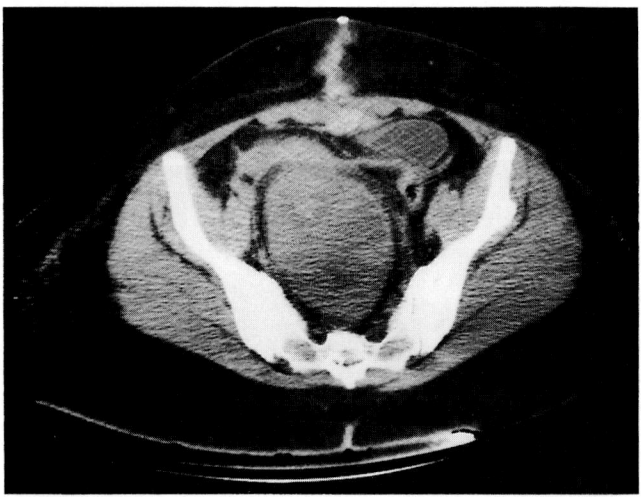

Fig. 63.3 Computed tomographic scan, showing a presacral mass distorting contiguous tissues.

increases the recurrence rate, and presacral abscesses and fistulas occur with significant frequency. A single exception may be the pediatric patient in whom needle biopsy permits accurate diagnosis and appropriate chemotherapy, which markedly decreases tumor size and facilitates safe operative resection later.

TREATMENT

Once a retroperitoneal tumor is diagnosed (even in an asymptomatic patient), the treatment of first choice (except with selected meningoceles) is surgical resection. The mortality with untreated anterior sacral meningocele is 30%, chiefly because of infection and meningitis. Neoplasms may be malignant or, with time, may undergo malignant transformation which obviates the need for a planned resection. Cystic lesions occasionally become infected, which leads to incomplete resection and a significant rate of recurrence. Repeated operations in the affected area may disrupt the neural function of bladder or bowel, leading to intractable incontinence.

Patients undergoing operation at our institution may be treated by various surgical specialties or, sometimes, by a team made up of several different specialties. In a previously reported[5] study of 70 patients, 60% were operated on by a pelvic surgeon (gynecologic-general surgeon), 8% by a neurosurgeon, 7% by an orthopedist, and 25% by a team composed of a combination of these specialties (Fig. 63.6). In our clinical experience, approximately one-half of the tumors are located at or above the midsacrum. An abdominal approach was selected in 56% of our patients, trans-sacral in 28%, abdominoperineal in 9%, and trans-

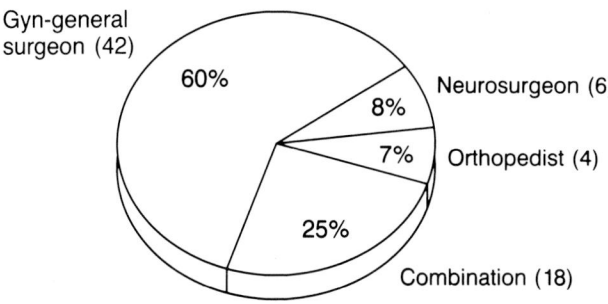

Fig. 63.6 Distribution of specialties in the care of patients with presacral tumors.

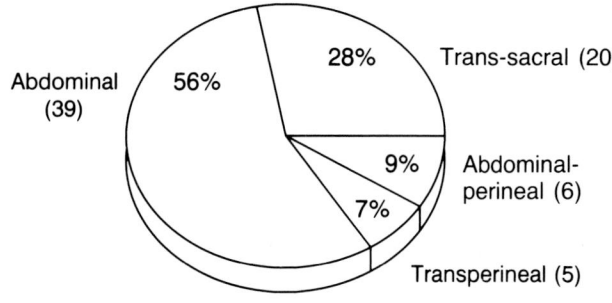

Fig. 63.7 Frequency of various operative approaches.

perineal in the lithotomy position in 7% (Fig. 63.7).

Benign presacral tumors can be managed surgically by one of several approaches, The choice is dictated by the size and location of the tumor and its relationship to contiguous structures. Generally, a trans-sacral approach (Fig. 63.8) is selected when the tumor is 8 cm or less in diameter and located over the lower 10 cm of the sacrum and coccyx. The patient is placed in the prone position with buttocks elevated and trunk and thighs tied (Kratske position). A midline incision is made over the sacrum down to the anal ring. The coccyx is excised, and the rectum is freed from the sacrum. Tumors that are fixed to the sacrum require sharp dissection with an osteotome and scissors – that is, dissection of the ligaments, muscles or portions of the sacrum lateral to the tumor margins. The nerves, especially the pudendal nerves, are protected. MacCarty et al[8] emphasized that urinary retention is avoided if the upper three sacral nerves can be preserved, at least unilaterally. Retention of urine occurs if the third, fourth and fifth sacral nerves or both pudendal nerves are cut bilaterally. If the tumor is not attached to the sacrum or is not invading the surrounding structures, it is freed from the sacrum by sharp dissection and the rectum is separated from the anterior surface of the tumor.

Tumors in a similar location can also be approached with the patient in the lithotomy position (Fig. 63.9). An incision that extends from the vagina, hooks around the rectum, and enters the presacral space is used, thus permitting the rectum and vagina to be elevated and displaced to the patient's right or left, depending on the location of the tumor.

An abdominal approach offers the advantage of a thorough evaluation of the abdomen and upper pelvis, with safe and accurate mobilization and displacement of the rectum and ureters from the upper and anterior surface of the tumor. Frequently, the anterior division of each internal iliac vessel is ligated as the perirectal and perivesical spaces are developed and the tumor is set up for excision. The tumor is usually excised *en bloc* but, occasionally, when the tumor is fixed against adjacent structures and the histologic diagnosis is known to be benign, we have found it expeditious to remove the center portion by morcellation, thus allowing a more accurate and safe dissection of the tumor from the upper vascular structures along the pelvic sidewall and from the sacral plexus. Similarly, a large cystic tumor (teratoma or epidermoid) may be entered (purposely or inadvertently) and its putty-like contents removed, thus collapsing the cyst. Placement of a hand within the cystic wall facilitates the dissection and complete excision of the tumor.

When the combined abdominoperineal approach is elected, the abdominal procedure is performed first. When the tumor is freed as completely as possible by this approach, the patient is turned, and a trans-sacral or transperineal dissection is performed to allow perineal

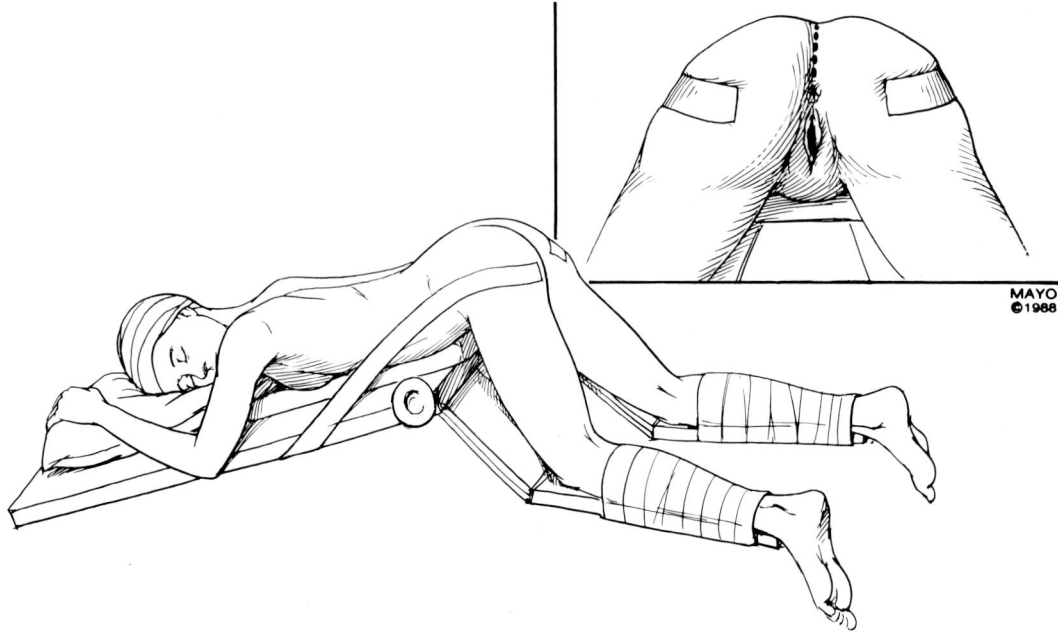

Fig. 63.8 Kratske position for excision of presacral tumors. (By permission of Mayo Foundation.)

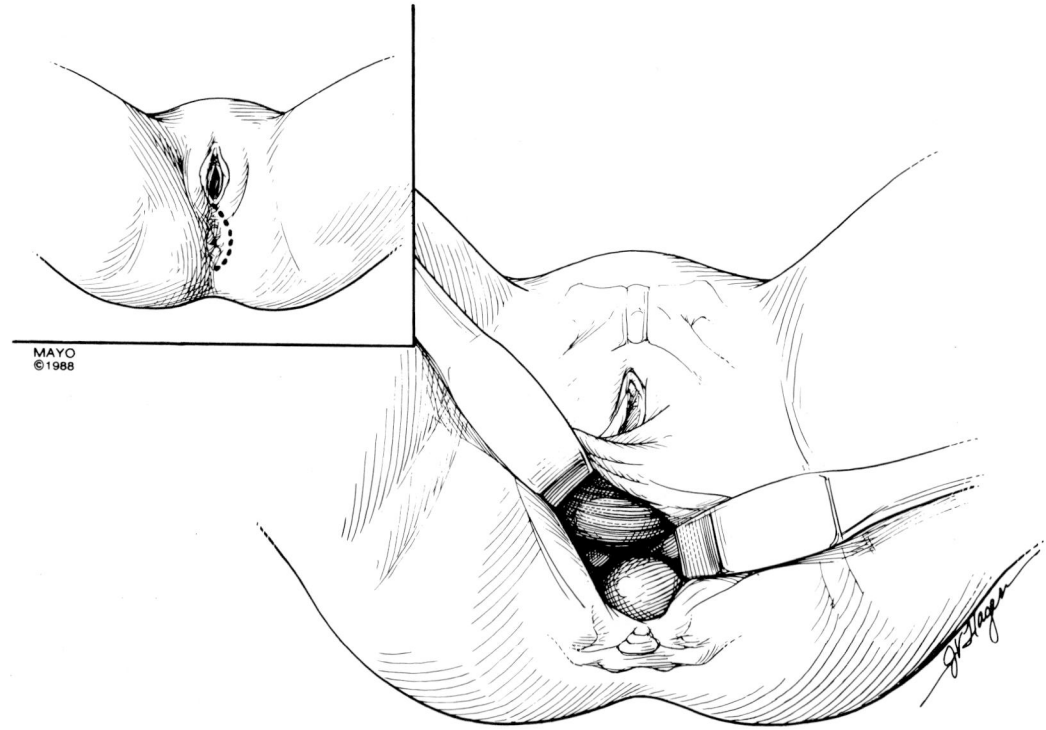

Fig. 63.9 Cephalad and lateral displacement of rectum from presacral space. *Inset.* Vaginal incision continued lateral to the rectum which is then lifted off the hollow of the sacrum. (By permission of Mayo Foundation.)

removal of the tumor. Occasionally, during a primary trans-sacral or transperineal approach, a concomitant abdominal dissection may be required for complete resection of the tumor. If the patient is in the lithotomy position (transperineal approach), a supplementary abdominal incision can be accomplished easily.

Localio et al[6] prefer a lateral synchronous abdominal-trans-sacral approach, noting that it provides maximal flexibility for tumors located in this rather inaccessible area and allows protection of the rectum, ureters and major vessels. The abdomen is entered through an oblique incision between the iliac crest and the costal margin, running parallel to the inguinal ligament. The colon and ureters are displaced, and the upper margin of the tumor is identified. Tapes are placed around the iliac vessels, a transverse incision is made over the sacrum, skin flaps are developed, and the gluteal muscles are detached from the sacral origin. The presacral space is entered and connected to the abdominal dissection. Sacral tuberous, sacrospinous and lower sacral iliac ligaments are divided, and the sacroiliac articulation is dissected via the abdominal incision.

Complete, preferably en bloc, excision should be performed to eliminate the possibility of recurrence or persistence of tumor. Benign tumors that displace contiguous structures can be removed safely and expeditiously with minimal risk of bleeding and postoperative complications. Treatment of invading malignant tumors along with their associated fixation, complications and frequent recurrence gives disappointing results. There is little apparent benefit from supplemental irradiation or chemotherapy.

COMPLICATIONS AND RESULTS

Complications occurred in approximately 25% of our patients. Bleeding occurred in 15% of cases (more than 1 unit [500 ml] of blood to a maximum of 17 units). Temporary urinary retention for 3 to 5 days was common, but decreased sensitivity to bladder filling or the need to apply suprapubic pressure was noted in 5% of the patients at the end of 6 months postoperatively. Wound infection occurred in 5% of patients; stool incontinence and retrorectal abscess occurred in 2%. We had no operative deaths.

REFERENCES

1. Cody H S III, Marcove R C, Quan S H 1981 Malignant retrorectal tumors: 28 years' experience at Memorial Sloan-Kettering Cancer Center. Dis Colon Rectum 24: 501
2. Ewing J 1940 Neoplastic Diseases. A Treatise on Tumors, 4th edn. Saunders, Philadelphia
3. Freier D T, Stanley J C, Thompson N W 1971 Retrorectal tumors in adults. Surg Gynecol Obstet 132: 681
4. Laird D R 1954 Presacral cystic tumors. Am J Surg 88: 793
5. Lee R A, Symmonds R E 1988 Presacral tumors in the female: clinical presentation, surgical management and results. Obstet Gynecol 71: 216
6. Localio S A, Eng K, Ranson J H C 1980 Abdominosacral approach for retrorectal tumors. Ann Surg 191: 555
7. Lovelady S B, Dockerty M B 1949 Extragenital pelvic tumors in women. Am J Obstet Gynecol 58: 215
8. MacCarty C S, Waugh J M, Mayo C W, Coventry M B 1952 The surgical treatment of presacral tumors: a combined problem. Proc Staff Meet Mayo Clin 27: 73
9. Oren M, Lorber B, Lee S H, Truex R C Jr, Gennaro A R 1977 Anterior sacral meningocele: report of five cases and review of the literature. Dis Colon Rectum 20: 492
10. Spencer R J, Jackman R J 1962 Surgical management of precoccygeal cysts. Surg Gynecol Obstet 115: 449
11. Stewart R J, Humphreys W G, Parks T G 1986 The presentation and management of presacral tumours. Br J Surg 73: 153
12. Teplick S K, Stark P, Clark R E, Metz J R, Shapiro J H 1978 The retrorectal space. Clin Radiol 29: 177
13. Uhlig B E, Johnson R L 1975 Presacral tumors and cysts in adults. Dis Colon Rectum 18: 581
14. Whittaker L D, Pemberton J de J 1938 Tumors ventral to the sacrum. Ann Surg 107: 96

PART XI

Trophoblastic tumors

64. Pathology and classification of trophoblastic tumors

F. J. Paradinas

INTRODUCTION

Trophoblastic tumors are fetal allografts in maternal tissues. As such, they present unique biological, immunological and pathological problems. Since one of the main functions of trophoblast is to gain access to the maternal circulation, normal trophoblast infiltrates, invades vessels and can even be transported to the lungs,[2] in a fashion which is otherwise only seen in malignant neoplasms. It follows, that histological criteria used to diagnose malignancy in other neoplasms are not applicable to trophoblast. In addition, trophoblastic tumors are relatively rare and likely to be unfamiliar to both physician and pathologist in non-specialized centers. This, and the frequent difficulties in obtaining adequate samples, can make pathological diagnosis difficult or impossible. The above facts fully justify the now well established approach of treating patients on the basis of clinical criteria and serological hCG estimations. It also means that some patients will be treated and cured without it ever being known whether the disease treated was an invasive hydatidiform mole or a choriocarcinoma. Terms such as *gestational trophoblastic disease (GTD)* and *persistent trophoblastic disease (PTD)* accurately describe this situation.[71]

The success of chemotherapy in gestational trophoblastic tumors has resulted in a marked reduction in the numbers of pathological specimens available for study, but the behavior of trophoblastic tumors unchecked by chemotherapy is well known from earlier accounts.[9,19,28,29,53,56,58] In recent years, genetic studies have provided additional information which has helped us both to understand the nature of these abnormalities and to test and improve the morphological criteria which have so far been the basis of pathological diagnosis.

Normal trophoblast

Two morphologically distinct trophoblastic populations are seen at the implantation site: villous and extravillous trophoblast.

Villous trophoblast covers chorionic villi (Fig. 64.1) and consists of cytotrophoblast and syncytiotrophoblast. The rather primitive mononuclear cytotrophoblastic cells have a clear cytoplasm (which reflects their paucity of cellular organelles) and a high mitotic rate. Syncytiotrophoblast differentiates from cytotrophoblast and is composed of multinucleated cells with abundant, dense cytoplasm. It secretes abundant hCG but has little capacity for further proliferation. The amount of villous trophoblast in relation to the amount of villous stroma gradually decreases as the pregnancy advances (Fig. 64.1).

Extravillous trophoblast forms the trophoblastic columns in the intervillous spaces and infiltrates decidua, spiral arteries and myometrium at the placental bed (placental-site trophoblast). It is composed of mononuclear and, less often, multinucleated cells with a dense eosinophilic cytoplasm (Fig. 64.2). It is morphologically different from villous cytotrophoblast and syncytiotrophoblast and is defined immunocytochemically by positive staining for human placental lactogen (hPL)[30] and cytokeratins,[42] scanty hCG and no placental alkaline phosphatase (PLAP).[72] The term *intermediate trophoblast* has been proposed for non-villous trophoblast. The possible functions and biological differences between the various types of trophoblast are under study.[12,57,73]

CLASSIFICATION OF TROPHOBLASTIC LESIONS

The common pathology of trophoblastic lesions (Table 64.1) is an excessive proliferation of trophoblast. In hydatidiform moles this essentially consists of chorionic villi covered by villous trophoblast and variable amounts of intermediate trophoblast. This is known to occur in association with at least two distinct genetic abnormalities: when all the diploid nuclear genome is derived from the father (complete mole)[36] and in association with triploidy

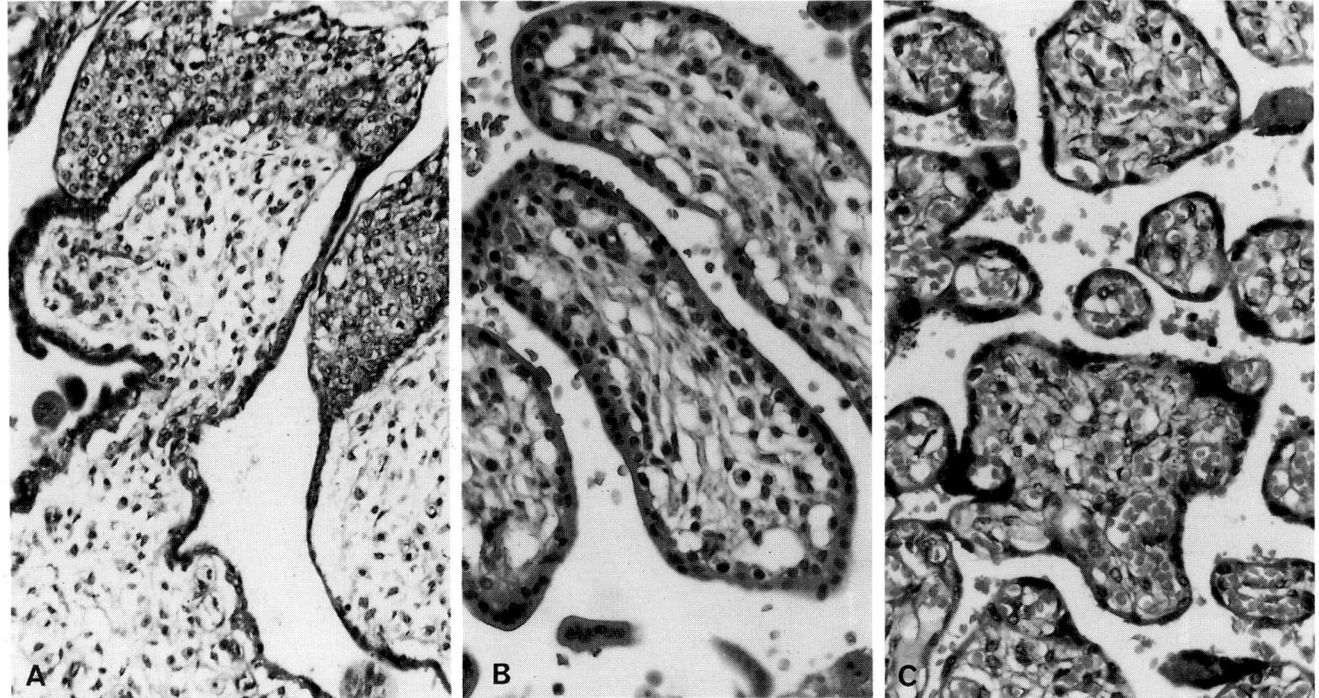

Fig. 64.1 Chorionic villi in a normal first trimester pregnancy (A), mid-trimester pregnancy (B) and at term (C). Note the abundant trophoblast and paucity of vessels in early pregnancy. In mid-trimester villi, there is thin but continuous syncytiotrophoblast covering an interrupted cytotrophoblastic layer. At term, there are numerous vessels, cytotrophoblastic cells are few and the nuclei of the syncytiotrophoblast cluster into syncytial knots. (H & E, ×210)

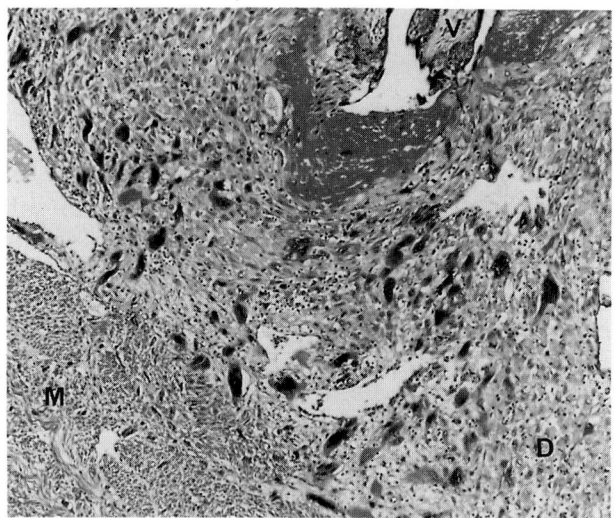

Fig. 64.2 Mononuclear and multinucleated intermediate trophoblast infiltrating decidua (D) and myometrium (M) in the placental bed of a normal pregnancy. A chorionic villus (V) is present at the top. (H & E, ×45)

contributed by both paternal and maternal chromosomes (partial mole).[36,62,69] In complete moles the disease can remit spontaneously or it can relentlessly progress, invade the myometrium and even perforate the uterus (invasive mole).

In the typical and most common form of choriocarcinoma the tumor is composed predominantly of cells resembling villous cyto- and syncytiotrophoblast without chorionic villi. The tumor invades and metastasizes in the most aggressive way and without treatment the disease was nearly always fatal.[9]

Placental site trophoblast can also proliferate excessively. Exaggerated forms of placental site reaction may remit spontaneously or be cured by simple curettage. Rarely, they progress unchecked, invade adjacent organs and metastasize in a neoplastic fashion; the term, placental site trophoblastic tumor (PSTT)[59] has been generally accepted for this rare disease. The name 'placental site nodule' has been recently suggested for exaggerated, but self-limiting proliferations of placental site trophoblast.[74]

HYDATIDIFORM MOLES

Complete hydatidiform mole

Cytogenetic studies have shown that the classical hydatidiform mole of previous classifications is the result of proliferation of a purely paternal conceptus;[36] this results either from fertilization of an egg by a single sperm bearing a 23X complement, consequent loss of maternal nuclear material

Table 64.1 Abnormal trophoblastic proliferations

Abnormality	Embryo	Villi	Trophoblast
Of villous trophoblast			
Hydropic abortion	Yes	Abnormal	No excess
Partial hydatidiform mole (HM)	Yes	Abnormal	Some excess
Complete and invasive HM	No	Abnormal	Marked excess
Choriocarcinoma	No	No	Neoplastic
Of placental-site trophoblast			
Placental-site trophoblastic nodule	No	No	Self-limiting
Placental-site trophoblastic tumor	No	No	Neoplastic

and duplication of paternal material to a 46XX homozygous complement, or, less frequently, from fertilization by two sperms resulting in 46XX or 46XY heterozygous complements.[33,35,47,55,69] As a rule, maternal DNA can be found only in mitochondria.[16,70] More recently, the androgenetic origin of complete mole has been confirmed by molecular genetic studies.[24]

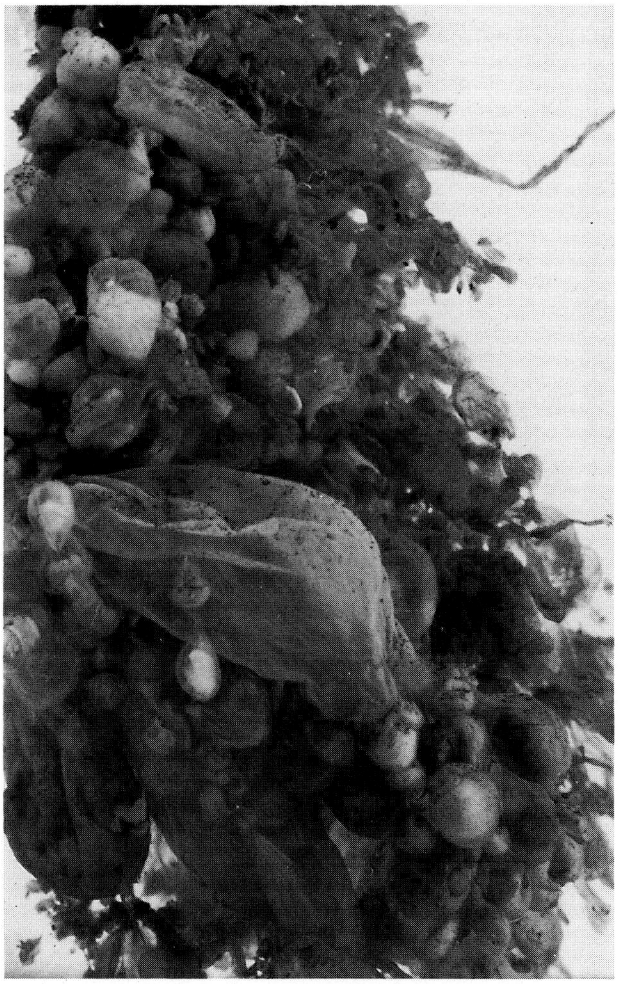

These genetic abnormalities result in trophoblastic differentiation in which cyto- and syncytiotrophoblast proliferate excessively around swollen chorionic villi, but neither an embryo nor, with possible exceptions, an amniotic cavity, are present. The swelling of villi is diffuse, and results in the characteristic 'bunch of grapes' of classical mole (Fig. 64.3).

Histological examination shows swollen villi, often completely surrounded by sprouts of villous trophoblast (Fig. 64.4) in which nuclear pleomorphism is often more intense than in normal pregnancy; clusters of similar cyto- and

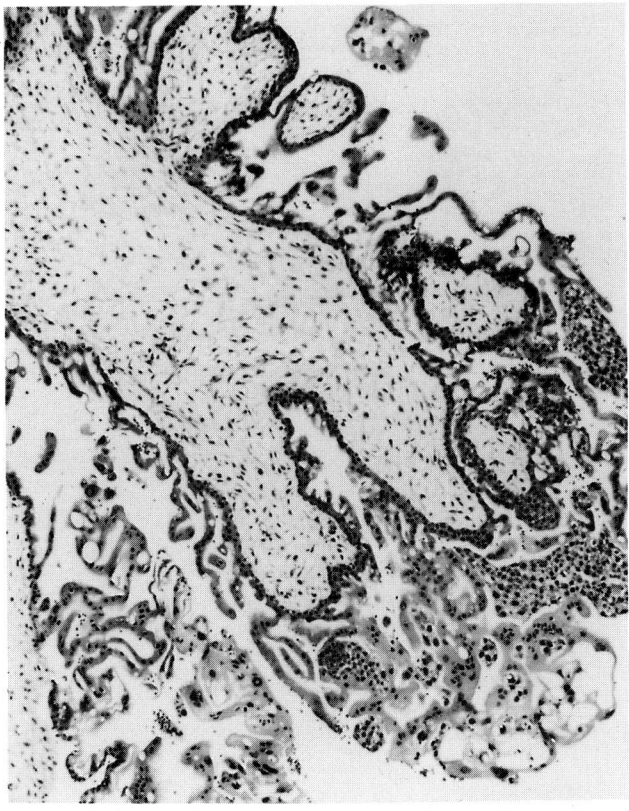

Fig. 64.3 Complete mole. Irregular mass of hydropic villi which affects the whole placenta. A fetus is absent and no amniotic cavity is usually discernible. (×1.8)

Fig. 64.4 Complete mole. Excessive amounts of cyto- and syncytiotrophoblast surround swollen villi which are also of a polypoid irregular shape. The stroma lacks patent vessels. (H & E, ×57)

syncytiotrophoblast and some intermediate trophoblast are often seen amongst villi.

Vessels are seen at the periphery of some villi; often collapsed and always empty, denoting the absence of a fetus and fetal circulation, but many villi are avascular. Fluid tends to collect in 'cisterns' in the middle of villi, resulting in compression of vessels and other components of villous stroma beneath the cytotrophoblastic layer (Fig. 64.5). Non-hydropic but irregularly shaped villi are also a feature of moles. No significant morphological differences have been observed between XX and XY complete moles, but pleomorphic villi and residual capillaries are more common in young moles and cisternae are more common in older moles.[35]

Ideally, a morphological diagnosis of complete mole based on these macroscopical and microscopical features should be confirmed by genetic studies, but this is seldom possible, or indeed, necessary. Additional support for a diagnosis of complete mole, rather than partial mole, can be derived from the finding of a diploid DNA complement by flow cytometry and by finding a hyperdiploid fraction significantly higher than that of normal placentas.[27] This can be done in fixed or paraffin-embedded material.

Invasive mole

The majority of complete moles remit after evacuation and curettage, but the tendency in some instances to invade the myometrium resulting in uterine perforation and extension to adjacent organs is well known. Histologically, the appearance of the chorionic villi is similar to that of other moles, but swelling of villi is less often seen in deeply implanted invasive moles, and histological diagnosis is based on the excessive trophoblastic proliferation, markedly irregular shape of villi and their invasive nature (Fig. 64.6). Some degree of myometrial invasion is probably present in most moles; indeed, myometrial invasion is not exclusive to molar pregnancies, and Hertig,[28] borrowing the terminology used for myometrial placentation, classified invasive moles into accreta, increta and percreta. Since hysterectomy is nowadays rarely necessary in the treatment of invasive moles the few specimens seen by the pathologist are, paradoxically, percreta moles (the rarest form). They present as acute abdomen due to uterine perforation, and consist of a hematoma with molar villi often implanted on a pelvic organ, such as the ovary, tube or broad ligament, or on a loop of intestine.

Molar metastases

Molar tissue can spread to the cervix, vaginal wall and

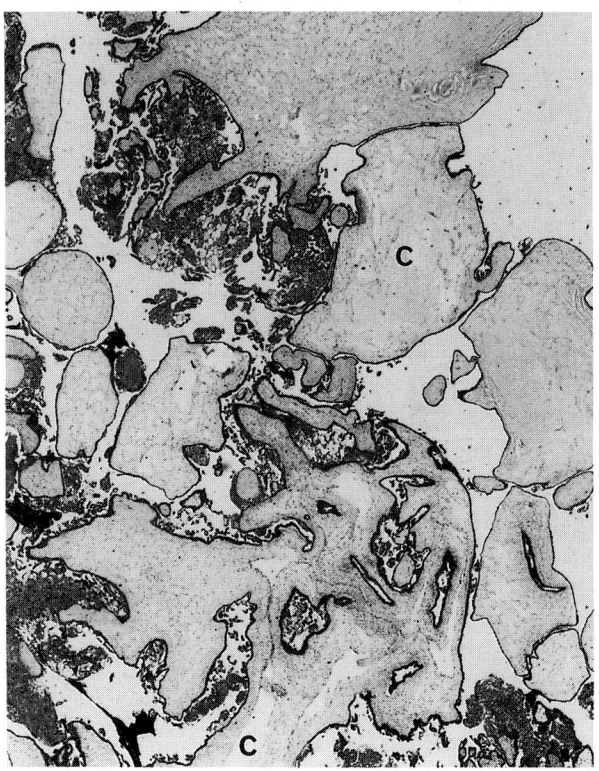

Fig. 64.5 Complete mole. Cisterns (C) are present in some villi; this change is usually more marked in older moles. (H & E, ×8)

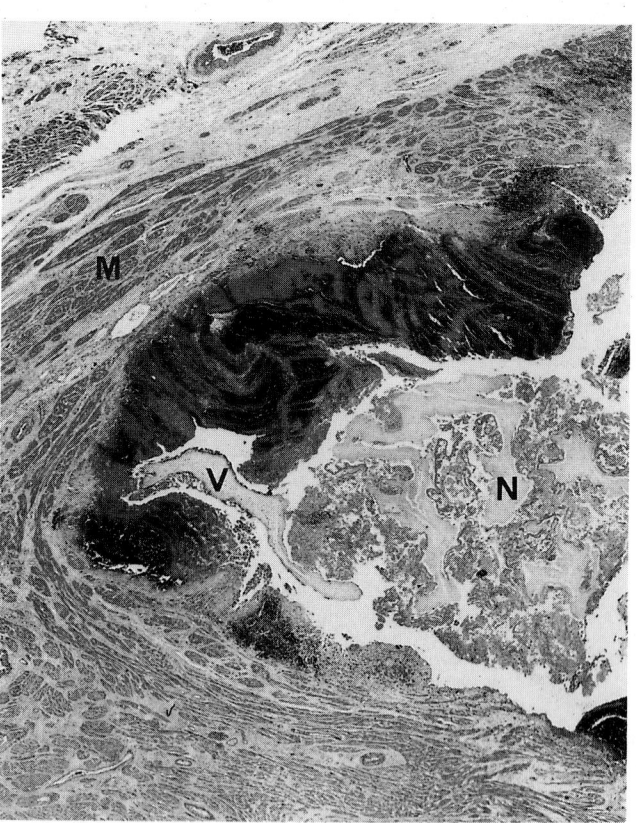

Fig. 64.6 Invasive mole. Viable (V) and necrotic (N) molar villi erode the myometrium (M). They are surrounded by a zone of dark hemorrhage. A thin myometrial layer (0.5 cm) separated the mole from the peritoneal cavity. (H & E, ×9.5)

vulva.[14,26] It has been estimated that 10% of patients with moles have radiological lung opacities which have been interpreted as metastases[4] and this has been confirmed histologically in some cases.[50,67] Exceptionally, molar tissue has been found in other sites, including brain, retroperitoneum and inguinal lymph nodes.[56] In pre-chemotherapy days lung metastases sometimes regressed after evacuation or eradication of the mole, but the appearance or persistence of metastases long after evacuation may indicate PTD or choriocarcinoma.

Prognosis of complete and invasive moles

It has proved impossible so far, to grow the trophoblast of moles in tissue culture or in nude mice,[37] whereas this can be readily done with choriocarcinomas. This supports the view that the excessive molar trophoblastic proliferation may be hyperplastic rather than neoplastic. Nevertheless, molar trophoblast can continue to grow and invade, needing active intervention to preserve the uterus or to avoid a catastrophic hemorrhage. It is doubtful whether molar trophoblast can survive more than 300 days, and most complications due to persistent or invasive moles occur in the 6 months following a molar evacuation. Although the incidence of moles needing treatment varies according to the criteria for selection and the lack of distinction between complete and partial moles in most series, they do not exceed 8%.[5]

Neoplastic transformation of a mole is recognized when villous stroma is no longer formed, but nothing is known about the factors which control this change in behavior. The degree of hyperplasia of molar trophoblast proposed by Hertig[29] has not, in the hands of others,[11,21,32] proven reliable in predicting the development of choriocarcinoma or PTD. Nuclear pleomorphism of trophoblast is more marked in moles than in non-molar pregnancies and this is reflected in a higher hyperdiploid fraction demonstrated by flow cytometry,[27] but this is similarly unreliable in predicting outcome. A higher incidence of persistent trophoblastic disease was initially reported in heterozygous moles, but this has not been supported by more recent studies.[22] Clearly, the problem requires further evaluation.

Ectopic moles

Ober & Maier[54] accepted only 4 of 22 cases reported in the literature[38] as possible examples of ectopic mole. It appears that tubal moles are considerably rarer than tubal choriocarcinoma, and no tubal mole appears to have been followed by choriocarcinoma.

Partial hydatidiform mole

The presence of swollen villi in triploid conceptuses has been known for a number of years[6] but, in a systematic

study, Vassilakos et al[69] pointed out that, characteristically, this change affected only part of the placenta (partial mole), a fetus, often with congenital malformations, was frequently found, and there was serological or morphological evidence of excessive trophoblastic proliferation. Subsequent studies[34,46,48,63] indicate that partial mole, defined as excessive trophoblastic proliferation in conceptuses with a maternal genetic contribution, is almost exclusively seen in triploid conceptuses with two chromosomal complements from the father and one from the mother. Fig. 64.7 demonstrates this focal hydropic change in a triploid conceptus.

The fetal malformations seen in triploid conceptuses include cranial, cardiac, urogenital and limb abnormalities,[15,51] but in some cases, particularly in live-born fetuses or those aborted late in pregnancy, both the fetus and the placenta may be apparently normal.[10]

In a typical case, the histological diagnosis of partial mole is favored by the finding of normal and swollen villi side by side (Fig. 64.8) and the presence of a fetus or, if a fetus is not found, a fetal circulation with vessels containing nucleated red cells (Fig. 64.9). Some villi show a curious scalloping or dentate outline (Fig. 64.10) which results in frequent trophoblastic pseudo-inclusions. Cisterns are formed in the same fashion as in complete mole. Trophoblastic proliferation is not as intense as in complete mole and, when present, consists predominantly of vacuolated syncytiotrophoblast. Often, the evidence of excessive trophoblastic proliferation is derived from unusually high serum hCG estimations rather than histologically detectable hyperplasia, which may be difficult to assess in some specimens. In some spontaneous triploid abortions, early fetal death precludes identification of a fetus or fetal red cells; in such cases, the presence of open blood vessels in villi (Fig. 64.11) or the presence of amniotic membranes (Fig. 64.12) suggests partial rather than complete mole.

Cytogenetic or molecular genetic studies would be helpful for accurate diagnosis. In their absence, DNA flow cytometry can usually distinguish between diploid complete moles and triploid partial moles, and also between triploid partial moles and non-molar diploid hydropic abortions.[23,43]

Although most instances of partial mole are triploid, a few cases of diploid partial moles have been reported.[66] In some of these cases, alternative explanations for the presence of a fetus, such as a complete mole coexisting with a non-molar pregnancy,[25] have not been excluded; there is, however, evidence that some trisomies and other chromosomal abnormalities may have trophoblastic hyperplasia and hydropic villi with cistern formation.[31,68]

Prognosis of partial mole

A few instances of partial moles followed by PTD have

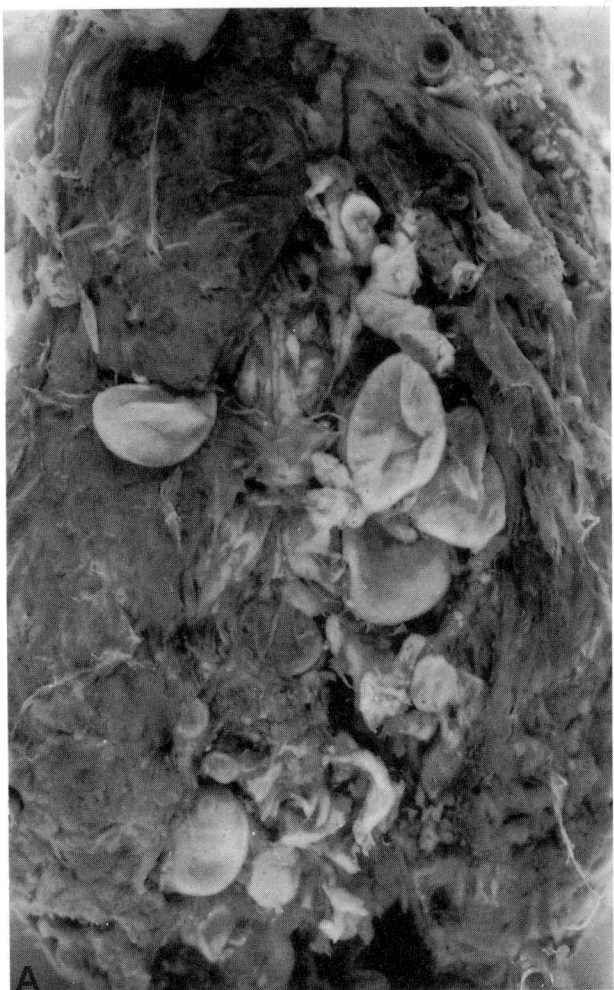 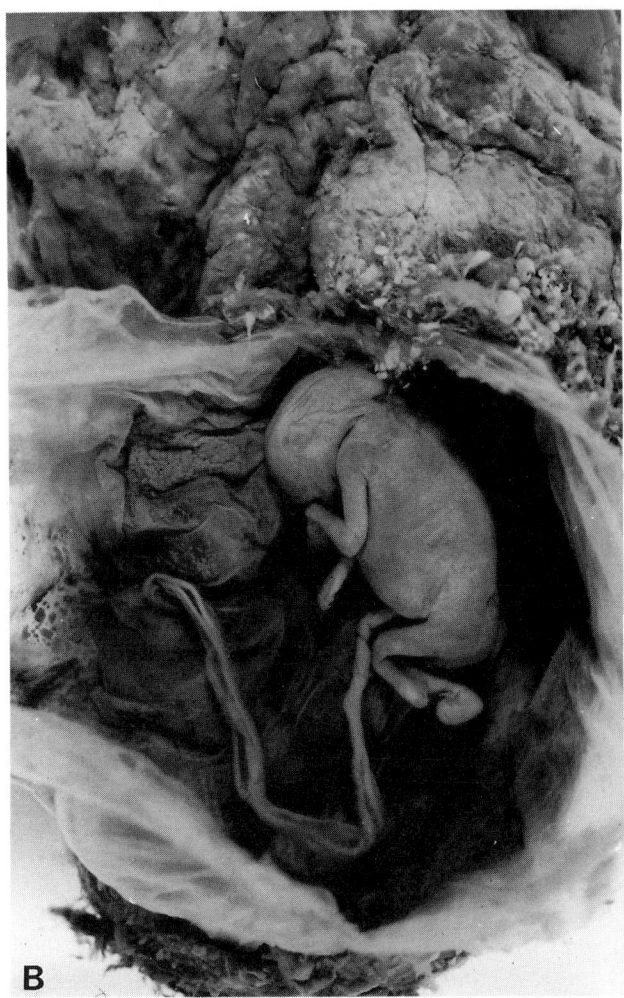

Fig. 64.7 Partial mole from a mid trimester abortion. **A** The maternal aspect of the placenta is shown with partial hydropic change. **B** The opposite aspect of the same specimen shows an amniotic cavity with a malformed fetus. (Natural size).

been reported,[8,64,65] as well as a choriocarcinoma.[49] In our experience, this undoubtedly occurs, but the incidence of PTD after triploid pregnancies, whether accompanied by excessive trophoblastic proliferation (partial moles) or not, is not known. If a parallel is drawn with complete moles, where the degree of trophoblastic proliferation is not a good predictor of the risk, it seems sensible to follow up women with any triploid pregnancies until this risk is better defined.

Further studies are also needed to ascertain the genetics, biological significance and nature of the risk of diploid partial moles.

Differential diagnosis of moles

Difficulties in diagnosis derive mainly from an inadequate sample, and from the fact that none of the histological features of moles is pathognomonic. The main problems encountered by the pathologist are:

1. *Is it early pregnancy or complete mole?* The intense trophoblastic proliferation of early pregnancy (Fig. 64.1) can be misinterpreted histologically as a mole. The problem is less likely to arise if the macroscopical appearances of the tissue have been clearly recorded and the likely age of the pregnancy is known. However, occasionally, early pregnancy has to be recognized by the polar, rather than circumferential, distribution of trophoblast around the villi, the rather less pleomorphic trophoblast, the relatively uniform size of villi, often radiating from a central cavity (Fig. 64.13) and the lack of well developed cisterns.

2. *Is it complete or partial mole?* The answer to this question is of crucial importance, given the different behavior and prognosis of these two diseases. When the sample is good, the differential diagnosis is easy, but a poor sample may not show the focal nature of the hydropic change in partial mole or the extent of trophoblastic proliferation in complete mole. Paucity of trophoblastic sprouts, scalloping of villi, and frequent trophoblastic inclusions favor partial

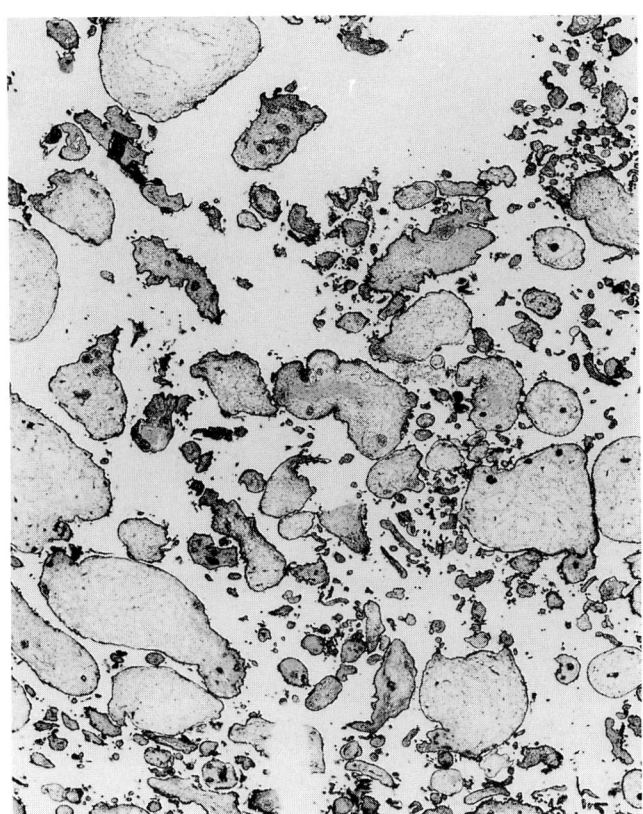

Fig. 64.8 Partial moles are so named, because the hydropic change is present in only some villi. (H & E, ×9.5)

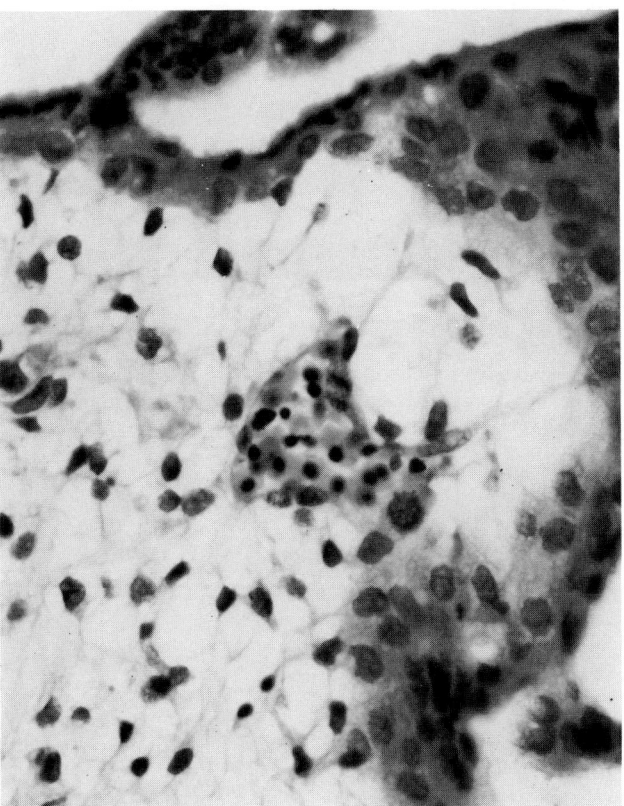

Fig. 64.9 Part of a hydropic villus in a partial mole showing a capillary vessel with a mixture of nucleated and non nucleated fetal red cells. Fetal erythroblasts are indirect evidence of the existence of a fetus and rule out a diagnosis of complete mole. (H & E ×425)

mole. The presence of fetal tissues or nucleated fetal red cells in the villi excludes a diagnosis of complete mole. The presence of recognizable amniotic membranes is also useful, since it is doubtful that amnios ever develops in complete moles. The problem of diploid partial moles has already been discussed, but in most cases DNA flow cytometry will differentiate between complete and partial moles.[23,43]

3. *Is it mole or are the hydropic changes due to other causes?* The observation of focal or generalized swelling of chorionic villi without excessive trophoblastic proliferation is common; occasionally, it turns out to be due to inadequate sampling of a complete or a partial mole, but more often no such diagnosis is possible. Early death of a normal embryo or an abnormal embryo in a variety of chromosomal defects, are possible explanations.[31,61] Examination of material from spontaneous abortions shows a high incidence of triploidy and we know that when triploidy is due to two maternal rather than two paternal chromosomal sets, trophoblastic proliferation is not excessive.[34,44,45] DNA flow cytometry in this group of hydropic abortions will therefore show a proportion of triploid conceptuses and some of them will not have the morphological features of a mole.[68] A better cytogenetic definition of these

cases and follow-up data are needed before we know whether there is an increased incidence of PTD in these abnormal conceptuses.

CHORIOCARCINOMA

Choriocarcinoma is a malignant neoplasm in which differentiation towards villous cytotrophoblast and syncytiotrophoblast is seen (Fig. 64.14). It can occur after normal pregnancy, stillbirth, abortion, ectopic pregnancy, complete or partial hydatidiform mole and possibly 'ab initio',[1] but the incidence of choriocarcinoma after complete hydatidiform mole is about a thousand times greater than after a normal pregnancy. The proportion of choriocarcinomas preceded by moles in reported series varies between 39 and 78%.[71] It has been shown, however, that the immediate antecedent pregnancy is not necessarily the pregnancy causing the tumor.

As in the case of hydatidiform mole, there are remarkable differences in the incidence of choriocarcinoma in various parts of the world. These are not always explained by an increase in preceding moles, but a serious epidemiological study of the problem is hindered by variations in the way in which the information is recorded, bias

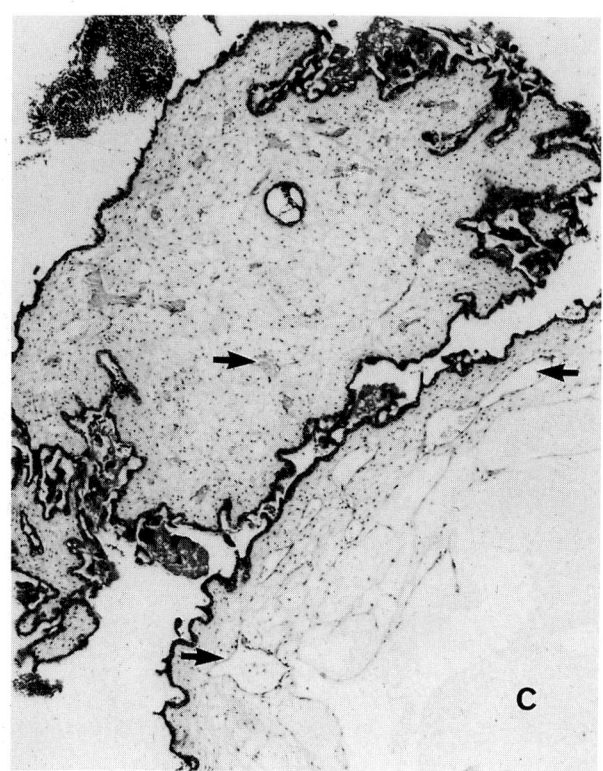 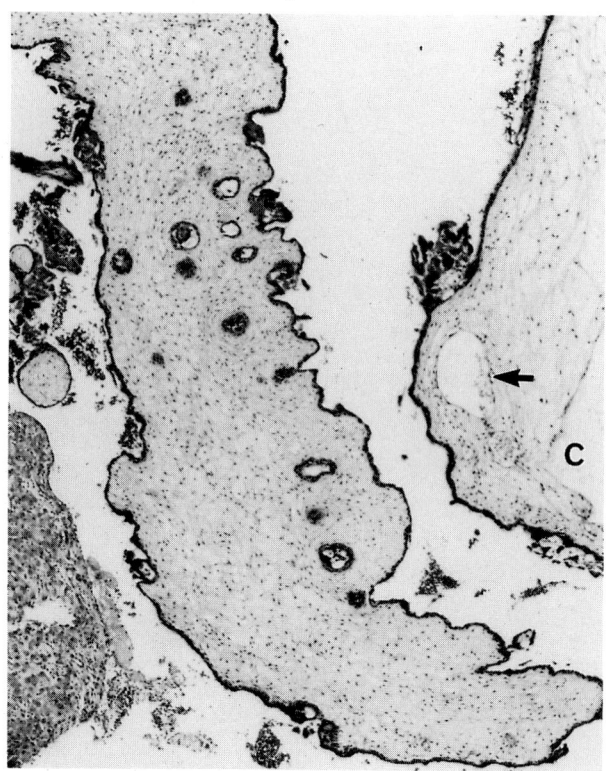

Fig. 64.10 Partial mole. Note the formation of cisterns (C), the scalloping outline of some villi and the presence of trophoblastic inclusions. No embryo was found, but the presence of numerous open vessels (arrows) suggest that an embryonic circulation and an embryo must have formed. (H & E, ×36)

in the selection of reported cases and the very success of therapy, which nowadays all too often precludes us from knowing the true nature of the trophoblastic disease treated.

Macroscopically, uterine choriocarcinoma appears as a hemorrhagic nodule which may be in contact with the lining of the uterine cavity or may lie in the myometrium (Fig. 64.15). Microscopically, viable tumor is usually seen only at the periphery of the nodule and within vascular spaces in the adjacent myometrium. The characteristic bilaminar structure of villous trophoblast is usually easily identifiable, but in some cases most of the tumor is either predominantly syncytiotrophoblastic (Fig. 64.16) or predominantly cytotrophoblastic (Fig. 64.17). In general, these histological variations are not associated with different behavior or prognosis but some predominantly cytotrophoblastic tumors secrete smaller amounts of hCG.[20] This is not surprising, since synthesis of hCG occurs mainly in syncytiotrophoblast. Some hPL is usually demonstrable in syncytiotrophoblast but, unlike placental-site trophoblast, villous cytotrophoblast does not contain significant amounts of hPL.

Choriocarcinoma metastasizes readily. It is not uncommon to find secondary nodules in the cervix or vagina. The lungs, brain and liver are the distant organs more often involved. In contrast, lymph nodes are rarely the site of

metastasis, and the finding of a tumor with apparent trophoblastic differentiation in lymph nodes without evidence of a gestational primary should raise doubts about the gestational origin of the tumor, which could be of germ cell origin or a carcinoma with trophoblastic metaplasia.

Heterotopic choriocarcinoma

Ober & Maier[54] found 58 acceptable examples of primary choriocarcinoma of the fallopian tube amongst 93 reported cases, and added 18 cases of their own. About 60% of patients presented with acute symptoms simulating an ectopic pregnancy and the rest had a pelvic mass indistinguishable from an ovarian tumor. In no case was there evidence of a preceding ectopic mole, but in two instances there were residual chorionic villi and evidence of an amniotic cavity. In all other aspects (distribution of metastases, mortality, response to chemotherapy) the tumors behaved like uterine choriocarcinomas. Only 5 of 47 patients survived after salpingectomy or salpingo-oophorectomy before the advent of modern chemotherapy; in contrast 15 of 16 patients treated with chemotherapy survived.

Although cases of gestational choriocarcinoma of the ovary and peritoneal cavity have been reported,[7,56] reliable evidence of their gestational rather than germ-cell origin

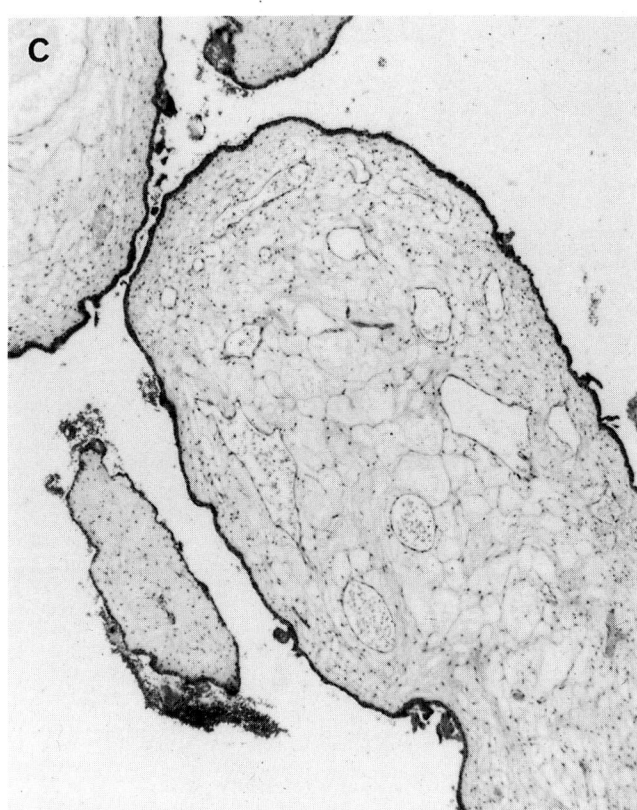

Fig. 64.11 Partial mole. These villi do not show significant trophoblastic hyperplasia but show cistern formation (C) and the presence of many dilated capillaries containing necrotic cellular debris. This appearance is common in partial mole after death of the fetus. (H & E, ×38)

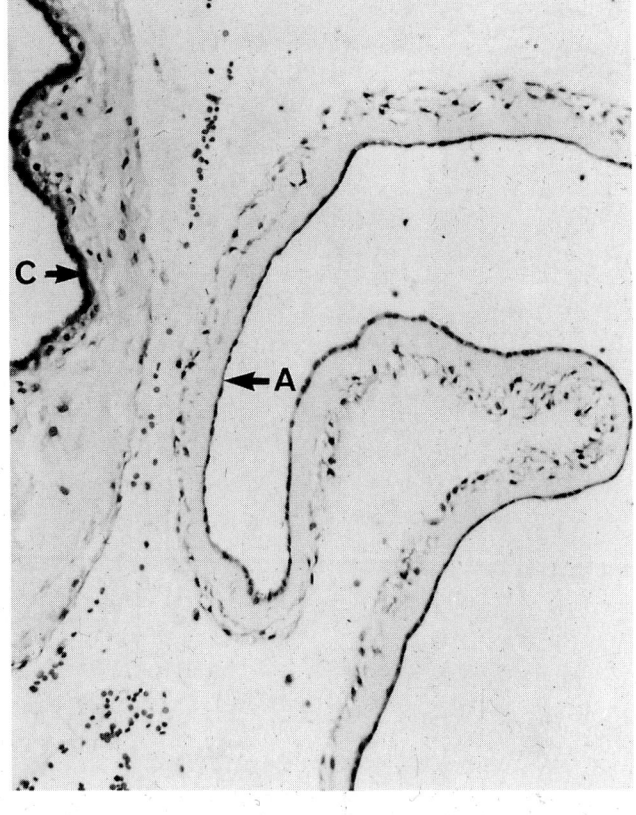

Fig. 64.12 Chorion (C) and amnios (A) from an aborted partial mole. The presence of amnios, even when a fetus or fetal circulation are not apparent, is against a diagnosis of complete mole. (H & E, ×143)

can only be obtained by genetic fingerprinting of the tumor, the patient and the patient's partner. Trophoblastic metaplasia and hCG production can occur in many carcinomas,[40] including ovarian and endometrial carcinomas.[3] Histological differentiation from choriocarcinoma is not always easy (see below) but carcinomas with trophoblastic metaplasia probably account for the majority of so called 'primary choriocarcinomas' reported in viscera, including the lungs, stomach, pancreas, bladder and kidney.

Differential diagnosis of choriocarcinoma

The main problems are as follows:

1. *Is it choriocarcinoma or trophoblast from an early pregnancy?* A curettage in an early pregnancy may yield abundant cyto- and syncytiotrophoblast only. As a rule, the trophoblast is less pleomorphic than in choriocarcinoma and its polar arrangement may still be discernible. It is exceptional to find villi when choriocarcinoma develops. The presence of villi in endometrial curettings is against a diagnosis of choriocarcinoma, but in a few cases residual, often degenerate villi were seen.[20] Ober[54] describes a choriocar-

cinoma in the fallopian tube with a blastocyst in the middle. The diagnosis was made on the basis of extensive trophoblastic infiltration of the wall without infiltration by the villi, and it was confirmed when the patient died with liver metastases.

2. *Is it choriocarcinoma or a complete mole?* Endometrial curettage weeks or months after evacuation of a mole may show pleomorphic trophoblast without villous stroma. Sometimes, this is not due to development of choriocarcinoma but to inadequate sampling of a mole. In these circumstances, a firm morphological diagnosis in endometrial curettings of choriocarcinoma, rather than mole, is seldom possible,[21] but the index of suspicion of choriocarcinoma increases with an increase in the period of time since evacuation of the mole and when the trophoblast is very abundant or very pleomorphic.

3. *Is it choriocarcinoma or carcinoma with trophoblastic metaplasia?* Anaplastic carcinomas of many organs, including the ovary and endometrium, can show hCG production and morphological trophoblastic metaplasia;[3,13,40] these tumors are usually less hemorrhagic and less necrotic than gestational choriocarcinoma, and viable tumor is often found in the middle of the masses. Immunostaining for

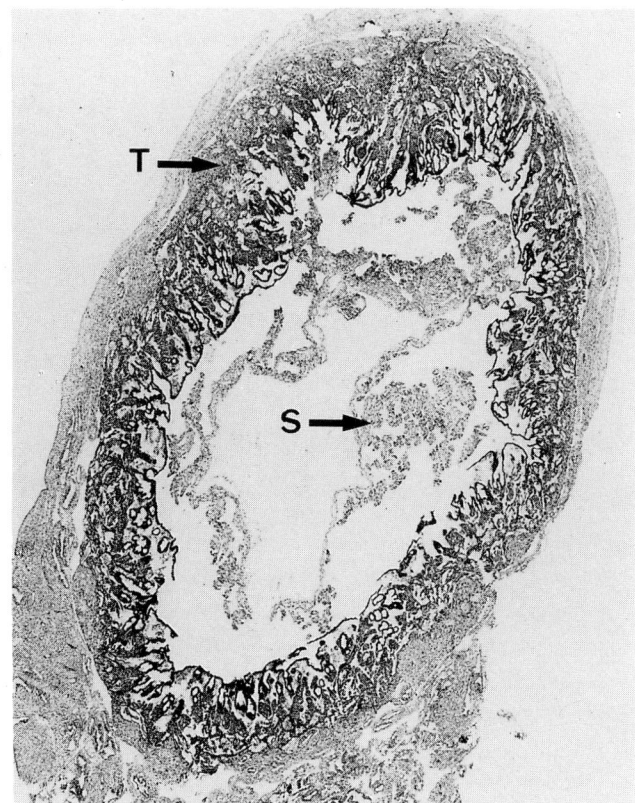

Fig. 64.13 Early implantation site from a normal pregnancy. Note the abundant villous trophoblast (T) and scanty villous stroma (S) which has artifactually shrunk within the central cavity. When large amounts of this villous trophoblast appear in fragmented endometrial curettings, they can be wrongly interpreted as part of a mole or as choriocarcinoma. (H & E, ×9.5)

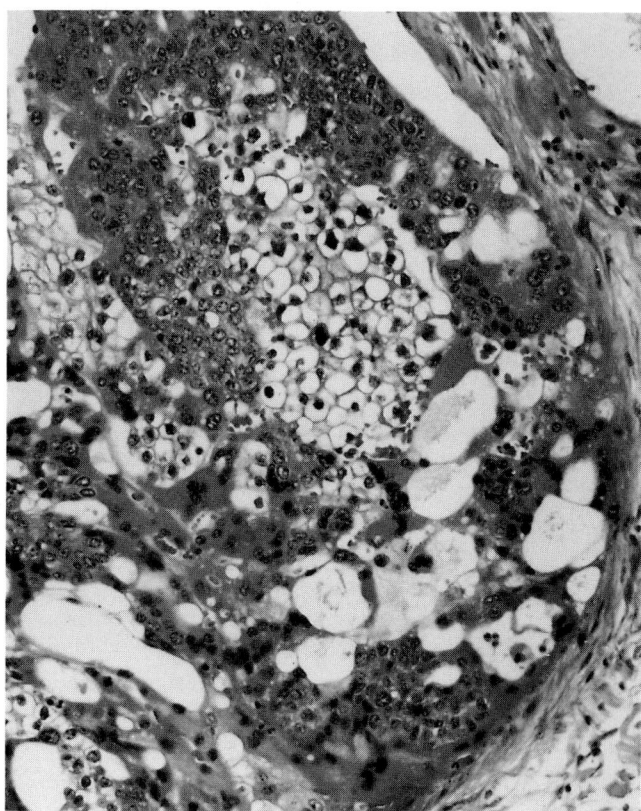

Fig. 64.14 Choriocarcinoma composed of a mixture of mononuclear cytotrophoblast and multinucleated syncytiotrophoblast. (H & E, ×143)

hCG is usually positive in carcinomas, but hPL is usually negative. The presence of a vascular stroma and the possible differentiation towards glands or other structures favor carcinoma with trophoblastic metaplasia but in some cases differentiation from gestational choriocarcinoma may be difficult and only confirmed by examination of genetic material from the tumor, the patient and her partner. The problem is of more than academic interest, since sustained remissions are seldom obtained in carcinomas with trophoblastic metaplasia.

4. *Is it choriocarcinoma or placental site trophoblastic tumor?* The histological distinction between these two neoplasms is usually easy, but in some cases the mononuclear component of a choriocarcinoma is a mixture of villous cytotrophoblast and cells resembling placental site trophoblast. Indeed, in the clinical course of some of these tumors there are sometimes great variations in the amounts of hCG present in the serum which are not explained by tumor regression alone, and it is relevant to ask whether tumors with mixed differentiation exist and whether the villous trophoblastic component of a mixed tumor is more easily eliminated by therapy, leaving behind a more resistant PST-like component. Predominantly

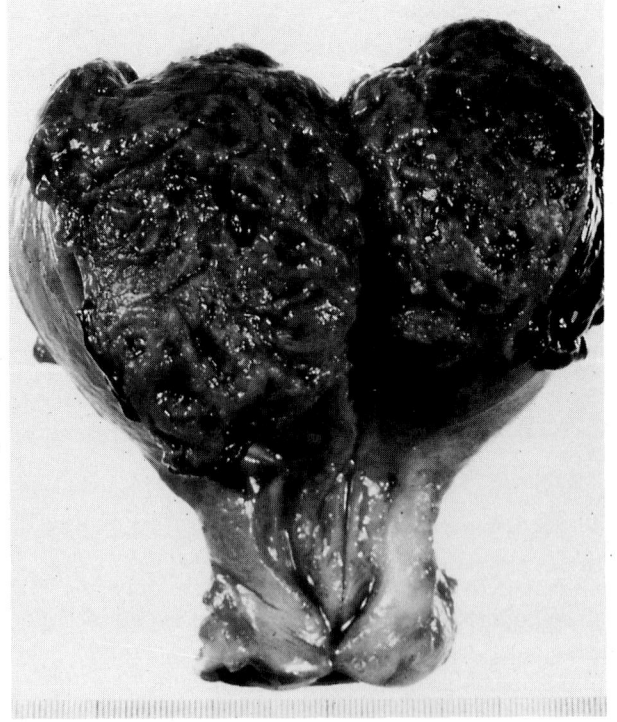

Fig. 64.15 Hemisected uterus showing hemorrhagic and necrotic choriocarcinoma replacing the uterine body.

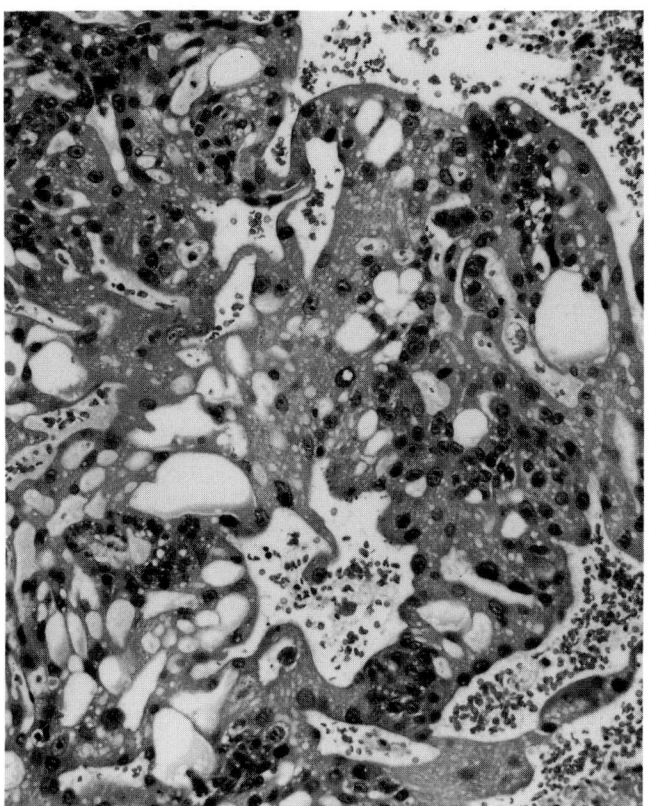

Fig. 64.16 Choriocarcinoma from an endometrial curettage. This example is predominantly syncytiotrophoblastic. (H & E, ×143)

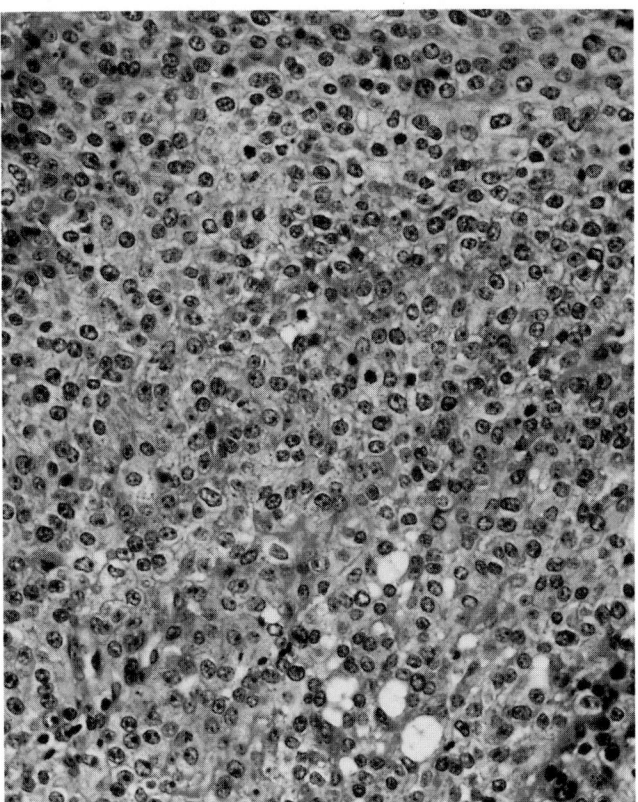

Fig. 64.17 Choriocarcinoma with predominant cytotrophoblastic pattern. The tumor showed typical syncytiotrophoblast in other areas. (H & E, ×143)

cytotrophoblastic choriocarcinomas differ from PSTT by the absence of hPL in villous cytotrophoblast.

PLACENTAL SITE TROPHOBLASTIC TUMOR

Placental site trophoblastic tumor (PSTT) is the tumorous counterpart of the non-villous trophoblast which infiltrates the placental site in normal pregnancy. Tumors of this type have been recognized for many years, and have been variously named 'atypical chorioepitheliomas', 'syncytiomas', and 'corionepitheliosis'.[19] More recently, Kurman, Scully & Norris,[41] described 12 cases in which the lesion remained localized and was sometimes eradicated by simple curettage. They proposed the term 'trophoblastic pseudotumor', but within a few years it was clear that, on occasions, this lesion behaved in a locally aggressive way and could metastasize.[17,59,75] Although recognizing that this tumor is an atypical form of choriocarcinoma, we prefer to use the name 'placental site trophoblastic tumor',[59] which reflects the morphological similarities with placental site trophoblast.

PSTT presents with amenorrhea or irregular vaginal bleeding months or years after a normal pregnancy, an abortion or, rarely, a hydatidiform mole.[17,18,75] The uterus is usually enlarged and serum levels of pregnancy proteins such as hCG, placental lactogen (hPL) and β1-glycoprotein

(SP-1) are elevated, although hCG is seldom as high as in choriocarcinoma. A curettage may yield decidua or myometrium infiltrated by trophoblastic cells with dense eosinophilic cytoplasm and pleomorphic nuclei (Fig. 64.18); they can be mononuclear or multinucleated and they often form clusters or cords and separate smooth muscle fibers. It may be difficult, or even impossible, to differentiate between an exaggerated placental site reaction and PSTT in endometrial curettings, since there may be scanty material or it may be extensively necrotic. The formation of large clusters of trophoblastic cells, and frequent mitoses, appear to be reliable criteria of neoplasia but, in many instances, it may only be possible to say that there is persistent placental site trophoblast and to judge whether it is physiological or pathological in the light of clinical and serological observations. In the few cases where DNA flow cytometry has been done, the tumor has been found to be diploid.[18,60]

Examination of hysterectomy specimens shows clear differences between PSTT and choriocarcinoma. PSTT forms masses in which necrosis is marked, but hemorrhage is less conspicuous (Fig. 64.19). This reflects a lesser tendency to vascular invasion, infiltration being predominantly interstitial. The process can nevertheless infiltrate relentlessly and extend into adjacent organs, such as the ovary and parametrium. Distant metastases can occur in peritoneum,

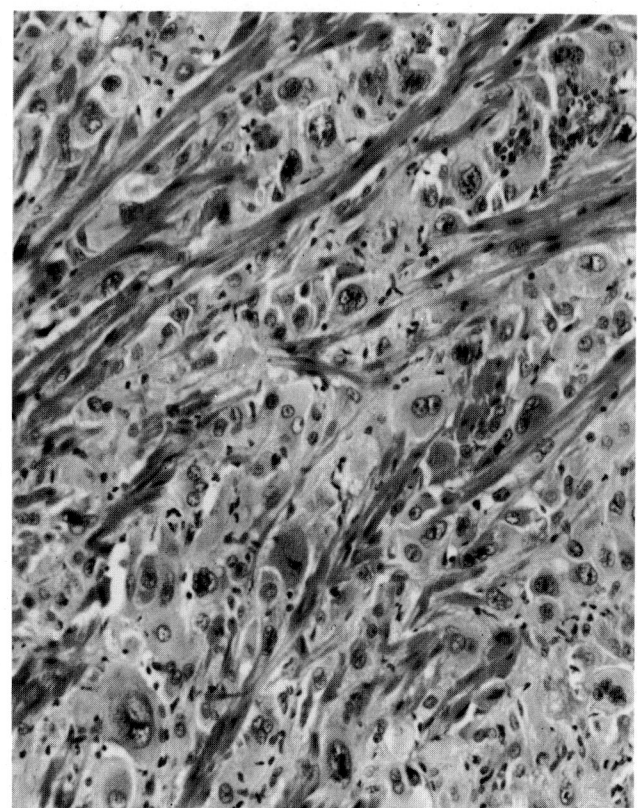

Fig. 64.18 Placental-site trophoblastic tumor. Note the interstitial infiltration of tumor cells amongst myometrial smooth muscle fibers. (H & E, ×143)

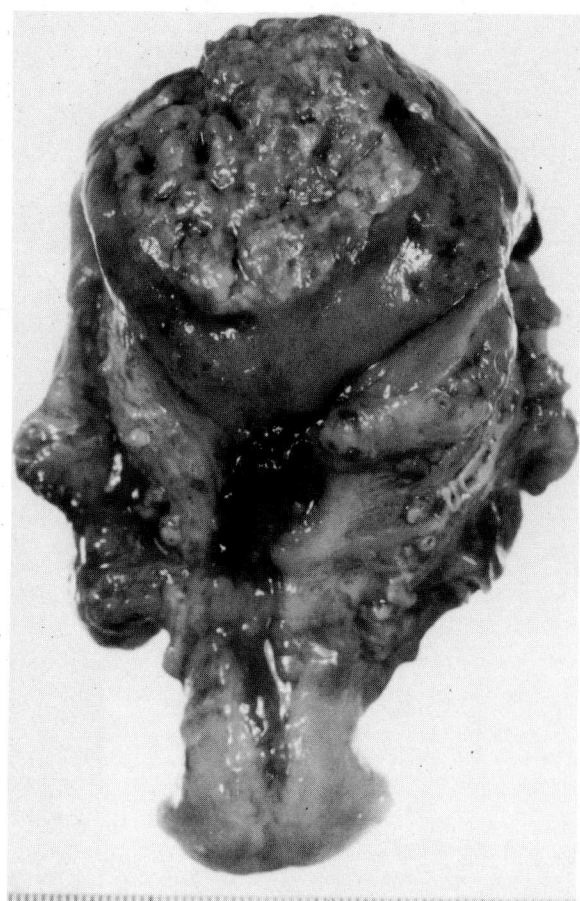

Fig. 64.19 Opened uterus with placental-site trophoblastic tumor. There is necrosis in the middle of the mass, but hemorrhage is less conspicuous than in choriocarcinoma (see Fig. 64.15).

liver, pancreas, lungs and brain. Since vascular invasion is not a reliable criterion of malignancy (physiological trophoblast can invade vessels) it appears that mitotic counts (more than 5 mitoses per 10 high power fields) may predict tumors with metastasizing potential.[75]

In four instances (about 10% of reported cases) PSTT has been associated with the nephrotic syndrome, which has remitted after eradication of the tumor.[17,76] Fibrin and IgM have been found in glomerular intracapillary deposits, and disseminated intravascular coagulation (DIC) postulated as the main pathogenetic mechanism. A report of virilization and testosterone production by a PSTT appears exceptional.[52]

The importance of recognizing this tumor type lies on the one hand in its lesser degree of metastasizing potential, which makes it amenable to surgery, and on the other hand in its great resistance to chemotherapy, which accounts for therapeutic failures when surgical resection is not possible. It has been pointed out that lesser degrees of placental site trophoblastic proliferation may regress spontaneously;[41,74] the term 'placental site trophoblastic nodule' has been proposed for these self-limiting lesions.[74] In our experience, regressing lesions often show marked hyalinization and, occasionally, there is difficulty in demonstrating cytoplasmic hPL, but the epithelial nature of the

trophoblastic cells can be demonstrated with cytokeratin antisera.

PATHOLOGICAL LESIONS ASSOCIATED WITH TROPHOBLASTIC TUMORS

Luteal ovarian cysts accompany hydatidiform mole and choriocarcinoma in a variable number of patients, and an incidence of 94% in one report is quoted by Park.[56] Luteinization of granulosa and theca cells occurs throughout both ovaries, but its intensity varies in different patients and does not appear to be related to hCG levels in serum. Rupture can occur[39] and needle aspiration of the cysts has been recommended to prevent this. It is important not to confuse these ovarian lesions with metastatic choriocarcinoma.

SUMMARY AND CONCLUSIONS

Recent genetic observations firmly link excessive trophoblastic proliferation in a conceptus to chromosomal abnormalities, particularly the presence of more than one chromosomal complement from the father. The most severe abnormality (two complements from the father and none from the mother) results in complete hydatidiform mole, a condition which may need treatment and can transform into choriocarcinoma. Triploidy, with two paternal complements, and possibly other chromosomal abnormalities are associated with partial mole, a condition in which a fetus develops and trophoblastic proliferation is less intense. This condition is not yet well characterized and we do not know how often it is followed by persistent trophoblastic disease or choriocarcinoma.

The differences in the behavior and response to therapy of the two well defined neoplasms arising from trophoblast: typical choriocarcinoma and placental site trophoblastic tumor, have stimulated research into the morphology and physiology of the various types of trophoblast, but the etiology and pathogenesis of trophoblastic neoplasia are still unknown.

ACKNOWLEDGMENTS

I am very grateful to Professor S. D. Lawler and Professor K. D. Bagshawe for their valuable help, advice and constructive criticism in the preparation of this manuscript.

REFERENCES

1. Acosta-Sison H 1959 Ab initio choriocarcinoma. Two unusual cases. Obstet Gynecol 13: 350
2. Attwood H D, Park W W 1961 Embolism to the lungs by trophoblast. J Obstet Gynaecol Br Commonw 68: 611
3. Azer P C, Braunstein G D, Van de Velde R L, Van de Velde S, Kogan R, Engwall E 1980 Ectopic production of pregnancy specific beta-1 glycoprotein by a nontrophoblastic tumour in vitro. J Clin Endocrinol Metab 50: 234
4. Bagshawe K D, Garnett E S 1963 Radiological changes in patients with trophoblastic tumours. Br J Radiol 36: 673
5. Bagshawe K D, Dent J, Webb J 1986 Hydatidiform mole in England and Wales 1973–1983. Lancet ii: 392
6. Beischer N A, Fortune D W, Fitzgerald M G 1967 Hydatidiform mole and coexistent foetus, both with triploid chromosome constitution, Br Med J iii: 476
7. Benjamin F, Rorat E 1978 Primary gestational choriocarcinoma of the ovary. Am J Obstet Gynecol 131: 343
8. Berkowitz R S, Goldstein D P 1981 Pathogenesis of gestational trophoblastic neoplasms. Pathobiol Annual 11: 391
9. Brewer J J 1959 The Albert F Mathieu Chorionepithelioma Registry. Ann NY Acad Sci 80: 140
10. Byrne J, Warburton D 1988 Triploidy in spontaneous abortion. Lab Invest 58: 2P
11. Coppleson M 1958 Hydatidiform mole and its complications. J Obstet Gynaecol Br Emp 65: 238
12. Dearden L, Ockleford C D, Gupta M 1983 Structure of human trophoblast: correlation with function. In: Whyte, Lake (eds) Biology of Trophoblast. Elsevier Science Publishers, p 69
13. Dehner L P 1980 Gestational and nongestational trophoblastic neoplasia. A historic and pathobiologic survey. Am J Surg Pathol 4: 43
14. Dinh-De T, Minh H N 1961 Hydatidiform mole with recurrent vaginal metastasis. Am J Obstet Gynecol 82: 660
15. Doshi N, Surti U, Szulman A E 1983 Morphologic anomalies in triploid liveborn fetuses. Hum Pathol 14: 716
16. Edwards Y H, Jeremiah S J, McMillan S L, Povey S, Fisher R A, Lawler S D 1984 Complete hydatidiform moles combine maternal mitochondria with a paternal nuclear genome. Ann Hum Genet 48: 119
17. Ekstein R P, Paradinas F J, Bagshawe K D 1982 Placental site trophoblastic tumour (trophoblastic pseudotumour): a study of four cases requiring hysterectomy including one fatal case. Histopathology 6: 211
18. Ekstein R P, Russell P, Friedlander M L, Tattersall M H N, Bradfield A 1985 Metastasizing placental site trophoblastic tumor: a case study. Hum Pathol 16: 632
19. Elston C W 1976 The histopathology of trophoblastic tumours. J Clin Pathol 29: (Suppl. Roy Coll Pathol 10), 111
20. Elston C W 1987 Gestational trophoblastic disease. In Fox H (ed) Haines & Taylor Obstetrical and Gynaecological Pathology, 3rd edn. Churchill Livingstone, Edinburgh, p 1045
21. Elston C W, Bagshawe K D 1972 The value of histological grading in the management of hydatidiform mole. J Obstet Gynaecol Br Commonw 79: 717
22. Fisher R A, Lawler S D 1984 Heterozygous complete hydatidiform moles: do they have a worse prognosis than homozygous complete moles? Lancet ii: 51
23. Fisher R A, Lawler S D, Ormerod M G, Imrie P R, Povey S 1987 Flow cytometry used to distinguish between complete and partial hydatidiform moles. Placenta 8: 249
24. Fisher R A, Povey S, Jeffreys A J, Martin C A, Patel I, Lawler S D 1989 Frequency of heterozygous complete hydatidiform moles estimated by locus-specific minisatellite and Y chromosome-specific probes. Human Genetics 82: 259
25. Fisher R A, Sheppard D M, Lawler S D 1982 Twin pregnancy with complete hydatidiform mole (46XX) and fetus (46XY): genetic origin proved by analysis of chromosome polymorphisms. Br Med J i: 1218
26. Haines M 1955 Hydatidiform mole and vaginal nodules. J Obstet Gynaecol Br Emp 62: 6
27. Hemming J D, Quirke P, Womak C, Wells M, Elston C W, Bird C C 1987 Diagnosis of molar pregnancy and persistent trophoblastic disease by flow cytometry. J Clin Pathol 40: 615
28. Hertig A T 1950 Hydatidiform mole and chorionepithelioma. In Meigs J B, Sturgis S H (eds) Progress in Gynecology, Vol. 2. Grune and Stratton, New York, p 372
29. Hertig A T, Mansell H 1956 Tumors of the female sex organs. Part 1. Hydatidiform mole and choriocarcinoma. In: Atlas of Tumor Pathology, Section 9, Fascicle 33. Armed Forces Institute of Pathology, Washington D C
30. Heyderman E, Gibbons A R, Rosen A W 1981 Immunoperoxidase localisation of human placental lactogen: a marker for the placental origin of the giant cells in 'syncytial endometritis' and pregnancy. J Clin Pathol 34: 303
31. Honoré L H, Dill F J, Poland B J 1976 Placental morphology in spontaneous human abortions with normal and abnormal karyotypes. Teratology 14: 155
32. Hunt W, Dockerty M B, Randall L M 1953 Hydatidiform mole: clinicopathologic study involving 'grading' as a measure of possible malignant change. Obstet Gynecol 1: 593
33. Jacobs P A, Wilson C M, Sprenkle J A, Rosenhein N B, Migeon B R 1980 Mechanism of origin of complete hydatidiform moles. Nature 286: 714
34. Jacobs P A, Szulman A E, Funkhouser J, Matsuura J S, Wilson C M 1982 Human triploidy: relationship between parental origin of the additional haploid complement and development of partial mole. Ann Hum Genet 46: 223
35. Kajii T, Kurashige H, Ohama K, Uchino F 1984 XY and XX complete moles: clinical and morphological correlations. Am J Obstet Gynecol 150: 57
36. Kajii T, Ohama K 1977 Androgenetic origin of hydatidiform mole. Nature 268: 633
37. Kato M, Tanaka K, Takeuchi S 1982 The nature of trophoblastic disease initiated by transplantation into immunosuppressed animals. Am J Obstet Gynecol 142: 497

38. Kika K, Matuda I 1957 Primary tubal hydatidiform mole. Obstet Gynecol 9: 227

39. Klein J 1963 Delayed appearance and rupture of lutein cysts with hydatidiform mole. Obstet Gynecol 21: 30

40. Kuida C A, Braunstein G D, Shintaku P, Said J W 1988 Human chorionic gonadotropin expression in lung, breast and renal carcinomas. Arch Pathol Lab Med 112: 282

41. Kurman R J, Scully R E, Norris H J 1976 Trophoblastic pseudotumor of the uterus. An exaggerated form of 'syncytial endometritis' simulating a malignant tumor. Cancer 38: 1214

42. Kurman R J, Young R H, Norris H J, Main C S, Lawrence W D, Scully, R E 1984 Immunocytochemical localization of placental lactogen and chorionic gonadotropin in the normal placenta and trophoblastic tumors, with emphasis on intermediate trophoblast and the placental site trophoblastic tumor. Int J Gynecol Pathol 3: 101

43. Lage J M, Driscoll S G, Yavner D L, Olivier A P, Mark S D, Weinberg D S 1988 Hydatidiform moles. Application of flow cytometry in diagnosis. Am J Clin Pathol 89: 596

44. Lawler S D 1984 Genetic studies on hydatidiform moles. In: Pattillo A, Hussa R O (eds) Human Trophoblast Neoplasms. Plenum Publishing, New York, p 147

45. Lawler S D, Fisher R A 1986 Genetic aspects of gestational trophoblastic tumours. In Ichinoe K (ed) Trophoblastic Diseases. Igaku-Shoin, Tokyo, p 23

46. Lawler S D, Fisher R A, Pickthall V J, Povey S, Wyn-Evans M 1982 Genetic studies on hydatidiform moles I. The origin of partial moles. Cancer Genet Cytogenet 5: 309

47. Lawler S D, Fisher R A, Pickthall V J 1982 Genetic studies on hydatidiform moles II. The origin of complete moles. Ann Hum Genet 46: 309

48. Lawler S D, Pickthall V J, Fisher R A, Povey S, Evans M W, Szulman A E 1979 Genetic studies of complete and partial hydatidiform moles. Lancet ii: 580

49. Looi L M, Sivanesaratnam V 1981 Malignant evolution with fatal outcome in a patient with partial hydatidiform mole. Aust NZ J Obstet Gynaecol 21: 51

50. Meyer J S 1966 Benign pulmonary metastasis from hydatidiform mole. Report of a case. Obstet Gynecol 28: 826

51. McFadden D E, Kaulosek D K 1988 Triploid phenotypes in embryos and fetuses. Lab Invest 58: 6P

52. Nagelberg S B, Rosen S W 1985 Clinical and laboratory investigation of a virilized woman with placental-site trophoblastic tumor. Obstet Gynecol 65: 527

53. Ober W B, Edgcomb J H, Price E B 1971 The pathology of choriocarcinoma. Ann N Y Acad Sci 172: 299

54. Ober W B, Maier R C 1981 Gestational choriocarcinoma of the fallopian tube. Diag Gynecol Obstet 3: 213

55. Ohama K, Kajii T, Okamoto E, Fukuda Y et al 1981 Dispermic origin of XY hydatidiform moles. Nature 292: 551

56. Park W W 1971 Choriocarcinoma. A Study of its Pathology. Heinemann, London.

57. Park W W 1975 Possible functions of nonvillous trophoblast. Europ J Obstet Gynecol Reprod Biol 5: 35

58. Park W W, Lees J C 1950 Choriocarcinoma. A general review, with analysis of 516 cases. Arch Pathol 49: 73 & 205

59. Scully R E, Young, R H 1981 Trophoblastic pseudotumor. A reappraisal. Am J Surg Pathol 5: 75

60. Sugimori H, Kashimura Y, Kashimura M et al 1978 Nuclear DNA content of trophoblastic tumors. Acta Cytol 22: 542

61. Szulman A E, Phillippe E, Boué J G, Boué A 1981 Human triploidy: Association with partial hydatidiform moles and nonmolar conceptuses. Hum Pathol 12: 1016

62. Szulman A E, Surti U 1978 The syndromes of hydatidiform mole. I Cytogenetic and morphological correlations. Am J Obstet Gynecol 131: 665

63. Szulman A E, Surti U 1978 The syndromes of hydatidiform mole. II Morphologic evolution of the complete and partial mole. Am J Obstet Gynecol 132: 20

64. Szulman A E, Surti U 1982 The clinicopathologic profile of the partial hydatidiform mole. Obstet Gynecol 59: 597

65. Szulman A E, Wong L C, Hsu C 1981 Residual trophoblastic disease in association with partial hydatidiform mole. Obstet Gynecol 57: 392

66. Teng N N H, Ballon S C 1984 Partial hydatidiform mole with diploid karyotype: report of three cases. Am J Obstet Gynecol 150: 961

67. Thiele R A, de Alvarez R R 1962 Metastasizing benign trophoblastic tumors. Am J Obstet Gynecol 84: 1395

68. Van Oven M W, Schoots C J F, Oosterhuis J W, Keij J F, Dam-Meiring A, Huisjes H J 1989 The use of DNA flow cytometry in the diagnosis of triploidy in human abortions. Hum Pathol 20: 238

69. Vassilakos P, Riotton G, Kajii T 1977 Hydatidiform mole: two entities. A morphologic and cytogenetic study with some clinical considerations. Am J Obstet Gynecol 127: 167

70. Wallace D C, Surti U, Adams C W, Szulman A E 1982 Complete moles have paternal chromosomes but maternal mitochondrial DNA. Hum Genet 61: 145

71. World Health Organization Scientific Group 1983 Gestational Trophoblastic Diseases. WHO Technical Report Series 692, WHO, Geneva

72. Yeh I, O'Connor D M, Kurman R J 1988 Further immunocytochemical characterization of intermediate trophoblast. Lab Invest 58: 106A

73. Yeh I, O'Connor D M, Kurman R J 1988 Vacuolated cytotrophoblast: a subpopulation of trophoblastic cells of the chorion leave. Lab Invest 58: 106A

74. Young R H, Kurman R J, Scully R E 1988 Placental site nodule. A report of 20 cases. Lab Invest 58: 107A

75. Young R H, Scully R E 1984 Placental-site trophoblastic tumor: current status. Clin Obstet Gynecol 27: 248

76. Young R H, Scully R E, McCluskey R T 1985 A distinctive glomerular lesion complicating placental site trophoblastic tumor: report of two cases. Hum Pathol 16: 35

65. Trophoblastic tumors: diagnostic methods, epidemiology, clinical features and management

K. D. Bagshawe

INTRODUCTION

The normal trophoblast possesses unique properties corresponding to its role as the fetal interface with the tissues of its genetically distinct host. The fact that it is not rejected as an allograft may be attributable to non-expression of major histocompatibility antigens (Class I and II) on villous trophoblast. Non-villous trophoblast of normal placenta and complete hydatidiform mole has been found to express Class I antigen, but only with antibodies directed at the monomorphic determinants.[49]

The ability of trophoblastic cells to penetrate the endometrium and vascular structures, thereby gaining access to the maternal circulation, and trophoblast's ability to evoke vascular proliferation to facilitate its own metabolic needs have led to parallels being drawn with the properties of malignant tumors. The identification of a factor promoting capillary growth from both normal placenta and various tumors strengthens this parallel.[22] The endocrinological repertoire of trophoblast is unique but changes during the course of pregnancy.

DIAGNOSTIC METHODS

Biochemical markers for trophoblastic tumors

Normal trophoblast's repertoire of synthesizing activity includes that of steroid hormones and glycoproteins. In the context of malignant trophoblast, the glycoproteins are important because of their utility in diagnosis and in monitoring the course of the disease. It is interesting that the substances useful for detecting malignant trophoblast are amongst those evident during early placental development when trophoblast is most invasive. Human chorionic gonadotrophin (hCG) remains the principal marker (see also Ch. 24).

Human chorionic gonadotrophin

Methods of measurement. In patients with clinically evident disease, pregnancy tests are usually positive and can therefore be used as a quick, though not necessarily the most sensitive, test for hCG. Quantitative measurement by sensitive radioimmunoassay (RIA) or enzyme immunoassay (EIA) is also required. The rate of increase of hCG in serum together with ultrasound constitute key elements in the diagnosis of pregnancy and trophoblastic tumors. Assays for hCG are performed with anti-sera raised against the β-subunit of hCG and, although these are often described as β-hCG assays, they measure both intact hCG and free β-hCG.[28] This is no disadvantage, and the important thing is that the assay should discriminate well between pituitary luteinizing hormone and hCG. A good assay detects down to 2 international units (WHO standard) per liter (5 iu/l or 1.0 μg/l) in normal serum. Assays on urine are useful in the long-term follow-up of patients, although the 'background noise' on urine assays tends to be higher than in serum so that values up to the equivalent of 30 iu/24 hours may not be significant. Urine estimations should be based on timed collections or be related to creatinine excretion; the preferred preservative for immunoassay is merthiolate (Thiomersal 100 mg per 24 hour collection). Sensitive assays can now be performed with very short incubation times, although for most purposes an overnight incubation giving a result within 24 hours of the specimen being received in the laboratory is satisfactory. Free β-subunit hCG assays which distinguish between intact hCG and β-hCG are now available in some centers and the free β/intact hCG ratio may be prognostically important. Assay of the various forms of hCG now known to exist is a complex subject[2] which cannot be reviewed here.

The 'background noise' in urine assays may be attributable to another hCG-related substance known as β core fragment.[30] Although assays for β core fragment seem unlikely to have any advantage over hCG for patients with invasive mole or choriocarcinoma, they may prove useful in placental site trophoblastic tumors (PSTT).

The markers play an important part in distinguishing between choriocarcinoma and PSTT.[45] Suspicion of PSTT may arise from finding relatively low serum hCG values for the size of the patient's tumor, since hCG values are usually in the hundreds, or at most in the low thousands, iu/l.[20] At the immunohistochemical level, hCG staining is scanty, and consistent with the scarcity of syncytiotrophoblastic cells in PSTT. More PSTT cells stain with specific monoclonal antibodies[29] for β core fragment and for human placental lactogen[31] than for intact hCG.

Interpretation of hCG values. Any excess of hCG not attributable to pregnancy or recent uterine evacuation is likely to be due to gestational trophoblastic neoplasm, a malignant teratoma or other malignancy. In many thousands of samples analysed at Charing Cross Hospital, only one exception to this has been found; this young woman has persistently elevated levels of hCG, alpha-fetoprotein (AFP) and CEA, but has not been found to have tumor of any sort during a 12 year follow-up.

Malignant teratomas arising in the ovary or in midline structures commonly produce hCG, although the site of origin, histology and the common finding of alpha-fetoprotein (AFP) in serum distinguishes them from gestational trophoblastic tumors. Production of hCG can be 'ectopic' by non-trophoblastic tumors. About 12 to 20% of tumors of various histological types produce detectable serum levels of hCG.[39] A high proportion of cancers of all histological types appears to be associated with urinary excretion of β core fragment, and this may account for many cases of ectopic hCG production. The DNA fingerprinting technique provides a basis for discriminating between ges-

tational and non-gestational tumors when other methods fail.[26] In general, in a young woman after a recent pregnancy, the presence of hCG in the body fluids is strongly suggestive of a gestational trophoblastic tumor when a new pregnancy has been excluded.

The range of concentrations of hCG in urine and serum following evacuation of hydatidiform mole is discussed in a later section (p. 1036), but we can consider here the relationship between the serum concentration of hCG and the number of cells in a choriocarcinoma or invasive mole. In vitro and in vivo studies suggest that when we can no longer detect hCG in serum or urine by the most sensitive tests, there may still be about 10^4 to 10^5 viable cells present. This undetectable amount of tumor has to be considered in treatment planning; it also accounts for 'relapse' after clinical and biochemical remission.

The broad quantitative relationship between hCG concentration or excretion rate and viable tumor mass is of particular value in monitoring the course of the disease. Rises and falls in these values provide a much more sensitive guide to the course of the disease than do radiographic findings (Fig. 65.1). However, allowance must be made for the plasma half-life of immunoreactive hCG, which is of the order of 24 to 30 hours and therefore clearance takes a finite time. Cessation of hCG production is not accompanied by instant fall in serum and urine values to zero. It has also to be recognized that cytotoxic agents often cause

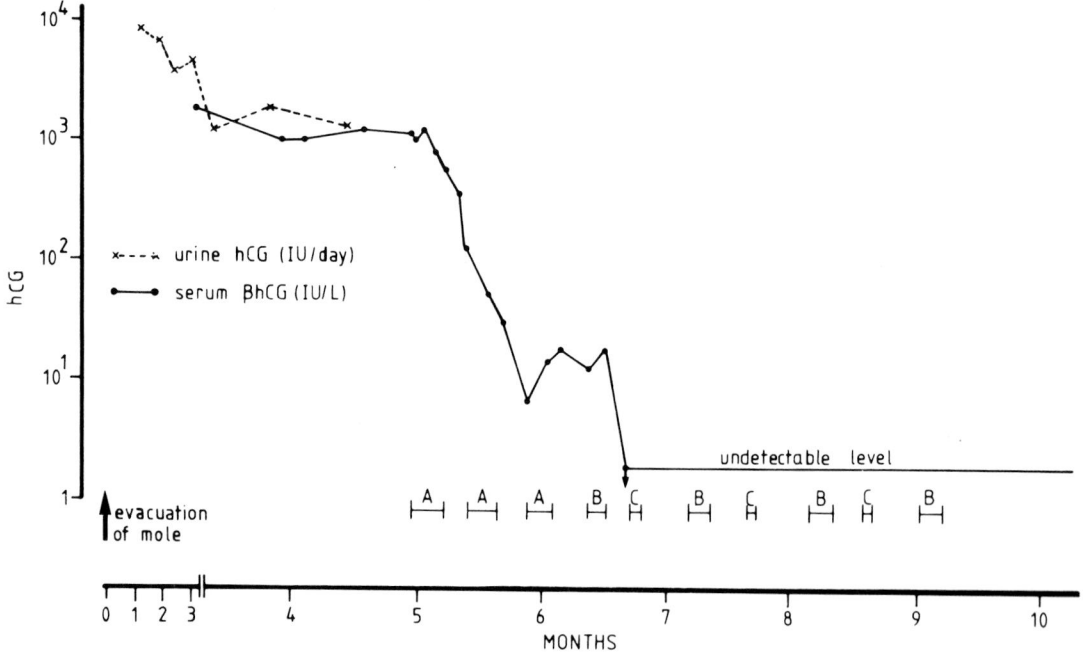

Fig. 65.1 Chart showing follow-up of hCG in a patient after evacuation of a hydatidiform mole. Chemotherapy was indicated because of persistently elevated hCG 4½ months after evacuation. The patient fell into the 'low risk' group and was initially treated with methotrexate and folinic acid. (A) Resistance to this regimen was shown by a levelling off of hCG levels which fell once more when treatment was changed to actinomycin-D (B) and vincristine and cyclophosphamide (C). In this patient, chemotherapy was continued until hCG had been undetectable in serum for 11 weeks.

an initial increase in serum and urine hCG values, and a significant fall may not be evident for 2 weeks after the start of an effective cytotoxic regimen. The clearance of hCG and its subunits proceeds at different rates.[50]

The rate of fall of hCG values during spontaneous regression of mole or therapeutically induced regression of choriocarcinoma varies substantially between patients, and often within the same patient from week to week. The rate of fall of hCG provides a guide to the minimum time for which treatment should be continued after hCG values have become normal. Thus, treatment needs to be continued longer if the slope is shallow than if it is steep. A graph can be used to extrapolate down to the theoretical 'zero cell' level to obtain an indication of the minimum length of treatment.

HCG remission may not coincide with radiological resolution. In general, hCG values remain elevated after radiological resolution has occurred. In cases with initially large tumors, hCG values may become normal whilst radiological opacities persist (Fig. 65.2). These persisting metastases may prove sterile if excised, and if left they may resolve spontaneously, but exceptions occur. Spontaneous radiological resolution may take a year or more to achieve.

Immunohistochemical studies on trophoblastic tumors indicate that synthesis of hCG is predominantly syncytial. Although the production of hCG by different tumors proceeds at different rates, we have no evidence that gestational choriocarcinomas ever fail to synthesize hCG; failure to find hCG in the presence of clinically detectable masses results either from incorrect histological diagnosis or from inadequate assay methodology for hCG. As already indicated, hCG serum and urine values are substantially lower in PSTT than for comparable volume of choriocarcinoma.

Frequency of estimation. In patients undergoing treatment, twice-weekly assays are adequate. After completion of treatment, assays should be performed every 1 to 2 weeks for 3 months and then progressively less frequently until, after 3 years, 3 to 6 monthly assays suffice. Rare relapses have occurred up to 8 years after terminating treatment.

Localization of brain metastases. Computerized axial tomography (CAT) has enabled a substantial advance in the localization of brain metastases and should be performed on all patients with pulmonary metastases; however, disturbance in the ratio of hCG in serum and spinal fluid (CSF) sometimes leads to detection of lesions not found by computerized axial tomography.[3] The CSF/serum ratio is greater than 1:60 in the absence of CNS metastases, and lower ratios strongly suggest CNS metastases.[10] However, where serum concentrations are falling rapidly, slow equilibration between CSF and serum may produce temporary disturbance. The CSF/serum ratio may also be normal when a small trophoblastic embolus or growth has produced cerebral hemorrhage or cerebral infarction. Papilledema or other evidence of raised intracranial pressure must be excluded. It is probably unnecessary to repeat these estimations during treatment of patients without lung metastases, but those who do have them should have the CSF/serum ratio value estimated,

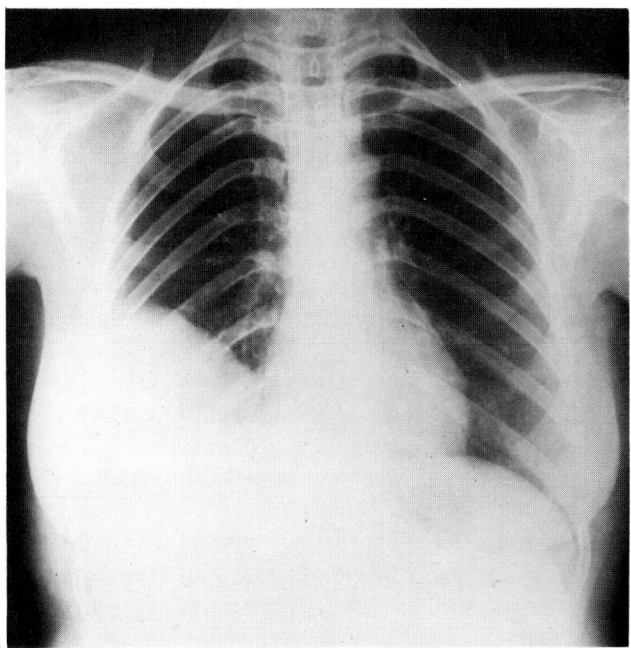
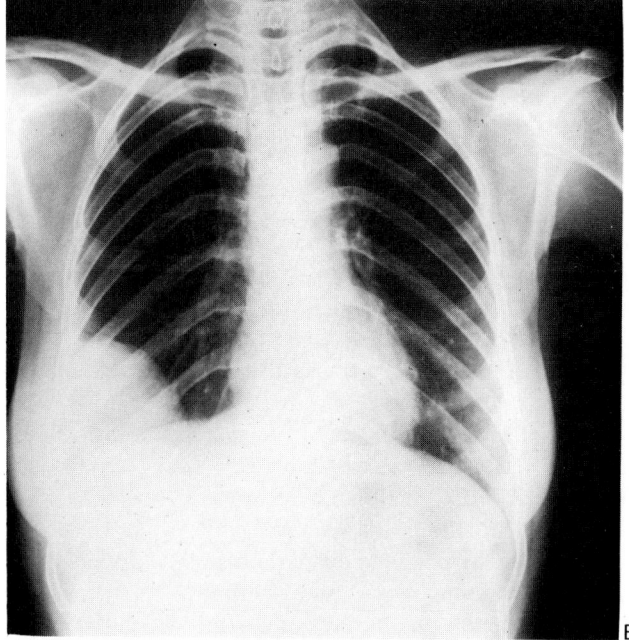

Fig. 65.2 (**A**) Chest X-ray of a patient with a single pulmonary metastasis in the right lower lobe. (**B**) After cytotoxic chemotherapy for 10 weeks, the opacity is smaller. When it was excised shortly after this radiograph was taken, histology showed necrotic tissue with no choriocarcinoma.

preferably every 2 weeks until hCG is undetectable in serum, or the lung fields are clear.

Other trophoblastic products

The pregnancy specific-β-glycoprotein (SP_1) is interesting in that it has a half-life similar to that of hCG and, like hCG, is actively synthesized by 'early' normal trophoblast. Prognostic significance has been attached to the SP_1/hCG ratio.[42] If it were not for β-hCG assays, SP_1 would provide an excellent marker for trophoblastic tumors. However, in practice, hCG is generally superior when the two markers are carefully compared.[46]

Human placental lactogen (HPL), which is a 'late' trophoblastic product, is detectable in the serum of some patients with trophoblastic tumors. Although it has been suggested that the ratio of HPL/hCG might provide a guide to the malignancy of trophoblastic lesions,[44] HPL measurements have not, in our experience, added anything useful to clinical assessment. HPL is a useful immunohistochemical marker for PSTT.

Alphafetoprotein (AFP) is not synthesized by gestational trophoblastic tumors. Levels of AFP can therefore be used to distinguish choriocarcinoma, invasive mole and classical hydatidiform mole from normal pregnancy.[47] Mole with fetus (partial mole) may cause both high hCG and high AFP values, as may malignant teratomas containing both trophoblastic and yolk sac elements. Prolonged treatment with chemotherapeutic agents, notably cisplatin, may cause elevation of AFP values, presumably through hepatic toxicity.[18]

Estrogen and progestogen levels in patients with malignant trophoblastic tumors tend to be much lower than in normal pregnancy. Measurement of these steroids has not found practical application in clinical management.

Special diagnostic procedures

Curettage

Although curettage occasionally reveals choriocarcinoma and gives a precise histological diagnosis, its limitations need to be recognized. Unless the lesion is close to the endometrial surface, which is by no means usual, curettage will be negative; thus, a negative result should not preclude other tests if a trophoblastic tumor is suspected. Myometrial invasion is necessary to establish a histological diagnosis. Placental site trophoblastic tumor seems to be more regularly detectable on curettings.

The interpretation of curettings is influenced by knowledge of the patient's obstetric history. Trophoblastic fragments without villi and without a history of hydatidiform mole in the previous 6 months are strongly suggestive of choriocarcinoma or PSTT. Where a hydatidiform mole has recently been removed, such fragments may be indicative of choriocarcinoma or persisting mole and often, in such patients, if hysterectomy is carried out, villi are found elsewhere in the uterus. In general, of course, hysterectomy is not necessary or desirable, except where placental site tumor is suspected.

Biopsy

Biopsy of choriocarcarcinoma can be a lethal act. Needle biopsy of a suspected hepatic metastasis in a woman of reproductive age should never be attempted without prior exclusion of choriocarcinoma by hCG test, and should certainly not be attempted if the patient is known to have choriocarcinoma.

Biopsy of a typical purplish lesion on the cervix may reveal classical infiltrating choriocarcinoma. Lesions in the vagina or vulva may be due either to choriocarcinoma or to invasive mole. Biopsy carries a considerable risk of severe bleeding, since vaginal metastases communicate with the greatly dilated arteriovenous network created in the pelvic tissues by invasive trophoblastic lesions.

Superficial lesions in the skin may be safely excised, but not lesions on the buccal mucosa.

Plain radiography of the chest

Chest X-ray is necessary for the identification of pulmonary metastases and for confirmation of their response to treatment.[9,11] Three forms of pulmonary metastatic lesion can be defined: (a) the classical opacity detectable at about 1 cm diameter, but which may be up to 15 or more cm, may be single or multiple and is usually, but not invariably, rounded (Figs 65.2 and 65.3), (b) the snowstorm appearance (Fig. 65.4) which is sometimes mistaken for miliary tuberculosis, viral or fungal infection and (c) pulmonary arterial obstruction resulting in multisegmental or unilateral loss of vascular marking and right ventricular enlargement and hypertrophy (Fig. 65.5).

Computerized axial tomography (CAT) and magnetic resonance imaging (MRI)

Computerized axial tomography (CAT) is more sensitive than plain radiography for detection of pulmonary metastases but need not be considered essential. Below the diaphragm, ultrasound is as satisfactory as CAT for liver metastases and much more useful in the pelvis. CAT or magnetic resonance imaging (MRI) examination is essential if brain metastases are suspected.

CAT and MRI are particularly useful when a patient has evidence from hCG values of persisting, drug resistant disease, and when plain radiography fails to reveal its location. The question then is whether a resection can be undertaken, and, clearly, the finding of multiple lesions in the lungs or elsewhere makes such procedures questionable.

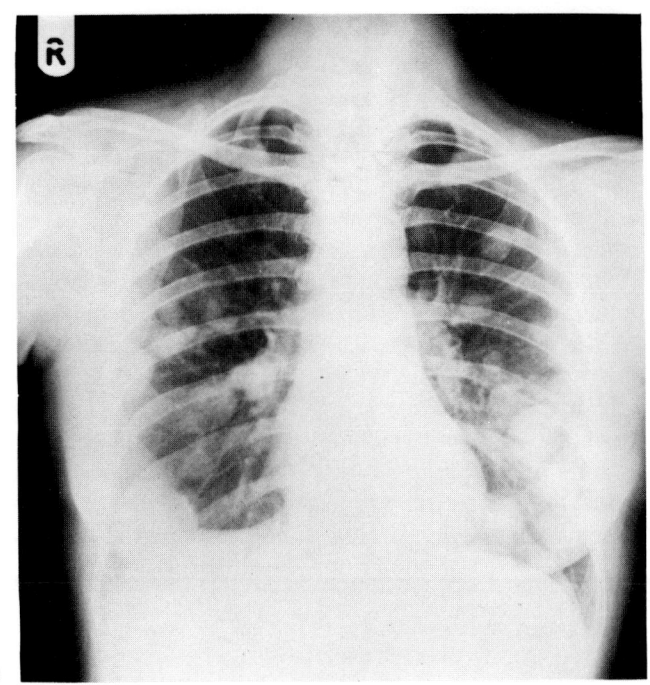
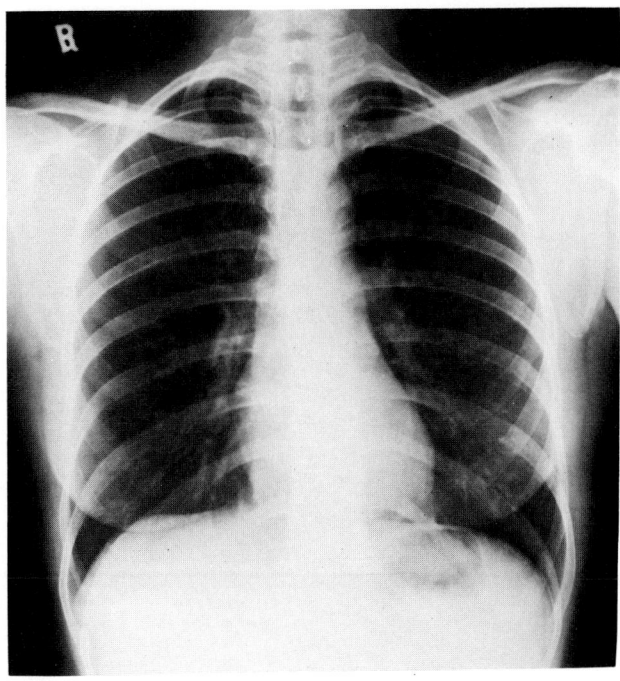

Fig. 65.3 (**A**) Chest X-ray showing multiple metastases of choriocarcinoma which resolved completely; (**B**) after 8 months of cytotoxic chemotherapy.

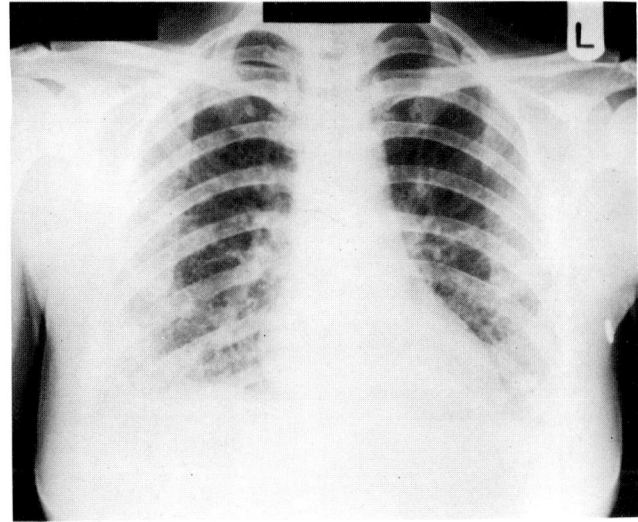
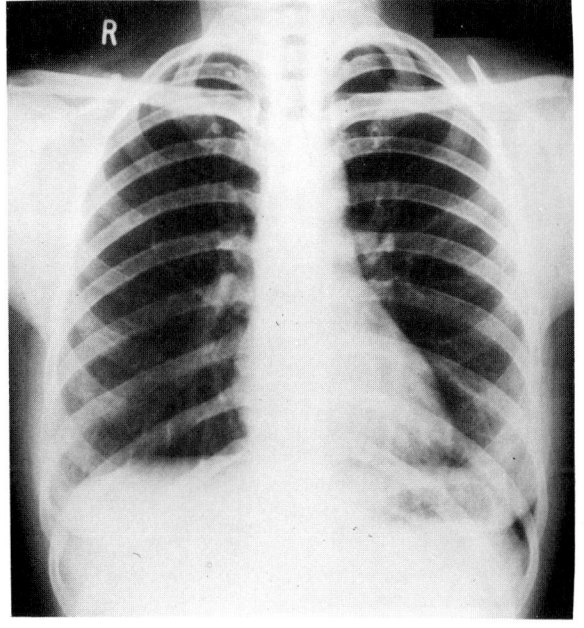

Fig. 65.4 (**A**) Chest X-ray showing a snowstorm appearance; (**B**) clearing completely after 3 months cytotoxic chemotherapy.

MRI is valuable in the pelvis and where vertebral body involvement is suspected.

Arteriography

Arteriography has taught us much about the vascular structure of trophoblastic tumors in the past 20 years. The vascular connections of vaginal metastases were previously unsuspected (Fig. 65.6). The extraordinary dilation of the ovarian arteries and veins, long reported by surgeons and sometimes resulting in surgical disasters, was revealed to all by this technique.[15]

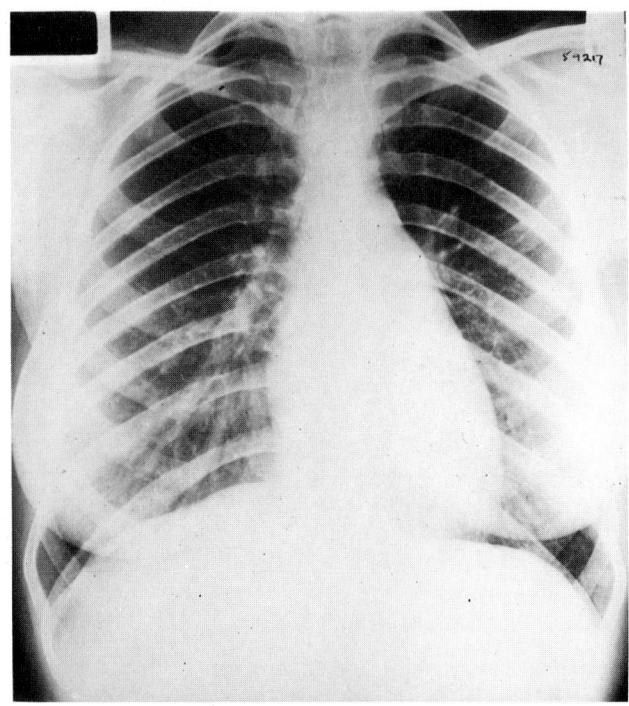

Fig. 65.5 Chest X-ray of a patient presenting with pulmonary hypertension caused by choriocarcinoma growing in the pulmonary arteries.

There is probably no longer any need to perform this investigation as a routine. It cannot be relied upon to confirm the presence or absence of a tumor in the uterus. However, if hysterectomy is contemplated and Doppler ultrasound is not available an extensive extra-uterine venous circulation may be demonstrated by arteriography and should be a deterrent unless hysterectomy is being undertaken for drug-resistant disease.

Pulmonary arteriography requires great caution in patients with evidence of choriocarcinomatous obstruction of the pulmonary arteries (Fig. 65.7). Pulmonary scintigraphy and gas studies can provide similar confirmation of obstruction more safely, but lack the precise anatomical definition of arteriography.

Immunoscintigraphy with ^{131}I anti-hCG antibodies has been used successfully to locate sites of residual choriocarcinoma after chemotherapy when CAT or MRI has failed. The main area of application is in patients with persisting drug-resistant disease, otherwise revealed only by serum hCG levels.[14]

Ultrasound

The contribution of ultrasound development to the diagnosis of pregnancy and hydatidiform mole[35,13] is widely recognized.

The usefulness of the technique is, of course, enhanced by its non-invasiveness, and it can reveal solid lesions in the uterus, elsewhere in the pelvis and in the liver, although the appearances are not pathognomonic and can be mimicked by retained products of conception, missed abortion and degenerating fibroids.[43] However, ultrasound has an established place in localizing tumor sites in

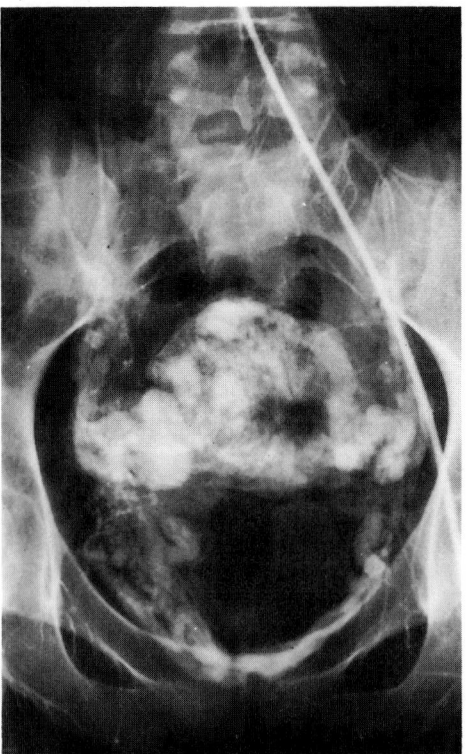

Fig. 65.6 Pelvic arteriogram showing vascular pattern in uterus which contains choriocarcinoma and a metastasis near the vaginal vault showing grossly enlarged vascular connections.

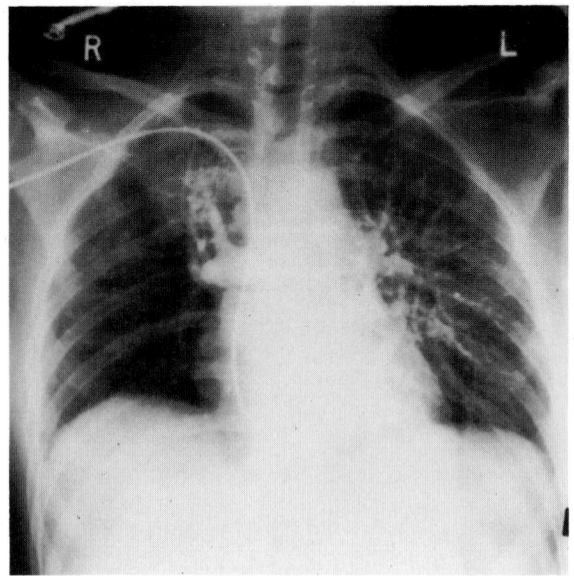

Fig. 65.7 Pulmonary arteriogram showing occlusion of pulmonary arteries to right lower and middle lobes.

choriocarcinoma. Uterine volume can also be determined by this technique. Doppler ultrasound readily demonstrates the increased vascularity of trophoblastic lesions.

Other investigations

Metastases in the kidneys and liver may be demonstrable by intravenous pyelography, by CT scan and, more dramatically, by arteriography (Fig. 65.8).

Whilst anemia in a patient with choriocarcinoma may be attributable to uterine or vaginal blood loss, it is important to remember that metastases in the gastrointestinal tract, particularly in the stomach and small intestine, may cause blood loss. The lesions are usually too small to be detectable by contrast studies. Anemia can also result from intrahepatic and intraperitoneal hemorrhage.

The ABO groups of the patient and her consort are relevant prognostic factors as discussed below.

The hematological indices need to be measured at least weekly during treatment. Weekly measurements of serum electrolytes, EDTA clearance and liver function tests are usually adequate, but individual patients may require close monitoring of renal or hepatic function. Disturbances of calcium and magnesium are rare problems, although cisplatin, actinomycin D and renal and gastrointestinal tract disturbances may contribute to low serum levels.

All patients should be tested for hepatitis B and HIV at the outset. Although antigen-positive serology does not preclude treatment, there is a hazard to the patient of

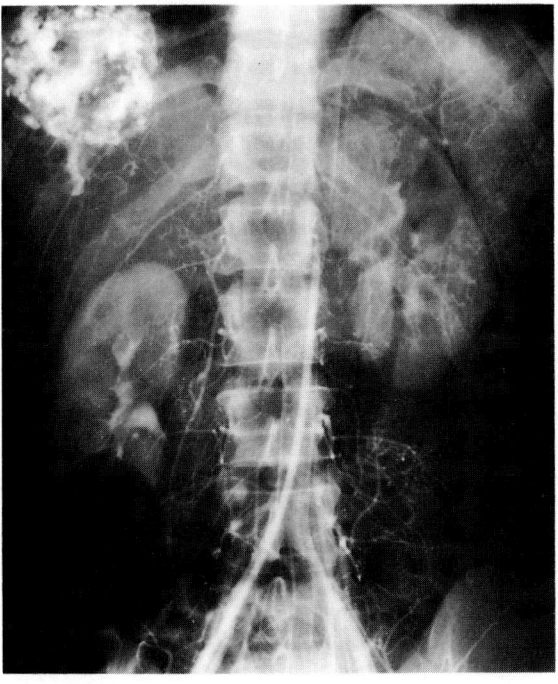

Fig. 65.8 Hepatic arteriogram in a patient with a moderate sized metastasis from choriocarcinoma.

active hepatitis as well as the hazard to laboratory staff. Hepatitis-B-antibody-positive subjects have converted to antigen-positive during cytotoxic chemotherapy, with consequent fatal active hepatitis.

Electrocardiography is appropriate in rare patients with heart disease, those with extensive pulmonary metastases and, particularly, those with pulmonary arterial obstruction. It should also be undertaken before using the cardiotoxic agents which have only a small place in treatment.

EPIDEMIOLOGY AND ETIOLOGY OF CHORIOCARCINOMA AND HYDATIDIFORM MOLE

Since choriocarcinoma is about 1000 times more common after hydatidiform mole than after term pregnancy, it is evident that variations in the incidence of mole worldwide could have a profound influence on the geographical distribution of cases of choriocarcinoma. Although there are many papers presenting data on the frequency of hydatidiform mole, invasive mole and choriocarcinoma in various parts of the world, comparisons are largely invalidated by problems of definition.[16] The variables which have to be considered in any attempt to collect valid data include the following: (1) definition of hydatidiform mole, i.e. complete or partial; (2) definition of invasive mole, i.e. morphological and/or clinical criteria; (3) definition of choriocarcinoma, i.e. morphological and/or clinical criteria; (4) relationship to pregnancy in a population, i.e. to live term births, to total pregnancies, to social abortion and to therapeutic abortion; (5) the population at risk, i.e. a total geographic or ethnic population, or subsets selected by various criteria for admission to hospital.

Reviewing the literature with these variables in mind, one may conclude that the incidence of hydatidiform mole is of the order of three to five times greater in Japan, Korea and, possibly, in some other populations in South East Asia than in populations of European origin, and that this is associated with a proportionately greater incidence of choriocarcinoma arising from hydatidiform mole. Beyond this, present evidence is too conflicting for reliable generalizations to be drawn.

Age and gravidity

It seems clear from all populations studied that the risk of a pregnancy resulting in complete hydatidiform mole increases steeply over the age of 40, and the risk continues to increase with age.[8] There is also an increased risk of complete mole in the under-16-year age group. Partial mole, in contrast to complete mole, does not show a significant association with age. Any effect from gravidity is difficult to distinguish from the effect of age.

Estrogens and progestogens

Suspicion that exogenous estrogens and progestogens might have adverse effects on trophoblastic tumors arose in the 1960's. Patients who took oral contraceptives (OC) immediately after completing treatment for choriocarcinoma appeared to have a higher relapse rate. Further, an increasing proportion of patients with postmolar trophoblastic neoplasia reported taking OC soon after evacuation of mole, and these had a greater risk of requiring chemotherapy.[48] A recent case control study in the Charing Cross data, matched 159 patients taking OC after mole and before hCG had fallen to normal, with 923 controls. They were matched for year of evacuation, interval between mole and start of OC and hCG values at the time of taking OC. 40 of the OC patients (25%) and 121 of the controls (13%) required chemotherapy.

Other workers[21] found no effect from OC on the frequency with which chemotherapy had to be given. However, the data are not comparable with UK data because of different criteria for chemotherapeutic intervention. In the USA series, 22.6% of all hydatidiform mole patients received chemotherapy, whereas in the UK series the overall figure was 8%. There is no evidence that women who have taken OC prior to conception have an increased risk of hydatidiform mole. There are numerous instances of hydatidiform mole occurring in pregnancies following clomiphene, but whether anti-estrogens increase the risk is unknown.

HLA factors

Early knowledge of the HLA system led some workers to suggest that choriocarcinoma could only occur when the patient conceived a child HLA-identical with herself, implying an accidental close match of patient and consort. However, systematic studies of the patients in the Charing Cross series,[32] their consorts and their children, and in the USA[34] have shown this hypothesis to be untenable. Although there is a slight excess of accidental matching for HLA factors between patient and consort, and between patient and child from a choriocarcinoma-associated pregnancy, most patients and their consorts are not more closely matched than patient/consort pairs selected at random.

Complete hydatidiform mole tends to be more immunogenic than normal pregnancy in evoking antibodies to paternal HLA antigens in maternal sera. It is not known whether this is due to the androgenetic nature of trophoblast, since mole also contains mesothelial elements. Antibodies to paternally-derived HLA factors have been used[33] to show that the immediate antecedent pregnancy is not necessarily the causal pregnancy of choriocarcinoma.

ABO groups

Data relating to ABO groups have been collected in various series, but they are often inadequate and the heterogeneity of the clinical material and of blood groups demands careful analysis of large series.

Earlier analysis of the present series showed no significant shift in the blood group distribution of patients with hydatidiform mole or of their consorts. In patients with choriocarcinoma, there was no significant shift towards Group A, but there was a significant trend for Group A patients to have Group O consorts.[12] An analysis of patients with choriocarcinoma after term or non-mole abortions showed:

$$\frac{(A \times O) + (O \times A)}{(O \times O) + (A \times A)} = 2.0$$

For the whole series of patients requiring chemotherapy for invasive mole or choriocarcinoma and for whom data were available, (328 patient/consort pairs) the ratio was 1.41. The effect of ABO group on prognosis is discussed in a later section (p. 1037).

HYDATIDIFORM MOLE

Diagnosis

The diagnostic problem of hydatidiform mole has been so much reduced by the introduction of ultrasound that it merits little space here. The classical feature of uterine enlargement in advance of dates occurs in about 50% of cases, and high hCG values, intermittent bright or brownish blood loss, nausea and vomiting and an approximately 10% incidence of toxemic features are well known. The mole which is small for dates and is unaccompanied by other abnormal features tends to be detected when the absence of fetal heart sounds arouses suspicion.

The formation of large unilateral or bilateral theca lutein cysts in patients with moles and choriocarcinoma is well recognized, and they are seen as trans-sonic areas of variable size adjacent to the uterus on ultrasound. They are, incidentally, unusual in patients presenting more than 18 months after the end of the antecedent pregnancy, and they have been attributed to prolonged stimulation by hCG. However, patients with high hCG values do not invariably have them and they have been reported in the absence of trophoblastic tumors (see Ch. 8). The appearance of the cysts at laparotomy is sometimes mistaken for metastasis, and leads to unnecessary oophorectomy. Large cysts may persist for several weeks during chemotherapy, but in our experience they invariably return to normal as the primary disease is eliminated. Rarely, patients develop pain requiring surgical intervention. Aspiration of the cyst fluid without oophorectomy has proved successful in the few patients in our series where symptoms necessitated intervention. (See Ch. 21.)

Serum AFP values are low in complete mole, but may be raised in cases of partial mole and in patients with twin pregnancies, one of which is complete mole.[47] Twin pregnancies in which there is one normal pregnancy and a complete or partial hydatidiform mole may present diagnostic problems and a dilemma in management.[27] Data are sparse, but whilst many abort, occasional cases go to successful term delivery.

Evacuation

Most complete moles are associated with invasion of the myometrium or other tissues, as indicated by the fact that hCG excretion persists long after curettage has ensured that there are no intracavity fragments of mole. In a study of data collected at Charing Cross Hospital,[48] it was found that vacuum extraction, curettage and spontaneous evacuation carried the smallest risk of sequelae requiring chemotherapy, whereas methods involving the manipulation of the uterus, such as medical induction and hysterotomy, carried a 2 to 3 fold greater risk. Vacuum extraction appeared the safest technique from this point of view, and has the added advantages that a large uterus can usually be evacuated and blood loss kept to a minimum. The uterus typically contracts well after vacuum extraction with control of bleeding, sharp curettage being reserved for patients in whom there is doubt about complete evacuation. Curettage is also indicated after spontaneous evacuation of a mole, to ensure that the uterus is empty and to obtain tissue for histological examination.

The greater risk of sequelae associated with uterine evacuation induced by oxytocin or prostaglandins is attributed to embolization of trophoblast by uterine contraction.[48] For the same reason, the administration of these drugs during or after evacuation by vacuum or sharp curettage should be avoided, except as a life-saving measure. However, the use of ergometrine to control bleeding after the evacuation of the mole is sometimes unavoidable. Hysterotomy is contraindicated. Hysterectomy for removal of mole, or soon after evacuation by other means, is no guarantee that all trophoblastic elements have been removed. One patient in our series had hysterectomy for mole at age 17, only to present at age 34 with advanced choriocarcinoma. If hysterectomy is indicated for a woman who has completed her childbearing, it is probably best performed after the mole has been evacuated by other means.

Follow-up after hydatidiform mole

The objective of follow-up after hydatidiform mole is to ensure that all patients who prove to require specific therapy receive it at a time when it is effective. It is no less important to ensure that it is not given to patients who do not need it. Although there is probably general agreement on the desirability of this objective, it is interesting that practice in different countries is so widely divergent.

There is no published evidence to indicate that the incidence of choriocarcinoma after mole (complete and partial) ever greatly exceeds the 3% level defined in studies antedating the introduction of chemotherapy. Nevertheless, the number of patients who require chemotherapy cannot sensibly be restricted to 3%, because at least as many require chemotherapy to avoid hysterectomy for invasive mole.

This said however, the percentage of patients receiving chemotherapy in the UK after mole is under 8%,[8] whereas in the USA the percentage ranges from 20 to 35% in different series. The high level of intervention in the USA arises from the practice of giving chemotherapy to patients with detectable hCG at 6 weeks post mole. It is argued that this early intervention is necessitated by the risk of litigation. It seems that the prospect of litigation on the grounds of unnecessary chemotherapy has not, so far, arisen.

The main threat in the early weeks after evacuation of mole is local invasion. The early dangers are from uterine hemorrhage, hemorrhage from vaginal metastases, and uterine perforation with hemoperitoneum. The latter event is generally heralded by persisting high levels of hCG in serum and urine. The threat from choriocarcinoma comes later, and arises from the fact that, if not treated with reasonable promptness, the risk of drug resistance increases. In more than 8000 cases followed up at Charing Cross Hospital since 1970, there have been 2 deaths from drug-resistant choriocarcinoma. One of these patients refused admission when treatment was suggested, the other proved drug resistant even though treatment started only 4 months post mole.

Indications for treatment

The indications for intervention with chemotherapy have been as follows:

1. High levels of hCG more than 4 weeks post-evacuation. (Serum >20 000 iu/l. Urine >30 000 iu/24 hours).
2. Persisting uterine hemorrhage.
3. Progressively increasing hCG values at any time post-evacuation.
4. Any detectable level of hCG not showing a tendency to extinction 4 to 6 months post evacuation.
5. At any level of hCG excretion, evidence of brain, renal, hepatic, gastrointestinal tract or pulmonary metastases (pulmonary metastases less than 2 cm in

diameter, not exceeding 3 in number and associated with falling hCG values when first seen may, however, regress spontaneously in the first few months following evacuation of the mole).

Using these criteria, the incidence of treatment has averaged 7.75%. Factors influencing the incidence of treatment probably include the mode of evacuation and the use of oral contraceptives. In the series at Charing Cross, the ratio of choriocarcinoma to invasive mole in the postmolar patients receiving chemotherapy has probably been in the range 1:1 to 1:3. In a series treating 30% of all mole patients, the corresponding ratio is about 1:10.

hCG and follow-up of mole patients

Estimations performed earlier than 3 weeks after evacuation of the mole are not highly informative. From 3 weeks post mole, they should be done every 2 weeks until hCG becomes undetectable. An analysis of over 5000 patients followed up after hydatidiform mole[8] has shown that 42% had normal serum hCG values (<5 mIu/l) by the 56th day post-evacuation. (A more recent analysis (unpublished) has shown that 60% of patients reach normal values by the 56th day.) Only one of these patients subsequently required chemotherapy. Where hCG normalized after the 56th day, there was still a risk of about 1% of recrudescence within 2 years. It is therefore recommended that, when serum hCG is normal by the 56th day post-evacuation, follow-up can subsequently be safely limited to monthly urine tests up to 6 months post evacuation. For the remainder, the 2 year follow-up is still advisable. For these patients, once serum hCG is normal, urine assays are performed monthly until 1 year post mole, and then 3-monthly during the second year of follow-up. There is a case for further hCG assay 3 weeks and 3 months after the end of any pregnancy subsequent to mole, because a few patients present with choriocarcinoma which follows subsequent pregnancies. Follow-up can usually be based on urine assays, which are more acceptable to the patient though less sensitive. Serum assays are used when doubt arises and as a routine check on reaching normality by urine testing.

Pregnancy after hydatidiform mole

The risks of malignant sequelae after mole have long been considered great enough to merit strongly advising patients against further pregnancy for 2 years.

For patients in the short follow-up category, there seems to be no reason why a further pregnancy should not be initiated once the 6 month follow-up has been completed. Those who fall into the 2 year follow-up category are likely to need a full explanation of the reason for the recommendation not to start a pregnancy during that period. Even

in this group, when hCG values have been normal for 6 months the risk of late choriocarcinoma falls to about 0.3%. In advising these patients there are conflicting issues. Whilst it is advisable to avoid a new pregnancy as long as there is a significant risk of developing choriocarcinoma, it may also seem reasonable to advise that if a further pregnancy be started 6 months after hCG values have become and remained persistently normal, then it may seem an acceptable risk, particularly if the patient is older. It also seems, on present evidence, that oral contraception should not be used until hCG values are known to be normal.

Women who have one hydatidiform mole have an increased risk of another in a subsequent pregnancy. The risk of second mole was 1:76 and for women who have had two moles the risk increases to 1:6.5.[8] After three hydatidiform moles few women have succeeded in having a normal pregnancy. Multiple moles do not appear to carry a greater risk than a single one of malignant sequelae.

INVASIVE MOLE AND CHORIOCARCINOMA

Diagnosis

The basis of diagnosis is recognition that a particular clinical picture can result from a trophoblastic tumor. It is fundamental to establish whether the patient has a hydatidiform mole, or an invasive trophoblastic tumor or some other disease process.

Invasive mole is seen in the early months following evacuation of hydatidiform mole and, since most women know when they have had a mole, it is only rarely recognized in the absence of such a history. Similarly, placental bed reaction is only a problem within 4 to 6 weeks of the end of a pregnancy and should no longer be confused with placental site trophoblastic tumor. Evidence for the persistence of trophoblast more than 6 months following a hydatidiform mole, or more than 2 months after any other pregnancy therefore constitutes prima facie evidence of choriocarcinoma.

Choriocarcinoma is one of the great mimics of other disease. As with invasive mole, irregular vaginal bleeding and low abdominal pain or discomfort are the commonest presenting features. The uterus may be enlarged, appear normal or be thought to be subinvoluted after the previous pregnancy. It may be irregular in contour. Bleeding vaginal metastases can be dealt with by suturing. Attempts at biopsy or excision can cause severe hemorrhage. Choriocarcinoma has a non-gynecological presentation in more than one-third of cases.[36] These include pleuritic type chest pain due to metastases on the pleural surface or due to pulmonary infarction by tumor emboli, as well as dyspnea, cough and, occasionally, hemoptysis.

Headaches may be due to raised intracranial pressure or cerebral hemorrhage. Loss of consciousness may result from cerebral hemorrhage or infarction. Spinal cord metastases also demand first time recognition if a permanent paraplegia is to be avoided. Anemia due to gastrointestinal blood loss, hematuria and hepatomegaly may all be presenting or associated features. Lymph node involvement is rare, and skin metastases are usually only present in late stage disease. Two of the 1100 patients in our treatment series have presented with retinal metastases.

Placental site trophoblastic tumor accounts for only about 1 to 2% of trophoblastic tumors and more commonly follows term delivery than mole (see also Ch. 64). It may be diagnosed on curettings, but clinical suspicion should be aroused if there is a uterine mass and hCG values are low.[20] A few patients with PSTT have had nephrotic syndrome. Since this tumor tends to be resistant to eradication by chemotherapy, it is generally advisable to perform hysterectomy at an early stage.

Another rare trophoblastic tumor is a form of choriocarcinoma which is confined to pelvic blood vessels and the pulmonary arterial bed. Presentation is with progressive dyspnea and evidence of pulmonary hypertension (Figs 65.5 and 65.7) and therefore to general physicians and cardiologists.[11,36] Our data suggest there may be between 100 and 200 cases per year worldwide to date, but there have been no cases reported in the literature diagnosed in life, apart from those at Charing Cross. It is no less curable than other forms of choriocarcinoma.

Unsuspected pregnancy complicating a non-trophoblastic tumor, particularly soft tissue sarcomas, can mimic choriocarcinoma, and the distinction may be difficult unless a histological diagnosis can be made or until events unfold.

Risk and prognosis

In the field of cancer generally, prognosis is largely a function of the natural history of the particular histological subtype and of the stage of the disease. In patients with trophoblastic tumors, the early occurrence of hematogenous spread and rapid growth rate means that disease progression to death may be rapid unless successful therapy intervenes. Given that early micrometastatic spread casts surgery in an adjuvant role, chemotherapy takes primary responsibility.

Two sets of factors affect prognosis and these can be defined as early and late risks. Early risks are a function of the site and bulk of the disease. Late risk is that of drug resistance.

Patients with brain metastases, large liver metastases, extensive pulmonary disease causing dyspnea or combinations of these features are at high risk from hemorrhage in brain and liver and from respiratory failure at the early stage of treatment.

The risk of a tumor becoming drug-resistant appears to depend on multiple factors. The various known factors ap-

pear to operate additively, so that a concept of overall risk of resistance has some reality and is one to which a crude numerical value can be ascribed to provide a guide to management. Also in contrast to many other tumors, the histological diagnosis *per se* is not readily taken into account in defining prognosis. This is not to say it is insignificant, since the morphological distinction between invasive mole and choriocarcinoma is the difference between a lesion which, in the present series of 1100 treated cases, has caused no deaths and one which has been present in all fatal cases. However, omission of the morphological distinction in the prognostic scoring system results firstly from the fact that a histological diagnosis may only be obtainable at the outset by a surgical procedure, which may disadvantage the patient. It is pertinent that no tumor was found in the uterus in about 10% of cases of metastatic choriocarcinoma in the pre-chemotherapy era. Also, the type of antecedent pregnancy and various other factors compensate for the lack of histological data consequent upon conservation of the uterus.

Risk factors for drug resistance

The Charing Cross series from 1957 to 73 consisted of 317 patients and was analyzed with respect to various factors for which there were data and which it was thought might influence prognosis.[4,5,19,24,51] It was found that survival was somewhat better overall in the younger age groups, but the effect was not statistically significant. Parity appeared to have a complex effect in the original analysis, but any effect was weak and it has been omitted in later scoring systems. Term antecedent pregnancies were less favorable than abortion or mole. The magnitude of the effect may have been underestimated in the past, and our more recent analyses suggest it should be scored more heavily. Genetically, post term choriocarcinoma differs from post mole choriocarcinoma. The effect of the ABO groups on predisposition for choriocarcinoma has been summarized in another section (p. 1034), but a different effect was observed in relation to survival. Patients in Groups B and AB had poorer survival rates, whereas patients with Group B or AB consorts had better survival rates.[5]

One of the two most powerful effects was of the time interval between the end of the antecedent pregnancy and the start of chemotherapy. This effect was not simply a measure of tumor burden, although this also proved to be a powerful effect as judged by hCG values at the start of treatment. The combined effect of 'tumor age' and hCG values are illustrated by the zero fatality rate in 72 patients whose initial hCG excretion rates were less than 10^4 iu/day when treated within 7 months of the antecedent pregnancy, compared with a fatality rate of 50% in 84 patients in whom the interval was >7 months and the hCG excretion rate was >10^4 iu/day. Metastases in the brain, gastrointestinal tract, liver or kidneys, large metastases or numerous metastases of moderate (>3 cm) size, or prior treatment were all adverse factors. Immunological unreactivity was found on testing for both cell-mediated and humoral immunity in some patients with advanced disease and appeared unfavorable, whereas a marked mononuclear cell reaction in the tumor[7] was a good prognostic factor. However, immune status and mononuclear invasion were relatively weak effects and could only be ascertained in a minority of patients; they have therefore been omitted from later versions of the scoring system.

Prognostic score

On the basis of the magnitude of effect of the various factors listed in the previous section, a scoring system was devised to predict the probability of drug resistance. Since it was first introduced in 1976, the Charing Cross scoring system has been simplified and the weighting of some factors modified (Table 65.1). Such a scoring system can also provide a basis for comparison of the effectiveness of treatment regimens used in different treatment centers. It now seems generally accepted by those treating trophoblastic tumors in most countries that a scoring system taking account of multiple factors affecting prognosis is much more relevant than a conventional staging system.

Chemotherapy strategy

A full discussion of the principles of cancer chemotherapy is not appropriate here, but certain principles of particular importance need to be considered.

It has been shown that most of the post-mole cases can be treated successfully with minimal toxicity using a methotrexate/folinic acid (MTX/FA) protocol.[7] Between 1962 and 1969, almost all patients in the Charing Cross series started treatment in this way, and those who showed resistance went on to other toxic drug schedules.[6] This approach had the advantage that even for advanced cases safe treatment was given at the beginning and considerable reduction in tumor bulk achieved. The risk inherent in this approach is that, with poor prognosis patients, such treatment may promote resistance to all available agents. Whilst this did not adversely affect the outcome for patients in the low risk category who proved to require more than the methotrexate/folinic acid regimen, the results in patients with high scores were less satisfactory than had been achieved in the early years with a more toxic methotrexate and 6-mercaptopurine regimen.

A further consideration is that, with about 10 effective drugs currently available, we have the problem of how best to deploy these drugs for higher risk patients. If all the best drugs are used together one may get the greater therapeutic response, but if resistance then develops only second line agents are left. It is an issue that can only be resolved in large series.

The use of high dose methotrexate in relation to brain metastases is also discussed later (p. 1041), but it is appropriate to indicate here that there is no evidence that multigram dosage of methotrexate has any advantage in systemic therapy. Unsuccessful attempts to prevent or overcome methotrexate resistance with dosages in the range 10 to 30 g over 24 hours have been recorded. In this unit, a trial of methotrexate in low risk patients at 35 mg/m^2 × 4 on alternate days with folinic acid on a 2 weekly cycle in comparison with 300 mg/m^2 given weekly, proved favorable to the former.

So long as cases of drug-resistant choriocarcinoma occur it will be necessary to experiment to find more effective

Table 65.1 Scoring system used in prognosis of invasive mole and choriocarcinoma

Prognostic factors	Score[a]			
	0	1	2	6
Age (years)	≤39	>39		
Antecedent pregnancy	HM[c]	Abortion	Term	
Interval[b]	4	4 to 6	7 to 12	>12
hCG (iu/liter)	<10^3	10^3 to 10^4	10^4 to 10^5	>10^5
ABO groups (female × male)		O × A / A × O	B / AB	
Largest tumor, including uterine tumor		3 to 5 cm	5 cm	
Site of metastases		Spleen, kidney	Gastrointestinal tract, liver	Brain
No. of metastases identified		1 to 4	4 to 8	8
Prior chemotherapy			Single drugs	Two or more drugs

[a] The total score for a patient is obtained by adding the individual scores for each prognostic factor. Total score: ≤ 5 = low risk
6 to 8 = middle risk
≥ 9 = high risk

[b] Interval: time (months) between end of antecedent pregnancy and start of chemotherapy
[c] HM = hydatidiform mole.

drugs and more effective ways of using them. It is very unlikely, however, that units seeing only a few cases can develop better treatments, and if they do it will be difficult to prove that they are better. Ideally, randomized trials should be carried out, but for rare tumors such as choriocarcinoma this has generally proved too difficult and therefore specialized treatment centers where expertise, facilities and experience can be developed are necessary. If a patient cannot be sent to such a center, it is better for the patient to be treated according to a major center's protocols rather than be subjected to 'one-off' chemotherapeutic experimentation which can at best make no contribution to knowledge and at worst contributes a fatal outcome.

The objective of treatment is cure, and this can only be achieved by obtaining a progressive reduction in the number of clonogenic trophoblastic cells. Cell numbers are reduced by each course of treatment, but regrowth occurs in the intervals between them. The intervals between treatments are critical. They need to be kept as short as possible but there should never be less than 5 days between successive courses and preferably not more than 7 to 8 days.

Stratification

The definition of low and high risk groups of patients has developed in several centers.[4,5,24] We have found it advantageous to use a three-level stratification, partly because, in the context of a research center, it is necessary to identify a group of patients suitable for the evaluation of new drugs such as etoposide. However, the introduction of etoposide[38] provided the basis for a more acceptable high risk protocol (EMA/CO) which eliminates the need for a middle risk protocol in a less specialized unit.

The prognostic scoring system described above and summarized in Table 65.1 provides a definable basis for matching a patient's treatment to the risk inherent in her disease. Patients with low risk of drug resistance can be safely treated with the MTX/FA protocol. Those with greater scores should start with EMA/CO.

On the basis of the scoring system already described, patients with total scores of 5 or less are defined as 'low risk', those with scores between 6 and 8 are 'middle risk' and those with scores of 9 or more are 'high risk'.

Duration of treatment

The number of courses of treatment is determined individually, and the principles have already been described in the section on hCG (p. 1028). If treatment of choriocarcinoma is discontinued as soon as hCG becomes undetectable, relapse occurs. In general, the worse the prognostic factors the longer the treatment needs to be continued after attaining zero hCG levels. Low risk cases generally need 2 to 3 courses lasting 3 to 6 weeks, whereas the highest risk cases need 3 to 4 months' treatment after reaching sustained

normal hCG values. Sometimes it is difficult to be sure whether eradication has been achieved; it may then be better to stop treatment and follow a watch-and-wait policy.

HCG values sometimes increase during a course of therapy and fall in the subsequent rest period. The peaking of hCG during therapy may be such that values do not reflect the full cytotoxic effect achieved by the time the next course of therapy is due. With this proviso, hCG values should fall to less than one-fifth of their pretreatment value by the start of the next course of treatment. In the later stages of treatment a lower rate of fall may be acceptable, but less than a halving of the pretreatment value indicates only a poor response.

Treatment methods

Patients in the 'low risk' category are treated with methotrexate 50 mg (or 35 mg/m²) followed by folinic acid (Fig. 65.9 and Table 65.2). The 8-day course is repeated after a 6-day rest period. Myelosuppression is generally slight. If mucositis is more than trivial, folinic acid dosage can be increased, but too much folinic acid will diminish the response. Alopecia does not occur. Occasional patients developed elevated hepatic enzymes and others have pleuritic pain; either of these responses may necessitate changing the protocol.

About 20% of low risk patients do not achieve complete remission with the MTX/FA protocol, or change protocols because of toxicity problems. If serum hCG levels are less than 500 iu/l, treatment with actinomycin-D 0.5 mg daily i.v. for 5 successive days alternating with vincristine 1.0 mg/m² and cyclophosphamide 400 mg/m² on day 1 and repeated on day 3 may be used. A treatment-free interval

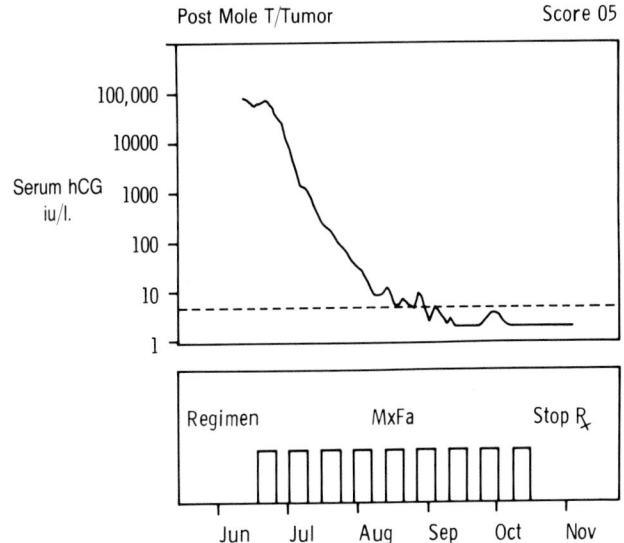

Fig. 65.9 Serum hCG values in a patient undergoing chemotherapy with methotrexate and folinic acid for an early post-mole trophoblastic tumor.

Table 65.2 Treatment of invasive mole and choriocarcinoma: low-risk regimen — methotrexate (MTX)/folinic acid (FA)

Day 1	Methotrexate 50 mg i.m. at noon
Day 2	Folinic acid 6 mg i.m. at 18.00 h or 30 h post MTX
Day 3	Methotrexate 50 mg i.m. at noon
Day 4	Folinic acid 6 mg i.m. at 18.00 h
Day 5	Methotrexate 50 mg i.m. at noon
Day 6	Folinic acid 6 mg i.m. at 18.00 h
Day 7	Methotrexate 50 mg i.m. at noon
Day 8	Folinic acid 6 mg i.m. at 18.00 h

Courses are repeated after an interval of 6 days. Each course is started on the same day of the week, unless toxicity contraindicates.

of 7 to 8 days is required between successive courses. In these patients severe alopecia may still be avoided, but if hCG levels do not fall promptly the patient should be transferred to the EMA/CO protocol (Table 65.3).

Patients in the 'high risk' category, or who fail to respond to the above regimen should be treated with the EMA/CO protocol[6] (Fig. 65.10 and Table 65.3) which has been widely used in many countries in recent years. It is easier to administer than our previous 'middle risk' and 'high risk' regimens, and, although treatment is given weekly, the protocol requires hospital admission for only 1 night every 2 weeks. This regimen causes alopecia in most patients, but mucositis and vomiting are variable and rarely severe. The interval between courses should not be extended for moderate degrees of myelosuppression.

Resistance to EMA/CO protocol

About 25% of patients with prognostic scores of greater than 8 fail to achieve complete remission on EMA/CO, as shown by a plateau in hCG values. It is important to make sure that it is a genuine plateau, but if confirmed two processes should be set in motion. The first is to introduce a protocol which includes cisplatin; the second is to initiate the search for sites of residual disease.

Cisplatin does not have the key role in controlling gestational choriocarcinoma that it occupies in germ cell tumors,[23,37] but it contributes to complete remission in about 30 to 40% of EMA/CO resistant tumors. EMA/CO resistance is usually relative, that is, hCG values fall but return to near pretreatment values before the next course. Cisplatin can be incorporated by substituting etoposide 200 mg/m² and cisplatin 100 mg/m² for the cyclophosphamide-vincristine (CO) part of the regimen. Resistance quickly develops when cisplatin is given alone. It must always be given with full hydration, magnesium supplements and only in the presence of adequate renal function. An alternative is to give cisplatin in the POMB regimen (Table 65.4) and, again, this should be alternated with the EMA protocol.

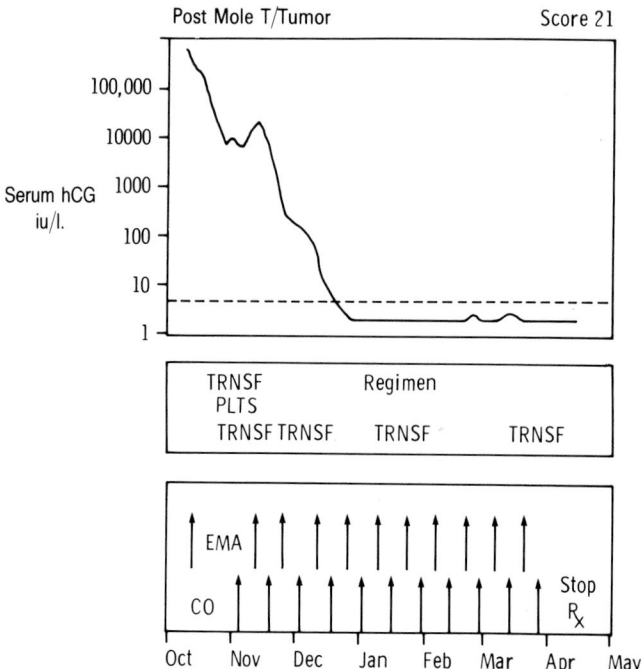

Fig. 65.10 Serum hCG values in an overseas patient with an advanced post-mole trophoblastic tumor and high prognostic score. The patient was treated with the EMA/CO regimen and required multiple blood and platelet transfusions for blood loss and myelosuppression. The interval of 3 weeks between the first and second courses of treatment was necessitated by respiratory distress commonly seen in patients who are breathless on presentation. The longer interval was accompanied by rising hCG values.

Table 65.3 Treatment of invasive mole and choriocarcinoma: the EMA/CO regimen

Course 1: EMA*

Day 1	Etoposide 100 mg/m² by i.v. infusion in 200 ml saline Actinomycin-D 0.5 mg i.v. stat Methotrexate 100 mg/m² i.v. stat Methotrexate 200 mg/m² by i.v. infusion over 12 hours
Day 2	Etoposide 100 mg/m² by i.v. infusion in 200 ml saline Actinomycin-D 0.5 mg i.v. stat Folinic acid 15 mg i.m. or orally every 12 h for 4 doses, beginning 24 hours after starting methotrexate

Course 2: Co*

Day 8	Vincristine (Oncovin) 1.0 mg/m² i.v. stat Cyclophosphamide 600 mg/m² i.v. in saline

* These courses can usually be given on Days 1 and 2, 8, 15 and 16, 22 etc. The intervals should not be extended without cause

Central nervous system metastases

Although some patients presenting with central nervous system metastases have survived from the earliest days of chemotherapy, brain metastases which developed during the course of their chemotherapy have generally proved resistant.[3] For this reason, prophylactic chemotherapy has been regarded as essential for any patient with lung metastases and for any patient in the medium- or high risk

Table 65.4 Treatment of EMA/CO-resistant tumors: the POMB regimen

Day 1	Vincristine (Oncovin) 1.0 mg/m² (max 2 mg) i.v. Methotrexate 300 mg/m² i.v. infusion over 12 h
Day 2	Bleomycin 15 mg i.v. as 24 h infusion Folinic acid 15 mg twice a day for 4 doses, 24 hours after the start of methotrexate
Day 3	Bleomycin 15 mg i.v. as 24 h infusion
Day 4	Cisplatin 120 mg/m² i.v. with forced diuresis and magnesium sulphate supplement

groups who does not have lung metastases on chest radiograph. Prophylaxis with intrathecal methotrexate 10 to 12.5 mg has been alternated weekly with systemic methotrexate as in the EMA regimen. Prophylactic intrathecal methotrexate should be continued until hCG has fallen to the limit of detection and lung fields are clear.

For the treatment of established metastases, intrathecal methotrexate is given in similar fashion to the above, but the alternating weekly systemic methotrexate is increased to 1 g/m². Intrathecal methotrexate cannot be given if there is raised intracranial pressure. An Omaya reservoir is an alternative route of administration for methotrexate. Antiepileptic drugs may be required.

Although radiation has proved only palliative in our experience, CNS neurosurgery can now make a valuable contribution, especially where CAT scan shows the lesion to be superficial. It is an alternative to chemotherapy for early lesions and may be effective in late drug-resistant lesions.

Results of treatment

Between 1964 and 1986, 348 patients in the low risk category were treated with methotrexate and folinic acid and only one of these patients died from choriocarcinoma (99.7% survival). Overall, 69 of 348 (19.8%) patients required additional drugs to achieve complete remission. A further 13 patients were treated as low risk patients, but retrospective analysis indicated they had been underscored. One of these patients died (92.3% survival) and 9 of the 13 (69%) had to change treatment.

The effectiveness of the EMA/CO regimen was assessed for 107 patients in the high risk category (Score >8). Thirteen of these patients died (88% survival). Seven of the deaths occurred in the first week after admission. Thirty required additional therapy with cisplatin regimen and/or surgery for residual disease.

Analysis of our series between 1957 and 1981[3] showed that 69 (8.8%) had CNS metastases; 37 presented with CNS metastases and 32 developed them during therapy. Survival rates were 49% and 6% respectively. After 1974, survival improved to 80% in the presentation group and

25% in the late CNS group. Of patients treated with the EMA/CO protocol, using methotrexate 1 g/m² and alternating intrathecal methotrexate with surgery where appropriate, 18 presented with CNS metastases, 3 of whom died in the first few days, 1 died with drug-resistant disease, 13 were disease free (72%) and 1 was alive with residual disease. Seven patients developed CNS metastases either on or after treatment with EMA/CO, 4 died from resistant disease, 1 was alive with resistant disease and 2 achieved sustained remission.

Surgery for residual drug resistant disease

It is not exceptional for high scoring tumors to respond incompletely to chemotherapy. As soon as an hCG plateau is observed, it is appropriate to start a search for sites of residual disease. Provided these are not inaccessible, multiple resection may be possible. In the earlier years of chemotherapy it was not uncommon to find residual disease in the uterus, but this has become infrequent as chemotherapy has improved. Even so, in a life saving situation hysterectomy carries the lowest penalty and should be the first procedure if a large uterine mass was present initially and if an alternative site of residual tumor is not evident.

Ultrasound, CAT, MRI and antibody scanning all have a place in the search for residual disease, which should include the CNS. Pulmonary lobectomy and partial lobe resections have been the commonest forms of intervention. One patient in our series had multiple metastases in one lung, whilst the other was radiologically clear. Pneumonectomy has been followed by remission now approaching 10-years duration.

The risk of dissemination of drug-resistant tumor by surgical procedures is difficult to evaluate, but it is our impression that this has been reduced by giving limited chemotherapy at the time of surgery even though the tumors are resistant. Preferred treatment is a single dose of etoposide, actinomycin-D or methotrexate, followed by folinic acid 24 hours later.

Sequelae

Pregnancies following chemotherapy for trophoblastic tumors have been reported since the early 1960's and, in general, fertility appears to be well preserved. A study of 445 long-term survivors treated between 1958 and 1978 showed that 86% of all those who wished for further pregnancies had one or more live births. Women who received three or more drugs were less likely to conceive than those who received only methotrexate.[40] Similar results have been reported from China.[25] The possibility that chemotherapy is responsible for early menopause in the older patients has not been excluded. A possible adverse effect of etoposide on ovarian function[17] was not confirmed as having an effect on fertility.[1] Data relating to the possible effects of platinum-containing protocols remain scanty at the present time.

The risk of second malignancies following chemotherapy for trophoblastic tumors has shown no statistically significant excess. The observed number of second neoplasms was less than that expected for the population at risk, totalling 3522 patient years.[41] However, amongst patients who have required prolonged intensive chemotherapy to achieve remission from choriocarcinoma, two developed acute myeloid leukemia subsequent to the 1983 report, and complacency in this matter is not justified.

ACKNOWLEDGEMENTS

I wish to thank my colleagues in the Department of Medical Oncology who have contributed much to the progress made against trophoblastic tumors. In particular, I thank Joan Dent who has run the hydatidiform mole follow-up scheme since its inception in 1973, and the immunoassay team led by Hugh Mitchell for unfailing service.

REFERENCES

1. Adewole I F, Rustin G J S, Newlands E S, Dent J, Bagshawe K D 1987 Fertility in patients with gestational trophoblastic tumors treated with etoposide. Eur J Cancer Clin Oncol 22: 1479
2. Amr S, Rosa C, Wehmann R, Birken S, Nisula B 1988 Unusual molecular forms of hCG in gestational trophoblastic neoplasia. Annales d'Endocrinologie (Paris) 45: 321
3. Athanassiou A, Begent R H J, Newlands E S, Parker D, Rustin G J S, Bagshawe K D 1983 Central nervous system metastases in choriocarcinoma. Twenty three years' experience at Charing Cross Hospital. Cancer 52: 1728
4. Azab M B, Pejovic M-H, Theodore C et al 1988 Prognostic factors in gestational trophoblastic tumors. Cancer 62: 585
5. Bagshawe K D 1976 Risk and prognostic factors in trophoblastic neoplasia. Cancer 38: 1373
6. Bagshawe K D 1987 From methotrexate to EMA/CO. In: Szulman A E, Buchsbaum H (eds) Gestational Trophoblastic Disease. Springer Verlag, New York, p 127
7. Bagshawe K D, Dent J, Newlands E S, Begent R H J, Rustin G J S 1989 The role of low dose methotrexate and folinic acid in gestational trophoblastic tumours. Br J Obstet Gynaecol 96: 795
8. Bagshawe K D, Dent J, Webb J 1986 Hydatidiform mole in the United Kingdom 1973–1983 Lancet ii 673
9. Bagshawe K D, Garnett E S 1963 Radiological changes in patients with trophoblastic tumors. Br J Radiol 36: 673
10. Bagshawe K D, Harland S 1976 Immunodiagnosis and monitoring of gonadotrophin producing metastases in the central nervous system. Cancer 38: 112
11. Bagshawe K D, Noble M M 1966 Cardio-respiratory aspects of trophoblastic tumors. Quart J Med 35: 39
12. Bagshawe K D, Rawlins G A, Pike M C, Lawler S D 1971 The ABO blood groups in trophoblastic neoplasia. Lancet i: 553
13. Baird A M, Beckly D E, Ross F G M 1977 The ultrasound diagnosis of hydatidiform mole. Clin Radiol 28: 637
14. Begent R H J, Bagshawe K D, Green A J, Searle F 1987 The clinical value of imaging with antibody to human chorionic gonadotrophin in the detection of residual choriocarcinoma. Br J Cancer 55: 657
15. Brewis R A L, Bagshawe K D 1968 Pelvic arteriography in invasive trophoblastic neoplasia. Br J Radiology 41: 481
16. Buckley J 1987 Epidemiology of gestational trophoblastic disease. In: Szulman A E, Buchsbaum H (eds) Gestational Trophoblastic Disease. Springer Verlag, New York
17. Choo Y C, Chan S Y W, Wong L C, Ma H K 1985 Ovarian dysfunction in patients with gestational trophoblastic neoplasia treated with short intensive courses of etoposide (VP 16–213) Cancer 55: 2348
18. Coppack S, Newlands E S, Dent J et al 1983 Problems of interpretation of serum concentrations of alpha-fetoprotein (AFP) in patients receiving cytotoxic chemotherapy for malignant germ cell tumour. Br J Cancer 48: 335
19. Deligdisch L, Driscoll S G, Goldstein D P 1978 Gestational trophoblastic neoplasms: morphologic correlates of therapeutic response. Am J Obstet Gynecol 130: 801
20. Eckstein R P, Paradinas F J, Bagshawe K D 1982 Placental site trophoblastic tumour (trophoblastic pseudotumour): a study of four cases requiring hysterectomy including one fatal case. Histopathology 6: 211
21. Eddy G L, Schlaerth J B, Nalick R H et al 1983 Postmolar trophoblastic disease in women using hormonal contraception with and without oestrogen. Obstet Gynecol 62: 736
22. Folkman J 1975 Tumor angiogenesis: a possible control point in tumor growth. Ann Intern Med 82: 96
23. Gordon A N, Kavanagh J J, Gershenson D M et al 1986 Cisplatin, vinblastine and bleomycin combination therapy in resistant gestational trophoblastic disease. Cancer 58: 1407
24. Hammond C B, Borchert L G, Tyrey L, Creasman W T, Parker R T 1973 Treatment of metastatic trophoblastic disease: good and poor prognosis. Am J Obstet Gynecol 115: 451
25. Hong-zhao Song, Pau-chen Wu, Yuan Wang, Shu-ying Dong 1988 Pregnancy outcome after successful chemotherapy for choriocarcinoma and invasive mole. Long term follow up. Am J Obstet Gynecol 158: 538
26. Jeffreys A J, Wilson V, Thein S L et al 1985 Individual-specific 'fingerprints' of human DNA. Nature 316: 76
27. Jones W B, Lauerson H H 1975 Hydatidiform mole with coexistent fetus. Am J Obstet Gynecol 122: 267
28. Kardana A, Bagshawe K D 1975 A rapid sensitive and specific immunoassay for human chorionic gonadotrophin. J Immunol Methods 9: 297
29. Kardana A, Taylor M E, Southall P J et al 1988 Urinary gonadotrophin peptide — isolation and purification and its immunohistochemical distribution in normal and neoplastic tissue. Br J Cancer 58: 281
30. Kato Y, Braunstein G D 1988 β-core fragment is a major form of immunoreactive urinary chorionic gonadotrophin in human pregnancy. J Clin Endocrinol Metab 66: 1197
31. Kurman R J, Young R H, Norris H J et al 1984 Immunocytochemical localisation of placental lactogen and chorionic gonadotrophin in the normal placenta and trophoblastic tumors, with emphasis on intermediate trophoblast and placental site trophoblastic tumor. Int J Gynecol Pathol 3: 101
32. Lawler S D 1978 HLA and trophoblastic tumors. Br Med Bull 34: 305
33. Lawler S D, Klouda P T, Bagshawe K D 1976 The relationship between HLA antibodies and the causal pregnancy in choriocarcinoma. Br J Obstet Gynaecol 83: 651
34. Lewis J L, Terasaki P I 1971 HLA leukocyte antigen studies in women with trophoblastic tumors. Am J Obstet Gynecol 111: 547
35. MacVicar J, Donald I 1963 Sonar in the diagnosis of early pregnancy and its complications. J Obstet Gynaecol Br Cwlth 70: 387
36. Magrath I T Golding P R, Bagshawe K D 1971 Medical presentation of choriocarcinoma. Br Med J ii: 633
37. Newlands E S 1982 New chemotherapeutic agents in the

management of gestational trophoblastic disease. Seminars in Oncology 9: 239

38. Newlands E S, Bagshawe K D 1982 The role of VP 16–213 (Etoposide; NSC 141540) in gestational choriocarcinoma. Cancer Chemother Pharmacol 7: 211

39. Papapetrou P D, Sakarelou Braouzi H, Fessas P H 1980 Ectopic production of human chorionic gonadotrophin (hCG) by neoplasms. Cancer 45: 2583

40. Rustin G J S, Booth M, Dent J et al 1984 Pregnancy after cytotoxic chemotherapy for gestational trophoblastic tumours. Br Med J 288: 103

41. Rustin G J S, Rustin F, Dent J et al 1983 No increase in second tumors after cytotoxic chemotherapy for gestational trophoblastic tumors. New Engl J Med 308: 473

42. Sakaragi N, Ohkubo H, Yamamoto R et al 1988 The serum pregnancy specific β_1-glycoprotein to beta human chorionic gonadotrophin ratio as an index of prognosis in patients with choriocarcinoma. Br J Obstet Gynaecol 95: 614

43. Sauvage J P, Crane J P, Kopta M M 1974 Difficulties in the ultrasonic diagnosis of hydatidiform mole. Obstet Gynecol 44: 546

44. Saxena B, Goldstein D P, Everson K, Selenkov H A 1968 Serum placental lactogen levels in patients with molar pregnancy or trophoblastic tumors. Am J Obstet Gynecol 102: 115

45. Scully R E, Young R H 1981 Trophoblastic pseudotumor. A reappraisal. J Surg Pathol 5: 75

46. Searle F, Leake B A, Bagshawe K D, Dent J 1978 SP$_1$ pregnancy-specific-β-glycoprotein in choriocarcinoma and other neoplastic disease. Lancet i: 579

47. Seppala M, Ruoslahti E, Bagshawe K D 1972 Radioimmunoassay of alpha-fetoprotein. A contribution to the diagnosis of choriocarcinoma and hydatidiform mole. Int J Cancer 10: 478

48. Stone M, Bagshawe K D 1979 An analysis of the influence of maternal age, gestational age, contraceptive method and the mode of primary treatment of patients with hydatidiform moles on the incidence of subsequent chemotherapy. Br J Obstet Gynaecol 86: 782

49. Sunderland C A, Redman W G, Stirrat G M 1985 Characterisation and localisation of HLA antigen on hydatidiform mole. Am J Obstet Gynecol 151: 130

50. Wehmann R E, Amr S, Rosa C, Nisula B C 1984 Metabolism, distribution and excretion of purified human chorionic gonadotrophin and its subunits in man. Annales d'Endocrinologie (Paris) 45: 291

51. World Health Organisation 1983 Gestational Trophoblastic Diseases. Technical Report Series 692 WHO, Geneva

PART XII

Miscellaneous malignant tumors of female genital tract

66. Genital tract malignancy in the prepubertal child

Sir John Dewhurst   J. H. Shepherd

INTRODUCTION

Prepubertal girls seldom suffer from malignant diseases of the genital tract and when they are affected the varieties of malignancy encountered do not resemble those seen in the adult. Certain cancers are so rare in childhood as to be mere curiosities; such are carcinoma of the vulva[22] and adenocarcinoma of the uterine body. Among the more common malignant tumors of the childhood period (although still rare when compared with incidence of adult diseases) are the embryonal rhabdomyosarcoma (botryoid sarcoma) and the clear cell adenocarcinoma of the vagina and cervix, the latter being associated in many instances with treatment of the girl's mother with estrogens in early pregnancy. A different pattern of ovarian tumor is also seen during childhood; in general, the epithelial tumors common in the adult are rare, and germ cell and sex cord stromal tumors preponderate.

EMBRYONAL RHABDOMYOSARCOMA

Embryonal rhabdomyosarcoma, a tumor of the vagina, is called by various names. Over many years it has been referred to as the botryoid sarcoma or mesodermal mixed tumor by gynecologists but more frequently as the rhabdomyosarcoma by surgeons. It is most commonly seen in the child of less than 2 years of age although cases may arise at any age during childhood or early adolescence and have even been present at birth.[23,28]

Pathology

To the naked eye, the tumor may take several forms. Classically, it resembles a bunch of grapes, as its name 'botryoid' implies, and has the form of a small group of soft pale polypi (Fig. 66.1) which project and quite frequently fill the vagina. At other times, the growth appears like a small simple polyp or as a dark hemorrhagic mass and, less often, as a fleshy bulbous swelling (Fig. 66.2). When the tumor looks like a simple polyp it is easy for the

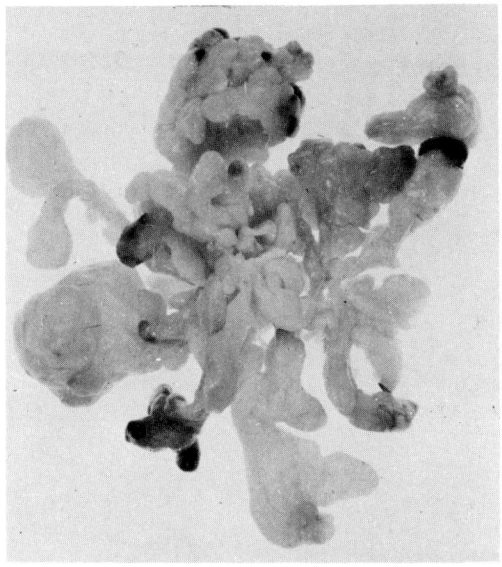

Fig. 66.1 A mass of white soft polypi representing a botryoid sarcoma. This material filled the vagina of a 3-year-old girl.

medical attendant to be lulled into a false sense of security and to believe it to be benign. Rare though these tumors of the vagina and cervix are in childhood, simple benign polypi are rarer still.

The histology shows many interesting and varied features. The stroma is loose and myxomatous (Fig. 66.3), and throughout fusiform cells may be seen which are sometimes collected into groups. Pleomorphism is always a marked feature. A characteristic finding is the presence of large cells with a vacuolated eosinophilic cytoplasm, the rhabdomyoblasts, which clearly indicate the embryonic nature of the growth. The most important distinguishing feature, however, is the presence of cross-striated muscle fibers (Fig. 66.3) which are few in number and may require careful search. The striations are often poorly defined and may be easily missed. Recognizable tissue, such as bone, cartilage or epithelial cells, which occasionally characterize this tumor in the older person, is rare in the prepubertal

1047

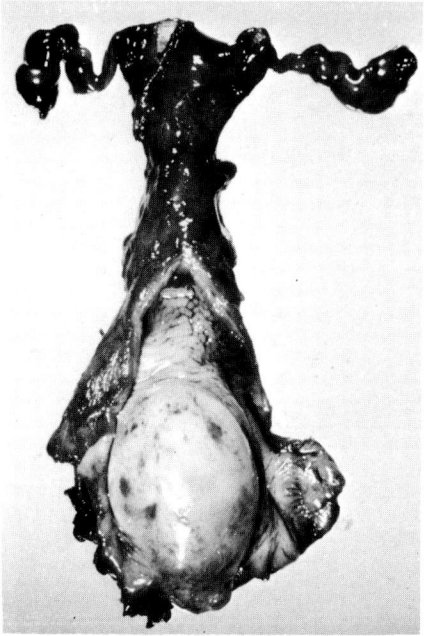

Fig. 66.2 A fleshy mass occupying the lower vagina of a 5 months old child. The mass on biopsy proved to be an embryonal rhabdomyosarcoma (sarcoma botryoides).

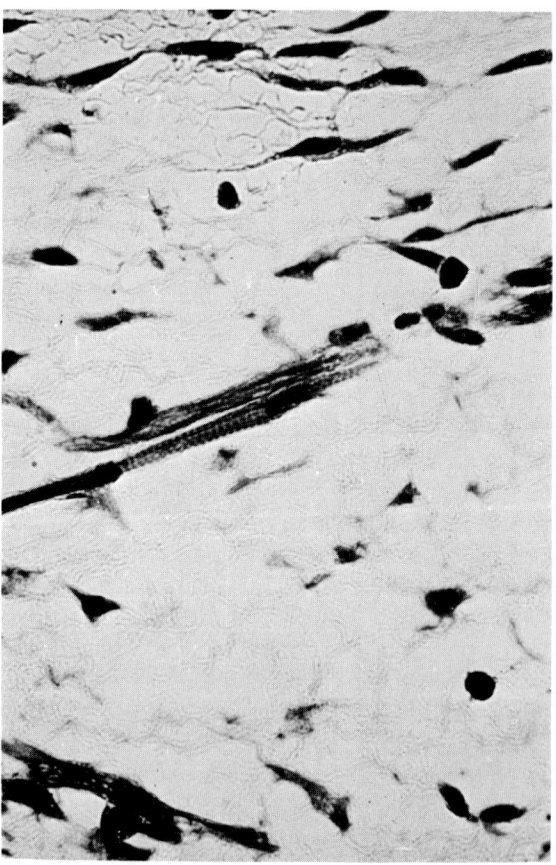

Fig. 66.3 Myxomatous stroma, fusiform cells and cross striated muscle fibers in an embryonal rhabdomyosarcoma.

child. It will be evident that many of these histological features do not strongly suggest malignancy and in many instances the appearances are those of a simple polyp, a diagnosis which has been made initially many times in the past and has been the reason for considerable delay in undertaking proper treatment.

Electronmicroscopy is of particular value in identifying the sinister features of the embryonal rhabdomyosarcoma. Rhabdomyoblasts and cross striated muscle fibers can more readily be recognized by this technique, so distinguishing these tumors from the so-called pseudosarcoma botryoides which has been described in young women, often in association with pregnancy.[26,27]

The tumor originates in and spreads rapidly through the subepithelial tissues, retaining a covering of stratified squamous epithelium over its surface until a comparatively late stage. The tumor mass bulges into the vagina giving it the characteristic macroscopic appearance described above. Local extension can be rapid. The tumor spreads first throughout the vagina and the pelvic tissues generally to involve nearby structures, and only later is there blood and lymph spread. So rapid however has been the early speed of growth, that many children in the past appear to have been overwhelmed by the tumor, death having been reported within a few months of the first appearance of the growth.

Clinical features

The important clinical feature of the vaginal embryonal rhabdomyosarcoma is bleeding. This bleeding may be minimal or occur as a sudden bright red loss or be associated with the passage of a clot or piece of tissue. The latter mode of presentation, when a small amount of the tumor sloughs and is passed per vaginam, may allow the histological examination to be made for certain without formal biopsy. In one such dramatic case, a child living in the desert near Benghazi in Libya passed a piece of tissue which was correctly identified as being a rhabdomyosarcoma; she was sent forthwith to London and successfully treated. Bleeding is always a serious symptom in a little girl, although not always due to a malignant lesion. Whenever bleeding occurs, it is imperative that investigation be undertaken immediately to confirm or refute the presence of malignancy. External examination will sometimes give a clue to the cause; if there are obvious signs of secondary sexual development in a 3 year old, for example, it is highly likely that the vaginal bleeding has originated from this cause. If a child has had an evil smelling, blood-tinged discharge for some weeks, a foreign body may be to blame. Unless there is clear evidence of precocious puberty as the sole cause of vaginal bleeding, examination under anesthesia is always advisable to be sure that no malignant tumor is present. Attention may here be drawn to the rare condition of premature menarche, in which a child with no secondary sexual development nonetheless develops more or less regular vaginal bleeding at monthly intervals without any evident explanation.[16] This diagnosis, however, cannot be made without vaginoscopy having first excluded an intravaginal cause for the bleeding.

Diagnosis

The technique of vaginoscopy in a small child is not always easy. Without an anesthetic it is not possible categorically to exclude a serious vaginal lesion. The whole lower genital tract should be carefully assessed. Initially, direct inspection within the introitus can be performed by digitally retracting the posterior part of the labia majora. A narrow retractor such as a Langenbech's retractor can then be gently inserted into the lower vagina, and moved in different directions to permit a satisfactory view of the lower half. Two such retractors side by side, gently pulled downwards at 4 and 8 o'clock will often expose a considerable amount of vagina and permit careful inspection. The upper half of the vagina and cervix cannot be visualized without an infant speculum or endoscope. Various speculae have been devised specifically for this purpose.[5,18] An infant's McGill laryngoscope gives illumination and a good view of the upper vagina. An adult 30° cystoscope or straight urethroscope introduced into the vagina with continuous running bladder irrigation fluid will distend the vagina allowing excellent visualization. Directed biopsies may be taken.

If an intravaginal tumor is found, in addition to taking a portion for biopsy, it is necessary to determine the extent and site of origin. This may be very difficult in a small patient. The tumor mass may be so large as almost to fill the vagina, and it is difficult to decide from which point the tumor is originating. A probe, gently inserted into the vagina and swept round its walls in a circular fashion, may help identify the probable attachment of the tumor. Rectal examination is also mandatory and gives valuable information concerning the possibility of extension of the tumor posteriorly in the region of the uterosacral ligaments. Cystoscopy must never be omitted since this gives valuable evidence of involvement or otherwise of the bladder. Every effort should be made to identify as precisely as possible the extent of the lesion, since an important part of the follow-up procedure may be to assess the response of the lesion to chemotherapy and radiotherapy. It is advisable to make careful diagrams which may be referred to on subsequent occasions. Other essential parts of the work up of the case will include chest X-ray, CAT scan and an intravenous pyelogram. In older children, lymphography may be of value though it is seldom helpful in the young. The possible value of magnetic resonance imaging is yet to be determined.

Treatment

Real progress has been made in the last few years in the management of embryonal rhabdomyosarcoma. In the past, only radical surgery instituted early in the course of the disease provided any real hope of cure. Not only was it generally necessary to carry out extended hysterectomy and total vaginectomy, but an anterior or posterior exenteration was often required. It is now realized that the response of tumors of this histological type, both in the vagina and elsewhere in the body, to appropriate chemotherapy and to a lesser extent to radiotherapy has been so promising that radical surgery of this nature may no longer be necessary. Grosfeld, Smith & Clatworthy,[14] for example, reported 13 cases of pelvic rhabdomyosarcomata with 6 survivors (46%); 5 of the patients were treated with a combination of operation, radiation and chemotherapy and all survived. Ghavimi et al[12] reported 17 survivors for periods of 18 months to 10 years out of 27 children with urogenital rhabdomyosarcomata. In their view, the combination of surgery, radiotherapy and multiple chemotherapy offered the best chance of prolonged survival and cure. Fleming et al[11] are of the same opinion; in their review of 10 girls with vaginal or cervical tumors, 8 were free from disease 1 to 14 years later. This has also been our experience in conjunction with the Paediatric Oncology Unit of St. Bartholomew's Hospital, London. We have employed a regime of chemotherapy with vincristine, actinomycin D and cyclophosphamide (VAC) given by intravenous injection every 2 to 3 weeks over a 6 month period. An alternate regime currently in use is bleomycin, etoposide, and cisplatin. Similar results occur and careful supervision is essential. After the first two or three courses of this treatment, a further reassessment under anesthesia is carried out. Further biopsy is taken to determine the response of the tumor to the treatment so far given and another assessment under anesthesia is made 6 months after the onset of chemotherapy. Generally, we have noticed shrinkage in the size of the tumor, and histological examination usually shows less cellular activity than was evident before. However the extent to which the tumor may still be viable is not easy to determine.

The place of radiotherapy is not yet completely defined. Encouraged by the response to VAC chemotherapy in our early cases, my colleagues and I eliminated this step in later ones in view of the depressive effect on the growth of the pelvic bones. Others,[11] however, still employ radiotherapy and claim improved results. Reynolds[30] reported that in a group of 44 patients with vaginal, bladder or prostate tumors, survival rates with VAC alone were 50%, with VAC and radiotherapy 68% and with VAC and surgery 67%; when all three were employed, 88% of patients were still alive. It should be remembered, however, that with small numbers like these, percentages magnify apparent advantages.

In a number of instances, the response of the primary growth to therapy has been most encouraging, leading us to hope that in certain circumstances complete disappearance of the tumor might render surgery unnecessary. Until now, it has been our rule nonetheless to embark upon surgery after this preliminary treatment. It is our aim to avoid an exenteration procedure if at all possible, but to carry out extended hysterectomy and total vaginectomy with lymph node dissection. Others[15] are of the same view.

The technique used differs significantly from the procedure in the adult. At the outset it is advisable to cut down onto a vein at the ankle and to tie in an intravenous line in order that suitable intravenous therapy can be maintained for a number of days postoperatively. Despite the small size of the patients the operation itself does not usually give rise to great difficulties. The uterus, tubes and ovaries are abdominal, not pelvic organs as in the adult and can be easily elevated into the wound permitting identification of the ureters and satisfactory dissection without undue difficulty. Most authorities favor preservation of the ovaries which can then become active at puberty in the usual way. Conservation is not difficult: the infundibulopelvic ligaments can be divided lateral to the fallopian tubes but medial to the ovaries, so preserving the ovarian blood supply. Oophoropexy may be considered if there is the possibility of pelvic radiotherapy. The gonads may be transposed by elevating them high into the paracolic gutter up to the level of the inferior pole of the kidney. They are fixed to the posterior abdominal wall with two or three interrupted 2/0 Proline sutures, and their position marked with a metal clip for radiological location. Retroperitoneal tissues can usually be opened up without difficulty and the operation generally proceeds in a satisfactory manner until the lower part of the vagina is reached when some difficulty may be encountered.

At this point it has been our practice to have the child's legs raised to the lithotomy position and to leave the assistant in charge of the abdominal-pelvic part of the operation. A circular incision is then made round the junction of the vagina and the vulva posteriorly from 9 o'clock to 3 o'clock which allows dissection upwards in the paravaginal tissues. This dissection is gently carried out until the fingers of the assistant are felt. Once the sides and the posterior part of the vagina are freed in this way, the incision may be carried anteriorly beneath the urethra and similar dissection is undertaken. The dissection in the suburethral area is less simple, however, and very gentle incision with a scalpel may be necessary before the urethra and vagina are fully separated from each other. The pelvic organs can then be lifted out en bloc and a drain inserted into the paravaginal tissues from below. The tissues need only be brought loosely together round the drain at this point. A return is then made to the abdominal part of the procedure where the abdominal lymph node dissection is completed, the pelvis reperitonized and the abdomen

closed. An indwelling catheter is placed in the bladder and left there for 4 to 6 days. Three to 4 weeks after operation, chemotherapy is recommended and continued at 2 to 3 weekly intervals for 6 months, or longer should the special circumstances of the case warrant it.

Special mention must be made of one exceptional case. This was a 14 year old child who completed her course of chemotherapy and radiotherapy in the usual fashion but when surgery was about to be undertaken, she was lost to surveillance to return 6 months later. Re-examination at that time showed no sign of any tumor nor indeed of any abnormality on vaginal examination, inspection and biopsy of the previously affected area. Chemotherapy was given for 6 more months and surgery has been withheld. A further case treated in similar fashion resulted in astonishing shrinkage of an enormous vagina filled with tumor. Not only was surgery, which had previously seemed almost impossible, practicable but it was possible to avoid exenteration.

Results

It is early days to make sweeping claims for the undoubted value of treatment of this nature. We are, however, encouraged by the results achieved. Over the last 10 years we have managed nine cases in which a combination of surgery, chemotherapy and radiotherapy has been employed. Our first use of chemotherapy was in a patient with recurrent tumor following treatment by anterior exenteration 4 years previously. She had an excellent response to the chemotherapy and radiotherapy, and is alive and apparently well $4\frac{1}{2}$ years later, that is, $8\frac{1}{2}$ years after the original surgery. Three further cases were given chemotherapy and radiotherapy alone. Although one child is alive and well, two have died of distal metastases. The other seven cases are still alive at the time of writing, with survival time varying from 2 to 10 years. At present, it would appear that surgical removal of the primary is still indicated, but the role of surgery will change and hopefully be more conservative in the future with more effective combination treatment alternatives.

CLEAR CELL ADENOCARCINOMA OF THE VAGINA AND CERVIX

Association with diethylstilbestrol

The association of clear cell adenocarcinoma of the vagina or cervix with prenatal treatment of the mother with diethylstilbestrol (DES) was first reported by Herbst & Scully in 1970.[17] By 1985, 497[33] examples of this tumor had been reported to the Registry (see also Ch. 32). The bulk of the patients are adolescent rather than prepubertal, but approximately 10% have not menstruated. The youngest patient so far recorded has been aged 7 years and the oldest 29 years, with the peak incidence at 19.5 years for those patients who have a positive history of DES exposure. About two-thirds of the cases in the Registry show a positive association with DES or other non-steroidal estrogen, but among the prepubertal patients fewer give a positive history of DES exposure. No case has apparently followed the use of a steroidal sex hormone in early pregnancy. The majority of mothers have been given comparatively large doses of DES, but some have received much less, even as little as 1.5 mg daily throughout pregnancy. Whenever there has been certainty about the regime employed, however, it is evident that treatment has always begun during the first trimester of pregnancy. Prolonged treatment is unnecessary for the establishment of the disease and on several occasions exposure for only 1 or 2 weeks during the first trimester has been reported.

Pathology

There has been considerable variation in the lesions. Some have been tiny, perhaps 3 mm or so in diameter, whilst others have been very extensive. Many growths are polypoid or nodular in character and firm or granular or indurated on palpation. Ulceration may be evident, whilst other tumors are flat and project little beyond the vaginal wall. Rarely, a covering of intact squamous epithelium over the tumor is found. Two-thirds of the tumors are confined to the vagina; some of the remainder affect the cervix alone whilst others appear to involve the nearby vagina as well. The latter are classed as cervical in origin although it seems more likely that they arise from the vagina.

In general, the histological appearance is not strikingly different from clear cell adenocarcinoma occurring elsewhere in the genital tract in older patients. The clear appearance of the cells is due to the presence of large amounts of glycogen in the cytoplasm. Although this glycogen is usually evident, it is not always present and a number of tumors simply appear to be adenocarcinomata without attracting the label 'clear-cell'. There is usually little difficulty in making the correct histological diagnosis, although Robboy et al[31] draw attention to problems which may occasionally arise in distinguishing what those authors call microglandular hyperplasia occurring in patches of vaginal adenosis.

Initial spread is local, but lymph node involvement has been reported very frequently even with small tumors. Both vaginal and cervical tumors may involve lymph glands at an early stage, despite the fact that the primary tumor does not seem to be invading deeply.

Clinical features and therapy

The first symptom, as with botryoid sarcoma of the vagina, is vaginal bleeding, which calls for immediate examination under anesthesia whether a history of DES exposure has been established or not. It is possible to make the diagnosis from exfoliated cells but this is not reliable, and most careful examination and biopsy similar to that described on page 1049 should be undertaken.

In Britain we have little experience of treatment of this condition. Judging from accounts from the United States, treatment should be radical, probably by extended hysterectomy and vaginectomy with lymph node dissection, as already described on page 1050. The use of radiotherapy will probably depend upon local custom but it is doubtful if there is clear evidence for or against. It certainly does not commend itself as primary treatment. Response to surgery, in general, has been good especially in early cases. Robboy et al[31] reported that nearly all patients with asymptomatic tumors, most of which were tiny and superficial, are alive and free from disease. One-quarter or so of the total cases have recurred, generally the larger and more deeply penetrating primary growths. Such recurrences have usually been local but metastases to supraclavicular nodes and to lung have been reported in one-third of the instances. Senekjian & Herbst[33] report a 5-year survival rate of 90% for Stage I vaginal and cervical lesions; for Stage IIa cervix and Stage II vagina the figure was 82%, for Stage IIb cervix lesions, 60%, and for Stage III cases, 37%. For all patients, 5-year survival has been 80%.

These encouraging results, especially for early lesions, have tempted some to employ less than radical treatment in attempts to preserve fertility. Twenty seven Registry patients received either local excision or partial vaginectomy for small tumors; although 5 of these later conceived, there were 6 recurrences and 2 deaths in the series indicating that such conservative management carries a decided risk.

Other cervical and vaginal lesions

Of particular interest is the likelihood that an exposed individual will develop adenocarcinoma of the vagina, and the relationship this bears to the other vaginal lesions which appear to be infinitely more common than carcinoma itself. Ulfelder[35] suggested that an incidence figure of 0.1% for exposed individuals developing adenocarcinoma might not be unreasonable; more recent figures quoted by the Registry are of a similar order — 0.14 to 1.4 per thousand for women up to 24 years of age. It is well known, however, that a variety of benign lesions is far more likely to affect the vagina and cervix in such exposed patients. The principal lesion is vaginal adenosis, but others include the transverse vaginal septum, the cockscomb cervix and the development of squamous metaplasia in which there may be dysplastic changes even amounting to carcinoma in situ.

Vaginal adenosis is the presence within the vagina of glandular areas lined by columnar-cell cervical-type

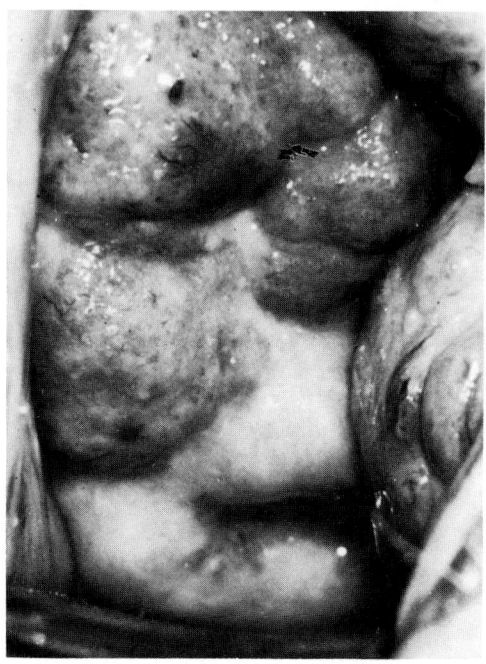

Fig. 66.4 Heaped up masses of vaginal adenosis in an adult (courtesy of the Editor, *British Journal of Obstetrics and Gynaecology*).

epithelium. Areas of adenosis may be heaped up as large glandular masses (Fig. 66.4) or be small and punctate; they may be confluent or discrete. They may be limited to a particular area of the vagina or extend almost throughout it. Some lesions open onto the surface, others are deep beneath intact squamous epithelium. The cervix itself may show similar lesions replacing the squamous epithelium on the portio vaginalis; at various points this columnar-type epithelium may extend to the fornices. When these changes are marked, one sees the appearance of pseudo-polyp formation on the cervix, sometimes described as the cockscomb cervix. Marked fibrosis which generally takes an annular form may be evident, and this may give rise to transvaginal septum formation which makes examination of the cervix and upper vagina very difficult.

The very extensive transformation zones in patients with extensive adenosis is viewed by some with great concern. Some observers have described atypical squamous metaplasia and even carcinoma in situ.[3,25,34] Although invasive squamous cell carcinoma has not yet been reported in such a case, the presence of in situ lesions and increased frequency of dysplasia suggests to some that there could be a considerable increase in the incidence of invasive cancer as the years go by. Reported incidences of intraepithelial neoplasia in DES-exposed patients have varied from 0 to 18%. In those exhibiting the higher incidence, it seems likely that the presence of immature squamous metaplasia, which bears a close resemblance to dysplasia, has been mis-

taken for the more serious condition[17,33] (see also Chs 32 and 33).

Evaluation of DES-exposed girls

There has been considerable discussion concerning the management of the patient at risk who as yet has not developed any symptoms suggestive of a vaginal or cervical lesion, innocent or malignant. In the early days of this disorder, when a great deal was to be learnt, we examined under anesthesia a number of prepubertal children who had been exposed in utero to DES. Adenosis was evident in some, but there is no doubt that the examination of the small child can be very difficult and it is not easy fully to evaluate what is seen. Because the difficulties are so great we now incline to the view promulgated by Herbst[17] that examination should be postponed until the age of 14 or until the patient menstruates, whichever is the earlier, unless there are clinical features which suggest that the examination should be made sooner. The initial examination may be under anesthetic. After a few years, once tampons are introduced for routine menstrual control, annual examination without sedation is feasible.

If the examination is made, it is essential to visualize the whole vagina very carefully. Mucus and vaginal debris, obscuring a good view, may be gently wiped away and smears taken for exfoliative cytology; these smears should be directed to specific areas — the cervix, the fornices and areas of the vagina with obvious adenosis lesions. It must be stressed again, however, that exfoliative cytology is fallible in this situation. The whole vagina should then be carefully palpated with special attention paid to those areas with an indurated or more granular consistency. Induration is a suspicious sign and biopsy of such an area may be required. Colposcopy is undoubtedly valuable in the assessment of the patient who has been exposed in utero to DES. It is, however, far from easy in the smaller child and it is most valuable when examining lesions at the vault of the vagina and on the cervix itself. Lesions beneath intact epithelium cannot properly be examined. Colposcopy may indicate areas from which biopsies can most helpfully be taken. The iodine staining technique has also been recommended as a guide to biopsy. It has been pointed out by Sandberg & Hebard[32] however, that neither metaplastic squamous epithelium nor benign endocervical-type epithelium take the iodine stain; in their words 'infinitesimally little which does not take the stain is cancer'.

All that can be done, however, is to examine the vagina very carefully and extensively throughout its length in this way and at a repeat examination perhaps a year later to note any changes. Senekjian & Herbst,[33] whose work is pre-eminent in this field, give an excellent account of the screening procedure to be adopted.

ENDODERMAL SINUS TUMORS OF THE VAGINA

Endodermal sinus tumor of the vagina, which is one of the rarest of the genital tract malignancies in children, is easily mistaken for a clear cell adenocarcinoma, to which it bears a histological resemblance. Allyn et al[1] however, clearly distinguished the two tumors, pointing out that the endodermal sinus tumor seldom occurs in patients over 2 years of age, whilst the clear cell adenocarcinoma does not arise in such young subjects. There are histological differences also, the endodermal sinus tumor showing glomeruloid formations of cells, hobnail patterns and PAS-positive hyaline globules. Alphafetoprotein levels are raised in the blood.

The tumor is highly malignant, and long-term survival is rare, although one of us treated a child aged 6 months by radical surgical excision of uterus and vagina and she is still alive and well more than 10 years later.[9] A review of the world literature by Goerzen et al[13] confirms the highly malignant nature of this tumor, which is best managed by radical excision followed by chemotherapy.

CARCINOMA OF CERVIX

Carcinoma of the cervix may rarely arise during childhood without a history of prior exposure to DES. In these cases, although the nature of the tumor is an adenocarcinoma, the cell pattern is not similar to the clear cell type just discussed. Huffman[18] describes these adenocarcinomas as 'mesonephric', believing that they arise in remnants of the mesonephric tissue. Undoubtedly their histological appearance supports this view, since they often show multiple gland-like spaces lined by neoplastic low columnar epithelium and at several points the gland is heaped up in projections in a sort of hob-nailed pattern. This pattern is variable, however, and as yet it is not certain that such tumors are of mesonephric origin.

The pattern of clinical presentation is similar to that of all other malignant disorders of the vagina and cervix already considered — vaginal bleeding. Any lesion visualized must be biopsied immediately and subjected to careful histological examination. If biopsy of the tumor shows unmistakable features of adenocarcinoma, immediate treatment is imperative. If such a lesion is discovered in a prepubertal child, a very rare event, the technical problems of radium insertion will probably be so great that radical surgery will be the treatment of choice. Extended hysterectomy and partial vaginectomy with lymph node dissection should be carried out as described on page 1050. Less of the vagina has to be removed than when an embryonal rhabdomyosarcoma is present and the operation is therefore simpler. It is not so easy to decide what part adjuvant radiotherapy should play in management. If the operation is successful and the lymph nodes on histological examination show no metastases, then radiotherapy may well be omitted; on the other hand, if there is doubt about the completeness of the surgical excision or the nodes are positive, external radiotherapy is probably advisable. The results of treatment have not been good in most cases of adenocarcinoma of the cervix in childhood, but this may have been mainly due to the fact that most were advanced cases with extensive involvement when the patient was first seen. In early cases much better results are possible; one of our own patients was well and free from disease 16 years after treatment, and another 8 years later. Both were treated with radiotherapy alone.[7]

OVARIAN TUMORS

Ovarian tumors are uncommon in children and frequently give rise to much clinical difficulty. Not all ovarian swellings in the prepubertal period are new growths and not all the new growths are malignant. In Breen & Maxson's series[4] there were 36% non-neoplastic swellings, the remainder being new growths of one kind or another. Huffman[18] reported that 30% of 999 tumors, and Breen & Maxson[4] 35% of 1309 tumors, in children were malignant. In other series malignancy rates have varied from 15 to 32%.[6]

Pathology

Comment has already been made about the differences in pattern that exist between the pathology of ovarian new growths in the prepubertal period and in the adult. When Breen & Maxson reviewed 648 cases collected from four series, they found that in the prepubertal group, germ cell tumors and sex cord stromal tumors clearly preponderated over epithelial and other growths.[4] Several tumors have a noted predilection for the young, particularly the dysgerminoma and the teratoma (Fig. 66.5). In the adolescent, however, the pattern of the tumors begins to relate more closely to that seen in the adult. In this respect, an interesting difference is seen in the different age groups in Breen & Maxson's collective series; epithelial tumors accounted for only 0.5% of new growths below the age of 9 years, but for 16% between the ages of 10 and 14 years, and 38% between the ages of 13 and 17 years.

Clinical features

In the prepubertal child, the clinical presentation of the ovarian tumor is somewhat different from that seen in the adult. The younger the patient, the more likely is laparotomy to be undertaken for undiagnosed abdominal pain when an ovarian tumor is discovered. Modes of clinical presentation are analyzed in detail in an interesting report by Linfors from Finland.[2] Of 81 cases of ovarian

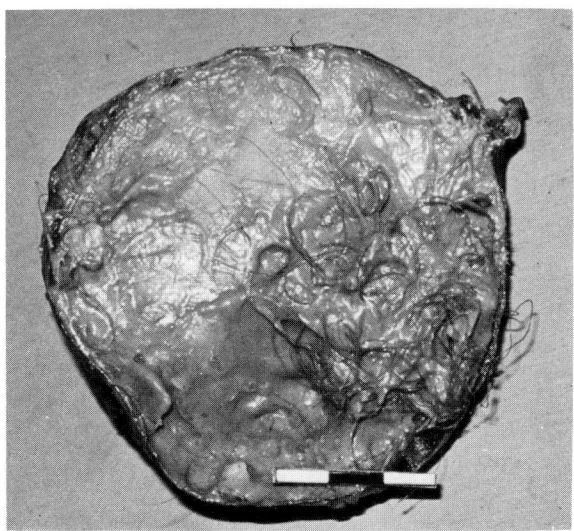

Fig. 66.5 An opened benign ovarian teratoma (dermoid cyst). The sebaceous type material and hair filling the tumor are clearly visible.

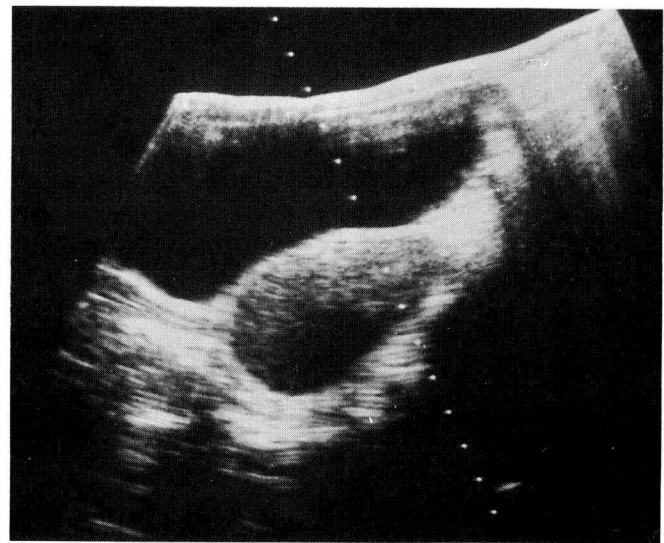

Fig. 66.6 An ultrasound scan of the pelvis in a child with precocious puberty. Behind the bladder, a semi-solid tumor can be seen which at operation proved to be a granulosa cell tumor.

tumor in the young, he found pain was easily the most common feature, present in 54% of cases. The reason for the pain was not always evident, although torsion of the tumor was recognized in 23% of the patients reviewed. The next most common clinical feature was abdominal distension which was present in only 18% of patients. It is easy to see why so many ovarian tumors in the child escape detection until some accident produces a series of symptoms. Recognition of a small tumor in the somewhat protruberant abdomen of a little girl can be quite difficult. If the tumor is big there should be no problem in recognizing it, although the precise nature may be more difficult to determine; Linfors reported a palpable mass in 76% of his cases. In the differential diagnosis, Wilms tumor, an enlarged spleen, a mesenteric cyst, a grossly distended bladder and, during the newborn period, hydrocolpos should be considered. On X-ray, a shadow of a probable tooth may sometimes be seen, suggesting the tumor is a benign teratoma.

The hormonally active tumors of the granulosa/theca cell group may present with signs of sexual precocity and vaginal bleeding. It is imperative to appreciate, however, that such tumors are relatively uncommon causes of precocious puberty, which is much more often either constitutional in origin or associated with an intracranial lesion, such as a third ventricle hamartoma, or with the McCune Albright syndrome. Moreover, in girls with precocious puberty which is not of ovarian tumor origin, the development of a follicular cyst of sufficient size to be clinically recognizable is not uncommon. Such a cyst is the *result* of the premature ovarian stimulation and *not the cause* of the condition. The distinction between them may be made by means of an ultrasound scan — an invaluable tool

in assessing the suspected ovarian lesion in a child — since the simple trans-sonic follicular cyst gives quite different appearances from those of a solid or semi-solid new growth (Fig. 66.6).

Operative findings

Once an ovarian new growth is suspected with confidence, the abdomen should be opened without delay. Serum should always be taken for tumor marker estimation, namely that of alphafetoprotein and hCG. The results may not necessarily be available prior to laparotomy, but may be useful as a baseline if further treatment is given and to monitor follow-up and possible recurrence. Certain physical features will help the surgeon to determine if the tumor is innocent or malignant. If the tumor wall is smooth, the swelling is unilateral, the contents are clearly cystic throughout and if there are no adhesions to other structures, nor papilliferous processes on the surface, then innocence can be assumed. If the tumor is bilateral the likelihood of it being malignant is much greater, although benign tumors, notably teratomata, are often bilateral. Linfors found a hard tumor was usually malignant.[21] Once the abdomen is open careful examination must be carried out; this may include bisection of the tumor to inspect its internal surface, very great care being taken not to spill any of the contents. If the tumor is a simple benign teratoma (dermoid cyst) this fact should be clearly evident on inspection when cystectomy, if necessary bilateral, can be performed preserving as much normal ovarian tissue as possible. If the tumor is bilateral and clearly not a benign cystic teratoma, the likelihood of it being malignant is much greater. In this circumstance, if possible, a frozen section should be cut and an attempt made to determine whether the tumors are innocent or malignant. The use of frozen section is, however, not without disadvantages. Assessment is not always easy and the portion taken for examination may not be representative of the tumor as a whole. Nonetheless, faced with a bilateral solid ovarian tumor the nature of which is uncertain in a prepubertal child, examination of a frozen section should, if at all possible, be the first step before any radical treatment is undertaken. It should be remembered that solid tumors may be either benign or malignant. A uniform solid fibrous-looking growth will probably be either a fibroma or, more rarely, a thecoma and benign; even a tumor with mixed solid and cystic areas may be innocent, although the presence of hemorrhage and necrosis suggests malignancy. In those instances where the clinical signs clearly indicate malignancy, such as spread to surrounding tissues, secondary deposits in omentum and peritoneum etc, there will be no doubt about the serious nature of the disorder.

Treatment

All the above considerations apply when making the decision on the precise method of treatment to be undertaken. If the ovarian tumor is clearly benign, ovarian cystectomy with ovarian preservation should be undertaken. The surgical procedure is simple. A benign solid tumor cannot be shelled out in this way and should be treated by an oophorectomy if possible preserving the fallopian tube. If there is doubt about the nature of a unilateral tumor, then our preference is still for unilateral removal and, if necessary, for a reappraisal of further treatment in the light of the histological report. If frozen section facilities are available they should be used, but unless there is unequivocal evidence of malignancy we prefer to perform salpingo-oophorectomy rather than a radical procedure at this stage. Should searching examination of the sections subsequently prove the tumor to be malignant, further operation, if necessary, can be undertaken without delay a week later. Such an approach, in the words of Carlson 'appears preferable to what may be unnecessary castration'.[6]

Many tumors are highly chemosensitive and, even with widespread metastatic disease, conservative surgery may now be carried out. It is essential to establish the diagnosis and accurately stage the patient. Cisplatin-based regimes such as the BEP regime (bleomycin, etoposide and cisplatin) may be successfully employed, with tumor marker estimation monitoring response.[29] Re-exploration to complete surgical removal of remaining masses may be carried out as an interval procedure after six courses. Often, necrotic, non-viable mature tumor tissue only is found. Fertility is conserved in these patients and pregnancy is possible in the future. Second-look surgery in the absence of remaining tumor masses is not necessary, but directed monoclonal antibody scanning may be helpful if tumor marker levels rise.

Certain tumors, notably the dysgerminoma are very radiosensitive. Should recurrence arise after chemotherapy and conservative surgery, pelvic clearance and then radiotherapy postoperatively may still cure the patient. However, radiotherapy would not be the primary method of treatment in view of the long-term sequelae in this young age group of patients.

It is better to undertake a laparotomy and biopsy a large, apparently inoperable metastatic tumor than attempt either difficult or inappropriate surgical extirpation. Re-exploration by a gynecological oncologist may always be carried out at a later date if necessary.

When the abdomen has been opened on a suspected diagnosis of a granulosa cell tumor, it must be remembered that, although such a tumor may well be discovered to have *caused* the condition, that which may be found may be a follicular cyst — or bilateral cysts — *resulting* from the condition. In the latter instance, the operation of ovarian cystectomy must be undertaken and all normal ovarian tissue preserved. If a new growth is found, unilateral removal in the first instance should be carried out unless there is undeniable evidence of spread of the growth. Although the granulosa cell tumor is, strictly speaking, malignant the degree of malignancy is low and the prognosis from unilateral removal good.

SPECIAL GONADAL TUMORS

For many years it has been recognized that intersexuality and malignant tumors of the gonads occasionally coexisted. Many of the circumstances of the association have now been elucidated, and an approach to treatment defined. Gonadal tumors in the child or adolescent may arise in two groups of patient.

1. In the ectopically situated testes of the genetic male whose phenotype is wholly or predominantly female.
2. In certain patients with gonadal dysgenesis.

The risk of gonadal malignancy is probably significantly greater in the latter group.

A genetic male (46XY) may be phenotypically female — wholly or predominantly — in three sets of circumstances:

1. When testosterone which is produced in normal amounts cannot be utilized (androgen insensitivity and 5-α-reductase deficiency).
2. In the presence of an enzyme defect preventing normal testosterone biosynthesis (enzymatic testicular failure).
3. When the testes have completely failed to differentiate and are replaced by useless streaks of tissue (pure gonadal dysgenesis).

In *androgen insensitivity*, the feminization is due to the failure of end organ to respond to normal male levels of testosterone which are circulating in the blood. The testes appear microscopically normal but are usually intra-abdominal, inguinal or, rarely, labial in position. The vulva is normal, the vagina short and blind and the uterus absent. Pubic and axillary hair is scanty or absent and the breasts are well formed. In 5-α-reductase deficiency a degree of external masculinization of the external genitalia is often present and patients are usually assigned initially to the male role. In the presence of a *biosynthetic defect of testosterone production*, the precise clinical features will depend upon the nature of the enzyme deficiency present. There may be some pubertal feminization or masculinization but the phenotype is likely to be predominantly female. Testosterone levels are fairly low. Again the testes are macroscopically normal but lie in a similar ectopic position to those in androgen insensitivity. Ectopically situated testes such as these are, however, at risk of malignancy although the risk is varyingly quoted. Jones & Scott[20] and Dewhurst, Ferriera & Gillett[8] suggest a malignancy rate of 5% at some time in a patient's life. The likelihood of a malignant tumor developing in a prepubertal child's testis is small although this risk probably increases after puberty with increasing age. Manuel, Katayama & Jones[24] suggest that the risk of gonadal malignancy in patients with androgen insensitivity is perhaps of the order of 3.6% up to the age of 25 years and increases thereafter. The youngest patient with a tumor in their series was 14 years. The histological varieties of tumor discovered, allowing for variations in terminology used by different authors, are predominantly of the seminoma/dysgerminoma group; the labels teratoma, arrhenoblastoma and the less specific 'alveolar cancer' and 'pelvic' cancer have occasionally been applied.

It is important to the proper management of the prepubertal child with one of these conditions to determine the likely form of secondary sexual development at puberty. If the child has typical features of androgen insensitivity and is likely to feminize without any suggestion of masculinization, the testes may be left in situ until breast development is complete, when they are removed and replacement estrogen therapy given. If there is doubt about the type of secondary sexual development which will appear at puberty, the testes should be removed in childhood and replacement estrogen therapy given at the appropriate time. The reason for this early removal, however, is not that the risk of malignancy is higher in such a patient, but to avoid the psychological disturbance of masculine changes occurring at puberty in a patient being brought up in the female role.

With regard to patients with *gonadal dysgenesis*, only those with a Y chromosome in their karyotype need be regarded as being at increased risk of gonadal malignancy. The great majority of gonadal dysgenesis patients are not

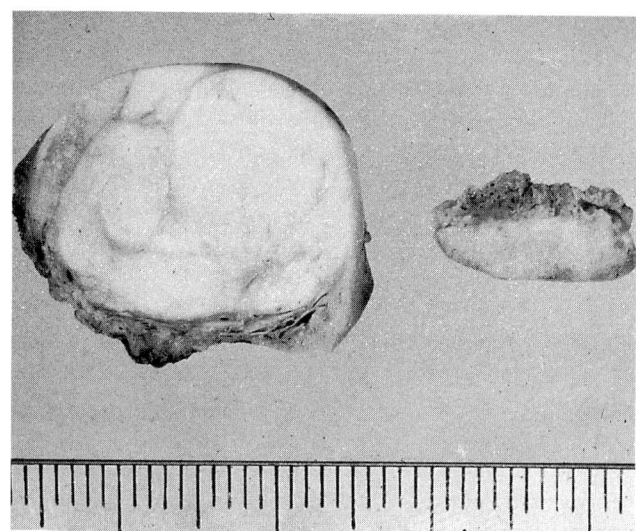

Fig. 66.7a Gross appearance of bilateral gonadal tumors in a 46XY child with precocious breast development. The scale is in inches.

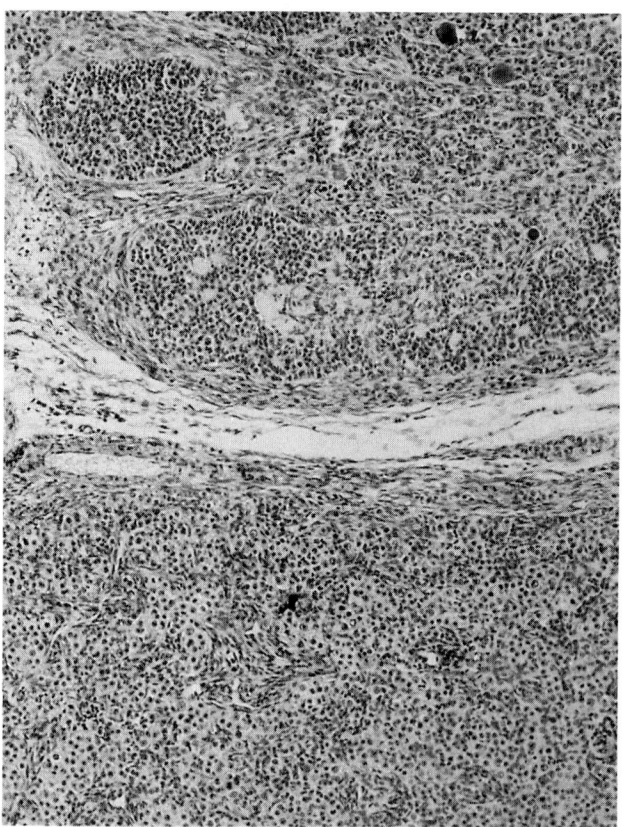

Fig. 66.7b Histological appearances of the tumors seen in Figure 66.7a. In its upper part, the tumor shows the characteristic pattern of a gonadoblastoma and in its lower part that of a dysgerminoma. (By courtesy of Marcel Dekker and Co.)

therefore at any greater risk since they do not possess a Y chromosome. If the Y is present, however, the risk of malignancy may be of the order of 30%.[2,8] Manuel et al[24] attempted to relate the risk of occurrence of malignancy to age. They concluded that in patients with gonadal dysgenesis, including those with some gonadal differentiation, the percentage of tumors rose appreciably after puberty and they therefore recommended gonadectomy before that time. Their series contained two patients aged 5 and 6 years with a gonadal tumor. This and other evidence clearly indicate that removal of the gonadal remnants is advisable and can be undertaken at any convenient time prior to puberty. The reason for early removal is not only that there is a significant prepubertal risk of malignancy but also the avoidance of psychological distress discussed above.

The type of tumor present in gonadal remnants is in most instances either gonadoblastoma or dysgerminoma or both (Fig. 66.7). In 41 cases of gonadal tumors in association with gonadal dysgenesis collected by Manuel et al,[24] the histological diagnosis was gonadoblastoma in 22, dysgerminoma in 11, gonadoblastoma and dysgerminoma in 3, gonadoblastoma and/or dysgerminoma with choriocarcinoma elements in 2, gonadoblastoma and dysgerminoma with embryonal elements in 1, Brenner tumor in 1, and unknown in 1. The pure gonadoblastoma is usually regarded as of low grade malignancy; indeed, some are circumscribed and microscopic in size and may have little significance. The dysgerminoma is another matter and must be regarded as malignant; it may need to be treated radically (see also Chs 57 and 58).

REFERENCES

1. Allyn D L, Silverberg S G, Salzberg A M 1971 Endodermal sinus tumor of the vagina. Cancer 27: 1231
2. Barr M L, Carr D H, Plunkett E R, Soltan H C, Wiens R G 1967 Male pseudohermaphroditism and pure gonadal dysgenesis in sisters. Am J Obstet Gynecol 99: 1047
3. Bibbo M, Gill W B, Azizi F et al 1977 Follow-up study of male and female offspring of DES-exposed mothers. Obstet Gynecol 49: 1
4. Breen J L, Maxson W S 1977 Ovarian tumors in children and adolescents. Clin Obstet Gynecol 20: 607
5. Capraro V J 1974 Vulvovaginitis and other local lesions of the vulva. Clinics Obstet Gynaecol 1: 553
6. Carlson J A 1985 Gynecological neoplasms. In: Lavery J P, Sanfilippo J S (eds) Pediatric and Adolescent Obstetrics and Gynecology. Springer Verlag, New York p 124
7. Dalley V M, Dewhurst C J, Flood C M 1971 Carcinoma of the cervix in childhood: (a report of two cases). J Obstet Gynaecol Br Commonw 78: 113
8. Dewhurst C J, Ferreira H P, Gillett P G 1971 Gonadal malignancy in XY females. J Obstet Gynaecol Br Commonw 78: 1077
9. Dewhurst J, Ferreira H P 1981 An endodermal sinus tumour of the vagina in an infant with 7 year survival. Br J Obstet Gynaecol 88: 859
10. Dewhurst J, Pryse-Davies J, Helm W, Stringer R 1985. Diagnosis and management of granulosa/theca tumors in childhood. Pediat Adol Gynecol 3: 131
11. Fleming I D, Etcubanas E, Patterson R et al 1984 The role of surgical resection when combined with chemotherapy and radiation in the management of pelvic rhabdomyosarcoma. Ann Surg 199: 509
12. Ghavimi F, Exelby P R, D'Angio G J et al 1973 Combination therapy of urogenital embryonal rhabdomyosarcoma in children. Cancer 32: 1178
13. Goerzen J L, Grant R M, Arthur K, Stuart G C E 1986 Primary endodermal sinus tumor of the vagina in childhood: case report and review of the results of treatment in the literature. Pediat Adol Gynecol 4: 47
14. Grosfeld J L, Smith J P, Clatworthy J R 1972 Pelvic rhabdomyosarcoma in infants and children. J Urol 107: 673
15. Hays D M, Raney R B, Lawrence W Jr 1981 Rhabdomyosarcoma of the female urogenital tract. J Pediat Surg 16: 828
16. Heller M E, Dewhurst J, Grant D B 1979 Premature menarche without other evidence of precocious puberty. Arch Dis Child 54: 472
17. Herbst A L, Scully R E 1970 Adenocarcinoma of the vagina in adolescence: a report of 7 cases including 6 clear-cell carcinomas (so-called mesonephromas). Cancer 25: 745
18. Huffman J W 1968 The Gynecology of Childhood and Adolescence. Saunders, Philadelphia
19. Huffman J W 1974 Tumors of the genitalia. Clin Obstet Gynecol 1: 663
20. Jones H W Jr, Scott W W 1971 Hermaphroditism, Genital Anomalies and Related Endocrine Disorders. Williams & Wilkins, Baltimore
21. Linfors O 1971 Primary ovarian neoplasms in infants and children: Study of 81 cases diagnosed in Finland and Sweden. Annal Chirurg Gynaecol Fenniae 60, Suppl 177: 7
22. Lister U M, Akinla O 1972 Carcinoma of the vulva in childhood. J Obstet Gynaecol Br Commonw 79: 470
23. McFarland J 1935 Dysontogenetic and mixed tumors of the urogenital region. Surg Gynecol Obstet 61: 42
24. Manuel M, Katayama K P, Jones H W Jr 1976 The age of occurrence of gonadal tumors in intersex patients with a Y chromosome. Am J Obstet Gynecol 124: 293
25. Mattingly R F, Stafl A 1976 Cancer risk in diethylstilbestrol-exposed offspring. Am J Obstet Gynecol 126: 543
26. Mitchell M, Talerman A, Sholl J S, Okagaki T, Cibils L A 1987 Pseudosarcoma botryoides in pregnancy. Obstet Gynecol 70: 522
27. Norris H J, Taylor H B 1966 A benign lesion resembling sarcoma botryoides. Cancer 19: 227
28. Ober W B, Smith J A, Rouillard F C 1958 Congenital sarcoma botryoides of the vagina. Cancer 11: 620
29. Pinkerton C R, Pritchard J, Spitz L 1986 High complete response in children with advanced germ cell tumors using cisplatin-containing combination chemotherapy. J Clin Oncol 4: 194
30. Reynolds V H 1984 In discussion on Fleming et al (1984) p 514
31. Robboy S J, Scully R E, Welch W R, Herbst A L 1977 Intrauterine diethylstilbestrol exposure and its consequences. Arch Pathol Lab Med 101: 1
32. Sandberg E C, Hebard J C 1977 Examination of young women exposed to stilbestrol in utero. Am J Obstet Gynecol 128: 364
33. Senekjian E L, Herbst A L 1985 Diethylstilbestrol exposure in utero. In: Lavery J P, Sanfilippo J S (eds) Pediatric and Adolescent Obstetrics and Gynecology. Springer Verlag, New York, p 149
34. Stafl A, Mattingly R F 1974 Vaginal adenosis: a precancerous lesion? Am J Obstet Gynecol 120: 666
35. Ulfelder H 1976 The stilbestrol-adenosis-carcinoma syndrome. Cancer 38: 426

67. Melanoma of female genital tract

J. P. Curtin   C. P. Morrow

INTRODUCTION

Melanoma is a malignant neoplasm of neuroectodermal origin characterized by production of the pigment melanin. It's capacity for bizarre, unpredictable behavior has been exaggerated, albeit well documented: long quiescent periods followed by rapid progression; mutiple recurrences over many years managed by local excision; spontaneous regression of both primary and metastatic disease; remission or exacerbation associated with pregnancy; and anomalous spread patterns. However, despite the peculiar behavior of a small number of cases, the behavior of malignant melanoma is generally predictable, based on thickness of the primary lesion, location and stage at diagnosis. The majority of patients with a thick lesion or lymph node metastases at the time of diagnosis will succumb to their disease within 2 years.

In the USA, malignant melanoma accounts for 1% of all cancers. The incidence of malignant melanoma has risen significantly over the past two decades. Risk factors for cutaneous melanoma are generally associated with pre-existing pigmented lesions (with or without dysplasia), congenital moles and caucasian race, especially sun-sensitive individuals (Table 67.1).[47] A small portion of melanomas are familial. These are characterized by early age at onset, multiple primary sites and a higher than usual survival rate. The anatomic distribution of malignant melanoma is: head and neck, 25%; lower extremity, 30%; trunk, 25%; and upper extremity 20%. Genital melanomas account for 1 to 5% of cases.[14,17,28] As the incidence of malignant melanoma increases worldwide, the distribution by anatomic site remains unchanged.[5] Recognition of risk factors in individuals who are disposed to the development of malignant melanoma may reduce the incidence by removal of potential precursors, or provide for early diagnosis of thinner, less invasive malignant melanomas, which are more favorable to successful therapy.

Melanomas arise from junctional nevi, the junctional component of compound nevi, or 'de novo' from epidermal melanocytes. Signs of malignant change in a nevus are

Table 67.1 Factors associated with an increased risk of developing melanoma*

Risk factor	Relative risk
1. Changing mole	Very high
2. Adulthood (≥ 15y)	88
3. One or more large or irregular pigmented lesions	
Dysplastic + familial	148
Dysplastic − familial	27
Lentigo maligna	10
4. Congenital mole	21
5. Caucasian	12
6. Previous melanoma	9
7. Melanoma in parents, siblings or children	8
8. Immunosuppression	4
9. Sun sensitivity	3
10. Excessive sun exposure	3

*From: Rhodes & Weinstock (1987)[47]

growth, color change, bleeding, ulceration, weeping and/or crusting. A surrounding erythematous flare may be associated with these changes. Nodular growth within the transformed nevus is an indicator of malignant change. Cutaneous melanoma occurs in three predominant forms:[16]

1. Superficial spreading melanoma (SSM) has a sharp margin which tends to form an arc. The surface is elevated and irregular and nodules may be present. SSM exhibits a haphazard combination of tan, brown, gray, black, pink, blue and white colors. SSM accounts for approximately 70% of cutaneous melanomas.
2. Nodular melanoma (NM) has a uniform dark, blue-black color. The surface may be smooth or irregular. NM accounts for 10 to 15% of cutaneous melanomas.
3. Lentigo maligna melanoma (LMM) often covers a large surface area with an irregular margin. The color

is a variable shade of brown. LMM is characterized by slow, radial growth and is usually diagnosed in the elderly.

Histologically, melanoma is characterized by three cell types (epithelioid, nevus cell and spindle cell) with varying degrees of melanin pigment present. Ten percent of melanomas are amelanotic. Immuno-histologic diagnosis by staining for S-100 protein aids in the dignosis in cases that are difficult to classify.[23]

The major determinants of survival are: stage at diagnosis, level of invasion, tumor thickness, sex and anatomic location. Stage I (local) versus Stage II (regional) or Stage III (distant) is the primary determinate of survival. In patients with Stage I disease, tumor thickness, described by Clark,[16] provides a reproducible prognostic indicator of survival. Favorable features include sex (female > male), anatomic location (extremity > trunk) and subtype (SSM, LMM > NM).

The vast majority of melanoma literature specifically deals with the cutaneous variety. The information obtained from this literature in regard to treatment and prognostic factors has been applied to malignant melanoma of the genital tract, although the validity of doing this has not been established. The cutaneous melanoma data are probably not directly applicable to the genital mucosal lesions, which have a more unpredictable lymphatic drainage. Development of a similar data base from patients with genital tract melanoma is hampered by the relative rarity of the condition and the reporting of small series of cases with non-uniform pathology review and microstage.

VULVAR MELANOMA

Incidence

The adult vulva occupies only 1 to 2% of the body surface area, but produces 3 to 5% of all melanomas in women.[1] This may be partly explained by the observation that nearly all vulvar nevi are junctional. Among vulvar cancers, malignant melanoma is second in frequency only to squamous carcinoma, accounting for 5 to 10% of all cases.[14,17] While relatively rare, more than 600 cases have been reported in the literature.

Melanoma of the vulva occurs most frequently in the sixth and seventh decades of life. The reported age range at diagnosis is 15 to 94 years. Almost all patients are caucasian; 2% of vulva melanomas occur in black or Asian females.

Symptoms

A vulvar mass is commonly the presenting complaint of the patient with vulvar melanoma, followed by pruritis and/or bleeding.[46] Ten percent arise in a pre-existing mole,[14,17,46] but the history of an antecedent mole is of no prognostic

significance. Bleeding tends to augur a poorer outcome, probably because it occurs secondary to ulceration of a larger, nodular lesion. Both patients and physicians contribute to the usual 6 to 12 month delay in diagnosis after onset of symptoms.

Pathology

The pigmented lesion of the vulvar melanoma most commonly has a brown to blue-black coloration. It may be flat, elevated or polypoid (Fig. 67.1). Ulceration, flare (Fig. 67.2) or satellite skin metastases may be present. The over-

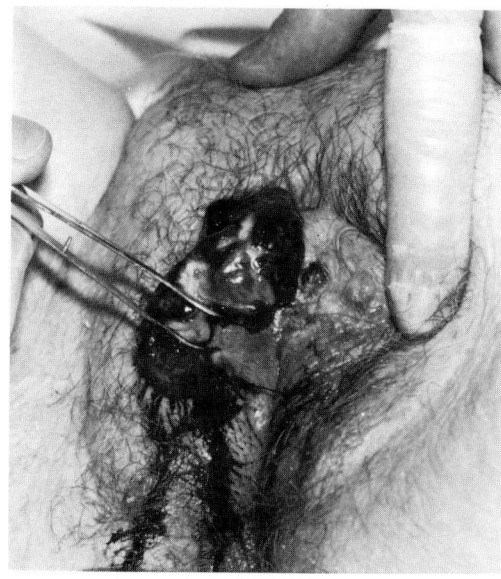

Fig. 67.1 Polypoid, deeply pigmented vulvar melanoma arising from the labium minus. Palpable, bilateral groin metastases were also present. (Reproduced from Byrne T K Jr, Banner E A, Pratt J H, Dockerty M B 1963 Polypoid malignant melanoma of the vulva. *Am J Obstet Gynecol* 86: 724, with permission.)

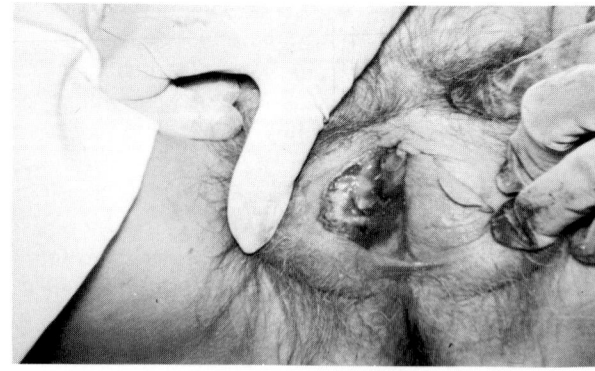

Fig. 67.2 Vulvar melanoma of the right labium minus with the clinical features of superficial spreading melanoma. Note the flare extending to the vagina. (Courtesy of F N Rutledge MD, Chief, Department of Gynecology, The University of Texas, M. D. Anderson Hospital and Tumor Institute, Houston, Texas.)

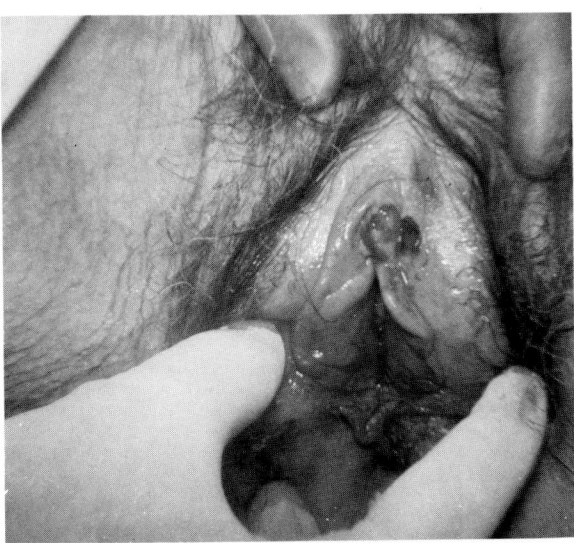

Fig. 67.3 Flat, circumscribed vulvar melanoma of the clitoral prepuce. The lesion is partially obscured by a keratinizing pseudoepitheliomatous hyperplasia of the epidermis. (Courtesy of F N Rutledge MD, Chief, Department of Gynecology, The University of Texas, M. D. Anderson Hospital and Tumor Institute, Houston, Texas.)

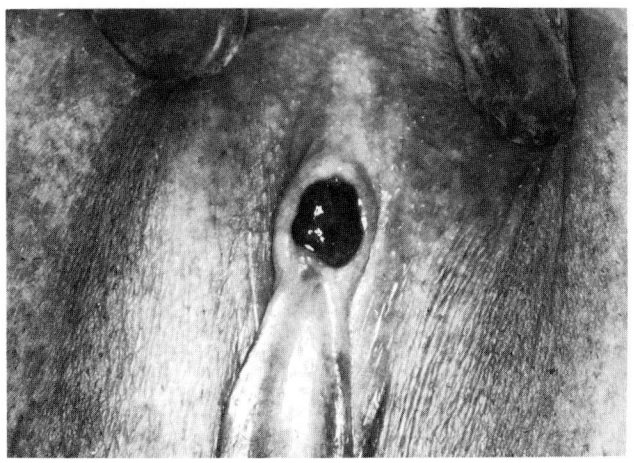

Fig. 67.4 Nodular melanoma arising directly from the glans clitoris. (Courtesy of J McL Morris, MD, John Slade Ely Professor of Gynecology, Yale University School of Medicine, New Haven, Connecticut.)

lying epidermis often develops a pseudo-epitheliomatous hyperplasia, producing a keratinized lesion (Fig. 67.3). An inflammatory reaction frequently accompanies the local tumor, producing an erythematous margin. Melanoma can arise anywhere on the vulva; however, most occur in the non-hair-bearing areas, specifically the labia minora and clitoris (Fig. 67.4). Melanomas tend to encroach on the urethral meatus and/or vagina which undoubtedly has led to misclassification of a small percentage of lesions. Approximately 10% are non-pigmented.

The differential diagnosis is extensive, covering a wide variety of benign and malignant conditions including urethral caruncle, labial furuncle, nevus, Paget's disease and Bowen's disease.[23] Biopsy and histologic review of pigmented lesions of the vulva is mandatory if the survival rate of patients with malignant melanoma at this site is to improve.

Staging

Traditional staging by FIGO standards has some predictive value and should be noted on all patients with a malignant melanoma of the vulva. An alternative is to use the simplified staging that is used for cutaneous melanoma: Stage I — local disease, with or without satellitosis; Stage II — regional spread to lymph nodes; Stage III — distant metastasis.

The most important prognostic factors are depth of invasion and thickness of the tumor. Experience in the surgical management of cutaneous melanoma has demonstrated that level of invasion as originally described by Clark,[16] and measurement of tumor thickness from the granular layer to the deepest invasion as described by Breslow,[12] are the most reliable predictors of local recurrence, regional lymph node metastasis and, ultimately, survival.

Chung, Woodruff & Lewis[14] reported the first review of melanoma of the vulva utilizing these microstaging techniques. They found that Clark's levels of invasion were unsuitable for use in microstaging melanoma of the vulva, due to the relative lack of a well defined papillary dermis. Their classification system modified Clark's definition of levels II, III and IV, utilizing tumor thickness, as measured by Breslow (Fig. 67.5). In their series of 44 patients, they were able to determine the level of invasion for 33. Survival was directly related to depth of invasion. Subsequent retrospective reviews of vulvar melanoma, using microstaging techniques, have confirmed the importance of depth of invasion and tumor thickness.[7,17,29,30,46,49] The distribution by microstage according to the methods of Breslow & Clark in these series combined is given in Tables 67.2 and 67.3. All vulvar melanomas should be classified by one or all of these techniques: preferably either Clark's, Chung's and/or Breslow's.

Diagnosis

Any pigmented lesion on the vulva should be viewed with suspicion. Most nevi of the vulva are junctional, and prophylactic removal is indicated. Any pigmented lesion with recent growth, change in color, bleeding or pruritis warrants immediate biopsy. Since 10% of melanomas are the amelanotic type, absence of pigment should not be a reason to postpone histologic diagnosis.

When the decision has been made to biopsy a lesion, an excisional biopsy with a margin of normal skin is the preferred method of biopsy. If the lesion is large or a more

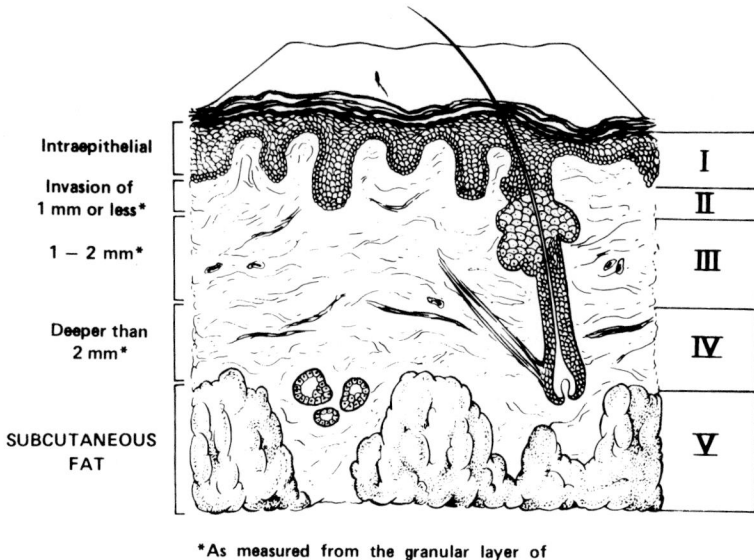

*As measured from the granular layer of surface epithelium

Fig. 67.5 Levels of invasion of vulvar melanoma. Level I (melanoma confined to the surface epithelium and pilar sheath) and level V (tumor extension into the underlying adipose tissue) are the same as Clark's[5] levels I and V. Levels II, III and IV are determined by measurements from the granular layer of the vulvar skin or outermost epithelial layer of the squamous mucosa. (Reproduced from Chung A F, Woodruff J M, Lewis J L Jr 1975 Malignant melanoma of the vulva. *Obstet Gynecol* 45: 638, with permission.)

extensive procedure is likely (e.g. radical vulvectomy), a wedge biopsy should be taken. There is no documentation that this type of biopsy alters the clinical behavior of melanoma. Any locally destructive measures (i.e. cryotherapy, laser, and/or hot cautery) must be condemned.

Evaluation

After establishing the diagnosis of malignant melanoma, the size and location of the primary lesion should be carefully examined, with the relationship of the lesion to the urethra, vulva and anus noted. Additionally, satellite lesions should be looked for and noted. Regional lymphadenopathy almost always indicates lymph node metastasis. Absence of palpable lymph nodes is a reason-

Table 67.3 Vulvar melanoma: distribution of cases by Clark's microstaging

Author	Total cases	Number of cases in each microstage				
		I	II	III	IV	V
Podratz[46]	48	—	6	7	11	24
Chung[14]	33[a]	—	8	5	15	5
Cleophax[17]	14	—	2	1	11	—
Benda[7]	14	1	2	6	4	1
Jaramillo[29]	16	1	2	6	6	1
Phillips[45]	14	—	2	4	8[b]	—
	139	2	22	29	55	31

[a] Modified Clark's
[b] 8 cases level IV or greater

Table 67.2 Vulvar melanoma: distribution of cases by Breslow's microstaging

Author	Total cases	Number of cases in each microstage			
		<0.75 mm	0.76 to 1.5 mm	1.51 to 3.0 mm	>3.0 mm
Podratz[46]	48	3	7	15	23
Rose[49]	22	7	4	4	7
Johnson[30]	14	1	1	1	11
Beller[6]	13	1	1	4	7
Benda[7]	14	1	3	3*	7
Jaramillo[29]	16	6	2	3*	5
	127	19	18	30	60

* Range 1.51 to 4.0 mm

ably sensitive predictor of the absence of lymph node metastasis. A chest X-ray and serum chemistry battery are a sufficient diagnostic survey to screen for distant metastasis, unless the patient has specific symptoms or there is an abnormal finding on physical examination.

Management

The surgical management of melanoma of the vulva without evidence of regional or distant spread is controversial. The controversy evolves around two key points of management and is similar to the controversy in management of cutaneous melanomas. Firstly, the optimal extent of excision of the primary tumor remains uncertain. Secondly, the curative value of prophylactic (elective) inguinal lymph node dissection (ELND) and whether unilateral or bilateral dissection should be done is still disputed by reasonable authorities. Unfortunately, information regarding the management of cutaneous melanomas can be a confusing factor rather than a guide to improved therapy. The positive aspect of the information regarding cutaneous melanoma is that the incidence is much higher and, therefore, a broader clinical population is available for study.

Several large cooperative groups have done prospective randomized studies to determine the optional or necessary extent of local excision[56] and the value of elective lymph node dissection.[51,55] The first study indicates that an excisional margin of 1 cm is adequate for local control of thin melanomas (<1.0 mm) when compared to a margin of 3 cm.[56] The value of elective lymphadenectomy in Stage I melanoma is more controversial. The results of the WHO melanoma group study (Veronesi et al)[55] and the Mayo Clinic study[51] (both prospective and randomized) demonstrate no survival benefit in extremity melanoma for immediate elective regional lymph node dissection compared to lymph node dissection performed when lymph nodes become clinically enlarged. Balch, in an excellent review article, examined the data from the WHO study.[4] He points out several faults in the stratification of patients (more patients with an ulcerative lesion in the ELND arm) and possible differences that are attendant with a multi-center, surgical study (higher incidence of occult positive lymph nodes).

Application of these data to vulvar melanoma is of uncertain validity. Further complicating the determination of proper management is the difficulty in interpreting the literature regarding vulvar melanoma. Although there are more than 600 cases reported, no single study has more than 50 patients, and all are retrospective, covering up to 60 years of patient care.[49] Fewer than one-third of all reported cases had microstaging carried out.

The most common site of recurrence is local, so any attempt at curative surgery must include a plan for an adequate surgical margin. Podratz reported a 32% local recurrence rate.[46] This compares to a 3 to 7% local recurrence rate in cutaneous melanoma. The mucosal margin is frequently the site of recurrence and therefore the planned surgical procedure must encompass an adequate mucosal margin. When the vagina is involved, vaginectomy (and hysterectomy) are recommended. Extension to the urethra or rectum should be managed by exenteration. Even with a thin lesion (0.76 mm) the margin must be adequate, as there are two reports of local recurrence in patients with thin lesions.[3,49]

The role of lymph node dissection remains uncertain. There are no reported cases of occult or overt inguinal lymph node metastasis in thin melanomas of the vulva (less than 0.76 mm or Clark's level II). Wide local excision (1 to 2 cm margin) without regional lymphadenectomy is, therefore, appropriate treatment for these lesions. Patients with lesions thicker than 0.76 mm (Clark's or Chung's level III), may benefit from prophylactic lymph node dissection, although when lesion thickness exceeds 3.0 to 4.0 mm this benefit may be out-weighed by the high incidence of distant metastasis. In a series from Iowa, Benda et al noted that of 10 patients with lesions >4 mm thick and histologically-negative regional lymph nodes, 7 died of disease.[7] To date, no series has stratified the benefit of ELND for intermediate (0.75 to 3.0 mm) lesions. Prospective, randomized trials, similar to the WHO and Mayo Clinic studies, are needed to define the proper role of ELND for patients with vulvar melanoma.

Survival

Overall survival for patients with vulvar melanoma and survival by Breslow's measurement and Clark's level are listed in Tables 67.4 and 67.5 respectively. While microstaging provides a reasonable guide to prognosis, as Table 67.6 indicates, the presence of regional node metastasis over-rides the prognostic significance of local factors. All authors reported corrected 5-year survival, with the exception of Phillips, who reported survival at 2 years. Even 5-year survival may be misleading, in that up to 20% of deaths due to melanoma occur more than 5 years after diagnosis. Podratz found that recurrence occurred from 3 months to 11 years after initial definitive operation. Among 24 patients with recurrence, 22 had died of disease, 1 was terminal with metastatic melanoma and 1 died without known disease 3 years after resection of a local recurrence. Fifty-six percent of patients died within 12 months of recurrence.[46]

Survival by histologic subtype favors superficial spreading melanoma (SSM) over nodular melanoma (NM). This survival advantage is dependent on the fact that SSMs are thinner and less invasive than NM.

VAGINAL MELANOMA

The vagina is the second most common site of malignant

Table 67.4   Vulvar melanoma: survival related to Breslow's microstaging

Author	5-yr survival (% all cases)	% survival by microstage			
		<0.75 mm	0.76 to 1.5 mm	1.51 to 3.0 mm	>3.0 mm
Podratz[46]	54	100	83	87	25
Rose[49]★	39	67	67	33	0
Johnson[30]	22	100	100	0	0
Beller[6]	71	100	100	50	43
Benda[7]	20	100	33	0	20
Jaramillo[29]	44	100	—	33	25

★ Reported as recurrence

Table 67.5   Vulvar melanoma: survival related to Clark's microstaging

Author	5-yr survival (% all cases)	% survival by microstage				
		I	II	III	IV	V
Podratz[46]	54	—	100	83	81	28
Chung[14]	30	—	87	0	19	25
Cleophax[17]	50	—	100	0	37	—
Benda[7]	20	100	50	0	33	0
Jaramillo[29]	44	—	100	50	40	0
Phillips[45a]	33	—	100	50	25[b]	

a Reported 2-year disease free
b Combined Levels IV and V

Pathology

Vaginal melanomas are usually large, polypoid lesions at presentation (Fig. 67.6). Ulceration and necrosis are often present. Chung et al found lateral junctional changes present in a majority of cases.[13] In half of the 18 reviewed cases, no melanin deposits were noted.

melanoma of the female genital tract;[28] it represents 0.7% of all melanomas and 2 to 5% of genital melanomas. A similar incidence was noted by Sulak et al, who reported 3 vaginal melanomas in a series of 48 primary vaginal carcinomas.[53] In an autopsy study, melanocytes, which are the presumed precursors of malignant melanoma, were found in the vagina in 3% of adult females.[41]

Presentation

The average age of presentation is in the sixth to seventh decade with a range of 37 to 84 years.[10,28,53] The most common location is the distal or lower one-third of the vagina. Typically, the patient presents with vaginal bleeding or discharge; less common is a complaint of a vaginal mass.

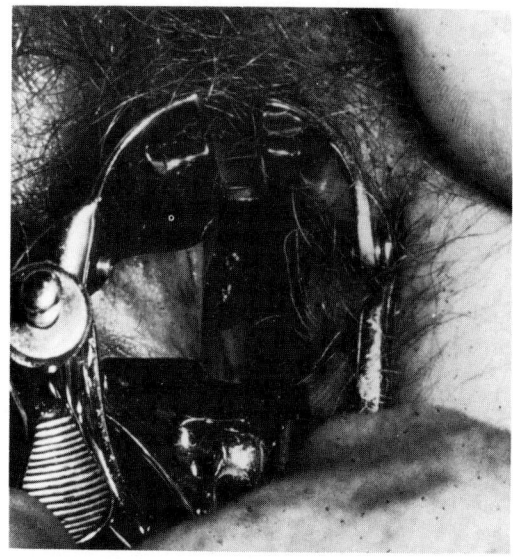

Fig. 67.6   Malignant melanoma of the vagina. The black, polypoid tumor mass occupies the vaginal wall just inside the introitus. (Courtesy of F N Rutledge MD, Chief, Department of Gynecology, The University of Texas, M. D. Anderson Hospital and Tumor Institute, Houston, Texas.)

Table 67.6   Vulvar melanoma: frequency of regional lymph node metastases and effect on survival

Author	Total cases	Lymph node metastases N (%)	Number with clinically positive nodes	5-year survival (%)
Podratz[46]	44	8 (18)	6	37
Chung[14]	31	15 (50)	13	13
Jaramillo[29]	16	4 (25)		0
Beller[6]	13	2 (15)		50
Benda[7]	13	3 (23)		0
Cleophax[17]	14	7 (50)	5	50
Phillips[45]	17	3 (18)	3	0
Rose[49]	13	2 (15)		0

Chung et al attempted to define thickness of the vaginal melanomas. Sixteen lesions were reviewed, and accurate measurements were obtained in 7 while the remaining 9 had an approximation of lesion thickness. Only one lesion was less than or equal to 1.0 mm thick. Two lesions were within the range of 1.0 to 2.0 mm and the remaining 13 were thicker than 2.0 mm.[13]

Survival

The survival prospect for the patient with malignant melanoma of the vagina is dismal (Table 67.7). Although approximately 10% of reported cases have survived for 5 years, there is only one documented 10-year survivor. This was the patient of Chung's with 1.0 mm of invasion. Even she had experienced recurrence treated by radical surgery.

Survival is probably unrelated to the skill and/or aggressiveness of the surgeon, but is more probably associated with tumor biology. In the series from the University of Michigan, 3 of 9 patients were treated with conservative therapy (wide local excision), 2 of whom were 5-year survivors; none of 6 patients treated by radical surgery survived. Of the 13 cases treated with radical surgery, 8 developed locoregional recurrences. Five of 6 patients with negative lymph nodes recurred, 4 of whom had locoregional recurrences.[10] It is probably true, however, that extent of disease may have influenced the radicalness of the treatment. Some lesions are not amenable to 'local' excision.

Management

Defining proper management of the patient with a melanoma of the vagina is difficult at best, since few of the published results were successful. Adding to the dilemma is the complex lymphatic drainage of the vagina, and the tendency for vaginal melanoma to be multifocal.[21] Bonner has suggested that high individual doses of preoperative radiotherapy (500 cGy × 3 days a week to a dose of 3000 cGy) followed by radical resection of gross disease may improve locoregional control, although this assumption is based on hypothesis alone. At the minimum, a wide

Table 67.7 Vaginal melanoma: reported 5-year survival

Author	Total cases	Survival (%)
Chung[13]	19	4 (21)
Bonner[10]	10	2 (20)
Iverson[28]	7	0
Sulak[53]	3	0
Davidson[19]	6	1 (16.6)
Liu[36]	7	1 (14.5)
	52	8 (15.4)

excision of the local tumor should be performed, but vaginectomy is probably better. If the tumor is large, more extensive surgery may be beneficial. Anterior, posterior or total exenteration should be considered. Removal of regional lymph nodes may be indicated and may provide prognostic information. Local or regional lymph node recurrence can be managed by re-excision. Occasionally, radiation treatment will result in long-term palliation.

MALIGNANT MELANOMA OF THE FEMALE URETHRA

At least 42 cases of malignant melanoma arising from the female urethra have been reported in the world literature. This represents 1 melanoma for every 25 squamous carcinomas, a ratio similar to that reported for vulvar and vaginal malignancies. The age at diagnosis has ranged from 32 to 80 years with an average of 64 years. Of the 42 collected cases only three were less than 50 years old.

Urethral melanomas invariably arise from the meatus and may be indistinguishable from a caruncle (Figs 67.7 and 67.8). They are blue-black to reddish-brown, pedunculated masses varying from 0.5 to 5 cm, but usually less than 3 cm in diameter. Often they are observed to protrude through the external meatus. The lesion spreads by destructive invasion of the vagina and vulva or it may involve these areas by superficial malignant flare. Urinary symptoms are present in over 80% of patients and consist of urinary frequency, dysuria and hematuria.[52] Other

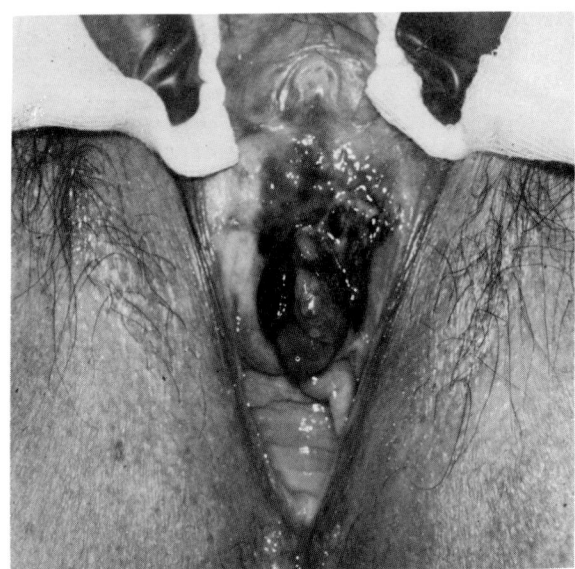

Fig. 67.7 Primary malignant melanoma of the urethra. The polypoid tumor mass is protruding from the urethral meatus. Extending toward the clitoris is a pigmented flare. (Reproduced from Ostergard D R, Townsend D E 1968 Malignant melanoma of the female urethra treated by cryosurgery with radical vulvectomy and anterior exenteration. *Obstet Gynecol* 31: 75, with permission.)

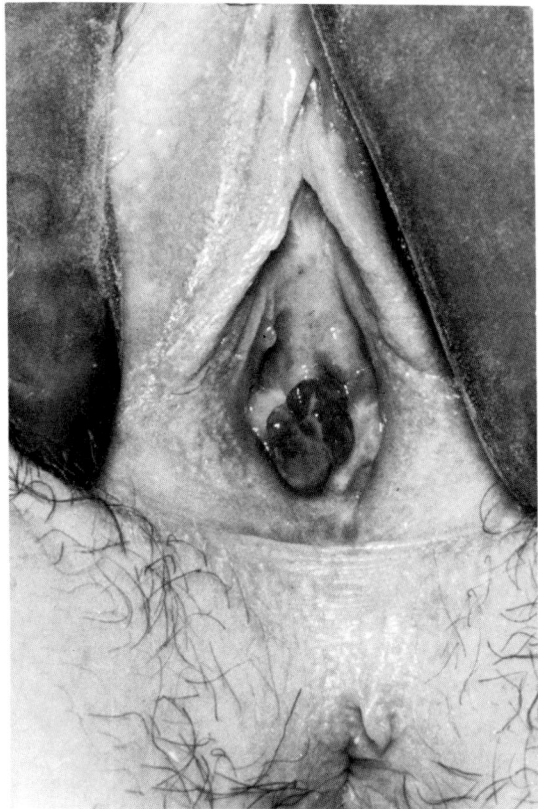

Fig. 67.8 Urethral caruncle. This benign, polypoid lesion arises from the posterior wall of the urethra and presents at the meatus. Clinically caruncles may be indistinguishable from malignant melanoma. (Reproduced from Morrow C P, DiSaia P J 1976 Malignant melanoma of the female genitalia: A clinical analysis. *Obstet Gynecol Surv* 31: 233, with permission.)

Table 67.8 Reported 5-year survival with urethral melanoma

Author	Treatment
Ruch et al[50a]	Radical vulvectomy and radiation
Glenn[24]	Subtotal urethrectomy and node dissection
Das Gupta & Grabstald[18]	Palliative cystectomy*
Block & Hotchkiss[8]	Cystectomy, urethrectomy; excision of left groin node metastasis 1 yr later
Katz & Grabstald[31]	Anterior exenteration and radiation therapy

* The patient surviving 5 years had pelvic node and hepatic metastases at diagnosis.

symptoms include vaginal spotting and/or discharge, usually indicative of advanced disease. Incontinence and obstruction are uncommon. The duration of symptoms is usually short, ranging from a few weeks to a few months.

It is difficult to develop a treatment plan for urethral melanoma based on the literature, because of the paucity of cases, the diversity of treatment and differences in disease extent at the time of diagnosis. There are 5 reported patients with 5-year survival (Table 67.8). Two were treated by radical surgery and radiation[18,31] and two were treated by urethrectomy with cystectomy. The 5-year survival of a patient reported by Das Gupta & Grabstald[18] provides an example of the difficulty of determining appropriate therapy for this rare tumor based on literature reports. Their patient was treated by palliative cystectomy because at her initial surgery positive pelvic lymph nodes were found as well as hepatic metastases. In spite of this, the patient survived for longer than 60 months before succumbing to her disease.

It seems reasonable from the general experience with cutaneous and vulvar melanomas that therapy needs to be tailored to the individual patient. In the constitutionally suitable cases in which the tumor is surgically resectable, an en bloc excision of the urethra and bladder plus surrounding organs, such as vagina, uterus and/or vulva should be performed. As is the case in vaginal melanoma, the therapeutic value of elective removal of regional lymph nodes is uncertain. If there is regional node metastasis, however, the operator may wish to scale down the extent of the operation if that is feasible. Radiation therapy may play a role either in preoperative treatment or as palliative therapy for advanced or recurrent melanoma.

MALIGNANT MELANOMA OF OTHER GENITAL ORGANS

Cervix

At least 21 cases of malignant melanoma arising in the cervix uteri have been reported in the literature.[26,38] While a few of these reports might be questioned, in at least five cases the specific junctional change associated with primary lesions was present.[32] The possibility of primary cervical melanoma was doubted for a long time because the organ was not believed to contain melanocytes. However, it is now documented that nevi do occur[20] and that a small proportion of normal cervices (3.5%)[15] have melanin containing cells.

The patients with primary cervical melanoma were 39 to 74 years of age. Most presented with vaginal bleeding or discharge of recent onset. Occasionally, symptoms of distant metastasis are the presenting complaint.[58] Several reports have described the cervical cytology findings associated with melanoma of the cervix. The smears demonstrated spindle-shaped cells with melanin pigment. The tumors are described as pigmented, exophytic or ulcerated, and usually involve one or more of the vaginal fornices. Only two patients have survived more than 3 years and, coincidentally, both died of their disease 13 years post diagnosis.[32] In three of the four cases treated surgically, recurrence was first manifested in the vagina.

A logical treatment for this rarity would seem to be radical hysterectomy with a large vaginal cuff or total vaginectomy with pelvic lymphadenectomy.

Endometrium

Apparently only one case of malignant melanoma arising in the endometrium has been reported.[34] Melanocytes have never been demonstrated in normal endometrium, but melanin (presumptive evidence of the melanocyte) has been identified in an endometrial polyp.[2] Melanoma metastatic to the endometrium may rarely present as a primary malignancy.[57] In a study of 63 patients with metastases to the uterine corpus from extragonadal cancers, only 2 patients had metastases from a cutaneous melanoma, and in both instances the metastases were identified at autopsy.[33] Three cases of a primary melanin-producing tumor of the endometrium similar to the retinal anlage tumor (melanotic progonoma) have been reported.[38] Although highly malignant and melanogenic, they are histologically quite distinct from malignant melanoma. All three women were postmenopausal and died with extensive disease within one year of diagnosis. The origin of these melanotic tumors of the endometrium has been postulated to be teratomatous; they might also be a form of mixed mesodermal tumor.

Ovary

Malignant melanoma arising in the female gonad is extraordinarily uncommon. Approximately 20 cases have been reported; 13 cases, with or without junctional activity, were associated with a cystic teratoma of the ovary.[11,54] The other 7 demonstrated neither teratoid elements nor evidence of an occult extra-ovarian primary.[27] The skin, meninges and ocular epithelium of dermoids may contain melanocytes, especially in blacks, and one instance of a pigmented nevus in the skin of a dermoid has been reported.[35]

It is widely held that malignant melanoma metastatic to the ovary is far more common than primary ovarian melanoma. Although metastasis to the ovary may occur in 18% of patients with disseminated melanoma, secondary ovarian involvement presenting as a primary lesion apparently occurs as infrequently as the primary tumor. In a review of 10 patients with malignant melanoma metastatic to the ovary, 8 had a history of cutaneous malignant melanoma.[22] The interval from diagnosis of melanoma to diagnosis of metastasis to the ovary ranged from 1 to 7 years.

The patients with primary ovarian melanoma reported in the literature range in age from 26 to 77 years. Their symptoms were generally related to the enlarging ovary causing pelvic discomfort and lower abdominal swelling. The longest reported survival is 2.5 years, but follow-up in most reports is very short. One patient was diagnosed during pregnancy. She had a superficial lesion confined to the ovary within a cystic teratoma (Clark's level II, Breslow's 0.24 mm invasion). After a successful completion of her pregnancy, she was alive without disease approximately 2 years later.[11]

The pattern of spread of ovarian melanoma encompasses that of the epithelial ovarian cancers plus the hematogenous route more characteristic of malignant melanoma. The surgical therapy should be that for any invasive ovarian malignancy. Patients with persistent and/or recurrent disease have been successfully treated with immunochemotherapy.[54]

CHEMOTHERAPY AND IMMUNOTHERAPY

The treatment of metastatic malignant melanoma has been the subject of extensive clinical trials utilizing cytotoxic chemotherapy and immunotherapy. However, in spite of the large number of trials, results are poor. Many responses to therapy are partial and duration of response is frequently reported in weeks. Dacarbazine (DTIC) used as a single agent remains the drug of choice for initial treatment of recurrence. Combination therapy may increase the overall response rate, but survival is unchanged and morbidity is significantly increased.[40]

The interest in immunotherapy for metastatic malignant melanoma is based on the reports of spontaneous regression of primary and metastatic tumor.[2] Initial studies utilized non-specific immunostimulants (BCG, C. parvum) with an occasional clinical response. Recent clinical trials have focused on two new approaches to immunotherapy (see also Ch. 7). Adoptive cellular therapy utilizes in vitro expansion of the patients lymphocytes. Two subsets of lymphocytes, lymphokine-activated killer (LAK) and tumor-infiltrating lymphocytes (TIL), have been expanded by interleukin 2 (IL-2) and reinfused into patients with metastatic melanoma, with some objective responses reported.[50] Active specific immunization, has also been reported to induce responses in patients with metastatic melanoma.[37] A key step in both of these clinical investigations is obtaining fresh tumor tissue. Therefore, prior to excision of a primary or metastatic lesion, the surgeon should consult with the pathologist and medical oncologist regarding proper processing of the specimen.

REFERENCES

1. Ariel I M 1981 Malignant melanoma of the female genital system: a report of 48 patients and review of the literature. J Surg Oncol 16: 371

2. Babes A 1927 Cellules pigmentaires rameuses dans un polype de la muqueuse uterine. Ann Anat Path 4: 373
3. Bailet J W, Figge D C, Tamimi H K 1987 Malignant melanoma of the vulva: a case report of distal recurrence in a patient with a superficially invasive primary lesion. Obstet Gynecol 70: 516

4. Balch C M 1988 The role of elective lymph node dissection in melanoma: Rationale, results and controversies. J Clin Oncol 6: 163

5. Balch C M, Soong S J, Milton G W et al 1982 Changing trends in cutaneous melanoma over a quarter century in Alabama, USA and New South Wales, Australia. Cancer 52: 1748

6. Beller U, Demopoulos R I, Beckman E M 1986 Vulvovaginal melanoma. A clinicopathologic study. J Reprod Med 31: 315

7. Benda J A, Platz C E, Anderson B 1986 Malignant melanoma of the vulva: a clinical-pathologic review of 16 cases. Int J Gynecol Pathol 5: 202

8. Block N L, Hotchkiss R S 1971 Malignant melanoma of the female urethra: report of a case with 5 year survival and review of literature. J Urol 105: 251

9. Bokun R, Perkovic M, Bakotin J, Milasinovic D, Mojsovic D 1985 Cytology and histopathology of metastatic malignant melanoma involving a polyp on the uterine cervix. A case report. Acta Cytol 29: 612

10. Bonner J A, Perez-Tamayo C, Reid G C, Roberts J A, Morley G W 1988 The management of vaginal melanoma. Cancer 62: 2066

11. Boughton R S, Hughmanick S, Marin-Padilla M 1987 Malignant melanoma arising in an ovarian cystic teratoma in pregnancy. J Am Acad Dermatol 17: 871

12. Breslow A 1970 Thickness, cross-sectional areas and depth of invasion in the prognosis of cutaneous melanoma. Ann Surg 172: 902

13. Chung A F, Casey M J, Flannery J T, Woodruff J M, Lewis J L 1980 Malignant melanoma of the vagina — report of 19 cases. Obstet Gynecol 55: 720

14. Chung A F, Woodruff J M, Lewis J L 1975 Malignant melanoma of the vulva. Obstet Gynecol 45: 638

15. Cid J M 1959 La pigmentation melanique de l'endocervix. Ann Anat Path 4: 617

16. Clark W H Jr, From L, Bernardino E A, Mihm M C 1969 The histogenesis and biologic behavior of primary human malignant melanomas of the skin. Cancer Res 29: 705

17. Cleophax J P, Pilleron J P, Durand J C, Laurent M 1976 Le melanome malin de la vulve. Gynecologie 27: 333

18. Das Gupta R, Grabstald H 1965 Melanoma of the genitourinary tract. J Urol 93: 607

19. Davidson T, Kissin M, Westbury G 1987 Vulvo-vaginal melanoma — should radical surgery be abandoned? Brit J Obstet Gynaecol 94: 473

20. Diaz de Molnar A M, Guralnick M, Ferenczy A 1978 Blue nevus of the endocervix: report of two cases and ultrastructure. Gynecol Oncol 6: 373

21. Ehrmann R L, Younger P A, Lerch V L 1962 The exfoliative cytology and histogenesis of an early primary malignant melanoma of the vagina. Acta Cytol 6: 245

22. Fitzgibbons P L, Martin S E, Simmons T J 1987 Malignant melanoma metastatic of the ovary. Am J Surg Path 11: 959

23. Glasgow B J, Wen D R, Al-Jetour S, Cochran A J 1987 Antibody to S-100 protein aids in separation of pagetoid melanoma from extramammary Paget's disease. J Cutan Pathol 14: 223

24. Glenn J F 1953 Malignancy of the female urethra: a report of 8 cases. N Carolina Med J 14: 201

25. Heslinga J M, Lycklama A, Nijeholt G A B, Ruiter D J 1986 Primary melanoma in the female distal urethra. Eur Urol 12: 446

26. Holmquist N D, Torres J 1988 Malignant melanoma of the cervix: report of a case. Acta Cytol 32: 252

27. Hsiu J G, Kemp G M, Given F T, D'Amato N A 1986 Malignant melanoma presenting as a unilateral ovarian neoplasm. Gynecol Oncol 24: 362

28. Iverson K, Roblins R E 1980 Mucosal malignant melanomas. Am J Surg 139: 660

29. Jaramillo B A, Ganjei P, Averette H E, Sevin B U, Lovecchio J L 1985 Malignant melanoma of the vulva. Obstet Gynecol 66: 398

30. Johnson T L, Kumar N B, White C D, Morley G W 1986 Prognostic features of vulvar melanoma: a clinicopathologic analysis. Int J Gynecol Pathol 5: 110

31. Katz J I, Grabstald H 1976 Primary malignant melanoma of the female urethra. J Urol 116: 454

32. Krishnamoorthy A, Desai M, Simanowitz M 1986 Primary malignant melanoma of the cervix. Case report. Br J Obstet Gynaecol 93: 84

33. Kumar N B, Hart W R 1982 Metastases to the uterine corpus from extragenital cancers. A clinicopathologic study of 63 cases. Cancer 50: 2163

34. Lamoureux C 1970 Melanome de l'uterus. L Union Med Du Canada 99: 282

35. Lewis M G 1968 Melanin-pigmented components in ovarian teratomas in Ugandan Africans. J Pathol Bacteriol 95: 405

36. Liu L Y, Hou Y J, Li J Z 1987 Primary malignant melanoma of the vagina: a report of seven cases. Obstet Gynecol 70: 569

37. Mastrangelo M J, Schultz S, Kane M, Berd D 1988 Newer immunologic approaches to the treatment of patients with melanoma. Semin Oncol 15: 589

38. Morrow C P, DiSaia P J 1976 Malignant melanoma of the female genitalia: a clinical analysis. Obstet Gynecol Surv 31: 233

39. McCarthy W H, Shaw H M, Milton G W 1985 Efficacy of elective lymph node dissection in 2,347 patients with clinical Stage I malignant melanoma. Surg Obstet Gynecol 161: 575

40. McClay E F, Mastrangelo M J 1988 Systemic chemotherapy for metastatic melanoma. Semin Oncol 15: 569

41. Nigogosyan G, De La Pava S, Pickren J W 1964 Melanoblasts in vaginal mucosa. Cancer 17: 912

42. Nissenkorn I, Servadio C, Avidor I, Marshak G 1987 Malignant melanomas of female urethra. Urol 29: 562

43. Novak P, Strmiska M 1980 Melanoblastoma of the female urethra. Int Urol Nephrol 12: 43

44. Owen O J, Pollard K, Khoury G G, Dyson J E D, Jarvis G J, Joslin C A F 1988 Case report: primary malignant melanoma of the uterine cervix. Clin Radiol 39: 336

45. Phillips G L, Twiggs L B, Okagaki T 1982 Vulvar melanoma. A microstaging study. Gynecol Oncol 14: 80

46. Podratz K C, Gaffey T A, Symmonds R E, Johansen K L, O'Brien P C 1983 Melanoma of the vulva: an update. Gynecol Oncol 16: 153

47. Rhodes A R, Weinstock M A, Fitzpatrick T B, Mihm M C, Sober A J 1987 Risk factors for cutaneous melanoma: a practical method of recognizing predisposed individuals. JAMA 258: 3146

48. Robutti F, Betta P G, Bellingeri D 1986 Primary malignant melanoma of the female urethral meatus. Sur Urol 16: 153

49. Rose P G, Piver M S, Tsukada Y, Lau T 1988 Conservative therapy for melanoma of the vulva. Am J Obstet Gynecol 159: 52

50. Rosenberg S A, Packard B S, Aebersold P M et al 1988 Use of tumor-infiltrating lymphocytes and interleukin-2 in immunotherapy of patients with metastatic melanoma. N Engl J Med 318: 1676

50a. Ruch R M, Frerichs J B, Arneson A N 1952 Cancer of the female urethra. Cancer 5: 748

51. Sim F H, Taylor W F, Pritchard D J et al 1986 Lymphadenectomy in the management of Stage I malignant melanoma: a prospective randomized study. Mayo Clinic Proc 61: 697

52. Stein B S, Kendall A R 1984 Malignant melanoma of the genitourinary tract. J Urol 132: 859

53. Sulak P, Barnhill D, Heller P et al 1988 Nonsquamous cancer of the vagina. Gynecol Oncol 29: 309

54. Tsukamoto N, Matsukuma K, Matsumura M, Kamura T, Matsuyama T, Kinjo M 1986 Primary malignant melanoma arising in a cystic teratoma of the ovary. Gynecol Oncol 123: 395

55. Veronesi U, Adamus J, Bandiera D C et al 1982 Delayed regional lymph node dissection in Stage I melanoma of the skin of the lower extremities. Cancer 49: 2420

56. Veronesi U, Cascinelle N, Adamus J et al 1988 Thin Stage I primary cutaneous malignant melanoma. Comparison of excision with margins of 1 or 3 cm. N Engl J Med 318: 1159

57. Wood C 1978 Metastatic melanoma simulating a primary endometrial tumor. Am J Obstet Gynecol 131: 820

58. Yu H C, Ketabchi M 1987 Detection of malignant melanoma of the uterine cervix from Papanicolaou smears. A case report. Acta Cytol 31: 73

PART XIII

Malignant tumors in pregnancy

68. Malignant disease in the pregnant woman

H. R. K. Barber

INTRODUCTION

Cancer complicating pregnancy is uncommon but occurs with a frequency of 1 in 1000 births. When it occurs it results in two diametrically opposing emotional reactions: pregnancy leads to a joyous elation while a diagnosis of cancer leads to a state of panic. The obstetrician and medical advisors are faced with a therapeutic dilemma involving surgical, perinatal, obstetrical, physiological, moral and ethical issues.

Cancer complicating pregnancy had special relevance at one time. The controversy surrounding the question whether an abortion was therapeutic in women with a cancer or was instead an unnecessary interference meant that the clinician was faced with a difficult decision. Each hospital had an abortion committee as well as a tumor board and, in order to perform an abortion, it was necessary to show that the mother's life was jeopardized by the continuance of the pregnancy. The conflicting reports in the literature made the decision difficult for the abortion committees. There were as many papers stating that pregnancy had no deleterious effects as there were those reporting on the dangers of cancer complicating pregnancy. However, with today's liberalized abortion laws, women are free to have an elective abortion whenever a diagnosis of cancer is made. The abortion committee no longer has to deal with the decision whether or not to abort. Faced with a life-threatening disease, women and their families may ask direct and specific questions about whether the pregnancy can have an adverse effect on the cancer and vice versa. If these women elect to continue the pregnancy, they seek help from physicians experienced in managing cancer complicating pregnancy. This clinical circumstance requires joint decisions among the obstetrician, surgeon, medical oncologist, social workers, clergy and other involved specialists.

The introduction of new concepts in preventative medicine, the enlightened use of antibiotics and the establishment of blood banks has brought about a sharp decline in heart disease, toxemia, hemorrhage and infectious diseases as killers of pregnant women. As a result, cancer is among those causes becoming increasingly important in maternal mortality studies.

Mortality for the five leading cancer sites in the major age groups for women are: *under 15*, leukemia, brain and central nervous system, kidney, bone and connective tissue; *15 to 34*, leukemia, breast, brain and the central nervous system, uterus and Hodgkin's disease; *35 to 54*, breast, lung, colon and rectum, cervix, endometrium and ovary.[15,34]

Since women are delaying childbearing for a variety of reasons, a greater number are having their children after the age of 35. Moreover, the incidence of breast, ovary, and endometrial cancer is more frequent below 40 years of age than previously recognized. It is anticipated that more cancer complicating pregnancy will be encountered.

The majority of cancers complicating pregnancy are breast cancer, lymphoma, malignant melanoma, gynecologic and bone cancers. The combination of a controlled growth (pregnancy) and an uncontrolled growth (cancer) in the same host provides a setting for answering important questions relating to both the pregnancy and cancer.[2]

The opinions expressed in the literature of the effects of pregnancy on the malignant process range from those stating that pregnancy increases resistance to cancer,[28,64] to, at the other extreme, those stating that pregnancy has a stimulating effect.[47,53] This lack of agreement makes it difficult, if not impossible, for the average physician to plan treatment.

A major reason for suspecting that pregnancy adversely affects the clinical course of cancer is the immunologic tolerance that characterizes both conditions. As Gleicher and associates[32] pointed out, normal pregnancy and cancer are the only two biologic conditions in which an antigenic tissue is tolerated by a seemingly intact system. It may be stated that the mechanisms that insure the survival of the fetus during pregnancy presumably also favor the progress of the neoplasia.

Cancer complicating pregnancy is best divided into pelvic and extrapelvic malignancy. In 1962, Barber &

Brunschwig[2] reviewed the former and, in 1964, Boronow, in a comprehensive article,[12] the latter. These reviews have served as models for numerous articles since that time. The division into pelvic and extrapelvic malignancy is followed in this chapter.

PELVIC CANCER COMPLICATING PREGNANCY

Pelvic cancer complicating pregnancy is most often treated by surgery. The rationale for this is based upon the fact that surgery can usually remove all the cancer rapidly.

In the past 35 years the improved results of therapy for cancer, particularly in younger patients, has led to more women becoming pregnant during treatment for cancer or during subsequent follow up. Improved cancer detection has also contributed to the increased discovery of cancer in pregnancy. It is important to establish a firm histologic diagnosis. Decidua changes in pelvic organs should be recognized so that these changes will not confuse the clinical and histologic diagnosis. Having established the diagnosis, the philosophy must be to treat the cancer and ignore the pregnancy. However, in certain instances, therapy may result in the interruption of pregnancy. Since there is no direct attack on the fetus in the management of cancer in the pelvis, and since this approach is medically sound, such therapy is accepted but not necessarily condoned by the clergy.

The pregnant state is divided into the standard three trimesters plus a fourth postpartum period which extends for 4 to 6 months.[54] There are now well established guidelines for treatment in each trimester, and principles should be adapted to patients on an individual basis. There is an increasing body of evidence appearing in the current literature that favors primary surgery as the preferred method of treatment for pelvic cancer complicating pregnancy.[9] Radiation therapy has its optimum effect in well oxygenated tissue that is growing rapidly. As soon as the pregnancy is damaged by radiation, involution follows and creates an anoxic environment which compromises the efficacy of radiotherapy.

Four questions constantly arise: Does pregnancy affect prognosis? What effect does cancer have on the fetus? What will treatment do to the fetus? Are future pregnancies possible?

The cancers that are included in the pelvic group are: cancers of the vulva, vagina, cervix, endometrium, ovary and rectum.

Cancer of the vulva

Cancer of the vulva accounts for only 1% of all cancers, and 3 or 4% of gynecologic cancers. It is a disease of the aged. It is rare in the young and extremely rare in as-sociation with pregnancy. When it does occur in pregnancy patients are often young.

With the current sexual revolution and start of intercourse at much earlier ages than previously recorded, the incidence of vulvar abnormal cytology and histology is increasing. The increasing incidence of vulvar intraepithelial neoplasia (VIN) may be due to a variety of reasons, such as increasing number of infections from human papillomavirus and viruses unnamed. Condyloma acuminata, which are frequent in the 20- and 30-year age group, are found in 7 to 31% of patients with vulvar carcinoma in situ. Human papillomavirus has become the prime suspect in vulvar neoplasms. Whatever the initial treatment, recurrences are common. In addition to the viral infection which contributes to an increase in carcinoma in situ and microinvasive lesions, and may herald an increase in invasive cancers, cigarette smoking is also undoubtedly playing a role. There are many carcinogens in cigarettes, and heavy smokers have an increased incidence of bladder cancer. It is conceivable that urine containing these carcinogens bathing the vulva may increase vulvar premalignant and malignant lesions. (See also p. 447.) Currently, in situ lesions and marked condyloma are being identified with increasing frequency in pregnant patients.

Barclay[4] in a review of the literature, found only 31 women with vulvar cancer associated with pregnancy. Of these cases, only two were actually diagnosed and treated during pregnancy, with another two being treated following termination of pregnancy.[19,20] Lutz et al[51] in 1977, reported five vulvar cancers associated with pregnancy, of which three were diagnosed and treated during pregnancy, and two within 6 months postpartum. The author reported on three others associated with pregnancy.[2] Two were diagnosed prior to pregnancy and one in the fifth month of pregnancy. Their average age was 27.3 years, and the age range reported in the literature is 25 to 35.[2]

Patients with condyloma, in situ carcinoma and very small microinvasive cancers can be treated during pregnancy by laser surgery. Since these lesions are often multifocal and multicentric, laser surgery is ideally suited to controlling them without mutilating the vulva. However, microinvasive lesions of greater than 1 cm in diameter or 1 mm depth of invasion should be considered for more aggressive treatment. It is acceptable during the pregnancy to perform wide local excision or unilateral vulvectomy and ipsilateral groin lymphadenectomy, if this is deemed necessary. Regardless of the pregnancy, more advanced disease should be treated by radical vulvectomy and bilateral groin lymphadenectomy.

The author's plan of management for patients who are pregnant with established, frankly invasive cancer of the vulva is as follows:

First trimester. Radical vulvectomy, bilateral superficial node dissection. A deep node dissection is only carried out if the highest node is positive (so called Cloquet node) or if the lowest external iliac node or several nodes in the groin are positive.

Second trimester. Same treatment as for the first trimester. However, it may be technically impossible to do an adequate node dissection. If so, a radical vulvectomy should be done and node dissection delayed until after delivery.

Third trimester. If the lesion is small, vaginal delivery should be permitted. Radical vulvectomy and node dissection should be carried out in the immediate postpartum period (2 to 4 weeks).

Postpartum. The conventional operation of radical vulvectomy and lymph node dissection should be performed. It must be pointed out that there has been a trend to scale down the operative procedure for all patients with invasive cancer of the vulva and even to irradiate the deep node area (see Chs 27, 28, 75 and 76).

Subsequent pregnancy. The patient should have a cesarean section only if obstetrically indicated.

Following radical vulvectomy, vaginal delivery should be allowed if there is suitable elasticity of the introitus, and aided by timely episiotomy to avoid scar tissue tearing. If there is significant vaginal stenosis or fibrosis, abdominal delivery is advisable. Should labor occur before the wound is healed, or if there has been a degree of dehiscence, then elective cesarean section would be advised. Pregnancy has no adverse effect on prognosis and termination is not indicated in such patients.

Cancer of the vagina

Cancer of the vagina is extremely rare, comprising less than 1% of all genital cancers. The ratio of cancer of the cervix to vaginal cancer is roughly 50 to 1. It is often difficult to tell if the tumor arises primarily in the vaginal epithelium or extends to it from a primary locus in the cervix. When both are involved together, the cervix is considered the primary site.

Cancer of the vagina has been found mainly in women over 50 years of age. The average age is 61 for white and 58 years for black women.[80]

Collins & Barclay[19] reported 10 vaginal carcinomas associated with pregnancy, collected from the literature. Lutz and his associates reported one such case. Among those reported with follow-up, the prognosis was poor.[51]

Carcinoma in situ of the vagina is becoming more common. This is probably related to the same epidemiologic and etiologic factors as reported for the vulva. These patients can either be carefully followed throughout their pregnancy or treated with laser surgery.

The lack of collected experience in managing vaginal cancer complicating pregnancy makes it difficult to recommend a plan for therapy. However, management in general should be similar to that which would apply if the patient were not pregnant. If the fetus is viable, delivery by a high vertical cesarean section should be performed and therapy started as if the pregnant patient were not recently pregnant. If the infant is not viable or near viable age, external radiation therapy should be started followed by intracavitary radium or cesium application. The application must take into consideration the location of lesion. In rare instances where the patient does not spontaneously abort following the external therapy, the uterus should be emptied before the cesium application is carried out. If the lesion is early (Stage I) and located in the upper part of the vagina, it can be managed by radical hysterectomy, vaginectomy and pelvic node dissection.

Herbst, Ulfelder & Poskanzer[37] reported seven young women of 15 to 22 years of age, with adenocarcinoma of the vagina (clear cell of müllerian type) between 1966 and 1969. The study revealed a highly significant association between the treatment of their mothers with diethylstilbestrol (DES) during pregnancy and the later development of adenocarcinoma in their daughters (see Ch. 32). The risk of clear cell carcinoma of the vagina and cervix is probably less than 0.1% in the female whose mother took stilbestrol. However, about 80 to 90% of these patients have vaginal adenosis or a congenital anomaly of the cervix and/or vagina. From these observations, it has been suggested that DES acts as a teratogen rather than as a primary carcinogen (see Ch. 33).

If adenocarcinoma is diagnosed during pregnancy in a DES-exposed patient, management should be the same as in the non-pregnant state, that is, radical hysterectomy, vaginectomy, and pelvic node dissection with the construction of a neovagina. If the diagnosis is made at viability, a cesarean section should be carried out, followed immediately by treatment as outlined above.

Cancer of the cervix

There have been approximately 2000 cases of invasive carcinoma of the cervix complicating pregnancy reported in the world literature. Most authors include patients diagnosed either during pregnancy or within 12 months of delivery.

Kistner, Gorbach & Smith[46] reviewed the world literature up to 1957 and found only 106 cases of invasive cervical cancer complicating pregnancy in which the duration of pregnancy, stage of disease and 5-year results were available for study; to these they added 30 more cases from three Boston hospitals. Kinch[45] in 1961 added 105 cases of cancer of the cervix not reported in Kistner's series. Kinch's cases were diagnosed during pregnancy or within 6 months postpartum from 1933 to 1953. Lutz and co-workers,[51] in 1977, reported 30 cases of invasive cancer of the cervix.

The average incidence from large centers is 1 in 2500

pregnancies, whereas the incidence of carcinoma in situ during pregnancy has been reported as 1 in 750. However, the increase in screening programs and the widespread availability of cervical smears at antepartum clinics have resulted in a substantial increase in the incidence of carcinoma in situ, and hopefully invasive cancers will be detected at a very early stage.

Often, the diagnosis is delayed in pregnancy. The youth of the patients and the accompanying pregnancy undoubtedly lead to reluctance on the part of the responsible physicians to examine them at the first sign of abnormal bleeding. Excessive discharge and vaginal bleeding during pregnancy should be investigated by a speculum examination. Cytologic screening should be carried out during pregnancy. Schmitz, Isaacs & Fetherston[74] identified 25 cases of cancer of the cervix by the use of smears in 10 369 pregnant women.

The consensus in the literature is that cancer of the cervix diagnosed in the latter part of pregnancy or immediately postpartum has a grave prognosis. This is probably more a function of stage of disease than gestational age. Creasman, Rutledge & Fletcher[22] found no difference in survival of women diagnosed during any of the three trimesters or postpartum, when corrected for stage of disease.

Approximately 10 to 15 abnormal smears are reported per 1000 pregnancies in the average large antenatal clinic, and these should be followed carefully. Expert colposcopic assessment should be carried out. During pregnancy, endocervical epithelium everts and the ectocervix is displaced so that the ectocervix and the lower endocervical canal can be viewed. It is important to exclude invasive carcinoma with colposcopically directed biopsy. Bleeding is controlled easily with Monsel's solution. If no invasion is present, the patient can be examined colposcopically in each trimester. If there is no change, there is no need for any treatment. However, any change should be followed by biopsy examination. There is no contraindication for these patients to deliver vaginally, and cesarean section is only required for an obstetrical complication. There is practically no indication for a cone biopsy during pregnancy; this procedure is fraught with danger due to abortion and infection as well as hemorrhage. (See Ch. 36.)

Although surgery is the preferred treatment[36] for invasive cancer of the cervix in pregnancy, radiation therapy is chosen by many physicians.[72] Both protocols of management are presented in outline form in Tables 68.1 and 68.2.

It is interesting to note the high frequency of squamous differentiation in tumors discovered in pregnancy. Glucksmann & Cherry[33] reported a similar high frequency of squamous differentiation in cervical tumors in pregnancy, perhaps related to the hormonal milieu.

Microinvasive disease requires careful assessment. Minimal lesions can be observed carefully during pregnancy

Table 68.1 Surgical treatment of clinical invasive cancer of the cervix in pregnancy

1. **First trimester and early part of second trimester**
   Radical hysterectomy and pelvic node dissection is performed with the fetus in utero.

2. **Late second trimester**
   Await viability of the fetus and then perform classical cesarean section followed immediately by radical hysterectomy and pelvic node dissection.

3. **Third trimester**
   Classical cesarean section is followed immediately by radical hysterectomy and pelvic node dissection.

4. **Postpartum**
   Radical hysterectomy and pelvic node dissection is performed.

Table 68.2 Radiation therapy of invasive carcinoma of the cervix in pregnancy

1. **Non-viable fetus — first and second trimesters**
   Treatment is given as if the pregnancy were not present. External therapy is given to the pelvis. Spontaneous evacuation is preferred to intervention.

2. **Viable fetus — third trimester**
   Classical cesarean section is immediately followed by external therapy and, on completion of this, a cesium implant.

3. **Postpartum**
   Radiate as in the non-pregnant patient, giving external therapy first followed by intravaginal and intra-uterine radiation.

and further biopsies should be carried out if there is any colposcopic change. In more extensive lesions, cone biopsy is required for adequate histological assessment. For patients who have lesions with less than 3 mm stromal invasion, the cone will suffice as therapy but will require re-evaluation following delivery. However, with multiple foci of invasion or vascular lymphatic space involvement, and if the penetration is greater than 3 mm, the patient must be treated as for invasive disease by either the surgical or radiation protocols of management (Tables 68.1 and 68.2).

In the presence of untreated invasive cancer of the cervix, vaginal delivery is fraught with danger. Hemorrhage, sepsis and cervical laceration may result. Whether malignant cells are spread by vaginal delivery is controversial. However, the complications that may arise give a strong impetus to carrying out cesarean section in the presence of anything but a very small invasive lesion.

Cancer of the endometrium

Cancer of the endometrium complicating pregnancy is extremely rare.[43,85] Sandstrom, Welch & Green[73] described one case and found 6 others reported in the literature. Four of the 7 tumors were adenoacanthoma. Follow up on 4 of the 6 previously reported patients indicates that 3 are well more than 5 years after diagnosis. Barber & Brunschwig[2] reported one case that was discovered after curettage for a spontaneous abortion. Karlen and associates,[43] in 1972, reported that there were 8 cases in the literature, 2 of which were incidental findings in conjunction with abortions, one being spontaneous, the other therapeutic. Of the other 6 cases, 4 were over 35 years of age. The treatment is total hysterectomy, bilateral salpingo-oophorectomy and node sampling with supplementary radiation therapy in high risk patients with poor prognostic features.

Cases of carcinoma of the endometrium coincident with pregnancy are too few to permit reliable evaluation of its biological behavior.

Cancer of the ovary

Cancer of the ovary accounts for approximately 5% of all cancers among women. Deaths from this disease have slowly increased over the last 40 years and the rate is now 2.5 times that of 1930. In 1991, it is anticipated that there will be more than 20 000 cases and more than 12 000 deaths from cancer of the ovary. It is now the leading cause of death from gynecologic cancer. Common epithelial ovarian cancer is usually seen over the age of 40, but increasing numbers of these tumors are now seen under 40 years of age. Germ cell tumors of the ovary are seen most commonly from birth to age 20. Gonadal stromal tumors are usually seen during the childbearing years. The germ cell and gonadal stromal tumors are more commonly unilateral than the common epithelial ovarian cancers; therefore, if they are confined to the ovary a unilateral salpingo-oophorectomy is an acceptable treatment.

Ovarian tumors are said to occur once in every 1000 pregnancies: 1 in 10 of these are normal physiological corpora lutea. Ovarian cancer occurs in about 1 in every 18 000 pregnancies. In the non-pregnant state about 20% of ovarian tumors are malignant, while in the pregnant state the rate drops to 5%. Beral[7] suggested that pregnancy may actually protect against the development of ovarian cancers, pointing out that ovarian cancer is rare in populations that do not practice birth control. Therefore, incessant ovulation is considered an epidemiologic risk factor.

Chung & Birnbaum[18] found that fewer than 40 cases of ovarian cancer complicating pregnancy had been reported between 1963 and 1972, and added an additional 10 cases during, and 4 after, pregnancy. Beischer and colleagues[6] recorded 164 ovarian tumors diagnosed during pregnancy or in the puerperium at the Royal Women's Hospital in Melbourne between 1947 and 1969. More than 50% were either adult cystic teratomas or mucinous cystadenomas, and only 4 (2.4%) were malignant. They commented on the difficulty of establishing a definite diagnosis during pregnancy, and concluded that the size of the tumor was not a reliable criterion of malignancy. This finding reflects the varied and favorable pathologic character of ovarian cancer in pregnancy. The overall 5-year survival rate for ovarian neoplasia in pregnancy is 76% as compared to a general figure for all age groups of 25%.

Novak, Lambrou & Woodruff[61] reported 100 cases of malignant ovarian neoplasia associated with gestation. Forty five were common epithelial ovarian tumors, 14 gonadal stromal tumors, 33 germ cell tumors, 2 sarcomas, 2 metastatic Krukenberg's type tumors, and 4 metastatic, of which 2 were unclassifiable. The absolute 5-year survival in these 100 cases was 76%. The excellent salvage is a reflection of the favorable pathologic state of these tumors.

The signs and symptoms of ovarian neoplasms in pregnant women are not basically different from those in the non-pregnant state. The presenting symptom may be a complication of the tumor, such as torsion, rupture, hemorrhage or infection.[87]

The pelvic findings are important in the decision whether to operate immediately or to observe the patient until the second trimester. The unilateral, seemingly well encapsulated, freely movable mass of uniform consistency and less than 10 cm in diameter can be kept under observation until the second trimester. If the mass decreases in size, it presumably represented a corpus luteum cyst. However, progressive growth requires exploration without further delay. On the other hand, a hard, knobbly, fixed mass of variegated consistency, or bilateral masses or signs of ascitic fluid are indications for surgical intervention whatever the trimester of pregnancy.

Fortunately, most ovarian malignancies in pregnancy are diagnosed at an early stage (Stage I). The survival rate is much the same as in the non-pregnant state and is determined by the type of tumor and its staging. If the tumor is diagnosed in the third trimester, surgery may be delayed until the fetus is viable, but to delay beyond that is not justifiable.

At all cesarean sections, routine inspection of tubes and

Table 68.3 Treatment of cancer of ovary in pregnancy

1. Treat as in the non-pregnant state

2. Undertake exploratory laparotomy

3. Aspirate fluid from the pelvis and the abdomen for cytologic assessment

4. If tumor is low grade, unilateral, encapsulated:
   a. unilateral salpingo-oophorectomy is performed
   b. biopsy the opposite ovary and, if negative, consider the treatment to be adequate
   c. allow the pregnancy to go to term

5. If tumor has extended beyond the ovary, undertake:
   a. aspiration for cytology
   b. total hysterectomy
   c. bilateral salpingo-oophorectomy
   d. appendectomy
   e. omentectomy
   f. chemotherapy as indicated
   g. node sampling

ovaries is mandatory. The management of cancer of the ovary complicating pregnancy is summarized in Table 68.3.

Cancer of the colon and rectum

The incidence of cancer of the rectum associated with pregnancy is extremely low; it is reported by McLean as 1 in 50 000 cases.[57] Less than 200 cases have been reported in the literature. Symptoms related to cancer may be overshadowed by those produced by pregnancy. Rectal bleeding, abdominal pain, changing bowel habits, weight loss, palpable abdominal mass and/or persistent nausea and vomiting in late pregnancy should alert the obstetrician to the possibility of a bowel lesion. Consideration of colonic cancer is particularly important in a patient with known factors predisposing to malignant change. Lesions have been discovered during all trimesters with equal frequency, as well as during labor, and a few patients have had obvious predisposing factors such as colitis, familial polyposis, Gardner's syndrome and villous tumors. Too often, symptoms related to the gastrointestinal tract are dismissed as side effects of pregnancy, with the result that bowel obstruction or perforation of the colon ultimately discloses the correct diagnosis. Consequently, the prognosis for carcinoma of the colon during pregnancy has generally been poor.[35]

Unless the symptoms improve, thorough investigation should be carried out. Harm to the fetus during barium studies must be weighed against the fatal outcome resulting from failure to diagnose cancer of the bowel in an early stage. The role of colonoscopy as a modality of management in these cases has not been reported, but its use would avoid the danger to the fetus from radiation exposure. Once the diagnosis has been established, it is important to proceed with treatment. The suggested plan of management is described below.[3]

First and second trimesters

An abdominal-perineal or an anterior resection is carried out, depending upon the position of the lesion. The pregnancy usually does not have to be interrupted unless there are technical difficulties. In most instances, the pregnancy is allowed to proceed unless the cancer has invaded the uterus.

Late second and third trimesters

If possible, management should be delayed until the fetus is viable. However, complications related to the cancer may require prompt treatment. Cesarean section is usually required to facilitate the bowel operation. An abdominal-perineal or an anterior resection are the procedures of choice. If there is any evidence of local spread, total hysterectomy and bilateral salpingo-oophorectomy may be required as well. In the presence of large bowel carcinoma, bilateral oophorectomy is frequently carried out in order to remove the ovary as a major site for later metastases.

The prognosis for pregnant women with colon cancer has been dismal. However, Barber & Brunschwig[3] reported a pregnancy that had occurred after an abdominal-perineal operation with the patient still surviving after more than 20 years. In general, the overall survival rate is comparable to the survival rate of non-pregnant women with rectal cancer. The stage of disease is the most important prognostic factor.

EXTRAPELVIC MALIGNANCY IN PREGNANCY

The obstetrician feels secure in managing the pregnant patient with pelvic cancer. However, he is less secure in management and control if the patient has an extrapelvic malignancy. If castration or termination of pregnancy is indicated, the obstetrician is the technician, and all too often the patient is then managed either by a medical or hematologic oncologist, or by a surgeon undertaking a radical approach to melanoma, breast or gastrointestinal cancer; the obstetrician becomes a bystander. This is neither ideal for management nor in the best interest of the patient. The obstetrician is the best qualified to serve as the primary care physician and to control and coordinate the care of the patient. If a specialist is called in, this should be as a consultant and not as physician in charge. The obstetrician must continue as the responsible physician and all orders and treatment should be controlled by him or her. The obstetrician has a particular relationship with the patient which has been established over several weeks if not months.[12]

Breast cancer

Breast cancer, the most frequent cancer in women, is also the second most frequent cause of all cancer deaths; breast cancer deaths now number more than 37 000 yearly in the United States. About 15% of the cases occur in women younger than 41 years of age; about 3% occur during pregnancy, complicating approximately one in every 3 000 pregnancies. Breast cancer has had considerable public attention because of its frequency, the controversy about management, and the importance of the breast to the woman in terms of body and sexual image.

There is a familial incidence of breast cancer, so that the risk of developing the disease is significantly increased if a first degree relative has had it. It is the leading site causing mortality from cancer in women between 39 and 44 years of age. When women delay their first pregnancy until the age of 35 or more, the risk of breast cancer increases by three times as compared to those women who first conceive prior to the age of 20. With changes in contraceptive practices, and more women delaying their pregnancies until their thirties, the incidence of breast cancer complicating pregnancy will increase. The dilemma for treatment is quite acute. Therapeutic abortion does not appear to improve the chances of a cure, even though this cancer is hormone sensitive. Hormone receptor studies are not available in any significant series, but may in the future give an indication as to which pregnancies should be terminated.

The diagnosis is often difficult, as physiologic changes continue throughout the pregnancy. However, if there is any suspicious change in the breast, the approach to diagnosis, including mammogram and biopsy, should be as in the non-pregnant patient.

Management of breast-cancer-associated pregnancy can be a severe test for the clinician.[25,40,70] In addition, non-clinical, religious, psychological and socioeconomic considerations will influence the choice of management.

In the United States, 3% of newly diagnosed breast cancers are accompanied by pregnancy, the concurrence being most common in the fourth decade of life. Holleb & Farrow[38] grouped patients into the following groups:

1. Simultaneous pregnancy
2. Postpartum pregnancy
3. Subsequent pregnancy.

The overall 5-year survival for these three major groups was 33%, 29% and 52% respectively. When there was metastasis to axillary nodes the 5-year survival was 21%, 15% and 30%. The frequency of axillary node metastases (70% of the cases) is somewhat higher than in the non-pregnant group. The outlook for such patients is less favorable than that of the non-pregnant, non-lactating woman, probably because the stage of the disease is more advanced when it is discovered. If age and stage of disease are taken into account, pregnancy itself seems to have a negligible influence on prognosis. Modified radical mastectomy can be expected to be as effective for pregnant patients with operable cancers as for others, and presents little chance for fetal loss.[84] The subject of whether a lumpectomy should be performed and the radiation delayed until the pregnancy is terminated is controversial.

The important questions in regard to pregnancy and lactating women with proven cancer of the breast are: How should the pregnant woman with breast cancer be treated? Is waiting for the termination of pregnancy indicated or even desirable before mastectomy is performed? Does accepted treatment by today's standards alter the life expectancy of women? If the woman is pregnant at the time of diagnosis or subsequent to mastectomy, is termination of pregnancy indicated? Should the surgeon plan to castrate surgically the women with treated breast cancer for therapeutic reasons or primarily to prevent future pregnancies?

Some of these questions have already been answered. The consensus of opinion from the literature is that patients presenting with early breast cancer in the first trimester should be treated in the same manner as the non-pregnant patient. However, this raises the question of whether lumpectomy should be chosen followed by radiation therapy at a later point, or whether the fetus can be adequately protected during radiotherapy of the breast. After a mastectomy there is no harm in allowing the pregnancy to continue. Termination, if elected, would then be based on social, economic and psychologic considerations. However, increasingly, patients with operable tumors and positive nodes are receiving adjuvant chemotherapy. If this policy is followed, there must be an argument for aborting the fetus if the disease is treated in the first trimester, because of the teratogenic risk of these drugs.

There are no special risks in treating patients with breast cancer in the second half of pregnancy rather than waiting for the postpartum period. A modest delay in therapy to allow for delivery probably has no deleterious effects.

Patients with Stage III and IV cancer have such a poor prognosis that a uniform plan of therapy is difficult to outline. After frank discussion with the patient, she may decide to accept treatment, knowing that there is a risk of teratogenesis, while others may elect termination of the pregnancy followed by therapy. There may be a place for castration in the treatment of disseminated disease, but its role is yet to be defined. Treatment should be undertaken with the expectations that, stage-for-stage, the outlook is as good as is that of the non-pregnant patient.

Subsequent pregnancy is permissible with a 3 year interval elapsing following treatment. This delay will identify patients who have a virulent tumor with early recurrence. If there is no sign of recurrence at 3 years, there is no evidence to suggest pregnancy alters the prognosis.

Breast feeding is a debatable issue, but most surgeons suggest that this should be discouraged. Lactation and consequent engorgement of the other breast would delay detection if a second occult primary was present.

Melanoma

Melanomas, or malignant melanomas, generally originate from pre-existing pigmented moles. The melanocyte is embryologically derived from neural crest cells and migrates to sites in the skin, eye, central nervous system and elsewhere during fetal development.

With a peak incidence in the third and fourth decades of life, melanoma occurs among women in their reproductive years. There is controversy concerning the effect of pregnancy on melanoma. In one updated series, the author reversed his previous opinion and reported a significant improvement in the prognosis of melanoma in some patients with associated pregnancy.[31,63] Although some authors advise termination of pregnancy, the consensus of opinion in the literature is that termination of pregnancy is not therapeutic.

It has been suggested that melanoma may be induced or exacerbated by pregnancy. The assumption is based on the following observations: pituitary gland melanocyte stimulating hormone (MSH) levels increase in pregnancy and result in increased pigmentation. Estrogen receptor proteins have been detected in melanomas. Metastatic spread appears to be more rapid in pregnancy, but stage-for-stage there may be no significant difference in the prognosis for the patient. At puberty, obvious pigmentation occurs in moles, genitalia and elsewhere. There is also increased pigmentation in pregnancy, as evidenced in the nipples, areola, vulva, linea nigra, occasionally in pre-existing nevi, and cases of chloasma. Melanocyte stimulating hormone (MSH) has been quantitated, and levels shown to increase after the second month of pregnancy. Furthermore, Bischitz & Snell[10] have demonstrated an effect of estrogen on melanocytes in guinea pig skin in ovariectomized animals given estrogen.

In 1951, Pack & Scharnagel[63] reported a poor prognosis in 32 cases of melanoma in pregnancy. In 1958, Shockett & Fortner[76] demonstrated that pregnancy and lactation stimulated neither the local development nor metastatic spread of transplantable hamster melanoma. Rather, growth of the local tumor appeared inhibited. In 1960, George, Fortner & Pack[31] reported on 115 cases of melanoma in pregnancy and 330 controls. They found that regional nodes appeared more rapidly in pregnant patients, but stage-for-stage there was little to support the prevailing opinion at that time that the outcome was influenced by pregnancy.[71,88] In 1976, Shiu and co-workers[75] reported that there was no statistical difference in disease free 5-year survival rates for Stage I melanoma between nulliparous, parous and non-pregnant, and pregnant women. For Stage II melanomas, however, a significantly lower survival rate was observed for pregnant women and parous women who had had activation of a lesion in a previous pregnancy, as compared to that of nulliparous patients and other patients in the parous group. They concluded an adverse influence of pregnancy on women with Stage II melanoma. However melanoma remains one of the most erratic cancers, and there is no conclusive evidence for either a beneficial or a deleterious effect of pregnancy on its clinical course.

It has been reported that women who had a pregnancy before the melanoma developed survived longer than women without a previous pregnancy. The explanation advanced is that exposure to fetal antigen protected against the dissemination of melanoma cells with similar fetal antigens. However, these findings were not confirmed by Elwood & Codman in Vancouver.[27] There remains a great deal of controversy surrounding melanoma complicating pregnancy.

The management of malignant melanoma is the same as in the non-pregnant patient. En bloc excision, with or without skin graft to close the defect, with regional node dissection is the treatment usually chosen. Nevi on the feet, hands and genitals should be excised, particularly in the pregnant patient. In our present state of knowledge, termination of pregnancy is not considered therapeutic.

Thyroid cancer

The incidence of thyroid cancer is low,[13] even though it occurs most often in young women. Apart from radiation, little is known of its cause.[1,23,26,86] There is a great deal of controversy as to whether it is stimulated by the pregnancy.[1,26,86] However, thyroid stimulating hormone (TSH) is elevated in pregnancy, and free thyroxin is decreased greatly by estrogen binding globulins so that the feedback mechanism to the pituitary is decreased. The protein-bound iodine (PBI) is elevated. About 10% of thyroid malignancies are functional and may respond to TSH stimulation.[14] Pregnancy subsequent to treatment for thyroid carcinoma is believed neither to cause recurrence in those who have been successfully treated earlier, nor to accelerate the tumor's growth in women who have not been cured.

The management is similar to that in the non-pregnant state. Total thyroidectomy and unilateral and/or bilateral dissection of lymph nodes in the neck is the treatment usually chosen. Thyroxine (100 to 300 μg daily) is given to control the output of TSH. Radioactive iodine is contraindicated in pregnancy.

Management is based on the trimester of pregnancy. If carcinoma is strongly suspected during the first or second trimester, the thyroid gland should be promptly explored. In the third trimester, exploration might be delayed until after delivery. Neck dissection, however, is obligatory for patients with histologically proven cervical lymph node metastases.

Although papillary and follicular cancer have a favorable prognosis, undifferentiated tumors are a highly lethal group and range from the giant and spindle cell variety to the small cell varieties. Abortion has not been found to be therapeutic.

Hodgkin's disease and non-Hodgkin's lymphoma

Non-Hodgkin's lymphoma is less common than Hodgkin's disease. Both types of lymphoma commonly affect young people and may be cured or controlled for long periods with irradiation and chemotherapy.[39,77] The majority of patients with Hodgkin's disease present with enlarged lymph nodes. The staging and comprehensive treatment are difficult to achieve during pregnancy without risk to the fetus. Evaluating the abdomen is an obvious difficulty. The liver-spleen scan and staging laparotomy should be avoided during pregnancy. Lymphangiography presents the same problem, though a single abdominal film 24 hours after the injection may be useful.

Most young women treated for Hodgkin's disease wish to maintain a normal lifestyle, marry, and have children. The mutagenicity of irradiation and chemotherapy with the possibility of long-term damage to the gonadal tissue is recognized. However, little is known regarding the magnitude of risk of fetal mortality and infant morbidity resulting from damaged gonadal tissue. If pelvic radiotherapy is planned, the gonads are usually placed out of the field of radiation at the time of staging laparotomy.

In patients treated for Hodgkin's disease with persisting disease 2 years after the start of treatment, the prognosis is poor. However, in patients free of disease for 3 or more years, the prognosis is good. Therefore, the patient should be told to wait for 3 years after treatment for Hodgkin's disease before attempting pregnancy. When relapse occurs in association with pregnancy, the patient is most vulnerable during the postpartum period. There are at least two documented cases of Hodgkin's disease in infants among 32 term deliveries.

When the patient is pregnant and found to have widespread Hodgkin's disease, the pregnancy usually has to be interrupted to give optimal therapy. It is accepted that the pregnant patient, except in highly selected instances, should be treated as in the non-pregnant state.[5,82]

There is no influence of pregnancy on the pattern or curability of Hodgkin's disease. Treatment should not be compromised because of pregnancy. Stage I and II disease above the diaphragm, frequently of the nodular sclerosing type in this youthful age group, can be treated with supradiaphragmatic irradiation with shielding of the abdomen. Fetal radiation exposure increases with the stage of pregnancy, as the uterus ascends in the abdomen. Fundal dose has been calculated at approximately 10.4 cGy at 16 weeks of pregnancy, with an increase to 100 cGy at 30 weeks.

If the abdominal nodes are unequivocally involved and the pregnancy is in its early months, the pregnancy should be terminated so that adequate treatment can be given.

In advanced stages of the disease, when chemotherapy is indicated, interruption of pregnancy should be considered because of the potentially teratogenic effects of chemotherapeutic agents. This risk is greatest in the first 10 weeks of pregnancy. Chemotherapy at later periods has been followed by delivery of normal infants. Cesarean section or induced labor can be used before beginning treatment if the fetus is viable.

The following protocol encompasses a variety of situations encountered in managing patients with Hodgkin's lymphoma complicating pregnancy. Women of childbearing age should not begin therapy for Hodgkin's disease unless a pregnancy test is negative; effective contraception should be used during therapy, and pregnancy should be avoided for at least 3 years following successful therapy. If the woman is pregnant at the time of diagnosis and desires the pregnancy, and the disease is not immediately life endangering, staging laparotomy should be avoided before 12 weeks and beyond 18 weeks of gestation, to minimize fetal jeopardy due to the technical difficulties that may be encountered. Treatment can be delayed until viability if the patient and her family recognize the fact that she is at risk and in some danger of developing a more advanced disease.

Both chemotherapy and irradiation used to treat Hodgkin's disease are potentially harmful to the growing fetus. Therefore, if therapy can be delayed without detriment to the patient, it should be postponed until after the fetus is viable and delivery is possible. McKeen and associates[55] investigated the results of pregnancy after treatment for Hodgkin's disease, and found that only 52% resulted in normal live births. Twenty-seven percent were either premature, stillborn or spontaneously aborted, and 15% of live births had malformation. As usual, there is controversy and Holmes & Holmes demonstrated no significant difference in spontaneous abortion or abnormal offspring in the subsequent pregnancies of patients treated for Hodgkin's disease and sibling controls.[39]

Non-Hodgkins lymphoma may complicate pregnancy, but this is less common than Hodgkin's disease. This group of diseases runs a variable course, and both radiotherapy and chemotherapy are effective treatments with chemotherapy being more widely used. Similar approaches to patients with non-Hodgkin's lymphoma and Hodgkin's disease are recommended in the pregnant patient.

Burkitt's lymphoma has been reported during pregnancy and lactation. Enlargement of the breast has been prominent in the gravid state, and the disease may run a rapidly fatal course. However, the disease is chemosensitive and chemotherapy may be combined with radiation to selected areas.

Acute leukemia

Leukemia is a cancer of the blood-forming tissues, which occurs in both sexes and all ages.[68] Acute lymphatic leukemia is the most common variety among children, while in adults the most common types are acute granulocytic and chronic lymphocytic leukemia.[11,48] Modern treatment has dramatically changed the survival rate of those with acute lymphatic leukemia.[50]

Leukemia complicates less than 1 in 75 000 pregnancies.[56] There is no evidence that pregnancy has a deleterious effect on leukemia and, therefore, terminating pregnancy has not proved to be therapeutic.[52]

Leukemia presents a problem in pregnancy in that there is a great susceptibility to infection, hemorrhage and spontaneous abortion.

The management is the same as in the non-pregnant patient. Although abortion is not considered therapeutic, if the leukemia occurs during the first trimester, abortion is usually advised since the rate of spontaneous abortion is high in the first trimester and fetal malformations are common, especially when aggressive chemotherapy is used. Acute leukemia can be treated in second and third trimesters with little effect on the pregnancy or fetus. If the fetus is viable, and amniocentesis reveals fetal lung maturity, delivery should be expedited before definitive therapy for the leukemia is started. In patients cured of acute leukemia, the potential for subsequent pregnancies exists with little likelihood of increase in fetal malformations. The long-term effects of chemotherapy on infants exposed in utero are not known.

Chronic leukemia

Chronic lymphatic leukemia is very rare in pregnancy; less than 100 cases have been reported.[48]

This malignant hematologic disorder is characterized by a persistent, absolute increase in morphologically mature lymphocytes in the peripheral blood and bone marrow. The disease may involve lymph nodes, spleen and liver, and cause no symptoms.

It is a rare disorder in persons less than 30 years of age and gradually increases in incidence with each decade.

Coincidence of a myeloproliferative disease, e.g. chronic granulocytic leukemia, in pregnancy is unusual. Pregnancy has no adverse effect on the course of the mother's hematologic disease. However, the myeloproliferative disease, especially if uncontrolled, results in increased fetal prematurity and mortality. Treatment of the pregnant patient should be conservative, and chemotherapy should be avoided until at least after the first trimester whenever possible.

Gastrointestinal tract tumors

A significant number of cases of cancer of the stomach associated with pregnancy have been reported. Almost all had an advanced stage of disease with secondary metastases to the ovaries (Krukenberg tumors). Most of these women delivered healthy children but have later died from the disease. A high index of suspicion and early diagnosis is the key to successful management of these patients. Progressive increase in symptoms over and above those seen in pregnancy, especially if accompanied by epigastric pain, requires careful investigation.

Liver tumors have been reported as a result of the use of the contraceptive pill.[44] The number of such cases of hepatic adenoma reported in the literature is increasing, and at least four have complicated pregnancy. All patients were symptomatic during pregnancy, and two were admitted with rupture of the adenoma. One subsequently died. Increased growth and vascularity of adenoma during pregnancy is highly likely. The potential for the development of lethal complications is considerable. Management is by surgical resection. Pregnancy is contraindicated in the presence of a non-resected liver adenoma or in one that has been partially resected.

Rectocolon cancer complicating pregnancy is the most commonly encountered gastrointestinal tumor (see p. 1076).

Central nervous system tumors

The tumors of the central nervous system that are most commonly affected adversely by pregnancy are pituitary adenomas, craniopharyngioma and meningioma. Pituitary tumors may or may not be associated with endocrinopathy.

Malignant brain tumors have a population incidence of 4.5 cases per 100 000, with a slightly higher frequency in men than in women. The age distribution of patients with brain tumor is biphasic, with the first peak between the ages of 6 and 9 years and accounted for by cerebellar astrocytomas, medulloblastomas, and ependymomas. The second peak appears in patients between 40 and 60 years of age, the principal lesions being malignant gliomas, meningiomas and adenomas. Malignant brain tumors complicating pregnancy are extremely rare.[17]

Pregnant women with malignant brain tumors are usually misdiagnosed, because many of the early symptoms are identical to the complaints encountered in normal pregnancy. Pregnancy is normally associated with an enlarged pituitary gland, mainly as a result of hyperplasia of the acidophilic cells concerned with prolactin secretion, and existent pituitary tumors may also increase rapidly in size in pregnancy. The resulting symptoms include headache and visual disturbances, decreased visual acuity and diminished visual fields.[8]

Early diagnosis offers the patient maximum chance of salvage. A high index of suspicion in patients with headache, visual disturbance or other cerebral symptoms that do not improve warrants investigation. A diagnosis may be established by complete physical and neurologic examination, CT scan, electroencephalography, testing visual acuity and visual fields, and angiography if indicated.[58,59] MRI is increasingly used for diagnosis.

Meningiomas predominate in women and have been reported to enlarge rapidly with pregnancy. They have been found to contain estrogen receptors. Meningiomas that are asymptomatic or do not enlarge can be observed until viability of the baby.

The treatment of malignant brain tumors during pregnancy is the same as that in the non-pregnant patient. Surgical excision with or without X-ray treatment is usually chosen.

Vaginal delivery is preferred, and cesarean section is reserved for obstetric indications or when instantaneous delivery is necessary. The increase in intra-abdominal pressure associated with bearing down markedly elevates cerebral spinal fluid pressure. This should be minimized by the use of outlet forceps. If the fetus has reached viability, delivery should be offered prior to surgical intervention or radiation therapy for the brain tumor.

Pituitary adenomas have recently received considerable attention in the literature. These are often micro-adenomas. As noted above, during pregnancy, there is a physiologic enlargement of the pituitary, and an asymptomatic patient with a small pituitary tumor in a non-pregnant state may develop acute neurologic symptoms during pregnancy.[81] Therefore, the question arises whether or not to treat patients with a known adenoma prior to pregnancy. In some patients, the tumor becomes apparent when they are pregnant. Since it is not possible to predict which tumors will enlarge and cause symptoms during pregnancy, it is probably safer to treat all patients with pituitary tumors before pregnancy is attempted.

Pheochromocytomas

Pheochromocytomas are extremely rare but very dangerous during pregnancy, with a 50% maternal and fetal mortality. Pheochromocytoma is a catecholamine-secreting tumor consisting of neuroectoderm or neural crest derived cells; it affects 1 in 200 000 members of the general population and is responsible for 0.1% of cases of diastolic hypertension. The presentation of pheochromocytoma in pregnancy is rare but well described, with approximately 150 cases reported in the literature.[21] The majority of these tumors occur sporadically; approximately 5% are familial and these are usually bilateral. Alpha blocker control, e.g. with phenoxybenzamine, is required, and surgical removal should be attempted only after localizing the tumor. It is preferable to do this postpartum.

If a pheochromocytoma is diagnosed during early pregnancy, phenoxybenzamine should be started and a therapeutic termination carried out. Attempts should then be made to localize the tumor using the radiologic technique that had been associated with its diagnosis, and the tumor should be removed surgically. Should the diagnosis not be made until the second or third trimester, the pregnancy should be allowed to continue until induction or cesarean section is indicated, under phenoxybenzamine control and with careful blood pressure monitoring. If progress is satisfactory, localizing investigations can be postponed until after delivery.

Sarcoma

Sarcoma complicating pregnancy is very rare. The management of the patient who is pregnant with a sarcoma depends on the type of lesion, its anatomic location, stage of disease and the age of the gestation. The question is asked whether or not pregnancy has an adverse effect on the growth rate of the tumor.

Cantin & McNeer[16] reported on 57 women who were pregnant simultaneously with, or subsequent to, the treatment of a variety of soft tissue tumors, and compared the 5- and 10-year survival rates both with those of premenopausal women without pregnancy and those of postmenopausal women. It was concluded that the survival rate compared favorably with rates for non-pregnant women of reproductive age.

Pack & Ariel[62] enumerate a list of soft tissue tumors that may be influenced by hormonal factors. One such is angiosarcoma. Cystosarcoma phylloides or, more specifically, giant intracanalicular myxoma arises from fibroadenomas, most frequently in women of multiparity and suppressed lactation. Desmoids frequently arise or recur during pregnancy. These should be treated as in women in the non-pregnant state.[41,67]

FETAL AND PLACENTAL TRANSMISSION OF MALIGNANCY

Metastases to the fetus and/or placenta have given rise to a great deal of interest and considerable controversy. When cancer complicates pregnancy, it is common for the woman and her family to ask whether the cancer will spread to the baby, and whether the baby is at risk from the later development of cancer.

Probably fewer than 40 cases of metastatic disease in the placenta have been reported. The most common primary tumors are melanoma, breast and leukemia-lymphoma. One of the best documented and often quoted cases is that of Holland, in which a melanoma metastasized to both placenta and fetus. This may rarely occur with other tumors, such as adenocarcinoma of the rectum.

Many theories have been advanced to explain the paucity of documented cases of placental and fetal metastases:

1. Most placentas are not carefully examined by both gross and histologic evaluation.
2. Active resistance by the trophoblast has been proposed.
3. The fetal environment may be unfavorable for the rare cancer cell that crosses the barrier established by the placenta.
4. Tumor cells have the potential to invade the chorionic villi and penetrate the intravillous capillaries, thus becoming blood-borne via the umbilical vein to the liver of the fetus.[63,69]

The sinuses around the villi are large and the circulation is sluggish. The presence of tumor cells in these sinuses does not truly represent metastases to the placenta. The term, metastasis should be reserved for the intravillous destruction and invasion of tumor cells. Using these criteria, few cases reported actually qualify as metastases to the placenta.

Metastases from the mother to the fetus are indeed rare. There are about two dozen cases reported in the literature. Criteria accepted include maternal and placental invasion, and the occurrence of the same cancer in the baby within 1 year of birth.

Despite the fact that the incidence is rare, routine gross and microscopic examination of the placenta of women who have, or have had, cancers is desirable, as is careful examination of the infant, particularly if the maternal tumor was a melanoma, leukemia or lymphoma.

RADIOTHERAPY AND CHEMOTHERAPY IN PREGNANCY

Surgery and radiation are effective forms of treatment for localized cancer. Chemotherapy, the treatment of cancer with drugs and hormones can be used for disseminated as well as localized tumors. The treatment of cancer with drugs is a relatively new development, dating from 1945 when nitrogen mustard was found to be effective against lymphomas. Since that time, many drugs have been added to the therapeutic armamentarium.

If employed in only the second and third trimester of pregnancy, single drug chemotherapy gives rise to few problems. Various problems may arise from use of anti-cancer drugs in the first trimester;[29,78] however, Nicholson[60] reported that the risk is small if a single drug is used.

There are very little data available on the use of newer combinations of drugs or agents during pregnancy. DeVita and coworkers[24] observed 10 women who became pregnant after MOPP (nitrogen mustard, oncovin, procarbazine, prednisone) therapy; all gave birth to normal children. However, the physician must be cautious, since the side effects of newer agents, especially in combination and particularly prior to organogenesis, are unknown.[30]

The delayed consequences of chemotherapy remain controversial. In women who have had chemotherapy, the fetus may be at risk in future pregnancies. In 96 later pregnancies in women who had had chemotherapy, approximately 16% terminated in abortion and 3% in still-births. Three of the pregnancies resulted in the birth of infants with significant general malformations.[83]

Fetal damage by radiation

Exposure of the developing embryo to ionizing radiation may cause abortion, malformation and, possibly, leukemia in the infant. Animal studies and follow-up after the atomic bomb clearly demonstrate the teratogenic and carcinogenic effects of radiation.[42,65,66] Radiation injuries sustained late in fetal life are less harmful than in the early stages, when organogenesis and differentiation are more active. Some abortions are not a direct effect of radiation, but may be indirectly produced by radiation-induced hormonal imbalance. Fetal structures, particularly the central nervous system, the eye and·mesenchymal tissues appear to be more radiosensitive than those of adults. It is strongly suggested that pregnant women be given no X-ray exposure during the first 16 weeks of pregnancy.

It has been shown that in utero exposure to X-rays in the diagnostic range leads to a higher mortality rate from neoplastic disease in the children.[79] The increase in childhood cancer is about 40% and includes acute leukemia, central nervous system neoplasms and other forms.

Embryos are exceedingly radiosensitive. The sensitivity changes with age; generally, older embryos are less sensitive than younger ones. According to the month, fetal damage results from the doses of radiation shown in Table 68.4.

Table 68.4 Dose of radiation causing fetal damage at various stages of pregnancy

Month of pregnancy	Radiation dose (cGy)
1st	40
2nd	90
3rd	140
4th	200
5th	250
6th	350
8th	500
10th	600

Irradiation of pregnant women should be restricted to necessary exposures; under all possible circumstances, exposures of the pelvis should be limited to emergency procedures.

No threshold for gene mutation has been established. Estimates for doubling of the spontaneous mutation rate in man run from 10 cGy to 14 cGy.

ACKNOWLEDGEMENTS

The author wishes to thank Ruzena Danek for her help in the preparation of this manuscript, and Mr Gilbert Lachow, Health Science Associate at Merck, Sharp & Dohme, for his help in compiling the bibliography.

REFERENCES

1. Asteris G T, DeGroot L J 1976 Thyroid cancer: relationship to radiation exposure and to pregnancy. J Reprod Med 17: 209
2. Barber H R K, Brunschwig A 1962 Gynecologic cancer complicating pregnancy. Am J Obstet Gynecol 85: 156
3. Barber H R K, Brunschwig A 1968 Carcinoma of the bowel: radiation and surgical management and pregnancy. Am J Obstet Gynecol 100: 926
4. Barclay D L 1974 Surgery of the vulva, perineum and vagina in pregnancy. In: Barber H R K, Graber E A (eds) Surgical Disease in Pregnancy. Saunders, Philadelphia, p 310

5. Barry R M, Diamond H D, Craver L F 1962 Influence of pregnancy on the course of Hodgkin's disease. Am J Obstet Gynecol 84: 445
6. Beischer N A, Buttery B W, Fortune D W, Macafee C A J 1971 Growth and malignancy of ovarian tumors in pregnancy. Aust NZ J Obstet Gynaecol 11: 208
7. Beral V 1980 The epidemiology of ovarian cancer. In: Newman C E, Ford C H J, Jordan J A (eds) Ovarian Cancer. Pergamon Press, New York
8. Bernard M H 1898 Sarcome cerebral a evaluation rapide au cours de la grossesse et pendant les suites des couches. Bull Soc d'Obstet de Paris 1: 296
9. Betson J R, Golden M L 1961 Cancer and pregnancy. Am J Obstet Gynecol 81: 719
10. Bischitz P G, Snell R S 1958 Effect of ovariectomy, oestrogen and progesterone on the activity of the melanocyte in the skin. Nature 181: 1413
11. Bitran J D, Roth D G 1976 Acute leukemia during reproductive life: its course, complications and sequelae for fertility. J Reprod Med 17: 225
12. Boronow R C 1964 Extrapelvic malignancy and pregnancy. Obstet Gynecol Surv 19: 1
13. Breese M W 1963 Cancer of the thyroid in women of childbearing age. Am J Obstet Gynecol 86: 616
14. Brunn T, Kristoffersen K 1978 Thyroid function during pregnancy with special reference to hydatidiform mole and hyperemesis. Acta Endocrinol 88: 383
15. Cancer — a Manual for Practitioners, 5th edn. 1978 American Cancer Society, Massachusetts Division, Boston
16. Cantin J, McNeer G P 1967 The effect of pregnancy on the clinical course of sarcoma of the soft somatic tissues. Surg Gynecol Obstet 125: 28
17. Carmel P W 1974 Neurologic surgery in pregnancy. In: Barber H R K, Graber E A (eds) Surgical Disease in Pregnancy. Saunders, Philadelphia, p 203
18. Chung A, Birnbaum S J 1972 Ovarian cancer associated with pregnancy. Obstet Gynecol 41: 211
19. Collins C G, Barclay D L 1973 Cancer of the vulva and cancer of the vagina in pregnancy. Clin Obstet Gynecol 6: 927
20. Collins J H, Birch H W, Pailet M, Avent J K 1960 Pregnancy and delivery following extensive vulvectomy. Am J Obstet Gynecol 80: 167
21. Coombes G B 1976 Phaeochromocytoma presenting in pregnancy. Proc Roy Soc Med 69: 224
22. Creasman W T, Rutledge F, Fletcher G H 1970 Carcinoma of the cervix associated with pregnancy. Obstet Gynecol 36: 495
23. DeGroot L J, Paloyan E 1973 Thyroid carcinoma and radiation: a Chicago endemic. JAMA 225: 487
24. DeVita V T, Ardeneau J D, Shevins R J Canellos G P, Young R C 1973 Intensive chemotherapy for Hodgkin's disease: long term complications. International Symposium on Hodgkin's Disease (DHEW Publication No. (NCI) 36), Washington DC., p 447
25. Donegan W L 1977 Breast cancer and pregnancy. Obstet Gynecol 50: 244
26. Duffy B J Jr, Fitzgerald P J 1950 Cancer of the thyroid in children: a report of 28 cases. J Clin Endocrinol Metabol 10: 1296
27. Elwood J M, Codman A P 1978 Previous pregnancy and melanoma prognosis. Letter. Lancet ii: 1000
28. Emge L A 1934 The influence of pregnancy on tumor growth. Am J Obstet Gynecol 28: 682
29. Finkbeiner J A 1974 Antineoplastic chemotherapy in pregnancy. In: Barber H R K, Graber E A (eds) Surgical Disease in Pregnancy. Saunders, Philadelphia, p 711
30. Garrett M J 1974 Teratogenic effects of combination chemotherapy. Ann Int Med 80: 667
31. George P A, Fortner J G, Pack G T 1960 Melanoma with pregnancy. Report of 115 cases. Cancer 13: 854
32. Gleicher N, Siegel L 1981 Common denominators of pregnancy and malignancy. In: Gleicher N (ed) Reproductive Immunology. Liss, New York, p 339
33. Glucksmann A, Cherry C P 1956 Incidence, histology and response to radiation of mixed carcinomas (adenoacanthomas) of the uterine cervix. Cancer 9: 971
34. Golomb H M, Ultmann J E 1976 An approach to general oncology: principles and procedures. J Reprod Med 17: 191
35. Green L K, Harris R E, Massey F M 1975 Cancer of the colon during pregnancy. A review of the literature and report of a case associated with ulcerative colitis. Obstet Gynecol 46: 480
36. Green T H Jr 1974 Carcinoma of the cervix in pregnancy. In: Barber H R K, Graber E A (eds) Surgical Disease in Pregnancy. Saunders, Philadelphia, p 354
37. Herbst A L, Ulfelder H, Poskanzer D C 1971 Adenocarcinoma of the vagina. Association of maternal stilbestrol therapy with tumor appearance in young women. N Engl J Med 284: 878
38. Holleb A I, Farrow J H 1962 The relation of carcinoma of the breast and pregnancy in 283 patients. Surg Gynecol Obstet 115: 65
39. Holmes G E, Holmes F F 1978 Pregnancy outcome of patients treated for Hodgkin's disease: a controlled study. Cancer 41: 1317
40. Hubay C A, Barry F M, Marr C C 1978 Pregnancy and breast cancer. Surg Clin N Am 58: 819
41. Jafari K, Lash A F, Webster A 1978 Pregnancy and sarcoma. Acta Obstet Gynecol Scand 57: 265
42. Jaffe H L, Reddi P R 1974 Radiation therapy in pregnancy. In: Barber H R K, Graber E A (eds) Surgical Disease in Pregnancy. Saunders, Philadelphia, p 727
43. Karlen J R, Sternberg L B, Abbott J N 1972 Carcinoma of the endometrium coexisting with pregnancy. Obstet Gynecol 40: 334
44. Kent D R, Nissen E D, Nissen S E, Ziehm D J 1978 Effect of pregnancy on liver tumor associated with oral contraceptives. Obstet Gynecol 51: 148
45. Kinch R A H 1961 Factors affecting the prognosis of cancer of the cervix in pregnancy. Am J Obstet Gynecol 82: 45
46. Kistner R W, Gorbach A C, Smith G V 1957 Cervical cancer in pregnancy. Review of the literature with presentation of thirty additional cases. Obstet Gynecol 9: 554
47. Kobak A J, Fitzgerald J E, Freda V C, Rudolph L 1945 Carcinoma of the cervix and pregnancy. Am J Obstet Gynecol 49: 307
48. Lessmann E M, Sokal J E 1959 Conception and pregnancy in a patient with chronic myelocytic leukemia under continuous colcemide therapy. Ann Int Med 50: 1512
49. Levin B 1976 Aspects of gastrointestinal tumors during the reproductive years. J Reprod Med 17: 233
50. Lilleyman J S, Hill A S, Anderton K J 1977 Consequences of acute myelogenous leukemia in early pregnancy. Cancer 40: 1300
51. Lutz M H, Underwood P B Jr, Rozier J C, Putney F W 1977 Genital malignancy in pregnancy. Am J Obstet Gynecol 129: 536
52. MacMahon B, Levy M A 1964 Prenatal origin of childhood leukemia. Evidence from twins. N Engl J Med 270: 1082
53. Martzloff K H 1933 In: Curtis H (ed) Textbook of Obstetrics and Gynecology. Saunders, Philadelphia
54. McDuff H C Jr, Carney W I, Waterman G W 1956 Cancer of the cervix and pregnancy. Obstet Gynecol 8: 196
55. McKeen E A, Mulvihill J J, Posner F et al 1979 Pregnancy outcome in Hodgkin's disease. Lancet ii: 590
56. McLain C R Jr 1974 Leukemia in pregnancy. Clin Obstet Gynecol 17: 185
57. McLean D W, Arminski T C, Bradley G T 1955 Management of primary carcinoma of the rectum diagnosed during pregnancy. Am J Surg 90: 816
58. Magyar D M, Marshall J R 1978 Pituitary tumors and pregnancy. Am J Obstet Gynecol 132: 739
59. Nabil H, Jewlewicz R, Van de Wiele R L 1977 Pregnancy in patients with pituitary tumors. Fertil Steril 28: 920
60. Nicholson H O 1968 Cytotoxic drugs in pregnancy. Review of reported cases. J Obstet Gynaecol Br Commonw 75: 307
61. Novak E R, Lambrou C D, Woodruff J D 1975 Ovarian tumors in pregnancy. An ovarian tumor registry review. Obstet Gynecol 46: 401
62. Pack G T, Ariel I M 1958 Tumors of the Somatic Soft Tissue. Hoeber, New York
63. Pack G T, Scharnagel I M 1951 The prognosis for malignant melanoma in the pregnant women. Cancer 4: 324

64. Peller S 1925 Karzinom und gravidität. Wien Klin Wchnschr 38: 892
65. Plummer G 1952 Anomalies occurring in children exposed in utero to the atom bomb on Hiroshima. Pediatrics 10: 687
66. Pizzarello D J, Witcofski R L 1972 Medical Radiation Biology. Lea & Febiger, Philadelphia
67. Pratt C B, Rivera G, Shanks E 1977 Osteosarcoma during pregnancy. Obstet Gynecol 50, No 1 (suppl): 24S
68. Raich P C, Curet L B 1975 Treatment of acute leukemia during pregnancy. Cancer 36: 861
69. Reynolds A G 1955 Placental metastasis from malignant melanoma. Report of a case. Obstet Gynecol 6: 205
70. Ribeiro G G, Palmer M K 1977 Breast carcinoma associated with pregnancy: a clinician's dilemma. Br Med J ii: 1524
71. Russell P, Laverty C R 1977 Malignant melanoma metastases in the placenta: a case report. Pathology 9: 251
72. Sablinska R, Tarlowska L, Stelmachow J 1977 Invasive carcinoma of the cervix associated with pregnancy. Correlation between patient age, advancement of cancer and gestation, and result of treatment. Gynecol Oncol 5: 363
73. Sandstrom R E, Welch W R, Green T H Jr 1979 Adenocarcinoma of the endometrium in pregnancy. Obstet Gynecol (Suppl) 53: 73S
74. Schmitz H E, Isaacs J H, Fetherston W C 1960 The value of routine cytologic smears in pregnancy. Am J Obstet Gynecol 79: 910
75. Shiu M H, Schottenfeld D, Maclean B, Fortner J G 1976 Adverse effect of pregnancy on melanoma. A reappraisal. Cancer 37: 181
76. Shockett E C, Fortner J G 1958 Melanoma and pregnancy: an experimental evaluation of a clinical impression. Surg Forum 9: 671
77. Smith H N Spaulding L 1978 Hodgkin's disease in pregnancy. South Med J 71: 374
78. Sokal J E, Lessmann E M 1960 Effects of cancer chemotherapeutic agents on the human fetus. JAMA 172: 1765
79. Stewart A, Kneale G W 1970 Radiation dose effects in relation to obstetric X-rays and childhood cancers. Lancet i: 1185
80. Survival for cancers of the genital organs. U.S. Department of Health, Education and Welfare, Public Health Service, National Institute of Health DHEW publication No. (NIH) 78–1543. Report No 5. Bethesda, Maryland.
81. Swanson J A, Chapler F K, Sherman B M, Crickard K 1978 Spontaneous pregnancy in women with a prolactin-producing pituitary adenoma. Fertil Steril 29: 629
82. Sweet D L Jr 1976 Malignant lymphoma: implications during the reproductive years and pregnancy. J Reprod Med 17: 198
83. Sweet D L Jr, Kinzie J 1976 Consequences of radiotherapy and antineoplastic therapy for the fetus. J Reprod Med 17: 241
84. Treves N, Holleb A I 1958 A report of 549 cases of breast cancer in women 35 years of age or younger. Surg Gynecol Obstet 107: 271
85. Wall J A, Lucci J A 1953 Adenocarcinoma of the corpus uteri and pelvic tuberculosis complicating pregnancy. Obstet Gynecol 2: 629
86. Werner S C 1962 The Thyroid. Harper & Row, New York
87. White K C 1973 Ovarian tumors in pregnancy. Am J Obstet Gynecol 116: 544
88. White L P, Linden G, Breslow L, Harzfeld L 1961 Studies on melanoma. The effect of pregnancy on survival in human melanoma. JAMA 117: 235

PART XIV

Surgical technique

69. Physical and surgical principles of carbon dioxide laser surgery in the lower genital tract

R. Reid   J. H. Dorsey

INTRODUCTION

The lower anogenital tract encompasses large areas of squamous mucosa and specialized hair-bearing skin, having a common origin from either the endodermal or ectodermal portions of the cloaca. Over the years, these elements are exposed to similar environmental carcinogens.[18,26,41] Hence, it is not surprising that squamous neoplasia is often *multicentric* (involving several distinct anatomic sites within the lower tract) and *multifocal* (originating at several discrete foci within each anatomic site). Such disease patterns pose therapeutic dilemmas, not easily solved by resective surgery. However, since most lesions are easily visualized, destructive techniques offer an easy way of removing large tracts of surface epithelium without sacrificing the underlying fibromuscular layers. Hence, for the gynecologist with sufficient training and discipline to exclude occult cancer, the carbon dioxide (CO_2) laser will produce results that cannot be attained with a cold knife.

LASER INSTRUMENTATION

What is a laser?

Lasers are devices in which an active medium is stimulated to emit an intense, narrow beam of coherent radiation (a series of monochromatic, highly parallel energy waves, each of which share the same spatial and temporal phase).[28,33] The generation of a laser beam is best explained in terms of the interaction of radiant energy with matter. Atoms and molecules can be thought of as quantum systems, wherein each of the electron orbits surrounding the nucleus represents a discrete energy level. When a quantity of transmitted energy impinges upon an atom or molecule, one of the orbiting electrons may be pushed into a more distant orbit. This process is called 'absorption', and corresponds to an increase in the kinetic energy carried by the displaced electron. When the electron drops back to its original orbit ('spontaneous emission'), the excess kinetic energy is emitted as a photon (packet) of electromagnetic radiation.

For a quantum system to emit *coherent radiation*, the lasing medium must be 'pumped' to a point of population inversion, by optical, radio frequency or electrical energy. 'Population inversion' refers to a situation in which there are more atoms or molecules in an upper level energy state than in one of the lower levels. Within a short time, some of these excited atoms or molecules will spontaneously return to the lower energy level, emitting photons that may strike atoms or molecules which are still at the higher level. The process stimulates the emission of a second photon that will be in the same phase and propagated in the same direction. Placing the laser medium in a cavity bounded at either end by mirrors having a common axis, causes the energy propagating back and forth between these mirrors to increase rapidly through an avalanche process. By making one of the mirrors partially transmissive, a portion of this energy will be emitted as a laser beam. The emitted radiation will have a wave length that is determined by the difference in energy levels responsible for the lasing action of that particular medium.

Space will not permit a fuller explanation of laser physics. However, to assist the reader, a glossary of relevant laser terminology is included at the end of the chapter.

Which laser is best?

Choosing the best laser for a given surgical application depends upon two things: (1) the absorptive characteristics of the tissue to be destroyed, and (2) the wavelength of the emitted radiation.

Absorptive characteristics

Electromagnetic radiation that impinges upon tissue can be reflected, scattered or absorbed. Absorption depends upon the presence of suitable chromophores (molecules capable of trapping the incident radiation and converting it to heat). The potential for therapeutic advantage depends upon the ratio of 'target' versus 'competing' chromophores. A high ratio will facilitate selective denaturation of diseased cells, while a low ratio will predispose to excessive damage within adjacent tissues.

The target chromophores for CO_2 lasers are water molecules. Hence, this wavelength offers a useful method for the photovaporization of any tissue which has a high aqueous content (epithelium, connective tissue, brain or muscle). In contrast, CO_2 laser energy is poorly absorbed by non-aqueous tissue (fat, bone), producing diffuse conduction burns or actual flaming, instead of a photovaporization crater. In the future, erbium YAG lasers may allow even more precise surgery upon aqueous tissues, with even less thermal damage to adjacent tissues.[63]

The target chromophores for Neodynium:YAG (Nd:YAG) radiation are proteins, and red or black pigment molecules. Hence, this instrument is an excellent tool for the deep destruction of diseased areas (e.g. endometrial ablation, treatment of superficial bladder cancers or coagulation of a vascular tumor bed), but is an atrocious choice for delicate surgery on an aqueous tissue.

Absorption of radiation from the visible portion of the electromagnetic spectrum (Argon, KTP and tunable dye lasers) is color-dependent, thus providing a potential for selective destruction of cells containing endogenous chromophores or light-sensitive drugs. Visible light lasers are generally used to selectively sclerose blood vessels. Hence, their usefulness depends upon the ratio of target (oxyhemoglobin) to competing chromophores (melanin or mitochondrial enzymes). Alternatively, red light from a tunable dye laser can be used to activate human porphyrin derivative (HPD), releasing toxic levels of singlet oxygen molecules.[27] Since HPD is selectively concentrated within malignant cells, this strategy could potentially destroy both non-resectable nodules and microscopic deposits within any area that can be adequately illuminated. The promise of new, more selective HPD derivatives may increase the therapeutic advantage to the point of making phototherapy a useful adjunct to any type of tumor debulking surgery.

Wavelength

The second consideration when choosing a laser is that of wave length, since this parameter defines both the type of tissue interaction and the volume of tissue that will be denatured by the incident radiation.

(1) **Tissue interactions.** Absorption of *high-energy* photons (gamma rays, X-rays, and ultraviolet light) produces electron excitations that may result in ionization, dissolution of covalent bonds and the formation of reactive molecular fragments. At the other end of the electromagnetic spectrum, radiation of increasingly *longer wavelength* exists as radio waves. Photons from the *middle* of the spectrum (visible light, infrared radiation, and microwaves) have insufficient energy to induce ionization. Rather, absorption of photons from this portion of the spectrum causes an increase in molecular vibration or molecular rotation, leading to heat production. Such phenomena are termed thermal interactions (Fig. 69.1).

Beam energy is inversely proportional to wavelength. Hence, wavelength determines whether a laser beam will

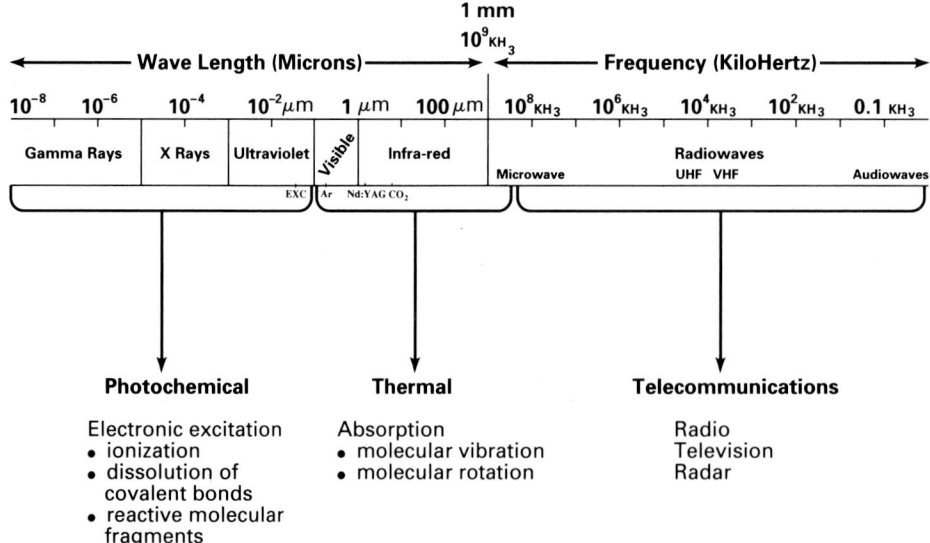

Fig. 69.1 A simplified diagram showing the different types of tissue interaction that occur with laser energy from various points in the electromagnetic spectrum. (Reproduced from Reid et al (1985),[42] with permission.)

produce ionization (excimer lasers) or thermal interactions (dye, argon, KTP, Nd:YAG and CO_2 lasers). In addition, wavelength also determines whether absorption will be color-dependent (dye and Nd:YAG) or color-independent (excimer and CO_2).

(2) Irradiance volume. The fraction of a given beam that will be absorbed within, or transmitted through, a given piece of tissue is also dependent upon wavelength. As described by Beer's law, the proportion of an incident beam that is transmitted through a tissue slab is determined from the equation:

$$I_t = I_0 . 10^{-\alpha x}$$

where I_t = transmitted intensity, I_0 = incident intensity, α = the absorption coefficient of the incident energy, as determined by the wavelength, and X = the thickness of tissue irradiated. If tissue thickness is set at $X = 1/\alpha$, Beer's law is reduced to the formula:

$$I_t = I_0 . 10^{-1}$$

Since 10^{-1} equates with one tenth, this simplified formula describes a distance from the tissue surface at which the incident beam has been reduced to 10% of its initial intensity. In other words, the *critical volume* of tissue needed to absorb 90% of the incident radiation is defined by the reciprocal of the absorption coefficient. This concept of critical volume is the major determinant of the type of surgical wound that will result at the impact site.[33] Photons of near infrared radiation (Nd:YAG laser emissions of wave length = 1.06 μm) display extensive scatter and relatively long extinction lengths. In contrast, mid infrared radiation (e.g., CO_2 laser emissions of wave length = 10.6 μm) have a very short extinction length and negligible scatter within tissues of high water content.

The surgical importance of these differences is best appreciated by considering the tissue effects of a small packet of photons from either a CO_2 or an Nd:YAG laser, each beam having an area of 1 mm^2. The very short extinction length (0.03 mm) of radiation from the *carbon dioxide* laser leads to absorption within a small critical volume (only 3×10^{-2} mm^3) (Fig. 69.2A). Such confined energy uptake results in (1) flash boiling of intracellular and extracellular water and (2) heating to incandescence of any anhydrous tissue remnants (mainly proteins and nucleic acids). Flash boiling results in steam formation, leading to explosive disruption of tissue at the impact site. In practice, this zone of vaporization is surrounded by a narrow, charred zone of thermal necrosis. Surrounding this is another zone of sublethal thermal injury. These effects are caused by thermal diffusion and the unequal energy distribution within the laser beam.

In contrast, the small packet of photons of Nd:YAG energy will display extensive lateral, backward and forward scatter, enlarging the effective diameter of irradiance to about 9 mm^2. In addition, the shorter wavelength will extend the extinction length to about 2 mm. Hence, the critical volume of tissue required to absorb a photon of Nd:YAG energy is approximated by a circular disc having a base area of about 9 mm^2, a height of about 2 mm and a volume of approximately 18 mm^3 (Fig. 69.2B). This dispersed pattern of energy absorption for Nd:YAG radiation results in the heating of relatively large tissue volumes to much lower temperatures. As a consequence of these spectral absorption differences, the CO_2 laser has become the 'workhorse' of modern laser surgery. Although it is surgically feasible to excise or ablate genital neoplasia by delivery of Nd:YAG energy through artificial sapphire tips, the laws of physics mandate that results must inevitably be inferior to that which could have been achieved through the skillful use of a CO_2 laser. Hence, as a rule of thumb, whenever an operation can be done with the CO_2 laser, this should be the automatic choice.

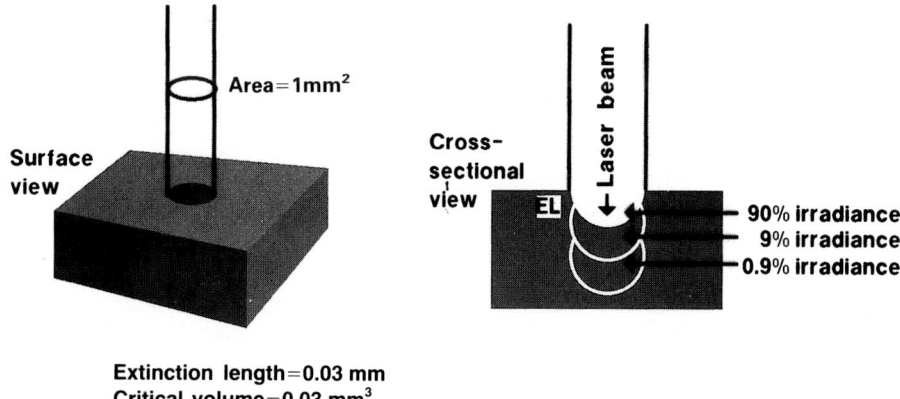

Fig. 69.2A The critical volume affected by a theoretic impact upon aqueous tissue by a single photon of CO_2 laser radiation having a perfectly uniform energy distribution. Because of the high affinity of this mid-infrared wavelength for water, 90% of the incident energy is absorbed within 0.03 mm^3. Moreover, because of negligible lateral scatter, the diameter of the resultant wound will correspond to the diameter of the incident beam.

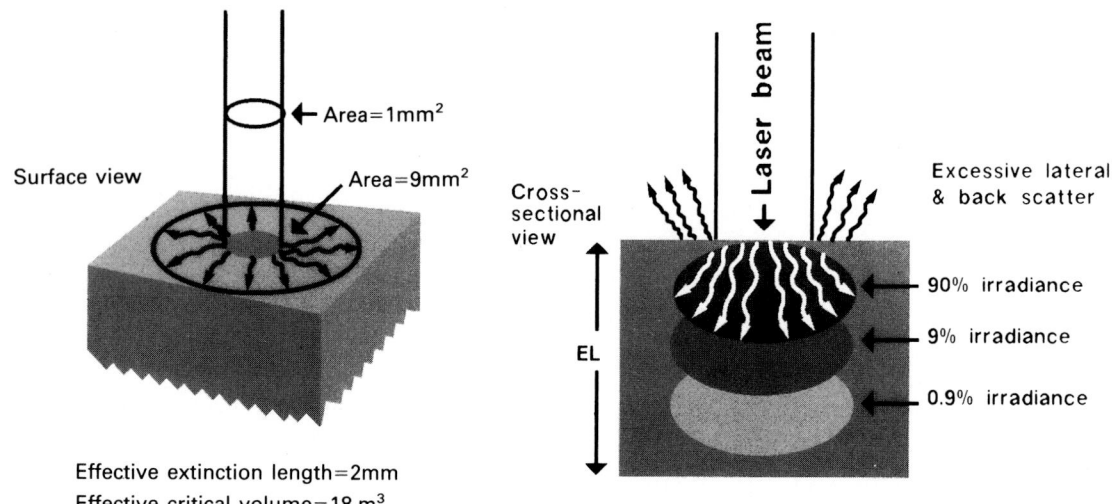

Fig. 69.2B The much larger critical volume affected by an impact from a single, uniformly distributed photon of Nd:YAG radiation. The higher energy and lower absorption coefficient of this near infrared would result in much deeper tissue penetration (say, 2 mm), and the dispersed pattern of absorption would destroy a much wider tissue volume (say, 18 mm³). Hence, the critical volume needed to absorb 90% of the incident Nd:YAG photon would be about 600 times larger than for the CO_2 photon. For artistic convenience, the Nd:YAG diagram is drawn to a smaller scale.

What advantages does the carbon dioxide laser offer?

Laser usage has expanded enormously over the last decade, particularly in the male and female genital tracts. Results are generally reported in glowing terms, and there is widespread belief that surgical success is essentially guaranteed by the technical sophistication of the CO_2 laser. Unhappily, but not unexpectedly, such beliefs are ill-founded.

Certainly, because of the affinity of water for mid-infrared radiation, optical energy from the CO_2 laser displays several unique surgical properties: (1) diseased volumes can be vaporized under precise visual control; (2) there need be little or no mechanical contact with the intended target; (3) heat propagation to adjacent tissue can be minimal; (4) microorganisms at the impact site will be automatically destroyed; and (5) vessels smaller than 0.5 mm (arterioles) will be thermally sealed. Unfortunately, these surgical advantages are easily dissipated by unskilled use.[43]

The CO_2 laser resembles the hot cautery, the electrodiathermy and the cryosurgical probe, in that all are instruments of thermal destruction. With conventional devices, lateral heat propagation declines down a slow, linear gradient. Adjacent tissues must recover from the ill effects of a diffuse conduction burn or frostbite before the healing response can begin. Moreover, collagen damaged by inept laser surgery can remain 'mummified' in the dermis for many months, where it acts to delay healing and promote cicatrization.[24] In contrast, if the laser is used skillfully, the heating of adjacent tissues will decline exponentially, allowing thermal injury to be confined to a very narrow (50 μm) and sharply defined band.[62] Hence,

healing will begin immediately, resulting in re-epithelialization before undue collagen deposition can occur.[45]

Lasers are like violins: an instrument of symphony in skilled hands, but otherwise productive of a rude cacaphony. Delusions born of a naive 'knowledge' of physics can lure ordinarily sensible physicians into the creation of devastating thermal injuries. The authors are aware of one ileal burn (during an inept laser conization), one rectovaginal fistula, two vesicovaginal fistulae, several third degree burns of vulvar or perianal skin (Fig. 69.3) and numerous serious cervical deformities (Fig. 69.4). In other words, the real hazards of lasers arise from the surgeon's lack of sophistication, rather than from the somewhat remote risk of accidental mishap.[43] Unless strategies are employed to restrict the diffusion of heat to adjacent tissues during photovaporization, the CO_2 laser can produce worse conduction burns than would seem possible with conventional instrumentation.

PHYSICAL PRINCIPLES GOVERNING SURGICAL CONTROL OF CARBON DIOXIDE LASERS

Laser surgery is defined as *tissue denaturation through the direct thermal effects of intense electromagnetic radiation*, as opposed to tissue denaturation by heat conduction from the laser crater. In expert hands, lateral heat conduction is kept to the bare minimum. Selective destruction of diseased foci is accomplished almost exclusively by radiant heat (which produces a sharply localized zone of thermal necrosis, in accordance with Beer's law),[62] rather than by thermal conduction (which produces a diffuse, poorly controllable burn

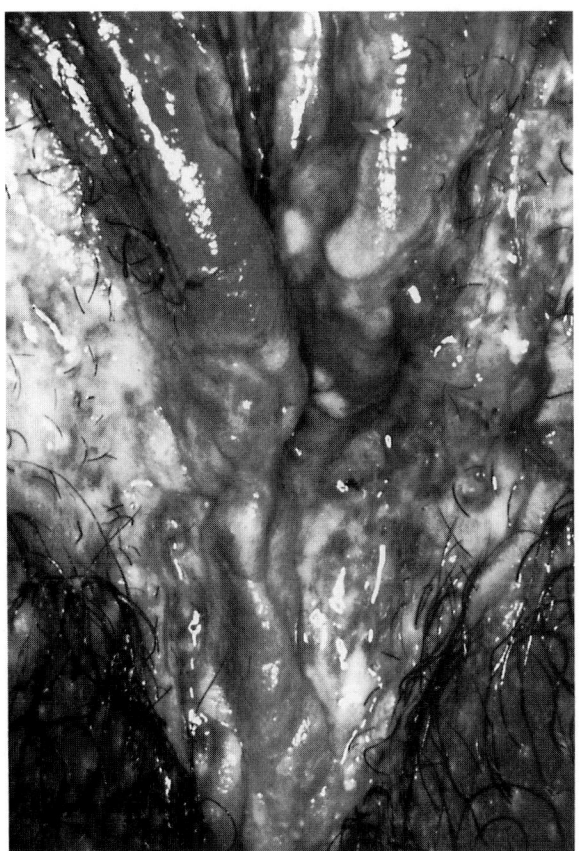

Fig. 69.3 A third degree burn of the vulva, produced by excessive heat conduction to the underlying tissues.

Table 69.1 The six physical principles underlying surgical expertise with the CO_2 laser

Parameters concerned with minimizing thermal diffusion
1. Use rapid superpulse or chopped wave, rather than continuous wave, thus preventing thermal relaxation between pulses.
2. Minimize duration of thermal diffusion, by using high power settings (to deliver the necessary energy as rapidly as possible).
3. Avoid carbonization of the impact crater, by keeping power density > 750 W/cm^2, wiping away debris, performing ablations with the operating microscope and not carmalizing extravasated blood.

Parameters influencing surgical control
4. Tailor pulse fluence or average power density to individual hand/eye speed.
5. Control beam geometry by incremental focus/defocus of the microslad, using tightly focused spots for incision and rounded beams for ablation.
6. Maintain high power in delicate situations, using shuttered pulses to maintain surgical control.

and a wide zone of sublethal injury). Achieving this objective depends upon the sophisticated (rather than simplistic) application of the laws of physics.

Of the six physical principles described in this section, the first three are concerned primarily with optimizing the distribution of the incident energy, and the last three with allowing the surgeon to control the extent of tissue destruction (Table 69.1).

Choice of an optimal temporal mode

In molecular terms, lateral heat conduction is a relatively slow event. For example, it takes about 600 μs for a col-

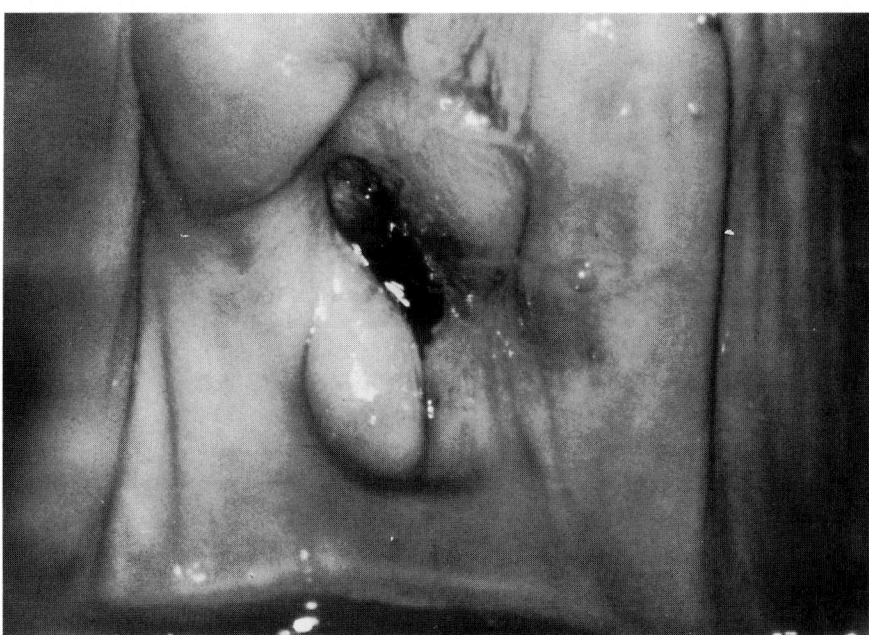

Fig. 69.4 Marked cervical deformity, produced by unskilled laser surgery.

SUPERPULSE

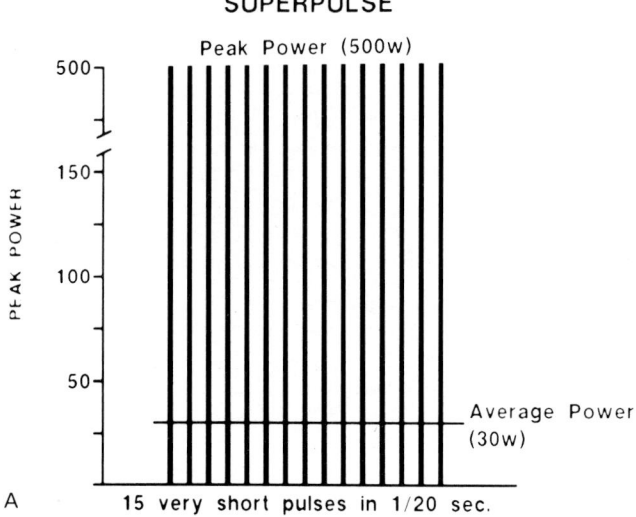

A

CHOPPED WAVE

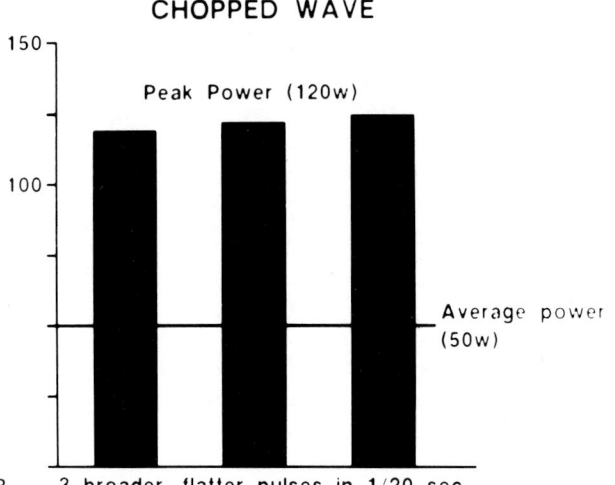

B

CONTINUOUS WAVE

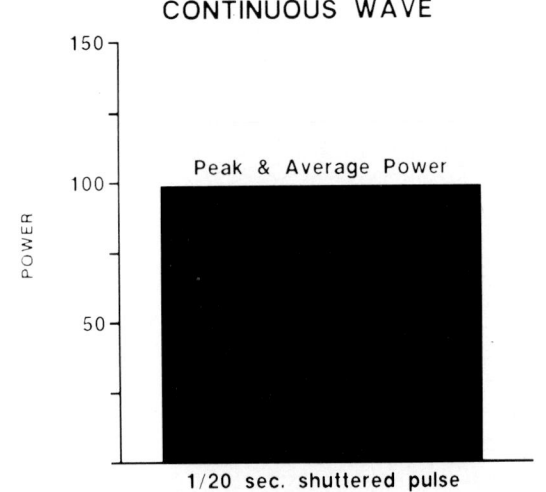

C

Fig. 69.5 A diagram showing the power/time characteristics of (A) a 1/20 s (0.5 ms) shuttered pulse of continuous wave laser energy, (B) a 1/20 s burst of superpulsed laser energy, comprising, say, 15 pulses of 300 μs duration, (C) a 1/20 s burst of chopped wave (duty cycle 6:12).

lagen matrix, suspended within an aqueous solution (i.e. dermis) to reach the critical temperature (65°C) for thermal denaturation.[62] Hence, if laser energy of sufficient fluence is supplied in pulses that are of shorter duration than this thermal relaxation time, the zone of coagulation at the crater base can be restricted to 70 μm or less. In contrast, if pulse duration is allowed to equal or exceed the thermal relaxation time of the target tissue, then the zone of coagulation necrosis will increase dramatically (e.g., 170 μm for a 2 μs pulse, 750 μm for a 1/20 second pulse).[62] To capitalize on this fact, modern lasers are now designed to operate in temporal modes other than continuous wave (Fig. 69.5).

For optimal tissue effects, a number of conditions must be fulfilled. (1) Pulse duration should be sufficiently short as to photovaporize a small volume with maximal efficiency. In contrast, if heat produced through the absorption of this same packet of photons is allowed to diffuse into adjacent tissues, then the proportion of photovaporization falls and the proportion of photocoagulation rises. Heat will accumulate between pulses, creating lateral heat conduction; (2) Interpulse intervals must be sufficiently broad as to allow cooling of the impact site (by radiation back into the atmosphere). A duty cycle (ratio of on:off time) of about 1:3 appears ideal. (3) The fluence (the rate of energy delivery) of each pulse must be significantly greater than the vaporization threshold (e.g. about 4 J/cm^2 for dermis). Under these circumstances, the distribution of tissue damage will conform to the optical penetration depth of the laser (i.e the critical volume of 1/α as described by Beer's law), rather than to a less perfect model dependent upon thermal diffusion.

Given a 100 W laser, optimal tissue effects would require a peak pulse of 500 to 700 W, a pulse duration of about 300 μs and an interpulse interval of about 3 ms. However, the choice of a narrow pulse width and low pulse frequency is not without disadvantage. Available power is reduced to about one-third of that attainable from the same laser tube in the continuous mode. Unfortunately, rapid superpulse has one major disadvantage: the choice of a short duty cycle will reduce power output by about two-thirds, making it impractical to treat large volumes of diseased epithelium with this temporal mode. Hence, in practice, rapid superpulse is generally reserved for situations in which small tissue volumes need to be treated with maximal precision.

A handy compromise between the high precision of rapid superpulse and the high power of continuous wave is obtained from the *chopped mode*, in which the laser tube is electrically pulsed to emit broader, flatter pulses with a shortened interpulse interval between pulses. Consider, for example, the electrical pulsing of a 120 W laser tube, governed such that the ratio of on:off time will never exceed 5:1. When used at the highest duty cycle, maximal output would be 100 W (i.e., 120 × 5/6). Conversely, selecting a 1:9 duty cycle would produce an output of only 12 W (i.e. 120 × 1/10). Because the peak power of each pulse is not amplified, an electrically pulsed laser tube does not have a refractory phase when used in chopped mode. Hence, repetition rate can be increased to virtually any frequency. However, as pulse frequency approaches a duty cycle of 2:1, heat will accumulate at the impact site, and the clinical effects will resemble those of a continuous wave laser. Thus, the best compromise is a duty cycle of about 1:1 producing 60 W of power output, while preserving about half of the interpulse cooling.

Rapid delivery of the required energy dose

Energy delivered to tissue is given by the formula:

$$\underset{\text{(J)}}{\text{Delivered energy}} = \underset{\text{(W)}}{\text{Beam power}} \times \underset{\text{(S)}}{\text{Exposure time}}$$

A given amount of energy will denature the same mass of tissue, regardless of the rate of energy delivery. In other words, irradiating with 100 W for 1 second or 10 W for 10 seconds will deliver 100 J of infrared energy in either instance. However, different rates of energy delivery produce profoundly different surgical effects.

With optimal equipment (i.e. a super-pulsed laser of adequate fluence, emitting pulses shorter than the thermal relaxation time and interspersed by sufficient cooling intervals), thermal damage is a function of the optical properties of the incident energy.[62] In contrast, when pulse duration exceeds thermal relaxation time, heat accumulates at the surface of the impact crater and lateral conduction begins. Tissue damage is now primarily a function of exposure time, such that low rates of energy delivery will unduly prolong exposure time (Fig. 69.6). Hence, it is surprising that surgeons should be so unaware of the dangers of using the laser at a low power setting, and so reluctant to employ high powers as a strategy for shortening exposure times. Experience from daily living teaches that, if a hot object be touched by flesh, the severity of burning is dependent upon the duration of contact. Why would it be different for heat conduction from the laser crater? In particular, if the expert cannot obtain good results with low rates of energy delivery, then surely it is indefensible to counsel the novice surgeon to begin operating at low wattages. Since tissue killed by conducted heat appears normal at the time of injury, such discrepancy between perception and reality can lead the unwary surgeon into error (Figs 69.3 and 69.4).

The magnitude of this error is reflected by an analysis of healing times, encountered at different phases during the evolution of the first author's present techniques. Up until

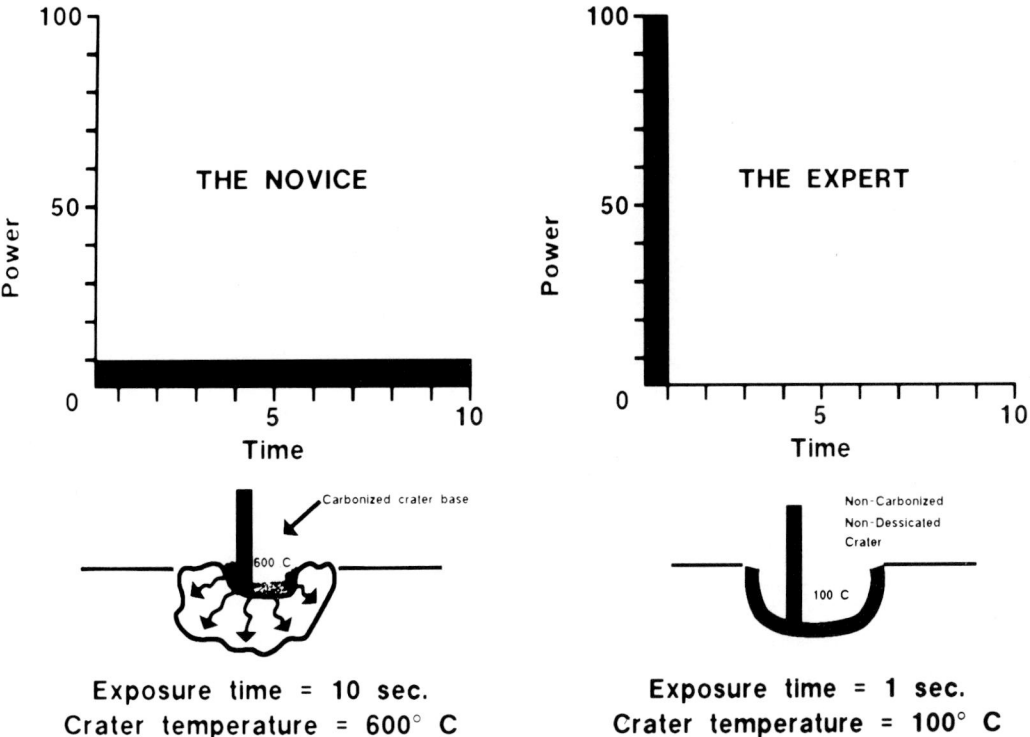

Fig. 69.6 Diagram showing how novice laser surgeons (left) erode the potential advantages of the CO$_2$ laser through the use of low rates of energy delivery, resulting in both prolonged durations of lateral heat conduction and higher crater temperatures. Only the expert (right), using maximal rates of energy delivery, is successful in minimizing thermal injury to adjacent tissues.

1984, there were no effective methods for reliably 'flattening' energy distribution within the incident laser beam. Hence, surgical control hinged upon the choice of low powers (<30 W of continuous wave energy), delivered at relatively low power densities (450 W/cm²).[42] However, as we learned to control surgical effects by manipulating beam geometry (see below), it was soon noticed that use of our continuous wave laser at maximal power (80 W) produced better results.[45] Healing times of vulvar epithelia were reduced by an average of 3 days (Fig. 69.7) and complication rates fell from 10.3% to 6.5%. With the purchase of a laser which delivered rapid superpulse and chopped wave, surgical morbidity was reduced even further. Healing times for patients treated to a shallow plane fell from 17 to 10 days, while healing from a deep plane was shortened from 22 to 16 days (Fig. 69.7). Postoperative pain was greatly ameliorated, and the incidence of heat related complications was quartered (from 10.3% to 2.7%).

Laser surgeons must weigh the intuitive fear of high power against the proven risks of using low powers. Unfortunately, the inappropriate use of low power outputs, arising out of the misdirected sense of caution, is still the most damaging error made by less skilled surgeons.[43] As a rule of thumb, effective photovaporization of a cervical lesion in the continuous wave requires at least 25 W of power. Paradoxically, because vulvar epithelia are more susceptible to untoward thermal effects, the safe photovaporization of vulvar and vaginal lesions requires at least 40 W of power in the continuous wave mode.

Avoiding carbonization within the laser crater

If surgical lasers emitted parallel beams of uniform intensity, power output would be the major factor in controlling tissue effects. However, CO_2 laser tubes used in medicine usually have diameters of 1 to 2 cm, producing beams that are too wide for direct surgical use. In order to limit incision width, the emergent beam must be focused to a small diameter, thereby increasing effective power ('power density') within the focal spot by as much as 10 000 times (Fig. 69.8). Although intensity varies substantially from point to point within the focal spot, the surgical effects of increasing effective beam power by focusing are best quantified by estimating average energy intensity within the central 86% of the incident beam.

Tissues irradiated at relatively low rates of irradiance (power density) tend to desiccate before the threshold for actual photovaporization is reached. Such desiccation produces areas of anhydrous protein which will carbonize, just as witnessed in the barbecuing of a steak. Continued irradiance of a carbonized impact surface will raise crater

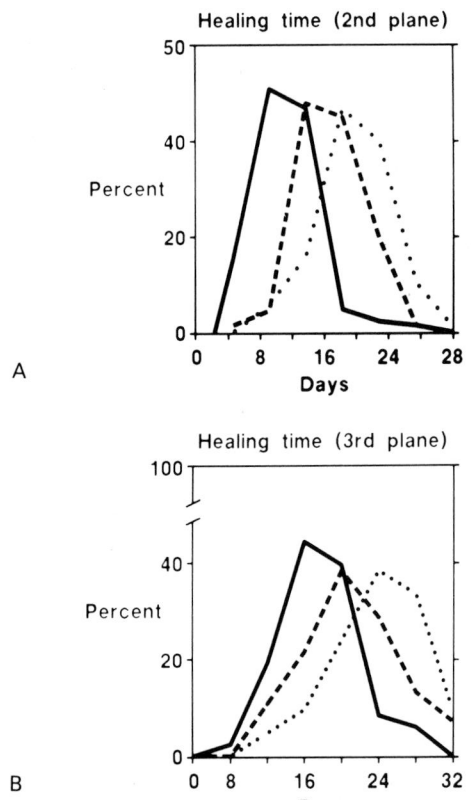

Fig. 69.7 Two graphs showing the reduction in healing time of vulvar epithelium attributable to improved heat control strategies. (A) Healing from a superficial level (second plane). (B) Healing from a deeper level (third plane). Superpulse and chopped wave are shown as the solid line, high power continuous wave as the slashed line and low power continuous wave as the dotted line. (Reproduced from Reid et al (1990),[45] with permission.)

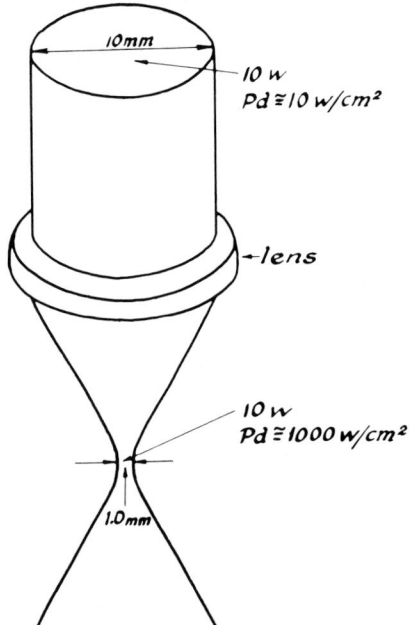

Fig. 69.8 The effect of focusing upon power density. A 10 W output from a 1 cm laser tube would have an average power density of 10 W/cm². By focusing this 10 W beam to a 1 mm spot, the effective beam power at the point of impact will be increased one hundred fold, to 1000 W/cm². (Reproduced from Fuller (1985),[16] with permission.)

temperatures from 100°C to more than 600°C, thereby increasing the conduction gradient (Fig. 69.9).

Allowing carbonization within the laser crater will inevitably produce a conduction burn, similar to (or worse than) that which would have followed the use of electrocautery or cryosurgery. This error generally arises in one of four ways:

1. Excessive defocus of the laser beam, such that average power density falls below 750 W/cm^2 and beam geometry assumes a 'watch glass' contour (see p. 1097).
2. Attempting ablative surgery with a hand probe (see p. 1101).

3. Failing to wipe accumulated debris from the laser crater (see p. 1103).
4. Irradiating a bleeding point at low power density, thus caramelizing hemoglobin at the surface but doing little to coagulate the underlying vessel wall (see p. 1101).

Tailoring power density to surgical requirements

When not using optimal superpulse, surgical control is closely tied to the effective power within the focal spot. Hence, tissue effects are dependent upon power density, rather than the level of raw power within the unfocused

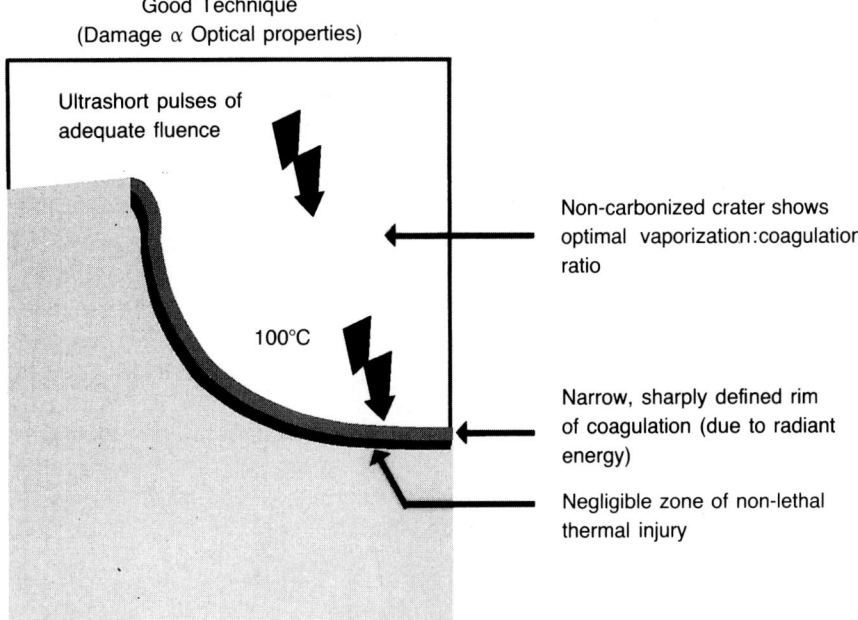

Good Technique
(Damage α Optical properties)

Ultrashort pulses of adequate fluence

100°C

Non-carbonized crater shows optimal vaporization:coagulation ratio

Narrow, sharply defined rim of coagulation (due to radiant energy)

Negligible zone of non-lethal thermal injury

A

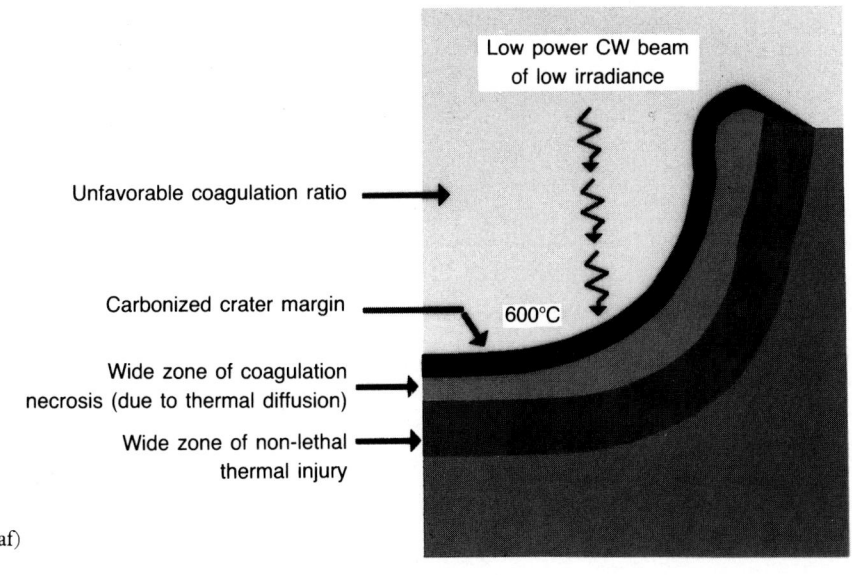

Poor Technique
(Damage α Thermal diffusion)

Low power CW beam of low irradiance

600°C

Unfavorable coagulation ratio

Carbonized crater margin

Wide zone of coagulation necrosis (due to thermal diffusion)

Wide zone of non-lethal thermal injury

B

Fig. 69.9 (caption overleaf)

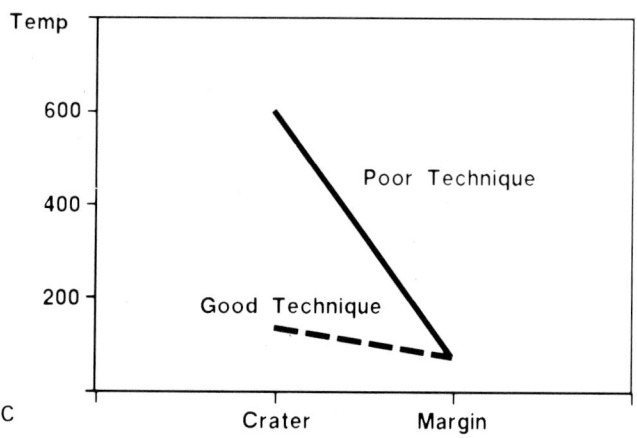

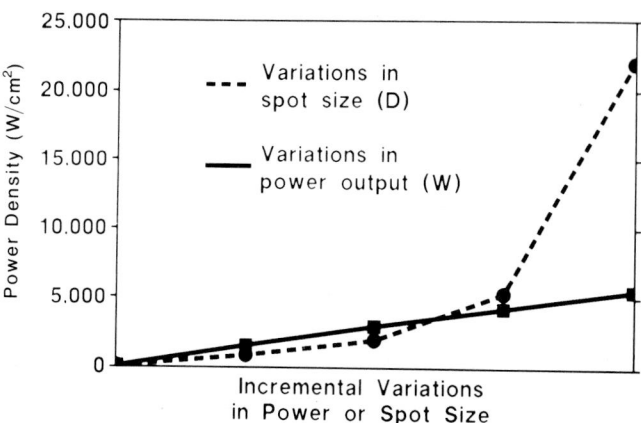

Fig. 69.9 A diagram comparing the thermal conduction gradients from (A) a non-carbonized (above) and (B) a carbonized (below) crater. With lower irradiance levels, there will be a relatively thick zone of tissue heated *above* the coagulation threshold, but *below* the vaporization threshold. Since such a coagulum is relatively anhydrous, this residue is no longer capable of vaporization. Rather, subsequent photons will carbonize and heat this residue to crater temperatures of the order of 600°C. (C) Effect of technique upon thermal conduction gradients.

Fig. 69.10 The different relative effects of increases in power output (a linear variable) versus reduction in spot size (a quadratic variable). Note that variations in spot size are plotted in an inverse direction, such that any reductions of spot diameter move the curve to the right side of the graph. Since average power density is a composite variable, power output can always be used at the maximum, by broadening the spot to compensate for any difficulties caused by turning up the power.

beam. Surgeons must be quite clear about this distinction. *Power output* (the speed of energy delivery from the laser tube) is a major factor in limiting thermal diffusion, but is irrelevant to surgical control or the qualitative nature of the resulting laser:tissue interaction. In contrast, *power density* (average power within the focal spot) is an important control variable. Irradiance levels determine both the qualitative interaction (tissue welding, photocoagulation, photovaporization or acoustic shock wave generation) and the speed of cut. However, provided that irradiance is maintained above the carbonization range, small changes in power density have little effect upon the degree of the diffusion to adjacent tissues.

Precise calculation of average power density is a complex exercise. However, for clinical purposes, a sufficiently accurate approximation is given by the formula:[16]

$$PD = \frac{100 \times W}{D^2} \ W/cm^2$$

where W = the power output shown by the in-line power meter on the laser console (in watts), and D = the measured diameter (in mm) of the imprint left by a 10 watt, 0.1 second pulse on a moistened tongue depressor. Since the area of a circle varies according to the square of its radius, any change in spot size will have a quadratic effect upon energy intensity within the focal spot. In contrast, increasing or decreasing the power output from the laser tube exerts only a linear effect upon power density (Fig. 69.10).

Despite the undoubted importance of average power density, the true influence of this parameter is poorly understood. Since minor variations are of no consequence,

power density is best seen as an essential concept rather than as an actual strategy for fine control. As a concept, power density is the key to two critical surgical effects:

(1) **Type of tissue interaction.** Different types of tissue interaction are produced by beams of different intensities (Fig. 69.11). Very low levels heat tissues just enough to denature proteins, thus permitting their use for tissue welding. Beams with an energy intensity of >100 W/cm² cause tissue removal by photovaporization, although carbonization limits the usefulness of this effect at the lower end of this range. Power densities >10 000 W/cm² cause ultra rapid photovaporization suited to thermal incision rather than shallow ablation. Finally, extremely high power densities (>10⁶ W/cm²) result in plasma formation and acoustic shock waves, producing mechanical tearing of tissues, rather than thermal denaturation.

(2) **Speed of cut.** Speed of cut is critical, since everyone's hand-eye coordination is governed by finite limits. When using the laser to make deep thermal incision, power densities of >50 000 W/cm² are easy to control, requiring about the same speed of movement as cutting with a sharp knife. When the objective is to ablate a wide field of epithelium to a shallow depth, average power density must be kept within the 750 to 2000 W/cm² range, since higher levels would require excessively rapid hand movements. Nonetheless, provided that a laser is equipped with a proper defocusing device, these limitations should seldom prevent the expert from capitalizing upon the full power attainable from any medical laser. Broadening spot diameter can make power outputs of 10 to 1000 W equally manageable. In contrast, focusing a 10 W beam to a spot diameter of 0.2 mm would produce an average power density of 25 000 W/cm², making it impossible for even the

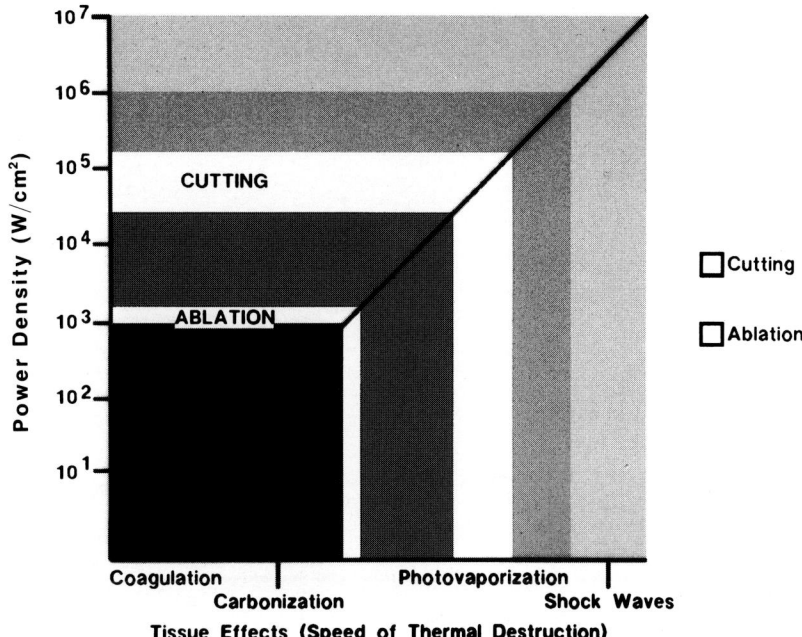

Fig. 69.11 Different qualitative effects (shown on the X axis), produced by different power densities (shown as a log scale on the Y axis). At low levels of irradiance (< 750 W/cm²) tissue heating is generally insufficient to reach the threshold of vaporization, hence, coagulation predominates over sublimation. However, at irradiance levels of 1000 to 500 000 W/cm², the rate of tissue heating is sufficient to ensure a predominance of vaporization. Beyond 500 000 W/cm², there will be electron stripping (analogous to a lightning bolt), resulting in acoustic shock waves and tissue tearing. Although photovaporization occurs across a wide range of irradiance levels, the clinical realities of beam control dictate that both ablation and incision be done within quite narrow limits.

most adroit surgeon to use such a beam for surface ablation.

Adjusting beam geometry to control crater shape

Because of the emphasis that has hitherto been placed upon the concept of average power density to describe the average intensity within the focal spot, there is a tendency to think of this value as being widely representative of energy intensity throughout the impact crater. In reality, even within an unfocused beam emitted from the laser tube, there is substantial variation in energy intensity from point to point within the focal spot. Obviously, these differences in energy intensity will affect the shape of the resultant crater at the point of impact. Points of higher energy intensity (usually the center of the beam) will vaporize more tissue per unit time than points of lower energy intensity (usually situated at the beam periphery). That is to say, the actual shape of the impact crater will be a mirror image of the energy profile of the incident beam.

The degree of variation in energy intensity within the raw beam is amplified many times by the focusing that occurs within the beam delivery system (Fig. 69.12). At points of extreme defocus, the energy profile will have an excessively flat geometry. Point Z therefore produces a 'watch-glass'-like defect crater characterized by excessive coagulation at the crater margin but minimal vaporization in the crater itself. Conversely, sharp focusing will concentrate the vast majority of incident photons at the center of the focal spot. That is to say, energy absorption at point X greatly exceeds the thresholds for both coagulation and vaporization, producing a narrow, deep crater shaped like a 'golf tee'. Between these two extremes (points X and Z in Fig. 69.12), there is a region of defocus (point Y) that will create a 'rounded' beam geometry. 'Rounding' means that the energy profile has been flattened to the point where beam amplitude is about half the spot diameter. The volume of tissue destruction therefore conforms to one-half of an imaginary sphere, crater depth approximating one radius and spot diameter approximating two radii. In defocusing to point Y, incident energy has to be balanced against the area of the focal spot. Ideally, if one is using rapid superpulse, fluence should approach or exceed the vaporization threshold, such that each pulse will sublimate a critical volume of target tissue. Alternatively, if using

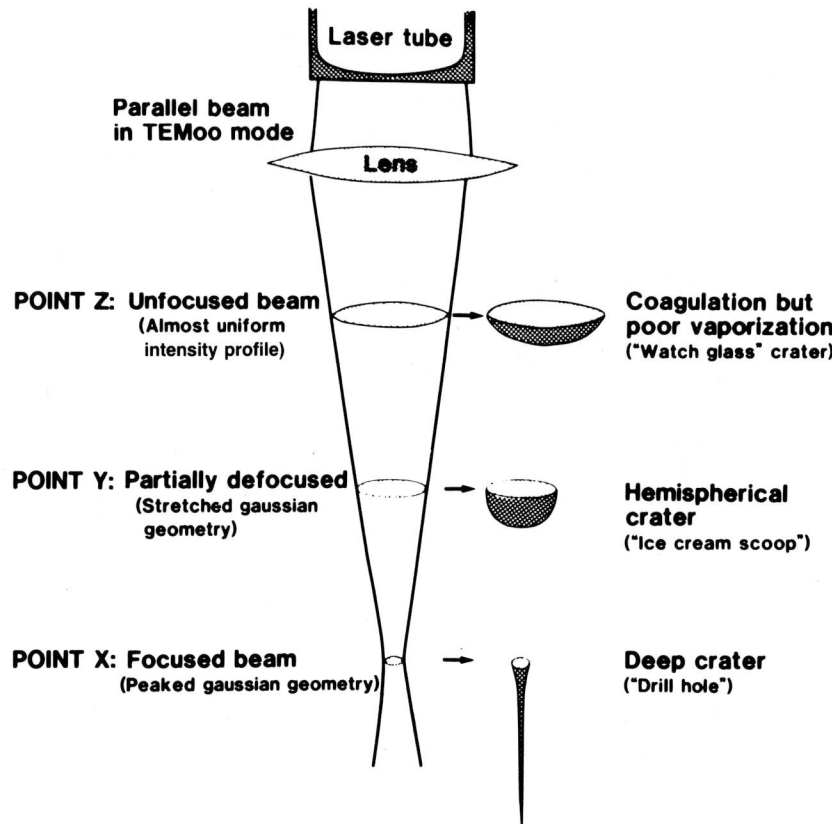

Fig. 69.12 The effect of defocusing on beam geometry. Whereas incisions are best made with a tightly focused beam (point X), surface ablation should always be done at a point of partial defocus (point Y). Fully defocused beams cause extensive char, with negligible penetration (point Z), and therefore have no surgical applications. (Redrawn from Reid et al (1985)[42].)

pulse durations longer than thermal relaxation time, irradiance must be sufficient to yield a favorable balance between sublimation and thermal coagulation. In either instance, rounding beam geometry will produce a shallow crater, like an 'ice cream scoop'. The ability to progressively defocus beam geometry until this hemispheric shape is reached is a crucial but neglected aspect of surgical control (Fig. 69.13). Incisions are always made with a tightly focused beam, and shallow photovaporization is always done with a beam defocused to the point of an hemispheric geometry. These considerations hold true at all anatomic sites and for all surgical situations. Any XY hybrid will be too blunt for optimal cutting (resulting in a three dimension incision), yet too sharp for controlled photovaporization (resulting in bleeding from the vessels transected at the base of the crater; Fig. 69.13B). Likewise, any YZ hybrid will have produced an excessive zone of coagulation necrosis (resulting in carbonization and excessive thermal injury; Fig. 69.13B).

In the past, beam geometry was controlled by mismatching the focal lengths of the optical and laser lenses (e.g. 300 mm visual and a 200 mm laser lens). However, modern lasers are now equipped with microslad defocusing devices, which contain both a converging and a diverging lens (Fig. 69.13C). Incisions are done at the point of 'zero defocus' wherein both lenses are in apposition and therefore behave like a single convex lens (Fig. 69.14A). Epithelial ablation is done by incrementally winding the microslad to progressive points of defocus, until a 1/10 second impact leaves an approximately hemispherical crater on the tongue blade (Fig. 69.14B).

BEAM GEOMETRY

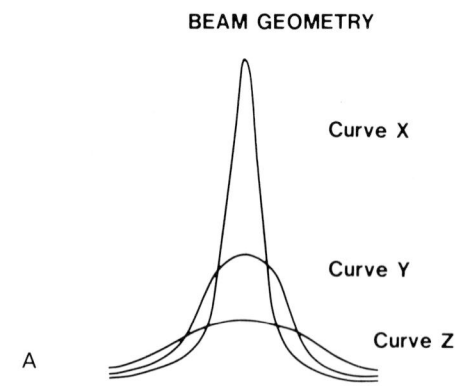

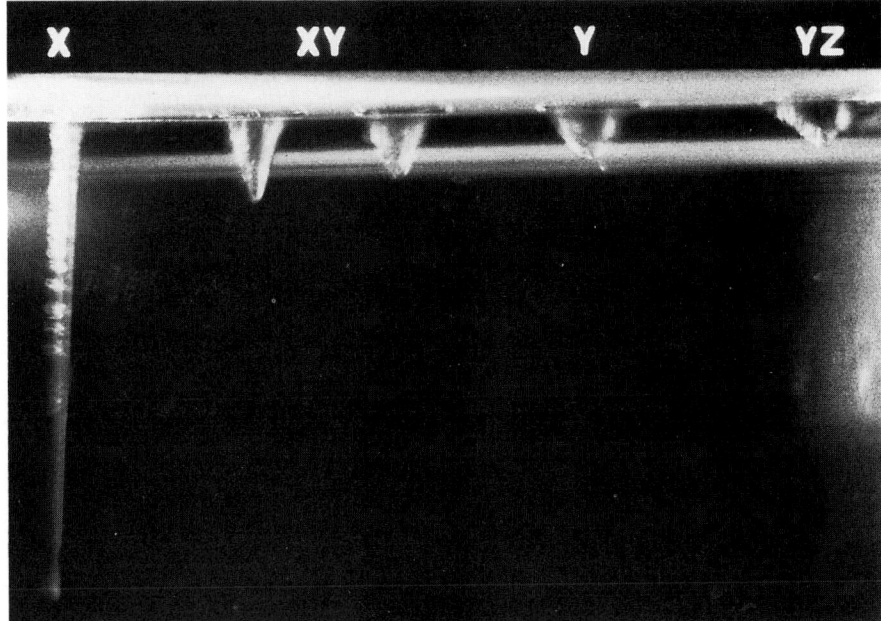

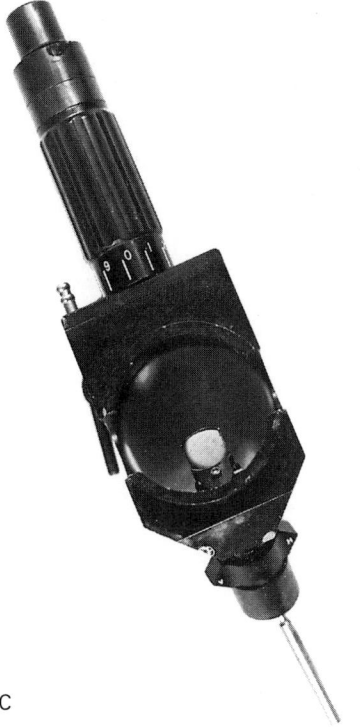

Fig. 69.13 (A) Three schematic intensity profiles showing beam geometry at sharp focus (point X), partial focus (point Y) and complete defocus (point Z). Craters corresponding to these points are shown in Figure 69.12. (Reproduced from R. Reid's teaching slides on 'Expert Laser Surgery'.) (B) Impact craters made by a laser beam at different points of focus, fired into the cross cut end of a plexiglass block. The craters are now viewed at right angles to the direction in which the laser beam traveled. Point X is the correct geometry for incision, and point Y is correct for shallow ablation. Hybrids XY and YZ are not suitable for surgical use. (Photograph courtesy of G. Absten, Columbus, Ohio.) (C) A photograph of an actual microslad defocusing device, used to create incremental defocus of the laser beam.

Shuttered pulses to improve delicate surgical control

Since quality of outcome is directly proportional to the speed of energy delivery, the surgeon must not turn the power down in delicate situations (for example, destruction of a lesion on the glans clitoris). Instead, the beam (whether continuous wave or superpulse) should be delivered in 1/10 to 1/20s bursts, by appropriate use of the internal shutter mechanism (Fig. 69.15). This strategy permits ample reaction time between pulses, thereby allowing the surgeon to maintain an optimal rate of energy delivery.

SURGICAL PRINCIPLES GOVERNING CONTROL OF THE CARBON DIOXIDE LASER

Simply observing optimal physical principles does not guarantee success. As in other forms of surgery, best results depend upon both sound theoretic principles and practical strategies for implementing the surgical objectives.[38]

Choice of an appropriate beam delivery system

Laser energy emerges from the optical resonance tube as a highly collimated beam. However, energy generated with medical lasers never reaches the tissue as a parallel beam. Rather, collimation is destroyed by the various delivery systems, either through beam divergence within a fiber-optic or through beam focusing within a lens system.[28]

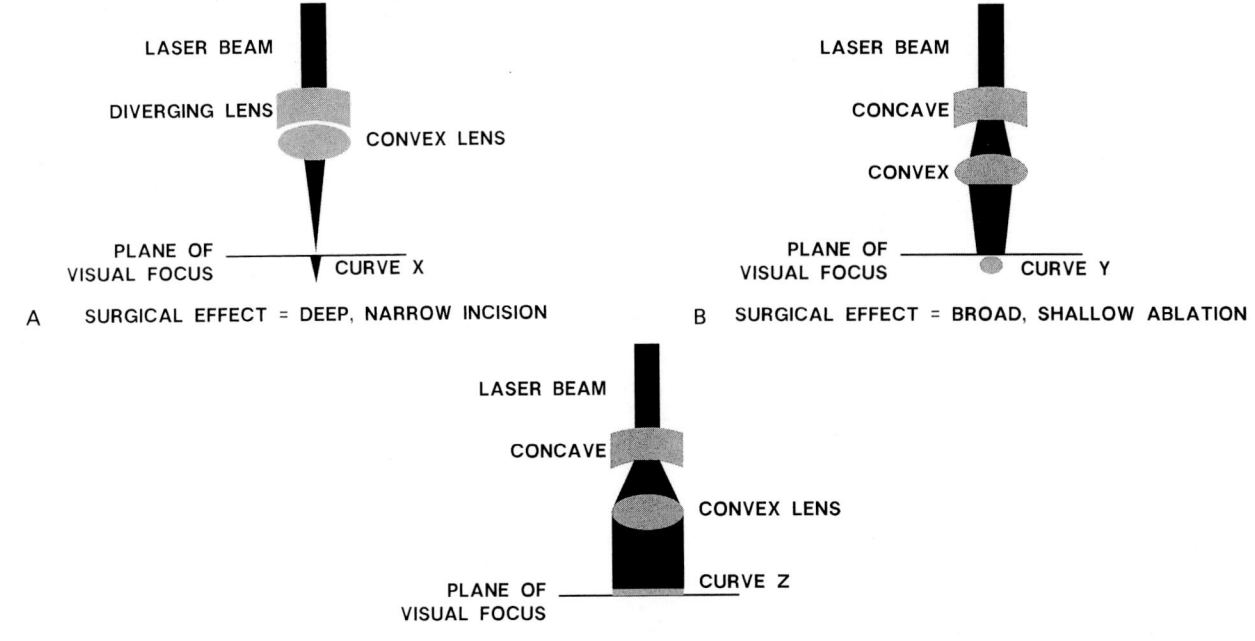

Fig. 69.14 (A) A diagram of the way the microslad can be used to produce a cutting beam geometry. At the point of 'zero defocus', the diverging and converging lenses are in apposition, thus behaving like a single convex lens. Hence, the laser energy reaches the plane of visual focus as a narrow beam which is also completely focused, thus producing a 'drill like' crater (corresponding to curve X in Figure 69.13A). (B) The manner in which the microslad can produce a beam geometry suitable for shallow ablation. Used at the point of partial defocus (say, 'position 4') the diverging lens is now separated from the converging lens, such that the laser beam reaches the visual plane in partial defocus. Whether such defocus reflects a laser beam that is still converging towards focus, or one that is diverging away from focus, is of no surgical importance. What does matter is that, for an incident power of 60 W, point 4 on this Sharplan Industries microslad will produce an approximately hemispherical impact crater on a tongue blade. Higher powers would require that the lenses be even further separated (e.g. point 5 for 100 W), while lower powers would require less separation (e.g. point 3 for 30 W). After using a tongue blade to find the beam geometry which approximately corresponds to curve 'Y' (In Figure 69.13A), the surgeon can now make some trial impacts on the tissues. If the tissue crater shows a tendency to carbonization, the microslad must be turned back to a position of tighter focus, thus raising power density to a safer level. In contrast, if the impact crater has a prominent central depression (corresponding to an XY hybrid shown in Figure 69.13B), then the beam geometry will need to be further 'flattened' by turning the microslad to a position of greater defocus. (C) The microslad turned to a position of excessive defocus (curve Z in Figure 69.13A). If a surgeon commits this error, he will nullify the advantages of rapid superpulsing, chopped wave or rapid energy delivery. Such excessive defocus will reduce effective power within the impact diameter, causing excessive coagulation but inefficient vaporization. Subsequent photons will carbonize this coagulated anhydrous tissue, creating an excessive thermal gradient for heat diffusion.

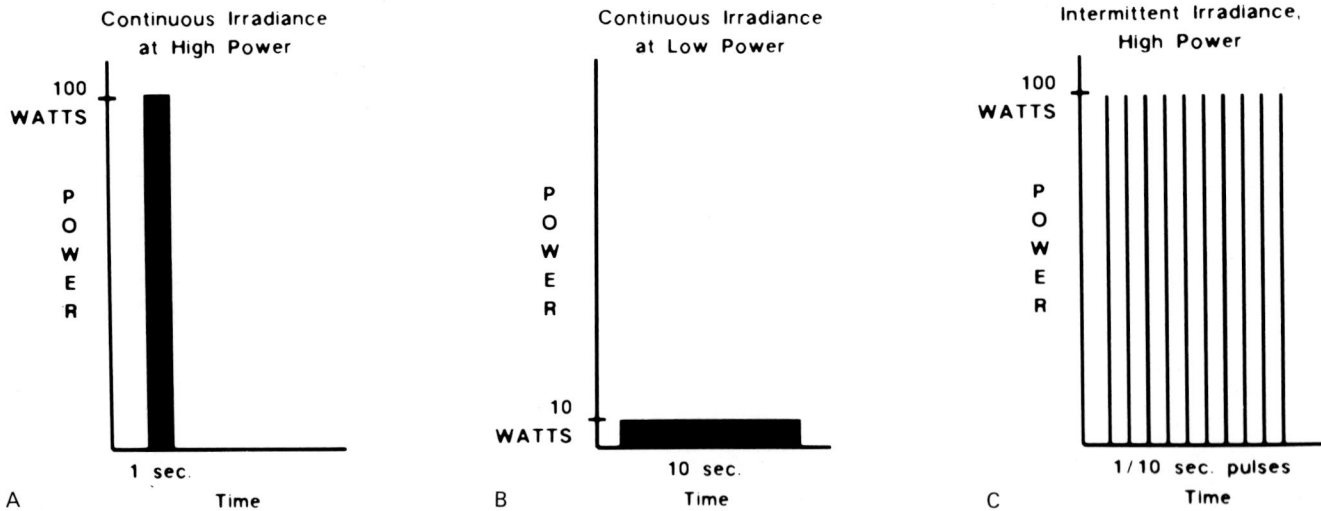

Fig. 69.15 The value of intermittent pulses as a means of maintaining surgical control in delicate situations. (A) 100 J delivered by irradiating with 100 W for 1 second satisfies the requirement of rapid energy delivery, but may be hard to control. (B) 100 J delivered as 10 W for 10 seconds will cause too much lateral heat conduction. (C) 100 J delivered by 10 shuttered pulses of an 100 W beam, each pulse lasting for 0.1 s. This approach satisfies both requirements: rapid energy delivery and easy beam control. (Reproduced from Reid (1987),[38] with permission.)

For energy of a given wavelength, both spot size and depth of field are directly proportional to the focal length of the objective lens. Operating microscopes generally use 300 to 400 mm objectives, thereby producing relatively large focal spots with an excellent depth of field. In contrast, hand held probes incorporate lenses of short focal length to attain very narrow spot diameters and correspondingly high power densities. Unfortunately, this amplification of power density is achieved as the cost of a marked diminution of focal depth.

Provided that the tip of the probe is kept in close focus, hand-held delivery systems are well suited to the creation of thermal incisions. However, attempting to perform surface ablation with a conventional hand probe is a mistake, for several reasons:

(1) The focal plane is so narrow that even slight variations in lens-to-target distance will dramatically spread spot diameter, causing an exponential fall in power density.

(2) If the probe is angulated to allow the surgeon to assume a comfortable 'pencil grip', the energy profile at the point of impact will have an oval (rather than circular) distribution. Creating an 'egg-shaped' crater adds a further dimension to the difficulty of trying to ensure uniformity of power density.

(3) Failure to use the operating microscope robs the surgeon of the benefit of anatomic landmarks, making depth control a very haphazard affair.

(4) The unaided eye has insufficient visual resolution to permit surgical control over beams of more than 750 W/cm^2.

In short, attempting to perform superficial ablation with a conventional hand-held probe generally condemns the surgeon to making a series of non-uniform, poorly localized cuts at a power density close to the carbonization range. However, equipping the hand probe with a microslad defocusing device will avoid many of the errors detailed above.

Minimizing thermal damage by tissue cooling

Despite the application of optimal physical principles, there will always be some heat conduction to adjacent tissues. Even with continuous wave, the amount of lateral heat propagation while using the laser as a thermal knife is relatively small. However, heat diffusion during vulvar laser ablation can be devastating. Hence, surgeons should limit thermal spread by chilling the tissues with iced saline. This strategy can reduce lateral heat conduction by about 25%,[62] thereby avoiding some postoperative pain and swelling, as well as contributing to more rapid healing.

Cooling is done with laparotomy packs soaked in a bowl of semi-frozen saline slush, to which a cephalosporin may be added. The tissues should be chilled prior to the initial laser impact and at frequent intervals during the operation.

Pre-cooling acts as a buffer against burning, in that diffused heat must first restore temperatures to the normal range before tissue injury can occur. Reapplication of the iced saline immediately following laser irradiation is also beneficial, probably because cooling antagonizes continued tissue damage by vasoactive peptides released at the time of the initial thermal injury.

Control of intraoperative bleeding

The easiest approach to this potentially frustrating problem is to prevent intraoperative bleeding by the use of vasoconstrictor injections. When hemorrhage is encountered, the surgeon must distinguish partial transection of a small vessel from laceration of a much larger artery or vein. Most intraoperative bleeding arises from a laser impact punching a hole in the side of a small vessel. Hence, tamponading the vessel with a *dry* Q tip and relasing through the cotton bundle is an effective strategy for trying to seal the vessel walls at the point of mechanical compression. However, if this maneuver is not successful, the surgeon should either insert a hemostatic suture or apply Monsel's solution (ferric subsulphate).[34]

Good exposure and perpendicular beam impact

Expert control over the CO_2 laser requires both good exposure and perpendicular beam delivery. Exposure on an external surface is generally simple. Although the need to continuously reposition either the laser or the target can be tedious, the surgeon should not trade the accuracy of the microscopically adapted laser for the easy maneuverability of the hand-held delivery system.

Exposure within body cavities depends upon having the correct instruments: a pediatric nasal speculum for the urethra, straight or angled Graves' speculae for the vagina, and suitable anoscope for the anus (Fig. 69.16). The angle of laser impact may be further improved by pressure with a cotton swab, traction with a Campion hook or manipulation with a tenaculum (perhaps applied lateral to the central aperture).

We have found the use of mirrors in treating difficult-to-expose areas of vaginal surface to be of limited usefulness. Visualization in a mirror is not as detailed as with direct colposcopic viewing. Moreover, the reflective surface is rapidly fogged by steam and particulate debris from laser plume, requiring constant wiping. The hand which holds the mirror is usually better utilized in either ironing out vaginal folds or maneuvering the vaginal speculum (see p. 1123).

Accurate depth control

Most gynecologists destroy the cervical transformation zone

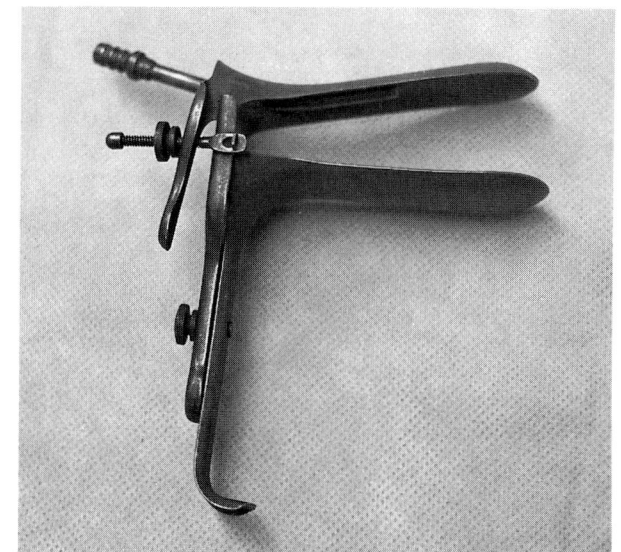

A

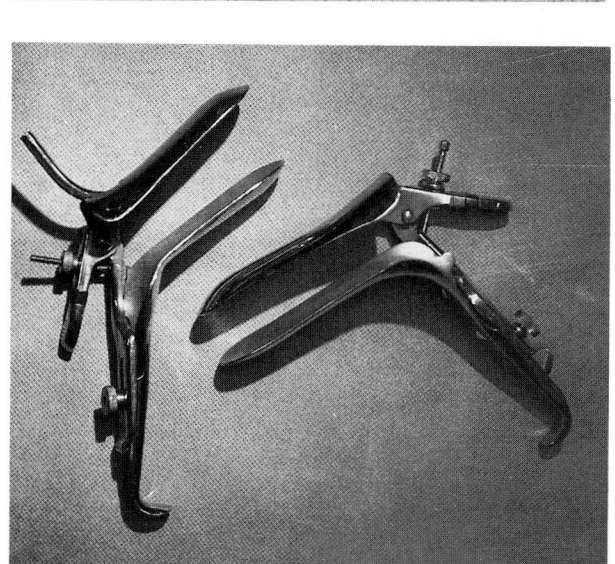

B

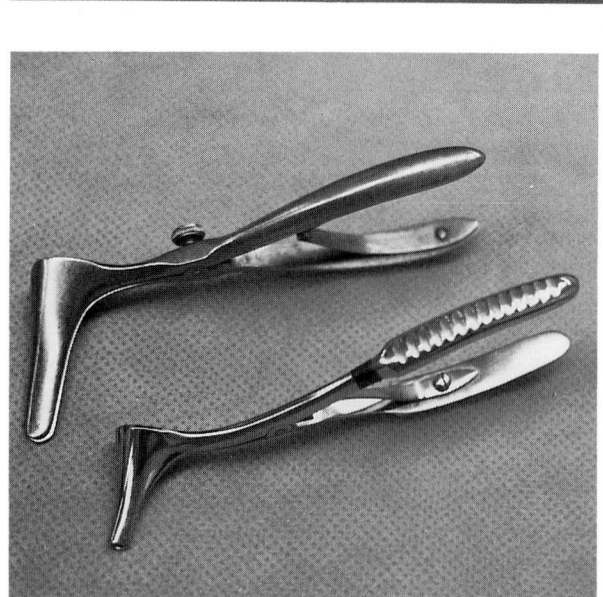

C

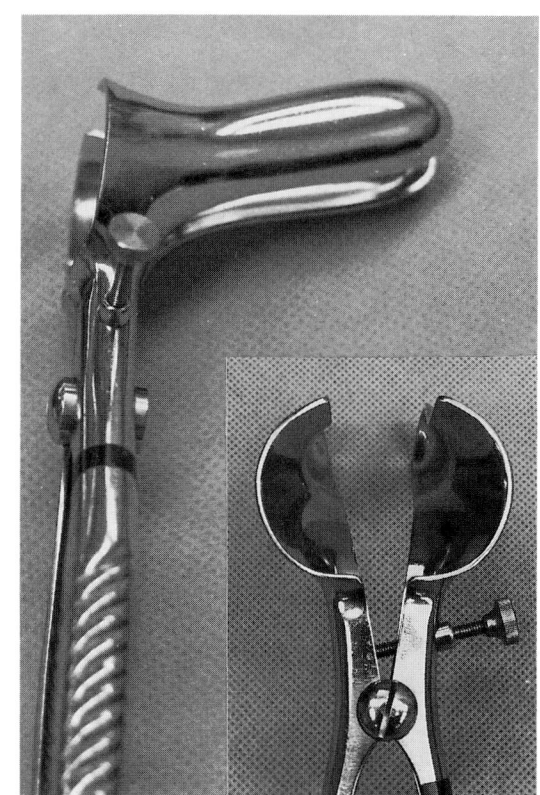

D

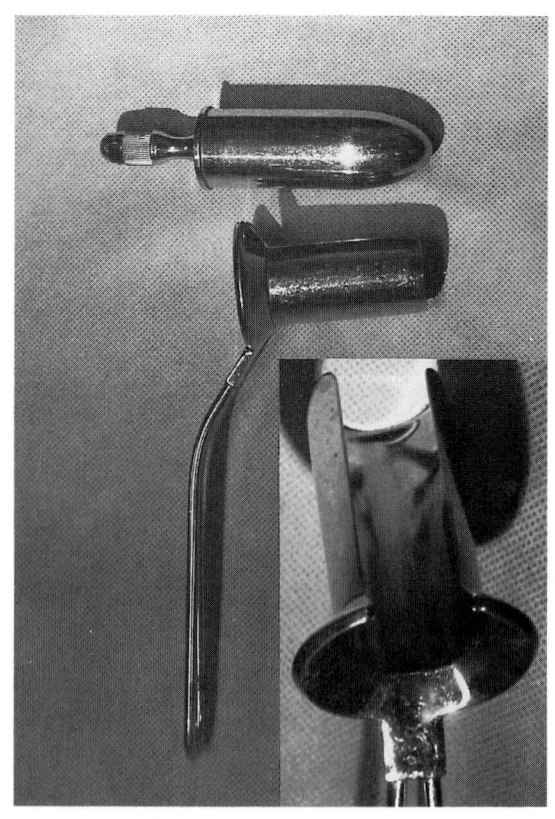

E

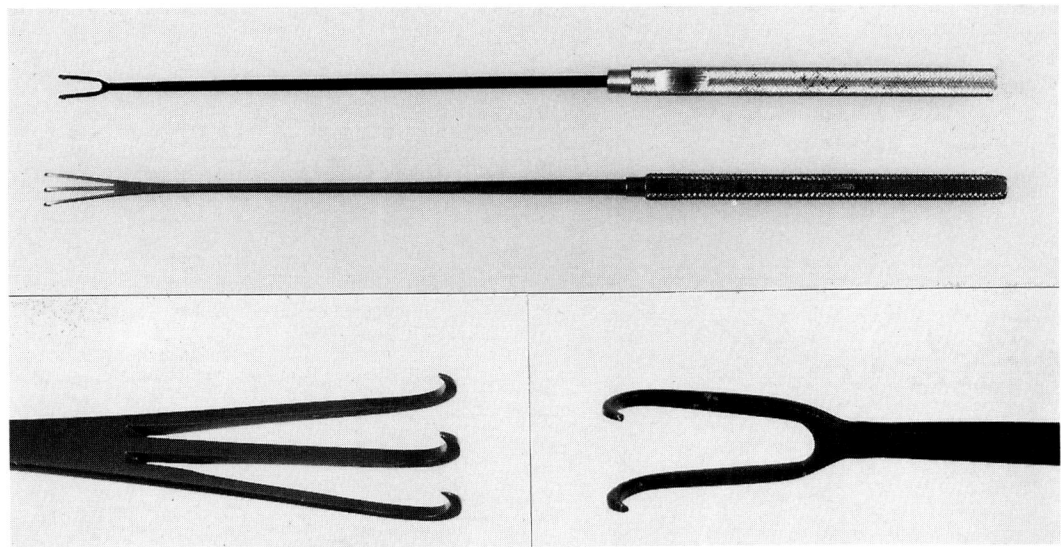

F

Fig. 69.16 Speculae used to secure exposure within the lower genital tract. (A) Graves speculum with suction port. (B) Pair of vaginal speculae, allowing easy access to the right and left vaginal walls. (C) Two pediatric nasal speculae for exposing the distal and proximal female urethra. (D) Bivalved anoscope, shown in side view and as seen by the surgeon's eye. (E) Fixed anoscope, shown with the obturator in place and removed. (F) Two pronged and three pronged Campion hooks.

to a depth of 7 mm[39] (see Ch. 70). The cylindrical nature of the resulting defect and the relatively large dimensions of the intended crater make it quite easy to control the depth of cervical ablation by actual measurements. Depth of destruction during vaginal and vulvar surgery is too shallow to control by measurement, particularly since the laser crater has no well defined sides to act as points of reference. What is more, satisfactory healing of vulvar wounds depends upon the preservation of the skin appendages, a task that is too delicate to trust to crude measurement. Hence, the surgeon must learn to control depth according to the visual characteristics at the site of impact.[42]

From the surgical viewpoint, tissue destruction occurs through two distinct mechanisms: immediate photo-vaporization and delayed coagulation necrosis.[16] The depth of the photovaporization crater is controlled by hand-eye coordination. In contrast, the thickness of the zone of coagulation necrosis is quite variable, depending upon whether the laser is used as a thermal cautery or a precise optical instrument.

Using a superpulsed laser of adequate fluence, coagulation necrosis is limited to a narrow, sharply defined zone at the crater margin, in which energy levels do not reach the vaporization threshold. Under these circumstances, crater depth conforms closely to the true level of thermal destruction.

In contrast, when pulse duration exceeds thermal relaxation time, the distribution of tissue damage bears little relation to the concept embodied in Beer's law. Rather, much of the normal appearing tissue on the wound surface will have suffered thermal denaturation, and will separate as an eschar after activation of the host inflammatory response. That is to say, if the surgeon does not adequately limit thermal diffusion, any structures visible within the crater base will be sloughed off over the succeeding week (Fig. 69.3).[42] Hence, under these circumstances, the art of expert CO_2 laser surgery is to judge crater depth such that the zone of thermal necrosis (rather than the zone of photovaporization) lies at the intended depth of penetration. Orientation is preserved by continuously wiping away the surface char, depth of destruction being inferred from anatomic landmarks in the crater base.[42] By means of this technique, four characteristic surgical planes[36] are identifiable (Fig. 69.17 and Table 69.2).

Accurate delineation of the treatment margins

In all forms of surgery, an ability to set accurate margins for the excision or destruction of diseased tissue is an essential ingredient of success. Failure to recognize the true extent of disease will adversely affect success rates. Strategies for setting operative margins within the lower genital tract vary according to anatomic site (for cervix, see Ch. 70).

Soaking the vulva with 5% acetic acid will usually produce prominent acetowhitening of skin that had appeared normal to naked eye examination (Fig. 69.18). In women without obvious condylomas, the true clinical significance of acetowhite changes and vestibular micro-papillae is presently shrouded in confusion;[40] (see also Ch. 16). Although biopsies from such areas will usually

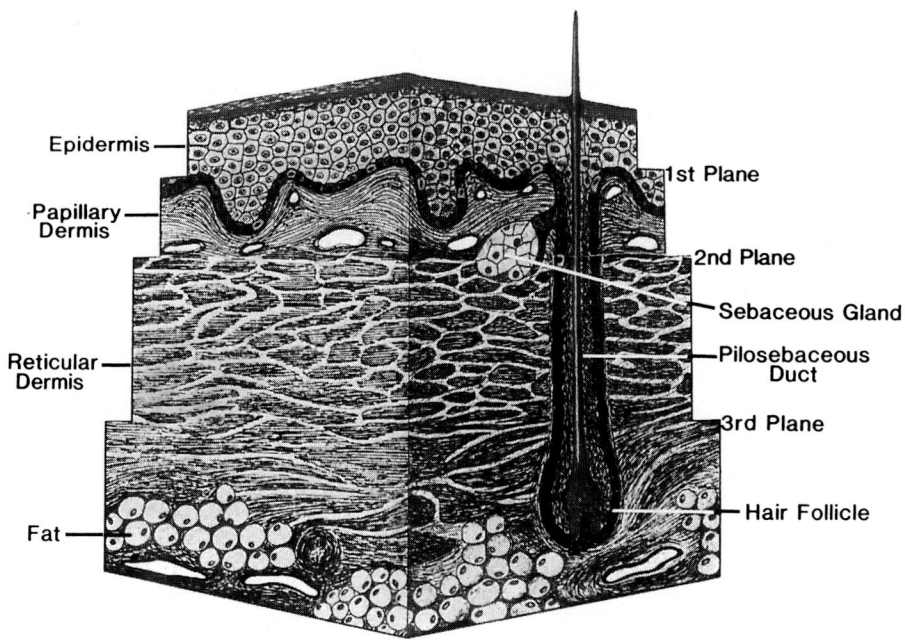

Fig. 69.17 A diagram of the first three surgical planes in vulvar laser surgery. Reading from surface to base, the points of reference for each plane are indicated as stepwise expansions. The first surgical plane corresponds to the basement membrane, the second to the papillary dermis, and the third to the mid-reticular dermis. (Reproduced from Reid (1985),[35] with permission.)

Table 69.2 Summary of the salient features of the four surgical planes in vulvar laser surgery

| Parameter | Surgical plane | | | |
	First	Second	Third	Fourth
Target tissue	Surface epithelium	Dermal papillae	Pilosebaceous ducts	Pilosebaceous glands
Zone of vaporization	Proliferating layer of epidermis	Superficial papillary dermis	Upper reticular dermis	Mid-reticular dermis
Zone of necrosis	Basement membrane	Deep papillary	Mid-reticular	Deep reticular
Type of healing	Rapid and cosmetic	Rapid and cosmetic	Slower but usually cosmetic	Needs grafting
Visual landmark	Opalescent epidermis debris (shiny pink after wiping)	Yellowish and non-reflectant (chamois cloth)	Stark white with arcuate vessels and fibrous 'grain'	Skin appendages visible as 'sand grains'

Reproduced from Reid et al (1985)[42] with permission

show low grade koilocytotic atypia, papillomaviral genomes are not generally detectable within these tissues.[44] In contrast, Southern blot hybridization of samples taken from acetowhite epithelium at the margins of exophytic condylomas or vulvar intraepithelial neoplasia (VIN) identify the same type of HPV DNA as found within the principal biopsies.[46] Ferenczy[12] correlated the risk of treatment failure with the presence of detectable HPV DNA at the lesion margin. Moreover, the Koebner phenomenon[3,53] (new warts arising at the treatment margins) is a well recognized manifestation of the proclivity for the conversion from latent HPV infection to active expression during tissue regeneration (Fig. 69.19). Hence, there is little doubt that these adjacent areas of acetowhite epithelium represent an important viral reservoir, at least among patients who present with classical disease stigmata.[22] As described on page 1111, destruction of the surrounding subclinical

HPV infection in difficult situations will produce higher surgical success rates.

LASER SAFETY

Sources of laser hazard

Faulty equipment. Several mishaps in the mid-1970's were attributable to equipment malfunction. With the addition of such safety features as covered foot pedals, safety shutters, and various interlocks, the laser has become a very reliable piece of equipment. However, as a safeguard against equipment failure, lasers should have regular (e.g. quarterly) maintenance by a laser technician or trained biomedical engineer.

The operator. The procedure established by the operator determines the safety of both patient and operat-

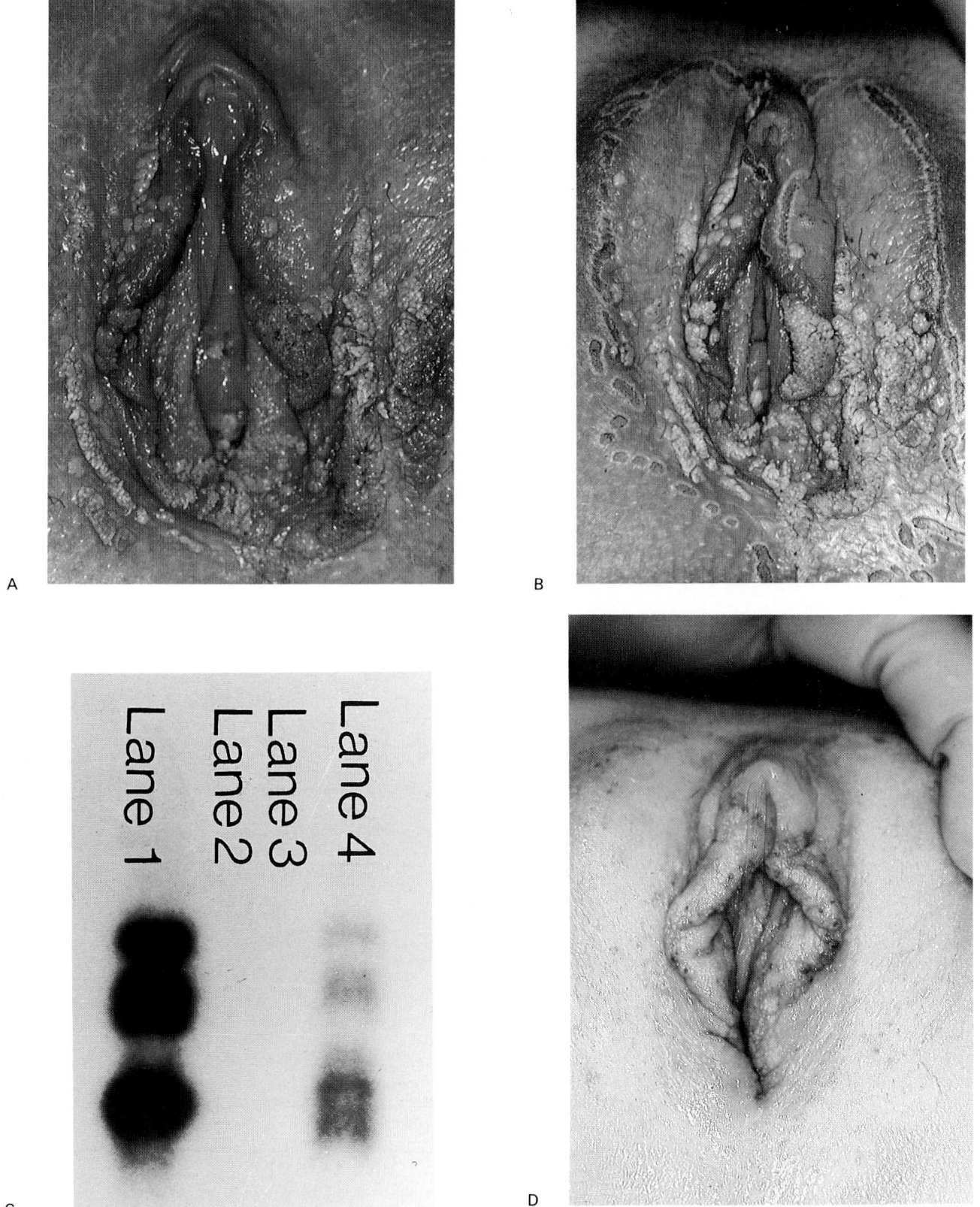

Fig. 69.18 (A) Extensive vulvar condylomas, prior to vinegar soaking. (B) The same patient after a 3-minute soak with 4.5% acetic acid, showing extensive subclinical HPV infection of the intervening skin. Biopsies from this area showed prominent histologic features of active (albeit subclinical) viral expression. (C) A Southern blot hybridization done under conditions of high stringency. (Courtesy of A. Lorincz, Ph.D.). Biopsies of an exophytic condyloma (lane 1) and an area of adjacent acetowhitening (lane 4) contain the typical banded pattern of HPV DNA, whereas biopsies of non-acetowhite skin and normal vaginal mucosa (lanes 2 and 3) had no detectable signal. (D) The extent of surgical destruction. Because healing occurs by epithelial regeneration from underlying skin appendages, healing time (and postoperative discomfort) are the same as that which follows focal destruction of the exophytic condylomas alone. (Reproduced from Reid et al (1990),[45] with permission.)

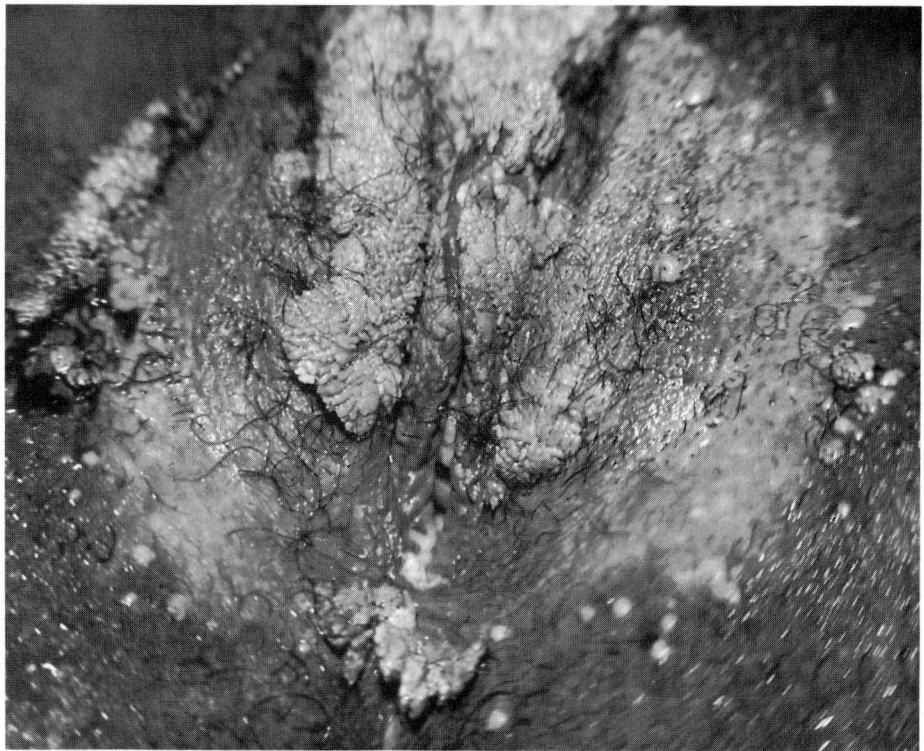

Fig. 69.19   A Koebner phenomenon, due to the active expression of latent HPV DNA during healing, resulting in condyloma formation at the treatment margins.

ing room staff. Hence, surgeons must be specifically credentialed for each type of laser and each type of operation. Laser privileges are granted after review by two sources:[7] (1) certification by the department chairman that the physician has knowledge of the disease being treated, and training in performance of the proposed operation and (2) certification by the laser committee that the physician has attained a knowledge of the relevant laser physics and the principles of the laser delivery system. In the United States, a plethora of laser training courses has arisen. Some offer excellent instruction and others are deficient. Hence, before granting privileges to the individual surgeon, hospital credentialing committees should scrutinize the content, duration and excellence of the training course from which the certificate of completion was obtained. Short courses teaching surgery for both upper and lower tract, using many types of lasers, should be regarded as a theoretic introduction, rather than a basis for credentialing.

Lack of awareness of safety rules. Training is the single most important factor in the safe use of the laser. For a complete explanation of laser safety rules, readers are directed to a reviews by Reid et al[43] & Martin.[31] Important practical considerations are summarized in Table 69.3.

Avoidance of laser injuries

Lasers are powerful but predictable surgical tools. Used with skill and discretion, they open new vistas in many medical specialties. However, despite their unique properties, careless or unskilled laser operations will yield un-

Table 69.3   Laser safety rules

1. Each program must appoint a laser safety officer to forestall hazards, educate staff and supervise protocol.

2. Surgical set-up should be checked by laser safety officer, to ensure correct coupling of laser tube to delivery device, placement of optical filters (if relevant) and coaxial gas flow to prevent burnout of laser mirrors.

3. To avoid electrical hazard, keep foot pedal clear of water and do not place liquids on laser console.

4. If visual precautions are relevant, spectators must don safety goggles *before* entering the room. No one should ever look directly into the laser beam, even with goggles.

5. Check beam alignment and power density on tongue blade *before* aiming at patient.

6. Fire only under direct vision, taking care that unintended targets do not fall within the path of the prefocused beam. Also ensure that the laser energy is terminated in the vicinity of the target, using wet gauze or a suitable backstop if necessary.

7. Remove foot from covered foot pedal during short pauses, and disarm the laser on longer breaks.

8. Prevent unauthorized laser access by key lock, master interlock and secure storage.

9. Ignitable drapes, Teflon or plastic instruments, and flammable solutions should not be used in the vicinity of laser surgery. If drapes are required, wet the perimeter with sterile saline, and have a bowl of liquid on hand (in case of flame-up).

desirable results. Misadventure may arise in several ways, as described below.

Errors of judgment

As with most forms of surgery, errors of judgment can be just as harmful as errors of technique. Judgment errors are of three main kinds: incorrect assessment of disease extent or severity, failure to exclude an underlying invasive cancer, and the choice of inappropriate laser settings. Avoidance of the first two errors depends on the surgeon's clinical competence and diligence. The major safeguard against the third error is an adequate understanding of laser physics and tissue interactions. That mishap may arise through the selection of too high a power is intuitively obvious. However, it is equally important to recognize that most bad outcomes follow the choice of unduly low output powers or power densities. Whether the surgical objective is to achieve cutting, ablation, or the coagulation of a bleeding vessel, the potential advantages of the various lasers are tied to their being able to accomplish the desired task without causing excessive thermal injury to neighboring tissues. Through failure to limit the extent of lateral heat conduction and through ignorance of surgical strategies for accurate depth control, unskilled laser surgeons can easily produce an unrecognized conduction burn extending well beyond the laser impact site. In such cases, the outcome will be no better than that which would have followed the use of hot cautery.

Optical hazard

The wavelength of the CO_2 laser corresponds to the mid-infrared region of the electromagnetic spectrum. This wavelength is well outside the retinal hazard range, but is rapidly absorbed by all water-containing cells, including those of the cornea or sclera. Hence, an impact of sufficient power density will produce intense ocular pain and acute ulceration. When using a focused CO_2 laser deployed through either a handpiece or an operating microscope, personnel at a distance of more than 4 feet from the focal spot are at negligible risk of ocular injury. If using a handpiece, the surgeon may elect to use safety glasses. However, when using an operating microscope, the surgeon's eyes are completely protected by the glass lens system. Spectators are afforded adequate optical protection by keeping at a safe distance (4 feet) and wearing either clear plastic safety glasses or their own corrective glass spectacles.

Skin hazards

From a safety standpoint, skin exposure is usually regarded as a minor hazard. Nonetheless, an inadvertent burn due to a misdirected beam striking either the patient or a staff member is probably the most common laser mishap.

Fire hazards

Any high-powered surgical laser, particularly if focused to a small spot of high power density, can ignite flammable materials or cause explosion of flammable gases. Theoretically, the methane in flatus could be ignited. However, the use of an efficient smoke evacuator will remove any flammable gas from the rectum, making it safe to lase within the anus without elaborate packing or bowel preparation.

If sponges and drapes are to be used in the operative field, they should be kept wet for protection. Cloth drapes should be moistened, and a bowl of sterile water or saline should be kept on the instrument table. Most paper drapes used in the United States are fire resistant and may be safely used during CO_2 laser surgery. If in doubt, a patch of material should be tested for flammability before the procedure is begun.

Chemical hazards

Laser radiation of flammable antiseptic solutions can cause fire, and radiation of water-based solutions can release irritant or noxious vapors. These risks are easily avoided because most laser surgery does not require preoperative antiseptic preparation. Where it is desired, cleansing of the intended operative site with a non-flammable antiseptic and drying of the target area are necessary.

It is especially important not to use Teflon-coated instruments or sutures in conjunction with laser surgery, since Teflon produces very toxic fumes when ignited.

Electrical hazards

The most lethal hazards associated with lasers are electrical hazards, and there have been at least three fatal accidents due to accidental electrocution by individuals working in breach of accepted safety procedures. Many lasers use high voltage and high amperage current. DC capacitors in some lasers can remain energized for an extended period of time after the laser has been unplugged from the wall outlet. Of course, these electrical hazards are adequately safeguarded by enclosure of high voltage devices within the laser cabinet, and danger only arises when an unauthorized person unscrews the laser console.

Because of the danger of internal short circuit in the event of spillage, liquids must not be placed on the laser cabinet, and the floor in the immediate vicinity must be kept dry.

BASIC TREATMENT PHILOSOPHY

Why the clinical consequences of papillomaviral infection

should be generalized in some patients, yet localized to differing anatomic sites in others, is a major puzzle.[37] In a study of 160 women presenting with papillomavirus-associated diseases, HPV DNA was detected in 69% of acetowhite epithelium surrounding florid vulvar lesions, 40% of the 'normal' vaginal mucosa and 25% of unremarkable squamous metaplasia from just proximal to a high grade CIN lesion.[46] These observations indicate that the presence of HPV genomic sequences is a necessary but insufficient cause for disease formation. Hence, HPV-induced diseases of the anogenital tract are best regarded as chronic, regional infections. After episomal infection is established, cell-virus interaction must thereafter be *regulated* by local factors.[30]

To reconcile this 'iceberg' concept with the realities of patient care, morphologic stigmata of HPV infection are best viewed as a cascade, in which disease expression ranges from minimal to florid (Table 69.4).[40] Lesions may be unicentric or multicentric, and disease extent ranges from minute to massive. Clinical course varies from trivial and self limiting to extensive and refractory. Since simple problems have simple solutions, it is reasonable to expect that the majority of patients will be managed by office methods.[45]

Aggressiveness of treatment must be counter-balanced against the degree of disease expression in the individual patient. Benign, asymptomatic, subclinical lesions of the vulva or vagina do not require any treatment. Hence, the first objective is to differentiate clinically important disease from the equivocal stigmata that are seen in at least one quarter of the normal population (Fig. 69.20). In particular, gynecologists must not be drawn into poorly considered therapy just because a biopsy of an area of asymptomatic acetowhitening is reported as 'condyloma' or 'HPV infection' by the pathologist. Rather, treatment must be tied to realistic objectives: the eradication of neoplastic foci, destruction of exophytic condylomas, control of infectivity or relief of symptoms. Treatment aimed at preventing 'to-and-fro' reinfection within a stable relationship is probably misguided,[50] and attempts to eradicate all HPV DNA from the genital tract are futile.[51]

Idiopathic vulvodynia

The only grounds for undertaking the destruction of low

Table 69.4 Varying levels of disease expression

Well developed papillomavirus infections
1. Vegetative viral replication (benign condylomas and subclinical papillomavirus infections)

2. Non-productive viral infection (intraepithelial neoplasia and invasive cancer)

Low grade papillomavirus infections
1. Normal cell phenotype ('true latency')

2. Minimal viral cytopathic effect

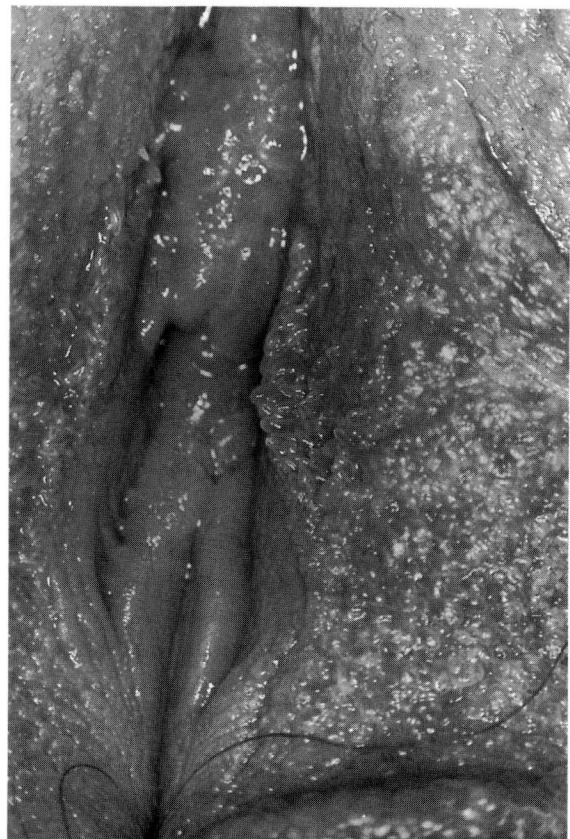

Fig. 69.20 Micropapillae seen in 25% of the normal population.

grade 'condylomatous' change within the vulvar vestibule is for the relief of symptoms. Over the last 10 years, there has been a dramatic rise in the prevalence of idiopathic vulvodynia,[14] an illness possibly related to genital tract colonization by a group of novel HPVs producing an asymptomatic micropapillary change in some patients and intractable sexual dysfunction in others. Physical examination has shown that this syndrome of idiopathic vulvodynia has three components:[44]

1. An irritative acetowhite reaction of the vulvar epithelium, seemingly attributable to chronic HPV infection.
2. A vascular ectasia affecting the dermal blood vessels within the entire vulvar vestibule.
3. Foci of painful erythema surrounding the minor vestibular glands, Skene's complex and the Bartholin's ducts.

Although the surface papillomaviral infection will often respond to topical 5-fluorouracil cream, the inflammation surrounding the minor vestibular glands is refractory to anti-inflammatory medication, including topical or injected steroids. The standard therapy has been an operation described by Woodruff,[66] in which the posterior three-quarters of the hymenal ring (including the minor vestibular glands) are excised and the defect closed by downward advancement of the posterior vaginal wall.

Woodruff's procedure is unsatisfactory for three reasons:[44] Firstly, excision of the minor vestibular glands will not cure chronic burning discomfort caused by the irritative epithelial changes. Secondly, since the cosmetic results are somewhat dismaying, hymenal resection should be a treatment of last resort, rather than an initial surgical approach. Thirdly, hymenal resection is no more than 50% successful. In some patients, scarring induced by the approximation of vaginal mucosa to perineal skin can exacerbate pre-existing incipient inflammation of Skene's and Bartholin's glands, resulting in a marked worsening of symptoms (Fig. 69.21A).[44]

Superficial CO_2 laser photovaporization of the irritative acetowhite epithelium can produce good results. However, the major role for the laser will probably be to photocoagulate the chronically hyperemic dermal blood vessels. This task will require laser energy within the visible portion of the electromagnetic spectrum, rather than from the infrared region. Argon lasers carry a severe risk of burning, because of the relatively poor affinity of blue and green light for oxyhemoglobin. However, we are presently getting promising results (Fig. 69.21B) from the more specific yellow light produced by the flash-pumped dye laser, allowing us to create selective photothermolysis within these target blood vessels while sparing the adjacent nonpigmented tissues (Reid: unpublished data).

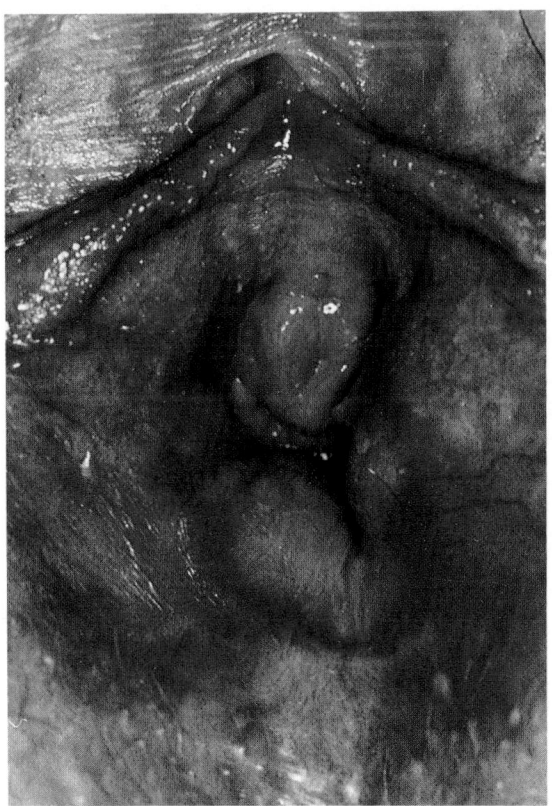

A

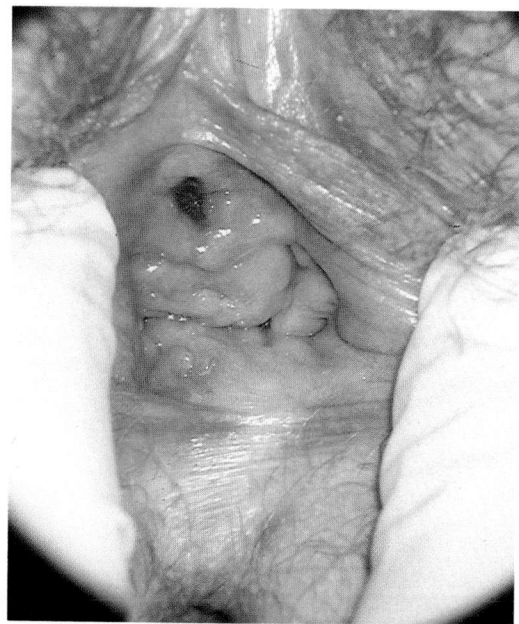

B

Fig. 69.21 (A) Vascular ectasia following CO_2 laser destruction of vestibular acetowhitening, in a patient presenting with mild vulvodynia. The patient now has incapacitating vulvar pain. (B) The same patient after selective thermolysis, using flash pumped dye laser.

Focal condylomas of recent onset

The modern gynecologist has to choose from an array of therapies for the management of the various HPV-associated diseases of the vagina, vulva and anus (Table 69.5). Despite the precision, hemostatic properties and ease of access afforded by the CO_2 laser, using this instrument as a simple 'spot welder', confers no special advantage in most patients. Of 1000 women referred with HPV-associated vulvar disease, 835 were controlled by traditional office therapies for the destruction of exophytic condylomas.[45]

Scissor excision is a useful means of obtaining tissue for histology or HPV typing, as well as for the treatment of a few isolated condylomas. However, the technique is impractical within the vaginal or anal canal, and carries a risk of tissue denudation if attempted in patients with extensive disease. Although wide excision with primary close can yield acceptable results in difficult situations, results attainable by the skilled laser surgeon will always be better.

For external condylomas, destruction with cytolytic chemicals is probably the best general strategy. Cytolytic chemicals do not require local anesthesia, and are therefore suited to any clinical setting (e.g. birth control and sexually transmitted disease clinics). Based upon an overly enthusiastic report in 1944,[5] which claimed control of penile warts in 96% of transient soldiers, 25% podophyllin resin has remained in common use. However, every subsequent trial of podophyllin has yielded disappointing results, cumulative success rates averaging 20 to 40% after 3 to 6 months of therapy.[19,56] Trichloracetic acid is just as effec-

Table 69.5   Treatment modalities for mucosal and cutaneous condylomas

Method	Advantage	Disadvantage	Clinical role
Traditional office methods for lesion eradication			
1. Scissor excision of isolated lesions	Obtains tissue for histology or viral typing. Removal of large papillomas may allow chemical destruction of remaining smaller lesions.	Cumbersome (local anesthesia, suture, instruments). Epithelial denudation and bleeding, if done to excess.	Baseline biopsy. Removal of large lesions.
2. Desiccant acids (85% trichloracetic acid in 70% alcohol; bichloracetic acid)	Quickest and easiest method. Sterile instruments not required. Can be used on mucosal surfaces (vagina, rectum, mouth).	Requires weekly or second weekly office visits. Less effective for cutaneous (rather than mucosal) warts. Safe during pregnancy.	Highly effective for localized mucosal papillomas. Moderately effective for localized cutaneous lesions.
3. Crude podophyllin extracts (e.g. 25% podophyllin in benzoin)	Nil	Crude, non-standardized mixture of toxins and active lignans. Rare but calamitous toxicity. No more effective than desiccant acids.	Obsolete.
4. Podophyllotoxin ('Podofilox')	Selective destruction of condylomatous areas, with sparing of normal epithelium. Self application regimens are more effective than single dose office therapies.	Cannot be used on highly absorptive surfaces (vagina, rectum). Contraindicated during pregnancy.	Highly effective for cutaneous condylomas. Effective for vulvar mucosal lesions of limited extent.
5. Localized physical destruction (hot cautery, liquid nitrogen, laser 'spot welding')	Immediate eradication of papillomas.	Cumbersome (local anesthesia, special equipment). Time-consuming for physician. Local infection or scarring more common than with chemical methods.	Destruction of isolated refractory papillomas.
6. Cytolytic 5-fluorouracil regimens	Non-surgical method of lesion eradication. Can forestall diffuse postoperative recurrence, if therapy begins before extensive papilloma formation.	Brutally painful alternative to skilled CO_2 laser photovaporization. Potentially teratogenic.	Effective for extensive, exophytic vaginal condylomas. Valuable postoperative 'rescue' strategy.
7. Alpha or gamma interferon (as primary therapy)	Biological substances with documented antiviral and immunomodulatory actions. Non-surgical method of lesion eradication.	Primary success rates have been disappointing and unpredictable. Intralesional regimens are slow, expensive and painful. Systemic regimens require high dosages, with corresponding frequency of side effects.	Value as primary therapy not established Valuable adjuvant (see below).
Destructive methods requiring operating room therapy			
1. Segmental excision and primary closure	Tissue available for histology, if genuine doubt exists.	Tissue removal is fundamentally undesirable.	Essentially outmoded by CO_2 laser surgery.
2. Extensive electrodiathermy ('Bovie' destruction)	Equipment readily available (e.g. Third World nations).	Morbid recovery and unacceptable scarring.	Outmoded in Western society.
3. Extended laser ablation	Can eradicate any volume of diseased epithelium, with negligible risk of scarring. Removes entire field of active HPV expression, irrespective of size, shape or location. Anatomic methods of depth control allow destruction of VIN 3 within pilosebaceous ducts.	Requires sophisticated laser instrumentation and highly developed physician skills. Not appropriate for simpler cases. Cannot prevent subsequent reactivation of latent viral reservoir. Not an appropriate alternative to simpler methods.	Very extensive condylomas (coalescent papillomas occupying $\geq$ 30% of vulva and perineum). Refractory condylomas (disease not controlled by $\geq$ 9 months of office therapy). High grade intraepithelial neoplasia (VIN* 2 to 3 and PAIN** 2 to 3).

*VIN = vulvar intraepithelial neoplasia
**PAIN = perianal intraepithelial neoplasia

Table 69.5 Treatment modalities for mucosal and cutaneous condylomas (cont'd)

Method	Advantage	Disadvantage	Clinical role
Method for controlling the residual viral reservoir			
1. Non-cytolytic 5-fluorouracil regimens	Relatively inexpensive. Minimal systemic absorption. Effective in immunosuppressed patients.	Limited efficacy (especially in simpler cases). Poorly tolerated in patients of fair complexion. Distressing side effects (vaginal scarring, vestibular ulceration, possible vulvodynia).	An essential ingredient for the control of HPV disease in immunosuppressed patients.
2. Low dose adjuvant interferon (IFN) regimens	Biological substance with documented antiviral and immunomodulatory actions. Adjuvant effect documented in controlled trial (IFN >> 5 FU or surgery alone).	Must monitor potential leukopenic and hepatotoxic effects. May not be effective in immunosuppressed patients. Theoretical risk of organ rejection in allograft recipients.	Probably indicated in immunocompetent patients with disease severe enough to warrant extended laser ablation

tive as podophyllin, but does not carry the same risks of neurologic, myocardial, hepatic, renal and embryologic toxicity. Moreover, since caustic agents are simple acid radicals which are not absorbed, their use in pregnancy or within the vagina is completely safe.[53]

Toxicology studies show that drugs in divided dose regimens are generally more effective than when used in a single dose. Hence, the purification of podophyllotoxin (the active lignin of crude podophyllin extracts) is a significant advance in the topical therapy of condylomas. The toxic effects of podophyllotoxin are relatively specific to diseased tissue, making this dosage sufficiently safe for self application, each course having a 3-day regimen and a 4-day rest period. Compared with crude podophyllin, self application of the purified derivative has yielded improved success rates (80% vs 40%), within shorter times.[61]

Focal destruction of condylomas (using electrocautery, cryosurgery or localized laser ablation) is another acceptable approach. On mucosal surfaces, cytolytic chemicals are just as effective as physical destruction. However, since surface keratin can impede access of topical medications to the reservoir of HPV infection at the basal layers, destructive techniques are sometimes needed for the removal of stubborn cutaneous lesions. Despite the inconvenience of needing infiltration with local anesthetic, thermal methods are more effective than freezing.[57] If cryosurgery is to be used on the vulva, liquid nitrogen is preferable to nitrous oxide cooled probes.

Very extensive, refractory and neoplastic disease

Although sexually transmitted HPV infections are remarkably common,[15,47,48] differences in host susceptibility produce enormous variability in clinical outcome. Clinical experience has taught that the overwhelming majority of patients will be cured by destruction of the macroscopically apparent papillomas alone, without regard to the adjacent areas of acetowhite epithelium.[45,50] However, significant management problems arise in: (1) women

with very extensive condylomas (coalescent lesions occupying >30% of the vulvar surface; Fig. 69.22), (2) women with refractory disease (unresponsive to >9 months of therapy; Fig. 69.23) and (3) women with multifocal, multicentric intraepithelial neoplasias (Fig. 69.24).

The rationale for using the laser in difficult cases is to destroy the entire field of HPV-infected epithelium (both clinically apparent and subclinical), thereby allowing the resurgent host immune response to establish lasting dominance over any residual viral reservoir. Done skill-

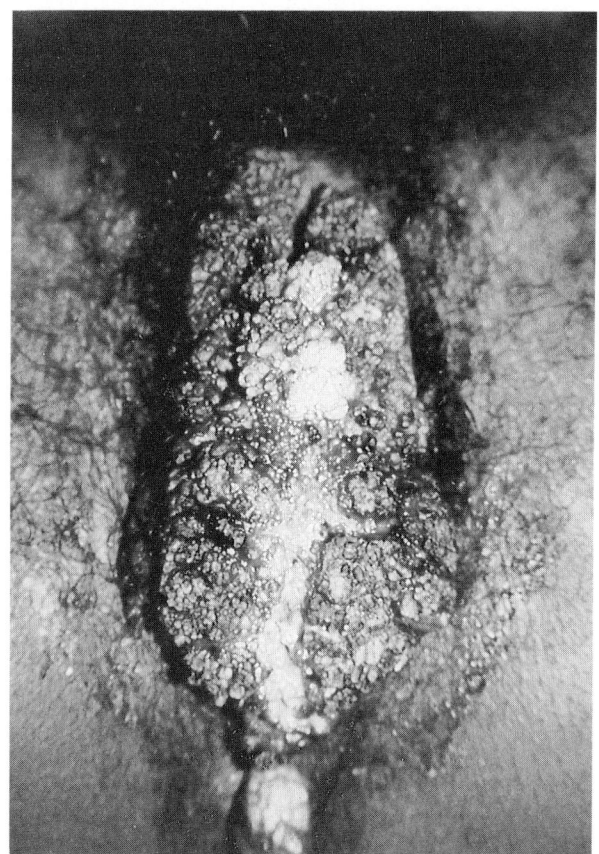

A
Fig. 69.22 (caption overleaf)

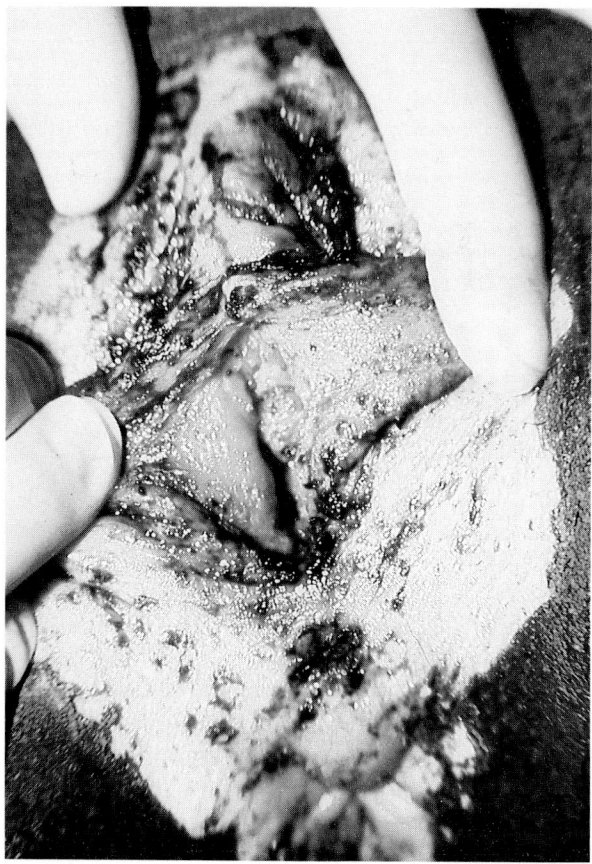

B

Fig. 69.22 (A) Massive coalescent condylomas of recent onset, occupying most of the vestibular and lateral vulvar surface. (Reproduced with permission from Schwartz et al (1987)[53]). (B) Immediately after destruction to the first surgical plane. (Reproduced from Schwartz et al (1987),[53] with permission).

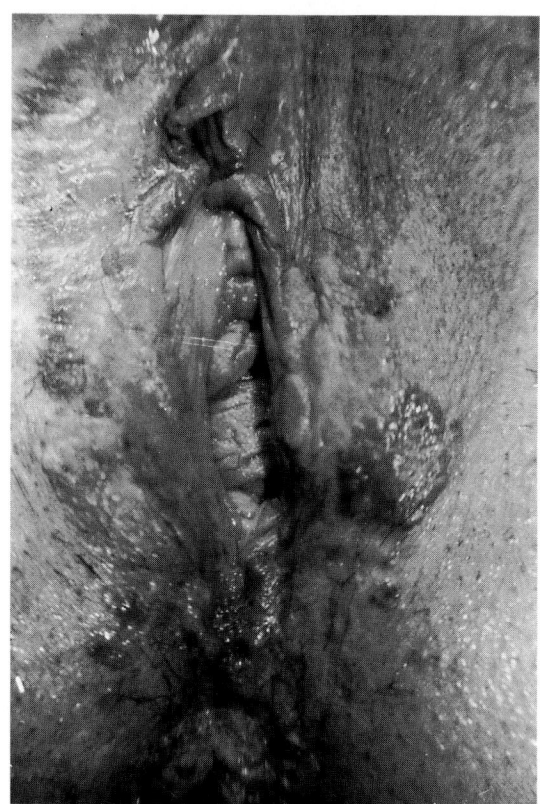

Fig. 69.23 Benign condylomata, refractory to multiple office and outpatient destructive therapies over the course of 23 years.

fully, healing will occur from unaffected keratinocytes in the underlying skin appendages, rather than by epithelial in-growth from the wound edges. Extended laser ablation is particularly helpful when there is extensive involvement of the 'sanctuary sites' (Fig. 69.25). Of course, such an aggressive method must be reserved for the small subset of women who present special management problems.

Factors that adversely affect treatment outcome are as follows:[50]

1. *Disease duration*. Because most individuals will mount an effective immune response, the treatment plan must take account of the various phases in the natural history of HPV infection; namely, inoculation, incubation, active expression, host containment and late stage disease (Fig. 69.26A).[32,40] Patients whose disease has been present for 10 months or longer have twice the failure rate of those with lesions of more recent onset.

2. *Very extensive disease volumes*. Patients with large coalescent disease volumes are inherently difficult to manage by office methods. The area of affected

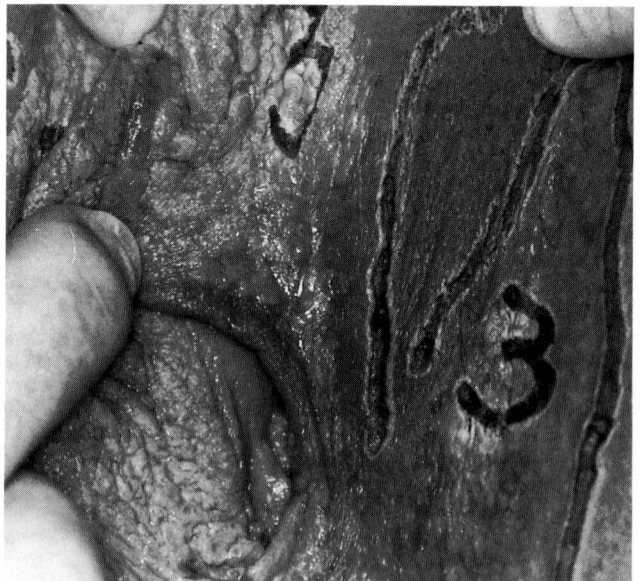

Fig. 69.24 Extensive vulvar intraepithelial neoplasia, Grade 3 (marked 3). Multiple biopsies showed no evidence of occult invasion. Hence, the patient was accepted as suitable for laser ablation.

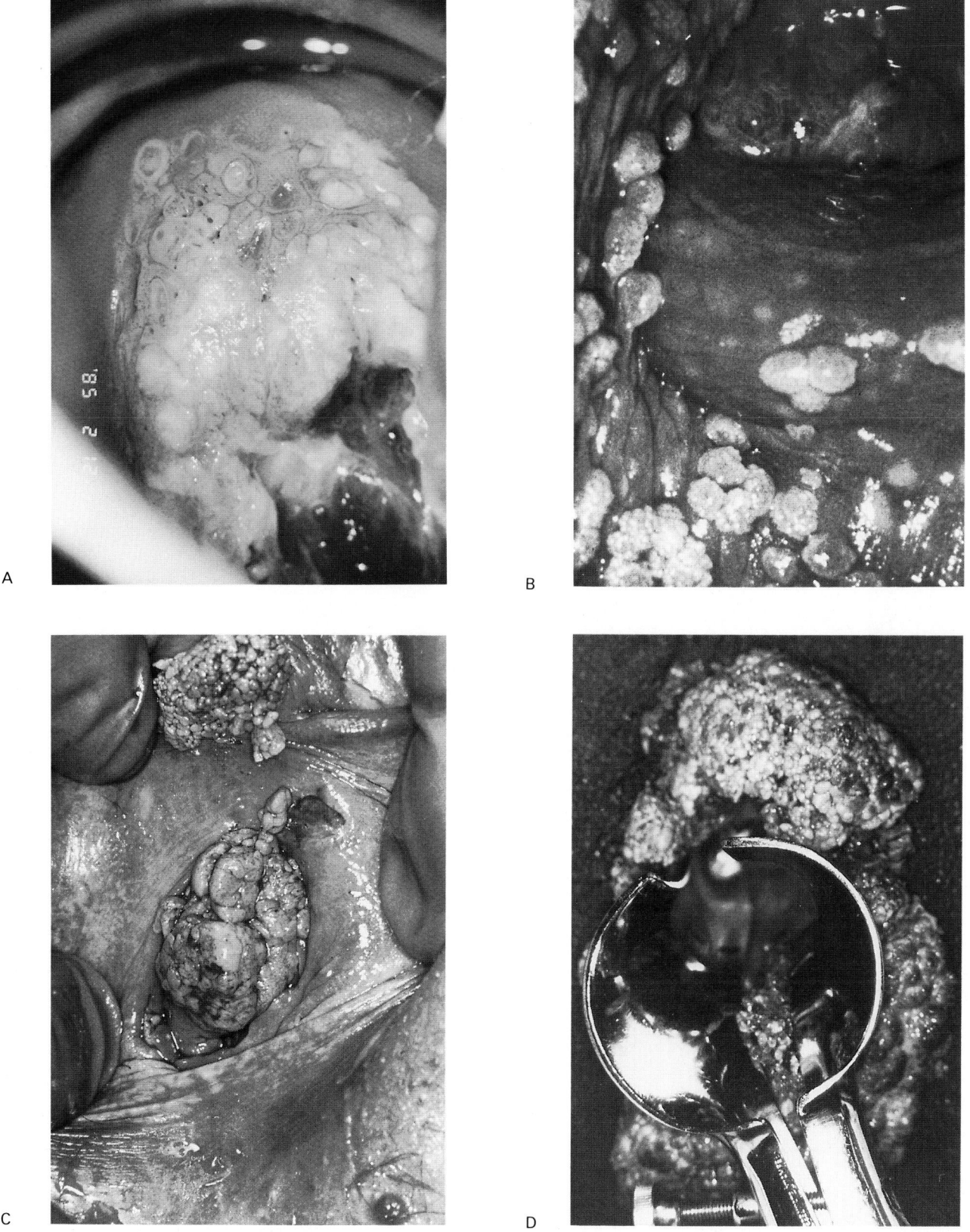

Fig. 69.25 'Sanctuary site' involvement beyond that which cannot be controlled by superficial 'spot welding'. (A) Cervix: a large condyloma replaced the entire transformation zone. (B) Vaginal walls: innumerable vaginal condylomas throughout the entire vagina. (C) Urethra: a large mass of condylomas distends and fills the external urethral meatus. A second papilloma occupies the entire surface of glans clitoris. (D) Anus: a large mass of perianal condylomas has occluded the anal canal.

epithelium is generally too large for satisfactory infiltration with local anesthesia, and such sensitive sites as the urethra, anus and lower vagina are frequently affected. Since these patients are usually scheduled for laser ablation under general or regional anesthesia, destruction of the adjacent areas of subclinical HPV infection adds nothing to patient morbidity.

3. *Smoking or other adverse host factors.* Patients who smoke, and those with immunosuppressive conditions, diabetes mellitis and chronic medical illnesses, have twice the failure rate of otherwise healthy women.

4. *Adverse viral factors.* Patients whose biopsies show high grade intraepithelial neoplasia, and those in whom oncogenic HPV types are detected, have also been found to have significantly higher failure rates.

5. *Refractory clinical course.* Patients who have failed previous, adequate therapy have significantly higher failure rates at any subsequent therapy.

That failure is not a random event is further supported by the fact that these adverse factors exert a cumulative effect (Fig. 69.26B). In contrast, outcome was not affected by either treating or not treating the male partner. Hence, it appears that success or failure ultimately depends upon whether the host immune response is able to prevent re-expression of the residual viral reservoir. Among patients who do not mount an early immune response, just continuing the strategy of local destruction is of little help. For example, a randomized trial comparing laser 'spot welding' with electrodiathermy reported control rates of only 9 of 21 in the laser group and 8 of 22 in the diathermy group.[10]

Experience gained in the treatment of large decorative tattoos on non-genital skin had shown that large expanses of epidermis could be safely removed by a rapid brushing technique, such that healing would occur by outgrowth

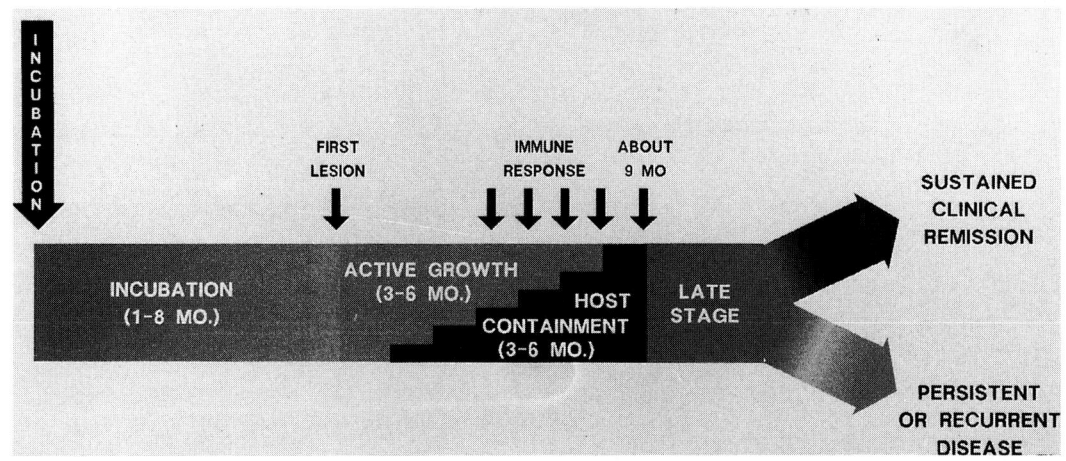

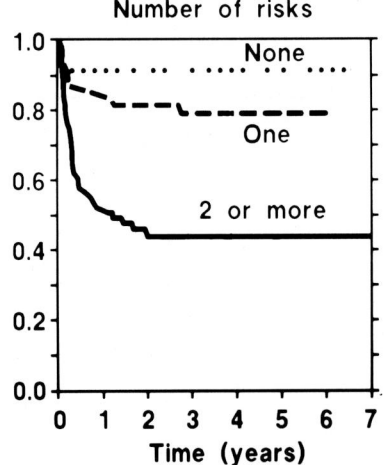

from the underlying skin appendages rather than by in-growth from the wound edges.[49] Clinical judgement suggested that, in difficult cases, the best hope for a resurgence of host immune dominance lay with the simultaneous destruction of both the macroscopic papillomas and the entire field of colposcopically recognizable HPV infection. Hence, in 1982, the first author began treating problematic patients by extended laser ablation.[35] Over the 6 succeeding years, 160 of the 1000 women referred with HPV-associated vulvar disease were found to have problems severe enough to warrant treatment in the operating room, using a surgical technique that would have a 2 to 3 week recovery time.[45]

Fig. 69.26 (A) Phases in the natural histology of HPV infection. (B) A Kaplan Meier survival curve, showing the cumulative effect of the various adverse factors upon treatment outcome. Two adverse factors shown as a solid line, one as a dashed line, and no factors as a dotted line. (Reproduced from Reid et al (1990),[45] with permission.)

VULVAR LASER TECHNIQUES

Destruction of exophytic condylomas

The surgeon should not attempt to remove condylomas by

undercutting them with the laser. Except for long-standing lesions (which can become quite pedunculated), most condylomas have a flat base (Fig. 69.27A). Attempts to undercut condylomas that are not required for histologic examination produce unnecessary dermal defects, and can be attended by troublesome bleeding (especially in pregnancy). Rather, the strategy should be to umbilicate the center of each lesion, debride the loosened epidermis, and relase to any residue.[36] Each condyloma should be umbilicated by lasing to the center and allowing tissue shrinkage at the laser impact site to pull the edge of the lesion into the operative field. It is unnecessary to laser to the edge of each condyloma; hence, the problem of unwanted damage to adjacent skin is easily avoided. The initial application of

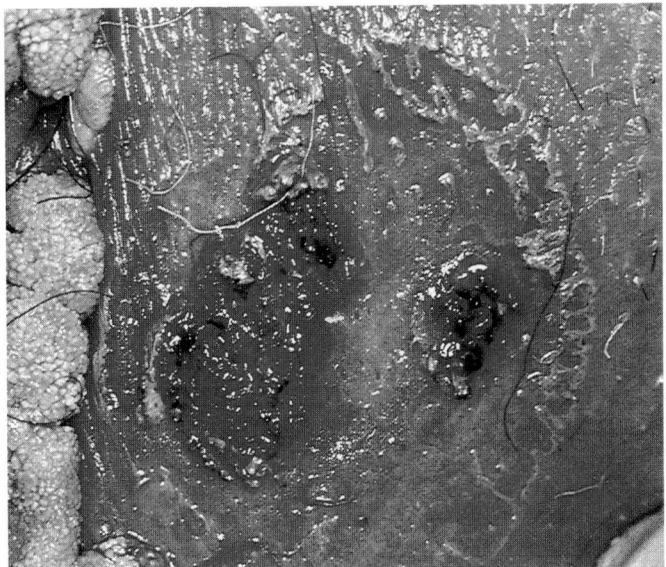

C

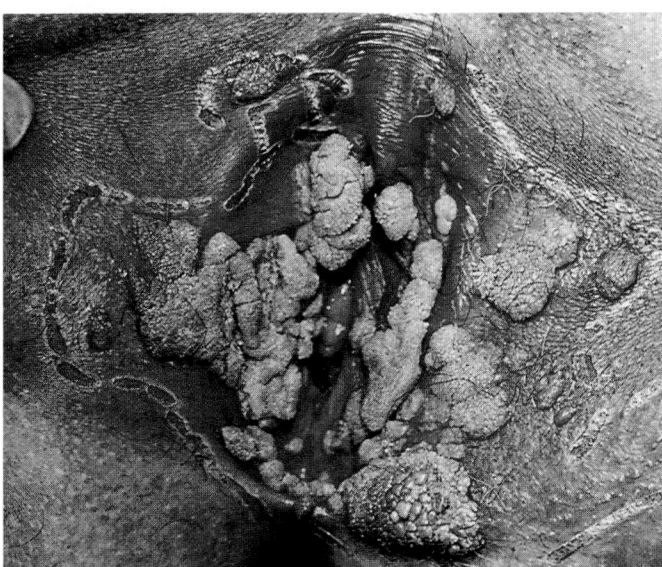

A

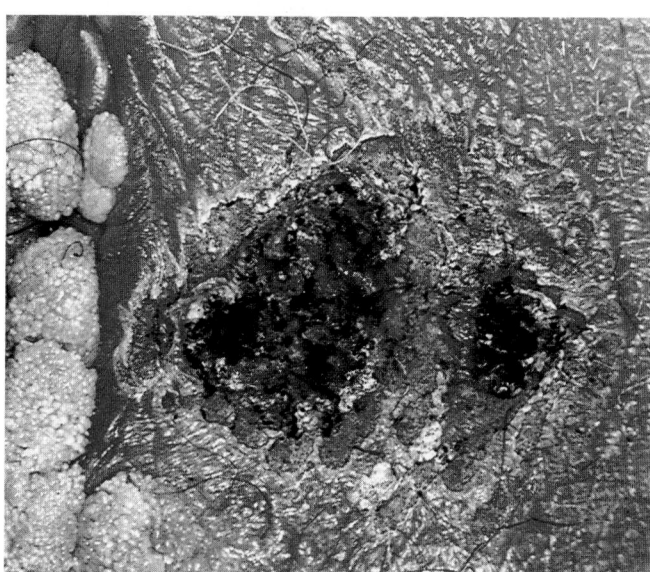

B

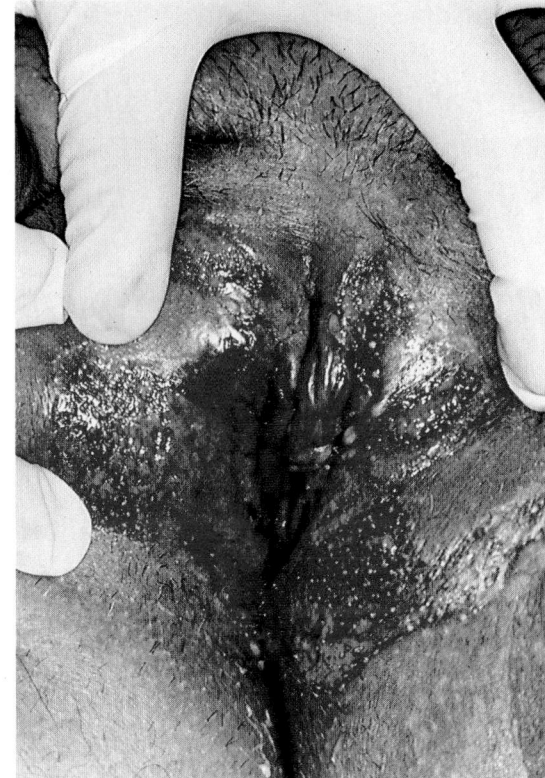

D

Fig. 69.27 (A) Chronic vulvar condylomas, after initial outlining, but prior to starting laser ablation. (B) Initial central vaporization of an exophytic condyloma, to about the level of the adjacent skin. (C) After wiping, the residual 'core' can easily be re-lased. (D) Six days post laser. Areas treated to the first plane are healed, while areas destroyed to the third plane show advanced regrowth of epithelial buds (originating from the skin appendages). Final cosmetic appearance will be indistinguishable from adjacent normal skin.

the laser should extend the vaporization crater to about the level of the surrounding skin (Fig. 69.27B), but there should be no penetration of the basement membrane at this point. Although it will be visually apparent that the zone of vaporization has not yet destroyed all of the abnormal keratinocytes at the base of the condyloma, lasing to this level will separate most of these cells from the basement membrane. Hence, this technique will minimize the extent of any unwanted thermal damage within the superficial dermis. Once the condylomas have been umbilicated, the area is easily debrided by gently wiping with a moist gauze swab. Any residual epithelial fronds or capillary spikes can then be accurately destroyed by spot lasing (Fig. 69.27C). Healing will then be both rapid and cosmetically indistinguishable from adjacent skin (Fig. 69.27D).

Extended laser ablation of vulvar intraepithelial neoplasia and problematic condylomas

After the induction of anesthesia, the perineum is carefully shaved (both to facilitate colposcopy and to simplify postoperative care; Fig. 69.18A). The use of antiseptic solutions is neither desirable (because it impairs response of tissue to acetic acid) nor necessary (because of the high temperatures attained at the site of laser impact). Rather, the vulva and anus are soaked for 3 minutes with 4 to 5% acetic acid. The perineum is then carefully examined with a colposcope. The borders of any foci of vulvar intraepithelial neoplasia and the outer margins of the surrounding subclinical papillomaviral infections are then outlined, before the acetic acid reaction fades (Fig. 69.18B). The viral reservoir (Fig. 69.18C) between this outer margin and the hymenal ring is then destroyed en bloc (Fig. 69.18D), using a microscopically controlled technique for depth control.

The frequency with which the epithelium of the skin appendages are colonized by HPV genomes is unknown. However, in the absence of neoplastic transformation, morphologic evidence of viral expression is usually limited to the surface epithelium.[35] Hence, for benign condylomas, destruction to just beneath the basement membrane is probably adequate. In contrast, vulvar intraepithelial neoplasia often extends into the pilosebaceous ducts. Involvement is generally limited to the superficial portions of the ducts, making laser ablation to the mid-reticular level an ideal treatment in most instances. Nonetheless, intended depth of destruction should be individualized by examining representative histologic sections. Foci of deep pilar exten-

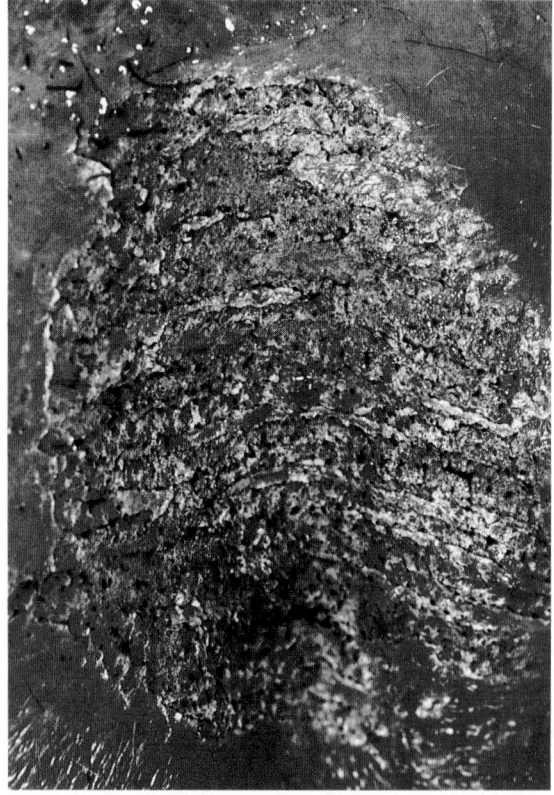

A   B

Fig. 69.28 (A) First surgical plane, as seen through the operating microscope, after the initial 'brushing' procedure. Beneath the charred remnants of the surface squames, one can see the refractile remnants of the plump keratinocytes that lie within the proliferating layers of the epidermis. (B) The first surgical plane, after this epithelial debris has been wiped away with a moist gauze. This maneuver exposes the intact surface of the underlying corium. The basement membrane is still intact, giving a shiny surface and a diffused pink color.

sion are rare. However, any areas of deep pilar extension must be managed by surgical excision, reserving the laser for the ablation of adjoining superficial disease.

First surgical plane

Destruction of the first plane removes only the surface epithelium to the level of the basement membrane. This plane is reached by placing the laser crater within the prickle cell layer. Penetration to the proper depth is accomplished by rapid oscillation of the micromanipulator, such that the helium-neon spot describes a roughly parallel series of lines. When done correctly, each pass of the laser beam will reveal bubbles of silver opalescence beneath the charred surface squames (Fig. 69.28A) and the maneuver will be accompanied by a distinctive crackling sound. Inadvertent penetration of the basement membrane is signaled by the loss of these two characteristic signs.

Lasing to the prickle cell layer shears the basal cells from the basement membrane, thereby producing a plane of cleavage. Hence, these detached basal cells are easily removed by wiping with a moistened gauze, thus exposing the smooth, intact surface of the papillary dermis (Fig. 69.28B). Such wounds heal completely within 5 to 14 days, depending upon the sophistication of energy delivery.[45] The cosmetic appearance and functional qualities of the healed wound are entirely indistinguishable from normal vulvar skin.

Second surgical plane

Destruction to the second surgical plane removes both the epidermis and the loose network of fine collagen and elastin fibers that compose the papillary dermis. This plane is reached by a similar set of rapid oscillations, moving the beam so quickly that the laser scorches (rather than craters) the exposed corium. When done correctly, the scorched surface should show a finely roughened contour and a yellowish color, somewhat reminiscent of a chamois cloth (Fig. 69.29A). This clinical appearance indicates that the zone of coagulation necrosis will lie within the papillary dermis, with only minimal thermal injury to the underlying reticular dermis (Fig. 69.29B). The second plane is the

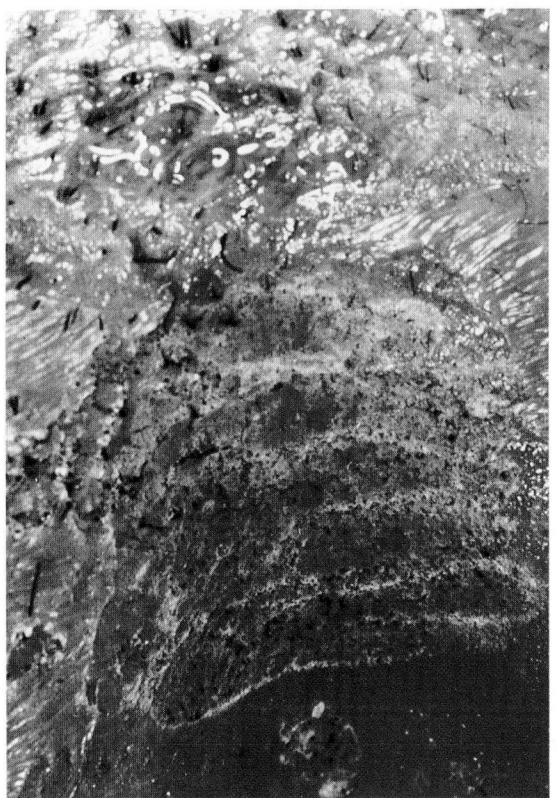
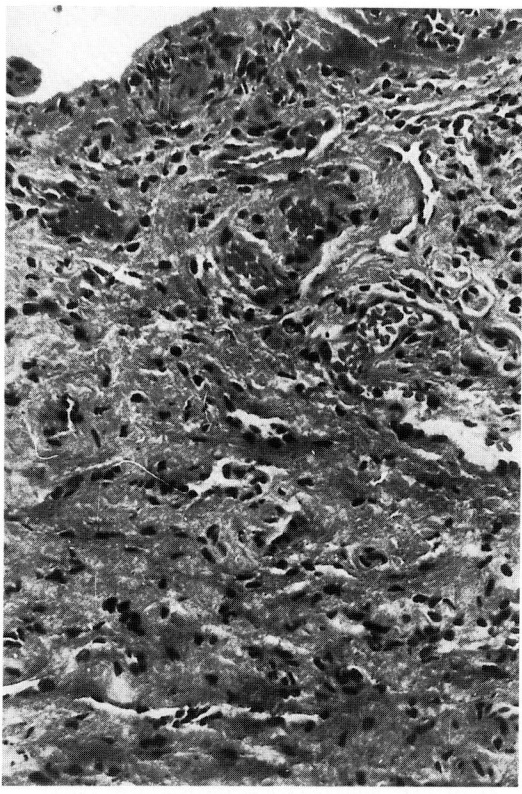

A

B

Fig. 69.29 (A) The second surgical plane. In the middle of the picture, exposed papillary dermis has been gently released, sufficient to scorch (but not cut) the dermal surface. Because the exposed dermal surface now consists of a myriad of transected collagen, elastin and reticulin fibrils (rather than a smooth mucopolysaccharide layer), light emanating from the underlying dermis is now heavily scattered, resulting in a dull appearance and a yellowish hue. Above this area is a field of third plane destruction, and below is an area of intact basement membrane, awaiting further destruction. (B) A biopsy from this wound shows coagulation necrosis within the upper papillary dermis (top), but no effect within the reticular dermis (bottom).

preferred level of ablation for extensive condylomas. Such wounds heal rapidly and also produce an end result indistinguishable from normal skin.

Third surgical plane

Destruction to the third surgical plane removes the epidermis, the upper portions of the pilosebaceous ducts, and a part of the reticular dermis. Correct depth control is tied to the recognition of three characteristic landmarks: (1) lasing to the mid-reticular layer uncovers coarse collagen bundles that can be seen through the operating microscope as gray-white fibers resembling water-logged cotton threads (Fig. 69.30A); (2) wiping with iced saline reveals the bright, alabaster white color of these basal collagen plates; (3) this maneuver also exposes a network of prominent arterioles and venules, running horizontal to the epithelial surface (Fig. 69.30B).

The technique of micromanipulator control for lasing to the third plane is a little different. Instead of a rapid, oscillating action, the surgeon uses slower, more deliberate movements. Speed of cut is coordinated to the visual recognition of a 'fibrous grain' within the crater base. Moving the beam too rapidly will not expose these collagen bundles, and moving the beam too slowly will uncover skin appendages within the deep reticular dermis. If uncovered, such hair follicles and sweat glands will be readily visible through the operating microscope, being seen as tiny refractile granules that resemble grains of sand. The rationale for limiting destruction to the third surgical plane is to allow re-epithelialization by regeneration from the keratinocytes within these skin appendages (Fig. 69.27D). Exposing these structures within the crater base signals the creation of a third degree burn in that area. Hence, the third surgical plane represents the deepest level from which optimal healing will occur.

Fourth surgical plane

Under rare circumstances, it may be necessary to produce a deliberate third degree burn in order to destroy abnormal keratinocytes within the hair follicles or sweat glands. Because of its precision, the CO_2 laser can destroy the adnexal epithelium while still preserving a layer of collagen fibers within the deep reticular dermis. Dermal regeneration produces a much better bed for skin grafting than either subcutaneous fat or granulation tissue. Hence, cosmetic and functional results are vastly superior to those attainable by skinning vulvectomy (Fig. 69.31).

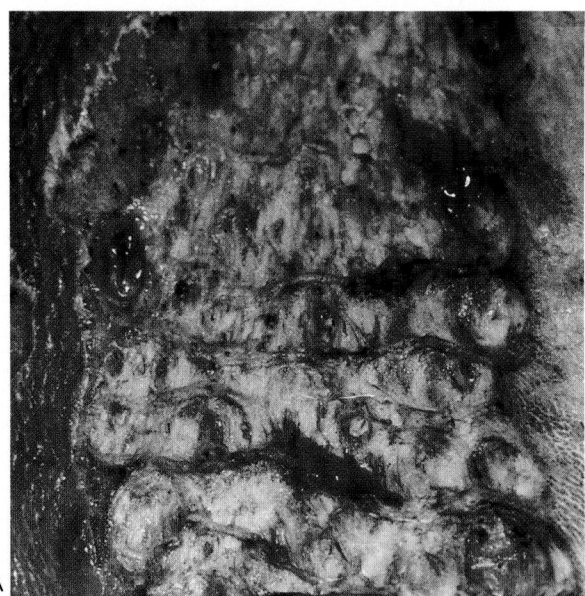

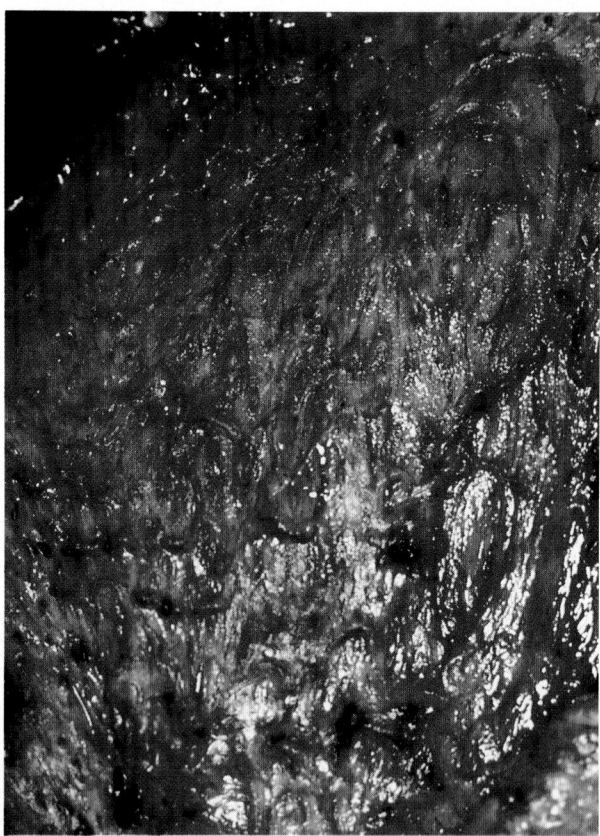

Fig. 69.30 (A) The third surgical plane. The upper half of the dermis has been vaporized by a series of slower, more deliberate movements of the laser beam (done in a transverse axis), revealing the dense collagen of the mid-reticular dermis. The stark white color is attributable to the high collagen content of the reticular dermis. The shiny reflectance is due to the fact that we are looking at collagen that has been condensed into dense bundles, running horizontal to the epithelial surface. That is to say, lasing to this deeper level exposes the long axis of these fibrous bundles, rather than the cut ends of the individual fibrils. Indeed, in this photograph, the direction of these collagen bundles is appreciable as a 'grain', that can be seen running beneath the transverse furrows made by the path of the laser beam. Vestiges of coagulated papillary dermis at the margin of each furrow are seen as residual traces of dull, yellowish debris. (B) After wipping, arcuate blood vessels at the base of the reticular dermis are visible against a background of starkly white collagen plates.

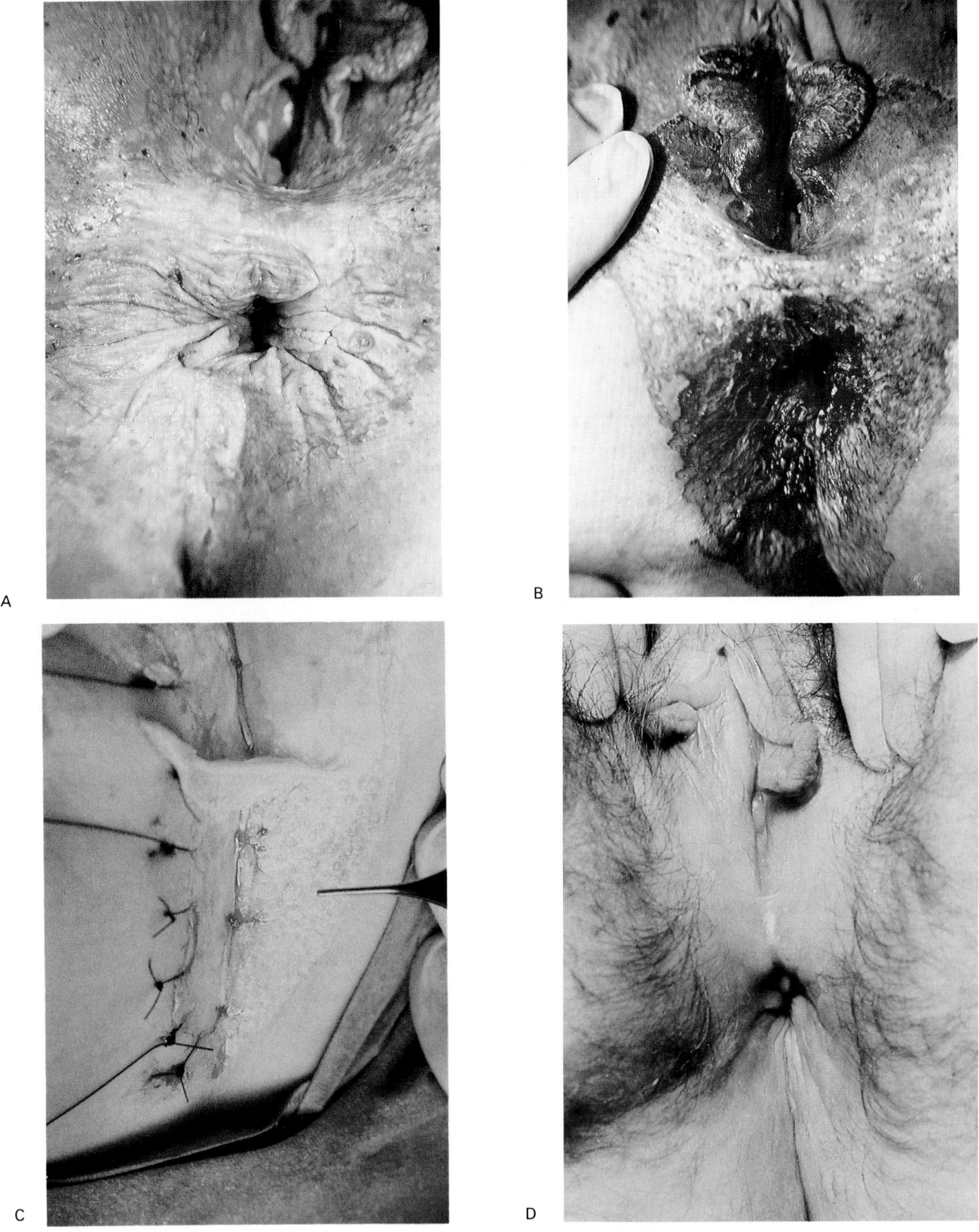

Fig. 69.31 The fourth surgical plane. (A) An area of refractory perianal dysplasia that has failed three prior superficial laser vaporizations. (B) Vaporization of the perianal skin to the fourth plane. Each of the craters represents a site at which a skin appendage was destroyed, whereas the intervening areas represent viable collagen bundles within the deep dermis. (C) The same area 10 days later, showing the extent of dermal regeneration at the time of skin grafting. (D) The final result is better than what would have been achieved by skinning vulvectomy. (Reproduced from Reid (1987),[38] with permission.)

Postoperative care

To prevent early postoperative pain, the treated areas are infiltrated with 0.25% bupivicaine in 1:100 000 adrenalin. Following the empiric observation that urinary diversion will prevent a great deal of anticipated postoperative pain, patients who require large areas of vulvar ablation are offered a suprapubic catheter with leg bag for 1 to 2 weeks (until healing is virtually complete). Malodor is prevented by the daily instillation of 1 ounce of white vinegar into the collecting bag. Safeguards against urinary infection include the prescription of prophylactic antibiotics and the daily cleansing of the collection system with household detergents. The catheter is removed at an office visit, when healing is well advanced.

Except in pregnant patients, treatments are performed as outpatient operations. Before discharge, patients also receive a prescription for narcotic analgesic, a complete set of postoperative instructions, a demonstration of how to care for the catheter and an appointment for office follow-up in 1 week.

The most important part of the postoperative regimen is to apply silver sulphadiazine cream or nitrofurazone soluble dressing as prophylaxis against conglutination of denuded surfaces. To prevent superinfection, the previous application of sulphadiazine or nitrofurazone cream must be washed off using a Sitz bath, at least three times per day. Except for prophylaxis against urinary infection, postoperative antibiotic therapy is not helpful. However, preoperative reduction of the vaginal flora by means of a course of vaginal suppositories (terramycin 100 mg b.i.d, clindamycin 100 mg in cocoa butter q.h.s or metronidazole 2 g in cocoa butter q.h.s).

Patients must be seen weekly for 3 weeks, to correct any early coaptation of adjacent raw surfaces. Healing should be virtually complete within 14 to 21 days. Thereafter, women with refractory condylomas should return every 2 to 4 weeks for the next 3 months, so that any focal recurrences can be controlled by caustic agent application. Provided that the diagnosis is made before the formation of large condylomatous aggregations, diffuse recurrence can also be forestalled by twice weekly applications of 5-fluorouracil cream. Because women with vulvar neoplasia or papillomaviral infections are at high risk for developing squamous neoplasia at other sites within the genital tract, surveillance by annual Papanicolaou smears is mandatory.

Complications

The adage that complication rates are a direct reflection of surgical skill is even more apparent for laser surgery than for conventional operative techniques. In the series of 160 patients treated by extended laser ablation,[45] the major complications were related to thermal damage in the adjacent tissues. The cumulative incidence of cellulitis, scarring or secondary hemorrhage was 10.3% among those treated with low power continuous wave, but fell to 2.7% with the use of high powers and pulsed temporal modes (Table 69.6). Likewise, recovery and postoperative pain were also dependent upon laser settings. Over a 6-year period, improvements in laser technique produced a 7-day reduction in mean healing times (see p. 1094).

Although there were no instances of non-healing or major scarring in this study, we have seen such problems among women treated elsewhere (Figs 69.3 and 69.4). Since the late cosmetic appearances of split skin grafting are suboptimal, the best approach to restoration of normal anatomy and adequate function depends upon the use of rotational flaps. For posterior defects, rhomboid skin flaps allow the surgeon to mobilize and transpose perianal or labial skin.[2,21,29] Small anterior or central defects are sometimes best repaired with a bulbo-cavernosus myocutaneous flap, using either an anterior or posterior pedicle.[20] However, if a larger volume of hairless skin is needed, the best choice is probably a pair of arterialized medial thigh flaps (based on the terminal branches of the pudendal arteries; Fig. 69.32). In the extreme case shown in Figure 69.33, we have a transverse rectus abdominus muscle ('TRAM') flap, allowing transposition of a large amount of abdominal skin, for the reconstruction of a vulva that had been totally destroyed by the reckless use of low powered laser surgery.

VAGINAL LASER TECHNIQUES

Ablation of vaginal intraepithelial neoplasia

The vaginal mucosa consists of a simple stratified

Table 69.6 Among 160 women having extended laser ablation of refractory vulvar condylomas or VIN 3, improved laser technique led to a significant reduction in complication rates

Laser setting	Number of patients	Cellulitis	Complications Scarring	Bleeding	Total
CW* < 35 watts	39	2 (5.1%)	2 (5.1%)	0	4 (10.3%)
CW 80 watts	46	1 (2.2%)	2 (4.3%)	0	3 (6.5%)
Chopped or rapid superpulse modes	75	2 (2.7%)	0	2 (2.7%)	4 (5.3%)

$X^2 = 0.98$; $P > 0.61$.
* CW = constant wave
Reproduced from Reid et al (1990),[45] with permission.

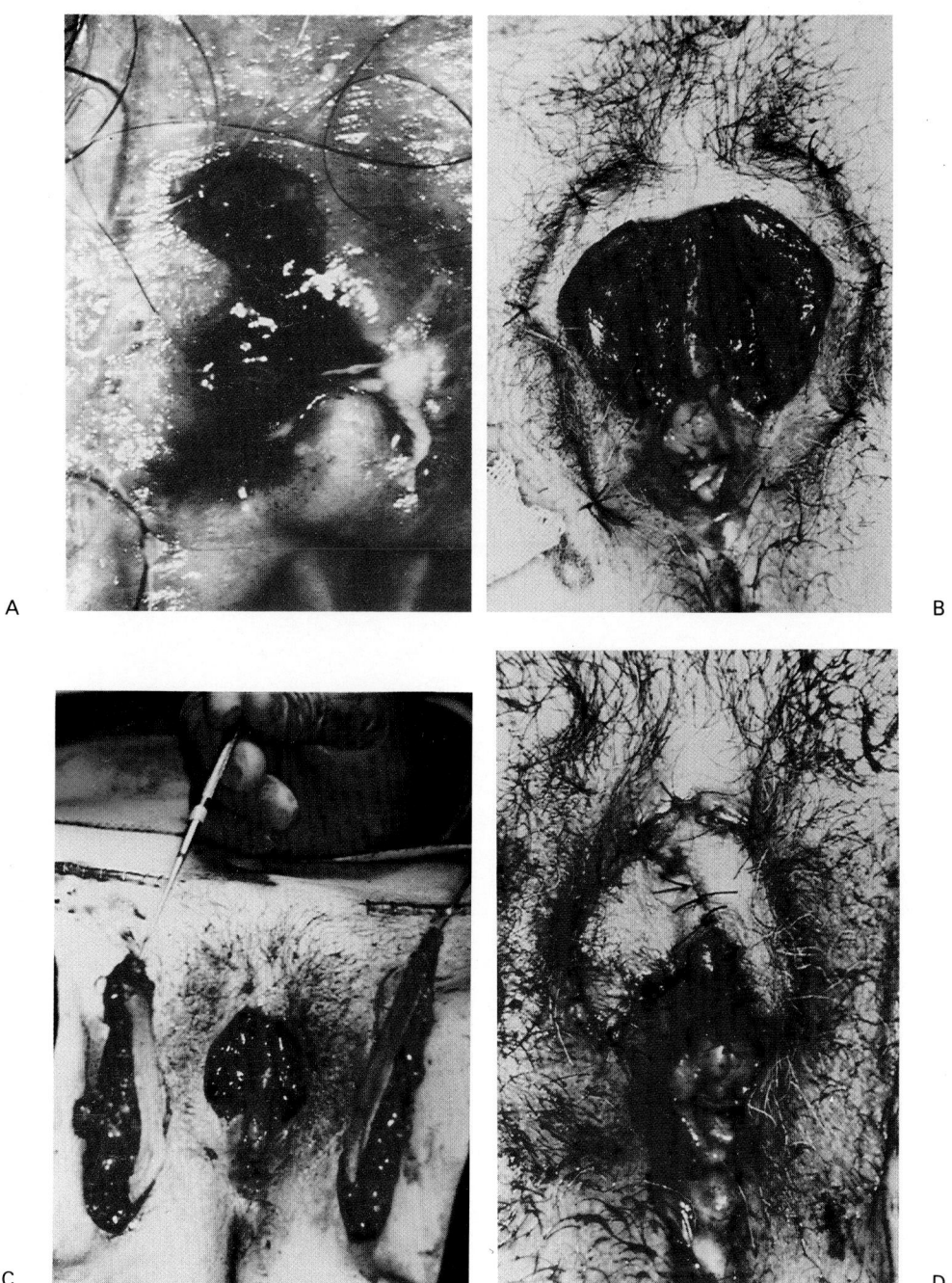

Fig. 69.32 The use of an arteriolized flap of medial thigh skin (based on the terminal branches of the pudendal artery) to allow clitoral conservation and restoration of normal anatomic appearance, after wide resection of this 0.5 mm deep, well differentiated, invasive squamous carcinoma arising in the skin overlying the shaft of clitoris. (A) A colpophotograph of the lesion, showing incipient ulceration and a bizarre mosaic vascular pattern. (B) Resection of the anterior vulva to the pilosebaceous lines exposing the crura and shaft of clitoris as they arise from the pubic bones. (C) Raising the flap of medial thigh and inguinal skin, by dissecting down to the fascia of adductor magnus. (D) Transposition of the flaps, to restore anatomic integrity. (Photographs courtesy of Dr. M. Gowda, Southfield, Michigan.)

squamous epithelium that is separated from the underlying muscularis by a loose layer of connective tissue, called the lamina propria. Although the mucosa is folded into a myriad of rugae, there are no deep epithelial clefts (as seen in the cervical transformation zone). Hence, the desired depth of destruction for VAIN 3 is relatively shallow.

Nonetheless, the authors are aware of two vesico-vaginal fistulas that followed destruction to just the level of the submucosa, because of poor surgical technique, permitting excessive heat conduction from a carbonized crater. Hence, high power outputs and adequate power densities are especially important for vaginal laser surgery. Since an

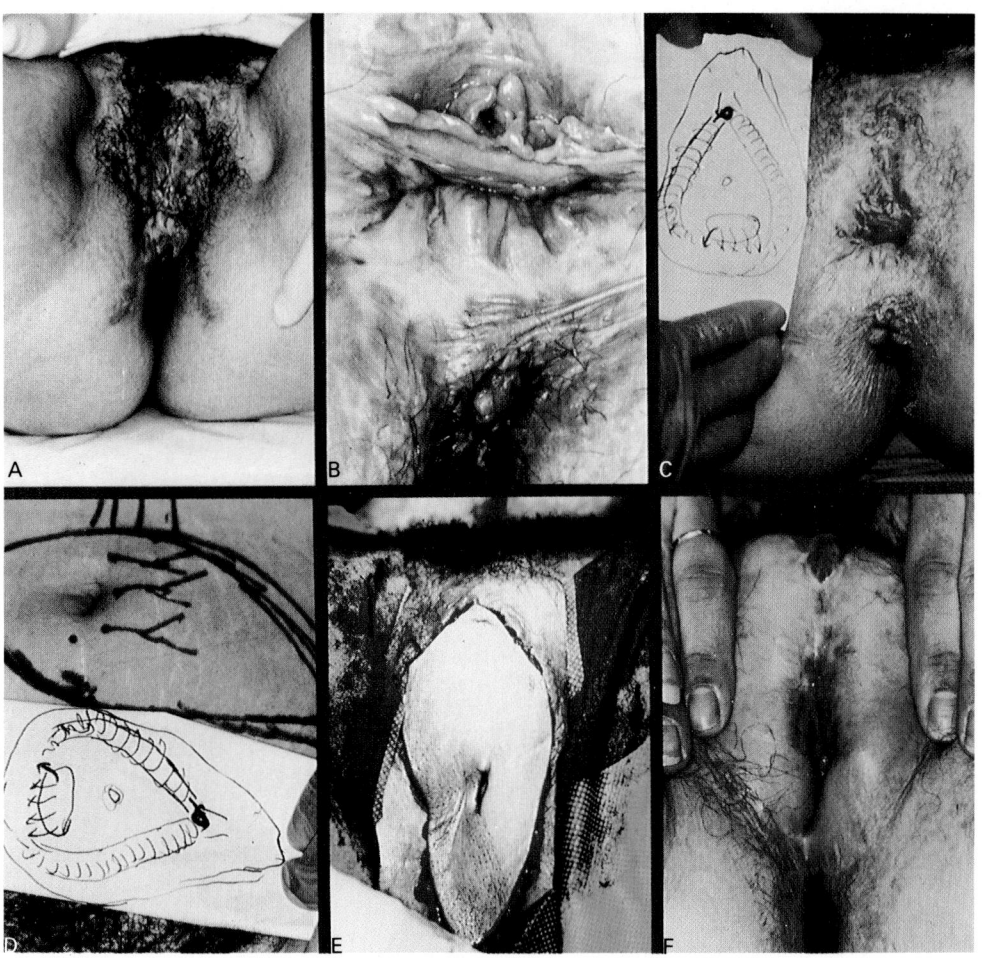

Fig. 69.33 The use of a transverse rectus abdominal myocutaneous ('TRAM') flap to reconstruct the vulva of a patient injured by poor laser technique. (A) A macroscopic view of the vulva, showing how the labia minora were sloughed off because of excessive thermal damage. The end result is a hideously deformed appearance, in which the vestibule has now undergone keratinization, because of the loss of the moistening labia minora. Moreover, dense scarring of the underlying connective tissue produced pain during any attempt at coitus, and even vigorous walking. (B) The exposed, keratinized, desensitized vaginal introitus. (C) Planning the area of skin needed to reconstruct the vulva. (D) Planning the 'TRAM' flap, to be based upon the left inferior epigastric artery. (E) Transposition of this myocutaneous flap through a tunnel to the left side of the glans clitoris. The flap has been rotated 90 degrees anticlockwise, such that the periumbilical defect is now positioned over the introitus and the left hypogastric skin is now at the apex of the vulva. (F) Appearances after a second operation 3 months later, during which the excess fat was removed from the center of the flap, thus giving better anatomic definition to the end result. If so desired, similar improvements could be made at the right and left lateral margins, to even more closely simulate the normal vulvar contour. (Photographs courtesy of Dr M. Gowda, Southfield, Michigan.)

oblique impact can inadvertently reduce effective power density to the carbonization range, extra care must be taken to manipulate the vaginal walls such that the beam impinges at right angles.

A number of anatomic and pathologic factors combine to complicate the management of VAIN. First, the vagina has a large surface area, much of which is obscured by the cervix, the speculum blades, and various rugose folds. Displaying lesions within the fornices can be especially difficult, because of the distensible nature of the upper vagina. Second, the colposcopic features of VAIN 3 are highly variable, such that significant lesions may not be recognized by less experienced eyes. Hence, the treatment of extensive, multifocal VAIN usually requires general anesthesia, both to avoid the pain of laser impact and to permit adequate manipulation of the vaginal speculum.

Staining with Lugol's iodine (diluted 1 in 3 with tap water) is another helpful aid to the identification and exposure of lesions that might otherwise escape detection.

Depth of destruction within the vagina cannot be controlled by actual measurement. Hence, vaginal laser surgery is always done through the operating microscope, controlling depth by a system of anatomic landmarks. Ablation is done in a stepwise fashion, removing a thin layer of tissue with each pass of the beam. Devitalization and shearing of the vaginal mucosa is denoted by a pearly opalescent color, admixed with a minimal amount of brownish char. Since the base of the laser crater is now obscured by debris, visual orientation depends upon repeated wiping with saline soaked swabs. Moreover, it will be found that such wiping will expose the intact surface of the lamina propria, still covered by the smooth, shiny basement membrane (Fig. 69.34). Although vaginal papillae are not as prominent as those of the vulvar skin, a pebble-like contour is readily appreciable.

In the vagina, islands of intact epithelium will often persist, due to the obscuring effect of the rugose folds. If it is desired to penetrate just to the first surgical plane, these epithelial remnants can be locally ablated. Alternatively, if destruction to the third plane is intended, the exposed lamina propria should be deliberately relased, such that the beam leaves a definite furrow. Fibrous bundles, similar to those visible in the vulvar dermis, can now be seen in the base of each furrow. Since the vaginal mucosa has neither crypts nor appendages, further destruction would be of no value. Healing will occur by ingrowth from the wound edge; nonetheless, re-epithelialization is relatively rapid, because this is a mucosal (rather than a cutaneous) surface.

Visualizing the vaginal vault always requires manipulation. If the uterus is in situ, the epithelial folds within each of the vaginal fornices can often be smoothed flat by pulling the cervix in an opposite direction. In easier cases, this will be accomplished by pressure in an opposite fornix, using a rectal swab held in place by pressure with the left thumb (Fig. 69.35A). Alternatively, the cervix can be grasped by a tenaculum (applied through the left side of

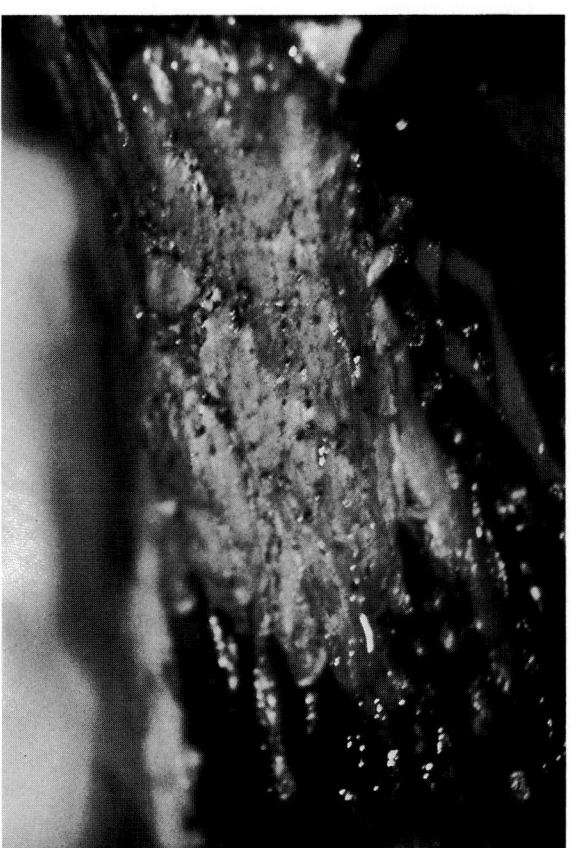

Fig. 69.34 The first vaginal plane. After the epithelial debris is wiped away, the surface of the lamina propria appears as a shiny, white layer.

the speculum), and used to expose the vaginal fornix by either pushing or pulling (Fig. 69.35B). In a patient who has had a prior hysterectomy, exposure of the lateral vaginal angles depends upon traction with a fine hook (Fig. 69.35C).

The lateral vaginal walls are exposed between the open blades of a bivalve speculum. Treatment of the anterior and posterior walls then proceeds by successive rotations and gradual withdrawal of the speculum. In the lower part of the vagina, a better angle of impact is obtained by aiming through the sides (rather than the central aperture) of the speculum (Fig. 69.35D). Once the entire circumference has been treated, the speculum is withdrawn and the epithelial debris wiped away by vigorous swabbing with a moist gauze square. When the speculum is reinserted, any untreated areas are easily identifiable, and can be ablated under direct vision.

Excision of vaginal intraepithelial neoplasia

The most important single factor in preventing the occurrence of invasive cancer following laser ablation is the exclusion of occult malignancy with absolute certainty, prior to any attempt at destructive surgery. In the observance of this dictum, we have used excisional techniques in the following circumstances: (1) if there is cytologic or colposcopic suspicion of invasion, (2) if a high grade lesion extends into a previous hysterectomy scar, and (3) if there remains a marked discrepancy between cytology and histology.

In performing this excision, the colposcope provides helpful magnification, irrespective of whether the actual surgery is done by CO_2 laser or cold knife.[8] For laser excision, the surgeon must use a tightly focused beam, rapid superpulse being preferable to continuous wave. If necessary, the wound can be closed by suturing, taking precautions not to invert any vaginal mucosa beneath the scar.

Combinations of excision and vaporization

Since VAIN is most often a multifocal problem, the surgeon may encounter instances where some portions require excision for proper diagnosis, while other portions are suited to ablation. By excising only the areas in doubt and vaporizing all others, the amount of normal tissue damaged in the surgical procedure is reduced to a minimum. For example, excisional cervical conization or excision of an obscured vaginal fornix is often combined with ablation of previously biopsied, multifocal areas of VAIN 3. Prior to the advent of laser surgery, treatment of such lesions would have necessitated resection of much of the vaginal mucosa. However, we have used laser combination procedures for a number of years, allowing treatment of very large areas by rather conservative methods.

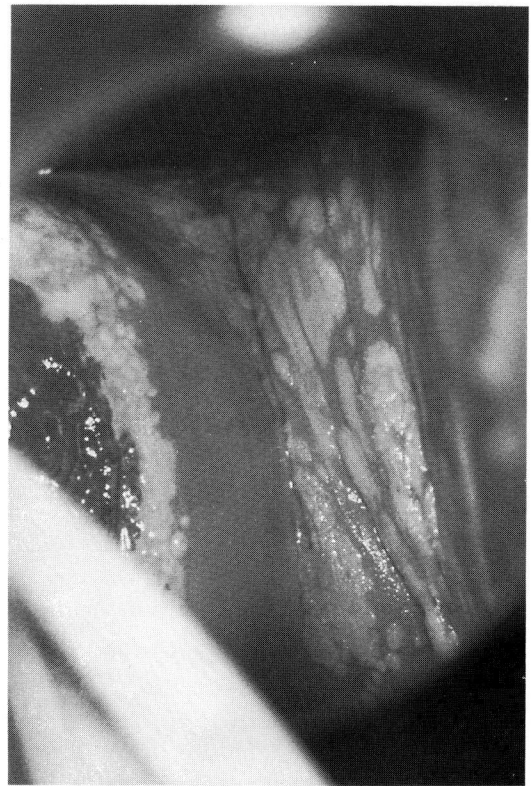

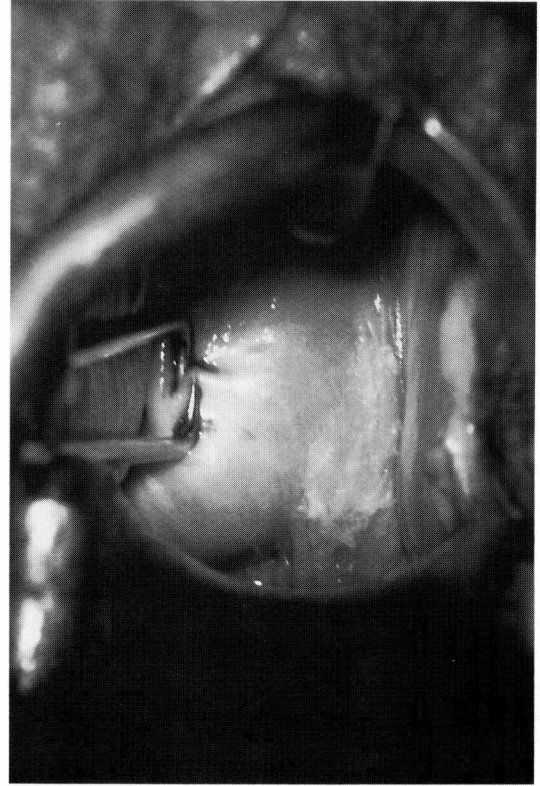

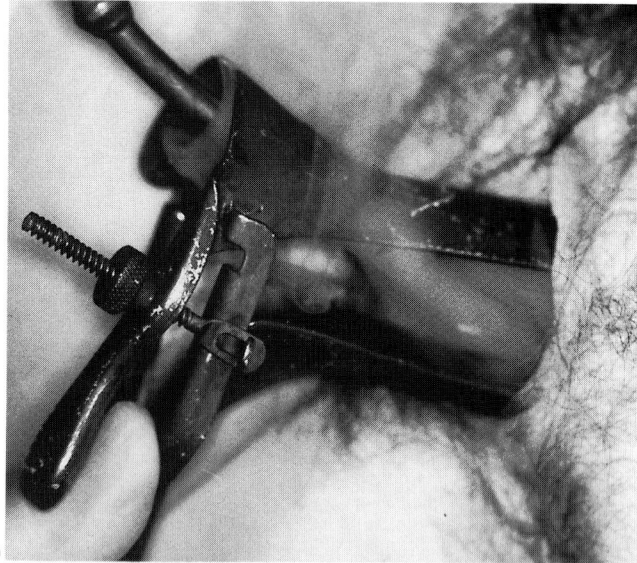

Fig. 69.35   Maneuvers for vaginal exposure. (A) Distending the vaginal fornix by pressure on the opposite fornix with a rectal swab, held in position by the thumb of the hand which controls the speculum. (B) Deviating the cervix by pushing or pulling with a tenaculum, applied lateral to the lateral blades of a Graves speculum. (C) Exposing the vaginal vault scar with a skin hook. (D) Improved exposure, by firing between lateral edges of the speculum blades.

Postoperative care

Because there are no skin appendages, the vagina is the slowest healing area within the lower genital tract. Nonetheless, provided that the lamina propria is not excessively burned by unskilled laser technique, complete re-epithelialization will usually occur within 4 to 6 weeks. Postoperative care of the vaginal wound is aimed primarily at preventing adhesions, vaginal shortening or postoperative scarring. To this end, it may be helpful to have the patient insert an applicator of estrogen or antibacterial cream every other day. Weekly vaginal examinations also help to prevent coaptation, as well as allowing an opportunity to treat early recurrence. Occasionally, squamous regrowth can be retarded by either persistent granulation tissue or areas of columnar metaplasia. Cauterizing with 85% trichloracetic acid or silver nitrate will reactivate the healing process.

RESULTS OF TREATMENT

Vaginal intraepithelial neoplasia

Although invasive carcinoma of the vagina remains one of the rarest of gynecologic malignancies, there has been a definite increase in the prevalence of VAIN over the last decade (see Ch. 29). In contrast to premalignant changes of the vulva, VAIN has a well-defined potential for malignant progression. Indeed, about one-third of the invasive cancers following therapy for cervical neoplasia have occurred in the original squamous epithelium of the vaginal vault.[18,39]

A number of different therapeutic techniques have been employed in the treatment of VAIN. However, because of the variation of etiology, pathology and the anatomic distribution and extent of the disease in the vagina, no single method has been universally endorsed. Although there are conflicting reports concerning the efficacy of ablative therapy for VAIN, this modality has one major advantage. The CO_2 laser is the only surgical method for destroying large areas of diseased epithelium without causing vaginal scarring or shortening.[6,59]

Although the primary success rates for vaginal laser surgery have been lower than for cervix or vulva, we are convinced that ablation or excision with the CO_2 laser remains the best option. Among 100 consecutive patients undergoing laser vaporization for VAIN 2 to 3, 61% were controlled by a single treatment.[7] Nine of the 29 primary laser failures were thereafter treated by excisional methods. However, of the 20 women who had a subsequent vaporization, 13 were controlled by this second procedure.

The vast majority of patients who have recurrences were diagnosed within the first 6 months following surgery. Moreover, 23 of the 29 primary laser failures occurred in patients with multifocal disease. This relationship held true, irrespective of whether surgery was done by excision or ablation. Some of these failures may represent failures to detect some disease foci even with the colposcope. However, it is also likely that patients who present with extensive multifocal disease represent more permissive hosts.

Although there are few risks to the use of the CO_2 laser when the uterus remains in situ, this is not true for the treatment of VAIN following hysterectomy.[58] In a series of 23 British women managed by laser vaporization of recurrent VAIN, Woodman et al[64,65] report that only six patients remained free of disease at 30 months after treatment. Of the 21 women in whom VAIN 2 to 3 involved the vault scar, three developed invasive cancer in islands of buried vaginal epithelium. Hence, recognizing the need for an excision or combined approach is the key to safety and efficacy under these circumstances.

Vulvar intraepithelial neoplasia and difficult condylomas

Over the last decade, there has been a dramatic increase in the prevalence of vulvar intraepithelial neoplasia (VIN) and perianal intraepithelial neoplasia (PAIN) in young women, particularly of the multifocal 'Bowenoid' variety.[4] Treatment of VIN is controversial, with recommendations ranging from wide excision to skinning vulvectomy;[52] (see also Ch. 26). Although the treatment originally proposed for 'carcinoma in situ' of the vulva was wide local excision, fears that the disease was preinvasive led to the widespread use of simple vulvectomy. However, most documented instances of invasion have occurred in immunosuppressed or elderly women.[4] In young patients, the risk of malignant progression is real (Fig. 69.36), but insufficient to justify such mutilating surgery. Moreover, recurrences following simple vulvectomy are common (Fig. 69.37).

Wide excision of small foci produces excellent results. However, multifocal or extensive lesions are difficult to treat by this method. Hence, in the past, the only reasonable alternative was skinning vulvectomy with grafting. Although a definite improvement over conventional vulvectomy, cosmetic and functional results are unpredictable. Fortunately, by providing an effective but non-mutilating treatment, the CO_2 laser offers an escape from this dilemma.[1,45]

Extended laser ablation

Of the 160 patients referred to above,[45] (p. 1114) 107 (67%) were controlled by a single laser ablation, and another 43 (27%) were controlled by either repeating this surgery or the use of therapeutic levels of topical 5-fluorouracil as soon as recurrence appeared inevitable (Fig. 69.38). Treatment of the remaining 10 (6%) required deep laser destruction with skin grafting (prior to 1986), or the use of adjuvant alpha interferon (after 1986). Even

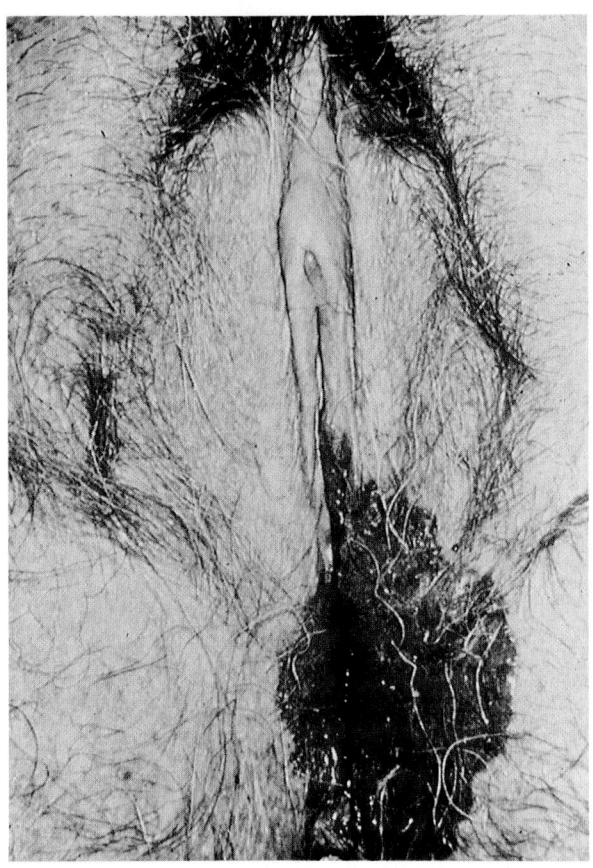
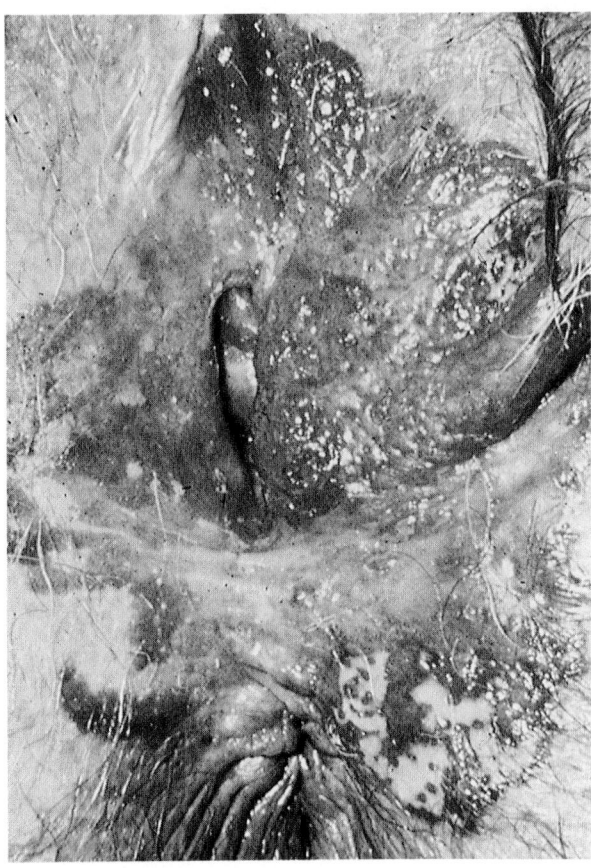

A

B

Fig. 69.36 (A) An extensive VIN 3 lesion, centered upon the left interlabial sulcus and extending both distal to the pilosebaceous line and proximal to the mucocutaneous line. (B) The same lesion after 3 years without treatment. A large area of invasive squamous carcinoma has now arisen in the left interlabial sulcus. (Reproduced with permission of R W Jones, M D, Auckland, New Zealand.)

so, two patients (1%) have never achieved lasting clinical remission.

Kaplan Meier cumulative survival analysis shows that recurrences continued for up to 1½ years. Thereafter, the tail of the survival curve becomes quite flat, indicating that these patients are in stable clinical control (Fig. 69.39). It is emphasized that these results refer to long-term freedom from clinical recurrence. In our opinion, the question of whether latent HPV DNA remains at the treatment site is of no practical relevance. Our primary control rate of 67% speaks to both the strength and weakness of the CO_2 laser. The strength is that, used skillfully, the laser can remove any volume of diseased tissue under fine control, with the assurance of rapid healing without scarring. However, the weakness is that the laser cannot prevent re-activation of the latent viral reservoir within surrounding areas of surface skin, and perhaps within the skin appendages themselves. Hence, the availability of an effective adjuvant would be a natural complement.

Non-cytotoxic doses of 5-fluorouracil

Although a 5 to 10 day course of topical 5-fluorouracil (5 FU) will slough cutaneous lesions,[55] such high dose regimens have been abandoned because they are inefficient, poorly controllable, and extremely painful. With the exception of isolated vaginal condylomas, disease destruction is best done with the laser, with 5 FU being used in non-cytotoxic doses in an attempt to prevent recurrence.

Sillman[54] has shown that, in patients with renal allografts or other immune deficiencies, the use of lifelong low dose 5 FU is a prerequisite to disease control. In 1986, Krebs[25] extended this concept to the treatment of immunologically competent women, reporting improved success (87% vs 62%) in the group randomized to use bi-weekly topical 5 FU for 6 months. In contrast, among the 160 women treated by extended laser ablation, we found that an adjuvant once-weekly regimen was better tolerated. Unfortunately, this low dose regimen did not provide any protection against postoperative recurrence in 53 of the women (Table 69.7).[45] 5 FU used on a once weekly schedule was only helpful in 50 of 76 women with two or more risk factors (88% vs 56%; see Fig. 69.26B and Table 69.8).

As opposed to the lack of efficacy of weekly 5 FU as a prophylaxis against laser failure, 22 (58%) of 38 patients

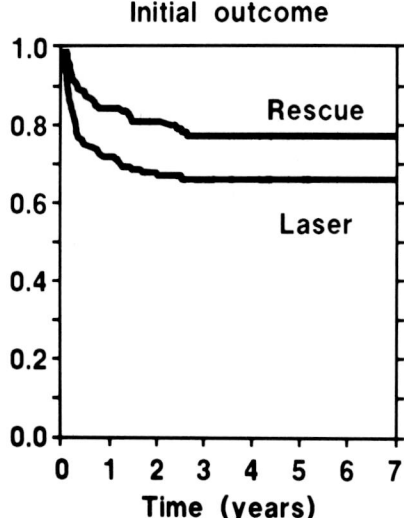

Fig. 69.39 A Kaplan-Meier survival curve, showing the curability obtained by the initial laser ablation in these 160 women. Fifty percent of failures occurred within 3 months and 95% within 18 months. The *lower* curve represents just the patients who had significant recurrences following their first surgery ('immediate successes'), while the *higher* curve ('eventual successes') represents both immediate successes plus those 'rescued' from a repeat laser ablation by various office therapies. As detailed in Figure 69.38, these initial failures were recycled for repeat laser ablation, resulting in the eventual control of all but two women. (Reproduced from Reid et al (1990),[45] with permission.)

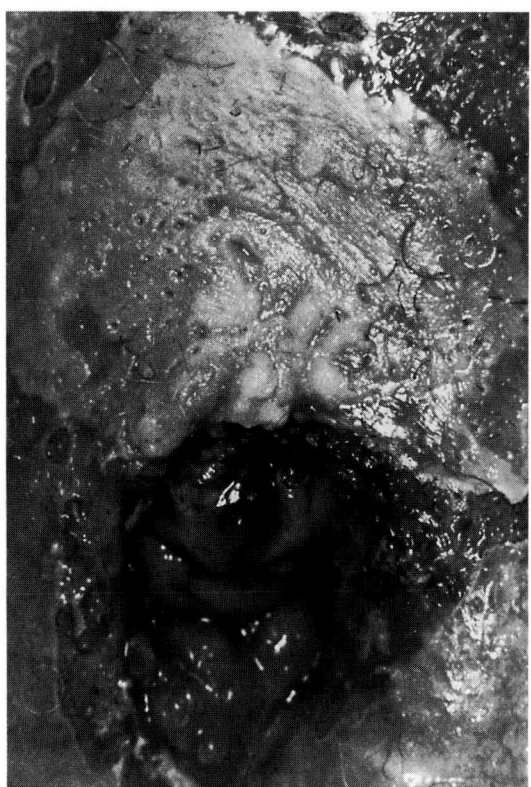

Fig. 69.37 Recurrence of VIN 3 after a simple vulvectomy.

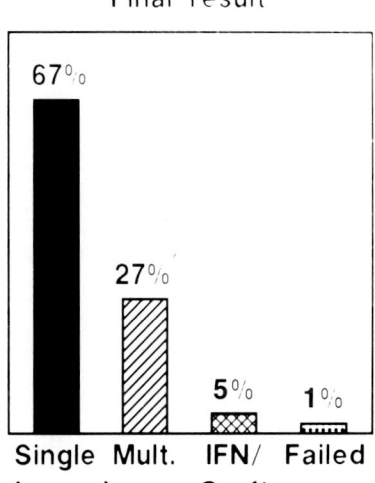

Fig. 69.38 A bar chart showing final outcome following 204 extended laser ablations among 160 women with extensive, refractory or neoplastic vulvar disease. Two-thirds (67%) were controlled by a single laser procedure. Among the one-third of patients in whom the initial laser surgery failed, the majority (27%) were controlled either by a subsequent extended ablation (the strategy prior to 1986), or by pushing topical 5 FU to the limits of patient tolerance (the strategy since 1986). Of the 6% of patients who failed repeated superficial laser ablation, 5% were eventually controlled by deep laser ablation and skin grafting (prior to 1986), or by high dose systemic alpha interferon (IFN) (since 1986). Two patients (1%) have failed all therapies to this point. (Reproduced from Reid et al (1990),[45] with permission.)

Table 69.7 The results of once-weekly topical 5 FU, used as prophylaxis against disease recurrence, within the entire sample of 160 women treated for significant vulvar disease between 1983 and 1987.

Adjuvant 5 FU usage	Controlled by a single laser surgery	Not controlled by the initial laser ablation	Total
Laser + 5 FU	28 (75.7%)	9 (24.3%)	37 (100%)
Laser alone	79 (64.2%)	44 (35.8%)	123 (100%)
Total	107	53	160

$X^2 = 1.68$; $P > 0.19$ (not significant)
Reproduced from Reid et al (1990),[45] with permission.

Table 69.8 The results of once-weekly topical 5 FU, used as prophylaxis against disease recurrence, within a subset of 76 patients who had two or more adverse factors.*

Adjuvant 5 FU usage	Controlled by a single laser surgery	Not controlled by the initial ablation	Total
Laser plus adjuvant 5 FU	21 (87.5%)	3 (12.5%)	24 (100%)
Laser alone	29 (55.8%)	23 (44.2%)	52 (100%)
Total	50	26	76

* For adverse factors see p. 1112.
$X^2 = 7.35$; $P < 0.01$
Reproduced from Reid et al (1990),[45] with permission.

with diffuse, impending failures were 'rescued' from the need for a second surgery by using therapeutic levels of this drug.[45] These patients were distinguished by diffuse, generally symptomatic subclinical or low volume recurrences which appeared to be rapidly evolving towards extensive, classical papilloma formation. In contrast to the disappointing results of trying to cure longstanding keratotic condylomas primarily with topical 5 FU, the balance between efficacy and morbidity is quite favorable in this specific subset of patients.

The role of interferon therapy

Interferons are a group of immunomodulatory proteins, produced by all mammalian species, which possess antiviral and antiproliferative properties.[60] Efficacy of alpha[17] and gamma[23] interferons against HPV infection has been documented. However, even when used in high doses by intramuscular injection, systemic interferons have proven to be disappointing primary therapies for significant HPV infections.[60]

In particular, the recently advocated regimen of intralesional injections appears to offer little to the practical gynecologist. Intralesional injections require two or three office visits per week over a several week course, produce substantial pain at the injection sites, and can only be expected to clear the lesions that are actually infiltrated.[11,13] Even for patients with only 3 to 5 warts (the maximum which can be injected in a course), such trivial disease should be readily amenable to simpler therapy.

In contrast, in a subsequent open labelled, randomized trial, systemic alpha interferon used at 1 Mu thrice weekly

(one-sixth of the usual therapeutic dose) conferred substantial protection against postoperative recurrence.[47] Initial success rate in the interferon arm was 27 of 33 (82%), versus 17 of 38 (44%) in the control arms ($X^2 = 10.31$; $P < 0.002$); see Figure 69.40. Moreover, 18 (86%) of 21 failures in the control arms and 3 of 6 failures in the study group were 'rescued' from a second laser surgery by crossover to either 1 Mu or 3 Mu of interferon, respectively.

GLOSSARY OF LASER TERMS

Absorption   The conversion of light energy into heat, during transmission through tissue (see Scattering).

Absorption coefficient   A factor describing the ease or difficulty with which a particular wave length of light will be absorbed, during passage through a given type of tissue.

Active medium   The material used to emit the laser (e.g. CO_2, Ar, Nd).

Aiming beam   A helium:neon (He:Ne) laser (or other light source), aligned coaxially with an otherwise invisible laser.

Amplitude   The maximum height of a wave.

Argon (Ar) laser   A gas laser using the rare element Argon as the active medium, emitting a blue (480 nm) and green (514 nm) band of visible light.

Articulated arm   A delivery device for CO_2 lasers, consisting of a series of hollow metal tubes fitted with joints (to move the 'arm') and mirrors (to reflect the beam).

Attenuation   A decrease in the intensity (power) of light, as it passes through an absorbent medium.

Beam geometry   Point-to-point variation of energy intensity across a cross section of the beam.

Carbon dioxide laser   A gas laser using carbon dioxide (CO_2) molecules as the active medium, emitting mid infra-red energy (= 10 600 nm or 10.6 μm).

Chopped wave   Electrical pulsing of a CO_2 laser, to produce relatively broad, flat pulses having the same peak power as when this tube is operated in continuous wave.

Chromophore   The optically active molecule responsible for light absorption in tissue.

Coagulation   Heating of tissue sufficient to denature structural and enzymatic proteins, but insufficient to sublimate the tissue into a vapor.

Coherence   Wave patterns traveling in the same temporal and spatial phases, thus allowing focusing to a spot of extremely high energy intensity.

Contact probe   A ceramic or other synthetic probe used to condense the energy emerging from a laser fiber, thus making it possible to produce irradiance levels sufficient to vaporize or coagulate tissues, even with relatively low power output.

Continuous wave (CW)   A temporal mode in which the

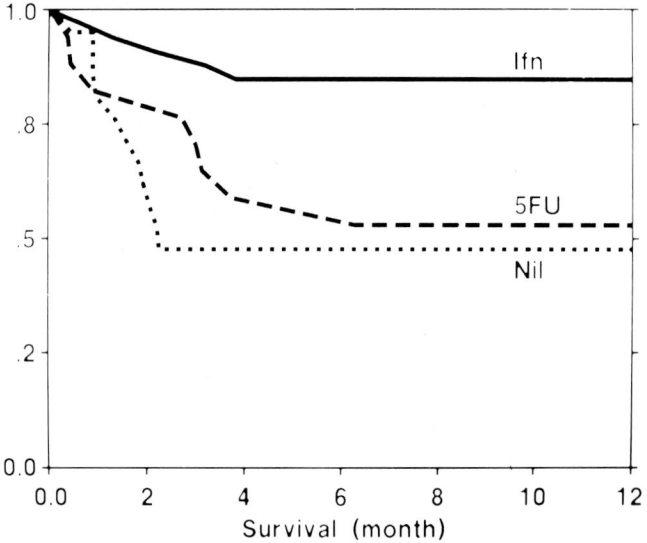

Cumulative proportion surviving

Fig. 69.40 A Kaplan Meier survival curve, showing the significantly improved rates for clinical control attending the use of adjuvant interferon (solid line), as compared to laser plus 5 FU (dashed line) or laser alone (dotted line) ($P < 0.002$).

laser emits a constant beam of energy, maximal power being a function of tube length.

Collimation The property of having emitted energy travel in parallel rays, thus conferring the ability of the laser beam to travel over long distances with minimal spread.

Critical volume The volume of tissue needed to absorb 90% of the photons contained within an incident beam.

Duty cycle The ratio of on:off time in a pulsed laser.

Electromagnetic radiation A series of energy waves, propagated by simultaneous variations in electric and magnetic intensity. This term includes the entire range of wavelengths from cosmic rays to radio waves.

Energy The ability to do work, expressed in Joules (J).

Erbium YAG Solid state lasers using the rare earth element erbium (Er) lasers 'doped' into a YAG crystal. This laser emits near infrared radiation of 2.94 μm, corresponding to the highest absorption peak for water.

Eximer lasers A family of gas lasers that use excited dimers to emit energy within the ultraviolet region of the electromagnetic spectrum.

Extinction length The depth of tissue needed to absorb 90% of an incident beam.

Fluence The rate of energy delivery expressed as Joules/cm^2.

Focal point The short distance over which a focused beam has its smallest diameter, and hence its greatest intensity.

Gaussian curve A family of curves, all of which show a central peak and an even distribution on either side of this peak. For a given Gaussian 'family', the area under the curve remains constant. Hence, narrowing the laser (i.e. spot diameter) will increase the amplitude (i.e. crater depth), while broadening the base (defocusing) will flatten the amplitude.

Ionizing radiation Radiation of sufficient energy (e.g. X-ray, gamma rays, cosmic rays) to cause DNA damage, without any accompanying thermal effect.

Irradiance Light intensity within the focal spot expressed in W/cm^2. This term is synonymous with 'average power density'.

Joule The unit of energy. 1 Joule = 1 watt × 1 second.

Laser Gaseous or solid state devices that convert electrical, light or radio frequency energy into a beam of intense, monochromatic, highly collimated electron magnetic radiation ('coherent light').

L-A-S-E-R An acronym for the process of Light Amplification by the Stimulated Emission of Radiation.

Laser beam The rod-like ray of light emitted from the laser tube.

Microslad The device which couples the articulated arm to the operating microscope. The microslad controls two key functions: the aiming of the laser beam, and the ability to obtain incremental defocus at the impact site.

Microsecond (μs) One millionth of a second (10^{-6} s).

Millisecond (ms) One thousandth of a second (10^{-3} s).

Nanosecond (nm) One billionth of a second (10^{-9} s).

Neodymium: YAG lasers A solid state laser in which a glass-like crystal of yttrium aluminum garnet (YAG) is 'doped' with a rare earth element called neodymium (Nd). This laser emits highly energized radiation in the near infra-red portion of the electromagnetic spectrum (= 1006 nm or 1.06 μm).

Population inversion A situation wherein there are more atoms or molecules in an excited state than in a resting state. Population inversion is a precondition for the lasing action of any material laser medium.

Power density Light intensity per unit area within the focal spot, expressed as W/cm^2 (see Irradiance).

Scattering Absorption and re-emission of energy in a different direction to that of the incident beam (e.g. lateral, backwards).

Selective thermolysis Photocoagulation of underlying blood vessels, with negligible photodamage to overlying epidermis and adjacent dermis, by the use of a flash lamp pumped tunable dye laser.

Spot size For a Gaussian beam, spot size is the area within which 86% of the laser beam falls.

Superpulse An adaptation of the CO_2 laser to produce fast pulses (>200 H^3) of energy, each pulse having a high peak power 5 to 10 times the normal maximum power attainable from that laser tube, when operated in a steady output (continuous wave) mode.

Thermal relaxation time The time required for a laser impact site to begin cooling itself by lateral heat conduction. Thermal relaxation varies with both wavelength and tissue type.

Transverse electromagnetic mode (TEM) The power distribution within a cross section of the laser beam.

Tunable dye laser Laser that can be adjusted for various color outputs.

Vaporization Sublimation of tissue into gases.

Watt The unit of power. A watt (W) is the work performed by one Joule in one second.

Wavelength The distance between peaks of an electromagnetic wave. Wavelength is a measure of the energy carried by the radiation. Radiation of extremely long wavelength is generally described by a reciprocal quantity, termed frequency; (see Fig. 69.1).

REFERENCES

1. Baggish M S, Dorsey J M 1980 CO_2 laser for the treatment of vulvar carcinoma in situ. Obstet Gynecol 57: 371
2. Barnhill D R, Hoskins W J, Metz P 1983 Use of the rhomboid flap after partial vulvectomy. Obstet Gynecol 62: 444
3. Bunney M H 1982 Viral Warts: Their Biology and Treatment. Oxford University Press, New York
4. Buscema J, Woodruff J D, Parmley T H, Genadry R 1980 Carcinoma in situ of the vulva. Obstet Gynecol 55: 225
5. Culp O S, Kaplan I W 1944 Condylomata acuminata: 200 cases treated with podophyllin. Ann Surg 120: 251
6. Dorsey J H 1986 Skin appendage involvement and vulval intraepithelial neoplasia. In: Sharp F, Jordan J A (eds) Gynaecologic Laser Surgery. Perinatology Press, New York, p. 193
7. Dorsey J H, Baker C H 1984 Credentialing of the gynecologic laser surgeon. Colpos Gynecol Laser Surg 1: 79
8. Dorsey J H, Baggish M S 1984 Vaginal intraepithelial neoplasia II. Indications and technique for total vaginectomy with split thickness graft replacement. Colpos Gynecol Laser Surg 1: 149
9. Dorsey J H, Baggish M S 1986 Multifocal vaginal and intraepithelial neoplasia with uterus in situ. In: Sharp F, Jordan J A (eds) Gynecologic Laser Surgery, Perinatology Press, New York, p. 173
10. Duus B R, Philipsen T, Christensen J D, Lunduam F, Sondergaard J 1985 Refractory condyloma acuminata: a controlled clinical trial of carbon dioxide laser versus conventional surgical treatment. Genitourin Med 61: 59
11. Eron L, Judson D, Tucker J et al 1986 Interferon therapy for condylomata acuminata. N Engl J Med 215: 1059
12. Ferenczy A, Mitao M, Nagai N, Silverstein S J, Crum C P 1985 Latent papillomavirus and recurring genital warts. N Engl J Med 313: 784
13. Friedman-Kien A E, Eron L J, Conant M et al 1988 Natural interferon alpha for treatment of condylomata acuminata. JAMA 259: 533
14. Friedrich E G Jr 1987 Vulvar vestibulitis syndrome. J Reprod Med 32: 110
15. Fuchs P G, Girardi F, Pfister H 1988 Human papillomavirus DNA in normal, metaplastic, preneoplastic and neoplastic epithelia of the cervix uteri. Int J Cancer 41: 41
16. Fuller T A 1985 Laser tissue interaction: the influence of power density. In: Baggish M (ed) Basic and Advanced Laser Surgery and Gynecology. Appleton-Century-Crofts, New York
17. Gall S A, Hughes C E, Mounts P, Segrit A, Weck P K, Whisnant J K 1986 Efficacy of human lymphoblastoid interferon in the therapy of resistant condyloma acuminata. Obstet Gynecol 67: 643
18. Graham J B, Meigs J V 1952 Recurrence of tumor after total hysterectomy for carcinoma in situ. Am J Obstet Gynecol 64: 1159
19. Hellberg D 1987 The female patient — clinical diagnosis and treatment. Proc Int Sym 17th World Congress Dermatol. Berlin, May
20. Hoskins W J, Park R C, Long R, Artman L E, McMahon E B 1984 Repair of urinary tract fistulas with bulbocavernosus myocutaneous flaps. Obstet Gynecol 63: 588
21. Jervis W, Salyer K E, Vargas-Busquests M A, Atkins R W 1974 Further applications of the Limberg and Dufourmentel flaps. Plast Reconstr Surg 54: 335
22. Jenson A B, Kurman R J, Lancaster W D 1987 Tissue effects of and host response to human papillomavirus infection. Obstet Gynecol Clin N Am 14: 397
23. Kirby P, Kiviat N, Beckman A, Wells D, Sherwin S, Corey L 1988 Tolerance and efficacy of recombinant human 'interferon' gamma in the treatment of refractory genital warts. Am J Med 85: 183
24. Kamat B R, Carney J M, Arndt K A, Stern R S, Rosen S 1986 Cutaneous tissue repair following CO_2 laser irradiation. J Invest Dermatol 87: 268
25. Krebs H B 1986 Prophylactic topical 5 fluorouracil following treatment of human papillomavirus-associated lesions of the vulva and vagina. Obstet Gynecol 68: 837
26. Lee R A, Symmonds R E 1975 Recurrent carcinoma in situ in the vagina in patients previously treated for in situ carcinoma of the cervix. Obstet Gynecol 48: 61
27. Lele S B, Piver M S, Mang T S, Dougherty T J, Tomczak M J 1989 Photodynamic therapy in gynecologic malignancies. Gynecol Oncol 34: 350
28. Lipow M 1986 Laser physics made simple. Curr Prob Obstet Gynecol Infert 9: 441
29. Lister G D, Gibson T 1972 Closure of rhomboid skin defects; the flaps of Limberg and Dufourmentel. Br J Plast Surg 25: 300
30. Lorincz A T, Reid R 1989 Association of human papillomavirus with gynecologic cancer. Curr Op Oncol 1: 123
31. Martin D C 1989 Laser safety. In Keye W (ed) Laser Surgery in Gynecology and Obstetrics. Yearbook Publishers, Chicago, p. 35
32. Oriel J D 1971 Natural history of genital warts. Br J Vener Dis 47: 1
33. Polanyi T G 1983 Laser physics: medical applications. Otolaryngol Clin North Am 16: 753
34. Reid R 1984 Symposium on cervical neoplasia. V. Carbon dioxide laser ablation. Colpo Gynecol Laser Surgery 1: 291
35. Reid R 1985 Superficial laser vulvectomy. I. The efficacy of extended superficial ablation for refractory and very extensive condylomas. Am J Obstet Gynecol 151: 1047
36. Reid R 1985 Superficial laser vulvectomy. III. A new surgical technique for appendage-conserving ablation of refractory condylomas and vulvar intraepithelial neoplasia. Am J Obstet Gynecol 152: 504
37. Reid R 1987 Human papillomaviral infection. The key to rational triage of cervical neoplasia. Obstet Gynecol Clin N Am 14: 407
38. Reid R 1987 Physical and surgical principles governing expertise with the carbon dioxide laser. Obstet Gynecol Clin N Am 14: 513
39. Reid R 1989 Preinvasive disease. In: Berek J S, Hacker N F (eds) Practical Gynecologic Oncology. Williams & Wilkins, Baltimore, p. 533
40. Reid R 1989 Laser therapy of human papillomavirus infections. In Keye W (ed) Laser Surgery in Gynecology and Obstetrics. Yearbook Publishers, Chicago, p. 46
41. Reid R, Campion M J 1988 The biology and significance of human papillomavirus infections in the genital tract. Yale J Biol Med 61: 307
42. Reid R, Elfont E A, Zirkin R M, Fuller T A 1985 Superficial laser vulvectomy. II. The anatomic and biophysical principles permitting accurate control of the depth of dermal destruction with the carbon dioxide laser. Am J Obstet Gynecol 151: 261
43. Reid R, Elson L, Absten G 1987 A practical guide to laser safety. Colpos Gynecol Laser Surg 2: 121
44. Reid R, Greenberg M D, Daoud Y, Husain M, Selvaggi S, Wilkinson E 1988 Colposcopic findings in women with vulvar pain syndromes. A preliminary report. J Reprod Med 33: 523
45. Reid R, Greenberg M D, Daoud Y et al 1990 Superficial laser vulvectomy. IV. Extended laser vaporization and adjuvant 5 fluorouracil therapy of human papillomavirus associated vulvar disease. Obstet Gynecol 76: 439
46. Reid R, Greenberg M, Jenson A B et al 1987 Sexually transmitted papillomaviral infections. I. The anatomic distribution and pathologic grade of neoplastic lesions associated with different viral types. Am J Obstet Gynecol 156: 212
47. Reid R, Greenberg M D, Pizzuti D et al 1990 Superficial laser vulvectomy. V. Surgical success rates are improved by the use of adjuvant alpha-interferon. Am J Obstet Gynecol (in press)
48. Reid R, Greenberg M D, Lorincz A T 1991 Should cervical cytology be augmented by cervicography or HPV typing? Am J Obstet Gynecol (in press)
49. Reid R, Muller S 1980 Tattoo removal by CO_2 laser dermabrasion. Plast Reconstr Surg 65: 717
50. Reid R, Pizutti D J, Stoler M et al 1990 Superficial laser vulvectomy. VI. Factors associated with an adverse treatment outcome. (In preparation)
51. Riva J M, Sedlacek T V, Cunnane M F, Mangan C E 1989 Extended carbon dioxide laser vaporization in the treatment of subclinical papillomavirus infection of the lower genital tract. Obstet Gynecol 73: 25

52. Rutledge F, Sinclair M 1968 Treatment of intraepithelial carcinoma of the vulva by skin excision and graft. Am J Obstet Gynecol 102: 806

53. Schwartz D B, Greenberg M D, Daoud Y, Reid R 1987 The management of genital condylomas in pregnant women. Obstet Gynecol Clin North Am 14: 589

54. Sillman F H, Sedlis A 1987 Anogenital papillomavirus infection and neoplasia in immunodeficient women. Obstet Gynecol Clin North Am 14: 537

55. Sillman F H, Sedlis A, Boyce J G 1985 A review of lower genital intraepithelial neoplasia and the use of topical 5 fluorouracil. Obstet Gynecol Survey 40: 190

56. Simmons P D 1981 Podophyllin 10% and 25% in the treatment of anogenital warts. Br J Vener Dis 57: 208

57. Simmons P D, Langlet F, Thin R N T 1981 Cryotherapy versus electrocautery in the treatment of genital warts. Br J Vener Dis 57: 273

58. Soutter W P 1988 The treatment of vaginal intraepithelial neoplasia after hysterectomy. Br J Obstet Gynaecol 95: 961

59. Stuart G C, Flagler E A, Nation J G, Duggan M, Robertson D I 1988 Laser vaporization of vaginal intraepithelial neoplasia. Am J Obstet Gynecol 15: 240

60. Trofatter K F 1988 Interferon. Obstet Gynecol Clin North Am 14: 569

61. von Krogh G 1982 Condylomata acuminata: an updated review. Semin Dermatol 2: 109

62. Walsh J T Jr, Flotte T J, Anderson R R, Deutsch T F 1988 Pulsed CO_2 laser tissue ablation: effect of tissue type and pulse duration on thermal damage. Lasers Surg Med 8: 108

63. Wolbarsht M L, Esterowitz L, Tran D, Levin K, Storm M 1986 A mid infrared (2.94 um) surgical laser with an optical fiber delivery system. Lasers Surg Med 6: 257

64. Woodman C, Jordan J A, Wade-Evans T 1984 The management of vaginal intraepithelial neoplasia after hysterectomy. Br J Obstet Gynaecol 91: 707

65. Woodman C, Mould J J, Jordan J A 1988 Radiotherapy in the management of vaginal intraepithelial neoplasia after hysterectomy. Br J Obstet Gynaecol 95: 976

66. Woodruff J D, Parmley T H 1983 Infection of the minor vestibular gland. Obstet Gynecol 62: 609

70. CO$_2$ laser surgery for intraepithelial neoplasia of cervix

·J. A. Jordan

INTRODUCTION

Most colposcopy centers accept that patients with pre-clinical carcinoma of the cervix can be treated safely by destructive techniques provided the following criteria are met:

1. The patient must be seen and assessed by a competent coloscopist.
2. The endocervical margin of the lesion and the transformation zone must be visible.
3. There must be no cytological suspicion of invasion.
4. There must be no colposcopic suspicion of invasion.
5. There must be no histological suspicion of invasion.
6. There must be no suspicion of atypical glandular cells in the cytology specimen, for this may suggest the coexistence of an underlying adenocarcinoma in situ. In this instance, an excision cone is obligatory.
7. The laser treatment should be performed by the colposcopist.
8. There must be every prospect of adequate follow-up.

Under these circumstances the lesion can be treated by destruction using either electrocoagulation diathermy under general anesthesia, cryocautery or laser (Ch. 36). Of these methods, laser is the most recent and although there is less information about the long term follow-up of patients than is available for those treated by diathermy or cryocautery, preliminary results from Bellina,[1] Stafl, Wilkinson & Mattingly,[8] and the author's team,[6] suggest that cure rates in excess of 95% can be expected.

THE LASER

The word laser is an acronym derived from the first letters of the words Light Amplification by Stimulated Emission of Radiation. The laser itself is a device for converting some form of energy, such as heat, light or electricity into radiant energy of a special kind at one or more discrete wavelengths. When the wavelength of radiant energy lies within the visible portion of the electromagnetic spectrum it is called light, with which we are all familiar. Not all lasers emit their radiant energy as light but the radiation emitted by all lasers has three special qualities. It is coherent (all the waves are exactly in phase with each other in both space and time); it is collimated (the rays are parallel to each other); it is monochromatic (all the waves are exactly the same wave length).

Lasers were first built in the late 1950's but the early instruments, such as the ruby lasers, were very inefficient, converting only a tiny fraction of their energy into coherent radiant energy. More recently the first practical gas lasers were developed, the most efficient of which is the carbon dioxide (CO$_2$) laser which converts about 15% of its energy into coherent output radiation. The primary radiant output of the CO$_2$ laser occurs at a wavelength of 10.6 μm which is in the infra-red portion of the spectrum where it is invisible to the naked eye. Since the surgeon cannot see the beam, he must have some means of knowing exactly where the beam is focused. The CO$_2$ laser therefore has a small helium-neon (He–Ne) laser built into the laser system which produces a red spot focused at the same point as the CO$_2$ laser beam, thus acting as a 'finder beam'. By a system of mirrors and a lens it can be directed and focused at a specific spot, where it is capable of releasing a tremendous amount of energy at its focal point. The size of the spot can be varied very simply according to whether the surgeon wishes to use it as a knife (requiring a small spot size) or for vaporization (requiring a large spot size). When used for the treatment of cervical disease, the laser is attached to a colposcope, with the laser and the colposcope having the same focal length. The diameter of the laser beam at its focal point can be varied from 0.1 to 2 mm, the smaller spot size being used as a knife and the larger for destruction of tissue; the beam is easily manipulated and is totally under the control of the surgeon, thereby allowing him to destroy tissue with great precision; (see also Ch. 69).

CERVICAL INTRAEPITHELIAL NEOPLASIA (CIN)

Patients are selected for treatment by either laser vaporization or excisional conization as outlined in the introduction. In both instances, the patient is placed in a modified lithotomy position (Fig. 70.1). No specific preoperative preparation of the vagina is necessary. Some surgeons use antibiotics, antiseptic pessaries or creams postoperatively, in the hope that this will minimize postoperative infection and thereby secondary hemorrhage, but there is no proof that these measures are beneficial.

Technique of laser vaporization

The depth of destruction is a function of two parameters, namely power density (W/cm^2) and time. The power density is controlled by a regulator on the laser console and will vary between machines and surgeons, but is usually between 500 and 1200 $W/cm.^2$

Most cases can be dealt with as an outpatient procedure without any form of anesthesia being necessary, although occasionally (less than 1% of cases) general anesthesia is advisable, usually where the disease process is extensive or where the patient is extremely apprehensive. Although it is usually possible to undertake treatment without any form of analgesia being used, operators are finding that some

form of pain relief is in the patient's interest. This being the case, local anesthetic can be injected directly into the cervix using a dental syringe and a fine gauge needle. The needle is inserted into the cervix at four points outside the lesion. If this technique is used, most surgeons find it beneficial to include a vasoconstrictor, both the analgesic agent and the vasoconstrictor being in the form of a combined preparation. The author now uses this technique routinely for all cases of laser vaporization for not only does it give adequate pain relief, but it minimizes bleeding problems significantly thereby allowing adequate depth of destruction to be achieved without discomfort to the patient. Other surgeons achieve analgesia by the use of a paracervical block, but usually local infiltration is better. The time for which the beam is released is controlled by the operator using a foot switch; the operator can preset the beam to release for a specific period of time, for example 0.1 seconds, or 0.5 seconds, or alternatively, the beam can be released in a continuous fashion and be controlled only by the foot switch. When beginning to use laser therapy the intermittent short bursts are safer, but very quickly the operator finds that the continuous beam is quicker and more effective. The laser destroys tissue by vaporizing the intracellular fluid at the speed of light. This produces a great deal of smoke which must be removed by some form of continuous suction device before vaporization

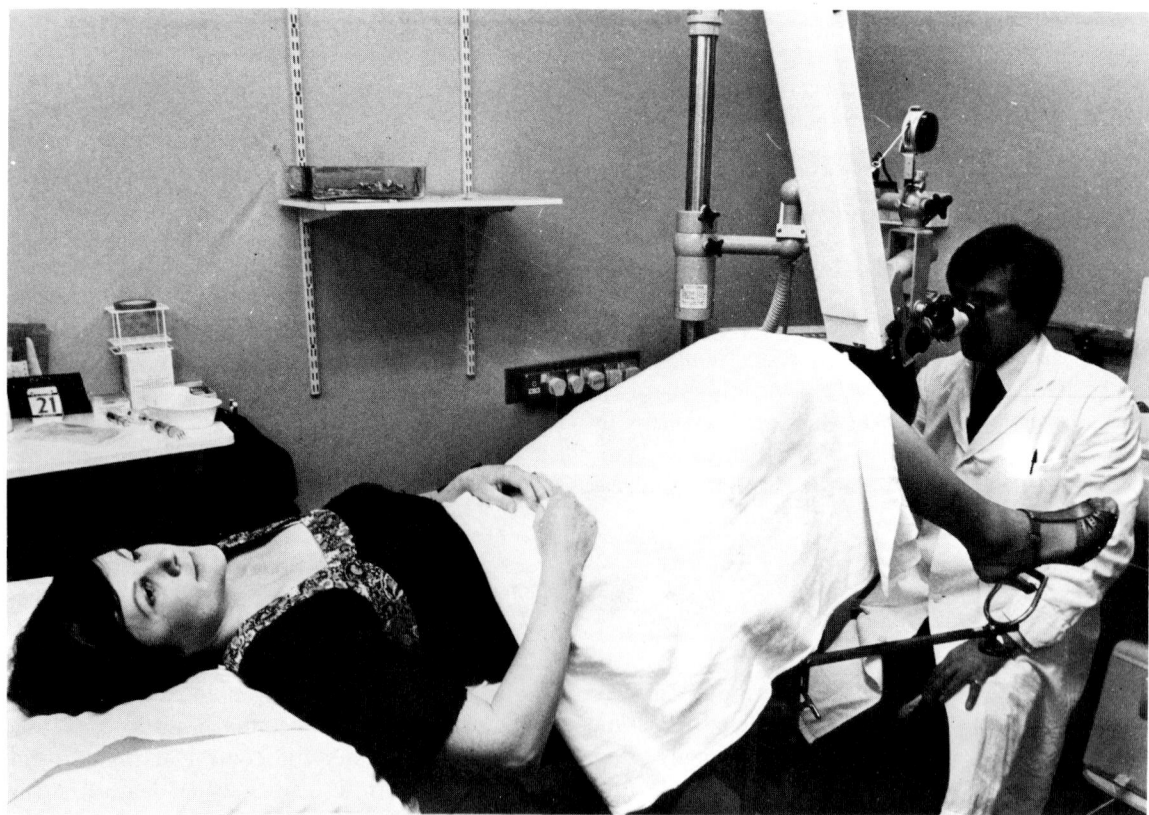

Fig. 70.1 The laser in use in the outpatient situation.

can continue. This is most easily achieved by using a specially designed speculum manufactured by most instrument makers for use with laser surgery. Underneath the upper blade of the speculum is a hollow metal tube which is open at its cervical end. This is then attached to a portable suction device; this must contain a charcoal-based filter which will allow the carbon particles in the vapor to be absorbed rather than released into the environment. Filters are not expensive and need to be changed regularly. The operator is cautioned against using those permanent suction devices which rely on fixed metal suction pipes usually built into the wall of the operating theater — the carbonization produced on the inside of these pipes will eventually block them leading to a major engineering problem in replacing them!

Many surgeons using laser surgery for the first time are disappointed with their results but, assuming that cases have been properly selected in the first instance, failures can be explained quite easily. The operator has not destroyed tissue to a great enough depth. The best results are obtained when tissue is destroyed to a depth of 5 to 7 mm (Fig. 70.2a and b) and destruction to a lesser depth inevitably leads to a high incidence of persistent disease.[6]

When attempting vaporization, the operator needs to use a spot size which is large enough to vaporize relatively quickly, while at the same time using a power density which is low enough to allow the beam to cause thermal destruction and vessel sealing at the edge of the vaporized area, thereby minimizing any bleeding. For example, a spot size between 1.6 and 1.8 mm in diameter will allow even large areas to be vaporized relatively quickly: the power density used with this spot size varies between 500 and 1500 W/cm^2 depending on the power output of the

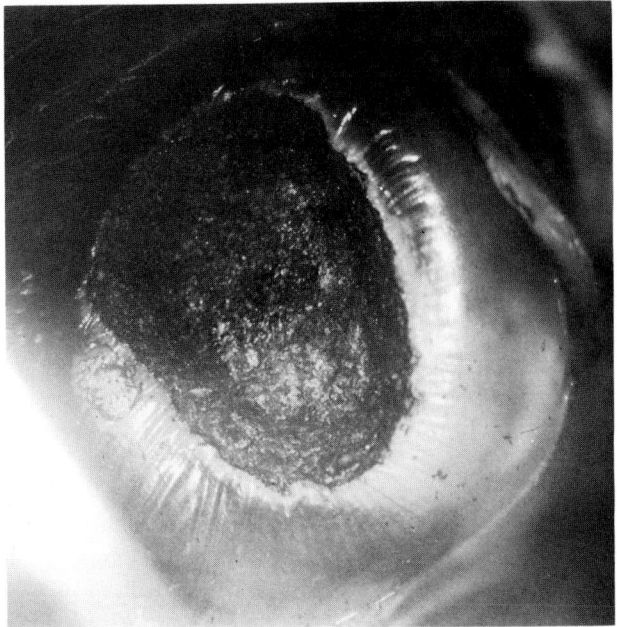

b

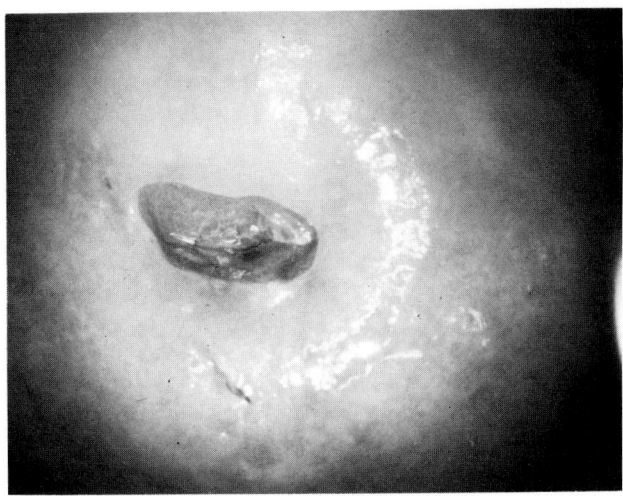

c

Fig. 70.2 (a) An area of CIN 3.
(b) The cervix immediately following laser vaporization to a depth of 5–7 mm.
(c) The same cervix 12 weeks following treatment: the squamocolumnar junction and gland openings are clearly seen.

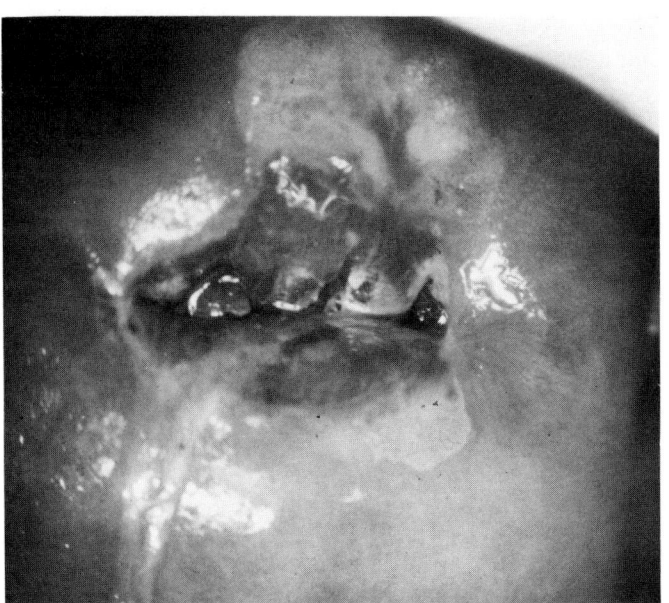

a

machine used. This will allow the tissue at the edge of the vaporization crater to undergo heat destruction which will, in turn, seal off all but the largest blood vessels in the area being vaporized. The surgeon will therefore achieve vaporization in the shortest possible time with minimal bleeding. On the other hand, a spot size of 0.1 mm is totally inappropriate for vaporization. Firstly, because the spot is small, it will act like a knife and vaporization will take a long period of time. Secondly, the power density will be so high (anything between 20 and 30 000 W/cm^2), that there will be minimal heat necrosis at the edge of the lasered tissue: subsequently there will be minimal sealing off of the vessels, with the result that hemorrhage is much more likely to occur.

With the chosen spot size the surgeon will then vaporize the tissue which has been identified colposcopically as being abnormal. The area to be vaporized should extend for 5 mm outside the abnormality. The outer margins of the area to be vaporized should be outlined with laser beam and the lesion then vaporized systematically. With small lesions the tissue can be vaporized very quickly, but with larger lesions it is useful to have some plan of action. The surgeon should remember that the end result is to destroy tissue to a depth of about 7 mm. It is sometimes helpful to mark a lesion into quadrants, i.e. draw a line with the laser from 12 o'clock to 6 o'clock and from 9 o'clock to 3 o'clock. The surgeon will then vaporize each quadrant in turn. It is best to start posteriorly so that any troublesome bleeding will not interfere with the vaporization of tissue later in the procedure. The spot should be moved relatively slowly until the desired depth has been reached. This can be ascertained by the use of a measuring stick, but with experience the surgeon will find that this is unnecessary. Ideally, the healed cervix should have the squamocolumnar junction at or just inside the new external os. To achieve this, the surgeon is advised to proceed as follows. Firstly, to destroy the lesion to a depth of about 7 mm. Secondly, when this stage has been completed, to destroy the lower part of the endocervical canal for a further 4 or 5 mm. In this way, the optimum end result is likely to be achieved.

Technique of laser excisional conization

Cold knife cervical conization is not without its problems, and bleeding has been reported in between 5.7%,[2] and 20.3%[5] of cases. There is often some degree of postoperative cervical stenosis which may lead to menstrual problems and may also restrict access to the squamocolumnar junction, thereby making adequate follow-up examination by colposcopy and cytology more difficult. Laser excisional conization allows an adequate cone to be removed with a reduction in hemorrhage[3] and a reduction in cervical stenosis with easy access to the squamocolumnar junction.[4]

The procedure is best carried out under general anesthesia with the patient in the lithotomy position, but in some instances can be performed under local anesthesia. The vasoconstrictor is injected into the cervical tissue using a fine gauge needle attached to a dental syringe. The cone is then cut by using a laser attached to the operating microscope. A small spot size (less than 0.5 mm) allows a very high power density to be used (in excess of 2500 W/cm^2) and in this way the cone can be cut easily and quickly. The lesion is first outlined colposcopically by the use of either acetic acid or Schiller's iodine solution. The ectocer-

vical limits of the cone are marked out using the laser beam, allowing approximately 5 mm of normal tissue between the edge of the lesion and the line of the incision. The operator then plans to remove a block of tissue the length of which will depend on how much of the endocervical canal has to be removed: this block of tissue will be more cylindrical than the traditional cone shape. After the edges of the cone have been demarcated, the surgeon needs a plan of excision which he should use each time and with which he feels comfortable. The easiest way is to cut the cylinder to the desired depth down the sides first, i.e. from 1 to 5 o'clock and then from 11 to 7 o'clock. While cutting, it is useful to use a skin hook to put the cut edge of the cylinder on traction. Having done the sides, the posterior incision should be made and finally the anterior incision. Having cut the cylinder to the desired depth, then the endocervical canal is cut with a scalpel or a pair of fine curved scissors, thereby allowing the pathologist to assess tissue at the upper margin of the cylinder which has not been damaged by laser. Following removal of the cone, an endocervical curettage is performed. The power density is then reduced by enlarging the spot size as in the vaporization cone, and the surgeon then lasers all of the cut surface of the defect to minimize hemorrhage. Most patients having this sort of procedure can be discharged home in 12 to 24 hours. Intra- and post-operative hemorrhage is uncommon. At the first postoperative visit the cervix will look totally different from the usual cold-knife conization cervix, in that there is minimal distortion, minimal cervical stenosis, and the squamocolumnar junction is usually visible or at least accessible for cytological assessment. Immediately postoperatively, the cone bed can be left open or alternatively packed with ribbon gauze soaked in Monsel's solution, which is removed 24 hours later. An alternative technique to minimize hemorrhage in the immediate postoperative period is to fill the cone bed with an antihemostatic material such as Surgicel (Johnson & Johnson). If this technique is to be used, then the patient should be warned that the deficit in the cervix has been filled with material which looks like fine gauze because, although this usually dissolves, occasionally it will fall out within a few days and the patient may be panicked into thinking that a gauze swab has been left in the vagina. Finally, antibiotic cover is favored by some surgeons.

Technique of combined vaporization and excisional conization

The technique of combined vaporization and excision conization is used when the circumstances are such that excision of the endocervical canal is thought to be necessary, but where that part of the lesion on the ectocervix involves most of the ectocervix or even some of the upper vagina. In this instance the surgeon combines the technique of laser vaporization with the technique of laser excisional conization. The central part of the lesion and the endocervical canal are first removed as described above. The peripheral part of the lesion is then vaporized to the required depth, leaving a deficit of anything up to 25 mm centrally but only 7 mm peripherally. This deficit has been described by Wright[9] as a 'cowboy hat procedure' because, seen in profile, the deficit looks rather like a hat with a wide brim. The alternative to this technique will often be either amputation of the cervix or even hysterectomy with removal of a cuff of vagina, so its advantages are obvious.

Complications

Most patients experience minimal discomfort, which is described variously as a warm feeling, a cramp-like feeling or tiny needles sticking into the cervix. Some patients feel nothing, while others (less than 1%) find that the discomfort is such that treatment cannot be completed without general anesthesia or paracervical block. Bleeding at the time of laser vaporization or laser conization is not usually a problem. However, it is more likely to occur in the presence of inflammatory changes so, if possible, any recognizable infective change should be eliminated before laser treatment takes place. If bleeding occurs during the laser treatment, then the operator should first remember one of the principal physical properties of CO_2 light, namely that it is absorbed totally by water. If the laser beam is directed at a pool of blood, then it will be unable to reach the underlying bleeding point and all that happens is that the blood becomes carbonized and bleeding continues. The surgeon should therefore identify the source of the bleeding and arrest it with a cotton tipped applicator. At this stage the laser beam must be used with a large spot size and low power density, as mentioned in the technique of laser vaporization. The spot should then be directed to the tissue at the side of the cotton tip applicator and, as the applicator is rolled away from the bleeding vessel, the laser energy will then coagulate the vessel tip. Occasionally, bleeding is so brisk that further measures are necessary, such as a suture. Even in the outpatient department, a suture with a small needle can be used without difficulty, particularly if the cervix has already been anesthetised. Other techniques which can control hemorrhage in an outpatient or an inpatient situation are to use silver nitrate, Monsel's solution, diathermy, cold coagulation or even cryocautery. Finally, it may be helpful to insert a further bolus of a vasoconstrictor.

Postoperative discharge is minimal and usually consists of a brown discharge for a period of 2 to 3 days; this is in marked contrast to the prolonged period of discharge, often offensive, which follows cryocautery and diathermy. Postoperative bleeding with the above procedures is uncommon. It may occur within a few hours of the laser treatment. Alternatively, there may be secondary hemorrhage at 7 to 10 days, usually because of an inflammatory change. If this happens, the patient should be seen by the colposcopist and any identifiable bleeding points treated by the application of Monsel's solution, silver nitrate, diathermy, cryocautery or cold coagulation. Usually a simple application of Monsel's solution is all that is required. A vaginal swab should be sent for culture and if there is any obvious inflammatory change the patient should be given an antibiotic.

Healing following laser treatment

Following laser destruction re-epithelialization of the cervix occurs very rapidly. In the series of patients studied by Mylotte, Jordan & Allen,[7] the regenerating tissue was studied by a combination of cytology, colposcopy and scanning electronmicroscopy. This revealed re-epithelialization occurred rapidly; within 8 to 10 days immature metaplastic cells were seen on the surface and in all cases the treated area was covered by mature squamous epithelium within 4 weeks. The appearance of squamous cells within days, even when extremely large areas have been vaporized, throws some light on the old argument as to the origin of new squamous epithelium. Following laser vaporization the new squamous cells can only come from the stroma and not from an ingrowth of mature squamous epithelium from the edge of the lesion. The new epithelium develops in an environment free of hemorrhage, necrosis or infection which explains the minimal discharge and the absence of fibrosis in the new epithelium — this is in contrast to the fibrosis which follows diathermy treatment. Furthermore, the squamocolumnar junction is almost always visible following laser vaporization (Fig. 70.2c), a factor which is very important when relying on colposcopy and cytology in follow-up.

The electronmicroscopic healing study has also revealed one other important factor. A constant criticism of destructive methods of treating cervical intraepithelial neoplasia has been the problem of inadequate destruction of tissue with the possibility of residual abnormality being covered with normal squamous epithelium and left to continue its natural history undetected. Following laser destruction of cervical intraepithelial neoplasia any abnormal tissue which has not been destroyed, either because surface epithelium has not been completely eradicated or because the abnormal epithelium extends into the depths of a crypt or gland beyond the depth of destruction, will remain on the surface during the healing process and be recognizable at follow up by colposcopy and/or cytology. Such residual abnormality will be visible at the first follow up visit in which case it can be readily destroyed by further laser vaporization.

CONCLUSION

It is now accepted that hysterectomy is over-treatment for

most patients with cervical intraepithelial neoplasia, and the increasing use of cervical diathermy and cryocautery under colposcopic direction has proved that cone biopsy too can be avoided in many instances. Recently, the laser has offered a new modality of treatment and is suitable for approximately 80% of patients. Under colposcopic direction, the CO_2 laser has the ability to destroy both extremely small and extremely large areas of tissue to any depth. Almost always it can be used as an outpatient procedure, and cure rates in the region of 95% are to be expected.[6] It must be stressed, however, that the success of vaporization treatment depends on careful patient selection by an expert colposcopist, and by destruction to a depth of 5 to 7 mm. Laser excisional conization is a technique which is easily learned and has advantages over the more traditional cold knife conization.

REFERENCES

1. Bellina J H 1977 Carbon dioxide laser in gynecology. Obstet Gynecol Annual 6: 371
2. Boutselis J G, Ullery J C 1964 Intraepithelial carcinoma of the cervix in pregnancy. Am J Obstet Gynecol 90: 593
3. Dorsey J H, Diggs E S 1979 Microsurgical conization of the cervix by carbon dioxide laser. Obstet Gynecol 54: 565
4. Fenton D W, Soutter W P, Sharp F, James C 1986 A comparison of knife and CO_2 laser excisional cone biopsies. In: Sharp F, Jordan J A (eds) Gynecologic Laser Surgery. Royal College of Obstetricians and Gynaecologists, London, p 77
5. Hollyock V E, Chanen W 1972 The use of the colposcope in selection of patients for cervical cone biopsy. Am J Obstet Gynecol 114: 185
6. Jordan J A, Woodman C B J, Mylotte M J et al 1985 The treatment of cervical intraepithelial neoplasia by laser vaporization. Br J Obstet Gynaecol 92: 394
7. Mylotte M J, Jordan J A, Allen J M 1979 Regeneration of cervical epithelium following laser destruction of intraepithelial neoplasia. Obstet Gynecol Surv 34: 859
8. Stafl A, Wilkinson E J, Mattingly R J 1977 Laser treatment of cervical and vaginal neoplasia. Am J Obstet Gynecol 128: 128
9. Wright V C 1984 Laser surgery for cervical intraepithelial neoplasia. Acta Obstet Gynecol Scand Suppl 125: 17

71. Cryosurgery

D. E. Townsend

INTRODUCTION

For the past two decades there has been an expansion in outpatient therapy for benign and premalignant disease of vulva, vagina and cervix through the introduction of cryosurgery. The principles of cryosurgery will be reviewed in this chapter together with its role in the treatment of patients with premalignant and malignant gynecological disease.

Cold as a therapeutic tool in medicine dates back to antiquity. It was used by the Egyptians as cold compresses for infected wounds and fractures, and by Hippocrates to reduce hemorrhage and swelling. Richardson,[23] in 1866, introduced ether spray as a freezing agent; ethyl chloride was substituted in 1891.

Cryotherapy was first used in gynecological cancer by Openchowski,[19] who circulated iced saline through the vagina of a woman with a large pelvic neoplasm and noted a marked tumor reduction. The first major study in gynecology was the treatment of chronic cervicitis with dry ice placed in the endocervical canal by Weitzner,[34] in 1940. Two years later, Hall[4] noted beneficial effects of cryosurgery with liquid freon delivered through probes in the treatment of benign cervical disease. Bobrow[2] repeated these studies with the addition of cytology; there was total healing after a single treatment session of 98% of women who completed follow-up, and there were no abnormal cells on cytological study.

From these modest beginnings, which spanned a period of about 20 years, gynecological cryosurgery attracted a sustained interest following the pioneering efforts of I.S. Cooper,[6] a neurosurgeon. In cooperation with industry, Cooper developed precise instrumentation which made the use of cold a therapeutic reality. Amongst the first to report safety and success of liquid nitrogen in the treatment of benign cervical disease was Collins,[4,5] as well as our own laboratory.[22,30] Crisp[9] was one of the first to point out the value of the technique for malignancy of the genital tract. These early studies were hampered by the size and expense of the apparatus delivering the refrigerant. The liquid nitrogen technique was impractical for the average physician. Thus, the burgeoning of the use of the technique in gynecology had to await the arrival of simpler and more economic systems in the mid-1960's. The first report on outpatient use of cryosurgery was from our laboratory in 1968, and emphasized the safety, simplicity and cost-saving aspects of the technique.[22]

Since this time, outpatient cryosurgery has been used to treat thousands of women with premalignant cervical disease,[8,13,29,32] so that now it is an accepted alternative and the most popular choice in the management of selected cases.

GENERAL PRINCIPLES AND EQUIPMENT

Hypothermia is achieved by two methods, the bases of which are:

1. Change of the cryogen phase (evaporation of liquid or solid) achieved by circulating liquid gas with a probe.
2. Adiabatic isentropic expansion of compressed gas through a small orifice (the Julius Thompson effect).

In both systems, the heat exchange occurs at the tip of the probe, which lies at the surface of the tissue to be frozen. Heat is withdrawn by the low temperature of the cryogen, so that ice forms in the tissues. This occurs in the range 0°C to −10°C. Cell death is caused primarily by dehydration, which increases the solute concentration and destroys protein. Water crystallizes, weakening the cell membrane and making it more prone to rupture. Singularly or collectively, such changes usually result in cell death. The rate of cooling determines whether ice forms in intracellular or extracellular water. Slow cooling of tissue temperature usually causes extracellular freezing and rapid cooling more frequently produces intracellular icing. Cell death is more readily produced by rapid cooling. Thawing rate also plays a part in cell death; slow thawing is the more injurious, and thus a rapid freeze and slow thaw sequence should be the most lethal combination. Tissue destruction

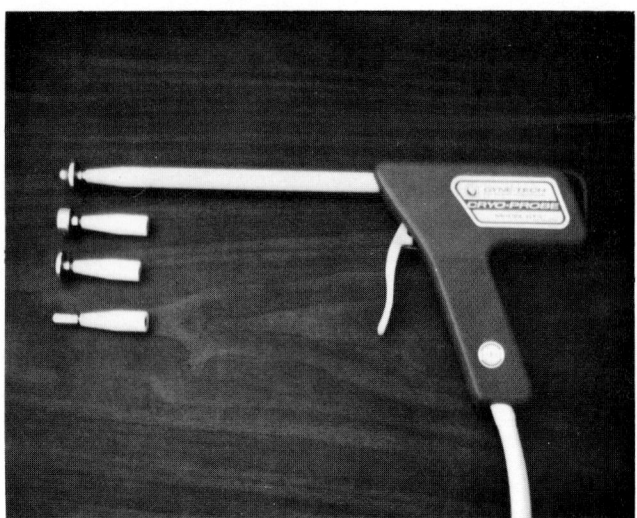

Fig. 71.1 Photograph of hand-gun type of cryosurgical unit with interchangeable tips. The handle is connected to a cylinder of nitrous oxide as refrigerant (not shown).

is also enhanced by repeated cycles of freeze–thawing, e.g. freeze, partial thaw, refreeze.[17]

Over the past 10 years, a number of cryosurgical instruments have been developed. Initially, the apparatus was bulky and required liquid nitrogen as the cryogen and electricity to power the probes. Modern units are more dependable and use the cryogen not only to freeze and destroy the tissue but also to defrost the probe tip. The most versatile units in current use are those with a gun-like configuration employing either carbon dioxide or nitrous oxide gas. These units have the advantage that the cryogen can be stored indefinitely, and they also avoid the use of electricity. They are highly reliable and almost indestructible, and their versatility is ensured by the availability of a wide range of probe tips (Fig. 71.1). In selecting a system for safe operation, it is best to ensure that all components are pressure-tested to twice the cryogen pressure, which varies between 700 and 900 PSI.

CERVICAL INTRAEPITHELIAL NEOPLASIA (CIN)

In the 1950s, conization of the cervix was virtually a routine procedure in women who had an abnormal Papanicolaou smear. This 'minor' high-risk procedure was used in women with abnormal Papanicolaou smears, i.e. Class III or worse, or suggestive of dysplasia or worse, because of the fear of missing invasive cancer. Moreover, many women, regardless of age and desire for childbearing were then subjected to hysterectomy if carcinoma in situ was found in the cone biopsy.

The extension of exfoliative cytology to women in the second and third decades of life disclosed 'dysplasia and carcinoma in situ with surprising frequency, and required that alternative diagnostic and therapeutic techniques be

developed in order to avoid the hazards, expense, and consequences of the traditional surgical attack.[33] Many studies clearly demonstrated that the vast majority of women with abnormal Papanicolaou tests can be safely evaluated without the need for hospitalization and conization.[1,7,10,14,15,20,27,31] Moreover, in most cases, a relatively minor office procedure will eradicate the lesion.[8,9,24,29]

The advent of colposcopy has permitted departure from the conventional evaluation and treatment techniques for cervical intraepithelial neoplasia (Chs 15 and 36). Although originally introduced as a means to detect invasive cervical neoplasia, colposcopy's greatest role lies in providing a route to more conservative and rational therapy for premalignant disease of the visible portion of the female genital tract, i.e. cervix, vulva and vagina.

Selection of patients

A scheme developed over 20 years ago in our own laboratory has been most effective when evaluating the individual with an abnormal Papanicolaou test (Table 71.1).

First, the cytology is repeated by ectocervical scrape and endocervical sample, since it has been shown that repeated cytological examination is extremely valuable in predicting the ultimate histologic diagnosis of the lesion[18,26] (Ch. 14). Colposcopy is then performed. The cervix is carefully cleansed with white vinegar (equal to 5% acetic acid). Initially we used 3% acetic acid, but changed to vinegar finding it less expensive, more dependable and, more importantly, that it rapidly accentuates the areas of abnormal epithelium. The surface topography is carefully inspected to locate abnormal areas. The squamocolumnar junction and the limits of the lesion are determined. After colposcopic inspection of the cervix, endocervical curettage is employed in all patients, except those who are pregnant or in whom invasive cancer is obviously present, regardless of whether the limits of the lesion can be seen. The curettage is mandatory because a surprisingly large number of endocervical invasive carcinomas have been reported, even though the colposcopist was under the impression that the limits of the lesion as well as the squamocolumnar junction had been defined.

After the endocervical curettage, which must include scraping from the internal os down to the upper limits of the lesion or to the external os if the lesion is confined to the ectocervix, directed colposcopic punch biopsies are taken. (Fig. 71.2) The number of biopsies taken in each patient will vary, depending upon the size and extent of the lesion. With large lesions up to 7 or 8 may be necessary (Fig. 71.3); with smaller lesions, a single biopsy may suffice (Fig. 71.4). Such proper tissue sampling coupled with curettage of the cervical canal is indispensible in order to detect or exclude invasive carcinoma. By carefully adhering to this scheme, we have never missed invasive cancer. With

Table 71.1 Evaluation of an individual with an abnormal Papanicolaou test.

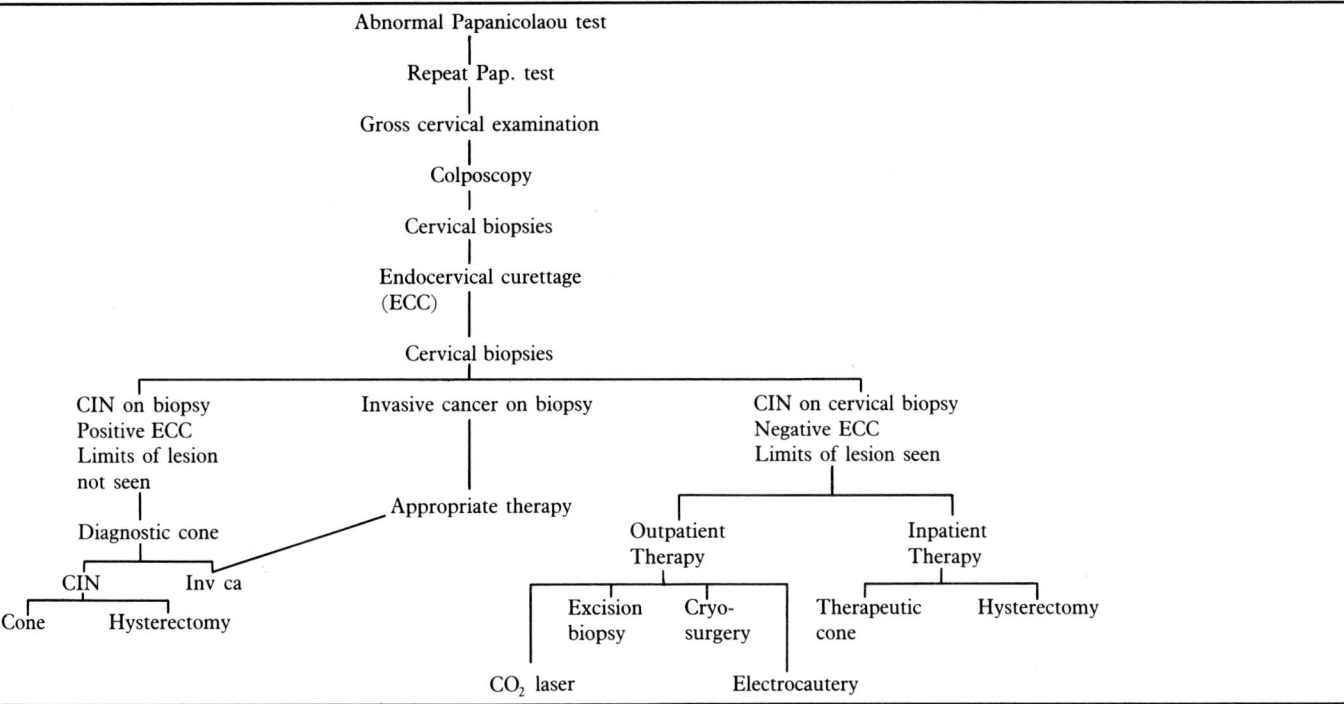

Abnormal Papanicolaou test

Repeat Pap. test

Gross cervical examination

Colposcopy

Cervical biopsies

Endocervical curettage (ECC)

Cervical biopsies

CIN on biopsy
Positive ECC
Limits of lesion not seen

Invasive cancer on biopsy

CIN on cervical biopsy
Negative ECC
Limits of lesion seen

Diagnostic cone

Appropriate therapy

Outpatient Therapy

Inpatient Therapy

CIN — Inv ca

Cone — Hysterectomy

Excision biopsy — Cryo-surgery

Therapeutic cone — Hysterectomy

CO₂ laser — Electrocautery

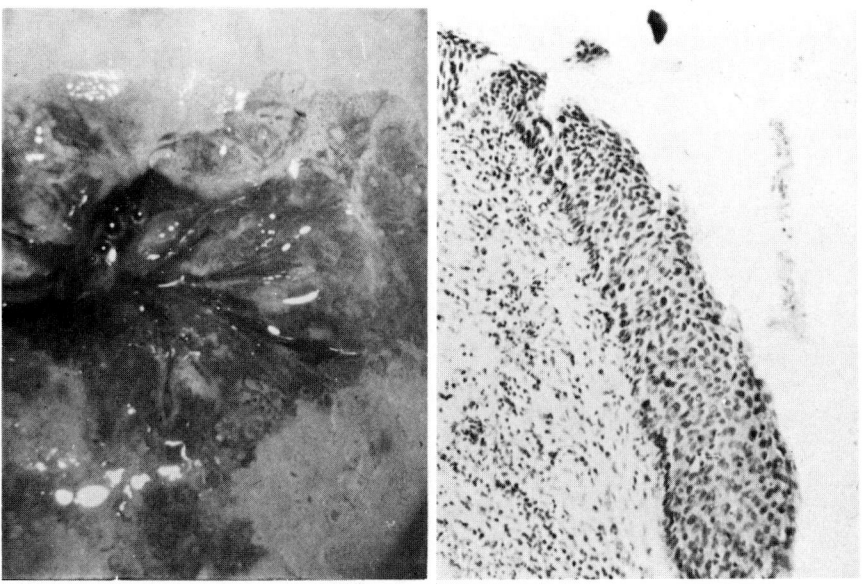

Fig. 71.2 Colpophotograph of cervix (left) in patient with a Pap smear suggestive of carcinoma in situ. Patchy areas of acetowhite epithelium are visible on both lips of the cervix beyond the physiological transformation zone around the cervical os. Directed biopsy (right) revealed carcinoma in situ. (×100).

deviation, especially the omission of the curettage of the canal, an occasional carcinoma has been missed.[28]

When invasive cancer has been excluded, and it is determined that the lesion is confined to the visible portion of the transformation zone, the woman is a candidate for outpatient therapy. Cryosurgery has merit because it has little or no effect on the patient's reproductive capacity, it is economical and because it can be performed in the clinic or office without the necessity of anesthesia or analgesia.

Prior to undertaking cryosurgery, a gynecological history is taken, with emphasis upon intermenstrual bleeding, menorrhagia, the quality and character of any discharge,

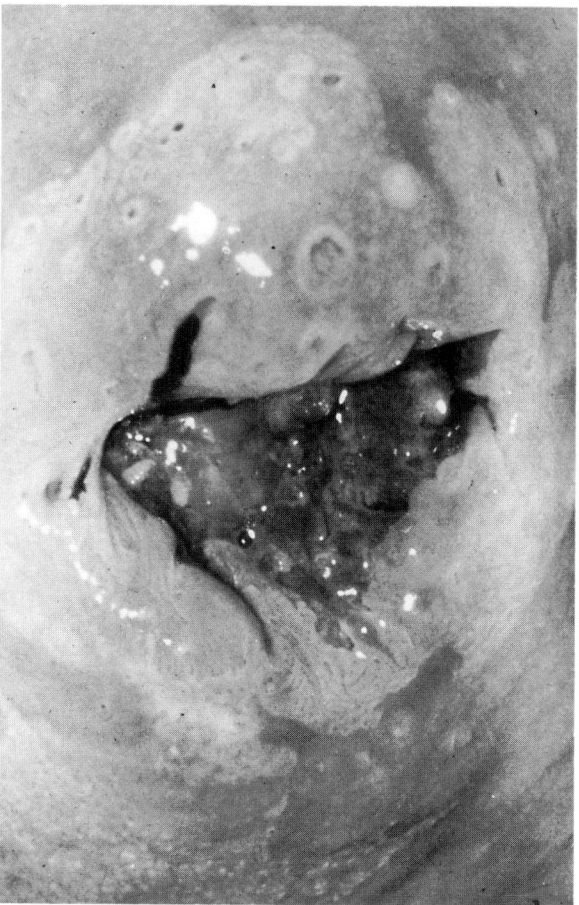

Fig. 71.3 Colpophotograph of large CIN II lesion. At least 4 to 5 biopsies are necessary for proper evaluation (×17). (Reproduced with permission of C.A.L. Inc.)

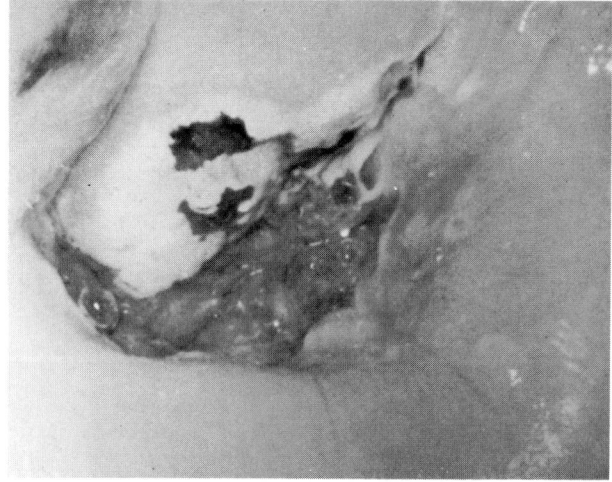

Fig. 71.4 Colpophotograph of small focal acetowhite lesion. Only a single biopsy is necessary (×17). (Reproduced with permission of C.A.L. Inc.)

previous salpingitis, and date of the last menstrual period. Cryosurgery is carried out within 1 week after the cessation of the last menstrual period. This will avoid freezing the cervix in a pregnant patient and permit the most active phase of regeneration to take place prior to the onset of the next menses.

Technique

The procedure is performed without anesthesia or analgesia. A speculum as large as can comfortably be tolerated is used. After insertion, the blades are fully extended. This provides optimum visualization of the cervix and reduces the chance of freezing vaginal epithelium. After the cervix is exposed, all mucus and cellular debris are removed from the cervix and vagina with gauze swabs or cotton balls soaked with a mucolytic agent such as vinegar or 3% acetic acid. The extent of the disease to be treated is carefully redetermined colposcopically. The cervical probe that best approximates the anatomical configuration of the cervix and maximally covers the area to be treated is attached to the unit. A thin film of lubricating jelly is then applied to the probe's surface to enhance the heat transfer from the tissue to the probe. The probe tip, at room temperature, is gently positioned onto the tissues and gentle pressure is applied. With large lesions, it is necessary to subdivide them so that each subdivision can be completely covered by the probe tip. Each subdivision is then individually frozen, making certain that the edges of the ice balls overlap one another.

After positioning the probe, the refrigerant is circulated. Crystallization first occurs on the back of the probe tip, and within 15 seconds spreads laterally from the edge of the probe onto the tissues. It is unnecessary to time the duration of freezing which, on average, lasts for about 2 to 5 minutes. A rapid lateral spread of the ice ball from the probe's edges indicates that the tissues are being adequately frozen. The freezing process is not terminated until the edge of the ice ball has extended 5 to 6 mm onto normal appearing epithelium (Figs 71.5 and 71.6). Probe-tip temperatures do not need to be monitored, since rapid lateral spread of ice from the probe means adequate tissue necrosis. If, during freezing, a portion of the vagina becomes attached to the probe, no complications result but the probe must be defrosted and reapplied to the cervix.

After treatment, the probe is defrosted and disengaged from the organ. Further inspection ensures that the iceball has extended the necessary 5 to 6 mm beyond the lesion. Any area not adequately frozen should then be treated again immediately. With overlapping freeze applications, it is important that the ice edges overlap. Generally we perform a single freeze–thaw application. An alternative recommendation is a freeze–partial thaw–refreeze technique. The cervix thaws after 10 to 15 minutes.

A recent discovery concerning successful cryosurgery is that the tank pressure should be maximum prior to the initiation of freezing. The rapidity of freezing depends on the rate of gas flowing into the probe tip. The more rapid the gas flow, which is directly related to the pressure

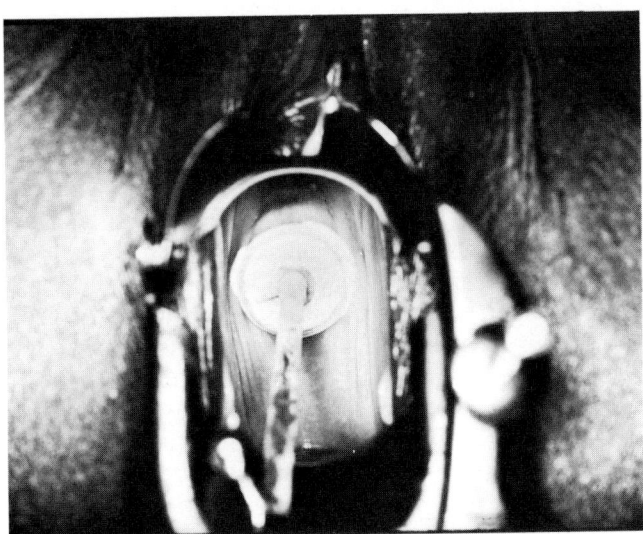

Fig. 71.5 Cryosurgical treatment being performed in office without anesthesia on cervix seen in Figure 71.2. The cervix has been exposed by a vaginal speculum. The circular portion of the tip applied to the cervix and the shaft of the probe appearing from the bottom of the photograph are shown. The iceball appears as a whiter rim around the edge of the probe-tip. The duration of freezing is determined by the extent of the iceball to 5–6 mm beyond this edge rather than by timing.

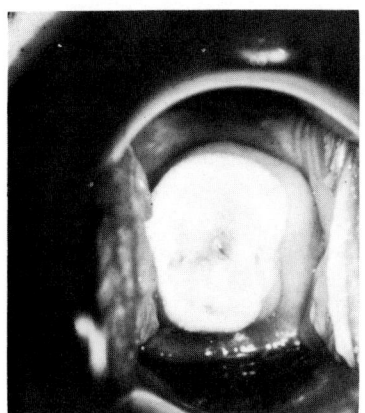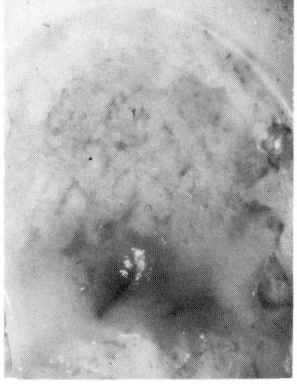

Fig. 71.6 Appearance of cervix immediately after cryosurgery. On the left the iceball is evident, on the right it has thawed.

within the tank, the greater will be the withdrawal of heat and subsequent formation of ice in the tissues. With a low tank pressure the rate of flow of gas is much slower, resulting in a slower freezing process which is less lethal to the tissues. The rate of thaw obtained from the body temperature is the ideal.

Post-treatment sequelae

The most common annoyance, which begins immediately after thawing, is the characteristic clear watery discharge which persists for at least 10 to 14 days and usually requires 2 to 5 sanitary napkins per day. The woman should

be informed as to the nature and extent of the discharge in order to alleviate anxiety. Any malodorous discharge is treated by douching and acidifying creams. The discharge becomes mucoid after 2 weeks and has usually disappeared by 5 weeks. The persistence of the discharge beyond 6 weeks generally indicates vaginal infection. Patients are requested not to use tampons and to refrain from sexual activity for the first 3 weeks after freezing, because of the risk of damage to the fragile regenerating epithelium and resultant contact bleeding. Mild, cramping, menstrual-like discomfort is common during the procedure, and in about one-half of patients persists for 24 to 48 hours. A mild analgesic is generally sufficient. More severe pain, either during or after cryosurgery, requiring more effective analgesics is rare. About one patient in four will show a vasomotor reaction, with flushing, headache and dizziness, just after freezing. This possibly vasovagal reaction rarely progresses to loss of consciousness. Vasomotor reactions are treated by 20 to 30 minutes rest, with analgesics. The unpredictability of these reactions obliges the patient to be accompanied to the freezing session. Spontaneous bleeding is rare, but a pinkish discharge occurs in half the patients probably due to a minimal ooze from the necrosed area. On the rare occasion bleeding is a problem, topical application of a caustic agent may be necessary, together with the packing of cotton balls for a few moments.

Healing is usually complete in 6 to 8 weeks (Fig. 71.7) although assessment as to the success or failure of therapy is delayed until 4 or 5 months. If a repeat freeze is necessary, a freeze–partial (2 to 5 minutes) thaw–refreeze cycle is used. Contraceptives, including intra-uterine devices, do not interfere with healing and the IUD string is not adversely affected by the freezing.

Even intense freezing does not interfere with fertility. Incompetence of the cervix is unknown as a sequel, and

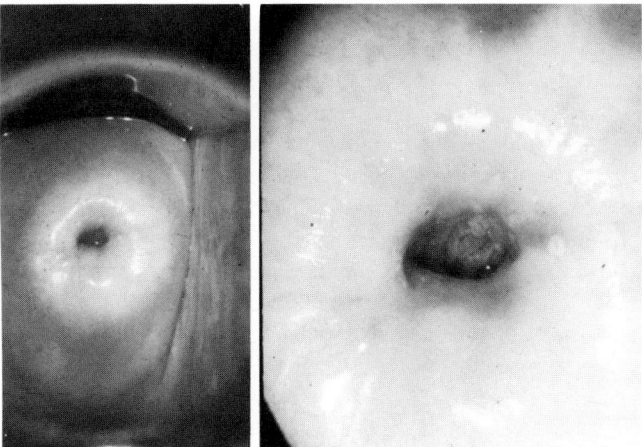

Fig. 71.7 Appearance of same cervix (as in Figs 71.2 & 71.3) 8 weeks after cryosurgery (left is macrophotograph, right is colpophotograph). Note the transformation zone has been replaced by normal regenerate squamous epithelium and that there is no stenosis.

labor and delivery are unaffected. After delivery, the cervix usually returns to its original post-freeze state. Cervical stenosis has not been reported, although there is occasionally reduction to a diameter of 2 mm in the cervical canal. Here, the probe tip shape may be important since most cases follow the use of the small cone-tipped probe. Simple dilatation or insertion of a laminaria tent as an office procedure suffices to control the condition. Rarely does stenosis produce dysmenorrhea.

Suitable antibiotics have been effective in the rare exacerbations of salpingitis where such a history exists.

Cytologic and histologic changes

Regeneration of squamous epithelium during the repair phases can occasionally mimic condyloma. At other times an abnormal Papanicolaou smear results, as the active regenerating epithelium can be mistaken for a mild to moderate dysplasia, especially when cervical biopsies, conization or hysterectomy are performed in the first 12 weeks after cryosurgery.[8,22] It is important that the pathologist be alerted to a history of recent cryosurgery. Unnecessary conization has been performed related to such misdiagnosis in patients due to lack of this clinical information. These cases should not be considered as freeze failures. The epithelial proliferation is usually self-limiting, with spontaneous disappearance or with removal by biopsy.

Follow-up

Patients who have been treated for CIN by outpatient cryosurgery are re-examined 4 to 6 weeks post-therapy to assess symptoms or untoward results. The first evaluation to determine the result of treatment is carried out at 18 to 24 weeks, when cytology and colposcopy are performed. These examinations are repeated again 36 to 40 weeks after therapy. The success of the procedure is assessed at this time.

When a patient had mild dysplasia (CIN I) prior to freezing and has two consecutive Papanicolaou tests of CIN 1 or worse, or biopsy reveals the same diagnosis, therapy is considered a failure. However, when the diagnosis pretreatment was CIN 2 or 3, the patient must have two consecutive Papanicolaou smears or a biopsy result indicating CIN 2 or 3 before treatment is considered a failure. Thus, keeping in mind the aberration of cell morphology which accompanies the repair (which can mimic CIN), the result of a single smear test, regardless of severity, does not necessarily mean failure. When the results of the surveillance are negative, the patient is seen every 6 months for the first 2 years and then yearly thereafter.

In our study we have treated over 1000 patients with CIN, with a distribution of approximately: one-third with CIN 1 (mild dysplasia); one-third with CIN 2 (moderate dysplasia); and one-third CIN 3 (severe dysplasia to carcinoma in situ). We have found cryosurgery to be effective for all degrees of intraepithelial neoplasia. Our overall success rate with a single freeze-thaw technique is 88%. Retreatment of the majority of the failures at a second cryosurgery session increased the cure rate to 95%.

First analysis of our data suggested that the patients with CIN 1 were more likely to be cured than those with CIN 3, the respective failure rates being 7% and 16%. However, when the data were evaluated with respect to lesion size, we noted that patients with a lesion less than 1 cm in surface area, regardless of the histologic diagnosis, had a 93% success rate, whereas those with lesions covering most of the ectocervix, regardless of histologic diagnosis, had a primary failure rate approaching 50%. Thus, it was evident that most of our failures occurred in patients with large lesions. Persistence following the initial treatment session was often less than 1 cm in size, so that re-treatment was possible in the majority of instances with a high success rate.

Patients forming our study group were a clinic population, so that follow-up has not been optimal. The majority were followed for 2 years, but thereafter the numbers lost to follow-up rapidly increased so that we have no data in respect to the long-term effects. However, Richart and colleagues[25] have surveyed over 2000 patients with CIN treated by cryosurgery. Individuals free of disease at 2 years and followed for up to 10 years had a very low risk of developing a new lesion. It is obvious that much longer follow-up, perhaps 20 years, is optimum for a true evaluation of results.

There is little doubt that the safe outpatient management of a large number of young women with CIN is possible, provided the gynecologist has expert colposcopic technique, experience and a sound knowledge of the natural history of CIN.

Unfortunately, some cases of invasive cancer have been reported following cryosurgery, CO_2 laser and electrocautery in the outpatient clinic.[13,32] Careful review has shown that the colposcopic evaluation has not always been above suspicion. Causes of failure include the absence of a repeat Papanicolaou test or of biopsy, and the failure to perform an endocervical curettage.[28] The latter may be forsaken in the mistaken belief that, should the limits of the lesion as well as the entire squamocolumnar junction be seen, endocervical curettage is unnecessary. In over one-half of the missed cancers, the examining physicians believed the lesion's epithelial limits to be visible, but it is just as obvious that they were wrong; the disease was in the canal and would have been detectable by endocervical curettage. Such curettage is thus obligatory unless the patient is pregnant or unless the presence of an invasive cancer is obvious.

INVASIVE CERVICAL CARCINOMA

Cryosurgery is not indicated as primary therapy for invasive cervical disease because of the inability to treat parametrial and lymph-node-bearing areas. However, it may be effective in the control of bleeding from cancerous areas while awaiting the initiation of conventional therapy.[16]

VULVA

Cryosurgery may be successfully used in carefully selected young patients with vulvar intraepithelial neoplasia (Ch. 26). In view of the multifocal nature of the disease, colposcopy with or without toluidine blue is mandatory to delineate abnormal areas. Each of several lesions must be biopsied to exclude an invasive component. Smaller lesions less than 2 cm in diameter are suitable for cryosurgery, leaving the larger lesions for treatment by surgical excision or by the CO_2 laser.

Treatment can be an outpatient procedure with supplemental local anesthetic usually necessary. During freezing, the ice ball should extend at least 3 mm onto tissue which appears normal colposcopically. Multifocal lesions require separate stages of therapy. Healing is usually complete by 4 to 6 weeks. Topical analgesics and sitz baths are used to relieve any discomfort. The more rapid freeze obtainable with nitrous oxide makes it the refrigerant of choice. Only a single freeze–thaw cycle is used in the treatment of vulvar disease.

Palliation of large, fungating, recurrent carcinoma of vulva and perineum has been achieved by Crisp[9] with the use of cryosurgery. He pointed out that, although life may not be prolonged, the procedure can relieve discomfort, control bleeding and reduce the malodorous discharge. Cryosurgery has been used as an adjunct to radical surgery in managing malignant melanoma of the urethra.[21]

VAGINA

Small vaginal intraepithelial lesions are suitable for cryosurgery. Experienced colposcopy is required for the location, evaluation and biopsy of each lesion (Chs 16 and 29). Freezing must be cautious in view of the proximity of bladder, urethra and rectum. A single freeze–thaw cycle is sufficient. The surface area of the lesions treated should approximate that of the probe tip. Larger lesions should be subdivided to achieve this approximation, the ice ball always extending up to 3 mm onto colposcopically normal appearing epithelium. No scarring or contracture is noted in the follow-up period of 6 years available to us in our studies.

UTERINE FUNDUS

Limited investigations have been carried out on the application of freezing for disease of the uterine cavity.[3,11] The inaccessibility, together with the lack of suitable outpatient and diagnostic techniques, probably accounts for the poor results obtained. Wider use of hysteroscopy in properly selected patients may encourage further use of the technique.

CRYOSURGERY AND THE CO_2 LASER

A few years following the introduction of cryosurgery, the carbon dioxide laser was introduced. The technique is now of extreme interest and, although this chapter is devoted primarily to cryosurgery, it is important to point out some of the major differences between the two techniques.

We have used the CO_2 laser on over 1500 patients with a variety of gynecologic conditions, primarily CIN. The procedure is performed in the office, although without local anesthesia, it does cause more discomfort than does cryosurgery. All patients experience some degree of unpleasant, mild cramp-like sensations, but occasionally they can be severe. With local anesthesia, discomfort is usually absent or minimal. Bleeding is more of a problem with laser than with cryosurgery, and in a few instances the bleeding can be brisk requiring vaginal packing. The discharge after laser is minimal compared to cryosurgery and, for that reason, the former is appealing to most patients.

Recently, Wetchler[35] carried out an extensive review of the utility of laser or cryosurgery for CIN. He compared the effectiveness as well as the costs of the two procedures. It was apparent that the two techniques are quite comparable in effectiveness. In our own experience, we noted that patients with large lesions tend to have a high failure rate with cryosurgery, whereas with laser they have a high cure rate. For this reason, we prefer to use laser vaporization with large CIN lesions when we are interested in having a single treatment session, although multiple freeze applications can be quite effective when using cryosurgery.

The cost of cryotherapy is considerably less than laser. Physician fees vary between US $50 to $150 and laser fees run between US $300 to $1000. When laser surgery is performed in the operating room, requiring anesthesia, the costs can be as high as US $4000. In those countries where physician reimbursement is controlled by the government, the laser reimbursement is slightly higher than cryosurgery. If a physician wishes to perform laser vaporization in the office, the least expensive equipment will run between US $25 000 to $35 000, with a maintenance cost as high as US $2000 per year. Cryosurgical equipment costs about US $1500 a year, with minimal maintenance cost.

Despite these differences, laser is still a very attractive modality since it gives the physician a sense of activity and accomplishment during the course of therapy. In addition, there is a sense of greater control of tissue destruction, since the physician is actually colposcopically viewing the treatment as it is taking place.

REFERENCES

1. Beller F K, Khatamee M 1966 Evaluation of punch biopsy of the cervix under direct colposcopic observation (Target punch biopsy). Obstet Gynecol 28: 622
2. Bobrow M L, Goldbaum A, Short V 1961 Treatment of cervicitis by the carbon dioxide snow cauterization method. Obstet Gynecol 18: 726
3. Cahan W G, Brockunier A, Jr 1967 Cryosurgery of the uterine cavity. Am J Obstet Gynecol 99: 138
4. Collins R J, Golab A 1966 Cryosurgical treatment of uterine cervicitis. Preliminary report. Bull Mill Fill Hosp 13: 47
5. Collins R J, Pappas H J 1972 Cryosurgery for benign cervicitis with follow up of six and one half years. Am J Obstet Gynecol 113: 744
6. Cooper I S, Lee A St J 1961 Cryothalamectomy-hypothermic congelation: a technical advance in basal ganglia surgery. Preliminary report. J Am Geriatr Soc 9: 714
7. Coppleson M, Pixley E C, Reid B L 1986 Colposcopy. A Scientific Approach to the Cervix, Vagina and Vulva in Health and Disease, 3rd edn. Thomas, Springfield.
8. Creasman W T, Weed J C Jr, Curry S L, Johnston W W, Parker R T 1973 Efficacy of cryosurgical treatment of severe cervical intraepithelial neoplasia. Obstet Gynecol 41: 501
9. Crisp W E, Asadourian L, Romberger W 1967 Application of cryosurgery to gynecologic malignancy. Obstet Gynecol 30: 668
10. Donohue L R, Meriwether W 1971 Colposcopy as a diagnostic tool in the investigation of cervical neoplasias. Am J Obstet Gynecol 113: 107
11. Droegemueller W, Greer B, Makowski E 1971 Cryosurgery in patients with dysfunctional uterine bleeding. Obstet Gynecol 38: 256
12. Hall F E 1942 The use of quick freezing methods in gynecologic practice. A preliminary report. Am J Obstet Gynecol 43: 105
13. Kaufman R H, Strama T, Norton P K, Conner J S 1973 Cryosurgical treatment of cervical intraepithelial neoplasia. Obstet Gynecol 42: 881
14. Kolstad P, Stafl A 1972 Atlas of Colposcopy. University Park Press, Baltimore.
15. Krumholz B A, Knapp R C 1972 Colposcopic selection of biopsy sites. Obstet Gynecol 39: 22
16. Lash A F 1972 The immediate control of hemorrhage from gynecologic malignancies by cryosurgery. Int J Gynecol Obstet 10: 72
17. Mazur P 1967 Factors affecting cell injury in cryosurgical freezing. Bull Mill Fill Hosp 14: 123
18. Miller E M, Von Haam E 1960 In symposium — Advantages and disadvantages of various techniques of obtaining material for routine cytological examinations. Acta Cytol 4: 236
19. Openchowski P H 1883 Sur l'action localisee du froid, applique a la surface de la region corticale du cervau. Compt rend Soc de biol 4: 38
20. Ostergard D R, Gondos B 1973 Outpatient therapy of preinvasive cervical neoplasia. Selection of patients with the use of colposcopy. Am J Obstet Gynecol 115: 783
21. Ostergard D R, Townsend D E 1968 Malignant melanoma of the female urethra treated by cryosurgery with radical vulvectomy and anterior exenteration. Report of a case. Obstet Gynecol 31: 75
22. Ostergard E, Townsend D E, Hiroze F M 1968 The treatment of chronic cervicitis by cryotherapy. Am J Obstet Gynecol 102: 426
23. Paloucek F P, Batayola W, Collins R H, Pappas H J 1968 Historical aspects of cryotherapy in gynecology. J Cryosurg 12: 148
24. Richart R M 1966 Influence of diagnostic and therapeutic procedures on the distribution of cervical intraepithelial neoplasia. Cancer 19: 1635
25. Richart R M, Townsend D E, Crisp W et al 1980 An analysis of 'long-term' follow-up results of patients with cervical intraepithelial neoplasia treated by cryotherapy. Am J Obstet Gynecol 137: 823
26. Richart R M & Vaillant H W 1965 Influence of cell collection techniques upon cytological diagnosis. Cancer 18: 1474
27. Stafl A, Mattingly R F 1973 Colposcopic diagnosis of cervical neoplasia. Obstet Gynecol 41: 168
28. Townsend D E, Richart R M 1981 Diagnostic errors in colposcopy. Gynecol Oncol (suppl 2): 259
29. Townsend D E, Ostergard D R 1971 Cryocauterization for preinvasive cervical neoplasia. J Reprod Med 6: 171
30. Townsend D E, Ostergard D R, Lickrish G M 1971 Cryosurgery for benign disease of the uterine cervix. J Obstet Gynaecol Br Commonw 18: 667
31. Townsend D E, Ostergard D R, Mishell D R, Jr, Hirose F M 1970 Abnormal Papanicolaou smears. Evaluation by colposcopy, biopsies and endocervical curettage. Am J Obstet Gynecol 108: 429
32. Tredway D R, Townsend D E, Hovland D N, Upton R T 1972 Colposcopy and cryosurgery in cervical intraepithelial neoplasia. Am J Obstet Gynecol 114: 1020
33. Villasanta U, Durkan J P 1966 Indications and complications of cold conization of the cervix. Observations on 200 consecutive cases. Obstet Gynecol 27: 717
34. Weitzer K 1940 The treatment of endocervicitis with carbon dioxide snow (dry ice). Am J Surg 48: 620
35. Wetchler S J 1984 Treatment of cervical intraepithelial neoplasia with the CO_2 laser: laser versus cryotherapy and review of effectiveness and cost. Obstet Gynecol Surv 39: 169

72. Electrocoagulation diathermy of cervix

W. Chanen

INTRODUCTION

Electrocoagulation diathermy is a most reliable and effective method of destroying those areas of abnormal change on the cervix that are precursors of invasive disease.[3,6] The method is simple, safe and requires no specialized or expensive equipment. Every operating theater possesses some type of electrosurgical diathermy apparatus. We believe this form of physical destruction is more effective in destroying larger areas and greater depths of abnormal tissue of the cervix than cryosurgery or CO_2 laser therapy. Its use in the treatment of vaginal lesions is limited. Generally under these circumstances, biopsy excision is preferred because of the ease of reconstruction of such excision. Electrocoagulation diathermy should not be confused with simple thermal or hot cautery. The method is of greatest advantage in the nulliparous and, in particular, women wanting further children.

CRITERIA FOR SELECTION OF PATIENTS

A rigid protocol for selection of patients is required to avoid the error of overlooking true invasive disease.[5] All patients with a cytologic smear report suggesting significant atypicality should be first examined with the colposcope either in the office or suitable 'dysplasia clinic'. As an additional safeguard, further cytologic smears can be taken from the endocervical canal with a cytobrush as well as a standard ectocervical smear. Both can be placed on the one slide and this provides the cytologist with additional and more accurate sampling. One or more directed biopsies are taken from the areas of maximal atypical colposcopic change. By integrating the findings of these three modalities — cytology, colposcopy and histology — it is possible to delineate the site, nature and extent of the cervical lesion responsible for the abnormal smear.

Patients in whom the *anatomic limits of the lesion can be exposed to the colposcope* are eminently suited for treatment by electrocoagulation. Under these circumstances, expert colposcopic assessment reinforced by the findings of cytology and histology will allow the exclusion of true invasive disease. It is now more fully understood that dysplasia and carcinoma in situ (cervical intraepithelial neoplasia; CIN) are simply part of a spectrum of a histologic change of the same biologic disease process, and that either are capable of progressing to true neoplastic disease (Ch. 35). The specific histologic label in that spectrum will frequently depend upon the subjectivity of the observer (p. 572). Therefore, once invasive cancer is excluded, the severity of the histologic change should never dictate the choice of treatment. The more important factor in management is the anatomic extent of the abnormal tissue to be eradicated. Thus, carcinoma in situ does not demand more extensive or radical treatment by cone biopsy or hysterectomy merely because the tissue has been histologically labelled as such.

In summary, the following criteria must be fulfilled:

1. Biopsy has been histologically confirmed as CIN (dysplasia and/or carcinoma in situ).
2. The anatomic extent of the atypical transformation zone (TZ) is 'in range'.
3. True invasive disease has been confidently excluded.

The term 'in range' means either that the whole of the TZ is readily within colposcopic view, or that the upper limits of the TZ may extend into the endocervical canal but can be assessed by (i) manipulation of the cervical lips or (ii) use of an appropriate endocervical speculum.

Where the lesion extends into the cervical canal apparently precluding adequate colposcopic evaluation the use of a suitably designed endocervical speculum[1] (Fig. 72.1), particularly with the advantage of examination under anesthesia, often permits the anatomic limits to be visualized for the first time (Fig. 72.2). Such patients, otherwise destined for diagnostic cone biopsy, are also suitable for electrocoagulation diathermy treatment.[4]

THE OPERATION

The aim of the operation is to destroy the whole area and depth of the abnormal transformation zone and adjacent

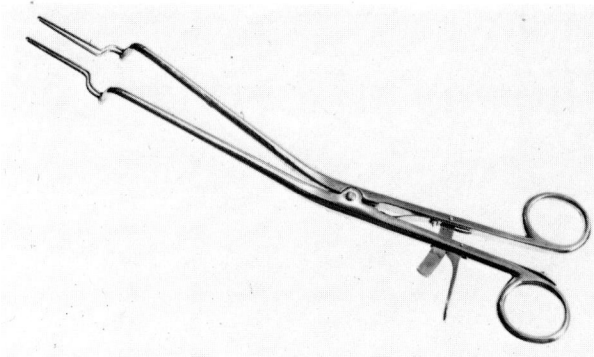

Fig. 72.1 Endocervical speculum as modified by the author.

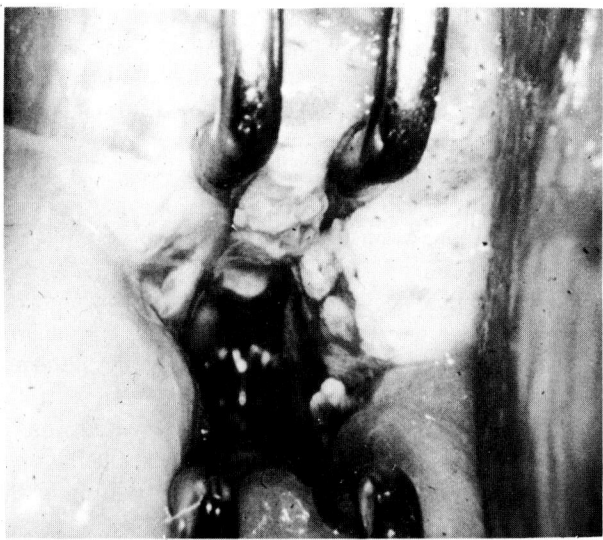

Fig. 72.2 Colpophotograph showing endocervical speculum opening up the cervical canal. Previously concealed anatomic boundaries of lesion on posterior cervical lip are now visible.

columnar epithelium extending into the lower canal. Destruction must include deep gland crypts which may extend for distances of at least 3 to 4 mm into the cervical stroma.

Anesthesia

The cervix is *not* an insensitive organ and therefore some form of anesthesia is required. In the past, because of the specific protocol advocated and the potential pain and discomfort likely to be involved in the procedure, general anesthesia was preferred. With expert anesthesia and suitable 'day care' or 'freestanding' theater facilities, no special preoperative preparation was required and the patient could be discharged as soon as she recovered from the anesthetic. At present, because of the increased pressure placed upon hospital facilities, with only minor modification of the protocol and technique, the electrodiathermy

can be effectively performed under local anesthetic infiltration as an 'office' type procedure.

General anesthesia

Treatment under general anesthesia can be reserved for those in whom the lesion is very extensive or who are very apprehensive. The risk of not having recognized an early invasive carcinoma is minimized by a further colposcopic assessment under the anesthetic prior to commencing the procedure. This is particularly valuable when the lesion appears to extend into the canal out of colposcopic range and the endocervical speculum has exposed the anatomic boundaries for the first time. It has been our practice to take additional colposcopically-directed biopsies for further histologic study. Under such circumstances, dilatation and fractional curettage has been part of the protocol. The endocervical curettage is performed prior to the dilatation and serves as a further 'fail safe' mechanism to avoid missing the diagnosis of unsuspected invasive carcinoma. Furthermore, this practice has helped to confirm the concept that CIN originates only within the anatomic confines of the transformation zone. 'Skip' lesions beyond these anatomical limits in the canal have not been demonstrated. Dilatation of the cervix to a number 6 or 7 Hegar's dilator may diminish the risk of subsequent cervical stenosis and facilitate the diathermy procedure to extend well into the cervical canal. Curettage of the uterine cavity is performed in order to exclude associated disease of the endometrium.

Local anesthesia (intracervical infiltration)

A Graves' bivalve speculum fitted with a smoke extraction device is inserted vaginally and the cervix is again examined with the colposcope to check the validity of the previous findings. When considered necessary, additional biopsies can be taken (after anesthetic infiltration) as a fail safe precaution. Where the limits of the lesion can be readily exposed, routine endocervical curettage has not been considered to be a necessary part of our protocol. This view is reinforced by our own historical data. A standard dental syringe and disposable cartridge (2.2 ml) with 27 gauge needle is used. (Fig. 72.3) For the more extensive lesion, a second cartridge provides more effective anesthesia. Nurocaine® (lignocaine with sympathin 1:50 000) or Xylocaine® 2% with adrenalin 1:80 000 are the most frequent local anesthetic combinations used. No significant side effects have been experienced with these preparations. Painting the cervix with Lugol's iodine solution provides a degree of antisepsis and also outlines the area to be destroyed. The syringe needle is inserted sequentially at the margin of the demarcation between the iodine-stained and iodine-negative tissue in at least four positions, 3, 6, 9 and 12 o'clock, angling the needle to-

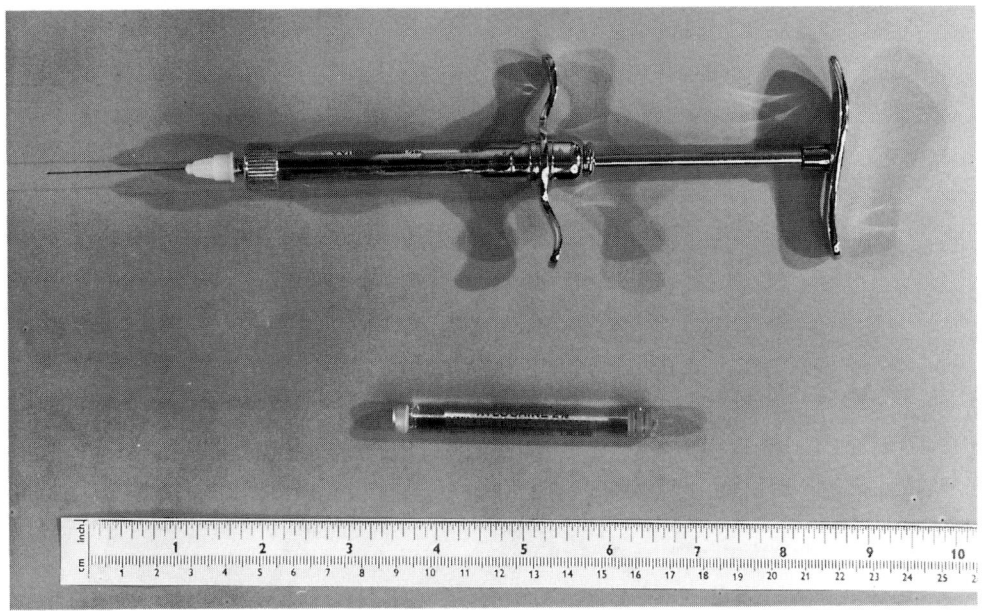

Fig. 72.3 Dental syringe with disposable fine gauge needle and cartouche of local anesthetic.

wards the endocervical canal. The momentary discomfort of the needle penetrating into the substance of the cervix can be blunted by requesting the patient to strain down, pushing the cervix onto the needle and injecting at the same time.

Technique, electrosurgical machine and electrodes

Preoperative staining of the cervix with Lugol's iodine solution will help demarcate the area that should be diathermied. A transistorized Valleylab unit (Boulder, Colorado) model SSE-2, with a coagulation setting of 3.5 to 4, is particularly useful for office work (Fig. 72.4). With the larger electrosurgical units, a digital reading of 35 to 40 W is used. The needle and ball electrodes, as illustrated in Figure 72.5, are employed to achieve the destruction. These two simple electrodes will cope with any size, shape or contour of cervix, irrespective of the area to be diathermied.

The *needle electrode* is inserted to a depth of approximately 7 to 10 mm into the long axis of the cervix. Multiple punctures are made over the whole of the transformation zone and adjacent columnar epithelium, and into all nabothian cysts. The number of insertions is purely empirical, and will depend on the area and extent of the lesion. Insertion and withdrawal of the needle is facilitated by keeping the current on at the time. Each insertion of the needle should last for at least 1 to 2 seconds at intervals of approximately 2 to 3 mm. The purpose of the needle insertions is to help destroy the deeper gland crypts and, in the process of postoperative healing, produce an in-

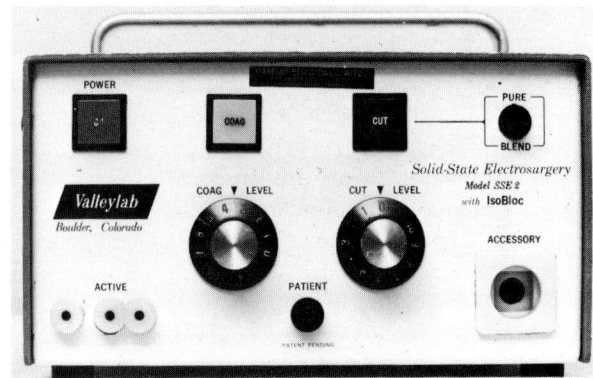

Fig. 72.4 Electrosurgical machine — a Valleylab (Boulder, Colorado) model SSE-2.

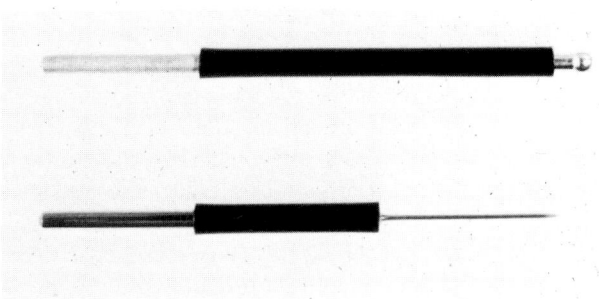

Fig. 72.5 Needle and ball electrodes employed in the technique of electrocoagulation diathermy.

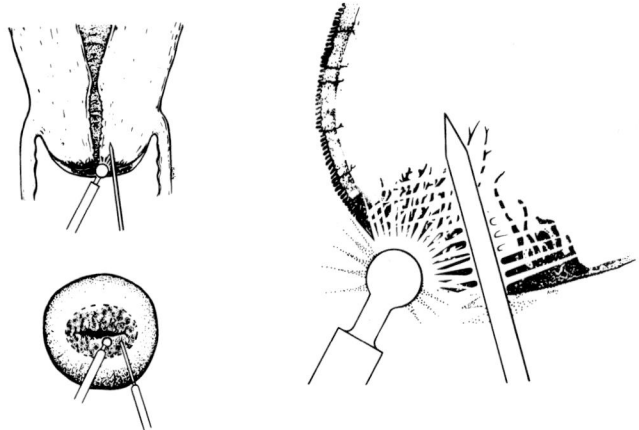

Fig. 72.6 Diagrammatic representation of the effect of a needle and ball electrocoagulation diathermy (only one electrode at a time is used). Superficial fulguration and deeper coagulation achieve destruction of CIN tissue both on the surface and in the gland crypts.

version effect on the cervix which will tend to limit the columnar epithelium to within the cervical canal. Following this the *ball electrode* is used, and by a process of fulguration and coagulation the whole surface area, already subjected to the needle electrode, is systematically diathermied (Fig. 72.6). The current may be applied continuously or periodically for 2 or 3 seconds duration. Rapid movement of the ball with continuous current tends to produce more spark or fulguration, whereas slower movement and direct contact on the tissue will produce a deeper coagulation effect. Destruction of abnormal tissue must be total and complete. The *end point of diathermy* is taken to be when the area is dessicated and no further mucus exudes, indicating the probable destruction of the deeper glands of the cervix. Cauterization by the traditional radial stroke method is not recommended because of the risk of leaving behind viable abnormal tissue between the radial strokes. Constant mopping of the cervix with dry gauze facilitates a better contact. The ball can be periodically cleansed of any adherent tissue; a scalpel blade or sterile abrasive material is suitable for this purpose. Diathermy should extend into the lower cervical canal. Inadequate electrocoagulation diathermy will result in failure to destroy the deeper crypts, which may be lined by the abnormal dysplastic epithelium. One should not be afraid of using the electrocoagulation diathermy too zealously, as there is really more risk in its under-use than over-use. When performing the procedure under local anesthetic infiltration, the ball electrode is utilized first, as it appears to provide some additional anesthesia due to diffused thermal destruction of the deeper layers. It is the deeper needle insertions that are more likely to produce pain. When the diathermy is performed under local infiltration, the use of a long chuck handle avoids working too close to the vulva and thereby gives more stable control of the end electrode.

Examples of successful eradication of carcinoma in situ (CIN 3) by electrocoagulation diathermy are illustrated in Figures 72.7 and 72.28.

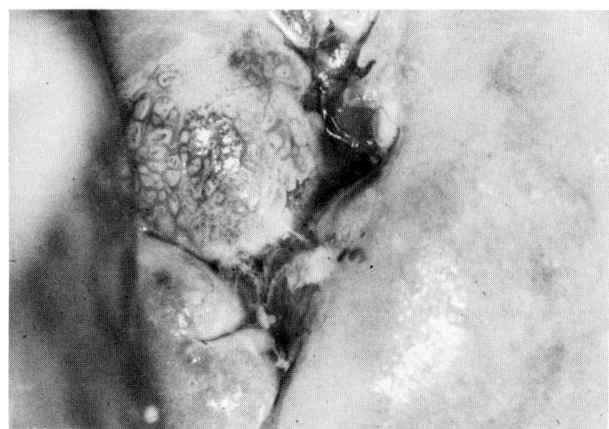

Fig. 72.7a Colpophotograph showing marked abnormal transformation zone (mosaic and punctation) confined to ectocervix. Biopsy reported as carcinoma in situ.

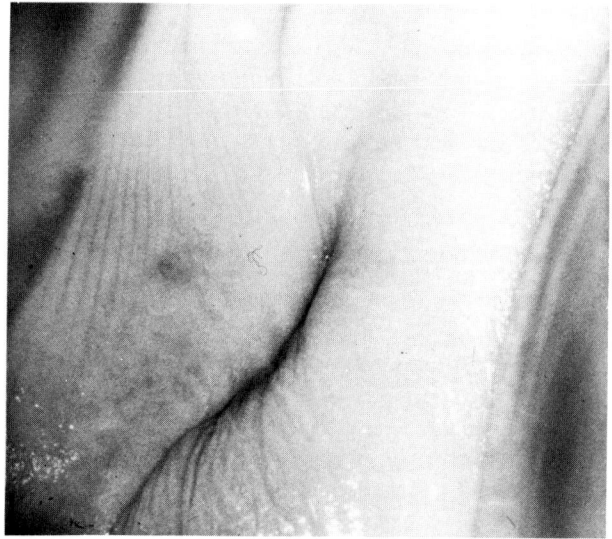

Fig. 72.7b Colpophotograph of same cervix as in Fig. 72.7a taken 18 months after electrocoagulation diathermy showing complete eradication of original lesion.

COMPLICATIONS

Early postoperative complications may be secondary infection and/or secondary hemorrhage, the two often being interrelated. In order to minimize these risks, specific printed instructions are issued to the patient, stressing the importance of avoiding coitus for at least 3 weeks, avoiding use of internal tampons for two cycles, and the nightly use of triple sulfa vaginal cream (Sultrin) for 12 to 14 days. After 3 weeks, cervical healing is well established. A course

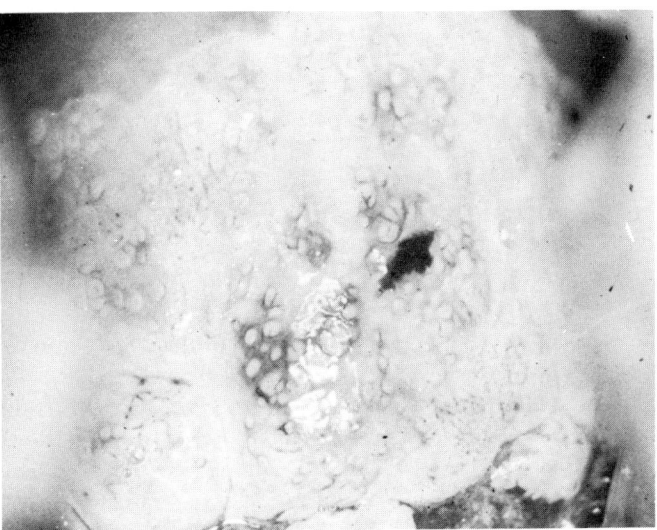

Fig. 72.8a Colpophotograph showing extensive area of abnormal transformation zone on the anterior lip of cervix (mosaic structure and punctation). Biopsy reported as carcinoma in situ.

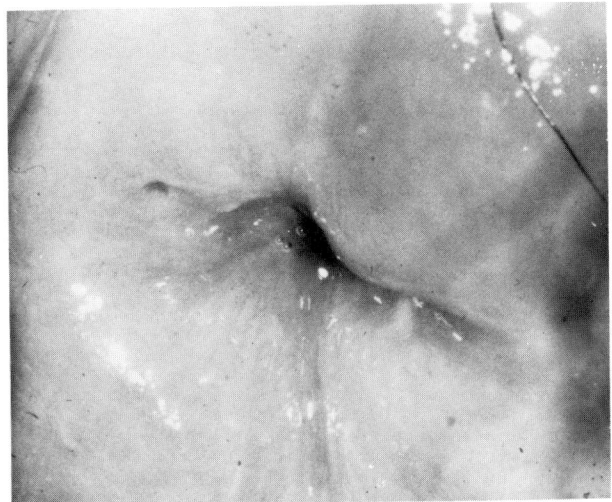

Fig. 72.8b Colpophotograph of same cervix as Fig. 72.8a taken 3 months after electrocoagulation diathermy showing complete eradication of carcinoma in situ.

of broad spectrum antibiotic is used at the first sign of, or in the event of a past history of, pelvic inflammatory disease. Because of less stringent aseptic conditions when performed as an office procedure, the tendency under such circumstances is to utilize routine prophylactic antibiotic cover. The postoperative instructions emphasize the likely occurrence of intermittent and sometimes annoying bleeding, and warn that it may persist for some weeks. Confusion can occur when this bleeding merges into a heavy menstrual period which may then be misconstrued as secondary hemorrhage. If the patient is using oral contraception, she should continue the regimen uninter-

rupted; otherwise, the increase in menstrual loss that occurs after ceasing oral contraception may be mistaken for secondary hemorrhage. On rare occasions, there may be severe secondary hemorrhage which requires hospitalization, necessitating the use of antibiotics, packing and, rarely, blood transfusion.

A later complication is cervical stenosis which may produce severe dysmenorrhea and prolongation of periods. Rarely, atresia or conglutination occur and produce amenorrhea. In view of the radical extent of the diathermy, this complication is surprisingly uncommon and readily rectified by dilatation of the cervix and insertion of an intra-uterine device for 6 to 12 weeks in order to keep the os open. Routine passage of a uterine sound or fine dilator at the first postoperative visit will diminish the risk of stenosis.

In our experience, long-term complications associated with subsequent pregnancy and labor are of little significance. There is no obvious impairment of fertility, but there may be some slight increase in incidence of cervical dystocia during labor due to slowness of dilatation if excess fibrosis has occurred. However, the incidence of subsequent cesarean section has been very low.[7]

The significant complication rate after electrocoagulation diathermy is approximately 2.0%.[8]

FOLLOW-UP

The first postoperative assessment is carried out 8 weeks after treatment. If the original lesion appears to have been eradicated at this visit, follow up examinations are performed at 6-month intervals for a period of 2 years, and yearly thereafter. Methods of detecting residual or recurrent disease are colposcopy, endocervical and ectocervical smears, and colposcopically directed biopsies of any suspicious tissue.

It is possible to achieve a 98% primary cure rate with the first treatment only.[8] Failures of primary eradication may be the result of inexperience of the operator, reticence with the use of electrodiathermy, technical reasons, such as inadequate current, or where the area involved is too extensive to be effectively treated on the one occasion. In many instances, eventual elimination of the residual disease can be achieved by re-diathermy. On occasions, the residual area of abnormality may even be small enough to be eliminated with a biopsy punch.

It is our belief that it is more important to eliminate cervical columnar epithelium from the vaginal environment than to be able to visualize colposcopically the squamocolumnar junction postoperatively. We have observed very few definitive recurrences of intraepithelial neoplasia in patients treated in this manner. In these instances, recurrence has been related either to persistent exposure of columnar epithelium to the vaginal environment due to inadequate diathermy, or to re-exposure of columnar epithelium by eversion in a subsequent pregnancy. The new squamocolumnar junction can still frequently be demonstrated, although well up the cervical canal, either by use of the endocervical speculum or by manipulation of the cervical lips with a swab stick. Difficulty with cytologic sampling due to a narrowed cervical canal can be overcome by use of the cytobrush.

SUMMARY

The described technique of electrocoagulation diathermy has successfully eradicated cervical intraepithelial neoplasia with *first treatment alone* in almost 98% of selected patients, with an overall very low incidence of cone biopsy and hysterectomy. Re-diathermy of any residual lesion has further enhanced the results. In recent years, even though more anatomically extensive lesions were tackled, results of effective eradication have been maintained.

To date, in a series of over 4000 patients treated in this fashion, there has been no known instance of invasive carcinoma of the cervix developing during the follow-up, in some cases the duration extending over 20 years. It is emphasized that in approximately 60% of those treated by electrocoagulation diathermy, the cervical lesion was histologically classified as major dysplasia or carcinoma in situ (CIN 3). The ectocervical extent of the lesion involved three or four segments in more than half of the group.[8]

Although other methods of physical destruction can be effective in destroying smaller areas of CIN, it is our belief that with one single treatment electrocoagulation diathermy

has the particular advantage of being able to eliminate extensive areas more effectively, especially where those changes are of major severity. This method destroys the abnormal tissue, ablating particularly the deeper gland crypts without any penalty of increased morbidity.

Capital expenditure and expensive maintenance of laser equipment is difficult to justify on a general basis outside highly specialized units, particularly when the results of eradication of extensive CIN 3 lesions by laser ablation or vaporization still fall short of those obtained with electrocoagulation diathermy. Furthermore, in developing countries in particular, or where finances are restricted, an electrosurgical unit will usually already be available from the operating theater suite or, at most, be relatively inexpensive to purchase and to maintain. In the past, the main criticism levelled against electrocoagulation diathermy has been the need for general anesthesia and hospitalization, albeit under day care facilities. This always had to be balanced against the security of a very high first time cure rate, particularly in a group of patients well known for their tendency to default from follow-up. More recently, with the advent of a technique of intracervical local anesthetic infiltration using a standard dental syringe, the feasibility of performing electrocoagulation diathermy either as an office procedure or on an ambulatory patient in a day care facility has been effectively demonstrated. The results obtained to date suggest the same low morbidity and high first treatment cure rate as previously achieved over a 20-year period of experience with general anesthesia.[2]

REFERENCES

1. Chanen W 1979 An endocervical speculum. Aust NZ J Obstet Gynaecol 19: 40
2. Chanen W 1989 The efficacy of electrocoagulation diathermy performed under local anaesthesia for the eradication of precancerous lesions of the cervix. Aust NZ J Obstet Gynaecol 29: 189
3. Chanen W, Hollyock V E 1971 Colposcopy and electrocoagulation diathermy for cervical dysplasia and carcinoma in situ. Obstet Gynecol 37: 623
4. Hollyock V E, Chanen W 1972 The use of the colposcope in the selection of patients for cervical cone biopsy. Am J Obstet Gynecol 114: 185
5. Chanen W, Hollyock V E 1974 Colposcopy and the conservative management of cervical dysplasia and carcinoma in situ. Obstet Gynecol 43: 527
6. Hollyock V E, Chanen W 1976 Electrocoagulation diathermy for the treatment of cervical dysplasia and carcinoma in situ. Obstet Gynecol 47: 196
7. Hollyock V E, Chanen W, Wein R 1983 Cervical function following treatment for intraepithelial neoplasia by electrocoagulation diathermy. Obstet Gynecol 61: 79
8. Chanen W, Rome R 1983 Electrocoagulation diathermy for cervical dysplasia and carcinoma in situ; a fifteen year survey. Obstet Gynecol 61: 673

73. Conization of cervix

W. Chanen

INTRODUCTION

Conization cannot be regarded as a minor surgical procedure. It has significant morbidity and may jeopardize future childbearing. The indications should be defined precisely, and the operation restricted to those patients in whom it is mandatory (see also Ch. 36).

CRITERIA FOR SELECTION OF PATIENTS

In general, the frequency of cone biopsy will be related to the experience, confidence and expertise of the colposcopist. Conization is always indicated when, colposcopically, the lesion is suspected of being true invasive disease but the target biopsy has not confirmed the diagnosis or has revealed suspected or 'minimal stromal' invasive disease.[2] The procedure is also obligatory if all of the endocervical portion of an apparent intraepithelial lesion cannot be exposed for colposcopic assessment, either by manipulation of the cervical lips or by the use of an endocervical speculum.[1] In some cases, more likely in the perimenopausal patient, the whole of the transformation zone may be located in the endocervical canal. Suspected adenocarcinomatous lesions based either on cytology report or target biopsy also require cone biopsy for their evaluation. It is now generally accepted that the Papanicolaou smear does not always faithfully reflect the underlying specific histologic pattern, and especially that the presence of an associated true invasive cervical lesion cannot be excluded by a 'negative' smear. The cone biopsy is therefore essential for accurate histologic evaluation of the concealed portion of the lesion, in particular to exclude associated invasive disease in that location.

When cone biopsy is indicated, one should aim for complete excision of the lesion so that the conization is therapeutic as well as diagnostic. On occasions, therefore, the cone may need to be quite extensive.

THE OPERATION

There are many opinions as to the best surgical method.

The technique described below attempts to deal with the following basic problems:

1. the extent, dimensions and shape of the cone specimen
2. the control of primary hemostasis
3. excision of the cone and avoidance of tissue trauma
4. the prevention of secondary infection and hemorrhage.

Extent, dimensions and shape of cone specimen

The size of the cone will be determined by the ectocervical extent of the lesion. In general terms, the broader the base of the lesion, the less extensive will be its spread into the cervical canal. Thus, if there is an appreciable ectocervical component, the shape of the cone will need to be broad and shallow in order to achieve total excision of the lesion. If the ectocervical involvement is small, and the major part of the lesion is located in the cervical canal, then a narrow and elongated cone specimen or narrow 'cylinder cone' will need to be fashioned.

Primary hemostasis

Intracervical injection of a hemostatic agent such as 30 ml of POR8® diluted 1 in 30, or neosynephrine diluted 1 in 10 000, provides excellent hemostatic control. Adrenaline is undesirable because of cardiovascular risks and incompatibility with certain anesthetic agents. The use of a large bore needle (16 to 18 gauge) and narrow bore syringe facilitates injection directly into the cervical stroma. The injected solution should evenly distend and blanch the cervix. A number of portals of entry are used, all outside the surface area to be examined histologically. The alleged risk of reactionary hemorrhage occurring after the effect of the hemostatic agent has worn off has not been a problem in our experience. The technique of securing descending branches of the uterine artery for hemostasis seems of dubious value, in view of the rich collateral blood supply of the cervix. It seems doubtful that complete obliteration of blood flow through these vessels can be achieved by such simple ligature.

Excision of cone and avoidance of tissue trauma

Preinvasive lesions of the cervix are notorious for the ease with which surface epithelium may be denuded. Hence, great care should be exercised to avoid epithelial damage in order to ensure accurate histologic evaluation. Routine vaginal preparation may be employed, providing the procedure is performed gently. It is important to ascertain the position of the uterus and cervix so that the incision outlining the margins of the cone is oriented in relation to the cervical canal, thereby avoiding the risk of perforating the neighboring tissues and pouch of Douglas. Dilatation and curettage must always be deferred until the cone specimen has been excised.

The exposed cervix is stained with Lugol's iodine solution demarcating the ectocervical portion to be excised. A length of either number 1 Dexon® or Vicryl® is inserted as a stay suture anteriorly and posteriorly, at the 6 and 12 o'clock positions, into the substance of the cervix just beyond this margin. These sutures will provide a means of traction to steady the cervix whilst making the initial circumscribed incision. A small, Bard-Parker size 15 scalpel blade is used to incise the cervix and outline the base of the cone. The incision is deepened sufficiently to allow the stromal surface of the base of the cone to pout. Two guy sutures of different colors of fine silk or linen are inserted with a fine cutting edge needle into the stromal surface, either at the 6 and 12 o'clock, or 3 and 9 o'clock positions. By tying these strands together, the sutures serve both as a tractor for the cone specimen, so that the surface to be examined histologically is not handled, and also to provide orientation for the pathologist. The incision is then deepened and extended, shaping the excised area into the desired proportions of the cone. This procedure is often facilitated by completing the anterior dissection first, identifying and exposing the cervical canal. After completing the excision of the cone posteriorly, the anterior lip of the cervix is secured by a tenaculum and the canal is dilated to facilitate curettage and reconstruction of the cervix. In addition to endometrial curettage, the remaining portion of the cervical canal is carefully curetted with a sharp curette and the tissue is examined separately from endometrium. This latter procedure provides additional information as to whether the excision of abnormal tissue has been complete. Diathermy cutting devices should not be used to excise the cone specimen, because of the risk of denudation and damage to the surface epithelium, and resultant coagulation destruction of tissue; all of those will interfere with the ability of the histologist to evaluate the specimen accurately.

Prevention of secondary infection and hemorrhage

In wide based cone specimens, healing by primary intention is the best prophylaxis. Sturmdorf-type sutures are employed to invert both anterior and posterior folds of epithelium as illustrated in Figure 73.1. In contrast to chromic catgut, the use of either Dexon® or Vicryl® sutures causes very little local reaction. These suture materials have proven a very satisfactory alternative to previously recommended monofilament nylon which, although producing minimal tissue reaction, has the disadvantage of requiring subsequent removal. Such suture materials decrease the risk of secondary infection. The suture, on a large trochar pointed needle, picks up the edge of epithelium with a transverse bite in the midline. Each strand in turn is directed well up into the cervical canal, both strands emerging through the ectocervical surface about 0.5 cm apart and approximately 2 cm from the newly constructed external os. The epithelial flaps will thus be drawn forward and cover the raw surface when the suture is firmly secured. A 'double throw' on the first throw of the tie ensures that the suture will not slip. A supplementary suture at each lateral angle will obliterate dead space and oppose epithelial margins. The patient may be discharged within 24 hours of operation providing there are no complications. Intercourse is not advised for 3 weeks. A broad spectrum antibiotic is used for 5 days.

'Open' cone method

The 'open' cone method, which involves no suturing and which leaves the raw area to granulate following hemostasis by diathermy of bleeding points and/or packing with gauze, is favored by some authors. Our experience suggests that the method is likely to be associated with a higher complication rate. Because of the greater risk of infection, secondary hemorrhage is more likely. As a result of an increased tendency of the opposing raw surfaces to adhere, the rate of cervical stenosis is likely to be greater. However, the open cone technique does have a role where the cervix is small and conical, as in many nulliparous or perimenopausal women, where only a small cone or cylindrical excision is technically feasible. Under these circumstances, the preoperative intracervical infiltration with hemostatic agent, as previously described, usually provides adequate hemostasis without the necessity for diathermy or to pack the area with gauze.

COMPLICATIONS

The list of complications is formidable. The most serious intraoperative risks are excessive bleeding, damage to adjacent organs, and inadvertent opening of the pouch of Douglas. Preoperative intracervical injection of a hemostatic agent, care in assessing the direction of the cervical

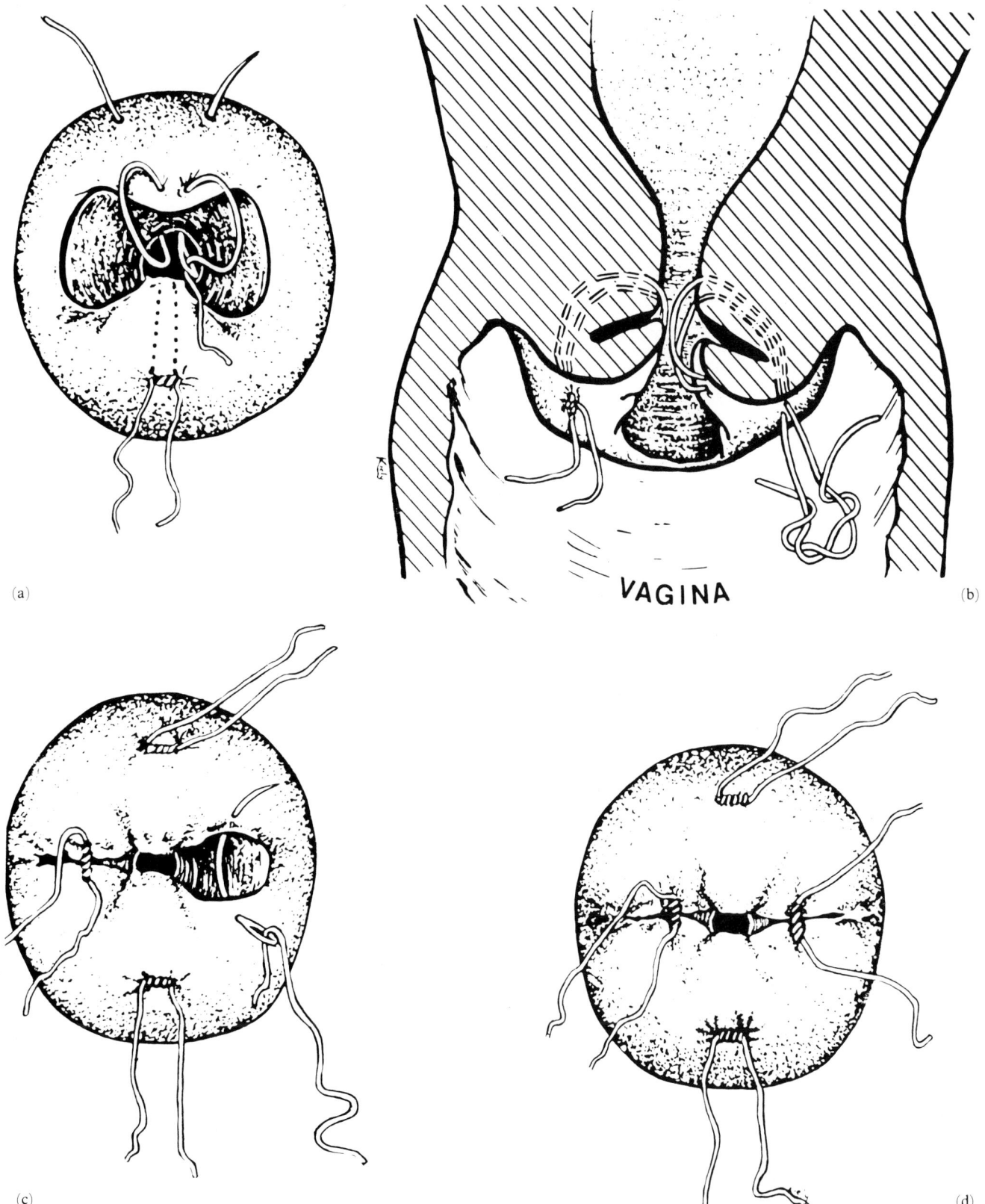

(a)

(b)

(c)

(d)

Fig. 73.1 Diagrammatic representation in which:
(a) Sturmdorf suture has inverted the posterior lip and been tied. Anterior lip suture is in the process of insertion.
(b) Side view of cervix showing the means whereby the cervical flaps are apposed and dead space obliterated. Anterior suture is being tied.
(c) and (d) Insertion of lateral sutures obliterating dead space and apposing epithelium. Monofilament nylon sutures are left long to facilitate removal.

canal prior to the incision and the use of a smaller scalpel blade, diminish these risks. Later complications are cervical stenosis and cervical incompetence. Accurate cervical reconstruction with accompanying hemostasis guards against stenosis. The risk of cervical incompetence is high, and probably proportional to the length of canal excised. Excision to the level of the internal os must predispose to a greater risk. Despite the most stringent precautions, cone biopsy still carries a significant complication rate. It would appear that the overall incidence of complications is in part related to the size of the cone excised. This factor, together with differences in actual technique, must account for the wide variations in incidence of complications in reported series. (See also Ch. 36.)

FOLLOW-UP

Follow-up is of paramount importance to detect the presence of residual or recurrent disease. Histologic appraisal as to whether cone biopsy has successfully excised the limits of atypical tissue is not always reliable. This may be due either to technical errors of histologic assessment, or to the fact that remaining adjacent areas of atypicality may be shed in the healing process. The practice of curetting the remaining portion of the endocervical canal after the excision of the cone specimen, and subsequent histologic assessment of these curettings, provides a further check on the 'completeness' of the cone biopsy. Cytology, colposcopy and target biopsy when indicated are the methods employed to ascertain the presence of residual or recurrent disease. At the 2-month postoperative visit, if the lesion appears to have been eradicated, the patient is then seen at 6-month intervals for 2 years, and yearly thereafter. Assessment of the ectocervix by the colposcope is no problem, but endocervical assessment may be made more difficult because of postoperative narrowing of the cervical os. However, the use of both an endocervical speculum for colposcopic inspection and a cytobrush for cytologic sampling will generally detect residual or recurrent disease of the endocervix.

SUMMARY

More extensive use of the endocervical speculum has considerably reduced the frequency of conization. Currently, in our hands, less than one in 10 of all patients with histologically proven intraepithelial cervical disease requires cone biopsy. Our indication for conization continues to be the need for histologic exclusion of invasive disease in the concealed portion of the cervical lesion, or when invasion is colposcopically suspected; but it is never performed on account of purported severity of cervical intraepithelial neoplasia (CIN). Where invasive carcinoma had been excluded, follow-up study indicates that conization successfully eradicated CIN in over 90% of cases in our series. Since most of our patients subjected to cone biopsy were over 35 years of age and had completed their family, persistence of CIN after conization usually resulted in subsequent hysterectomy. Repeat cone biopsy was very rarely indicated.

REFERENCES

1. Chanen W 1979 An endocervical speculum. Aust NZ J Obstet Gynaecol 19: 40

2. Hollyock V E, Chanen W 1972 The use of the colposcope in the selection of patients for cervical cone biopsy. Am J Obstet Gynecol 114: 185

74. Abdominal incisions and sutures in gynecologic oncological surgery

P. Scheidel   M. K. Hohl

GENERAL CONSIDERATIONS

Many gynecologists feel that a transverse incision, predominantly the Pfannenstiel incision, is perfectly adequate for all kinds of gynecological surgery. However, cosmetic and functional aspects are poor excuses for inadequate exposure of suspected malignancies. With improved diagnostic imaging techniques and tumor markers there is no excuse today for faulty incisions. In the Department of Obstetrics and Gynecology in Munich, we have treated 168 patients with ovarian cancer from 1984 to 1986 (Table 74.1). 98 patients were operated on primarily in our department and 70 have been referred after initial surgery in another hos-

Table 74.1 Type of abdominal incision in 168 patients with carcinoma of the ovary (Jan. 1984 to Dec. 1986)*

Primary surgery	University patients	Referral patients	Total
Vertical incision	94 (96%)	43 (62%)	137 (82%)
Transverse incision	4 (4%)	27 (38%)	31 (18%)
	98	70	168

* Department of Obstetrics and Gynecology, Klinikum Großhadern, Munich (FRG).
Mean age x = 56.3 years (min. 9 years, max. 85 years)

Table 74.2 Correlation of radical treatment to initial surgery (Jan. 1984–Dec. 1986)*

Tumor debulking	University patients	Referral patients
Incomplete (> 2 cm residual tumor)	49 (50%)	54 (77%)
Complete (< 2 cm residual tumor)	49 (50%) 98	16 (23%) 70
Additional surgery		
Bowel resection	9 (9%)	2 (3%)
Colostomy	10 (10%)	3 (4%)
Bladder/ureter resection	4 (4%)	1 (1%)
Lymph node dissection	13 (13%)	3 (4%)

* Department of Obstetrics and Gynecology, Klinikum Großhadern, Munich

pital. The incidence of transverse incisions in the referred patients was 39%. The type of incision correlates excellently with the radicality of cancer surgery (Table 74.2).

OPENING THE ABDOMEN

The ideal abdominal incision should fulfill the following requirements:

1. Sufficient exposure of the operative field
2. Simplicity and speed
3. Ease of extension
4. Low incidence of wound healing complications (wound disruption, infection, sinus formation, incisional hernia)

No incision can satisfy all of the above criteria; perhaps that is why so many exist. There are several techniques which are equal, at least as far as the more important requirements are concerned. Our present knowledge about wound healing, suture technique and materials should allow us, however, to make a choice based more on facts than on impressions.

Most often, the gynecological surgeon will select a lower midline (with the advantages of: simplicity, good access and flexibility) or transverse incision (the advantages being good wound healing and cosmetics). If we consider wound healing, we are most concerned to avoid serious complications, e.g. eviscerations and incisional hernia. There are no prospective clinical trials which compare the incidence of these complications in gynecological patients after lower vertical or transverse abdominal incisions. Retrospective data can be summarized as follows:

1. The overall reported incidence of evisceration is lower in patients undergoing gynecological, compared with general surgical, operations.
2. In gynecology, eviscerations and incisional hernias are observed almost without exception after vertical incisions, although recent studies in upper abdominal surgery question this.[90] The earlier studies may have

1157

been biased, because vertical incisions, which can be performed faster, might have been used more often in more seriously ill patients. It is possible, therefore, that healing is related more to the type of suture and surgical technique than to the type of incision.[49]

3. Several series including thousands of patients report a very low incidence of burst abdomen after transverse incisions independent of suture techniques and material.[69,44,47]

The anatomy of the abdominal wall offers an explanation which is independent of all other factors known to influence the incidence of severe wound healing complications (patient, technique, materials). In the lower abdominal wall, all muscles or aponeuroses (except for the rectus muscle) run more or less in a transverse direction. Thus, there is always tension on vertical incisions. This is much less in transverse incisions because the direction of muscle fibers does not deviate more than 30° from the horizontal. Thus, tension will rather appose the wound edges. The rectus muscles, on the other hand, exert only a little transverse tension through their tendinous intersections. With the advent of better suture materials and improved suture techniques, these mechanical factors have become less important. Today, the primary consideration in selecting an incision should always be adequate exposure for the planned operation. If there is any uncertainty about the type or extent of surgery to be done, one should choose a low midline, vertical incision because of the ease with which it can be extended.

Location and direction

Where the abdominal incision should lie and in which direction it may be extended has been the subject of long debates. In principle, vertical (midline), paramedian and transverse incisions (interiliacal) are used for gynecological oncology (Fig. 74.1). If lower abdominal incisions have to be extended into the upper abdomen, transverse incisions should be avoided. A 'hockey-stick' incision provides good access to the left or right upper abdomen. Obviously, care should be taken not to circle the umbilicus at the side of a planned stoma (e.g. colostomy). Poole[77] found that vertical midline wounds are more likely to rupture in the upper third than in the middle or lower third. This difference is thought to be due to the relative fixation of the upper abdominal musculo-aponeurotic layers to the narrow angle between the ribs, which limits wound elongation and consequently causes greater tension at the fascia-suture interface.

Vertical incisions

Besides their ease of extension, vertical incisions have the advantage of speed of entry. The midline incision, called

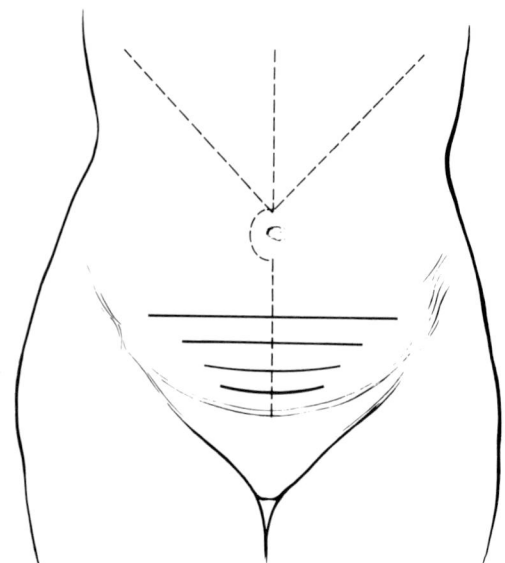

Fig. 74.1 Location of abdominal incisions in gynecological surgery.

the 'maid for all purposes' in abdominal surgery[25] has a definite place in gynecology. In emergency operations where time is critical, for example in hemorrhagic shock, this is the incision of choice. It is mandatory in malignant ovarian neoplasia or when a transperitoneal para-aortic lymphadenectomy is planned. As far as wound healing complications are concerned, a conventional paramedian incision does not seem to offer any advantages.[8,25]

Recently, an important and interesting modification, the lateral paramedian incision has been described.[35] The advantage is that a very wide shutter mechanism is provided by the rectus muscle, resulting in a diminished risk of burst abdomen and incisional hernia. However, access is more restricted, it is not easy to perform and takes longer to carry out and close. Therefore its application seems to be limited in gynecological surgery.

Transverse incisions

Low transverse incisions in the lower abdomen have a reduced incidence of wound breakdown. Another advantage is that these incisions leave an almost invisible scar which in some instances is even hidden by the pubic hair. They should only be used when the surgeon is certain that only pelvic surgery is necessary.

There are several modifications of the widely used Pfannenstiel incision. For radical pelvic surgery we prefer a transverse (interiliacal) muscle-splitting incision.[64] Here, in contrast to the Pfannenstiel incision, all layers are cut transversely (Fig. 74.2). Excellent exposure of the lateral pelvic wall is gained. In obese patients, access is definitely better than in a vertical incision where the cut must curve its way through the panniculus. A further advantage is that it can be closed 'en masse'.

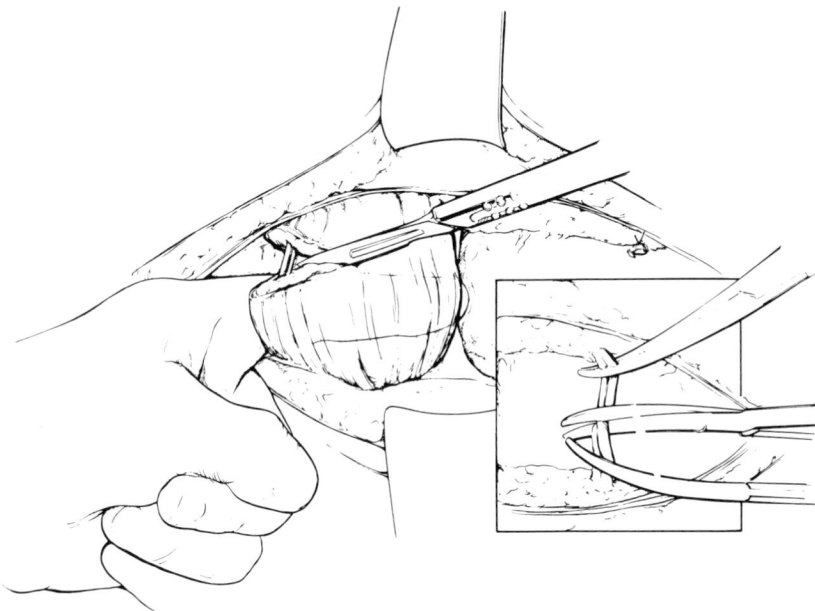

Fig. 74.2 Transverse (interiliacal) incision, cutting all layers transversely (clamping of the superior epigastric vessels).

Access can be greatly improved in extremely obese patients when a wedge resection of the panniculus is performed at the same time.[79] Excellent exposure of the fascial layers allows them to be cut either transversely or vertically. In this situation, a vertical incision can even be extended above the umbilicus. At the same time, any rectus muscle diastasis can be surgically repaired.

CHOICE OF SUTURES

Tradition and personal experience can no longer be accepted as arguments for the use of catgut or chromic catgut in gynecology, because modern synthetic absorbable sutures have changed the situation dramatically.

Absorbable sutures

Catgut is a natural material with many problems involved in its processing. The standards of catgut vary widely. If a surgeon asks for 2-0 catgut he may receive an 0 or a 3-0 suture, which differ in tensile strength between 4 kg (3-0) and 11 kg (0). It is unfair to ask the manufacturers for greater accuracy in this respect, because this is an unavoidable problem caused by variations in the quality of the basic material and the difficulties of the production process. Many people believe that catgut is constantly and rapidly integrated in the body. Both beliefs are untrue. The loss of tensile strength after implantation is not predictable, and sutures of the same diameter (2-0) may have 30% of their initial strength after 28 days, whereas others are down to zero after 21 days. Postlethwait et al[78] could demonstrate that catgut in a post mortem investigation was more or less

unchanged 8 and even 11 years after implantation. It has been known for a long time that catgut may cause toxic and allergic reactions through the by-products of collagen degradation.[3,53] The strongest argument against the use of catgut, and especially chromic catgut, is the fact that this material causes and sustains infection, thus providing a negative effect on wound healing. Additionally, in infected wounds there is a decrease in the pH. Under these circumstances, catgut loses more than 50% of its initial tensile strength in half of the usual time.[67] Because of this, it is clear that there is a strong association between the incidence of postoperative infections, wound dehiscence and hernias, and the use of catgut sutures. The inclusion of glycerine in the processing of chromic catgut did facilitate the knotting,[90] but the detrimental effects of chromic catgut have not been altered.

Polyglycolic acid and polyglactin 910 are now clear alternatives. Both materials are hydrolysed and do not require enzymatic degradation, thus causing less tissue reaction.[12,78] When compared to catgut resorption, the loss of tensile strength and histological reactions are not as erratic, and the initial tensile strength is also superior (Fig. 74.3). A comparison of tensile strength, knot breaking strength and knot holding capacity also reveals the superiority of synthetic absorbable sutures.[60] There are some differences in coated and uncoated material with respect to knot holding capacity, but because of the more comfortable handling, coated sutures are commonly used.

In this respect one has to be aware of the fact that the coating of polyglycolic acid (third generation Dexon) is partly removed when gliding through tissue, whereas the coating of polyglactin 910 (Vicryl) remains on the suture.

The differences can be seen in clinical handling, and selection has to be made on personal preferences and knowledge of this fact.

A very important factor is the influence of the suture material on infected tissue. In bacterial[21] as well as in viral infections,[6] synthetic absorbable sutures are not likely to potentiate infection in a contaminated wound, and may even partially inhibit bacterial multiplication. In contrast to catgut, the tensile-strength loss patterns are not altered by infection, i.e. pH changes.

For clinical use, it is especially important that the diameter of the suture is chosen correctly; by this means the amount of suture material implanted can be reduced dramatically. Therefore, the negative effect on wound healing can be reduced qualitatively as well as quantitatively.

The advantages and disadvantages of catgut and synthetic absorbable suture materials are summarized in Tables 74.3 and 74.4. It should be mentioned that monofilament synthetic absorbable sutures are used more frequently. Polydioxanon (PDS) represents a new substance for suture materials, and retains its strength for twice as long as comparable sutures (see Fig. 74.3). In vivo comparison of monofilament absorbable sutures (PDS and Maxon) demonstrated that absorbable sutures are initially equal or superior to non-absorbables in terms of tensile

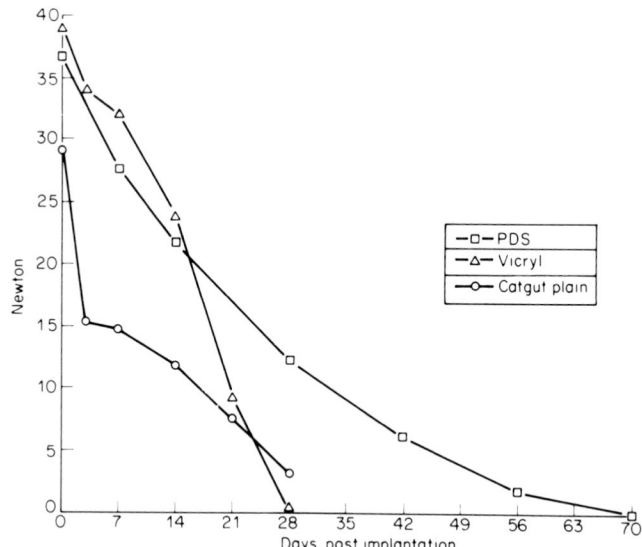

Fig. 74.3 Comparison of tensile strength after implantation of catgut (size 3-0), polyglactin (Vicryl) and PDS (Polydioxanon) from Ethicon Research Laboratory.

strength, but are absorbed at variable rates by the action of hydrolysis.[5] When wound healing cannot take place within 2 weeks (e.g. fascia), non-absorbable or monofilament absorbable sutures should be chosen.

Sufficient suture tensile strength with PDS can be expected to last about 5 to 6 weeks more than other absorbable suture material. Knot security and tensile strength of the knot have to be considered carefully. PDS is not the suture material requiring the fewest throws to achieve security. Five or six throws are recommended by experimental surgeons. Slippery gloves in the operating room may result in knots of less than optimal security.[61]

PDS is a monofilament suture with sufficient flexibility and is absorbed completely after 6 months. It retains its breaking strength long enough for fascial closure (58% at 4 weeks) and foreign-body reactions are minimal (Fig. 74.4).

Table 74.3 Properties, advantages and disadvantages of catgut (reabsorbable)

Ground substance	Serosa (cattle) Submucosa (sheep)
Production form	Twisted, ground, conditioned, plain, iodized, chromized
Advantages	Short time resorption High flexibility Hardly traumatic to tissue Good knotting characteristics
Disadvantages	Considerable but not permanent tissue reaction Allergic reactions with repeated use Varying tensile strength Moderate knotting security due to swelling

Table 74.4 Properties, advantages and disadvantages of polyglycolic acid and polyglactin (absorbable)

Ground substance	Fully synthetic polyglycolic acid Fully synthetic polyglycolic acid 90% and lactic acid 10%
Production form	Monofilament, woven, coated
Advantages	Good flexibility No bacterial transport between filaments due to anti-bacterial action of the ground substance. Initial low risk of ligature breakage Initial high tensile strength Linear reduction in tensile strength Minimal tissue reaction, fibrous tissue reaction can be ignored
Disadvantages	If uncoated, relatively high tissue drag Special knot-tying technique required

Non-absorbable sutures

Very few non-absorbable sutures are used in gynecological surgery (Table 74.5). The most important ones are those used for skin closure, preferably polypropylene with atraumatic needles. To prevent scarring, the smallest diameter which allows skin closure should be used (usually 3-0 or 4-0). If intradermal sutures are preferred, 2-0 sutures can be used to avoid rupture when taking out the running suture. Polypropylene is the suture of choice for skin closure because of its mild tissue reaction and tensile strength. It is also monofilament and thus inhibits capillarity and possible bacterial transport. Because of their capillarity, silk and other sutures should not be used in skin closures. Monofilament nylon is an alternative, especially in the closure of the abdomen when mass closure of the abdominal incision is attempted.[100] Polypropylene and nylon have also been used in microsurgery with little tissue reaction.[19] Finally, sutures made from polyester should be mentioned. They are available as mono- and polyfilament sutures. The pseudomonofilament suture (polyfilament with coating) provides reduced capillarity and high tensile strength. These sutures are ideal when tensile strength is required to be longstanding, e.g. it can be used in colposuspension in combination with a special

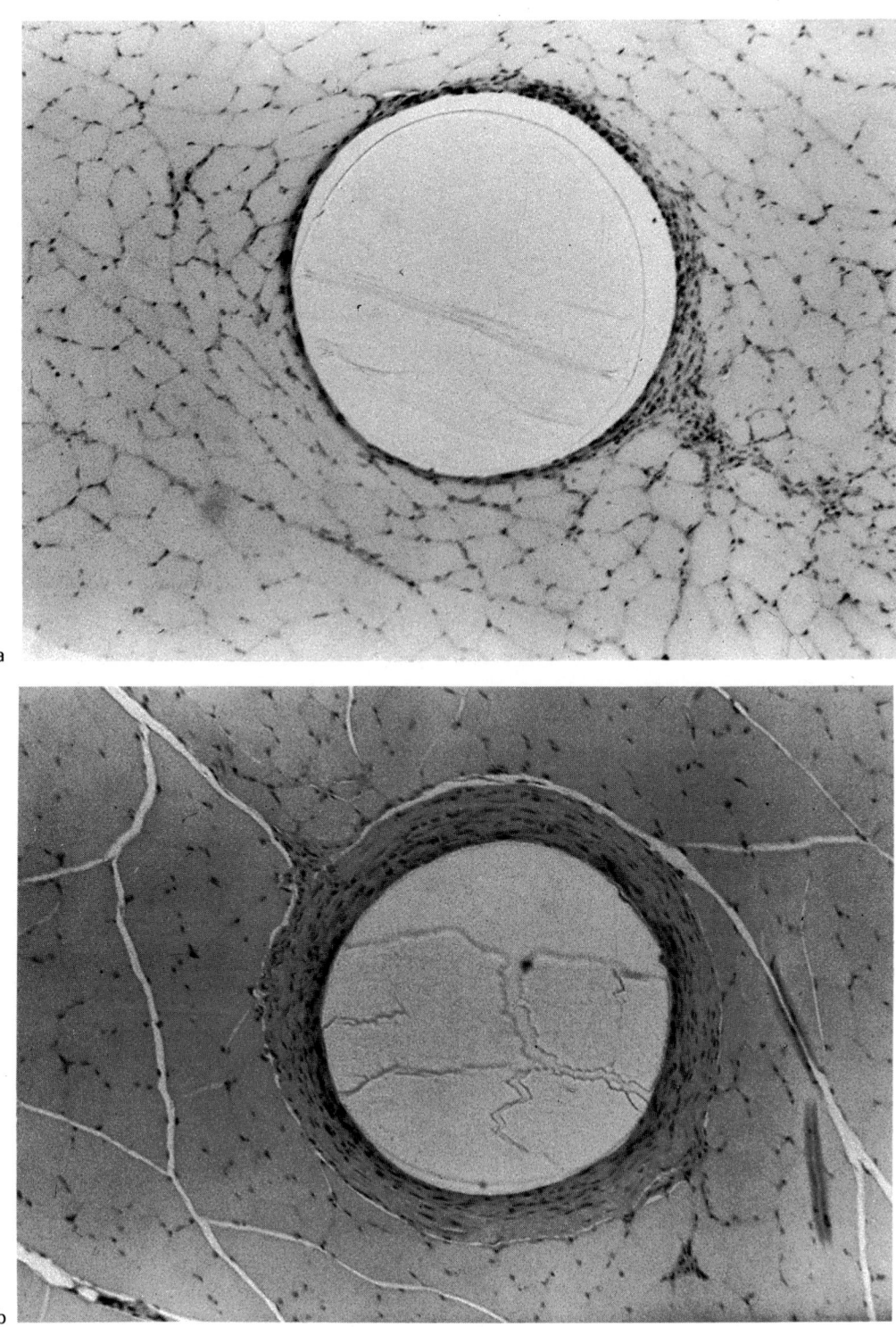

a

b

Fig. 74.4   (caption overleaf)

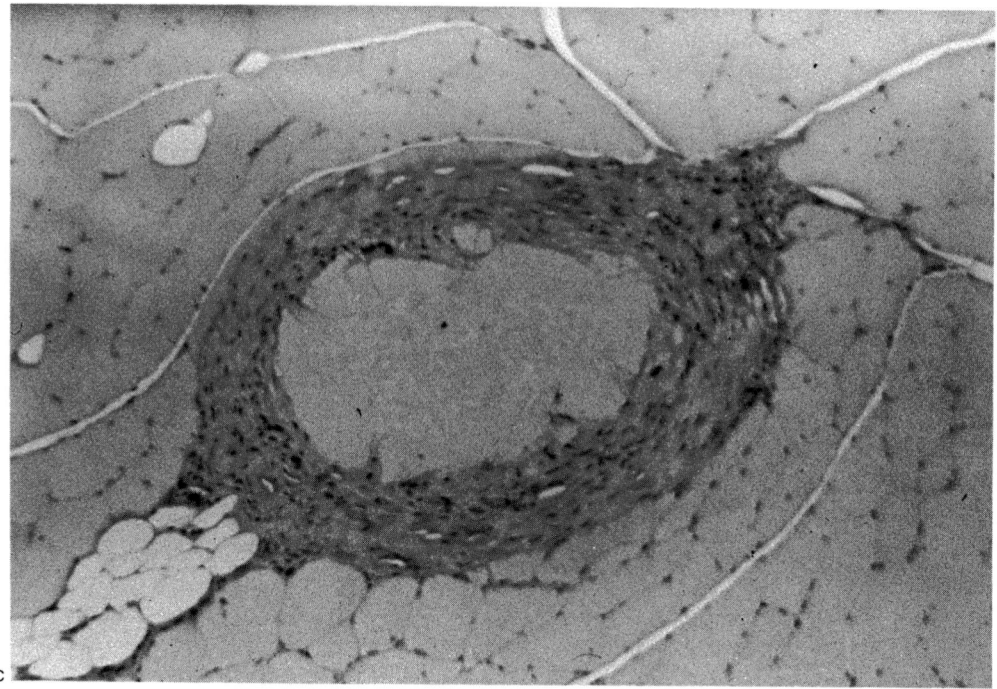

Fig. 74.4 (a) Polydioxanon (PDS) 14 days after implantation (×24). (b) Polydioxanon (PDS) 63 days after implantation (×24). (c) Polydioxanon (PDS) 168 days after implantation (×24).

Table 74.5 Properties, advantages and disadvantages of polyamide sutures, polypropylene sutures and polyethylene sutures (permanent)

Ground substance	Fully synthetic polyamide (nylon) Fully synthetic polyolefine: polypropylene and polyethylene
Production form	Monofilament pseudomonofilament (polyamide)
Advantages	No capillarity No bacterial carriage between filaments Low coefficient of friction (glides well) Minimal but permanent tissue reaction
Disadvantages	Low flexibility in the higher strength (monofilament) Moderate knotting ability Danger of knot breakage Possibility of surface damage in pseudomonofilament sutures

5/8 circular needle with a sharp tip.[83] These sutures, however, cause more tissue reaction, and foreign body granulomas can be observed.[95]

Few experimental data are available on the clinical use of different suture materials in gynecological surgery. Most reports are more or less personal experiences and opinions. It appears that clinical trials are almost impossible because of the multiple factors involved in the outcome of surgery. Personal series will never provide numbers sufficient for statistical evaluation. Therefore we have to rely on experimental data, published mostly by microsurgeons. These have been summarized recently.[82] In general, one should keep in mind that functional sequelae of the various sutures are difficult to determine. Bad surgery is not improved by good suture material; good surgery with inadequate suture material can, however, be optimized.

Needle choice

More attention should be given to the selection of atraumatic needles. In gynecology, often needles with only two or three different diameters or features are used. There is a wide variety of needles on the market in addition to the normal semicircular needle with various tips, rounded or sharp. The selection of the appropriate needle is of considerable importance in making the life of the gynecological surgeon easier.

WOUND DRAINAGE

The history of drains is as old as surgery, but their postoperative use, indications and efficacy remain controversial. The reader is referred to several excellent reviews of the history, current use and perspectives of drains.[16,68,87]

Therapeutic drainage in the presence of serous or purulent material is less controversial than its prophylactic use. Halsted's dictum in 1898 that 'No drainage at all is better than the ignorant employment of it'[68] holds true today.

The facts on which the decision to drain *prophylactically* should be based are discussed below.

Type of drain

There is no place today for prophylactic passive 'open'

drains like the traditional Penrose drains. These not only serve as a portal of entry for bacteria, but often drain inefficiently because they are mostly not dependent and working against gravity in their attempt to remove fluid. It comes as no surprise, therefore, that their use in upper abdominal surgery was associated with increased intraperitoneal and wound sepsis.[14,68] Erosion into the bladder and intestine, producing fistulas, has also been seen.[68] Open passive drains in the subcutaneous spaces have promoted wound sepsis instead of preventing it.[39]

Closed active (suction) drains have become almost synonymous with wound drainage in current surgical practice.[40] Modern, non-reactive, soft silicone drains (e.g. Jackson-Pratt silicone drains) are flexible enough to allow free patient movements, and soft enough not to erode blood vessels or intestinal organs, while maintaining the internal lumen thus reducing the incidence of catheter occlusion.

Indications for drainage

When large skin flaps are developed, as in radical vulvectomy or mastectomy, and after a wedge resection of the panniculus in obese patients, closed wound suction eliminates dead spaces. Thus, tension on the wound edges through fluid accumulation is prevented and better approximation of skin flaps and grafts is facilitated. Reduced hematoma formation, necrosis of wound edges, and wound infections have been reported after its use.[68]

Prophylactic closed suction drainage of the vaginal vault has reduced febrile morbidity after vaginal or abdominal hysterectomy.[88]

After radical surgical procedures with lymphadenectomy, fluid volumes of over 200 ml per 24 hours can accumulate.[70] Suction drainage has been said to decrease the risk of febrile morbidity, fistula and lymphocyst formation.[70,89] There is no doubt that suction drainage effectively drains the retroperitoneal dead space when the peritoneum is closed. Less attention has been given to the large capacity of peritoneal surfaces to reabsorb fluid containing electrolytes and proteins. When pelvic peritonization with suction drainage after radical pelvic surgery (66 patients) was compared with non-peritonization combined with omentoplasty (20 patients), lymphocele developed in 23% of the former compared with none in the latter group.[101] One of us (MKH) has used non-peritonization without omentoplasty successfully in a consecutive series of 24 patients undergoing radical pelvic surgery.

CLOSING THE ABDOMEN

The major goal of laparotomy closure is to minimize wound-healing complications. One must understand that usually not one but several factors together will ultimately lead to severe wound failure (evisceration, incisional hernia). Besides the patients' primary and associated disease, nutritional status, age, bodyweight, sex and use of corticosteroids, the type of incision and closure technique as well as the choice of suture materials are all contributory factors.[1,7,23,37,48] The patient at risk (Table 74.6) requires special attention. Antibiotic prophylaxis in high-risk patients has been shown to be very effective in patients undergoing intestinal, and also some types of gynecological, operations.[75] Measures to prevent postoperative pneumonia and abdominal distension are also important. The lower incidence of risk factors in gynecological, compared to general surgical, patients partly explains why severe wound-healing complications are observed less frequently in the former.

Table 74.6 Risk factors for the occurrence of evisceration and incisional hernia

General factors	Local factors
Advanced age	Wound infection
Male sex	Factors compromising fascial closure
Anemia	(stomas and drains through
Hypoproteinemia	wounds)
Malnutrition	
Obesity	
Malignant disease	
Intestinal surgery	
Pneumonia	
Distension	
Jaundice	
Azotemia	
Treatment with steroids	

Peritoneal and musculofascial layers

Does the peritoneum need to be sutured? According to a prospective randomized study by Ellis & Heddle[27] there is no difference in wound-healing failures whether the peritoneal layer is sutured or not. Neither was there a difference in adhesion formation to the abdominal wall in experimental animals.[27,46]

The integrity of the abdominal wound depends almost entirely on the strength of the musculofascial layers. Earlier, it was believed that technical factors played a minor role in the pathogenesis of wound disruption;[1,23,37] today, we know that suture materials and technique are of central importance.

There are many ways to close a laparotomy wound. Valuable information about the contribution of suture technique and materials can therefore be obtained only through carefully planned prospective randomized clinical trials. If we consider the abundance of different materials and techniques available, it is no surprise that in no two trials are all variables the same. However, some definite statements based on hard data can be made:

1. Four properly controlled studies have proven beyond any doubt that catgut is associated with an unacceptably high risk of evisceration and incisional hernia, independent of suture technique.[32,50,59,93] This material

should therefore no longer be used to close musculo-fascial layers.

2. Mathematical calculations and experimental data have shown that mass closure to include all layers apart from skin increases extrinsic wound strength provided that wide bites of tissue on either side of the incision line are incorporated.[20,43] Because abdominal circumference increases up to 30% postoperatively,[43] the sutures should not be tied too tightly and stitches should lie about 1 to 1.5 cm apart. This results in a total suture length measuring about four times the length of the incision.

3. Clinical use of mass closure of the abdominal wall using non-absorbable materials, such as nylon or wire, used either in a continuous fashion[8,50,52,63,76,84] or as interrupted sutures (Smead-Jones sutures)[4,42,58,99] has led to a low complication rate (eviscerations in 0 to 1% of cases). These results were achieved at the expense of a higher risk of sinus formation and postoperative wound pain, which was reported in almost all trials using these materials.

4. According to experimental results, non-absorbable braided materials (silk, multi-filament nylon) should not be used since these sutures provide a continuing nidus for infection within their fibrin meshes.[10]

5. Suture-related wound pain is almost completely eliminated, and sinus formation rarely occurs with synthetic absorbable sutures (polyglycolic acid, polyglactin 910). Whether they are as safe as non-absorbable sutures remains somewhat controversial. In three trials, the incidence of incisional hernias was significantly higher with polyglycolic acid compared to nylon sutures.[2,7,45] In seven others, however, no significant difference was found.[11,13,41,51,54,58,96] Polyglycolic acid sutures lose 90% of their strength within 3 weeks,[10] whereas 120 days are required for the fascial layer to regain its initial strength.[18]

6. Among absorbale sutures, Polydioxanon (PDS) is now the center of interest. The value of PDS, which retains its strength longer (40% at 6 weeks), has been shown in prospective clinical trials involving large numbers of patients.[55,94] There was no difference in the incidence of evisceration or defective wounds one year after operation, when compared with non-absorbable material. However, in 1.7% of patients the non-absorbable sutures had to be removed due to persistent pain or sinus formation.

In our hands the following approach has proven to be satisfactory in gynecological patients:

1. In low-risk patients, a vertical abdominal incision is closed using a double absorbable Polydioxanon (PDS) suture strength 1, applied as a continuous over-and-over mass closure suture (Fig. 74.5).

2. In high-risk patients where a complicated postoperative course is expected, non-absorbable nylon is used. An

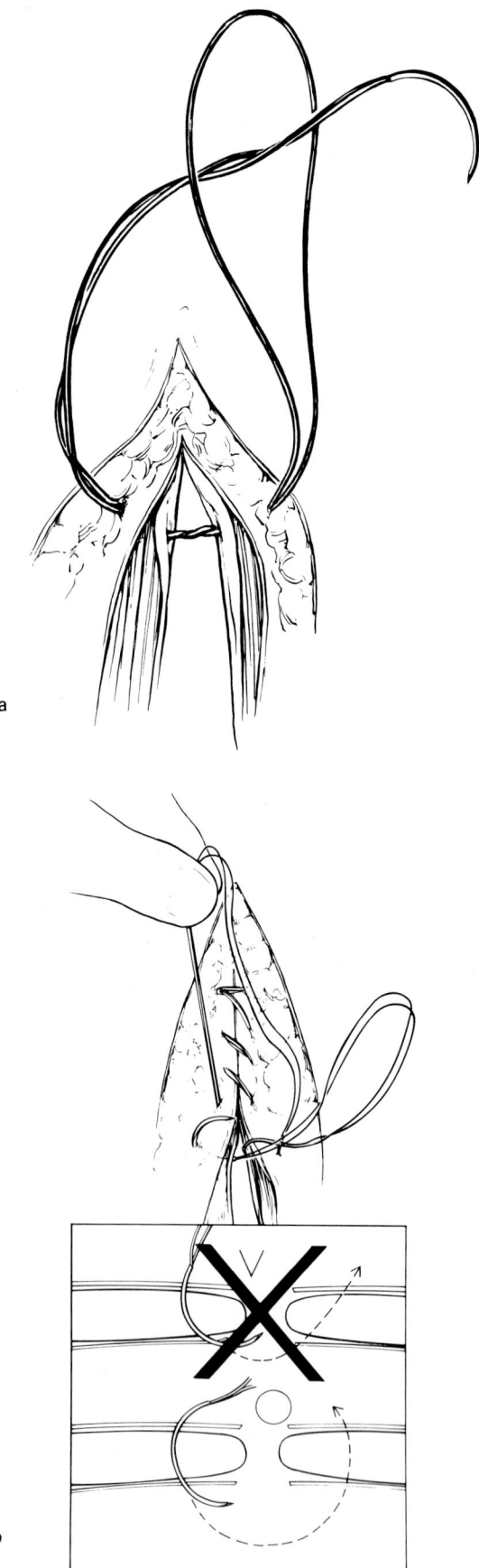

a

b

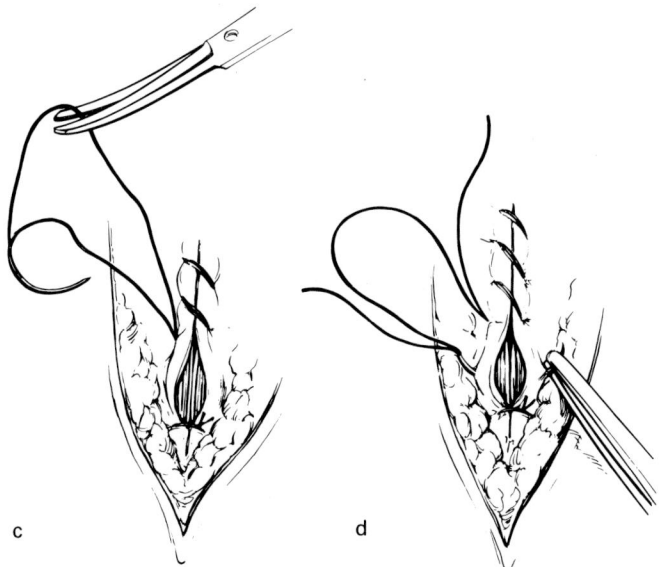

c   d

Fig.74.5 (a) Abdominal wound closure by a loop suture. The needle passes through all layers of the abdominal wall (1 to 2 cm of fascia) and through the loop (according to W. G. Everett). (b) The wound edges are *loosely* approximated with continuous suture taking large bites of tissue. (c) At the end of the wound, the needle is passed through the wound edges and the loop is cut and held. (d) The needle is then passed backwards through the wound edges. This leaves two suture strands. The final knot should be tied with a double reef knot.

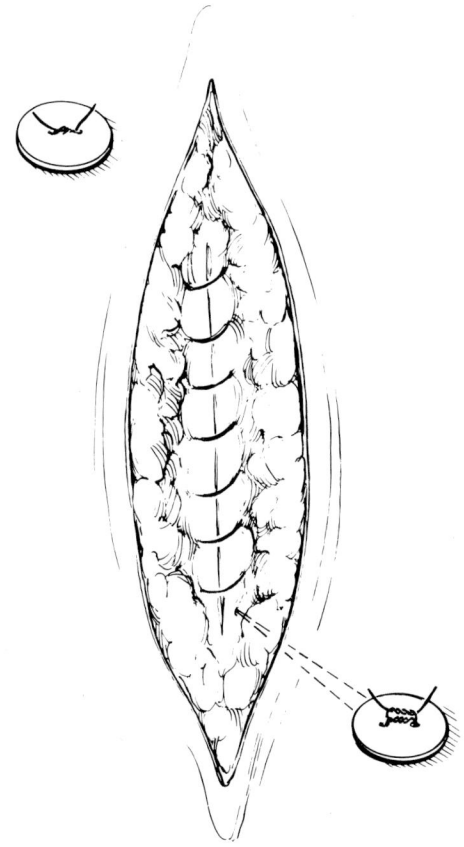

Fig. 74.6 Mass closure of abdominal wound with a double suture tied outside the skin over small teflon plates.

alternative technique (Fig. 74.6) allows the removal of the suture after about 6 to 8 weeks. The ends of the double suture are tied outside the skin over small teflon plates.

Thanks to better materials and improved surgical technique, the most serious of wound complications, evisceration, has been reduced to a very low incidence. The same cannot be said about postoperative incisional hernia. Long-term follow-up studies revealed that even years after operation new hernias were observed. Ellis et al[26] examined 363 patients in whom incisional hernia could not be found after one year. Two-and-a-half and 5 years later, 21 patients (5.8%) were found to have developed incisional hernia. These hernias, however, were small and none of them required surgical repair or a supporting corset. Harding et al[38] observed hernias in 28 of 564 patients (5%) after one year, an additional 14 of 482 patients after 3 years (2.9%), 6 of 431 after 5 years (1.4%) and 4 of 376 (1%) after 7 years. It may be that incisional hernias are 'undiscovered' rather than occurring late. Playforth et al[74] applied metal clips to the edges of the aponeuroses and found when these were shown on X-ray, that if they were together one month after operation, they did not subsequently separate and neither did the wound herniate. On the other hand, when early postoperative X-rays showed clip separation, incisional hernia was not found until months or years later.

Recently, late complications of abdominal wound closure with continuous non-absorbable suture have been described.[56] These late complications are difficult to explain on a mechanical basis. Some late hernias may, according to these authors, be the result of persistence of continuous suture material with the hernias developing at the sites where the suture material penetrated fascia, muscle and peritoneum.

A very low incidence of incisional hernia has been reported when stainless steel staples were applied in addition to conventional continuous sutures.[15]

The staple closure of midline incision of the upper part of the abdomen has successfully been used in nearly 800 patients[81]. Future development of absorbable clips for fascial staple closure is promising.

When all layers have been incised transversely (muscle-splitting incision), mass closure is feasible and should be performed as in a midline incision.

Mass closure by continuous or interrupted sutures

Equally good results (low incidence of wound dehiscence, incisional hernia) have been obtained with either continuous or interrupted far-near-suturing. This near-far-far-near technique (Smead-Jones) was also applied very success-

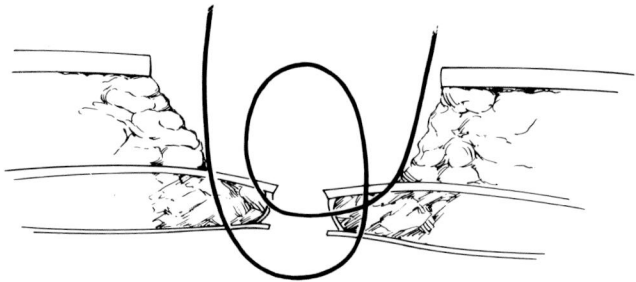

Fig. 74.7 Far-near-near-far mass closure suture.

fully in the repair of dehiscent wounds.[80] Smead-Jones type stitches serve as tension sutures, and may also be applied in high-risk patients for primary closure (Fig. 74.7). However, closure technique (e.g. adequate tissue bites) seems to be more important than the method of closure (interrupted or continuous).[49]

Subcuticular layers

Again there are many options in closing the subcuticular layers. Should the subcutaneous fat layer be sutured? Certainly it adds nothing to the strength of the abdominal scar. We recommend that Scarpa's fat fascia be approximated by a few single resorbable sutures to prevent depression of the suture line later on. Closed suction drainage will help in some instances to prevent an unwanted accumulation of blood and serous fluid, and thus add to a tension-free apposition of wound edges. Numerous trials have shown the efficacy of antibiotic prophylaxis in reducing the incidence of postoperative wound infections after intestinal surgery.[75] The data for abdominal gynecological surgery are controversial, however.[92] The value of wound irrigation with topical antiseptics or antibiotics is questionable.[17,29,75,86] Povidone iodine, in particular, appears not to be beneficial in clean or so-called clean contaminated wounds.

Skin closure

In cases where the wound is grossly contaminated, antibiotics prophylaxis cannot significantly reduce a very high wound infection rate.[91,98] These cases are best managed by delayed primary closure of the wound. Skin sutures are placed but not tied initially. The wound is covered with saline-soaked dressings which are changed two or three times per day. About 3 days later the sutures are tied.[65] An alternative method uses adhesive tapes (Steristrip®, Opsite®, Micropore®) instead. If problems arise in achieving accurate apposition of the wound edges, skin staples may do the job.

The cosmetic appearance of the final scar is a concern of many gynecological patients. The surgeon, on the other hand may particularly wish to avoid infection and the use of time-consuming techniques of wound closure. Detailed

knowledge about how to achieve these goals will allow the surgeon to choose the most appropriate method for the individual case. A prerequisite to return skin incisions to as near normal a state as possible, is to appose epithelial edges accurately without undue tension while controlling any tendencies to inversion and eversion. An incision which is in, or parallel to, the natural skin creases and lines will create a wound with the least possible tension. Skin tension is caused by elastic fibres in the skin and the effect of gravity. Since both vary, tension also varies everywhere on the body surface.

Excellent apposition of the skin is achieved by interrupted simple loop sutures. If the path of the needle is selected according to Figure 74.8, skin edges are slightly everted and an optimal adaptation of the wound edges is achieved (Fig. 74.9). Wound edema usually develops within 48 hours after closure. Sutures tied too tightly may strangulate a wound and lead to ischemic necrosis and disfiguring cross-hatched scars later on. A disadvantage of

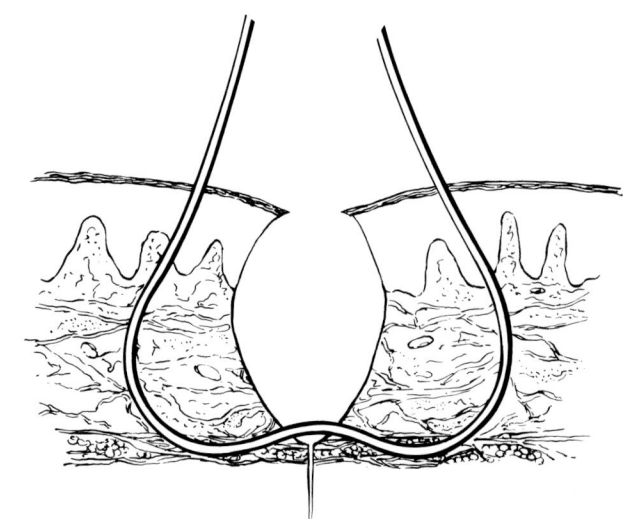

Fig. 74.8 An everting loop suture is made by going wider as one goes deeper. Thus, more tissue is included on the bottom.

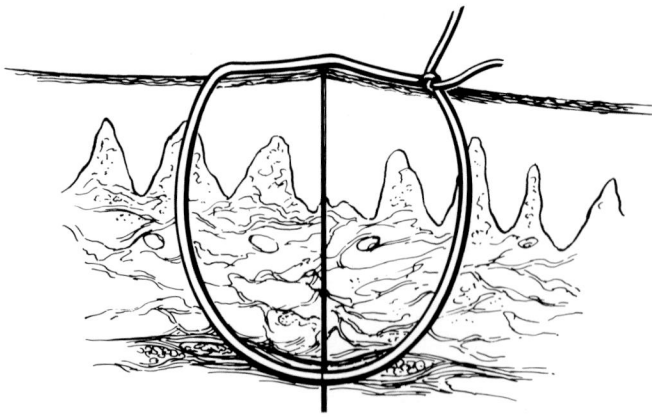

Fig. 74.9 When the suture is tied, the wound edges, despite a tendency to invert, are forced to evert resulting in accurate alignment.

full-thickness skin sutures is their potential for propagation of infection in the subcutaneous tissues along the suture track. Down-growth of epithelium along the suture usually starts on the fourth postoperative day.[31] The intensity of epithelialization and puncture mark formations depends on the size of the suture and the amount of tissue reaction it provokes. Because of their low reactivity, very thin (gauge 4-0) monofilament, non-absorbable materials are preferred.

Continuous intradermal or subcuticular sutures do not have these disadvantages and will give the best cosmetic results. Depending on the thickness of the epidermis, a two-layer technique is sometimes advisable. The subcuticular suture will align the deeper layers of the epidermis. Skin has only about 10% of its original tensile strength at 14 days, whereas most skin sutures are removed at 7 to 10 days when the wound is still very weak. There is no wound breakdown, probably because of the protective action of elastin,[28] but a widening of the scar can often be observed. If there is tension on the suture line, as in midline incisions, intradermal and subcuticular sutures can be left for several weeks until the scar has obtained sufficient strength. Again, monofilament, non-absorbable material should be used, because absorbable synthetic suture (polyglycolic acid) causes hypertrophic scarring in paramedian and inguinal wounds.[85]

Clips have been used for many years. Currently, disposable automatic skin staplers are enjoying a vogue. Basically, an incomplete rectangular steel staple secures the edges of the skin wound with little or no invasion of the subcutaneous tissue (Fig. 74.10). Thus, there is less chance for bacterial migration into the wound, resulting in a lower infection rate in clean[9] and in clean-contaminated as well as contaminated wounds as compared with conventional skin sutures.[73] The greatest advantage lies in their speed and convenience.[24,30,66] The cosmetic results are at least as good as those with conventional sutures[66] or even better.[9] In one trial, wound pain was more frequent after stapling,[24] but the only real disadvantage is possibly the substantial cost of disposable staplers.

Another sutureless type of skin closure uses sterile adhesive cloth rayon tapes or polyurethane membranes. The porous nature of the materials prevents fluid accumulation and bacterial growth on the wound surface.[62] Usually, these wounds heal with a better cosmetic result than wounds closed with conventional sutures.[22,71] We routinely use a microporous adhesive tape (Steristrip®) in combination with a subcuticular suture or clips which helps to accurately appose wound edges.

MANAGEMENT OF ABDOMINAL WOUND DEHISCENCE

In cases of abdominal wound dehiscence, frequently associated with re-exploration and/or peritonitis, an individual approach to the clinical problem is needed.

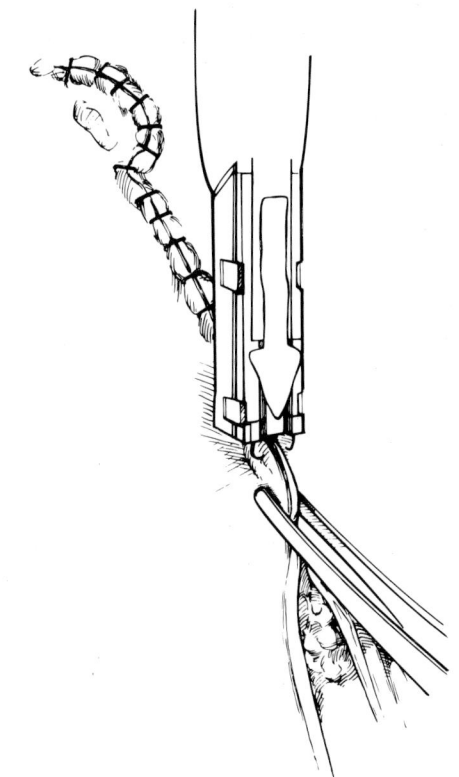

Fig. 74.10 Disposable skin stapler — fast and easy approximation of wound edges.

The fact that tension sutures are used to repair dehisced wounds that were initially closed with tension sutures, and the fact that the second closure usually succeeds when the first one failed, would indicate that the surgeon's technique in placing the 'retention sutures' was the key factor.[80] Although fascial deshiscence may not be eliminated, its incidence can certainly be reduced with proper attention to the mechanics of fascial closure. In most cases of wound dehiscence, secondary closure is successfully achieved. Sometimes, local skin flaps[97] or even myocutaneous flaps[72] have been used to cover a large defect in the abdominal wall. These techniques may be reserved for extreme cases. Primary reclosure, however, is only seldom a wise procedure. The patients suffer from peritonitis, and ventilation may often be impaired by high tension on the abdominal wound edges. The aim in these patients is a decrease in intra-abdominal pressure and effective drainage of the abdominal cavity.

This can be achieved by the use of synthetic material (Mersilene, Marlex or Vicryl mesh) or by an open treatment of the abdominal wall. Recently, Vicryl mesh has been used frequently with excellent results.[34] In the open treatment, all layers of the wound edges are approximated without tension by sutures guarded with polyethylene tubing. To stabilize the abdomen, silicone drains cover the abdominal defect allowing continuous drainage of the wound and protection of the intestines from the sutures.[36]

As in primary closure, skin and subcutaneous layers should be left open in all cases when contamination is suspected.

SUMMARY

The introduction of modern synthetic suture materials, and an individualized approach to wound closure techniques in gynecological surgery, has created new options. Although many issues remain open to debate, we have no doubt that catgut and chromic catgut can be declared obsolete in gynecological surgery. The choice of synthetic absorbable suture materials has to be made on personal preferences and clinical experience. If the use of non-absorbable sutures is desired, with few exceptions monofilament suture material is clearly the first choice.

Transverse wounds are equally strong, whether closed in layers or by a mass technique. For vertical wounds, incorporation of all layers within each stitch ('mass closure') has been shown many times to be superior to closure of each fascial layer individually ('layered closure'). When retention sutures are added to layered closure, the incidence of wound failure is diminished and is equivalent to that of mass closure. Continuous sutures are as reliable as interrupted sutures for wound closure.

Abdominal opening and closure techniques, and the selection of appropriate suture materials, have to be considered as important factors in minimizing wound healing complications. The decision-making process is based on knowledge of anatomy, wound healing and possible risk factors.

REFERENCES

1. Alexander H C, Prudden J F 1966 The causes of abdominal wound disruption. Surg Gynecol Obstet 122: 1223
2. Askew A R 1983 A comparison of upper abdominal wound closure with monofilament nylon and polyglycolic acid. Aust NZ J Surg 53: 353
3. Babcock W W 1935 Catgut allergy with a note on the use of alloy steel wire for sutures and ligatures. Am J Surg 27: 67
4. Baggish M S, Lee W K 1975 Abdominal wound disruption. Obstet Gynecol 46: 530
5. Bourne R B, Bitar H, Andreae P R, Martin L M, Finlay J B, Marquis F 1988 In-vivo comparison of four absorbable sutures: Vicryl, Dexon Plus, Maxon and PDS. Canad J Surg 31: 43
6. Brückner W L, Loeweneck H, Mahnel H, Fonkalsrund E W 1982 Nahtmaterial in virusinfizierten Wunden. In: Thiede A, Hamelmann H (eds) Moderne Nahtmaterialien und Nahttechniken in der Chirurgie, Springer-Verlag, Berlin
7. Bucknall T E, Ellis H 1981 Abdominal wound closure — a comparison of monofilament nylon and polyglycolic acid. Surgery (back) 89: 672
8. Bucknall T E, Cox P J, Ellis H 1982 Burst abdomen and incisional hernia: a prospective study of 1129 major laparotomies Br Med J 282: 931
9. Bucknall T E, Ellis H 1982 Skin closure. Comparison of nylon, polyglycolic acid and staples. Eur Surg Res 14: 96
10. Bucknall T E, Teare L, Ellis H 1983 The choice of a suture to close abdominal incisions. Eur Surg Res 15: 59
11. Cameron A E P, Gray R C F, Talbot R W, Wyatt A P 1980 Abdominal wound closure: a trial of Prolene and Dexon. Br J Surg 67: 487
12. Conn J Jr, Beal J M 1980 Coated vicryl synthetic absorbable sutures. Surg Gynecol Obstet 150: 843
13. Corman M L, Veidenheimeri M C, Coller J A 1981 Controlled clinical trial of three suture materials for abdominal wall closure after bowel operations. Am J Surg 141: 510
14. Cruse P J F, Foord R 1973 A five year prospective study of 23 649 surgical wounds. Arch Surg 107: 206
15. Danto L A, Albertazzi V J, Elliot T E 1981 The stapled abdominal wall closure revisited. Am J Surg 142: 391
16. Day T G 1988 Drainage in gynecologic surgery. Clin Obstet Gynecol 31: 744
17. De Jong T E, Vierhout R J, Van Vroonhoven T J 1982 Povidone-iodine irrigation of the subcutaneous tissue to prevent surgical wound infections. Surg Gynecol Obstet 155: 221
18. Douglas D M 1952 The healing of aponeurotic incisions. Br J Surg 40: 79
19. Driscoll G L, Baird P J, Merkelbach P J, Smith D H 1982 Synthetic absorbable and nonabsorbable microsutures: a histological comparison. Clin Reprod Fert 1: 151
20. Dudley H A F 1970 Layered and mass closure of the abdominal wall. A theoretical and experimental analysis. Br J Surg 57: 664
21. Dudley H A F, Kapadia C R 1982 Sutures and infection: studies of conventional materials and new synthetic absorbables. In: Thiede A, Hamelmann H (eds) Moderne Nahtmaterialien und Nahttechniken in der Chirurgie. Springer-Verlag, Berlin
22. Eaton A C 1980 A controlled trial to evaluate and compare a sutureless skin closure technique (Op-site skin closure) with conventional skin suturing and clipping in abdominal surgery. Br J Surg 67: 857
23. Efron G 1965 Abdominal wound disruption. Lancet i: 1287
24. Eldrup J, Wied U, Andersen B 1981 Randomized trial comparing Proximate stapler with conventional skin closure. Acta Chirurg Scand 147: 501
25. Ellis H 1984 Midline abdominal incisions. Br J Obstet Gynaecol 91: 1
26. Ellis H, Gajraj H, George C D 1983 Incisional hernias: when do they occur? Br J Surg 70: 290
27. Ellis H, Heddle R 1977 Does the peritoneum need to be closed at laparotomy? Br J Surg 64: 733
28. Forrester J 1972 Suture materials and their use. Br J Hosp Med 11: 578
29. Galle P C, Homesley H D 1980 Ineffectiveness of povidone-iodine irrigation of abdominal incisions. Obstet Gynecol 55: 744
30. Gatt D, Quick C R G, Owen-Smith M S 1982 Staples for wound closure: a controlled trial. Ann Roy Coll Surg Eng 67: 318
31. Gillmann T, Penn J 1956 Studies on the repair of wounds with reference to epidermal reaction to sutures and pathogenesis of carcinoma in scars. Medical Proc 2: 121
32. Goligher J C, Irvin T T, Johnston D et al 1975 A controlled trial of three methods of closure of laparotomy wounds. Br J Surg 62: 823
33. Greenburg G A, Saik R P, Peskin G W 1979 Wound dehiscence. Pathophysiology and prevention. Arch Surg 114: 143
34. Gross E, Erhard J, Eigler F W 1984 Kunststoffnetze als Hilfsmittel zum Bauchdeckenverschluß bei postoperativer Peritonitis, post-operativer Bauchdeckendehiszenz und zur Rekonstruktion der Bauchwand. Zentralb Chirurg 109: 1238
35. Guillon P J, Hall T J, Donaldson D R, Broughton A C, Brennan T G 1980 Vertical abdominal incisions — a choice? Br J Surg 67: 395
36. Guthy E 1984 Taktik und Technik des Bauchverschlusses bei Relaparotomie, Platzbauch und Peritonitis. Zentralb Chirurg 109: 524
37. Hampton J R 1963 The burst abdomen. Br Med J ii: 1032

38. Harding K G, Mudge M, Leinster S J, Hughes L E 1983 Late development of incisional hernia: an unrecognized problem. Br Med J 286: 519
39. Higson H I, Kettlell M G W 1978 Parietal wound drainage in abdominal surgery. Br J Surg 65: 326
40. Hilton D 1988 Surgical wound drainage: a survey of practices among gynaecologists in the British Isles. Br J Obstet Gynaecol 95: 1063
41. Irvin T T, Koffmann C G, Duthie H L 1976 Layer closure of laparotomy wounds with absorbable and non-absorbable suture material. Br J Surg 63: 793
42. Irvin T T, Stoddard C J, Greaney M G, Duthie H L 1977 Abdominal wound healing: a prospective clinical study. Br Med J ii: 351
43. Jenkins T P N 1976 The burst abdominal wound: a mechanical approach. Br J Surg 63: 873
44. Joel-Cohen S J 1978 The place of the abdominal hysterectomy. Clin Obstet Gynaecol 501: 525
45. Johnson C D, Bernhardt L W, Bentley P G 1982 Incisional hernia after mass closure of abdominal incisions with Dexon and Prolene. Br J Surg 69: 55
46. Karipineni R C, Wilk P J, Danese C A 1976 The role of the peritoneum in the healing of abdominal incisions. Surg Gynecol Obstet 142: 729
47. Käser O, Iklé F A, Hirsch H A 1983 Atlas der gynäkologischen Operationen (4th edn) Thieme, Stuttgart
48. Keill R H, Keitzer F, Nichols W K, Henzel J, Deneese M S 1973 Abdominal wound dehiscence. Arch Surg 106: 573
49. Kenady D E 1984 Management of abdominal wounds. Surg Clin Nth Am 64: 803
50. Kirk R M 1972 Effect of method of opening and closing the abdomen on incidence of wound bursting. Lancet ii: 352
51. Kjaergaard J, Laursen N P, Madsen C M, Tilma A, Zimmermann-Nielsen C 1976 Comparison of Dexon and Mersilene sutures in the closure of primary laparotomy incisions. Acta Chirurg Scand 142: 315
52. Knight C D, Griffen D F 1983 Abdominal wound closure with a continuous monofilament polypropylene suture. Arch Surg 118: 1305
53. Kraissl C J 1936 Suture material: a review of recent literature. Surg Gynecol Obstet 62: 417
54. Kronborg O 1976 Polyglycolic acid (Dexon) versus silk for fascial closure of abdominal incisions. Acta Chirurg Scand 142: 9
55. Krukowski Z H, Cusick E L, Engeset J, Matheson N A 1987 Polydioxanone or polypropylene for closure of midline abdominal incisions: a prospective comparable clinical trial. Br J Surg 74: 828
56. Krukowski Z H, Matheson N A 1987 Button hole incisional hernia: a late complication of abdominal wound closure with continuous non-absorbable sutures. Br J Surg 74: 824
57. Leaper D J, Allan A, May R E, Corfield A, Kennedy R H 1985 Abdominal wound closure: a controlled trial of polyamide (nylon) and polydioxanone suture (PDS). Ann Roy Coll Surg Engl 67: 273
58. Leaper D J, Pollock A V, Evans M 1977 Abdominal wound closure: a trial of nylon, polyglycolic acid and steel sutures. Br J Surg 64: 603
59. Leaper D J, Rosenberg I L, Evans M, Pollock A V 1976 The influence of suture materials in abdominal wound healing assessed by controlled clinical trials. Eur Surg Res 8: 75
60. Lünstedt B, Thiede A 1982 Standardisierung der Nachweisverfahren zur Objektivierung der linearen Fadenzug-, Knotenbruch- und Knotensitzfestigkeit verschiedener absorbierbarer und nichtabsorbierbarer Nahtmaterialien. In: Thiede A, Hamelmann H (eds) Moderne Nahtmaterialien und Nahttechniken in der Chirurgie. Springer Verlag, Berlin
61. Lynch M O, Berry R E 1987 Knot security and breaking stress of polydioxanone and other suture materials. Health Care Instrument 2: 141
62. Marples R R, Klingman A M 1969 Growth of bacteria under adhesive tapes. Arch Dermatol 99: 107
63. Martyak S N, Curtis L E 1976 Abdominal incision and closure. A systems approach. Am J Surg 131: 476
64. Maylard A E 1907 Direction of abdominal incisions. Br Med J ii: 895
65. McLachlin A D, Wall W 1976 Delayed primary closure of the skin and subcutaneous tissue in abdominal surgery. Canad J Surg 19: 37
66. Meiring L, Cilliers K, Barry R, Nel C J C 1982 A comparison of a disposable skin stapler and nylon sutures for wound closure. Sth Afric Med J 62: 371
67. Morrill W P 1936 Surgical catgut. Hospital 34: 39
68. Moss J P 1981 Historical and current perspectives on surgical drainage. Surg Gynecol Obstet 152: 517
69. Mowat J, Bonnard J 1971 Abdominal wound dehiscence after cesarean section. Br Med J ii: 256
70. Orr J W, Barter J F, Kilgore L C, Soong S J, Shingleton H M, Hatch K D 1986 Closed suction pelvic drainage after radical pelvic surgical procedures. Am J Obstet Gynecol 155: 867
71. Pedersen V M, Jensen B S, Hansen B 1981 Skin closure in abdominal incisions. Acta Chirurg Scand 147: 619
72. Pfandlsteiner G 1984 Der muskulokutane Lappen beim Körperhöhlenverschluß nach erweiterter Tumorresektion. Handchirurg, Mikrochirurg, Plastische Chirurg 2: 127
73. Pickford I R, Rennan S S, Evans M, Pollock A V 1983 Two methods of skin closure in abdominal operations: a controlled clinical trial. Br J Surg 70: 226
74. Playforth M J, Sauven P, Evans M, Pollock A V 1986 The prediction of incisional hernias by radio-opaque markers. Ann Roy Coll Surg Eng 68: 82
75. Polk H C, Simpson C J, Simmons B P, Alexander J W 1983 Guidelines for prevention of surgical wound infections. Arch Surg 118: 1213
76. Pollock A V, Greenall M J, Evans M 1979 Single layer mass closure of major laparotomies by continuous suturing. J Roy Soc Med 72: 889
77. Poole G V, Meredith J W, Kon N D, Martin M B, Kawamoto E H, Meyer R F 1984 Suture technique and wound bursting strength. Ann Surg 50: 569
78. Postlethwait R W, Willigan D A, Ulin A W 1975 Human tissue reaction to sutures. Ann Surg 181: 144
79. Pratt J H, Irons G B 1978 Panniculectomy and abdominoplasty. Am J Obstet Gynecol 132: 165
80. Sanders R J, Di Clementi D 1977 Principles of abdominal wound closure II. Prevention of wound dehiscence. Arch Surg 112: 1188
81. Sapala J A, Brown T E, Sapala A 1986 Anatomic staple closure of midline incisions of the upper part of the abdomen. Surg Gynecol Obstet 163: 282
82. Scheidel P, Hohl M K 1987 Modern synthetic suture materials and abdominal wound closure techniques in gynaecological surgery. In: Monaghan J M (ed) Gynaecological Surgery. Baillière Tindall, London
83. Schüssler B, Wiedemann R 1985 Die Blasenhalssuspension — anatomische und funktionelle Grundlagen für die Wahl von Nahtmaterialien und Implantation. In: Hepp H, Scheidel P (eds) Nahtmaterialien und Nahttechniken in der operativen Gynäkologie. Urban & Schwarzenberg, München
84. Shepherd J S, Cavanagh D, Riggs D, Praphat H, Wisniewski B J 1983 Abdominal wound closure using a nonabsorbable single layer technique. Obstet Gynecol 61: 248
85. Simpson J E P, Ornstein M, Spicer C C, Cox A G 1979 Hypertrophic scarring: Dexon suture in a randomized trial. Br J Surg 66: 281
86. Sindelar W F, Mason G R 1979 Irrigation of subcutaneous tissue with povidone-iodine solution for prevention of surgical wound infections. Surg Gynecol Obstet 148: 227
87. Smith S R G, Gilmore O J A 1985 Surgical drainage. Br J Hosp Med 33: 308
88. Swartz W H, Tanaree P 1975 Suction drainage as an alternative to prophylactic antibiotics for hysterectomy. Obstet Gynecol 45: 305
89. Symmonds R E, Pratt J H 1961 Prevention of fistulas and lymphocysts in radical hysterectomy: preliminary report of a new technique. Obstet Gynecol 17: 57
90. Stone I K, von Fraunhofer J A, Masterson B J 1985 A comparative study of suture materials: chromic gut and chromic gut treated with glycerin. Am J Obstet Gynecol 151: 1087
91. Stone H H, Hester T R 1972 Topical antibiotic and delayed

primary closure in the management of contaminated surgical incisons. J Surg Res 12: 70

92. Sweet R L, Gibbs R S 1985 Infectious Diseases of the Female Genital Tract. Williams & Wilkins, Baltimore, p 355

93. Tagart R E B 1967 The suturing of abdominal incisions. A comparison of monofilament nylon and catgut. Br J Surg 54: 952

94. Taylor T V 1985 The use of polydioxanone suture in midline incisions. J Roy Coll Surg Edinb 30: 191

95. Thiede A 1985 Moderne synthetische Nahtmaterialien und aktuelle Nahtverfahren in der gastrointestinalen Chirurgie. In: Hepp H, Scheidel P (eds) Nahtmaterialien und Nahttechniken in der operative Gynäkologie. Urban & Schwarzenberg, München, p. 11

96. Ullrich F, Henningen B, Böttcher W 1982 Polyglykolsäure-(Dexon-) oder Polyesterfäden, eine Alternative beim Faszienverschluß medianer Laparotomien? In: Thiede A, Hamelmann H (eds) Modern Nahtmaterialien und Nahttechniken in der Chirurgie. Springer-Verlag, Berlin, p 179

97. Valesky A, Nissen R, Vatankhah M 1985 Chirurgische Versorgung von Narbenhernien und akuten Bauchwanddefekten. In: Hepp H & Scheidel P (eds) Nahtmaterialien und Nahttechniken in der operativen Gynäkologie. Urban & Schwarzenberg, München

98. Verrier E D, Bossart K J, Heer F W 1979 Reduction of infection rates in abdominal incisions by delayed wound closure techniques. Am J Surg 138: 22

99. Wallace D, Hernandez W, Schlaerth J B, Nalick R N, Morrow C P 1980 Prevention of abdominal wound disruption utilizing the Smead-Jones closure technique. Obstet Gynecol 56: 226

100. Wissing J, van Vroonhoven T H, Schattenkerk, Veen H F, Posent R J G, Jeekel J 1987 Fascia closure after midline laparotomy: results of randomized trial. Br J Surg 74: 738

101. Zamora A, Balladur A, Rolet F, Salet-Lizee D, Lefranc J P, Blondon J 1987 Un traitement préventif des lymphocèles après Lymphadéno-colpo-hysteréctomie élargie (L.C.H.E.). J Chir 124: 323

75. Surgery for invasive carcinoma of vulva

J. M. Monaghan

INTRODUCTION

Vulvar carcinoma is rare, representing 5 to 8% of genital cancers.[29] It is a problem mainly affecting the aged, the average age at presentation being in the late seventh decade. However, the age range is wide, occasionally being reported in girls in their teens and not infrequently in women in their twenties and thirties.

Younger patients show a tendency to develop multifocal disease on the vulva and perianal region and also have a higher incidence of cancer and precancer elsewhere in the lower genital tract.[33] Older patients often have significant medical problems, including hypertension, obesity, diabetes and heart and lung disease. It is important that these complicating factors are taken into account prior to any decision about the type of operative procedure to be performed. The patient should be assessed both by the surgeon and his anesthetist. The judgement must be made in the light of their experience; if they work closely together in a department dealing with a large number of such cases, then the operability rate will be high, increasing further with the use of spinal and epidural anesthesia. Reports from major centers commonly quote operability rates of the order of 96%.[43,51]

THE DEVELOPMENT OF SURGICAL TREATMENT

Traditionally, carcinoma of the vulva has been treated by radical vulvectomy with groin and pelvic node dissection. This belief was founded on the work of Basset,[7] Stoeckel,[54] Taussig[57] and Way,[59] who each demonstrated the very much improved overall survival when patients were treated in this manner. In spite of these advances, critics have been unhappy about the extent of these mutilating radical procedures. Little, if any, evidence was available to show that this standard approach could be modified or tailored to the individual patient until the early 1970s.

Rutledge et al,[53] suggested that those patients with small tumors, (T1 N0 M0, 2 cm in diameter), with a depth of invasion of less than 5 mm may not require a groin node dissection, as there was little evidence of metastases in this group of patients. Wharton et al,[61] reported on a series of 25 patients who met these criteria, 15 of whom were treated with radical vulvectomy alone, and 10 of whom had additional groin node dissection. They reported a 100% 5-year survival rate. These reports stimulated a considerable amount of study and interest. Unfortunately, it rapidly became clear that parallels with microinvasive carcinoma of the cervix could not be drawn. Many authorities reported individual cases and series showing nodal metastases and deaths in patients with T1 N0 M0 (Stage I, FIGO) tumors with less than 5 mm of invasion.[22,38,44,45,63] These reports confirmed that before individualization of treatment can be achieved a number of factors must be considered in order to identify those patients at risk of nodal metastases in carcinoma of the vulva.

When surgery for carcinoma of the vulva is limited to vulvectomy alone, the results are very poor. The extremely high survival rates recorded in major series for patients with negative nodes (Table 75.1) frequently tempt less experienced operators to adopt a more conservative technique, dispensing with the groin node dissection. The usual end result is a disastrous recurrence. It is clear that the groin node dissection not only deals with gross metastases in the nodes, but also effectively removes micrometastases which are not detectable. These are usually dealt with when the groin nodes are removed in direct continuity with the vulvar dissection. There are no large series comparing the results of dissection in continuity with those of separate incisions. The success of procedures using separate groin incisions will depend on the hypothesis that squamous carcinoma of the vulva spreads primarily by embolization and not by permeation.[62]

The author believes that small tumors spread by embolization primarily and only later spread by permeation to fill the lymphatic channels. It is frequently seen that, in large tumors, the groin lymphatics become obstructed and then retrograde lymphatic permeation occurs, especially down the lymph channels running alongside the saphenous

Table 75.1 Results of radical surgical treatment of cancer of the vulva

Study	Patients	Rad V GND*		Rad V GND+PND**	
		Node status	5-yr survival	*Node status*	5-yr survival
Monaghan personal series (1989)	345	Negative	95%	Negative	89%
		Positive	62%	Positive	26.5%
Benedet et al (1979)	204	Negative	86%	Negative	81.8%
		Positive	55.6%	Positive	50%

* Rad V GND = Radical vulvectomy and groin node dissection.
** Rad V GND+PND = Radical vulvectomy and groin node dissection + pelvic node dissection.

vein. It is important that the relative merits of separate groin incisions versus the traditional en bloc dissection in continuity with the vulva should be fully evaluated. In the meantime, separate incisions should be reserved for small tumors. Since 1985, the author has carried out 72 procedures where separate groin node incisions have been performed. One patient subsequently developed a groin recurrence with metastatic nodules in the pubic area. Her lymph nodes had been reported as negative, and it must be concluded that the cause of the recurrence was a residue of tumor left in the skin bridge. Christopherson et al[14] have reported a case of recurrence in the skin bridge between the groin and vulvar incisions following excision of a Stage I carcinoma. Therefore, at the present time, it is important that any deviation from an en bloc dissection to separate incisions be critically assessed and not routinely practised.

The main cause of failure of treatment of cancer of the vulva is an inability to control lymphatic and distant metastases. Control of local disease is relatively simple. A fundamental and detailed knowledge of the lymphatic drainage and anatomy of the regional lymph nodes is essential if the diagnosis and treatment of vulvar carcinoma is to be improved. Lymphatic spread occurs in approximately 30 to 40% of patients, and is primarily to the inguinal nodes and then sequentially to the pelvic nodes. Bloodborne spread is extremely rare.

FACTORS DETERMINING EXTENT OF SURGERY

Tumor staging

Clinical staging of carcinoma of the vulva remains unsatisfactory and has had limited use as a guide to extent of surgery required.

Errors in clinical staging of vulvar squamous carcinoma can be unacceptably high, reaching 25%,[50] and in a series of malignant melanomas from the same institution, 31% inaccurate assessments were noted.[52] The TNM system has particularly serious limitations in the staging of malignant melanoma, in that many tumors are less than 2 cm in diameter but are extremely aggressive and tend to have widespread metastatic patterns.[43,52]

The disease clearly requires an operative staging system.[27] Staging, including the new FIGO surgical staging classification, is discussed in detail in Chapter 28.

Histopathology

There are potential variations in treatment according to the histological pattern of the primary tumor, therefore it is vital to provide an adequate biopsy prior to determining definitive treatment.

Squamous carcinoma

Among the squamous carcinomas, which constitute 85% of vulvar cancers, are included basal cell carcinomas and verrucous carcinomas, both of which are relatively benign and do not warrant radical surgical treatment. Both basal cell and verrucous carcinomas have a very low propensity for lymphatic metastases,[39] therefore a vulvectomy or a wide local excision is usually sufficient. The verrucous carcinoma is similar to the giant condyloma of Buschke-Lowenstein. It should not be treated by radiotherapy, as there is a theoretical risk of transformation of the tumor into a poorly differentiated and highly malignant carcinoma.

In squamous cell carcinomas, the degree of differentiation is closely related to the metastatic potential. In 1960, Way[60] showed an almost two-fold increase in metastases when anaplastic squamous carcinomas were compared with well differentiated tumors. Iversen et al[36] found no difference in the two groups. Andreasson et al[3] found a lower metastatic rate in better differentiated tumors only where these were less than 4 cm in diameter. The author, however, has found a statistically significant difference, with squamous carcinoma of poor differentiation showing a higher rate of nodal metastases.[42]

Melanoma

Malignant melanoma is the second most common malignancy of the vulva, constituting about 5% of cases.[25] It is an extremely aggressive tumor, widespread metastases developing even when the primary is small. A progressive decrease in survival is seen as the melanoma penetrates the lower levels of the epithelium (levels II to IV),[15] and when the disease reaches the subcutaneous level (level V), survival drops rapidly,[10] and the recurrence rate reaches 78%.[52] Only patients with disease in levels IV and V appear to exhibit nodal metastases (see also Ch. 67).

There has been general acceptance that an en bloc dissection of the inguinal and/or pelvic lymph nodes with radical vulvectomy is the optimum management for lesions reaching these deeper levels. In recent times, Davison et al[20] have questioned the need for such radicality. In a retrospective review of 32 patients, they found no advantage in using the radical approach, and advocated dealing with nodal metastases as and when they arose. In the author's series of 14 patients, groin node metastases occurred in 50% whereas none had involvement of the pelvic nodes.

Carcinoma of Bartholin's gland

Primary carcinoma of Bartholin's gland is rare, representing approximately 1 to 3% of all vulvar tumors. This disease is characterized by a high groin node metastasis rate of between 37%[41] and 47%;[46] in the former series there was also 18% pelvic node involvement. Even those patients with negative groin nodes have a poor 5-year survival of 52%.[42] This compares very badly with squamous carcinoma of the vulva, where similar node-negative patients can expect to have a 94% chance of surviving 5 years.[44] However, Copeland et al[16] demonstrated a high 5-year survival of 84% in their series of Bartholin's gland cancer, where management was individualized and consisted of surgery plus or minus radiotherapy. Pelvic node dissection as part of the basic management is not necessary, unless four or more groin nodes are involved.[17] Although it is commonly written that carcinoma of the Bartholin's gland has a capacity for direct spread to the pelvic lymph nodes, the only case reported is that of Barclay et al.[6]

Sarcoma

These rare tumors are predominantly leiomyosarcomas and can present difficult diagnostic and management problems. The histological appearance may not be that of a malignant tumor, but any lesion with more than 10 mitoses per high power field must be regarded as such. They tend to grow rapidly, and frequently give the appearance of arising from the Bartholin's gland; the center of the tumor becomes necrotic and can be scooped out at surgery. Radical surgery is the basis of management, but because of the tendency to both local recurrence and widespread bloodborne metastases, this may have to be supported by electron beam therapy and chemotherapy.

Secondary carcinoma

The vulva is the site of secondary cancers from a variety of primary sites, including cervix and vagina, the ovary, the gastrointestinal tract, the renal tract, and even distant sites such as the breast and thyroid. Before embarking on local radical treatment, it is important to determine whether there are other metastases in other sites, and to evaluate the prospect of long-term survival from the primary disease.

Size of tumor

Podratz et al[51] showed that the larger the tumor the greater the chance of both groin and pelvic lymph node metastases. In the author's experience of over 200 groin, or groin and pelvic node dissections, there is a clear cut-off point at 4 cm diameter between those with pelvic node metastases (>4 cm), and those without (<4 cm).[43] A similar observation was noted by Andreasson & Nyboe.[4] Thus, by reserving pelvic node dissection for only those patients with tumors greater than 4 cm, a small but significant salvage might be achieved without subjecting all patients to the extended surgical procedure. The author recommends dissection of the pelvic nodes only where the vulvar carcinoma exceeds 4 cm.

Site of tumor

Clitoris

The lymphatics of the clitoris are said to communicate directly with the pelvic lymphatics[46] and it is usually recommended that clitoral tumors should be treated aggressively. However, direct communication has never been satisfactorily demonstrated. Recent work,[33] showing no evidence of such a communication, demonstrated frequent bilateral flow of the clitoral lymphatics as well as evidence of contralateral flow following laterally placed injection of a radionuclide (Technetium) into the labia (28 of 42 patients, 67%). Higher lymph flow rates were not apparent from any particular part of the vulva. However, care must be used in interpreting these findings since the patients examined were suffering from *carcinoma of the cervix* and no allowance was made or could be made for any disturbance of lymphatic drainage which might occur in the presence of *vulvar carcinoma*. It is possible that a cancer of the vulva could obstruct the normal routes of drainage, allowing secondary routes through the perineal membrane to open up causing direct spread to the pelvic lymph nodes.

In the author's earlier series, the clitoris was involved in 54 out of 200 cases, 47 of whom had nodal dissections. Twenty five (53%) had metastases to the groin nodes, but only 2 (4.2%) had metastases to the pelvic nodes, thus giving little support for the routine dissection of pelvic nodes. Piver & Xynos[49] in a similar sized series came to the same conclusion. However others[4] consider that the clitoris is a high risk site giving a poorer overall prognosis. The author believes that the pelvic nodes should not be routinely dissected simply because the clitoris or any other particular site on the vulva is involved.

Laterally placed tumors

It has been proposed that when Stage I vulvar carcinoma affects the labia alone and does not impinge on the clitoris, urethra, vagina, fourchette or perianal region, it may be reasonable to carry out a local excision or vulvectomy plus an ipsilateral groin node dissection, the contralateral nodes being preserved. This proposal is based on the belief that contralateral spread alone and bilateral spread from a laterally placed tumor is extremely rare. Hacker et al[31] stated that they had never seen positive contralateral nodes with negative ipsilateral nodes; they developed their argument further by stating that if ipsilateral nodes are found to be negative, then a contralateral dissection is unnecessary (see Ch. 76).

In a recent analysis of 296 vulvar cancers in the author's series, 71 patients with Stage I carcinomas had groin node dissection. Of the 40 patients where the tumor was laterally placed, only six (14%) had positive nodes. Five of the six patients had positive nodes on the *same* side as the carcinoma. Thus, this particular group may well benefit from a more limited approach. It is of interest that contralateral alone and bilateral spread did occur in those carcinomas which affected midline structures and in Stage II and III disease, as has been found elsewhere.[34]

Therefore, in those cases where Stage I tumors are laterally placed, there appears to be a place for the performance of an ipsilateral node dissection alone, but caution should still be exercised.

ASSESSMENT OF GROIN NODE STATUS

Preoperative identification of lymphatic spread and nodal involvement

The techniques available to the clinician for preoperatively diagnosing metastatic disease include the following:

Palpation of groin nodes. This is notoriously inaccurate,[8] with error rates of between 13% and 39%.

Computerized axial tomography (CAT) scan. This non-invasive technique has a relatively high false positive and false negative rate plus an unacceptably high limit of resolution, particularly in the pelvis. The method is reasonably accurate in the para-aortic region.

Magnetic resonance imaging (MRI). This non-invasive technique may have a place in diagnosis, as recent modifications using tissue subtraction techniques have shown great promise in differentiating cancer tissue from normal, opening the way to identification of metastatic

cancer at an early stage. Unfortunately, this facility is not widely available due to its high capital cost.

Lymphography. Although some authorities regard this technique as of value an equal number have highlighted its pitfalls and traps, which include the difficulty of identifying micrometastases, and equivocal lymphograms due to fatty infiltration and hyperplasia.

Fine needle aspiration (FNA). Fine needle aspiration of lymph nodes or suspicious areas is a frequently used technique, often saving major operative procedures or biopsies and commonly modifying management. The morbidity is low, even in potentially dangerous areas such as the posterior thorax. False positives are virtually nil. The specificity of the investigation is close to 100% and the sensitivity may reach 90%. (See Ch. 22.)

Open biopsy. This can now be restricted to those patients with negative or unsatisfactory results.

In summary, preoperative assessment of groin node status remains inaccurate. At the present time, complete groin node dissection should be performed for all invasive tumors except where there is less than 1 mm of invasion. The degree of involvement of the groin nodes by metastases will determine further action.

Intraoperative sampling

This procedure has been used to determine whether to proceed to removal of deep inguinal nodes, or to carry out pelvic node dissection. Curry et al[17] stated that where four or more nodes were involved in the groin, then pelvic node dissection should be carried out. DiSaia et al[24] have recommended dissection of the superficial nodes initially and then removing a sentinel node which is submitted to frozen section. If the node demonstrates metastases, then the remainder of the groin dissection should be performed. However, there is no single superficial node which can be confidently identified as a 'sentinel node'. A random sampling technique is thus fraught with potential inaccuracies. In the author's view, a full groin node dissection is the basic procedure which should be advocated.

PLAN OF MANAGEMENT

From the information now available, it is clear that a high degree of individualization of surgical management can be achieved for patients with carcinoma of the vulva. The following methods of management are proposed.

For patients with Stage I laterally placed tumors, radical vulvectomy with ipsilateral groin node dissection may be performed through separate incisions.

For Stage I disease encroaching on midline structures, radical vulvectomy with bilateral groin node dissection may be performed through separate incisions.

For later stage disease with carcinomas up to 4 cm in diameter, radical vulvectomy and bilateral groin node dissection either through separate incisions or by use of a 'butterfly' incision should be carried out.

For carcinomas greater than 4 cm in diameter, a pelvic node dissection should be added to the groin node dissection and the groins should be dissected en bloc in direct continuity with the radical vulvectomy using the 'butterfly' incision. Radiotherapy to the groin and pelvic nodal areas is an alternative or adjunct in those patients in whom it is thought that the surgery may not have been curative, or where two or more groin nodes are shown to contain metastases.[35] Other roles for radiotherapy would appear to be as a palliative in the few patients who are deemed inoperable, as a tumor reductive agent preoperatively and in those patients whose cancers affect the anus.[1,26,32] Where the cancer extends onto the anus or lower rectum, an anovulvectomy with colostomy or a posterior exenteration may be performed together with groin and pelvic node dissection. (See also Ch. 28.)

THE OPERATION

Patient preparation

The patient should be admitted two days prior to surgery, for intensive cleansing of the vulvar region by antiseptic bathing as well as routine preoperative preparation. Occasionally, if the patient has significant medical problems earlier admission may be necessary, for stabilization of diabetes for example. It is important not to bring the patient into hospital for too long a preoperative period, since idleness may initiate venous stasis with an increased risk of thromboembolic disease developing during and following the operation.

Thromboembolic prophylaxis. This group of patients is at high risk of developing thromboembolic disease. These women are often old, obese, suffer from degenerative diseases of the cardiovascular, respiratory and joint systems and already have major difficulties in mobility. Adequate prophylactic measures are essential. The choices are many, the author preferring low dose subcutaneous heparin, (5000 units twice daily). Special stockings and intraoperative muscle pumps are of value. However, a reduction of preoperative immobility and early postoperative mobilization remain the cornerstone of efforts to reduce the thromboembolic risk.

Prophylactic antibiotics. Wound infections can be reduced if intraoperative prophylactic antibiotics are used. The patient's personal allergies should be noted, and an appropriate antibiotic regimen employed which will cover both anaerobic and aerobic bacteria.

The anesthetic

It is the author's view that all radical surgery is better performed under either spinal or epidural anesthesia. The advantages are two-fold: firstly, the intraoperative blood pressure can be lowered with small vessel oozing reduced and a concomitant reduction in intraoperative blood loss; and secondly, the patient requires either minimal or no general anesthetic, a matter of particular benefit when the patient is old and infirm.

Patient position

The patient is positioned lying supine, with the feet approximately 25 cm apart and supported by an ankle rest to elevate the calves from the table. Some authorities recommend the 'ski' position,[55] so that two and even three teams can operate simultaneously. In the author's view, this is a recipe for confusion and does not significantly speed up the operation. Slight Trendelenburg is sometimes necessary to facilitate access to the groins, especially if the patient is fat.

The skin incision

Over the years the original 'butterfly' skin incisions have been modified in many ways, generally aimed at removing less and less skin. In some centers, a linear incision in the groin is recommended. However, the author continues to remove a narrow (less than 1 cm wide) band of skin, as this can be grasped with tissue forceps and the entire block of tissue containing the groin nodes manipulated with ease. If tissue forceps are applied to fat after using a linear incision, the forceps tend to 'cut through', often resulting in a loss of orientation. The trainee surgeon, and even more experienced colleagues, may become disorientated during this operation if the first incisions are incorrectly placed. Bony landmarks should be identified, and natural skin folds, which may be very variable, ignored, particularly in the obese patients.

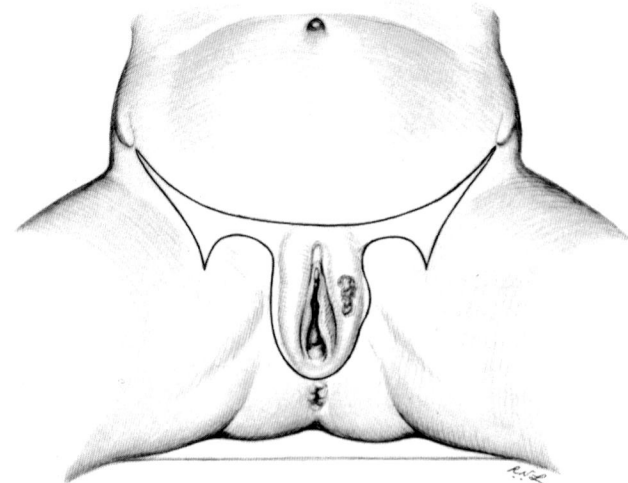

Fig. 75.1 The incisions for the groin node dissection.

The initial incision, curving down towards the groin, is made from the inferio-medial aspect of the anterior superior iliac spine, over the medial border of the origin of the sartorious muscle down to a midpoint low over the symphysis pubis. This is followed by an incision from the same point on the anterior superior iliac spine to a point 4 cm below the pubic tubercle, with its curve towards the groin fold. A third incision is then made from this last point, curving upwards and medially to terminate close to the lower border of the crural fold (Fig. 75.1). This third incision will function as a releasing incision facilitating closure of the wound. The skin removed from the groin will be minimal, a narrow band less than 1 cm wide, with a narrow releasing incision over the line of the upper part of the saphenous vein.

Defining the fascial planes in the lower and upper incisions

The band of skin in the groin is elevated by the assistant using Lane's tissue forceps. By exerting slight tension with the left hand on the upper edge of the skin incision, undercutting can be carried out by the surgeon down to aponeurosis of the external oblique muscle above the groin (Fig. 75.2). The fascia over the medial part of the sartorious muscle forming the lateral boundary of the femoral triangle can now be identified in a similar manner. This fascia is now incised longitudinally from the anterior superior iliac spine to the apex of the femoral triangle (Fig. 75.3). Small arteries and veins in the fat and fascial surfaces will be cut during these incisions; they should be meticulously identified and ligated or diathermied.

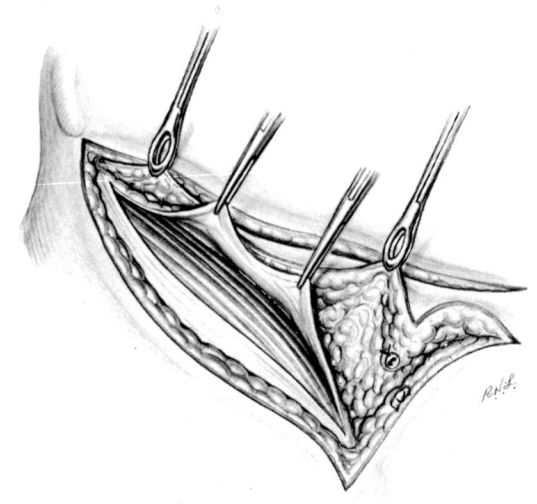

Fig. 75.3 The fascia over sartorious muscle is incised close to the medial edge of the muscle.

Dividing the saphenous vein

The saphenous vein is identified in the lower part of the releasing incision. The vein is isolated where it lies above the fascia lata, then divided and ligated at the apex of the releasing incision. At this point, the dissection can be deepened down to the fascia over the adductor muscles. The fascia is incised transversely medial to the femoral artery (Fig. 75.4).

The medial edge of the incised fascia covering the sartorious muscle is now picked up using two small Spencer

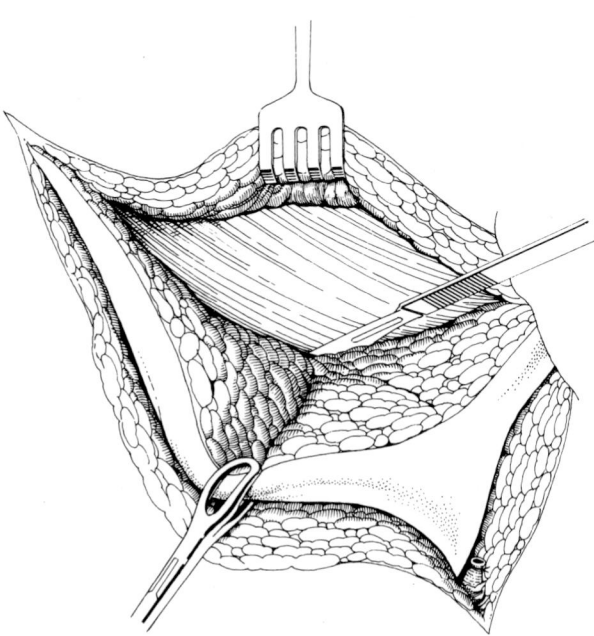

Fig. 75.2 The aponeurosis of the external oblique muscle is exposed in the upper part of the incision.

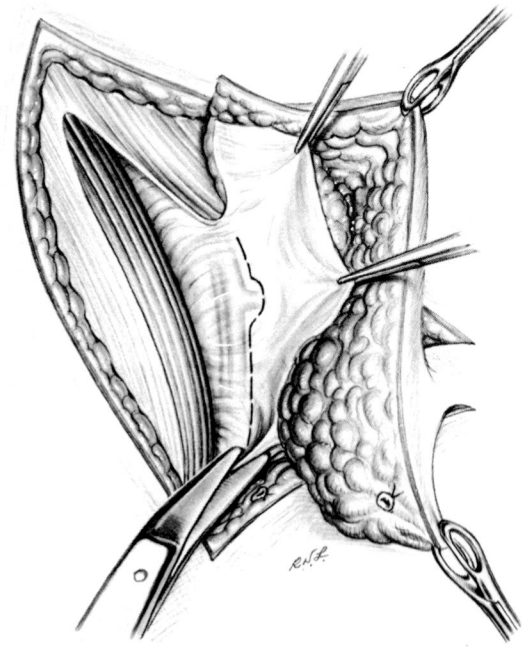

Fig. 75.4 After dividing the saphenous vein, the lower part of the incision is carried down to the adductor fascia.

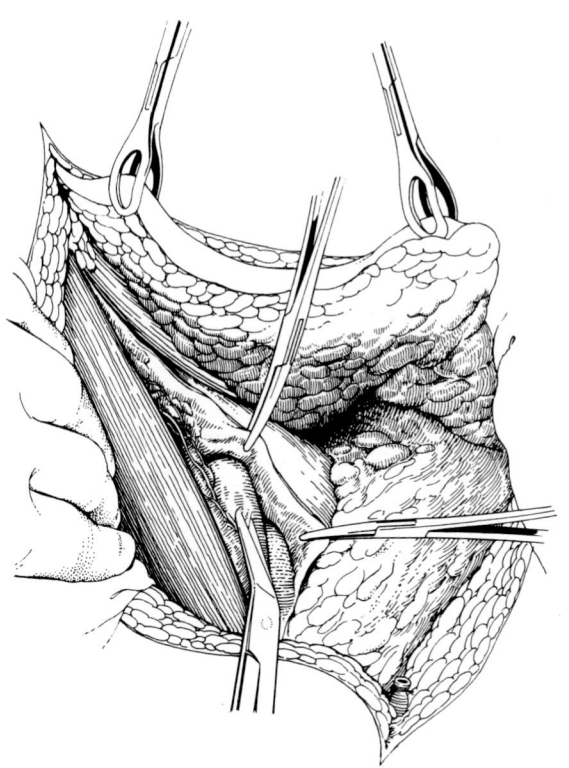

Fig. 75.5 The medial edge of the sartorious muscle fascia is elevated using two clips. The femoral artery and vein are cleaned.

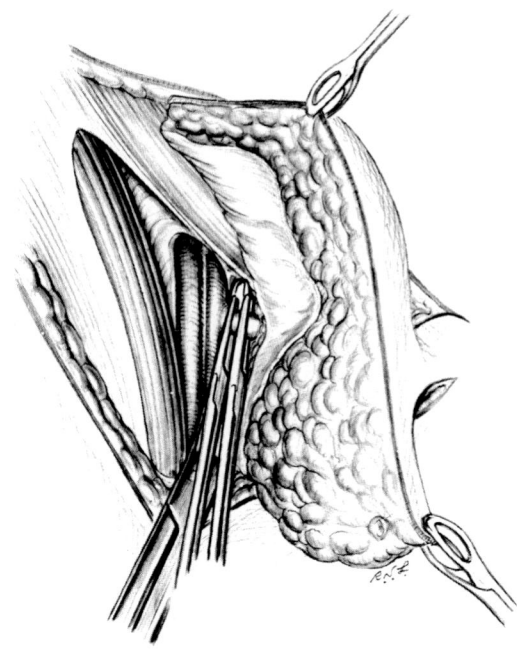

Fig. 75.6 The saphenous vein is isolated and divided below the cribriform fascia as it enters the femoral vein.

Wells clips and elevated (Fig. 75.5). The strands of nerve which can now be seen in the soft tissue at the medial side of the sartorious muscle are the branches of the femoral and the genito-femoral nerves. Some of these fibers may be cut as the femoral artery is defined and cleaned by incising the fascia of the lateral wall of the femoral sheath. The artery should be meticulously cleaned from the apex of the femoral triangle to the inguinal ligament. The author uses fine modifications of 'Bonney's' scissors for this cleansing. It is important to identify the tissue plane on the artery surface so that all fascia and lymphatics can be removed. The condensation of fascia lateral to the artery along the inguinal ligament is divided with scissors to leave the external oblique aponeurosis clean. It is here that the superficial circumflex iliac artery will be encountered and may be cut two or three times as it wanders laterally below the inguinal ligament. If the surgeon exercises patience, this vessel together with the superficial external pudendal and superficial external epigastric arteries will all be picked up as they originate from the anterior surface of the femoral artery.

Removing the groin nodes from the femoral vessels

On the medial side of the femoral artery, the femoral vein can be seen and it is cleaned from the inguinal ligament distally. The saphenous vein can now be isolated as it enters the femoral vein (Fig. 75.6). When the fascia is lifted and rotated medially by the assistant, it has the effect of opening the saphenous opening (the fossa ovalis). The loose cribriform fascia which fills the fossa can be separated and the edges of the opening defined. The saphenous vein is now clamped, cut and ligated as it enters the femoral vein. The author simply single ties the saphenous vein using either 1 Dexon or Vicryl; there is no need to make a ritual of this particular part of the operation. Thus, by elevating this fascia, all the superficial nodes and lymphatic tissue lying above the fascia will be automatically removed. These are variable in distribution, therefore it is essential that a wide block of tissue is removed by undercutting the skin.

Cleaning the adductor muscles

The whole block of tissue containing the groin nodes is turned medially. On the medial side of the femoral vein, the fascia over the adductor muscles is incised as close to the vein as possible. Small veins which enter the muscles may require ligating at this point. The releasing incision at the apex of the femoral triangle is now joined and the fascia is stripped from the adductor muscles as far medially as the gracilis tendon aponeurosis. In the upper part of this dissection, the round ligament is picked up, divided and ligated as it leaves the inguinal canal (Fig. 75.7). The subfascial dissection is then completed through to the pubic symphysis. The entire superficial and deep inguinal nodes have been removed en bloc through a small groin incision.

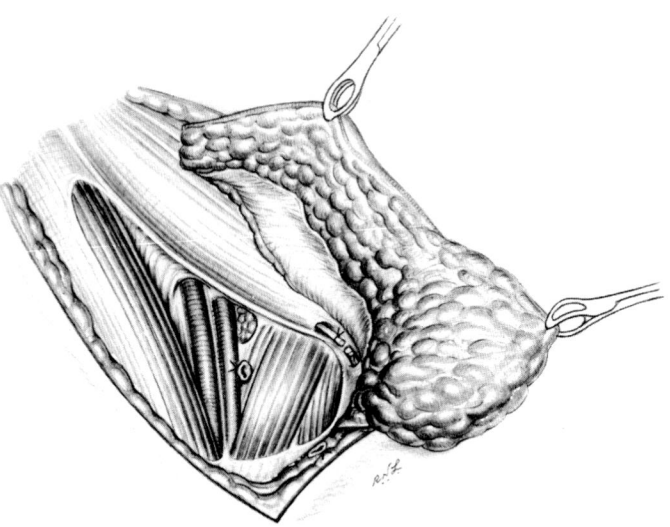

Fig. 75.7 The complete block of lymph nodes is elevated from the medial part of the dissection and the round ligament divided.

Pelvic node dissection

The pelvic nodes may now be approached by incising through the external oblique muscle approximately 2 cm above the inguinal ligament, beginning above the femoral canal and extending superolaterally for 8 cm (Fig. 75.8). The internal oblique is then incised along the line of its fibers, exposing the transversalis fascia and peritoneum. Using the fingers, the peritoneum is swept from the outer pelvis exposing the iliacus muscle and then the external iliac vessels. The exposure is completed by extending the medial end of the wound through the muscles of the anterior abdominal wall down to the femoral canal, applying large clips to the inferior epigastric arteries (Fig. 75.9).

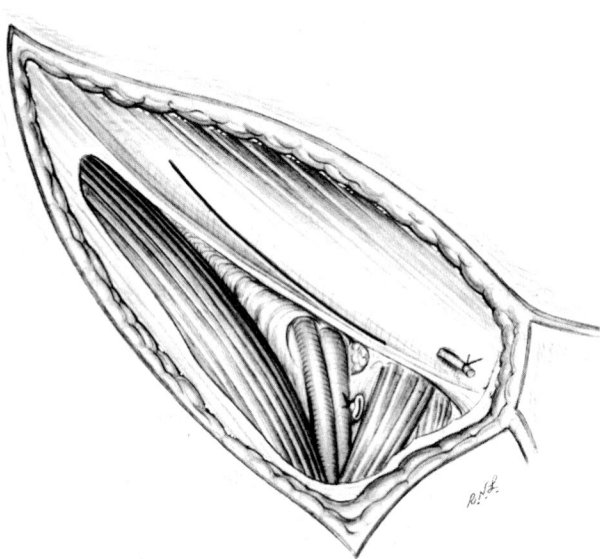

Fig. 75.8 The incision in the external oblique muscle allowing access to the pelvic lymph nodes.

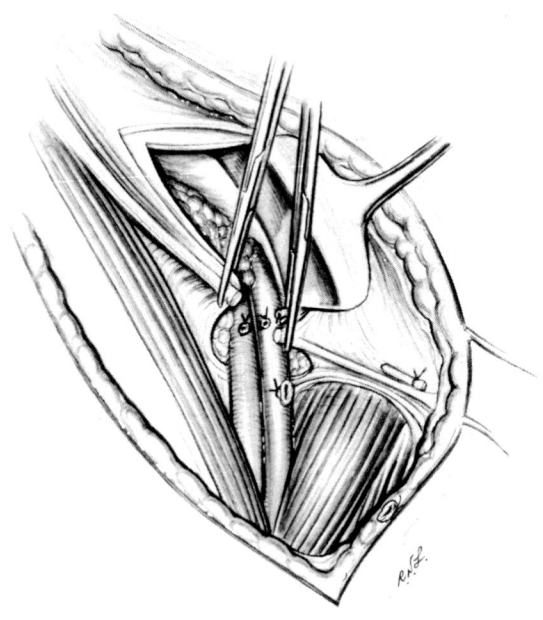

Fig. 75.9 The inferior epigastric arteries are clipped.

Through this incision, the external iliac vessels can be cleaned of nodes as far up as the common iliac vessels; the ureter is usually visible in the upper part of the dissection. This dissection is thus performed in direct continuity with the groin node dissection (Fig. 75.10). Although Cloquet's or Rosenmuller's node is said to be constant in the femoral canal, the lateral and medial external iliac nodes

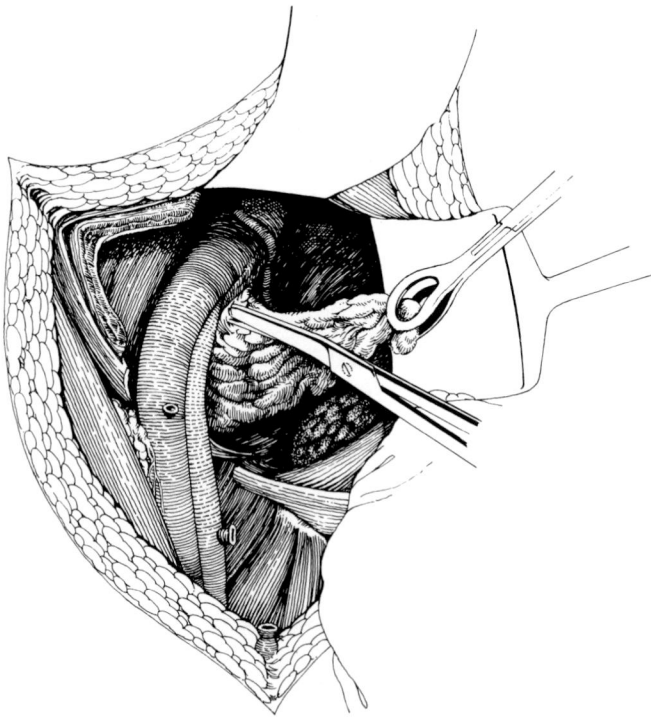

Fig. 75.10 Removal of the pelvic lymph nodes.

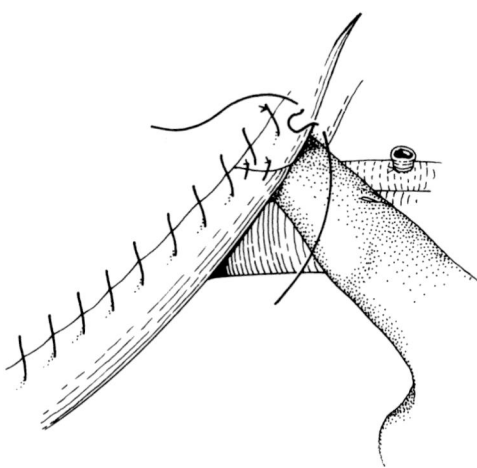

Fig. 75.11 Repair and closure of the inguinal ligament defect.

lying above the inguinal ligament are a more regular feature.

Closure of the abdominal wall and inguinal ligament defect

This is achieved by a continuous Dexon or Vicryl suture, beginning with the internal oblique muscles at the medial end of the incision over the femoral canal, travelling laterally, and then returning to the medial end, completing the closure of the external oblique muscles. At this point, the femoral canal is reconstituted by suturing the medial part of the external oblique incision to the fascia of the pectineal line (Cooper's ligament), so that the femoral canal admits a finger tip and pressure is not put on the femoral vein (Fig. 75.11).

Drainage of the groin and closure of the skin incision

Drainage of the space left in the groin is mandatory, as up to 300 ml of fluid can collect on each side per day. Drainage is carried out by either vacuum or low pressure continuous suction drainage through large diameter drains. Using the modern narrow skin and releasing incisions, closure of the skin presents no problems and can be carried out without tension using either interrupted Dexon or skin staples for extra speed. No attempt is usually made to close the fascia, as the defect is usually too large. The author feels that the old practice of sartorious muscle transplant to cover the femoral vessels is not necessary, as the risk of disruption appears to be more theoretical than real.

A similar procedure is now performed on the opposite side.

Radical vulvectomy

The patient is now placed in the lithotomy position.

The vulvar incision must be varied according to the size and position of the cancer. The basic principles of removal are:

1. A wide margin of normal skin surrounding the cancer must be removed.
2. The margin must be adequate both laterally and medially. It is very tempting to pass very close to a cancer which lies close to the urethra or anus. It is in these circumstances that a desire to preserve such structures will increase the risk of local recurrence.
3. All dystrophic skin must be removed with the specimen.

In parts of Europe and North America, cutting electrodiathermy is used for this part of the procedure as there is a theoretical reduction in small vessel bleeding. Most of the hemorrhage, however, arises from three sites, the two pudendal vessels and the clitoral base; electrodiathermy cannot cope with vessels of this size. The author therefore prefers a standard knife technique, picking up the major bleeding sites with clips.

The incision that was carried into the crural fold is now extended inferiorly lateral to the vulva to end alongside the anus. If the cancer is large, it may be necessary to extend the incision onto thigh skin. The anus is skirted by a

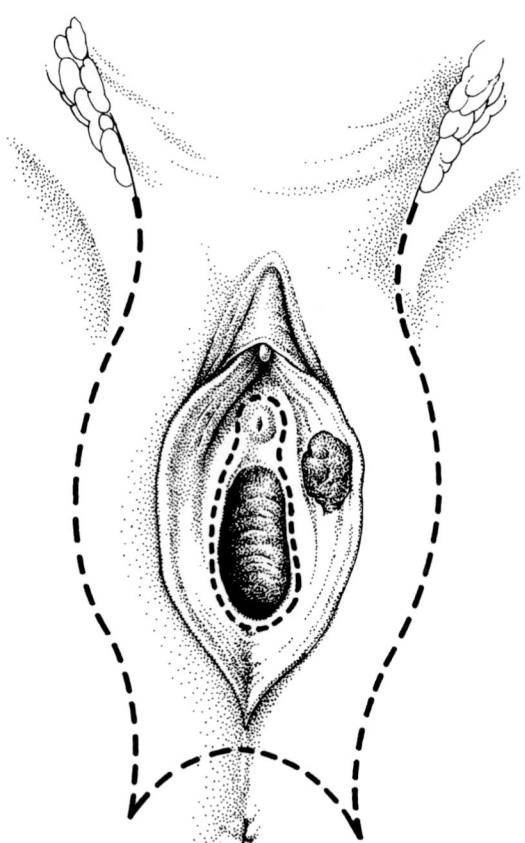

Fig. 75.12 The incisions for the vulvar part of the dissection.

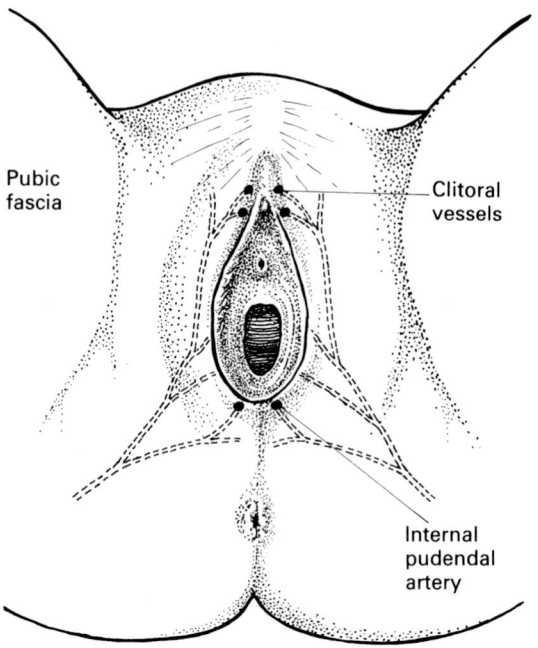

Fig. 75.13 Blood vessels encountered during vulvectomy.

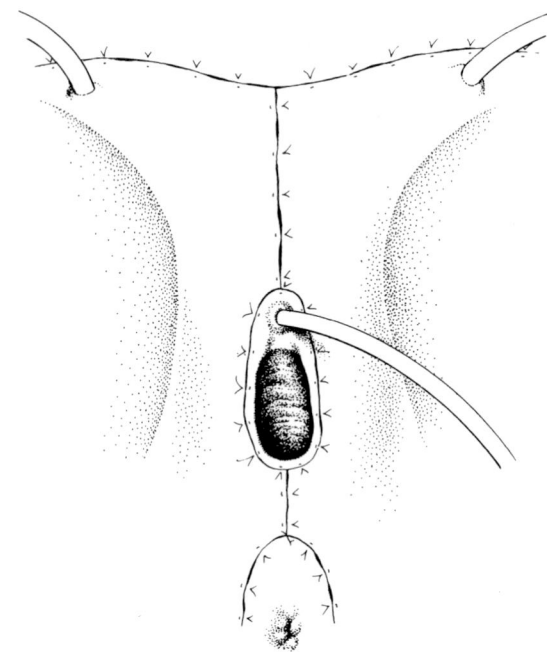

Fig. 75.14 Completed repair of the vulvar wound.

curved incision. A similar incision is made on the opposite side. The curved incision may be modified so that posterior releasing incisions are made to facilitate closure. These lateral incisions are carried down to muscle fascia. The urethra and vagina are now encircled by the inner incision, so as to clear the cancer medially (Fig. 75.12). If the lesion extends close to the urethra, it may be necessary to remove its lower half. Occasionally, if the cancer extends into the lower vagina, it is easier to cut vertically down to open the anterior part of the vagina, and then drop the whole tumor mass down to make the vaginal incision under direct vision thus reducing the risk of a compromised margin.

The lateral incisions are now deepened down to the deep fascia and periosteum and the entire vulva is removed. Free bleeding occurs at this time from three main sites; the ends of the two internal pudendal arteries, and the vascular erectile tissue around the base of the clitoris (Fig. 75.13). Square mattress sutures are of great value in dealing with these bleeding points.

Primary closure of these wounds is usually easily achieved, and the patient leaves theater lying flat, with suction drains in the groins and a three way catheter in her bladder (Fig. 75.14). If closure of the vulvar wound cannot be achieved without tension, either a flap may be swung from the thigh or the area left open and packed with an antiseptic gauze which can be replenished in the post-operative period.

VARIATIONS IN TECHNIQUE

In recent years, there have been many moves towards individualization of treatment for patients with cancer of the

vulva. DiSaia, in 1987,[23] put a case against the traditional surgical concept of an 'en bloc' dissection for a number of cancers, including vulva. There is no doubt that at times this operation may be carried out without the need for continuity of tissue between the vulva and the groin. Indeed, Stoeckel,[54] in some of his early writings commented on the use of separate incisions, as have others,[7,11,12] Hacker discusses this procedure using separate incisions in Chapter 76. Since 1985, the author has carried out 72 operations using a three incision technique. The lines of incision are shown in Figure 75.15. The technique is very simply performed and gives the same access to the groins as the butterfly incision. The groin dissection is performed as described in this chapter, and the dissection is completed by removing the block of tissue at the point where the

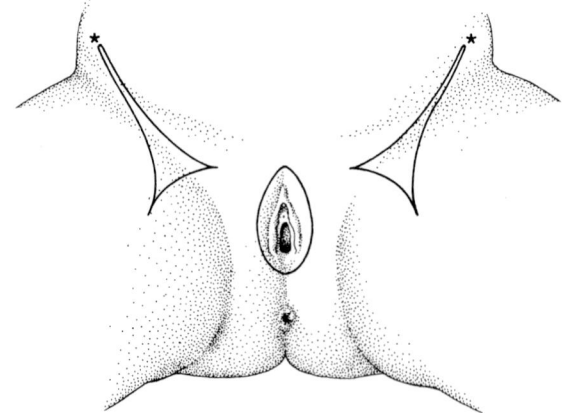

Fig. 75.15 The three incision technique used for radical vulvectomy and groin node dissection.

round ligament appears from the inguinal canal. The skin may be closed as a Y using a Dexon suture to bring the midpoints together, and the remainder is apposed using a stapling device. If the skin to be removed is kept to a minimum, then the arrow shaped incision can be closed as a single line. There is no tension in the wounds and the primary healing rate is excellent. Drainage of the space is essential.

Variations of the basic butterfly incision

Separate incisions

Stoeckel,[54] Ballon,[5] Hacker,[30] and Taussig[56] all used separate incisions for selected cases. Christopherson, in 1985,[14] reported a case with a recurrence in the skin bridge; however, this appears to be a rare complication.

Rotational flaps and grafting

Chafe,[13] Trelford,[58] Wheeless,[64] Achauer[2] and Knapstein[40] have all demonstrated various rotational flaps to cover the inguinal and vulvar defect. Lifshitz has used porcine grafts.

Delayed closure

Although this technique is old, Daly[18] has demonstrated a reduced hospitalization rate using this method. Final healing took almost 7 weeks on average.

Incision modifications

There have been many modifications of the original 'butterfly' incisions,[1,28] and the groin nodes have been removed using a 'sneak' technique burrowing under the crural and groin skin.[42]

This wide variety of techniques reflects on man's inventiveness. However, the basic principle of surgery remains. For the best results, the groin nodes must be completely removed and a radical resection of all the vulva tumor must be performed, including a satisfactory margin of normal tissue.

POSTOPERATIVE CARE AND COMPLICATIONS

Radical surgery has the potential to produce major complications. Probably because the procedures performed for vulvar cancer do not involve entering the abdomen or seriously compromising fluid and electrolyte balance, the complications experienced tend not to be life threatening, but they do require careful and often prolonged nursing to produce satisfactory recovery.

The epidural catheter is removed at the end of the procedure. Subcutaneous heparin 5000 units b.d. is administered for 10 days. As the patient's legs are no longer immobilized, she is encouraged to commence active movements at a very early stage. It is probably this factor, as much as the subcutaneous heparin or anti-embolism stockings, which has contributed to the reduction of thromboembolic disease in the postoperative period.

Prophylactic antibiotics are not routinely used to supplement the intraoperative regimen, although they should be rapidly prescribed if there is any sign of systemic infection.

Primary healing is now achieved in the majority of patients. Wound breakdown, however, remains the major complication for approximately 20% of patients. It should be treated by meticulous local cleansing using Eusol and hydrogen peroxide or one of the commercially available debriding agents. Thereafter, wound healing can be promoted by the use of honey dressings and artificial sea water baths. Silastic foam dressings have improved the healing rate after wound breakdown, but are now banned in some countries. The mainstay of good wound healing is meticulous nursing care.

It is often found that the wounds are completely healed before drainage has stopped; in these circumstances, the patient may have to suffer a small lymphatic fistula or even the development of a tense femoro-inguinal lymphocyst before drainage ceases. Piver et al[48] postulated that prophylactic heparin anticoagulation may be a possible cause of femoro-inguinal lymphocyst. The author has not been able to confirm any association.

Leg edema is a frequent problem which may arise in the postoperative period or may develop slowly in the months following operation It is more frequent following groin infection, particularly when associated with cellulitis of the thigh. It is important that lymphangitis be actively treated with antibiotics. For the patient with established edema, exercises, massage (both manual and mechanical) and elevation will help to reduce the problem.

Osteitis pubis can be a seriously debilitating complication. In the author's series, four patients out of 345 have developed the problem. It is characterized by intense pubic pain, particularly on weight bearing or walking. Often, X-ray and bone scan may not show any evidence of bone damage for a long period after symptoms begin. The diagnosis should be made on clinical grounds and the patient started on long-term antibiotics suitable for bony infections.

Occasionally, groin herniae, especially after pelvic node dissection and vaginal prolapse, may occur and require surgical correction.

POSTOPERATIVE MANAGEMENT OF NODAL METASTASES

Positive groin nodes

There appears to be general agreement that if fewer than four groin nodes are involved the patient's prognosis is excellent, since the chance of extension to the pelvic nodes is negligible and surgery is adequate. However, the results of purely surgical treatment when the groin nodes are extensively involved, would suggest that surgery alone is not the answer.

There is clearly a place for an extended study of the use of adjunctive treatment for those patients with two or more involved groin nodes.[35] In such cases, the author recommends radiotherapy in fields to cover the groins and the pelvic lymph nodes along the external iliac vessels. In the past, such a study has been difficult because of accrual problems and the prolonged healing time involved when traditional incisions are used. The healing time can be considerably reduced by performing separate groin incisions, thus the patient may begin her adjunctive treatment earlier.

Positive pelvic nodes

For the patient with involved pelvic lymph nodes, the prospects of survival are poor, with a 5-year rate around 20%. A recent report by Homesley et al[35] showed that there is a significant survival advantage over surgery alone when radiotherapy is used postoperatively to treat the groin and pelvic areas, with a significant associated reduction in groin recurrences.

Systemic chemotherapy for the management of the patient with positive pelvic nodes appears to be of limited value, however. This may be because of the relatively poor condition of such patients, and the low response rate of carcinoma of the vulva.

LOCAL RECURRENCE

Approximately 15% of patients will develop local recurrence. The most common sites are close to the urethra and around the anus and fourchette. One of the main reasons for these central recurrences is that the margin of normal tissue removed is often reduced on the medial aspect because of the closeness of vital structures, such as the urethra and the anal musculature. It is particularly important not to sacrifice these margins in the interest of saving such structures.

Management

If the recurrence is recognized early, further surgery can be performed so as to satisfactorily remove the affected area with a margin of normal tissue. However, many recurrences are extremely close to or involve the urethra or anal margin. Since surgery would involve the removal of, or severe damage to, these structures, radiotherapy, usually in the form of local implantation, has been used extensively to treat these areas. External beam irradiation has also been used with some success, particularly using electron beam techniques. With further recurrence after radiotherapy, more extensive surgery in the form of exenteration with an appropriate bypass procedure may be necessary.

As with all patients with vulvar cancer, a high degree of individualization is essential.

IN CONCLUSION

The surgical management of cancer of the vulva should be carried out in departments with a considerable surgical, anesthetic and nursing experience of the disease. This centralization will result in high operability rates (97% in the author's current series), and excellent long-term survivals. In a series of over 345 cases, the author has an overall actuarial 5-year survival of 72%. When the groin nodes are negative, this rate rises to 94.7%; it falls to 62% when they are positive. The operative mortality is 2%.

ACKNOWLEDGEMENT

Figures 75.1 to 75.12 and Figures 75.14 and 75.15 are reproduced with permission from Monaghan J M (ed) (1985) Bonney's Gynaecological Surgery. Baillière Tindall, London.

REFERENCES

1. Abitol M M 1973 Carcinoma of the vulva: improvements in the surgical approach. Am J Obstet Gynecol 117: 483
2. Achauer B M, Braly P, Berman M L, DiSaia P J 1984 Immediate vaginal reconstruction following resection for malignancy using the gluteal flap. Gynecol Oncol 19: 79
3. Andreasson B, Bock J E, Visfeldt J 1982 Prognostic role of histology in squamous cell carcinoma in the vulvar region. Gynecol Oncol 14: 373
4. Andreasson B, Nyboe J 1985 Value of prognostic parameters in squamous cell carcinoma of the vulva. Gynecol Oncol 22: 341
5. Ballon S C, Lamb E J 1975 Separate inguinal incisions in the treatment of carcinoma of the vulva. Surg Gynecol Obstet 140: 81
6. Barclay D L, Collins C R, Macey A B 1964 Cancer of the Bartholin gland: a review and report of 8 cases. Obstet Gynecol 24: 329
7. Basset A 1912 Traitement chirurgical operatoire de l'epithelioma primitif de clitoris. Rev Chir Paris 46: 546
8. Benedet J L, Turko M, Fairey R N, Boyes D A 1979 Squamous carcinoma of the vulva: results of treatment, 1938 to 1976. Am J Obstet Gynecol 134: 201
9. Boronow R C 1982 Combined therapy as an alternative to exenteration for locally advanced vulvo-vaginal cancer. Cancer 49: 1085
10. Breslow A 1970 Thickness, cross sectional areas and depth of invasion in the prognosis of cutaneous melanoma. Annal Surg 172: 902
11. Byron R L, Lamb E J, Yonemoto R H, Kase S 1962 Radical inguinal node dissection in the treatment of cancer. Surg Obstet Gynecol 114: 401
12. Byron R L, Mishell D R, Yonemoto R H 1965 The surgical treatment of invasive cancer of the vulva. Surg Obstet Gynecol 121: 1243
13. Chafe W, Fowler W C, Walton L A, Currie J L 1983 Radical vulvectomy with use of tensor fascia lata flap. Am J Obstet Gynecol 145: 207
14. Christopherson W, Buchsbaum H J, Voet R, Lifschitz S 1985

Radical vulvectomy and bilateral groin lymphadenectomy utilising separate groin incisions: report of a case with recurrence in the intervening skin bridge. Gynecol Oncol 21: 247

15. Clark W H, From L, Bernadino E A, Mihm M C 1969 The histogenesis and biologic behavior of primary human malignant melanomas of the skin. Cancer Research 29: 705

16. Copeland L J, Nour Sneige, Gershenson D M, McGuffie V B, Abdul-Karim F, Rutledge F N 1986 Bartholin gland carcinoma. Obstet Gynecol 67: 794

17. Curry S L, Wharton J T, Rutledge F N 1980 Positive lymph nodes in vulvar squamous carcinoma. Gynecol Oncol 9: 63

18. Daly J W, Pomerance A J 1979 Groin dissection with prevention of tissue loss and postoperative infection. Obstet Gynecol 53: 395

19. Daseler E H, Anson B J, Reimann A F 1948 Radical excision of the inguinal and iliac lymph glands. Surg Gynecol Obstet 87: 679

20. Davison T, Kissin M, Westbury G 1987 Vulvo-vaginal melanoma – should radical surgery be abandoned? Br J Obstet Gynaecol 94: 473

21. Deppe G, Cohen C J, Bruckner H W 1979 Chemotherapy of squamous cell carcinoma of the vulva: a review. Gynecol Oncol 7: 345

22. DiPaolo G R, Gomez-Rueda N, Arrighi L 1975 Relevance of microinvasion in carcinoma of the vulva. Obstet Gynecol 45: 647

23. DiSaia P J 1987 The case against the surgical concept of en bloc dissection for certain malignancies of the reproductive tract. Cancer 60: 2025

24. DiSaia P J, Creasman W T, Rich W M 1979 An alternate approach to early cancer of the vulva. Am J Obstet Gynecol 133: 825

25. Edington P T, Monaghan J M 1980 Malignant melanoma of the vulva and vagina. Br J Obstet Gynaecol 87: 422

26. Fairey R N, Mackay P A, Benedet J L, Boyes D A, Turko M 1985 Radiation treatment of carcinoma of the vulva, 1950–1980. Am J Obstet Gynecol 151: 591

27. Friedrich E G, DiPaolo G R 1977 Postoperative staging of vulvar carcinoma: a retrospective study. Int J Gynecol Obstet 15: 270

28. Goldberg M I, Belinson J L, Ford J H, Averette H E 1979 Surgical management of invasive carcinoma of the vulva utilizing a lower midline incision. Gynecol Oncol 7: 296

29. Green T H 1978 Carcinoma of the vulva; reassessment. Obstet Gynecol 52: 462

30. Hacker N F, Leuchter R S, Berek J S, Castaldo T W, Lagasse L D 1981 Radical vulvectomy and bilateral inguinal lymphadenectomy through separate groin incisions. Obstet Gynecol 58: 574

31. Hacker N F, Berek J S, Lagasse L D, Nieberg R K, Leuchter R S 1984 Individualisation of treatment for Stage I squamous cell vulvar carcinoma. Obstet Gynecol 63: 155

32. Hacker N F, Berek J S, Juillard G J F, Lagasse L D 1984 Preoperative radiation therapy for locally advanced vulvar cancer. Cancer 54: 2056

33. Hammond I G, Monaghan J M 1983 Multicentric carcinoma of the female genital tract. Br J Obstet Gynaecol 90: 557

34. Hoffman J S, Kumar N B, Morley G W 1983 Microinvasive squamous carcinoma of the vulva: search for a definition. Obstet Gynecol 61: 615

35. Homesley H D, Bundy B N, Sedlis A, Adcock L 1986 Radiation therapy versus pelvic node resection for carcinoma of the vulva with positive groin nodes. Obstet Gynecol 68: 733

36. Iversen T, Abeler V, Aalders J 1981 Individualised treatment of Stage I carcinoma of the vulva. Obstet Gynecol 57: 85

37. Iversen T, Aas M 1983 Lymph drainage of the vulva. Gynecol Oncol 16: 179

38. Jafari K, Cartnick E N 1976 Microinvasive squamous cell carcinoma of the vulva. Gynecol Oncol 4: 158

39. Japaze H, Van Dinh T, Woodruff J D 1981 Verrucous carcinoma of the vulva: study of 24 cases. Obstet Gynecol 60: 462

40. Knapstein P G, Friedberg V 1987 Plastische Chirurgie in der Gynakologie. Georg Thieme Verlag, Stuttgart, p 90

41. Leuchter R S, Hacker N F, Voet R L, Berek J S, Townsend D E, Lagasse L D 1982 Primary carcinoma of the Bartholin gland: a report of 14 cases and review of the literature. Obstet Gynecol 60: 361

42. Monaghan J M 1985 Management of carcinoma of the vulva. In: Shepherd J S, Monaghan J M (eds) Clinical Gynaecological Oncology. Blackwells, Oxford

43. Monaghan J M, Hammond I G 1984 Pelvic node dissection in the treatment of vulval carcinoma – is it necessary? Brit J Obstet Gynaecol 91: 270

44. Nakao C Y, Nolan J F, DiSaia P J, Futoran R 1974 'Microinvasive' epidermoid carcinoma of the vulva with an unexpected natural history. Am J Obstet Gynecol 120: 1122

45. Parker R T, Duncan I, Rampone J, Creasman W 1975 Operative management of early invasive epidermoid carcinoma of the vulva. Am J Obstet Gynecol 123: 349

46. Parry-Jones E 1963 Lymphatics of the vulva. Br J Obstet Gynaecol 70: 751

47. Patsner B, Mann W J 1988 Radical vulvectomy and 'sneak' superficial inguinal lymphadenectomy with a single elliptical incision. Am J Obstet Gynecol 158: 464

48. Piver S M, Malfetano J H, Lele S B, Moore R H 1983 Prophylactic anticoagulation as a possible cause of inguinal lymphocyst after radical vulvectomy and inguinal lymphadenectomy. Obstet Gynecol 62: 17

49. Piver M S, Xynos F P 1977 Pelvic lymphadenectomy in women with carcinoma of the clitoris. Obstet Gynecol 49: 592

50. Podratz K C, Symmonds R E, Taylor W F, Williams T J 1980 Treatment of invasive squamous cell carcinoma of the vulva at the Mayo Clinic 1955–1975. (Abstract) Gynecol Oncol 10: 362

51. Podratz K C, Symmonds R E, Taylor W F 1982 Carcinoma of the vulva: analysis of treatment failures. Am J Obstet Gynecol 143: 340

52. Podratz K C, Gaffey T A, Symmonds R E, Johansen K L, O'Brien P C 1983 Melanoma of the vulva: an update. Gynecol Oncol 16: 153

53. Rutledge F N, Smith J P, Franklin E W 1970 Carcinoma of the vulva. Am J Obstet Gynecol 106: 1117

54. Stoeckel W 1930 Zur Therapie des Vulvakarzinoms. Zentralblatt fur Gynakologie 1: 47

55. Symmonds R E, Webb M J 1981 Pelvic exenteration. In: Coppleson M (ed) Gynecologic Oncology, 1st edn. Churchill Livingstone, London, p 896

56. Taussig F J 1935 Primary cancer of the vulva, vagina and female urethra: five year results. Surg Gynecol Obstet 60: 477

57. Taussig F J 1940 Cancer of the vulva: an analysis of 155 cases (1911–1940). Am J Obstet Gynecol 40: 764

58. Trelford J D, Deer D A, Ordorica E, Franti C E, Trelford-Suader M 1984 Ten year prospective study in a management change of vulvar carcinoma. Am J Obstet Gynecol 150: 288

59. Way S 1948 The anatomy of the lymphatic drainage of the vulva, and its influence on the radical operation for carcinoma. Ann Roy Coll Surg Engl 3: 187

60. Way S 1960 Carcinoma of the vulva. Am J Obstet Gynecol 79: 692

61. Wharton J T, Gallagher S, Rutledge F N 1974 Microinvasive carcinoma of the vulva. Am J Obstet Gynecol 118: 159

62. Wheeless C R, McGibbon B, Dorsey J H, Maxwell G P 1979 Gracilis myocutaneous flap in the reconstruction of the vulva and female perineum. Obstet Gynecol 54: 97

63. Yasigi R, Piver S M, Tsukada Y 1978 Microinvasive carcinoma of the vulva. Obstet Gynecol 51: 368

76. Conservative surgery for Stage I carcinoma of vulva

N. F. Hacker

INTRODUCTION

The modern management of Stage I carcinoma of the vulva is based on individualization of treatment.[1,2] There is no standard operation which is applicable to every patient. The emphasis is on performing the most conservative operation consistent with cure of the disease.

In considering the most appropriate operation, it is necessary to determine independently the best approach to (1) the primary tumor and (2) the groin lymph nodes. By definition, patients with Stage I vulvar cancer do not have clinically suspicious (N2) groin nodes, so such patients have virtually no risk of pelvic lymph node metastases.

MANAGEMENT OF THE PRIMARY LESION

Radical local excision is usually the most appropriate operation for the primary tumor in patients with Stage I vulvar cancer. The procedure is called a radical local excision to imply both a wide and a deep resection of the primary tumor.

In an elderly patient with extensive vulvar dystrophy or vulvar intraepithelial neoplasia (VIN) in addition to an invasive lesion, radical vulvectomy will still usually be the most appropriate operation. However, the groin dissection(s) may be performed through a separate incision or incisions, so primary healing should be achieved.

In younger patients with VIN and invasive carcinoma, it will be more appropriate to treat the VIN with laser therapy or superficial local excision(s), and the invasive focus with radical local excision, thereby achieving the best cosmetic result possible.

Technique for radical local excision

Labial lesions

A marking pen is used to outline the surgical resection margins. The lateral margin should be the labiocrural fold, and the medial margin the introitus. Anteriorly and posteriorly, the incision is shaped elliptically, to allow satis-

factory closure. A margin of at least 1 cm of normal skin should be left around the invasive disease (Fig. 76.1).

After incising the skin with a scalpel or the cutting mode of the electrosurgical unit, the coagulation mode is used for

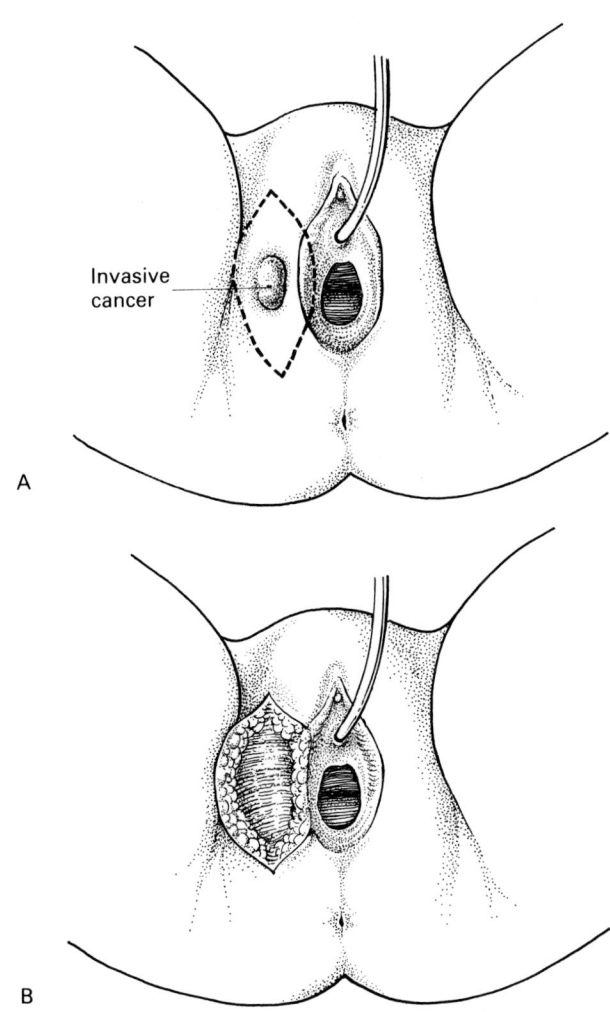

Fig. 76.1 Radical local excision of a lateral lesion. Note that the incision is carried down to the deep fascia. Margins of resection should be at least 1 cm.

the remainder of the procedure, as this will significantly decrease blood loss.

The dissection is commenced anteriorly and carried down to the level of the deep fascia. The inferior fascia of the urogenital diaphragm is coplanar with the fascia lata of the thigh and the fascia overlying the pubic symphysis. Once this plane is reached, a finger or artery forceps can be passed along the deep fascia to define the deep margin of resection and to elevate the tissue to be resected. Dissection of the medial and lateral margins is facilitated by grasping the edges with Allis forceps to keep the tissues on traction.

After securing hemostasis, the defect is closed in two layers.

Perineal lesions

For perineal or posterior fourchette lesions, the lateral margins are less clearly defined anatomically, but it is important to ensure at least 1 cm of normal skin around the invasive focus if possible (Fig. 76.2). This may be difficult for posterior lesions which are close to the anus, and preoperative or postoperative radiation to the vulva may be useful in such cases.

The deep margin of resection will be the anal sphincter and distal rectum. The correct rectovaginal space is best defined by sharp dissection with Metzenbaum scissors. The index finger of the left hand is placed in the rectum, while the assistant keeps upward traction on the perineal specimen with two pairs of Allis forceps. As with labial lesions, it is usually possible to close the defect primarily in two layers (Fig. 76.3). If the perineal defect is too large for primary closure, bilateral rhomboid flaps may be advanced (Fig. 76.4).

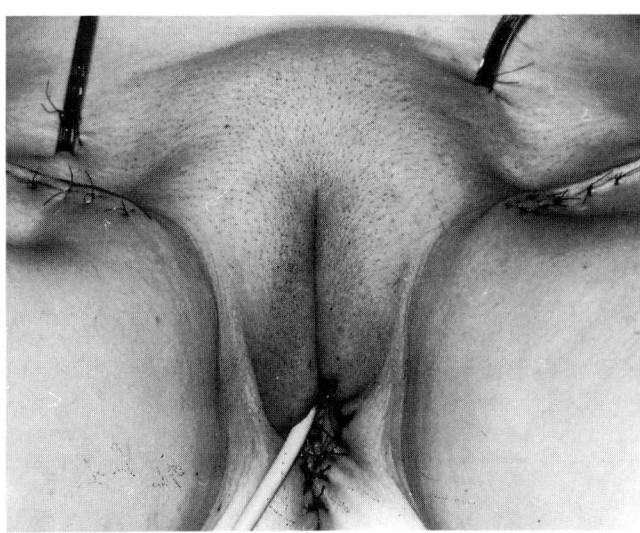

Fig. 76.3 Radical local excision and bilateral groin dissection. The lesion shown in Figure 76.2 has been excised, and primary closure achieved. Note that the groin nodes have been removed bilaterally through separate skin incisions.

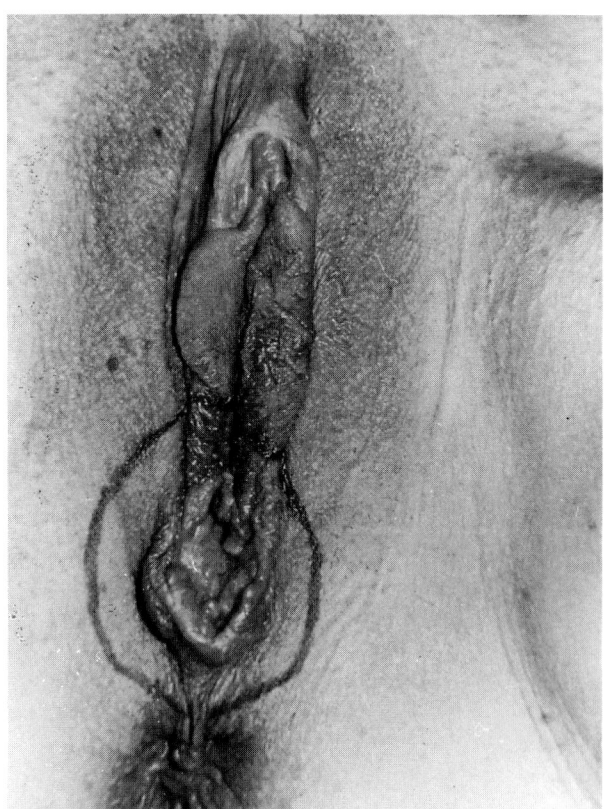

Fig. 76.2 Small carcinoma at the posterior fourchette. The closest margin in posterior lesions is always at the anus. Note that most of the labia can be spared in this case, as the remainder of the vulva is entirely normal.

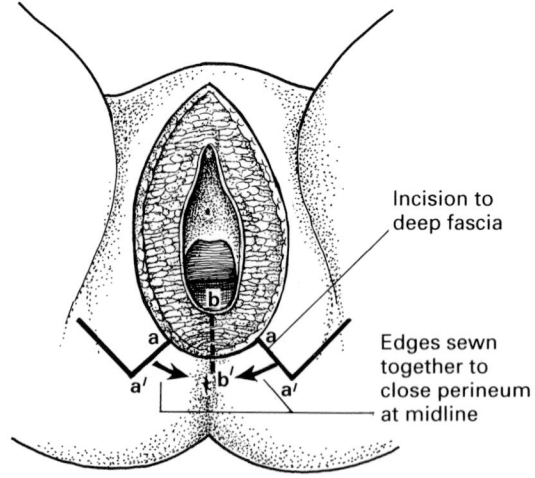

Incision to deep fascia

Edges sewn together to close perineum at midline

Fig. 76.4 Bilateral rhomboid flaps. The incisions are carried down to the deep fascia. The length a–a' should equal the diameter of the perineal defect b–b'.

Clitoral lesions

In elderly women, the simplest procedure is to perform a radical vulvectomy. If a radical local excision is performed and the labia are left, they may become very edematous and uncomfortable because of the interruption of lymphatic channels which are passing forward from the vulva prior to deviating laterally to the inguinal lymph nodes. This may become so uncomfortable that resection of residual labia has to be subsequently performed. In younger patients, radiation therapy may be considered in order to preserve the clitoris.

Technique for radical vulvectomy

To perform the vulvectomy, an elliptical lateral incision is made, commencing anteriorly on the mons pubis, passing posteriorly along each labiocrural fold, and ending at the perineal body. The medial incision passes around the introitus, anterior to the urethra. If the tumor encroaches close to the urethra, it may be necessary to sacrifice the distal 1 cm of urethra in order to achieve satisfactory clearance. With this elliptical incision, primary closure in two layers should be achieved without tension. If the perineum is normal, it is easier to leave it intact, removing

a horseshoe-shaped piece of tissue extending from the mons pubis anteriorly to the posterior aspect of each labium majus.

MANAGEMENT OF THE GROIN LYMPH NODES

Groin dissection may be omitted in patients with Stage I vulvar cancer whose tumor penetrates the stroma 1 mm or less, as such patients have virtually no risk of lymph node metastases. All other patients should ideally have a unilateral groin dissection if the tumor is laterally located, or a bilateral dissection if it is centrally located.

Technique for groin dissection

With a marking pen, a line is drawn 1 cm below and parallel to the groin crease. The line should be 10 to 12 cm long, and should start laterally at the medial border of the sartorius muscle and extend to the lateral border of the adductor longus (Fig. 76.5). This line defines the incision, which may be linear in most patients. If there is a possibility of impaired vascularity (e.g. in an elderly or diabetic patient), it is preferable to remove an ellipse of skin based on this line. This will improve the likelihood of primary healing.

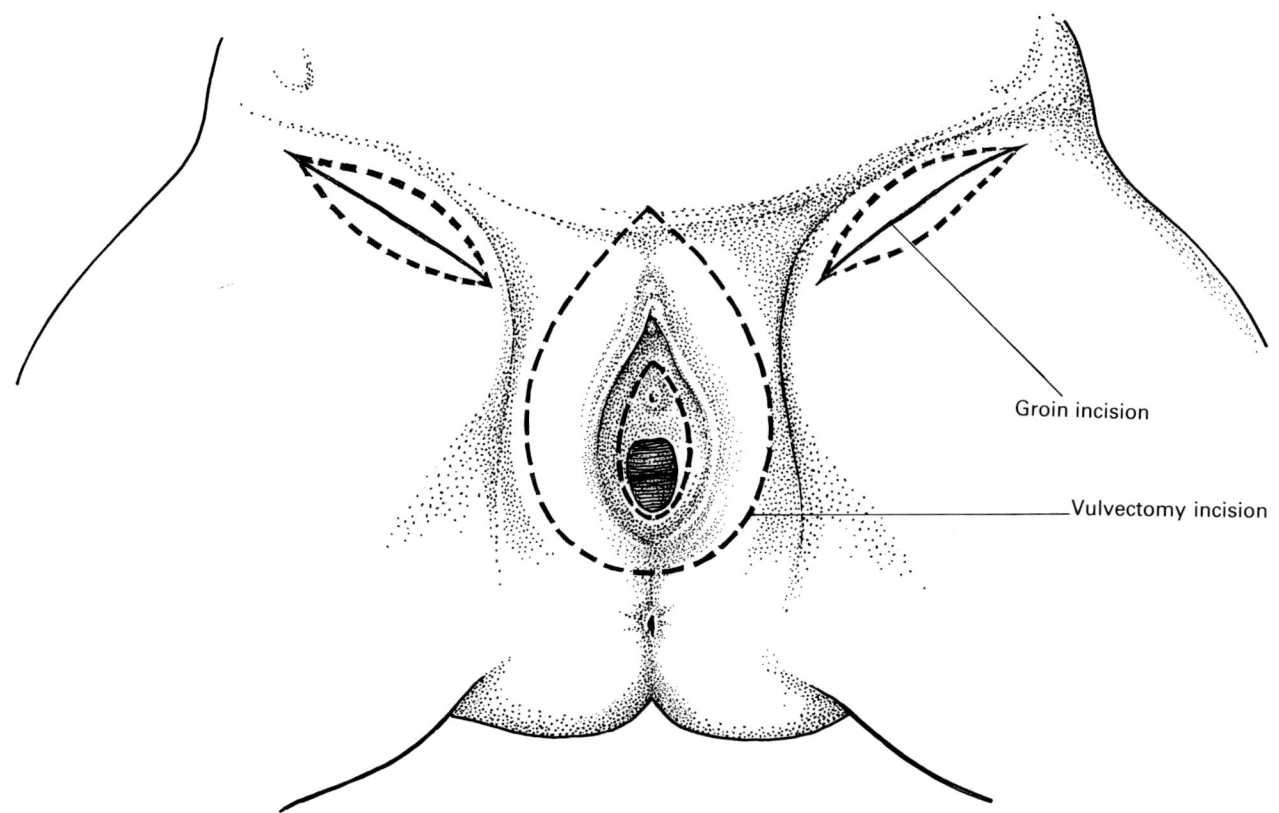

Fig. 76.5 The skin incision for groin dissection through a separate incision. If there is a likelihood of skin necrosis (e.g. elderly or diabetic patients) it is desirable to make an elliptical rather than a linear incision.

The incision is carried through the skin and sub-cutaneous tissues to the superficial (Camper's) fascia (Fig. 76.6). The inguinal lymph nodes lie between this superficial fascia and the fascia lata. There are no lymph nodes in the subcutaneous fat, and this layer of fat must be carefully preserved if primary healing is to be achieved.

The superficial fascia is incised along the length of the skin incision. This fascia is then grasped with two artery forceps and traction applied, to define the level for the dissection of the skin flaps (Fig. 76.7). The upper skin flap

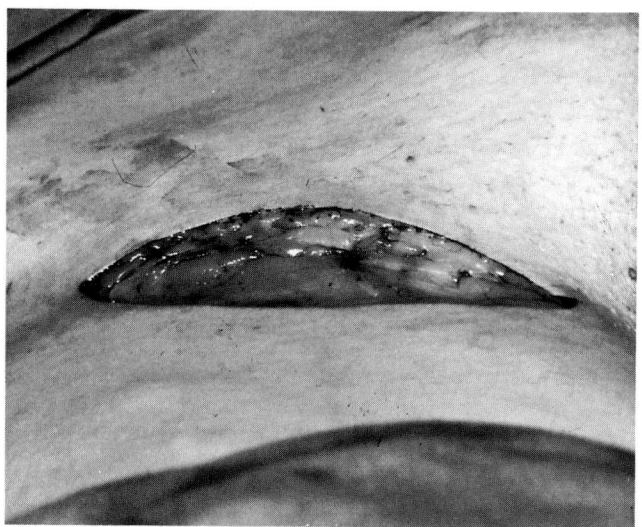

Fig. 76.6 The groin incision. An ellipse of skin has been excised, down to Camper's fascia. Note the subcutaneous fat on the superior skin edge. This fat must be preserved to avoid wound necrosis.

is developed initially. While an assistant keeps traction on the superficial fascia, the surgeon keeps traction on the node-bearing fatty pad with a small sponge, while using Metzenbaum scissors to dissect this fatty pad off the overlying superficial fascia. The dissection extends about 2 cm above the inguinal ligament. The inferior skin flap is developed in a similar fashion, the dissection extending to the apex of the femoral triangle.

Having raised the skin flaps, the inguinal node-bearing fatty pad is then ready to be removed from the fascia lata and external oblique aponeurosis. Inferiorly and medially, the saphenous vein is tied off at the apex of the femoral triangle. Similarly, it is tied off at its entry into the femoral vein. Using the coagulation mode of the electrosurgical unit, the dissection is carried down to the fascia lata around the borders of the femoral triangle, and the fatty pad is then stripped off the fascia lata using traction and some sharp dissection. Preservation of the fascia lata minimizes femoral nerve injury.

Having removed the inguinal nodes, the fascia lata is then incised longitudinally over the femoral vessels from the inguinal ligament to the apex of the femoral triangle. The fatty femoral node-bearing tissue is then dissected off the femoral artery and vein, particularly medially between the femoral artery and the adductor longus muscle (Fig. 76.8). Cloquet's node is removed from the femoral canal. If any significant defect is present in the region of the femoral canal, the inguinal ligament is sutured to Cooper's ligament with 0 black-silk to prevent a femoral hernia.

Unless the patient is at high risk for infection (e.g. is obese or diabetic) there is no need to release the sartorius

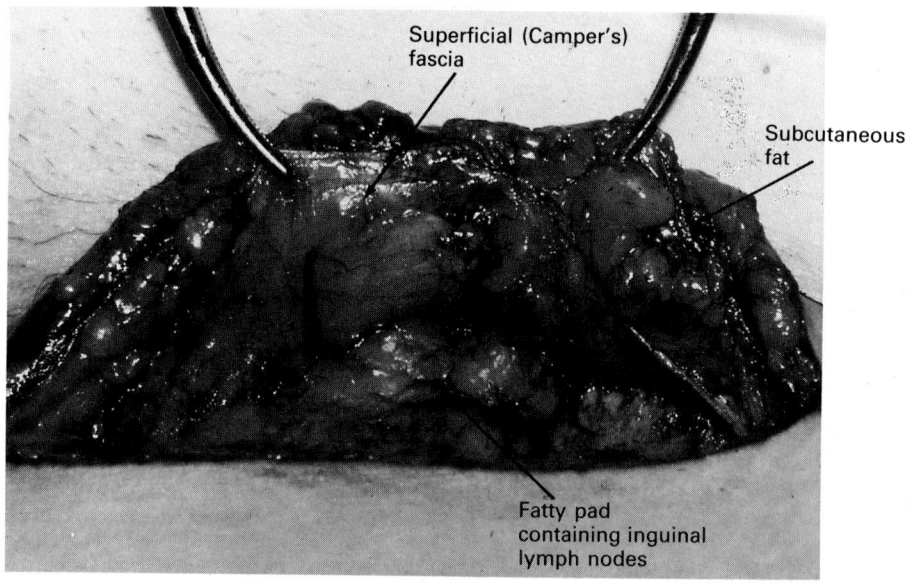

Fig. 76.7 Elevation of the superior skin flap. The Camper's fascia is grasped by two artery forceps so that it can be elevated and placed on traction. The fatty pad to the right contains the inguinal lymph nodes and lies between Camper's fascia and the fascia lata.

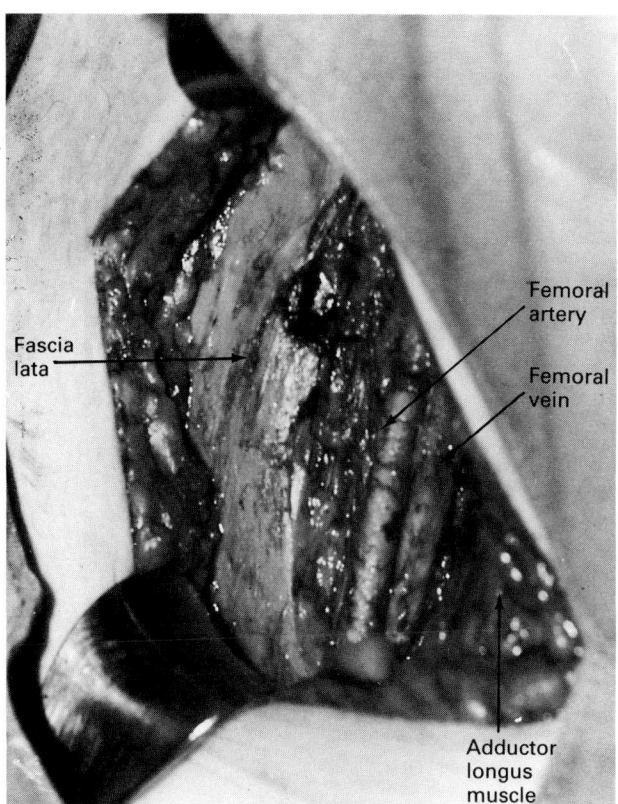

Fascia lata

Femoral artery

Femoral vein

Adductor longus muscle

Fig. 76.8 Inguinal-femoral lymphadenectomy. Note the femoral artery and vein have been dissected out. The fascia lata seen to the left has been preserved, as has the subcutaneous fat.

muscle from the anterior superior iliac spine and transpose it across to cover the femoral vessels.

A negative suction drainage tube is inserted and brought out in the iliac fossa, and the incision closed in two layers.

POSTOPERATIVE CARE

The patient is kept in bed for four days, leg movement is actively encouraged, and subcutaneous heparin is given to help prevent deep venous thrombosis. The groin and vulvar wounds receive routine care. When the patient mobilizes fully on the fifth day, sitz baths are given twice daily, following which the vulva and perineum are dried with a hair dryer if necessary. The groin suction continues for about 10 days, to help prevent a groin seroma. The patient is usually ready for discharge about the 10th to 14th day. If there has been any breakdown of the groin or vulvar incisions, daily wound care by home nurses will ensure adequate granulation and epithelialization.

REFERENCES

1. Hacker N F, Berek J S, Lagasse L D, Nieberg R K, Leuchter R S 1984 Individualisation of treatment for Stage I squamous cell vulvar carcinoma. Obstet Gynecol 63: 155
2. Iversen T, Abeler V, Aalders J 1981 Individualised treatment for Stage I carcinoma of the vulva. Obstet Gynecol 57: 85

77. Radical vaginal operations: I. Schauta radical vaginal hysterectomy, II. Vaginectomy

Sir Rustam Feroze

I. SCHAUTA RADICAL VAGINAL HYSTERECTOMY

The radical vaginal hysterectomy was developed by Schauta[20] at the turn of the century at about the same time as Wertheim[23] was promoting the radical abdominal hysterectomy. The operation has since been modified by Amreich[1] and by Stoeckel[22] and it is their techniques that are usually described today. The basic principles are constant but there are variations in the sequence of the steps of the operation all of which may be applicable under varying circumstances. The operation has never had the popularity amongst British and American gynecologists that it has amongst the Europeans and in particular the German school of surgeons. Today it is probably regarded more as of historical interest than of practical use.

In the early days of surgery the advantages of a vaginal approach to hysterectomy considerably outweighed those of an abdominal one. There was no abdominal wound, no transgression of abdominal peritoneum, little disturbance of the intestines and in the early days of anesthesia the pelvic surgeon could supplement relatively light general anesthesia with local anesthesia. As a result the morbidity and mortality compared very favorably indeed with the abdominal operations. The considerable improvements in anesthesia, preoperative techniques and postoperative care have obviated the advantages once held by the vaginal route.

There probably still is an advantage as regards mortality and morbidity especially in regard to injury of the urinary tract. Navratil[16] had an operative mortality of 0.85% in 724 cases with a general fistula rate of 1.2% and only 0.27% ureteric fistula and he and Lirmberger[17] declared a ureteric fistula rate of 0.5% in 1003 cases. Despite the remaining advantages of the vaginal approach it is faulted irretrievably in the eyes of most by failure to remove the lymph nodes draining the cervix. Mitra[14] overcame this disadvantage by combining the operation with extraperitoneal lymphadenectomy either in stages or concomitantly; today such a procedure seems illogical in the face of the modern Wertheim operation. Chowdhury[4] has persisted with the Mitra operation. Starting with the bilateral extraperitoneal dissection he also ligates the ovarian and uterine vessels with partial mobilization of the parametria, he then proceeds to the radical vaginal procedure. If the lymph nodes show malignant involvement; postoperative external irradiation is

Table 77.1 Results of Mitra operation. 5-year survival rate (%).*

Stage	Number of cases (%)	5-year survival (%)
I	21.0	76.2
II	69.5	54.3
III	9.5	40.0
I, II, III		60.9

* From: Chowdhury (1976)[4]: 270 cases

used. His results in 230 cases are shown in Table 77.1. The primary mortality for the series was 1.8%. De Graff[5] is also an exponent of what he calls the Mitra-Schauta operation. His regime is quite a marathon for the patient. First a preoperative dose of intracavitary radium for 42 hours is placed; 4 weeks later bilateral extraperitoneal lymphadenectomy and radical vaginal hysterectomy with bilateral Schuchardt incisions is performed and then if the lymph nodes are involved the patient receives external irradiation. A fistula rate of 2.9% is recorded as low! 5-year survival rates (%) for Stages Ib, IIa, IIb are given as 83.9, 72.2, 68.9% respectively. In the last 20 years there has been a steady decline in reports of the operation in the treatment of carcinoma of the cervix to the extent that Nelson[18] did not see fit to include it in his *Atlas of Radical Pelvic Surgery*. There are a number of reasons for this decline — firstly there has been a great increase in the use of radiotherapy to the detriment of radical surgery in general. Even when surgery is preferred many surgeons feel confident in attempting the radical abdominal procedure but only a few are prepared to undertake the vaginal equivalent largely from lack of training and experience. Another and more important factor is that the whole concept of what is a radical operation has changed. In the past surgeons were concerned to remove as much parametrial tissue as possible and there is no doubt that this can be done with far greater effect from the vagina where the ligaments are within closer reach and vision of the surgeon. Now that only early cases are subjected to surgery this wide excision is thought to be less important than the lymphadenectomy. It might then be considered that the vaginal approach would be ideal for the very early stages but microinvasive carcinoma has been shown to be associated with virtually no lymph node involvement so that total hysterectomy either vaginal or abdominal, should be adequate treatment. Kudo et al[12] propose a modified radical vaginal procedure for microinvasive disease; they dissect the lower end of the ureter to allow excision of the parametria to a distance of 2 cm. Kovacic et al[11] still advocate the radical vaginal operation for Stage Ia disease and report a 5-year survival of 97.3% in 147 cases. They also advocate it for women aged over 40 who have cervical intraepithelial neoplasia where they find a higher incidence (14.4%) of associated microinvasion than is found in younger women. Occult invasion requires a more extensive procedure and as the incidence of lymph node involvement must be low the radical vaginal operation would suit the majority of cases. Because many of the patients are young, most surgeons prefer Wertheim's hysterectomy, modified as to the extent of the parametrial excision and with conservation of the ovaries but inclusive of pelvic lymphadenectomy (Ch. 42).

So it appears that all the advantages once attributed to the Schauta operation have been whittled away. However, before casting the procedure into limbo it is only fair to examine its record in practice as opposed to theory. On theoretical grounds the value of lymphadenectomy does not stand too well. It has been generally accepted that not less than 10% of Stage I cancers of the cervix have involved pelvic lymph nodes at operation and it has been shown that 25 to 50% of such patients treated survive 5 years or more, so that it could be argued that for every 100 women with Stage I lesions only 5 at the most are salvaged as a result of lymphadenectomy and that 95 undergo unnecessarily a procedure which considerably increases mortality and morbidity. Morley & Seski[15] found 12.6% involved nodes in 143 cases of Stage I carcinoma of cervix of whom 55% were alive at 5 years. This suggests that the Schauta operation is not so illogical and the results of treatment reported by its advocates support this contention.

Table 77.2 shows the results obtained by those expert in

the technique and it must be admitted that they compare favorably with figures for other methods of treatment. Inguilla & Stocker[8] treated some of their patients with postoperative radiotherapy and noticed an improvement in their Stage II results. It has been shown[19] that external radiation can destroy tumor in pelvic lymph nodes so that this adjunctive treatment could be used to counterbalance the declared inadequacy of the vaginal operation. Schwarz & Büttner[21] reporting on 234 radical vaginal hysterectomies performed with low morbidity and no mortality found that where the tumor was greater than 20×20 mm at the surface or extended more than 10 mm in depth the 5-year survival was 75% but where the tumor was less than this three dimensional measurement the 5-year survival was 91%. This suggests a method of selection and implies lymphatic involvement in the more advanced cases as would be expected. These more advanced cases would benefit from postoperative external radiation.

More recently, Carenza & Villani[3] have selected cases for radical vaginal hysterectomy with preoperative assessment of the lymph nodes using CT scanning, for which they claim an accuracy of 89%. They advocate the operation for cervical stump carcinoma in all stages up to IIa with negative lymphography; Stages Ia, Ib with negative lymphography and IIa with negative lymphography in patients unfit for abdominal surgery. They report results before and after selection by lymphography, showing an improvement with selection, as seen in Table 77.3. If the parametrium is involved histologically then external irradiation is used.

One of the major problems in any radical procedure for cancer of the cervix is damage to the urinary system and whilst today fistula formation has been reduced to an acceptable minimum there still remains a number of patients who suffer from loss of bladder sensation and control. This physiological damage follows both the abdominal and vaginal operations but is more common following the latter because the parametrial excision tends to be more extensive; Barclay & Roman-Lopez[2] found that the mean duration of postoperative catheter drainage in 68 patients treated by radical vaginal hysterectomy was 33 days. The problem for the bladder lies in the excision of the uterosacral ligaments to which the pelvic plexus is closely related. Kobayashi & Matsuzawa[10] have described a method in the abdominal approach of preserving the nervi erigentes which allows rapid return of bladder function

Table 77.2 Radical vaginal hysterectomy results of treatment: 5-year survival rate (%)

Authors	Inguilla & Stocker	Navratil	Navratil & Lirmberger
No. of cases	327	426	1003
Stage I	81.5	87.4	86.5
Stage II	56.1	59.2	55.4
	63.1 (I & II)		74.3 (I–III)

Table 77.3 Schauta-Amreich operation 5-year survival (%) before and after selection by lymphography.*

Stage	1968 to 71 (no selection)	1972 to 76 (selection).
Ia	90.4	100.
IIb	85.4	89.6
IIa	72.7	72.7

* From: Carenza & Villani (1982)[3]

postoperatively and does not reduce the radicality of the procedure (see Ch. 79) but in the vaginal approach the resection of the ligaments is a very necessary preliminary to the excision of the cardinal ligaments and no such niceties of dissection are possible.

SURGICAL ANATOMY

Before considering the techniques of the operation it is useful to consider the anatomy of the pelvis as it appears in the vaginal approach. As in the abdominal operation it is necessary to dissect the lower ureter so that it shall not be damaged whilst extending the limits of clearance of the pelvic fascia. In approaching the ureter the vaginal surgeon becomes aware of the existence and importance of the bladder pillars to an extent less obvious to the abdominal surgeon. The pillars invest the ureters and during the dissection a medial and lateral wall is artificially created; these are divided as far from the cervix as possible but this cannot be achieved with safety until the ureter has been dissected free and retracted out of the way (Fig. 77.1).

The altered relationship of the ureter and the uterine artery is another important variant in the vaginal approach. Under normal circumstances the uterine artery crosses medially in the roof of the ureteric tunnel before turning upwards to supply the uterus. The ureter runs forward in a tunnel of loose connective tissue in the upper part of the cardinal ligament to reach the side of the cervix above the vaginal angle before turning medially through the vesicocervical ligament to enter the bladder angle obliquely. This is the situation familar to the abdominal surgeon. In the vaginal operation the uterus is pulled downwards and the bladder retracted upwards with the result that the uterine vessels now run downwards and medially whilst the ureter runs downwards and then upwards to enter the

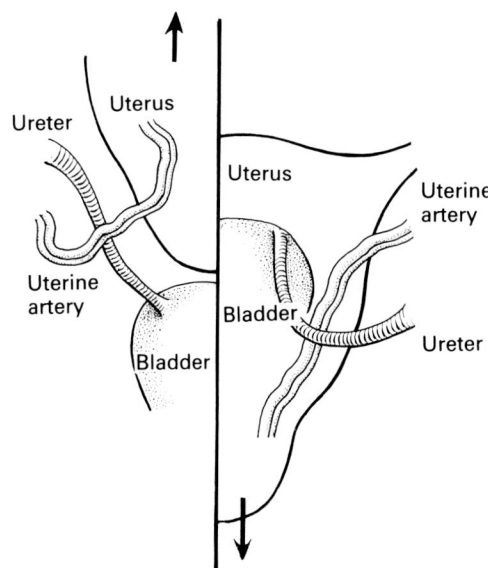

Fig. 77.2 Relation between ureters and uterine arteries with bladder displacement downwards in abdominal operation on left of figure and upwards in vaginal operation on right of figure.

bladder. There is thus created a ureteric loop, the bend of which is called the ureteric knee; through this loop run the uterine vessels passing first above and then beneath the ureter (Fig. 77.2).

Thus in order to ligate the uterine artery at as high a level as possible it is necessary to dissect and reflect the ureter. The ureteric branch of the uterine artery must be sacrificed so as to free the ureter completely; this artery is seen and divided in the performance of simple vaginal hysterectomy but then it is not necessary to dissect the ureters which however can always be palpated in the bladder pillars prior to reflecting the lateral angles of the bladder.

To free the bladder and demarcate the medial wall of the bladder pillars it is necessary to divide the posterior cervicovesical ligament or supravaginal septum. Because the initial dissection is between the bladder and vagina there is a tendency to dissect too close to the vagina and then too close to the cervix and so beneath the ligament. This must be avoided so as not to cut into the growth and so as not to make the further steps of the operation more difficult (Fig. 77.3).

The Schuchardt incision is essential to the operation in that it allows the necessary access. Bilateral incisions have been recommended and in cases of exceptional difficulty can be employed but are seldom necessary. The incision is quite vascular and in the course of a long operation an appreciable amount of blood may be lost, also for the patient this is the most painful part of the postoperative period. Most authorities recommend the performance of the Schuchardt incision prior to the formation of the vaginal cuff, but if, as is usual, there is sufficient room I prefer to make the cuff first as it allows dissection of the

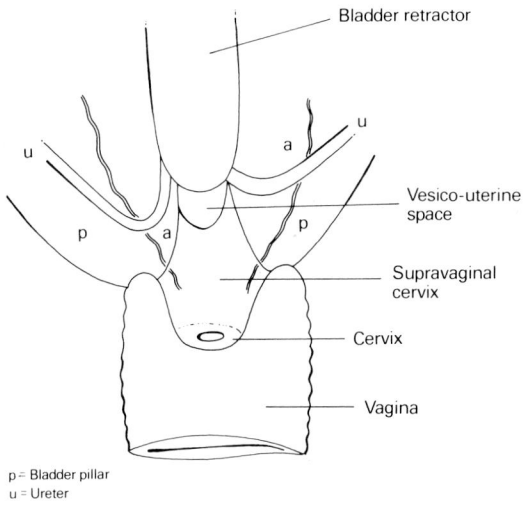

p = Bladder pillar
u = Ureter
a = Uterine artery

Fig. 77.1 Bladder pillars showing position of ureters and uterine arteries with vesico-uterine space.

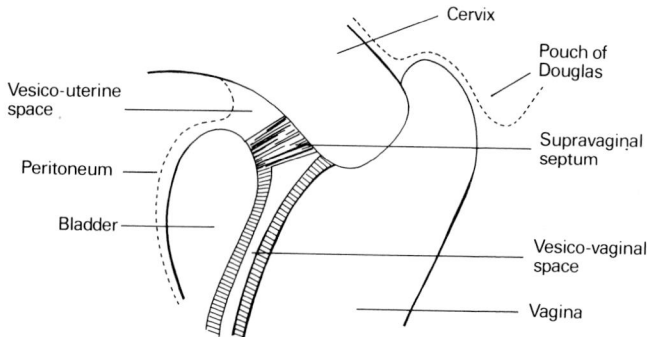

FIg. 77.3 Disposition of vesico-uterine space, supravaginal septum and vesicovaginal space.

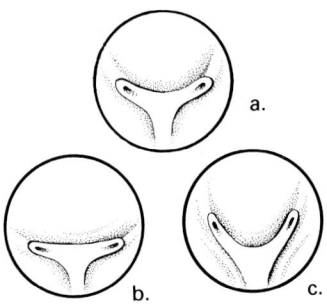

Fig. 77.4 Ureteric orifices as seen on cystoscopy in the different positions of the ureter. (a) trigone, normal anatomy, (b) trigone, lateral ureteral situation, (c) trigone, medial ureteral situation.

rectum from the posterior vaginal wall and the uterosacral ligaments or rectal pillars prior to performing the Schuchardt incision which is thus made safer. Where access is limited the incision must of course precede the formation of the cuff.

To display the lateral wall of the bladder pillars which is a crucial step in the dissection of the ureters it is necessary to open up the paravesical spaces; similarly development of the pararectal spaces precedes the division of the rectal pillars. The spaces are seen clearly in the abdominal operation and are developed on the side of the Schuchardt incision quite easily but on the opposite side they have to be dissected out more formally as will be described.

PREOPERATIVE REQUIREMENTS

The usual investigations for any major gynecological procedure such as hemoglobin estimation, blood group and cross matching of blood are required. Particular attention has to be paid to the urinary system, infection must be excluded or treated if present, and the blood urea should be estimated. Intravenous pyelography is mandatory to exclude renal pathology, congenital or acquired, and to demonstrate the course of the ureters.

Whilst bladder invasion by carcinoma of the cervix is uncommon, preoperative cystoscopy should be performed and is usually done at the preliminary examination under anesthesia for staging and biopsy. The disposition of the ureteric orifices relative to the interureteric bar is noted to give an indication of the site of the terminal portion of the ureters in the bladder pillars as described by Högler[6] (Fig. 77.4) who points out that occasionally the ureter is fixed in an abnormally medial position by inflammation, tumor or post radiation fibrosis and because of its unexpected course is in danger of being damaged during the dissection. Conversely, prolapse may cause a more lateral displacement of the ureters which are then more difficult to locate. Lymphography would today be particularly valuable when considering treatment by radical vaginal

hysterectomy; lymph nodes clearly involved by malignant disease would be a contraindication unless lymphadenectomy or external irradiation were to be included in the treatment. On the other hand an early, small tumor with no apparent lymph node involvement would be a more suitable case for the operation. It is important to ensure that the lower bowel is empty before the patient comes to operation. Pre- and postoperative cover with metronidazole is probably an advantage but antibiotics should be reserved for use if infection arises.

Preoperative intracavity radium has become popular with surgeons treating cancer of the cervix and is particularly valuable in connection with the Schauta operation if the tumor to be treated is large, exophytic and infected; a preoperative radium application will render the cervix clean and of normal size or at least diminish the size of the tumor, thus obviating the necessity to destroy the growth by fulguration at the time of operation, a procedure which used to be advocated in the early days of radical vaginal hysterectomy.

THE OPERATION

Anesthesia

No particular requirements are mandatory in the type of anesthesia employed for the operation but a supplementary epidural or caudal anesthetic does help to conserve blood loss and provide a drier operative field.

Position of patient on the operating table

The routine lithotomy position with legs outside the stirrups is usually adequate so long as the buttocks are well over the end of the table but improved access is achieved if the thighs are hyperflexed by advancing the poles towards the head of the table, but care must be taken that the calves are not compressed.

Assistants

There must be two assistants, one on each side. They should have a good knowledge of the procedure and know how best to use the instruments special to the operation. Good retraction to display the various steps is essential to the success of the operation. This is much more the case than with the abdominal approach.

Instruments

There are a number of special instruments described as useful in the performance of this operation but the important principles to be met are that most of the instruments are longer than in routine procedures and this applies particularly to ligature carriers, needle holders, scissors and forceps. Also required are flat bladed retractors of varying widths but with long blades which are directed at just less than 90 degrees to the handles which must be strong as the assistants have, on occasion, to retract with considerable force.

Preparation of the vaginal cuff

Access to the upper vagina is obtained by the use of an Auvard or Sims speculum and two narrow lateral vaginal retractors. Four Kocher's forceps are placed, two on the anterior wall and two on the posterior to demarcate the amount of vagina to be removed; usually about half the vagina is taken but in very early stage disease the excision may be restricted to the upper third (Fig. 77.5a). Phenylephrine 1: 200 000 in saline is injected under the vaginal skin all round the cuff and extending from the distal margin up as far as the cervix. This injection will balloon the vaginal skin off the underlying tissues, make dissection easier and diminish oozing from small blood vessels.

The cuff is now circumcised with the diathermy cutting needle (Fig. 77.5b). Anteriorly the bladder is dissected from the vagina with blunt scissors angled on the flat (Fig. 77.5c). It is important that the dissection is made in the vesicovaginal space between bladder and vaginal fascia and not too close to the vaginal wall which is the natural tendency. If the dissection is carried too close to the vagina the wall may be perforated or the cuff may be too thin and tear when traction is applied or, if there is vaginal extension of the growth, it may not be cleared by the dissection. Furthermore, if the plane is too superficial when the supravaginal cervix is reached, there is a danger of dissecting underneath the vesicocervical ligament or supravaginal septum and into the superficial layer of the cervix (Fig. 77.3).

At this stage it is as well not to dissect too far laterally as troublesome bleeding may be encountered; it is sufficient to form enough cuff to close over a swab. Posteriorly the dissection is rendered particularly easy by the injection

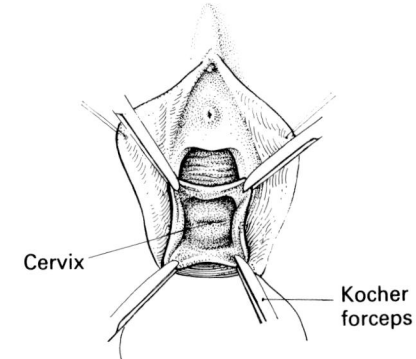

Fig. 77.5a–d Formation of vaginal cuff.
Fig. 77.5a Demarcation of vaginal cuff.

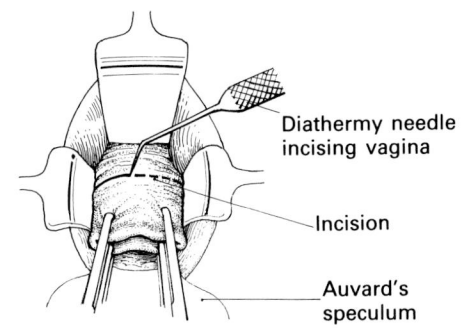

Fig. 77.5b Anterior incision.

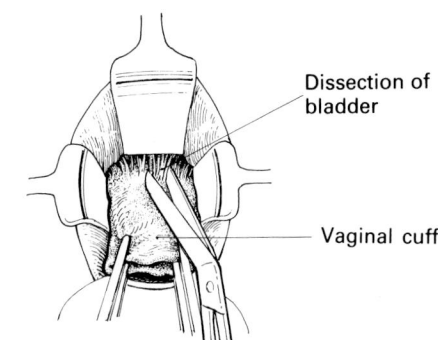

Fig. 77.5c Bladder dissection.

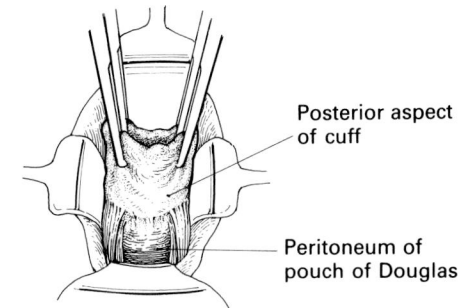

Fig. 77.5d Posterior dissection.

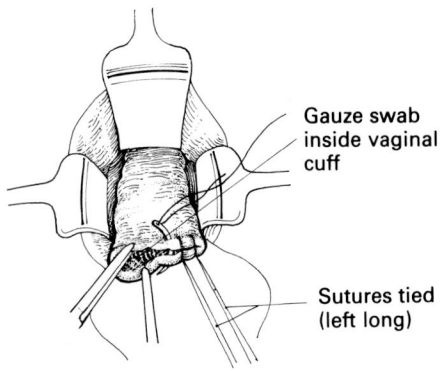

Fig. 77.6 Closure of vaginal cuff.

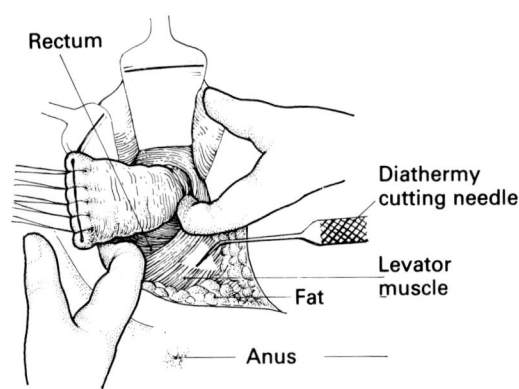

Fig. 77.7 Schuchardt incision.

of phenylephrine; using the blunt scissors still, the plane of cleavage between vaginal wall and rectum is easily found, the blade of the Auvard speculum is inserted into the vaginal wound and can be used to reflect the rectum from the vagina by blunt dissection, usually quite bloodlessly. A combination of blunt scissor and swab dissection completes the reflection of the rectum off the medial aspects of the uterosacral ligaments on each side. The posterior dissection is carried up as far as the peritoneum of the pouch of Douglas (Fig. 77.5d).

A gauze swab soaked in 1: 2000 perchloride of mercury is wrung out and packed firmly into the prepared cuff and the anterior and posterior skin edges approximated over it with silk interrupted sutures, the ends being kept long for traction (Fig. 77.6). Continental surgeons favor special clamps for occluding the cuff but although these give good traction they are more cumbersome and take up more space.

The Schuchardt incision

This is usually made on the patient's left side and so the cuff is retracted towards the surgeon's left by the assistant. The surgeon inserts his left index finger into the vagina posterolaterally, reaching above the levator ani muscle and the cut edge of the distal vagina and towards the left ischial spine. The assistant similarly places his right forefinger into the vagina above and laterally. The vagina is now stretched by these two forefingers. An injection of phenylephrine in saline is made under the perineal skin, under the vagina up as far as the vaginal incision and through the underlying tissues and into the pararectal space in the region of the ischial spine. This will reduce the amount of blood lost by oozing from the incision.

With the tissues still on the stretch, an incision is made with the diathermy cutting needle through vaginal and perineal skin. Extending from the cut edge of the vagina above, well out on to the lateral perineum, the subcutaneous tissues are divided and as the incision reaches higher and deeper some muscle fibers of the levator ani

will be divided, the rectum is protected by the surgeon's finger in the vagina and because it has already been reflected off the vagina in the formation of the cuff (Fig. 77.7).

It is not necessary to divide totally the levator muscle; once the pararectal fossa is opened up the four fingers of the surgeon's right hand can be inserted to open up the pararectal space posteriorly and the paravesical space above so that they are continuous. This must be done gently to avoid brisk venous bleeding. A pack is now placed over the incision after any obvious bleeding points have been arrested, either by diathermy coagulation or by ligature.

In cases where access to the vault is restricted by narrowing of the vagina, it is necessary to make the Schuchardt incision prior to the formation of the cuff and most authorities in fact recommend this but in my experience the cuff can usually be made first and this is safer in regard to the rectum and makes it easier to prepare the pararectal and paravesical spaces.

Division of the vesicocervical ligament

The Auvard speculum is replaced and helps to apply pressure on the pack overlying the Schuchardt incision. The cuff is retracted downwards and the vagina retracted upwards and laterally by two vaginal retractors. The

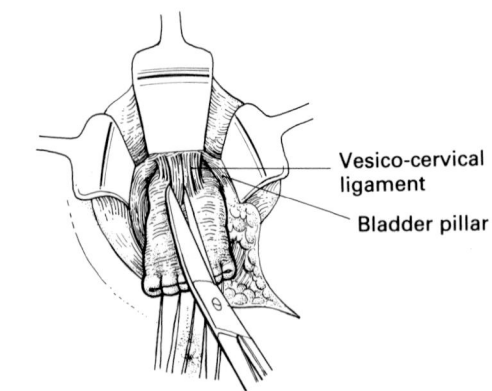

Fig. 77.8 Division of supravaginal septum.

dissection between bladder and vagina is continued in the midline with blunt scissors angled on the flat. If the dissection is proceeding in the correct layer when the supravaginal cervix is reached, the vesicocervical ligament will be displayed and after being put on the stretch can be divided with the scissors to open up the vesicocervical space leading to the uterovesical pouch of peritoneum. The tissue lateral to the vesicocervical space must not be divided as they are the bladder pillars (Fig. 77.8). This is a critical step in the operation for without it the bladder pillars will not be clearly delineated and dissection of the ureters will be rendered difficult. If the dissection between bladder and vagina is too close to the vagina, it will be carried up under the cervicovesical ligament and into the cervical tissues which is undesirable because of the malignant condition.

Dissection of the ureters

By retracting the cuff downwards, the bladder upwards and the vaginal walls laterally, the two bladder pillars connecting bladder to cervix are exposed. In these pillars the ureter curves downwards and then upwards to enter the bladder; it can easily be palpated between either forefinger and thumb or fore- and mid-fingers placed on either side of the pillar; the right ureter is situated at a higher level than the left. Högler[3] points out that the position of the ureters can be predicted at cystoscopy carried out preoperatively. The relative proximity of the orifices and the disposition of the interureteric bar indicates whether the ureters will lie medially, laterally or in the more normal position in the bladder pillars (Fig. 77.4).

Käser, Ikle & Hirsch[9] advocate transilluminating the bladder pillar from the uterovesical space to delineate the ureter. Usually there is no difficulty in finding the ureters but if there is growth or, more likely, inflammatory reaction in the tissues, difficulty can be encountered and then Högler's predictive cystoscopic findings will be valuable.

The cuff is now retracted downwards and to the surgeon's left, the bladder being retracted upwards and the lateral vaginal wall laterally; then having identified the left ureter, the lateral wall of the pillar is carefully snipped away with blunt scissors below the ureter and laterally until by a mixture of blunt and sharp dissection it is exposed lying in its bed of loose areolar tissue. This fatty layer when encountered is the key to the proximity of the ureter when identification is difficult (Fig. 77.9).

Before proceeding further and dividing the bladder pillar it is advisable to expose the right ureter. In order to do this, the right paravesical fossa must be opened up so as to display the lateral wall of the right bladder pillar. The cuff is retracted downwards and to the patient's left, the bladder is similarly retracted upwards and to the left. The right labiae are retracted laterally and the surgeon then

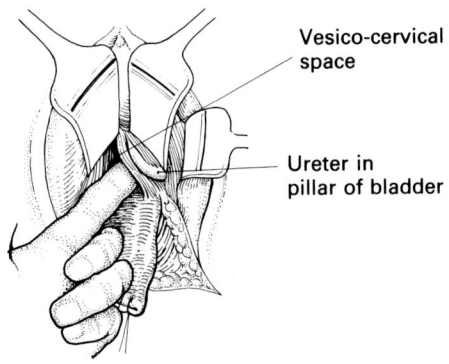

Fig. 77.9 Dissection of left ureter in bladder pillar.

Vesico-cervical space

Ureter in pillar of bladder

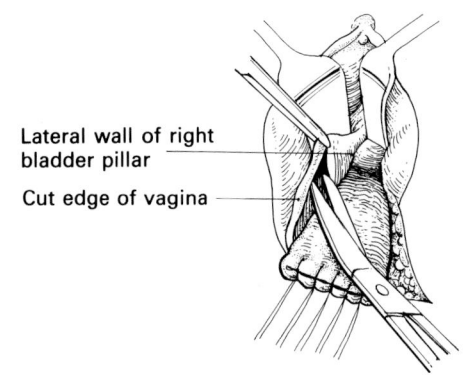

Fig. 77.10 Opening the right paravesical fossa.

Lateral wall of right bladder pillar

Cut edge of vagina

dissects between the vagina and the lateral wall of the bladder pillar. The dissection is best carried out with blunt scissors inserted closed and withdrawn slightly opened (Fig. 77.10).

Once the correct plane has been reached, the space can be opened up by retracting the vaginal skin laterally and the bladder pillar medially, inserting first the fingers and then the half hand; the surgeon can open up the paravesical space and join it to the pararectal space posteriorly; any intervening connective tissue strands can be divided between clamps and ligated.

The right bladder pillar is now exposed and the ureter can be palpated and dissected out in the same manner as on the left side. The right ureter usually lies higher and more lateral in relation to the cervix than the left and in cases where exposure is difficult, it is best to dissect out this ureter first because as the ureteric dissection proceeds the bladder and ureters are retracted further upwards.

Once the ureter has been clearly exposed, the surgeon's forefinger is inserted into the distal part of the ureteric tunnel following the ureter cephalad. If necessary the entry to the tunnel can be achieved by advancing the closed blunt scissors and opening them slightly, working lateral to and below the ureter (Fig. 77.11). Once the tunnel has been entered the lateral wall can be divided between ligatures

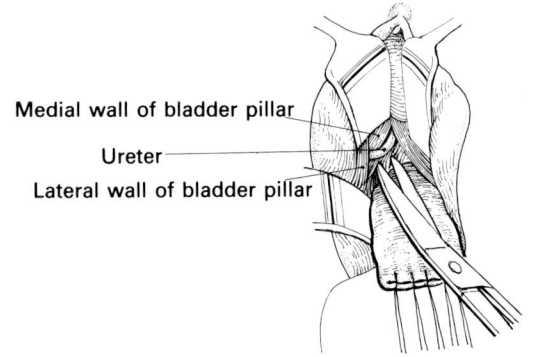

Fig. 77.11   Dissecting lateral wall of bladder pillar before ligation.

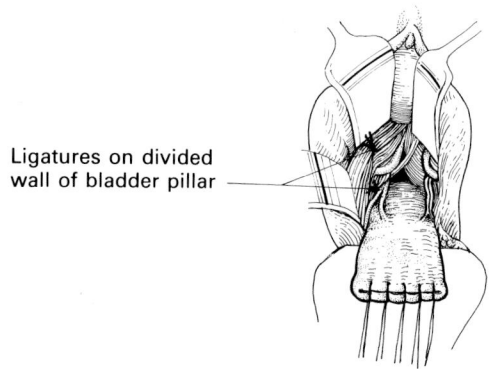

Fig. 77.12   Division of medial wall of bladder pillar to display uterine vessels. Lateral wall ligated and divided.

passed with a long pedicle needle (Dechamps); it should be divided as far laterally as possible.

Ligation of the uterine vessels

The bladder and ureters are now retracted upwards and the medial wall of the bladder pillar can be divided with scissors close to the ureter and away from the uterine vessels which will be seen coursing down medially under the ureter (Fig. 77.12).

The uterine vessels are now underun with the pedicle needle and doubly ligated, the ligatures being kept long for traction: the vessels are not transected. By applying traction downwards to the vessels and reflecting the ureter upwards, the ureteric branch of the uterine artery becomes visible and is divided between ligatures passed on the pedicle needle. The ureter is now free to be retracted upwards and the uterine vessels are displayed at a higher level. They are now divided at as high a level as possible between ligatures passed on the pedicle needle; the proximal uterine bundle must be contained within a double ligature (Fig. 77.13).

Some care must be exercised in passing these high ligatures as the vessels are lying close to the peritoneum and this should not be perforated for fear of damaging the bowel; on the other hand the whole bundle of vessels must be included because if one is divided inadvertently whilst unligated it will retract and the subsequent bleeding will be difficult to control. The right ureter is now quite free and can be retracted out of the way during the further steps in the operation. The left ureter and uterine vessels are now treated in the same manner.

Ligation of infundibulopelvic ligaments

The uterovesical pouch of peritoneum is now opened in the midline and the opening enlarged laterally to the origins of the round ligaments.

The fundus of the uterus is grasped with a tenaculum and drawn forwards through the opening in the uterovesical pouch. By drawing it to the patient's right and inserting retractors to lift up the bladder superiorly and retract the lateral margin of the wound, the round ligament on the left can be doubly ligated using the pedicle needle; the ligament should not be divided. The opposite ligament is similarly treated. The ovary and tube are now grasped with ring forceps and drawn through the opening in the uterovesical peritoneum towards the contralateral side and using the pedicle needle the vessels contained in the infundibulopelvic ligament are underun and doubly ligated; they are then divided (Fig. 77.14). When the vascular

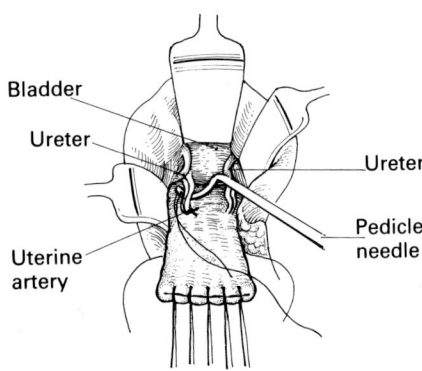

Fig. 77.13   Ligation of uterine vessels.

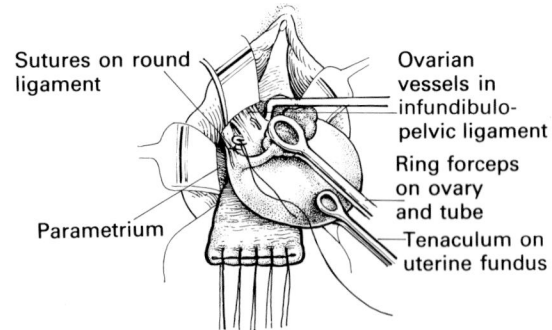

Fig. 77.14   Ligation of round ligament, not divided, and infundibulopelvic ligament, to be divided.

bundle on both sides has been divided, the two round ligaments are also divided and the ligatures kept long and held with artery forceps. Retaining the round ligaments before dividing the infundibulopelvic ligaments prevents the latter tearing during the traction required for their ligation. In early stage disease, if the patient is young and has not been treated with preoperative radiotherapy, the ovaries can be conserved.

It may be necessary to insert a swab on a forceps or a gauze roll if the intestines bulge through the peritoneal opening during this stage of the operation. If access to the infundibulopelvic ligaments is difficult, their ligation can follow the division of the uterosacral ligaments and if necessary the cardinal ligaments but a better exposure of the cardinals is achieved if the adnexae are dealt with first.

Division of the uterine ligaments

The cuff enclosing the cervix is now drawn upwards to expose the peritoneum of the pouch of Douglas which is opened in the midline and the opening extended laterally to the uterosacral ligaments. The rectum is retracted downwards, making sure that it is free from the medial aspects of the uterosacral ligaments. A pack is inserted into the peritoneal cavity to hold back the intestines and the uterosacral ligament is displayed with retractors and using the pedicle needle, the ligament is ligated and divided as close to the rectum as possible, the surgeon's fingers protecting the rectum by enclosing the rectal pillars during this step (Fig. 77.15).

After both uterosacral ligaments have been divided, the uterus is held solely by the two cardinal ligaments. The peritoneum on the posterior surface of each ligament is raised off the ligament with blunt scissors and divided laterally away from the cervix; this reduces the size of the ligamentous bundle and allows a more radical excision.

By drawing the uterus in the opposite direction the ligament is put on the stretch and can either be ligated in sections with the pedicle needle or clamped, the method depending on the thickness of the ligament and the access, and the extent to which the ligament requires resection (Fig. 77.16).

After resection of one side, the opposite ligament is similarly treated. The uterus and appendages are now removed. A search is made for any obvious bleeding points which are seized and ligated.

Closure of the peritoneal cavity

A degree of head-down tilt of the operating table is now helpful and the intestines are packed away with a gauze roll. The lateral angles of the peritoneal opening are now seized with long forceps. The retained round ligament ligatures are a useful guide here. A purse-string suture is passed around each lateral angle to close it and leave all

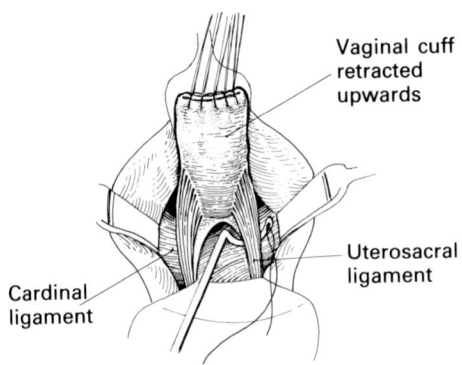

Fig. 77.15 Ligation of rectal pillars.

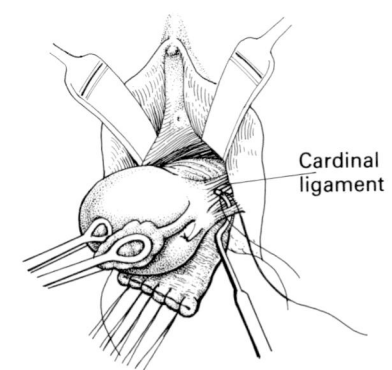

Fig. 77.16 Ligation of cardinal ligament.

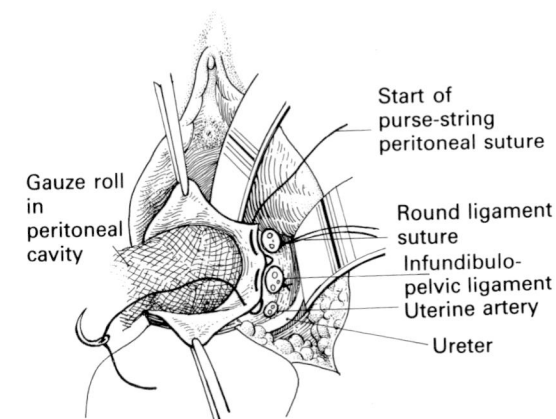

Fig. 77.17 Closure of peritoneum.

stumps extraperitoneal; care is needed at this stage because both the ureter and the uterine vessels are in close proximity to the peritoneum of the lateral angle (Fig. 77.17). When both angles are secured, the peritoneum is closed anteroposteriorly with a continuous suture after removal of the gauze roll.

Many Continental surgeons favor inserting Kelly type urethropexy sutures or some form of bladder wall plication at this stage, in the belief that it will help to prevent sub-

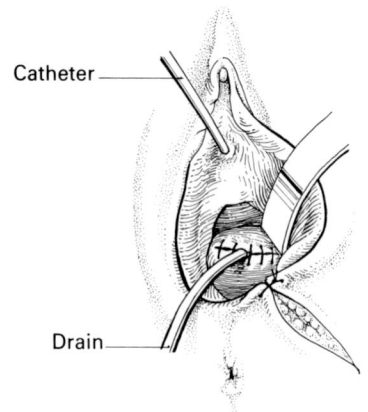

Fig. 77.18 Closure of vagina and Schuchardt incision.

sequent bladder dysfunction, but as this is nearly always neurogenic when it occurs, such a step is of little practical value unless there is an associated anterior vaginal wall prolapse. The round ligament is now attached to the ipsilateral angle of the vagina for support, using the ligature which has been left long.

A T-tube drain is inserted into the space between peritoneum and vagina and the vagina closed with interrupted sutures around the extruding limb of the drain. If there is persistent oozing which cannot be arrested by hemostats or diathermy coagulation, then it is better to insert a gauze roll pack instead. The Schuchardt incision is closed in layers with interrupted catgut sutures for the levator muscle and the subcutaneous tissues and with interrupted silk sutures for skin closure (Fig. 77.18). A self retaining catheter is necessary in all cases.

Variations

As has been mentioned, if access is limited so that formation of the vaginal cuff is inhibited, then the Schuchardt incision is made first and the cuff secondarily. The procedures are the same but more care must be taken to protect the rectum during the Schuchardt incision as it will not have been reflected from the vagina.

If difficulty is experienced in reaching the infundibulopelvic ligaments in removal of the adnexae, the uterus will descend more readily if the uterosacral ligaments are divided prior to this step. If further descent is required, then the cardinal ligaments also can be divided.

Again, with difficulty of access, the adnexae may be removed more easily if the uterus is removed first and the adnexae secondarily.

POSTOPERATIVE CARE

Postoperative care varies from routine mainly in respect of the bladder, the drain and the Schuchardt incision.

Trouble with bowel distension is uncommon as the intestines are little disturbed. Absence of an abdominal wound improves early ambulation but the perineal wound makes sitting uncomfortable.

The indwelling catheter is left on closed continuous drainage for 7 days, followed by 3 days of intermittent drainage. Regular bacteriologic checks are made and any infection promptly treated. After removal of the catheter, a close watch on residual urine must be made until it is certain that the bladder is functioning normally. This can be the most troublesome part of the postoperative phase for patient and attendants. The patient often suffers from loss of bladder sensation and must be encouraged to void regularly every 4 hours at least, and to aid voiding if necessary by manual abdominal compression. During the phase of residual urine estimations, infection becomes a real danger and must be very carefully controlled. Overdistension of the bladder must be prevented at all costs as it will prolong considerably the time before resumption of normal bladder tone.

The drain should be kept on continuous suction and removed after 24 hours if bleeding has ceased, but maintained for 48 hours if drainage persists. If a pack has been inserted, half should be removed after 24 hours and the remainder at 48 hours, being left longer only if there has been severe hemorrhage at operation uncontrolled other than by the pack. If packs are left in longer than 48 hours, prophylactic antibiotic cover is indicated.

The Schuchardt incision is the main source of pain for the patient and requires ample pain relief early on. The skin sutures are removed on the seventh postoperative day.

II. VAGINECTOMY

Total vaginectomy is an operation for which there is probably less indication than there is for the Schauta procedure. The main indications are primary carcinoma of the middle third of the vagina, carcinoma of the cervix extending into the lower third of the vagina, and recurrent carcinoma of the corpus uteri at the vaginal vault extending downwards. It is unlikely that vaginectomy would be preferred in these situations unless radiotherapy was not available or had failed, and in the case of corpus carcinoma that intensive hormone therapy had also failed.

Whilst Howkins[7] advocated combined synchronous abdominoperineal hysterocolpectomy to extend the scope of surgery in some cases of cervical or vaginal cancer, the procedure has not become popular particularly as the tendency today is to reserve surgery for the earlier stages of malignant disease of the cervix. It is in advanced cases which are considered suitable for exenteration procedures that the combined synchronous technique is invaluable and it renders the removal of bladder or rectum or both with the vagina a simpler and less traumatic procedure. The very close proximity of bladder and rectum to the vagina renders suspect the operation of total vaginectomy as being adequate for cancer surgery in this area.

Vaginal adenosis and carcinoma in situ of the vagina present special problems in that both can be extensive and both are potentially premalignant conditions; where malignancy supervenes vaginectomy becomes necessary but where it is thought not to be imminent then more conservative measures are to be considered (see Chs 29, 30, 32 and 33). Colposcopic control is vital in this type of case and helps the conservative approach.

The most valuable adaptation of radical vaginal surgery is in the formation of a vaginal cuff as a preliminary step in the operations of radical abdominal hysterectomy and extended abdominal hysterectomy. The procedure is easy, does not add to the length of the operation and has certain advantages:

1. The level of vaginal excision is accurately determined.
2. Prevention of spill of viable malignant cells into the cut edge of the vagina which is the probable mechanism of vault recurrence in endometrial cancer.
3. Easy and relatively atraumatic reflection of rectum from vagina and uterosacral ligaments.
4. The cardinal and uterosacral ligaments are clearly defined and the precise extent of their excision more easily determined.
5. A Williams[24] vulvovaginoplasty can be quickly and simply performed where the vagina has to be unduly shortened thereby restoring adequate length for coital function (Ch. 87).

TECHNIQUE

Total vaginectomy

A subvaginal injection of phenylephrine, 1 in 200 000 in saline, is inserted all around the introitus of the vagina and throughout its length. A circular incision is made around the introitus (Fig. 77.19) and four short Kocher forceps applied to the vaginal edges. The posterior wall is dissected first as this is the easiest and any bleeding will not obscure

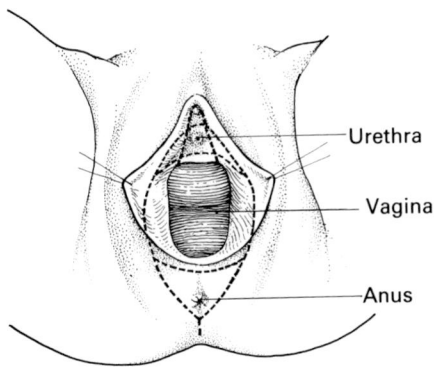

Fig. 77.19 Incisions for vaginectomy and exenteration procedures.

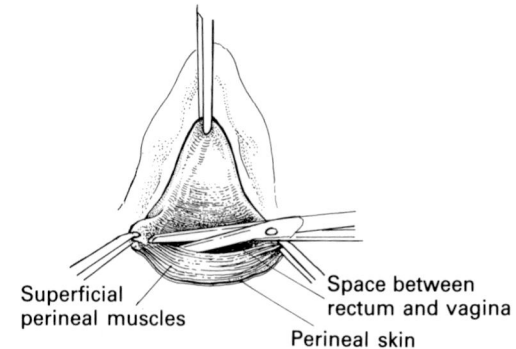

Superficial perineal muscles — Space between rectum and vagina — Perineal skin

Fig. 77.20 Lateral perineal dissection from vagina.

the anterior dissection. If the perineum is well clear of growth and is not entirely deficient, the procedure is simplified by excising the skin at the junction of vagina and perineum together with 1.5 cm of underlying tissue as in most parous women this is scar tissue and its removal allows access to deeper normal tissues. By raising the vaginal wall and dissecting against the surgeon's two fingers in the vagina with blunt scissors the superficial muscles are easily freed from the vagina and the space between rectum and vagina quickly reached. The dissection proceeds in the midline and once the space has been reached, the lateral dissection of vagina from perineal body is easily achieved by inserting one blade of the blunt scissors into the space and then cutting laterally (Fig. 77.20).

Further separation of vagina from rectum is by swab dissection and is carried up as far as the peritoneum of the pouch of Douglas. The anterior vaginal wall must now be separated from the bladder and the initial dissection between urethra and lower vaginal wall must be done with the scalpel, but the vesicovaginal plane of cleavage is soon reached and dissection proceeds relatively easily, especially when the phenylephrine solution is correctly injected. At this point it is usual to pack the vagina with gauze and close its edges anteroposteriorly over the pack (Fig. 77.6). The dissection is carried up as far as the cervicovesical ligament which must then be divided as described for the Schauta operation (Fig. 77.8).

Separation of the anterior and posterior vaginal walls is not difficult where the tissues are normal but if there is malignant involvement or postradiation fibrosis then there is risk of damaging either bladder or rectum. The use of a bladder sound and of a finger in the rectum helps considerably in such cases. If the bladder wall is thinned unduly the area should be oversewn and if inadvertently the lumen is opened, it should be repaired immediately. If the rectum is involved with malignant disease, it is more difficult to maintain its integrity and a fistula is a very likely complication. The very close proximity of bladder and rectum to vagina puts the rationale for vaginectomy in question.

Most gynecologists will not have much difficulty in the

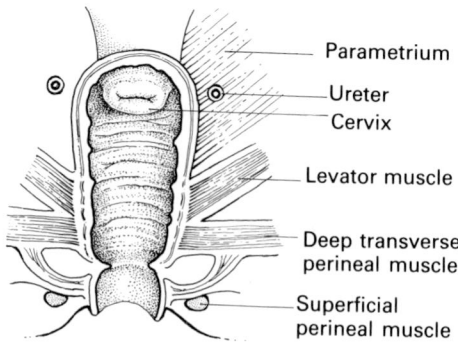

Fig. 77.21 Lateral relations of vagina.

separation of the anterior and posterior vaginal walls as they will be on familiar territory and all that is required is an extension of normal colporrhaphy procedures. The main problem in total vaginectomy arises with the lateral attachments which are unfamiliar ground to the general gynecologist (Fig. 77.21).

In the lower vagina the lateral relation is the posterior part of the urogenital diaphragm which is a relatively feeble structure in the female and can be divided without fear of much bleeding. In the middle third of the vagina the lateral relation is the medial border of the puborectalis which requires sharp dissection of fibers attaching to the fascial coat of the vagina. Obviously if growth is in proximity, sacrifice of muscle fibers themselves will be required to obtain adequate clearance. In the upper third is to be found the vaginal insertion of the inferior part of the cardinal ligament and posterolaterally the vaginal insertions of the uterosacral ligaments. These can be divided between ligatures passed on a pedicle needle. However, if radical excision of the area around the vault is indicated, as is likely, either as part of a combined abdominoperineal operation or solely for excision of the residual vagina, then the territory involved in the radical vaginal hysterectomy has now been reached and further steps are those of that operation with obligatory display of the ureters.

Vaginectomy with pelvic exenteration

More logical but more heroic procedures are involved in types of exenteration (Ch. 81). Either the bladder or the rectum or both may require removal with the vagina. Such operations are today rare because primary therapy is usually maximal and does not allow much subsequent opportunity for further treatment.

The vaginal part of total urethrocystectomy is easy; the anterior incision advances forwards around the urethra (Fig. 77.19), and by cutting with scissors upwards and backwards behind the pubic symphysis, the urethra is freed with only venous bleeding which soon ceases. The lateral attachments of the pelvic diaphragm are easily separated from the descending pubic rami by finger dissection,

again with little bleeding. Perineal resection of the rectum requires more effort. The incision must circumscribe the anus and be continued backward over the coccyx (Fig. 77.19). The anus is occluded with a strong purse-string suture over a gauze swab placed in the canal and the suture ends are kept long and held in an artery forceps. The incision is deepened posteriorly until the firm attachment of iliococcygeus muscle and fascia of Waldeyer to the sacrococcygeal junction is reached. This raphe is divided by sharp dissection with strong scissors to open up the space between rectum and the hollow of the sacrum. It is probably easier to extend the incision backwards over the coccyx and deepen it until either a coccygeal joint or the sacrococcygeal joint itself is reached. The coccyx is now bent forward and the point of the scalpel is inserted into the appropriate joint and the relevant piece of bone displaced (Fig. 77.22a). The fascia of Waldeyer is now exposed and by passing a finger forwards and laterally, the iliococcygeus can be divided together with the overlying

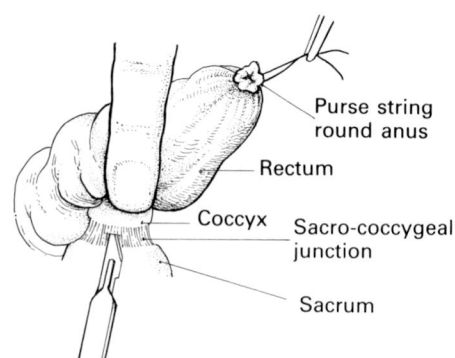

Fig. 77.22a–c Perineal excision of rectum.
Fig. 77.22a Excision of coccyx which is flexed and the scalpel inserted into a joint space.

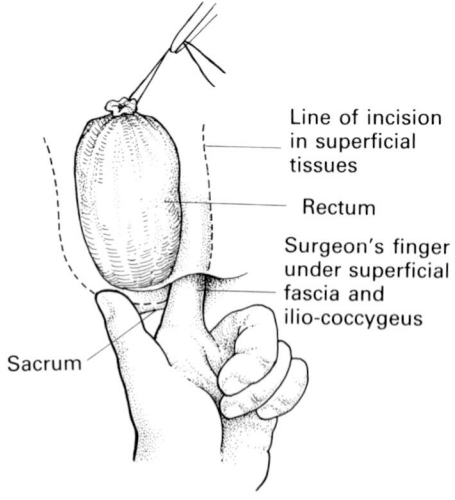

Fig. 77.22b Incisions in fascia of Waldeyer (see text).

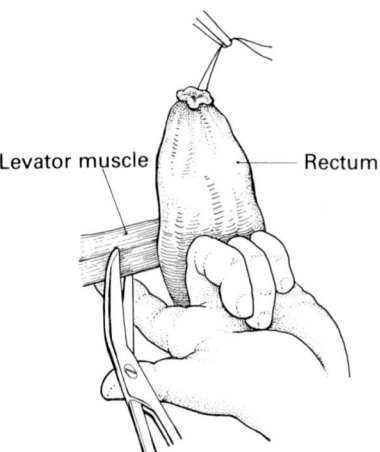

Fig. 77.22c Division of levator ani muscle.

fat and the inferior hemorrhoidal vessels. The main portion of the fascia of Waldeyer is now displayed and is incised in a horseshoe fashion (Figs 77.22b and c). By inserting his fingers into the space thus opened up, the surgeon can separate the rectum from the sacrum by breaking down the loose areolar connections. The lateral relationship of the lower rectum is the levator ani or pelvic floor at the lower end and loose areolar tissue or paraproctium at the upper end. The middle hemorrhoidal (rectal) vessels run above the pelvic floor into the lateral aspect of the rectal pillars (Fig. 77.23). Sharp dissection of the muscle sufficient to clear growth adequately is required and the middle hemorrhoidal vessels must be secured in order to prevent brisk bleeding.

In the upper lateral rectal region, finger dissection is appropriate until the inferior aspect of the cardinal liga-

ments is reached. If a Schuchardt incision has been performed, the dissection on that side is simplified by being under more direct vision.

The problem with combined synchronous abdominoperineal operations is that each of the two surgeons is pulling the pelvic viscera in opposing directions and there must be good cooperation by each to allow his partner to perform his part of the procedure satisfactorily. It is probably easier for the abdominal surgeon to be responsible for the dissection of the ureters in toto and for the ligation of the uterine vessels, but the radical excision of the parametrium is strictly the province of the vaginal surgeon.

Where vaginectomy alone is being undertaken the rectal pillars must not be resected too close to the sacrum and the excision should remain just anterior to the rectum for fear of damaging the branches of the middle hemorrhoidal arteries. If these vessels are damaged and if the anastomosis with the superior hemorrhoidal vessels be inadequate, avascular necrosis and fistula formation may occur (Fig. 77.23).

Formation of vaginal cuff

The technique is the same as in the formation of the cuff in the radical vaginal hysterectomy (Fig. 77.5). The amount of vagina to be removed will depend on the case, being less for extended hysterectomy for carcinoma corpus uteri (see also Ch. 80). The dissection anteriorly and laterally proceeds only as far as is necessary to form a satisfactory cuff; posteriorly the dissection should be carried up to the peritoneum of the pouch of Douglas and should separate the rectum from the vagina and the medial aspects of the uterosacral ligaments. The perchloride of mercury in the small pack in the cuff is cytotoxic to any malignant cells spilt during operation for corpus carcinoma. It is, of course, not necessary in cases of cervical carcinoma but the cuff should still be packed to make a firm structure against which the bladder dissection can be made in the abdominal part of the operation. Because the vaginal operation is limited in extent and does not reach up to the cervicovesical ligament or supravaginal septum, this structure will be encountered beneath the bladder in the abdominal dissection of that organ and will have to be penetrated before the opening in the vagina below the cuff is entered from above.

Having made the cuff and oversewn its edges with a continuous locking suture, the rest of the vagina is packed with a dry gauze roll, the free end of which is brought over the foot of the operating table to enable it to be removed at the end of the abdominal operation. Attaching the distal limb of a T-tube drain to the abdominal end of the pack prior to removal will draw the drain into position. Lees[13] recommends opening the peritoneum of the posterior cul-de-sac and dividing the uterosacral ligaments as part of the vaginal approach (p. 1272), and indeed the procedure is

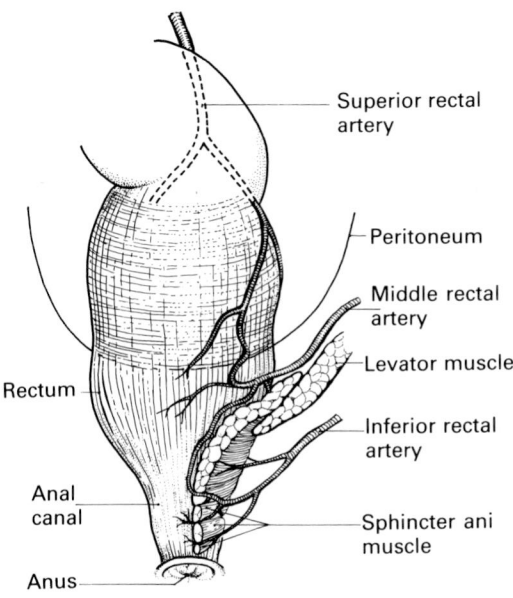

Fig. 77.23 Vascular supply and lateral relations of rectum.

capable of much variation as to the extent of the vaginal part of the operation.

REFERENCES

1. Amreich A I 1943 Bericht über die Gefahren und Erfolge der erweiterten vaginalen Total extirpation auf Gund von 1505 Operationen. Wien Klin Wschr 56: 162
2. Barclay D L, Roman-Lopez J J 1975 Bladder dysfunction after Schauta hysterectomy. One year follow-up. Am J Obstet Gynecol 123: 519
3. Carenza L, Villani C 1982 Schauta radical vaginal hysterectomy. Clin Obstet Gynecol 25: 913
4. Chowdhury N N 1976 Mitra operation for cancer of the cervix. Indian J Cancer 13: 234
5. de Graff J 1980 The Mitra Schauta operation in combination with preoperative irradiation as treatment for carcinoma of the cervix. Gynecol Oncol 10: 267
6. Högler H 1963 Schauta-Amreich's Radical Vaginal Operation of Cancer of the Cervix. Thomas, Springfield
7. Howkins J 1959 Synchronous combined abdominovaginal hysterocolpectomy for cancer of the cervix. A report of fifty patients. J Obstet Gynaecol Br Emp 66: 212
8. Inguilla W, Rey-Stocker I 1965 On radical vaginal operation in cervical carcinoma using the Schauta-Amreich method. Analysis of series of 327 cases. Gerburtch u Frauenheilk 25: 855
9. Käser O, von, Ikle F A, Hirsch H A 1973 Atlas der Gynakologischen Operationen. Thieme, Stuttgart
10. Kobayashi T, Matsuzawa M 1967 In: Wood C, Walters W A W (eds) Proceedings of Fifth World Congress of Gynecology and Obstetrics. Butterworth, Sydney
11. Kovacic J, Novak F, Stucin M, Cavic M 1976 The place of Schauta's radical vaginal hysterectomy in the therapy of cervical carcinoma. Gynecol Oncol 4: 33
12. Kudo R, Ito E, Kusanagi T, Hashimoto M 1984 Vaginal semi-radical hysterectomy: a new operative procedure for microinvasive carcinoma of the cervix. Obstet Gynecol 64: 810
13. Lees D H, Singer A 1978 Colour Atlas of Gynaecological Surgery Vol III. Wolfe Medical, London
14. Mitra S 1954 In: Meigs J V (ed) Surgical Treatment of Carcinoma of the Cervix. Grune and Stratton, New York
15. Morley G W, Seski J C 1976 Radical surgery versus radiation therapy for Stage I carcinoma of the cervix. Am J Obstet Gynecol 126: 785
16. Navratil E 1965 Radical vaginal hysterectomy (Schauta-Amreich operation). Clin Obstet Gynecol 8: 676
17. Navratil E, Lirmberger M 1969 Results of vaginal radical hysterectomy within the scope of selective therapy for invasive cervix carcinoma. Wien Klin Wschr 81: 760
18. Nelson J H Jr 1977 Atlas of Radical Pelvic Surgery. Appleton-Century-Crofts, New York
19. Rutledge F N 1962 Cancer of the Uterine Cervix, Endometrium and Ovary. Year Book Medical Publishers, Chicago
20. Schauta F 1908 Die erweiterte vaginale Total extirpation beim Collum-Karzinom. Safar, Wein und Leipzig
21. Schwarz R, Büttner H H 1976 Vaginal radical surgery using the Schauta-Amreich method. Zbl Gynäk 98: 1162
22. Stoeckel W 1956 Typische Gynäkol. Operationen. Urban und Schwartzenberg, München–Berlin
23. Wertheim A 1905 A discussion on the diagnosis and treatment of cancer of the uterus. Br Med J ii: 689
24. Williams E A 1964 Congenital absence of the vagina: a simple operation for its relief. J Obstet Gynaecol Br Commonw 71: 511

78. Extensive abdominal hysterectomy and bilateral pelvic lymphadenectomy

J. D. Thompson

INTRODUCTION

Worldwide, cervical cancer continues to be a major public health concern. In some developing countries, cervical cancer is the leading cause of death among adult women because of a high prevalence rate and inadequate early detection and treatment programs. In other countries, such as the Peoples Republic of China, great strides have been made in reducing the mortality rate from cervical cancer by a national commitment to early detection through mass population screening with cervical cytology. In the United States, it is estimated that 7000 women will die of cervical cancer in 1989. This is a dramatic decrease from the much larger number who died each year in previous decades. However, since it can be said that each death could be prevented if cervical cancer detection programs were universally available and utilized by all adult women in the country, 7000 deaths annually is a regrettably large number. Thus, in the United States, this potentially curable cancer has not been eliminated and remains an important and potentially lethal disease. In the absence of early detection, it is still necessary to treat women for invasive cervical cancer with methods that provide the best hope of cure with as little interference with function as possible.

The comments in this chapter are derived from the author's relatively modest background of experience in the management of over 2500 patients with invasive cervical cancer in three institutions, but primarily and most recently in the hospitals affiliated with the Woodruff Health Science Center of Emory University, Atlanta, Georgia. Some parts of this chapter are reproduced from Chapter 68, 'Radical Hysterectomy with Pelvic Lymphadenectomy' written for the 1981 edition of this text by the late Dr. Richard F. Mattingly. His comments are still useful and pertinent today. Much of this same information and illustrations have also been published in *TeLinde's Operative Gynecology*, 6th and 7th edns.[83]

Extensive hysterectomy and pelvic lymphadenectomy is occasionally used to treat patients with adenocarcinoma of the endometrium with involvement of the endocervical canal; and also patients who have a small cervical cancer that persists or recurs in the cervix following primary radiation therapy. In this chapter, emphasis will be given to the use of extensive abdominal hysterectomy and pelvic lymphadenectomy as primary treatment for invasive cervical cancer.

It will be noticed by the reader that the author has a preference for the term 'extensive' rather than 'radical' when referring to this operation. There are unfortunate and undesirable connotations in using the word 'radical' that may be disturbing to the patient and to others. An operation that needs to be 'extensive' in order to cure the disease is not a 'radical' operation, in the sense of being an 'extreme' measure, nor is it necessary that it be done by a 'radical' surgeon.

SOME HISTORICAL POINTS IN THE DEVELOPMENT OF EXTENSIVE SURGERY FOR TREATMENT OF CERVICAL CANCER

Surgical removal of cervical cancer was suggested by Osiander and Wrisberg in the 18th century. In 1821, Sauter did a vaginal hysterectomy on a patient with a '6 months bleeding tumor'.[117] This was a remarkable achievement, in that the patient survived the operation, but she died of intercurrent disease 4 months later, as reported by Zweifel.[148] However, there was very little that could be done for patients with this dreadful disease until basic discoveries in medical and surgical therapy (anesthesia, for example) had been made. The primary surgical treatment of carcinoma of the cervix began in Europe over 100 years ago, when Freund (1878) in Germany developed a technique for removal of the uterus in patients with cervical cancer.[33,34] This operative procedure was not adequate for cervical cancer, and the operative mortality was 50%. A more extensive operation was proposed by Reis of Chicago who, in 1895, demonstrated the technique of lymph gland removal at the autopsy table, although he apparently never performed lymphadenectomy with extensive hysterectomy.[107] J. G. Clark, while still a resident trainee at the

Johns Hopkins Hospital in 1895, performed extensive abdominal operations for cancer of the cervix.[23] His operations did not include lymphadenectomy, but did include removal of the broad ligament to the lateral pelvic wall and removal of the upper vagina with the surgical specimen.

In 1898, Wertheim of Vienna performed his first radical extended abdominal hysterectomy and partial lymphadenectomy, and thereby began his monumental work of systematically investigating the surgical treatment of cervical cancer. His initial operative mortality was 30%.[140] In 1911, when Wertheim reported his series of 500 cases, the operative mortality was reduced to 10%.[142]

Because of the high mortality associated with the abdominal approach, Schauta, also of Vienna, developed an extensive vaginal operation in 1902. The surgical mortality was approximately 10% with a 5-year survival rate of 40%.

In the several decades which followed, the technique of the original Schauta operation was modified and further developed by Amreich, Navratil, Mitra, van Bastiaanse and others.[87,95] The technique of Wertheim's original operation was modified and further extended by Wertheim's pupil, Werner, and by other outstanding pelvic surgeons in Europe. Latzko & Schiffmann offered important modifications to extend the abdominal approach.[73] Okabayashi, in Japan, described his radical abdominal hysterectomy in 1921 and this operation was developed further by technically skilled Japanese surgeons to include a more extensive dissection of the parametrium.[97] Competition developed between the abdominal (Wertheim) and vaginal (Schauta) approaches, and this has continued almost to the present.

In the early 20th century, extensive pelvic surgery by either the vaginal or abdominal route prior to the advent of antibiotics and blood transfusions was accompanied by an unacceptably high surgical mortality in the hands of even the most skilful surgeons. Also, operability by either method was less than satisfactory. The original enthusiasm for surgery waned because of these problems and also because of the discovery of radium by the Curies in Paris in 1898. In 1907, Klein irradiated carcinoma of the cervix. In the United States during the first half of the 20th century, more attention was given to radiation as the primary therapy in carcinoma of the cervix, because of greater applicability, lower mortality rates and good survival rates with radiation treatment. Patients were treated with central radium applications according to the Paris, the Stockholm, or the Manchester techniques plus additional external pelvic radiation with 200 or 400 kilovolt X-ray machines. It was soon realized that the 5-year cure rate for all cases treated with radiation therapy was only about 40%. As the dose of radiation therapy was increased in an attempt to achieve a better cure, the rate of complications also increased. In 1949, Morton reported complications in 90.5% of patients treated with radiation therapy, including colitis, proctitis, bowel obstruction and even death.[91] In spite of the popularity of radiation therapy, interest in surgery as primary treatment for invasive cervical cancer had fortunately continued, mostly in Europe and by pupils of Wertheim and Schauta.

Victor Bonney, in England, was another advocate of the Wertheim hysterectomy. In 1941, Bonney reported his series of 500 patients who received primary surgical treatment for invasive cervical cancer.[14] The 5-year cure was 42%, comparable to cure rates achieved with radiation therapy. However, the operative mortality was 14%. Stallworthy, a disciple of Bonney, continued to use the Wertheim hysterectomy and pelvic lymphadenectomy. Although Stallworthy modified the approach with the use of preoperative central radiation, the extensive parametrial and lymph node dissection remained an integral part of his operative technique with good results.[125]

Full credit for the American renaissance of extensive pelvic surgery belongs to Joe V Meigs.[85,86] In the early 1930s, Meigs, a surgeon from Boston, visited Vienna and was impressed with the logic of Wertheim's original operative procedure and the potential for surgical control of cervical cancer by this technique. Meigs returned to Boston and championed the Wertheim operation as primary treatment of cervical cancer. To the Wertheim operation he added a more extensive pelvic lymphadenectomy. The Wertheim-Meigs procedure resulted in an estimated increase in survival of 30%. The first report of his primary surgical treatment of invasive cervical cancer appeared in 1944 and included 344 cases. It set the stage for the subsequent use of this operative procedure by others. Many outstanding gynecologic surgeons in the United States (Parsons, Ulfelder, Green, Brunschwig, Barber, Morton, Pratt, Symmonds, Rutledge, Morley, Nelson, Averette, Shingleton, and many others) have made contributions and modifications in an attempt to decrease the incidence of urinary tract and other complications, while preserving the necessity of extensive parametrial dissection and complete pelvic lymphadenectomy. Some gynecologic surgeons have extended the lymphadenectomy to include the para-aortic nodes. In spite of obvious advances in the surgical treatment of cervical cancer, however, radiation has remained the main line of treatment for most patients. After all, advances and improvements in the technique of radiation therapy have also been made, especially the availability of new megavoltage equipment. It is to be admitted that most patients who are cured with primary surgery could also be cured with radiation. By and large, the gynecologic surgeon is privileged to treat the most favorable patients. In some clinics, this may constitute as many as 50% of all patients referred with invasive cervical cancer since, thankfully, a larger and larger percentage of patients are being diagnosed in the earliest stages of the disease.

PATIENT SELECTION FOR EXTENSIVE HYSTERECTOMY

In most clinics throughout the United States, most patients with Stage Ib and Stage IIa cervical cancer are offered extensive abdominal hysterectomy and bilateral pelvic lymphadenectomy as primary treatment (see also Ch. 42). Patients with Stage IIb invasive cervical cancer are usually excluded from primary treatment with surgery, and treated instead with radiation therapy. Admittedly, it is somewhat difficult to be certain about extension of disease into the parametrium based on pelvic examination alone. The clinical significance of parametrial involvement dates from the early studies of Kundrat[69] and of Sampson.[114] Kundrat, working in Wertheim's clinic, found in a careful study of over 21 000 serial microscopic sections of the parametrium that in 44 of 80 patients, the parametrium of one or both sides was involved. In a similar study at the Johns Hopkins Hospital, Sampson pointed out that the parametrium may feel indurated and yet show no evidence of cancer in it.[114] Also, the parametrium may feel normal and yet contain cancer. Sampson emphasized that only by the microscope can one exclude cancer from the parametrium. More recently, Inoue & Okumura found parametrial extension in 7% of Stage Ib patients and in only 34% of Stage IIb patients.[55] Burghardt & Pickel found true parametrial involvement in only 19% of Stage IIb patients.[20] Matsuyama, et al found no parametrial cancer in 58% of Stage IIb patients.[82] These studies were based on careful examination of microscopic sections, and emphasize again the difficulty of being certain about parametrial extension from pelvic examination alone. However, if there is reasonable suspicion of spread into the parametrial tissues by examination, by CT scan or by magnetic resonance imaging (Stage IIb), we prefer to offer radiation therapy as primary treatment sometimes following initial laparotomy with selective pelvic lymphadenectomy for staging. When tumor has broken through the fibrous 'capsule' in which it is contained in the cervix, the percentage of lymph nodes involved with metastatic disease more than doubles, and rates of persistent disease following surgery with or without postoperative radiation increase. Inoue & Okumura studied 628 operative specimens from patients treated with radical hysterectomy and lymphadenectomy and found that parametrial extension is an important factor in the number of positive lymph nodes found, and in patient survival.[55]

We are also somewhat reluctant to treat with primary surgery patients with large, bulky (>4 cm in diameter) endophytic tumors invading the cervix and lower uterine segment. Such patients are probably best treated with radiation therapy plus extrafascial hysterectomy, as suggested by Fletcher in 1979.[31] Gallion et al, and others, have reported good results with combined radiation therapy and extrafascial hysterectomy in the treatment of Stage Ib barrel-shaped cervical cancer.[38] We have occasionally been very successful in shrinking large, predominantly exophytic cervical lesions with preoperative transvaginal radiation, thus rendering such patients more acceptable candidates for extensive surgery. Six patients in our series at Emory University received planned preoperative, transvaginal radiation in variable doses to control bleeding or to shrink large, bulky tumors. None of these patients had extensive disease in their surgical specimen and they required no further radiation therapy postoperatively. None of the patients in this small group has developed a recurrence. We have had no experience in using preoperative chemotherapy, as suggested by Kim et al, and by others, especially in patients with large lesions limited to the cervix, in order to reduce the size of the central tumor mass so that operability is facilitated and possibly survival improved.[62] Preliminary results of these studies sound promising, however (see Ch. 44).

The major point to be emphasized, however, is that the gynecologic surgeon should not attempt to treat a patient with a large cervical tumor with primary extensive surgery unless there is reasonable assurance that the operation will result in the removal of the central tumor with an adequate margin of tumor-free tissue around it. One should not operate on patients with the idea that radiation can always be used postoperatively to eliminate residual fragments of tumor tissue left behind after incomplete resection. Such patients are better treated with primary complete radiation therapy from the beginning, possibly after staging laparotomy is done first.

If a patient has had an adequate cervical conization with only minimal invasive disease found on thorough pathological examination of the cone tissue, an extensive hysterectomy and pelvic lymphadenectomy is not usually done (see Ch. 38). Such patients are treated adequately with simple extrafascial hysterectomy, with or without partial vaginectomy. No attempt is made to remove parametrial tissue. It is important to emphasize that the extent of the disease must be accurately determined by thorough examination of an adequate cone specimen. There must be no question or indefiniteness about this. The disease must be microscopic and must not invade deeper than 3 mm into the cervical stroma. We believe the presence of a confluent pattern of stromal invasion or lymphovascular channel involvement does not contraindicate a conservative hysterectomy, as long as the invasion is not deeper than 3 mm. Very, very few such patients have been shown to have persistent disease following simple extrafascial hysterectomy, as shown by Kolstad,[67] by Maiman et al,[77] and many others.

TeLinde developed a 'modified Wertheim hysterectomy' which included a conservative resection of the most medial parametrium and upper vagina (Fig. 78.1). Although originally designed for patients with carcinoma in situ of the cervix, it is no longer used for this purpose. It is now

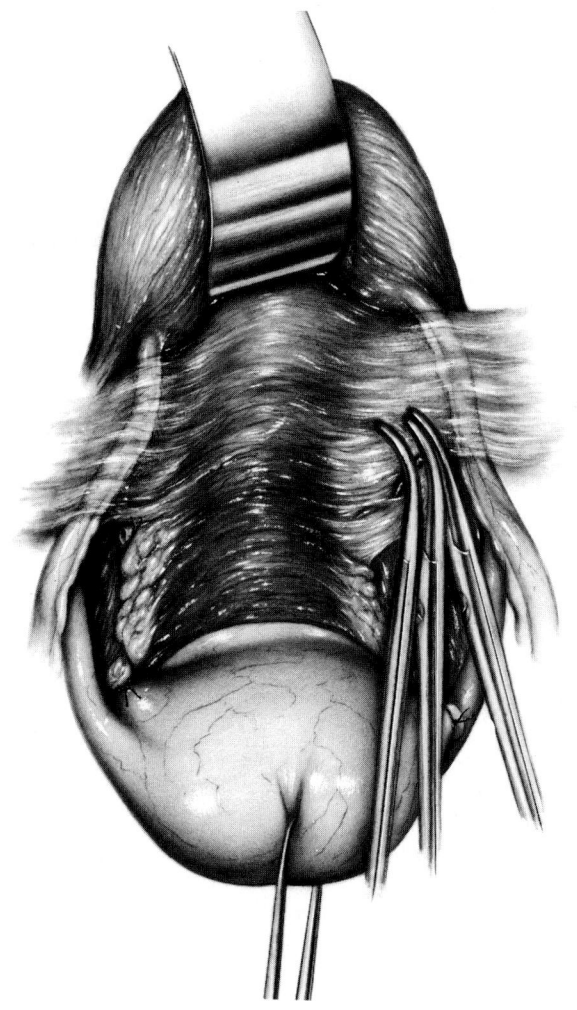

Fig. 78.1 TeLinde's modified Wertheim hysterectomy. The parametrium has been dissected widely by deep displacement of the bladder and terminal ureter. The uterine vessels have been clamped medial to the ureter, removing the medial one-third of the cardinal ligament with the uterus.

used for patients with microinvasive cancer with less than 3 mm invasion into the stroma. It is also used in patients with barrel-shaped bulky tumors of the cervix who have been treated with radiation. Since clamps are placed close to the ureters but the ureters are not dissected sufficiently to allow their identification, it is advisable to place ureteral catheters preoperatively to facilitate dissection without ureteral injuries.

There is no histologic type of cervical cancer which will contraindicate primary surgical treatment. Indeed, there is some evidence that the survival of patients with Stage I adenocarcinoma of the cervix is better with surgery than with radiation, as suggested by Brand et al.[16] Patients with Stage I adenosquamous cancer, clear-cell cancer, and undifferentiated adenocarcinoma have a poorer prognosis regardless of the method of treatment chosen, and should be considered for adjuvant radiation therapy or chemotherapy after primary surgery (see Chs. 43 and 44).

Experience in the management of 203 patients with gland cell carcinoma of the cervix at the University of Michigan Medical Center indicated no difference in survival according to histologic type, but considerable difference in survival according to degree of differentiation (well-differentiated, 57%, poorly differentiated, 29%). Another study from the same clinic compared the pattern of metastatic spread of squamous cell cancer and adenocarcinoma of the cervix as determined by autopsy findings of 21 patients with each tumor type. Patients dying of adenocarcinoma were found to have a higher incidence of tumor involvement of para-aortic nodes, uterine corpus, and adrenal glands. Ascites and hydrothorax were also significantly more common. The findings imply that adenocarcinoma of the cervix does behave differently in regard to pattern of metastatic spread and response to treatment, according to the authors.

Of course, patients must be acceptable candidates for operation and free of serious medical problems that might contraindicate extensive surgery. In former years, we limited extensive surgery as primary treatment to premenopausal women in order that ovarian function might be conserved. As experience accumulated, it was apparent that the operation was also well tolerated by older women, but patients older than around age 70 years are usually treated with radiation therapy. In 1988, Kinney et al from the Mayo Clinic reported their experience with the Wertheim operation in a geriatric population.[63] Thirty-eight selected patients between 65 and 89 years of age (median age 69 years) were compared to 320 patients younger than 65 years of age. The survival rates were almost identical in the two groups. Perioperative morbidity was minimally increased in the geriatric group. In order to achieve such excellent results in older women, the authors point out that 'meticulous surgical technique, high quality ancillary services, and support from internal medicine and anesthesia services' are required. Such high quality care is obviously not available in every hospital.

Extreme obesity (especially morbid obesity) presents especially difficult technical problems when extensive surgery is chosen for primary treatment. Not only is the performance of the operation less satisfactory, but there is an increased risk of wound dehiscence and evisceration, postoperative infection, intraoperative hemorrhage, pulmonary embolus, pulmonary atelectasis, and anesthesia and other problems. Unfortunately, primary treatment with radiation therapy is also less satisfactory in extremely obese patients. Quite honestly, the result of treatment for the extremely obese patient is likely to be poor regardless of the method of treatment chosen.

In our experience, primary treatment with extensive surgery is, paradoxically, also more risky in very thin patients. The incidence of fistula formation is higher. Perhaps in his/her enthusiasm for curing the cancer and removing the usual adequate specimen from an operative field with superb exposure, the gynecologic surgeon may strip the ureters, the bladder, the rectum and the major blood vessels too cleanly, thereby removing essential vasculature from essential places. Ischemic necrosis may result. A thin patient has less fat around the pelvic vessels and in the lymph fields; thus, the gynecologic surgeon should be satisfied to remove less tissue in an operation that is still adequate in a thin patient. Special care must be taken to leave vital circulation intact, especially around the ureters.

Pregnancy is not a contraindication to primary treatment of Stage Ib or IIa carcinoma of the cervix with extensive surgery, as experience reported from our clinic indicates. Extensive abdominal hysterectomy and pelvic lymphadenectomy was performed in 26 selected obstetric patients in the antepartum (22), intrapartum (1), and postpartum period (3) with no operative deaths, five major complications, and a good survival rate. A larger series was reported by Sall, Rini & Pineda in 1974.[113] Twenty-nine patients with Stage Ib invasive carcinoma of the cervix in pregnancy were treated with extensive abdominal hysterectomy and pelvic lymphadenectomy. Twenty-eight patients were alive and well, and 23 patients had been followed for more than 5 years. There were no fistulas or major complications. In our experience, it is difficult to accurately judge the tolerance of pelvic tissue to radiation during or following a recent pregnancy. Fifty percent of our patients radiated for Stage Ib and IIa cancer of the cervix had major complications of radiation treatment. On the other hand, extensive hysterectomy and pelvic lymphadenectomy is only slightly more difficult and is associated with slightly greater blood loss in pregnant patients.

In select expectant patients desiring to maintain their pregnancy, Greer and associates also recommend a delay in delivery until fetal lung maturity can be definitely documented.[44] We subscribe to the dictum that once invasive carcinoma of the cervix is diagnosed in a pregnant patient, a decision should be made to go either for the pregnancy or for the cancer and, regardless of which way it is, one should go all the way. A compromise could yield tragic results, possibly losing the mother because of delaying treatment for several weeks or months, or losing the baby from premature delivery by cesarean section, or both. We have made an exception to this dictum only in some carefully selected patients with Stage Ia carcinoma of the cervix. It should be emphasized that such an exception is made only if an adequate examination of an adequate cervical conization specimen shows only minimal microscopic stromal invasion limited to the superficial 3 mm of stroma beneath the surface. In such patients, a planned delay in definitive treatment until delivery at term may be recommended without undue risk. Our experience with this carefully selected group of pregnant patients has been uniformly satisfactory. All other patients should either be treated promptly in an attempt to cure the cancer, or be

allowed to continue their pregnancy to term in an attempt to deliver by cesarean section a mature infant whose chance of survival is optimal. Obviously, the patient makes the final decision whether to go for the cancer now, or delay treatment and go for the baby with delivery at term. She will need to be carefully informed of the risks involved to enable her to make a proper choice (see also Ch. 68).

ADVANTAGES OF EXTENSIVE SURGERY AS PRIMARY TREATMENT FOR INVASIVE CERVICAL CANCER

The most important considerations in choosing a method of therapy for any cancer are, firstly, effectiveness of the treatment in curing the disease; and secondly, mortality and morbidity rates associated with the treatment plan. For the indications listed previously, the cure rates of primary radiotherapy and primary extensive surgery are approximately equal. The modern mortality rates are also approximately equal. Both modalities of therapy have a list of complications unique to each, that seem to have about equal potential to be serious complications when they occur. However, there are important major and minor advantages of primary extensive surgery over radiation, some of which will be discussed (see also Ch. 42).

1. The findings at operation and from careful pathological examination of the surgical specimen can be immensely helpful in selection of patients for adjuvant postoperation radiation therapy and/or chemotherapy. The majority of patients operated upon will not need either, but some (about 20%) will.

2. The findings at operation and by careful pathological examination of the surgical specimen can be helpful in prognosis and in the identification of those patients who are at greatest risk for persistence of disease. Such high risk patients may require special diagnostic procedures and follow-up examinations at more frequent intervals.

3. When primary radiation therapy is used to treat invasive cervical cancer in premenopausal women, premature loss of ovarian function is an unfortunate and inevitable result. When primary surgery is used instead, the function of normal ovaries can be conserved. In 1981, Zander et al reported that 53% of 1092 patients operated on for invasive cervical cancer had one or both ovaries conserved.[147] As pointed out by McCall, Keaty & Thompson, conservation of ovaries does not interfere with the completeness of an extensive operation.[84] Ovarian function, including cyclic production of estrogen and progesterone, will continue until the usual age of the menopause in most patients, even when an extensive operation has been done, as indicated by Thompson et al,[131] by Webb,[137] and by Ellsworth et al.[29] There is no evidence that continued ovarian function will interfere with the rate of cancer cure in such patients. Finally, the adnexal organs (the tube and ovary are usually

conserved together, in order not to interfere with ovarian blood supply) are an infrequent site of metastasis from primary carcinoma of the cervix, even in late stages of the disease, and are very rarely involved in patients with Stages I and II, as pointed out by Henriksen.[46] The 'residual adnexal syndrome' seems to be reasonably infrequent in patients who have had ovaries conserved at the time of extensive hysterectomy. Re-operation for pathologic conditions of the adnexa was necessary in one of 20 patients reported by Ellsworth et al[29] (peritoneal inclusion cyst adherent to an ovary), in 10 of 183 patients reported by Langley et al[70] (nine for 'cystic degeneration' and one for ovarian carcinoma), and two of 61 patients in our series at Emory University (one for benign cystic teratoma and one for benign cystadenoma of the ovary).

Podczaski et al transposed ovaries into the paracolic gutters in 30 patients who had pre-treatment laparotomy.[102] Some patients experienced periodic cysts that could be felt by abdominal palpation. No patient required re-exploration for a persistent mass, but four patients had vasomotor symptoms and elevated gonadotropins after radiation therapy. The technique used for ovarian transposition was described by Husseinzadeh and associates.[53]

Mann has warned that the incidence of ovarian metastasis may be higher in women with adenocarcinoma of the cervix as compared with squamous cell carcinoma, and has advised that ovarian conservation is not indicated in these young women.[78,79] Nahhas et al reported ovarian metastases in a postmenopausal patient whose deeply invasive glassy cell carcinoma was treated with extensive surgery including bilateral salpingo-oophorectomy.[93] A glassy cell cancer is the most undifferentiated form of adenosquamous cancer, with a greater risk for metastases and poor survival rates. Most patients with ovarian metastases from cervical adenocarcinoma will also have metastases to pelvic lymph nodes, as reported by Tabata et al.[129] On the other hand, Berek & Brand report no ovarian metastases in over 60 patients with adenocarcinoma of the cervix treated with extensive surgery.[10,16] Greer and associates treated 55 patients with Stage Ib adenocarcinoma of the cervix with radical hysterectomy and pelvic lymphadenectomy.[45] 91% had ovarian preservation and there was no evidence that this contributed to tumor recurrence. Hopkins et al found the best cumulative 5-year survival (93%) with cervical adenocarcinoma was in those patients treated by radical hysterectomy without bilateral salpingo-oophorectomy, and concluded that 'ovarian conservation seems to be an acceptable alternative to bilateral salpingo-oophorectomy' in young patients.[51]

Although we have no hesitation about ovarian conservation in a young woman with a small, well differentiated adenocarcinoma limited to the cervix, there may be reason for concern about spread to the ovaries in the presence of large and/or undifferentiated gland cell tumors, or when positive pelvic lymph nodes and/or parametrial extension are found at operation.

Of course, all patients who are postmenopausal should have tubes and ovaries removed when extensive hysterectomy and pelvic lymphadenectomy are done for cervical cancer. But, in premenopausal patients, ovarian conservation has important health benefits especially in protection against osteoporosis and heart disease, and in maintenance of healthy vaginal tissues. In addition, there is the important psychological benefit to the young patient who has just learned that she has cervical cancer, when she is also told that it may be possible to conserve ovarian function. As gynecologic surgeons strive to eradicate cervical cancer with extensive surgery, they should also strive to modify their treatment so that as many as possible of those cured may live with bodies more nearly normal.

4. Studies on the effect of surgical and radiation treatment for cervical carcinoma on sexual function have been published by Seibel, Freeman and Graves from Emory University,[119,120] and by others (see also Ch. 89). Among patients treated with radiation, there is a decrease in sexual enjoyment, the ability to attain orgasm, frequency of intercourse, and desire for intercourse. Marked alterations can be seen and felt in the upper vagina and paravaginal tissues. The vagina is usually shorter from stenosis. The upper vagina is less pliable. Tissues are fixed and firm. The vaginal mucosa is thin and smooth and dry, with a tendency to split and bleed with slight trauma. Some of these changes are made more pronounced in young women because of hypoestrogenism from radiation-induced premature menopause. However, they are not reversed completely by intravaginal or oral administration of estrogen. These functional and anatomic changes are not seen nearly as frequently in patients treated with primary extensive surgery. Even if the vagina has been shortened by several centimeters with primary surgery, it remains soft, pliable, healthy and functional. Unfortunately, in those patients who must receive postoperative adjuvant pelvic radiation, some of this advantage will be lost.

5. Primary surgical treatment allows first and foremost an accurate assessment of the extent of the cervical cancer. However, it also allows discovery of the other, entirely unrelated, intra-abdominal incidental conditions and diseases which may or may not be important to the overall health of the patient. For example, in the last 100 patients in our series, significant pelvic pathology in addition to primary disease was found in four patients (Stage Ia ovarian cystadenocarcinoma in one patient, early endometrial carcinoma in two patients, and pelvic tuberculosis in one patient). Any number of other patients will be found to have sigmoid diverticulitis, cholelithiasis, and other conditions.

6. Late recurrences after treatment for cervical cancer are almost never seen following primary extensive surgery.

Late recurrences occur more often when patients are treated with primary radiation therapy. The same can be said for complications of treatment (see Chs 41, 85 and 86). Because of the gradual and progressive obliterative endarteritis produced by radiating tissue, complications resulting from ischemic changes (cystitis, proctitis, enteritis, colpocliesis, etc.) can be seen many years after the treatment was given. Late onset of complications following primary extensive surgery are very unusual. These points are especially important when selecting a method of primary treatment for young patients.

7. There are probably important psychological benefits of primary treatment with extensive surgery compared to radiation. Most patients prefer to have the tumor removed, and are especially encouraged when the surgeon can report that no evidence of metastatic disease was found at operation. Radiation therapy carries an unfortunate connotation to some patients, who feel that it is the treatment of last resort, that the treatments are actually 'cooking' the tissues in the pelvis, or that radiation can cause other cancers. All gynecologic surgeons have heard patients express disappointment when they are told that they cannot be treated with an operation. Some patients will continue to request an operation even after they have completed radiation therapy.

JUSTIFICATION FOR PELVIC LYMPHADENECTOMY

For many years, there was competition between those gynecologic surgeons who advocated extensive vaginal hysterectomy without lymphadenectomy, and those who advocated extensive abdominal hysterectomy with lymphadenectomy. The advocates of extensive vaginal hysterectomy without lymphadenectomy (the Schauta-Amreich-Navratil operation) pointed out that their patients had fewer postoperative complications (especially urinary fistulas), a lower operative mortality rate, and a cure rate that was almost equal to that achieved by an abdominal operation that included lymphadenectomy. Furthermore, they pointed out that pelvic lymphadenectomy is an incomplete operation at best, in that removal of all pelvic lymph nodes that may possibly be involved with metastatic tumor is technically impossible. This is especially true of those inferior gluteal nodes which are located in the region of the ischial spine, as pointed out by Reiffenstuhl.[106] Of course, it has also been known since Henriksen's work that involvement of para-aortic lymph nodes may also be present in a significant number of patients with metastasis to pelvic nodes, and that para-aortic nodes cannot be completely removed and are not routinely sampled by gynecologic surgeons in abdominal operations for cervical cancer.[46] However, even Navratil stated in 1965 that 'indications for the Schauta operation must take the lymph node problem into account'.[83] He performed extraperitoneal pelvic lymphadenectomy with the Schauta operation in all cases of Stage I and II which were locally advanced. So did Mitra.[87]

In recent years, the operative mortality and rate of complications in patients with extensive abdominal hysterectomy and bilateral pelvic lymphadenectomy has decreased significantly (see Ch. 42). Currently, operative mortality and fistulas occur in only 1% of patients. Therefore, this disadvantage of lymphadenectomy has essentially been removed, and one can now concentrate on the question of whether or not lymphadenectomy adds anything to the possibility of cure.

It is the opinion of some that pelvic lymphadenectomy is of no value in 80 to 90% of patients who have negative lymph nodes. We disagree with this view. We feel that lymphadenectomy is helpful in achieving an adequate central dissection around the cervical tumor, the most important part of the operation. This is especially true of that part of the lymphadenectomy that involves removal of tissue from around the hypogastric vessels, from the obturator fossa, and from the lower presacral region. Admittedly, dissection of lymph nodes from the common iliac vessels and from the para-aortic region does not add to the completeness of the central dissection. However, removal of these and other nodes is helpful in prognosis and in identifying those patients at greater risk of persistent disease, who should receive adjuvant postoperative radiation therapy to the pelvis and perhaps to extended fields along the aorta (see also Chs 23, 40 and 42). Although we rarely dissect and remove the highest para-aortic lymph nodes, the lowest para-aortic nodes around and just above the aortic bifurcation are usually removed. If pelvic lymph nodes involved with tumor are found during the operation, a concerted effort is made to do a more complete para-aortic dissection. Although it is possible for para-aortic nodes to be involved directly without involvement of pelvic nodes, this does not happen very often. For the group of patients who would usually be chosen for treatment with primary extensive surgery, routine para-aortic lymph node dissection would not result in therapeutic benefit very often. Podczaski and associates found positive para-aortic lymph nodes in 7 of 52 patients (13.4%) with Stages Ib and IIa disease.[102] However, 28 of the 52 patients had 'bulky' tumors greater than 5 cm in greatest diameter. Such patients are not considered by us to be appropriate candidates for treatment with primary extensive surgery. It is our estimate that only about 1% of patients who are appropriate candidates for treatment with primary extensive surgery would benefit from routine para-aortic node dissection, and, therefore, it is not done routinely, but selectively in patients who appear to have positive pelvic nodes at operation. The para-aortic region should always be carefully palpated, and any enlarged or firm nodes removed, but the gynecologic surgeon should be aware of the added morbidity attendant upon routine para-aortic lymphadenectomy.

A contrary view of the value of para-aortic lymphadenectomy has been expressed by Lovecchio and associates from the University of Miami.[75] Three hundred and forty patients with clinical Stage Ib and IIa cervical cancer were explored for probable radical hysterectomy. A complete para-aortic lymphadenectomy in all patients showed histologically documented metastatic disease in 36 patients (10.6%). In all cases, clinically suspicious pelvic lymph nodes were histologically positive for carcinoma. Radiation therapy was extended to the para-aortic region with no increase in complications. The 5-year actuarial survival rate was 50% with a median survival of 29 months. Cancer recurred in 80% of patients, two of whom remained clinically free of disease after chemotherapy. Thus, para-aortic lymphadenectomy in 340 patients with early invasive cervical cancer benefited nine patients (2.6%). The authors believe 'these data demonstrate that survival may be favorably influenced by employing extended-field radiotherapy in those patients with early-clinical stage cervical cancer and para-aortic nodal metastases' (see also Ch. 23).

If pelvic lymphadenectomy is not done in patients who have extensive hysterectomy for invasive cervical cancer, approximately 15 to 20% of patients with positive nodes will be inadequately treated for their disease (unless perhaps all patients received postoperative pelvic radiation). In our judgement, it is better to do pelvic lymphadenectomy in all patients and give postoperative radiation selectively, than to avoid lymphadenectomy and give postoperative radiation to all patients.

In 1978, Tulzer & Kupka of the First University Women's Clinic in Vienna discussed the effectiveness of obligatory lymphadenectomy in treating carcinoma of the cervix.[133] They reported a significant reduction in mortality rates from persistent disease when complete lymphadenectomy was made an obligatory part of extensive hysterectomy. When lymphadenectomy was selective (only suspicious nodes were removed) there was a 71% mortality rate in patients with positive nodes. When lymphadenectomy was made obligatory and complete, the mortality rate in patients with positive nodes was reduced to 39%.

If one does extensive hysterectomy and bilateral pelvic lymphadenectomy in 100 patients with Stages I and IIa cervical cancer, theoretically one might find positive nodes in 20 and negative nodes in 80. Of the 80 patients without positive nodes, maybe 74 (93%) will be cured. Of the 20 patients with positive nodes, about 12 (60%) will be cured by a combination of extensive hysterectomy and pelvic lymphadenectomy plus postoperative pelvic radiation. In other words, pelvic lymphadenectomy is done in 100 patients to cure an additional 12 patients in this theoretical exercise. We believe the risk of doing the lymphadenectomy in all patients is worth the benefit of additional cures.

Of course, one must presume that all patients with untreated positive pelvic lymph nodes would eventually die of their disease.

A recent study from the University of Minnesota Hospital and Clinics provides indirect evidence that postoperative pelvic radiation is more effective in controlling disease after pelvic lymphadenectomy has removed lymph nodes containing metastatic tumor.[27] The amount of radiation required to eliminate tumor in lymph nodes is directly related to the volume of tumor present. Thus, removing the larger nodes involved with tumor increases the probability of control of tumor with radiation. Despite a 44% rate of para-aortic node metastases, patients in this study who underwent resection of large positive pelvic nodes followed by postoperative extended-field radiation had a surprisingly high 5-year survival rate (51%) without evidence of persistent disease.

COMMENTS ON RADIATION THERAPY IN COMBINATION WITH EXTENSIVE SURGERY

Experience has shown that a planned treatment program consisting of complete pelvic irradiation followed by extensive abdominal hysterectomy and pelvic lymphadenectomy yields a prohibitively high rate of complications, especially as regards fistulas and urinary tract difficulties. Such a combination has been abandoned in almost all clinics. Routine preoperative treatment with central radium, followed by extensive surgery followed by selective external irradiation therapy is still used in some clinics (see Ch. 43). The good results of such a program in 612 patients with Stage Ib cancer of the cervix treated at the Norwegian Radium Hospital were reported in 1983. The crude 5-year survival was 81%. The authors concluded that no significant increase in complications could be attributed to the use of preoperative intracavitary irradiation.[65] Since there has been no clinical trial that conclusively proves that preoperative central radium treatments improve the cure rates (and results seem equally good without it), we have chosen to use it in only a few selected patients, as described above, to shrink large, bulky exophytic and/or bleeding cervical tumors.

Radiation therapy is used most often in the postoperative period, as an adjunct to extensive abdominal hysterectomy and bilateral pelvic lymphadenectomy (see also Ch. 43). It is given selectively to patients considered to be at high risk of persistent disease, based on operative findings and a careful study of the surgical specimen. If only one or two lymph nodes show micrometastases, postoperative radiation may not be given. However, when several nodes are involved, the risk of persistent disease is greater. In such cases, postoperative radiation is given and may be extended to include the para-aortic nodes as high as T-12.

Justification for using postoperative pelvic radiation selectively in high risk patients is difficult to find. In 1989,

Barter and associates reported on 50 patients who were treated with extensive hysterectomy and lymphadenectomy followed by postoperative radiation therapy for high risk factors (nodal metastases, lymph-vascular space invasion, close or involved margins) at the University of Alabama at Birmingham Medical Center.[8] Thirty percent of patients had serious complications, some requiring re-operation, and one patient died as a result of the combined treatment. The overall 5-year survival for the group was 66%. These authors reviewed a list of studies that show no evidence that survival rates are improved by administering postoperative pelvic irradiation to patients at high risk for persistent disease.[5,35,49,112,147] Russell and associates reported on 37 patients who received combined therapy.[96] Fourteen patients (38%) demonstrated persistent disease, 10 of whom showed persistent tumor within the field of radiation treatment.[111]

In a collected series, Morrow reported a 50% 5-year survival in patients with positive nodes treated with surgery alone, and a 61.5% 5-year survival in patients treated with surgery plus adjuvant radiation therapy.[90] The difference approached, but did not attain statistical significance. In a more recent report from the University of Texas M. D. Anderson Hospital, Larson and associates suggest that adjuvant postoperative radiotherapy may reduce pelvic recurrences and improve survival in patients with pelvic node metastases treated with extensive abdominal hysterectomy and lymphadenectomy.[72] Five of 20 patients who received adjuvant radiotherapy had persistent disease, compared with five of 10 patients who did not receive radiotherapy. The radiation therapy treated group contained all the patients with four or more metastases. Postoperative radiation therapy caused only one serious complication.

In our modest series, 15 patients had invasive lesions close to the margins of resection, or extensive involvement of lymphatic or vascular channels in the cervical stroma, and/or positive pelvic nodes, and were, therefore, treated with 4500 to 5800 cGy (rads) from combined vaginal ovoids and whole pelvis irradiation. Two patients died of persistent disease, but 13 patients are living without evidence of tumor. Most, but not all, have been followed for 5 years. Radiation therapy was well tolerated by all 15 patients. The only complaints were of temporary diarrhea and gastroenteritis. One patient did develop a progressive hydronephrosis due to ureteral stenosis beginning 6 months postoperatively. This patient required complete pelvic irradiation following her surgical procedure, because of extensive tumor in the cervix and positive pelvic nodes. She underwent a ureteroneocystotomy and lymphocyst removal.

Because of this favorable experience, we continue to give postoperative pelvic radiation to patients at greater risk for persistent disease. As reported by Hatch, most gynecologic oncologists in the United States use adjuvant postoperative radiation therapy in high risk patients.[8]

More and more often, patients are selectively treated with extended-field irradiation to include the para-aortic lymph chain, especially in patients who have several positive pelvic nodes. To numerous previous studies can be added two recent studies from Japan, which describe the results of para-aortic node irradiation in the treatment of cervical cancer. Inoue & Morita administered extended field irradiation after extensive surgery to 76 patients with nodal metastases.[54] The 5-year disease-free survival rates were 95% for 27 patients with one positive node, 64% for 37 patients with multiple positive nodes, and 44% for 12 patients with unresectable nodes. Two patients developed severe intestinal complications requiring re-operation. Postoperative extended field irradiation improved the survival of patients with four or more positive nodes from 39% to 69% as well as the survival of patients with unresectable nodes from 0% to 44%. The authors concluded that postoperative extended field irradiation can both control the distant spread via lymphatic routes and increase the survival time of patients with nodal metastases from cervical carcinoma in Stages Ib to IIb.

Eighty-six patients with cervical cancer were treated with para-aortic node irradiation by Horii and associates.[52] None of the patients developed severe complications of the treatment, although this is certainly not the usual experience. Based on their selection criteria for para-aortic node irradiation, the authors found a statistically significant improvement in the prognosis for the treated group. If complications of para-aortic irradiation can be kept to a minimum by further refinements in technique, lymphadenectomy will be essential in the management of patients with cervical cancer.

In 1987, Jones reported a collected series of 332 patients with para-aortic lymph node metastases who received extended field irradiation.[57] Twenty-six percent were long-term survivors. Although it is true that the majority of patients with positive para-aortic lymph nodes will die of their disease (probably because systemic disease is already present), it is also clear that some patients are curable with extended field irradiation, especially if the nodes are involved with only microscopic disease. One must anticipate a 10% incidence of enteric complications, even with doses limited to 5000 cGy (rads). Again, micrometastatic disease is more likely to be eradicated by a dose of para-aortic irradiation that can be tolerated by the patient. Patients with para-aortic nodes that contain a large volume of tumor are not likely to be cured even with a dose of para-aortic irradiation that exceeds 5000 cGy.

PREOPERATIVE EVALUATION AND PREPARATION

After the initial history and physical examination have indicated the possibility of primary treatment with extensive hysterectomy and pelvic lymphadenectomy, there are a number of additional tests and procedures that may be appropriate before the operation is actually performed (see also Ch. 40). The list may include the following:

1. Medical evaluation and treatment
2. Anesthesia consultation
3. CT scan of chest, abdomen, and pelvis
4. Intravenous pyelography
5. Magnetic resonance imaging of the abdomen and pelvis
6. Cystoscopy
7. Sigmoidoscopy and/or barium enema
8. Pelvic examination under anesthesia

Contrary to the frequent practice of doing all possible tests on every patient, it is the present author's practice to be selective and to do only those tests and procedures that are expected to yield useful information. It is not necessary (and indeed may be inappropriate) to subject every patient to a long list of preoperative procedures that are expensive, exhausting, and have very little, if any, expectation of providing useful information. Indeed, it is most unfortunate when a test or procedure yields 'questionable' or 'suspicious' findings that require that the test be repeated over and over before a 'negative' or 'indeterminant' answer is finally given, when the test or procedure was not indicated or needed to begin with. A young, healthy patient with a small cervical lesion may need an admission history and physical examination, chest X-ray and routine laboratory studies, and anesthesia consultation on the day of admission. In the evening, she receives a bath and vaginal douches with hexachlorophene and prep for intravenous pyelogram (IVP). The IVP is done early the next morning, with the operation to begin shortly after it is completed. A careful pelvic examination is always done as the initial step after anesthesia is induced. Cystoscopy and whatever shaving is necessary may also be done. Then the operation begins. If the patient is older, or has medical complications or has a larger or undifferentiated cervical lesion, the preoperative work-up and preparation may be more involved and thorough. As much as possible should be done as an outpatient before admission to the hospital.

If the patient has a large or undifferentiated cervical cancer, computed tomography studies of the chest may be more valuable than simple chest X-ray. CT scans may be used to look for enlarged para-aortic lymph nodes, which may need further study with fine needle aspiration (see also Chs 19 and 22). Matsukuma and associates evaluated the accuracy of abdominopelvic CT scans in the diagnosis of para-aortic and pelvic lymph node metastases from carcinoma of the cervix.[81] CT scan was positive in 71.4% of patients with para-aortic lymph node metastases. In two patients, the CT scan was falsely positive. These authors found CT scan more useful in evaluating para-aortic than pelvic lymph nodes. Only a small number of metastatic pelvic nodes were diagnosed by CT scan as enlarged nodes.

Vercamer and associates studied computed tomography and bipedal lymphography in 62 patients, and concluded that only limited information was added to the routine presurgical staging of patients with cancer of the cervix.[136] Bandy et al used computed tomography for detecting metastatic tumor in the common iliac and para-aortic lymph nodes in 44 patients with cervical carcinoma.[6] The sensitivity for detection of metastatic nodes was 75%, the specificity was 91%, the negative predictive value was 91% and the positive predictive value was 75%. Fine needle aspiration of nodes 1.5 cm or greater in size detected 67% of metastatic nodes. Camilien and associates studied the preoperative abdominopelvic CT scans of 61 patients and compared the findings with gross and microscopic surgical findings.[22] For para-aortic nodes, the CT scan had a specificity of 100% and a sensitivity of 67%. Histologically positive pelvic nodes were often missed by CT scan. Our clinical experience would agree with these findings. However, since computed tomography scanning is a non-invasive procedure with no significant contraindications, it is often done as a part of the preoperative evaluation of Stage Ib and IIa patients with larger and/or undifferentiated cervical tumors. If a double urinary collecting system can be ruled out by a combination of CT scan and cystoscopy (finding only one ureteral orifice on each side), then an intravenous pyelogram may not be needed in the preoperative evaluation.

Magnetic resonance imaging (MRI) can be helpful in the preoperative evaluation of patients with cervical cancer (see Ch. 19). Burghardt and associates have used MRI to determine exactly the in vivo measurements of the volume of the tumor in the cervix.[19] The measurements of tumor volume correlated extremely well (r = 0.983) with those obtained by histomorphometric analysis of surgical specimens. On the other hand, the correlation with clinical examination was poor. The authors concluded that, in the future, MRI could provide a basis for more precise classification of cervical cancer than the current staging system based on clinical examination. It might also provide a more accurate means of predicting the likelihood of parametrial spread and metastatic tumor in pelvic and para-aortic nodes. It is to be expected that, in the future, further advances in imaging techniques will provide additional useful information to the gynecologic surgeon in selecting the best primary treatment for his patients with cervical cancer.

In order to evaluate the extent of a very early lesion, cervical conization is occasionally required (see Ch. 38). If simple extrafascial hysterectomy is subsequently chosen as the correct surgical treatment, the operation should be done within 48 hours of the conization, or delayed until the cervix has healed, usually about 6 weeks later. If the hysterectomy is done after 48 hours and before the cervix has healed, the risk of serious postoperative infectious morbidity is increased (see p. 597). However, we have found that an extensive abdominal hysterectomy and bilateral pelvic lymphadenectomy can be done at any time after cervical conization, even before the cervix is healed, without increasing the risk of serious postoperative infectious morbidity. The reason for this difference is not clear, but may be related to the fact that indurated and possibly infected paracervical and parametrial tissue is actually removed when an extensive hysterectomy is done. Whenever possible, one should avoid doing diagnostic cervical conization in a patient with deeply invasive cervical cancer. Cervical conization is unavoidable in some patients, when it is necessary to confirm a depth of invasion limited to the superficial 3 mm of cervical stroma so that a more conservative extrafascial hysterectomy may be correctly chosen as adequate primary treatment.

Bowel preparation ordinarily required for intestinal resection is not usually needed for extensive abdominal hysterectomy. The usual preparation for intravenous pyelogram or CT scan (without oral contrast) is usually sufficient preoperative bowel preparation. An intestinal tube for suction is also not usually necessary.

PERTINENT PELVIC ANATOMY

Arterial and venous anatomy

Although the lower portions of the aorta and vena cava are frequently incorporated into the operative field of the pelvic lymphadenectomy, the major operative dissection includes the common iliac, external iliac and hypogastric arteries and veins, and their various branches and tributaries. The abdominal aorta emerges through the aortic hiatus of the diaphragm at the lower border of the last thoracic vertebra, and descends along the ventral surface of the vertebral column where it bifurcates into the left and right common iliac artery at the fourth lumbar vertebra (Fig. 78.2). This is an important anatomic landmark, as the bifurcation at L4 lies directly beneath the umbilicus in most cases. Therefore, an abdominal midline incision that would provide surgical exposure to the lower aorta would need to be extended somewhat above the umbilicus. As demonstrated in Figure 78.2, the right common iliac artery crosses the upper portion of the left common iliac vein at the aortic bifurcation. This segment of the venous drainage of the left side of the pelvis joins with the right common iliac vein to form the vena cava, which lies directly along the right side of the aorta and on the right lateral side of the bodies of the lumbar vertebrae in its retroperitoneal course through the abdomen.

Both common iliac arteries continue along the medial border of the psoas muscle to the pelvic brim, where they divide into external iliac and hypogastric vessels. As shown in Figure 78.3, this important vascular division marks the site where the ureters enter the pelvis from the abdomen, usually overlying the terminal end of the common iliac artery on the left, and commonly crossing the actual bifur-

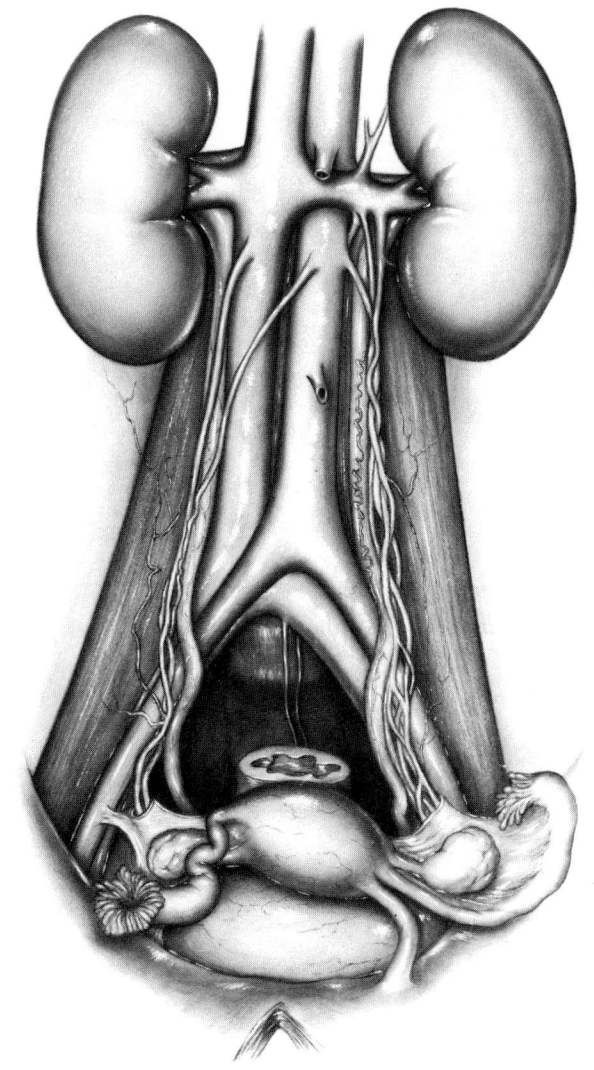

Fig. 78.2 Abdominal and pelvic anatomy, showing the anatomic relationships of the aorta, vena cava, iliac vessels, and ureters. Note the arterial-venous crossing of the right common iliac artery and the left iliac vein.

cation of the artery on the right. Both external iliac arteries pass beneath the inguinal ligament to proceed into the leg as the femoral artery. The external iliac artery makes no direct vascular contribution to the pelvis. There is a fairly consistent arterial branch to the ureter from the mid portion of the common iliac artery.

The external iliac vein emerges from beneath the inguinal ligament, where it courses along the lateral pelvic brim on the medial side of the artery until it reaches the proximal segment. Here, the vein passes directly beneath the artery at the bifurcation of the common iliac artery and then passes along the lateral side of the upper half of the artery. It then joins the left common iliac vein to become the inferior vena cava at the fifth lumbar vertebra. In dissecting the lymph nodes along the external iliac vessels, these anatomic landmarks are important, in order to avoid

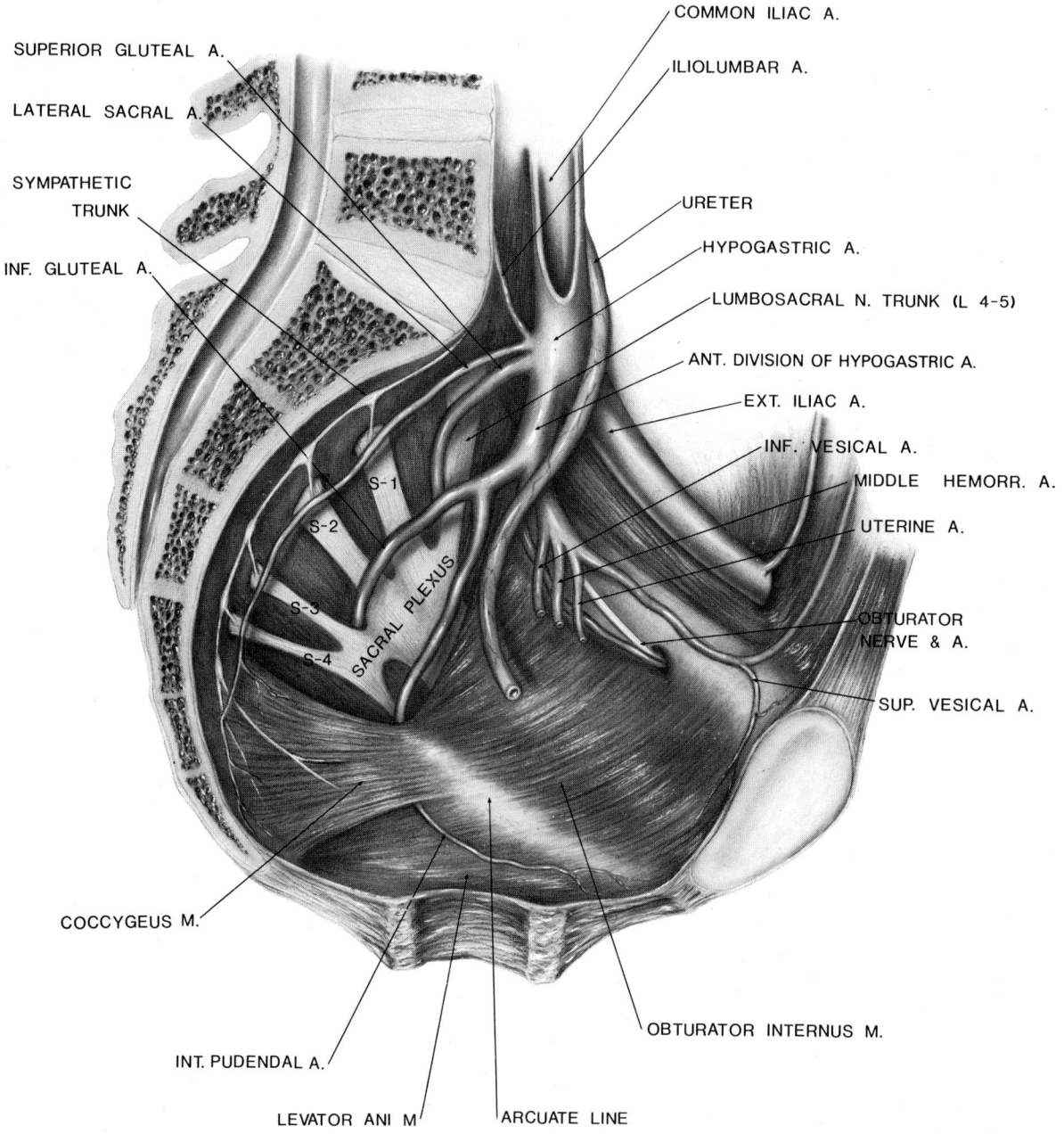

Fig. 78.3 Anatomy of the arterial blood supply to the female pelvis showing relationships of pelvic musculature, divisions of hypogastric artery, and lumbosacral and sacral nerve plexes. Note that the anterior division of the hypogastric artery provides the blood supply to the pelvic viscera.

trauma to the wall of the vein as it deviates from the medial to the lateral side of the arterial tree.

The hypogastric artery provides the major blood supply to the pelvic viscera and, for descriptive purposes, it is conveniently divided into an anterior and posterior division. The important branches of the hypogastric artery are shown in Figure 78.3 and are outlined in Table 78.1.

A fairly consistent arterial branch to the ureter arises from the hypogastric artery near the common iliac bifurcation. This vessel passes medially to the ureter and should

be preserved, if possible, during the dissection of the hypogastric vessels. The hypogastric artery continues beneath the coccygeus muscle and through the ischiorectal fossa, where it becomes the internal pudendal artery to supply the perineum and vulva.

It is important to understand that the major blood supply to the pelvic viscera is derived from the anterior division of the hypogastric artery. As shown in Figure 78.3, the anterior division gives off the uterine artery prior to continuing along the posterolateral pelvic wall to give off the

Table 78.1 Branches of the hypogastric artery

Anterior division	Posterior division
Visceral branches	**Parietal branches**
Uterine	Iliolumbar
Superior vesical	Lateral sacral
Middle vesical	Superior gluteal
Inferior vesical	
Middle hemorrhoidal	
Inferior hemorrhoidal	
Vaginal	
Parietal branches	
Obturator	
Inferior gluteal	
Internal pudendal	

superior and inferior vesical branches to the bladder. The anterior division then continues as the obliterated umbilical artery as it passes cephalad along the inferior surface of the rectus muscle to the umbilicus. In dissecting along the hypogastric artery in a caudad direction, the uterine artery is the first vessel that one encounters which emanates from the medial side of the vessel. Passing more inferiorly and medially is the middle hemorrhoidal artery which supplies a major segment of the rectum and communicates with the superior hemorrhoidal (from the inferior mesenteric) and the inferior hemorrhoidal (from the internal pudendal) arteries.

The hypogastric vein and its tributaries course along the pelvic floor and medial side of the artery to drain the pelvis in close relationship to the arterial blood supply. However, its extensive anatomical variations and its location along the pelvic sidewall and floor place these tortuous thin-walled veins in a precarious and vulnerable position for trauma during deep dissection of the pelvis. As shown in Figure 78.4, the delicate tributaries of the trunk of the hypogastric vein extend into sacral foramina, and pass beneath nerve fibers and muscles within the pelvis such that their identity during the dissection of the pelvis is frequently obscured. The continuation of the hypogastric vein, in association

with the artery, beneath the coccygeus muscle is a troublesome site of bleeding when dissection is undertaken along the pelvic floor. When this occurs, it is difficult to identify the vessel, as it retracts beneath the margins of the muscle.

The collateral blood supply to the ureter is an important anatomical safeguard that protects its pelvic segment from ischemic necrosis as a result of the extensive hysterectomy. As shown in Figure 78.5, the ureter has the advantage of a multiple source blood supply. This favorable collateral circulation permits interruption of small arteries and veins deep in the pelvis during extensive dissection of the base of the broad ligament, without producing a significant incidence of ischemic necrosis and fistula formation. The freely anastomosing arterial and venous network that courses along the longitudinal surface of the ureter in its adventitial layer is supplied in its superior segment by branches from the renal and ovarian arteries. The middle segment of the ureter derives its blood supply directly from aortic branches and from a vessel from the common iliac artery. As the ureter enters the pelvis and courses along the lateral pelvic wall, it receives arterial branches from the uterine, vaginal, middle hemorrhoidal and vesical arteries. As it approaches the trigone of the bladder, it has a rich arterial and venous collateral circulation from the arterial branches to the vagina and base of the bladder. Protection of this important vascular network is important for the integrity of the terminal ureter during extensive dissection of the cardinal ligament. Preservation of the lateral aspect of the posterior segment of the vesicouterine ligament has been recommended to insure adequate vascularity to the terminal segment of the ureter, but we have encoun-

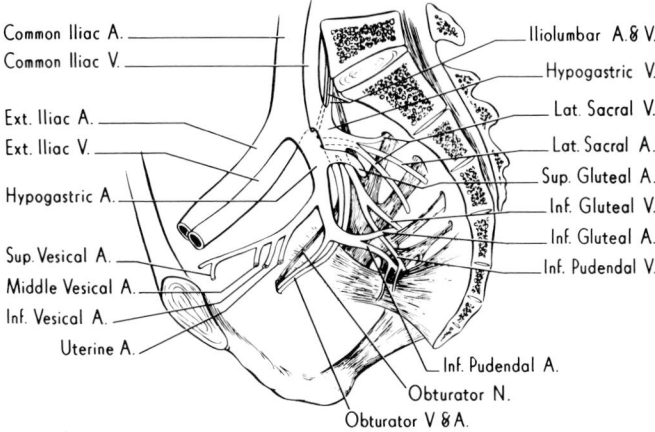

Fig. 78.4 Anatomy of hypogastric vein.

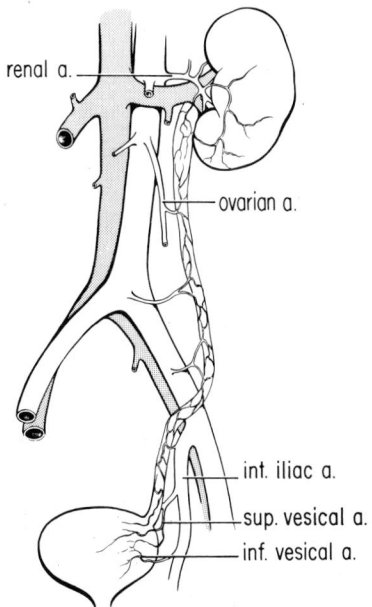

Fig. 78.5 Blood supply of the ureter showing multiple source of collateral arterial circulation.

tered no difficulty in removing this tissue and have no hesitation in doing so to enhance the adequacy of the central dissection.

Lymphatic anatomy

The lymphatic drainage of the pelvis follows the course of the arterial and venous blood supply. Although there are multiple variations in the lymphatic anatomy of the pelvis, in general there are lateral, superior, medial and inferior lymph nodes and communicating lymphatic channels that surround the common iliac, external iliac and hypogastric vessels (Fig. 78.6). One of the important pathways of the pelvic nodes and thin-walled lymphatics that drain the upper vagina, cervix and uterus courses along the posterior aspect of the endopelvic fascia. Here, they pass through the uterosacral ligament area and terminate in lymph nodes along the lateral aspect of the sacrum. These nodes communicate freely with lymphatic channels from the bifurcation of the common iliac artery near the lateral sacral and ischiosacral fossae. These may be difficult nodes to resect, as they are closely attached to the thin-walled tributaries of the hypogastric vein. In dissecting the nodes from the bifurcation of the common iliac vessels, care must be taken to avoid injury to the hypogastric vein, which extends from beneath the artery on the medial side in this area.

The most direct lymphatic drainage of the cervix and upper vagina is through the lateral parametrium (cardinal ligament) to the hypogastric and obturator lymphatics. Due to the presence of obscure obturator veins and multiple venous tributaries from the hypogastric vein along the pelvic floor, the obturator dissection may be associated with troublesome venous bleeding. Injury may also occur to the obturator nerve, which arises from the anterior division of the second, third, and fourth lumbar nerves, enters the pelvis through the psoas muscle and runs along the lateral pelvic wall in the obturator fossa to exit the pelvis through the obturator foramen along with the obturator vessels. It is a motor nerve to the adductor muscles of the thigh, and is the only motor nerve that arises from the lumbar plexus without innervating any of the pelvic structures. Damage to the obturator nerve will not only produce motor impairment to the adductor muscles, but will also cause sensory loss along the medial aspect of the thigh. Deep dissection beneath the obturator nerve may be complicated by bleeding from the tributaries of the hypogastric and obturator veins. Many clinics omit this portion of the pelvic lymph node dissection along the floor of the obturator space, in order to avoid this complication. It is our position however, that such a conservative dissection provides a sanctuary for occult metastatic tumor and can give false assurance of the absence of tumor spread from the cervical cancer. It is on this point that gynecologic surgeons can be divided into two groups: those who do a rather timid removal of pelvic lymph nodes, taking counsel from Wertheim's own modifications to limit the procedure; and those who do an extensive lymphadenectomy, insisting that all removable pelvic nodes that are potential sites for tumor metastasis be removed.

Reiffenstuhl, in his classic study of the lymphatics of the female genital organs, describes efferent lymph channels from the cervix to the interiliac lymph nodes, to the lateral and medial external iliac lymph nodes, to the lateral and medial common iliac lymph nodes, to the sacral lymph nodes, to the subaortic lymph nodes, to the aortic lymph nodes, to the superior gluteal lymph nodes, to the inferior gluteal lymph nodes and to the rectal lymph nodes.[106] Of these, the inferior gluteal nodes are not technically possible to remove. This is because the nodes lie around the ischial spine in close proximity to the inferior gluteal artery and pudendal artery and nerve. An imposing network of veins also surrounds the inferior gluteal nodes. They are thin-walled, easy to damage, difficult to expose, and difficult to control when damaged. Admittedly, this is a weak point in the performance of pelvic lymphadenectomy, and in attempting to remove all nodes that represent a primary station to which cancer from the cervix may metastasize.

Reiffenstuhl 's concepts of the lymphatic drainage of the cervix are partially illustrated in Figures 78.7 to 78.10.

CONCEPT OF EXTENSIVE ABDOMINAL HYSTERECTOMY AND BILATERAL PELVIC LYMPHADENECTOMY

Various modifications of the extensive hysterectomy and pelvic node dissection are practiced at the M. D. Anderson Hospital in Houston, Texas, where five classes of extended hysterectomy are used for the treatment of cervical cancer. The Class I hysterectomy is a slight extension of the total hysterectomy with removal of a small amount of parametrium. It is used primarily for microinvasive carcinoma and for removal of the uterus with a barrel-shaped endocervical adenocarcinoma after preoperative irradiation.

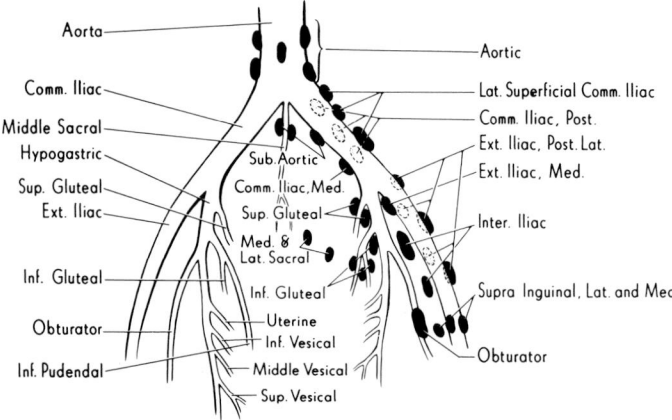

Fig. 78.6 Lymphatic drainage of the pelvis.

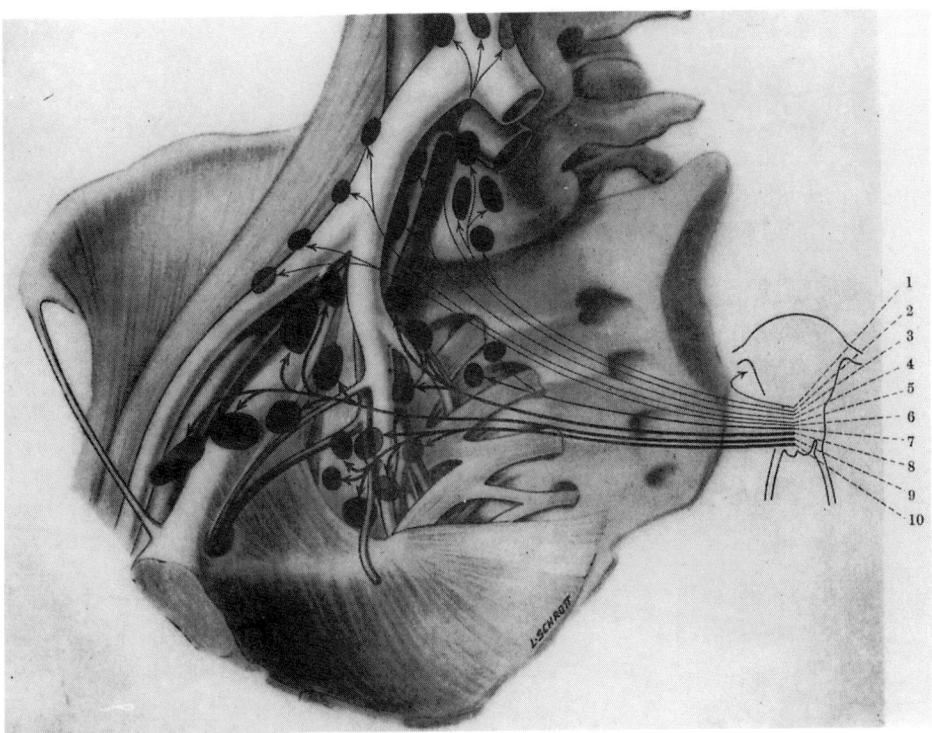

Fig. 78.7 The regional lymph node stations of the uterine cervix. Channels 8, 9 and 10 (indicated by especially heavy lines) lead to those regional lymph node stations most frequently reached by the efferent lymph vessels of the cervix. Nonetheless, it is necessary to remember that carcinoma cells can also reach the pelvic lymph nodes by way of channels 1 to 7, without previous interruption.

To (1) rectal, (2) subaortic (promontorial), (3) aortic, (4) medial common iliac, (5) lateral common iliac, (6) lateral external iliac, (7) sacral, (8) superior gluteal, (9) interiliac and (10) inferior gluteal lymph nodes.

(Reproduced from Reiffenstuhl G 1964 *The Lymphatics of the Female Genital Organs*. Lippincott, Philadelphia, with permission.)

The Class II extended hysterectomy (TeLinde modified Wertheim) removes a more generous parametrial cuff, ligates the uterine artery on the medial side of the ureter, but does not dissect the ureter from the vesico-uterine ligament. The Class III operation is the classical Meigs' procedure, with removal of all of the parametrium and paravaginal tissue in addition to some of the pelvic lymph nodes. A more extensive procedure is performed in the Class IV radical hysterectomy, whereby the ureter is completely dissected from the cardinal and vesico-uterine ligaments; the superior vesical artery is sacrificed and three-fourths of the vagina is removed, as well as the uterus and parametria, along with a complete lymphadenectomy. A far more extensive procedure is done with the Class V radical hysterectomy, whereby the terminal ureter or a segment of the bladder and/or rectum are removed along with the uterus, parametria, adnexa and pelvic lymph nodes.

While many techniques emphasize a more or less extensive dissection in one phase of the operation or another, the management of the parametria and the dissection of the pelvic lymph nodes appear relatively uniform. Since the most serious complication of this procedure is related to ureteral fistulae and stenosis, many modifications have been undertaken in recent years to insure an adequate blood supply to the terminal ureter. We agree that the terminal ureter must have a good blood supply, and feel that this can be accomplished without jeopardizing the adequacy of the central dissection. The classical Wertheim hysterectomy, with wide resection of the parametrium, dissection of the terminal ureter from the vesico-uterine ligament, and wide resection of the uterosacral ligaments, upper 3 to 4 cm of vagina and paravaginal tissues, along with a thorough pelvic lymphadenectomy, constitutes the procedure that is traditionally used in this clinic.

The major focus of the operation is the adequacy of the central dissection. The central cervical tumor must be removed with an adequate margin of uninvolved normal tissue around it. This is the most crucial point in the success of the operation and has been emphasized by many of the famous pelvic surgeons of former years, including Parsons and Navratil, and many others. The central dissection can be facilitated by developing the pelvic spaces and utilizing proper planes for dissection. Correct dissection along natural, rather than artificial connective tissue planes, and correct development of the pelvic spaces (paravesical, pararectal, vesicocervical and rectovaginal), will avoid unnecessary injury to pelvic vessels, keep blood loss to a minimum and facilitate an adequate central dissection. These connective tissue planes and pelvic spaces are beautifully described by Reiffenstuhl.[105] The central

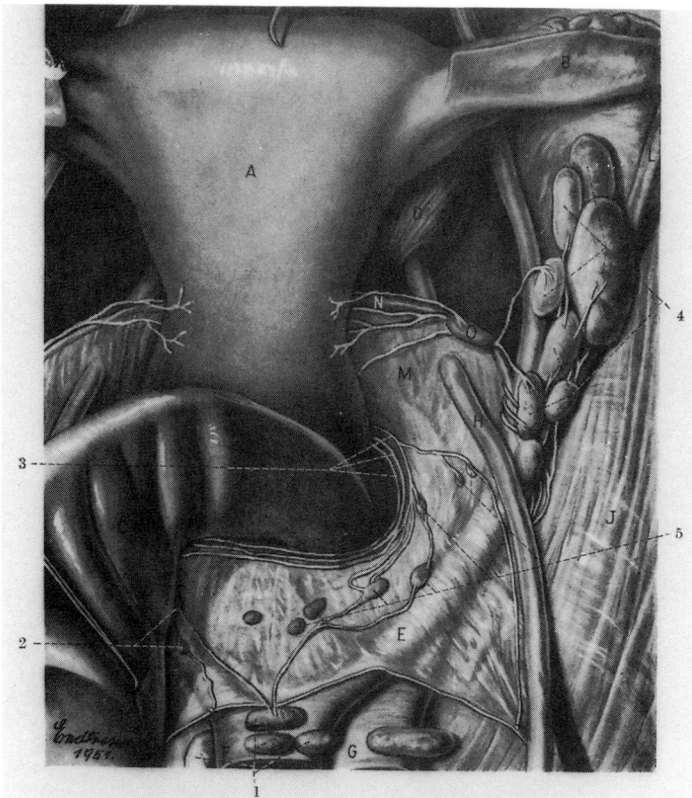

Fig. 78.8 Lymphatic drainage of the cervix along the uterine artery and the sagittal rectal pillar (recto-uterine ligament). The uterus is drawn markedly upward. View of the posterior surface of the uterus (A).

Several lymph vessels from the cervix twine about the uterine artery (N), pass the uterine-ureteral nodule (O), which is located on the right side of the specimen at the lateral edge of the ureter (H), and, after crossing over the lateral umbilical ligament (K), empty into the uppermost interiliac lymph nodes (4). A few lymph channels from the cervix (3) run dorsally at the base of Mackenrodt's ligament (M) in the sagittal rectal pillar and reach the superior rectal lymph nodes (2) which lie along the likenamed artery on the posterior surface of the rectum. The lymph vessels in the ureteral leaf, coming from the cervix, first run dorsally in the sagittal rectal pillar for some distance and then, before reaching the rectum, turn upward to the nodes in the ureteral leaf (5). The ureteral leaf is a continuation of the sagittal rectal pillar cranially. The lymph channels then empty directly into the lowest aortic lymph nodes (1).

One lymph vessel from the cervix runs upward on the medial edge of the right ureter (variant).

(A) Uterus (intestinal surface); (B) right ovary; (C) rectum; (D) urinary bladder (posterior surface); (E) common iliac artery; (F) aorta; (G) inferior vena cava; (H) ureter; (J) psoas muscle; (K) lateral umbilical ligament; (L) external iliac artery; (M) Mackenrodt's ligament; (N) uterine artery; (O) lymph node. (1) Aortic lymph nodes; (2) rectal lymph nodes; (3) lymphatic vessels; (4) interiliac lymph nodes; (5) lymph nodes. (Reproduced from Reiffenstuhl G 1964 *The Lymphatics of the Female Genital Organs.* Lippincott, Philadelphia, with permission.)

dissection is also facilitated by a complete removal of the contents of the obturator fossa (except the obturator nerve, of course) so that branches of the hypogastric artery and vein in the cardinal ligament are clearly visible and can be dissected away from their attachment to the lateral pelvic sidewall.

The importance of an adequate central dissection was emphasized recently by Girardi and associates.[41] By studying surgical specimens processed according to the giant section technique of Burghardt & Pickel, parametrial lymph nodes were found in 280 (78%) of the 359 surgical specimens from extensive hysterectomies.[20] Metastatically involved parametrial nodes were found in 63 (22.5%) of these 280. The lymphatic drainage from the cervix to the pelvic lymph nodes runs through the parametrium, and deposits of tumor often are found there. An adequate central dissection must include removal of a wide margin

of parametrial tissue around the central tumor, and total removal of the parametria from the bladder, the rectum and the lateral pelvic wall, since positive lymph nodes can be found in the lateral, as well as medial parametrium.

When a large vaginal cuff must be removed because of a bulky cervical tumor and/or involvement of adjacent vaginal mucosa, starting the operation from below will facilitate the central dissection. A bulky lesion is sometimes excised and fulgurated transvaginally. The formation of the vaginal cuff is done in a manner similar to the Schauta-Amreich procedure. The vaginal incision is made around the entire circumference of the vagina, mobilizing the vaginal cuff from paravaginal tissue. Further dissection from below into the paravesical space, vesicocervical space and rectovaginal space, will sometimes be easier than from above. (See also Chs 77 and 80.)

Above the mid-common iliac arteries and in the para-

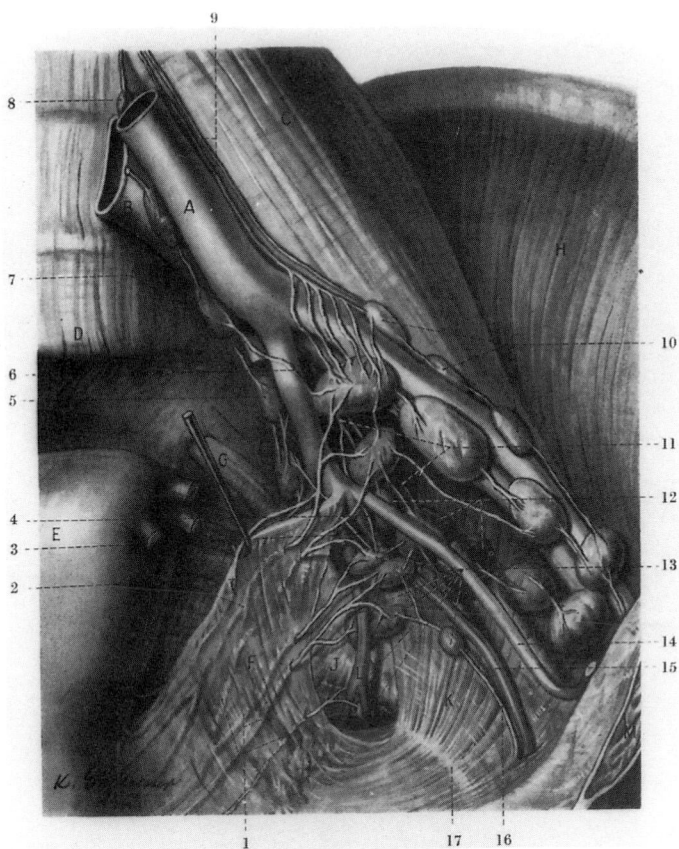

Fig. 78.9 Inflow and outflow of the inferior gluteal lymph nodes. View of the anterior surface of Mackenrodt's ligament (F). The uterine artery is drawn upward by means of a hook. The lateral portion of the pelvic origin of Mackenrodt's ligament was removed to bring the deep nodes of the group on the sacral plexus (J) into view. Furthermore, the veins of the vesico-utero-vaginal plexus, which hide the nodes, were not drawn in. The lateral umbilical ligament (14) was left in place.

Cervical lymphatic channels (1), which run to the pelvic wall in the basal portions of the parametrium and then empty into the inferior gluteal lymph nodes (13) predominate. These nodes extend along the inferior gluteal — internal pudendal artery down as far as the infrapiriform foramen and, in part, lie behind the parietal blood vessels. From the inferior gluteal lymph nodes (a) efferent vessels (3) run to the superior gluteal lymph nodes (5), (b) vessels turn as deep channels (4, then 11) to the posterior side of the parietal blood vessels, and (c) connections run to those interiliac lymph nodes on the obturator artery (12), which, on their part, send their deep channels (11) upward to the deep lateral common iliac lymph nodes. From the uppermost interiliac lymph nodes lying in the hypogastric angle, one lymph channel (6) reaches the medial common iliac lymph nodes (7) by crossing over the stem of the internal iliac artery. Note also the numerous efferent vessels of the uppermost interiliac nodes which cross over the initial portion of the external iliac artery and then run upward on the lateral edge of the common iliac artery as a cable (9).

(A) Common iliac artery; (B) common iliac vein; (C) psoas muscle; (D) promontory; (E) uterus; (F) Mackenrodt's ligament; (G) 1st sacral nerve; (H) iliac muscle; (J) sacral plexus; (K) internal obturator muscle; (L) internal pudendal-inferior gluteal artery; (M) internal oblique and transverse abdominal muscles. (1 & 2) Cervical lymph vessels; (3 & 4) efferent vessels; (5) superior gluteal lymph nodes; (6) efferent vessel; (7) medial common iliac and (8) deep lateral common iliac lymph nodes; (9) lymphatic vessels; (10) lateral external iliac lymph nodes; (11) efferent vessels; (12) interiliac (obturator) and (13) inferior gluteal lymph nodes; (14) lateral umbilical ligament; (15) obturator artery; (16) lymphatic vessel; (17) tendinous arch of the levator ani muscle.
(Reproduced from Reiffenstuhl G 1964 *The Lymphatics of the Female Genital Organs.* Lippincott, Philadelphia, with permission.)

aortic region, lymph nodes are sampled and a special effort is made to remove any nodes that look or feel suspicious. A serious effort is made to do a very complete lymphadenectomy below the level of the mid-common iliac artery. This includes the tissue around the major vessels down to the inguinal ligament. Special attention is given to removal of lymph nodes that are located between the lower common iliac vessels and the psoas muscle (lateral common iliac nodes) at the point where the obturator nerve enters the obturator fossa through the belly of the psoas muscle. Complete removal of these nodes will expose the

roots of the lumbo-sacral nerve plexus. The obturator nerve is dissected free from its entrance into the superior obturator fossa through the psoas muscle, to its exit through the obturator foramen inferiorly. The anterior division of the hypogastric artery is routinely ligated at a point just distal to the origin of the posterior trunk. According to Roberts and associates, it cannot be proved that ligation of the anterior division of the hypogastric artery increases the risks of urinary tract fistulas.[108] The dissection leaves the hypogastric vein and its branches exposed and intact. The various vessels that compose the cardinal

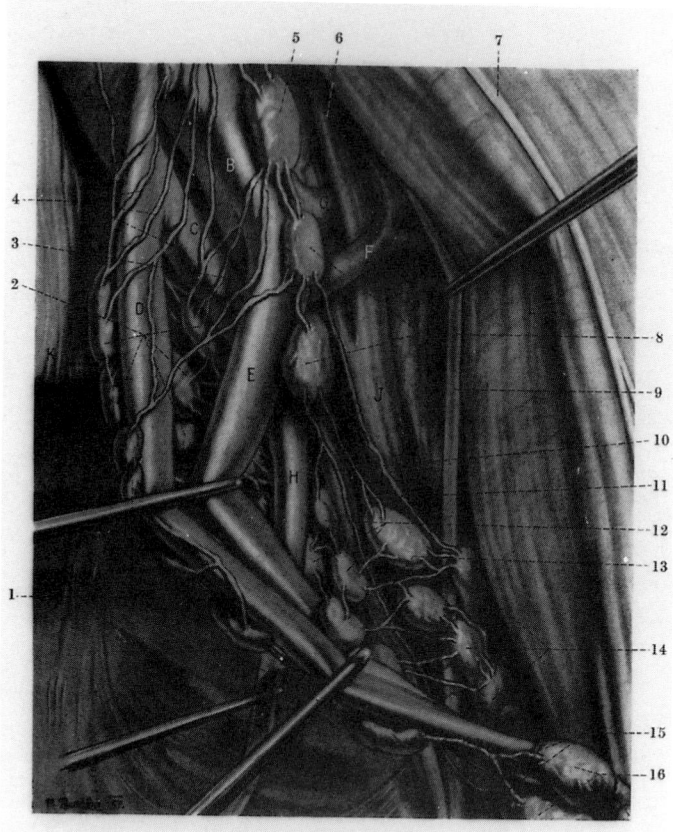

Fig. 78.10 View into the niche between the psoas muscle and the external iliac vessels, representing a continuation of Figure 78.9, down to the femoral ring. The blood vessels (C, D, E, H) were drawn medially by a hook (view of their posterior side), and the psoas muscle (L) with the obturator nerve (9) was forced laterally. The lumbosacral trunk (J) appears at the bottom of the niche.

The efferent channels of the uppermost interiliac lymph nodes climb over (4) the outer edge of the external and the common iliac arteries and reach the deep lateral common iliac lymph nodes (see Fig. 78.9). However, the deep efferent channels (3) of the uppermost interiliac lymph nodes also open into the deep nodes located on the posterior side of the parietal blood vessels, after crossing under the internal iliac artery (C). The nodes (12) lying at the cranial edge of the obturator artery (13) and the nodes (14) of this group (interiliac lymph nodes) found laterally to the obturator nerve (9) send efferent vessels to the deep lateral external iliac lymph nodes (8). From the great nodes on the femoral ring (16) two primary lymphatic paths lead upward. One path (15) runs along the outer edge of the external iliac artery where several superficial lateral external iliac lymph nodes (1) are located. The other, in the form of numerous lymph nodes (14, 12), which in part lie lateral and in part medial to the obturator nerve, and their connecting lymph vessels lead upward.

(A) Common iliac artery; (B) common iliac vein; (C) internal iliac artery (posterior aspect); (D) external iliac artery (posterior aspect); (E) external iliac vein (posterior aspect); (F) iliolumbar artery; (G) iliolumbar vein; (H) lateral umbilical ligament; (J) lumbosacral trunk; (K) promontory; (L) psoas muscle. (1) lateral external iliac and (2) interiliac lymph nodes; (3) deep efferent vessels; (4) efferebt vessels; (5) deep lateral common iliac lymph node; (6) half of 4th lumbar nerve; (7) genitofemoral nerve; (8) deep lateral external iliac lymph nodes; (9) obturator nerve; (10 & 11) efferent vessels; (12) interiliac lymph nodes; (13) obturator artery; (14) interiliac lymph nodes; (15) efferent vessels; (16) femoral ring lymph nodes. (Reproduced from Reiffenstuhl G 1964 *The Lymphatics of the Female Genital Organs.* Lippincott, Philadelphia, with permission.)

ligament are individually clipped or ligated at the lateral pelvic sidewall and an attempt is made to remove as much of the cardinal ligament as possible. No attempt is made to do an en bloc removal of the nodes. Suspicious nodes may be sent for frozen section and various parts of the specimen are marked for identification. The ureters are left intact until the lymphadenectomy is completed. The surgeon is cognizant of the closeness of the dissection to the central tumor throughout the remainder of the operation. The plane of dissection usually comes closest to the cervix in development of the vesicocervical space. The ureter is freed from its passage through the 'tunnel' and the anterior and posterior parts of the vesico-uterine ligament are

ligated as close to the bladder as possible without injury. The peri-ureteral sheath is carefully preserved, but the ureter is otherwise usually completely detached for a distance of 4 to 5 cm above its entrance into the bladder wall. The development of the posterior rectovaginal space allows identification of the posterior parametrium including the uterosacral ligaments. This tissue is clamped and dissected away as close to the rectum as possible. The only remaining tissue to be clamped and removed is paravaginal, following which the specimen is removed by an incision in the vaginal wall at an appropriate distance from the cervix. Several biopsies are taken from the margin of the vaginal apex left remaining.

Two different approaches to performing an extensive abdominal hysterectomy and bilateral pelvic lymphadenectomy will be described. The traditional transperitoneal approach has been used in our clinic for many years with satisfactory results. The transverse Maylard incision is preferred for this approach, but lower midline incisions have also been used in selected patients. In recent years, encouraged by the experience of doing extraperitoneal lymphadenectomies following the Schauta-Amreich extensive vaginal hysterectomy, and by the experience of Breen[17] and others, our preferred technique is to first perform the bilateral pelvic lymphadenectomy extraperitoneally through an elliptical transverse Maylard incision across the lower abdominal wall that is extended upward and laterally to the level of the anterior superior iliac spine or above if necessary. Exposure of the pelvic sidewall is superb and removal of lower para-aortic lymph nodes can be accomplished with proper retraction. Reflection of the intact peritoneum away from the pelvic sidewalls greatly assists in retraction of the bowel with less trauma to the serosa. Thus unnecessary and prolonged exposure of intraperitoneal organs is avoided during extraperitoneal lymphadenectomy. It is our impression that intestinal function returns more promptly in the postoperative recovery period and postoperative adhesion formation may be less.

There are a few disadvantages of this approach, related to the fact that exploration of the abdomen and pelvis, ordinarily done first, is delayed. The transperitoneal central dissection is delayed until the extraperitoneal lymphadenectomy is completed, and is the last stage of the operation. Theoretically, there could be findings from exploration that might alter the treatment plan, but we have thus far not encountered a situation in which we regretted having done the bilateral extraperitoneal lymphadenectomy first before exploring the abdomen and pelvis transperitoneally.

In a study of 284 patients from Gynecologic Oncology Group institutions, a comparison of extraperitoneal and transperitoneal selective para-aortic lymphadenectomy was made.[139] Although the difference in the two approaches was not great, the authors concluded that selective para-aortic lymphadenectomy should be performed by the extraperitoneal approach rather than the transperitoneal approach, to minimize certain post-irradiation enteric complications. Gallup et al have favored extraperitoneal pelvic lymphadenectomy for pre-radiation surgical staging and also extensive hysterectomy, although their preference is for a midline incision.[39] Extraperitoneal pelvic lymphadenectomy has been done for many years in patients with advanced vulvar cancer, for urologically related cancers, and following the Schauta-Amreich extensive vaginal hysterectomy for cervical cancer. It is a familiar technique to most gynecologic surgeons.

At present, we use the combined extraperitoneal-transperitoneal extensive hysterectomy and pelvic lymphadenectomy technique for all patients selected for primary surgical treatment, with few exceptions. If, in addition to cancer of the cervix, there also exists a large pelvic tumor (leiomyomata uteri, ovarian cysts, intra-uterine pregnancy, etc.), the removal of which will improve exposure, then the entire operation is done through a transperitoneal approach using the extended Maylard incision. If there is good reason to suspect para-aortic node metastases or other significant upper abdominal or intraperitoneal disease, the entire operation is done through a transperitoneal approach. Otherwise we feel there is an advantage to performing the bilateral lymphadenectomy extraperitoneally and the extensive hysterectomy transperitoneally through the same extended transverse Maylard incision.

Teamwork is needed to do the operation correctly, and no member of the team is more important than the anesthesiologist. With prior planning and cooperation between the surgeon and the anesthesiologist, a safe and effective technique of anesthesia can be chosen which will not only provide pain relief and relaxation, but will also deliberately induce hypotension and reduce circulation to the operative field. A reduction in arteriolar resistance will lower blood pressure and reduce, to a certain degree, bleeding in the operative field. However, the main mechanism for control of operative field bleeding by anesthesia lies in reduction of venous tone, which reduces ventricular filling and cardiac output, the major determinant of blood pressure. The desired reduction in venous tone is achieved by one or more of the following anesthetic techniques: ganglionic blockage; spinal or epidural anesthesia; specific venodilating agents, such as sodium nitroprusside or glyceryl trinitrate; and by the effect of some anesthetic agents. The use of induced hypotension is more effective if the operative field is raised above the level of the heart in order to encourage local venous emptying by gravity. Therefore, a modest Trendelenburg position should be used.

Deliberate hypotension is now an established practice, although some anesthesiologists are more enthusiastic about its use than others, and must be trained in the technique to use it safely. Our experience with its use in extensive pelvic dissections for malignant disease has been uniformly favorable. The blood loss in extensive hysterectomy can be reduced by 50% or more, and the need for blood replacement reduced by a corresponding amount. In a report by Powell and co-workers, a deliberate hypotensive anesthetic technique utilizing nitroglycerin and general anesthesia decreased the blood loss in extensive abdominal hysterectomy with pelvic lymphadenectomy by 70% when compared to a control group. The percentage of patients requiring blood transfusion was reduced from 81% to 11.5%.[103] Favorable experience with induced hypotensive anesthetic techniques to reduce blood loss during extensive hysterectomy and pelvic lymphadenectomy was also reported by Bithal et al[11] and by Wong et al.[146]

Unnecessary bleeding in the area of dissection stains tissues, obscures visibility, restricts technical freedom, increases the possibility of unnecessary injury to other structures, and gradually adds up to a significant amount of blood loss that may require replacement. We have no doubt that deliberate hypotension is a valuable technique, but it cannot substitute for a lack of technical skill or careful surgical hemostasis. 'Reactionary hemorrhage' bleeding after blood pressure returns to normal, will occur until hemostasis is meticulous.

After anesthesia is induced, the patient is placed comfortably in Allen Universal stirrups with the buttocks brought to the edge of the 'broken' table. The knees are separated about 90°. The thighs are elevated only 15 to 20° relative to the abdomen. Care is taken to avoid pressure on the peroneal nerve. This position has several advantages. There is less strain on the patient's lumbosacral spine when the thigh is slightly flexed; this is especially important for patients with lumbosacral back problems. It is possible to have a second assistant stand at the foot of the table between the patient's legs; his/her participation in the operation is greatly facilitated by being closer to the operative field. Lastly, in this position, the urethral orifice, vaginal introitus and anal orifice are all available for instrumentation should this be necessary.

After the patient is positioned on the operating table, the bladder is emptied with a catheter and a careful rectovaginal-abdominal pelvic examination is done. This may be followed by cystoscopy and/or sigmoidoscopy if desired. It may be necessary to shave a small amount of the escutcheon, but vulvar hair is not shaved. The skin is prepped from the rib margin to the midthigh, with special attention given to the umbilicus and vagina. The patient is draped, a transurethral Foley catheter is inserted into the bladder, and the operation begins.

When operating abdominally, the exposure achieved will depend on the choice of incision, the method(s) of retracting, the placement and intensity of overhead lights, and the participation of willing and skilful assistants. Suction should be available to keep the field as dry as possible, and is preferred over sponges for two reasons. Firstly, sponges are more traumatic to delicate serosal surfaces and other tissues. And secondly, a determination of the amount of blood lost can be more accurate if the largest percentage has actually been suctioned from the operative field into a calibrated bottle and measured. Unfortunately, patients undergoing extensive hysterectomy and lymphadenectomy are not considered appropriate candidates for intraoperative autologous transfusion unless the need is desperate.

It is usually possible (and always desirable) to keep the number of clamps in the operative field to an absolute minimum. If the field is cluttered with clamps, the operator cannot see as well to operate. There is an unfortunate tendency for gynecologic surgeons to use instruments that are too short. Pedicle clamps, tissue forceps, dissecting scissors, needle holders and all other instruments must be longer when operating deep in the pelvis and when operating on obese patients. The handles of the instruments must come all the way out and above the level of the incision, so as not to interfere with the operator's vision.

After the incision is made, the lymphadenectomy is done first. A right-handed surgeon will usually stand on the patient's right side to dissect the left pelvic sidewall. He/she will usually change positions several times during the course of the operation. One should choose to dissect that side of the pelvis first which corresponds to the side of the cervix with the greatest tumor involvement.

SURGICAL TECHNIQUE OF TRANSPERITONEAL APPROACH

Evaluation at laparotomy

The operation is initiated through an extended Maylard or low midline incision. In most cases, the umbilicus identifies the location of the bifurcation of the aorta, and therefore, extension of the incision approximately 2 to 3 cm above the umbilicus is recommended for adequate exposure. The bladder is decompressed by an indwelling catheter throughout the procedure, in order to maintain an accurate record of urinary output. The incision is protected by a moist pack beneath each arm of the self-retaining retractor, in order to avoid excessive compression of the epigastric vessels that course beneath the rectus muscles. In case of a lengthy operative procedure, the mechanical retractors are released at periodic intervals in order to improve circulation through the abdominal musculature.

Prior to initiating the pelvic procedure, the abdominal viscera and parietal peritoneum of the abdominal cavity are evaluated meticulously for possible evidence of metastatic tumor. The superior and inferior surfaces of the liver are carefully inspected, as well as the region of the celiac plexus. The undersurface of the diaphragm is particularly vulnerable for metastases, especially the right hemidiaphragm where the para-aortic lymphatics pass from the abdominal cavity into the mediastinum. The mesentery of the large and small bowel, and the serosal surface of the bowel, along with the omentum, should be carefully examined for evidence of metastatic tumor. The kidneys are examined and the retroperitoneal space along the aorta and vena cava is palpated repeatedly, as these are the major sites of extrapelvic spread of cervical cancer. It is well known that 15% or more of para-aortic node metastases are occult, so that even the most unsuspecting node should be removed and evaluated histologically by frozen section study for possible metastatic tumor. It is our practice, therefore, to sample any para-caval or para-aortic node that is identifiable prior to initiating the procedure. Should there be histopathologic evidence of unsuspected, metastatic tumor in several para-aortic lymph nodes, the operation is abandoned and the disease is considered technically inoperable. In such cases, the patient is treated with full pelvic and para-aortic irradiation.

Although considered unnecessary by some, we take peritoneal washings routinely for cytological examination. The significance of a positive result may be difficult to determine, however.

Evaluation of the extent of the pelvic tumor is carried out at this time by examining the course of the lymphatic drainage of the pelvis, which is carefully palpated along the pelvic vessels. When enlarged or clinically suspicious nodes are found, they are removed and immediately sent for frozen section study while further evaluation of the pelvis is undertaken. The paravesical and pararectal spaces are important anatomic landmarks, as they provide an area for thorough exploration of the intervening base of the broad ligament (Fig. 78.11). Tumor will extend into the base of the broad ligament without anatomic evidence of disease being detected prior to operation. This step is therefore a safeguard in determining the possible extension of tumor beyond the cervix and into the immediate paracervical tissues. When there is evidence of extracervical disease, we may abandon the surgical procedure unless there is clear evidence that the disease can be cleanly removed. In either case, full pelvic irradiation is indicated. Certainly, the lateral pelvic wall must be free of tumor. When the central tumor is clearly resectable, we do not hesitate to complete the operation even if there is evidence of metastatic disease in the pelvic lymph nodes.

Development of paravesical space

The anterior leaf of the broad ligament forms the roof of the paravesical space and blends with the bladder peritoneum medially and with the parietal peritoneum laterally. This deep fossa beneath the peritoneal covering is composed of loose connective tissue and fat. It occupies the area between the bladder and retropubic space medially, with the pelvic sidewall and obturator muscle forming the lateral boundaries. The superior boundary is formed by the cardinal ligament, while the floor is composed of the levator ani muscle. After clamping, ligating and excising the round ligament approximately midway along its course, the anterior leaf of the broad ligament is opened in an inferior direction, passing well into the pelvis before diverting the incision medially to reflect the bladder peritoneum from the lower uterine segment (Fig. 78.12). With gentle digital pressure, the paravesical space can be entered without difficulty, making certain that the dissection is initiated on the lateral side of the obliterated hypogastric artery (lateral umbilical ligament), and carried all the way down to the levator ani muscle (Fig. 78.13). The hypogastric artery gives off the superior vesical artery in this area and continues onto the undersurface of the rectus muscle where it becomes the obliterated umbilical artery. There are no major blood vessels in this potential space, although occasionally an aberrant obturator vessel may emerge from the inferior epigastric artery and course along the posterior aspect of the pubic bone to the obturator space. With gentle digital dissection, the pelvic floor can be palpated and the posterior aspect of the space can be identified, including the anterior margin of the cardinal ligament.

Development of pararectal space

The pararectal space lies beneath the pelvic peritoneum and extends between the cardinal ligament laterally and the uterosacral ligament medially. It can be entered by extend-

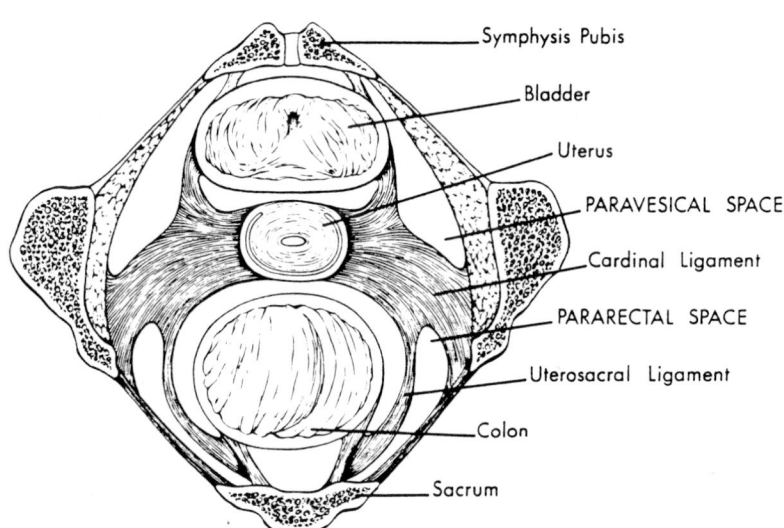

Fig. 78.11 Cross section of pelvis showing paravesical and pararectal space. The base of the broad ligament (cardinal ligament) extends to the lateral pelvic wall and contains the major lymphatics draining the cervix.

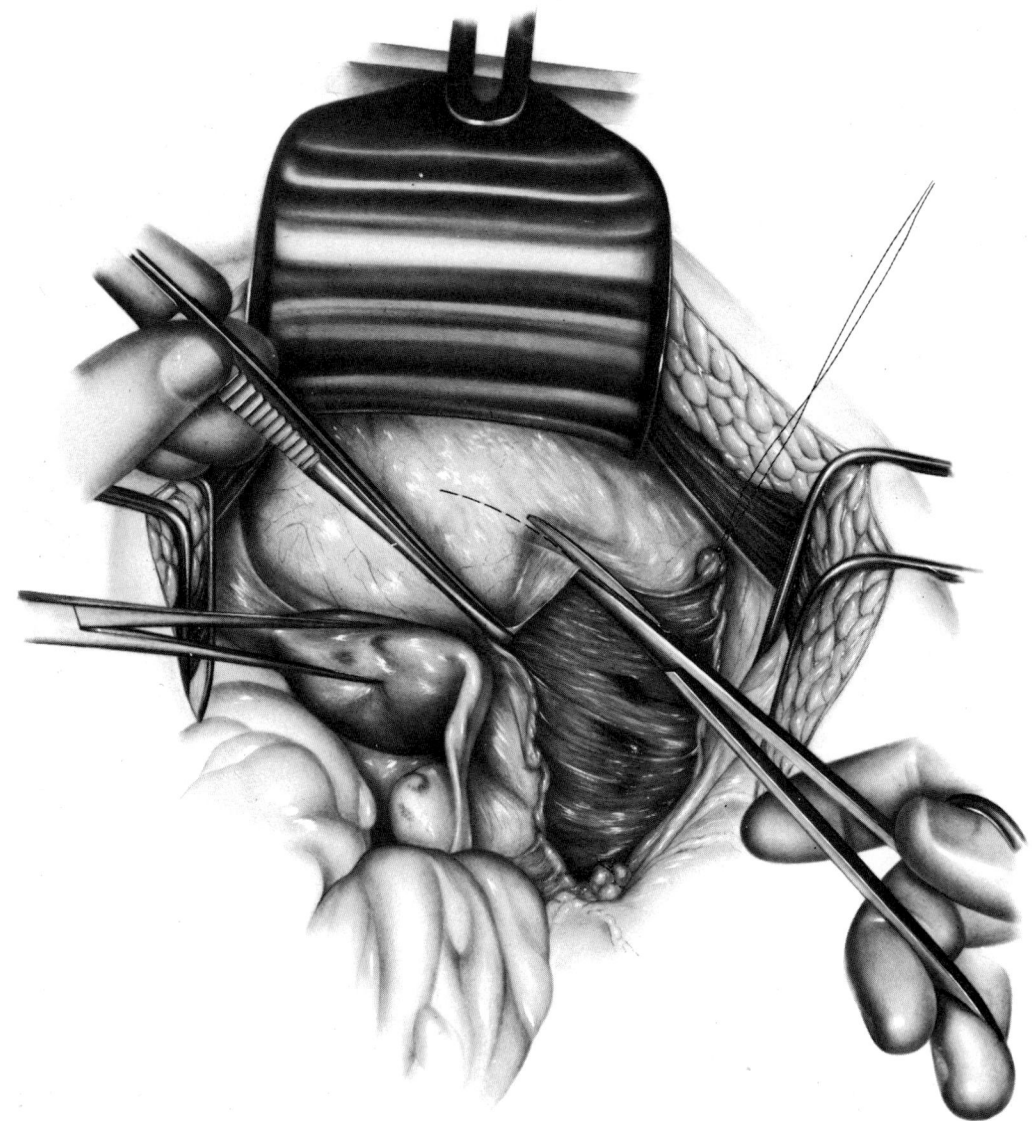

Fig. 78.12   Opening the anterior leaf of the broad ligament after ligating the round ligament and infundibulopelvic ligament.

ing the incision in the anterior leaf of the broad ligament in a cephalic direction along the lateral margin of the infundibulopelvic ligament (Fig. 78.14A). By retracting the infundibulopelvic ligament and displacing the uterus medially, the uterosacral ligament is placed on a stretch and the pararectal space is widened. Dissection of this space is much more precarious than that of the paravesical space. Unskilled dissection in this area is frequently associated with troublesome bleeding. The medial border of the fossa is bounded by the uterosacral ligament and rectum, while the lateral border is formed superiorly by the piriformis muscle and inferiorly by the levator muscle. The sacrum forms the posterior margin of the space and the ureter is attached to the peritoneum along the roof of the space, before entering the medial aspect of the cardinal ligament.

The hypogastric artery and vein are located in the deeper aspect of the pararectal space along the levator ani muscle. The cardinal ligament forms the caudal and lateral border of this important area. Entry into the pararectal space must be made cautiously (Fig. 78.14A), with medial displacement of the ureter and its attached peritoneum. A point between the ureter, which is attached to the medial leaf of peritoneum, and the hypogastric artery is selected. Blunt dissection should be used in this area, and careful handling of tissue is imperative to avoid unnecessary damage to small veins deep in this fossa. When the examining finger reaches the pelvic floor and levator ani muscle, the fossa narrows, and care must be taken to avoid damage to the lateral sacral and hemorrhoidal vessels in this area. The dissection is carried vertically downward for a short distance. The direction of development of the space then

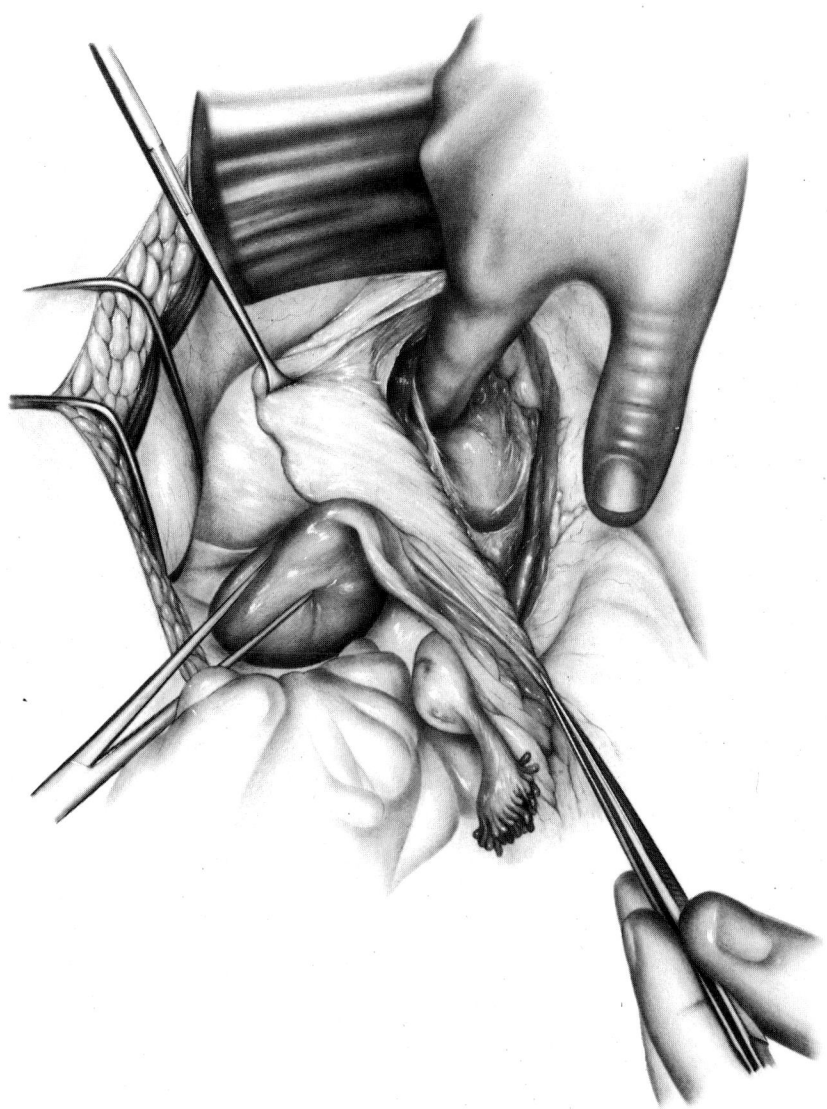

Fig. 78.13 Development of paravesical space.

changes to an inferior and caudal direction lateral to the rectum. If the development of the space is difficult, it should be delayed until a later time in the operation. When the paravesical and pararectal spaces have been developed (Fig. 78.14B), the pelvic floor and cardinal ligament can be easily identified and inspected. In the absence of demonstrable tumor extension, the case is considered operable and the lymph node dissection is initiated at this time.

Pelvic lymphadenectomy

Dissection of the lymphatic tissue along the iliac vessels may begin in the region of the bifurcation of the common iliac artery and extend superiorly to the bifurcation of the aorta and inferiorly to the inguinal ligament, or it may begin at another point along the course of the iliac vessels. The opening of the posterior peritoneal leaf of the broad ligament must be extended to the area of the pelvic brim, where the ureter is easily identified as it enters the pelvis at the bifurcation of the common iliac artery. This dissection is made easier if the infundibulopelvic ligament has been ligated and divided; however, the ligament and ovarian vessels can be retracted medially if the adnexa are preserved. In dissecting the presacral area in the angle of the bifurcation of the aorta, care must be taken to avoid bleeding from the middle sacral vessels, as well as from the proximal part of the left external iliac vein which courses through this retroperitoneal space. It is best to occlude the middle sacral vessels with smaller vascular clips as they are identified; if traumatized, the venous bleeding can be controlled with positive pressure against the sacrum and with

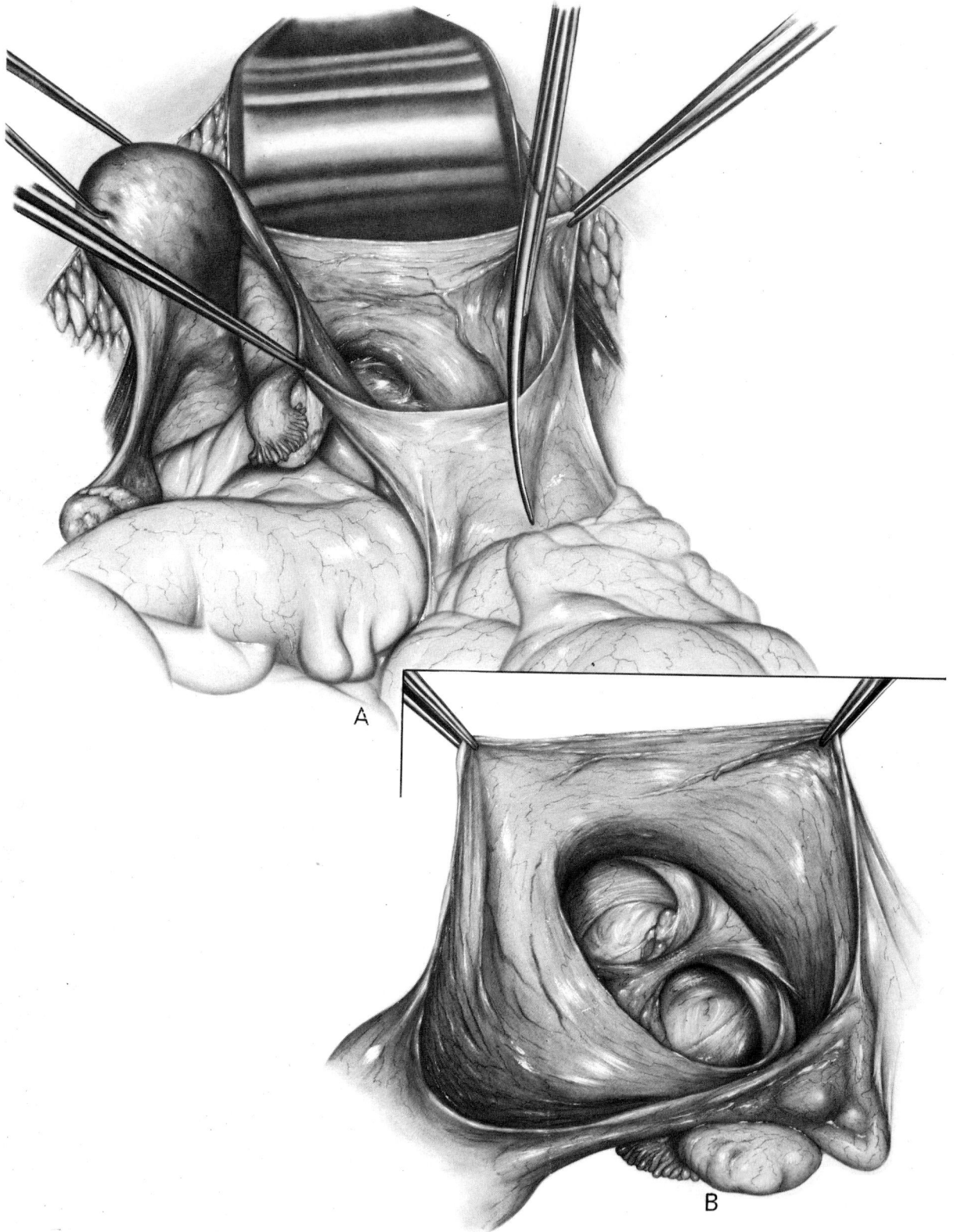

Fig. 78.14 (A) Opening the posterior leaf of the broad ligament for development of the pararectal fossa. (B) Paravesical and pararectal fossae with intervening base of broad ligament attached to pelvic floor and lateral pelvic wall.

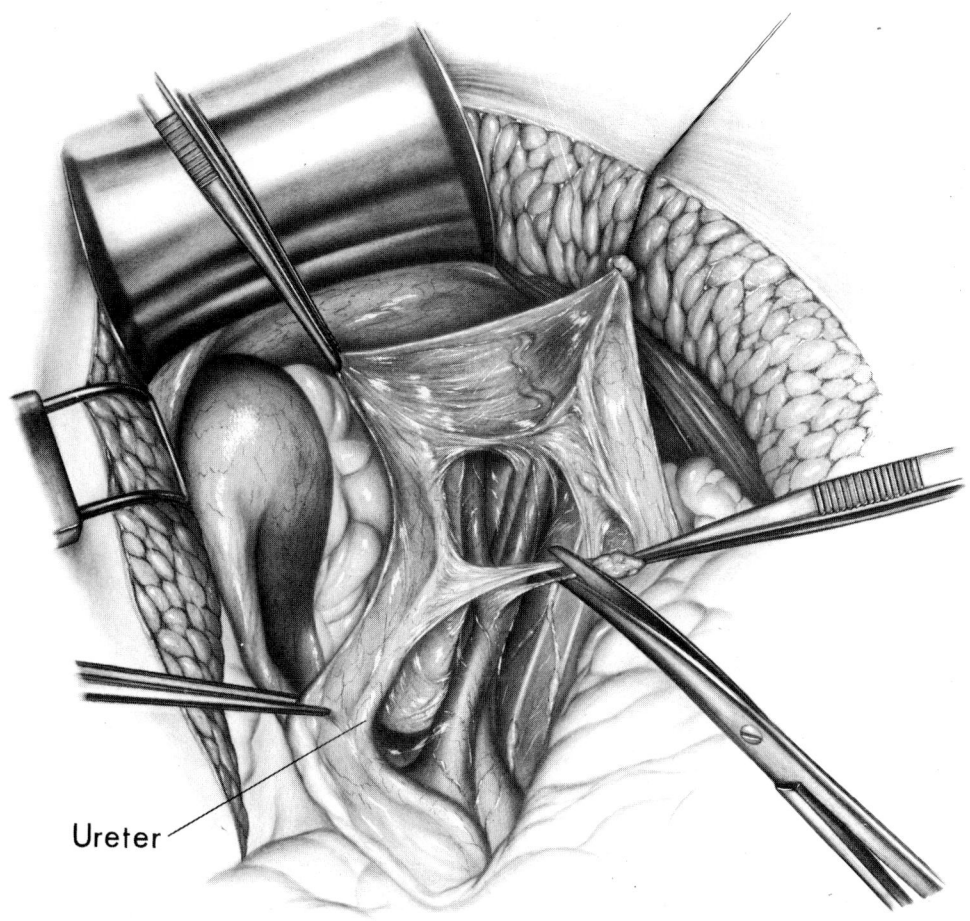

Ureter

Fig. 78.15   Pelvic lymphadenectomy with dissection of right common iliac vessels and their branches, including the external iliac and hypogastric artery and vein. Note attachment of ureter to parietal peritoneum. Genitofemoral nerve courses along psoas muscle.

vascular clips. The lymphatic tissue along the common iliac vessels is removed by sharp dissection with the points of the Metzenbaum scissors directed upward, while special care is taken to avoid trauma to the ureter (Fig. 78.15). The ureter is reflected medially during the dissection of the common iliac vessels, and left attached to the parietal peritoneum in order to maintain its blood supply.

It is important to remove the loose areolar tissue and fascial sheath from the iliac vessels, but, in order to avoid trauma to the intima or wall of the vessels, particularly the veins, one should not attempt to skeletonize the pelvic vessels to the point of producing a pearl-white, vascular tree. If there is tumor in the adventitia of the vessel wall, the patient will probably not be cured by this procedure; consequently, such compulsive surgical efforts produce far more complications than benefits. It is important to rotate the vessels medially and laterally with a vein retractor during the dissection of the common and external iliac trunks, in order to obtain the posterior lymphatic chain behind the vessels along the psoas muscle. The genitofemoral nerve, which is seen lateral to the external

iliac vessels, should be preserved, as damage to this peripheral nerve will produce postoperative discomfort in the groin and medial aspect of the thigh.

The external iliac vessels are carefully dissected until they are seen to pass beneath the inguinal ligament. At this point, care must be taken to avoid injury to the inferior epigastric artery and vein, which arise from the anterior and medial side of the iliac vessels and course along the anterior peritoneum onto the lower abdominal wall. One must also be cognizant of the anomalous obturator artery and vein, which may arise from the lower portion of the external iliac or inferior epigastric vessels and course over the pelvic sidewall into the obturator space. If accidentally traumatized, they should be ligated at their point of origin from the artery or vein. In order to avoid bleeding in the obturator space, these vessels are frequently occluded with small vascular clips as they pass through the obturator space, regardless of their origin. The clips can also be used to occlude the lymphatic channels coming into the pelvis from the leg.

The obturator space is entered by reflecting the external

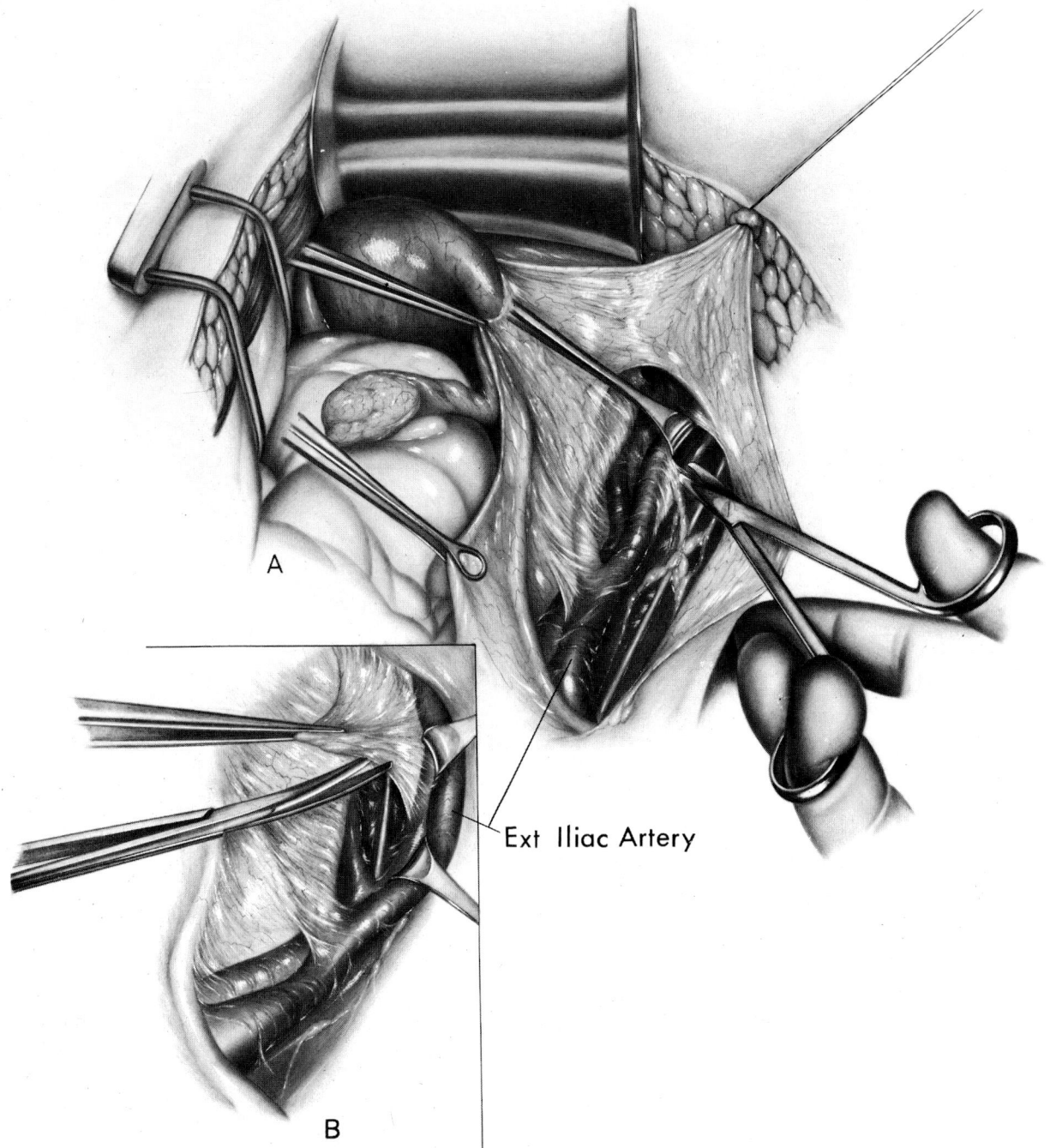

Fig. 78.16 (A) Entry into obturator space by medial reflection of external iliac vessels. (B) Dissection of obturator fossa demonstrating obturator nerve with areolar tissue attachment superiorly to external iliac vessels.

iliac vessels medially away from the psoas muscle and freeing the areolar tissue that lies directly between these vessels and the lateral pelvic wall (Fig. 78.16A); this is usually done with the index finger. Once the space has been entered and the adjacent tissue cleaned from the external iliac vessels, the artery and vein are released and gently retracted laterally with a vein retractor, and the obturator space is clearly exposed. The lymphatic and areolar tissue is dissected from the obturator space to the region of the

pelvic floor, with particular care taken to avoid trauma to the obturator nerve (Fig. 78.16B) and vessels. The dissection is continued by removing all of the nodes below the bifurcation of the iliac vessels, including the hypogastric nodes and the nodes in the obturator fossa. A lymph node may be encountered in the angle formed by the external iliac and hypogastric arteries and must be carefully dissected out, avoiding trauma to the adjacent hypogastric vein.

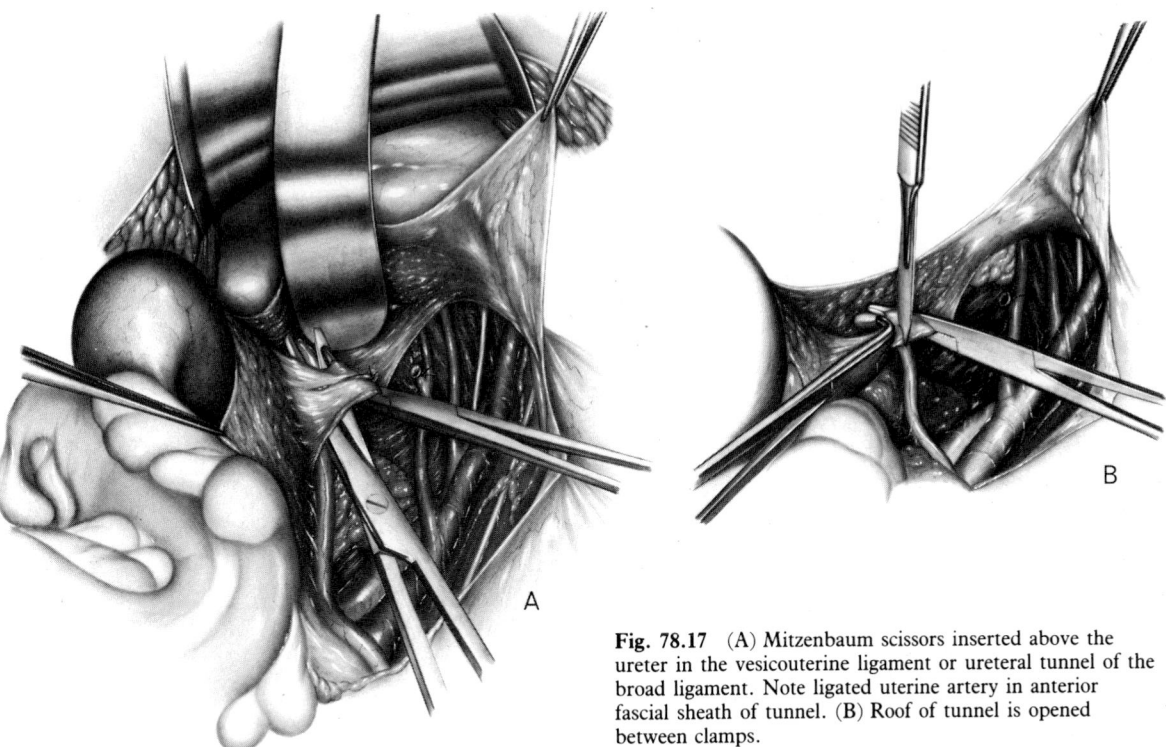

Fig. 78.17 (A) Mitzenbaum scissors inserted above the ureter in the vesicouterine ligament or ureteral tunnel of the broad ligament. Note ligated uterine artery in anterior fascial sheath of tunnel. (B) Roof of tunnel is opened between clamps.

Retraction of the common iliac artery and vein medially will expose a group of lymph nodes that should be carefully removed. These lymph nodes are the lateral common iliac nodes. There is danger of venous bleeding in this area. When this area has been cleared, one can see the obturator nerve entering the obturator fossa through the belly of the psoas muscle. The nerve roots of the lumbosacral plexus will also be exposed. Particular care must be exercised in the dissection of the lateral sacral and sacroiliac plexus just medial to the hypogastric artery and vein, near their origin. The rich arcade of small arteries and veins increases the risk of bleeding in this area. When the vessels retract into the sacral foramen, control of bleeding becomes quite difficult.

The obturator artery can be identified as it courses along the lateral pelvic wall adjacent to the obturator nerve (Fig. 78.16B). The nerve, artery, and vein advance toward the obturator foramen, through which they leave the pelvis. Care must be taken to avoid trauma to all of the structures, particularly the obturator veins, which have a rich anastomotic network against the lateral pelvic wall and communicate freely with the adjacent hypogastric veins. It is best to ligate or clip the obturator vessels, but in the event that uncontrolled bleeding should occur in this area, hemostasis is best obtained by packing the space tightly with a hot pack and providing adequate time for a fibrin clot to develop. If excessive bleeding occurs on one side of the pelvis, dissection may continue on the opposite side in the interim after pressure packing.

Dissection of hypogastric artery and ureter

The hypogastric artery is dissected with identification of the visceral branches of the anterior trunk; these include the uterine, superior, middle and inferior vesical, vaginal, and middle hemorrhoidal arteries. The anterior division of the hypogastric artery continues along the paravesical fossa to become the obliterated lateral umbilical ligament beneath the anterior abdominal wall. Should the superior vesical artery be damaged, it can be ligated without serious compromise to the blood supply of the bladder. In patients who have a small volume tumor in the cervix, the uterine artery may be ligated at its origin from the hypogastric artery. However, rather than ligating the uterine artery individually, we feel that a more adequate central dissection is achieved by ligating the anterior division of the hypogastric artery just distal to the point of origin of its posterior division. The vessel is doubly ligated. The distal branches traversing the cardinal ligament are removed with the specimen or are ligated again distally. No attempt is made to remove the hypogastric vein. The other adjacent veins should be ligated to avoid brisk bleeding in this area.

The bladder is now reflected off the lower uterine segment by incising the bladder peritoneum from its attachment to the uterus. The fascial adhesions of the base of the bladder are released from the cervix and upper vagina by sharp scissor dissection and the vesico-cervical space is developed inferiorly and laterally. The ureter tunnels between the anterior fascial bundles of the base of the

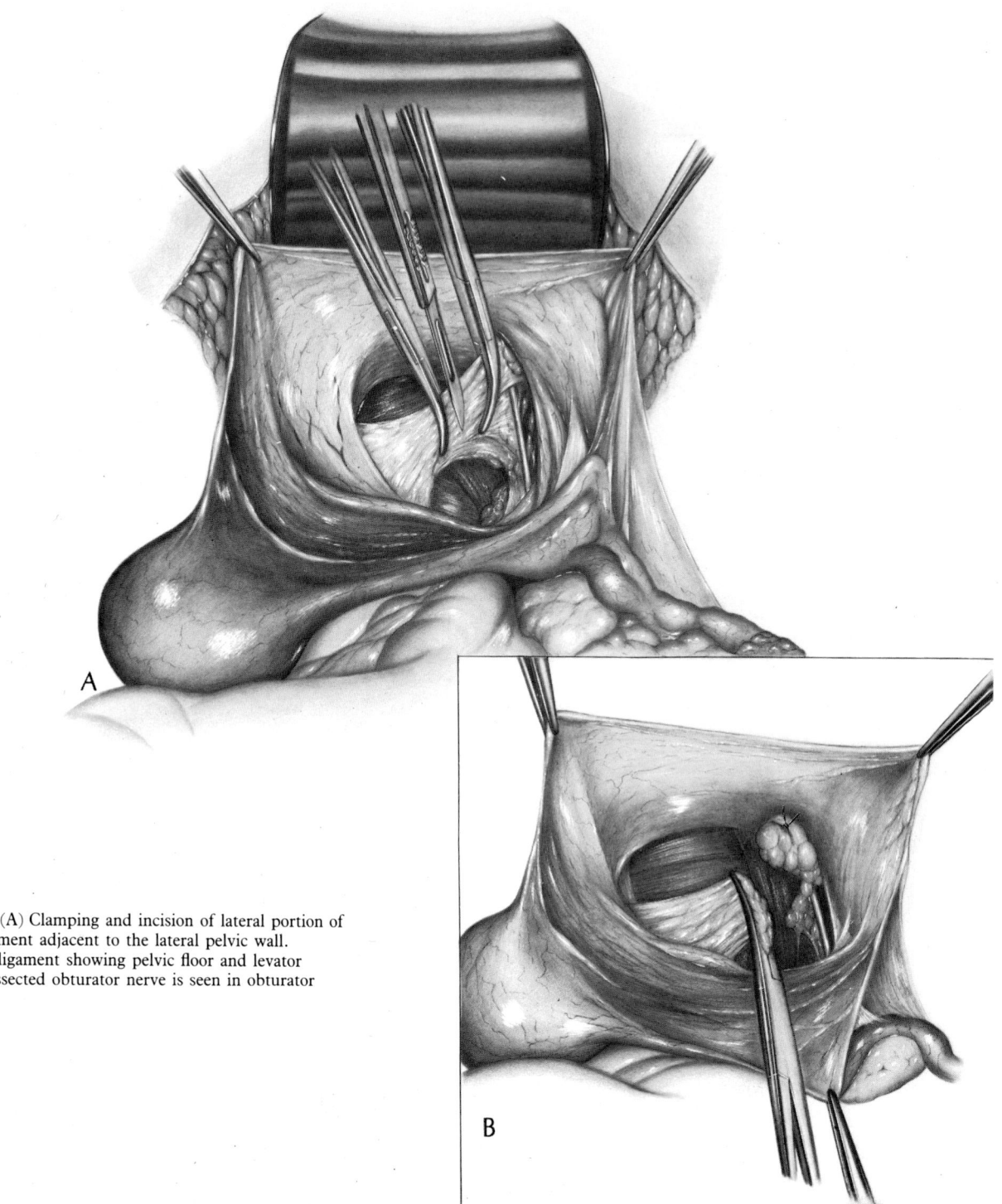

Fig. 78.18 (A) Clamping and incision of lateral portion of cardinal ligament adjacent to the lateral pelvic wall. (B) Excised ligament showing pelvic floor and levator muscles. Dissected obturator nerve is seen in obturator space.

broad ligament, commonly called the vesico-uterine ligament. This fascial tunnel is carefully opened by sliding the Metzenbaum scissors, with concave surface pointed upward, along the anterior and medial surface of the ureter, and by gently spreading the blades, as demonstrated in Figure 78.17A. The uterine artery and vein(s) course along the fascial roof of this ligament. Adson clamps are used in

dissecting the tunnel, as these long-handled instruments have delicate points that are relatively atraumatic when placed adjacent to the ureter and bladder. As demonstrated in Figure 78.17B, the anterior sheath of the vesico-uterine ligament is opened by doubly clamping and incising this tissue. Each of the fascial bundles is suture ligated for control of bleeding, and the ureter is dissected free of its

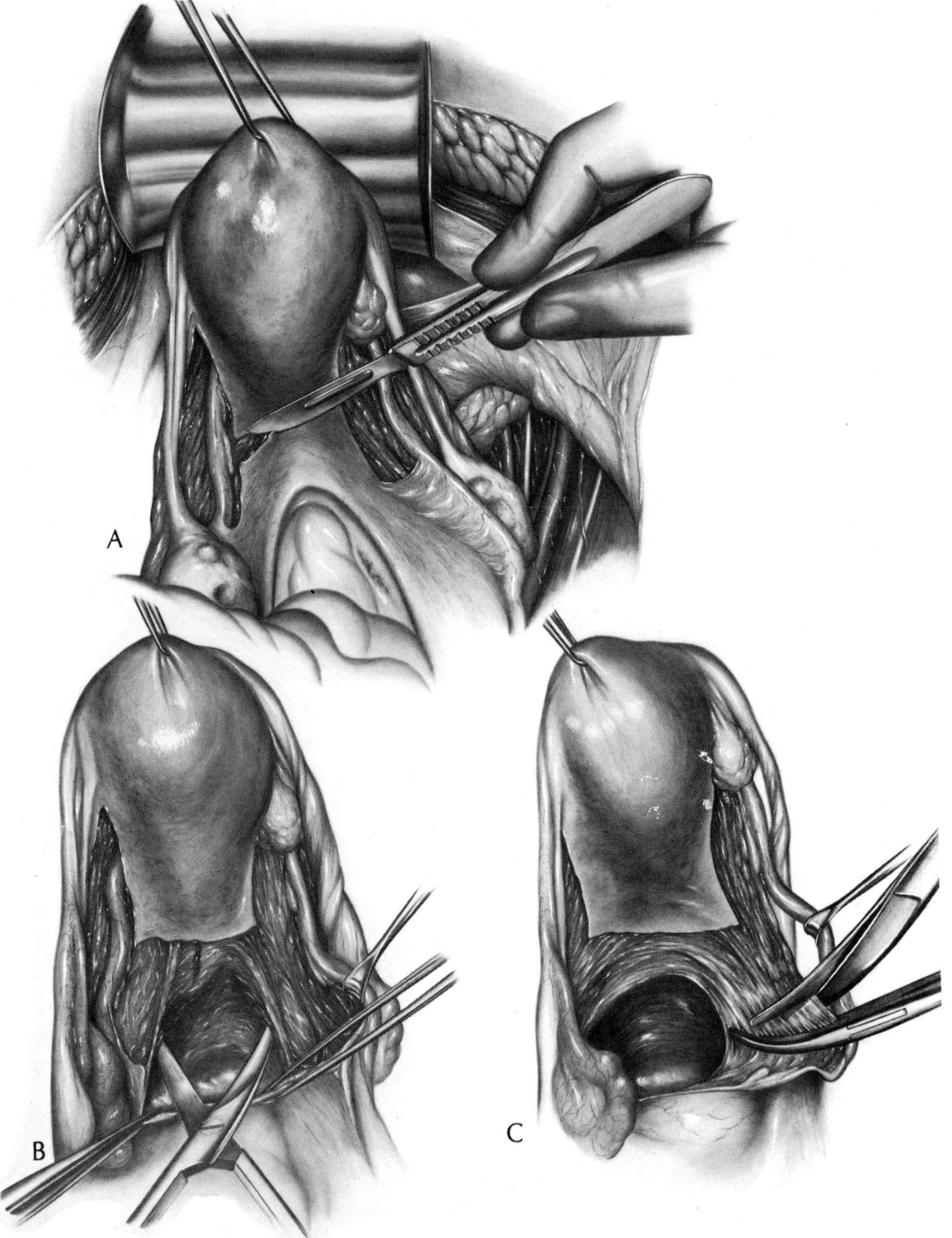

Fig. 78.19 (A) Cutting the cul-de-sac peritoneum as it reflects onto the rectum. Ureters course laterally, devoid of peritoneum. (B) Dissection of the rectovaginal septum with development of rectal stalks (uterosacral ligaments) laterally. (C) Clamping the uterosacral ligament. Ureter is gently retracted to avoid trauma.

attachment to the posterior leaf of the vesicouterine ligament. Care must be taken to prevent damage to the adventitia and muscular wall of the ureter, which contain nutrient vessels from the collateral circulation. In the event that the blood supply to the ureter is compromised by thrombosis or trauma to the veins, fistula formation is a serious and frequent complication. The ureter is retracted gently with an umbilical tape or vein retractor. Forceps should not be used in handling the ureter.

Dissection of cardinal ligament

The base of the broad ligament (the cardinal ligament) may now be excised from its attachment at the lateral pelvic wall. The technique of clamping and ligating the vascular cardinal ligament will vary depending on the circumstances. Sometimes, a part of the ligament can be included in a single clamp. Sometimes, it is better to ligate or clip individual vessels. The ligament is excised with sharp scissor dissection and ligated with No. 1 delayed absorbable suture. A series of clamps are placed until the dissection is completed to the pelvic floor and along the paravaginal tissues (Fig. 78.18A and B). Should serious bleeding occur in this region due to trauma to the pelvic floor veins, hemostatic control is best obtained by firm packing of the pelvis and shifting the dissection temporarily to the opposite side.

The uterosacral ligaments, commonly called the pararectal stalks, are placed on a stretch by sharply withdrawing the uterus forward. The peritoneal reflection of the cul de sac of Douglas is now incised, leaving a small segment of peritoneum attached to the anterior surface of the rectum. Care must be taken to avoid injury to the ureters, which are attached to the peritoneum just lateral to the uterosacral ligament (Fig. 78.19A). The rectovaginal space is opened by sharp scissor dissection, and deepened by blunt and sharp dissection (Fig. 78.19B). This procedure separates the posterior reflection of the endopelvic fascia from the lateral wall of the rectum, which includes the more superficial uterosacral ligaments. The entire fascial bundle of the uterosacral ligament is identified, clamped as far posteriorly as possible and excised (Fig. 78.19C). Continuation of this plane of dissection along the posterior endopelvic fascia will free the posterior aspect of the cervix from the pelvic floor. It is important to dissect the paravaginal fascia in order to obtain all of the microlymphatic channels that communicate between the cervix and upper vagina (Fig. 78.20A). The bladder is then dissected further from the upper portion of the vagina by sharp and blunt dissection, making certain to avoid trauma to the blood supply of this organ. It is important, therefore, that sharp dissection, rather than blunt trauma, be used to free the base of the bladder, in order to avoid forceful tearing of the blood vessels and musculature of the bladder. The specimen is removed by the open technique, as shown in Figure 78.20B, applying long, right-angle clamps in front of the cervix (not shown) along the proximal surgical margins of the vagina to avoid spillage of tumor cells into the pelvis.

Closure

Several biopsies are taken from the margin of the vaginal apex. The vaginal margins are sutured with a continuous locking 2–0 delayed absorbable suture and the vagina is left open to obtain adequate pelvic drainage (Fig. 78.20C). No additional attempt is made to support the vaginal vault, since all of the fascial support of the uterus and vagina has been removed. The remaining vagina, which has been shortened by approximately 3 cm, is well supported by its attachments to the levator ani muscles and urogenital diaphragm and, mainly, by the effects of postoperative fibrosis during the healing phase. Suction catheters are placed in the obturator fossae and along the lateral pelvic walls, and brought out through stab wounds in the lower abdomen. These catheters are later connected to intermittent, low suction drainage units, and are effective in preventing lymphocyst formation and ureteral damage.

No attempt is made to suspend the ureters to the hypogastric artery, as suggested by Green,[43] or to place the terminal ureter on the inside of the peritoneal surface, as recommended by Novak.[96] In view of the fact that the pelvis is well-drained and the blood supply of the terminal ureter is preserved, we have had little difficulty with stenosis or fistula formation of the terminal ureter. In contrast to the methods of Novak from Yugoslavia, Green from Boston, and Ohkawa from Japan, our technique, adopted from Symmonds & Pratt, is to leave the pelvic ureters in their normal retroperitoneal position, and to place retroperitoneal suction drains along the pelvic walls.[13,43,96,128] If the operative field remains dry postoperatively, it has been our experience that pelvic cellulitis and lymphocysts can be avoided, and ureteral complications are infrequent (1%).

Prior to reperitonizing the pelvis, the free margin of the bladder peritoneum is sutured to the anterior cuff of the vagina for additional protection to the denuded bladder base. In essence, this provides an extra layer of tissue between the denuded pelvis and the base of the bladder and terminal ureters. This is an added step which is useful in decreasing both vesicovaginal and ureterovaginal fistulae. The edge of peritoneum over the rectum is sutured to the posterior vaginal cuff. The peritoneum is then closed across from one side to the other with a continuous suture. This method of closure was first described by Symmonds & Pratt and has, we feel, been helpful in preventing fistulas and lymphocysts.[128]

If the tubes and ovaries are to be preserved, a tunnel is dissected beneath the peritoneum laterally and superiorly toward each lateral gutter. An incision in the peritoneum is made as high as possible at the top of the tunnel. The adnexal structures are guided through the tunnel and through the incision at the top of the tunnel, making absolutely certain that the ovarian vessels in the infundibulopelvic ligament are not twisted. Permanent suture

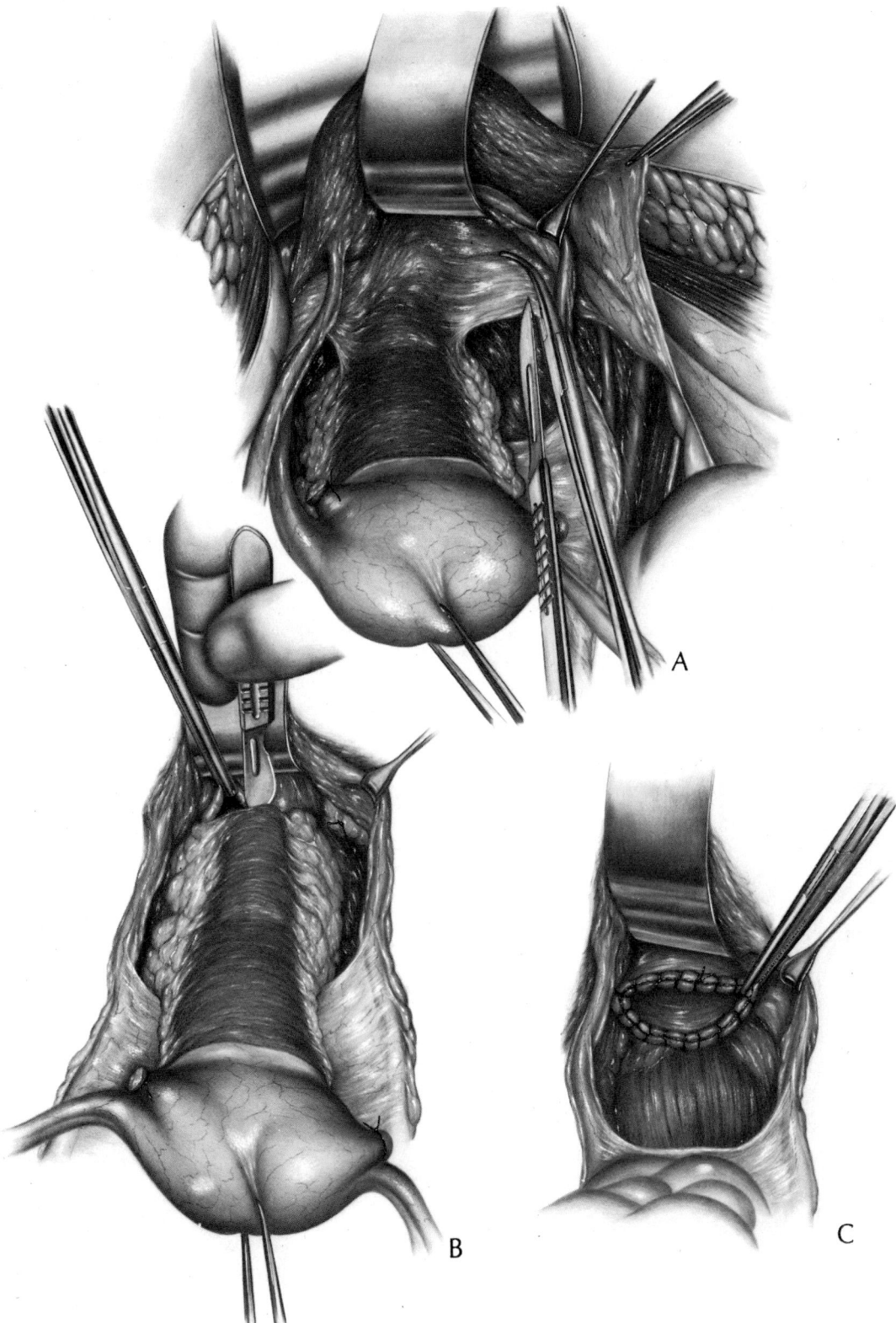

Fig. 78.20 (A) Dissection and retraction of bladder and terminal ureter from vagina and excising the paravaginal fascia from the lateral pelvic wall. (B) Opening of vagina and securing lower vaginal cuff. Upper 3 cm of vagina are removed with surgical specimen. (C) Closure of open vaginal cuff with continuous locking suture for hemostasis. Ureters are seen laterally and denuded rectum posteriorly.

material is used to suture the tubo-ovarian pedicle as high as possible to the peritoneum and underlying muscle. Two large metal clips are also placed across the pedicle in order to later identify the location of the ovaries with an abdominal X-ray. This ovarian suspension is done when there is a reasonable chance that a patient will need postoperative pelvic irradiation. Otherwise, the tubes and ovaries may be left in their natural position in the pelvis.

Prior to closure of the peritoneum over the pelvis, a careful inspection for bleeding points should be made, preferably after the patient's blood pressure has been returned to normal. In closing the peritoneum, one should carefully avoid constriction, compression, or kinking of the ureter beneath.

DESCRIPTION OF TECHNIQUE OF EXTRAPERITONEAL/TRANSPERITONEAL APPROACH

The preparation of the patient is the same as for the previously described approach. After preparation and draping, an operator standing on the patient's right side will make a transverse elliptical incision that begins just above the left anterior superior iliac spine and continues medially about 2 cm above the inguinal ligament, across the midline about 3 cm above the symphysis pubis, turning upwards on the right side toward the right anterior superior iliac spine (Fig. 78.21). Only about two-thirds of the length of the incision need be made at this point. The rectus muscles are transected transversely. The incision is extended laterally and superiorly on the left through the external abdominus, transverse abdominus, and internal abdominus muscles. With sharp and blunt dissection beneath the inferior edge of the muscles, the peritoneum is carefully reflected superiorly and medially. Three structures must be clamped and ligated in order to accomplish this: the

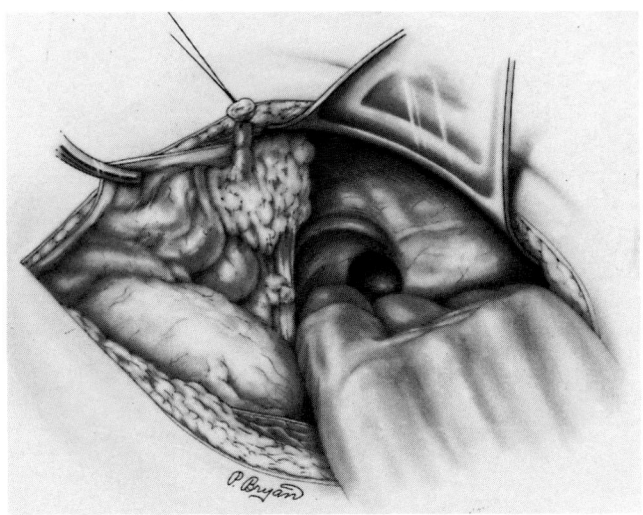

Fig. 78.22 The peritoneum is reflected from the left lateral pelvic sidewall, and the left paravesical space is entered.

inferior epigastric artery and vein, the round ligament and the obliterated hypogastric artery. Once these have been ligated, dissection usually proceeds without difficulty, attempting to preserve the integrity of the peritoneum. The psoas muscle, the external iliac artery and vein, and the lateral bladder wall come easily into view. The left paravesical space is developed down to the levator muscle (Fig. 78.22). The peritoneum is peeled away from the vessels. After identification of the lateral femoral cutaneous and genitofemoral nerves, dissection of the lymphatic and fatty tissue may begin at any point along the external iliac artery and vein (Fig. 78.23). Further reflection of the peritoneum will identify the ureter attached to the peritoneum as it is peeled away, and will identify the uterine artery crossing over the ureter. Between the bifurcation of the common iliac artery and vein and the reflected peritoneum, a point to begin the dissection of the pararectal space is selected. The space is developed by sharp and blunt dissection posteriorly, and then changed to an inferior direction. The development of the pararectal space usually goes easily, but it should not be forced if difficulty is encountered. The tissue between the paravesical space and the pararectal space is the cardinal ligament or 'web' (Fig. 78.24). As dissection proceeds, the tissue must be removed from the peritoneal attachments medially and also from the pelvic sidewall. The obturator fossa can be entered between the psoas muscle and the external iliac artery and vein, or medially and beneath these vessels. The small lateral perforating vessels are clipped. The obturator nerve is identified along with the obturator artery and vein (Fig. 78.25). These vessels must be securely ligated before they traverse the obturator foramen. All lymph nodes and fat are removed from the obturator fossa (Fig. 78.26). After the retroperitoneal reflection of the rectum and sigmoid further medially it is usually helpful to put a

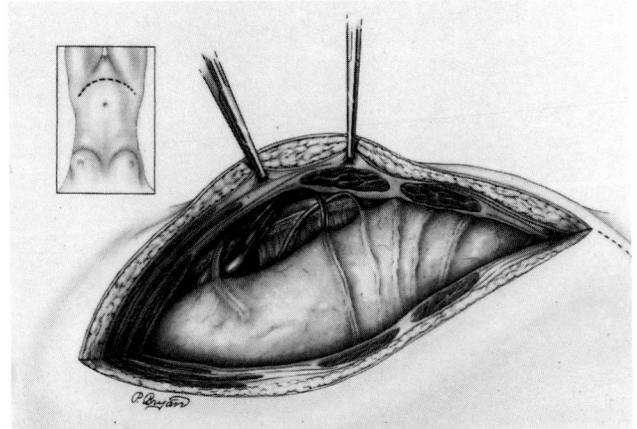

Fig. 78.21 A transverse incision demonstrating the round ligament, the inferior epigastric artery and vein, and the obliterated hypogastric artery.

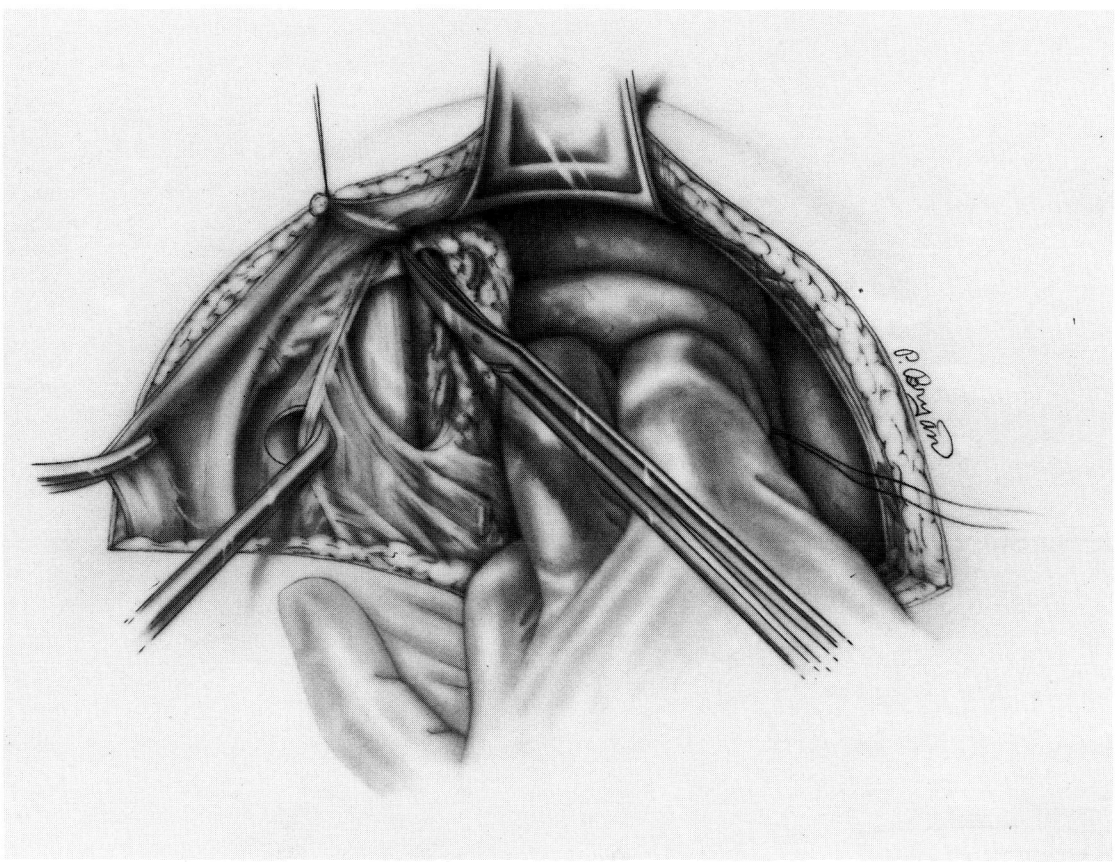

Fig. 78.23 After identification and retraction of the genitofemoral and lateral femoral cutaneous nerves, the lymphadenectomy begins along the external iliac artery and nerves.

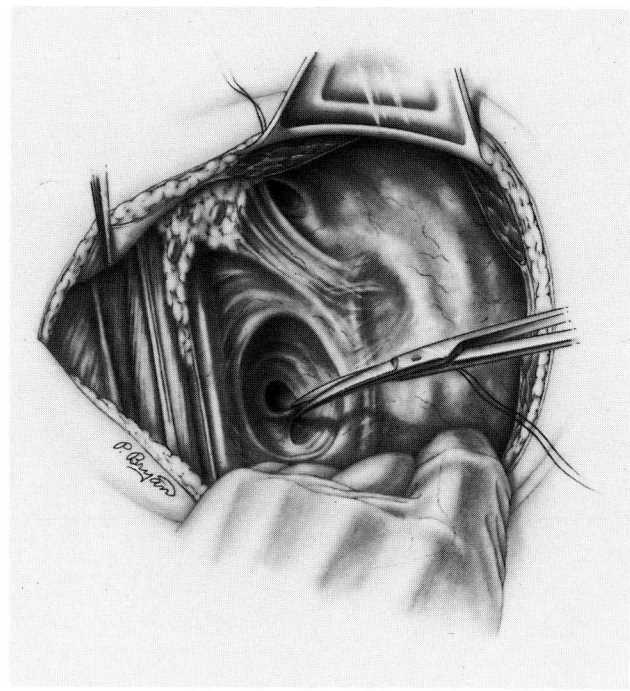

Fig. 78.24 The ureter is peeled away from the lateral pelvic wall with the peritoneum. The pararectal space is developed.

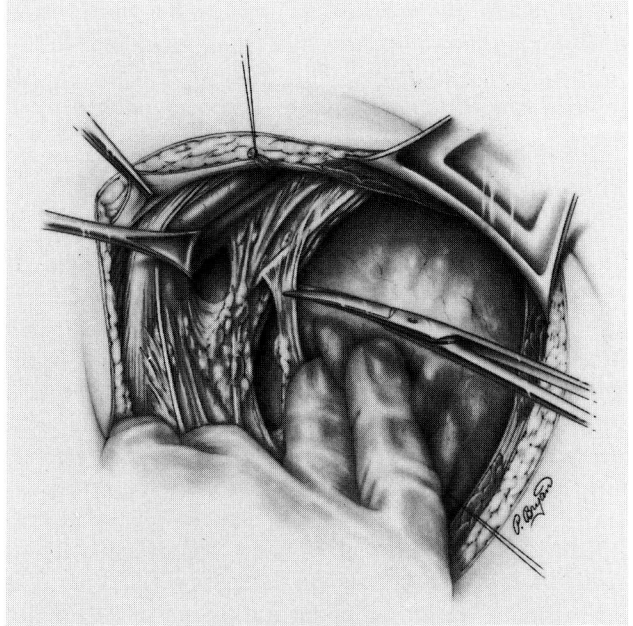

Fig. 78.25 The external iliac artery and vein are retracted laterally, and dissection of the obturator fossa begins.

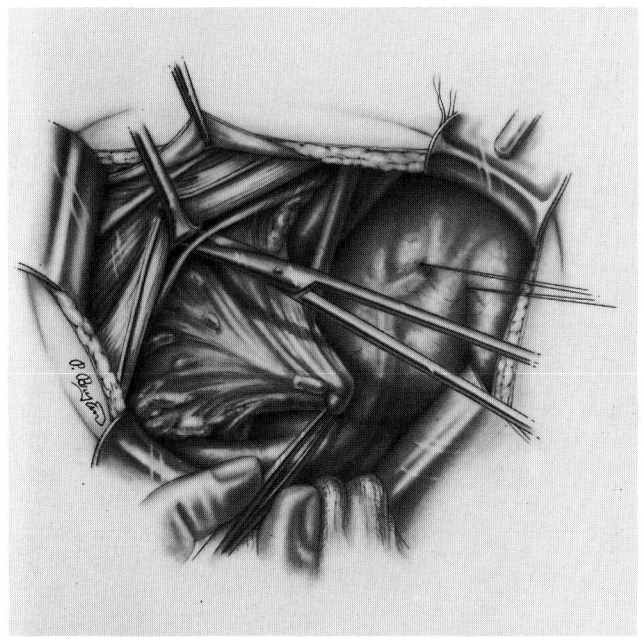

Fig. 78.26 With careful identification of the obturator nerve, the contents of the obturator fossa are removed.

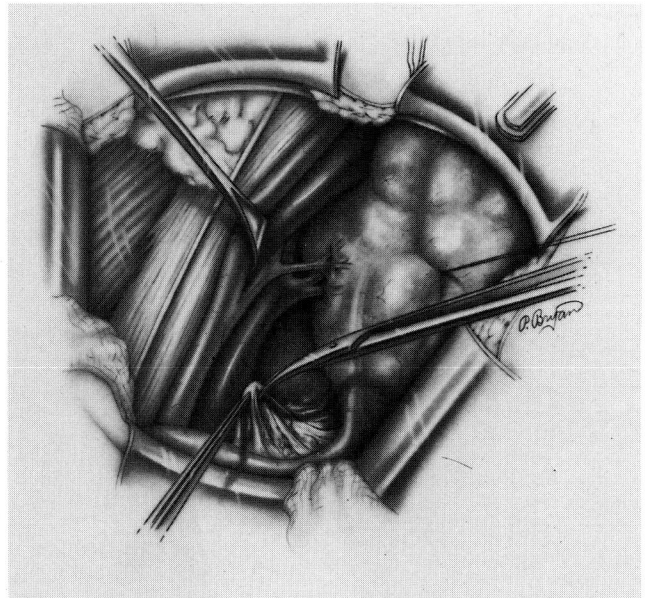

Fig. 78.27 Lymphatic tissue is removed from the presacral area and from the common iliac artery and veins.

self-retaining retractor in place. A Bookwalter retractor has multiple blades of various sizes and configurations that can be assembled around the operative field to provide optimum exposure. A retractor blade should not be placed beneath the inguinal ligament just lateral to the external iliac vessels pressing against the psoas muscle. Although not visible without further dissection, the femoral nerve is located here and can be damaged by pressure from a retractor.

With the excellent exposure provided by the incision, the retractor, and the extraperitoneal approach, the dissection continues. Lymphatic tissue is removed from the presacral area between the sigmoid medially and the common iliac vein (Fig. 78.27). A small artery to the ureter will be seen and will usually be sacrificed in order to accomplish a clean dissection. Lymphatic tissue is then removed up to the level of the mid-common iliac vessels, but, if necessary, the dissection can be extended to the lower para-aortic nodes with proper retraction and lighting. The anterior division of the hypogastric artery is identified just distal to the origin of the posterior trunk. Thorough cleaning of this vessel will allow its safe ligation, usually first with a free tie followed by a transfixation suture distally. One must be careful to avoid injury to the hypogastric vein (Fig. 78.28). In the dissection of the cardinal ligament which follows, the branches of the anterior division of the hypogastric artery are removed and ligated distally. For example, the uterine artery is traced to its point of crossing over the ureter and is secured with a clip. Ligation or clipping individual arteries and veins in the cardinal ligament involves a meticulous and tedious dissec-

tion to avoid unnecessary bleeding, which may be difficult to control (Fig. 78.29). Removal of some superior gluteal nodes is usually accomplished if the most inferior portion of the cardinal ligament is removed. However, it is not possible to remove the inferior gluteal nodes, as this is an extremely dangerous and inaccessible area for dissection in the region of the ischial spine. This is probably the weakest point in performing pelvic lymphadenectomy for cervical

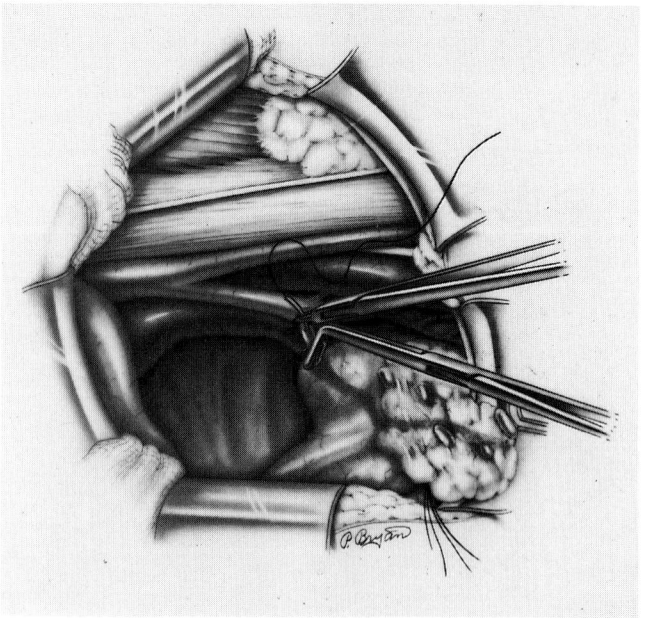

FIg. 78.28 The anterior trunk of the hypogastric artery is first ligated with a free tie and then suture ligated.

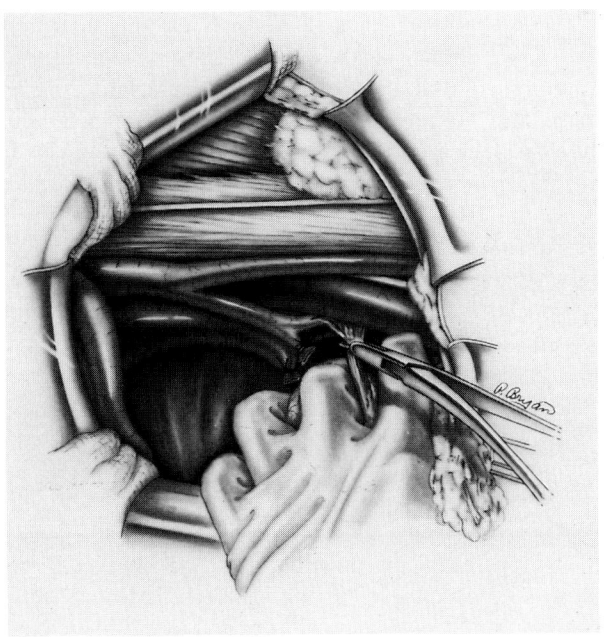

Fig. 78.29 Cardinal ligament vessels along the lateral pelvic wall are clipped or ligated.

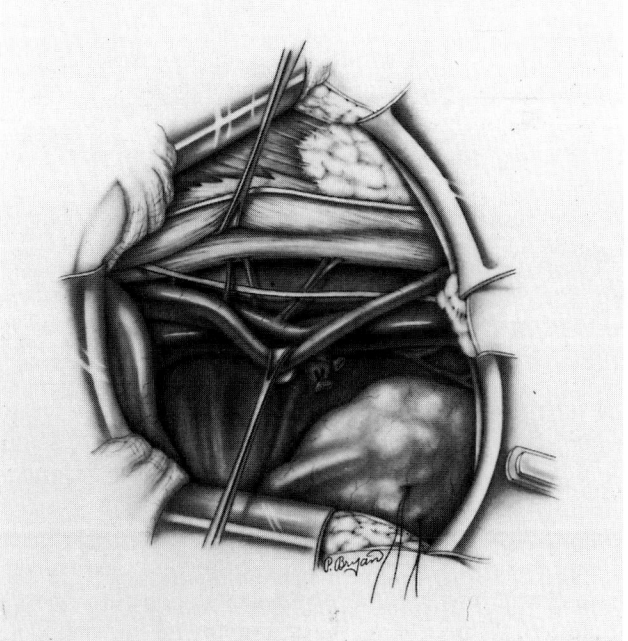

Fig. 78.30 The lateral common iliac nodes are removed completely, thus exposing the entire course of the obturator nerve.

cancer, since superior and inferior gluteal nodes are among those most frequently involved with metastatic disease from cervical cancer.

Finally, the extraperitoneal lymphadenectomy is completed by removing all tissue around the bifurcation of the common iliac artery and vein, the region called the 'axilla of the pelvis' by Leitch.[74] Retraction of the distal common iliac artery and vein medially away from the psoas muscle will expose the lateral common iliac lymph nodes. We insist that these nodes be removed completely (Fig. 78.30). Dissection must be done carefully to avoid injury to the common iliac vein and its branches, and the iliac branches of the iliolumbar artery and vein. Clean removal of the lipolymph node tissue will expose the obturator nerve as it enters the obturator fossa through the psoas muscle, and also the 4th and 5th lumbar nerves and nerve roots of the lumbosacral plexus. It has been suggested that the lateral common iliac nodes should be preserved in order to reduce the incidence of postoperative edema of the lower extremities. We insist that they be removed in an effort to achieve a complete lymphadenectomy.

The operative field is carefully inspected for bleeding. When hemostasis is achieved, the retractor is removed, the abdominal incision is extended to the right anterior superior iliac spine, and the right extraperitoneal pelvic lymphadenectomy is done in a similar fashion. Upon completion of the bilateral pelvic lymphadenectomy, the remainder of the operation, the central dissection, is carried out through a transverse incision in the peritoneum (Fig. 78.31). Exploration of the upper abdomen is followed by placement of the self-retaining retractor. Peritoneal

washings are taken for cytological study. The round ligaments have already been ligated extraperitoneally; their medial portions still attached to the uterus can be easily retrieved into the peritoneal cavity. Depending on whether the tubes and ovaries are conserved or removed, the clamps are placed across the infundibulopelvic ligaments or

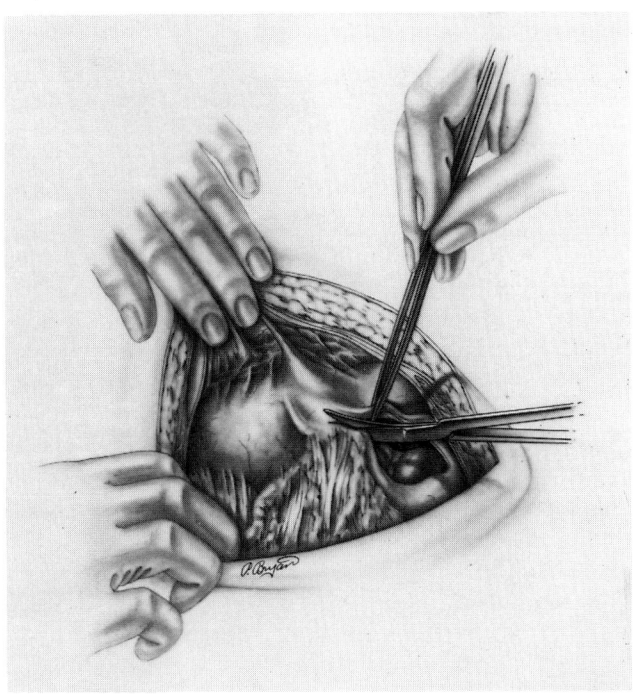

Fig. 78.31 Following bilateral extraperitoneal lymphadenectomy, a transverse incision is made in the peritoneum.

the utero-ovarian ligaments. Dissection of the ureters from the tunnel is done as described in the transperitoneal approach. The remainder of the central dissection is carried out as previously described and illustrated. The exposure provided by the incision described is unsurpassed. The suction catheters are placed, the ovaries are suspended, and the peritoneum is closed in the manner previously described (Figs 78.32 to 78.42).

PATHOLOGICAL EXAMINATION OF THE OPERATIVE SPECIMEN

Considerable useful information about the extent of the disease can be obtained by a careful pathological examination of the operative specimen. This will be helpful in determining prognosis, but is also absolutely essential in the identification of patients at greater risk of persistent disease in order that additional therapy and close surveillance can be provided. Even though the operator may be exhausted at the end of the operation, he/she should accompany the specimen to the pathology laboratory where it should be examined with the pathologist before it is placed in fixative and sectioned. The gynecologic surgeon can point to worrisome parts of the specimen; such information will assist the pathologist in taking sections. Critical margins of dissection can be pointed out and stained with India ink so that they can be seen on the microscopic slides. The primary cervical tumor should be measured as accurately as possible in order that at least an estimate of its size and volume can be recorded. Numerous microscopic sections of the cervix with adjacent vaginal cuff, lower uterine segment, and paravaginal, paracervical and parametrial tissue should be examined to show the cell type, the degree of differentiation, depth of stromal invasion, the presence or absence of invasion of lymphatic and vascular spaces, and the stromal reaction to the tumor. Not only is it important to know the depth of invasion, but it is also important to know the thickness of the uninvolved fibromuscular stroma of the cervix, as pointed out by Kishi and co-workers.[64] These authors found that the nodal metastasis and 5-year cancer death rates were 7% and 8%, respectively, in patients with uninvolved fibromuscular stroma thickness above 3 mm, and 37% and 26%, respectively, in patients with the thickness below 3 mm. The thickness of the cancer-unaffected cervical fibromuscular stroma may be as useful as other parameters in determining the biological behavior of invasive cervical cancer.

Unfortunately, the exquisite giant section technique of pathological examination employed by Burghardt and co-workers is not available in all laboratories.[21] These authors measured ratio of tumor size to the size of the cervix. The

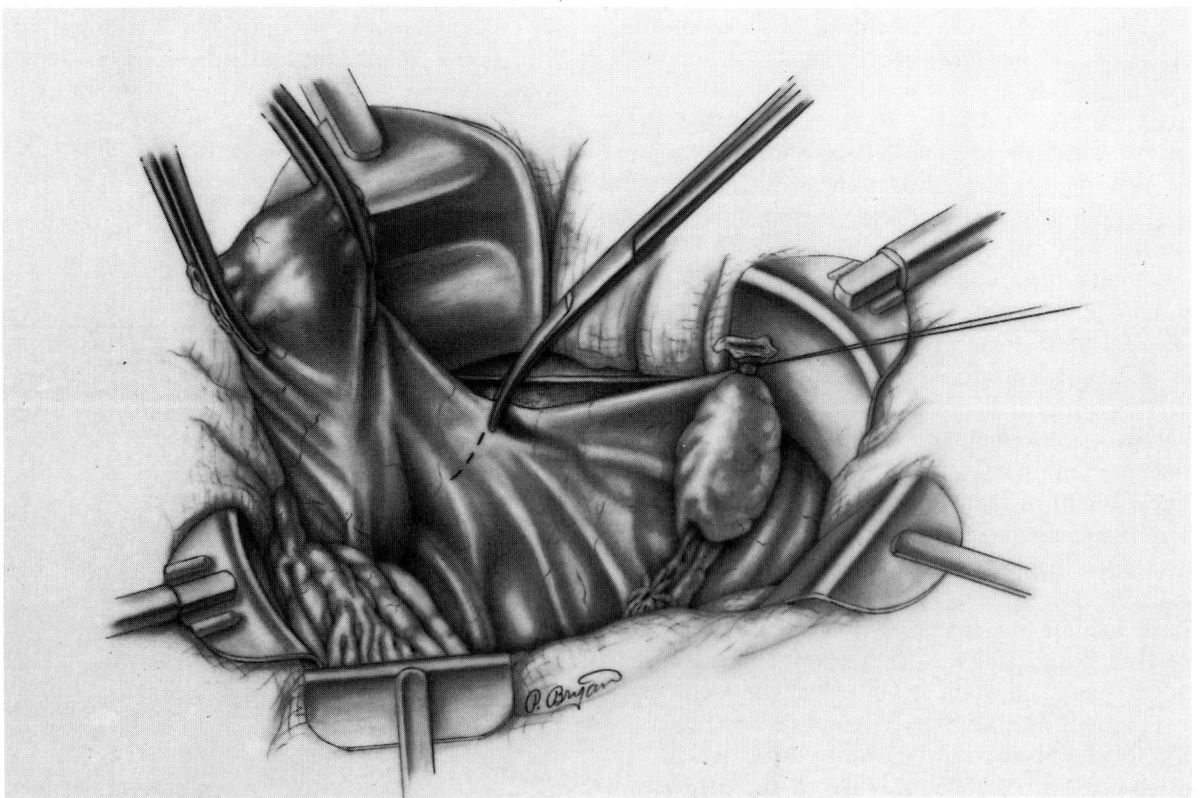

Fig. 78.32 An incision is made in the anterior and posterior leaves of the right broad ligament. The round ligament was previously ligated extraperitoneally.

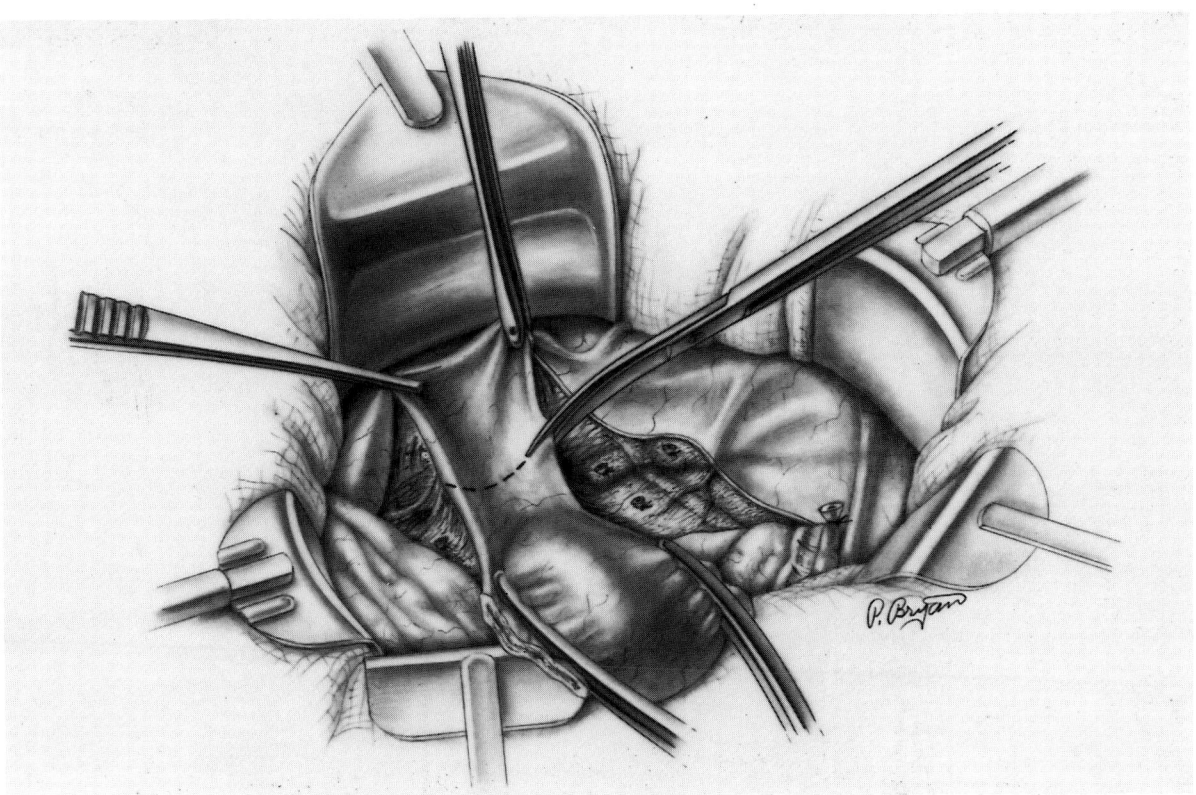

Fig. 78.33   The vesicocervical peritoneum is incised to mobilize the bladder inferiorly.

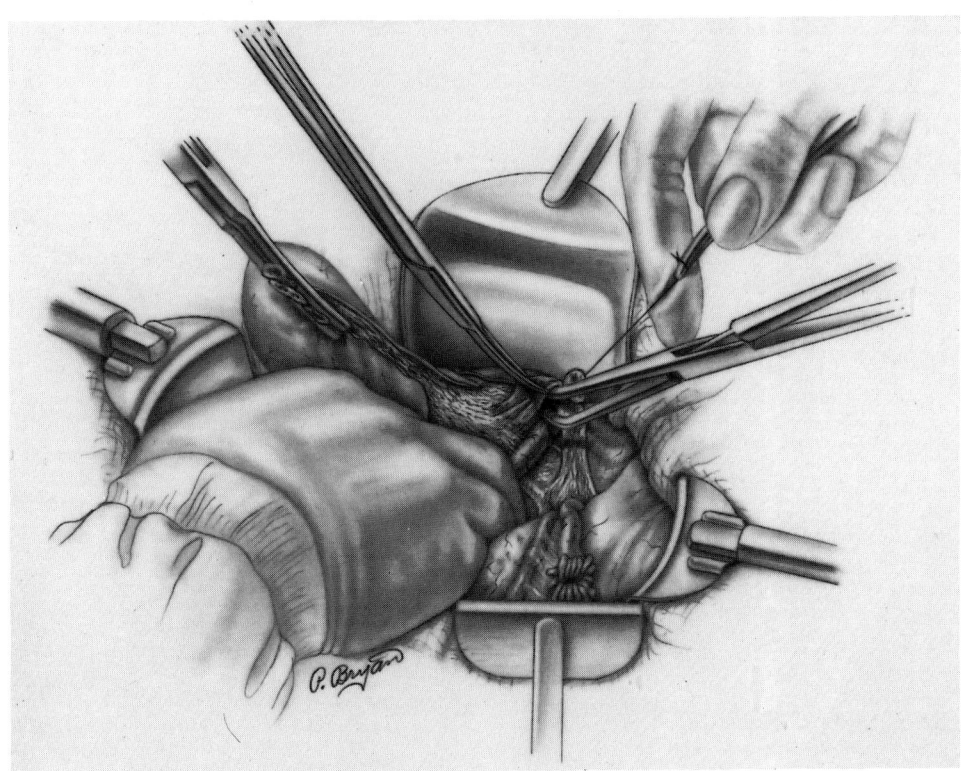

Fig. 78.34   The ureter is dissected completely free from its tunnel in the cardinal ligament.

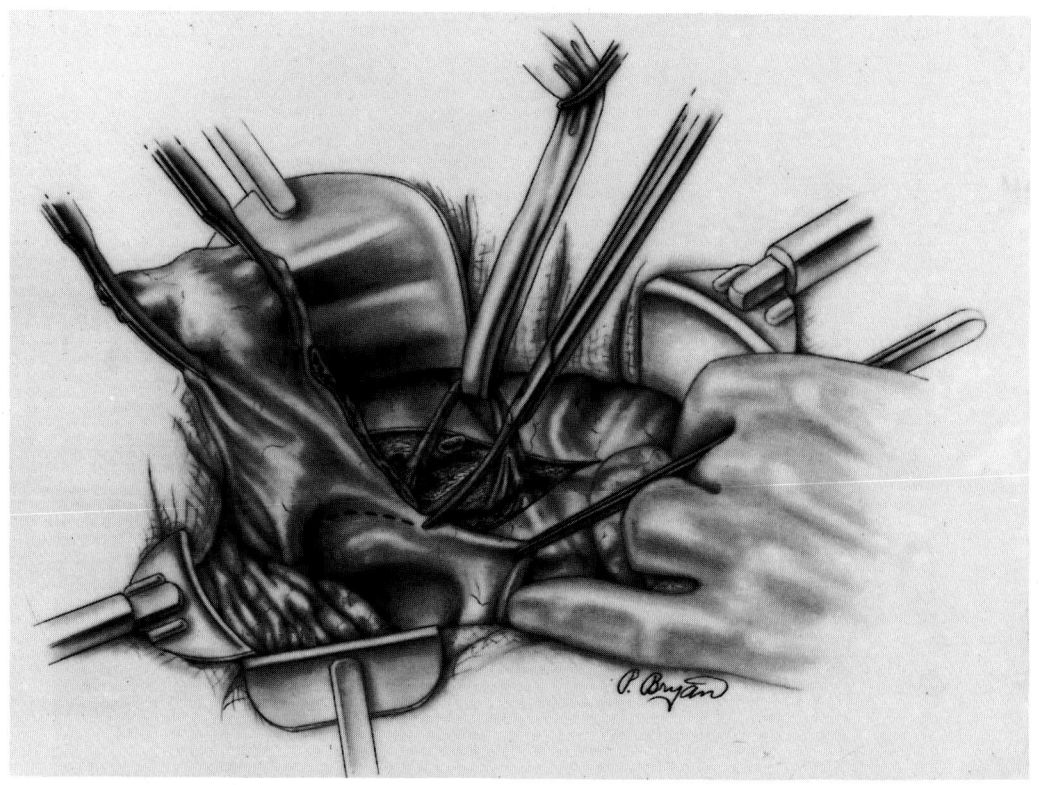

Fig. 78.35   An incision is made in the cul-de-sac peritoneum below the cervix if possible, to allow development of the rectovaginal space.

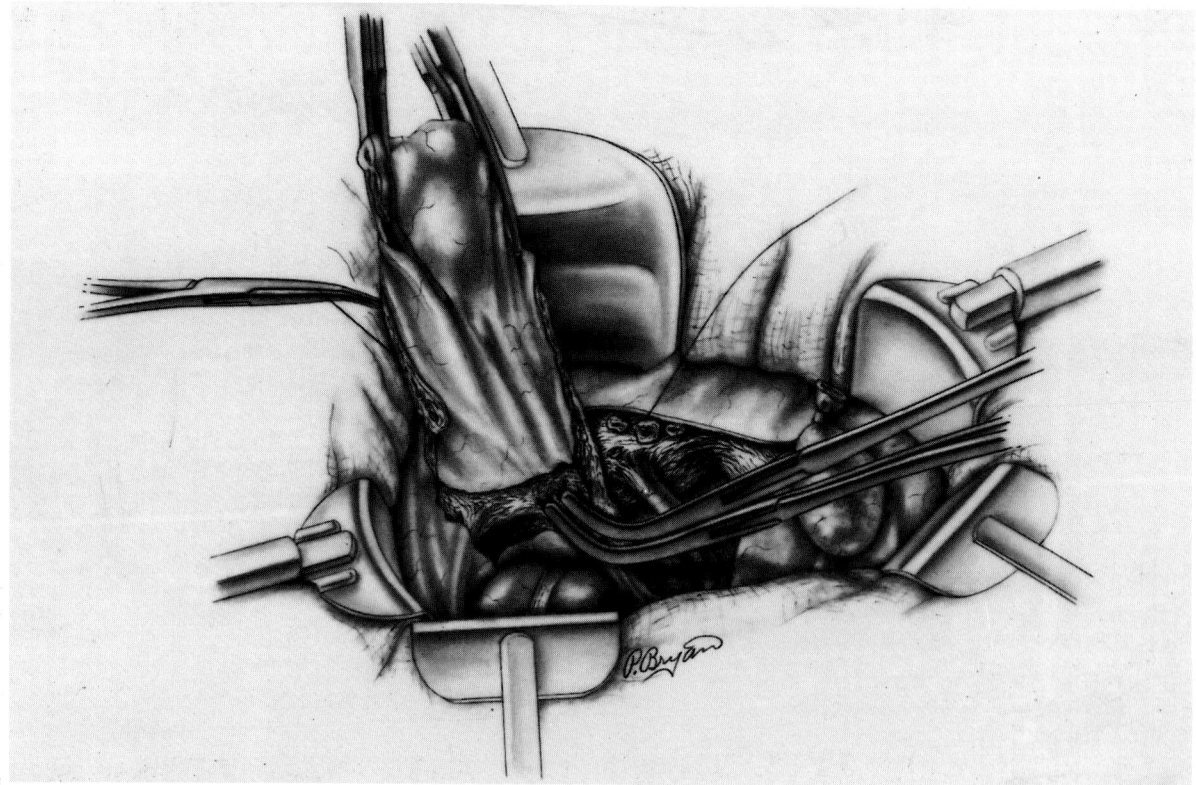

Fig. 78.36   The posterior parametrium and uterosacral ligaments are clamped adjacent to the rectum.

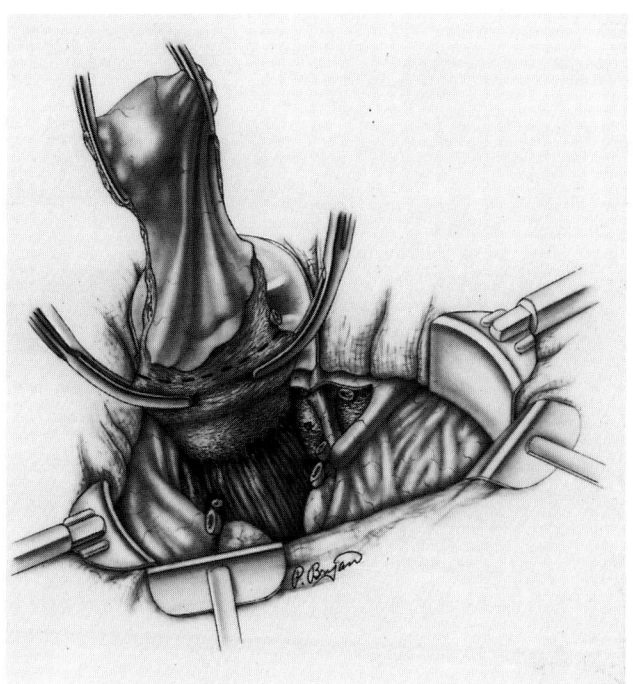

Fig. 78.37 After clamping and ligating paravaginal tissue laterally, an incision is made in the vagina several centimeters below the cervix.

incidence of lymph node involvement increased with tumor size, reaching a maximum of 68.3% in the group with a ratio from 70 to 80%. Surprisingly, direct spread into the parametrium was rarely found, even when large tumors were found to occupy the entire cervix. This finding is contrary to that of Bleker et al who found 16.8% unrecognized parametrial tumor involvement in patients with Stage Ib and IIa lesions.[12] The 5-year survival fell with parametrial involvement.

Thorough examination of the lymphadenectomy specimens must be done. Tumor metastasis to lymph nodes adversely affects patient survival. Among patients with positive nodes, the pathological examination should report whether the metastatic disease is microscopic or macroscopic, single or multiple, unilateral or bilateral. The location of lymph nodes positive for tumor should also be reported, since the prognosis is especially poor in patients with positive common iliac and/or para-aortic nodes. The usual standard technique of pathological examination of lymphadenectomy specimens involves removal of visible and palpable nodes from fatty tissue, with bisection of each node for microscopic examination. This technique may not be adequate. A significant increase in positive findings can be obtained if special pathological examination techniques are used, as demonstrated by To et al,[132] Ahrens & Tschoke[1] and Wilkinson & Hause.[144] With their technique of dissection of lymph nodes at multiple levels before paraffin embedding, To and associates showed that 9% of patients originally reported to have negative nodes actually had positive nodes.

An accurate assessment of the extent of disease by a

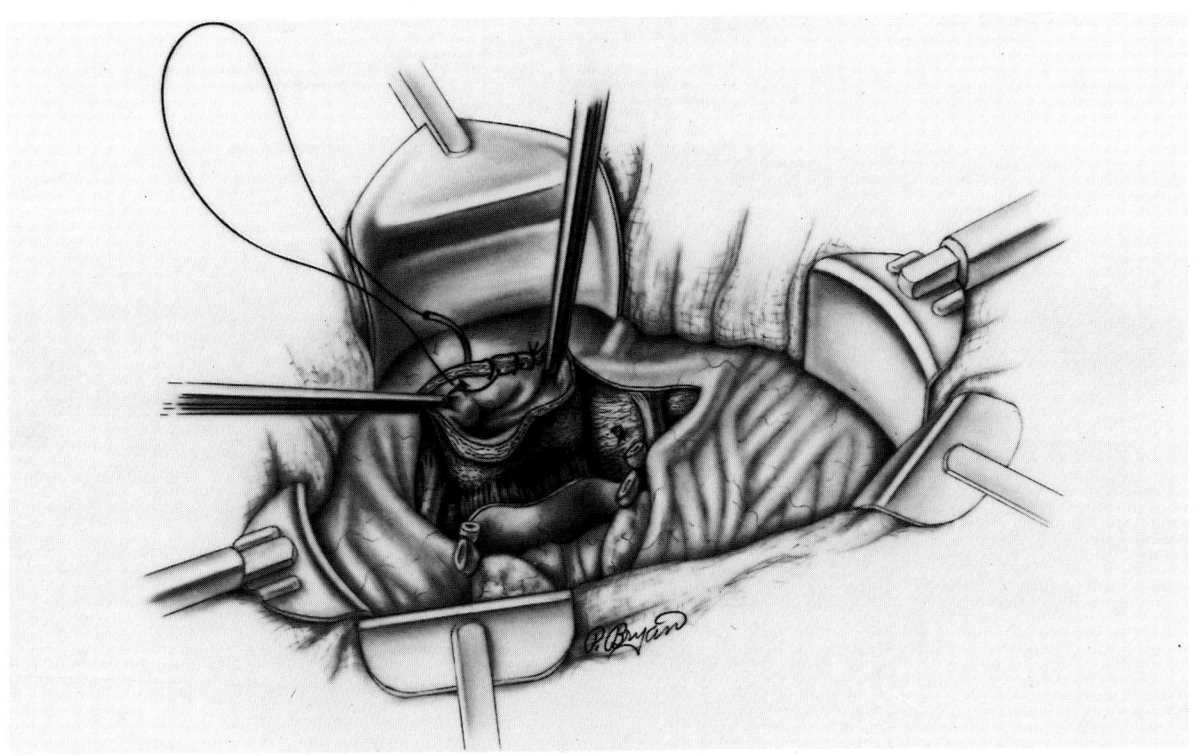

Fig. 78.38 A continuous hemostatic suture is placed in the vaginal cuff.

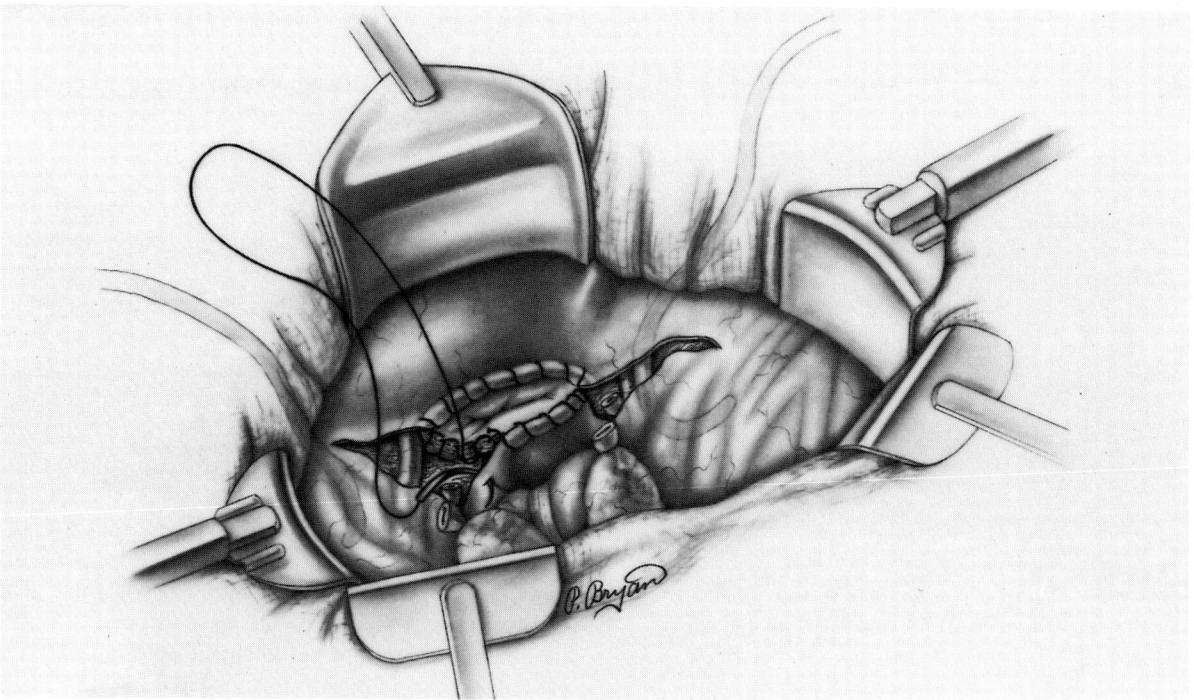

Fig. 78.39 Suction catheters are placed in the retroperitoneal spaces bilaterally. The bladder peritoneum is sutured to the anterior vaginal cuff and the cul-de-sac peritoneum is sutured to the posterior vaginal cuff.

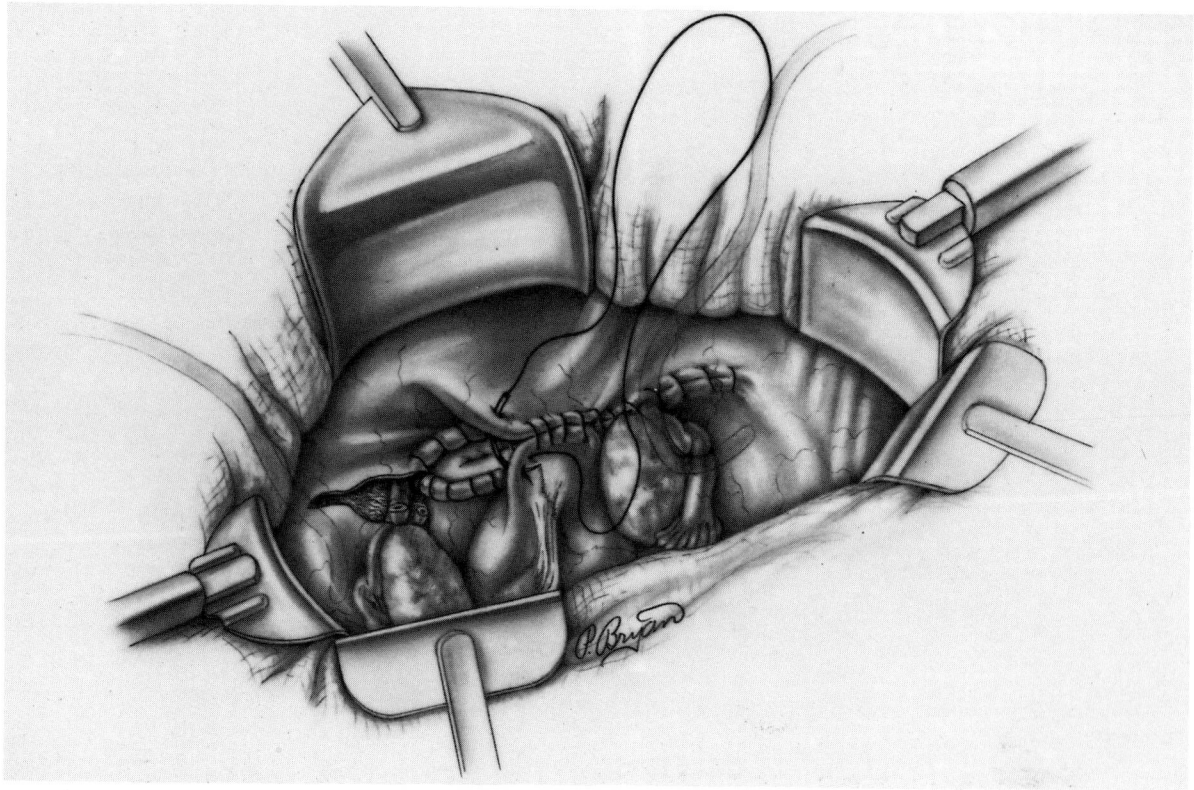

Fig. 78.40 The remainder of the peritoneum is closed across the pelvic floor.

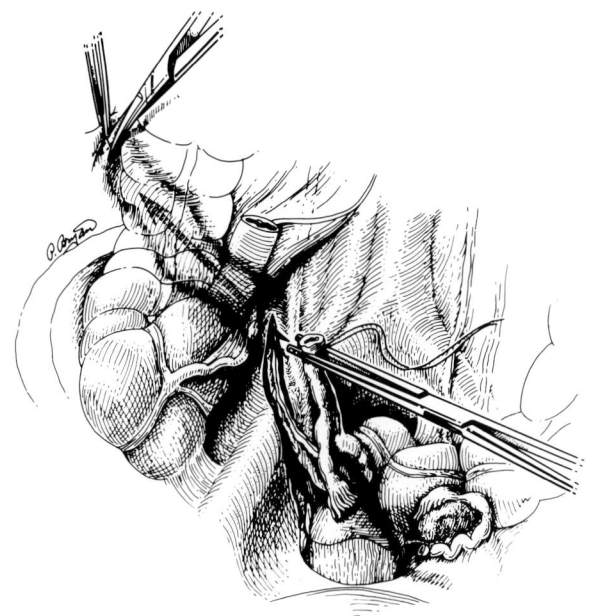

Fig. 78.41 If the ovaries are to be suspended, a tunnel can be made under the peritoneum and the cecum on the right. The tube and ovary are guided through the tunnel to the new position in the right colic gutter above the pelvis.

careful pathology examination of the operative specimen is imperative in deciding whether or not additional treatment is needed. Indeed, it is such an important component in the surgical management of patients with cervical cancer that such patients should be operated upon only in hospitals where expert pathologists also work.

POSTOPERATIVE COMPLICATIONS

Bladder

Fistula

In the absence of prior pelvic irradiation, bladder ischemia and vesicovaginal fistula are infrequent complications of this procedure. In our experience, suture of the bladder peritoneum to the margins of the anterior vaginal wall has protected the bladder and terminal ureter from secondary infection and subsequent fistula formation. It is our view that this has significantly decreased the incidence of vesicovaginal and ureterovaginal fistula.

Neurogenic bladder dysfunction

An extensive abdominal hysterectomy effectively denervates the bladder and upper urethra. The more extensive

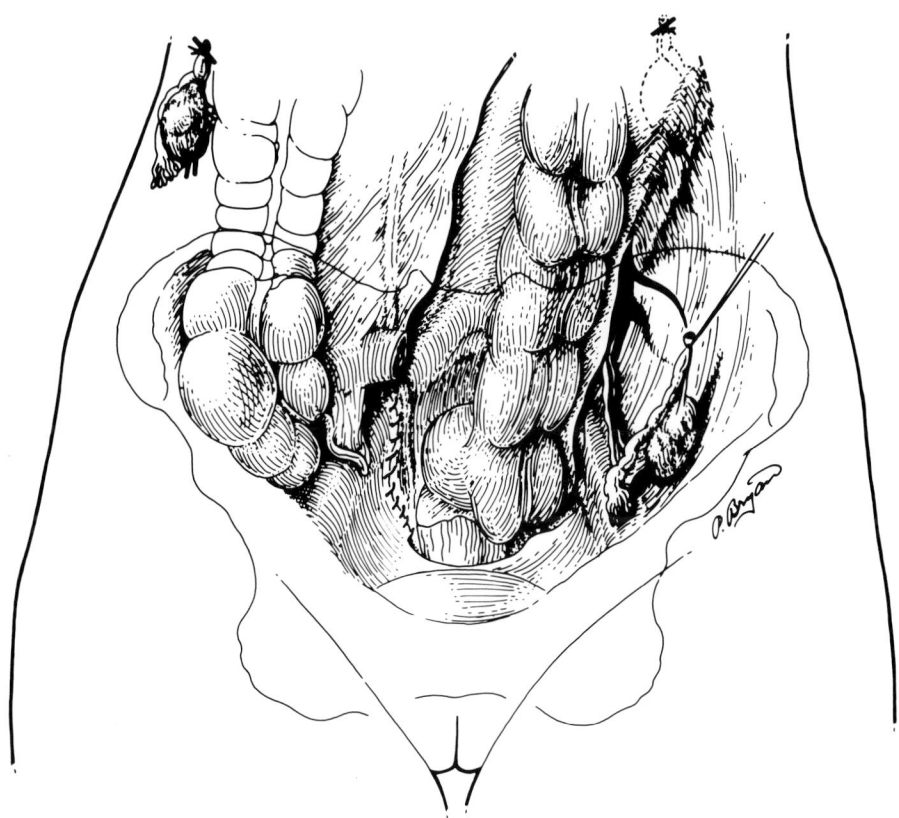

Fig. 78.42 A similar procedure can be done on the left. The ovarian vessels should not be twisted. Metal clips are placed on the pedicles to allow later identification with abdominal X-ray.

the dissection, the greater the degree of interference with their function. Parasympathetic and sympathetic nerve fibers to and from the bladder and urethra are removed along with paracervical, paravaginal, cardinal ligament tissues and pelvic lymph nodes. All patients will have some degree of bladder dysfunction; the incidence of significant bladder dysfunction may be as high as 50%.

Mundy[92] and Sasaki et al[116] have suggested that the posterior part of the cardinal ligament (pars nervosa) contains the major part of the parasympathetic and sympathetic nerve supply to the bladder and urethra, and that its removal is responsible for postoperative bladder dysfunction. Sasaki et al demonstrated that removal of the anterior cardinal ligament (pars vasculosa) with preservation of the pars nervosa will reduce the difficulty of postoperative bladder dysfunction.[116] The work of Kadar et al[58] and Asmussen & Ulmsten[3] suggests that the nerve supply to the bladder and urethra can be spared without compromising the necessary extensive dissection and tissue removal around the central disease, thus sparing many patients the loss of urethrovesical function. This suggestion has not been widely adopted by gynecologic surgeons, presumably because of a concern that this same cardinal ligament tissue also carries lymph channels draining the cervix, and should be removed in a complete central dissection. It would seem to us, therefore, that some degree of bladder dysfunction is inevitable with a technique of extensive hysterectomy that emphasizes adequacy of the central dissection and complete lymphadenectomy.

Studies have demonstrated that the bladder may initially be hypertonic with decreased bladder capacity, increased resting pressure, and increased residual urine volume. Patients often have difficulty initiating micturition and there is a loss of sensation of bladder fullness. Using sensitive urodynamic instrumentation, Scotti et al found a variety of abnormalities, including obstructive voiding patterns, immediate and delayed loss of compliance, sensory losses and genuine stress incontinence.[118] Some patients had complete absence of bladder contractions during voiding.

Techniques of managing the postoperative bladder have varied widely. Duration of catheter drainage, suprapubic versus transurethral drainage, the value of self-catheterization and the value of cystometric studies have all been debated, as described by Bandy et al.[7] These authors also found that patients receiving postoperative adjunctive pelvic radiation had significantly more contracted and unstable bladders than patients treated with surgery alone. Proper management of the bladder in the first few weeks after operation is essential to avoid over-distension. Our preference is for continuous catheter drainage, either transurethral or suprapubic, for seven days, followed by intermittent clamping and release of the catheter for several more days. A postoperative intravenous pyelogram is performed on the tenth postoperative day. If only the usual mild ureteral dilatation is seen, the catheter is removed and the patient is taught intermittent self-catheterization. She must be thoroughly schooled in the importance of not allowing her bladder to become over-distended. Allowing the bladder to over-distend, especially in the early postoperative recovery period, may result in a flaccid bladder from stretching and decompensation of the detrusor muscle, prolongation of bladder dysfunction with high residual urine volumes, and the likelihood of urinary infections. Patients are asked to void by the clock and to catheterize themselves three times each day after voiding. When bladder sensations return and residual urine volumes are consistently below 50 to 75 ml, then self-catheterization can be cautiously discontinued, to be reinstituted whenever there is a suggestion of incomplete bladder emptying. Those patients who are unwilling or unable to perform these tasks assiduously are best managed with prolonged indwelling catheter drainage for several weeks before attempting to remove it. If a serious episode of over-distension of the bladder ever occurs, continuous indwelling catheter drainage should be reinstituted, sometimes for several weeks, with the hope that permanent impairment of bladder function can be avoided. Urinary tract infections may occur in conjunction with bladder dysfunction; they should be looked for with periodic urinalysis and culture, and treated with appropriate antibiotics. Patients should be encouraged to maintain a urinary output above 2000 ml per day to avoid urinary tract infection.

In most patients, a satisfactory voiding pattern will be established within several months. However, urodynamic studies may show some evidence of slight and persistent chronic bladder dysfunction for several years. Fraser stated that 20% of his patients continued to report changes in bladder sensation as long as 5 to 15 years after operation.[32] In many patients who have had properly performed extensive abdominal hysterectomy and pelvic lymphadenectomy, it is inevitable that the bladder function will never be completely normal again. However, with proper postoperative bladder care and rehabilitation, function should be satisfactory in most patients at the end of the first year. According to Fishman et al 35% of patients continued to express unhappiness at the extent and effect of their postoperative urinary dysfunction.[30]

Ureter

Clark, working at the Johns Hopkins Hospital, published one of the first descriptions of extensive hysterectomy for cervical cancer in 1895.[23] Sampson, working in the same institution during the same period, recognized that injury to the ureter was the most serious problem associated with primary extensive surgery for this disease. His publications on ureteral anatomy and blood supply, and the relationship between the ureter and gynecologic disease are classic and pertinent today. Devascularization and ischemic necrosis of the wall of the terminal ureter has proven to be one of the more serious complications of this operation. Wertheim, himself, found this complication to be one of the more serious sequelae. In Meig's clinic, there was a 12.5% significant ureteral complication rate, including an 8.5% incidence of ureterovaginal fistulae and a 4% incidence of ureteral stricture. As recently as 1965, Talbert et al reported that nine of 112 patients (8%) who had extensive hysterectomy developed ureterovaginal fistulas, two of which were bilateral.[130] Seven kidneys were lost. The incidence of ureteral stricture was also high. The high percentage of ureteral complications may have been related to a large number of patients with pelvic cellulitis, and also to a large number of patients (71%) who received preoperative radiation. It is well known that these two factors increase the risk of ureteral complications. In a recent report of 111 patients undergoing extensive hysterectomy and lymphadenectomy for cervical cancer in the same institution, only two minor ureteral injuries and no fistulas occurred (see also Ch. 42).

For many years, gynecologic surgeons have attempted to lower the rate of ureteral complications with special techniques. Novak, from Yugoslavia, reduced the incidence of ureteral fistula following primary extensive surgery to 2% by placing the dissected pelvic ureter on the inside (peritoneal surface) of the pelvic peritoneum and by preservation of the lateral mesentery to the terminal ureter.[96] Green suggested that the terminal ureter should be lifted out of the accumulated fluid in the retroperitoneal space by suturing it to the obliterated hypogastric artery.[43] Ohkawa developed a procedure which attempted to elevate and isolate the ureter from the infected retroperitoneal fluid, and also to develop a new blood supply to the terminal ureter by placing it in a peritoneal envelope from the pelvic brim to the bladder. Blythe and associates[13] compared this technique with simple retroperitoneal suction drainage first advised by Symmonds & Pratt.[128] They found that ureteral obstruction and ureterovaginal fistulas occurred twice as often, and that the operative time was extended 45 minutes to one hour with the Ohkawa technique.

Given a normal, unirradiated ureter, we believe the incidence of ureteral fistula and permanent stenosis can be kept below 1% with meticulous intraoperative management of the ureter by a technically skilful operator, who can prevent vascular trauma to the peri-ureteral sheath and injury to the muscularis of the ureter, and by postoperative removal of retroperitoneal space fluid by constant suction.

Some temporary postoperative changes in ureteral function are an almost inevitable result of extensive hysterectomy, as pointed out by Gal & Buchsbaum.[37] Using special static and cinefluoroscopic intravenous pyelogram techniques, these authors found ureteral dilatation in 87% of patients in the first week following surgery. Usually 6 weeks after surgery, the dilatation had regressed and the pyelograms returned to normal. Peristalsis was altered in the distal ureter, which appeared as a rigid conduit during the first postoperative week. Peristalsis had returned one month later. These changes may explain the increased frequency of urinary tract infections following extensive hysterectomy, and the possibility of permanent ureteral stenosis if radiation, serious infection or lymphocyst formation is superimposed.

Retroperitoneal spaces

A closed system of constant suction must be used in the retroperitoneal spaces on each side. The purpose is to remove the potentially enormous accumulation of fluid that normally collects in these spaces after a complete and thorough lymphadenectomy. The fluid composition is similar to that of the fluid which exudes from the surface of a third degree burn; it consists of blood components, lymph and tissue fluid, and contains a high percentage of protein. The drains should be irrigated with sterile saline as often as necessary to ensure their patency and continued function. The amount of drainage varies, but may be as much as several hundred milliliters per day for as long as a week, before the amount begins to decrease. Obviously, such a large amount of fluid loss must be replaced intravenously until the patient is able to take adequate oral fluids and food. A drain may be removed if it produces less than 50 ml in a 24 hour period for two consecutive days.

Prolonged closed drainage of the retroperitoneal spaces is probably responsible for a reduction in the incidence of ureterovaginal fistulas. The lower ureter, which has been dissected free of its surrounding attachments is not constantly bathed in a large accumulation of retroperitoneal fluid under pressure and probably heals better. Likewise, the incidence of lymphocyst formation has been reduced by suction drainage of retroperitoneal spaces to less than 5% of patients. The use of antibiotics, and attempts to ligate or clip lymphatic channels may also contribute to a reduced incidence of postoperative lymphocysts. The few patients who develop lymphocysts today are usually those whose retroperitoneal suction catheters did not function properly to provide adequate drainage.

A lymphocyst will become obvious by symptoms and examination several months after extensive hysterectomy and pelvic lymphadenectomy. It may be small and asymptomatic. Patients with large lymphocysts usually complain of lower abdominal discomfort on the same side with radiation to the back, hip and/or thigh. Some edema of the lower extremity on the same side may be present. Evidence of ureteral obstruction may be found on intravenous pyelogram.

Small asymptomatic lymphocysts that do not cause ureteral obstruction may be observed. Large symptomatic lymphocysts that cause ureteral obstruction should be aspirated either vaginally or abdominally with a needle. As much as 500 ml of clear yellow fluid may be obtained. CT-directed needle aspiration may be done with local anesthesia, and may be repeated as needed. The fluid should be submitted for cytological examination. It is rarely necessary to perform open drainage of a lymphocyst. Mann et al have reported successful sclerosis of a recurrent lymphocyst by injection of a solution of tetracycline.[80]

Infection

The occurrence of pelvic cellulitis has been greatly diminished following radical pelvic surgery with the use of adequate abdominal drainage of the operative site. Further, the prophylactic use of broad spectrum antibiotics, including both aerobic and anaerobic coverage, has proven to be a useful addition to the surgical armamentarium. Previously, patients were treated with antibiotics only if postoperative infection occurred. At the present time, it is our practice to initiate broad spectrum antibiotic coverage for both aerobic (Gram-positive and Gram-negative) and anaerobic bacteriological coverage immediately before surgery. This treatment is maintained for 72 hours postoperatively and has resulted in a markedly reduced incidence of pelvic cellulitis to less than 5% of the cases. When secondary infection does occur in spite of the use of prophylactic antibiotics, the vaginal vault is cultured, drainage from the abdominal suction catheters is cultured, and bacterial-specific, high-dose antibiotic therapy is utilized at that time. Rarely is it necessary to drain a pelvic abscess where there has been accumulation of serum, blood with secondary infection. In our experience, this has occurred in less than 0.5% of patients.

It must be admitted that only a few studies have been done on the use of peri-operative prophylactic antibiotics in extensive hysterectomy patients. The rates of postoperative infectious morbidity appeared to be reduced in studies by Orr et al,[98] by Rosenshein et al,[109] and by Sevin et al.[121] However, Bendvold & Kjorstad were unable to find justification for prophylactic antibiotics, since patients undergoing extensive hysterectomy in the Norwegian Radium Hospital had a very low incidence of postoperative infectious morbidity.[9] Indeed, there were no instances of surgical site-related infections observed among 35 patients who had extensive abdominal hysterectomy.

Venous thrombosis and pulmonary embolus

The patient who undergoes extensive pelvic surgery is at the highest risk for the development of venous thrombosis of the lower extremity, as compared to patients who have other types of gynecological surgery (see also Ch. 84). Virchow's classic triad of etiological factors, as described more than 125 years ago, are relevant today in the patient who has undergone extensive pelvic surgery. Such factors as postoperative alteration of blood coagulation, trauma to the vein wall and venous stasis are recognizable features of this type of surgery. In particular, pelvic lymphadenectomy invariably produces some trauma to the vein wall during the mobilization of the vessel and resection of the adherent lymphatic tissue. One of the biologic effects of extensive surgery is the occurrence of local tissue necrosis during the process of healing. This results in the release into the circulation of tissue thromboplastin, which contributes to venous thrombosis by acceleration of the clotting mechanism. The release of thromboplastin from the intima of the vein wall itself will also provide an excellent nidus for the formation of fibrin, particularly an area of the venous system where there is alteration in venous flow with stagnation of blood. This is frequently seen behind the valves of the veins of the lower extremity, where silent thrombosis is common. In studies utilizing I[125]-labeled fibrinogen scanning of the lower extremity, as many as 20% of gynecologic patients having a hysterectomy have been found to have venous thrombosis by this technique. Prolonged immobilization of the lower extremities during a lengthy operative procedure is responsible for intraoperative venous stasis and clot formation.. There is now good evidence to document the fact that patients who develop postoperative thrombosis of the lower extremity have the origin of this complication during the surgical procedure in more than 50% of cases. Efforts to decrease the frequency of this complication include prophylactic low-dose heparin, using 5000 units subcutaneously, 3 times daily, beginning 2 hours before surgery and given every 8 hours thereafter for the subsequent 5 postoperative days. By using this regimen alone, the incidence of deep vein thrombosis in Kakkar's study was decreased from 24.6% in the untreated control group to 7.7% in the heparin treated group of surgical cases.[59,60,61] More impressive was the observation in the latter study that 16 patients in the control group, as compared to only 2 patients in the heparin treated group, were found on autopsy study to have died from acute, massive pulmonary embolism. Clarke-Pearson et al on the other hand, were unable to demonstrate a significant difference in the incidence of venous thrombosis or pulmonary emboli when comparing a low-dose heparin and control group.[24] Perioperative heparin has the potential of increasing intraoperative blood loss and the incidence of postoperative hematoma. Currently, we are not using perioperative mini-dose heparin (see also p. 1307) but favor instead the use of intermittent compression hose on the lower extremity, beginning in the recovery room, especially in high risk patients, as advocated by Clarke-Pearson. For another viewpoint, see pages 701 and 1346.

Recent clinical evidence, as shown by I[125] fibrinogen scans, demonstrates that approximately 3 to 5% of patients with occult venous thrombosis of the lower extremities will develop a pulmonary embolus. Unfortunately, more than

50% of the cases of fatal pulmonary embolism occur in patients with silent venous thrombosis and without any clinical evidence of this complication prior to the acute pulmonary catastrophe. When evidence of venous thrombosis of the lower extremity is verified, full anticoagulation therapy is required for prevention of pulmonary embolism. Should a pulmonary embolus occur after full anticoagulation has been achieved, it is necessary in such rare cases to prevent further migration of clot to the lung, either by inferior vena cava ligation or by the use of an intracaval silastic umbrella. Such complications are rare, but the sinister effects of thromboembolism must be carefully evaluated on a daily basis in this high risk group of patients.

Hemorrhage

In spite of the surgeon's adequate technical skills and careful dissection, serious hemorrhage may suddenly appear especially during retroperitoneal dissections on the lateral pelvic sidewalls and around the sacrum. When this happens, hopefully the operative field will not be cluttered with clamps, exposure will be adequate, the patient's condition will be stable, and anesthesia will be sufficient to maintain good relaxation. If the bleeding vessel cannot be clamped quickly, the simplest and most effective method of controlling the bleeding is provided by pressure applied by the index finger of the gloved hand. With cessation of bleeding, the operative site can be cleared of accumulated blood by suctioning, exposure of the area can be improved, and the surgeon can gain a few moments to evaluate the situation and choose the best possible course of action. Arterial bleeding is easy to identify and control with clips and clamps and ligatures. The difficult problem with hemorrhage in the pelvis comes from lacerations of deep pelvic veins that are fragile, tortuous, distended, sometimes hidden or retracted from view, and sometimes held open by attachment of the vein wall to surrounding tissue. Blood returning through the lacerated vein may come from multiple sources unavailable for ligation. Placing clamps or sutures blindly is dangerous and may even make the problem worse. Digital pressure for at least seven minutes is sometimes the most effective procedure to control venous bleeding. Sometimes, additional careful dissection in the area will be required to free the vessel above and below the bleeding point to allow more precise clipping or suture ligation. A cardinal rule in dissecting in the pelvis is to avoid creating a deep hole, the bottom of which cannot be exposed, in case a deep vein is lacerated. This is the reason why dissection of the pararectal space should not be forced if it does not develop easily.

Whenever an extensive pelvic dissection is anticipated, preparations should be made in advance just in case severe intraoperative bleeding is suddenly encountered. Obviously, adequate quantities of blood should be available to replace lost volume. More blood should be requested in advance of its need. A responsible member of the operating or anesthesia team should be assigned the task of monitoring blood loss, blood replacement and urine output. In the excitement of the moment, it is possible to lose count of the number of units of whole blood, blood components, crystalloids and other fluids that have been given, and how much blood has been lost. A dependable route for administering blood must be maintained. Without it, rapid blood replacement is not possible. If massive hemorrhage occurs or even a possibility of its occurrence exists, a Swan-Ganz or similar catheter should be placed for better monitoring of physiologic functions and blood replacement. In extreme cases, where no other vessels are available for rapid intraoperative blood volume replacement, transfusions may be given under pressure directly into the common iliac artery, with the needle pointed in the direction of the heart.

Intraoperative bleeding

The most frequent site of troublesome intraoperative bleeding during extensive hysterectomy occurs from the pelvic floor veins in the dissection of the cardinal ligament and the hypogastric vessels. The collateral venous circulation of the hypogastric veins is an ever-present source of troublesome bleeding, due to difficulty in identification of these vessels as they course among muscle bundles and fascial planes on the pelvic floor. The pararectal fossa, cardinal ligament, presacral and para-aortic areas are frequent sites of venous bleeding. Therefore, meticulous dissection is important to avoid such complications. When venous bleeding does occur, it may be difficult to identify the site of the lacerated vein. In such circumstances, it is important to use compression of the pelvic floor veins by either a sponge stick or finger held in place for no less than seven minutes, or the use of an abdominal pack placed firmly against the site of bleeding for a similar length of time. In such cases, it is advisable to keep pressure on the vein until full control of the bleeding has been established, while in the meantime dissecting in other places in the pelvis. Only when the wall of a major pelvic vein has been severely traumatized and has retracted out of the operative field, is there a serious problem in re-establishing hemostasis. In contrast to arterial bleeding, hemorrhage from deep pelvic veins is rarely benefited by hypogastric artery ligation, due to the extensive collateral venous circulation to the pelvis from the lower extremity and vena cava. It is occasionally beneficial to ligate the anterior division of both hypogastric arteries to determine whether interruption of the major arterial blood supply to the pelvis will reduce the venous bleeding. When more extensive trauma to the wall of the external or common iliac vein has occurred, it is necessary to place vascular clamps above and below the area of injury and to repair the defect with fine vascular sutures.

Postoperative hemorrhage

This condition is a rare complication of extensive pelvic surgery. Due to the fact that all of the blood supply to the pelvis has been skeletonized as a part of the operative procedure, it is exceedingly rare for secondary hemorrhage to occur unless there has been uncontrolled bleeding at the completion of the operation. In such cases, the pelvis is usually packed with multiple gauze packs with one end exteriorized through the open vagina. Tamponade of the pelvis by means of an umbrella gauze pack and external ring has been used in many clinics where there has been persistent venous oozing in the pelvis at the completion of the operation. Pelvic packs should be advanced within 24 to 48 hours and removed shortly thereafter, in order to avoid ascending infection from the vagina by aerobic and anaerobic bacteria.

Neuropathies

Nerve injury with extensive hysterectomy was reviewed by Hoffman et al who reported its infrequent occurrence.[47] The most important injuries are to the femoral, obturator, peroneal, sciatic, genitofemoral, ilioinguinal, iliohypogastric, lateral femoral cutaneous and pudendal nerves. An awareness of the anatomic location of these nerves in the operative field, careful surgical technique in dissection and securing hemostasis, careful placement of self-retaining retractors and careful positioning of patients in stirrups will prevent most nerve injuries. Fortunately, most nerve injuries are not associated with serious or permanent disability; a few, however, are.

FOLLOW-UP AFTER EXTENSIVE SURGERY FOR CERVICAL CANCER

In spite of carefully planned and executed extensive surgery for Stage I and IIa cervical cancer, 5 to 20% of patients in various series will show evidence of recurrent or persistent tumor. Approximately one-half will occur in the first year following treatment. Almost all will occur within the first 3 years. Very few will occur later. Very, very late recurrences are extremely rare following primary surgical treatment, and are more likely to be seen in patients treated with primary radiotherapy (see Ch. 45).

Persistent or recurrent disease after primary extensive surgery may represent incomplete resection of the central tumor undetected at operation or by the pathologist's examination of the surgical specimen. Microscopic metastatic involvement of lymph nodes may be undetected by incomplete pathology examination, or left behind by incomplete lymphadenectomy. Viable tumor cells may escape in small numbers via lymphatics or vascular channels to distant sites and overcome host resistance. Probably in as many as 10% of patients with persistent disease, it may result from continued growth of unrecognized intraperitoneal spread of tumor. Cytologic study of peritoneal fluid and washings may have been overlooked or may have been falsely negative.

After the immediate postoperative recovery is completed, patients are scheduled for regular follow-up examinations which will vary depending on circumstances. Patients who are at greater risk for recurrence should be followed especially closely at frequent intervals. These will usually be the same patients who have been given postoperative radiotherapy, and will include patients with metastatic disease in lymph nodes, close surgical margins, large volume cervical tumors, lymph-vascular channel involvement, highly undifferentiated tumors, adenosquamous and glassy cell tumors, and those patients with positive peritoneal cytology. The frequency of examination will vary somewhat from patient to patient. However, in general, patients are seen every 2 to 3 months during the first and second years after primary treatment, every 3 to 4 months during the third and fourth years, and every 6 months to a year thereafter. Patients are instructed to report unusual signs or symptoms (vaginal bleeding or discharge, leg swelling, discomfort in the pelvis, discomfort in the legs, difficulty with urination or defecation, enlarged nodes, etc.), at any time they appear. However, Krebs et al reported that 25% of their patients were asymptomatic when persistent disease was diagnosed.[68] In the study reported by Larson et al 37% were asymptomatic.[71]

A follow-up examination should include palpation of the neck for enlarged lymph nodes, abdominal and leg examination, and a speculum and bimanual rectovaginal abdominal examination. A vaginal cytology smear is performed with each visit. Chest X-ray, CT scan of the abdomen and pelvis, proctosigmoidoscopy, cystoscopy, intravenous pyelography, and biopsy (needle and/or punch) of any suspicious lesions may be required, depending on the patient's symptoms and examination findings. These special diagnostic procedures are not done routinely as a part of postoperative follow-up surveillance in asymptomatic patients. Positive findings are rare unless the patient is symptomatic. For example, intravenous pyelogram rarely shows ureteral obstruction in a patient who does not also have symptoms of pelvic sidewall persistent disease and is, therefore, not routinely done at specific intervals. It is in the patient's best interest to have follow-up examinations done in the same center in which her treatment was administered. Current findings at each visit must be compared to previous information all the way back to her original presentation.

Regular pelvic examinations and vaginal cytology smears may detect a central pelvic recurrence early. This may be a great advantage. Just as it is important to detect the original cancer in the earliest stage possible in order that the patient may have the best possible chance of cure, so also it is important to detect persistent disease at the earliest possible moment, and for the same reason. For example, Jobsen et al have recently reported on the use of radiotherapy to treat 'locoregional recurrence' of carcinoma of the cervix after primary surgery.[56] The overall 5-year survival was 44%. Response to radiotherapy was strongly correlated with tumor volume, providing additional supportive evidence for the idea that persistent disease should be diagnosed as early as possible and hopefully when the volume of persistent tumor is still small and responsive.

Tumor ulceration in the upper vagina may produce vaginal discharge and spotting, a palpable tumor mass, and induration and nodularity of tissue extending to the pelvic sidewalls. Pain may not be present unless the tumor involves nerve roots. Symptoms related to urination and defecation may result from pressure, infection, or tumor involvement of the bladder and rectum. Either unilateral or bilateral edema of the lower extremities, or unilateral or bilateral hydroureter and hydronephrosis may be an ominous sign of persistent disease, but may also be the result of a combination of the effects of extensive surgery and postoperative radiation treatment. When initially diagnosed, recurrences may be central in approximately one-fourth of patients, involve the pelvic sidewall(s) in one-fourth, and involve distant sites in one-fourth, with the remaining one-fourth of patients showing multiple sites of involvement.

About 20 to 25% of patients with recurrence following primary extensive surgery may still be cured. The best chance of cure is in patients who had no postoperative radiation treatment and no metastatic disease to pelvic lymph nodes, and whose persistent disease is limited to the central pelvis. A combination of total pelvic irradiation to 5000 cGy central pelvis plus vaginal brachytherapy may be effective in controlling the disease (Ch. 41). When there is evidence of unresectable persistent disease in the pelvis in patients who have already received postoperative pelvic radiation, or when there is persistent disease in distant sites, chemotherapy may be given for palliation but is not often effective in eradication of the disease (Chs. 44 and 45). Fuller et al analyzed the experience at the Memorial Sloan-Kettering Cancer Center and reported that 'none of the 29 patients with recurrent carcinoma and positive nodes at the time of their initial lymphadenectomy was successfully treated'.[36]

Although the early detection of persistence is the primary purpose of, and justification for, follow-up visits, assessment of urinary tract function is also important. Particular attention should be paid to bladder function and maintaining a satisfactory voiding pattern. Urinary tract infection should be diagnosed and treated promptly. If ureteral stenosis impairs renal function, early intervention may be successful in avoiding nephrectomy. This is more likely to be seen in patients who receive a combination of extensive surgery and irradiation as primary treatment (see Ch. 85).

Rehabilitation of sexual function after surgical therapy for cervical cancer is usually easily done by the patient and her partner, but is more difficult if the vagina and paravaginal tissues have received heavy doses of radiation or if the patient has lost ovarian function as a result of treatment (see Ch. 90). The gynecologic surgeon should inquire about sexual problems and give advice and permission when needed. Counseling, including instruction in the technique of alternative means of sexual gratification (interfemoral intercourse, etc.) may be needed. If ovarian function has been lost as a result of treatment, estrogen replacement therapy should be provided even though symptoms of hypo-estrogenism are not present. If normal ovaries were conserved, their function should be monitored with periodic FSH and estrogen levels, in order that estrogen replacement may be provided when ovaries cease functioning in future years. There may be other contraindications to estrogen replacement therapy in patients treated for cervical cancer, but a history of treatment for cervical cancer is not one of them.

Finally, patients who have been treated for cervical cancer are at greater risk of developing other primary cancers at different sites, especially if the treatment included radiation. Detection of other primary malignancies should be a part of post-treatment follow-up. This subject has been studied by Hoffman et al,[48] by Buchler[18] and by others. Axelrod et al reported that 3.9% of patients with invasive cervical cancer had second primaries.[4] In 1987, Arneson & Kao reported that there were 61 new primary cancers detected among 718 patients with invasive cervical cancer who had been studied from 1955 to 1979.[2]

SUMMARY

There have been many improvements in the operative technique of the extensive hysterectomy and lymphadenectomy since its original description. The incidence of complications following this procedure has decreased during the past 75 years and the survival rates have increased. The operation has achieved its peak of clinical usefulness during this period of time and is now considered to be the principal method of treatment of early invasive carcinoma of the cervix. In the better surgical clinics, the meticulous execution of this operative procedure has reduced the incidence of complications to an acceptable and infrequent occurrence. The operation affords very little additional surgical risk to the patient than is associated with a hysterectomy performed for benign disease. In surgical clinics where the operation is performed well, the 5-year cure rate of Stage Ib carcinoma of the cervix varies between 85 to 90% of cases. When its use is extended for the treatment of Stage IIa lesions, the 5-year cure rate varies between 70 to 75%. Comparative studies with primary radiation therapy demonstrate an equal cure rate with primary radical surgery, although the complications of irradiation are far more difficult to manage than are those of primary surgery. In young women, where preservation of ovarian function is important, primary surgery is a preferable choice of treatment.

The major limiting factor in the long-term surgical cure of this tumor is related to the spread of the disease at the time of initiation of treatment. In cases where pelvic lymph nodes are positive for metastatic tumor, the 5-year cure rate is reduced to about 60%. The use of postoperative radiation in these cases is highly controversial, as there seems to be difficulty in showing statistically significant improvement of cure rates in long-term follow-up studies, as compared to control studies, in those cases where supplemental pelvic radiation therapy is given. Since this question remains unanswered, it is our preference to give megavoltage irradiation therapy postoperatively to cases that have histologic evidence of pelvic lymph node metastases and/or close surgical margins, since this additional treatment is generally well tolerated. The indications have not been firmly established for extended-field postoperative radiation to include para-aortic lymph nodes.

It is important to understand that it is the individual surgical expertise that offers the highest cure rate and lowest incidence of complications to the patient with invasive carcinoma of the cervix. One of the greatest errors in clinical judgement is made by the gynecologist who attempts an extensive hysterectomy and pelvic lymph node dissection without adequate surgical experience. Unless the pelvic surgeon is performing this type of surgery regularly, in a well-staffed medical center with trained assistants, he/she would be well advised to refer the patient to an established oncology center. From the patient's point of view, the initial treatment, whether primary surgery or irradiation, provides the best chance for long-term cure of this disease. It would be to her advantage to have the treatment conducted in the most expert hands, since secondary treatment for recurrent disease offers only limited long-term cure.

The gynecologic surgeon who becomes thoroughly familiar with the pathology and natural history of cervical cancer, who appreciates the history of the development of extensive hysterectomy and pelvic lymphadenectomy as primary treatment of the disease, and then thoroughly masters the technical details of performing the operation can feel enormous pride in his/her achievement. There is no greater challenge in gynecologic surgery and no greater personal satisfaction than that which comes to those who are able to perform the operation correctly and save a woman from the intense suffering and undignified death that cervical cancer can cause.

ACKNOWLEDGEMENTS

Figures 78.1–78.3, 78.5, 78.6, 78.11–78.20 are reproduced from Mattingly R F 1977 *TeLinde's Operative Gynecology*, 5th edn, Figures 78.21–78.42 are reproduced from Thompson J D 1991 Cancer of the cervix. In: Thompson J D, Rock J A (eds) *TeLinde's Operative Gynecology*, 7th edn. Lippincott, Philadelphia by permission of the publishers, Lippincott/Harper & Row. Figures 78.7, 78.8, 78.9, 78.10 are reproduced from Reiffenstuhl G 1964 *The Lymphatics of the Female Genital Organs*. Lippincott, Philadelphia by kind permission of the publishers Lippincott/Harper & Row.

REFERENCES

1. Ahrens C A, Tschoke S 1961 Lymphknotenbefunde nach Wertheim-Meigscher Operation. Geburtshilfe Frauenheilkd 21: 219
2. Arneson A, Kao M S 1987 Long-term observations of cervical cancer. Am J Obstet Gynecol 156: 614
3. Asmussen M, Ulmsten U 1975 Simultaneous urethrocystometry and urethra pressure profile measurement with a new technique. Acta Obstet Gynecol Scand 54: 385
4. Axelrod J H, Fruchter R, Boyce J G 1984 Multiple primaries among gynecologic malignancies. Gynecol Oncol 18: 359
5. Baltzer J, Kopcke W, Lohe K J, Kaufmann C, Ober K G, Zander J 1984 Die operative behandlung des zervixkarzinoms. Geburtsh Frauenheilk 44: 279
6. Bandy L C, Clarke-Pearson D L, Silverman P M, Creasman W T 1985 Computed tomography in evaluation of extrapelvic lymphadenopathy in carcinoma of the cervix. Obstet Gynecol 65: 73
7. Bandy L C, Clarke-Pearson D L, Soper J T, Mutch D G, MacMillian J, Creasman W T 1987 Long-term effects on bladder function following radical hysterectomy with and without postoperative radiation. Gynecol Oncol 26: 160
8. Barter J F, Soong S J, Shingleton H M, Hatch K D, Orr J W Jr 1989 Complications of combined radical hysterectomy — postoperative radiation therapy in women with early stage cervical cancer. Gynecol Oncol 32: 292
9. Bendvold E, Kjorstad K E 1987 Antibiotic prophylaxis for radical abdominal hysterectomy. Gynecol Oncol 28: 201
10. Berek J S, Brand E 1988 Controversies in the management of cervical adenocarcinoma. (Reply to Letter to the Editor). Obstet Gynecol 72: 289
11. Bithal P K, Vijayaraghavan S, Shahani J M, Oberoi G S 1987 Blood loss in Wertheim's hysterectomy: Comparison of three anaesthetic techniques. Indian J Med Sci 41: 78
12. Bleker O P, Ketting B W, van Wayjen-Eecen B, Kloosterman G J 1983 The significance of microscopic involvement of the parametrium and/or pelvic lymph nodes in cervical cancer stages Ib and IIa. Gynecol Oncol 16: 56
13. Blythe J G, Hodel K A, Wahl T P 1988 A comparison between peritoneal sheathing of the ureters (Ohkawa technique) and retroperitoneal pelvic suction drainage in the prevention of ureteral damage during radical abdominal hysterectomy. Gynecol Oncol 30: 222
14. Bonney V 1941 The results of 500 cases of Wertheim's operation for carcinoma of the cervix. J Obstet Gynaecol Br Emp 48: 421
15. Bonney V 1949 Wertheim's operation in retrospect. Lancet 1: 637
16. Brand E, Berek J S, Hacker N F 1988 Controversies in the management of cervical adenocarcinoma. Obstet Gynecol 71: 261
17. Breen J A 1989 Personal communication
18. Buchler D A 1975 Multiple primaries and gynecologic malignancies. Am J Obstet Gynecol 123: 376
19. Burghardt E, Hoffmann H M H, Ebner F, Haas J, Tamussino

K, Justich E 1989 Magnetic resonance imaging in cervical cancer: a basis for objective classification. Gynecol Oncol 33: 61

20. Burghardt E, Pickel H 1978 Local spread and lymph node involvement in cervical cancer. Obstet Gynecol 52: 138

21. Burghardt E, Pickel H, Haas J, Lahousen M 1987 Prognostic factors and operative treatment of Stages Ib to IIb cervical cancer. Am J Obstet Gynecol 156: 988

22. Camilien L, Gordon D, Fruchter R G, Maiman M, Boyce J G 1988 Predictive value of computerized tomography in the presurgical evaluation of primary carcinoma of the cervix. Gynecol Oncol 30: 209

23. Clark J G 1895 A more radical method of performing hysterectomy for cancer of the uterus. Bull Johns Hopkins Hosp 6: 120

24. Clarke-Pearson D L, Jelovsek F R, Creasman W T 1983 Thromboembolism complicating surgery for cervical and uterine malignancy: incidence, risk factors, and prophylaxis. Obstet Gynecol 61: 87

25. Crawford J S, Harisiadis L, McGowan L, Rogers C C 1987 Para-aortic lymph node irradiation in cervical carcinoma without prior lymphadenectomy. Radiology 164: 255

26. Creasman W T, Fetter B F, Clarke-Pearson D L, Kaufman L, Parker R T 1985 Management of Stage Ia carcinoma of the cervix. Am J Obstet Gynecol 153: 164

27. Downey G O, Potish R A, Adcock L L, Prem K A, Twiggs L B 1989 Pretreatment surgical staging in cervical carcinoma: therapeutic efficacy of pelvic lymph node resection. Am J Obstet Gynecol 160: 1055

28. Drescher C W, Hopkins M P, Roberts J A 1989 Comparison of the pattern of metastatic spread of squamous cell cancer and adenocarcinoma of the uterine cervix. Gynecol Oncol 33: 340

29. Ellsworth L R, Allen H H, Nisker J A 1983 Ovarian function after radical hysterectomy for Stage Ib carcinoma of the cervix. Am J Obstet Gynecol 145: 185

30. Fishman I J, Shabsigh R, Kaplan A L 1986 Lower urinary tract dysfunction after radical hysterectomy for carcinoma of the cervix. Urology 28: 462

31. Fletcher G H 1979 Predominant parameters in the planning of radiation therapy of carcinoma of the cervix. Bulletin of Cancer 66: 561

32. Fraser A C 1966 Late effects of Wertheim's hysterectomy on the urinary tract. J Obstet Gynaecol Br Commw 73: 1002

33. Freund W A 1878 Eine neue Methode der Exstirpation des ganzen Uterus. Zentralb Gynaekol 10: 222

34. Freund W A 1879 Method of complete removal of the uterus. Am J Obstet Gynecol 7: 200

35. Fuller A F Jr, Elliott N, Kosloff C, Hoskins W J, Lewis J L 1989 Determinants of increased risk for recurrence in patients undergoing radical hysterectomy for Stage Ib and IIa carcinoma of the cervix. Gynecol Oncol 33: 34

36. Fuller A F Jr, Elliott N, Kosloff C, Lewis J L Jr 1982 Lymph node metastases from carcinoma of the cervix, Stage Ib and IIa: implications for prognosis and treatment. Gynecol Oncol 13: 165

37. Gal D, Buchsbaum H J 1983 A cinefluoroscopic study of ureteral function following radical hysterectomy. Obstet Gynecol 61: 82

38. Gallion H H, van Nagell J R Jr, Donaldson E S, Hanson M B, Powell D E, Maruyama Y, Yoneda J 1985 Combined radiation therapy and extrafascial hysterectomy in the treatment of Stage Ib barrel-shaped cervical cancer. Cancer 56: 262

39. Gallup D G, Jordan G H, Talledo O E 1986 Extraperitoneal lymph node dissections with use of a midline incision in patients with female genital cancer. Am J Obstet Gynecol 155: 559

40. Gallus A S, Hirsh J, Tuttle R J et al 1973 Small subcutaneous doses of heparin in prevention of venous thrombosis. New Engl J Med 228: 545

41. Girardi F, Lichtenegger W, Tamussino K, Haas J 1989 The importance of parametrial lymph nodes in the treatment of cervical cancer. Gynecol Oncol 34: 206

42. Gordon-Smith I C, Grundy D J, LeQuesne L P, Newcombe J F, Bramble F J 1972 Controlled trial of two regimens of subcutaneous heparin in prevention of postoperative deep vein thrombosis. Lancet i: 1133

43. Green T H Jr, Meigs J V, Ulfelder H, Curtin R R 1962 Urologic

complications of radical Wertheim hysterectomy; incidence, etiology, management and prevention. Obstet Gynecol 20: 293

44. Greer B E, Easterling T R, McLennan D A et al 1989 Fetal and maternal considerations in the management of Stage Ib cervical cancer during pregnancy. Gynecol Oncol 34: 61

45. Greer B E, Figge D C, Tamimi H K, Cain J M 1989 Stage Ib adenocarcinoma of the cervix treated by radical hysterectomy and pelvic lymph node dissection. Am J Obstet Gynecol 160: 1509

46. Henriksen E 1949 Lymphatic spread of carcinoma of the cervix and of body of uterus: study of 420 necropsies. Am J Obstet Gynecol 58: 924

47. Hoffman M S, Roberts W S, Cavanagh D 1988 Neuropathies associated with radical pelvic surgery for gynecologic cancer. Gynecol Oncol 31: 462

48. Hoffman M S, Roberts W S, Cavanagh D 1985 Second pelvic malignancies following radiation therapy for cervical cancer. Obstet Gynecol Surv 40: 611

49. Hogan W M, Littman P, Griner L, Miller C L, Mikuta J J 1982 Results of radiation therapy given after radical hysterectomy. Cancer 49: 1278

50. Hopkins M P, Schmidt R W, Roberts J A, Morley G W 1988 Gland cell carcinoma (adenocarcinoma) of the cervix. Obstet Gynecol 72: 789

51. Hopkins M P, Schmidt R W, Roberts J A, Morley G W 1988 The prognosis and treatment of Stage I adenocarcinoma of the cervix. Obstet Gynecol 72: 915

52. Horii T, Mitsumoto T, Noda K 1988 Significance of para-aortic node irradiation in the treatment of cervical cancer. Gynecol Oncol 31: 371

53. Husseinzadeh N, Nahhas W A, Velkley D E, Whitney C W, Mortel R 1984 The preservation of ovarian function in young women undergoing pelvic radiation therapy. Gynecol Oncol 18: 373

54. Inoue T, Morita K 1988 5-year results of postoperative extended-field irradiation on 76 patients with nodal metastases from cervical carcinoma Stages Ib to IIIb. Cancer 61: 2009

55. Inoue T, Okumura M 1984 Prognostic significance of parametrial extension in patients with cervical carcinoma Stages Ib, IIa, and IIb: a study of 628 cases treated by radical hysterectomy and lymphadenectomy with or without postoperative irradiation. Cancer 54: 1714

56. Jobsen J J, Leer J W H, Cleton F J, Hermans J 1989 Treatment of locoregional recurrence of carcinoma of the cervix by radiotherapy after primary surgery. Gynecol Oncol 33: 368

57. Jones W B 1987 Surgical approaches for advanced or recurrent cancer of the cervix. Cancer 60: 2094

58. Kadar N, Saliba N, Nelson J H 1983 The frequency, causes, and prevention of severe urinary dysfunction after radical hysterectomy. Br J Obstet Gynaecol 90: 858

59. Kakkar V V, Corrigan T P, Fossard D P 1975 Prevention of fatal postoperative pulmonary embolism by low dose heparin. Lancet ii: 45

60. Kakkar V V, Corrigan T, Spindler J et al 1972 Efficacy of low doses of heparin in prevention of deep-vein thrombosis after major surgery. Lancet ii: 101

61. Kakkar V V, Field E S, Nicholaides A N, Flute P T 1971 Low dose of heparin in prevention of deep-vein thrombosis. Lancet ii: 669

62. Kim D S, Moon H, Kim K T, Hwant Y Y, Cho S H, Kim S R 1989 Two-year survival: preoperative adjuvant chemotherapy in the treatment of cervical cancer Stages Ib and II with bulky tumor. Gynecol Oncol 33: 225

63. Kinney W K, Egorshin E V, Podratz K C 1988 Wertheim hysterectomy in the geriatric population. Gynecol Oncol 31: 227

64. Kishi Y, Hashimoto Y, Sakamoto Y, Inui S 1987 Thickness of uninvolved fibromuscular stroma and extrauterine spread of carcinoma of the uterine cervix. Cancer 60: 2331

65. Kjorstad K E, Martimbeau P W, Iversen T 1983 Stage Ib carcinoma of the cervix, the Norwegian Radium Hospital: results and complications. Gynecol Oncol 15: 42

66. Knapp R C, Donahue V C, Friedman E A 1973 Dissection of paravesical and pararectal spaces in pelvic operations. Surg Gynecol Obstet 137: 758

67. Kolstad P 1989 Follow-up study of 232 patients with Stage Ia1

and 411 patients with Stage Ia2 squamous cell carcinoma of the cervix (microinvasive carcinoma). Gynecol Oncol 33: 265

68. Krebs H B, Helmkamp B F, Sevin B-U, Poliakoff S R, Nadj M, Averette H E 1982 Recurrent cancer of the cervix following radical hysterectomy and pelvic node dissection. Obstet Gynecol 59: 422

69. Kundrat R 1903 Uber die Ausbreitung des Karzinoms in parametranen Gewebe beim krebs des collum uteri. Arch Gynaekol 69: 355

70. Langley I I, Moore D W, Tarnasky J W, Roberts P H R 1980 Radical hysterectomy and pelvic lymph node dissection. Gynecol Oncol 9: 37

71. Larson D M, Copeland L J, Malone J M Jr, Stringer C A, Gershenson D M, Edwards C L 1988 Diagnosis of recurrent cervical carcinoma after radical hysterectomy. Obstet Gynecol 71: 6

72. Larson D M, Stringer C A, Copeland L J, Gershenson D M, Malone J M Jr, Rutledge F N 1987 Stage Ib cervical carcinoma treated with radical hysterectomy and pelvic lymphadenectomy: role of adjuvant radiotherapy. Obstet Gynecol 69: 378

73. Latzko W, Schiffmann J 1919 Klinisches und anatomisches zur radikaloperation des gebarmutterkrebses. Zentralb Gynaekol 43: 715

74. Leitch A 1910 On the pathological bases of operations for cancer of the uterus. Trans Roy Soc Med 4: 69

75. Lovecchio J L, Averette H E, Donato D, Bell J 1989 5-year survival of patients with periaortic nodal metastases in clinical stage Ib and IIa cervical carcinoma. Gynecol Oncol 34: 43

76. Low J A, Mauger G M, Carmichael J A 1981 The effect of Wertheim hysterectomy upon bladder and urethral function. Am J Obstet Gynecol 139: 826

77. Maiman M A, Fruchter R G, DiMaio T M, Boyce J G 1988 Superficially invasive squamous cell carcinoma of the cervix. Obstet Gynecol 72: 399

78. Mann W J 1988 Controversies in the management of cervical adenocarcinoma (Letter to the Editor). Obstet Gynecol 72: 289

79. Mann W J, Chumas J, Amalfitano T, Westermann C, Patsner B 1987 Ovarian metastases from Stage Ib adenocarcinoma of the cervix. Cancer 60: 1123

80. Mann W J, Vogel F, Patsner B, Chalas E 1989 Management of lymphocysts after radical gynecologic surgery. Gynecol Oncol 33: 248

81. Matsukuma K, Tsukamoto N, Matsuyama T, Ono M, Nakano H 1989 Preoperative CT study of lymph nodes in cervical cancer – its correlation with histological findings. Gynecol Oncol 33: 168

82. Matsuyama T, Inoue I, Tsukamoto N et al 1984 Stage Ib, IIa, and IIb cervical cancer, postsurgical staging and prognosis. Cancer 54: 3072

83. Mattingly R F, Thompson J D 1985 TeLinde's Operative Gynecology, 6th edn. Lippincott, Philadelphia

84. McCall M L, Keaty E C, Thompson J D 1958 Conservation of ovarian tissue in the treatment of carcinoma of the cervix with radical surgery. Am J Obstet Gynecol 75: 590

85. Meigs J V 1944 Carcinoma of the cervix: the Wertheim operation. Surg Gynecol Obstet 78: 195

86. Meigs J V 1945 The Wertheim operation for carcinoma of the cervix. Am J Obstet Gynecol 49: 542

87. Mitra S 1951 Radikale vaginale hysterektomie und extraperitoneale lymphadenektomie bei zervixkrebs. Zentralb Gynaekol 73: 574

88. Moore D H, Fowler W C Jr, Walton L A, Droegemueller W 1989 Morbidity of lymph node sampling in cancers of the uterine corpus and cervix. Obstet Gynecol 74: 180

89. Morley G W, Seski J C 1976 Radical pelvic surgery vs. radiation therapy for Stage I carcinoma of the cervix (exclusive of microcarcinoma). Am J Obstet Gynecol 126: 785

90. Morrow C P 1980 Panel report: Is pelvic radiation beneficial in the postoperative management of Stage Ib squamous cell carcinoma of the cervix with pelvic node metastases treated by radical hysterectomy and pelvic lymphadenectomy? Gynecol Oncol 10: 105

91. Morton D G, Kerner J A 1949 Reactions to X-ray and radium therapy in the treatment of cancer of the uterine cervix. Am J Obstet Gynecol 57: 625

92. Mundy A R 1982 An anatomical explanation of bladder dysfunction following rectal and uterine surgery. Br J Urol 54: 501

93. Nahhas W A, Abt A B, Mortel R 1977 Stage Ib glassy cell carcinoma of the cervix with ovarian metastases. Gynecol Oncol 5: 87

94. Natsume M 1973 Systematic Radical Surgery for Carcinoma of Uterine Cervix. NanKodo, Tokyo

95. Navratil E 1965 Indications and results of the vaginal and abdominal radical operation in the treatment of carcinoma of the cervix. J Int Coll Surg 43: 82

96. Novak F 1978 Gynakologische Operationstechnik. Springer-Verlag, Berlin

97. Okabayashi H 1921 Radical abdominal hysterectomy for cancer of the cervix uteri. Surg Gynecol Obstet 33: 335

98. Orr J W, Shingleton H M, Hatch K D, Mann W J, Austin J M, Soong S-J 1982 Correlation of perioperative morbidity and conization to radical hysterectomy interval. Obstet Gynecol 59: 726

99. Parsons L, Cesare F, Friedell G H 1959 Primary surgical treatment of invasive cancer of the cervix. Surg Gynecol Obstet 109: 279

100. Piver M S, Rutledge F, Smith J P 1974 Five classes of extended hysterectomy for women with cervical cancer. Obstet Gynecol 44: 265

101. Plentl A A, Friedman E A 1974 Lymphatic system of the female genitalia. Saunders, Philadelphia

102. Podczaski E S, Palombo C, Manetta A, Andrews C, Larson J, Degeest K, Mortel R 1989 Assessment of pretreatment laparotomy in patients with cervical carcinoma prior to radiotherapy. Gynecol Oncol 33: 71

103. Powell J L, Mogelnicki S R, Franklin III E W, Chambers D A, Burrell M O 1983 A deliberate hypotensive technique for decreasing blood loss during radical hysterectomy and pelvic lymphadenectomy. Am J Obstet Gynecol 147: 196

104. Rampone J F, Klem F V, Kolstad P 1973 Combined treatment of Stage Ib carcinoma of the cervix. Obstet Gynecol 41: 163

105. Reiffenstuhl G 1982 The clinical significance of the connective tissue planes and spaces. Clin Obstet Gynecol 25: 811

106. Reiffenstuhl G 1964 The Lymphatics of the Female Genital Organs. Lippincott, Philadelphia

107. Reis E 1895 Modern treatment of carcinoma of the uterus. Chicago Med Res 9: 284

108. Roberts W S, Cavanagh D, Marsden D E, Roberts V C 1985 Urinary tract fistulas following ligation of the internal iliac artery during radical hysterectomy. Gynecol Oncol 21: 359

109. Rosenshein N B, Ruth J C, Villar J, Grumbine F B, Dillon M B, Spence M R 1983 A prospective randomized study of doxycycline as a prophylactic antibiotic in patients undergoing radical hysterectomy. Gynecol Oncol 15: 201

110. Rubin S C, Brookland R, Mikuta J J, Mangan C, Sutton G, Danoff B 1984 Para-aortic nodal metastases in early cervical carcinoma: Long-term survival following extended field radiotherapy. Gynecol Oncol 18: 213

111. Russell A H, Tong D Y, Figge D C, Tamimi H K, Greer B E, Elder S J 1984 Adjuvant postoperative pelvic radiation for carcinoma of the uterine cervix: pattern of cancer recurrence in patients undergoing elective radiation following radical hysterectomy and pelvic lymphadenectomy. Int J Radiat Oncol Biol Phys 10: 211

112. Rutledge F N, Fletcher G H, MacDonald R J 1965 Pelvic lymphadenectomy as an adjunct to radiation therapy in treatment for cancer of the cervix. Am J Roentgenol Radium Ther Nucl Med 93: 607

113. Sall S, Rini S, Pineda A 1974 Surgical management of invasive carcinoma of the cervix in pregnancy. Am J Obstet Gynecol 118: 1

114. Sampson J A 1906 A careful study of the parametrium in twenty-seven cases of carcinoma cervicis uteri and its clinical significance. Am J Obstet Gynecol 54: 433

115. Sardi J, Sananes C, Giaroli A et al 1989 Is subradical surgical

treatment for carcinoma of the cervix uteri Stage Ib logical? Gynecol Oncol 32: 360

116. Sasaki H, Yoshida T, Noda K, Yachiku S, Minami K, Kaneko S 1982 Urethral pressure profiles following radical hysterectomy. Obstet Gynecol 59: 101

117. Sauter J N 1822 Die ganzliche Exstirpation der carcinomatosen Gebarmutter obne Vorfall Konstanz

118. Scotti R J, Bergman A, Bhatia N N, Ostergard D R 1986 Urodynamic changes in urethrovesical function after radical hysterectomy. Obstet Gynecol 68: 111

119. Seibel M M, Freeman M G, Graves W L 1980 Carcinoma of the cervix and sexual function. Obstet Gynecol 55: 484

120. Seibel M M, Freeman M G, Graves W L 1982 The effect of surgical and radiation treatment for cervical carcinoma on sexual function. South Med J 75: 1195

121. Sevin B-U, Ramos R, Lichtinger M, Girtanner R E, Averette H E 1984 Antibiotic prevention of infections complicating radical abdominal hysterectomy. Obstet Gynecol 64: 539

122. Silverberg E, Lubera J A 1989 Cancer statistics 1989 Ca-A Cancer Journal for Clinicians 39 Jan–Feb: 3

123. Speert H 1956 Obstetrical-gynecological eponyms: Ernst Wertheim and his operation for uterine cancer. Cancer 9: 859

124. Stallworthy J 1964 Radical surgery following radiation treatment for cervical carcinoma. Ann Roy Coll Surg Engl 34: 161

125. Stallworthy J 1976 Pelvic cancer priorities. Am J Obstet Gynecol 126: 777

126. Symmonds R E 1966 Morbidity and complications of radical hysterectomy with pelvic lymph node dissection. Am J Obstet Gynecol 94: 663

127. Symmonds R E 1975 Some surgical aspects of gynecological cancer. Cancer 36: 646

128. Symmonds R E, Pratt J H 1961 Prevention of fistulas and lymphocysts in radical hysterectomy: preliminary report of a new technique. Obstet Gynecol 17: 57

129. Tabata M, Ichinoe K, Sakuragi N, Shiina Y, Yamaguchi T, Mabuchi Y 1987 Incidence of ovarian metastases in patients with cancer of the uterine cervix. Gynecol Oncol 28: 255

130. Talbert L M, Palumbo L, Shingleton H, Bream C A, McGee J A 1965 Urologic complications of radical hysterectomy for carcinoma of the cervix. South Med J 58: 11

131. Thompson J D, Caputo T A, Franklin E W III, Dale E 1975 The surgical management of invasive cancer of the cervix in pregnancy. Am J Obstet Gynecol 121: 853

132. To A C W, Gore H, Shingleton H M, Wilkerson J A, Soong S J, Hatch K D 1986 Lymph node metastasis in cancer of the cervix: a preliminary report. Am J Obstet Gynecol 155: 388

133. Tulzer H, Kupka S 1978 The effectiveness of obligatory lymphadenectomy in treating carcinoma of the cervix. Int J Gynaecol Obstet 16: 197

134. Uyttenbroeck F 1987 Verleden en heden van de radicale chirurgie in de gynecologische oncologie. Verhandelingen-Koninklijke Academie voor Geneeskunde van Belgie 49(1): 5

135. van Nagell J R Jr, Greenwell N, Powell D F, Donaldson E S, Hanson M B, Gay E C 1983 Microinvasive carcinoma of the cervix. Am J Obstet Gynecol 145: 981

136. Vercamer R, Janssens J, Usewils R et al 1987 Computed tomography and lymphography in the presurgical staging of early carcinoma of the uterine cervix. Cancer 60: 1745

137. Webb G A 1975 The role of ovarian conservation in the treatment of carcinoma of the cervix with radical surgery. Am J Obstet Gynecol 122: 476

138. Webb M J, Symmonds R E 1979 Wertheim hysterectomy: a reappraisal. Obstet Gynecol 54: 140

139. Weiser E B, Bundy B N, Hoskins W J et al 1989 Extraperitoneal versus transperitoneal selective para-aortic lymphadenectomy in the pretreatment surgical staging of advanced cervical carcinoma. (A Gynecologic Oncology Group Study). Gynecol Oncol 33 :283

140. Wertheim E 1900 Zur Frag der Radikaloperation beim Uteruskrebs. Arch Gynaekol 61: 627

141. Wertheim E 1905 Discussion on the diagnosis and treatment of carcinoma of the uterus. Br Med J 2: 689

142. Wertheim E 1911 Die erweiterte abdominale Operation bei Carcinoma Colli Uteri (Auf Grund Von 500 Fallen). Urban, Berlin

143. Wertheim E 1912 The extended abdominal operation for carcinoma of the cervix. Am J Obstet Gynecol 66: 169

144. Wilkinson E J, Hause L 1974 Probability in lymph node sectioning. Cancer 33: 1269

145. Williams H T 1971 Prevention of postoperative deep-vein thrombosis with perioperative subcutaneous heparin. Lancet ii: 950

146. Wong C-H, Tso H-S, Ho E S, Mok M S 1985 Induced hypotension during radical hysterectomy and bilateral pelvic lymphadenectomy. Anesth Sinica 23: 181

147. Zander J, Baltzer J, Lohe K J, Ober K G, Kaufmann C 1981 Carcinoma of the cervix: an attempt to individualize treatment. Results of a 20 year cooperative study. Am J Obstet Gynecol 139: 752

148. Zweifel P 1922 Zum Anclenken an die erste Totalexstirpation des Karzinomatosen uterus. (Ausgefuhrt von Dr. Joh Neb Sauter in Konstanz) Munch Med Wochem 69: 19

79. Radical hysterectomy with pelvic lymphadenectomy — the Tokyo method

S. Sakamoto

INTRODUCTION

There is no doubt that the elaboration by Shuichi Okabayashi of methods of greater radicality than the conventional Wertheim operation marked a milestone in the history of radical hysterectomy. After Okabayashi introduced his method, a number of surgeons introduced numerous improvements so that today there exists no unified method that can be distinctively labeled the Japanese method. Roughly classified, two groups of methods are used in Japan: one embraces techniques of the original Okabayashi approach; the other, called the Tokyo University method was improved and revised by Ogino,[2] Kobayashi[3] and Sakamoto.[4]

In the Okabayashi method, the surgeon first ligates and cuts the uterine arteries, isolates the ureters, then severs the sacrouterine ligaments, exposes widely the area posterior to the uterus and severs the cardinal ligaments. The lymphadenectomy is conducted after the hysterectomy.

In this chapter, I introduce the method I am at present using which includes the following steps:

1. First, the surgeon widens the paravesical and pararectal spaces on either side of the cardinal ligament (retinaculum uteri) and broadens visibility in order both to make clear the pelvic anatomy and facilitate dissection and hemostasis.
2. Pelvic lymphadenectomy is then performed in retrograde order to prevent centripetal cellular spread.
3. The pelvic autonomic nerve bundle under the cardinal ligament is preserved (except in advanced cases).
4. A wall is formed to protect the ureter using the walls of the rectum and bladder lateral to the ureter. The aim of this maneuver is to prevent adhesion of the ureter to the pelvic wall.
5. Exudate is removed from the parametrial deadspace with a vaginal drain.

This method makes radical hysterectomy easier especially for the untrained, lessens bleeding during the operation and considerably reduces postoperative complications related to the urinary tract.

Patients should not be older than 70 years of age and the lesion should be, by FIGO classification, Stage I or Stage II. In case of adenocarcinoma, the radical operation can be performed even in Stage III.

THE OPERATION

Positioning of the team (Fig. 79.1)

The surgeon, if right-handed, begins the operation standing on the right side of the patient (A) and maintains this position until the left cardinal ligament is severed. He then shifts to the left side of the patient (B) and continues the operation until its completion.

Special instruments

The following instruments have been specially designed for the operation (Fig. 79.2). (1) Self-retaining retractor with a third rubber blade, (2) rectum retractor, (3) bladder retractor (4) right angled retractor, (5) ureter hook, (6) horizontally curved forceps, (7) membrane forceps.

Incision of abdominal wall

The abdomen is opened through a midline incision extending from the mons veneris to above the umbilicus. The specially designed self-retaining retractor is particularly useful in major gynecological operations such as radical hysterectomy as it serves the additional purpose of holding back the intestines with the aid of rubber plates.

Incision of pelvic peritoneum (Fig. 79.3)

Kocher's forceps with long, straight jaws are applied to the round ligament and the fallopian tube, on each side, close to the uterus in order to hold it and to prevent the spreading of cancer cells. Triple ligatures are applied on the left

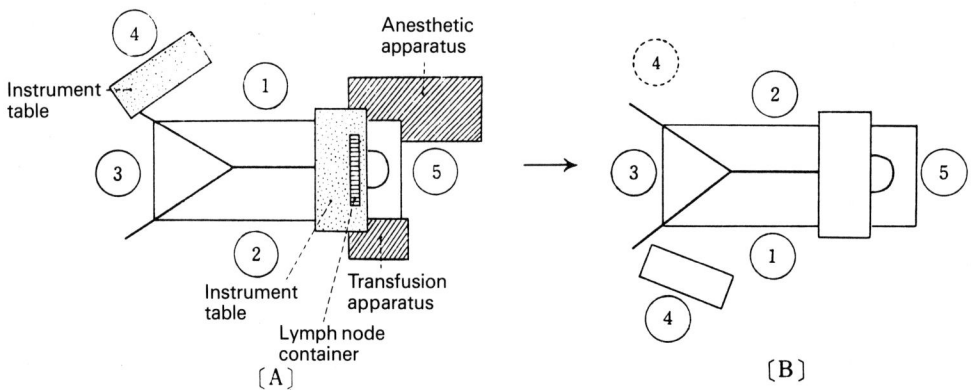

Fig. 79.1   Positioning of operation team
1. Operator
2. 1st assistant
3. 2nd assistant
4. Nurse
5. Anesthesiologist.

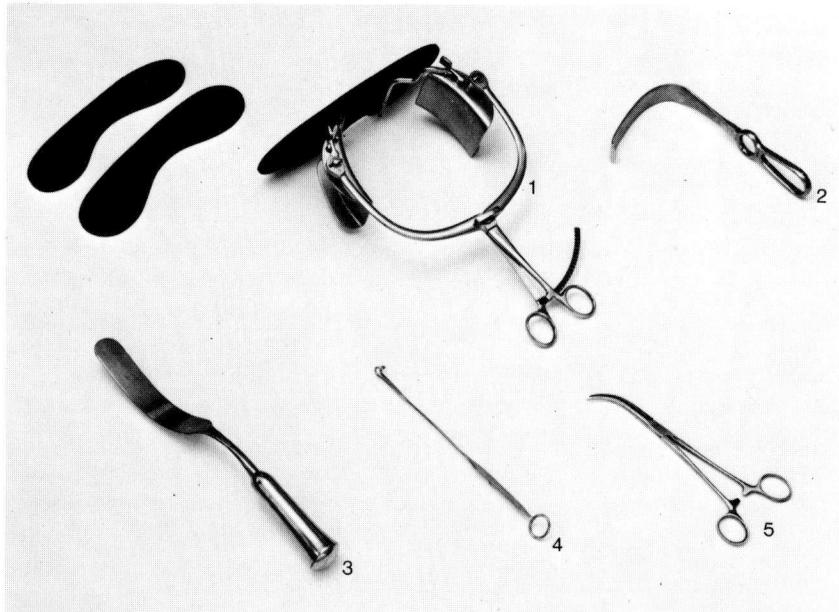

Fig. 79.2   Operation instruments designed for our method
1. Self-retaining retractor
2. Right angled retractor
3. Rectum retractor
4. Ureter hook
5. Horizontally curved forceps.

round and infundibulopelvic ligaments which are then severed between the medial and two lateral ligatures. Each end of the medial member of the lateral ligature pair is left long enough to serve afterward for retraction. It is advisable to cut the round ligament before the infundibulopelvic ligament as it enables a better direct view of the ureter and its direction. After the round ligament is divided, the peritoneum of the medial aspect of the iliac fossa is cut in the direction of the psoas muscle. The

peritoneum of the vesicouterine pouch is incised at the same time. A similar operation is carried out on the left side.

After the peritoneum of the vesicouterine pouch is incised on both sides the anterior peritoneal flap is sutured to the abdominal wall with one stitch. The bladder is then separated from the cervix as a preliminary in order to exclude bladder involvement with tumor and so ensure operability. The adnexae on both sides are then sutured

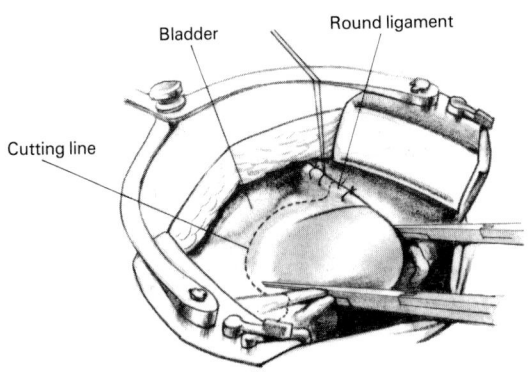

Fig. 79.3 Incision of pelvic peritoneum.

together to prevent hindrance to vision. The next stages of the operation are performed first on the left side.

Preliminary opening of paravesical and pararectal spaces

The stump of the infundibulopelvic ligament is pulled up by the bladder retractor for a wider view of the operative field, and the paravesical space and the pararectal space are opened by the fingers so that the anatomical relationship between organs in the pelvic cavity can be better determined. Figure 79.4 shows the inlet of the pararectal space and the paravesical space.

The pararectal space can be opened easily by separating the ureter from the pelvic vessels in a medial direction. The space is cleared until the posterior side of the cardinal ligament is seen. A gauze swab is inserted to soak up blood and is left at this site until a late stage of the lymphadenectomy.

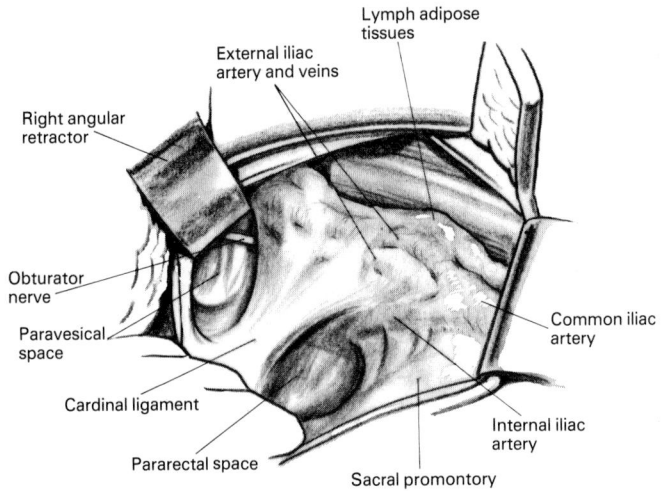

Fig. 79.4 Preliminary opening of paravesical and pararectal spaces.

Lymphadenectomy

Separation of left external iliac vessels from psoas muscle (Fig. 79.5)

Prior to lymphadenectomy, it is advisable to prepare the field with the operator's fingers to disclose the anatomical relationships of pelvic blood vessels in the following order. First the external iliac vessels are isolated from the psoas muscle with a swab and fingers and then the pelvic wall is exposed to sufficient depth as to reveal the obturator nerve. Continuing this procedure the entire lengths of both the external iliac artery and vein are laid bare and all the branches of the hypogastric veins are exposed. Hemorrhage during lymphadenectomy can now be readily controlled. A gauze swab is placed lateral to the obturator node group to push it medially. It is also useful to absorb blood during lymphadenectomy.

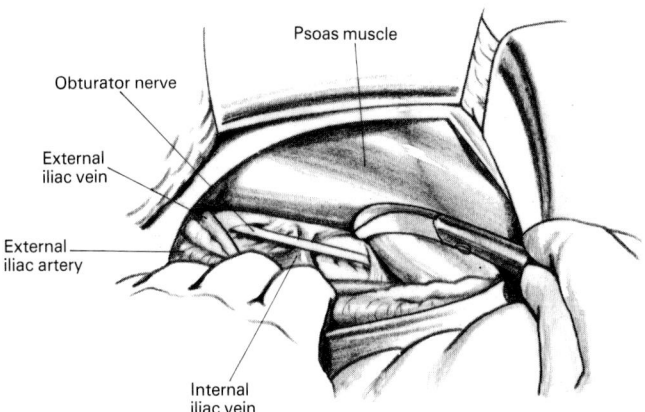

Fig. 79.5 Separation of external iliac vessels from psoas muscle.

Retrograde dissection of lymph nodes on left side

Next, the lymph nodes are dissected distally along the pelvic wall in the order shown (Fig. 79.6). A recommended technique for removal of nodes is to dissect the perivascular sheet from the vessels, lifting the nodes with the sheet by membrane forceps and pressing down the vessels at the same time by means of a swab or scissors. As observed by lymphography, the pelvic lymph vessels converge to a main trunk at the common iliac vessels. To prevent centripetal spreading of cancer cells, the main trunk should be ligated first.

The order of dissection is aortic nodes followed by common iliac nodes followed by external iliac nodes. The lymph nodes and adipose tissues are isolated together with the perivascular sheet. The upper end of the common iliac nodes is picked up with membrane forceps and the main lymph trunk is then clamped. Thereafter, it is not necessary to dissect the lymph nodes en bloc. The common iliac lymph nodes should be removed carefully on their deep aspect, protecting the venous wall with the fingertips.

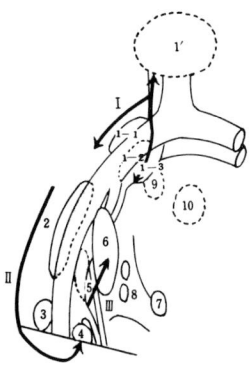

Fig. 79.6 Order of lymphadenectomy and names of pelvic lymph nodes 1–1.2.3. Common iliac nodes
1. Abdominal aortic nodes
2. External iliac nodes
3. Lateral suprainguinal nodes
4. Medial suprainguinal nodes
5. Obturator nodes
6. Internal iliac nodes
7. Uterine artery nodes
8. Cardinal ligament nodes
9. Lateral sacral nodes
10. Medial sacral nodes.

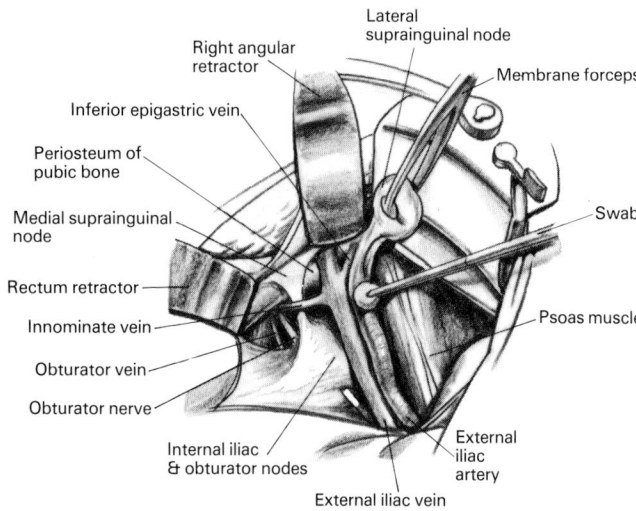

Fig. 79.7 Lymph node dissection with the swab (right suprainguinal lymph node).

Now the order becomes lateral suprainguinal nodes followed by medial suprainguinal nodes (Fig. 79.7). After dissecting the external iliac nodes, the retractor is raised to permit removal of the suprainguinal nodes. There are many nutrient vessels here which can be easily damaged, but hemorrhage can be readily arrested by simple compression. First the lateral part of these nodes is removed, then the medial part. Care should be taken not to damage the inferior epigastric vein at this time. The medial suprainguinal nodes are removed to a point where the periosteum is exposed. The appearance of the periosteum of the pubic bone in the field means that the nodes have been completely

removed. Extreme care should be taken not to damage the innominate vein (pubic vein) communication. To prevent hemorrhage the lymph nodes are lifted and dissected while the surrounding vessels are pushed with the swab.

Next the obturator nodes are dissected followed by the internal iliac nodes. Take out the gauze previously inserted in the paravesical space, pararectal space and lateral to the obturator nodes. Since the lateral part of the node mass has already been completely isolated from the pelvic wall the nodes can be removed from the surface of the cardinal ligament with a swab, pulling the mass medially. The nodes can be removed easily only in this way. When removing the obturator nodes the obliterated umbilical artery is exposed. This facilitates the following part of the operation. If the sacral nodes are enlarged they are also cleared.

The lymph nodes are identified for the pathologist according to their respective location.

Ligation and cutting of left uterine artery (Fig. 79.8)

The obliterated umbilical artery is lifted up and hooked with a right angled retractor, and the uterine artery is isolated. Double ligatures are then applied and the artery is severed between ligatures. About 5 cm of thread are left on the side of the uterus as a marker, and the remainder is cut off. If uterine veins are found running along with the uterine artery, they should be carefully separated from the uterine artery and managed independently.

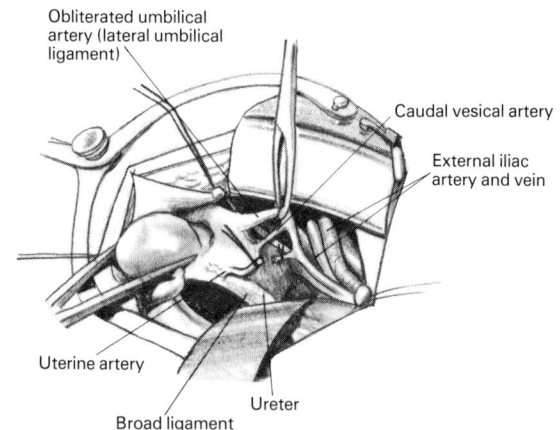

Fig. 79.8 Ligation and section of the uterine artery.

Isolation of left ureter (Fig. 79.9)

The posterior leaf of the broad ligament is grasped and stretched with two pairs of membrane forceps. The ureter is isolated from the peritoneum pulling it laterally with a ureter hook and leaving as much of the mesoureter intact as possible. The isolation should progress in a downward direction until the ureter enters the tunnel which is formed

sacrouterine ligament. A sheet of sympathetic nerve fibers is first separated from the lateral surface of the sacrouterine ligament with scissors and can be severed without risk of bleeding. Then the rectovaginal ligament will appear like a membrane below the sacrouterine ligament. Sheets of tissue containing sympathetic nerve fibers are easily recognized as they run along the rectum.

3. *Preservation of vesical branches of parasympathetic nerves* (Fig. 79.13). The branches of the pelvic nerves supplying the uterus are divided, extreme care being taken not to sever the vesical branches. By pushing up the caudal end of the sympathetic nerve plate the pelvic nerve plexus is usually preserved automatically and no special manipulation is needed.

Severing and suturing the rectovaginal ligament (Fig. 79.14)

Two curved Pean's forceps are applied to the rectovaginal ligament which is then cut between the forceps and ligated. Sometimes repetition of the procedure is necessary to get as deep a separation as possible. The forceps near the uterus will prevent hemorrhage from the anastomosis of blood vessels between the paracolpium and the cardinal ligament. If there is no hemorrhage on removal of this forceps, ligature will not be necessary.

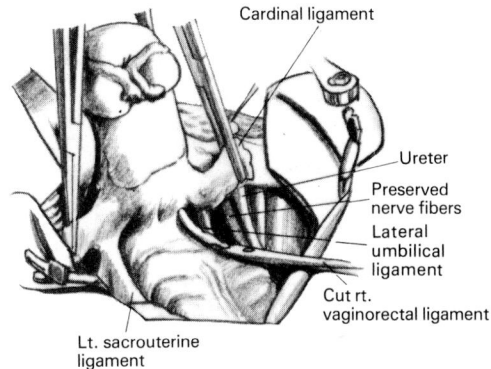

Fig. 79.14 Dissection of sacrouterine ligament.

Dissection of contralateral sacrouterine ligament

The same procedure is made on the other side.

Dissection of vesicouterine ligament (right side)

Extensive separation of bladder from cervix and vagina (Fig. 79.15)

The bladder must be separated adequately from the anterior wall of the vagina to the same extent that the rectum is separated from its posterior wall. The separation is started first at the medial portion and then at the lateral portion. The latter separation is set forward with the

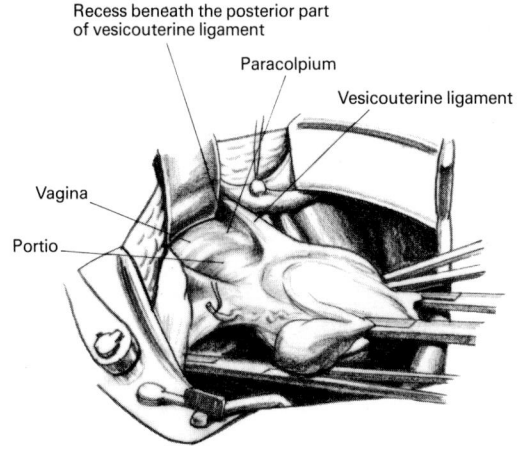

Fig. 79.15 Extensive separation of bladder from vagina.

anterior layer of the vesicouterine ligament pressing laterally enough to reach the surface of the paracolpium. It is important to ascertain the proper layer for separation so that the vesicouterine ligament can be separated from the paracolpium without hemorrhage.

Preparation of anterior layer of vesicouterine ligament

In manipulating the vesicouterine ligament the utmost care based on the anatomy of the part is necessary to prevent ureteral fistula formation. First, the ureter is separated from the uterine artery and its entry into the ligament is confirmed (Fig. 79.16). The uterine artery is lifted up with the thread previously left as a marker and drawn medially and the ureter is displaced to the lateral side with the cardinal ligament. In this way, anatomical relationships are clarified. Next, the capsule (or perisheath) of the ureter is separated from the uterine artery revealing, between both layers of the vesicouterine ligament, the tunnel into which the ureter enters.

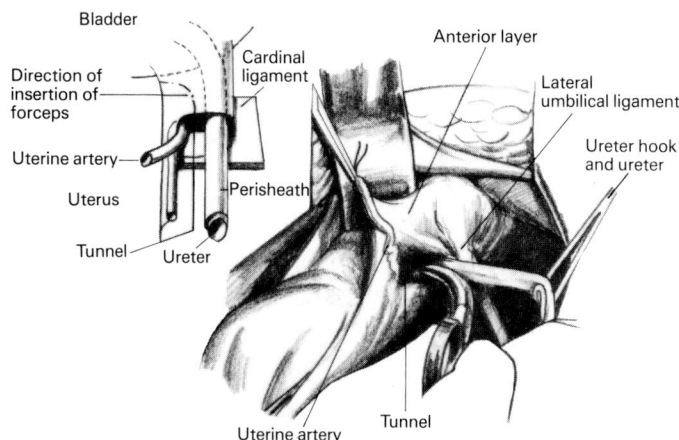

Fig. 79.16 Separation of anterior layer of vesicouterine ligament with curved forceps and its direction of insertion.

Separation, cutting and suturing of anterior layer (Fig. 79.17)

Curved Pean's forceps are inserted into the tunnel. In passing Pean's forceps through the tunnel, their tip must be directed medially or they may injure the juxtavesical portion of the ureter or the paracolpium. The anterior layer is lifted by opening the tips of the inserted forceps. Two horizontally curved forceps are then applied. The part between the forceps is cut and ligated with absorbable materials. To prevent the kinking of the ureter, it is highly advisable to carry out this procedure in two or three steps. Almost the entire length of the ureter between the ligaments can now be seen. Cutting the entire anterior part clearly shows the ureter connected to the posterior part.

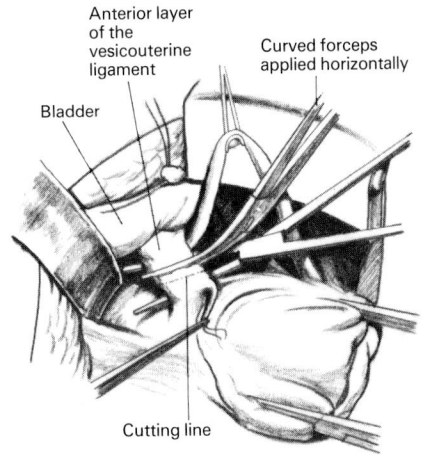

Fig. 79.17   Dissection of anterior layer of the vesicouterine ligament.

Preparation of posterior layer of vesicouterine ligament (Fig. 79.18)

The ureter is partially isolated from the surface of the posterior part by cutting the connective tissue (Fig. 79.18). It is then pushed laterally, widely exposing the posterior layer.

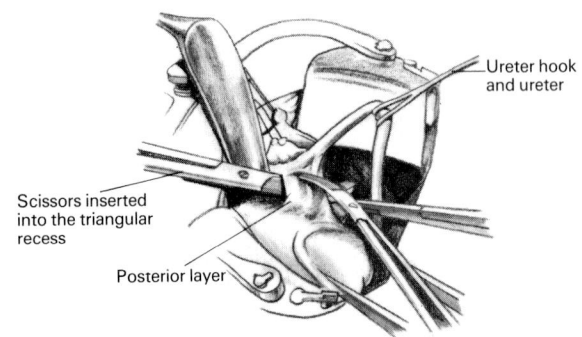

Fig. 79.18   Separating and pushing the ureter on the surface of posterior layer of the vesicouterine ligament.

Isolation and severing of posterior layer (Fig. 79.19)

With the bladder pressed downward and the ureter retracted laterally, a triangular-shaped recess surrounded by the bladder, the paracolpium and the caudal margin of the posterior layer is seen. Curved Pean's forceps are next inserted into the recess, the least resistant part by palpation with two fingertips, below the posterior part of the ligament. The forceps are turned and the posterior layer of the ligament is lifted in front of the cardinal ligament. After opening the blades of the inserted forceps, two horizontally curved forceps are applied onto the ligament at the part between the opened blades. The part between the forceps is cut and ligated. At this time, the ureter should be carefully separated laterally again so that the forceps can be applied about 5 mm from the ureter to avoid damage. Next, both parts of the vesicouterine ligament are severed and the ureter is completely separated from the vagina and the uterus.

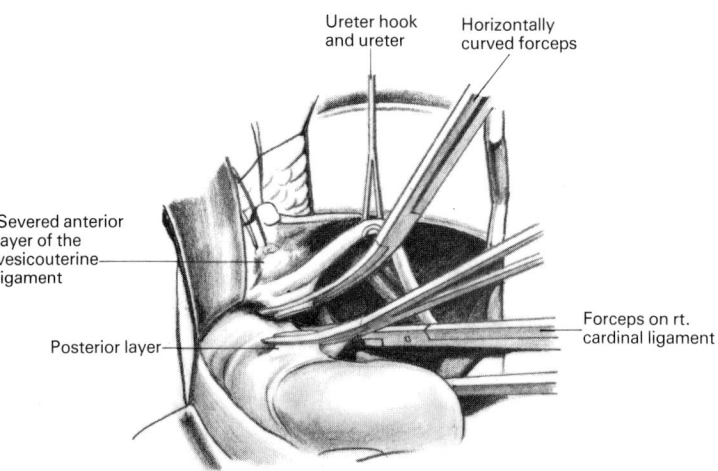

Fig. 79.19   Clamping and cutting posterior layer of the right vesicouterine ligament.

Double suturing and cutting of paracolpium (right side) (Fig. 79.20)

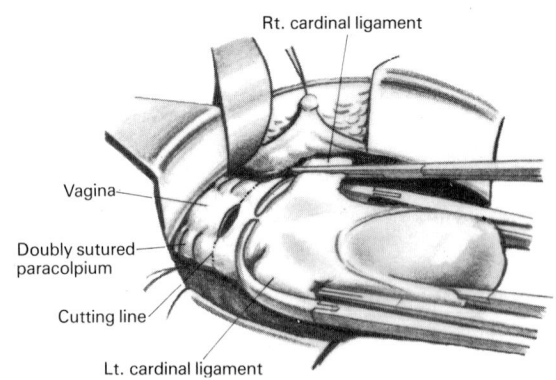

Fig. 79.20   Double suturing of paracolpium on both sides and opening the vagina.

The upper part of the vagina and the paracolpium are clamped with strongly curved forceps to prevent the loss of uterine secretions. The bladder is further separated from the vaginal wall and paracolpium to a required level. The paracolpium should be ligated and cut as deeply as possible at the level required to obtain a generous cuff of vagina to protect against vault recurrence. Utmost care should be taken not to cut any remaining autonomic nerve fibers. Double ligatures are applied to the paracolpium and the part between the ligature and the forceps is severed.

Repeat procedures on the left side

The left vesicouterine ligament is now dissected and sutures are inserted into the left paracolpium.

Cutting of vagina and suturing of vaginal stump (Fig. 79.21)

Gauze is spread on the surface of the rectum. The anterior wall of the vagina is cut and the vaginal canal sterilized. The cut end of the vagina is now clamped with Kocher's forceps, and the posterior wall of the vagina is incised. Thus the uterus is completely extirpated.

To prevent a tear between the upper end of the paracolpium and the vaginal wall, Z-sutures are applied at the corner of the vaginal stump with chromicized catgut. This is followed by partial closure of the vaginal canal. A favorable hemostatic effect can be obtained by now suturing the cut end of the rectovaginal ligament to the vaginal angle. A thorough check should now be made inside the pelvis for confirmation of hemostasis.

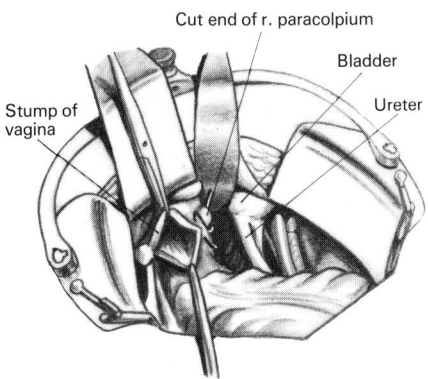

Fig. 79.21 The incised vagina with Z-suture between vaginal stump and cut end of paracolpium.

Drainage

Two polyethylene Salan sump tube drains are inserted into the dead space on each side of the pelvis and brought through the vagina. A Y-shaped tube is convenient for this purpose. Both tubes are fixed with one suture, on the internal surface of each thigh. The secretion in the dead space is drained with an aspirator. The drain is removed after 3 or 4 days.

Construction of protecting wall of juxtavesical portion of the ureter with the rectal wall and the bladder wall (Figs 79.22 and 79.23)

Lateral or backward displacement and kinking of the ureter is one of the serious postoperative problems that occurs and may result in hydroureter and hydronephrosis with eventual impairment of renal function. To guard against this complication the following step is introduced. Two sutures are applied on the outside of each ureter between the external walls of the rectum and bladder to prevent the juxtavesical portion of the ureter both from being immersed in secretion in the pelvic dead space and from adhering to the pelvic wall. These may cause unexpected kinking of the ureter. The polyethylene tube drains should be inserted beneath these protecting walls to avoid difficulty with their removal.

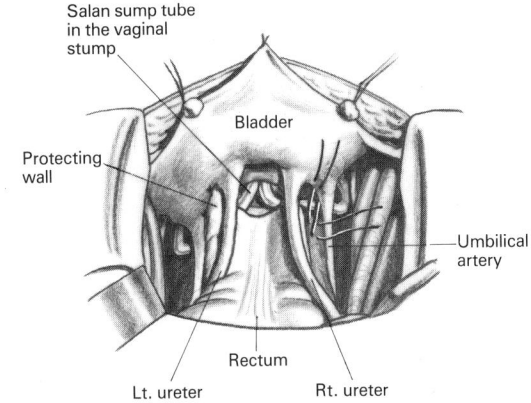

Fig. 79.22 Formation of protecting wall of the juxtavesical part of the ureter.

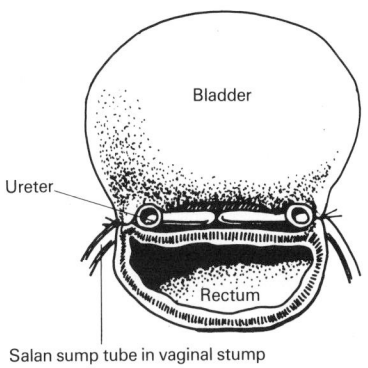

Fig. 79.23 Protecting wall of the ureter and the new location of the ureter.

Closure of pelvic peritoneum and abdominal wall

The pelvic peritoneum is sutured with interrupted sutures and the abdominal wall is closed to complete the operation.

Application of cavitron ultrasonic aspiration system for lymphadenectomy

In advanced cases with adherent and enlarged metastatic lymph nodes, the node dissection may be very difficult, especially for young and less experienced surgeons. Heavy bleeding and incomplete lymphadenectomy are usually encountered when normal techniques are used.

Since 1980, we have introduced a new ultrasonic surgical technique and recommend usage of this procedure in difficult cases. The cavitron ultrasonic aspiration (CUSA) system (Cavitron Corporation, USA) has three functions: tissue fragmentation, aspiration and tissue incision with dissection. The handpiece of CUSA which the surgeon applies to the tissues is shown in Figure 79.24. The tip of the handpiece is composed of a rod of ultrasonicator and two opened canals, one for irrigation by saline solution to produce tissue suspension, and the other for suction of fragmented tissue. An acoustic vibrator in the handpiece gives the rod-tip 23 000 vibrations per second and softens parenchymal tissue, with the exception of blood vessels, into fragments. Maximum power is 100 W and vibration amplitude 300 μm.

The CUSA device in the process of aspirating fatty tissue around lymph nodes on the pelvic sidewall is shown in Figure 79.25. For this purpose, I prefer the power to be less than 50 W and vibration amplitude less than 150 μm to avoid damage to small capillary vessels. CUSA will not damage even the thin blood vessels when applied with 40% of its full energy. The range of power should be changed depending upon the state of the surrounding tissue.

CUSA is highly recommended in the dissection of obturator nodes, internal iliac nodes, sometimes para-aortic nodes, and the lymph nodes at the base of the cardinal ligament that are usually embedded in deep adipose tissue with a plexus of thin-walled blood vessels. The technique is remarkably simple. CUSA is also of special use for dissecting metastatic lymph nodes tightly adherent to the major pelvic vessels, because it can preserve the thin nourishing branch to the node and reduce bleeding. In Figure 79.26 a large metastatic lymph node is being isolated by CUSA step-by-step, without bleeding.

POSTOPERATIVE TREATMENT

1. A Foley catheter inserted before the surgery is left in the bladder for 7 days following the operation. Patients are asked to urinate by their own efforts every 4 hours. After every urination, residual urine volume is measured and recorded until the residual volume decreases to less than 50 ml and remains at this level for 3 days.
2. Urinary infection should be carefully avoided.
3. The drain through the vaginal vault may be removed 3 or 4 days after operation.
4. Other postoperative management is similar to that of total hysterectomy.

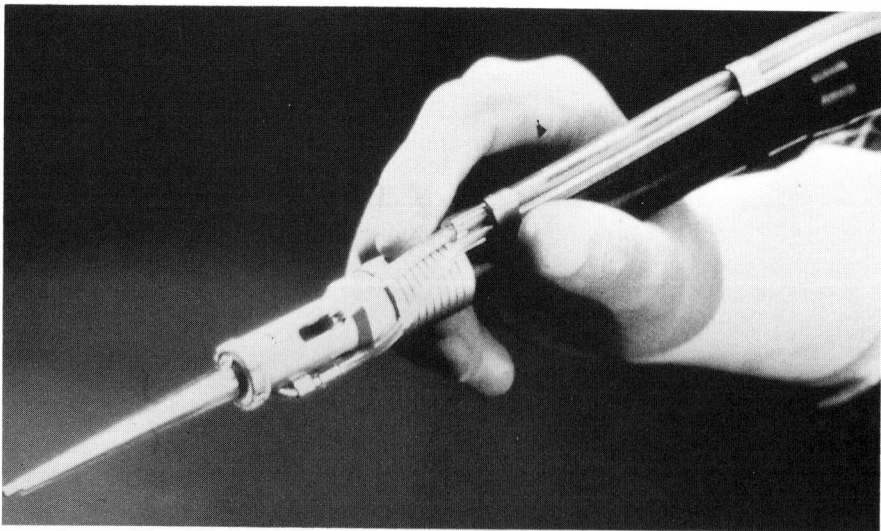

Fig. 79.24 Handpiece of the cavitron ultrasonic surgical aspiration (CUSA) system. The tip contains an ultrasonicator and two open channels, one for irrigation, the other for suction of fragmented tissue. The acoustic vibrator within the handpiece permits 23 000 vibrations of the rod-tip per second.

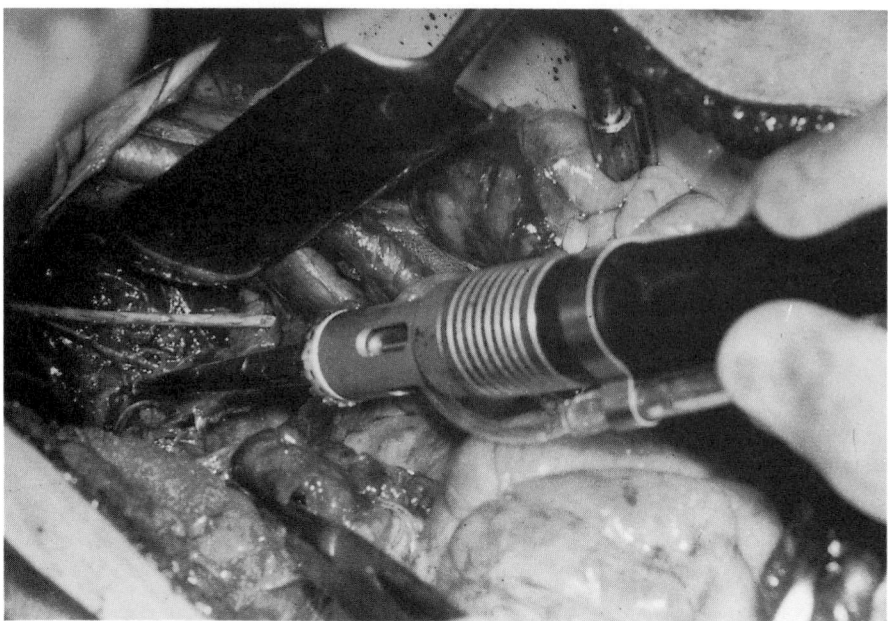

Fig. 79.25 The CUSA handpiece is aspirating fatty tissue from the pelvic sidewall. Immediately superior to the device is the obturator nerve. The dissected external iliac vessels are partly obscured by the speculum blade.

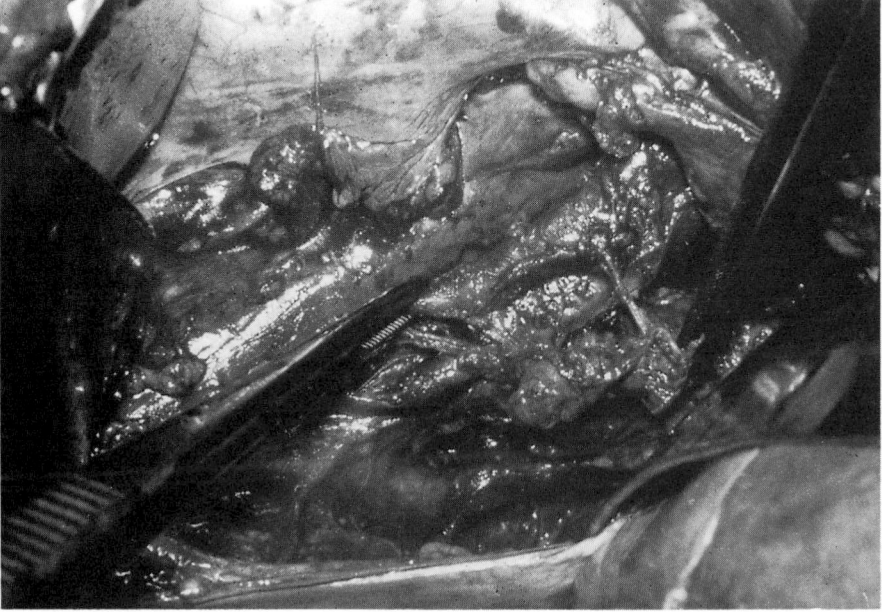

Fig. 79.26 Metastatic lymph nodes (between the two tissue forceps) have been almost dissected free from the external iliac vessels by CUSA, without bleeding.

COMMENT

1. Operation time occupies 2 to 3 hours. The amount of blood loss averages 600 to 700 ml with a minimum of 270 ml. In some cases, blood transfusions are thought to be unnecessary.
2. By preservation of the pelvic nerves, 87.2% of patients had no residual urine 1 month after surgery as compared with 63.8% treated by routine methods.
3. By the construction of a protecting wall about the ureter the incidence of functional stenosis of the ureter due to adhesion is reduced to 13.8% as assessed 1 month after surgery and 5.7% 6 months after surgery. No severe stenosis was found.
4. The frequency of ureteral fistula is reduced from 11.1% to 0.8% by preservation of the capsule (periureteral sheath) of the ureter and careful dissection of the vesicouterine ligament.

REFERENCES

1. Okabayashi S 1921 Radical abdominal hysterectomy for cancer of the cervix uteri. Surg Gynecol Obstet 33: 335
2. Ogino K 1950 Modified Okabayashi method by Ogino. Surgery 4: 4 (Jap)
3. Kobayashi T 1961 Abdominal Radical Hysterectomy with Pelvic Lymphadenectomy for Cancer of the Cervix, 1st edn. Nanzando (Jap), Tokyo
4. Sakamoto S 1970 & 1972 Abdominal radical hysterectomy with pelvic lymphadenectomy for beginners. Obstet Gynecol Ther 20: 81, 259, 369, 497, 611 and 24: 6 (Jap)

80. Hysterectomy for carcinoma of endometrium

A. Singer

INTRODUCTION

Current views on the management of endometrial cancer, including the extent of the operation and the place and timing of adjuvant radiotherapy, are considered elsewhere (see Ch. 49). The most common surgical approach has been the standard total hysterectomy with bilateral salpingo-oophorectomy. Over the past 40 years however, certain authorities have modified the operation to increasing radicality. This chapter will consider whether this modification is justified, and also the alternative techniques of hysterectomy. In the corresponding chapter in the first edition of this book, much prominence was given to the individualization of surgical techniques in management. This was particularly relevant with respect to excision of the vaginal vault to prevent recurrence. In this edition, the relevance of vaginal vault excision will be examined in the light of recent surgical studies.

HYSTERECTOMY TECHNIQUES INCORPORATING VAGINAL VAULT REMOVAL

The vaginal vault was considered to be a prime site for recurrence of endometrial cancer after surgical extirpation.[14] This led to the development of various techniques designed to remove the area of risk, which included the upper part of the vagina.[2] To satisfactorily and safely accomplish such a removal, ureters usually have to be displaced laterally out of their respective tunnels, allowing the safe clamping and removal of the vaginal angle and upper vagina. The basic hysterectomy techniques which are used in treating endometrial cancer and which specifically deal with the vaginal vault, will be considered. Because of the present widespread use of these procedures, a description is given of each, as also is the evidence for and against their use.

Total abdominal hysterectomy with bilateral salpingo-oophorectomy with cuff of vagina

In the simplest of hysterectomy procedures, suited for

Stage 0 (endometrial carcinoma in situ) or Stage I, Grade 1 endometrial cancer, no ureteric dissection is undertaken.

The technique involves securing the upper uterine attachments and opening the broad ligament with definition of the uterine vessels, and then division, ligation and subsequent detachment of these vessels (Fig. 80.1). The uterosacral ligaments are clamped postero-laterally to the uterus, and then divided and ligated. The bladder anteriorly and the rectum posteriorly are stripped off the cervix as deeply as possible (Fig. 80.2). Transverse incisions are made into the vagina not less than 3 cm from the cervix

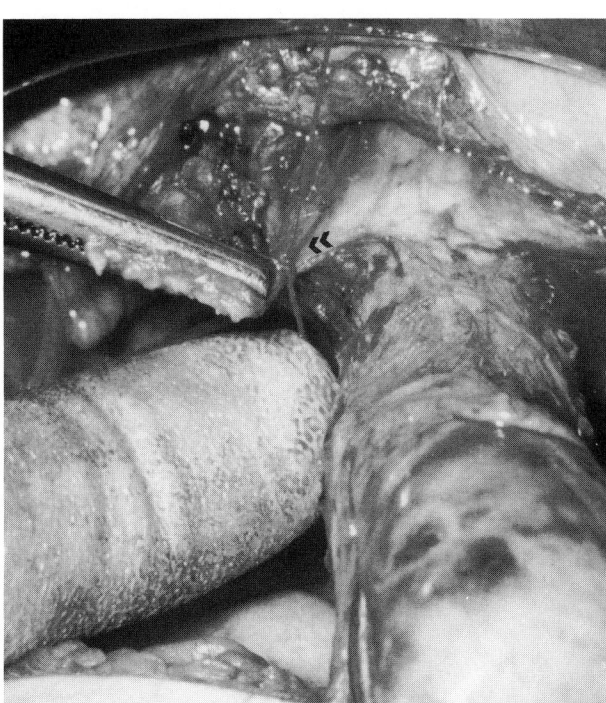

Fig. 80.1 Ligation of uterine vessels. Left uterine vascular pedicle has been transfixed by a needle carrying a No. 1 suture material. The stitch is tied under the point of the forceps, where there is seen to be adequate length of free pedicle (arrowed), with no opportunity for slipping.

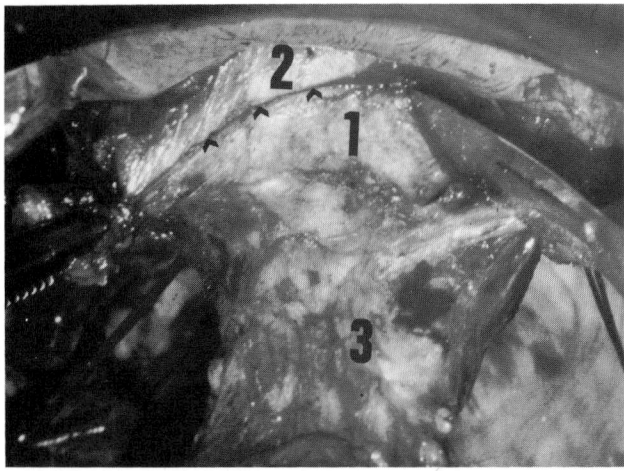

Fig. 80.2 Separation of bladder from uterus. The bladder is completely separated in a downward direction off the cervix, so freeing the vagina in the region of the anterior fornix (1). In the photograph, the scalpel blade is being stroked across the upper part of the vagina, to divide any remaining fibers of the pubocervical fascia from the bladder (2), which is then pushed away from the uterus (3) along the line of the arrows.

(Fig. 80.3). To this point in the procedure there has been no danger to the ureters. The vaginal vault is excised by joining the ends of the anterior and posterior vaginal incisions laterally with the scissors under direct vision (Fig. 80.3). Cutting close in against the cervix with the scissors, the right lateral cardinal ligament is detached from it and

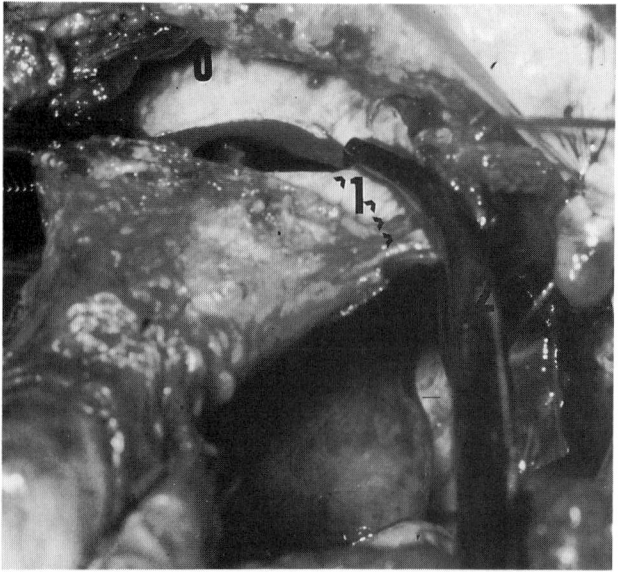

Fig. 80.3 Opening into the vagina and clamping vaginal angles. The scalpel has cut boldly into the anterior vaginal fornix, just clear of the bladder edge and moved the maximum amount of the vaginal skin anteriorly. The cavity of the vagina is obvious (0). The vaginal angles are now clamped; the right angle (1) is being clamped in this photograph, with one limb of the forceps (2) within the vagina and the other external to it. The incision to detach the vaginal skin is indicated by the path of the arrows.

retracts laterally, carrying the right ureter with it to leave only the stretched vaginal skin of the right lateral fornix. It is the vaginal skin that the surgeon wishes to remove, and this can now be incised sufficiently lateral to the cervix to give a wide cuff without endangering the ureter. The same procedure is then carried out on the other side.

Extended (modified radical) hysterectomy with ureteric dissection

In this more complex operation, sometimes employed for Stage I endometrial cancer (G2, G3), the ureters are dissected laterally out of their tunnel, allowing safe clamping of the vaginal angle and excision of a wider area of the vaginal vault and parametrial tissue.

The first step in the procedure involves freeing and elevating the uterus from the pelvis by separation of any adhesions of the sigmoid colon and infundibular pelvic folds, and traction on heavy forceps applied to the medial side of the broad ligament beside the uterus.

By elevation of the uterus upwards and forwards, the ureters are exposed extra-peritoneally as they lie medial to the corresponding ovarian pedicles. The ureter is steadied with dissecting forceps while the peritoneal incision is made just lateral to it, after which scissors are used to free it up (Fig. 80.4). Tapes are used to under-run the ureter for identification. Once exposed, the ureters are not further disturbed at this stage.

After division of the upper uterine attachments, (i.e. the round ligament and ovarian pedicle) the broad ligament is opened anteriorly, after which the vesico-uterine peritoneal fold is incised, allowing the separation of the bladder from the uterus. The posterior peritoneal leaf of the broad ligament has already been opened when exposing the ureter, and now the lower part of this leaf is opened down to the attachment of the uterosacral ligament. The bladder is pushed well off the cervix in front, and the peritoneum is swept laterally to expose the ureteric tunnel on each side; within the roof of the ureteric tunnel the uterine vessels run to and from the uterus (Figs 80.5 and 80.6).

Displacement of the ureters from the ureteric tunnels is achieved by passing a pair of long, straight Spencer-Wells forceps along the line of the ureter as it passes through the tunnel (Figs 80.5 and 80.6). When opened, they demonstrate the roof of the tunnel with the vessels, as shown in Figure 80.6. The long Spencer-Wells forceps are gently and gradually advanced along the surface of the ureter, the closed jaws being partially opened from time to time to free the ureter in its tunnel. The forceps traverse the complete tunnel, i.e. a distance of approximately 1.5 cm. Closed points emerge at the distal limit. The roof of the tunnel is at the same time steadied and held up by non-toothed dissecting forceps; it is preserved as a one-piece bridge of tissue and is subsequently dealt with as such. The same Spencer-Wells forceps pick up the liga-

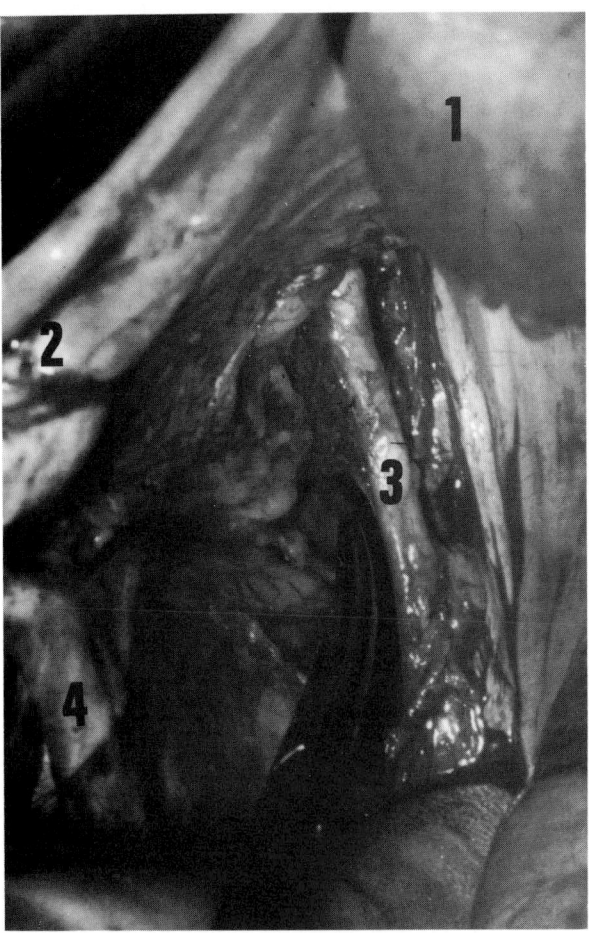

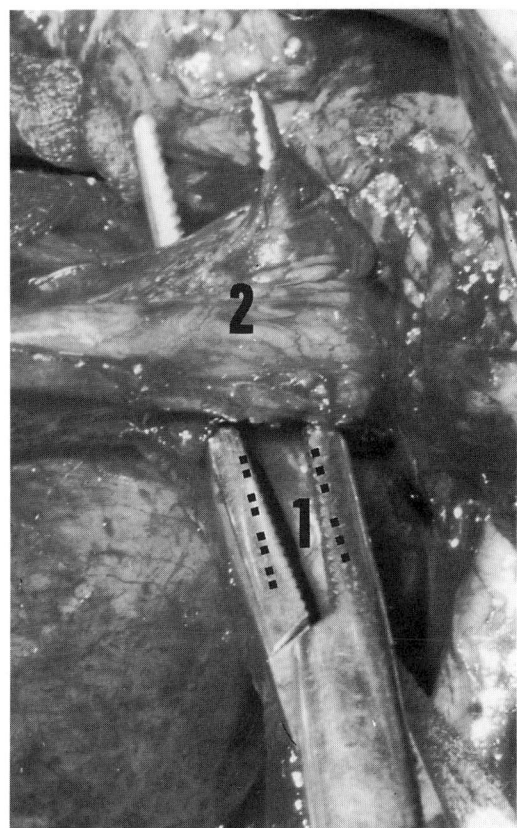

Fig. 80.5

Fig. 80.4 Exposure of left ureter. The left ureter is exposed after the posterior aspect and the base of the left broad ligament have been opened. The uterus is at (1), the left appendage at (2), the ureter (3) and the ovarian pedicle (4).

tures and pull them back beneath the bridge or roof of the tunnel. The ligatures are tied at a distance of 1.5 cm from each other (Fig. 80.6), ensuring that the ureter is not caught up in either suture. The jaws of the forceps are now partially opened as they lie on top of the ureter; the roof of the tunnel is cut precisely midway between the ligatures, leaving a cuff of 0.75 cm beyond each ligature.

With scissors or with forceps carrying a cotton pledget, the ureter is then easily displaced laterally without separation from its mesentery or damage to its blood supply (Fig. 80.7). With the lower ureters displaced laterally and their intra-pelvic course clearly visible, the way is clear to remove the uterus, the cervix and a sizeable cuff of the vagina.

In securing the lower uterine attachments, it must be remembered that the uterus is still attached by the uterosacral ligaments. Part of each cardinal ligament forms the roof of the parametrial (ureteric) tunnel and was divided when exposing the ureters; any remaining fibers of the cardinal ligament will be clamped and divided with the vaginal angle pedicle when the uterus is removed. The uterosacral ligaments are now clamped at least 2 cm clear

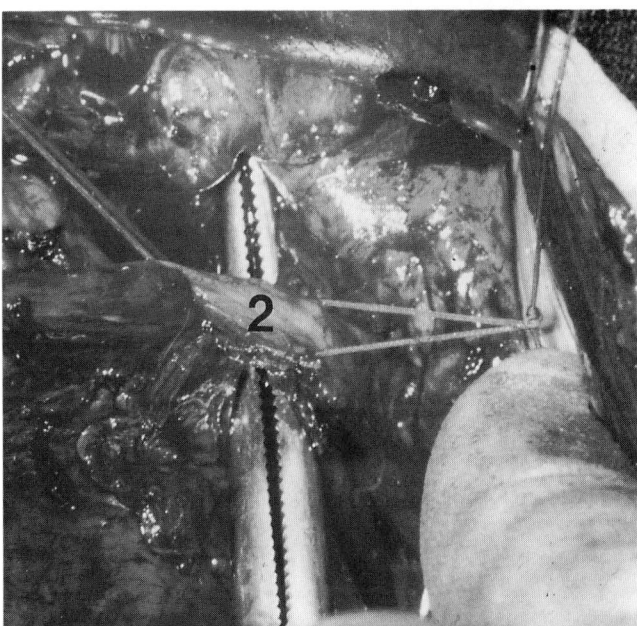

Figs 80.5 and 80.6 Exposure of ureters in the ureteric tunnel. The line of the right ureter [outlined (---) at (1)], is followed into the ureteric tunnel by large Spencer Wells forceps. The roof of the tunnel with its uterine vessels (2) is then defined and doubly ligated (Fig. 80.6).

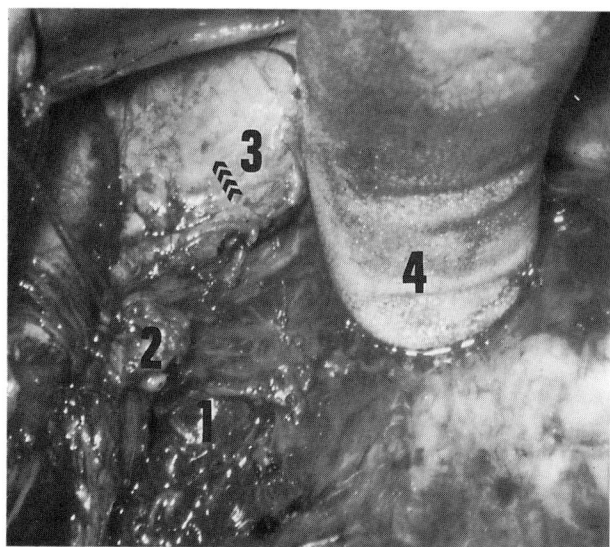

Fig. 80.7 Displacement of left ureter. The photograph shows the left ureter (1) lying medial to the ligated uterine pedicle (2) and being displaced along with the angle of the bladder (3) from the outer vaginal angle with the finger (4), in the direction of the arrow.

of the uterus, and detached medial to the forceps with scissors. The peritoneum of the posterior aspect of the cervix between these points is then divided with a scalpel and the lower leaf pushed downwards, so that the whole uterus is released posteriorly (Fig. 80.8). By blunt dissection and

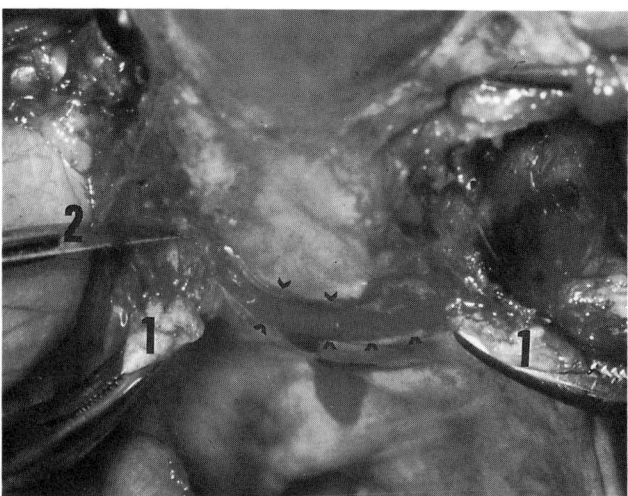

Fig. 80.8 Freeing the uterus posteriorly. Both uterosacral ligaments have been separated off the uterus and are held by forceps (1) and (1). The scalpel (2) has completed a stroke across the posterior aspect of the cervix at the level of its inferior border, to divide the peritoneum (arrowed) where it is attached to the posterior aspect of the cervix and also to divide any superficial fibrous tissue which is still anchoring the uterus. Immediately this is done, the uterus can be lifted from the pelvic floor, and the uterosacral ligaments and the peritoneal edge between them fall back to expose the posterior fornix of the vagina. By blunt dissection and leverage on the forceps, it is simple to strip the peritoneal covering from the upper third of the posterior vaginal wall.

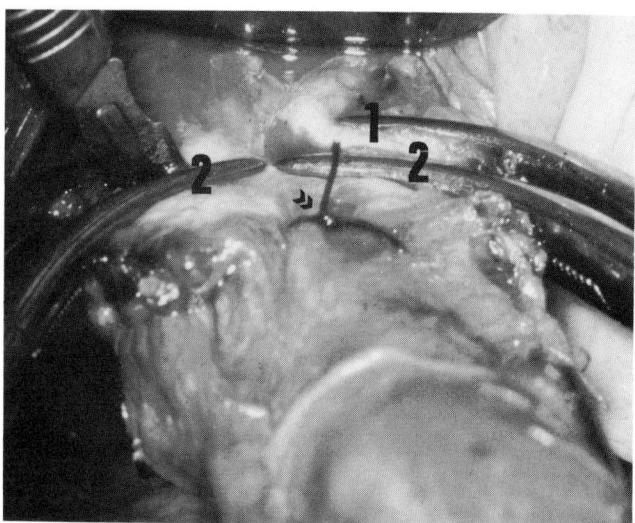

Fig. 80.9 Removal of vaginal cuff. The level of the external cervical os is indicated by the stitch (arrowed) and shows that the cuff is adequate in length. Above the two clamps already in place (1) and (1), two further occluding forceps are applied across the vagina (2) and (2). The scalpel now divides the vagina between the two sets of forceps, removing the uterus and vaginal cuff and leaving the original clamps (1) and (1) and open vaginal vault.

leverage on the forceps, the tissues are stripped sufficiently far distally to ensure that the uterus is free.

The vaginal vault is now widely excised. With the uterus being pulled to the opposite side and in a cephalad direction (Fig. 80.9), the upper vagina is clamped first on one, and then on the other side at the junction of its upper and middle thirds. The clamps also include in their grasp any remaining fibers of the cardinal ligament and related paravaginal tissue. The aim of the operation is to take a substantial portion of vagina. The vaginal angles are then secured on each side and the vault closed centrally by three mattress sutures. The free ends of the detached uterosacral ligaments are incorporated when tying the two lateral vaginal vault mattress stitches. The pelvis is then reperitonized in the usual manner, a continuous suture being used from the round and ovarian ligaments on one side to the same structures on the other side. Drains may be placed below this peritoneal suture. By performing this type of closure, the risk of kinking the ureter when the peritoneum is gathered together by separate anchor stitches on each side is avoided.

Extended hysterectomy with hemivaginectomy

In this operation, devised by Lees, preliminary steps are made by the vaginal route prior to embarking on the abdominal hysterectomy. The vagina is circumscribed above its midpoint, and the whole of the vault skin is raised from its underlying tissues as a pouch (Figs 80.10 and 80.11). The mouth of this pouch is closed by a purse-string suture.

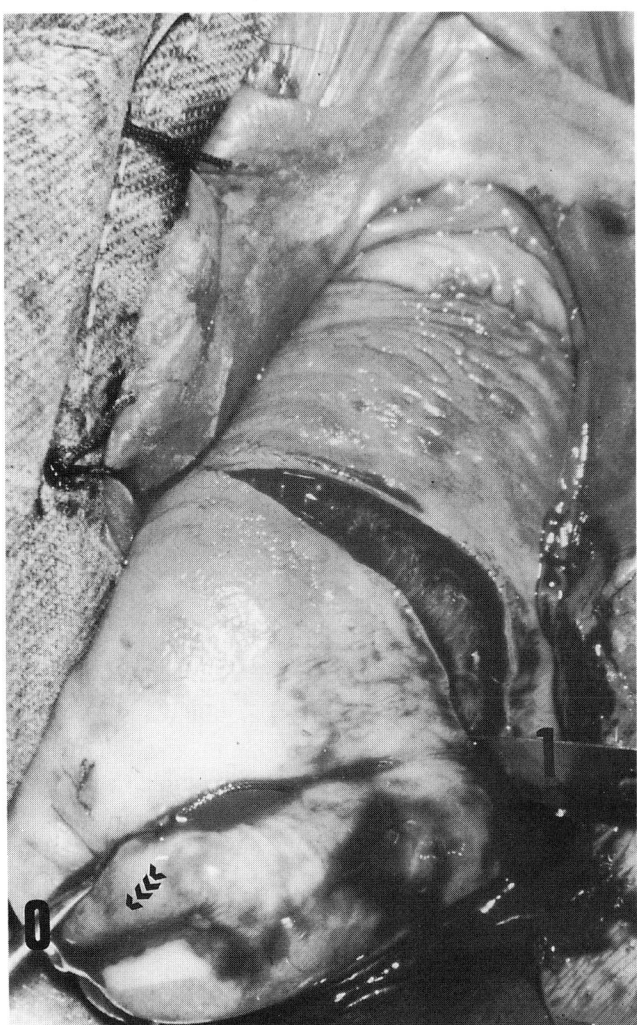

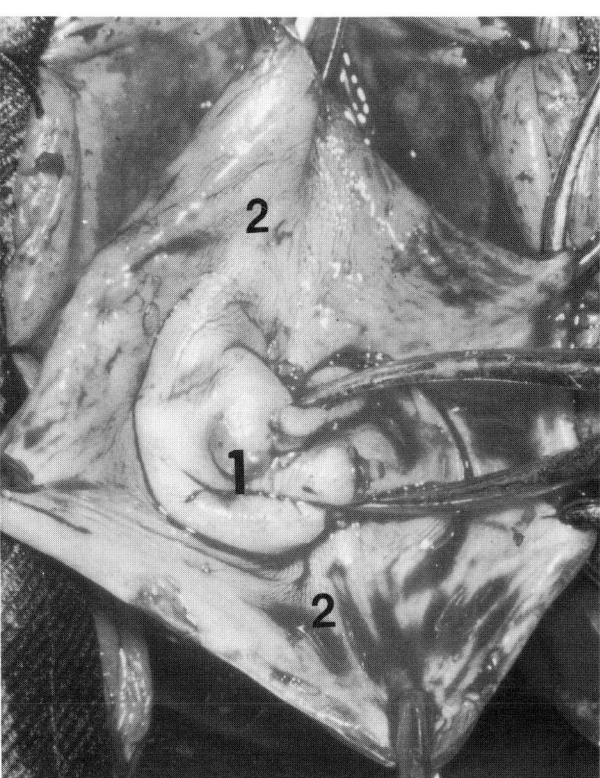

Fig. 80.11 Freeing sac of upper vaginal skin. The skin of the upper vagina is raised from the underlying structures in the form of a pouch. The stitch in the cervix (1) and the midpoints of the detached anterior and posterior vaginal skin flaps (2) and (2) are shown.

Fig. 80.10 Incision of vaginal skin. The anterior lip of the cervix is held in Littlewoods' forceps (0) and the arrow indicates the direction in which it is being held. The scalpel (1) cuts through the full thickness of the skin of the anterior wall at about its midpoint, beginning on the right side. The incision continues in the same plane across the left side.

Is removal of the vaginal vault necessary?

At least five studies have concerned the use of preoperative radiation to the vaginal vault in an attempt to prevent vaginal recurrence.[2,3,10,13] The control groups were treated by standard total hysterectomy with bilateral salpingo-oophorectomy, *without* any additional excision of the vaginal vault. In all reports, there was very little difference in the mortality in the two groups. In the Gynecology Oncology Group (GOG) study[3] involving 222 women who received preoperative or postoperative radiation, they appeared to have a lower incidence overall of vaginal vault recurrences than those treated by surgery alone. However, this difference was not evident in those with Grade 1 or 2 lesions. When sites of recurrence were analysed, only two (1%) patients had an isolated vaginal vault recurrence; one patient had been treated with surgery only and the other with surgery plus radiation. It would appear from this study and others[2,13] that the vaginal vault is not at high risk for recurrence.

In a large Italian study, Candiani et al[1] reviewed 971 patients with Stage I endometrial cancer. The operability rate was 96%. One group, treated by a modified radical hysterectomy in which a significant amount of tissue in the upper vagina was taken, was compared with another group

The uterovesical peritoneum anteriorly is opened as in a vaginal hysterectomy. The pouch of Douglas is then opened, giving access to the uterosacral ligaments which are clamped, divided and sutured. The whole uterus is now pushed up into the pelvic peritoneal cavity and the vaginal vault closed transversely by a series of interrupted vertical mattress sutures.

The abdominal total hysterectomy is then performed through a transverse incision; the dissection of the ureters is as described in the preceding section. Since the uterosacral ligaments are already detached, only the cardinal ligaments remain to be clamped and cut well laterally before the uterus is removed. The vaginal vault has already been closed during the vaginal part of the procedure.

of women submitted to standard total abdominal hysterectomy with bilateral salpingo-oophorectomy. In the former group, the vault recurrence was 1.3%, and in the latter, 2.1%. This was not a statistically significant difference, and suggests that the former operation may have been too radical.

RADICAL (WERTHEIM'S) HYSTERECTOMY WITH BILATERAL SALPINGO-OOPHORECTOMY AND LYMPHADENECTOMY — IS IT NECESSARY?

The realization that a significant lymph node metastasis rate occurs in less differentiated (i.e., Grades 2 and 3) Stage I endometrial cancers led to the understandable belief that either complete removal of pelvic and para-aortic nodes, or at least the pelvic nodes, was necessary to achieve satisfactory rates of survival. The history of this development and the case for and against such radical surgery for endometrial cancer has already been discussed in Chapter 49 (see p. 782). In summary, there does not seem to be sufficient evidence to warrant lymphadenectomy in all such cases, many of whom are obese and poor surgical risks.

Lees treated 102 patients by radical hysterectomy and partial vaginectomy.[11] In 76 patients, bilateral lymphadenectomy following preoperative intracavity radiation was performed; in the other 26 women, formal lymphadenectomy was omitted in preference to biopsy of the three major lymph node groups on each side of the pelvis. Node-positive cases received adjunctive radiotherapy to the pelvic side wall by linear accelerator. The 5-year survival rate for the first group was 74%, and for the second group, 80%. Nothing had been added by these extensive operative procedures with their associated increased morbidity. These results support the view that extensive removal of both pelvic and para-aortic glands is unnecessary, and that only a biopsy of those reckoned to be clinically enlarged or suspicious should be undertaken.

RECOMMENDED SURGICAL TECHNIQUE — TOTAL HYSTERECTOMY WITH BILATERAL SALPINGO-OOPHORECTOMY (with nodal sampling of enlarged or suspicious nodes)

The patient's general medical condition may well dictate the extent of surgical treatment. Patients with endometrial cancer are predominantly elderly, and often suffer from obesity, hypertension or cardiopulmonary disease; many, indeed, have more than one disease. Most, however, are able to have at least a simple and expeditious hysterectomy after careful preparation in hospital.

Pre- and postoperative measures

Anesthesia

General anesthesia is preferred. However, in recent times the use of epidural anesthesia in radical pelvic surgery, either exclusively or in conjunction with general anesthesia, has been shown to offer many advantages. It reduces blood pressure, lessens the risk of neurogenic shock, and the epidural catheter can be retained to control pain postoperatively by the instillation of either local anesthetic or narcotic agents.

Care of bladder and ureters

Since ureters are not dissected out during this operation, it is not essential to obtain a preoperative intravenous urogram unless clinical conditions dictate, such as in the presence of broad ligament fibroids or pelvic endometriosis. The bladder is emptied by catheter prior to commencement of the operation; an indwelling catheter is left in situ if significant vault resection is planned. The subject of bladder function after radical pelvic surgery is discussed in Chapters 78, 84 and 85.

Prevention of venous thrombosis and embolism

Patients with endometrial cancer constitute a group exceptionally prone to venous thrombosis and embolism, and it is prudent to anticipate such complications.[8] Subcutaneous heparin should be administered to all women over age 40, and especially in high risk cases (see Chs 78 and 84). The dose is 5000 units subcutaneously twice or three times daily. Early ambulation is mandatory, and meticulous physiotherapy and use of pressure antiembolism stockings are considered essential.[7]

Antibiotics

The use of prophylactic antibiotics in the postoperative period is controversial. However, recent studies[7,8] using combinations of antibiotics indicate a beneficial effect in reducing morbidity following pelvic surgery.

Sexual rehabilitation

Many women with endometrial cancer are postmenopausal and may be sexually inactive. However, it is still important to enquire and to counsel especially the younger women as regards the long-term effect of the operation on subsequent sexual intercourse. This subject is considered in Chapter 90.

Surgical technique

The basic surgical technique for abdominal hysterectomy and bilateral salpingo-oophorectomy, the mainstay operation for Stage I endometrial carcinoma, involves four stages. These are:

Stage 1: separation of the upper uterine attachments

Stage 2: defining and securing uterine vessels

Stage 3: dividing lower uterine attachments and removal of uterus

Stage 4: reconstruction of vaginal vault.

Separation of the upper uterine attachments

The abdomen is opened through a transverse incision situated in line with the anterior superior iliac spines. This incision is higher than that usually employed for routine hysterectomy. The incision can be made below the apron of fat in obese patients.

Packing of the abdominal contents is usually facilitated by releasing fine peritoneal adhesion attachments to the lateral sigmoid with scalpel or scissors. It also ensures better access to the left infundibulo-pelvic ligament. Prior to packing, a full manual examination is made by the surgeon of the abdominal organs, particularly liver and spleen, and then the lymph node chains in the abdomen and pelvis. The main purpose is to detect any extrapelvic spread of growth. Also at this point, if either ovary is attached to the side wall of the pelvis or the pelvic floor, it is freed with scissors. Peritoneal cytological washings are taken using 50 to 75 ml of saline solution.

The first part of the operation involves the clamping of the left broad ligament with curved forceps close to the cornu of the uterus. By retraction laterally, the round ligament and broad ligament are easily seen (Fig. 80.12). The round ligament is ligated and detached from the uterus. In Figure 80.13, the clamping of the left ovarian pedicle is seen, a defect having been made by the finger through the base of the posterior layer of the broad ligament opposite the gap in the anterior layer where the round ligament was

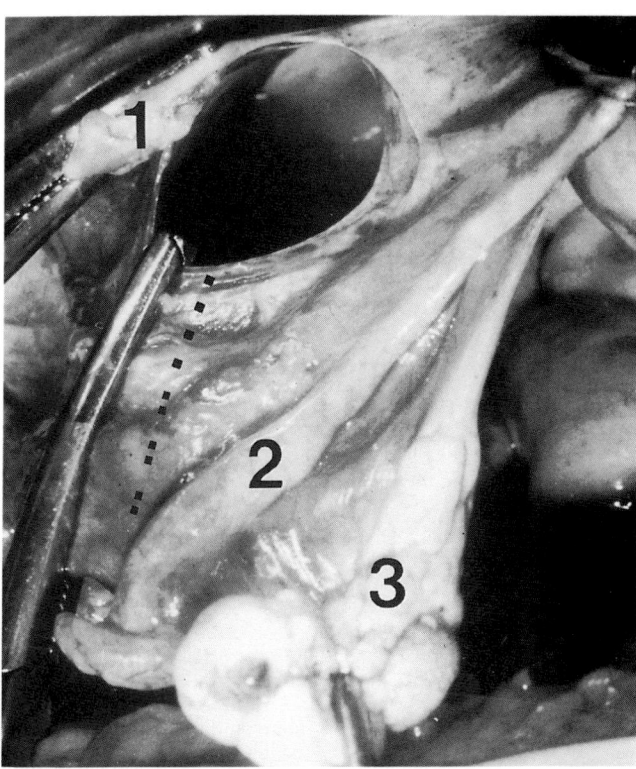

Fig. 80.13 Securing the left ovarian pedicle. Safe clamping of the left broad ligament involves the forefinger being introduced through the posterior layer of the broad ligament opposite the gap in the anterior layer where the round ligament (1), was divided. The tube is at (2) and ovary at (3). Detachment of the pedicle is along the dotted line.

divided. The round ligament and the ovarian pedicle are then ligated in similar fashion on the right (Fig. 80.14).

The next step is separation of bladder from cervix. Curved scissors are inserted under the loose peritoneum

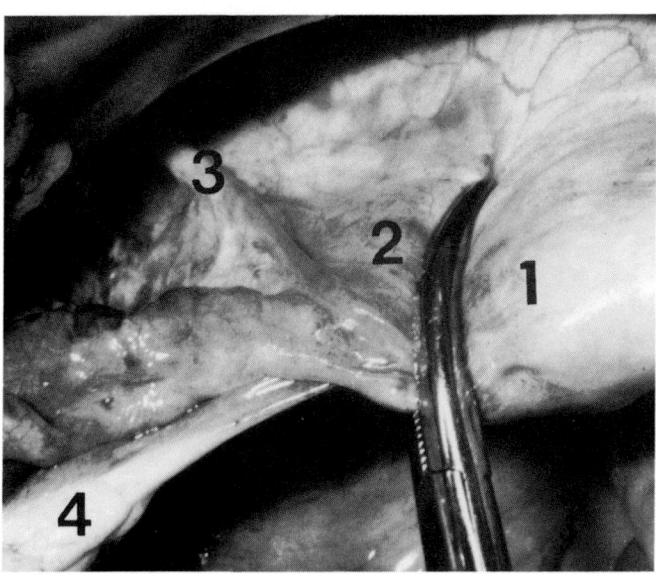

Fig. 80.12 Upper uterine ligaments. Retraction of the uterus (1) laterally displays the broad ligament (2) and round ligament (3), and ovary (4).

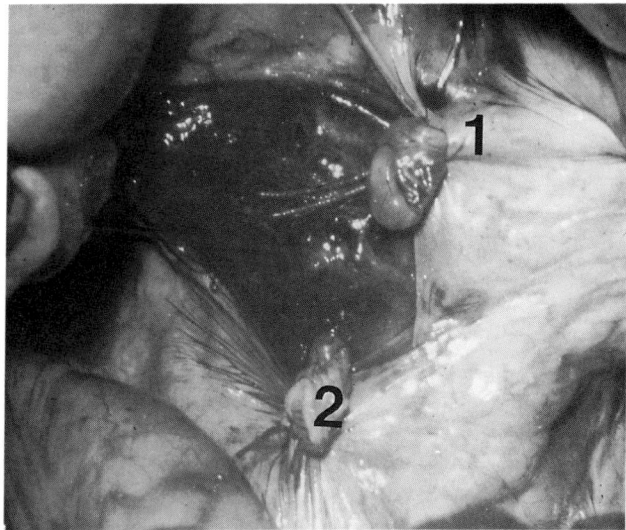

Fig. 80.14 Ligation of right round ligament (1) and right ovarian pedicle (2).

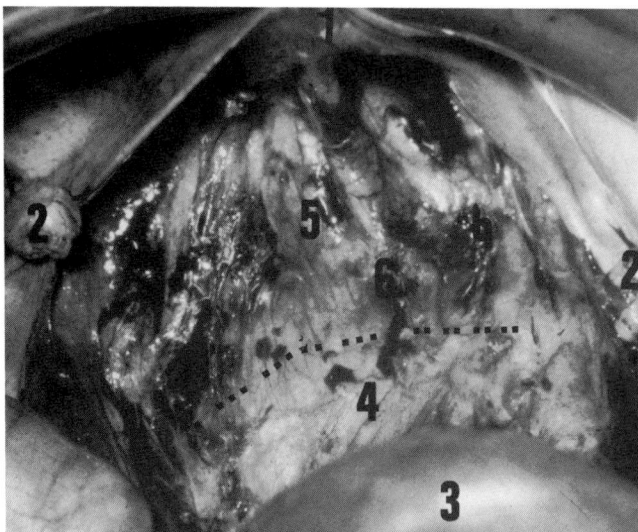

Fig. 80.15 Separation of bladder from the cervix completed. The pelvic peritoneum is held by forceps and retracted upwards to show the superior and part of the posterior aspect of the bladder separated off the front of the uterus. This has been done by sharp dissection, taking care to avoid the larger veins and sealing off any smaller vessels with diathermy. Further separation will in fact be required when the lower uterine attachments have been divided. The various structures are numbered; and the dotted line indicates the vesico-vaginal junction; (1) peritoneum held by forceps, (2) round ligament pedicles, (3) fundus uteri, (4) cervix, (5) bladder, (6) diathermy fulguration area.

between the bladder and the uterus, and the blades opened to form a tunnel. The uterovesical peritoneum is then incised. Once separated, the bladder can then be dissected downwards off the cervix, either with curved scissors or the use of a gauze swab on the finger. However, this latter procedure carries the risk of tearing a weak bladder wall, especially in an elderly woman. In Figure 80.15, the pelvic peritoneum is held up by forceps, showing the superior, and part of the posterior aspect of the bladder that has been separated off the front of the lower uterus and cervix. Care should be taken to avoid the larger veins and to seal off any small vessels with diathermy.

Defining and securing the uterine vessels

The uterine vessels are now defined, by firstly opening up the posterior leaf of the broad ligament, as shown in Figure 80.16. The vessels, now clearly isolated, are carefully stripped of loose fat and light adhesions by gentle snips with the scissors and then clamped with straight forceps. The point of the posterior limb of the forceps presses against the uterus, just above the attachment of the uterosacral ligament, and as the jaws close, the line of the forceps is nearly at right angles to the vertical axis of the uterus (Fig. 80.17). With straight scissors (Fig. 80.18) the uterine pedicle is divided between the straight forceps and small curved forceps, which have been applied to

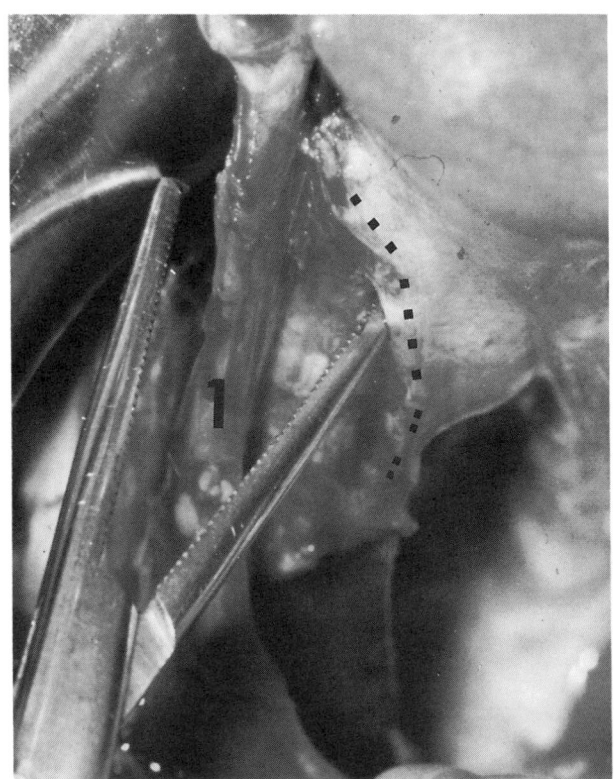

Fig. 80.16 Defining and dividing posterior layer of broad ligament prior to clamping left uterine pedicle. To gain access to the uterine vessels (1), it is necessary to open up both leaves of the broad ligament. In this illustration, the procedure has been done posteriorly and is shown by the dotted line.

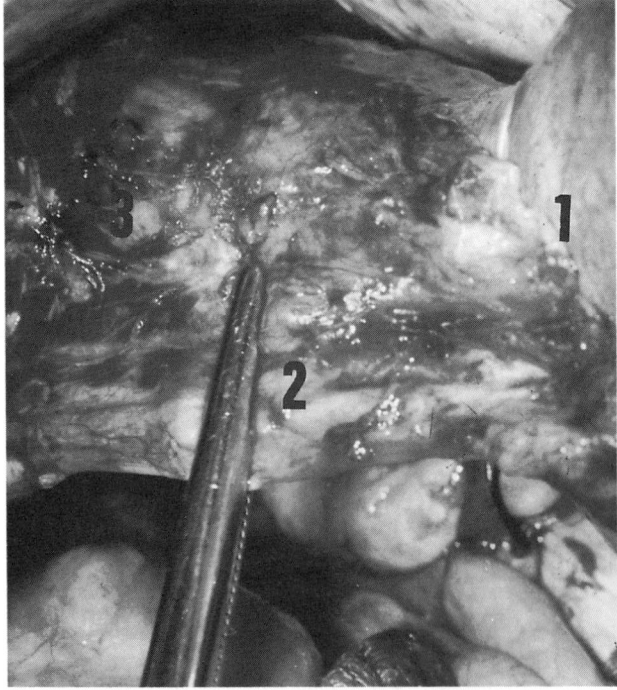

Fig. 80.17 The anterior limb of the forceps is closed on the uterus marked (1) so that no branch of the artery (2) is missing; the outline of the ectocervix is at (3).

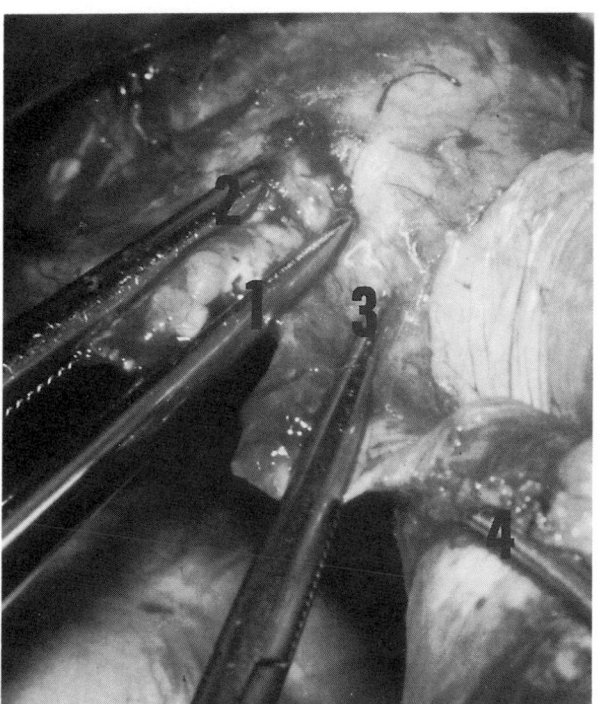

Fig. 80.18 Detachment of uterine pedicle. Straight scissors (1) divide the uterine pedicle between the straight forceps just applied (2) and small Spencer Wells forceps applied to prevent backflow of blood from the uterine body (3). The cut is made parallel to the larger forceps, leaving a good cuff of tissue, and is carried right up to the uterine wall. Holding forceps on the left cornu of the uterus are at (4).

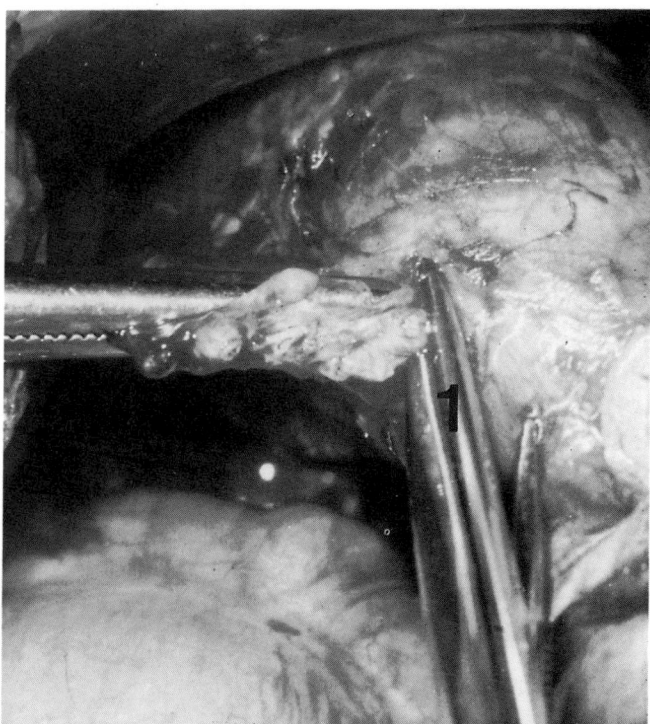

Fig. 80.19 Further detachment of left uterine pedicle. The uterine pedicle is further freed from the uterus by making a short cut (1) at right angles to the first, just beyond the point of the forceps. Subsequent to this, the forceps are used as a lever to strip the pedicle off the side of the uterus by a controlled rolling and pushing movement. The pedicle is then free and can be safely tied without fear of it slipping from the ligature.

prevent back flow of blood from the uterine body. After the parallel cut has been made, leaving a good cuff of tissue right up to the uterine wall, the pedicle is then further freed from the uterus by making a short cut at right angles to the first, just beyond the forceps (Fig. 80.19). The forceps are then used as a lever to strip the pedicle off the side of the uterus by a controlled rolling and pushing movement in a downward direction. The pedicle is then ligated, after transfixion at its midpoint.

Dividing lower uterine attachments and removal of uterus

With the uterine vessels secured, the uterus is held up and forward, but it is still firmly attached to the floor of the pelvis by the uterosacral ligaments. These are detached from the uterus after having been first clamped and then ligated, and the intervening peritoneum is then divided where it is attached to the posterior aspect of the cervix. At this stage, the bladder is further separated from the cervix, after which the vaginal angles are clamped. The operator holds the uterus in one hand, and checks by palpation by the forefinger and thumb of the other that the vagina can be entered below the level of the cervix. Curved clamps are then applied medial to and clear of the ligated uterine pedicles, and also, obviously, clear of the bladder

edge anteriorly. When closed, this clamp includes the whole vaginal angle and the medial part of the cardinal ligament. This is shown in Figure 80.20 (anterior view) and Figure 80.21 (posterior view).

The incision into the vaginal angle is the next step, and is performed by cutting at a distance of 0.5 cm beyond the forceps. The vaginal edge curls back to show the cavity, as air is audibly drawn in. The same maneuver is repeated on the other side. Curved scissors divide the anterior and posterior vaginal walls, and the uterus is removed (Fig. 80.22).

Reconstruction of the vaginal vault

With the uterus removed and the vaginal vault open, the next stage is to ensure a closure that will make the vault at least as firm as previously. This is aided by attaching the ends of the uterosacral ligaments to the vault during closure. Some surgeons prefer to leave the vault open in vascular or infected cases, to ensure adequate drainage. Others do so as a routine. If the vault is left open, then steps must be taken to prevent bleeding from the cut edge. An effective method is to insert a running stitch all around the edge of the vault that is drawn sufficiently tight to con-

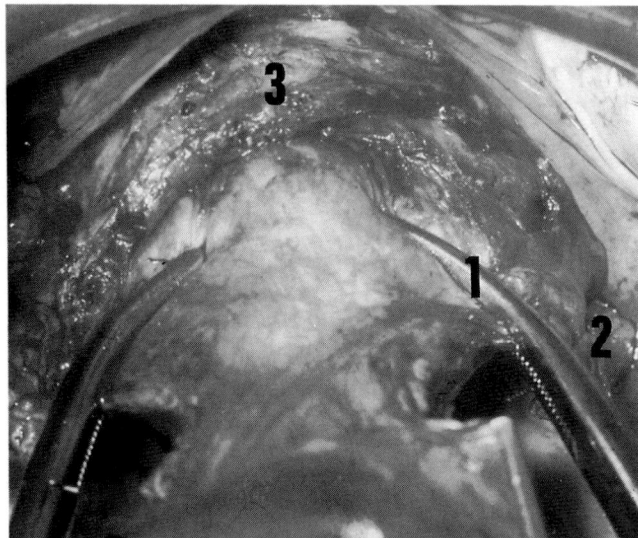

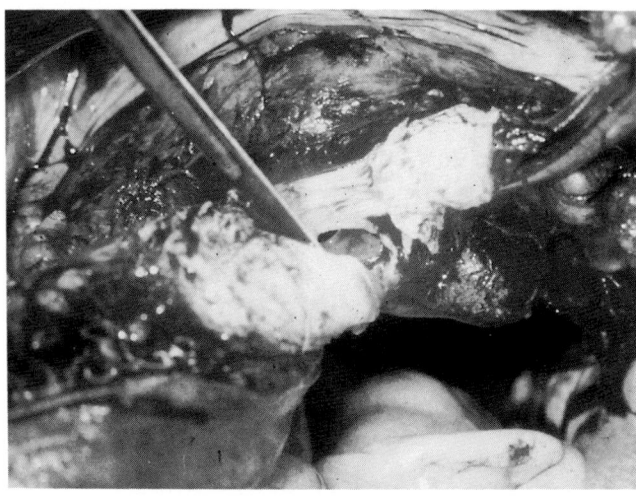

Fig. 80.22   Separation of uterus from vagina.

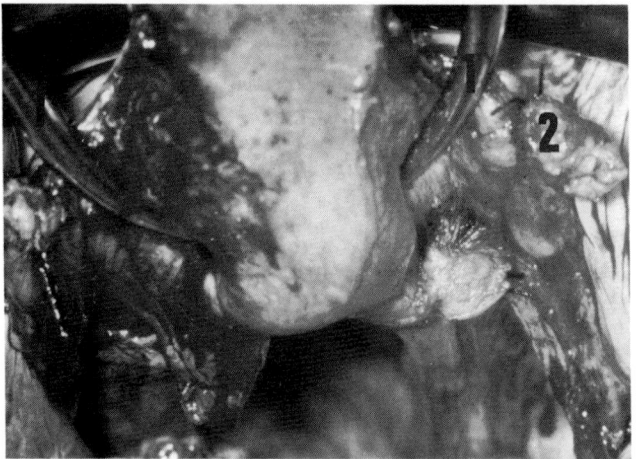

Figs 80.20 and 80.21   Securing the vaginal angles. Both vaginal clamps (1) have been applied clear of the uterine pedicle (2). In Figure 80.20, the anterior view is seen and in Figure 80.21, the uterus is lifted forward to show the posterior aspect.

trol the bleeding or oozing. The completed stitch draws the vault together in purse-string fashion, so that the opening becomes quite small. In Figure 80.23, the vault is open, and sutures are about to be placed at the vaginal angles; three interrupted mattress sutures will then close the central vault's defect, the lateral ones transfixing the respective uterosacral ligaments.

Nodal biopsy procedure

The risk of nodal spread with Stage I, Grade 2 to 3 lesions is significant and, when feasible, lymph nodes should be sampled. As mentioned above, recent evidence suggests that biopsy of enlarged or clinically suspicious nodes, a less traumatic procedure, gives essentially the same results as the more formal and thorough lymphadenectomy.

The first step in sampling nodes involves the lateral extension of the peritoneal opening into the broad ligament

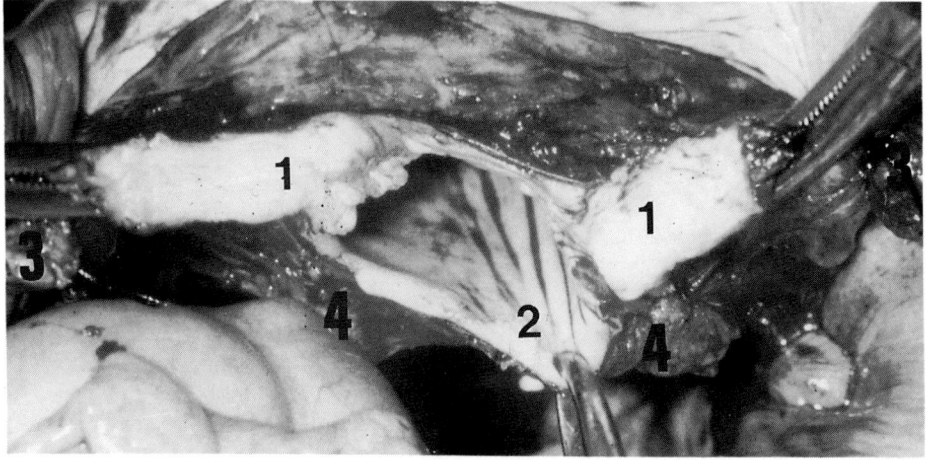

Fig. 80.23   Vaginal vault ready for suture. The uterus has now been separated and the vaginal vault is seen displayed and open with the forceps on the vaginal angles in place (1); the posterior wall is now held by a Littlewoods forceps (2), the uterine pedicles are now seen at (3) and uterosacrals can just be made out at (4).

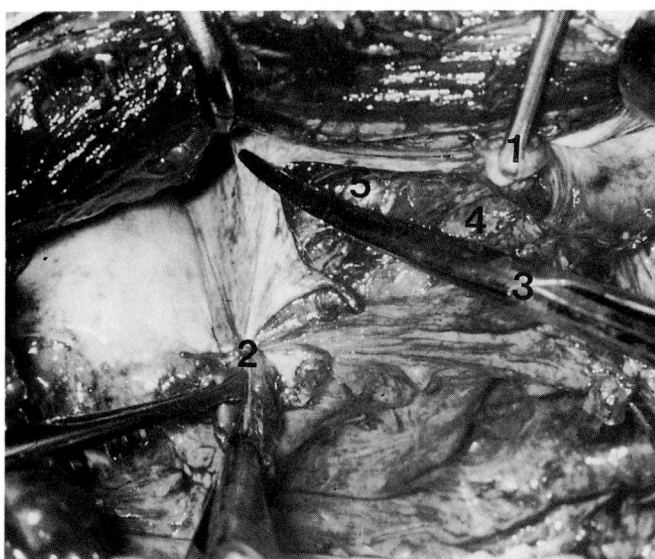

Fig. 80.24 Lateral extension of opening into broad ligament. Access to the large vessels in the pelvic sidewall; the round ligament and ovarian pedicles are held in tissue forceps (1) and (2) respectively, while the scissors (3) divide the peritoneum to expose the external iliac artery (4) and the psoas muscle (5). Genito-femoral nerve is usually seen on the muscle.

(Fig. 80.24). This permits access to the large vessels on the pelvic side wall. Digital examination is made of the major lymph chains on the pelvic side walls (Fig. 80.25). These are: (a) external iliac group, (b) common iliac group, (c) internal iliac group and (d) obturator fossa group. In Figure 80.26, a large group of nodes covering the external iliac vessels has been sampled. In this instance, the three groups of nodes — lateral, middle and medial — are conglomerated in a suspicious mass. After removal of the largest and most obvious nodes from the internal iliac chain, the finger examines the obturator fossa and a collection of suspicious nodes in this area is removed (Fig. 80.27).

The author's preference for nodal removal involves the extensive use of small metal (aneurysm) clips. These are applied on the afferent and efferent vessels (vascular and lymphatic) running into the nodes. The nodes are elevated by a pair of Allis or Babcock forceps, permitting easy application of the metal clips.

Suction drains (e.g. Redivac) are placed extraperitoneally. If the vault is left open, insertion of a T-tube drain into the vagina with the two arms lying across the vaginal vault is an option. The peritoneum is closed in the traditional manner. Care must be taken not to encircle the ureter as it crosses the pelvic brim.

Recent evidence[15] suggests that the parietal peritoneum very quickly covers the denuded pelvic vault surface, and many surgeons now leave the pelvic and parietal peritoneum unsutured. However, the author feels that, especially in infected or very vascular cases, the effective use of the pelvic drain is aided by a peritoneal closure.

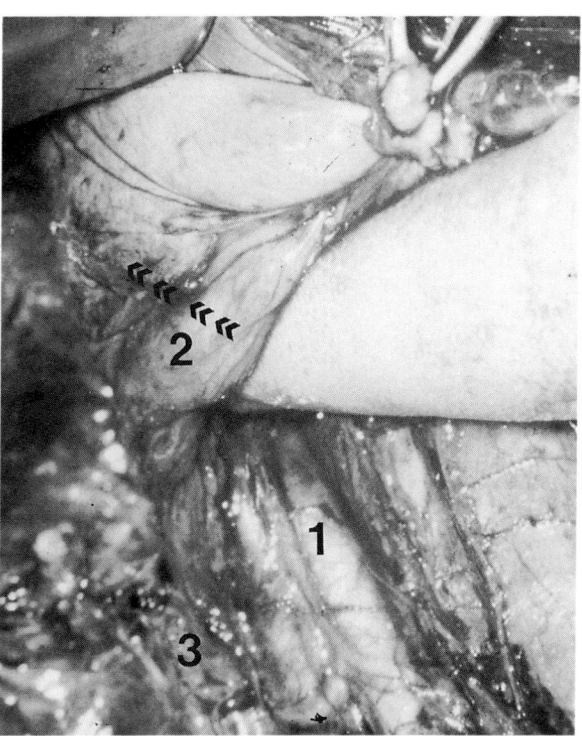

Fig. 80.25 Digital examination of right sidewall glands. The forefinger is hooked under the anterior leaf of the lateral extension and tunnels forward along the line of the external iliac artery (1) in the direction of the arrow as far as the obturator fossa. The finger then sweeps the peritoneum, extraperitoneal fat and the glands medially, from the surface of the great vessels on the pelvic sidewall, to open up the paravesical space (2). In a similar fashion, the finger hooks under the posterior leaf of the upper peritoneal incision and tunnels upwards along the external and common iliac arteries before sweeping the tissue medially from the pelvic sidewall. The ureter (3) is always immediately apparent on the extraperitoneal surface during this maneuver.

SURGERY FOR STAGE II ENDOMETRIAL CARCINOMA

Stage II carcinoma of the endometrium involves extension of the disease into the endocervix, and a greater propensity for lymph node metastasis. Extension can either be in the form of endocervical glandular involvement of occult disease (Stage IIa, G1, 2 and 3), or invasion into the actual cervical stroma (Stage IIb, G1, 2 and 3). In the latter case, it seems rational to use therapy that would encompass likely metastatic sites. Several options are available, and choice will depend partly on the patient's medical status. Surgery is usually performed using radical hysterectomy and pelvic lymphadenectomy, and if pelvic node metastasis is present, adjuvant radiation therapy is added. Alternatively, preoperative external irradiation or brachytherapy can be used, followed by simple hysterectomy and bilateral salpingo-oophorectomy as described in the previous section. The recommended external radiation dosage is between 40 and 50 Gy (4000 to 5000 rads) to the whole pelvis. The surgery is usually performed 6 weeks after radiation therapy has been completed.

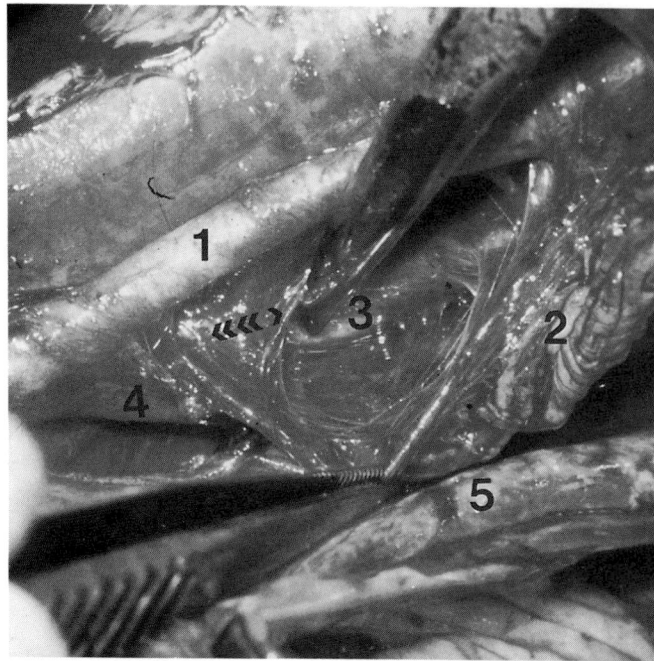

Fig. 80.26 Dissection of glands from external and common iliac arteries. The scissors have cleared the lateral and middle chain of external iliac artery glands and continue proximally to separate common iliac glands (1) from the artery. The most medial chain of the glands (2) has been separated in the plane (arrowed) between the external iliac artery (1) and vein (3). The internal iliac artery is at (4) and the ureter at (5).

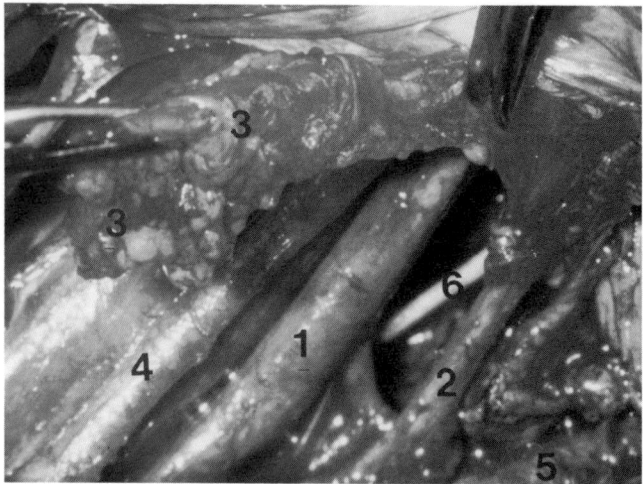

Fig. 80.27 Removal of glands from iliac vessels and obturator fossa. The photograph shows the angle between the external iliac vein (1) and the internal iliac artery (2). The area is seen to be quite clear of glands and fat (3). The external iliac artery is at (4), the ureter at (5) and the obturator nerve at (6).

It must always be remembered that a firm diagnosis of Stage II disease based purely on endocervical curettings, can be difficult. However, with occult Stage II disease, when no visible disease is present on the cervix and no suspicion exists of parametrial disease, the treatment recommended is that outlined above for use with patients presenting with Stage I, Grade 2 or Grade 3 disease, an approach also preferred by DiSaia and Creasman.[4] It is well recognized that patients with endocervical involvement have a higher risk for extra-uterine disease than those who have disease limited to the fundus. Postoperative radiation therapy is given in selected cases, especially those with node metastases.

SUMMARY

Many techniques are employed by surgeons using hysterectomy as the primary surgical method of treating Stage I endometrial carcinoma. On present evidence, it would seem that the formal removal of a large area of vaginal vault may well be over-treatment. A simple hysterectomy delivers the specimen for thorough histopathological examination to assess various risk factors, such as depth of penetration into myometrium, grade of lesion and obvious spread to the endocervix. It would seem that in Stage 1, Grade 2 and 3 lesions which have a significant nodal involvement rate, lymph node sampling is warranted.

ACKNOWLEDGEMENT

The photographs in this chapter have been produced from Lees D H, Singer A (eds) (1979) *The Colour Atlas of Gynaecological Surgery*, Vols II and III with kind permission of the publishers, Wolfe Medical Publications Limited, London.

REFERENCES

1. Candiani G B, Mangioni C, Marzi M M 1978 Surgery in endometrial cancer. Age, route and operability state in 854 Stage 1 and 2 fresh consecutive cases, 1955–1976. Gynecol Oncol 6: 363
2. de-Waal J C, Lochmuller H 1982 Pre-operative radium insertion in the management of endometrial cancer. Odurshilfe Fraunheilkd 42: 394
3. DiSaia P J, Creasman W T, Boronow R C, Blessing J A 1985 Risk factors in recurrent patterns in Stage I endometrial cancer. Am J Obstet Gynecol 151: 1009
4. DiSaia P J, Creasman W T 1989 Clinical Gynecologic Oncology, 3rd edn. Mosby, St Louis, p 189
5. Editorial 1988 Management of venous thromboembolism. Lancet i: 275
6. Editorial 1989 Diagnosis of deep-vein thrombosis. Lancet ii: 23
7. Hemsell D L 1989 Infections after gynecologic surgery. Obstet Gynecol Clinic North Am 16: 381
8. Hemsell D L, Heard M C, Hemsell P G 1988 Alteration in lower reproductive tract flora after single dose piperacillin and triple dose cifoxitrin at vaginal and abdominal hysterectomy. Obstet Gynecol 72: 875
9. Javert C, Douglas R 1956 Treatment of endometrial cancer. Am J Roentgenol 75: 580
10. Jones H W 1975 Treatment of adenocarcinoma of the endometrium. Obstet Gynecol Surv 30: 147

11. Lees D H 1978 Surgery of endometrial cancer. Clinics Obstet Gynaecol 5: 675
12. Lees D H, Singer A (eds) 1979 Colour Atlas of Gynaecological Surgery, Vol III. Wolfe Medical Publishers, London
13. Onsrud M, Kolstad P, Norman T 1976 Postoperative external pelvic irradiation in carcinoma of the corpus Stage I: a controlled clinical trial. Gynecol Oncol 4: 222
14. Rutledge F N 1974 The role of radical hysterectomy in adenocarcinoma of the endometrium. Gynecol Oncol 2: 331
15. Tulandi T, Hun H S, Gelfand M 1988 Closure of laparotomy incisions with or without peritoneal laparoscopy. Am J Obstet Gynecol 158: 536

81. Pelvic exenteration

R. E. Symmonds   M. J. Webb

GENERAL CONSIDERATIONS

A survey of the literature suggests that exenterative operations have not been widely accepted, or at least not commonly reported, procedures other than within the United States. The reason for this is obscure. It is apparent that the operation can provide a significant salvage rate in patients with recurrent genital malignancy (30 to 40%);[6,11,13,22,25] no other equally curative form of therapy exists for this distressing condition. Although central recurrence of cervical malignancy represents the most suitable lesion for exenterative operation, the procedure can provide salvage in some cases of resectable primary or recurrent neoplasms of other types and origins: endometrial, vesical, urethral, vulvar, rectal and, rarely, ovarian epithelial tumors, in addition to melanomas and sarcomas of various types. Rather than relegating patients with recurrent malignancy to the scrap heap of repeated irradiation and chemotherapy, which are rarely curative, one should consider exenteration, regardless of the origin of the cell type of the tumor (see also Ch. 45).

From the technical standpoint at least, the extirpative phase of the operation represents a less demanding dissection than, for instance, a radical hysterectomy, which requires rather meticulous preservation of the bladder, ureters and rectum, organs that are simply sacrificed with an exenteration procedure.

The operation can now be accomplished with a low and acceptable mortality (2 to 3%).[22] Despite this, it is important to appreciate that the operation can be taxing and stressful, for the patient and for the surgeon. It is essential for the operation to be accomplished expeditiously and accurately; the surgeon must be completely familiar with all aspects of pelvic surgery and with various techniques of bowel and ureteral surgery in particular. Even more imperative, if excessive blood loss is to be avoided, is an accurate knowledge of the pelvic anatomy, especially the rather complex fascial planes of the pelvis and their relationship to the pelvic organs, the internal iliac vessels, the sacral plexus, the levator muscles and the pelvic

sidewall.[18] The prompt and accurate identification of the fascial planes and the vascular landmarks will not only determine the resectability of the lesion, but also allow the dissection to proceed and to be completed rapidly with relatively little blood loss. Nevertheless, as a rule, the administration of 2 to 4 units of blood will be required. In addition, there will be considerable loss of fluid from the extensively dissected surfaces, which extend from above the aortic bifurcation down to the perineum.

It has been well documented that there is a direct correlation between an operative time of more than 7 hours and increased morbidity and mortality.[13] Actually, it should seldom be necessary for the operation to require more than 4 to 5 hours. In order to conserve operative time, some surgeons have advised the use of a two-team technique, with simultaneous dissections through the abdomen and via the perineum. However, the levator muscle attachments to the pelvic sidewalls can be more accurately divided from the abdominal approach; when this is accomplished properly, the perineal phase of the exenteration either can be avoided or will require so little time that it does not justify the operating room 'clutter' that results from the use of two teams.

Similarly, it has been suggested that the various phases of the operation should be accomplished by three operating teams: general surgeon, urologist and gynecologist and their assistants. This results in considerable crowding and, undoubtedly, a cumbersome scheduling problem for the various surgeons; apparently, it does not diminish the operative time and may even prolong it. Exenteration is most commonly required for a gynecologic lesion. The operability of the patient's lesion should be determined by a gynecologic surgeon — one who is familiar with the biologic behavior of the disease entity, and who has had sufficient training and experience with abdominal-pelvic surgery to ensure the operative dissection and the complex pelvic reconstruction can be accomplished with dispatch.

Any discussion of exenterative operative technique must represent a simplified overview; a stereotyped, systematic operation is rarely possible. It is essential for the surgeon

1283

to exercise considerable ingenuity and to develop considerable judgment regarding the type of operation required, the type of pelvic sidewall dissection that is best suited for the individual lesion, and the best and safest methods for restoring bowel, urinary and sexual function for each patient. Very infrequently are any two operations accomplished in the same manner.

It is important for the pelvic surgeon to be flexible in the surgical approach to the recurrent lesion. The type of radical surgical approach to be used will vary not only with the size and location of the lesion, but also with the degree of fibrosis and devascularization and with the dosage of any previous irradiation. For instance, with a small central recurrent lesion, it may be that the fascial planes have not been destroyed, that dissection of bladder, ureters and rectum is possible, and that a radical hysterectomy will provide good clearance of the malignancy, with a relatively low and acceptable risk of fistula formation. Similarly, with a lesion that is predominantly anteriorly located, anterior exenteration may represent the operation of choice when the rectum can be dissected easily from the posterior vaginal wall.

Nevertheless, it is most difficult after a high dosage of irradiation to determine accurately the distribution of malignancy in the pericervical tissues. Histologic study of exenteration specimens has disclosed bladder and rectal involvement in 40 to 50% of the cases, even though there is no gross evidence of the disease involving these organs. In addition, even when it is possible to dissect and preserve the bladder or the rectum, the relative devascularization of these organs by operation, when superimposed on the endarteritic obliteration produced by previous irradiation, can lead to ischemia and an unacceptable fistula rate of 20 to 25%. Most often, to prevent this morbidity and to provide the best opportunity of cure, total exenteration is required.

Similarly, the exenteration and the technique used to accomplish the pelvic sidewall dissection may vary with the size and fixation of the lesion. In many instances, a relatively simple and safe ligation of the medially directed visceral branch of the hypogastric artery and vein will provide adequate clearance of the malignancy. Resection of the entire hypogastric (internal iliac) arterial and venous system, including the gluteal vessels, which was advocated in the early description of the operation and which proved to be potentially hazardous, is no longer considered essential. Even so, this step still becomes necessary in certain patients because of the size of the lesion or the presence of lymph node metastasis fixed to these vessels.

PREOPERATIVE PREPARATION

The patient should be admitted to the hospital 1 to 2 days before the scheduled operation. This allows sufficient time for additional discussion of the operation with the patient and her family, and consultation with the stomal therapists — an important and integral part of the therapy team required in the management of these patients. The therapist can additionally reassure, instruct and support the patient, who often feels insecure regarding the various stomas and appliances that will be required. In addition, the therapists mark the most appropriate spot on the abdominal wall for the creation of the various stomas; particularly in the obese patient, the areas should be marked with the patient in a standing position. Early admission of the patient also permits the necessary mechanical and antibiotic preparation of the colon, and it allows additional evaluation of the patient, pulmonary preparation, metabolic improvement, blood transfusions or fluid replacement if needed. The bowel preparation is set out in Table 81.1.

Table 81.1 GoLYTELY lavage (1 day prep)

Day prior to operation	Day of operation
Clear liquid diet beginning at noon; no laxatives	Weigh patient at 6 a.m. Nothing by mouth from midnight
GoLYTELY lavage	
Drink 4–6 liters of GoLYTELY from noon to 6 p.m. (need not drink all 6 liters if bowel return is clear and remains clear before 6 p.m.) (feeding tube may need to be used)	
Neomycin 2 g 6 p.m. to 11 p.m. Metronidazole 2 g 6 p.m. to 11 p.m. (after GoLYTELY is finished)	

The anesthesiologist is responsible for the patient's supportive management, including the blood and electrolyte requirements, throughout the lengthy procedure. A general endotracheal anesthetic supplemented by muscle relaxants is considered preferable; accurate monitoring of the patient is essential. A cardiac monitor, Swan-Ganz catheter, and intravenous catheters in both arms represent standard preparation. Blood loss is determined by a weighed-sponges method. Before division of the ureters, the urinary output can be evaluated; thereafter, the urinary excretion can be observed from the cut end of the ureters. For this reason, it is important not to ligate the ureters, as some have suggested. The prompt and accurate volume-for-volume replacement of blood and electrolytes is essential. It is better to be a little ahead rather than behind in this replacement, in case unanticipated and rapid blood loss occurs.

A standard operating table is used when the patient will not require a perineal phase of the operation, or when vaginal reconstruction is not planned; when that phase is necessary, the patient may be placed in a 'ski' position, with the legs separated and slightly flexed laterally on well-padded leg braces. If a complete radical vulvectomy is essential, the patient is placed in the lithotomy position at the proper time. Snug elastic stockings, extending up to the knees, are worn, and the table is placed in a medium Trendelenburg position to promote venous drainage during the operation. Sequential positive pressure leg compression devices are also used.

Pelvic examination under anesthesia is done to re-evaluate the extent of the lesion. A small Foley catheter is inserted in the bladder; the vagina, perineum and thighs are prepared with povidone-iodine solution, and a pack soaked in 90% alcohol is inserted in the infected and, per-haps, necrotic malignant cavity in the upper vagina. The abdomen is prepared up to the xiphoid and draped widely so that the stomas can be created without rearranging the drapes. When the patient is in the ski position, secondary drapes may be used to exclude the perineal field; these are applied in such a manner that they can be readily removed at the proper time to expose both operative fields without disturbing the abdominal exposure.

EVALUATION OF OPERABILITY

Although various elaborate diagnostic techniques (such as lymphography, venography, ultrasonography, magnetic resonance imaging and computed tomography) can be ap-plied in an effort to determine the operability of the individual patient, none has been reliably accurate. As a rule, abdominal exploration provides the most prompt, inexpensive, and accurate method of determining the operability of the recurrent lesion. Unilateral leg edema and sciatic nerve pain are the only relatively reliable indicators of inoperability, short of exploration.

Initially, only a short midline incision should be made just below the umbilicus; it should be large enough to allow a cursory abdominal exploration by palpation. Attention is directed to palpation of the aortic and pelvic lymph nodes, celiac area, liver and all peritoneal surfaces. When obvious gross extrapelvic malignancy is noted, either a direct biopsy or the passage of a Tru-cut needle or fine needle aspir-ation through the abdominal wall (guided by the intra-abdominal hand) can be used to secure sufficient tissue for an immediate pathologic study and histologic confirmation of the distant metastases. (See Ch. 22.)

Extrapelvic lymph node, peritoneal or distant metastasis represents the only absolute indication that the lesion is inoperable. Peritoneal involvement by direct extension of the malignancy into an adjacent, adherent structure (sigmoid, ileum, tube or ovary) does not contraindicate proceeding with the operation; significant salvage has been obtained in patients with this rather ominous-appearing situation. When the lesion is deemed inoperable, the small diagnostic abdominal incision is quickly closed; this ap-proach produces minimal morbidity, avoids the time and expense required for many of the elaborate 'closed' diag-nostic techniques, and requires only brief hospitalization.

When nothing has been detected that would indicate absolute inoperability, the midline incision is extended around and well above the umbilicus and down to the pubic symphysis. Wide exposure and considerable deep

pelvic sidewall dissection will be required in order to determine the local resectability of the recurrent pelvic malignancy. Although some surgeons prefer to use a long transverse lower abdominal incision, we continue to prefer the midline: (1) it provides better access to the upper ab-domen if that is required for assessment of metastasis; (2) the mobilization of omentum, which is often used to cover the denuded pelvis or the newly constructed vagina, can be more readily accomplished; (3) it may be necessary to use the transverse colon to create the urinary conduit; and (4) the stomas can be created more readily, especially if previous irradiation has made the skin of the lower ab-domen unsuitable for acceptance of the appliances that will be required.

In most of the patients considered for exenteration, preceding irradiation and inflammation have produced a variable degree of pelvic fibrosis and fixation of all struc-tures. Simple inspection and palpation of the pelvic node-bearing areas, even by the experienced surgeon, may provide little information other than to indicate that large, matted and fixed areas of metastasis are present. If such metastatic masses are securely fixed to the major vessels, this may well indicate that resection is not feasible or that a resection will be palliative at best.

As a rule, the resectability of lymph node metastasis and the possibility of complete removal of a central pelvic recurrent lesion can be determined only after the peritoneum has been opened to expose the various fascial planes of the pelvis and broad ligaments. It is important at this early stage in the operation to obtain accurate assess-ment of pelvic involvement by developing the paravesical, pararectal, and presacral spaces to a deep level in the pel-vis. Familiarity with these fascial spaces allows rather complete evaluation of resectability without division of any of the major vessels, without significant blood loss, and with minimal trauma to the bladder, ureters and rectum. Because no major structure has been divided, a simple retreat remains possible when a non-resectable area of malignancy is encountered. Evaluation of the pelvic sidewall should be attempted first on the side that appears to be most extensively involved, and then on the other side. Punch biopsy and needle biopsy specimens may be ob-tained from deep points of fixation to the pelvic sidewall or levator fascia and can provide valuable additional information.

Retreat becomes quite difficult once the ureters and colon have been divided. It is apparent that these struc-tures should be avoided until the decision has been made to proceed with the operation. This decision can be ex-cruciatingly difficult; frequently, it is based to a major extent on the experience and judgment of the surgeon. This will not be infallible even in the best of hands, and occasionally one will proceed beyond the point of easy return before finding a non-resectable area.

Malignant involvement of the fascia covering the

puborectalis or pubococcygeus portion of the levator muscle can be easily resected en bloc with the specimen; extensions of malignancy into sacrum, sacral plexus, iliopsoas muscle and sidewall of pelvis, even though they may be 'technically resectable', are usually considered 'inoperable' because significant salvage and cures have not been obtained. Histologic evidence of resectable, recurrent malignancy is a requisite for proceeding with operation; rarely, exenteration will be essential for a patient who has incapacitating, painful irradiation necrosis producing rectovesicovaginal fistula.

OPERATIVE TECHNIQUE

Initial dissection

The round ligament, a relatively constant landmark even in a pelvis obliterated by irradiation fibrosis and adhesions, is divided and ligated near the internal abdominal ring.

The peritoneal incision extends upward just lateral to the ovarian vessels to the pelvic brim, and medially toward the bladder. Blunt dissection of the areolar tissue in the lateral portion of the broad ligament exposes the external iliac vessels. Tracing these in a cephalad direction, one can quickly identify the bifurcation of the iliac artery and the internal iliac artery (Fig. 81.1A). The ureter is attached to the peritoneum just medial to the iliac bifurcation. The ovarian vessels are elevated, and the infundibulopelvic ligament is ligated and divided just above the pelvic brim (Fig. 81.1B).

Development of paravesical space

Using firm traction on the uterus and on the medial leaf of the broad ligament peritoneum toward the opposite side, one can dissect downward on the internal iliac artery to identify the obliterated hypogastric artery (umbilical), which extends anteriorly as a white fibrous cord along the lateral edge of the bladder. Blunt dissection immediately

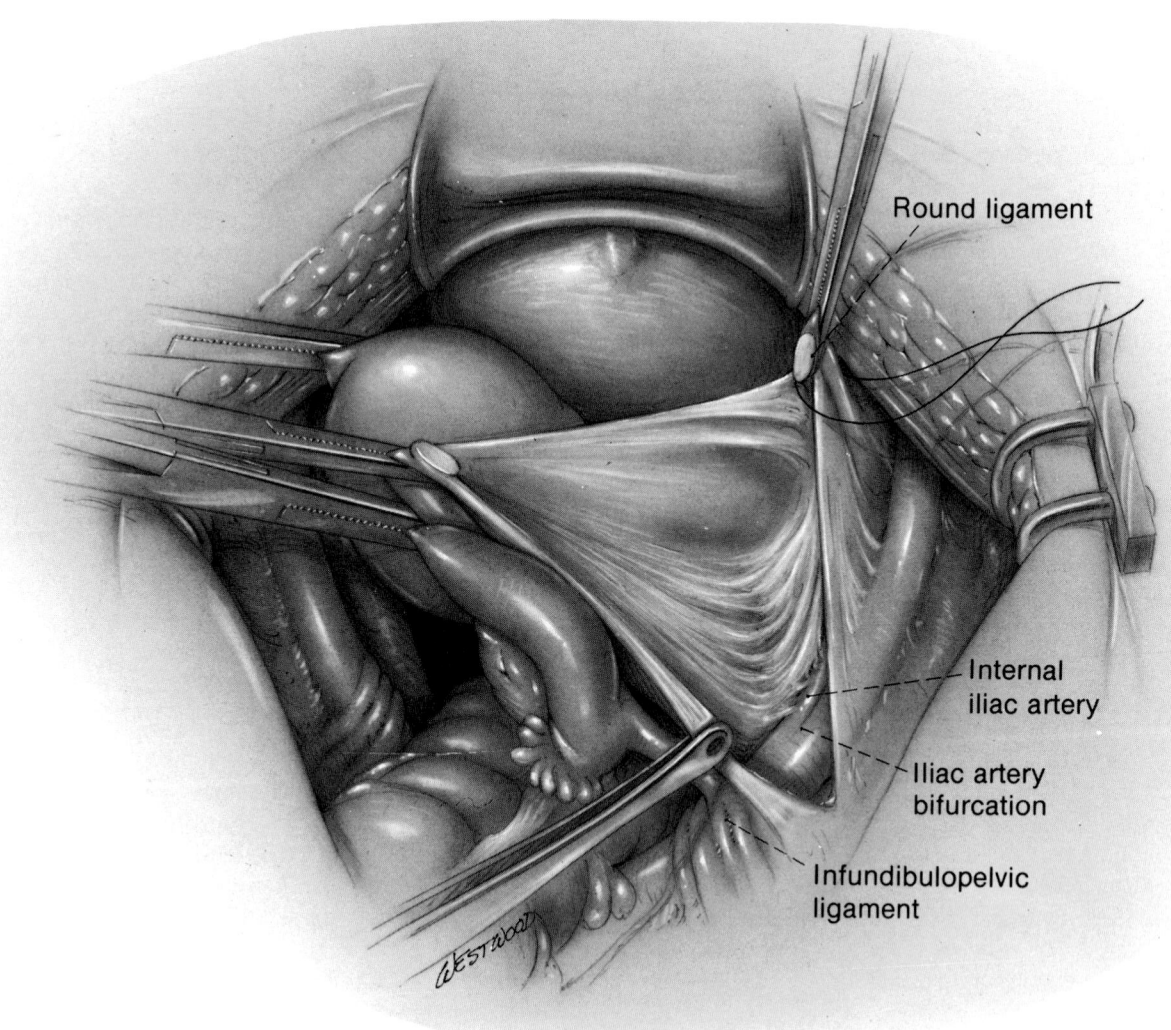

Round ligament

Internal iliac artery

Iliac artery bifurcation

Infundibulopelvic ligament

A

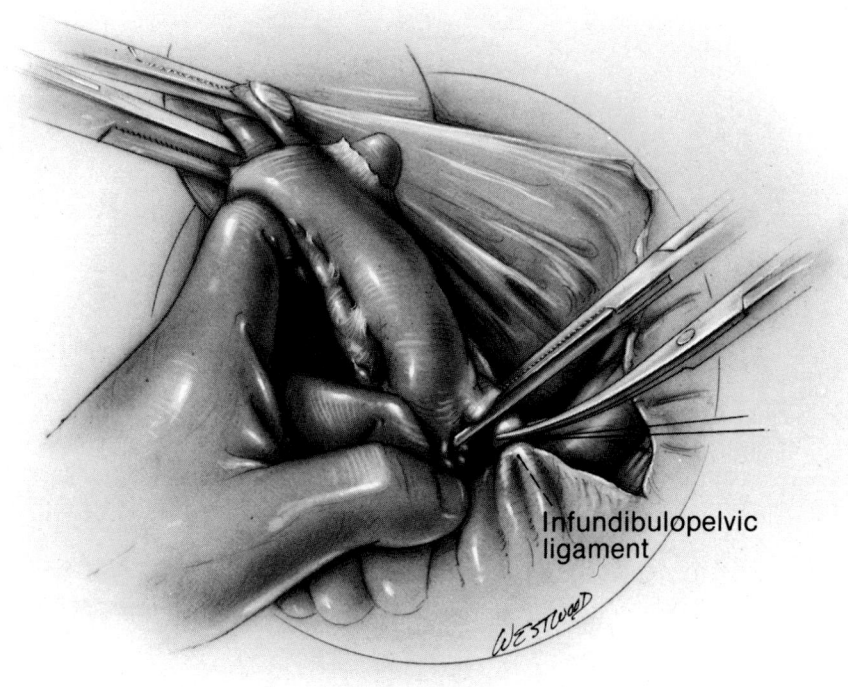

B

Fig. 81.1 (A) The round ligament is divided; the uterus and adnexa are pulled firmly to the opposite side. Dissection of the broad ligament areolar tissue exposes the iliac artery bifurcation and ovarian vessels at the pelvic brim. The ureter is located just medial to the ovarian vessels in the infundibulopelvic ligament. (B) Elevation of the tube and ovary displaces the ovarian vessels and allows their ligation at the pelvic brim adjacent to the ureter.

lateral to this 'white cord' allows it to be displaced medially along with the bladder, and permits entry into the avascular paravesical space (Fig. 81.2). With progressive blunt downward dissection and with medial displacement of the bladder, the latter is completely mobilized from the anterior pubic ramus, exposing the lower end of the obturator vessels, nerves and lymph nodes in the obturator space (which have been displaced laterally); the fascial surface of the obturator internus muscle; and the anterior portion of the levator muscles. Even in the presence of previous high-dosage pelvic radiation therapy, this paravesical fascial plane can be easily developed down to the anterior pelvic floor (levator muscle) without encountering any significant bleeding. A wide Deaver or Harrington retractor is inserted into this space to hold the bladder and vagina medially (Fig. 81.2).

Development of presacral and pararectal space

Similarly, with medial and upward traction on the medial leaf of peritoneum containing the ureter, blunt dissection progressing downward and medially from the internal iliac artery allows identification of the presacral and pararectal spaces. If the risk of heavy venous bleeding is to be avoided, this dissection must be directed medially toward

the hollow of the sacrum and away from the internal iliac vessels and the lateral sacral veins (Fig. 81.3). When the proper fascial plane has been identified, blunt dissection by hand can develop the presacral and pararectal spaces to a low, almost coccygeal, level. Once again, this is a bloodless tissue plane that, as a rule, has not been obliterated by previous irradiation fibrosis. It can be identified and dissected quickly and expeditiously. A second Harrington retractor can be inserted in this presacral space and pulled carefully toward the opposite side.

Evaluation of resectability of lesion

With the paravesical and pararectal dissection established, and with the bladder, uterus, vagina and rectosigmoid retracted toward the opposite side, the entire lateral 'web' of tissue extending from these organs to the pelvic sidewall and the pelvic floor has been exposed (Fig. 81.3). This web contains all of the visceral branches of the internal iliac vessels, the parametrial, paracervical and paravaginal supporting tissues (cardinal ligament), and the postrectal pillars and pararectal tissues. With these lateral tissues thus displayed, careful palpation of them between opposing thumb and fingers will disclose the lateral extent of the central malignancy and the degree of fixation, and will

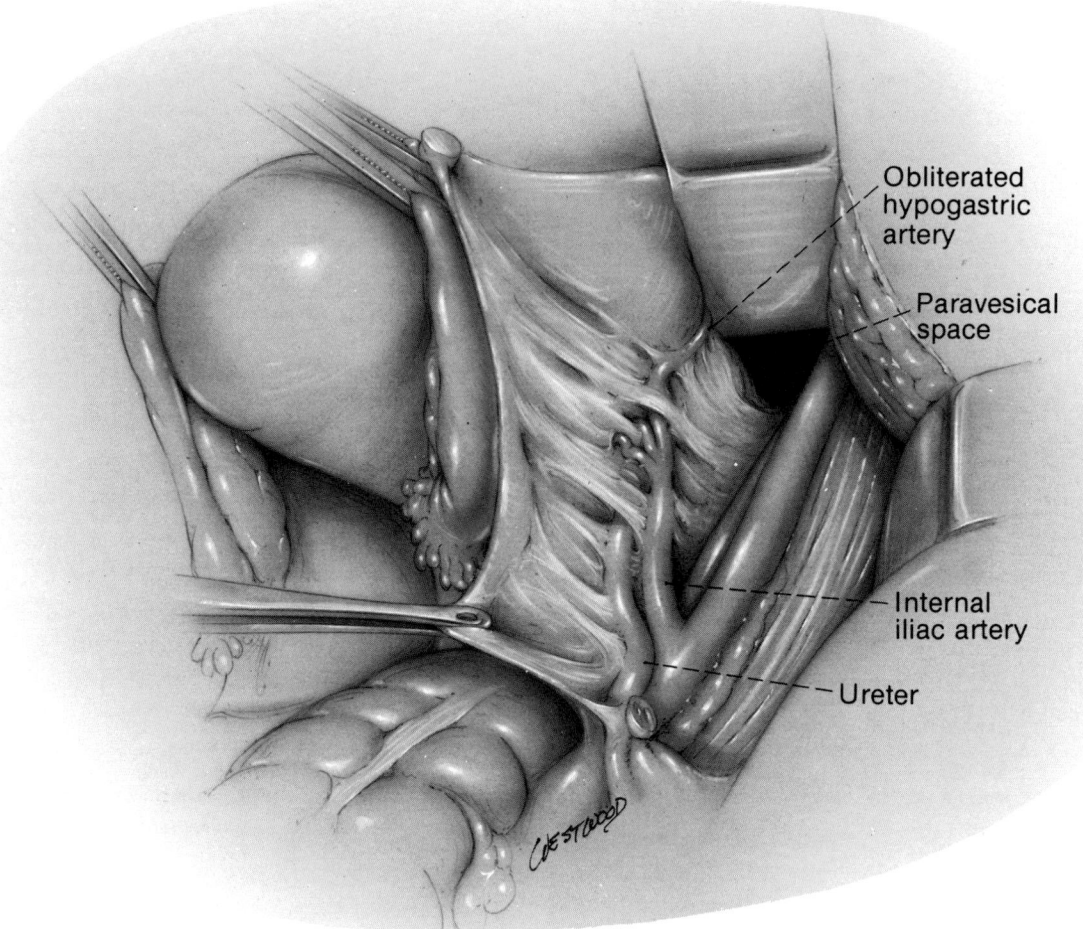

Fig. 81.2 Blunt dissection downward along the course of the internal iliac artery allows identification of the obliterated hypogastric artery; its medial displacement will permit identification of the paravesical space through an avascular field.

allow an estimate of resectability. To this point, as a rule, the node-bearing tissue in the area of the external iliac vessels and obturator fossa has been allowed to remain in place. These regions are carefully palpated to detect the presence and resectability of lymph node metastasis.

Occasionally, to determine the resectability of large and relatively fixed lymph node metastasis before proceeding with a dissection of the paravesical and pararectal spaces, one is safer in starting the dissection by proceeding downward between the external iliac vessels (which are displaced medially) and the iliopsoas muscle, which is retracted laterally. This allows one to enter the obturator space laterally and expose the obturator nerve as it emerges from beneath the iliopsoas muscle (Fig. 81.4). Usually, the nerve can be displaced laterally from any obturator lymph node involved by metastasis; however, the nerve can be sacrificed with little resulting disability whenever it appears to be incorporated into the malignant process. Similarly, it may be found that the node metastases are securely fixed to the external iliac vein (usually to the inferior surface) and to the anterior surface of the internal iliac vein and

artery. Because all of these vessels can be removed without producing significant sequelae, one can still proceed with the operation when it appears that their sacrifice will permit complete clearance and medial displacement of the metastatic mass.

A word of caution is necessary; the dissection should not proceed too far into this deep area along the lateral pelvic wall, where venous bleeding from gluteal branches of the internal iliac vein can be critical. When cursory evaluation of the lateral obturator space suggests resectability of a direct extension or nodal metastasis, the efforts of the surgeon should be directed elsewhere and additional dissection of this difficult region deferred until later, after dissection of the opposite and more favorable side of the pelvis and after the entire specimen has been 'teed-up,' so to speak.

Serious bleeding is invariably of venous origin with this operation. When this is encountered in a deep and difficult area, it is advisable merely to insert a pack, perhaps with compression of the pack with a deep Harrington retractor held by an assistant, rather than to waste time and effort in trying to control it. One then proceeds with the dissec-

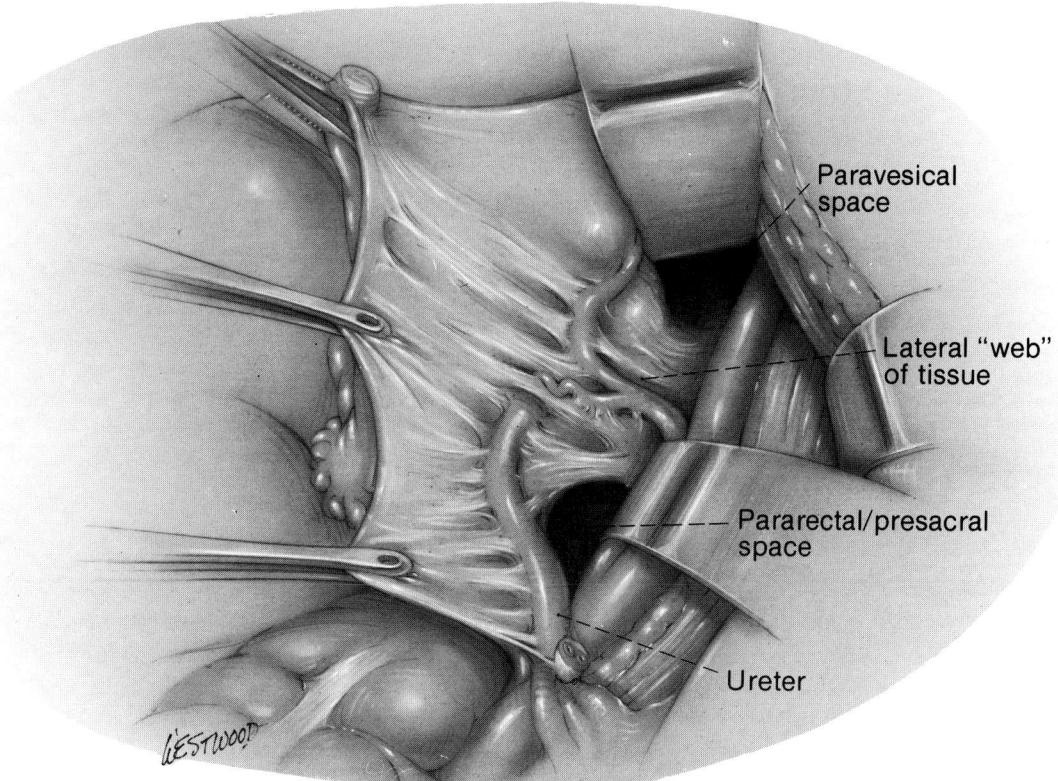

Paravesical space

Lateral "web" of tissue

Pararectal/presacral space

Ureter

Fig. 81.3 Firm upward and medial traction on the uterus and medial leaf of peritoneum allows blunt dissection of the pararectal and presacral spaces. With a retractor inserted in the paravesical space and another in the pararectal space, the lateral 'web' of tissue extending to the pelvic side-wall will be displayed. This contains all of the visceral branches of the internal iliac artery and veins.

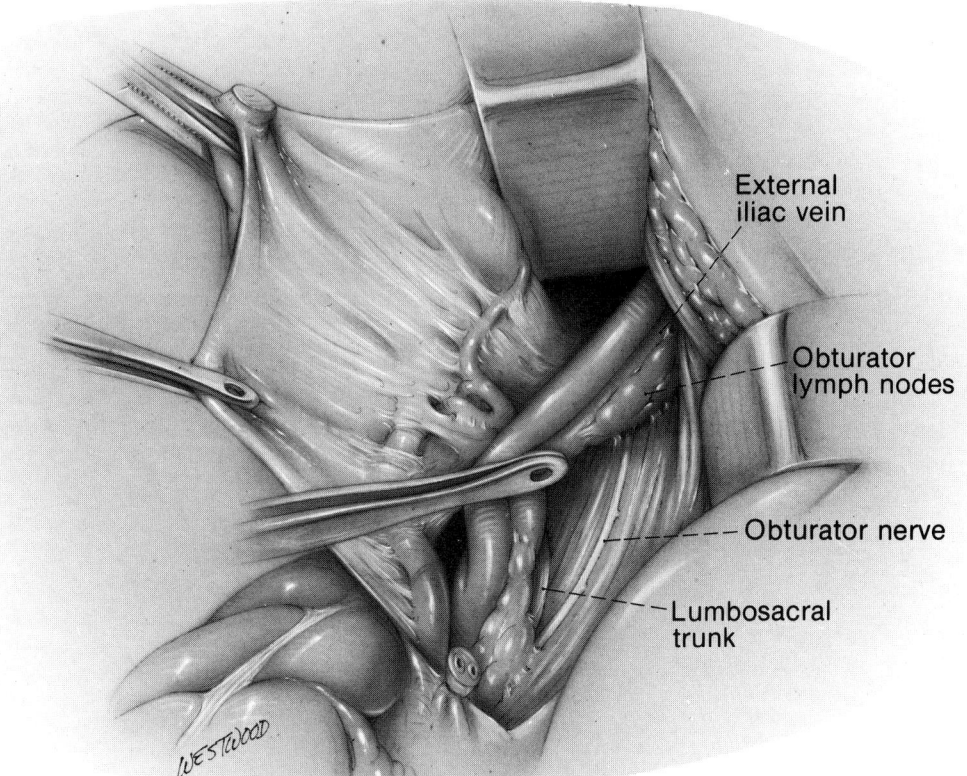

External iliac vein

Obturator lymph nodes

Obturator nerve

Lumbosacral trunk

Fig. 81.4 In the presence of a large fixed mass in the cardinal ligament 'web' (or dense postradiation fibrosis), a lateral approach to the area may be essential to determine operability. The external iliac vessels are displaced and retracted medially; this will permit dissection down through for identification of the obturator nerve, lumbosacral trunk, and parietal branches of the internal iliac vessels (not shown) that perforate posteriorly. Dissection should proceed very cautiously in this deep area, for serious bleeding can occur and its control can be difficult.

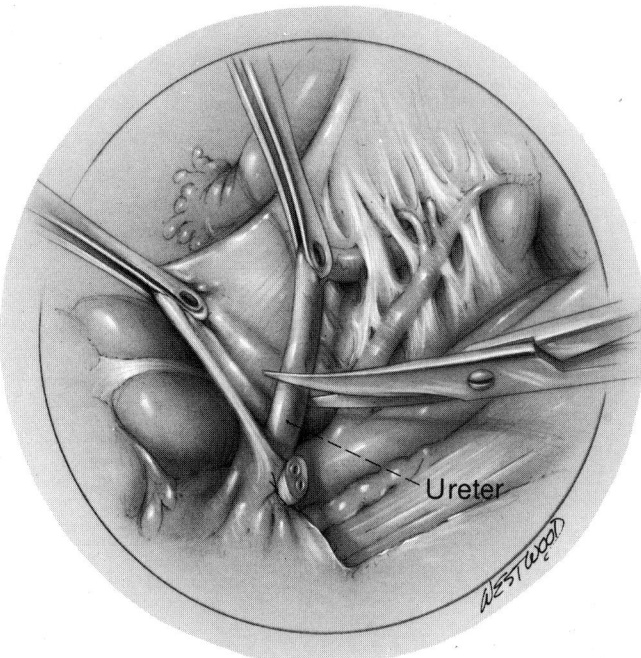

Fig. 81.5 When both sides of the pelvis have been evaluated and the lesion appears to be resectable, the ureters can be divided near the pelvic brim and the incision can be carried medially across the posterior pelvic peritoneum to the lower sigmoid area.

tion in another and, one hopes, more favorable area. Biopsy specimens can be taken of any suspicious areas, which, if positive, might influence the decision to continue with the operation.

Mobilization of rectum and bladder

When it is apparent that the lesion is resectable, the operation can proceed to the point of commitment. The ureters are divided about 2 cm below the pelvic brim, approximately where they cross the bifurcation of the iliac artery (Fig. 81.5). The pelvic peritoneum is incised medially to the lower sigmoid on each side. The superior hemorrhoidal vessels are ligated and divided; the colon is divided between clamps at the appropriate level (Figs 81.6 and 81.7).

At this time, if a colostomy is to be created, the bowel can be brought through the left lower abdominal wall at the proper position (marked preoperatively); however, when a sigmoid conduit is planned for urinary diversion — the conduit that we favor with total exenteration — the sigmoid is merely wrapped in a laparotomy pad and displaced out onto the abdominal wall at the upper end of the incision.

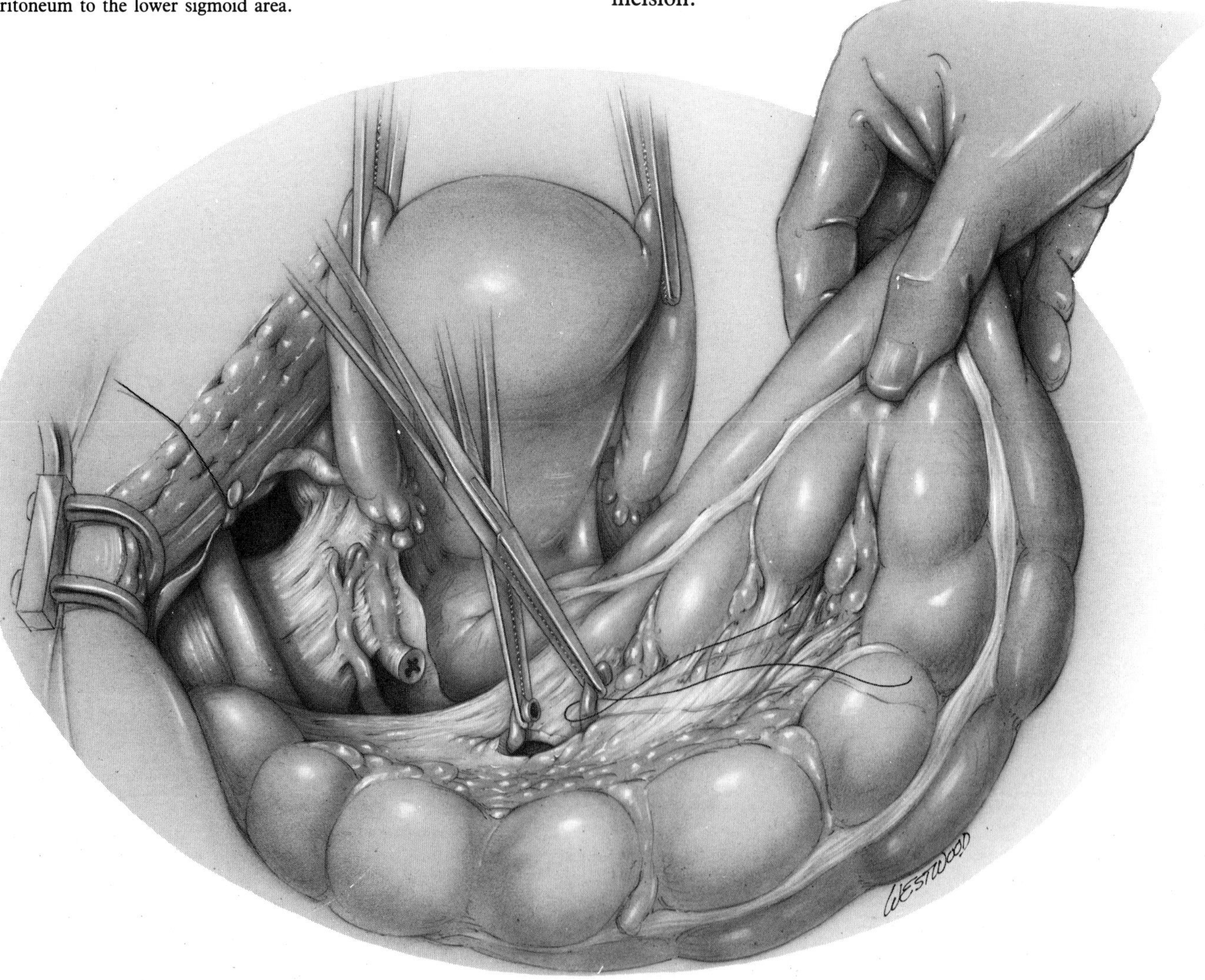

Fig. 81.6 The superior hemorrhoidal vessels are ligated and divided at the low-sigmoid level.

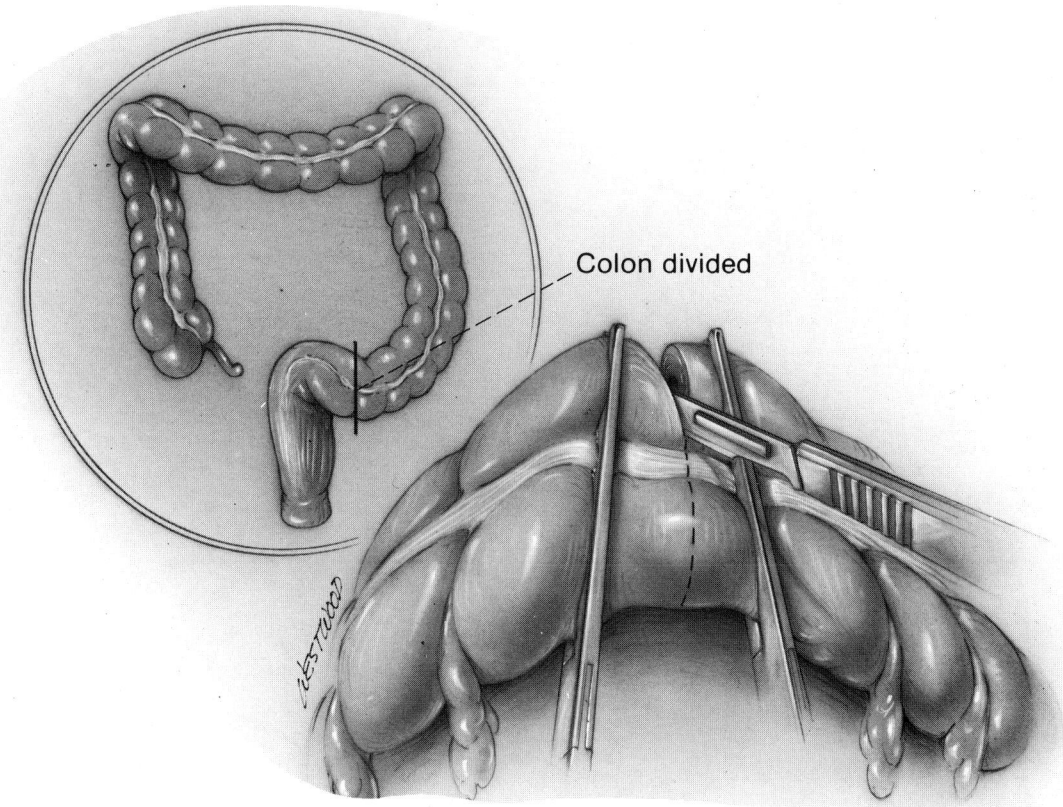

Colon divided

Fig. 81.7 The sigmoid is divided between clamps at a low level, with preservation of as much of the colon as possible since it may be used later for a sigmoid conduit urinary diversion. The clamp on the distal end of the divided bowel can remain in place to be used for traction on the specimen; as an alternative method, the distal end of the bowel can be closed with a single row of hemostatic stitches.

The advent of the intraluminal stapling device has allowed low re-anastomosis of the descending colon to the anus in a significant number of instances. Usually, the previous pelvic irradiation has not extended to the region of the anus, and a stapled anastomosis avoids a permanent colostomy. If the perianal area has been fully irradiated, then a temporary defunctioning colostomy may be indicated to protect the anastomosis. (See Ch. 88.)

The clamp on the distal end of the divided bowel remains in place, to be used for traction and manipulation of the specimen during the remainder of the dissection; however, when a wide perineal resection is anticipated and the entire specimen will be delivered from below, the distal end of the bowel should be oversewn or stapled and dropped back into the pelvis.

Going anteriorly, the distal end of the obliterated hypogastric artery is ligated near the anterior abdominal wall, and the parietal peritoneum is incised medially over the dome of the bladder (Fig. 81.8). Downward pressure on the bladder completely mobilizes it down to the subpubic arch and urethral region. As much vesical peritoneum as possible is preserved to cover the denuded pelvic floor. Once again, this is an avascular plane. With the bladder thus freed up, and the rectum mobilized from the hollow of the sacrum, the tissues can be retracted to the opposite side of the pelvis by means of two deep Harrington retractors placed lateral to the organs. This permits exposure of the lateral web so that the individual branches of the internal iliac vessels can be accurately ligated and divided (Fig. 81.8).

Dissection and management of internal iliac vessels

The internal iliac vessels are managed in one of several ways, depending on the extent of the malignancy and their degree of fixation by irradiation fibrosis. When the lesion is centrally located, it may be possible to obtain wide clearance of the malignancy merely by individually ligating all of the visceral branches of the internal iliac vessels. The anterior division (uterine artery, vesical and obliterated hypogastric artery) of the internal iliac artery is ligated and divided initially; this is followed by individual ligation and division, as far laterally as possible, of the more deeply located minor visceral branches that course medially (vaginal, vesical and obturator arteries and veins; Fig. 81.9). The pudendal artery, which is located more laterally and extends directly inferiorly, should be ligated when a perineal phase of the operation is planned. This is a relatively simple and safe dissection, for it avoids the sacral plexus and the gluteal vessels. Unfortunately, it is not always

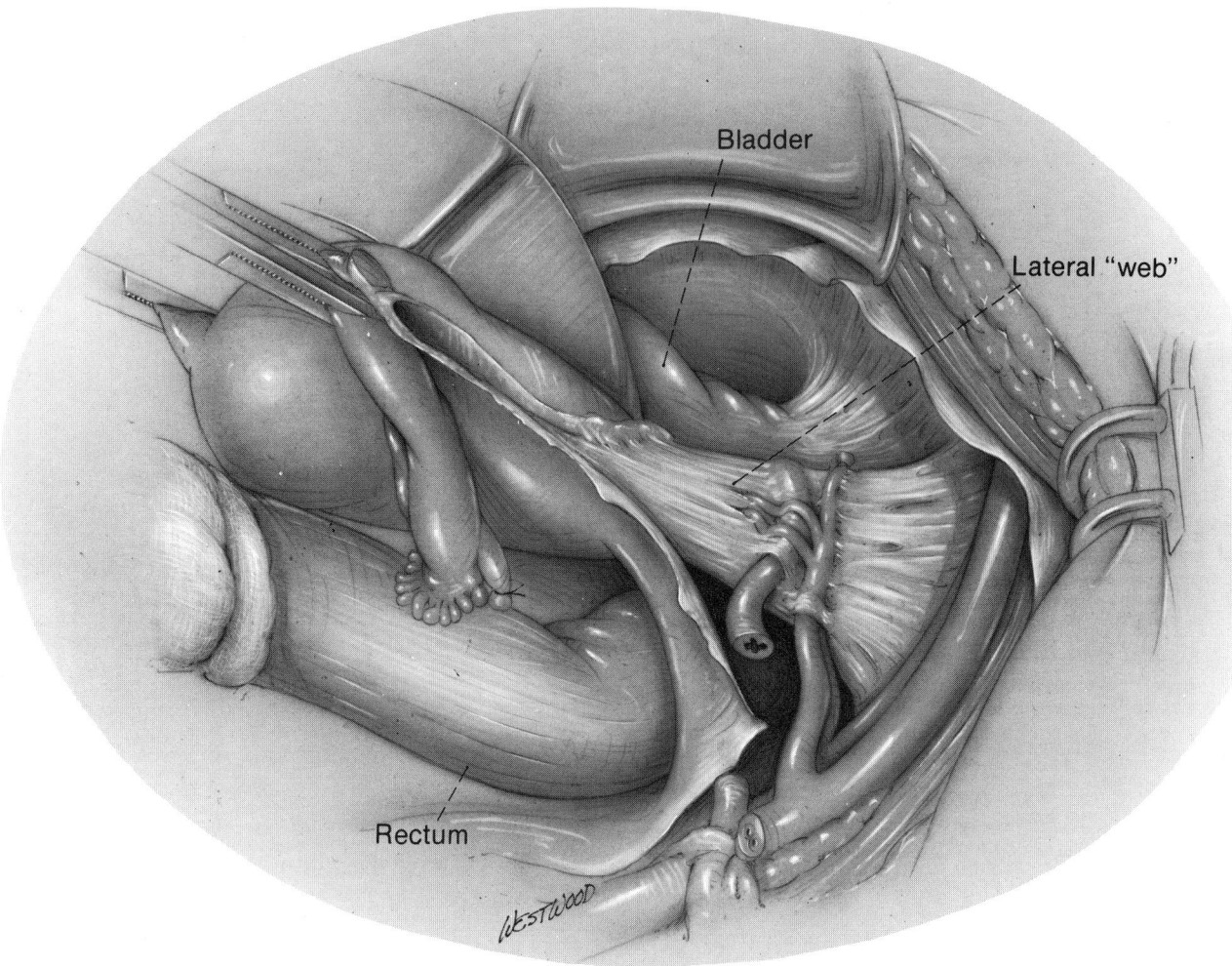

Fig. 81.8 After the distal end of the obliterated hypogastric artery has been divided and the anterior parietal peritoneum has been incised on each side, the bladder can be easily displaced posteriorly from the pubic rami and pubic symphysis. The rectum is additionally mobilized with blunt dissection from the hollow of the sacrum down to the sacrococcygeal level. Firm traction upward and to the opposite side on the specimen will allow accurate dissection of the lateral web of tissue and ligation of the individual branches of the internal iliac vessels flush with the pelvic side wall and sacral plexus.

possible. There may be relatively little space between the tumor and the pelvic sidewall, or the area may be so densely fibrotic that the identification of individual branches is impossible.

In most instances, after ligation and diversion of the anterior division of the internal iliac artery, it is advisable from the standpoint of time and risk of blood loss merely to cross-clamp the entire cardinal ligament 'web' of tissue as far laterally as possible without injuring the sacral plexus. Even with a large and fixed tumor, it should be possible to insert a large-curve Kelly clamp down across this relatively broad, fibrous and vascular web (Fig. 81.10). When the tissue is divided, the entire specimen can be displaced medially; backbleeding from the visceral (specimen) side will not be excessive, or it can be covered with a laparotomy pad and compressed with a Harrington retractor. The rather thick, linear mass of fibrotic tissue engaged by the Kelly clamp, which contains all of the remaining visceral branches of the internal iliac artery and vein, is too large and dense for it to be merely ligated. It must be controlled by undersewing the clamp. After removal of the clamp, traction on the suture prevents retraction of the vessels. As a rule, hemostasis is satisfactory; nevertheless, a second row of continuous locking sutures is advisable for this rather large and vascular stump (Fig. 81.11). Absorbable suture material should be used for this purpose because it is possible that the suture may be close to, or even engage, some of the underlying fibers of the sacral plexus. The 'mass ligature' method described can save considerable operative time; in addition, it avoids or diminishes the hazard of severe bleeding from the underlying gluteal veins.

In still other patients, depending on the size and location of the malignancy, it may be necessary to remove the entire internal iliac artery and vein. If possible, the artery is ligated just below the origin of the superior gluteal artery;

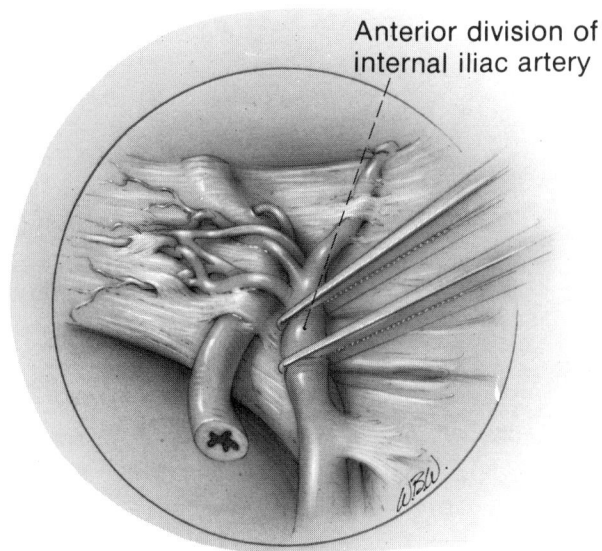

Anterior division of
internal iliac artery

Fig. 81.9 With some vascular configurations, the ligation of the 'anterior division' of the internal iliac artery may include not only the uterine artery but most of the vaginal and vesical arterial branches as well; this leaves little arterial supply to the specimen below this level. Control of arterial bleeding is rarely a problem with this operation; however, serious, even critical, bleeding of venous origin can commonly occur below this level.

one can then ligate and divide the large internal iliac vein, which lies just posterolaterally. By gentle retraction of the distal stumps of artery and vein medially, the dissection can proceed deep to the fascial plane covering the sacral plexus, and the posteriorly perforating parietal vessels (gluteal and pudendal vessels and lesser branches) can be identified and ligated individually for gradual exposure of the roots of the sacral plexus (Fig. 81.12).

In some patients, the internal iliac vein is located more laterally — almost on the pelvic brim with the lumbosacral trunk — and can be left undisturbed. In others, after division of the internal iliac artery, a lateral approach to the internal iliac vein through the obturator space may be safer. The external iliac artery and vein are retracted medially, and the iliopsoas muscle is retracted laterally for better exposure of the individual venous trunks. The upper end of the obturator fossa is exposed; the obturator nerve emerges from beneath the medial edge of the iliopsoas (Fig. 81.12). The fatty node-bearing tissue is carefully displaced downward from this area. Immediately underlying the obturator nerve, approximately 1 cm deeper and slightly medial, the lumbosacral trunk courses downward across the pelvic brim to join the roots of the sacral plexus in

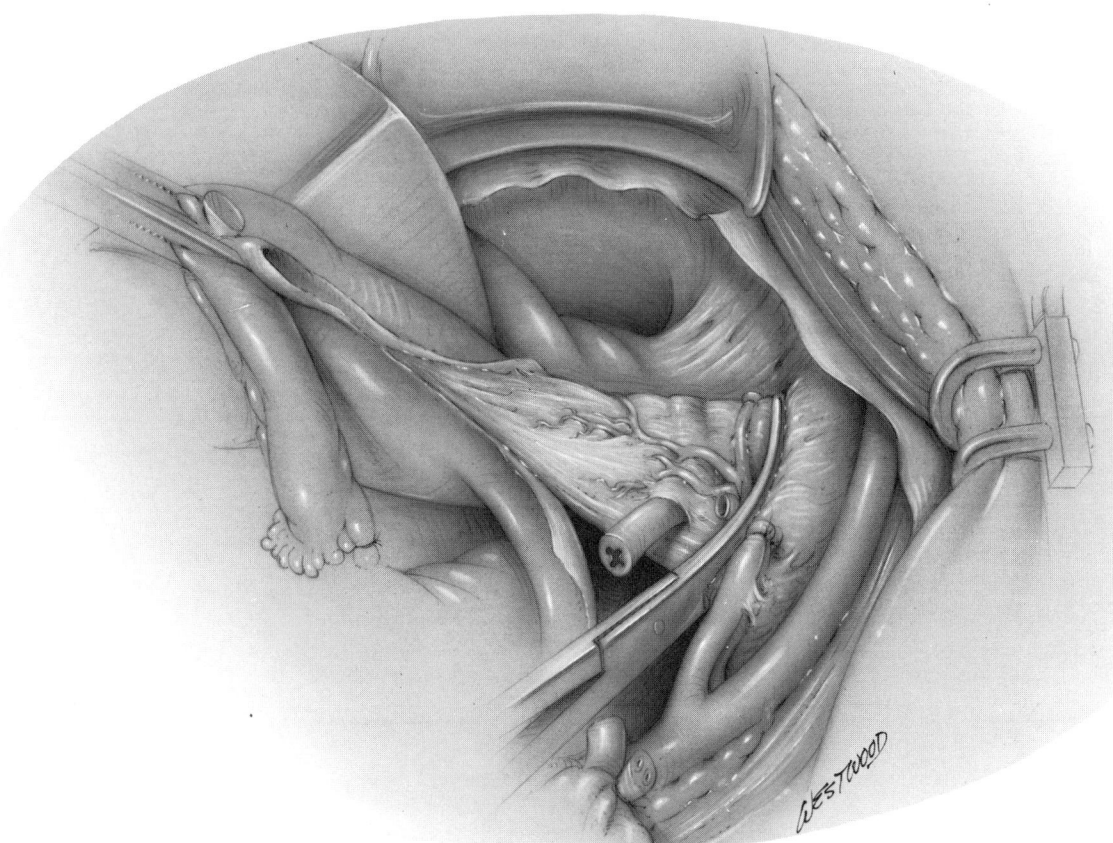

Fig. 81.10 Particularly in the postirradiation patient, efforts to dissect the individual branches may be associated with excessive blood loss. Rather than a tedious dissection of the individual large venous branches in the lower portion of the cardinal 'web', it may be safer to cross-clamp the tissue en mass as far lateral as possible without damage to the roots of the underlying sacral plexus.

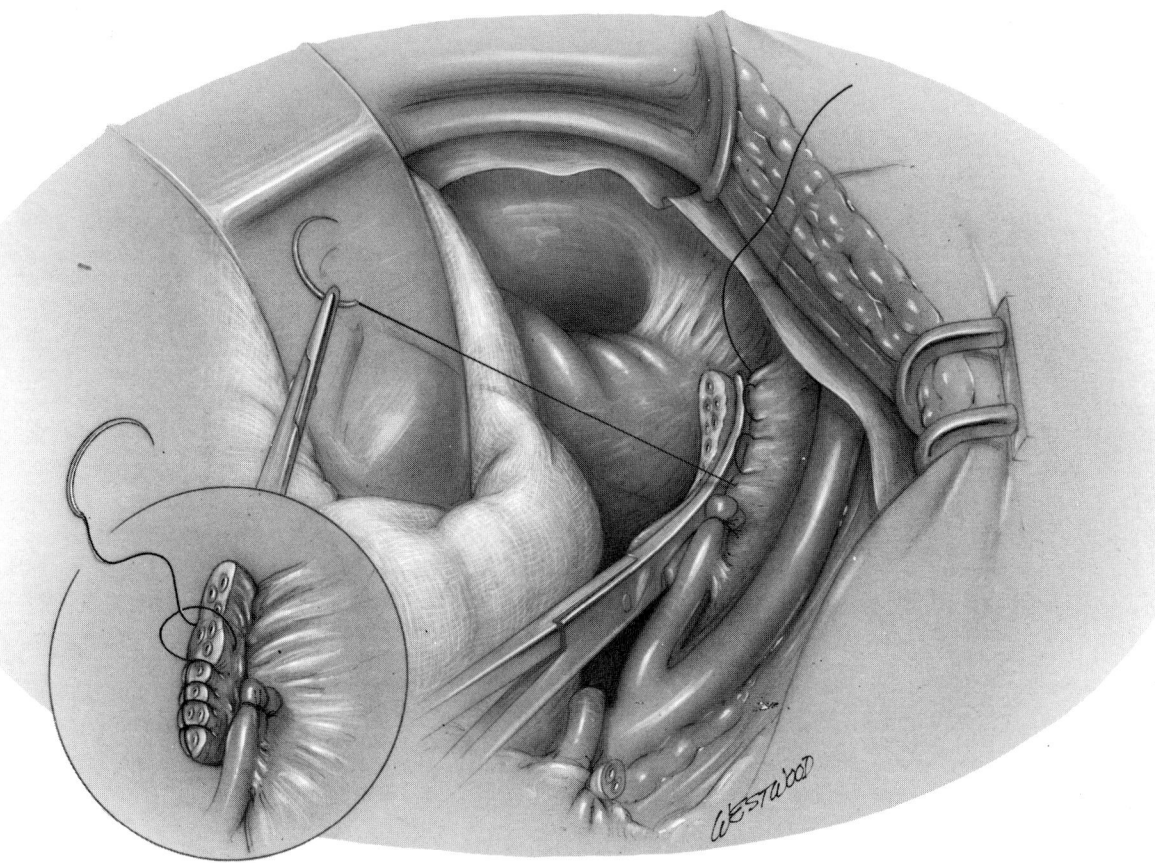

Fig. 81.11 Hemostasis can be obtained most securely and safely merely by undersewing the clamp with heavy suture material (no. 1 chromic catgut). With traction on the two ends of the suture material, good hemostasis is provided when the clamp is removed. The suture prevents retraction of vessels between roots of the sacral plexus. The same suture can be carried as a running lock stitch back down the ligament stump to provide additional hemostasis.

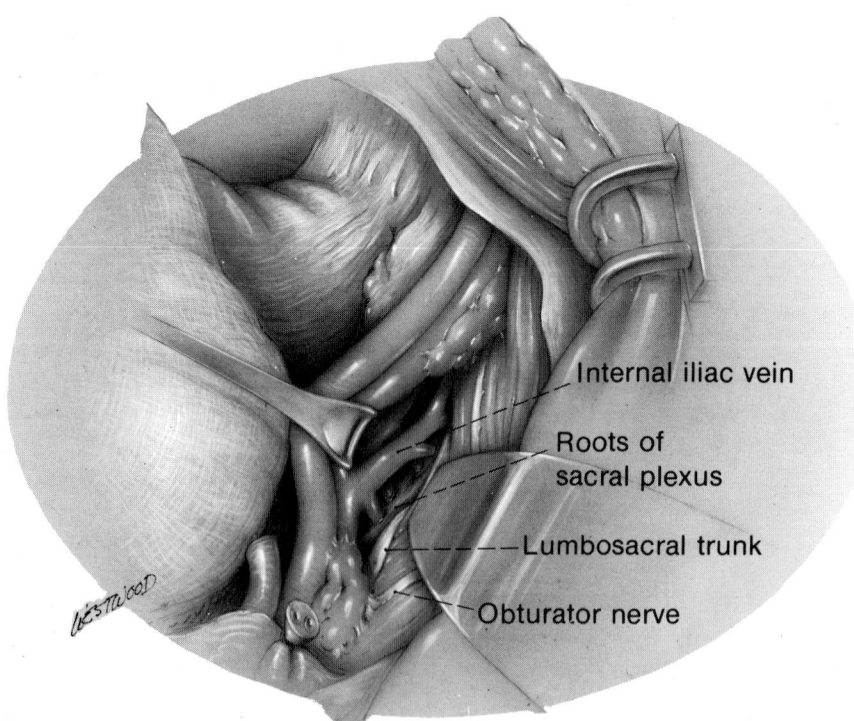

Fig. 81.12 When it is essential to remove the entire internal iliac artery and vein, accurate identification of the short, perforating posterior gluteal branches may be best obtained in some patients by a lateral approach through the obturator area. In other situations, lateral retraction of the external iliac vessels may allow better exposure for individual ligation of the gluteal and pudendal branches of the internal iliac vessels.

forming the sciatic nerve. Extreme care must be taken in this area to avoid the iliolumbar vein and the smaller iliolumbar artery, which branch posteriorly from the internal iliac vessels; bleeding can be difficult to control in this deep crevice without producing injury to the lumbosacral trunk (L-4 and L-5), the source of fibers of the common peroneal nerve. With the use of a right-angle gallbladder forceps (Shallcross) passed down either lateral or medial to the external iliac vessels (whichever gives the best access), the superior and inferior gluteal veins and the pudendal artery and vein can be clamped and ligated on the pelvic sidewall, flush with the exposed roots of the sacral plexus (Fig. 81.12). Either manual or retractor pressure on the vessels on the specimen side prevents significant backbleeding.

The inferior gluteal vessels perforate downward between the roots of the sacral plexus (S-2 and S-3). Before efforts are made to ligate and divide the critical vessels, it is imperative to have the viscera vigorously retracted medially to maintain good exposure of this deep area. It is wise to anticipate blood loss and to administer blood transfusions, or at least to have the supply hooked up at this critical point of the dissection.

When the gluteal veins are lacerated or they escape from the clamp or ligature and perhaps retract under the sacral plexus, vigorous bleeding can ensue that can be most difficult to control. Serious, even fatal, venous bleeding can occur from this area.

Finger compression of the bleeding source followed by undersewing of the fingertip with a fine absorbable suture may provide the best means of control; a small atraumatic needle is used for this purpose. As the finger compression is slightly relaxed, the needle is dipped under the fingertip and down between the sacral roots in the hope of engaging a portion of the retracted vein (Fig. 81.13). In some instances, rather than make a prolonged effort to obtain hemostasis, it is best to insert a small, free patch of rectus muscle into the area; this is a good and quickly available hemostatic agent. A laparotomy pad is placed over the area and compressed with a deep Harrington retractor while one proceeds with the dissection in a more favorable region. When it is necessary to remove the pack later in the operation, minimal bleeding may be noted, or at least the area will be more readily exposed and the bleeding controlled after the viscera have been removed.

Division of levator muscles

When the recurrent malignancy does not involve the lower one-third of the vagina, and the patient is not grossly

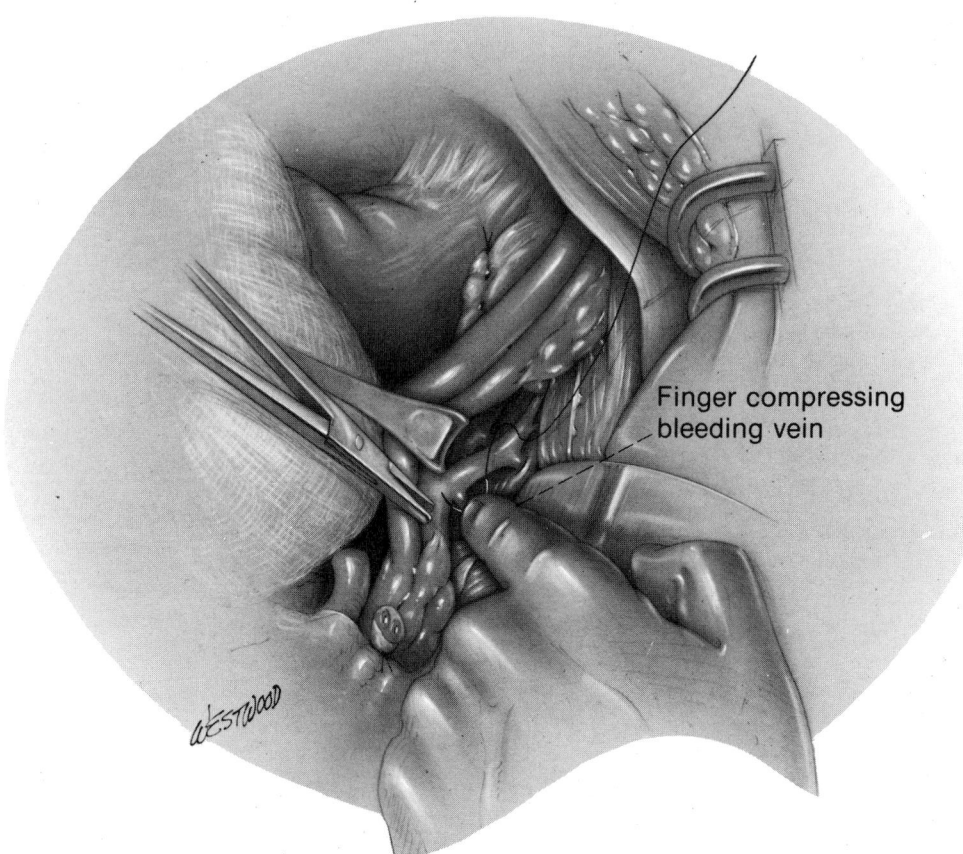

Finger compressing bleeding vein

Fig. 81.13 When vigorous bleeding occurs from a venous sinus or a gluteal vein, finger compression from either a lateral (obturator) or a medial (not shown) approach can provide the most rapid control. It may be possible to undersew the fingertip to catch the walls of the gluteal vein and prevent its retraction; gentle traction on the suture will provide sufficient hemostasis to allow the remainder of the damaged vessel to be oversewn.

obese, the exenteration can be completed entirely from the abdominal approach. The viscera have been completely mobilized from the pelvic sidewall and are free except for the inferior attachment of the pelvic organs to the levator muscles and the low sacrococcygeal area. With firm traction on the specimen in a cephalad direction, long scissors or a long-handled knife can be used to divide the deep tissues (Fig. 81.14). The anterior and lateral attachments of the levator muscles to the pubic rami and to the obturator internus fascia, are inside the pelvis and are easily exposed; they can be divided most accurately from above under direct vision. The anterior portion of the levator muscles is incised at the pelvic sidewall where these muscles attach at the arcus tendineus to the fascia of the obturator internus muscle. This exposes the underlying fatty tissue within the ischiorectal fossa. The pubic arch attachment of the pubococcygeus muscle, the pubourethral ligaments, and the urogenital diaphragm are divided. Less bleeding occurs if the levator muscles are incised directly on the pubic bone and as close to the arcus tendineus as possible (Fig. 81.14). Blunt finger dissection under the pubic arch separates the tissues above the external urethral meatus. Firm anterior and upward traction on

the rectum and on the specimen permits division of the posterior rectal pillars and the levator muscle from their sacral and coccygeal attachments (Fig. 81.15).

Resection of organs

With all of the rectal, vaginal and urethral musculofascial attachments divided, vigorous cephalad traction on the entire specimen now elevates the entire urethra, vagina, portions of labia, perineal body and anal canal inside the pelvis. With the use of a long-handled knife, the mucous membrane is divided just above and laterally on each side of the external urethral meatus. The left hand grasps the specimen anteriorly at a low level, and one or two fingers are passed out under the pubic arch and through the aperture above the urethra (Fig. 81.16). With traction and finger palpation to identify the proper external landmarks, the skin can be divided with long scissors or a knife and the specimen can be removed. This should include, in addition to the bladder, uterus, vagina and rectum, the entire urethral area, vaginal introitus, perineum and anal canal (Figs 81.17A and B). The labia minora and clitoris are preserved. Minimal bleeding occurs from the perineal

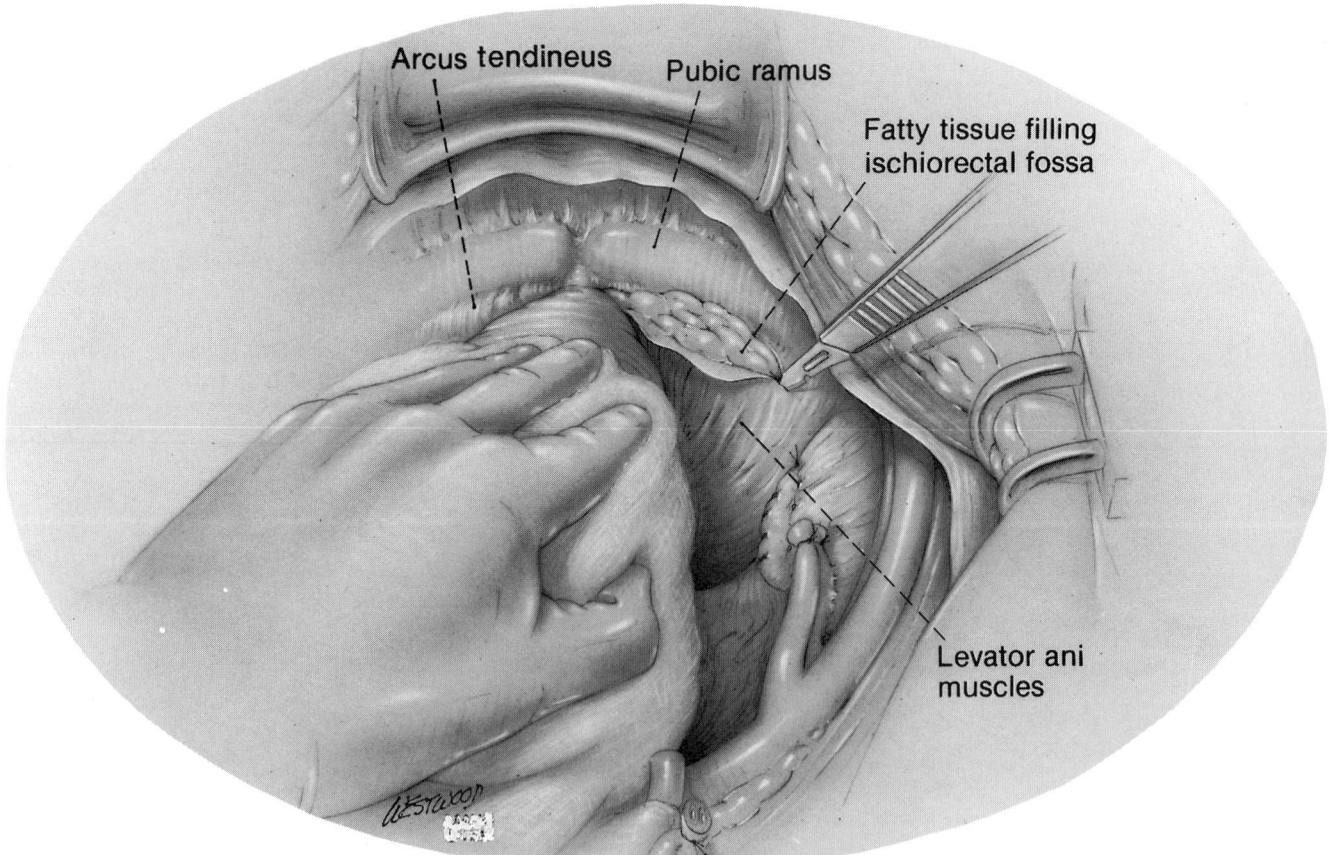

Fig. 81.14 With all of the visceral branches of the internal iliac vessels ligated and divided on each side, the entire specimen has been mobilized except for its attachment to the pelvic floor. The anterior and lateral attachments of the levator muscles to the pubic rami and to the obturator internis fascia are divided with a long-handled knife. This exposes the underlying fatty tissue within the ischiorectal fossa.

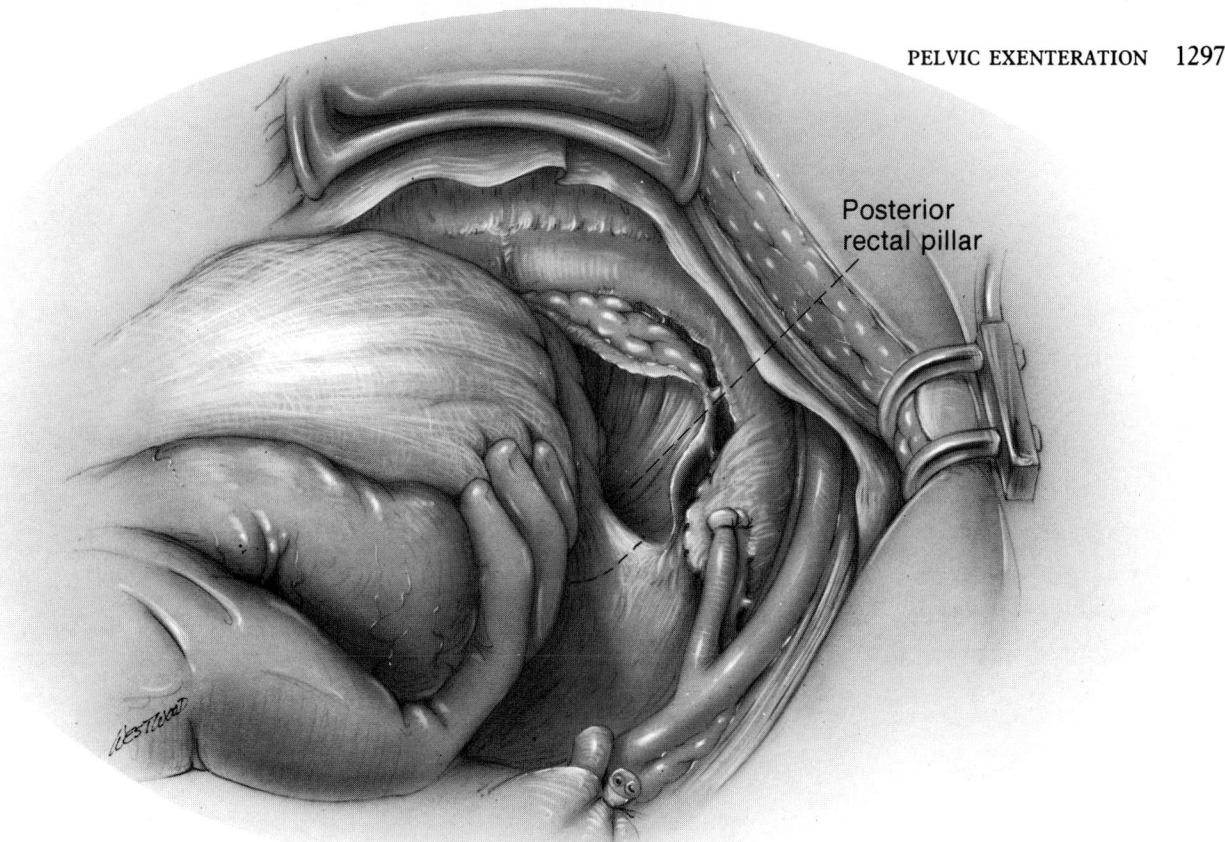

Posterior
rectal pillar

Fig. 81.15 Firm anterior and upward traction on the specimen and on the rectum will permit direct division of the posterior rectal wall pillars and the posterior portion of the levator muscle attachments; this is best accomplished with long scissors.

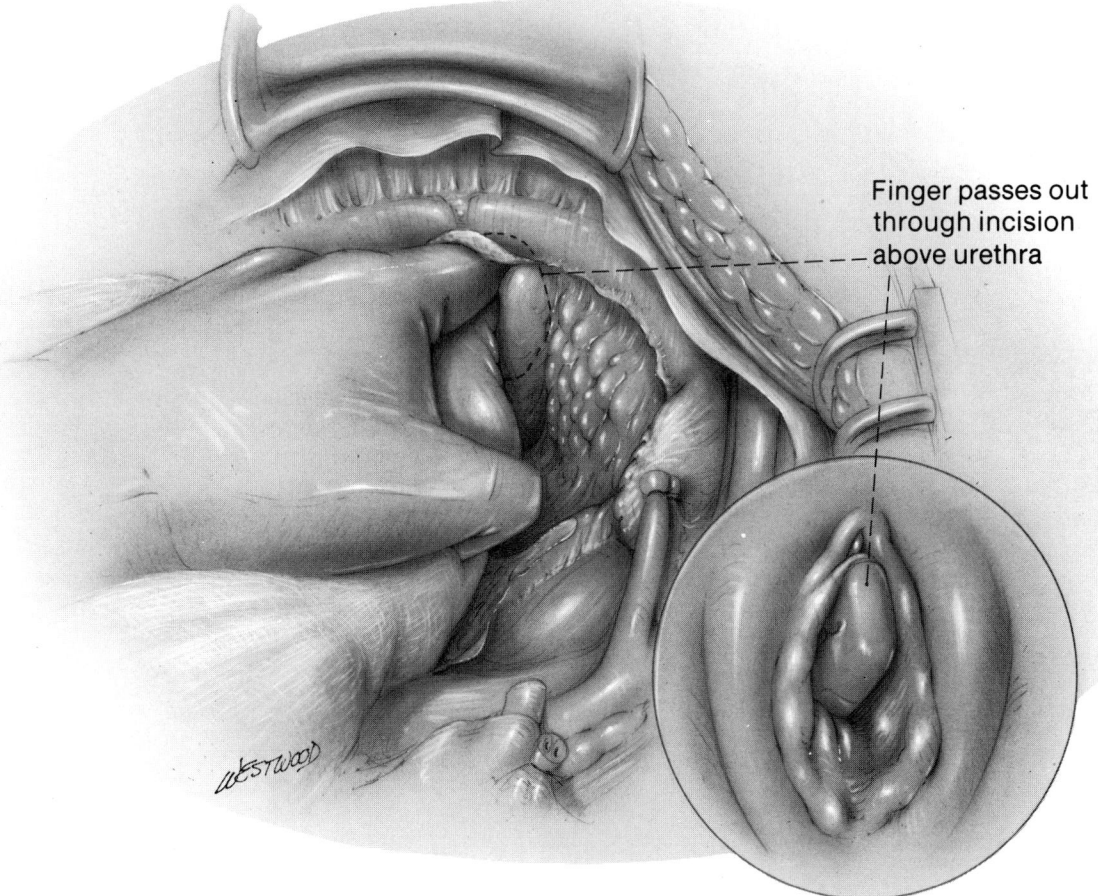

Finger passes out
through incision
above urethra

Fig. 81.16 Left-hand traction on the specimen with the index finger passed outside the pelvis just above the urethra allows identification of the vagina or vaginal and rectal margins of the excision with either a long-handled knife or long scissors.

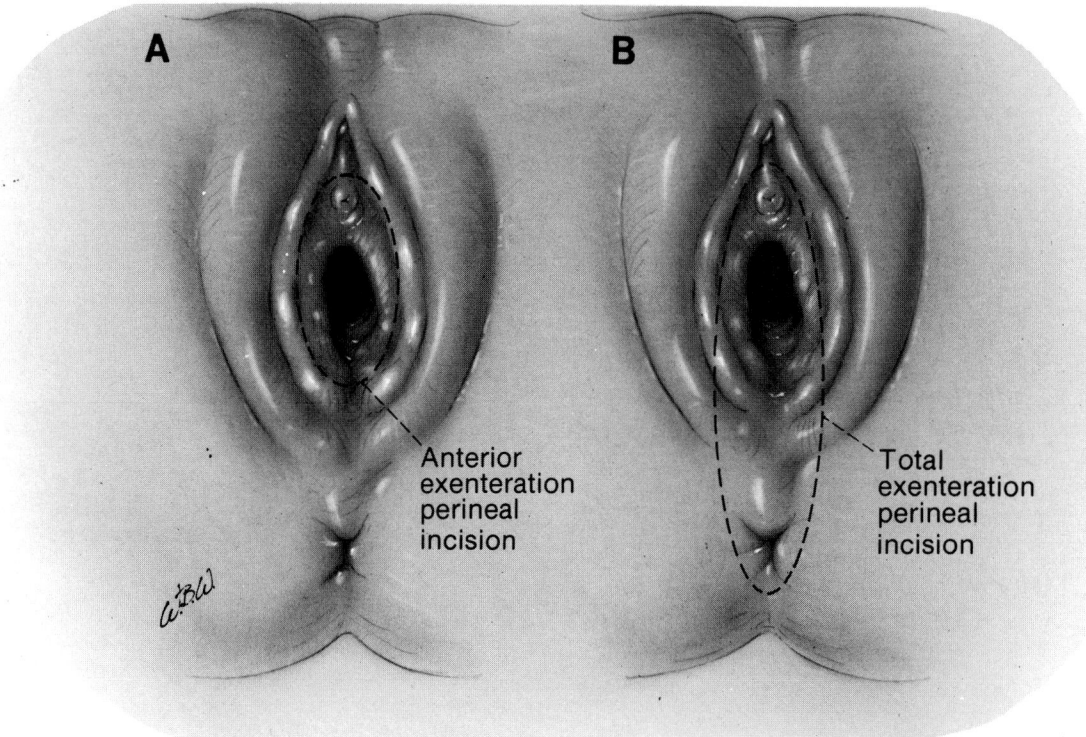

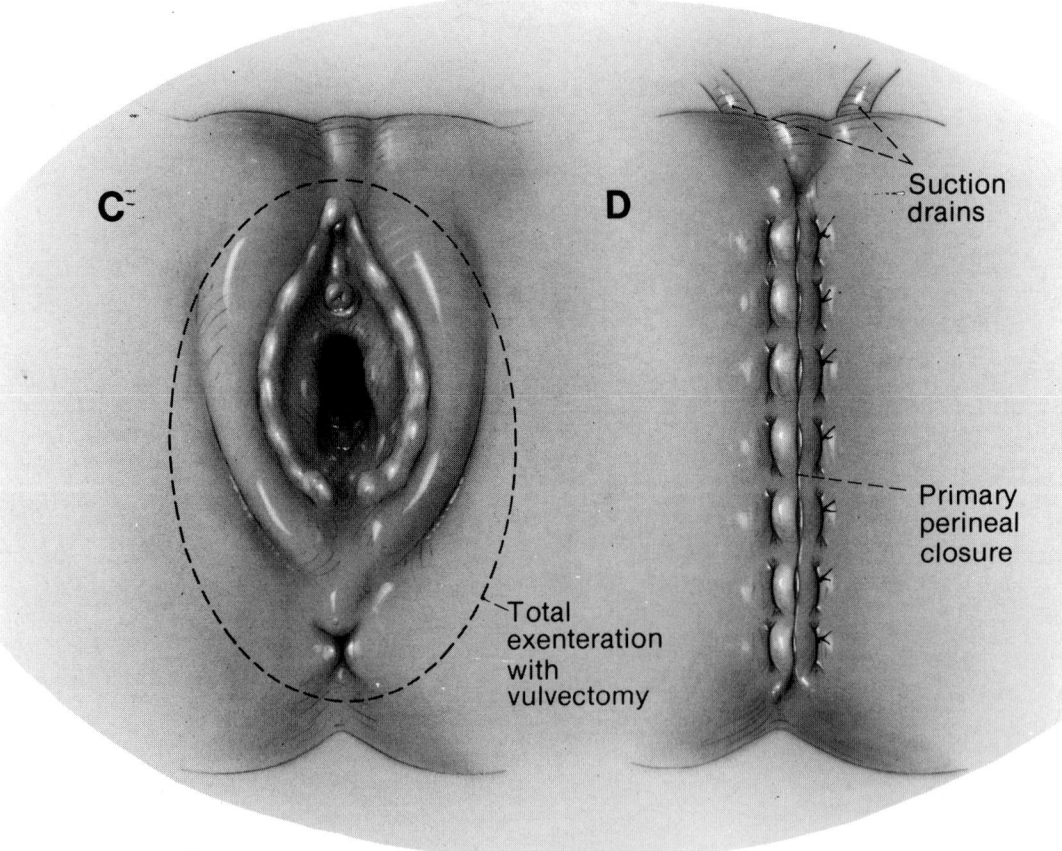

Fig. 81.17 Various incisions depending on extent of malignancy. (A) Perineal incision for anterior exenteration. (B) Perineal incision for total exenteration. (C) Total exenteration with vulvectomy. (D) Perineum is closed with vertical mattress sutures.

wound. If some blood loss is noted from the inferior hemorrhoidal vessels or from the ischiocavernosus muscles on the inferior pubic rami, it can be easily controlled by transfixing with absorbable suture material or merely by inserting a laparotomy pad deep in the perineal wound and compressing it with a deep retractor.

When the exenteration is accomplished in this fashion, one can proceed with the pelvic 'clean-up' (additional node dissection, meticulous pelvic sidewall hemostasis) and the extensive, time-consuming reconstructive aspects of the operation, without any delay for a perineal phase. After all of the abdominal portion of the operation has been completed and the incision has been closed, the patient's legs are elevated. Then, depending on individual requirements, the perineal skin margins are trimmed and the skin is closed with mattress sutures or vaginal reconstruction is performed.

When the lower one-third of the vagina is involved by malignancy, the patient is placed in a modified lithotomy (ski) position on the operating table at the beginning of the operation, and the drapes are applied to provide perineal access when it becomes appropriate. Because the levator muscle attachments have already been divided from above, the perineal operation involves little more than a wide elliptical skin incision to mobilize anal canal, perineum, and labia (Fig. 81.17C). The presacral space is entered just anterior to the tip of the coccyx. With a finger passed through this opening to identify landmarks (ischiorectal fossa, pubic rami), the excision can be rapidly accomplished and the viscera are then delivered. Once again, bleeding is relatively trivial. If a neovagina is not required, the subcutaneous tissues are closed with absorbable sutures, and the skin is closed with mattress sutures to provide accurate epithelial approximation (Fig. 81.17D). Pelvic packs are not used for hemostasis, and perineal drainage is not necessary; suction drainage of the pelvis is provided by inserting catheters through the lower abdominal wall on each side. Attention can now return to the abdominal field of operation.

With increasing experience, familiarity with the anatomy allows rapid and safe dissection of the internal iliac vessels and the sacral plexus; serious blood loss occurs infrequently, and the extirpative aspects of the operation may require not more than 45 to 60 minutes. The reconstructive efforts, however, may require several hours.

Pelvic lymph node dissection

In most instances, exenteration is accomplished for recurrent malignancy following previous irradiation; extensive fibrosis may have replaced the fatty tissues in the customarily easily dissected node-bearing areas. Unless involved by metastasis, the lymph nodes may be quite sparse or unidentifiable. Once the paravesical and pararectal spaces have been established, most of the potential node-containing tissue that remains has been mobilized from the external iliac, obturator and internal iliac region, and displaced medially with the specimen, as these vessels are exposed, ligated and divided. Once the extirpative phase of the operation has been completed, a pelvic 'clean-up' is appropriate. This includes careful inspection of the node-bearing areas and of the major vessels that have been ligated and removal of the lymph nodes from the common iliac vessels and front of the lower vena cava, which have been relatively undisturbed to this point. If frozen-section histologic study has shown that pelvic lymph nodes are involved by metastasis, an aortic node dissection is accomplished.

It is generally conceded that the primary objective of the exenteration should be the wide clearance of the central malignancy.[2] Certainly, the survival after exenteration of patients with lymph node metastasis (12 to 15% at 5 years) leaves much to be desired; nevertheless, some survival may be obtained, even though one or more lymph node metastases are present. Because the outcome remains unpredictable for the individual patient, we continue to consider node dissection worthwhile (see also Ch. 45).

Urinary conduit diversion

The diversion can be accomplished by means of either an ileal[5] or a sigmoid[21] conduit or rarely, in the face of severe irradiation damage of these structures, a transverse colon conduit. More recently, continent urinary pouches are being used in exenteration patients. (See Ch. 88.) Usually constructed from the detubularized ileum or cecum, the continent stoma allows the patient to intermittently self-catheterize rather than wear an appliance.

With total exenteration, the distal sigmoid has already been divided. The sigmoid conduit represents the simplest method of diversion because it obviates a small bowel anastomosis. The function of sigmoid and ileal segments is quite comparable.[21] By transillumination of the sigmoid mesentery, the arcades of sigmoidal vessels are identified that supply the distal 20 to 30 cm of the sigmoid. The mesentery of the sigmoid is divided just proximal to these vessels, and the bowel is transected. The proximal end of the conduit segment is closed with a row of continuous absorbable sutures and a second row of interrupted silk sutures (Fig. 81.18).

With anterior exenteration, an ileal conduit is considered the diversion method of choice. This is isolated by transilluminating the mesentery and making an appropriate incision to preserve one or two vascular arcades that supply a segment of ileum about 20 cm long, located about 20 cm above the ileocecal valve. In the obese individual, a longer ileal segment (25 to 30 cm) may be necessary; the additional length is necessary to allow the distal end to reach the skin level without tension. In addition, it is necessary to place the urinary stoma at a higher abdominal wall level (above

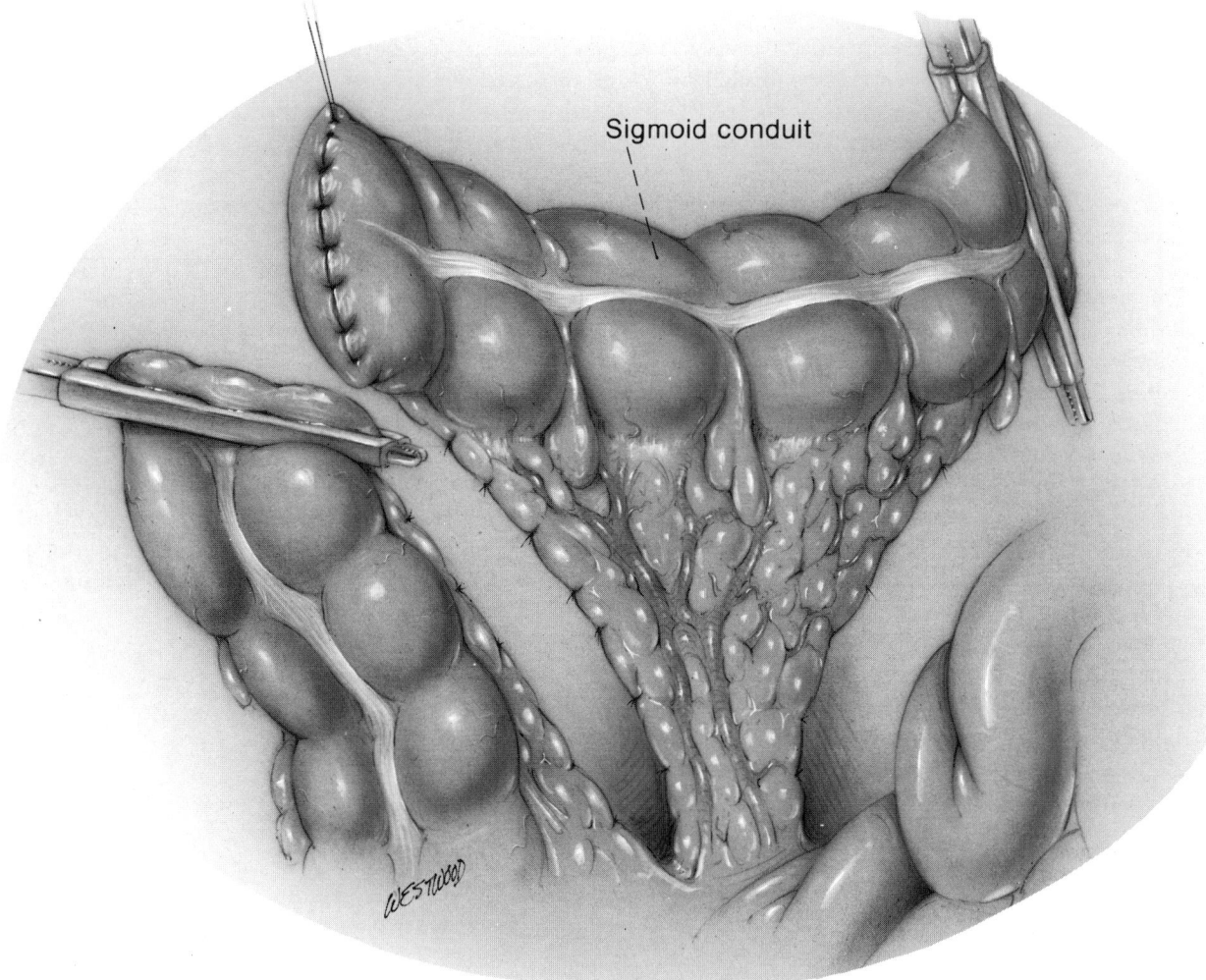

Sigmoid conduit

Fig. 81.18 With total exenteration, a sigmoid conduit is created; transillumination will reveal the appropriate sigmoidal branches of the inferior mesenteric artery which are to be preserved.

the prolapsing panniculus) to enable the patient to see the stoma for accurate placement of the appliance. For the same reason, it may be necessary to select a segment of ileum at a higher level where the mesentery and vascular arcades are longer.

If re-anastomosis to the anus is not possible, the end of the proximal sigmoid is brought through the abdominal wall at a previously marked site to provide a colostomy. This is accomplished through a lateral portion of the rectus muscle just below the level of the umbilicus. A 3 to 4 cm circle of the skin is excised; the opening through the fascia, muscles and peritoneum is enlarged without excision of any tissue, so that two or three fingers can be readily admitted without tension. Care must be exercised to avoid any shearing effect on the bowel by the fascial edges, which may 'slide' when the midline abdominal incision is closed. This can be tested by placing Kocher forceps on the edges of the peritoneum, posterior and anterior rectus fascia, and subcutaneous tissue in the abdominal incision, and pulling

these structures toward the opposite side. When a finger is placed within the colostomy site, one can detect and appropriately divide any sharp fascial edge that might compress the blood supply of the conduit, or compromise the bowel lumen. The full thickness of bowel wall is sutured securely to the skin margins with interrupted absorbable sutures. No effort is made interiorly to attach the bowel wall to the peritoneal gutter lateral to the colostomy. Peristomal hernia or bowel obstruction related to the lateral openings has not presented a significant clinical problem.

Uretero-intestinal anastomosis

Uretero-intestinal anastomosis is accomplished in the same fashion, whether with an ileal or a sigmoid conduit. A simple end-to-side, mucosa-to-mucosa anastomosis is established. It has been suggested that an 'anti-reflux procedure' (placing the distal centimeter or so of ureter in a muscular tunnel within the bowel wall) is advisable to prevent urinary reflux up the ureter, with subsequent infection and deterioration of renal function. However, if the conduit is not excessively long, and if the conduit stoma is not stenotic, the pressure within the conduit should be considerably lower than the intra-ureteral pressure, and rapid runoff of urine should occur; there should not be any urinary reflux, and no significant reabsorption of urinary constituents. In long-term follow-up of postexenteration patients, reflux has not been a problem of clinical significance. However, if a continent pouch is constructed, an anti-reflux procedure is mandatory. (See Ch. 88.)

A small incision is made in the serosa and muscularis of the midlateral bowel wall (equidistant from the mesenteric and antimesenteric borders) and on the inferior surface of the conduit segment (Fig. 81.19). This is located about 2.5 cm from the end of the conduit. This small opening should be spread with the tip of a curved forceps to a size no larger than the ureter that is to be transplanted. A button of submucosa will bulge up through the opening; this is grasped with a small curved intestinal forceps (Bainbridge). Small scissors are used to divide the mucosa immediately under the tip of the instrument; this produces a small opening in the mucosa (Fig. 81.19 inset). Effort should be made to make this opening quite small; invariably, it will be larger than anticipated, and this can make the anastomosis difficult.

The left ureter is always anastomosed initially. The distal end of the ureter is freshened by excising a few millimeters, and a small, 0.5 to 1 cm, linear incision is made in the side of the lumen to increase the diameter and to facilitate the anastomosis; obviously, with a dilated ureter, this step is unnecessary.

The anastomosis is accomplished with 6 to 8 interrupted sutures of fine absorbable material (4–0) on a small atraumatic needle. These are placed so that the full thickness of the ureter is anastomosed in a mucosa-to-mucosa fashion to the full thickness of the bowel wall. Each suture is placed from outside to inside on the ureter, and from inside to outside on the bowel; this arrangement places the suture knot outside the lumen (Fig. 81.20A). To provide a secure one-layer anastomosis, one must take care to include a portion of the ureteral sheath (adventitia) with each suture. After the posterior row of 3 or 4 sutures has been placed and tied, the ends of the lateral pair of sutures should be tagged with an instrument to maintain good exposure (Fig. 81.20B).

At this point, one may elect to insert a splinting ureteral catheter. This is more commonly performed now using a J stent or number 8 ureteral stent. It is advisable in patients who have severe irradiation changes involving bowel, ureters and other retroperitoneal structures. The stent is passed up the ureter to the renal pelvis, and the distal end of the stent is inserted into the bowel lumen, where it is grasped and retrieved by passing a long, curved Kelly instrument through the distal end of the conduit. It

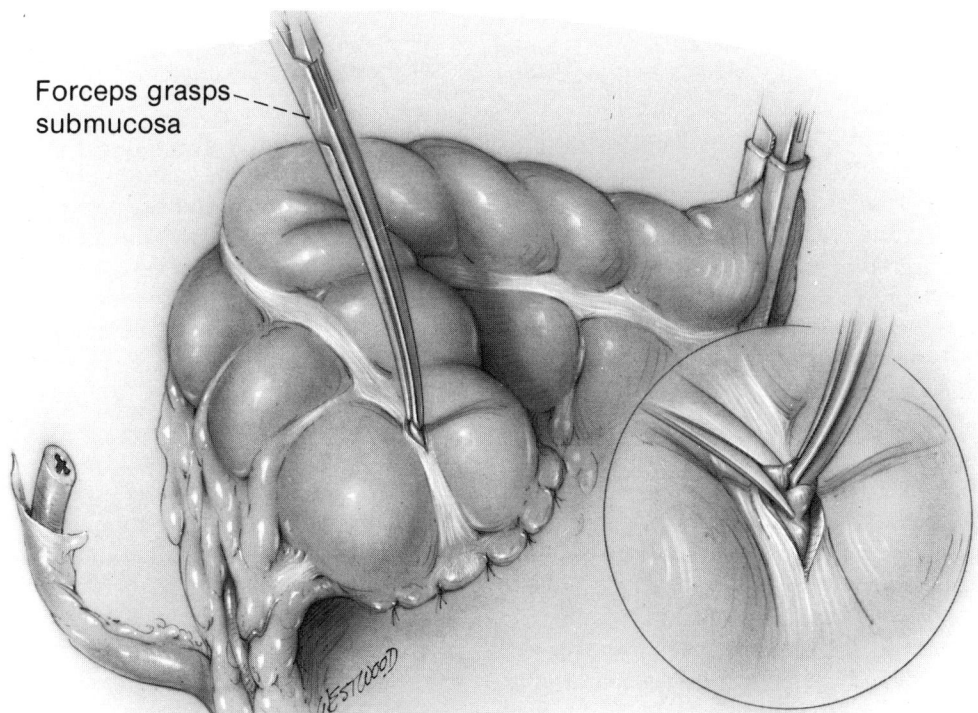

Forceps grasps submucosa

Fig. 81.19 A simple end-to-side ureterosigmoid anastomosis is accomplished on the posterior surface of the bowel segment; the opening into the bowel should be quite small, no larger than the ureter that is to be transplanted.

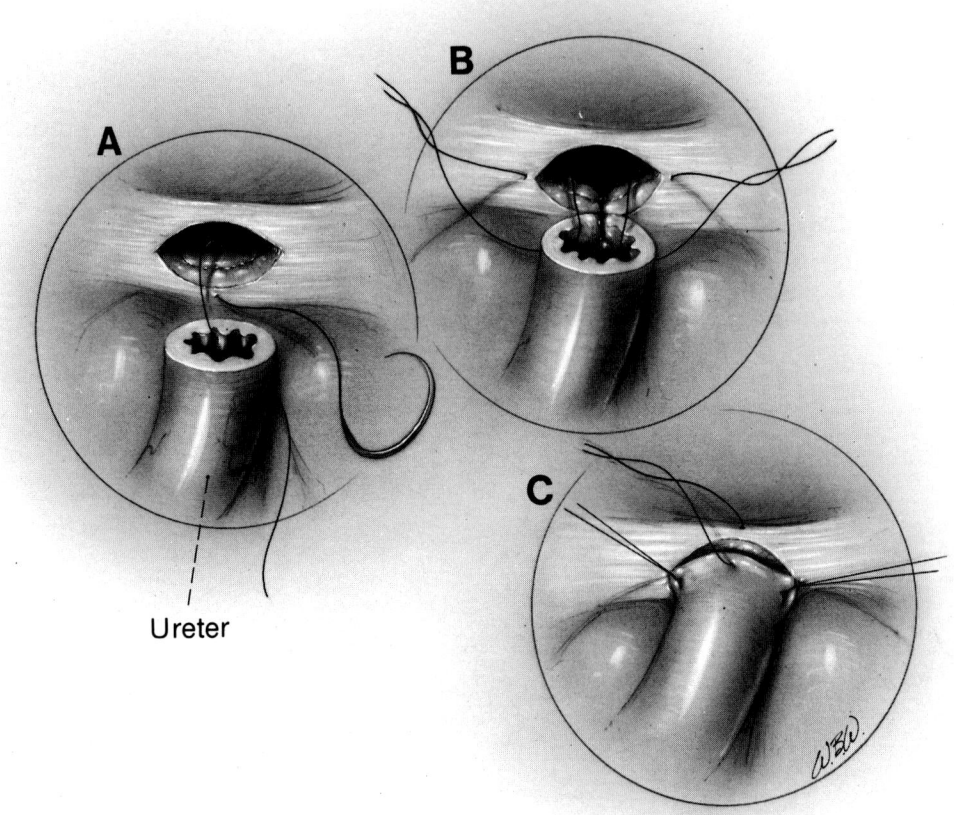

Fig. 81.20 **A** to **C**, The ureterointestinal anastomosis is accomplished with 4–0 chromic catgut sutures, so placed that the knots are outside the lumen; the full thickness of ureter (including adventitia) and of bowel wall are approximated (**A**). After the lateral pair of sutures have been tied and tagged, gentle traction on these will maintain good exposure (**B**) and allow accurate placement of the anterior row of sutures (**C**). Obstruction of the anastomosis is avoided by not tying the sutures in the anterior row until all sutures are in place.

is not necessary to transfix the ureteral stents in position. The stents are removed in 7 to 10 days, depending on the patient's condition.

The anterior 3 or 4 interrupted sutures can now be inserted, and this completes the anastomosis (Fig. 81.20C). Some authorities suggest a second reinforcing anastomotic row of fine 4–0 silk sutures to approximate ureteral adventitia and bowel serosa; others advocate the placement of 1 or 2 sutures at a higher level, between the ureteral adventitia and the bowel wall at the mesenteric border, to relieve any tension on the anastomosis. These additional measures appear to be unnecessary; excessive suture material may lead to obstructive edema, distortion and kinking, or even to tissue necrosis.

At the time the ureter is initially divided, early in the course of the exenteration, it is most often possible to preserve a patch of peritoneum attached to the ureteral sheath; the peritoneal tissue can be attached to bowel wall with 3 or 4 sutures placed lateral to the anastomosis (Fig. 81.21). This procedure will relieve any 'pull' on the anastomosis, and the serosal approximation should promote rapid healing and a watertight seal.

The right ureter is anastomosed in an identical fashion to the inferior surface of the bowel segment about 2.5 to 5 cm distal to the left anastomosis. A hiatus will exist between the left ureter and the proximal end of the conduit; theoretically, small bowel can herniate through this site. The aperture can be closed by fixing with a few sutures the proximal end of the conduit to the peritoneum at the base of the mesentery of the sigmoid used to create the colostomy. The peri-ureteral aperture on the right side is less likely to be the site of a hernia, because it is protected by the conduit mesentery.

With an anterior exenteration, and thus with an ileal conduit, the left ureter must be brought to the right side of the patient's abdomen through an avascular opening made in the sigmoid mesentery just above (ventral) the superior hemorrhoidal vessels; partial ureteral obstruction can occur when it passes through the mesentery under (dorsal) the vessels. To avoid the hiatus under the ureter and the end of the ileal conduit, one must fix the proximal end of the ileal segment and its pedicle, with several sutures, to the opening in the sigmoid mesentery and to the posterior peritoneum on the right side of the pelvis.

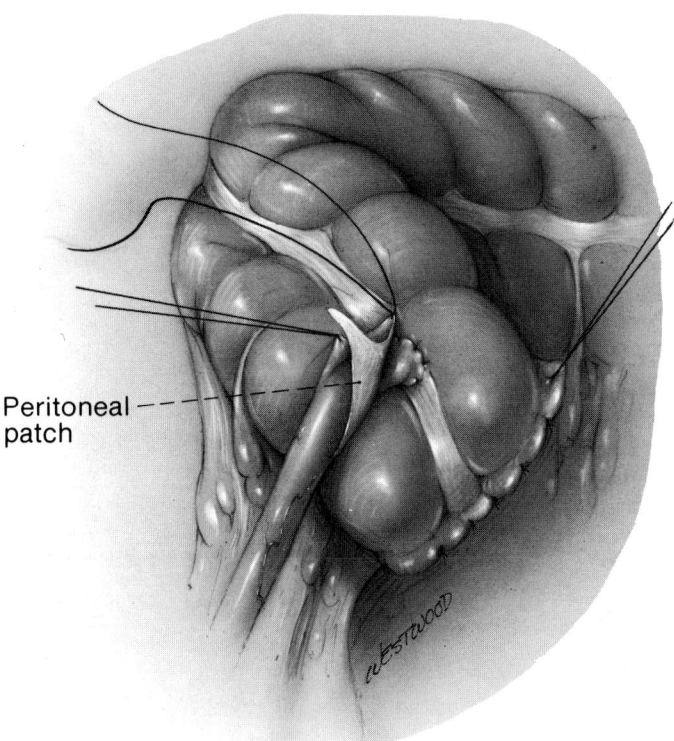

Peritoneal patch

Fig. 81.21 A peritoneal flap (preserved on the ureter when it was divided at the level of the pelvic brim) is now attached to the bowel wall to 'seal' and relieve any 'pull' on the anastomosis.

If the conduit has been properly envisioned, created and fixed in position by the surgeon, it should now fold down into its proper, final position and create a smooth arch across the pelvis at about the level of L-5, without dropping far down into the pelvis; in this way, any tension or pull on the uretero-intestinal anastomosis is avoided. There should be no redundancy of the ureters that could lead to a kinking type of obstruction; in addition, there should be no redundancy of the conduit. Although the conduit should be as short as possible, it is always comforting to have too much, rather than too little conduit! After the external stomal aperture has been produced, the length of the conduit can be governed merely by delivering any redundant portion through the stoma and excising it before attaching the mucosa to the cutaneous margins.

The external stoma for the distal end of the conduit should now be established. This is done on the right side, at the site selected before operation, at a level a few centimeters higher than the colostomy site on the left. As a rule, this is through the lateral edge of rectus muscle. It should be positioned almost equidistant between the anterior-superior iliac spine and the costal margin, and sufficiently lateral to the umbilicus to allow room for application of the faceplate of the watertight appliance that will be necessary. As noted in relation to the colostomy, it is necessary to vary the position of the stomas somewhat in the presence of obesity or of severe changes due to cutaneous

irradiation. In addition, a previous appendectomy or upper right rectus operative incision may modify the position selected, for a scarred, irregular cutaneous surface will interfere with the secure attachment of the appliance.

As with the colostomy stoma, a button of skin (3 to 4 cm) is excised, and an underlying opening, two or three fingers wide, is made through all layers of the abdominal wall. So that it can accept the larger sigmoidal conduit, the aperture must be larger than that required for an ileal conduit. Furthermore, with a thick abdominal wall, the opening must be made considerably wider (three to four fingers) to allow acceptance of the longer segment of bowel and the thicker mesenteric pedicle that must be delivered through it to the skin level, without tension on the anastomosis and without compression of the blood supply. The stoma is established with interrupted sutures that fix the full thickness of the bowel to the subcuticular margins. Sutures placed through the full thickness of the skin eventually may 'cut through' and leave small, linear scars around the stoma which prevent a good seal of the appliance. When the ileum is used, the sutures are placed through the edge of skin and substantially into the tough subcuticular layer, then into bowel serosa about 2 or 3 cm down from the end, and finally through the edge of the bowel (Fig. 81.22). This will produce a 1 or 2 cm nipple or 'rosebud' eversion of the ileal mucosa. Mucosal eversion is more difficult to achieve with the thicker-walled, muscular sigmoid. Fortunately, with the very efficient present-day materials that are available to provide watertight attachments of the appliances, the nipple eversion of the bowel mucosa is no longer an essential feature. Most patients can wear the urinary appliance for 4 to 8 days without skin irritation, accidental leaks or any necessity to change the faceplate of the appliance.

Management of the pelvic floor

Bowel obstruction has been one of the most frequent and most serious complications of the operative procedure.[15,22] In the past, various methods of managing the denuded pelvic basin have been tried in an effort to prevent adherence and fixation of the small bowel, including a pelvic pack to keep bowel out of the pelvis, a pelvic 'lid' of tantalum mesh or other synthetic material, replacement of the pelvic peritoneum with frozen preserved amnionic membrane, and pouches of omentum or parietal peritoneum.[15,26] None of the techniques reported has been entirely successful. In our experience, the obstruction has most commonly been mechanical, and secondary to adhesions deep in the pelvis.

In recent years, the incidence of bowel obstruction has been significantly diminished by the use of either a free patch of peritoneum, or an omental pedicle to cover the pelvic floor. The peritoneal 'patch' is obtained by excising a segment of parietal peritoneum from the low-anterior abdominal wall just lateral to the bladder area; in fact, an

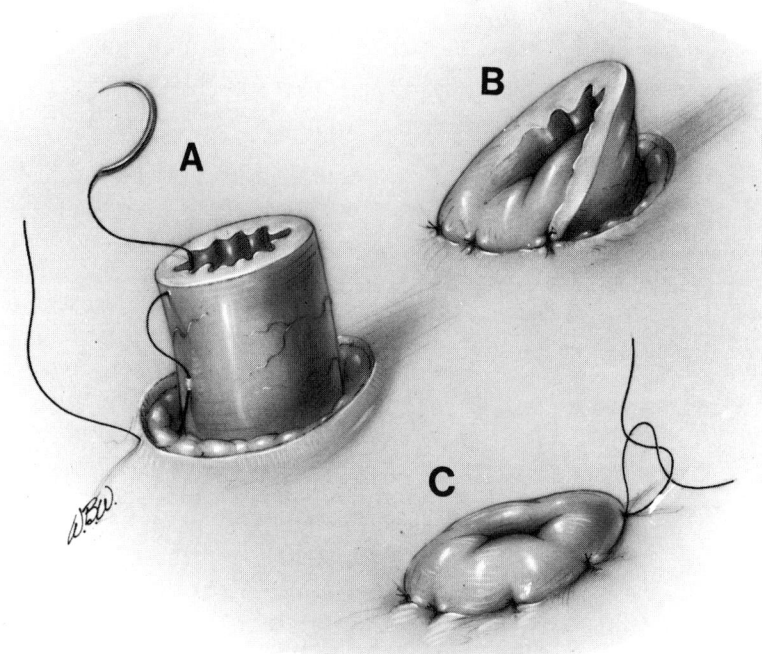

Fig. 81.22 In creating an ileal conduit stoma, the sutures are placed to include the subcuticular skin margins, the bowel wall 2 to 3 cm from the end, and full-thickness of bowel at the end of the segment; this produces an everted 'rose bud' of bowel mucosa.

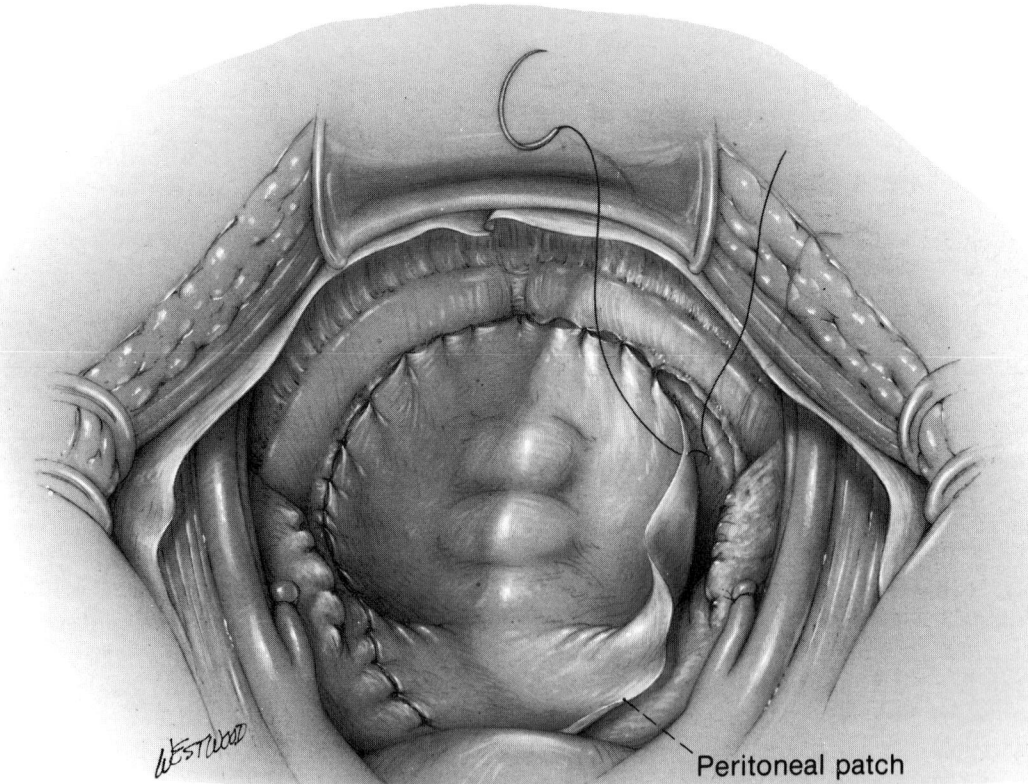

Peritoneal patch

Fig. 81.23 The pelvic floor can be covered with a free peritoneal 'patch' obtained from the lower anterior abdominal wall and the lateral vesical area. This is attached with interrupted or continuous absorbable sutures to the symphysis pubis, obturator internis fascia, margins of excised levator muscles, and presacral fascia to prevent prolapse of small bowel.

effort is made early in the operation to preserve the peritoneum covering the lateral portion of the bladder, to be used for this purpose. The peritoneal patch is attached with interrupted catgut sutures to the obturator internus muscle (at the level of the levator muscle attachments), to the back of the pubic symphysis, and to the fascia covering the sacrococcygeal area (Fig. 81.23).

For the most part, the peritoneal patch is used in patients who do not have any adequate fatty omentum, or in whom the omentum has been so fixed and scarred into the upper abdomen by previous upper abdominal surgery that it is difficult to mobilize. When the omentum appears to be adequate, a viable omental pedicle can be created in a simple fashion and without including the gastro-epiploic artery. This is accomplished merely by dividing omentum on the right side at the level of its attachment to transverse colon, almost over the midline, and then making a secondary incision down through the omentum (Fig. 81.24). By careful inspection and transillumination, one can avoid the distally located circulation coming from the left side of the omentum and provide a long, viable segment of omentum. The omental pedicle can be led down the midline, anterior to the small intestine between the two stomas, and immediately beneath the abdominal incision. It is sutured to the obturator internus muscles and the pubic rami and symphysis anteriorly, and a few sutures attach it to presacral fascia posteriorly. This provides a serosal cover for most of the pelvic floor, and presents a clean peritoneal surface for the small bowel to prolapse upon. Synthetic absorbable mesh made of polyglactin 910 may be used when omentum is not available, to form a lid or sling to exclude the small bowel from the pelvis[7] (Fig. 81.25). The mesh is sutured across the pelvis at the pelvic brim. If any omentum is present, it can be laid across the mesh. The cavity beneath the mesh must be drained using suction catheters. Freeze-dried human dura mater has also been used in a similar fashion.[12] The advantage of these absorbable materials is that they are not associated with the high incidence of chronic sepsis associated with non-absorbable meshes. Nevertheless, with an operative procedure of this magnitude, some degree of postoperative adhesions will develop and some bowel obstructions will occur. Vaginal reconstruction with myocutaneous flaps has the additional advantage of filling the denuded pelvis with viable tissue,

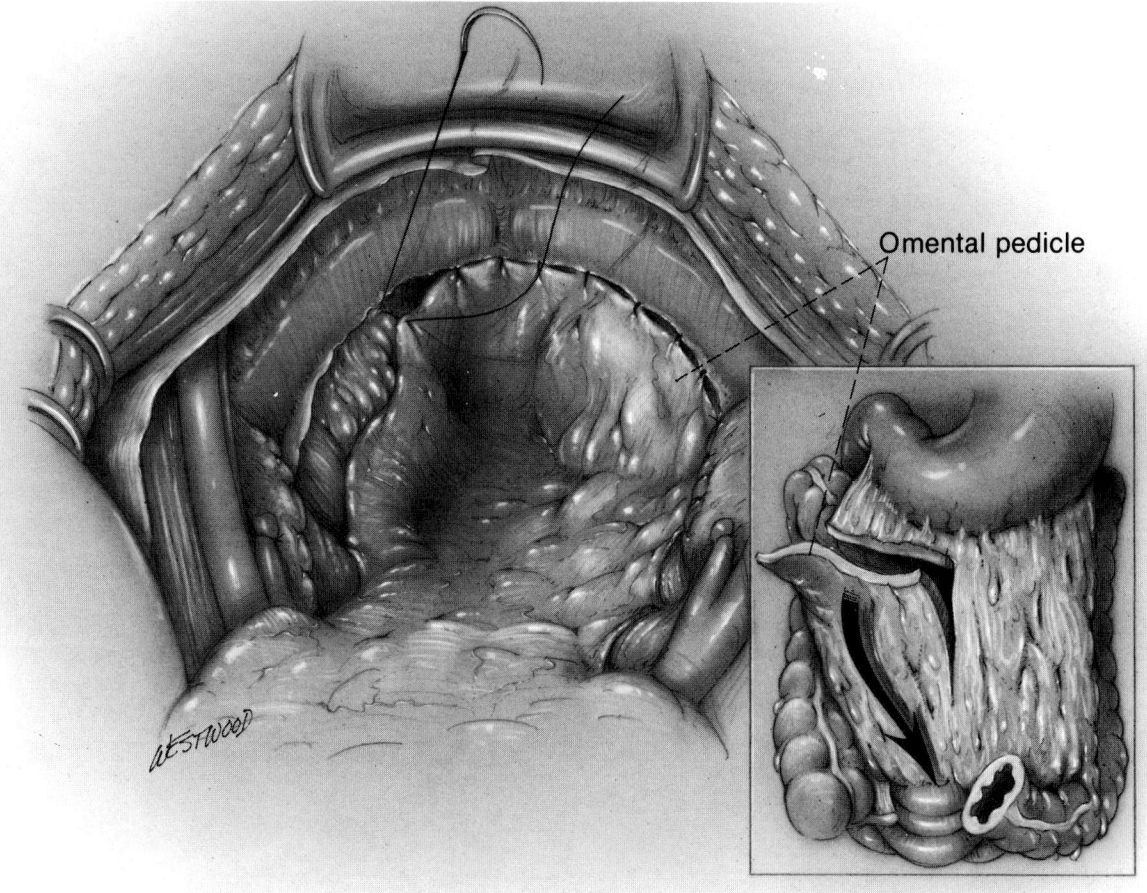

Omental pedicle

Fig. 81.24 When the omentum is adequate, the pelvic floor can be covered with a simple omental pedicle; careful inspection and transillumination will reveal whether the entire gastroepiploic artery must be mobilized to maintain the vascular integrity of the pedicle.

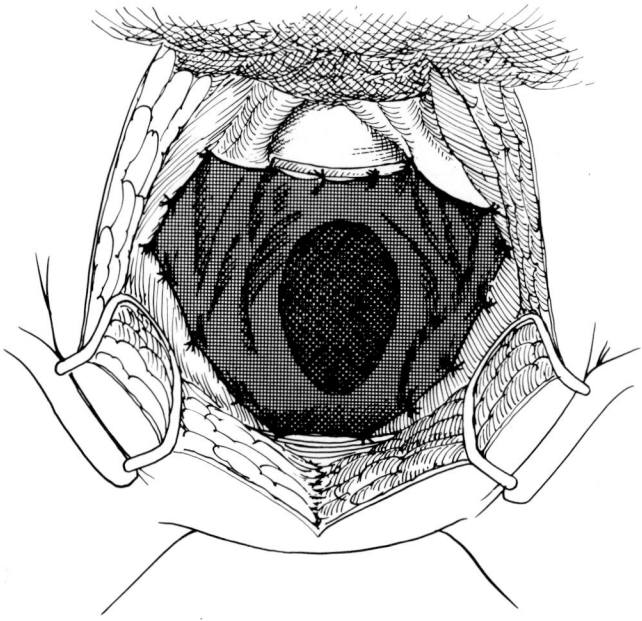

Fig. 81.25   Synthetic absorbable mesh sutured to pelvic sidewalls as a pelvic lid.

helping to prevent bowel adhesion to the denuded pelvic floor. Dura mater, absorbable and non-absorbable mesh, muscle flaps and myocutaneous flaps have all been successfully used to repair the uncommon postoperative complication of perineal herniation.[3,4,8,14]

VAGINAL RECONSTRUCTION

With improved survival rates in patients having pelvic exenteration, there has been an increasing emphasis on quality-of-life issues.[1,24] Sexual rehabilitation with vaginal reconstruction has assumed a more important role.

Many techniques have been used to reconstruct the vagina after pelvic exenteration. It is important that vaginal reconstruction be discussed with the patient preoperatively, as the most advantageous time to perform the reconstructive surgery is at the time of exenteration. Attempting to reconstruct a vagina in the fibrotic pelvis years after pelvic exenteration is fraught with risk and seldom effective.

Most of the patients in this series who had vaginal reconstructive surgery had a pack placed in the pelvic cavity to maintain a space into which a skin graft on a mold was inserted 8 to 12 days later, using the McIndoe technique. Many had a sigmoid neovagina constructed, using one segment of sigmoid colon for the conduit and another for the neovagina and bringing the descending colon out as a colostomy. It is important in these cases that the entire vagina is removed; otherwise, a stricture develops at the anastomotic junction between sigmoid and vagina.

These techniques are not as effective if a total exenteration has been performed, either because the resultant

cavity is too large or because the neovagina becomes rigid and fixed to the front of the sacrum. The split-thickness skin graft neovagina requires use of a mold to maintain the vaginal cavity, and the sigmoid neovagina has the disadvantage of producing copious mucus and occasionally prolapsing.

In patients who have required levator muscle or vulvoperineal excision, myocutaneous pedicle flaps provide an alternative technique. We have favored bilateral gracilis myocutaneous flaps to construct a neovagina.[10] These pedicle flaps help close the perineal defect, and also fill the pelvic cavity by effectively covering the denuded pelvic floor.

Unfortunately, the procedure does add some morbidity to the operation, with long thigh scars and prolongation of operating time. Necrosis of part or all of the flaps can also occur. Unfortunately, even with an excellent anatomic result, patient satisfaction with, and use of, the neovagina are not high.

Rectus abdominis myocutaneous flaps,[23] fasciocutaneous thigh flaps,[25] and bulbocavernosus myocutaneous flaps[9] have also been used with varying success.

More recently, we have favored inserting a split-thickness, skin-graft-covered mold at the time of exenteration, wrapping the graft in the omental pedicle. This eliminates one operative procedure from the old technique of inserting the graft 8 to 13 days after exenteration. (See also Ch. 87.)

PALLIATIVE EXENTERATION

Although widely thought that if an exenteration is likely to be palliative only, then it should not be performed, a review of the exenterative operations done at the Mayo Clinic showed that 18% were in fact palliative in nature because of pelvic or aortic nodal metastases, pelvic peritoneal or sidewall involvement, bone involvement or distant metastases. A 17% 5-year survival was obtained in this group of patients.[19] Certainly, the presence of regional lymph node metastases is not a contraindication to surgery, as 25% or more of these patients can expect to survive 5 years.[17] It is difficult, however, to predict whether quality of life will be improved in situations in which resection is likely to be only palliative.

Recurrent tumors fixed to the presacral area were formerly regarded as inoperable, but reports are appearing in the literature regarding sacral resection for recurrent anorectal cancer,[16] and this technique may be applicable to an occasional gynecologic cancer patient for palliation.

POSTOPERATIVE CARE

The postoperative care of the patients subjected to pelvic exenteration is quite similar to that for any major abdominal operation (Ch. 84). However, special emphasis must be placed on several areas because of the extent of the operation. The patient should be placed in an intensive-care unit where the necessary monitoring facilities are available. After the acute postoperative phase is over, the patient will need aggressive care, preferably managed by a respiratory service, to promote the elimination of pulmonary secretions and to prevent static congestion and pneumonia.

During the operation, the patient receives blood replacement on the basis of measured and estimated losses. It is important to realize that the loss of erythrocytes and plasma into the operative area from the extensive denuded surfaces, which extend from the promontory to the perineum, will be continuous over several days, even in the absence of obvious active bleeding. If the perineum has been closed, one can get some estimate of the extent of this loss of serosanguineous fluid by the output through the suction catheters placed in the depths of the pelvis. From 200 to 800 ml of sanguineous fluid may be obtained through the suction drains for 4 to 6 days. The invasive hemodynamic monitoring, urinary output, hemoglobin, hematocrit and other measures of blood volume should be obtained periodically. It is not unusual for the patient to require an additional unit or so of blood at some time during the first week of hospitalization after the operation.

The most satisfactory replacement fluid has been a balanced crystalloid solution (Ringer's lactate). During the early postoperative period, the need for this type of replacement can best be determined by the Swan Ganz catheter and the hourly output of urine. Ideally, a urinary output of 30 to 50 ml per hour should be maintained from the completion of the operation and thereafter. Any significant decrease in urinary output is an indication of inadequate replacement therapy, hypovolemia being the most frequent cause of diminished or absent urinary output in the early postoperative period. When correction of hypovolemia followed by a trial of loading the kidneys together with the use of a diuretic does not improve the urine flow, some other cause of the oliguria or anuria must be considered.

Although there is a chance that one ureter may be mechanically obstructed because of technical inadequacy of the uretero-intestinal anastomosis, the possibility of bilateral mechanical obstruction of the ureters would be extremely unlikely. In fact, it has not occurred in our experience with exenterative operations. If only a single ureter is obstructed, as a rule it will not be recognized and will not result in any diminution in urinary output. If the patient is definitely oliguric or anuric, one should evaluate the external stoma of the conduit to ensure its patency. One can do this by inserting a finger or a Foley catheter into the conduit stoma to determine whether there is any retention of urine.

Early in our experience with exenteration, particularly when ureterosigmoidostomies into the intact bowel represented the method of urinary diversion, it was relatively frequent that patients would be encountered who had little or no urinary output for rather lengthy periods in the immediate postoperative period. It was our practice in this situation merely to avoid overloading the patient with fluids, and to observe the situation for from 2 to as many as 5 or 6 days with the expectation that the ureters would eventually 'open up'. In all instances, urinary output suddenly improved and remained adequate thereafter. Whether such temporary obstruction represents edema, ureteral dyskinesia or a plug of mucus in the ureteral stoma, or whether it is simply that some time is required for the pressure of urinary excretion to force open the anastomosis, remains open to question.

Naturally, if bilateral ureteral obstruction with complete anuria persisted for a longer time, reoperation would become essential in order to establish urinary output. It may be quite hazardous to reoperate on the previously irradiated and operated bowel and ureters at a time when the tissues would be extremely friable. Somewhat depending on the patient's condition, a unilateral or bilateral percutaneous nephrostomy may represent the preferable temporizing procedure. At a later date, when the patient is in a satisfactory condition, reoperation could be accomplished much more safely and effectively if the mechanical ureteral obstruction has persisted.

The color of the visible portion of the urinary and colostomy stomas should be observed carefully every day. Some necrosis of the terminal mucosa is not unusual as many as 7 or 8 days after the operation. Late necrosis of this type occurs particularly in obese persons, even when the aperture through the abdominal wall has apparently been of adequate size. Prolapse of the patient's panniculus in the erect position may still instigate some shearing or fascial compression of the terminal stoma, and result in necrosis. As a rule, inserting a curved clamp into the stoma and spreading it slightly will indicate that deeper within the abdominal wall the mucosa of the conduit is quite pink and healthy. Necrosis of the entire conduit has not been experienced. When viable tissue can be observed within the abdominal wall, there is no urgency about revising the necrotic area; urinary output should remain adequate. In 10 to 20 days, when the patient's condition is suitable, one can mobilize the conduit stoma with a circular incision around the stoma. After the fascia opening has been enlarged, it has always been possible to pull the conduit up through the abdominal wall sufficiently to re-establish skin continuity.

Vigorous efforts should be made to prevent venous thrombosis and embolism. Because of the extensive raw surfaces and oozing and the multiple drain sites, we have not advocated prophylactic anticoagulant therapy. Other measures are vigorously pursued. These include elastic stockings, sequential calf compression devices, leg exercises, frequent turning of the patient, and early ambulation. Early ambulation is accomplished beginning on the morning after operation (12 to 24 hours), even though it is difficult with exenteration patients because of the multiple tubes, drains and dressings. It is almost impossible for the patient to sit because of the perineal wound; nevertheless, with assistance, the patient can be walked about the room three times a day.

The major nursing problem during the postoperative period consists of care of the ileostomy and colostomy stomas. A stomal therapist, available in most hospitals where operations of this type are accomplished, is an invaluable and essential aid in the management of these patients during the postoperative period. The stomal therapist consults the patient daily. When the patient is capable and her postoperative condition permits, she is carefully instructed in the accurate placement of the appliance so that she will feel competent in her ability to manage the bag when dismissed from the hospital.

All postexenteration patients have a relatively long period of intestinal ileus; as noted, there is a high incidence of intestinal obstruction. Many of the patients should be started on some type of total parenteral nutrition early in the postoperative period, if not preoperatively. A nasogastric tube or, even better, a long intestinal tube should be inserted before or during the operative procedure. In recent years, a long intestinal tube has commonly been inserted through either a gastrostomy or jejunostomy at the time of operation. This is passed down through the entire length of small bowel with the hope that postoperative ileus and postoperative obstruction, in particular, can be prevented. Oral feedings are never started before the fifth or sixth postoperative day, or until the patient is passing flatus. When the patient is able to take a diet orally, the tube is simply clamped off and left in place for several days. If there is recurrence of the ileus or abdominal distention, the tube is irrigated and again put on suction.

RESULTS

A total of 198 pelvic exenterations were performed at the

Table 81.2 Sites of origin of malignant lesions

Site	No. of patients
Cervix	117
Vagina	27
Endometrium	13
Colon	12
Vulva	8
Urethra	6
Bladder	4
Ovary	4
Other	6
Unknown	1
Total	198

Mayo Clinic between 1950 and 1971. The site of origin of the malignant lesions is shown in Table 81.2. In only 37 cases (19%) was the exenteration performed as a primary treatment for the malignancy. Of the 198 tumors, 126 (64%) were squamous cell carcinoma, 45 (23%) were adenocarcinoma, 6 were melanomas, 5 were transitional tumors, and 16 were other types of tumors.

In this series, 57% of patients had anterior exenteration, 9% had posterior exenteration, and 34% had total exenteration. However, in 15 of the cases of anterior exenteration, a low-anterior resection of rectosigmoid was also accomplished, followed by a low-rectal anastomosis; in some reports, these are included in the total exenteration category.

Operative morbidity and mortality

Dismissal from the hospital in less than 4 weeks occurred in 68%. A total of 16 patients died within 60 days of their surgery, and this represents an operative mortality of 8.1% overall. However, in the last 9 years of the series (102 patients), the operative mortality has been only 3%. This improved survival is thought to reflect better techniques of urinary diversion, better management of fluid balance and the availability of better antibiotics.

Postoperative complications

Table 81.3 shows the incidence of postoperative complications occurring both before and after dismissal from the hospital. Metabolic problems accounted for the great majority of the postoperative complications. This problem has been almost abolished by the use of conduit urinary diversion, instead of ureterosigmoidostomy.

The incidence of urinary fistula and obstruction is low; the number of bowel fistulas has been greatly diminished in recent years by performing low colonic anastomosis with irradiated bowel, by using the intraluminal stapler, and by protecting the anastomosis by means of a proximal diverting colostomy. Unfortunately, the incidence of bowel obstruction remains at a disturbingly high level. Bowel obstruction occurred in 23 patients (11.6%), and intestinal fistula formation in 25 patients (12.6%). In six of these patients, a combination of obstruction and fistula developed. In 70% of the patients who experienced postoperative obstruction, a technique to reperitonealize the pelvis had not been used; this would appear to be the most important causative factor in the development of the obstruction. Of the 13 patients who required surgery for bowel obstruction, 12 had obstruction from non-malignant adhesions of small bowel to the denuded pelvic sidewall; only one had an adherent loop of small bowel above the pelvic brim. (See also Chs 85 and 86.)

Similarly, previous irradiation seemed to play an important role in the development of intestinal fistula (23 of the

Table 81.3 Postoperative complications in 198 patients

Complication	Before dismissal No.	%	After dismissal No.	%
Metabolic	42	21	18	9
Wound				
Infection	29	15	1	<1
Evisceration	2	1	—	—
Urinary				
Infection	14	7	7	4
Fistula	2	1	6	3
Obstruction	2	1	3	2
Bowel				
Fistula	10	5	15	8
Obstruction	13	7	10	5
Pelvis				
Abscess	8	4	—	—
Perineal evisceration	4	2	—	—
Chest				
Infection	6	3	—	—
Embolism	4	2	—	—
Phlebitis	9	5	1	<1
Peritonitis or septicemia	8	4	—	—
Cardiac or cerebrovascular event	7	4	2	1
Psychosis, convulsions, coma	6	3	1	1
Hemorrhage	3	2	2	1
Other	13	7	14	7

25 patients) and bowel obstruction (16 of the 23 patients). The survival curves for patients with intestinal complications after pelvic exenteration are shown in Figure 81.26; there was no significant difference in overall survival except for borderline significance ($P = 0.053$) when the obstruction group was compared with the fistula group. However, a comparison of patients with bowel fistulas and those without fistulas at 1 year after surgery showed a lower survival for the fistula group ($P = 0.15$).

Survival

The overall 5-year survival was 32% in the series, and the 10-year survival was 23% (Fig. 81.27). In each instance, the normal survival curves derived from the 1960 survival probability tables for women in the upper midwestern United States are given. No significant difference was demonstrated according to the site of origin of the cancer in relation to survival; there was no significant difference according to the type of treatment the patient had received previously for the primary cancer.

Survivorship by grade of tumor (Broders' classification) showed a significant difference in survival ($P < 0.05$) at 1 year between patients with lesions of Grade 1 (82%) and those with lesions of Grade 4 (47%). No significant difference could be demonstrated between adenocarcinoma and squamous cell carcinoma as far as survival was con-

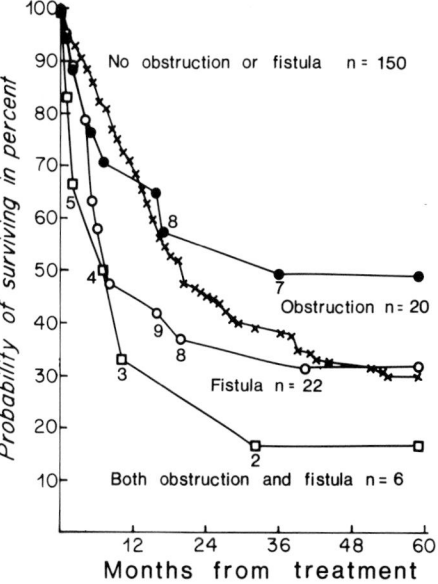

Fig. 81.26 Survival curves for patients with intestinal complications after pelvic exenteration. x — x No obstruction or fistula (n = 150); ● — ● obstruction (n = 20); ○ — ○ fistula (n = 22); □ — □ both obstruction and fistula (n = 6). (Reproduced from Webb M J, Symmonds R E 1977 Management of the pelvic floor after pelvic exenteration. *Obstet Gynecol* 50: 166, with permission of American College of Obstetricians and Gynecologists.)

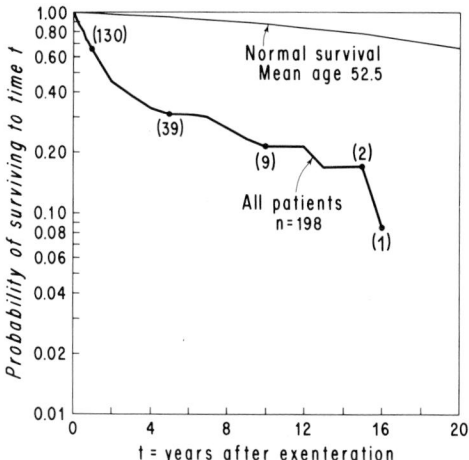

Fig. 81.27 Survivorship of all patients. (Reproduced from Symmonds R E, Pratt J H, Webb M J 1975 Exenterative operations: experience with 198 patients. *Am J Obstet Gynecol* 121: 907, with permission of C. V. Mosby Company.)

cerned. There was, however, a statistically significant ($P < 0.05$) difference in survival rates at 5 years when patients with metastatic involvement of lymph nodes were compared with those in whom the nodes were not involved with tumor (Fig. 81.28).

When patients with squamous cell carcinoma of the cervix were compared, the survival curves for anterior and total exenterations did not show any significant difference between the two operations.

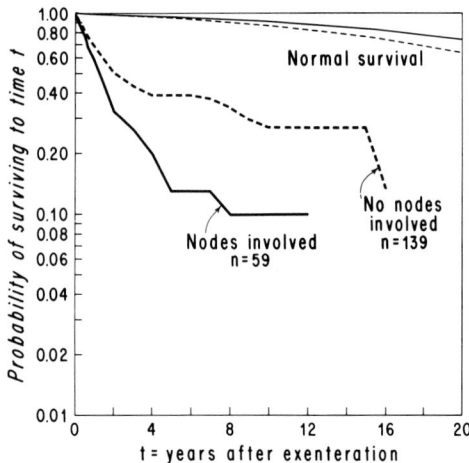

Fig. 81.28 Survivorship by lymph node involvement. (Reproduced from Symmonds R E, Pratt J H, Webb M J 1975 Exenterative operations: experience with 198 patients. *Am J Obstet Gynecol* 121: 907, with permission of C. V. Mosby Company.)

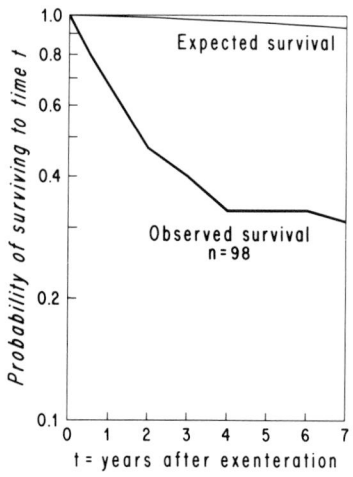

Fig. 81.29 Squamous cell carcinoma of cervix: survival of all patients. (Reproduced from Symmonds R E, Pratt J H, Webb M J 1975 Exenterative operations: experience with 198 patients. *Am J Obstet Gynecol* 121: 907, with permission of C. V. Mosby Company.)

Figure 81.29 shows the survival of 98 patients with squamous cell carcinoma of the cervix. The 5-year survival in this group was 33%, and the 10-year survival was 23%. Involvement of lymph nodes with metastases resulted in a significant decrease in survival in the patients with squamous cell carcinoma of the cervix. At 5 years, only 15% of the patients who had squamous cell carcinoma of the cervix with metastases to the lymph nodes were alive, compared with 42% of those in whom lymph nodes were negative at operation.

When we analyzed patients eligible for 5-year survival in relation to the disposition of the ureters, it was evident that use of a urinary conduit as the method of diversion gave a far superior 5-year survival rate compared with the use of diversion directly into the fecal stream (Table 81.4).

An analysis of 218 urinary diversions using either ileal (156) or sigmoid (62) conduits performed at the Mayo Clinic showed no significant difference between the two groups as far as survival and morbidity were concerned. Ureteral obstruction occurred in 20 patients (9.2%) and fistula in 8 (3.7%).[20]

Table 81.4 Disposition of ureters

Type	No. of patients	Total eligible 5-yr survival	Percent surviving 5 yr
Sigmoid conduit	39	19	47
Ileal conduit	55	26	38
Wet colostomy	13	12	25
Rectal reservoir	19	19	21
Ureterosigmoidostomy	54	50	12

REFERENCES

1. Andersen B L, Hacker N F 1983 Psychosexual adjustment following pelvic exenteration. Obstet Gynecol 61: 331
2. Barber H R K, Jones W 1971 Lymphadenectomy in pelvic exenteration for recurrent cervix cancer. JAMA 215: 1945
3. Barnhill D, Hoskins W, Heller P, Repka M, Park R 1985 Repair of vaginal prolapse and perineal hernia after pelvic exenteration. Obstet Gynecol 65: 764
4. Bell J G, Weiser E B, Metz P, Hoskins W J 1980 Gracilis muscle repair of perineal hernia following pelvic exenteration. Obstet Gynecol 56: 377
5. Bricker E M 1957 The technique of ileal segment bladder substitution. Prog Gynecol 3: 695
6. Brunschwig A 1948 Complete excision of pelvic viscera for advanced carcinoma: a one-stage abdominoperineal operation with end colostomy and bilateral ureteral implantation into the colon above the colostomy. Cancer 1: 177
7. Clarke-Pearson D L, Soper J T, Creasman W T 1988 Absorbable synthetic mesh (polyglactin 910) for the formation of a pelvic 'lid' after radical pelvic resection. Am J Obstet Gynecol 158: 158
8. Delmore J E, Turner D A, Gershenson D M, Horbelt D V 1987 Perineal hernia repair using human dura. Obstet Gynecol 70: 507
9. Hatch K D 1984 Construction of a neovagina after exenteration using the vulvobulbocavernosus myocutaneous graft. Obstet Gynecol 63: 110
10. Heath P M, Woods J E, Podratz K C, Arnold P G, Irons G B Jr 1984 Gracilis myocutaneous vaginal reconstruction. Mayo Clin Proc 59: 21
11. Ingersoll F M, Ulfelder H 1966 Pelvic exenteration for carcinoma of the cervix. N Engl J Med 274: 648
12. Jarrell M A, Malinin T I, Averette H E, Girtanner R E, Harrison C R, Penalver M A 1987 Human dura mater allografts in repair of pelvic floor and abdominal wall defects. Obstet Gynecol 70: 280
13. Ketcham A S, Deckers P J, Sugarbaker E V, Hoye R C, Thomas L B, Smith R R 1970 Pelvic exenteration for carcinoma of the uterine cervix: a 15-year experience. Cancer 26: 513
14. Leuchter R S, Lagasse L D, Hacker N F, Berek J S 1982 Management of postexenteration perineal hernias by myocutaneous axial flaps. Gynecol Oncol 14: 15
15. Massee J S, Symmonds R E, Dockerty M B, Hallenbeck G A 1962 Use of fetal membranes as replacement for pelvic

peritoneum after pelvic exenteration in the dog. Surg Forum 13: 407

16. Pearlman N W, Donohue R E, Stiegmann G V, Ahnen D J, Sedlacek S M, Braun T J 1987 Pelvic and sacropelvic exenteration for locally advanced or recurrent anorectal cancer. Arch Surg 122: 537

17. Rutledge F N, McGuffee V B 1987 Pelvic exenteration: prognostic significance of regional lymph node metastasis. Gynecol Oncol 26: 374

18. Spratt J S Jr, Butcher H R Jr, Bricker E M 1973 Exenterative surgery of the pelvis. Major Probl Clin Surg 12: 1

19. Stanhope C R, Symmonds R E 1985 Palliative exenteration — what, when, and why? Am J Obstet Gynecol 152: 12

20. Stanhope C R, Symmonds R E, Lee R A, Williams T J, Podratz K C, O'Brien P C 1986 Urinary diversion with use of ileal and sigmoid conduits. Am J Obstet Gynecol 155: 288

21. Symmonds R E, Jones I V 1975 Sigmoid conduit urinary diversion after exenteration. Prog Gynecol 6: 729

22. Symmonds R E, Pratt J H, Webb M J 1975 Exenterative operations: experience with 198 patients. Am J Obstet Gynecol 121: 907

23. Tobin G R, Day T G 1988 Vaginal and pelvic reconstruction with distally based rectus abdominis myocutaneous flaps. Plast Reconstr Surg 81: 62

24. Vera M I 1981 Quality of life following pelvic exenteration. Gynecol Oncol 12: 355

25. Wang T-N, Whetzel T, Mathes S J, Vasconez L O 1987 A fasciocutaneous flap for vaginal and perineal reconstruction. Plast Reconstr Surg 80: 95

26. Webb M J, Symmonds R E 1977 Management of the pelvic floor after pelvic exenteration. Obstet Gynecol 50: 166

82. Surgery for carcinoma of ovary

C. N. Hudson   J. H. Shepherd

INTRODUCTION

Surgical treatment for cancer of the ovary should be individually tailored for every patient (Chs 55 to 61). Factors which are relevant are age, general medical condition, reproductive status, stage of disease and histological classification. In addition, the compassionate surgeon should give careful consideration to the patient's wishes, to the likely quality and expectancy of her life and to her ability to tolerate the rigors of treatments currently available.

Age

The age of the patient should influence primary management, because the pathology may be different. Tumors of germ cell origin are relatively more common in young patients; and in most instances radical surgery would be inappropriate. Aggressive chemotherapy has entirely altered the outlook and for many such patients there would seem to be no virtue in performing hysterectomy or removing the contralateral ovary.

Reproductive status

Conservative surgery (retention of uterus and one ovary) is appropriate only in selected instances of young women desirous of preserving reproductive function. With the exception of young patients with the possibility of a germ cell tumor, ovarian conservation is not generally recommended whenever there is clinical evidence at operation of actual or likely spread beyond the single ovary involved, or in the postmenopausal patient. If at laparotomy in a young patient the disease appears confined to one ovary, a decision for ovarian and uterine conservation may be made, but it should be made in the full knowledge and appreciation that a second-stage more radical ablation may be required in the light of histopathology. Adequate samples for histopathology should be provided including slice biopsy of the apparently normal contralateral ovary whose retention is contemplated, and peritoneal biopsy from the pelvis, omentum and elsewhere as indicated, together with peritoneal fluid for cytological evaluation. Frozen section may be helpful if malignancy of an ovarian tumor is in doubt (see Chs 56, 58 and 60).

Histopathology

Ideally the histopathology of malignant ovarian tumors should influence the extent and nature of appropriate surgery. Unfortunately this information is rarely available to the surgeon at the time of an initial exploratory laparotomy. Surgeons should nevertheless have a considerable understanding of the intricate pathology of malignant ovarian disease so that an intelligent guess may be made, even if frozen section is not available (see Chs 55, 57, 59 and 61).

The ways in which histopathology should influence the extent and nature of surgery may be summarized as follows:

Germ cell tumors

1. Immature teratoma, nongestational choriocarcinoma and endodermal sinus tumor (yolk sac tumor): There is little place for radical surgery as primary therapy. (See Ch. 58.)
2. Dysgerminoma: Although these tumors are in general extremely radiosensitive, combinations of (usually platinum-based) chemotherapy are proving just as effective. This allows conservative surgery to be undertaken even with more advanced disease. There is an incidence of bilateral disease and an association with gonadal dysgenesis. In both these instances bilateral ovarian ablation should be performed. When postoperative radiotherapy is contemplated, it may be possible to preserve the residual ovary on a vascular pedicle outside the radiation field. As oocyte donation is now feasible, there may be virtue in retention of the uterus even if bilateral ovarian ablation is required. Abdominal and pelvic lymphography with or without

computerized axial tomography (CAT scan) may provide an important guide to management. Some cases of dysgerminoma are of mixed histology and tumor marker secretion occurs. Together with medical imaging further surveillance is now more precise.

Secondary surgery may be indicated for evidence of recurrence or residual masses. The possibility of the teratoma maturation syndrome thus must not be overlooked.

3. Malignant change in previously benign cystic teratoma (dermoid cyst): This change, most often squamous carcinoma, is more likely in the older age group of patients. Once spread has occurred beyond the ovary results of treatment in this group are extremely poor. Radical surgery is therefore advocated for any dermoid cyst with local adhesion in whom the possibility of malignant change is suspected.

Gonadal stromal tumors

Patients with granulosa cell carcinoma often run an extremely protracted course, and metastases may appear at extended intervals. For this reason aggressive primary and repeated surgery should be considered. The value of radiotherapy is debatable and its use may compromise subsequent surgery. The possibility that estrogen production may stimulate malignant change in uterus or even the breast, should not be overlooked. (See also Ch. 60.)

Malignant (surface) epithelial tumors

The great majority of malignant ovarian tumors arise from the surface epithelium. Histological subdivisions within this group can influence the natural history and hence the management. (See Ch. 56.)

Serous papillary cystadenocarcinoma. This is the commonest variety of epithelial carcinoma with the greatest tendency towards bilateral origin. Its propensity for surface exfoliation or transcapsular extension enhances the likelihood of early transperitoneal dissemination. It would be imprudent, in early stage disease, to retain an apparently normal other ovary unless the woman wished to have a future pregnancy. After such a pregnancy prophylactic residual oophorectomy should be considered. In all other cases bilateral oophorectomy should be advised.

Endometrioid tumors. These tumors form a continuum in the histological spectrum between the mucinous and serous papillary tumors. There is a risk of bilateral disease, not necessarily synchronous, and an additional hazard of associated endometrial cancer. Both these risks need to be evaluated if conservation of uterus and second ovary is planned. If the uterus is retained, diagnostic curettage is mandatory.

Mucinous tumors. Compared with the preceding groups a greater percentage of mucinous tumors is well differentiated and of low-grade malignancy. Many will come into the specific group considered to be of low potential malignancy. There is a lower incidence of bilateral ovarian involvement and a conservative approach may more readily be justified. Mucinous tumors spread locally and metastasize late so that a surgical approach to locally extensive disease is potentially rewarding. This may apply equally to local recurrence, particularly as some authorities regard this group of tumors as relatively radioresistant.

Clear cell tumors. Although classed separately, these are commonly regarded as being a variant of the endometrioid tumor. The histologic appearance sometimes belies their malignant potential. It is most important that they should be distinguished from the 'endodermal sinus tumor' of germ cell origin whose natural history is so different.

Undifferentiated or anaplastic tumors. The most malignant features of the above groups are illustrated in these tumors and there is little place for conservative management even in early stage disease.

Stage of disease

Prognosis is most clearly related to the stage of disease at presentation, and this factor must influence the extent and nature of surgery. International staging has been slightly simplified but nevertheless the staging information is unfortunately commonly inaccurate. Inadequate staging leading to understaging is probably responsible for some of the poor results currently reported in early stage disease. Accurate determination of stage may possibly influence prognosis by determining the need for adjuvant therapy which is as yet of unproven long term value in those cases in which there is no evidence of spread beyond the ovary.

From the surgeon's point of view the initial operative treatment may be determined by grouping patients in three categories, namely, those with disease apparently confined to one or both ovaries, those with local extension or metastasis generally confined to the pelvis or immediately adjacent lower abdomen, and those with widespread intraabdominal or extra-abdominal dissemination.

Disease confined to the ovaries

The surgical treatment is simple and traditional, namely hysterectomy and bilateral salpingo-oophorectomy. The modern emphasis is on accurate staging at this time, with limited application of a more conservative approach. The staging procedure should include inspection with cytology or biopsy of subphrenic peritoneum, pouch of Douglas, contralateral normal ovary (if retained), omentum and paracolic peritoneum. It is very important specifically to consider the possibility that ovarian malignancy is secondary to an occult gastrointestinal primary. Thus, the stomach, and small and large intestines must be inspected. In addition, the lymph node status should be carefully assessed and any suspicious nodes sampled from the pelvic or para-aortic regions.

For primary treatment of early encapsulated malignant ovarian disease, hysterectomy is not an essential requirement, provided that concomitant endometrial tumor is excluded. In all cases in which retention of the uterus is contemplated, it is wise to perform a preliminary curettage so that an associated endometrial cancer will be known to the surgeon at the time of laparotomy. Removal of the uterus as a secondary procedure should be entertained if the pathology of the ovarian malignancy turns out to be endometrioid.

Disease with local extension

The traditional approach was a 'piecemeal' or intraperitoneal resection often transgressing malignant adhesions or cutting across frank tumor. Such local surgery is often incomplete (see 'debulking' below). The preferred alternative is a primary extraperitoneal radical oophorectomy. Adjuvant therapy is almost always required, either chemotherapy, radiotherapy or both. The best results are likely to follow macroscopic clearance of visible disease. If therefore, a surgeon unexpectedly finds locally extensive malignant ovarian disease, and is not prepared to carry out radical oophorectomy, it is better to obtain a tissue diagnosis, document the stage and close the abdomen pending re-operation by a subspeciality colleague.

Advanced intraperitoneal disease

In the past the majority of such patients at laparotomy were closed after biopsy alone. Nearly all were dead within less than a year, unless the tumor histology was particularly low grade. Discomfort from large abdominal masses and recurrent malignant effusions are two of the features leading to an unhappy physical state for such patients and 'piecemeal' removal of the main tumor masses, including any large omental 'cake', has a place as a purely palliative procedure only when it is clear that cytoreduction to residual lesions less than 1.5 cm in diameter cannot be achieved. The philosophy of an attempt to reduce the residual tumor volume at the end of a primary incomplete surgical procedure to an absolute minimum depends on the widely held belief that the kinetics of chemotherapy are such that the chances of prolonged remission are greatest when the residual tumor volume is minimal (Ch. 9). The truth of this 'article of faith' has not definitely been established when visible tumor is left behind, but certainly several studies have shown that the bulk of residual tumor is an independent variable for survival, even allowing that maximal cytoreduction is more easily achieved in somewhat earlier cases. Patient comfort is temporarily improved by a major reduction of bulk disease, provided always that surgery itself does not carry an increased morbidity and complication rate. For instance, breach of the bowel wall in a semi-obstructed patient almost inevitably leads to intractable fistula formation which makes her last days considerably more miserable. Fine judgement as to the extent of surgery is required.

Hysterectomy is an integral part of the radical removal of locally extensive disease. Hysterectomy per se probably adds little benefit to grossly-incomplete removal of widespread intraperitoneal disease although it may well facilitate removal of an adherent pelvic mass and control some of the afferent blood supply. Under such circumstances the subtotal operation may occasionally be preferred as the risk of subsequent vault ulceration, fistula and bleeding may thereby be reduced.

There is no place for ovarian conservation in women with advanced local or intraperitoneal extension nor in any postmenopausal patient.

General medical status

Although this must of course be taken into consideration, most patients derive some benefit, even if only temporary, from an operation for ovarian cancer. Operation should not be withheld lightly.

The association of a malignant ovarian tumor with cancer in another site needs to be constantly borne in mind. The presence of an ovarian tumor may be the first clue to a primary gastrointestinal or breast lesion (Ch. 62). Adequate clinical examination should have detected the latter but the former may not be apparent if the history has been nonspecific and misleading. If another primary malignancy is found, both tumors should be dealt with on their respective merits, bearing in mind that almost always the ovarian tumor is found to be a secondary deposit and therefore represents metastatic disease for which surgical treatment should be regarded as palliative. A gastrointestinal primary tumor should preferably be submitted at least to palliative resection, provided continuity of the bowel can be restored. It would be wrong to raise a colostomy for a symptomless rectosigmoid lesion in the presence of widespread peritoneal disease.

SIMPLE BILATERAL SALPINGO-OOPHORECTOMY WITH OR WITHOUT HYSTERECTOMY (tumor apparently confined to one or both ovaries)

The standard technique need not be described but the following points are relevant to all operations for malignant or potentially malignant ovarian tumors.

Malignant ovarian cysts are best removed intact and this may be extremely difficult if a transverse incision has been used. Under these circumstances, the surgeon who encounters an ovarian cyst whose removal is likely to be difficult, should not hesitate to divide the rectus abdominis muscles transversely to improve both access and ease of delivery of the cyst. Deliberate puncture and aspiration should be condemned, as should translaparoscopic puncture and aspiration for diagnostic purposes. Should rupture occur, by definition the case is upstaged and the need for adjuvant therapy increased.

An adequate staging procedure should always be carried out (see p. 896). This is likewise very difficult through a small transverse incision.

Prophylactic removal of the infracolic omentum is recommended in early disease as it may well provide the only evidence of extra-ovarian disease.

STANDARD HYSTERECTOMY AND BILATERAL SALPINGO-OOPHORECTOMY (for tumors with local spread to the uterus alone)

This restricted procedure is appropriate to local extension involving only the uterus, oviducts or back of broad ligament. The major difficulty arises from intraligamentary extension between the leaves of the broad ligament. Such extension is not necessarily of sinister import, but does imperil the ureter. Early identification of the ureter and ligation of the ovarian vessels above the pelvic brim (as in radical oophorectomy) will facilitate the procedure. Small bowel and omental adhesions should be carefully examined. If these are more than flimsy the advisability of bowel resection and anastomosis should be assessed.

This operation is incorrectly used with a 'debulking' procedure when there is more advanced local extension or metastasis within the pouch of Douglas. Tumor involving the cul de sac and possibly anterior rectal wall is, therefore, left behind, which is suboptimal surgery if the disease is otherwise operable.

RADICAL OOPHORECTOMY

The objective is the monobloc removal of an adherent tumor and its local metastases by operating in planes not infiltrated by tumor.

Preoperative preparation

The standard preparation appropriate to pelvic surgery for malignant disease should be carried out including intravenous urography and screening for occult metastatic disease. Adequate blood should be cross-matched. Formal bowel sterilization is not required provided careful attention has been paid to mechanical cleansing with oral laxatives and enemas. Metronidazole or tinidazole is advocated. Sigmoidoscopy should have been carried out prior to anesthesia if there is a possibility of a colorectal primary.

Positioning and preparation

The Lloyd Davies position with legs apart is preferred. The bladder is catheterized. Dilatation and curettage is carried out (and cystoscopy) if necessary.

Incision and laparotomy

An extended lower midline incision is made to as high a level above the umbilicus as is necessary. This allows adequate access to the whole abdomen for thorough exploration, staging and resection of whatever tumor bulk is present. Any ascites found is aspirated for cytology. If none is present, peritoneal washings are taken by instilling 300 ml of normal saline into the abdomen and tilting the patient from side to side and up and down, enabling exfoliated malignant cells to be sampled. The upper abdomen is explored, commencing with the subdiaphragmatic peritoneum, liver, gall bladder, spleen, kidneys, stomach, small intestine including terminal ileum, appendix, mesentery and omentum. The paracolic gutters are inspected and then the pelvis. The side walls and lymph nodes are assessed, followed by the pelvic mass, ovaries, uterus, rectosigmoid and bladder. Now the patient should have been surgically staged, but definitive histopathological staging will be required to confirm this.

Surgical clearance of the upper abdomen

Clearance of upper abdominal tumor masses is normally advisable first, to allow adequate access to the pelvis for definitive pelvic clearance. Often an omental cake of tumor is present, making it impossible to separate the peritoneal layers of the omentum. Separate pedicles are taken, therefore, close to the transverse colon thereby mobilizing the omentum from the hepatic flexure to the splenic flexure. Hemostasis is secured by 00 black silk or linen ties. If the supracolic omentum is involved, this may be similarly removed, care being taken to secure adequate hemostasis on the greater curve of the stomach. Occasionally, tumor extension onto the spleen necessitates this organ being removed also. Division of the lieno-colic and lieno-phrenic ligaments make this relatively simple. When the splenic vessels are secured, care is taken to avoid the tail of the pancreas. The lesser sac may be carefully palpated to ensure there is no pancreatic pathology. If there is significant small bowel or mesenteric involvement, then preliminary intestinal resection with reanastomosis is required. More than 20% of cases have required a non-gynecological procedure.[1] The upper abdominal contents may then be packed away and attention centered on the pelvic pathology. (See also Ch. 83.)

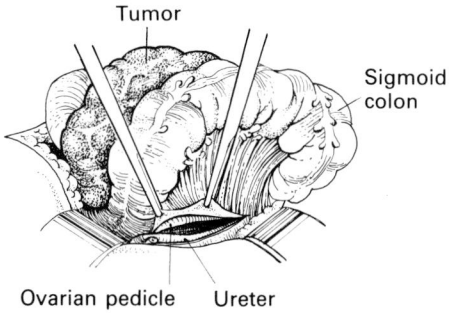

Fig. 82.1 The left paracolic region has been opened exposing the ureter and ovarian vessels above the pelvic brim away from the tumor site.

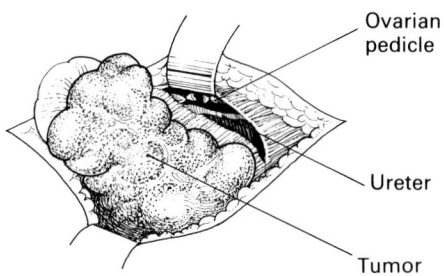

Fig. 82.2 The right side of the pelvic peritoneum has been incised to expose the right ureter and right ovarian vessels. It may be necessary to mobilize the cecum to achieve this exposure.

Ligation of the ovarian vessels and identification of the ureters

The junction of the sigmoid colon and descending colon should be held by the assistant and drawn over to the patient's right. The 'white line' marking the attachment of the mesosigmoid to the posterior parietal peritoneum is incised exposing the retroperitoneal space (Fig. 82.1). This space should be developed by the fingers pushing the left colon medially away from the posterior abdominal wall, and within it the left ureter and left ovarian vessels become apparent; the ureter commonly remains adherent to the medial flap of the peritoneum. The ovarian vessels should be divided and ligated. The distal ligature should be left long to permit ease of identification as the vascular pedicle requires mobilization towards the tumor. The space may be further developed digitally as far as the promontory of the sacrum where the retrorectal space may be entered. The peritoneal incision is extended anteriorly around the left side of the pelvic brim as far as the round ligament.

The approach to the right side is not so easy. The upper rectosigmoid must be deflected towards the patient's left and the right aspect of the pelvic brim exposed. If the terminal ileum and cecum are adherent they need either to be mobilized or resected still attached to the tumor. Anastomosis may then be deferred until later in the operation. Once the brim is clear the pelvic peritoneum is incised from the base of the sigmoid mesentery around to the right. This incision should be carried out carefully because it crosses the course of both the right ureter and ovarian vessels which need to be identified. Thereafter the incision may be continued round as far as possible towards the right round ligament (Fig. 82.2). The right ovarian vessels are divided between ligatures well clear of the pelvic brim, the distal ligature likewise being left long for identification.

Mobilization of the distal ovarian vascular pedicle will display the ureter as it passes over the division of the common iliac vessels eventually to disappear behind the tumor impacted in the pelvis. The retroperitoneal space may be developed over the brim of the pelvis into the retrorectal space to join the area developed from the earlier explor-

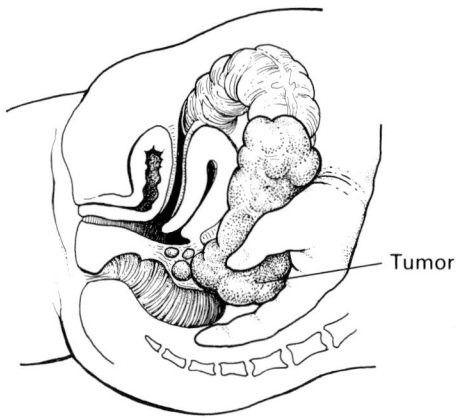

Fig. 82.3 Development of the retroperitoneal space by insertion of the operator's hand behind the rectum and within the presacral Waldeyer's fascia. This elevates the pouch of Douglas and starts mobilization of the pelvic contents.

ation posterior to the superior hemorrhoidal vessels (Fig. 82.3).

Exposure of the uterovesical pouch

Exposure of the uterovesical peritoneum can be difficult because of anterior displacement of the uterus by the pelvic mass. If there is any suspicion of peritoneal seedling or involvement in this pouch, the peritoneal incision should be continued round the pelvic brim just below the lower limit of the vertical abdominal incision. The peritoneum may then be stripped back towards its reflection on the front of the uterus by using sharp dissection from the dome of the bladder. If there is obvious metastasis or infiltration in this area it is a simple matter to enter the bladder and remove a disk of bladder wall, which may be subsequently closed using absorbable sutures. Otherwise if this area is clear the peritoneal reflection may be divided in front of the uterus using the standard technique.

Further mobilization

At this stage an attempt should be made to increase the

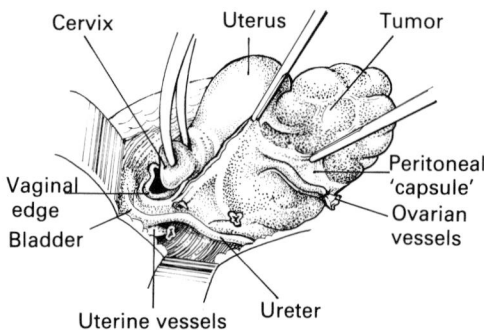

Fig. 82.4 Retrograde hysterectomy has commenced. Partial elevation has brought the ureter into view but the base of the peritoneal sac is still obscured.

retroperitoneal mobilization of the tumor starting on the side where the tumor is least adherent and therefore the approach is easier. This involves mobilization of the ureter from the peritoneal sac of the pouch of Douglas up to the point where the ureter enters its tunnel in the cardinal ligament. The uterine artery can now be exposed and clamped using the classical Wertheim technique. This area however is only rarely infiltrated in carcinoma of the ovary so that it may be simpler and quicker to divide the uterine artery above and medial to the ureter once the latter has been freed from the peritoneum and its position within its tunnel in the cardinal ligament identified (Fig. 82.4).

Retrograde hysterectomy

It may be convenient next to attempt ureteric mobilization and division of the uterine vessels on the other side. However, access to the cardinal ligament and uterine artery may be difficult if the main mass of the ovarian tumor is adherent on this side. Further mobilization may be achieved by freeing the uterus from the vagina which allows the anterior part of the pelvic mass to be pulled upwards. The vagina is entered by a stab incision in the anterior fornix without mobilization of the uterus from the tumor bed (Fig. 82.4). Once the vagina has been opened in the midline it is incised circumferentially with scissors; if one uterine artery has already been ligated and divided the circumcision is relatively easy. On the opposite side however, if the uterine vessels are still intact they can be clamped by insertion of a Moynihan (cholecystectomy) clamp through the vaginal incision or alternatively they have to be cut blindly and picked up later with a Moynihan clamp. At this stage the anesthetist should be prepared for an increase in local blood loss.

Mobilization of the posterior leaf of the broad ligament from the back of the vagina and pelvic side wall

When the posterior part of the vaginal wall circumference

is divided, care must be taken not to 'buttonhole' the overlying peritoneum. It is usually possible to enter a loose space containing areolar tissue over the posterior fornix. If however this space is infiltrated with tumor or metastasis, it may be better to cut along the posterior vaginal wall on each side thereby removing a disk of vaginal wall adjacent to the posterior fornix. The postero-inferior limit of this space is the attachment of the peritoneum to the front of the rectum. The appearance of the longitudinal muscle fibers of the rectum, as encountered during the mobilization of an enterocele sac, is characteristic and familiar to gynecologists.

Elevation of the pouch of Douglas

Once the posterior surface of the broad ligament has been freed from the pelvic sidewall and posterior vaginal wall, the pelvic tumor and its 'false capsule' of pelvic peritoneum are only held down by the anterior rectal wall. Full visualization of this area can be achieved by mobilization of the rectum down to the anorectal ring and, if necessary, division of the lateral ligaments of the rectum. The necessity for the latter maneuver will depend on the depth of the pouch of Douglas and the degree of impaction of the pelvic tumor. Rectal mobilization is achieved by finger and scissor dissection anterior to Waldeyer's fascia in the hollow of the sacrum. Once fingers have been insinuated into a space below and behind both rectum and tumor, air will be allowed to enter with a characteristic sucking noise. Full mobilization of the pelvic contents can then gradually be achieved. It is necessary to break down fine adhesions across the retroperitoneal space on either side in the pararectal areas but in general there are no major vascular communications and mobilization is relatively bloodless. Once mobilization is complete, the entire tumor mass consisting of uterus, ovarian tumor, false capsule of pouch of Douglas and adherent rectosigmoid may be elevated to the level of the anterior abdominal wall (Fig 82.5).

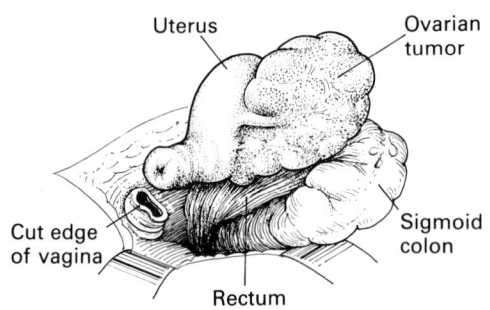

Fig. 82.5 This diagram shows the extent of mobilization of the tumor mass achieved by rectal mobilization after detachment of the uterus from the vagina. Note that the uterus and tumor have not been separated.

Separation of tumor from anterior rectal wall

A decision now has to be made between a limited anterior rectal resection with colorectal anastomosis and a painstaking dissection of the adherent peritoneum from the anterior rectal wall. In many cases a limited restorative resection of the rectum is quicker and seems to give very satisfactory results. There is always sufficient distal rectum for the intrapelvic anastomosis to be relatively easy. The technique will be described later. As soon as a decision is taken to proceed to large bowel resection, perioperative intravenous broad spectrum antibiotic therapy should be instituted.

Preliminary closure of vaginal vault

The open vaginal vault should be closed with interrupted absorbable sutures and any resected part of the bladder is repaired, preferably with polyglycollic acid sutures. Once hemostasis has been secured, the wound is closed, preferably with suction drainage through a separate stab incision using a wide lumen tube. It is the practice of one of us (C.N.H.) to irrigate the raw area with mercuric chloride (1 in 500) mopping it out after a few minutes. This agent should never be flushed around the general peritoneal cavity.

ANTERIOR RECTAL RESECTION

Two techniques of rectal resection and reanastomosis are described for those cases where its use is desirable.

Division of the mesocolon

The rectosigmoid mesentery is divided in the vascular arcade at an appropriate interval from the bowel. Preferably artery forceps are applied to mesenteric vessels easily demonstrable by transillumination. Because one is not dealing with intrinsic rectal disease, high ligation of the arterial supply is unnecessary and the superior hemorrhoidal artery can be tied on the promontory of the sacrum. The vein may be secured separately.

Preparation of the proximal loop

At this stage the level of viability of the rectosigmoid may be delineated by a cyanotic color change in the distal segment brought about by interruption of the blood supply. Once an appropriate area for division is selected, the bowel is prepared for severance. Appendices epiploicae are removed from the immediate area so that a clean area is presented for the insertion of the seromuscular suture layer. The bowel is severed between two closely applied Parker-Kerr clamps, following which both clamps are covered by an appropriate cap. The proximal loop is then lifted out of the wound.

Distal resection

A Finch's right angle clamp is placed across the rectum below the peritoneal reflection of the pouch of Douglas. An assistant now passes a proctoscope through the anal canal and irrigates and cleans the distal rectum and anus until all fecal material has been removed.

The tumor mass is still attached by the distal rectum which has been occluded by the Finch's clamp. Two Babcock forceps are applied to the distal rectum above the lateral ligaments on either side below the Finch's clamp. The anal canal and rectum should by now be clean and the bowel may be severed below the Finch's clamp with scissors, any soiling being immediately mopped with gauze pledgets. The whole mass en bloc is now removed.

Preparation for anastomosis

The two intestinal ends are then prepared for intrapelvic anastomosis. If there is any tension on the proximal loop further mobilization of the peritoneum and lateral attachment of the descending colon should be carried out, if necessary up to and including the splenic flexure; in ovarian cases this is very rarely necessary. The bowel must lie easily without twisting or distortion, and anastomosis is effected with one or two layers of continuous or interrupted sutures. We prefer polyglycollic acid or polyglactin (Fig. 82.6). A second layer of interrupted black silk sutures is optional.

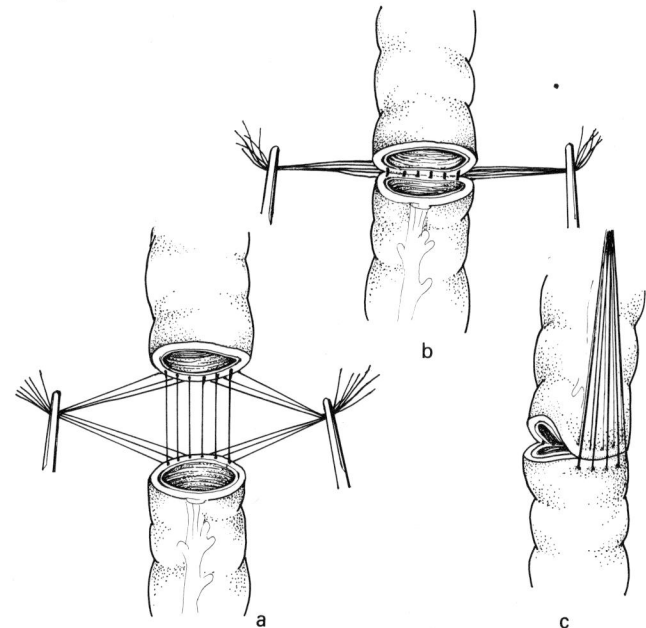

Fig. 82.6 Colorectal anastomosis. (a) Interrupted black silk seromuscular sutures have been inserted as a posterior layer. They are kept taut until the proximal bowel is 'railroaded' down to a comfortable adjacent position. (b) A continuous 'all-coat' layer of polyglycollic acid sutures. (c) The anterior seromuscular layer is completed.

Insertion of posterior layer of interrupted black silk sutures

Five to seven interrupted sutures are placed with a single bite through the seromuscular layer of the upper loop of bowel picking up the sacral aspect of the muscle of the inferior loop. Suture ends should be attached to artery forceps, to be tied later.

Approximation of bowel ends

Now the Parker-Kerr clamp is removed by excision to leave a viable proximal edge of bowel exhibiting fresh bleeding. Care must be taken to remove any fecal contamination during the subsequent open anastomosis. With the assistants holding the previously inserted ligatures reasonably taut using two Babcock forceps, the proximal loop of bowel is 'railroaded' down the sutures into the pelvis. At this stage the individual posterior wall black silk sutures are tied and cut short, the exception being the two sutures at either end of the line which are left long as markers.

Suturing

Two sutures of 00 polyglycollic acid or polyglactin to be used as markers are inserted right through the now adjacent posterior walls of the two loops of bowel. The cut edges of the two loops are now approximated when the two sutures are lightly tied in the middle with care to avoid necrosis of the underlying tissue. One needle is selected and an over-and-over suture is inserted away from the operator until the corner of the anastomosis is reached, at which stage the suture procedure is changed to a Connell suture in which the individual loops lie on the mucosa of the bowel. Connell sutures are inserted alternately above and below the anastomosis until the anterior wall is closed almost to the midline. At this juncture the other needle from the double ended posterior wall suture is picked up and the posterior part of the anastomosis completed by continuous suture through all coats until the anastomotic angle nearest to the surgeon is reached when once again reversion to Connell sutures takes place. This form of suture is carried across the anterior wall of the bowel

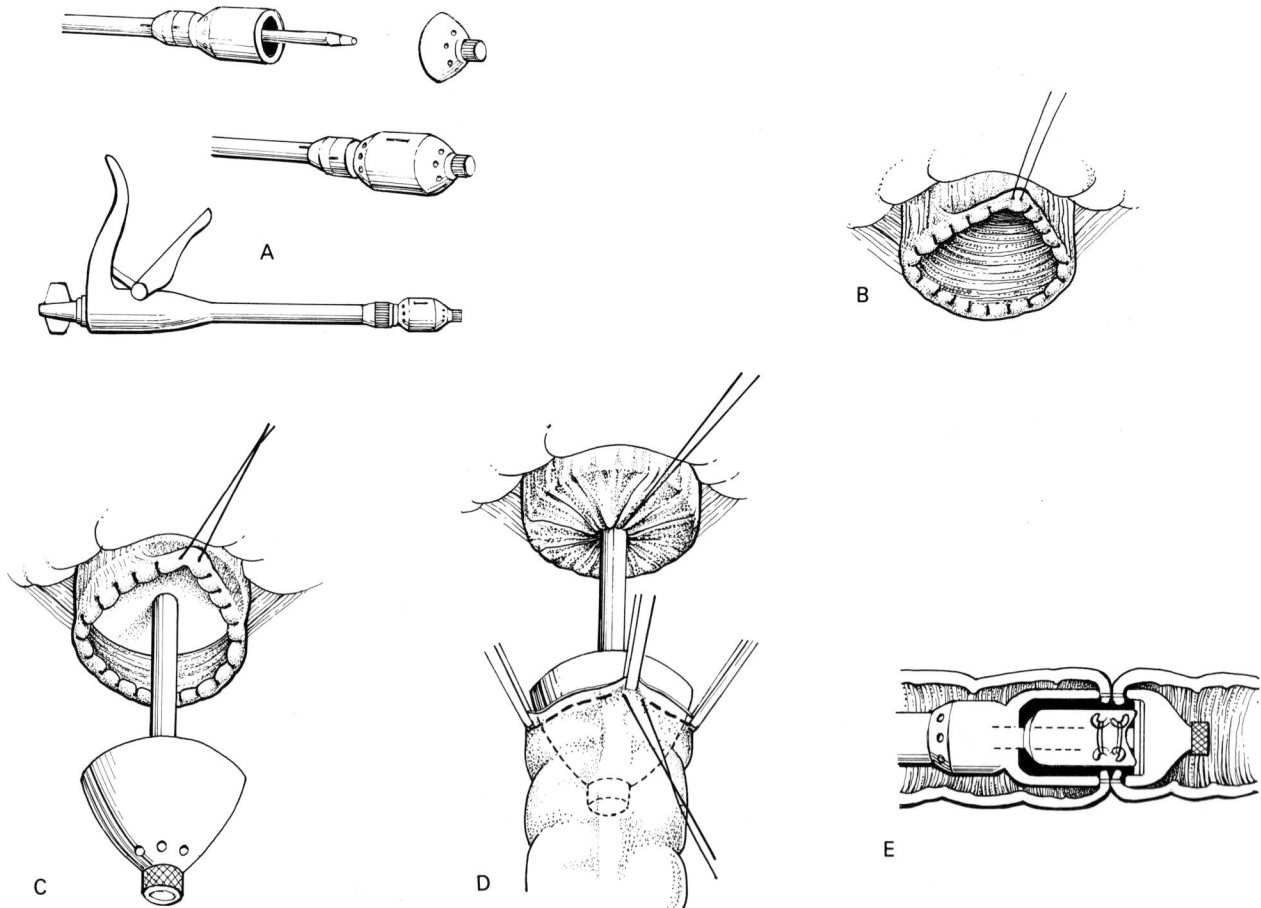

Fig. 82.7 (A) End-to-end stapling (EEA) instruments. (B) Preparation of the distal anastomotic limb. (C) EEA advanced from the perineum through the anus in distal limb. (D) Distal limb closed and proximal limb drawn down to meet anastomotic site. (E) Anastomosis complete with EEA in situ prior to closing the instrument and removing it with a 'doughnut' of colon tissue at the anastomosis site.

until the fellow suture from the other side is met and the 'all coats' layer is complete. The two are tied together and cut; this type of suture must not be cut flush.

Completion of anastomosis

The black silk interrupted seromuscular layer of Lembert sutures is then completed between the two marker sutures covering in the previous layer just inserted. The distal rectal stump will be completely without a peritoneal investment and care must be taken that these sutures do not cut out. The peritoneal covered proximal loop will tend to hold the sutures very much better and adjacent appendices epiplöicae may be brought down across the suture line if appropriate. The anastomosed bowel should rest easily in the pelvis without tension, rotation or distortion.

Stapling technique

Alternatively, a stapling technique can be used. Transanal use of the end-to-end anastomotic stapler (EAA) would be the most appropriate. Such an instrument facilitates very low colo-anal anastomoses, particularly in males. It would be rare for this to be a special advantage in the primary resection of ovarian cancer by radical oophorectomy, however. (See also Ch. 88.)

Assessment of cartridge size is required before assembly of the instrument — in most instances a 31 mm cartridge will be appropriate. The initial phases of resection are as described above, with preparation of the anastomotic sites. The next step is the insertion of a monofilament purse string suture, approximately 2 mm from the cut margins of the proximal and distal bowel. A purse stringing clamp is sometimes used for this purpose. The assembled instrument is lubricated, carefully inserted through the anus and manipulated to the cut end of the rectum. The anvil is manipulated through the aperture and the distal purse string is tied below the anvil. The proximal bowel is then gently eased over the anvil so that its purse string can be tied in turn. The instrument is then closed until the bowel becomes closely approximated. There is a vernier scale which has to be aligned before correct apposition of the cartridge and anvil has been achieved. After a final inspection of the anastomosis by rotation of the instrument, the safety catch is released and the instrument fired. The wing nut is opened and the instrument can then be withdrawn from the rectum. The anvil should then be removed and two 'doughnut rings' removed from the shaft of the instrument and checked for completeness (Fig. 82.7).

Termination of the procedure and closure

Individual preferences will dictate closure technique. 'Sump' drainage to the hollow of the sacrum and nasogastric aspiration are considered desirable by the authors.

'SECOND-LOOK' SURGERY

The role of 'second-look' operations is still debatable. (See also p. 907.) Although originally precisely defined, the term now covers several classes of reoperation.

Immediate reoperation

Definitive radical surgery by a subspecialist oncologist should be carried out at the earliest convenient opportunity after exploration and biopsy by a generalist. This will equally apply in early disease if adequate staging and documentation has not been carried out.

Interval reoperation

This may be recommended in the middle of a course of chemotherapy if operability has been improved. There is little to commend this approach as superior to primary surgery.

Residual disease difficult to evaluate while receiving chemotherapy

Some patients with known minimal residual disease recorded at primary surgery offer no physical signs for the subsequent evaluation of adjuvant treatment including chemotherapy. In the absence of an acceptable tumor marker for most ovarian cancers, a 'second-look' procedure may be advocated prior to discontinuing chemotherapy. This can be by laparoscopy although many surgeons believe that the extent of the previous disease and the effects of previous surgery render this procedure unsatisfactory and hazardous. (See also Ch. 21.) Alternatively a formal laparotomy may be carried out. The timing of this 'second-look' procedure is determined either by arrival at the cumulative dose of the prescribed agent, or by waiting up to 2 years postoperatively. By such time the majority of patients with progressive disease will have become obvious and thus will be spared unrewarding surgery. This type of procedure should be confined to treatment centers with investigational protocols.

Gross residual disease left at primary operation subsequently responding with major remission to chemotherapy

A few such patients will be found at 'second-look' laparotomy to have no detectable evidence of residual disease. Often, however, islands of viable carcinoma cells may be found in selected biopsy sites. Other patients may merely have had diagnostic biopsy performed at the primary operation and for them there exists the possibility of definitive ablative surgery at a 'second-look' operation.

Bilateral oophorectomy with removal of the omentum may now be quite easy.

Inoperable disease with partial reduction only after chemotherapy

Significant improvement in operability is most unlikely unless the clinical tumor mass has almost disappeared. The decision to reoperate in these cases may only reflect the willingness or ability of a second surgeon to undertake major surgical ablation which should have been carried out on the first occasion. This type of 'second-look' operation should not be undertaken unless a change of chemotherapy is contemplated which would thus justify a preliminary 'debulking' procedure in its own right. Within these guidelines 'second-look' surgery has a place but the temptation to perform it too early, or to satisfy the curiosity of an attendant physician should be resisted.

SURGERY OF COMPLICATIONS

Fistula

Fecal fistulae are not uncommon in the terminal stages of this disease and add considerably to the distress of the patient. An immediate resort to colostomy may not be the correct answer, and technically the procedure can be extremely difficult. An attempt must be made to identify the loop of bowel involved and also to determine whether the distal bowel is obstructed. Sigmoidoscopy and contrast radiography of the fistula are required.

Ileovaginal fistula. The terminal ileum frequently becomes adherent in the pelvis or right iliac fossa following surgery for malignant ovarian disease, and may be perforated by recurrent growth or radiotherapy reaction, or both. It is often a mistake to attempt to resect the damaged loop in such cases. The ideal operation is a side-to-side enterocolic anastomosis using the transverse colon.* High polymer sutures should be used as wound healing is protracted in such patients.

Colovaginal fistula. The apex of the sigmoid colon may adhere to the pelvis in much the same way. In late ovarian cancer, fistulae of large bowel origin are more commonly colonic than rectal although they are often incorrectly referred to as rectovaginal fistulae. They may be managed by performing a transverse colostomy. This procedure is not easy if the infracolic and supracolic omentum are involved with growth but almost always left iliac colostomy will be difficult or impossible. Occasionally, even if the fistula has followed irradiation, a modified posterior pelvic exenteration may be considered, provided there is no evidence of

* For other approaches see Ch. 86.

extrapelvic metastatic disease. After radiotherapy however, there is a definite risk of producing an additional urinary fistula where one did not exist before (see Ch. 85).

Alternatives to colostomy should certainly be considered in patients who do not have significant life expectation as well as those with a better prognosis. Colpocleisis may be used for genital fistulae even in the presence of pelvic malignant disease. Unfortunately this is not applicable to a colovaginal fistula as there is almost always concomitant distal obstruction and a fecal mass will build up and burst out through the closed off vagina. A measure which may be tried under these circumstances is the construction of a rectal fenestration or aperture between the posterior vaginal fornix and upper rectum. This can usually be carried out using a Parks or Eisenhammer speculum through the anus by attempting to make an aperture at least 2 cm in diameter. The cut edges of the rectum should be oversewn with a high polymer suture as there is a risk of troublesome hemorrhage. Palliative procedures of this sort may relieve some of the distress of a dying patient, many of whom are grateful that something is being done to relieve terminal distress, without the addition of an abdominal stoma.

Intestinal obstruction

This is a common complicating event in carcinomatosis peritonei. It may be related to progressive disease, postoperative adhesions, intraperitoneal instillations (especially of radioactive gold) and even to systemic chemotherapy which on occasions can produce a massive reaction from peritoneal metastases resulting in a plastic peritonitis. Alternatively, the complication may be the result of whole abdominal radiotherapy without active disease being present. In most instances exploratory laparotomy should be carried out, the incision being sited over the area of maximum distension which usually corresponds with that in the diagnostic plain film. The patient should have been sigmoidoscoped prior to operation so that the condition of the distal colon may be determined. It is often unwise to attempt dissection of adherent loops within the pelvis. The chances of buttonholing the bowel during dissection are extremely high and if the distal obstruction is not relieved, the sequel of abdominal-fecal fistula is almost inevitable. If soiling occurs there may be little option but to proceed to resection, and ileostomy. Fine judgment is required to avoid overtreating a patient with progressive disease.

The obstructed loops should be well packed off and decompressed through the site chosen for subsequent anastomosis, preferably using a Savage decompressor. Enteral anastomosis should be carried out side-to-side in two layers, either between two loops of ileum or, more commonly, between the obstructed ileum and the transverse colon. A dilated distal colon is an absolute indication for colostomy. Other procedures will result in an uncontrolled abdominal-fecal fistula. On occasion, a defunctioning ileostomy with a distal mucus fistula may be necessary.

For the nursing care of gynecological patients with fistula or artificial stoma, the assistance of a trained stomatherapist is invaluable. If the prognosis is reasonable, consideration should be given to total parenteral nutrition (p. 1349) but in these circumstances, the compassionate surgeon must not lose sight of the fact that his maneuvers are palliative and the objective should be to relieve rather than to cause distress in the days remaining to the patient.

The majority of patients still die from their ovarian cancer, and most from cachexia associated with progressive sub-acute intestinal obstruction. This often may, and should be, managed medically but actively, with adequate analgesia, antiemetics and a suitable diet. This may be liquid and of low roughage with stool softeners. Support services for palliative care both at home and in the hospital or hospice must be utilized. (See also Ch. 92.)

CONCLUSION

Within the past two decades, the role of surgery in malignant disease of the ovary has been transformed from a uniform standard procedure in operable cases and total defeatism in the inoperable majority, to a wide range of surgical procedures, some of which are the most testing in gynecological practice. Such procedures can offer palliation and sometimes a measure of hope to an increasing number of patients with this unpleasant malignancy.

REFERENCES

1. Hudson C N (ed) 1986 Ovarian Cancer. Oxford University Press, Oxford
2. Shepherd J H 1990 Surgical management of ovarian cancer. In: Shepherd J H, Monaghan J M (eds) Clinical Gynaecological Oncology, 2nd edn. Blackwell, Oxford

83. Surgery for carcinoma of ovary: extrapelvic cytoreduction

C. T. Griffiths   N. J. Finkler

INTRODUCTION

With few exceptions, extrapelvic surgical procedures for advanced ovarian carcinoma are limited to the abdominal cavity and retroperitoneum. In our experience, a surgical approach similar to that described in the previous chapter has always enabled us to clear the pelvic cavity of gross tumor in primary cases. Consequently, the completion of a successful cytoreductive operation has depended on the size and anatomic site of metastatic deposits in the upper abdomen. Although we have defined successful cytoreduction as the excision of all tumor masses exceeding 1 cm in diameter, survival time has correlated inversely with decrements in residual mass size below this upper limit (p < 0.0001). We now attempt to remove all masses excepting widespread miliary implants 2 to 3 mm in diameter. Once again, the degree of operability will be determined by the largest residual mass size in the upper abdomen. Consequently, the abdominal procedures are undertaken prior to pelvic resection.

OPERABILITY

In reference to cytoreductive operations, operability can be defined as the feasibility of safely excising all masses larger than a designated size limit below which chemotherapeutic sensitivity and survival of the patient will be enhanced. In most instances, operability is determined during the course of a multiphased cytoreductive operation. Inoperability should be determined as early as possible, thereby sparing the patient extensive dissection and organ resection beyond the scope of palliation.

In our prospective clinical series of 77 consecutive patients in whom aggressive cytoreductive operations were attempted, residual mass size was the strongest prognostic factor, eliminating the factors of stage and histologic grade on multivariant analysis. On the other hand, the adverse prognostic effect of specific organ involvement by metastases greater than 1 cm was not always mitigated by extirpation. Our studies indicate that the following conditions render a patient inoperable:

1. parenchymal liver metastases
2. pancreatic metastases
3. splenic metastases in the presence of Stage IV disease
4. involvement of suprarenal para-aortic lymph nodes
5. penetrating lesions of the diaphragm (Stage IV disease)
6. dense tumor involvement of the porta hepatis
7. infiltration of the abdominal wall.

With extensive upper abdominal tumor, inoperability based on retroperitoneal, splenic or diaphragmatic involvement may not be determined until excision of tumor bulk has been sufficient to expose the upper abdominal organs. As soon as access to the areas in question is gained, careful examination must be carried out with biopsy as needed.

OPERATIVE PROCEDURES

Omentectomy and splenectomy

The initial presentation at laparotomy may be a lobulated, multi-hued, friable and hemorrhagic fixed slab of tumor tissue which completely obscures the remaining abdominal contents. These omental cakes, particularly when adherent to surrounding parietal and visceral peritoneum, may seem to present a formidable, or even insurmountable problem. Despite their vascularity, large, friable masses can be removed by gentle and systematic dissection without losing more than one unit of blood (Fig. 83.1).

In the absence of ascites, which seems to inhibit serosal adhesions, tumor cakes are usually adherent to anterior and lateral parietes and upper abdominal organs. Entry into the peritoneal cavity is best accomplished at the cephalad extremity of an incision that extends from the symphysis pubis to the xyphoid process. Anterior wall peritoneum is best left on the tumor mass when an avascular plane cannot otherwise be found. Blunt dissection and traction on the cake itself can result in persistent and diffuse bleeding from the tumor surface or its attachment. The electrosurgical unit may help with hemostasis, but the dial must be set at the highest output level.

Typically, omental caking results from confluent nodular

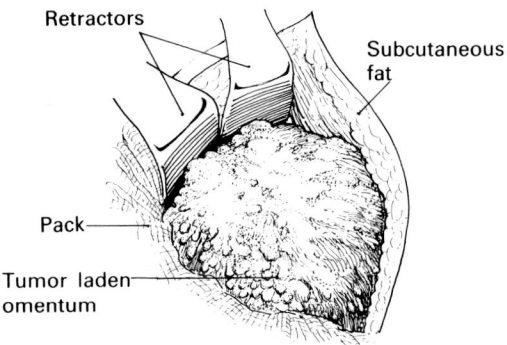

Fig. 83.1A Omentum caked with tumor that extended to the greater curvature of the stomach and the splenic hilum.

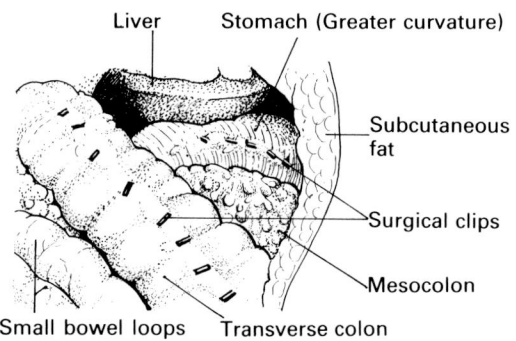

Fig. 83.1B Anterior abdominal contents after total omentectomy and splenectomy.

tumor growth within the omentum that extends cephalad, crossing the transverse colon to the greater curvature of the stomach and then along the gastrocolic ligament into the left upper quadrant. Tumor progression into the gastro-splenic ligament leads to tumor involvement of the splenic pedicle. The blood supply is derived from the three major omental arteries and veins which, in turn, are branches of the left and right gastro-epiploic vessels that form an arcade 2 cm below the greater curvature of the stomach. Control of this blood supply should be obtained prior to further manipulation of the tumor cake. The initial step is entry into the lesser sac (omental bursa) through a clear space in the gastrocolic ligament at the greater curvature between the small gastric branches of the gastro-epiploic arcade. At this level, the lesser sac may be a potential space only and lies between the gastrocolic ligament (the anterior two of four omental lamellae) and the anterior portion of

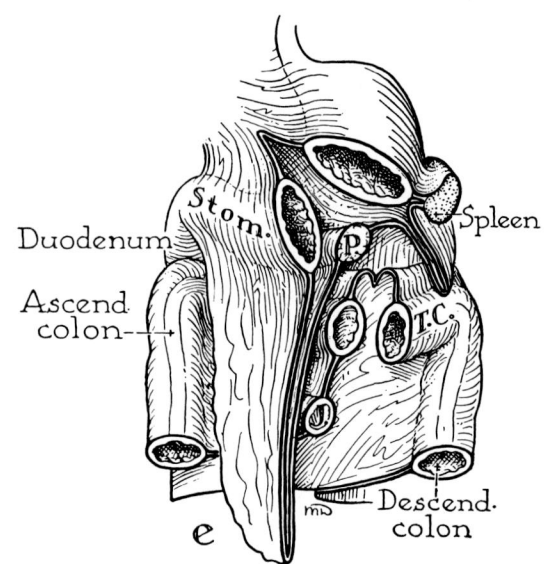

Fig. 83.2 Interrelation of the bilaminar serous supports of the upper abdominal viscera. Textual references to omental lamellae are in anterior to posterior sequence, i.e. first through fourth. (Reproduced from Anson & Maddock (1952),[1] with permission.)

the transverse mesocolon which is fused with the third and fourth omental lamellae (Fig. 83.2). Identification of the proper space can be difficult, but is facilitated by placing a forefinger into the lesser sac via the epiploic-foramen of Winslow, and by selecting a point of entry to the left of midline rather than at the antral margin of the stomach (Fig. 83.3). Once the gastrocolic ligament can be clearly separated from the transverse mesocolon, the former is detached from the stomach by careful isolation, ligature and division of gastro-epiploic branches using either fine ties or hemoclips for speed. Although early isolation and ligation of the gastro-epiploic arteries will immediately decrease vascularity of the omental cake, collateral flow through the delicate gastric branches increases considerably and makes their ligation difficult. The gastro-epiploic vessels are easily identified once detached from the stomach, and both sides of the arcade are ligated, artery before vein.

When the tumor extends into the gastrosplenic ligament and splenic hilum, splenectomy is usually necessary. Isolated implants on the splenic capsule greater than 1 cm in diameter also require splenectomy, but smaller lesions, if few in number, can be destroyed by thorough fulguration. With contiguous tumor involvement of the splenic pedicle, the dissection is carried along the greater curvature toward the fundus until the stomach can be retracted upward, thus exposing the lesser sac and the pancreas (Fig. 83.4). The parietal peritoneum at the superior margin of the tail of the pancreas is incised, and the splenic artery and vein, readily found in this location, are ligated in that sequence (Fig. 83.5). In most instances, the short gastric artery can be seen as it courses from the splenic artery to the upper, lesser curvature of the stomach, and is ideally ligated at this time (Fig. 83.4).

The dissection into the left upper quadrant is facilitated if the omental cake is freed from the right transverse colon by dissection within the avascular cleavage plane between the third and fourth lamellae (Fig. 83.2). On rare occasions, the tumor mass will invade the wall of the transverse colon and require resection and anastomosis of this organ. After vascular control has been obtained, downward

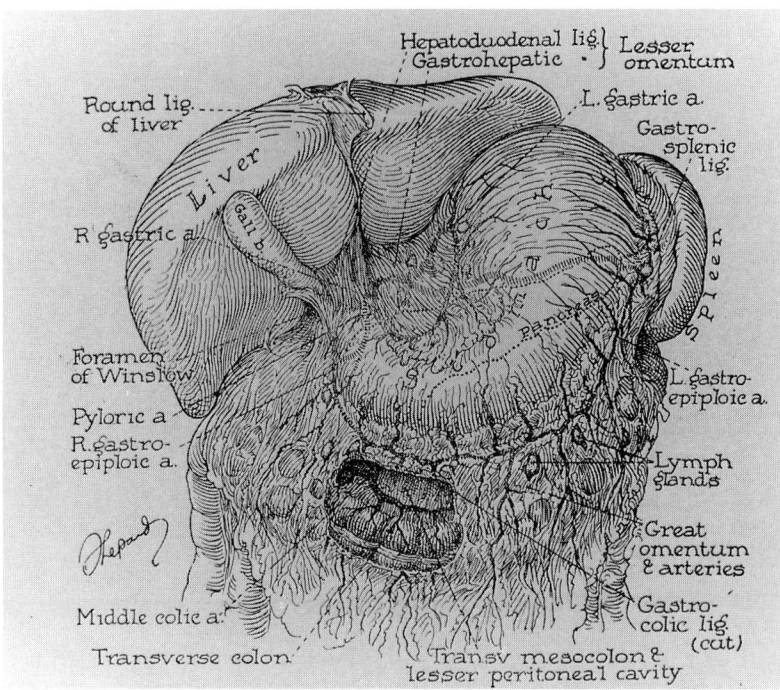

Fig. 83.3 Anterior view of the upper abdominal viscera with exposure of the lesser sac below the gastro-epiploic arcade. (Reproduced from Black & Exelby (1980),[2] with permission.)

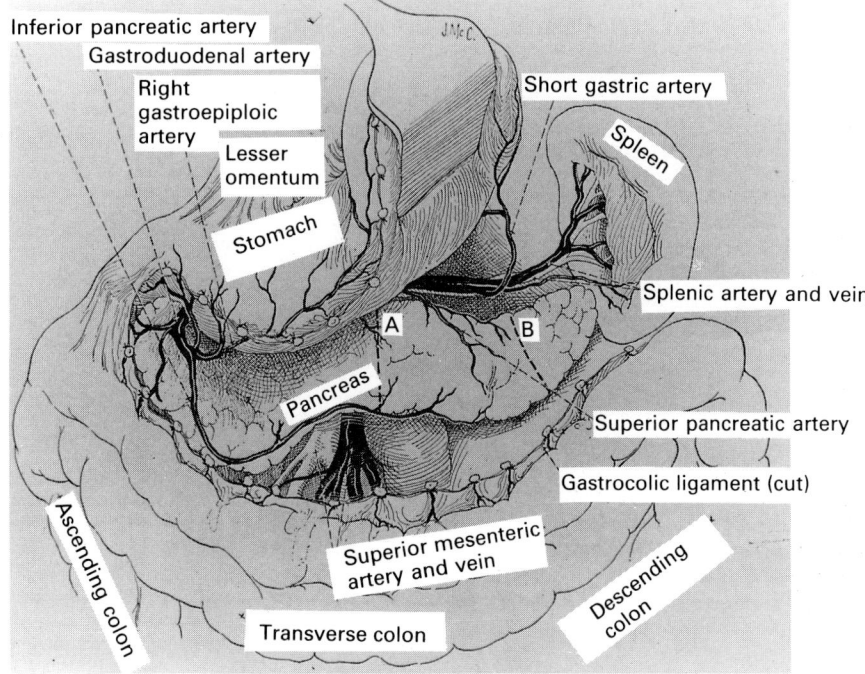

Fig. 83.4 Vascular supply to the spleen, pancreas and stomach. The origin of the short gastric artery is proximal to the splenic pedicle but the distal portion is easily injured when clamping the pedicle. (Reproduced from Anson & Maddock (1952),[1] with permission.)

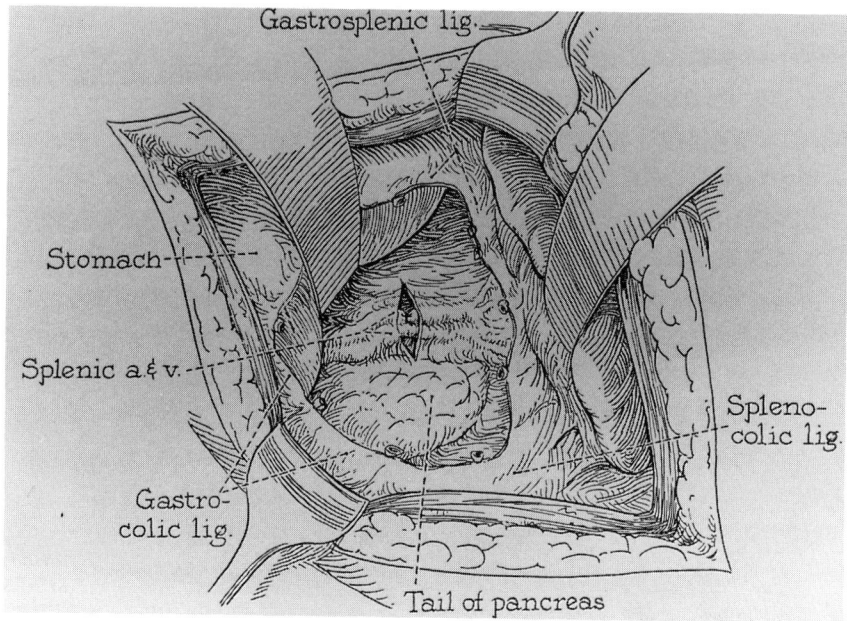

Fig. 83.5 Ligation of the splenic artery at the superior border of the pancreas. (Reproduced from Black & Exelby (1980),[2] with permission.)

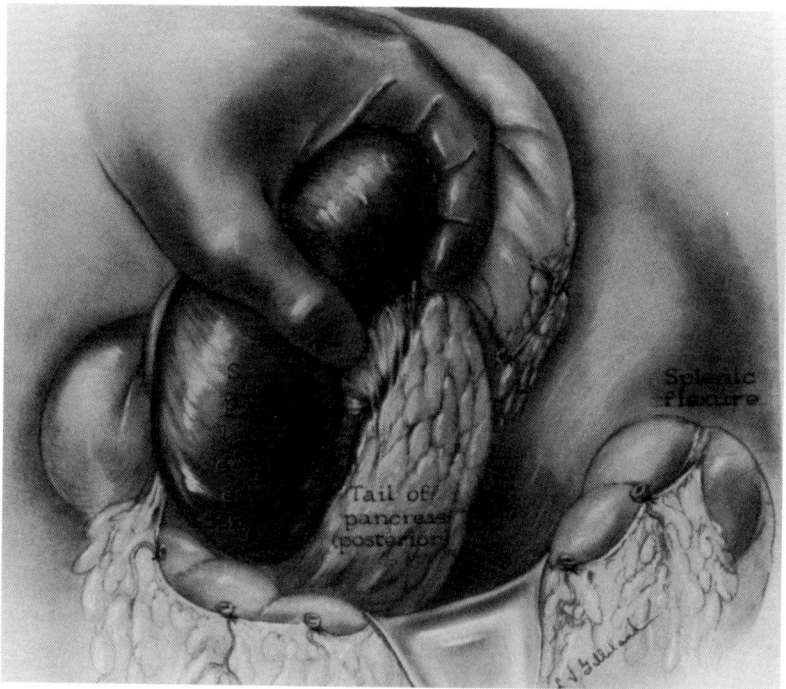

Fig. 83.6 Mobilization of the tail of the pancreas prior to clamping of the splenic pedicle. (Reproduced from Silen (1964),[5] with permission.)

traction on the omental mass may now be applied and will aid in completing the left upper quadrant dissection. An incision is made in the peritoneum in the upper left paracolic gutter and is carried across the diaphragm, thus mobilizing the splenic flexure of the colon and the superior pole of the spleen. Tumor extension in this area can adhere these structures to the diaphragm, but mobilization can still be accomplished by dissecting in the avascular plane between the diaphragmatic serosa and muscle. The lieno-renal attachment is then incised, as well as the remaining gastrosplenic ligament. The tail of the pancreas, which is in juxtaposition to the splenic pedicle, may be obscured by tumor nodules and must be carefully dissected from the pedicle prior to its ligation (Fig. 83.6). After ensuring that the short gastric artery is ligated, the splenic pedicle is clamped, divided and doubly ligated with 0 silk suture.

The final step in the omentectomy-splenectomy procedure is the dissection of the specimen from the left transverse colon, unless colonic invasion requires bowel resection. Even within the usually avascular plane, a number of small vessels from colonic serosa or mesocolon may penetrate the tumor mass and cause troublesome bleeding. They can be managed by closure with closely approximated horizontal mattress sutures of 3–0 silk. Drainage is, of course, mandatory.

Total omentectomy augmented by splenectomy has been described in detail, although we have found lesser procedures adequate in 50% of our cases and splenectomy has been necessary in only 50% of the remainder. Obviously, gross tumor that does not extend above the transverse colon can be removed simply by infracolic omenectomy. When the tumor nodules in the gastrocolic ligament do not extend to the stomach, the gastro-epiploic vessels may be spared. We recommend initial entry into the lesser sac, however, because we prefer retrograde dissection of the mass off the transverse colon following vascular control. In addition, exposure of the lesser sac permits direct palpation of suprarenal para-aortic nodes. We have had no gastric complications following ligation of the gastro-epiploic and short gastric vessels.

Excision of diaphragmatic tumor masses

In our experience, the diaphragm is involved by metastases greater than 1 cm in diameter in 18% of patients with Stage III disease, and in 41% of patients with Stage IV disease. Diaphragmatic implantation does not in itself worsen prognosis, and excision of these masses improves survival consistent with the degree of cytoreduction afforded. On the other hand, in a subsequent trial, diaphragmatic resection necessitated by full thickness penetration by the tumor in putative Stage III patients (occult Stage IV) was associated with a markedly shortened median survival time compared to that of other Stage IV patients. Although tumor penetration was discernible only after entering the chest cavity, all of the individual masses exceeded 5 cm in diameter. None of the masses that could be excised from the underlying muscle exceeded 4 cm in diameter and this difference was significant ($p < 0.01$). Consequently, we no longer attempt removal of adherent masses exceeding 4 cm in diameter.

Access to the diaphragm is gained by downward traction on the liver after mobilization by transection of supporting ligaments. The ligamentum teres is divided and ligated, thus exposing the falciform ligament. This avascular structure can be incised without clamping, except for the superior portion where the diaphragm and liver come together. The left triangular ligament is easily clamped and divided (Fig. 83.7), providing exposure of the diaphragm to the coronary ligament, i.e. the anterior peritoneal sulcus between the liver and diaphragm. Nodules 4 cm or less in

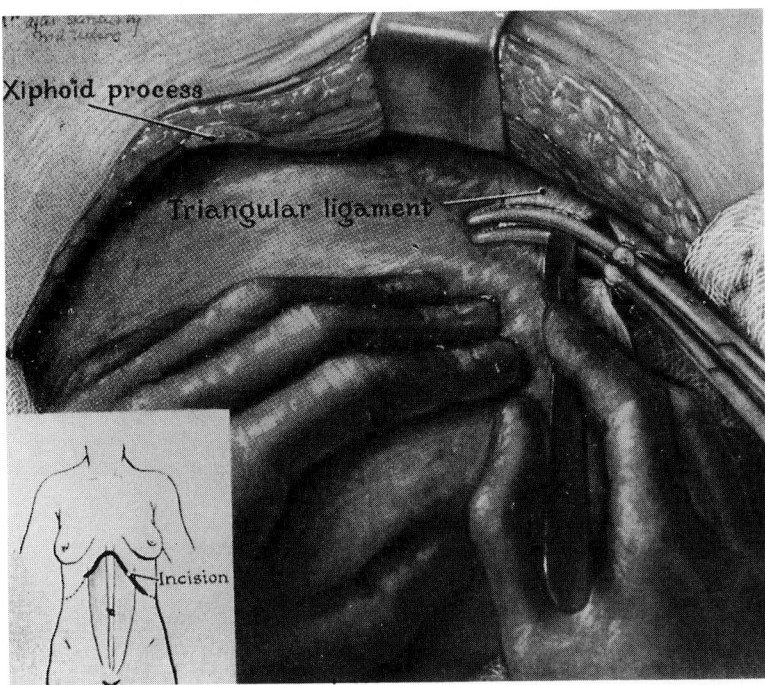

Fig. 83.7 Division of the left triangular ligament for hepatic mobilization. (Reproduced from Longmire & Sanford (1948),[4] with permission.)

diameter can usually be dissected from the underlying muscle, and excised without entry into the chest cavity. A small incidental pleural defect can be managed by passing a soft rubber catheter through the defect and encircling it with a purse string suture. During simultaneous aspiration through the catheter and inflation of the lung, the catheter is withdrawn as the suture is tightened. Larger defects require insertion of a chest tube through the chest wall under direct vision for continuous suction postoperatively.

Excision of liver nodules

Although parenchymal metastases are considered inoperable Stage IV disease, implanted surface nodules can be removed easily. Some degree of liver mobilization may be required, depending on the location of the tumor implants. Implanted nodules that are partially compressed below the liver surface are almost invariably encapsulated. By incising Glisson's capsule at the tumor margin, the nodules can usually be shelled out with minimal blood loss. Bleeding can be controlled by high-frequency electrocautery at the highest setting. Rarely, horizontal mattress sutures with blunt 'liver' needles are required to approximate the raw surfaces, between which strips of absorbable gelatin sponges soaked in topical thrombin are placed. Occasionally, strips of Teflon are required to act as bolsters, thereby preventing the mattress sutures from pulling through the soft liver tissue.

Mid-abdominal procedures

On completion of the upper abdominal procedures, the largest residual mass above the transverse colon sets the standard for the extent of tumor resection required in the lower abdomen and pelvis.

Mid-abdominal procedures are directed at tumor involvement of the small bowel, parietal peritoneum and para-aortic lymph nodes. Tumor implants on small bowel serosa may be few and superficial, and readily excised without entering the lumen; an edematous plane beneath tumor-bearing serosa permits excision without disturbing the muscularis. Serosal defects can be left alone, but seromuscular defects must be repaired transversely with interrupted inverting sutures of fine silk. Any compromise of the lumen by closure of these defects necessitates immediate resection and anastomosis before the problem is forgotten.

Since the density of tumor implantation is greatest in proximity to the primary tumor, the terminal ileum, with its propensity to dip into the pelvis, may be massively involved. Consequently, resection of the terminal ileum is almost as common as resection of the rectosigmoid colon. In many instances, the distal 5 cm of ileum is completely tumor-free, and end-to-end ileoileostomy is permissable. Tumor involvement at or near the ileocecal valve requires an end-to-end or side-to-side ileo-ascending colostomy, and inversion closure of the distal ileal stump. Dense implantation of the cecum and ileocecal junction necessitates resection of terminal ileum and proximal colon in continuity.

Fistulization of the small intestine is a common complication of end-stage carcinoma of the ovary and, unfortunately, is not a rare complication of primary operations for this disease. The tendency toward leaking anastomoses results from both nutritional compromise and microscopic serosal involvement at the bowel resection margin. Nutritional compromise may be managed only by a sustained program of preoperative hyperalimentation. The avoidance of suture-line tumor is not always possible. We have found that patients with more than two small bowel anastomoses are particularly prone to anastomotic leaks, probably because multiple anastomoses reflect both extensive serosal involvement and the surgeon's concern for preservation of small bowel length. The resection of the entire ileum or a short small bowel overall can be easily managed, unlike the serious complications that follow anastomotic disruption; the surgeon must act accordingly. Apparent 'skip areas' of tumor involvement may best be included in a longer excised segment. Intestinal stapling techniques, with their rapidity and efficiency, have been a welcome addition to prolonged operative procedures for ovarian carcinoma. On the other hand, every anastomotic leak outside of the pelvic cavity that we have had in the past 15 years among patients with ovarian carcinoma has been through a stapled anastomosis. For this reason, we have reverted to double-layered sutured anastomoses in the belief that the inverted serosa-to-serosa technique provides greater security, particularly if microscopic tumor is present (Fig. 83.8). Certainly, in patients who are not nutritionally compromised and in whom anastomotic tumor is highly unlikely, stapled anastomoses are reasonable.

Isolated tumor implants on bowel mesentery can almost always be excised without interference with the vascular supply. With infiltrating lesions involving large segments of mesentery, bowel resection becomes necessary. Patients with tumor infiltrating the root of the small bowel mesentery must be considered inoperable.

The excision of parietal peritoneal implants is uncomplicated, but may be tedious and time consuming. The anterior wall peritoneum, and that of the paracolic gutters, are likely to be most heavily involved, but sheets of tumor-bearing peritoneum can be excised en bloc. Careful search of peritoneum overlying the kidneys and behind the right lobe of the liver may reveal larger masses that are difficult to excise because of inaccessibility and a more luxuriant blood supply. When the surgical goal is to remove all gross tumor, multiple parietal peritoneal implants of 1 to 5 mm in diameter may be electrocoagulated.

Other than excluding the presence of grossly enlarged suprarenal lymph nodes at the beginning of the procedure,

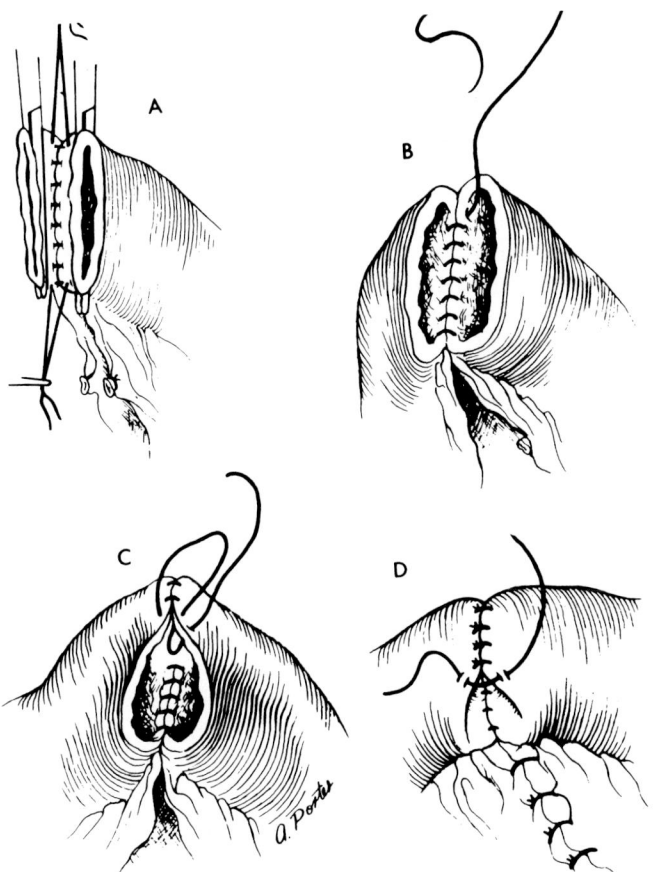

Fig. 83.8 Technique of standard sutured small bowel anastomosis. (A) Posterior row of interrupted seromuscular (Lembert) sutures of intestinal silk. (B) Posterior full thickness row of continuous chromic catgut. (C) Continuation of posterior layer anteriorly with continuous Connell suture. (D) Anterior row of interrupted seromuscular (Lembert) sutures of intestinal silk. (Reproduced from Halverson, Harper & Ballinger (1980),[3] with permission.)

para-aortic nodes are best dealt with at the conclusion of the other upper abdominal procedures. Exposure is not usually difficult, since the abdominal incision is long and the bowel has been well mobilized. We incise the peritoneum overlying the aorta in order to undertake careful palpation of the para-aortic and paracaval fat and to excise any palpable nodes. In the presence of multiple enlarged or matted nodes, a standard node dissection is carried out from the left renal vein to the bifurcation of the aorta. We prefer the exposure afforded by mobilization of the right colon and the ileal mesentery prior to undertaking the dissection.

PERIOPERATIVE MANAGEMENT

Preoperative care

The first priority in overall management is the acquisition of a histologic diagnosis. Although laparotomy is usually required, biopsy of enlarged inguinal or cervical lymph nodes, or cytologic examination of aspirated peritoneal or pleural fluid can obviate the need for laparotomy in those patients unsuitable for a primary cytoreductive operation. Patients with moderate to severe cardiac or pulmonary disease and ascites or pleural effusion will be best managed by one or two courses of combination chemotherapy and 2 to 4 weeks of hyperalimentation prior to a major extirpative procedure. Similarly, patients without comorbid disease but with evidence of moderate to severe protein-calorie malnutrition are best served by the more conservative initial approach. The disordered gastrointestinal motility and metabolic demands of an enlarging tumor bulk may result in a barely compensated state of subclinical protein malnutrition that can be converted into florid malnutrition by the imposition of a surgical burden. We consider patients with serum albumin of less than 2.5 g per dl or weight loss in excess of 15% of their usual body weight (making allowances for the positive effect of ascites) poor candidates for early surgical cytoreductive procedures.

For those patients who are candidates for an extended primary procedure, we have tried to limit the preoperative studies to those that provide information not readily obtained at laparotomy. Barium enema, although overused in the past, is the most convenient method for ruling out the colon as the primary site of the neoplasm. A high quality CT scan of the abdomen may be used for identifying primary sites when a clinical diagnosis of ovarian carcinoma is in doubt. Particularly important is the identification of a pancreatic primary tumor or a retroperitoneal lymphoma. A high quality ultrasound may reveal ureteral obstruction and the cystic nature of the neoplasm, but this information can usually be obtained at the time of laparotomy.

Routine chest roentgenograms are, of course, mandatory, and preoperative aspiration of pleural fluid may be necessary for adequate staging. With significant pleural effusions, the evacuation of as much pleural fluid as possible is important in improving pulmonary function. Pulmonary function studies should be carried out on all candidates for these procedures, and if either obstructive or restrictive lung disease is detected, arterial blood gases must be obtained prior to operation.

Finally, the frequency of coagulation disorders with advanced ovarian carcinoma can lead to an intraoperative or postoperative disseminated intravascular coagulation, or aggravate the consumption coagulopathy of intraoperative bleeding. We recommend at least a partial thromboplastin time and prothrombin time as a screen. A bleeding time is advisable for patients with a history of non-steroidal anti-inflammatory drug ingestion.

The single most important preoperative procedure is adequate preparation of the bowel. The necessity for bowel resection cannot be predicted preoperatively, and must be anticipated in all patients with advanced disease. Our regimen calls for 2 days of clear liquids and mechanical cleansing of the gastrointestinal tract using polyethelyne glycol and electrolyte solution (GoLYTELY) during the morning of the day prior to operation. This preparation must be administered by a strict schedule, i.e. 240 ml every 10 minutes without any other oral intake. Patient compliance has generally been poor, because insufficient encouragement and attention to detail have accompanied its administration. In some instances, administration by means of nasogastric tube is required. The advantage of this physiologic flushing of the gastrointestinal tract is the avoidance of intravascular fluid or electrolyte deficit incurred by purging and repetitive enemas. These deficits are often unrecognized and lead to hypotension during the surgical procedure. Erythromycin, 1 g and neomycin, 1 g are administered at 1 p.m, 2 p.m and 11 p.m. of the day prior to operation. Nausea from the combination of these two drugs may be offset by administering each in a staggered fashion, i.e. one hour apart, or by the concurrent administration of prochlorperazine. Because of the length and extent of these procedures, we use a systemic cephalosporin, a single dose preoperatively and immediately postoperatively.

Intraoperative management

Either general endotracheal or continuous epidural anesthesia may be used singly or in combination. With inhalational anesthesia, we have tried to avoid nitrous oxide which causes intraoperative bowel distension. The combination of light inhalational and continuous epidural anesthesia plus narcotic provides excellent relaxation and permits rapid recovery. In addition, the epidural catheter can be retained for postoperative pain relief.

Hemodynamic instability is common during these operations. Hypovolemia brought on by intraoperative fluid and blood loss is aggravated by serous effusions and a low serum albumin that permit volume shifts from intravascular to extravascular spaces. Consequently, the infusion of large volumes of crystalloid in response to hypotensive episodes tends to rapidly expand the extracellular compartment.

Considerable controversy exists over preference of crystalloid solutions over colloidal solutions as replacement. We have experienced a high frequency of pulmonary edema and massive peripheral edema during the postoperative phase as a result of crystalloid overload. For this reason, we prefer replacement with colloid solutions, as far as possible, in these patients with a low oncotic pressure and a leaky vascular tree. Administered red blood cells are an excellent volume expander, and are important in avoiding flow-dependent oxygen delivery. Although blood loss may be difficult to estimate when admixed with ascites, blood replacement should approximate loss. Replacement of coagulation components with fresh frozen plasma must also begin early when a protracted operation is anticipated.

A triple lumen central line is advisable in all operative cases of advanced ovarian cancer. In addition to vascular access and monitoring of central venous pressure, the third lumen can be preserved for postoperative hyperalimentation.

The insertion of a cordis sheath and Swan Ganz catheter is indicated for underlying cardiopulmonary disease, unexplained hypotension or central venous pressures that do not accurately reflect volume status and cardiac function. Placement of a Swan Ganz catheter with a thermistor enables measurement of:

1. cardiac index
2. pulmonary artery wedge pressure
3. systemic vascular resistance
4. oxygen delivery and consumption
5. mixed venous oxygen saturation.

Postoperative management

During the first 48 hours, shifts in fluid volume and varying degrees of hemodynamic instability may persist. Exudation of fluid into the peritoneal cavity will continue, but can be monitored if intraperitoneal suction catheters have been inserted. Continued monitoring of central venous pressure may be necessary to avoid congestive heart failure, and permit the use of diuretics as volume overload becomes apparent. (See Ch. 84.)

The potential for coagulopathies remains during the early postoperative phase, and a postoperative determination of prothrombin and partial thromboplastin times is recommended. As a prophylaxis against thromboembolic complications, we routinely apply pneumatic boots preoperatively and allow them to remain until the patient is ambulatory. We have not used postoperative heparin for this purpose. In the event of preoperative thrombophlebitis of the lower extremities, the inferior vena cava is clipped as early as possible during the procedure.

Postoperative nasogastric suction is used for several days to prevent gastric dilatation in those patients who have undergone small bowel resection or excision of the gastro-epiploic or short gastric vessels.

The only significant sequelae to splenectomy in the adult is decreased resistance to infection by encapsulated bacteria. Consequently, a single intramuscular injection of 0.5 ml of polyvalent pneumococcal vaccine should be given in the early postoperative period.

At laparotomy, the solution to a seemingly insurmountable anatomic problem may assume paramount importance. On the other hand, precedent physiologic derangements induced by a heavy tumor burden can be both relieved and aggravated in different ways by the procedure. Awareness of physiologic derangements, therefore, must be uppermost in the surgeon's mind throughout the perioperative period. With compromised patients, only meticulous monitoring as described above will permit immediate correction of adverse physiologic effects that can lead to an irreversible downhill course. The surgical intensive care unit (SICU) should be freely utilized and its need anticipated. Rather than as a measure of desperation, the SICU must be viewed as an integrated phase in the patient's overall management.

REFERENCES

1. Anson B J, Maddock W G 1952 Callanders Surgical Anatomy, 3rd edn. Saunders, Philadelphia.

2. Black G E, Exelby P R 1980 The spleen. In: Nora P F (ed) Operative Surgery. Principles and Technique. Lea & Febiger, Philadelphia

3. Halverson J D, Harper F B, Ballinger W F 1980 Small intestine. In: Nora P F (ed) Operative Surgery. Principles and Technique. Lea & Febiger, Philadelphia.

4. Longmire W P Jr, Sanford M C 1948 Intrahepatic cholangio-jejunostomy with partial hepatectomy for biliary obstruction. Surgery 24: 264

5. Silen W 1964 Surgical anatomy of the pancreas. Surg Clin Nth Am 44: 1253

PART XV

Management of complications of radical therapy (surgery and radiotherapy)

84. Postoperative care and complications

R. C. Wright   R. Lee

PREDICTION OF POSTOPERATIVE PROBLEMS

The factors which influence the outcome from major surgery include: the preoperative status, the nature and extent of the surgery, and the quality of operative and postoperative care. The operative skills of the surgeon are most important. A poor surgeon can be a source of disaster to the fittest patient despite the best postoperative care. But even the best surgeon will be unable to compensate for errors in selection of patients for surgery, or poor postoperative management.

A full preoperative assessment is essential to anticipate and prevent major problems. With some conditions, the predicted immediate postoperative mortality approaches 50% after major surgery. Thus, the risk of the surgery may outweigh any benefit. Most problems should be detected in the initial office consultation, but may then require specialist referral and complex investigation for quantification of risk and therapy.

General assessment

Particular clues which alert the gynecologist to an increased risk include:

General — recent weight loss[81]
Cardiac — angina, murmur, previous coronary bypass grafting, previous infarct
Respiratory — dyspnea particularly on minor exertion, heavy smoking, chronic airways disease, asthma
Central nervous system — stroke or transient ischemic attacks
Renal — sallow complexion, lethargy
Endocrine — tachycardia/agitation (thyrotoxicosis)
Hematology — anemia, bleeding tendency

Basic simple screening investigations should be performed especially before major surgery and in the elderly:

Hematology — hemoglobin, platelet count, coagulation screen
Biochemistry — full screen is justified as multiple analysis is cheap and efficient. It should include electrolytes, creatinine and serum albumin (an indicator of malnutrition or protein loss)
Electrocardiograph — to detect arrhythmias, previous infarction or ischemia
Chest X-ray — to detect cardiomegaly, pulmonary congestion, pulmonary fibrosis or chronic airflow limitation

Complex investigations should be undertaken only on specialist advice.

Heart disease

From the Framingham study, we know that approximately 20% of women will have severe cardiovascular disease by the age of 65. These patients are at risk from infarction, arrhythmia and cardiac failure. Patients with suspected cardiac disease should not undergo elective surgery without a complete assessment. With emergency surgery, the risks of waiting or delaying surgery must be weighed against the risks of proceeding. The risk of suffering a perioperative infarction is about 5% if the patient has suffered a previous infarction. If the infarct was within the last 3 months, the risk rises to about 25% (Table 84.1).[67,71] More recent work suggests that aggressive hemodynamic therapy and monitoring has reduced this rate in recent times (Table 84.2).[58] If perioperative infarct does occur, the mortality is 50% in most series.[70]

Other *cardiac risk factors* were prospectively investigated by Goldman.[22] In a multivariate analysis of 1001 patients over 40 years of age, he identified and scored nine adverse

Table 84.1 Reinfarction rate following anesthesia in patient with myocardial infarction (%)

| Study | Number | Previous infarct (months) | | |
		<3	4 to 6	>6
Tarhan[71]	32 877	37	16	3
Steen et al[67]	73 321	27	11	6

1337

Table 84.2 Reinfarction rate following anesthesia in patient with myocardial infarction (%)*

	Number	Group	Previous infarct (months)	
			<3	4 to 6
Group I				
(1973 to 1976)	364	7.7	36	26
Group II				
(1977 to 1982)	733	1.9	5.7	2.3

* From: Rao, Jacobs & El-Etr (1983)[58]

Table 84.3 Multifactorial index of cardiac risk in non-cardiac surgical procedures*

Risk factors	Score (pts)
S$_3$ gallop, raised JVP	11
AMI <6/12	10
Non-sinus rhythm	7
>5 VEBS/min	7
Age >70	5
Aortic stenosis	3
Operation — emergency	4
— thoracic, aortic	3
Poor condition: P$_{O_2}$ > 60 P$_{CO_2}$ > 50	3

* From: Goldman et al (1977)[22]

Table 84.4 Cardiac risk in non-cardiac surgical procedures.*

Class	Risk factor score (pts)**	Complications (%)		
		Nil or minor	Serious	Cardiac deaths
I	0 to 5	99	0.7	0.2
II	6 to 12	93	5	2
III	13 to 25	86	11	2
IV	>25	22	22	56

* Based on Goldman et al (1977)[22]
** See Table 84.3

risk factors (Table 84.3). Patients with high total scores had corresponding high complication rates (Table 84.4).

Certain principles of management are evident. Patients with valvular heart disease should be assessed by a cardiologist, as some may warrant valve replacement before undertaking major surgery. All patients with valve or congenital heart lesions require antibiotic[48] cover perioperatively until intravenous cannulae and drains have been removed. Medications are considered on an individual basis, but most should be continued perioperatively.

Chronic lung disease

Chronic lung disease is associated with a greatly increased risk of respiratory failure after abdominal surgery.[47] Chest X-ray, respiratory function tests and arterial blood gas (ABG) should be considered in consultation with a respiratory physician. The patients most at risk are those with (a) breathlessness at rest, (b) a chronic hypoxia or (c) a forced vital capacity less than 1 liter. In all patients with chronic lung disease, bronchodilator therapy should be optimized and sputum cleared by physiotherapy preoperatively. A sputum culture should be performed if there is any evidence of respiratory infection.

Obesity

Obesity is associated with an increased perioperative morbidity and mortality. Hypertension, cardiac failure and lung impairment are common in this group. Technical problems in monitoring, intubation and venous access compound the risks. If the surgery is not urgent then weight reduction is mandatory.

Increased age

Increased age is associated with increasing severity of heart and lung disease as well as disturbed physiology.[14,16,64] There is a great variability in the response of the elderly to surgical stress. The most important indicator is the preoperative functional status assessed by lifestyle, degree of independence and exercise tolerance. The survival of independently active patients is much better than that of nursing home patients of the same age.

Medications

Medications may provide a source of problems. Assessment is on an individual basis.

Beta-blockers should be continued perioperatively as they reduce myocardial strain and may help to control angina, blood pressure and rhythm. Sudden withdrawal leads to tachycardias and may precipitate infarction.[51]

Aspirin blocks platelet function for 7 to 10 days (irreversibly) and may increase the incidence of postoperative bleeding. Unless contraindicated, aspirin should be withdrawn 1 week preoperatively.

Antihypertensives should be continued to facilitate perioperative blood pressure control.

Diuretics should be maintained. Serum electrolytes should be checked for electrolyte disorders, (e.g. hypokalemia, hyponatremia).

Digoxin is used for control of atrial fibrillation and, less commonly nowadays, for cardiac failure. Toxicity (anorexia, visual disturbance, ECG changes) should be excluded preoperatively.

Corticosteroids must be continued preoperatively if the patient is on long-term steroid treatment or is believed to have been on steroids for more than 2 weeks within the last month. Dosage is increased at the time of surgery (e.g. dexamethasone 4 mg IVI 8-hourly) to cover the period of stress.

Insulin/hypoglycemics require specialist supervision. Blood glucose levels should be monitored closely. If insulin or oral hypoglycemics have been given then intravenous glucose is required while the patient is 'nil by mouth'.

ROUTINE POSTOPERATIVE CARE

The aims of postoperative care are to maintain physiological homeostasis and to correct the disturbances caused by operative trauma, thus enabling the patient to make a rapid uncomplicated recovery.

To achieve these goals, the organs must be adequately supplied with oxygen and nutrients via the blood stream, the cellular environment maintained within normal limits, and various toxins and micro-organisms prevented from damaging the tissues.

Monitoring

The continued assessment of the patient is primarily by physical examination, but this may be guided by specific monitoring and tests.

Physical examination

Skin perfusion. This gives a good indication of peripheral resistance and, indirectly, of cardiac output. The patient with cold periphery, poor capillary return and peripheral cyanosis is greatly shocked and is compensating for low cardiac output with sympathetic stimulation. On the other hand, the patient with low blood pressure but warm vasodilated periphery possibly has shock with vasodilatation due to such causes as sepsis, anaphylaxis, or excessive sedative drugs.

Pulse. The majority of patients with shock have tachycardia indicative of the sympathetic response to decreased systemic blood pressure. In a young patient with good compensatory mechanism, tachycardia and vasoconstriction may be the only indications of the shock state. An inappropriately slow pulse may occur in old age, β-blocker therapy, myxedema, spinal shock or ischemic heart disease (particularly acute inferior myocardial infarction).

Blood pressure. This may be high, 'normal' or low in shocked patients. It is important to observe trends from the patients usual blood pressure. It may be slow to fall in young patients who have efficient compensatory mechanisms, and hypotension then indicates severe shock.

Jugular venous pressure (JVP). Observed with the patient at 45°, JVP gives a clue to right heart function. JVP is dependent on venous tone, blood volume, intrathoracic pressure, right ventricular compliance and function and

pulmonary vascular resistance, so all these factors should be taken into account when following the trends. JVP is usually low in hypovolemic shock and elevated in some forms of cardiogenic shock.

Rectal temperature. This gives the clue to infection. The majority of septic patients have a temperature greater than 38°C, although patients who are immunocompromised, or have hepatic failure, renal failure or myxedema may have low or normal core temperatures. Oral and axillary temperatures are both misleading and useless in sick, hyperventilating and vasoconstricted patients.

Special monitoring after major surgery

Hourly urine output. This is a crucial measure of renal function and renal perfusion. It must be kept above 0.5 ml/kg per hour (see section on postoperative oliguria, p. 1366).

Continuous EKG monitoring. EKG monitoring using leads II or V5 is indicated for patients with a history of recent myocardial infarction, severe ischemic heart disease (IHD) or unstable arrhythmias.

Strict fluid balance. This gives a guide to fluid replacement. Losses may be occult, so fluid replacement should be guided by full clinical assessment of thirst, tissue turgor, pulse, blood pressure and JVP.

Central venous pressure. Inspection of the neck for the JVP can be misleading or impossible, therefore direct measurement of CVP by central line may be indicated.[72,78]

An isolated reading may be difficult to interpret (a patient with pulmonary hypertension secondary to chronic obstructive airways disease (COAD) and hypovolemia may have elevated CVP), so response of the CVP to fluid challenge is more helpful. The CVP will rise markedly in the patient who is volume replete or overloaded.

A line is inserted via the basilic, external jugular, internal jugular or subclavian veins into the superior vena cava, and is attached to a simple manometer to record the CVP. The patient is placed horizontally, and if the measurement is taken with the baseline at the sternal angle, the normal central venous pressure varies between +2 and −2 cm of H_2O (Fig. 84.1). If the midaxillary line is used, the normal range is 8 to 12 cm of H_2O. The factors that effect central venous pressure are (1) right ventricular (RV) function. (2) blood volume, (3) venous tone, (4) intrapleural pressure. As the great veins traverse the pleural cavity, a rise in intrapleural pressure (as occurs with mechanical ventilation or tension pneumothorax) will also raise the venous pressure.

Left atrial pressure. The main pumping chamber of the heart is the left ventricle, hence the best index of left ventricular (LV) function is the left ventricular end diastolic pressure (LVEDP) or left atrial (LA) pressure.[26,41,50,57]

The advent of the Swan Ganz catheter has simplified this measurement. It consists of a fine catheter which is inserted into the superior vena cava in the same fashion as a

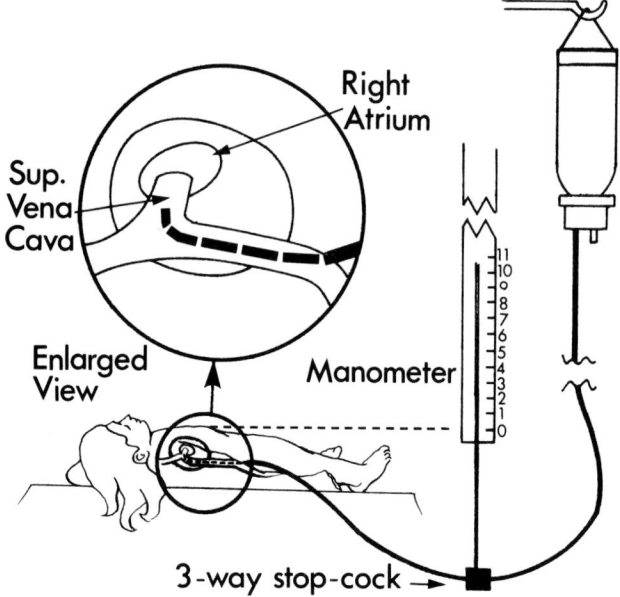

Fig. 84.1 A catheter is placed in the superior vena cava and connected to a simple saline manometer via a 3-way stop-cock. With the patient supine and the sternal angle as baseline, the normal venous pressure lies between +2 and −2 cm of water.

CVP catheter. A small balloon situated near the tip is inflated, and the catheter then becomes flow directed and passes through the right atrium (RA), right ventricle (RV) and pulmonary artery (PA), until it becomes wedged in a small pulmonary artery, the so-called pulmonary capillary wedge (PCW) position (Fig. 84.2). There is no need for

fluoroscopic control, as the position of the catheter is determined by observation of the pressure wave forms on an oscilloscope. The most important pressure recording is the PCW, which corresponds closely to LA pressure. In the wedged position there is no flow, and theoretically a static column of blood exists from the pulmonary capillaries to the pulmonary veins and thence to the LA. As the pressure in any system equalizes when there is absence of flow, the PCW pressure equals LA pressure. The normal PCW pressure is 5 to 13 mm/Hg. Low PCW pressures indicate hypovolemia and high PCW pressures indicate LV failure.

Postoperative investigations

Erect chest X-ray gives a guide to fluid status and the presence of respiratory complications such as atelectasis and pneumonia. It should be performed erect to detect heart size, fluid status, effusions and pneumothoraces.

12 lead EKG should be checked daily in patients with ischemic heart disease or a history of arrythmias.

Hemoglobin estimation should be checked after major surgery associated with major blood loss to guide the necessity for transfusion.

Electrolytes, urea and creatinine should be checked daily in patients with pre-existing renal disease, patients on diuretics and those who require prolonged intravenous fluids.

Routine fluid and electrolyte therapy

Body compartments

Water comprises 60% of the body weight of the average adult. This water is distributed in the intracellular (40%

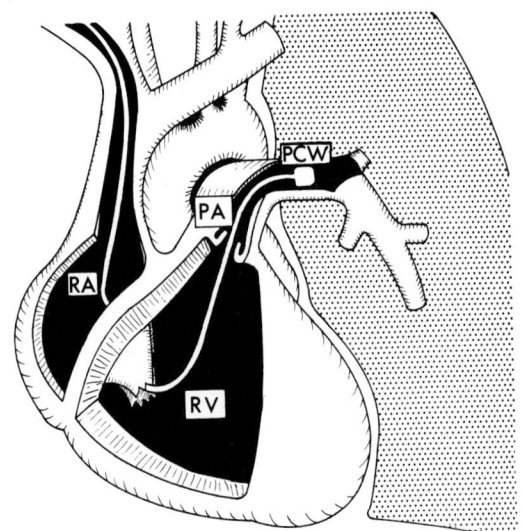

Fig. 84.2 Swan Ganz catheter. The catheter is introduced into the superior vena cava and the balloon inflated. It then becomes flow directed and passes through the chambers of the heart until it wedges in a pulmonary artery. The pulmonary capillary wedge (PCW) pressure, which closely approximates left atrial pressure can then be measured.

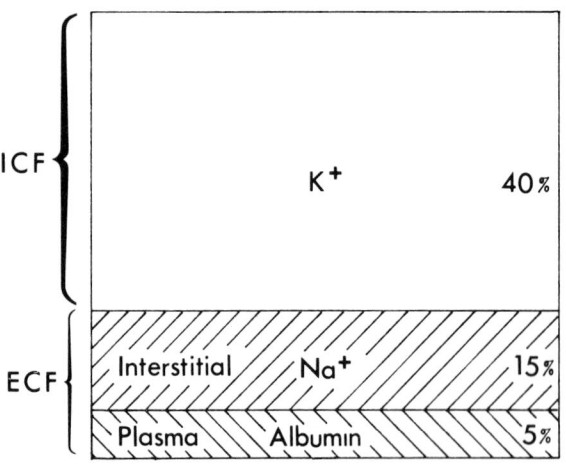

Fig. 84.3 Body water is subdivided into various compartments. Intracellular fluid (ICF) is 40% of body weight and contains most of the body potassium. Extracellular fluid (ECF) is 20% of body weight and contains most of the body sodium. Plasma represents a quarter of the ECF and has a high albumin content.

of body weight) and the extracellular (20% of body weight) fluid compartments. The latter compartment can be further subdivided into interstitial fluid (15%) and plasma (5%) (Fig. 84.3).

Intracellular fluid contains most of the body potassium, extracellular fluid contains most of the body sodium, and plasma has a high albumin content.

The distribution of intravenous fluids

From the foregoing, the volume of distribution of various intravenous fluids can be predicted.

5% dextrose

5% dextrose is composed of glucose and water. The glucose is metabolized to form carbon dioxide, water and energy. The remaining water is distributed throughout the total body water and thus expands both the intracellular and extracellular compartments. Hence, it is a poor plasma volume expander and is therefore useful in the patient with heart failure who requires fluids for the continuous intravenous infusion of drugs such as catecholamines, anti-arrhythmics or heparin.

Crystalloid solutions

These comprise the common sodium-containing solutions such as normal saline and Rigner's lactate (Hartmann's solution), both of which have a sodium content approximating that of normal extracellular fluid. As a consequence, they are distributed throughout the sodium space of the body, the extracellular fluid compartment, and expand both the interstitial fluid and the plasma. Since plasma volume is 25% of the extracellular volume, crystalloid solutions have only a 25% efficiency in expanding plasma volume and are therefore not the solutions of choice in hypovolemic shock. If large volumes of crystalloids are used for this purpose 75% of the volume administered enters the interstitial space resulting in skin edema and, more importantly, in interstitial pulmonary edema with serious impairment of oxygenation.

Plasma expanders

These include blood and colloid solutions. The latter contain large molecules which have difficulty crossing the capillary membrane and are confined predominantly to the plasma volume. Colloid solutions include albumin, dextrans, hetastarch, and gelatin preparations such as Haemaccel. Their efficiency as plasma volume expanders varies. Blood is entirely confined to the intravascular space, whereas Haemaccel contains molecules of degraded gelatin (molecular weight 35 000) some of which diffuse out of the capillaries into the interstitial space. As a result, Haemaccel has a 50% efficiency as a plasma volume expander.

Albumin solutions. Albumin, a physiological colloid, with a half life of approximately 18 days is a very efficient plasma volume expander. Its side effects are few and include a small incidence of allergic reactions. However, certain albumin preparations contain bradykinin-like substances which have both a vasodilator effect and constrict smooth muscle.[30] If these preparations are given rapidly they can cause reactions such as flushing, headache, nasal stuffiness and backache. More importantly vasodilatation can give rise to marked hypotension.

Dextrans. Dextran solutions of varying molecular weights, (commonly 70 000 and 40 000) are available. While these agents are efficient plasma volume expanders, their clinical usefulness is limited by their interference with coagulation mechanisms, particularly platelet function. As plasma volume expanders are most commonly indicated in hemorrhagic shock, it is probably unwise to infuse a substance which itself has anticoagulant properties. In addition, the dextrans can occasionally produce allergic reactions and renal failure.

Haemaccel. This is a solution containing degraded gelatin (molecular weight 35 000) dissolved in normal saline, to which is added small amounts of potassium and calcium. It is excreted by the kidneys with a half-life of 2 to 4 h, so it allows the patient to be rapidly resuscitated. While the gelatin is being excreted, cross-matched blood may be administered. The main side effects of Haemaccel are allergic reactions causing urticaria, laryngeal edema, bronchospasm and, occasionally, anaphylactic shock.

Balance of body components

When the body is in balance, the amount of any substance entering the body equals the amount leaving, thus the body composition stays constant and there is no net loss or gain.

Table 84.5 Water balance—24 hours

Intake	Fluid	1500 ml
	Food	750 ml
	Water of oxidation	250 ml
Output	Urine	1500 ml
	Stool	0–250 ml
	Lungs and skin	750 ml

Table 84.6 Sodium balance—24 hours

Intake	Diet	50–90 mmoles
Output	Urine	10–80 mmoles
	Gastrointestinal	0–20 mmoles
	Sweat	10–60 mmoles

Note: With sodium restriction urinary Na$^+$ losses can fall to less than 1 mmole per day.

Table 84.7 Potassium balance—24 hours

Intake	Diet	60–80 mmoles
	Cell breakdown	variable
Output	Urine	50–70 mmoles
	Gastrointestinal	
	and sweat	10 mmoles

Note: Potassium excretion cannot fall below a minimum of 5–10 mmoles a day. There is always a compulsory potassium loss.

As far as fluids and electrolytes are concerned, it is possible to construct tables of average figures for water, sodium and potassium balance (Tables 84.5 to 84.7).

Fluid regime

There are three essential components to the proper restoration and maintenance of fluid status:

1. replace pre-existing deficit
2. provide maintenance fluid
3. replace continuing abnormal losses.

Pre-existing deficits

The assessment of a pre-existing deficit, for example in a patient with intestinal obstruction and vomiting, can be very difficult. A number of clinical signs should be noted, and the basic aim is to administer fluids until these parameters are restored to normal. The tissue turgor is a useful clinical parameter. If the skin of the chest or upper arms remains as a fold after gentle pinching, a deficit exists in interstitial fluid volume. Conversely, edema of the skin indicates an expanded interstitial volume. Pulse, blood pressure and CVP are indicators of plasma volume, and reduction of plasma volume is reflected by tachycardia, hypotension and low central venous pressure. With progressive hypovolemia and dehydration, the urinary output falls and the specific gravity rises. Body weight is the most accurate method of detecting large changes in body salt and water balance. However, unless the patient is being regularly weighed this information is frequently unavailable. Perusal of a carefully recorded fluid balance chart gives a good indication of whether the patient has been in positive or negative fluid balance over the preceding days. Laboratory tests may also be of value. With severe losses of body water, there is a rise in the hemoglobin and packed cell volume. Changes in electrolytes will be discussed in a succeeding section, however the urea and creatinine give a good index of renal perfusion and with hypovolemia or dehydration there is a progressive rise in both. The osmolality of the serum and urine can also be useful. The type of fluid chosen for replacement may be guided by the known fluid lost (Table 84.8).

Maintenance fluid

Having replaced the existing deficit the normal adult requires 40 ml/kg per 24 hours of water for maintenance of total body water to replace usual urine, gastrointestinal tract, lung and skin losses. This may be reduced to the replacement of only insensible losses in renal failure (about 15 ml/kg per 24 hours), or less in congestive cardiac failure.

Electrolytes required daily are:

Na^+ – 1 to 2 mmol/kg
K^+ – 1 mmol/kg
Cl^- – 1 to 2 mmol/kg.

Electrolytes required after an intermediate period are:

Mg^{2+} – 0.1 mmol/kg (small body stores depleted by diarrhea, diabetic polyuria, diuretics)
Ca^{2+} – (large body stores, important to measure ionized serum Ca^{2+})
Po_4^{3-} – 0.1 mmol/kg (falls rapidly with glucose infusion)

Requirements are increased to cover extra losses (e.g. diarrhea, polyuria).

Table 84.8 Fluid losses and replacement

Site	Volume (l/day)	Na^+ (mmol/l)	K^+ (mmol/l)	Cl^- (mmol/l)	HCO_3^- (mmol/l)	pH	Replacement
Saliva	1.5	40	20	40	—	8	Glucose/saline
Gastric juice	1 to 2	40	5 to 10	140	—	1 to 5	Normal saline
Bile	1	150	5 to 10	100	30	8	Hartmann's solution
Pancreatic	1 to 2	120	5 to 10	50	90	8	Hartmann's alternating with 5% glucose
Small bowel	1 to 2	140	5 to 10	100	30	8	Hartmann's alternating with 5% glucose
Diarrhea		40	35	40	45	9	Glucose/saline + KCl
Sweat (acclimatized)		10		10			5% glucose
(non-acclimatized)		60		60			0.45% saline
Lungs	0.5	—	—	—	—	—	5% glucose

Fit young people are able to compensate, within limits, by appropriate renal retention or excretion of Na^+ and H_2O. Plasma volume takes priority over electrolyte concentrations in body homeostatic mechanisms. The average 70 kg person therefore requires approximately 2.5 to 3 liters per day of fluid, which may be administered as a liter of glucose saline with added KCl every 8 hours. Extra losses of 1 liter of nasogastric aspirate (Table 84.8) per day may be replaced with an extra liter of normal saline during the day. An elderly patient is unable to compensate for water and electrolyte excess or deprivation, so should be commenced on a lower rate (e.g. 30 ml/kg of water per 24 h) and titrated according to physical signs, urine output and biochemical investigation (e.g. 50 kg patient: 1 liter of glucose saline + 500 ml of normal saline per 24 hours).

Abnormal losses

Abnormal losses are replaced according to measurement of losses and clinical assessment. Table 84.8 shows expected volume and electrolyte content of some losses and possible replacement fluid.

Where exact site of loss is not apparent (e.g. upper gastrointestinal tract fistula) electrolyte content should be measured.

Postoperative pain relief

Adequate pain relief is of great importance in postoperative care.[27,74] (See also Ch. 89.) The amount of pain experienced by patients undergoing the same procedure using

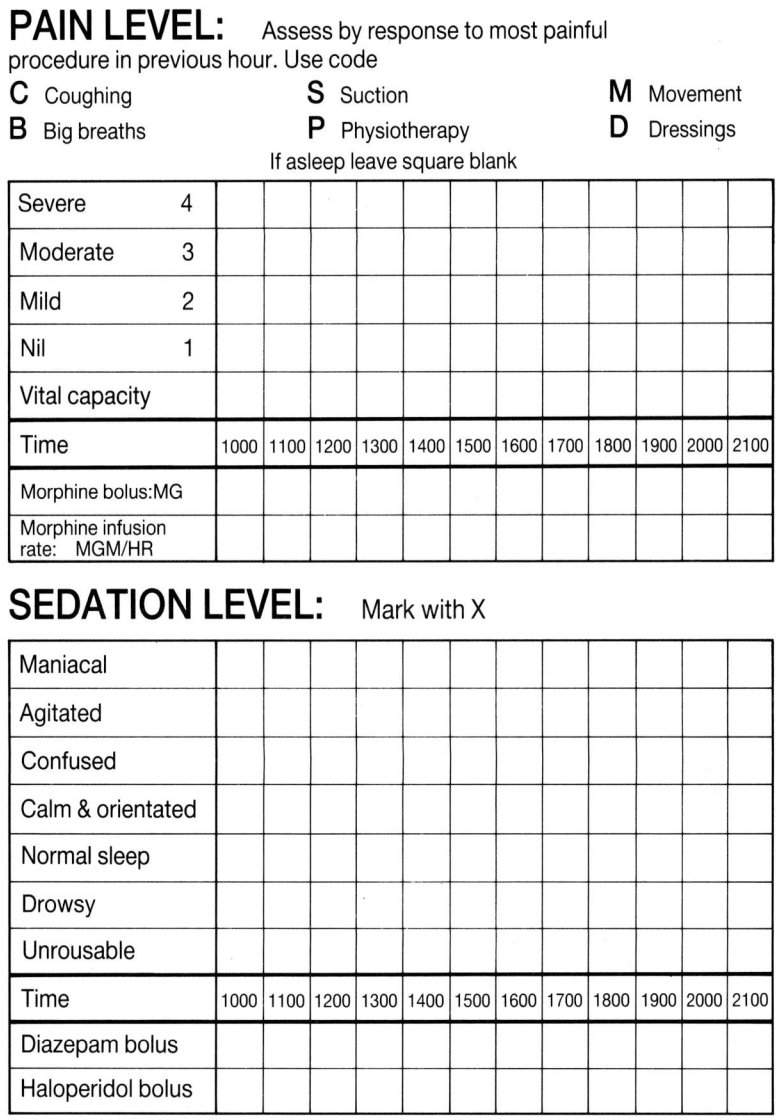

Fig. 84.4 Pain and sedation chart. By graphing a patient's response to maneuvers such as physiotherapy it is possible to accurately assess the adequacy of analgesia.

the same techniques varies enormously. Unfortunately, the deliverers of care are often conditioned by tradition and routine practice to provide a set amount of pain relief. The amount of pain relief given should be titrated to an assessment of the discomfort induced by levels of activity, and this can be guided by the use of a chart which requires the deliverer to assess the patient's response (Fig. 84.4).

Narcotic analgesics

The traditional method whereby the patient is given intermittent injections of a narcotic analgesic, such as morphine, is most unsatisfactory due to the varying blood level of the analgesic agent. Shortly after the injection, a high blood level is achieved during which time there is adequate pain relief often accompanied by considerable cerebral depression with obtundation of protective reflexes and hypoventilation. After 2 to 4 hours, the analgesic level falls and pain returns. Thus, the patient can alternate between a pain-free comatose state and severe pain.

For this reason it is preferable to administer the drug by continuous infusion. When using morphine or meperidine (pethidine), the rule is to start with half the dose that one would administer by intermittent injection; for example, if a patient is receiving 15 mg of morphine 4 hourly intramuscularly, this dose can be infused in a liter of maintenance fluid over a period of 8 hours. To prevent a rapid intravenous overdose, the infusion should be given through a pediatric microdrip, preferably with a burette or via an infusion pump.

In this way, a constant level of analgesia is achieved which can be titrated against the patient's response by increasing or decreasing the amount of morphine in the flask and the infusion rate. By this means it is possible to give the patient adequate analgesia and still retain her cooperation for physiotherapy and other treatment.

Local anesthetic techniques

Local anesthetic techniques for postoperative gynecological pain relief emanate from the extensive experience of epidural analgesia in obstetric practice. The lower abdominal operative site is very suitable for epidural analgesia. A catheter is inserted into the lumbar epidural space, and a local anesthetic agent such as 0.5% bupivicaine is injected. This gives rapid pain relief which lasts up to 3 to 4 hours when further increments must be given.

The main complications of this technique are hypotension, inadequate analgesia, infection, inadvertent subarachnoid puncture and convulsions from intravenous injection. Hypotension is due to sympathetic blockade and depends upon the level at which the catheter is placed and also the volume of local anesthetic agent injected. The pulse and blood pressure must be continuously monitored, and if serious hypotension occurs, this can be counteracted by tilting the patient's head down and infusing a plasma expander. Inadequate analgesia can be due to malpositioning of the catheter. In some cases it is remedied by pulling the catheter back slightly; in other situations it may have to be replaced. Infection in the epidural space is a feared complication, which is rarely seen and must be prevented by scrupulous attention to aseptic technique and by the use of bacterial filters in the epidural catheter. Inadvertent subarachnoid puncture can be followed by severe low pressure headache due to leakage of cerebrospinal fluid. Also, if a large dose of a local anesthetic drug is injected into this space, a 'total spinal anesthetic' with severe hypotension and paralysis can result.

Regional narcotic technique

More recently, very small doses of opiates such as morphine or meperidine have been administered into the subarachnoid or extradural space, resulting in prolonged analgesia with retention of both motor power and sympathetic tone. This produces intense analgesia in the effected dermatome by placing narcotic in close proximity to spinal receptors.

Intrathecal administration precludes the use of a catheter for repeated administration, but good analgesia may be obtained for up to 24 hours by small doses of morphine. However, a few patients remain in pain and others occasionally develop delayed severe respiratory depression of rapid onset. Use of the technique mandates admission to intensive care for observation.

Extradural administration of morphine, fentanyl and buprenorphine has been used extensively with success by intermittent catheter doses or constant infusions. The problems associated include pruritus, nausea, vomiting and respiratory depression and, again, intensive care admission is mandatory.

Inhalational analgesia

In the postoperative phase, procedures such as physiotherapy, examinations, removal of sutures etc. may have to be performed. Rather than give a large dose of narcotic analgesic, it is often more expedient to use a rapidly acting inhalational analgesic agent such as 'Entonox', which is a mixture of equal parts of oxygen and nitrous oxide. This gas is self-administered via a demand valve; the effect is rapid, and within 2 to 3 minutes a considerable level of analgesia is achieved. Following cessation of breathing the mixture, the offset of analgesia is equally rapid.

Continuous inhalation for long periods (e.g. 24 hours) may lead to megaloblastic marrow changes, agranulocytosis and a syndrome similar to subacute combined degeneration of the cord. Inhalation should therefore be restricted to short intermittent periods, as with dressings or removal of packs.

Postoperative bladder care

Following gynecological surgery, catheterization may be required if there has been surgical trauma to the bladder or if monitoring of urinary output is necessary for any reason, such as postoperative shock or monitoring fluid status. Other indications include postoperative urinary retention due to pain or interference with the mechanical or neurological functions of the bladder which may follow radical pelvic surgery, obese patients who have difficulty sitting on a bed pan, and incontinent patients who may develop decubitus ulceration from a wet bed.

In any of these circumstances a urinary catheter is passed either transurethrally or suprapubically. The choice depends upon individual preference, but with the latter method there is less chance of urinary infection and less patient discomfort. If a transurethral catheter is to be left indwelling for longer than 24 hours, it is essential to use a silastic catheter which is less toxic to the urethra than latex. The catheter should be placed on continuous drainage as this is preferable to intermittent clamping with its consequent risk of over distension and generation of an atonic

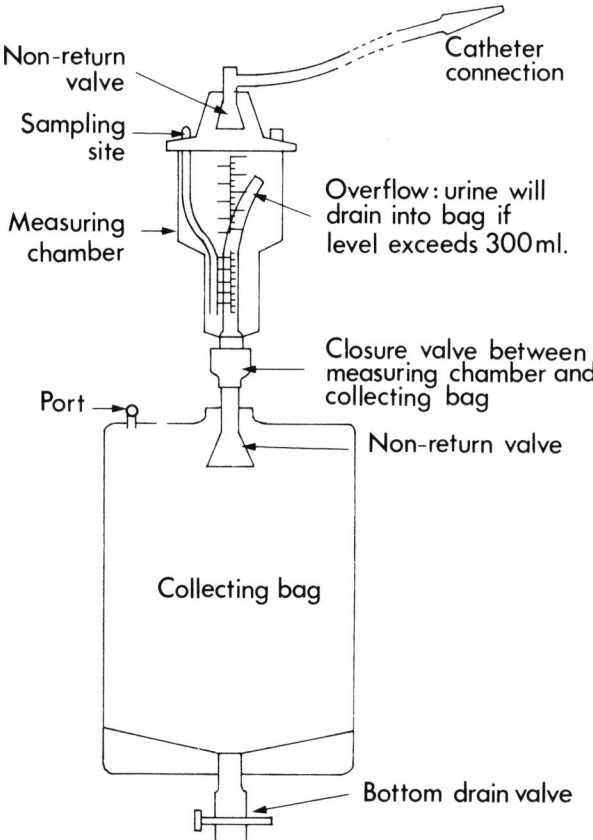

Non-return valve

Sampling site

Measuring chamber

Catheter connection

Overflow: urine will drain into bag if level exceeds 300 ml.

Port

Closure valve between measuring chamber and collecting bag

Non-return valve

Collecting bag

Bottom drain valve

Fig. 84.5 Urinary drainage system. To prevent urinary tract infection the catheter and drainage system must constitute a closed system. The above system allows measurement of hourly urine volumes and intermittent sampling without having to disconnect the catheter.

bladder. In shocked patients the urine output should be measured hourly.

The drainage system

The choice of drainage system is important in the prevention of urinary tract infection. The catheter and its drainage system should be a totally closed unit, as the incidence of urinary tract infection is proportional to the number of times the catheter is disconnected from the drainage system. As shown in Figure 84.5, the ideal system should have three components. Firstly, a one-way valve to prevent reflux of potentially infected urine from the collecting system back into the bladder. Secondly, a measuring chamber so that accurate hourly urinary volumes can be determined. It should be possible to collect aseptic samples of urine from this chamber for bacteriological culture, urinalysis for sugar etc. The chamber should have a valve which permits it to empty into the collecting bag and also an overflow system to prevent overfilling. Finally, there should be a collecting bag or bottle with a stopcock to allow drainage of urine without disconnection.

The use of this system allows the patient to be catheterized for several days without developing a urinary tract infection. During the period of catheterization, periodic urine samples should be taken for culture. Provided the patient is asymptomatic, it is probably preferable not to treat asymptomatic bacteriological evidence of infection until the catheter is removed. With a catheter in situ, infection will persist and the use of antibiotics often results in the generation of antibiotic resistant organisms. When the catheter is to be removed, the urine should be examined microscopically, cultured and any infecting organisms treated vigorously with appropriate antibiotics.

Prevention of deep venous thrombosis and pulmonary embolus

In gynecological surgery, the prophylaxis of postoperative deep venous thrombosis and pulmonary embolism is of great importance.[8,12,13,44,59] Table 84.9 lists the individual risk factors. Indeed, all patients who undergo gynecological operations are at risk, and active prophylactic measures are

Table 84.9 Risk factors for thromboembolism

Immobility

Age — patients over 60 years of age are at greater risk

Previous thromboembolism — indicates high risk

Obesity

Malignancy — particularly uterus and breast

Surgery — prolonged

Oral contraceptive

Cardiac failure

warranted according to the guidelines listed in Table 84.10. To be effective, the measures must be started preoperatively, maintained intraoperatively and then continued postoperatively, because contrary to popular opinion, deep venous thrombosis is not a 10-day postoperative phenomenon but commonly occurs during the operation. Prophylactic measures may be mechanical and chemical.

Table 84.10 Guidelines for thromboembolism prophylaxis (bedbound surgical or medical patients)

All patients:	Calf muscle exercise Graded compression stockings Early ambulation
Usual risk:	Add heparin 5000 units S.C. q8hr

High risk:	Add intermittent pneumatic calf compression
	and heparin 7500 units S.C. q8hr
	— Check APTT* 4 h after heparin
	    if APTT <35 s increase dose
	    if APTT >50 s decrease dose
	— Check platelet count twice weekly

* APTT = activated partial thromboplastin time; the best coagulation test for heparin monitoring

Mechanical

1. Sustaining the action of the muscle pump in the legs by encouraging the patient to move her legs continuously whilst in bed. Early ambulation is of obvious assistance, and the provision of a footboard so that the patient can sit up in bed, helps utilize the muscle pump.

2. Elastic stockings are recommended to compress the legs and divert blood from the superficial to the deep veins, thus accelerating flow and reducing stasis. I-labeled fibrinogen studies have shown the efficacy of this technique. It is necessary to have well-fitting elastic stockings which are applied only from toe to the knee, as larger stockings, particularly in the obese, may clump and obstruct at the groin. The use of non-shaped stockings which are of uniform diameter all the way up the leg is counter productive, as they exert a tourniquet effect on the thigh, cause stasis and increase the risk of deep venous thrombosis.

3. Two devices are available for accelerating venous flow in the intraoperative period: electrical calf stimulators and intermittent calf compressors. With the former, which is only suitable for anesthetised patients, electrical contacts are applied to the calf muscle and connected to a pulse generator so that the calf muscles periodically contract and accelerate venous flow. The latter consist of devices which envelope the lower limb in a circumferential pneumatic stocking which is intermittently inflated and deflated. This also accelerates venous flow through the lower limb.

Chemical

1. Numerous trials have shown the efficacy of anticoagulants in preventing deep venous thrombosis provided they are administered preoperatively and continued throughout the postoperative phase. The most popular regime is low dose heparin given in a dose of 5000 units 8 to 12 hourly, by subcutaneous injection. This has been shown to decrease the incidence of deep venous thrombosis from approximately 30% to below 10% with only a minor increase in the incidence of wound hematoma.

2. Oral anticoagulants, such as phenindione or coumadin, have been used in some centers and are also effective. However, their use is more complicated and carries a greater risk of excessive anticoagulation and consequent hemorrhage than does the subcutaneous low dose heparin regime.

Physiotherapy

A combination of coughing, percussion and vibration aid in the clearance of secretions. Early mobilization and assuming the erect posture also facilitate sputum clearance.

Sputum clearance is not the only problem, because the abdominal wound, muscle splinting and supine posture will decrease lung volumes and lead to atelectasis.[52] This loss of lung volume may be counteracted by encouraging deep breathing, which will increase the functional residual capacity (FRC) and expand lung bases. Incentive spirometry has the advantages of giving the patient an endpoint to aim for and being frequently repeatable. The technique of continuous positive airway pressure (CPAP) by mask aims to elevate FRC and re-expand collapsed alveoli by maintaining a positive pressure in the airway at the end of expiration. It is less painful.[4,68]

Oxygen therapy

Some postoperative patients require oxygen by mask or nasal prongs for a minimum of 1 to 2 hours postoperatively. Oxygen may be required beyond this time after major surgery if the patient is elderly or obese, or has pre-existing lung disease. Arterial blood gases should be checked in these patients before removing O_2 therapy.

Oxygen may be administered by several methods.[49] The concentration of oxygen that the patient receives from *nasal prongs* or *ordinary mask* is dependent on the oxygen flow rate, the size and shape of the mask and the patient's inspiratory flow pattern.

Nasal cannulae provide low added oxygen (particularly low to mouth breathers) with unpredictable inspired O_2 concentration from 0.25 to 0.35 at gas flows of 2 to 4 liters per minute. They are useful for patients with minor V/Q abnormality who cannot tolerate a mask because of confusion or claustrophobia. The flow of dry gas to the nasopharynx may irritate the mucosa but the main advantage is the simple provision of continuous O_2.

General use masks (Hudson, Puritan, etc.) provide

inspired O_2 concentration varying from 0.30 to 0.50 depending upon oxygen flow (4 to 12 l/min), and factors as above. They are useful for patients with more severe lung problems. Patients with severe respiratory complications who require the most oxygen usually have high respiratory rate and inspiratory flow, therefore they entrain air around the mask and receive relatively low inspired O_2 concentration. These patients should have arterial blood gas analysis checked regularly and be considered for continuous positive airways pressure (CPAP) or intubation if hypoxia persists.

High concentration masks (non re-breathing mask) possess a reservoir bag on the inspiratory line and one-way valves at the bag outlet and over the expiratory holes, so that the patient breathes undiluted oxygen from the bag and breathes out through the one-way valves at the side of the mask, not into the bag. Inspired O_2 concentration may approach 0.8 with this system. Patients who require this amount of oxygen have large shunts, are at risk of decompensation and should be considered for other measures (intubation and mechanical ventilation).

Venturi masks (e.g. Ventimask) use the air entrainment principle through a fixed orifice to deliver high flows of oxygen (approximately 75 liters) at low inspired oxygen concentration, usually 0.24 to 0.28. These masks should only be used in patients with *documented* severe chronic lung disease with oxygen sensitivity. If Venturi masks are used to provide oxygen fractions around 0.3 to 0.4, total flow falls and the patient's inspired O_2 concentration again depends on mask fit and inspiratory flow pattern.

NUTRITION

In developed countries, malnutrition is mainly seen in hospitalized patients. With any sickness, appetite decreases and metabolic expenditure increases. When this is compounded by periods of prolonged fasting for hospital tests, postoperative complications such as vomiting and infection, wasting from neoplastic disease[19] and unappetizing hospital food, various degrees of malnutrition occur.

Nutritional support can improve the tolerance for surgery,[25] chemotherapy or radiotherapy.

Metabolic pathways

The three major body nutrients are carbohydrates, fat and protein.[66] As can be seen in Figure 84.6, glucose is converted to pyruvate and then metabolized via the Krebs cycle to generate energy. Fat and protein can be either generated or utilized by these metabolic pathways, and glucose can be converted into glycogen.

In starvation, endogenous body stores must be used as sources of energy (Fig. 84.7). Glycogen is rapidly broken down to form glucose, and liver glycogen stores are depleted within 24 hours. Once the glycogen is gone, then

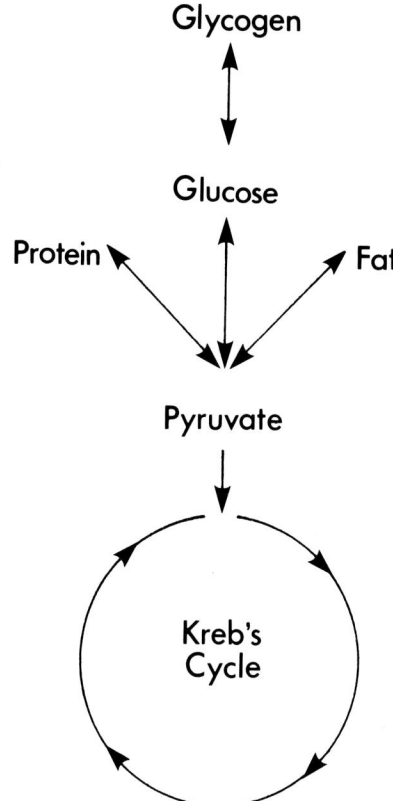

Fig. 84.6 The three major foodstuffs — carbohydrate, protein and fat can be metabolized to provide energy via the Krebs cycle, be stored as fat and glycogen or else synthesized into body components.

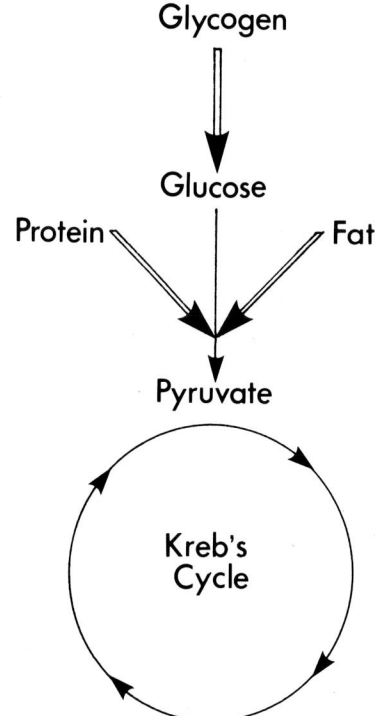

Fig. 84.7 During starvation the body stores of glycogen are rapidly depleted and then body fat and protein are catabolized to form energy. Loss of protein is a serious disability as it represents loss of body function.

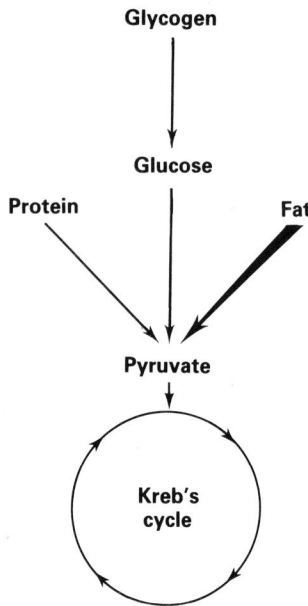

With adaption, starvation leads to slower loss of protein for fuel

Fig. 84.8 With adaption to starvation, a slower loss of protein for fuel occurs. Ketone bodies are generated from the metabolism of free fatty acids from adipose tissue. These ketone bodies can be used for energy by muscle and brain.

body fat and protein are catabolized to generate energy. Loss of fat is of little consequence. It is an excellent store of energy but its main role in the body is insulation. However, the loss of protein, or negative nitrogen balance, is a serious disability. Protein is a constituent of vital structures such as cell walls, muscle, hormones, enzymes, etc, and loss of protein implies loss of function. In fact, this is the major cause of death in malnutrition, as it leads to muscle wasting, hypoproteinemia with edema, and susceptibility to infection with poor immune response and poor wound healing. Every effort must be made to prevent negative nitrogen balance and, if possible, induce a state of positive nitrogen balance with synthesis of new protein.

Starvation eventually leads to a process of adaption which slows the loss of protein by slowing metabolism and using mainly adipose tissue as a fuel source (Fig. 84.8). In the critically ill (stressed, septic) patient, the catabolic process dictates continued breakdown of muscle protein for acute phase protein (e.g. immunoglobulin, fibrinogen) genesis and maintenance of high blood energy (glucose) levels.

Postoperative requirements are often greater than those of normal body activity, both because there may be pre-existing malnutrition and because there is an increased metabolic rate in the postoperative period, especially if complicated by fever and sepsis.

Oral/enteral nutrition

Patients who have a normally functioning gastrointestinal tract should be fed by mouth, nasogastric tube or ostomy[54,62] (Table 84.11).

Table 84.11 Nutrition: Why prefer the gastrointestinal tract (GIT)?

	Oral enteral nutrition	Total parenteral nutrition
Cost	Oral ward diet, $6/day Nasogastric feed, $10/day	>$100/day (solutions alone)
Labor	Simple	Intensive, costly
Complications	Few, short lived (e.g. diarrhea and cramping)	Many and serious
Monitoring	Basic	Complex, expensive
GIT integrity	Enteral mass and immunity preserved	Enteral mass lost, immunity disturbed
Physiology	Normal GIT hormone response (e.g. insulin)	Bypass GIT
Nutritional quality	Complete diet, 1 to 2 kcal/ml	Incomplete, <1 kcal/ml

Oral feeding is preferable if the patient has a reasonable appetite, can swallow and has a functional gastrointestinal tract. Dietetic consultation should be sought for calorie counting and opinion of oral supplements if there is doubt about adequacy of the diet. Many palatable, commercial liquid supplements (e.g. Sustagen®) are available if intake is inadequate due to chewing difficulty or anorexia.

Enteral feeding is necessary if the patient has poor appetite or swallowing difficulty but has a functional bowel. This may be undertaken by nasogastric tube or via ostomy. For long term feeding, fine-bore silicone catheters are preferred if the nasal route is chosen, as PVC tubes become hard and rigid after 10 days in situ. Constant round the clock infusion of the feed (by gravity or pump) is preferable to bolus feeding, because of the lesser incidence of diarrhea and cramping and the larger potential input.

Feed choice is dependent on the individual patient's requirements:

1. Whole protein, whole fat, glucose polymer feeds with milk (Compleat®, Sustain®, Sustagen®). These are well tolerated by patients with normal gastrointestinal function. They are low in osmolality, inexpensive, provide usually 1 kcal/ml and a complete diet, and are usually very palatable for oral intake.

2. Intact nutrients without milk. (Ensure®, Isocal®, Osmolite® and Precision®). These feeds are generally well tolerated and suitable for feeding most patients. They are preferred in postoperative or critically ill patients who may have lactose intolerance. Being mostly isotonic, there is no need to dilute with water. Hypertonic feeds are irritating and initially cause cramping and diarrhea; they should be diluted 1:2 milk with water for the first 1 to 2 days. Hyponatremia may develop if half-strength feeds are prescribed for too long.

3. Special feeds. 'Elemental diets' consist of the food elements (amino acids, oligosaccharides and medium chain triglycerides) which require no digestion and have no residue. They are hypertonic, expensive, unpalatable and more likely to cause diarrhea but are indicated in some specific conditions such as short bowel syndrome, malabsorption, fistula or following prolonged starvation after which the digestive capacity or enzyme function is disturbed. High calorie feeds (Isocal HCN®, Ensure Plus®) may be indicated for patients on fluid restriction (e.g. congestive cardiac failure).

Requirements

The aim is to provide 40 kcal/kg per 24 h with 1 g protein/kg per 24 h to satisfy basic requirements. The feeds are introduced slowly, perhaps 30 ml/h for 12 h, then 60 ml/h. Full strength feed is used if the feed is isotonic (Isocal®/Osmolite®), or half-strength if the feed is hypertonic (elemental diet such as Flexical® or Vivonex®). Strict monitoring of clinical hydration and fluid balance is essential.

Complications

Diarrhea and cramping may occur. Factors such as bolus feeding, pseudomembranous colitis, and spurious diarrhea should be excluded. Reintroduction of the feed at a slower rate and perhaps diluted with water will usually settle the diarrhea.

Parenteral nutrition

Parenteral nutrition (PN) is an attempt to provide a complete diet via the intravenous route.[15,40,46,53] It is expensive, labor intensive and associated with complications.

Indications

1. *The patient who cannot eat.* This usually implies a disorder of the gastrointestinal tract preventing normal oral intake. It should be stressed that normal oral intake, either by swallowing or gastric tube, is the best means of feeding, and that intravenous alimentation should only be initiated if this is not possible. A common example is the postoperative patient with paralytic ileus or intestinal obstruction, in whom nutrients cannot be absorbed from the gut.

2. *The patient who should not eat.* This group mainly comprises patients with gastrointestinal fistulae (e.g. postoperative, Crohn's disease). It has been shown that gastrointestinal rest is important to accelerate healing of fistulae.

3. *The patient who will not eat.* This may be due to stomatitis secondary to chemotherapy, and conditions such as anorexia nervosa.

4. *Supplementation.* If, for various reasons the oral intake is inadequate and tube feeding has proved to be unsuccessful, or energy requirements are very high, it may be necessary to supplement oral feeding with intravenous nutrition.

Typical gynecological cases include: (a) Prolonged postoperative ileus (b) Radiation enterocolitis, short bowel syndrome (c) Fistulae (d) Major bowel surgery with multiple anastomoses.

Requirements

The basic needs of the starved patients are for water, electrolytes, protein, energy source, vitamins and trace elements (Table 84.12).

1. **Water.** The usual requirement is 30 to 50 ml/kg per 24 h to replace urinary and insensible losses. This may be reduced to less than 1000 ml/24 h in the case of renal failure, or less in congestive cardiac failure. Extra fluid is added to cover pre-existing deficits plus continuing losses in patients with *vomiting, diarrhea, polyuria* and *fistula* (See fluids/electrolytes section, p. 1368). Maintenance fluid is given as the vehicle for the PN but, since extra PN produces problems with glucose tolerance and nitrogen loading, additional fluid to replace losses is given separately.

2. **Electrolytes.** See fluids/electrolytes section (p. 1369).

3. **Protein.** Crystalline amino acids are administered as the source of building blocks for body proteins. To make sure that the administered nitrogen is used for protein synthesis, an energy source must be administered simultaneously. Approximately 1.5 g/kg of protein or amino acids should be administered daily. Calories are provided at a ratio varying from 1 g N_2:160 kcal in stable patients to 1:80 kcal in critically ill, catabolic patients.

4. **Energy.** Energy in the form of carbohydrate and/or fat is given to meet the metabolic needs of the patient. The

Table 84.12 Basic needs of starved patients

Water	40 ml/kg
Calories	40 calories/kg
Protein	1 to 2 g/kg
Sodium	1 mmol/kg
Potassium	1 mmol/kg
Magnesium	0.2 mmol/kg
Phosphate	0.4 mmol/kg
Calcium	0.15 mmol/kg
Trace elements: 　Vitamins 　Essential fatty acids 　Albumin and blood	

Caloric values of common nutrients
Carbohydrate: 4 calories/g
Amino acid: 4 calories/g
Fat: 9 calories/g

non-catabolic patient requires approximately 40 kcal/kg per 24 h.

Carbohydrate is the major energy source. It provides 4 kcal/g. It is cheap and essential to brain, kidney and red cells with a mandatory requirement of 400 to 500 kcal/24 h. It is administered as a concentrated solution of glucose, 12.5%, 25% or 35%, in combination with the amino acid solution. Being hypertonic, the solutions are very irritating to veins and must be administered via central catheter. The glucose infusion is slowly increased to induce insulin response and to observe the patient's response in terms of blood glucose level and urinalysis. When ceasing the high glucose solutions it is important to wean over 24 hours with decreasing glucose loads, and ensure enteral diet is tolerated.

Fat (lipid) is available as 10 to 20% emulsions and provides 9 kcal/g. The emulsions are isotonic and well tolerated via peripheral veins, but are expensive. They are a concentrated source of calories as well as providing phosphorous and essential fatty acids. They should be given at least weekly, but serum cholesterol, triglycerides and turbidity require monitoring in patients with hyperlipidemia. Tolerance and clearance should be checked by measuring serum triglyceride level 6 hours after infusion, or observing the serum for abnormal milkiness indicating lipemia.

5. Vitamins. Water-soluble vitamins (B group, C, folate) in general have small labile stores and must therefore be given early when enteral intake ceases. Hypervitaminoses are uncommon. Fat soluble vitamins (A,D,E,K) have larger stores with slower turnover. Except for vitamin K, which is given immediately to prevent coagulation disorders, they are given for specific deficiencies or after 1 month of poor oral intake. Hypervitaminoses can occur (e.g. vitamin D excess → severe hypercalcemia). Many commercial products which meet WHO or American Society of Parenteral and Enteral Nutrition guidelines are available.

6. Trace elements. Zinc deficiency produces mental apathy, depression, tremor, diarrhea, immune dysfunction and delayed wound healing. Zinc is required early. Moni-

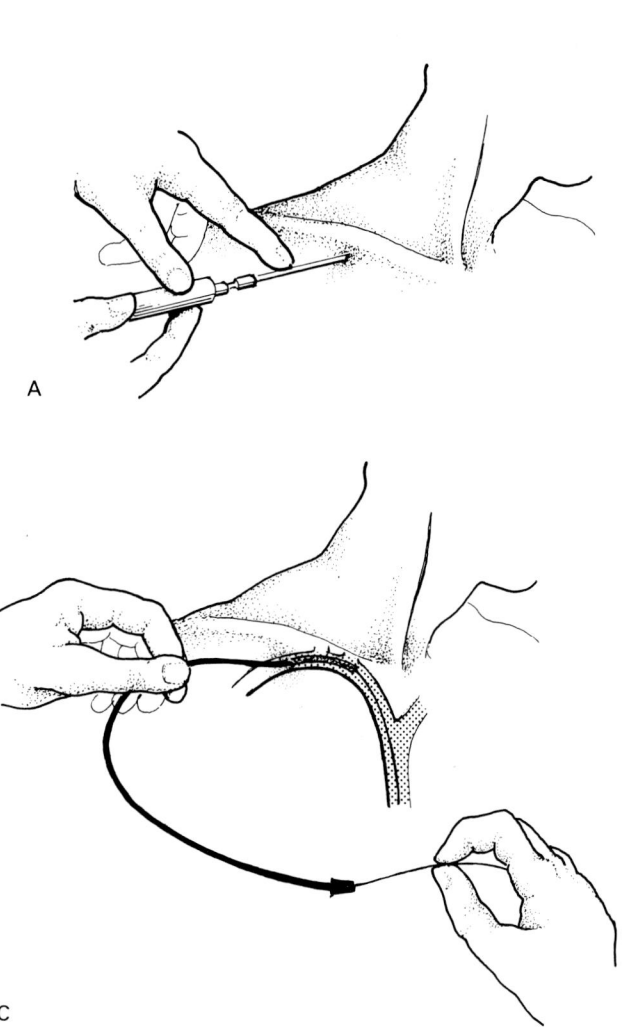
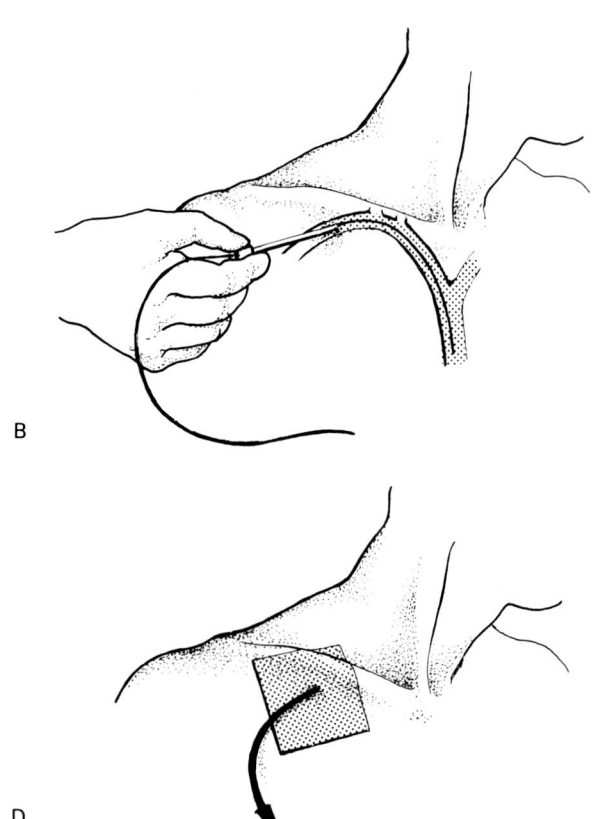

Fig. 84.9 Seldinger technique for insertion of a subclavian catheter (A) A small bore needle is inserted into the subclavian vein via the infraclavicular route. The patient is supine and slightly head down. (B) Through the small needle a guidewire is fed into the subclavian vein and the needle is withdrawn. (C) The catheter is fed over the wire into the vein while keeping control of the wire at all times. (D) The wire is removed, the infusion is connected and the catheter is secured to the skin by stitch and then covered with transparent dressing.

toring, though inexact, is by regular estimation of serum levels or balance studies. Other trace elements, iodine, cobalt, chromium, copper and manganese, are only a problem with prolonged PN. Deficiency is difficult to diagnose, and serum or tissue levels are difficult to monitor.

Venous access

PN solutions must be infused via a catheter with its tip in a central vein, specifically the superior vena cava at the level of the aortic knob as demonstrated on chest X-ray. Long lines from the cubital fossa should be left in situ for no longer than 5 days, as the incidence of thrombophlebitis and thrombosis increases greatly after this time. Catheters directly inserted into central veins via the subclavian (Fig. 84.9) or internal jugular route are maintained for longer periods. Polyurethane catheters (e.g. Cavafix®) may remain in situ for up to a month if inserted with meticulous sterile technique and if carefully maintained. If it is anticipated from the outset that a catheter will need to be maintained for longer than 1 month, then a silicone catheter (Hickman or Broviac) should be inserted by cutdown or percutaneous introducer technique in the operating theater.

Administration technique

PN solutions are administered via constant infusion pump into the central catheter.

Preparation of solutions

Additions to the PN solution should be made under laminar flow conditions. The PN solution (amino acids + glucose + electrolytes and possibly lipid) may be premixed in a single bag by the manufacturer.

Catheter care and line changes

The most common and serious complication of PN is infection. Meticulous care of the insertion site and sterile handling of all connections will help to prevent life-threatening septicemia. The infusion set should be changed every 48 hours.

Monitoring

Monitoring for early detection of complications (such as fluid overload, dehydration, hyperglycemia, etc) consists of regular bedside and laboratory assessment.

Bedside: 6-hourly pulse and *rectal* temperature; 6-hourly fingerprick for blood glucose and urinalysis for sugar and ketones; strict fluid balance of all intake and output; daily weight; check central line dressing for loss of seal, inflammation or discharge.

Laboratory tests: daily biochemical screen and blood glucose until stable, thence second daily; twice weekly serum magnesium and liver function tests; weekly serum zinc, coagulation screen and full blood count; nitrogen balance (24 h urine collection), amino acid profile, trace element levels, serum transferrin and pre-albumin, and arterial blood gases are measured when indicated.

Special situations

Depending on their problems, patients tolerate fluid, protein, carbohydrate, electrolytes and vitamins differently.

a) Critically ill patients. Stressed patients have high circulating levels of endogenous corticosteroids, glucagon and adrenaline. Skeletal muscle protein is preferentially broken down as a source of glucose. There is a persistently high blood sugar level, and intolerance to exogenous carbohydrate. Feeding these patients with PN can lead to progressive hyperglycemia and glycosuria. The catabolic process is not reversed. Treatment should be aimed at reversing the underlying disease (e.g. infection), and restoring blood volume and serum electrolytes before commencing PN. Small amounts of protein, glucose and fat may be given parenterally and increased as glucose tolerance improves.

b) Renal failure. Renal failure requires adjustment of (1) fluid volume (2) protein intake (3) sodium intake (4) potassium intake and (5) magnesium intake. If the patient is on dialysis, then adjustments can be made for nutritional input by increasing dialysis frequency.

c) Anesthesia. PN is usually reduced because of anticipated glucose intolerance due to surgical stress. But it is imperative to make sure that the PN is not stopped suddenly, particularly if insulin has been given, as unobserved hypoglycemia may occur. Fingerprick blood glucose level and urinalysis should be strictly observed.

d) Diabetes. Glucose solutions are introduced slowly to check glucose tolerance. The insulin regimen given depends on the severity of the diabetes, the degree of stress and whether the patient is taking medication with anti-insulin effects (e.g. steroids). Patients who are receiving insulin are at risk of *hypoglycemia* if glucose infusion is interrupted for any reason. Insulin may be provided by: (1) intermittent subcutaneous sliding scale guided by fingerprick blood glucose; (2) addition to PN solution (50% of insulin is lost by binding to glass); (3) separate continuous insulin infusion (e.g. 2 units/hour guided by fingerprick).[33]

Weaning

PN can be rapidly decreased and discontinued over 12 to 24 hours, provided the patient is absorbing sufficient oral nutrients. If PN is suddenly stopped in the starved patient (blocked or infected line), then 5% glucose should be commenced via a peripheral line as a matter of urgency to prevent hypoglycemia.

Complications and emergencies

These are summarized in Table 84.13. The most important are:

Table 84.13 Complications of central venous catheters

1. Failure of cannulation.
2. Hemorrhage in the upper mediastinum especially in patients with bleeding disorders.
3. Thrombosis of the superior vena cava.
4. Infection and septicemia.
5. Pneumothorax and hemothorax.
6. Malposition of catheter
    a. other veins e.g. arm veins, internal jugular
    b. pleura with infusion of fluid into the pleural cavity
    c. mediastinum
    d. heart with danger of arrhythmias and perforation of the heart
    e. pericardium following perforation of the right ventricle.
7. Embolism
    a. air
    b. catheter due to the catheter being severed during insertion.
8. Perforation or damage to structures
    a. pleura with resultant pneumothorax or hemothorax
    b. arteries, especially the carotid or subclavian artery
    c. trachea
    d. thoracic duct
    e. heart
    f. brachial plexus
    g. phrenic nerve
    h. recurrent laryngeal nerve.
9. Cardiac arrhythmias.
10. Catheter knotting.

(a) Air embolism. The patient and all staff must be aware of this devastating emergency. Air can be sucked into the heart if the central line becomes disconnected. The air obstructs the right heart outflow tract, causing severe hypotension, hypoxia and frequently death. Therefore, prevention is paramount. All connections must be securely Luer-Loked and the lines must not be allowed to pull on connections or positioned so as to allow entanglement during sleep. When the giving set is being changed or removed, the patient must lie flat and hold her breath. If air embolism is suspected, the patient should immediately be placed in left lateral head down position. The line must be immediately clamped. Oxygen is administered via mask at maximum flow rate, and CPR is commenced if respiration or pulse disappear. An attempt to aspirate air via the line should be made.

(b) Septicemia. The indwelling catheter provides a direct route of access for bacteria and fungi to the bloodstream. In addition, the sleeve of thrombus that covers the intravascular portion of the catheter soon after insertion can be seeded by bacteremia from infection elsewhere in the body. PN solutions are bacteriostatic but will support the growth of fungi. The common organisms to cause catheter-related sepsis are *Staphylococcus epidermis* and *Diphtheroids* from the skin or connection site of the catheter, and Gram-negative organisms seeded from other sites of infection. Fever that cannot be explained by infection elsewhere dictates immediate removal and culture of the catheter and blood cultures. If systemic symptoms develop or fever persists, then antibiotics are indicated.

(c) Hyperglycemia. Hyperglycemia is a consequence of administration of high dextrose concentration solution, bypassing normal gastrointestinal tract insulin stimulation, pre-existing diabetes and/or stress-induced insulin resistance. It produces glycosuria, polyuria and dehydration associated with a hyperosmolar state. Prevention is by slowly increasing glucose input and closely monitoring blood sugar levels and urine analysis. Treatment consists of decreasing the glucose input, diagnosing the cause of glucose intolerance and, if necessary, providing insulin according to a sliding scale.

(d) Hypoglycemia. If the high concentration glucose infusion is suddenly ceased, then the circulating insulin will cause a rapid fall in blood sugar level. Prevention is by tapering off TPN solutions over 24 hours and ensuring either an adequate oral intake or administering peripheral infusion of 5% glucose.

(e) Fluid overload. Regular clinical assessment, strict fluid balance and daily weighing will give warning of retained excess fluid which may lead to pulmonary and peripheral edema, particularly in elderly patients with congestive cardiac failure or renal failure, and during refeeding after a period of prolonged malnutrition.

(f) Metabolic complications. These are hyper/hyponatremia, hyper/hypokalemia, hyperchloremic acidosis, hypophosphatemia and hypomagnesemia. They are common consequences of PN in complex patients with extra fluid losses and malnutrition. Close monitoring is required and treatment is on an individual basis.

CARDIAC ARREST

Every doctor, no matter how senior, no matter what position, should be able to perform *basic life support* and, when equipment arrives, assist with *advanced life support*. Cardiac or respiratory arrest can occur anywhere or anytime, but particularly in the operating theater or recovery room. Prompt, appropriate action is imperative to give the patient a chance of functional survival.

Basic life support (BLS)

When a person collapses, his/her life may depend on the successful application of the principles of the ABC of resuscitation:[3,24] A = Airway, B = Breathing, C = Circulation.

If someone collapses in your presence, or you find someone collapsed, take the following steps (Table 84.14):

Table 84.14 Immediate action with collapsed patient

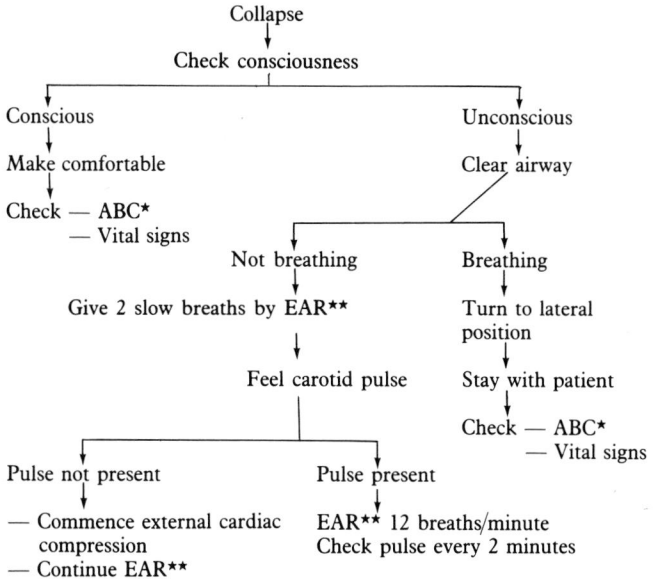

* ABC = airway, breathing, circulation
** EAR = expired airway resuscitation

(1) *Determine consciousness*, shake gently and speak to the patient. (2) If the patient is *unconscious*, stay with patient, shout for help, commence resuscitative measures. (3) *Clear the airway* — manually remove solids and loose fitting dentures, drain fluids by turning the patient to the side. *Open the airway* — apply head-tilt and chin lift. (4) *Observe for breathing* — look, listen and feel. If *breathing is present* — position patient on left side, monitor pulse, blood pressure and respiration, stay with the patient. If *breathing is absent* — commence expired airways resuscitation (EAR) (mouth-to-mouth, mouth-to-nose, mouth-to-stoma or mouth-to-mask). Deliver two breaths of 1 to 1.5 seconds each, observe the chest for rise and fall. (5) *Check circulation* — feel for the carotid pulse at the angle of the jaw (4 s). If *pulse is present*, continue EAR (12 breaths/minute; 800 ml/breath). If *pulse is absent*, commence external cardiac compressions, position the patient flat on a firm surface, use arrest board if necessary and available. *Locate the middle of the lower half of the sternum.* Position yourself so that your shoulders are over the patient's sternum and your arms are straight. Place the heel of one hand on the midline, not across the sternum, and use your other hand for additional force. Keep fingers raised and compress the sternum, 4 to 5 cm and 80 to 100 times/minute. During compressions do not lift your hands from the sternum. *One operator* provides 2 breaths then 15 compressions; *two operators*, 1 breath then 5 compressions. Pause to allow breath. Feel carotid pulse every 2 minutes. (6) *Do not stop resuscitation until either the patient recovers or someone of appropriate skill and authority takes over.*

The *prognosis* of the surviving patient who has sustained cardiopulmonary arrest depends on early initiation of basic life support measures followed by effective advanced life support. Therefore obtain *help and emergency equipment quickly* without interrupting basic life support.

Advanced life support

BLS provides a cardiac output of 10 to 20% of pre-arrest output, and mouth-to-mouth resuscitation produces ventilation with 15 to 18% inspired oxygen, so these are only temporary substitutes for normal circulation and respiration. Advanced life support aims to produce return of spontaneous circulation (ROSC) with adjunctive equipment as soon as possible. Table 84.15 illustrates the sequence of actions to be undertaken once this equipment is available. The most important intervention strategies that give the patient best chance of survival are: (a) defibrillation, (b) adrenaline, (c) intubation plus ventilation. If a full cardiac arrest team is present, then several tasks in the flow chart may be undertaken concurrently.

Electrical therapy

Direct current (DC) shock is indicated for ventricular fibrillation (VF) and pulseless ventricular tachycardia (VT). It is also the initial management in the event of apparent asystole or undetermined rhythm. This can be due to either fine or isoelectric VF masquerading as asystole dependent on lead placement, or to technical problems, such as inappropriate lead selection, broken lead or sensitivity turned down. Technical problems are identified by the absence of electrical artifact during external cardiac massage.

The rationale of electrical therapy is the simultaneous depolarization of the mass of myocardial cells. This will enable resumption of organized electrical activity. Paddles are placed apex to right parasternal area. With refractory VF, anterior/posterior placement may be used so that the maximum amount of current traverses the myocardium. Defibrillation pads are used for maximum electrical contact. Care should be taken to ensure that they are not in contact with each other. Don't defibrillate over ECG leads and don't defibrillate over a pacemaker.

Drugs

Adrenaline. This is the first-line drug of cardiopul-

Table 84.15 Advanced life support protocol

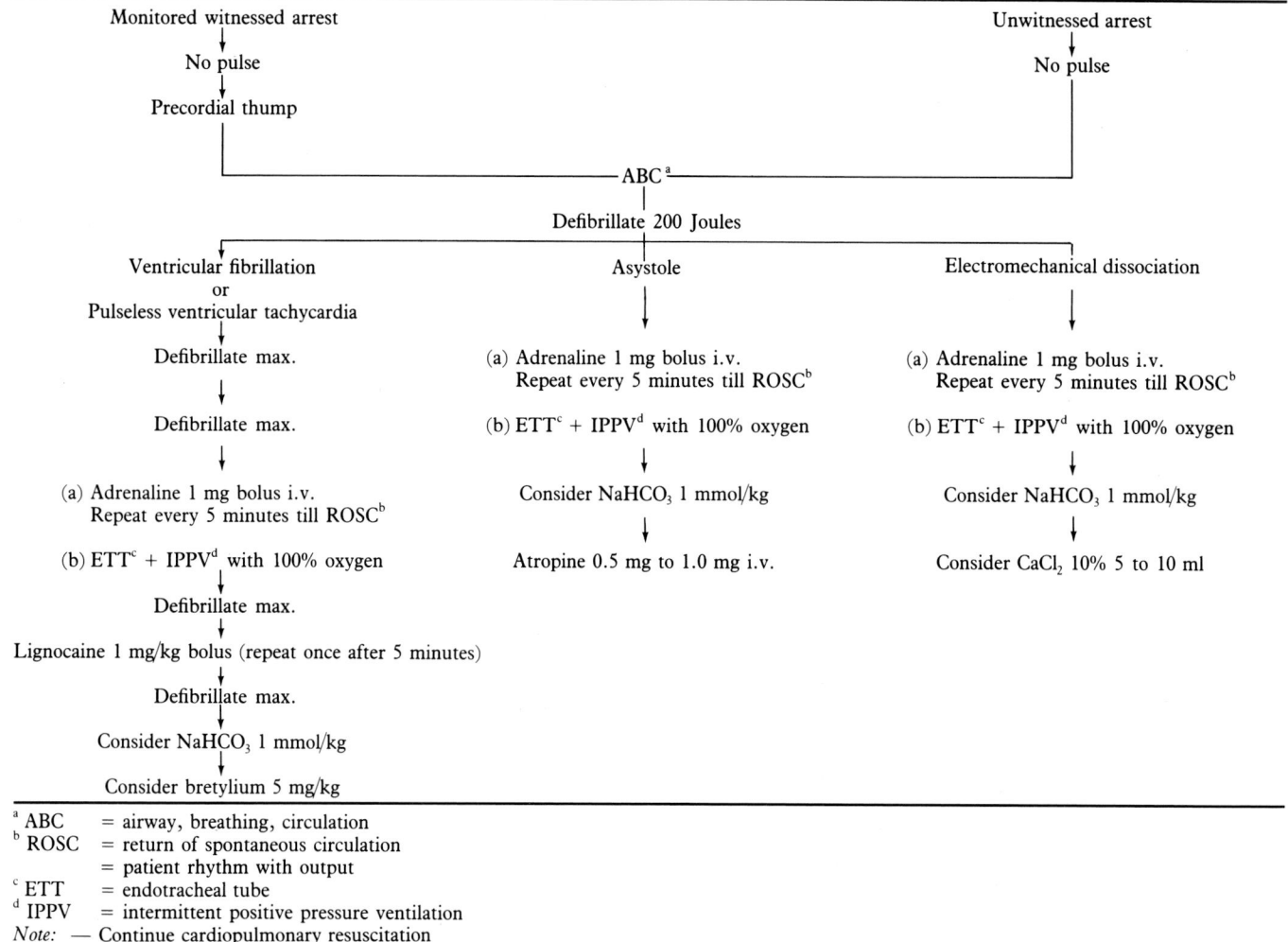

^a ABC   = airway, breathing, circulation
^b ROSC   = return of spontaneous circulation
            = patient rhythm with output
^c ETT   = endotracheal tube
^d IPPV   = intermittent positive pressure ventilation
Note: — Continue cardiopulmonary resuscitation
       — If no ROSC move to next step
       — After initial steps, seek cause.
Consider: hypovolemia, cardiac tamponade, hypoxemia, tension pneumothorax, acidosis, pulmonary embolus.

monary resuscitation (CPR). Via its adrenergic action, it produces peripheral vasoconstriction and directs available cardiac output to myocardium and brain. It also facilitates defibrillation by improving myocardial blood flow during CPR. The initial adult dose is 1 mg and this should be repeated at regular intervals (every 5 minutes) during CPR. Adrenaline may be required in continued increments or by infusion after ROSC to produce an adequate blood pressure.

Lignocaine. Is given after multiple DC shocks and i.v. adrenaline have failed to defibrillate ventricular fibrillation. It is also the first-line anti-arrhythmic for prophylaxis of ventricular fibrillation after successful defibrillation or treatment of ventricular ectopic beats and ventricular tachycardia. It is given initially as a 1 mg/kg bolus. During resuscitation, the bolus is repeated once after 5 minutes. When an infusion pump is available, a maintenance infusion is commenced.

Sodium bicarbonate. Is indicated for the treatment of severe metabolic acidosis, hyperkalemia, especially in the setting of protracted arrest and at the discretion of the team leader. It is initially given as a bolus of 1 mmol/kg, then as guided by arterial blood gases. $NaHCO_3$ is *no longer routine therapy*, because of the risk of alkalosis, hypernatremia, hyperosmolality and cellular acidosis secondary to generation of CO_2 which enters the cell. In most cardiac arrests, hyperventilation and early CPR negate the need for $NaHCO_3$.

Calcium. May be used in the treatment of hyperkalemia or arrhythmias associated with hypocalcemia or hypotension associated with Ca-channel blocking drugs. There is some evidence it may aid ROSC in patients with resistant electromechanical dissociation (EMD), particularly with broad QRS complexes. The usual bolus dose is 5 to 10 ml of 10% calcium chloride.

Atropine. May be useful in bradycardias and in asystole

resistant to standard treatment. The aim is to remove high vagal tone. Atropine is given as a bolus of 1 mg in asystole, or increments of 0.5 mg for bradycardias which may be associated with increased vagal tone.

Equipment

Mouth to mask ventilation should be used as an aid as soon as possible. Mouth to mask ventilation is a safe, efficient and easily taught technique of ventilation. All staff should be adept. Insertion of a Guedel airway will facilitate ventilation. *Bag mask* (e.g. Laerdal Bag/Air Viva) does not efficiently provide ventilation unless used by the most experienced operator. It is not recommended unless the patient is intubated. If the patient is unconscious and has no gag reflex and no trismus, the airway should be secured by *intubation* by an experienced operator at first opportunity, and the patient *ventilated* with 100% oxygen. The patient should be on a firm surface for effective external cardiac compression (ECC). Patients in ward beds should have a rigid *arrest board* placed at the first opportunity, under the patient, and not under the mattress.

Intravenous access. In most hands, this is reliably and quickly achieved by a peripheral cannula. The external jugular approach should be considered if access is difficult and the patient has been intubated. Central access has no advantages in the initial stages and has major risks. Endotracheal administration of adrenaline may be necessary if i.v. access is impossible. Adrenaline dosage via endotracheal tube is approximately 10 × i.v. dose.

Post arrest therapy

The aims are to: (1) determine and treat the cause of arrest, (2) continue respiratory support, (3) maintain cerebral perfusion and (4) treat and prevent cardiac arrhythmias. Causes to be excluded include: hypovolemia, cardiac tamponade, tension pneumothorax, hypoxemia, acidosis, pulmonary embolus, hypo/hyperkalemia and drug overdose (chloral hydrate, tricyclic antidepressants, etc).

Respiration is supported until the patient is awake, alert and cooperative. The patient must be able to protect her own airway and have a stable cardiovascular system. It is imperative to restore the systemic BP after return to normal electrical function. Aim for a BP equal to the patient's usual BP or at least a systolic greater than 100 mmHg. If the BP falls, adrenaline is given by small increments (0.1 mg) or infusion, until fluid status can be assessed by JVP, CVP and CXR. As soon as possible, all vasoconstrictor drugs are given by dedicated central lines. Hypo/hyperglycemia and electrolyte disorders such as hypo/hypernatremia may produce continuing cerebral damage. Blood glucose level, biochemical screen and arterial blood gases are checked. There is no evidence that steroids are beneficial and they may be harmful. Antiepileptics may be indicated.

SHOCK

Shock is best defined as 'a state of inadequate tissue blood flow' producing an acute nutritional insufficiency at the level of the cell.[32,65] In septic shock, there may also be cellular failure and inability to use available substrate. Shock is manifest as a failure of vital organ function, e.g.

brain — confusion, depressed level of consciousness
heart — ischemia, arrhythmias, pump failure
kidneys — oliguria (polyuria early in sepsis)
lungs — tachypnea.

Blood flow is proportional to blood pressure and inversely proportional to peripheral resistance. In the past, too much emphasis has been placed on blood pressure alone. Shock may be associated with what is apparently a 'normal' blood pressure or it may be associated with hypotension. Accepting a set value of blood pressure as normal (e.g. 120/80 mmHg) is dangerous, because blood pressure may be misleading. Flow to the core tissues is the key. As examples, the patient's usual blood pressure may be much higher as in pre-existing systemic hypertension, or a young patient, in shock, may compensate by large increase in peripheral resistance and heart rate and maintain blood pressure. The shock state is manifest by pallor, and cold and clammy periphery, with restlessness, tachycardia and oliguria.

Classification of causes

In its most simplistic form, the circulation of blood can be reduced to three components; the blood volume, the vascular bed and the pump (Fig. 84.10). Derangements of any one or a combination of these can produce inadequate flow and hence:

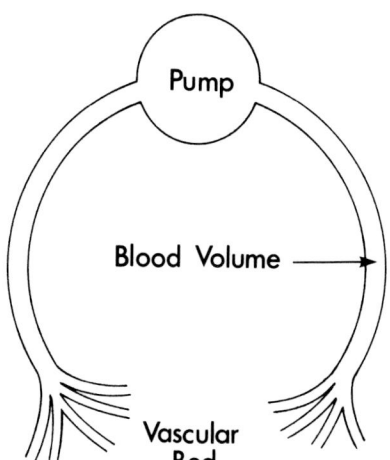

Fig. 84.10 Shock can be due to pump failure (cardiogenic), loss of blood volume (absolute hypovolemia), or dilatation of the vascular bed (relative hypovolemia) or septic (combination).

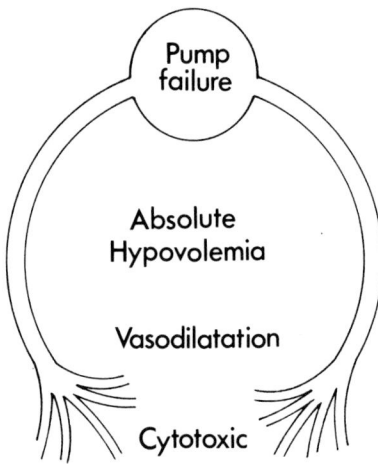

Fig. 84.11 In infective shock, 4 mechanisms may be operative. These include pump failure, absolute hypovolemia, vasodilatation and possibly a 'cytotoxic effect' in which the tissues fail to utilize oxygen.

1. Hypovolemic shock — absolute (loss of blood or components)
   — relative (vasodilatation)
2. Pump failure (cardiogenic shock)
3. Septic shock (a combination of both; see Fig. 84.11).

In terms of pathophysiology, there may be overlap between the individual causes (e.g. anaphylaxis is associated with vasodilatation, absolute hypovolemia and eventually myocardial depression). Consideration of this classification permits a logical approach to the problem when one is confronted by shock of unknown origin (Table 84.16).

Table 84.16 Causes of shock

Hypovolemic	
Absolute	Due to loss of fluid from the vascular space. — plasma (burns, peritonitis, pancreatitis) — blood (trauma, melena, hematemesis) or — water and electrolytes (vomiting, diarrhea, polyuria)
Relative	Due to increase in size of the vascular space (anaphylaxis, drug overdose, spinal or epidural anesthetic).
Pump failure	Lumen — pulmonary embolus Endocardium — valve stenosis or rupture, acute VSD Myocardium — infarct, cardiomyopathy, contusion Conducting tissue — arrhythmias (SVT, VT) Pericardium — tamponade Extrapericardial — tension pneumothorax
Septic	A dynamic combination of absolute and relative hypovolemia, pump failure and mitochondrial failure

VSD = ventricular septal defect
SVT = supraventricular tachycardia
 VT = ventricular tachycardia

Clinical assessment

Definitive diagnosis is concurrent with resuscitation and based on history, examination and investigations.

History

The history gives the first and important clues to the type of shock.

1. Absolute hypovolemia is suggested by a visible source of bleeding or hematoma, or fluid loss such as vomiting, diarrhea or polyuria.
2. Relative hypovolemia is suggested by drug exposure, epidural or spinal anesthesia
3. Cardiogenic shock is suggested by chest pain, deep venous thrombosis (DVT), hemoptysis.
4. Septic shock is suggested by presence of *fever*, rigors, cough, sputum, dysuria, urinary catheter, abdominal pain, CVP catheter, previous splenectomy, tampon use.

A full system review should follow. Trends in vital signs are checked, particularly if the patient has been in hospital (pulse, blood pressure, temperature).

Physical examination

Special attention must be directed to five key parameters; skin perfusion, pulse, blood pressure, jugular venous pressure (JVP) and rectal temperature. Skin perfusion gives a good indication of peripheral resistance. If two patients have blood pressures of 90 systolic, and one has cold white or cyanotic skin whilst the other has warm pink skin, the former is obviously more shocked. The majority of patients with shock have tachycardia. A slow pulse indicates cardiac disease or else the patient is on beta-blocker therapy for hypertension or has ischemic heart disease. The degree of hypotension usually parallels the severity of shock, but it must always be interpreted in combination with peripheral resistance as evidenced by skin perfusion. The jugular venous pressure is assessed with the patient momentarily raised to an angle of 45°. All shocked patients must have their temperature recorded rectally, as vasoconstriction and hyperventilation make axillary and oral temperatures useless and misleading. Neglect of this simple measurement may lead to delay in the diagnosis of septicemia. The vast majority of patients with septicemia have rectal temperatures in excess of 38.5°C. Reports of normothermic or hypothermic septicemia usually emanate from centers where rectal temperatures are not measured.

General examination

A complete and thorough physical examination with special

emphasis on the cardiovascular and respiratory systems must be performed.

Special investigations

Urine output. As the central problem in shock is a lack of blood supply to the tissues, it is important to have an *objective* measurement of blood flow. Only two organs are available for clinical measurement: the skin, where blood flow can be assessed by inspection, palpation and skin temperature measurement; and the kidney, where in the absence of diuretics or kidney disease the urinary output parallels renal blood flow. Provided the urine output is in excess of 0.5 ml/kg per hour (i.e. 30 ml/hour in an adult) renal perfusion is adequate and, by inference, other vital organs are well perfused. An indwelling urinary catheter should be routinely inserted in all shocked patients to monitor progress.

Central venous pressure (CVP) and left atrial pressure (LAP). See section on monitoring (p. 1339).

Chest X-ray. Performed at regular intervals, serial X-rays provide a useful index of how the heart is responding to a fluid load. Problems of interpretation can arise if the patient has respiratory complications such as infection, shock lung, etc.

Acid-base and blood gases. Pa_{O_2}, Pa_{CO_2}, and base excess should be measured early in shock. Common abnormalities which may require correction are: (1) Low Pa_{O_2} — this is usually due to pulmonary shunting and aggravated by the low cardiac output which causes decreased oxygen saturation of the venous blood. It is corrected by adding more oxygen to the inspired gas. (2) Low Pa_{CO_2} — this is due to hyperventilation in response to shock and also as compensation for metabolic acidosis. (3) Low pH with negative base excess — this indicates metabolic acidosis usually secondary to lactic acid accumulation from anaerobic metabolism in poorly perfused tissues (see also p. 1372). If the pH falls below 7.25 with a pure metabolic acidosis, it is wise to correct this with $NaHCO_3$ solution. Metabolic acidosis depresses cardiac contractility and potentiates arrhythmias.

Routine laboratory tests. Depending on the clinical circumstances, these would include full blood count, coagulation profile, electrolytes, urea, creatinine, glucose, liver function tests and cultures of blood, body fluids, pus, etc.

Treatment of the shocked patient

Treatment revolves around three principles; general measures, hemodynamic correction and specific therapy.

1. General measures

Posture. The majority of shocked patients are best man-aged in the supine position. However, with severe hypovolemia there is considerable advantage in elevating the foot of the bed or operating table to obtain an auto-transfusion of blood from the venous system into the central circulation. Occasionally a patient with a large mobile pelvic mass who is laid flat can develop 'supine hypotension' due to compression of the inferior vena cava by the mass. This is relieved by placing the patient in the left lateral position.

Conversely, with cardiogenic shock and pulmonary edema the supine posture hinders breathing and these dyspneic patients benefit from a semi-sitting position.

Oxygen therapy. The main problem in shock is failure to deliver oxygen to the tissues and in some cases the Pa_{O_2} is low due to intrapulmonary shunting. High concentration oxygen therapy should be routinely administered via an efficient oxygen mask.

Pain relief. In most situations, pain itself does not cause shock. In rare situations, pain may stimulate vasovagal reflexes leading to bradycardia and vasodilatation with poor perfusion or, conversely, sympathetic reflexes causing excessive vasoconstriction and poor perfusion. Severe pain must be relieved if only for humane reasons. Usually a narcotic analgesic, such as morphine etc, is favored. The drug must be given directly intravenously in small increments repeated every 2 to 3 minutes, whilst carefully observing the response. An average aliquot of morphine would be 2.5 mg. The narcotic analgesic must never be given by intramuscular injection, as absorption from muscle during shock is poor. As a consequence, large doses may be given which can constitute an overdose once the circulation is restored. When a narcotic analgesic is given, the circulation must be closely monitored, as vasodilatation may occur and aggravate the shock state. In addition, the level of consciousness may be depressed leading to respiratory insufficiency. Inhalation agents such as Entonox, a mixture of equal parts of oxygen and nitrous oxide may be useful for these critically ill patients.

Reversal of metabolic acidosis. Metabolic acidosis depresses myocardial contractility, potentiates arrhythmias and causes peripheral vasoconstriction. If the pH is less than 7.25, and the acidosis is metabolic and not respiratory, then it should be reversed with $NaHCO_3$. An 8.4% solution containing 1 millimole of HCO_3 per ml is used and, depending on the severity of the acidosis, is administered in 50 to 100 ml aliquots. Following each aliquot, the acid base status is remeasured and the need for further alkali determined. This is preferable to relying on formulae based on in vitro measurements which do not allow for in vivo variation. Respiratory acidosis causes release of catecholamines, stimulates the circulation and does not require correction with $NaHCO_3$, but it may require artificial ventilation.

2. Hemodynamic correction

It is imperative to determine whether the shock is hypovolemic or cardiogenic in nature, as the treatment of each is diametrically opposed. The key parameters in hypovolemic shock are low CVP or PCW pressure with a clear chest X-ray, and in cardiogenic shock a high CVP or PCW pressure with a congested chest X-ray.

Hypovolemic shock. Restoration of circulating blood volume is the first priority, and fluids that stay in the vascular space should be used for resuscitation. This implies the use of plasma expanders or blood. The volume and rate at which plasma expanders are administered depend upon the degree of hypovolemia. In general, plasma expanders are administered until the key signs of shock are reversed, that is, skin vasoconstriction has disappeared, the pulse rate has slowed below 100, the blood pressure has risen to normal, the central venous pressure has normalized and an adequate urinary output has been restored. With severe hypovolemia, fluids should be given rapidly via a large-bore intravenous cannula using a pressure pump set. By this means, it is possible to administer 500 ml every 3 to 5 minutes. With severe exsanguination two intravenous routes may be necessary. Cold blood should be passed through a blood warming coil to prevent hypothermia with its associated problems, such as cardiac depression and arrhythmias.

Cardiogenic shock. The first prerequisite is to exclude all reversible causes of cardiogenic shock, e.g. arrhythmias, hypoxia, acidosis, pericardial tamponade, major pulmonary embolism and valvular disruption. Usually, however, the problem is a poorly contracting left ventricle. Treatment basically consists of fluid restriction and administration of an inotropic agent. This is further discussed in the specific management of cardiogenic shock.

3. Specific treatment of shock

Four common types of shock require specific measures. These are: hemorrhagic shock, septic shock, cardiogenic shock and anaphylactic shock. Each will be discussed in turn.

Hemorrhagic shock

Hemorrhagic shock is due to either external or internal blood loss.[45,55,61] Physiological compensation for hemorrhage includes vasoconstriction in arterioles and veins to decrease the size of the vascular bed, increased heart rate and increased cardiac contractility. The ability to compensate depends upon many factors, but the main ones are the age and physical fitness of the patient. Obviously the young fit patient can withstand hemorrhage much better than the older patient with heart and lung disease, anemia, etc.

In adults, the normal blood volume is 70 ml/kg, hence, a 70 kg woman has a total blood volume of approximately 5000 ml. Clinical assessment of the amount of blood lost can be quite difficult, particularly if the bleeding is internal or if external loss cannot be accurately measured. With 10% blood volume loss (500 ml in an adult) one usually detects no changes in the patient. With 20% loss, the main signs are those of pallor due to vasoconstriction, together with an elevation of pulse rate above 100. With 30% loss, the body is unable to compensate and the systolic blood pressure falls below 100. By the time 60% of the blood volume has been lost (3 liters in an adult), the systolic blood pressure is usually 60 mmHg or lower. Another useful sign is that a tissue swelling or hematoma the size of an open or closed adult fist is equivalent to 500 ml of blood.

Treatment of hemorrhage

Whilst resuscitation is proceeding, primary treatment consists of stopping the hemorrhage. With exsanguinating hemorrhage where the patient is intensely shocked and in danger of imminent death, a life-saving measure can be the application of the medical anti-shock trouser (mast suit). This ingenious suit, devised prior to 1900 by Dr. George Crile of the Cleveland Clinic and used for the treatment of hypovolemic shock, has undergone a resurrection in the last decade. The garment consists of three compartments (Fig. 84.12) which envelope the legs and the abdomen up to the diaphragm. The garment is applied, the three compartments are inflated by means of a foot pump, and circumferential pressure is applied to the lower half of the body. This has two beneficial effects: the direct pressure tamponades the internal bleeding site, and the external pressure reduces the size of the vascular bed, allowing the reduced blood volume to be distributed to the brain and heart. There is also said to be some autotransfusion, but this is small. The effect of application of the mast trousers can be miraculous. A pulseless, comatose, exsanguinated

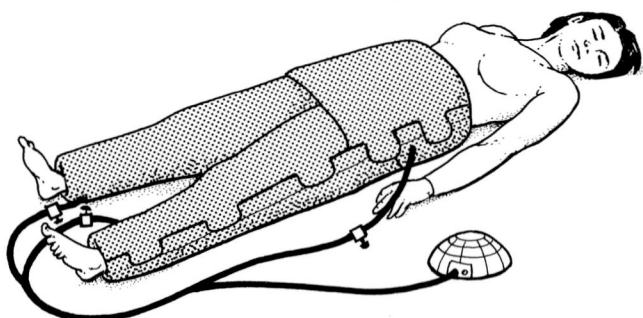

Fig. 84.12 The medical anti-shock trouser is used in hypovolemic shock and consists of a pneumatic suit with 3 separate compartments that are inflated to compress both lower limbs and the abdomen.

patient can be immediately restored to consciousness, with a palpable pulse and a blood pressure of 80 to 100 mmHg systolic. A further benefit is that veins suddenly appear, making intravenous cannulation simpler.

The next step is to restore circulating blood volume by infusion of colloid solutions or blood.[29] Once the blood volume has been restored and the vital signs normalized, a decision must be made regarding release of the suit. If there is internal hemorrhage and surgery is indicated, the suit should be left inflated until the patient is in the operating theater, the surgeon is gowned and gloved and the patient is anesthetized, then the abdominal section of the suit is gradually deflated, leaving the legs inflated. Once the bleeding site has been ligated and blood volume restored, the suit can be removed.

Septic shock

Septic shock is a state of evolving signs and pathology that develops as a complication of overwhelming infection.[11,17,39] The majority of cases are secondary to Gram-negative bacteria, with a smaller significant proportion being due to Gram-positive bacteria. Viruses, fungae, rickettsiae and protozoa have also been reported to produce a clinical picture of septic shock.

The genitourinary tract is the most common site of infection, as instrumentation of this area can initiate bacteremia and shock. The gastrointestinal tract (diverticular disease, trauma, perforated peptic ulcer) and respiratory tract (pneumonia) are the next most common. Wound infections, infected intravenous lines, pelvic infections and septic abortions may lead to septic shock. In the immunocompromised woman, (due to cancer, chronic illness or immunosuppressive therapy) no primary site may be obvious. Other conditions which depress host defenses and make patients more susceptible to infection are previous splenectomy, cirrhosis, trauma, acute renal failure, and neoplastic disease.

Early non-specific symptoms include anorexia, nausea, vomiting and diarrhea, accompanied by mild confusion and restlessness. Hyperventilation and respiratory alkalosis are early signs. Fever, often associated with rigors, is almost invariable. Hypothermia can occur late with overwhelming infection in the elderly, or in the presence of liver or renal failure, hypothyroidism or drugs, such as phenothiazines. Reports of normothermic septic shock usually indicate that oral or axillary temperatures were recorded instead of rectal. An inappropriate polyuria occurs initially, perhaps related to a tubular concentrating defect (nephrogenic diabetes insipidus). In immunosuppressed patients, the only clue may be confusion, diarrhea, tachycardia or being 'unwell'. Non-specific changes in laboratory tests may include leukocytosis, leukopenia, hypoglycemia or hyperglycemia.

Pathophysiology

There is initially a failure of normal cellular metabolism (mitochondrial oxidative failure), associated with peripheral vasodilatation, and high cardiac output. This combination of vascular dilatation and loss of fluid via capillary leak leads to hypovolemia (relative and absolute). Myocardial depression occurs but is initially masked by the peripheral vasodilatation (low afterload) leading to high cardiac output. With time (if treatment is delayed) a low flow state supervenes, with vasoconstriction, worsening metabolic acidosis and worsening hypotension. Organisms, bacterial exotoxins and endotoxins have been implicated in causing direct injury or triggering destructive cascades to produce the septic shock syndrome.

Endotoxin, one of the historical culprits, is a complex lipopolysaccharide which forms part of the cell wall of many organisms, particularly Gram-negative. It contains a cytotoxic portion, lipid A and an antigen handle. Lipid A has the ability to damage all cells. Some of the actions of endotoxins are mediated via release of interleukin-1, cachectin and TNF from circulating and tissue macrophages. These actions include: (1) pyrogen production, (2) activation of coagulation and fibrinolysis, (3) release of complement, kinins, prostaglandins and histamine, (4) aggregation of polymorphonuclear cells.

Multiple organ effects can result due to a combination of hypoperfusion, direct toxin and mediator effects in any of these forms of septic shock:

Lung — adult respiratory distress syndrome.
Heart — arrhythmias (atrial fibrillation 40 to 60%), pump failure
Brain — septic encephalopathy
Kidney — acute tubular necrosis
Liver — jaundice, intrahepatic cholestasis
Blood — disseminated intravascular coagulation (DIC), thrombocytopenia, leukopenia/cytosis
Stomach — stress ulceration

Toxic shock syndrome. This distinctive disorder is due to the effects of an *exotoxin* from the *Staphylococcus aureus*. Over 90% of the cases occur in menstruating women. It is characterized by an abrupt onset of high fever, conjunctival and mucosal suffusion, erythematous rash with subsequent desquamation, hypotension and multisystem features (including renal impairment, DIC, vomiting, diarrhea, confusion and hepatic dysfunction). The classical association is the presence of vaginal staphylococcus and tampon use, although the syndrome has occurred in other settings. Management includes removal of the source of infection, antibiotics and supportive treatment.[56]

Diagnosis

History. Dysuria, cough, sputum, abdominal pain, vaginal discharge, cellulitis.

Physical examination. Involves complete assessment of

the patient from head to toes, front and back, including skin, (e.g. scalded skin in staphylococcal septicemia or exotoxemia) looking for a source of infection or signs of systemic illness.

Investigations. Should include: full blood count to check leukocytosis/leukopenia/thrombocytopenia; biochemical profile, coagulation screen to check for disseminated intravascular coagulants (DIC); cultures of urine, sputum, blood, wound, central lines, sinuses, (if specimens are available, urgent Gram stains should be performed to guide initial antibiotic therapy); chest X-ray; and determination of acid base status and arterial blood gases.

Management of septic shock

Hemodynamic correction. Circulation is restored by initially normalizing the circulating volume with either plasma volume expanders or blood transfusion if anemia exists. If there are signs or symptoms of fluid overload or cardiac failure (increasing dyspnea, raised JVP, gallop rhythm) or if hypoxia due to ARDS (p. 1364), or 'shock lung' supervenes, then fluid loading may be limited. If shock persists in the presence of normal or high plasma volume, inotropic agents are necessary to elevate the cardiac output, to increase peripheral resistance and to restore vital organ perfusion.

Atrial arrhythmias (fibrillation and flutter) are common in this setting, particularly in the older age groups so prophylactic digitilization is indicated (15 μg/kg i.v. over 2 to 3 hours) once hypokalemia is excluded.

Treat the cause. Remove infected intravenous lines, drain the pus (intra-abdominal, perinephric abscess), excise necrotic tissue (necrotizing fascitis), repair leaking viscus, remove foreign body, decompress obstruction.

Antibiotics. In the early stages, the infecting organism is usually unknown. The backbone of the 'shotgun' approach, necessary until results of cultures are known, is an aminoglycoside (e.g. gentamicin)[69] for Gram-negative cover, plus a penicillin (e.g. ampicillin) for Gram-positive cover and metronidazole if bowel anaerobes are suspected. If thrombophlebitis, infected intravenous lines, scalded skin syndrome or typical pneumonia implicate *Staphylococcus aureus*, then flucloxacillin (or vancomycin if methicillin resistant *Staphylococcus aureus* is a local problem) should be added.

The commonly used aminoglycosides are gentamicin and tobramycin, both of which have a wide spectrum. The usual dose of gentamicin is 1 mg/kg; in severe infections, this can be increased to 1.5 mg/kg. If 1 mg/kg of gentamicin is infused intravenously over an hour or given intramuscularly, a peak level of 4 μg/ml is reached at 1 hour. As the drug is excreted by glomerular filtration, this level gradually falls so that by 7 hours the trough level is approximately 1 μg/ml, the rate of fall depending upon renal

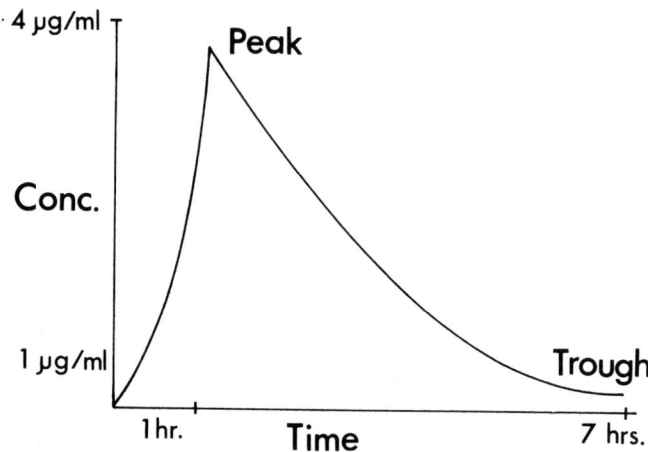

Fig. 84.13 Following the intramuscular injection of 1 mg/kg of gentamicin a peak level of 4 μg/ml is obtained at 1 hour. The drug is eliminated by the kidney and with normal renal function a trough level below 1 μg/ml is reached at 7 hours.

function (Fig. 84.13). As a consequence, the time interval between doses has to be titrated according to renal function. The serum creatinine is a useful clinical guide. The serum creatinine expressed in mmol/l is multiplied by 80 to determine the frequency of administration in hours. For example, with a normal serum creatinine of 0.1 mmol/l, the dose of gentamicin is given every 8 hours; with moderate renal dysfunction and a creatinine of 0.3 mmol/l, the dose is given every 24 hours; with the patient on regular hemodialysis, the dose is administered after each dialysis. Gentamicin toxicity usually occurs when the serum level exceeds 10 μg/ml. The two target organs are: the eighth nerve, causing both vestibular and auditory disability which may be permanent; and the kidney, causing tubular damage, especially when the drug is used in combination with a cephalosporin antibiotic. With renal failure, trough levels of gentamicin should be measured to ensure that the drug does not accumulate and reach toxic levels.

In situations where the causative organism is unknown, gentamicin or tobramycin alone is insufficient, as there are two serious gaps in its spectrum. Firstly, it is ineffective against streptococcus, pneumococcus and meningococcus, and an antibiotic such as ampicillin 1 g 6-hourly, or a cephalosporin needs to be added to the therapeutic regime. Secondly, anaerobes are insensitive to gentamicin, hence a drug effective against anaerobes, such as clindamycin 300 to 600 mg 6-hourly, or metronidazole 500 mg 8-hourly, must be exhibited. Situations where anaerobic organisms can be anticipated are infections involving the upper airway, the gut and the genital tract. If clostridial infection is suspected, then penicillin is administered in a dose of 20 million units daily. Aminoglycoside and clindamycin combination may be substituted if penicillin allergy is suspected or status unknown.

When culture results and sensitivities are available from

blood secretions, pus, etc the most appropriate antibiotics are administered. Negative blood cultures in septicemia may be due to (a) commencement of antibiotics before taking the cultures, (b) poor technique in taking the cultures, or (c) the presence of endotoxemia (absorbed from abscess or bowel lumen) which may produce the sepsis syndrome in the absence of micro-organisms in the circulation.

Immunotherapy. Nutrition is important in the maintenance of normal immunity. The catabolic response of the critically ill leads to peripheral muscle breakdown in an attempt to sustain the acute phase response. Unfortunately, exogenous fuel at this time will not turn off the catabolic process and may lead to metabolic complications (hyperglycemia, fatty liver, etc). Therefore the plan should be to attack the underlying disease, provide small amounts of glucose/amino acids/fat as tolerated, and increase feeding as the stress response settles.

Corticosteroids are contraindicated. Early reports suggested that if given early, they increased survival by stabilization of lysozymal membranes, maintenance of capillary integrity and inhibition of endotoxin and complement activation. These impressions were not confirmed by clinical trials[7,75] and current practice is to *avoid steroids* because of potential immunosuppression, unless the patient has Addisons disease or has recently been on steroid therapy.

Therapy to boost the patient's own immune reponse is a field of future interest. Suggested modalities include: fresh frozen plasma (contains opsonins, fibronectin, immunoglobin), gammaglobulin and anti-endotoxin serum (so far a research tool).

Cardiogenic shock

The main priority in cardiogenic shock is to exclude correctable factors, such as arrhythmias, hypoxia, acidosis, pericardial tamponade, acute valvular or septal disruption and massive pulmonary embolism.[18,23] Having excluded these potentially correctable factors, the diagnosis is 'poorly contracting heart'. The prognosis is usually poor. This is particularly so following acute myocardial infarction, when cardiogenic shock indicates that greater than 40% of the myocardium is necrotic.

Management

The treatment of cardiogenic shock, as opposed to that of hypovolemic shock, involves the restriction of fluid and the use of drugs to improve vascular and myocardial contractility. The majority of these drugs are catecholamines, for example epinephrine, norepinephrine, dobutamine and dopamine.[60] The choice of drug depends on individual preference, but their properties can be summarized by subdividing them into alpha and beta adrenergic effects (Table 84.17). The alpha effect refers to constriction of arterioles,

Table 84.17 Cardiogenic shock. Drug therapy: Sympathomimetic effects

Drug	Receptor effect			
	Alpha	Beta 1	Beta 2	Dopaminergic
Norepinephrine	+++	+++	+	−
Epinephrine	++	+++	++	−
Dopamine	++	++	+	+++
Dobutamine	+	++	++	−
Isoprenaline	+	+++	+++	−

with a consequent increase in peripheral vascular resistance and rise in systemic blood pressure. Beta effects are subdivided into beta 1 and beta 2. Beta 1 refers to increased cardiac contractility and conductivity. Beta 2 effect refers to bronchodilatation and metabolic effects, together with vasodilatation of blood vessels in skeletal muscle.

Dopamine. Is currently a popular inotropic and vasopressor drug. Apart from possessing both alpha and beta effects similar to epinephrine, in low dosage it stimulates dopaminergic receptors in the renal and visceral circulation which increase the blood supply to the kidney, liver and gut.

Dobutamine. A newer inotropic agent, dobutamine has found a place particularly in moderate forms of cardiogenic hypotension. In doses around $5\mu g/kg$ per minute, it produces an increase in cardiac output with minimal change in heart rate or vascular resistance. In higher dose it produces tachycardias and peripheral vasodilatation.

Epinephrine. Has mixed alpha and beta effects, depending on the dose. As the dose is increased, the alpha effect starts to predominate. Epinephrine and dopamine are the most common inotropic agents for general use.

Norepinephrine. Has predominantly an alpha effect. Hence, it causes widespread vasoconstriction with a rise in systemic blood pressure. This drug is sometimes used for severe resistant hypotension associated with sepsis or following pulmonary embolus. Coronary perfusion is very dependent upon diastolic blood pressure, and norepinephrine raises this pressure and improves coronary perfusion. In this situation, it is also important to minimize the beta 1 effect which, by increasing myocardial oxygen consumption, may compromise the viability of areas of partially ischemic myocardium.

These catecholamines are dissolved in 5% dextrose and given by continuous intravenous infusion observing several precautions: (1) an infusion pump should be used to prevent either under or overdosage with their obvious dangers; (2) the intravenous route must be a dedicated line to which no other infusions or drugs are added, to prevent a surge or a bolus effect; (3) a large central vein should be utilized, as norepinephrine in particular will cause tissue gangrene if it extravasates.

Typical doses of these drugs would be 2 ml of 0.1% norepinephrine, 1 mg of epinephrine, or 200 mg of dopamine dissolved in 100 ml of 5% dextrose. The diluted drug is administered by infusion pump until the desired effect is obtained; usually this is a systolic blood pressure greater than 100 mmHg. An indwelling arterial line is essential to constantly monitor arterial blood pressure. An overdose of catecholamines will give rise to tachycardia, arrhythmias and hypertension.

Digoxin. Of little use in acute cardiogenic shock, as it is a relatively weak inotropic agent and, even if given intravenously, there is a delay of 1 to 2 hours before any effect is noted. Hence, rapidly acting powerful agents such as dopamine or epinephrine are preferred.

Counterpulsation. Mechanical circulatory support using devices such as intra-aortic balloon counterpulsation is utilized in certain special centers.[63]

Anaphylactic shock

Anaphylaxis can occur as an adverse response to various antigens such as penicillin, plasma expanders, blood products, X-ray contrast media and anesthetic agents.[20,21] A typical story is the sudden onset of shock associated with erythema and urticaria of the skin, bronchospasm and laryngeal edema. This reaction is due to the antigenic substance reacting with IgE antibodies, which in turn cause sensitized basophils to release chemical mediators. This gives rise to generalized vasodilatation with leaking capillaries and hypotension due to a combination of relative and absolute hypovolemia. The specific therapy for anaphylactic shock is epinephrine, as it corrects both the vasodilatation and the leaking capillaries. Epinephrine should be given without delay, either as 0.5 mg subcutaneously or, if an intravenous line is available, in intravenous infusion of 1 ml of 1 in 10 000 epinephrine per minute up to a maximum dose of 10 ml. The epinephrine should preferably be given under EKG control monitoring for arrhythmias. In addition, urgent volume expansion is required and plasma expanders are rapidly infused to elevate the blood pressure. If there is a poor response to fluids and epinephrine, then norepinephrine infusion should be used to correct the hypotension. Other drugs, such as antihistamines and steroids, play a secondary role in treatment and it must be stressed that epinephrine is the specific treatment of anaphylaxis.

Complications of shock

Common complications include acute renal failure, 'shock lung' (acute respiratory distress syndrome, ARDS) and disseminated intravascular coagulation.

Acute renal failure. This may result from decreased cortical perfusion secondary to hypotension or direct effects of endotoxin release. It is further discussed in the section on oliguria (see p. 1366).

Acute respiratory distress syndrome ('ARDS'). A term used for acute pulmonary edema that develops in a shocked patient. Its etiology is usually multifactorial, and includes alveolocapillary membrane damage from such factors as release of endotoxin and other vasoactive substances, embolism of transfusion debris, acid aspiration, oxygen toxicity and disseminated intravascular coagulation, and also cardiogenic factors, such as myocardial ischemia, overtransfusion of blood or crystalloids. The management is that of acute pulmonary edema, and includes oxygen, fluid restriction, diuretics and mechanical ventilation with positive end expiratory pressure (PEEP) (see p. 1366).

Disseminated intravascular coagulation (DIC). This can occur with any type of shock but is more common with infective shock. Initially, there is widespread thrombosis throughout the microcirculation giving rise to ischemic lesions in various organs, especially the skin and kidneys. A hemorrhagic state then develops secondary to the consumption of coagulation factors and platelets. Thus, the patient usually presents a combination of thrombotic and hemorrhagic lesions. Coagulation tests may show depletion of coagulation factors, thrombocytopenia and elevated fibrin degradation products. The most important principle of management is to vigorously treat the primary cause of the shock; in many cases the DIC will then cease. The use of heparin and fresh frozen plasma plays a secondary role and requires expert hematological supervision.

POSTOPERATIVE RESPIRATORY FAILURE

The oxygen transport chain

To understand postoperative respiratory failure, it is necessary to examine the mechanisms by which oxygen is carried from the ambient air to the tissues.[28] This involves a number of factors; the oxygen concentration in the inspired air, pulmonary ventilation, proper matching of ventilation to perfusion in the lung, hemoglobin and a circulation to carry oxygen to the tissues (Fig. 84.14).

Hypoxia

Hypoxia is defined as deficiency of oxygen at tissue level, whereas hypoxemia is a deficiency of oxygen in the blood. The clinical detection of hypoxia is not easy. The main clue to the diagnosis is the presence of confusion. This is the first sign of tissue hypoxia and occurs long before the patient becomes cyanosed; indeed, the presence of central cyanosis implies gross hypoxemia. It is now known that moderate degrees of hypoxemia can only be recognized by the performance of blood gas estimations. The causes of hypoxia, shown diagrammatically in Figure 84.15 are discussed below.

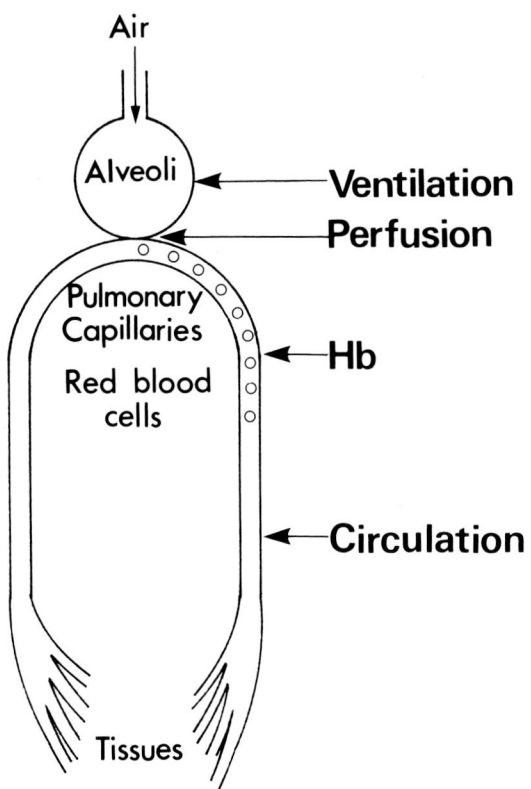

Fig. 84.14 Oxygen enters the alveoli by the process of ventilation and provided there is adequate perfusion with pulmonary capillary blood enters the blood stream where it is bound to hemoglobin. It is then carried in the circulation to the tissues.

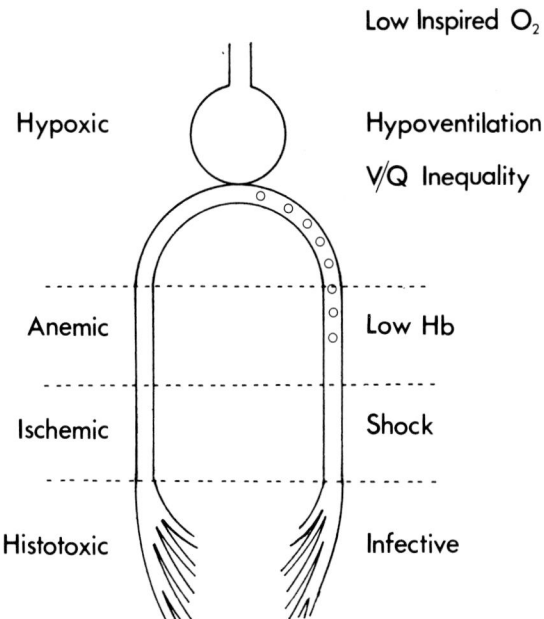

Fig. 84.15 There are 4 classic types of hypoxia. Hypoxic hypoxia characterized by a low P_aO_2 is due to a low inspired O_2, hypoventilation or V/Q inequality. Anemic hypoxia is due to a low or altered Hb e.g. carboxyhemoglobin, methemoglobin. Ischemic hypoxia occurs with shock states. Histotoxic hypoxia is due to interference with cellular cytochromes and may occur with infective shock.

Table 84.18 Causes of hypoventilation

a. Brain: Anything that depresses the brain and causes coma will lead to hypoventilation. For example, drugs, strokes, space occupying lesions etc.
b. Spinal cord: High spinal anesthesia, cord trauma etc.
c. Nerves: Polyneuritis.
d. Neuromuscular junction: Overdose of neuromuscular relaxants, myasthenia gravis etc.
e. Chest wall: Fractured ribs, gross obesity, large breasts.
f. Pleural cavity: Pneumothorax, hemothorax.
g. Airway: Upper or lower airway obstruction.

Low inspired oxygen concentration

Although common at high altitudes, this is a rare occurrence in hospital situations and usually only occurs when a patient is connected to an anesthetic machine and the oxygen supply fails.

Hypoventilation

For ventilation to be adequate, one must have a normal respiratory rate, tidal volume and minimal dead space. If the respiratory rate is too slow, the tidal volume too small, or the dead space increased, then hypoventilation results. As a consequence, there is a failure of oxygenation and, because carbon dioxide is excreted via the lung, CO_2 retention occurs. Thus, the blood gas profile is a low Pa_{O_2} and high Pa_{CO_2}. The causes of hypoventilation are shown in Table 84.18. In the postoperative period, the commonest causes are upper airway obstruction, excessive sedation from anesthetic or analgesic agents and residual paralysis from neuromuscular blocking drugs.

Ventilation perfusion inequality

The ventilation (V) of alveoli must be accompanied by an adequate perfusion (Q) of blood to the capillaries surrounding the alveoli. If this balance is impaired, then VQ inequality is said to exist. There are two main types of VQ inequality. The first is an impairment of ventilation to some alveoli whilst the perfusion remains normal which results in the venous blood failing to take up oxygen so that deoxygenated blood passes into the arterial circulation. This is termed an 'intrapulmonary shunt' and causes hypoxia (Fig. 84.16A). On the other hand, (Fig. 84.16 A and B) if the ventilation of alveoli is adequate but there is a block of perfusion, as for example in pulmonary embolism or shock, wasted ventilation of these alveoli results. This is called increased 'alveolar dead space' (Fig. 84.16B).

Intrapulmonary shunting is the major cause of postoperative hypoxia and must be considered in more detail. As previously explained, portions of the lung receive little

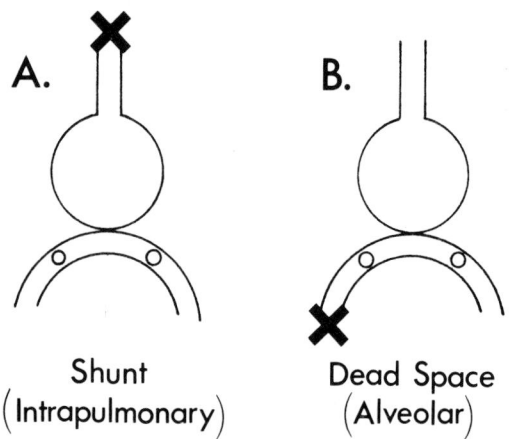

Fig. 84.16 There are 2 types of V/Q inequality.
A. Interference with alveolar ventilation leading to intrapulmonary shunting with impairment of pulmonary capillary O_2 uptake and a low P_aO_2.
B. Interference with pulmonary capillary perfusion causing wasted ventilation by increasing the alveolar dead space. Hyperventilation is required to prevent CO_2 accumulation.

or no ventilation and yet are adequately perfused with blood.[76] There are three mechanisms by which this can occur.

The first mechanism involves increased closing volume. During expiration, as the intrathoracic pressure rises, there is a gradual narrowing of the airways and eventually some airways close completely, particularly those in the basal parts of the lung. Whenever this occurs, these alveoli are no longer ventilated and shunting of blood occurs (Fig. 84.17A). With increasing age and with lung diseases which lead to airway obstruction or loss of elastic support of the lungs, airway closure occurs earlier in expiration than it

does in young healthy people. Thus, with increasing age and chronic obstructive airways disease, there is a progressive increase in closing volume and increased intrapulmonary shunting. The normal partial pressure of oxygen in the arterial blood of a patient breathing room air varies between 70 to 100 mmHg and is related to age; teenagers having a Pa_{O_2} of 100 mmHg, whilst 70 year olds have a Pa_{O_2} of 70 mmHg. This fall with age is due to increased intrapulmonary shunting secondary to the gradual increase in closing volume.

Secondly, if the functional residual capacity (FRC) — that is the amount of air left in the lungs at the end of a normal expiration — falls, there is decreased overall lung volume with collapse of basal alveoli and intrapulmonary shunting (Fig. 84.17B). The commonest cause of a low FRC is any factor causing the diaphragm to move upwards into the chest. These include the supine posture commonly adopted in the post anesthetic period, obesity with the weight of the abdominal contents pushing the diaphragm upwards, painful upper abdominal incisions,[35] abdominal distension, diaphragmatic irritation and residual effects of muscle relaxants.

Thirdly, with intrapulmonary pathology, the alveoli may collapse or become filled with fluid or cells (Fig. 84.17C). Examples include atelectasis from secretions, pulmonary edema, pneumonia and ARDS.[1]

Anemia

Patients are frequently anemic postoperatively due to unreplaced operative blood loss. Modest degrees of anemia are well tolerated provided the patient is fit and has no other interference with the oxygen transport chain. However, if a patient has respiratory complications or cardiac disease with a diminished cardiac output, the presence of

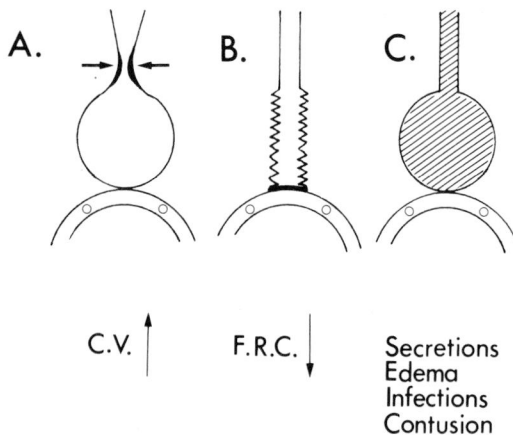

Fig. 84.17 Intrapulmonary shunting is due to three mechanisms:
A. Increased closing volume (CV) with premature airway closure occurring during expiration at the lung bases.
B. Decreased functional residual capacity (FRC) leading to atelectasis of alveoli especially at the lung bases.
C. Lung pathology where the alveoli become filled with fluid or cells thus interfering with gas exchange.

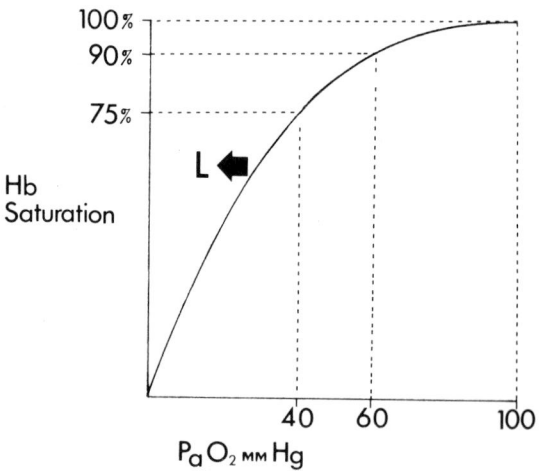

Fig. 84.18 Oxygen hemoglobin dissociation curve. When the P_aO_2 falls below 60 mmHg the amount of oxygen carried by the Hb rapidly diminishes. Certain conditions such as alkalosis, hypothermia and a low 2–3 DPG level cause the curve to shift to the left (see arrow). The Hb then binds the O_2 more tightly and less is released to the tissues.

anemia can lead to significant hypoxia. In these circumstances, it is wise to maintain a hemoglobin of approximately 12 gm or a hematocrit of 36%.

In certain circumstances, there is a shift of the oxygen hemoglobin dissociation curve to the left; consequently the hemoglobin does not readily dissociate and deliver its oxygen to the tissues. Common causes of this left shift of the curve are hypothermia, alkalosis and a low red cell 2,3-diphosphoglyceric acid (2,3DPG) level following blood transfusion (Fig. 84.18).

Shock

This is discussed previously in the section on shock (p. 1357).

Histotoxic

This type of hypoxia occurs when oxygen is delivered to the tissues but the cytochrome chain is damaged and the tissues are unable to utilize it. It occurs with cyanide poisoning and in some types of septic shock.

Management of respiratory failure

The management of postoperative respiratory insufficiency revolves around eight principles; oxygen administration, posture, physiotherapy, analgesia, intubation, respiratory support, fluid therapy and drugs.

Oxygen therapy

In the postoperative period, hypoxemia is virtually universal; the main mechanism being VQ inequality secondary to increased closing volume and/or diminished FRC in the recumbent postanesthetic patient. Postoperative hypoxemia persists for varying periods of time: following minor extremity operations it may only last minutes; however, following major upper abdominal procedures it may last several days.

Once the Pa_{O_2} falls below 60 mmHg, because of the shape of the oxyhemoglobin dissociation curve, the amount of oxygen carried in the red cells starts to drop markedly and supplemental oxygen therapy is urgently required (Fig. 84.18).

All postoperative patients should have routine oxygen therapy. Common methods of oxygen administration include nasal cannulae and oxygen therapy masks, such as the MC and Hudson masks. The main factor which determines the inspired oxygen concentration is the oxygen flow rate. With these methods, 4 liters of oxygen gives an inspired oxygen concentration of 35%, 8 liters 50%, and 14 liters 65%. These figures represent average values and there may be major differences between individual patients, depending on mask fit and breathing patterns. Low concentration oxygen masks, such as the 24% and the 28% Ventimask, should not be used for routine postoperative therapy. These masks are designed exclusively for the rare patient with chronic obstructive airways disease who has CO_2 retention and depends upon hypoxia to stimulate her respiratory center. If this patient is given high concentration oxygen, the 'hypoxic drive' is removed leading to hypoventilation with further CO_2 retention and, ultimately, CO_2 narcosis.

Posture

Sitting the patient upright in bed facilitates breathing. Gravity prevents the diaphragm being pushed up, increases the functional residual capacity and decreases intrapulmonary shunting. The main impediment to maintaining this posture is the poor design of hospital beds. It is advisable to have special postoperative beds with an adjustable footboard so that the patient can be sat upright and brace her legs against the footboard to prevent slipping down. A further advantage is that continual exercise of the muscle pump of the legs helps prevent postoperative venous thrombosis.

Physiotherapy

The main role of physiotherapy in the postoperative period is to assist the patient to cough up secretions. The principles are simple and are basically the same as those used for extracting the remnants of sauce from a near empty bottle. Firstly, the patient is positioned so that the secretions are uppermost, thus utilizing gravity. The secretions are then expelled by a combination of coughing, percussion and vibration. Other useful roles of physiotherapy are to encourage the patient to take deep breaths and expand the lung bases, thereby increasing functional residual capacity and decreasing intrapulmonary shunting. Devices such as incentive spirometers which encourage deep breaths, and CPAP masks which increase FRC[4] may be of value.

Analgesia

With operations involving the upper part of the abdomen, pain often limits respiratory excursions and prevents coughing, leading to retention of secretions with atelectasis and superimposed infection. Pain relief is necessary to allow the patient to breathe and cough normally.

Intubation

There are four main indications for tracheal intubation: (1) to relieve upper airway obstruction from the tongue falling back, and from secretions and swellings including laryngeal edema; (2) to protect the airway in states of unconsciousness where the patient has lost her gag or cough reflex, and aspiration of pharyngeal or gastric contents is possible; (3) to facilitate respiratory support whenever the patient requires mechanical ventilation or high concentrations of oxygen; and (4) to allow tracheal toilet in circumstances where the patient has profuse bronchial secretions and is unable to cough.

Nowadays, non-irritating polyvinylchloride endotracheal tubes with large volume low pressure cuffs can be inserted by the oral or nasal route and left in situ for some days. The indications for tracheostomy are decreasing, and it is usually reserved for a patient who requires an artificial airway for a period exceeding one week.

Mechanical respiratory support

In certain circumstances, the patient's respiratory function is so poor that mechanical respiratory support with a ventilator is required. The two main indications are hypoventilation, and severe intrapulmonary shunting with gross hypoxia due to such conditions as severe pulmonary edema, marked atelectasis and overwhelming pneumonia. The details of respiratory support with the use of mechanical ventilators and newer modes of respiratory therapy, such as positive end expiratory pressure (PEEP) and intermittent mandatory ventilation, are outside the scope of this discussion.

Fluid therapy

The prime essentials of early postoperative fluid replacement are to maintain plasma volume to prevent shock, and to maintain the hemoglobin level so that oxygen carriage is adequate. The inappropriate use of large volumes of crystalloids in an attempt to maintain plasma volume is inefficient and leads to interstitial pulmonary edema with intrapulmonary shunting and hypoxia.

Drugs

A number of drugs are of value in treating respiratory complications:

Antibiotics. The common organisms causing postoperative respiratory infection in patients with chronic bronchitis are pneumococcus and *Hemophilus influenzae*. Both of these pathogens respond to either augmentin 500 mg 6-hourly, or a combination of trimethoprim 160 mg and sulphamethoxazole 800 mg 12-hourly. Other pathogens which are encountered less frequently are *Staphylococcus aureus* and Gram-negative organisms, such as Klebsiella and Pseudomonas. In these circumstances, sensitivities should be determined from sputum culture and the appropriate antibiotic administered.

Bronchodilators. In patients with asthma or chronic bronchitis who have reversible airways obstruction, a bronchodilator such as salbutamol administered by inha-

lation is of great benefit. The usual dose is 1 ml administered every 4 hours by nebulizer, or 2 puffs every 4 hours from a pressurized aerosol.

Heparin. Low dose heparin is useful in the prevention of deep venous thrombosis and pulmonary embolism. The usual dose is 5000 units every 8 to 12 hours by the subcutaneous route.

POSTOPERATIVE OLIGURIA

The patient who passes little or no urine is a common postoperative problem.[9,42,43,79] The three most important steps are to exclude retention by catheterizing the patient, to exclude a blocked catheter by irrigating it under sterile conditions and ensuring that the injected volume of fluid is returned and to be certain there is no obstruction to the ureters as a result of surgery. If, having excluded retention and a blocked catheter, the patient is passing less than 0.5 ml of urine per kg body weight per hour (30 ml in a normal adult), she is said to be oliguric.

Oliguria may be an early sign of impending renal failure. It should be remembered, however, that renal failure can occur in the presence of normal urine output (non-oliguric renal failure).

Oliguria can be conveniently subdivided into three types; prerenal, renal and postrenal.

Prerenal oliguria

The urinary output is an excellent guide to renal perfusion. If renal perfusion is impaired as a consequence of shock, either hypovolemic or cardiogenic, oliguria will occur. Shock must be vigorously treated otherwise renal damage called acute tubular necrosis may occur.[6] Raised intraabdominal pressure (IAP) should be excluded. It causes oliguria and, eventually, acute renal failure by compressing renal veins and parenchyma. IAP may be measured by instilling 100 ml of saline into the bladder and connecting a CVP line to the catheter (Fig. 84.19). Pressures above 25 cm H_2O necessitate urgent abdominal decompression.[10,37]

It is useful to distinguish between prerenal oliguria and established acute tubular necrosis. This can be done by examination of the urine; with prerenal oliguria, the urinary specific gravity and osmolality are raised and the urinary sodium is very low as renal mechanisms are operating to conserve volume. Once acute tubular necrosis has occurred, the urine specific gravity and the ability to concentrate the urine is lost; osmolality becomes the same as the serum, and the ability to retain sodium is lost so that the urinary sodium concentration rises.

When confronted with prerenal oliguria, the first step is to detect hypovolemia and correct this with a plasma expander. If there is no immediate response to this fluid load, dopamine is commenced in low dose (2 to 3 mg/kg per

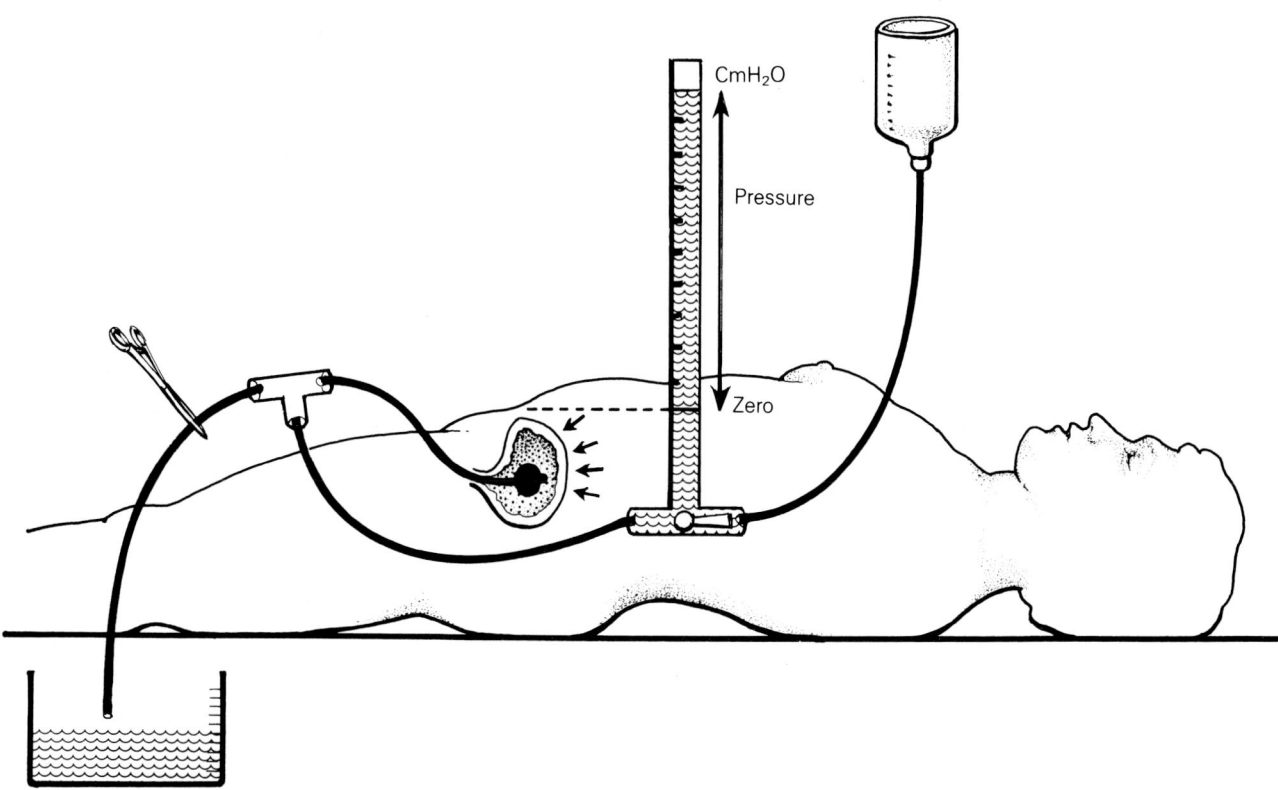

Fig. 84.19 Measurement of intra-abdominal pressure. 100 ml of normal saline is instilled into the bladder via a CVP catheter giving set. The stopcock on the CVP set is then turned so that the manometer column is in continuity with the bladder. The height of the fluid in the manometer column above the symphysis pubis after equilibration is then equal to the intra-abdominal pressure.

minute) to selectively dilate renal arterioles, and it is useful to give a dose of 100 ml of 20% mannitol, an osmotic agent which has a number of beneficial effects. It expands plasma volume and decreases viscosity, it may decrease the intra-renal vascular spasm which precedes the onset of acute tubular necrosis, it reduces ischemic swelling of renal tubular cells and, by inducing a diuresis, it may prevent blockage of the tubules with casts.

If mannitol is ineffective, then 40 mg of frusemide is given slowly intravenously in an attempt to generate a urinary output. If this dose is ineffective, then larger doses can be given. The use of mannitol with or without frusemide is thought to be beneficial in that it may prevent the development of acute tubular necrosis or it may convert low urinary output acute tubular necrosis into a high output renal failure. The latter state is more easily managed as there are less problems with hyperkalemia and fluid overload.

Renal oliguria

There are many renal causes of oliguria, including all the common renal diseases such as glomerulonephritis, pyelonephritis, nephrosclerosis and vascular occlusion of the kidney.

In the immediate postoperative period, the main renal cause is acute tubular necrosis. This is due to spasm or maldistribution of the cortical blood supply of the kidney, giving rise to a lack of glomerular filtration and tubular damage. The major causes of acute tubular necrosis are: renal ischemia and hypoxia, septicemia, pigments such as bilirubin, hemoglobin and myoglobin, and drugs such as the nephrotoxic antibiotics, aminoglycosides in particular.

As mentioned above there are two clinical types of acute tubular necrosis. The commonest is the 'oliguric', in which the patient passes very small quantities of urine with a high sodium content and a specific gravity and osmolality the same as that of serum. Oliguria usually persists for days to weeks, the average period being approximately 2 weeks. If the patient survives, this phase is followed by gradual restoration of urinary volume; only rarely is the so called 'classic' polyuric phase seen. The second type of acute tubular necrosis is the 'non-oliguric' type, in which the urinary output is well maintained or may even be greater than normal. However, the urine is dilute and of poor quality, and there is a progressive rise in the blood urea and creatinine. This type of acute tubular necrosis is thought to result from a milder insult to the kidney than occurs in the oliguric type.

Management of oliguric acute tubular necrosis (established renal failure)

The principles of management are:

1. Once blood volume is adequately restored, salt and water must be restricted. Ill advised attempts to induce a diuresis by the administration of large volumes of fluids cause acute pulmonary edema. The temptation to drown the patient with fluid must be resisted.

2. Control the serum potassium. With oliguria, potassium excretion diminishes and breakdown of cells and acidosis leads to release of intracellular potassium. As a consequence, the serum potassium gradually rises. Regular serum potassium estimations must be performed, and the patient should have continuous EKG monitoring looking for premonitory signs of hyperkalemia. The treatment of hyperkalemia is discussed on page 1371.

3. Infection must be prevented and treated vigorously when detected.

4. Calories and essential amino acids must be provided. Recent studies have shown that attention to nutrition and, especially, the judicious use of essential amino acids results in a decreased mortality and a shorter period of oliguria. If oral intake is impossible, parenteral feeding is required (see p. 1349).

5. Beware of certain drugs. The dose of drugs which are directly nephrotoxic, such as aminoglycosides, or excreted by the kidney, such as digoxin, must be adjusted.

Dialysis

The indications for dialysis are:

1. Clinical (i.e. uremic symptoms with disordered level of consciousness, hemorrhage, nausea, vomiting, etc.)
2. Elevated blood urea, usually greater than 30 mmol/l
3. Hyperkalemia with levels greater than 7 mmol/l
4. Metabolic acidosis
5. Fluid overload.

The modern trend with acute renal failure is towards early dialysis.[38] As a consequence, patients are maintained in better clinical status and the overall results are better. The two common forms of dialysis are peritoneal and hemodialysis. In the former method, a plastic catheter is placed in the peritoneal cavity and fluid is instilled. This fluid has a composition similar to that of normal extracellular fluid with osmotic particles such as glucose or mannitol added. The fluid is allowed to equilibrate, and as a consequence the serum electrolytes are normalized and urea and other retained toxins pass into the peritoneal fluid which is allowed to run out prior to the next cycle. As a general rule, 2 liters of fluid are instilled every hour and this sequence is maintained for periods of 48 to 72 hours. Hemodialysis requires the formation of an arteriovenous shunt. Arterial blood is pumped through an external system where the blood is dialyzed against a solution of composition similar to that of extracellular fluid, and urea, toxic substances and potassium are removed. The blood is then returned to the patient's venous system.

Postrenal oliguria

Provided retention has been excluded by insertion of a catheter, postrenal anuria is due to ureteric obstruction by such conditions as stones, necrotic papillae and tumors, or by inadvertent ligation or hyperangulation at operation. The main clue to postrenal oliguria is the presence of complete anuria. If this is suspected, the diagnosis must be confirmed by the passage of retrograde ureteric catheters.

ABNORMALITIES OF EXTRACELLULAR FLUID AND ELECTROLYTES

The common abnormalities can be summarized into four groups: changes in extracellular fluid volume, changes in serum sodium, changes in serum potassium and acid base abnormalities.[36]

Changes in extracellular fluid volume

The extracellular fluid consists of interstitial fluid and plasma.

Interstitial fluid excess. This is characterized by edema of all tissues. It is most easily recognized in the skin and also in the lungs, where it causes interstitial pulmonary edema and interferes with oxygenation.

Interstitial fluid deficit. Characterized by poor tissue turgor.

Plasma volume excess. Characterized by raised blood pressure, elevated venous pressure, basal crepitations and a chest X-ray showing pulmonary vascular congestion which precedes pulmonary edema.

Plasma volume deficit. Characterized by signs of shock with poor skin perfusion, tachycardia, hypotension, low central venous pressure, low pulmonary capillary wedge pressure and a chest X-ray showing oligemic lung fields.

Table 84.19 Extracellular fluid volume deficit

Cause	An isotonic loss of $Na^+ + H_2O$
	1. External loss
	    gastrointestinal
	    renal
	2. Internal loss
	    ascites
	    3rd space

Signs	1. Low plasma volume 2. Low interstitial volume
Treatment	Expand plasma volume and administer an isotonic Na^+ solution

Table 84.20 Extracellular fluid volume excess

Cause	An isotonic gain of Na^+ + H_2O
	1. Excessive intake of Na^+ + H_2O either oral or intravenous
	2. Decreased loss of Na^+ + H_2O
	  a. renal disease
	  b. congestive cardiac failure
	  c. low albumin states

Signs	1. High plasma volume 2. High interstitial volume

Treatment	1. Treat the cause
	2. Decrease intake of Na^+ + H_2O
	3. Increase loss of Na^+ + H_2O
	  a. diuretics
	  b. dialysis
	  c. venesection

Table 84.21 Decrease in ECF H_2O (dehydration)

Causes	1. Decreased water intake
	  a. poor oral intake with anorexia, stomatitis
	  b. inadequate parenteral fluid administration
	2. Increased water losses
	  a. skin
	  b. lungs
	  c. gastrointestinal
	  d. renal

Signs	1. Low ECF volume 2. Low ICF volume
Treatment	1. Oral H_2O 2. Intravenous water as 5% dextrose (avoiding osmotic diuresis)

Table 84.22 Gain in ECF sodium

Causes	Administration of hypertonic Na^+ either orally or intravenously e.g. excessive $NaHCO_3$ administration
Signs	1. High ECF volume 2. Low ICF volume
Treatment	1. Administer H_2O to lower the osmolality and diuretics such as frusemide to increase Na^+ excretion 2. Dialysis

Table 84.23 Depletional hyponatremia

Cause	The replacement of high Na^+ losses (e.g. vomiting, diuresis etc.), with water.
Signs	1. Low ECF volume 2. High ICF volume
Treatment	Sodium replacement either orally or intravenously. May need hypertonic saline.

The causes, clinical signs and treatment of extracellular fluid volume deficit and extracellular fluid volume excess are set out in Tables 84.19 and 84.20 respectively.

Changes in serum sodium concentration

Serum sodium concentration is the ratio of extracellular sodium to extracellular water. Hence, it can be altered by quantitative changes in either the extracellular sodium or the extracellular water. The normal serum sodium concentration is 140 mmol/l.

Sodium is the main contributor to extracellular fluid osmolality; hence, any change in serum sodium concentration is accompanied by changes in osmolality of the extracellular fluid, with resultant shifts of water between the intracellular and the extracellular spaces. For example, when the serum sodium concentration is elevated, this causes a shift of water out of cells in an attempt to maintain osmotic equilibrium. As a result, extracellular fluid volume is increased and intracellular fluid volume falls. Conversely, if the serum sodium concentration is low, the drop in extracellular fluid osmolality causes a shift of water into the cells. Thus, low sodium states are accompanied by cellular swelling leading to dysfunction of many organs, particularly the brain.

High serum sodium concentration (hypernatremia). This is due to either a decrease in extracellular water, i.e. dehydration, or a gain in extracellular sodium, i.e. hypertonic sodium gain. The causes, clinical signs and treatment of each condition are summarized in Tables 84.21 and 84.22.[21,22]

Low serum sodium concentration (hyponatremia). This is a common clinical problem. There are basically three types:

1. ***Artifactual hyponatremia***. The commonest cause is an elevated blood sugar which causes water to be drawn out of the cells diluting the sodium in the extracellular fluid space and giving rise to 'pseudohyponatremia'. A similar problem occurs in situations where the serum lipids or serum proteins are greatly raised, because in laboratory practice the serum sodium concentration is determined by a formula in which the sodium content of the sample is divided by the plasma water plus the volume of the lipids and protein. Thus, if lipid or protein concentration is raised the apparent sodium concentration will fall, displaced by the lipid etc. Hyperlipidemia therefore produces an apparent, not real, hyponatremia.

2. ***Depletional hyponatremia*** i.e. a decrease in the extracellular sodium (Table 84.23).

Table 84.24 Dilutional hyponatremia

Cause	$Na^+ + H_2O$ overload with H_2O excess predominating
	1. Excessive intake of H_2O either oral or intravenous
	2. Decreased loss of H_2O
	a. renal disease
	b. antidiuretic hormone excess
	(i) appropriate
	hypovolemia
	heart failure
	low albumin states
	(ii) inappropriate (SIADH)
	(iii) exogenous
	c. adrenal insufficiency.
Signs	1. High ECF volume
	2. High ICF volume
Treatment	1. Restrict H_2O intake
	2. Increase H_2O losses with diuretics or dialysis.

3. **Dilutional hyponatremia** i.e. an increase in the extracellular water (Table 84.24).

In artifactual hypernatremia, the serum osmolality will be normal or high, while the osmolality will be low in dilutional or depletional hyponatremia. The differentiation between depletional and dilutional hyponatremia is possible on simple clinical grounds. With depletional hyponatremia, patients show evidence of sodium depletion with a decreased extracellular fluid volume, that is, a low plasma volume with signs of shock, and a low interstitial volume with poor tissue turgor. With dilutional hyponatremia, there is an excess of extracellular salt and water, with the water excess predominating. Hence, there is increased interstitial volume and these patients are always edematous, sometimes grossly so. The only exception to this rule is the patient with the syndrome of inappropriate antidiuretic hormone (SIADH), in whom the salt and water overload is less marked and the edema less obvious.

The syndrome of inappropriate antidiuretic hormone (SIADH). This is seen in the following states; intracranial lesions, pulmonary disease, malignant disease, certain drugs, such as diuretics, and also in myxedema. The patient presents with a low serum sodium concentration, and some degree of fluid retention which falls short of frank tissue edema. Normally in situations like this where the serum osmolality is low, one would expect the body to compensate by turning off antidiuretic hormone (ADH) secretion and generating dilute urine with a low osmolality. However, with inappropriate ADH secretion the urine is less than maximally dilute.

The hallmarks for the diagnosis of inappropriate ADH are: (1) the serum sodium and osmolality are low; (2) the osmolality of the urine is usually higher than that of the serum, that is, it is inappropriately high. To make the diagnosis, there must be normal renal and adrenal function and no evidence of volume depletion. Treatment is to restrict the oral intake to less than 1 liter/day and allow continuing obligatory losses of water to raise the serum sodium gradually towards normal. If the serum sodium is very low and the patient has cerebral edema with coma and fitting, hypertonic saline should be administered. This raises the osmolality of the extracellular fluid and sucks water out of the neurons allowing them to regain normal function. If given together with frusemide, which induces a diuresis of H_2O in excess of Na^+, the problems of fluid overload are minimized.

Changes in serum potassium concentration

Potassium is the main intracellular electrolyte, and 98% of the body potassium is contained inside cells. The normal serum potassium concentration is approximately 4 mmol/l, and since the plasma volume is 3 liters, the amount of potassium circulating in the plasma is only 12 mmol. Great care must therefore be taken when administering potassium intravenously. If a 12 mmol bolus of potassium were to be instantaneously injected into the blood stream, the serum potassium would double from 4 to 8 mmol/l with consequent risk of cardiac arrhythmias and sudden death. Hence, intravenous potassium must be given slowly, with frequent monitoring of serum levels.

Potassium derangements are more complex than those of sodium because potassium has both an external balance, with potassium gain and loss from the body as a whole, and an internal balance, where the potassium moves in and out of a large intracellular reservoir. The factors which control intracellular potassium concentration are:

1. *pH.* With acidosis, there is an excess of hydrogen ions outside the cell, hydrogen ions then enter the cell and potassium moves out causing hyperkalemia. Conversely, with alkalosis, hydrogen ions move out of the cell allowing potassium to move in. This is the mechanism underlying the use of sodium bicarbonate to lower serum potassium.

2. *Aldosterone.* This is essential for the sodium pump that expels sodium from, and maintains potassium within the cell.

3. *Cellular hypoxia and cellular destruction.* In these situations, the permeability of the cell membrane is impaired and potassium leaks out.

4. *Insulin.* Insulin causes glucose and potassium to enter cells.

5. *Autonomic nervous system.* Sympathetic overactivity via its B_2 effect causes potassium to enter cells.

The symptoms and signs of hyper- and hypokalemia are summarized in Table 84.25.

Hyperkalemia can be a medical emergency. When the serum potassium exceeds 7 mmol/l, fatal arrhythmias can occur. With hyperkalemia, there are progressive EKG

Table 84.25 Signs of hyper- and hypokalemia

	K$^+\uparrow$	K$^+\downarrow$
Neuromuscular	Weakness Paralysis	Weakness Paresthesiae
Gastrointestinal tract	Anorexia Nausea, Vomiting, Diarrhea, Colic	Ileus
Cardiovascular system	Peaked T waves QRS widening Ventricular arrhythmias	U waves ST-T changes Digoxin sensitivity Ventricular arrhythmias

Table 84.26 Causes of hyperkalemia

External balance
1. Excessive gain of K$^+$
   a. oral administration
   b. intravenous supplementation

2. Decreased urinary loss of K$^+$
   a. renal failure
   b. adrenal failure
   c. spironolactone

Internal balance
   Movement of K$^+$ out of cells
   a. acidosis
   b. adrenal insufficiency
   c. cellular hypoxia and breakdown

changes. Initially, there is peaking of the T wave followed by prolongation of the PR interval and widening of the QRS complex. Finally, a sine wave pattern occurs, culminating in ventricular fibrillation or asystole.

The causes of hyperkalemia are shown in Table 84.26. Care should be taken that laboratory samples are not hemolysed, as this causes artifactual hyperkalemia.
The treatment of hyperkalemia is as follows:

1. Treat the cause and stop any potassium administration.

2. If the situation is urgent, with EKG changes reflecting an impending fatal arrhythmia, rapid measures must be utilized. 100 ml of 8.4% sodium bicarbonate (NaHCO$_3$) is administered to drive the potassium temporarily into the cell, together with 10 ml of 10% calcium chloride which is a specific antagonist to the cardiac effects of potassium.

3. In less urgent circumstances, the serum potassium can be lowered by the infusion of glucose and insulin in a ratio of 5 g of glucose to one unit of actrapid insulin to drive potassium into cells, by the administration of ion exchange resins to bind potassium in the gut, and by the use of dialysis, either peritoneal or hemodialysis.

Hypokalemia is a common electrolyte abnormality in postoperative patients. Unlike the case of sodium, in situations of potassium restriction there is a sizable obligatory daily loss in the urine. Consequently, all postoperative patients with a normal urinary output require potassium supplementation of at least 1 mmol/kg per day. Failure to do so results in the patient developing muscle weakness, paralytic ileus and cardiac arrhythmias, especially if digitalis is being administered.

The causes of hypokalemia are shown in Table 84.27.

Table 84.27 Causes of hypokalemia

External balance
1. Insufficient intake of K$^+$
2. Excessive losses of K$^+$
   a. gastrointestinal with vomiting, suction and diarrhea
   b. renal with renal disease, diuretics, osmotic diuresis, steroids and alkalosis.

Internal balance
   Movement of K$^+$ into cells
   a. NaHCO$_3$ administration
   b. glucose and insulin therapy
   c. sympathetic overactivity

The treatment of hypokalemia includes:

1. Treatment of the cause, for example, excessive diuresis, gastrointestinal losses, etc.

2. Potassium replacement using the chloride salt, because metabolic alkalosis frequently coexists and requires the chloride ion for correction. In non-urgent circumstances, oral potassium chloride supplements as either tablets or liquid can be used. Some oral potassium supplements contain little or no chloride ion and are unsuitable. If oral replacement is not possible, then potassium chloride should be added to the intravenous fluid and infused slowly. In a normal postoperative patient, 20 to 30 mmol KCl are added to each liter of 4% dextrose and fifth normal saline and administered over 8 hours. If the patient has a serum potassium below 3 mmol/l, larger amounts are required. The safest way to do this is to use a constant infusion pump. 5 mmol KCl are added to 40 ml of 5% dextrose in the burette and infused slowly hourly. In severe cases, the hourly increment of KCl may have to be increased to 10 mmol. This should be done with continuous EKG monitoring and frequent measurements of serum potassium.

3. Renal potassium loss can sometimes be minimized by using aldosterone antagonists, such as spironolactone, or potassium sparing diuretics, such as amiloride and triamterene.

4. Whenever hypokalemia occurs, there is usually coexistent magnesium deficiency which needs correction with 50% magnesium sulphate in a dose of 10 to 20 ml infused slowly every 24 hours.

Acid-base abnormalities

The blood gas and acid base status of the patient is determined by the measurement of P_{O_2}, P_{CO_2}, pH, standard bicarbonate (HCO_3) and base excess in arterial blood. Normal figures are:

1. P_{O_2} between 70 and 100 mmHg depending on the age of the patient and provided that 21% oxygen is being breathed
2. P_{CO_2} 40 mmHg
3. pH 7.4 pH expresses the acidity or hydrogen ion concentration of the body. With acidosis the pH falls, and with alkalosis it rises.
4. standard bicarbonate 24.
5. base excess, +2 to −2. Base excess is a complex method of expressing the metabolic and base status, but the more negative the base excess the less bicarbonate there is in the blood stream, and vice versa.

The abnormalities of acid-base balance can be termed either respiratory or metabolic. Respiratory refers to changes in carbon dioxide level, whereas metabolic is used to indicate changes in the non-respiratory component, particularly the hydrogen ion and bicarbonate concentration. There are four major abnormalities; (1) respiratory acidosis characterized by a low pH and a high P_{CO_2}, (2) respiratory alkalosis characterized by a high pH and a low P_{CO_2}, (3) metabolic acidosis characterized by a low pH, low bicarbonate and a negative base excess, (4) metabolic alkalosis characterized by a high pH, high bicarbonate and a positive base excess. Whenever there is a primary acid base disturbance, compensation occurs to return these parameters towards normal. The first is respiratory compensation. With metabolic disorders, such as metabolic acidosis or alkalosis, the respiratory center acts to either excrete or retain carbon dioxide and thus return the pH towards normal. For example, with metabolic acidosis, the respiratory center is stimulated and the P_{CO_2} drops. This explains the classic Kussmaul's breathing with diabetic ketoacidosis. Conversely, with metabolic alkalosis, the respiratory center is depressed and the consequent CO_2 retention helps restore normal pH. Respiratory compensation is rapid and occurs within minutes. The second compensation is renal. With acidosis, renal compensation causes excretion of an acid urine and returns the pH towards normal. Conversely, with alkalosis, the kidney retains acid and secretes an alkaline urine. Renal compensation takes several days to reach its maximum.

In interpreting acid-base status, three questions should be asked:

1. What is the primary acid base abnormality? This is determined by looking at the pH. If it is below 7.4 the primary abnormality is acidosis; if above 7.4 it is alkalosis.
2. Is the primary abnormality respiratory or metabolic?

The P_{CO_2} and standard HCO_3 are examined with regard to pH. For example, if the pH indicates primary acidosis and the P_{CO_2} is raised, this is a respiratory acidosis; on the other hand if the HCO_3 is low, it is a metabolic acidosis.

3. Is there any respiratory or renal compensation? The P_{CO_2} and HCO_3 are examined to determine if they have moved to return the primary pH abnormality towards normal. For example, consider the following figures: pH 7.25, HCO_3 12, Pa_{CO_2} 20. As the pH and HCO_3 are low, this represents a primary metabolic acidosis; the low P_{CO_2} indicates respiratory compensation to raise the pH towards normal. Thus, the final diagnosis is primary metabolic acidosis with respiratory compensation.

Respiratory acidosis. Whenever the level of carbon dioxide in the blood rises, it combines with water to form carbonic acid which dissociates to give hydrogen ions and, hence, an acidosis. Thus an excess of carbon dioxide causes the equation,

$$CO_2 + H_2O \rightarrow H_2CO_3 \rightarrow H^+ + HCO_3$$

to move to the right. As CO_2 is excreted by the lungs, the commonest cause of respiratory acidosis is hypoventilation (see Table 84.28). The management of respiratory acidosis is to treat the cause and consider ventilation.

Table 84.28 Respiratory acidosis

1. Increased production of CO_2
   a. pyrexia, shivering and convulsions
   b. thyrotoxicosis

2. Decreased excretion of CO_2
   i.e. alveolar hypoventilation
   a. low respiratory rate
   b. small tidal volume
   c. large dead space either apparatus or alveolar

Respiratory alkalosis. When the carbon dioxide level in the blood falls, the equation

$$CO_2 + H_2O \leftarrow H_2CO_3 \leftarrow H^+ + HCO_3$$

moves to the left and the hydrogen ion level falls. A low carbon dioxide level is due to increased excretion from the body via the lungs. Common causes of hyperventilation are hypoxia, compensation for metabolic acidosis, excessive mechanical ventilation, shock, central nervous system disease, psychogenic, septicemia and salicylates. Respiratory alkalosis can give rise to paresthesia and tetany resembling hypocalcemia. The treatment is that of the cause. With psychogenic hyperventilation, the patient is allowed to rebreathe carbon dioxide from a paper bag.

Metabolic acidosis. Metabolic acidosis is a non-respiratory acidosis due to the gain of acid (other than H_2CO_3) or the loss of alkali. The common causes of this are summarized in Table 84.29.

The treatment of metabolic acidosis is:

Table 84.29 Metabolic acidosis

Gain of Acid
1. lactic acid, e.g. hypoxia
2. ketoacids, e.g. diabetes
3. renal acids, e.g. uremia
4. exogenous acids, e.g. ammonium chloride, salicylates

Loss of Alkali
1. gastrointestinal loss
   small bowel or colonic losses
   ureterocolic anastomosis
2. renal loss
   renal tubular acidosis
   acetazolamide

1. Treat the cause; for example, diabetic hyperglycemia, shock, etc.

2. If the pH is below 7.25, and particularly if the acidosis has developed acutely and is depressing cardiac function, rapid correction of acidosis by the administration of sodium bicarbonate may be indicated. The active part of sodium bicarbonate is the bicarbonate ion, which combines with hydrogen ion to form carbonic acid which then dissociates to form CO_2 to be excreted by the lungs. This results in a net loss of hydrogen ions. There are many formulae for the administration of sodium bicarbonate, but the best practice is to give intravenous increments of 50 to 100 mmol of sodium bicarbonate (usually in the form of 8.4% sodium bicarbonate which contains 1 mmol per ml) and then remeasure the acid-base status. These increments are given until the pH is restored towards normal.

3. Monitor P_{CO_2}, potassium and calcium. If the patient is on a ventilator, the P_{CO_2} must be adjusted by the clinician to compensate for metabolic derangements; for example, with metabolic acidosis the ventilator should be set to hyperventilate the patient and lower the P_{CO_2}. With metabolic acidosis, there is a loss of potassium from the cells and the serum level rises. With the administration of sodium bicarbonate, potassium re-enters the cell and may produce symptomatic hypokalemia. In addition, the ionized calcium increases with acidosis, and as sodium bicarbonate is given, the ionized calcium falls. This may have a deleterious effect upon cardiac function, and calcium replacement should be given empirically whenever large amounts of sodium bicarbonate are being infused.

Metabolic alkalosis. The causes of metabolic alkalosis are (1) gain of alkali, (2) loss of acid and (3) correction of a chronically raised P_{CO_2}.

1. *Gain of alkali* may result from excessive sodium bicarbonate administration, absorbable antacids and citrated blood in which the citrate anticoagulant is metabolized to bicarbonate.

2. *Loss of acid* may result from loss of gastric juice and from renal losses of hydrogen ion due to potassium and chloride depletion. It is imperative to understand the complex interrelation between hydrogen, potassium and chloride ions, as with metabolic alkalosis there is usually coexistent hypokalemia and hypochloremia. Potassium depletion causes alkalosis by two mechanisms. In the renal mechanism, sodium is reabsorbed in the distal tubule in exchange for hydrogen ion and potassium which are excreted. If there is a body deficit of potassium, hydrogen ion is therefore preferentially excreted in exchange for sodium, giving rise to alkalosis. The other mechanism involves all cells of the body. In states of potassium depletion, hydrogen ion enters the cells to preserve ionic equilibrium. As a consequence, a paradoxical situation results with an extracellular alkalosis and an intracellular acidosis. Chloride depletion is closely related to potassium and hydrogen ion depletion. It is most simply understood through the renal reabsorption of sodium. 90% or more of the filtered sodium is reabsorbed from the proximal tubule accompanied by chloride ion. In situations where there is a deficit of chloride, the amount of proximal reabsorption of sodium is decreased leaving more sodium to be reabsorbed in the distal tubule. This occurs at the cost of increased potassium and hydrogen loss. Hence, to repair a metabolic alkalosis, adequate amounts of chloride ion, either as potassium chloride or sodium chloride, are essential.

The causes of potassium and chloride depletion are shown in Table 84.30.

Table 84.30 Causes of low serum potassium and chloride

1. *Loss* of K^+ and Cl^- from the body
   a. gastrointestinal
      vomiting
      suction drainage
      diarrhea
   b. renal
      renal disease
      diuretics
      steroids
      Na depletion

2. *Movement* into cells (applies to K^+ only)
   a. $NaHCO_3$ administration
   b. sympathetic overactivity
   c. glucose and insulin therapy

3. *Compensated respiratory acidosis.* Patients with chronic obstructive airways disease and CO_2 retention have chronic renal compensation with retention of bicarbonate. If the patient's respiratory status improves or she is mechanically ventilated, the P_{CO_2} is decreased while the bicarbonate level, which has been generated by renal compensation, is left elevated. Hence, the resultant acid base and blood gas profile is that of metabolic alkalosis.

The treatment of metabolic alkalosis is:

1. Treat the cause, e.g. renal potassium loss by stopping diuretics, etc.

2. Administer sodium chloride if volume depleted. This diminishes the distal tubule mechanism where sodium is reabsorbed in exchange for potassium and hydrogen ion which are excreted in the urine.

3. Give copious quantities of potassium as the chloride salt, either orally or intravenously.

4. With severe, life-threatening metabolic alkalosis, intravenous administration of dilute hydrochloric acid may be indicated. Occasionally, acetazolamide may be given to generate an alkaline urine.

POSTOPERATIVE ABDOMINAL COMPLICATIONS

In gynecological surgery, the main postoperative abdominal complications are hemorrhage, sepsis, paralytic ileus, small bowel obstruction, injury to adjacent organs and stress ulceration. Stress ulceration will be dealt with separately (see p. 1379).

The first four complications commonly coexist. The classical presentation is the patient who bleeds extraperitoneally and develops a pelvic hematoma. If the vagina has been opened, the field is contaminated, infection supervenes and the hematoma is converted into a pelvic abscess. Paralytic ileus occurs and small bowel adhesions may form and cause mechanical obstruction. Some days later, the abscess may rupture into the vagina, thus being drained, and the ileus and small bowel obstruction then usually resolve.

Hemorrhage

Postoperative gynecological hemorrhage may present in three ways: extraperitoneal hemorrhage, intraperitoneal hemorrhage and vaginal bleeding (see also p. 1249.)

Extraperitoneal hemorrhage

In the broad ligament, the vessels are encased in fibrous tissue and hemostasis may be difficult to achieve. Serious hemorrhage may occur after radical surgical procedures, due to retraction of uterine or ovarian vessels causing ligatures to slip. This type of hemorrhage may present (1) acutely with shock, or (2) subacutely with episodic hypotension and progressive anemia, both of which respond to blood transfusion. In addition, there may be distension and lower abdominal tenderness. It may be difficult to decide whether to reoperate or to treat the patient conservatively. In general terms, if there is shock or if blood loss has been sufficient to merit blood transfusion, reoperation is indicated to secure hemostasis and avoid the complications of a pelvic hematoma with secondary abscess formation and prolonged ileus.

Intraperitoneal hemorrhage

The signs are those of hypovolemic shock with abdominal distension and peritonism. This usually requires urgent operation. After appropriate suction, it may be difficult to identify the specific bleeding point. It may sometimes be necessary to ligate the anterior division of the internal iliac artery in order to control hemorrhage, although the effectiveness of this measure is limited by the extensive collateral supply from the opposite side, and from the gluteal vessels. Temporary control of the common iliac artery on both sides may be helpful, and on occasions manual compression of the aorta may allow the bleeding site to be identified. The anterior division of the internal iliac artery is approached by a peritoneal incision lateral to the common iliac artery leaving the ureter on the medial peritoneal aspect. Having identified that the ligation site is distal to the posterior division of the vessel, the artery may be tied in continuity with vascular clamps.

Vaginal bleeding

Hemorrhage may occur from the small arteries and large venous channels at the top of the resected vagina. Such hemorrhage may occur at any stage in the postoperative period, especially within 24 hours (reactionary hemorrhage) and again at about the 10th to 12th day (secondary hemorrhage). The latter is usually associated with local sepsis. There is vaginal blood loss and sometimes shock. Firm packing is immediately undertaken and at times may be successful in controlling the hemorrhage. If unsuccessful it is necessary to examine the patient under an anesthetic preparatory to ligation of the vessel concerned, if possible by the vaginal route.

Sepsis

Infection in gynecologic operations is nearly always endogenous and caused by the release of vaginal bacteria into the pelvis or wound at the time of operation. The presence of a pelvic hematoma further increases the risk of abscess formation. Septic thrombophlebitis can occur and may lead to septic pulmonary emboli or septicemia.

The vaginal flora vary with ovarian activity. In premenopausal patients, anaerobic organisms such as bacteroides and anaerobic streptococci predominate, especially in the first half of the menstrual cycle, and are the commonest cause of pelvic sepsis. In postmenopausal patients, aerobic organisms are more frequent, and pelvic sepsis is less common unless there is advanced malignant disease.

In operations such as abdominal or vaginal hysterectomy where the vagina is opened, there is a 25 to 35% risk of pelvic or wound sepsis. Several controlled studies have shown this can be reduced to between 0 and 13% by the use of prophylactic antibiotics. To be effective, the antibiotic must be administered so that an effective tissue level is present at the time of contamination. For premenopausal patients in whom anaerobic infection is common, metronidazole is given intravenously in a dose of 500 mg 8-hourly. Following the menopause, a cephalosporin such as cephalothin 1 g 6-hourly is more appropriate, as anaerobic infections are less common. There is no rationale for antibiotic administration beyond 24 hours in routine, uncomplicated surgery.

Paralytic ileus and small bowel obstruction

When the postoperative patient develops abdominal distension, vomiting and copious gastric aspirate, the differentiation between paralytic ileus and small bowel obstruction may be difficult. In many instances both conditions may coexist, particularly in the presence of pelvic abscess. In addition, paralytic ileus may not be generalized but may be segmental adjacent to an area of inflammation. The differential diagnosis relies upon three key features.

History. The presence of small bowel colic is indicative of mechanical obstruction, but this can be difficult to interpret in a postoperative patient with pain in the operative site.

Physical examination. The absence of bowel sounds suggests paralytic ileus, whilst the presence of hyperactive bowel sounds associated with colic is indicative of small bowel obstruction.

Plain X-ray of the abdomen, with both supine and erect or decubitus lateral views. With paralytic ileus, the gaseous distension affects the large as well as the small bowel, whereas with mechanical small bowel obstruction, distension is maximal in the small bowel. With ileus, the loops of distended bowel and fluid levels are smaller and more diffusely scattered than with mechanical obstruction.

Management. If mechanical small bowel obstruction is suspected, then laparotomy is indicated, and may incorporate the draining of abscesses. On the other hand, the management of paralytic ileus requires treatment of the cause, continuous nasogastric suction and intravenous fluids. Treatment of the cause may require drainage of hematomas and abscesses, the use of antibiotics and correction of hypokalemia. The aim of nasogastric suction is to keep the stomach empty of gas, secretions and saliva, to prevent further distension of the small and large, bowel. Continuous nasogastric suction with a sump tube to minimize gastric mucosal damage is more efficient than intermittent suction; however, it is wise to aspirate the tube manually every hour to detect blockage. Signs of a resolving ileus include diminishing gastric aspirate, decreasing abdominal distension and the appearance of bowel sounds, and the passage of flatus. When these occur, continuous suction should be ceased, the patient given 30 ml of water

hourly, and the tube aspirated 4-hourly. If the fluid load is tolerated the tube can then be removed.

Injury to adjacent organs

The ureter may be inadvertently divided, ligated, clamped or hyperangulated. If one ureter is affected, this may present with the signs of acute hydronephrosis and backache; however, it may be silent, without any notable clinical features. If both ureters are ligated there is complete anuria. On the other hand, if a ureter is divided, urine leaks into the peritoneal or extraperitoneal tissues giving rise to local peritonitis, and may appear through a drain or as a ureterovaginal fistula. (See Ch. 85.)

When copious quantities of yellow fluid drain from a wound it may be difficult to determine whether or not a urinary leak is present, as a yellow serous effusion may be associated with small bowel obstruction due to leakage of fluid from loops of small bowel proximal to the obstruction. The diagnosis is resolved by measuring the urea level of the fluid. Levels similar to those in plasma indicate a serous effusion, whereas levels several times higher indicate urine.

The bladder may be injured giving rise to either hematuria or a urinary fistula.

The bowel may be injured with fecal contamination of the pelvis. This may lead to pelvic, and sometimes generalized, peritonitis from mixed organisms in which anaerobes predominate. Fistulae may also result, especially when the surgery follows irradiation. (See Ch. 86.)

DEEP VENOUS THROMBOSIS AND PULMONARY EMBOLISM

Pathology of deep venous thrombosis

Clotting occurring in the veins of the lower limb and pelvis is a common complication of gynecological surgery. The causes of clotting were enumerated many years ago by Virchow in his classical triad of stasis, hypercoagulable state and endothelial damage. Stasis is the major cause of venous clotting, and occurs with bed rest especially in the presence of obesity, varicose veins and heart failure. A hypercoagulable state can occur in the postoperative period when there is an elevation of platelet count and a change in clotting factors. It also accompanies polycythemia and thrombocytosis. Endothelial damage occurs secondary to pressure on veins, from lithotomy stirrups and from surgical procedures adjacent to veins.

Most commonly, venous thrombosis starts in the area behind a venous valve. Here, stasis is maximal, a clot forms, starts to propagate and may occlude the whole vessel. Hours later the clot retracts and a small channel of blood flow may be restored. Then, as time proceeds, fibrinolysis occurs and the clot may be totally removed leaving no residual damage to the vein. On occasions, the clot is resistant to fibrinolysis and becomes replaced by fibrous tissue. When fibrosis occurs in relation to a venous valve, the valve may be destroyed, with resultant postphlebitic syndrome and venous engorgement of the limb.

Pathology of pulmonary embolism

When a clot has formed in the leg or pelvis, it may break off and be carried in the venous circulation to the heart and lungs.[31] This can occur especially with movement, exertion and straining. When the clot reaches the lungs there are four possible sequelae: no effect on the lung, obstruction of pulmonary arteries, pulmonary infarction or atelectasis and superinfection.

No effect on the lung

This is the commonest consequence of pulmonary embolism. The clot reaches the pulmonary circulation, occludes a vessel, retracts, undergoes fibrinolysis and disappears. This filtering and removal mechanism is thought to operate in normal people in whom small amounts of clot may periodically reach the lung, and explains the commonly observed phenomenon of an absence of physical signs together with a normal chest X-ray and EKG.

Obstruction of pulmonary arteries

This varies from massive obstruction of the outflow tract of the right ventricle with acute right ventricular failure and sudden death, to a situation where a number of pulmonary arteries may be obstructed with the development of pulmonary hypertension.

Pulmonary infarction

It is not appreciated that pulmonary infarction is a rare event. Indeed, less than 10% of pulmonary emboli give rise to pulmonary infarction.
There are two types of pulmonary infarction:

1. *Incomplete infarction* is the commonest type, and occurs when the alveoli in the area supplied by the embolized vessel become filled with red cells and fibrin. However, the alveolar walls remain alive, phagocytes enter the area, the red cells and fibrin are digested and the lung is restored to normality.
2. *Complete infarction* is uncommon and usually occurs only in patients with heart failure. Here, the alveoli are filled with red cells and fibrin and the alveolar walls necrose due to deficient pulmonary and bronchial circulation secondary to chronic venous congestion of the lungs.

As a consequence, the infarcted area can never return to normal and either heals, leaving a fibrous scar, or else becomes infected and gives rise to abscess formation. A pulmonary infarct is never the classic wedge shape which is traditionally described. Due to collateral vessels supplying the lung tissue adjacent to the embolus, an infarct is 'hump shaped', with its base abutting on a pleural surface and the hump directed towards the hilum of the lung.

Atelectasis and superinfection

Whenever a pulmonary artery is obstructed, in order to preserve ventilation/perfusion balance, the ventilation to that segment of lung decreases, atelectasis may occur and this tissue in turn may become secondarily infected. Normally, atelectasis secondary to sputum retention is visible on the chest X-ray as an opaque area, the radio-dense area being due to crowding of the blood vessels. In contrast, atelectasis following pulmonary embolism is not seen as a radiopaque area, as there is no blood supply to the embolized segment; elevation of the diaphragm may be the only abnormality.

Diagnosis of deep venous thrombosis

The traditional description of deep venous thrombosis of the leg is that of a swollen, warm, tender limb. Unfortunately, studies involving postmortem dissection of legs and, more recently, radioactive iodine tagging of fibrinogen have shown that the majority of patients with deep venous thrombosis do not have this classic finding. There is a spectrum of signs ranging from the swollen, warm, tender leg, through a tender leg, to a completely normal leg. In approximately two-thirds of cases, the legs are normal to physical examination. Hence, lack of clinical evidence of deep venous thrombosis, such as edema, pain and Homan's sign, does not negate the diagnosis of pulmonary embolism.

The diagnostic yield can be increased by the use of special tests. These include: lower limb venography demonstrating venous clots, Doppler studies showing decreased flow through the major venous channels, and radioactive iodine labelled fibrinogen which, if given preoperatively, becomes incorporated in clots and is detected by scanning the legs.

Diagnosis of pulmonary embolism

No disease is more underdiagnosed than pulmonary embolism, and this is due to lack of knowledge of the main diagnostic criteria. It must be appreciated that pulmonary embolism is a disease characterized by symptoms and a lack of physical signs.

Symptoms

As the majority of emboli reach the lung and undergo rapid dissolution, symptoms relevant to the respiratory tract are the clue to the diagnosis. Dyspnea is the commonest symptom, particularly if it is episodic. Any patient with a predisposing factor, such as bed rest, postoperative state, varicose veins or heart failure, who experiences attacks of dyspnea must be suspected as having had a pulmonary embolus. It is particularly dangerous to label as hysterical postoperative patients with hyperventilation attacks.

Pulmonary embolism gives rise to two forms of pain: pleuritic pain usually due to infarction with pleural irritation, and central chest pain similar to that of ischemic heart disease, probably due to a low cardiac output and poor coronary perfusion. Hemoptysis usually indicates incomplete or complete infarction. Cough and sputum are secondary to atelectasis with superinfection and usually there is fever. Finally, 'faints and funny turns' can result from embolic episodes causing transient decreases in the cardiac output and hence in cerebral perfusion.

Signs

The only consistent sign is tachypnea. Others, less commonly present, are signs indicating pulmonary hypertension, such as tachycardia, hypotension, elevated jugular venous pressure, right ventricular gallop rhythm and split second sound, and respiratory abnormalities, including cyanosis, atelectasis, consolidation, pleuritis, effusion and, occasionally, bronchospasm.

Chest X-ray

In the majority of cases, the chest X-ray is either normal or shows only minor abnormalities. This fact should be utilized in the differential diagnosis. Any patient with severe respiratory distress and a relatively normal chest X-ray should be suspected of having pulmonary embolism. This particularly applies with massive pulmonary embolism, in which case the chest X-ray commonly shows only minor abnormalities. X-ray signs which occur include: elevation of the diaphragm due to atelectasis of the lung, enlargement of the pulmonary artery, vascular cut-off with distal oligemia (Westermarks's sign), linear atelectases, pleural effusions and hump-shaped shadows ('Hampton's hump'), which are characteristic of pulmonary infarction.

EKG signs

The EKG is usually normal or shows only sinus tachycardia. With severe embolism, one may see right ventricular strain pattern with S_1Q_3-T_3 pattern, T wave inversion over the right ventricle, clockwise rotation, partial or complete right bundle branch block and right ventricular hypertrophy. Additional changes include any arrhythmias, particularly atrial, and ischemic changes due to poor coronary perfusion secondary to a fall in cardiac output.

Blood gases

The typical blood gas abnormality is that of hypoxia with hyperventilation leading to a low Pa_{O_2} and low Pa_{CO_2}. Unfortunately, this profile is seen in many other respiratory diseases, such as pneumonia, pulmonary edema and atelectasis, and it is therefore unhelpful in the differential diagnosis.

Radioisotope lung scan

This is the most useful test for the diagnosis of pulmonary embolism, and utilizes the principle of embolization of the lung with intravenously administered radio-isotope tagged particles which lodge in the pulmonary capillaries. The particles fail to reach any area of lung which has been embolized, and hence a defect shows on the lung scan. Unfortunately, other lung pathology, such as lung cysts, pneumonia and atelectasis, can also give rise to decreased perfusion, and thus this test is not by itself diagnostic. However, if it is interpreted in conjunction with the chest X-ray, the diagnostic yield is high. For example, if the chest X-ray is clear with no area of atelectasis or lung cysts and there is a large defect in the scan, this is highly suggestive of pulmonary embolism. Conversely, if there is an opacity in a chest X-ray which could be infective or embolic, the presence of a corresponding defect in lung scan does not help clarify the diagnosis. In many cases of shock due to massive pulmonary embolism, the chest X-ray is fairly normal. In this circumstance, the presence of defects of 50% or more of the lung is highly indicative of massive pulmonary embolism.

Pulmonary arteriography

This is the most specific diagnostic test for pulmonary embolism and involves right heart catheterization and injection of contrast medium into the pulmonary artery. The signs of embolism include: obstruction of pulmonary arteries with distal oligemia, filling defects in the pulmonary arteries, obliteration of the normal vascular bed with vascular cut-off, pruning of side branches and enlargement of the artery proximal to the obstruction. Pulmonary arteriography is more invasive than lung scanning, and is usually reserved for circumstances in which the diagnosis is unclear, or prior to emergency embolectomy.

Treatment of deep venous thrombosis and pulmonary embolism

The treatment of deep venous thrombosis and pulmonary embolism consists of specific and supportive measures.

Specific treatment is directed at the thrombus or embolus and includes: anticoagulants to prevent extension of the thrombus, fibrinolytic agents to dissolve thrombus in the legs or embolic material in the lungs, inferior vena caval plication to prevent further embolism and pulmonary embolectomy to remove massive emboli from the pulmonary arteries.

Supportive treatment consists of bed rest, elastic stockings, oxygen, diuretics and digoxin for heart failure, and antibiotics for secondary infection. In the shocked patient, an isoproterenol infusion is of particular value to increase the cardiac output and dilate the pulmonary arteries. In the severely shocked patient, noradrenaline infusion may be the only measure to restore blood pressure.

Anticoagulants

Heparin. This is the drug of choice for the immediate management of the patient with either deep venous thrombosis or pulmonary embolism. It should be clearly understood that heparin only prevents further clotting and does nothing to dissolve clot which has already formed. It may prevent the release of chemical mediators from platelets which cause pulmonary vasoconstriction and bronchoconstriction.

When pulmonary embolism is diagnosed, an immediate bolus dose of 5000 units of intravenous heparin is administered. In situations of massive pulmonary embolism with shock, some authorities recommend an initial dose of 15 000 units for its postulated effect in diminishing pulmonary vasoconstriction. Following the bolus, anticoagulation is maintained by a continuous intravenous infusion of heparin, preferably utilizing an infusion pump. Thus, a constant level of heparinization is achieved without the fluctuations inherent in an intermittent intravenous administration regime. The dose of heparin for a normal sized adult would be 30 000 units over 24 hours. However, this must be titrated against her response, as measured by the activated partial thromboplastin time or thrombin time; ideally either time should be doubled. On occasions, particularly with larger patients, the dose of heparin may have to be increased to 40 000 units every 24 hours. Particular care should be taken with small, elderly female patients as this is the group most prone to bleeding complications; generally, a lower dose should be prescribed. Heparin is usually administered for approximately 10 days. If further embolic episodes occur early in therapy, this does not necessarily mean that heparin has been ineffective, as the clots may have formed prior to heparin administration.

One should be alert to the occurrence of the *heparin induced thrombotic thrombocytopenic syndrome (HITTS)*[5] in which both thrombosis and bleeding problems are seen due to an antibody induced by the heparin. The platelet count should be checked every 2 days in patients on heparin. If the count falls, then a specialist hematologist should be consulted.

Oral anticoagulants. Most authorities do not use oral anticoagulants for the immediate treatment of pulmonary embolism, as they take 5 days to achieve adequate anticoagulation and their action is more difficult to reverse than that of heparin. As a consequence, oral agents are usually reserved for long-term anticoagulation after a course of heparin. Five days overlap of therapy is allowed for oral anticoagulants to take effect before ceasing the heparin. The use of long-term anticoagulation following an embolic episode is controversial. It is recommended by a number of authorities provided there are no contraindications, such as lesions that may cause lethal hemorrhage, e.g. peptic ulcer, unreliability in follow-up, and severe hepatic or renal disease. Oral anticoagulation should be maintained for a period of 3 to 6 months. This recommendation is based on the clinical impression that these patients have an increased risk of further embolism for a period of some months. Certainly, any patient who has suffered a postoperative pulmonary embolus will have a high risk of recurrence with any future operation, and it is imperative that effective prophylaxis be instituted.

Fibrinolytic agents

Fibrinolytic agents such as streptokinase or urokinase have been advocated for deep venous thrombosis and pulmonary embolism. These agents have a different mode of action to that of anticoagulants, and lyse clots in the legs and pulmonary arteries. The main indications for their use are: (1) deep venous thrombosis associated with massive leg swelling in an attempt to dissolve the clot and prevent valve damage leading to the postphlebitic syndrome, and (2) major pulmonary embolism with significant obstruction of the pulmonary arteries causing acute severe pulmonary hypertension.

Fibrinolytic agents are very effective in dissolving clot provided it is fresh, and studies have shown accelerated lysis when compared with patients on heparin therapy alone. However, they are associated with considerable risk of hemorrhage and *cannot be used within 10 days of an operation*, as they dissolve the clot responsible for hemostasis in the operative site and postoperative hemorrhage will result. In addition, the patient must not have intramuscular injections, as massive hematomas can occur. With streptokinase, allergic reactions are common and may be ameliorated by pretreatment with steroids. Because of the risks inherent in this therapy, and the close monitoring and skill required to titrate the dose, fibrinolytic therapy is confined to major centers with particular expertise in this area.

Inferior vena cava plication

On occasions, despite the use of anticoagulants, patients continue to embolize. This may be due to clots that were formed prior to the administration of anticoagulants, or clotting which has occurred despite anticoagulation. In this circumstance, if major embolic episodes are occurring, inferior vena cava plication should be considered. This is usually performed by a retroperitoneal route and a clip is placed on the inferior vena cava. Plication affords temporary relief from further major embolic episodes; however, with the passage of time, large collaterals may develop and the patient is then subject to the risk of further embolism.

Pulmonary embolectomy

If a patient is shocked with massive pulmonary embolism, and the diagnosis has been confirmed by lung scan or pulmonary arteriography, there is a definite place for emergency pulmonary embolectomy. The mortality rate for patients with massive pulmonary embolism and severe shock is extremely high, and although streptokinase has been advocated, better results are achieved by the use of cardiopulmonary bypass and removal of clot from the outflow tract of the right ventricle. At the conclusion of the operation, the inferior vena cava should be plicated to prevent further embolic phenomena in the immediate postoperative period.

STRESS ULCERATION

In patients who have a complicated postoperative course (particularly if they are anxious), have a history of previous peptic ulceration, are taking ulcerogenic drugs such as salicylates, phenylbutazone or indomethacin, or have renal failure, there is an appreciable risk of stress ulceration occurring either in the stomach or the duodenum.[34,37] There are currently three main techniques for the prevention of stress ulceration: (1) intravenous H_2 antagonists, (2) antacids orally or by nasogastric tube, and (3) cytoprotective agents (e.g. Sucralfate) orally or by nasogastric tube.

For ulceration to occur, the gastric juice must be acidic. Provided the gastric pH is kept above 5, by the administration of antacids or H_2 antagonists, stress ulceration will not occur. Parenteral H_2 antagonists (e.g. Ranitidine 50 mg IVI 8-hourly) block histamine-induced acid secretion, and thus decrease the risk of stress ulceration. Antacid therapy is achieved by passing a nasogastric tube and administering 30 ml of an antacid preparation, such as a combination of magnesium and aluminum hydroxide, every 4 hours if the pH is less than 5. If antacid prophylaxis is commenced immediately after surgery or the stressful event, bleeding from stress ulceration can be completely prevented. More recently, cytoprotective agents have been introduced which bind with damaged mucosa, prevent the action of acid but retain the normal gastric environment.

HYPERTENSION

Patients with hypertension should have their antihypertensive therapy continued throughout the preoperative period. Therapy often consists of various combinations of diuretics, beta blockers, sympatholytics and direct vasodilator drugs. In the postoperative period, hypertensive episodes must be prevented as they may cause bleeding in the operative site, cerebral hemorrhage, pulmonary edema or myocardial ischemia. These patients must be closely monitored, and significant rises in blood pressure, for example diastolic pressures greater than 110 mmHg, should be lowered immediately by the use of rapidly acting agents. One such drug in common usage is *diazoxide* which is given initially as a small intravenous dose of 75 mg and then, if necessary, in further increments up to a total of 300 mg. This drug is a potent vasodilator and causes a rapid fall of the blood pressure to normal levels which may be maintained for some hours. In closely monitored situations, the vasodilator of choice is sodium nitroprusside in a dose of 100 mg dissolved in 500 ml of 5% dextrose and given by continuous infusion. The blood pressure is carefully monitored by means of an intra-arterial line.

Other factors may exacerbate hypertension. Pain increases sympathetic activity and may cause vasoconstriction and hypertension. If pain is present, the patient must be given adequate analgesia. Certain patients, particularly those with pre-existing hypertension, may respond to hypovolemia by excessive vasoconstriction, thus generating a rise in blood pressure. This paradoxical hypertension can be cured by the rapid infusion of a plasma expander. A particular danger is the antihypertensive drug, clonidine, which can cause severe rebound hypertension when it is abruptly withdrawn. Any patient taking clonidine requires special precautions. Ideally, the drug should be suspended preoperatively and the patient placed on alternative antihypertensive therapy. If this is not possible, the patient should be given intramuscular clonidine immediately prior to surgery and throughout the postoperative period. Should a hypertensive crisis occur, it is treated with either diazoxide or sodium nitroprusside.

POSTOPERATIVE CONFUSION

The easiest approach to the problem of postoperative confusion is to consider the neuron and the factors that are necessary for it to function normally. These are: oxygen; glucose; a normal chemical environment with regard to sodium, potassium, hydrogen ions and osmolality; an absence of toxins, drugs or drug withdrawal states; and an absence of neurological disease or injury.

Causes

Alterations in any of these six essential factors may result in confusion, coma and fitting. These factors are considered in more detail below.

Hypoxia. This is the commonest cause of postoperative confusion and should be considered in any patient who is confused. The hypoxic episode may have occurred preoperatively, during the anesthetic or in the postoperative period. The causes of cellular hypoxia can be summarized by consideration of the oxygen transport chain. The main cause is a low partial pressure of oxygen in the arterial blood due to a low inspired oxygen, hypoventilation/ventilation perfusion inequality. Other causes are anemia and an inadequate cerebral blood supply secondary to shock or localized cerebrovascular disease.

Alterations in the glucose level. Hypoglycemia is always a danger with diabetics, especially during anesthesia when the signs are obscured. Any patient who has received either insulin or oral hypoglycemic and is on 'nil-by-mouth' should receive glucose by constant infusion. It is imperative to monitor these patients closely and to avoid hypoglycemia which can lead to permanent brain damage. Hyperglycemia induces a hyperosmolar state with cerebral dysfunction.

Alterations in blood chemistry. Either hyper- or hyponatremia reflecting hyperosmolar and hypo-osmolar states or changes in pH can adversely affect neuronal function.

Toxic states. These include bacterial endotoxemia, uremia and hepatic coma.

Drugs. Many drugs, including anesthetic agents, sedatives, analgesics, and psychotropic drugs, can lead to confusion. Conversely, if patients are habituated to drugs such as benzodiazepines, alcohol, barbiturates and narcotics, sudden withdrawal can lead to confusion and agitation.

Specific neurological diseases. These include cerebral tumors, cerebrovascular disease, intracranial infection, trauma, epilepsy and psychiatric conditions. Critical care units, with their lack of differentiation between day and night and continuous treatment leading to lack of sleep, may cause a confusional state which has been referred to as 'intensive care psychosis'.

Management

The first priority is to discover the cause of the confusion. Cerebral oxygenation; glucose level, electrolytes, urea, liver function and presence of drugs must be checked. While oxygen therapy and treatment of the specific cause is proceeding, symptomatic therapy may be required. If the patient is very confused, aggressive and uncontrollable, sedation is necessary. In this circumstance, the drugs which are of most benefit are intravenous diazepam and haloperidol. The aim when administering tranquillizers is to decrease excessive activity while avoiding their serious side effects such as coma, respiratory depression and hypotension. The dose of these drugs varies enormously from patient to patient. Diazepam is usually administered to robust patients in increments of 5 mg every 2 to 3 minutes until adequate sedation is achieved. If, however, the patient is aged, debilitated or gravely ill with compromised cardiovascular function, smaller increments of 1 to 2 mg should be cautiously administered. Haloperidol can be given in increments of 2.5 mg and is less prone to cause hypotension than phenothiazines such as chlorpromazine.

REFERENCES

1. Alexander G, Spence A, Parikk R, Stuart B 1973 The role of airway closure in postoperative hypoxaemia. Br J Anaesth 45: 34
2. Alverdy J, Chi H S, Sheldon G F 1985 The effect of parenteral nutrition on gastrointestinal immunity. Ann Surg 202: 6
3. American Heart Association 1986 Standards and guidelines for cardiopulmonary resuscitation (CPR) and emergency cardiac care (ECC). JAMA 244: 453
4. Anderson J B, Olesen K P, Eikard B, Jansen E, Qvist J 1980 Periodic continuous positive airway pressure, CPAP, by mask in the treatment of atelectasis. Eur J Respir Dis 61: 20
5. Arthur C K, Isbister J P, Aspery E M 1985 The heparin induced thrombosis — thrombocytopenia syndrome (HITTS): a review. Pathology 17: 82
6. Badr K F, Ichikawa I 1988 Prerenal failure: a deleterious shift from renal compensation to decompensation. N Engl J Med 319: 10
7. Bone R C, Fisher C J, Clemmer T P, Slotman G J, Metz C A, Balk R A 1987 A controlled clinical trial of high-dose methylprednisolone in the treatment of severe sepsis and septic shock. N Engl J Med 317: 653
8. Browne N L 1988 Prevention of postoperative deep vein thrombosis. Br J Surg 75: 835
9. Cameron S J 1986 Acute renal failure — the continuing challenge. Quart J Med 59: 337
10. Celoria G, Steingrub J, Dawson J A, Teres D 1987 Oliguria from high intra-abdominal pressure secondary to ovarian mass. Critical Care Med 15: 78
11. Clarke G M 1987 Septic shock. Med Internat 1582
12. Collins R, Scrimgeour A, Yusef S, Peto R 1988 Reduction in fatal pulmonary embolism and venous thrombosis by perioperative administration of subcutaneous heparin. N Engl J Med 318: 1162
13. Consensus Conference 1986 Prevention of venous thrombosis and pulmonary embolism. JAMA 256: 744
14. Craig D B, McLeskey C H, Mitenko P A, Thomson I R, Janis K M 1987 Geriatric anesthesia. Can J Anesth 34: 156
15. D'Attellis N P, Bursztein S, Askanazi J, Kvetan V 1988 Tailoring nutritional support: what, when and why? J Crit Illness 3: 49
16. Desmeules H, Fournier L, Tremblay P 1985 Systemic changes in the elderly patient and their anesthetic implications. Can Anesth Soc J 32: 184
17. Ellrodt A G 1986 Sepsis and septic shock. Emergency Med Clin Nth Am 4: 809
18. Ewer M S, Ali M K 1988 Critical cardiologic considerations in the cancer patient. Critical Care Clin. Jan, p 41
19. Fearon K C H, Carter D C 1988 Cancer cachexia. Ann Surg 208: 1
20. Fisher M M 1987 Anaphylaxis. Disease of the Month, August,

21. Fisher M M, Baldo B A 1988 Acute anaphylactic reactions. Med J Aust 149: 34
22. Goldman L, Caldera D L, Samuel R N et al 1977 Multifactorial index of cardiac risk in noncardiac surgical procedures. N Engl J Med 297: 845
23. Handler C E 1985 Cardiogenic shock. Postgrad Med J 61: 705
24. Hands M E, Rutherford J D 1987 Cardiopulmonary resuscitation: new concepts and strategies. Aust NZ J Med 17: 543
25. Haydock D A, Hill G L 1986 Impaired wound healing in surgical patients with varying degrees of malnutrition. J Parent Enter Nut 10: 6
26. Hopkinson R 1985 Using pulmonary artery catheters. Care of the Critically Ill 1: 15
27. Hull C J 1988 Control of pain in the perioperative period. Br Med Bull 4: 341
28. Ingbar D H, White D A 1988 Acute respiratory failure. Critical Care Clin. Jan, p 11
29. Isbister J P 1984 Haemotherapy for acute haemorrhage. Anaesth Intens Care 12: 217
30. Isbister J P, Biggs J 1976 Reactions to rapid infusions of 5% stable plasma protein solutions (SPPS) during large volume plasma exchange. Anaesth Intensive Care 4: 105
31. Jones R, Sabiston D 1976 Pulmonary embolism. Surg Clin Nth Am 56: 891
32. Kahn R C 1988 Shock as a complication of cancer. Critical Care Clin Jan, p 129
33. Kidson W, Casey J, Kraegen E, Lazarus L 1974 Treatment of severe diabetes mellitus by insulin infusion. Br Med J 2: 691
34. Kleiman R L, Adair C G, Ephgrave K S 1988 Stress ulcers: current understanding of pathogenesis and prophylaxis. Drug Intell Clin Pharm 22: 452
35. Knudsen J 1970 Duration of hypoxemia after uncomplicated upper abdominal and thoraco-abdominal operations. Anaesthesia 25: 372
36. Kopec I, Groeger J S 1988 Life-threatening fluid and electrolyte abnormalities associated with cancer. Critical Care Clin Jan, p 81
37. Kron I L, Harman P K, Nolan S P 1984 The measurement of intra-abdominal pressure as a criterion for abdominal re-exploration. Ann Surg 199: 28
38. Lazarus J M 1986 Acute renal failure. Intensive Care Med 12: 61
39. Ledingham I McA, Messmer K, Thijs L 1988 Report on the European Conference on Septic Shock of the European Society of Intensive Care Medicine and the European Shock Society, Brussels, Belgium, March 1–2 1987. Intensive Care Med 14: 181
40. Lemoyne M, Jeejeebhoy K N 1986 Total parenteral nutrition in the critically ill patient. Chest 89: 568
41. Lipman J 1985 Pitfalls in the interpretation of pulmonary capillary wedge pressure. SAMJ 67: 174
42. Mann H J, Fuhs D W, Hemstrom C A 1986 Acute renal failure. Drug Intell Clin Pharm 20: 421
43. Mazze R 1977 Critical care of the patient with acute renal failure. Anaesthesiology 47: 138
44. Merli G J, Martinez J 1987 Prophylaxis for deep vein thrombosis and pulmonary embolism in the surgical patient. Med Clin North Am 71: 377
45. More D G 1984 Initial assessment of acute haemorrhage. Anaesth Intens Care 12: 206
46. Muller J M, Keller H W, Brenner U, Walter M, Holzmuller W 1986 Indications and effects of preoperative parenteral nutrition. World J Surg 10: 53
47. Nunn J F, Milledge J S, Chen D, Dore C 1988 Respiratory criteria of fitness for surgery and anaesthesia. Anaesthesia 43: 543
48. Oakley C M 1987 Controversies in the prophylaxis of infective endocarditis: a cardiological view. J Antimicrob Chemother 20 (suppl A): 99
49. Oh T E, Duncan A W 1988 Oxygen therapy. Med J Aust 149: 141
50. Pace N 1977 A critique of flow-directed pulmonary arterial catheterisation. Anaesthesiology 47: 455
51. Pasternack P F, Imparato A M, Bauman F G et al 1987 The haemodynamics of B-blockade in patients undergoing abdominal aortic aneurysm repair. Circulation 76 (Suppl III): 1
52. Paul W L, Downs J B 1981 Postoperative atelectasis. Arch Surg 116: 861
53. Phillips G D 1985 Total parenteral nutrition in acute illness. Anaesth Intens Care 13: 288
54. Phillips P J, Fazio V A 1985 Enteral feeding — a practical approach. Anaesth Intens Care 13: 283
55. Raper R F, Fisher M McD 1984 Resuscitation in acute haemorrhage. Anaesth Intens Care 12: 212
56. Raper R F, Ibels L S 1982 Toxic shock syndrome. Mod Med Aust, p 31
57. Raper R, Sibbald W J 1986 Misled by the wedge? The Swan-Ganz catheter and left ventricular preload. Chest 89: 427
58. Rao R L K, Jacobs K H, El-Etr A A 1983 Reinfarction following anaesthesia in patients with myocardial infarction. Anaesthesiology 59: 499
59. Ruckley C V 1985 Protection against thrombo-embolism. Br J Surg 72: 421
60. Runciman W B 1980 Sympathomimetic amines. Anaesth Intens Care 8: 289
61. Runciman W B, Skowronski G A 1984 Pathophysiology of haemorrhage shock. Anaesth Intens Care 12: 193
62. Russell R I 1986 Enteral nutrition. Hospital Update, p 261
63. Scheidt S 1978 Preservation of ischemic myocardium with intraaortic balloon pumping: modern therapeutic intervention or primum non nocere. Circulation 58: 211
64. Seymour D G, Vaz F G 1987 Aspects of surgery in the elderly: Preoperative medical assessment. Br J Hosp Med, p 102
65. Skowronski G A 1988 The pathophysiology of shock. Med J Aust 148: 576
66. Shaw J H F 1986 Recent advances in the nutritional and metabolic management of critically ill surgical patients. NZ Med J 99: 665
67. Steen P, Tinker J, Tarhan S 1978 Myocardial reinfarction after anesthesia and surgery. JAMA 239: 2566
68. Stock M C, Downs J B, Gauer P K, Alster J M, Imrey P B 1985 Prevention of postoperative pulmonary complications with CPAP, incentive spirometry, and conservative therapy. Chest 87: 2
69. Stone H, Kolb L, Geheber C, Dawkins E 1976 Use of aminoglycosides in surgical infection. Ann Surg 183: 660
70. Symposium 1988 Anaesthesia and myocardial ischaemia. Br J Anaesth 61: 1
71. Tarhan S 1972 Myocardial infarction after general anesthesia. JAMA 220: 1451
72. Teplick R S 1987 Measuring central vascular pressures: a surprisingly complex problem. Anaesthesiology 67: 3
73. Thomson A D 1988 Cytoprotection: the new era. Update: J Postgrad G P 6: 29
74. Veselis R A 1988 Sedation and pain management for the critically ill. Critical Care Clinics Jan, p 167
75. Veterans Administration System Sepsis Cooperative Study Group 1987 Effect of high-dose glucocorticoid therapy on mortality in patients with clinical signs of systemic sepsis. N Engl J Med 317: 659
76. West J 1979 Respiratory Physiology, 2nd edn. Williams and Wilkins, Baltimore
77. Wheeler A P, Jaquiss R D B, Newman J H 1988 Physician practices in the treatment of pulmonary embolism and deep venous thrombosis. Arch Intern Med 148: 1321
78. Wiedemann H P, Matthay M A, Matthay R A 1984 Cardiovascular-pulmonary monitoring in the intensive care unit (Part 1). Chest 85: 537
79. Wilkes B, Melloux L 1986 Acute renal failure. Am J Med 80: 1129
80. Windsor J A 1988 Risk factors for postoperative pneumonia. Ann Surg 208: 209
81. Windsor J A, Hill G L 1988 Weight loss with physiologic impairment: a basic indicator of surgical risk. Ann Surg 207: 290

85. Urological complications of radical pelvic surgery and radiation therapy

C. P. Morrow   J. P. Curtin

INTRODUCTION

In many forms of gynecologic cancer the malignant disease itself may extend to involve the lower urinary tract and complicate the overall plan of management. This chapter, however, is devoted to urological complications that result from the therapy itself, whether this be by radical pelvic surgery alone, by primary radiation therapy alone, or by a combination of surgery and irradiation. The intimate anatomic proximity of the female reproductive and lower urinary tracts accounts for the fact that urological complications following treatment of pelvic malignancies are relatively common. Both the bladder and ureters figure prominently in the extended dissection of most radical pelvic operations, and both are also in the direct line of fire when the radiotherapist uses either intracavitary or external radiation to treat pelvic cancer. Hence, both radical surgery and radiation therapy have the intrinsic potential for causing anatomic or functional impairment of the lower urinary tract. The various urological complications may be under three broad headings: intraoperative, postoperative and post-radiation, rather than simply according to anatomic sites. It is apparent that there are fundamental differences between those that occur after radical surgery and those that follow irradiation with respect to etiologic mechanisms, preventive measures, time of occurrence and clinical manifestations, and above all the overall plan and technique of management. Although the main emphasis is on diagnosis and management of each complication, it seems important to include also a brief discussion of specific methods that have proved valuable in its prevention. General preventive measures are noted in the introduction, while more specific ones are presented in the appropriate sections that follow.

GENERAL CONSIDERATIONS

Urological complications following radical pelvic surgery are seldom the result of direct surgical trauma to the ureters or bladder. In fact, accidental direct injury to these structures should rarely occur in the hands of the well-trained and experienced pelvic surgeon completely familiar with the regional anatomy and proper techniques of dissection. Rather, ureteral and vesical complications of either an anatomic (e.g. fistula and stricture) or a functional (e.g. bladder dysfunction) nature more commonly result from extensive pelvic dissection which may damage the vascular bed and autonomic nerve supply to these structures. In addition extensive dissection also sets the stage for postoperative wound healing problems secondary to a collection of serum or blood and/or bacterial cellulitis, either of which can lead to excessive fibrosis and impaired blood supply to ureters and bladder. Thereafter, avascular necrosis may ensue causing fistula or stricture formation. Division or resection of the autonomic nerve fibers to the lower ureters and bladder impairs peristalsis and may contribute to ureteral dilation, obstruction, and fistulization. In the case of the bladder, a diminished sensation of fullness and prolonged voiding difficulty may be encountered.

With the above mechanisms in mind, it is clear that a careful, minimally traumatic dissection, preserving the longitudinal and the segmental blood supply to the ureters, meticulous hemostasis and postoperative drainage of the pelvis when indicated are general measures useful in avoiding urological complications after radical pelvic surgery. In addition, a few specific intraoperative techniques as well as postoperative maneuvers during the early weeks of convalescence are especially valuable in preventing these complications and will be detailed later.

Radiation-induced urological complications do not appear immediately, as is the case with the majority of postoperative urological problems. Rather, they tend to occur in the 6 to 18 month interval after treatment when the radiation reaction tends to reach its peak and then commences to subside slowly over the next few years. This is because of the nature of the tissue injury created by radiation, which biologically consists of varying combinations of direct mucosal necrosis, submucosal fibrosis, regional devascularization, ischemia and fibrosis of the surrounding connective tissue. Brachytherapy tends to produce localized injury while teletherapy effects are more homogeneous and tend to involve the entire treatment field. With either absolute overdosage or relative overdosage, it is easy to understand why these forms of radiation-induced tissue damage may lead to urological complications such as vesicovaginal fistula, ureterovaginal fistula, ureteral stricture, periureteral fibrosis with secondary obstruction, and contracted bladder.

With these radiobiologic mechanisms in mind, general measures of importance in avoiding tissue damage that might lead to urological complications following radiotherapy for pelvic malignancies include correction of nutritional deficits and treating pelvic infection. Careful local and external radiation dosimetry to avoid 'hot spots' or generalized overdosage are even more important. Proper vaginal packing and constant bladder drainage to maintain the bladder, lower ureters, and rectum at the greatest possible distance from the radioactive sources are critical to proper brachytherapy.

UROLOGICAL COMPLICATIONS OF RADICAL HYSTERECTOMY

The Wertheim procedure, or radical hysterectomy with bilateral pelvic lymphadenectomy, is one of the most commonly performed radical surgical procedures for gynecologic cancer. (See Chs 42, 78 and 79.) The incidence of urological complications following the Wertheim procedure has remained as a significant cause of morbidity associated with the procedure, although the rate has decreased substantially over the past 50 years. While it is our impression that urologic complications are more often associated with radical debulking procedures for epithelial ovarian tumors, the Wertheim procedure serves as a paradigm for management of urologic complications. Therefore, post-Wertheim urological complications will be presented in great detail, to be followed by brief supplementary coverage of the similar or related urinary tract problems that may occasionally follow some of the other radical pelvic operations.

Ureteral complications

General comments

Ureteral complications were formerly the most frequent and serious of the postoperative problems following radical hysterectomy, with ureterovaginal fistulas occurring in 5 to 10% of all reported series.[6,16,30] In a series of 623 radical Wertheim procedures performed from 1939 to 1961 by the gynecologic surgical staff of the Massachusetts General and Pondville State Cancer Hospitals, Green et al[16] reported 78 patients with ureteral complications, a 12.5% overall incidence, with ureterovaginal fistula occurring in 8.5% and ureteral stricture in 4.0%. Factors demonstrated to increase the risk of ureteral complications in that series included the presence of pelvic endometriosis (1.5 × the baseline risk), pelvic inflammatory disease (3 ×), coexisting pregnancy (4 ×), or preoperative irradiation (a full course doubled the risk). Known operative injury to the lower ureters had occurred in only 14 of the 623 patients. Beginning in the 1960s, improvements in operative technique with emphasis on preservation of the sheath with its longitudinal blood supply, gentle atraumatic handling of the ureter, use of retroperitoneal suction drainage and a

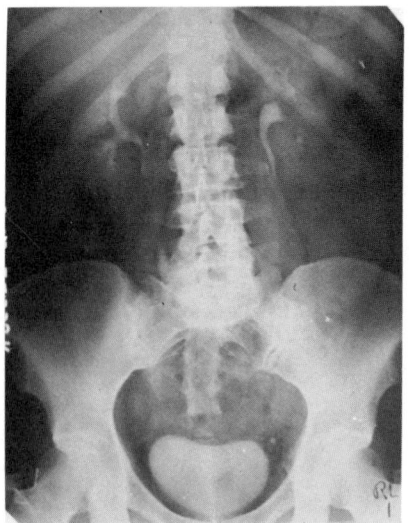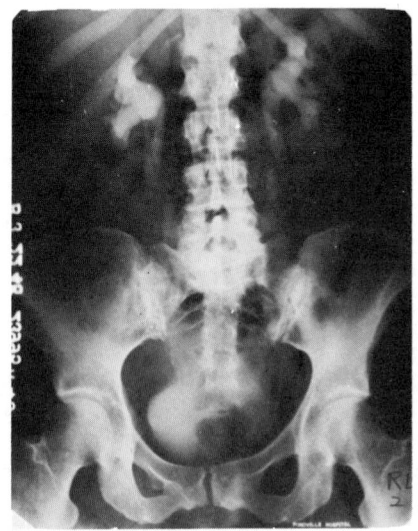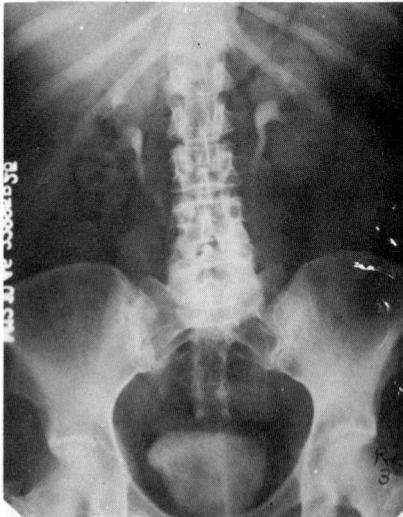

Fig. 85.1 Intravenous pyelogram illustrating temporary, asymptomatic, spontaneously reversible hydroureter and hydronephrosis frequently observed during the early postoperative weeks. Left: Preoperative pyelogram. Center: First postoperative pyelogram, 16th postoperative day. Right: Subsequent pyelogram 1 year later, showing spontaneous return to normal appearances. (Reproduced from: Green T H Jr 1981 Urological complications of radical pelvic surgery and radiation therapy. In: Coppleson M (ed) Gynecologic Oncology. Churchill Livingstone, Edinburgh.)

decrease in pelvic infections has led to a reduction in the injury rate to 0.5–2.0% in modern series.[22]

A significant observation pertinent to a discussion of ureteral complications and their prevention and treatment concerns the development to some extent in all patients, of a transient hydroureter and hydronephrosis, unaccompanied by any urinary tract infection or renal impairment (Fig. 85.1). Spontaneous clearance occurs usually within 3 or 4 months[15,31] after radical hysterectomy. This temporary postoperative hydroureter with its accompanying mild hydronephrosis presumably represents a transient functional obstructive effect of the extensive dissection around the lower ureter and ureterovesical junction, with the resulting edema and impaired peristaltic action.

It seems likely that this temporary physiologic impairment and dilatation of the ureters may be an important factor in the development of ureteral fistulas. In the presence of varying degrees of impaired blood supply and injury of the periureteral adventitia and supporting tissue, dilatation and thinning out of the ureteral wall, as well as increased intraluminal pressure, tend to favor the occurrence of 'blow-outs' and fistula formation in the critical lower 4 to 6 cm of the dissected ureters.

Careful, atraumatic handling of the ureter and preservation of the adventitia and segmental blood supply consistent with the removal of all potential routes of cancer spread are of great importance in avoiding subsequent complications. The routine use of preoperative intravenous pyelography (IVP) provides little protection against ureteral injury. Double ureter, pelvic kidney and/or ureteral obstruction are rarely found and should be recognized during the course of the surgical procedure. The routine use of inlying ureteral catheters during the Wertheim dissection has little to recommend it. The necessary skill and experience required of the operator performing radical pelvic surgery and the exposure afforded by the dissection itself are such that inlying catheters should not be needed to delineate the course of the ureter. Furthermore, their presence within the lumen of the ureter during the latter's extensive mobilization impedes the dissection, a potential predisposition to ureteral injury.

The avoidance of postoperative hematomas and serous collections as well as pelvic sepsis (either cellulitis or infected hematomas) beneath the pelvic peritoneal closure is also important in preventing postoperative ureteral fistulas and strictures. Postoperative pelvic sepsis and hematomas especially tend to compromise the blood supply, distort the anatomy, and interfere with efficient function of the lower ureters. Optimal hemostasis and retroperitoneal suction catheters, together with prophylactic antibiotic therapy, are indicated in an effort to avoid or minimize these complications.

A 3 to 6 week period of postoperative bladder drainage has traditionally proven helpful in reducing the incidence of ureteral complications. By keeping the bladder continuously empty during this period postoperatively, the lower, most vulnerable portion of the dissected ureters is kept at rest while local healing and revascularization proceed.

Intraoperative injury

Recognition of a ureteral injury intraoperatively allows for prompt surgical repair, placement of ureteral stents and close postoperative monitoring of the urinary tract, all of which minimize the likelihood of permanent injury and the necessity of a second surgery. Broadly speaking, the types of injuries are devascularization of the ureteral adventitia, crush injury (ligature and/or clamp) and transection. If there is a doubt regarding whether the lumen of the ureter has been entered, intravenous indigo carmine may be given, or retrograde stents passed through a cystotomy.

The female distal ureter receives its blood supply primarily from the uterine artery with additional supply from the internal iliac, superior vesical and vaginal arteries. The ureter is invested by an adventitia, carrying a longitudinal network of blood vessels. Atraumatic dissection of the ureter, especially in the area of the vesicouterine 'tunnel' will avoid injury to the blood supply. However, occasionally, due to the presence of fibrosis, inflammation and/or tumor, a portion of the ureter can have its blood supply compromised during dissection, as manifested by poor color. If the length of the involved segment is only a few mm, placement of a double-J stent[41] along with closed drainage may be adequate. If a longer segment is involved, or there are other confounding medical problems (previous irradiation, diabetes, vascular disease) resection with neoureterocystostomy should be performed.

Crush injury to the distal ureter rarely occurs during a radical hysterectomy due to the excellent exposure. Where the ureter may be at risk is at the pelvic brim near the infundibulopelvic pedicle. A crush injury related to suture ligature, if promptly recognized, can usually be managed by releasing the stitch. Crush injury by a clamp is usually more traumatic. Stenting and drainage suffice if the injury on inspection is not severe. Otherwise a uretero-ureterostomy at or above the pelvic brim or neoureterocystostomy more distally should be performed.[51]

Transection of the ureter may occur as part of tumor resection or inadvertently. When it occurs in the distal ureter, neoureterocystostomy is the proper method of repair, as reported by Green et al.[16] In their review of 14 ureteral injuries recognized intraoperatively, 6 underwent neoureterocystostomy and none had complications. Eight had repair by uretero-ureterostomy and all 8 had complications: 5 fistulas and 3 strictures. Granted these injuries and repairs occurred in the days before broad-spectrum antibiotics, suction drainage and stents were in common usage; however, the difference in outcome still favors reimplantation, which should be the procedure of choice.

Postoperative complications

Diagnosis. The sudden appearance of profuse watery discharge, often with characteristic uriniferous odor, 7 to 14 days after operation is strongly suggestive of the presence of a ureterovaginal fistula. The most common signs and symptoms of ureteral injury are abdominal pain and tenderness along with fever.[32,54] The presence of a ureteral rather than a vesical fistula should be rapidly established. This can readily be done by first instilling methylene blue or indigo carmine into the bladder. If the dye does not appear on a dry sponge inserted into the vagina, then indigo carmine is given intravenously. The appearance of dye on the vaginal sponge makes the diagnosis of a ureteral fistula.

If a patient with closed suction drainage should have a marked increase in output with or without concomitant drop in urine flow, the creatinine level of the suction fluid is determined. If it is greater than the serum level, most likely there is a ureteral leak.

Intravenous pyelography may be helpful, both in establishing the presence of ureteral fistula and the side involved, as well as in determining whether or not obstruction exists (Fig. 85.2). However, at times, the intravenous pyelogram is misleading with the intact ureter exhibiting slight, transient dilatation, and the ureter and renal pelvis on the side of the fistula actually showing better drainage. CT scanning with intravenous contrast medium may demonstrate extra-urinary tract contrast enhancement of fluid collections.[21]

Cystoscopy with attempted retrograde catheterization with pyelography should be done promptly, first, because it will precisely reveal the side and site of the fistula, and second, in the hope that a polyethylene or silastic catheter can be inserted past the fistula into the renal pelvis. If the attempt is successful, the splinting ureteral catheter is left in place to gravity drainage until the fistula is healed, usually 14 to 21 days. The placement of a stent by retrograde catheterization is successful in fewer than half of patients with a ureteral fistula, however. Ureteroscopy utilizing a flexible 3.7 mm fiberoptic scope has been reported to be more effective in retrograde catheterization.[22]

In the case of a ureteral stricture, the symptoms and signs are those of impaired drainage with secondary infection. (Bilateral strictures produce uremia.) Strictures usually are manifested much later than fistulas and definitive therapy can be undertaken as soon as the diagnosis is made. The diagnosis is readily established by intravenous pyelography, and the initial evaluation should include cyst-

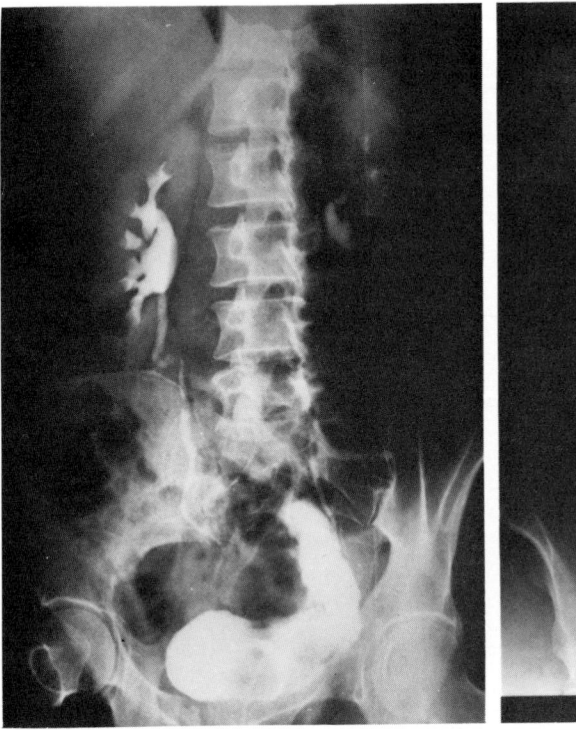
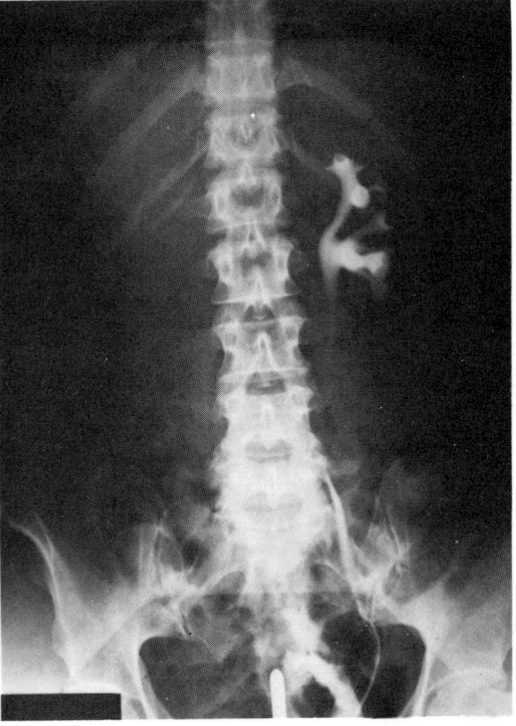

Fig. 85.2 Left: Intravenous pyelogram on the 13th postoperative day following radical Wertheim hysterectomy revealing essentially normal kidneys and ureters but demonstrating an extravasation of dye arising in the region of the left ureterovesical junction and draining into the vagina. Right: Left retrograde pyelogram on 14th postoperative day at time of attempted passage of ureteral catheter by the ureterovaginal fistula, confirming the presence and location of the fistula and revealing no proximal obstruction of the left ureter. (Reproduced from: Green T H Jr 1981 Urological complications of radical pelvic surgery and radiation therapy. In: Coppleson M (ed) Gynecologic Oncology. Churchill Livingstone, Edinburgh.)

oscopy and retrograde catheterization, both to confirm the diagnosis as well as to attempt dilatation of the strictured area and passage of a stent. In the earlier series of patients treated at the Massachusetts General and Pondville State Cancer Hospitals, retrograde dilatations with ultimate permanent restoration of normal function and anatomy were successful in 9 of 25 patients who had developed ureteral strictures.[16]

Management. When retrograde stent placement, for either ureteral fistula or stenosis is unsuccessful, percutaneous nephrostomy should be the next option. This procedure has become increasingly the preferred method of management of ureteral injuries. The procedure may be an adjunct to therapy or a definitive treatment. Dowling et al[9] reported a series of 23 patients with a delayed diagnosis of a ureteral injury. Percutaneous nephrostomy was attempted in 17 patients and was successful in 15. Of the 15 patients with nephrostomy placement, 11 (5 ureteral fistulas and 6 ureteral ligations) were successfully managed. During treatment, normal renal function was maintained and for patients with a fistula, urinary leakage was controlled. The mean treatment time was 53 days.

If the trans-nephrostomy placement of the ureteral stent is unsuccessful in treatment of ureteral fistula, an obstructing ureteral catheter may be inserted and the affected kidney drained via the nephrostomy tube. This will allow time for the fistula to heal or time to ready the patient for surgery.

If a nephrostomy cannot be established and/or maintained, the ureterovaginal fistula usually remains open, renal function and drainage invariably are excellent, infection will be absent, and there will be no significant dilatation of the ureter or renal pelvis above the fistula. A period of 3 to 6 or more several months should elapse to allow restoration of optimal tissue conditions before operative repair is undertaken. Although some patients prefer to simply change perineal pads frequently, many can be kept reasonably dry and far more comfortable when fitted with a plastic cup-like vaginal receptacle that can be connected by plastic tubing to a collecting bag worn on the thigh.

If drainage ceases spontaneously, the patient should be followed carefully by intravenous pyelograms, since healing with stricture and eventual silent renal atrophy can also occur. If healing with stricture does take place, periodic ureteral dilatation may restore normal drainage, prevent recurrent pyelonephritis, and avoid progressive decline in renal function. If this type of conservative approach is unsuccessful, definitive operative repair is indicated to preserve renal function on the side of the healed fistula.

As in the case of primary repair of the lower ureter inadvertently injured or subjected to elective partial resection during radical hysterectomy, the most successful definitive

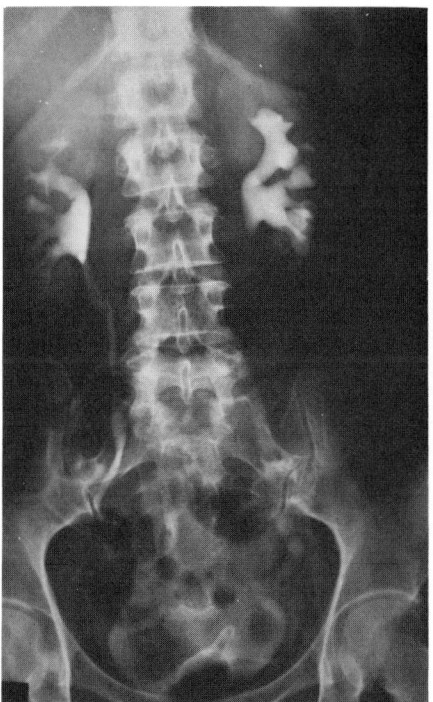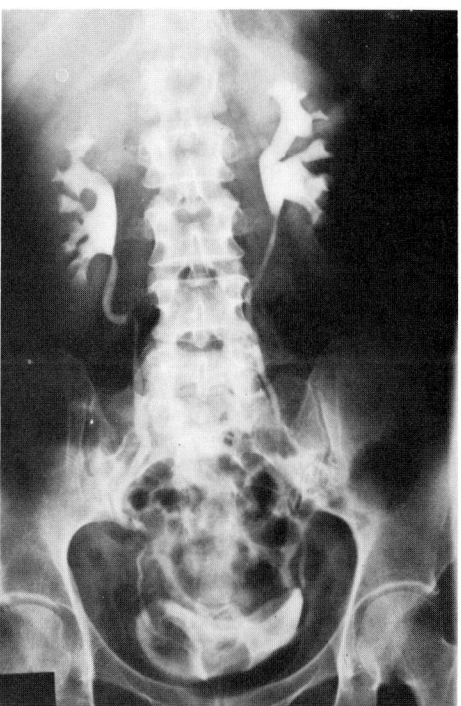

Fig. 85.3 Same patient as in Figure 85.2. Left: Intravenous pyelogram done 9½ weeks following radical Wertheim hysterectomy and 24 hours prior to operative repair of left ureterovaginal fistula, revealing slight narrowing of the distal left ureter with mild proximal dilatation and again demonstrating drainage into the vagina on the same side. Right: Intravenous pyelogram on 14th postoperative day following reimplantation of the left ureter into bladder (ureteroneocystostomy), demonstrating completely normal function and anatomy of both upper and lower urinary tracts bilaterally and absence of any fistula. (Reproduced from: Green T H Jr 1981 Urological complications of radical pelvic surgery and radiation therapy. In: Coppleson M (ed) Gynecologic Oncology. Churchill Livingstone, Edinburgh.

repair of the postoperative ureteral fistula or stricture is by implantation into the bladder (ureteroneocystostomy) (Fig. 85.3). A transabdominal, transperitoneal approach through a midline lower abdominal incision affords excellent exposure. Preliminary placement of a three-way drainage catheter in the bladder permits it to be distended later to facilitate cystotomy. Starting near the pelvic brim, the ureter is mobilized and followed carefully along the pelvic side wall toward the bladder and vaginal apex. Just above the point of fistula formation or stricture, the ureter is divided and the distal end securely ligated. Both the proximal normal ureter and the corresponding bladder wall are mobilized sufficiently so that there will be no tension on the anastomosis. The bladder is then filled with sterile saline via the three-way catheter, a suprapubic cystotomy carried out and the incision extended to expose the trigone. A small circular opening is made just above the old ureteral orifice, excising a piece of the mucosa, and then a short 1–2 cm submucosal tunnel is established, running obliquely laterally and posteriorly on the floor of the bladder. A Kelly clamp is introduced into this tunnel and the tip guided through the muscularis at the end of the tunnel to penetrate the bladder wall at that point. The Kelly clamp is used to grasp a suture placed through the cut end of the ureter. The ureter is then pulled through the posterior bladder wall opening, through the submucosal tunnel and into the bladder. After the cut end of the ureter has been freshened and spatulated, the ureter is sutured to the bladder mucosa using interrupted 4–0 or 5–0 chromic catgut sutures. (Some authors also recommend ureteral stents.) When it is obvious that the ureter is draining freely and that a water-tight closure has been attained, the cystotomy is closed in two layers. The periureteral adventitia is sutured to the adjacent bladder wall to further anchor the ureter and minimize tension at the mucosal reimplantation site. The entire region is then reperitonized, using the peritoneal flap created by the preliminary dissection to expose the lower ureter. The retroperitoneal area is drained by closed suction, and a transurethral catheter is left in place for 10 days.

When the transected proximal ureter is within 3–4 cm of the bladder, there is often enough mobility to directly reimplant the ureter without tension into the bladder. However, when a portion of the ureter must be excised due to tumor, radiation, and/or fibrosis, mobilization of the bladder and fixation to the psoas muscle above the iliac vessels, the so-called vesicopsoas hitch, is indicated. Often with complete mobilization of the bladder attachments, the vesicopsoas hitch may be able to compensate for loss of most of the pelvic ureter.[10]

In the case where additional length is required for the ureteroneocystostomy, there are several techniques for bridging the gap between bladder and ureter including various bladder flaps and also the use of an ileal segment.[42]

Bladder complications

Intraoperative injury

The frequency with which bladder injury occurs during radical hysterectomy is seldom reported, but it is presumably greater than the frequency of vesicovaginal fistula which, on the average, is less than 1% of cases (Hansen found 1 instance of bladder and 2 ureteral repairs among 211 cases[19]). The most common site of injury is the trigone, which is adherent to the anterior vagina just distal to the cervix. The thin trigone is susceptible to injury from dissection and ischemia as the experience with simple hysterectomy has repeatedly demonstrated. Predisposing factors are prior cesarean section, anterior colporrhaphy, conization, hysterectomy (complete or supracervical) and pelvic cellulitis. The bladder may be entered while dissecting it from the cervix, but this is readily repaired since this part of the bladder is mobile, well vascularized, accessible and relatively remote from the ureters.

The recognition of bladder injury may be apparent if the mucosa is visible and not mistaken for vaginal epithelium or peritoneum. If the dissection has been difficult, or bloody, it is prudent to test for a bladder defect, especially if there has been an injury to the muscularis. This is done by distending the bladder with methylene blue solution via the transurethral catheter. If a defect is present, the bladder wall needs to be mobilized to achieve good exposure and determine the complete dimensions of the defect. After placing opposing stay sutures, the defect is closed water tight with a running, through and through chromic suture. A second layer of uninterrupted, inverting chromic or PGA suture is inserted. The integrity of the suture line is tested by again distending the bladder with the methylene blue solution.

Measures to prevent bladder injury include the use of bladder drainage during surgery (transurethral Foley), and good surgical technique. If the patient has had a hysterectomy, packing the vagina with gauze may be helpful to identify the anatomic planes. Occasionally, opening the bladder in the space of Retzius will assist in accurately identifying the bladder wall and permit dissection of very firm adhesions, or to localize an area involved by tumor which needs to be resected. In the usual case, sharp dissection of the trigone area is needed to achieve adequate mobilization of the bladder so the vaginal cuff can be closed without putting sutures into the muscularis. This will reduce the likelihood of postoperative ischemic necrosis and fistulization.

The bladder is easily opened in the space of Retzius by grasping the Foley bulb and dissecting down on it with a hemostat. If one simply wants to check the integrity of the bladder mucosa a laparoscope can be introduced and the bladder distended with water or CO_2. In the same manner ureteral patency can be observed. If urine is not seen spurting from the ureteral orifices, indigo carmine can be given intravenously. Otherwise, the bladder is opened longitudinally in the midline to provide access for visual examination. This defect is closed in two layers as previously described. For retropubic incisions, the Foley catheter can be removed in 2 to 3 days postoperatively. For a dependent suture line it is recommended that bladder drainage be continued 7 to 10 days in the non-irradiated patient, depending upon the quality of the tissues, the postoperative course, and the surgeons judgement regarding the quality of the repair.

Postoperative complications

Detrusor dysfunction and incontinence. Numerous adverse effects on the lower urinary tract consequent to radical hysterectomy may be manifested postoperatively. Among these are incontinence, cystocele, shortened urethra, inability to void, high residual urine volume, loss of bladder sensation, detrusor instability, hypotonic detrusor and vesico-ureteric reflux. Most of these abnormalities result from interruption of the parasympathetic and sympathetic nerves to the lower urinary tract, loss of anatomic vesical neck support and overdistension of the bladder. These phenomena have been studied by numerous investigators.[3,7,13,14,23,27,29,43,45,46]

The autonomic nerve supply to the bladder, distal ureters and urethra consists of sympathetic and parasympathetic components, the former derived from T-11 to L-1 spinal cord segments, and the latter from the S2–4 spinal cord segments. The sympathetic branches from the hypogastric plexus join the pelvic visceral (parasympathetic) nerves to form the pelvic plexus on the antero-lateral pelvic wall. The pelvic plexus traverses the lower (posterior) portion of the cardinal ligament, thence to the bladder, ureter and urethra via the bladder pillar.[45,48] Thus, it is inevitable that, in the course of performing a radical hysterectomy, some of the autonomic innervation to the lower urinary tract is interrupted. The degree to which the nerves are disrupted, the severity of dysfunction and the extent of recovery are reported to vary widely and presumably depends upon the radicalness of the operation, postoperative management, and, perhaps, to individual anatomic variations.

Early postoperative urodynamic studies after radical hysterectomy are in general agreement that, in the absence of overdistension, complete transection of the cardinal ligaments produces in nearly every case marked reduction in bladder sensation, increased intravesical pressure, decreased volume and decreased urethral closing pressure. Incontinence is observed in 10–70% of patients who had normal bladder function preoperatively. If only the anterior portion of the cardinal ligament is divided, a hypertonic bladder is reported in about 30%, while incontinence and a decreased urethral pressure are reported in 10%.[14,45]

It is clear that the frequency of most adverse effects of radical hysterectomy on lower urinary tract function is increased by complete bilateral transection of the cardinal ligaments. Thus, for early cancers, preservation of the posterior cardinal ligament through which the main trunk of the pelvic plexus passes is highly desirable. As noted by many authors,[3,14,20] however, a major complicating factor in post radical hysterectomy bladder dysfunction is overdistension which results because the patient does not have the sensation of fullness. This converts the hypertonic bladder into a hypotonic bladder which the patient is unable to empty well, if at all, even with the Valsalva, Credé and other maneuvers to increase intravesical pressure.

The first measure then to avoid postoperative bladder complications is adequate drainage. Our protocol is to leave a size #16F transurethral catheter to continuous drainage until 3 weeks post operation. At this time, the bladder is filled with 250 ml of sterile water, the catheter is removed and the patient instructed to void. If the calculated residual is >75 ml, the catheter is replaced and the patient checked again in 3 weeks. Around 75–95% of the patients will be able to void successfully at 3 weeks depending on the extent of surgery.

Preoperative urodynamics cannot predict which patients among those with a normal study will have postoperative bladder problems. However, those with detrussor instability are very likely to be made somewhat worse by radical hysterectomy, as are those patients with diminished anatomic support of the vesical neck. In the latter group, especially if the patient already has stress incontinence, a Burch procedure should be performed at the time of surgery.

Management of the hypertonic bladder which functions adequately is expectant. If frequency is excessive or incontinence develops, medical measures are indicated. Estrogens, in the woman with absent or failed ovaries, are recommended in managing post radical hysterectomy urinary incontinence. Ostergard[39] has reviewed the role of drugs in treating lower urinary tract problems. Anticholinergic agents (e.g. bethanechol 25 mg qid) are indicated to inhibit spontaneous bladder contractions; cholinergic agents (e.g. oxybutynin 5 mg 2–3 × daily; propantheline 7.5–15 mg 3–4 × daily) which stimulate bladder contraction are useful if the patient is unable to void because of a hypotonic bladder. Incontinence associated with a low urethral pressure may be ameliorated by the administration of alpha adrenergic stimulating agents (ephedrine 15–50 mg 3–4 × daily; phenylpropanolamine 25–50 mg 3–4 × daily) which increase urethral tone. Inability to void may also reflect high proximal urethral pressure or loss of the reflex urethral relaxation during detrussor contraction. In this situation alpha adrenergic blockade which lowers urethral pressure (phenoxybenzamine 10–50 mg 3–4 × daily) may be of value. Some patients may require combination drug therapy, e.g. if spontaneous bladder contractions are associated with low urethral pressure. Incontinence may require surgical correction if it is associated with a loss of anatomic bladder neck support (retropubic suspension) or low urethral proximal pressure (plication of proximal urethra; Ball procedure). Occasionally, inability to void necessitates management by intermittent self-catheterization on a temporary or longterm basis. The Valsalva and/or Credé maneuvers are often effective in these cases.

In our experience, which reflects the reported experience in general, patients who undergo radical hysterectomy with preservation of the posterior cardinal ligament on at least one side, seldom encounter serious voiding problems provided they are kept on continuous bladder drainage until effective voiding occurs, a minimum of 2 to 3 weeks postoperatively. If both cardinal ligaments are completely transected, serious voiding problems are common. While improvement occurs with time, the loss of sensation, various degrees of incontinence or the need to employ the Valsalva/Credé maneuvers to assist voiding may persist for years or the lifetime of the patient. Rarely a hypertonic, contracted bladder with uncorrectable severe incontinence has required urinary diversion.

Vesicovaginal fistula. Despite the extensive dissection and mobilization of the bladder required for radical hysterectomy, postoperative vesicovaginal fistulas are reported in less than 1% of patients who undergo surgery as the primary therapy.[1,2,24,28,35,44,53] Predisposing factors are seldom reported but conditions which tend to obliterate the cervico-vesico-vaginal plane making dissection difficult are obvious candidates — prior cone biopsy, anterior repair, pelvic cellulitis, low transverse cesarean section. The minority of fistulas result from unrecognized entry into the bladder at the time of surgery. These can be prevented by distending the bladder with methylene blue solution to identify and correct the defect before closing, a prudent procedure in any difficult dissection. Fistulas consequent to trauma, ischemia, sutures, local infection, hematoma, etc. appear 2 to 10 days postoperatively as a rule. Adequate bladder drainage, prophylactic antibiotics and suction drainage of the pelvis (when hemostasis is not tight) may diminish the risk for fistula formation.

The presence of a vesicovaginal fistula rather than a ureterovaginal fistula is readily established by instillation of methylene blue dye solution into the bladder and its immediate appearance on a dry sponge placed in the vagina. Since occasionally both types of urinary tract fistulas may be present, intravenous pyelography and cystoscopy with intravenous indigo carmine or retrograde catheterization of the ureters may be necessary to exclude the additional presence of a ureteral fistula.

Once the diagnosis has been established, it is well to continue catheter drainage, because in an occasional patient spontaneous healing of a tiny fistula may occur (almost always within 30 days), and also to keep the patient as dry and comfortable as possible. When an inlying Foley catheter fails to keep the patient reasonably dry, a plastic vaginal collecting cup is sometimes effective. In general a minimum waiting period of 2 to 3 months will be necessary before local tissue conditions favorable for healing and successful repair are reestablished. While the waiting interval for repair of a fistula after simple hysterectomy is somewhat controversial, it is surely prudent to wait the 2 to 3 months until full recovery of the tissues after radical hysterectomy. Recovery is indicated by absence of infection, necrosis, sutures and minimal evidence of inflammation and edema. The blood supply in these cases is usually good. In this situation, with the typical small fistula at the vaginal apex above the intraureteric ridge, repair can be accomplished in the standard fashion using the Latzko procedure. The occasional case with a pin hole fistula may be cured by fulguration. An abdominal approach is indicated when the vagina will not provide good exposure, for fistulas too near the ureters and for repair of complex fistulas.[25,26,55] For recurrent or large fistulas, as in the case of the post radiation fistulas, more complex repair techniques are required such as use of omentum, bulbocavernosus fat pad or Marshall procedure employing the transperitoneal bladder splitting approach.[12,33,37] Antibiotics, postoperative continuous bladder drainage for 6 to 8 weeks and estrogens are recommended.

UROLOGICAL COMPLICATIONS OF PELVIC EXENTERATION

The types of urologic complications following posterior pelvic exenteration are similar to, but presumably more common, than those occurring after radical hysterectomy. With anterior and total pelvic exenteration, however, the bladder and lower ureters are resected. Thus, the urologic complications are related entirely to the urinary diversion. The most common methods of diversion employ a distal ileal, sigmoid colon or transverse colon segment as a conduit to carry the urine from the ureters to the skin where it is collected in a bag. (See Ch. 81.) Continent urinary diversion, which is becoming more widely used, is discussed in Chapter 88.

Complications of urinary diversion by means of an intestinal conduit are numerous. The most frequently encountered in the postoperative period are pyelonephritis (10%), stomal retraction/necrosis (10%) and conduit leaks (4.5%) based upon 527 cases reported from three institutions.[17,38,49] None of these authors reported an infarction of the conduit. Clearly the most serious of the common complications is the conduit leak which usually develops from the ureteral-intestinal segment anastomosis within 3 weeks postoperatively. It is not clear that the choice of intestinal segment per se is related to the risk of the anastomotic failure, but such a complication is undoubtedly more common when irradiated ureters are implanted into an irradiated intestinal segment. For this reason some authors recommend the transverse colon conduit since the transverse colon is unlikely to have been in the pelvic field of radiation. It is, of course, important to resect the ureters proximal enough to assure good vascularity. Other steps in minimizing the risk of a postoperative conduit leak are the use of ureteral stents, stabilizing the conduit to prevent tension on the anastomosis and performing a technically exact, leak free ureteral anastomosis with minimal trauma to the ureters. A leaking conduit can result in urinary-perineal fistula, urinary-bowel fistula or intraperitoneal retention of urine.

Stoma complications can be minimized by careful attention to certain technical details. Most important is to have sufficient length and mobility of the intestinal segment that it can be brought through the abdominal wall without tension. This is more likely to be a problem in the obese or irradiated patient. A useful technique if the ileal segment is chosen is the loop stoma of Turnbull. Skinner et al[47] recommend this for all ileal conduits. The stoma itself should be everted to form a nipple which protrudes 1–2 cm above the skin. The skin opening and opening through the abdominal wall must not obstruct the free flow of urine, or compromise the mesenteric blood supply. A conduit leak usually presents as low urine output. Management of conduit leak depends upon the patient's condition and the extent of urine loss. In the post-exenteration patient the urine usually makes its way out the perineum so maneuvers to achieve external drainage are unnecessary. Conservative management by catheter drainage of the conduit to intermittent suction often suffices. Radiologic contrast studies (IVP; loopogram) and/or fiberoptic investigation should be undertaken to assess the leak because a detached or infarcted ureter will not respond to conservative therapy. Antegrade stenting by percutaneous nephrostomy has been used successfully.[50]

Operation is required in about half the patients with a post exenteration conduit leak and the mortality rate is over 50%. Thus, the corrective surgery should be the simplest effective procedure. Simple closure of the leak is seldom possible because of the edema, inflammation and friability of the tissues. Ureteral re-implantation may work but temporary proximal diversion and delayed repair are usually preferable.

Late complications increase with duration of follow-up. Reported frequencies are: ureteral stenosis (7%), stomal stenosis requiring repair (5%), recurrent pyelonephritis (12%, including the patients with a history of pyelonephritis), loss of a kidney (3%), kidney and conduit stones, renal failure, and metabolic acidosis.

UROLOGICAL COMPLICATIONS OF RADICAL VULVECTOMY

Significant bladder and ureteral complications are rarely encountered following radical vulvectomy. When the vulvar carcinoma is close enough to the urethral meatus to require resection of the meatus along with 1–2 cm of distal urethra, varying degrees of incontinence can develop, and urethral prolapse may occur. Not uncommonly cystourethrocele and/or rectocele develop to a degree requiring operative repair.

UROLOGICAL COMPLICATONS OF PELVIC RADIATION

General comments

The Patterns of Care Study[18] was carried out under the auspices of the National Cancer Institute to establish a profile of the practice of radiation therapy in the United States. In all, 163 facilities were randomly selected and sample records of cervical cancer patients were reviewed from each institution. Among 706 patients studied, 86 (12%) experienced 159 major complications (defined as requiring hospitalization and or surgery). Thirty (49%) of the major complications were urological, including 8 vesicovaginal fistulas (1.1%), 8 patients with hemorrhagic cystitis, 9 patients with chronic radiation cystitis, one patient with a contracted bladder and four unnamed complications. The rate of complications in this survey most strongly correlated with young age, total central radiation dose and the daily dose of external beam therapy. At institutions treating large numbers of patients, the overall complication rate increased with clinical stage (I = 8%, II = 15%, and III = 25%). (See also Ch. 41.)

Numerous papers have reported individual series of radiation related complications[11,36,52] after therapy for cervical cancer. Perez et al[40] analyzing their experience with 811 patients noted 5% experienced significant (grade 2, 3) urologic injury. The more common were ureteral stricture (1.7%), vesicovaginal fistula (1.1%) and bladder ulcer (0.2%). The most important factor associated with the risk for complications was total dose of irradiation (external beam plus intracavitary). It is generally recognized that the majority of radiation induced bowel injuries appear between 6 and 18 months post therapy. Urologic complications, especially hemorrhagic cystitis, are more likely to appear after a longer interval, even 15 to 20 years post therapy. The average time in the Perez study was 48 months.

Radiation cystitis

Immediate reaction to pelvic irradiation includes the mild cystitis that patients almost uniformly experience during and for a few weeks following therapy. This is due to temporary mucosal inflammation, often with a low-grade secondary infection, and is manifested by urinary frequency, urgency, dysuria, and sometimes acute bacterial cystitis. Symptomatic management employing urinary tract antiseptics or antibiotics and bladder antispasmodics is usually all that is required, but routine periodic urine culture during radiation therapy may be warranted.[4]

Severe radiation cystitis characteristically becomes apparent 6 to 18 months following treatment, by which time deep mucosal ulcerations and submucosal fibrosis are frequently present. These changes are often associated with constant, deep-seated pelvic pain as well as dysuria, hematuria, and secondary bacterial infection. The rigidity of the bladder wall accompanying the mucosal and submucosal changes may also produce disabling urgency and frequency due to the reduced vesical capacity.

Careful urologic investigation by intravenous pyelography and cystoscopy will often be necessary to be certain the symptoms are not due to persistent or recurrent disease rather than radiation cystitis. However, bladder biopsies should be done only when absolutely necessary and then with great care, in order to avoid an iatrogenic fistula. When hematuria is insignificant, moderate degrees of pain, dysuria, frequency, and urgency can usually be managed conservatively with bladder antispasmodics and vigorous antibiotic control of any secondary urinary tract infection.

DeVries & Freiha[8] have recently reviewed the management of hemorrhagic cystitis. Initially, bladder irrigations using water, saline, silver nitrate, alum or aminocaproic acid are employed. When repeated episodes of heavy bleeding occur, more aggressive therapy may become necessary. Transurethral clot evacuation and careful ful-

guration of bleeding sites is occasionally effective. When this and bladder irrigations fail and serious bleeding continues, intravesical instillation under general anesthesia of 10% formalin solution (after excluding reflux) for a period of 4–10 minutes followed by thorough water irrigation and catheter drainage for 3 to 4 days is often effective. Another alternative is selective embolization of branches of the hypogastric arteries, which may, however, in the irradiated patient result in necrosis of the bladder and other pelvic organs. If these maneuvers fail to arrest the hemorrhage, permanent urinary tract diversion, with cystectomy, is usually necessary and may be lifesaving.

For selected patients with a chronically contracted bladder, augmentation cystoplasty is sometimes applicable. Anastomosis between the fundus of the bladder and an isolated segment of ileum or nearby colon with its mesentery intact is carried out to increase the capacity or reservoir function of the damaged bladder. Other alternatives are urinary conduit diversion or continent urostomy. (See Chs 81 and 88.)

Vesicovaginal fistula

Unfortunately, severe radiation cystitis with mucosal and submucosal ulcerations often progresses to vesicovaginal fistula formation. This results from the development of a permanent ischemic fibrosis of the submucosa and mus-

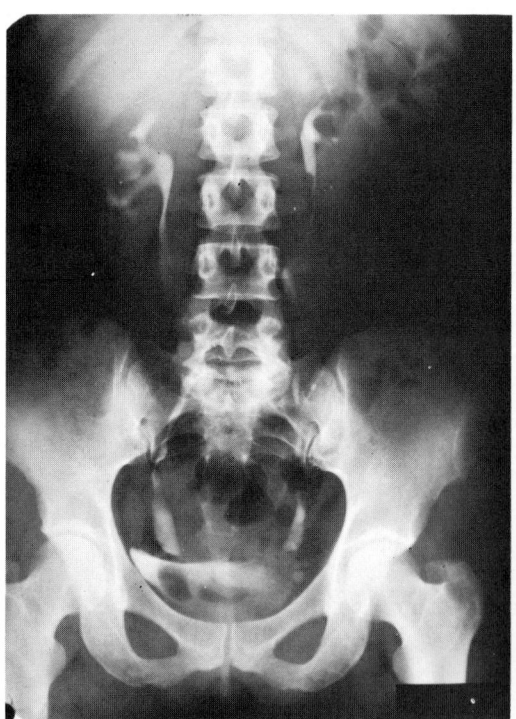
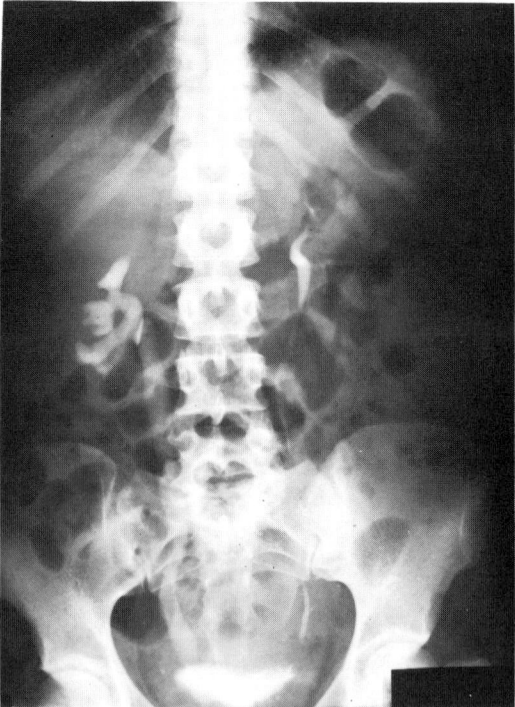

Fig. 85.4 Left: Pretreatment intravenous pyelogram revealing prompt bilateral excretion but slight to moderate bilateral hydronephrosis and hydroureter, most marked on the right. Right: Intravenous pyelogram about 2 years post-radiation therapy and 10 days after the sudden development of vesicovaginal fistula, showing essentially normal function and antomy in the left kidney and ureter, but persistence of and slight increase in the right-sided hydroureter with slight hydronephrosis. (Reproduced from: Green T H Jr 1981 Urological complications of radical pelvic surgery and radiation therapy. In: Coppleson M (ed) Gynecologic Oncology. Churchill Livingstone, Edinburgh.)

cular layers of the organs involved, often accompanied by local areas of deep ulceration or even complete necrosis of the entire bladder wall and vagina in the area where the maximal amount of radiation was absorbed. Fistulas, like hemorrhagic cystitis, may occur as early as 3 to 6 months from the time therapy is completed, or may be delayed for many years (Fig. 85.4). The diagnosis is usually immediately obvious, but once again it is important to rule in or out the possibility of persistent or recurrent malignancy, since its presence and extent would have an important bearing on the manner in which the fistula would best be handled. A significant number, perhaps 25 to 30%, of patients with radiation-induced vesicovaginal fistulas will also develop a rectovaginal fistula, the latter appearing either simultaneously or within a few months of the former (Fig. 85.5).

Because of their usual large size, the poor blood supply and limited mobility of adjacent tissues, radiation-induced vesicovaginal fistulas can rarely be managed by standard techniques of simple closure, even after an interval of several years. Our own experience is in agreement with that reported by Boronow,[5] to the effect that, at best, it is ultimately possible to achieve closure in properly selected radiation-induced vesicovaginal fistulas only 30 to 50% of the time. This can most often be accomplished in the patient with a brachytherapy injury. Even in this fortunate group, closure usually can be accomplished only by complete colpocleisis. However, small fistulas, especially those

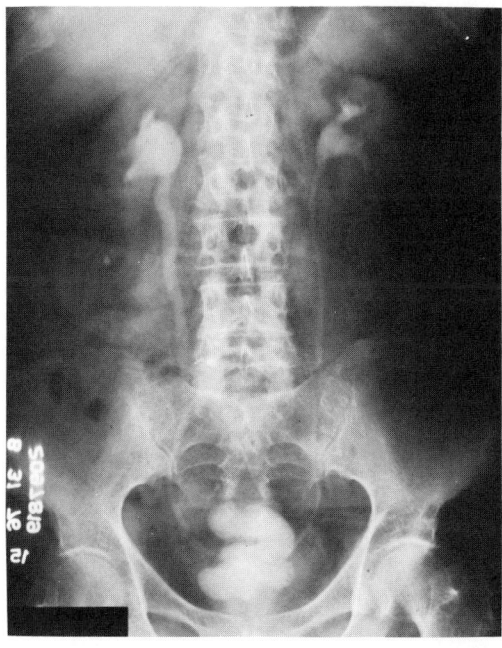

Fig. 85.5   Intravenous pyelogram showing contrast material filling the rectum as well as draining into the vagina; there is also mild dilatation of the right ureter. (Reproduced from: Green T H Jr 1981 Urological complications of radical pelvic surgery and radiation therapy. In: Coppleson M (ed) Gynecologic Oncology. Churchill Livingstone, Edinburgh.)

arising after combined radiation and surgery, can sometimes be closed. A much longer time interval must elapse before optimal tissue conditions prevail, and attempted repair should be delayed a minimum of 6 to 8 months, and sometimes much longer. Usually urinary diversion is required to alleviate pain and stop the necrosis. Because the local tissues are poorly vascularized and fibrotic, the repair must be buttressed by well-vascularized tissue such as a Martius bulbocavernosus pedicle graft from beneath the labium majus. When necessary, bilateral Martius grafts can be done, and for larger defects, or when the bulbocavernosus fat pads have also been damaged by radiation, gracilis, rectus abdominis or other muscles can be employed. Another option is an omental segment which can be mobilized transabdominally and then brought down to reinforce the fistula repair.

In the remaining 50 to 70% of women with radiation induced vesicovaginal fistulas, the defects are just too large and local tissue conditions so hopelessly poor that closure is impossible. Urinary tract diversion is the proper treatment for these patients and for those in whom fistula repair is unsuccessful. The serious morbidity of the diverting procedure is low, the long-term results in terms of preservation of normal renal function are excellent, and the patients are extremely grateful for the complete and permanent relief from the fistulous drainage and pain.

Even in the presence of known recurrence of malignant disease, urinary tract diversion for radiation-induced vesicovaginal fistula should be strongly considered, since it provides such worthwhile and often long-term comfort and convenience for the patient. Many of these patients come to surgery in the hope that cure by pelvic exenteration can still be accomplished. If the findings are such that even total pelvic exenteration would not be potentially curative, a palliative ileal loop should nevertheless be done.

Ureteral complications

Ureteral injury may be due to localized intrinsic damage to the mucosa and muscular wall, or more often it may be secondary to a more diffuse periureteral fibrosis resulting from extensive postinflammatory scarring of the retroperitoneal connective tissue with subsequent constriction of the ureter (Figs 85.6 and 85.7). Periureteral fibrosis following radiotherapy appears to occur with greatest frequency in patients who also have had pelvic inflammatory disease. Ureteral obstruction due to radiation fibrosis may appear as early as 5 to 6 months after treatment or be delayed as long as 5 years, but most commonly develops 18 to 24 months after completion of therapy. The usual site of obstruction is about 4–6 cm above the ureterovesical junction where the ureter lies closest to the cervix. Less often submucosal fibrosis in the region of the bladder trigone may affect only the intramural portion of the ureter.

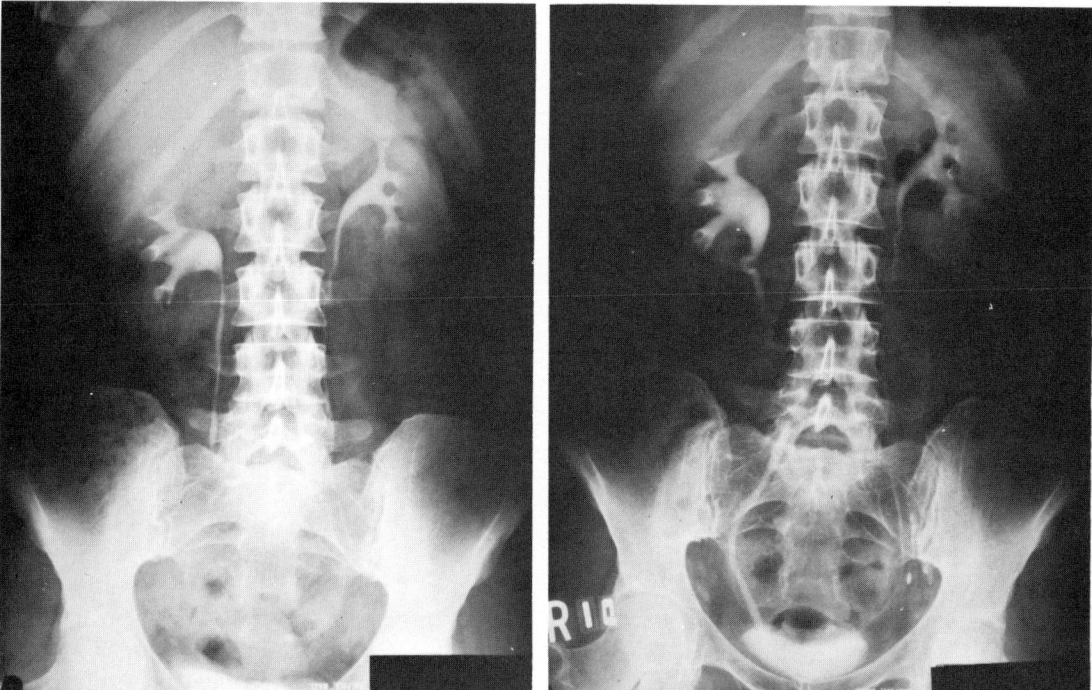

Fig. 85.6 Left: Pretreatment intravenous pyelogram showing normal kidneys, ureters, and bladder. Right: Intravenous pyelogram 5½ months following completion of radiotherapy, revealing a partially obstructed right ureter with slight dilatation above the point of obstruction. (Reproduced from: Green T H Jr 1981 Urological complications of radical pelvic surgery and radiation therapy. In: Coppleson M (ed) Gynecologic Oncology. Churchill Livingstone, Edinburgh.)

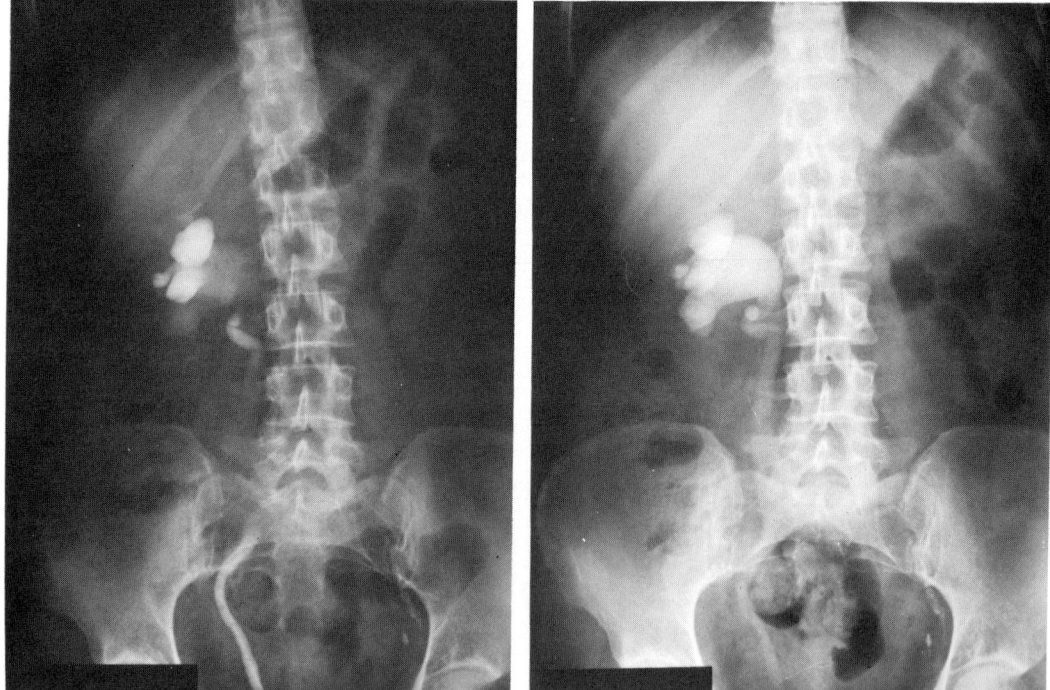

Fig. 85.7 Same patient as in Figure 85.6. Léft: Right retrograde pyelogram demonstrating obstruction just proximal to the right ureterovesical junction with resulting moderate ureteral dilatation and mild hydronephrosis. Right: Post-drainage 75 minutes after completion of right retrograde pyelography, showing marked delay in the drainage of contrast material and moderate hydronephrosis and hydroureter. (Reproduced from: Green T H Jr 1981 Urological complications of radical pelvic surgery and radiation therapy. In: Coppleson M (ed) Gynecologic Oncology. Churchill Livingstone, Edinburgh.)

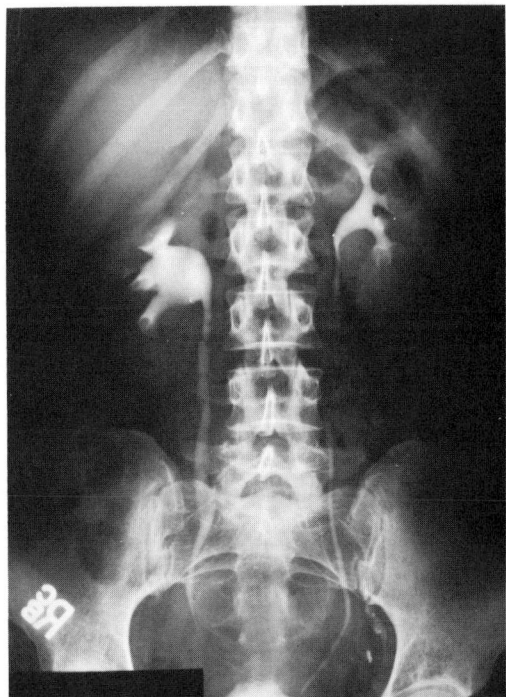 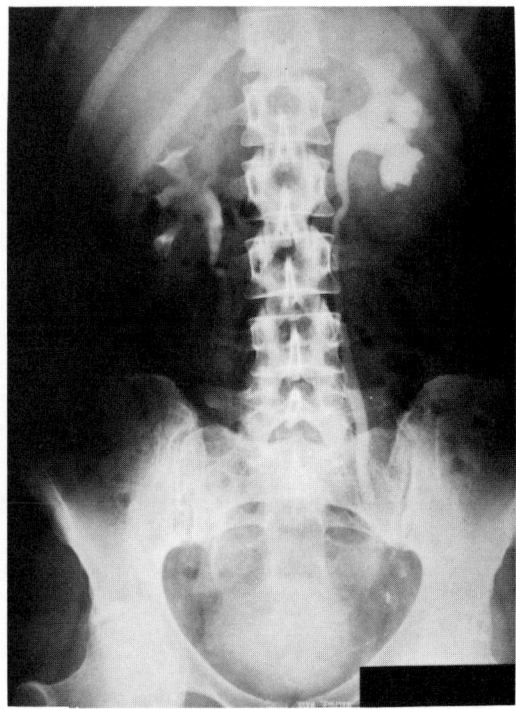

Fig. 85.8 Same patient as in Figures 85.6 and 85.7. Left: Intravenous pyelogram 9 days following right ureteroneocystostomy, revealing prompt excretion on the right side with no residual ureteral narrowing, hydroureter, or hydronephrosis. Right: Most recent intravenous pyelogram 21 months following right ureteroneocystostomy, revealing normal anatomy and function on the right, but narrowing of the lower left ureter with moderate proximal hydroureter and slight hydronephrosis consistent with periureteral fibrosis on the left side. Because she is completely asymptomatic at present, the patient has so far been reluctant to undergo any further investigation, but the situation is being followed closely. (Reproduced from: Green T H Jr 1981 Urological complications of radical pelvic surgery and radiation therapy. In: Coppleson M (ed) Gynecologic Oncology. Churchill Livingstone, Edinburgh.)

Mild to moderate ureteral obstruction during or early after radiation therapy may improve spontaneously, but progressive stenosis should be treated by double-J stents. Surgical exploration is often indicated to determine if the ureteral obstruction is secondary to recurrent disease or to radiation-induced fibrosis. The former is nearly always the cause unless the patient had previous surgery or an unusually high radiation dose.

In the presence of ureteral obstruction due to relatively localized fibrosis, mobilization of the involved segment of ureter and wrapping it in omentum may correct the problem. More often, however, reimplantation of the proximal normal ureter by ureteroneocystostomy or ileal interposition will be the procedure of choice (Fig. 85.8). In the case of bilateral ureteral obstruction not amenable to ureteroneocystostomy or ileal interposition, ileal loop urinary diversion may be the best alternative.

Note

The authors are indebted to Thomas H. Green, Jr. who wrote this chapter for the first edition of this book. Much of his chapter has been retained as the basis for this revision. R.I.P.

C. Paul Morrow, M.D.
John P. Curtin, M.D.

REFERENCES

1. Allen H H, Nisker J A, Anderson R J 1982 Primary surgical treatment in 195 cases of Stage Ib carcinoma of the cervix. Am J Obstet Gynecol 143: 581
2. Artman L E, Barnhill D R, Bibro M C, Heller P B, Hoskins W J, Park R C, Weiser E B 1987 Radical hysterectomy and pelvic lymphadenectomy for Stage Ib carcinoma of the cervix: 21 years experience. Gynecol Oncol 23: 8
3. Barclay D L, Roman-Lopez J J 1975 Bladder dysfunction after Schauta hysterectomy. Am J Obstet Gynecol 123: 519
4. Bialas I, Bessel E M, Sokal M, Slack R 1989 A prospective study of urinary tract infection during pelvic radiotherapy. Radiotherapy Oncology 16: 305
5. Boronow R C 1986 Repair of the radiation-induced vaginal fistula utilizing the Martius technique. World J Surgery 10: 237
6. Brunswick A, Frick H C II 1956 Urinary tract fistulas following radical surgical treatment of carcinoma of the cervix. Am J Obstet Gynecol 72: 479
7. Carenza L, Nobili F, Giacobini S 1982 Voiding disorders after radical hysterectomy. Gynecol Oncol 13: 213
8. DeVries C R, Freiha F S 1990 Hemorrhagic cystitis: A review. J Urol 14: 1

9. Dowling R A, Corriere J N Jr, Sandler C M 1986 Iatrogenic ureteral injury. J Urol 135: 912

10. Ehrlich R M, Melman A, Skinner D G 1978 The use of vesico-psoas hitch in urologic surgery. J Urol 119: 322

11. Einhorn N, Patek E, Sjoberg B 1985 Outcome of different treatment modalities in cervix carcinoma Stage Ib and IIa. Cancer 55: 949

12. Elkins T E, Delancey J O L, McGuire E J 1990 The use of modified Martius graft as an adjunctive technique in vesicovaginal and rectovaginal fistula repair. Am J Obstet Gynecol 75: 727

13. Farquharson D I M, Shingleton H M, Orr J W Jr, Hatch K D, Hester S, Soong S-J 1987 The short-term effect of radical hysterectomy on urethral and bladder function. Br J Obstet Gynaecol 94: 351

14. Forney J P 1980 The effects of radical hysterectomy on bladder physiology. Am J Obstet Gynecol 138: 374

15. Gal D, Buchsbaum H J 1983 A cinefluoroscopic study of ureteral function following radical hysterectomy. Obstet Gynecol 61: 82

16. Green T H Jr, Meigs J V, Ulfelder H, Curtin R R 1962 Urologic complications of radical Wertheim hysterectomy: Incidence, etiology, management and prevention. Am J Obstet Gynecol 20: 293

17. Hancock K C, Copeland L J, Gershenson D M, Saul P B, Wharton J T, Rutledge F N 1986 Urinary conduits in gynecologic oncology. Obstet Gynecol 67: 680

18. Hanks G E, Herring D F, Kramer S 1983 Patterns of care outcome studies: Results of the national practice in cancer of the cervix. Cancer 51: 959

19. Hansen M K 1980 Surgical and combination therapy of cancer of the cervix uteri: Stages Ib and IIa. Obstet Gynecol 11: 275

20. Hinman F 1976 Postoperative overdistension of the bladder. Surg Gynecol Obstet 142: 901

21. Hirsh M 1985 Enhanced ascites: CT sign of ureteral fistula. J Computer Assisted Tomography 9: 825

22. Hoskins W J, Ford H J, Lutz M H, Averette H E 1976 Radical hysterectomy and pelvic lymphadenectomy for management of early invasive cancer of the cervix. Gynecol Oncol 4: 272

22a. Huffman J L, Bagley D H, Lyon E S 1982 Ureteroscopy. Saunders, Philadelphia

23. Kadar N, Nelson J H 1984 Treatment of urinary incontinence after radical hysterectomy. Obstet Gynecol 64: 400

24. Kajanoja P, Raisanen I, Lehtovirta P 1985 Wertheim radical hysterectomy. Obstet Gynecol 74: 94

25. Latzko W 1942 Postoperative vesicovaginal fistulas. Am J Surg 58: 211

26. Lee R A, Symmonds R E, Williams T J 1988 Current status of genitourinary fistula. Obstet Gynecol 72: 313

27. Lee R B, Park R C 1981 Bladder dysfunction following radical abdominal hysterectomy. Gynecol Oncol 11: 304

28. Lerner H M, Howard W J, Hill E C 1980 Radical surgery for the treatment of early invasive cervical carcinoma (Stage Ib): Review of 15 years' experience. Obstet Gynecol 56: 413

29. Low J A, Mauger G M, Carmichael J A 1981 The effect of Wertheim hysterectomy upon bladder and urethral function. Am J Obstet Gynecol 139: 826

30. Macasaet M A, Lu T, Nelson J H Jr 1976 Ureterovaginal fistula as a complication of radical pelvic surgery. Am J Obstet Gynecol 124: 757

31. Malik M K B 1960 A study of the ureters following Wertheim's hysterectomy. J Obstet Gynaecol Br Emp 67: 556

32. Mann W J, Arato M, Patsner B, Stone M L 1988 Ureteral injuries in an obstetrics and gynecology training program: Etiology and management. Obstet Gynecol 72: 82

33. Marshall V F 1979 Vesicovaginal fistulas on one urological service. J Urol 121: 25

34. Marziale P, Atlante G, Le Pera V, Marino T, Pozzi M, Iacovelli 1981 A combined radiation and surgical treatment of Stages Ib and IIa and IIb carcinoma of the cervix. Gynecol Oncol 11: 175

35. Mattsson T 1975 Frequency and management of urological and some other complications following radical surgery for carcinoma of the cervix uteri, Stages I and II. Acta Obstet Gynecol Scand 54: 271

36. Montana G S, Fowler W C, Varia M A, Walton L A, Mack Y 1985 Analysis of results of radiation therapy for Stage II carcinoma of the cervix. Cancer 55: 956

37. O'Connor V J Jr 1980 Review of experience with vesicovaginal fistula repair. J Urol 123: 367

38. Orr J W Jr, Shingleton H M, Hatch K D, Taylor P T, Austin J M Jr, Partridge E E, Soong S J 1982 Urinary diversion in patients undergoing pelvic exenteration. Am J Obstet Gynecol 142: 883

39. Ostergard D R 1979 The effect of drugs on the lower urinary tract. Obstet Gynecol Surv 34: 424

40. Perez C A, Breaux S, Bedwinek J M, Madoc-Jones H, Camel H M, Purdy J A, Waltz B J 1984 Radiation therapy alone in the treatment of carcinoma of the uterine cervix. Cancer 54: 235

41. Pettit P D 1989 Double-J ureteral catheters in gynecologic surgery. Obstet Gynecol 73: 536

42. Podratz K C, Angerman N S, Symmonds R E 1982 Complications of ureteral surgery in the nonradiated patient. In: Delgado G, Smith J P (eds) Management of Complications in Gynecologic Oncology. Wiley & Sons, New York, p 113

43. Roman-Lopez J J, Barclay D L 1973 Bladder dysfunction following Schauta hysterectomy. Am J Obstet Gynecol 115: 81

44. Sall S, Pineda A A, Calango A, Heller P, Greenberg H 1979 Surgical treatment of Stages Ib and IIa invasive carcinoma of the cervix by radical abdominal hysterectomy. Am J Obstet Gynecol 135: 442

45. Sasaki H, Yoshida T, Noda K, Yachiku S, Minami K, Kaneko S 1982 Urethral pressure profiles following radical hysterectomy. Obstet Gynecol 59: 101

46. Seski J C, Diokno A C 1977 Bladder dysfunction after radical abdominal hysterectomy. Am J Obstet Gynecol 128: 643

47. Skinner D G, Lieskovsky G, Skinner E C, Boyd S D 1987 Urinary diversion. Current Problems in Surgery 24: 407

48. Smith P H, Ballantyne B 1968 The neuroanatomical basis for denervation of the urinary bladder following major pelvic surgery. Br J Surg 55: 929

49. Stanhope C R, Symmonds R E, Lee R A, Williams T J, Podratz K C, O'Brien P C 1986 Urinary diversion with use of ileal and sigmoid conduits. Am J Obstet Gynecol 155: 288

50. Stern J L, Maroney T P, Lacey C 1987 Treatment of urinary conduit fistula by antegrade ureteral stent catheter. Obstet Gynecol 70: 276

51. Symmonds R E 1976 Ureteral injuries associated with gynecologic surgery: Prevention and management. Clin Obstet Gynecol 19: 623

52. Unal A, Hamberger A D, Seski J C, Fletcher G H 1981 An analysis of the severe complications of irradiation of carcinoma of the uterine cervix: Treatment with intracavitary radium and parametrial irradiation. Int J Radiat Oncol Biol Phys 7: 999

53. Webb M J, Symmonds R E 1979 Wertheim hysterectomy: A reappraisal. Obstet Gynecol 54: 140

54. Witters S, Cornelissen M, Vereecken R 1986 Iatrogenic ureteral injury: Aggressive or conservative treatment. Am J Obstet Gynecol 155: 582

55. Tancer M L 1980 The post-total hysterectomy (vault) vesicovaginal fistula. J Urol 123: 839

86. Intestinal complications of radiation therapy of pelvic malignancy

C. R. Wheeless Jr

INTRODUCTION

When pelvic malignancy is treated by irradiation, the incidence of intestinal injury is 15 to 25%. About 1 to 5% of irradiated patients have injuries severe enough to require surgical treatment.[3,6,7,13,15] This type of intestinal injury is unique, and is associated with high morbidity and mortality. Its successful therapy demands a thorough understanding of its pathophysiology, special clinical presentation, and surgical features.

PATHOPHYSIOLOGY

Several factors are involved in the pathophysiology of these injuries. These include: (1) altered anatomical position of the small bowel, and (2) encasement of intestines within a tumor mass. These factors are present in many gynecologic oncology patients requiring radiation therapy. Ionizing radiation alters both the macro- and the microcirculation of irradiated tissues. Photons passing through the nucleus of a cell produce free radicals of $H+$ and $OH-$ and disrupt the orderly mitosis of the nucleus and ultimate division of the cell. Severe endarteritis (Fig. 86.1) is common, producing ischemia and extensive tissue fibrosis both of which retard the basic chemistry and physiology of wound healing.[3,6,7] Irradiation damage to the intestine occurs most often in the rectosigmoid colon, and the terminal ileum. Clinically these injuries present as inflammatory disease in these sites. Enterovaginal fistulae, and intestinal obstruction may occur in extreme cases. While fistulae occur most frequently in the rectum, bowel obstruction appears more often in the terminal ileum. However, fistulae may occur

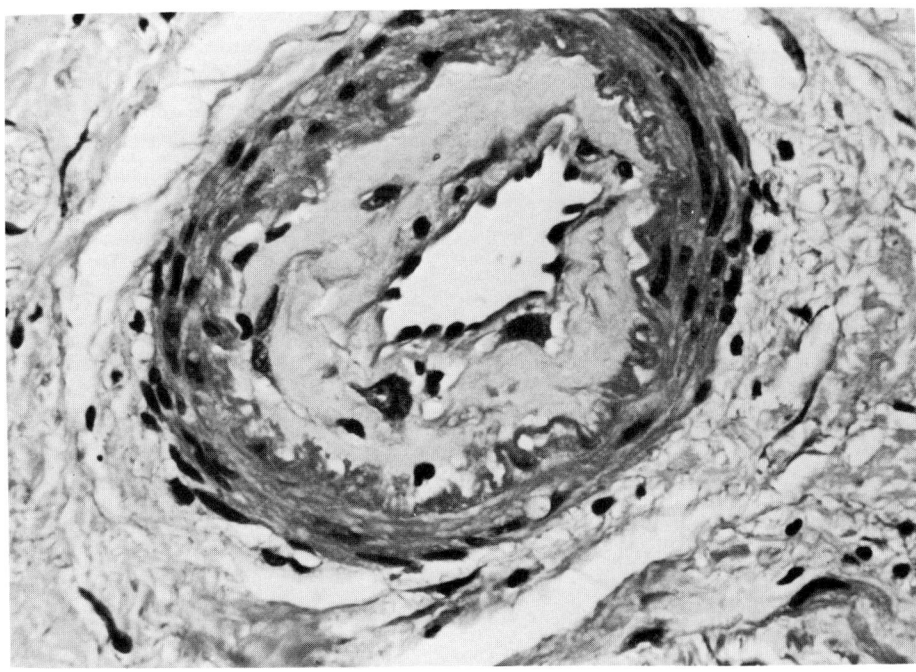

Fig. 86.1 Photograph of irradiation endarteritis showing subendothelial fibrosis and partial obliteration of the arterial lumen.

between the terminal ileum, vagina, bladder or rectum (compound fistulae).

PREVENTION

Prevention of radiation therapy injuries to the intestine demands a thorough knowledge of radiation biology and of the unique clinical and physical presentation of these patients. A past history of severe pelvic infections and/or multiple pelvic laparotomies should alert the gynecologist and radiation oncologist to the potential for high risk of bowel injury from pelvic irradiation. A history of inflammatory bowel disease (IBD) or diverticulitis signals possible added risk for ileal, colonic, or rectal injury from pelvic irradiation.

Once the gynecologic oncology patient has been identified as high risk for radiation intestinal injury, prevention may follow three routes: (1) imaging the small bowel through an X-ray upper gastrointestinal (G.I.) series with small bowel follow through while planning irradiation ports; (2) adjusting daily fractionalization doses through each selected port to minimize intestinal irradiation; (3) in extreme cases the use of other strategies to minimize intestinal irradiation injury including (a) exploratory laparotomy and lysis of adhesions with instillation of chemical compounds that reduce adhesion formation such as low density dextran (Hiscon), and, at laparotomy, suspension of the small bowel by 'slings' of synthetic absorbable mesh, (b) administration of radioprotective drugs such as free radical scavengers such as glutathione and WR 2721.[8] Prospective randomized trials are needed to demonstrate scientific efficacy of these procedures and drugs.

DIAGNOSIS

Early and accurate diagnosis of irradiation injury to the bowel is important. Fistulae can be multiple, and an erroneous diagnosis can lead to improper management. The most common presenting complaint of a patient with a fistula of the terminal ileum is a yellow watery vaginal discharge that produces excoriation of and extreme pain in the vulva secondary to the digestive enzymes in small bowel secretions. The pH of this discharge is alkaline (Fig. 86.2). X-ray examination of the small intestine, using dilute barium solution, can often delineate the fistula, and it may demonstrate other fistulae of the colon or rectum.

Patients with an enterovaginal fistula of the rectum or the sigmoid colon complain of passing flatus through the vagina and a brownish vaginal discharge mixed with stool. The pH of this discharge is usually neutral, but is sometimes acid. These patients have little if any pain from digestion of the vulva as there are few digestive enzymes in the stool of the rectum. Accurate diagnosis can be ob-

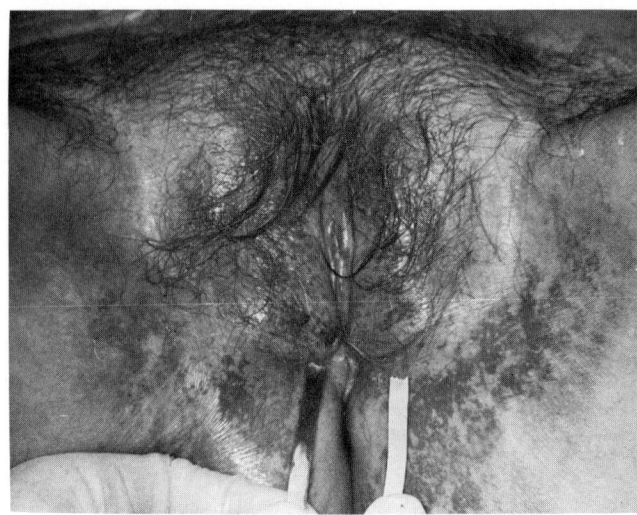

Fig. 86.2 Photograph of vulvar excoriation with alkaline pH of the vaginal discharge with a small bowel vaginal fistula.

tained by sigmoidoscopy and X-ray examination using an enema of dilute barium solution.

If the fistulous tract of the small or large bowel can be visualized per vagina, a small catheter can be inserted and injected with radiologic contrast medium to give roentgenographic evidence of the fistula and possible involvement of other loops of bowel or bladder (compound fistulae).

Obstruction of the terminal ileum is often only a partial obstruction, giving postprandial crampy abdominal pain and mild to moderate nausea and some vomiting, but allowing most patients to take a liquid or semi-solid diet. These patients often have diarrhea rather than obstipation. Abdominal distension is intermittent and depends upon the degree of obstruction. Complete intestinal obstruction of the terminal ileum gives the classical signs of nausea, vomiting, abdominal distension, and obstipation. Obstruction in the rectosigmoid colon generally produces a watery diarrhea, abdominal distension and, later, fecal vomiting.

Diagnostic aids in demonstrating obstruction of the terminal ileum include: supine and upright X-rays of the abdomen and instillation of a small amount of water soluble X-ray contrast medium through a long nasointestinal tube (Cantor tube).[2,16] Barium should be avoided. Water soluble X-ray contrast media may demonstrate not only the site of partial obstruction but will frequently identify that portion of irradiated bowel most likely to become obstructed in the future. Passage of a long tube (Cantor) is helpful in those patients in whom there is enough intestinal peristalsis to advance the tube into the jejunum or proximal ileum. Cases of mild partial obstruction will often be temporarily resolved by decompression with a Cantor tube. Although this decompression of the small bowel may sometimes postpone surgery and allow better metabolic and nutritional stabilization of the patient, rarely does it eliminate the need for operative treatment because of the unique progressive pathophysiology of irradiation injuries as opposed to obstruction secondary to operative adhesions.

TREATMENT OF IRRADIATION INJURIES OF THE ILEUM

The management priority for patients with intestinal obstruction or fistula should first be medical and then surgical. These patients rarely have bowel necrosis that demands immediate surgical exploration. The patients are often in a debilitated state with anemia, acid-base and electrolyte abnormalities, and malnutrition, making them poor surgical risks. Their therapy should start with the correction of as many of these abnormalities as possible. In patients with fistula of the terminal ileum, time spent in correcting nutritional and metabolic deficiencies will improve the postoperative course. A long (Cantor) nasointestinal tube should be passed. The patient's serum electrolytes should be corrected, and blood transfusions administered if anemia is present. A central venous catheter should be inserted for the administration of an intravenous hyperalimentation diet (TPN) (see p. 1349). Prior to the availability of such diets, these patients were operated upon as soon as the anemia, electrolytes, and the acid-base problems were corrected. Today, surgery is delayed for 1 to 3 weeks in patients without evidence of intestinal necrosis and who are nutritionally debilitated to allow intravenous hyperalimentation therapy to improve their nutritional status.

In some patients an ileovaginal fistula from irradiation

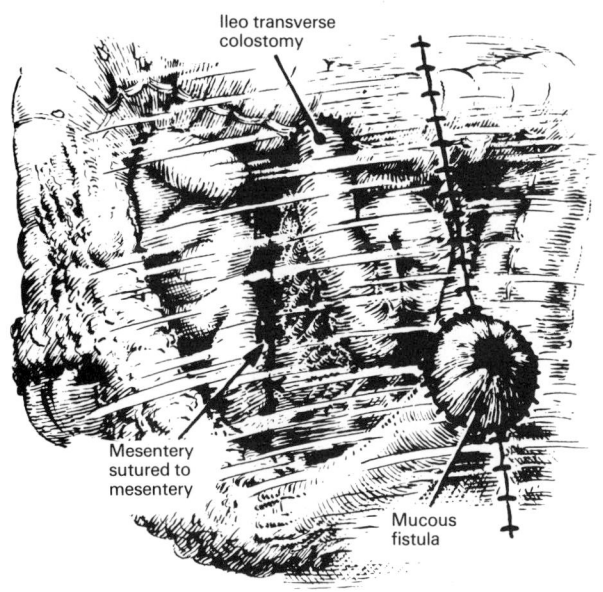

Ileo transverse colostomy

Mesentery sutured to mesentery

Mucous fistula

Fig. 86.3 Drawing of small bowel bypass procedure leaving the pathology (fistula-obstruction, etc.) within the pelvis, exteriorizing an ileal mucous fistula and performing an ileo-transverse colostomy. (Courtesy, Wheeless C R *Atlas of Pelvic Surgery*. Lea & Febiger, 1980.)

will spontaneously close following intestinal suction with a long (Cantor) tube and an intravenous hyperalimentation diet. However, among five cases of spontaneous fistula closure in our clinic, two reopened within 3 to 5 weeks after discontinuance of intestinal suction, and resumption of a regular diet. The intestinal wall in these cases was severely compromised by a combination of irradiation, inflammation, and scarring from fistula formation. Moreover, many patients with an ileovaginal fistula have some degree of partial intestinal obstruction distal to the site of fistula. Therefore, it is not surprising that a number of them do not respond to this conservative medical therapy.

Surgical correction of a small intestine fistula should involve intestinal bypass or radical resection rather than segmental intestinal resection and end-to-end anastomosis.[1,6,7,16] These fistulae are frequently deeply embedded in the true pelvis, with dense adhesions of the bowel to the irradiated fibrotic pelvic walls. Dissection and mobilization of such intestinal adhesions frequently result in multiple enterotomies and spillage of intestinal contents. In addition, intestinal suture lines become adherent to the irradiated pelvic walls resulting in recurrence of fistula formation and obstruction. The bypass procedure can often avoid these problems.

The bypass procedure of choice is ileo-transverse colostomy (Fig. 86.3). No attempt is made to dissect the fistula site or to resect the multiple loops of adherent bowel in the pelvis. The ileum is divided above the fistula taking care to allow enough mobility of the distal fistula bearing segment of ileum to permit its exteriorization as a mucous fistula.

Frequently, with extensive irradiation, the proximal ileum and the transverse colon are the only available non-irradiated intestine with unquestionable vascular integrity.

A second strategy may be used if the patient is in excellent health and a good candidate for surgery. It consists of radical terminal ileectomy, right colectomy, and enterotransverse colostomy. This procedure is aided by construction of an omental 'carpet' to the pelvic floor as an omentopexy. Advantages of this approach include (a) removal of all diseased bowel; (b) no mucous fistula-ostomy on the abdominal wall; (c) anastomosis of non-irradiated proximal ileum or distal jejunum to non-irradiated transverse colon. Disadvantages of this technique are (a) large denuded, irradiated area in the pelvis, in spite of the omental 'carpet' in the pelvis, with the possible increased chance of recurrent intestinal obstruction; (b) increased length of operating time compared to the bypass procedure in a compromised patient; (c) loss of terminal ileum for absorption of fat soluble vitamins, vitamin B-12 and bile salts, resulting in loose watery stools.

Either of these two options is superior to segmental resection of the irradiated bowel with attempted ileo-ileal anastomosis embedded deep in the pelvis.[14]

Surgical technique — general

Few situations in the practice of pelvic surgery demand more attention to detail, surgical expertise, and delicate surgical technique than the operative correction of intestinal complications of pelvic irradiation.

A lower midline abdominal incision usually extended around the umbilicus is preferred for all cases because a lower transverse abdominal incision does not afford adequate access to the ascending and transverse colon. Occasionally, the safest and easiest place for entry into the abdomen after extensive pelvic irradiation, and previous radical surgery, is the upper midline with extension of the incision downward as far as needed.

Because the majority of intestinal abnormalities associated with gynecologic disease occur in the terminal ileum, this is the area to explore first. However exploration of the entire bowel from the ligament of Treitz to the rectum is desirable unless the patient is medically compromised and a bypass with enterotransverse colostomy is indicated. Dilated loops of small intestine are usually found proximal to the area of obstruction or fistula, and defunctionalized loops of terminal ileum with a smaller diameter are likely distal to the site of bowel injury.

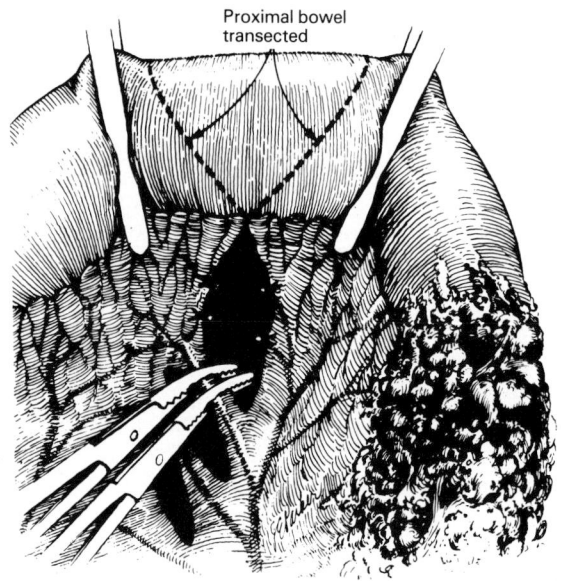

Fig. 86.4 Drawing of small bowel transection technique. The small bowel is transected in an oblique manner to ensure maximum vascular supply to the antimesenteric border. The segment of bowel on the right containing the pathology will be exteriorized as the mucous fistula. (Courtesy, Wheeless C R *Atlas of Pelvic Surgery*, Lea & Febiger, 1980.)

Technique for small bowel bypass

After satisfactory sites for division of the ileum have been selected, a healthy free piece of proximal ileum is elevated. The mesentery is transilluminated and the arcade of vessels is identified. The peritoneum overlying the mesentery is incised on both sides with a sharp scalpel.[18] Small hemostats are used to open avascular spaces in the mesentery. One centimeter segments of mesentery are cross clamped and tied with number 4/0 synthetic absorbable suture. Linen shod intestinal clamps are placed across the intestine 6 to 8 cm on each side of the intended point of transection (Fig. 86.4). Crushing clamps should not be used on irradiated bowel with its compromised microcirculation for fear of further injuring the blood supply to the anastomosis. The jaws of the linen shod clamps are closed just enough to block the lumen of the bowel but never more than one notch of the ratchet handles for fear of damaging the delicate intestinal blood supply. The bowel is transected in an oblique manner (Fig. 86.4). Transection is made by a scalpel or scissors rather than by electric cautery to avoid thermal injury at the site of the anastomosis.[18]

Anastomosis of the proximal ileum to the transverse colon can be accomplished by two acceptable techniques in irradiated bowel; the Gambee single layer technique or the surgical stapler technique. Both have been shown to have greater blood flow to the anastomosis than the standard two layer technique. The Gambee through-and-through anastomosis technique is a more physiologic method of bowel anastomosis than the classical multi-layer tech-

niques.[4,5,7,9,10,18] We prefer 3/0 synthetic absorbable suture on an atraumatic needle. The anastomosis is begun on the mesenteric border (Fig. 86.5 (3)) with a Lembert inverting suture into the submucosa of each side of the ileum and transverse colon. The anastomosis is inverted as the suture is tied (Fig. 86.5 (4)). Gambee sutures are placed at 3 to 5 mm intervals around the entire circumference of the anastomosis (Fig. 86.5 (5)). The Gambee suture starts on the mucosa, perforates all layers of the bowel and exits the serosa. It re-enters the serosa of the opposite bowel and exits the mucosa. When tied it inverts the bowel. The last suture on the antimesenteric border is a near-far inverting suture (Fig. 86.6 (a and b)). This is begun on the serosal surface approximately 7 to 8 mm from the edge of the anastomosis and passes through the entire bowel wall. The needle then re-enters the mucosal surface of the same-side approximately 2 to 3 mm from the edge, traverses the entire bowel wall, and emerges on the serosal surface. It is then passed through the serosal surface of the opposite side approximately 3 mm from the edge and through the entire bowel wall into the bowel lumen. It is returned through the mucosal surface approximately 7 to 8 mm from the edge and passes through the entire bowel wall to emerge on the serosal surface (Fig. 86.6 (b)). When tied, this near-far suture creates further inversion of the intestine.[17]

After the anastomosis is complete, the diameter is checked by placing the forefinger and thumb on opposite sides of the anastomosis and palpating the opening. Several Lembert sutures may be placed through the serosa and

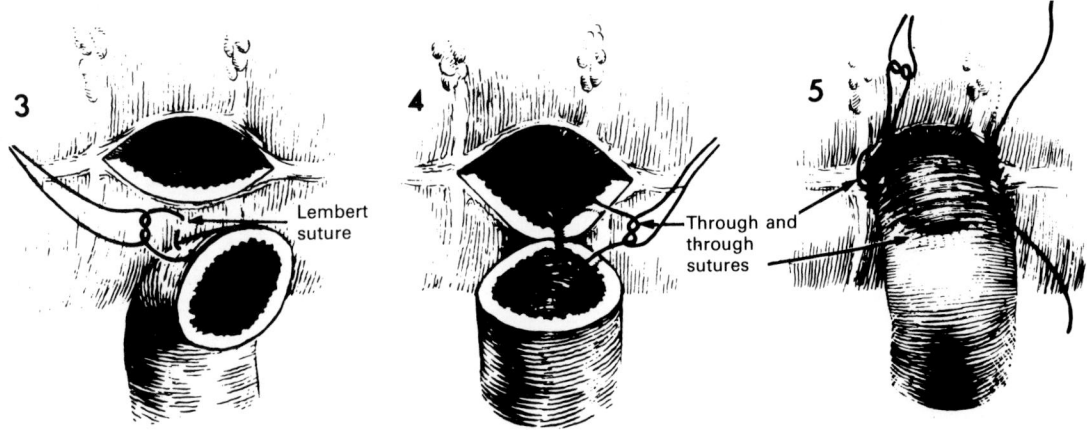

Fig. 86.5 A drawing of the Gambee technique (3–4–5) for intestinal anastomosis using a single layer through and through 3/0 chromic stitch. (3) A Lembert suture is placed 5–6 mm from the edge of the intestine. (4) The Gambee suture is passed through all layers of intestine, and the knot is tied within the lumen of the bowel. (5) Gambee sutures are placed every 3–4 mm around the intended anastomosis. (Courtesy, Wheeless C R *Atlas of Pelvic Surgery*, Lea & Febiger, 1980.)

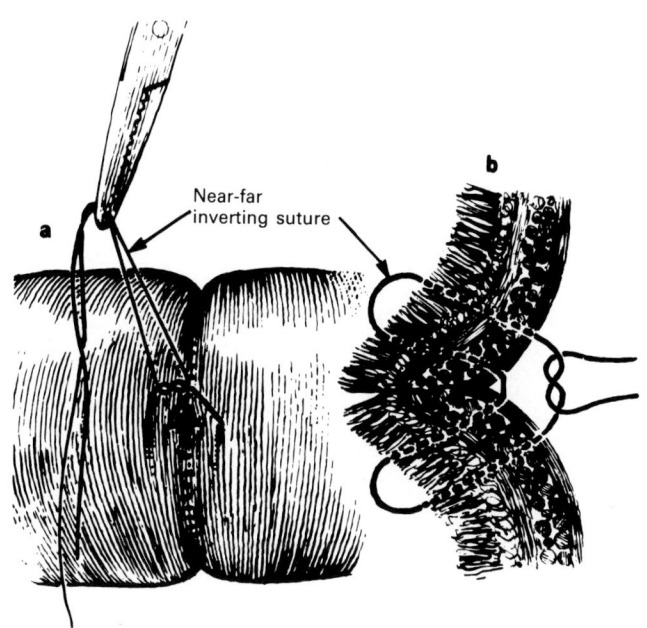

Fig. 86.6 A drawing of the 'near-far inverting suture'. (Courtesy, Wheeless C R *Atlas of Pelvic Surgery*, Lea & Febiger, 1988.)

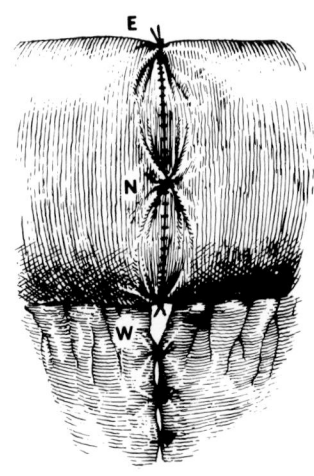

Fig. 86.7 A drawing of the completed Gambee anastomosis. Several Lembert sutures have been placed N-E-W and S to take tension off the suture line. (Courtesy, Wheeless C R *Atlas of Pelvic Surgery*, Lea & Febiger, 1980).

muscularis around the anastomosis, 3 cm apart, to further invert the anastomosis and take tension off the Gambee suture line (Fig. 86.7). The mesentery is closed with interrupted fine sutures to prevent internal hernia.

A contemporary method of intestinal anastomosis that has become popular is the use of autosuture stapling devices.[12] The stapled anastomosis may have the advantage in heavily irradiated bowel of allowing a more vascular anastomosis than the traditional suture technique. Thus it may be a more physiological anastomosis. In addition there is less handling of the intestine and therefore less likelihood of injury from repeated application of thumb and forceps.[12]

Although our experience with the Gambee suture anastomosis has been satisfactory, we feel the autosuture staple anastomosis may have two advantages. First, as previously stated, a more vascular anastomosis and, second, the saving of valuable operative time in these critically ill patients.[19]

In a vascular flow study completed in our laboratory[19] using dog intestine, three separate techniques of end-to-end anastomosis, (i) the classic two layer catgut and silk, (ii) the Gambee single layer with synthetic absorbable suture, and (iii) the surgical stapler, were evaluated. Blood flow through the anastomosis on the 4th postoperative day was measured by iodine 125. The blood flow was greatest after

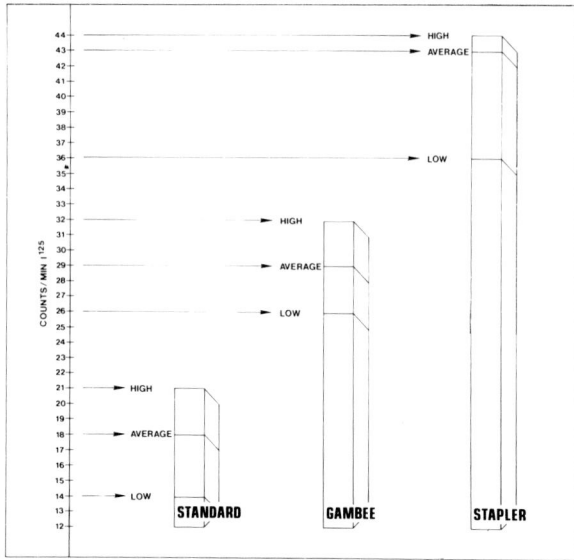

Fig. 86.8 Drawing comparing iodine 125 flow through three types of anastomoses in dogs.

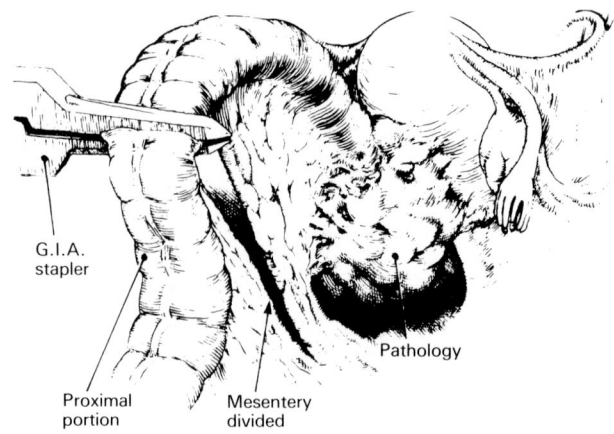

Fig. 86.9 A drawing of the GIA stapler placed across the intestine. When activated it will staple-close each segment of bowel and transect the bowel between the rows of staples. (Courtesy, Wheeless C R *Atlas of Pelvic Surgery*, Lea & Febiger, 1980.)

the stapler technique and least after the classic two layer anastomosis (Fig. 86.8).

The technique of autostaple anastomosis in small bowel bypass requires the use of a GIA (Gastrointestinal Anastomosis) stapler. After the appropriate segment of ileum is selected, the mesentery is opened and divided as previously described, and the GIA stapler is placed across the bowel in an oblique fashion to ensure maximum vascular supply to the antimesenteric border of the incised loop of bowel[18] (Fig. 86.9). The stapler is activated and the bowel stapled and transected at the same time.

The technique for functional end-to-end enterotransverse colostomy using stapler anastomosis is now described. The antimesenteric corner of the ileum is transected with curved Mayo scissors. One half of the GIA stapler is inserted into the small defect in the bowel along the antimesenteric border. The other half of the GIA stapler is inserted into the small enterotomy in the transverse colon. The stapler is articulated and closed. The stapler is activated, transecting and stapling an 8 cm segment of the antimesenteric borders of the small bowel and colon (Fig. 86.10). After removing the stapler, the anastomosis is carefully inspected for hemorrhage and integrity. The opened portions of the two segments of bowel are elevated with three Allis clamps. The TA-55 4.8 mm stapler is then placed across this open defect and activated (Fig. 86.11). The redundant portion of bowel outside the TA-55 stapler is trimmed away with curved Mayo scissors. Small bleeders are lightly touched with the electrocautery. A small amount of capillary bleeding through the stapled suture line is an asset in surgery on irradiated bowel rather than a liability because it demonstrates the vascular in-

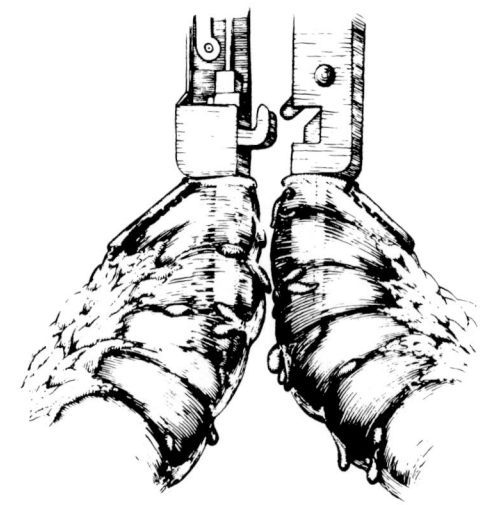

Fig. 86.10 A drawing of the functional end-to-end small bowel anastomosis using the GIA stapler. The segments of bowel are positioned side to side with the antimesenteric borders approximated for the anastomosis. (Courtesy, Wheeless C R *Atlas of Pelvic Surgery*, Lea & Febiger, 1980.)

tegrity of the anastomosis. Such oozing is easily controlled with light needlepoint and cautery.

Over 1800 anastomoses have been performed in our clinic with the autostapler device in the treatment of irradiated bowel injury since 1970. We continue to be impressed by the saving of operative time but more so by the quality of the anastomoses achieved.

The mucous fistula of distal ileum should be exteriorized through a convenient area of the anterior abdominal wall (Fig. 86.3). The margins in the defect in the rectus fascia and the submucosal layer of the bowel should be sutured with several 4/0 synthetic absorbable sutures to prevent herniation. The mucosa of the bowel is sutured to the skin

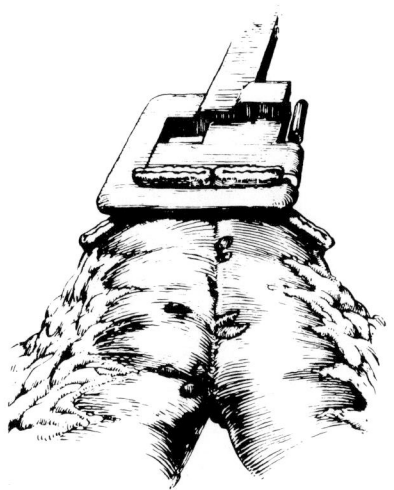

Fig. 86.11 A drawing of the closure of the remaining defect in the bowel anastomosis using the TA-55 stapler. (Courtesy, Wheeless C R *Atlas of Pelvic Surgery*, Lea & Febiger, 1980.)

with interrupted synthetic absorbable sutures, thus creating a defunctionalized ileostomy. Drainage from the mucous fistula may at first be copious. Generally, within a month after operation, most patients require nothing more than a small gauze pad to cover the stoma. There appears to be little difference in the volume of drainage whether the fistulous segment of the bowel is surgically isolated or left connected to the cecum and right colon.

We have found no advantage in exteriorizing both proximal and distal ends of a mucous fistula. Double exteriorization adds another stoma to the abdomen and achieves no surgical or physiological benefit; however, the patient has to manage two stomas.

The question of subsequent removal or takedown of the mucous fistula requires mature judgment. Re-operation and exploratory laparotomy carry significant hazards for morbidity and mortality in patients who have been heavily irradiated and who, therefore, have low resistance to infection and poor wound healing capacity. Because of the potential complications, it is desirable in most cases to avoid repeat laparotomy for resection of the mucous fistula. Few patients actually request such corrective surgery. Most do not complain of the small skin stoma of the mucous fistula which usually has minimal drainage after several months.

The small bowel bypass may produce the 'short intestine syndrome' when the bypassed segment of bowel includes most of the ileum. Patients with this disorder may have diarrhea and poor absorption of the fat soluble vitamins. They require low fat diet, antidiarrheal medications, and administration of fat soluble vitamins and vitamin B12 injections.

Technique of radical terminal ileectomy, right colectomy and ileo-transverse enterocolostomy

After the abdomen has been opened through an extended midline incision, the small bowel is dissected from the ligament of Treitz to the ileocecal junction. This may produce a number of enterotomies, especially in those loops of small bowel adherent deep in the pelvis.

After dissection of the entire small intestine the proximal site for transection is carefully selected. All irradiated intestine including the multiple enterotomies should be resected (Figs 86.12 and 86.13). Liberal use of frozen section to determine the proximal level of non-irradiated bowel is used.

The proximal small bowel, usually the proximal ileum or the distal jejunum, is cross clamped with the GIA surgical stapler, stapled and transected. Blood vessels in the mesentery, branches of the ileojejunal arteries arising from the superior mesenteric artery, are clamped distal rather than proximal to preserve as much collateral circulation to the proximal small bowel as possible. Transection of the small bowel mesentery proceeds to the avascular plane of Treves and is carried up to the ileocolic branch of the right colic artery. The ileocolic artery is clamped at its junction with the right colic artery.

The right colon is mobilized by transecting the peritoneum in the right colonic gutter along the line of Holts up to the hepatic flexure of the colon. All irradiated right colon is removed.

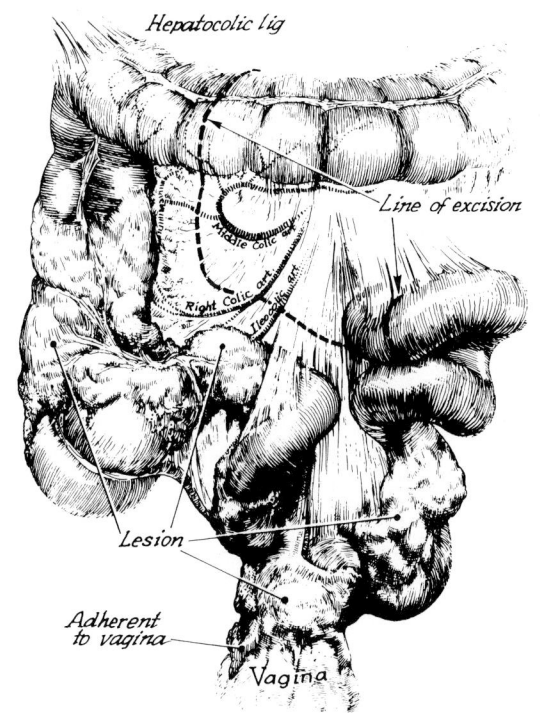

Fig. 86.12 Drawing demonstrating sites of transection of ileum and transverse colon for radical resection.

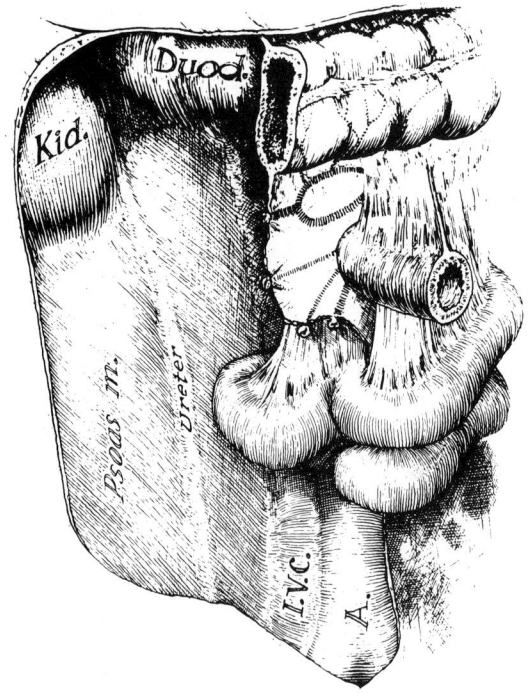

Fig. 86.13   The terminal ileum and the right colon have been removed.

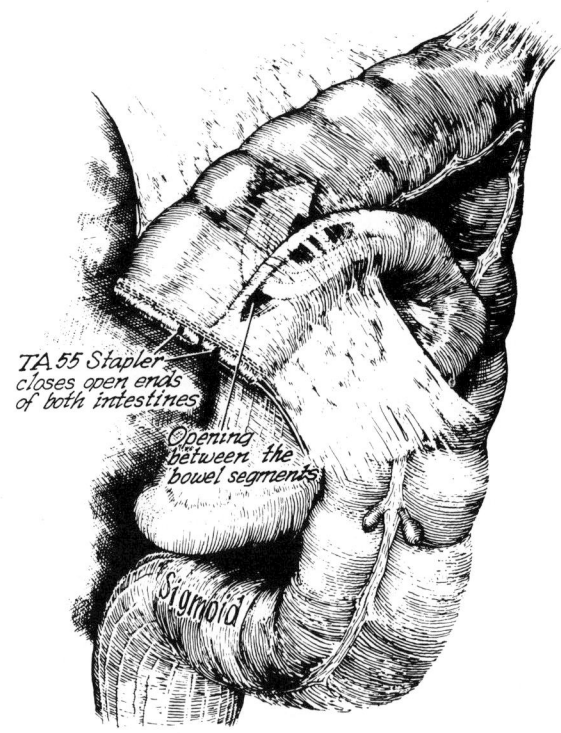

Fig. 86.14   The ileo-transverse colostomy has been performed with the stapler functional end-to-end anastomosis technique.

The right ureter is identified and protected. Ureteral catheters are rarely indicated.

The proximal ileum is anastomosed to the proximal transverse colon at the hepatic flexure using the functional end-to-end technique with the surgical staplers, first the GIA, then the TA55–4.8 mm (Fig. 86.14).[18]

The mesentery of the ileum and the transverse colon are sutured to reduce the incidence of internal herniae. The two mesenteries can be stapled with a skin closure staple gun to reduce operative time. The omentum is mobilized from the transverse colon and stomach and brought into the large defect to be sutured as an omental carpet or omentopexy.

After extensive intestinal surgery for irradiation complications benefit may be obtained from a surgical feeding gastrostomy until normal intestinal function returns.

TREATMENT OF RECTOSIGMOID COMPLICATIONS

The most frequent sites of intestinal complication from irradiation therapy for a pelvic malignancy are the colon and rectum. The majority of these complications involve a mild to moderate proctosigmoiditis that can be managed by medical therapy with cortisone preparations (suppositories, enemas), antidiarrheal medication and low residue diets. A small percentage (1–4%) develop serious complications, the most common of which are rectovaginal fistula and rectocolonic stricture with obstruction. In all postirradiation patients who manifest a significant degree of bloody diarrhea, it is desirable to perform cautious sigmoidoscopy and a barium enema X-ray study. If proctoscopy shows the mucosa of the anterior rectal wall to be ulcerated or necrotic, a diverting colostomy should be performed promptly to reduce the incidence of formation of a rectovaginal fistula.

Fortunately, modern techniques of irradiation therapy have lowered the incidence of rectovaginal fistula. However, it continues to occur in approximately 1 to 5% of patients who receive pelvic irradiation.[15] Successful closure has been reported in 20 to 60% of cases attempted.[13] All too often, however, the patient is advised to tolerate a diverting colostomy and not to seek repair of the fistula. This may be sound advice for elderly and poor risk patients, but in younger patients in good medical condition, fistula repair should be attempted.

When a rectovaginal fistula develops following irradiation therapy, a diverting colostomy should be performed. There are three areas of the colon that may be used, right transverse, left transverse, or sigmoid. One of three types of colostomy can be employed: loop colostomy leaving the posterior mesenteric wall of the bowel intact, a double barrel colostomy dividing the posterior mesenteric wall, or an end colostomy with closure and intraperitoneal replacement of the distal colon into the peritoneal cavity as a Hartman's pouch.[18] For patients who are to have a temporary colostomy that will be closed in 1 to 3 months, loop transverse colostomy in the left upper quadrant leaving the posterior mesenteric wall intact, is generally preferred. It leaves the marginal artery of the colon intact. This may be very important in irradiated bowel. The loop type of colostomy is easier to close and closure is associated with less morbidity than when the posterior wall of the colon and the mesentery have been divided. However, if fecal spill into the distal non-functioning loop of bowel must be avoided, a double barrel left transverse colostomy, dividing the posterior bowel wall, should be used. If the colostomy is to be permanent, the procedure of choice is a low sigmoid end colostomy, with closure of the distal segment of colon (Hartman's pouch) and its replacement into the peritoneal cavity. The woman is far more comfortable with low end sigmoid colostomy, and the bowel content is better formed, permitting easier colostomy training. A left transverse colostomy is preferable to a right transverse colostomy because of the possibility, in the presence of intestinal complications from the pelvic irradiation or malignancy, of the development of a small bowel fistula or obstruction which would require ileo-right transverse enterocolostomy bypass as previously described.

Technique of transverse loop colostomy

For a transverse loop colostomy, the abdomen is entered through a 7.5 to 10 cm transverse incision slightly above and to the left of the umbilicus, leaving the rectus muscle intact. Careful identification of the transverse colon is essential to avoid confusion with the stomach. The three most reliable anatomical landmarks are the omentum, the haustral markings, and the taenia coli. A loop of left transverse colon is selected and the omentum is carefully dissected off its surface. A small hole is made in an avascular portion of the omentum and a loop of transverse colon is brought through the opening in the mesentery. The mesentery of the transverse colon is transilluminated and an avascular portion selected, avoiding the marginal artery and vein. A small opening is made in the mesentery and a soft rubber drain is passed. The loop of colon is exteriorized through a defect in the abdominal wall; a glass rod is inserted through the mesentery defect. The peritoneum and fascia are closed in layers, allowing one finger-space between the bowel wall and the fascia to prevent strangulation and ischemia of the intestinal loop.[18] If the intestine has been mechanically cleansed and prepared with antibiotics, the loop colostomy should be sutured to the skin. The wall of the intestine sutured to the peritoneum or fascia reduces peristomal herniae. For closure of the fascia, a strong monofilament suture such as o-prolene or nylon suture is used. The skin is closed with fine monofilament sutures or steel staples. Monofilament

suture material avoids bacteria becoming embedded between the fibers of the suture and continually seeding the surrounding tissue with bacteria. A colostomy bag is applied to the exteriorized portion of the colon. Low suction is applied to a nasogastric tube passed into the patient's stomach if the bowel has not been properly prepared and the loop colostomy is not sutured. On the 3rd postoperative day, the anterior wall of the colon is divided. On the 5th postoperative day the glass rod is removed and a permanent colostomy bag applied. The skin surrounding the colostomy stoma should be inspected daily and protected from excoriation and inflammation. The stoma is carefully measured and a bag applied that fits snugly, to allow as little exposure of the skin as possible. Should the skin become excoriated, the bag should be removed each day, the skin bathed with antiseptic soap, painted with Maalox or aluminum paste, dusted with Karaya gum powder, and the Karaya gum ring replaced. If the skin surrounding the stoma becomes infected with monilia, dusting with nystatin powder each day is necessary. In severe cases the patient can be given nystatin tablets by mouth to reduce the level of Candida albicans in the intestinal flora.

Technique of end colostomy

If an end colostomy is to be performed, the lowest segment of sigmoid colon outside the irradiation port is selected. The distal segment to be left in the peritoneal cavity (Hartman's pouch) is closed by a running inverting suture or stapled with the TA-55 4.8 mm autosuture stapler (Fig. 86.15). The proximal stoma is brought through an incision in the lower abdominal wall at a point to the left of the umbilicus and slightly below the waistline.[18]

In obese patients the proposed stomal site is marked by skin tattoo preoperatively with the patient in the standing position to avoid subsequent displacement of the stoma under a large panniculus.

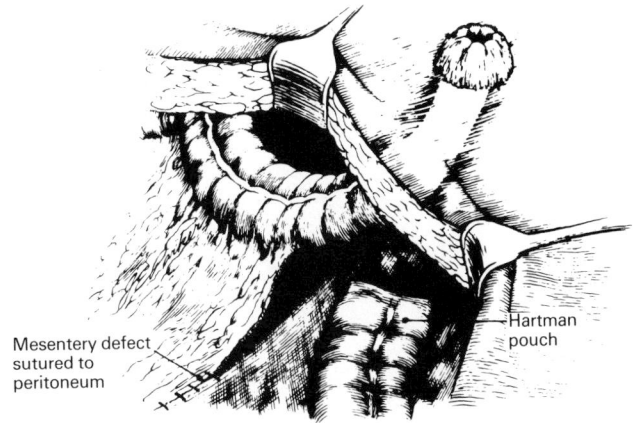

Mesentery defect sutured to peritoneum

Hartman pouch

Fig. 86.15 A drawing of an end sigmoid colostomy with a Hartman's pouch. (Courtesy, Wheeless C R *Atlas of Pelvic Surgery*, Lea & Febiger, 1980.)

After the proximal loop of the end colostomy is brought through the abdominal wall, several 3/0 synthetic absorbable sutures are placed between the abdominal fascia and the serosal layer of the intestine to prevent prolapse of the colon. The stoma is secured by suturing it to the skin of the lower abdomen by a 'rosebud' technique using 3/0 synthetic absorbable suture on a small intestinal needle. This suture starts in the margin, anchors the serosa of the intestinal wall approximately 3–4 cm from the free end of the bowel, and is passed through the free edge of the intestine. When tied, it brings the edge of the intestine out over the skin in a 'rosebud' fashion and prevents retraction of the mucosa below the skin edge[18] (Fig. 86.16). Before replacing a temporary loop colostomy, a barium enema X-ray examination and an endoscopic examination of the distal colon and rectum are required to ascertain that healing of this irradiated wound is complete. Ordinarily, closure of a colostomy is not done for 6 to 8 weeks following the initial low bowel anastomosis or closure of a rectovaginal fistula in irradiated colon. Bowel preparation prior to surgery is essential before closure. The defunctionalized segment of distal colon is cleansed with enemas and irrigated with a 1% neomycin solution shortly before surgery.

Closure requires an adequate abdominal incision to allow visualization of the rectus fascia that circumscribes the colostomy stoma. Before the peritoneal cavity is entered, the edges of the bowel wall are trimmed away, and the proximal and distal margins of the bowel are closed by means of a standard Gambee anastomosis with 3/0 synthetic absorbable sutures on intestinal needles or steel staples using the TA55 4.8 mm autosuture. This technique prevents accidental spillage of feces into the peritoneal cavity.[18] After the bowel is closed, the dissection is continued until the peritoneal cavity is entered, and the colon is replaced. The peritoneum and fascia are often closed together using strong monofilament sutures such as 0-

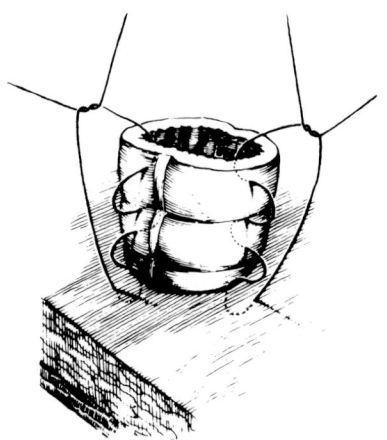

Fig. 86.16 A drawing of the 'rosebud' suture technique of colostomy stoma to the skin. (Courtesy, Wheeless C R *Atlas of Pelvic Surgery*, Lea & Febiger, 1980.)

prolene. The wound is irrigated copiously with sterile saline. The subcutaneous tissue is drained with a small closed suction drain. The skin is closed with 4/0 prolene sutures or skin staples. Prolene sutures or steel staples are preferred in the skin because they have the least tissue reactivity, and can be left in place longer if wound infection occurs. The delayed closure technique for these incisions is no longer used since the above technique has proven to be satisfactory. All patients are given preoperative antibiotics such as cephalosporin or doxycycline.

Repair of rectovaginal fistula and rectocolonic stricture

In most cases of rectovaginal fistula from irradiation, successful repair has required grafting of non-irradiated tissue with a good blood supply onto the sutured fistulous area.[2,6,13] Omentum, bulbocavernosus muscle, gracilis muscle, and even a colonic flap[2] have been successful in attaining closure. The adjunctive techniques may be added to the standard rectovaginal fistula repair described below or the contemporary technique of a colonic flap "patch" advocated by Bricker[2] or very low resection of the rectum and very low coloproctostomy with the EEA stapler gun.

Adequate preoperative bowel preparation prior to surgery is needed irrespective of the technique of fistula repair. Regardless of technique selected the fistula site must be adequately exposed. For the vaginal approach this frequently requires the use of a posterolateral relaxing incision in the vagina extended into the right or left ischiorectal fossa.[18] The dense fibrous tissue surrounding the fistula must be excised until distinct layers of bowel mucosa, submucosa, and vagina can be separated. In addition, wide mobilization of the bowel from the vagina must be obtained to prevent tension on the suture lines. This may require a laparotomy in order to mobilize the rectosigmoid colon from above, making the operation an abdominoperineal procedure. If there is any tension on the suture lines, healing will not occur and the fistula will reopen shortly after repair.

After wide mobilization of the fistula site has been achieved, the edges of the rectal mucosa are closed transversely with inverting interrupted 3/0 synthetic delayed absorbable sutures. A second layer is placed. At this point, a vascular pedicle graft is needed to add blood supply to the suture lines (Figs 86.17 and 86.18). The decision to use omentum, bulbocavernosus or gracilis muscle must be made according to the conditions encountered at the operation. If omentum is used it must be dissected from the transverse colon to form a 'J' pedicle flap. The flap must be long enough to reach the vagina without tension. The omentum is sutured into place over the fistula with interrupted 3/0 synthetic absorbable sutures.[18] If the bulbocavernosus fat pad or gracilis muscle is used, it is carefully mobilized, preserving the vascular and nerve supply. The vaginal mucosa must be mobilized adequately

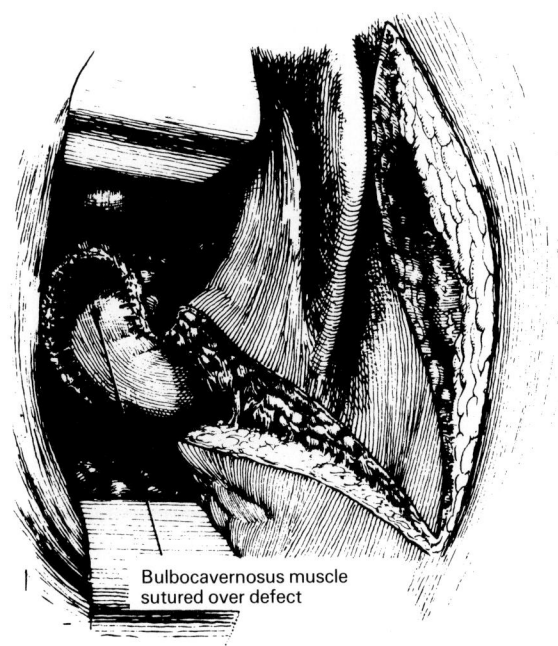

Fig. 86.17 A drawing of the rectovaginal fistula closure. Adequate exposure to the fistula is achieved by a mediolateral episiotomy. The bulbocavernosus muscle has been mobilized and sutured over the fistula closure as a vascular pedicle flap. (Courtesy, Wheeless C R *Atlas of Pelvic Surgery*, Lea & Febiger, 1980.)

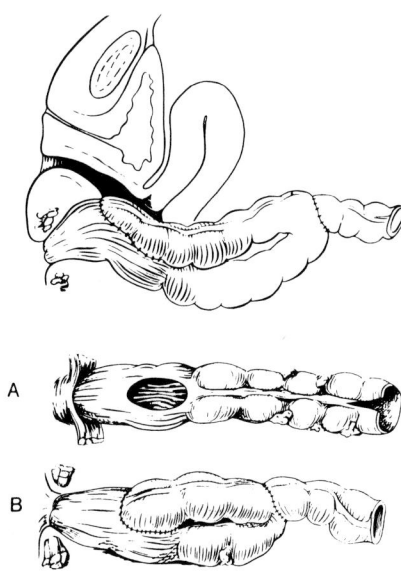

Fig. 86.19 A drawing of the colonic vascular flap used to 'patch' the rectovaginal fistula. (A) shows a rectovaginal fistula. (B) shows a segment of descending colon folded over to cover the fistula. The remaining descending colon is anastomosed to the dome of the new pouch. The top drawing shows the completed operation from a sagittal view of the pelvis. (Courtesy, Bricker E M and Johnston W D (1979) Surg Gynecol Obstet 148: 499.)

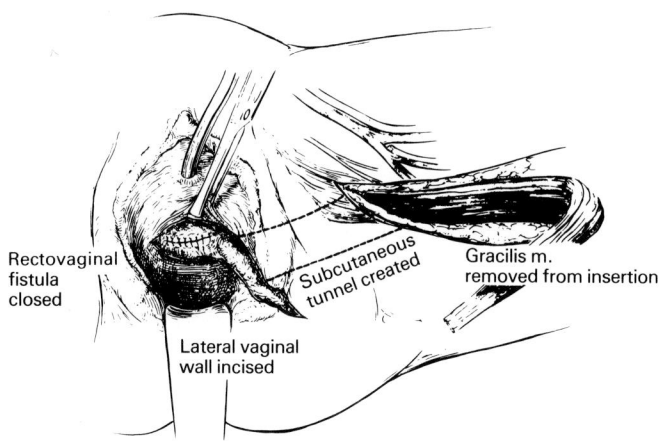

Fig. 86.18 A drawing of a vascular pedicle flap to cover the closure of the rectovaginal fistula using the gracilis muscle.

to permit closure of the vagina without tension over the vascular graft. These procedures often obliterate much of the vaginal cavity.

Recently Bricker and Johnston[2] have described a technique of rectovaginal fistula closure and rectal stricture repair using a vascular colonic flap. The left colon is divided proximal to the fistula and distal to the left loop colostomy and folded upon itself to cover or "patch" the defect or provide circumference to the strictured rectosigmoid colon. The colostomy is mobilized and anastomosed to the dome of the pouch (Fig. 86.19).

In patients with rectal stricture, the colon proximal to and including the stricture can be 'filleted' along its antimesenteric border and the 'colonic flap' sutured onto itself creating a rectocolonic pouch with adequate diameter. Proximal colon is again anastomosed to the dome of the pouch and protected by a diverting proximal colostomy. The diverting protective colostomy is performed proximal to the reconstruction and later closed after healing and rectal continence is demonstrated.

With the advent of the end-to-end anastomosis stapler (EEA) surgical interest has been awakened to the efficacy of extremely low coloproctostomies, often 2–3 cm from the anal verge but frequently below 6 cm. This new technology has dramatically reduced the incidence of permanent colostomy. It has added another technique for repair of rectovaginal fistulae. The technique often requires an abdominoperineal approach. The vagina and rectum are transected below the lower margin of the fistula. The vagina is separated from the lower rectum. Purse-string sutures are placed in the margin of the lower rectum and in the proximal sigmoid colon. The purse-string sutures secure the colon and rectum around the shaft of the EEA stapler. The stapler is activated and the anastomosis is completed. An omental flap is secured around the anastomosis and wedged between the vaginal mucosa and the rectum. A protective proximal diverting loop colostomy is left in place for approximately 8 weeks until healing has been demonstrated.

Surgery for intestinal complications following radiation therapy for gynecologic malignancy is a difficult and dangerous area. The surgeon must have the discipline to perform staged operations utilizing Halstedian techniques of wound management and accept the fact that irradiated wounds are not competitive with non-irradiated wounds in a statistical analysis of success or failure.

REFERENCES

1. Bricker E M 1970 Pelvic exenteration. Advances in Surgery. Yearbook Medical Publishers, Chicago, p 13
2. Bricker E M, Johnston W D 1979 Repair of post irradiation rectovaginal fistula and stricture. Surg Gynecol Obstet 148: 499.
3. DeCose J J, Rhodes R S, Wentz W B, Reagan J W, Dworken H J, Holden W D 1969 The natural history and management of radiation into the gastrointestinal tract. Ann Surg 170: 369
4. Gambee L P 1951 A single-layer open intestinal anastomosis applicable to the small as well as the large intestine. West J Surg Obstet Gynecol 59: 1
5. Gambee L P, Garnjobst W, Harwick C E 1956 Ten years' experience with a single-layer anastomosis in colon surgery. Am J Surg 92: 222.
6. Graham J B 1965 Vaginal fistulas following radiotherapy. Surg Gynecol Obstet 120: 1019
7. Graham J B, Villalba R J 1963 Damage to the small intestine in radiotherapy. Surg Gynecol Obstet 116: 665.
8. Hall E J 1988 Radioprotectors, Chapter 10, Radiobiology for the Radiologist. 3rd Edn, Lippincott, Philadelphia, PA.
9. Halsted W S 1887 Circular suture of the intestine: An experimental study. Am J Med Sci 94: 436.
10. Hamilton J E 1967 Reappraisal of open intestinal anastomosis. Ann Surg 165: 917.
11. Ketcham A S, Joye R C, Pilch Y H, Morton D L 1970 Delayed intestinal obstruction following treatment for cancer. Cancer 25: 406.
12. Ravitch M, Steichen F M 1972 Technics of staple suturing in gastrointestinal tract. Ann Surg 175: 815.
13. Smith J P, Golden P E, Rutledge F 1969 The surgical management of intestinal injuries following irradiation for carcinoma of cervix. Cancer of the Uterus and Ovary. M.D. Anderson Hospital. Yearbook Medical Publishers, Chicago, p. 241
14. Swan R W, Fowler W C Jr, Boronow R C 1976 Surgical management of radiation injury to small intestine. Surg Gynecol Obstet 142: 325.
15. Villasanta U 1972 Complications of radiotherapy in carcinoma of the uterine cervix. Am J Obstet Gynecol 114: 717.
16. Wheeless C R 1973 Small bowel bypass for complications related to pelvic malignancy. Obstet Gynecol 42: 661.
17. Wheeless C R 1975 The Gambee intestinal anastomosis in gynecologic surgery. Obstet Gynecol 46: 448.
18. Wheeless C R 1988 Atlas of Pelvic Surgery, 2nd edn. Lea & Febiger, Philadelphia
19. Wheeless C R, Smith J J 1983 A comparison of the flow of iodine 125 through three different intestinal anastomoses: Standard, Gambee, and stapler. Obstet Gynecol 62: 513.

PART XVI

Surgical reconstruction of the gynecologic oncology patient

87. Vulvar-vaginal reconstruction

C. R. Wheeless Jr

INTRODUCTION

For the past 2 decades there has been a definite trend among pelvic surgeons to immediately reconstruct the large defects created by deforming radical cancer surgery in the female pelvis and perineum. Extensive en bloc removal of more tissue has enhanced the probability of increased 5-year survival.[13] At the same time, however, the quality of life following radical surgery has been a great concern to both patient and surgeon. Recent advances have been made in techniques for reconstruction of the vulva and vagina. These techniques, hopefully, will stimulate consideration among gynecological oncologists toward the design of other techniques for reconstruction and rehabilitation of the gynecological cancer patient.

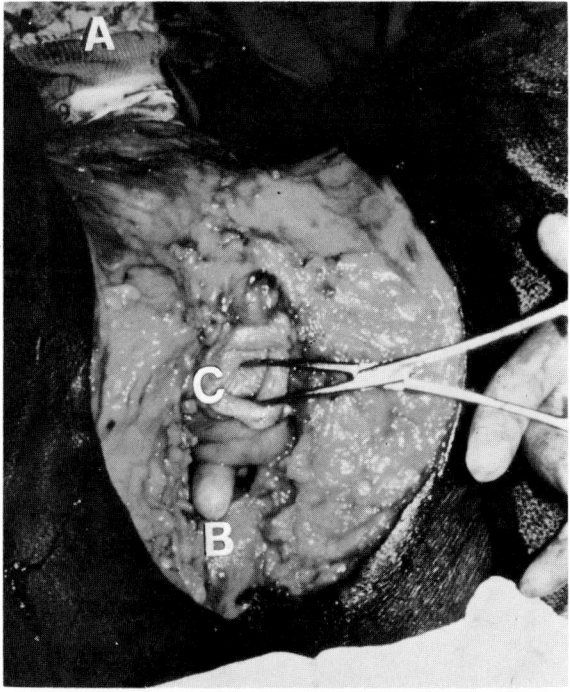

Fig. 87.1 Photo of large vulvar defect after resection for carcinoma of the vulva. (Courtesy of Wheeless C R 1979)[15]

The work of Way[13] with patients with squamous cell carcinoma of the vulva has demonstrated the efficacy of en bloc removal of the vulva, mons pubis and inguinal lymph nodes from the anterior-posterior iliac spine to the adductor canal. By using a more extensive dissection, pelvic surgeons have been able to remove more tissue and, thereby, enhance the probability of increased 5-year survival (Fig. 87.1). This type of radical excision, however, has been complicated by problems associated with closure of such large wounds involving postoperative necrosis of the suture line over the mons pubis and the inguinal areas. Attempts have been made to redesign the incision for a radical vulvectomy to allow an adequate cancer operation and, at the same time, provide better primary healing of the incision with reduced necrosis.[7,15] Although slight modifications of the original Way incision have allowed some improvements in the incidence of necrosis and pelvic contracture, many patients have had significant wound breakdown requiring split thickness skin grafts to cover areas that have become necrotic during the postoperative period. The hospital stay of these patients has been prolonged awaiting acceptable healing of the wound. In addition, patients have developed severe perineal contractions with significant distortion of the bladder resulting in total incontinence of urine, perineal pain, pressure and, in some cases, difficulty in walking.[15]

Total vaginectomy, whether in conjunction with a simple hysterectomy, radical hysterectomy, or total exenteration, represents a significant physical as well as psychological loss to the patient particularly if she is sexually active.

The ability to reconstruct a functional vagina provides the contemporary woman with a tremendous source of psychological contentment in approaching her cancer therapy and alleviates some of the fears that she has toward her future psychosexual well being as well as the domestic relationship with her husband. In addition to the psychosexual factors (see Ch. 90), reconstruction of the vagina after total pelvic exenteration by the myocutaneous flap technique has a significant beneficial effect from the point of view of wound healing.[7] The insertion of the myocutaneous tissue in the true pelvis obliterates a great deal of dead space and provides a healthy vascular pedicle in an area usually ischemic from heavy pelvic irradiation. Currently, there appear to be five functional and very acceptable methods for restoring the vagina. They are (1) the McIndoe vaginoplasty[8,9] using a split thickness skin graft over a mold following nonradical procedures, (2) the same split thickness skin graft over a mold applied to an omental flap cylinder anastomosed to the introitus,[17] (3) the gracilis myocutaneous flap,[7,15] (4) the sigmoid neovagina,[3,6] and (5) the Williams operation for neovaginal reconstruction using the skin of the labia majora.[18]

The ideal method of perineal reconstruction following a radical resection of the vulva or vagina should provide an immediate anatomic restoration and primary healing at the time of tumor resection. The new vulva or vagina should have as many of the anatomic characteristics of the original vulva or vagina as possible. The donor tissue should ideally be expendable and transferable with minimal patient morbidity. It should be emphasized that most radical vulvectomy operations can be closed primarily. Others can be closed with the assistance of Z-plasty pedicle flaps advocated by Julian & Woodruff[5] (Fig. 87.3). However, there are occasional perineal resections that are so extensive that neither of the above techniques is adequate for primary closure. In these patients myocutaneous flap is a means of primary closure.

TECHNIQUES FOR VULVAR RECONSTRUCTION

The discussion of reconstruction of the perineum-vulva will consist of a review of those methods currently available to the pelvic surgeon for these procedures. That is, split thickness skin graft, Z-plasty flap, and gracilis myocutaneous flap.

The concept that skin can be nutritionally maintained by its underlying muscle was pioneered by Owens[11] in his early work with compound myocutaneous flaps. The work of Orticochea[10] using the gracilis myocutaneous flap in reconstruction of the penis following radical orchidectomy and penectomy led McGraw and colleagues to use the gracilis myocutaneous flap for vaginal reconstruction following total pelvic exenteration.[7] McGraw reported 22 cases of successful vaginal reconstruction with this technique. In addition, others have reported the use of the gracilis myocutaneous flap to cover large defects in the perineum as well as reconstruction of the vagina.[4,7,15]

Split thickness skin graft

The use of the split thickness skin graft for reconstruction of the vulva will not be extensively described here. The technique for taking the graft is available in multiple standard surgical texts.[4,17] It involves taking a 0.35 mm split

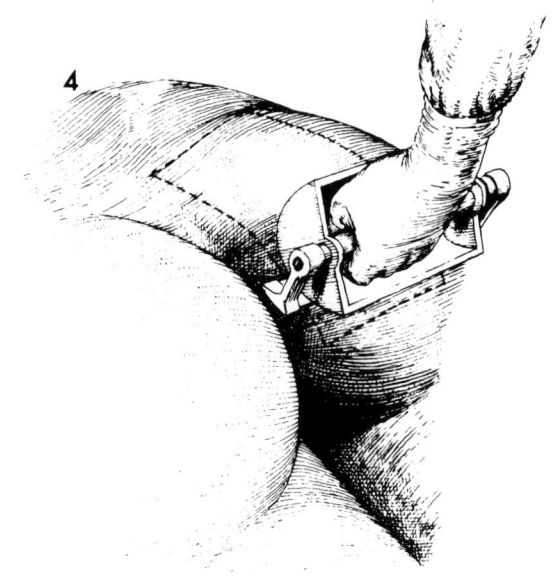

Fig. 87.2 A drawing of the Reese dermatome taking a split thickness skin graft from the buttocks.

thickness skin graft from an acceptable donor site with either the Reese (Fig. 87.2), Padgett, or Brown dermatome and applying these split thickness grafts to the denuded area. The margin of the graft is sutured to the margin of the defect with fine sutures and a moist stint-pack is used to ensure that the split thickness skin graft is adequately pressed against the wound. Small pockets of serum can be aspirated by needle to allow the graft to lie flat over the entire denuded area. We have found the use of meshed grafts to be of particular value in large wounds with the potential of infection and subgraft serum collection. The small defects in the mesh allow adequate drainage of the wound while epithelialization takes place. After complete epithelialization of such a large wound, contraction takes place for months. Experience has shown that many of these wounds eventually contract after 4 to 6 months to a linear scar along the path of the original incision as Way noted without skin grafting. However, the physiological and logistical advantages of covering and closing large open wounds is well documented and is preferable to the long costly process of granulation.

Z-plasty full thickness pedicle flap

In cases where primary closure of the vulvar wound cannot be performed without tension, the use of a Z-plasty full thickness pedicle flap, as advocated by Julian & Woodruff,[5] has proven efficacious. The flap is relatively easy to perform, but must be well designed prior to making the incision for the Z-plasty. Particular attention should be given to the width of the base of the Z-flap to ensure an adequate blood supply to the point of each flap in the Z

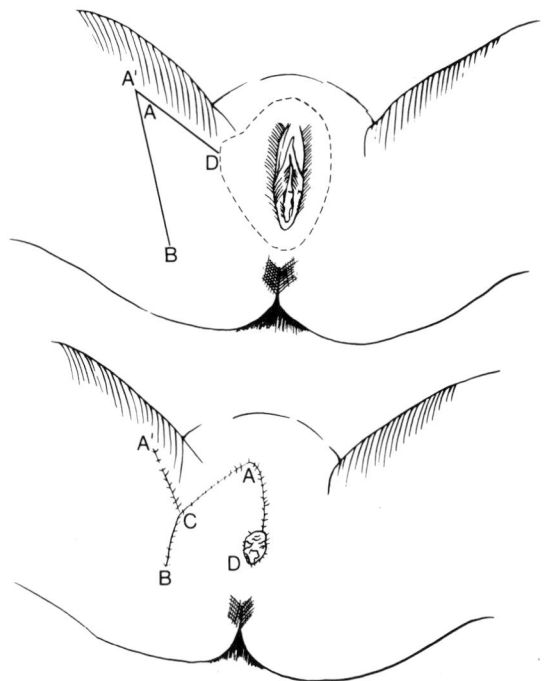

Fig. 87.3 A drawing of the Z-plasty full thickness skin flap to cover vulvar-perineal defects. The area to be excised is marked with the dotted line. The flap is marked off with points A & A'–B, D and line C as shown. The flap is used to cover the defect in such a manner that points A & D cover the new medial margin of the vulva. The flap defect is closed along line A'–C. (Julian C G *Obstet Gynecol* 38: 193.)

pedicle (Fig. 87.3). A general rule to follow is that 1 cm of base should be present for each 2 cm of length of the flap. After measuring the defect, and translating these measurements into the appropriate size of flap needed, the future flap is marked with brilliant green solution before incisions are made along the designated lines. The incision should be full thickness including epidermis, dermis, and subcutaneous fat. The flap is rotated into position and sutured to the midline of the perineum without tension. Generally, it is difficult to rotate the flap beyond the mid-perineal line. If additional tissue is needed to close the vulvar incision from the opposite side, a Z-plasty flap should be raised from that side and sutured in the midline. The flap should be sutured to the underlying fascia covering the pubic rami and to the incision line on the opposite side. Generally, this is carried out with 3/0 polyglycolic acid suture (Dexon). The suture in the skin margin is usually fine prolene or nylon. The medial margin of the flap should be sutured to the margin of the vaginal mucosa with interrupted 2/0 polyglycolic acid sutures. Generally, we have avoided bringing the polyglycolic acid suture through the cutaneous skin and have preferred to suture the vaginal mucosa edge to the subcuticular margin of the skin flap. A soft, silastic, closed suction drain is placed under the flap, sutured into place with 4/0 polyglycolic acid

suture and connected to low suction. The remaining flap of the Z-plasty is brought into position to close the donor site and is usually sutured with a subcutaneous row of interrupted 3/0 polyglycolic acid sutures and 4/0 nylon in the skin. The cardinal feature of successful healing of these flaps is that they must be brought into position without tension. If they are under tension, they will separate and not heal properly.

Gracilis myocutaneous flap for reconstruction of the vulva

Gracilis myocutaneous flap operation is started with the patient in the dorsal supine position with the hips abducted at 45 degrees and flexed 30 degrees for exposure of the vulva. The knees are extended in the gynecologic stirrups (Fig. 87.4).[3]

The size of the perineal defect is carefully measured in width and length. The approximate upper limit for flap viability is 24 cm × 7 cm. After determining the length and width of the flap needed, the gracilis muscle is palpated from its origin on the pubic ramus to its insertion on the medial aspect of the knee (Fig. 87.5). Extension of the knee aids in the palpation of the gracilis muscle and reduces the possibility of mistaking the sartorius muscle for the gracilis muscle. A line is drawn along the length of the

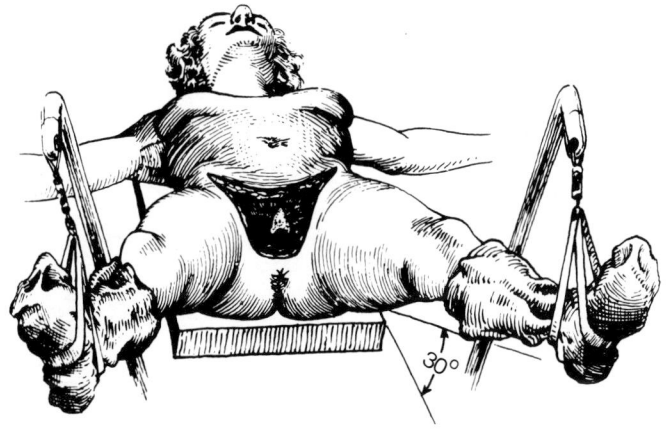

Fig. 87.4 A drawing of the position for the gracilis myocutaneous flap. The hips are abducted 45 degrees and flexed 30 degrees. The knees are extended. (Courtesy of Wheeless C R (1988).[16])

gracilis muscle. The flap is drawn in a 'paddle' shape originating at the lateral margin of the perineal defect. An incision is made through the skin and subcutaneous tissue down to the adductor longus fascia along the length of the superior margin of the outlined 'paddle-shaped flap'. The vascular pedicle of the gracilis muscle is invested by the fascial layer which separates the adductor longus and adductor magnus muscles (Fig. 87.6). It has been found that the best surgical approach to the gracilis vascular

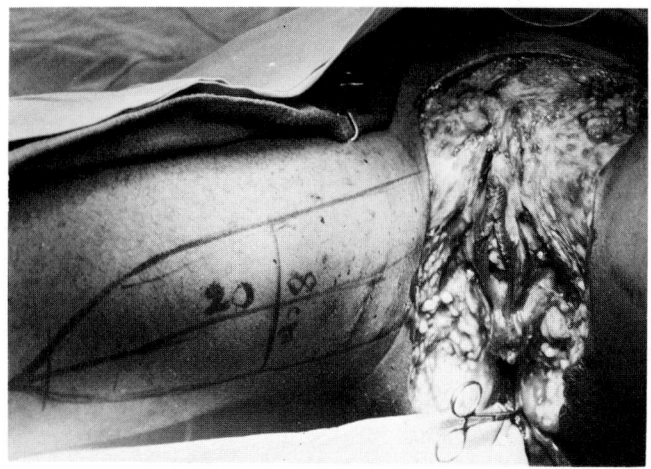

Fig. 87.5 Photo of a large perineal defect from a resection of extensive benign adenitis. The gracilis muscle is marked by a line down the length of the muscle. The proposed flap 20 cm × 8 cm is outlined.

the dominant vascular pedicle using the sterile ultrasound Doppler monitor. Repeated use of the sterile ultrasound Doppler monitor confirms the location of the blood supply and ensures its protection (Fig. 87.8). When the flaps on both sides have been adequately dissected and are ready for rotation, 1 to 3 g of intravenous fluorescein is administered. The dose depends on the size and race of the patient. The flaps are exposed to an ultraviolet Woods' lamp in a dark room. Nonviable areas of the flaps are demonstrated by their failure to fluoresce, and these areas are excised. Each flap is rotated into position covering one half of the defect (Fig. 87.9). The subcutaneous tissue of the defect is sutured to the subcutaneous tissue of the flap with interrupted 3/0 Dexon sutures. The skin of the flap is sutured to the skin of the defect. The medial portion of the flap is sutured to the vaginal mucosa with interrupted 3/0 Dexon sutures. The opposite flap is rotated into position and sutured to the margin of the perineal defect (Fig. 87.10).

TECHNIQUES OF VAGINAL RECONSTRUCTION

Ideally, vaginal reconstruction should be performed at the time of the vaginal resection except for the Williams operation which uses the skin of the labia majora. Dissection into the pelvis through the perineum following radical pelvic surgery, especially radical surgery after pelvic

bundle is attained by reflecting the fascia to the adductor longus muscle. When the fascia is reflected, the adductor longus and the gracilis muscles are identified, exposing the proximal vascular bundle of the gracilis muscle approximately 10 cm from the pubic ramus (Fig. 87.7). The gracilis muscle is isolated and divided at its origin on the pubic ramus. Care is taken at this point to locate

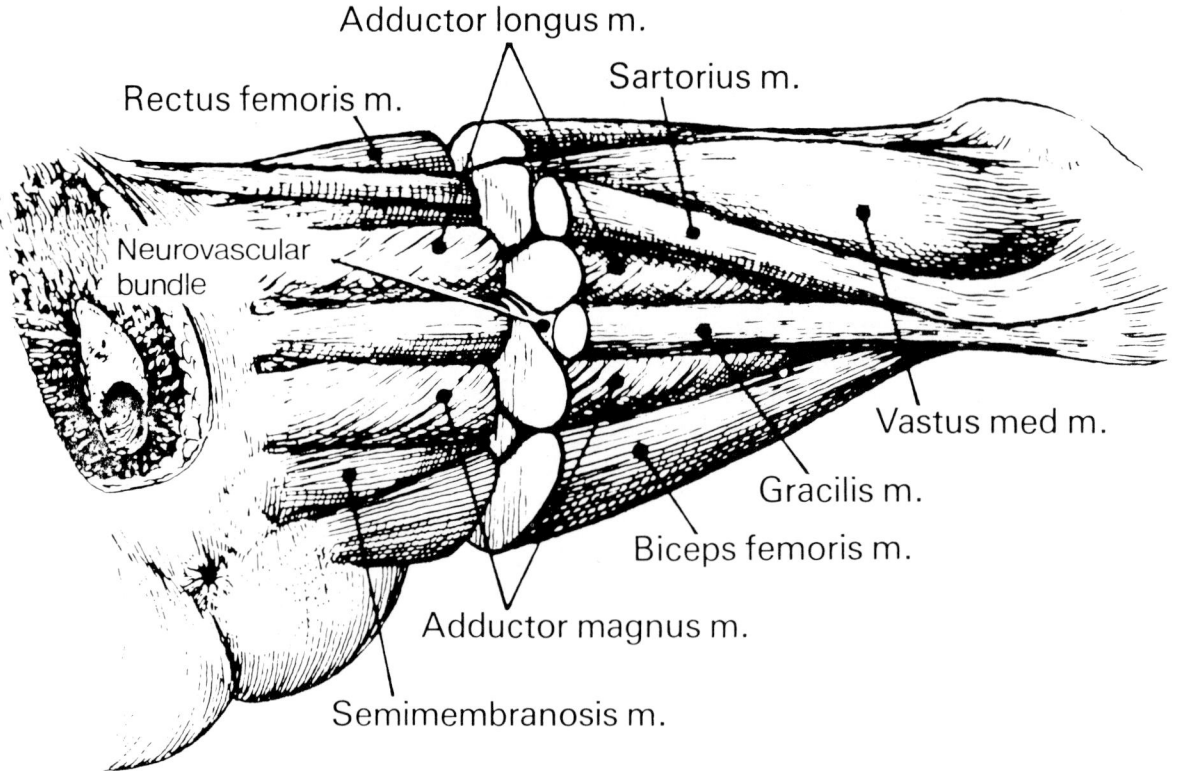

Fig. 87.6 The anatomy of the gracilis muscle. The relationship of the vital gracilis neurovascular bundle to the adductor longus and adductor magnus muscle is shown. (Courtesy of Wheeless C R (1988).[16])

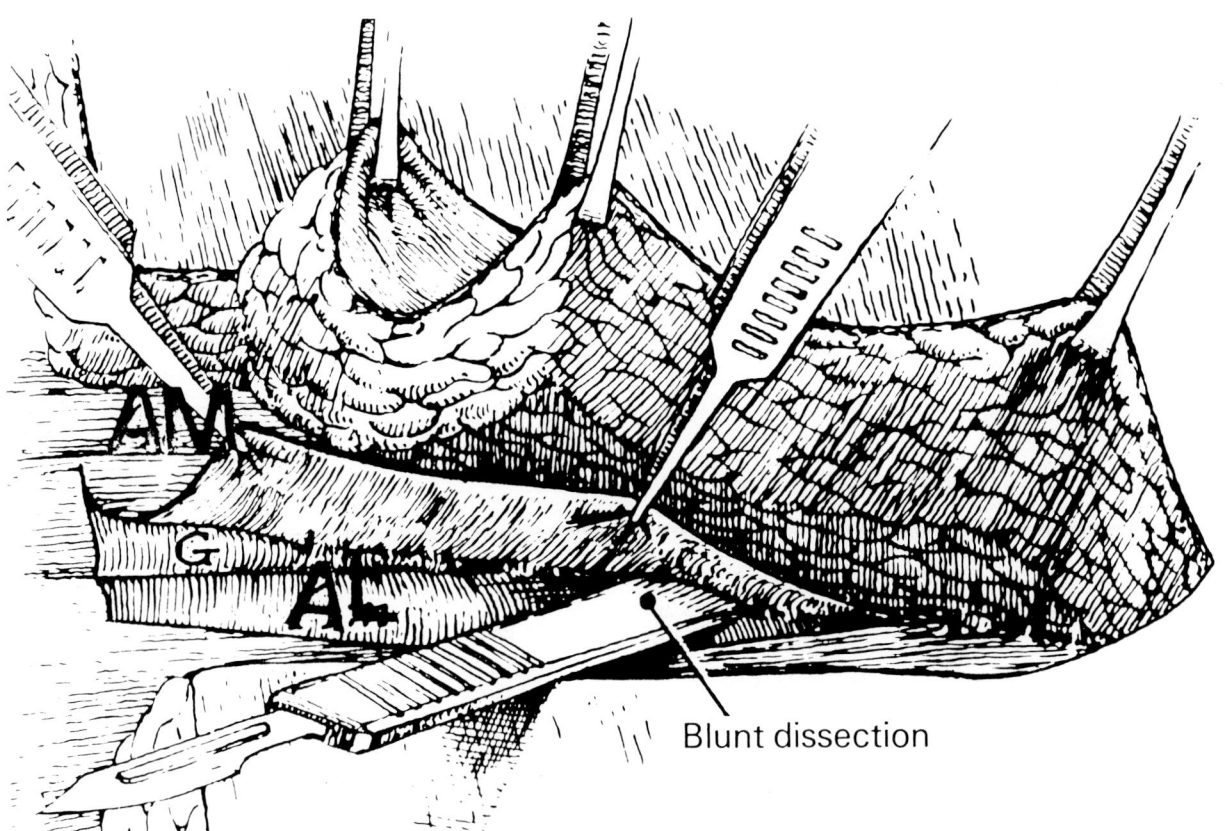

Fig. 87.7   A drawing demonstrating the reflection of the fascia separating the adductor longus (AL) and the adductor magnus (AM). (Courtesy of Wheeless C R (1988).[16])

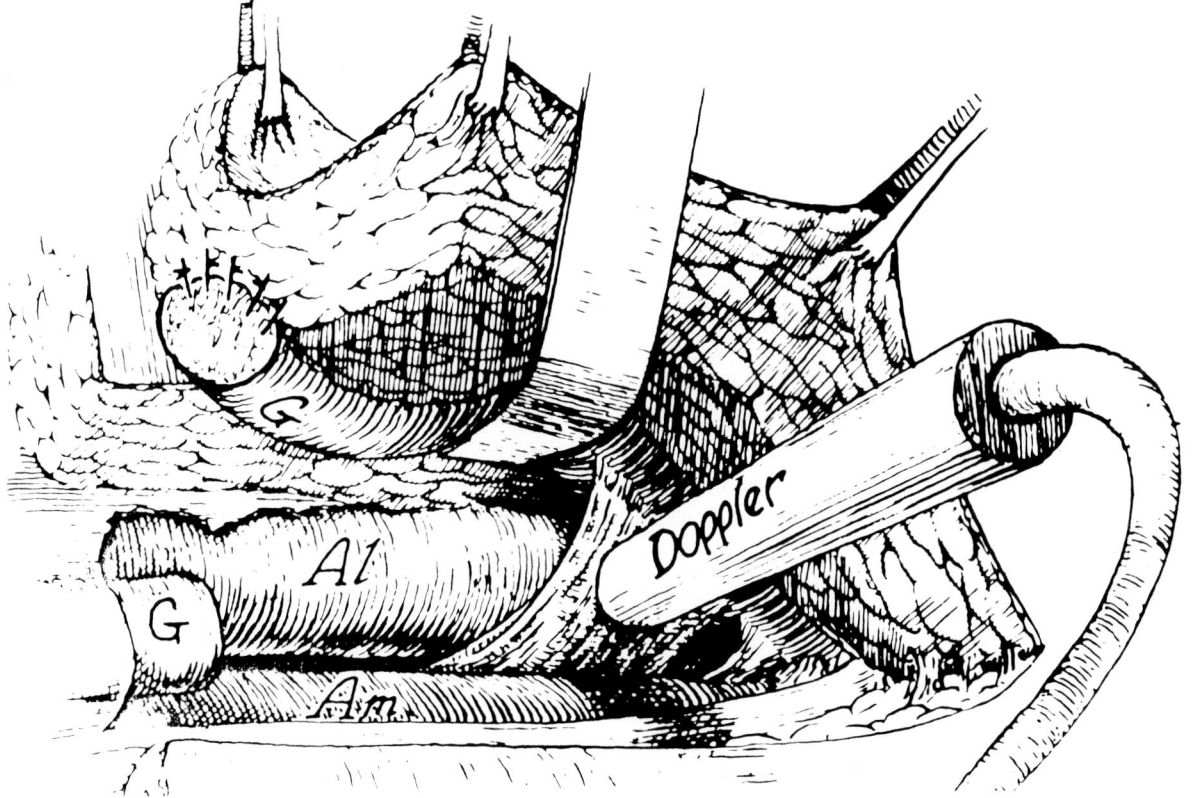

Fig. 87.8   A drawing demonstrating the isolated neurovascular bundle of the gracilis muscle. The small ultrasound Doppler is used to confirm the presence of the pulsating artery. Al = adductor longus, G = gracilis, Am = adductor magnus. (Courtesy of Wheeless C R (1988).[16])

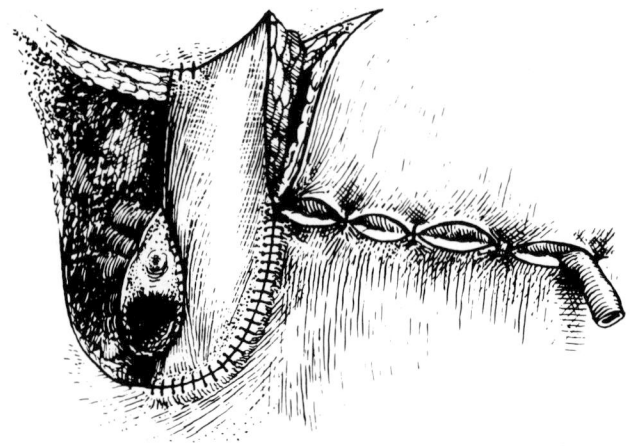

Fig. 87.9 A drawing showing the gracilis myocutaneous flap rotated into position. The leg closure of the wound has begun over a Penrose drain. (Courtesy of Wheeless C R (1988).[16])

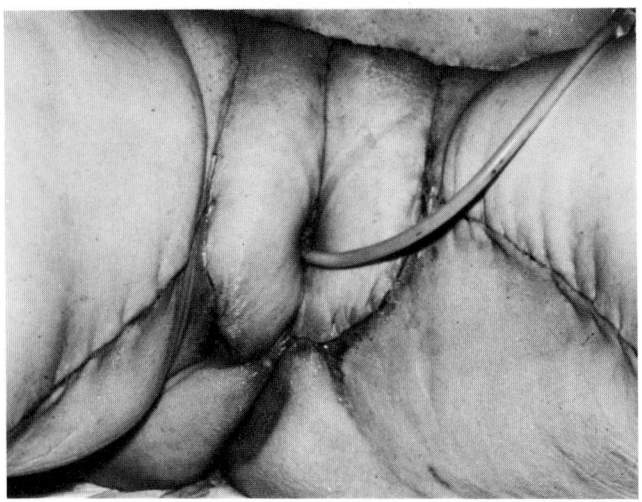

Fig. 87.10 A photograph of a completed vulvar reconstruction.

irradiation, can be hazardous from the point of view of injuring the gastrointestinal tract and/or bladder. If surgical conditions do not permit reconstruction at the time of the original vaginal resection, it is probably preferable to perform the Williams operation rather than the McIndoe split thickness graft or the gracilis myocutaneous flap procedure.[18] The discussion of reconstruction of the vagina will consist of a review of those methods currently available to the pelvic surgeon for these procedures, i.e. the McIndoe split thickness skin graft, the skin graft to an omental cylinder, the gracilis myocutaneous flap, the sigmoid neovagina and the Williams operation.

McIndoe split thickness skin graft

The McIndoe split thickness skin graft was described in 1950.[8,9] It was originally intended for use in congenital ab-

sence of the vagina. Its use in gynecological oncology has been usually reserved for those cases where vaginectomy was performed for early carcinoma of the vagina. It is ideal in those cases where length and diameter are desirable in the sexually active younger patient. A variant of the McIndoe operation, the Wharton operation,[14] which consists of placing a vaginal form in the stump of vagina remaining after pelvic exenteration allows epithelialization from the vaginal margin upward and around the form. This process takes several months, but has produced surprisingly satisfactory results, and has avoided a second surgical procedure. However, this type of vagina is usually shortened, and is not always sexually satisfactory particularly in younger patients.

The technique of McIndoe vaginoplasty consists of first selecting the donor site for split thickness skin graft.[4,17] In the past, this site has been chosen from an area generally covered by bathing suits such as the buttocks, or lower abdomen (Fig. 87.2). However, the ever shrinking fashion of the feminine bathing suit makes an ideal site difficult in modern times. We prefer to take the split thickness skin graft prior to the radical resection procedure. This avoids repreparing and draping the patient in order to obtain a graft from an appropriate donor site. The chosen donor site is prepared with a surgical antiseptic solution and care is taken to remove as much soap as possible using ether or an acetone preparation. The Reese drum type dermatone or the Brown electrical scissor type dermatone is acceptable. While hand-excised split thickness skin grafts have been used, their thickness is variable and their quality relies on the experience of the surgeon taking the graft. We prefer the Padgett dermatone. It gives a precise thickness of graft and the configuration and size of the graft is controllable. Ideally, a split thickness skin graft should be thin enough to allow transudate to penetrate the graft by osmosis which must nourish the graft for the first 48 to 72 hours prior to microcapillary ingrowth and, at the same time, be thick enough to withstand the wear and tear of the vaginal form. A split thickness skin graft of 0.35 mm (12 one thousandths of an inch) has proven successful over the years for this purpose.

After the vagina has been excised, meticulous care should be made to ensure that hemostasis is complete. Obviously, small hematomas will not allow the graft to remain flat on its bed and thus those segments of the split thickness skin graft may not survive.

Various vaginal forms have been used over the years ranging from balsa wood covered with foam rubber to soft silastic. Because hard metallic and wooden forms can produce pressure necrosis and fistula formation into the bladder or rectum, we have preferred to use soft foam rubber molded into a tubular shape and covered with a contraceptive condom as a vaginal form (Fig. 87.11). These materials are easy to obtain and the tubular configuration can be easily carved in the operating room from a block of

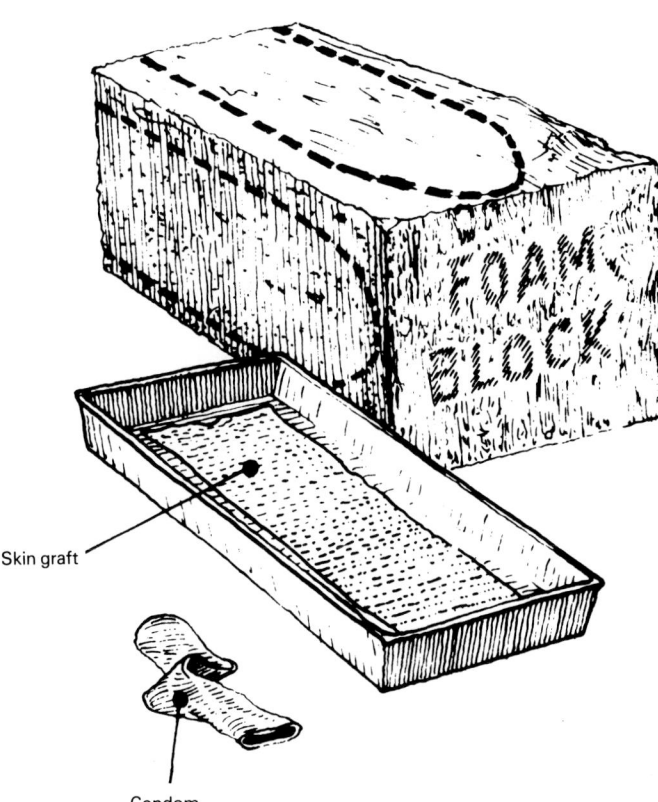

Fig. 87.11 A drawing of foam rubber block used to carve the vaginal form. The split thickness skin graft is left in a saline solution. A contraceptive condom is used to cover the foam rubber vaginal form. (Courtesy of Wheeless C R (1988).[16])

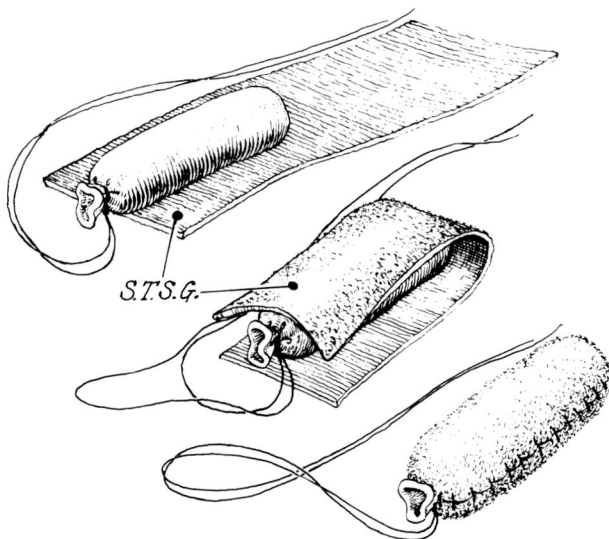

Fig. 87.12 A drawing of foam rubber vaginal mold covered with a condom. The split thickness skin graft (STSG) is sutured over the mold.

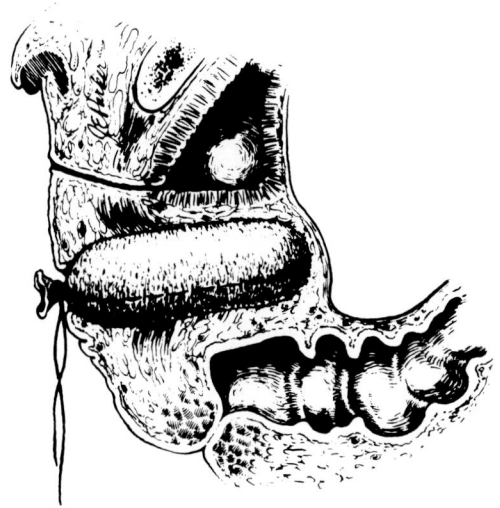

Fig. 87.13 A drawing of the vaginal form covered with a split thickness skin graft placed into the new vaginal canal. The pelvic perineum has been closed. (Courtesy of Wheeless C R (1988).[16])

foam rubber with a pair of curved Mayo scissors. The previously sterilized foam rubber form is compressed and inserted into a double layer of contraceptive condoms. By compressing the foam rubber inside the condoms the appropriate size can be achieved. The ends of the condoms can be tied with a 2/0 silk suture and the form will remain the desired size. It is an excellent idea to check the size of the form by placing it into the vagina several times prior to covering the vaginal form with the split thickness skin graft to ensure that the vaginal form is adequate in both length and diameter. If it is too large, the condoms can be removed and additional foam rubber can be trimmed away with scissors. The split thickness skin graft is then sutured around the form (Fig. 87.12) taking care that the epidermal surface is adjacent to the rubber condom and that the lower layer of dermis is adjacent to the recipient bed (Fig. 87.13). The vaginal form is held in place by suturing the labia closed with 2 or 3 interrupted 2/0 black silk sutures. The graft and the dressing over the donor site are left in place undisturbed for 10 to 12 days. We prefer to perform a dressing change and graft inspection in the operating room under general anesthesia. After inspection, the new vagina is irrigated with saline solution and then measured, and a soft silastic vaginal form is selected for use in the postoperative period. Care must be taken that no portion

of the vaginal form protrudes through the hymenal ring otherwise labial ulceration may result. The form should be used continuously for 4 to 6 months postoperatively unless the patient engages in regular sexual intercourse. If the form is left out for 24 to 48 hours it will be difficult to reinsert and, frequently, reinsertion has to be performed under general anesthesia. This is a particular problem in young and/or immature females. McIndoe vaginoplasty is almost universally successful except in those cases where the patient has failed to wear her form for the appropriate length of time. We encourage the patient to remove the form each day, douche the vagina, and then replace the form.

Omental J flap neovagina with split thickness skin graft

The classic McIndoe[8,9] technique for construction of a neovagina is not available when the bladder and rectum have been removed after total pelvic exenteration. After total pelvic exenteration, when the colon has been reconnected to a preserved rectum, Berek & Hacker[1,2] have demonstrated that the neocolon-rectal anastomosis serves as a posterior wall of a proposed neovagina. The anterior and lateral walls could be made from an omental flap.

By modifying the omental flap which is normally used to close off the pelvic inlet after total pelvic exenteration[12] (Fig. 87.14), with or without low coloproctostomy, the surgeon can create a cylinder providing anterior, posterior and lateral walls for the neovagina. When the cylinder is sutured to the introitus and lined with a split thickness skin graft of 0.35 mm (12 one thousandths of an inch), and expanded in the postoperative period by a soft vaginal form, a satisfactory functional neovagina can be created[16,17] (Figs 87.12, 87.15, 87.16). It is interesting that the omentum, innervated by the vagus nerve, forms the wall of the neovagina. Normally, tugging or pulling on the omentum does not produce the sensation of pleasure that one would associate with sexual intercourse. However, approximately 40% of the patients who have undergone this operation report that they experience sexual orgasm. Another interesting physiological change is the development of estrogen hormone receptors in the split thickness skin graft. Derived from skin on the buttocks or thigh that normally has no demonstrable hormonal receptors, the skin graft eventually becomes indistinguishable from normal vaginal mucosa on histological examination. If the original split thickness skin graft has been taken at a thickness greater than 12 one thousandths of an inch, hair follicles may be preserved and therefore a biopsy can distinguish between normal vagina and skin by the presence of hair follicles. At present, it is unknown whether the maturation index of the graft can be influenced by the administration of systemic estrogen as can occur in normal vaginal mucosa.

If construction of the neovagina immediately follows total pelvic exenteration, it is important to ensure hemostasis in the pelvic wound before applying the split thickness skin graft. If hemostasis is uncertain, the omental pocket for the neovagina should be packed with gauze or foam rubber covered by a contraceptive condom. When hemostasis and serous drainage has been secured, a split thickness skin graft can be taken from the thigh or buttocks and applied to the vaginal form.

After the split thickness skin graft has been inserted, the neovagina must remain dilated with a vaginal form until healing is complete. Thereafter, a soft silastic vaginal form

should be worn at all times, except during intercourse, for a period of 6 months. After this time, the soft silastic vaginal form is worn only at night if sexual intercourse is not part of the patient's life style.

A sagittal section illustrating a patient who has undergone a total pelvic exenteration is shown in Figure 87.14. In this patient, the rectal stump was left and the descending colon was brought down for a very low coloproctostomy. The urethral meatus and a small vaginal stump below the levator sling remain in place. The omentum has been brought down as a flap based on the left gastro-epiploic artery, and sutured to the sacral promontory posteriorly and the pubic symphysis anteriorly.

In patients who have insufficient omentum to form both the pelvic lid and walls of the neovagina, the omentum making the pelvic lid is supplemented by the use of a sheet of polyglycolic acid mesh.

The upper part of the drawing in Figure 87.15 shows the omental flap with the intestines lying in the pelvic lid sling. In the lower part of the drawing, the distal portion of the flap has been rolled into a cylinder. The lateral walls of the cylinder have been sutured with interrupted 3/0 polyglycolic acid sutures.

A split thickness skin graft is laid out in a vaginal form

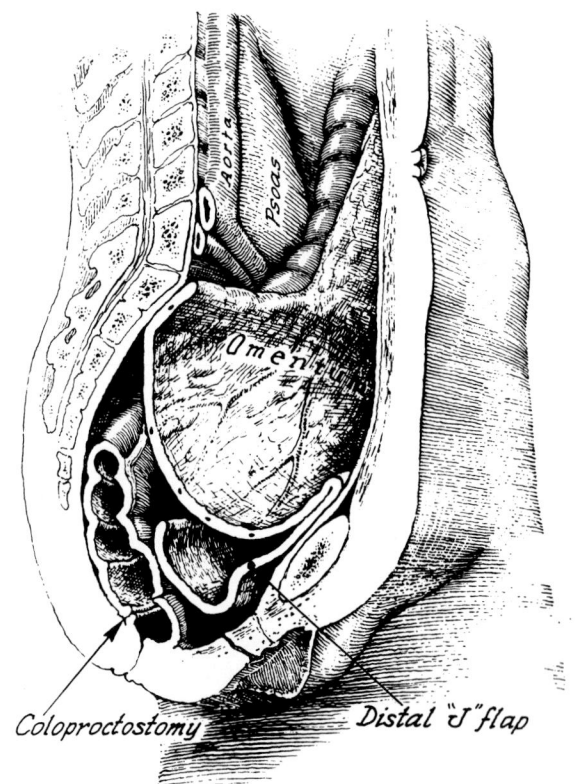

Fig. 87.14 A sagittal drawing after total exenteration. The colon has been re-anastomosed to the rectum. The omentum has been taken off the stomach and brought into the pelvis as a flap for a pelvic lid. The distal omentum is available for the walls of the neovaginal cylinder.

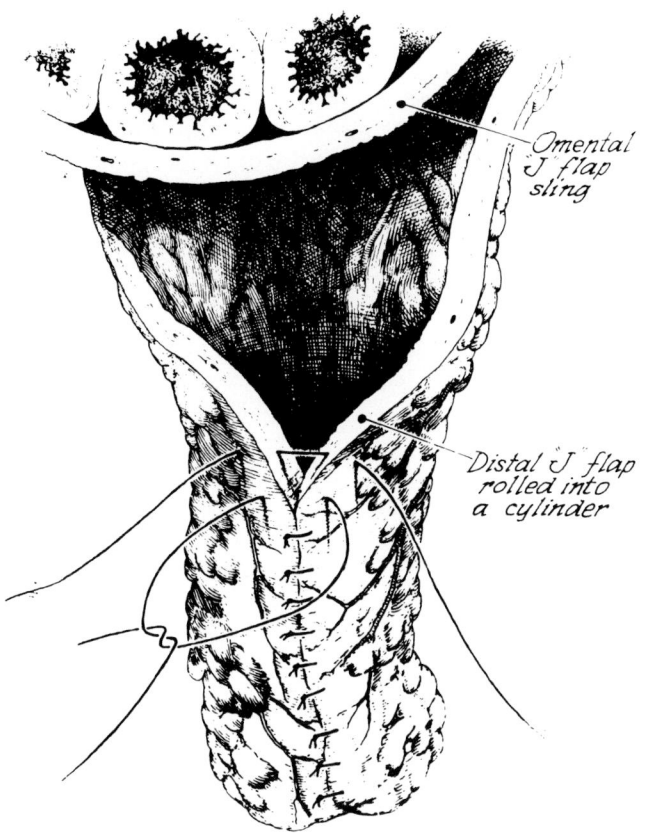

Fig. 87.15 The distal omentum is rolled into a cylinder to be lined with a split thickness skin graft.

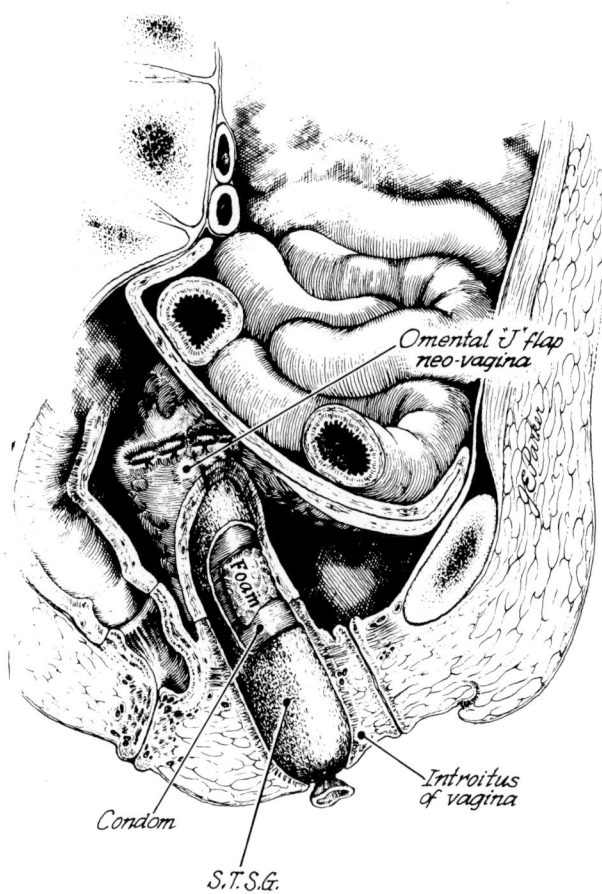

Fig. 87.16 A sagittal drawing of the omental flap neovagina, lined with a split thickness skin graft (STSG) fashioned over a foam rubber vaginal mold covered with a condom.

as fashioned from foam rubber stuffed into a contraceptive latex condom as previously demonstrated in Figures 87.11 and 87.12. The split thickness skin graft is folded over the vaginal form, and edges of the graft are sutured with interrupted 4/0 polyglycolic acid sutures.

The completed operation is illustrated in Figure 87.16. A sagittal section is shown with the omental J flap as the pelvic lid, and the residual of the omental flap that forms the walls of the neovaginal cylinder. The split thickness skin graft covered vaginal form has been introduced into the neovagina.

Gracilis myocutaneous flap for reconstruction of the vagina

The gracilis myocutaneous flap, suggested by McGraw et al[7] not only offers the advantage of reconstruction of an adequate vagina but gives the physiological advantage of filling the pelvic defect with a nonirradiated vascular pedicle that serves as an internal pelvic lid and fills the pelvic deadspace promoting wound healing and reducing infection.

The technique for gracilis myocutaneous flap reconstruction is as follows. Two 15 × 10 cm paddle shaped flaps are marked over the gracilis muscle. The technique for

making the flap is the same as stated previously under construction of the vulva[16] (Fig. 87.17). After both flaps have been made, and their vascular integrity demonstrated, a tunnel is dissected under the skin bridge from the proximal margin of the flap incision on the thigh, under the labia majora and minora, into the vaginal canal (Fig. 87.18). Care must be taken not to damage the artery and nerve to the flap during this maneuver. The flaps are placed along the side of each other symmetrically (Fig. 87.19A). They are coiled into the desired tubular shape and sutured together with 3/0 Dexon sutures in a subcuticular fashion (Fig. 87.19B). A second layer of 3/0 Dexon subcutaneous interrupted sutures is placed for additional support on three of the four sides of the paddle shaped flap. The fourth side remains open as an entrance to the new vagina.

Through the abdominal incision a Babcock or Allis clamp is used to gently pull the tubular shaped flaps through the introitus and into the true pelvis. Multiple interrupted 2/0 Dexon sutures are placed between the subcutaneous tissue of the flap and the available fascia of the sacrum, pelvic side walls and pubic symphysis.

The pointed distal ends of the paddle shaped flap at the entrance to the new vagina can be trimmed away until it

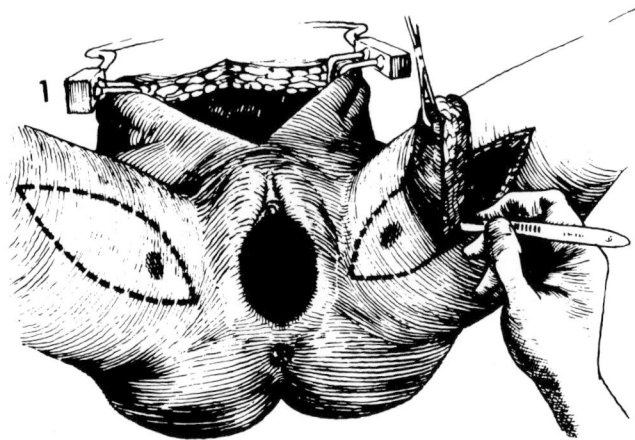

Fig. 87.17 A drawing at the completion of a pelvic exenteration. The gracilis myocutaneous flap is being taken from the left thigh. The shaded area marks the location of the neurovascular bundle. (Courtesy of Wheeless C R (1988).[16])

conforms with the shape of the introitus. Interrupted 3/0 Dexon sutures are used to suture the distal margin of the flap to the introitus.

Several sump-type suction drains are placed under the flap and brought out through the introitus and placed on continuous low suction (Fig. 87.20). No vaginal packing or forms are used.[16]

The flaps should be inspected daily for vascular integrity. Any small necrotic areas should be removed. Sexual intercourse is allowed after 6 weeks. However, because of the extensiveness of the cancer surgery, most patients do not attempt intercourse for 4 to 6 months.

Sigmoid neovagina

The use of intestine lumen, both small bowel as well as large bowel, has been an intriguing concept for construction of neovagina.[3,6] Recently Kindermann[6] from Munich has published his experience with this technique. In selected cases we find it very useful. The cardinal feature of the use of an isolated segment of rectosigmoid colon is the integrity of the vascular supply of the colon via the superior hemorrhoidal artery (Fig. 87.21). The essential feature of this technique is to ensure the integrity of the superior hemorrhoidal branch of the inferior mesenteric artery at the time of surgical resection. Unlike small bowel, the secretions of an isolated small (10 to 12 cm) segment of sigmoid colon are not so copious as to inconvenience the patient with troublesome discharge from the neovagina. An additional anatomical advantage of the rectosigmoid colon over the use of isolated segments of small bowel is the unique anatomical feature of the marginal artery of the colon (marginal artery of Drummond). This allows the surgeon to reverse the peristaltic direction of the colon in order to obtain greater mobility, by transecting the mesentery proximal to the marginal artery with the sigmoid branches of the hemorrhoidal artery, and allowing the superior hemorrhoidal artery to provide the appropriate vascular supply to the colonic segment via the marginal artery. Thus, by bringing down the proximal segment of the isolated colon, it will reach the desired vaginal introitus without tension (Fig. 87.22). The margins of the colon are sutured to the vaginal introitus with interrupted 3/0 polyglycolic acid sutures.

The technique first requires transection of a segment of

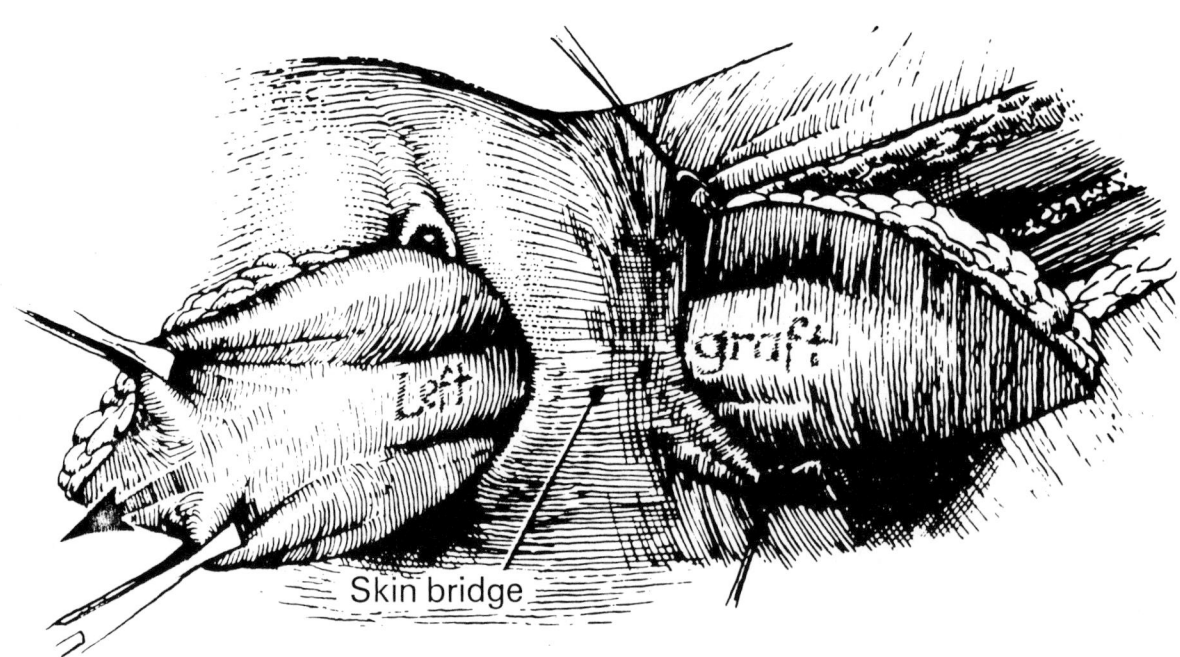

Fig. 87.18 A drawing of the left gracilis myocutaneous flap pulled under the skin bridge. (Courtesy of Wheeless C R (1988).[16])

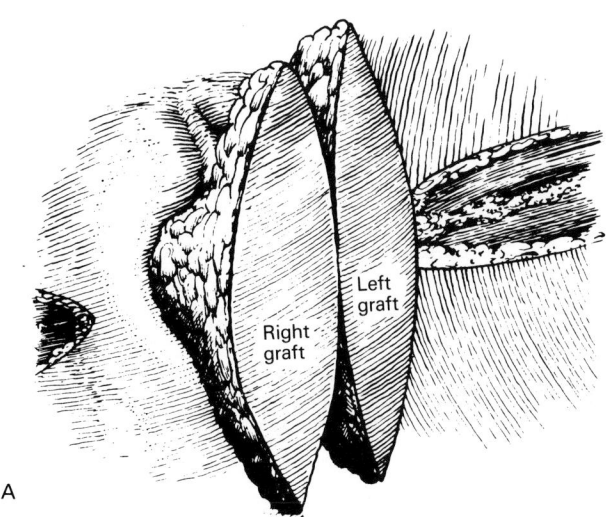

A

Fig. 87.19A A drawing of the two myocutaneous flaps lined up in front of the vaginal opening. (Courtesy of Wheeless C R (1988).[16])

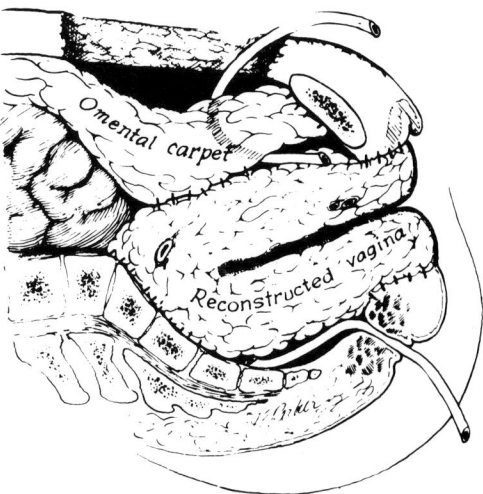

Fig. 87.20 A drawing of the new vagina in place in the pelvis. Suction drains have been placed and an omental carpet has been brought down to complete the closure of the pelvic inlet. (Courtesy of Wheeless C R (1988).[16])

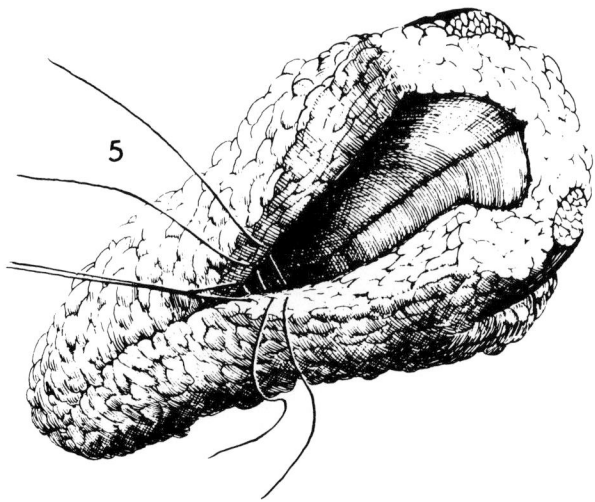

B

Fig. 87.19B A drawing of the flaps sutured together making the new vagina. (Courtesy of Wheeless C R (1988).[16])

rectosigmoid colon in routine manner (Fig. 87.21). It is vital to insure the integrity of the superior hemorrhoidal artery. In most cases, the isolated rectosigmoid segment will not reach the vaginal introitus in its normal peristaltic direction. Greater mobility can be achieved by transecting the mesentery back to the superior hemorrhoidal artery and vein, and bringing down the proximal segment of the rectosigmoid colonic segment. As seen in Figure 87.22, this segment is sutured to the vaginal introitus, and a soft foam rubber mold is inserted to keep the isolated rectosigmoid segment dilated in the postoperative period.

Williams operation for vaginal reconstruction

The Williams operation for vaginal reconstruction is ideal

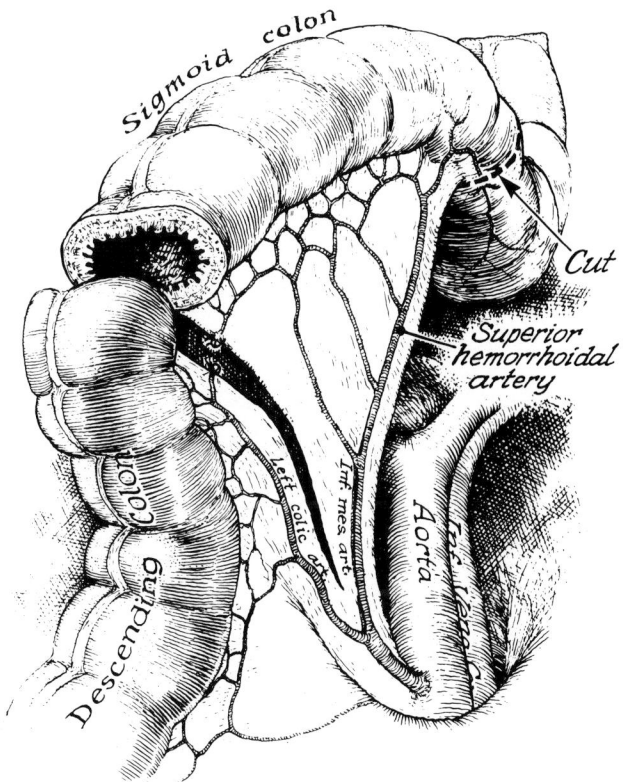

Fig. 87.21 A 12 to 14 cm segment of rectosigmoid colon is removed based on the superior hemorrhoidal artery.

in those cases where the pelvic surgeon does not wish to invade the perineum following radical resection and/or irradiation of the pelvis.[18] Obviously, such a dissection could be hazardous because numerous loops of small bowel have frequently descended into the true pelvis. Therefore, a noninvasive technique creating a vaginal pouch

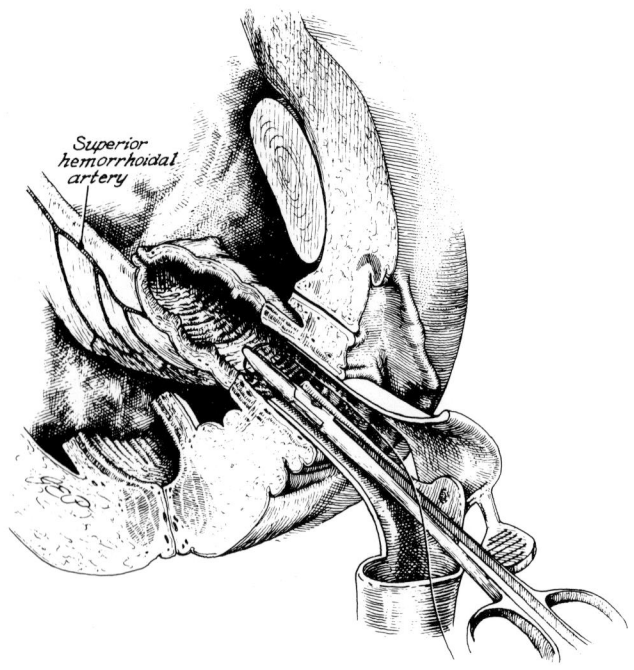

Fig. 87.22 The proximal segment of rectosigmoid colon based on the superior hemorrhoidal artery is sutured to the vaginal introitus.

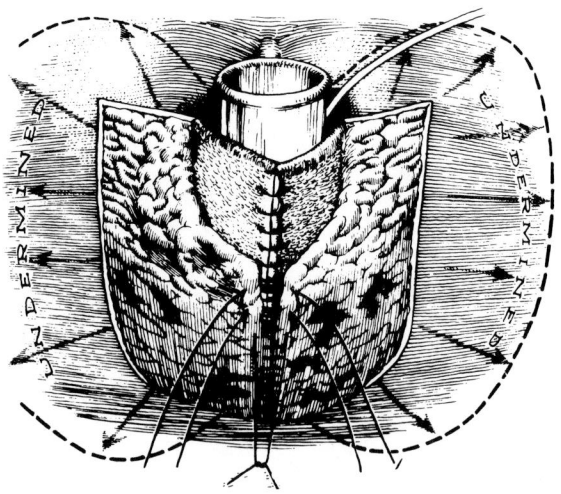

Fig. 87.24 A drawing showing the skin flap closed over a cylinder. A second layer of subcutaneous fat is closed over the flap. The peripheral skin has been undermined for mobilization and closure. (Courtesy of Wheeless C R (1988).[16])

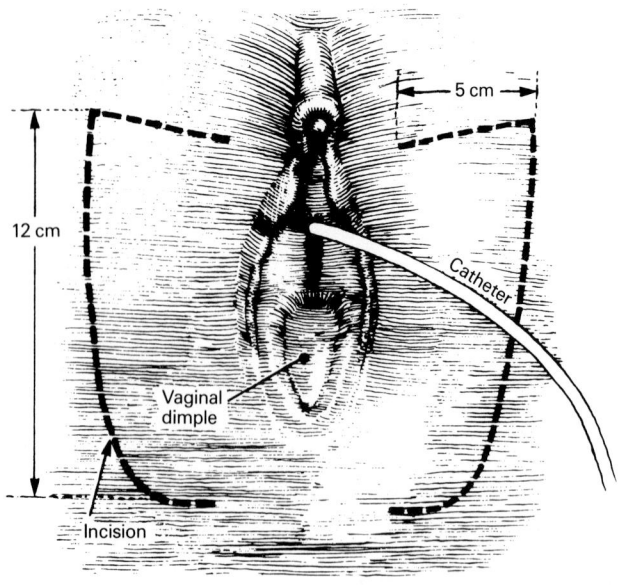

Fig. 87.23 A drawing of the outline of proposed vulvar skin flap to be used for the new vagina. (Courtesy of Wheeless C R (1988).[16])

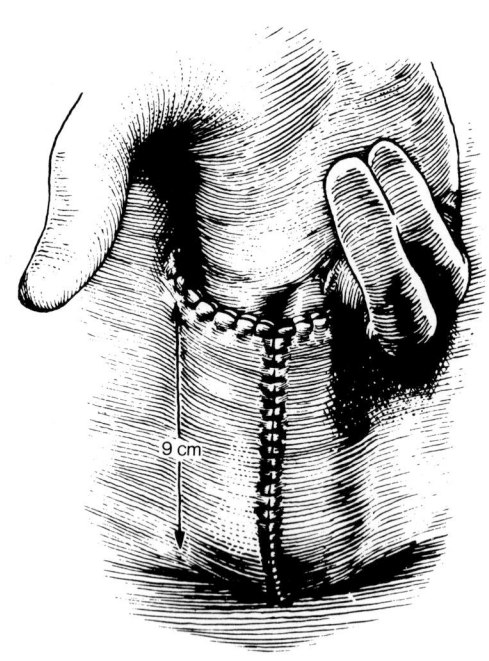

Fig. 87.25 A drawing of the completed new vagina. (Courtesy of Wheeless C R (1988).[16])

exteriorly is desirable in these cases. The Williams operation has proven efficacious. Although the vertical direction of the newly constructed vaginal pouch initially may seem awkward, the axis of the new pouch, with use, becomes progressively more horizontal. The key to the success of the operation is to design the skin flaps adequately prior to making the initial incision and to adequately mobilize the skin of the perineum so that it covers the skin

flaps without tension. If adequate mobilization is not performed and the margins are brought together under tension, they will necrose and separate producing an undesirable result.

The operation is begun by placing the patient in the dorsal lithotomy position.[16,18] A metal ruler is used to carefully ascertain the length and width of the desired skin flap. This is determined after measuring the amount of 'normal vagina' remaining after the radical procedure. In many cases, in women with redundant and large labia minora and majora, the initial flap of skin can be quite conservative. Ideally, the new vaginal pouch should be 5 cm in diameter and 10 cm long. To achieve this, the skin over the labia majora is marked in a U-shaped fashion, 3 cm lateral to the introitus and for a distance of 10 to 12 cm along the vertical axis over the labia majora and across the perineal body, preceding a U shaped incision (Fig. 87.23). The incision is then made full thickness 'dermis and epidermis' and the medial skin is mobilized toward the vagina taking care not to injure its vascular supply at its base along the introitus. This skin flap is rolled into position and sutured together with interrupted 3/0 Dexon sutures. The bridge of skin over the perineal body is elevated and sutured to the bottom of the vaginal pouch.

The skin lateral to the initial incision over the labia majora is mobilized for a distance of approximately 5 cm in all directions. This is then brought together in the midline with interrupted subcutaneous sutures of 3/0 Dexon (Fig. 87.24). Thus, this forms a second layer to the newly constructed vaginal pouch and gives support to the new vagina. Skin margins of this second layer brought together in the midline are closed with interrupted nylon sutures. The opening to the new vagina is sutured to the second skin flap with interrupted 3/0 Dexon sutures.

After completing the new vagina it should admit two fingers for a depth of approximately 8 to 9 cm. A tubular shaped soft silastic vaginal form 8 cm long and 4 cm in diameter is inserted into the new vagina each day (Fig 87.25). This should be carried out until active sexual intercourse is achieved. Sexual intercourse is allowed after 6 weeks.

REFERENCES

1. Berek J S, Hacker N F, Lagasse L D 1983 Delayed vaginal reconstruction in the fibrotic pelvis following radiation or previous reconstruction. Obstet Gynecol 61: 331
2. Berek J S, Hacker N F, Lagasse L D 1984 Vaginal reconstruction performed simultaneous with pelvic exenteration. Obstet Gynecol 63: 318
3. Burger R A, Riedmiller H, Friedberg V, Hohenfellner R 1987 The ileocecal vagina. Geburtshilfe Frauenheilkd 47: 644
4. Franklin E W, Bostwick J, Burrell M O 1977 Reconstructive techniques in radical pelvic surgery. Am J Obstet Gynecol 129: 285
5. Julian C G, Woodruff J D 1974 Surgery of the vulva: vulvectomy. In: Ridley J H (ed) Gynecologic Surgery. Errors, Safeguards, Salvage. Williams & Wilkins, Baltimore, p 256
6. Kindermann G 1987 The sigmoid vagina: experiences in the treatment of congenital absence or later loss of vagina. Geburtshilfe Frauenheilkd 47: 650
7. McGraw J B, Massey F M, Shanklin K D, Horton C E 1976 Vaginal reconstruction with gracilis myocutaneous flap. Plast Reconstr Surg 58: 176
8. McIndoe A H 1950 Treatment of congenital absence and obliterative conditions of vagina. Br J Plast Surg 2: 254
9. McIndoe A H, Bannister J B 1938 An operation for the care of congenital absence of the vagina. J Obstet Gynaecol Br Emp 45: 490
10. Orticochea M 1972 Musculo-cutaneous flap method: an immediate and heroic substitute for the method of delay. Br J Plast Surg 25: 106
11. Owens N 1955 Compound neck pedicle designed for repair of massive facial defects. Plast Reconstr Surg 15: 369
12. Valle G, Ferraris G 1969 Use of the omentum to contain the intestines in pelvic exenteration. Obstet Gynecol 33: 772
13. Way S 1948 The anatomy of the lymphatic drainage of the vulva and its influences on the radical operation for carcinoma. J Obstet Gynaecol Br Commonw 73: 594
14. Wharton L R 1938 A simple method of constructing a vagina: report of four cases. Am J Surg 107: 842
15. Wheeless C R 1979 Gracilis myocutaneous flap in reconstruction of the vulva and female perineum. Obstet Gynecol 54: 97
16. Wheeless C R 1988 Atlas of Pelvic Surgery. Lea & Febiger, Philadelphia
17. Wheeless C R 1989 Neovagina constructed from an omental J flap and a split thickness skin graft. Gynecol Oncol 35: 224
18. Williams E A 1964 Congenital absence of the vagina: A simple operation for its relief. J Obstet Gynaecol Br Commonw 71: 511

88. Urinary and rectal continence saving operations

C. R. Wheeless Jr

INTRODUCTION

Fecal and urinary diversion have been an essential part of total pelvic exenteration (TPE) surgery. The early pioneer work of Brunschwig[2] in TPE surgery utilized uretero-sigmoidostomy for urinary diversion. Reflux of fecal contaminated urine resulted in unaccepted rates of pyelonephritis and progressive renal deterioration. Bricker,[1] in 1950, introduced isolated ileal loop urinary diversion. Later, the colonic loop modification was preferred by some.[20] These two techniques have been preferred for urinary diversion for over 30 years. However, long-term follow-up of patients with intestinal loop urinary diversion revealed a high incidence of ureteral stenosis and upper renal tract deterioration, especially in those who have had total pelvic irradiation associated with therapy for gynecologic malignancies.[4,14,18] In addition, negative quality of life issues secondary to the required urostomy bag; its odor, reduced self image, and impaired sexuality make an alternative technique without a bag desirable if surgically and physiologically feasible.[10,21]

Resection of the rectosigmoid colon in the surgical management of the patient with primary or recurrent gynecologic malignancy may be required. In the past, very low anastomosis of the colon to the rectum was rarely performed and most patients were left with a permanent end sigmoid colostomy.[3,11] Renewed interest in very low anastomosis of colon to the rectum was rekindled with the introduction of the EEA stapler.[6,17]

CONTINENT UROSTOMY OPERATIONS

There are unique pathologic and physiologic changes in the pelvic organs following the application of irradiation treatment for gynecologic malignancies. These high levels of pelvic irradiation are not required for the treatment of most urologic malignancies, such as carcinoma of the prostate and bladder; and the pathophysiological changes of irradiation induced endarteritis, ischemia, and fibrosis are clearly not present in urinary diversions required for congenital anomalies.

Therefore, in selecting the physiological requirements for a continent non-refluxing urostomy several features must be considered. The ureteral-intestinal anastomosis must be as free as possible from potential stricture formation that would result in hydronephrosis and eventual upper renal unit deterioration. Careful choice of non-irradiated bowel and ureter is ideal, as irradiation changes in bowel can be progressive and chronic. Techniques which require burying the irradiated ureter in the muscular layers of irradiated colon to achieve the non-refluxing feature of some of the continent urostomy operations may be associated with a risk for stenosis and secondary hydronephrosis that is higher than acceptable. This remains to be evaluated in prospective randomized trials comparing the Kock pouch-type continent urostomy and the ileo-ascending colonic variety of these operations. The continent urostomy pouch should have a low pressure, less than 40 ml of water, to reduce the chance of ureteral reflux but also to reduce the incidence of incontinence. The incorporation of large bowel may lead to unacceptable levels of pressure as its properties of compliance are less than small bowel.[10] A larger segment of denervated colon, i.e. the entire ascending and proximal transverse colon, may overcome this problem and allow pressures within the pouch to remain at acceptable levels.[16] The pouch should maintain a low pressure even at volumes of urine greater than 500 ml. The patient should catheterize her continent pouch about 3 to 4 times per day.

Our motivation in gynecologic oncology for using the continent urostomy has been 85% for medical reasons, i.e., to prevent contaminated reflux and thus deterioration of the upper renal units which are commonly associated with ileal or colonic loops followed more than 5 years post pelvic exenteration; and 15% of our motivation has been for the improvement in quality of life. These percentages will vary in different geographical areas. The elimination of the urinary bag with its attendant problems of awkwardness and odor has been a positive effect on the quality of the cancer patient's life, the rebuilding of her self image, and the improvement of her sexuality. (See Ch. 90.)

As gynecologic oncologists, we felt unbiased and free to review all the available data from continent urostomies, i.e., Kock,[10] Mentz,[24] and Indiana[19] pouches, and utilize different available techniques to meet our needs and accomplish our goal of surgical rehabilitation of the patient.

Continent urostomy with ileal reservoir (Kock pouch)

The Kock pouch, developed by Kock[10] in 1982, was devised as a continent non-refluxing urostomy. Modifications by Skinner[22] improved the surgical technique and reduced the postoperative complications of the original Kock technique. This alternative to ileal or colonic loop urinary diversion deserves the consideration of gynecologic oncologists. Skinner et al[23] have shown that construction of an internal reservoir suitable for urinary bladder replacement must provide: (1) retention of 500 to 1000 ml of fluid; (2) maintenance of low pressure after filling; (3) elimination of intermittent pressure spikes; (4) true continence; (5) ease of catheterization; and (6) prevention of reflux.

The ileal mucosa of the pouch appears to adapt well to urine; villus height decreases and, in time, the mucosa becomes nearly flat, thereby reducing the absorption of electrolytes from the urine.

Prerequisites to construction of the Kock pouch include: reasonable renal function (creatinine less than 3.0 mg/dl); adequate length of small bowel so that utilization of 80 cm of ileum taken out of the digestive tract will not result in a significant short bowel syndrome; and a patient and her surgeon who are motivated for the procedure and who understand the inherent risks (a 20% incidence of malfunction of the continent valve mechanism requiring additional surgery).

A midline incision is preferred for the construction of a continent urostomy. The site of the stoma can be determined preoperatively. For young, slim women we prefer to place the opening of the stoma below the underwear line immediately above the pubic hair. For older and/or obese patients, the stoma is often placed higher to facilitate catheterization. However, the surgeon should not feel bound by the preoperative selected stomal site if the mesentery of the efferent bowel limb does not allow the pouch to reach

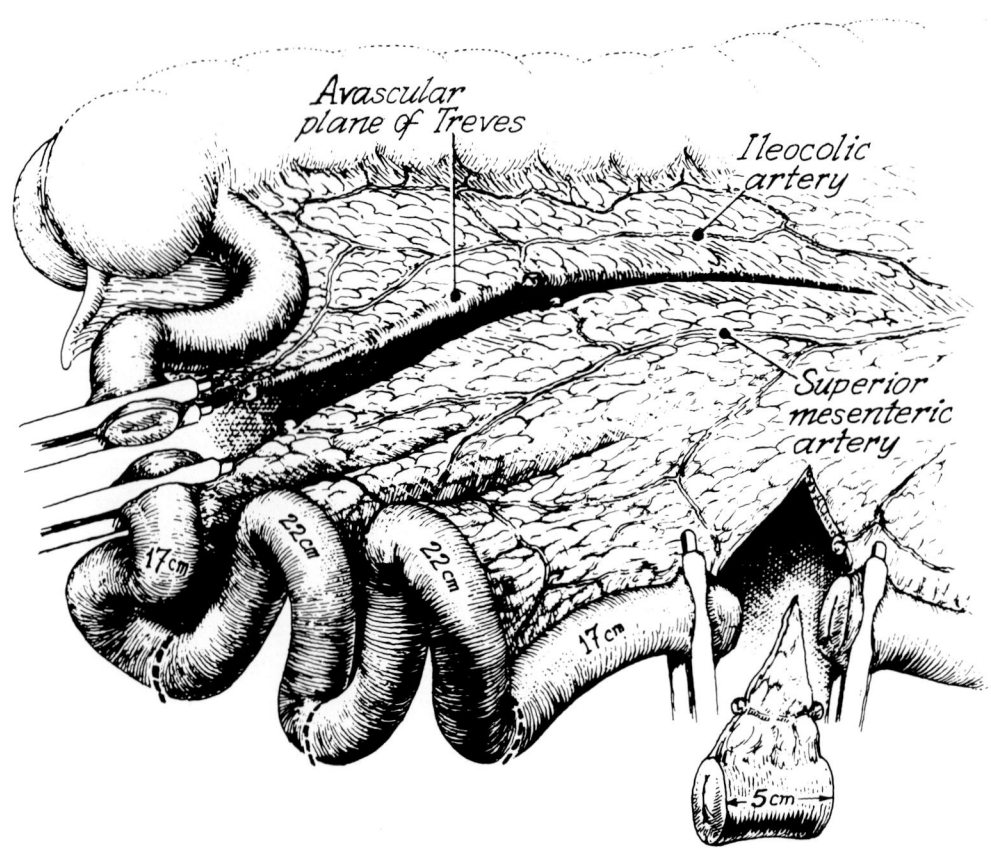

Fig. 88.1 Anatomical drawing of terminal ileum illustrating the avascular plane of Treves, the ileocolic artery and the superior mesenteric artery. Note that the efferent system requires 17 cm of bowel, Kock pouch requires two 22 cm segments of bowel, and afferent system requires 17 cm of bowel. Five centimeters of intestine are resected to give additional mobility to the completed Kock pouch.

that location without tension. Since no applicance bag is worn for the collection of urine, one need not worry about skin folds. When the pouch procedure is done in conjunction with total pelvic exenteration or cystectomy, pelvic resection is performed first. For conversion of an existing ileal conduit, all the intra-abdominal wall adhesions to the intestine must be taken down prior to initiating the Kock pouch continent urostomy.

Follow-up from the Kock and Skinner series has been approximately 7 years. Follow-up from our series of irradiated patients has been 2 years. Longer follow-up and greater numbers of patients with continent urostomies following gynecologic oncology procedures, especially after the unique levels of irradiation required in gynecologic oncology, must be evaluated and published.

Technique for Kock pouch continent urostomy: Skinner modification

As seen in Figure 88.1, a clear knowledge and understanding of the anatomy of the terminal ileum, ascending colon and the blood supply to these structures is vital for the success of the operation. The terminal ileum is transected approximately 16 cm from the ileocecal junction in the area of the avascular plane of Treves.[26] To insure mobility of the pouch, an incision is carried up the avascular plane of Treves for 25 to 30 cm. The ileocolic artery must be lateral and the branches of the superior mesenteric artery medial to this incision.

The continent urostomy pouch requires 17 cm of ileum for the efferent nipple valve and bowel limb, two 22 cm segments of ileum for the pouch itself, and a 17 cm segment of ileum for the afferent bowel limb and non-refluxing nipple. As seen in Figure 88.1, 5 cm of proximal ileum is sacrificed to allow greater mobility of the completed pouch. The anterior wall of the pouch is opened with electrocautery. The posterior wall is sutured with two layers of polyglycolic acid suture[26] (Fig. 88.2).

The nipples are constructed by intussusception of the small intestine. Stapling the nipple intussusception with a TA55 4.8 mm stapler to prevent dessusception is a vital step in this procedure (Figs 88.3 and 88.4). The walls of the pouch are folded over and sutured in place to complete the pouch (Fig. 88.5).

The ureters are anastomosed to the afferent bowel limb over silastic stents (Fig. 88.6). The efferent bowel limb is brought through a defect in the abdominal wall. The afferent bowel limb with non-refluxing nipple and ureters anastomosed over silastic stents is positioned near the promontory of the sacrum. The pouch itself is positioned in the pelvic inlet. The efferent system of the pouch requires a 30 French Medena catheter placed through the stoma and passed through the efferent nipple into the pouch for drainage of intestinal mucus[26] (Fig. 88.7).

During the postoperative phase, all continent urostomies

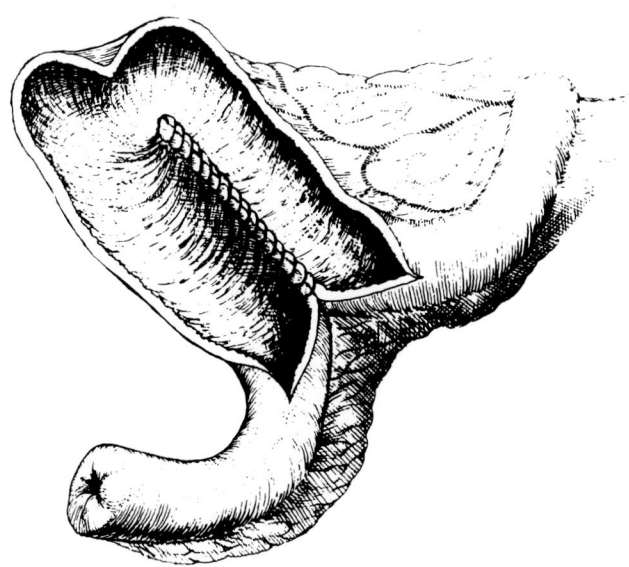

Fig. 88.2 A drawing of the Kock pouch opened, the posterior wall of the Kock pouch has been sutured with two layers of running synthetic absorbable sutures.

are drained by a closed suction drain placed in the area of the pouch. Leakage has been frequent and if not drained a uroma with septic abscess may occur. The efferent catheter and the closed suction drain can be removed 3 weeks postoperatively. Thereafter the patient is trained by the enterostomal therapist in the technique for catheterizing her pouch. She will empty the pouch less frequently until the 8th postoperative week when the pouch should be emptied three times a day.[7] Three weeks postoperatively the pouch is endoscoped, the silastic stents are removed from the ureters, and the pouch is tested for ureteral reflux as well as continence by filling the pouch with several hundred ml of radiopaque saline. Intravenous pyelogram should be obtained at this time for assessment of the renal status; slight pyelocaliectasis is not unusual for 6 to 8 weeks.

For the first 3 weeks postoperatively, the patient is placed on an antibiotic sensitive to pseudomonas, such as ciprofloxacin or noroxin. After this initial 3 week period the patients are given prophylactic urosepsis for 2 additional months by oral triple sulfa antibiotics.

Early results from this procedure have been very encouraging. In highly irradiated bowel there will always be a higher percentage of nipple valve fistulas, as compared to the Kock and Skinner series predominately using non-irradiated patients. There has been little doubt as to the efficacy of this procedure in the re-establishment of quality of life in these cancer patients. The elimination of the urine bag with its undesirable odor and problems of leakage has resulted in improved self-image. Long-term evaluation of upper renal tract deterioration as compared to ileal and colonic loops awaits further evaluation. Early results as reported by Skinner indicate a protective effect on the upper

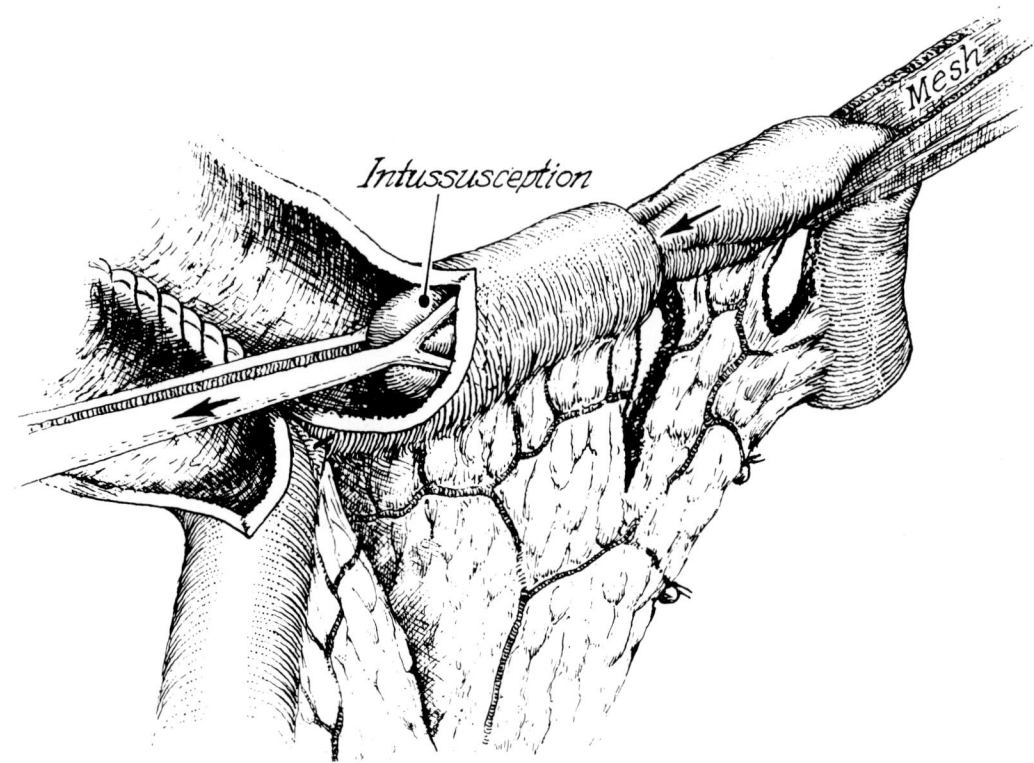

Fig. 88.3 The nipples are constructed by intussusception of the small intestine.

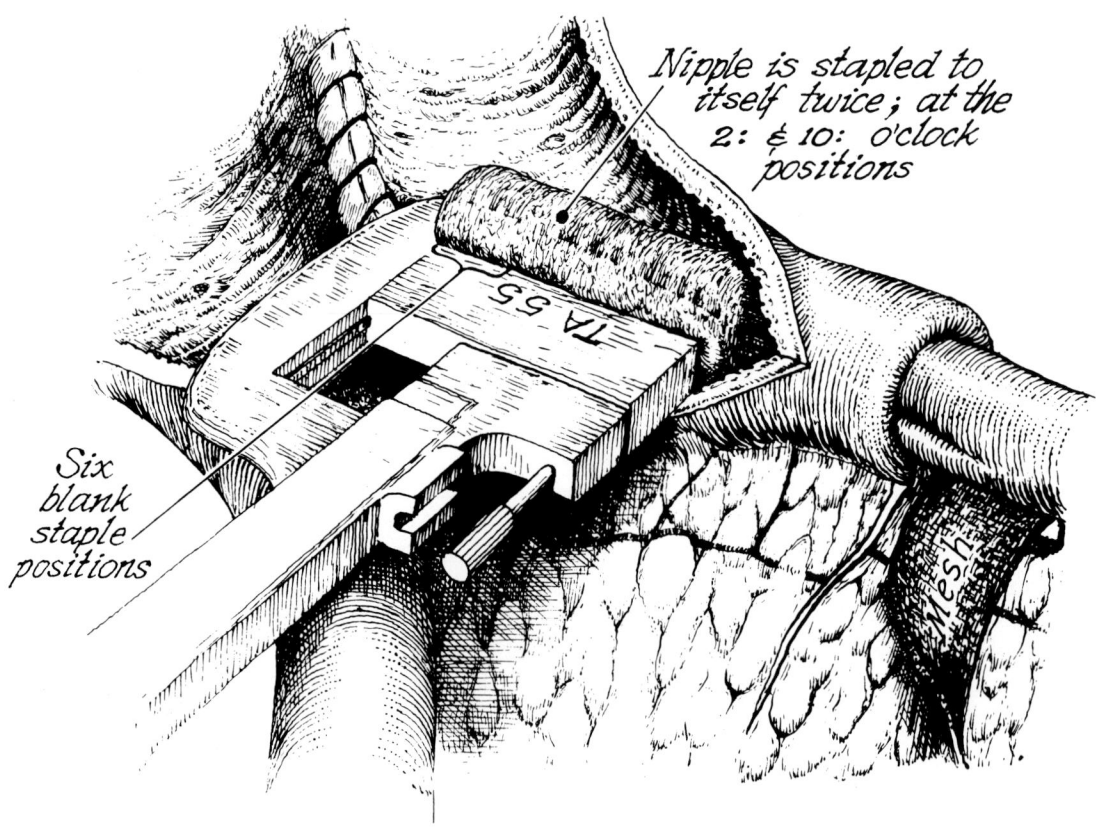

Fig. 88.4 The TA55 4.8 stapler is used to staple the nipples at the 2 and 10 o'clock positions to prevent dessusception.

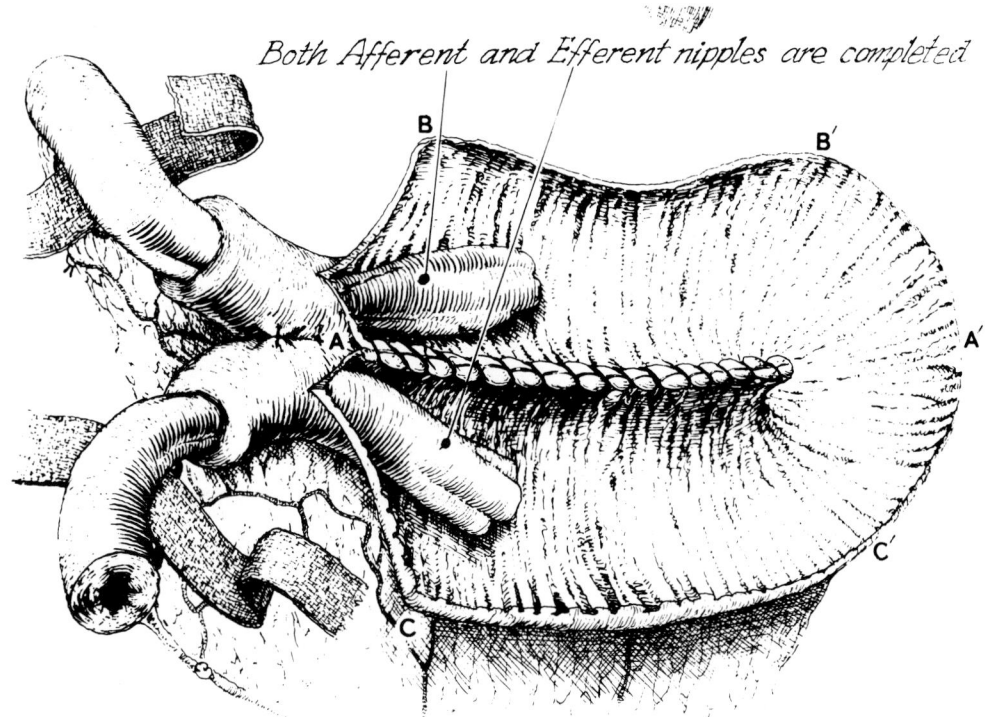

Both Afferent and Efferent nipples are completed

Fig. 88.5 Drawing of the completed pouch showing the efferent and afferent nipples having been constructed with their respective efferent and afferent bowel limbs. Strips of polyglycolic acid mesh have been inserted through the mesentery to be sutured adjacent to the intussusception to further reduce the incidence of dessusception. The walls of the pouch have been labeled B, B', A, A', C, C'. These letters will obviously be connected forming the pouch.

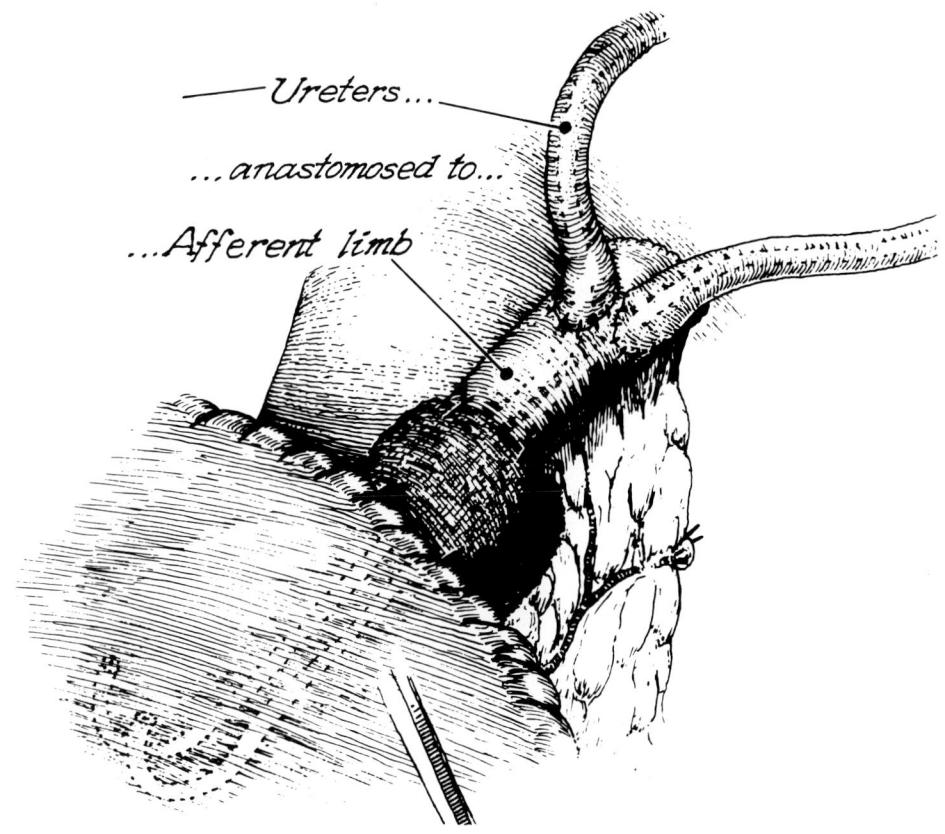

——Ureters...——

...anastomosed to...

...Afferent limb

Fig. 88.6 The ureters are anastomosed to the afferent bowel limb over silastic stents.

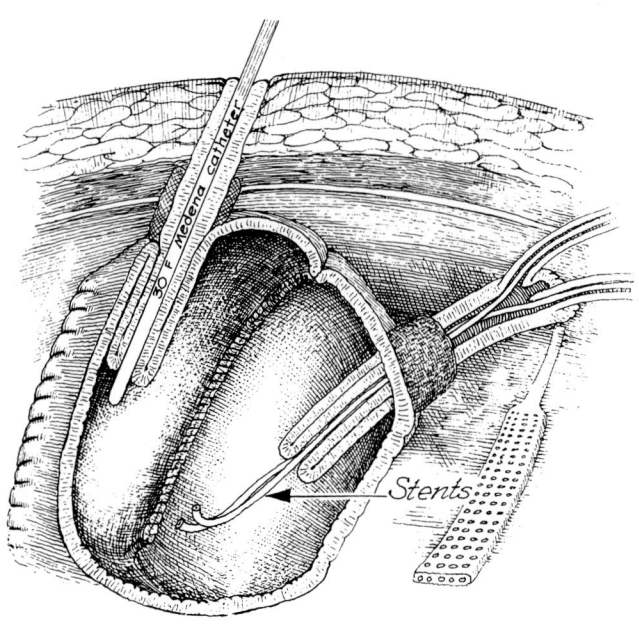

Fig. 88.7 The completed pouch is positioned in the pelvic inlet. The efferent system of the pouch requires a 30 French Medena catheter placed through the stoma and passed through the efferent nipple into the pouch for drainage of urine.

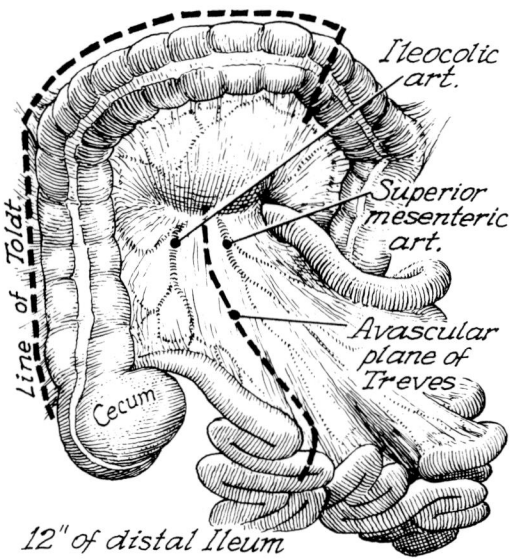

Fig. 88.8 The ileocolonic pouch requires a larger volume of colon. The small bowel is transected approximately 16 cm from the ileocecal bowel. Incision is carried up the avascular plane of Treves. The transverse colon is transected to provide an equal segment of transverse colon to the right colon. Care is taken to preserve the middle colic artery.

renal tracts secondary to a reduction of contaminated urinary reflux and subclinical chronic pyelonephritis.[13]

Ileocolic continent urostomy

A second procedure for continent urostomies following removal of the bladder has been the use of a small portion (12 to 14 cm) of terminal ileum, the ascending colon, and the proximal transverse colon.[16] Early series using this procedure were discouraging because the amount of colon utilized was small (ascending colon only). The small segment of colon resulted in higher pouch pressures and therefore greater ureteral reflux. Modifications at the University of Miami utilized a larger segment of colon that included the entire ascending colon as well as the proximal portion of the transverse colon.[16] Thus, the larger pouch resulted in reduced pouch pressure (Fig. 88.8).

The ileocolonic continent urostomies do not require the intussusception of bowel to create the continent mechanism for the efferent system. A combination of the ileocecal valve as well as reduction in the diameter of the lumen of the terminal ileum elevates the pressure in the efferent system to approximately 80 to 90 cm of water. The efferent pressure is higher than the pressure in the pouch which is less than 40 cm of water. It is unclear at present whether patients who are continent after an ileocolonic continent urostomy are those who have a competent ileocecal valve. A question yet to be answered is whether, in those patients with incompetent ileocecal valves demonstrated preoperatively, this technique, which reduces the lumen of the

ileum, will result in continence of the urostomy after construction? A second question with the ileocolonic technique concerns the mechanism for achieving a non-refluxing anastomosis of the ureters to the colon. Further data are required to show whether the traditional technique for achieving non-reflux, i.e. imbedding the ureter in the wall of the colon, will be free of stenosis at the anastomotic site. Stenosis will inevitably result in hydroureter and hydronephrosis.

An advantage of the ileocolonic continent urostomy technique is elimination of the need for intussusception of the bowel to produce the continent afferent and efferent systems. The surgical construction of the ileocolonic continent urostomy is surgically simpler. It also lends itself to the use of the polysorb (PGL) automatic surgical staplers for closure of the margins of the pouch walls. Use of the absorbable automatic stapler reduces the overall operative time.

Technique

Technique for ileocolonic continent urostomy requires that two loops of colon (ascending and proximal transverse) be placed adjacent to each other and opened near the antimesenteric border with a cautery[16] (Fig. 88.9).

The opened pouch utilizes the TA55 0.60 mm polysorb stapler to close the posterior wall (Fig. 88.10). The technique for anastomosing the ureters to the pouch uses a modified Leadbetter ureterocolonic anastomosis to create the non-refluxing feature of this operation[13] (Fig. 88.11). The continent feature of the efferent system is constructed

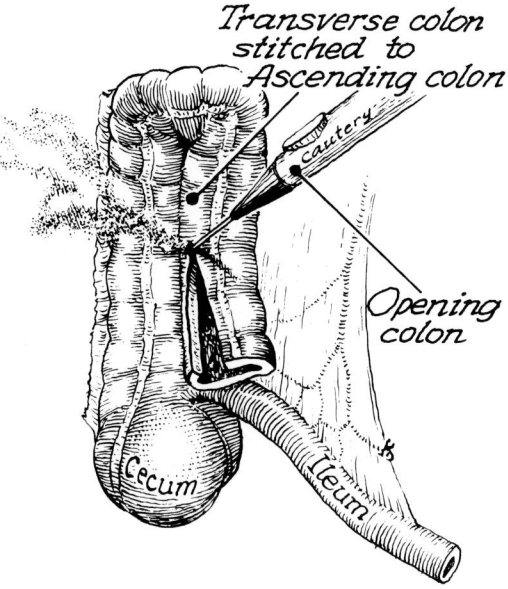

Fig. 88.9 The transverse colon is brought alongside the right colon. Interrupted sutures are placed in the adjacent segments of colon. A cautery is used to open the transverse colon around to the cecum.

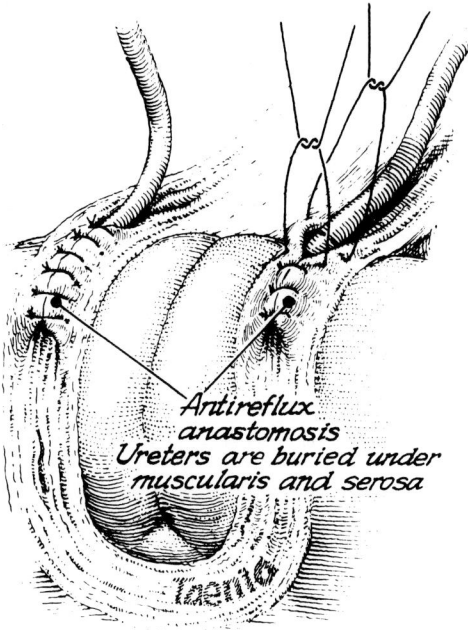

Fig. 88.11 The technique for anastomosing the ureters to the pouch using the modified Leadbetter ureterocolonic anastomosis to create the non-refluxing feature of the operation.

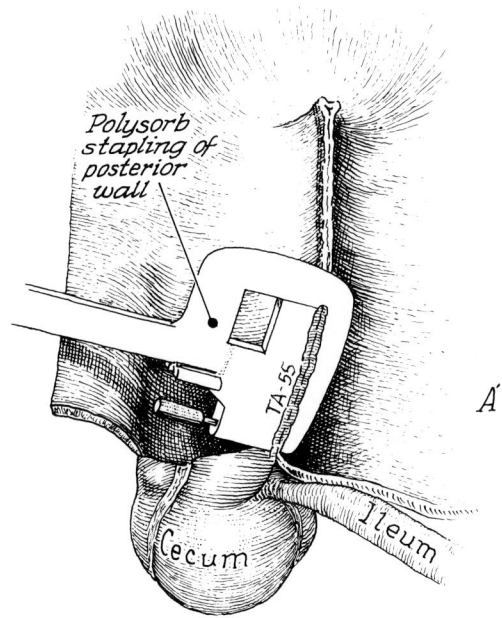

Fig. 88.10 The opened pouch utilizes the TA55 0.60 mm polysorb stapler to close the posterior wall.

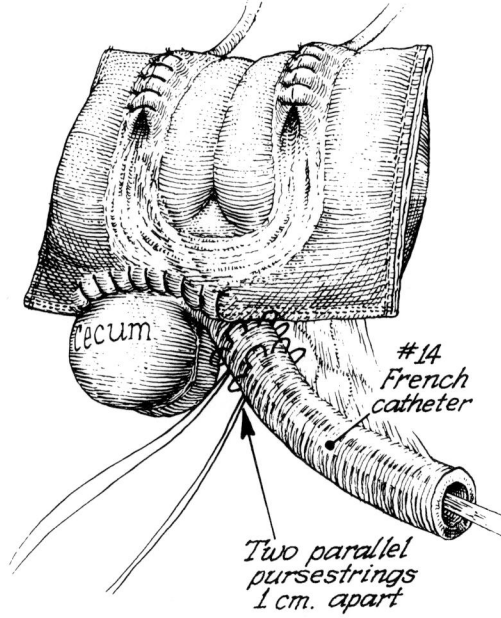

Fig. 88.12 The continent feature of the efferent system is constructed by two separate surgical techniques. This drawing illustrates the two purse-string sutures being placed adjacent to the ileocecal junction. Note there is a 14 French catheter used as a sizer inserted through the ileum into the pouch.

by two separate surgical techniques: (1) two purse-string sutures are placed at the ileocecal junction (Fig. 88.12), and (2) the diameter of the lumen of the terminal ileum is reduced by applying the GIA stapler over a 14 French catheter used as a sizer (Figs 88.13 A and B). After completion of the continent urostomy, the efferent system is brought through the right lower quadrant of the abdomen (Fig. 88.14).

The same postoperative techniques, as described above in the Kock pouch, for closed suction drainage, urosepsis prophylaxis, and catheterization of the pouch are used in the ileocolonic pouch.

Although this technique has potential promise, prospec-

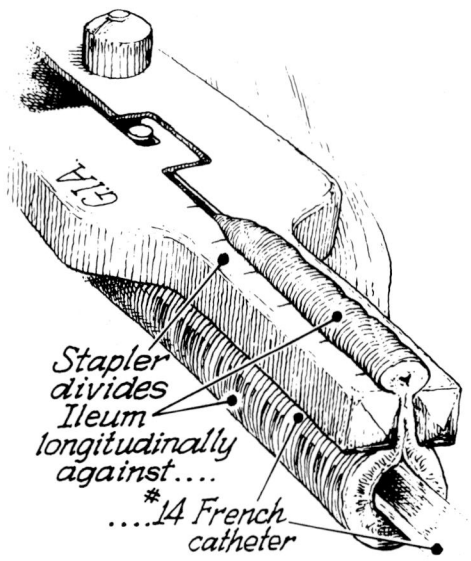

Fig. 88.13A Diameter of the lumen of the terminal ileum was reduced by applying the GIA stapler over a 14 French catheter used as a sizer.

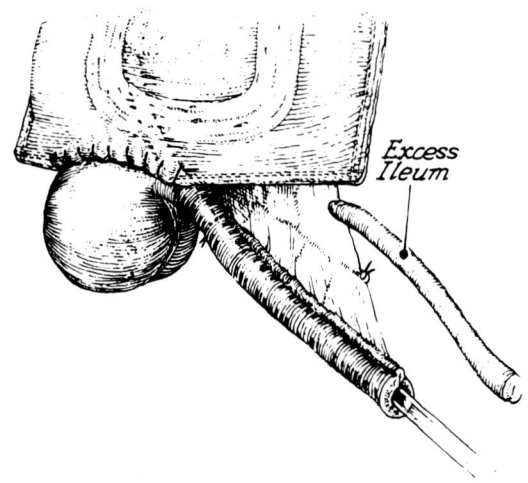

Fig. 88.13B Completed pouch stapled with the TA55 0.60 mm staples and the completed efferent arm of the pouch with a 14 French catheter going through the efferent terminal ileum into the pouch.

tive randomized trials comparing Kock and ileocolonic pouches are needed before the efficacy of these techniques is known.

RECTAL CONTINENCE SAVING OPERATIONS

Rectal J pouch reservoir for very low coloproctostomy

Renewed interest in very low (<6.0 cm above the anal verge) anastomosis of the colon to the rectum was rekindled with the introduction of the automatic end-to-end anastomosis (EEA) stapler.[17] The efficacy of this instrument in re-establishing the continuity of the colon has been well documented.[8] The patient with a traditional

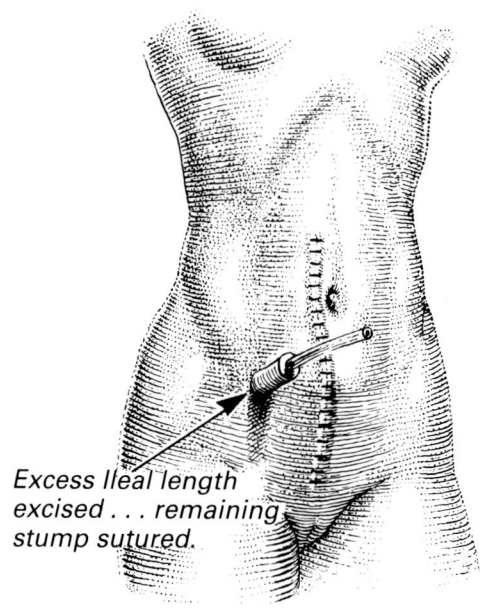

Fig. 88.14 Shows the efferent arm after completion of the pouch being brought through the right lower quadrant of the abdomen.

end-to-end, very low anastomosis of colon to rectum (<6.0 cm) was frequently left with increased tenesmus that resulted in unacceptable fecal frequency.[25]

Reports from the literature indicate that re-establishment of the rectal bulb or reservoir by performance of a rectal J pouch coloproctostomy significantly reduces tenesmus and thus fecal frequency with no significant increase in fecal incontinence.[12,15] The use of this technique in patients operated upon for gynecologic malignancy, and particularly those who have been previously treated by total pelvic irradiation and brachytherapy, has not been extensive.

A pilot study of 11 patients in whom rectal J pouch coloproctostomy was performed following low anterior resection of the colon as part of the treatment for either primary or recurrent gynecologic malignancy was reported[27] (Table 88.1).

Ten patients underwent total pelvic exenteration, and one patient underwent extensive surgical cytoreduction for advanced Stage III, Grade 3 epithelial ovarian cancer with invasion of the rectosigmoid mesentery. In all patients, continuity of the fecal stream was re-established by construction of a rectal J pouch reservoir with Strasbourg-Baker end-to-side coloproctostomy[26] (Figs 88.15, 88.16, 88.17). Eight of the 11 patients who underwent rectal J pouch reconstruction had received total pelvic irradiation. In the patients who had been previously irradiated, a diverting loop colostomy was performed to protect the anastomosis. This colostomy was closed 6 to 8 weeks following the primary surgical procedure.[25]

Patients were monitored for the development of fecal frequency, tenesmus, and fecal incontinence.

Results of this pilot series are outlined in Table 88.2.

Table 88.1 Rectal J pouch colpoproctostomy

Patient	Age	Disease	Operation
EH	54*	Squamous cell carcinoma cervix Stage IIb recurrent	Total pelvic exenteration
SP	34*	Squamous cell carcinoma cervix Stage Ib recurrent	Total pelvic exenteration
DC	58*	Squamous cell carcinoma cervix Stage IIa recurrent	Total pelvic exenteration
DT	64*	Adenocarcinoma colon recurrent	Total pelvic exenteration
LT	73	Stage III, Grade 3 papillary serous cystoadenocarcinoma ovary	Cytoreduction
PG	67	Mixed mesodermal sarcoma uterus recurrent	Total pelvic exenteration
HP	39*	Adenocarcinoma colon recurrent	Total pelvic exenteration
RP	40	Mesothelioma pelvic recurrent	Total pelvic exenteration
BJ	35*	Squamous cell carcinoma cervix Stage IIb	Total pelvic exenteration
HS	45*	Squamous cell carcinoma cervix Stage IIIb recurrent	Total pelvic exenteration
DY	68*	Clear cell carcinoma cervix Stage IIIb recurrent	Total pelvic exenteration

* Patient previously treated with radiation therapy. A diverting colostomy was performed to protect anastomosis at initial surgery. It was closed 6 to 8 weeks after primary surgery.

The distance of the anastomosis from the anal verge ranged from 4 to 6 cm. No patient reported having more than three stools per day or symptoms of tenesmus or episodes of fecal incontinence. There were no postoperative complications attributable to the rectal J pouch reservoir.[27]

Low anterior resection of the colon in patients with pelvic malignancy is a common gynecologic oncology pro-

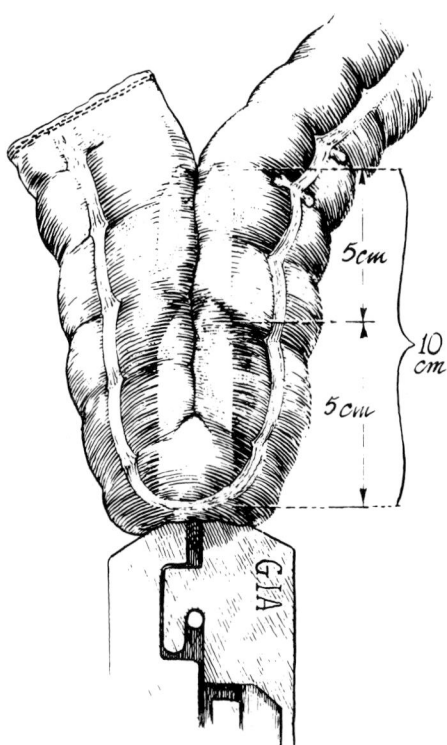

Fig. 88.15 Shows the terminal sigmoid colon folded upon itself for a distance of 10 cm and the GIA stapler placed through an enterotomy in the inferior portion of this pouch and the septums are cut and stapled at the same time. The terminal end of the sigmoid colon has been previously stapled with a TA55 4.8 mm stapler.

cedure. Historic attempts to re-establish continuity of the fecal stream in patients requiring very low anastomosis of the colon to the rectum at or below the level of the levator sling met with discouraging results.[3,11] Accordingly, patients in whom very low anterior resection of the colon was performed were frequently left with an end sigmoid colostomy.

The development of the EEA stapler[17] renewed interest in sphincter-saving operations and very low anastomosis of the colon to the rectum.

It is known that metastasis of cervical cancer to the anus and lower rectum is rare. Javert,[9] in 1954, reported that metastases of cervical carcinoma to the anus and rectum occurred in less than 1% of cases. Survival rates from sphincter-sparing pelvic exenteration procedures were not statistically different from those in which the rectum was removed.[5]

In 1986 and 1987, our institution reviewed a series of patients who underwent end-to-end, low anastomosis of the colon to the rectum. The data were quite encouraging and reaffirmed the efficacy of the procedure. Nevertheless, in this series of patients the troublesome side effects of tenesmus, and fecal frequency (> four bowel movements per day) were reported in more than 70% of patients. Forty-two percent of patients were still having 4 to 6 bowel movements per day up to 2 years following surgery.[25] The need for opiates to control tenesmus and fecal frequency reduces the improved quality of life afforded by the low end-to-end anastomosis and elimination of the colostomy.

The problem of tenesmus and fecal frequency has been addressed by Lazorthes et al[12] in a study of 65 patients who underwent low anterior resection of the colon for rectal carcinoma. Forty of the 65 patients underwent end-to-end anastomosis at a mean distance of 2.3 cm from the anal verge, and 20 had construction of a rectal J pouch reservoir with anastomosis to rectum at a mean distance of 1.4 cm from the anal verge. A statistically significant dif-

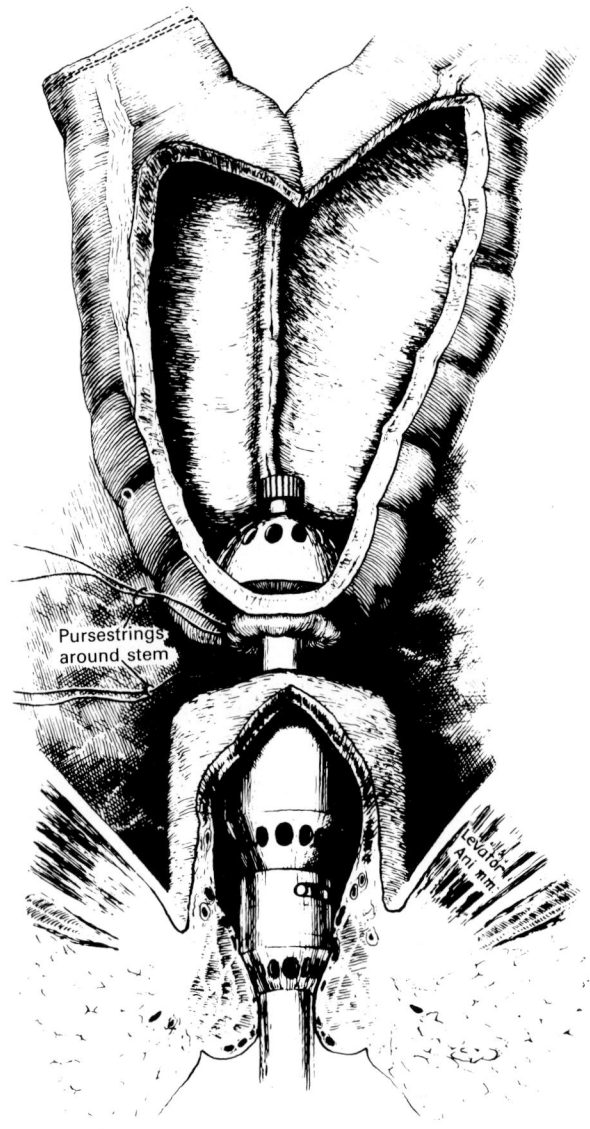

Fig. 88.16 The completed rectal J pouch positioned over the anus and rectal stump with an EEA stapler inserted through the anus up the rectum. The anvil of the stapler has been inserted into the pouch and two adjacent purse-string sutures are applied and tied. The stapler is closed and activated creating an end-to-side Strasbourg-Baker anastomosis.

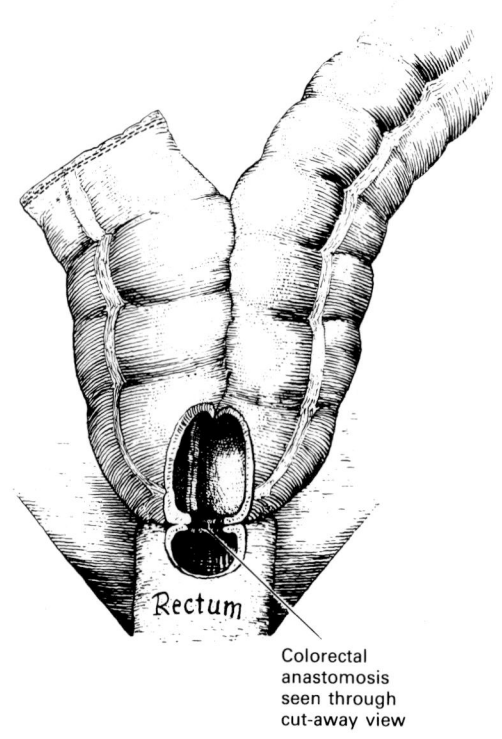

Fig. 88.17 The completed rectal J pouch anastomosed to the rectum.

ference in the number of patients having 1 to 2 stools per day was noted between the group with end-to-end anastomosis versus those having construction of a J pouch reservoir. Sixty percent of those with a reservoir had 1 to 2 bowel movements per day versus 33% of those with end-to-end anastomosis. This improvement was ascribed to a manometrically confirmed and statistically significant higher maximum pressure and tolerable fecal volume in the neorectum of those patients with a neoreservoir versus those having direct end-to-end anastomosis.

A confirmatory study was published by Parc et al.[15] He reported on 30 patients who underwent low anterior resection. The mean number of bowel movements in his

Table 88.2 Results of rectal J pouch colpoproctostomy

Patient	Anastomosis level (cm)	No. of stools per day	Months post-op	Fecal incontinence	Tenesmus
EH	4	1 to 3	12	—	—
SP	5	1 to 3	3	—	—
DC	5	1 to 3	6	—	—
DT	5	1 to 3	7	—	—
LT	6	1 to 3	3	—	—
PG	5	1 to 3	3	—	—
HP	4	1 to 3	3	—	—
RP	6	2 to 3	6	—	—
BJ	4	1 to 3	3	—	—
HS	4	1 to 3	6	—	—
DY	4	2 to 3	12	—	—

group following surgery was 1.1, and no patient reported tenesmus.[27]

Our series of patients with heavily irradiated bowel reported from 1 to 3 bowel movements per day. No patient required opiate medication or reported tenesmus.[27]

Tenesmus and fecal frequency are not uncommon side effects of very low end-to-end coloproctostomy following rectosigmoid resection. The creation of a rectal J pouch reservoir, even in irradiated colon and rectum, appears to be an effective method of substantially decreasing these troublesome symptoms.

Further evaluation of this technique in irradiated patients with a larger multiple institution randomized study design needs to be performed.

REFERENCES

1. Bricker E M 1950 Symposium on clinical surgery: bladder substitution after pelvic evisceration. Surg Clin North Am 30: 1511
2. Brunschwig A 1948 Complete excision of the pelvic viscera for advanced carcinoma. Cancer 1: 177
3. Coliger J C 1951 Functional results from sphincter saving resection of the rectum. Ann Roy Coll Surg Eng 8: 42
4. Cordonnier J J, Nicolai C H 1972 An evaluation of the use of an isolated segment of ileum as a means of urinary diversion. J Urol 83: 834
5. DiSaia P J, Creasman W T 1984 Invasive cervical cancer. Clinical Gynecologic Oncology, 2nd edn. Mosby, St Louis, p 61
6. Fegiz G, Angelini L, Bezzi M 1983 Rectal cancer: restorative surgery with the EEA stapling device. Int Surg 68: 13
7. Greig B 1986 Intervention of the ET nurse with the continent urinary Kock pouch patient. J Enterostomal Ther 13: 226
8. Harris W J, Wheeless C R 1986 Use of the end-to-end anastomosis stapling device in low colorectal anastomosis associated with radical gynecology surgery. Gynecol Oncol 23: 350
9. Javert C T 1954 Lymph nodes and lymph channels of the pelvis. In: Meigs J V (ed) Surgical Treatment of Cancer of the Cervix. Grune & Stratton, New York
10. Kock N G, Nilsson A E, Nilsson L O, Nolan L J, Philipson B M 1982 Urinary diversion via continent ileal reservoir: clinical results in 12 patients. J Urol 128: 469
11. Lahey F H 1951 Disadvantages of sphincter preserving operations for cancer of the rectum. JAMA 149: 626
12. Lazorthes F, Fages P, Chiotasso P, Lemozy T, Bloom E 1986 Resection of the rectum with construction of a colonic reservoir and colo-anal anastomosis for carcinoma of the rectum. Br J Surg 73: 136
13. Lieskovsky G, Skinner D G, Boyd S D 1986 Late complications of the continent ileal reservoir (Kock pouch). Read before the American Urological Association. New York, NY
14. Orr J W, Shingleton H M, Hatch K D, Taylor P T, Austin J M 1982 Urinary diversion in patients undergoing pelvic exenteration. Am J Obstet Gynecol 142: 883
15. Parc R, Tiret E, Frileaux P, Moszkowski E, Loygue J 1986 Resection and colo-anal anastomosis with colonic reservoir for rectal carcinoma. Br J Surg 73: 139
16. Penalver M, Bejany D E, Averette H E et al 1989 Continent urinary diversion in gynecologic oncology. Gynecol Oncol 34: 274
17. Ravitch M, Steichen F M 1979 A stapling instrument for end to end inverting anastomosis in the gastrointestinal tract. Ann Surg 189: 791
18. Richie J P, Skinner D G, Waisman J 1974 The effect of reflux on the development of pyelonephritis in urinary diversion: an experimental study. J Surg Res 16: 256
19. Rowland R G, Mitchell M E, Bihrle R, Kahnoski R J, Piser J E 1987 Indiana continent urinary reservoir. J Urol 137: 1136
20. Schmidt J D, Buchsbaum H J, Jacoby E C 1976 Transverse colon conduit for supravesical urinary tract diversion. Urology 8: 542
21. Skinner D G, Boyd S D, Lieskovsky G 1985 Ongoing experiences with the Kock continent ileal reservoir for urinary diversion. World J Urol 3: 155
22. Skinner D G, Lieskovsky G, Boyd S D 1984 Technique of creation of a continent internal ileal reservoir (Kock Pouch) for urinary diversion. Urol Clin Nth Am 11: 741
23. Skinner D G, Lieskovsky G, Boyd S D 1986 Continuing experience in continent urinary diversion — the Kock pouch in 250 patients. Read before the American Urological Association. New York, NY
24. Thuroff J W, Alken P, Engelmann U et al 1985 Der Mainz-Pouch zur Blasenerweiterungsplastik und kontinenten Harnableitung. Akt Urol 16: 1
25. Wheeless C R 1987 Incidence of fecal incontinence after coloproctostomy below 5 cm in the rectum. Gynecol Oncol 27: 373
26. Wheeless C R 1988 Atlas of Pelvic Surgery. Lea & Febiger, Philadelphia, PA
27. Wheeless C R, Hempling R E 1989 Rectal J pouch reservoir to decrease the frequency of tenesmus and defecation in low coloproctostomy. Gynecol Oncol 34: 379

PART XVII

After care

89. Gynecologic pain

W. G. Brose   M. J. Cousins

INTRODUCTION

The importance of treating chronic pain due to cancer is beginning to be appreciated by increasing numbers of health care providers throughout the world. The establishment of the guidelines for cancer pain treatment by the World Health Organization (WHO) in 1982, which were distributed over a world wide network of the WHO in 1986, has helped to focus attention on treatment and research of cancer pain. The WHO estimates that approximately 6 million people are diagnosed as having cancer each year. In addition, more than 4 million people suffering from cancer die each year. 70% of patients with advanced cancer relate pain as a major complaint.[83] Approximately 50% of patients undergoing treatment for cancer experience pain.[33] On a world wide scale it is estimated that approximately 3.5 million people are suffering from cancer pain.[83] Pain in patients with cancer appears to progress, and the prevalence of pain increases as the disease progresses. Moderate to severe pain is reported by 50% of patients and 30% report excruciating pain.[26]

This chapter deals mainly with *chronic* pain in patients with gynecologic cancer. (See also Ch. 92.) However, the mechanisms listed in Table 89.1 may also result in *acute* pain similar to post-traumatic pain, in terms of severity and requirements for analgesia. Postoperative pain relief after surgery for gynecologic cancer also requires discussion, in view of recent editorials calling for improved management of all forms of postoperative pain.

CHRONIC PAIN ETIOLOGY IN GYNECOLOGIC CANCER

There are a large number of potential causes of pain in patients with cancer, either directly due to the cancer (Table 89.1A), due to its therapy, or due to psychological and/or other factors (Tables 89.1B to 89.1D). The true incidence of cancer pain requiring referral to a specialized unit is not currently known; however, the following data indicate that it lies between 1 and 40%, depending upon

Table 89.1A Pain syndromes in patients with cancer: pain directly caused by cancer (primary or metastatic)*

Mechanism	Common sites and characteristics of pain
Infiltration of bone by tumor	Dull, constant aching; ± muscle spasm
Base of skull (jugular foramen, clivus, sphenoid sinus)	Early onset pain in occiput, vertex, frontal areas respectively
Vertebral body (subluxation atlas, metastases C7 to T1, L1, sacral)	Early onset pain in neck and skull, neck and shoulders, midback, lower back, and coccyx, respectively ± neurologic deficit
Metastatic fracture close to nerves	Acute onset pain + muscle spasm
Infiltration or compression of nerve tissue by tumor Peripheral nerve (± peripheral and perivascular lymphangitis)	Burning constant pain in area of peripheral sensory loss ± dysesthesia and hyperalgesia ± signs of sympathetic overactivity
Plexus, e.g. lumbar	Radicular pain to anterior thigh and groin (L1 to L3) or to leg and foot (L4 to S2)
Plexus, e.g. sacral	Dull aching midline perianal pain + sacral sensory loss and fecal and urinary incontinence.
Plexus, e.g. brachial	Radicular pain in shoulder and arm ± Horner's syndrome (superior pulmonary sulcus or Pancoast syndrome)
Meningeal carcinomatosis	Constant headache ± neck stiffness or low back and buttock pain
Epidural spinal cord compression (± vertebral body infiltration)	Severe neck and back pain locally over involved vertebra, or radicular pain
Obstruction of hollow viscus	Poorly localized, dull, sickening pain, typical visceral pain often associated with nausea and vomiting
Occlusion of arteries and veins by tumor	Ischemic pain, e.g. rest pain (skin) or claudication (muscle), or pain due to venous engorgement

1439

Stretching of periosteum or fascia, in tissues with tight investment by tumefaction	Severe localized pain (e.g. periosteum) or typical visceral pain (e.g. ovary)
Inflammation owing to necrosis and infection of tumor (± superficial ulceration)	Severe localized pain (e.g. perineum), visceral pain (e.g. cervix)
Soft tissue infiltration	Localized pain; unsightly and foul smelling if ulcerated
Raised intracranial pressure	Severe constant headache, behavioral changes, confusion, etc.

the stage of the cancer and the experience in pain management of the referring gynecologist. A study, of 36 500 cancer *inpatients* at the Sloan-Kettering Cancer Center, New York reported in 1979 that 9% of patients with cancer were referred to the pain unit with difficult pain problems.[15] An overall referral rate to the Oxford Pain Unit of 1% was reported from the regional population of approximately 21 000 patients with cancer, as reported to the Oxford Regional Health Authority.[48] A more limited study was carried out on two occasions at the Sloan-Kettering Center on all patients with cancer in the hospital during a 1 week period (540 and 420 patients respectively). Patients with pain were estimated to be 29% on the first occasion and 38% on the second. Of the patients with terminal cancer, a surprising 60% had pain. The latter figure has been supported by studies at St. Christopher's Hospice in London where 80% of terminal cancer patients required pain relief.[15] It should be recognized that both the Sloan-Kettering and the St. Christopher's manage patients with difficult cancer problems. In the Oxford study, gynecologic cancer was at the top of the list with a referral rate of over 4%. A total of 44 cases per 1000 diagnoses of gynecologic cancer comprised 38 cervix, 5 uterine and 1 ovarian cancer per 1000. In comparison, 12 cases per 1000 breast cancer diagnoses were referred.

Cancer of the cervix was not only the most common cancer to require referral (3.8% with pain) but these patients also had the longest median survival of 8 months after referral.[48] This group clearly requires methods of pain relief which keep them ambulatory and yet cause minimal morbidity.

It is sometimes difficult to separate cancer treatment from pain relief; for example, pituitary adenolysis relieves pain but may also cause metastatic cancer to regress. The incidence of severe cancer pain can be reduced if full use is made of the wide range of measures now available to treat cancer and its complications, as described in previous chapters in this book on radiotherapy, surgery, cytotoxic drugs, immunotherapy, hormonal therapy or ablation of endocrine glands and CO_2 laser therapy. It is important to remember that cancer therapy may also sometimes cause pain (Table 89.1B).

The cardinal rule of 'pain clinics' is that pain is not treated symptomatically unless treatable causes of the underlying disease have been identified. Unfortunately, patients with gynecologic cancer who do not have a

Table 89.1B Pain syndromes in patients with cancer: pain associated with cancer therapy*

Mechanism	Common sites and characteristics of pain
Following surgery	
Acute postoperative pain	Wound or referred pain; back or other sites (owing to positioning during surgery)
Nerve trauma	Neuralgic pain in area of peripheral nerve or spinal nerve
Entrapment of nerves in scar tissue	Superficial wound scar hypersensitivity of area supplied by scarred nerves (e.g. perineum)
Amputation of limb or other area (breast)	Localized stump pain (neuroma) or phantom pain referred to absent region
Following radiotherapy	
Acute lesions or inflammation of nerves or plexuses	Pain associated with motor and sensory loss
Radiation fibrosis of nerves or plexuses	e.g. brachial plexus, lumbar plexus; diffuse limb pain, 6 months to many years after radiation ± lymphedema and local skin changes ± sensory loss ± motor loss (difficult to distinguish from tumor recurrence)
Myelopathy of spinal cord	Brown-Sèquard syndrome (ipsilateral motor and touch with contralateral loss of pain and temperature) with pain at level of spinal cord damage or referred pain
Peripheral nerve tumors owing to radiation	Painful enlarging mass in area of radiation along line of peripheral nerve or plexus
Following chemotherapy	
Vinca alkaloids (vincristine>vinblastine)-induced peripheral neuropathy	Burning pain in hands and feet associated with symmetrical polyneuropathy
Steroid pseudorheumatism owing to slow as well as rapid withdrawal of steroid treatment	Diffuse joint and muscle pain with associated tenderness to palpation but no inflammatory signs. Pain resolves when steroid reinstituted
Aseptic necrosis of bone (femoral or humoral head) with chronic steroid therapy	Pain in knee, leg, shoulder with limitation of movement; bone scan changes delayed after pain onset
Postherpetic neuralgia, following herpes zoster infection in area of tumor or area of radiotherapy with onset during chemotherapy	Continuous burning pain in area of sensory loss, painful dysesthesia, intermittent shock-like pain

* Tables 89.1A–D are modified from: Cousins M J, Bridenbaugh P O (eds) (1988) *Neural Blockade in Clinical Anesthesia and Management of Pain*, 2nd edn. Lippincott, Philadelphia, with permission.

treatable cause of their pain are amongst the most difficult problems requiring pain management. Still, up to the present time, too few of these patients are referred to specialized pain management units, and as a result the success rate and quality of pain relief for patients in other settings has often been poor. Two reasons for this may be: (1) unfamiliarity with recent major changes in knowledge of pain conduction, and thus continued reliance on approaches which in many cases have proved erroneous and (2) lack of experienced personnel and/or slow acceptance of their role in pain diagnosis and management.

In addition to pain, patients with gynecologic cancer often complain of diverse areas of discomfort (Table 89.1C)

Table 89.1C Pain syndromes in patients with cancer: pain unrelated to cancer or cancer therapy, but probably exacerbated by cancer.*

Mechanism	Common sites and characteristics of pain
Neuropathy (e.g. diabetic)	Burning pain in hands, feet
Degenerative disc	Back pain ± radicular pain
Rheumatoid arthritis	Joint pain on movement
Diffuse osteoporosis	Back pain, limb pain (may be like causalgia)
Posture abnormalities after surgery	Back pain and muscle spasm ± radicular pain
Myofascial syndromes owing to anxiety	Local pain in muscle with muscle spasm ± referred pain; trigger areas in muscle
Headache	Typical migraine or tension type

and are commonly subject to anguish and suffering (Table 89.1D). The latter terms are not easy to define but are all too familiar to those who treat cancer patients. Such symptoms require palliation whether or not they are associated with a lesion which also results in severe pain. The term palliation is appropriate, since it derives from the 'pallium' or large cloak (or 'pall', archbishop's cloak) and involves alleviating symptoms without curing the underlying illness. Psychologic aspects of these problems and their treatment are discussed in Chapters 90 to 93. The Hospice concept has contributed greatly to treating the 'total pain' problems of patients with terminal cancer;[4] it should be remembered that up to 60% of these patients will have pain.[68] Depression, anxiety and sleep disturbance are common in all forms of cancer and may require drug treatment. It is worth emphasizing that attention to the problem of helping the patient and family to cope with dying (Table 89.1D) is quite frequently far more important than attempting to treat pain, which may be wrongly assumed to be entirely due to the patient's cancer. Destructive neurolytic or neurosurgical procedures should not be considered unless attention to the factors discussed above still leaves the patient with pain which is unrelieved by less invasive measures.

Table 89.1D Pain syndromes in patients with cancer: pain exacerbated by or entirely due to psychological factors*

Psychological factor	Possible causes
Anxiety**	Sleeplessness, fear of death, loss of dignity (loss of self control), fear of surgical mutilation, uncontrollable pain, fear of the future, loss of social position and work, confused understanding of disease due to poor communication, family and financial problems
Depression**	Sleeplessness, loss of physical abilities, sense of helplessness, disfigurement, loss of valued social position
Anger**	Frustration with therapeutic failures, resentment of sickness, irritability caused by pain and general discomfort

** A vicious circle usually develops:

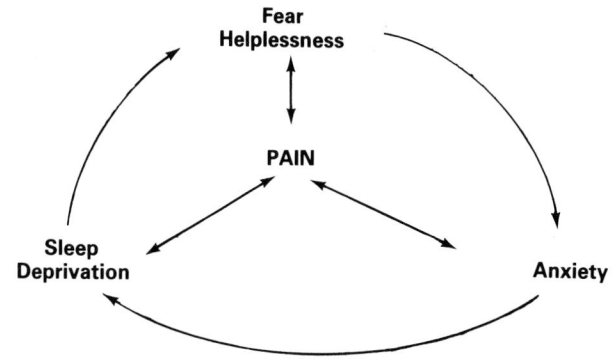

Cancer has usually been thought to produce pain by a variety of assaults on pain receptors or primary afferent nerve fibers (Table 89.1A). Unfortunately, convincing confirmatory studies are not available. Indeed, postmortem review often reveals surprisingly minimal pathology where pain has been severe and vice versa. This serves to emphasize the potential for mechanisms noted in Tables 89.1B to 89.1D to cause pain in patients with cancer. New knowledge of pain transmission has expanded the understanding of how interference with spinal cord neurons and afferent tracts as well as brain, descending influences, *and* efferent activity via muscle spasm and reflex sympathetic effects may contribute to pain.

The proposed etiologic factors in Table 89.1 emphasize the potential for palliative procedures to relieve pain by controlling the cause. For example, palliative *surgical* bypass procedures frequently relieve pain when tumor obstructs a hollow viscus. Fungating surface lesions may be painful, and often have offensive odors and discharges which lower the patient's morale. They should be removed or, when this is impossible, necrotic tissue removed and dressings changed frequently.

Palliative *radiotherapy* will often shrink tumor tissue with subsequent pain relief. However, initially pain may increase so that special pain relief should be arranged for this period. The discomforts of systemic toxicity may be reduced and dyspnea and cough may improve if pulmonary metastases are reduced in size by radiotherapy. Pain relief appears to be best for bone metastases from glandular organs (e.g. 90% for breast cancer). Unfortunately, painful bone metastases from well differentiated cancer (e.g. uterine) may be difficult to relieve with radiotherapy. Pain from inoperable cancer of the cervix is perhaps the most difficult problem and, although radiotherapy helps, other forms of treatment often are also needed (vide infra).

OTHER CAUSES OF PAIN IN GYNECOLOGIC CANCER

Metastases from pelvic cancer may result in pain in widespread areas of the body, as indicated in preceding chapters. It is important to remember that patients with cancer may also develop some of the pain syndromes which are only indirectly related to the cancer. For example, poor muscle tone, surgery and/or depression may lead to postural changes and resultant low back pain (see Tables 89.1B to 89.1D). Anxiety about the cancer may cause muscle spasm and a variety of musculoskeletal pain syndromes similar to acute back strain. These problems may be diagnosed and treated with appropriate local anesthetic blocks of trigger points or muscle nerve supply.[74] Surgical trauma to somatic nerves may result in neuralgic pain which may be relieved by transcutaneous nerve stimulation (TNS). Increased sympathetic activity may lead to limb pain which is similar to causalgic pain (burning pain, hyperesthesia, and trophic changes). It is also worth emphasizing that even patients with cancer pain may report pain relief following placebos approximately 30% of the time; usually, the response to placebos is not sustained.

ADVERSE EFFECTS OF ACUTE PAIN

Is acute pain harmful to the patient? From a subjective point of view, patients are unanimous in their continued reports of postoperative pain as a major unpleasant experience during surgical care. Acute pain may be of considerable diagnostic value in various surgical conditions; however, once the diagnosis is made there is no reason to delay in relieving the pain. Data concerning the harmful physiologic effects of severe pain continue to be reported.[43] The role of pain stimuli in evoking various aspects of the stress response has not been completely evaluated. The general impression is that severe pain intensifies reflex responses, leading to metabolic changes which mediate complications such as pulmonary and gastrointestinal problems, thromboembolism and increased demands on the heart. When attention is focused on improving pain relief, recent data suggest that outcome is also improved.[90]

Respiratory effects

It has been widely held that severe abdominal or thoracic pain impairs respiratory function. Recent studies with postoperative and post-traumatic pain indicate that effective pain relief improves several parameters of pulmonary function. Outcome studies providing conclusive data about any commensurate decrease in postoperative pulmonary infections are needed.

Endocrine and renal effects

There is marked increase in secretion of various hormones in response to trauma and surgery, which results in hyperglycemia, water and salt retention, oliguria and other deleterious effects. These may be favorably influenced by blockade of noxious impulses from the operative area.

Cardiovascular effects

Severe pain results in increased sympathetic activity with possible adverse effects on the cardiovascular system, such as: severe tachycardia interfering with diastolic time available for coronary blood flow and increasing oxygen demand of the myocardium; and increased peripheral resistance with further increase in myocardial oxygen demand. This imbalance of myocardial oxygen supply and demand is most dangerous in patients with pre-existing myocardial disease. Studies following coronary artery surgery indicate that severe postoperative pain was associated with marked hypertension and signs of myocardial hypoxia. In this instance, relief of pain by thoracic epidural block resulted in signs of greatly improved myocardial oxygenation.[66]

Effects during parturition

During labor, severe unrelieved pain may increase gastrointestinal stasis, increase oxygen consumption and maternal acidosis, exaggerate the increase in plasma cortisol, inhibit uterine contraction and decrease uterine blood flow. All of these changes may be modified or prevented by effective epidural blockade. This beneficial effect is reflected in improved fetal acid-base status. This is perhaps one of the most convincing demonstrations of the adverse effects of severe unrelieved pain.[17]

ADVERSE EFFECTS OF CHRONIC PAIN

The International Association for the Study of Pain has laid the foundation for more consistent and rational approaches to pain diagnosis and management. A taxonomy of terms to be used in pain management was published in 1979 (Appendix 1).[40] In addition, a classification system for chronic pain syndromes was introduced in 1986.[41]

Pain is now defined as:

'An unpleasant sensory and emotional experience associated with actual or potential tissue damage, or described in terms of such damage'.[41]

It is clear that even acute pain has some emotional or psychological component. Beecher referred to a 'perceptive' and 'affective' component of pain.[9] When pain becomes longstanding or chronic, psychological and pathophysiological changes occur and these may complicate diagnosis of the cause of pain and may also act as positive feedback increasing the pain. The patient with chronic pain manifests a gradual change in attitude to the environment, with a gradual withdrawal and restriction of activities. These changes, in addition to poor sleeping habits, often make patients depressed. In addition, patients also experience increasing amounts of anxiety, anger, and frustration. Each of these individual problems combines to form a self-perpetuating pain cycle. In time the patient's whole life may be centered around the pain (see Table 89.1D).[15] This situation is of course quite different from acute pain, and it would be naive to expect that the techniques used for acute pain would be successful for chronic pain if used by themselves. Because of the possibility of contributing factors from a number of specialty areas of medicine, Collaborative Pain Management Units have been established in many major hospitals.

MODERN CONCEPTS OF NEUROLOGIC MECHANISMS OF PAIN

The classical teaching of a simple pathway for pain transmission still exists in the minds of many practicing medical professionals. The understated sophistication of a dedicated spinothalamic tract which relayed all pain messages received from peripheral nerves arising on the contralateral side of the body, supported the concepts of pain and analgesia prevalent even in the mid to later twentieth century. An ever increasing body of knowledge has now displaced this simple model of pain transmission. Very complex interactions of many different peripheral and central nervous system structures, from the skin surface to the cerebral cortex, are now known to be involved in the processing of pain. Blockade of any of these pathways and/or antagonism of involved neurotransmitters may now be rationally considered to treat specific pain problems. Chemical or electrical recruitment of endogenous modulation of pain sensation at multiple different sites along the afferent pathway has also been employed to relieve pain. Presentation of these various treatment options is best preceded by a brief discussion of certain established parts of this complex pathway for pain transmission. Yaksh summarized the detailed neurophysiological and neuropharmacological findings from 1913 until 1986 in his review which referenced over 700 papers.[87]

Peripheral sensory receptors

Each individual can appreciate that when a potentially tissue-damaging stimulus is applied to a sensitive area of the body, such as the skin, a chain of signals is initiated which will result in the identification of the stimulus as painful. Early descriptions of peripheral nerves indicated that each nerve fiber was modality specific, and that each class of nerve fiber was responsible for only one sensory modality.[58] This concept was not supported by anatomical studies of skin surface, which demonstrated that each class of nerve ending is not present in all skin areas. More recent neurophysiologic work has established the existence of specific primary afferent nerves for signaling noxious stimulation. These nerves are termed nociceptors.

Nociceptors are activated by some form of energy (mechanical, thermal or chemical). They transduce that energy into an electrical impulse which is conducted through the nerve axon towards the brain. The reflex response and subjective report of pain associated with a noxious stimulus is the result of spinal cord, brain stem, midbrain and higher cortical processing of signals from the numerous primary afferent nociceptors which were activated by the stimulus. Nociceptors are characterized by:

1. High threshold to all naturally occurring stimuli compared with other receptors in the same tissue.
2. Progressively augmenting response to repeated or increasingly noxious stimuli (sensitization).

Cutaneous pain sensation

Mechanosensitive nociceptors respond when the pressure to produce tissue damage has been achieved. Most of these receptors initiate impulses carried by thinly myelinated fibers (Aδ). The responses increase in proportion to magnitude of the pressure applied. In the trunk, these receptors have fairly large receptive fields while those in the face have smaller fields. *Thermoreceptive* nociceptors respond to normal heating/cooling, with sensitivity near 1°C when the temperature is between 30 and 40°C; they also respond to noxious thermal stimuli with an increasing frequency of discharge. High frequency discharge can be seen in C-fiber afferents following application of intense heat (47 to 51°C) to the small receptive fields near these receptors. *Mechanothermal* nociceptors are activated by high intensity heat or pressure sensation. They have small receptive fields and are likely to be responsible for the 'first pain' transmitted by small myelinated Aδ-fibers. *Polymodal* C-fiber nociceptors respond to many different noxious stimuli and are the most common of all nociceptors. These receptors are activated by pressure, temperature and chemical stimuli supplied to their small receptive fields.

Skeletal muscle pain

Group III and Group IV nociceptors found in skeletal muscle respond to chemical agents that are released locally during muscle contraction. Metabolic by-products alone do not trigger these receptors. There appears to be a need for other algogenic agents, perhaps prostaglandins released during intense muscle contraction, to be present as well.

Cardiac muscle pain

Cardiac muscle afferents are activated by high intensity mechanical stimulation, heat and chemical agents. Humoral agents released locally may be responsible for the pain seen with angina. Prostaglandins are released following myocardial hypoxia. Prostaglandins, histamine, bradykinin or serotonin have all been shown to stimulate these receptors.

Joint pain

Group III nociceptors activated by deformation or expansion within the joint will relay pain messages via Aδ-fiber afferents. These receptors also appear to be sensitized by certain chemical substances injected into the joint (e.g. urate crystals, endotoxin, prostaglandins).

Visceral pain

These nociceptors have not been well identified. Pain is seen in response to both mechanical (distension), as well as thermal and chemical stimuli. These receptors also appear to be sensitized by the presence of certain chemicals (e.g. prostaglandins).

As indicated in the previous discussion, nociceptors respond to particular types of stimuli and not to others. While the precise pathways involved in the transduction of noxious information by nociceptors have not yet been elucidated, it appears that the peripheral terminal of the Aδ mechanical nociceptor is sensitive to pain.[31] Whether this is true for other nociceptors remains the subject of speculation.

The presence of vesicles in primary nociceptive afferent terminals has been determined by electronmicroscopy. These vesicles probably provide the substrate for various peripherally active agents. Substance P (sP) is an undecapeptide found in small-diameter primary afferent neurons. This peptide has been shown to be transmitted to the periphery by these nerves, and stimulation of these primary afferents leads to the release of sP from the distal terminus of the nerve. However, local application of exogenous sP to these nerve terminals does not induce a painful response. So, while sP is not likely to be the peripheral agent responsible for pain transduction, it does appear to activate local vasculature promoting extravasation of fluid into the tissues. Certain chemicals present in the blood and tissues have been demonstrated to be algesic. Serotonin, histamine, acetylcholine, bradykinin and potassium all excite primary noxious afferents. Prostaglandins alone do not excite pain fibers; however, they

do appear to sensitize primary afferents to painful substances.

Direct tissue trauma results in potassium release, synthesis of bradykinin in plasma and synthesis of prostaglandins in the region of damaged tissue (Fig. 89.1A).

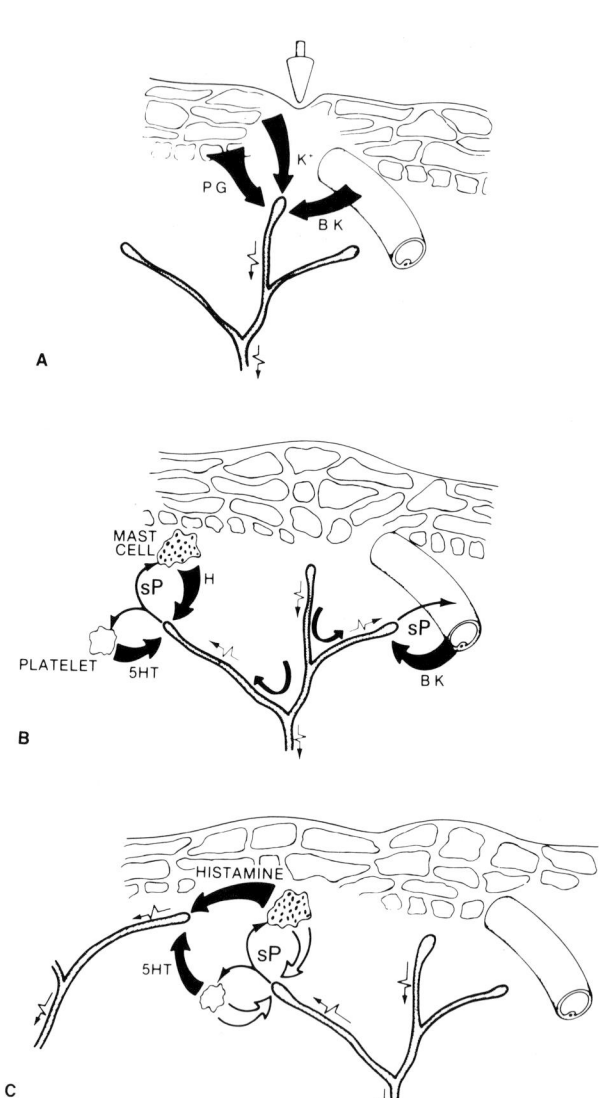

Fig. 89.1 Events leading to activation, sensitization, and spread of sensitization of primary afferent nociceptor terminals. (**A**) Direct activation by intense pressure and consequent cell damage. Cell damage leads to release of potassium (K$^+$) and to synthesis of prostaglandins (PG) and bradykinin (BK). Prostaglandins increase the sensitivity of the terminal to bradykinin and other pain-producing substances. (**B**) Secondary activation. Impulses generated in the stimulated terminal propagate not only to the spinal cord but into other terminal branches, where they induce the release of peptides including substance P (sP). Substance P causes vasodilation and neurogenic edema with further accumulation of bradykinin. Substance P also causes the release of histamine (H) from mast cells and serotonin (5HT) from platelets. (**C**) Histamine and serotonin levels rise in the extracellular space, secondarily sensitizing nearby nociceptors. This leads to a gradual spread of hyperalgesia and/or tenderness. (Reproduced from Fields (1987),[31] with permission.)

Antidromic impulses in primary nociceptor afferents result in an increase in sP from nerve endings. This is associated with an increase in vascular permeability, and this in turn results in very marked release of bradykinin. There is also an increase in histamine production from mast cells, and an increase in serotonin production from platelets; both of these are capable of powerful activation of nociceptors (Fig. 89.1B) Histamine release combines with sP release to increase vascular permeability. Local increases in histamine and serotonin, via activation of nociceptors, result in a further increase in sP, so that a self-perpetuating cycle can be seen to develop at each region of a nociceptive afferent nerve fiber in the damaged tissue. In surrounding extracellular fluid, increases in histamine and serotonin result in activation of nearby nociceptors and this is one reason for secondary hyperalgesia (Fig. 89.1C). Superimposed on all of these events are the effects of increased release of catecholamines from sympathetic nerve endings, which result in sensitization of nociceptors. Evidence from animal models of arthritis, and various human data point to the sympathetic postganglionic neuron as being integral in the changes seen in vascular permeability in response to activation of primary afferent nociceptors.[46]

Primary afferent transmission

After a noxious stimulus has been detected by a nociceptor, the resultant impulse travels away from the point of origin via the primary afferent nerve. The primary afferent nerves which carry pain impulses are almost exclusively unmyelinated C-fibers and finely myelinated Aδ-fibers. Most C-fiber afferents originate from polymodal nociceptors, which are activated by mechanical, chemical and thermal noxious stimuli. The conduction velocity of these C-fibers is approximately 1 m/s, which likely explains the 'slow pain' which is felt one to two seconds following the application of a noxious stimulus. The finely myelinated Aδ-fibers also transmit pain impulses, but the conduction velocity of these neurons is much faster, at 12 to 30 m/s. Aδ-fibers are particularly sensitive to stimulation with sharp instruments. In addition, 20 to 50% of Aδ-fibers respond to heat as well as mechanical stimulation. These fibers likely carry the impulses that initially report a noxious stimulus. These primary afferent nociceptors make up the majority of fibers in any peripheral nerve.

Peripheral nerve injuries can lead to pain. The proposed pathways for such an injury to evoke a pain response include:

1. Increased activity in sympathetic fibers near the damaged area.
2. Neuroma formation due to sprouting from damaged axons.
3. Collaterals sprouting from intact neighboring fibers.
4. Changes in dorsal root ganglion cells or in central terminals of damaged axons which have lost part of their normal input.
5. Stimulation of nociceptive nervi nervorum of peripheral nerves.
6. Damage to myelin sheaths, producing a localized area of spontaneous electrical activity.

While certain nerve injuries are associated with pain, clearly others are not. Lesion of a peripheral nerve does not necessarily correlate with presence or absence of pain. The incidence of phantom pain reported by amputees is an example of the variability that can be seen in pain-reporting after a peripheral nerve injury. The gate theory of pain proposed by Melzack & Wall[53] introduced a construct which supported the variability of pain experience seen across all humans. Individuals injured during sporting events or in battle often report little or no pain, while similar or even less potent stimuli will often evoke pain at another time. The gate, which Melzack & Wall proposed, has multiple modulating influences, including decreased perception of small fiber activity by the presence of large fiber input. The loss of large fiber input in some cases leads to an open gate that allows transmission of all noxious stimuli which might otherwise be blocked by large fiber afferent transmission closing the gate. This gate theory introduced the concept of pain modulation by endogenous systems. Since that time, multiple sites of endogenous modulation have been described throughout the nervous system.

Spinal cord terminals of primary afferents

Dorsal and ventral roots

The cell bodies of all somatic primary afferent fibers are in the dorsal root ganglia adjacent to the spinal cord. The only primary afferent cell body outside this position is the trigeminal ganglia, which is the rostral continuation of the dorsal root ganglia. Fibers from the dorsal root are organized within the root according to diameter. The large diameter afferents enter the spinal cord in the dorsal region of the entry zone, while the small diameter afferents enter into the lateral region of the cord. Having entered the spinal cord, the nociceptive primary afferent fibers (Aδ- and C-fibers) bifurcate into both cephalad and caudad projecting branches travelling in the Lissauer tract. These fibers terminate primarily in the ipsilateral dorsal gray matter, but a small number of the fibers will cross dorsal to the central canal to terminate in the dorsal gray matter of the contralateral side. While the majority of sensory afferents enter the spinal cord through the dorsal root entry zone, a significant number of non-myelinated C-fibers have been delineated which travel in the ventral root to terminate in the superficial dorsal horn. The clinical relevance of the fibers which cross, and those which enter, the ventral root is not known. This heterogeneity in the pathway of the primary afferents associated with pain transmission helps explain the incomplete pain relief that is seen following ablation of a unilateral dorsal root entry zone.

Dorsal horn

Once the impulses have entered the spinal cord via the dorsal or ventral roots, they terminate in the ipsilateral dorsal horn of the spinal cord. The dorsal horn is organized into distinct laminae with specific primary afferent terminals found in individual lamina (Fig. 89.2). Aδ-fibers terminate primarily in lamina I, ventral portions in lamina II, and lamina V. Unmyelinated C-fibers terminate primarily in lamina II. Individual dorsal horn neurons then project the noxious information to higher centers in the nervous system. Each dorsal horn cell may be subject to information from several different primary afferents.

The convergence of somatic nociceptive afferents and visceral nociceptive afferents on the same dorsal horn

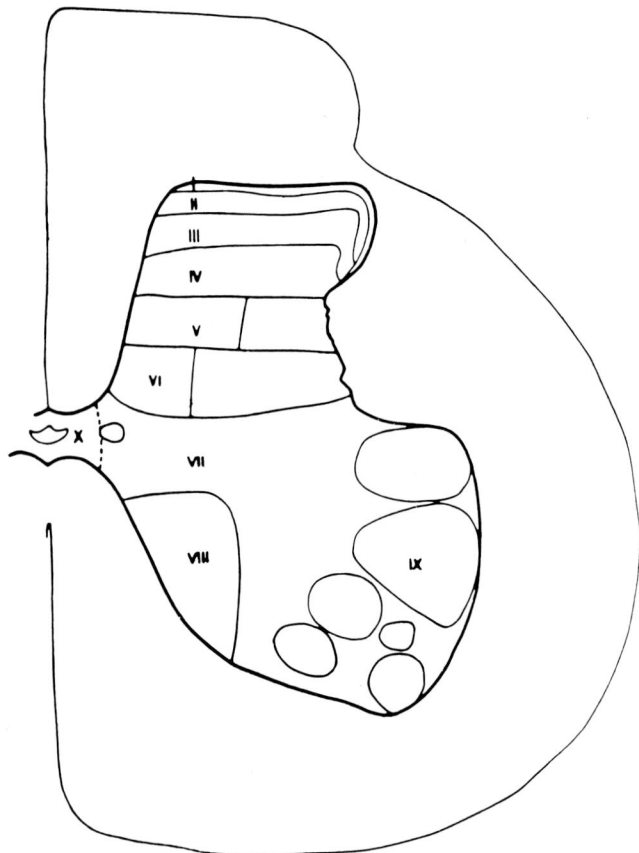

Fig. 89.2 Schematic drawing of the lamination of the ventral cell column of the 7th lumbar spinal cord segment in the full-grown cat. Lamina I is also known as the marginal zone. Lamina II is also known as the substantia gelatinosa, while laminae III and IV combine to make up the nucleus proprius. (Reproduced from Rexed B J 1952 *Comp Neurol* 96: 415, with permission.)

neuron probably explains the phenomena of referred pain. The presence of viscero/somatic, muscle/somatic and viscero/viscero convergence seen in the various lamina of the dorsal horn, and the development of fairly large receptive fields in some of these second order neurons, also help to explain some of the peculiar characteristics of nonsomatic pain. These are shown schematically in Figure 89.3.

Ascending sensory pathways

The second order neurons that arise in the respective laminae of the dorsal horn of the spinal cord subsequently use several specific routes to carry noxious impulses to higher brain centers (Fig. 89.4). The specific routes are characterized as tracts and systems, which include the spinothalamic, spinoreticular system, spinomesencephalic and spinosolitary tracts. The names given to these nociceptive pathways are derived from the point of origin and termination of their respective fibers.

Axons from lamina I, IV, V, VI and VII ascend predominantly in the contralateral ventral quadrant of the spinal cord, where they form the spinothalamic and spinoreticular tracts. The spinothalamic and spinoreticular systems represent the most important tracts associated with pain transmission in humans. Fibers from these tracts make up the anterolateral funiculus. Crossed fibers predominate, but neuro-anatomic studies indicate that perhaps 25% of all fibers ascend in the ipsilateral ventral quadrant. The spinothalamic fibers divide into lateral (neospinothalamic) and medial (paleospinothalamic) components in the posterior portions of the thalamus. The medial fibers terminate in the nucleus parafascicularis, and the intralaminar and paralaminar thalamic nuclei. The larger lateral group of fibers terminate in several different thalamic nuclei, including the nucleus ventralis, posterolateralis, the posterior nucleus and the intralaminar nuclei.

Numerous other systems are also involved in the rostral projection of nociceptive information. Important among these other systems are the dorsal funicular systems, and intersegmental systems which are probably involved in descending inhibitory transmission as well.

Brain stem processing

The brain stem is involved in transmission of all ascending and descending information. Nociceptive afferent fibers relay to projection neurons in the dorsal horn which ascend in the anterolateral funiculus to end in the thalamus. During the rostral conduction of these impulses, collaterals activate the nucleus reticularis gigantocellularis, which in turn sends projections to the thalamus as well as the periaqueductal gray matter (Fig. 89.4). The periaqueductal

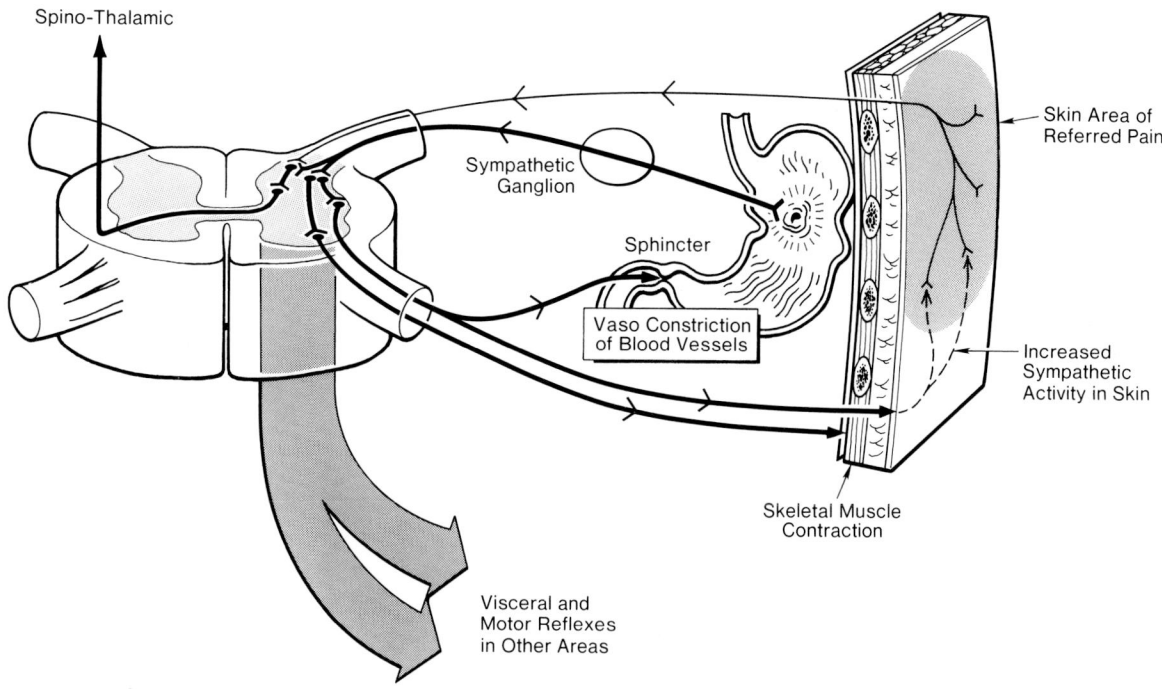

Fig. 89.3 Visceral pain: convergence of visceral and somatic nociceptive afferents. Visceral sympathetic afferents converge on the same dorsal horn neuron as do somatic nociceptive afferents. Visceral noxious stimuli are then conveyed, together with somatic noxious stimuli, by means of the spinothalamic pathways to the brain. Note the following: (1) Referred pain is felt in the cutaneous area corresponding to the dorsal horn neurons upon which visceral afferents converge. This is accompanied by allodynia and hyperalgesia in this skin area. (2) Reflex somatic motor activity results in muscle spasm, which may stimulate parietal peritoneum and initiate somatic noxious input to the dorsal horn. (3) Reflex sympathetic efferent activity may result in spasm of sphincters of viscera over a wide area causing pain remote from the original stimulus. (4) Reflex sympathetic efferent activity may result in visceral ischemia and further noxious stimulation. Also, visceral nociceptors may be sensitized by norepinephrine release and microcirculatory changes. (5) Increased sympathetic activity may influence cutaneous nociceptors, which may be at least partly responsible for referred pain. (6) Peripheral visceral afferents branch considerably, causing much overlap in the territory of individual dorsal roots. Only a small number of visceral afferent fibers converge on dorsal horn neurons compared with somatic nociceptive fibers. Also, visceral afferents converge on the dorsal horn over a wide number of segments. Thus dull, vague visceral pain is very poorly localized. This is often called 'deep visceral pain'. (Reproduced from Cousins M J 1988 Introduction to acute and chronic pain: implications for neural blockade. In: Cousins M J, Bridenbaugh P O (eds) *Neural Blockade in Clinical Anesthesia and Management of Pain*, 2nd edn. Lippincott, Philadelphia, with permission.)

gray matter also receives direct input from the spino-mesencephalic tract.

Thalamic relays

Several nuclear groups of the thalamus are associated with the relay of nociceptive afferent impulses (Fig. 89.5). Included among these are the posterior nuclear complex, the ventrobasilar complex and the medial intralaminar nuclear complex. In the thalamus, spinothalamic neurons terminate largely on the ventral posterior lateral and the central lateral nuclei. The ventral posterior lateral nucleus projects to areas 1, 2 and 3 of the parietal lobe, but these areas have not been found to be involved with aversive or emotional aspects of nociception. Consequently, it is currently believed that the ventral posterior lateral nucleus is involved with localization of the impulse, rather than its qualitative aspects.[10,82] The central lateral nucleus is believed to be involved in the qualitative aspects of nociception, in that stimulation of this region triggers the unpleasantness associated with tissue damage.[10] The

projections of the central lateral nucleus are poorly understood at present, but presumably they activate the aversive centers in the limbic system. The nucleus submedius has also been implicated in nociceptive processing, as it receives all of its input from terminals of marginal projection neurons in the spinal cord. However, the physiologic functions and connections of this nucleus are unknown.

Cerebral cortex

The somatosensory cortex receives processed input from spinothalamic, spinoreticular and dorsal column systems, as outlined earlier. The majority of attention has been focused on SII as the principal cortical region involved with the reception and perception of noxious information. The anterior portion of SII receives input from the ventrobasal thalamus, while the posterior portion of SII receives input from the posterior thalamus. Berk & Palmer demonstrated that bilateral ablation of the posterior region of SII produces an increase in nociceptive threshold.[11]

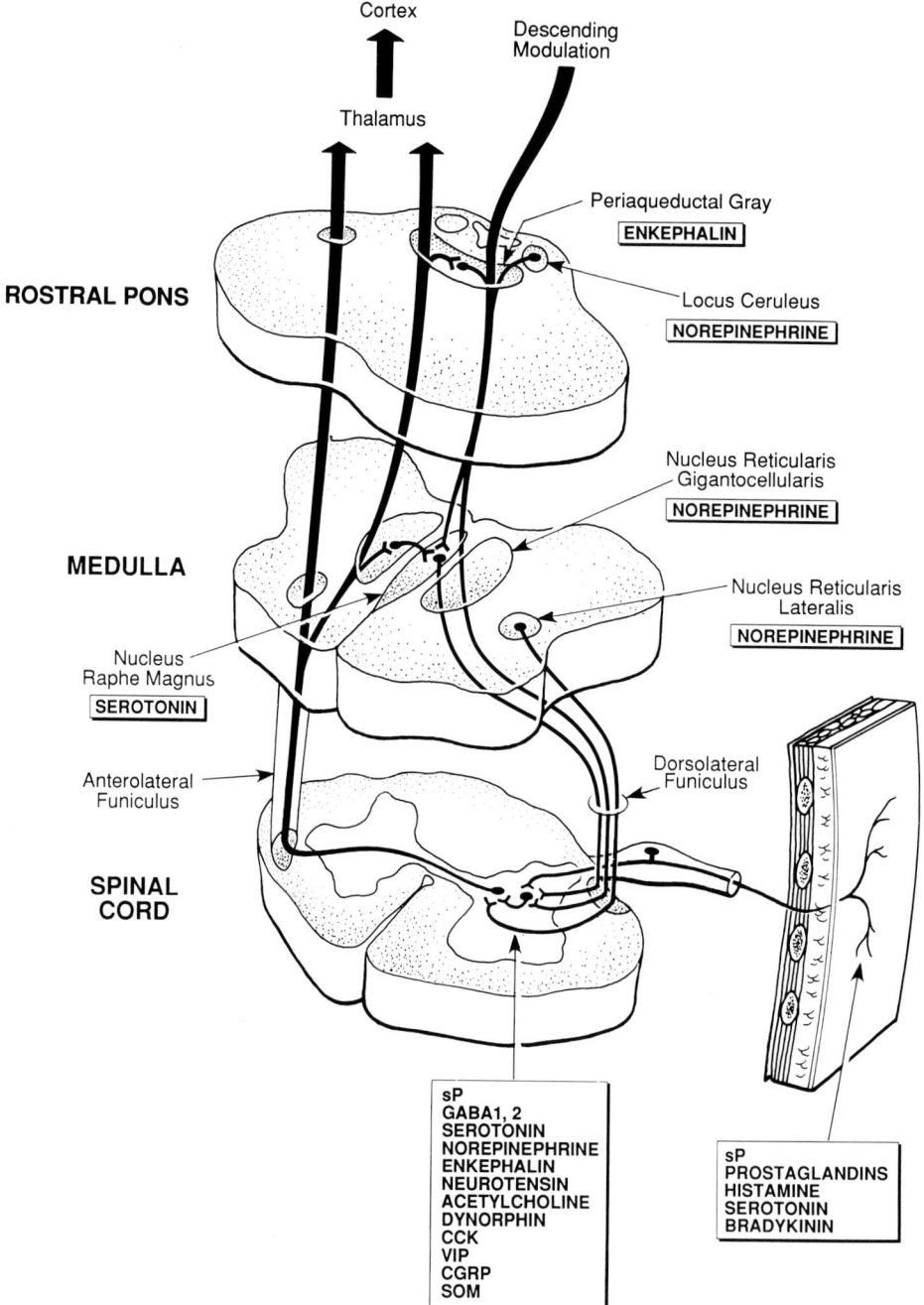

Fig. 89.4 Schematic drawing of nociceptive processing outlining ascending (left side of drawing) and descending (right side of drawing) pathways. Stimulation of nociceptors in the skin surface leads to impulse generation in the primary afferent. Concomitant with this impulse generation, increased levels of various endogenous algesic agents (substance P, prostaglandins, histamine, serotonin, bradykinin) are detected near the area of stimulation in the periphery. The noxious impulse is conducted to the dorsal horn of the spinal cord where it is subjected to local factors and descending modulation. Primary nociceptive afferents relay to projection neurons in the dorsal horn which ascend in the anterolateral funiculus to end in the thalamus. En route, collaterals of the projection neurons activate multiple higher centers, including the nucleus reticularis gigantocellularis (NRG). Neurons from the NRG project to the thalamus and also activate the periaqueductal gray (PAG) of the midbrain. Enkephalinergic neurons from the PAG and noradrenergic neurons from the NRG activate descending serotonergic neurons of the nucleus raphe magnus (NRM). These fibers join with noradrenergic fibers from the locus ceruleus and nucleus reticularis lateralis to project descending modulatory impulses to the dorsal horn via the dorsolateral funiculus. Multiple endogenous peptides which have been identified to be involved with processing or modulation of noxious information at the dorsal horn are listed in the figure: Substance P (sP), gamma amino butyric acid (GABA), serotonin (5-HT), norepinephrine (NE), enkephalin (ENK), neurotensin, acetylcholine (ACH), dynorphin (DYN), cholecystokinin (CCK), vasoactive intestinal peptide (VIP), calcitonin-gene-related peptide (CGRP), somatostatin (SOM), (Modified from Brose W G, Cousins M J (in press) Physiology and the relief of pain. In: Shaw R, Soutter W, Stanton S (eds) *Gynaecology.* Churchill Livingstone, Edinburgh, with permission.)

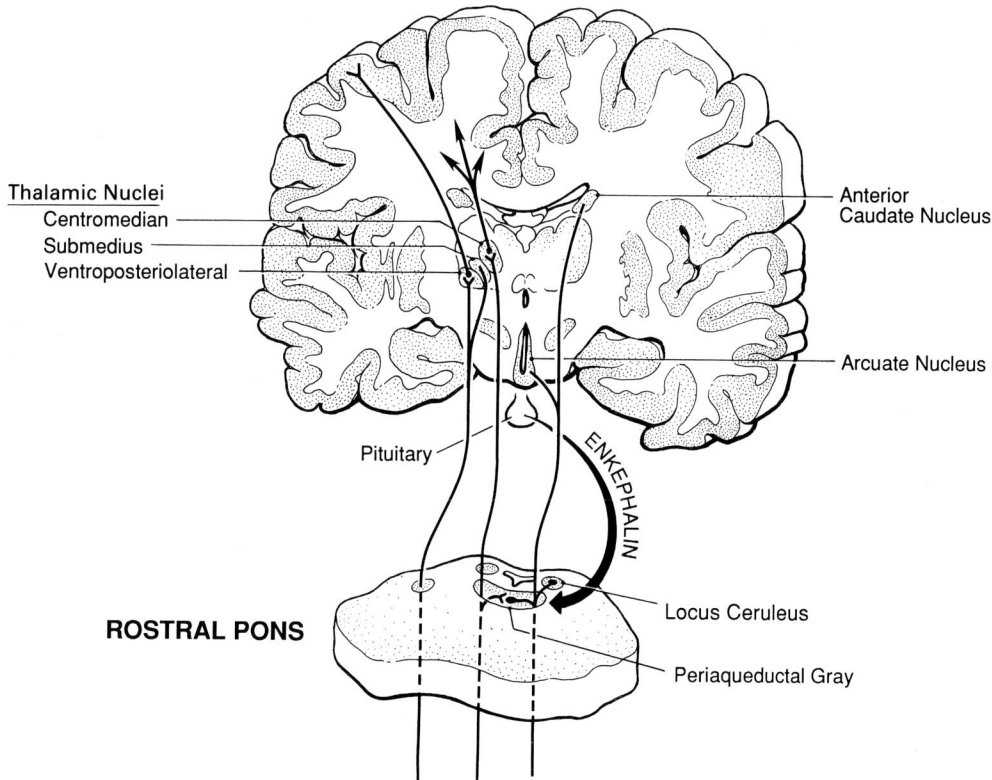

Fig. 89.5 Rostral projections of nociceptive processing. Ascending stimuli (left side of diagram) traveling in the anterolateral funiculus as well as impulses relayed from the medulla, pons and midbrain are projected to the thalamic nuclear complex. The ventroposterior lateral (VPL), centromedian, and submedian nuclei receive nociceptive information. The VPL projects discretely to the cortex. The centromedian nucleus projects more diffusely, particularly to the limbic region. The descending fibers (right side of diagram) inhibit the transmission of nociceptive information between primary afferents and the projection neurons in the dorsal horn. The periaqueductal gray (PAG) is controlled by projections from the anterior caudate, midline limbic nuclei, and the arcuate nucleus of the hypothalamus. In addition to direct neural connections, endorphins synthesized in the pituitary are released into the CSF and blood, where they can exert an inhibitory effect at multiple centers including the PAG.

Descending modulation

Up to this point, the discussion of pain pathways has primarily been limited to the rostral projection of primary noxious stimuli. In addition, modulation of painful stimuli occurs at many different levels in the pathway. The failure of a particular painful stimulus to provoke given pain behavior over different individuals points out the uncoupling of a simple stimulus — response concept of pain processing. The uncoupling of pain stimulus and response is perhaps best identified by observing the absence of pain in some individuals that are injured in battle or in association with a sporting event. One of the primary focuses of research over the last two decades has been to delineate the physiological explanations for these observed differences in pain response. Through this investigation, it has become apparent that the discussion of the afferent limb of the pain pathway mandates consideration of the modulating influences on that pain transmission.

As mentioned earlier, Melzack & Wall proposed the gate control theory to explain the variability in pain response. They predicted modulation of small fiber activity by the presence of large fiber activity in the same region of the dorsal horn. Cutaneous activation of large fiber afferents by counter-irritation, acupuncture and transcutaneous nerve stimulation supports this peripheral modulation at the dorsal horn.

In addition, the stimulation of dorsal columns which mimics the activation of descending inhibition has also been shown to inhibit the discharge of dorsal horn interneuron nociceptors. Early work by Hagbarth & Kerr demonstrated the existence of descending long tract systems to modulate spinal evoked activity.[37] Virtually every pathway carrying nociceptive information, including the spinothalamic and spinoreticular tracts, is under modulatory control from supraspinal systems. Experimental evidence of this supraspinal influence includes inhibition of nociceptive reflexes by electrical stimulation or microinjections of opioid at brain stem sites, both of which are naloxone-reversible. Various nuclei of the medulla oblongata and the pons project caudally to the spinal gray matter and the spinal nucleus of the trigeminal nerve. Serotonergic neurons in the nucleus raphe magnus, as well as catecholaminergic neurons of the lateral reticular formation and the locus ceruleus, are all believed to play a role in descending modulation.[6,10,32] Axons from these centers project to all levels of the spinal cord through the dorsolateral funiculus (Fig. 89.4). Stimulation of these centers within the brainstem inhibits nociceptive second order neurons in the dorsal horn or trigeminal gray matter.[6,10,32] The exact mechanism of this descending inhibition has not been characterized, but several models have been proposed (Fig. 89.6).[5,27] There is evidence of additional descending inhibitory influences that have yet to be fully characterized. The inhibition of spinothalamic neurons by cortical and pyramidal stimulation is an example of such an uncharacterized pathway. Continued research in this area will help to unravel the complex relation between pain stimulus and response, and perhaps suggest additional therapeutic modalities that may be applied to the treatment of pain.

NEUROPHARMACOLOGY

Pharmacology of pain

Basic research on the processing of nociceptive information by the central nervous system has led to an improved understanding of pain and pain treatment. Figure 89.4 summarizes the site of action of several of the chemical substances that have been identified with nociceptive processing. By using this simplified model of nociceptive processing, we can focus on pharmacologic intervention at different points in the pathway and determine a clinical effect on the relief of pain.

Peripheral desensitization

A rough schematic drawing of the local circuitry involved

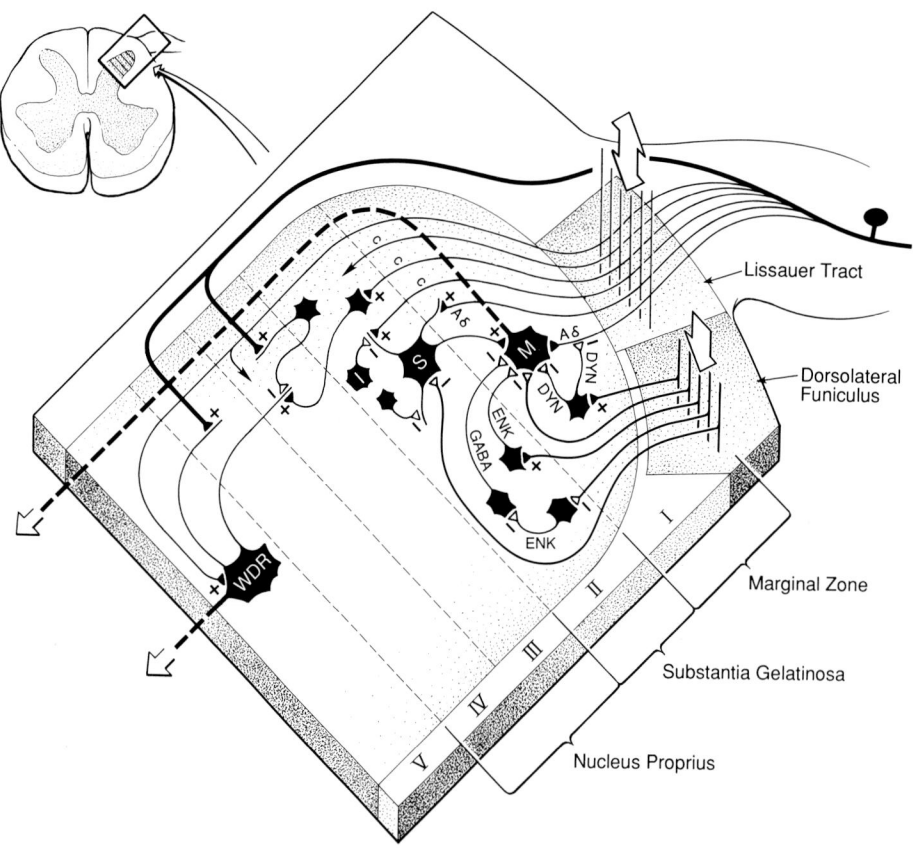

Fig. 89.6 Dorsal horn processing. Large and small diameter primary afferent neurons have their cell bodies in the dorsal root ganglia. These fibers segregate as they approach the spinal cord. Large diameter afferents (shown as a thickened solid line) travel in the medial portion, while small diameter afferents (thin solid lines marked C and Aδ) segregate to the lateral portions of the entry zone. The spinal terminals of the small fibers enter the cord, where they may ascend or descend for several segments in the dorsolateral tract (Lissauer) and subsequently terminate throughout the dorsal horn of the spinal cord. Aδ-fiber afferents terminate primarily in lamina I (marginal zone), while C afferents terminate in lamina II (substantia gelatinosa). In lamina I, nociceptive fibers synapse on dendrites of the large marginal neurons (M). Smaller neurons in lamina I may exert presynaptic inhibition of the small diameter afferent and post synaptic inhibition of the marginal neuron. Other nociceptive fibers (Aδ) synapse with stalked cells (S) in lamina II. These stalk neurons stimulate marginal neurons in lamina I. The relay between primary afferent fibers and stalk cells is also subject to modulation by inhibitory islet neurons (I) in lamina II. Central transmission is accomplished by marginal neurons (M) directly, wide dynamic range neurons (WDR) directly or stalk cells (S) indirectly. Marginal neurons are subject to inhibition by neurons in lamina II. Descending serotonergic neurons from the nucleus raphe magnus, which travel in the dorsolateral funiculus, are also shown. These neurons terminate throughout the spinal cord on interneurons (GABA, ENK), to provide inhibition of nociceptive transmission.

in the detection of noxious stimuli from the periphery is shown in Figure 89.7. As discussed previously, following trauma to a peripheral site, an inflammatory reaction including the activation of complement and coagulation/fibrinolytic pathways will begin. Local release of histamine, serotonin, prostaglandins and substance P occurs. Subsequent changes in the local environment, such as decreased tissue pH, changes in the microcirculation and an increase in efferent sympathetic activity all appear to increase the response of peripheral nociceptors.

Numerous drug therapies have been tried to interrupt these peripheral processes. Blockade of pain by aspirin-like drugs is such a peripheral action. Aspirin, indomethacin, ibuprofen, phenylbutazone and diclofenate are all cyclo-oxygenase inhibitors. Cyclo-oxygenase is the enzyme responsible for the synthesis of prostaglandins, prostacyclins and thromboxanes. All of these endogenous substances have been proposed as mediators of the local pain response.[42] Clinical trials with topical capsaicin are also focused on peripheral action. This drug has been shown to deplete substance P from cutaneous nerve endings and central terminals of primary afferents.[86] Initially, the effect is a burning pain, which is then followed by insensitivity to subsequent painful stimuli.

The involvement of the sympathetic nervous system is also suspected. It is known that sympathetic fibers are present in large numbers near cutaneous nociceptors. Blockade of these sympathetic fibers can eliminate the pain of causalgia in some patients. The burning dysesthetic pain and hyperalgesia that are seen with this syndrome and which may be eliminated by sympathetic blockade can be made to reappear with local application of norepinephrine, the sympathetic neurotransmitter.

Neural blockade

In 1902, Cushing presented his theory that nerve block could prevent the pain and shock of amputation.[25] Later in 1910, Crile proposed that disruption of the pain pathway might improve outcome from trauma.[24] Indeed, a multitude of investigations have proven the beneficial effect of neural blockade with respect to neuroendocrine function following trauma and/or surgery.[43]

Neural blockade can occur at any point along the pain pathway. The most common sites of neural block would be peripheral nerves, somatic plexi and dorsal roots. These blocks can be performed with relatively short-acting agents, such as local anesthetics for acute pain, whereas long-acting (permanent) blockade with alcohol or phenol may be more appropriate for cancer pain. Surgical lesions at any of these points have also been suggested to provide long-lasting interruption of specific pain pathways. The disadvantage with permanent techniques is that they are neither specific for pain fibers nor reliable for protracted pain problems. The lack of anatomical separation of fibers carrying pain, motor and other sensory information obligates the patient, in whom neural blockade is employed, to varying amounts of sympathetic, somatic and, perhaps motor dysfunction. While these side effects may be well tolerated in certain acute pain situations where the patient is expected to rapidly improve, or in the chronic cancer pain where the life expectancy is less than

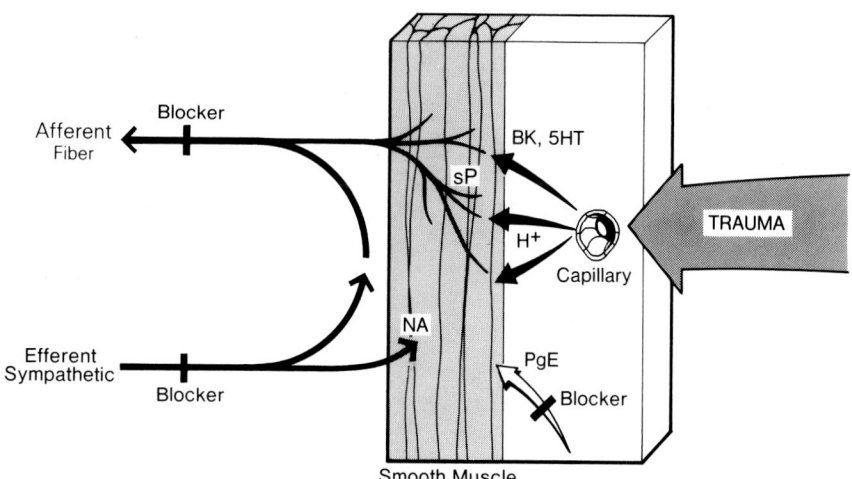

Fig. 89.7 Local tissue factors and peripheral pain receptors. The physical stimuli of 'trauma', the chemical environment (e.g., H^+), algesic substances (e.g., serotonin[5-HT], bradykinin [BK]), and microcirculatory changes may all modify peripheral receptor activity. Efferent sympathetic activity may increase the sensitivity of receptors by means of noradrenalin (NA, norepinephrine) release. Substance P may be the peripheral pain transmitter. Points of potential blockade of nociception are shown as 'blocker'. Other potential sites involve BK, 5HT, NA, and sP. (Reproduced from Phillips G D, Cousins M J 1986 Neurologic mechanisms of pain and the relationship of pain, anxiety, and sleep. In: Cousins M J, Phillips G D (eds) *Acute Pain Management*. Churchill Livingstone, London, with permission.)

12 months, the use of these techniques in most chronic pain management situations is inappropriate.

Opioid analgesia

In recent years, researchers have identified multiple endogenous opioid peptides that have analgesic effects. Included among these are the enkephalins, dynorphin, and β-endorphin. These peptides bind to at least four different types of opioid receptors which have been demonstrated in the brain and spinal cord.[60] Table 89.2 summarizes the pharmacodynamic effects achieved when each of these receptors is stimulated. In 1976, Yaksh & Rudy reported long-lasting analgesia following the introduction of intrathecal opioids.[89] The discovery that spinally administered opioids produced dose-dependent, stereospecific, naloxone-reversible analgesia has led to development of an important clinical tool to combat pain.

Brain receptors

Opium has been known for centuries to possess analgesic properties. Despite this being a well recognized phenomenon, the location of the active sites for opium was not known. Microinjection techniques utilized in the 1960's have identified the periaqueductal gray matter of the midbrain, and midline medullary nuclei to be the most sensitive sites. Through descending serotonergic and/or noradrenergic links with the spinal cord, morphine microinjections into these centers have been shown to inhibit spinal reflexes. This analgesic effect has also been shown to be similar to the effect achieved by systemically administered morphine. Further research has documented dose dependency, stereospecificity, naloxone-reversibility, and well defined structure activity relationships of these centers to other opiate agonists.

Spinal cord receptors

Equally interesting to the delineation of descending inhibition of nociception initiated by centrally administered opioids is the growing appreciation of opioid systems in spinal function. Opioids administered systemically will produce inhibition of nociceptive reflexes in spinal transected animals.[81,84] Also, administration of opioids to the dorsal horn of the spinal cord will inhibit the discharge of nociceptive neurons.[20,29] Multiple discrete populations of opioid receptors have been identified. Stimulation of mu, kappa, and delta systems present in the spinal cord are able to depress the response to noxious stimulation.

Opioid systems appear to be active in the modulation of noxious impulses presented to the substantia gelatinosa via both direct action and indirect descending inhibition via serotonergic and noradrenergic systems. In addition, other non-opioid systems appear to be functioning at this level to produce analgesic effects. Baclofen [β-(p-chlorophenyl) GABA] produces a dose-dependent, stereospecific analgesic action when it is injected intrathecally in cats. This analgesia was not effected by naloxone. Yaksh has reported that a preparation of morphine, serotonin and baclofen demonstrated synergistic analgesia when administered intrathecally. This finding suggested that these analgesic actions were not via a common final pathway.

In summary, it appears that the substantia gelatinosa receives collaterals from nociceptive primary afferents and this information is subject to extensive modulation at the spinal level. Chemical mediators that have been shown to be associated with analgesia at this level include:

Table 89.2 Pharmacodynamic effects obtained when an opioid agonist interacts with the various types of opioid receptor.*

Effect	Receptor subtype			
	Mu	Kappa	Sigma	Delta
Pain relief	Yes	Yes, especially at spinal cord level	Yes	Yes
Sedation	Yes	Yes	–	–
Respiratory effects	Depression	Depression but not as much as for mu (may reach plateau)	Stimulation	Depression
Affect	Euphoria	–	Dysphoria	–
Physical dependence	Marked	Less severe than with mu	–	Yes
Prototype agonist (other drugs with predominantly agonist activity)	Morphine (Pethidine) (Methadone) (Fentanyl) (Heroin) (Codeine) (Propoxyphene) (Buprenorphine)	Ketocyclazocine (Nalbuphine) (Dynorphine) (Butorphanol) (Nalorphine) (Pentazocine)	SKF 10,0 47	Enkephalins

* Modified from: Gourlay G K, Cousins M J, Cherry D A 1987 Drug therapy. In: Burrows, Elton & Stanley (eds) *Handbook of Chronic Pain Management*. Elsevier Science, Amsterdam, with permission.

Table 89.3 Spinal neurotransmitters, receptors and ligands

Neurotransmitter systems	Proposed receptor	Endogenous ligand	Exogenous ligand
Opioid	Mu	β-endorphin; met/leu-enkephalin	Morphine
	Delta	Met/leu-enkephalin	DADL
	Kappa	Dynorphin	U50488H
Adrenergic	Alpha 1	Norepinephrine	Methoxamine
	Alpha 2	Norepinephrine	Clonidine
	Beta	Epinephrine	Isoproterenol
Serotonergic	5-HT	Serotonin	Serotonin
Gabaergic	A	GABA	Baclofen
	B	GABA	Muscimol
Neurotensin	–	Neurotensin	Neurotensin
Cholinergic	Muscarinic	Acetylcholine	Oxotremorine

* Modified from Yaksh T L (1988)[87] with permission.

1. opioids
2. serotonin
3. norepinephrine
4. GABA
5. neurotensin
6. cholinergic.

Some of the proposed endogenous and exogenous ligands for these neurotransmitter systems are shown in Table 89.3.

Electrical stimulation

Electrical currents modulate pain via entirely different mechanisms depending on the anatomical site which is stimulated. The prediction that large-fiber activity could block certain noxious information at the level of the dorsal horn was shown to have clinical utility in 1967, when transcutaneous electrical nerve stimulation (TCS, TENS) was introduced. The success of TENS in certain pain problems has provided enthusiastic support for development of newer treatment modalities based on research theory. Dorsal column stimulation (DCS) excites descending inhibitory pathways with electricity to provide analgesia. The success of DCS has been mixed, but it does appear to have a place in certain deafferentation pain syndromes.

The success of central morphine microinjection techniques to provide analgesia may have prompted Reynolds[67] to demonstrate similar results in animals, using electrical stimulation of the periaqueductal gray. Hosobuchi has subsequently demonstrated naloxone-reversible analgesia in humans following implantation of brainstem electrodes.[15] Each of these applications of electrical stimulation was predicted on the basis of improved understanding of pain mechanisms. Electrical stimulation seems to have found a place in pain management by exciting intrinsic mechanisms used for the modulation of nociceptive information.

ACUTE PAIN MANAGEMENT

General

The previous section of this chapter has discussed the intricate relationships involved in the rostral processing of noxious stimuli. This complicated system has developed phylogenetically to aid in perpetuation of the human species. The importance of acute pain in signaling potential damage to the organism cannot be overlooked. Acute pain serves to inform an individual that action needs to be taken to avoid injury. Indeed, the process of symptom-oriented diagnosis relies on acute pain to suggest an accurate diagnosis. For example, the pain of a bone fracture leads to voluntary and involuntary immobilization of a fracture site to prevent further damage. This well localized stimulus also directs the orthopedist to the injured area. Similarly, diagnosis and treatment of acute appendicitis, ruptured viscus, and ureterolithiasis are all aided by the presence of acute pain. While the diagnostic advantage provided by an unmedicated patient seems desirable, it is interesting to note that the one study which has been performed to assess the effect of medication on masking diagnosis revealed no difference. In this prospective randomized blinded study, only 12% of patients displayed changes in physical signs and none had altered diagnosis.[91] Certainly, once any warning signs have been heeded and the proper diagnosis and treatment initiated, acute pain no longer serves a useful purpose. While intervention at the point of injury may abolish the painful stimulus (e.g. drainage of an abscess, reduction of a dislocation), at other times the pain will not resolve for some time.

These persistent or refractory pain impulses are a focus of attention in both acute and chronic pain management. The most common forms of treatment for such pain are analgesic drugs and regional blockade.

ANALGESIC DRUGS FOR ACUTE PAIN AND CANCER PAIN

Analgesic ladder

The World Health Organization (WHO) in 1986 published a small booklet with guidelines for drug treatment of patients with cancer pain.[83] These guidelines are formulated around the concept of an analgesic ladder (Table 89.4). It should be emphasized that there is now overwhelming evidence that oral opioids are just as effective as parenteral opioids, if proper dosing regimens are utilized. This analgesic ladder has now been tested in many developing and developed countries. Published data indicated that the use of the analgesic ladder was successful in treating over 80% of patients, without the need for other measures.[75] In developed countries, the challenge lies in education and the implementation of the simple principles behind the analgesic ladder.

Non-steroidal anti-inflammatory drugs (NSAIDs)

As discussed earlier, prostaglandins are formed in damaged tissue and appear to be involved in sensitizing the peripheral nociceptors to painful stimuli. The effect of NSAIDs to inhibit the synthesis of prostaglandins is currently thought to be the explanation of their pain-relieving properties. The prostaglandins, leukotrienes and also the thromboxanes, are all oxygenated derivatives of arachadonic acid, an essential polyunsaturated fat. The term 'eicosanoids' is often used to describe all of the products of arachadonic acid metabolism. NSAIDs inactivate cyclo-oxygenase, which catalyses the formation of cyclic endoperoxides from arachadonic acid. Anti-inflammatory steroids act at an earlier step by the formation of a polypeptide with an anti-phospholipase effect.[63]

The indications for NSAIDs range from the treatment of aches, sprains and dysmenorrhea, to long-term therapy for rheumatoid and osteoarthritis, as well as degenerative joint diseases (ankylosing spondylitis, gout, etc.) Their anti-inflammatory activity has also been shown to relieve pain in cancer patients with bone metastases. In contrast to the opioid drugs, there has not been a clear demonstration of a relationship between blood levels of NSAIDs and pain relief. The majority of NSAIDs can be classified into one of two groups based on their elimination half-lives (Table 89.5). The NSAIDs in group one have half-lives between 2 and 4 hours. Paracetamol is also included with group one drugs, despite the lack of anti-inflammatory properties. The drugs in group two have longer half lives ranging from 6 to 60 hours. Patients with renal insufficiency are thought to be at risk for toxicity due to these agents, because they are excreted through the kidney. However, pharmacokinetic studies have not indicated that major dose adjustments are needed for these patients.

The use of NSAIDs alone has been supported through years of clinical practice. However, the different sites of action found with NSAIDs and opioids would also suggest additive, or possibly even synergistic, effects. Trials with a relatively new NSAID, Ketorolac, indicate that this drug has strong analgesic properties and that it will significantly reduce opioid requirements. Ketorolac has been shown to be as effective as low dose morphine in treating postoperative pain. Ketorolac will likely find a place particularly in the acute management of postoperative pain, as it is available in a parenteral form.

Dosing of the individual agents is covered in Table 89.5. These doses have been derived from long-term therapy of rheumatologic disease, and represent near maximal anti-inflammatory activity. While these doses are considered safe for long-term therapy, careful monitoring of side effects is appropriate. Side effects of NSAIDs include gastric irritation, salt and fluid retention, platelet inhibition and tinnitus. The gastric damage occurs due to decreased prostaglandin levels. This causes less gastric mucus production, increased acid secretion and decreased gastric mucosal blood supply. Paracetamol does not share the potential for these prostaglandin-mediated side effects, but carries the potential for liver damage with excessive doses.

Antidepressants

Earlier in the chapter the involvement of serotonin and catecholaminergic neurotransmitters in the modulation of nociception was discussed. Many of the antidepressant drugs act by blocking the uptake of noradrenalin and serotonin in the CNS. This effect may also occur in the medulla and increase the concentrations of these neurotransmitters at the synapses involved in descending inhibition of dorsal horn cells. Table 89.6 lists the names and properties of some of these antidepressants. Secondary

Table 89.4 Analgesic ladder in cancer pain[+]

Step 1:	Paracetamol,* aspirin or other NSAIDs** ± adjuvants*** (co-analgesics)
Step 2:	Codeine, dextropropoxyphene (or ? oxycodone) ± NSAIDs ± adjuvants***
Step 3:	Morphine, methadone, ± NSAIDs ± adjuvants***

* Paracetamol = acetaminophen
** NSAIDs = non-steroidal anti-inflammatory drugs.
*** Psychotropics (anxiolytics, antidepressants), anticonvulsants, steroids, etc.
[+] Reproduced from Cousins M J 1988 Introduction to acute and chronic pain: implication for neural blockade. In: Cousins M J, Bridenbaugh P O (eds) *Neural Blockade in Clinical Anesthesia and Management of Pain*, 2nd edn. Lippincott, Philadelphia, with permission.

Table 89.5 Terminal half-life, recommended dose, influence of food on absorption and incidence of gastric erosion from NSAIDs.†

Drug	Terminal half-life (h)	Oral dose and frequency (mg/h)	Effect of food on absorption*	Incidence of gastric erosion**
Aspirin	0.2 to 0.3	600 to 900/4	a	+++
Salicylate	2 to 3	600/4	a	++
Difusinal	8 to 12	500/12	a	+
Diclofenac	1.5 to 2	25 to 50/8	a	+
Ibuprofen	2 to 3	200 to 400/8	a	+
Naproxen	12 to 15	250 to 375/12	c	+
Fenoprofen	2 to 3	400 to 600/6	b	+
Indomethacin	6 to 8	50 to 75/8	a	++
Sulindac	6 to 8	100 to 200/12	b	+
Piroxicam	30 to 60	20 to 30/24	a	+
Flufenamic acid	8 to 10	500/6	a	−
Mefanamic acid	3 to 4	250/6	a	++
Ketoprofen	1 to 4	50/6	a	+
Ketorolac***	5	10 to 30/6	?	?

* a = decrease in rate of absorption, no change in oral bioavailability; b = decrease in rate of absorption and oral bioavailability; c = no change in rate of absorption or oral bioavailability
** + = low incidence of gastritis; ++ = intermediate gastritis; +++ = high incidence of gastritis
*** = not currently available for clinical use, doses based on review of scientific literature.
† Modified from Gourlay G K, Cousins M J, Cherry D A 1987 Drug therapy. In: Burrows, Elton, Stanley (eds) *Handbook of Chronic Pain Management*. Elsevier Science, Amsterdam, with permission.

amines are thought to be more effective blockers of norepinephrine, while the tertiary amines appear more effective in blocking serotonin re-uptake.

Oral tricyclic antidepressants are well absorbed from the gastrointestinal tract. There is conflicting information regarding the existence of therapeutic ranges for antidepressants. All of the currently available pharmacodynamic information refers to the antidepressant activity of these drugs. The time taken for the perception of pain relief following the institution of these drugs is only 2 to 7 days, as compared with the accepted time for antidepressant effect of 3 to 4 weeks. This observation suggests that different mechanisms may be involved in their analgesic effect compared with their antidepressant action.

Side effects from tricyclic antidepressant use include autonomic anticholinergic and adrenergic effects. Dry mouth is the most common, and can be relieved by increased fluid intake, and salivary stimulants such as sugarless candy. Blurring of vision is also common and may interfere with reading. Constipation has also been described in association with these agents.

Co-analgesics

Review of the analgesic ladder promoted by the WHO (Table 89.4) demonstrates the application of co-analgesic compounds. A multitude of agents has been purported to have analgesic properties. The majority of these agents are thought to potentiate analgesia provided by opioid and non-opioid analgesics. While the data in support of the use of such compounds may be anecdotal, a small number of these drugs do appear to have clinical utility in the management of cancer pain. Table 89.7 summarizes some of the currently available co-analgesics.

Corticosteroids are the first group of drugs to be considered as co-analgesics. These drugs have been utilized successfully for the management of neuropathic pain from direct neural compression, and also from pain due to increased intracranial pressure. Systemic steroids are thought to reduce perineural edema, and lymphatic edema that may be contributing to pain by compressing individual nerves. This treatment appears to be especially helpful in cases of spinal cord compression. Treatment of such neural compression involves relatively high doses of dexamethasone, near 30 mg/day. Steroids are best employed on a trial basis. A single morning dose or twice daily dose of 2 to 4 mg/day of dexamethasone can be utilized over a 10 to 14 day period.[63] If no improvement in pain is noted during this period of time, the dose can be tapered off over 3 to 5 days. An additional benefit of corticosteroids is that they often stimulate appetite; this may aid in the nutritional support of patients with malignancy. The use of steroids is not without problems, however. Attention needs to be

Table 89.6 Terminal half-life, recommended daily doses and other properties of antidepressant drugs.[††]

Drug	Amine group[*]	Terminal half-life (h)	Inhibitor concentration[**] NA	5-HT	Recommended daily dose (mg)[†]
Amitriptyline	3	20 to 30	4.6	4.4	50 to 150
Nortriptyline	2	18 to 36	0.9	17	50 to 150
Protriptyline	2	50 to 90	—	—	10 to 50
Clomipramine	3	20 to 30	4.6	0.5	50 to 75
Imipramine	3	20 to 30	4.6	0.5	50 to 75
Desipramine	2	12 to 24	0.2	35	75 to 150
Doxepin	3	10 to 25	6.5	20	75 to 150
Dothiapen	3	20 to 30	—	—	50 to 100
Mianserin	3	10 to 20	20	130	20 to 50
Nomifensine	1,3	2 to 4	2	120	75 to 150
Zimelidine	3	5 to 10	630	14	200 to 300

[*] 1 = primary amine group; 2 = secondary amine group; 3 = tertiary amine group.
[**] Inhibitor concentration (IC50) represents the antidepressant concentration ($\times 10^{-8}$ M) required to inhibit the uptake of either noradrenalin (NA) or serotonin (5-HT) by 50% using rat mid-brain synaptosomes. [Adapted from Maitre et al (1982)]
[†] It is generally recommended that the antidepressant be administered as a single dose at night, unless significant side effects occur where a night and morning dose (divided dose) may be appropriate.
[††] Reproduced from Gourlay G K, Cousins M J, Cherry D A 1987 Drug therapy. In: Burrows, Elton, Stanley (eds) *Handbook of Chronic Pain Management*. Elsevier Science, Amsterdam, with permission.

Table 89.7 Co-analgesic medications

Drug	Classification	Indication	Comments
Amitriptylline Imipramine Mianserin Clomipramine Doxepin	Antidepressant	Chronic pain, neuropathic pain associated with neuropathy and headache	Improves sleep, may improve appetite
Dexamethasone Prednisolone Fludrocortisone	Corticosteroid	Neuropathic pain secondary to direct neural compression, pain secondary to increased intracranial pressure	May stimulate appetite, limit trial to 2 weeks and recesses efficacy
Carbamazepine Phenytoin Valproate Clonazepam	Anticonvulsant	Neuropathic pain with paroxysmal character	Start slowly, increase gradually while observing for side effects
Lidocaine 2-Cloroprocaine Tocainide Mexiletine	Membrane stabilizer	Neuropathic pain associated with peripheral neuropathy	Efficacy of oral preparations is not established
Levomepromazine	Phenothiazine	Insomnia unresponsive to antidepressant or short-acting benzodiazepine	Increase dose slowly to achieve desired effect
Haloperidol	Butyrophenone	Acute confusion, nausea, vomiting	Prolonged use may be complicated by tardive dyskinesia
Hydroxyzine	Antihistamine	Nausea, pruritis, anxiety	Anticholinergic side effects
Dexamphetamine Cocaine Caffeine	CNS stimulant	Opioid induced sedation, potentiation of NSAID, potentiation of opioid analgesia not proven in cancer	Should only be employed as short term therapeutic trial

focused on the possible development of oral and vaginal candidiasis. In addition, this treatment may worsen peripheral edema.

Anticonvulsants are also often advocated as analgesic adjuvants. They suppress neuronal firing and have been successfully employed for treatment of neuropathic pain states, including trigeminal neuralgia and peripheral neuropathies. Carbamazepine has been helpful in managing cancer pain with dysesthetic components.[76] Sodium valproate, clonazepam and phenytoin may also demonstrate similar utility. These drugs need to be started at low doses, and increased gradually to avoid possible side effects, such as dizziness, ataxia, drowsiness, blurred vision and gastrointestinal irritation. In addition, carbamazepine has been associated with bone marrow toxicity, while sodium valproate is known to produce hepatic toxicity.

The use of lidocaine and 2-chloroprocaine in the treatment of certain peripheral neuropathies that have been refractory to other analgesic medications has led to the investigation of another group of drugs which may be loosely classified as membrane stabilizers. In addition to intermittent i.v. infusion of these two local anesthetics, oral administration of the lidocaine congeners, mexiletine and tocainide, has been reported to be useful in certain patients. Typically, these patients are thought to have neuropathic components to their pain. In comparison to patients with episodic lancinating neuropathic pain, who benefit from anti-epileptics, those patients who benefit from membrane stabilizers may have a more constant pain.

Antipsychotics have long been purported to potentiate the analgesic effect of opioids. However, most studies employing these drugs are uncontrolled, and the enthusiasm for their continued use is actually in contrast to the available literature. The phenothiazines are the most commonly employed antipsychotics for analgesia. Dundee has published data regarding the analgesic potency of 14 different phenothiazines in an uncontrolled trial of experimental pain.[28,55,56] The results of these studies suggest that the action of a few potentially analgesic phenothiazines was initially anti-analgesic, and only after 2 to 3 hours mildly analgesic.[1] Review of phenothiazines in both experimental and clinical pain reveals that only levomepromazine (methotrimeprazine) has established analgesic properties. Levomepromazine appears to have analgesic potency about one-half that of morphine in patients with cancer pain.[8] Haloperidol is a butyrophenone antipsychotic. This drug has found a useful role in the management of acute confusional states associated with terminal cancer. Haloperidol also has useful anti-emetic properties which can be helpful in the management of cancer pain. Animal studies have reported haloperidol to potentiate opioid analgesia in some species, but this has not been confirmed in humans. The appropriate utilization of antipsychotics in the chronic management of cancer pain has not been established. Care must be utilized in the long-term administration of these drugs, because of the potential for developing tardive dyskinesia.

Benzodiazepines are often discussed as co-analgesics. These drugs actually do not have any demonstrated analgesic effect. Diazepam has been studied extensively with respect to analgesic activity, and it does not alter sensitivity to pain or potentiate the analgesic activity of opioids. These drugs do, however, decrease the affective responses to acute pain, and may produce extended relief in chronic pain due to musculoskeletal disorders associated with muscle spasm.[39] Judicious use of benzodiazepines in cancer pain is appropriate for short-term relief of anxiety, but superior analgesic effects and night time sedation can be achieved by employing a tricyclic agent.

Hydroxyzine is an anti-histaminic agent. It has proven analgesic properties at high doses. It does not consistently improve analgesia obtained with opioids, but it does potentiate the effect of opioids on the affective components of pain. It appears that hydroxyzine administered intramuscularly has analgesic properties similar to low doses of morphine.[7] In addition, the sedative and antipruritic properties of this drug are useful in the setting of chronic cancer pain.

The final group of analgesic adjuvants to be considered are the CNS stimulants. This group includes amphetamines, cocaine and caffeine. Chronic cancer pain has been treated for nearly a century with combinations of opioid and stimulant in Brompton's cocktail. This mixture contains morphine, cocaine and a phenothiazine. Despite years of clinical experience with such a mixture, controlled studies have not demonstrated superior analgesia with this combination as compared to opioid alone. Potentiation of analgesia by sympathomimetics has been well described. Caffeine is known to increase the analgesic effects of aspirin and paracetamol, and one study suggests that dextro-amphetamine doubled the analgesic potency of morphine.[34] The long-term use of these stimulants in cancer pain has not been systematically evaluated. The use of these drugs should probably be limited to a therapeutic trial period of several days, to determine efficacy for individual patients.

Opioids

Opioids are extremely effective agents in treating nociceptive components of acute pain. Many misconceptions surround the use of opioid drugs, and result in a marked tendency for inadequate doses at inappropriately long dosing intervals. Once a decision has been made to use opioid medications, it is both logical and essential to use an effective dosage regimen. (See also Ch. 92.)

While vasts sums of money have been invested into development of new opioids over the last decade, an increased understanding of the pharmacokinetics and pharmacodynamics involved in opioid administration has done more to improve the treatment of pain than any new drug. The introduction of concepts such as MEC (the minimum effective analgesic concentration) have helped health care providers conceptualize the association between blood opioid concentrations and analgesic effect. Equally as important to effective pain treatment has been the realization that there may be as much as a five to six fold interpatient variability in the value of MEC for any one agent. MEC is influenced by a number of psychological and physical factors. It is impossible to predict the value of MEC for any patient/opioid combination. Therefore, it is necessary that the dose for each individual be titrated to the desired effect. While MEC and other pharmacokinetic variables cannot be used ahead of time to predict exact analgesic doses of opioids necessary to obtain analgesia, these concepts do provide a good starting point, and also allow the prediction of the effect of certain disease states on opioid requirements.

A list of the currently available pure opioid agonists and partial agonists is given in Table 89.8. The pure opioid agonists all share in common high affinity for the mu receptor, which is associated with pain relief, sedation, euphoria and respiratory depression. The partial agonists typically have kappa receptor affinity and were developed to provide pain relief without significant respiratory depression and also with less tendency towards physical dependency. The clinical results seen with the partial agonists have been unimpressive in terms of analgesia; in addition, respiratory depression and physical dependence remain important concerns. The drugs listed in Table 89.8 range from drugs with a high oral bioavailability and long half-life, such as methadone, which may be ideal for daily oral therapy, to ultrashort acting alfentanil, which is effective primarily as a continuous intravenous infusion. In either case, the correlation between analgesia and blood concentration of opioids is an essential key to the planning of opioid dosing.

In addition to planning effective analgesic therapy with opioids individualized to a particular patient, the use of opioids often involves management of side effects. The major side effects which limit the effectiveness of opioid therapy are nausea, vomiting, sedation and respiratory depression. Long-term opioid therapy is also complicated by constipation. The incidence and severity of the side effects seen with the different mu agonists are probably similar at equi-analgesic doses. Rather than restrict the dose of opioids to the point where a patient is free from side effects but experiencing pain, one should administer other medications to treat these side effects.

Nausea and vomiting are frequently responsive to drugs such as metoclopramide, phenothiazines or butyrophenones. Figure 89.8 illustrates a logical progressive approach to the treatment of nausea and vomiting. Adherence to such a treatment program can usually allow a patient to continue using the oral analgesic until tolerance to the side effects develops. Practical experience shows that tolerance to the emetic effects of opioids usually occurs over the first 2 weeks of use.[78] Respiratory depression is immediately reversible with naloxone, but should be monitored in patients receiving opioids.

Delivery systems

The continued reports of inadequate pain relief, despite use of vast numbers of newly developed opioids, points to the problems associated with opioid delivery rather than to any defect in the individual drugs per se. Depending on the clinical situation, there are many different delivery systems and dosing regimens that can provide good pain relief when

Table 89.8 Doses, pharmacokinetic parameters, minimum effective concentration and duration of pain relief for various opioid drugs.*

Opioid	Dose (mg)		Pharmacokinetic parameters		MEC** (ng/ml)	Duration of pain relief (h)	Comments
	i.m/i.v.	Oral	Terminal half-life (h)	Bioavailability (%)			
Codeine	130	250	2 to 3	50	—	3 to 4	Weak opiate, frequently combined with aspirin. Useful for pain with visceral and integumental components.
Propoxyphene	240	500	8 to 24	40	—	4 to 6	Weak opioid. Unacceptable incidence of side effects.
Oxycodone	10	30	–	30 to 50	—	4 to 6	Suppository (30 mg) can provide pain relief for 8 to 10 hours.
Diamorphine	5	15	0.05	0	—	2 to 3	Very soluble, rapidly converted to 6-mono-acetyl morphine and morphine in vivo. Zero oral bioavailability.
Morphine	10	40	2 to 4	10 to 40	10 to 40	3 to 4	Standard opiate to which new opioids are compared. New sustained release formulation available in some countries of considerable benefit in chronic cancer pain.

Table 89.8 Cont'd

Opioid	Dose (mg)		Pharmacokinetic parameters		MEC** (ng/ml)	Duration of pain relief (h)	Comments
	i.m./i.v.	Oral	Terminal half-life (h)	Bioavailability (%)			
Methadone	10	10 to 15	10 to 80	70 to 95	20 to 80	10 to 60	Duration of pain relief ranges from 10 to 60 hours both postoperatively and for cancer pain. Variable half-life. Requires initial care to establish dose for each patient to avoid accumulation. Otherwise of great value.
Hydromorphone	2	4 to 6	2 to 3	50 to 60	4	3 to 4	More potent but shorter acting than morphine.
Levorphanol	2	4	12 to 16	40 to 60	—	4 to 6	Good oral availability but long half-life compared to analgesia may lead to accumulation
Phenazocine	3	10 to 20	—	20 to 30	—	4 to 6	Similar to morphine, more potent
Oxymorphone	1	6	—	10 to 40	—	3 to 4	Similar to morphine, more potent
Meperidine	100	300	3 to 5	30 to 60	200 to 800	2 to 4	Not as effective in relieving anxiety as morphine. Suppositories (200 to 400 mg) have slow onset (2 to 3 hrs) but can last for 6 to 8 hours. Normeperidine toxicity.
Dextromoramide	7.5	10	—	75	—	2 to 3	Methadone-like chemical structure. Short acting. Useful in covering exacerbation pain. Supposed good oral bioavailability (oral compared to parenteral doses)
Fentanyl	0.1	—	3 to 6	—	0.6 to 2	0.5 to 1	Potent opioid. Usually administered by i.v. injection. Short duration of pain relief. Therefore repeated doses on the basis of pain relieving effects may cause accumulation and respiratory depression. Transdermal patch under evaluation.
Alfentanil	0.5	—	1 to 3	—	250	0.1 to 0.3	Rapid and short acting opioid with small initial volume of distribution. Pharmacokinetic characteristics make this drug suitable primarily for continuous i.v. infusion.
Sufentanil	0.02	—	2 to 5	—	—	0.5 to 1	More potent drug similar to fentanyl. Small doses utilized make the determination of MEC from blood extremely difficult. Only available as i.v. form.
Buprenorphine	0.3	0.2 to 1.2	2 to 3	30	—	6 to 8	Available as a sublingual tablet in many countries which appears useful in treatment of cancer pain. Ceiling in analgesic effect at dose near 5 mg/day. Should not be utilized with a pure opioid agonist.
Butorphanol	2	—	2.5 to 3.5	—	—	3 to 6	Oral form unavailable in many countries. Value in treatment of chronic pain not established.
Nalbuphine	10	40	4 to 6	20	—	3 to 6	Oral form unavailable in many countries. Value in treatment of chronic pain not established.

Data presented are estimates obtained from the literature.

* Modified from: Gourlay G K, Cousins M J & Cherry D A 1987 Drug therapy. In: Burrows, Elton, Stanley (eds) *Handbook of Chronic Pain Management*. Elsevier Science, Amsterdam, with permission.

** MEC = minimum effective analgesic concentration

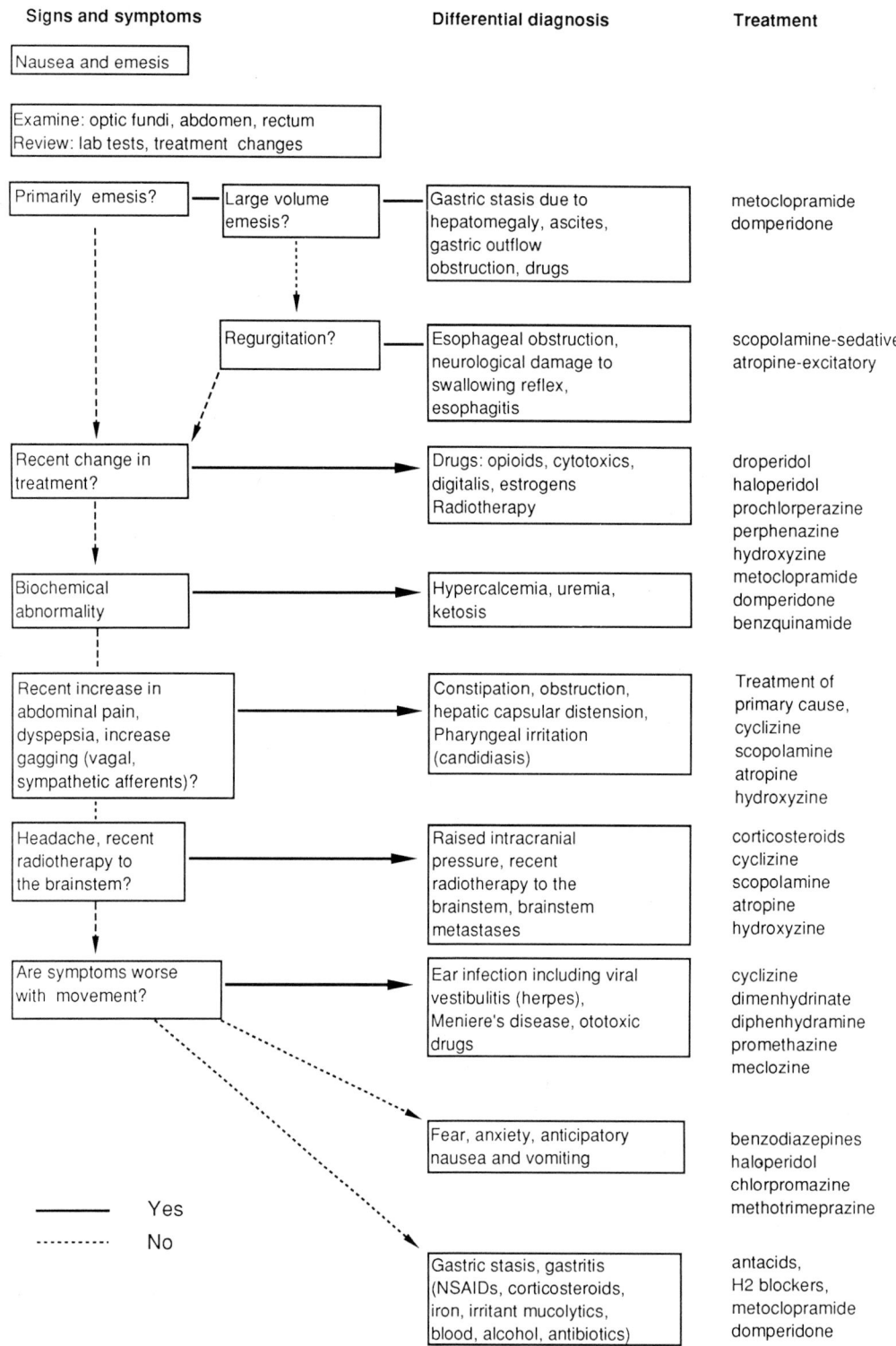

Fig. 89.8 Nausea and vomiting treatment algorithm.

utilized properly. The association between stable blood levels of opioids and continuous analgesia must be remembered when planning any systemic opioid therapy. The effective dose of opioid medication is the minimum dose which provides acceptable pain relief with a low incidence of side effects.

Oral opioids

The clearance of the majority of opioids combined with the extensive hepatic metabolism has implications when choosing oral dosing. Drugs are absorbed from the gastrointestinal tract directly into the portal circulation where they travel to the liver. Therefore, following oral dosing, a significant percentage of the dose is metabolized to inactive products prior to the opioids reaching the systemic circulation.[52] This phenomenon is referred to as the hepatic 'first pass effect'. This effect, and poor oral bioavailability seen with certain opioids, leads to perceptions that oral administration of opioids is ineffective.

Oral bioavailability ranges from zero for heroin to 80% for methadone. Morphine oral bioavailability ranges from 10 to 40%, leading to very wide fluctuations in oral dosing requirements between different patients. Similar variability is seen in meperidine (pethidine) and other opioids (Table 89.8). The high bioavailability of methadone and the long terminal half-life suggest that stable blood levels of the drug could be obtained from oral dosing.

Much attention has also been focused on the development of effective sustained release preparations of morphine. While the concept of sustained release is fairly simple, obtaining a pharmacologic preparation that maintains a steady dose release without dose dumping which can lead to bolus effect has proven more difficult. At present, sustained release morphine products are available in many countries. The actual changes in pharmacokinetics of these sustained release preparations with regards to food intake, activity, and posture have not been evaluated. As continued progress is made in this area, a reliable sustained release preparation should become available.

In summary, satisfactory analgesia with oral dosing can be obtained if attention is focused on the pharmacokinetics of the particular opioid to be administered, the oral bioavailability of the drug and titration of the drug to achieve adequate analgesia in each individual patient.

Sublingual administration

Ongoing interest in the improved pain management of patients with terminal malignancy has led to the investigation of sublingual administration. The sublingual route is particularly useful in patients who complain of nausea, vomiting and dysphagia, who cannot tolerate oral medication. This method of administration has theoretical advantages in that the oral cavity is well perfused providing rapid onset of action, and subsequent absorption results in systemic rather than portal drug delivery. Sublingual absorption of the lipid-soluble drugs, methadone, fentanyl and buprenorphine from alkaline solution was shown to provide analgesic concentrations very quickly in a recent study.[80] The utility of this technique in comparison with other methods of administration still needs to be assessed.

Rectal administration

Rectal administration of opioids has been advocated for patients who cannot swallow, or who have a high incidence of nausea or vomiting following oral administration. The studies of rectal administration of meperidine indicate a bioavailability similar to that seen following oral dosing (50%). Prolonged pain relief of 6 to 8 hours was observed following large doses (400 mg) of rectal meperidine, but a significant latency of 2 to 3 hours following administration can be seen. Rectal oxycodone has also been shown to have clinical utility providing pain relief for up to 8 hours.

Intramuscular

The most commonly used approach for managing postoperative pain is intramuscular administration of morphine or meperidine. The typical prescription would read: 'morphine 10 mg (or meperidine 100 mg) intramuscularly every three to four hours as needed for pain'. This approach has been shown to have many reasons for providing inadequate analgesia: the patient may not request medication despite experiencing severe pain; the nurse may not administer the medication; the dose may not be adequate for the patient's needs. Even withstanding all of these potential problems, the variable blood levels seen following intramuscular dosing, usually result in periods of pain, alternating with periods of toxicity.[3]

Subcutaneous

Subcutaneous administration of opioids has been used for decades to provide analgesia. More recent attention has been focused on this technique with the availability of small infusion pumps for delivering continuous opioids to ambulatory patients. Recent applications include subcutaneous infusion for cancer pain and subcutaneous patient controlled analgesia (PCA). Bruera and colleagues recently presented data confirming the efficacy of subcutaneous infusion in treating patients with severe pain due to malignancy, both at home and in the hospital.[18] The pharmacokinetic information available for subcutaneous administration of opioids is very limited. Continuous infusion of subcutaneous morphine has been demonstrated to provide equivalent analgesia and blood levels to intravenous infusion in postoperative patients.[79] Other drugs have been delivered by this route, but no definitive information is available of blood levels achieved. Subcutaneous infusion appears to act clinically like a continuous intravenous infusion, but more carefully controlled trials need to be carried out to determine if this similarity is true for all opioids.

Intravenous

The use of intravenous opioids, by intermittent injection

as well as continuous infusion, has been known to provide more rapid and effective analgesia for years. The clinical utility of this technique in the management of cancer pain was recently reviewed by the Sloan Kettering Group.[62] The pharmacokinetic support for this clinical observation has been developed over the last few years. Intravenous administration of opioid can maintain analgesia as long as the blood opioid concentration is kept above the minimum effective concentration (MEC) in a given patient. Knowledge of the systemic clearance of a drug will allow close approximation of the MEC value for a specific opioid to be delivered via continuous infusion. Using an infusion alone, however, will require approximately four times the terminal half-life to achieve stable concentrations. The clinical analgesia from continuous infusion opiates is best provided with a loading dose followed by a continuous infusion. The amount of the loading dose and the initial infusion can be predicted if the MEC, volume of distribution (Vd), and clearance (Cl) are known. The practical steps in calculating such an analgesic infusion are as follows:

1. Loading dose = $Vd \times MEC$
2. Maintenance infusion = $Cl \times MEC$

Providing the loading dose as an infusion over 10 to 15 minutes, followed by the maintenance rate, will allow good analgesia to be rapidly established with a minimum of toxicity. Subsequently, the maintenance rate should be titrated to patient comfort (see Ch. 92).

Patient-controlled analgesia (PCA)

The wide interpatient variability of the pharmacokinetic parameters discussed thus far is a primary reason that individual titration of opioid dosing is required to achieve adequate analgesia. While the physician can do this by evaluating patients at a given time after the therapy has been initiated, the option of patient-controlled analgesia (PCA) is well suited to accommodate the differences between the theory and practice of pain relief. Using PCA, the physician decides the drug to be employed, and the dose to be given. The patient can decide when a dose should be administered and the timing between doses.

While there are several variants of PCA, the one most commonly employed is a bolus demand form. With this type of PCA, the physician prescribes the drug based on his/her own personal preferences. The usual practice is to prescribe a bolus dose range that can be adjusted if inadequate analgesia or toxicity develops from a single demand. In addition, the minimum time between doses ('lock-out interval') is also prescribed by the physician, to avoid potential toxicity from repeated demands being provided before the peak effect of each bolus has been seen.

The majority of pharmacokinetic information applied to PCA has been inferred from single dose or continuous infusion of opioids. The applicability of this information to the multiple dose system of PCA has yet to be investigated. Despite this theoretical uncertainty, the clinical practice of PCA is successful. Several investigators have reported higher patient satisfaction and lower pain scores when this therapy is compared with other forms of parenteral opioid analgesia in acute pain management. Recently, the efficacy of short-term subcutaneous PCA was also demonstrated in cancer pain management.[19]

Spinal

The use of spinal opioids for acute pain management dates back only to the last decade. As compared with all of the previous delivery systems that we have discussed, which utilize indirect delivery of the opioid to the receptor site via the systemic circulation, spinal opioids are a direct system. Spinal opioids are delivered directly to the receptors in the spinal cord via local transportation from the epidural or subarachnoid space. The presence of opioid receptors in the dorsal horn of the spinal cord was suggested by Calvillo in 1974.[20] The localization of high concentrations of opioid receptors in the substantia gelatinosa followed in 1977.[2] Behavioral analgesia from intrathecal administration of morphine in rats was reported by Yaksh & Rudy in 1976.[89] Large numbers of clinical reports of long-lasting analgesia obtained with spinal opioids followed, but these were also accompanied by frequent reports of side effects. These side effects included nausea, vomiting, sedation, pruritis, urinary retention and respiratory depression. Fortunately, the identification of these side effects tempered the rampant application of this new technique. Meanwhile, fundamental knowledge about the use of spinal opioids was obtained through extensive animal studies.[85,88]

The term spinal opioid as applied in this section is used to describe intrathecal, and epidural administration of opioids. In an effort to present some of the data concerning spinal opioids, the remainder of the section will relate to epidural opioids, except where specifically stated.

The pharmacokinetics of epidurally administered morphine applied in the lumbar epidural space are still incompletely studied. It appears that after epidural injection of morphine, only low concentrations of lipid soluble, un-ionized drug will be present in the epidural space. Movement of the drug into the cerebrospinal fluid (CSF) by diffusion across the dura mater, transfer across the arachnoid granulations, as well as vascular uptake by spinal arteries and the epidural venous system all regulate the distribution of epidural morphine (Fig. 89.9). Because only small concentrations of the morphine present in the CSF will be un-ionized, the transfer across the spinal cord to the dorsal horn receptors will be slow. Morphine will also be available to move upward with the flow of CSF towards the brain. This explanation of epidural morphine distribution correlates well with the delayed onset of analgesia, and the late respiratory depression seen.

EPIDURAL: Hydrophilic Narcotic

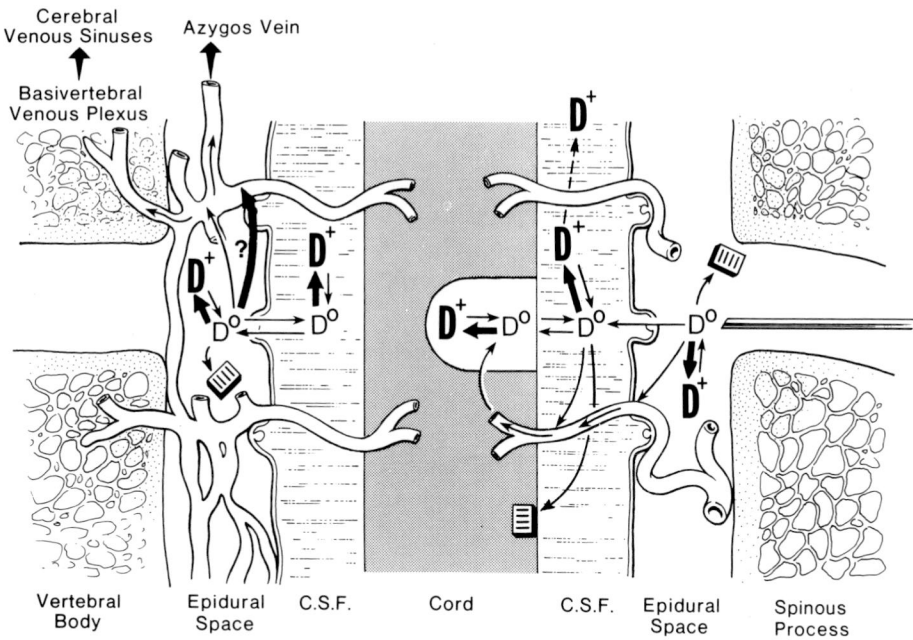

Fig. 89.9 Pharmacokinetic model: epidural injection of a hydrophilic opioid such as morphine. $D°$ = un-ionized, lipophilic drug; D^+ = ionized, hydrophilic drug. An epidural needle is shown delivering drug to the epidural space. The role of absorption by way of the radicular arteries remains speculative. The shaded squares represent non-specific binding sites. (Reproduced from Cousins M J, Cherry D A, Gourlay G K (1988),[22] with permission.)

While some of the physical principles governing the interaction of opioids with their receptors at the spinal level are similar to those seen with spinal local anesthetics, the drug effects obtained are quite different. Table 89.9 details the comparative effects of spinal administration of opioids and local anesthetics. The selective analgesia obtained from spinal administration of opioids without motor weakness or sympathetic blockade has promoted more widespread acceptance.

There are no data in humans indicating differences in efficacy among different opioids at equivalent doses. The latency and clinical duration of effect for some spinal opioids are presented in Table 89.10. The long duration of action seen following the administration of morphine epidurally has led to the increased use of this approach. The toxicity that was reported early in the clinical use of spinal opioids has been evaluated in several studies.

The sedation that was seen early in the use of spinal morphine appears to be a dose-related phenomenon. In fact, most clinical observations report that appropriate doses of spinal morphine result in less sedation than analgesic doses of parenteral opioids. Nausea, vomiting, pruritus and urinary retention were also reported early in the use of spinal opioids. While the incidence of these side effects seems to vary between patient groups, no factor has been identified that predicts patients who are likely to experience these problems. Some studies have again suggested that the severity of side effects may be dose-related, and there are conflicting reports of successful treatment of each of these side effects with the opioid antagonist, naloxone. It appears that the analgesia obtained from spinal morphine is unaffected by intravenous administration of small doses of naloxone. This advantage has led to the successful treatment of spinal opiate-induced side effects with systemic naloxone.[65]

Much of the concern about the utilization of spinal opioids has focused on the issue of respiratory depression. This can be early, associated with the peak blood levels following epidural administration, or later, perhaps due to the rostral migration of morphine within CSF into sensitive respiratory centers. Outcome studies generated from large groups of patients in Sweden who received spinal opioids indicate that the incidence of severe delayed respiratory depression following epidural morphine is approximately 1:1000 patients.[64] While certain demographic characteristics of at risk populations have been identified,[64] the inability to predict the occurrence of delayed respiratory depression in healthy patients highlights the need for increased surveillance of all patients receiving opioid analgesia.[16]

The spinal administration of opioids is appropriate for pain in virtually any region of the body. Spinally administered morphine has been shown to migrate over the entire length of the spinal cord, even when injected in the

Table 89.9 Comparison of actions and efficacy of spinally administered opioids and local anesthetics[†]

Property	Opioids	Local anesthetics
Actions		
Site of action	Substantia gelatinosa of dorsal horn of spinal cord★	Nerve roots (long tracts in spinal cord)
Types of blockade	Presynaptic and postsynaptic inhibition of neuron cell excitation	Blockade of nerve impulse conduction in axonal membrane
Modalities blocked	'Selective' block of pain conduction	Blockade of sympathetic and pain fibers, often also loss of sensation and motor function
Efficacy		
Type of pain/efficacy		
Surgical pain	Partial relief	Complete relief possible
Labor pain	Partial relief	Complete relief
Postoperative pain★★		
Early, first 24 hours	Partial to complete relief (high dose)	Complete relief
After first 24 hours	Complete relief (low dose)	Complete relief
Chronic pain	Complete relief	Impractical (usually)

★ And/or other sites where opioid receptors are present
★★ Pain after major surgery requires higher doses than after minor surgery
[†] Adapted from Cousins M J, Cherry D A, Gourlay G K (1988),[22] with permission.

Table 89.10 Epidural opioids: latency and duration of postoperative analgesia★

Drug	Dose (mg)	Detectable onset (min)	Complete pain relief (min)	Duration (h)
Pethidine	30 to 100	5 to 10	12 to 30	6
Morphine	5 to 10	23	60	20
Methadone	5	13	17	7
Hydromorphone	1	13	23	11
Fentanyl	0.1	5	20	3
Diamorphine	5	15	30	8

★ Adapted from Cousins M J, Cherry D A, Gourlay G K (1988),[22] with permission.

lumbar epidural space.[35,36] Initially, spinal opioids were promoted for use in acute pain management and temporary epidural catheters were used to provide access to the neuraxis. As the acceptance of this technique has grown, more permanent delivery systems have been devised to allow treatment of chronic pain. Figure 89.10 illustrates the technical aspects of epidural portal placement. Pain relief from such spinal opioid systems has been shown for pain in cervical dermatomes and even the trigeminal system. The shortcomings of this therapy include: fibrous sheath formation around the catheter, development of hyperesthesias in a minority of patients who receive high doses of spinal morphine, eventual loss of efficacy due to opioid tolerance, and resistance of certain neuropathic pains.[22,30] These shortcomings may be less than the same effects seen with other therapies. Spinal opioids may also be administered via the subarachnoid route with such a portal system. Alternatively, a continuous implantable subarachnoid or epidural pump system has been employed. In addition, the access to the epidural or subarachnoid space allows the utilization of local anesthetic medication to provide reversible neural blockade.

Continued efforts to refine and evaluate spinal opioids should help to determine the appropriate utilization of this therapy. The high quality of analgesia and the enthusiastic reports of patient satisfaction following epidural morphine analgesia provide ample justification for research in this field.[22]

As mentioned previously, multiple endogenous chemicals have been identified in the region of the dorsal horn of the spinal cord which are thought to modulate nociceptive processing. The clinical success of opioids to provide selective spinal analgesia has prompted the evaluation of other proposed analgesic agents. Intrathecal and epidural administration of clonidine has been shown to provide analgesia both in acute and chronic pain states. This drug is thought to mediate analgesia by facilitating alpha 2 adrenergic transmission in the spinal cord. The activity of GABA in nociceptive processing at the dorsal horn has also promoted the evaluation of intrathecally administered Baclofen. While these and many other drugs have been demonstrated to be effective when administered spinally, the appropriate role for them in the treatment of pain has not been determined. These and other spinally active drugs may prove useful in patients who develop tolerance to spinal opioids. Alternatively, as more characterization of the neuropharmacology of the dorsal horn becomes available, these drugs may be applied to particular clinical situations where spinal opioids have not been successful.

Intracerebroventricular opiates have also been employed in cases of advanced malignancy to achieve analgesia with very small doses of opioid. Further investigation of the potential risks and benefits of this technique versus spinal opioids or other, less invasive, treatment options is needed.

ELECTRICAL STIMULATION

Transcutaneous nerve stimulation

The origins of transcutaneous nerve stimulation (TENS) in western medicine dates back to the Roman times, when use of electric fish was ascribed analgesic properties. The publication of the gate control theory of pain by Melzack

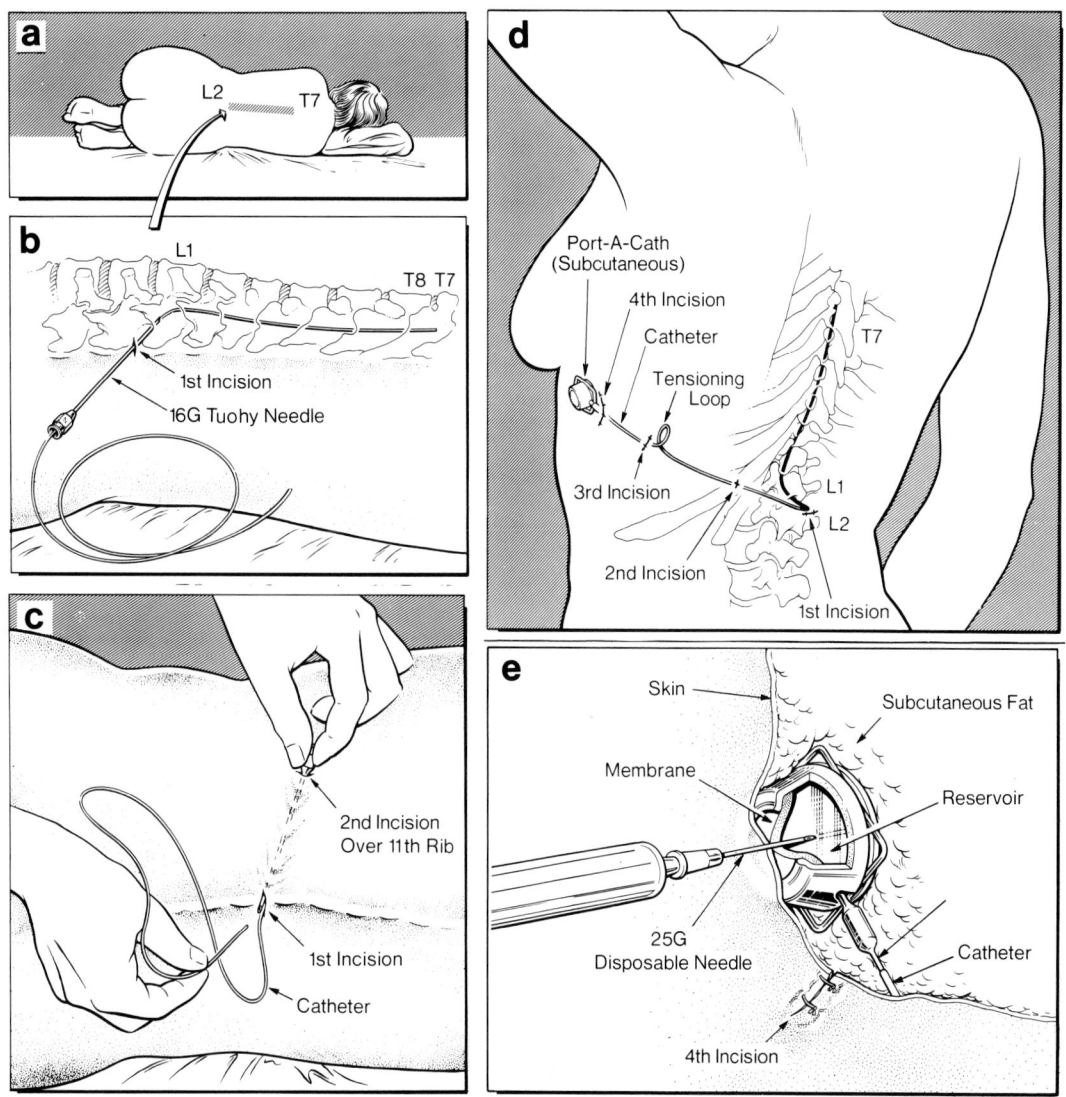

Fig. 89.10 Implantation of epidural portal system. (a) Position of patient before implantation. (b) Insertion of 16-gauge epidural catheter through a Tuohy needle. (c) Tunneling technique used to relocate the end of the epidural catheter to the anterior chest wall. (d) Portal attached to the inserted epidural catheter. (e) Injection technique and exposed view of the epidural portal. (Reproduced from Cousins M J, Cherry D A, Gourlay G K (1988),[22] with permission.)

& Wall renewed interest in electrical stimulation to produce analgesia. Excitation of large fiber peripheral afferents by electrical stimulation at the periphery has been successful in treating nociceptive and neuropathic pain.[44,49] TENS is a low-intensity stimulation of skin and muscle afferents in a specific segmental distribution. Numerous studies have documented the efficacy of TENS in certain pathologic pain states.[59,69,71] In addition, TENS has been shown to decrease opioid requirements seen following surgery, when used as an adjunct for postoperative analgesia.[61,72]

Acupuncture

Classical acupuncture differs from modern concepts of acupuncture analgesia in that the techniques evolved initially for the management of disease. Acupuncture analgesia uses stimulation of designated body sites by manual rotation of needles to produce a sensation known as 'teh chi'. The classic acupuncture stimulation has been modernized more recently by the application of low frequency (less than 5 Hz) stimulation of the needles which also produces powerful muscle contractions. Acupuncture produces a high intensity stimulation that is believed to induce a chemical modulation of pain, which explains why the relief is not confined to a local segmental distribution.

Dorsal column stimulation

Many patients with deafferentation pain are candidates for

dorsal column stimulation. This technique utilizes percutaneously positioned electrical leads that deliver a high frequency current over the dorsal spinal cord in an effort to stimulate descending analgesic pathways. Effective electrical stimulation induces analgesic paresthesias in the painful area. Successful trial stimulation suggests that implantation of a self-contained, battery powered device may be efficacious in selected patients. There have been no prospective trials of this therapy in the management of neuropathic terminal cancer pain, but the responses achieved with other deafferentation pain syndromes point to possible efficacy in this difficult circumstance.

NEURAL BLOCKADE

Patients who develop toxicity problems from analgesics may benefit from techniques of neurolytic blockade. The most common approach is to proceed from the least invasive, to the more invasive techniques, as required for pain management. In one major study undertaken in a comprehensive cancer care center, only 20% of patients required treatment with neurolytic blocks or other neurodestructive techniques. The continued advancement of spinal opioid techniques, as well as the success of continuous subcutaneous opioid infusions, will probably continue to decrease the need for neurodestructive techniques in the future.

There are many potential sites for neural blockade. (Table 89.11). In cancer pain, local anesthetics may be used for:

1. diagnostic blocks
2. prognostic blocks
3. therapeutic blocks.

Diagnostic blocks are used to localize the specific neuroanatomical structures, and to pharmacologically differentiate the fiber type, involved in mediating the pain. It is difficult to be certain that only a specific fiber type will be blocked by using differing concentrations of local anes-

Table 89.11 Classification of neural blockade procedures

Infiltration anesthesia	Extravascular (subcutaneous) Intravascular (intravenous) – Local anesthetic – Guanethidine, Bretylium (sympathetic block)
Peripheral nerve block	Minor nerve (e.g. pudendal) Paravertebral spinal nerve (e.g. intercostal) Major nerve or plexus (e.g. lumbar)
Central neural blockade	Epidural (extradural, peridural) Subarachnoid (spinal)
Sympathetic block	Stellate, celiac, lumbar ganglia
Topical anesthesia	Epidermal Mucous membrane

thetics. Thus, many pain clinicians prefer to block at sites where the fibers are anatomically separated (e.g lumbar sympathetic block, individual somatic nerve blocks). The interpretation of diagnostic neural blockade is both difficult and crucial to the appropriate utilization of these techniques. This interpretation is discussed in detail by Cousins & Boas.[13] *Prognostic blocks* should always be carried out at least twice prior to neurolytic or surgical ablation. This permits confirmation that the pain is relieved, and also gives the patient an opportunity to decide if any side effects are acceptable. *Therapeutic blocks* with local anesthetic cannot be expected to permanently relieve pain directly due to the processes depicted in Table 89.1A. Nevertheless, pain in cancer patients may be due to muscle spasms, postoperative neuralgia, denervation phenomena, neuroma formation, etc. In some of these cases, a series of long-acting local anesthetic blocks will produce long-lasting or permanent pain relief.

Local anesthetics

Cocaine was the first local anesthetic introduced into clinical use. It is a naturally occurring compound that was discovered in South America during the 1850's by German scientists. Cocaine is an ester local anesthetic and is used today primarily as a topical anesthetic, especially of the nose and throat. Unlike other local anesthetics, cocaine causes vasoconstriction by inhibiting the re-uptake of norepinephrine locally in vascular smooth muscle. Mood elevation is a much sought after property of cocaine, and accounts for the high rate of dependency seen in recreational use of this drug. The deaths associated with the high toxicity of cocaine were identified even in the late 19th century, and promoted the search for a safer alternative local anesthetic.

Procaine was introduced into clinical practice just prior to the first world war. Procaine is also an ester local anesthetic; however, unlike cocaine, this drug was rapidly metabolized and provided no mood elevation. The inherent safety of procaine led to widespread acceptance of this drug for regional anesthesia, but the long latency and short duration of action necessitated the development of other agents.

The other local anesthetics derived from procaine were numerous. 2-chloroprocaine and tetracaine represent the currently used ester local anesthetics which developed from procaine. 2-chloroprocaine is a rapid acting local anesthetic with low systemic toxicity. It is used widely in epidural anesthesia for labor and cesarean section; it is also used clinically for peripheral nerve block when the expected duration of operation will not exceed 60 minutes. Tetracaine remains a popular drug for spinal anesthesia, but the onset of neural blockade is too slow for it to be used for other regional techniques; the onset in spinal anesthesia is within 5 minutes.

The remaining local anesthetics are primarily amide local anesthetics. This difference is conferred by the presence of an amide linkage replacing the ester linkage seen with procaine and its congeners. The first amide local anesthetic was lidocaine; this was soon followed by mepivacaine, prilocaine, bupivacaine and etidocaine. These drugs all share in common the amide linkage which confers a greater stability on the drug.

Lidocaine is the most versatile and widely used of all local anesthetics. It has a short latency and an intermediate duration of action. Lidocaine is employed for peripheral nerve block, topical anesthesia, local infiltration and, plexus anesthesia, as well as epidural and spinal anesthesia.

Mepivacaine is similar to lidocaine in terms of onset and duration. Its uses are similar to lidocaine, except that mepivacaine is not effective as a topical agent. In addition, the metabolism of mepivacaine is prolonged in the newborn, so that the usefulness of this agent in obstetric analgesia is limited.

Prilocaine is also similar to lidocaine in terms of anes-

thetic profile. It is utilized for local infiltration, peripheral block and epidural anesthesia. In addition, prilocaine is the least toxic of all amide local anesthetics. This characteristic has led to the wide acceptance of this drug for intravenous regional anesthesia. It should be noted, however, that doses in excess of 600 mg of prilocaine may result in methemoglobinemia.

Bupivacaine has had a prominent influence on the practise of regional anesthesia. This agent has an intermediate latency and a long duration of action, but seems to have its main benefit by producing significant sensory blockade without dominant motor block. This differential sensory blockade has led to the wide acceptance of bupivacaine in labor analgesia and postoperative pain relief. The toxicity of bupivacaine compared to an equianalgesic dose of lidocaine is approximately four to one; this indicates the need for great caution when utilizing this agent.

Etidocaine is the most recent local anesthetic released for clinical use. It has rapid onset and prolonged duration of action. The anesthetic profile of etidocaine provides rela-

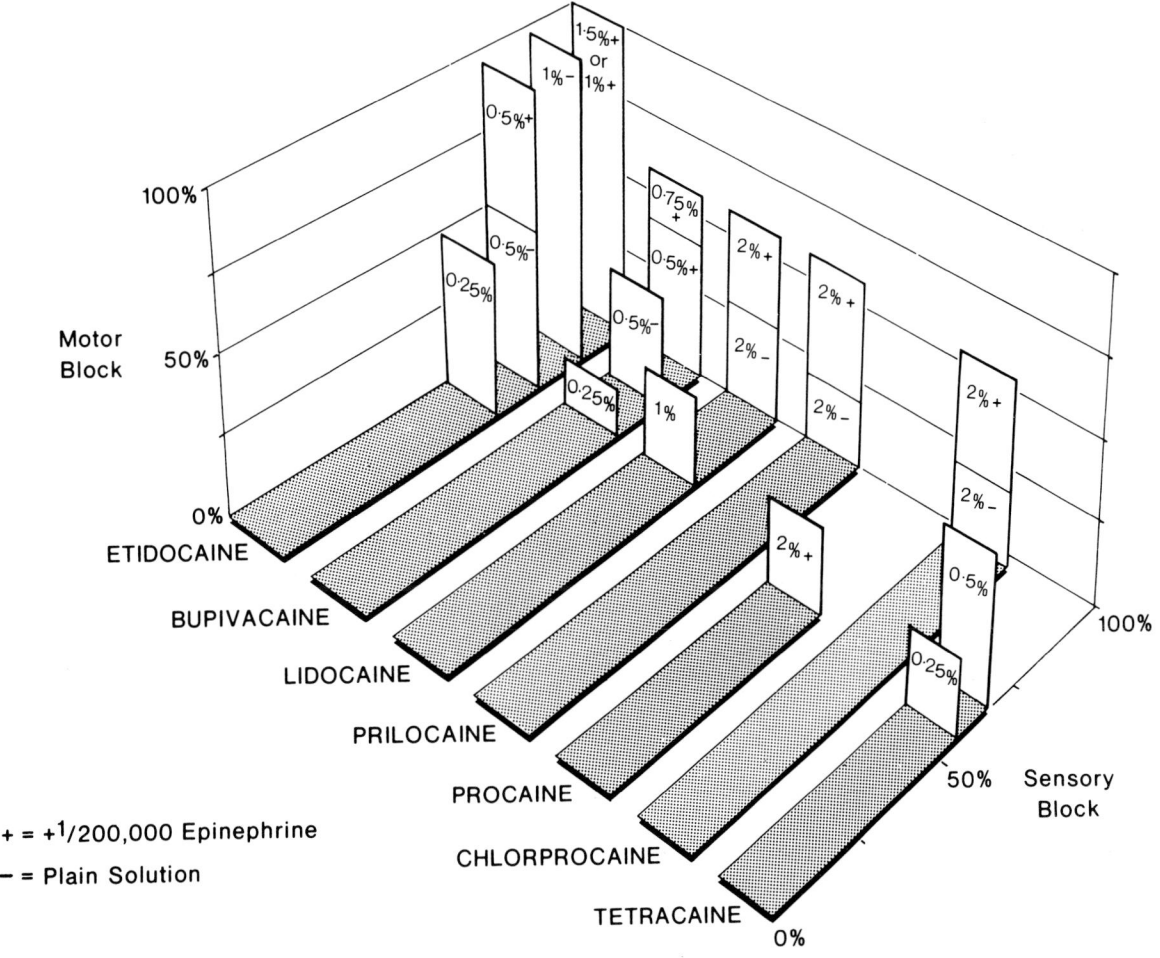

Fig. 89.11 Comparison of agents in epidural block. The percentage of motor blockade and the percentage of success of sensory blockade are illustrated for each agent. This illustration is based on subjective clinical data, and thus only approximate comparisons can be drawn. (Reproduced from Covino (1988),[23] with permission.)

tively greater motor block as compared with sensory blockade. This has limited the utilization of this agent in obstetric anesthesia and postoperative analgesia.

Choice of local anesthetic

The differential somatic blockade obtained with the use of low concentrations of bupivacaine makes it the most logical choice of agent for acute and chronic pain management (Fig. 89.11). Lidocaine is also employed in some situations because of the shorter latency, but the prolonged action of bupivacaine is usually preferred. It must be noted that there is considerable variation between duration of action of a local anesthetic and the particular block for which it is employed. For example, peripheral nerve block with bupivacaine may last 10 hours, while epidural blockade rarely lasts more than 3 hours. The reasons for this difference are multifactorial. While higher concentrations of a given agent will typically increase the duration of effect by a small amount, the change to higher concentrations will also increase the degree of motor block. For bupivacaine this difference is marked; the use of 0.25% bupivacaine provides good sensory analgesia and minimal motor block,

whereas 0.50% bupivacaine provides only slightly improved sensory analgesia with much greater motor block (Fig. 89.11). In addition to this undesirable change in the differential blockade seen with more concentrated solutions, higher concentrations also increase the potential of toxicity developing with each block. Prior to initiating any use of local anesthetic neural blockade, one should have thorough knowledge of the potential toxicity of local anesthetic agents. Local anesthetics are known to cause CNS excitation followed by CNS depression at higher blood levels. Cardiac toxicity is also a concern with high doses of local anesthetics. The reader is referred to the detailed discussion by Covino for a review of local anesthetic toxicity.[23]

Anatomy of neural blockade

Knowledge of the neuroanatomy of the pelvic organs is essential to appropriately employ local anesthetic or permanent neural blockade. The knowledge of pain transmission from pelvic structures in humans is primarily derived from detailed studies of patients with labor pain or cancer pain. These pathways are summarized in Figures 89.12 A and B and Table 89.12. The most common error

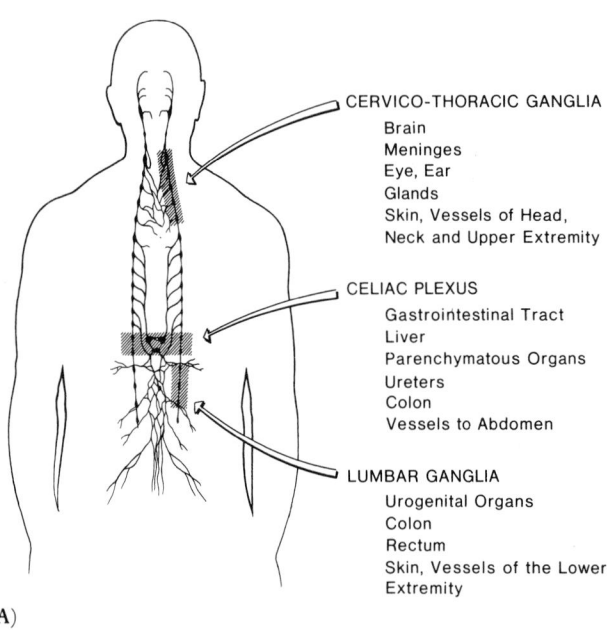

(A)

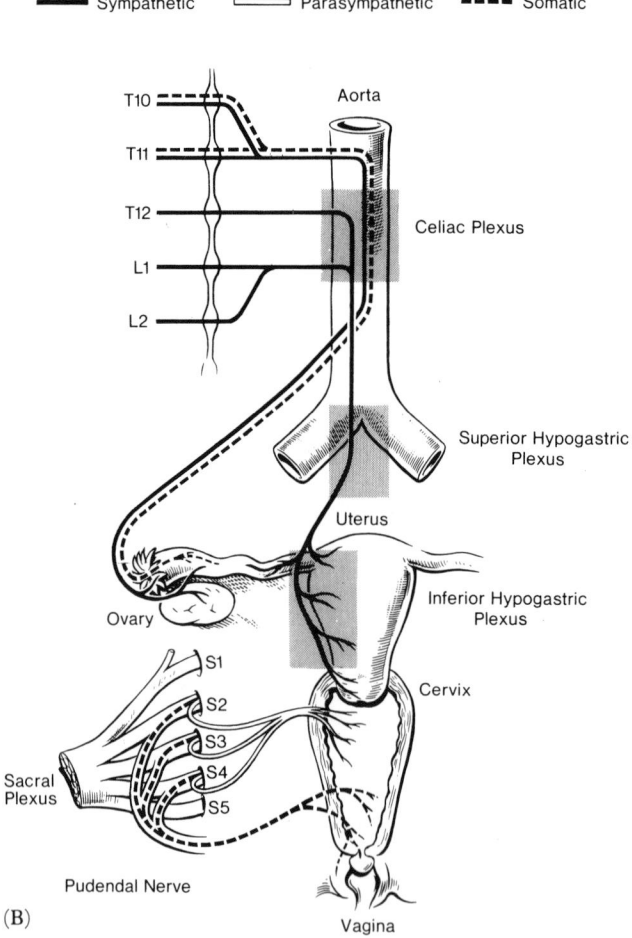

(B)

Fig. 89.12 (A) Sympathetic chain. The three main levels of potential local anesthetic or neurolytic blockade are shown and the areas supplied with sympathetic pain fibers are indicated. Neurolytic block of celiac plexus and lumbar ganglia is now highly effective and safe (see also Fig. 89.18). Cervicothoracic (stellate ganglion) ganglia are more suited anatomically to local anesthesia blockade or surgical removal since somatic nerves are not shielded by an intervening muscle layer in neck and thorax. (Reproduced from Cousins M J, Bridenbaugh P O (eds) 1980 *Neural Blockade in Clinical Anesthesia and Management of Pain.* Lippincott, Philadelphia, with permission.) (B) Gynecologic pain, internal and external genitalia. Note pain from cervix is via sympathetic fibers (see also Table 89.12).

Table 89.12 Nerve supply of pelvic structures and pain patterns

Structure	Predominant afferent modality	Afferent nerves	Resulting pain
Internal genitalia			
Cervix and uterus, medial part of fallopian tube	Sympathetic T_{10} to L_2	Sympathetic fibers via pelvic, inferior, middle and superior hypogastric plexi, to lumbar sympathetic chain, to white rami, to spinal nerves T_{10} to L_2	Low back pain (upper sacrum, below anterior superior iliac spines). Referred pain to dorsal rami of T_{10} to L_4, since the lateral branches of these rami descend 10 cm before becoming superficial.
Ovary and lateral tube	Sympathetic T_{10} to T_{11} ? Somatic	Sympathetic, with ovarian vessels to celiac plexus to T_{10} to T_{11}	Lower abdominal pain[a] (below iliac crests) in one or both iliac fossae. May extend to thigh (see Fig. 89.15)
Adjacent ligaments and roots of lumbosacral plexus	Somatic L_2 to S_4	Somatic nerve roots, L_2 to S_4	Pain in thighs and legs
Upper half of vagina	Parasympathetic S_2 to S_4	Parasympathetic fibers via sacral plexus to S_2 to S_4	Local pain in upper vagina referred pain to lower sacrum.
External genitalia			
Labia, clitoris, perineum, lower half of vagina	Somatic S_2 to S_4	Perineal nerve via pudendal nerve to spinal nerves S_2 to S_4[b] (supplies posterior 2/3 of labia majora, perineum and anus)	Localized perineal pain, and/or vulvar pain and/or sacrococcygeal pain.
		Ilioinguinal nerve (L_1) (contributes to area around clitoris and base of perineum).	Sometimes referred pain to upper thigh and lower back and abdomen.
		Posterior femoral cutaneous nerve (S_1 to S_3) (perineum and labium majus)	
		Genitofemoral nerve (L_1 to L_2)	

[a] Sometimes referred epigastric pain occurs, possibly because of proximity of superior hypogastric plexus to celiac plexus.
[b] Sensory supply to bladder and rectum, also S_2 to S_4

made in many texts is the innervation of the cervix. There is no doubt that pain relief is obtained by blockade of the sympathetic fibers travelling via lumbar ganglia to spinal cord segments T10 to L2 rather than somatic nerves S2 to S4. The anatomy of the somatic innervation of the pelvic and perineal region is summarized in Figure 89.13. Successful blockade of these areas peripherally requires precise placement of the local anesthetic. In addition to knowledge of specific pathways associated with the primary afferent transmission of pain from pelvic structures, the utilization of appropriate neural blockade requires knowledge of the different somatic referral patterns of pain from abdominal viscera. Figure 89.14 and Tables 89.12 and 89.13 depict the common referral areas from the female reproductive organs.

Somatic blockade

The innervation of the lower abdominal wall is via somatic nerve fibers travelling in the tenth, eleventh, and twelfth thoracic nerves, as well as the ilio-inguinal, iliohypogastric and genitofemoral nerves. Pain states characterized by nociceptive sensations from this region can be diagnosed, and possibly treated, by utilizing local anesthetic blockade of this region. The thoracic nerves can be blocked with a solution of 0.25% bupivacaine administered just below the border of the costal margin. This is most successfully ac-

complished when the nerve is blocked proximally to the angle of the rib, where the nerve lies in close approximation to the rib. The ilio-inguinal, genitofemoral, and iliohypogastric nerves are best blocked by the administration of local anesthetic around the anterior superior iliac crest. This technique, known as the iliac crest block, uses 30 to 40 ml of 0.25% bupivacaine administered in a fan-like distribution along the course of these nerves as they

Table 89.13 Internal genitalia: other possible pain patterns

Structure	Site of pain
Cervix, uterus, tube, ovary	Lower abdomen, slightly above iliac crest★ Lower sacrum★ (both uncommon)
Tube and ovary	Sometimes above anterior and posterior superior iliac spines
Cervix and uterus	Referred pain to anterior aspect of upper thigh
Cervical cancer spread to sacral plexus	Radicular pain in posterior thigh and leg

★ Pain of gynecologic cancer origin is usually continuous and not relieved by rest; it should be differentiated from episodic pain due to benign causes. However, continuous pain may sometimes be due to benign causes such as adhesions, neuroma formation, postoperative neuralgia, musculoskeletal abnormalities, etc.

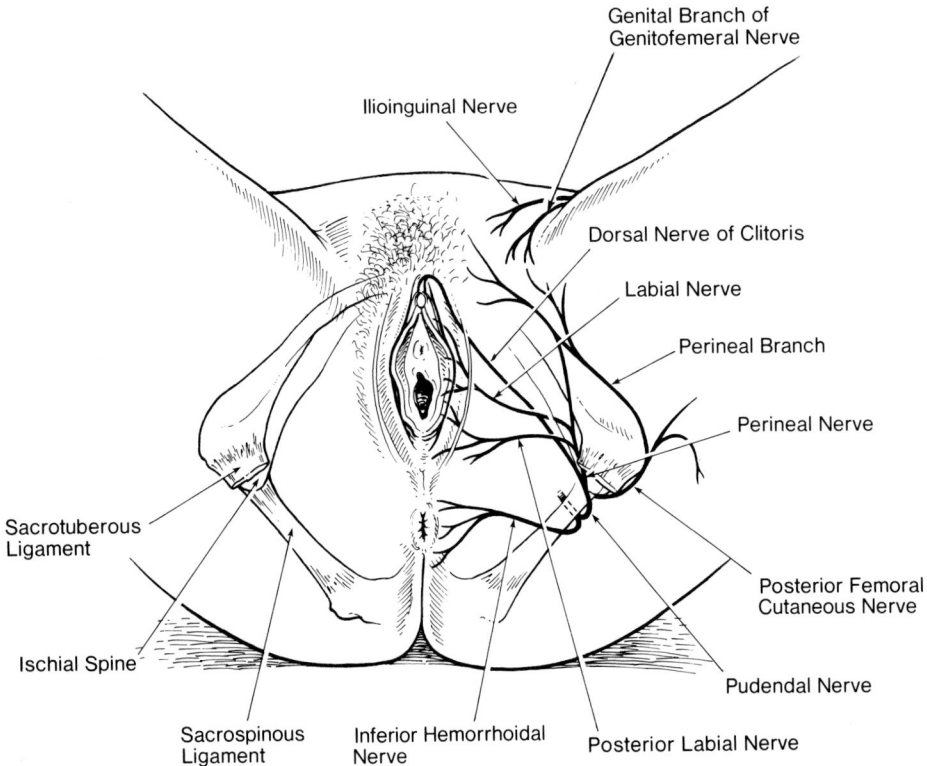

Fig. 89.13 Cutaneous innervation of the perineal region. (Redrawn from Brownridge & Cohen (1988),[17] with permission.)

pass near the iliac crest. Figure 89.15 illustrates the technique utilized to block the ilio-inguinal, iliohypogastric and genitofemoral nerves. Transvaginal or transperineal blockade of the pudendal nerve near the sacrospinous ligament will provide regional anesthesia over all but the anterior portion of the vaginal introitus. This technique is familiar to many obstetricians due to its utility in labor analgesia (Fig. 89.16).

Sympathetic blockade

The motor innervation of the major intra-abdominal organs, including the gonads, is via the sympathetic postganglionic fibers extending from the celiac plexus, and the inferior hypogastric plexus. Visceral sensory fibers travel from these organs along with the sympathetic efferents. Effective blockade of the celiac fibers can be obtained from administration of local anesthetic directly adjacent to the celiac plexus in the upper abdomen. Utilization of 30 to 40 ml of 0.25% bupivacaine for celiac plexus block will be followed by many hours of analgesia to the abdominal viscera. The lumbar sympathetic ganglia can be blocked with local anesthetic applied adjacent to the vertebral bodies of lumbar vertebrae 1,2,3 and 4 providing analgesia to the cervix.

Central neural blockade

Epidural, caudal and spinal administration of local anesthetic can be utilized to provide central blockade of the nociceptive fibers of both the body wall and the viscera if the level of blockade is carried throughout the lower thoracic, lumbar, and sacral dermatomes. The utilization of continuous techniques employing indwelling catheters either in the caudal or lumbar epidural space have found wide acceptance in the treatment of postoperative pain. Utilization of dilute solutions of bupivacaine can provide dominant sensory blockade minimizing the effect on motor function.

NEURODESTRUCTIVE PROCEDURES

The continued progress in management of cancer pain with opioids and opioid/co-analgesic combinations has decreased utilization of neurodestructive procedures. The more recent success of continuous subcutaneous infusion and spinal opioid techniques in managing severe pain has allowed patients to maintain good functional capacity without subjecting them to the risk of neurolysis. Despite the continued success of less invasive and non-destructive techniques, neurolytic blockade still provides valuable adjunctive treatment of nociceptive and neuropathic pain in

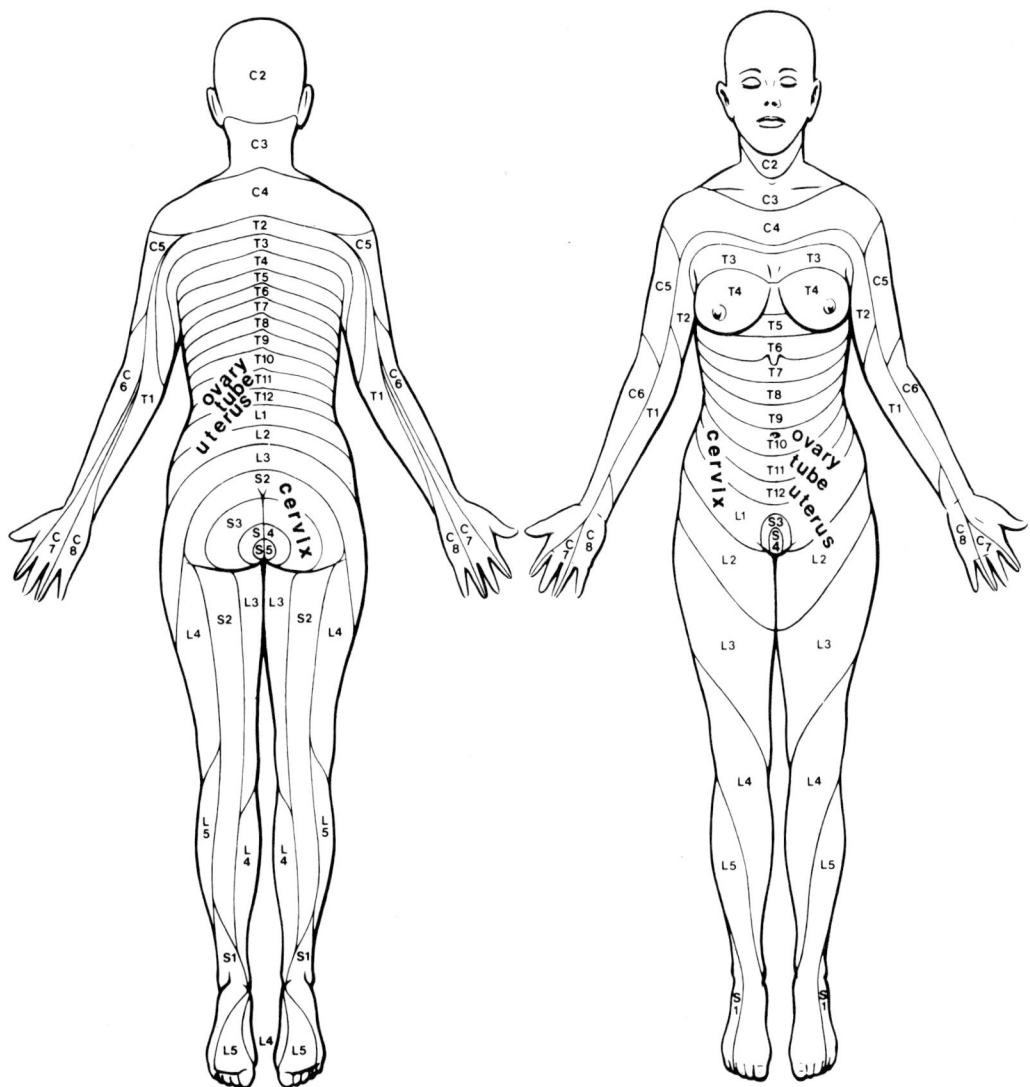

Fig. 89.14 Dermatomal chart. Also shown are surface areas where pain from pelvic viscera are commonly referred.

terminal cancer patients. Often, a properly performed neurodestructive procedure can markedly decrease medication use and avoid the unwanted side effects associated with high doses of analgesics. Virtually all neurodestructive techniques should be confined to the treatment of nociceptive pain. The central and peripheral changes seen associated with neuropathic pain are often not relieved by neurodestructive techniques, and may be aggravated by such procedures. Neurolytic blocks are mainly indicated for localized unilateral pain, except for pituitary adenolysis, which is suitable for diffuse areas of pain.

Neurolytic agents

Although not strictly a neurolytic agent, cold has been increasingly employed for somatic nerve block using a cryoprobe.[47] Cryoanalgesia refers to the destruction of peripheral nerves by extreme cold to achieve analgesia.

This technique was developed to provide destructive blockade of peripheral nerves that had responded favorably to somatic blockade. The alternative destructive techniques, which include cutting, crushing and burning, are each associated with development of neuralgia. There is complete functional loss after a cryolesion, but recovery is usually seen over a period of weeks. The lesion created by freezing of a nerve is classified as a second degree nerve injury under Sunderland's classification.[73] This is demonstrated by Wallerian degeneration with axonal disintegration, but minimal disruption of the endoneurium. The clinical limitation of cryoanalgesia is that the duration of analgesia is determined by the time for normal peripheral nerve regeneration. Figure 89.17 illustrates the equipment employed for cryoanalgesia. Successful utilization of cryoanalgesia requires precise localization of the needle tip to the peripheral nerve. This localization is facilitated by the incorporation of a peripheral nerve

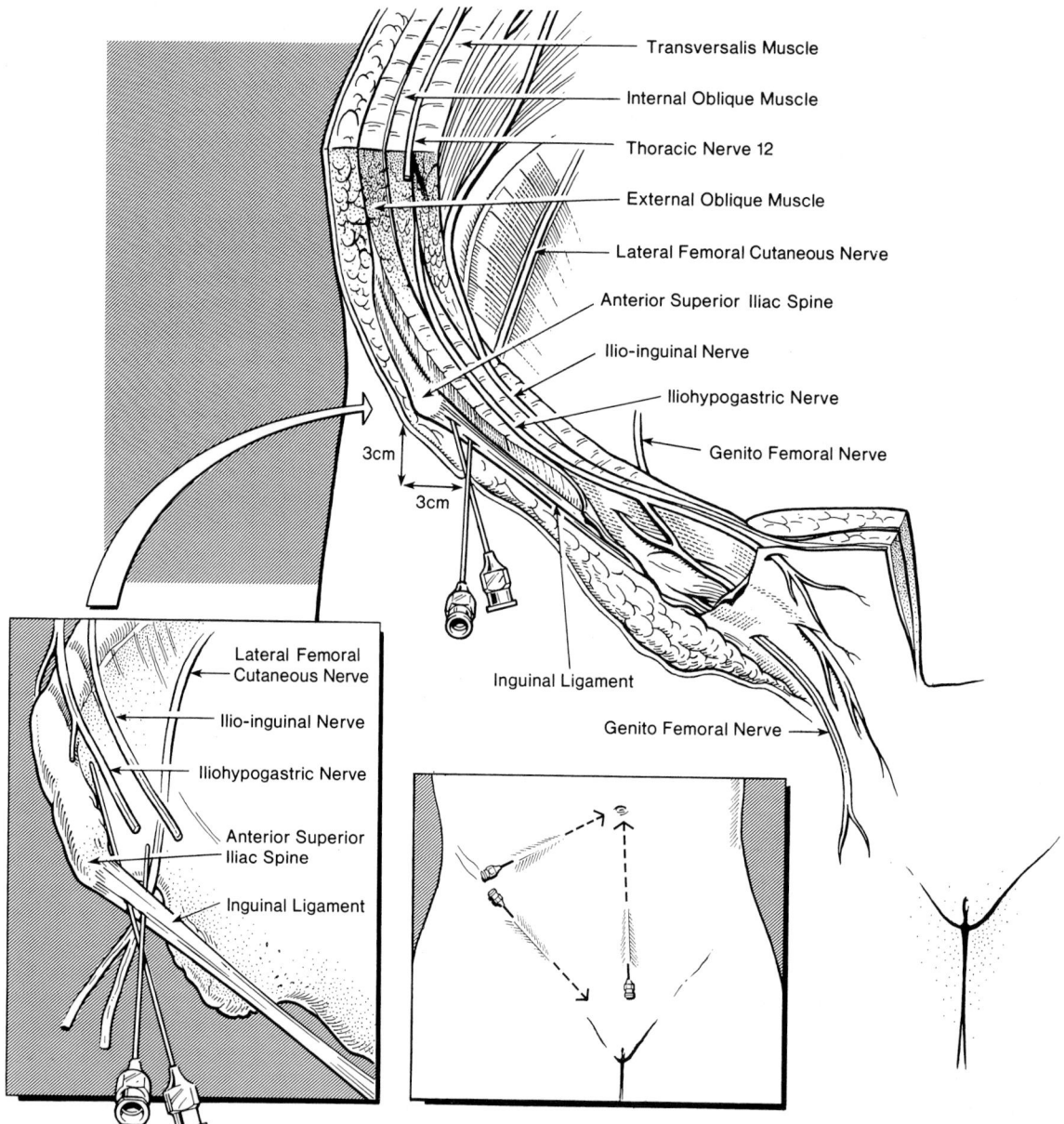

Fig. 89.15 Cutaneous innervation of the lower abdomen. Iliac crest block pictured allows the simultaneous blockade of the ilioinguinal, iliohypogastric, and lateral femoral cutaneous nerves. **Upper panel**. Note the point of needle insertion 3 cm caudad and 3 cm medial to the anterior superior iliac spine (ASIS). Initial direction of the needle is superolateral to reach the inner aspect of the iliac bone, then the needle is redirected approximately perpendicular to the long axis of the body. Note the relation of the nerves to the muscles of the anterior abdominal wall. An alternative approach is to insert the needle along a line from the ASIS to the umbilicus. **Lower panel**. (Left) Bone and ligamentous landmarks in relation to the nerves. (Right) Superficial infiltration for right lower quadrant anesthesia. (Redrawn from Thompson G E, Moore D C 1988 Celiac plexus, intercostal, and minor peripheral blockade. In: Cousins M J, Bridenbaugh P O (eds) *Neural Blockade in Clinical Anesthesia and Management of Pain*, 2nd edn. Lippincott, Philadelphia, with permission.)

stimulator in the tip of the cryoneedle. The ice ball which forms around the tip of the needle must incorporate the nerve to achieve complete neurolysis.

The neuropathology of neurolytic agents is now better documented.[54] Table 89.14 summarizes various neurolytic techniques currently available. Absolute alcohol is hypobaric and is used mainly for thoracic chemical posterior rhizotomy (Fig. 89.18A) as well as celiac plexus

block (Fig. 89.18C). Phenol is used as a 6% solution in water or glycerine; the latter is hyperbaric and is very useful when administered for hyperbaric subarachnoid saddle block to treat midline perineal pain (Fig. 89.18B). Cold saline injected in the subarachnoid space is claimed to have selective action on C-fibers, but the relief obtained is short lived and the procedure very painful. Ammonium salts were utilized very early to provide neurolysis. Initial claims

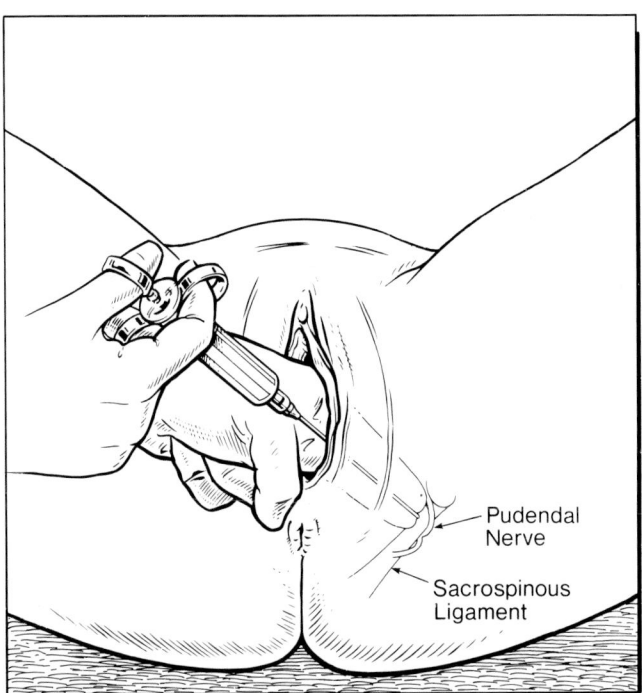

Fig. 89.16 Pudendal nerve block by the transvaginal approach. (Reproduced from Brownridge & Cohen (1988),[17] with permission.)

were of selective antinociceptive effect. The clinical studies which have tried to document this selective effect have failed to support this early claim.[14,38,50]

Specific techniques

Subarachnoid neurolytic block can be performed either with absolute alcohol as a hypobaric technique or with phenol in glycerine as a hyperbaric solution. Meticulous attention is paid to positioning of the patient to localize the spread of neurolytic solution. It is most commonly employed for thoracic posterior rhizotomy, but also is of great use in unilateral limb or pelvic pain due to malignancy. Unfortunately, there is a significant risk of bladder incontinence, although careful 'lateralizing' techniques can still avoid this complication in a majority of patients. Good results are obtained in approximately 50% of patients with terminal malignancy treated with this technique.[51]

Trans-sacral neurolytic block can be utilized for perineal pain associated with vulvar malignancy. Perineal sensation is primarily from S4 and this can be blocked fairly selectively through the fourth sacral foramen with low volume of 6% phenol. If after 24 hours the block appears inadequate, it can be repeated with extension to the third sacral root via the corresponding sacral foramen. This technique avoids the complication of urinary or fecal incontinence.[21]

Neurolytic lumbar sympathectomy is a well established technique with low incidence of morbidity and mortality

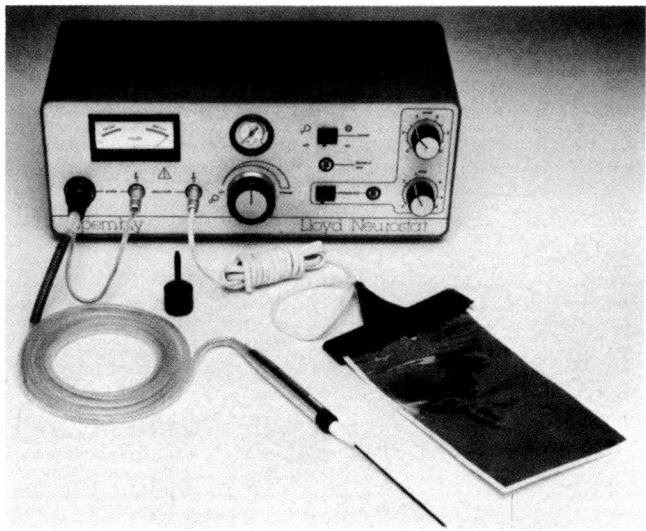

(A)

Fig. 89.17 (A) Cryoanalgesia apparatus for somatic nerve blockade. (B) Cryoprobe tip. The needle is 15 gauge. Nitrous oxide at about 700 p.s.i. is ejected through into the needle and cools to −75°C as it expands. Excess gas is exhausted via a separate channel back up the needle. The needle also has a thermocouple to confirm the temperature achieved at the tip and an electrical connection to permit stimulation to confirm needle placement next to the nerve. (Reproduced from Lloyd J W, Barnard J D W, Glynn C J (1976),[47] with permission.)

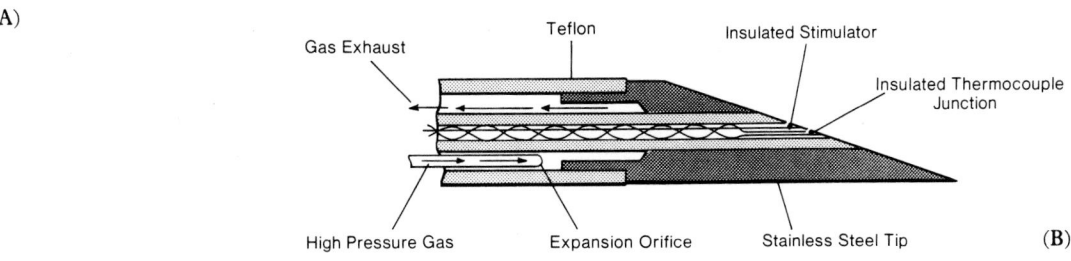

(B)

Table 89.14 Neurolytic agents, techniques, results and comparisons

Agent	Technique	Results	Complications
Cold	Cryoprobe block for somatic nerves	Pain relief for 10 days to several months	Skin slough (prevented by use of infrared)
	Intrathecal hypertonic cold saline	Very variable results	Nil (care with blood pressure response)
10% ammonium sulfate	Somatic nerve block Caudal nerve block	No controlled study Effects probably due to hypotonicity	Neuralgia if incomplete block
Hypertonic and hypotonic solutions (distilled water, hypertonic saline)	Subarachnoid block	Pain relief for 2 days to 2 to 3 weeks	Hypertension during injection of hypertonic solution
Alcohol 100%, 6% phenol in water	Celiac plexus block	70% of patients with upper abdominal cancer (or metastases), pain relief 3 to 6 months	Segmental sensory loss (T_{10} to L_2) (8%) Postural hypotension (2%) Urinary retention (1%) Lower chest pain (3% transient)
Alcohol 100% Phenol 6% in glycerine, 5 to 8% in iophendylate	Subarachnoid (hypobaric[a]) Subarachnoid (hyperbaric[b])	50 to 60% of patients with upper abdominal or pelvic pain, pain relief 3 to 4 months	Sensory loss (3 to 10%), paresthesia (0.3 to 3%); bladder paresis (1 to 10%) depending on extent of block. Rectal dysfunction (1%)
10% phenol in Conray 420	Lumbar sympathetic block	80% of patients with pain mediated by lumbar ganglia, pain relief approximately 6 months	L_1 neuralgia (3 to 7.5%) — transitory Sensory loss and limited motor deficit (5%)

[a] Hypobaric = solution with specific gravity less than CSF, thus affected side placed uppermost.
[b] Hyperbaric = solution with specific gravity greater than CSF, thus affected area placed below point of needle entry.

when performed under image intensifier guidance. Ten percent phenol with Conray allows visualization of the spread of the neurolytic solution (Fig. 89.19). This has been used extensively for occlusive peripheral vascular disease, but often finds applicability in patients with malignancy of the rectum and sigmoid colon. Some patients with cervical cancer also obtain relief from this block until the malignancy spreads to involve the lumbosacral plexus.

Nociceptive stimuli for the majority of the uterus as well as the ovaries and fallopian tubes is carried predominantly in the visceral afferents that traverse the celiac plexus. In order to obtain good relief, most authorities would suggest bilateral blockade of the celiac plexus. Figure 89.18C illustrates the desired needle placement in a prone bilateral celiac block. Multiple different techniques have been presented in which 50 to 75% alcohol with contrast medium have been used. Injection performed under image intensifier guidance allows confirmation of adequate spread and correct localization of the neurolytic solution. While specific studies of efficacy in gynecologic malignancy have not been performed, one could expect a similar response to that seen with other abdominal malignancy, 70% of patients reporting good effect.[12] Such techniques will not relieve pain if the parietal peritoneum is involved; however, they deserve more consideration prior to embarking on subarachnoid blocks, with attendant risks of incontinence,

or percutaneous cordotomy with risks of respiratory and other neurologic complications.

Chemical hypophysectomy was introduced in 1963 by Morrica as a technique to manage widespread pain.[57] This technique involves the percutaneous placement of a destructive agent into the sella turcica via the nasal passage and sphenoid sinus. The lytic agent is administered through a specialized needle that is positioned with X-ray guidance. The analgesic mode of action of pituitary ablation has not been established. In a series of 82 cancer patients presented by Levin,[45] 84% of these patients treated with chemical hypophyesectomy reported good pain relief. The reader is referred to the discussion by Cousins[21] for a critical review of the procedure.

Neurosurgical techniques

Percutaneous cordotomy is an effective treatment modality for nociceptive pain below the level of C4. This technique is minimally invasive and has relatively low morbidity and mortality. The procedure employs a radiofrequency lesion performed under neurolept anesthesia which allows the patient to confirm localization of the spinothalamic tract. The high cervical (C1 to 2) approach offers high somatic levels of analgesia and precision in manipulating the electrode within the cord.[77] Figure 89.20 depicts a schematic of percutaneous cordotomy. Successful cordo-

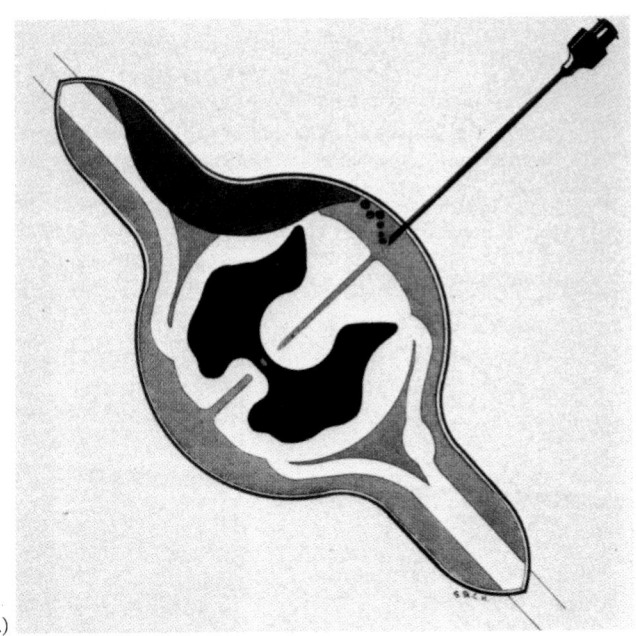

(A)

Fig. 89.18 (A) Neurolytic posterior rhizotomy with hypobaric subarachnoid alcohol. Positioning in the semi-prone position with affected side uppermost permits blockade of only posterior roots, leaving anterior roots (motor function) and spinal cord long tracts intact. (B) Neurolytic subarachnoid block with hyperbaric phenol in glycerine. The heavy solution falls to the sacral nerve roots if the patient is kept sitting. More selective block can be achieved by supporting the patient tilted towards the more affected side and also sitting at about 60° to the horizontal. (C) Celiac plexus block. (Reproduced from Dwyer B D, Gibb D 1980 Chronic pain and neurolytic neural blockade. In: Cousins M J, Bridenbaugh P O (eds) *Neural Blockade in Clinical Anesthesia and Management of Pain.* Lippincott, Philadelphia, with permission.)

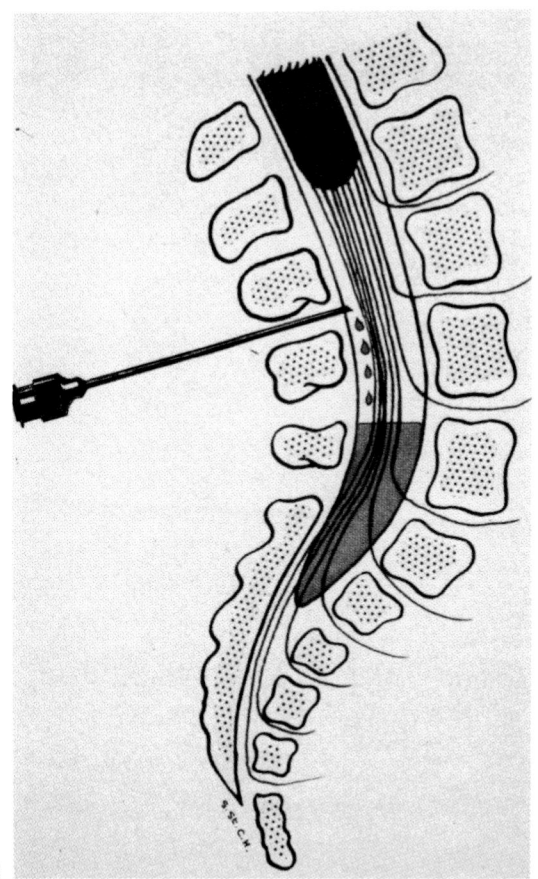

(B)

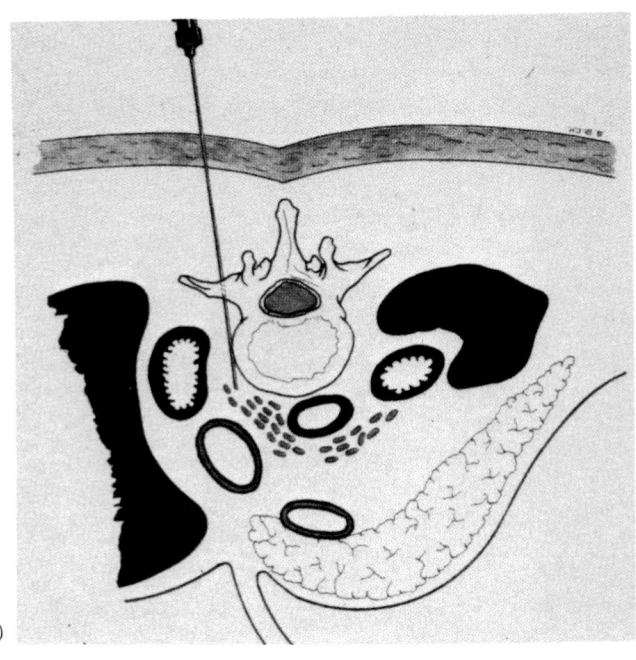

(C)

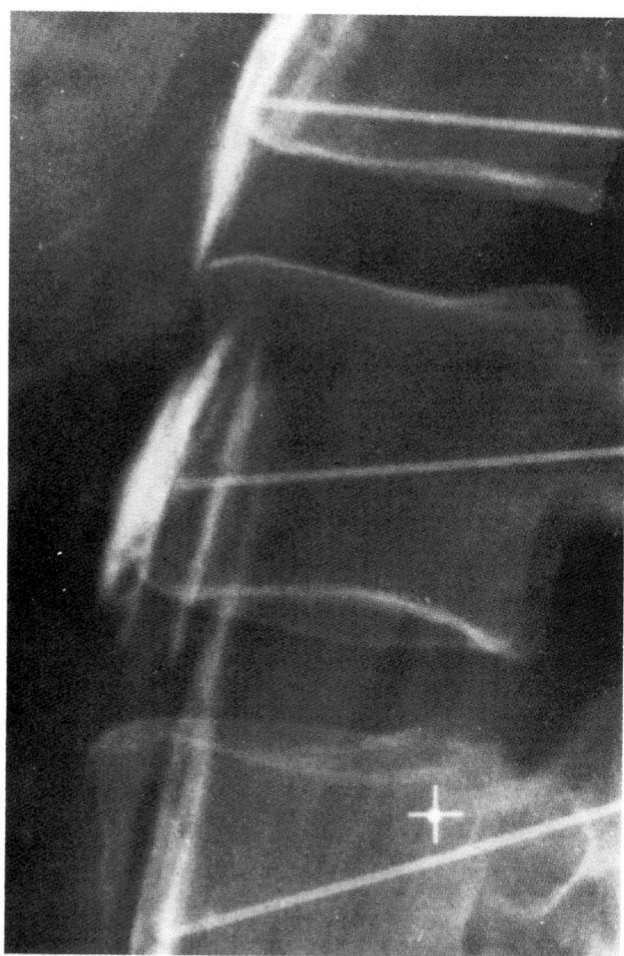

Fig. 89.19 Lumbar sympathetic neurolytic block. Needles are placed at L_2, L_3, L_4 and 10% phenol in Conray 420 injected under image intensifier. As little as 1 ml at each level may result in effective coverage of sympathetic chain. (Reproduced from Cousins M J et al 1979 Neurolytic lumbar sympathetic blockade: duration of denervation and relief of rest pain. *Anaesth Intens Care* 7: 121, with permission.)

tomy will disrupt the anterolateral funiculus and interfere with the rostral processing of the crossed nociceptive projection neurons. This technique is best used to treat refractory unilateral pain that may be very widespread. Bilateral cordotomy can also be performed, but the risk of respiratory and autonomic dysfunction is significantly higher. A review of the literature in cancer pain patients indicates that it provides effective pain relief in 75% of patients during the first 6 months, dropping to 40% effectiveness at one year.[70]

Extralemniscal myelotomy is a percutaneous procedure aimed at the ascending pain fibers travelling near the central canal. This technique involves radiofrequency ablation of the center of the spinal cord at the level of the cervico-medullary junction. The indications for this procedure appear to be midline or bilateral trunk pain.[77] The number of cases reported in the literature is fairly small, but extralemniscal myelotomy has been successful in obtaining good, transient pain relief in approximately 75 to 80% of patients treated.[70] Further evaluation of this technique needs to be performed before the appropriate role in cancer pain management can be established.

Commissural myelotomy is an open procedure which has been reported to be effective in patients with advanced malignancy. The technique involves disrupting the nociceptive and thermoreceptive fibers which decussate from both sides of the body in the anterior white commissure, over the spinal cord area corresponding to the pain. Opening of the dorsal fissure and disruption of the commissures with a blunt object, CO_2-laser or ultrasound has been reported. This has been performed most often at the thoraco-lumbar level for pain in the abdomen and pelvis. The pain relief provided has been transient but effective for well localized pain, even if bilateral or midline.[70]

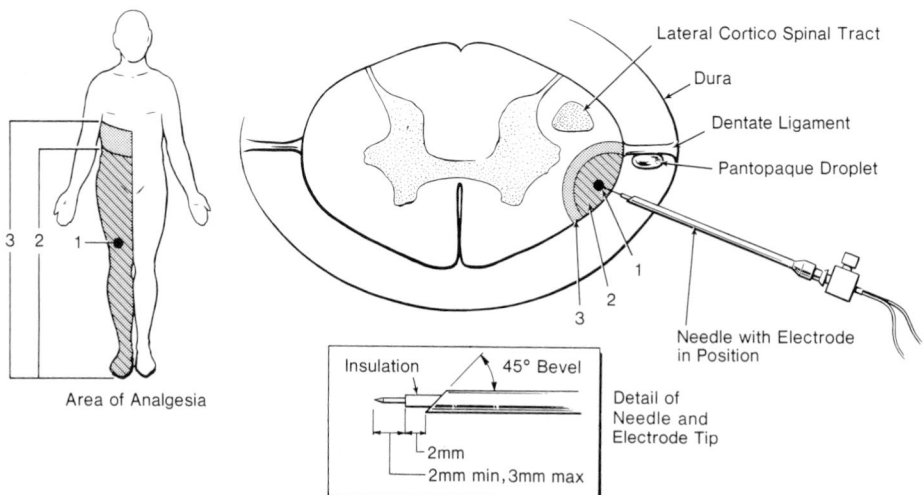

Fig. 89.20 Percutaneous anterolateral cordotomy. The needle with inner electrode is placed through the dura at the C_1-C_2 level. Its position anterior to the dentate ligament is confirmed by injecting a small amount of radiopaque medium (e.g. Pantopaque). The electrode is then advanced into the spinal cord aided by impedance monitoring. The lesion is gradually extended as shown (1–3), until it covers the patient's area of pain.

Dorsal root entry zone lesion (DREZ) is the newest of the neuroablative procedures suggested for pain management. The procedure is an open approach to the dorso-lateral region of the spinal cord at the level corresponding to the entry of the primary afferent neurons. DREZ sections the central portion of the dorsal roots, Lissauer's tract and laminae 1 to 5 of the dorsal horn. This disrupts rostral processing of noxious information by destroying primary afferents as well as projecting neurons. DREZ is promoted as a therapy for the management of focal neuropathic as well as nociceptive pain. A small number of surgeons have reported success in using this therapy to tract brachial plexus avulsion, which is one of the most refractory pain problems yet identified. The use of DREZ has been understandably small because of the novelty of the technique. While the appropriate utilization of this technique in cancer pain management has yet to be determined, initial results suggest that it will be an effective modality to treat topographically limited carcinomas.[70]

The introductory paragraph to this section on neurosurgical treatment of pain mentioned that the above techniques were best employed in managing nociceptive pain. The management of neuropathic pain remains very difficult. While nociceptive pain is the most common type presenting in patients with malignancy, neuropathic pain is also frequently described. The use of electrical stimulation has been focused on the treatment of neuropathic pain. The techniques of TENS and DCS were presented earlier in this chapter. These techniques have been applied to different types of neuropathic pain but the results are not very favorable.[77] The appropriate use of neurostimulation in management of neuropathic components of malignant pain has yet to be addressed.

physical intervention to ablate these noxious impulses has direct application to control of gynecologic cancer pain. The options now available are dramatically wider than those presented in the first edition of this book. The physical methods outlined in this chapter must be used in concert, with attention being focused on the psychologic aspects of each patient's pain to provide optimal patient care.

The concept of 'total pain' is important in treating cancer pain; thus, attention should be focused not only on the somatic source of pain, but also psychologic and environmental factors affecting the patient and family. This type of care can be best organized in a multidisciplinary pain clinic. The integration of medical, nursing, psychological and palliative care, physical therapy, social work and the attention of other health professionals will provide a well balanced treatment plan.

The initiation of medical therapy with simple analgesics according to the analgesic ladder can be escalated as required by changing components of the patients pain. The addition of co-analgesics to the therapy of cancer patients will result in adequate analgesia by the oral route in the vast majority of cases. Patients who suffer severe ongoing pain will require more invasive treatment than the analgesic ladder provides. These patients will often benefit from subcutaneous opioid administration or the use of spinal opioids. The placement of a percutaneous epidural portal system or an intrathecal totally implanted pump system will allow the utilization of both opioids and local anesthetics either by continuous infusion or intermittent boluses to control refractory pain. The appropriate utilization of neurodestructive procedures in concert with these other treatment options can provide analgesia in virtually all patients suffering with cancer pain.

CONCLUSIONS

A major increase in the knowledge of neurologic mechanisms of pain and research into pharmacologic and

REFERENCES

1. Atkinson J H, Kremer E F, Garfin S R 1985 Current concepts review: Psychopharmacologic agents in the treatment of pain. J Bone Joint Surg (Am) 67: 337
2. Atweh S F, Kuhar M J 1977 Autoradiographic localization of opiate receptors in rat brain. I. Spinal cord and lower medulla. Brain Res 124: 53
3. Austin K L, Stapleton J V, Mather L E 1980 Multiple intramuscular injections: a major source of variability in analgesic response to pethidine. Pain 8: 4
4. Baines M J 1981 The principles of symptom control. In: Saunders C M, Summers D H, Teller N (eds) Hospice: The Living Idea. Edward Arnold, London, p 93
5. Basbaum A I 1985 Functional analysis of the cytochemistry of the spinal dorsal horn. In: Fields H L, Dubner R, Cervero F (eds) Advances in Pain Research and Therapy, Vol 9. Raven Press, New York, p 149
6. Basbaum A I, Fields H L 1978 Endogenous pain control mechanisms: review and hypothesis. Ann Neurol 4: 451
7. Beaver W T, Feise G 1976 Comparison of the analgesic effects of morphine, hydroxyzine, and their combination in patients with postoperative pain. In: Bonica J J, Albe-Fessard D G (eds) Advances in Pain Research and Therapy, Vol 1. Raven Press, New York, p 553
8. Beaver W T, Wallenstein S L, Houde R W, Rodgers A 1966 A comparison of the analgesic effects of methotrimeprazine and morphine in patients with cancer. Clin Pharmacol Ther 7: 436
9. Beecher H K 1946 Pain in men wounded in battle. Ann Surg 123: 96
10. Beeson J M, Chaouch A 1987 Peripheral and spinal mechanisms of nociception. Physiol Rev 67(1): 67
11. Berkley K J, Palmer R 1974 Somatosensory cortical involvement in response to noxious stimulation in the cat. Exp Brain Res 20: 363
12. Black A, Dwyer B 1973 Coeliac plexus block. Anaesth Intensive Care 1: 315
13. Boas R A, Cousins M J 1988 Diagnostic neural blockade. In: Cousins M J, Bridenbaugh P O (eds) Neural Blockade in Clinical

Anesthesia and Management of Pain, 2nd edn. Lippincott, Philadelphia, Pa, p 885

14. Bonica J J 1953 The Management of Pain. Lea and Febiger, Philadelphia

15. Bonica J J, Venatifrida V 1979 Advances in pain research and therapy: International Symposium on Pain of Advanced Cancer. Raven Press, New York

16. Brose W G, Cohen S E 1989 Arterial oxygen saturation following cesarean section in patients receiving epidural morphine, PCA or IM meperidine analgesia. Anesthesiology 70: 948

17. Brownridge P, Cohen S E 1988 Neural blockade for obstetrics and gynecologic surgery. In: Cousins M J, Bridenbaugh P O (eds) Neural Blockade in Clinical Anesthesia and Management of Pain, 2nd edn. Lippincott, Philadelphia, Pa, p 593

18. Bruera E, Brenneis C, Michaud M, Bocovsky R, Chadwick S, Emeno A, MacDonald N 1988 Use of subcutaneous route for the administration of narcotics in patients with cancer pain. Cancer 62: 407

19. Bruera E, Brenneis C, Michaud M, MacMillan K, Hanson J, MacDonald N 1988 Patient controlled subcutaneous hydromorphone versus continuous subcutaneous infusion for the treatment of cancer pain. J Natl Cancer Inst 80: 1152

20. Calvillo O, Henry J L, Newman R S 1974 Effects of morphine and naloxone on dorsal horn neurones in the cat. Can J Physiol Pharmacol 52: 1207

21. Cousins M J 1988 Chronic pain and neurolytic neural blockade. In: Cousins M J, Bridenbaugh P O (eds) Neural Blockade in Clinical Anesthesia and Management of Pain, 2nd edn. Lippincott, Philadelphia, Pa, p 1053

22. Cousins M J, Cherry D A, Gourlay G K 1988 Acute and chronic pain: use of spinal opioids. In: Cousins M J, Bridenbaugh P O (eds) Neural Blockade in Clinical Anesthesia and Management of Pain, 2nd edn. Lippincott, Philadelphia, Pa, p 955

23. Covino B G 1988 Clinical pharmacology of local anesthetic agents. In: Cousins M J, Bridenbaugh P O (eds) Neural Blockade in Clinical Anesthesia and Management of Pain, 2nd edn. Lippincott, Philadelphia, Pa, p 111

24. Crile G W 1910 Phylogenetic association in relation to certain medical problems. Boston Medical and Surgical Journal 163: 893

25. Cushing H 1902 On the avoidance of shock in major amputations by cocainization of large nerve-trunks preliminary to their division. Ann Surg 36: 321

26. Daut R L, Cleeland C S 1982 The prevalence and severity of pain in cancer. Cancer 50: 1913

27. Dubner R 1985 Specialization of nociceptive pathways: sensory discrimination, sensory modulation, and neural connectivity. In: Fields H L, Dubner R, Cervero F (eds) Advances in Pain Research and Therapy, Vol 9. Raven Press, New York, p 111

28. Dundee J W, Love W J, Moore J 1963 Alterations in response to somatic pain associated with anesthesia. XV: Further studies with phenothiazine derivatives and similar drugs. Br J Anaesth 35: 597

29. Duggan A W, Hall J G, Headley P 1977 Suppression of transmission of nociceptive impulses by morphine: selective effects of morphine administered in the region of the substantia gelatinosa. Br J Pharmacol 61: 65

30. Durant P A, Yaksh T L 1986 Epidural injections of bupivacaine, morphine, fentanyl, lofentanil, and DADL in chronically implanted rats: a pharmacologic and pathologic study. Anesthesiology 64: 43

31. Fields H L 1987 Pain. McGraw-Hill, New York, p 13

32. Fields H L, Basbaum A I 1984 Endogenous pain control mechanisms. In: Wall P D, Melzack R (eds) Textbook of Pain. Churchill-Livingstone, Edinburgh, p 142

33. Foley K M 1979 The management of pain of malignant origin. In: Tyler H R, Dawson D M (eds) Current Neurology, Vol 2. Houghton Mifflin, Boston, p 279

34. Forrest W H, Brown B W, Brown C R et al 1977 Dextroamphetamine with morphine for the treatment of postoperative pain. N Engl J Med 296: 712

35. Gourlay G K, Cherry D A, Cousins M J 1985 Cephalad migration of morphine in CSF following lumbar epidural administration in patients with cancer pain. Pain 23: 317

36. Gourlay G K, Cherry D A, Plummer J L, Armstrong P J, Cousins M J 1987 The influence of drug polarity on the absorption of opioid drugs into the CSF and subsequent cephalad migration following lumbar epidural administration: application to morphine and pethidine. Pain 31: 297

37. Hagbarth K E, Kerr D I B 1954 Central influences on spinal afferent conduction. J Neurophysiol 17: 295

38. Hand L V 1944 Subarachnoid ammonium sulfate therapy for intractable pain. Anesthesiology 5: 354

39. Hollister L E, Conley F K, Britt R H, Shuer L 1981 Long term use of diazepam. JAMA 246: 1568

40. International Association for the Study of Pain, Subcommittee on Taxonomy 1979 Pain terms: a list with definitions and notes on usage. Pain 6: 249

41. International Association for the Study of Pain. Subcommittee on Taxonomy 1986 Classification of chronic pain; description of pain terms. In: Merskey H (ed) Pain suppl 3: S1

42. Juan H 1978 Prostaglandins as modulators of pain. Gen Pharmacol 9: 403

43. Kehlet H 1988 Modification of responses to surgery by neural blockade: clinical implications. In: Cousins M J, Bridenbaugh P O (eds) Neural Blockade in Clinical Anesthesia and Management of Pain, 2nd edn. Lippincott, Philadelphia, Pa, p 145

44. Langley G B, Sheppard M, Johnson M, Wigley R D 1984 The analgesic effect of transcutaneous electrical nerve stimulation and placebo in chronic pain patients. Rheumatol Int 4: 119

45. Levin A B, Ramirez L L 1984 Treatment of cancer pain with hypophysectomy: surgical and chemical. In: Benedetti C, Chapman C R, Moricca G (eds) Advances in Pain Research and Therapy, Vol 7. Raven Press, New York, p 631

46. Levine J D, Coderre T J, Basbaum A I 1988 The peripheral nervous system and the inflammatory process. In: Dubner R, Gebhart G F, Bond M R (eds) Proceedings of the Vth World Congress on Pain. Elsevier Science Publishers, Amsterdam, p 33

47. Lloyd J W, Barnard J D W, Glynn C J 1976 Cryoanalgesia: a new approach to pain relief. Lancet ii: 932

48. Lloyd J W, Glynn C J, Adams C B T, Durant K R 1978 The pain of cancer. Practitioner 220: 453

49. Loeser J D, Black A A, Christman A 1975 Relief of pain by transcutaneous stimulation. J Neurosurg 29: 48

50. Lund P C 1971 Principles and Practice of Spinal Anesthesia Thomas, Springfield, Ill

51. Mark V H, White J C, Zervas N T, Ervin F R, Richardson E P 1962 Intrathecal use of phenol for the relief of chronic severe pain. N Engl J Med 267: 589

52. Mather L E, Gourlay G K 1984 The biotransformation of opioids. In: Nimmo W S, Smith G (eds) Opioid Agonist/Antagonist Drugs in Clinical Practice. Excerpta Medica, Amsterdam.

53. Melzack R, Wall P D 1965 Pain mechanisms: a new theory. Science 150: 971

54. Meyers R R, Katz J 1988 Neuropathy of neurolytic and semidestructive agents. In: Cousins M J, Bridenbaugh P O (eds) Neural Blockade in Clinical Anesthesia and Management of Pain, 2nd edn. Lippincott, Philadelphia, Pa, p 1031

55. Moore J, Dundee J W 1961 Alterations in response to somatic pain associated with anaesthesia. V: the effect of promethazine. Br J Anaes 33: 3

56. Moore J, Dundee J W 1961 Alterations in response to somatic pain associated with anaesthesia. VII: the effects of nine phenothiazine derivatives. Br J Anaes 33: 422

57. Morrica G 1974 Chemical hypophysectomy for cancer pain. In: Bonica J J (ed) Advances in Neurology, Vol 4, Pain. Raven Press, New York

58. Müller J 1844 Von den Ergentumlichkeiten der ein zelnen Nerve. In: Kobling L (ed) Handbuch der Physiologie des Menschen. Holscher, Coblenz

59. Nathan P W, Wall P D 1974 Treatment of postherpetic neuralgia by prolonged electrical stimulation. Br Med J 14: 645

60. Pert C B, Snyder S H 1973 Opiate receptors: demonstration in nervous tissue. Science 179: 1011

61. Pike P M 1978 Transcutaneous electrical stimulation: its use in management of post-operative pain. Anaesthesia 33: 165

62. Portenoy R K, Moulin D E, Rodgers A, Inturrisi C E, Foley

K M 1986 IV infusion of opioids for cancer pain: clinical review and guidelines for use. Cancer Treat Rev 70: 575

63. Raja S N, Meyer R A, Campbell J N 1988 Peripheral mechanisms of somatic pain. Anesthesiology 68: 571

64. Rawal N, Arner S, Gustaffson L L, Allvin R 1987 Present state of extradural and intrathecal opioid analgesia in Sweden. A nationwide follow-up survey. Br J Anaesth 59: 791

65. Rawal N, Schött U, Dahlström B et al 1986 Influence of naloxone infusion on analgesia and respiratory depression following epidural morphine. Anesthesiology 64: 194

66. Reiz S, Balfors E, Sorensen M B et al 1982 Coronary hemodynamic effects of general anesthesia and surgery: modification by epidural analgesia in patients with ischemic heart disease. Regional Anesthesia 7: S8

67. Reynolds D V 1969 Surgery in the rat during electrical analgesia induced by focal brain stimulation. Science 164: 444

68. Saunders C M 1967 The Management of Terminal Illness. Hospital Medicine Publications, London

69. Sindou M 1978 L'électro-analgésies transcutanée dans les syndromes de déafférentation périphérique. Ann Anesthesiol Fr 19: 409

70. Sindou M, Daher A 1988 Spinal cord ablation procedures for pain. In: Dubner R, Gebhart G F, Bond M R (eds) Proceedings of the Vth World Congress on Pain. Elsevier Science, Amsterdam, p 477

71. Sindou M, Keravel Y 1980 Analgésie par al méthodee d'électrostimulation transcutanée. Neurochirurgie 26: 153

72. Solomon R A, Viernstein M C, Long D M 1980 Reductions of postoperative pain and narcotic use by transcutaneous electrical nerve stimulation. Surgery 87: 142

73. Sunderland S 1978 Nerves and Nerve Injuries 2nd edn. Churchill-Livingstone, Edinburgh

74. Symposium on Pain 1973 Postgrad Med J 53: 56

75. Takeda F 1986 Preliminary report from Japan on the results of field testing of WHO draft interim guidelines for relief of cancer pain. The Pain Clinic Journal 1: 83

76. Tanelian D L, Cousins M J 1989 Combined neurogenic and nociceptive pain in a patient with Pancoast tumor managed by epidural hydromorphone and oral carbamazepine. Pain 36: 85

77. Tasker R R 1988 Neurostimulation and percutaneous neural destructive techniques. In: Cousins M J, Bridenbaugh P O (eds) Neural Blockade in Clinical Anesthesia and Management of Pain, 2nd edn. Lippincott, Philadelphia, Pa, p 1085

78. Twycross R G, Lack S A 1984 Therapeutics in Terminal Cancer. Pitman, London

79. Waldeman C, Eason J, Rambohui E et al 1984 Serum morphine levels: a comparison between continuous subcutaneous and intravenous infusions in post-operative patients. Cancer Treat Rev 71: 953

80. Weinberg D S, Inturrisi C E, Reidenberg B et al 1988 Sublingual absorption of selected opioid analgesics. Clin Pharmacol Ther 44: 335

81. Wilker A 1950 Sites and mechanisms of action of morphine and related drugs in the central nervous system. Pharmacol Rev 2: 385

82. Willis W D 1985 Thalamocortical mechanisms of pain. In: Fields H L, Dubner R, Cervero F (eds) Advances in Pain Research and Therapy Vol 9. Raven Press, New York

83. World Health Organization 1986 Cancer Pain Relief. Australian Government Publishing Service, Canberra

84. Yaksh T L 1978 Inhibition by etorpine of the discharge of dorsal horn neurons: effects on the neuronal response to both high and low threshold sensory input in the decerebrate spinal cat. Exp Neurol 60: 23

85. Yaksh T L 1981 Spinal opiate analgesia: characteristics and principles of action. Pain 11: 293

86. Yaksh T L 1986 The central pharmacology of primary afferents with emphasis on the disposition and role of primary afferent substance P. In: Yaksh T L (ed) Spinal Afferent Processing. Plenum Press, New York

87. Yaksh T L 1988 Neurologic mechanisms of pain. In: Cousins M J, Bridenbaugh P O (eds) Neural Blockade in Clinical Anesthesia and Management of Pain, 2nd edn. Lippincott, Philadelphia, Pa, p 79

88. Yaksh T L, Noueihed R 1985 The physiology and pharmacology of spinal opiates. Annu Rev Pharmacol Toxicol 25: 443

89. Yaksh T L, Rudy T A 1976 Narcotic analgesia produced by a direct action on the spinal cord. Science 192: 1357

90. Yeager M P, Glass D D, Neff R K, Brink-Johnsen T 1987 Epidural anesthesia and analgesia in high risk surgical patients. Anesthesiology 66: 729

91. Zoltie N, Cust M P 1986 Analgesia in the acute abdomen. Ann Roy Coll Surg Engl 68: 209

90. Sexual morbidity following gynecologic cancer

B. L. Andersen   J. van der Does   B. Anderson

INTRODUCTION

Sexuality and sexual functioning are the most probable areas of life disruption for the sexually active woman treated for gynecologic cancer. Coital difficulties may begin with the signs/symptoms of the disease and continue, although with a different clinical picture, when intercourse is resumed following treatment.[5,6] Attention to sexual morbidity is not unique to gynecologic cancer patients, as both the American Cancer Society,[2] and the National Institutes of Health[51] have examined research and clinical issues in the study and prevention/treatment of sexual functioning morbidity for all cancer patients.

The earliest concern for the sexual problems of cancer patients was raised for breast[15] and colon cancer[64] patients. Issues centered on disruption of sexual activity, impairment of sexual responsiveness, emotional responses to the body changes, and secondary marital disruption. Forty years later, these issues remain relevant. We are, however, closer to specifying the disease and treatment contexts, the specific sexual difficulties, the time course, and the etiologies of the sexual problems. As these issues are clarified, we will eventually be able to provide preventive and/or rehabilitative sexual therapy tailored to the needs of gynecologic cancer patients.

The chapter includes three main sections. In the first, we overview our conceptualization of sexual functioning and dysfunction, including the sexual behavior and the sexual response cycle aspects. We overview the hallmarks of sexual dysfunction among gynecologic cancer patients, and note the differences between the sexual problems of cancer patients and the sexual difficulties of healthy individuals. We discuss the etiology of sexual dysfunction for women with gynecologic cancer. Data suggest, for example, that the severity of sexual dysfunction is directly related to the 'magnitude' of cancer treatment and resulting pelvic and hormonal disruption. These factors produce a particular pattern of sexual behavior and response cycle change.

The second section critically reviews the international literature on sexual morbidity for preinvasive and invasive cervical and vulvar disease. There have been no investigations of sexual outcomes for endometrial or ovarian cancer patients; however, the difficulties for those with early stage disease would be expected to be similar to those for cervical cancer patients. We have summarized the findings from these investigations so as to distinguish the sexual behavior changes, sexual response cycle disruptions, and the sexual dysfunctions. We have also, unabashedly, highlighted our own research on the etiology and prevention of sexual difficulties in gynecologic cancer patients. We will briefly note the sexual concerns of women with disseminated cancer. We include in this group, for example, patients diagnosed with distant metastases or Stage III ovarian cancer failing first treatment courses. For these women, sexual concerns, per se, are often not pre-eminent, although the need for interpersonal intimacy may be acute.[44]

The final section provides an overview of current directions for the prevention of sexual morbidity. An important context is the provision of the least 'radical' cancer treatment which is also comparably curative. Following this consideration, psychological interventions will be described, including the provision of sexuality information and specific suggestions to the women for resuming sexual activity and enhancing responsiveness. Complementary medical interventions (e.g. hormonal replacement therapy) will also be noted.

A CONCEPTUALIZATION OF FEMALE SEXUAL FUNCTIONING AND SEXUAL MORBIDITY FOR WOMEN WITH GYNECOLOGIC CANCER

Appreciation of the sexual difficulties of women with gynecologic cancer begins with an understanding of sexual functioning in normal, healthy women. We have conceptualized sexual functioning as including three areas: sexual behavior, the sexual response cycle, and sexual dysfunction.

In the United States, the first large scale study of sexual

behavior was that by Alfred Kinsey and colleagues.[38,39] For women, they included the following types of sexual activity: pre-adolescent heterosexual and homosexual play, masturbation, nocturnal sex dreams, premarital petting, marital and extra-marital coitus, homosexual contacts and, finally, the 'total sexual outlet', defined as the sum of the various types of sexual activity culminating in orgasm. As Figure 90.1 illustrates, our own studies of sexual behavior have identified five empirical groupings of sexual behavior among heterosexual, sexually active women.[8] Of these activities, the most important is intercourse, as the frequency is significantly related to other sexual activities[8] and to sexual satisfaction and adjustment.[9]

The second and third components of sexual functioning are phases of the sexual response cycle (including desire, excitement, orgasm and resolution) and the corresponding sexual dysfunctions for each phase. Of the phases, *sexual desire* is the least understood. It is most often thought of as a biologic drive or urge for sexual activity. Some hypothesize that for male sexual desire adequate testosterone is needed, with androgen providing the hormonal basis for female sexual desire. Other conceptualizations view sexual desire as a subjective feeling which may be triggered by internal (e.g. fantasy, erection, vaginal lubrication) or external (e.g. pornography, the presence of an interested partner) cues.[45]

The diagnosis of inhibited sexual desire or hypoactive sexual desire includes individuals that are generally uninterested in sexual activity. Such an attitude can be manifest by avoidance of sexual contexts or refusal of sexual activity, but these behaviors are not presumed to be due to negative responses (e.g. aversions) to genital or interpersonal contact. Instead, individuals with a desire

disorder are believed to be indifferent or neutral towards sexual activity; sexual drive or urging is not blocked, but instead seems not to occur.[45] They report no sexual fantasies or other pleasant, arousing sexual cognitions. Emotionally, they describe themselves as not feeling 'sexy' or sexual, and behaviorally they do not initiate or respond to a partner's initiative for sexual activity. Disruption in the focus, intensity or duration of sexual activity is probable, and secondary disruption of subsequent response cycle phases is common.

The phase of *sexual excitement* begins with physical or psychologic sexual stimulation. The physiologic responses are widespread vasocongestion, either superficial or deep, and myotonia, with either voluntary or involuntary muscle contractions. Other changes include heart rate and blood pressure increases, and respiration becoming deeper and more rapid. For women, sexual excitement is also characterized by the appearance of vaginal lubrication, produced by vasocongestion in the vaginal walls leading to transudation of fluid. Other changes include a slight enlargement of the clitoris and uterus with engorgement. The uterus also rises in position, with the vagina expanding and ballooning out. Maximal vasocongestion of the vagina produces a congested orgasmic platform in the lower one-third of the vaginal barrel.

Psychological descriptions of sexual arousal may yield reports of the woman's awareness of the physiologic sensations (e.g. vaginal lubrication, pelvic warmth or 'heaviness') and a feeling of excitement or being 'turned on'. We have studied the organization of sexual activites and behaviors to which women can potentially become aroused.[9] Women make distinctions in their arousability to the following activities: erotica (e.g. pornographic literature or photography) and masturbation; seductive activities (e.g. passionate kissing, being undressed); body caressing by a male partner; oral-genital and genital stimulation; and intercourse. On the basis of other data,[8] anal stimulation and anal intercourse would likely represent a sixth area.

Among healthy women, inhibited sexual excitement involves disruption of the predominant physiologic responses (i.e. insufficient vaginal engorgement and/or lubrication), such that activities such as penetration would be difficult and/or painful. For example, the woman may report that her genitals feel 'dry' to the touch and that her body is not responding. She does not feel psychologically aroused or excited (e.g. her thoughts are not characterized by positive, arousing sexual content). Thus, for some women arousal may not occur, occur only at low levels, or occur for some responses and not others (e.g. lubrication may be present, but the woman reports little psychological arousal). For other women, arousal may be blocked or disrupted due to inhibitory affects or circumstances. A salient example of the former is sexual anxiety, producing interfering physiologic (i.e. sympathetic rather than parasympathetic activation), psychologic (i.e. fears rather

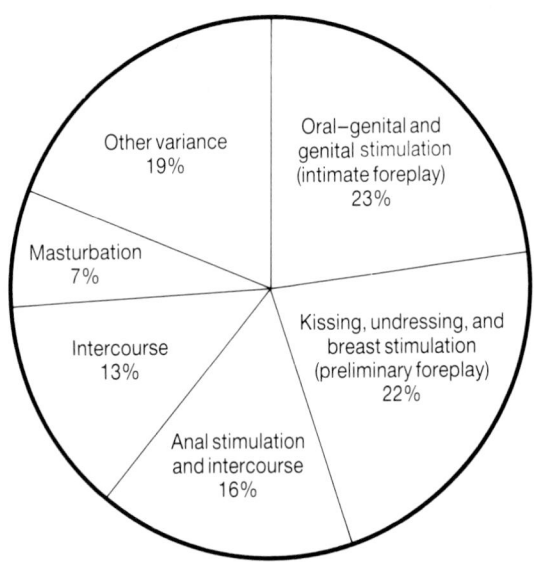

Fig. 90.1 A factor analytic study of sexual behavioral activities among heterosexual women. The percentages indicate the relative emphasis of the particular item on the inventory. (See reference 8 for details.)

than sexually arousing cognition) and behavioral (i.e. withdrawal or avoidance rather than approach) responses. Disruptive circumstances can, for example, include fatigue or pain. As with desire phase difficulties, arousal deficits can lead to disruption of other phases. For example, with longstanding arousal problems, a woman may eventually lose her desire for engaging in sexual activity; even when desire is maintained, it is difficult for a woman to be orgasmic when arousal is low.

Masters & Johnson[46] proposed that *orgasm* occurs via a reflex-like process once a plateau of excitement has been reached or exceeded, although the specific neurophysiologic mechanisms are not known. Orgasm is marked by rhythmic contractions of the uterus, the orgasmic platform and the rectal sphincter, beginning at 0.8-second intervals and then diminishing in intensity, duration, and regularity. Orgasm has also been regarded as a total body response, including facial grimacing, generalized myotonia, carpopedal spasms, and contractions of the gluteal and abdominal muscles. The subjective experience includes feelings of intense pleasure with a peaking and rapid, exhilarating release. Attention is usually focused on internal bodily sensations (usually concentrated in the clitoris, vagina, and uterus), and awareness of competing environmental stimuli is lessened. These sensations are reported to be singular, regardless of the manner in which orgasm is achieved.[52] Women are unique in their capability to be multi-orgasmic — that is, capable of a series of distinguishable orgasmic responses — without a lowering of excitement between them.

After orgasm occurs, the anatomic and physiologic changes of excitement reverse. The orgasmic platform disappears as blood is pumped away. The uterus moves back into the true pelvis, and the vagina shortens and narrows. When these responses follow orgasm, they are generally accompanied by subjective feelings of tension release, relaxation, and contentment. If orgasm has not occurred, the same physiologic processes occur at a much slower rate, and the psychologic responses are usually either neutral or negative (e.g. continued sexual tension, disappointment at having not experienced orgasm). The clinical presentation of orgasmic dysfunction typically takes one of two forms. Primary orgasmic dysfunction includes women who have never experienced orgasm under any circumstances (the possible exception might be an occasional orgasm during sleep with erotic dreams). If the woman has experienced orgasm but expresses concern with its frequency or circumstances of occurrence (e.g. orgasm may occur on a random basis or not with desired activities, such as coitus), the difficulty is labeled secondary. Cases of healthy women who have experienced sexual orgasm becoming non-orgasmic are rare. As noted above, orgasmic dysfunction more commonly occurs secondary to excitement difficulties, such that a woman is insufficiently aroused to even 'get close' to experiencing orgasm.

The final phase of the sexual response cycle, *resolution*, refers to the immediate postorgasm period. A filmy sheet of perspiration covers the body and the elevated heart rate and respiration from orgasm gradually return to normal; there are concomitant psychological sensations of bodily relaxation, and feelings of release and sexual contentment/satisfaction. Resolution dysfunctions have not been previously defined. This is due in part to infrequent complaints with resolution following unimpaired excitement and orgasm; when complaints occur, they typically are prompted by inhibitory affects, such as guilt, marital discord, fear of impregnation, etc., associated with sexual activity in general. Sexual distress during the resolution period commonly occurs secondary to dysfunction of prior phases (e.g. individuals complain of pelvic vasocongestion, sexual tension, lack of satisfaction, negative affect, etc. following orgasmic dysfunction).

The scientific literature on sexuality in normal, healthy women is central to understanding the qualitative and quantitative similarities and differences between the sexual difficulties of healthy women and those of gynecologic cancer patients. These eight aspects, from the appearance of the first difficulties to determination of their prognosis, are described below and summarized in Table 90.1.

It is appropriate to begin this discussion with the observation that, prior to the appearance of her disease, the woman with gynecologic cancer had, in all likelihood, a normal *premorbid sexual adjustment*. That is, the base rate of sexual problems and difficulties in this population is no higher (or lower) than that for other healthy women. For example, in our study of the pretreatment sexual functioning of early stage endometrial and cervical cancer patients, we found no difference in the base rate of sexual behavior (e.g. frequency of sexual intercourse) or dysfunction with an age-matched sample of healthy women.[52] Interestingly, we hypothesize that this history of a normal sexual functioning may heighten post-treatment sexual distress. That is, if a woman has never had to cope with significant sexual problems, their appearance is distressing[7] and she (and her partner) may have few skills to cope with sexual problems, particularly when they are severe and persistent.

The *timeline* for the appearance of sexual difficulties for cancer patients differs from that for healthy individuals. The onset of difficulties for women with cancer is acute, appearing immediately post-treatment/recovery as intercourse is resumed.[7] The immediacy and, if patients have not been forewarned about the likelihood or nature of the problem, unexpectedness of sexual difficulty contribute to the stressfulness of the problem. In contrast, healthy individuals often come to sexual therapy either with longstanding sexual difficulties that may have worsened or become more distressing, or with a history of satisfactory sexual functioning that is only recently situationally dysfunctional (e.g. coital inorgasmia with a new partner).

Table 90.1 Similarities and differences in sexual dysfunction(s) between healthy women and women with gynecologic cancer.

Aspect	Healthy women	Women with cancer
Premorbid sexual adjustment	Normal	Normal; sexual difficulties may occur with disease appearance
Timeline for onset	Longstanding sexual difficulties or acute situational dysfunction	Acute, with resumption of intercourse post-treatment
Clinical pattern of dysfunction	None notable	Arousal deficits are central; desire, orgasm and/or resolution disruption may be secondary
Accompanying deterrents	Marital disruption possible	Disease/treatment side effects (e.g. pain, fatigue)
Extent of difficulty	Phasic dysfunction with no to moderate disruption of other phases	Pervasive disruption across phases
Etiologic factors	Relationship factors for desire problem; anxiety is hypothesized for difficulties with arousal and orgasm	Treatment induced dyspareunia and/or nerve disruption; estrogen deprivation for premenopausal women
Treatment	Behavioral sex therapy	None presently documented Current possibilities: behavioral sex therapy medical intervention
Prognosis	Good	Guarded; possibly refractory to treatment

For the majority of women, there is a specific *clinical pattern* to the sexual difficulties. This pattern has two components: sexual behavior changes and sexual response cycle changes. For heterosexual women with gynecologic cancer, the primary sexual behavior disruption is the frequency of intercourse. For example, our controlled longitudinal study of early stage cervix and endometrial cancer patients revealed a reduction in intercourse frequency from 9 or 10 occasions per month pretreatment, to 6 per month at 1 year post-treatment (roughly a 33% reduction).[7] Despite this, a change in the frequency of other sexual behaviors (e.g. body caressing, genital stimulation) did not occur. That is, although the patients had intercourse less often, when they did have intercourse they reported the same sexual activities as occurring. If intercourse becomes too difficult (e.g. extremely painful) or impossible (e.g. following vaginectomy), the typical pattern is for all sexual activity between partners to cease.[10,11] The single exception to the latter might be continued (but low frequency) 'friendly' kissing. In contrast, a common pattern of behavioral disruption for healthy women has not been identified, although it appears that much of the behavioral change may be due to the particular type of sexual dysfunction (e.g. non-orgasmic women may report little change in the frequency of intercourse per se, whereas a woman with desire problems may be insufficiently interested to engage in any sexual behavior, and so dramatic reductions in intercourse frequency might be found).

The second component of the clinical pattern is changes in the sexual response cycle, including desire, excitement, orgasm and resolution. Disruption of sexual desire can occur as the primary problem, but more typically the loss is concomitant with disruption of other phases. In fact, for many women treated for gynecologic cancer, desire remains intact despite significant disruption in their responsiveness; further, sexual intercourse continues even when there are significant deterrents (e.g. dyspareunia, see below).[7] This fact underscores the importance accorded to the maintenance of a sexual life for the majority of women successfully treated for gynecologic cancer. Difficulty with sexual excitement, both bodily responses (e.g. lubrication, pelvic vasocongestion) and subjective feelings of arousal, is the most common and the most central sexual problem faced by gynecologic cancer patients. Our controlled longitudinal study[7] of Stage I and II cervix and endometrial cancer patients revealed a post-treatment incidence of inhibited sexual excitement diagnoses of 58%, in contrast to 25% for women treated for benign gynecologic disease and 15% for healthy women. In general, women treated for disease (whether benign or malignant) reported fewer signs of sexual arousal, and lower arousability for a variety of sexual activities; independent, trained interviewers rated the responses as dysfunctional, which also confirmed the evaluations from the women. The significantly greater incidence of excitement diagnoses, however, suggests that the added burden of a malignant diagnosis and the more radical treatment it imposes results in an arousal deficit of significantly greater severity, which makes the woman feel quite dysfunctional and distressed.

In view of the decline in sexual excitement, disruption of orgasm would be expected. Also, orgasmic dysfunction for gynecologic cancer patients is usually complete rather than situational, unlike the case for healthy women who have a higher frequency of secondary orgasmic dysfunction. For example, a woman who was regularly orgasmic during intercourse prior to cervical cancer discovers that she is non-orgasmic following treatment. Also, she may report not feeling sufficiently aroused to even 'get close' to orgasm. In this context, it is not surprising that many women report resolution disruption, including the possibility of residual sexual tension (if arousal is experienced), but more commonly residual pain from dyspareunia and/or concerns about the possibility of permanently changed sexual functioning occurs.

To summarize, the clinical pattern of sexual difficulty for the women with gynecologic cancer includes the following components: (1) If sexual activity continues, a lowered frequency of intercourse is the primary behavioral change. (2) Disruption of sexual desire is seldom a primary problem. When it occurs, it is secondary to arousal deficits. (3) Disruption of sexual excitement is central, with the etiology due primarily to treatment-related factors (e.g. pelvic/genital disruption from surgery and/or radiotherapy), and secondarily to treatment side effects (e.g. diminution of vaginal lubrication from premature menopause). For women with gynecologic cancer, these outcomes are salient and distressing. They contribute to the impairment of the psychological aspects of sexual arousal and are specifically disruptive to intercourse. (4) If orgasmic disruption occurs, it may be primary and complete (i.e. the woman is non-orgasmic following treatment) or it may be secondary to arousal deficits or significant disruptors to arousal (e.g. dyspareunia). (5) Disruption of resolution is common and occurs secondary to arousal and/or orgasm dysfunctions.

In addition to the direct effects of cancer treatment, there are usually *accompanying deterrents* which may also contribute to the greater severity of sexual problems. Specifically, disease/treatment side effects may also produce sexual dysfunction, and, unfortunately, the most common ones are difficult to treat. After recovery many cancer patients report residual, activity-disrupting fatigue,[10,11] with low sexual desire as a concomitant. Nongenital pain can be a common outcome for women who have had extensive pelvic and/or genital surgery. Coital pain (see Tables 90.2 and 90.4 for summaries of relevant data) is a deterrent to desire for, and arousal during, sexual activity.[7] In contrast, healthy women usually do not have significant accompanying deterrents, the notable exceptions might be women in troubled marital relationships or other difficulties (e.g. psychopathology; substance abuse) which might be generally disruptive to sexual functioning.

The *extent of the sexual difficulty* for cancer patients is pervasive, with major reductions in the frequency of intercourse and disruption of more than one phase of the sexual response cycle, as noted above. With problems of this magnitude, maintaining any sexual activity can be a concern. For some women, the fear is realistic and, unfortunately, realized. The classic examples are pelvic exenteration and radical vulvectomy patients. Women treated for cervix or vaginal cancer with radiotherapy, which may result in severe dyspareunia, may also serve as examples. In contrast, sexual dysfunction for healthy individuals is usually

most severe for a particular phase of the sexual response cycle with little to moderate impairment of the other phases (e.g. unimpaired arousal with primary orgasmic dysfunction). Also, unless a particular dysfunction makes intercourse impossible (e.g. vaginismus, erectile failure), most healthy couples continue to have intercourse despite their sexual dysfunction(s).

A likely *etiology* for the clinical pattern of difficulty, specifically the decline in sexual excitement, is the appearance of significant dyspareunia. The incidence of dyspareunia in the healthy female population is low (e.g. 1 to 2%). Our prospective study of women treated with either surgery (e.g. radical hysterectomy) or radiation therapy found that 47% of the sample was diagnosed with dyspareunia at some point during the post-treatment year. The estimates from the retrospective studies range from 6 to 50% (see Table 90.2). While intercourse pain does lessen in severity across time, 29% of the women with cancer and 13% of the women treated for benign disease followed longitudinally were diagnosed at 12 months.

Knowledge of the effects of the treatments for benign and malignant gynecologic disease, and our medical data, would indicate that dyspareunia among early stage cervix and endometrial patients is due to diminution in vaginal lubrication during sexual activity. For example, many cancer patients experience a surgical menopause, and a notable effect of the decline in estrogen levels is general changes to the genitals and atrophic vaginitis. For women with benign disease or gynecologically healthy women, hormone replacement therapy is usually available. In contrast, women with estrogen-sensitive endometrial tumors may not receive such therapy. Other women eligible for replacement therapy may receive radiation to the pelvis and/or vagina. For them, the vasocongestion and lubrication capacity of their vaginal tissues is completely halted, and topical estrogen therapy, even when it can be used, has a limited effect.[59] Thus, the case is strong for differential rates of treatment-induced dyspareunia.

Regarding *treatment*, behavioral sex therapy has been extremely effective for healthy sexually dysfunctional individuals (see reference 4 for a review); however, it is likely that these techniques will be insufficient for the sexual problems of women with cancer. Particularly for women with genital disease, the problems have the potential of being refractory due to the direct disruption of the organs or innervation. This situation, coupled with the many other reasons that interventions may not succeed, some specific to the context of cancer and others not, requires that future intervention efforts include both behavioral and medical (e.g. more effective treatments of dyspareunia) components. Sexual therapy techniques with documented effectiveness among healthy individuals do, however, stand as the important starting point (see discussion below).

Unlike the positive *prognosis* for the treatment of sexual difficulties among healthy individuals (see reference 4, for

Table 90.2 Summary of retrospective studies of sexual outcome (percentage of sample with significant sexual behavior changes or sexual difficulties) following cervix cancer.

Treatment Author	Country	Year	N	Sexual behavior (%)		Sexual dysfunction (%)			
				Not active	Decrease in frequency	Desire	Excitement	Orgasm	Dyspareunia
Surgery									
Decker	US	1962	32	12	12				
Abitbol	US	1974	32	6	13	6			6
Heiss	Austria	1954	30			53		47	
Froewis	Austria	1955	333	7		22		29	33
Lau	E. Germany	1967	314	22	32				32
Tamburini	Italy	1984	22		36	15	19		
O'Hoy	Hong Kong	1985	40		30	41	28	23	30
Ngan	Hong Kong	1988	28		25	43			
Radiation therapy									
Vasicka	US	1958	16	6	44				25
Decker	US	1962	29	31	24				
Abitbol	US	1974	28	25	53	43		43	
Seibel	US	1980	22		72		45		
Heiss	Austria	1954	20		25	60		40	
Picha	Austria	1957	156		26	25		21	
Lasnik	Austria	1986	57	16	54	58			50
Tamburini	Italy	1984	15	7	27	24	33		
O'Hoy	Hong Kong	1985	10		40	50	80	60	
Ngan	Hong Kong	1988	28		25	36			
Lau	E. Germany	1967	43	35	36				
Bertelsen	Denmark	1983	45	4	36	62			26
Combination therapy									
Abitbol	US	1974	15		33				
O'Hoy	Hong Kong	1985	53		77	64		58	
Ngan	Hong Kong	1988	17		10	55			17
Bertelsen	Denmark	1983	22		16	50			
Tamburini	Italy	1984	61	8	38	17	24		

example), the outlook for the prevention or remediation of sexual difficulties for cancer patients is guarded. However, the most important step would be the selection of the least sexually disruptive (but comparably curative) cancer treatment. Psychological and behavioral techniques would likely result in significant reductions in morbidity if provided prior to and immediately following therapy. As noted above, modification of existing behavioral strategies and the development of others will be necessary. Finally, we reiterate that medical treatments must also be available to treat the physical/somatic components of the sexual difficulties (e.g. dyspareunia, lubrication problems).

REVIEW OF SEXUAL MORBIDITY FOLLOWING CERVICAL CANCER

Much is known about the sexual outcome for cervical cancer patients. In fact, sufficient retrospective and prospective data exist for the design of interventions to prevent sexual functioning morbidity. Prior to review of the investigations, it is important to note the methodology for the retrospective studies and its weaknesses and contributions. These studies have used surveys of a single patient group, and patient self-selection is a potential problem. Participation rates are generally low, with a resultant oversampling of 'adjusted' patients. The follow-up interval is not controlled and, thus, a variety of factors (e.g. general health of the women or partner; the occurrence of major life stresses, such as job loss, moving, death of a relative, etc.), in addition to the direct or indirect effects of cancer or its treatment, may influence sexual functioning. Comparison groups (e.g. healthy women) have not been included. Finally, the assessment of sexual functioning has been modest, consisting mainly of verbal reports to an interviewer, who has often been the patient's own physician.

Despite these methodological weaknesses, the data have generally been consistent in the incidence and type of sexual morbidity. This observation is more compelling in that this consistency has been found across nationalities. We have presented the data according to the conceptualization described above, highlighting changes in sexual behavior, disruption of the sexual response cycle and the occurrence of sexual dysfunction. The retrospective data for cervix cancer is grouped according to treatment regimen: radical hysterectomy, radiotherapy or combined treatment for localized disease, and pelvic exenteration for recurrent disease. Table 90.2 summarizes the findings for the localized disease patients. We conclude the section with controlled longitudinal studies which provide important data on the timeline for difficulties, their nature, and their etiology.

Retrospective studies

In situ disease: conization

Preinvasive lesions are common. While the specter of cancer can be raised in a woman's mind, and the diagnostic process and treatment can be frightening,[49] the lesions can be treated effectively. Kilkku, Grönroos & Punnonen[36] reported on the sexual outcomes for 64 Finnish women who underwent conization of the cervix for diagnosis and treatment. There was no decline in the frequency of sexual intercourse and no increase in sexual dysfunction. In fact, reports of dyspareunia declined significantly at the 6- and 12-month post-treatment assessments.

Radical hysterectomy

Historically there have been conflicting reports on the sexually disruptive effects of hysterectomy per se (see reference 18 for a methodological discussion), and our data[7] confirm that even simple hysterectomy for benign disease produces significant sexual disruption. Thus, the vaginal shortening with radical hysterectomy (approximately one-third of the upper vagina is removed) can contribute to subjective feelings for the woman that the vagina is 'too short' for intercourse. Reports of coital discomfort are common. Nerve and vascular disruption to the pelvis may also result in loss of sensitivity and orgasmic disruption. For some women, it is possible that the ovaries may be preserved; however, this is not the case for all, and premature menopause, with the direct effects of atrophic vaginitis from estrogen deprivation, can also result in sexual difficulties.

There have been two retrospective investigations from the US and both are reports of approximately 30 patients each. The first, by Decker & Schwartzman,[25] included 32 patients with Stage I, II or III disease who were treated with hysterectomy (including removal of adnexa). Unfortunately, an unreported number of patients also received postoperative radiation therapy, which makes the interpretation in terms of the effects of hysterectomy per se, difficult. Patients were interviewed at least 6 months post-treatment and were asked to recall their pretreatment sexual behavior and provide a global evaluation of the changes in the frequency of sexual contact, interest and gratification. Twelve percent of the women reported that the frequency of sexual activity had declined, and another 12% reported the end of all sexual activity. In 1974, Abitbol & Davenport[1] provided additional data. At least 30 of the 32 women they studied were diagnosed with Stage I disease and treated with a Wertheim hysterectomy. The remaining two patients had Stage II disease, but their sur-

gical treatment is not described. Women were asked to recall their sexual functioning both prior to the appearance of the disease and approximately one year after treatment. Thirteen percent of the women reported a lower coital frequency, and intercourse was abandoned for 6%. Additionally, 6% of the women reported no sexual desire and the same percentage also reported discomfort during intercourse, presumably due to inadequate vaginal length.

In 1954, Heiss[32] provided the first of two reports from Austria. Thirty patients, aged 23 to 40 years, who had normal and frequent sexual activity prior to the hysterectomy, were studied. Unlike other studies which survey all patients, this investigation describes the sexual problems of a premenopausal sample who had any type of sexual problem. In this context, 63% noted 'strong' (unfortunately, 'strong' was not defined) sexual dysfunction due to vaginal shortening. In addition, 53% mentioned a decrease or complete loss of sexual desire and 47% a loss of orgasm. Finally, a majority of the sample, 86% of the women, mentioned that the loss of their inner genitals had negatively affected their body image. In this same period, Froewis & Picha[30] studied a large sample of patients (333) treated with Wertheim hysterectomy. Description of subject characteristics (e.g., stage of disease, time between treatment and study, etc.) or the assessment methods used is not provided. Of the women who had a sexual partner at the time of the study, 33% (74 of 223) noted difficulties with intercourse (e.g., pain) and 7% reported that intercourse was no longer possible. Also, 22% (73 of 223) of the women mentioned a decrease or loss of desire, and 29% (61 of 207) delayed or loss of orgasm. These two studies provide complementary methodologies; the Froewis & Picha survey provides an estimate of the 'base rate' of sexual difficulties among Austrian women, whereas the Heiss study provides an estimate specifically for a younger, premenopausal sample, a group at greater risk for sexual disruption due to their greater level of sexual activity.

Two reports from the same research group have described the sexual outcomes for Chinese women.[55,56] In these reports, 40 and 28 Chinese patients, respectively, were studied 6 months or longer following radical hysterectomy for in situ or Stage I disease. As 75% of the patients had their ovaries preserved, lower rates of sexual morbidity would be expected. Women were interviewed to assess changes in coital frequency, ability to attain orgasm and enjoyment of sex. In the two reports, 13% and 29%, respectively, noted a minor decrease in coital frequency, and an additional 30% and 25%, respectively, noted a significant decrease (greater than a 50% reduction). In terms of the sexual response cycle, approximately 40% of the women in both reports experienced a decreased sexual desire. In the first report, 28% had decreased sexual enjoyment/excitement and 23% a decrease in orgasm frequency (for 3% of the sample there was a complete loss of orgasm). One-third of the patients reported dyspareunia.

The two remaining studies each come from two different countries. Lau[43] studied a large sample (N = 314) of East German women following 'vaginal radical' hysterectomy. Women at all stages of disease were included. Of the women sexually active prior to treatment (N = 250), 32% experienced significant (type unspecified) difficulties during coitus, and for another 22% coitus was no longer possible. It may be important to note that both in the Froewis & Picha[30] and the Lau[43] investigations, the decision of 'coitus not possible' and the reason(s) for this difficulty are not specified. Tamburini et al[65] studied 22 Italian patients who had been treated at least 6 months previously for Stage Ia (N = 13) or Ib (N = 9) disease. Results indicated that 36% of the patients reported a decline in the frequency of sexual activity, 15% reduced sexual desire, and 19% noted reduced sexual enjoyment/excitement.

Radiation therapy

Radiation destroys ovarian function for the premenopausal woman, thereby inducing menopausal symptomatology; it also causes scarring, vaginal atrophy and stenosis. These outcomes are most severe for women treated with vaginal irradiation (intracavitary radium/cesium implants; see reference 12 for a discussion of the psychological aspects of this difficult treatment) when it is used alone or in combination with external beam irradiation.[7] Estrogen therapy following treatment can control such symptoms· as 'hot flushes' and aid in the healing of the vaginal epithelium,[59] but due to the magnitude of the vaginal changes, dyspareunia still occurs. Further, it has been estimated that radiation-induced tissue changes continue for 36 months or longer following the completion of therapy.

In the United States, there have been four reports on the sexual outcome for women following radiotherapy. The studies are similar in strategy, in that the sample sizes are in the range of 20 patients, individual interviews were usually conducted at least one year following treatment, and patients with Stage I, II, or III disease were included. The first was reported by Vasicka, Popovich & Brausch[67] in 1958. Sixteen patients with Stage I or II disease were interviewed 1 to 10 years post-treatment. In addition to an interview, a pelvic examination was performed. The gynecologic findings indicated that for 10 women the vaginal barrel was markedly shortened, and only minimally functional for another 5 patients. For one woman, the vagina was completely closed. Seven of the patients (44%) reported a decrease in sexual activity following treatment and 4 (25%) reported dyspareunia. Four years later, Decker & Schwartzman[25] provided data for 29 patients with Stage I, II, or III disease. Twenty-four percent of the women indicated that their sexual functioning was diminished following treatment, and an additional 31% reported stopping intercourse following treatment. Abitbol

& Davenport[1] interviewed 28 women with Stage I or II disease. Sexual activity was markedly reduced for 53% of the women, and completely halted for 25% of the women. Accompanying physical examination data indicate that major vaginal changes (i.e., narrowing or obliteration of the vagina) were noted in 78% of the patients. Forty-three percent of these latter women also reported declines in sexual desire and the disappearance of orgasm. Finally, Seibel et al[61] reported outcomes for 22 patients with Stage I, II, or III disease. Medical records described 72% of the patients as having shortening and/or stenosis of the vagina. The majority of the women (72%) reported a decrease in coital frequency. Estimates that sexual enjoyment was diminished after treatment were reported by 45% of the patients, and the percentage of coital instances in which orgasm was attained declined from a mean of 61% pretreatment to 39% post-treatment.

There have been three reports of sexual outcomes for Austrian women following radiotherapy. The first report by Heiss[32] is similar in strategy to the US reports, but the latter two[42,58] are distinguished by their large sample sizes. Heiss[32] studied 20 patients. Physical examination data indicated that for 25% of the patients the upper portion of the vagina was coapted, and 25% showed a high degree of stenosis. In this context, 25% of the women complained of 'strong' sexual dysfunction on anatomical grounds. Hormonal failure symptoms (e.g., hot flushes, night-sweats, nervousness, depression) were reported by 60% of the patients. Also, 60% noted a decrease or loss of desire and 40% a loss of orgasm. In this same period, Picha[58] studied the sex life of 156 women following radiation therapy. Patients were interviewed and examined one month or longer after treatment for Stage I to IV cervical cancer. Anatomical impossibility to have coitus post-treatment was reported for 3% (2 of 70) of the sexually active women. For 23% (16 of 70) disturbances during coitus due to unspecified anatomic reasons were reported. The estimates of a complete loss or decrease in desire was 25% (39 of 156). Eighteen percent (12 of 68) of the sexually active women experienced a loss of orgasm, and 3% (2 of 68) a delayed orgasm. The most recent study comes from Lasnik & Tatra[42]. Fifty-seven patients were interviewed 18 months or longer after treatment for Stage I, II, or III disease. All women were sexually active prior to treatment, but 16% were not after treatment. Of the 84% of the sample who maintained some sexual activity, coital frequency was reduced for more than half (54%) of the women. Also, 50% reported discomfort during coitus. These latter patients all complained of deficient lubrication, in addition to pain from a shortened or narrowed vagina. For 39% (22 of 57), sexual desire was absent, and another 19% (11 of 57) reported a decline in sexual desire.

There have been two reports of sexual outcomes for Chinese women. O'Hoy & Tang[56] and Ngan & Tang[55] reported 10 and 28 Chinese women, respectively, treated for Stage I, II, or III disease. A significant decrease in coital frequency (greater than 50%) post-treatment was reported by 40% and 25% of the women, respectively. Fifty percent and 36% of the patients, respectively, noted a decrease in desire. Also, 80% of the Chinese women noted that they did not enjoy sex as much as before treatment. In both reports, the majority of the women attributed their sexual problems to fatigue and physical weakness.

The three remaining studies come from different countries. In a small sample report from Italy, Tamburini et al[65] provided data on 15 radiation therapy patients with Stages I (N = 14) or II (N = I) disease. A decrease in sexual activity was reported by 27% of the patients, and 7% reported that activity had ceased. Twenty-four percent of these Italian women noted a reduction in desire, and 33% a reduction in sexual enjoyment/excitement. In East Germany, Lau[43] interviewed 83 radiation therapy patients with Stage I, II, or III disease, 43 of whom were sexually active prior to treatment. Of these latter women, 36% experienced 'strong' difficulties during coitus, and for 35% coitus was no longer possible.

Finally, in Denmark, Bertelsen[19] interviewed 45 radiation therapy patients with Stage Ib (N = 44) and IIa (N = 1) disease. Subjects were interviewed 3 years or longer post-treatment. It is noteworthy that 62% of the sample described their sexual life as 'radically changed' after the treatment. Estimates that coital frequency was reduced (by 25% or less) were obtained from 36% of the women, and 4% of the patients reported stopping coital activity because of their disease and treatment. Sixty-two percent noted a decrease or loss of desire. Regarding physical disruptors to intercourse, 26% of the patients complained of pain, 16% of bleeding, 58% of dryness, and 28% of tightness of the vagina. Examinations in 62% of the patients indicated vaginal agglutination. A relationship between the severity of vaginal fibrosis and sexual function was found: two-thirds of the patients who stopped coitus or experienced sexual dysfunction had a moderate to severe fibrosis, whereas moderate to severe fibrosis was present in 50% of those reporting unchanged sexual functioning. Similar relationships were also found with the severity of vaginal mucosa atrophy and/or pelvic fibrosis and sexual functioning.

Combined treatment

Rather than receive surgery or radiation therapy alone, some cervix (or endometrial) cancer patients receive combination therapy, typically in one of two ways. Radiation therapy can follow a (radical) hysterectomy if the pelvic lymph nodes are positive for malignancy or if a recurrence of the disease occurs post-hysterectomy. In contrast to this strategy, the radiation can be given first, followed by an extrafascial hysterectomy. Patients treated with combination therapy usually receive a lower total dose of radiation than those treated with radiotherapy only. In addition, depending on the surgical procedure, the apex of the vagina, which is exposed to the largest dose of radiation when intracavitary treatment is included, is removed during surgery. Thus, the remaining portion of the vagina is less affected and, perhaps, less vulnerable to problems of dyspareunia. Only four studies on the sexual outcomes of combined treatment have been reported, and all come from different countries. Unfortunately, the authors do not always mention the sequence of the combined treatment, making interpretation difficult and comparison of sequences impossible.

In the US, Abitbol & Davenport[1] interviewed 15 patients, 1 year or longer following combined treatment. Six of these patients were diagnosed with Stage II disease and received external radiation followed by a Wertheim hysterectomy. Of the nine Stage I patients, some received radiation therapy following a Wertheim hysterectomy, and others underwent a simple hysterectomy after completion of radiation therapy. Taken together, 33% reported a marked reduction in sexual activity. Also, in 60% of these patients, major vaginal changes were found.

From Denmark, Bertelsen[19] also provided data for 22 Danish patients with Stage Ib (N = 18) and IIa (N = 4) disease interviewed 1 to 4 years after completion of treatment. Patients received intracavitary radiation therapy followed by radical hysterectomy (including removal of adnexa). Estimates that coital frequency was lower (at least by 25%) were obtained from 16% of the patients. Fifty percent of the women also reported a decrease or loss of desire. Of the 32% of the sample reporting sexual dysfunction, 17% complained of dryness, and 4% of tightness of the vagina.

From Italy, Tamburini et al[65] provided data. Sixty-one patients with Stage Ia (N = 2), Ib (N = 56), and IIa (N = 3) were interviewed. Estimates of a decrease in sexual activity were obtained from 38% of the patients, and an additional 8% reported that sexual activity had stopped. A reduction in desire was reported by 17% of the women, and 24% noted a decrease in sexual enjoyment/excitement.

Finally, two reports provide data for 53 and 17 Chinese patients, respectively, treated with combined therapy for Stage I and II disease.[55,56] Patients first received radiation therapy then surgery. Of the women who were still sexually active post-treatment, 81% and 65%, respectively, had minor or major decreases (more than 50%) in coital frequency. Estimates of a decrease in libido were obtained from 64% and 54% of the women, respectively. Additional data from the larger sample report indicated that 23% noted a decrease in the ability to attain orgasm, 35% a loss of orgasm, and 50% reported a decrease in sexual enjoyment/excitement.

Pelvic exenteration

This surgery is considered for some women with recurrent disease or with extensive but resectable disease at diagnosis. It is a disfiguring operation, involving removal of the uterus, tubes, ovaries, urinary bladder, rectum and vagina. Clinical reports, not surprisingly, have commonly reported the cessation of sexual activity for the majority of women (80 to 90% of those surveyed). This discouraging scenario has been replicated with data from several investigators in the United States.[11,20,27,41,68] For the majority of women and couples, the prospect of ending their sexual life (as most couples cease all sexual activity when intercourse becomes impossible) is distressing and may be a source of continuing marital discord, particularly among younger couples (e.g. less than 60 years; see reference 11 for a discussion).

Vaginal reconstruction (e.g., with a loop of bowel, myocutaneous flaps, etc.) is a possibility for some, and enables a woman to maintain sexual activity that includes intercourse; however, sexual difficulties often remain. Some women have difficulties with the physical characteristics of the new vagina (e.g., the cavity is too large or too narrow), others have general problems with arousal, orgasm, pain or bleeding with intercourse. Regardless of whether or not women with pelvic exenteration undergo vaginal reconstruction, these women face the greatest disruption to their sexual body and functioning of any female cancer group.

Prospective studies

Sexual disruption at diagnosis

Clinical studies and texts (e.g. reference 17) have noted that signs and symptoms, such as postcoital bleeding or pelvic pain, may alert a woman to her gynecologic disease and need for medical care. The sexually disruptive effects of these early signs was reported, and the concurrent sexual dysfunction described, by Andersen, Lachenbruch, Anderson & deProsse.[13] Forty-one women recently diagnosed with early stage cervical or endometrial cancer, and a matched group (i.e., age, menopausal and sexually active status) of healthy women in no gynecologic distress provided data on the range and frequency of sexual behavior, level of sexual responsiveness and the presence of sexual dysfunction. Analyses indicated that prior to the onset of cancer signs and symptoms, the gynecologic cancer patients reported similar patterns of sexual activity and responsiveness to those of the healthy sample. With the appearance of disease signs/symptoms (i.e., fatigue, postcoital bleeding, vaginal discharge, pain), the women who would subsequently receive a cancer diagnosis reported experiencing significant sexual dysfunctions. The data in Table 90.3 display the comparability in the frequency of sexual dysfunction between the women with gynecologic cancer and the gynecologically healthy women

Table 90.3 Frequency of sexual dysfunction diagnoses prior to and following the appearance of early stage cervical or endometrial cancer for 41 women, and comparative data for 41 age-matched gynecologically healthy women.

Dysfunction	Healthy women (%)	Women with cancer	
		Prior to symptoms (%)	After symptoms (%)
Inhibited desire	17	12	56
Inhibited excitement	7	10	49
Inhibited orgasm	10	7	37
Dyspareunia	0	5	37

(see columns 1 and 2) and the 4- to 5-fold increase in the frequency of sexual dysfunctions from pre to post appearance of cancer signs/symptoms (see columns 2 and 3). Since 75% of the women with cancer experienced a substantial change in sexual functioning, it is likely that such obvious and disruptive sexual problems influenced the women to negatively interpret their gynecologic disease signs/symptoms and seek medical consultation (see reference 21 for a complete discussion of the psychological processes involved in symptom interpretation and delay).

Longitudinal studies

The only experiment to be conducted which examined differential sexual outcomes was reported by Vincent, Vincent, Greiss & Linton[69] in 1975. Fifty women with early stage cervical disease were randomly assigned to receive either radical hysterectomy or radiotherapy. The groups were matched for such important factors as age, education, socioeconomic status, marital status, parity, race and disease stage. Unlike the results from the retrospective studies, the changes in sexual desire and activity from pretreatment to 6 months post-treatment were comparable: estimates of diminished desire were obtained from 24% of the radiation therapy and 20% of the surgical patients. Decreased frequency of intercourse was reported by 29% of the radiation and 33% of the surgical patients. The experiment provides convincing evidence that, in general, the rates of sexual behavior disruption and dysfunction are comparable for the two major treatment options.

Our research has examined the nature and timing of sexual difficulties for women with early stage disease.[7] Forty seven women with Stage I or II cervical or endometrial disease were assessed prior to treatment and at 4, 8, and 12 months post-treatment. The sexual behavior, sexual response cycle, sexual dysfunction and medical outcomes for the women with cancer were compared with data from two matched comparison groups: women diagnosed and treated for benign disease (e.g. uterine fibroids treated with simple hysterectomy), and gynecologically healthy women. The former group provides an estimate of sexual disruption due to disease in and treatment to the pelvis, and the latter estimates the base rate of sexual difficulties due to normal life circumstances.

Analyses indicated that the primary sexual behavior disrupted by the disease and treatment process for women with malignant or benign disease was the frequency of intercourse, declining from an average of 9.5 occasions per month to 6 to 7 occasions per month during the post-treatment period. The absence of change in sexual behavior variables (e.g. range of current sexual activities) other than intercourse would appear to indicate that disruption of the couples behavioral repertoire during sexual activity did not occur. That is, when couples engaged in intercourse, albeit less often, the women reported the same sexual activities (e.g. body caressing, oral-genital stimulation) as having occurred.

It is important to note that there were no significant differences between groups in the percentage of women becoming sexually inactive, with the estimates ranging from 5 to 15% across the assessments. However, half of the sexually inactive cases in the cancer group (i.e. 2 of 4 women) were due to disease-related causes. Specifically, two women stopped intercourse after two failed attempts. In both cases, the male partners had histories of prior erectile difficulties, the onset of which was correlated with the diagnosis and treatment of hypertension. It was also the case, however, that both women reported dyspareunia with the two intercourse attempts. On the basis of the interviews with the women, it appeared that their complaints of intercourse pain likely contributed to the men's erectile capabilities becoming additionally vulnerable, as both husbands lost erections during the attempts. As they recovered, the women indicated a preference to continue intercourse but, by their reports, the partners were unwilling to consult their physician regarding their hypertension

medication. By 12 months, both women felt that it was unlikely that they would resume intercourse. Longitudinal data such as these underscore the need for the careful interpretation of findings on failure to resume intercourse.

The difficulty with sexual excitement for both disease groups was substantial. Following treatment, women with disease reported awareness of fewer signs of sexual excitement (lower arousability for sexual activities) with their partner, and the evaluators and the women themselves felt that significant arousal problems were experienced. This consistency in the excitement data, and the absence of any change on a measure of sexual anxiety, would appear to indicate that the arousal problems for the women with disease were not anxiety based. In contrast, anxiety is hypothesized to play a central role in arousal difficulties for healthy women (see reference 16 for a review). As noted above, a likely source of the arousal deficits was the co-occurrence of significant disruptors (e.g. dyspareunia, due in part to radiation effects and/or induced menopause).

Table 90.4 summarizes the percentage of sexual dysfunction diagnoses for each group and their duration during the post-treatment year. The diagnoses were made by trained evaluators who conducted structured interview assessments with the subjects both pretreatment and on four occasions during the first year post-treatment. It is important to note the following: (a) The healthy group provides estimates of sexual dysfunction frequencies comparable to those obtained by other investigators.[29] (2) The 'continuing dysfunction' cases (e.g. sexual dysfunction which continued from 4 to 12 months post-treatment) would represent the numbers of women who had chronic problems and who are at greatest risk for permanently impaired sexual functioning. (3) The 'new late' (i.e. no dysfunction reported at 4 months but difficulties at 12 months) represent cases which could potentially be

Table 90.4 Percentage of sexual dysfunction diagnoses by group at 12 months post-treatment considering diagnoses at 4 months post-treatment.

Dysfunction	Status at 12 months post-treatment			
	Never dysfunctional	Continuing dysfunction	New late dysfunction	Resolved dysfunction
Inhibited desire				
Cancer	47	16	16	21
Benign	60	0	13	27
Healthy	82	2	7	9
Inhibited excitement				
Cancer	47	16	13	27
Benign	67	0	20	13
Healthy	87	0	9	4
Inhibited orgasm				
Cancer	58	18	11	13
Benign	73	7	7	13
Healthy	91	2	4	2
Dyspareunia				
Cancer	53	21	8	18
Benign	67	7	7	20
Healthy	93	0	2	4

prevented with therapy during the immediate post-treatment period. (4) The 'resolved' cases are heterogeneous. They include cases which resolved (e.g. cases of dyspareunia which improved with continued recovery) as well as women who adapted (i.e. reported lower levels of emotional distress) to their changed sexual responsiveness.

REVIEW OF SEXUAL MORBIDITY FOR VULVAR DISEASE

Vulvar cancer typically occurs late in life; the average age of onset is 65 years. Data suggest that the incidence for in situ disease is increasing and that the age at diagnosis is lower and occurs in the third or fourth decade rather than the sixth or seventh.[72] Attention to the sexual outcomes for women with vulvar disease is recent. The absence of prior data may have been due to attitudes that sexuality in latter life is unimportant, inappropriate or expendable. However, the constancy of sexual needs through the lifespan has been demonstrated; there is a natural decline in the frequency of sexual behavior with age; however, the presence of a healthy and interested partner, rather than age, is the variable of greatest importance to the maintenance of female sexual activity.[53,57] In view of the recency of attention, all of the studies are retrospective, although comparison data from matched samples of healthy women are available.

In situ disease

The original treatment for carcinoma in situ advocated by Knight[40] was wide local excision, but many gynecologists have preferred to remove the entire vulva (i.e. total or radical vulvectomy), arguing that the disease is preinvasive and frequently multicentric. Surgical alternatives have included wide local excision of the lesion or skinning vulvectomy. The primary non-surgical approaches have included the topical use of chemotherapy (5-fluorouracil) or laser vaporization (CO_2 laser).

We conducted a collaborative retrospective investigation of 83 sexually active patients treated at eight medical centers in the United States from 1 to 10 years previously.[14] Patients' sexual functioning was compared to that of 57 age- and menopausal status-matched healthy women. Analyses revealed that there were differences in sexual functioning among the women treated for in situ disease, and the healthy women. Analyses examining the extent of treatment found no differential disruption for women treated with limited (e.g. wide local excision) vs. extended (e.g. skinning procedure) surgery. Also, when treatment options are available, such as wide local excision vs. laser vs. combined treatment, these data indicate no differential disruption between the groups. Sexual partners reported that the treatments had not adversely affected their sexual relationship. Thus, these data suggest that the

risk for sexual disruption may be limited for women treated for in situ disease.

Invasive disease

Treatment typically involves radical vulvectomy (removal of all labial tissue, often including the clitoris) and bilateral groin lymph node removal, with or without pelvic lymph node removal, although there has been encouragement of individualization of treatment for patients with early disease, with particular emphasis on vulvar conservation if appropriate.[31,33] An early survey highlighted the considerable emotional and sexual cost of radical surgery for women.[28] Eighteen patients treated with wide excision of the lesion rather than vulvectomy for microinvasive disease indicated that all women continued to be orgasmic during sexual activity, in contrast to two patients treated with radical vulvectomy who reported loss of orgasmic ability and dyspareunia.

Our retrospective study of women who received radical surgery indicates a limited capacity for sexual arousal in these patients, but little diminution in sexual desire.[10] Interestingly, orgasmic responsiveness is reported by women who had, as well as those who had not, undergone clitoral excision at the time of vulvectomy. As many as 60 to 90% of women may stop all sexual activity. For some this is due to negative feelings (by the woman or her partner) about the physical changes to the body, and for others it may be due to severe dyspareunia, such as may occur with a narrowed introitus. Our findings have been replicated by investigators in the United States,[63] Denmark,[50] the Netherlands[60] and Italy.[66]

INTERVENTION FOR SEXUAL DIFFICULTIES

The above reviews indicate that sufficient data have accumulated to begin controlled outcome research to prevent or remediate sexual difficulties. However, there have been few studies of sexual therapy for female cancer patients. Two investigations provided information on brief counseling on a variety of topics (e.g., causes of cancer, relaxation training, diet and exercise), including sexuality.[22,23] Sexual functioning was significantly less disrupted in comparison to the outcomes for untreated control patients or patients receiving standard care from physicians, nurses or social workers. These data and those indicating that sexual functioning is a major source of concern for the woman with gynecologic cancer suggest that intervention can enhance sexual functioning and reduce treatment-related sexual morbidity.

The easiest route to reduce the incidence and severity of sexual problems would be to identify and use cancer treatments which produce the lowest level of morbidity with no compromise in cure rate. The emergence of segmental mastectomy and radiotherapy (or, previously, modified radical mastectomy rather than radical mastectomy) for localized breast cancer is a salient example. Our data suggest, for example, that either surgery or radiotherapy, rather than combined therapy, for localized cervical or endometrial cancer results in significantly less sexual dysfunction. Thus, if less radical treatments are available and utilized, sexual morbidity, on average, will be reduced.

If psychological intervention is needed, it is more cost effective and of greater benefit to patients to provide preventive rather than rehabilitative therapy. The former would involve, for example, intensive information about, and teaching of, sexual 'problem-solving' skills pretreatment and during the immediate post-treatment period, with a gradual decrease in therapeutic efforts during early recovery. As sexual difficulties are manifest as soon as intercourse resumes, this would provide the woman with an educated perspective for understanding the sexual changes that have occurred, the foresight for anticipating, minimizing or averting sexual difficulties, and specific suggestions for enhancing sexual functioning during the recovery period. Considering the context for delivery, interventions to enhance sexual functioning for healthy women have been successfully conducted within women-only formats (e.g. reference 3). For some women it may be advantageous to include the sexual partner, as even greater gains in sexual functioning might be realized; clinical reports of women with cancer have noted the importance of the partner's reaction in the prediction of the couple's post-treatment sexual adjustment.[44,48,50]

To design a preventive intervention, at least three components appear essential. Firstly, sexuality information (e.g. male and female sexual anatomy, the sexual response cycle, sexual dysfunctions and potential sources of difficulty) is needed. This is an important first step in sexual therapy to enhance function and decrease sexual anxiety (e.g. reference 37). Further, explication of the specific sexual changes following cancer treatment is essential. For example, the woman with cervical disease treated with radiotherapy who experiences a diminution of vaginal lubrication needs to be aware that this is a normal circumstance and not, for example, an indication of a loss of desire for her partner. Although the sexual problems of gynecologic cancer patients will be more difficult to treat than those of healthy individuals, and not responsive to information only, such intervention may prevent problems due to ignorance or misconceptions, or decrease the severity of problems that arise from other factors.

Secondly, medical intervention is an important part of prevention. Several examples can be cited. Hormonal medication, which can have positive effects on enhancing sexual desire and, possibly, arousal,[71] can be prescribed (unless contraindicated by the disease). Estrogen therapy also aids in the healing of the vaginal epithelium (and thereby reducing the severity of dyspareunia) following radiotherapy. Patients receiving radiotherapy need to be instructed on the use of dilators to reduce adhesions. Finally, reconstructive surgery may be necessary for some patients.

Thirdly, the delivery of specific suggestions for the enhancement of post-treatment sexual functioning and responsiveness are necessary. Behavioral sex therapy used with healthy individuals stands as a starting point. The effectiveness of sex therapy has been found to be stable over lengthy (e.g., 5 year) follow-up periods.[26,47] With greater precision in defining the sexual difficulties of women with cancer, interventions can be developed for phase- or behavior-specific sexual difficulties. We will now turn to a discussion of current sexual therapy techniques which may be appropriate for use with gynecologic cancer patients.

Of all sexual difficulties, interventions for desire phase problems are the least articulated. Important in their treatment, however, is careful determination of etiology. As discussed above, desire problems in healthy individuals often occur secondary to other response cycle disruptions. That is, individuals may lose desire for sexual activity after repeated failure or disruption of excitement or orgasm. In these cases, the focus of intervention is not on desire per se, but remedying the other sexual difficulties with the expectation that sexual desire will occur naturally once sexual activity becomes arousing or fulfilling again. For women with cancer who may experience direct disruption of excitement or orgasm from their treatments, it is not surprising that many will also report loss of sexual desire. Women may report that their body does not respond, or they may not experience the bodily sensations of arousal. Unfortunately, intervention to first enhance arousal or orgasm may be met with only limited success for women with cancer; the desire problems may remain and require direct treatment.

Interventions for desire problems can include, among others: (1) determining what conditions for sexual activity are more or less appealing, with encouragement that sexual activity occur under the most desirable circumstances; (2) increasing the frequency of a range of intimate activities (not only sexual behaviors) which the woman might find pleasurable; (3) increasing the frequency and variety of the woman's sexual fantasies during sexual activity and on other occasions. Such suggestions come from interventions for desire problems among healthy individuals (e.g. reference 34) and basic research on the behavioral characteristics of individuals seeking treatment for desire-related problems.[54,73] All interventions are designed to increase the frequency of positive sexual cognitions, intimate occasions with the partner, and optimal times and circumstances for sexual activity for the woman.

Many of the desire phase interventions described have also been used to enhance arousal. Additional efforts have included the use of individual and couple body touching exercises (i.e., sensate focus). A series of graduated steps are suggested to the woman or couple with each successive stage employing more intimate touching and higher levels of arousal expected. For example, couple sensate focus could involve steps which include caressing of: (1) hands, arms and face; (2) whole body without genitals, breasts, or buttocks; (3) whole body without genital stimulation; (4) whole body; and (5) whole body with focused stimulation (masturbation). Individual activities can be designed according to the same principles.

A graduated series of sexual activities has several benefits. Firstly, they reintroduce relaxing and enjoyable sexual activity for a woman or couple. Secondly, the activities are not strenuous, a particular aid for the woman not yet recovered. Thirdly, exercises do not focus on a particular body part or area, and new areas for stimulation can be discovered. Fourthly, touching and examination of an affected area (e.g. the pelvis, the vagina) can be eliminated or can be introduced gradually. This strategy facilitates anxiety reduction for both the woman and her partner. She has a way to discover what sensitivity, if any, remains; some areas will have similar sensations to those prior to cancer treatment, whereas other areas may feel unpleasant to the touch (e.g., numb, odd tingling sensations at the site of an incision). As noted, some women or couples may prefer not to explore/touch certain areas. When done in the context of sensate focus exercises such as those described above, other body areas remain for touching and the context remains loving and sexual, rather than rejecting or anxiety provoking.

Instances of women reacting negatively to their body after cancer treatment have been described (e.g. references 35, 62). Such reactions have been described following radical surgery — mastectomy, vulvectomy, or pelvic exenteration — although such reactions can occur for any woman with cancer. Extreme responses have included anxiety or disgust at looking at the site or fear of being seen by one's spouse, among others. While these responses are difficult, they are not unique, as many healthy women with sexual difficulties report similar feelings. For such women, anxiety reduction techniques, systematic desensitization or individual sensate focus exercises, have proven effective. While such activities may not change a woman's negative body feelings to positive, they may achieve neutrality or no longer be disruptive of the woman's sexual activity or mood.

Orgasmic dysfunction is common for women treated for pelvic or genital disease. The dysfunction is typically pervasive, with the woman who was regularly orgasmic with coital activity prior to treatment, subsequently non-orgasmic. For a smaller subset, orgasm remains but is difficult to achieve. The majority of these difficulties are probably due to altered structure or innervation. However, it is important to consider other etiologies, such as insufficient arousal or dyspareunia. Once these latter sources are ruled out or treated, the important question is, 'Under op-timal arousing circumstances, can orgasm be achieved by any means?'

The most successful treatment programs for healthy, non-orgasmic women include a series of individual sexuality and masturbation exercises. Analogous to the strategy for couples, the sequence of such programs includes body examination, identification of genital anatomy, tactile body and genital self-examination to identify pleasurable whole-body and genital sensations, and focused genital stimulation. Such steps can be important in identifying what familiar or new body areas respond to stimulation. Even though pelvic or genital anatomy is changed, it is possible that orgasm can still be experienced through other means, since women can experience orgasm without genital stimulation[39] or without specific organs (e.g., clitoris) believed critical to the response.[10] If such a treatment program is completed satisfactorily (i.e., the woman is motivated, the exercises were completed with conscientious effort, etc.) and orgasm still does not occur, then this may provide convincing diagnostic evidence that the change in orgasmic ability may be longstanding. Even if this is the case, the exercises provide other beneficial effects, such as the woman taking a more active role in her sexuality, an improved body concept, discovery of new modes of sexual pleasuring, etc. (e.g. references 24, 70).

As discussed above, sexual dysfunction during resolution is common for women treated for gynecologic cancer. Sources of difficulty include residual pain if there has been dyspareunia or continued arousal and/or frustration due to lack of orgasm. The straightforward remedy to such problems is improving sexual functioning during earlier phases so that resolution is satisfactory. However, for those women with permanent sexual changes (e.g. intervention fails to renew orgasm), efforts may focus on the woman's feelings of 'let down', continued tension, or discouragement about her sexual life. Cognitive restructuring may be helpful in assisting the woman to focus on remaining, positive aspects, such as continued ability to engage in sexual activity, feelings of physical closeness and intimacy with her partner, or the sharing of alternative sexual activities with her partner, and others.

CONCLUSIONS

Vigorous concern for the sexual problems of women treated for gynecologic cancer is recent. Within the last 10 years, however, research has progressed beyond descriptive clinical reports to, in some cases, controlled prospective longitudinal investigations tracing the development of sexual problems. Models for conceptualizing and assessing the sexual difficulties of cancer patients have been proposed and tested. Further, sufficient reliability and validity data have been published such that any gynecologic oncology program could implement a program to assess and monitor the sexual behavior and sexual responses of its patients. Thus, many of the significant impediments to assessing and understanding sexual outcomes for gynecologic cancer patients have been addressed.

An extensive literature exists on the sexual outcomes for women with early stage cervix, endometrial, or ovarian cancer treated with hysterectomy, radiotherapy or combination procedures. Although there are significant methodological weaknesses with the retrospective designs, the summary in Table 90.2 provides an estimate, albeit flawed, of the base rate of sexual difficulties. The prospective longitudinal data provides (e.g. Table 90.4) the first important perspectives on the course, specific nature and etiology of the difficulties. When the international literature and prospective data are considered, the following conclusions emerge: (1) The frequency of women abandoning sexual activity following treatment is higher than the 'normal' base rate for healthy women in the same age group; the latter is in the range of 10 to 15%. The hypothesized mechanism for this higher base rate is that the cancer-related sexual difficulties for couples may provide a sufficient, added vulnerability if sexual intercourse is already problematic for other reasons (e.g. couples in which the male has erectile difficulties due to declining health). (2) A significant decrease in the frequency of intercourse occurs beyond that which would normally occur with advancing age. Frequency of intercourse is an important 'barometer' of the sexual health of intimate relationships. Thus, any decline that is noticeable and extends in time will, necessarily, burden a woman and potentially threaten the stability and satisfaction of her intimate sexual relationships. (3) Arousal deficits play a central role in influencing the incidence and severity of other response cycle disruptions. Further, dyspareunia is an important moderator of arousal. Thus, to the extent that interventions can directly address the problems of dyspareunia, rates of sexual dysfunction can be significantly lowered. (4) Vigorous medical efforts to treat dyspareunia are needed. For example, the rates of sexual dysfunction and dyspareunia in the Andersen, Anderson & deProsse investigation[7] occurred in a context of vigorous monitoring and encouragement to use vaginal dilators, lubricants and estrogen therapy, when possible. These data represent the 'best case' scenario, and the rates of dyspareunia and other dysfunctions are exceedingly high. Thus, other medical treatments for dyspareunia must be developed. (5) Review of the international literature reinforces the strength of these conclusions as the data in Table 90.2 reveal consistencies across investigators, time, measurement strategies, nationality, and the important role that cultural factors may play in influencing sexual behavior. (6) Study of the sexual morbidity in early stage cervix, endometrial or ovarian patients will not be significantly advanced by further retrospective study; sufficient data exist to begin investigations to prevent sexual morbidity.

In contrast to the latter extensive literature, fewer data are available on the sexual outcome for women with vulvar disease. Again, however, consistency of findings is emerging and preliminary observations can be made. (1) Sexual morbidity is directly correlated with the radicality of treatment, such that genital-preserving treatments will, necessarily, be more preserving of sexual functioning. Continued efforts to empirically examine the suitability of such conservative surgeries is potentially the most important effort that can be taken to reduce sexual morbidity. (2) The sexual difficulties of women with vulvar disease will be the most difficult to prevent or treat with psychological intervention. A realistic goal may be, for example, to reduce the incidence and severity of sexual morbidity for women with vulvar disease to the range of that for the cervix patient described above (i.e. reduction of 80 to 90% morbidity to 40 to 50%).

Despite the high incidence and severity of sexual morbidity for women with gynecologic cancer, we are much closer to addressing the difficulties of these women. Increasingly, issues of quality of life are being raised.[2,51] The international community of oncologists (e.g. International Union Against Cancer) and gynecologic oncologists (e.g. International Gynecologic Cancer Society) have taken significant steps, for example, to include sexuality data in the scientific programs of its meetings. As with most issues, further commitment, attention, education and action is needed, but important forward steps have begun.

ACKNOWLEDGEMENT

Research in and preparation of this chapter was supported by Grant I R23 GA 35702-01A1 from the National Institutes of Health — National Cancer Institute, and Grant PRB-27 from the American Cancer Society awarded to Barbara L. Andersen.

REFERENCES

1. Abitbol M M, Davenport J H 1974 Sexual dysfunction after therapy for cervical carcinoma. Am J Obstet Gynecol 119: 181
2. American Cancer Society 1987 Workshop on psychosexual and reproductive issues of cancer patients. January, 1987, San Antonio, Texas
3. Andersen B L 1981 A comparison of systematic desensitization and directed masturbation in the treatment of primary orgasmic dysfunction in females. J Consult Clin Psychol 49: 568
4. Andersen B L 1983 Primary orgasmic dysfunction: diagnostic considerations and review of treatment. Psychol Bull 93: 105
5. Andersen B L 1985 Sexual functioning morbidity among cancer survivors: present status and future research directions. Cancer 55: 1835

6. Andersen B L (ed) 1986 Women with Cancer: Psychological Perspectives. Springer-Verlag, New York
7. Andersen B L, Anderson B, deProsse C 1989 Controlled prospective longitudinal study of women with cancer: I. Sexual functioning outcomes. J Consult Clin Psychol 57: 683
8. Andersen B L, Broffitt B 1988 Is there a reliable and valid self report measure of sexual behavior? Arch Sex Behav 17: 509
9. Andersen B L, Broffitt B, Karlsson J A, Turnquist D C 1989 A psychometric analysis of the Sexual Arousability Index. J Consult Clin Psychol 57: 123
10. Andersen B L, Hacker N F 1983 Psychosexual adjustment after vulvar surgery. Obstet Gynecol 62: 457
11. Andersen B L, Hacker N F 1983 Psychosexual adjustment following pelvic exenteration. Obstet Gynecol 61: 331
12. Andersen B L, Karlsson J A, Anderson B, Tewfik H H 1984 Anxiety and cancer treatment: Response to stressful radiotherapy. Health Psychol 3: 535
13. Andersen B L, Lachenbruch P A, Anderson B, deProsse C 1986 Sexual dysfunction and signs of gynecologic cancer. Cancer 57: 1880
14. Andersen B L, Turnquist D, LaPolla J P, Turner D 1988 Sexual functioning after treatment of in situ vulvar cancer: preliminary report. Obstet Gynecol 71: 15
15. Bard M, Sutherland A M 1952 Adaptation to radical mastectomy. Cancer 8: 656
16. Barlow D H 1986 Causes of sexual dysfunction: the role of anxiety and cognitive interference. J Consult Clin Psychol 54: 140
17. Berek J S, Hacker N F (eds) 1985 Practical Gynecologic Oncology. Williams & Wilkins, Baltimore
18. Bernard L 1986 Methodology issues in studies of sexuality and hysterectomy. J Sex Res 22: 108
19. Bertelsen K 1983 Sexual dysfunction after treatment of cervical cancer. Dan Med Bull 30: 31
20. Brown R S, Haddox V, Posada A, Rubio A 1972 Social and psychological adjustment following pelvic exenteration. Am J Obstet Gynecol 114: 162
21. Cacioppo J T, Andersen B L, Turnquist D C, Petty R E 1986 Psychophysiological comparison processes: interpreting cancer symptoms. In Andersen B L (ed) Women with Cancer: Psychological Perspectives. Springer-Verlag, New York, p 141
22. Cain E N, Kohorn E I, Quinlan D M, Latimer K, Schwartz P E 1986 Psychosocial benefits of a cancer support group. Cancer 57: 183
23. Capone M A, Good R S, Westie K S, Jacobsen A F 1980 Psychosocial rehabilitation of gynecologic oncology patients. Arch Phys Med Rehabil 61: 128
24. Cotten-Huston A L, Wheeler K A 1983 Preorgasmic group treatment: assertiveness, marital adjustment, and sexual function in women. J Sex Marital Ther 9: 296
25. Decker W H, Schwartzman E 1962 Sexual function following treatment for carcinoma of the cervix. Am J Obstet Gynecol 83: 401
26. Dekker J, Everaerd W 1983 A long term follow-up study of couples treated for sexual dysfunctions. J Sex Marital Ther 9: 99
27. Dempsey G M, Buchsbaum H J, Morrison J 1975 Psychosocial adjustment to pelvic exenteration. Gynecol Oncol 3: 325
28. DiSaia P J, Creasman W T, Rich W M 1979 An alternate approach to early cancer of the vulva. Am J Obstet Gynecol 33: 825
29. Frank E, Anderson C, Rubenstein D 1978 Frequency of sexual dysfunction in 'normal' couples. N Engl J Med 299: 111
30. Froewis J, Picha E 1955 Der Einfluss der Radikaloperationen bei Carcinoma colli uteri auf das Sexualleben der Frau mit besonderer Berucksichtigung der Wertheimschen Operation (The influence of radical operations upon the sexual activity of women with special regards to Wertheim surgery). Geburtshilfe Frauenheilkd 15: 806
31. Hacker N F, Berek J S, Lagasse L D et al 1984 Individualization of treatment for Stage I squamous cell vulvar carcinoma. Obstet Gynecol 63: 155
32. Heiss M 1954 Ueber Sexualstorungen nach Radikalbehandlung des Collumcarcinoms und ihre Therapie (Sexual disturbances following radical treatment for collumcarcinoma and their therapy). Med Klin 25: 992
33. Iversen T, Abeler V, Aalders J 1981 Individualized treatment of Stage I carcinoma of the vulva. Obstet Gynecol 57: 85
34. Kaplan H S 1979 Disorders of Sexual Desire. Brunner/Mazel, New York
35. Kemp M 1979 Dealing with depression after radical surgery. Nursing, February p 47
36. Kilkku P, Gronroos M, Punnonen R 1982 Sexual function after conization of the uterine cervix. Gynecol Oncol 14: 209
37. Kilmann P R, Mills K H, Bella B et al 1983 The effects of sex education on women with secondary orgasmic dysfunction. J Sex Marital Ther 9: 79
38. Kinsey A C, Pomeroy W B, Martin C E 1948 Sexual Behavior in the Human Male. Saunders, Philadelphia
39. Kinsey A C, Pomeroy W G, Martin C E, Gebhard P H 1953 Sexual Behavior in the Human Female. Saunders, Philadelphia
40. Knight R V D 1943 Bowen's disease of the vulva. Am J Obstet Gynecol 46: 514
41. Knorr N J 1967 A depressive syndrome following pelvic exenteration and ileostomy. Arch Surg 94: 258
42. Lasnik E, Tatra G 1986 Sexualverhalten nach primarer Strahlentherapie des Zervixkarzinoms (Sexual behavior after primary radiotherapy of cervical carcinoma). Geburtshilfe Frauenheilkd 46: 813
43. Lau H U 1967 Rehabilitation bei Kollumkarzinomen (Rehabilitation for cervical carcinoma). Zentralbl Gynakologie 89: 1649
44. Leiber L, Plumb M, Gerstenzang M, Holland J 1976 The communication of affection between cancer patients and their spouses. Psychomet Med 38: 379
45. Lieblum S R, Rosen R C (eds) 1988 Sexual Desire Disorders. Guilford Press, New York
46. Masters W H, Johnson V E 1966 Human Sexual Response. Little Brown, Boston, Ma
47. Masters W H, Johnson V E 1970 Human Sexual Inadequacy. Little Brown, Boston, Ma
48. Metzger L F, Roberts T F, Bauman L J 1983 Effects of age and marital status on emotional distress after mastectomy. J Psychosoc Oncol 1: 17
49. Miller S M, Mangan G E 1983 Interacting effects of information and coping style in adapting to gynecologic stress: should the doctor tell all? J Pers Soc Psychol 45: 223
50. Moth I, Andreasson B, Jensen S B, Bock J E 1983 Sexual function and somatopsychic reactions after vulvectomy. Dan Med Bull 30: 27
51. National Institutes of Health 1987 International Conference on Reproduction and Human Cancer. Bethesda, Md
52. Newcomb M D, Bentler P M 1983 Dimensions of subjective female orgasmic responsiveness. J Pers Soc Psychol 44: 862
53. Newman G, Nichols C R 1960 Sexual activities and attitudes in older persons. JAMA 173: 33
54. Nutter D E, Condron M K 1983 Sexual fantasy and activity patterns of females with inhibited sexual desire versus normal controls. J Sex Marital Ther 9: 276
55. Ngan H Y S, Tang G 1988 Further study of sexual functioning following treatment of carcinoma of the cervix in Chinese patients. J Psychosom Obstet Gynaecol 9: 117
56. O'Hoy K M, Tang G W K 1985 Sexual functioning following treatment for carcinoma of the cervix. J Psychosom Obstet Gynaecol 4: 51
57. Pfeiffer E, Davis G 1972 Determinants of sexual behavior in middle and old age. J Am Gerontol Society 20: 151
58. Picha E 1957 Uber das Sexualleben von Frauen nach Radiumbehandlung gynakologischer Erkrankungen. (The sex life of women after radiation therapy for gynecologic cancer). Geburtshilfe Frauenheilkd 17: 81
59. Pitkin R M, Van Voorhis L W 1971 Post-irradiation vaginitis: an evaluation of prophylaxis with topical estrogen. Therapeutic Radiology 99: 417
60. Schultz W C M, Weijmar M, Wimja K, Van de Wiel H B M, Bouma J, Janssens J 1986 Sexual rehabilitation of radical vulvectomy patients: a pilot study. J Psychosom Obstet Gynaecol 5: 119

61. Seibel M M, Freeman M G, Graves W L 1980 Carcinoma of the cervix and sexual function. Obstet Gynecol 55: 484

62. Steinberg M D, Juliano M A, Wise L 1985 Psychological outcome of lumpectomy versus mastectomy in the treatment of breast cancer. Am J Psychiatry 142: 34

63. Stellman R E, Goodwin J M Robinson J M, Dansak D, Hilgers R D 1984 Psychological effects of vulvectomy. Psychosom 25: 779

64. Sutherland A M, Orbach C F, Dyk R B, Bard M 1952 The psychological impact of cancer and cancer surgery. I. Adaptation to the dry colostomy. Cancer 5: 857

65. Tamburini M, Filiberti A, Ventafridda V, Bianchi F, Volterrani F 1984 Emotional status, sexuality and quality of life in patients treated for carcinoma of uterine cervix. The Cervix 2: 261

66. Tamburini M, Filiberti A, Ventafridda V, DePalo G 1986 Quality of life and psychological state after radical vulvectomy. J Psychosom Obstet Gynaecol 5: 263

67. Vasicka A, Popovich N R, Brausch C C 1958 Post-irradiation course of patients with cervical carcinoma. Obstet Gynecol 11: 403

68. Vera M I 1981 Quality of life following pelvic exenteration. Gynecol Oncol 12: 355

69. Vincent C E, Vincent B, Greiss F C, Linton E B 1975 Some marital-sexual concomitants of carcinoma of the cervix. Southern Med J 68: 552

70. Wallace D H, Barbach L G 1974 Preorgasmic group treatments. J Sex Marital Ther 1: 146

71. Walling M K, Andersen B L, Johnson S R 1989 Hormonal replacement therapy for postmenopausal women: Sexual outcomes and related gynecologic effects. Arch Sex Behav. 19: 119

72. Woodruff J D 1985 Carcinoma in situ of the vulva. Clin Obstet Gynecol 28: 230

73. Zimmer D, Borchardt E, Fischle C 1983 Sexual fantasies of sexually distressed and non-distressed men and women: an empirical comparison. J Sex Marital Ther 9: 38

91. The psychological processes of recovery from gynecologic cancer

L. J. Thompson   B. L. Andersen   A. D. DePetrillo

INTRODUCTION

Cancer is not a single event or time limited crisis. Rather, the experience can include a series of threats and challenges to the physical, psychological, sexual and social integrity of patients and their families. These threats may vary in intensity and duration, and thus the impact of cancer and the problems it imposes may change. Some women with gynecologic cancer surmount their difficulties and adjust, 'while others move from crisis to crisis, causing themselves and their families much anguish'.[30] For decades, descriptions of adjustment to cancer and its treatment were largely clinical, and focused on the general effects or outcome of a particular event, such as diagnosis or beginning treatment. More recently, controlled research describing the specific difficulties that cancer patients may face, the etiologic mechanisms for adjustment, and the methods for coping with the experiences has appeared. In much of this research, breast cancer patients have been studied (see reference 52 for a review) and these findings can be applied, in part, to the experiences of other cancer patients. Also, some research programs now focus specifically on gynecologic cancer patients.[2] With early diagnosis and aggressive therapy, approximately two-thirds of women with gynecologic cancer will survive at least 5 years. The quality of that survival, however, needs to be examined.

The present chapter provides an overview of the psychological processes of adjustment to gynecologic cancer, from first symptom to cure (or an extended disease-free interval). Mullen[57] has suggested that survival from cancer begins at the point of diagnosis, as patients are forced to confront their own mortality and make transitions or changes in their lives that may become permanent. According to this model, individuals go through some relatively predictable stages called 'seasons of survival', including acute, extended and permanent survival. Data on the psychological processes of adjustment to gynecologic cancer will be reviewed within this framework, to enhance our understanding of the many challenges facing women with gynecologic cancer.

SYMPTOM APPEARANCE

Efforts have recently begun in the area of tertiary cancer prevention in an effort to shorten the delay in seeking a diagnosis once symptom awareness has occurred.[69] Unlike many medical problems, the development of malignancy and the appearance of symptoms is usually protracted, and a complex and changing symptom experience can be typical. The psychological and behavioral aspects of illness representation[47] and symptom interpretation[16] have been offered as theoretical frameworks for understanding illness interpretation and patient delay in seeking medical advice. Recent studies indicate that the lion's share of cancer delay (i.e. from symptom/sign awareness to appearing before a physician for consultation) is accounted for by the time necessary for the patient to decide that the symptoms indicate 'illness' rather than a normal and/or non-serious health condition; (e.g. a 45-year-old woman eventually decides that her irregular vaginal bleeding may indicate cancer, rather than menopause). In addition, unexpected symptoms, such as sexual dysfunction,[7] can add to the complexity of symptom interpretation for gynecologic cancer patients.

ACUTE SURVIVAL

This stage begins with diagnosis and continues into the primary treatment course of surgery, radiation and/or chemotherapy. Emotional reactions to the initial diagnosis of cancer may include shock, sadness (depression), fear (anxiety), guilt, disbelief, anger, confusion and helplessness.[3,17,57,62,66,70] Each emotion is important for understanding the process patients undergo when learning of their diagnosis, completing tumor evaluation and beginning treatment.

Diagnosis

Comparison of studies examining the incidence and prevalence of emotional distress and psychiatric sequelae among people with cancer is difficult, because of the variety of research designs, assessment strategies and diagnostic criteria used. Most studies cite depression as the most prevalent affective problem, but estimates of unipolar diagnosis are in the order of 5 to 6%.[25,45] When major depression and adjustment disorder with depressed mood are considered, prevalence rates are higher.[25]

In a study of 83 women with gynecologic cancer, Evans et al[29] reported that 23% of the women had a major depression, 24% had an adjustment disorder with depressed mood, and 14% had other psychiatric illnesses. Depressive reactions of 60 women with cervical, ovarian or endometrial cancer were classified by Cain et al[17] as mild in 30%, moderate in 35% and severe in 35% of patients. In general, higher rates of depression are found in patients in active treatment rather than in follow-up, receiving palliative rather than curative treatment, with pain or other disturbing symptoms rather than not, and with a history of an affective disorder. The latter attributes may represent risk factors for depression among women with gynecologic cancer. Among patient samples not having these characteristics, the base rate of major depression is likely to be in the range of 5 to 6%, comparable to that of the general population.

It is difficult to make a diagnosis of depression in cancer patients, as it is for patients with other serious illnesses. Vegetative symptoms, i.e. poor appetite or weight loss, insomnia or hypersomnia, loss of energy or fatigue, and loss of sexual desire or interest, may provide important initial clues. The diagnostician must determine if such symptomatology is representative of depression, disease-related events, or some combination of factors. When depression does occur, it is often reactive, i.e. it occurs soon after the diagnosis and the content of the ruminations reflect the diagnostic event.[61] Depressive symptoms include dysphoric mood, loss of interest, loss of energy or fatigue and difficulty in thinking or concentrating.

Anxiety disorder is the affective problem second in frequency among cancer patients. Derogatis et al[25] estimated the prevalence to be 7% among outpatient cancer patients currently undergoing treatment. In a study of 44 breast cancer patients interviewed at the time of diagnosis, Hughes[40] estimated that 25% of the sample had severe anxiety reactions. Anxiety-related problems are typically manifested by the symptoms of generalized anxiety; in addition to the classic fear, worry and rumination, other symptoms include motor tension (e.g. feeling shaky, muscle tension, restlessness and easy fatigability), autonomic hyperactivity (e.g. abdominal distress, frequent urination), and/or indications of vigilance and scanning (e.g. difficulty concentrating, trouble falling asleep or staying asleep, feeling on edge). Much of the content of the anxiety-provoking thought is focused on medical examinations and fear of the cancer treatment effects. Other targets include the life disruption and change that may occur because the individual

has cancer. The common spheres of worry include family, money, work and illness[12] (e.g. Who will take care of the children when I am in hospital? What if our insurance does not cover the bills? Will I be able to go back to work? What if I never get well?).

Silberfarb & Greer[66] maintain that it is the factors of helplessness and uncertainty that set the cancer experience apart from other illnesses, and influence how patients respond to their illness. Patients' inability to control much of what happens to them in this acute survival stage increases dependency on health care professionals and reduces one's sense of mastery. For patients and physicians alike, the eventual outcome of the disease and its treatment may be uncertain. Among women with gynecologic cancer, such uncertainties and feelings of helplessness may be most common and troublesome for those with ovarian cancer.[23] With this type of disease, multiple treatment protocols may be used with limited certainty offered as to their benefits. Treatment success is often evaluated by additional difficult procedures, such as a second look operation.

Treatment

A certain component of the emotional distress occurring at diagnosis is the anticipation of undergoing difficult treatment(s). The strength of a patient's belief in her ability to cope with the adverse effects (e.g. pain, nausea, anorexia) of those treatments, may determine the amount of distress experienced.[68,69] Data consistently portray more distress (particularly fear and anxiety), slower rates of emotional recovery and, perhaps, additional behavioral difficulties (e.g. conditioned anxiety reactions) than are found with relatively healthy women also undergoing medical treatment (e.g. hysterectomy, cholecystectomy).

There have been few investigations of cancer surgery, and no studies of women facing gynecologic cancer surgery. However, there are numerous descriptive and intervention studies of the reactions of healthy women undergoing surgery for benign conditions such as uterine fibroids.[9] The latter studies are consistent in their portrayal of high levels of self-reported preoperative anxiety predictive of lowered postoperative anxiety, and postoperative anxiety predictive of recovery (e.g. time out of bed, pain reports). What may distinguish cancer surgery patients are higher overall levels of distress and slower emotional rebound. Gottesman & Lewis,[32] for example, found greater and more lasting feelings of crisis and helplessness among cancer patients in comparison to benign surgery patients for as long as 2 months following discharge.

Considering the latter data, findings on the interaction patterns of physicians and cancer patients on morning surgical rounds is disturbing. Blanchard et al[13] found attending physicians on a cancer unit to be less likely to engage in supportive behavior and address patients needs than physicians treating general medical patients. The heavier volume of more seriously ill patients common to cancer units may be a source of this unfortunate relationship. Related findings indicate that oncology nurses may find their job significantly more stressful than other assignments (e.g. cardiac, intensive care or operating room nursing).[67] Taken together, these findings suggest that the interactions between oncologists, oncology nurses and gynecologic cancer patients may be even more important to patient adjustment than is commonly acknowledged.

While radiation therapy can be used for all gynecologic sites of disease, the majority have either cervical or endometrial disease. For empirical understanding of radiation fears, the surgical anxiety studies described above have been used as a paradigm. Here, again, high levels of anticipatory anxiety are found, and if interventions to reduce distress are not conducted,[63] heightened post-treatment anxiety is also found[6,8] and may be maintained for as long as 3 months post-therapy, particularly when treatment symptoms, such as diarrhea or fatigue, linger.[43] When subacute side effects resolve (usually by 12 months post-treatment), there appears to be no higher incidence of emotional difficulties for patients receiving radiation therapy than for patients undergoing surgery.[41] A clinical description of women's concerns and fears while receiving radiation therapy is provided in Table 91.1.

Of all the treatment modalities, the greatest progress has been made toward understanding the psychological reactions to chemotherapy, particularly the side effects of nausea and vomiting. Research has progressed from prevalence estimates[59] and single-subject and large sample descriptive studies, to controlled investigations focused on eliminating or reducing the disruptive side effects of nausea and vomiting through hypnosis,[64] progressive muscle relaxation with guided imagery,[18] systematic desensitization,[56] attentional diversion or redirection[34] and biofeedback.[15] Research has also targeted individual (i.e high pretreatment anxiety or general distress, severity of post-treatment vomiting in the early cycle, age) and situational (i.e. more emetogenic regimens, higher doses or greater amounts of chemotherapy) differences which place patients at risk.[10]

As an example of investigations in this area, Nerenz et al[58] studied 61 patients receiving chemotherapy, and found that the vague, diffuse side effects such as fatigue or pain, resulted in higher levels of distress than did specific symptoms, such as nausea and vomiting. The variations in

---

Table 91.1 Common misconceptions and concerns about radiotherapy for gynecologic cancer patients.*

Misconceptions
Treatment results in permanent radiation contamination and, during treatment, one is radioactive.
Radiation attacks only malignant cells and leaves other cells/tissues/structures unaffected.
Radiation is reserved for poor prognosis or terminal patients.

Concerns regarding external beam treatment
It is difficult for many patients to manage transportation and scheduling in order to receive a daily treatment during a 4 to 6 week period.
Many patients waiting for their daily treatment are visibly ill and/or in pain. This waiting room experience is depressing and anxiety-provoking to the less debilitated or ambulatory patients.
Disrobing and exposing the pelvis and genitals for treatment is embarrassing.
Field markings and tattoos are visible reminders of a diseased body.
The treatment machines are imposing; lying under one is threatening and can feel dangerous.
For patients 'in house' during treatment, isolation and boredom may characterize the non-treatment hours.
Once treatment side effects of fatigue, loss of appetite, and bowel irritation begin, they are debilitating and worsen with continued treatment.
For the woman who was premenopausal at diagnosis, hot flushes may signal the unexpected and regretted loss of fertility.
With perineal fields, the skin becomes irritated and painful.
With extended fields, nausea, vomiting, food aversions and anorexia are difficult to tolerate and, on occasion, self-perpetuating.
As side effects worsen over the course of treatment, they are convincing reminders to a woman that she is ill and her life threatened by cancer.
Most patients are unaware that physical recovery following treatment, particularly energy level, requires months.
Post-treatment follow-up reminds patients of their cancer, prompt recollections of the difficulties of diagnosis and treatment, and generate fears that a recurrence will be found.

Concerns regarding intracavitary radiotherapy
Unlike external radiotherapy, most patients have never heard of, and/or know nothing about, intracavitary treatment.
Being radioactive during placement is a realistic, fear-producing circumstance.
The treatment is uncomfortable and painful: e.g. the vaginal packing produces pain and/or a sensation of bloating; gas pains are common; achiness, particularly in the back, is common.
The isolation required for treatment produces loneliness and fear (e.g. 'Will someone come or stay with me if I need help?').
From a self-care perspective, the treatment experience is annoying (e.g. minimal bathing, dependence on others who are only present for minutes at a time) and frustrating (e.g. the difficulty of eating while on one's back).
Removal of the intracavitary radioactive applicator is keenly anticipated and delay, whether minutes or hours, occurs when patients have the least tolerance and energy to cope.
The time needed to remove the packing and instruments can be brief, but women describe it as extremely painful.
From the patient's perspective, these experiences are worsened for any second application, although medical staff may mistakenly believe that the second treatment should be easier. Women are usually more debilitated prior to their second treatment and less tolerant of the anxiety-provoking and painful experiences.

* Adapted from Karsson J A, Andersen B L 1986 Radiation therapy and psychological distress: outcomes and recommendations for enhancing adjustment. *J Psychosom Obstet Gynaecol* 5: 283

distress may reflect the different meanings ascribed to the symptoms. For example, to patients, fatigue may be a clearer marker of disease progression or recurrence, and thus fear and distress may increase. Nerenz and colleagues[58] suggest that patients should be given detailed information during their treatment so that they interpret symptoms more accurately. When possible, they should also be encouraged to monitor and interpret objective signs of treatment effectiveness, such as the shrinking of palpable nodes or reduction of ascites, to reduce some of the distress associated with uncertainty of outcome.

In addition to those discussed above, there are other distressing side effects of cancer treatment in general that remain for patients to cope with. Appetite and weight loss are significant clinical problems for gynecologic cancer patients, particularly for women with ovarian disease receiving chemotherapy, women treated with extended field abdominal radiation, and/or individuals susceptible to tumor-induced adverse effects. Cosmetic side effects of cancer treatment (e.g. loss of scalp and pubic hair, skin changes, and distorted features) are also problematic, as they can affect the woman's body image, sexuality and self-esteem. Patient resources, such as the book 'Beauty and Cancer',[60] can offer very practical solutions to help overcome some of the fear, intimidation and isolation women may feel during and after cancer therapies.

As the literature on adjustment during the acute survival period is examined, it is important to question why some patients are more effective than others in coping with this crisis period. Prior levels of psychological stability, patterns of past coping, the presence of supportive persons and, of course, disease and treatment variables have all been identified as important predictors.[24,27,29,37,49,54,55,66,70] It has been hypothesized that psychological difficulties do not spontaneously occur because of cancer. Instead, prior difficulties are believed to recur or worsen during the cancer crisis and complicate a patient's adjustment.[50] There is no evidence to suggest that cancer precipitates additional or more severe psychiatric episodes than would otherwise occur.

EXTENDED SURVIVAL

The next period, of 'extended survival' begins as the woman attempts to resume previous activities, re-establish her social role(s), and renew her relationships following initial treatment. There is an effort to re-establish normality in her life, and challenges associated with re-entering the home, workplace, and other environments must be met. The earliest writings (from the 1950's to the 1980's) suggested that the psychological trajectory of adjustment for women was, at best, difficult, with somatic problems, psychological distress,[11,51] impaired relationships,[28,71] preoccupation with death,[33] and/or general life disruption,

such as reduced employment or career opportunities.[65] Many of these pioneering reports of primarily breast cancer patients were clinical in focus and, in general, uncontrolled for disease variables now recognized as moderators of adjustment. By the end of this same period, cancer had become more public, more survivable for some (e.g. there has been a 63% decline in the age-adjusted death rate for uterine cancer from 1950 to 1980–82),[1] and clinical trials were able to examine treatment toxicity following the establishment of effective therapy (e.g. extent of surgery for breast disease). These important changes account, in part, for the positive findings emerging in the study of long-term adjustment.

If the disease is controlled, and recovery from treatment proceeds unimpaired, longitudinal data indicate that by one year post-treatment the severe distress of diagnosis has dissipated and emotions have stabilized. One controlled, prospective longitudinal study indicates no differences between the levels of emotional distress of women with Stage I or II gynecologic cancer and either benign disease or healthy comparison subjects.[3] Similar data by other investigators,[36] and longitudinal study of breast cancer patients compared with subjects who have benign disease, reveals the same pattern of positive long-term adjustment.[14] Similar decreased levels of distress have been found in retrospective[21] and longitudinal[26] studies of Hodgkin's disease and non-Hodgkin's lymphoma patients. This consistency of findings for the studies conducted during the 1980's is important, because they represent replications across gender, site and, to some degree, treatment toxicity, and would reflect the base rate estimates for emotional distress due to disease and treatment factors.

Data on the interpersonal relationships of cancer patients suggest that, in general, satisfaction predominates. The majority of relationships remain intact, satisfactory and, on occasion, stronger.[48,53] When problems do occur, they include estrangement and distress.[71] For example, a female cancer patient may wish to discuss her feelings in an attempt to cope with the cancer, but her husband may be more inclined to advise his wife to 'put the experience behind you'.[48] For other couples, the distress of kin (e.g. spouse) may approach that of the patient.[20] Particularly for the mother with young children in the home, the mother and the family is at heightened risk for emotional distress.

Special adjustment difficulties may be encountered by women of childbearing age who are infertile following treatment. They may experience feelings of loss, grief and further lack of control. As one patient remarked, 'it's not that I can't have children so much, but that the choice is taken away from me. It's one more way in which this cancer is stripping me of the things I value'. For most women, this loss may be made manifest as they socialize with friends or family who are pregnant or who have young children, or as they consider adoption. Acceptance may not come for months, and well-intended comments of others (e.g. 'You should just be thankful you are alive') may not be helpful.

Sometimes, treatment for gynecologic cancer requires an extended recovery period. Further, the emotional impact of genital disfigurement, pelvic scarring or hair loss may not occur until the woman is in the privacy of her own home. Retrospective reports from women who underwent radical gynecologic treatment indicate that the magnitude of post-treatment physical complications, such as leg edema or chronic fatigue, are predictive of continuing or new emotional distress. Feelings of depression, social isolation and body dissatisfaction have all been reported by patients as they recover from extensive surgery such as radical vulvectomy or pelvic exenteration.[4,5,44]

Dealing with the possibility of recurrence is a challenge to all who have been treated for cancer; however, few data have documented the impact of this concern on the day-to-day functioning of former patients. Anecdotal reports suggest that individuals may be reluctant, for example, to purchase investments for their retirement or make long range commitments in their personal or professional lives, because of their own uncertainty about the future. Data appear to indicate that such fear of disease progression or recurrence is common to patients and their partners, whether or not their disease is early or advanced.[33]

Psychological reactions to disease recurrence can produce higher levels of distress than were experienced at the time of initial diagnosis, probably because the patient realizes that the treatment with the greatest likelihood of cure has failed. Data indicate that the initial diagnosis of gynecologic cancer is characterized by a significant depressive effect, whereas recurrence may be characterized by even greater depression and anger.[3] Patients with ovarian cancer often have to cope with multiple treatments and failures during the course of their illness, and consequently may be at higher risk of prolonged emotional distress.[23]

PERMANENT SURVIVAL

During this stage, the likelihood of disease recurrence is reduced, and the disease is regarded as arrested or 'cured'. This may be the point at which the long-term effects of cancer and its treatment are realized. Literature on adjustment during the permanent survival period is limited, and the need for research documenting the experience of long-

term cancer survivors has been emphasized only recently.[19,39] Although studies of adults at 5, 10 or 15 years or longer after their treatment are few, research suggests that long-term effects may not always be negative. This may be due in part to some of the factors previously mentioned as contributing to positive findings in studies of long-term adjustment, e.g. advances in effective treatment with reduced toxicity. Descriptions of a greater appreciation of life and a more positive attitude toward living following an experience with cancer[22,31,42,50] may also reflect a shift in values, a reprioritization of worries and concerns, and an increased awareness of people, nature and relationships. Cancer is not a devastating and permanently debilitating experience for all.[20] As women search for the meaning of illness to them, they may begin to describe its positive, life-enriching aspects. The attempt to find a silver lining may be seen as both a coping strategy and a positive outcome of the cancer experience.

SUMMARY

Significant progress has been made in the understanding of the psychological and behavioral aspects of cancer. While more is known about the adjustment of breast cancer patients, men, children and women with diseases of other sites, such as gynecologic cancer, are becoming more commonly studied. Future research will likely test the generality of these descriptive data, and formulate general principles of adjustment to illness. Also, the rich descriptive data base is providing a foundation for developing and testing clinical interventions designed to prevent and treat psychological and/or behavioral morbidity. With this knowledge, we can move more effectively toward the ultimate goal of cancer care as described by Magnes & Mendelson[50] a decade ago. That is, 'to minimize the discontinuity between a patient's life before and after cancer and to support those transitions that maximize a patient's sense of self-determination, usefulness, satisfaction and self-esteem'.

ACKNOWLEDGEMENT

This effort was supported in part by Grant 1 R23 CA35702 from the National Institutes of Health — National Cancer Institute and Grant PBR-27 from the American Cancer Society awarded to Barbara L. Andersen.

REFERENCES

1. American Cancer Society 1986 Facts and Figures. American Cancer Society, New York
2. Andersen B L, Anderson B 1986 Psychosomatic aspects of gynecologic oncology: present status and future research directions. J Psychosom Obstet Gynaecol 5: 233
3. Andersen B L, Anderson B, deProsse C 1989 Controlled

prospective longitudinal study of women with cancer: II Psychological outcomes. J Consul Clin Psychol 57: 692
4. Andersen B L, Hacker N F 1983 Psychosexual adjustment after vulvar surgery. Obstet Gynecol 62: 457
5. Andersen B L, Hacker N F 1983 Psychosexual adjustment following pelvic exenteration. Obstet Gynecol 61: 331
6. Andersen B L, Karlsson J A, Anderson B, Tewfik H H 1984

Anxiety and cancer treatment: response to stressful radiotherapy. Health Psychol 48: 1024

7. Andersen B L, Lachenbruch P A, Anderson B, deProsse C 1986 Sexual dysfunction and signs of gynecologic cancer. Cancer 57: 1880

8. Andersen B L, Tewfik H H 1985 Psychological reactions to radiation therapy: reconsideration of the adaptive aspects of anxiety. J Pers Soc Psychol 48: 1024

9. Anderson K O, Masur F T 1983 Psychological preparation for invasive medical and dental procedures. J Behav Med 6: 1

10. Andrykowski M A, Redd W H, Hartfield A K 1985 Development of anticipatory nausea: a prospective analysis. J Consult Clin Psychol 53: 447

11. Bard M, Sutherland A M 1952 Adaptation to radical mastectomy. Cancer 8: 656

12. Barlow D H 1986 Causes of sexual dysfunction: the role of anxiety and cognitive inference. J Consult Clin Psychol 54: 140

13. Blanchard C G, Ruckdeschel J C, Labreque M S, Frisch S, Blanchard E B 1987 The impact of a designated cancer unit on house staff behaviors toward patients. Cancer 60: 2348

14. Bloom J R 1987 Psychological aspects of breast cancer study group. Psychological response to mastectomy. Cancer 59: 189

15. Burish T G, Shartner C D, Lyles J N 1981 Effectiveness of multiple muscle site EMG feedback and relaxation training in reducing the aversiveness of cancer chemotherapy. Biofeedback and Self Regulation 6: 523

16. Cacioppo J T, Andersen B L, Turnquist D C, Petty R E 1986 Psychophysiological comparison processes: interpreting cancer symptoms. In: Andersen B L (ed) Women with Cancer: Psychological Perspectives. Springer-Verlag, New York p 141

17. Cain E N, Kohorn E, Quinlan D, Schwartz P, Latimer K, Rodgers L 1983 Psychological reactions to the diagnosis of gynecological cancer. Obstet Gynecol 62: 635

18. Carey M P, Burish T G 1988 Etiology and treatment of the psychological side effects associated with cancer chemotherapy. Psyc Bull 104: 307

19. Carter B 1989 Cancer survivorship: A topic for nursing research. ONF 16: 435

20. Cassileth B R, Lusk E J, Strouse T B et al 1984 Psychological status in chronic illness: a comparative analysis of six diagnostic groups. New Engl J Med 311: 506

21. Cella D F, Tross S 1986 Psychological adjustment to survival from Hodgkin's disease. J Con Clin Psyc 54: 616

22. Danoff B, Kramer N, Irwin P, Gottlieb A 1983 Assessment of quality of life in long term survivors after definitive radiotherapy. Am J Clin Oncol 6: 339

23. DePetrillo A D, Thompson L J 1989 The experience of ovarian cancer: a quality of life perspective. In: Sharp F, Soutter W (eds) Ovarian Cancer: Proceedings of the Second International Forum on Ovarian Cancer. Chameleon Press, London

24. Derogatis L R, Feldstein M, Morrow G R et al 1979 A survey of psychotropic drug prescriptions in an oncology population. Cancer 44: 1919

25. Derogatis L R, Morrow G R, Fetting J et al 1983 The prevalence of psychiatric disorders among cancer patients. JAMA 249: 751

26. Devlen J, Maguire P, Phillips P, Crowther D, Chambers H 1987 Psychological problems associated with diagnosis and treatment of lymphomas I: Retrospective study, and II: Prospective study. Br Med J 195: 953

27. Dobkin P L, Morrow G R 1986 Long term side effects in patients who have been treated successfully for cancer. J Psychosocial Oncology 34: 23

28. Dyk R B, Sutherland A M 1956 Adaptation of the spouse and other family members to the colostomy patient. Cancer 9: 123

29. Evans D W, McCartney C F, Nemeroff C B et al 1986 Depression in women treated for gynecologic cancer: clinical and neuroendocrine assessment. Am J Psychiatry 143: 447

30. Fitch M I 1986 The Construction and Initial Psychometric Evaluation of a Self-Report Questionnaire Designed to Predict Psychological Distress in Newly Diagnosed Cancer Patients. University of Toronto Press, Toronto

31. Frank Strongberg M, Wright P 1984 Ambulatory cancer patients perception of physical and psychosocial changes in their lives since the diagnosis of cancer. Cancer Nursing 7: 17

32. Gottesman D, Lewis M 1982 Differences in crisis reactions among cancer and surgery patients. J Consul Clin Psychol 50: 381

33. Gotay C 1984 The experience of cancer during the early and advanced stages. Soc Sci Med 18: 605

34. Green P G, Seime R J, Smith M E 1985 Distraction and relaxation training in the treatment of anticipatory nausea and vomiting: a single subject intervention. (Unpublished manuscript)

35. Gullo V, Cherico J, Shadick R 1974 Suggested stages and response styles in life threatening illness: a focus on the cancer patient. In: Schoenberg, Carr, Kutscher, Peretz, Golding (eds) Anticipatory Grief. Columbia University Press, New York

36. deHaes J C J M, van Oostrom M A, Welraart K 1986 The effect of radical and conserving surgery on quality of life of early breast cancer patients. Europ J Surg Oncol 12: 337

37. Holland J C 1981 The humanistic side of cancer care: changing issues and challenges. In American Cancer Society Proceedings of the 3rd National Conference on Human Values and Cancer. ACS, Washington

38. Holland J C 1982 Psychological aspects of cancer. In: Holland J F, Frei E (eds) Cancer Medicine. Lea & Febiger, Philadelphia

39. Holland J C 1988 Directions for the future. In: American Cancer Society Proceedings of the 5th National Conference on Human Values and Cancer. ACS, New York

40. Hughes J 1981 Emotional reactions to the diagnosis and treatment of early breast cancer. J Psychosom Res 26: 277

41. Hughson A V M, Cooper A F, McArdle C S, Smith D C 1987 Psychological effects of radiotherapy after mastectomy. Br Med J 294: 1515

42. Kennedy B J, Tellegen A, Kennedy S, Havernich N 1976 Psychological response of patients cured of advanced cancer. Cancer 38: 2184

43. King K B, Nail L M, Kreamer K, Strohl R A, Johnson J E 1985 Patients descriptions of the experience of receiving radiation therapy. ONF 12: 55

44. Knorr N J 1967 A depressive syndrome following pelvic exenteration and ileostomy. Arch Surg 94: 258

45. Lansky D B, List M A, Merrmann C A et al 1985 Absence of major depressive disorders in female cancer patients. J Clin Oncol 3: 1553

46. Levin P M, Silberfarb P M, Lipowski S J 1978 Mental disorders in 100 cancer patients. Cancer 42: 1385

47. Leventhal H, Meyer D, Nevenz D 1980 The common sense representation of illness danger. In Rachman S (ed) Contributions to Medical Psychology, Vol 2. Pergamon, Oxford

48. Lichtman R R, Taylor S E 1986 Close relationships and the female cancer patient. In: Andersen B L (ed) Women with Cancer: Psychological Perspectives. Springer-Verlag, New York, p 141

49. Magnes N L, Castro J R, Fobair P et al 1981 Patterns of psychosocial response to cancer: can effective adaptation be predicted? Radiation Oncology Biol Phys 7: 385

50. Magnes N L, Mendelson G A 1979 Effects of cancer on patients lives: a personological approach. In: Stone G C, Cohen F, Adler N E (eds) Health Psychology. Jossey-Bass Pub, San Francisco, p 280

51. Maguire G P, Lee E G, Bevington D J, Kuchermann C S, Crabtree R J, Cornell C E 1978 Psychiatric problems in the first year after mastectomy. Br Med J 1: 963

52. Meyerowitz B E 1980 Psychosocial correlates of breast cancer and its treatments. Psychol Bull 87: 108

53. Meyerowitz B E, Watkins I K, Sparks F C 1983 Psychological implications of adjuvant chemotherapy. A two year follow up. Cancer: 1541

54. Mishel M H, Hostetter T, King B, Graham V 1984 Predictors of psychosocial adjustment in patients newly diagnosed with gynecologic cancer. Cancer Nursing 7: 291

55. Morris T, Greer S, White P 1977 Psychological and social adjustment to mastectomy. Cancer 40: 2381

56. Morrow G R 1984 Appropriateness of taped versus live relaxation in the systematic desensitization of anticipatory nausea and vomiting in cancer patients. J Consult Clin Psychol 52: 1098

57. Mullen F 1981 Seasons of survival: reflections of a physician with cancer. New Engl J Med 313: 270

50. Nerenz D R, Leventhal H, Love H 1982 Factors contributing to emotional distress during cancer chemotherapy. Cancer 50: 1020

59. Nicholas D R 1982 Prevalence of anticipatory nausea and emesis in cancer chemotherapy patients. J Behav Med 5: 461

60. Noyes D D, Mellody P 1988 Beauty & Cancer: A Womans Guide to Looking Great While Experiencing the Side Effects of Cancer Therapy. AC Press, Los Angeles

61. Noyes R, Kathol R G 1986 Depression and cancer. Psychiatr Developments 2: 77

62. Peck A 1972 Emotional reactions to having cancer. Ca-A Cancer Journal for Clinicians 22: 284

63. Rainey L C 1985 Effects of preparatory education for radiation oncology patients. Cancer 56: 1056

64. Redd W H, Andersen G V, Minagawa R Y 1982 Hypnotic control of anticipatory emesis in patients receiving cancer chemotherapy. J Consult Clin Psychol 50: 14

65. Schonfield J 1972 Psychological factors related to delayed return to an earlier life-style in successfully treated cancer patients. J Psychosom Res 16: 41

66. Silberfarb P M, Greer S 1982 Psychological concomitants of cancer: clinical aspects. Am J Psychother 36: 470

67. Stewart B E, Meyerowitz B E, Jackson L E, Yarkin K L, Harvey J H 1982 Psychological stress associated with outpatient oncology nursing. Can Nur October: 383

68. Telch C, Telch M 1985 Psychological approaches for enhancing coping among cancer patients: a review. Clin Psychol Rev 5: 325

69. Temoshok L, DiClemente R J, Sweet D M, Blois M S, Sagebiell R W 1984 Factors related to patient delay in seeking medical attention for cutaneous malignant melanoma. Cancer 54: 3048

70. Thompson L J 1987 A pilot study examining the use of self-efficacy theory as applied to the problem of anorexia in patients with cancer who are receiving chemotherapy. University of Toronto Press, Toronto

71. Weisman A D 1974 Coping with Cancer. McGraw-Hill, New York

72. Wortman C B, Dunkel-Schetter C 1979 Interpersonal relationships and cancer: a theoretical analysis. J Soc Iss 35: 120

92. Palliative care: the care of the patient with far advanced gynecologic cancer

J. N. Lickiss

INTRODUCTION

Good clinicians have always focused not on diseases in patients but on patients with diseases. There is nothing new about comprehensive care of patients with far advanced irreversible gynecological cancer: indeed, it is the increased possibility of cure or at least control of gynecological cancer which has been the advance of recent decades. Yet the closing years of this century are witnessing a focusing of clinical efforts on the care of those women with irreversible and progressing disease.

There appears to be a concurrence of; *clinical realism* (more than half of the women who develop gynecological cancer will eventually die from this disease and, in many, therapy is clearly palliative from the time of diagnosis); the influence of *20th century psychology and personalist philosophies* (so manifest in the arts) at last impinging on medical practice; and the fruitfulness in such a milieu of the ideas and praxis generated within the *hospice movement* in the United Kingdom in the 1960s and 70s, with now international consequences. Whatever the reasons are, rigorous gynecological oncology includes, increasingly, within mainstream practice, a renewed focus on the care of patients in the final phase of their lives, with due regard for the care also of those most closely bonded with them and affected by their disease, notably their families.[29]

It is the concept of the *patient-as-subject* which has come into focus: the patient-as-person, center of her own activity, with capacities to know, understand, to love and receive love, to formulate objectives, to prepare to close her life (as an artist completes an artwork, a speaker a sentence, a musician a symphony) and to do all this in a unique ecological context, in time and space, with a unique personal history, on the foundation of a unique biological and cultural inheritance. An adequate anthropology must be at the basis of adequate human medicine, and each age, and indeed each person, redefines what it means to be human in the face especially of crisis, whether societal or personal.

There is evidence of a paradigm shift, in Kuhnian terms,[21] with respect to cancer medicine: vigorous new ideas are surviving and flourishing — and are influencing practice. The burgeoning of writing, both popular and scientific, concerning subjective aspects of illness, especially with respect to cancer, bares witness to the unease with which therapeutic endeavors, however brilliant, are being perceived. It is increasingly recognized that the stress that a cancer diagnosis places upon a patient and her family may be aggravated by treatment unless sufficient attention is paid to profoundly personal issues.[15] Suffering may actually be increased, not relieved, by poorly conceived and executed medical efforts: iatrogenic suffering is a reality.[7]

Trials of various antitumor measures have focused on response rates, and the improvements in survival and, often, quality of life of the responders are recognized as welcome advances: however, the situation of non-responders has had inadequate attention.

The woman whose tumor progresses or relapses rapidly may not only have failed to gain benefit, but may have lost a great deal in terms of quality and, especially, time, when time has become most precious. Non-responders (or even temporary responders) to direct anti-tumor measures (surgery, chemotherapy, radiotherapy) are occasionally not only sad but angry, even with the very doctors who have carefully and ethically tried well researched strategies. The issue of not only living well but also of dying with dignity has become prominent in public debate as well as in private discussion.[30] Indeed, the goal of medicine is, at least in part, being redefined in relation to the relief of suffering, whatever else is done.

It is not surprising that there is a movement towards a redefinition of good quality care, not merely in the minds of patients but also in the work of clinicians, including clinical investigators. Wholly objective measures of outcome (survival time, tumor response) have been recognized as being on their own inadequate, and they should not merely be supplemented by, but even yield priority to, measures based upon the patient-as-subject. Such measures may include measures of symptom alleviation (especially related to pain), activity facilitation (including performance status and achievement of personal objectives), and relief of suffering (including not merely measures of mood but of suffering) as conceptualized by Cassell in terms of a sense of disintegration of the self. The concept of quality of life, as a subjective evaluation of the overall character of a person's life, addresses some of these dimensions[17] and there is a clear need for conceptual and practical advances in this area of enquiry.

Clinical studies in cancer are beginning to take some of these matters into account[43] but subjective measures may not yet be given adequate weight as outcome variables; a major scientific task lies ahead in the development of more adequate measures and in their application.

CLINICAL PROCESSES IN PALLIATIVE THERAPEUTICS

The care of a woman with far advanced gynecological malignancy involves several components: diagnosis, delineation of therapeutic possibilities, treatment decisions and implementation, monitoring of treatment, and a further diagnostic effort as the patient develops new problems with the passage of time. Care of the patient also involves care of those caring for her, especially her family.

It is to be stressed that diagnosis is, in fact, a continuous process; the human patient who is host to advancing irreversible cancer is, in a sense, a continuously changing ecosystem. The pathological mechanisms causing problems today may yield to a new set of circumstances tomorrow. It is not only the pathological processes that may change but also the patient's response to her situation, which may change quite dramatically over even short periods of time, even while personal development is proceeding rapidly. The art and science of diagnosis must be continually refined to take note of this dynamic.

Comprehensive diagnosis involves at least: (1) ascertainment of the patient's symptoms or problems, in her order of priority; (2) clarification of the nature and extent of the neoplastic process with the careful consideration of other pathology which may be contributing to the present problems; (3) delineation of the personal and social context within which this patient is living and from which she may draw support; and (4) some elucidation of her personal objectives at this time. In the course of this clinical encounter, the opportunity should be sought whilst listening to the patient's narration of her own illness experience, to understand what she has found to be most distressing and how she has responded to situations of stress, including various forms of loss.

The pursuit of an adequate diagnosis may well involve not only interaction with the patient and with medical information available, but may also, if the patient gives consent, involve seeking information from family members or friends. In this, as in all components of the care of a very ill patient, privacy must be safeguarded — the more powerless she becomes the more onerous is the charge.

On the basis of a comprehensive diagnosis it is normally possible to delineate the therapeutic possibilities. Palliative medicine is concerned with the facilitation of freedom, and the choice among therapeutic options should reflect this. In general, the least restrictive alternative, involving least dependence on medical facilities and least use of her time, resources and personal energy, should be selected, all other things being reasonably equal. Careful consideration of other relevant anti-tumor measures is mandatory (surgery, radiotherapy or chemotherapy), since control of the neoplastic process offers the best chance for alleviating symptoms unless access to, or use of, such measures would be so burdensome that benefits would not be proportionate to the efforts in having treatment.

In any case, other non-tumor-directed symptomatic measures are usually essential: palliative care, adequately conceived, is not an alternative to appropriate antitumor therapy but, rather, involves antitumor measures as well as other palliative therapeutic measures as components of the comprehensive care of the patient. The field of palliative therapeutics is developing so rapidly that reference to specialist literature is often essential, but some matters are considered briefly in this chapter (see below).

Decisions concerning treatment — the choice between options — should normally involve the patient, who should be adequately informed concerning the foreseeable cost (personal as well as material), gains and consequences of the various treatment options. Whilst the patient should share in decision-making so far as she wishes, it is also true that her doctor should, on the whole, clearly indicate the course of action he or she favors and, in the end, take the responsibility for the decision for an intervention, though not necessarily for an omission if the patient clearly prefers not to have an advised intervention.

The burden of decision making is considerable, and ways of reaching decisions vary according to social, cultural, economic and medical contexts. However, the doctor has the duty to bear a part of the burden so that distressing outcomes should not engender guilt in the patient or family; this being said, the doctor should not act positively against his or her better judgement or conscience, despite patient or family pressure.

Decision making in all these circumstances, whether collective or individual, involves not merely information, communication and experience, but also wisdom and integrity; there is no opting out of this task. Indecisiveness may add to the suffering of the patient, but on the other hand, waiting as a situation unfolds may in some circumstances be the wiser course. Ethical issues abound and are considered briefly elsewhere.

Monitoring of interventions is best performed by the informed patient — there is no better monitoring device — although observation of carers and some physical and behavioral indices should have due place. Monitoring in some form is essential, since time, often the patient's most precious possession, should not be wasted by ineffective interventions if other options are open or modifications possible. The more restricted the life expectancy, the more grave is the misuse of time. Formal outcome measures based on subjective criteria, as indicated above, should ideally be introduced into routine clinical practice; certainly, a symptom profile and some measures of quality of life should be routine.

This clinical process, although the overall responsibility of medical practitioner, involves, as does other clinical activity (for example, surgery) participation of appropriately skilled nurses especially, and under some circumstances also other professions. The care of the family throughout the whole process, especially at times of uncertainty, must remain constantly in focus.

SYMPTOM RELIEF

If it is the task of each person to explore the limits of his or her own possibilities even in the final phase of life, it is surely the task of the doctor to free a very ill patient from obstacles, such as pain, to such an exploration. There is now an abundant literature concerning the understanding and therapy of major symptoms.[4,10,37,48,51]

In general, in oncology practice, pain and other symptoms may arise directly or indirectly from the tumor itself, or from treatment and/or concurrent unrelated causes. Whatever the cause, symptom relief is essential and usually possible with relatively simple measures if a logical and precise approach is taken. In gynecological cancer, these symptoms tend to cluster, and it may be useful to delineate, as a conceptual tool, some major and relatively common symptom complexes, each of which can logically be dealt with on the basis of rational palliative therapeutics:

1. *Pelvic mass syndromes*, with various manifestations of pressure and infiltration effects on hollow viscera, blood vessels, ureters, lymphatics, nerves (including lumbosacral plexopathy)
2. *Abdominal mass syndromes*, especially with interference with bowel function causing obstructive patterns, liver syndromes or ascites, or various combinations of these
3. *Perineal syndromes*, especially with ulceration as major source of discomfort
4. *Lung syndromes*, with dyspnea due to pleural effusion, diffuse lung involvement or bronchial occlusion, or to pulmonary emboli
5. *Radiation- and chemotherapy-induced syndromes*, involving emesis, pain from mucositis, myelopathy, bone marrow depression, fibrosis, neural damage, ischemia of bowel and other bowel damage (stricture, perforation, ulceration or radiation proctitis).

Other symptoms, such as those arising from paraneoplastic manifestations, coagulopathy or metabolic disturbances often as consequence of renal tract obstruction, also need to be recognized. Discussion will be limited mainly to the relief of the more common major symptoms.

Pain management

Pain has been defined by the International Association for the Study of Pain as, 'An unpleasant sensory and emotional experience associated with actual or potential tissue damage or described in terms of such damage'. Pain is a subjective phenomenon, an experience. It is not surprising, therefore, that there are difficulties both in measuring pain and in pain management. Nevertheless, the advances of the last decade in pain management should be readily available to all patients with advanced gynecological cancer. Improvements have been based on a more adequate understanding of pain physiology and classification as well as precise research, especially with respect to drug management (see also Ch. 89).

It is essential to recognize that pain in a patient with cancer may arise directly or indirectly from the cancer (affecting soft tissues, bones or neural structures), from treatment (notably radiotherapy or chemotherapy), or from quite unrelated causes. Whatever the etiology, the pain requires attention, precise diagnosis and precise management. Since pain is a subjective experience, the *patient* is always correct in her appraisal of the severity of the pain.

Cautious optimism is justified, and many approaches to pain management have been published.[8,14,22,34,46,52] The following simple schema may provide some guidelines in the face of complexity of recent research and practice. Pain management may be considered as having four steps (see Table 92.1).

Step one — always reduce the noxious stimulus at the periphery

This step demands a careful and adequate understanding of the mechanisms for the noxious stimulus in the individual patient, on the base of carefully focused history, examination and, if necessary, investigation. A precise history (of the mode of onset, characteristics, distribution, aggravating factors and trends over time, including response to therapeutic endeavors) is the fundamental guide to the likely mechanism or mechanisms (in the case of several different pains). Pain caused by treatment, for example radiotherapy, requires as close attention as that due directly to tumor.

Consideration should then be given to specific therapeutic measures, for example, radiotherapy, chemotherapy or antibiotics (if infection is playing a part), regional neural blockade or, occasionally, surgical approaches,

Table 92.1 Principles of pain management

1. **Always: reduce pain stimulus**
   Treat lesion if possible
   — Antibiotics?
   — Radiation therapy? etc
   Consider regional nerve block
   Appropriate drugs
   — Aspirin . . . . NSAID*
   Paracetamol
2. **Always: raise pain threshold**
   Concern, comfort, care
   Relaxation
   — ? Special techniques
   Diversion
   Antidepressant *or* anxiolytic (occasionally)
3. **Maybe also: use opioid drugs (for opioid responsive pain)**
   Choose:
   — correct opioid
   — correct dose
   — correct dose interval
   Usually prescribe laxatives to prevent constipation
   Do not prescribe morphine p.r.n.
   Watch for renal failure
4. **If neuropathic pain (neural irritation or destruction)**
   Tricyclic antidepressant
   and/or
   Anticonvulsants
   and/or
   Corticosteroid
   (Use in minimum effective doses with due regard to drug hazards)

* Non steroidal anti-inflammatory agents.

whether or not peripherally acting analgesic drugs are also used.

Bone metastases frequently cause inflammatory changes and prostaglandin production: prostaglandins may sensitize the tissues to other noxious stimuli. When the pain is arising clearly from bone metastases and has the characteristics of bone pain (and not nerve root pain which may also occur in the same patient), then the use of drugs interfering in some way with prostaglandin synthesis, for example various non-steroidal anti-inflammatory drugs (NSAIDs) is logical. These drugs should be avoided or used with caution in patients with a history of peptic ulceration, excessive alcohol consumption or bleeding states (including notably thrombocytopenia), and in patients with known idiosyncratic reactions to aspirin or related drugs. Where the use of NSAIDs is precluded, then paracetamol (aminoacetophen) is useful although the mechanism of action of this drug is obscure; it may have central effects as well as some peripheral action. Whilst paracetamol is fairly well tolerated and safe, the drug needs to be used with caution, in reduced dosage (less than 2 g per day), in patients with extensive liver damage, especially alcoholic cirrhosis.

Peripherally acting drugs such as the above are also useful in relation to other tumor sites, including soft tissue masses, and in postoperative pain; indeed, they should rarely be omitted from drug analgesic regimens, even in moribund patients, although route changes may be necessary. Rectal preparations of NSAIDs and paracetamol

(aminoacetophen) prove most useful in these circumstances as an adjunct to rectal or parenteral (preferably subcutaneous) morphine, in patients unable to take oral drugs.

Step two — always raise the pain threshold

It is clear that the threshold for pain perception is varied by many factors: it may well be raised significantly by comfort, care and concern, and by diversion and various forms of relaxation; and lowered by depression, extreme anxiety, loneliness and isolation. Although, occasionally, anxiolytic drugs or antidepressants may help, it needs to be stressed that threshold problems are best not approached by drug measures; other issues are at stake. A wide range of strategies exists for facilitating coping with pain, and the wise clinician will recognize the place of at least simple non-drug measures.

Step three — sometimes also reduce pain perception by the careful and precise use of opioid drugs

There is abundant literature on opioid use,[19,24,45] with a range of opioids available. In practice, weak opioids, such as codeine or dextraproproxyphene, or stronger opioids, typically morphine, are usefully combined with peripherally acting drugs, such as paracetamol or aspirin, with due regard to the contraindications. It is now widely recognized that opioids should be given regularly, at precisely determined doses, at fixed intervals in accord with the half-life of the drug concerned, rather than haphazardly in response to a severe pain stimulus.

The most commonly used morphine preparation, morphine sulphate solution, is best used 4-hourly with a double dose (or one-and-a-half standard dose in the frail) on retiring, and a break for approximately 8 hours overnight to permit sleep of both patient and carers.

A reasonable starting dose of oral morphine in a patient not already on an opioid drug, in whom an opioid is considered necessary in addition to a peripherally acting drug, would be 5 to 10 mg in a patient of average size, and 3 to 5 mg in the frail or elderly, with repetition of the original dose in 1 to 2 hours if there has been no pain relief. Over the next 24 to 48 hours, dose-finding is undertaken by prescription of regular 'by the clock' 4-hourly doses, with the provision of one or two breakthrough or rescue doses equal to the standard dose between the standard doses until the correct dose is apparent. This may range from 2 mg to over 100 mg 4-hourly, but the majority of patients will need less than 50 mg 4-hourly. Twycross & Lack[48] provide detailed directions for the institution and use of oral morphine in pain management.

If significant drowsiness (after the first 24 hours) or any other suggestion of morphine toxicity occurs without relief of pain, the morphine level is probably above the therapeutic range for that patient. The morphine dose should not be raised — the pain therapy usually requires another approach. It is clear that some types of pain are relatively unresponsive to opioids, notably pain arising in bone metastases and from nerve irritation or damage.

Controlled release morphine tablets represent a significant advance in convenience of administration, with the proviso that dose finding should be undertaken by use of morphine sulphate solution with administration thereafter of the total 24-hour dose in two fractions (12-hourly) or, occasionally, in three fractions (8-hourly) in the controlled release form (tablets); it is also essential that the tablets are not crushed.[6,18]

It is of interest that the efficacy of the regular dosing approach to morphine administration may depend on the contribution of an active metabolite (morphine 6-glucuronide) which is a more powerful analgesic than morphine.[20] Hepatic impairment, if severe, interferes with morphine metabolism to glucuronides; renal impairment interferes with excretion of these metabolites. In both of these circumstances, but especially in the latter, dose reduction is essential.

Whether or not an opioid is effective is not often significantly dependent on route of administration but, rather, on the etiology of the pain.

The oral route is most usually available for opioids, and the rectal route is a useful alternative in some patients. If parenteral drugs are essential, the subcutaneous route has proved satisfactory, either with an indwelling butterfly needle using 4-hourly morphine sulphate or tartrate, or by use of a subcutaneous infusion using a battery driven syringe driver.[49] In general, a parenteral dose of approximately one-half or one-third of the oral requisite dose appears equi-analgesic in the case of morphine in a patient on a regular dosing regimen.

In patients in whom morphine is clearly efficacious, but in whom side effects are especially troublesome, the epidural route is very occasionally advantageous. The intravenous route, especially intravenous infusion of morphine, although logical and sometimes satisfactory, has been shown to be somewhat hazardous, one risk being the development of acute tolerance which may not always be overcome by the addition of further morphine.[33] Heroin offers virtually no advantages over morphine and is best regarded as a pro-drug: its efficacy depends on metabolism to morphine.

When morphine is to be commenced, counselling is usually necessary with regard to three issues in order to counteract widely held fears in many communities. Firstly, it needs to be stressed that the use of morphine with careful dose-finding and monitoring does not, in the vast majority of patients, lead to addiction (although physical dependence does, of course, occur). Secondly, it needs to be stressed that the introduction of morphine does not mean that the patient is actually dying, but, rather, that morphine is the most appropriate opioid at this time; it is the type of pain and its severity which dictates whether or not an opioid should be introduced, not the prognosis of the patient. Thirdly, patients and families may need to be reassured that the introduction of morphine will not mean that there will be no adequate analgesic available at a later stage in the illness, when the situation may be worse.

Although morphine is currently the most useful strong opioid in widespread use, other strong opioids are occasionally preferable to morphine: availability varies, as does the availability of morphine. Oxycodone (available as tablet and suppository) provides a convenient intermediate level opioid. If more than 10 mg 4-hourly of oxycodone is inadequate, morphine in general is more satisfactory for the patient. Pethidine (meperidine) is of very little value in palliative care; certainly at high doses the drug is clearly neurotoxic and can add much to the distress of dying patients. Methadone is occasionally useful, but its long half-life is sometimes disadvantageous, and the complex and unpredictable changes in pharmacokinetics make the drug difficult to use. Opioids such as codeine, often combined with aspirin, paracetamol or dextraproproxyphene, are useful for mild pain, but these opioids should not be combined with morphine. Care should be taken to use only one opioid at a time; a combination of two opioids is unwise, unnecessary and hazardous.

The side effects of opioid drugs are in large part avoidable by precise prescribing. For example, as already noted, drowsiness after the first day, and not attributable to other causes, usually means that the drug is being used above the therapeutic range for that patient. Predictable side effects, such as constipation, can be almost wholly prevented by concomitant use of a laxative which combines softening and stimulant properties.

Nausea is in fact uncommon, except in highly anxious patients, or in patients in whom morphine is introduced in such a manner that serum morphine levels rise rapidly, or without careful counselling. Morphine-induced nausea may have several mechanisms including gastric stasis, stimulation of the chemo-trigger zone (CTZ) and, rarely, stimulation of the vestibular centers, in addition to anxiety. For this reason, metaclopramide may be of assistance with respect to the former mechanism, whereas centrally acting anti-nauseants as discussed below (including prochlorperazine, haloperidol, or antihistamines) will be more useful with respect to the last two mechanisms. Metaclopramide, 10 to 20 mg 6-hourly, or haloperidol, 3 mg at night, are in practice useful anti-nauseants, the former having action on both the gastrointestinal center and CTZ, the latter being specific for CTZ. Routine prescription of anti-nauseant drugs is not necessary for patients on morphine.

If fecal impaction has occurred as a result of the use of opioids without laxative, pelvic and abdominal pain may ensue (or be worsened) and nausea be made more likely. Such patients are in preventable misery, and the diagnosis should always be suspected and excluded in a patient with diarrhea, nausea, abdominal distension or pain and, in the case of an elderly patient, confusion.

Step four — recognize neuropathic pain and treat correctly

Neuropathic pain may be due to irritation or destruction of peripheral nerves; it may be neuralgic or have an unpleasant burning quality, and may be felt in an anesthetic area.[44] Such pain is a feature of plexopathies caused by tumor infiltrating the pelvic soft tissues, or radiation damage.

When pain is neuropathic in origin with severe neuralgia or burning pain in a segmental distribution, as can occur if the lumbosacral plexus is injured or destroyed, morphine and peripherally active drugs need to be supplemented by other drugs.[26] Such supplements are usually low doses of tricyclic antidepressant drugs, (notably amitriptyline, clomipramine, dothiapin, imipramine, 10 to 25 mg daily), or anticonvulsants (e.g. sodium valproate 200 mg to 1 g daily), or corticosteroids (e.g. dexamethasone 2 to 4 mg mane initially, with dose reduction as soon as possible). Other drugs, such as clonazepam or flecainide, may be of value.

In general, the management of neuropathic pain is difficult. The drugs used, including the above and also some less frequently used, have significant side effects, and specialist assistance may well be necessary. Regional blockade with local anesthetic techniques may be worthy of consideration.

It is essential to recognize that, whilst pain is a subjective experience (and therefore the patient is always the arbiter of its severity), it is usually possible to differentiate pain from suffering. Occasionally, anxiety and depression are so clearly pathological that the patient is being impeded in her attempts to relate to her loved ones and to come to terms with her disease: in such circumstance, a formal psychiatric consultation may be of assistance and, occasionally, anxiolytics or antidepressants may be used in the usual fashion. However, on the whole, threshold issues, including extreme anguish, issues concerning futility, loss of sense of meaning, personal guilt and other forms of spiritual pain require a different approach, with help from skilled counsellors, pastors and, above all, from those persons who are so close to the patient that admission even into the private space of suffering is welcome.

Human suffering is not a matter for morphine, but for sharing, for walking alongside, albeit in silence, when all that can be done to alleviate physical, emotional and spiritual distress is done, and done well.

Alimentary symptoms

Nausea, vomiting, colic and constipation are common in advanced gynecological cancer. Each symptom requires precise diagnosis in order that rational therapy may be applied.[2,47]

Nausea, with or without vomiting, is mediated finally by the vomiting center situated in the reticular formation of the medulla oblongata, an area rich in histamine receptors. This vomiting center is influenced by several connections, each of which can be the causal pathway for nausea:

1. cortical pathways (e.g. anxiety-conditioned responses)
2. vestibular center — rich in histamine receptors (e.g. some forms of morphine-induced nausea, occasionally cerebral metastases)
3. chemosensitive trigger zone (CTZ) — rich in dopamine receptors (e.g. nausea induced by some drugs, chemical, hypercalcemia, uremia)
4. alimentary (e.g. gastric stasis, intestinal obstruction, fecal impaction, abnormalities of gut motility).

Once a careful history and clinical examination (with investigations if necessary, especially biochemical) permits a working clinical diagnosis of the likely mechanism, knowledge of the mechanism of action of anti-nauseant drugs influences the choice of drug used.

Nausea related clearly to the CTZ requires a drug with high affinity for dopamine receptors, notably haloperidol: 3 to 5 mg at night, oral or s.c. may be sufficient.

Nausea arising from stimuli in the alimentary tract associated with slowing of the gut should respond to gastrokinetic anti-nauseants, such as metaclopramide or domperidone, which promote gastric emptying and increase gut motility in general. However, these very actions will, of course, be disastrous in a patient with high gastrointestinal obstruction, and vomiting will be aggravated. Metaclopramide also has some central action on the CTZ, and is therefore useful in premedication for chemotherapy. However, it should be avoided even in chemotherapy patients if gastrointestinal obstruction is suspected or even threatening (a common situation in ovarian cancer).

When anxiety dominates the scene, anxiolytics may be crucial in reduction of nausea. When vestibular mechanisms are suspected (uncommon) or when there appears to be a need to use drugs acting directly on the vomiting center, rather than using a more specific approach on the relevant nausea pathway, then antihistamines, especially cyclizine and meclozine, are useful.

Drugs such as prochlorperazine have some affinity for both muscarinic and histamine receptors and are moderately useful, though less specific. Clearly, drugs available by more than one route are advantageous — especially oral, subcutaneous and rectal routes. Metaclopramide and haloperidol may both be used subcutaneously as well as orally, but some other useful drugs (notably prochlorperazine) may not be used subcutaneously.

Many other drugs have useful anti-nauseant activity through various mechanisms, including, for example, amitriptyline which has a useful central action.

In addition to the established anti-nauseant drugs, it has been noted that dexamethasone, acting by a mechanism unknown, is also useful in suppressing nausea. For this reason, dexamethasone is used in some premedication programs prior to chemotherapy, but it is also useful in some patients with far advanced disease, used however in the lowest possible doses and as an adjunct to other therapy. Caution must obviously be exercised if the patient has a history of active peptic ulceration or tuberculosis, or is diabetic. If the risks of corticosteroids are acceptable, then small doses (e.g. 2 mg dexamethasone mane) may reduce nausea associated with tumors involving the alimentary tract, especially hepatic metastases or motility disturbances.

Constipation, a common symptom, may be due simply to changing diet, inactivity, or opioids used without laxatives, or to varying degrees of tumor-induced intestinal obstruction. Opioid-induced fecal impaction is almost always avoidable, but if present requires initially vigorous local treatment, such as glycerine, stimulant suppositories or careful enemas, or (unfortunately still occasionally necessary) manual removal, with some analgesia. Laxatives, including large bowel stimulants and softeners and, occasionally, small bowel flushers (such as lactulose), are also essential. Constipation due to intestinal obstruction as a direct effect of tumor or adhesions requires either relief of the obstruction by medical or surgical means, or acceptance as an end stage manifestation.

Medical management of intestinal obstruction

Obstruction may occur at any and several levels of the alimentary tract in gynecological cancer, and is a common late stage problem.[41]

In general, the first episode of obstruction in a patient not yet exposed to reasonable chemotherapy justifies very active measures, including nasogastric suction, maintenance of fluid and electrolyte balance by intravenous therapy, and surgery if these measures fail and the obstruction persists.

In patients who have exhausted reasonable chemotherapy options, the approach to such a situation may be more conservative. Obstruction of one or two sites may still justify a surgical approach in fairly fit patients with relatively slowly progressing tumors, or when there is suspicion of adhesions. Another alternative may be the trial of a short course (over a few days) of corticosteroids (e.g. dexamethasone 4 mg orally or parenterally daily for 3 to 5 days): the obstruction may be relieved and the maneuver may be repeated in the future. There is special need for caution in the use of corticosteroids in patients with diabetes, a history of psychiatric disorder, of active peptic ulceration in recent years, or of tuberculosis at any stage, recent infection, or impending perforation.

In a situation of end stage obstruction, when the above measures have failed to relieve the problem, note should be taken of the wholly symptomatic approach developed at St Christopher's Hospice.[3] In brief, this approach avoids the use of both nasogastric tube and i.v. line, allows the patient to be a little dehydrated (this benefits the patient considerably), and relies on exquisite mouth care with a little food and drink as desired, careful use of centrally acting anti-nauseants, sometimes in combination, and, if necessary, low doses of analgesics.

Hyoscine hydrobromide serves multiple purposes in patients with bowel obstruction, since it acts not only on the vomiting center but also relaxes the gut and increases the gut reservoir, enabling the patient with complete obstruction to avoid multiple vomiting, although having infrequent (2 to 3 per day), large emeses. Hyoscine butyl bromide is similar, but lacks the central effects.

A subcutaneous butterfly needle with or without a battery driven syringe driver can be used to deliver appropriate doses of anti-nauseants, such as haloperidol, 2 to 6 mg per day, as well as hyoscine hydrobromide or butyl bromide, 0.1 to 0.2 mg, 6-hourly. A hyoscine transdermal patch may also be useful, changed every 2 to 3 days.

Morphine may be given in the same syringe if necessary, but pain other than colic is rarely a problem. If colic is not controlled by a little morphine, additional hyoscine may be useful. Rectal prochlorperazine, 25 to 75 mg per day, may be tried instead of haloperidol, but is less useful than cyclizine (oral, parenteral, rectal) which is, however, not available everywhere.

This treatment implies the virtual abolition of nausea but the acceptance of vomiting two or three times a day, and most patients prefer bouts of even feculant vomiting with the ability to drink tea or coffee and so on, to a continuous nasogastric tube. If the obstruction is very high, intermittent insertion of a nasogastric tube for a few minutes to relieve pressure may be undertaken in the last days of life, but is very rarely advantageous. Under all these circumstances, electrolytes are neither monitored nor corrected; electrolyte imbalance becomes inevitable and should, in general, be allowed to take its course. Although requiring considerable medical and nursing experience, this approach has much improved the last phase (weeks, days or hours) of a large number of women dying with intestinal obstruction: it represents a major advance in palliative therapeutics.

Diarrhea in a patient with advanced gynecological cancer is probably best considered as a sign of fecal impaction until proved otherwise. True irritative diarrhea can occur by involvement of the bowel wall. Loperamide is an advance in the management of such a patient, but corticosteroids may occasionally be used for short periods with few side effects and considerable benefit to relieve such diarrhea. Tenesmus usually responds to rectal anticholinergic derivatives, e.g. hyoscine butyl bromide suppositories, and also to corticosteroids in addition to analgesics.

When diarrhea is associated with a rectovaginal fistula, and when surgical procedures are not possible, the emphasis in management is on nursing procedures calculated to keep the vagina clean and comfortable, and to support the patient in her quite extreme distress. Antibiotics, especially metronidazole, locally as well as systemically, may be of much value in reducing some of the distressing odor where much necrosis has occurred.

Abdominal distension due to intractable ascites can be a major cause of distress. Recurrent paracentesis has a limited but definite place; shunting procedures have severe limitations also. Initially at least, diuretics, especially spironolactone, 50 to 150 mg per day, may prove helpful. Occasionally, corticosteroids in very low dose may reduce fluid production and are worthy of trial. The actual discomfort is readily controlled with a combination of a peripherally acting drug, such as paracetamol, and maybe a little opioid.

Respiratory symptoms

Dyspnea is common,[9] and the dominant cause can usually be clarified by history taking, clinical examination and very simple investigations. It should be possible to differentiate a major pleural effusion, mediastinal obstruction, bronchial obstruction, diffuse lung involvement, reduced excursion due to massive ascites or other condition such as bronchial asthma, chronic airways limitation, cardiac failure or respiratory infection, and to treat accordingly.

Especially where the dyspnea is due to diffuse lung involvement, the careful use of morphine, with or without a small dose of corticosteroids, may improve the situation dramatically. Oral morphine, 2 to 5 mg 4-hourly, beginning with the lower dose in frail or very dyspneic patients with or without corticosteroids in low dose, may improve dyspnea not only through central mechanisms but possibly also due to peripheral effects. Morphine by inhalation has been tried in some subjects but its place is as yet unclear. Laxatives are essential if the morphine dose is not trivial.

If medical management of dyspnea is optimal, oxygen is rarely necessary or truly advantageous, even in widespread pulmonary metastases. Anxiolytics, however, may be very valuable and essential in modest doses: small doses of benzodiazepines, for example 2 mg of diazepam orally or 0.5 mg of lorazepam sublingually, may significantly improve the comfort of the patient.

Urinary tract symptoms

Urinary tract symptoms are common in women with far advanced gynecological cancer. Hydronephrosis, with infection, pain and even obstructive nephropathy as consequences, may justify mechanical measures such as nephrostomy or stent insertion if prognosis for life on other grounds is at least some good months (see also Ch. 45). Whilst some patients clearly benefit, complications are frequent and the costs (personal and financial) to the patient can be considerable; fine judgement is required in the individual case.

In the short term, patency of ureters may be achieved by short courses (a few days) of modest doses of corticosteroids, e.g. oral dexamethasone 4 mg daily for 3 to 5 days, with quite dramatic reduction in serum creatinine and improved quality of life. Bladder symptoms may yield to the use of NSAIDs to reduce detrusor irritability, or of drugs with anticholinergic action, such as tricyclic antidepressants, flavoxate or propantheline, to reduce bladder contractility. Catheterization may be unavoidable in some circumstances.

Edema

Leg swelling can be distressing due to venous or lymphatic obstruction, and may respond to small doses of diuretics (with care not to induce hypotension), or to careful massage towards the trunk beginning at the top of the leg, or to mechanical means such as support hosiery, or very occasionally by the application of various pump devices or intermittent compression apparatus. Systematic bandaging of the legs, by nurses or occupational therapists skilled in this technique, when the edema is minimal may improve comfort in some patients. Careful use of low doses of corticosteroids may also improve the situation without leading to side effects, and should probably be tried if leg swelling is a dominant symptom unrelieved by more simple measures.

Weakness

Weakness can be a dominant symptom where there is a large tumor mass, but there are many reversible causes of weakness in women with far advanced cancer. These include nutritional deficiencies, hypotension, hypokalemia, hypo- or hyperglycemia, hypoadrenalism, hypercalcemia, renal failure, infections and severe anemia. A glance indicates that at least some of these may be either easily excluded or readily treated in appropriate circumstances. Nutritional deficiencies may aggravate the sense of debility associated with advanced cancer through many mechanisms; careful attention is necessary.

Anemia is not in itself an indication for transfusion; benefit may be short-lived, maybe even a few days, and not proportionate to the expenditure of resources involved. If the hemoglobin is very low, and weakness is a dominant symptom, transfusion may however be justified.

Wisdom is needed with respect to undertaking the treatment of hypercalcemia; it may not be justified very close to death, but otherwise may justify vigorous treatment, normally with specialist assistance.

CARE OF THE MORIBUND PATIENT

Once this state is recognized, the goal is dignity and peace; this is best served by precise control of major symptoms, usually by continuing with the indicated drugs in correct dose by either subcutaneous or rectal route, and not usually by the i.v. route. Sometimes it is justified to offer direct sedation when, after precise control of pain, distress is extreme and opportunities for verbal communication are over. Phenothiazines such as chlorpromazine may cause distressing dissociation, and direct anxiolytics are preferable. In such circumstances sublingual lorazepam 0.5 to 1 mg, or even 2.5 mg 4- or 6-hourly may be of much value. Alternatively, parenteral midazolam, for example 2 to 5 mg by subcutaneous or intramuscular injection, may assist in achieving appropriate sedation, with the use of a subcutaneous infusion, 30 mg per 24 hours, if the situation is protracted. Large doses of opioids are not appropriate for sedation of the dying.

If possible, avoidance of complex equipment is of importance, and it is consoling to both patient and family to avoid tubes of all sorts wherever possible to facilitate maximum physical contact with loved ones. The latter, in turn, should be well supported in their anticipatory grieving, as well as subsequently, during their bereavement.[35,53]

Space, time, privacy and peacefulness are the essence of good care and these are facilitated by therapeutic clarity in the face of imminent death, whilst also recognizing the difficulty of a situation fraught with uncertainties. Respect for individual religious and cultural customs is mandatory.[28]

It is essential that there be acceptance of the value and personal significance of the final phase of life, even the last days, with an articulated personal view of the meaning of dying and with fear of dying articulated.[27] If the clinician and other professional staff regard dying as a battle failure, the patient may understandably feel like a battlefield (and some do); if dying is regarded as 'a master test of our journeyman years' (as articulated by Bloch),[5] there is implied the need for space, time and privacy to undertake such a test; if dying is regarded rather as a mysterious (even sacred) personal drama in which the doctor and the patient and the rest are all actors, or as a rite of passage, a prelude taking place in a foyer, then there is, indeed, implied the need for a sense of awe in the face of unique personal mystery.

In any case, and irrespective of philosophical and/or religious systems, there is entrenched in human history the awareness that the dying are involved in a mystery and justify respect — even if this respect has been denied in some circumstances, with blame falling at times on doctors.[1]

ETHICAL ISSUES

Whatever is of human concern is also of ethical concern. In the care of patients in the final phase of life, at whatever age, and carried out by whomsoever, certain issues emerge which justify some attention.

1. The issue of the availability of care when tumor control is no longer possible is paramount

In situations of scarce health resources there is a danger that patients who have progressive, irreversible disease or who are dying may not have even the fundamental core of the care needed, and certainly not a just proportion of resources available, for cancer care. There is surely a basic right to reasonable and adequate control of major symptoms, but the exercise of this right will involve widespread shifts in both attitudes and competence within the medical profession, as well as vast improvements on a global scale in the availability of crucial drugs, such as morphine, as well as knowledge, a matter of major concern to the World Health Organization.[52]

The principles of pain management have been widely disseminated in prestigious journals and in national documents, but, as far as can be ascertained, pain management remains patchy indeed even in affluent societies, and a dominant cause of suffering.[23] The management of other symptoms is also dependent on the availability of interested and competent health professionals in locations where needy patients are found. Good palliative therapeutics can involve the minimum of equipment and very few drugs, and is not dependent on a favorable context for care. If hospital facilities are needed (whether in a special care unit or a general acute hospital), these facilities should be available for the dying irrespective of political pressures or funding mechanisms, especially in circumstances where home care is encouraged and diligently undertaken.

What will guide health policy concerning the distribution of scarce resources (in the form of knowledge, skills, personnel and supplies) with impact on the care of the dying in our communities? Difficulties in allocating resources raise ethical issues and currently cause much stress, even or especially in affluent circumstances where personal (and familial) expectations are high and a communal sense is weak. Even in respect of palliative care advances, these tensions are perceptible.

John Rawls,[36] according to the general principles he expressed, would have all concerned (patients, nurses, politicians, families, doctors of various types, administrators, etc) decide on social policy and methods of implementation under a 'veil of ignorance', not knowing their individual social situation along the above spectrum of possibilities — whatever the issue be at stake.

Should resources available for palliative care be expended on creating centers of excellence where comprehensive palliative care can be made available? Or should one as a matter of policy seek not to optimize the best, but to minimize the worst (as Karl Popper might have advised[32]) by, for example, at the very least trying to ensure that *all* the gravely and incurably ill members of the community have basic pain relief? There is an issue of justice at stake as well as benevolence. It may be that centers of excellence can only be justified if knowledge is diffused from them (by education) and increased within them (by research).

How then shall care be organized?

McKeown,[3] towards the end of his thoughtful tome written at the end of a long and distinguished career as Professor of Social Medicine of Birmingham (1945 to 1977), actually cautioned against the divorce of the care of those in their final illness from the rest of medical practice.

'Some centres are concerned with terminal care, and a few devote themselves entirely to patients who face extreme physical and mental distress in their last illness . . . . Their work is beyond praise; but it should be taken as an example rather than a model, for the size and character of the problem is such that it cannot be divorced from the rest of medical care. Doctors need to regard prolonged and terminal care as an important and rewarding part of their task which should not be transferred to other people or to special institutions.'

In the past, sometimes and in some places, palliative care, at least in some forms, has been seen as an alternative to 'conventional' care,[16] but this concept is outmoded. Palliative care is increasingly recognized as an essential component of comprehensive cancer practice, and the therapeutic and conceptual advances generated within the hospice movement should be manifest in mainstream clinical practice, whether or not specialist palliative care staff are involved.

Palliative care is independent of context; care of high quality can be given anywhere, albeit more easily in favorable circumstances, provided appropriate knowledge, skills and attitudes are applied. It is not merely a matter of kindness.[38] A hospice is defined, after all, as a place of rest on the way to a sacred place; there is a challenge to ensure that such peacefulness is the context of care for every patient everywhere.

The dilemma is painful; how can it be resolved? It may be that where special centers for palliative care exist, they must recognize that their educational role is of equal importance to their service role and needs to be planned from the beginning; otherwise the pursuit of such excellence in a community where other patients are in very grave need could be unjustified. Further, such centers should be closely associated with teaching hospitals and academic medicine in general. Consultative services within major hospitals clearly have a catalytic and educational role in fostering the integration of contemporary concepts of palliative practice with mainstream gynecological oncology.

There are many ways to develop policy concerning various types of patients, and value judgements are inevitable;

but, however scarce the resources, the need of such patients should be clearly recognized. In fact, a society can be judged by the way it approaches the needs of the non-rehabilitatable sick, its weakest members.

2. *Precise and appropriate clinical decision making, as free as possible from ambiguity, is an ethical requirement*

Medical decision making is made in a pro-life context, but that very context demands that life be considered wholly, not partially, with the recognition that human persons are mortal and that dying is not defeat but a human process and personal act, whatever its significance may be (and each age reconsiders the meaning of death).[50] Where there is an adequate anthropology, there is likely to be an adequate ethic.

Decision making with respect to treatment options normally involves the patient, who is as fully informed as possible, whilst also (if she consents) taking into account the views of those closest to her; there should be great care taken that there is due proportion between the rigors, risk or costs of a treatment proposed and its likely benefit. In the case of the 'incompetent' patient, the ethical requirement is that the decision be made in the patient's best interests[11] with due recognition that it is rare (though not impossible) that it be in a patient's best interests to die.

Caution always remains essential with respect to decisions likely to permit the death of the patient; however, the most correct course in many circumstances is, with the patient's informed consent in so far as this is possible, to allow natural processes to take their course whilst maintaining optimum control of distressing symptoms.

The availability of health resources to patients with far advanced irreversible disease can itself be facilitated by more precise clinical medicine and less ambiguous clinical decision making. Indeed, wastefulness of resources can be encouraged, as well as the suffering of patients magnified, by lack of clarity concerning goals. In fact, if clear decision making can be undertaken with respect to the goals of therapy — despite all the difficulties of uncertainty of outcome and the desire to ensure that an adequate and appropriate value is placed on life itself, however poor in quality, but with acceptance of death — then maybe there will in fact be sufficient resources for all.

Wasteful and excessive use of very expensive resources in a situation where there is virtually no hope of tumor control or recovery of the patient, followed by an almost immediate reversal towards an attitude approaching active euthanasia, is not only a distressing indictment of medical practice, but is also harmful to ethical decision-making regarding resource distribution.

The wisest course in the care of a patient close to death is to manage as precisely as possible the major symptoms present by careful and appropriate medical means, and to support the patient, by walking with her the last few steps of life as she plays out the last notes of what is her symphony.

It is, at this stage, often of comfort to the patient to be assured gently that the doctor she trusts is doing nothing to prolong her life at this point, or to shorten it, but is concentrating on improving the quality of her life for whatever time she has by the best of his or her clinical ability. Taking active steps to truncate that final process is not only unfitting but inappropriate in the perspective of what the mystery of human life is at its core; it is also unnecessary if medical skills are precisely and calmly harnessed in the patient's best interest. As Pollard notes, 'By any criteria it must be ethically superior to attend to the elimination of the human distress before the elimination of the human in distress', and he further comments that, 'it is a bitter paradox that euthanasia is being promoted, primarily because of poor medical care, at a time when we know better than ever before, how to care well for the dying. The medical profession has in its hands the best social answer to the call for euthanasia. It is at once the partial cause of the problem and the best hope for the effective remedy.[31] Discussion of these difficult issues calls for a climate of wisdom, integrity and respect for the mystery of humanness and life as gift.

3. A further ethical consideration is the issue of the focusing of hope; if hope is given a false focus some of the problems with regard to resource allocation may be aggravated.

From the onset of palliative treatment, which in fact begins as soon as incurability is recognized, care needs to be taken to understand the processes of personal development and the value of appropriately based hope.

Erikson saw human growth as taking place by negotiation of developmental tasks through the resolution of crises.[12,13] The growing human being is continually faced with options, each life stage being characterized by its own options which, while they confront one throughout life, do come to a point of ascendancy in a given stage. Where the life process is characterized by the embracing of favorable options, the personality becomes characterized by trust, reasonable autonomy, initiative, capacity for effort, a sense of identity, intimacy instead of isolation, fruitfulness rather than stagnation and, finally, a sense of integrity or wholeness of life, rather than despair.

Erikson's analysis of personal growth is sensitive indeed in its consideration of the developmental task of the elderly and, by analogy, of those of any age approaching death.[12] He conceives that task as the development of a sense of wholeness, integrity:

'Only he who in some way has taken care of things and people and has adapted himself to the triumphs and disappointments of being, by necessity, the originator of others and the generator of things and ideas — only he may gradually grow the fruit of the seven stages. I know no better word for it but

integrity .... It is the acceptance of one's own and only life cycle and of the people who have become significant to it as something that had to be ... an acceptance of the fact that one's life is one's own responsibility. It is a sense of comradeship with men and women of distant times and of different pursuits, who have created orders and objects and sayings conveying human dignity and love.'

On the other hand, Erikson notes further:

'... the lack or loss of this accrued ego integration is signified by despair and an often unconscious fear of death: the one and only life cycle is not accepted as the ultimate of life.

Despair expresses the fear that the time is short, too short for the attempt to start another life and to try out alternate roads to integrity. Such a despair is often hidden behind a show of disgust, a misanthropy, or a chronic contemptuous displeasure with particular institutions and particular people — a disgust and displeasure which (where not allied with constructive ideas and a life of co-operation) only signify the individual's contempt of himself.'

The magnitude and shape of this developmental task needs to be understood by those in contact with patients who are approaching death. Patients may well vacillate between wholeness and despair and need to be supported gently. They may long and need to try to express their internal states, explore the threat of despair and, through dialogue with significant others, reach out again towards the wholeness which is possible.

Erikson's sensitive portrayal of the developmental task of the final phase of life as being the movement towards integrity and away from despair calls for a consideration of the doctor's role in the sustaining and reconstructing of *hope*. No one can live without hope, but in what may hope be anchored, if it is not doomed to fail?

No person should die in despair, and it is clear that the doctor should surely assist the patient to center hope not on what will in the end probably fail (for example chemotherapy, radiotherapy, surgery) but in what will not fail, such as the doctor's commitment to care and the control of pain and other symptoms, and the intrinsic value of the patient as a unique irreplaceable subject of existence. No patient should die with hope wholly centered on the next chemotherapy course, or another surgical intervention. These matters call for much pondering if medical practice is not to add to the despair of women dying in complex hospital contexts — or anywhere — when the medical task is meant to be the relief, not cause, of suffering.

It is surely the doctor's responsibility and privilege to help the patient to cope with the stresses laid on her; to trust the wisdom of careful decisions made with her real good as a total person at heart, even if she herself is incompetent; to be confident that she will not be left to suffer pain and other major symptoms; and to provide care, support and concern no matter what ensues. She should feel that all the effort she applies to combating her cancer is encouraged against that backdrop, and that if she prefers to die 'raging against the dying of the light' and not in peaceful acquiescence, that too is respected. Such concepts assist the patient to walk, even run, in realistic hope, rooted in what will not fail, whilst giving all that is empirical and even ephemeral every chance.

Nothing, then, should be said or done by doctors to induce despair, and all should be said and done to facilitate the emergence of a final integrity and wholeness, a feeling that life has been lived as it should, albeit with a sense of self-forgiveness. This is real hope, rooted in reality, which is abiding. Good palliative care is concerned with enrichment of life, even when facing the human task common to all at the end, of dying.

IN CONCLUSION

In conclusion, doctors are called on to exercise leadership, to be agents in the healing process with a new appraisal of what cancer medicine needs in order to be truly scientific, and to be unfailing advocates of the weak. Leadership involves many tasks including the capacity to grasp the central anxieties of our time and of our present context and 'at midnight to be confident of the dawn'.[5] However, it is as advocates of the weak that the gynecological oncologist may surely be most tested, with the dignity of woman, even when utterly bereft, being the value most assiduously guarded. There may be no greater trust.

REFERENCES

1. Alexander L 1949 Medical science under dictatorship. N Engl J Med 241: 39
2. Allan S G 1988 Emesis in the patient with advanced cancer. Palliat Med 2: 89
3. Baines M, Oliver D J, Carter R L 1985 Medical management of intestinal obstruction in patients with advanced malignant disease: a clinical and pathological study. Lancet ii: 990
4. Billings J A 1985 Outpatient Management of Advanced Cancer: Symptom Control, Support and Hospice-in-the-Home. Lippincott, Philadelphia
5. Bloch E 1970 Man On His Own, (trans Ashton E B). Herder & Herder, New York, p 47
6. Brescia F J, Walsh M K, Savarese J J, Kaiko R F 1987 A study of controlled-release oral morphine (MS contin) in an advanced cancer hospital. J Pain Symptom Manag 2: 193
7. Cassell E J 1982 The nature of suffering and the goals of medicine. N Engl J Med 306: 639
8. Cleeland C S, Rotondi A, Brechner T et al 1986 A model for the treatment of cancer pain. J Pain Symptom Manag 1: 209
9. Cowcher K C, Hanks G 1990 Long term management of respiratory symptoms in advanced cancer. (In press)
10. Doyle D 1984 Palliative Care: The Management of Far Advanced Illness. Croom Helm, London
11. Emanuel E J 1988 What criteria should guide decision makers for incompetent patients? Lancet i: 170
12. Erikson E H 1968 Identity and the Life Cycle, Psychological Issues Monograph. International Universities Press, New York, p 52
13. Erikson E H 1982 The Life Cycle Completed. Norton, London
14. Foley K M, Inturrisi C E 1987 Analgesic drug therapy in cancer pain: principles and practice. Med Clin Nth Am 71: 207
15. Freidenbergs I, Gordon W, Hibbard M, Levine L, Wolf C, Diller L 1982 Psychosocial aspects of living with cancer: a review of the literature. Int J Psyc Med 11: 4
16. Greer D S, Mor V, Morris J N, Sherwood S, Kidder D, Birnbaum H 1986 An alternative in terminal care: results of the National Hospice Study. J Chron Dis 39: 9
17. de Haes J C J M, Van Knippenberg F C E 1985 The quality of life of cancer patients: a review of the literature. Soc Sci Med 20: 809
18. Hanks G W, Twycross R G, Bliss J M 1987 Controlled release morphine tablets: a double-blind trial in patients with far advanced cancer. Anaesthesia 42: 840
19. Hanks G W, Hoskins P J 1987 Opioid analgesics in the management of pain in patients with cancer: a review. Palliat Med 1: 1
20. Hanks G W, Hoskins P J, Aherne G W, Turner P 1987 Explanation for potency of repeated oral doses of morphine. Lancet ii: 723
21. Kuhn T S 1970 The Structure of Scientific Revolutions, 2nd edn. Univ Chicago Press, Chicago
22. Levy M H 1985 Pain management in advanced cancer. Semin Oncol 12: 394
23. Lickiss J N, McCosker C, Best M 1989 Suffering and cancer: self rated chief causes of suffering in 100 consecutive patients referred to the Royal Prince Alfred Hospital Palliative Care Service, Sydney. (Unpublished observations)
24. Lipman A G 1989 Opioid analgesics in the management of cancer pain: pharmacokinetic considerations. Am J Hospice Care, Vol 6
25. McKeown T 1979 The Role of Medicine. Blackwell, Oxford
26. McQuay H J 1988 Pharmacological treatment of neuralgic and neuropathic pain. In: Franks L M, Hanks G W (eds) Pain and Cancer: Cancer Surveys: Advances and Prospects in Clinical Epidemiology and Laboratory Oncology. 7: 1
27. Mount B M 1986 Dealing with our losses. J Clin Oncol 4: 1127
28. Neuberger J 1987 Caring for Dying People of Different Faiths. The Lisa Sainsbury Foundation Series
29. Northouse L 1984 The impact of cancer on the family: an overview. Int J Psyc Med 14: 3
30. Parliament of Victoria, Social Development Committee 1987 Upon the Inquiry into Options for Dying with Dignity, Second and Final Report. (232 pages) Parliament of Victoria, Melbourne
31. Pollard B 1989 Euthanasia: Should We Kill The Dying? Little Hills Press, Bedford
32. Popper K 1966 The Open Society and its Enemies, Vols 1 & 2. Routledge, London
33. Portenoy R K, Dwight E M, Rogers A, Inturrisi C E, Foley K M 1986 IV infusion of opioids for cancer pain: clinical review and guidelines for use. Cancer Tr Rep 70: 575
34. Portenoy R K 1988 Practical aspects of pain control in the patient with cancer. CA-A Canc J for Clin 38: 327
35. Raphael B 1985 The Anatomy of Bereavement. Hutchinson, London
36. Rawls J 1972 A Theory of Justice. Oxford University Press, Oxford
37. Saunders C M 1985 The Management of Terminal Malignant Disease, 2nd edn. Edward Arnold, London.
38. Saunders C 1987 The philosophy of terminal cancer care. Ann Acad Med 16: 151
39. Seravalli E P 1988 The dying patient, the physician and the fear of death. N Engl J Med 319: 1728
40. Stjernswärd J 1988 The WHO cancer pain relief programme. In: Franks L M, Hanks G W (eds) Pain and Cancer. Cancer Surveys: Advances and Prospects in Clinical Epidemiological and Laboratory Oncology. 7: 1
41. Solomon H J, Atkinson K H, Coppleson M et al 1983 Bowel complications in the management of ovarian cancer. Aust NZ J Obstet Gynaecol 23: 65
42. Stedeford A 1984 Facing Death: Patients, Families and Professionals. Heinemann, London
43. Stuart Harris R, Simes R J, Coates A A S, Raghavan D, Devine R, Tattersall M H N 1987 Patient treatment preference in advanced breast cancer: a randomised crossover study of doxyrubicin and mitozantrone. Eur J Cancer Clin Oncol 23: 557

44. Tasker R R 1984 Deafferentation. In: Wall P D, Melzack R (eds) Textbook of Pain. Churchill Livingstone, London, p 119
45. Twycross R G 1988 Opioid analgesics in cancer pain: current practice and controversies. Cancer Surv 7: 29
46. Twycross R G, Lack S A 1983 Symptom Control in Far Advanced Cancer: Pain Relief. Pitman, London
47. Twycross R G, Lack S A 1986 Control of Alimentary Symptoms in Far Advanced Cancer. Churchill Livingstone, Edinburgh
48. Twycross R G, Lack S A 1990 Therapeutics in Terminal Cancer, 2nd edn. Churchill Livingstone, London
49. Ventafridda V, Spoldi E, Caraceni A, Tamburini M, DeConno F 1986 The importance of continuous subcutaneous morphine administration for cancer pain control. Pain Clin 1: 47
50. Von Balthazar U 1982 Greatness and limitation of the human being. In: Kehl M, Loser W (eds) The Von Balthazar Reader, (trans Daly R J and Lawrence F). Clark, Edinburgh, p 83
51. Walsh T D 1988 Symptom Control. Blackwell, London
52. World Health Organization 1991 Cancer Pain Relief, 2nd edn. WHO, Geneva, in preparation
53. Worden W J 1982 Grief Counselling and Grief Therapy. Tavistock, London

93. Attitudes to dying

W. Middleton   B. Raphael

INTRODUCTION

There is no reason to believe that, in general, gynecologists deal differently with death than do other specialists, or that the issues confronting the terminally ill gynecology patient aren't those common to many with terminal illness.

If we can accept, at least in part, Feifel's hypothesis[4] that physicians enter medicine because of their own above average fears of death, then it is in keeping with the more general hypothesis that the majority of the literature in this area deals eventually with mechanisms of coping with information or situations that are uncomfortable, painful or even terrifying.

Vaillant[16] listed some of the inferred 'purposes' of ego defense mechanisms as including: the keeping of affects within bearable limits during sudden alterations in one's emotional life; obtaining 'time-out' to master changes in self-image that cannot be immediately integrated; the handling of unresolvable conflict with important people living or dead of whom one cannot bear to take leave; and the restoration of psychological 'homeostasis'.

With respect to those dying with terminal illness, the three key principal groups forced to make some accommodation to it are the patient, the patient's spouse and relatives, and the doctor and other health staff. The issues vary for each group and for each group common coping or defensive styles emerge, with consequences that range from helpful through to pathological. The responses of each group can have a marked impact on the facilitating or obstructing adaptive functioning of the other groups.

THE DYING PATIENT

Some patients suspect they have terminal illness long before it is confirmed, some find out in the course of having symptoms or signs investigated, while for others the diagnosis may come as a result of some routine investigation performed without any expectation of the likelihood of serious illness.

While all patients manifest a degree of denial, virtually all will acknowledge their terminal illness in time. In 1969, Kubler-Ross[10] reported that in interviews with over 200 patients dying in hospital, only three maintained denial to the end. Community surveys, such as that of Blumenfield et al,[1] support the view that the vast majority (90%) express the wish to be informed should they develop a terminal illness.

Just how devastating the news of terminal illness can be when presented suddenly to someone who thought they were well is illustrated in Goldie's[6] account of a patient who, not suspecting anything amiss, had gone for 'blood tests'. Because of the results, an appointment was made with a specialist who without preamble told the unsuspecting patient that he had a very serious form of leukemia. The patient collapsed and was incontinent of urine and feces.

In 1969 Kubler-Ross[10] drew a great deal of attention to the psychological processes of the dying. Her model of conceptualizing the process of dying, by describing five stages of response on the part of the terminally ill, as being stages characterized by denial, anger, bargaining, depression and acceptance, is in keeping with the utilization of ego-defense mechanisms.

The issues that the dying patient confronts are multiple. Aside from anxieties about death itself, frequently construed in ways congruent with the woman's social, cultural and religious upbringing, concerns include:

1. Fear of pain. Patients may have vivid memories of relatives dying in pain. They may be concerned with being able to cope if pain does indeed progressively worsen.
2. Concern for spouse/family. Frequently, the major stated concern is for the surviving spouse or children. There is regret that the children won't be seen to grow into adults, that grandchildren won't be met, that the patient's husband will have to cope alone.
3. Fear of becoming physically dependent. Some

patients state they would rather be dead than have to rely on others to complete the basic tasks of life for them.

4. Fear of loss of function. Many express major concerns about the processes of physical deterioration, such that the possibility of reaching a stage where they could not go to the toilet, or where their cognitive processes become impaired, hold major anxieties.

5. Fear of physical deformity or of becoming physically repugnant to others. Many have concerns that physical debilitation, or ugly or odorous lesions will be difficult for themselves or others to accept and, in turn, add to feelings of isolation. Additional to concerns regarding the effects of disease, are concerns regarding the side effects of treatment, e.g. hair loss due to chemotherapy, nausea and drowsiness due to opiates, or enteritis secondary to radiation therapy.

For many, to find that they are dying, is the most momentous crisis of their life, and unlike many other crises it has an irrevocable conclusion. Little wonder that it induces a range of defensive measures that need to be seen against the background of the course and time span of the particular terminal illness. It should be emphasized that in attaining the status of dying, not all patients approximate each other; those that were immature, intolerant and prone to use a primitive defensive style prior to their terminal illness will, as a rule, manifest exaggerated primitive defenses after being confronted with their prognosis. Also, as illustrated in the example already quoted, the lack of any opportunity to be prepared for the diagnosis can induce the instantaneous overwhelming of defenses that in other contexts may service the individual well.

Kubler-Ross' model of staging the dying process is useful in highlighting common defensive patterns in the dying. Some patients do not fit well into the popularized version of her model. The subsequent orientation of her work has had her described in the role of a charismatic religious leader.[9]

The variable emergence of defenses is illustrated by the care of a 35-year-old married mother of two whose uterine malignancy was diagnosed a little later than it might have been. The patient had a hysterectomy only to be readmitted several months later with metastatic disease. She expressed some anger, stating that she had been told that her operation was curative. She acknowledged the terminal nature of her illness and talked abstractly about her family's response to it. She was discharged after a course of chemotherapy and radiotherapy, only to be admitted again with further progression of her illness. A crisis occurred when she was unable, due to illness, to leave hospital and travel interstate to attend a wedding that she had been looking forward to. She no longer acknowledged

the terminal nature of her disease and spoke of 'cure'. She described her pain as 'unbearable' and criticized doctors for not doing enough. There was further anger expressed about her late diagnosis and the failed 'promise' of cure. Whilst relatives visited frequently, central issues of conversation became the pain and the wish for further radiotherapy, despite her limited improvement with it.

Her responses are typical of many. Her early intellectual acceptance of dying gave way to denial and anger as her illness progressed. In a sense, the conflicts she had about dying were displaced onto the issue of pain. Staff were criticized for not curing her pain. Offered a palliative neurosurgical procedure for her pain, she did not want to discuss it, much less consider it. The fact that it was an irreversible palliative procedure rather than radiotherapy which she equated with 'cure' challenged her denial too much.

Dying forces on the patient a number of radical changes that can profoundly affect their self-image. There is a marked revision of the power dynamics and a marked increase in the dependency needs.[15] Powerful, driven, self-reliant personalities may regress to a state of marked dependency, to the point where they may not wish to be left alone and want others to do things for them that they are capable of doing themselves. The dying person is confronted by a world in which they have little control over their own destiny and are suddenly forced to rely on others for treatment, for pain relief, for information about life expectancy, for nursing care, etc.

Some patients maintain an outward persona of coping to their doctor and colleagues, whilst those closest to them bear the brunt of their regressive behavior and anger.

Depending on her personality, some feeling of control can be given back to the patient by addressing those areas in which something can be done, e.g. by giving the patient access to as much information about her condition as she requests, by discussing management options, by accommodating specific requests/wishes, e.g. arranging leave from hospital to attend an important function, or by providing symptomatic relief in such a way that the patient is not cast in the demeaning role of having to ask for it.

THE DOCTOR

Confronted with the discovery of terminal illness in a patient, the patient's doctor/gynecologist has also to make accommodation with issues that are not necessarily easily dealt with and to which the doctor can mobilize his/her own defenses.

In the cultural context of medicine, death is not infrequently consciously or unconsciously equated with failure, and in most walks of life dwelling too long on issues that remind one of failure is uncomfortable. Take the issue of telling the patient about her terminal illness. There are scenarios that relate far more to the doctor's anxieties than to the patient's clinical state, including:

1. The blunt statement, graphically giving the patient details of her illness and prognosis, as if by so doing a certain duty has been fulfilled. This gives that patient little opportunity to mobilize her defenses. It may be rationalized that such a statement is useful, in that it penetrates the denial that the patient might mobilize to less direct communication. However this fails to appreciate the protective role that denial plays, or the responsibility for providing an alternative for defenses that have been stripped away. Goldie[6] points out that one should not set out to tell the patient without undertaking to remain with her while she digests and assimilates it. 'To do otherwise would be like performing a skilful surgical operation and then leaving the skin unsutured, the wound uncovered, and the patient deteriorating.'
2. The converse of the above, is where the doctor never gets 'around' to telling the patient precisely what the clinical situation is. The subject may be approached obliquely and euphemisms employed to draw attention away from the seriousness of the condition. Whilst it is frequently stated that not telling the patient is protective, this is frequently a rationalization of the doctor's discomfort.
3. The doctor's difficulty may be such that he/she formally, or more frequently informally, delegates the task.
4. The doctor may be induced into giving an overly optimistic prognosis, unconsciously colluding with what the patient may wish to hear.
5. The doctor, through identification with a particular patient, finds his/her objectivity compromised, resulting in either a denial of the seriousness of the illness or, alternatively, embarking on an overly zealous treatment approach.

The doctor's defenses are of course frequently adaptive and, as Freeman[5] points out, some degree of intellectualization, distancing and isolation of affect promotes objectivity and protects against depression or anxiety, enabling a position of 'compassionate detachment' to be adopted.

In many ways, the 'sick role'[12] is invalidated for the dying patient. Patient's adherence to the constraints of that role are predicated on cooperation with treatment in order to get well. Similarly, doctors whose role traditionally is to expect patients to cooperate with treatment in the expectation of cure or at least improvement, frequently find difficulty in treating patients for whom they cannot offer cure but, at best, only time-limited improvement.

Again, a number of defenses can be demonstrated by

consideration of the sorts of responses that can occur:

1. Therapeutic impotence can be compensated for by persisting with investigations and treatment regimes to a degree that is out of keeping with likely benefit, and which may indeed be harmful. This may reflect compromised objectivity.
2. Alternatively, overly zealous or overly invasive treatment may represent a protective mechanism for the doctor whereby he/she isolates the physical component from the emotional aspects of treatment.
3. Where the doctor feels that he/she has little to offer, it is all too easy to withdraw from the dying patient. In the hospital setting, ward rounds may become less frequent or more perfunctory; new physical complaints may not be investigated and simply be assumed to be part of a deteriorating picture. The patient may be moved from acute to progressively less acute settings, with each stage characterized by a further withdrawal of medical contact. (A survey by Herman[7] showed that a majority of medical house staff members believed that the patient with terminal disease has no place in an acute teaching hospital.)
4. The patient may be blamed. For example, a patient's complaints of pain may be construed as excessive, or out of keeping with physical findings. The patient may be subtly criticized for denying early signs and symptoms and presenting late; alternatively, she may be criticized for reluctance to pursue unpleasant palliative treatments, as if the 'sick role' and its obligations could be fairly assigned to such a patient.
5. The patient may be referred to another specialty in such a way as to rationalize withdrawal, with an assumption along the lines of, 'We've done all we can, the patient's major problem is now pain/depression/nausea etc.'.
6. Some doctors may encourage or participate in a process of subtly enforcing some form of 'counselling', frequently designed to challenge the patient's defenses in accordance with some model of what a 'good death' should be. They may overlook a patient's obvious reluctance or discomfort, or describe it as yet another manifestation of the patient's denial.
7. The doctor may show an apparent willingness to respect the views of the patient's relatives, to withdraw from the necessity of taking responsibility for management decisions.

The physician finds his/her position a complex one. Often the object of displaced anger and unrealistic idealization of the patient and her family, the physician embodies tremendous power and is a frame of reference for one who has little power. In such a context, even the most innocuous comment by the physician may embody particular significance to the dying patient. As an example, a terminally ill woman ruminated for days concerning the possible meaning of the fact that two different specialists on separate occasions had both said to her, 'Let me know if anything happens . . .'. She construed this as some sort of covert message about some complication that was going to happen but about which she had not been told.

The medical profession is criticized for the under-utilization of drugs for the treatment of pain in the terminally ill.[11] Ignorance of the types of pain, the spectrum of use of available analgesics, and a misguided concern about addicting a patient are cited as contributory factors.

Indicative of an overall trend towards denial of death in our society are: criticisms of the lack of importance attached to including courses on treating the dying in medical school syllabuses;[2] criticisms about the standard of care for the terminally ill;[18] and the high status afforded branches of medicine dedicated to saving life.

Interestingly, whilst the establishment of hospices has become a major source of alternative terminal care over the last two decades, the assignment of patients to a different treatment setting does not necessarily change medical practices. Perkins & Jonsen,[13] in a comparison between hospices and a conventional hospital, found that hospice physicians noted non-medical effects of illness on patients, and families' ability to cope emotionally or to give care, as infrequently as conventional hospital physicians did.

As Eissler[3] observed in 1955, a vast literature has accumulated regarding death induced by disease, implying situations of a potentially preventable nature, but there had been little emphasis on seeing death in the context of being an unavoidable or logical process, the ultimate consummation of life, as it were.

THE DYING PATIENT'S FAMILY

Many of the same responses and defenses that characterize the dying patient's adjustment are shared by the patient's spouse and close family. For the spouse the diagnosis of his wife's terminal illness may be the most major stress of his lifetime.

An oft quoted issue is that pertaining to situations where the family is aware of the diagnosis and requests that the patient not be told. Not infrequently, the relative's request that the patient not know is a projection of their own wish not to know, and must be seen in the context of other adjustments. For example, whilst repressed rage might be present, related to the patient's imminent abandonment of her family, the expression of such rage is unacceptable and may be displaced onto others, such as health care professionals.

The nature of progressive terminal illness is such that the time course allows for the dying person and those close to her to go through anticipatory mourning,[14] a difficult process of relinquishing bonds at the same time as being

party to a situation in which the dying person may need close support. With the patient's death, the grieving process seen in acute loss may be modified. Much of the shock, the acute pangs of grief, numbness etc. may already have been experienced.

With sudden death, close relatives lack the opportunity to make any final farewells; indeed, the time of death may coincide with a period of temporary dispute, leaving residual feelings of guilt on the part of spouse or children. Terminal illness does at least provide time for efforts to be made to make appropriate farewells.

Hinton,[8] discussed three common circumstances in which the degree of communication between the patient and spouse concerning the terminal illness was limited. The first instance was where, based on 'an almost automatic response to communicate hope and encourage the patient to fight the disease', the patient and spouse colluded in voicing no pessimism. In the second case, there was a more conscious avoidance of discussion in order to prevent distress, with both partners acknowledging their avoidance of the topic — but not to each other. A corollary to this is the situation where the dying person can speak of dying to a son or daughter, but finds it too distressing to discuss it with her spouse. The third example was where the lack of discussion of dying was but another example of a couple's longstanding pattern of discussing little of emotional significance.

CONCLUSION

Advances in medical science have led to another problematical area for terminally ill patients, their physicians, and their families, namely the debated issue of the patient's right to die in circumstances where the withdrawal of life-sustaining procedures would hasten the death of the already terminally ill patient. As Wanzer et al[17] infer, it is not possible to formulate any universal recommendations with respect to the justification for either prolonging or ceasing active life-support. 'Some patients want every possible day of life, regardless of how limited the quality, whereas others apparently prefer early death to prolongation of a very limited life on a day-to-day basis.' As is the case with much technology applied to medicine, its use engenders ethical or legal conflicts as society finds existing precedents unsatisfactory.

What is hard for us, as physicians, is that when it comes to the care of the terminally ill, technological advances may be used as a rationale by patients or their families for voicing hopes of survival, while for the physician they may provide a means of distancing him/herself from the patient. We have to decide what the issues of patient care are for the individual, and be mindful of the ways in which the defenses of the patient, the patient's family and of ourselves can both help and hinder the process.

REFERENCES

1. Blumenfield M, Levy N B, Kaufman D 1978 The wish to be informed. Omega 4: 323
2. Dickinson G E 1981 Death education in US medical schools: 1975–1980. J Med Educ 56: 111
3. Eissler K 1955 The Psychiatrist and the Dying Patient. International Universities Press, New York
4. Feifel H 1963 Death. In: Faberow L (ed) Taboo Topics. Atherton Press, New York
5. Freeman A 1987 The dying patient. Psychiatric Clin Nth Am 10: 101
6. Goldie L 1982 The ethics of telling the patient. J Med Ethics 8: 128
7. Herman T A 1980 Terminally ill patients: assessment of physician attitudes within teaching institutions. N Y State J Med 80: 200
8. Hinton J 1981 Sharing or withholding awareness of dying between husband and wife. J Psychosom Res 25: 337
9. Klass D, Hutch R A 1985 Elizabeth Kubler-Ross — religious leader. Omega 16: 89
10. Kubler-Ross E 1969 On Death and Dying. Macmillan, London
11. McGivney W T, Crooks G M 1984 The care of patients with severe chronic pain in terminal illness. JAMA 251: 1182
12. Parsons T 1950 Illness and the role of the physician. Am J Orthopsych 21: 452
13. Perkins H S, Jonsen A R 1985 Dying right in theory and practice — What do we really know of terminal care? Arch Intern Med 145: 1459
14. Raphael B 1984 The Anatomy of Bereavement. Hutchinson, London
15. Raphael B, Middleton W 1987 Whose life and whose death. Quality Assurance & Utilization Review 2: 22
16. Vaillant G E 1971 Theoretical hierarchy of adaptive ego mechanisms. Arch Gen Psychiat 24: 107
17. Wanzer S H, Adelstein S J, Cranford R E et al 1984 The physician's responsibility toward hopelessly ill patients. N Engl J Med 310: 955
18. Wilkes E 1984 Dying now. Lancet i: 950

Index

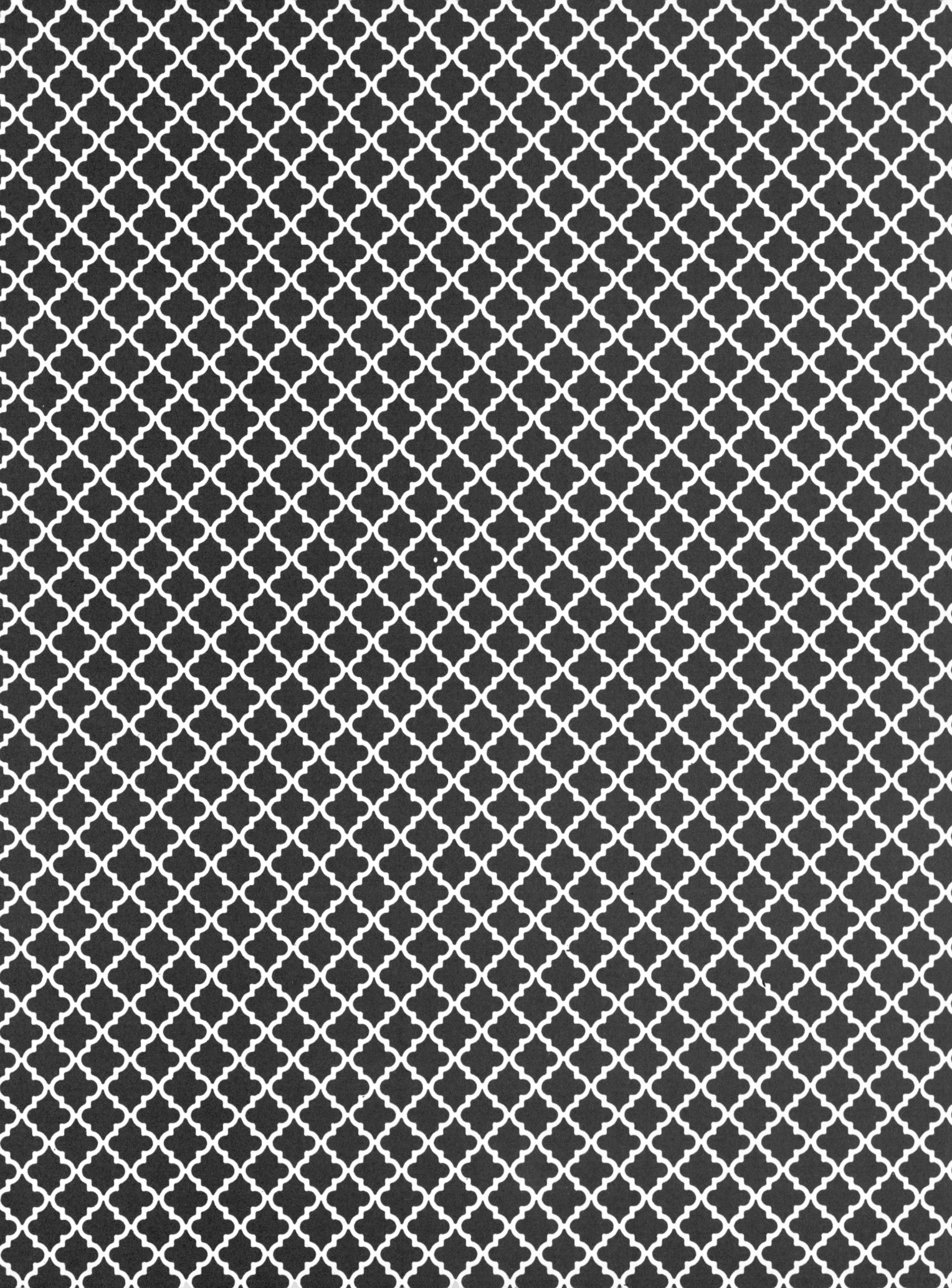